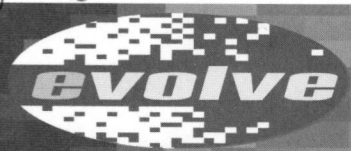

The Latest *Evolution*...

Evolve provides online access to free resources designed specifically for you. The resources will provide you with information that enhances the material covered in the book and much more.

Visit the Web address listed below to start today!

▶▶ **LOGIN:** *http://evolve.elsevier.com/millerkeane/*

Evolve Resources for *Miller-Keane Encyclopedia & Dictionary of Medicine, Nursing, & Allied Health,* 7th edition, offer the following features:

- **Crossword Puzzles**
  Challenge your knowledge of medical, nursing, and allied health vocabulary.

- **Word of the Day**
  Learn a new term and definition each day.

- **Specialty Word Lists**
  Review lists of terms applicable to specific areas of study.

- **PDA Downloads**
  Expand your portable database with handy inf

- **WebLinks**
  Access links to places of interest on th

Think outside the book... *evolve.*

ENCYCLOPEDIA
& DICTIONARY *of*
MEDICINE,
NURSING, &
ALLIED HEALTH

ENCYCLOPEDIA
&DICTIONARY *of*
MEDICINE,
NURSING,&
ALLIED HEALTH

SEVENTH EDITION

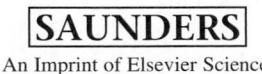

SAUNDERS
An Imprint of Elsevier Science

SAUNDERS
An Imprint of Elsevier Science (USA)

The Curtis Center
Independence Square West
Philadelphia, Pennsylvania 19106-3399

MILLER-KEANE ENCYCLOPEDIA AND DICTIONARY OF
MEDICINE, NURSING, AND ALLIED HEALTH ISBN 0-7216-9791-7

NOTICE

Nursing and Allied Health are ever-changing fields. Standard safety precautions must be
followed, but as new research and clinical experience broaden our knowledge, changes in
treatment and drug therapy may become necessary or appropriate. Readers are advised to
check the most current product information provided by the manufacturer of each drug to be
administered to verify the recommended dose, the method and duration of administration, and
contraindications. It is the responsibility of the licensed prescriber relying on experience and
knowledge of the patient, to determine dosages and the best treatment for each individual
patient. Neither the Publisher nor the editor assumes any liability for any injury and/or damage
to persons or property arising from this publication.

The Publisher

Previous editions copyrighted 1997, 1992, 1987, 1983, 1978, 1972

Library of Congress Cataloging-in-Publication Data

Miller-Keane encyclopedia & dictionary of medicine, nursing, and allied health–7th ed.
Editor: Marie O'Toole
p. cm.
Some previous eds. published as: Encyclopedia & dictionary of medicine, nursing,
and allied health/by Benjamin F. Miller and Claire Brackman Keane.
ISBN 0-7216-9791-7
1. Medicine—Dictionaries. 2. Nursing—Dictionaries. 3. Allied health personnel–
Dictionaries. I. Title: Miller-Keane encyclopedia and dictionary of medicine, nursing,
and allied health. II. Title: Encyclopedia & dictionary of medicine, nursing, and allied
health. III. Title: Encyclopedia and dictionary of medicine, nursing, and allied health.
IV. Miller, Benjamin Frank, 1907–1971. Encyclopedia & dictionary of medicine,
nursing, and allied health.
R121.M65 2003
610′.3–dc21   2003041542

Executive Publisher: Darlene Como
Senior Developmental Editor: Barbara Watts
Senior Project Manager: Peter Faber
Book Design Manager: Gail Morey Hudson
Cover Design: Liz Rohne Rudder
Lexicographers: Douglas M. Anderson, Michelle A. Elliott, Jeff Keith,
            Patricia D. Novak, PhD
CE/RDC
Printed in the United States of America.

Last digit is the print number: 9 8 7 6 5 4 3 2 1

v

Consultants and Contributors

Marie A. Abate, BS, PharmD
Director, West Virginia Drug
  Information Center
Professor of Clinical Pharmacology
School of Pharmacy
West Virginia University
Morgantown, West Virginia

Elaine Auld, MPH, CHES
Executive Director
Society for Public Health Education
Washington, DC

Karen Baldwin, MS, CNM, RN
Adjunct Instructor
College of Nursing
Rutgers, The State University of
  New Jersey
Newark, New Jersey

Peter A. Blasco, MD
Director, Neurodevelopmental Program
Child Development and Rehabilitation
  Center
Oregon Health and Science University
Portland, Oregon

Gloria M. Bulechek, PhD, RN, FAAN
Professor
College of Nursing
The University of Iowa
Iowa City, Iowa

**Stewart C. Bushong, ScD,
FACR, FACMP**
Professor of Radiologic Science
Baylor College of Medicine
Houston, Texas

Caroline Camuñas, EdD, RN
Adjunct Associate Professor
Teachers College
Columbia University
New York, New York

Jorge Camuñas, MD
Associate Clinical Professor of
  Cardiothoracic Surgery
Division of Thoracic Surgery
The Mount Sinai Medical Center
New York, New York

Beverly Christie, RN, BSN
Program Manager
Hemophilia & Thrombosis Center
Fairview-University Medical Center
Minneapolis, Minnesota

Glen E. Combs
Physician Assistant Program
The Bowman-Gray School of
  Medicine of Wake Forest
  University
Winston-Salem, North Carolina

Ramona Connor, RN, BSN, MA
Perioperative Nursing Specialist
AORN Center for Nursing Practice
Denver, Colorado

Michele L. Darby, MS, BSDH
Eminent Scholar, University Professor
Graduate Program Director
School of Dental Hygiene
Old Dominion University
Norfolk, Virginia

**Joanne McCloskey Dochterman,
PhD, RN, FAAN**
Distinguished Professor
Director, Center for Nursing
  Classification and Clinical
  Effectiveness
Chairperson, Organizations,
  Systems, and Community Health
College of Nursing
The University of Iowa
Iowa City, Iowa

Steven B. Dowd, EdD, RT(R)
Program Director, Radiographer
  Program
Associate Professor
University of Alabama at Birmingham
Birmingham, Alabama

Judith Felson Duchan, PhD, CCC
Emeritus Professor
Department of Communicative Disorders
  and Sciences
University at Buffalo, The State
  University of New York
Buffalo, New York

David Duffy, PhD, MBBS
Epidemiologic Unit
The Queensland Institute of Medical
Research
Brisbane, Queensland, Australia

Lucille Sanzero Eller, PhD, RN
Assistant Professor
College of Nursing
Rutgers, The State University of
New Jersey
Newark, New Jersey

Thomas Elwood, DrPH
Executive Director
Association of Schools of Allied Health
Professions
Washington, DC

Claire Fagin, PhD, RN
Leadership Professor Emeritus and
Dean Emeritus
School of Nursing
University of Pennsylvania
Philadelphia, Pennsylvania

Phyllis Fineberg, COMT
Program Director
Ophthalmic Medical Personnel Training
Program
Georgetown University Medical Center
Washington, DC

**Dorothy L. Gordon, DNSc,
RN, FAAN**
Associate Professor
School of Nursing
University of Texas at Austin
Austin, Texas

**Davina J. Gosnell, PhD,
RN, FAAN**
Dean and Professor
College of Nursing
Kent State University
Kent, Ohio

Beth Herrera, BA, RN
School Nurse
Haddonfield Board of Education
Haddonfield, New Jersey

Tracey Hergert, RN, MS, FNP-C
Family Physicians of Windsor
Windsor, Colorado

Carlton Hogan
Community Programs for Clinical
Research on AIDS Statistical Center
Coordinating Center of Biometric
Research
Division of Biostatistics, School of
Public Health
University of Minnesota
Minneapolis, Minnesota

Chris Keegan, MS, CST
Assistant Professor
Department of Surgical Technology
Vincennes University
Vincennes, Indiana

Nancy Kelly, MHS
Executive Director
Health Volunteers Overseas
Washington, DC

Imogene King, EdD, RN, FAAN
Professor Emeritus
S. Pasadena, Florida

Lisa Lippincott, BSN, RN
University of Pennsylvania Health
System
Philadelphia, Pennsylvania

Karen S. Martin, MSN, RN, FAAN
Health Care Consultant
Martin Associates
Omaha, Nebraska

Ruth McCorkle, PhD, RN, FAAN
Chair, Doctoral Program
School of Nursing
Yale University
New Haven, Connecticut

Donna L. MacIntyre, PhD
Associate Professor, Physical Therapy
School of Rehabilitation Sciences
University of British Columbia
Vancouver, British Columbia,
Canada

Yvonne McHugh, PhD
Rabies Medical Education Consultant
Chiron Vaccines
Emeryville, California

Brent McNeill, DipT, MA Aud(c)
McNeill Audiology
Victoria, British Columbia, Canada

Denise Moffa, BSN, RN
Kidney/Pancreas Transplant Coordinator
University of Pennsylvania Health System
Philadelphia, Pennsylvania

Paul Montenegro, MA, RN, ANP
Wound Care Specialties
Wound Healing Solutions, LLC
Marlton, New Jersey

**Margaret A. Newman,
PhD, RN, FAAN**
Professor Emeritus
School of Nursing
University of Minnesota
Minneapolis, Minnesota

Obesity Education Initiative
National Heart, Lung, and Blood Institute
Bethesda, Maryland

Amie N. Osborn, BS
Houston, Texas
www.treachercollins.org

Karl M. Peters, DVM
Program Director
Veterinary Technology Program
Foothill College
Los Altos Hills, California

**Judith Barberio Pollachek,
PhD, ANPC, GNPC, SNC**
Clinical Assistant Professor
College of Nursing
Rutgers, The State University of
New Jersey
Newark, New Jersey

Robert Rakel, MD
Professor and Chairman
Department of Family Medicine
Baylor College of Medicine
Houston, Texas

**Virginia K. Saba,
EdD, RN, FAAN, FACMI**
Distinguished Scholar
School of Nursing
Georgetown University
Washington, DC

Deborah Sansoucie, EdD, RN
Clinical Associate Professor
Director, Neonatal Nurse Practitioner
Program
State University of New York at Stony Brook
Stony Brook, New York

**Sharan L. Schwartzberg,
EdD, OTR, FAOTA**
Professor and Chair
Boston School of Occupational Therapy
Tufts University
Medford, Massachusetts

Janice Selekman, DNSc, RN
Professor and Chair
Department of Nurisng
University of Delaware
Newark, Delaware

**Rose Ann G. Soloway,
RN, MSEd, DABAT**
Associate Director
American Association of Poison
Control Centers

Edward R. Stapleton, EMT-P
Director of Prehospital Care and Education
University Hospital
Assistant Clinical Professor
Department of Emergency Medicine
School of Medicine
State University of New York at
Stony Brook
Stony Brook, New York

Walt A. Stoy, PhD, EMT-P, CCEMT-P
Associate Professor and Chair
Emergency Medicine Program
School of Health and Rehabilitation Sciences
Research Associate Professor of Emergency
Medicine
Department of Emergency Medicine
School of Medicine
University of Pittsburgh
Director, Office of Education and
International Emergency Medicine
Center for Emergency Medicine
Pittsburgh, Pennsylvania

John Suler, PhD
Professor of Psychology
Science and Technology Center
Rider University
Lawrenceville, New Jersey

Richard B. van Breeman, PhD
Professor of Medicinal Chemistry and
Pharmacognosy
College of Pharmacy
University of Illinois
Chicago, Illinois

**Anne Robin Waldman,
MSN, RN, AOCN, BC**
Clinical Nurse Specialist
Oncology Nursing Society
Albert Einstein Cancer Center
Philadelphia, Pennsylvania

Elisabeth R. Warner, MSLS, AHIP
Education Services Librarian
Scott Memorial Library
Thomas Jefferson University
Philadelphia, Pennsylvania

Jean Watson, PhD, RN, HNC, FAAN
Distinguished Professor of Nursing
Endowed Chair in Caring Science
School of Nursing
University of Colorado Health Sciences
    Center
Denver, Colorado

Jeffrey L. Weaver, OD, MS
Director, Clinical Care Group
American Optometric Association
St. Louis, Missouri

Sharon Walker-Brown, MS, RN
Administrative Nursing Supervisor
South Jersey Hospital System
Bridgeton, New Jersey

**Jo Anne Zerwekh,
EdD, RN, FNP, CS**
Nursing Education Consultants
Dallas, Texas

Publisher's Foreword

Today's health professionals face the challenge of an evolving, multidisciplinary knowledge base. Innovations, research findings, new technologies, and new products drive the continual changes in all health science fields. As a result, new terms are introduced and existing terms take on new or modified meanings. Understanding the new language as it develops is essential to communicating effectively within the health care arena. The *Miller-Keane Encyclopedia & Dictionary of Medicine, Nursing, & Allied Health* provides a current and authoritative guide to this dynamic vocabulary.

Editorial Board, Consultants, and Contributors

Once again, we have assembled an outstanding group of Editorial Board members, Consultants, and Contributors. This group represents the major nursing specialties and the allied health professions in the United States and Canada. Their contributions to the revision of the vocabulary, and the addition of new terms, have been invaluable. We also owe our thanks to numerous professional organizations in the health sciences for their assistance in reviewing entries.

Revision of the Vocabulary

In keeping with the dictionary's reputation as an authoritative, current, and comprehensive vocabulary source for the health sciences, thousands of new entries have been added to this edition, and archaic or obsolete terms have been deleted. The dictionary now contains more than 40,000 terms, including 3,900 new terms. The existing entries have been thoroughly reviewed and revised to keep terminology up to date in even the most rapidly changing fields. In particular, the latest changes for diagnosis-related groups, nursing diagnoses and the other key nursing taxonomies have been included. The number of cross-references has been increased to help readers find related entries and additional information and gain a fuller understanding of a term. Tables and illustrations have been revised, and several hundred new ones have been added.

Encyclopedic Entries

Our hallmark encyclopedic entries present detailed descriptions with extensive background information on topics of special significance to health professionals. We have given these entries special attention to ensure they remain complete, up-to-date, and relevant. Many changes have therefore been made to those entries that appeared in the previous edition, and new ones have been added for major topics.

Format

In our ongoing efforts to improve the usefulness of the dictionary, we have changed its format and dimensions to increase its portability. We worked closely with our design and lexicographic staff to develop a new format that achieves this goal without compromising the dictionary's comprehensiveness or the readability of the type.

Windows

As a unique feature of this dictionary, we have included "windows" boxes throughout the vocabulary section. In the "windows," distinguished leaders in the health sciences expand on our entries and provide valuable insights into topics of interest to today's health professionals. New "windows" have been added to this edition to expand coverage of key topics across the spectrum of health-related professions.

Color Plates

We have completely updated our color atlas of human anatomy and function. It provides a tool for reviewing and understanding anatomical structures. In addition, our expanded section of color plates greatly illuminates the understanding of the disorders we have depicted. Many new illustrations have been added, often drawing from those used in *Dorland's Illustrated Medical Dictionary*.

Appendices

In this edition, our extensive Appendices have been reorganized according to topic areas to make them easier to use. They have been rigorously updated to include the latest information.

Spellchecker

As an added benefit to our readers, this edition includes spellchecker software on the mini-CD-ROM inserted inside the back cover. Derived from *Dorland's Medical Speller* 3.0, this software enables users to check the spelling of more than 275,000 medical terms. This spellchecker, along with the new edition of *Miller-Keane's*

Dictionary, provides a powerful tool for building and using a complete and accurate health science vocabulary.

Website

To further enhance the value of this edition, we have developed a companion website. The website includes an exciting collection of supplemental material, as well as links to a carefully selected list of websites that provide reliable and authoritative information of major interest to students and practitioners in the health sciences. Updates will be posted to the website when major changes occur in specialized health professional vocabularies.

Preface

There is a dynamic and vibrant vocabulary for health care professionals that is both descriptive and normative. It is descriptive because it assists the health care provider to narrate patient care situations. It is normative because it communicates a standard or model of care. Research and new developments mandate the addition of new terms to the health care lexicon. Studies can modify the meaning of existing terms. Additionally, patient records and other historic documents often prompt health care professionals to access terms not in current use. The *Miller-Keane Encyclopedia & Dictionary of Medicine, Nursing, & Allied Health* has always been committed to serving as an exemplary reference tool to assist users to understand the health care vocabulary. It is not merely a collection of words and explanations of their meanings in alphabetical order, but rather the organization of words, phrases, and vocabularies in a manner that assists all users to decode the complex, interdisciplinary world of health science.

The goal of the *Miller-Keane Encyclopedia & Dictionary of Medicine, Nursing, & Allied Health* is to be the premier reference work for practical, accurate, and interdisciplinary health care terms. It is not possible, nor even advisable, to include every word or phrase in the corpus of English language health care terms in a printed text. The decisions about what to include and what to omit can be difficult. The *Miller-Keane Encyclopedia & Dictionary* is fortunate to have an outstanding interdisciplinary editorial board to assist in the selection and review of entries. Additionally, consultants representing a wide variety of students, educators, researchers, scholars, and clinicians provide specific suggestions for entries. Moreover, the lexicographical research for this, as well as previous editions of the *Miller Keane Encyclopedia & Dictionary*, is supported by a superb team of lexicographers. It is the collaboration of all of these individuals that has led to the creation of the seventh edition—a reference tool of which we are all proud.

The language of health care is a powerful tool in the care of patients. The interdisciplinary nature of the development of the *Miller-Keane Encyclopedia & Dictionary of Medicine, Nursing, & Allied Health* is reflected in its entries. It has been designed to supplement texts and journals, as well as to assist its users to employ the vocabulary of health care with confidence.

Marie O'Toole Ed.D, RN, FAAN
Editor

Acknowledgments

There are many individuals and groups to acknowledge and to thank for their contributions to the Seventh Edition of the *Miller-Keane Encyclopedia & Dictionary of Medicine, Nursing, & Allied Health*. It continues to be an honor to work with so many talented and dedicated people.

Elsevier Science supported and extended the tradition of excellence established in previous editions. Access to primary sources in the Elsevier Science catolog dramatically expanded the database for text and illustrations in this edition. Darlene Como, Executive Editor for the Nursing Division, has been a champion for this edition. She has provided expert guidance in the development of a Seventh Edition that is responsive to the needs of its users. Barbera Watts, the Developmental Editor, has been a joy to work with. Her attention to detail has been tremendous in every phase of assembling a work of this magnitude.

Douglas Anderson, Chief Lexicographer, and his team of lexicographers—Jeff Keith, Patricia Novak, and Michelle Elliot—provide a resource that is invaluable in the compilation of the *Miller-Keane Encyclopedia & Dictionary of Medicine, Nursing, & Allied Health*. They maintain a database that establishes the gold standard as a corpus of health care terms. A special acknowledgment is extended to Jeff Keith, who is a dedicated and precise guardian of the definitions included in *Miller-Keane*.

An outstanding editorial board and numerous consultants continue to play an important role in refining the language of health care. Professional and governmental organizations also share their expertise through the development of standards and controlled vocabularies that assist health care providers in the advancement of research and the evaluation of patient care. A special thank-you is extended to the Association of Operating Room Nurses, The Oncology Nurses Society, The Centers for Disease Control and Prevention, The American Diabetes Association, and The American Physical Therapy Association.

Finally, I wish to acknowledge the support and encouragement of my colleagues and family. I am truly fortunate to work in a scholarly environment. My colleagues and former students at Teachers College, Columbia University, and my colleagues and current students at Rutgers, The State University of New Jersey are extraordinary individuals. They inspire me, inform me, and always remind me of the importance of collaboration. Moreover, my family and extended family support the intense concentration required to undertake a project the magnitude of a dictionary/encyclopedia.

To all the members of the team that created a new edition of the *Miller-Keane Encyclopedia & Dictionary of Medicine, Nursing, & Allied Health*—a sincere and enthusiastic thank-you.

Marie O'Toole, RN, FAAN
Editor

Contents

Notes on the Use of This Book

STRUCTURE OF ENTRIES

Entries in this book are either main entries or subentries.

Main Entries

Headword. Main entries begin with the term being defined, set in **boldface** type, known as the headword. If an abbreviation for a term is included, it is often given in the headword, enclosed in parentheses.

For Example: **hiatus**
                deoxyribonucleic acid (DNA)

Pronunciation. In most main entries the headword is followed by the pronunciation, enclosed in parentheses (see "Indication of Pronunciation," below).

For Example: **hiatus** (hi-a′tus)

Plural. If the plural of the main entry is not an ordinary English plural, the plural form is given following the pronunciation, set in *italic* type, with the position of the stress indicated.

For Example: **hiatus** (hi-a′tus), pl. *hia′tus*

Derivation. If the main entry is a foreign word (Latin, for example), the language from which the word comes is given in brackets; in the case of Latin, this would be [L]. (For the abbreviations used, see below.)

For Example: **hiatus** (hi-a′tus), pl. *hia′tus* [L.]

Definition. The definition of the term follows, set in regular type. The definition may contain a number of subsections, indicated by headings set in SMALL CAPITALS; these subsections help to organize the information in the definition and include information on topics such as SYMPTOMS, TREATMENT, and PATIENT CARE.

Adjectival Forms. An adjective that goes with an entry may be given within the definition, set in **boldface** type, with the position of the stress indicated; it is usually placed at the end of the entry, although it may be placed at the end of the first sentence or the first paragraph if the structure of the entry so dictates.

Synonyms. Synonyms for a term may occur at the end of the definition and are identified by the words "Called also."

The following main entry illustrates how a number of these elements are combined to make up a complete entry:

hiatus (hi-a′tus), pl. *hia′tus* [L.] a gap, cleft, or opening, adj., **hia′tal.**

Subentries

Subentries are used for compound terms (see below). Subentries usually consist of a **boldface** headword set off by a comma from the definition, which is set in regular type. In the headword for each subentry, the main entry under which it is placed is represented by the initial letter only, or by the initial letter followed by an 's if the subentry is plural but the main entry is singular (in the case of foreign or irregular plurals, the plural form is spelled out in full). For subentries that are Latin phrases (usually terms used in anatomy), the positions of the stresses are given. The following examples of subentries with their main entries will illustrate the possibilities:

crus (main entry)   **fiber** (main entry)
  c. cer′ebri   **A f′s**
  c. of clitoris   **association f′s**
  crura of diaphragm   **dietary f.**
                                     motor f′s
                                     muscle f.

Elements that occur in main entries, such as abbreviations, pronunciations, and synonyms, may also occur in subentries.

INDICATION OF PRONUNCIATION

The pronunciation of words is indicated by a simple phonetic respelling. Long and short vowels are marked only when necessary.

1. An unmarked vowel ending a syllable is long *(ba′be).*
2. An unmarked vowel in a syllable ending with a consonant is short *(ab-dukt′).*
3. A long vowel that is a syllable that ends with a consonant is marked with a macron *(be-hāv′yer).*
4. A short vowel at the end of a syllable is marked with a breve *(lip″ĭ-do′sis).*
5. In stressed syllables, *ah* represents the sound heard in f*a*ther. In unstressed syllables, it represents the sound (called "schwa") heard in sof*a*. In the pronunciations used by many people, vowels marked short in this dictionary are pronounced as schwa (as the *o* in ŏ-kl$\overline{oo}$d′).
6. The following vowel combinations are used in the phonetic respellings: *au* (paw), *oi* (oil), *oo* (foot, bruise), *ow* (ounce).

The primary stress in a word is marked with a single boldface accent (′). The secondary stress is marked with a double lightface accent (″).

ENCYCLOPEDIC ENTRIES

One of the features of this book is the presentation of some topics in entries that are longer and more comprehensive than ordinary dictionary entries. These are termed *encyclopedic entries*. Such entries allow for the presentation of more detail or of some background information, the integration of various facets of a topic, and the inclusion of material that may be of particular interest to members of the various health care specialties. Many of the entries in this dictionary contain cross-references to the encyclopedic entries, to which the user should turn for a fuller discussion of the term cross-referenced or for related information. For the placement of encyclopedic entries in the dictionary, see "Order of Entries."

ORDER OF ENTRIES

Entries appear in alphabetical order according to the sequence of their letters, regardless of spaces or hyphens that may occur between them. This is illustrated by the following sequences of entries:

carbon	heart
carbonate	heartbeat
carbon dioxide	heart block
carbon dioxide-oxygen therapy	heartburn
carbonic acid	heart failure
carbon monoxide	heart-lung machine
	heart murmur

An exception to this rule occurs in terms containing proper names, where only the name itself counts for alphabetical order. An *'s* (if one occurs) and any following words are not counted. (However, if several terms begin with the same name, then the terms are put in order on the basis of what follows the name.) Thus *Fried's rule* precedes *Friedländer's rule*, *Gram's stain* precedes *gramicidin*, and *Parkinson's disease* and *Parkinson's facies* precede *parkinsonian*.

Subentries appear in alphabetical order as determined by the modifying words or phrases, regardless of whether they are singular or plural. Prepositions, whether English or foreign, are ignored. In the following sequences of entries, the words that determine the order are italicized:

(main entry **crus**)	(main entry **fragility**)
c. *cerebri*	f. of *blood*
c. of *clitoris*	*capillary* f.
crura of *diaphragm*	*erythrocyte* f.
crura of *fornix*	
c. of *penis*	

Placement of Compound Terms

Terms composed of a noun modified by an adjective or by a proper name (the latter are called eponymic entries) are generally placed under the noun as subentries. In some cases, exceptions to this rule have been made. For example, acids are given in straight ahead order, so that *hydrochloric acid* is defined at *hydrochloric*, not at *acid*. Diseases and syndromes are handled in the same way, so that *Parkinson's disease* appears under *P*. For the most part, this is done to avoid long strings of subentries. In some cases, such as the names of theories or of organizations, it has seemed more logical to give compound terms as main entries, so that *American Type Culture Collection* appears under *A*. It is hoped that this system will help save time and effort by giving the entry where the user is most likely to look for it.

Placement of Encyclopedic Entries

Encyclopedic entries that are compound terms are generally given in straight ahead order. They may be given as main entries or (when the first word of the term is itself a main entry) as subentries. At times, this results in the placement of an encyclopedic entry in a place that would not be expected according to the ordinary rules for the order of entries (for example, the encyclopedic entry *ileal conduit* falls under *I*, not *C*). In such cases a brief entry is given at the place that the entry would be expected (here at *conduit*) and a cross reference is given to the encyclopedic entry.

CROSS REFERENCES

Words set in SMALL CAPITALS denote cross references. They are used liberally, and the reader is advised to turn to the entry for that term, because important additional information will be found there.

ABBREVIATIONS

Abbreviations used in the entries are few and fairly obvious. They include:

adj. (adjective)	It. (Italian)
Fr. (French)	L. (Latin)
Ger. (German)	pl. (plural)
Gr. (Greek)	sing. (singular)

In the elaboration of entries that are themselves abbreviations, the words "abbreviation for" have been omitted.

Combining Forms in Medical Terminology*

The following is a list of combining forms encountered frequently in the vocabulary of medicine. A dash or dashes are appended to indicate whether the form usually precedes (as *ante-*) or follows (as *-agra*) the other elements of the compound or usually appears between the other elements (as *-em-*). Following each combining form, the first item of information is the Greek or Latin word, or both a Greek and a Latin word, from which it is derived.

Greek words have been transliterated into Roman characters. Latin words are identified by [L.], Greek words by [Gr.]. Information necessary to an understanding of the form appears next in parentheses. Then the meaning or meanings of the words are given, followed, where appropriate, by reference to a synonymous combining form. Finally, an example is given to illustrate the use of the combining form in a compound English derivative.

a-   *a-* [L.] (*n* is added before words beginning with a vowel) negative prefix. Cf. in-³. *a*metria

ab-   *ab* [L.] away from. Cf. apo-. *ab*ducent

abdomin-   *abdomen, abdominis* [L.] abdomen. *abdomin*oscopy

ac-   See ad-. *ac*cretion

acet-   *acetum* [L.] vinegar. *acet*ometer

acid-   *acidus* [L.] sour. *acid*uric

acou-   *akouō* [Gr.] hear. *acou*ethesia. (Also spelled acu-)

acr-   *akron* [Gr.] extremity, peak, *acro*megaly

act-   *ago, actus* [L.] do, drive, act. re*act*ion

actin-   *aktis, aktinos* [Gr.] ray, radius. Cf. radi-. *actin*ogenesis

acu-   See acou-. osteo*acu*sis

ad-   *ad* [L.] (*d* changes to *c, f, g, p, s,* or *t* before words beginning with those consonants) to. *ad*renal

aden-   *adēn* [Gr.] gland Cf. gland-. *aden*oma

adip-   *adeps, adipis* [L.] fat. Cf. lipand stear-. *adip*ocellular

aer-   *aēr* [Gr.] air. an*aer*obiosis

aesthe-   See esthe-. *aesthe*sioneurosis

af-   See ad-. *af*ferent

ag-   See ad-. *ag*glutinant

-agogue   *agōgos* [Gr.] leading, inducing, galact*agogue*

-agra   *agra* [Gr.] catching, seizure. pod*agra*

alb-   *albus* [L.] white. Cf. leuk-. *alb*ocinereous

alg-   *algos* [Gr.] pain. neur*alg*ia

all-   *allos* [Gr.] other, different. *all*ergy

alve-   *alveus* [L.] trough, channel, cavity. *alve*olar

amph-   See amphi-. *amph*eclexis

amphi-   *amphi* [Gr.] (*i* is dropped before words beginning with a vowel) both, doubly. *amphi*celous

amyl-   *amylon* [Gr.] starch. *amylo*synthesis

an-¹   See ana-, *an*agogic

an-²   See a-. *an*omalous

ana-   *ana* [Gr.] (final *a* is dropped before words beginning with a vowel) up, positive. *ana*phoresis

ancyl-   See ankyl-. *ancyl*ostomiasis

andr-   *anēr, andros,* [Gr.] man. gyn*andr*oid

angi-   *angeion* [Gr.] vessel. Cf. vas-. *angi*emphraxis

ankyl-   *ankylos* [Gr.] crooked, looped. *ankylo*dactylia. (Also spelled ancyl-)

ant-   See anti-. *ant*ophthalmic

ante-   *ante* [L.] before. *ante*flexion

anti-   *anti* [Gr.] (*i* is dropped before words beginning with a vowel) against, counter. Cf. contra-. *anti*pyogenic

antr-   *antron* [Gr.] cavern. *antr*odynia

ap-¹   See apo-. *ap*heter

ap-²   See ad-. *ap*pend

-aph-   *haptō, haph-* [Gr.] touch. dys*aph*ia. (See also hapt-)

apo-   *apo* [Gr.] (*o* is dropped before words beginning with a vowel) away from, detached. Cf. ab-. *apo*physis

arachn-   *arachnē* [Gr.] spider. *arach*nodactyly

arch-   *archē* [Gr.] beginning, origin. *arch*enteron

arter(i)-   *arteria* [Gr.] windpipe, artery. *arteri*osclerosis, peri*arter*itis

*Compiled by Lloyd W. Daly, A.M., Ph.D., Litt. D., Allen Memorial Professor of Greek Emeritus, University of Pennsylvania.

arthr-   *arthron* [Gr.] joint. Cf. articul-. syn*arthr*osis

articul-   *articulus* [L.] joint. Cf. arthr-. dis*articul*ation

as-   See ad-. *as*similation

at-   See ad-. *at*trition

aur-   *auris* [L.] ear. Cf. ot-. *aur*inasal

aux-   *auxō* [Gr.] increase. enter*aux*e

ax-   *axōn* [Gr.] or *axis* [L.] axis. *ax*ofugal

axon-   *axōn* [Gr.] axis. *axon*ometer

ba-   *bainō, ba-* [Gr.] go, walk, stand. hypno*ba*tia

bacill-   *bacillus* [L.] small staff, rod. Cf. bacter-. actino*bacill*osis

bacter-   *bactērion* [Gr.] small staff, rod. Cf. bacill-. *bacter*iophage

ball-   *ballō, bol-* [Gr.] throw, *ball*istics. (See also bol-)

bar-   *baros* [Gr.] weight. pedo*ba*rometer

bi-¹   *bios* [Gr.] life. Cf. vit-. aero*bi*c

bi-²   *bi-* [L.] two (see also di-¹). *bi*lobate

bil-   *bilis* [L.] bile. Cf. chol-. *bil*iary

blast-   *blastos* [Gr.] bud, child, a growing thing in its early stages. Cf. germ-. *blast*oma, zygoto*blast*

blep-   *blepō* [Gr.] look, see. hemia*blep*sia

blephar-   *blepharon* [Gr.] (from *blepō*; see blep-) eyelid. Cf. cili-. *blephar*oncus

bol-   See ball-. em*bol*ism

brachi-   *brachiōn* [Gr.] arm. *brachi*ocephalic

brachy-   *brachys* [Gr.] short. *brachy*cephalic

brady-   *bradys* [Gr.] slow. *brady*cardia

brom-   *brōmos* [Gr.] stench. podo*brom*idrosis

bronch-   *bronchos* [Gr.] windpipe. *bronch*oscopy

bry-   *bryō* [Gr.] be full of life. em*bry*onic

bucc-   *bucca* [L.] cheek. disto*bucc*al

cac-   *kakos* [Gr.] bad, abnormal. Cf. mal-. *cac*odontia, arthro*cace*. (See also dys-)

calc-¹   *calx, calcis* [L.] stone (cf. lith-), limestone, lime. *calc*ipexy

calc-²   *calx, calcis* [L.] heel. *calc*aneotibial

calor-   *calor* [L.] heat. Cf. therm-. *calor*imeter

cancr-   *cancer, cancri* [L.] crab, cancer. Cf. carcin-. *cancr*ology. (Also spelled chancr-)

capit-   *caput, capitis* [L.] head. Cf. cephal-. de*capit*ator

caps-   *capsa* [L.] (from *capio*; see cept-) container. en*caps*ulation

carbo(n)-   *carbo, carbonis* [L.] coal, charcoal. *carbo*hydrate, *carbo*nuria

carcin-   *karkinos* [Gr.] crab, cancer. Cf. cancr-, *carcin*oma

cardi-   *kardia* [Gr.] heart. lipo*cardi*ac

cary-   See kary-. *cary*okinesis

cat-   See cata-. *cat*hode

cata-   *kata* [Gr.] (final *a* is dropped before words beginning with a vowel) down, negative. *Cata*batic

caud-   *cauda* [L.] tail. *caud*ad

cav-   *cavus* [L.] hollow. Cf. coel-. con*cav*e

cec-   *caecus* [L.] blind. Cf. typhl-. *cec*opexy

cel-¹   See coel-. amphi*cel*ous

cel-²   See –cele. *cel*ectome

-cele   *kēlē* [Gr.] tumor, hernia. gastro*cele*

cell-   *cella* [L.] room, cell. Cf. cyt-. *cell*iferous

cen-   *koinos* [Gr.] common. *cen*esthesia

cent-   *centum* [L.] hundred. Cf. hect-. Indicates fraction in metric system. [This exemplifies the custom in the metric system of identifying fractions of units by stems from the Latin, as centimeter, decimeter, millimeter, and multiples of units by the similar stems from the Greek, as hectometer, decameter, and kilometer.] *cent*imeter, *cent*ipede

cente-   *kenteō* [Gr.] to puncture. Cf. punct-. entero*cente*sis

centr-   *kentron* [Gr.] or *centrum* [L.] point, center. neuro*centr*al

cephal-   *kephalē* [Gr.] head. Cf. capit-. en*cephal*itis

cept-   *capio, -cipientis, -ceptus* [L.] take, receive. re*cept*or

cer-   *kēros* [Gr.] or *cera* [L.] wax. *cer*oplasty, *cer*omel

cerat-   See kerat-. a*cerat*osis

cerebr-   *cerebrum* [L.] brain. *cerebr*ospinal

cervic-   *cervix, cervicis* [L.] neck. Cf. trachel-. *cervic*itis

chancr-   See cancr-. *chancr*iform

cheil-   *cheilos* [Gr.] lip. Cf. labi-. *cheil*oschisis

cheir-   *cheir* [Gr.] hand. Cf. man-. macro*cheir*ia. (Also spelled chir-)

chir-   See cheir-. *chir*omegaly

chlor-   *chlōros* [Gr.] green. a*chlor*opsia

chol-   *cholē* [Gr.] bile. Cf. bil-. hepato*chol*angeitis

chondr-   *chondros* [Gr.] cartilage. *chondr*omalacia

chord-   *chordē* [Gr.] string, cord. peri*chord*al

chori-   *chorion* [Gr.] protective fetal membrane. endo*chori*on

chro-   *chrōs* [Gr.] color. poly*chro*matic

chron-   *chronos* [Gr.] time. syn*chro*nous

chy-   *cheō, chy-* [Gr.] pour. ec*chy*mosis

-cid(e)   *caedo; -cisus* [L.] cut, kill. infanti*cid*e, germi*cid*al

cili-   *cilium* [L.] eyelid. Cf. blephar-. super*cili*ary

cine-   see Kine-. auto*cine*sis

-cipient   See cept-. in*cipient*

circum-   *circum* [L.] around. Cf. peri. *circum*ferential

-cis-   *caedo, -cisus* [L.] cut, kill. ex*cis*ion

clas-   *klaō* [Gr.] break. cranio*clast*

clin-   *klinō* [Gr.] bend, incline, make lie down. *clino*meter

clus-   *claudo, -clusus* [L.] shut. malo*cclus*ion

co-   See con-. *co*hesion

cocc-   *kokkos* [Gr.] seed, pill. gono*cocc*us

coel-   *koilos* [Gr.] hollow. Cf. Cav-. *coel*enteron. (Also spelled cel-)

col-¹   See colon-. *col*ic

col-²   See con-. *col*lapse

colon-   *kolon* [Gr.] lower intestine. *colon*ic

colp-   *kolpos* [Gr.] hollow, vagina. Cf. sin-. endo*colp*itis

com-   See con-. *com*masculation

con-   *con-* [L.] (becomes co- before vowels or *h*; col- before *l*; com- before *b, m,* or *p*; cor- before *r*) with, together. Cf. syn-. *con*traction

contra-   *contra* [L.] against, counter. Cf. anti, *contra*indication

copr-   *kopros* [Gr.] dung, Cf. sterc-. *copr*oma

cor-¹   *korē* [Gr.] doll, little image, pupil. iso*cor*ia

cor-²   See con-. *cor*rugator

corpor-   *corpus, corporis* [L.] body. Cf. somat-. intra*corpor*al

cortic-   *cortex, corticis* [L.] bark, rind. *cortic*osterone

cost-   *costa* [L.] rib. Cf. pleur-. inter*cost*al

crani-   *kranion* [Gr.] or *cranium* [L.] skull. peri*crani*um

creat-   *kreas, kreato-* [Gr.] meat, flesh, *creat*orrhea

-crescent   *cresco, crescentis, cretus* [L.] grow. ex*crescent*

cret-¹   *cerno, cretus* [L.] distinguish, separate off. Cf. crin-. dis*cret*e

cret-²   See-crescent, ac*cret*ion

crin-   *krinō* [Gr.] distinguish, separate off. Cf. cret-¹. endo*crin*ology

crur-   *crus, cruris* [L.] shin, leg. brachio*crur*al

cry-   *kryos* [Gr.] cold. *cry*esthesia

crypt-   *kryptō* [Gr.] hide, conceal. *crypt*orchism

cult-   *colo, cultus* [L.] tend, cultivate. *cult*ure

cune-   *cuneus* [L.] wedge. Cf. sphen-. *cune*iform

cut-   *cutis* [L.] skin. Cf. derm(at)-. sub*cut*aneous

cyan-   *kyanos* [Gr.] blue. antho*cya*nin

cycl-   *kyklos* [Gr.] circle, cycle. *cycl*ophoria

cyst-   *kystis* [Gr.] bladder. Cf. vesic-. nephro*cyst*itis

cyt-   *kytos* [Gr.] cell. Cf. cell-. plasmo*cyt*oma

dacry-   *dakry* [Gr.] tear. *dacry*ocyst

dactyl-   *daktylos* [Gr.] finger, toe, Cf. digit-. hexa*dactyl*ism

de-   *de* [L.] down from. *de*composition

dec-¹   *deka* [Gr.] ten. Indicates multiple in metric system. Cf. dec-². *dec*agram

dec-²   *decem* [L.] ten. Indicates fraction in metric system. Cf. dec-¹ *dec*ipara, *dec*imeter

dendr-   *dendron* [Gr.] tree. neuro*dend*rite

dent-   *dens, dentis* [L.] tooth. Cf. odont-. inter*dent*al

derm(at)-   *derma, dermatos* [Gr.] skin. Cf. cut-. endo*derm, dermat*itis

desm-   *desmos* [Gr.] band, ligament. syn*desm*opexy

dextr-   *dexter, dextr-* [L.] right-hand. ambi*dextr*ous

di-¹   *di-* [Gr.] two. *di*morphic. (See also bi-²)

di-²   See dia-. *di*uresis

di-³   See dis-. *di*vergent

dia-   *dia* [Gr.] (*a* is dropped before words beginning with a vowel) through, apart. Cf. per-. *dia*gnosis

didym-   *didymos* [Gr.] twin. Cf. gemin-. epi*didym*al

digit-   *digitus* [L.] finger, toe. Cf. dactyl-. *digiti*grade

diplo-   *diploos* [Gr.] double. *diplo*myelia

dis-   *dis-* [L.] (*s* may be dropped before a word beginning with a consonant) apart, away from. *dis*location

disc-   *diskos* [Gr.] or *discus* [L.] disk. *disc*oplacenta

dors-   *dorsum* [L.] back. ventro*dor*sal

drom-   *dromos* [Gr.] course. hemo*drom*ometer

-ducent   See -duct. ad*ducent*

-duct   *duco, ducentis, ductus* [L.] lead, conduct, ovi*duct*

dur-   *durus* [L.] hard. Cf. scler-. in*dur*ation

dynam(i)-   *dynamis* [Gr.] power. *dyna*moneure, neuro*dynam*ic

dys-   *dys-* [Gr.] bad, improper. Cf. mal-. *dys*trophic. (See also cac-)

e-   *e* [L.] out from. Cf. ec- and ex-. *e*mission

ec-   *ek* [Gr.] out of. Cf. e-. *ec*centric

-ech-   *echō* [Gr.] have, hold, be. syn*ech*otomy

ect-   *ektos* [Gr.] outside. Cf. extra-. *ect*oplasm

ede-   *oideō* [Gr.] swell. *ede*matous

ef-   See ex-. *ef*florescent

-elc-   *helkos* [Gr.] sore, ulcer. enter*elc*osis. (See also helc-)

electr-   *ēlectron* [Gr.] amber. *electro*therapy

em-   See en-. *em*bolism, *em*pathy, *em*phlysis

-em-   *haima* [Gr.] blood. an*em*ia. [See also hem(at)-]

en-   *en* [Gr.] (*n* changes to *m* before *b, p*, or *ph*) in, on. Cf. in-². *en*celitis

end-   *endon* [Gr.] inside. Cf. intra-. *end*angium

enter-   *enteron* [Gr.] intestine. dys*enter*y

ep-   See epi-. *ep*axial

epi-   *epi* [Gr.] (*i* is dropped before words beginning with a vowel) upon, after, in addition, *epi*glottis

erg-   *ergon* [Gr.] work, deed, en*erg*y

erythr-   *erythros* [Gr.] red. Cf. rub(r)-. *erythr*ochromia

eso-   *esō* [Gr.] inside. Cf. intra-. *eso*phylactic

esthe-   *aisthanomai, aisthē-* [Gr.] perceive, feel. Cf. sens-. an*esthe*sia

eu-   *eu* [Gr.] good, normal. *eu*pepsia

ex-   *ex* [Gr.] or *ex* [L.] out of. Cf. e-. *ex*cretion

exo-   *exō* [Gr.] outside. Cf. extra-. *exo*pathic

extra-   *extra* [L.] outside of, beyond. Cf. ect- and exo, *extra*cellular

faci-   *facies* [L.] face. Cf. prosop-. brachio*faci*olingual

-facient   *facio, facientis, factus, -fectus* [L.] make. Cf. poie-. cale*facient*

-fact-   See facient-. arte*fact*

fasci-   *fascia* [L.] band. *fasci*orrhaphy

febr-   *febris* [L.] fever. Cf. pyr-. *febr*icide

-fect-   See facient. de*fect*ive

-ferent   *fero, ferentis, latus* [L.] bear, carry. Cf. phor-. ef*ferent*

ferr-   *ferrum* [L.] iron. *ferro*protein

fibr-   *fibra* [L.] fiber. Cf. in-¹. chondro*fibr*oma

fil-   *filum* [L.] thread. *fil*iform

fiss-   *findo, fissus* [L.] split. Cf. schis-. *fiss*ion

flagell-   *flagellum* [L.] whip. *flagell*ation

flav-   *flavus* [L.] yellow. Cf. xanth-. ribo*flav*in

-flect-   *flecto, flexus* [L.] bend, divert. de*flect*ion

-flex-   See -flect-. re*flex*ometer

flu-   *fluo, fluxus* [L.] flow. Cf. rhe-. *flu*id

flux-   See flu-. af*flux*ion

for-   *foris* [L.] door, opening, per*for*ated

-form   *forma* [L.] shape. Cf. -oid. ossi*form*

fract-   *frango, fractus* [L.] break. re*fract*ive

front-   *frons, frontis* [L.] forehead, front. naso*front*al

-fug(e)   *fugio* [L.] flee, avoid. vermi*fuge*, centri*fug*al

funct-   *fungor, functus* [L.] perform, serve, function. mal*funct*ion

fund-   *fundo, fusus* [L.] pour. in*fund*ibulum

fus-   See fund-. dif*fus*ible

galact-   *gala, galactos* [Gr.] milk. Cf. lact-. dys*galact*ia

gam-   *gamos* [Gr.] marriage, reproductive union. a*gam*ont

gangli-   *ganglion* [Gr.] swelling, plexus. neuro*gangli*itis

gastr-   *gastēr, gastros* [Gr.] stomach. cholangio*gastr*ostomy

gelat-   *gelo, gelatus* [L.] freeze, congeal. *gelat*in

gemin-   *geminus* [L.] twin, double. Cf. didym-. quadri*gemin*al

gen-   *gignomai, gen-, gon-* [Gr.] become, be produced, originate, or *gennaō* [Gr.] produce, originate. cyto*gen*ic

germ-   *germen, germinis* [L.] bud, a growing thing in its early stages. Cf. blast-. *germ*inal, ovi*germ*

gest-   *gero, gerentis, gestus* [L.] bear, carry, con*gest*ion

gland-   *glans, glandis* [L.] acorn. Cf. aden-. intra*gland*ular

-glia   *glia* [Gr.] glue. neuro*glia*

gloss-   *glōssa* [Gr.] tongue. Cf. lingu-. tricho*gloss*ia

glott-   *glōtta* [Gr.] tongue, language. *glott*ic

gluc-   See glyc(y)-. *gluc*ophenetidin

glutin-   *gluten, glutinis* [L.] glue. a*glutin*ation

glyc(y)-   *glykys* [Gr.] sweet. *glyc*emia, *glyc*yrrhizin. (Also spelled gluc-)

gnath-   *gnathos* [Gr.] jaw. orthog*nath*ous

gno-   *gignōsiō. gnō-* [Gr.] know, discern. dia*gno*sis

gon-   See gen-. anphi*gon*y

grad-   *gradior* [L.] walk, take steps. retro*grad*e

-gram   *gramma* [Gr.] letter, drawing. cardio*gram*

gran-   *granum* [L.] grain, particle, lipo*gran*uloma

graph-   *graphō* [Gr.] scratch, write, record. histo*graph*y

grav-   *gravis* [L.]. heavy. multi*grav*ida

gyn(ec)-   *gynē, gynaikos* [Gr.] woman, wife. andro*gyn*y, *gynec*ologic

gyr-   *gyros* [Gr.] ring, circle. *gyro*spasm

haem(at)-   See hem(at)-. *haem*orrhagia, *haemat*oxylon

hapt-   *haptō* [Gr.] touch, *hapt*ometer

hect-   *hekt-* [Gr.] hundred. Cf. cent-. Indicates multiple in metric system. *hect*ometer

helc-   *helkos* [Gr.] sore, ulcer, *helc*osis

hem(at)-   *haima, haimatos* [Gr.] blood. Cf. sanguin-. *hem*angioma, *hemat*ocyturia. (See also -em-)

hemi-   *hēmi-* [Gr.] half. Cf. semi-. *hemi*ageusia

hen-   *heis, henos* [Gr.] one. Cf. un-. *hen*ogenesis

hepat-   *hēpar, hēpatos* [Gr.] liver. gastro*hepat*ic

hept(a)-   *hepta* [Gr.] seven. Cf. sept-[2]. *hept*atomic, *hepta*valent

hered-   *heres, heredis* [L.] heir. *here*doimmunity

hex-[1]   *hex* [Gr.] six. Cf. sex-. *hex*yl-. An *a* is added in some combinations

hex-[2]   *echō, hex-* [Gr.] (added to *s* becomes *hex-*) have, hold, be. ca*hex*ia

hexa-   See hex-[1]. *hexa*chromic

hidr-   *hidros* [Gr.] sweat. hyper*hidr*osis

hist-   *histos* [Gr.] web, tissue. *histo*dialysis

hod-   *hodos* [Gr.] road, path. *hodo*neuromere. (See also -od- and -ode[1])

hom-   *homos* [Gr.] common, same. *hom*omorphic

horm-   *ormē* [Gr.] impetus, impulse. *horm*one

hydat-   *hydōr, hydatos* [Gr.] water. *hydat*ism

hydr-   *hydōr, hydr-* [Gr.] water. Cf. lymph-. anclor*hydr*ia

hyp-   See hypo-. *hyp*axial

hyper-   *hyper* [Gr.] above, beyond, extreme. Cf. super-. *hyper*trophy

hypn-   *hypnos* [Gr.] sleep. *hypn*otic

hypo-   *hypo* [Gr.] (*o* is dropped before words beginning with a vowel) under, below. Cf. sub-. *hypo*metabolism

hyster-   *hystera* [Gr.] womb, colpo*hyster*opexy

iatr-   *iatros* [Gr.] physician. ped*iatr*ics

idi-   *idios* [Gr.] peculiar, separate, distinct. *idi*osyncrasy

il-   See in-[2,3]. *il*linition (in, on), *il*legible (negative prefix)

ile-   See ili- [ile- is commonly used to refer to the portion of the intestines known as the ileum]. *ile*ostomy

ili-   *ilium* (ileum) [L.] lower abdomen, intestines [ili- is commonly used to refer to the flaring part of the hipbone known as the ilium]. *ili*osacral

im- See in-.[2,3] *im*mersion (in, on), *im*perforation (negative prefix)

in-[1] *is, inos* [Gr.] fiber. Cf. fibr-. *in*osteatoma

in-[2] *in* [L.] (*n* changes to *l, m,* or *r* before words beginning with those consonants) in, on. Cf. en-. *in*sertion

in-[3] *in-* [L.] (*n* changes to *l, m,* or *r* before words beginning with those consonants) negative prefix. Cf. a-. *in*valid

infra- *infra* [L.] beneath. *infra*orbital

insul- *insula* [L.] island *insul*in

inter- *inter* [L.] among, between. *inter*carpal

intra- *intra* [L.] inside. Cf. end- and eso-. *intra*venous

ir- See in-.[2,3] *ir*radiation (in, on), *ir*reducible (negative prefix)

irid- *iris, iridos* [Gr.] rainbow, colored circle. kerato*irid*ocyclitis

is- *isos* [Gr.] equal. *is*otope

ischi- *ischion* [Gr.] hip, haunch, *ischi*opubic

jact- *iacio, iactus* [L.] throw. *jact*itation

-ject *iacio, -iectus* [L.] throw, in*ject*ion

jejun- *ieiunus* [L.] hungry, not partaking of food. gastro*jejun*ostomy

jug- *iugum* [L.] yoke. con*jug*ation

junct- *iungo, iunctus* [L.] yoke, join. con*junct*iva

kary- *karyon* [Gr.] nut, kernel, nucleus. Cf. nucle-. mega*kary*ocyte. (Also spelled cary-)

kerat- *keras, keratos* [Gr.] horn. *ker*atolysis. (Also spelled cerat-)

kil- *chilioi* [Gr.] one thousand. Cf. mill-. Indicates multiple in metric system. *Kil*ogram

kine- *kineō* [Gr.] move. *kine*matograph. (Also spelled cine-)

labi- *labium* [L.] lip. Cf. cheil-. gingivo*labi*al

lact- *lac, lactis* [L.] milk. Cf. galact-. gluco*lact*one

lal- *laleō* [Gr.] talk, babble. glosso*lal*ia

lapar- *lapara* [Gr.] flank. *lapar*otomy

laryng- *larynx, laryngos* [Gr.] windpipe, *laryng*endoscope

lat- *fero, latus* [L.] bear, carry. See -ferent. trans*lat*ion

later- *latus, lateris* [L.] side. ventro*later*al

lent- *lens, lentis* [L.] lentil. Cf. phac-. *lent*iconus

lep- *lambanō, lēp-* [Gr.] take, seize. cata*lep*tic

leuc- See leuk-. *leuc*inuria

leuk- *leukos* [Gr.] white. Cf. alb-. *leuk*orrhea. (Also spelled leuc-)

lien- *lien* [L.] spleen. Cf. splen-. *lien*ocele

lig- *ligo* [L.] tie, bind. *lig*ate

lingu- *lingua* [L.] tongue. Cf. gloss-. sub*lingu*al

lip- *lipos* [Gr.] fat. Cf. adip-. glyco*lip*in

lith- *lithos* [Gr.] stone. Cf. calc-.[1] nephro*lith*otomy

loc- *locus* [L.] place. Cf. top-. *loc*omotion

log- *legō, log-* [Gr.] speak, give an account. *log*orrhea, embry*olog*y

lumb- *lumbus* [L.] loin, dorso*lumb*ar

lute- *luteus* [L.] yellow. Cf. xanth-. *lute*oma

ly- *lyō* [Gr.] loose, dissolve. Cf. solut-. kerato*ly*sis

lymph- *lympha* [Gr.] water. Cf. hydr-. *lymph*adenosis

macr- *makros* [Gr.] long, large. *macr*omyeloblast

mal- *malus* [L.] bad, abnormal. Cf. cac- and dys-. *mal*function

malac- *malakos* [Gr.] soft, osteoma*lac*ia

mamm- *mamma* [L.] breast. Cf. mast-. sub*mamm*ary

man- *manus* [L.] hand. Cf. cheir-. *man*iphalanx

mani- *mania* [Gr.] mental aberration. *mani*graphy, klepto*mani*a

mast- *mastos* [Gr.] breast. Cf. mamm-. hyper*mast*ia

medi- *medius* [L.] middle. Cf. mes-. *medi*frontal

mega- *megas* [Gr.] great, large. Also indicates multiple (1,000,000) in metric system. *mega*colon, *mega*dyne. (see also megal-)

megal- *megas, megalou* [Gr.] great, large, acro*megal*y

mel- *melos* [Gr.] limb, member. sym*mel*ia

melan- *melas, melanos* [Gr.] black. hippo*melan*in

men- *mēn* [Gr.] month. dys*men*orrhea

mening- *mēninx, mēningos* [Gr.] membrane. encephalo*mening*itis

ment-   *mens, mentis* [L.] mind. Cf. phren-, psych-, and thym-. de*ment*ia

mer-   *meros* [Gr.] part. poly*mer*ic

mes-   *mesos* [Gr.] middle. Cf. medi-. *mes*oderm

met-   See meta-. *met*allergy

meta-   *meta* [Gr.] (*a* is dropped before words beginning with a vowel) after, beyond, accompanying, *meta*carpal

metr-¹   *metron* [Gr.] measure. stereo*metr*y

metr-²   *metra* [Gr.] womb. endo*metr*itis

micr-   *mikros* [Gr.] small. photo*micr*ograph

mill-   *mille* [L.] one thousand. Cf. kil-. Indicates fraction in metric system. *mill*igram, *mill*ipede

miss-   See -mittent. intro*miss*ion

-mittent   *mitto, mittentis, missus* [L.] send. inter*mittent*

mne-   *mimnērcō, mnē-* [Gr.] remember. pseudoa*mne*sia

mon-   *monos* [Gr.] only, sole. *mon*oplegia

morph-   *morphē* [Gr.] form, shape. poly*morph*onuclear

mot-   *moveo, motus* [L.] move. vaso*mot*or

my-   *mys, myos* [Gr.] muscle. ino*my*leio*my*oma

-myces   *mykēs, mykētos* [Gr.] fungus. myelo*myces*

myc(et)-   See -myces. asco*mycet*es, strepto*myc*in

myel-   *myelos* [Gr.] marrow. polio*myel*itis

myx-   *myxa* [Gr.] mucus. *myx*edema

narc-   *narkē* [Gr.] numbness. topo*narc*osis

nas-   *nasus* [L.] nose. Cf. rhin-. palato*nas*al

ne-   *neos* [Gr.] new, young. *ne*ocyte

necr-   *nekros* [Gr.] corpse. *necr*ocytosis

nephr-   *nephros* [Gr.] kidney. Cf. ren-. para*nephr*ic

neur-   *neuron* [Gr.] nerve. esthesio*neur*e

nod-   *nodus* [L.] knot. *nod*osity

nom-   *nomos* [Gr.] (from *nemō* deal out, distribute) law, custom. taxo*nom*y

non-   *nona* [L.] nine. *non*acosane

nos-   *nosos* [Gr.] disease. *nos*ology

nucle-   *nucleus* [L.] (from *nux, nucis* nut) kernel. Cf. kary-. *nucle*ide

nutri-   *nutrio* [L.] nourish. mal*nutri*tion

ob-   *ob* [L.] (*b* changes to *c* before words beginning with that consonant) against, toward, etc. *ob*tuse

oc-   See ob-. *oc*clude

ocul-   *oculus* [L.] eye. Cf. ophthalm-. *ocul*omotor

-od-   See -ode¹. peri*od*ic

-ode¹   *hodos* [Gr.] road, path. cath*ode*. (See also hod-)

-ode²   See -oid. nemat*ode*

odont-   *odous, odontos* [Gr.] tooth. Cf. dent-. orth*odont*ia

-odyn-   *odynē* [Gr.] pain, distress. gastr*odyn*ia

-oid   *eidos* [Gr.] form. Cf. -form. hy*oid*

-ol   See ole-. cholester*ol*

ole-   *oleum* [L.] oil. *ole*oresin

olig-   *oligos* [Gr.] few, small. *olig*ospermia

omphal-   *omphalos* [Gr.] navel. peri*omphal*ic

onc-   *onkos* [Gr.] bulk, mass. hemat*onc*ometry

onych-   *onyx, onychos* [Gr.] claw, nail. an*onych*ia

oo-   *ōon* [Gr.] egg. Cf. ov-. peri*oo*thecitis

op-   *haraō, op-* [Gr.] see. erythr*op*sia

ophthalm-   *ophthalmos* [Gr.] eye. Cf. ocul-. ex*ophthalm*ic

or-   *os, oris* [L.] mouth. Cf. stom(at)-. intra*or*al

orb-   *orbis* [L.] circle. sub*orb*ital

orchi-   *orchis* [Gr.] testicle. Cf. test-. *orchi*opathy

organ-   *organon* [Gr.] implement, instrument. *organ*oleptic

orth-   *orthos* [Gr.] straight, right, normal. *orth*opedics

oss-   *os, ossis* [L.] bone. Cf. ost(e)-. *oss*iphone

ost(e)-   *osteon* [Gr.] bone. Cf. oss-. en*ost*osis, *oste*anaphysis

ot-   *ous, ōtos* [Gr.] ear. Cf. aur-. par*ot*id

ov-   *ovum* [L.] egg. Cf. oo-. syno*v*ia

oxy-   *oxys* [Gr.] sharp. *oxy*cephalic

pachy(n)-   *pachynō* [Gr.] thicken. *pachy*derma, myo*pachyn*sis

pag-   *pēgnymi, pag-* [Gr.] fix, make fast. thoraco*pag*us

par-¹   *pario* [L.] bear, give birth to. primi*par*ous

par-²   See para-. *par*epigastric

para-   *para* [Gr.] (final *a* is dropped before words beginning with a vowel) beside, beyond, *para*mastoid

part-   *pario, partus* [L.] bear, give birth to. par*turition*

path-   *pathos* [Gr.] that which one undergoes, sickness. psycho*path*ic

pec-   *pēgnymi, pēg-* [Gr.] (*pēk-* before *t*) fix, make fast. sym*pec*tothiene. (See also pex-)

ped-   *pais, paidos* [Gr.] child. ortho*ped*ic

pell-   *pellis* [L.] skin, hide. *pell*agra

-pellent   *pello, pellentis, pulsus* [L.] drive. re*pellent*

pen-   *penomai* [Gr.] need, lack, erythrocyto*pen*ia

pend-   *pendeo* [L.] hang down. ap*pend*ix

pent(a)-   *pente* [Gr.] five. Cf. quinque-. *pent*ose, *penta*ploid

peps-   *peptō, peps-* [Gr.] digest. brady*peps*ia

pept-   *peptō* [Gr.] digest. brady*pept*sia

per-   *per* [L.] through. Cf. dia-. *per*nasal

peri-   *peri* [Gr.] around. Cf. circum-. *peri*phery

pet-   *peto* [L.] seek, tend toward. centri*pet*al

pex-   *pēgnumi, pēg-* [Gr.] (added to *s* becomes *pēx*), fix, make fast. hepato*pex*y

pha-   *phēmi, pha-* [Gr.] say, speak. dys*pha*sia

phac-   *phakos* [Gr.] lentil, lens. Cf. lent-. *phac*osclerosis. (Also spelled phak-)

phag-   *phagein* [Gr.] eat. lipo*phag*ic

phak-   See phac-. *phak*itis

phan-   See phen-. dia*phan*oscopy

pharmac-   *pharmakon* [Gr.] drug. *pharmac*ognosy

pharyng-   *pharynx, pharyng-* [Gr.] throat, glosso*pharyng*eal

phen-   *phainō, phan-* [Gr.] show, be seen. phos*phen*e

pher-   *pherō, phor-* [Gr.] bear, support. peri*pher*y

phil-   *phileō* [Gr.] like, have affinity for. eosino*phil*ia

phleb-   *phleps, phlebos* [Gr.] vein. peri*phleb*itis

phleg-   *phlogō, phlog-* [Gr.] burn, inflame, adeno*phleg*mon

phlog-   See phleg-. anti*phlog*istic

phob-   *phobos* [Gr.] fear, dread. claustro*phob*ia

phon-   *phōne* [Gr.] sound. echo*phon*y

phor-   See pher-. Cf. -ferent. exo*phor*ia

phos-   See phot-. *phos*phorus

phot-   *phōs, phōtos* [Gr.] light. *phot*erythrous

phrag-   *phrassō, phrag-* [Gr.] fence, wall off, stop up. Cf. sept-[1]. dia*phrag*m

phrax-   *phrassō, phrag-* [Gr.] (added to *s* becomes *phrax-*) fence, wall off, stop up. em-*phrax*is

phren-   *phrēn* [Gr.] mind, midriff. Cf. ment-. meta*phren*ia, meta*phren*on

phthi-   *phthinō* [Gr.] decay, waste away. *phthi*sis

phy-   *phyō* [Gr.] beget, bring forth, produce, be by nature. noso*phy*te

phyl-   *phylon* [Gr.] tribe, kind. *phyl*ogeny

-phyll   *phyllon* [Gr.] leaf. xantho*phyll*

phylac-   *phylax* [Gr.] guard. pro*phylac*tic

phys(a)-   *physaō* [Gr.] blow, inflate. *phys*ocele, *physa*lis

physe-   *physaō, physē-* [Gr.] blow, inflate. em*physe*ma

pil-   *pilus* [L.] hair. epi*pil*ation

pituit-   *pituita* [L.] phlegm, rheum. *pituit*ous

placent-   *placenta* [L.] (from *plakous* [Gr.]) cake. extra*placent*al

plas-   *plassō* [Gr.] mold, shape. cine*plas*ty

platy-   *platys* [Gr.] broad, flat. *platy*rrhine

pleg-   *plēssō* [Gr.] strike. di*pleg*ia

plet-   *pleo, -pletus* [L.] fill. de*plet*ion

pleur-   *pleura* [Gr.] rib, side. Cf. cost-. peri*pleur*al

plex-   *plēssō, plēg-* (added to *s* becomes *plēx-*) strike, apo*plex*y

plic-   *plico* [L.] fold. com*plic*ation

pne-   *pneuma, pneumatos* [Gr.] breathing. traumato*pne*a

pneum(at)-   *pneuma, pneumatos* [Gr.] breath, air. *pneum*odynamics, *pneumat*othorax

pneumo(n)-   *pneumōn* [Gr.] lung. Cf. pulmo(n)-. *pneumo*centesis, *pneumon*otomy

pod-   *pous, podos* [Gr.] foot. *pod*iatry

poie-   *poieō* [Gr.] make, produce. Cf. -facient. sarco*poie*tic

pol-   *polos* [Gr.] axis of a sphere. peri*pol*ar

poly-   *polys* [Gr.] much, many. *poly*spermia

pont-   *pons, pontis* [L.] bridge, *pont*ocerebellar

por-[1]   *poros* [Gr.] passage. myelo*por*e

por-²   *pōros* [Gr.] callus. *por*ocele

posit-   *pono, positus* [L.] put, place. re*posit*or

post-   *post* [L.] after, behind in time or place. *post*natal, *post*oral

pre-   *prae* [L.] before in time or place. *pre*natal, *pre*vesical

press-   *premo, pressus* [L.] press. *press*oreceptive

pro-   *pro* [Gr.] or *pro* [L.] before in time or place. *pro*gamous, *pro*cheilon, *pro*lapse

proct-   *prōktos* [Gr.] anus. entero*proct*ia

prosop-   *prosōpon* [Gr.] face. Cf. faci-. di*prosop*us

pseud-   *pseudēs* [Gr.] false. *pseudo*paraplegia

psych-   *psychē* [Gr.] soul, mind. Cf. ment-. *psych*osomatic

pto-   *piptō, ptō-* [Gr.] fall. nephro*pto*sis

pub-   *pubes* and *puber, puberis* [L.] adult. ischio*pub*ic. (See also puber-)

puber-   *puber* [L.] adult. *puber*ty

pulmo(n)-   *pulmo, plumonis* [L.] lung. Cf. pneumo(n)-. *pulmo*lith, cardio*pulmon*ary

puls-   *pello, pellentis, pulsus* [L.] drive. pro*puls*ion

punct-   *pungo, punctus* [L.] prick, pierce. Cf. cente-. *puncti*form

pur-   *pus, puris* [L.] pus. Cf. py-. sup*pur*ation

py-   *pyon* [Gr.] pus. Cf. pur-. nephro*py*osis

pyel-   *pyelos* [Gr.] trough, basin, pelvis, nephro*pyel*itis

pyl-   *pylē* [Gr.] door, orifice. *pyl*ephlebitis

pyr-   *pyr* [Gr.] fire. Cf. febr-. galacto*pyr*a

quadr-   *quadr-* [L.] four. Cf. tetra-. *quadr*igeminal

quinque-   *quinque* [L.] five. Cf. pent(a)-. *quinque*cuspid

rachi-   *rachis* [Gr.] spine. Cf. spin-. encephalo*rachi*dian

radi-   *radius* [L.] ray. Cf. actin-. ir*radi*ation

re-   *re-* [L.] back, again. *re*traction

ren-   *renes* [L.] kidneys. Cf. nephr-. ad*ren*al

ret-   *rete* [L.] net. *ret*othelium

retro-   *retro* [L.] backwards. *retro*deviation

rhag-   *rhēgnymi, rhag-* [Gr.] break, burst. hemor*rhag*ic

rhaph-   *rhaphē* [Gr.] suture. gastror*rhaph*y

rhe-   *rhaphē* [Gr.] flow. Cf. flu-. diar*rhe*al

rhex-   *rhēgnymi, rhēg-* [Gr.] (added to *s* becomes *rhēx*) break, burst, metror*rhex*is

rhin-   *rhis, rhinos* [Gr.] nose. Cf. nas-. basi*rhin*al

rot-   *rota* [L.] wheel. *rot*ator

rub(r)-   *rubber, rubri* [L.] red. Cf. erythr-. bili*rub*in, *rubr*ospinal

salping-   *salpinx, salpingos* [Gr.] tube, trumpet. *salping*itis

sanguin-   *sanguis, sanguinis* [L.] blood, Cf. hem(at)-. *sanguin*eous

sarc-   *sarx, sarkos* [Gr.] flesh. *sar*coma

schis-   *schizō, schid-* [Gr.] (before *t* or added to *s* becomes *schis*-) split. Cf. fiss-. *schis*torachis, rachi*schis*is

scler-   *sklēros* [Gr.] hard. Cf. dur-. *scler*osis

scop-   *skopeō* [Gr.] look at, observe. endo*scope*

sect-   *seco, sectus* [L.] cut. Cf. tom-. *sect*ile

semi-   *semi* [L.] half. Cf. hemi-. *semi*flexion

sens-   *sentio, sensus* [L.] perceive, feel. Cf. esthe-. *sens*ory

sep-   *sepō* [Gr.] rot, decay. *sep*sis

sept-¹   *saepio, saeptus* [L.] fence, wall off, stop up. Cf. phrag-. naso*sept*al

sept-²   *septem* [L.] seven. Cf. hept(a)-. *sept*an

ser-   *serum* [L.] whey, watery substance. *sero*synovitis

sex-   *sex* [L.] six. Cf. hex-¹. *sex*digitate

sial-   *sialon* [Gr.] saliva. poly*sial*ia

sin-   *sinus* [L.] hollow, fold. Cf. colp-. *sin*obronchitis

sit-   *sitos* [Gr.] food. para*sit*ic

solut-   *solvo, solventis, solutus* [L.] loose, dissolve, set free. Cf. ly-. dis*solut*ion

-solvent   See solut-. Dis*solvent*

somat-   *sōma, somatos* [Gr.] body. Cf. corpor-. psycho*somat*ic

-some   See somat-. dictyo*some*

spas-   *spaō, spas-* [Gr.] draw, pull. *spas*m, *spas*tic

spectr-   *spectrum* [L.] appearance, what is seen. micro*spectr*oscope

sperm(at)-   *sperma, spermatos* [Gr.] seed. *sperma*crasia. *spermat*ozoon

spers-   *spargo, -spersus* [L.] scatter. di*spers*ion

sphen-   *sphēn* [Gr.] wedge. Cf. cune-. *sphen*oid

spher-	*sphaira* [Gr.] ball. hemi*sphere*
sphygm-	*sphygmos* [Gr.] pulsation. *sphygm*omanometer
spin-	*spina* [L.] spine. Cf. rachi-. cerebro*spin*al
spirat-	*spiro, spiratus* [L.] breathe. in*spirat*ory
splanchn-	*splanchna* [Gr.] entrails, viscera. neuro*splanchn*ic
splen-	*splēn* [Gr.] spleen. Cf. lien-. *splen*omegaly
spor-	*sporos* [Gr.] seed. *spor*ophyte, zygo*spor*e
squam-	*squama* [L.] scale. de*squam*ation
sta-	*histēmi, sta-* [Gr.] make stand, stop. genesi*sta*sis
stal-	*stellō, stal-* [Gr.] send. peri*stal*sis. (See also stol-)
staphyl-	*staphylē* [Gr.] bunch of grapes, uvula. *staphyl*ococcus, *staphyl*ectomy
stear-	*stear, steatos* [Gr.] fat. Cf. adip-. *stear*odermia
steat-	See stear-. *steat*opygous
sten-	*stenos* [Gr.] narrow, compressed. *sten*ocardia
ster-	*stereos* [Gr.] solid. chole*ster*ol
sterc-	*stercus* [L.] dung. Cf. copr-. *sterc*oporphyrin
sthen-	*sthenos* [Gr.] strength. a*sthen*ia
stol-	*stellō, stol-* [Gr.] send. dia*stol*e
stom(at)-	*stoma, stomatos* [Gr.] mouth, orifice. Cf. or-. ana*stom*osis, *stomat*ogastric
strep(h)-	*strephō, strep-* (before *t*) [Gr.] twist. Cf. tors-. *streph*osymbolia. *strep*tomycin. (See also stroph-)
strict-	*stringo, stringentis, strictus* [L.] draw tight, compress, cause pain. con*strict*ion
-stringent	See strict-. a*stringent*
stroph-	*strephō, stroph-* [Gr.] twist. ana*stroph*ic. (See also strep(h)-)
struct-	*struo, structus* [L.] pile up (against). ob*struct*ion
sub-	*sub* [L.] (*b* changes to *f* or *p* before words beginning with those consonants) under, below. Cf. hypo-. *sub*lumbar
suf-	See sub-. *suf*fusion
sup-	See sub-. *sup*pository
super-	*super* [L.] above, beyond, extreme. Cf. hyper-. *super*motility
sy-	See syn-. *sy*stole
syl-	See syn-. *syl*lepsiology
sym-	See syn-. *sym*biosis, *sym*metry, *sym*pathetic, *sym*physis
syn-	*syn* [Gr.] (*n* disappears before *s*, changes to *l* before *l*, and changes to *m* before *b, m, p,* and *ph*) with, together. Cf. con-. myo*syn*izesis
ta-	See ton-. *ta*ectasis
tac-	*tassō, tag-* [Gr.] (*tak*-before *t*) order, arrange. a*tac*tic
tact-	*tango, tactus* [L.] touch. con*tact*
tax-	*tassō, tag-* [Gr.] (added to *s* becomes *tax*-) order, arrange. a*tax*ia
tect-	See teg-. pro*tect*ive
teg-	*tego, tectus* [L.] cover. in*teg*ument
tel-	*telos* [Gr.] end. *tel*osynapsis
tele-	*tēle* [Gr.] at a distance. *tele*ceptor
tempor-	*tempus, temporis* [L.] time, timely or fatal spot, temple. *tempor*omalar
ten(ont)-	*tenōn, tenontos* [Gr.] (from *teinō* stretch) tight stretched band. *ten*odynia, *tenon*itis, *tenont*agra
tens-	*tendo, tensus* [L.] stretch. Cf. ton-. ex*tens*or
test-	*testis* [L.] testicle. Cf. orchi-. *test*itis
tetra-	*tetra-* [Gr.] four. Cf. quadr-. *tetra*genous
the-	*tithēmi, thē-* [Gr.] put, place. syn*the*sis
thec-	*thēkē* [Gr.] repository, case. *thec*ostegnosis
thel-	*thēlē* [Gr.] teat, nipple. *thel*erethism
therap-	*therapeia* [Gr.] treatment. hydro*therap*y
therm-	*thermē* [Gr.] heat. Cf. calor-. dia*therm*y
thi-	*theion* [Gr.] sulfur. *thi*ogenic
thorac-	*thōrax, thōrakos* [Gr.] chest. *thorac*oplasty
thromb-	*thrombos* [Gr.] lump, clot. *thromb*openia
thym-	*thymos* [Gr.] spirit. Cf. ment-. dys*thym*ia
thyr-	*thyreos* [Gr.] shield (shaped like a door *thyra*). *thyr*oid
tme-	*temnō, tmē-* [Gr.] cut. axonot*me*sis
toc-	*tokos* [Gr.] childbirth. dys*toc*ia
tom-	*temnō, tom-* [Gr.] cut. Cf. sect-. appendec*tom*y
ton-	*teino, ton-* [Gr.] stretch, put under tension. Cf. tens-. peri*ton*eum

top- *topos* [Gr.] place. Cf. loc-. *top*esthesia

tors- *torqueo, torsus* [L.] twist. Cf. strep-. ec*tors*ion

tox- *toxicon* [Gr.] (from *toxon* bow) arrow poison, poison. *tox*emia

trache- *tracheia* [Gr.] windpipe. *tra-cheo*tomy

trachel- *trachēlos* [Gr.] neck. Cf. cervic-. *trachel*opexy

tract- *traho, tractus* [L.] draw, drag. pro*tract*ion

traumat- *trauma, traumatos* [Gr.] wound. *traumat*ic

tri- *treis, tria* [Gr.] or *tri-* [L.] three. *tri*gonid

trich- *thrix, trichos* [Gr.] hair. *trich*oid

trip- *tribō* [Gr.] rub. en*trip*sis

trop- *trepō, trop-* [Gr.] turn, react. sito*trop*ism

troph- *trepō, troph-* [Gr.] nurture. a*troph*y

tuber- *tuber* [L.] swelling, node. *tuber*cle

typ- *typos* [Gr.] (from *typto* strike) type. a*typ*ical

typh- *typhos* [Gr.] fog, stupor. adeno*typh*us

typhl- *typhlos* [Gr.] blind. Cf. cec-. *typhl*ectasis

un- *unus* [L.] one. Cf. hen-. *uni*oval

ur- *ouron* [Gr.] urine. poly*ur*ia

vacc- *vacca* [L.] cow. *vacc*ine

vagin- *vagina* [L.] sheath. in*vagi-n*ated

vas- *vas* [L.] vessel. Cf. angi-. *vas*cular

vers- See vert-. in*vers*ion

vert- *verto, versus* [L.] turn. di*vert*iculum

vesic- *vesica* [L.] bladder. Cf. cyst-. *vesic*ovaginal

vit- *vita* [L.] life. Cf. bi-[1]. de*vit*alize

vuls- *vello, vulsus* [L.] pull, twitch. con*vuls*ion

xanth- *xanthos* [Gr.] yellow, blond. Cf. flav- and lute-. *xantho*phyll

-yl- *hyle* [Gr.] substance. cacod*yl*

zo- *zoē* [Gr.] life, *zōon* [Gr.] animal. micro*zo*aria

zyg- *zygon* [Gr.] yoke, union. *zyg*odactyly

zym- *zymē* [Gr.] ferment. en*zym*e

THE HUMAN BODY
Highlights of Structure and Function
SKELETAL SYSTEM

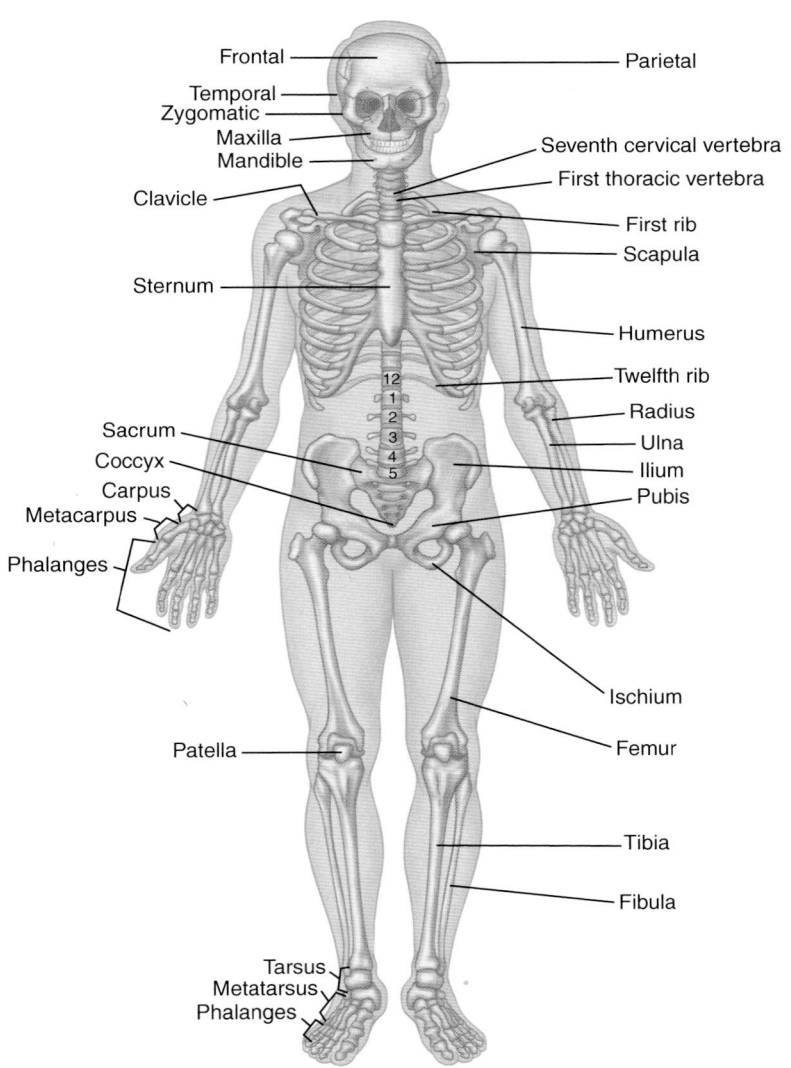

Frontal — Parietal

Temporal —
Zygomatic —
Maxilla —
Mandible —

Seventh cervical vertebra
First thoracic vertebra

Clavicle —
First rib
Scapula

Sternum —
Humerus
Twelfth rib

12
1
2
3
4
5

Sacrum —
Coccyx —
Carpus —
Metacarpus —
Phalanges —

Radius
Ulna
Ilium
Pubis

Ischium
Femur

Patella —
Tibia
Fibula

Tarsus —
Metatarsus —
Phalanges —

PLATE 1 ■ ANTERIOR VIEW OF THE HUMAN SKELETON

SKELETAL SYSTEM Continued

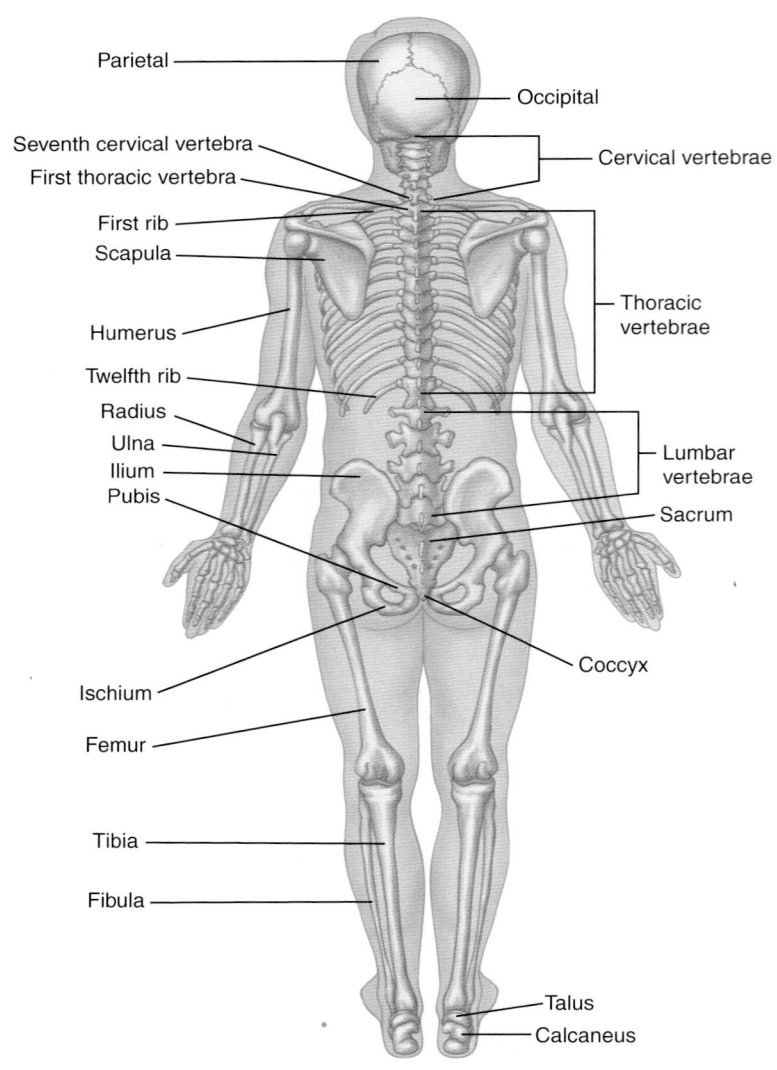

Parietal

Occipital

Seventh cervical vertebra

First thoracic vertebra

Cervical vertebrae

First rib

Scapula

Humerus

Thoracic vertebrae

Twelfth rib

Radius

Ulna

Ilium

Lumbar vertebrae

Pubis

Sacrum

Ischium

Coccyx

Femur

Tibia

Fibula

Talus

Calcaneus

PLATE 2 ■ POSTERIOR VIEW OF THE HUMAN SKELETON

SKELETAL SYSTEM Continued

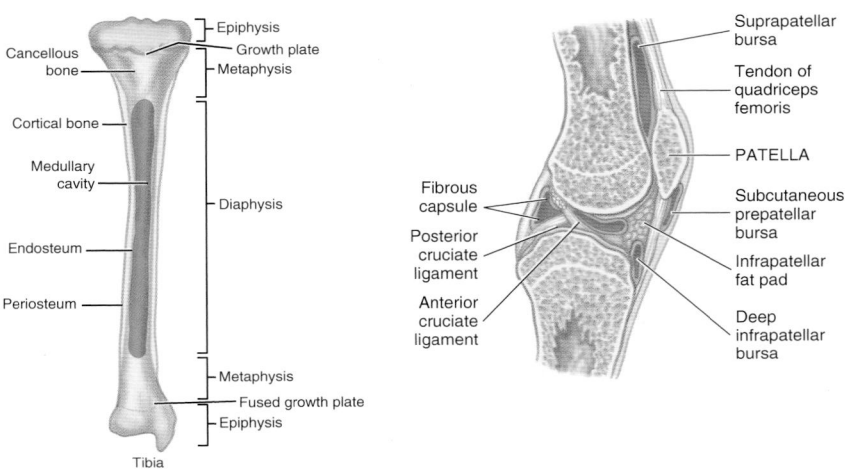

Epiphysis
Growth plate
Metaphysis
Cancellous bone
Cortical bone
Medullary cavity
Endosteum
Periosteum
Diaphysis
Metaphysis
Fused growth plate
Epiphysis
Tibia

Suprapatellar bursa
Tendon of quadriceps femoris
PATELLA
Fibrous capsule
Subcutaneous prepatellar bursa
Posterior cruciate ligament
Infrapatellar fat pad
Anterior cruciate ligament
Deep infrapatellar bursa

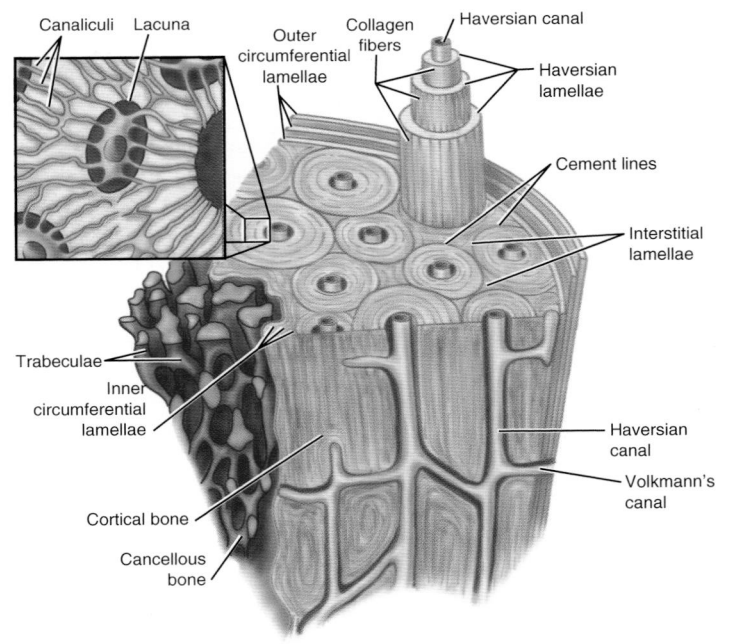

Canaliculi   Lacuna
Outer circumferential lamellae
Collagen fibers
Haversian canal
Haversian lamellae
Cement lines
Interstitial lamellae
Trabeculae
Inner circumferential lamellae
Haversian canal
Volkmann's canal
Cortical bone
Cancellous bone

Sector of the shaft of a long bone,
showing cortical and cancellous bone

PLATE 3 ■ STRUCTURE OF THE BONE

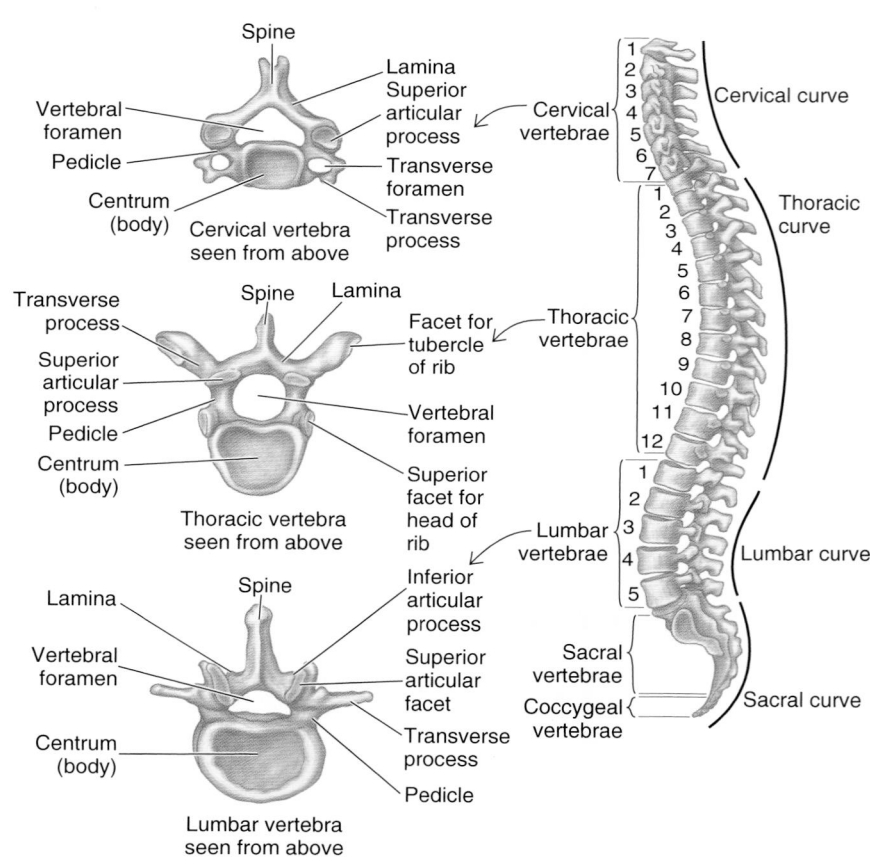

Spine

Lamina
Superior
articular
process

Vertebral
foramen

Pedicle

Centrum
(body)

Transverse
foramen

Transverse
process

Cervical vertebra
seen from above

Cervical
vertebrae

Cervical curve

Transverse
process

Superior
articular
process

Pedicle

Centrum
(body)

Spine   Lamina

Facet for
tubercle
of rib

Vertebral
foramen

Superior
facet for
head of
rib

Thoracic vertebra
seen from above

Thoracic
vertebrae

Thoracic
curve

Lamina

Vertebral
foramen

Centrum
(body)

Spine

Inferior
articular
process

Superior
articular
facet

Transverse
process

Pedicle

Lumbar vertebra
seen from above

Lumbar
vertebrae

Sacral
vertebrae

Coccygeal
vertebrae

Lumbar curve

Sacral curve

PLATE 4 ▪ STRUCTURE OF THE SPINE

INTEGUMENTARY SYSTEM

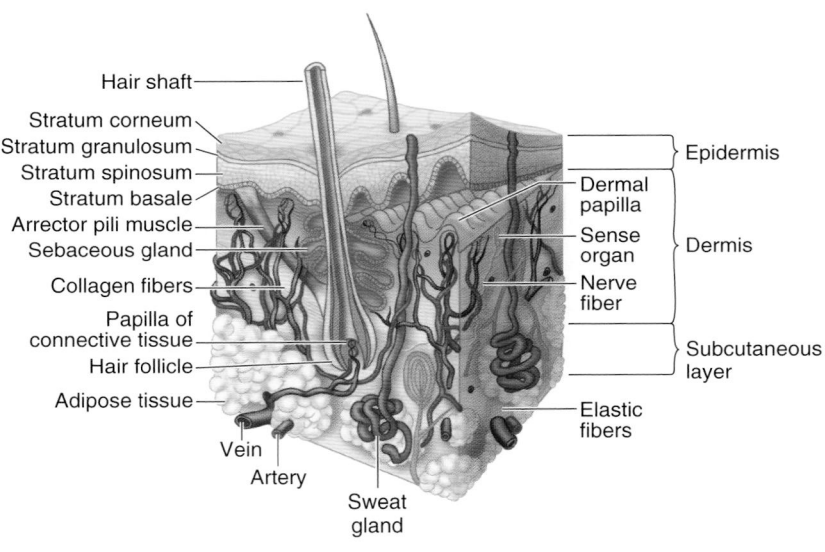

Hair shaft

Stratum corneum
Stratum granulosum
Stratum spinosum
Stratum basale
} Epidermis

Arrector pili muscle
Sebaceous gland

Dermal papilla
Sense organ
Nerve fiber
} Dermis

Collagen fibers

Papilla of connective tissue
Hair follicle

Adipose tissue

} Subcutaneous layer

Vein
Artery

Elastic fibers

Sweat gland

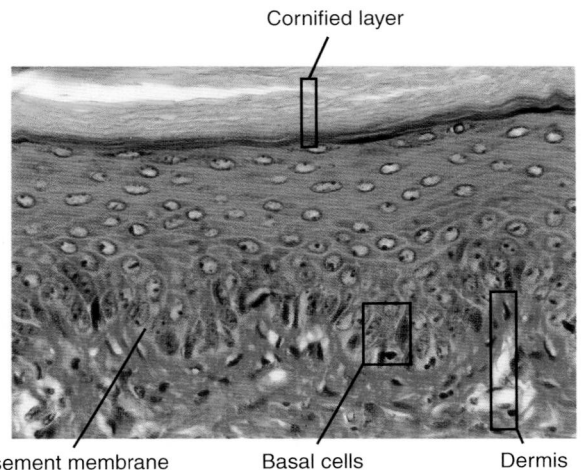

Cornified layer

Basement membrane   Basal cells   Dermis

PLATE 5 ■ SKIN

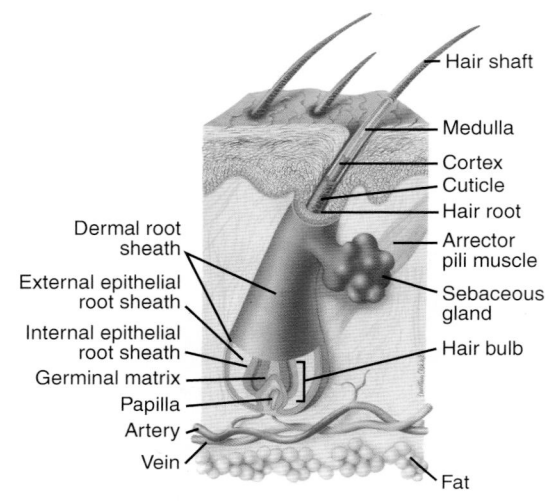

Hair shaft
Medulla
Cortex
Cuticle
Hair root
Arrector pili muscle
Sebaceous gland
Hair bulb
Fat

Dermal root sheath
External epithelial root sheath
Internal epithelial root sheath
Germinal matrix
Papilla
Artery
Vein

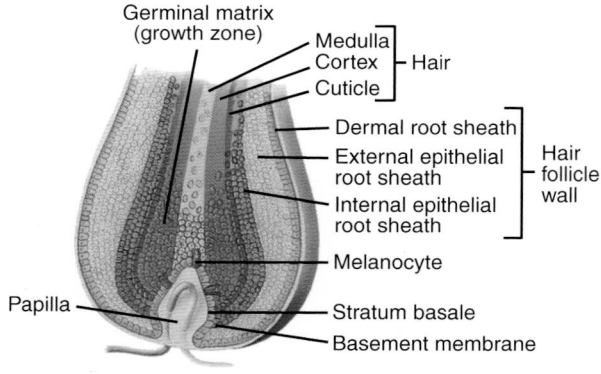

Germinal matrix (growth zone)

Medulla
Cortex } Hair
Cuticle

Dermal root sheath
External epithelial root sheath
Internal epithelial root sheath
} Hair follicle wall

Melanocyte

Papilla
Stratum basale
Basement membrane

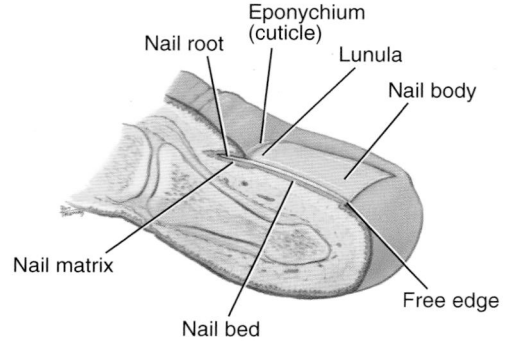

Eponychium (cuticle)
Nail root
Lunula
Nail body
Nail matrix
Free edge
Nail bed

PLATE 6 ■ HAIR AND NAIL

MUSCLE SYSTEM

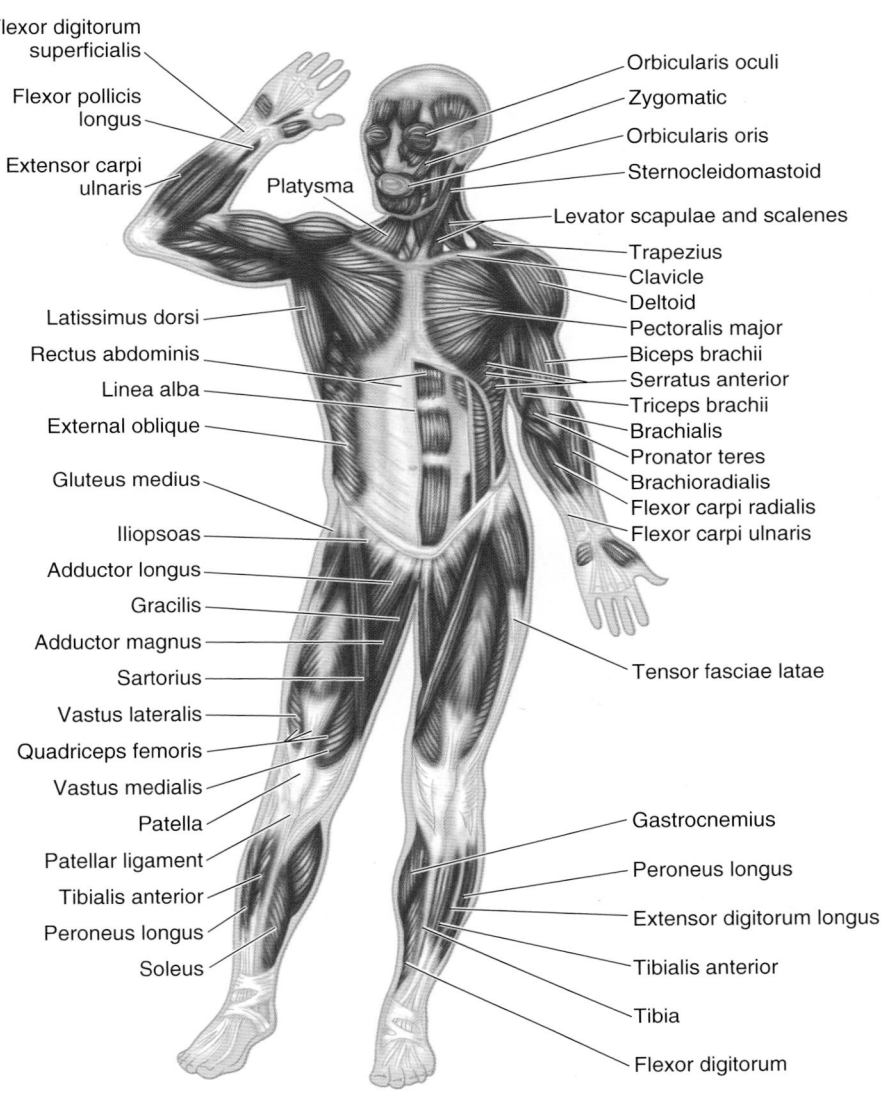

Flexor digitorum superficialis
Flexor pollicis longus
Extensor carpi ulnaris
Platysma
Latissimus dorsi
Rectus abdominis
Linea alba
External oblique
Gluteus medius
Iliopsoas
Adductor longus
Gracilis
Adductor magnus
Sartorius
Vastus lateralis
Quadriceps femoris
Vastus medialis
Patella
Patellar ligament
Tibialis anterior
Peroneus longus
Soleus

Orbicularis oculi
Zygomatic
Orbicularis oris
Sternocleidomastoid
Levator scapulae and scalenes
Trapezius
Clavicle
Deltoid
Pectoralis major
Biceps brachii
Serratus anterior
Triceps brachii
Brachialis
Pronator teres
Brachioradialis
Flexor carpi radialis
Flexor carpi ulnaris
Tensor fasciae latae
Gastrocnemius
Peroneus longus
Extensor digitorum longus
Tibialis anterior
Tibia
Flexor digitorum

PLATE 7 ■ ANTERIOR SUPERFICIAL MUSCLES

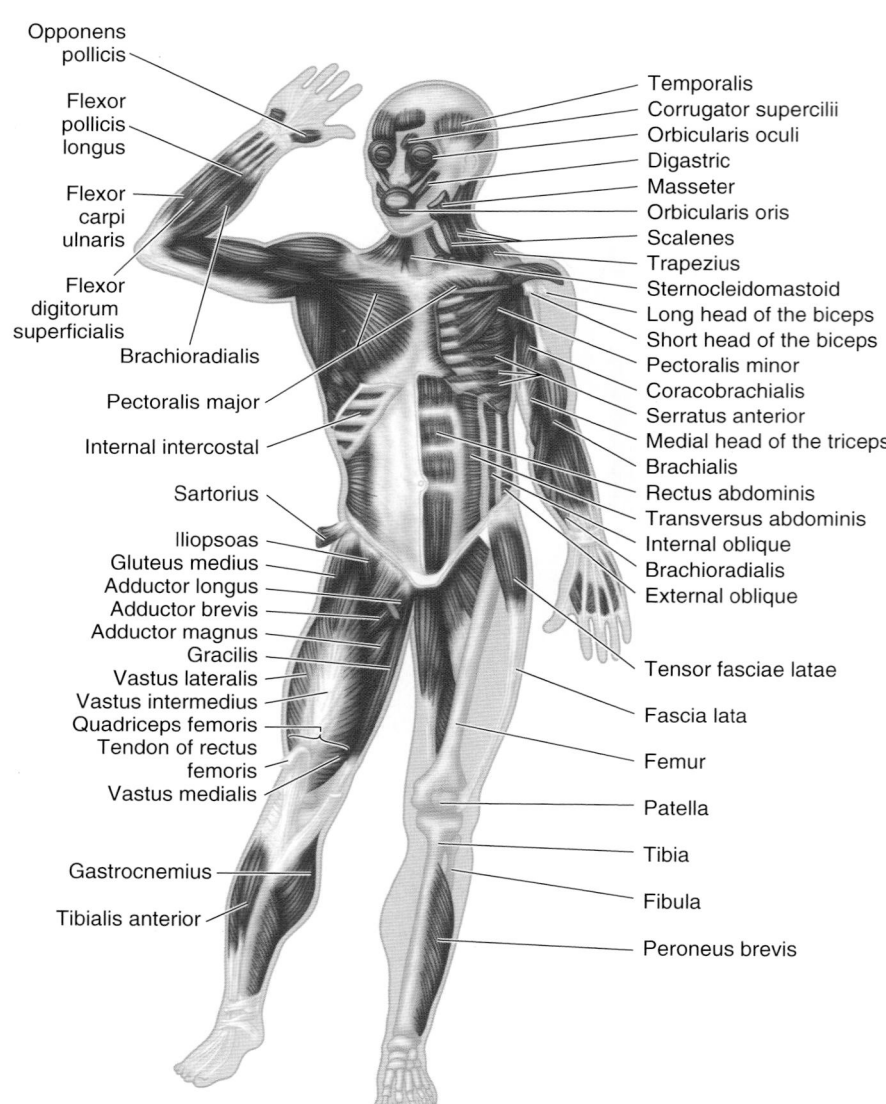

Opponens pollicis

Flexor pollicis longus

Flexor carpi ulnaris

Flexor digitorum superficialis

Brachioradialis

Pectoralis major

Internal intercostal

Sartorius

Iliopsoas

Gluteus medius

Adductor longus

Adductor brevis

Adductor magnus

Gracilis

Vastus lateralis

Vastus intermedius

Quadriceps femoris

Tendon of rectus femoris

Vastus medialis

Gastrocnemius

Tibialis anterior

Temporalis

Corrugator supercilii

Orbicularis oculi

Digastric

Masseter

Orbicularis oris

Scalenes

Trapezius

Sternocleidomastoid

Long head of the biceps

Short head of the biceps

Pectoralis minor

Coracobrachialis

Serratus anterior

Medial head of the triceps

Brachialis

Rectus abdominis

Transversus abdominis

Internal oblique

Brachioradialis

External oblique

Tensor fasciae latae

Fascia lata

Femur

Patella

Tibia

Fibula

Peroneus brevis

PLATE 8 ■ ANTERIOR DEEP MUSCLES

MUSCLE SYSTEM Continued

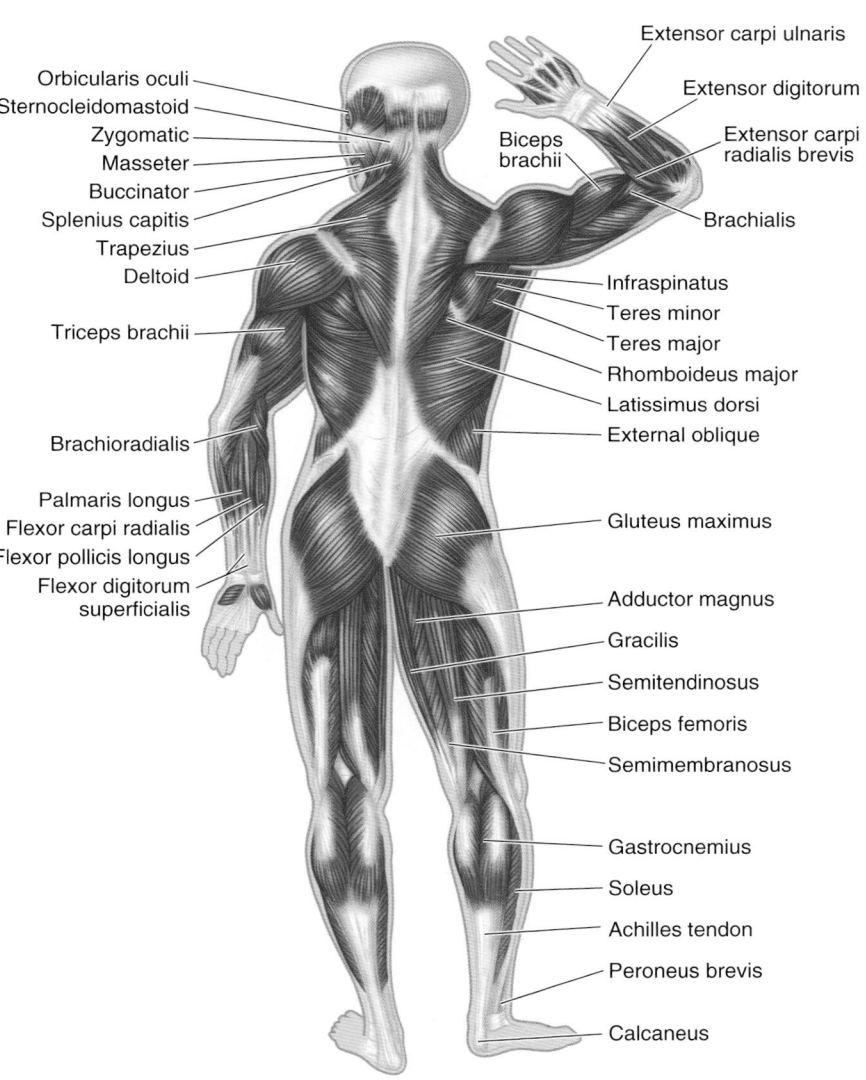

Orbicularis oculi
Sternocleidomastoid
Zygomatic
Masseter
Buccinator
Splenius capitis
Trapezius
Deltoid

Triceps brachii

Brachioradialis

Palmaris longus
Flexor carpi radialis
Flexor pollicis longus
Flexor digitorum
superficialis

Extensor carpi ulnaris
Extensor digitorum
Extensor carpi
radialis brevis
Biceps
brachii
Brachialis

Infraspinatus
Teres minor
Teres major
Rhomboideus major
Latissimus dorsi
External oblique

Gluteus maximus

Adductor magnus
Gracilis
Semitendinosus
Biceps femoris
Semimembranosus

Gastrocnemius
Soleus
Achilles tendon
Peroneus brevis
Calcaneus

PLATE 9 ■ POSTERIOR SUPERFICIAL MUSCLES

MUSCLE SYSTEM Continued

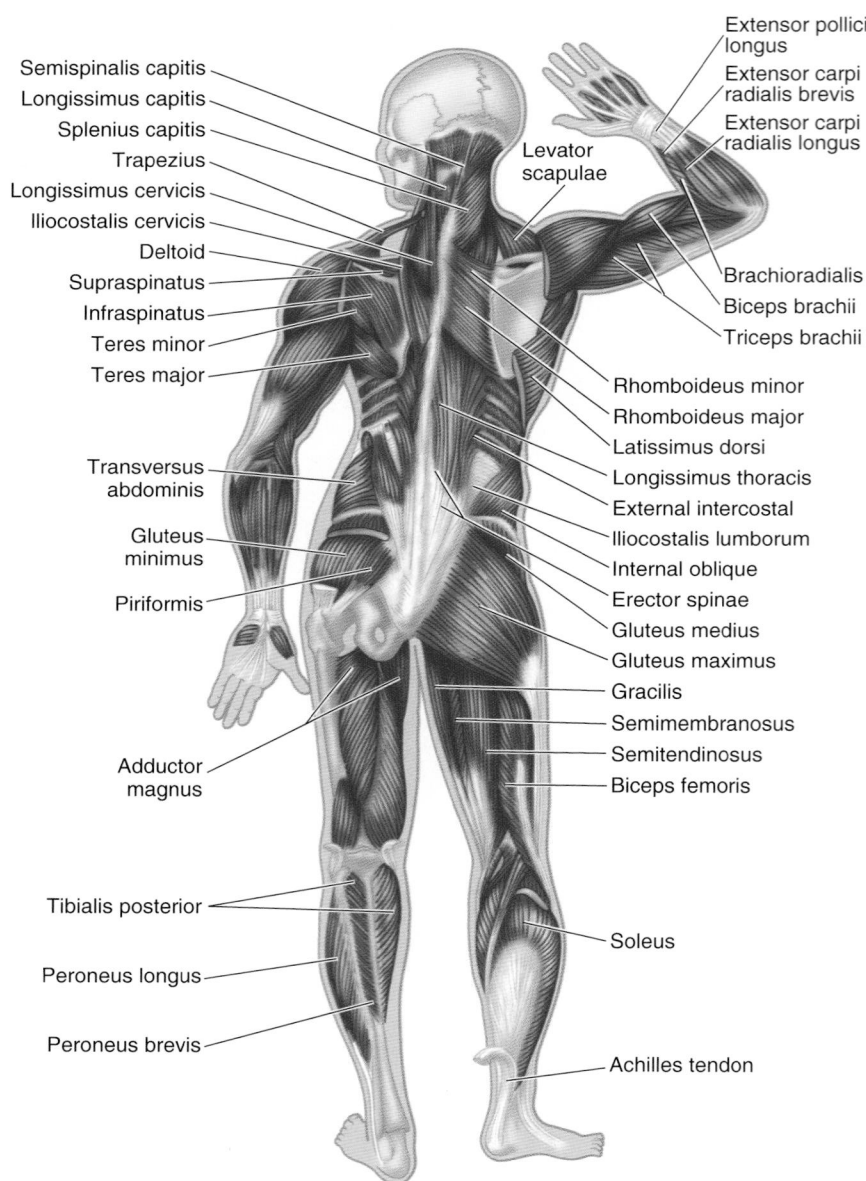

Semispinalis capitis
Longissimus capitis
Splenius capitis
Trapezius
Longissimus cervicis
Iliocostalis cervicis
Deltoid
Supraspinatus
Infraspinatus
Teres minor
Teres major

Transversus abdominis
Gluteus minimus
Piriformis

Adductor magnus

Tibialis posterior
Peroneus longus
Peroneus brevis

Levator scapulae

Extensor pollicis longus
Extensor carpi radialis brevis
Extensor carpi radialis longus

Brachioradialis
Biceps brachii
Triceps brachii

Rhomboideus minor
Rhomboideus major
Latissimus dorsi
Longissimus thoracis
External intercostal
Iliocostalis lumborum
Internal oblique
Erector spinae
Gluteus medius
Gluteus maximus
Gracilis
Semimembranosus
Semitendinosus
Biceps femoris

Soleus

Achilles tendon

PLATE 10 ■ POSTERIOR DEEP MUSCLES

STRUCTURE OF THE HEART

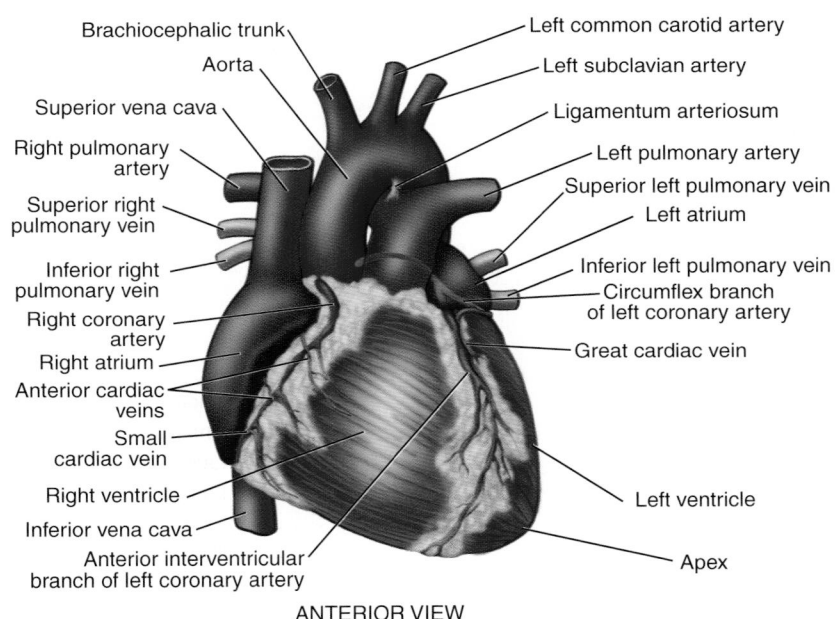

Brachiocephalic trunk
Aorta
Superior vena cava
Right pulmonary artery
Superior right pulmonary vein
Inferior right pulmonary vein
Right coronary artery
Right atrium
Anterior cardiac veins
Small cardiac vein
Right ventricle
Inferior vena cava
Anterior interventricular branch of left coronary artery

Left common carotid artery
Left subclavian artery
Ligamentum arteriosum
Left pulmonary artery
Superior left pulmonary vein
Left atrium
Inferior left pulmonary vein
Circumflex branch of left coronary artery
Great cardiac vein
Left ventricle
Apex

ANTERIOR VIEW

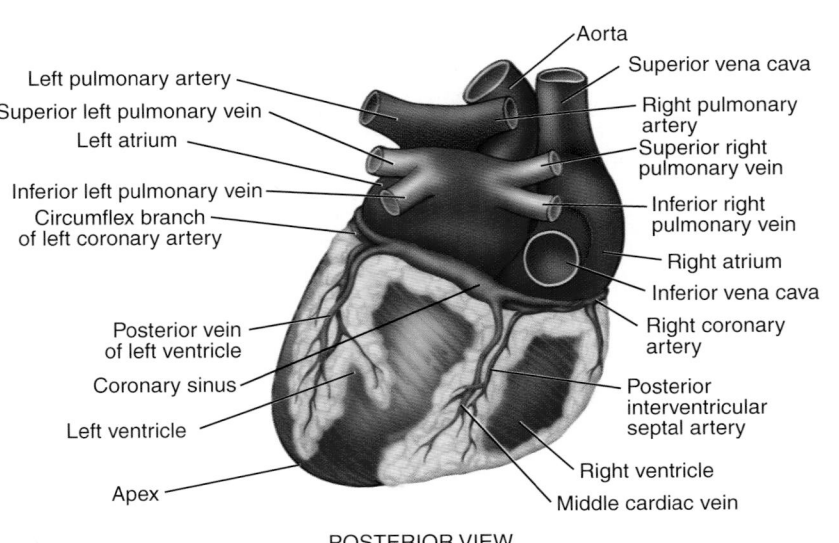

Left pulmonary artery
Superior left pulmonary vein
Left atrium
Inferior left pulmonary vein
Circumflex branch of left coronary artery
Posterior vein of left ventricle
Coronary sinus
Left ventricle
Apex

Aorta
Superior vena cava
Right pulmonary artery
Superior right pulmonary vein
Inferior right pulmonary vein
Right atrium
Inferior vena cava
Right coronary artery
Posterior interventricular septal artery
Right ventricle
Middle cardiac vein

POSTERIOR VIEW

PLATE 11 ■ ANTERIOR AND POSTERIOR VIEW OF THE HEART

RESPIRATORY SYSTEM

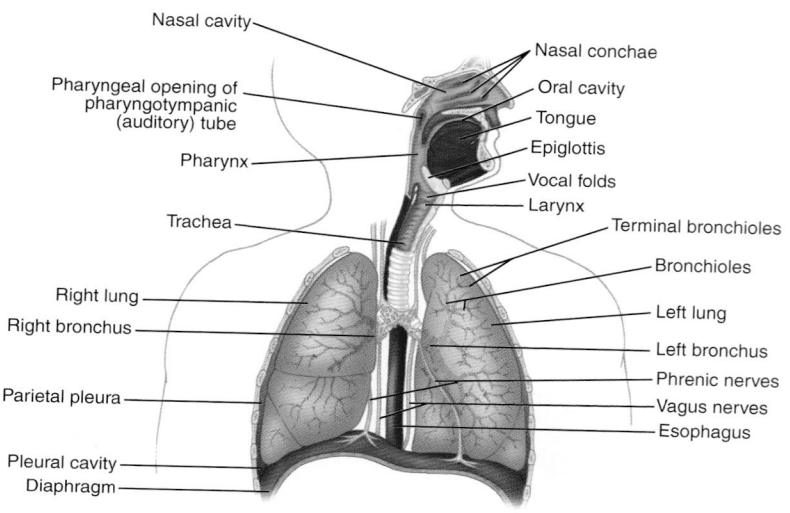

Nasal cavity
Nasal conchae
Pharyngeal opening of pharyngotympanic (auditory) tube
Oral cavity
Tongue
Epiglottis
Pharynx
Vocal folds
Larynx
Trachea
Terminal bronchioles
Bronchioles
Right lung
Left lung
Right bronchus
Left bronchus
Phrenic nerves
Parietal pleura
Vagus nerves
Esophagus
Pleural cavity
Diaphragm

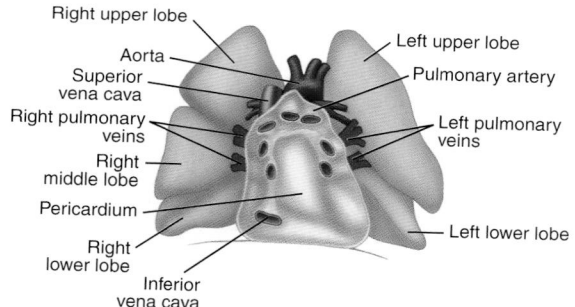

Right upper lobe
Left upper lobe
Aorta
Pulmonary artery
Superior vena cava
Right pulmonary veins
Left pulmonary veins
Right middle lobe
Pericardium
Left lower lobe
Right lower lobe
Inferior vena cava

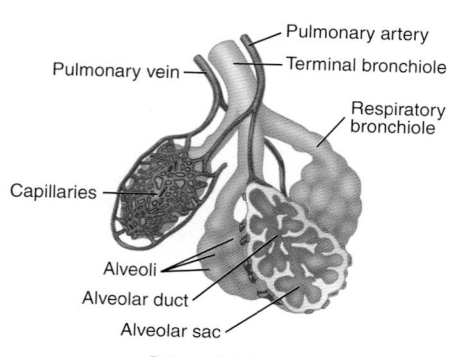

Pulmonary artery
Pulmonary vein
Terminal bronchiole
Respiratory bronchiole
Capillaries
Alveoli
Alveolar duct
Alveolar sac

Primary lobule of lung
(terminal respiratory unit)

PLATE 12 ■ ORGANS OF THE RESPIRATORY SYSTEM

CIRCULATORY SYSTEM

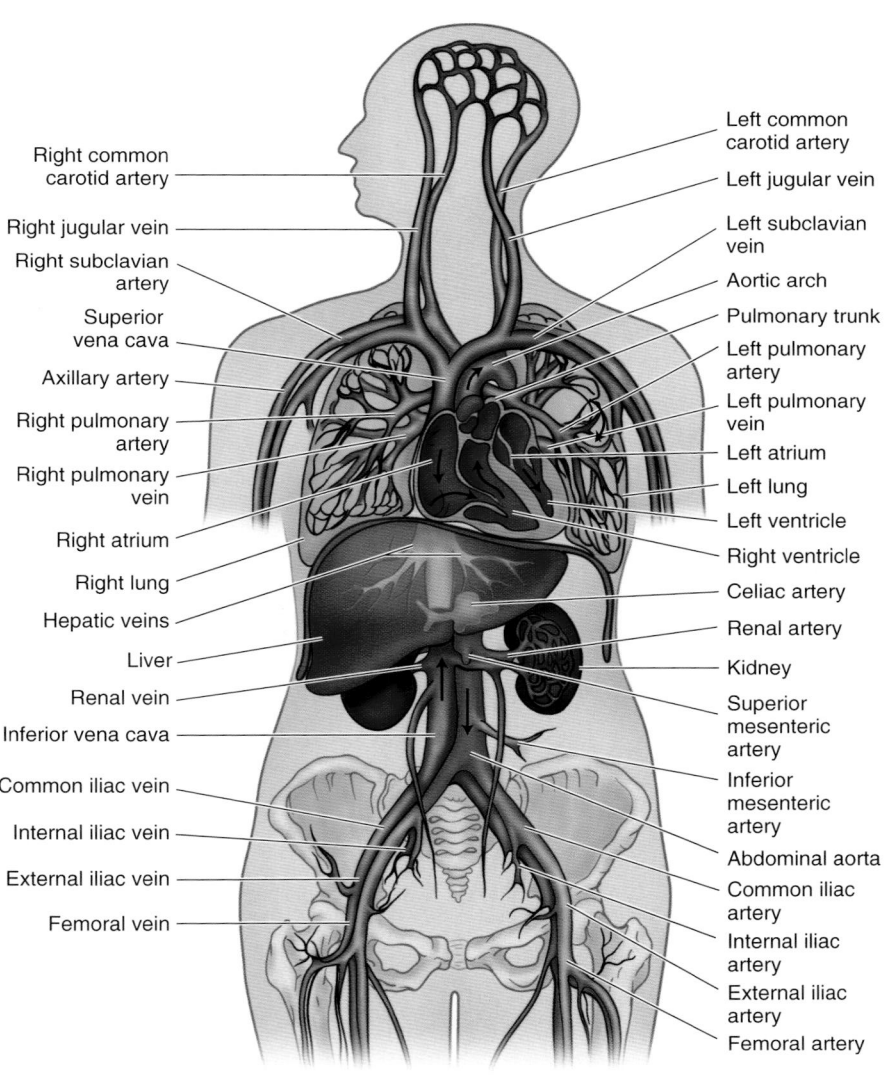

Right common carotid artery

Right jugular vein

Right subclavian artery

Superior vena cava

Axillary artery

Right pulmonary artery

Right pulmonary vein

Right atrium

Right lung

Hepatic veins

Liver

Renal vein

Inferior vena cava

Common iliac vein

Internal iliac vein

External iliac vein

Femoral vein

Left common carotid artery

Left jugular vein

Left subclavian vein

Aortic arch

Pulmonary trunk

Left pulmonary artery

Left pulmonary vein

Left atrium

Left lung

Left ventricle

Right ventricle

Celiac artery

Renal artery

Kidney

Superior mesenteric artery

Inferior mesenteric artery

Abdominal aorta

Common iliac artery

Internal iliac artery

External iliac artery

Femoral artery

PLATE 13 ■ BLOOD

LYMPHATIC SYSTEM

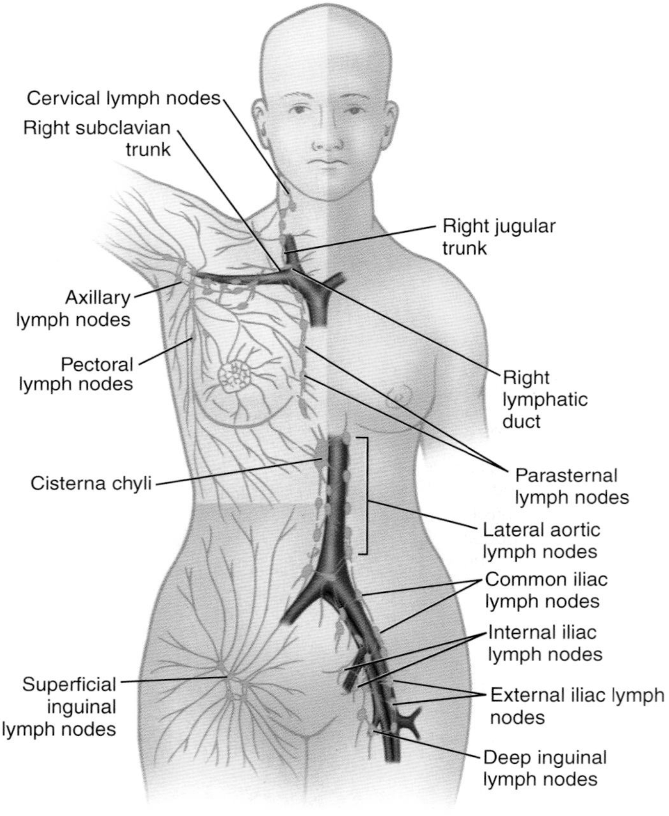

Cervical lymph nodes

Right subclavian trunk

Right jugular trunk

Axillary lymph nodes

Pectoral lymph nodes

Right lymphatic duct

Cisterna chyli

Parasternal lymph nodes

Lateral aortic lymph nodes

Common iliac lymph nodes

Internal iliac lymph nodes

Superficial inguinal lymph nodes

External iliac lymph nodes

Deep inguinal lymph nodes

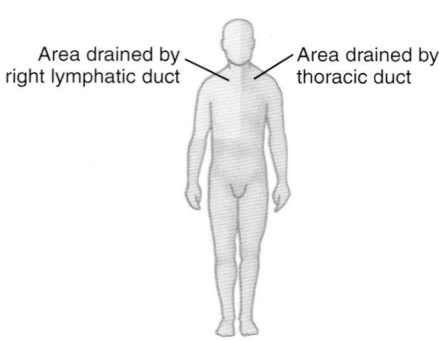

Area drained by right lymphatic duct

Area drained by thoracic duct

PLATE 14

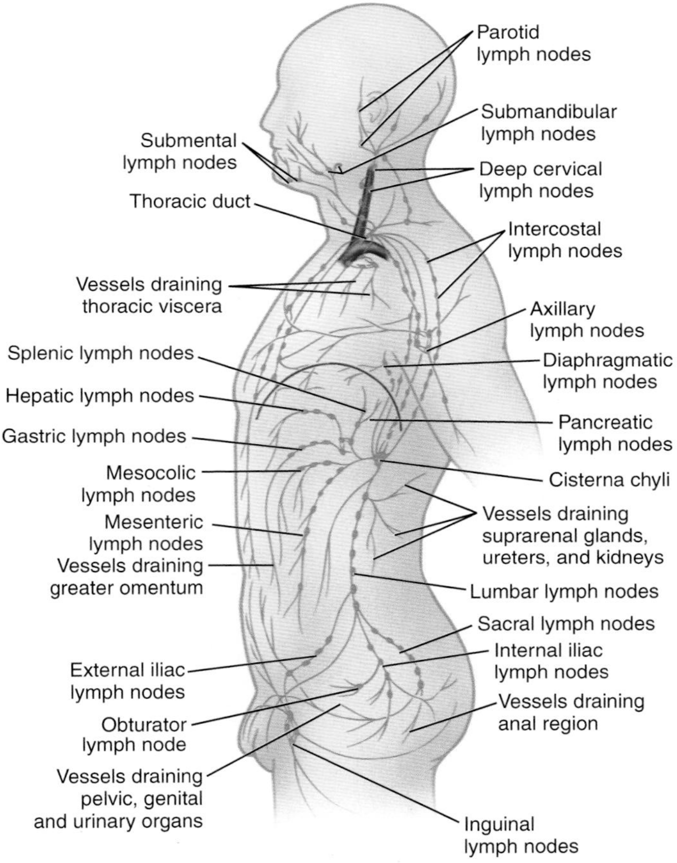

LYMPHATIC SYSTEM Continued

Parotid
lymph nodes

Submandibular
lymph nodes

Submental
lymph nodes

Deep cervical
lymph nodes

Thoracic duct

Intercostal
lymph nodes

Vessels draining
thoracic viscera

Axillary
lymph nodes

Splenic lymph nodes

Diaphragmatic
lymph nodes

Hepatic lymph nodes

Gastric lymph nodes

Pancreatic
lymph nodes

Mesocolic
lymph nodes

Cisterna chyli

Mesenteric
lymph nodes

Vessels draining
suprarenal glands,
ureters, and kidneys

Vessels draining
greater omentum

Lumbar lymph nodes

Sacral lymph nodes

Internal iliac
lymph nodes

External iliac
lymph nodes

Vessels draining
anal region

Obturator
lymph node

Vessels draining
pelvic, genital
and urinary organs

Inguinal
lymph nodes

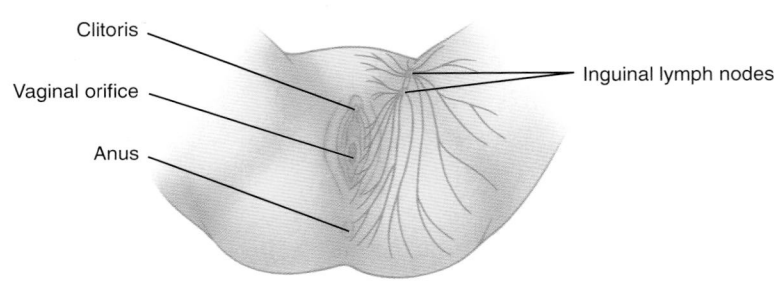

Clitoris

Inguinal lymph nodes

Vaginal orifice

Anus

PLATE 15

ENDOCRINE SYSTEM

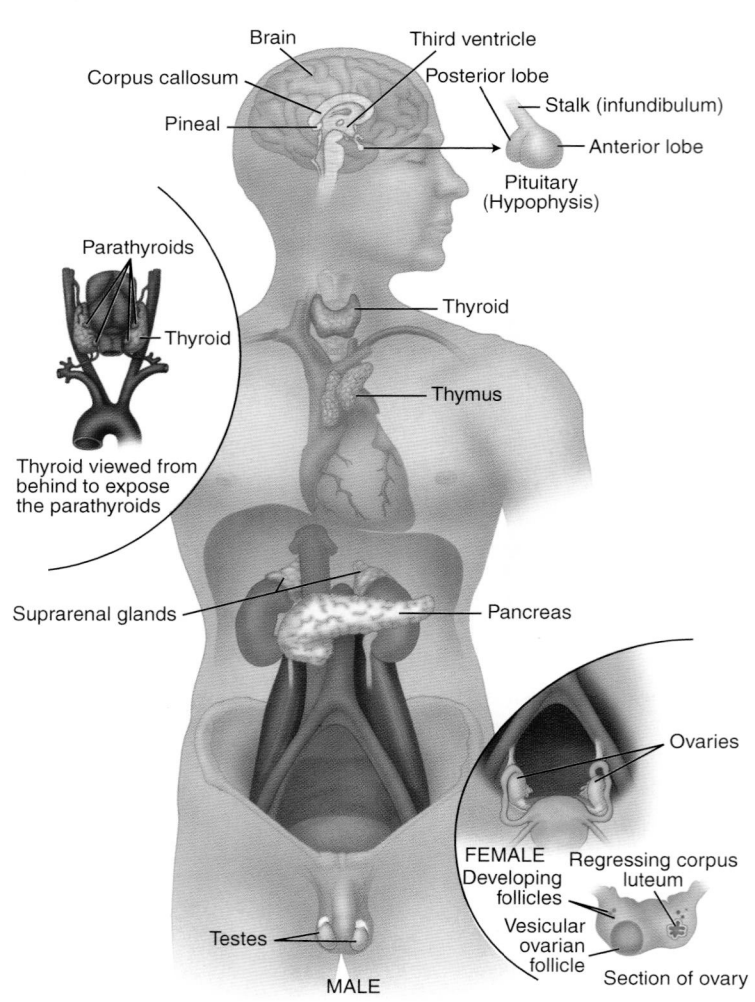

Brain
Third ventricle
Corpus callosum
Posterior lobe
Pineal
Stalk (infundibulum)
Anterior lobe
Pituitary
(Hypophysis)

Parathyroids
Thyroid
Thyroid

Thymus

Thyroid viewed from
behind to expose
the parathyroids

Suprarenal glands
Pancreas

Ovaries

FEMALE
Developing
follicles
Regressing corpus
luteum

Testes
Vesicular
ovarian
follicle
Section of ovary
MALE

PLATE 16 ■ THE ENDOCRINE GLANDS

DIGESTIVE SYSTEM

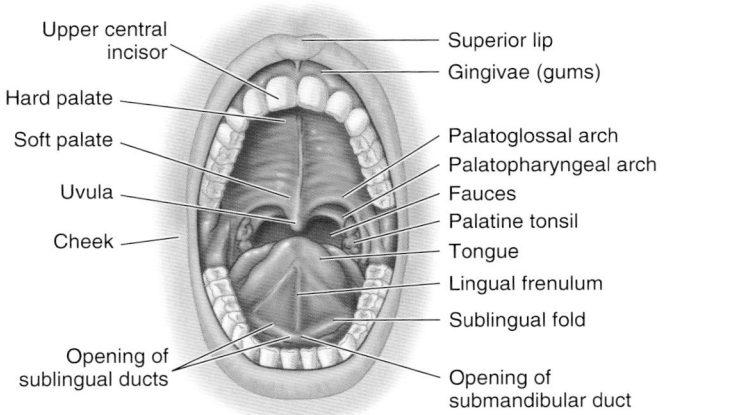

Crown

Neck

Root

Enamel

Pulp cavity

Gingiva

Pulp

Dentin

Ligament

Cementum

Root canal

Spongy bone of alveolar process

Nerve

Vein

Artery

Upper central incisor

Hard palate

Soft palate

Uvula

Cheek

Opening of sublingual ducts

Superior lip

Gingivae (gums)

Palatoglossal arch

Palatopharyngeal arch

Fauces

Palatine tonsil

Tongue

Lingual frenulum

Sublingual fold

Opening of submandibular duct

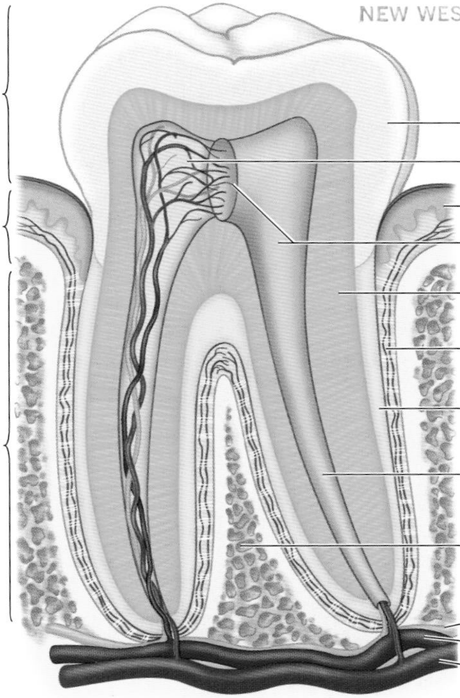

PLATE 17 ■ TOOTH AND ORAL CAVITY

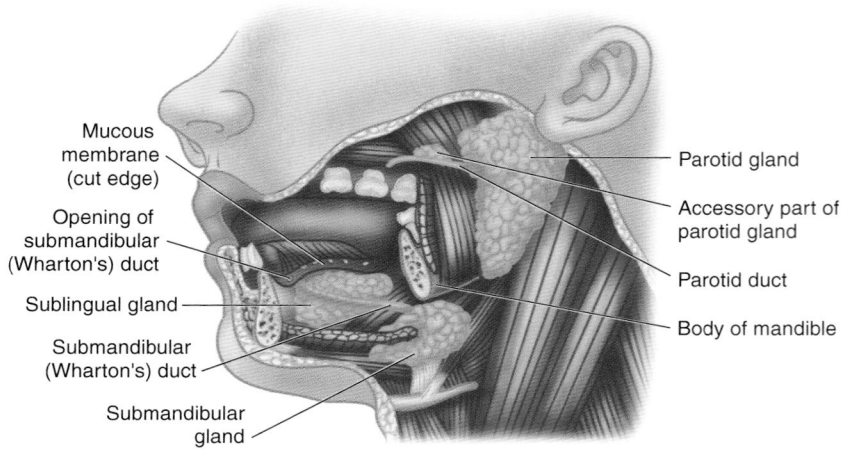

Mucous membrane (cut edge)

Opening of submandibular (Wharton's) duct

Sublingual gland

Submandibular (Wharton's) duct

Submandibular gland

Parotid gland

Accessory part of parotid gland

Parotid duct

Body of mandible

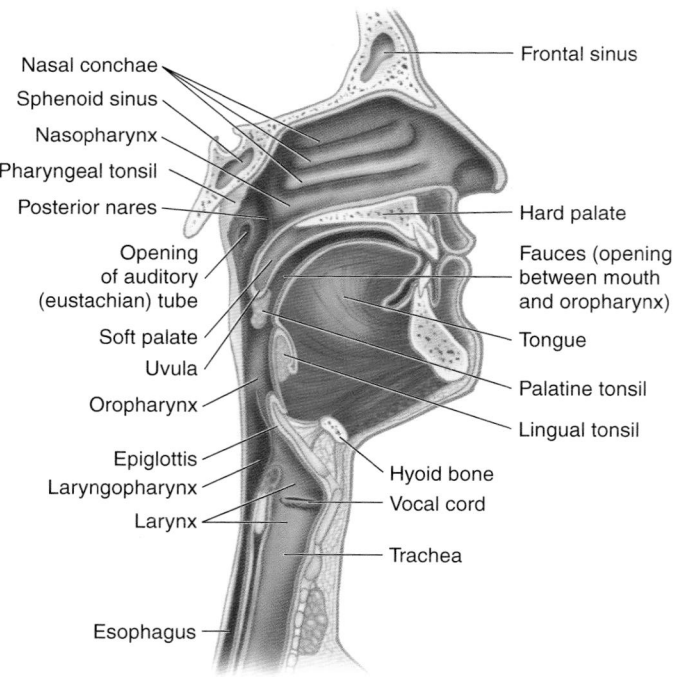

Nasal conchae

Sphenoid sinus

Nasopharynx

Pharyngeal tonsil

Posterior nares

Opening of auditory (eustachian) tube

Soft palate

Uvula

Oropharynx

Epiglottis

Laryngopharynx

Larynx

Esophagus

Frontal sinus

Hard palate

Fauces (opening between mouth and oropharynx)

Tongue

Palatine tonsil

Lingual tonsil

Hyoid bone

Vocal cord

Trachea

PLATE 18

DIGESTIVE SYSTEM Continued

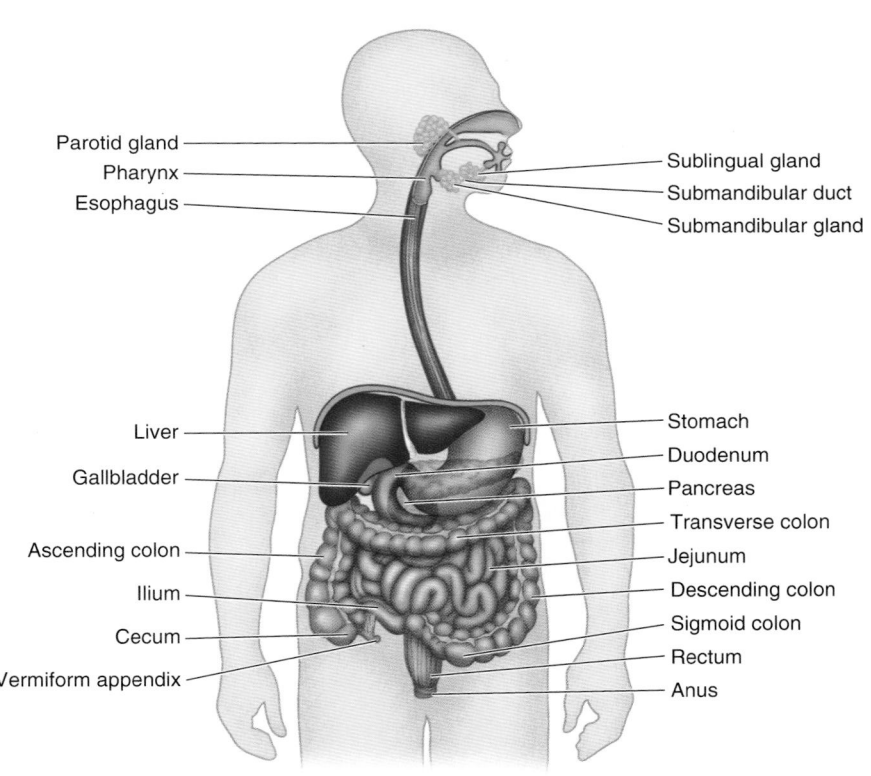

Parotid gland
Pharynx
Esophagus
Sublingual gland
Submandibular duct
Submandibular gland
Liver
Gallbladder
Ascending colon
Ilium
Cecum
Vermiform appendix
Stomach
Duodenum
Pancreas
Transverse colon
Jejunum
Descending colon
Sigmoid colon
Rectum
Anus

PLATE 19

GENITOURINARY SYSTEM

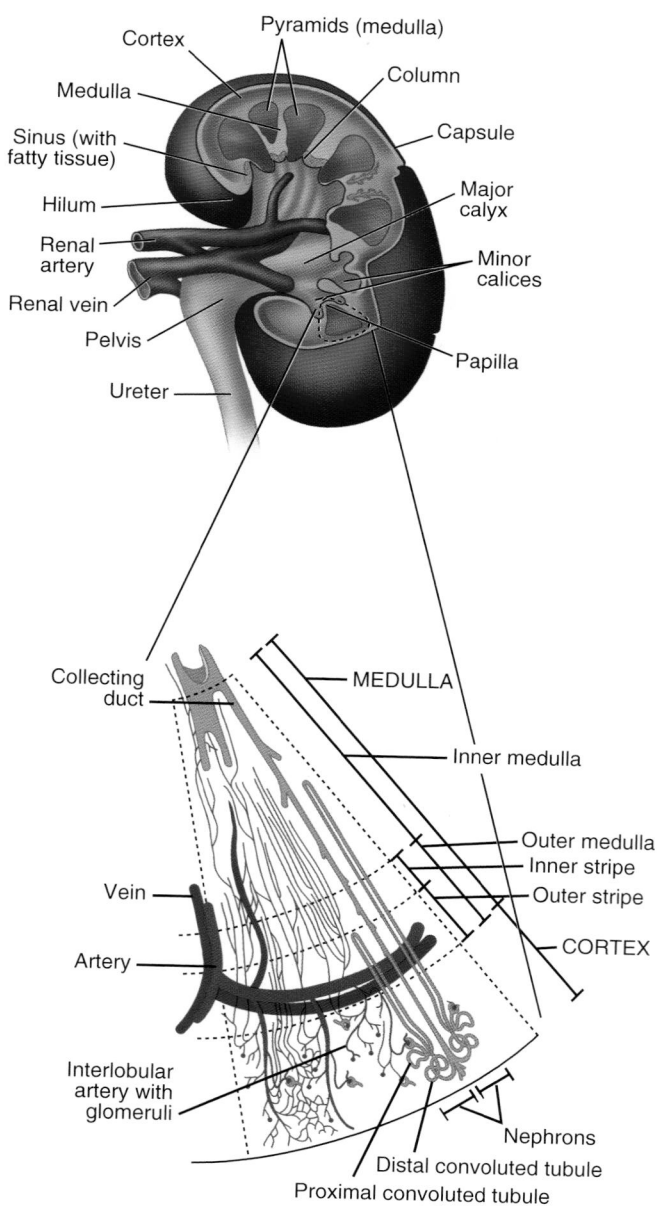

PLATE 20 ■ STRUCTURE OF THE KIDNEY

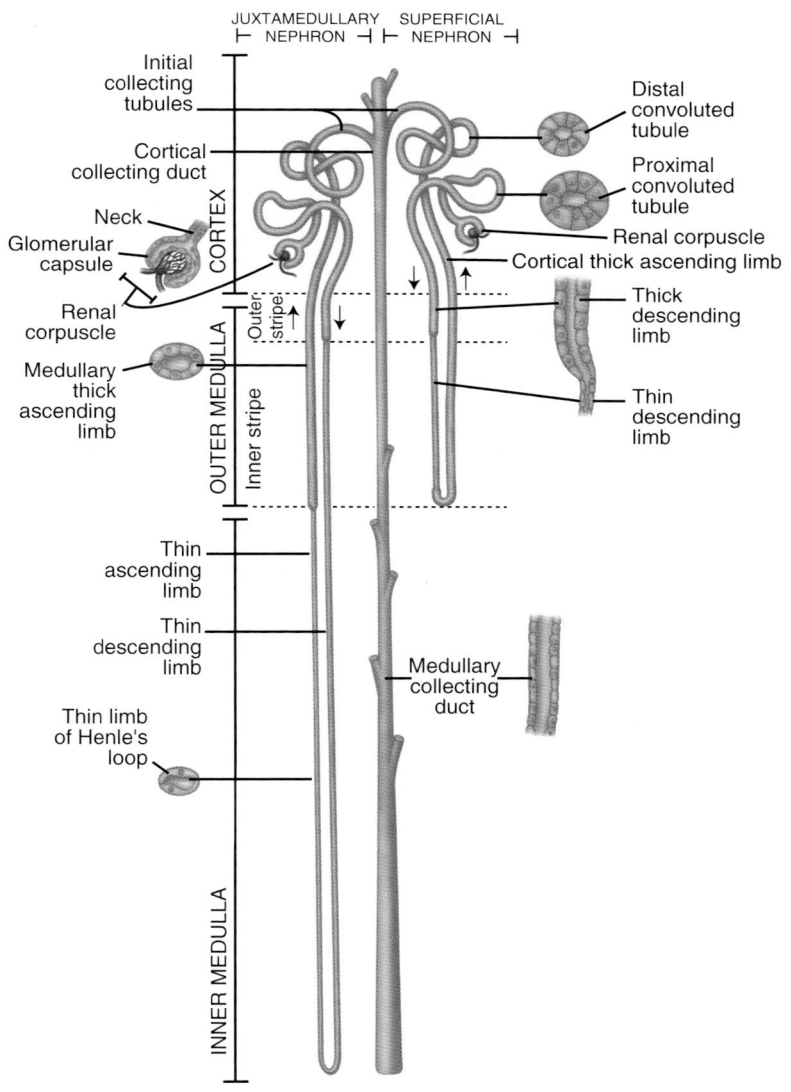

JUXTAMEDULLARY SUPERFICIAL
⊢ NEPHRON ⊣ ⊢ NEPHRON ⊣

Initial
collecting
tubules

Cortical
collecting duct

Neck

Glomerular
capsule

Renal
corpuscle

Medullary
thick
ascending
limb

CORTEX

OUTER MEDULLA

Outer stripe

Inner stripe

Distal
convoluted
tubule

Proximal
convoluted
tubule

Renal corpuscle

Cortical thick ascending limb

Thick
descending
limb

Thin
descending
limb

Thin
ascending
limb

Thin
descending
limb

Thin limb
of Henle's
loop

INNER MEDULLA

Medullary
collecting
duct

PLATE 21 ■ STRUCTURE OF THE NEPHRON

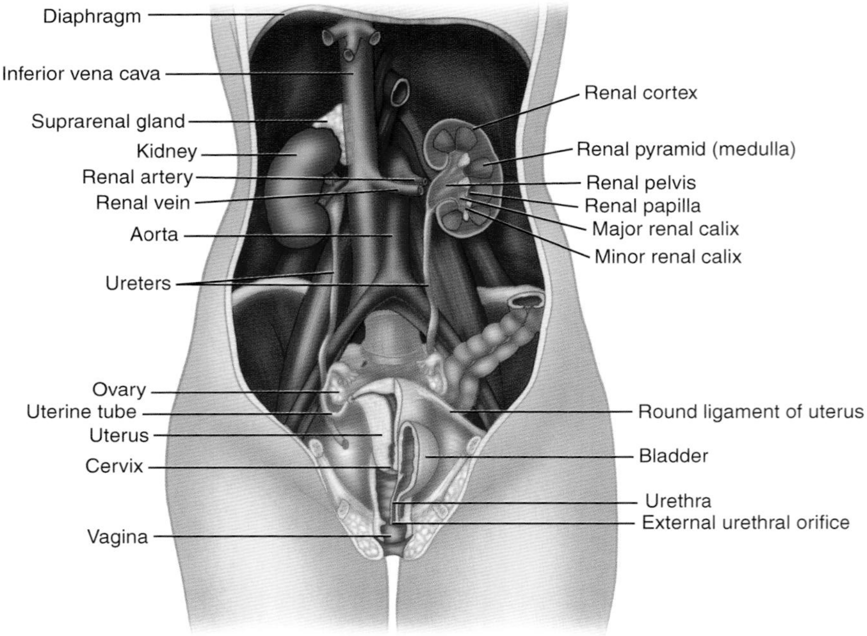

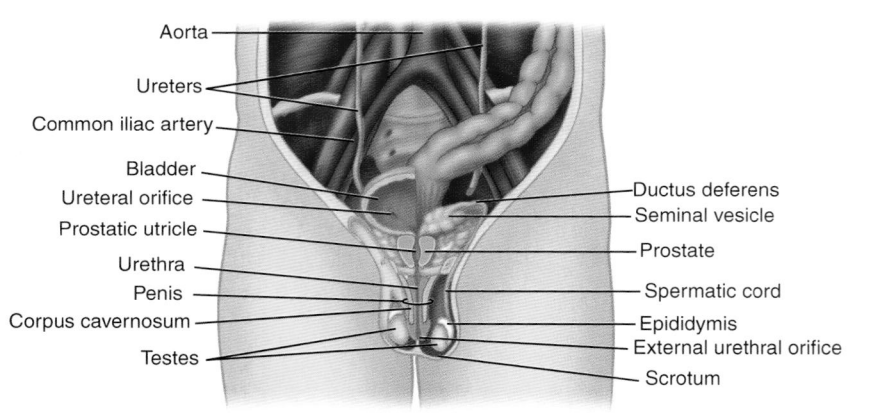

Diaphragm

Inferior vena cava

Suprarenal gland

Kidney

Renal artery

Renal vein

Aorta

Ureters

Renal cortex

Renal pyramid (medulla)

Renal pelvis

Renal papilla

Major renal calix

Minor renal calix

Ovary

Uterine tube

Uterus

Cervix

Vagina

Round ligament of uterus

Bladder

Urethra

External urethral orifice

Aorta

Ureters

Common iliac artery

Bladder

Ureteral orifice

Prostatic utricle

Urethra

Penis

Corpus cavernosum

Testes

Ductus deferens

Seminal vesicle

Prostate

Spermatic cord

Epididymis

External urethral orifice

Scrotum

PLATE 22

STRUCTURE OF THE BRAIN

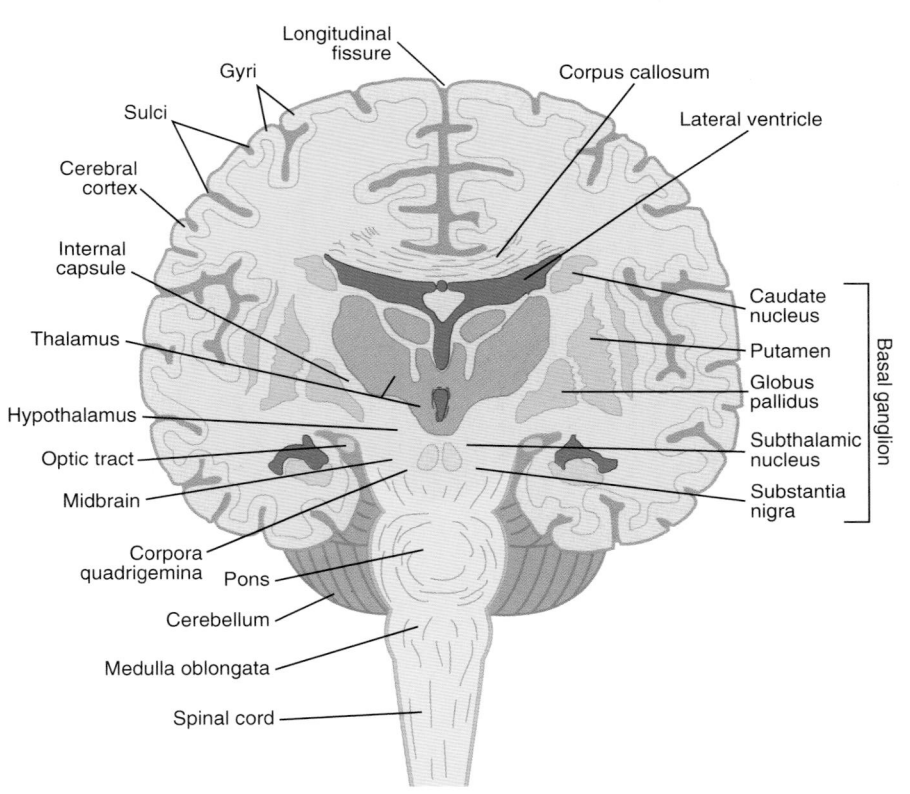

PLATE 23 ■ CORONAL SECTION OF THE BRAIN

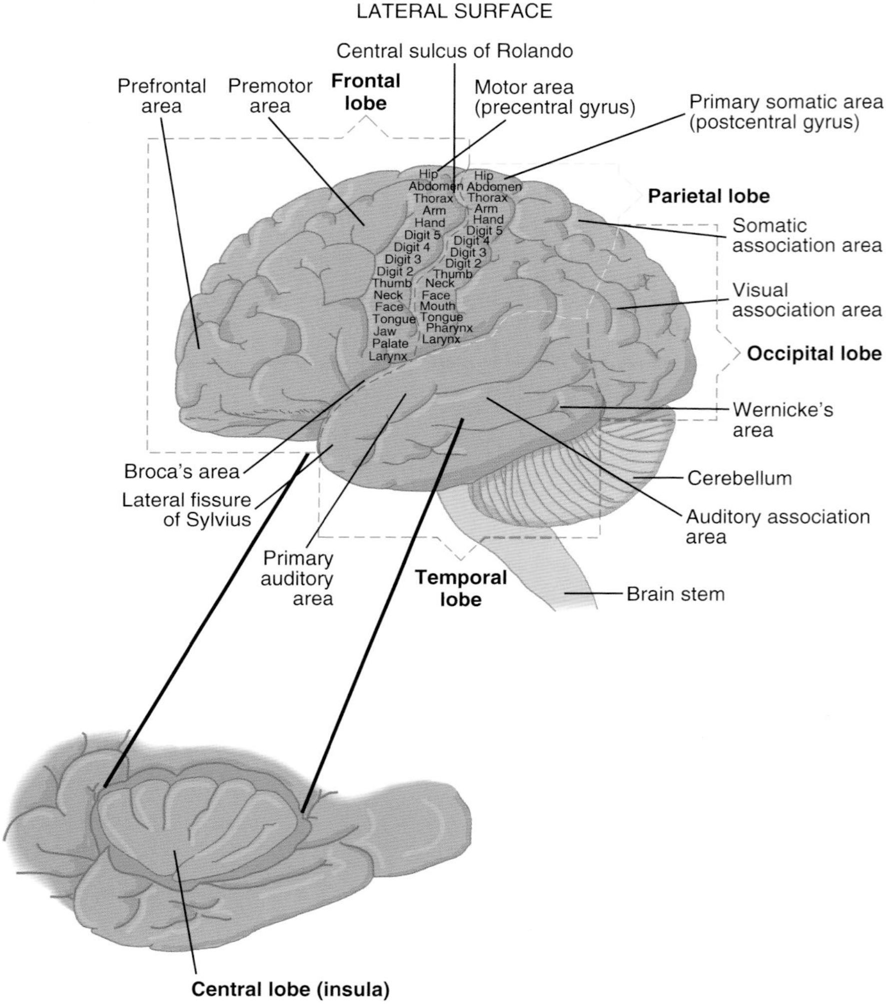

LATERAL SURFACE

Central sulcus of Rolando

Prefrontal area

Premotor area

Frontal lobe

Motor area (precentral gyrus)

Primary somatic area (postcentral gyrus)

Hip
Abdomen Abdomen
Thorax Thorax
Arm Arm
Hand Hand
Digit 5 Digit 5
Digit 4 Digit 4
Digit 3 Digit 3
Digit 2 Digit 2
Thumb Thumb
Neck Neck
Face Face
Tongue Mouth
Jaw Tongue
Palate Pharynx
Larynx Larynx

Parietal lobe

Somatic association area

Visual association area

Occipital lobe

Wernicke's area

Broca's area

Lateral fissure of Sylvius

Cerebellum

Auditory association area

Primary auditory area

Temporal lobe

Brain stem

Central lobe (insula)

PLATE 24 ■ LATERAL SURFACE OF THE BRAIN

STRUCTURE OF THE BRAIN Continued

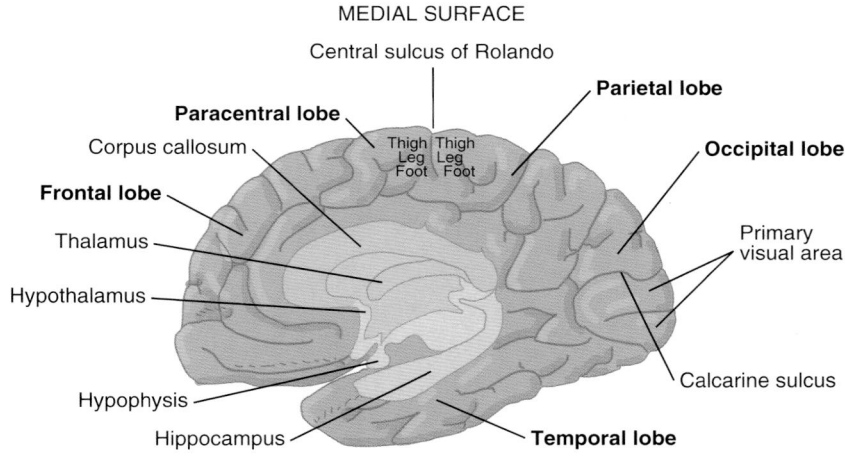

MEDIAL SURFACE

Central sulcus of Rolando

Paracentral lobe

Parietal lobe

Corpus callosum

Thigh Thigh
Leg Leg
Foot Foot

Occipital lobe

Frontal lobe

Thalamus

Primary
visual area

Hypothalamus

Hypophysis

Calcarine sulcus

Hippocampus

Temporal lobe

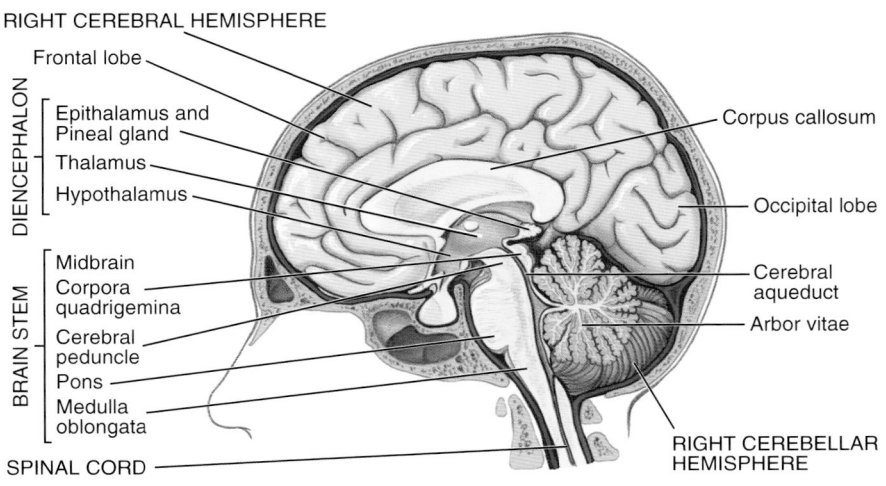

RIGHT CEREBRAL HEMISPHERE

Frontal lobe

DIENCEPHALON

Epithalamus and
Pineal gland

Thalamus

Hypothalamus

Corpus callosum

Occipital lobe

BRAIN STEM

Midbrain

Corpora
quadrigemina

Cerebral
peduncle

Pons

Medulla
oblongata

Cerebral
aqueduct

Arbor vitae

SPINAL CORD

RIGHT CEREBELLAR
HEMISPHERE

**PLATE 25 ■ MEDIAL SURFACE AND
MIDSAGITTAL SECTION OF THE BRAIN**

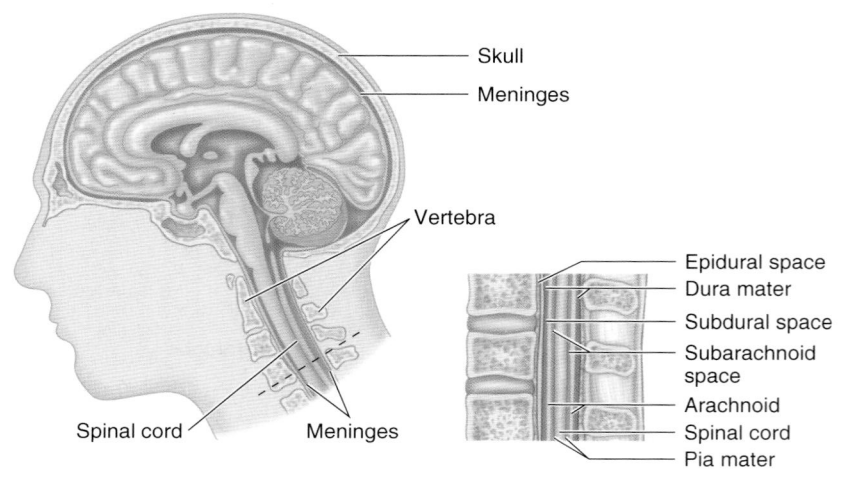

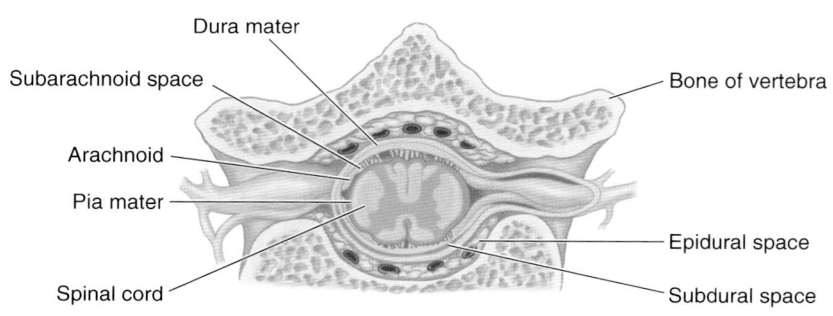

PLATE 26

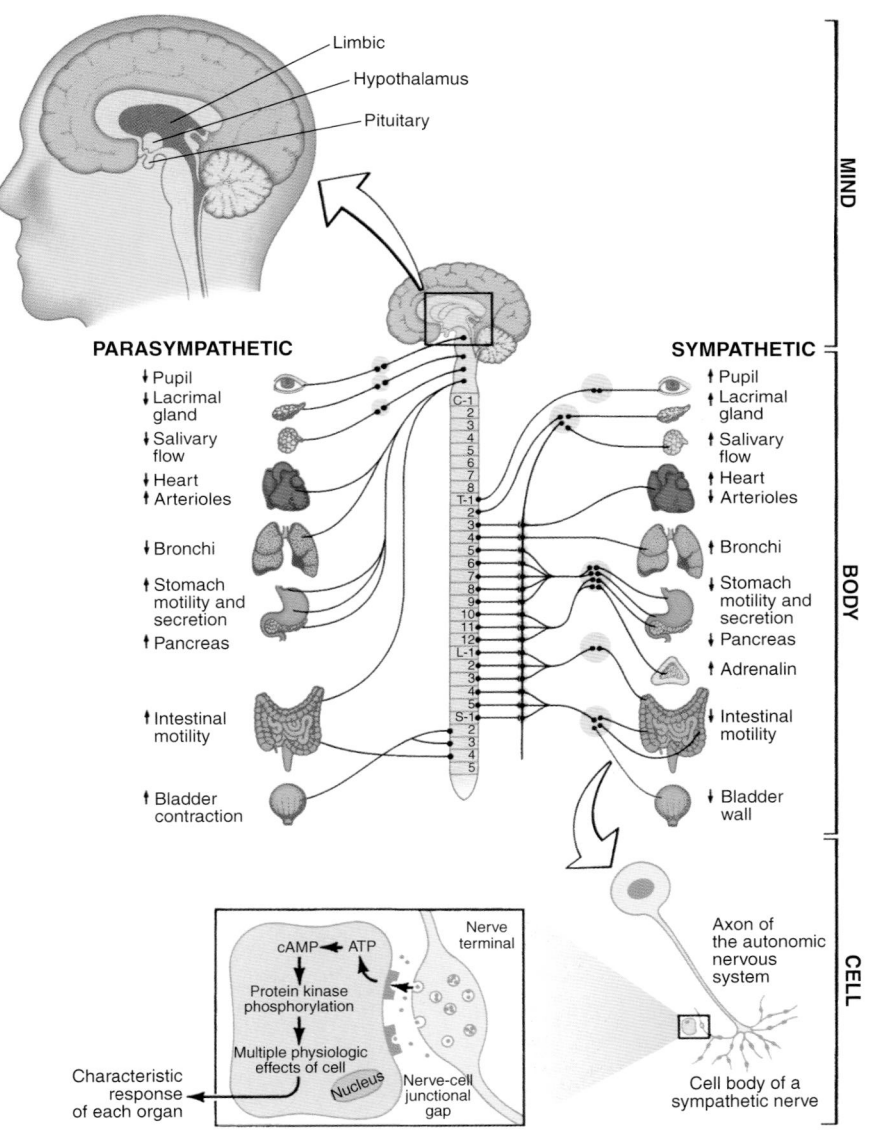

Limbic
Hypothalamus
Pituitary

MIND

PARASYMPATHETIC

↓ Pupil
↓ Lacrimal gland
↓ Salivary flow
↓ Heart
↑ Arterioles

↓ Bronchi

↑ Stomach motility and secretion
↑ Pancreas

↑ Intestinal motility

↑ Bladder contraction

C-1
2
3
4
5
6
7
8
T-1
2
3
4
5
6
7
8
9
10
11
12
L-1
2
3
4
5
S-1
2
3
4
5

SYMPATHETIC

↑ Pupil
↑ Lacrimal gland
↑ Salivary flow
↑ Heart
↓ Arterioles

↑ Bronchi

↓ Stomach motility and secretion
↓ Pancreas

↑ Adrenalin

↓ Intestinal motility

↓ Bladder wall

BODY

cAMP ← ATP

Protein kinase phosphorylation

Multiple physiologic effects of cell

Characteristic response of each organ

Nucleus

Nerve terminal

Nerve-cell junctional gap

Axon of the autonomic nervous system

Cell body of a sympathetic nerve

CELL

PLATE 27

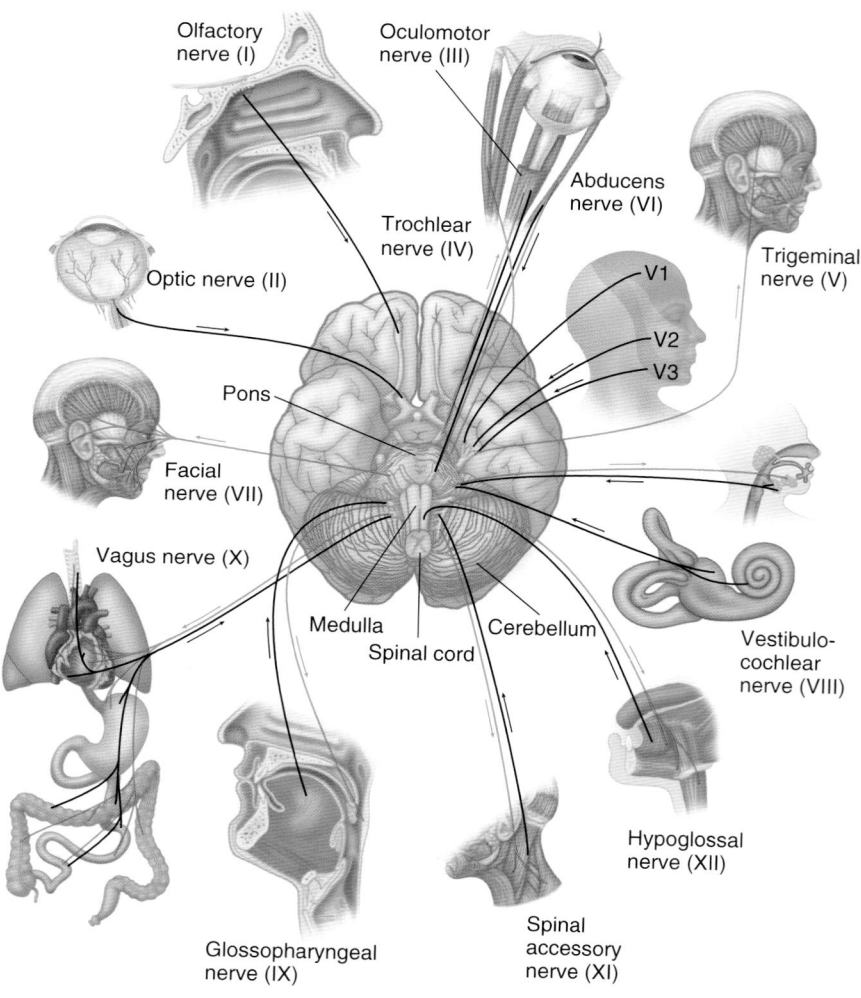

Olfactory nerve (I)

Oculomotor nerve (III)

Abducens nerve (VI)

Trochlear nerve (IV)

Trigeminal nerve (V)

Optic nerve (II)

V1

V2

V3

Pons

Facial nerve (VII)

Vagus nerve (X)

Medulla

Cerebellum

Spinal cord

Vestibulo-cochlear nerve (VIII)

Hypoglossal nerve (XII)

Glossopharyngeal nerve (IX)

Spinal accessory nerve (XI)

PLATE 28

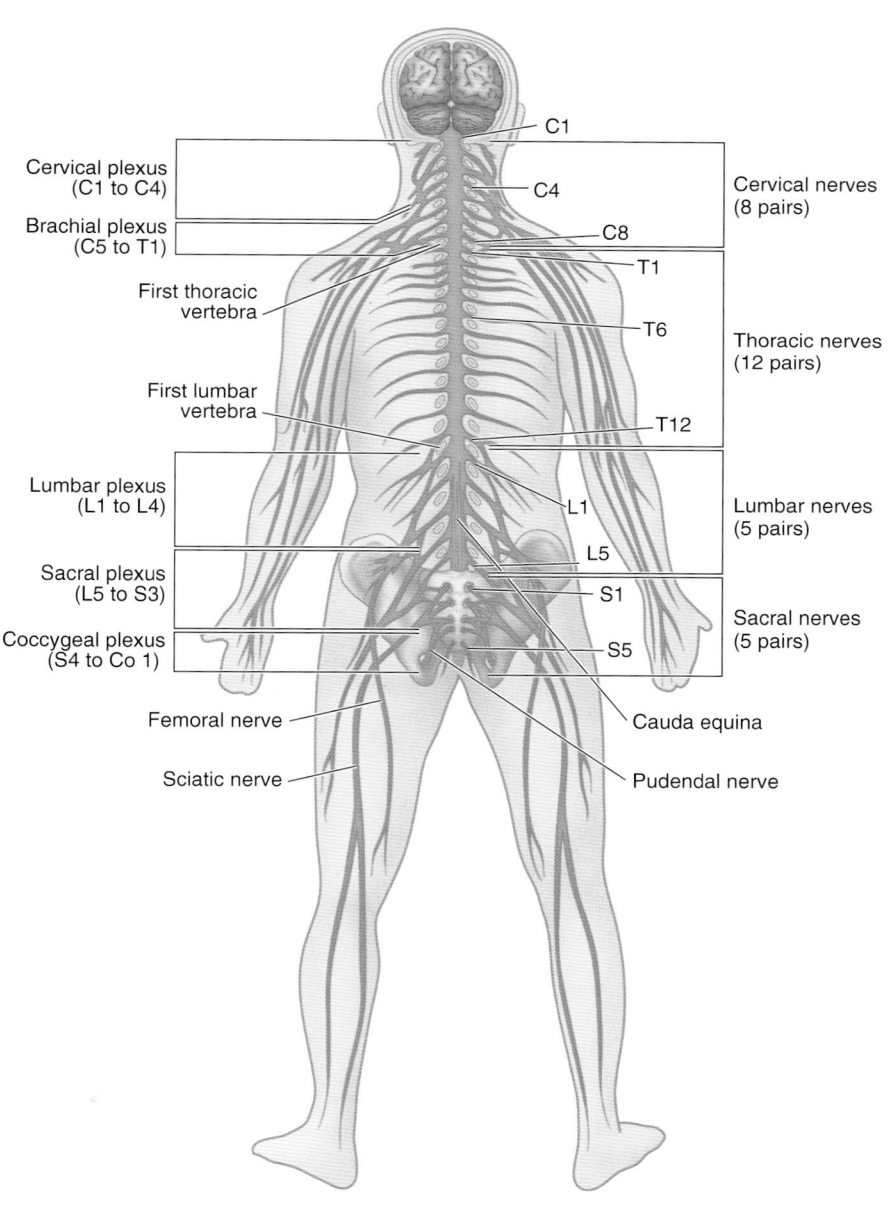

Cervical plexus (C1 to C4)

Brachial plexus (C5 to T1)

First thoracic vertebra

First lumbar vertebra

Lumbar plexus (L1 to L4)

Sacral plexus (L5 to S3)

Coccygeal plexus (S4 to Co 1)

Femoral nerve

Sciatic nerve

C1

C4

C8

T1

T6

T12

L1

L5

S1

S5

Cervical nerves (8 pairs)

Thoracic nerves (12 pairs)

Lumbar nerves (5 pairs)

Sacral nerves (5 pairs)

Cauda equina

Pudendal nerve

PLATE 29 ■ AUTONOMIC NERVES

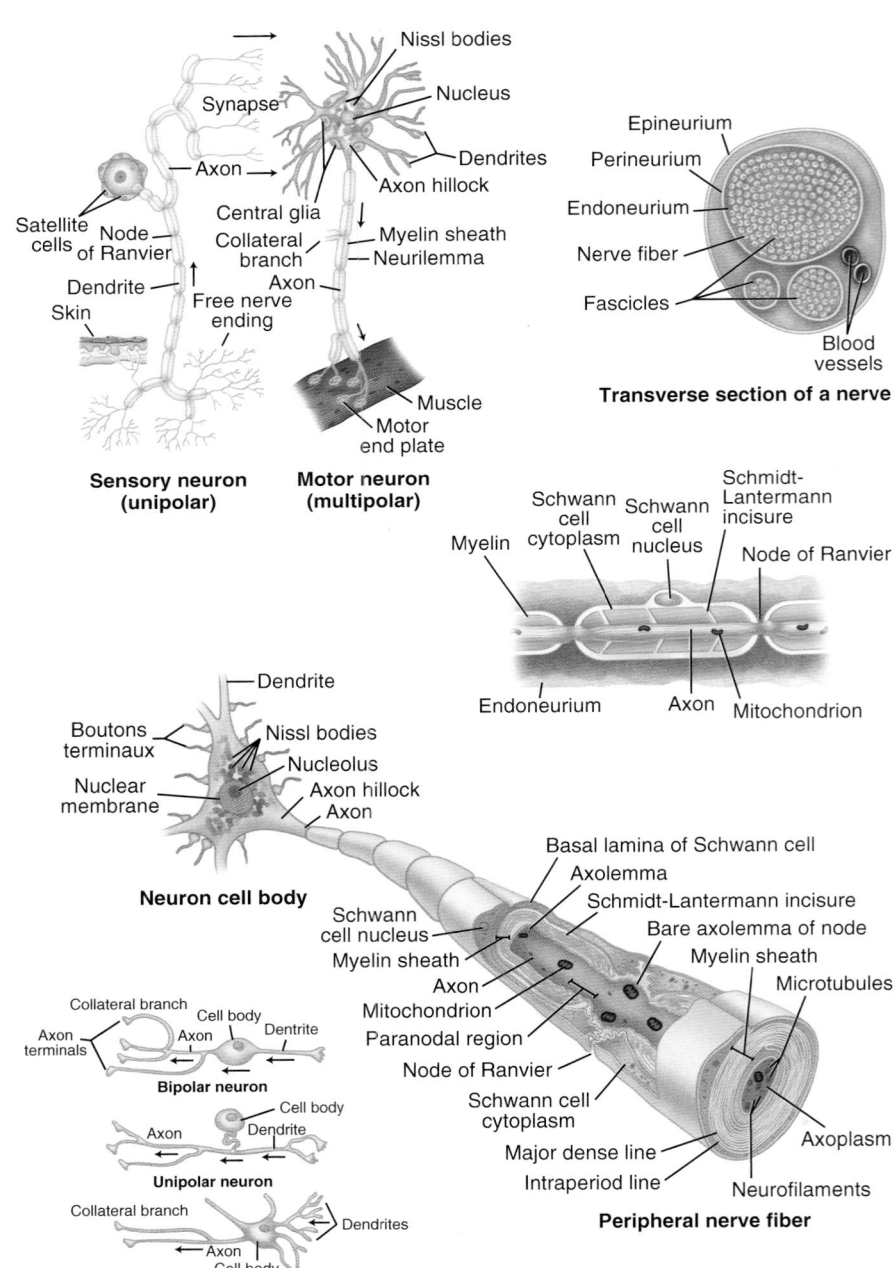

Nissl bodies
Nucleus
Synapse
Dendrites
Axon
Axon hillock
Central glia
Satellite cells
Node of Ranvier
Myelin sheath
Collateral branch
Neurilemma
Dendrite
Axon
Free nerve ending
Skin

Epineurium
Perineurium
Endoneurium
Nerve fiber
Fascicles
Blood vessels

Transverse section of a nerve

Muscle
Motor end plate

Sensory neuron (unipolar)

Motor neuron (multipolar)

Schmidt-Lantermann incisure
Schwann cell cytoplasm
Schwann cell nucleus
Node of Ranvier
Myelin
Endoneurium
Axon
Mitochondrion

Dendrite
Boutons terminaux
Nissl bodies
Nucleolus
Nuclear membrane
Axon hillock
Axon

Neuron cell body

Basal lamina of Schwann cell
Axolemma
Schmidt-Lantermann incisure
Bare axolemma of node
Myelin sheath
Microtubules
Schwann cell nucleus
Myelin sheath
Axon
Mitochondrion
Paranodal region
Node of Ranvier
Schwann cell cytoplasm
Major dense line
Intraperiod line
Axoplasm
Neurofilaments

Peripheral nerve fiber

Collateral branch
Cell body
Axon terminals
Axon
Dentrite
Bipolar neuron

Cell body
Axon
Dendrite
Unipolar neuron

Collateral branch
Dendrites
Axon
Cell body
Multipolar neuron

PLATE 30 ■ NERVOUS TISSUE

ORGANS OF SPECIAL SENSE

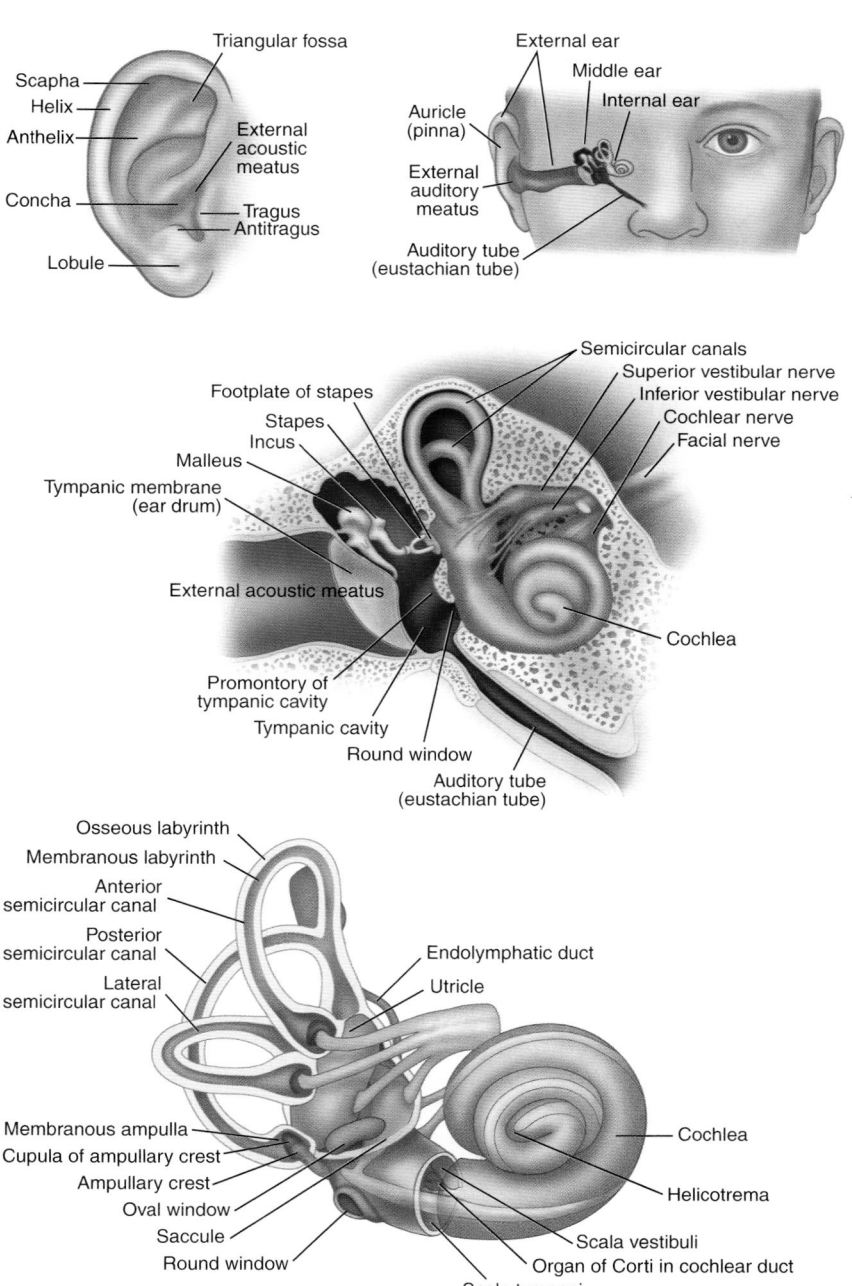

Triangular fossa

Scapha
Helix
Anthelix
Concha
Lobule

External acoustic meatus
Tragus
Antitragus

External ear
Middle ear
Internal ear
Auricle (pinna)
External auditory meatus
Auditory tube (eustachian tube)

Footplate of stapes
Stapes
Incus
Malleus
Tympanic membrane (ear drum)

Semicircular canals
Superior vestibular nerve
Inferior vestibular nerve
Cochlear nerve
Facial nerve

External acoustic meatus

Cochlea

Promontory of tympanic cavity
Tympanic cavity
Round window
Auditory tube (eustachian tube)

Osseous labyrinth
Membranous labyrinth
Anterior semicircular canal
Posterior semicircular canal
Lateral semicircular canal

Endolymphatic duct
Utricle

Membranous ampulla
Cupula of ampullary crest
Ampullary crest
Oval window
Saccule
Round window

Cochlea
Helicotrema
Scala vestibuli
Organ of Corti in cochlear duct
Scala tympani

PLATE 31 ■ EXTERNAL AND INTERNAL STRUCTURES OF THE EAR

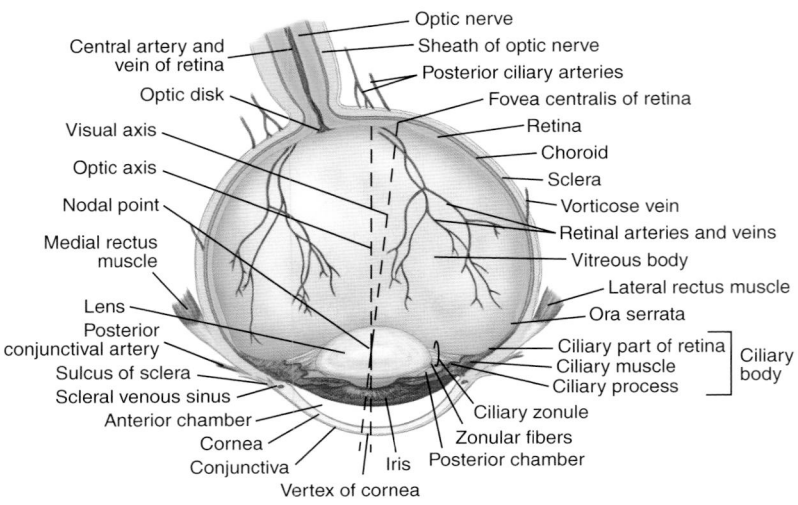

Optic nerve
Central artery and vein of retina
Sheath of optic nerve
Posterior ciliary arteries
Optic disk
Fovea centralis of retina
Visual axis
Retina
Optic axis
Choroid
Nodal point
Sclera
Medial rectus muscle
Vorticose vein
Retinal arteries and veins
Vitreous body
Lateral rectus muscle
Lens
Ora serrata
Posterior conjunctival artery
Ciliary part of retina
Sulcus of sclera
Ciliary muscle
Ciliary body
Scleral venous sinus
Ciliary process
Anterior chamber
Ciliary zonule
Cornea
Zonular fibers
Conjunctiva
Iris
Posterior chamber
Vertex of cornea

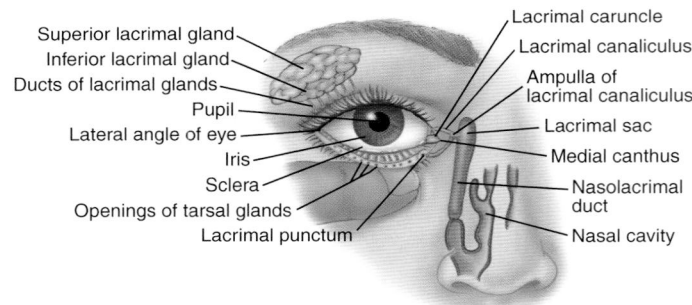

Superior lacrimal gland
Lacrimal caruncle
Inferior lacrimal gland
Lacrimal canaliculus
Ducts of lacrimal glands
Ampulla of lacrimal canaliculus
Pupil
Lateral angle of eye
Lacrimal sac
Iris
Medial canthus
Sclera
Nasolacrimal duct
Openings of tarsal glands
Lacrimal punctum
Nasal cavity

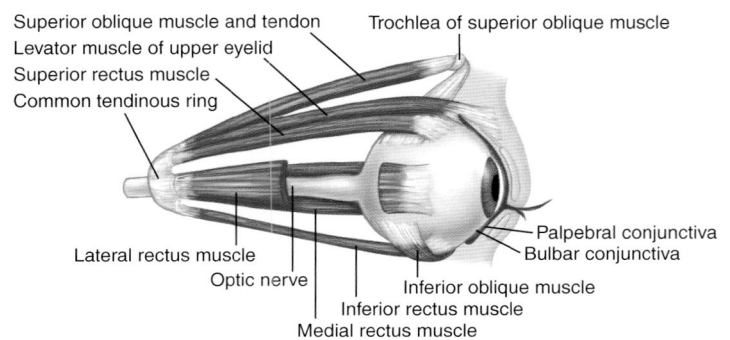

Superior oblique muscle and tendon
Trochlea of superior oblique muscle
Levator muscle of upper eyelid
Superior rectus muscle
Common tendinous ring
Lateral rectus muscle
Palpebral conjunctiva
Bulbar conjunctiva
Optic nerve
Inferior oblique muscle
Inferior rectus muscle
Medial rectus muscle

PLATE 32 ■ STRUCTURE OF THE EYE

ATLAS 1 ■ Atlas of Children With Distinctive Physical Features*

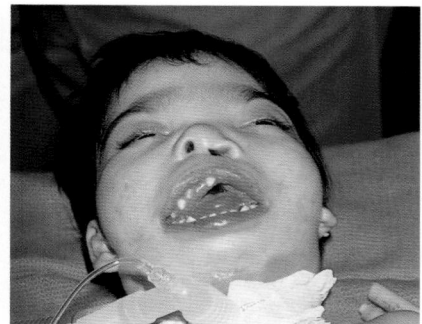

Child with cleft lip and palate.*

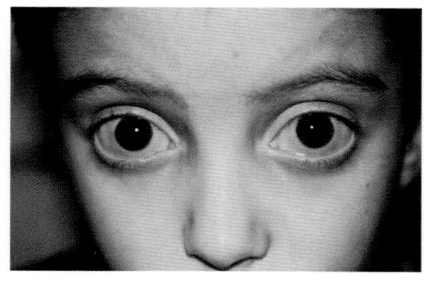

Child with osteogenesis imperfecta, displaying the characteristic blue sclera.**

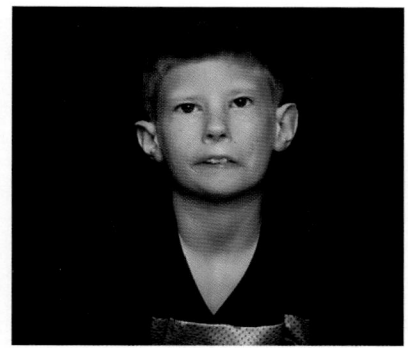

Child with Mobius syndrome, displaying facial paralysis.*

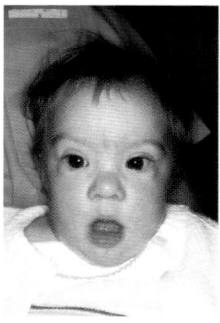

Infant with Down syndrome, with the characteristic wide-set eyes and flat-bridged nose.**

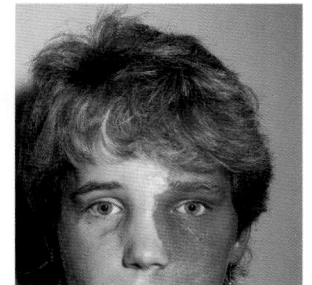

Child with Nevus flemmeus (port-wine stain).**

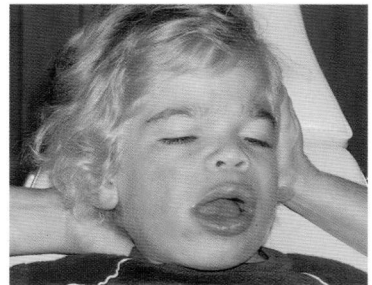

Child with Sanfilippo syndrome.*

*Illustrations courtesy of Dr. Burton Nussbaum.
**Kanski, 2001.

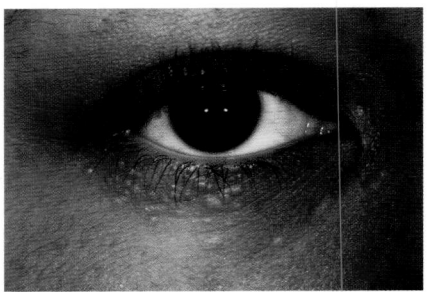

Syringomas are small, firm, flesh-colored dermal papules that occur on the lower lids and less commonly, on the forehead, chest, and abdomen. (From Habif et al., 2001.)

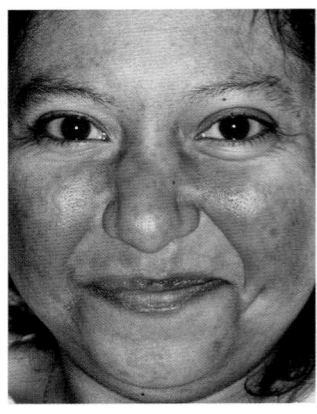

A woman with the butterfly rash of systemic lupus erythematosus. Reprinted from the ARHP Arthritis Teaching Slide Collection. (Used with permission of the American College of Rheumatology.)

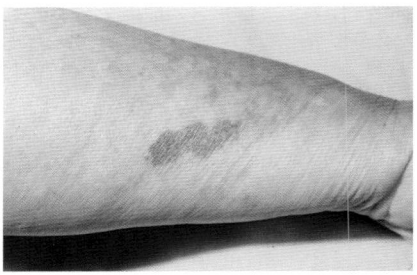

Actinic purpura. (From Lookingbill and Marks, 1993.)

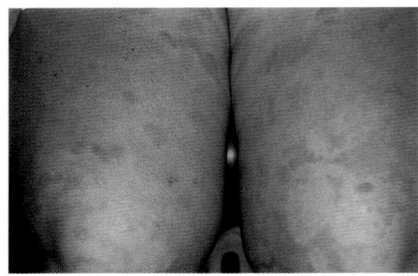

Urticaria. (From Murphy and Herzberg, 1996.)

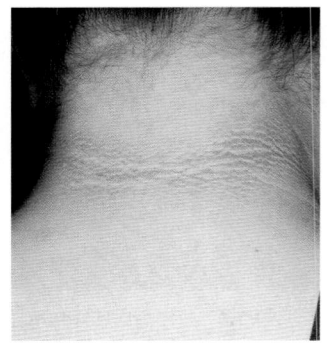

Acanthosis Nigrans. (From Habif et al., 2001.)

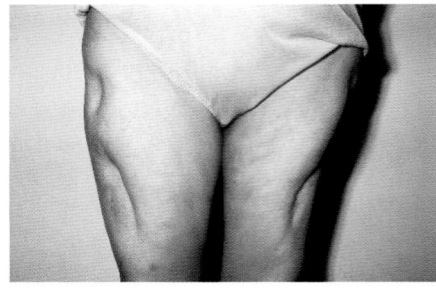

Lipodystrophy at sites of insulin injection. (From Kanski, 2001.)

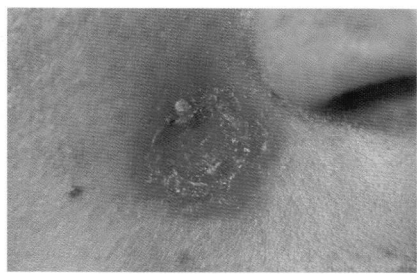

Impetigo on the face. (From Murphay and Herzberg, 1996.)

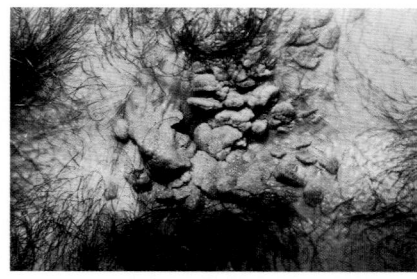

Condyloma acuminatum, with elevated wartlike lesions. (From Murphy and Herzberg, 1996.)

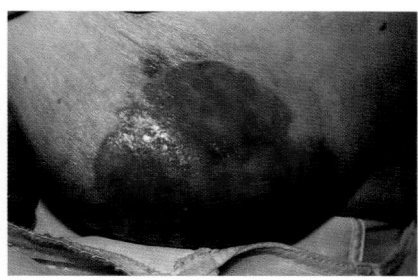

Paget's disease of the breast. (From Murphy and Herzberg, 1996.)

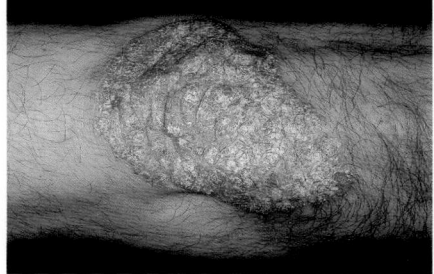

Plaque psoriasis. The classic presentation. Thick red plaques have a sharply defined border and an adherent silvery scale. (From Habif et al., 2001.)

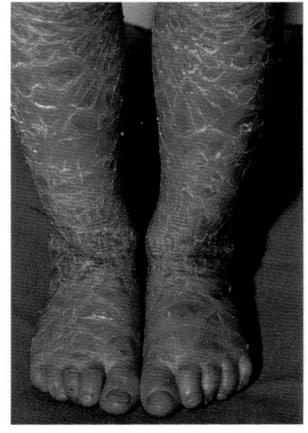

Lamellar ichthyosis, with characteristic "fishlike" scales. (From Murphy and Herzberg, 1996.)

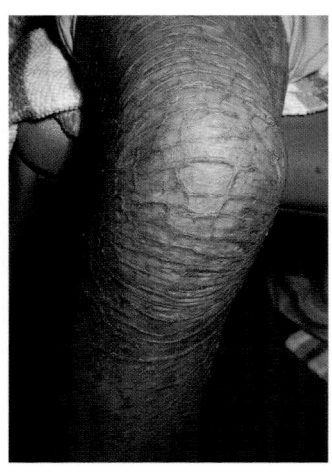

Ichthyosis. (From Kanski, 2001.)

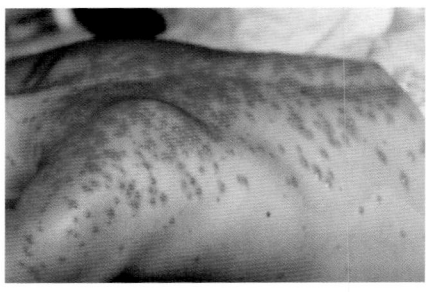

Chicken pox rash distribution. (From Moschella and Hurley, 1992.)

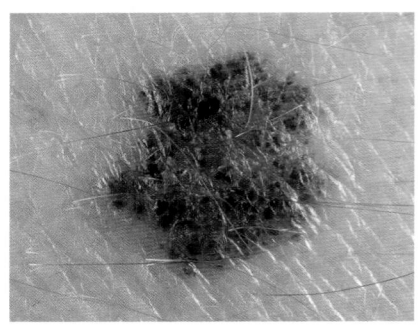

Junction nevi are flat or slightly raised, brown-tan papules. (From Habif et al., 2001.)

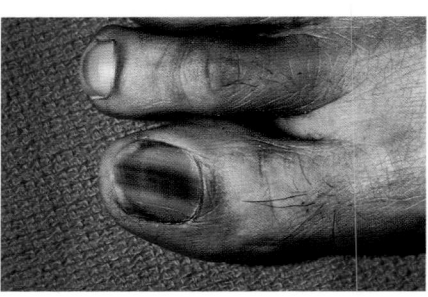

Lentigo of nail bed. (From Murphy and Herzberg, 1996.)

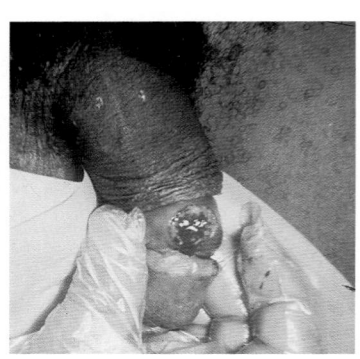

Primary syphilis. The lesion begins as a papule that undergoes ischemic necrosis and erodes, forming a 0.3- to 2.0-cm, painless to tender, hard, indurated ulcer; the base is clean, with a scant, yellow, serous discharge. (From Habif et al., 2001.)

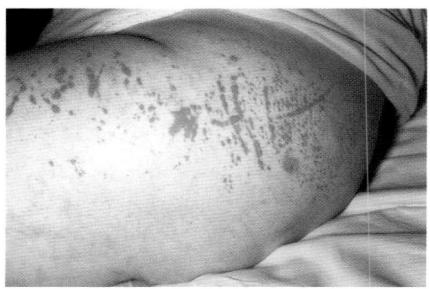

Purpura is a small cutaneous extravasation of blood. (From Kanski, 2001.)

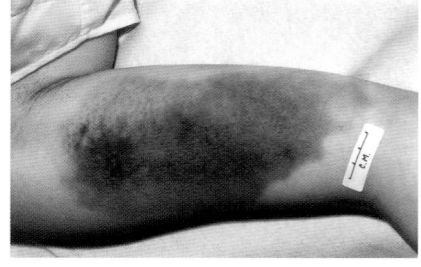

Echymosis or bruising is more extensive cutaneous bleeding. (From Kanski, 2001.)

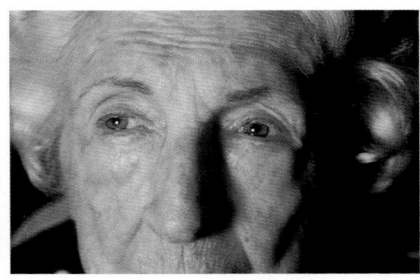

A characteristic change associated with aging is deepening of orbit. (From Ignatavicius et al., 1995, Transparencies and Slides.)

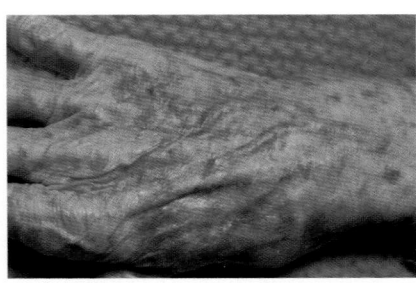

Paperlike or transparent skin is a common physical manifestation of the aging process. (From Ignatavicius et al., 2002.)

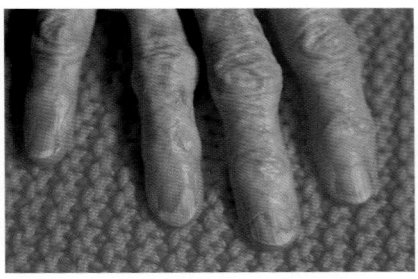

Nail changes: Longitudinal ridges and thickening occur as the individual ages. (From Ignatavicius et al., 2002.)

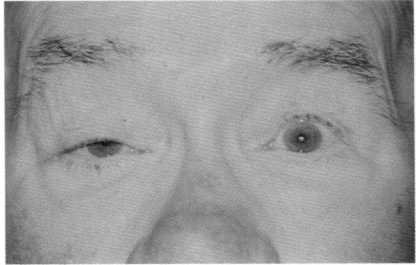

Ptosis of the upper eyelid can occur with aging and may be associated with cerebrovascular accidents, cranial nerve damage, or a variety of other neurologic problems. (Courtesy of Heather Boyd-Monk and Wills Eye Hospital, Philadelphia, PA.)

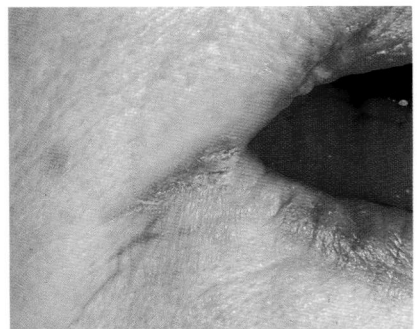

Chelitis. This elderly patient experiences recurrent inflammation from saliva flowing into the deep skinfold at the angle of the mouth. (From Habif et al., 2001.)

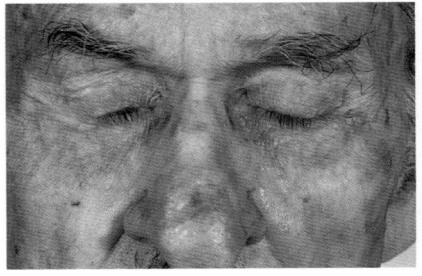

Older adult with actinic keratosis. (From Murphy and Herzberg, 1996.)

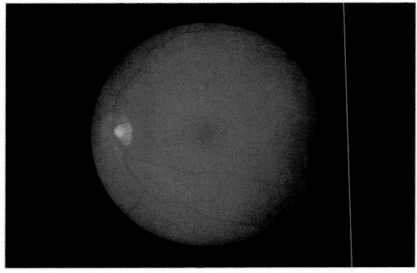

A normal optic fundus. (Courtesy of Dr. Harry Kaplan and Dr. Lawrence P. Roach, Philadelphia, PA.)

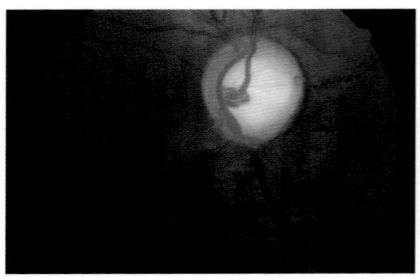

Optic fundus with glaucoma. (From Swartz, 1994.)

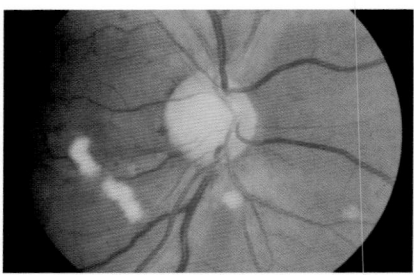

Optic fundus with hypertension; note the cotton-wool exudate. (From Swartz, 1994.)

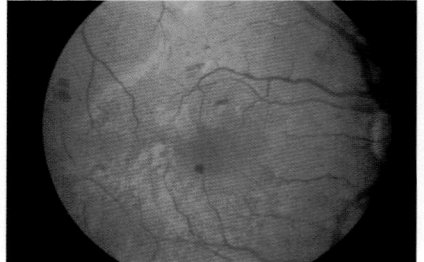

Optic fundus with diabetes. (From Swartz, 1994.)

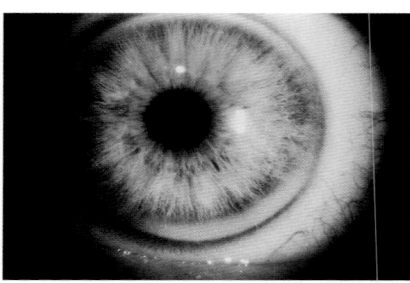

Arcus senilis of the iris. (Courtesy of Dr. John Costin, Lorain, OH.)

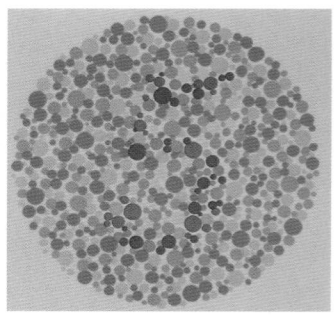

Ishihara chart for testing color vision. (From Ignatavicius et al., 2002.)

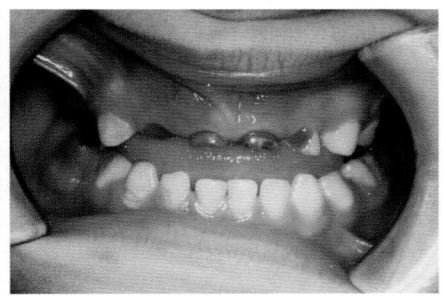

Baby bottle mouth caries. (From Jarvis, 2000.)

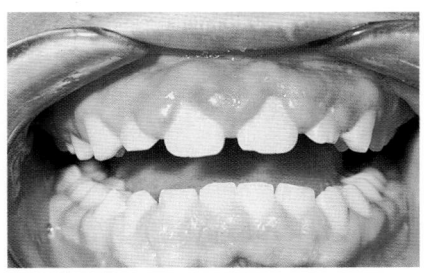

Dilantin gingivitis. (From Daniel and Harfst, 2002.)

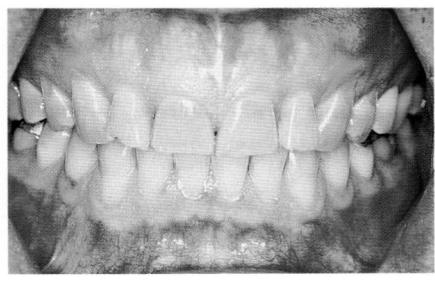

Intrinsic stain—This patient was treated with tetracycline medication during infancy. (From Daniel and Harfst, 2002.)

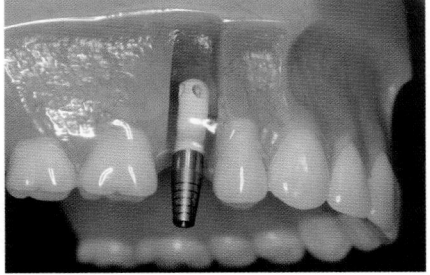

Dental implant—Clean area around the implant demonstrates how it fits into the bone. (From Christensen, 2002.)

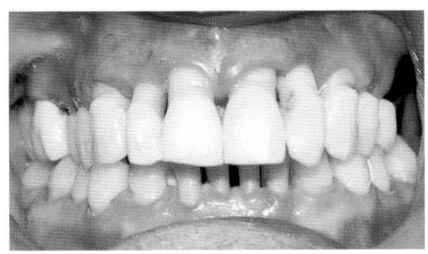

Periodontal disease—Loose teeth caused by bone and gum degeneration. (From Christensen, 2002.)

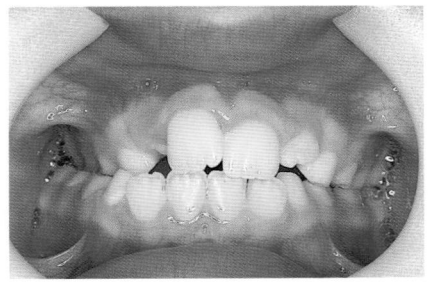

Crossbite—Right side. (From Millett and Welbury, 2000.)

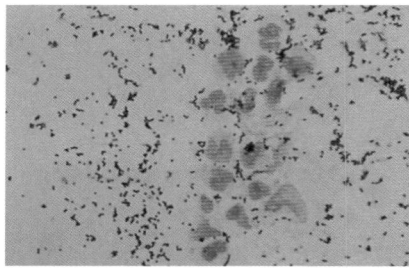

Staphylococcus aureus—Gram stain of pustular wound material.*

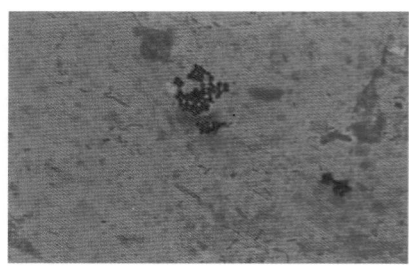

Pseudomonas aeruginosa—Gram stain of sputum.*

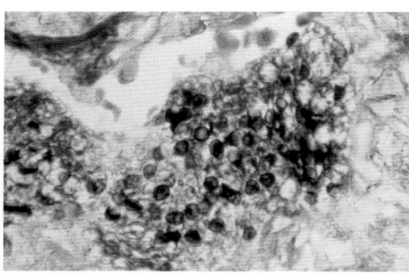

Pneumocystis carinii—Silver impregnation stain of lung with cysts of *P. carinii.**

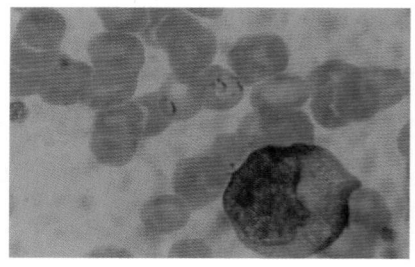

Epstein-Barr virus (HHV-4)—Peripheral blood film from a patient with infectious mononucleosis due to Epstein-Barr virus.*

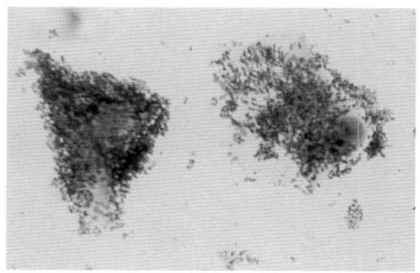

Gardnerella vaginalis—Gram stain of *G. vaginalis* attached to periphery of epithelial cells, sometimes called "clue cells."*

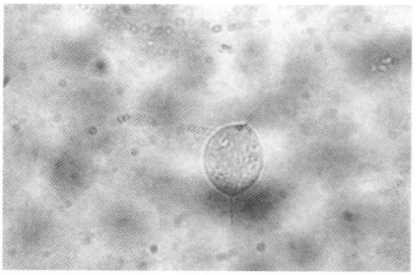

Trichomonas vaginalis—Wet preparation of *T. vaginalis* by phase-contrast microscopy.*

*From Hart and Shears, 1997.

A accommodation; adenine or adenosine; alanine; ampere; anode; anterior; (as a subscript) alveolar gas. See also POINT A.

A absorbance, activity (radioactivity), area, mass number.

A₂ aortic second sound (the aortic component of the second heart sound); see HEART SOUNDS.

Å angstrom.

a atto-.

a. [L.] a′qua (water); arte′ria (artery).

a- word element [L.], *without; not.*

ā [L.] an′te (before).

α alpha, the first letter of the Greek alphabet, often used to indicate the first member of a series, such as the α chain of HEMOGLOBIN. See also terms beginning ALPHA.

AA achievement age; Alcoholics Anonymous.

A̅A̅ [Gr.] a̅a̅.

aa. [L.] arte′riae (arteries).

a̅a̅ an′a (of each), in prescriptions.

AAAS American Association for the Advancement of Science.

AABB American Association of Blood Banks.

AACE American Association of Clinical Endocrinologists.

AACN American Association of Colleges of Nursing; American Association of Critical-Care Nurses.

AAFP American Academy of Family Physicians.

AAGP American Academy of General Practice.

AAIN American Association of Industrial Nurses.

AAMRL American Association of Medical Record Librarians.

AAN American Academy of Nursing.

AANN American Association of Neuroscience Nurses.

AAO American Association of Orthodontists; American Academy of Ophthalmology.

AAO-HNS American Academy of Otolaryngology-Head and Neck Surgery.

AAOS American Academy of Orthopaedic Surgeons.

AAP American Academy of Pediatrics; American Academy of Periodontology; American Association of Pathologists.

AAPA American Academy of Physician Assistants.

AAPMR American Academy of Physical Medicine and Rehabilitation.

AARC American Association for Respiratory Care.

Aaron sign (ar′un) a sensation of pain or distress in the epigastric or precordial region on pressure over the McBurney point in appendicitis.

AARP American Association of Retired Persons.

Ab antibody.

ab [L.] preposition, *from.*

ab- word element [L.], *from; off; away from.*

abacavir (ah-bak′ah-vir) a non-nucleoside reverse transcriptase INHIBITOR used as an ANTIRETROVIRAL in treatment of human immunodeficiency VIRUS infection; administered orally as the sulfate salt.

Abadie's sign loss of feeling in the ACHILLES TENDON, associated with TABES DORSALIS.

abaptiston (a-bap-tis′ton) a saw used to remove a circular area of the skull, constructed so as to avoid slippage with damage to the brain.

abarognosis (ah-bar″og-no′sis) loss of sense of weight.

abasia (ah-ba′zhah) inability to walk. adj., **aba′sic, abat′ic.**

   a.-asta′sia astasia-abasia.

   a. atac′tica abasia with uncertain movements, due to a defect of coordination.

   choreic a. abasia due to chorea of the limbs.

   paralytic a. abasia due to paralysis.

   paroxysmal trepidant a., spastic a. abasia due to spastic stiffening of the legs on attempting to stand.

   trembling a., a. tre′pidans abasia due to trembling of the legs.

abatement (ah-bāt′ment) decrease in severity of a pain, symptom, or disorder.

abciximab (ab-sik′sĭ-mab) a human-murine monoclonal ANTIBODY FAB fragment that inhibits the aggregation of platelets, used in prevention of THROMBOSIS in percutaneous transluminal coronary ANGIOPLASTY; administered by intravenous infusion.

ABC 1. argon beam coagulator; aspiration biopsy cytology. 2. airway, breathing, circulation; acronym used to recall the basics of support for a critically ill patient.

ABCDE an expansion of the ABC's to include airway, breathing, circulation, disability, and exposure.

ABCs airway, breathing, circulation, and cervical spine; these are a priority assessment that is critical in nature. See also ABCDE.

abdomen (ab′dah-men, ab-do′men) the anterior portion of the body between the

THORAX and the PELVIS; it contains the abdominal CAVITY, which is separated from the chest area by the DIAPHRAGM. The cavity, which is lined with a membrane known as the PERITONEUM, contains the stomach, large and small intestines, liver, spleen, pancreas, kidneys, gallbladder, urinary bladder, and other structures. Called also belly and venter. adj., **abdom'inal.** (See accompanying illustration.)

acute a., surgical a. an acute intra-abdominal condition of abrupt onset, usually associated with severe pain due to inflammation, perforation, obstruction, infarction, or rupture of abdominal organs, and usually requiring emergency surgical intervention.

abdomin(o)- word element, *abdomen.*

abdominocentesis (ab-dom″ĭ-no-sen-te′-sis) abdominal PARACENTESIS.

abdominocystic (ab-dom″ĭ-no-sis′tik) pertaining to the abdomen and gallbladder.

abdominohysterectomy (ab-dom″ĭ-no-his″tĕ-rek′-tah-me) abdominal hysterectomy.

abdominohysterotomy (ab-dom″ĭ-no-his″ter-ot′ah-me) abdominal hysterotomy.

abdominoscopy (ab-dom″ĭ-nos′kah-pe) examination of the abdominal cavity, especially direct examination of its organs by endoscopy.

abdominovaginal (ab-dom″ĭ-no-vaj′ĭ-n'l) pertaining to the abdomen and vagina.

abducens (ab-du′senz) [L.] abducent.

a. nerve the sixth CRANIAL NERVE; it arises from the pons and supplies the lateral rectus muscle of the eyeball, allowing for motion. Paralysis of the nerve causes DIPLOPIA (double vision). See anatomic Table of Nerves in the Appendices.

abducent (ab-du′sent) serving to ABDUCT something.

abduct (ab-dukt′) to draw away from an axis or the median plane.

abduction (ab-duk′shun) the act of abducting; the state of being abducted.

abductor (ab-duk′ter) that which abducts; see also anatomic Table of Muscles in the Appendices.

aberratio (ab″er-a′she-o) [L.] aberration.

aberration (ab″er-a′shun) 1. deviation from the normal or usual. 2. imperfect refraction or focalization of a lens.

chromatic a. unequal refraction by a lens of light rays of different lengths passing through it, producing a blurred image and a display of colors.

dioptric a., spherical a. inability of a spherical lens to bring all rays of light to a single focus.

ventricular a. aberrant ventricular conduction.

abetalipoproteinemia (a-ba″tah-lip″o-pro″te-ne′me-ah) a rare autosomal recessive syndrome marked by a lack of low-density LIPOPROTEINS (β-lipoproteins) in the blood and by ACANTHOCYTOSIS, HYPERCHOLESTEROLEMIA, progressive ataxic neuropathy, atypical retinitis pigmentosa involving the macula, and malabsorption. Called also Bassen-Kornzweig syndrome.

abfraction (ab-frak′shun) pathological loss of tooth structure owing to biomechanical

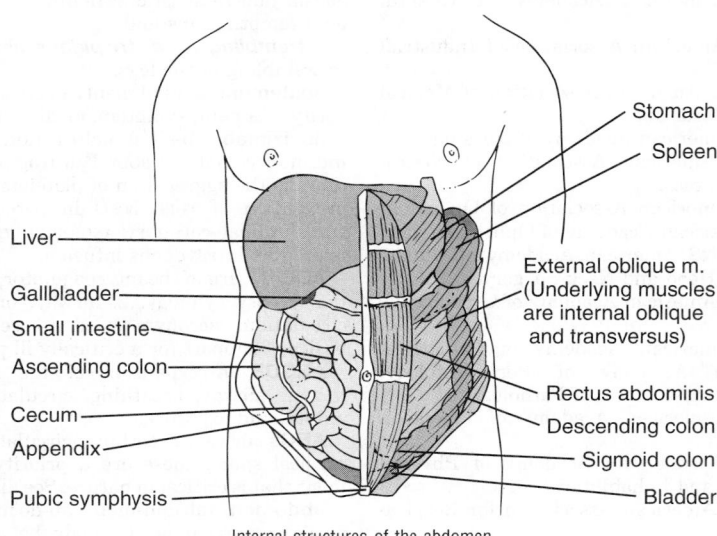

Liver
Gallbladder
Small intestine
Ascending colon
Cecum
Appendix
Pubic symphysis

Stomach
Spleen
External oblique m. (Underlying muscles are internal oblique and transversus)
Rectus abdominis
Descending colon
Sigmoid colon
Bladder

Internal structures of the abdomen.

forces (flexion, compression, or tension) or chemical degradation; it is most visible as V-shaped notches in the cervical area of a tooth.

ABGs arterial blood gases.

abiosis (a″bi-o′sis) absence of life. adj., **abiot′ic.**

abiotrophy (a″bi-ot′rah-fe) progressive loss of vitality of certain tissues or organs leading to disorders or loss of function; applied especially to degenerative hereditary diseases of late onset, such as HUNTINGTON'S CHOREA. adj., **abiotroph′ic.**

ablate (ab-lāt′) to remove, especially by cutting, usually with a laser or electrocautery.

ablatio (ab-la′she-o) [L.] detachment.

   a. re′tinae retinal DETACHMENT.

ablation (ab-la′shun) 1. separation or detachment; extirpation; eradication. 2. removal, especially by cutting with a laser or electrocautery.

   catheter a. radiofrequency ablation.

   endometrial a. removal of the ENDOMETRIUM; methods used include radiofrequency, electrical energy, lasers, and hot and cold liquids.

   radiofrequency a., radiofrequency catheter a. destruction of an accessory conduction PATHWAY or other troublesome area of DYSRHYTHMIA by means of unmodulated high frequency alternating current delivered by a bipolar or unipolar catheter. The current causes heat with tissue destruction and formation of scar tissue to block the pathway or dysrhythmic area. Transvenous radiofrequency ablation has been successful in treatment of supraventricular TACHYCARDIA and is an attractive option to surgery. Called also catheter ablation.

ablepharia (a″blĕ-far′e-ah) congenital absence, partial or complete, of the eyelids. adj., **ableph′arous.**

ablepharon (a″blef′ah-ron) ablepharia.

ablepsia (a″blep′se-ah) blindness.

abluent (ab′loo-ent) 1. detergent; cleansing. 2. a cleansing agent.

abnormality (ab″nor-mal′ĭ-te) 1. the state of being unlike the usual condition. 2. a malformation.

   left atrial a. an atrial conduction abnormality accompanied by an enlarged left atrium; on the electrocardiogram it is seen as notched upright P waves in leads I, II, and V4 to V6, and a deep broad terminal trough in V1. See also P-MITRALE.

aborad (ab-or′ad) away from the mouth.

aboral (ab-or′al) opposite to, or remote from, the mouth.

abort (ah-bort′) to arrest prematurely a disease or developmental process; to expel the products of conception before the fetus is viable.

abortifacient (ah-bor″tĭ-fa′shent) 1. causing abortion. 2. an agent that induces abortion.

abortion (ah-bor′shun) termination of pregnancy before the fetus is viable. In the medical sense, this term and the term MISCARRIAGE both refer to the termination of pregnancy before the fetus is capable of survival outside the uterus. The term *abortion* is more commonly used as a synonym for *induced abortion,* the deliberate interruption of pregnancy, as opposed to miscarriage, which connotes a spontaneous or natural loss of the fetus. Because of this distinction made by the average layperson, care should be exercised in the use of the word abortion when speaking of a spontaneous loss of the fetus.

The technique chosen to terminate pregnancy depends on the stage of pregnancy and the policies of the institution and patient needs. It is rare for a fetus to survive if it weighs less than 500 g, or if the pregnancy is terminated before 20 weeks of gestation. These factors are, however, difficult to determine with a high degree of accuracy while the fetus is still *in utero;* survival of the fetus delivered near the end of the second trimester often depends to a great extent on the availability of personnel and equipment capable of supporting life until the infant develops sufficiently.

Viability of the fetus outside the uterus is frequently used as the determining factor in deciding the legality and morality of induced abortion. Whether this is a valid criterion is essentially based on whether one believes that the fetus is human from the moment of conception or that it achieves humanity at some point during physical development. Those who oppose abortion on moral grounds believe that the fetus is human or potentially human and that destruction of the fetal body is tantamount to murder. Many others have equally strong beliefs that abortion is a woman's right.

The liberalization of abortion laws has resulted in a dramatic increase in the number of abortions performed in physicians' offices, clinics, and hospitals. While this has diminished the occurrence of septic abortions performed at the hands of unscrupulous abortionists and has improved the possibility of safe and uneventful physical recovery from an induced abortion, the issue remains controversial and charged with emotion. The health care provider who strongly objects to abortion is legally and morally free to choose not to participate in the procedure and is advised to avoid situations involving responsibility for the care of patients who have chosen abortion as a means of ending an unwanted pregnancy. Women who have made a decision to have an abortion need a safe, non-judgmental environment to recover physically and emotionally from the procedure.

The patient should know that other alternatives are available and that an abortion after 20 weeks is inadvisable for medical and other reasons. Preabortion counseling in the psychological, religious, and legal aspects of abortion should be readily available, with immediate referral to the proper resources. Although delay in carrying out the procedure may increase the risk of complications, no patient should be encouraged to go through with an abortion until she has had time and sufficient counseling to reach a rational decision. During postabortion counseling there should be a discussion of various methods of CONTRACEPTION. The client will need information on the advantages and disadvantages of each method, her responsibilities in preventing future unwanted pregnancies, and available help in initiating and following through on a program of effective contraception. She should be informed that women who have had two or more abortions run a greatly increased risk of miscarriage or spontaneous abortion in the first six months of subsequent pregnancies.

Patient Care. The type of care required and the complications to be avoided in abortion will depend on the stage of pregnancy at the time of termination and whether the abortion is spontaneous, is induced under sterile conditions, or is performed by an unskilled abortionist or the patient herself. Many women who choose to have an abortion are anxious and confused about the physical and psychological outcomes of the procedure. Therefore both pre- and postabortion counseling are recommended.

In cases of spontaneous or habitual abortion, patient care is directed toward emotional support of the patient and acceptance of her feelings of bitterness, grief, guilt, relief, and other emotions associated with the loss of the fetus. The patient should be able to express her feelings in an open, nonjudgmental, and nonthreatening environment.

complete a. complete expulsion of all the products of conception.

criminal a. termination of pregnancy by illegal interference, usually undertaken when legal induced abortion is unavailable.

The most frequent complications are severe hemorrhage and sepsis, and for those who delay seeking medical attention the mortality rate is high.

early a. abortion within the first 12 weeks of pregnancy.

elective a. induced abortion done at the request of the mother for other than therapeutic reasons.

habitual a. spontaneous ABORTION in three or more consecutive pregnancies before the 20th week of gestation.

incomplete a. abortion in which parts of the products of conception are retained in the uterus.

induced a. abortion brought on intentionally by medication or instrumentation.

inevitable a. a condition in which vaginal bleeding has been profuse, membranes usually show gross rupturing, the cervix has become dilated, and abortion is almost certain.

infected a. abortion associated with infection of the genital tract from retained material, with a febrile reaction.

missed a. retention of dead products of conception in utero for more than 8 weeks.

septic a. abortion associated with serious infection of the products of conception and endometrial lining of the uterus, leading to generalized infection; it is usually caused by pathogenic organisms of the bowel or vagina.

spontaneous a. termination of pregnancy before the fetus is sufficiently developed to survive; called *miscarriage* by laypersons. In the United States this definition is confined to the termination of pregnancy before 20 weeks' gestation (based upon the date of the first day of the last normal menses). Chromosomal abnormalities cause at least half of spontaneous abortions.

therapeutic a. abortion induced legally by a qualified physician to safeguard the health of the mother.

threatened a. a condition in which vaginal bleeding is less than in inevitable abortion, the cervix is not dilated, and abortion may or may not occur; this is the presumed diagnosis when any bloody vaginal discharge or vaginal bleeding occurs in the first half of pregnancy.

abortionist (ah-bor'shun-ist) one who performs abortions; usually refers to criminal abortions.

abortive (ah-bor'tiv) 1. incompletely developed. 2. abortifacient.

abortus (ah-bor'tus) a dead fetus or one that is nonviable (defined as one weighing less than 500 g at birth).

ABPANC American Board of Post Anesthesia Nursing Certification.

ABR auditory brainstem response.

abrachia (ah-bra′ke-ah) a developmental ANOMALY consisting of absence of the arms.

abrachiocephalia (ah-bra″ke-o-sĕ-fa′le-ah) acephalobrachia.

abrasion (ah-bra′zhun) 1. the wearing away of a substance or structure, such as the skin or teeth, through some unusual or abnormal process. 2. a wound caused by rubbing or scraping the skin or a mucous membrane; a "skinned knee" and a "floor burn" are common examples. To treat the injury, the wound should be washed, a mild antiseptic or antibiotic ointment applied, and the wound covered with sterile gauze.

    air a. a type of MICROABRASION in which a jet of air blows tiny particles against the tooth or cavity surface.

abrasive (ah-bra′siv) 1. causing abrasion. 2. an agent that produces abrasion.

abreaction (ab″re-ak′shun) the expression of emotions associated with repressed material, usually of an anxiety-provoking or conflictual nature, which is brought into a person's awareness and relived. See also CATHARSIS.

abruptio (ab-rup′she-o) [L.] separation.

    a. placen′tae premature separation of a normally situated but improperly implanted PLACENTA; it usually occurs late in pregnancy, but may take place during labor. Separation of the placenta before the 24th week of pregnancy is considered a spontaneous ABORTION if the abruption is so severe that the pregnancy is lost.

Contributing factors include multiple pregnancies (grand multiparity), chronic hypertensive disease, direct trauma to the uterus, or sudden release of amniotic fluid.

Premature separation of the placenta is classified from Grade 0 to Grade 3 according to the degree of separation. In *Grade 0* mother and fetus are asymptomatic. Diagnosis is made after delivery when the placenta is examined and a clot is found adhering to the maternal surface. *Grade 1* is minimal separation that causes some vaginal bleeding and changes in maternal vital signs. Fetal distress and hemorrhagic shock are absent. *Grade 2* is moderate separation in which there is evidence of fetal distress and maternal symptoms of a tense uterus and pain on palpation. *Grade 3* is the most serious. There is extreme separation which, without prompt intervention, can lead to maternal shock and fetal death. (See accompanying illustration.)

Patient Care. Treatment and patient care are based on the grade of separation and maternal and fetal status. Maternal vital signs are monitored and blood loss is assessed. The uterus is assessed for any tenderness, tension, or rigidity. The location and nature of pain reported by the mother are noted; for example, a sharp stabbing pain high in the fundus can occur when separation begins. Pain that is in addition to the pain of contractions is also significant.

Oxygen may be administered to the mother to limit fetal anoxia. Fetal heart sounds are monitored for signs of fetal distress. The patient is kept in a lateral rather than supine position during labor to prevent pressure on the vena cava and further inhibition of fetal blood supply. Vaginal or pelvic examinations and an enema are restricted lest the placenta be disturbed further.

Grade 2 and Grade 3 separations require delivery as soon as possible, either vaginally

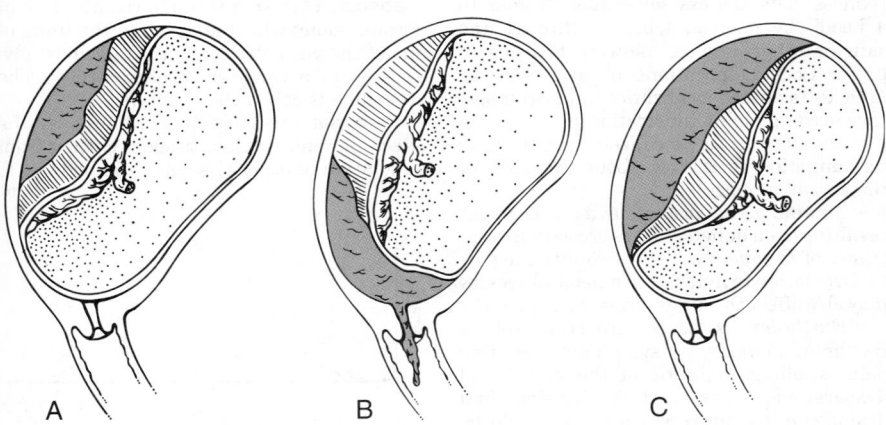

Abruptio placentae. *A,* Mild abruption with concealed hemorrhage. *B,* Severe abruption with external hemorrhage. *C,* Complete separation with concealed hemorrhage.

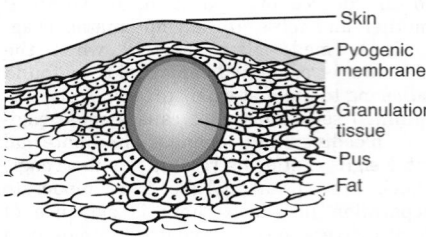

Abscess, cross section.

Skin
Pyogenic membrane
Granulation tissue
Pus
Fat

or by cesarean section. Without prompt and effective intervention, abruptio placentae can lead to maternal death from hemorrhage, shock, and circulatory collapse. Fetal prognosis depends on the extent of hypoxia suffered by the fetus during labor and delivery.

abscess (ab′ses) a localized collection of pus in a cavity formed by the disintegration of tissue. Abscesses are usually caused by specific microorganisms that invade the tissues, often by way of small wounds or breaks in the skin. An abscess is a natural defense mechanism in which the body attempts to localize an infection and wall off the microorganisms so that they cannot spread throughout the body. As the microorganisms destroy the tissue, an increased supply of blood is rushed to the area. The cells, bacteria, and dead tissue accumulate to form a clump of cream-colored liquid, which is the pus. The accumulating pus and the adjacent swollen, inflamed tissues press against the nerves, causing pain. The concentration of blood in the area causes redness. The abscess sometimes "comes to a head" by itself and breaks through the skin or other tissues, allowing the pus to drain. Local applications of heat may be used to facilitate localization and drainage. (See accompanying illustration.)

alveolar a. a localized suppurative inflammation of tissues about the apex of the root of a tooth.

amebic a. an abscess cavity of the liver resulting from liquefaction necrosis due to entrance of *Entamoeba histolytica* into the portal circulation in amebiasis; amebic abscesses may also affect the lungs, brain, and spleen.

Bartholin a. acute infection of a Bartholin gland with symptoms including pain, swelling, cellulitis of the vulva, and dyspareunia. Treatment is incision and drainage of the abscess. Cultures should be obtained to rule out infections by *Neisseria gonorrhoeae* or *Chlamydia*.

Bezold's a. one deep in the neck resulting from a complication of acute mastoiditis.

brain a. see BRAIN ABSCESS.

Brodie's a. a circumscribed abscess in bone, caused by hematogenous infection, that becomes a chronic nidus of infection.

cold a. one of slow development and with little inflammation, usually tuberculous.

diffuse a. an uncircumscribed abscess whose pus is diffused in the surrounding tissues.

gas a. one containing gas, caused by gas-forming bacteria such as *Clostridium perfringens*. Called also Welch's abscess.

miliary a. one composed of numerous small collections of pus.

pancreatic a. one that occurs as a complication of acute pancreatitis or postoperative pancreatitis caused by secondary bacterial contamination.

perianal a. one beneath the skin of the anus and the anal canal.

periapical a. inflammation with pus in the tissues surrounding the apex of a tooth.

periodontal a. a localized collection of pus in the periodontal tissue.

peritonsillar a. a localized accumulation of pus in the peritonsillar tissue subsequent to suppurative inflammation of the tonsil; called also quinsy.

phlegmonous a. one associated with acute inflammation of the subcutaneous connective tissue.

stitch a. one developed about a stitch or suture.

thecal a. one in the sheath of a tendon.

wandering a. one that burrows into tissues and finally points at a distance from the site of origin.

Welch's a. gas abscess.

abscissa (ab-sis′ah) the horizontal line in a graph along which are plotted the units of one of the variables considered in the study, as time in a time-temperature study. The other line is called the ORDINATE.

abscopal (ab-sko′p'l) pertaining to the effect on nonirradiated tissue resulting from irradiation of other tissues of the body.

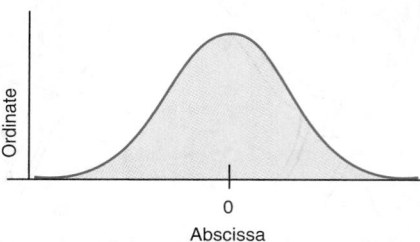

Ordinate
0
Abscissa

Axes of graph showing normal distribution curve.

Absidia a genus of perfect fungi; the species *A. ramo′sa* is found on decaying plants and baked goods and can cause MUCORMYCOSIS.

absorb (ab-sorb′) 1. to take in or assimilate, as to take up substances into or across tissues, e.g., the skin or intestine. 2. to stop particles of radiation energy so that their energy is totally transferred to the absorbing material. 3. to retain specific wavelengths of radiation incident upon a substance, either raising its temperature or changing the energy state of its molecules.

absorbance (ab-sor′bans) in radiology, a measure of the ability of a medium to absorb radiation, expressed as the logarithm of the quotient of the intensity of the radiation entering the medium divided by that leaving it.

absorbefacient (ab-sor″bĕ-fa′shent) 1. causing absorption. 2. absorbent (def. 3).

absorbent (ab-sorb′ent) 1. able to take in, or suck up and incorporate. 2. a tissue structure involved in absorption. 3. a substance that absorbs or promotes absorption.

absorptiometry (ab-sorp″she-om′ĕ-tre) in radiology, the measurement of the degree to which the radiation emitted by a radioisotope is completely dissipated within a tissue.

dual energy a. **(DEXA)** an imaging technique that uses two low-dose x-ray beams with different levels of energy to produce a detailed image of body components; used primarily to measure bone mineral density.

dual photon a. measurement of bone mineral content in the axial skeleton, particularly the lumbar spine, by comparing transmission of the two separate photoelectric energy peaks emitted by GADOLINIUM 153 through both soft and bone tissues.

absorption (ab-sorp′shun) 1. the act of taking up or in by specific chemical or molecular action; especially the passage of liquids or other substances through a surface of the body into body fluids and tissues, as in the absorption of the end products of DIGESTION into the villi that line the intestine. 2. in psychology, devotion of thought to one object or activity only. 3. in radiology, uptake of energy by matter with which the radiation interacts. It can vary with the mass (density) subjected to x-radiation and the penetrability of the x-rays. A thin lead plate might absorb 100 per cent of an x-ray beam, while several centimeters of tissue might attenuate it only slightly, even at low voltages. 4. in chemistry, the penetration of a substance within the inner structure of another; see also ADSORPTION.

chemical a. any process by which one substance in liquid or solid form penetrates the surface of another substance.

digestive a. the passage of the end products of DIGESTION from the gastrointestinal tract into the blood and lymphatic vessels and the cells of tissues. Absorption of this kind can take place either by diffusion or by active transport.

radiation a. the dissipation of radiant energy as it passes through matter. This phenomenon is of particular importance in diagnostic and therapeutic radiology, which depends on the interaction between ionizing radiations and matter. As radiation passes through matter, it is absorbed by an amount dependent on the atomic and molecular structure and thickness of the substance, and the energy of the primary photons. If radiations pass through a medium of living or nonliving material without absorption (loss of energy), no biologic or photographic effects can occur. In true absorption the photons of radiation waves give up or transfer all of their energy to electrons within the atoms of the matter through which they are passing.

absorptive (ab-sorp′tiv) having the power of absorption; involving absorption.

absorptivity (ab″sorp-tiv′ĭ-te) a measure of the amount of light absorbed by a solution.

abstinence (ab′stĭ-nens) a refraining from the use of or indulgence in food, stimulants, or coitus.

periodic a. natural family planning; see CONTRACEPTION.

a. syndrome withdrawal (def. 2).

abstract (ab′strakt) 1. a short description of a scientific presentation or article. 2. a thought process that is oriented toward the development of an idea without application to, or association with, a particular instance. This type of thinking is independent of time and space.

abstraction (ab-strak′shun) 1. the mental process of forming ideas that are theoretical or representational rather than concrete. 2. the withdrawal of any ingredient from a compound. 3. malocclusion in which the occlusal plane is farther from the eye-ear plane, causing lengthening of the face.

abulia (ah-bu′le-ah) 1. lack of will or willpower; inability to make decisions. adj. **abu′lic.** 2. akinetic mutism.

abuse (ah-būs′) misuse, maltreatment, or excessive use.

child a. see CHILD ABUSE.

domestic a. abuse of a person by another person with whom the victim is living, has lived, or with whom a significant relationship exists. The abuse may take the form of verbal abuse, sexual abuse, physical battering, or psychological (emotional) unavailability. Abuse is a learned behavior and has an escalating cycle; abusive behavior cuts across all racial, ethnic, educational, and socioeconomic boundaries.

drug a. see DRUG ABUSE.

elder a. maltreatment of an older adult, ranging from passive neglect of needs to overt mental, physical, or sexual assault.

physical a. any act resulting in a non-accidental physical injury, including not only intentional assault but also the results of unreasonable punishment.

psychoactive substance a. substance abuse.

sexual a. any act of a sexual nature performed in a criminal manner, as with a child or with a nonconsenting adult, including RAPE, INCEST, oral copulation, and penetration of genital or anal opening with a foreign object. The term also includes lewd or lascivious acts with a child; any sexual act that could be expected to trouble or offend another person when done by someone motivated by sexual interest; acts related to sexual exploitation, such as those related to pornography, prostitution involving minors, or coercion of minors to perform obscene acts.

substance a. a substance use disorder characterized by the use of a mood or behavior-altering substance in a maladaptive pattern resulting in significant impairment or distress, such as failure to fulfill social or occupational obligations or recurrent use in situations in which it is physically dangerous to do so or which end in legal problems, but without fulfilling the criteria for substance DEPENDENCE. Specific disorders are named for their etiology, such as alcohol abuse and anabolic steroid abuse. DSM-IV includes specific abuse disorders for alcohol, amphetamines or similar substances, cannabis, cocaine, hallucinogens, inhalants, opioids, PCP or similar substances, and sedatives, hypnotics, or anxiolytics. See also DRUG ABUSE.

abutment (ah-but′ment) the anchorage tooth for a bridge. (See accompanying illustration.)

Ac actinium.

a.c. [L.] an′te ci′bum (before meals).

acalculia (a″kal-ku′le-ah) inability to solve mathematical calculations.

acampsia (ah-kamp′se-ah) rigidity of a part or limb.

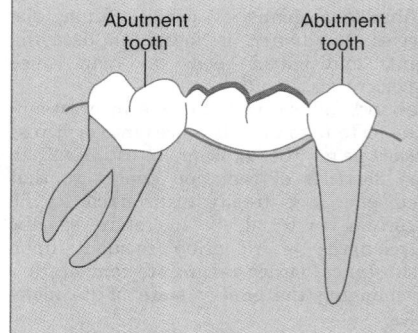

Abutment tooth. From Darby and Walsh, 1995.

acanth(o)- word element [Gr.], *sharp spine; thorn.*

acantha (ah-kan′thah) 1. spine (def. 1). 2. spinous process of vertebra.

Acanthamoeba (ah-kan″thah-me′bah) a genus of free-living ameboid protozoa found usually in fresh water or moist soil. Certain species, such as *A. castella′ni, A. poly′phaga, A. astronyx′is,* and *A. culbert′soni,* may occur as opportunistic human pathogens, causing an acute fatal or chronic infection of the eye, brain, liver, kidney, lung, pancreas, and skin in patients with underlying disease or in immunocompromised patients.

acanthesthesia (ah-kan″thes-the′zhah) a sensation of a sharp point pricking the body.

acanthion (ah-kan′the-on) a point at the tip of the anterior nasal spine.

Acanthocephala (ah-kan″tho-sef′ah-lah) a phylum of elongate, mostly cylindrical organisms (thorny headed worms) parasitic in the intestines of all classes of vertebrates.

acanthocephaliasis (ah-kan″tho-sef″ah-li′ah-sis) infection with worms of the phylum Acanthocephala.

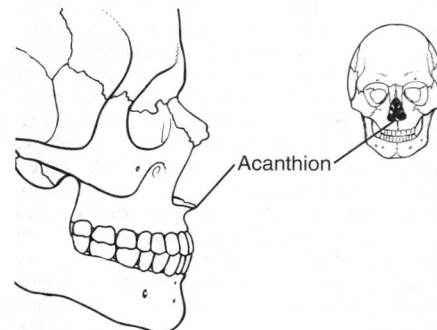

Acanthion. From Dorland's, 2000.

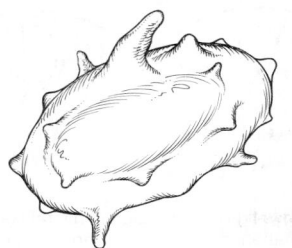

Acanthocyte. From Dorland's, 2000.

acanthocyte (ah-kan'tho-sīt) an irregularly spiculated erythrocyte of normal or slightly reduced size, with 3 to 12 spicules of varying lengths along the periphery of the cell membrane; seen in congenital ABETALIPOPROTEINEMIA, CIRRHOSIS, HEMOLYTIC ANEMIA, hepatitis of the newborn, vitamin E deficiency, and HYPERCHOLESTEROLEMIA. Called also spur cell.

acanthocytosis (ah-kan″tho-si-to'sis) the presence in the blood of acanthocytes.

acantholysis (ak″an-thol'ĭ-sis) disruption of the intercellular connections between keratinocytes of the epidermis, caused by lysis of intercellular cement substance. It is associated with the formation of epidermal vesicles in such conditions as pemphigus vulgaris, pemphigus foliaceus, and other skin disorders.

acanthoma (ak″an-tho'mah), pl. *acanthomas, acantho'mata* a tumor in the prickle cell layer of the skin.

acanthosis (ak″an-tho'sis) diffuse hypertrophy or thickening of the prickle cell layer of the skin. adj., **acanthot'ic.**

a. ni'gricans diffuse acanthosis with gray, brown, or black pigmentation, chiefly in the axillae and other body folds, occurring in an adult form, often associated with an internal carcinoma (called *malignant acanthosis nigricans*) and in a benign, nevoid form, more or less generalized. A benign form associated with obesity, which is sometimes due to endocrine disturbance, is called *pseudo-acanthosis nigricans.* (See Atlas 2, Part E).

acarbia (ah-kahr'be-ah) decrease of bicarbonate in the blood.

acarbose (a'kahr-bōs) an α-glucosidase inhibitor used to combat HYPERGLYCEMIA in treatment of type 2 DIABETES MELLITUS.

acardia (ah-kahr'de-ah) a developmental ANOMALY consisting of absence of the heart.

acardiacus (a″kahr-di'ah-kus) [L.] having no heart.

acardius (a-kahr'de-us) a parasitic twin fetus that lacks a heart and uses the circulation of its twin. See also HEMIACARDIUS and HOLOACARDIUS.

acariasis (ak″ah-ri'ah-sis) infestation with mites.

acaricide (ah-kar'ĭ-sīd) an agent that destroys mites.

acarid (ak'ah-rid) a tick or a mite of the order Acarina.

Acarina (ak″ah-ri'nah) an order of arthropods (class Arachnoidea), including mites and ticks.

acarinosis (ah-kar″ĭ-no'sis) any disease caused by mites; acariasis.

acarodermatitis (ak″ah-ro-der″mah-ti'tis) skin inflammation due to bites of parasitic mites (acarids).

acarophobia (ak″ah-ro-fo'be-ah) irrational fear of mites or of other minute objects, which may be animate (insects, worms) or inanimate (pins, needles). Sometimes there is also a fear of parasites crawling beneath the skin.

acaryote (ah-kar'e-ōt) 1. non-nucleated. 2. a non-nucleated cell.

acatalasemia (a″kat-ah-la-se'me-ah) acatalasia.

acatalasia (a″kat-ah-la'zhah) a rare hereditary disease seen mostly in Japan and Switzerland, marked by congenital absence of catalase; it may be asymptomatic but is usually associated with recurrent infections of oral structures. A variety in Japan is characterized by oral ulcerations and gangrene and is known as TAKAHARA'S DISEASE.

acatamathesia (ah-kat″ah-mah-the'zhah) 1. loss or impairment of the power to understand speech. 2. impairment of any one of the perceptive faculties, due to a central lesion.

acceleration (ak-sel″er-a'shun) 1. a quickening, as of the pulse rate. 2. in physics, the time rate of change of velocity.

psychomotor a. generalized physical and emotional overactivity in response to internal and external stimuli, such as that seen in the manic phase of BIPOLAR DISORDER.

ACC American College of Cardiology.

accelerator (ak-sel'er-a″ter) [L.] an agent or apparatus that increases the rate at which something occurs or progresses.

serum prothrombin conversion a. **(SPCA)** factor VII, one of the COAGULATION FACTORS.

acceptor (ak-sep'ter) a substance that unites with another substance.

hydrogen a. the molecule accepting hydrogen in an oxidation-reduction reaction.

access (ak'ses) a means of approaching something.

arteriovenous a. the usual type of vascular ACCESS, connecting an artery and a vein, usually in the arm.

hemodialysis a., vascular a. the means by which HEMODIALYSIS apparatus is connected to blood vessels; the most common type is arteriovenous ACCESS. Other types include venovenous ACCESS and types of FISTULAS and SHUNTS.

venovenous a. vascular ACCESS via a tube that begins at a vein and ends at a vein, used in HEMODIALYSIS and continuous venovenous HEMOFILTRATION.

accessory (ak-ses′ah-re) supplementary or affording aid to another similar and generally more important thing.

a. nerve the eleventh CRANIAL NERVE (called also spinal accessory nerve); it originates in the medulla oblongata and provides motion for the sternocleidomastoid and trapezius muscles of the neck. See anatomic Table of Nerves in the Appendices.

accident (ak′sĭ-dent) an unforeseen occurrence, especially one of an injurious nature.

cerebral vascular a., cerebrovascular a. (CVA) stroke syndrome.

accipiter (ak-sip′ĭ-ter) a facial bandage with tails like the claws of a hawk.

acclimation (ak″lĭ-ma′shun) physiological or psychological adjustment to a new environment.

accommodation (ah-kom″ah-da′shun) adjustment, especially adjustment of the eye for seeing objects at various distances. This is accomplished by the ciliary muscle, which controls the LENS of the eye, allowing it to flatten or thicken as is needed for distant or near vision. (See accompanying illustration.)

absolute a. the accommodation of either eye separately.

amplitude of a. range of accommodation.

histologic a. changes in morphology and function of cells following changed conditions.

negative a. adjustment of the eye for long distances by relaxation of the ciliary muscle.

positive a. adjustment of the eye for short distances by contraction of the ciliary muscle.

accouchement (ah-kōōsh-maw′) [Fr.] 1. childbirth. 2. delivery.

a. forcé rapid forcible delivery by one of several methods (such as forceps or a vacuum extractor); originally, rapid dilatation of the cervix with the hands, followed by version and extraction of the fetus.

accountability (ah-kown″tah-bil′ĭ-te) responsibility for one's own actions; this is a principle of professional practice that is obligatory for health care providers.

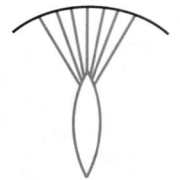 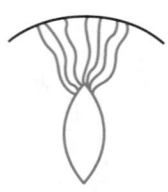

Ligaments tight—lens flattened   Ligaments relaxed—lens more rounded

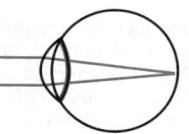 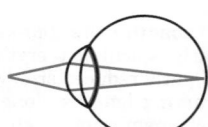

Rays from a *distant* object are focused on the retina by a flattened lens   Rays from a *nearby* object are focused on the retina by a more rounded lens

Flattening and rounding of lens during accommodation.

ACCP American College of Chest Physicians.

accreditation (ah-kred″ĭ-ta′shun) a process that a health care institution, provider, or program undergoes to demonstrate compliance with standards developed by an official agency. Accreditation for institutions and agencies in the United States and Canada is voluntary.

Accredited Record Technician (ART) see MEDICAL RECORD ADMINISTRATOR.

accretion (ah-kre′shun) 1. growth by addition of material. 2. accumulation. adherence of parts normally separated.

acculturation (ah-kul″cher-a′shun) the process of adapting or learning to take on selected behaviors of another group; change generally occurs between both cultures that are in contact.

ACE angiotensin-converting enzyme.

acebutolol (as″ĕ-bu′to-lol) a cardioselective β₁-adrenergic blocking agent with intrinsic sympathomimetic activity; used in the form of the hydrochloride salt for treatment of hypertension, angina pectoris, and arrhythmias; administered orally.

acellular (a-sel′u-ler) lacking cells or not cellular in structure.

acelomate (a-se′lah-māt) having no coelom or body cavity.

acentric (a-sen′trik) 1. not central; not located in the center. 2. lacking a centromere, so that the chromosome will not survive cell divisions.

ACEP American College of Emergency Physicians.

acephalobrachia (a-sef″ah-lo-bra′ke-ah) congenital absence of the head and arms.

acephalocardia (a-sef″ah-lo-kahr′de-ah) congenital absence of the head and heart.

acephalocardius (a-sef″ah-lo-kahr′de-us) a fetus without a head or heart.

acephalochiria (a-sef″ah-lo-ki′re-ah) congenital absence of the head and hands.

acephalogaster (a-sef″ah-lo-gas′ter) a fetus without a head or stomach.

acephalogastria (a-sef″ah-lo-gas′tre-ah) congenital absence of the head, chest, and stomach.

acephalopodia (a-sef″ah-lo-po′de-ah) congenital absence of the head and feet.

acephalopodius (a-sef″ah-lo-po′de-us) a fetus without a head or feet.

acephalorhachia (a-sef″ah-lo-ra′ke-ah) congenital absence of the head and vertebral column.

acephalostomia (a-sef″ah-lo-sto′me-ah) congenital absence of the head, with the mouth aperture on the upper aspect of the body.

acephalothoracia (a-sef″ah-lo-tho-ra′se-ah) congenital absence of the head and thorax.

acephalous (a-sef′ah-lus) headless.

acephalus (a-sef′ah-lus) a headless fetus.

acervuline (ah-ser′vu-līn) occurring in clusters; aggregated; said of certain glands.

acervulus (ah-ser′vu-lus) [L.] sandy matter in or about the pineal body and other parts of the brain.

acetabular (as″ĕ-tab′u-ler) pertaining to the acetabulum.

acetabulectomy (as″ĕ-tab″u-lek′to-me) excision of the acetabulum.

acetabuloplasty (as″ĕ-tab′u-lo-plas″te) plastic repair of the acetabulum.

acetabulum (as″ĕ-tab′u-lum), pl. *aceta′-bula* [L.] the cup-shaped cavity on the lateral surface of the hip bone in which the head of the femur articulates. (See accompanying illustration.)

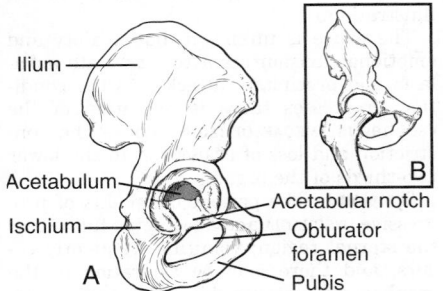

Acetabulum, showing the cup-shaped cavity *(A)*, and its articulation with the femur *(B)*. From Dorland's, 2000.

acetal (as′ĕ-t′l) 1. any of a class of organic compounds formed by combination of an aldehyde molecule with two alcohol molecules. 2. $CH_3CH(OC_2H_5)_2$, a colorless volatile liquid used as a solvent and in cosmetics.

acetaldehyde (as″et-al′de-hīd) a colorless volatile liquid used in the manufacture of acetic acid, perfumes, and flavors, which is irritating to mucous membranes and has a general narcotic action. It is also an intermediate in the metabolism of alcohol.

acetaminophen (ah-se″tah-min′o-fen) an ANALGESIC and ANTIPYRETIC commonly used instead of ASPIRIN, particularly for patients who are allergic to aspirin, are taking ANTICOAGULANTS, or have PEPTIC ULCER or GASTRITIS. Unlike aspirin, it has only weak antiinflammatory effects and is not used to treat the inflammation associated with rheumatoid ARTHRITIS.

Acute acetaminophen overdosage can cause severe and potentially fatal hepatic necrosis, when a large amount of the drug is accidentally ingested. One of the ways that the liver detoxifies the drug is by conjugation of a metabolite with glutathione, and when the glutathione stores are used up, the metabolite attacks the liver tissues. Treatment is symptomatic and supportive. Two drugs, methionine and acetylcysteine, can reduce the liver damage by serving as substitutes for glutathione.

acetate (as′ĕ-tāt) a salt or ester or the conjugate base of acetic acid.

acetazolamide (as″et-ah-zol′ah-mīd) a carbonic anhydrase INHIBITOR used in treatment of glaucoma, petit mal epilepsy, familial periodic paralysis, and acute mountain sickness, and as a urinary alkalyzer in prophylaxis and treatment of uric acid renal calculi. Side effects are minor but an electrolyte imbalance with potassium depletion may occur. Administered orally, intravenously, and intramuscularly.

Acetest (as′ĕ-test) trademark for a reagent tablet containing sodium nitroprusside, aminoacetic acid, dibasic sodium phosphate, and lactose, turning a purple color in the presence of ketone bodies in urine, blood, plasma, or serum; the intensity of the color reaction indicates the acetoacetate or acetone concentration, ranging from a pale lavender through a dark purple as the concentration increases.

acetic (ah-se′tik, ah-set′ik) pertaining to vinegar or its acid; sour.

acetic acid (ah-se′tik) the two-carbon carboxylic acid, the characteristic component of vinegar; used as a SOLVENT, MENSTRUUM, and pharmaceutic NECESSITY. *Glacial* *acetic acid* (anhydrous acetic acid) is used as a solvent, vesicant and caustic, and pharmaceutic necessity.

acetoacetic acid (ah-se″to-ah-se′tik) one of the KETONE BODIES formed in the body in metabolism of certain substances, particularly in the liver in the combustion of fats. It is present in the body in increased amounts in abnormal conditions such as uncontrolled DIABETES MELLITUS and starvation.

acetohexamide (as″ĕ-to-heks′ah-mīd) a SULFONYLUREA administered orally to treat hyperglycemia in patients with type 2 diabetes mellitus whose blood glucose cannot be controlled by diet and exercise alone.

acetohydroxamic acid (as″ĕ-to-hi″droks-am′ik) an inhibitor of bacterial UREASE used in prophylaxis and treatment of struvite KIDNEY STONES whose formation is favored by urease-producing bacteria and as an adjunct in treatment of URINARY TRACT INFECTIONS caused by urease-producing bacteria; administered orally.

acetone (as′ĕ-tōn) a compound, $CH_3 \cdot CO \cdot CH_3$, with a characteristic odor; it is used as a solvent and as an antiseptic. Acetone is one of the KETONE BODIES produced in abnormal amounts in uncontrolled DIABETES MELLITUS and metabolic ACIDOSIS. See also KETOSIS.

acetonemia (as″ĕ-to-ne′me-ah) ketonemia.

acetonuria (as″ĕ-to-nu′re-ah) ketonuria.

acetrizoate sodium (as″ĕ-tri-zo′āt) the sodium salt of acetrizoic acid, used as a contrast medium in hysterosalpingography.

acetyl (as′ĕ-til, as′ĕtēl″) the monovalent radical $CH_3CO—$, a combining form of acetic acid.

acetylator (ah-set″ĭ-la′ter) an organism capable of metabolic acetylation. Individuals that differ in their inherited ability to metabolize certain drugs, e.g., isoniazid, are termed fast or slow acetylators.

acetylcholine (ACh) (as″ĕ-til-ko′lēn) the acetic acid ester of choline, normally present in many parts of the body and having important physiologic functions. It is a neurotransmitter at cholinergic synapses in the central, sympathetic, and parasympathetic nervous systems. Used in medicine as a miotic.

acetylcholinesterase (as″ĕ-til-ko″lin-es′-ter-ās) an enzyme present in nervous tissue, muscle, and red blood cells that catalyzes the hydrolysis of ACETYLCHOLINE to choline and acetic acid. This enzyme is present throughout the body, but is particularly important at the myoneural JUNCTION, where the nerve fibers terminate. Acetylcholine is released when a nerve impulse reaches a myoneural junction. It diffuses across the synaptic cleft and binds to cholinergic receptors on the muscle fibers, causing them to contract. CHOLINESTERASE splits acetylcholine into its components, thus stopping stimulation of the muscle fibers. The end products of the metabolism of acetylcholine are taken up by nerve fibers and resynthesized into acetylcholine. The drugs NEOSTIGMINE, PHYSOSTIGMINE, and PYRIDOSTIGMINE inhibit acetylcholinesterase and are used to treat MYASTHENIA GRAVIS, a disease in which the cholinergic receptors are attacked by autoantibodies. The drug extends the effect of acetylcholine on the muscle fiber. Called also true cholinesterase

acetylcoenzyme A (as″ĕ-til-ko-en′zīm a) acetyl-CoA, an important biochemical intermediate in the tricarboxylic acid CYCLE and the chief precursor of lipids; it is formed by the attachment to coenzyme A of an acetyl group during the oxidation of pyruvate, fatty acids, or amino acids.

acetylcysteine (as″ĕ-til-sis′te-ēn) a MUCOLYTIC agent used by instillation or nebulization to reduce the viscosity of respiratory tract secretions and orally or intravenously as an antidote to acetaminophen poisoning.

acetylene (ah-set′ĭ-lēn) $HC{\equiv}CH$, a colorless, combustible, explosive gas, the simplest alkyne (unsaturated, triple-bonded hydrocarbon).

acetylsalicylic acid (ASA) (ah-sēt′il-sal-ĭ-sil′ik) aspirin.

ACG American College of Gastroenterology.

AcG accelerator globulin (COAGULATION FACTOR V).

ACh acetylcholine.

achalasia (ak″ah-la′zhah) failure to relax of the smooth muscle FIBERS of the gastrointestinal tract at any junction of one part with another. Especially failure of the lower esophagus to relax with swallowing, due to degeneration of ganglion cells in the wall of the organ. (See accompanying illustration.)

The cause is unknown, but anxiety and emotional tension seem to aggravate achalasia and precipitate attacks. As the condition progresses there is dilatation of the esophagus (MEGAESOPHAGUS) above the constriction and loss of PERISTALSIS in the lower two-thirds of the organ.

Symptoms. The patient complains of progressive DYSPHAGIA and a feeling of fullness in the sternal region; vomiting frequently occurs, and there may be aspiration of the esophageal contents into the respiratory passages. As a result of this aspiration the patient may develop pneumonia or

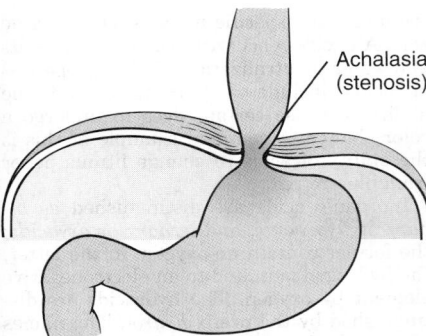

Achalasia (stenosis)

Achalasia. From Damjanov, 2000.

atelectasis. Diagnosis is confirmed by manometric readings, which document motor dysfunction.

Treatment. Conservative treatment of mild cases consists of advising the patient to eat a bland diet that is low in bulk. Very large meals should be avoided and all foods should be eaten slowly with frequent drinking of fluids during the meal. To reduce the possibility of aspiration of esophageal contents during sleep, the patient is instructed to sleep with the head and shoulders elevated.

A nonsurgical method for treating resistant cases is repeated dilation of the esophageal sphincter by means of a bougie or by a pneumatic bag that is guided into place under x-ray visualization.

As a last resort surgical intervention may be necessary. An incision, which includes the lower esophagus and upper stomach wall, is made down to but not through the intestinal mucosa. This allows for stretching of the mucosa to accommodate food passing through. Approach is made through an incision into the chest; thus, preoperative care and postoperative care are the same as for elective chest surgery (see THORACIC SURGERY).

AChE acetylcholinesterase.

ache (āk) 1. continuous pain, as opposed to sharp pangs or twinges. An ache can be either dull and constant, as in some types of backache, or throbbing, as in some types of headache and toothache. 2. to suffer such pain.

acheilia (ah-ki´le-ah) a developmental ANOMALY consisting of absence of the lips. adj., **achei´lous.**

acheiria (ah-ki´re-ah) 1. a developmental ANOMALY consisting of absence of one hand or both hands. 2. a sensation of loss of the hands or a feeling of their absence, seen in CONVERSION DISORDER.

acheiropodia (ah-ki´´ro-po´de-ah) a developmental ANOMALY characterized by absence of both hands and feet.

Achilles tendon (ah-kil´ēz) the strong tendon at the back of the heel that connects the calf muscles (triceps surae muscle) to the heel bone. The name is derived from the legend of the Greek hero Achilles, who was vulnerable only in one heel. Tapping this tendon normally produces the reflex called the Achilles or ankle jerk. Failure or exaggeration of this reflex indicates disease or injury to the nerves of the leg muscles or of a part of the spinal cord.

achillobursitis (ah-kil´´o-bur-si´tis) inflammation of the bursae about the Achilles tendon.

achillodynia (ah-kil´´o-din´e-ah) pain in the Achilles tendon or its bursa.

achillorrhaphy (ak´´il-or´ah-fe) suturing of the Achilles tendon.

achillotenotomy (ah-kil´´o-ten-ot´ah-me) surgical division of the Achilles tendon.

achlorhydria (a´´klor-hi´dre-ah) absence of HYDROCHLORIC ACID from gastric juice; associated with PERNICIOUS ANEMIA, stomach cancer, and pellagra. adj., **achlorhy´dric.**

achloropsia (a´´klor-op´se-ah) inability to distinguish green colors.

ACHNE Association of Community Health Nurse Education.

acholia (a-ko´le-ah) absence or failure of secretion of bile. adj., **acho´lic.**

achondrogenesis (ah-kon´´dro-jen´ĕ-sis) a hereditary disorder characterized by hypoplasia of bone, resulting in markedly shortened limbs; the head and trunk are normal.

achondroplasia (ah-kon´´dro-pla´zhah) a disorder of cartilage formation in the fetus, leading to achondroplastic DWARFISM. adj., **achondroplas´tic.** See accompanying illustration.

achromasia (ak´´ro-ma´zhah) 1. achromia. 2. the inability of tissues or cells to be stained.

achromat (ak´ro-mat´´) 1. achromatic OBJECTIVE. 2. monochromat.

achromate (ah-kro´māt) monochromat.

achromatic (ak´´ro-mat´ik) 1. producing no discoloration, or staining with difficulty. 2. refracting light without decomposing it into its component colors. 3. monochromatic (def. 2).

achromatism (ah-kro´mah-tizm) 1. the quality or the condition of being ACHROMATIC. 2. monochromatic VISION.

achromatophil (ak´´ro-mat´o-fil) 1. not easily stainable. 2. an organism or tissue that does not stain easily.

achromatosis (ah-kro´´mah-to´sis) 1. deficiency of pigmentation in the tissues. 2. lack of staining power in a cell or tissue.

achromatous (ah-kro´mah-tus) colorless.

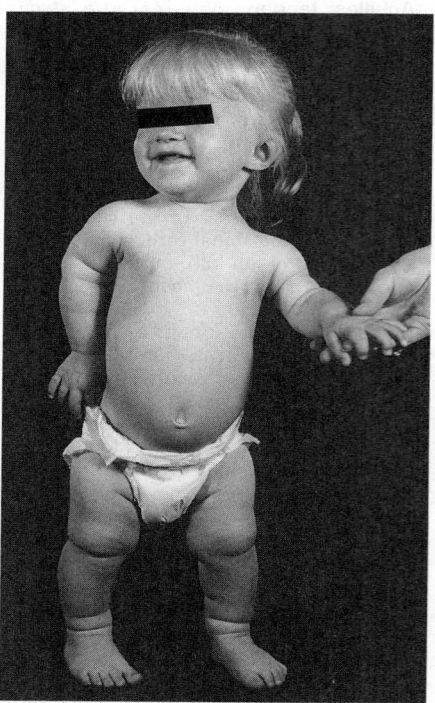

A young child with achondroplasia. From Mueller and Young, 2001.

achromaturia (ah-kro"mah-tu're-ah) the excretion of colorless urine, such as from HYPERHYDRATION.

achromia (ah-kro'me-ah) the lack or absence of normal color or pigmentation, as of the skin. adj., **achro'mic.**

a. parasi'tica a variant of tinea versicolor occurring in dark-skinned infants, particularly in the tropics, which begins in the diaper region and spreads rapidly, causing marked depigmentation of the skin.

achromophil (ah-kro'mo-fil) achromatophil.

Achromycin (ak"ro-mi'sin) trademark for preparations of TETRACYCLINE hydrochloride, a broad-spectrum ANTIBIOTIC.

achylia (ah-ki'le-ah) absence of HYDROCHLORIC ACID and enzymes in the gastric secretions.

achylous (ah-ki'lus) deficient in chyle.

achymia (ah-ki'me-ah) deficiency of chyme.

acicular (ah-sik'u-ler) needle-shaped.

acid (as'id) 1. sour. 2. a substance that yields hydrogen ions in solution and from which hydrogen may be displaced by a metal to form a salt. For the various acids,

see under the specific name, such as ACETIC ACID. All acids react with bases to form salts and water (neutralization). Other properties of acids include a sour taste and the ability to cause certain dyes to undergo a color change. A common example of this is the ability of acids to change litmus paper from blue to red.

Inorganic acids are distinguished as *binary* or *hydracids,* and *ternary* or *oxyacids;* the former contain no oxygen; in the latter, the hydrogen is united to an electronegative element by oxygen. The hydracids are distinguished by the prefix *hydro-.* The names of acids end in *-ic,* except in the case in which there are two degrees of oxygenation. The acid containing the greater amount of oxygen has the termination *-ic,* the one having the lesser amount has the termination *-ous.* Acids with the termination *-ic* form the salts ending in *-ate;* those ending in *-ous* form the salts ending in *-ite.* The salts of hydracids end in *-ide.* These rules are demonstrated by the acids and salts: hydrochloric acid (HCl), sodium chloride ($NaCl$), sulfuric acid (H_2SO_4), sodium sulfate (Na_2SO_4), sulfurous acid (H_2SO_3), sodium sulfite (Na_2SO_3). Acids are called *monobasic, dibasic, tribasic,* and *tetrabasic,* respectively, when they contain one, two, three, or four replaceable hydrogen atoms.

The most common organic acids are carboxylic acids, containing the carboxyl group (—COOH); examples are acetic acid, citric acid, amino acids, and fatty acids. Their salts and esters end in *-ate,* e.g., ethyl acetate. Other organic acids are phenols and sulfonic acids.

Acids play a vital role in the chemical processes that are a normal part of the functions of the cells and tissues of the body. A stable balance between acids and bases in the body is essential to life. See also ACID-BASE BALANCE.

a. elution test air-dried blood smears are fixed in 80 per cent methanol and immersed in a pH 3.3 buffer; all hemoglobins are eluted except fetal hemoglobin (HbF), which is seen in red blood cells after staining.

inorganic a. an acid containing no carbon atoms.

a. perfusion test Bernstein test.

a. phosphatase a lysosomal enzyme that hydrolyzes phosphate esters liberating inorganic phosphate and has an optimal pH of about 5.0. Serum activity of the prostatic isoenzyme is greatly increased in metastatic cancer of the prostate and is used to monitor the course of the disease.

acid-base balance a state of equilibrium between acidity and alkalinity of the body fluids. An acid is a substance capable of giving up a hydrogen ion during a chemical exchange, and a base is a substance that can accept it. The positively charged hydrogen ion (H^+) is the active constituent of all acids.

Most of the body's metabolic processes produce acids as their end products, but a somewhat alkaline body fluid is required as a medium for vital cellular activities. Therefore chemical exchanges of hydrogen ions must take place continuously in order to maintain a state of equilibrium. An optimal pH (hydrogen ion concentration) between 7.35 and 7.45 must be maintained; otherwise, the enzyme systems and other biochemical and metabolic activities will not function normally.

Although the body can tolerate and compensate for slight deviations in acidity and alkalinity, if the pH drops below 7.30, the potentially serious condition of ACIDOSIS exists. If the pH goes higher than 7.50, the patient is in a state of ALKALOSIS. In either case the disturbance of the acid-base balance is considered serious, even though there are control mechanisms by which the body can compensate for an upward or downward change in the pH. Shifts in the pH of body fluids are controlled by three major regulatory systems, which may be classified as *chemical* (the buffer systems), *biologic* (blood and cellular activity), and *physiologic* (the lungs and kidneys).

Chemical Controls. The chemical buffer systems are dependent on the capability of certain substances to either combine with or release hydrogen ions. In the plasma and the intracellular and interstitial fluids there are three major buffer systems that regulate hydrogen ion activity: the carbonic acid–bicarbonate system, the protein buffer system, and the phosphate buffer system.

Of these three, the *carbonic acid–bicarbonate system* is the most important in fluids outside the cell. It is the most extensive and is the first to react to an acid-base imbalance. Carbonic acid and bicarbonate are both derived from water and carbon dioxide and therefore exist in large quantities in the body. Carbonic acid is, however, weakly ionized and needs to coexist with its salt in order to effectively remove excess hydrogen or hydroxyl ions from the extracellular fluids. Hence it is actually the *carbonic acid and sodium bicarbonate* buffer system that works to maintain normal levels of hydrogen ion concentrations in the extracellular fluids. It is important to remember that these two chemical components must be in the ratio of 1:20; that is, for every one part of carbonic acid (H_2CO_3) there must be twenty parts of sodium bicarbonate (NaHCO$_3$). It is not the absolute amount of each

component that is crucial in the control of acid-base balance, but the ratio of the one substance to the other. The carbonic acid–bicarbonate buffer system is capable of either accepting or releasing hydrogen ions without forcing the pH to dangerous levels.

The *protein buffer system* is especially remarkable because proteins are powerful buffers that can function as either acid or base, depending on the state of the body fluids. This system is active in the plasma and in intracellular and extracellular fluids.

The *phosphate buffer system* operates in much the same way as the carbonic acid–bicarbonate system but is more active within the cell than in extracellular fluids.

Although the chemical buffer systems react almost instantaneously to a change in the pH of the body fluids, they cannot provide sustained regulation of the pH because they are absorbed rapidly and cannot be replaced immediately. The hydrogen ions that are not handled by the chemical buffer systems become the responsibility of other regulatory controls which respond less rapidly but are not less important.

Biologic Regulators. This type of control is concerned with the shifting of excess acid or alkali in and out of the cell. As excess ions cross over the cell membrane they must do so in combination with ions of the opposite charge, or in exchange for ions of the same charge. Sodium and potassium are the two cations most often exchanged for the positively charged hydrogen ion.

The hemoglobin-oxyhemoglobin system is another regulatory control. As chloride leaves the oxygenated blood cells and enters the plasma, the bicarbonate moves from the plasma and crosses over into the cellular fluid. This reciprocal exchange between bicarbonate and chloride is a continuous process.

Physiologic Regulators. The lungs begin to compensate for a metabolic acid-base imbalance within minutes of its onset. They do this by regulating the retention or the excretion of carbon dioxide. If acidosis is present, respiratory activity is increased so that the arterial CO_2 concentration falls. If alkalosis is present, respiratory activity is automatically decreased, and CO_2 is retained, thus producing a compensatory respiratory acidosis.

The kidneys act as regulators by reabsorbing bicarbonate when it is needed to control excess acidity and by excreting it when there is a deficit of acid in the body. The kidneys also facilitate the excretion of excess hydrogen ions in combination with phosphate ions (in the form of phosphoric acid), or in combination with ammonia (excreted in the form of ammonium).

Imbalances of the acid-base ratio are discussed under ACIDOSIS and ALKALOSIS. Diagnosis and monitoring of either of these conditions are greatly enhanced by periodic determination of the pH and by BLOOD GAS ANALYSIS.

acidemia (as″ĭ-de′me-ah) abnormal acidity of the blood.

acid-fast (as′id-fast) not readily decolorized by acids after staining; said of bacteria, especially *Mycobacterium tuberculosis.*

acidic (ah-sid′ik) of or pertaining to an acid; acid-forming.

acidifier (ah-sid′ĭ-fi″er) an agent that causes acidity, especially in the stomach.

acidity (ah-sid′ĭ-te) 1. the quality of being acid; the power to unite with positively charged ions or with basic substances. 2. excess acid quality, as of the gastric juice.

acidophil (as′id-o-fil″) 1. a histologic structure, cell, or other element staining readily with acid dyes. 2. one of the hormone-producing acidophilic cells of the adenohypophysis; types include CORTICO-TROPHS, LACTOTROPHS, LIPOTROPHS, and SOMA-TOTROPHS. Called also alpha cell. 3. an organism that grows well in highly acid media. 4. acidophilic.

acidophilic (as″ĭ-do-fil′ik) 1. easily stained with acid dyes. 2. growing best on acid media.

acidosis (as″ĭ-do′sis) 1. the accumulation of acid and hydrogen ions or depletion of the alkaline reserve (bicarbonate content) in the blood and body tissues, resulting in

a decrease in pH. 2. a pathologic condition resulting from this process, characterized by increase in hydrogen ion concentration (decrease in pH). The optimal ACID-BASE BALANCE is maintained by chemical buffers, biologic activities of the cells, and effective functioning of the lungs and kidneys. The opposite of acidosis is ALKALOSIS. adj., **acidot′ic.** Acidosis usually occurs secondary to some underlying disease process; the two major types, distinguished according to cause, are *metabolic acidosis* and *respiratory acidosis* (see accompanying table). In mild cases the symptoms may be overlooked; in severe cases symptoms are more obvious and may include muscle twitching, involuntary movement, cardiac arrhythmias, disorientation, and coma.

In general, treatment consists of intravenous or oral administration of sodium bicarbonate or sodium lactate solutions and correction of the underlying cause of the imbalance. Many cases of severe acidosis can be prevented by careful monitoring of patients whose primary illness predisposes them to respiratory problems or metabolic derangements that can cause increased levels of acidity or decreased bicarbonate levels. Such care includes effective teaching of self-care to the diabetic so that the disease remains under control. Patients receiving intravenous therapy, especially those having a fluid deficit, and those with biliary or intestinal intubation should be watched closely for early signs of acidosis. Others predisposed to acidosis are patients with shock, hyperthyroidism, advanced circulatory failure, renal failure, respiratory disorders, or liver disease.

ACIDOSIS				
	Causes	Pathophysiology	Assessment Findings	Blood Gas Findings
Metabolic Acidosis	Starvation, uremia, diabetic keto-acidosis, renal tubular acidosis, diarrhea, gastrointestinal fistulas, lactic acidosis, poisoning	A deficit of base bicarbonate, increased concentration of fixed acids	Weakness, lethargy, headache, disorientation, tremors, nausea and vomiting, convulsions, coma	Decreased pH, decreased bicarbonate, decreased base excess, decreased Pco_2 (if lung compensation)
Respiratory Acidosis	Upper airway obstruction, acute infections and inflammation of the lung, ventilatory impairment as in drug overdose, chronic airway limitation	Carbon dioxide retention, excess of carbonic acid	Confusion, weakness, headache, tachycardia, tachypnea, drowsiness, visual disturbances, coma	Decreased pH, increased Pco_2, normal or slightly decreased base excess, elevated bicarbonate (if renal compensation)

compensated a. a condition in which the compensatory mechanisms have returned the pH toward normal.

diabetic a. a metabolic ACIDOSIS produced by accumulation of ketones in uncontrolled DIABETES MELLITUS.

hypercapnic a. respiratory acidosis.

hyperchloremic a. renal tubular acidosis.

lactic a. a metabolic acidosis occurring as a result of excess LACTIC ACID in the blood, due to conditions causing impaired cell RESPIRATION. It occurs most commonly in disorders in which oxygen is inadequately delivered to tissues, such as SHOCK, SEPTICEMIA, or extreme HYPOXEMIA, but it can also result from exogenous or endogenous metabolic defects. Initially manifesting as HYPERVENTILATION, it progresses to mental confusion and coma.

metabolic a. any of the types of acidosis resulting from accumulation in the blood of KETO ACIDS (derived from fat metabolism) at the expense of bicarbonate; this diminishes the body's ability to neutralize acids. This type is contrasted with respiratory ACIDOSIS. It occurs when there is either an acid gain (as in diabetic ketoacidosis, lactic acidosis, poisoning, or failure of the renal tubules to reabsorb bicarbonate) or a bicarbonate loss (as in diarrhea or a gastrointestinal fistula).

The symptoms of metabolic acidosis include weakness, malaise, and headache. As the acid level goes up these symptoms progress to stupor, unconsciousness, coma, and death. The breath may have a fruity odor owing to the presence of acetone, and the patient may experience vomiting and diarrhea. Loss of fluids can deplete body fluid content and aggravate the acidosis. Hyperventilation may occur as a result of stimulation of the hypothalamus. BLOOD GAS ANALYSIS will reveal a lowered pH and an elevated Pa_{CO_2}. (See accompanying table.)

Treatment and Patient Care. Treatment of metabolic acidosis is primarily concerned with control of the underlying causes. Diabetic ketoacidosis may be corrected by the administration of insulin and fluids. In acute renal failure the patient requires dialysis, and in chronic uremic acidosis the condition is controlled by restricting sodium intake and buffering with bicarbonate. The patient's vital signs should be checked frequently to assess the progress of compensation. A rising pulse rate and a drop in blood pressure frequently occur as a result of hypovolemia in the diabetic-acidotic patient, and cardiac arrhythmias can be caused by increased calcium levels in the blood. A careful recording of intake and output provides a means of determining the kidneys' ability to regulate

the ACID-BASE BALANCE. Safety measures to avoid injury during involuntary muscular contractions should be carried out. (See also CONVULSIONS.) Nursing measures to relieve discomfort from vomiting and to avoid the hazards of aspiration of vomitus are required. Education of the patient and family in the prevention of acute episodes of metabolic acidosis, particularly diabetic ketoacidosis, is of primary importance.

renal tubular a. (RTA) a metabolic ACIDOSIS resulting from impairment of the reabsorption of bicarbonate by the renal tubules, characterized by low plasma bicarbonate and high plasma chloride; the urine is alkaline.

respiratory a. acidosis resulting from ventilatory impairment and subsequent retention of CARBON DIOXIDE, in contrast to metabolic ACIDOSIS. The respiratory system has an important role in maintaining ACID-BASE BALANCE. In response to an increase in the hydrogen ion concentration in body fluids, the respiratory rate increases, causing more carbon dioxide to be released from the lung. When either an acute obstruction of the airways or a chronic condition involving the organs of respiration causes interference with the exhalation of the carbon dioxide produced by metabolic activity, carbon dioxide accumulates in the blood and unites with water to form carbonic acid.

Acute respiratory acidosis occurs when there is a relatively sudden malfunction of respiratory activities, as in upper airway obstruction, acute infections and inflammation of the lung and bronchial tissues, and pulmonary edema. In acute respiratory acidosis the compensatory chemical buffer systems are of limited benefit in restoring the acid-base balance because they depend on normal blood circulation and tissue perfusion for optimal effect. The physiologic regulators, the lungs and kidneys, are of little help because the lungs are malfunctioning and the kidneys require more time to compensate than the acute condition permits.

Chronic respiratory acidosis results from gradual and irreversible loss of ventilatory function, as in CHRONIC OBSTRUCTIVE PULMONARY DISEASE (COPD). Although the patient in this condition does have an increased retention of CO_2, there is time for the kidneys to compensate by retaining bicarbonate and thereby maintaining a pH within tolerable limits. If, however, even a minor respiratory infection develops, the patient is subject to a rapidly developing state of acute acidosis because the lungs cannot be depended upon to remove more than a minimal amount of CO_2.

Treatment and Patient Care. The initial treatment for acute respiratory acidosis is to establish an airway immediately and maintain adequate ventilation and hydration. Acute cases may require the use of an ENDOTRACHEAL TUBE or TRACHEOSTOMY tube. Some form of INTERMITTENT POSITIVE PRESSURE BREATHING is applied through a machine-driven ventilator, essentially to force adequate O_2 delivery and concomitant CO_2 removal from the lungs, thereby avoiding further rises in CO_2 levels to the point that CO_2 narcosis will develop. Beyond a certain point the respiratory center may cease responding to the higher CO_2 levels, and breathing will stop abruptly. Drugs that further depress the respiratory center (narcotics, hypnotics, and tranquilizers) must be avoided. Patients in the acute stage are watched for cessation of breathing and cardiac arrest. CARDIOPULMONARY RESUSCITATION may be required to revive the patient.

It is recommended that oxygen administration be limited in patients with chronic obstructive pulmonary disease (COPD). In COPD the stimulus to breathe is a hypoxic state, therefore administration of high concentrations of O_2 will remove this needed stimulus. The rate of oxygen flow should be closely correlated with blood gas studies. In patients with acute lung diseases the stimulus to breathe is still dependent on CO_2 concentrations, so that O_2 can be supplied without fear of inhibiting the stimulus to breathe.

Measures that facilitate breathing are essential to patient care during respiratory acidosis. Frequent turning, coughing, and deep breathing exercises to encourage oxygen–carbon dioxide exchange are beneficial, as is suctioning when needed to remove secretions obstructing the airway. POSTURAL DRAINAGE, unless contraindicated by the patient's condition, may be effective in promoting adequate ventilation.

starvation a. a metabolic ACIDOSIS due to accumulation of ketones following a severe caloric deficit.

acid-proof (as′id-prōōf) acid-fast.

acidulous (ah-sid′u-lus) moderately sour.

aciduria (as″ĭ-du′re-ah) the excretion of acid in the urine. There are many specific forms, such as AMINOACIDURIA, OROTIC ACIDURIA, and so on.

aciduric (as″ĭ-du′rik) capable of growing in extremely acid media.

acinar (as′ĭ-ner) pertaining to or affecting an acinus or acini.

acinetic (as″ĭ-net′ik) akinetic.

aciniform (ah-sin′ĭ-form) shaped like a cluster of grapes.

acinitis (as″ĭ-ni′tis) inflammation of the acini of a gland.

acinose (as′ĭ-nōs) 1. made up of acini. 2. acinar.

acinous (as′ĭ-nus) 1. resembling a grape. 2. acinar.

acinus (as′ĭ-nus), pl. *a′cini* [L.] any of the smallest lobules of a compound gland.

liver a. the smallest functional unit of the liver, a mass of liver parenchyma that is supplied by terminal branches of the portal vein and hepatic artery and drained by a terminal branch of the bile duct. See accompanying illustration.

pulmonary a. terminal respiratory unit.

acitretin (as″e-tret′in) a second generation RETINOID used in treatment of severe PSORIASIS; administered orally.

aclasia (ah-kla′zhah) aclasis.

aclasis (ak′lah-sis) pathologic continuity of structure, as in dyschondroplasia.

diaphyseal a. hereditary multiple exostoses.

ACLS advanced cardiac life support.

acme (ak′me) the critical stage or crisis of a disease.

acne (ak′ne) a disorder of the skin with eruption of papules or pustules; more particularly, ACNE VULGARIS.

a. congloba′ta, conglobate a. severe acne, seen almost exclusively in males, with many comedones, marked by suppuration, cysts, sinuses, and scarring.

cystic a. acne with the formation of cysts enclosing a mixture of keratin and sebum in varying proportions.

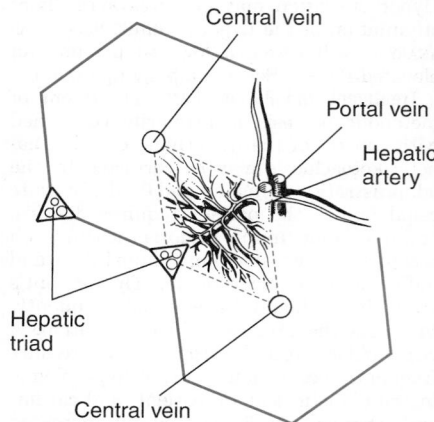

Liver acinus: Hepatic lobules are represented by hexagons *(solid lines);* liver acinus is represented by rhombus *(dotted line).* From Dorland's, 2000.

a. ful'minans a rare form of severe cystic acne seen in teenage boys, characterized by highly inflammatory nodules and plaques that undergo suppurative degeneration leaving ulcerations, fever, weight loss, anemia, leukocytosis, elevated erythrocyte sedimentation rate, and polyarthritis.

a. indura'ta a progression of papular acne, with deep-seated and destructive lesions that may produce severe scarring.

keloid a. keloid folliculitis.

a. necro'tica milia'ris a rare and chronic form of folliculitis of the scalp, occurring principally in adults, with formation of tiny superficial pustules that are destroyed by scratching. See also ACNE VARIOLIFORMIS.

a. neonato'rum ACNE VULGARIS in infants, usually in males before 3 months of age, chiefly characterized by papules, pustules, and open and closed comedones on the face; it is thought to be due to hormonal stimulation of sebaceous glands. The affected child may be predisposed to more severe acne in adolescence.

a. papulo'sa acne vulgaris with the formation of papules.

a. rosa'cea a form of acne in which the skin around each pustule is a rosy red; it is usually seen in persons over 25 years of age and is often psychogenic.

tropical a., a. tropica'lis a severe type of ACNE VULGARIS seen in the tropics when the weather is hot and humid, characterized by large painful cysts, nodules, and pustules that lead to the formation of rounded abscesses and frequent scarring and tend to localize on the back, nape of the neck, buttocks, thighs, and upper arms and usually sparing the face. It tends to affect those who have had acne vulgaris at an earlier age.

a. variolifor'mis a rare condition with reddish-brown, papulopustular umbilicated lesions, usually on the brow and scalp; probably a deep variant of acne necrotica miliaris.

a. venena'ta acne produced by contact with any of numerous chemicals, including those used in cosmetic and grooming agents and in industry.

a. vulga'ris a chronic skin disorder usually seen in adolescents and young adults, in which there is increased production of sebum (oil) from the sebaceous glands and formation of COMEDONES (BLACKHEADS and WHITEHEADS) that plug the pores. Noninflammatory acne produces plugged follicles and a few pimples. Inflammatory acne is characterized by many pimples, pustules, nodules, and inflamed cysts. The lesions are found on the face, neck, chest, back, and shoulders.

Treatment. The noninflammatory lesions often respond to over-the-counter creams and lotions, but inflammatory lesions may require intensive and individualized medical treatment under the direction of a dermatologist. Acne is treated by both topical and systemic drugs; the one most frequently recommended is BENZOYL PEROXIDE in a 5 or 10 per cent concentration. It is applied to the skin daily or as frequently as necessary to produce mild dryness of the skin. A mainstay for treatment of inflammatory acne continues to be oral TETRACYCLINE, which is effective for most cases and safe even when taken for years. A relatively new systemic drug for severe, treatment-resistant acne is ISOTRETINOIN (13-*cis*-retinoic acid). It inhibits the secretion of sebum and alters the lipid composition of the skin surface. Isotretinoin is a teratogen; hence it is not given to pregnant women. It can also cause bone changes. Minor side effects include dry mouth and dry eyes. Another agent used against acne is TRETINOIN (all-*trans*-retinoic acid), which is applied topically to reduce the number of comedones and to prevent formation of inflammatory lesions.

Acne therapy can continue for months and even years. Patients who conscientiously follow the prescribed regimen greatly increase their chances for improvement and the prevention of permanent scarring and pitting of the skin.

When acne has left permanent, disfiguring scars, there are medical techniques that can remove or improve the blemishes. One method is planing with a rotary, high-speed brush. This removes the outer layer of pitted skin, leaving the growing layer and the layers containing the glands and hair follicles. New epithelium grows from the layers underneath; it is rosy at first and gradually becomes normal in color. The technique has also been used successfully in removing some types of disfigurations resulting from accidents. This so-called "sand-paper surgery" or dermabrasion is recommended only for selected cases of acne and results are not always satisfying.

Patient Care. Because patients with acne often have a lack of knowledge about the nature of their skin disorder, patient education is a major component of care. Additionally, the disorder often affects young people at a time when they are deeply concerned about their appearance and acceptance by their peers. Adolescents need to know that their concerns are taken seriously. Even though the disorder is not life-threatening, it can adversely affect one's self-image and self-esteem.

Laypersons often are misinformed about the cause and effects of acne. It is not a contagious disease, nor is it due to uncleanliness or poor personal hygiene. It is not caused or made worse by lack of sleep, constipation, masturbation, venereal disease, or by anger or hostility. Dietary indiscretion can sometimes contribute to the appearance of lesions, but there are very few people who can find a cause-effect relationship between certain foods they have eaten and the appearance of acne lesions. In general, cola drinks, chocolate, and fried foods need not be restricted or eliminated from the diet in hopes that acne can be avoided or cured. A well-balanced diet is all that is recommended for the management of acne.

Scrubbing the skin and using harsh soaps is not recommended because this only serves to damage the skin and predispose it to breakdown. A mild soap is as effective as special medicated soaps. If the hair is excessively oily, it may help to shampoo regularly and keep the hair off the face.

Pimples and pustules should not be squeezed. This can press the sebum and accumulated debris more firmly into the clogged duct and increase the chance of inflammation and the spread of infection. Blackheads and whiteheads are best removed by applying a prescription medication that causes peeling of the skin.

Since the management of acne can go on for years, requiring periodic evaluation by a dermatologist, patients and their families will need continued support and encouragement. Patients taking prescription medications will need to know the expected results, any adverse reactions that might occur, their symptoms, and to whom they should be reported.

acnegenic (ak″ne-jen′ik) producing acne.

acneiform (ak-ne′ĭ-form) resembling acne.

ACNHA American College of Nursing Home Administrators.

ACNM American College of Nurse-Midwives.

acoelomate (a-se′lah-māt) 1. without a coelom or body cavity. 2. an acoelomate animal.

aconative (ah-kon′ah-tiv) without conation; lacking any desire or impulse to act.

aconite (ak′ah-nīt) an extremely toxic substance from the dried root of *Aconitum napellus* (monkshood or wolfsbane), containing several closely related alkaloids, principally aconitine. It has variable effects on the heart leading to heart failure and it also affects the central nervous system;

poisoning can be fatal, and with large doses death may be instantaneous. It was formerly used as an antipyretic and cardiac and respiratory depressant and topically as a counterirritant and local anesthetic.

acorea (ah″kor′e-ah) absence of the pupil.

acoria (ah-kor′e-ah) insatiable appetite.

acoustic (ah-koos′tik) pertaining to sound or hearing.

a. reflex test measurement of the acoustic reflex threshold; used to differentiate between conductive and sensorineural deafness and to diagnose acoustic neuroma.

acoustics (ah-koos′tiks) the science of sound and hearing.

ACP American College of Physicians.

ACPS acrocephalopolysyndactyly.

acquired (ah-kwīrd′) incurred as a result of factors acting from or originating outside the organism or individual; not inherited.

a. cystic kidney disease, a. cystic disease of kidney development of cysts in a formerly noncystic kidney during END-STAGE RENAL DISEASE.

a. immune deficiency syndrome (AIDS), a. immunodeficiency syndrome suppression or deficiency of cellular IMMUNITY, acquired by exposure to the human immunodeficiency VIRUS (HIV), which attacks the T LYMPHOCYTE subgroup known as the CD4 CELLS. The World Health Organization estimates that in the year 2000 there were over 10 million people infected with the virus worldwide. AIDS is a global epidemic with no cure at the present time; health promotion through education is imperative. Infection by the virus and the consequent suppression of immunity predisposes the infected person to opportunistic INFECTIONS and malignancies. One or more of the diseases from the CDC surveillance case definition must be present for a patient to be diagnosed with AIDS. (See table.)

Routes of Transmission. Human immunodeficiency virus has been found in blood, semen, cerebrospinal fluid, and cervical/vaginal secretions; there is no evidence of transmission by saliva, tears, or urine. The number one means of transmission in the United States is as a sexually transmitted disease. Factors that increase the route of sexual transmission include multiple sexual partners, receptive anal intercourse, the presence of lesions in the genital area, and sexual exposure without some form of barrier protection such as a condom.

Users of intravenous drugs compose a significant percentage of reported cases of AIDS. The sharing of needles and equipment and poor or nonexistent precautions against transmission by needle are the major reasons persons in this group are at high risk.

The HIV-infected mother can also transmit the virus to her infant in utero. HIV has been transmitted via breast milk, and the CDC recommends that mothers infected with the virus not breastfeed their babies.

Treatment. A wide variety of treatments are now available, including nucleoside ANALOGUES and HIV protease INHIBITORS Multiple agents are often given in a "cocktail" to forestall resistance. Short-course therapy with ZIDOVUDINE for pregnant women with the virus is now included in clinical guidelines.

ACR American College of Radiology.

acr(o)- word element [Gr.], *extreme; top; extremity.*

acral (ak′ral) pertaining to or affecting a limb or apex.

acrania (ah-kra′ne-ah) partial or complete absence of the cranium. adj., **acra′nial.**

CLASSIFICATION SYSTEM FOR ACQUIRED IMMUNODEFICIENCY SYNDROME (AIDS)

The Centers for Disease Control and Prevention issued a revised classification system for HIV-infected adolescents and adults in 1993. It emphasizes the importance of CD4+ lymphocyte testing in the clinical management of HIV infected clients. There are laboratory and clinical categories. According to this system, HIV infected clients would be classified on the basis of both of these categories.

Laboratory Categories:*

Category 1: 500 or more

Category 2: 200 to 499 CD4+ cells

Category 3: Less than 200 CD4+ cells

Clinical Categories:

Category A: One or more of the following conditions occurring in an adolescent or adult with documented HIV infections (conditions listed in Categories B and C must not have occurred):

Asymptomatic HIV infection
Persistent generalized lymphadenopathy
Acute (primary) HIV infection with accompanying illness, or history of acute HIV infection

Category B: Symptomatic conditions, occurring in an HIV-infected adolescent or adult, that are not included among the conditions listed in clinical category C and that meet at least one of the following criteria:

1. The conditions are attributed to HIV infection and/or are indicative of a defect in cell-mediated immunity.
2. The conditions are considered by physicians to have a clinical course or management that is complicated by HIV infection.

Category C: Any of the following conditions in an adolescent or adult:[†‡]

Candidiasis of bronchi, trachea, or lungs
Candidiasis, esophageal
Cervical cancer, invasive
CD4+ T-lymphocyte count less than 200 per mm^3
Cocciodioidomycosis, disseminated or extrapulmonary
Cryptococcosis, extrapulmonary
Cryptosporidiosis, chronic intestinal (over 1 month in duration)
Cytomegalovirus disease (other than liver, spleen, or nodes)
Cytomegalovirus retinitis (with loss of vision)
Encephalopathy, HIV related
Herpes simplex: chronic ulcer(s) (over 1 month in duration) or bronchitis, pneumonitis, or esophagitis
Histoplasmosis, disseminated or extrapulmonary
Isosporiasis, chronic intestinal (over 1 month in duration)
Kaposi's sarcoma
Lymphoma, Burkitt's (or equivalent term)
Lymphoma, immunoblastic (or equivalent term)
Lymphoma, primary, of brain
Mycobacterium avium complex or *Mycobacterium kansasii*, disseminated or extrapulmonary
Mycobacterium tuberculosis, pulmonary or extrapulmonary
Mycobacterium, other species or unidentified species, disseminated or extrapulmonary
Pneumocystis carinii pneumonia
Pneumonia, recurrent
Progressive multifocal leukoencephalopathy
Salmonella septicemia, recurrent
Toxoplasmosis of brain
Wasting syndrome caused by HIV

---

*The lower accurate CD4+ count is used, whether or not it is the most recent.
[†]The most severe clinical condition diagnosed is used, regardless of the client's current condition.
[‡]Data from Morbidity and Mortality Weekly Report (1992).

acranius (ah-kra′ne-us) a fetus in which the cranium is absent or rudimentary.

Acremonium (ak″rĕ-mo′ne-um) a genus of Fungi Imperfecti of the form-class Hyphomycetes, formerly called *Cephalosporium*. Some species produce CEPHALOSPORIN ANTIBIOTICS.

acridine (ak′rĭ-dēn) an alkaloid from anthracene, the basis of certain dyes and drugs.

acritical (a-krit′ĭ-k′l) having no crisis.

acrivastine (ak″rĭ-vas′tēn) an ANTIHISTAMINE used in treatment of HAY FEVER; administered orally.

ACRM American Congress of Rehabilitative Medicine.

acroagnosis (ak″ro-ag-no′sis) lack of sensory recognition of a limb.

acroanesthesia (ak″ro-an″es-the′zhah) anesthesia of the limbs.

acrobrachycephaly (ak″ro-brak″e-sef′ah-le) abnormal height of the skull, with shortness of its anteroposterior dimension.

acrocentric (ak″ro-sen′trik) having the centromere toward one end of the replicating chromosome.

acrocephalia (ak″ro-sĕ-fa′le-ah) oxycephaly.

acrocephalopolysyndactyly (ACPS) (ak″ro-sef″ah-lo-pol″e-sin-dak′tĭ-le) any of several inherited disorders characterized by ACROCEPHALOSYNDACTYLY (head deformity and webbed FINGERS and TOES) and POLYDACTYLY (extra fingers or toes). *Type I* (or ACPS I) is PFEIFFER'S SYNDROME; *type II* (or ACPS II) is CARPENTER'S SYNDROME; *type III* (or ACPS III) is SAKATI-NYHAN SYNDROME.

acrocephalosyndactyly (ak″ro-sef″ah-lo″-sin-dak′tĭ-le) any of a group of autosomal dominant disorders in which CRANIOSTENOSIS is associated with ACROCEPHALY (conical deformity of the head) and SYNDACTYLY (webbed FINGERS and TOES), sometimes occurring with additional anomalies. *Type I* is APERT'S SYNDROME; *type III* is CHOTZEN'S SYNDROME; and *type V* is PFEIFFER'S SYNDROME.

acrocephaly (ak″ro-sef′ah-le) oxycephaly. adj., **acrocephal′ic.**

acrochordon (ak″ro-kor′don) a pedunculated skin tag occurring principally on the neck, upper chest, and axillae in women of middle age or older.

acrocinesis (ak″ro-si-ne′sis) acrokinesia.

acrocyanosis (ak″ro-si″ah-no′sis) persistent cyanosis of the fingers and hands or the toes and feet, with mottled blue or red discoloration, coldness, and profuse sweating of the digits. It may be seen in newborn infants or during the first weeks of life in response to exposure to cold.

acrodermatitis (ak″ro-der″mah-ti′tis) inflammation of the skin of the limbs, especially the hands or feet.

chronic atropic a., a. chro′nica atro′-phicans 1. chronic inflammation of the skin of the extremities, leading to atrophy. 2. a diffuse chronic skin disease usually confined to the limbs, seen mainly in women in Northern, Central, and Eastern Europe, and characterized initially by an erythematous, edematous, pruritic phase followed by sclerosis and atrophy. It is caused by infection with *Borrelia burgdorferi*. See also LYME DISEASE.

a. conti′nua, continuous a. chronic inflammation of the skin of the limbs, in some cases becoming generalized.

enteropathic a., a. enteropa′thica a hereditary disorder of infancy due to defective zinc uptake, characterized by dermatitis with vesicles and pustules, usually around the mouth or anus and on the head, elbows, knees, hands, and feet; there are also gastrointestinal disturbances such as diarrhea, as well as total ALOPECIA.

a. per′stans acrodermatitis continua.

acrodermatosis (ak″ro-der″mah-to′sis), pl. *acrodermato′ses.* Any disease of the skin of the limbs.

acrodynia (ak″ro-din′e-ah) a disease of infancy and early childhood marked by pain and swelling in, and pink coloration of, the fingers and toes and by listlessness, irritability, FAILURE TO THRIVE, profuse perspiration, and sometimes scarlet coloration of the cheeks and tip of the nose. It is due to absorption of MERCURY. Called also erythredema polyneuropathy and pink disease.

acroesthesia (ak″ro-es-the′zhah) 1. exaggerated sensitiveness. 2. pain in the limbs.

acrognosis (ak″rog-no′sis) sensory recognition of the limbs.

acrohypothermy (ak″ro-hi′po-ther″me) abnormal coldness of the hands and feet.

acrokeratosis verruciformis (ak″ro-ker″-ah-to′sis vĕ-roo″sĭ-for′mis) a hereditary dermatosis characterized by flat wartlike papules on the dorsal aspect of the hand, foot, elbow, and knee.

acrokinesia (ak″ro-kĭ-ne′zhah) abnormal motility or movement of the limbs.

acromegaly (ak″ro-meg′ah-le) excessive enlargement of the limbs due to thickening of bones and soft tissues, caused by hypersecretion of GROWTH HORMONE, usually from a tumor of the PITUITARY GLAND. In adults whose bone growth has stopped, the bones most affected are those of the face, jaw, hands, and feet (see accompanying illustration). Gradual enlargement of paranasal sinuses,

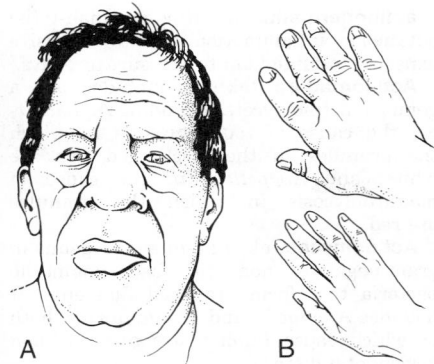

Appearance in acromegaly: *A,* facial appearance; *B,* acromegalic hand *(upper)* and normal hand *(lower).* From Dorland's, 2000.

prominence of nose and supraorbital ridges, prognathism, widely separated teeth, and an underbite are part of the coarsening of facial features. Early signs include increased metabolism and strength and profuse sweating. Later joint pain, weakness, and sometimes diabetes mellitus and visual disturbances are seen. In children overproduction of growth hormone stimulates growth of long bones and results in GIGANTISM. Surgical treatment includes removal of the tumor or the pituitary gland (transsphenoidal HYPOPHYSECTOMY), pituitary irradiation, or a combination of the two. Drug therapy with the dopamine receptor agonist bromocriptine may be used as adjuvant therapy in conjunction with either surgery or radiation.

acromelalgia (ak″ro-mel-al′jah) bilateral vasodilation, particularly of limbs, with burning pain, increased skin temperature, and redness. Called also erythromelalgia.

acromi(o)- word element [Gr.], *acromion.*

acromicria (ak″ro-mi′kre-ah) abnormal smallness of the limbs, including hands and feet, and sometimes the nose and jaws, due to a deficiency in pituitary function after puberty.

acromiohumeral (ah-kro″me-o-hu′mer-al) pertaining to the acromion and humerus.

acromion (ah-kro′me-on) the lateral extension of the spine of the scapula, forming the highest point of the shoulder. adj., **acro′mial.**

acromionectomy (ah-kro″me-on-ek′tah-me) resection of the acromion.

acromioplasty (ah-kro′me-o-plas″te) surgical removal of the anterior hook of the ACROMION to relieve mechanical compression of the rotator cuff during movement of the glenohumeral joint; called also anterior acromioplasty.

acromiothoracic (ah-kro″me-o-tho-ras′ik) pertaining to the acromion and thorax.

acromphalus (ah-krom′fah-lus) 1. bulging of the navel; sometimes a sign of umbilical hernia. 2. the center of the navel.

acroneurosis (ak″ro-noo-ro′sis) any neuropathy of the limbs.

acropachy (ak′ro-pak″e) clubbing of the fingers.

acropachyderma (ak″ro-pak″e-der′mah) thickening of the skin of the limbs, as seens in ACROMEGALY and PACHYDERMOPERIOSTOSIS.

acroparalysis (ak″ro-pah-ral′ĭ-sis) paralysis of the limbs.

acroparesthesia (ak″ro-par″es-the′zhah) an abnormal sensation, such as tingling, numbness, pins and needles, in the hands and fingers.

acropathy (ah-krop′ah-the) any disease of the limbs.

acrophobia (ak″ro-fo′be-ah) irrational fear of heights.

acroposthitis (ak″ro-pos-thi′tis) inflammation of the prepuce.

acroscleroderma (ak″ro-skle″ro-der′mah) acrosclerosis.

acrosclerosis (ak″ro-sklĕ-ro′sis) a combination of RAYNAUD'S DISEASE and SCLERODERMA of the distal parts of the limbs, especially the digits, and of the neck and face, particularly the nose.

acrosome (ak′ro-sōm) the caplike, membrane-bound structure covering the anterior portion of the HEAD OF A SPERMATOZOON; it contains enzymes involved in penetration of the ovum. (See illustration.)

a. reaction changes in the spermatozoon that result in development of perforations in the ACROSOME, allowing release of enzymes that facilitate FERTILIZATION.

acrotism (ak′ro-tizm) absence or imperceptibility of the pulse. adj., **acrot′ic.**

acrylic (ah-kril′ik) pertaining to polymers of acrylic acid, methacrylic acid, or

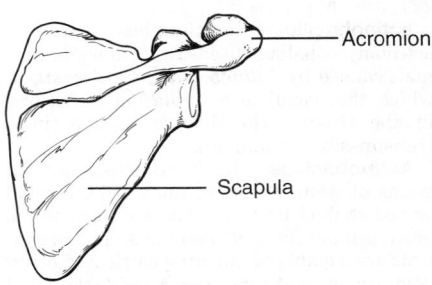

Posterior (dorsal) surface of the scapula, showing the acromion. From Dorland's, 2000.

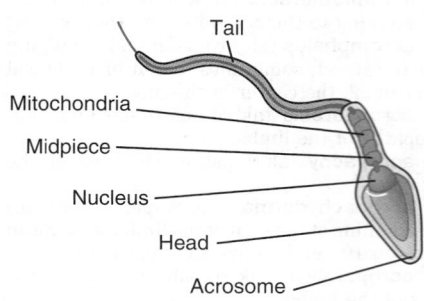

Acrosome of a spermatozoon. From Applegate, 2000.

acrylonitrile, such as acrylic RESINS used in making dental restorations, prostheses, and appliances.

ACS acute confusional state; American Cancer Society; American Chemical Society; American College of Surgeons.

ACTH adrenocorticotropic hormone; see CORTICOTROPIN.

actin (ak′tin) a muscle protein localized in the I band of MYOFIBRILS; acting along with MYOSIN particles, it is responsible for the contraction and relaxation of muscle FIBERS.

actin(o)- word element [Gr.], *ray; radiation.*

acting out (ak′ting owt) the habitual expression of unconscious feelings through nonverbal behavior as a means of avoiding the direct experiencing of them; reacting to present situations as if they were the childhood situation that gave rise to the feelings and fantasies, as the acting out of a transference. Often applied imprecisely to any sort of disapproved impulsive behavior.

actinic (ak-tin′ik) producing chemical action; see under RAY.

actinium (Ac) (ak-tin′e-um) a chemical element, atomic number 89, atomic weight 227. (See Appendix 6.)

actinobacillosis (ak″tĭ-no-bas″ĭ-lo′sis) an actinomycosis-like disease of domestic animals caused by *Actinobacillus ligniere′sii,* in which the bacilli form radiating structures in the tissues; the disease is sometimes transmissible to humans.

Actinobacillus (ak″tĭ-no-bah-sil′us) a genus of gram-negative, nonmotile, coccoid or rod-shaped bacteria that are part of the normal microflora of mammals. The organisms are capable of infecting cattle and other domestic animals and, rarely, are associated with human infection; *A. ligniere′sii* is the causative agent of ACTINOBACILLOSIS.

actinodermatitis (ak″tĭ-no-der″mah-ti′tis) cutaneous inflammation due to excessive exposure to sunlight or to exposure to x-rays.

Actinomadura (ak″tĭ-no-mah-doo′rah) a genus of actinomycetes including *A. madu′r-ae,* the cause of MADUROMYCOSIS in which the granules in the discharged pus are white, and *A. pelletier′ii,* the cause of maduromycosis in which the granules are red.

Actinomyces (ak″tĭ-no-mi′sēz) a genus of gram-negative, non–acid fast, nonmotile bacteria that form branched filaments. It includes *A. israe′lii* and *A. naeslun′dii,* both of which cause human ACTINOMYCOSIS and periodontal disease.

actinomyces (ak″tĭ-no-mi′sēz) an organism of the genus *Actinomyces.* adj., **actino-mycet′ic.**

actinomycete (ak″tĭ-no-mi′sēt) a moldlike bacterium (order Actinomycetales) occurring as elongated, frequently filamentous cells, with a branching tendency. adj., **acti-nomycet′ic.**

actinomycin (ak″tĭ-no-mi′sin) a family of ANTIBIOTICS from various species of *Streptomyces,* which are active against bacteria and fungi; it includes the antineoplastic AGENT DACTINOMYCIN (actinomycin D).

actinomycoma (ak″tĭ-no-mi-ko′mah) a tumorlike reactive lesion due to *Actinomyces.*

actinomycosis (ak″tĭ-no-mi-ko′sis) an infection involving the deeper tissues of the skin and mucous membranes, most often of the head and neck, caused by bacteria of the genus *Actinomyces.* The lesions begin as painless tumorlike masses around the jaw and neck that later break down and begin to suppurate with a discharge through a network of sinuses extending through the skin. Intraperitoneal abscesses and lung abscesses may also occur. The source of infection is unknown, although the mouth is thought to be the portal of entry because the organisms are often found in decayed teeth and in the tonsillar crypts of persons who are otherwise normal.

The infection progresses slowly, without remission, and without at first seeming to affect the general health of the patient. If it is not treated successfully the condition may eventually be fatal.

Diagnosis is established by identifying the causative microorganisms in anaerobic culture from a lesion. The usual treatment is with penicillin, the drug of choice. In cases of allergy to this drug, tetracycline, clindamycin, or chloramphenicol can be used. Surgical measures include resection, incision, and drainage of chronic abscesses and sinuses.

action (ak'shun) the accomplishment of an effect, whether mechanical or chemical, or the effect so produced.

cumulative a. the sudden and markedly increased action of a drug after administration of several doses.

independent nursing a. NURSING CARE that can be provided without the direction of other health care providers.

reflex a. an involuntary response to a stimulus conveyed to the nervous system and reflected to the periphery, passing below the level of consciousness; see also REFLEX.

action potential the electrical activity developed in an excitable CELL when stimulated; it may be elicited by electrical, chemical, or mechanical stimulation, by temperature change, and so on.

On an ELECTROCARDIOGRAM, action potential is seen as the cardiac cycle of a single cell, produced by a rapid sequence of changes at the cell membrane, and consists of phase 0 to phase 4, with phases 0 to 3 representing electrical SYSTOLE and phase 4 representing electrical DIASTOLE. The characteristics of action potentials vary in different parts of the heart; for example, the cells of the sinoatrial and atrioventricular nodes and the atrial cells do not have phases 1 or 2 and are shorter in duration than those of the His-Purkinje system and the ventricles.

depressed fast response a. p. an action potential produced when some but not all of the fast sodium channels are available to depolarize the fiber; on an electrocardiogram, it signifies the presence of slow conduction.

fast response a. p. the action potential produced by a cell when all of the fast sodium channels are available for depolarization; on an electrocardiogram, it signifies rapid upstroke velocity and maximal amplitude for phase 0, with consequent optimal conduction velocity.

slow response a. p. the action potential produced when only slow channels are available to depolarize the fiber; it is normal only in the sinoatrial and atrioventricular nodes and results in very slow conduction.

activator (ak'tĭ-va″ter) a substance that makes another substance active or reactive, induces a chemical reaction, or combines with an enzyme to increase its catalytic activity.

plasminogen a. a substance that activates PLASMINOGEN and converts it into PLASMIN; see t-plasminogen ACTIVATOR and u-plasminogen ACTIVATOR.

tissue plasminogen a.* (TPA, t-PA), *t-plasminogen a. a serine endopeptidase synthesized by endothelial cells, the

major physiologic activator of PLASMINOGEN; when bound to FIBRIN clots it catalyzes the conversion of plasminogen to PLASMIN by hydrolysis of a specific arginine-valine bond. It can be produced by recombinant technology for use in thrombolytic THERAPY. It acts directly on blood clots and therefore presents a small risk of systemic bleeding; occasionally allergic reactions may occur.

u-plasminogen a., urinary plasminogen a. a serine endopeptidase that acts as a plasminogen activator by catalyzing the preferential cleavage of plasminogen at the same arginine-valine bond where t-plasminogen ACTIVATOR cleaves. It is produced in the kidney and excreted in the urine and is used in thrombolytic THERAPY (when used as a pharmaceutical, it is usually called UROKINASE). Unlike t-plasminogen activator or prourokinase, it does not require FIBRIN for activity. Called also urokinase.

active transport (ak'tiv trans'port) the movement of ions or molecules across cell MEMBRANES and epithelial layers, usually against a concentration GRADIENT, as a direct result of the expenditure of metabolic energy. For example, under normal circumstances more potassium ions are present within the cell and more sodium ions are present extracellularly. The process of maintaining these normal differences in electrolytic composition between the intracellular and extracellular fluids is active transport. The process differs from passive TRANSPORT, simple DIFFUSION, and OSMOSIS in that it requires the expenditure of metabolic energy.

activity (ak-tiv'ĭ-te) 1. the quality or process of exerting energy or of accomplishing an effect. 2. a thermodynamic quantity that represents the effective concentration of a solute in a non-ideal solution. Symbol a. 3. the number of disintegrations per unit of a radioactive material. Symbol A. 4. the presence of recordable electrical energy in a nerve or muscle. 5. optical activity.

***a's of daily living* (ADL)** activities that are necessary for daily care of oneself and independent community living. It includes using the toilet and grooming, dressing, and feeding oneself; independent community living includes driving, shopping, homemaking, care of family, work activities, and so on. See also self CARE, self care DEFICIT, and self care ASSISTANCE. (See accompanying table.)

deficient diversional a. a NURSING DIAGNOSIS approved by the North American

ACTIVITIES OF DAILY LIVING

Grooming
  Obtain and use supplies to shave
  Apply and use cosmetics
  Wash, comb, style, and brush hair
  Care for nails
  Care for skin
  Apply deodorant

Oral Hygiene
  Obtain and use supplies
  Clean mouth and teeth
  Remove, clean, and reinsert dentures

Bathing
  Obtain and use supplies
  Soap, rinse, and dry all body parts
  Maintain bathing position
  Transfer to and from bathing position

Toilet Hygiene
  Obtain and use supplies
  Clean self
  Transfer to and from bedpan, toilet, and
    commode
  Main toileting position on bedpan, toilet, and
    commode

Dressing
  Select appropriate clothing
  Obtain clothing from storage area
  Dress and undress in sequential fashion
  Fasten and adjust clothing and shoes
  Don and doff assistive or adaptive equipment,
    prostheses, or orthoses

Feeding and Eating
  Set up food
  Use appropriate utensils and tableware
  Bring food or drink to mouth
  Suck, masticate, cough, and swallow

Medication Routine
  Obtain medication
  Open and close containers
  Take prescribed quantities as scheduled

Socialization
  Interact in appropriate contextual and cultural
    ways

Functional Communication
  Use equipment of systems to enhance or provide
    communication, such as writing equipment,
    telephones, typewriters, communication
    boards, call lights, emergency systems, braille
    writers, augmentative communication systems,
    and computers

Functional Mobility
  Move from one position or place to another
  Perform in-bed mobility, wheelchair mobility, and
    transfers (bed, car, tub, toilet, chair)
  Perform functional ambulation with or without
    adaptive aids
  Drive
  Use public transportation

Sexual Expression
  Recognize, communicate, and perform desired
    sexual activities

Nursing Diagnosis Association, defined as the experiencing by an individual of decreased stimulation from, interest in, or engagement in recreational or leisure activities. Formerly called diversional activity deficit. Possible causes include prolonged hospitalization or immobility at home, frequent and lengthy treatments such as renal dialysis, and a monotonous, nonstimulating environment. The patient usually gives subjective evidence that this condition exists by verbalizing a feeling of boredom or stating a desire for something to do or gives objective evidence by acting depressed or restless.

Nursing interventions that could be appropriate for diversional activity deficit include interviewing the patient to assess the current situation and to assist in developing plans for activities that provide interest and stimulation. These activities could include music, games, reading, handwork, or any other pastimes enjoyed by the patient. Patients may need assistance in identifying available resources and motivation to take advantage of the activities they provide.

enzyme a. the catalytic effect exerted by an enzyme, expressed as units per milligram of enzyme (*specific activity*) or molecules of substrate transformed per minute per molecule of enzyme (*molecular activity*).

malignant ventricular ectopic a. ventricular FIBRILLATION or ventricular TACHYCARDIA with syncope, heart failure, myocardial ischemia, or hypotension.

optical a. the ability of a chemical compound to rotate the plane of polarization of plane-polarized light.

physical a. bodily movements, such as those accompanying ACTIVITIES OF DAILY LIVING.

pulseless electrical a. (PEA) continued electrical rhythmicity of the heart in the absence of effective mechanical function; it may be due to uncoupling of ventricular muscle contraction from electrical activity or may be secondary to cardiac damage with respiratory failure and cessation of cardiac venous return. Called also electromechanical dissociation.

purposeful a. in OCCUPATIONAL THERAPY, tasks or experiences in which the individual actively participates that require and elicit coordination between the sensory, motor, cognitive, and psychological systems. Each person has a unique set of purposeful activities, influenced by his or her life roles, and, when doing one of them, directs attention to the task itself rather than to the internal processes involved. Activities may yield immediate results or may require sustained effort and repetition, and they may either represent new responses or be part of complex, longstanding patterns of behavior.

sustained rhythmic a. the continuous generation of ACTION POTENTIALS within the heart in the absence of artificial or external stimulation.

triggered a. activity in which non-driven ACTION POTENTIALS arise from AFTER-POTENTIALS that were caused by the previous action potential.

actomyosin (ak″to-mi′o-sin) the complex of ACTIN and MYOSIN constituting muscle fibers and responsible for the contraction and relaxation of muscle. (See accompanying illustration.)

acuity (ah-ku′ĭ-te) 1. Acuteness (see ACUTE [def. 2]); the level of severity of an illness. This is one of the parameters considered in patient classification systems that are designed to serve as guidelines for allocation of nursing staff, to justify staffing decisions, and to aid in long-range projection of staffing and budget. 2. clearness of the visual perception of an image.

visual a. the ability to discriminate visually between forms. See accompanying illustration.

acuminate (ah-ku′mĭ-nāt) sharp-pointed.

acupressure (ak′u-presh″er) 1. the application of digital pressure on parts of the body in a therapeutic way so as to relieve pain or produce anesthesia. 2. in the NURSING INTERVENTIONS CLASSIFICATION, a nursing INTERVENTION defined as application of firm, sustained pressure to special points on the body to decrease pain, produce relaxation, and prevent or reduce nausea.

acupuncture (ak′u-pungk″cher) the Chinese practice of inserting needles into specific points along the "meridians" of the body to relieve the discomfort associated with painful disorders, to induce surgical ANESTHESIA, and for preventive and therapeutic purposes. Acupuncture is generally used to treat functional disorders rather than organic diseases that bring about severe tissue changes. It may be used in combination with other therapies for treatment of degenerative diseases. Use of it as a form of anesthesia is considered by traditional Chinese practitioners to be a minor part of acupuncture practice.

Advocates of acupuncture speak of the concept of a vital energy flow or life force (*c'hi*) which circulates through the body along meridians similar to the blood, lymphatic, and neural circuits. It is believed that there are two energy flows, which are in everything in the universe. *Yang,* the positive principle, tends to stimulate and to contract; *yin,* the negative principle, tends to sedate and to expand. Health depends upon the equilibrium of yang and yin, first in the body and secondly in the universe.

The therapeutic objective of acupuncture is to rectify an imbalance in the energy flow. This is accomplished by the insertion of needles at specific points along the meridians. The needles are inserted in the skin to varying depths according to the point of insertion and the condition being treated. They may be left in place for varying lengths of time and are vibrated manually or electrically.

Traditionally an East Asian practice, acupuncture is becoming accepted in Western countries as a valid form of therapy.

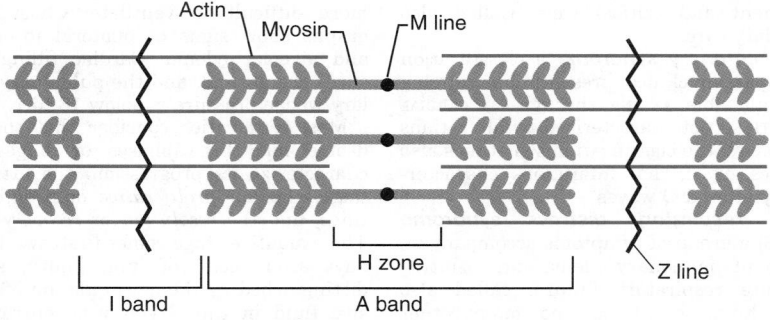

Actomyosin in muscle fibers. From Applegate, 2000.

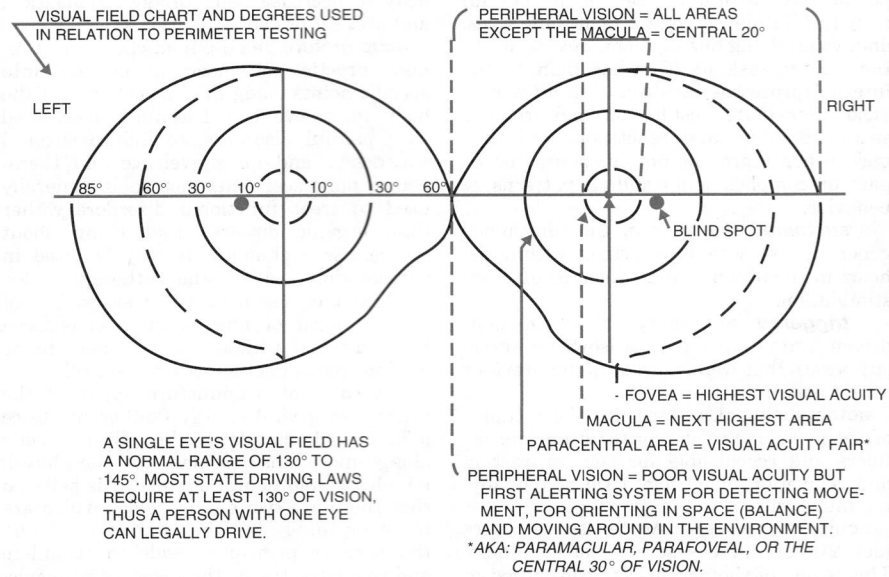

VISUAL FIELD CHART AND DEGREES USED IN RELATION TO PERIMETER TESTING

PERIPHERAL VISION = ALL AREAS EXCEPT THE MACULA = CENTRAL 20°

LEFT

RIGHT

85° 60° 30° 10° 10° 30° 60°

BLIND SPOT

- FOVEA = HIGHEST VISUAL ACUITY
MACULA = NEXT HIGHEST AREA
PARACENTRAL AREA = VISUAL ACUITY FAIR*

A SINGLE EYE'S VISUAL FIELD HAS A NORMAL RANGE OF 130° TO 145°. MOST STATE DRIVING LAWS REQUIRE AT LEAST 130° OF VISION, THUS A PERSON WITH ONE EYE CAN LEGALLY DRIVE.

PERIPHERAL VISION = POOR VISUAL ACUITY BUT FIRST ALERTING SYSTEM FOR DETECTING MOVE-MENT, FOR ORIENTING IN SPACE (BALANCE) AND MOVING AROUND IN THE ENVIRONMENT.
*AKA: PARAMACULAR, PARAFOVEAL, OR THE CENTRAL 30° OF VISION.

Visual field chart illustrating the divisions of the visual field related to visual acuity. (Courtesy of Josephine C. Moore, PhD, OTR.) From Pedretti and Early, 2001.

There is some research support for the idea that the procedure produces an analgesic effect because it causes the release of enkephalin, a naturally occurring ENDORPHIN that has opiate-like effects.

acus (a′kus) a needle or needle-like process.

acute (ah-kūt′) 1. sharp. 2. having severe symptoms and a short course. Some serious illnesses that were formerly considered acute (such as myocardial infarction) are now recognized to be acute episodes of chronic conditions.

a. care the level of care in the HEALTH CARE SYSTEM that consists of emergency treatment and critical care. Called also secondary care.

a. coronary syndrome a classification encompassing clinical presentations ranging from unstable ANGINA through MYOCARDIAL INFARCTIONS not characterized by alterations in Q WAVES; the classification sometimes also includes myocardial infarctions characterized by altered Q waves.

a. respiratory distress syndrome **(ARDS)** a group of symptoms accompanying fulminant pulmonary edema and resulting in acute respiratory failure; called also shock lung, wet lung, and many other names descriptive of etiology or clinical manifestations. Many etiologic factors have been associated with ARDS, including shock, fat embolism, fluid overload, oxygen toxicity, fluid aspiration, narcotic overdose, disseminated intravascular coagulation, multiple transfusions, inhalation of toxic gases, diffuse pulmonary infection, and systemic reactions to sepsis, pancreatitis, and massive trauma or burns.

ARDS is characterized clinically by DYSP-NEA, TACHYPNEA, TACHYCARDIA, CYANOSIS, and HYPOXEMIA. Pa_{O_2}/FI_{O_2} remains low (below 2 cc) even with oxygen therapy at high oxygen concentrations. The lung compliance is decreased so that the lung is stiffer and more difficult to ventilate. Chest radiographs show signs of bilateral interstitial and alveolar edema. Cardiac filling pressures are normal, and the pulmonary capillary wedge pressure is below 18 torr.

Most authorities consider that the syndrome has three phases or stages that characterize its progression: the *exudative stage,* the *fibroproliferative* or *proliferative stage,* and the *resolution* or *recovery stage.* The exudative stage comes first, two to four days after onset of lung injury, and is distinguished by the accumulation of excessive fluid in the alveoli with entrance of protein and inflammatory cells from the alveolar capillaries into the air spaces. The fibroproliferative stage comes second and is characterized by an increase in connective tissue and other structural elements in the lungs in response to the initial injury. It begins between the first and third weeks after the initial injury and may last up to ten weeks. Microscopic examination reveals lung tissue that appears densely cellular. The patient is at risk for PNEUMONIA, SEPSIS, and PNEUMOTHORAX at this time. The third stage is the resolution or recovery stage. During this stage the lung reorganizes and recovers, although it continues to show signs of FIBROSIS. Lung function may continue to improve for as long as six to twelve months or even longer, depending on the precipitating condition and severity of the injury. It is important to remember that there are often different levels of pulmonary recovery in patients with ARDS.

Some authorities refer to a fourth phase or stage of ARDS, the period after the resolution or recovery stage. Some patients continue to experience health problems caused by the acute illness, such as coughing, limited exercise tolerance, and fatigue. Anxiety, depression, and flashback memories of the critical illness may also occur and be similar to POSTTRAUMATIC STRESS DISORDER.

Treatment and Patient Care. Mechanical VENTILATION must be begun at the first signs of HYPERVENTILATION and HYPOXEMIA, before obvious signs of respiratory distress develop. A cuffed ENDOTRACHEAL TUBE or TRACHEOSTOMY tube is used to maintain an airway. The patient is ventilated at the lowest oxygen concentration that maintains the arterial oxygen saturation (Sa$_{O_2}$) at 90 per cent. POSITIVE END-EXPIRATORY PRESSURE (PEEP) or CONTINUOUS POSITIVE AIRWAY PRESSURE (CPAP) may be used to increase the number of alveoli that remain open at the end of exhalation and thus decrease pulmonary shunt. HEMODYNAMIC MONITORING, using a SWAN-GANZ CATHETER, is done to measure cardiac output, pulmonary capillary wedge pressure, and right atrial wedge pressure. An arterial line is placed to continuously monitor BLOOD PRESSURE and measure arterial BLOOD GASES. A diuretic such as FUROSEMIDE (Lasix) may be administered to reduce fluid volume overload and pulmonary edema. If infection develops, antibiotics are administered. Hemodynamic parameters, arterial blood gas levels, intake and output, breath sounds, vital signs, inspiratory pressure, tidal volume, inspired oxygen concentration, and end-expiratory pressure are all continuously monitored.

a. situational reaction a transient, self-limiting acute emotional reaction to severe psychological stress. See ACUTE STRESS DISORDER, ADJUSTMENT DISORDER, POSTTRAUMATIC STRESS DISORDER, and brief reactive PSYCHOSIS.

a. stress disorder an ANXIETY DISORDER characterized by development of ANXIETY, DISSOCIATION, and other symptoms within one month following exposure to an extremely traumatic event, the symptoms including reexperiencing the event, avoidance of trauma-related stimuli, anxiety or increased arousal, and some or all of the following: a subjective sense of diminished emotional responsiveness, numbing, or detachment, derealization, depersonalization, and amnesia for aspects of the event. If persistent, it may become POSTTRAUMATIC STRESS DISORDER.

a. stress reaction acute situational reaction.

acyanotic (a-si″ah-not′ik) not characterized or accompanied by cyanosis.

acyclovir (a-si′klo-vir) a synthetic acyclic purine nucleoside with selective antiviral activity against the human HERPESVIRUSES, used in treatment of genital and mucocutaneous herpesvirus infections in both IMMUNOCOMPROMISED patients and those who are not. Administered orally, topically, or intravenously.

acyesis (a″si-e′sis) 1. sterility in a woman. 2. absence of pregnancy.

acyl (a′sil) an organic radical derived from an organic acid by removal of the hydroxyl group from the carboxyl group.

acylation (a″si-la′shun) introduction of an acyl radical into the molecule of a compound.

acystia (a-sis′te-ah) congenital absence of the bladder.

AD [L.] au′ris dex′tra (right ear).

AD alcohol dehydrogenase.

ad [L.] preposition, *to*.

ADA American Dental Association; American Diabetes Association; American Dietetics Association.

ADAA American Dental Assistants' Association.

adactylia (a″dak-til′e-ah) adactyly.

adactyly (a-dak′til-e) a developmental anomaly characterized by the absence of fingers or toes or both. adj., **adac′tylous**.

Adam's apple (ad′amz) popular name for the laryngeal PROMINENCE.

adamantine (ad″ah-man′tin) pertaining to the enamel of the teeth.

adamantinoma (ad″ah-man″ti-no′mah) ameloblastoma.

ADAMHA Alcohol, Drug Abuse, and Mental Health Administration, a former agency of the United States Department of Health and Human Services.

Adams' disease (ad′amz) Adams-Stokes disease.

Adams-Stokes disease (ad′amz stōks) a condition characterized by sudden attacks of unconsciousness, with or without convulsions, which frequently accompanies heart block; called also Stokes-Adams disease.

adapalene (ah-dap′ah-lēn) a synthetic analogue of RETINOIC ACID used topically in the treatment of ACNE VULGARIS.

adaptation (ad″ap-ta′shun) 1. a dynamic, ongoing, life-sustaining process by which living organisms adjust to environmental changes. 2. adjustment of the pupil to light.

    biological a. the adaptation of living things to environmental factors for the ultimate purpose of survival, reproduction, and an optimal level of functioning.

    color a. 1. changes in visual perception of color with prolonged stimulation. 2. adjustment of vision to degree of brightness or color tone of illumination.

    dark a. adaptation of the eye to vision in the dark or in reduced illumination.

    light a. adaptation of the eye to vision in the sunlight or in bright illumination (photopia), with reduction in the concentration of the photosensitive pigments of the eye.

    physiological a. the ongoing process by which internal body functions are regulated and adjusted to maintain homeostasis in the internal environment.

    psychological a. the ongoing process, anchored in the emotions and intellect, by which humans sustain a balance in their mental and emotional states of being and in their interactions with their social and cultural environments.

    social a. adjustment and adaptation of humans to other individuals and community groups working together for a common purpose.

adaptation model a CONCEPTUAL MODEL of nursing, formulated by Sister Callista ROY, concerned with problems of adaptation to the changing environment. The *person* is an adaptive system that includes regulator and cognator coping mechanisms. The individual or group that has actual or potential adaptation problems is the recipient of care. The *environment* is all the internal and external stimuli that affect an individual or group. Environmental stimuli include the conditions, circumstances, and influences that surround and affect the development and behavior of an individual or group. *Health* is a state of being and a process of becoming an integrated and whole

person. Adaptive behavior in four modes (physiological, self-concept, role function, and interdependence) is termed wellness; illness is ineffective adaptation in one or more of these modes. *Nursing* is a theoretical system of knowledge that prescribes a systematic process related to the care of the ill or potentially ill person.

The goal of nursing is to promote patient adaptation in all four adaptive modes during wellness and illness. The nursing process component of the adaptation model involves six steps. In step one, assessment of behaviors, data regarding the client's physiological, self-concept, role function, and interdependence behaviors are collected. Once the data have been collected, the nurse must judge whether the behaviors are adaptive or ineffective. Thus the primary question is: To what extent is the person adapting to environmental stimuli? In step two, assessment of influencing factors, priorities are set for further assessment and identification of the environmental stimuli that influence the client's behavior and so contribute to the adaptive or ineffective responses. Step three, nursing diagnosis, involves a behavioral description of the client's adaptive or ineffective responses and identification of the most relevant influencing factors, as well as establishment of a hierarchy of importance for the nursing diagnoses. In step four, goal setting, the goals for nursing care are formulated. These goals are stated as behaviors expected as the outcome of nursing intervention. Step five, intervention, involves management of environmental stimuli, which takes the form of an increase, decrease, modification, maintenance, or removal of internal or external stimuli. The intervention with the highest probability of reaching the desired goal is selected. In step six, evaluation, the effectiveness of the nursing intervention is judged. The criterion for effectiveness is whether the desired behavioral goal was attained. The outcome of this step is updating of the nursing care plan.

adaptometer (ad″ap-tom′ĕ-ter) an instrument for measuring the time required for retinal adaptation, i.e., for regeneration of the visual purple; used in detecting night blindness, vitamin A deficiency, and retinitis pigmentosa.

ADA Seal of Acceptance an approval given by the American Dental Association to oral care products that are supported by adequate research evidence as to their safety and efficacy.

adder any of numerous venomous elapid and viperine snakes; the *death adder* is found in Australia and New Guinea and the *puff adder* is found in Africa and Arabia. See also SNAKEBITE.

ADC average daily census.

ADCC antibody-dependent cell-mediated cytotoxicity.

addict (ad′ikt) a person exhibiting ADDICTION.

addiction (ah-dik′shun) 1. the state of being given up to some habit or compulsion. 2. strong physiological and psychological dependence on a drug or other agent; see ALCOHOLISM and DRUG DEPENDENCE.

   drug a. a state of heavy dependence on a drug; sometimes defined as physical dependence but usually also including emotional dependence, i.e., compulsive or pathological drug use. It is often used synonymously with DRUG DEPENDENCE.

Addis test (method) (ad′is) after the patient is given a dry diet for 24 hours, the specific gravity of the urine is determined.

Addison's disease (ad′ĭ-sunz) a rare syndrome resulting from chronic adrenocortical INSUFFICIENCY. If there is normal function of the testes and ovaries, the physiologic effects from decreased production of the adrenal sex hormones are minor. The disease may occur as either a primary or a secondary deficit in hormone production. Primary insufficiency is thought to be due to AUTOIMMUNE DISEASE involving the ADRENAL GLANDS. Causes include tubercular infection, fungal infections, amyloidosis, and nonsecreting tumors of the adrenal cortex. Secondary causes are related to deficient production of adrenocorticotropic HORMONE (ACTH), the hormone that triggers the release of hormones from the adrenal cortex, which itself is secreted by the PITUITARY GLAND. Underfunctioning of the pituitary, its surgical removal, and certain pituitary tumors can eventually result in a decrease or total absence of ACTH.

Serious and potentially life-threatening problems associated with Addison's disease are fluid and electrolyte imbalance and profound HYPOGLYCEMIA. Deficiency of MINERALOCORTICOIDS leads to depletion of sodium (HYPONATREMIA), resulting in depletion of extracellular fluid and potassium retention (HYPERKALEMIA). The patient experiences generalized malaise and muscular weakness, muscle pain, orthostatic hypotension, and vulnerability to cardiac arrhythmias.

Deficiency of CORTISOL adversely affects blood sugar levels, causing hypoglycemic reactions. Anorexia, nausea, vomiting, flatulence, and diarrhea can also occur. These symptoms, as well as anxiety, mental depression, and loss of mental acuity, are believed to be related to absence of the

cyclic peaks of cortisol output that normally occur every 24 hours. Hyperpigmentation of certain areas of the skin occurs only in primary adrenal insufficiency. An insufficient supply of cortisol signals the pituitary gland to secrete more ACTH, which has the effect of increasing the coloration of scars, skin folds, pressure areas, and the areolae of the nipples. Diagnosis of Addison's disease also includes synthetic ACTH stimulation testing.

Patient Care. Treatment of Addison's disease is focused on replacement of the deficient hormones; that is, on administration of exogenous glucocorticoids and mineralocorticoids. Replacement therapy usually brings about a rapid recovery.

Acute nursing care is concerned with intensive support of the patient should there be an addisonian CRISIS, prevention of problems related to HYPOGLYCEMIA and orthostatic HYPOTENSION, alleviation of gastrointestinal problems, and instruction of the patient in self-care. It includes providing regular feedings throughout the day and providing for adequate rest. When fasting is required for diagnostic studies or surgery, the patient probably will need intravenous feedings of GLUCOSE to avoid profound hypoglycemia. Maintenance doses of exogenous glucocorticoids are especially important during fasting. Gastrointestinal problems require attention to adequate nutrition and avoidance of foods that are irritating to the gastrointestinal mucosa and difficult to digest.

The patient's intake and output are measured regularly, and postural blood pressure is checked periodically. The apical-radial pulse is taken along with other vital signs to identify early symptoms of HYPERKALEMIA. Cardiac monitoring may be indicated if cardiac arrhythmias develop. Safety measures must be taken to prevent falls during spells of weakness and fainting that may occur.

Stress, even relatively mild physical and emotional stress, can quickly bring on an addisonian CRISIS. When this occurs, the physiologic defense provided by cortisol is no longer operating, and the patient suffers from HYPOTENSION and eventual circulatory collapse. Absence of mineralocorticoids compounds the problem by depletion of extracellular fluids and impairment of cardiac function. Treatment should be immediately initiated if addisonian crisis is suspected.

A person with Addison's disease usually can lead a fairly normal life with exogenous hormone THERAPY. Patient education includes instruction in the signs and symptoms of inadequate or excess steroid replacement (which require return to the health care provider or clinic), in the importance of avoiding stressful situations whenever possible, and in the ideal regimen of diet and rest to avoid hypoglycemic reactions. The patient should carry an injectable form of cortisol when traveling for emergency treatment. Anyone with Addison's disease should wear a medical identification tag stating that he or she has the condition and is receiving steroid therapy.

addisonism (ad′ĭ-sun-izm″) symptoms seen in pulmonary tuberculosis, consisting of debility and pigmentation, resembling ADDISON'S DISEASE.

additive (ad′ĭ-tiv) 1. characterized by addition. 2. a substance added to another, such as to improve its appearance or increase its nutritive value.

adduct (ah-dukt′) to draw toward an axis or median line.

adduction (ah-duk′shun) the act of adducting; the state of being adducted. (See accompanying illustration.)

adductor (ah-duk′ter) that which adducts; see also anatomic Table of Muscles in the Appendices.

aden(o)- word element [Gr.], *gland.*

adenalgia (ad″ĕ-nal′jah) pain in a gland; called also adenodynia.

adendritic (a″den-drit′ik) without dendrites.

adenectomy (ad″ĕ-nek′tah-me) surgical excision of a gland.

adenectopia (ad″ĕ-nek-to′pe-ah) displacement of a gland.

adeniform (ah-den′ĭ-form) gland-shaped.

adenine (ad′ĕ-nēn) a purine base present in nucleoproteins of cells of plants and animals; adenine and GUANINE are essential components of NUCLEIC ACIDS. The end product of

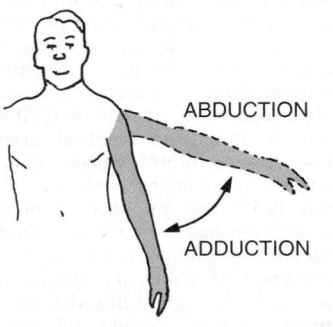

ABDUCTION

ADDUCTION

Adduction versus abduction of arm. From Chabner, 1996.

the metabolism of adenine in humans is URIC ACID. A preparation of adenine is used to improve the preservation of whole blood. Symbol A.

a. arabinoside **(ara-A)** vidarabine.

adenitis (ad″ĕ-ni′tis) inflammation of a gland.

cervical a. a condition characterized by enlarged, inflamed, and tender lymph nodes of the neck; seen in certain infectious diseases of children, such as acute infections of the throat. Called also cervical lymphadenitis.

cervical a., tuberculous tuberculous cervical LYMPHADENITIS.

adenoacanthoma (ad″ĕ-no-ak″an-tho′-mah) adenocarcinoma in which some of the cells exhibit squamous differentiation.

adenoameloblastoma (ad″ĕ-no-ah-mel″o-blas-to′mah) an odontogenic tumor with formation of ductlike structures in place of or in addition to a typical ameloblastic pattern.

adenoblast (ad′ĕ-no-blast″) 1. an embryonic forerunner of gland tissue. 2. any tissue that produces secretory or glandular activity.

adenocarcinoma (ad″ĕ-no-kahr″sĭ-no′-mah) carcinoma derived from glandular tissue or in which the tumor cells form recognizable glandular structures. The World Health Organization recognizes four categories of adenocarcinoma: acinar, papillary, bronchioalveolar, and solid carcinoma with mucus formation; it can be further subclassified into well, moderate, and poorly differentiated forms.

alveolar a., bronchioalveolar a., bronchiolar a., bronchioloalveolar a., bronchoalveolar a. bronchioloalveolar carcinoma.

clear cell a. a rare malignant tumor of the female genital tract, resembling a renal cell carcinoma and containing tubules or small cysts with some cells that are hobnail-shaped and others whose cytoplasm is clear, containing abundant glycogen and inconspicuous stroma. It may occur in the ovary, uterus, cervix, or vagina. One form has been linked to in utero exposure to DIETHYLSTILBESTROL. Called also clear cell carcinoma and mesonephroma.

a. of the lung a type of bronchogenic CARCINOMA made up of cuboidal or columnar cells in a discrete mass, usually at the periphery of the lungs.

adenocele (ad′ĕ-no-sēl″) a cystic adenomatous tumor.

adenocellulitis (ad″ĕ-no-sel″u-li′tis) inflammation of a gland and the cellular tissue around it.

adenochondroma (ad″ĕ-no-kon-dro′mah) a tumor containing both glandular and cartilaginous elements.

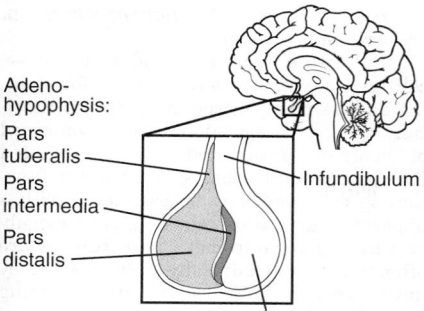

Adeno-
hypophysis:
Pars
tuberalis
Pars
intermedia
Pars
distalis

Infundibulum

Neurohypophysis

Adenohypophysis. From Dorland's, 2000.

adenocystoma (ad″ĕ-no-sis-to′mah) adenoma in which there is cyst formation.

adenodynia (ad″ĕ-no-din′e-ah) adenalgia.

adenoepithelioma (ad″ĕ-no-ep″ĭ-the″le-o′mah) a tumor composed of glandular and epithelial elements.

adenogenous (ad″ĕ-noj′ĕ-nus) originating from glandular tissue.

adenohypophysis (ad″ĕ-no-hi-pof′ĭ-sis) the anterior or glandular portion of the PITUITARY GLAND. adj., **adenohypophys′eal.**

adenoid (ad′ĕ-noid) 1. pharyngeal TONSIL. 2. pertaining to the pharyngeal tonsils or to hypertrophy of them. 3. resembling a gland. 4. (in the plural) hypertrophy of the pharyngeal tonsils, usually seen in children; adenoids may cause obstruction of the outlet from the nose so that the child breathes chiefly through the mouth, or the eustachian tube may be blocked, with pain in the ear or a sense of pressure resulting. It also may prepare the way for infections of the middle ear and occasionally interferes with hearing. Prolonged obstruction by enlarged adenoids produces a typical adenoid FACIES. The child appears to be dull and apathetic, and has some degree of nutritional deficiency and hearing loss, and some delay in growth and development. Surgical excision of the enlarged tissue is called ADENOIDECTOMY. (See accompanying illustration.)

adenoidectomy (ad″ĕ-noid-ek′tah-me) surgical excision of the adenoids. The operation is usually performed in conjunction with tonsillectomy since both the adenoids and palatine tonsils tend to become enlarged after repeated infections of the throat. It may be combined with the placement of ear ventilation tubes in cases of recurrent ear infections. The preoperative and postoperative care in adenoidectomy is similar to that in TONSILLECTOMY and is described under that heading.

adenoiditis (ad″ĕ-noid-i′tis) inflammation of the adenoids.

adenolipoma (ad″ĕ-no-lĭ-po′mah) a tumor composed of both glandular and fatty tissue elements.

adenolipomatosis (ad″ĕ-no-lip″o-mah-to′-sis) the formation of numerous adenolipomas in the neck, axilla, and groin.

adenology (ad″ĕ-nol′ah-je) the sum of knowledge regarding glands.

adenolymphitis (ad″ĕ-no-lim-fi′tis) lymphadenitis; inflammation of lymph nodes.

adenolymphoma (ad″ĕ-no-lim-fo′mah) a cystic salivary-gland tumor containing epithelial and lymphoid tissue, affecting almost exclusively the parotid gland.

adenoma (ad″ĕ-no′mah) a benign epithelial tumor in which the cells form recognizable glandular structures or in which the cells are derived from glandular epithelium.

acidophilic a. in a classification system formerly used for pituitary adenomas, an adenoma whose cells stain pale pink with acid dyes; most adenomas that secreted excessive amounts of growth hormone were in this group

ACTH-secreting a., adrenocorticotrophic hormone–secreting a. corticotroph adenoma.

basophilic a. in a classification system formerly used for pituitary adenomas, an adenoma whose cells stain pale blue with

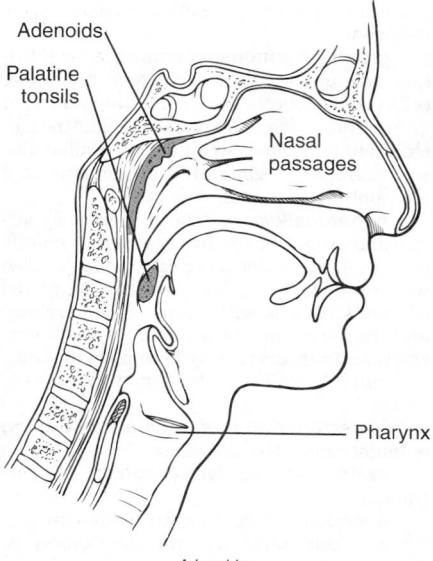

Adenoids

Palatine
tonsils

Nasal
passages

Pharynx

Adenoids.

basic dyes; most adenomas that secreted excessive amounts of adrenocorticotrophic hormone were in this group.

chromophobe a., chromophobic a. a pituitary adenoma composed of cells that lack acidophilic or basophilic granules; this is the same entity as the more precisely named null-cell a.

corticotrope a., corticotroph a. a pituitary adenoma made up predominantly of corticotrophs; excessive corticotropin secretion may cause Cushing's disease or Nelson's syndrome. Called also ACTH-secreting or adrenocorticotropic hormone–secreting adenoma and corticotropinoma.

endocrine-active a. a pituitary adenoma that secretes excessive amounts of a hormone; see PROLACTINOMA, corticotroph adenoma, gonadotroph adenoma, growth hormone–secreting adenoma, and thyrotroph adenoma. Called also hyperfunctional or hyperfunctioning adenoma.

endocrine-inactive a. a pituitary adenoma that does not secrete excessive amounts of any hormone; many null-cell adenomas are of this type. Called also nonfunctional or nonfunctioning adenoma and nonsecreting or nonsecretory adenoma.

eosinophilic a. growth hormone–secreting adenoma.

gonadotrope a., gonadotroph a. a rare type of pituitary adenoma made up of GONADOTROPH-like cells that secrete excessive amounts of follicle-stimulating hormone or luteinizing hormone or both; it may cause precocious puberty, visual disturbances, or hypogonadism.

growth hormone–secreting a. a pituitary adenoma made up of SOMATOTROPH-like cells that secrete excessive amounts of growth hormone; it may cause gigantism in children or acromegaly in adults. Called also somatotrope or somatotroph adenoma and eosinophilic adenoma.

hepatocellular a. a large, fleshy, hypervascular tumor of the liver occurring chiefly in women of childbearing age and associated with oral contraceptive use. It is composed of sheets of cells with areas of hemorrhage and necrosis and has a tendency to hemorrhage and rupture; it may become malignant.

Hürthle cell a. a benign HÜRTHLE CELL TUMOR.

hyperfunctional a., hyperfunctioning a. endocrine-active adenoma.

lactotrope a., lactotroph a. prolactinoma.

liver cell a. hepatocellular adenoma.

nonfunctional a., nonfunctioning a. endocrine-inactive adenoma.

nonsecreting a., nonsecretory a. endocrine-inactive adenoma.

null-cell a. a pituitary adenoma whose cells give negative results on tests for staining and hormone secretion; although classically they were considered to be composed of sparsely granulated or degranulated (nonfunctioning) cells, some contain functioning cells and may be associated with a hyperpituitary state such as acromegaly or Cushing's syndrome. These tumors are often discovered clinically only when they have grown large and are pressing on surrounding structures. Called also chromophobic adenoma.

pituitary a. a benign neoplasm of the anterior pituitary gland; some contain hormone-secreting cells (endocrine-active adenomas) but some are not secretory (endocrine-inactive adenomas).

plurihormonal a. an endocrine-active adenoma that secretes more than one kind of hormone.

prolactin cell a., prolactin-secreting a. prolactinoma.

sebaceous a. hypertrophy or benign hyperplasia of a sebaceous (oil-secreting) GLAND.

a. seba'ceum nevoid hyperplasia of sebaceous glands, forming multiple yellow papules or nodules on the face. See also NEVUS.

somatotrope a., somatotroph a. growth hormone–secreting adenoma.

thyroid-stimulating hormone–secreting a. thyrotroph adenoma.

thyrotrope a., thyrotroph a. TSH-secreting a. a rare type of pituitary adenoma made up of THYROTROPH-like cells that secrete excess THYROTROPIN and cause hyperthyroidism; called also thyroid stimulating hormone–secreting adenoma.

villous a. a large soft papillary polyp on the mucosa of the large intestine.

adenomalacia (ad″ĕ-no-mah-la′shah) undue softness of a gland.

adenomatosis (ad″ĕ-no″mah-to′sis) the formation of numerous adenomatous growths.

adenomatous (ad″ĕ-nom′ah-tus) pertaining to ADENOMA or to nodular HYPERPLASIA of a gland.

adenomere (ad′ĕ-no-mēr″) the blind terminal portion of the glandular cavity of a developing gland, being the functional portion of the organ.

adenomyoma (ad″ĕ-no-mi-o′mah) 1. a benign tumor consisting of smooth muscle and glandular elements. 2. see ADENOMYOSIS.

adenomyometritis (ad″ĕ-no-mi″o-mĕ-tri′tis) adenomyosis of the uterus.

adenomyosarcoma (ad″ĕ-no-mi″o-sahr-ko′mah) ADENOSARCOMA containing striated muscle.

adenomyosis (ad″ĕ-no-mi-o′sis) invasion of the muscular wall of an organ (e.g., uterus) by glandular tissue.

adenopathy (ad″ĕ-nop′ah-the) 1. enlargement of a gland. 2. lymphadenopathy.

adenopharyngitis (ad″ĕ-no-far″in-ji′tis) inflammation of the adenoids and pharynx, usually involving the tonsils.

adenosarcoma (ad″ĕ-no-sahr-ko′mah) adenoma blended with sarcoma.

adenosclerosis (ad″ĕ-no-sklĕ-ro′sis) hardening of a gland.

adenosine (ah-den′o-sēn) 1. a nucleoside composed of the pentose sugar D-ribose and adenine. It is a structural subunit of RIBONUCLEIC ACID (RNA). Adenosine nucleotides are involved in the energy metabolism of all cells. Adenosine can be linked to a chain of one, two, or three phosphate groups to form *adenosine monophosphate* (AMP), *adenosine diphosphate* (ADP), or *adenosine triphosphate* (ATP). The bond between the phosphate groups in ADP or the two bonds between phosphate groups in ATP are called *high-energy bonds,* because hydrolysis of a high-energy bond provides a large amount of free energy that can be used to drive other processes that would not otherwise occur. The energy that is derived from the breakdown of carbohydrates, fats, or proteins is used to synthesize ATP. The energy stored in ATP is then used directly or indirectly to drive all other cellular processes that require energy, of which there are four major types: (1) the transport of molecules and ions across cell membranes against concentration gradients, which maintains the internal environment of the cell and produces the membrane potential for the conduction of nerve impulses; (2) the contraction of muscle fibers and other fibers producing the motion of cells; (3) the synthesis of chemical compounds; (4) the synthesis of other high-energy compounds. (See accompanying illustration.) 2. a preparation of adenosine, which acts as a cardiac depressant of automaticity in the sinus node and conduction in the atrioventricular node and as a VASODILATOR. It is used as an ANTIARRHYTHMIC and is also used to cause coronary vasodilation during myocardial perfusion imaging in patients who cannot exercise adequately to perform an exercise stress test, administered intravenously.

cyclic a. monophosphate a cyclic nucleotide, adenosine 3′,5′-cyclic monophosphate, involved in the action of many hormones, including catecholamines, ACTH,

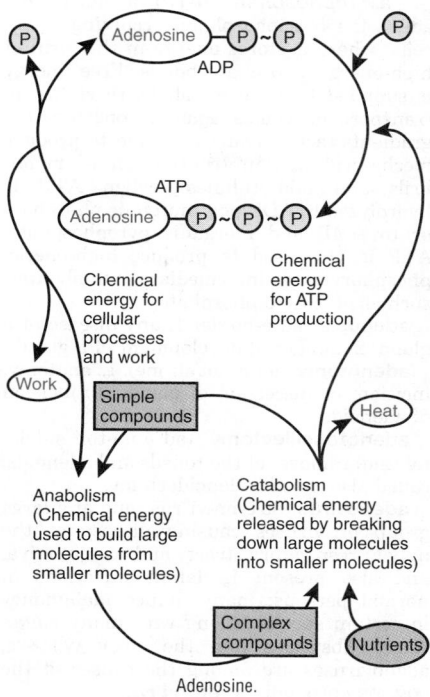

Adenosine.

and vasopressin. The hormone binds to a specific receptor on the cell membrane of target cells. This activates an enzyme, adenylate cyclase, which produces cyclic AMP from ATP. Cyclic AMP acts as a second messenger activating other enzymes within the cell. Abbreviated 3′,5′-AMP, cAMP, and cyclic AMP.

a. diphosphate (ADP) a nucleotide, adenosine 5′-pyrophosphate, produced by the hydrolysis of adenosine triphosphate (ATP). It is then converted back to ATP by the metabolic processes oxidative phosphorylation, glycolysis, and the tricarboxylic acid CYCLE.

a. monophosphate (AMP) a nucleotide, adenosine 5′-phosphate, involved in energy metabolism and nucleotide synthesis. Called also adenylic acid.

a. triphosphatase (ATPase) a term used to refer to the enzymatic activity of certain intercellular processes that split ATP to form ADP and inorganic phosphate, when the energy released is not used for the synthesis of chemical compounds. Examples are the splitting of ATP in muscle contraction and the transport of ions across cell membranes.

a. triphosphate (ATP) a nucleotide, adenosine 5′-triphosphate, occurring in all cells, where it stores energy in the form of high-energy phosphate bonds. Free energy is supplied to drive metabolic reactions, to transport molecules against concentration gradients (active transport), and to produce mechanical motion (contraction of myofibrils and microtubules), when ATP is hydrolyzed to ADP and inorganic phosphate or to AMP and inorganic pyrophosphate. ATP is also used to produce high-energy phosphorylated intermediary metabolites, such as glucose 6-phosphate.

adenosis (ad″ĕ-no′sis) 1. any disease of a gland. 2. abnormal development of a gland.

adenotomy (ad″ĕ-not′ah-me) 1. anatomy, incision, or dissection of glands. 2. incision of adenoids.

adenotonsillectomy (ad″ĕ-no-ton″sĭ-lek′-tah-me) removal of the tonsils and adenoids; called also tonsilloadenoidectomy.

adenovirus (ad′ĕ-no-vi″rus) any of a large group of viruses causing disease of the upper respiratory tract and conjunctiva, and also present in latent infections in normal persons; many induce malignancy in certain species. Along with many RHINO-VIRUS subspecies and the PICORNAVIRUSES, adenoviruses are among the causes of the COMMON COLD. adj., **adenovi′ral.**

adenylate (ah-den′ĭ-lăt) a salt, anion, or ester of adenylic acid.

adenylate cyclase (ah-den′ĭ-lăt si′clās) an enzyme that catalyzes the conversion of adenosine triphosphate (ATP) to cyclic adenosine monophosphate (cAMP) and inorganic pyrophosphate (PP_i). It is activated by the attachment of a hormone or neurotransmitter to a specific membrane-bound receptor.

adenylic acid (ad″ĕ-nil′ik) adenosine monophosphate; a component of nucleic acid, consisting of adenine, ribose, and phosphoric acid.

adequate (ad′ĕ-kwit) sufficient in quantity, quality, or amount to achieve a desired therapeutic effect.

adermia (ah-der′me-ah) congenital defect or absence of the skin.

ADH antidiuretic hormone (see VASOPRESSIN).

ADHA American Dental Hygienists' Association.

adhesion (ad-he′zhun) 1. a fibrous band or structure by which parts abnormally adhere. 2. union of two surfaces that are normally separate, such as in wound healing or in some pathological process. Surgery within the abdomen sometimes results in

adhesions from scar tissue; as an organ heals, fibrous scar tissue forms around the incision and may cling to the surface of adjoining organs. Adhesions are usually painless and cause no difficulties, but occasionally they produce pain, with or without obstruction or malfunction, by distorting the organ. They can also occur following peritonitis and other inflammatory conditions. They may occur in the pleura, in the pericardium, and around the pelvic organs, in addition to the abdomen. Surgery is sometimes required to release symptomatic adhesions. 3. artificial joining of two things, such as the bonding of materials to a tooth.

adhesiotomy (ad-he″ze-ot′ah-me) surgical division of adhesions.

adhesive (ad-he′siv) 1. pertaining to, characterized by, or causing close adherence of adjoining surfaces. 2. a substance that causes close adherence of adjoining surfaces.

adiadochokinesia (ah-di″ah-do″ko-kĭ-ne′-zhah) inability to perform fine, rapidly repeated, coordinated movements.

adiaphoria (ah-di″ah-for′e-ah) nonresponse to stimuli as a result of previous exposure to similar stimuli.

Adie's syndrome (a′dēz) a syndrome consisting of a pathologic pupil reaction (Adie's PUPIL) whose most important element is MYOTONIA on accommodation; the affected pupil contracts to near vision more slowly than does the opposite one, and also dilates more slowly. The affected pupil does not usually react to light (direct or indirect), but it may do so in an abnormal fashion. Certain tendon reflexes are absent or diminished, but there are no motor or sensory disturbances or other demonstrable changes indicative of disease of the nervous system.

adip(o)- word element [L.], *fat.*

adipic (ah-dip′ik) pertaining to fat.

adipocele (ad′ĭ-po-sēl″) a hernia containing fat.

adipocellular (ad″ĭ-po-sel′u-ler) composed of fat and connective tissue.

adipocyte (ad′ĭ-po-sīt″) fat cell.

adipofibroma (ad″ĭ-po-fi-bro′mah) a fibrous tumor with fatty elements.

adipogenic (ad″ĭ-po-jen′ik) lipogenic.

adipogenous (ad″ĭpoj′ĕ-nus) lipogenous.

adipokinesis (ad″ĭ-po-kĭ-ne′sis) the mobilization of fat in the body.

adipokinin (ad″ĭ-po-ki′nin) a factor from the anterior pituitary that accelerates mobilization of stored fat.

adipolysis (ad″ĭ-pol′ĭ-sis) the digestion of fats. adj., **adipolyt′ic.**

adiponecrosis (ad″ĭ-po-nĕ-kro′sis) necrosis of fatty tissue.

a. neonato′rum, a. subcuta′nea subcutaneous fat NECROSIS of newborn.

A

adipopexis (ad″ĭ-po-pek′sis) the fixation or storing of fat.

adipose (ad′ĭ-pōs) fatty.

adiposis (ad″ĭ-po′sis) 1. obesity. 2. abnormal deposits or degeneration of fatty tissue.

a. cerebra′lis fatness from cerebral pituitary disease.

a. doloro′sa a painful condition due to pressure on nerves caused by fatty deposits.

a. hepa′tica fatty degeneration of liver.

a. tubero′sa simplex adiposis dolorosa in which the fatty degeneration occurs in nodular masses.

adiposity (ad″ĭ-pos′ĭ-te) obesity.

adiposogenital dystrophy (ad″ĭ-po-so-jen′ĭ-t′l dis′trah-fe) increased body fat (obesity) accompanied by underdevelopment of the genitalia and altered secondary sex characteristics, caused by damage to certain parts of the HYPOTHALAMUS, with a decrease in the secretion of gonadotropic hormones from the anterior lobe of the PITUITARY GLAND. Treatment depends on the primary cause of the condition, usually a tumor or infection involving the hypothalamus. Called also adiposogenital syndrome and Fröhlich's syndrome.

adiposuria (ad″ĭ-po-su′re-ah) lipiduria.

adipsia (ah-dip′se-ah) absence of thirst; abnormal avoidance of drinking.

aditus (ad′ĭ-tus), pl. *a′ditus* [L.] an OPENING or entrance; used in anatomic nomenclature for various passages in the body.

adjunct (ad′junkt) an accessory or auxiliary agent or measure.

adjustment (ah-just′ment) the changing of something to improve its relationship to something else.

a. disorder a mental disorder characterized by a maladaptive reaction to identifiable stressful life events, such as divorce, loss of job, physical illness, or natural disaster; this diagnosis assumes that the condition will remit when the stress ceases or when the patient adapts to the situation. Called also adjustment reaction.

impaired a. a NURSING DIAGNOSIS accepted by the North American Nursing Diagnosis Association, defined as inability to modify lifestyle or behavior in a manner consistent with a change in health status.

adjuvant (aj′ah-vant, ă-joo′vant) 1. assisting or aiding. 2. a substance that aids another, such as an auxiliary remedy.

ADL activities of daily living.

Adler (ad′ler) Alfred (1870–1937). Austrian psychiatrist who dissented from Freud's emphasis on the role of infantile sexuality in personality development. He started a psychological movement called *individual psychology* to indicate that the individual is viewed as a unified personality and an indivisible unit. He introduced the terms *inferiority feelings* and *overcompensation* and taught that the child has inferiority feelings in relation both to parents and to other people. This sense of inadequacy stems from the child's physical immaturity, uncertainty, dependence upon parents and society, and a painful feeling of subordination to others. This leads to compensatory reactions and a striving for significance, achievement, and superiority. In cases in which the feelings of inferiority are overpowering and a child fears never being able to compensate for perceived weakness and inadequacy, he or she may develop an exaggerated striving for power and dominance (overcompensation), characterized by great haste and impatience, violent impulses, lack of consideration for others, and grandiose goals; a different manner of overcompensation is to become passive and dependent. Many of Adler's views have been adopted by other schools of psychiatry.

administration (ad-min″is-tra′shun) the giving or application of a pharmacologic or other therapeutic agent.

analgesic a. in the NURSING INTERVENTIONS CLASSIFICATION, a nursing INTERVENTION defined as the use of pharmacologic agents to reduce or eliminate pain.

analgesic a.: intraspinal in the NURSING INTERVENTIONS CLASSIFICATION, a nursing INTERVENTION defined as the administration of pharmacologic agents into the epidural or intrathecal space to reduce or eliminate pain.

anesthesia a. in the NURSING INTERVENTIONS CLASSIFICATION, a nursing INTERVENTION defined as the preparation for and administration of anesthetic agents and monitoring of patient responsiveness during administration.

blood products a. in the NURSING INTERVENTIONS CLASSIFICATION, a nursing INTERVENTION defined as administration of blood or blood products and monitoring of a patient's response.

medication a. in the NURSING INTERVENTIONS CLASSIFICATION, a nursing INTERVENTION defined as preparing, giving, and evaluating the effectiveness of prescription and nonprescription drugs.

medication a.: ear in the NURSING INTERVENTIONS CLASSIFICATION, a nursing INTERVENTION defined as preparing and instilling OTIC medications.

medication a.: enteral in the NURSING INTERVENTIONS CLASSIFICATION, a nursing

INTERVENTION defined as delivering medications through an intestinal tube.

medication a.: epidural in the NURSING INTERVENTIONS CLASSIFICATION, a nursing INTERVENTION defined as preparing and administering medications via the EPIDURAL route.

medication a.: eye in the NURSING INTERVENTIONS CLASSIFICATION, a nursing INTERVENTION defined as preparing and instilling OPHTHALMIC medications.

medication a.: inhalation in the NURSING INTERVENTIONS CLASSIFICATION, a nursing INTERVENTION defined as preparing and administering inhaled medications.

medication a.: interpleural in the NURSING INTERVENTIONS CLASSIFICATION, a nursing INTERVENTION defined as the administration of medication through an interpleural catheter for reduction of pain.

medication a.: intradermal in the NURSING INTERVENTIONS CLASSIFICATION, a nursing INTERVENTION defined as preparing and giving medications via the INTRADERMAL route.

medication a.: intramuscular in the NURSING INTERVENTIONS CLASSIFICATION, a nursing INTERVENTION defined as preparing and giving medications via the INTRAMUSCULAR route.

medication a.: intraosseous in the NURSING INTERVENTIONS CLASSIFICATION, a nursing INTERVENTION defined as the insertion of a needle through the bone cortex into the medullary cavity for the purpose of short-term, emergency administration of fluid, blood, or medication.

medication a.: intravenous in the NURSING INTERVENTIONS CLASSIFICATION, a nursing INTERVENTION defined as preparing and giving medications via the INTRAVENOUS route.

medication a.: oral in the NURSING INTERVENTIONS CLASSIFICATION, a nursing INTERVENTION defined as preparing and giving medications by mouth and monitoring patient responsiveness.

medication a.: rectal in the NURSING INTERVENTIONS CLASSIFICATION, a nursing INTERVENTION defined as preparing and inserting rectal suppositories.

medication a.: skin in the NURSING INTERVENTIONS CLASSIFICATION, a nursing INTERVENTION defined as preparing and applying medications to the skin.

medication a.: subcutaneous in the NURSING INTERVENTIONS CLASSIFICATION, a nursing INTERVENTION defined as preparing and giving medications via the SUBCUTANEOUS route.

medication a.: vaginal in the NURSING INTERVENTIONS CLASSIFICATION, a nursing INTERVENTION defined as preparing and inserting vaginal medications.

medication a.: ventricular reservoir in the NURSING INTERVENTIONS CLASSIFICATION, a nursing INTERVENTION defined as administration and monitoring of medication through an indwelling catheter into the lateral ventricle.

total parenteral nutrition a., TPN a. in the NURSING INTERVENTIONS CLASSIFICATION, a nursing INTERVENTION defined as the preparation and delivery of nutrients intravenously and monitoring of patient responsiveness; see also PARENTERAL NUTRITION.

adnerval (ad-ner′val) near or toward a nerve.

adneural (ad-noor′al) adnerval.

adnexa (ad-nek′sah) [L.] appendages; accessory organs, as of the eye (*adnex′a oc′uli*) or uterus (*adnex′a u′teri*). adj., **adnex′al.**

adolescence (ad″o-les′ens) the period between the onset of puberty and the cessation of physical growth; roughly from 11 to 19 years of age. adj., **adoles′cent.** Adolescents vacillate between being children and being adults. They are adjusting to the physiologic changes their bodies are undergoing and are working to establish a sexual identification and to use these changes for their personal benefit and for the benefit of society. They are searching for personal identity and wanting freedom and independence of thought and action, but they continue to have a strong dependence on their parents and suffer feelings of loss in separating from them. In reaction to this they identify with their peers and tend to yield to peer pressure and conform to peer group values, behavior, and tastes in such things as clothing, food, and entertainment.

Developmental Tasks. During the period of time between childhood and adulthood, as for other life stages, there are certain developmental tasks to be accomplished before one can move on to the next stage of maturity. The developmental tasks of adolescents include (1) becoming comfortable with their own bodies, (2) working toward independence from parents and other adult authority figures, (3) building new and meaningful relationships with others of the same and opposite sexes, (4) seeking economic and social stability, (5) developing a personal value system, and (6) learning to verbalize conceptually.

Health Care Needs. Young people in today's society have special needs related to their lifestyle and health habits. About half of those between the ages of 15 and 19 years are sexually active, predisposing them to sexually transmitted diseases and pregnancy. Approximately 10 per cent of the girls in this age group do become pregnant, and many of their newborns are born prematurely or have difficulty at birth. The major causes of injury and death in adolescents are motor vehicle and other accidents, homicide, and suicide. Obesity, substance abuse, and nutritional deficiency also are common health problems in adolescents.

A major goal in the health care of today's youth is education so that adolescents can become knowledgeable about the relationship between their lifestyle and their physical and mental health. They also need help in achieving the maturity essential to choosing a healthy lifestyle and accepting responsibility for their personal health.

Adolescents need health care providers who are able to communicate with them in a manner they can understand, and who respect them as unique individuals. In surveys of adolescents and their health care needs as they perceive them, adolescents have said they want health care providers who are warm and compassionate, have a sense of humor and are able to show emotional responsiveness, can be objective and nonjudgmental when dealing with adolescent health problems, are able to demonstrate flexibility, tolerance, and enjoyment in working with young people, can maintain their adult identity and serve as role models, and are knowledgeable about the special needs of adolescents.

adoral (ad-or'al) 1. situated near the mouth. 2. directed toward the mouth.

ADP adenosine diphosphate.

ADPKD autosomal dominant POLYCYSTIC KIDNEY DISEASE.

adren(o)- word element [L.], *adrenal glands.*

adrenal (ah-dre'nal) 1. pertaining to one of the small glands just above each kidney. Called also suprarenal. 2. an ADRENAL GLAND. 3. paranephric.

a. gland a small triangular endocrine gland situated in the retroperitoneal tissues at the cranial pole of each kidney; it is the result of fusion of two organs, one forming the inner core or *medulla,* and the other forming an outer shell, or *cortex.* These two structures are different in both their anatomy and the kinds of hormone they synthesize and secrete. Called also suprarenal gland. (See accompanying illustration.)

Adrenal Medulla. This is actually a glandular extension of sympathetic effector fibers or postganglionic neurons. It releases the hormones EPINEPHRINE and NOREPINEPHRINE in response to stimulation of the sympathetic nervous system. These hormones enter the blood stream and are carried throughout the body where they indirectly act as stimulants to the various organs. Their production and distribution by the blood usually occur at the same time that the organs are being stimulated by the sympathetic nerves. In this way, the adrenal

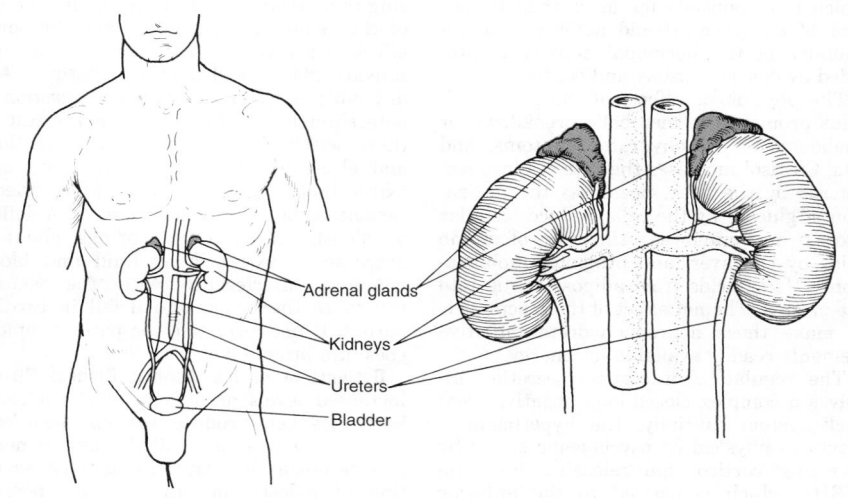

Adrenal glands.

medulla and the sympathetic nerves support each other and can act as substitutes for each other. Epinephrine and norepinephrine both constrict blood vessels (except in muscle tissue) and are released in anticipatory states and other times of increased emotion, causing such changes as elevated BLOOD PRESSURE; release of GLUCAGON, INSULIN, and FATTY ACIDS into the blood; and increases in heart rate, sweating, metabolic rate, and peristaltic activity. Epinephrine is important in initiating the physiological changes in the "fight or flight" response (see ALARM REACTION) and has a more prolonged effect than norepinephrine because of being removed more slowly from the blood.

Adrenal Cortex. The adrenal cortex synthesizes and secretes more than 30 different steroids and is responsible for the maintenance of several life-sustaining physiological activities. The steroids are divided into three major groups: GLUCOCORTICOIDS, MINERALOCORTICOIDS, and ANDROGENS. The glucocorticoids get their name from the fact that they cause an increase in blood glucose levels (*gluco-*), are produced by the adrenal cortex (*corti-*), and are synthesized from cholesterol, which is a steroid (*-oid*). The mineralocorticoids, as their name implies, are chiefly concerned with the concentration of electrolytes (minerals) in the extracellular fluid. The adrenal cortex also secretes small amounts of androgens and is the major source of these hormones in females.

Glucocorticoids. The principal glucocorticoid is CORTISOL (also known as hydrocortisone), which is responsible for more than 95 per cent of all glucocorticoid activity. The remainder of the hormonal activity is provided by CORTICOSTERONE and CORTISONE.

The physiologic effects of the glucocorticoids promote the metabolic breakdown or anabolism of carbohydrates, proteins, and fats. Cortisol increases the rate of gluconeogenesis by the liver, decreases the utilization of glucose by the cells, reduces cellular protein and enhances utilization of amino acids by the liver, and promotes mobilization of fatty acids from adipose tissue into the plasma. The net effect of these actions is to make these noncarbohydrate nutritive elements readily available for energy.

The regulation of cortisol secretion involves a complex closed-loop negative feedback system. Initially, the hypothalamus reacts to physical or psychogenic stress by secreting corticotropin-releasing hormone (CRH), which is carried to the anterior pituitary gland (adenohypophysis) via the hypothalamic-hypophyseal portal system. In response to the presence of CRH, the adenohypophysis secretes adrenocorticotropic hormone (ACTH), which stimulates the adrenal cortex to release cortisol. Cortisol then initiates a series of metabolic activities which help to relieve the physiologic effects of stress. Cortisol inhibits both release of CRH from the hypothalamus and of ACTH from the adenohypophysis. This exerts a negative feedback effect; high serum cortisol levels inhibit further production of cortisol. Thus, during times of relative calm when the body is not experiencing abnormal stress, the cortisol level returns to normal.

Another factor that influences the secretory rates of CRH, ACTH, and cortisol is a biologic clock mechanism that establishes a cyclic pattern of signals from the hypothalamus. This is a 24-hour cycle that has its peak right after completion of the major portion of a night's sleep, usually around 4 or 5 AM. About 12 hours later, the blood level of cortisol is at its lowest. This cycle is dependent on sleeping patterns; therefore, if a person changes the pattern and sleeps in the daytime, the cycle of hormonal levels changes accordingly. This information is significant in testing for cortisol levels as a means of diagnosing a disorder of the endocrine system. When blood is drawn for testing, the specimen should be clearly labeled as to the precise time it was taken.

Mineralocorticoids. The principal mineralocorticoid is ALDOSTERONE. This and other mineralocorticoids prevent excessive loss of sodium and chloride in the urine by enhancing their reabsorption from the distal ends of the renal tubules. They have the same effect to a lesser degree on the sweat and salivary glands and on the intestines. Additionally, aldosterone promotes excretion of potassium in the urine. The net result of these activities is the maintenance of fluid and electrolyte balance in the blood and extracellular fluid, which, in turn, affects cardiac output and blood pressure. A deficit of aldosterone secretion brings about a decrease in extracellular fluid and blood volumes, interference with the venous return to the heart, and a fall in cardiac output. If not corrected, the patient rapidly goes into profound shock.

Dysfunction of the Adrenal Glands. Either increased levels or deficits of the adrenal hormones can produce various disorders. CUSHING'S SYNDROME, called also primary aldosteronism, is related to excessive secretion of aldosterone. In ADDISON'S DISEASE there is an overall hypofunction of the adrenal cortex, resulting in insufficient production of all three groups of adrenocortical hormones. ADRENOGENITAL SYNDROME, which is usually caused by a tumor of the adrenal cortex, results from excessive secretion of androgens. Since androgens have a masculinizing effect, the symptoms are primarily those of changes in the secondary sex characteristics.

adrenalectomy (ah-dre″nah-lek′tah-me) surgical excision of an adrenal gland, done when a disorder of the adrenal gland, such as CUSHING'S SYNDROME, PHEOCHROMOCYTOMA, or adrenal adenoma or carcinoma causes an overproduction of adrenal hormones. In some instances of severe Cushing's syndrome, total bilateral adrenalectomy is done.

Adrenalin (ah-dren′ah-lin) trademark for preparations of EPINEPHRINE, an adrenergic agent.

adrenaline (ah-dren′ah-lin) epinephrine.

adrenalism (ah-dren′al-izm) any disorder of adrenal function, whether of decreased or of heightened function.

adrenergic (ad″ren-er′jik) 1. activated by, characteristic of, or secreting EPINEPHRINE or other substances with similar activities; see also adrenergic FIBERS and adrenergic RECEPTORS. See also SYMPATHOMIMETIC. 2. an agent that acts like epinephrine.

a. blocking agent a drug that blocks the secretion of EPINEPHRINE and NOREPINEPHRINE at the postganglionic nerve endings of the sympathetic nervous system. (See also ALPHA-ADRENERGIC BLOCKING AGENTS and BETA-ADRENERGIC BLOCKING AGENTS.) By blocking these adrenergic substances, which cause constriction of blood vessels and increased cardiac output, adrenergic blocking agents produce dilatation of the blood vessels and a decrease in cardiac output, causing an ANTIHYPERTENSIVE effect. During therapy with these drugs, patients should avoid strenuous exercise, which is likely to produce a sudden drop in blood pressure. They also can cause postural hypotension.

adrenocortical (ah-dre″no-kor′tĭ-k'l) pertaining to or arising from the adrenal CORTEX; called also corticoadrenal.

adrenocorticoid (ah-dre″no-kor′tĭ-koid″) corticosteroid.

adrenocorticomimetic (ah-dre″no-kor″tĭ-ko-mĭ-met′ik) having effects similar to those of hormones of the adrenal cortex.

adrenocorticotrophic (ah-dre″no-kor″tĭ-ko-trof′ik) adrenocorticotropic.

adrenocorticotrophin (ah-dre″no-kor″tĭ-ko-tro′fin) corticotropin.

adrenocorticotropic (ah-dre″no-kor″tĭ-ko-trop′ik) having a stimulating effect on the adrenal cortex; called also adrenocorticotrophic and corticotropic.

adrenocorticotropin (ah-dre″no-kor″tĭ-ko-tro′pin) corticotropin.

adrenogenital syndrome (ah-dre″no-jen′ĭ-t'l) a group of symptoms associated with alterations of secondary sex characters, due to abnormally increased production of androgens by the adrenal glands. The term most commonly applies to the development of masculine traits in the female or premature puberty in male children. The condition may be congenital, in which case it is due to an inherited defect of the adrenal gland, or acquired, developing as a result of a tumor or hyperplasia of the adrenals.

Symptoms. Females with the congenital form may be reared as boys because of masculinization of the external genitalia. Males may show sexual precocity, with development of the reproductive organs, appearance of pubic hair, and excessive body growth in early childhood. In acquired adrenogenital syndrome there is appearance of masculine secondary sex characters in the female, and precocious puberty in the male.

Treatment. When an adrenal tumor is the underlying cause of the disorder, it is removed surgically. Estrogen therapy is successful in some cases.

adrenoleukodystrophy (ah-dre″no-loo″-ko-dis′trah-fe) an X-linked recessive disease of childhood, closely related to SCHILDER'S DISEASE, marked by diffuse abnormality of the cerebral white matter and adrenal atrophy with abnormal adrenal functioning; characteristics include mental deterioration progressing to dementia, with aphasia, apraxia, dysarthria, and loss of vision in about a third of patients.

adrenolytic (ah-dre″no-lit′ik) inhibiting the action of the adrenergic nerves or of epinephrine.

adrenomedullary (ah-dre″no-med′u-ler″e) pertaining to or originating in the adrenal medulla; called also medulloadrenal.

adrenomegaly (ah-dre″no-meg′ah-le) enlargement of the adrenal gland.

adrenomimetic (ah-dre″no-mi-met′ik) having actions similar to those of adrenergic compounds; sympathomimetic.

adrenopathy (ad″ren-op′ah-the) any disease of the adrenal glands.

Adriamycin (a″dre-ah-mi′sin) trademark for preparations of DOXORUBICIN, an antineoplastic ANTIBIOTIC.

Adson's test (ad′sunz) a test for THORACIC OUTLET SYNDROME; with the patient in a sitting position, the hands resting on the thighs, the examiner palpates both radial pulses as the patient rapidly fills the lungs by deep inhalation and, holding the breath, hyperextends the neck and turns the head toward the affected side. If the radial pulse on that side is decidedly or completely obliterated, the result is positive.

adsorb (ad-sorb′) to attract and retain other material on the surface; to conduct the process of adsorption.

adsorbent (ad-sorb′ent) 1. pertaining to or characterized by adsorption. 2. a substance that attracts other materials or particles to its surface.

gastrointestinal a. a substance, usually a powder, taken to adsorb gases, toxins, and bacteria in the stomach and intestines. Examples include activated CHARCOAL and KAOLIN.

adsorption (ad-sorp′shun) 1. the action of a substance in attracting and holding other materials or particles on its surface; see also ABSORPTION. 2. attachment (def. 2).

adtorsion (ad-tor′shun) a turning inward of both eyes.

adult (ah-dult′) having attained full growth or maturity, or an organism that has done so.

a. respiratory distress syndrome acute respiratory distress syndrome.

adulteration (ah-dul″ter-a′shun) addition of an impure, cheap, or unnecessary ingredient to cheat, cheapen, or falsify a preparation.

advance directives instructions about a person's wishes, goals, and values regarding what will be done in case he or she becomes incapable of making decisions about medical care; called also living will, durable power of attorney for health care, and sometimes advance health care directives or health care advance directives.

A *proxy directive* designates another person to make decisions; an *instruction directive* provides instructions about the person's values and goals or treatment preferences; a *combined directive* can do both. An instruction directive should focus on goals and values more than on specific medical interventions; interventions can be good in some situations and undesirable in others.

Formal directives are signed and legally authorized written documents. *Informal directives* are oral communications with family, significant other, or health care provider. Advantages of formal directives are: (1) they are preferences and values more likely to have been carefully considered; (2) they reflect more accurately a person's preferences; (3) they invoke legal practice that commits health care providers to a course of action; and (4) they provide legal enforcement for a person's preferences. Disadvantages

include: (1) relatively few people make them or leave explicit directions; (2) identified decision makers might not be available, might be incompetent to make good decisions, or might have a conflict of interest; (3) some people change their preferences regarding treatment but fail to change their directives (and a few, when legally incompetent, protest a surrogate's decision); (4) state laws often severely restrict the use of advance directives; (5) professionals have no basis to overturn instructions that are against the patient's best medical interests, even though the patient might have formulated the instructions without foreseeing a given situation; and (6) some patients do not have an adequate understanding of the decision making needed, or even with an adequate understanding, cannot foresee all clinical situations. Because of inadequate counseling or imprecise language, documents may reflect uninformed preferences.

People often have difficulty identifying decisions and questions delineating adequately the full range of situations that may occur. Because of this, designation of surrogates has become more prevalent. The document can be used for refusal of life sustaining treatment.

advancement (ad-vans′ment) detachment of a portion of tissue, especially muscle or tendon, and reattachment at a point further forward than the original attachment, as is done with an eye muscle for correction of strabismus.

capsular a. attachment of Tenon's capsule in front of its normal position.

adventitia (ad″ven-tish′e-ah) tunica adventitia. adj., **adventi′tial.**

adventitious (ad″ven-tish′us) not normal to a part.

adverse reactions (ad′vers) unexpected, serious symptoms coinciding with the administration of a drug; see also SIDE EFFECT.

adynamia (a″dĭ-na′me-ah) lack of normal or vital powers. adj., **adynam′ic.**

A-E, AE above-elbow; see under AMPUTATION.

AEC Atomic Energy Commission.

aec- for words beginning thus, see those beginning *ec-*.

AED automatic external defibrillator.

Aedes (a-e′dēz) a genus of mosquitoes, including approximately 600 species. *A. aegyp′ti* transmits the causative organisms of YELLOW FEVER and DENGUE. *A. triseria′tus* transmits La Crosse ENCEPHALITIS.

aeg- for words beginning thus, see those beginning *eg-*.

aer(o)- word element [Gr.], *air; gas.*

aeration (ār″a′shun) 1. the exchange of carbon dioxide for oxygen by the blood in the lungs. 2. the saturation of a liquid with air or gas.

Aerobacter (a″er-o-bak′ter) in former systems of classification, a genus of the family Enterobacteriaceae, consisting of gram-negative facultatively anaerobic motile rods; individual species have been assigned to the genus *Enterobacter*.

aerobe (ār′ōb) a microorganism that lives and grows in the presence of free oxygen. adj., **aero′bic.**

facultative a. one that can live in the presence of oxygen, but does not require it.

obligate a. one that cannot live without oxygen.

AeroBid (ār′o-bid″) trademark for preparations of FLUNISOLIDE, an ANTIINFLAMMATORY agent administered by inhalation to treat ASTHMA.

aerocele (ār′o-sēl) pneumatocele (def. 1).

aerodermectasia (ār″o-der″mek-ta′zhah) subcutaneous or surgical EMPHYSEMA; an accumulation of air in the subcutaneous tissues.

aerodontalgia (ār″o-don-tal′jah) toothache experienced at lowered atmospheric pressures, as in aircraft flight or in a decompression chamber, caused by the expansion of air in the maxillary sinuses.

aerodynamics (ār″o-di-nam′iks) the science of air or gases in motion.

aeroembolism (ār″o-em′bo-lizm) obstruction of a blood vessel by air or gas.

aerogen (ār′o-jen″) a gas-producing bacterium.

aerogenesis (ār″o-jen′ĕ-sis) formation or production of gas.

aerohydrotherapy (ār″o-hi″dro-ther′ah-pe) therapeutic use of air and water.

Aeromonas (a″er-o-mo′nas) a genus of gram-negative, facultatively anaerobic, rod-shaped bacteria. *A. hydro′phila* causes CELLULITIS, wound infections, diarrhea, septicemia, and urinary tract infections. *A. ca′viae* and *A. so′bia* are found in fresh water and sewage and on fish, and cause gastroenteritis and wound infections in humans.

aeropathy (ār″op′ah-the) bends (decompression sickness).

aerophagia (ār″o-fa′jah) excessive swallowing of air, usually an unconscious process associated with anxiety, resulting in abdominal distention or belching; these are often interpreted by the patient as signs of a physical disorder.

aerophilic (ār″o-fil′ik) requiring air for proper growth.

aerophilous (ār-of′ĭ-lus) aerophilic.

aerosinusitis (ār″o-si″nŭ-si′tis) barosinusitis.

aerosol (ār′o-sol″) a colloid system in which solid or liquid particles are suspended in a gas, especially a suspension of a drug

or other substance to be dispensed in a cloud or mist. See also AEROSOL THERAPY.

a. clearance removal of particles that have been deposited in the respiratory tissues. Clearance may occur by ciliary transport, by phagocytosis, by encapsulation and immobilization in a deposit of fibrous tissue (in which case the particles remain in the body), and by dissolving in tissue fluid and subsequently diffusing into the general circulation where the particles are metabolized.

a. deposition the depositing of aerosol particles onto a nearby surface, especially deposition or retention of the particles within the respiratory system. Closely related to aerosol penetration and affected by the same factors.

a. penetration the maximum distance aerosol particles can be carried into the respiratory tract by inhaled air. Depth of penetration increases as particle size decreases. Factors affecting where aerosol particles will be deposited and how deeply they can penetrate are: gravity, kinetic activity of gas molecules, inertial impaction, physical nature of the particle, and the ventilatory pattern.

a. therapy use of an aerosol for RESPIRATORY CARE in the treatment of bronchopulmonary disease. The major purpose of this is the delivery of medications or humidity or both to the mucosa of the respiratory tract and pulmonary alveoli. Agents delivered by aerosol therapy may act in a number of ways: (1) to relieve spasm of the bronchial muscles and reduce edema of the mucous membranes, (2) to render bronchial secretions more liquid so that they are more easily removed, (3) to humidify the respiratory tract, and (4) to administer antibiotics locally by depositing them in the respiratory tract.

Physical and chemical substances used as medical aerosols include drugs that act as BRONCHODILATORS and DECONGESTANTS, such as EPINEPHRINE, EPHEDRINE, ISOPROTERENOL, ATROPINE, and the STEROIDS. Wetting AGENTS administered as aerosols to render the bronchial secretions more liquid include TYLOXAPOL and ACETYLCYSTEINE. The choice of antibiotics to be given as aerosol therapy is determined by the patient's specific condition and the preference of the health care provider. Most standard antibiotic drugs are available in aerosol form.

In general, the RESPIRATORY THERAPIST is concerned with factors that affect how deeply aerosol particles can penetrate into the bronchial tract and the locations at which these particles are deposited on the bronchial mucosa and alveolar tissues. Depth of penetration is affected by particle size. Particles as large as 100 μm and as small as 5 μm are trapped in the nose. Those 2 to 5 μm in size are deposited somewhere in the respiratory tract proximal to the alveoli. Deposition in the alveoli is 90 to 100 per cent for particles 1 to 2 μm in size.

Because aerosol particles are so small, they present the phenomenon of brownian MOVEMENT as they are bombarded by the molecules of the gas in which they are carried. The velocity with which these particles move about directly affects their diffusion and deposition onto nearby surfaces. Thus the type of aerosol generator used in aerosol therapy is of primary importance.

Another factor affecting penetration and deposition of aerosol particles that should be of concern to respiratory therapists and other members of the health team who are teaching patients the techniques of effective aerosol therapy is that of ventilatory pattern. The ideal pattern of breathing for optimum delivery of aerosol particles is that of slow, moderate deep breathing with breath holding at the end of each inhalation.

Aerosporin (a″er-o-spōr′in) trademark for a preparation of POLYMYXIN B sulfate, an ANTIMICROBIAL.

aerotitis (ār″o-ti′tis) barotitis.

aerotolerant (ār″o-tol′er-ant) surviving and growing in small amounts of air; said of anaerobic microorganisms.

aes- for words beginning thus, see those beginning *es-*.

Aesculapius (es″cu-la′pe-us) the god of healing in Roman mythology. The staff of Aesculapius, a rod or staff with a snake entwined around it, is a symbol of medicine and is the official insignia of the American Medical Association.

aet- for words beginning thus, see those beginning *et-*.

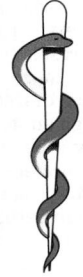

Staff of Aesculapius.

AFCR American Federation for Clinical Research.

afebrile (a-feb′rīl) without fever.

affect (af′ekt) the external expression of emotion attached to ideas or mental representations of objects. see also MOOD.

blunted a. severe reduction in the intensity of affect; a common symptom of schizophrenic disorders.

constricted a. restricted affect.

flat a. lack of emotional expression.

inappropriate a. affect that is incongruent with the situation or with the content of a patient's ideas or speech.

labile a. that characterized by rapid changes in emotion unrelated to external events or stimuli.

restricted a. reduction in the intensity of affect, to a somewhat lesser degree than is characteristic of blunted affect.

affection (ah-fek′shun) a morbid condition or diseased state.

affective (ah-fek′tiv) pertaining to affect.

a. congruency consistency between the self-concept of an individual and the related behaviors and responses of others.

a. disorders mood disorders.

afferent (af′er-ent) 1. conveying toward a center; called also centripetal. See also EFFERENT and CORTICIPETAL. 2. something that so conducts, as an afferent fiber or nerve.

a. loop syndrome chronic partial obstruction of the proximal loop (duodenum and jejunum) after gastrojejunostomy, resulting in duodenal distention, pain, and nausea following ingestion of food.

affinity (ah-fin′ĭ-te) 1. attraction; a tendency to seek out or unite with another object or substance. 2. in chemistry, the tendency of two substances to form strong or weak chemical bonds forming molecules or complexes. 3. in immunology, the thermodynamic bond strength of an antigen-antibody complex.

afibrinogenemia (a″fi-brin″o-jĕ-ne′me-ah) absence or deficiency of FIBRINOGEN in the circulating blood. *Congenital afibrinogenemia* (complete absence of fibrinogen) is a rare anomaly that is inherited. *Acquired afibrinogenemia* is actually a deficiency of fibrinogen *(hypofibrinogenemia)* and often is a serious complication in obstetrics, the primary cause being excessive maternal use of fibrinogen during an abnormal pregnancy. The condition may be seen in association with malignancies of the bone and prostate and with leukemia. It also may follow transfusion of incompatible blood and sometimes may complicate thoracic and abdominal surgery.

Symptoms. As would be expected in a deficiency of fibrinogen, which plays an important role in the blood clotting mechanism, the chief symptom is generalized bleeding, external or internal. In obstetric or surgical patients suffering from this condition there is frequently sudden and uncontrollable hemorrhage.

Treatment. Fibrinogen is administered intravenously to supply the body with this essential substance; transfusions of fresh frozen PLASMA or CRYOPRECIPITATE may also be indicated. In patients with cancer of the prostate the fibrinogen level often returns to normal after administration of estrogens. In obstetric patients the fibrinogen level returns to normal after the uterus has been emptied.

AFP alpha-fetoprotein.

African sleeping sickness African TRYPANOSOMIASIS.

AFS American Fertility Society.

afterbirth (af′ter-berth″) the PLACENTA and fetal membranes expelled from the uterus after childbirth. Called also secundines.

afterbrain (af′ter-brān) metencephalon.

afterdepolarization (af″ter-de-po″lah-rĭza′shun) an oscillation in membrane POTENTIAL that is dependent upon a preceding ACTION POTENTIAL for its initiation, and which upon reaching threshold POTENTIAL can induce arrhythmias that are said to be "triggered." Early afterdepolarizations occur during phases 2 and 3 of REPOLARIZATION; delayed afterdepolarizations follow full repolarization.

afterimage (af′ter-im″ij) a visual impression persisting briefly after cessation of the stimuli causing the original image. In a *positive* afterimage the brights, darks, and colors remain unchanged; in a *negative* afterimage the brights and darks are reversed, and the colors are complementary.

afterload (af′ter-lōd) the tension developed by the heart during contraction; it is an important determinant of myocardial energy consumption, as it represents the resistance against which the ventricle must pump and indicates how much effort the ventricles must put forth to force blood into the systemic CIRCULATION. Factors that increase afterload include aortic and pulmonarySTENOSIS, systemic and pulmonary HYPERTENSION, and high peripheral RESISTANCE.

afterpain (af′ter-pān″) pain that follows expulsion of the placenta, due to contraction of the uterus, seen particularly in multiparas due to vigorous periodic contractions of the puerperal uterus. It is noticeable particularly when the infant nurses, and may be severe; the intensity usually decreases to become mild by the third day postpartum.

afterperception (af″ter-per-sep′shun) perception of aftersensations.

afterpotential (af″ter-po-ten′shul) an electrical event that follows and is caused by preceding ACTION POTENTIALS. Also written *after-potential*.

aftersensation (af″ter-sen-sa′shun) sensation persisting after cessation of the stimulus that caused it.

aftertaste (af′ter-tāst″) sensation of taste continuing after the stimulus has ceased.

Ag silver (L. *argen′tum*); antigen.

AGA 1. appropriate for GESTATIONAL AGE. 2. American Gastroenterological Association.

agalactia (ag″ah-lak′she-ah) absence or failure of secretion of milk.

agammaglobulinemia (a″gam-ah-glob″u-lin-e′me-ah) absence or severe deficiency of the plasma protein GAMMA GLOBULIN. There are three main types: transient, congenital, and acquired. The *transient* type occurs in early infancy, because gamma globulins are not produced in the fetus and the gamma globulins derived from the maternal blood are soon depleted. This temporary deficiency of gamma globulin lasts for the first 6 to 8 weeks, until the infant begins to synthesize the protein. *Congenital agammaglobulinemia* is a rare condition, occurring in males, and resulting in decreased or absent production of antibodies. *Acquired agammaglobulinemia* is secondary to other disorders and is usually a hypogammaglobulinemia, that is, a deficiency rather than total absence of this plasma protein. It is often secondary to malignant diseases such as leukemia, myeloma, and lymphoma, and to diseases associated with hypoproteinemia such as nephrosis and liver disease. Some patients have a family history of rheumatoid arthritis or allergies. This seems to indicate the presence of genetic factors in the development of agammaglobulinemia.

Symptoms. Because gamma globulin is so important in the production of antibodies and thus in the body's ability to defend itself against infection, it follows that a deficiency or absence of gamma globulin would result in severe and recurrent infections. The infections are usually bacterial rather than viral in origin and are extremely difficult to eliminate. The condition is often complicated by local damage to tissues because of scarring and repeated infection. Disorders of connective tissue such as scleroderma, arthritis, and lupus erythematosus are also frequent complications.

Treatment. Replacement therapy with human gamma globulin is effective in preventing severe infections. The aim is to maintain the gamma globulin level above 150 mg per 100 mL of blood. The optimal dose is determined by the patient's response. Antibiotics are also given and are continued until all signs of infection have disappeared. The prevention and management of infections requires close collaboration between all members of the health care team. The administration of live vaccines is contraindicated.

common variable a. common variable IMMUNODEFICIENCY.

X-linked a. a primary X-linked immunodeficiency disorder characterized by absence of circulating B lymphocytes, plasma cells, or germinal centers in lymphoid tissues, very low levels of circulating immunoglobulins, susceptibility to bacterial infection, and symptoms resembling rheumatoid arthritis. Pre-B cells apparently fail to differentiate into mature B cells, express surface immunoglobulins, and produce antibody.

aganglionic (a-gang″gle-on′ik) lacking ganglion cells.

aganglionosis (ah-gang″gle-on-o′sis) congenital absence of parasympathetic ganglion cells, such as in congenital MEGACOLON.

agar (ag′ahr) a dried hydrophilic, colloidal substance extracted from various species of red algae. It is used in cultures for bacteria and other microorganisms, in making emulsions, and as a supporting medium in procedures such as immunodiffusion and electrophoresis. Because of its bulk it is also used in medicines to promote peristalsis and relieve constipation.

agastric (ah-gas′trik) having no stomach.

age (āj) 1. the duration, or the measure of time of the existence of a person or object. 2. to undergo change as a result of passage of time. developmental age.

achievement a. a measure of achievement expressed in terms of the chronologic age of a normal child showing the same degree of attainment.

chronologic a. the actual measure of time elapsed since a person's birth.

developmental a. 1. age estimated from the degree of anatomical development. 2. in psychology, the age of an individual determined by degree of emotional, mental, anatomical, and physiological maturation.

gestational a. see GESTATIONAL AGE.

mental a. the age level of mental ability of a person as gauged by standard intelligence tests.

aged (a′jed) 1. of advanced age. 2. persons of advanced age; called also ELDERLY. Improvements in public health, nutrition,

surgery, drugs, and health care since 1900 have added years to life expectancy, resulting in an ever larger elderly population.

According to the National Institute on Aging, the number of Americans over 65 is expected to grow from 26 million to 66.6 million by the year 2040. Data from the Bureau of the Census show that in 1900 the percentage of Americans over 65 was 3.8 per cent, in 1970 it was 9.1 per cent and by 2030 it is expected to be 18.2 per cent. Because elderly persons are more likely to suffer from chronic illnesses, decreased mobility, and sensory losses, they are the most intensive users of health care resources. Their ever-increasing numbers are having a tremendous impact on health care, the economy, and political action as the elderly strive to keep physically active and independent.

The Aging Process. The many changes that take place as one grows older are highly individual and can be attributed to a host of physiological, psychological, social, and environmental factors. Physiologically the body replaces worn-out cells by the millions every day of our lives. As the years pass, this replacement slows down very gradually, beginning at about the time the body has reached its full growth. The part of the body that typically ages least and maintains its vigor into later years is the brain.

Hereditary factors play a part in determining how durable a person may be. It is known, for example, that persons born to long-living parents and grandparents tend to be longer-lived themselves. It is also evident that the capacity to withstand or adapt to stresses of living such as disease-producing agents, difficult social interactions, and psychological stressors comes in part from one's hereditary makeup.

The process of aging may be hastened by physical and social environment, ineffective mechanisms for coping with conflict and stress, and an unhealthy style of living. In fact, many of the choices of lifestyle made before the age of 30 can and do have a direct bearing on one's state of health later in life.

Effects of Aging. Old age brings certain physical changes as a normal aspect of aging. The body has less strength and less endurance as it ages. Its speed of reaction and its agility are slowed. The basal metabolism, or rate of energy production in the body cells, is gradually lowered, so that people tire more easily, and are more sensitive to weather changes. Sexual desire and ability decline although they need never entirely end for either sex. The capacity to bear children ends in women with MENOPAUSE, but many men retain their reproductive function into the late years. Those who never used eyeglasses usually need them in later years, or their regular glasses will need changing to BIFOCALS (see also PRESBYOPIA). Hearing changes also come with greater age. Older people hear low tones fairly well, but their ability to perceive the high tones declines. The capacity of tissue and bone to repair itself is slowed, as is cellular growth and division. Bones are more brittle. Skin becomes drier and loses some of its elasticity. However, much of the disability and discomfort that used to be considered a part of normal aging can now be delayed with proper health care and health habits.

Disorders of Old Age. No disease is specifically caused by old age, but the expected changes that occur with aging increase the possibility that illness will occur. For example, the cardiovascular system undergoes many structural and functional changes that predispose a person to some pathological conditions. The three heart diseases that occur most commonly in older persons are coronary artery disease, congestive HEART FAILURE, and defects in the heart's conduction system, including HEART BLOCK.

DIABETES MELLITUS, CANCER, and pulmonary diseases such as EMPHYSEMA and CHRONIC AIRFLOW LIMITATION are more prevalent in the elderly. Arthritic changes and other musculoskeletal disorders also are typical of the aging process. All of these disorders can predispose the elderly person to loss of mobility and increased dependence on others. Visual impairment in the elderly often is the result of CATARACTS, GLAUCOMA, and AGE-RELATED MACULAR DEGENERATION. Early recognition of these conditions and prompt treatment can significantly reduce loss of vision or restore useful sight. Other sensory losses that accompany aging include changes in the senses of taste, touch, and smell.

Health Needs of the Elderly. A major goal of health care for the aged is to help them remain as physically, mentally, and socially active as they can for as long as they can. Most aged persons want to remain in their homes and live independently. In order to do this they need help in devising ways to keep mobile. For example, physical handicaps associated with arthritis and other musculoskeletal disorders can be minimized with creative use of self-care devices that allow the elderly person to continue doing daily household chores such as cooking, housekeeping, and laundry.

Developmental Tasks. Developmental tasks of persons over 65 include redirection of their available energy and talents to new roles and activities after retirement, acceptance

of life as it is with its joys and limitations, and development of a personal view of death and preparation for this final stage of life.

Psychosocial Needs. Attention to the psychosocial needs of the aged is important to the integrity of their self-esteem and sense of worth. Older persons have much to offer in terms of wisdom and life experiences. They can enhance the self-image of younger persons in their families and society by giving them a sense of belonging and an awareness of their personal history and family traditions. Opportunities to do volunteer work for others in the community and to be involved in maintaining the well-being of the society in which they live can do much to help elderly persons meet their need for love and a sense of belonging.

Health Maintenance. Older persons will need some assistance in achieving and preserving a maximum level of health. They should be taught good health habits and allowed to continue caring for themselves and making decisions about their own lifestyles as long as possible. It is recommended that persons over the age of 60 have a comprehensive assessment of health status at least once a year. Medical care is an essential part of their health maintenance because of the normal physiological changes and chronic illnesses they are likely to have. Older persons comprise the largest group of health-care consumers in the United States.

Nutrition plays an important role in health maintenance of the elderly. Poor eating habits may originate in younger years, but they have profound effects as one grows older. Some older persons may subsist on poor diets because they live alone. Preparing meals for oneself and eating alone can take the joy out of cooking and eating. Other factors that can affect nutrition include poorly fitting or absent dentures, periodontal disease, and changes in the sense of taste. Unfortunately the sweet and salty taste buds are lost first, while ability to discern bitter and sour tastes remain. This could account for an aged person's complaints about food tasting bitter, the habit of using excessive amounts of salt and pepper, or a craving for sweets.

The aged need the same vitamins and minerals that are necessary to the good health of anyone at any age. Calcium from milk and dairy foods is especially important to combat osteoporosis and maintain sound bones and teeth. Because of decreased physical activity the caloric intake of elderly persons probably should be reduced. This might not be true of all aged persons; the important goal is maintenance of ideal body weight to avoid either obesity or emaciation. Reduction of fat in the diet as one grows older is necessary because of a gradual decrease in the production of fat-digesting enzymes in the intestinal tract.

Exercise. Regular exercise promotes good circulation and respiration, improves appetite, gives a sense of well-being, and helps maintain mobility and coordination. Whatever the health status of the elderly person, and regardless of whether the elderly person is confined to a bed or wheelchair or able to be up and about, there are some simple exercises that can be done without exhaustion and overexertion. The exercises should be performed once or twice daily, starting slowly at first and gradually building up to the maximum capabilities of the individual.

ageism (āj′izm) prejudice against an individual because of his or her age; see also AGED.

agency (a′jen-se) an organization that performs actions for other people, particularly of a service nature.

home health a. a public agency or private organization that is primarily engaged in providing skilled or paraprofessional HOME HEALTH CARE to individuals in out-of-hospital settings, such as private homes, boarding homes, hospices, shelters, and so on. Its policies must be established and supervised by professional personnel, including one or more physicians and one or more registered nurses. It must maintain clinical records on all patients. In states with laws licensing such agencies, it must be licensed pursuant to such laws and approved as meeting the standards established for such licensing. It must also meet certain other requirements as specified in the Social Security Act, section 1861 (o).

Agency for Health Care Policy and Research (AHCPR) former name of the AGENCY FOR HEALTHCARE RESEARCH AND QUALITY.

Agency for Healthcare Research and Quality (AHRQ) a governmental agency of the United States Department of Health and Human Services; its mission is to support research "to improve the outcomes and quality of healthcare, reduce its costs, address patient safety and medical errors, and broaden access to effective service." The agency systematically develops statements and recommendations to help individuals, institutions, and agencies make better decisions about healthcare based on research that provides evidence-based information. It publishes scientific information for other agencies and organizations on which to base clinical guidelines, performance measures,

and other quality improvement tools through its evidence-based practice centers, outcomes research findings for clinicians, and technology reviews. It provides access to scientific evidence, recommendations on clinical preventive services, and information on how to implement recommended preventive services in clinical practice. Copies of the reports may be obtained free from the Publications Clearinghouse by calling 1-800-358-9295 or consulting the agency's web site at http://www.ahcpr.gov. The agency was formerly called the Agency for Health Care Policy and Research.

Agency for Toxic Substances and Disease Registry (ATSDR) an agency of the United States Department of Health and Human Services, charged with performing specific functions concerning the effect on public health of hazardous substances in the environment. These functions include public health assessments of waste sites, health consultations concerning specific hazardous substances, health surveillance and registries, emergency responses to release of hazardous substances, applied research in support of public health assessments, information development and dissemination, and education and training concerning hazardous substances.

agenesis (a-jen′ĕ-sis) absence of an organ due to nonappearance of its primordium in the embryo.

agenitalism (a-jen′ĭ-tal-izm″) absence of the genitalia, or a condition due to lack of secretion of the testes or ovaries.

agenosomia (ah-jen″o-so′me-ah) a developmental ANOMALY consisting of imperfect development of reproductive organs, usually with protrusion of intestines through an imperfectly developed abdominal wall.

agent (a′jent) a person or substance by which something is accomplished.

adrenergic blocking a. see ADRENERGIC BLOCKING AGENT.

adrenergic neuron blocking a. one that inhibits release of NOREPINEPHRINE from postganglionic adrenergic nerve endings.

alkylating a's see ALKYLATING AGENTS.

alpha-adrenergic blocking a., alpha-blocking a. see ALPHA-ADRENERGIC BLOCKING AGENT.

antianxiety a. see ANTIANXIETY AGENT.

anticholinergic a. cholinergic blocking agent.

antidiabetic a. an agent that prevents or alleviates DIABETES, such as a hypoglycemic AGENT.

antifungal a. an agent that destroys or checks the growth of fungi, such as AMPHOTERICIN B or FLUCYTOSINE (5-FC). Called also antifungal and antimycotic.

antihyperglycemic a. an agent that counteracts high levels of glucose in the blood. See also hypoglycemic AGENT.

antihypertensive a. see ANTIHYPERTENSIVE AGENT.

antimalarial a. an antiprotozoal AGENT particularly effective against the MALARIA parasite.

antimicrobial a. see ANTIMICROBIAL AGENT.

antineoplastic a. a compound that inhibits the maturation or proliferation of neoplastic cells. See also ANTINEOPLASTIC THERAPY.

antiprotozoal a. an agent that destroys PROTOZOA or checks their growth or reproduction. Antimalarial AGENTS are one type.

antipsychotic a. see ANTIPSYCHOTIC AGENT.

beta-adrenergic blocking a. see BETA-ADRENERGIC BLOCKING AGENT.

blocking a. an agent that inhibits a biological action, such as movement of an ion across the cell membrane, passage of a neural impulse, or interaction with a specific receptor.

calcium channel blocking a. see CALCIUM CHANNEL BLOCKING AGENT.

chelating a. 1. a compound that combines with metal ions to form stable ring structures. 2. a substance used to reduce the concentration of free metal ion in solution by complexing it. 3. a medication used to remove toxic metals from the body.

cholinergic blocking a. one that blocks the action of ACETYLCHOLINE at nicotinic or muscarinic RECEPTORS of nerves or effector organs.

contrast a. contrast medium.

Eaton a. *Mycoplasma pneumoniae.*

emulsifying a. emulsifier.

ganglionic blocking a. one that blocks nerve impulses at autonomic ganglionic synapses; used for initial control of blood pressure in patients with acute dissecting aortic aneurysm, production of controlled hypotension during surgery, and treatment of autonomic dysreflexia.

hypoglycemic a. any of various synthetic drugs that lower the blood GLUCOSE level and are used to treat type 2 DIABETES MELLITUS. They may stimulate synthesis of INSULIN by pancreatic beta CELLS, inhibit glucose production, facilitate transport of glucose to muscle cells, and sometimes increase the number of receptor sites where insulin can be bound and can initiate the process of breaking down glucose. Most are SULFONYLUREAS, including ACETOHEXAMIDE, CHLORPROPAMIDE, GLIPIZIDE, TOLAZAMIDE, and TOLBUTAMIDE. Patients should be advised that these drugs are not a cure for diabetes

but only a means of controlling it, and that it is important to continue to comply with dietary and exercise prescriptions.

inotropic a. any of a class of agents affecting the force of muscle contraction, particularly a drug affecting the force of cardiac contraction; positive inotropic agents increase, and negative inotropic agents decrease the force of cardiac muscle contraction.

luting a. lute (def. 1).

neuromuscular blocking a. a compound that causes paralysis of skeletal muscle by blocking neural transmission at the neuromuscular JUNCTION.

nonsteroidal antiinflammatory a. nonsteroidal antiinflammatory drug.

oral hypoglycemic a. see hypoglycemic AGENT.

A. Orange a toxic herbicide consisting of equal quantities of 2,4,5-T and 2,4-D, sometimes with the contaminant DIOXIN; so named because drums of it were marked with orange bands during the war in Vietnam. It is suspected of being CARCINOGENIC and TERATOGENIC.

oxidizing a. a substance that acts as an electron acceptor in a chemical oxidation-reduction reaction.

potassium channel blocking a. any of a class of ANTIARRHYTHMIC agents that inhibit the movement of potassium ions through potassium CHANNELS, thus prolonging repolarization of the cell membrane. Called also potassium channel blocker.

progestational a. any of a group of hormones that induce formation of a secretory ENDOMETRIUM and help start the luteal phase of the MENSTRUAL CYCLE. They are secreted by the CORPUS LUTEUM and PLACENTA, and in small amounts by the adrenal CORTEX. The most important of the group is PROGESTERONE. Agents having progestational activity are also produced synthetically and are most commonly used in CONTRACEPTIVES and in hormone replacement THERAPY. Called also gestagen, progestational hormone, progestin, and progestogen.

psychoactive a., psychotropic a. psychoactive SUBSTANCE.

reducing a. a substance that acts as an electron donor in a chemical oxidation-reduction reaction.

sclerosing a. a chemical irritant injected into a vein in SCLEROTHERAPY. Called also sclerosant.

sodium channel blocking a. any of a class of ANTIARRHYTHMIC agents that prevent ectopic beats by acting on partially inactivated sodium CHANNELS to inhibit abnormal depolarizations. Called also sodium channel blocker.

surface-active a. a substance that exerts a change on the surface properties of a liquid, especially one that reduces its surface tension, such as a DETERGENT. Called also surfactant.

TRIC a. an agent that causes TRACHOMA and inclusion CONJUNCTIVITIS.

tubulin binding a's a group of medications that bind TUBULIN and arrest cell MITOSIS; abnormal blood vessels in tumors are particularly sensitive to these agents.

tumoricidal a. an agent that is destructive to cancer cells; see also antineoplastic AGENT.

wetting a. a substance that lowers the surface tension of water to promote wetting.

ageusia (ah-gu′ze-ah) absence or impairment of the sense of taste.

agger (aj′er), pl. *ag′geres* [L.] an elevation.

a. na′si ridge of nose: an elevation at the anterior free margin of the middle nasal CONCHA.

agglutinable (ah-gloo′ti-nah-b'l) capable of agglutination.

agglutinant (ah-gloo′ti-nant) 1. acting like glue. 2. a substance that holds parts together during healing.

agglutination (ah-gloo″ti-na′shun) 1. the action of an agglutinant substance. 2. the clumping together in suspension of antigen-bearing cells, microorganisms, or particles in the presence of specific antibodies (AGGLUTININS). (See accompanying illustration.) 3. the process of union of the surfaces of a wound. adj., **agglutina′tive.**

cross a. the agglutination of particulate antigen by an antibody raised against a different but related antigen; see also group AGGLUTINATION.

group a. agglutination, usually to a lower titer, of various members of a group of biologically related organisms by an agglutinin specific for one of that group. For instance, the specific agglutinin of typhoid

bacilli may agglutinate other members of the colon-typhoid group, such as *Escherichia coli* and *Salmonella enteritidis*.

intravascular a. clumping of particulate elements within the blood vessels; used conventionally to denote red blood cell agglutination.

platelet a. the clumping together of platelets owing to the action of platelet AGGLUTININS; such agglutinins are important in platelet typing.

a. test any test based on an agglutination reaction, as serologic tests for specific antibodies.

agglutinin (ah-gloo′ti-nin) any substance causing AGGLUTINATION (clumping together) of cells, particularly a specific antibody formed in the blood in response to the presence of an invading agent. Agglutinins are proteins (IMMUNOGLOBULINS) and function as part of the immune mechanism of the body. When the invading agents that bring about the production of agglutinins are bacteria, the agglutinins produced bring about agglutination of the bacterial cells. Erythrocytes also may agglutinate when agglutinins are formed in response to the entrance of noncompatible blood cells into the bloodstream. A transfusion reaction is an example of the result of agglutination of blood cells brought about by agglutinins produced in the recipient's blood in response to incompatible or foreign cells (the donor's blood). Anti-Rh agglutinins are produced in cases of Rh incompatibility and can result in a condition known as ERYTHROBLASTOSIS FETALIS when the maternal blood is Rh negative and the fetal blood is Rh positive. (See also RH FACTOR.)

cold a. antibody that agglutinates erythrocytes or bacteria more efficiently at temperatures below 37°C than at 37°C.

group a. one that has a specific action on certain organisms, but will agglutinate other species as well.

H a. one that is specific for flagellar antigens of the motile strain of an organism.

immune a. a specific agglutinin found in the blood after recovery from the disease or injection of the microorganism.

incomplete a. one that at appropriate concentrations fails to agglutinate the homologous antigen.

O a. one specific for somatic antigens of a microorganism.

platelet a. an antibody capable of agglutinating platelets; these may be associated with a variety of disorders, with and without frank thrombocytopenia.

warm a. an incomplete antibody that sensitizes and reacts optimally with erythrocytes at 37°C.

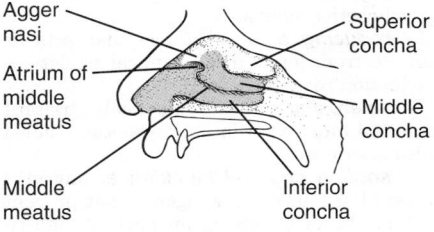

Agger nasi. Superior concha. Atrium of middle meatus. Middle concha. Middle meatus. Inferior concha.

Agger nasi. From Dorland's, 2000.

A

Type A blood of donor | "Anti-B" agglutinins of type A recipient | No agglutination

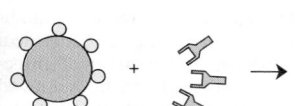 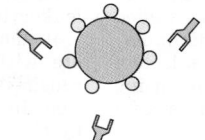

B

Type B blood of donor | "Anti-B" agglutinins of type A recipient | Agglutination | Hemolysis

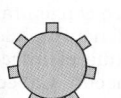 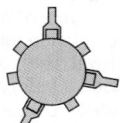 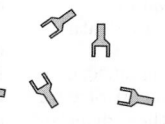 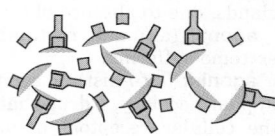

Agglutination reactions. From Applegate, 2000.

agglutinogen (ag″loo-tin′o-jen) a substance (antigen) that stimulates the animal body to form agglutinin (antibody).

aggravate (ag′rah-vāt″) to cause a patient's condition to deteriorate.

aggregate (ag′rĕ-gat) individuals, families, or other groupings who are associated because of similar social, personal, health care, or other needs or interests.

aggregation (ag″rĕ-ga′shun) 1. massing or clumping of materials together. 2. a clumped mass of material.

familial a. the occurrence of more cases of a given disorder in close relatives of a person with the disorder than in control families.

platelet a. platelet agglutination.

aggression (ah-gresh′un) a form of physical or verbal behavior leading to self-assertion; it is often angry and destructive and intended to be injurious, physically or emotionally, and aimed at domination of one person by another. It may arise from innate drives and/or be a response to frustration, and may be manifested by overt attacking and destructive behavior, by covert attitudes of hostility and obstructionism, or by a healthy self-expressive drive to mastery.

aging (āj′ing) the gradual changes in the structure of any organism that occur with the passage of time, that do not result from disease or other gross accidents, and that eventually lead to the increased probability of death as the individual grows older. See also AGED and SENESCENCE, and see the Atlas on Aging.

agitation (aj″ĭ-ta′shun) extreme restlessness, as manifested in depression and other mental disorders. Called also psychomotor agitation.

Agkistrodon (ag-kis′trŏ-don) a genus of venomous pit VIPERS. *A. contor′trix* is the COPPERHEAD and *A. pisci′vorus* is the water MOCCASIN. See also SNAKEBITE.

aglossia (ah-glos′e-ah) congenital absence of the tongue.

aglossostomia (ah″glos-o-sto′me-ah) congenital absence of the tongue and the mouth opening.

aglutition (ag″loo-tish′un) inability to swallow.

aglycemia (a″gli-se′me-ah) absence of sugar from the blood; see also HYPOGLYCEMIA.

aglycon (a-gli′kon) the noncarbohydrate group of a glycoside molecule.

aglycone (a-gli′kōn) aglycon.

aglycosuric (ah-gli″ko-su′rik) free from GLYCOSURIA.

agnathia (ag-na′the-ah) congenital absence of the lower jaw.

agnogenic (ag″no-jen′ik) of unknown origin.

agnosia (ag-no′zhah) inability to recognize the import of sensory impressions; the varieties correspond with several senses and are distinguished as auditory (acoustic), gustatory, olfactory, tactile, and visual.

finger a. loss of ability to indicate one's own or another's fingers.

tactile a. inability to recognize familiar objects by touch. See also ASTEREOGNOSIS.

time a. loss of comprehension of the succession and duration of events.

visual a. inability to recognize familiar objects by sight, usually due to a lesion in one of the visual association areas. Called also object blindness and psychic blindness.

visual-spatial a., visuospatial a. lack of the ability to analyze and orient using visual representations and their spatial relationships.

-agogue word element [Gr.], *something that leads or induces.*

agonad (ah-go′nad) an individual having no sex glands (gonads).

agonadal (ah-gon′ah-dal) having no sex glands; due to absence of sex glands.

agonal (ag′o-nal) pertaining to death or extreme suffering.

agonist (ag′o-nist) 1. agonistic MUSCLE. 2. in pharmacology, a drug that has affinity for the cellular receptors of another drug or natural substance and that produces a physiological effect.

agony (ag′ah-ne) severe pain or extreme suffering.

agoraphobia (ag″or-ah-fo′be-ah) an ANXIETY DISORDER characterized by intense, irrational fear of open spaces, especially a marked fear of being alone or of being in public places where escape would be difficult or help might be unavailable. It may be associated with panic attacks (see PANIC DISORDER) or may occur independently (officially called *agoraphobia without history of panic disorder*).

a. without history of panic disorder agoraphobia with fear of having an attack of one or only a few incapacitating or embarrassing symptoms, which the person may or may not have had in the past, rather than a full panic attack.

-agra word element [Gr.], *attack; seizure.*

agrammatism (a-gram′ah-tiz′m) inability to speak grammatically because of brain injury or disease, usually with simplified sentence structure (telegraphic SPEECH) and errors in tense, number, and gender.

agranulocyte (a-gran′u-lo-sīt″) nongranular LEUKOCYTE.

agranulocytosis (a-gran″u-lo-si-to′sis) an acute disease in which there is a dramatic decrease in the production of granulocytes, so that a pronounced neutropenia evolves, leaving the body defenseless against bacterial invasion. A great majority of cases are caused by sensitization to drugs or chemicals that affect the bone marrow and depress the formation of granulocytes. Called also malignant or pernicious leukopenia and idiopathic or malignant neutropenia.

Symptoms. The first manifestations are usually produced by a severe infection and include high fever, chills, prostration, and ulcerations of mucous membranes such as in the mouth, rectum, or vagina. Laboratory tests reveal a profound leukopenia (low leukocyte count).

Treatment. Treatment is aimed at immediate withdrawal of the drug or chemical causing the disorder, and control of infection. In most cases control can be achieved by the administration of antibiotics. If the bone marrow is not irreparably damaged, the prognosis is good with proper treatment, and the patient will recover as the production of granulocytes resumes. Occasionally the leukocyte-producing tissues are damaged beyond repair and death ensues.

infantile genetic a. a severe congenital condition of virtual absence of neutrophils from the blood; most patients die of infection before reaching adulthood. Called also congenital neutropenia and Kostmann's syndrome or neutropenia.

agranuloplastic (a-gran′′u-lo-plas′tik) forming only nongranular cells.

agraphia (a-graf′e-ah) loss of ability to express thoughts in writing.

AGS American Geriatrics Society.

agyria (ah-ji′re-ah) a malformation in which the gyri of the cerebral cortex are not normally developed; called also lissencephaly.

AHA American Heart Association; American Hospital Association.

AHCPR Agency for Health Care Policy and Research, former name of the Agency for Healthcare Research and Quality.

AHF antihemophilic factor (factor VIII, one of the COAGULATION FACTORS).

AHG 1. antihuman globulin (test). 2. antihemophilic globulin (factor VIII, one of the COAGULATION FACTORS).

AHIMA American Health Information Management Association.

AHRQ Agency for Healthcare Research and Quality.

AI aortic incompetence; aortic insufficiency; apical impulse; artificial insemination; artificial intelligence.

AICC anti-inhibitor coagulant complex.

AICD activation-induced cell death; automatic implantable cardioverter-defibrillator.

AID artificial INSEMINATION by donor.

aide (ād) a worker who is an assistant to another.

home health a. a paraprofessional worker with specified training and certification to provide unskilled HOME HEALTH CARE under the direction of a registered nurse.

AIDS acquired immunodeficiency syndrome.

AIH artificial INSEMINATION by husband.

ailurophobia (i-loor″o-fo′be-ah) irrational fear of cats.

ainhum (ān′hum, i′num, or [Portuguese] īn-yoom′) a condition of unknown origin, seen chiefly in dark-skinned people, consisting of a linear constriction that causes spontaneous amputation of the fourth or fifth toe.

airway (ar′wa) 1. the passage by which air enters and leaves the lungs. 2. a mechanical device used for securing unobstructed respiration when the patient is not breathing or is otherwise unable to maintain a clear passage, such as during general ANESTHESIA or respiratory arrest.

Oropharyngeal Airway. This device is inserted into the mouth to prevent the tongue from obstructing the pharynx. (See accompanying illustration.) It should not be used on alert or semiconscious patients, as it invariably stimulates the gag reflex and causes vomiting or injury to the jaw unless the patient is deeply unconscious.

Selection of proper size is essential because an airway that is too short cannot lift the tongue away from the oropharynx. The airway should be gently inserted so as to avoid trauma to the mucous membranes. It must be inserted with the tip up and rotated 180 degrees when it reaches the back of the throat so that the tongue is not displaced back into the pharynx, where it will obstruct

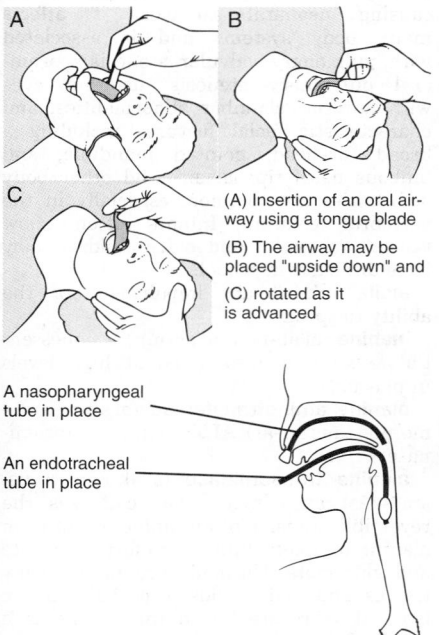

(A) Insertion of an oral airway using a tongue blade

(B) The airway may be placed "upside down" and

(C) rotated as it is advanced

A nasopharyngeal tube in place

An endotracheal tube in place

Esophageal airway.

the air passage. The proper size is the distance from the earlobe to the edge of the mouth.

Esophageal Obturator Airway. This is a hollow tube inserted into the esophagus to maintain airway patency in unconscious persons and to permit positive-pressure ventilation through the face mask connected to the tube. It was designed to be used by trained pre-hospital medical personnel to establish an airway. Its use has declined because of training of pre-hospital medical personnel in the insertion of endotracheal tubes, and because studies have suggested poor performance.

Esophageal Gastric Tube Airway. This is a hollow tube with a balloon at the end, which is blindly inserted into the esophagus, obstructing the esophagus and theoretically forcing air into the trachea, thus decompressing the stomach and alleviating abdominal distention; it represents an improvement in the design of the esophageal obturator airway. Ventilation occurs in the oropharynx.

Nasopharyngeal Airway. This is a hollow tube placed through the nose into the nasopharynx to bypass upper airway obstruction or to decrease trauma from nasotracheal suctioning.

Endotracheal Tube (or Airway). This inflatable tube is inserted into the mouth or nose and passed into the trachea to provide mechanical ventilation, to provide a suction route, to prevent aspiration of stomach contents, and to bypass upper airway obstruction.

Tracheostomy. This involves a surgical incision into the trachea and insertion of a metal or plastic tube through the incision. (See also TRACHEOSTOMY.)

a. clearance, ineffective a NURSING DIAGNOSIS accepted by the North American Nursing Diagnosis Association, defined as inability by an individual to clear secretions or obstructions from the respiratory tract to maintain a clear airway. Etiologic factors include decreased energy and fatigue; infection, obstruction, or excessive secretions in the tracheobronchial tree; perceptual/cognitive impairment associated with decreased oxygenation to brain cells; and trauma to the respiratory tract.

Defining characteristics presented by a person with ineffective airway clearance are likely to include abnormal breath sounds, alterations in respiratory rate or depth, cough (effective or ineffective and with or without sputum), cyanosis, dyspnea, and possibly fever.

Patient Care. Goals and outcome criteria for planning and interventions to prevent, minimize, or alleviate ineffective airway clearance will depend on the patient's medical diagnosis, specific nursing diagnoses, and related pathophysiology. In general, the goals are to promote the movement of air in and out of the lungs; prevent development of infection, atelectasis, and accumulations of stagnant secretions in the lungs; and encourage preventive and therapeutic pulmonary hygiene to maintain good ventilation.

Some appropriate nursing interventions to accomplish these goals might include teaching the patient effective coughing practices, assisting with postural drainage and other techniques used by the respiratory therapist to remove secetions from the respiratory tract, helping the patient to stop smoking, helping the patient identify and avoid allergens in the environment, maintaining a clean and infection-free environment, repositioning and encouraging early ambulation in post-surgical patients, and providing instruction in ways to avoid extreme fatigue in patients with chronic obstructive pulmonary disease.

conducting a. the lower and upper airways together, from the nares to the terminal bronchioles.

lower a. the airway from the lower end of the larynx to the ends of the terminal bronchioles.

upper a. the airway from the nares and lips to the larynx.

AIUM American Institute of Ultrasound in Medicine.

AJCC American Joint Committee on Cancer.

A-K, AK above-knee; see transfemoral AMPUTATION.

akaryocyte (ah-kar′e-o-sīt″) a non-nucleated cell, e.g., an erythrocyte.

akaryote (ah-kar′e-ōt) 1. non-nucleated. 2. a non-nucleated cell.

akathisia (ak″ah-thĭ′zhah) a condition of motor restlessness in which there is a feeling of muscular quivering, an urge to move about constantly, and an inability to sit still, a common side effect of neuroleptic drugs.

akinesia (a″ki-ne′zhah) 1. absence or loss of the power of voluntary movement. 2. the temporary paralysis of a muscle by the injection of procaine.

a. al′gera a condition characterized by generalized pain associated with movement of any kind.

akinesthesia (ah-kin″es-the′zhah) absence of the perception of movement.

akinetic (a″ki-net′ik) affected with akinesia.

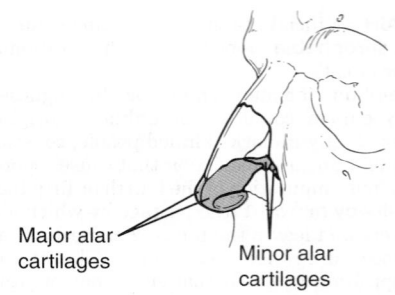

Ala nasi with major and minor alar cartilages. From Dorland's, 2000.

Major alar cartilages
Minor alar cartilages

Akineton (a″ki-ne′ton) trademark for preparations of BIPERIDEN, an ANTIDYSKINETIC.

Al aluminum.

ala (a′lah), pl. a′lae [L.] a winglike process. adj., **a′lar, a′late.**

a. na′si the cartilaginous flap on the outer side of each nostril. (See accompanying illustration.)

alacrima (ah-lak′rĭ-mah) deficiency or absence of the secretion of tears. It may be inherited as an autosomal dominant trait, or it may occur in association with other disorders or as an isolated congenital defect.

Alagille syndrome (ah-lah-zhēl′) a syndrome caused by the stoppage or suppression of BILE flow because of absence or paucity of intrahepatic bile ducts. Besides causing neonatal JAUNDICE, it affects many body systems and is associated with pulmonary valvular stenosis, peripheral pulmonary stenosis, deep-set eyes with anterior chamber abnormalities, and characteristic facial features including a broad forehead, pointed mandible, and bulbous nasal tip. RICKETS and other bony deformities are common, especially in the vertebral column. Infants often show FAILURE TO THRIVE and older children may have difficulty in school.

alalia (ah-la′le-ah) impairment of the ability to speak.

alanine (al′ah-nēn, al′ah-nin) a nonessential AMINO ACID, also found at high levels in plasma.

alanine aminotransferase (al′ah-nēn ah-me″no-trans′fer-ās) ALT; alanine transaminase.

alanine transaminase (al′ah-nēn trans-am′ĭ-nās) an enzyme that catalyzes the reversible transfer of an amino group from alanine to α-ketoglutarate to form pyruvate and glutamate. Normally present in many tissues and body fluids, especially in the liver, it is released into the serum as a result of tissue injury; the serum concentration is increased particularly when there is acute damage to hepatic cells, as in viral or toxic hepatitis, infectious mononucleosis, and obstructive jaundice. Called also alanine aminotransferase and glutamic-pyruvic transaminase.

Al-Anon (al'ah-non) a resource and support group for adult relatives and close friends of alcoholics. Al-Anon is available to interested individuals even if the alcoholic does not participate in ALCOHOLICS ANONYMOUS.

alar (a'lahr) pertaining to or like a wing.

alarm reaction the first stage of the GENERAL ADAPTATION SYNDROME; the response of the sympathetic nervous system to either physical stress or a strong emotional state (see also STRESS REACTION). It is an automatic and instantaneous response that increases the body's capability to cope with a sudden emergency. The physiologic changes that occur increase physical strength and mental activity. The blood pressure is elevated, the blood glucose level is raised for additional energy, the blood coagulates more readily, and the flow of blood to muscles needed for activity is increased, while those organs not needed for "fight" or "flight" receive a diminished blood supply. One of the most striking manifestations of this reaction is the involution of lymphoid tissues due to the action of adrenal hormones. Called also sympathetic stress reaction and fight-or-flight reaction.

Alateen (al'ah-tēn) a self-help program sponsored by AL-ANON for children (ages 12 to 20) of alcoholics. Alateen provides a forum for the discussion of the problems of living in a family affected by alcohol abuse and the opportunity to develop healthy coping skills.

alatrofloxacin (ah-lat″ro-flok'sah-sin) a broad-spectrum ANTIBACTERIAL that is the PRODRUG of TROVAFLOXICIN, to which it is rapidly converted after intravenous infusion; used in the form of the mesylate salt.

alba (al'bah) [L.] white.

albendazole (al-ben'dah-zōl) a broad-spectrum ANTHELMINTIC used against many parasites, including in treatment of HYDATID DISEASE and CYSTICERCOSIS.

Albers-Schönberg disease (al'berz shān'-berg) osteopetrosis.

albicans (al'bĭ-kans) [L.] white.

albiduria (al″bĭ-du're-ah) the discharge of white or pale urine.

albinism (al'bĭ-nizm) a hereditary disorder, usually transmitted as an autosomal recessive trait, in which there is partial or total absence of pigment in the skin, hair, and eyes (*oculocutaneous albinism*) or in the eyes alone (*ocular albinism*), caused by defective or absent function of the enzyme

tyrosinase. It is imperative that individuals affected with albinism be taught how to protect themselves from the harmful effects of the sun.

albino (al-bi'no) a person affected with ALBINISM.

albinuria (al″bĭ-nu're-ah) albiduria.

Albright's syndrome (hereditary osteodystrophy) (awl'brĭts) a group of symptoms of unknown cause, including distortion of bone with fibrous changes in the bone marrow spaces, brownish pigmentation of the skin, and precocious puberty in females. The bones may become bowed or shortened, resulting in susceptibility to fractures and difficulty in walking. Treatment is concerned with the resulting fractures and deformities; corrective orthopedic surgery is often indicated. See also fibrous DYSPLASIA of bone.

albuginea (al″bu-jin'e-ah) a tough whitish layer of fibrous tissue investing a part or organ, such as the testicle or ovary. See also TUNICA ALBUGINEA.

albumin (al-bu'min) 1. any protein that is soluble in water and moderately concentrated salt solutions and is coagulable by heat. 2. serum albumin; the most abundant plasma protein, formed principally in the liver and constituting up to two thirds of the 6 to 8 per cent protein concentration in the plasma. (See accompanying table.) Albumin is responsible for much of the colloidal osmotic pressure of the blood, and thus is a very important factor in regulating the exchange of water between the plasma and the interstitial compartment (space between the cells). Because of hydrostatic pressure, water is forced through the walls of the capillaries into the tissue spaces. This flow of water continues until the osmotic pull of protein (albumin) molecules causes it to stop. A drop in the amount of albumin in the plasma leads to an increase in the flow of water from the capillaries into the interstitial compartment. This results in an increase in tissue fluid which, if severe, becomes apparent as edema. Albumin serves also as a transport protein carrying large organic anions, such as fatty acids, bilirubin, and many drugs, and also

SERUM ALBUMIN LEVELS	
Newborn:	2.8–4.4 g/dl
Child:	3.2–5.4 g/dl
Adult under 60:	3.5–5 g/dl
Adult over 60:	3.4–4.8 g/dl

hormones, such as cortisol and thyroxine, when their specific binding globulins are saturated.

The presence of albumin in the urine (albuminuria) indicates malfunction of the kidney, and may accompany kidney disease or heart failure. A person with severe renal disease may lose as much as 20 to 30 g of plasma proteins in the urine in one day.

A decrease in the serum albumin level may occur with severe disease of the kidney. Other conditions such as liver disease, malnutrition, and extensive burns may result in serious decrease of plasma proteins.

a.-globulin ratio the ratio of albumin to globulin in blood serum, plasma, or urine.

a. human a preparation of human serum albumin, used as an artificial plasma extender and to increase bilirubin binding in hyperbilirubinemia.

iodinated I 125 a. a radiopharmaceutical used in blood and plasma volume, circulation time, and cardiac output determinations, consisting of albumin human labeled with iodine-125.

iodinated I 131 a. a radiopharmaceutical used in blood pool imaging and plasma volume determinations, consisting of albumin human labeled with iodine-131.

normal human serum a. albumin human.

serum a. albumin of the blood.

albuminoid (al-bu′mĭ-noid) 1. resembling albumin. 2. an albumin-like substance; the term is sometimes applied to insoluble substances known as scleroproteins.

albuminoptysis (al-bu″mĭ-nop′tĭ-sis) albumin in the sputum.

albuminuria (al-bu″mĭ-nu′re-ah) 1. the most common kind of PROTEINURIA, characterized by presence of ALBUMIN in the urine. adj. **albuminu′ric.** 2. sometimes used as a synonym for PROTEINURIA in general.

Albumisol (al-bu′mĭ-sol) trademark for a preparation of ALBUMIN HUMAN.

albuterol (al-bu′ter-ol) a relatively selective beta₂-adrenergic RECEPTOR agonist used as the base or sulfate salt as a BRONCHODILATOR.

Alcaligenes (al″kah-lij′ĕ-nēz) a genus of gram-negative, aerobic, rod-shaped bacteria, found in the intestines of vertebrates, as part of the normal skin flora, and in dairy products. Occasionally it causes opportunistic infections, *A. faeca′lis* being a cause of nosocomial septicemia in immunocompromised patients.

alclometasone (al-klo-met′ah-sōn″) a synthetic CORTICOSTEROID used topically in the dipropionate form for the relief of inflammation and pruritus.

alcohol (al′kah-hol) 1. any organic compound containing the hydroxy (—OH) functional group except those in which the OH group is attached to an aromatic ring, which are called *phenols*. Alcohols are classified as *primary, secondary,* or *tertiary* according to whether the carbon atom to which the OH group is attached is bonded to one, two, or three other carbon atoms and as *monohydric, dihydric,* or *trihydric* according to whether they contain one, two, or three OH groups; the latter two are called *diols* and *triols,* respectively. 2. ethanol. 3. an official preparation of ETHANOL, used as a disinfectant, solvent, and preservative, and applied topically as a rubbing compound, disinfectant, astringent, hemostatic, and coolant.

absolute a. dehydrated a.

benzyl a. a colorless liquid used as a bacteriostatic in solutions for injection and as a topical local anesthetic.

dehydrated a. an extremely HYGROSCOPIC, transparent, colorless, volatile liquid used as a solvent and injected into nerves and ganglia for relief of pain. Called also absolute a.

denatured a. ethanol made unfit for human consumption by the addition of substances known as denaturants. Although it should never be taken internally, denatured alcohol is widely used on the skin as a disinfectant.

ethyl a., grain a. ethanol.

isopropyl a. a transparent, volatile colorless liquid used as a solvent and disinfectant and applied topically as an antiseptic; called also isopropanol. Diluted with water to approximately 70 per cent strength, it is called *isopropyl rubbing alcohol* and is used as a rubbing compound.

methyl a. methanol.

pantothenyl a. 1. dexpanthenol. 2. panthenol.

phenethyl a., phenylethyl a. a colorless liquid used as an antimicrobial agent in pharmaceuticals.

rubbing a. a preparation of ACETONE, methyl isobutyl ketone, and ETHANOL, used as a rubefacient.

wood a. methanol.

Alcohol, Drug Abuse, and Mental Health Administration (ADAMHA) a former agency of the United States Department of Health and Human Services; in 1992 its services were divided between the SUBSTANCE ABUSE AND MENTAL HEALTH SERVICES ADMINISTRATION, the National Institute on Alcohol Abuse and Alcoholism, and the National Institute on Drug Abuse.

alcoholic (al″kah-hol′ik) 1. containing or pertaining to alcohol. 2. a person suffering from alcoholism.

Alcoholics Anonymous a self-help group of recovering alcoholics who provide support to each other in understanding and overcoming alcohol abuse. From their own experiences, group members learn how to motivate and encourage others in their desire to stop drinking. Meetings and discussions give the alcoholic an opportunity to air his or her problems and learn from the experiences of others who have similar problems. Hundreds of thousands of alcoholics and their families have been helped by AA since it was founded in 1935. Help in locating local groups and information about AA and ALCOHOLISM can be obtained from Alcoholics Anonymous, Inc., 475 Riverside Dr., New York, NY 10115.

alcoholism (al′kah-hol″izm) a term used to denote a variety of conditions involving abuse of or dependence on ALCOHOL; see also DRUG ABUSE, DRUG DEPENDENCE, and SUBSTANCE-RELATED DISORDERS. Alcoholism in its many forms is a major drug problem in almost all Western societies. Problems related to it are both immediate and long-term; alcohol abuse adversely affects the physical, spiritual, social and mental health of the individual as well as the integrity of the society in which he or she lives. Once viewed as a moral problem, alcoholism has now been redefined as a disease.

Alcoholism may be associated with other diagnoses: it may be associated with MOOD DISORDERS; it may occur in both manic and depressive episodes of BIPOLAR DISORDERS; and individuals with ANTISOCIAL PERSONALITY DISORDER often consume excessive amounts of alcohol (although it is uncertain how many are actually alcoholics).

Etiology. There is no universally accepted explanation of why one person becomes an alcoholic while another does not. There are a number of theories. There has been increasing research focusing on a biologic explanation for alcoholism, particularly on genetic predispositions. To date this has not been confirmed. Other theories suggest that alcoholism is related to psychological issues, is a learned behavior, or perhaps is a combination of numerous different factors.

Associated Pathologies. Alcohol is a toxic drug that is harmful to all of the body tissues. Protracted use can lead to a host of pathologic changes in the central nervous system, the liver (which detoxifies the drug), and the heart, kidney, and gastrointestinal tract. Although CIRRHOSIS of the liver is the most recognized complication of alcoholism, recent research indicates that

intellectual impairment can arise in the early stages of the disease, and permanent and disabling brain damage can eventually occur. Prolonged and abusive intake of alcohol coupled with nutritional depletion and thiamine deficiency can produce WERNICKE-KORSAKOFF SYNDROME. Newborn infants of mothers who drink heavily during pregnancy are susceptible to FETAL ALCOHOL SYNDROME.

Abuse and Dependence. Substance use disorders result in DRUG DEPENDENCE and DRUG ABUSE. The criteria for alcohol abuse include a maladaptive pattern of use either by continued use despite knowledge of having a persistent or recurrent social, occupational, psychologic, or physical problem that is caused by the alcohol, or by recurrent use in situations in which use is physically hazardous, with the pattern continuing for one month or more or recurring over time.

Alcohol dependence is characterized by the following symptoms occurring for at least one month or repeatedly over time: taking the substance in larger amounts or over a longer period than intended; lack of desire or attempt to cut or control intake; much time devoted to getting alcohol or recovering from its effects; frequent intoxication or withdrawal symptoms when expected to fulfill major role obligations; social, occupational, or recreational activities being given up or reduced; continued use despite evidence of harm; marked tolerance; withdrawal symptoms; and the taking of alcohol to avoid withdrawal symptoms. Dependence is classified as mild, moderate, or severe or in partial or full remission, depending on the severity and number of symptoms.

Effects of Alcohol. Alcohol is a SEDATIVE that is absorbed in the small intestine. About 95 per cent is broken down by the liver. Usually a person can metabolize 10 mL of alcohol (1 ounce of whiskey) every 90 minutes. If taken in high enough doses, alcohol can depress respiration and cause death. INTOXICATION is defined legally according to a person's blood alcohol level; the definition is 0.10 per cent or more in most states in the U.S. and 0.8 per cent or more in Canada. Symptoms include irritability, mood swings, short attention span, talking loudly, slurred speech, lack of coordination, unsteady gait, nystagmus, and flushed face.

Simple intoxication lasts less than twelve hours and is usually followed by a HANGOVER, defined as the unpleasant symptoms that occur about 4 to 6 hours after alcohol ingestion. Symptoms include nausea, vomiting, headache, gastritis, fatigue, sweating, thirst, and vasomotor instability. These are attributed to HYPOGLYCEMIA and accumulation of LACTIC ACID and ACETALDEHYDE in the blood.

Physical dependence is manifested most strikingly when the person is deprived of the drug and WITHDRAWAL symptoms appear. These symptoms are manifestations of neurologic impairment and range from mild tremors of the hands to seizures (DELIRIUM TREMENS).

Alcohol withdrawal refers to withdrawal without delirium. Tremulousness may occur while drinking or as long as 2 hours afterwards; hallucinations may begin 12 to 48 hours after cessation of drinking. Grand mal seizures resulting from withdrawal of alcohol may occur 2 to 3 days after cessation of drinking. There is usually neither the forewarning nor aura characteristic of epilepsy. Residual twitching in specific areas of the body or a stuporous condition sometimes follows the seizure. About one third of those having seizures associated with alcohol withdrawal may develop the potentially fatal condition called DELIRIUM TREMENS, which is an emergency situation.

Medical Treatment and Patient Care During Withdrawal. A patient experiencing DETOXIFICATION and withdrawal from alcohol requires coordinated care by the health care team. Symptoms of the withdrawal syndrome can last from 2 to 4 days or longer. During this time, the patient probably will exhibit problems related to fluid and electrolyte imbalance; acid-base imbalance; anxiety and psychomotor agitation; nausea, vomiting, and possibly gastrointestinal bleeding; and potentially severe nutritional deficits.

Fluid and electrolyte status should be assessed and any imbalance corrected, preferably by oral rather than intravenous therapy. Some alcoholic patients are dehydrated, and others are overhydrated and therefore need a diuretic to restore fluid balance. Transient hyperventilation associated with anxiety may produce respiratory ALKALOSIS, an increase in blood pH, and a decrease in magnesium levels.

Extreme irritability, restlessness, and insomnia can be relieved by the administration of a mild TRANQUILIZER such as CHLORDIAZEPOXIDE, and by SEDATIVES that help the patient achieve adequate rest and sleep without interfering with normal daily activities. The agitated patient will benefit from a quiet, nonstimulating environment and calm assurance of being safe and cared for. If hallucinating, the person may or may not be frightened (not all hallucinations are

unpleasant) but will probably be confused and disoriented at times. Safety measures are necessary to prevent unintentional or intentional self-injury. There is always the possibility that an alcoholic patient will be suicidal; therefore expressions of depression and feelings of remorse should be taken seriously.

PHENOBARBITAL is usually prescribed to prevent and control seizures. (Care for and protection of the patient before, during, and after a convulsive seizure is discussed under CONVULSION.)

Nausea and vomiting should be controlled with medication and nursing measures in order to prevent upper GI tract trauma and hemorrhaging. If the patient has esophageal VARICES (which are fairly common in conjunction with cirrhosis of the liver), the varices could rupture during an episode of strenuous vomiting and create an emergency situation.

The nutritional status of the alcoholic patient should be evaluated before therapy is begun. Many alcoholics have a vitamin deficiency, especially a deficiency of THIAMINE. Vitamin therapy (B complex and C) of some kind usually is a valuable adjunct to other measures intended to improve the overall health status and produce a sense of well-being in the alcoholic patient.

Finally, it should be remembered that symptoms of withdrawal from alcohol may be seen in an accident victim, surgical patient, or other patient with a medical problem unrelated to alcohol who has a hidden drinking problem and is being deprived of alcohol. When early symptoms of withdrawal first appear in the hospitalized patient, assessment should include a history of drinking patterns as well as an appraisal of health status with respect to physiologic changes attributable to alcoholism. Once the assessment is done, a plan is developed to help meet specific needs.

Because of the denial of alcoholism, the patient and family may not readily acknowledge and confront the problem. All members of the health care team should be prepared to help individuals who abuse alcohol get appropriate treatment. Delay in treatment of early signs of withdrawal sets the stage for more serious and sometimes fatal progression of the withdrawal syndrome.

Treatment of Chronic Alcoholism. Alcohol abuse and dependence are complex behavior disorders for which there is no simple remedy. This is not to say that alcoholism is a hopeless condition. Many people are able to bring their destructive drinking patterns under control when given the support and care they need.

There are several approaches to the treatment of alcoholism in addition to those that focus on correction of the patient's medical problems. Behavior techniques are aimed at helping the individual find more acceptable and healthier ways to cope with the stresses of everyday living. Group therapy has been found to be particularly helpful when conducted under the direction of clinical psychologists, psychiatrists, and psychiatric nurse specialists who plan a program of activities in conjunction with their clients and assist them in implementing it. If the patient drinks to cope with depression, the underlying depression must also be treated.

Self-help groups such as ALCOHOLICS ANONYMOUS have a good record of success in helping alcoholics conquer their habitual drinking. Another resource for materials helpful to the patient and family is the National Council on Alcoholism and Drug Dependence, 20 Exchange Place, Suite 2902, New York, NY 10005.

alcuronium (al-ku-ro′ne-um) a nondepolarizing skeletal muscle relaxant used in general anesthesia for surgical procedures; used in the form of the chloride salt.

Aldactazide (al-dak′tah-zīd) trademark for a preparation of SPIRONOLACTONE and HYDROCHLOROTHIAZIDE, a diuretic.

Aldactone (al-dak′tōn) trademark for a preparation of SPIRONOLACTONE, an aldosterone antagonist used as a diuretic.

aldehyde (al′dĕ-hīd) 1. an organic compound containing the aldehyde functional group (—CHO); that is, one with a carbonyl group (C═O) located at one end of the carbon chain. 2. acetaldehyde.

aldesleukin (al″des-loo′kin) a recombinant INTERLEUKIN-2 used as an antineoplastic AGENT and biological response MODIFIER in treatment of metastatic renal cell carcinoma and malignant melanoma.

Aldomet (al′do-met) trademark for preparations of METHYLDOPA, an ANTIHYPERTENSIVE AGENT.

aldopentose (al″do-pen′tōs) any one of a class of sugars that contain five carbon atoms and an aldehyde group (—CHO).

Aldoril (al′do-ril) trademark for a preparation of METHYLDOPA and HYDROCHLOROTHIAZIDE, an ANTIHYPERTENSIVE AGENT.

aldose (al′dōs) one of the two main types of MONOSACCHARIDE SUGARS; those that contain an aldehyde group (—CHO), such as GLUCOSE, GALACTOSE, or MANNOSE.

aldosterone (al-dos′ter-ōn, al′do-ster-ōn″) the main MINERALOCORTICOID hormone secreted by the adrenal cortex, the principal biological activity of which is the regulation of electrolyte and water balance by promoting the retention of sodium (and, therefore,

of water) and the excretion of potassium; the retention of water induces an increase in plasma volume and an increase in blood pressure. Its secretion is stimulated by ANGIOTENSIN II.

a. antagonist a compound that blocks the action of aldosterone; the group includes potassium sparing DIURETICS such as SPIRONOLACTONE that compete with aldosterone for receptor sites, thus blocking the aldosterone-dependent exchange of sodium and potassium in the distal tubule.

aldosteronism (al-dos′ter-ōn-izm″, al″doster′ōn-izm) an abnormality of electrolyte metabolism produced by excessive secretion of ALDOSTERONE, it may be primary or occur secondarily in response to extra-adrenal disease. There may be hypertension, hypokalemia, alkalosis, muscular weakness, polyuria, and polydipsia. Called also hyperaldosteronism.

primary a. that arising from oversecretion of aldosterone, characterized typically by hypokalemia, alkalosis, muscular weakness, polyuria, polydipsia, hypertension, cardiac irregularity, and tetany. The most common etiologic factors are adrenal adenoma, idiopathic hyperplasia of the adrenal cortex, and occasionally carcinoma of the adrenal gland. Most adenomas affect only one of the two glands and therefore can be removed surgically without depriving the patient of a sufficient supply of adrenal cortical hormones. If removal of both glands is necessary, this creates a serious and potentially fatal insufficiency of the hormones. Called also Conn's syndrome.

pseudoprimary a. that caused by bilateral adrenal hyperplasia and having the same signs and symptoms as primary aldosteronism.

secondary a. that due to extra-adrenal stimulation of aldosterone secretion; it is commonly associated with edematous states, as in nephrotic syndrome, hepatic cirrhosis, heart failure, and accelerated hypertension.

Aldrich syndrome (awl′drich) Wiskott-Aldrich syndrome.

alecithal (ah-les′ĭ-thal) having no distinct yolk.

alemtuzumab (al″em-tuz′u-mab″) a recombinant, DNA-derived, humanized monoclonal ANTIBODY directed against the CD antigen CD52; administered intravenously as an ANTINEOPLASTIC in the treatment of B-cell chronic lymphocytic LEUKEMIA.

alendronate (ah-len′dro-nāt) a calcium-regulating agent used in the form of the sodium salt to inhibit resorption of bone in the treatment of osteitis deformans, osteoporosis, and hypercalcemia related to malignancy; administered orally.

aleukemia (a″loo-ke′me-ah) 1. leukopenia. 2. aleukemic leukemia.

aleukia (a-loo′ke-ah) leukopenia.

aleukocytosis (a-loo″ko-si-to′sis) leukopenia.

alexia (ah-lek′se-ah) a form of receptive aphasia in which there is inability to understand written language. adj., **alex′ic.**

alexithymia (ah-leks″ĭ-thi′me-ah) inability to recognize or describe one's emotions.

aleydigism (ah-li′dig-izm) absence of secretion of the interstitial cells of the testis (Leydig cells).

alfacalcidol (al″fah-kal′sĭ-dol) a synthetic analogue of CALCITRIOL, to which it is converted in the liver; used in the treatment of hypocalcemia, hypophosphatemia, rickets, and osteodystrophy associated with various medical conditions including chronic RENAL FAILURE and HYPOPARATHYROIDISM, administered orally or intravenously.

alfentanil (al-fen′tah-nil) an opioid ANALGESIC of rapid onset and short duration derived from FENTANYL; the hydrochloride salt is used as a primary agent for induction of general anesthesia, as an adjunct in maintenance of general anesthesia, and as an adjunct to regional or local anesthesia.

ALG antilymphocyte globulin.

alg(o)- word element [Gr.], *pain; cold.*

algae (al′je) a group of plants living in the water, including all seaweeds, and ranging in size from microscopic cells to fronds hundreds of feet long.

blue-green a. former name for members of the group now called CYANOBACTERIA.

algefacient (al″jĕ-fa′shent) cooling or refrigerant.

algesia (al-je′zhah) 1. nociception. 2. excessive sensitivity to pain, a type of HYPERESTHESIA. adj., **alge′sic, alget′ic.**

algesimeter a device for measuring sensitivity to painful stimuli; called also algometer.

algesimetry (al″jĕ-sim′ĕ-tre) measurement of sensitivity of pain; called also algometry.

algesthesia (al-jes-the′zhah) nociception.

-algia word element [Gr.], *pain.*

algicide (al′jĭ-sīd) 1. destructive to algae. 2. an agent that destroys algae.

algid (al′jid) chilly; cold.

alginate (al′jĭ-nāt) a salt of alginic acid, a colloidal substance from brown seaweed; used, in the form of calcium, sodium, or ammonium alginate, for dental impression materials.

alginic acid (al-jin′ik) a hydrophilic colloidal carbohydrate obtained from seaweed,

used as a tablet binder and emulsifying agent.

alglucerase (al-gloo′ser-ās″) a modified form of the enzyme lacking in GAUCHER'S DISEASE, used in treatment of the adult form of the disease.

algodystrophy (al″go-dis′tro-fe) a combination of pain and dystrophic changes in bone.

algogenic (al″go-jen′ik) dolorific.

algometer (al-gom′ĕ-ter) algesimeter.

algometry (al-gom′ĕ-tre) algesimetry.

algophobia (al″go-fo′be-ah) irrational dread of pain.

algorithm (al′go-rithm) 1. a series of algebraic equations. 2. a logical progression that is programmed for a computer. 3. a model for making decisions. (See accompanying illustration.)

Alidase (al′ĭ-dās) trademark for a preparation of HYALURONIDASE for injection, used as a spreading agent to promote diffusion and hasten absorption.

alienation (āl″yen-a′shun) 1. estrangement from society; feelings of being an outsider, foreigner, or outcast. 2. estrangement from one's self; feelings of unreality or depersonalization. 3. alienation of affect; isolation of ideas from feelings, avoidance of emotional situations, and other efforts to estrange one's self from one's feelings.

alienia (a″li-e′ne-ah) absence of the spleen.

aliform (al′ĭ-form) shaped like a wing.

aliment (al′ĭ-ment) food; nutritive material.

alimentary (al″ĭ-men′tah-re) pertaining to or caused by food or nutritive material.

a. canal, a. tract the portion of the DIGESTIVE SYSTEM consisting of the organs making up the route taken by food as it passes through the body from mouth to anus; this includes the ESOPHAGUS, STOMACH, and small and large INTESTINES. (See accompanying illustration and Plate 9.) Called also digestive tract.

alimentation (al″ĭ-men-ta′shun) giving or receiving of nourishment.

parenteral a. administration of nutrients intravenously.

alinasal (al″ĭ-na′zal) pertaining to either of the cartilaginous flaps of the nose.

aliphatic (al″ĭ-fat′ik) pertaining to any member of the group of organic compounds having a branched or straight chain structure.

aliquot (al′ĭ-kwot) 1. a sample that is representative of the whole. 2. a number that will divide another without a remainder; e.g., 2 is an aliquot of 6.

alitretinoin (al″ĭ-tret′ĭ-noin″) a topical antineoplastic used in the treatment of AIDS-related cutaneous Kaposi's sarcoma.

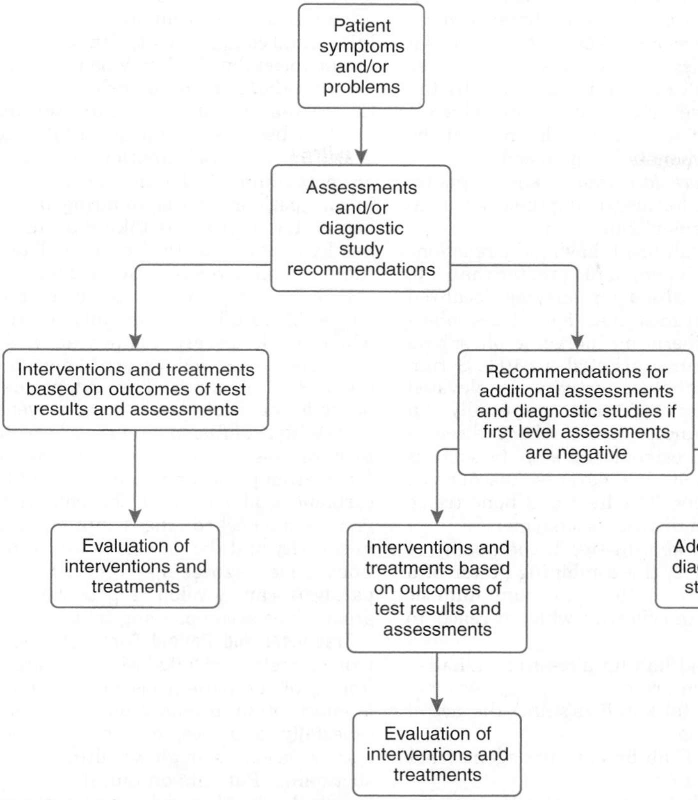

```
        ┌─────────────┐
        │   Patient   │
        │  symptoms   │
        │   and/or    │
        │  problems   │
        └──────┬──────┘
               │
               ▼
        ┌─────────────┐
        │ Assessments │
        │   and/or    │
        │ diagnostic  │
        │    study    │
        │recommendations│
        └─────────────┘
```

Interventions and treatments based on outcomes of test results and assessments

Recommendations for additional assessments and diagnostic studies if first level assessments are negative

Evaluation of interventions and treatments

Interventions and treatments based on outcomes of test results and assessments

Additional diagnostic studies

Evaluation of interventions and treatments

Algorithm. Model of a decision algorithm. ACC/AHA Guidelines for the Management of Patients with Unstable Angina and Non-ST Segment Elevation Myocardial Infarction. JACC 2000, 36: 970-1062. Copyright 2000, by the American College of Cardiology and American Heart Association. Permission granted for one time use. Further reproduction is not permitted without permission of the ACC/AHA.

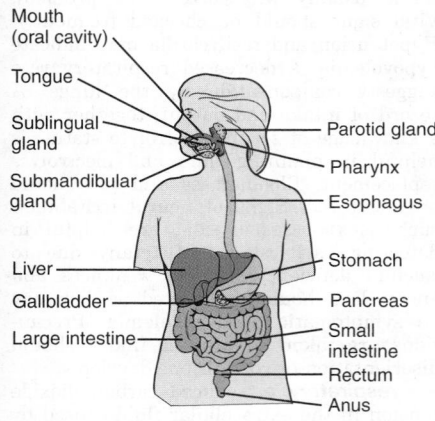

Mouth (oral cavity)
Tongue
Sublingual gland
Submandibular gland
Liver
Gallbladder
Large intestine
Parotid gland
Pharynx
Esophagus
Stomach
Pancreas
Small intestine
Rectum
Anus

Organs of the alimentary canal. From Applegate, 2000.

alkalemia (al″kah-le′me-ah) abnormal alkalinity, or increased pH, of the blood.

alkali (al′kah-li) any of a class of compounds such as sodium hydroxide that form salts with acids and soaps with fats; a BASE, or substance capable of neutralizing acids. Other properties include a pH value greater than 7.0, a bitter taste, and the ability to turn litmus paper from red to blue. Alkalis play a vital role in maintaining the normal functioning of the body chemistry. See also ACID-BASE BALANCE.

a. reserve the ability of the combined buffer systems of the blood to neutralize acid. The pH of the blood normally is slightly on the alkaline side, between 7.35 and 7.45. Since the principal buffer in the blood is bicarbonate, the alkali reserve essentially is represented by the plasma bicarbonate concentration. However, hemoglobin, phosphates, and other bases also act as buffers. A lowered alkali reserve means a state of acidosis; increased reserve indicates alkalosis. Alkali reserve is measured by the combining power of carbon dioxide, which is the amount of carbon dioxide that can be bound as bicarbonate by the blood.

a. denaturation test a spectrophotometric method for measuring the concentration of fetal hemoglobin (Hb F).

alkaline (al′kah-līn) 1. having the reactions of an alkali. 2. having a pH greater than 7.0.

a. phosphatase an enzyme localized on cell membranes that hydrolyzes phosphate esters liberating inorganic phosphate and has an optimal pH of about 10.0. Serum alkaline phosphatase activity is elevated in hepatobiliary disease, especially in obstructive jaundice, and in bone diseases with increased osteoblastic activity such as HYPERPARATHYROIDISM, OSTEITIS DEFORMANS, and bone cancer. The liver and bone tissue each produce a distinct isoenzyme.

alkalinity (al″kah-lin′ĭ-te) 1. the quality of being alkaline. 2. the combining power of a base, expressed as the maximum number of equivalents of acid with which it reacts to form a salt.

alkalinuria (al″kah-lin-u′re-ah) an alkaline condition of the urine.

alkalization (al″kah-lĭ-za′shun) the act of making alkaline.

alkalizer (al′kah-līz″er) an agent that causes alkalization.

alkaloid (al′kah-loid) one of a large group of organic, basic substances found in plants. They are usually bitter in taste and are characterized by powerful physiologic activity. Examples are morphine, cocaine, atropine, quinine, nicotine, and caffeine. The term is also applied to synthetic substances that have structures similar to plant alkaloids, such as procaine.

vinca a's see VINCA ALKALOIDS.

alkalosis (al″kah-lo′sis) a pathologic condition resulting from accumulation of base, or from loss of acid without comparable loss of base in the body fluids, and characterized by decrease in hydrogen ion concentration (increase in pH). Alkalosis is the opposite of ACIDOSIS. See also ACID-BASE BALANCE.

compensated a. a form in which compensatory mechanisms have returned the pH toward normal.

hypochloremic a. a metabolic alkalosis in which gastric losses of chloride are disproportionately greater than sodium loss because of corresponding increase in potassium loss.

hypokalemic a. a metabolic alkalosis associated with a low serum potassium level; retention of alkali or loss of acid occurs in the extracellular (but not intracellular) fluid compartment, although the pH of the intracellular fluid may be below normal.

metabolic a. a disturbance in which the ACID-BASE BALANCE shifts toward the alkaline because of uncompensated loss of acids, ingestion or retention of excess base, or potassium depletion. This can occur in any patient who is vomiting frequently, has gastric suction, is taking a diuretic, or has hyperadrenocortical disease. The condition is characterized by a blood serum pH above 7.45, an increase of serum CO_2 above 32 mEq/L, and an unchanged PCO_2 when the lungs are compensating for the alkalosis. These values are determined by BLOOD GAS ANALYSIS. The symptoms may be mild at first, with muscle weakness, irritability, confusion, and muscle twitching. Respirations are shallow and slow as the lungs attempt to compensate by building up carbonic acid stores. If the condition progresses unchecked, the symptoms increase in severity and the patient lapses into coma. Convulsive seizures may occur. Respiratory paralysis can develop if potassium loss is great. (See accompanying table.)

Treatment and Patient Care. The best control of metabolic alkalosis is careful monitoring of the patient because the condition is most often brought on by medication, especially diuretics, and by postoperative loss of acids through vomiting or gastric suctioning. Patients on diuretic therapy are taught to be alert for, and to report, the signs of potassium depletion and alkalosis. The primary aim of treatment is to reestablish fluid and electrolyte balance. Administration of potassium chloride and normal saline usually will correct the problem. Vital signs should be checked frequently. Hypotension and tachycardia may indicate hypovolemia; a decreased respiratory rate suggests compensation by the lungs. A record of intake and output, together with a knowledge of serum electrolyte status, is helpful in planning fluid and electrolyte replacement. Blood gases and pH should be monitored. Signs of neural irritability, such as TROUSSEAU'S SIGN, are helpful in detecting early stages of tetany due to calcium deficiency. Muscle weakness and energy loss should be reported, as they may be symptomatic of hypokalemia. Precautions are taken to prevent injury should disorientation or convulsions develop.

respiratory a. reduced carbon dioxide tension in the extracellular fluid caused by excessive excretion of carbon dioxide

ALKALOSIS				
Metabolic Alkalosis	Severe vomiting, nasogastric suctioning, diuretic therapy, excessive ingestion of bases (sodium bicarbonate)	Excess of base bicarbonate, or loss of hydrogen and chloride	Diarrhea, numbness and tingling of extremities, nausea and vomiting, bradycardia and a decreased respiratory rate	Increased pH (> 7.45), increased bicarbonate, increased base excess, increased Pco$_2$ (if lung compensation)
Respiratory Alkalosis	Hyperventilation, fever, anxiety, pain, pulmonary emboli, mechanical overventilation, early pulmonary edema, high environmental temperature	Deficit of carbonic acid, increased carbon dioxide loss due to alveolar hyperventilation	Inability to concentrate, dizziness, lightheadedness, numbness and tingling of mouth and extremities, blurred vision, diaphoresis, dry mouth, muscle cramps	Increased pH (> 7.5), increased Pco$_2$, normal or slightly decreased base excess, decreased bicarbonate (if renal compensation)

through the lungs (HYPERVENTILATION). This is commonly associated with conditions such as anxiety, hysteria, pain, hypoxia, fever, high environmental temperature, poisoning, early pulmonary EDEMA, pulmonary EMBOLISM, STROKE SYNDROME, central nervous system disease, and overuse of a mechanical VENTILATOR. Characteristics include dizziness or lightheadedness, inability to concentrate, tingling and numbness in the limbs and around the mouth, blurred vision, heavy sweating, dry mouth, muscle cramps, carpopedal spasms, and, in uncontrolled alkalosis, convulsions and syncope. Arterial BLOOD GAS values typically show a pH greater than 7.5 and a Pa$_{CO_2}$ below 35 mm Hg. The Pa$_{O_2}$ may be normal except in cases in which hyperventilation is caused by ANOXIA. (See also BLOOD GAS ANALYSIS.)

Acute respiratory alkalosis is typified by the HYPERVENTILATION SYNDROME. The chronic form usually is manifested by few symptoms except those associated with CHRONIC OBSTRUCTIVE PULMONARY DISEASE (COPD). (See accompanying table.)

Treatment and Patient Care. Treatment is primarily aimed at removal of the underlying cause, particularly in cases of hyperventilation due to hysteria. The patient who has ANOXIA caused by pulmonary infection or congestive HEART FAILURE should be given oxygen to reduce respiratory effort and the resultant blowing off of carbon dioxide. If there is involvement of the central nervous system, sedation to suppress activity of the respiratory center may be indicated.

alkalotic (al″kah-lot′ik) pertaining to or characterized by alkalosis.

alkane (al′kān) a saturated hydrocarbon, i.e., one that has no carbon-carbon multiple bonds.

alkapton (al-kap′ton) a class of substances with an affinity for alkali, sometimes found in the urine and causing the condition known as alkaptonuria. The urinary formation of alkaptons results from the incomplete oxygenation of tyrosine and phenylalanine. The compound commonly found, and most commonly referred to by the term, is homogentisic acid.

alkaptonuria (al-kap″to-nu′re-ah) an autosomal recessive AMINOACIDOPATHY characterized by accumulation of HOMOGENTISIC ACID. It is manifested by elevated concentrations of homogentisic acid in the urine (which darkens on standing or with alkalinization), a peculiar discoloration of body tissues known as ochronosis, and arthritis.

alkene (al′kēn) an aliphatic hydrocarbon containing a double bond.

alkyl (al′kil) the radical that results when an aliphatic hydrocarbon loses one hydrogen atom.

alkylate (al′kĭ-lāt) to cause the substitution of an alkyl group for an active hydrogen atom in an organic compound; see also ALKYLATING AGENTS.

alkylating agents (al′kĭ-lāt-ing) a group of synthetic compounds containing alkyl groups that combine readily with other molecules. Their action seems to be chiefly on the DNA in the nucleus of the cell, so that they are cell cycle phase nonspecific.

They cross-link the strands of DNA, preventing its replication and the transcription of RNA; the major site of action is on the base guanine. They are primarily used in CHEMOTHERAPY of cancer (see ANTINEOPLASTIC THERAPY). However, they do not damage malignant cells selectively, but also have a toxic action on normal cells; all killing occurs primarily in rapidly proliferating tissue. Locally they cause blistering of the skin and damage to the eyes and respiratory tract. Systemic toxic effects are nausea and vomiting, reduction in both leukocytes and erythrocytes, hemorrhagic tendencies, amenorrhea or impaired spermatogenesis, damage to the intestinal mucosa, and alopecia. Among the agents of this group used in therapy are BUSULFAN, CYCLOPHOSPHAMIDE, IFOSFAMIDE, and THIOTEPA; the NITROGEN MUSTARDS CHLORAMBUCIL, MELPHALAN, and MECHLORETHAMINE; and the NITROSOUREAS CARMUSTINE, LOMUSTINE, and STREPTOZOCIN. They may be carcinogenic in humans; some have been linked to bladder cancer and acute leukemia. However, the major benefits obtained in treating diseases such as lymphoma, Hodgkin's disease, breast cancer, and multiple myeloma far outweigh the risks of developing a second malignancy.

alkyne (al′kīn) an aliphatic hydrocarbon containing a triple bond.

ALL acute lymphoblastic leukemia.

all(o)- word element [Gr.], *other; deviating from normal.*

allachesthesia (al″ah-kes-the′zhah) allesthesia.

optical a. visual allesthesia.

allantochorion (ah-lan″to-kor′e-on) the allantois and chorion as one structure.

allantoid (ah-lan′toid) 1. sausage-shaped. 2. pertaining to the allantois.

allantoin (ah-lan′to-in) a crystalline substance from allantoic fluid and fetal urine, also produced synthetically; used as an ASTRINGENT and KERATOLYTIC, often as a component in multi-ingredient dermatological medications.

allantoinuria (ah-lan″to-ĭ-nu′re-ah) allantoin in the urine.

allantois (ah-lan′to-is) a small sausage-shaped outpouching from the caudal wall of the yolk sac of the early embryo, associated with early blood formation and development of the urinary bladder; its blood vessels become the umbilical arteries and veins. adj., **allanto′ic.**

allele (ah-lēl′) one of two or more alternative forms of a gene at the same site in a chromosome, which determine alternative characters in inheritance. adj., **allel′ic.**

silent a. one that produces no detectable effect.

allelotaxis (ah-le″lo-tak′sis) development of an organ from several embryonic structures.

Allen's law (al′enz) the more carbohydrates a diabetic takes, the less he or she utilizes.

Allen's test (al′enz) a test for occlusion of radial or ulnar arteries: the patient makes a tight fist so as to express the blood from the skin of the palm and fingers; the examiner makes digital compression on either the radial or ulnar artery. Failure of blood to return to the palm and fingers when the hand is opened indicates obstruction of the blood flow in the artery that has not been compressed. Either this test or a DOPPLER ULTRASOUND examination should always be performed prior to insertion of a radial artery line.

allergen (al′er-jen) 1. a substance, protein or nonprotein, capable of inducing allergy or specific hypersensitivity. 2. a purified protein of a food (such as milk, eggs, or wheat), bacterium, or pollen. adj., **allergen′ic.** Allergens are used to test a patient for HYPERSENSITIVITY to specific substances (see SKIN TEST). They are also used to desensitize or hyposensitize allergic individuals (see IMMUNOTHERAPY).

Almost any substance in the environment can be an allergen. The list of known allergens includes plant pollens, spores of mold, animal dander, house dust, foods, feathers, dyes, soaps, detergents, cosmetics, plastics, and drugs. Allergens can enter the body by being inhaled, swallowed, touched, or injected. Once the allergen comes in contact with body cells it sets off a series of IMMUNE RESPONSES that can range from localized inflammation to a fatal systemic ANAPHYLAXIS.

allergic (al-ler′jik) pertaining to or having an ALLERGY.

a. reaction a local or general reaction characterized by altered reactivity of the animal body to an antigenic substance; see also ALLERGY.

allergist (al′er-jist) a physician specializing in the diagnosis and treatment of allergic conditions.

allergization (al″er-jĭ-za′shun) active sensitization by introduction of allergens into the body.

allergy (al′er-je) a state of abnormal and individual HYPERSENSITIVITY acquired through exposure to a particular substance called an ALLERGEN; reexposure reveals a heightened capacity to react. (See accompanying illustration.)

Allergies can be divided into three major types: (1) delayed-reaction allergies caused

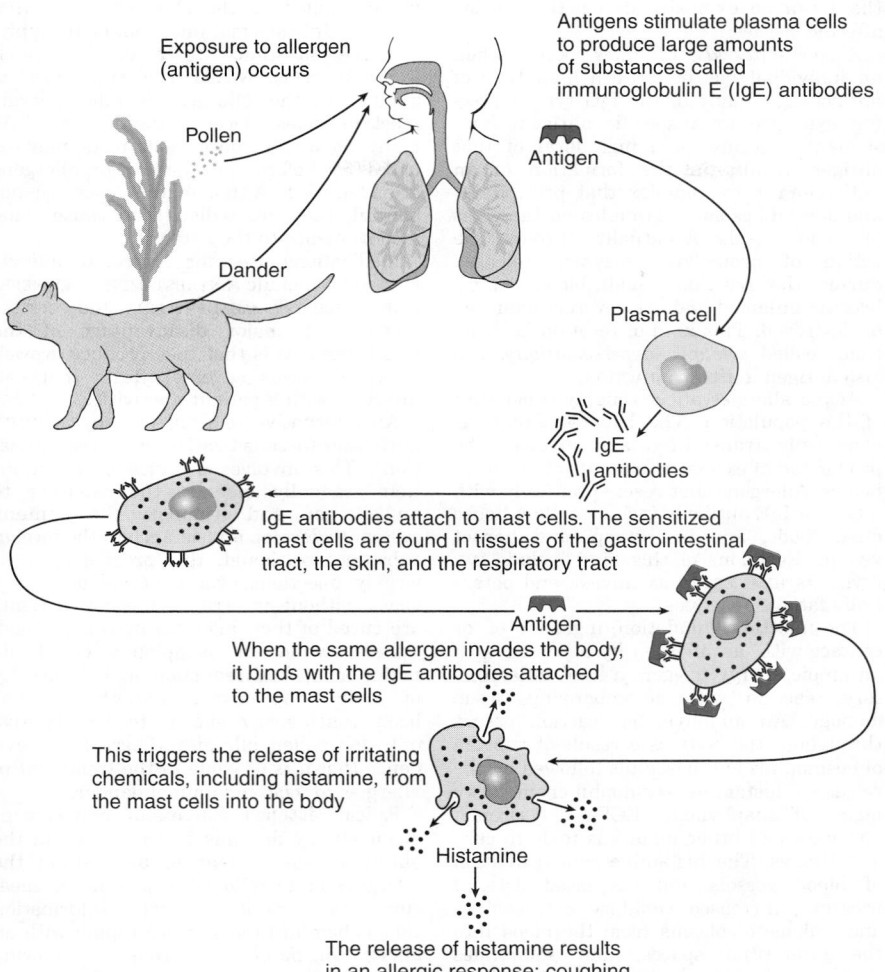

Exposure to allergen (antigen) occurs

Antigens stimulate plasma cells to produce large amounts of substances called immunoglobulin E (IgE) antibodies

Pollen

Antigen

Dander

Plasma cell

IgE antibodies

IgE antibodies attach to mast cells. The sensitized mast cells are found in tissues of the gastrointestinal tract, the skin, and the respiratory tract

Antigen

When the same allergen invades the body, it binds with the IgE antibodies attached to the mast cells

This triggers the release of irritating chemicals, including histamine, from the mast cells into the body

Histamine

The release of histamine results in an allergic response: coughing, sneezing, wheezing, rash, diarrhea

Mechanisms of allergic reaction. From Frazier et al., 2000.

by sensitized LYMPHOCYTES; (2) ANTIGEN-ANTI-BODY allergies caused by a reaction between gamma immunoglobulin (IgG) antibodies (IMMUNOGLOBULINS) and antigens; and (3) atopic or inherited allergies, which are characterized by the presence of large amounts of sensitizing antibodies called *IgE antibodies.*

Examples of *delayed-reaction* allergies (also called cell-mediated hypersensitivity) include CONTACT DERMATITIS or skin eruptions resulting from exposure to certain drugs, to chemicals, such as those in cosmetics and household cleansers, or to the toxins of POISON IVY, OAK, and SUMAC. On first contact with the allergen there is no response, but with repeated exposure some lymphocytes become sensitized. Once these lymphocytes are activated they remain in the body until a subsequent contact with the allergen to which they are sensitized. Then they diffuse into the skin and bring about a cell mediated IMMUNE RESPONSE. During this reaction toxins are released from the sensitized lymphocytes, and macrophages invade the tissues. If this process continues unchecked, there can be extensive destruction of the affected tissues.

Antigen-antibody allergies occur when an individual has built up a high titer of antibodies, usually of the IgG type, following exposure to a specific antigen. Subsequent exposure to a high level of that antigen results in the formation of an antigen-antibody complex that precipitates and deposits as small granules on the walls of blood vessels. Eventually, through the action of proteolytic enzymes released during the reaction, small blood vessels become inflamed and are severely damaged or destroyed. This kind of reaction is sometimes called *cytotoxic hypersensitivity*. See also antigen-antibody REACTION.

Atopic allergies affect roughly 9 per cent of the population. The hypersensitivity is genetically transmitted and involves the production of excessive amounts of IgE antibodies. Allergens that react specifically with a type of IgE antibody include pollen, house dust, foods, and bee, wasp, and hornet venom. Reactions of this kind include HAY FEVER, ASTHMA, URTICARIA (hives), and potentially fatal ANAPHYLAXIS.

The injection, inhalation, ingestion of, or contact with, an allergen by a person with an atopic allergy triggers a local inflammatory reaction with accompanying tissue damage. An anaphylactic reaction occurs throughout the body as a result of rupture of eosinophils and basophils followed by the release of histamine, eosinophil chemotactic factor of anaphylaxis (ECF-A), lysosomal enzymes, and other materials toxic to cells and tissues. The histamine causes dilation of blood vessels and decreased arterial pressure, increased capillary permeability and leakage of plasma from the blood into the interstitial spaces, and sometimes spasms of the bronchioles. These pathologic changes produce circulatory shock that can be fatal in a matter of minutes. If the bronchioles are affected, the individual becomes dyspneic and has a wheezing type respiration.

Prevention and Treatment. The most successful means of preventing the symptoms of allergy is, of course, identification and avoidance of the offending allergen. In some instances, a cause and effect relationship can be clearly established, as in drug reactions, insect stings, and food allergies. In other cases, good detective work is needed to identify the allergen.

One diagnostic method that is fairly successful is the SKIN TEST. A minute quantity of various suspected allergens is applied to the skin of the person's inner forearm, either by means of a saturated adhesive patch applied to the skin surface (PATCH TEST), by intradermal injection, or by applying the substance to a small scratch (SCRATCH TEST). When the substance so applied is the allergen, a mild allergic reaction takes place at the test site. As many as 30 or more such tests may be necessary before the allergen or allergens are identified. Although the tests are not painful, they are tedious and cause some inconvenience to the patient.

Medications used for control of allergic reactions include ANTIHISTAMINES, EPINEPHRINE, EPHEDRINE, AMINOPHYLLINE, and CORTICOSTEROIDS. A major disadvantage of the antihistamines is that they produce drowsiness and other adverse effects that can interfere with a patient's activities.

An alternative to drug therapy is IMMUNOTHERAPY (desensitization or hyposensitization). This involves a series of injections that gradually increase the exposure to an allergen and stimulate the immune system to develop a resistance to the foreign substance. Although this process requires weekly injections over a period of 3 to 5 years without interruption, some patients are cured of their allergies by this method. Others, while not completely cured, do notice a marked reduction in the severity of their symptoms. Immunotherapy has been conclusively shown to be effective only for pollen allergies. There is no evidence that it is of value in the treatment of allergies to food and animal dander.

Patient Education. Successful management of an allergy depends in large part on the ability of the patient to understand the allergy and to follow the preventive measures and prescribed therapy. Information that is helpful to laypersons coping with an allergy can be obtained from the following sources: Allergy Foundation of America, 1233 20th Street NW, Suite 402, Washington, DC 20036; and National Institutes of Allergy and Infectious Disease, National Institutes of Health, Bethesda, MD 20814.

atopic a. atopy.

bacterial a. a specific hypersensitivity to a particular bacterial antigen, such as *Mycobacterium tuberculosis.*

bronchial a. asthma.

cold a. any condition in which signs and symptoms of allergy are produced by exposure to cold, such as cold urticaria.

contact a. CONTACT DERMATITIS.

delayed a. an allergic response which appears hours or days after application or absorption of an allergen. It includes CONTACT DERMATITIS and bacterial allergy.

drug a. an allergic reaction as a result of unusual hypersensitivity to a drug.

food a., gastrointestinal a. allergy produced by ingested antigens, such as food or drugs; strawberries, milk, and eggs are the most common offenders. The organ affected usually is the skin.

hereditary a. atopy.

insulin a. see INSULIN ALLERGY.

latent a. allergy that does not have overt symptoms but may be detected by tests.

latex a. allergy to natural rubber latex, a type IV HYPERSENSITIVITY REACTION; see also LATEX (def. 1). Additional information about latex allergy is available from the National Institute for Occupational Safety and Health (NIOSH); on their web site at http://www.cdc.gov/niosh, or by calling 1-800-35-NIOSH.

physical a. a condition in which the patient is sensitive to the effects of physical agents, such as heat, cold, or light.

pollen a. hay fever.

spontaneous a. atopy.

allesthesia (al″es-the′zhah) the experiencing of a sensation, e.g., pain or touch, as occurring at a point remote from where the stimulus is actually applied.

visual a. the transposition of visual images from one-half of the visual field to the other. Called also optical allachesthesia.

alleviate (ah-le′ve-āt) to cause the lessening or disappearance of a patient's problem.

allied health any of diverse health care professions, including clinical laboratory personnel, physical therapy, occupational therapy, dietetic services, medical record personnel, radiologic services, speech-language pathology and audiology, and respiratory therapy. It does not include physicians, nurses, dentists, or podiatrists. Schools of Allied Health exist at the collegiate level to prepare health care practitioners, generate and disseminate research in allied health disciplines, promote interdisciplinary communication and collaboration, and increase the efficient use of resources by a variety of health care providers in order to improve health care.

Allis' sign (al′is) relaxation of the fascia between the crest of the ilium and the greater trochanter; a sign of fracture of the neck of the femur.

alloantibody (al″o-an′tĭ-bod″e) isoantibody.

allobarbital (al″o-bahr′bĭ-tal) diallylbarbituric acid, a BARBITURATE used as an intermediate- to long-acting SEDATIVE and HYPNOTIC.

allocentric (al″o-sen′trik) focused on the thoughts and feelings of others; not egocentric.

allocheiria (al″o-ki′re-ah) allesthesia.

allochromasia (al″o-kro-ma′zhah) change in color of hair or skin.

allodynia (al″o-din′e-ah) pain produced by a non-noxious stimulus.

alloeroticism (al″o-ĕ-rot′ĭ-siz-em) 1. sexual feeling directed to another person, as opposed to AUTOEROTICISM. 2. a state of maturity characterized both by direction of erotic energies to another and also by the ability to form a love relationship with that other. adj., **alloerot′ic.**

alloerotism (al″o-er′o-tiz-em) alloeroticism.

allogeneic (al″o-jĕ-ne′ik) denoting individuals of the same species but of different genetic constitution (antigenically distinct); called also homologous.

allograft (al′o-graft) 1. homologous GRAFT. 2. a graft of tissue between individuals of the same species but of disparate genotype; types of donors are cadaveric, living related, and living unrelated (see under TRANSPLANTATION). Called also allogeneic graft and homograft.

allolalia (al″o-la′le-ah) any defect of speech of central origin.

alloplasty (al′o-plas-te) in psychoanalytic theory, adaptation by alteration of the external environment (alloplastic change). adj., **alloplas′tic.**

allopurinol (al″o-pūr′ĭ-nol) a drug that inhibits uric acid production and reduces serum and urinary URIC ACID levels; used for treatment of HYPERURICEMIA of GOUT and prophylaxis and treatment of hyperuricemia secondary to blood dyscrasias or cancer chemotherapy and of uric acid nephropathy, as well as for prophylaxis of KIDNEY STONE formation.

allorhythmia (al″o-rith′me-ah) irregularity of the pulse.

allosteric (al″o-ster′ik) pertaining to an effect produced on the biological function of a protein by a compound not directly involved in that function (an allosteric effector) or to regulation of an enzyme involving cooperativity between multiple binding sites (allosteric sites).

a. site that subunit of an enzyme molecule which binds with a nonsubstrate molecule, inducing a change in form or shape that results in inactivation of the enzyme for its substrate.

allotherm (al′o-therm) an organism whose body temperature changes with its environment.

WINDOW ON ALLIED HEALTH

The term "allied health" is used to classify more than 100 professions. Practitioners encompassed by this rubric provide all kinds of services, including primary care, and they work in all types of settings, including clinics, hospitals, laboratories, long-term care facilities, schools, and homes. Their responsibilities include: delivery of health or related services pertaining to the identification, evaluation, and prevention of diseases and disorders; dietary and nutrition services; rehabilitation; and health system management. A wide range of disciplines that are commonly identified as being part of allied health are: audiology, dental hygiene, dietetics, health information management, clinical laboratory science, nutrition, occupational therapy, physical therapy, radiologic technology, respiratory therapy, speech-language pathology, and surgical technology.

Many types of allied health professionals play vital roles in the acute care setting. For example, from the moment of admission to a health care facility, medical records will be generated and integrated with other types of patient data by individuals who specialize in health information management. Once admitted, patients typically will experience medical laboratory testing and diagnostic radiologic procedures as a means of aiding in the determination of treatment regimens. Following the acute phase of care, long-term rehabilitation therapy services typically will have to be provided.

Educational preparation in allied health is as diverse as the services provided. Some individuals enter their respective professions through hospital-based educational programs and spend one or two years in clinical training. Others attend college/university-based programs that culminate in associate, baccalaureate, master's, or doctorate degrees, depending on the profession involved.

As society in the United States continues to undergo demographic and epidemiological shifts, the education of these professionals has changed accordingly. An increased emphasis has been placed on enabling practitioners to work effectively with older segments of the population. The same holds true for enhancing the skills required to address the needs of minority and underserved groups that reside in both urban and rural areas. Simultaneously, efforts continue at these educational institutions to increase the amount of diversity among those entering the allied health workforce so that it will be more reflective of society at large.

THOMAS W. ELWOOD, Dr PH

allotransplantation allogeneic transplantation.

allotriogeustia (ah-lot″re-o-goos′te-ah) abnormal sense of taste or appetite.

allotropic (al″o-trop′ik) 1. exhibiting allotropism. 2. more preoccupied with the ideas, actions, and feelings of others than with oneself.

allotropism (ah-lot′ro-pizm) existence of an element in two or more distinct forms, sometimes with different physical properties.

allotropy (ah-lot′ro-pe) allotropism.

allowance (ah-low′ans) something permitted or allowed.

recommended daily a. term popularly used as a synonym for recommended dietary allowance.

recommended dietary a. **(RDA)** the amount of nutrient and calorie intake per day considered necessary for maintenance of good health, calculated for males and females of various ages and recommended by the Food and Nutrition Board of the National Research Council. See Appendices 4 and 5. Popularly called recommended daily allowance.

alloxan (ah-lok′san) an oxidized product of uric acid that tends to destroy the islet cells of the pancreas, thus producing diabetes. It has been obtained from intestinal mucus in diarrhea and has been used in nutrition experiments and as an antineoplastic AGENT.

alloy (al′oi) a solid mixture of two or more metals, or of one or more metals and certain metalloids, that are mutually soluble in the molten condition.

almotriptan (al″mo-trip′tan) a selective serotonin receptor agonist used as the malate salt in the acute treatment of migraine; administered orally.

aloe (al′o) 1. a succulent plant, of the genus *Aloe.* 2. the dried juice of leaves of various species of *Aloe,* used in various dermatologic and cosmetic preparations.

alopecia (al″o-pe′shah) loss of hair; baldness. The cause of simple baldness is not yet fully understood, although it is known that the tendency to become bald is limited almost entirely to males, runs in certain families, and is more common in certain racial groups than in others. Baldness is often associated with aging, but it can occur in younger men. MINOXIDIL has been approved as a topical treatment for male pattern baldness. Approximately one-third of the men undergoing this therapy have experienced hair regrowth. The effects of the drug take several months to develop and new hair growth may be limited; the hair is lost if treatment is discontinued. Hair transplants are also available to selected patients. Many men opt for no treatment.

Alopecia as an outcome of chemotherapy for a malignancy can be very distressing. The loss of hair usually is temporary and the hair will grow back after the course of treatment is completed. Male patients may feel more comfortable wearing a hat or cap when out in public. Female patients who wish to wear a wig are encouraged to obtain one that is lightweight and the same color as their hair. Having a hairdresser cut the wig to the patient's usual hair style can increase self-esteem. A kerchief or head scarf can be worn around the house if it is more comfortable than a wig. Receipts for wigs, hairpieces, and other headcovering should be saved; they are tax-deductible medical expenses when related to chemotherapy.

androgenetic a., a. androgene′tica a progressive, diffuse, symmetric loss of scalp hair. In men it begins in the twenties or early thirties with hair loss from the crown and the frontal and temple regions, ultimately leaving only a sparse peripheral rim of scalp hair *(male pattern alopecia* or *male pattern baldness)*. In females it begins later, with less severe hair loss in the front area of the scalp. In affected areas, the follicles produce finer and lighter terminal hairs until terminal hair production ceases, with lengthening of the anagen phase and shortening of the telogen phase of hair growth. The cause is unknown but is believed to be a combination of genetic factors and increased response of hair follicles to androgens.

a. area′ta hair loss in sharply defined areas, usually the scalp or beard.

a. ca′pitis tota′lis loss of all the hair from the scalp.

cicatricial a., a. cicatrisa′ta irreversible loss of hair associated with scarring, usually on the scalp.

congenital a., a. congenita′lis congenital absence of the scalp hair, which

may occur alone or be part of a more widespread disorder.

a. limina′ris hair loss at the hairline along the front and back edges of the scalp.

male pattern a. see ANDROGENETIC A.

moth-eaten a. syphilitic alopecia involving the scalp and beard and occurring in small, irregular scattered patches, resulting in a moth-eaten appearance.

symptomatic a., a. symptoma′tica loss of hair due to systemic or psychogenic causes, such as general ill health, infections of the scalp or skin, nervousness, or a specific disease such as typhoid fever, or to stress. The hair may fall out in patches, or there may be diffuse loss of hair instead of complete baldness in one area.

a. tota′lis loss of hair from the entire scalp.

a. universa′lis loss of hair from the entire body.

Alpers' disease (al′perz) polydystrophia cerebri.

alpha (al′fah) the first letter of the Greek alphabet, α; used to denote the first position in a classification system; as, in names of chemical compounds, to distinguish the first in a series of isomers, or to indicate the position of substituent atoms or groups; also used to distinguish types of radioactive decay, brain waves or rhythms, adrenergic receptors, and secretory cells that stain with acid dyes, such as the alpha cells of the pancreas.

a.-adrenergic blocking agent, a.-blocker, a.-blocking agent any of a group of drugs that selectively inhibit the activity of alpha RECEPTORS in the sympathetic nervous system. As with BETA-ADRENERGIC BLOCKING AGENTS, alpha-blocking agents compete with the CATECHOLAMINES at peripheral autonomic receptor sites. This group includes ERGOT and its derivatives, and PHENTOLAMINE.

a. chain disease the most common HEAVY CHAIN DISEASE, occurring predominantly in young adults in the Mediterranean area, and characterized by plasma cell infiltration of the lamina propria of the small intestine resulting in malabsorption with diarrhea, abdominal pain, and weight loss, or, exceedingly rarely, by pulmonary involvement. The gastrointestinal form is immunoproliferative small intestine disease.

a.-fetoprotein (AFP) a plasma PROTEIN produced by the fetal liver, yolk sac, and gastrointestinal tract and also by hepatocellular CARCINOMA, germ cell neoplasms, and other cancers in adults; elevated levels may also be seen in benign liver disease such as CIRRHOSIS and viral HEPATITIS. The serum AFP level is used to monitor the effectiveness of cancer treatment.

During pregnancy some AFP crosses from the amniotic fluid to the mother's blood. If the fetus has a NEURAL TUBE DEFECT, large amounts of AFP will be found in the amniotic fluid and maternal blood. Blood screening tests for serum AFP can thus be done as a first step in the screening process; if test results are positive, further testing is indicated to diagnose the defect.

a. particles a type of emission produced by the disintegration of a radioactive substance. The atoms of radioactive elements such as uranium and radium are very unstable, continuously breaking apart with explosive violence and emitting particulate and nonparticulate types of radiation. The alpha particles, consisting of two protons and two neutrons, have an electrical charge and form streams of tremendous energy when they are released from the disintegrating atoms. These streams of energy (alpha RAYS) can be used in treatment of various malignancies. See also RADIATION and RADIATION THERAPY.

alpha₂-antiplasmin (al″fah-an″tĭ-plaz′min) see ANTIPLASMIN.

alpha₁-antitrypsin (al″fah-an″tĭ-trip′sin) a member of the SERPIN group, a plasma protein (α₁-globulin), produced primarily in the liver. It inhibits the activity of elastase, cathepsin G, trypsin, and other proteolytic enzymes. Congenital deficiency of this protein is associated with development of emphysema in young adulthood. Written also α₁-antitrypsin. Called also alpha₁-proteinase inhibitor.

Alpha Eta (al′fah a′tah) the honor society for allied health professions.

alpha₂-macroglobulin (al″fah-mak′ro-glob″u-lin) α₂-macroglobulin.

alpha₁-proteinase inhibitor alpha₁-antitrypsin.

Alport's syndrome (al′ports) an autosomal dominant disorder marked by progressive nerve deafness, progressive pyelonephritis or glomerulonephritis, and occasionally ocular defects.

alprazolam (al-pra′zo-lam) a benzodiazepine ANTIANXIETY AGENT.

alprostadil (al-pros′tah-dil) name for PROSTAGLANDIN E₁ when used pharmaceutically as a vasodilator and platelet aggregation inhibitor; used for treatment of PATENT DUCTUS ARTERIOSUS and for diagnosis and treatment of impotence.

ALS antilymphocyte serum; amyotrophic lateral sclerosis.

Alström's syndrome (al′stromz) an autosomal recessive syndrome usually occuring after age 10, consisting of retinitis pigmentosa with nystagmus and early loss of central vision, deafness, obesity, and diabetes mellitus.

ALT alanine transaminase.

alteplase (al′tĕ-plās) a tissue plasminogen ACTIVATOR produced by recombinant DNA technology; used in therapy for acute MYOCARDIAL INFARCTION, acute ischemic STROKE, and acute pulmonary EMBOLISM, administered intravenously.

alteration change.

alternation (awl″ter-na′shun) interrupted occurrence, being interspersed with different or opposite events.

a. of generations metagenesis.

altitude sickness (al′tĭ-tūd) a syndrome caused by exposure to altitude high enough to cause significant HYPOXIA (lack of oxygen). At high altitudes the atmospheric pressure, and thus arterial oxygen content, are decreased. Called also high-altitude sickness and mountain sickness.

Acute altitude sickness may occur after a few hours' exposure to a high altitude. Mental functions may be affected; there may be lightheadedness and breathlessness; and eventually headache and prostration may occur. Older persons and those with pulmonary or cardiovascular disease are most susceptible. After a few hours or days of acclimation the symptoms will subside.

Chronic altitude sickness (called also Monge's disease and Andes disease) occurs in those living in the high Andes above 15,000 feet. It resembles POLYCYTHEMIA, but is completely relieved if the patient is moved to sea level.

altretamine (al-tret′ah-mēn) an antineoplastic AGENT used in the palliative treatment of ovarian carcinoma. It is structurally related to an ALKYLATING AGENT but does not act as one; its exact mechanism is unknown. Administered orally.

alum (al′um) a local astringent and styptic, prepared as an ammonium *(ammonium a.)* or potassium *(potassium a.)* compound; also used as an adjuvant in adsorbed vaccines and toxoids.

alumina (ah-loo′mĭ-nah) 1. aluminum oxide. 2. (in pharmaceuticals) aluminum hydroxide.

aluminosis (ah-loo″mĭ-no′sis) a form of PNEUMOCONIOSIS caused by aluminum-bearing dust in the lungs

aluminum (Al) (ah-loo′mĭ-num) a chemical element, atomic number 13, atomic weight 26.982. (See Appendix 6.) It occurs naturally in many foods in low concentrations and is also present in many pharmaceuticals and drinking water. High levels in the body can be toxic; see ALUMINUM POISONING.

a. acetate solution Burow's solution.

basic a. carbonate gel an aluminum hydroxide–aluminum carbonate gel, used as an antacid, for treatment of hyperphosphatemia in renal insufficiency, and to prevent phosphate urinary calculi.

a. chloride a topical astringent solution and antiperspirant.

a. chlorohydrate an antiperspirant; called also aluminum hydroxychloride.

a. hydroxide the hydroxide of aluminum, used as an ANTACID and phosphate BINDER; the official preparation is ALUMINUM HYDROXIDE GEL.

a. hydroxide gel a preparation of ALUMINUM HYDROXIDE in suspension or dried form, used as an ANTACID in the treatment of peptic ulcer and gastric hyperacidity and as a phosphate BINDER in treatment of phosphate nephrolithiasis.

a. hydroxychloride aluminum chlorohydrate.

a. oxide Al_2O_3, occurring naturally as various minerals; used in the production of abrasives, refractories, ceramics, catalysts, to strengthen dental ceramics, and in chromatography.

a. phosphate gel a water suspension of aluminum phosphate and some flavoring agents; used as a gastric antacid, astringent, and soothing agent.

a. poisoning the toxic effects of high levels of aluminum or its compounds in the body. In the gastrointestinal tract aluminum inhibits absorption of electrolytes; inhalation of aluminum fumes may cause pulmonary FIBROSIS; and aluminum in the bloodstream may lead to serious neurological symptoms, such as in dialysis ENCEPHALOPATHY.

a. silicate the silicate salt of aluminum, found in nature in several different hydrated forms that have pharmaceutical or dental uses; see ATTAPULGITE, FULLER'S EARTH, and KAOLIN.

a. subacetate a compound used as an astringent, diluted with water.

a. sulfate a compound used as an astringent solution and antiperspirant.

alveolalgia (al″ve-o-lal′jah) pain in the alveolus of a tooth after extraction; see also dry SOCKET.

alveolectomy (al″ve-o-lek′to-me) surgical excision of part of the alveolar process.

alveolitis (al″ve-o-li′tis) inflammation of a dental or pulmonary alveolus.

allergic a., extrinsic allergic a. hypersensitivity pneumonitis.

a. sic′ca doloro′sa dry socket.

alveolodental (al-ve″o-lo-den′tal) pertaining to teeth and the alveolar process.

alveolotomy (al″ve-ah-lot′ah-me) incision of the alveolar process.

alveolus (al-ve′o-lus), pl. *alve′oli* [L.] a little hollow, as the socket of a tooth, a follicle of an acinous gland, or a pulmonary alveolus. adj., **alve′olar.**

dental alveoli the cavities or sockets of either jaw, in which the roots of the teeth are embedded.

pulmonary alveoli small outpouchings along the walls of the alveolar sacs and alveolar ducts; through them, gas exchange takes place between alveolar gas and pulmonary capillary blood.

alveus (al′ve-us), pl. *al′vei* [L.] a canal or trough.

alymphia (ah-lim′fe-ah) deficiency or absence of lymph.

alymphocytosis (a-lim″fo-si-to′sis) deficiency of lymphocytes in the blood.

alymphoplasia (a-lim″fo-pla′zhah) failure of development of lymphoid tissue.

Alzheimer's disease (altz′hi-merz) irreversible DEMENTIA characterized by intellectual deterioration, disorganization of the personality, and functional disabilities in carrying out ACTIVITIES OF DAILY LIVING. The official name is now DEMENTIA OF THE ALZHEIMER TYPE. It is categorized as either *presenile (early onset)* or *senile (late onset)* depending on whether or not it begins by the age of 65, and is subcategorized on the basis of accompanying features, including delirium, delusions, depressed mood, behavioral disturbances, or none (uncomplicated).

Diagnosis is tentatively made on the basis of the symptoms presented and their progression over a period of time. Confirmation of the diagnosis of Alzheimer's disease can be made only by postmortem examination of brain tissue. The defining characteristics noted on autopsy are neurofibrillary tangles in the cytoplasm of neurons, neuritic plaques or deposits resulting from degeneration in the neural processes, and granulovacuolar degeneration in the neurons.

Etiology. The cause or causes of Alzheimer's disease are under investigation. Postmortem studies have revealed below normal levels of choline acetyltransferase; altered levels of the neurotransmitters acetylcholine, somatostatin, substance P, and norepinephrine; and higher than normal deposits of aluminum in cerebral tissue. It is hypothesized that there is no single cause of the disease. Age is the most important risk factor. Many researchers believe that genetics plays a role. APOLIPOPROTEIN e is also being actively studied as having a possible role.

Symptoms. Alzheimer's disease can progress slowly over a period of ten to fifteen years or it can become steadily worse in a matter of only a few years. In the early stages there are forgetfulness, especially of recent events, inability to learn or remember new information, impaired concentration, and deterioration in personal hygiene. Later as symptoms worsen, memory, language, and motor functions become increasingly impaired and the patient becomes more intellectually and physically disabled.

Perseveration, or continuous repetition of words or gestures, is characteristic of Alzheimer's disease in its later stages. Personality changes, incontinence, voracious appetite, and a compulsion to put everything in the mouth are other manifestations of the disease.

Treatment. At present there is no cure for Alzheimer's disease; therapies are aimed at relieving symptoms and managing behavior problems. There has been limited success in the use of drugs. TACRINE, DONEPEZIL, RIVASTIGMINE, or GALANTAMINE may slow progression of symptoms in the early stages. Research in this area is ongoing.

Patient Care. As cognitive and psychomotor functions become more impaired, the impact on family members or other caregivers becomes more profound. They will need continued guidance and support as physical care of the patient escalates from a part-time to a full-time responsibility. In the early stages the patient may be able to handle basic self-care functions and can live in the community and take care of personal financial and marketing chores with minimal help. However, the forgetfulness that accompanies Alzheimer's disease places the patient at a safety risk because of the tendency to wander and get lost. Later, assistance with activities of daily living such as eating, grooming, and toileting will be required. Eventually the patient will be unable to handle the most basic tasks of personal care, and all motor abilities and forms of communication will be lost.

Family members and other caregivers encounter emotional outbursts and progressive intellectual and physical deterioration that make the tasks of care even more challenging. Part-time or full-time help in the home usually is needed to give some respite to caregivers. They will also need guidance in the management of incontinence and help in coping with role reversals and their own feelings about the loss they have suffered

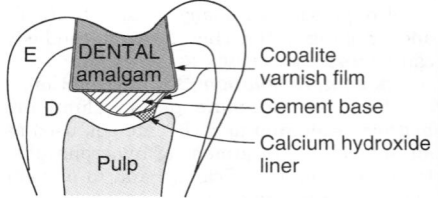

Varnish, liner, and base applications for use with dental amalgam that is not bonded to the cavity preparation walls. *E,* enamel; *D,* dentin. From Darby and Walsh, 1995.

and the burden of care that they bear. Eventually, it may be necessary to institutionalize the person with Alzheimer's disease. This can bring on feelings of guilt and a sense of failure on the part of the caregiver.

Educational materials and information on clinical trials are available from the Alzheimer's Disease Education and Referral Center (ADEAR) by writing them at P.O. Box 8250, Silver Spring MD 20807-8250, calling them at 1-800-272-3900, or consulting their web site at http://www.alzheimer.org.

Am americium.

AMA American Medical Association.

amacrine (am′ah-krĭn) without long processes.

amalgam (ah-mal′gam) an alloy of mercury with other metals; used in dental restorations. (See accompanying illustration.)

amalgamation (ah-mal″gah-ma′shun) trituration.

Amanita (am″ah-ni′tah) a genus of mushrooms, several species of which are poisonous. *A. phalloi′des,* the destroying angel or death cup, and the similar species *A. ver′na* and *A. viro′sa* produce a hemolysin and a mixture of peptide toxins such as PHALLOIDIN that cause irreversible damage to cardiac muscle, liver, and kidney cells. Symptoms are often delayed from six to 20 hours, and mortality ranges from 50 to 90 per cent. *A. musca′ria,* fly agaric, causes a drunkenlike intoxication and loss of consciousness but is rarely fatal. Initial signs of toxicity mimic those of parasympathetic stimulation and can be treated with atropine.

amantadine (ah-man′tah-dēn) an antiviral compound used as the hydrochloride salt to treat influenza A; also used as an antidyskinetic in the treatment of parkinsonism and drug-induced extrapyramidal reactions.

amastia (ah-mas′te-ah) congenital absence of one or both mammary glands.

amaurosis (am″aw-ro′sis) loss of sight without apparent lesion of the eye, as from disease of the optic nerve, spine, or brain. ***a. conge′nita, a. congenita of Leber, congenital a.*** hereditary blindness occurring at or shortly after birth, associated with an atypical form of diffuse pigmentation and commonly with optic atrophy and attenuation of the retinal vessels.

a. fu′gax sudden temporary or fleeting blindness.

Leber's congenital a. amaurosis congenita.

amaurotic (am″aw-rot′ik) pertaining to, or of the nature of, amaurosis.

a. familial idiocy former name for neuronal ceroid LIPOFUSCINOSIS.

ambenonium (am″be-no′ne-um) a cholinesterase INHIBITOR used to increase muscular strength in patients with MYASTHENIA GRAVIS.

ambidextrous (am″bĭ-deks′trus) able to use either hand with equal dexterity.

ambilateral (am″bĭ-lat′ter-al) pertaining to or affecting both sides.

ambilevous (am″bĭ-le′vus) unable to use both hands with equal dexterity.

ambisexual (am″bĭ-sek′shoo-al) denoting sexual characteristics common to both sexes, e.g., pubic hair.

ambivalence (am-biv′ah-lens) simultaneous existence of conflicting emotions, attitudes, ideas, or wishes toward a goal, object, or person. adj., **ambiv′alent.**

amblyaphia (am″ble-a′fe-ah) dullness of the sense of TOUCH.

amblygeustia (am″ble-go͞os′te-ah) hypogeusia.

Amblyomma (am″ble-om′ah) a genus of ticks, comprising approximately 100 species, which are vectors of various disease-producing organisms. *A. america′num* is the Lone Star tick, a species widely distributed from the southern United States to South America and is a vector of ROCKY MOUNTAIN SPOTTED FEVER. *A. cajennen′se* is found in many parts of the Americas and is a vector of São Paulo fever, a form of TYPHUS. *A. macula′tum* is the Gulf Coast tick, which mainly infests cattle and is widely distributed in the Americas; its bite causes painful sores that serve as sites of screwworm infections and secondary bacterial and fungal infections.

amblyopia (am″ble-o′pe-ah) impairment of vision not due to organic defect or refractive errors. adj., **amblyop′ic.**

color a. impairment of color vision due to toxic or other influences.

nutritional a. central or centrocecal scotomata due to poor nutrition; seen in persons with a history of ALCOHOL abuse and those with severe nutritional deprivation or vitamin B_{12} deficiency, as in PERNICIOUS ANEMIA. Complete recovery is possible with good diet and B vitamins; prolonged deficiency results in permanent loss of central vision.

amblyoscope (am′ble-o-skōp″) an instrument for measuring binocular vision or for training an amblyopic eye to take part in vision.

ambon (am′bon) the fibrocartilaginous edge of the socket in which the head of a long bone is lodged.

ambulant (am′bu-lant) ambulatory.

ambulatory (am′bu-lah-to″re) 1. walking or able to walk; not confined to bed. 2. of a condition or procedure, not requiring admission to a hospital for an overnight stay.

amcinonide (am-sin′o-nīd) a synthetic CORTICOSTEROID used for topical application in treatment of dermatoses.

amdinocillin (am-de′no-sil″in) a semisynthetic penicillin effective against many gram-negative bacteria and used in the treatment of urinary tract infections.

ameba (ah-me′bah), pl. *ame′bae, amebas* [L.] a minute, one-celled protozoan. The common laboratory example is *Amoeba proteus.* The usual cause of human amebic infection is *Entamoeba histolytica.*

amebiasis (am″e-bi′ah-sis) infection with amebae, especially *Entamoeba histolytica.* See illustration.

a. cu′tis cutaneous manifestation of amebiasis usually manifested as painful ulcers with distinct undermined borders surrounded by erythematous rims, principally seen in patients with active intestinal or hepatic disease.

intestinal a. amebic dysentery.

amebic (ah-me′bik) pertaining to, caused by, or of the nature of, an ameba.

a. dysentery a form of dysentery caused by *Entamoeba histolytica* and spread by contaminated food, water, and flies; it was formerly thought to be a purely tropical disease, but it is now known that many cases occur throughout the United States. It is usually less acute and virulent than BACILLARY DYSENTERY, but it frequently becomes chronic. Symptoms are diarrhea, fatigue, and intestinal bleeding. Complications include involvement of the liver, liver abscess, and pulmonary abscess. For treatment several drugs are available, for example, emetine hydrochloride and chloroquine, which may be used singly or in combination. Called also intestinal amebiasis.

amebicide (ah-me′bĭ-sīd) destructive to amebas.

ameboid (ah-me′boid) resembling an ameba.

ameboma (am″e-bo′mah) a tumorlike mass caused by granulomatous reaction in the intestines in AMEBIASIS.

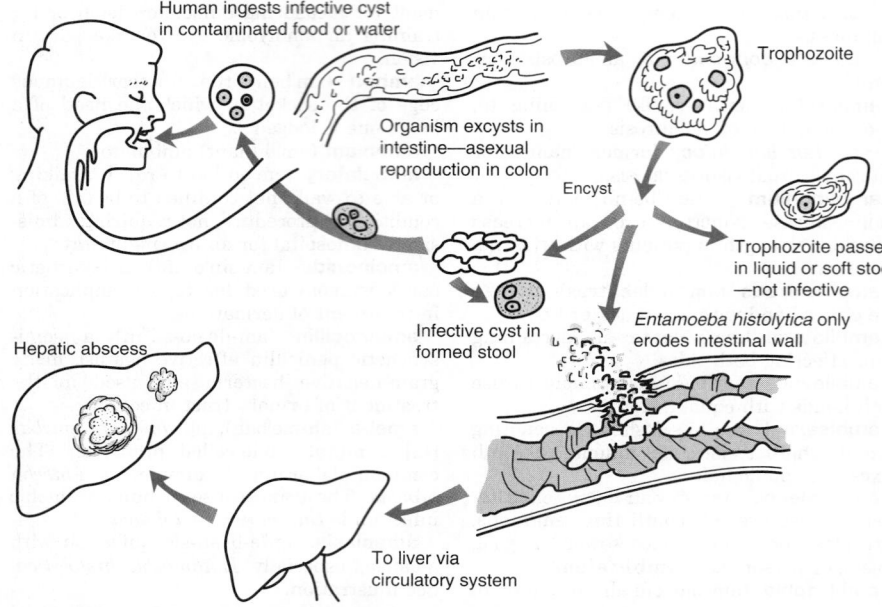

Human ingests infective cyst
in contaminated food or water

Trophozoite

Organism excysts in
intestine—asexual
reproduction in colon

Encyst

Trophozoite passed
in liquid or soft stool
—not infective

Entamoeba histolytica only
erodes intestinal wall

Infective cyst in
formed stool

Hepatic abscess

To liver via
circulatory system

Generalized life cycle of intestinal amebae. From Mahon and Manuselis, 2000.

amelanosis (ah-mel″ah-no′sis) complete lack of melanin in the tissues.

amelia (ah-me′le-ah) a developmental ANOMALY consisting of absence of one or more limbs.

amelification (ah-mel″ĭ-fĭ-ka′shun) the development of ameloblasts into enamel.

ameloblast (ah-mel′o-blast) a cell that takes part in forming dental enamel.

ameloblastoma (ah-mel″o-blas-to′mah) a locally invasive, highly destructive tumor of the jaw; called also adamantinoma.

pituitary a. craniopharyngioma.

amelodentinal (am″ĕ-lo-den′tĭ-nal) pertaining to dental enamel and dentin.

amelogenesis (ah-mel″o-jen′ĕ-sis) formation of dental enamel.

a. imperfec′ta a hereditary disease in which there is imperfect formation of enamel, resulting in brownish coloration and friability of the teeth.

amelogenic (am″ĕ-lo-jen′ik) forming enamel.

amelus (am′ĕ-lus) an individual exhibiting amelia.

amenorrhea (a-men″o-re′ah) absence of the menses. adj., **amenorrhe′al.** *Primary amenorrhea* refers to absence of the onset of menstruation at puberty or before age 18; it may be caused by underdevelopment or

malformation of the reproductive organs or by endocrine disturbances. When menstruation has begun and then ceases, the term *secondary amenorrhea* is used. The most common cause of this is pregnancy, but if that is excluded, there is usually a disturbance of the endocrine glands concerned with the menstrual process. General ill health, a change in climate or living conditions, emotional shock or, frequently, either the hope or fear of becoming pregnant can sometimes stop the menstrual flow.

dietary a. cessation of menstruation accompanying loss of weight due to dietary restriction, the loss of weight and of appetite being less extreme than in ANOREXIA NERVOSA and unassociated with psychological problems.

hypogonadotropic a. cessation of menstruation due to failure to maintain a critical body fat-to-lean ratio, resulting in hypothalamic suppression; seen in women who engage in strenuous exercise, such as athletes, dancers, and those who are excessively weight conscious.

lactation a. absence of the menses in association with lactation.

nutritional a. dietary a.

amensalism (a-men′sal-izm) interaction between coexisting populations of different species, one of which is adversely affected and the other unaffected.

amentia (a-men'shah) former term for profound mental retardation.

American Academy of Nursing (AAN) a working body of nursing leaders and scholars in education, practice, administration, and research. Fellows are elected to membership in the Academy based on their contributions to the nursing profession and health care. The Academy identifies emerging nursing and health care issues, promotes their scholarly exploration, challenges the status quo, and proposes creative solutions.

American Association of Colleges of Nursing (AACN) an organization founded in 1969 to improve the practice of professional nursing and its delivery in the public interest through advancing the quality of academic nursing education and strategic leadership in nursing. It has institutional membership rather than individual membership.

American Association of Retired Persons (AARP) the largest organization for older people in the United States. It serves the elderly through extensive lobbying at the federal level, maintaining a high-volume pharmaceutical service, publishing a variety of printed materials, and performing other services.

American Health Information Management Association (AHIMA) an organization founded in 1928 for individuals interested in health systems information management, biostatistics, classification systems, and systems analysis. An important function is the certification of medical record personnel as *registered record administrators* and *accredited record technicians* (see MEDICAL RECORDS ADMINISTRATOR). It also publishes the *Glossary of Health Care Terms* to standardize health care terminology. The address is 233 North Michigan Avenue, Suite 2150, Chicago, Illinois 60601-5800.

American Joint Committee on Cancer (AJCC) a nonprofit organization that creates and publishes systems of classification for CANCER staging, such as the TNM STAGING system and Collaborative Stage Data collection systems.

American Law Institute Formulation a section of the American Law Institute Model Penal Code: "A person is not responsible for criminal conduct if at the time of such conduct as a result of mental disease or defect he lacks substantial capacity either to appreciate the criminality [wrongfulness] of his conduct or to conform his conduct to the requirements of the law...the terms

'mental disease or defect' do not include an abnormality manifested only by repeated criminal or otherwise antisocial conduct [antisocial personality]." This test of criminal responsibility or closely related rules have been adopted by many state and federal jurisdictions.

American Nurses' Association (ANA) the national organization and official spokesperson for registered nurses. It was founded in 1896 and exists for the purposes of improving the standards of nursing and promoting the general welfare of professional nurses. The association is a federation of local organizations in the 50 states, the District of Columbia, Puerto Rico, and the Virgin Islands. The local organizations serve to implement the goals and carry out the functions of the national organization. The official publication of the ANA is the *American Nurse*. Offices of the organization are located at 600 Maryland Ave. SW, Suite 100 West, Washington, DC 20024. Information on ANA programs and services can be obtained by calling (800) 274– 4ANA.

American Occupational Therapy Association (AOTA) the professional association for OCCUPATIONAL THERAPISTS. The bylaws of the AOTA identify its purpose as "acting as an advocate for occupational therapy in order to enhance the health of the public in its medical, community, and educational environments through research, education, action, service, and the establishment and enforcement of standards." The address of the American Occupational Therapy Association is 4720 Montgomery Lane, P.O. Box 31220, Bethesda MD 20824-1220.

American Organization of Nurse Executives (AONE) the national organization for nurse executives and nurse managers, a subsidiary of the American Hospital Association. It provides direction and leadership for the advancement of nursing practice and patient care in organized health care systems, for achievement of excellence in nursing practice, and for shaping of policies affecting health care delivery from the perspective of the nurse executive.

American Society of Allied Health Professionals (ASAHP) an association of ALLIED HEALTH professionals dedicated to the improvement of health care by enhancing the effectiveness of education for allied health professionals and the public's appreciation and support of the professions. The expertise of allied health professionals spans every facet of the health care system, including such specialties as audiology, dental hygiene, dietetics, medical, radiological, and microbiological technology, nutrition, occupational and physical therapy, respiratory care, speech-language pathology, and other health care professions. ASAHP is located at 1101 Connecticut Avenue N.W., Suite 700, Washington D.C. 20036.

American Type Culture Collection (ATCC) an organization in Rockville, Maryland, established as a depository for reference cultures. It maintains and distributes authentic reference strains of algae, bacteria, fungi, protozoa, bacteriophages, and viruses, as well as cell lines of animal tissues.

americium (Am) (am″er-ish′e-um) a chemical element, atomic number 95, atomic weight 243. (See Appendix 6.)

Ames test (āmz) a test for mutagenic substances, in which a strain of *Salmonella typhimurium* that lacks the enzyme necessary for histidine synthesis is cultured in the absence of histidine and in the presence of the suspected mutagen. If the substance causes DNA damage resulting in mutations, some of the bacteria will regain the ability to synthesize histidine and will proliferate to form colonies.

ametria (ah-me′tre-ah) congenital absence of the uterus.

ametropia (am″ĕ-tro′pe-ah) an ocular disorder in which parallel rays fail to come to a focus on the retina. adj., **ametrop′ic.**

AMI acute myocardial infarction.

amiculum (ah-mik′u-lum), pl. *ami′cula* [L.] a dense surrounding coat of white fibers, as the sheath of the inferior olive and of the dentate nucleus.

amide (am′īd) any compound derived from ammonia by substitution of an acyl radical for hydrogen, or from an acid by replacing the —OH group by —NH₂.

amido (am′ĭ-do) the monovalent radical NH₂ united with the radical CO.

amifostine (am″ĭ-fos′tēn) a CHEMOPROTECTANT used to prevent renal toxicity in CISPLATIN chemotherapy and to reduce ESOPHAGITIS, XEROSTOMIA, and loss of taste in patients receiving radiation THERAPY for head, neck, or lung cancer.

Amigen (am′ĭ-jen) trademark for a protein HYDROLYSATE preparation for intravenous injection as a fluid and nutrient replenisher.

amikacin (am″ĭ-ka′sin) a semisynthetic AMINOGLYCOSIDE antibiotic derived from KANAMYCIN, used as the sulfate salt in the treatment of a wide range of infections due to susceptible gram-negative organisms.

amiloride (ah-mil′o-rīd) a potassium sparing DIURETIC, used as the hydrochloride salt, usually in combination with HYDROCHLOROTHIAZIDE, in the treatment of edema and hypertension and the prevention and treatment of hypokalemia.

amiloxate (am″il-ok′sāt) an absorber of ultraviolet B radiation, used topically as a SUNSCREEN.

amimia (a-mim′e-ah) loss of the power of expression by the use of signs or gestures.

amine (am′in, ah′mēn) an organic compound containing nitrogen.

biogenic a. bioamine.

sympathomimetic a's amines that mimic the actions of the sympathetic nervous system, the group includes the CATECHOLAMINES and drugs that mimic their actions.

vasoactive a's amines that cause VASODILATION and increase small vessel permeability, such as HISTAMINE and SEROTONIN.

amino (ah-me′no, am′ĭ-no) the monovalent radical NH₂, when not united with an acid radical.

a. acid any of a class of organic compounds containing the amino (NH₂) and the carboxyl (COOH) groups, occurring naturally in plant and animal tissues and forming the chief constituents of PROTEIN. Twenty amino acids are necessary for protein synthesis. Eleven (the *nonessential amino acids*) can be synthesized by the human body and thus are not specifically required in the diet: ALANINE, ARGININE, ASPARAGINE, ASPARTIC ACID, CYSTEINE, GLUTAMIC ACID, GLUTAMINE, GLYCINE, PROLINE, SERINE, and TYROSINE. Nine (the *essential amino acids*) cannot be synthesized by humans and thus are required in the diet: HISTIDINE, ISOLEUCINE, LEUCINE, LYSINE, METHIONINE, PHENYLALANINE, THREONINE, TRYPTOPHAN, and VALINE. (See accompanying illustration.) Protein foods that provide the essential amino acids are known as *complete proteins;* these include proteins from animal sources, such as meat, eggs, fish, and milk. Proteins that cannot supply the body with all the essential amino acids are known as *incomplete proteins;* these are the vegetable proteins most abundantly found in LEGUMES (peas and beans), as well as certain grains. Because different incomplete proteins lack different amino acids, specific combinations can provide all of the essential amino acids.

In certain inherited or acquired disorders of metabolism, specific amino acids accumulate in the blood (AMINOACIDEMIA) or are excreted in excess in the urine (AMINOACIDURIA). Urinary amino acid levels are increased in liver disease, muscular dystrophies, phenylketonuria (PKU), lead poisoning, and folic acid deficiency.

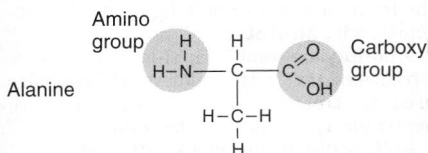

Structural formulas for some representative amino acids. From Applegate, 2000.

aminoacetic acid (ah-me′no-ah-se′tik) glycine.

aminoacidemia (ah-me″no-as″ĭ-de′me-ah) an excess of amino acids in the blood.

aminoacidopathy (ah-me″no-as″ĭ-dop′ah-the) any inborn ERROR of metabolism of AMINO ACIDS that produces a metabolic block that results in accumulation of one or more amino acids in the blood (AMINOACIDEMIA) or excess excretion in the urine (AMINOACIDURIA), or both.

aminoaciduria (ah-me″no-as″ĭ-du′re-ah) an excess of AMINO ACIDS in the urine; it may be either the *overflow type* caused by excessive levels in the blood, or the *renal type* caused by defective transport mechanisms in the renal tubules. Many types are called by the name of the amino acid plus the suffix -*uria,* such as CYSTINURIA, LYSINURIA, and TRYPTOPHANURIA.

aminobenzoate (ah-me″no-ben′zo-āt) *p*-aminobenzoate, any salt or ester of *p*-AMINOBENZOIC ACID; the potassium salt is administered orally as an antifibrotic in some dermatologic disorders and various substituted esters, such as PADIMATE O are used as topical sunscreens.

***p*-aminobenzoic acid (PAB) (PABA)** (ah-me″no-ben-zo′ik) a substance required for the synthesis of FOLIC ACID by many organisms; it is included in the B vitamin complex, although it is not an essential nutrient for humans. It is synthesized by many bacteria; sulfonamides act by blocking its synthesis; it also absorbs ultraviolet light, specifically UVB rays, and is used as *aminobenzoic acid* as a topical sunscreen.

γ-aminobutyric acid (GABA) (gam″ah-ah-me″no-bu-tēr′ik) an amino acid that is one of the principal inhibitory neurotransmitters in the central nervous system.

ε-aminocaproic acid (ep′sĭ-lon-ah-me″no-kah-pro′ik) an amino acid that is a potent inhibitor of plasminogen and plasmin and indirectly of fibrinolysis; used for treatment (as *aminocaproic acid*) of acute bleeding syndromes due to fibrinolysis and for the prevention and treatment of postsurgical hemorrhage.

aminoglutethimide (ah-me″no-gloo-teth′ĭ-mīd) an ANTIHORMONE that inhibits conversion of cholesterol to pregnenolone, thus reducing adrenocortical steroid synthesis; administered orally in treatment of CUSHING'S SYNDROME. It also inhibits conversion of androstenedione to estrone in peripheral tissues and is sometimes used as a component of hormonal THERAPY for advanced breast carcinoma.

aminoglycoside (ah-me″no-gli′ko-sīd) any of a group of antibacterial ANTIBIOTICS derived from species of *Streptomyces;* they interfere with the function of bacterial ribosomes. They contain an inositol moiety substituted with two amino or guanidino groups and with one or more sugars or aminosugars. The group includes AMIKACIN, GENTAMICIN, KANAMYCIN, NEOMYCIN, STREPTOMYCIN, and TOBRAMYCIN. They are used to treat infections caused by gram-negative organisms and are classified as bactericidal agents because of their interference with bacterial replication. All are highly toxic, requiring frequent monitoring of blood serum levels and careful observation of the patient for early signs of toxicity, particularly OTOTOXICITY and NEPHROTOXICITY.

***p*-aminohippurate** (ah-me″no-hip′u-rāt) a salt, conjugate base, or ester of *p*-aminohippuric acid; the sodium salt is used to measure effective renal plasma flow and to determine the functional capacity of the tubular excretory mechanism.

p-aminohippuric acid (PAH) (PAHA) (ah-me″no-hĭ-pūr′ik) a derivative of *p*-AMINOBENZOIC ACID, secreted primarily by renal tubular secretion; see also *p*-AMINOHIPPURATE.

aminolevulinic acid (ALA) (ah-me″no-lev″u-lin′ik) δ-aminolevulinic acid; a precursor of PORPHYRINS and HEMOGLOBIN; serum levels of this acid are elevated in LEAD POISONING and urinary levels are increased in some PORPHYRIAS. The hydrochloride salt is used as a topical photosensitizer in the treatment of nonhyperkeratotic actinic KERATOSES.

aminophylline (am″ĭ-no-fil′in) a mixture of THEOPHYLLINE and ETHYLENEDIAMINE, acting as a respiratory stimulant, smooth muscle relaxant, myocardial stimulant, and diuretic. It is used as a bronchodilator and also as an antidote to dipyridamole toxicity. Administration may be oral, intramuscular, intravenous, or rectal. If intravenous administration is too rapid it can cause circulatory collapse. Intramuscular administration should be done with caution because aminophylline is very irritating to the tissues. Oral administration must also be cautious because there could be gastric or urinary irritation.

aminoquinoline (ah-me″no-kwin′o-lēn) a heterocyclic compound derived from QUINOLINE by the addition of an amino group; the *4-aminoquinoline* and *8-aminoquinoline* derivatives are groups of antimalarial AGENTS.

aminosalicylate (ah-me″no-sah-lis′ĭ-lāt) any salt of *p*-aminosalicylic acid; they are antibacterials effective against mycobacteria and the sodium salt is used orally as a tuberculostatic.

aminosalicylic acid (-sal-ĭ-sil′ik) official pharmaceutical name for *p*-AMINOSALICYLIC ACID.

5-aminosalicylic acid (ah-me″no-sal″ĭ-sil′-ik) mesalamine.

p-aminosalicylic acid (PAS) (PASA) (ah-me″no-sal-ĭ-sil′ik) an analogue of *p*-aminobenzoic acid that inhibits folic acid synthesis in *Mycobacterium tuberculosis,* used in the treatment of TUBERCULOSIS, administered orally. In pharmacy it is officially called aminosalicylic acid. It enhances the potency of streptomycin and delays the development of bacilli resistant to streptomycin. Gastrointestinal irritation accompanied by anorexia, nausea, and vomiting may be reduced by administering the drug with food at mealtime.

Aminosol (ah-me′no-sol) trademark for an AMINO ACID preparation for intravenous injection.

aminotransferase (ah-me″no-trans′fer-ās) transaminase.

aminuria (am″ĭ-nu′re-ah) an excess of amines in the urine.

amiodarone (ah-me′o-dah-rōn″) a potassium channel blocking AGENT used orally or by intravenous infusion as the hydrochloride salt in treatment of ventricular ARRHYTHMIAS.

amitosis (am″ĭ-to′sis) direct cell division; simple cleavage of the nucleus without the formation of a spindle figure or chromosomes. adj., **amitot′ic.**

amitriptyline (am″ĭ-trip′tĭ-lēn) a tricyclic ANTIDEPRESSANT with sedative effects; also used in treating enuresis, chronic pain, peptic ulcer, and bulimia nervosa.

AML acute myelogenous leukemia.

amlexanox (am-lek′sah-noks) a topical antiulcerative agent used in treatment of recurrent aphthous STOMATITIS.

amlodipine (am-lo′dĭ-pēn) a CALCIUM CHANNEL BLOCKING AGENT administered orally in the form of the besylate salt in treatment of hypertension and chronic stable and vasospastic ANGINA.

ammeter (am′me-ter) an instrument for measuring in amperes the strength of a current flowing in a circuit.

ammonia (ah-mo′nyah) a colorless alkaline gas, NH_3, with a pungent odor and acrid taste, and soluble in water.

a. N 13 ammonia in which a portion of the molecules are labeled with ^{13}N; used in positron emission TOMOGRAPHY of the cardiovascular system, brain, and liver.

ammoniate (ah-mo′ne-āt) to combine with ammonia.

ammoniemia (ah-mo″ne-e′me-ah) hyperammonemia.

ammonium (ah-mo′ne-um) a hypothetical radical, NH_4, forming salts analogous to those of the alkaline metals.

a. carbonate a mixture of ammonium compounds used as a liquefying expectorant in the treatment of chronic bronchitis and similar lung disorders. It is sometimes used as a reflex stimulant in "smelling salts" because of the strong ammonia odor it gives off.

a. chloride colorless or white crystals, with a cool, salty taste, used as an expectorant because it liquefies bronchial secretions. In the body it is changed to UREA and HYDROCHLORIC ACID, and thus is useful in acidifying the URINE and increasing the rate of urine flow. Excessive dosage may produce ACIDOSIS.

a. lactate lactic acid neutralized with ammonium hydroxide, applied topically in the treatment of ichthyosis vulgaris and xerosis.

ammoniuria (ah-mo″ne-u′re-ah) hyperammonuria.

amnesia (am-ne′zhah) pathologic impairment of memory. Amnesia is usually the result of physical damage to areas of the brain from injury, disease, or alcoholism. Psychologic factors may also cause amnesia; a shocking or unacceptable situation may be too painful to remember, and the situation is then retained only in the subconscious mind. The technical term for this is REPRESSION. (See also DISSOCIATIVE DISORDERS.)Rarely is the memory completely obliterated. When amnesia results from a single physical or psychologic incident, such as a concussion suffered in an accident or a severe emotional shock, the victim may forget only the incident itself; the victim may be unable to recall events occurring before or after the incident or the order of events may be confused, with recent events imputed to the past and past events to recent times. In another form, only certain isolated events are lost to memory.

Amnesia victims usually have a good chance of recovery if there is no irreparable brain damage. The recovery is often gradual, the memory slowly reclaiming isolated events while others are still missing. Psychotherapy may be necessary when the amnesia is due to a psychologic reaction.

anterograde a. impairment of memory for events occurring after the onset of amnesia. Unlike RETROGRADE AMNESIA, it is the inability to form new memories.

circumscribed a. loss of memory for all events during a discrete, specific period of time. Called also localized amnesia.

continuous a. loss of memory for all events after a certain time, continuing up to and including the present.

dissociative a. the most common of the DISSOCIATIVE DISORDERS; it is usually a response to some stress, such as a threat of injury, an unacceptable impulse, or an intolerable situation. The patient suddenly cannot recall important personal information and may wander about without purpose and in a confused state.

Persons with a dissociative disorder may at times forget what they are doing or where they are; when they regain self-awareness, they cannot recall what has taken place. A less severe form than amnesia is sleepwalking. Dissociative disorders are very likely an attempt by the mind to shield itself from the anxiety caused by an unresolved conflict. The patient, upon encountering a situation that may be symbolic of this inner conflict, goes into a form of trance to avoid experiencing the conflict.

generalized a. loss of memory encompassing the individual's entire life.

lacunar a. partial loss of memory; amnesia for certain isolated experiences.

localized a. 1. circumscribed amnesia. 2. lacunar amnesia.

post-traumatic a. amnesia resulting from concussion or other head trauma. Called also traumatic amnesia. See also AMNESTIC SYNDROME.

psychogenic a. dissociative amnesia.

retrograde a. inability to recall events that occurred prior to the episode precipitating the disorder. Unlike ANTEROGRADE AMNESIA, it is the loss of memories of past events.

selective a. loss of memory for a group of related events but not for other events occurring during the same period of time.

transient global a. a temporary episode of short-term memory loss without other neurological impairment.

traumatic a. post-traumatic amnesia.

amnestic (am-nes′tik) characterized by or pertaining to amnesia.

a. disorders mental disorders characterized by acquired impairment in the ability to learn and recall new information, sometimes accompanied by inability to recall previously learned information, and not coupled to dementia or delirium. The disorders are subclassified on the basis of etiology as amnestic disorder due to a general medical condition, substance-induced persisting amnestic disorder, and amnestic disorder not otherwise specified.

a. syndrome a mental disorder characterized by impairment in short- and long-term memory, with anterograde and sometimes retrograde AMNESIA, occurring in a normal state of consciousness. Disorientation, confabulation, and a lack of insight into the memory deficit may be present. The most common cause is thiamine deficiency associated with chronic alcohol abuse (alcohol amnestic disorder, KORSAKOFF'S SYNDROME), but the syndrome may result from any pathologic process causing bilateral damage to certain structures in the medial temporal lobe and diencephalon, including head trauma, brain tumors, infarction, cerebral hypoxia, carbon monoxide poisoning, and herpes simplex encephalitis.

amniocentesis (am″ne-o-sen-te′sis) transabdominal perforation of the amniotic sac in order to obtain a sample of amniotic fluid, which contains cells shed from the skin of the fetus as well as biochemical substances. Analyses of changes in chemical and cellular

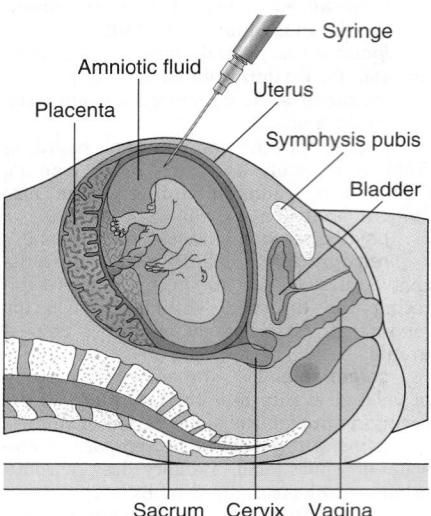

Syringe
Amniotic fluid
Uterus
Placenta
Symphysis pubis
Bladder
Sacrum   Cervix   Vagina

A diagram of the technique of amniocentesis. From Mueller and Young, 2001.

composition of the fluid are helpful in assessing the maturation and viability of the fetus. Amniocentesis also provides for prenatal diagnosis of certain genetically transmitted errors of metabolism, congenital abnormalities, and chromosomal disorders. It is feasible to detect by amniocentesis the presence of over 40 different types of inherited disorders in embryos and fetuses as young as 16 weeks' gestation. (See accompanying illustration.) A common indication for amniocentesis is the suspected presence of ERYTHROBLASTOSIS FETALIS, which results from incompatibility of Rh factors in the fetal and maternal blood. Samples of amniotic fluid are analyzed for concentrations of protein and bilirubin. The higher the concentration, the stronger the evidence that erythrocytes are being destroyed, and measures must be taken to forestall the effects of the disorder on the fetus.

Another biochemical study involves measuring the level of ALPHA-FETOPROTEIN (AFP) in the amniotic fluid. Abnormally high levels indicate an open defect of the spine, e.g., spina bifida or anencephaly.

Because of the ability to determine fetal maturation by amniotic fluid studies, it is possible to predict whether an infant will suffer from HYALINE MEMBRANE DISEASE at birth. A favorable ratio of lecithin to sphingomyelin indicates sufficient lung maturity.

Patient Care During and After Amniocentesis. While the procedure for removal of amniotic fluid has minimal risk for the fetus and mother, there are slight risks of bleeding, leakage of fluid, or infection. There also is a remote chance of miscarriage.

When being performed for prenatal diagnosis, amniocentesis is usually offered to women 35 years or older, women with a child with a chromosomal abnormality, parents with a child with neural tube defect, and women with elevated serum alpha-fetoprotein, or when one parent has a chromosomal abnormality or is a carrier for a metabolic disease. Parents who agree to amniocentesis must be prepared to make a decision whether or not to abort the fetus if the laboratory tests indicate the presence of a birth defect. Frequently, however, parents who have a high risk for having an abnormal child find that the developing fetus is normal and the prognosis for delivery of a healthy baby is excellent.

During the procedure, the physician inserts a long pudendal needle into the mother's abdomen and into the amniotic cavity, avoiding the fetus and the placenta (which is located via ultrasonography). Local anesthesia is used to minimize discomfort. The patient is cautioned not to move during the procedure lest the needle become displaced. A syringe is attached and fluid is withdrawn. It is sometimes necessary to repeat the procedure because of an insufficient sample or unsuccessful laboratory testing. The repeat procedure is done several days after the first.

Following amniocentesis the patient is observed for changes in blood pressure, excessive leakage of fluid, and signs of infection. Hemorrhage from the placenta must be considered a possibility if the blood pressure begins to drop. Increased fetal activity or other signs of fetal distress such as changes in the fetal heart rate must be reported to the physician at once as they may warrant immediate measures such as delivery of the infant if it is considered to be viable. The Centers for Disease Control and Prevention publish a useful patient education booklet on amniocentesis titled "Amniocentesis for Prenatal Chromosomal Diagnosis," which can be obtained by request from the CDC: Chronic Disease Division, Bureau of Epidemiology, Atlanta, GA 30333.

amniochorial (am″ne-o-kor′e-al) pertaining to amnion and chorion.

amniogenesis (am″ne-o-jen′ĕ-sis) the development of the amnion.

amniography (am″ne-og′rah-fe) radiography of the pregnant uterus after injection of an opaque contrast medium into the amniotic fluid.

amnioinfusion (am″ne-o-in-fu′zhun) 1. injection of solutions into the amniotic fluid, usually to induce abortion. 2. infusion of normal saline to increase intra-amniotic fluid in cases of oligohydramnios or rupture of the membranes; this may reduce the number and severity of variable decelerations due to cord compression during labor; see also FETAL MONITORING. 3. in the NURSING INTERVENTIONS CLASSIFICATION, a nursing INTERVENTION defined as the infusion of fluid into the uterus during labor to relieve umbilical cord compression or to dilute meconium-stained fluid.

amnion (am′ne-on) the innermost fetal membrane, which forms a sac filled with AMNIOTIC FLUID that surrounds the embryo and later the fetus; as it enlarges it gradually obliterates the chorionic cavity and enfolds the umbilical cord. Called also bag of waters. (See accompanying illustration.)

a. nodo′sum a nodular condition of the fetal surface of the amnion, usually appearing near the insertion of the cord; it may be associated with multiple congenital abnormalities, especially hypoplastic kidneys and oligohydramnios.

amnionitis (am″ne-o-ni′tis) inflammation of the amnion, a manifestation of an intra-uterine infection, often associated with prolonged membrane rupture and long labor.

amniorrhea (am″ne-o-re′ah) escape of the amniotic fluid.

amniorrhexis (am″ne-o-rek′sis) rupture of the amnion.

amnioscope (am′ne-o-skōp″) an endoscope that, by introduction into the cervical canal, permits direct visualization of the fetus and amniotic fluid.

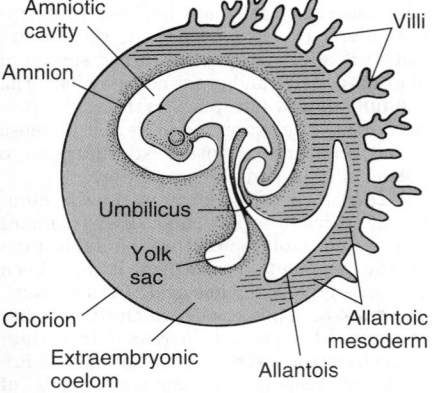

Amnion, chorion, and other embryonic membranes surrounding the embryo of a placental mammal. From Dorland's, 2000.

amniote (am′ne-ōt) any animal that develops an AMNION.

amniotic (am″ne-ot′ik) pertaining to the amnion.

a. band syndrome a condition characterized by isolated or multiple constriction defects of the fingers, toes, limbs, and less frequently the skull, face, or viscera. It results from a tear of unknown etiology in the amnion, which allows amniotic fluid and fetal parts to escape from the amnion into the chorion. When the amnion and chorion are separated, strands from either the maternal amnion or the fetal chorion may entangle fetal parts. As the fetus grows the strands become more constrictive, causing defects.

a. fluid the albuminous fluid contained in the amniotic sac; called also liquor amnii and, informally, waters. The fetus floats in this fluid, which serves as a cushion against injury from sudden blows or movements and helps maintain a constant body temperature for the fetus. Normally the fluid is clear and slightly alkaline; discoloration or excessive cloudiness may indicate fetal distress or disease, as in erythroblastosis fetalis in which fluid is usually greenish yellow. The amount varies from 500 to 1500 ml.

An excessive amount of amniotic fluid (more than 2000 ml) is called *hydramnios*; the amount may be as much as several gallons. The cause of this condition is unknown but it frequently accompanies multiple pregnancy or some congenital defect of the fetus, especially hydrocephalus and meningocele.

An abnormally small amount of amniotic fluid is referred to as *oligohydramnios*; there may be less than 100 ml of fluid present. The cause is unknown. The condition may produce pressure deformities of the fetus, such as clubfoot or torticollis. Adhesions may result from direct contact of the fetus with the amnion.

Removal of a sample of amniotic fluid from the pregnant uterus is called AMNIOCENTESIS.

amniotome (am′ne-o-tōm) an instrument for puncturing the fetal membranes.

amniotomy (am″ne-ot′ah-me) surgical rupture of the fetal membranes.

Patient Care. Amniotomy results in drainage of the amniotic fluid and thus hastens labor by allowing the head to fit more snugly into the dilating cervix. There is little or no discomfort accompanying the procedure; the patient will require only an explanation of what is to be done, and proper draping and cleansing of the perineum.

Labels in illustration: Amniotic cavity, Amnion, Villi, Umbilicus, Yolk sac, Chorion, Allantoic mesoderm, Extraembryonic coelom, Allantois

After amniotomy the expelled fluid is carefully observed for color. A yellow or green color indicates fetal distress. The fetal heart rate is monitored for signs of fetal distress because amniotomy increases the risk of a prolapsed cord.

amobarbital (am″o-bahr′bĭ-tal) a BARBITURATE used as a short-acting SEDATIVE and HYPNOTIC. Effects develop rapidly and the drug is eliminated more quickly than other barbiturates.

amodiaquine (am″o-di′ah-kwin) an antimalarial, administered orally as the hydrochloride salt in the treatment of MALARIA, especially falciparum malaria.

Amoeba (ah-me′bah) a genus of ameboid protozoa, most of which are free-living. Those parasitic in humans and once included in this genus have been assigned to other genera.

amoric (ah-mo′rik) without particles.

amorph (a′morf) an inactive mutant gene, i.e., one that produces no detectable product.

amorphia (ah-mor′fe-ah) the state of being amorphous.

amorphism (ah-mor′fizm) amorphia.

amorphous (ah-mor′fus) having no definite form; shapeless.

amoxapine (ah-mok′sah-pēn) a tricyclic ANTIDEPRESSANT of the dibenzoxazepine class; administered orally.

amoxicillin (ah-moks″ĭ-sil′in) an ANTIBIOTIC that is a PENICILLIN analogue similar in action to AMPICILLIN but more efficiently absorbed from the gastrointestinal tract and therefore requiring less frequent dosage and not as likely to cause diarrhea.

Amoxil (ah-mok′sil) trademark for preparations of AMOXICILLIN, an ANTIMICROBIAL.

AMP adenosine monophosphate.

3′,5′-AMP, cyclic AMP cyclic adenosine monophosphate.

amp. ampere, ampule.

ampere (A) (am′pēr) the base SI UNIT of electric current strength, defined in terms of the force of attraction between two parallel conductors carrying current.

ampere-hour a unit of electric charge, being the amount of charge that passes a given point as a current of one ampere in one hour.

amperemeter (am′pēr-me″ter) ammeter.

amphetamine (am-fet′ah-mēn) 1. a white crystalline powder used as a central nervous system stimulant. It is odorless and has a slightly bitter taste. 2. any of a group of drugs closely related to this substance and having similar actions, such as METHAMPHETAMINE and DEXTROAMPHETAMINE. See also DRUG ABUSE and DRUG DEPENDENCE.

amphi- word element [Gr.], *both; on both sides.*

amphiarthrosis (am″fe-ahr-thro′sis) a joint in which the surfaces are connected by disks of fibrocartilage, as between vertebrae.

Amphibia (am-fib′e-ah) a class of animals that breathe by means of gills in the larval state but after metamorphosis breathe by means of lungs.

amphicentric (am″fĭ-sen′trik) beginning and ending in the same vessel.

amphidiarthrosis (am″fĭ-di′ahr-thro′sis) a joint having the nature of both ginglymus and arthrodia, as that of the lower jaw.

amphitrichous (am-fit′rĭ-kus) having flagella at each end.

amphophil (am′fo-fil) a cell or element that is amphophilic.

amphophilic (am″fo-fil′ik) staining with either acid or basic dyes.

amphoric (am-for′ik) pertaining to a bottle; resembling the sound made by blowing across the neck of a bottle.

amphoteric (am″fo-ter′ik) capable of acting as both an acid and a base; capable of neutralizing either bases or acids.

amphotericin B (am″fo-ter′ĭ-sin) an antifungal AGENT and antibiotic used to treat deep-seated fungal infections, especially HISTOPLASMOSIS, and also to treat cutaneous and mucocutaneous CANDIDIASIS. It may be applied topically or administered intravenously or by intracavitary instillation. Anorexia, chills, fever, and headache may occur as side effects. Renal damage with evidence of renal tubular acidosis occurs, but usually clears when the drug is discontinued.

amphotony (am-fot′o-ne) hypertonia of the entire autonomic nervous system.

ampicillin (am″pĭ-sil′in) a broad-spectrum ANTIBIOTIC, a PENICILLIN of synthetic origin, adminsistered orally as the base or intramuscularly or intravenously as the sodium salt. It is effective against a broad spectrum of gram-positive and gram-negative bacteria.

amplification (am″plĭ-fĭ-ka′shun) the process of making larger, such as the increase of an auditory or visual stimulus, as a means of improving its perception.

DNA a. artificial increase in the number of copies of a particular DNA fragment into millions of copies through replication of the segment into which it has been cloned, a type of nucleic acid AMPLIFICATION.

gene a. a process by which the number of copies of a gene is increased in certain cells because extra copies of DNA are made in response to certain signals of cell development or of stress from the environment. In humans this process is seen most often in malignant cells.

nucleic acid a. amplification of a specific NUCLEIC ACID sequence, such as to test for presence of a given virus or bacteria in a sample. Types include DNA AMPLIFICATION, LIGASE CHAIN REACTION, and POLYMERASE CHAIN REACTION.

amplitude (am′plĭ-tōōd) 1. largeness, fullness; wideness or breadth of range or extent. 2. in conventional TOMOGRAPHY, the motion of the x-ray tube (with the cassette moving in the opposite direction) during the x-ray exposure.

amprenavir (am-pren′ah-vir) an HIV protease INHIBITOR used in the treatment of human immunodeficiency VIRUS (HIV) infection; administered orally.

ampule (am′pūl) a small, hermetically sealed flask or container made of glass or polyethylene, e.g., one containing medication for parenteral administration.

ampulla (am-pul′ah), pl. *ampul′lae* [L.] a flasklike dilatation of a tubular structure, especially of the expanded ends of the semicircular canals of the ear.

   a. chy′li cisterna chyli.

   a. duc′tus deferen′tis, Henle's a. the enlarged and tortuous distal end of the ductus deferens.

   hepatopancreatic a. ampulla of Vater; a flasklike cavity in the major duodenal papilla into which the common bile duct and pancreatic duct open. (See accompanying illustration.)

   Lieberkühn's a. the blind termination of the lacteals in the villi of the intestines.

   ampul′lae membrana′ceae membranous ampullae: the dilatations at one end of each of the three semicircular ducts.

   ampul′lae os′seae the dilatations at one of the ends of the semicircular canals.

   phrenic a. the dilatation at the lower end of the esophagus.

   a. of rectum the dilated portion of the rectum just proximal to the anal canal.

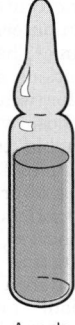

Ampule.

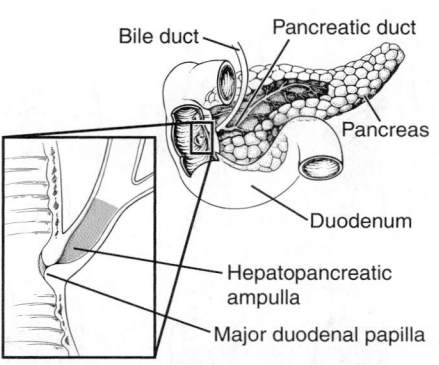

Hepatopancreatic ampulla, receiving the common bile and pancreatic ducts and entering the duodenum at the major duodenal papilla. From Dorland's, 2000.

   a. of Thoma one of the small terminal expansions of an interlobar artery in the pulp of the spleen.

   a. of uterine tube the longest and widest portion of the fallopian (uterine) tube between the infundibulum and the isthmus of the tube.

   a. of Vater hepatopancreatic ampulla; the term "ampulla of Vater" is often mistakenly used instead of "papilla of Vater," or major duodenal papilla.

amputation (am″pu-ta′shun) the removal of a limb or other appendage or outgrowth of the body. The most common indication for amputation of an upper LIMB is severe trauma. Blood vessel disorders such as ATHEROSCLEROSIS, often secondary to DIABETES MELLITUS, account for the greatest percentage of amputations of the lower LIMB. Other indications may include malignancy, infection, and gangrene.

   There are two general types of surgical procedure for amputation: (1) the closed or "flap" amputation and (2) the open or "guillotine" amputation. The latter is often required when infection is present and there is a need for free drainage from the operative site. A second surgical procedure involving stump (or residual limb) revision or closure is needed after the guillotine procedure. This is done only after the infection has been eliminated.

   Patient Care. The goal of patient care for the amputee is total rehabilitation with attainment of full function and normal active life. Such total rehabilitation is not always possible because of physical and mental limitations of the patient. It requires that the patient be physically and psychologically able to accept and adapt to a PROSTHESIS and

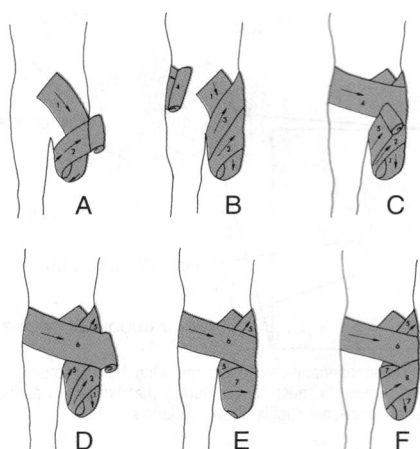

Amputation. Bandaging on above-knee amputation stump. *A,* Use 6" elastic bandage. Enclose medial, distal end of stump. Apply pressure via bandage to end of stump. Use diagonal, not circular turns. *B,* Turn No. 3 must be high in groin and then turn made around waist to hold No. 3 in place. Do not pull hip into flexion. (A second 6" roll may be needed.) *C,* Turn No. 5 must be high in groin and a loop made around waist again. *D,* See diagram. *E,* Enclose lateral, distal end of stump. (A 4" roll may be needed.) Continue diagonal and figure-of-8 turns around stump. *F,* Continue turns to shape end of stump. (Courtesy of University of Washington Department of Prosthetics, from booklet Prosthetics-Orthotics.)

that each member of the health care team fulfill his or her responsibilities in preventing complications and in preparing the patient for optimum use of an artificial limb. Some patients, because of age or disease, do not have the necessary energy, muscular coordination, or mental capacity to undertake prosthetic training.

Preoperative Care. Unless time is a factor, as in emergency cases demanding immediate surgery, the preoperative care of the potential amputee should include emotional and vocational aspects as well as the physical. If patients are fully involved in plans for their rehabilitation, understand what is expected of them, and know the regimen of exercise and skills they will need to develop, their chances of full recovery and achievement of independence will be greatly enhanced. Much emotional support and encouragement can be offered by other amputees who are successfully mastering their prosthesis and making progress toward their goal of total rehabilitation.

Patients undergoing amputation will need help in dealing with the changes in body image as they adjust to the loss of a limb. They should be encouraged and given the opportunity to express feelings of anxiety, grief, anger, and depression, and given guidance in working toward a healthy acceptance of their handicap.

In general, physical preparation of the patient undergoing surgical amputation includes measures to promote optimum health and well-being, to establish nutritional and fluid balances, and to increase muscular strength and endurance levels. A program of exercises may be started to help the patient develop skill in using an overhead trapeze, crutches, and a walker and transferring from wheelchair to bed.

Postoperative Care. The residual limb is watched for hemorrhage, edema, infection, and ischemia. Some bleeding is not unusual but should rarely be more than a modest red stain on the dressing. Ischemia may be caused by a constricting dressing or the development of edema. Ischemia is recognized by the presence of excessive pain.

Traction was formerly commonly used after guillotine amputations but is rarely used nowadays. Generally such stumps are closed by delayed primary closure on the fourth or fifth day after amputation to save time in the hospital and accelerate rehabilitation.

Fitting of a prosthesis may be *delayed* or *immediate* depending on the condition of the patient and the reason for the amputation. Immediate fitting of a prosthesis involves the application of a rigid plastic dressing which serves to protect the stump and prevent edema. The dressing is similar to a cast and the patient will require cast CARE. The temporary prosthetic device is applied at the time of surgery and includes a pylon and foot-ankle assembly.

Early ambulation is a major advantage of immediate fitting of a prosthesis. Other benefits arise from the local compression exerted by the dressing. This serves to inhibit bleeding, to mold and help shrink the stump, and to reduce phantom sensations, pain, and contractures. Unfortunately, not all amputees are candidates for immediate fitting. The technique is not advised for amputations above the knee or above the elbow, for weak and debilitated patients, or for those who are mentally or emotionally unable to cooperate with efforts at rehabilitation. The procedure also requires the services of prosthetic experts.

The more conventional, and probably more frequently chosen, technique of delayed prosthetic fitting requires special care of the stump and a gradual preparation of the patient for weight-bearing and ambulation. During the immediate postoperative period the stump dressings are changed or reinforced as ordered. The stump usually is wrapped with elastic bandages or covered with stump socks. The bandages are checked frequently for signs of bleeding and for slippage, which may lead to a tourniquet effect and the occlusion of blood supply. Exercises are started as soon as possible, regardless of the surgical approach, in order to strengthen the muscles and prevent contractures.

The patient with amputation of an upper limb also may receive immediate or delayed fitting of a prosthesis. When the surgeon has chosen the delayed fitting technique, the patient requires stump care similar to that for the lower limb except that an upper limb stump is bandaged more loosely, especially when amputation was the result of trauma. Exercises are begun the day after surgery and within ten to fourteen days the patient is fitted with a temporary prosthesis.

above-elbow (A-E) a. amputation of the upper limb between the elbow and the shoulder.

above-knee (A-K) a. transfemoral amputation.

below-elbow (B-E) a. amputation of the upper limb between the wrist and the elbow.

below-knee (B-K) a. transtibial amputation

Chopart's a. amputation of the foot, with the calcaneus, talus, and other parts of the tarsus being retained.

cineplastic a. kineplasty.

closed a. one in which flaps are made from skin and subcutaneous tissue and sutured over the bone end of the stump; called also flap amputation.

congenital a. absence of a limb at birth, attributed to constriction of the part by an encircling band during intrauterine development.

a. in contiguity amputation at a joint.

a. in continuity amputation of a limb elsewhere than at a joint.

Dupuytren's a. amputation of the upper LIMB at the shoulder joint.

flap a. closed amputation.

flapless a. guillotine amputation.

Gritti-Stokes a. amputation of the lower LIMB at the knee through condyles of the femur.

guillotine a. one in which the entire cross-section is left open (flapless) for dressing; called also flapless or open amputation.

Hey's a. amputation of the foot between the tarsus and metatarsus.

interpelviabdominal a. amputation of the lower LIMB with excision of the lateral portion of the pelvic girdle.

interscapulothoracic a. amputation of the upper LIMB with excision of the lateral portion of the shoulder girdle.

kineplastic a. kineplasty.

Lisfranc's a. amputation of the foot between the metatarsus and tarsus.

major a. amputation of the lower limb above the ankle or of the upper limb above the wrist.

minor a. amputation of a hand or foot, or of a part thereof.

open a. guillotine amputation.

pulp a. pulpotomy.

racket a. one in which there is a single longitudinal incision continuous below with a spiral incision on either side of the limb.

root a. excision of the root of a tooth; amputation of the root of a single-rooted tooth is called APICOECTOMY, and that of one root of a two-rooted mandibular tooth is HEMISECTOMY. Called also radectomy and radiectomy.

spontaneous a. loss of a part without surgical intervention, as in LEPROSY, AINHUM, and certain other conditions.

Syme's a. disarticulation of the foot with removal of both malleoli.

transfemoral a. amputation of the lower leg between the knee and the hip. Called also above-knee (A-K) amputation.

transtibial a. amputation of the lower leg between the ankle and the knee. Called also below-knee (B-K) amputation

traumatic a. the sudden, accidental removal of a limb or appendage. A limb that is properly cared for may be reimplanted. It should be placed in a plastic bag, and if ice is available the bag containing the limb should be placed in a larger one that contains ice and water.

Tripier's a. amputation of the foot through the calcaneus.

amrinone (am'rĭ-nōn) inamrinone.

amsacrine (am'sah-krēn) an antineoplastic AGENT that inhibits DNA synthesis; used to treat some forms of leukemia.

amusia (a-mu'ze-ah) loss of ability to produce (motor amusia) or to recognize (sensory amusia) musical sounds.

AMWA American Medical Writers' Association.

amyelia (a″mi-e'le-ah) congenital absence of the spinal cord.

amyelinic (ah-mi″ĕ-lin'ik) without myelin.

amyelonic (ah-mi″ĕ-lon'ik) 1. having no spinal cord. 2. having no marrow.

amyelus (ah-mi'ĕ-lus) a fetus with no spinal cord.

amygdala (ah-mig'dah-lah) 1. an almond-shaped structure. 2. CORPUS AMYGDALOIDEUM.

amygdalin (ah-mig′dah-lin) a glycoside from kernels and pits of bitter almonds, apricots, cherries, peaches, and apples, as well as certain other plant parts. Crushed and moistened residues release an enzyme that catalyzes a chemical reaction leading to release of HYDROGEN CYANIDE, so that excessive ingestion can be toxic. Preparations of amygdalin have been alleged to be anticancer agents, but this has never been scientifically proven. See also LAETRILE.

amygdaline (ah-mig′dah-lin) 1. like an almond. 2. tonsillar.

amyl nitrite (am′il ni′trīt) a volatile, flammable liquid with a pungent ethereal odor. It is administered by inhalation for the treatment of CYANIDE POISONING, producing methemoglobin which binds cyanide, and as a diagnostic aid in tests of reserve cardiac function and diagnosis of certain HEART MURMURS. It is abused to produce euphoria or sexual stimulation.

amyl(o)- word element [Gr.], *starch.*

amylaceous (am″ĭ-la′shus) composed of or resembling starch.

amylase (am′ĭ-lās) an enzyme that catalyzes the hydrolysis of starch into simpler compounds. The α-amylases occur in animals and include pancreatic and salivary amylase; the β-amylases occur in higher plants. Measurement of serum α-amylase activity is an important diagnostic test for acute and chronic pancreatitis.

amylogenesis (am″ĭ-lo-jen′ĕ-sis) the formation of starch. adj., **amylogen′ic.**

amyloid (am′ĭ-loid) 1. resembling starch; characterized by starchlike staining properties. 2. the pathologic extracellular proteinaceous substance deposited in amyloidosis; it is a waxy eosinophilic material. Amyloid deposits are composed primarily of straight, nonbranching fibrils arranged either in bundles or in a feltlike meshwork; each fibril is composed of identical polypeptide chains in stacked sheets. There are two major biochemical types of amyloid protein: *amyloid light chain protein* and *amyloid A protein,* as well as others seen less often.

amyloidosis (am″ĭ-loi-do′sis) the deposition in various tissues of AMYLOID. This protein is almost insoluble and once it infiltrates the tissues they become waxy and nonfunctioning. Primary, or immunocyte-derived, amyloidosis is thought to be due to some obscure metabolic disturbance in which there is an abnormal protein in the plasma; the tissues most often affected are cardiac and smooth and skeletal muscle tissue. Secondary, or reactive systemic, amyloidosis is related to chronic suppuration, especially those types associated with tuberculosis, lung abscess, osteomyelitis, or bronchiectasis; it may also occur in association with chronic noninfectious inflammatory disease, such as rheumatoid arthritis. The most common sites of deposition are the spleen, kidney, liver, and adrenal cortex.

The symptoms of amyloidosis appear insidiously and progress slowly. They depend on the specific organ affected, and frequently in secondary amyloidosis they are overshadowed by symptoms of the disease causing the disorder. Primary systemic amyloidosis is treated symptomatically; there is no cure, and death usually occurs within 3 years of the onset. Heart failure is the most common cause of death. Secondary amyloidosis is best treated by eliminating the underlying cause. This includes control of suppuration by effective use of antibiotic drugs.

dialysis a., hemodialysis-associated a. that occurring in patients on long-term HEMODIALYSIS, caused by the deposition of beta$_2$-microglobulin, which cannot be removed from the blood by dialysis, in the joints, synovial membranes, and tendon sheaths. Manifestations include CARPAL TUNNEL SYNDROME and ARTHRITIS.

amylopectin (am″ĭ-lo-pek′tin) the insoluble constituent of starch; the soluble constituent is amylose.

amylopectinosis (am″ĭ-lo-pek′tĭ-no′sis) glycogen storage disease (type IV), a condition in which deficiency of the brancher enzyme amylo-1:4,1:6-transglucoside results in cirrhosis of the liver, hepatosplenomegaly, and progressive hepatic failure and death. Called also Andersen's disease.

amylophagia (am″ĭ-lo-fa′jah) the habit of eating starch, such as laundry starch, a form of PICA.

amylorrhea (am″ĭ-lo-re′ah) the presence of an abnormal amount of starch in the feces.

amylose (am′ĭ-lōs) 1. any carbohydrate other than a glucose or saccharose. 2. the soluble constituent of starch, as opposed to amylopectin.

amyoplasia (ah-mi″o-pla′zhah) lack of muscle formation or development.

a. conge′nita generalized lack in the newborn of muscular development and growth, with contracture and deformity at most joints.

amyostasia (ah-mi″o-sta′zhah) a tremor of the muscles.

amyotrophia (ah-mi″o-tro′fe-ah) amyotrophy.

amyotrophic lateral sclerosis a progressive neurologic disease characterized by degeneration of cell bodies of the lower motor NEURONS in the gray matter of the anterior horns of the spinal cord, some brainstem motor neurons, and the pyramidal tracts. Called also Lou Gehrig's disease.

The disease presents in adulthood, usually between the ages of 40 and 70, and affects men two to three times more often than women. The initial symptom is weakness of skeletal muscles, especially in the limb. As the disease progresses the patient has difficulty swallowing and talking, with dyspnea as the accessory muscles of respiration are affected. Eventually muscles atrophy and the patient becomes a functional quadriplegic. Mentation is not affected, so that the patient remains alert and aware of functional loss and the inevitable outcome. Although there may be periods of remission, the disease usually progresses rapidly, with death in 2 to 5 years. The cause of ALS is not known and there is no cure. Treatment is intended to provide symptomatic relief, prevent complications, and maintain optimal function as long as possible.

Patient Care. For the most part, ALS patients are cared for at home and are hospitalized only for diagnosis, when severe dysphagia demands an esophagostomy or gastrostomy for feeding, or when medical treatment is necessary for acute respiratory problems.

Intervention is planned and implemented according to each patient's needs at specific times during the course of the illness. In general, the major problems encountered are those related to (1) dysphagia and the need to meet nutritional requirements and avoid aspiration, (2) dyspnea and maintenance of blood gases within normal range, (3) aphasia and impaired verbal communication, (4) weakness, impaired mobility, and activity intolerance, (5) constipation, (6) pain and discomfort due to muscle cramps, and (7) alteration in self-concept and body image.

The patient and family also will need assistance in managing home care, coping with the effects of the illness, and maintaining optimal functioning in the patient. Community health nurses and home health care professionals and paraprofessionals should be available to provide a variety of services including physical therapy, occupational therapy, social services, mental health care, and medical and nursing care.

A resource agency that can provide assistance and information to ALS patients and their families is the Amyotrophic Lateral Sclerosis Association, 21021 Ventura Blvd., Suite 321, Woodland Hills, CA 91364-2206, (800) 782–4747; http://www.alsa.org.

amyotrophy (a″mi-ot′ro-fe) a painful condition with wasting and weakness of muscle, commonly involving the deltoid muscle.

Amytal (am′ĭ-tal) trademark for preparations of AMOBARBITAL, a short-acting SEDATIVE and HYPNOTIC.

amyxia (ah-mik′se-ah) absence of mucus.

amyxorrhea (ah-mik″so-re′ah) absence of mucous secretion.

An anode.

ANA antinuclear antibody; American Nurses Association.

ana (an′ah) [Gr.] of each, used in prescription writing; abbreviated $\overline{AA}$.

ana- word element [Gr.], *upward; again; backward; excessively.*

anabiosis (an″ah-bi-o′sis) restoration of life processes after their apparent cessation.

anabolism (ah-nab′o-lizm) the constructive phase of METABOLISM, in which the body cells synthesize protoplasm for growth and repair; the opposite of CATABOLISM. The manner in which this synthesis takes place is directed by the genetic code carried by the molecules of deoxyribonucleic acid (DNA). The "building blocks" for this synthesis of protoplasm are obtained from amino acids and other nutritive elements in the diet. adj., **anabol′ic.**

anacidity (an″ah-sid′ĭ-te) abnormal lack or deficiency of acid.

gastric a. achlorhydria.

anaclisis (an″ah-kli′sis) physical and emotional dependence on another for protection and gratification; used to refer to the normal dependence of an infant on its mother or to excessive leaning on others for emotional support by an older individual. adj., **anaclit′ic.**

anacrotism (ah-nak′rŏ-tizm) a pulse anomaly evidenced by a prominent notch on the ascending limb of the pulse tracing. adj., **anacrot′ic.**

anadipsia (an″ah-dip′se-ah) intense THIRST; see HYPERDIPSIA and POLYDIPSIA.

anadrenalism (an″ah-dre′nal-izm) absence or failure of adrenal function.

anaerobe (an′er-ōb) an organism that lives and grows in the absence of molecular oxygen. (See accompanying table.) adj., **anaero′bic.**

facultative a. a microorganism that can live and grow with or without molecular oxygen.

obligate a. an organism that can grow only in the complete absence of molecular oxygen.

anagen (an′ah-jen) the first phase of the hair CYCLE, during which synthesis of the HAIR takes place.

ANAEROBES AT VARIOUS ANATOMICAL SITES	
Anaerobe	Site
Bacteroides spp.	Oral Cavity Upper Respiratory Tract Urethra Vagina Colon
Clostridium spp.	Colon
Fusobacterium spp.	Oral Cavity Upper Respiratory Tract Urethra
Peptostreptococcus spp.	Upper Respiratory Tract Skin Urethra Vagina Colon
Veillonella spp.	Oral Cavity Upper Respiratory Tract

anagrelide (an-ag′rĕ-līd) an agent used in the form of the hydrochloride salt to reduce elevated platelet counts and the risk of THROMBOSIS in treatment of hemorrhagic THROMBOCYTHEMIA; administered orally.

anakatadidymus (an″ah-kat″ah-did′ĭ-mus) a deformed twin fetus, separated above and below, but united in the trunk.

anakusis (an″ah-ku′sis) total DEAFNESS.

anal (a′nal) relating to the anus.

analbuminemia (an″al-bu″mĭ-ne′me-ah) absence or deficiency of serum albumins.

analeptic (an″ah-lep′tik) 1. a drug that acts as a stimulant to the central nervous system, such as CAFFEINE or AMPHETAMINE. 2. a restorative medicine.

analgesia (an″al-je′ze-ah) absence of sensibility to pain, particularly the relief of pain without loss of consciousness; absence of pain or noxious stimulation.

   continuous epidural a. continuous injection of an anesthetic solution into the sacral and lumbar plexuses within the epidural space to relieve the pain of childbirth, in general surgery to block the pain pathways below the navel, or to relieve chronic unremitting pain.

   epidural a. analgesia induced by introduction of the analgesic agent into the epidural space of the vertebral canal.

   infiltration a. infiltration ANESTHESIA.

   patient controlled a. **(PCA)** an apparatus used to relieve acute pain. It consists of a pump attached to an intravenous or subcutaneous injection site and filled with multiple doses of medication that are available when the system is activated by the patient. The pump is programmed to "lock-out" the patient for specified intervals making overdosage unlikely.

   patient controlled epidural a. patient controlled ANALGESIA in which a narcotic or local anesthetic is administered into the epidural space via a catheter.

   relative a. in dental anesthesia, a maintained level of conscious sedation short of general anesthesia, usually induced by inhalation of nitrous oxide and oxygen.

   transdermal a. a method of pain control in which a patch with a rate-controlling membrane is applied to the skin; the medication is deposited in the upper layers of the skin where it is absorbed into the systemic circulation.

analgesic (an″al-je′zik) 1. relieving pain. 2. pertaining to analgesia. 3. an agent that relieves pain without causing loss of consciousness.

   narcotic a. opioid analgesic.

   nonsteroidal antiinflammatory a. **(NSAIA)** nonsteroidal antiinflammatory drug.

   opiate a., opioid a. any of a class of compounds that bind with a number of closely related specific receptors (opioid RECEPTORS) in the central nervous system to block the perception of pain or affect the emotional response to pain; such compounds include OPIUM and its derivatives, as well as a number of synthetic compounds, and are used for moderate to severe pain. Chronic administration or abuse may lead to dependence.

analgia (an-al′jah) painlessness. adj., **anal′gic.**

anality (a-nal′ĭ-te) the psychic organization of all the sensations, impulses, and personality traits derived from the anal stage of psychosexual development.

analog (an′ah-log) 1. pertaining to an electronic system in which a continuous electrical signal is used to carry nonelectrical information (such as sound), which is represented by variations in the voltage or current that are in direct correlation to the information carried. See also DIGITAL. 2. analogue.

analogous (ah-nal′o-gus) resembling or similar in some respects, as in function or appearance, but not in origin or development.

analogue (an′ah-log) 1. a part or organ having the same function as another, but of different evolutionary origin. 2. a chemical compound having a structure similar to that of another but differing from it in respect to a certain component; it may have similar or opposite action metabolically. Also spelled analog.

nucleoside a. a structural analogue of a nucleoside, a category that includes both purine analogues and pyrimidine analogues.

purine a. a structural analogue of one of the purine BASES (PURINE, ADENINE, or GUANINE); MERCAPTOPURINE and THIOGUANINE are used as ANTINEOPLASTICS and AZATHIOPRINE is an IMMUNOSUPPRESSIVE. The antiviral agent VIDARABINE is an analogue of the ADENINE nucleoside ADENOSINE.

pyrimidine a. a structural analogue of one of the pyrimidine BASES (CYTOSINE, THYMINE, or URACIL); FLUOROURACIL and CYTARABINE are important ANTINEOPLASTIC agents.

analogy (ah-nal′o-je) the quality of being analogous; resemblance or similarity in function or appearance, but not in origin or development.

analysand (ah-nal′ĭ-sand) a person undergoing psychoanalysis.

analysis (ah-nal′ĭ-sis), pl. *anal′yses* 1. separation into component parts. 2. psychoanalysis. adj., **analyt′ic.**

activity a. the breaking down of an activity into its smallest components for the purpose of assessment.

bivariate a. statistical procedures that involve the comparison of summary values from two groups on the same variable or of two variables within a group.

blood gas a. see BLOOD GAS ANALYSIS.

chromosome a. see CHROMOSOME.

concept a. examination of the attributes of a concept as it occurs in ordinary usage in order to identify the meanings attached to the concept.

content a. a systematic procedure for the quantification and objective examination of qualitative data, such as written or oral messages, by the classification and evaluation of terms, themes, or ideas; for example, the measurement of frequency, order, or intensity of occurrence of the words, phrases, or sentences in a communication in order to determine their meaning or effect.

correlational a. a statistical procedure to determine the direction of a relationship (positive or negative correlation) between two variables and the strength of the relationship (ranging from perfect correlation through no correlation to perfect inverse correlation and expressed by the absolute value of the correlation coefficient).

a. of covariance (ANCOVA) a variation of analysis of variance that adjusts for confounding by continuous variables.

data a. the reduction and organization of a body of data to produce results that can be interpreted by the researcher; a variety of quantitative and qualitative methods may be used, depending upon the nature of the data to be analyzed and the design of the study.

ego a. in psychoanalytic treatment, the analysis of the strengths and weaknesses of the EGO, especially its DEFENSE MECHANISMS against unacceptable unconscious impulses.

gait a. see GAIT ANALYSIS.

gastric a. see GASTRIC ANALYSIS.

multiple-locus variable number of tandem repeat a. (MLVA) a laboratory tool designed to recognize tandem REPEATS and other qualities in the GENOME of an individual to provide a high resolution DNA FINGERPRINT for the purpose of identification.

multivariate a. statistical techniques used to examine more than two variables at the same time.

power a. a statistical procedure that is used to determine the number of required subjects in a study in order to show a significant difference at a predetermined level of significance and size of effect; it is also used to determine the power of a test from the sample size, size of effect, and level of significance in order to determine the risk of Type II ERROR when the null HYPOTHESIS is accepted.

qualitative a. the determination of the nature of the constituents of a compound or a mixture of compounds.

quantitative a. determination of the proportionate quantities of the constituents of a compound or mixture.

SNP a. analysis of single nucleotide POLYMORPHISMS to assess artificially produced genetic modifications or identify different strains of an organism.

transactional a. a type of psychotherapy based on an understanding of the interactions (transactions) between patient and therapist and between patient and others in the environment; see also TRANSACTIONAL ANALYSIS.

a. of variance ANOVA; a statistical test used to examine differences among two or more groups by comparing the variability between the groups with the variability within the groups.

variance a. the identification of patient or family needs that are not anticipated and the actions related to these needs in a system of managed CARE. There are four kinds of origin for the variance: patient-family origin, system-institutional origin, community origin, and clinician origin.

vector a. analysis of a moving force to determine both its magnitude and its direction, e.g., analysis of the scalar electrocardiogram to determine the magnitude and direction of the electromotive force for one complete cycle of the heart.

analyst (an′ah-list) 1. one who performs analysis. 2. psychoanalyst.

analyte (an′ah-līt) a substance or material determined by a chemical analysis.

anamnesis (an″am-ne′sis) [Gr.] 1. recollection. 2. a medical or psychiatric patient case history, particularly using the patient's recollections. Compare CATAMNESIS.

anamnestic (an″am-nes′tik) 1. pertaining to anamnesis. 2. aiding the memory.

anamniotic (an″am-ne-ot′ik) having no AMNION.

ANA-PAC the political action committee of the American Nurses' Association.

anaphase (an′ah-fāz) the third stage of division of the nucleus of a cell in either MEIOSIS or MITOSIS.

anaphia (an-a′fe-ah) lack or loss of the sense of touch.

anaphoresis (an″ah-fo-re′sis) movement of charged particles toward the positive pole (anode) in electrophoresis.

anaphoria (an″ah-for′e-ah) the tendency to tilt the head downward, with visual axes deviating upward, on looking straight ahead.

anaphrodisiac (an″af-ro-diz′e-ak) 1. repressing sexual desire. 2. a drug that represses sexual desire.

anaphylactic (an″ah-fi-lak′tik) pertaining to or affected by ANAPHYLAXIS.

 a. reaction anaphylaxis.

 a. shock a serious and profound state of shock brought about by hypersensitivity (ANAPHYLAXIS) to an ALLERGEN such as a drug, foreign protein, or toxin. Sometimes it occurs upon second injection of a patient with a previously injected serum or protein.

anaphylactogen (an″ah-fi-lak′to-jen) a substance that produces ANAPHYLAXIS.

anaphylactogenesis (an″ah-fi-lak′to-jen′ĕ-sis) the production of anaphylaxis. adj., **anaphylactogen′ic.**

anaphylactoid (an″ah-fi-lak′toid) resembling ANAPHYLAXIS.

 a. reaction a reaction resembling generalized anaphylaxis but not caused by IgE-mediated allergic reaction but rather by a nonimmunologic mechanism.

anaphylatoxin (an″ah-fil′ah-tok″sin) a substance produced by complement activation that causes the release of histamine and other mediators of immediate hypersensitivity from basophils and mast cells, thereby producing signs and symptoms of immediate hypersensitivity (anaphylaxis) without involvement of IgE.

anaphylaxis (an″ah-fi-lak′sis) an unusual or exaggerated allergic REACTION of an organism to foreign protein or other substances. Substances most likely to cause this include drugs such as antibiotics, local anesthetics, and codeine; drugs prepared from animals, such as insulin, adrenocorticotropic hormone, and enzymes; diagnostic agents, such as iodinated x-ray contrast media; biologicals used to provide immunity, such as vaccines, antitoxins, and gamma globulin; protein foods; the venom of bees, wasps, and hornets; and pollens, molds, and animal dander. The latex in gloves or Foley catheters may cause a reaction in sensitive individuals.

 Physiologic Basis. Anaphylaxis is an allergen-reagin reaction brought about by large quantities of IgE antibodies (IMMUNOGLOBULINS) that respond to the presence of foreign agents. Individuals who have an anaphylactoid type of IMMUNE RESPONSE have a familial predisposition to overreact in the presence of an allergen because of their tendency to produce an overabundance of IgE antibodies. When an allergen enters the body *reagins* (IgE antibodies), which are attached to cells throughout the body, interact with the allergens. This interaction is destructive to some of the body's cells. If the interaction is severe, the outcome can be fatal.

 During the interaction mast cells and eosinophils release histamine, slow-reacting substance of anaphylaxis (SRS-A), bradykinin, and enzymes. Histamine brings about bronchospasm, widespread peripheral vasodilation, and increased permeability of the capillaries. SRS-A causes increased constriction of the bronchioles and bronchi. Bradykinin has effects similar to those of histamine. Together they promote collapse of the vascular network by permitting the loss of fluid from the blood vessels into the interstitial fluid compartment.

 Clinical Manifestations. If the allergen comes into contact with cell-bound IgE in the respiratory tract, the tissues of the mucosa release chemical mediators that produce the symptoms of ASTHMA and HAY FEVER. An insect bite or sting can produce localized swelling, redness, and itching, or a more severe systemic reaction.

 Local anaphylactic reactions usually produce mildly irritating symptoms, which should not be ignored because the reaction can rapidly escalate into a systemic response involving cells throughout the body. The patient may then experience generalized itching, swelling, and urticaria. As the process continues, respiration is impaired because of bronchospasm and laryngeal edema. If an airway is not maintained and supplemental oxygen provided, the person will die of respiratory failure.

Another life-threatening series of events is related to vascular collapse resulting from a shift in body fluid. The symptoms are hypotension, decreasing levels of consciousness, tachycardia, and diminished production of urine. Without effective treatment these symptoms progress to profound shock and death.

Treatment and Patient Care. Mild anaphylaxis can be treated with ANTIHISTAMINES, local applications of cold to minimize swelling, and topical applications of medications to relieve itching and soothe the skin. *All* anaphylactic reactions require careful assessment and monitoring, and the patient should be instructed to seek additional help if he or she experiences dizziness, heart palpitations, or prolonged or spreading edema anywhere in the body. The drug of choice in the initial treatment of severe anaphylaxis is EPINEPHRINE, administered intravenously, subcutaneously, sublingually, or by intermittent positive pressure breathing. The mode of administration is governed by the urgency of the situation and the presenting symptoms. Epinephrine causes bronchodilation, reduces laryngeal spasm, and elevates the blood pressure.

Steroid therapy is initiated to counteract the effects of histamine by decreasing capillary permeability. Acting as ANTIINFLAMMATORY agents, steroids also stabilize mast cells and prevent further release of chemical mediators.

Supportive measures include administration of intravenous fluids and plasma to restore intravascular fluid volume. Pressor agents, such as DOPAMINE, NOREPINEPHRINE, and ISOPROTERENOL, are given to increase and maintain blood pressure.

The best way to control anaphylaxis is by preventing it from happening in the first place, but this is not always possible. A person engaging in normal activities outside the clinical setting can accidentally come in contact with an allergen. An allergic individual should be prepared for such an event by understanding his or her allergy and knowing what actions to take. Those with known atopic allergies should wear a medical identification necklace or bracelet, and those who undergo systemic reactions should carry with them at all times a kit containing DIPHENHYDRAMINE (BENADRYL), a syringe and needle, and vials of epinephrine. These kits require a written prescription from a primary health care provider.

In the clinical setting, all health care personnel should be alert to the need for identifying patients with known allergies and communicating this information to their co-workers. Emergency equipment should be readily available in all places where drugs or diagnostic agents with a risk of provoking anaphylaxis are administered.

active a. that produced by injection of a foreign protein.

antiserum a., passive a. that resulting from injection of serum of a sensitized person into a normal person.

passive cutaneous a. PCA; localized anaphylaxis passively transferred by intradermal injection of an antibody and, after a latent period (about 24 to 72 hours), intravenous injection of the homologous antigen and Evans blue dye; blueing of the skin at the site of the intradermal injection is evidence of the permeability reaction. Used in studies of antibodies causing immediate hypersensitivity reactions.

reverse a. that following injection of antigen, succeeded by injection of antiserum.

anaplasia (an″ah-pla′zhah) loss of differentiation of cells and their orientation to each other, a characteristic of tumor cells; called also dedifferentiation and undifferentiation.

anaplastic (an″ah-plas′tik) characterized by anaplasia.

anapophysis (an″ah-pof′ĭ-sis) an accessory vertebral process.

Anaprox (an′ah-proks) trademark for a preparation of NAPROXEN sodium, a NONSTEROIDAL ANTIINFLAMMATORY DRUG used in treatment of ARTHRITIS, acute attacks of GOUT and CALCIUM PYROPHOSPHATE DEPOSITION DISEASE, pain, dysmenorrhea, vascular HEADACHES, and BURSITIS and TENDINITIS.

anaptic (an-ap′tik) pertaining to or characterized by loss of the sense of touch.

anarithmia (an″ah-rith′me-ah) inability to count, due to a lesion of the brain.

anarthria (an-ahr′thre-ah) severe dysarthria resulting in speechlessness.

anasarca (an″ah-sahr′kah) generalized massive edema.

anastomosis (ah-nas″to-mo′sis), pl. *anastomo′ses* [Gr.] 1. communication between two tubular organs. 2. surgical, traumatic, or pathologic formation of a connection between two normally distinct structures. adj., **anastomot′ic.**

arteriovenous a. 1. anastomosis between an artery and a vein. (See accompanying illustration.) 2. arteriovenous shunt.

crucial a. an arterial anastomosis in the upper part of the thigh, formed by the anastomotic branch of the sciatic artery, the internal circumflex artery, and the first perforating and transverse portions of the external circumflex artery.

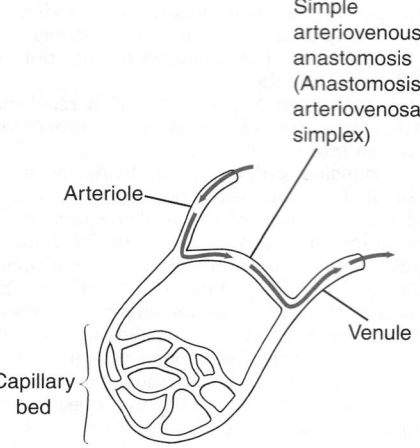

Simple arteriovenous anastomosis (Anastomosis arteriovenosa simplex)

Arteriole

Venule

Capillary bed

Simple arteriovenous anastomosis. From Dorland's, 2000.

end-to-end a. 1. an anastomosis connecting the end of an artery and that of some other vessel, either directly or with a synthetic graft. 2. anastomosis of two sections of colon, such as with partial colectomy or when an ileostomy is closed.

end-to-side a. an anastomosis connecting the end of one vessel with the side of a larger one.

heterocladic a. one between branches of different arteries.

ileorectal a. surgical anastomosis of the ileum and rectum after total colectomy, as is sometimes performed in the treatment of ulcerative colitis.

intestinal a. establishment of a communication between two formerly distant portions of the intestine.

anastrozole (ah-nas′trah-zōl″) an aromatase INHIBITOR used for treatment of advanced breast carcinoma in postmenopausal women; it inhibits conversion of circulating ANDROGENS into ESTROGENS.

anat. anatomy.

anatomic (an″ah-tom′ik) anatomical.

anatomical (an″ah-tom′ĭ-k'l) pertaining to anatomy or to the structure of the organism.

anatomist (ah-nat′o-mist) one skilled in anatomy.

anatomy (ah-nat′o-me) the science dealing with the form and structure of living organisms. (See accompanying illustration.)

clinical a. anatomy as applied to clinical practice.

comparative a. description and comparison of the form and structure of different animals.

developmental a. the field of EMBRYOLOGY concerned with the changes that cells, tissues, organs, and the body as a whole undergo from a germ cell of each parent to the resulting offspring; it includes both prenatal and postnatal development.

gross a., macroscopic a. that dealing with structures visible with the unaided eye.

microscopic a. histology.

morbid a., pathologic a. anatomy of diseased tissues.

radiologic a. x-ray anatomy.

special a. anatomy devoted to study of particular organs or parts.

topographic a. that devoted to determination of relative positions of various body parts.

x-ray a. study of organs and tissues based on their visualization by x-rays in both living and dead bodies.

anatropia (an″ah-tro′pe-ah) upward deviation of the visual axis of one eye when the other eye is fixing. adj., **anatrop′ic.**

anchorage (ang′kŏ-rij) 1. fixation (def. 1), especially surgical fixation of a displaced VISCUS. 2. in operative dentistry, fixation of fillings, or of artificial crowns or bridges. In orthodontics, the support used for a regulating apparatus. 3. in orthodontics, the support used for a regulating apparatus. 4. in tissue cell culture, the attachment of proliferating cells to a solid surface.

ancipital (an-sip′ĭ-tal) two-edged or two-headed.

anconad (ang′ko-nad) toward the elbow or olecranon.

anconal (ang′ko-nal) cubital.

anconeal (ang-ko′ne-al) cubital.

anconitis (ang″ko-ni′tis) inflammation of the elbow joint.

ANCOVA analysis of covariance.

ancrod (ang′krod) a proteinase obtained from the venom of the Malayan pit viper *Agkistrodon rhodostoma,* acting specifically on fibrinogen; used as an ANTICOAGULANT in the treatment of retinal vein occlusion and deep vein thrombosis and to prevent postoperative rethrombosis.

ancyl(o)- for words beginning thus, see those beginning ANKYL(O)-.

Ancylostoma (an″sĭ-los′to-mah) a genus of parasitic HOOKWORMS.

A. america′num *Necator americanus.*

A. brazilien′se a species parasitic in dogs and cats in tropical and subtropical regions; its larvae may cause a creeping ERUPTION in humans.

A. cani′num the common hookworm of dogs and cats.

A. duodena′le a common HOOKWORM parasitic in the human small intestine.

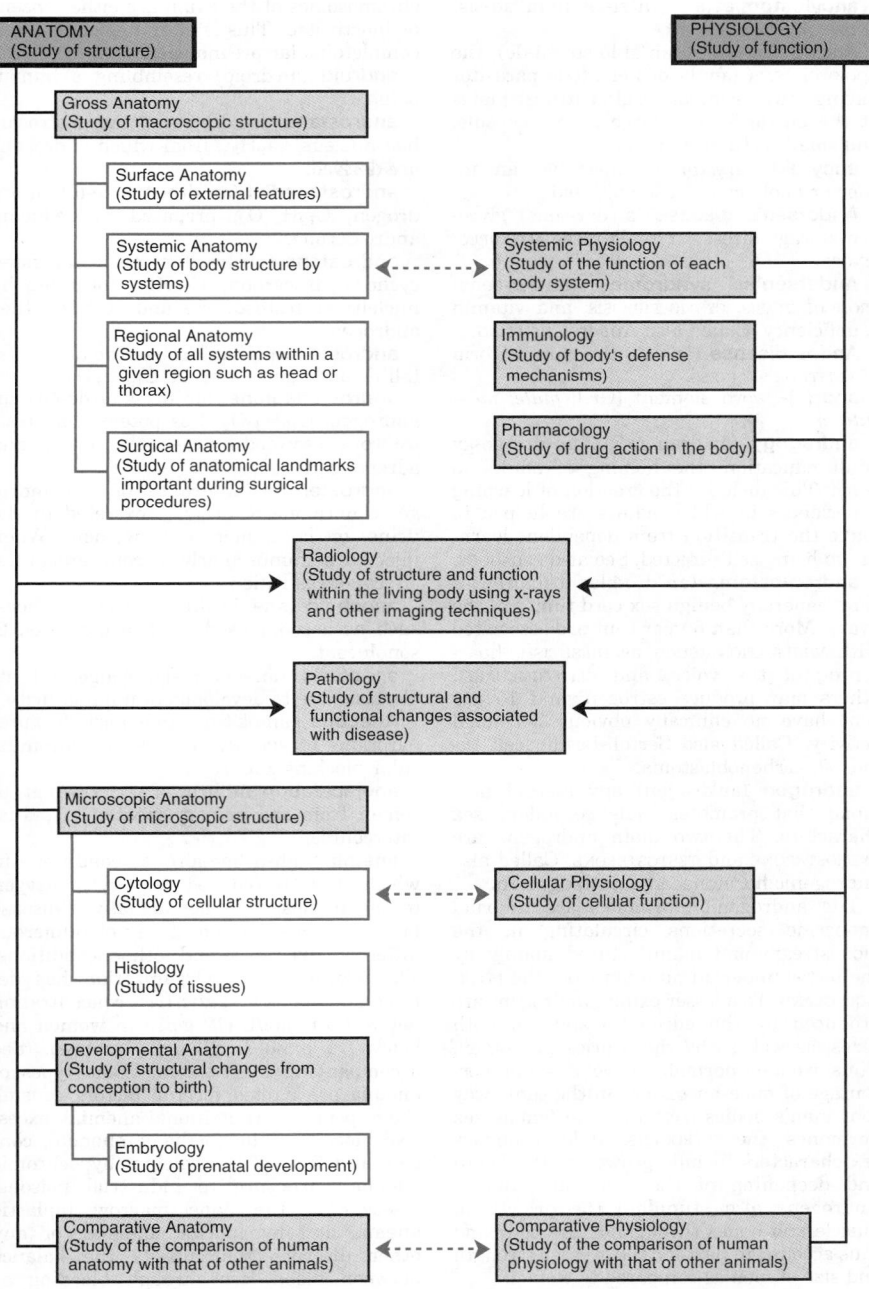

Examples of specialty areas of anatomy and physiology. From Applegate, 2000.

ancylostomiasis (an″sĭ-los″to-mi′ah-sis) HOOKWORM DISEASE.

Ancylostomidae (an″sĭ-lo-sto′mĭ-de) the HOOKWORMS, a family of nematode parasites having two ventrolateral cutting plates at the entrance to a large buccal capsule, and small teeth at its base.

ancyroid (an′sĭ-roid) shaped like an anchor or hook; called also ankyroid.

Andersen's disease (an′der-senz) glycogen storage disease (type IV); see AMYLOPECTINOSIS.

Andersen's syndrome (an′der-senz) BRONCHIECTASIS, CYSTIC FIBROSIS, and vitamin A deficiency. Called also Andersen's triad.

Andes disease (an′dēz) the chronic form of ALTITUDE SICKNESS.

andr(o)- word element [Gr.], *male; masculine.*

andragogy (an′drah-go″je), an·dra·go·gy adult education; the helping of adults to learn. This includes the creation of learning experiences in which adults are helped to make the transition from dependent learning to being self-directed. See also PEDAGOGY.

androblastoma (an″dro-blas-to′mah) 1. a rare, generally benign sex cord tumor of the ovary. More than 60 per cent are associated with VIRILIZATION (such as HIRSUTISM, hoarsening of the voice, and CLITORIMEGALY); others may produce estrogen; and 15 per cent have no clinically obvious hormonal activity. Called also Sertoli-Leydig cell tumor. 2. arrhenoblastoma.

androgen (an′dro-jen) any steroid hormone that promotes male secondary sex characters. The two main androgens are ANDROSTERONE and TESTOSTERONE. Called also androgenic hormone. adj., **androgen′ic.**

The androgenic hormones are internal endocrine secretions circulating in the bloodstream and manufactured mainly by the testes under stimulation from the PITUITARY GLAND. To a lesser extent, androgens are produced by the adrenal glands in both sexes, as well as by the ovaries in women. Thus women normally have a small percentage of male hormones, in the same way that men's bodies contain some female sex hormones, the ESTROGENS. Male secondary sex characters include growth of the beard and deepening of the voice at puberty. Androgens also stimulate the growth of muscle and bones throughout the body and thus account in part for the greater strength and size of men as compared to women.

a. insensitivity syndrome complete androgen RESISTANCE.

androgenesis (an″dro-jen′ĕ-sis) a phenomenon in which an ovum is fertilized by a haploid sperm, which then duplicates its own chromosomes after meiosis; the chromosomes of the ovum are either absent or inactivated. This is often associated with complete molar pregnancies.

android (an′droid) resembling a human being.

androstane (an′dro-stān) the hydrocarbon nucleus, $C_{19}H_{32}$, from which androgens are derived.

androstanediol (an″dro-stān′de-ol) an androgen, $C_{19}H_{32}O_2$, prepared by reducing androsterone.

androstene (an′dro-stēn) an unsaturated cyclic hydrocarbon, $C_{19}H_{30}$, forming the nucleus of testosterone and certain other androgens.

androstenediol (an″dro-stēn′de-ol) a crystalline androgenic steroid, $C_{19}H_{30}O_2$.

androstenedione (an″dro-stēn′de-ōn) an androgen, $C_{19}H_{30}O_2$, less potent than testosterone, secreted by the testis, ovary, and adrenal cortex.

androsterone (an-dros′ter-ōn) an androgenic hormone, $C_{19}H_{30}O_2$, excreted in the urine of both men and women. When injected intramuscularly, it counteracts the effects of castration.

anechoic (an-ĕ-ko′ik) 1. without echoes, such as a room used for hearing tests. 2. sonolucent.

anectasis (an-ek′tah-sis) congenital atelectasis due to developmental immaturity.

Anectine (an-ek′tin) trademark for preparations of SUCCINYLCHOLINE, a neuromuscular blocking AGENT.

anejaculation failure of EJACULATION of semen from the urinary meatus in sexual intercourse.

anemia (ah-ne′me-ah) a condition in which there is reduced delivery of oxygen to the tissues; it is not actually a disease but rather a symptom of any of numerous different disorders and other conditions. The World Health Organization has defined anemia as a HEMOGLOBIN concentration below 7.5 mmol/L (12 g/dL) in women and below 8.1 mmol/L (13 g/dL) in men. (See accompanying illustration.) Some types of anemia are named for the factors causing them: poor diet (nutritional anemia), excessive blood loss (hemorrhagic anemia), congenital defects of hemoglobin (hypochromic anemia), exposure to industrial poisons, diseases of the bone marrow (aplastic anemia and hypoplastic anemia), or any other disorder that upsets the balance between blood loss through bleeding or destruction of blood cells and production of blood cells. Anemias can also be classified according to the morphologic characteristics of the erythrocytes, such as size (microcytic,

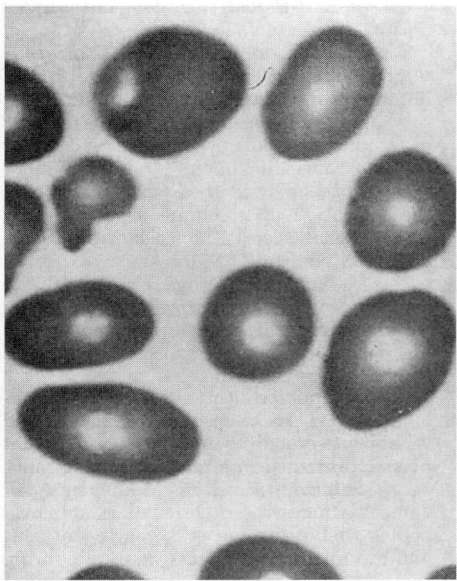 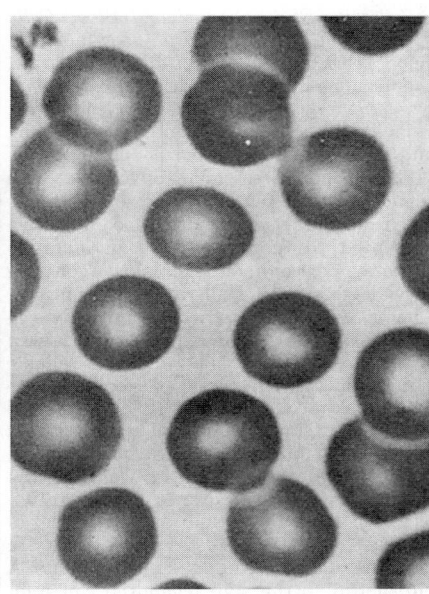

Peripheral blood smears from a patient with megaloblastic anemia (left) and from a normal subject (right), both at the same magnification. The smear from the patient shows variation in the size and shape of erythrocytes and the presence of macro-ovalocytes. From Goldman and Bennett, 2000.

macrocytic, and normocytic anemias) and color or hemoglobin concentration (hypochromic anemia). A type called *hypochromic microcytic anemia* is characterized by very small erythrocytes that have low hemoglobin concentration and hence poor coloration. Data used to identify anemia types include the erythrocyte indices: (1) mean corpuscular volume (MCV), the average erythrocyte volume; (2) mean corpuscular hemoglobin (MCH), the average amount of hemoglobin per erythrocyte; and (3) mean corpuscular hemoglobin concentration (MCHC), the average concentration of hemoglobin in erythrocytes. adj., ane'mic.

Symptoms. Mild degrees of anemia often cause only slight and vague symptoms, perhaps nothing more than easy fatigue or a lack of energy. As the condition progresses, more severe symptoms may be experienced, such as shortness of breath, pounding of the heart, and a rapid pulse; these are caused by the inability of anemic blood to supply the body tissues with enough oxygen. Pallor, particularly in the palms of the hands, the fingernails, and the conjunctiva (the lining of the eyelids), may also indicate anemia. In very advanced cases, swelling of the ankles and other evidence of heart failure may appear.

Common Causes of Anemia. *Loss of Blood (Hemorrhagic Anemia):* If there is massive bleeding from a wound or other lesion, the body may lose enough blood to cause severe and acute anemia, which is often accompanied by shock. Immediate transfusions are generally required to replace the lost blood. Chronic blood loss, such as excessive menstrual flow, or slow loss of blood from an ulcer or cancer of the gastrointestinal tract, may also lead to anemia. These anemias disappear when the cause has been found and corrected. To help the blood replenish itself, the health care provider may prescribe medicines containing iron, which is necessary to build hemoglobin, and foods with high iron content, such as kidney and navy beans, liver, spinach, and whole wheat bread.

Dietary Deficiencies and Abnormalities of Red Blood Cell Production (Nutritional Anemia, Aplastic Anemia, and Hypoplastic Anemia): Anemia may develop if the diet does not provide enough iron, protein, vitamin B_{12}, and other vitamins and minerals needed in the production of hemoglobin and the formation of erythrocytes. The combination of poor diet and chronic loss of blood makes for particular susceptibility to severe anemia. Anemias associated with folic acid deficiency are very common.

Excessive Destruction of Red Blood Cells (hemolytic anemia): Anemia may also develop related to HEMOLYSIS due to trauma, chemical agents or medications *(toxic hemolytic anemia),* infectious disease, isoimmune hemolytic reactions, autoimmune disorders, and the paroxysmal HEMOGLOBINURIAS.

Patient Care. Assessment of patients with some form of anemia will depend to some extent on the specific type of blood dyscrasia presented. In general, these patients do share some common problems requiring special assessment skills and interventions. Anemia can affect many different body systems (see table). Although pallor of the skin is a sign of anemia, it is not the most reliable sign; many other factors can affect complexion and skin color. Jaundice of the skin and sclera can occur as a result of hemolysis and the release of bilirubin into the blood stream, where it eventually finds its way into the skin and mucous membranes. (See also JAUNDICE.) Bleeding under the skin and bruises in response to the slightest trauma often are present in anemic and leukemic patients. A bluish tint to the skin (cyanosis) can indicate hypoxia due to inadequate numbers of oxygen-bearing erythrocytes.

ACTIVITY INTOLERANCE is a common problem for patients with anemia. Physical activity increases demand for oxygen, but if there are not enough circulating erythrocytes to provide sufficient oxygen, patients become physically weak and unable to engage in normal physical activity without experiencing profound fatigue. This can result in some degree of self-care DEFICIT as the fatigue interferes with the patient's ability to carry on regular or enjoyable activities.

acute posthemorrhagic a. hemorrhagic anemia.

aplastic a. see APLASTIC ANEMIA.

autoimmune hemolytic a. (AIHA) an acquired disorder characterized by hemolysis due to the production of autoantibodies against one's own red blood cell antigens.

Blackfan-Diamond a. congenital hypoplastic anemia (def. 1).

congenital hypoplastic a. 1. idiopathic progressive anemia occurring in the first year of life, without leukopenia and thrombocytopenia; it is due to an isolated defect in erythropoiesis and is unresponsive to hematinics, requiring multiple blood transfusions to sustain life. For those responding to steroid therapy the prognosis is good. Called also Blackfan-Diamond anemia or syndrome, Diamond-Blackfan anemia or syndrome, and erythrogenesis imperfecta. 2. Fanconi's syndrome (def. 1).

Cooley's a. tthalassemia major.

deficiency a. nutritional anemia.

Diamond-Blackfan a. congenital hypoplastic anemia (def. 1).

drug-induced hemolytic a., drug-induced immune hemolytic a. a form of immune hemolytic anemia induced by the taking of drugs, involving one of four different mechanisms: *Immune complex problems:* Ingestion of any of a large number of drugs is followed by immunization and the formation of a soluble drug–anti-drug complex that adsorbs nonspecifically to the erythrocyte surface. *Drug absorption:* Drugs bind firmly to erythrocyte membrane proteins, inducing the formation of specific antibodies; the drug most commonly associated with this mechanism is penicillin. *Membrane modification:* A nonimmunologic mechanism whereby the drug involved is able to modify erythrocytes so that plasma proteins can bind to the membrane. *Autoantibody formation:* Methyldopa (Aldomet) induces the production of autoantibodies that recognize erythrocyte antigens and are serologically indistinguishable from those seen in patients with warm autoimmune hemolytic anemia.

Fanconi's a., Fanconi's hypoplastic a. Fanconi's syndrome (def. 1).

hemolytic a. see HEMOLYTIC ANEMIA.

hemorrhagic a. anemia caused by the sudden and acute loss of blood; called also acute posthemorrhagic anemia.

hypochromic a. anemia in which the decrease in hemoglobin is proportionately much greater than the decrease in number of erythrocytes.

hypochromic microcytic a. any anemia with microcytes that are hypochromic (reduced in size and in hemoglobin content); the most common type is iron deficiency anemia.

hypoplastic a. anemia due to incapacity of blood-forming organs.

immune hemolytic a. an acquired HEMOLYTIC ANEMIA in which a hemolytic response is caused by isoantibodies or autoantibodies produced on exposure to drugs, toxins, or other antigens. See also autoimmune hemolytic ANEMIA, drug-induced immune hemolytic ANEMIA, and ERYTHROBLASTOSIS FETALIS.

iron deficiency a. a type of hypochromic microcytic anemia that results from the presence of greater demands on stored IRON than can be met, usually because of chronic blood loss, dietary deficiency, or defective absorption; it is characterized by low or absent iron stores, low serum iron concentration, low TRANSFERRIN saturation, elevated transferrin (total iron-binding

BLOOD VALUES IN ANEMIA

	RBC (per mm³)	Hb (g/dl)	Hct (%)	MCV (per μm³)	MCH (pg)	MCHC (g/dl)	WBC (per mm³)	Reticulocyte Count (per mm³)	Platelet Count (per mm³)
Normal	Male: 4.7–6.1, female: 4.2–5.4	Male: 14–18, female: 12–16	Male: 42–52, female: 37–47	80–90	27–31	32–36	5000–10,000	0.5–2	150,000–400,000
Acute hemorrhagic anemia	Initial increase, latent decrease	Initial decrease, latent decrease	Normal initially, latent decrease	Increase	Decrease	Normal	Increase	Increase	Decrease
Chronic hemorrhagic anemia	Decrease	Decrease	Decrease	Slight decrease	Slight decrease	Slight decrease	Normal	Decrease	Normal
Iron deficiency anemia	Decrease	Decrease	Decrease	Decrease	Decrease	Decrease	Normal	Decrease	Normal to increase
Aplastic anemia	Gross decrease	Gross decrease	Gross decrease	Moderate decrease	Gross decrease	Gross decrease	Gross decrease	Decrease	Gross decrease
Pernicious anemia	Decrease	Gross decrease	Gross decrease	Increase	Increase	Increase	Slight decrease	Decrease	Slight decrease
Folic acid deficiency anemia	Decrease	Gross decrease	Gross decrease	Increase	Increase	Increase	Slight decrease	Decrease	Slight decrease
Sickle cell anemia	Decrease	Decrease	Decrease	Decrease	Normal	Normal	Increase	Increase	Normal
Hemolytic anemia	Decrease	Decrease	Decrease	Increase	Slight decrease	Normal	Normal	Increase	Normal to increase

Hb, hemoglobin; Hct, hematocrit; MCV, mean corpuscular volume; MCH, mean corpuscular hemoglobin; MCHC, mean corpuscular hemoglobin concentration. RBC, red blood cells; WBC, white blood cells.
From Frazier et al., 2000.

capacity), and low HEMOGLOBIN concentration or HEMATOCRIT. Iron deficiency anemia is the most common nutritional disorder in the United States.

macrocytic a. anemia characterized by MACROCYTES (erythrocytes much larger than normal).

Mediterranean a. thalassemia major.

megaloblastic a. any of various anemias characterized by the presence of MEGALOBLASTS in the bone marrow or blood; the most common type is PERNICIOUS ANEMIA.

microangiopathic hemolytic a. thrombotic thrombocytopenic purpura.

microcytic a. anemia characterized by MICROCYTES (erythrocytes smaller than normal); see also *hypochromic microcytic anemia* and *microcythemia*.

myelopathic a., myelophthisic a. leukoerythroblastosis.

normochromic a. that in which the hemoglobin content of the red blood cells is in the normal range.

normocytic a. anemia characterized by proportionate decrease in hemoglobin, packed red cell volume, and number of erythrocytes per cubic millimeter of blood.

nutritional a. anemia due to a deficiency of an essential substance in the diet, which may be caused by poor dietary intake or by malabsorption; called also deficiency anemia.

pernicious a. see PERNICIOUS ANEMIA.

sickle cell a. see SICKLE CELL ANEMIA.

sideroachrestic a., sideroblastic a. any of a heterogenous group of acquired and hereditary anemias with diverse clinical manifestations, commonly characterized by large numbers of SIDEROBLASTS in the bone marrow, ineffective erythropoiesis, variable proportions of hypochromic erythrocytes in the peripheral blood, and usually increased levels of tissue iron.

spur cell a. anemia in which the erythrocytes are ACANTHOCYTES (spur cells) and are destroyed prematurely, primarily in the spleen; it is an acquired form occurring in severe liver disease in which there is increased serum cholesterol and increased uptake of cholesterol into the erythrocyte membrane, causing the abnormal shape.

anemic (ah-ne′mik) pertaining to anemia.

anencephaly (an″en-sef′ah-le) congenital absence of the cranial vault, with the cerebral hemispheres completely missing or reduced to small masses. adj., **anencephal′ic.**

anephric (a-nef′rik) without kidneys.

anergy (an′er-je) 1. lack of energy; extreme passivity. 2. diminished reactivity to specific antigen(s). adj., **aner′gic.**

anesthecinesia (an-es″thĕ-sĭ-ne′zhah) combined sensory and motor paralysis.

anesthesia (an″es-the′ze-ah) 1. lack of feeling or sensation. 2. artificially induced loss of ability to feel pain, done to permit the performance of surgery or other painful procedures. It may be produced by a number of agents (ANESTHETICS) capable of bringing about partial or complete loss of sensation. (See accompanying table.)

Patient Care. Interventions of the health care team will be individualized based on the type of procedure the patient has undergone and the type of anesthesia administered. Patients recovering from general anesthesia must be assessed constantly until they have reacted. The vital signs and blood pressure are checked regularly; any sudden change is reported immediately. They must be observed to see that the airway is clear at all times. The observation is in specialized recovery rooms called *postanesthesia care units* that are equipped with a variety of monitors to measure such variables as blood pressure, respiratory and pulse rates, cardiac output, body temperature, fluid balance, and oxygenation. When necessary, patients are initially managed with ventilators that inflate the lungs mechanically through endotracheal tubes. Changes in breathing pattern, eye movements, lacrimation, and muscle tone are indicators for the depth of anesthesia. Breathing patterns are the most sensitive of these.

When patients are awakening from general anesthesia they may be restless, attempting to get out of bed or even striking out at those around them because they are afraid and disoriented. This state is called *emergence delirium* and should be assessed, as it can indicate hypoxia. Retrograde amnesia may be associated with the administration of anesthesia and adjuncts, causing the patient to forget events occurring in the immediate postoperative period.

ambulatory a. anesthesia performed on an outpatient basis for ambulatory surgery.

balanced a. anesthesia that uses a combination of drugs, each in an amount sufficient to produce its major or desired effect to the optimum degree and to keep undesirable effects to a minimum.

basal a. a reversible state of central nervous system depression produced by preliminary medication so that the inhalation of anesthetic necessary to produce surgical anesthesia is greatly reduced.

block a. regional anesthesia.

caudal a. a type of regional anesthesia that was used in childbirth between the 1940s and the 1960s. The anesthetizing solution, usually PROCAINE, was injected into

STAGES OF ANESTHESIA*

(These stages are seen in reverse order on emergence from anesthesia.)

Stage I: Stage of Analgesia
  Begins with the initiation of anesthesia and ends with the loss of consciousness. Characterized by sensory and mental depression. Patients can open their eyes on command, breathe unassisted, maintain protective reflexes, and tolerate mild painful stimuli.

Stage II: Stage of Delirium
  Begins with the loss of consciousness and ends with onset of a regular pattern of breathing and the disappearance of the lid reflex. It is characterized by excitement and during this period vomiting, laryngospasm, and cardiac arrest are possible.

Stage III: Stage of Surgical Anesthesia
  Begins with the onset of a regular breathing pattern and ends if there is cessation of respiration. Absence of response to a surgical incision. This state is divided into four planes:

  Plane 1—Lid reflex is abolished and respiration is regular. The vomiting reflex is abolished. Swallowing, retching, and vomiting reflexes usually disappear in that order during induction and reappear during emergence from anesthesia.
  Plane 2—Lasts from the time the eyeball ceases to move (becoming concentrically fixed) to the beginning of a decrease in activity of the intercostal muscles. The laryngospasm reflex disappears during this plane.
  Plane 3—Intercostal muscle activity begins to decrease. Complete intercostal muscle paralysis occurs in this plane, and respiration is carried on solely by the diaphragm.
  Plane 4—Lasts from the time of paralysis of the intercostal muscles to any occurrence of cessation of spontaneous respiration.

Stage IV: Stage of Overdose
  From the cessation of respiration to failure of the circulatory system. An emergency situation.

---

*Modern anesthetic agents make the stages of anesthesia of little value during the induction of anesthesia. They are of some help in the assessment of the postoperative patient since some adjuncts to anesthesia have been reversed (or their effects minimized) over time.

---

the caudal area of the spinal canal through the lower end of the sacrum and affected the caudal nerve roots, rendering the cervix, vagina, and perineum insensitive to pain. Called also caudal block.

  central a. lack of sensation caused by disease of the nerve centers.

  closed circuit a. that produced by continuous rebreathing of a small amount of anesthetic gas in a closed system with an apparatus for removing carbon dioxide.

  compression a. loss of sensation resulting from pressure on a nerve.

  crossed a. loss of sensation on one side of the face and loss of pain and temperature sense on the opposite side of the body.

  dissociated a., dissociation a. loss of perception of certain stimuli while that of others remains intact.

  electric a. anesthesia induced by passage of an electric current.

  endotracheal a. anesthesia produced by introduction of a gaseous mixture through a tube inserted into the trachea.

  epidural a. regional anesthesia produced by injection of the anesthetic agent into the epidural space. It may be performed by injection of the agent between the vertebral spines in the cervical, thoracic, or lumbar regions. An old method was caudal ANESTHESIA, which involved injecting the agent into the sacral hiatus. Called also epidural block.

  general a. a state of unconsciousness produced by anesthestic agents, with absence of pain sensation over the entire body and a greater or lesser degree of muscular relaxation; the drugs producing this state can be administered by inhalation, intravenously, intramuscularly, or rectally, or via the gastrointestinal tract.

  gustatory a. loss of the sense of taste.

  hysterical a. loss of tactile sensation occurring as a symptom of conversion disorder, often recognizable by its lack of correspondence with nerve distributions.

  infiltration a. local anesthesia produced by injection of the anesthetic solution directly into the area of terminal nerve endings. Called also infiltration analgesia.

  inhalation a. anesthesia produced by the respiration of a volatile liquid or gaseous anesthetic agent.

  insufflation a. anesthesia produced by introduction of a gaseous mixture into the trachea through a tube.

  local a. that produced in a limited area, as by injection of a local anesthetic or by freezing with ethyl chloride.

  open a. general inhalation anesthesia in which there is no rebreathing of the exhaled gases.

paraneural a. perineural block.

paravertebral a. regional anesthesia produced by the injection of a local anesthetic around the spinal nerves at their exit from the spinal column, and outside the spinal dura. Called also paravertebral block.

perineural a. perineural block.

peripheral a. lack of sensation due to changes in the peripheral nerves.

rectal a. anesthesia produced by introduction of the anesthetic agent into the rectum.

refrigeration a. cryoanesthesia.

regional a. insensibility caused by interrupting the sensory nerve conductivity of any region of the body; the two primary types are *field block,* the encircling of an operative field by means of injections of a local anesthetic and *nerve block,* the making of injections in close proximity to the nerves supplying the area. Called also block.

saddle block a. saddle BLOCK.

segmental a. loss of sensation in a segment of the body due to a lesion of a nerve root.

spinal a. 1. anesthesia due to a spinal lesion. 2. regional anesthesia produced by injection of the agent beneath the membrane of the spinal cord. Called also spinal block.

surgical a. that degree of anesthesia at which operation may safely be performed.

tactile a. loss of the sense of TOUCH.

topical a. that produced by application of a local anesthetic directly to the area involved.

anesthesiologist (an″es-the″ze-ol′o-jist) a physician who specializes in anesthesiology.

anesthesiology (an″es-the″ze-ol′o-je) the branch of medicine concerned with administration of ANESTHETICS and the condition of the patient while under ANESTHESIA.

anesthetic (an″es-thet′ik) 1. pertaining to, characterized by, or producing ANESTHESIA. 2. a drug or agent used to abolish the sensation of pain, to achieve adequate muscle relaxation during surgery, to calm fear and allay anxiety, and to produce amnesia for the event.

Inhalational anesthetics are gases or volatile liquids that produce general anesthesia when inhaled. The commonly used inhalational agents are HALOTHANE, ENFLURANE, ISOFLURANE, and NITROUS OXIDE. Older agents, such as ETHER and CYCLOPROPANE, are now used infrequently. The mechanism of action of all inhalational anesthetics is thought to involve uptake of the gas in the lipid bilayer of cell membranes and interaction with the membrane proteins, resulting in inhibition of synaptic transmission of nerve impulses. For surgical anesthesia, these agents are usually used with preanesthetic medication, which includes SEDATIVES or OPIATES to relieve preoperative and postoperative pain and TRANQUILIZERS to reduce ANXIETY. Neuromuscular blocking agents are used as muscle RELAXANTS during surgery. They include TUBOCURARINE, METOCURINE, SUCCINYLCHOLINE, PANCURONIUM, ATRACURIUM, and VECURONIUM.

Intravenous anesthetics are sedative hypnotic drugs that produce anesthesia in large doses. The most common of these are the phenol derivative PROPOFOL and ultra–short acting BARBITURATES such as THIOPENTAL and METHOHEXITAL; these can be used alone for brief surgical procedures or for rapid induction of anesthesia maintained by inhalational anesthetics.

Other intravenous methods of anesthesia are NEUROLEPTANALGESIA, which uses a combination of the butyrophenone tranquilizer DROPERIDOL and the opioid FENTANYL; NEUROLEPTANESTHESIA, which uses neuroleptanalgesia plus NITROUS OXIDE; and *dissociative anesthesia,* which uses KETAMINE, a drug related to the hallucinogens that produces profound analgesia.

Local anesthetics are drugs that block nerve conduction in the region where they are applied. They act by altering permeability of nerve cells to sodium ions and thus blocking conduction of nerve impulses. They may be applied topically or injected into the tissues. The first local anesthetic was COCAINE. Synthetic local anesthetics are all given names ending in -*caine;* examples are PROCAINE and LIDOCAINE.

anesthetist (ah-nes′the-tist) a person trained in administering anesthetics.

anesthetization (ah-nes″the-ti-za′shun) production of anesthesia.

anetoderma (an″e-to-der′mah) localized elastolysis producing circumscribed areas of soft, thin, wrinkled skin that often protrude as small outpouchings. It may be a primary condition or it may be secondary to some other condition involving the skin, such as syphilis, leprosy, or tuberculosis.

aneuploidy (an″u-ploi′de) the state of having chromosomes in a number that is not an exact multiple of the haploid number. adj., **an′euploid.**

aneurysm (an′u-rizm) a sac formed by the localized dilatation of the wall of an artery, a vein, or the heart. (See illustration.) adj., **aneurys′mal.** The chief signs of an *arterial* aneurysm are the formation of a pulsating tumor, and often a bruit (aneurysmal bruit) heard over the swelling. Sometimes there are symptoms from pressure on contiguous parts.

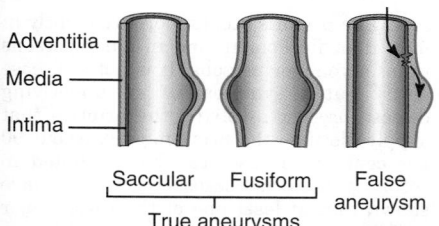

Adventitia — Media — Intima —

Saccular   Fusiform   False aneurysm

True aneurysms

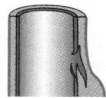

Dissecting aneurysm

Classification of aneurysms. All three tunica layers are involved in true aneurysms (fusiform and saccular). In false aneurysms, blood escapes between tunica layers and they separate. If the separation continues, a clot may form, resulting in a dissecting aneurysm. From Copstead and Banasik, 2000.

The most common site for an arterial aneurysm is the abdominal aorta. A *true* aneurysm results from formation of a sac by the arterial wall with at least one unbroken layer. It is most often associated with ATHEROSCLEROSIS. A *false* aneurysm usually is caused by trauma. In this case, the wall of the blood vessel is ruptured and blood escapes into surrounding tissues and forms a clot. Because of pressure within the clot arising from the heart's contractions, the clot often pulsates against the examiner's hand as does a true aneurysm.

Although atherosclerosis is responsible for most arterial aneurysms, any injury to the middle or muscular layer of the arterial wall *(tunica media)* can predispose the vessel to stretching of the inner and outer layers of the artery and the formation of a sac. Other diseases that can lead to an aneurysm include syphilis, cystic medionecrosis, certain nonspecific inflammations, and congenital defects in the artery.

It is possible for a person to be unaware of a small aneurysm for years. About 80 per cent of all abdominal aneurysms are palpable and may be noticed on a routine physical examination. One should be particularly alert to the possibility of an aneurysm in persons with a history of cardiovascular disease, hypertension, or peripheral vascular disease.

Aneurysms tend to increase in size, presenting a problem of increasing pressure against adjacent tissues and organs and a danger of rupture. When an aneurysm ruptures, a critical situation ensues. The patient with a ruptured aortic aneurysm exhibits severe pain and blood loss, leading to shock. A ruptured cerebral aneurysm produces neurologic symptoms and can resemble the clinical picture of STROKE SYNDROME.

Treatment of aneurysm depends on the vessel involved, size of the aneurysm, and general health status of the patient.

arteriosclerotic a. an aneurysm arising in a large artery, most commonly the abdominal aorta, as a result of weakening of the wall in severe atherosclerosis; called also atherosclerotic aneurysm.

arteriovenous a. an abnormal communication between an artery and a vein in which the blood flows directly into a neighboring vein or is carried into the vein by a connecting sac.

atherosclerotic a. arteriosclerotic aneurysm.

bacterial a. an infected aneurysm caused by bacteria.

berry a., brain a. a small saccular aneurysm of a cerebral artery, usually at the junction of vessels in the circle of Willis; such aneurysms frequently rupture, causing subarachnoid hemorrhage. Called also cerebral aneurysm.

cardiac a. thinning and dilatation of a portion of the wall of the left ventricle, usually a consequence of myocardial infarction.

cerebral a. berry aneurysm.

cirsoid a. dilatation and tortuous lengthening of part of an artery; called also racemose aneurysm.

compound a. one in which some of the layers of the wall of the vessel are ruptured and some merely dilated; called also mixed aneurysm.

dissecting a. one resulting from hemorrhage that causes lengthwise splitting of the arterial wall, producing a tear in the inner wall (intima) and establishing communication with the lumen of the vessel. It usually affects the thoracic aorta (see aortic DISSECTION) but can also occur in other large arteries. See illustration.

false a. 1. one in which the entire wall is injured and the blood is contained by the surrounding tissues, with eventual formation of a sac communicating with the artery (or heart). See illustration. 2. pseudoaneurysm.

fusiform a. a spindle-shaped aneurysm; see illustration.

infected a. one produced by growth of microorganisms (bacteria or fungi) in the vessel wall, or infection arising within a preexisting arteriosclerotic aneurysm.

mixed a. compound aneurysm.

mycotic a. an infected aneurysm caused by fungi.

racemose a. cirsoid aneurysm.

saccular a., sacculated a. a saclike aneurysm; see illustration.

spurious a. 1. false aneurysm (def. 1). 2. pseudoaneurysm.

varicose a. one formed by rupture of an aneurysm into a vein.

aneurysmectomy (an″u-riz-mek′to-me) surgical excision of an aneurysm.

aneurysmoplasty (an″u-riz′mo-plas″te) plastic repair of an artery for aneurysm.

aneurysmorrhaphy (an″u-riz-mor′ah-fe) suture closure of an aneurysm.

ANF atrial natriuretic factor.

anger (ang′ger) a feeling of tension and hostility, usually caused by anxiety aroused by a perceived threat to one's self, possessions, rights, or values.

angi(o)- word element [Gr.], *vessel (channel).*

angiectasis (an″je-ek′tah-sis) abnormal, often extreme, dilatation of a blood or lymphatic vessel. See also LYMPHANGIECTASIS and VASODILATION. adj., **angiectat′ic.**

angiectomy (an″je-ek′to-me) surgical excision of part of a blood or lymph vessel.

angiitis (an″je-i′tis), pl. *angii′tides* vasculitis.

allergic granulomatous a. CHURG-STRAUSS SYNDROME.

angina (an-ji′nah, an′ji-nah) spasmodic, choking, or suffocative pain; now used almost exclusively to denote ANGINA PECTORIS. adj., **an′ginal.**

agranulocytic a. agranulocytosis.

crescendo a. old term for unstable angina.

a. cru′ris intermittent claudication.

herpes a., a. herpe′tica herpangina.

intestinal a. generalized cramping abdominal pain occurring shortly after a meal and persisting for one to three hours, due to ischemia of the smooth muscle of the bowel.

Ludwig's a. see LUDWIG'S ANGINA.

a. pec′toris acute pain in the chest resulting from myocardial ISCHEMIA (decreased blood supply to the heart muscle); the condition has also been called *cardiac pain of effort and emotion* because the pain is brought on by physical activity or emotional stress that places an added burden on the heart and increases the need for blood being supplied to the myocardium. Some patients can predict the kinds of events that will precipitate an attack while others are unaware of any relationship between onset of an attack and any particular situation in their lives.

Angina pectoris occurs more frequently in men than in women, and in older persons than in younger persons. It is not a disease entity but a symptom of an underlying disease process involving the arteries that supply blood to the heart muscle. About 90 per cent of all cases can be attributed to coronary ATHEROSCLEROSIS. Studies have shown that at least one of the three major coronary arteries usually is stenosed before angina develops. In most cases, all of the major coronary arteries are involved.

Angina pectoris also can result from stenosis of the aorta, pulmonary stenosis and ventricular hypertrophy, or connective tissue disorders such as systemic lupus erythematosus and periarteritis nodosa that affect the smaller coronary arteries.

Symptoms. The chief symptom is chest pain, usually unmistakably distinguished by the patient as different from other types of pain such as that caused by indigestion. It is generally described as a feeling of tightness, strangling, heaviness, or suffocation and is usually concentrated on the left side, beginning just under the sternum; it sometimes radiates to the neck, throat, and lower jaw and down the left arm, and occasionally to the stomach, back, or across to the right side of the chest. The pain seldom lasts more than 15 minutes and is usually relieved by rest and relaxation or by administration of nitrates. If it is not relieved in 10 to 15 minutes, the physician should be notified and the patient taken to a cardiac care unit. The decreased blood supply to the heart makes it especially vulnerable to ARRHYTHMIAS and MYOCARDIAL INFARCTION, which are the cause of death in about one third of all cases.

Coronary arteriography and ventriculography are valuable in determining the prognosis for angina pectoris. The mortality rate for patients having a narrowing of all three main coronary arteries is higher than for those who have only one vessel involved. Severity of pain is not a good prognostic indicator; some patients with severe discomfort live for many years, while others with mild symptoms die suddenly. An enlarged heart, a third heart sound, ECG abnormalities at rest, and hypertension are all indicative of a poor prognosis.

Treatment and Patient Care. Relief from pain by rest and prevention of attacks by avoiding situations which precipitate them are the first steps in the care of the patient with angina. In most cases patients are eager to learn about the disease process causing the pain and want to know how they can participate in control of their attacks. However, compliance with the prescribed regimen usually requires a change in life style and the breaking of some lifelong habits. The known risk factors for coronary heart disease are explained to the patient, and a regimen designed to avoid further damage to the arteries is prescribed.

Organic nitrates may be administered orally or sublingually for relief from anginal pain. They act by dilating the arteries and may be used to treat acute attacks, for long-term prophylaxis and management, or for prophylaxis in situations likely to provoke an attack. Commonly used nitrates are ERYTHRITYL TETRANITRATE, ISOSORBIDE dinitrate, and NITROGLYCERIN.

BETA-ADRENERGIC BLOCKING AGENTS, such as PROPRANOLOL, are used to treat patients who do not respond to weight control and treatment with vasodilators and whose angina significantly limits their activities. These agents decrease the heart rate, blood pressure, and myocardial oxygen consumption and increase the patient's exercise tolerance.

The CALCIUM CHANNEL BLOCKING AGENTS (NIFEDIPINE, VERAPAMIL, DILTIAZEM, and others) are drugs that are particularly beneficial in relieving pain in patients whose angina is the result of coronary artery spasm or constriction. They act by selectively inhibiting the transport of calcium across the cell membrane of myocardial cells and also by reducing myocardial oxygen utilization. Patients most likely to obtain dramatic relief from drugs of this kind are those who experience chest pain while resting or sleeping, upon exposure to cold, or during emotional stress.

Surgical procedures involving arterial BY-PASS and ANGIOPLASTY have become fairly common as a form of treatment of certain types of ischemic heart disease and resulting angina pectoris. The surgical procedures attempt to bypass the diseased portion of the coronary artery by suturing a vein graft or the internal mammary artery from the aorta to one or more coronary arteries beyond the area of obstruction. In most instances the graft is obtained from the patient's saphenous vein. Angioplasty reestablishes patency of the vessels; in most cases, it is now accompanied by insertion of a stent to help prevent restenosis.

An attitude of calmness and efficiency is most important when caring for a person suffering from an attack of angina pectoris. The pain produces emotional reactions and the strongest of these is fear. Most of these patients know that their pain is resulting from an insufficient supply of oxygen to the heart and they frequently have a feeling of impending death. It usually helps to raise the patient to a sitting position so that breathing is less difficult. The prompt administration of nitroglycerin or the specific drug ordered by the physician should shorten the attack and relieve pain. Above all, the calm presence of someone who knows how to care for them can do much to reassure patients and help them relax, thus lessening the severity of the attack.

Plaut's a. necrotizing ulcerative gingivostomatitis.

preinfarction a. angina that lasts longer than 15 minutes; it is a symptom of worsening cardiac ischemia.

Prinzmetal's a. a variant of angina pectoris in which the attacks occur during rest, exercise capacity is well preserved, and attacks are associated electrocardiographically with elevation of the ST segment. It is cyclic in nature and is believed to be caused by coronary artery spasm.

pseudomembranous a. necrotizing ulcerative gingivostomatitis.

stable a. chest pain of cardiac origin that has not changed in character, frequency, intensity, or duration for 60 days.

unstable a. chest pain of cardiac origin that is variable, usually increasing in frequency and intensity and with irregular timing.

variant a. Prinzmetal's angina.

Vincent's a. see VINCENT'S ANGINA.

anginoid (an′jĭ-noid) resembling angina.

angioblast (an′je-o-blast″) 1. the earliest formative tissue from which blood cells and blood vessels arise. 2. an individual vessel-forming cell. adj., **angioblast′ic.**

angioblastoma (an″je-o-blas-to′mah) 1. hemangioblastoma. 2. a blood vessel tumor arising from the meninges of the brain or spinal cord; called also angioblastic meningioma.

angiocardiogram (an″je-o-kahr′de-o-gram″) a radiograph made during cardiac catheterization or coronary arteriography.

angiocardiography (an″je-o-kahr″de-og′rah-fe) a radiographic diagnostic study of the heart in which valves and vessels are examined via x-ray and fluoroscopy following the introduction of contrast media. See CARDIAC CATHETERIZATION.

equilibrium radionuclide a. a form of radionuclide angiocardiography in which images are taken at specific phases of the cardiac cycle over a series of several hundred cycles, with image recording set, or gated, by the occurrence of specific electrocardiographic waveforms. The data can be used to determine average activity during specific cardiac cycles or can be accumulated and displayed in rapid sequence, as a movie. Called also MUGA or multiple gated acquisition scanning and gated cardiac blood pool imaging.

first pass radionuclide a. a form of radionuclide angiocardiography in which a rapid sequence of images is taken immediately after administration of a bolus of radionuclide, recording only the initial transit of the isotope through the central circulation.

gated equilibrium radionuclide a. equilibrium radionuclide angiocardiography.

radionuclide a. a form in which the contrast medium is radioactively labeled, usually with technetium Tc 99m.

angiocardiokinetic (an″je-o-kahr″de-o-kĭ-net′ik) pertaining to dilation and contraction of the heart and blood vessels.

angiocarditis (an″je-o-kahr-di′tis) inflammation of the heart and blood vessels.

angiodermatitis (an″je-o-der-mah-ti′tis) inflammation of the vessels of the skin; when it is associated with arteriovenous fistula it is known as pseudo–Kaposi's SARCOMA.

angiodysplasia (an″je-o-dis-pla′zhah) small vascular abnormalities, such as of the intestinal tract.

angioedema (an″je-o-ĕ-de′mah) a localized edematous reaction of the deep dermis or subcutaneous or submucosal tissues appearing as giant wheals; URTICARIA is the same physiologic reaction occurring in the superficial portions of the dermis.

hereditary a. an autosomal dominant disorder of the complement system manifested as recurrent episodes of edema of the skin, upper respiratory tract, and gastrointestinal tract. It may be mediated by such factors as minor trauma, sudden changes in environmental temperature, and sudden emotional stress. adj., **angioede′matous.**

angioendothelioma (an″je-o-en″do-the″le-o′mah) hemangioendothelioma.

angiofibroma (an″je-o-fi-bro′mah) an ANGIOMA containing fibrous tissue.

juvenile nasopharyngeal a. a benign tumor of the NASOPHARYNX composed of fibrous connective tissue with abundant endothelium-lined vascular spaces, usually occurring during puberty in boys. Nasal obstruction may become total, with adenoid-type speech, discomfort in swallowing, obstruction of the EUSTACHIAN TUBE, and EPISTAXIS.

angiofollicular (an″je-o-fŏ-lik′u-lar) pertaining to a lymphoid follicle and its blood vessels.

angiogenesis (an″je-o-jen′ĕ-sis) 1. development of blood vessels in the embryo. 2. any formation of new blood vessels; see also NEOVASCULARIZATION (def. 2) and REVASCULARIZATION. Called also angiopoiesis and vasculogenesis. adj., **angiogenic.**

tumor a. the induction of the growth of blood vessels from surrounding tissue into a tumor by a diffusible protein factor released by the tumor cells.

angioglioma (an″je-o-gli-o′mah) a form of vascular GLIOMA.

angiogram (an′je-o-gram″) a radiograph of a blood vessel.

angiogranuloma (an″je-o-gran″u-lo′mah) an ANGIOMA containing granulation tissue, which represents a vasoproliferative inflammatory RESPONSE. When the epithelial surface is ulcerated and suppuration is evident, the lesion is referred to as pyogenic GRANULOMA.

angiography (an″je-og′rah-fe) radiography of vessels of the body after injection of contrast material; see also ARTERIOGRAPHY, LYMPHANGIOGRAPHY, and PHLEBOGRAPHY. Called also vasography.

digital subtraction a. radiographic visualization of blood vessels, with images produced by subtracting background structures and enhancing the contrast of those areas that change in density between a preliminary "mask" image and subsequent images.

angiohemophilia (an″je-o-he″mo-fil′e-ah) von Willebrand's disease.

angiohyalinosis (an″je-o-hi″ah-lĭ-no′sis) hyaline degeneration of the walls of blood vessels.

angioid (an′je-oid) resembling blood vessels.

angiokeratoma (an″je-o-ker″ah-to′mah) a dermatosis marked by telangiectasia with secondary epithelial changes, including acanthosis and hyperkeratosis. (See accompanying illustration.)

a. cor′poris diffu′sum an inborn ERROR of metabolism of GLYCOLIPIDS characterized by purpuric skin lesions (ANGIOKERATOMAS); see also FABRY'S DISEASE.

angiokinetic (an″je-o-kĭ-net′ik) vasomotor.

angioleiomyoma (an″je-o-li″o-mi-o′mah) a LEIOMYOMA arising from vascular smooth muscle, usually a solitary, nodular, sometimes painful, tumor on the lower limb in middle-aged women; it is often more deeply situated than ordinary leiomyoma and is usually subcutaneous.

angiolipoma (an″je-o-lĭ-po′mah) ANGIOMA containing fatty tissue.

angiology (an″je-ol′o-je) scientific study or description of the blood and lymph vessels.

angiolupoid (an″je-o-loo′poid) a tuberculous skin lesion consisting of small, oval, red plaques, chiefly on the side of the nose.

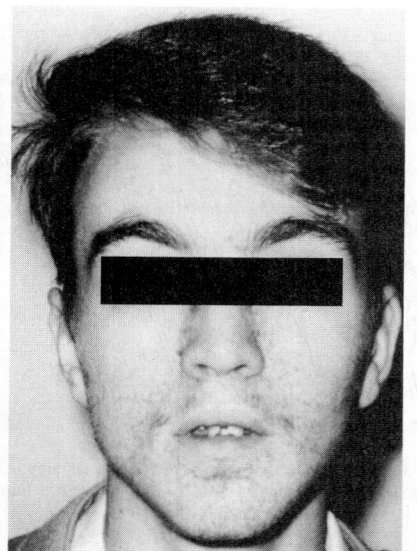

Facial rash of angiokeratoma in a male with tuberous sclerosis. From Mueller and Young, 2001.

angiolysis (an″je-ol′ĭ-sis) retrogression or obliteration of blood vessels, as in embryologic development.

angioma (an″je-o′mah) a benign tumor made up of blood vessels (HEMANGIOMA) or lymph vessels (LYMPHANGIOMA). adj., **angiom′-atous.**

    a. **caverno′sum, cavernous** ***a.*** cavernous hemangioma.

    a. **serpigino′sum** a skin disease marked by minute vascular points arranged in rings on the skin.

    telangiectatic a. an angioma made up of dilated blood vessels.

angiomatosis (an″je-o-mah-to′sis) the presence of multiple ANGIOMAS.

    a. of retina diseased retinal blood vessels with subretinal hemorrhages.

angiomegaly (an″je-o-meg′ah-le) enlargement of blood vessels, especially a condition of the eyelid marked by great increase in its volume.

angiomyolipoma (an″je-o-mi″o-lĭ-po′mah) a benign tumor containing vascular, adipose, and muscle elements, occurring most often in the kidney with smooth muscle elements.

angiomyoma (an″je-o-mi-o′mah) angioleiomyoma.

angiomyosarcoma (an″je-o-mi″o-sahr-ko′-mah) ANGIOMA blended with MYOMA and SAR-COMA.

angioneurectomy (an″je-o-noo-rek′to-me) surgical excision of vessels and nerves.

angioneuropathy (an″je-o-noo-rop′ah-the) any neuropathy affecting primarily the blood vessels; a disorder of the vasomotor system, as angiospasm or angioparalysis. adj., **angioneuropath′ic.**

angioparalysis (an″je-o-pah-ral′ĭ-sis) paralysis of blood vessel walls.

angiopathy (an″je-op′ah-the) any disease of the blood vessels or lymphatics.

angioplasty (an′je-o-plas″te) an angiographic procedure for elimination of areas of narrowing in blood vessels.

    balloon a. angioplasty in which a balloon CATHETER is inflated inside an artery, stretching the intima and leaving a ragged interior surface after deflation, which triggers a healing response and breaking up of plaque.

    percutaneous transluminal a. a type of balloon angioplasty in which the catheter is inserted through the skin and through the lumen of the vessel to the site of the narrowing.

    percutaneous transluminal coronary a. **(PTCA)** percutaneous transluminal angioplasty to enlarge the lumen of a sclerotic coronary artery (see accompanying illustration). This provides an alternative to cardiac BYPASS surgery for selected patients with ischemic heart disease. See also HEART.

angiopoiesis (an″je-o-poi-e′sis) angiogenesis. adj., **angiopoiet′ic.**

angiorrhaphy (an″je-or′ah-fe) suture of a blood vessel.

angiosarcoma (an″je-o-sahr-ko′mah) a malignant tumor of vascular tissue; called also hemangiosarcoma.

angiosclerosis (an″je-o-sklĕ-ro′sis) hardening of the walls of blood vessels.

angioscope (an′je-o-skōp″) 1. a fiberoptic catheter for viewing the inside of a blood vessel. 2. a microscope for observing capillary blood vessels.

angioscopy (an″je-os′kah-pe) 1. use of a fiberoptic angioscope to visualize the lumen of a blood vessel. 2. visualization of capillary blood vessels with a special microscope (angioscope).

angioscotoma (an″je-o-sko-to′mah) a defect in the visual field caused by the shadow of the retinal blood vessels.

angiospasm (an′je-o-spazm″) vasospasm. adj., **angiospas′tic.**

angiostrongyliasis (an″je-o-stron″jĭ-li′ah-sis) infection by nematodes of the genus *Angiostrongylus.*

Angiostrongylus (an″je-o-stron′jĭ-lus) a genus of nematode parasites. *A. cantonen′sis* has been reported in cases of human MENINGOENCEPHALITIS in the Pacific and eastern

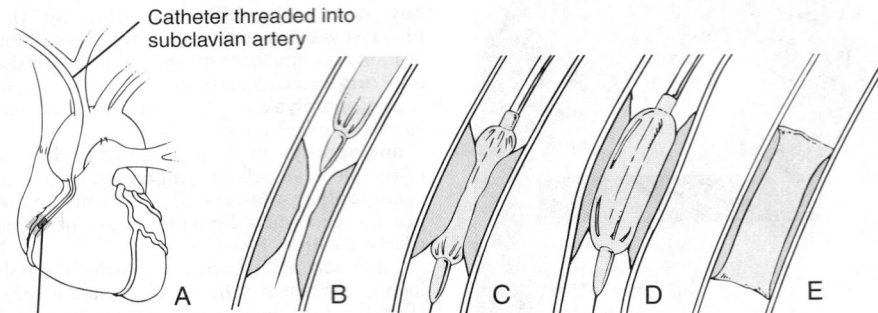

Catheter threaded into subclavian artery

Balloon in position in right coronary artery

A B C D E

Percutaneous transluminal coronary angioplasty (PTCA). *A,* Balloon-tipped catheter positioned in blocked artery. *B,* Balloon is centered. *C,* Balloon expands to *(D)* compress blockage. *E,* Artery diameter opened. From Polaski and Tatro, 1996.

Asia. *A. vaso'rum* parasitizes the pulmonary arteries of dogs.

angiotelectasis (an″je-o-tel-ek′tah-sis), pl. *angiotelec'tases.* dilation of minute arteries or veins.

angiotensin (ACE) (an″je-o-ten′sin) a vaso-constrictive substance formed in the blood when RENIN is released from the juxtaglo-merular apparatus in the kidney. The enzymatic action of renin acts on ANGIOTEN-SINOGEN to form the decapeptide angiotensin I, which is relatively inactive. It in turn is acted upon by peptidases (converting enzymes), chiefly in the lungs, to form the octapeptide angiotensin II, a powerful vasopressor and a stimulator of aldosterone secretion by the adrenal cortex. By its vasopressor action, it raises blood pressure and diminishes fluid loss in the kidney by restricting blood flow. Angiotensin II is hydrolyzed in various tissues to form hepta-peptide angiotensin III, which has less vasopressor activity but more effect on the adrenal cortex.

a.-converting enzyme (ACE) an enzyme of the hydrolase class that catalyzes cleavage of a dipeptide from the C-terminal end of angiotensin I to form activated angiotensin II; called also PEPTIDYL-DIPEPTIDASE A.

a.-converting enzyme inhibitors com-petitive inhibitors of ANGIOTENSIN-CONVERTING ENZYME, which converts angiotensin I to angiotensin II and inactivates bradykinin. ACE inhibitors, such as CAPTOPRIL, are an-tagonists of the RENIN-ANGIOTENSIN-ALDOSTE-RONE SYSTEM and potentiators of the kinin system and are used for treatment of hypertension, usually in conjunction with

a diuretic. They are also used as vasodila-tors in the treatment of congestive heart failure.

angiotensinogen (an″je-o-ten′sin-o-jen) a serum α_2-globulin secreted in the liver which, on hydrolysis by renin, gives rise to angiotensin.

angiotomy (an″je-ot′ah-me) incision of a blood vessel or lymphatic channel.

angiotonic (an″je-o-ton′ik) increasing vas-cular tension.

angiotrophic (an″je-o-trof′ik) vasotrophic.

Angle's classification (ang′g′lz) a classifi-cation of dental malocclusion based on mesiodistal (anteroposterior) position of the mandibular dental arch and teeth relative to the maxillary dental arch and teeth.

angle (ang′g′l) the space or figure formed by two diverging lines, measured as the number of degrees one would have to be moved to coincide with the other.

acromial a. that between the head of the humerus and the clavicle.

alpha a. that formed by intersection of the visual axis with the optic axis.

buccal a's 1. the tooth angles between the buccal surface and the other surfaces of a posterior tooth; see accompanying illustra-tion. 2. the cavity angles between the buccal wall of a tooth cavity and other walls.

cardiodiaphragmatic a. that formed by the junction of the shadows of the heart and diaphragm in posteroanterior radio-graphs of the heart.

cavity a's the angles formed by the junction of two or more walls of a tooth cavity, named according to the walls partic-ipating in their formation.

cavosurface a. the angle formed by the junction of a wall of a tooth cavity preparation and a surface of the crown of the tooth.

costovertebral a. the angle formed on either side of the vertebral column between the last rib and the lumbar vertebrae.

distal a's 1. the tooth angles formed between the distal surface and the other surfaces of a tooth; see accompanying illustration. 2. the cavity angles between the distal wall of a tooth cavity and other walls.

filtration a., a. of the iris the angle between the iris and cornea at the periphery of the anterior chamber of the eye, through which the aqueous humor readily permeates.

a. of jaw the junction of the lower edge with the posterior edge of the lower jaw.

lingual a's 1. the tooth angles formed between the lingual surface and the other surfaces of a tooth; see accompanying illustration. 2. the cavity angles between the lingual wall of a tooth cavity preparation and other walls.

a. of Louis an anatomical landmark located on the sternum; it can be felt as a notch or ridge at the top of the sternum.

mesial a's 1. the tooth angles formed between the mesial surface and other surfaces of a tooth; see accompanying illustration. 2. the cavity angles between the mesial wall of a tooth cavity and other walls.

meter a. the angle formed by intersection of the visual axis and the perpendicular bisector of the line joining the centers of rotation of the two eyes when viewing a point one meter distant (small meter angle) or the angle formed by intersection of the visual axes of the two eyes in the midline at a distance of one meter (large meter angle).

optic a. visual angle.

a. of pubis that between the pubic bones at the symphysis.

sternoclavicular a. that between the sternum and the clavicle.

tooth a's the angles formed by the junction of two or more surfaces of a tooth, named according to the surfaces participating in their formation (see accompanying illustration).

visual a. the angle between two lines passing from the edges of an object seen, through the nodal POINT of the eye, to the corresponding edges of the image of the object seen.

angology (ang-gol′o-je) the study of pain.

angstrom (Å) (ang′strom) a unit of length used for atomic dimensions and light wavelengths; it is nominally equivalent to 10^{-10} meter.

angulation (ang″gu-la′shun) 1. formation of a sharp obstructive angle as in the

intestine, the ureter, or similar tubes. 2. deviation from a straight line, as in a poorly set bone.

angulus (ang′gu-lus), pl. *an′guli* [L.] angle; used in names of anatomic structures or landmarks.

anhedonia (an″he-do′ne-ah) inability to enjoy what is usually pleasurable.

anhidrosis (an″hĭ-dro′sis) absence of SWEATING.

anhidrotic (an″hĭ-drot′ik) 1. pertaining to ANHIDROSIS. 2. antiperspirant.

anhydrase (an-hi′drās) an enzyme that catalyzes the removal of water from a compound.

carbonic a. an enzyme that catalyzes the decomposition of carbonic acid into carbon dioxide and water, facilitating transfer of carbon dioxide from tissues to blood and from blood to alveolar air.

anhydremia (an″hi-dre′me-ah) diminution of the fluid content of the blood; see also DEHYDRATION and HYPOVOLEMIA.

anhydride (an-hi′drīd) a compound derived from a substance, usually an acid, by removal of a molecule of water.

anhydrous (an-hi′drus) containing no water.

anideus (ah-nid′e-us) a parasitic fetus consisting of a shapeless mass of flesh.

anidrosis (an″ĭ-dro′sis) anhidrosis.

anileridine (an″ĭ-ler′ĭ-dēn) a synthetic opioid ANALGESIC used for the relief of moderate to severe pain, as premedication for general anesthesia, as a postoperative sedative, and as an obstetric analgesic; administered orally or parenterally. Abuse of this drug may lead to dependence.

aniline (an′ĭ-lin) an oily liquid from coal tar and indigo or prepared by reducing nitrobenzene; the parent substance of colors or dyes derived from coal tar. Aniline and its derivatives are an important cause of serious industrial poisoning. Household items such as indelible ink, shoe dye, and some wax crayons have been associated with poisonings. Routes of exposure include the respiratory tract, the mouth, and percutaneous absorption. Aniline from the mother can cross the placental barrier to poison a fetus. The predominant acute toxic effect is methemoglobinemia.

anilingus (a″nĭ-ling′gus) sexual stimulation of the anus with the lips or tongue.

anilism (an′ĭ-lizm) aniline poisoning.

anility (ah-nil′ĭ-te) 1. the state of existing as or like an old woman. 2. senility.

anima (an′ĭ-mah) [L.] 1. the soul. 2. in jungian psychology, the soul or inner being of a person, as opposed to the persona, the

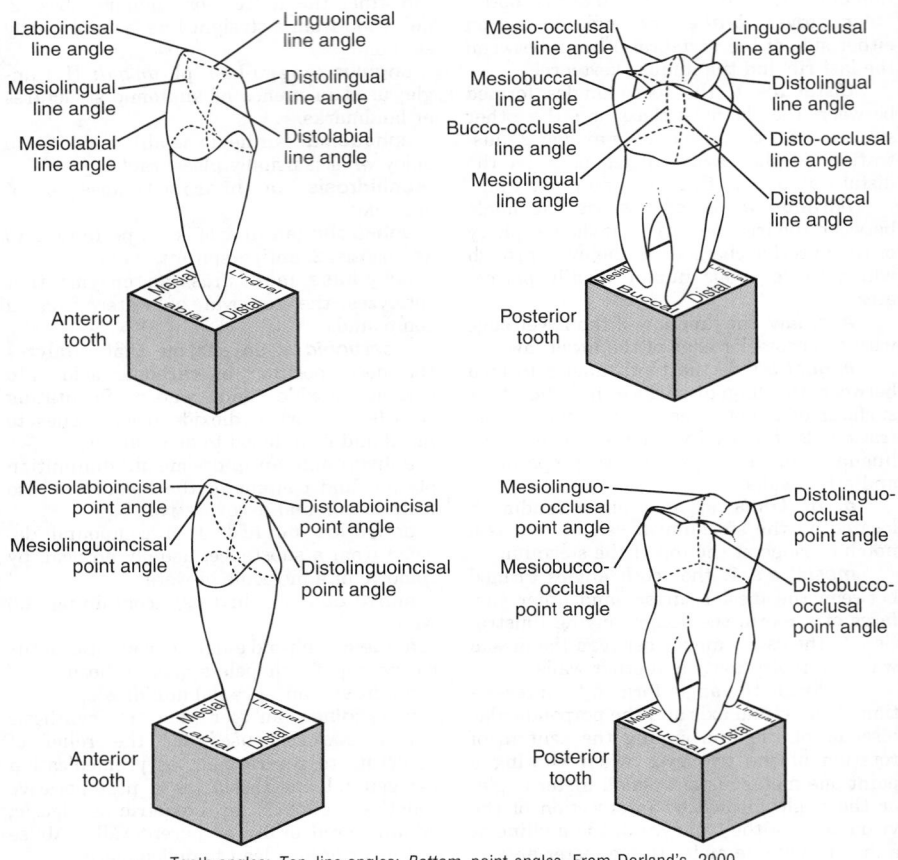

Tooth angles: *Top,* line angles; *Bottom,* point angles. From Dorland's, 2000.

social facade presented to the world. Because the inner and outer facades are often opposing, Jung also used the term to refer to the feminine aspect of a man's soul. See also ANIMUS.

animal (an′ĭ-mal) 1. a living organism having sensation and the power of voluntary movement and requiring for its existence oxygen and organic food; animals comprise one of the five KINGDOMS in the most widely used classification of living organisms. 2. any member of the animal kingdom other than a human being. 3. of or pertaining to such an organism.

control a. an untreated animal otherwise identical in all respects to one that is used for purposes of experiment; used for checking results of treatment.

animation (an″ĭ-ma′shun) the quality of being full of life.

suspended a. temporary suspension or cessation of the vital functions, with loss of consciousness.

animus (an′ĭ-mus) [L.] 1. disposition. 2. ill will or hostility; animosity. 3. in jungian psychology, the masculine aspect of a woman's soul or inner being. See also ANIMA.

anion (an′ĭ-on) an ION carrying a negative charge. adj., **anion′ic.**

aniridia (an″ĭ-rid′e-ah) congenital absence of the iris.

anis(o)- word element [Gr.], *unequal.*

anisakiasis (an″ĭ-sah-ki′ah-sis) infection with the third-stage larvae of the roundworm *Anisakis marina,* which burrow into the stomach wall, producing an eosinophilic granulomatous mass. Infection is acquired by eating undercooked marine fish.

Anisakis (an″ĭ-sa′kis) a genus of nematodes that parasitize the stomachs of marine mammals and birds.

aniseikonia (an″is-i-ko′ne-ah) inequality of the retinal images of the two eyes.

anisindione (an″is-in′de-ōn) an INDANEDIONE ANTICOAGULANT; used when a coumarin derivative can not be used.

anisochromatic (an-i″so-kro-mat′ik) not of the same color throughout.

anisocoria (an-i″so-kor′e-ah) inequality in size of the pupils of the eyes.

anisocytosis (an-i″so-si-to′sis) the presence in the blood of erythrocytes showing abnormal variations in size; see also MACROCYTHEMIA and MICROCYTHEMIA.

anisokaryosis (an-i″so-kar″e-o′sis) inequality in the size of the nuclei of cells.

anisomastia (an-i″so-mas′te-ah) inequality in size of the breasts.

anisometropia (an-i″so-mĕ-tro′pe-ah) inequality in the refractive power of the two eyes, of considerable degree. adj., **anisometrop′ic.**

anisopiesis (an-i″so-pi-e′sis) difference in blood pressure recorded in corresponding arteries on the right and left sides of the body.

anisosthenic (an-i″sos-then′ik) not having equal power; said of muscles.

anisotonic (an-i″so-ton′ik) 1. varying in tonicity or tension. 2. having different osmotic pressure; not isotonic.

anisotropic (an-i″so-trop′ik) 1. having unlike properties in different directions. 2. doubly refracting, or having a double polarizing power. 3. in cardiac physiology, having nonuniform conduction; used to describe the nonuniform characteristics of the myocardium in the direction perpendicular to the conduction direction of a fiber. See also ISOTROPIC.

anisotropine (an-is″o-tro′pēn) an ANTICHOLINERGIC drug that produces relaxation of visceral smooth muscle and is used as an ANTISPASMODIC in gastrointestinal disorders.

anisotropy (an″i-sot′ro-pe) the quality of being ANISOTROPIC.

anistreplase (an″is-trep′lās) a THROMBOLYTIC agent primarily used to clear coronary vessel occlusions associated with MYOCARDIAL INFARCTION; administered intravenously.

anisuria (an″i-su′re-ah) alternating oliguria and polyuria.

ankle (ang′k'l) 1. the joint between the leg and foot. 2. the area around this joint (see illustration). The ankle is a hinge joint formed by the junction of the TIBIA and FIBULA with the TALUS (ankle bone). The bones are cushioned by cartilage and connected by a number of ligaments, tendons, and muscles that strengthen the joint

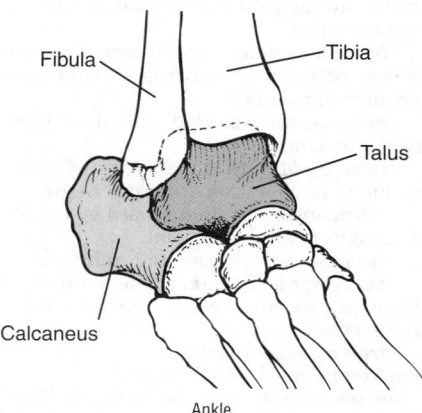

Ankle.

and enable it to be moved. Because it is in almost constant use, the ankle is particularly susceptible to injuries, such as SPRAIN and FRACTURE. It is also often one of the first joints to be affected by ARTHRITIS or GOUT. 3. tarsus (def. 2). 4. talus.

a. **cuff** a weighted strip wrapped around the ankle and closed with a Velcro band; used during exercise.

ankyl(o)- word element [Gr.], *bent; crooked; in the form of a loop; adhesion.*

ankyloblepharon (ang″kĭ-lo-blef′ah-ron) adhesion of the eyelids to each other.

ankylocheilia (ang″kĭ-lo-ki′le-ah) adhesion of the lips to each other.

ankyloglossia (ang″kĭ-lo-glos′e-ah) abnormal shortness of the FRENULUM OF THE TONGUE, resulting in limitation of its motion; called also tongue-tie.

a. **superior** extensive adhesion of the tongue to the palate, sometimes with limb deformities.

ankylopoietic (ang″kĭ-lo-poi-et′ik) producing ankylosis.

ankylosed (ang′kĭ-lōsd) affected with ankylosis.

ankylosis (ang″kĭ-lo′sis), pl. *ankylo′ses* [Gr.] immobility and consolidation of a joint due to disease, injury, or surgical procedure. adj., **ankylot′ic.** Ankylosis may be caused by destruction of the membranes that line the joint or by faulty bone structure. It is most often a result of chronic rheumatoid arthritis, in which the affected joint tends to assume the least painful position and may become more or less permanently fixed in it. Other causes include infection and traumatic injury to the joint. *Artificial ankylosis* (arthrodesis), fusion of a joint by surgical operation, is sometimes done to ameliorate the pain experienced in a severe joint condition.

bony a. union of the bones of a joint by loss of articular cartilage, resulting in complete immobility.

extracapsular a. that caused by rigidity of surrounding parts.

false a., fibrous a. reduced joint mobility due to proliferation of fibrous tissue.

intracapsular a. that caused by rigidity of structures within the joint.

spurious a. extracapsular ankylosis.

stapedial a. fixation of the footplate of the stapes in otosclerosis, causing conductive HEARING LOSS.

true a. bony ankylosis.

ankyroid (ang′kĭ-roid) ancyroid.

anlage (ahn′lah-geh), pl. *anla′gen* [Ger.] primordium; the first beginnings of an organ or part in the developing embryo.

ANNA American Nephrology Nurses' Association.

anneal (ah-nēl′) 1. to heat a material, such as glass or metal, followed by controlled cooling to remove internal stresses and induce a desired degree of toughness, temper, or softness of the material. 2. to homogenize an amalgam alloy ingot by heating it in an oven. 3. to heat a material, such as gold foil, to volatilize and drive off impurities from its surface, and to increase its cohesive properties.

annectent (ah-nek′tent) connecting; joining together. Also spelled *annectant.*

Annelida (ah-nel′ĭ-dah) a phylum of metazoan invertebrates, the segmented worms, including leeches.

annular (an′u-ler) ring-shaped.

annuloplasty (an′u-lo-plas″te) plastic repair of a cardiac VALVE by shortening the circumference of its annulus.

annulus (an′u-lus), pl. *an′nuli* [L.] alternate spelling of ANULUS.

anococcygeal (a″no-kok-sij′e-al) pertaining to the anus and coccyx.

anode (an′ōd) the electrode at which oxidation occurs and to which anions are attracted. adj., **ano′dal.**

anodontia (an″o-don′she-ah) congenital absence of some or all of the teeth; called also edentia.

anodyne (an′o-dīn) analgesic.

anomalad (ah-nom′ah-lad) a term proposed to designate a single, localized anomaly occurring during morphogenesis, together with the pattern of subsequent morphologic defects that stem from it.

anomaloscope (ah-nom′ah-lo-skōp″) an apparatus used to detect anomalies of color vision.

anomaly (ah-nom′ah-le) marked deviation from normal. adj., **anom′alous.**

Axenfeld's a. a developmental anomaly characterized by a circular opacity of the posterior peripheral cornea, and caused by an irregularly thickened, axially displaced Schwalbe's ring.

congenital a., developmental a. absence, deformity, or excess of body parts as the result of faulty development of the embryo.

Ebstein's a. see EBSTEIN'S ANOMALY.

May-Hegglin a. a rare dominantly inherited disorder of blood cell morphology, characterized by RNA-containing cytoplasmic inclusions (similar to Döhle bodies) in granulocytes, by large, poorly granulated platelets, and by thrombocytopenia.

anomia (ah-no′me-ah) loss of the ability to name objects or recognize names.

anonychia (an″o-nik′e-ah) absence of the nail(s).

anonymity (an″o-nim′ĭ-te) protection of the subjects in a research study so that their identity cannot be linked with their individual responses, even by the researcher; see also CONFIDENTIALITY.

Anopheles (ah-nof′ĕ-lēz) a widely distributed genus of mosquitoes, comprising over 300 species, many of which are important vectors of MALARIA.

anophthalmia (an″of-thal′me-ah) a developmental ANOMALY consisting of complete absence of the eyes or presence of only rudimentary eyes.

anophthalmos (an″of-thal′mos) anophthalmia.

anoplasty (a′no-plas″te) plastic repair of the anus.

anopsia (ah-nop′se-ah) suppression of vision in one area only; see also QUADRANTANOPIA.

anorchia anorchism.

anorchid (an-or′kid) 1. lacking testes. 2. a male who lacks testes.

anorchidism (an-or′kĭ-dizm) anorchism.

anorchism (an-or′kizm) congenital absence of one or both testes.

anorectic (an″o-rek′tik) 1. pertaining to ANOREXIA. 2. without appetite. 3. an agent that diminishes or suppresses the appetite for food. Most of the drugs used for this purpose are central nervous system stimulants (the amphetamines and similar sympathomimetic amines). These drugs should not be used in a lifelong weight-control program. Abuse of them, which is frequent, can lead to tolerance and psychological dependence.

anorectum (a″no-rek′tum) the distal portion of the digestive tract, including the entire anal canal and the distal 2 cm of the rectum. adj., **anorec′tal.**

anorexia (an″o-rek′se-ah) lack or loss of APPETITE; appetite is psychological, dependent on memory and associations, as compared with HUNGER, which is physiologically aroused by the body's need for food. Anorexia can be brought about by subjectively unpleasant food, surroundings, or company, or emotional states such as anxiety, irritation, anger, or fear; it may also be a symptom of a physical disorder or emotional disturbance.

a. nervo′sa an EATING DISORDER consisting of loss of appetite due to emotional states, such as anxiety, irritation, anger, and fear. In true anorexia nervosa there is no real loss of appetite, but rather a refusal to eat or an aberration in eating patterns; hence, the term anorexia is probably a misnomer. The clinical picture is usually that of a young woman who is obsessed with the idea of being thin and restricts her food intake to the point of danger; she may alternate fasting with periods of bingeing (BULIMIA). She often may be described as "a model child" with perfectionistic tendencies. A personal crisis often triggers the disorder.

The syndrome was first described more than 300 years ago and was once thought to be exceedingly rare. However, in recent years its incidence has been rapidly increasing throughout the world in developed countries as diverse as Russia, Japan, Australia, and the United States. The condition occurs mainly in girls after the age of puberty, and the prevalence may be as high as one in a hundred.

Cause. The cause of anorexia nervosa is unknown, but it is thought to be a complex of psychological, social, and biological factors. There are numerous theories, such as that the victim is attempting to control some aspects of life in an environment where it is difficult to exert control; that it is an attempt to manipulate others and gain attention; and social pressures, conflicting roles, and family disorders that serve as stimuli. Other theorists hypothesize that the disorder is a defense against sexual maturation, related to a fear of sexual intimacy. Society's obsession with physical appearance is also thought by some to play a role. Researchers are studying whether there could be a genetic component, as well as whether malfunction of the hypothalamus might play a role.

Symptoms. Criteria for diagnosis of anorexia nervosa identified by the American Psychiatric Association are as follows: (1) intense fear of becoming obese that does not diminish as weight loss progresses; (2) disturbance of body image, such as claiming to

feel fat even when emaciated; (3) refusal to maintain body weight over a minimal normal weight for age and height; (4) no known physical illness that would account for the weight loss; and (5) amenorrhea in postmenarchal females. It is often accompanied by self-induced vomiting or use of laxatives and/or diuretics (see also BULIMIA NERVOSA) and extensive exercise. Accompanying physical signs in addition to profound weight loss include hypotension, bradycardia, edema, lanugo, metabolic changes, and endocrine disturbances.

Treatment. The treatment of anorexia nervosa is difficult and lengthy. The primary goals are restitution of normal nutrition and resolution of underlying psychological problems. Modes of therapy that can be used include behavior therapy, behavioral contracts, psychoanalysis, group therapy, insight-oriented therapy, and family therapy.

Nutritional counseling, social services and support, health education, and health care are all components in the physical and psychological recovery from an eating disorder. The physical sequelae, as well as the social and cultural aspects, require a multidisciplinary approach individualized to the unique needs of the victim and family. Inpatient treatment, either partial or complete, is required when the individual's problems warrant intensive services or if outpatient treatment is not successful. Some hospitals have special units for patients with eating disorders, providing an environment for treatment that emphasizes the simultaneous treatment of physiologic and psychological problems by professionals trained in the management of these patients. The American Psychological Association has identified numerous areas for research related to eating disorders.

Information and support for professionals as well as persons affected by the disorder can be obtained from the National Association of Anorexia Nervosa and Associated Disorders by writing to them at P.O. Box 7, Highland Park IL 60035 or calling their hotline at 1-847-831-3438.

anorexia-cachexia a systemic response to cancer occurring as a result of metabolites which may be produced by the tumor cells and released into the blood stream, stimulating the satiety center in the hypothalamus and producing appetite loss, gross alterations of metabolic patterns, and a profound systemic confusion which may result in further anorexia. This leads to malnutrition, weight loss, muscular weakness, and a negative nitrogen balance that contributes to the development of cachectic wasting.

anorexic (an″o-rek′sik) anorectic.

anorexigenic (an″o-rek″sī-jen′ik) 1. producing anorexia. 2. anorectic (def. 3).

anormalization (a-nor″mal-ī-za′shun) the possessing of expectations that differ from those originally anticipated.

anorthography (an″or-thog′rah-fe) loss of the ability to write.

anorthopia (an″or-tho′pe-ah) 1. distorted vision in which straight lines appear as curves or angles, and symmetry is incorrectly perceived. 2. strabismus.

anoscope (a′no-skōp) a speculum or endoscope used in direct visual examination of the anal canal.

anoscopy (a-nos′kah-pe) examination of the anal canal with an anoscope.

anosigmoidoscopy (a″no-sig-moi″dos′-kah-pe) endoscopic examination of the anus and sigmoid.

anosmia (an-oz′me-ah) absence of the sense of SMELL. adj., **anosmat′ic, anos′mic.**

anosmic (an-oz′mik) 1. having no sense of smell. 2. odorless.

anosognosia (an-o″so-no′zhah) unawareness or denial of a neurological deficit, such as hemiplegia.

anospinal (a″no-spi′nal) pertaining to the anus and spinal cord.

anostosis (an″os-to′sis) defective formation of bone.

anotia (an-o′she-ah) congenital absence of one or both external ears.

anovaginal (a″no-vaj′ĭ-nal) pertaining to or communicating with the anus and vagina.

anovarism (an-o′vah-rizm) absence of the OVARIES; see also HYPOGONADISM and TURNER'S SYNDROME.

anovesical (a″no-ves′ĭ-kal) pertaining to the anus and bladder.

anovular (an-ov′u-lar) not accompanied by OVULATION.

anovulation absence of OVULATION.

anovulatory (an-ov′u-lah-tor″e) anovular.

anoxia (an-ok′se-ah) absence of oxygen in the tissues; formerly used interchangeably with HYPOXIA to mean a reduction of oxygen in body tissues below physiologic levels. adj., **anox′ic.**

ansa (an′sah), pl. *an′sae* [L.] a looplike structure.

a. cervica′lis a nerve loop in the neck attached in front and above to the hypoglossal nerve and behind to the upper cervical spinal nerves. Its hypoglossal attachment is misleading since this part of the loop ultimately rejoins the upper spinal nerves. Called also ansa hypoglossi.

a. of Henle Henle's loop.

a. hypoglos′si ansa cervicalis.

a. lenticula′ris a small nerve fiber tract arising in the globus pallidus and joining the anterior part of the ventral thalamic nucleus.

a. nephro′ni Henle's loop.

an′sae nervo′rum spina′lium loops of spinal nerves joining the anterior spinal nerves.

a. peduncula′ris peduncular loop: a complex grouping of nerve fibers connecting the amygdaloid nucleus, piriform area, and anterior hypothalamus, and various thalamic nuclei.

Antabuse (an′tah-būs) trademark for a preparation of DISULFIRAM, used in the treatment of ALCOHOLISM; it causes nausea and other distressing symptoms in persons who ingest alcohol while taking it.

antacid (ant-as′id) 1. counteracting acidity. 2. an agent that counteracts acidity; antacids are often used in the treatment of PEPTIC ULCER. Substances that act as antacids include SODIUM BICARBONATE, ALUMINUM HYDROXIDE GEL, CALCIUM CARBONATE, MAGNESIUM HYDROXIDE, MAGNESIUM OXIDE, and MAGNESIUM TRISILICATE. Since many substances used as medications are weak acids or weak bases, there is a high potential for drug-drug interaction involving antacids. Antacids can form insoluble complexes, interfere with drug absorption, and affect renal excretion of drugs by changing the pH of urine.

In the most commonly used antacids the main active agents are magnesium hydroxide and aluminum hydroxide. Magnesium hydroxide, or "milk of magnesia," can produce diarrhea. Aluminum hydroxide and calcium carbonate are constipating. It may be necessary to alternate types of antacids when they are taken on a long-term basis. The sodium content varies; some antacids may contain as much as ten times more sodium than others. The sugar content of antacids must also be taken into account, particularly for patients with diabetes mellitus or those on a low-calorie diet. Some have no sugar, whereas others have a considerable amount.

antagonist (an-tag′o-nist) 1. antagonistic MUSCLE. (see illustration.) 2. a substance that tends to nullify the action of another, as a drug that binds to a cellular receptor for a hormone, neurotransmitter, or another drug blocking the action of that substance without producing any physiologic effect itself. See also blocking AGENT. 3. a tooth in one jaw that articulates with one in the other jaw.

α-adrenergic a. alpha-adrenergic blocking agent.

β-adrenergic a. beta-adrenergic blocking agent.

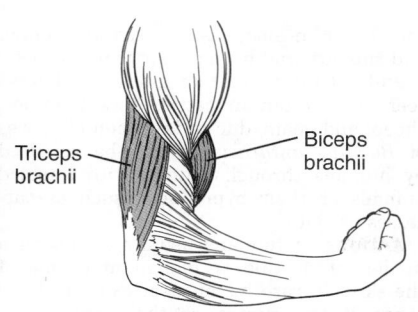

Triceps brachii

Biceps brachii

Antagonists: the triceps brachii extends the forearm at the elbow and the biceps brachii flexes the elbow. From Dorland's, 2000.

folic acid a. see FOLIC ACID ANTAGONIST.

H₁ receptor a. any of a large number of agents that block the action of histamine by competitive binding to the H₁ receptor. Such agents also have sedative, anticholinergic, and antiemetic effects, the exact effect varying from drug to drug, and are used for the relief of allergic symptoms and as antiemetics, antivertigo agents, sedatives, and antidyskinetics in parkinsonism. This group is traditionally called the ANTIHISTAMINES.

H₂ receptor a. an agent that blocks the action of histamine by competitive binding to the H₂ receptor; used to inhibit gastric secretion in the treatment of PEPTIC ULCER.

antalgic (ant-al'jik) 1. counteracting or avoiding pain, as a posture or gait assumed so as to lessen pain. 2. analgesic.

antarthritic (ant"ahr-thrit'ik) antiarthritic.

antazoline (an-taz'o-lēn) a derivative of ETHYLENEDIAMINE, used as an ANTIHISTAMINE; the phosphate salt is applied topically to the eyes in treatment of allergic CONJUNCTIVITIS.

ante (an'te) [L.] preposition, *before.*

ante- word element [L.], *before* (in time or space).

antebrachium (an"te-bra'ke-um) the forearm. adj., **antebra'chial.**

antecedent (an"te-se'dent) a precursor.

plasma thromboplastin a. (PTA) factor XI, one of the COAGULATION FACTORS.

ante cibum (a.c., AC) (an'te si'bum) before meals.

antecubital (an"tĭ-ku'bĭ-t'l) pertaining to the surface of the arm in front of the elbow.

antecurvature (an"te-kur'vah-chur) a slight anteflexion.

anteflexion (an"te-flek'shun) 1. the bending of an organ so that its top is thrust forward. 2. anterior displacement of a tooth or teeth or of the mandible.

ante mortem (an'te mor'tem) [L.] before death.

antemortem (an"te-mor'tem) performed or occurring before death.

antenna (an-ten'ah), pl. *anten'nae* one of the appendages on the head of arthropods.

Antepar (an'te-pahr) trademark for preparations of PIPERAZINE citrate and piperazine phosphate, ANTHELMINTICS.

antepartal (an"te-pahr't'l) antepartum.

antepartum (an"te-pahr'tum) occurring before CHILDBIRTH, with reference to the mother. Spelled also ante partum. Called also antepartal and prepartal.

antepyretic (an"te-pi-ret'ik) before the onset of fever.

anter(o)- word element [L.], *anterior; in front of.*

anterior (an-tēr'e-or) situated at or directed toward the front; opposite of posterior.

anterior cord syndrome localized injury to the anterior portion of the spinal cord, characterized by complete paralysis and hypalgesia and hypesthesia to the level of the lesion, but with relative preservation of posterior column sensations of position and vibration. (See accompanying illustration.)

anterograde (an'ter-o-grād") extending or moving forward.

anteroinferior (an"ter-o-in-fēr'e-or) situated in front and below.

anterolateral (an"ter-o-lat'er-al) situated in front and to one side.

anteromedian (an"ter-o-me'de-an) situated in front and toward the midline.

anteroposterior (an"ter-o-pos-tēr'e-or) directed from the front toward the back.

anterosuperior (an"ter-o-soo-pēr'e-or) situated in front and above.

anteversion (an"te-ver'zhun) the tipping forward of an entire organ.

anteverted (an"te-vert'ed) tipped or bent forward.

anthelix (ant'he-liks) antihelix.

anthelmintic (ant"hel-min'tik) 1. destructive to parasitic worms; called also antihelmintic and vermifugal. 2. an agent destructive to worms; examples include PIPERAZINE and HEXYLRESORCINOL for the roundworm *Ascaris lumbricoides;* QUINACRINE for TAPEWORMS; OXYTETRACYCLINE and EMETINE for protozoan infections such as AMEBIC DYSENTERY; and MEBENDAZOLE for several different intestinal worms. Many anthelmintic drugs are toxic and should be given with care; the toxic effects of a specific drug should be known prior to administration and the patient observed carefully for such effects after the drug is given. Called also vermicide, and vermifuge

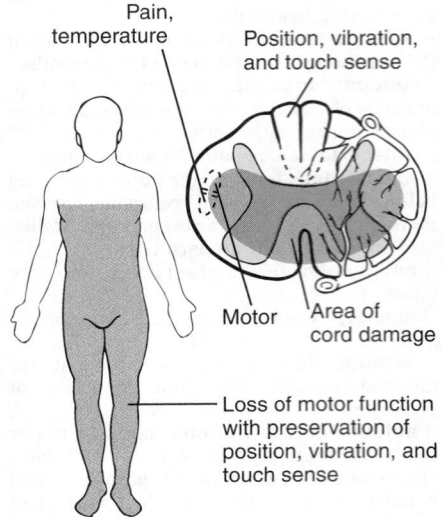

Pain, temperature

Position, vibration, and touch sense

Motor

Area of cord damage

Loss of motor function with preservation of position, vibration, and touch sense

Anterior cord syndrome. Redrawn from Ignatavicius and Workman, 2002.

anthracene (an'thrah-sēn) 1. a crystalline hydrocarbon, $C_{14}H_{10}$, from coal tar, used in making dyes.

anthracenedione (an"thrah-sēn-di'ōn) any of a class of derivatives of ANTHRAQUI-NONE; some have antineoplastic properties; the group includes MITOXANTRONE hydrochloride.

anthracoid (an'thrah-koid) resembling anthrax.

anthracosilicosis (an"thrah-ko-sil"ĭ-ko'-sis) PNEUMOCONIOSIS in coal workers caused by inhalation of coal dust (ANTHRACOSIS) and fine particles of silica (SILICOSIS). Called also silicoanthracosis.

anthracosis (an"thrah-ko'sis) a type of coal workers' PNEUMOCONIOSIS due to inhalation of coal dust not containing silica.

anthracycline (an"thrah-si'klēn) a class of ANTIBIOTICS isolated from cultures of *Streptomyces peucetius;* it includes the antineoplastic AGENTS DAUNORUBICIN and DOXORUBICIN. The use of these drugs is limited by a chronic, cumulative, dose-related toxicity resulting in irreversible congestive HEART FAILURE. (See accompanying illustration.)

anthralin (an'thrah-lin) an ANTHRAQUINONE used topically in treatment of psoriasis.

anthraquinone (an"thrah-kwin'ōn) 1. a derivative of ANTHRACENE, used in dye manufacture. 2. any of the usually highly colored derivatives of this compound which may be yellow, orange, red, red-brown, or violet;

they occur in aloe, cascara sagrada, senna, and rhubarb and have cathartic properties.

anthrax (an'thraks) an infectious disease seen most often in cattle, horses, mules, sheep, and goats, due to ingestion of spores of *Bacillus anthracis.* It can be acquired by humans through contact with infected animals or their byproducts, such as carcasses or skins.

Anthrax in humans usually occurs as a malignant pustule or malignant edema of the skin. In rare instances it can affect the lungs if the spores of the bacillus are inhaled, or it can involve the intestinal tract when infected meat is eaten. The condition often is accompanied by hemorrhage, as the EXOTOXINS from the bacillus attack the endothelium of small blood vessels. The condition is treated by the use of antibiotics such as penicillin and the tetracyclines. The malignant edema can be treated with intravenous hydrocortisone. The disorder is also known by a variety of names, including woolsorters' disease, ragpickers' disease, and charbon.

  cutaneous a. anthrax due to lodgment of the causative organisms in wounds or abrasions of the skin, producing a black crusted pustule on a broad zone of edema.

  gastrointestinal a. anthrax due to ingestion of poorly cooked meat contaminated with *Bacillus anthracis,* with deposition of spores in the submucosa of the intestinal tract, where they germinate, multiply, and produce toxin, resulting in massive edema, which may obstruct the bowel, hemorrhage, and necrosis.

  inhalational a. a usually fatal form of anthrax due to inhalation of dust containing anthrax spores, which are transported to the regional lymph nodes where they germinate, multiply, and produce toxin, and characterized by hemorrhagic edematous mediastinitis, pleural effusions, dyspnea, cyanosis, stridor, and shock. It is usually an

Anthracycline. For daunorubicin, $R_1 = $ ——CH_3; for doxorubicin, $R_1 = $ ——$CHOH$.

occupational disease, such as in persons who handle or sort contaminated wools and fleeces. Antimicrobial prophylaxis is used to prevent the condition. The Centers for Disease Control and Prevention has published interim guidelines for investigation and response to *Bacillus anthracis* infection. The evaluation of risk for exposure to aerosolized spores is of highest priority. Obtaining adequate samples, avoiding cross-contamination, and insuring proficient testing and evaluation of test results are all recommended.

meningeal a. a rare, usually fatal form of anthrax resembling typical hemorrhagic meningitis due to spread through the bloodstream of *Bacillus anthracis* from a primary focus of infection; manifestations include cerebrospinal fluid that is hemorrhagic and neurological signs and symptoms.

pulmonary a. inhalational anthrax.

anthrop(o)- word element [Gr.], *man (human being).*

anthropocentric (an″thro-po-sen′trik) with a human bias; considering humans the center of the universe.

anthropoid (an′thro-poid) resembling a human being; the anthropoid apes are tailless apes, including the chimpanzee, gibbon, gorilla, and orangutan.

Anthropoidea (an″thro-poi′de-ah) a suborder of Primates, including monkeys, apes, and humans, characterized by a larger and more complicated brain than the other suborders.

anthropology (an″thro-pol′o-je) the study of human beings and their development, including their customs and practices, that is based on an understanding of the contexts from which observations about human activities are derived. adj., **anthropolog′ical.**

applied a. the use of anthropological approaches and knowledge to influence human behavior or encourage change (including economic development) in the living patterns of different cultural groups.

physical a. the field of anthropology that focuses on human physical characteristics.

sociocultural a. the field of anthropology that focuses on shared patterns of behavior and on customary, agreed-upon solutions that influence behavior; it also includes the study of interactions between individuals.

anthropometry (an″thro-pom′ĕ-tre) the science that deals with the measurement of the size, weight, and proportions of the human body. adj., **anthropomet′ric.**

anthropomorphism (an″thro-po-mor′-fizm) the attribution of human characteristics to nonhuman beings and objects.

anthropophilic (an″thro-po-fil′ik) preferring human beings to animals; said of parasites such as fungi or mosquitoes.

anti- word element [Gr.], *counteracting; effective against.*

antiadrenergic (an″te-ad″ren-er′jik) sympatholytic.

antiagglutinin (an″te-ah-gloo′tĭ-nin) a substance that opposes the action of an agglutinin.

antiamebic (an″te-ah-me′bik) 1. destroying or suppressing the growth of AMEBAS. 2. a type of antiprotozoal AGENT that particularly destroys or suppresses the growth of amebas.

antianaphylaxis (an″te-an″ah-fĭ-lak′sis) a condition in which the anaphylaxis reaction does not occur because of free antigens in the blood; the state of desensitization to antigens.

antiandrogen (an″te-an′dro-jen) any substance capable of inhibiting the biological effects of androgens.

antianemic (an″te-ah-ne′mik) 1. counteracting ANEMIA. 2. an agent that so acts.

antiantibody (an″te-an′tĭ-bod″e) an antibody directed against antigenic determinants on other antibody molecules.

antianxiety (an″ti-ang-zi′ĕ-te) dispelling ANXIETY; called also anxiolytic.

a. agent a PSYCHOTROPIC medication that dispels anxiety; the group includes the BENZODIAZEPINES such as DIAZEPAM (VALIUM) and CHLORDIAZEPOXIDE (LIBRIUM) and a few less widely used nonbenzodiazepines such as MEPROBAMATE (MILTOWN or EQUANIL) and HYDROXYZINE (ATARAX or VISTARIL). Called also anxiolytic and minor tranquilizer.

antiarrhythmic (an″te-ah-rith′mik) 1. preventing or alleviating cardiac arrhythmias. 2. an agent that has this effect.

antiarthritic (an″te-ahr-thrit′ik) 1. effective in treatment of arthritis. 2. an agent used in treatment of arthritis.

antiasthmatic (an″te-az-mat′ik) 1. relieving ASTHMA. 2. an agent that has this effect.

antibacterial (an″te-, an″ti-bak-tēr′e-al) 1. destroying or suppressing the growth or reproduction of bacteria. 2. an agent having such properties.

antibiosis (an″te-, an″ti-bi-o′sis) 1. an association between two populations of organisms that is detrimental to one of them. 2. a relationship between an organism and an ANTIBIOTIC produced by another.

antibiotic (an″te-, an″ti-bi-ot′ik) 1. destructive of life. 2. a chemical substance produced by a microorganism that has the capacity, in dilute solutions, to kill other microorganisms or inhibit their growth. Antibiotics that are sufficiently nontoxic to the host are used as chemotherapeutic agents in the treatment of infectious diseases. See also ANTIMICROBIAL AGENT.

antineoplastic a's, antitumor a's a class of antineoplastic AGENTS that apparently affect the function or the synthesis, or both, of nucleic acids and thus are cell cycle nonspecific. See also ANTINEOPLASTIC THERAPY.

broad-spectrum a. one that is effective against a wide range of bacteria, both gram-positive and gram-negative.

β-lactam a. any of a group of antibiotics, including the cephalosporins and the penicillins, whose chemical structure contains a β-lactam ring.

antibody (an'tĭ-bod"e) an IMMUNOGLOBULIN molecule having a specific amino acid sequence that gives each antibody the ability to adhere to and interact only with the ANTIGEN that induced its synthesis. This antigen-specific property of the antibody is the basis of the antigen-antibody REACTION that is essential to an IMMUNE RESPONSE. The antigen-antibody reaction begins as soon as substances interpreted as foreign invaders gain entrance into the body. See also IMMUNITY. Abbreviated Ab.

Antibodies are synthesized by the plasma cells formed when antigen-specific groups (CLONES) of B LYMPHOCYTES respond to the presence of antigen. The developmental process of antibody production begins when stem cells are transformed into B lymphocytes; this transformation usually is completed a few months after birth, at which time the lymphocytes migrate to lymphoid tissue primarily located in the lymph nodes, although they are also found in the spleen, gastrointestinal tract, and bone marrow.

Antibody production, its interaction with a specific antigen, and the activation of complement (C), an interrelated group of eleven proteins, are the major components of the *humoral system of immunity.* (See accompaning illustration.) Fortunately, the immune response of antibody and complement can be transferred passively from one individual to another, as for example the transfer of maternal antibody across the placental barrier to the fetus, who has not yet developed a mature immune system. An antibody present in an individual without known prior exposure to the corresponding red cell antigen is termed an ISOAGGLUTININ. (Examples are the ABO antibodies anti-A, anti-B, and anti-A,B.)

Antibodies can be classified according to their mode of action as they react to and set about defending the body against foreign invaders. Some cause clumping together of bacterial cells (AGGLUTINATION) and are called AGGLUTININS. Those antibodies that cause bacterial cells to dissolve or liquefy are called BACTERIOLYSINS. This activity is assisted by COMPLEMENT, which interacts with the antigen-antibody complex in such a way that the cell ruptures and there is dissolution (LYSIS) of the cell body. OPSONINS coat the outside of bacteria, making them more attractive to phagocytes. Other types of antibodies include those that neutralize the toxins of antigens (ANTITOXINS) and those that cause precipitation of antigens in a fluid medium (PRECIPITINS).

anaphylactic a. a substance formed as a result of the first injection of a foreign anaphylactogen and responsible for the anaphylactic symptoms following the second injection of the same anaphylactogen.

antinuclear a's (ANA) autoantibodies directed against components of the cell nucleus, e.g., DNA, RNA, and histones; they may be detected by immunofluorescence. A positive ANA test is characteristic of systemic lupus erythematosus. Antinuclear antibodies also occur in patients with rheumatoid arthritis, Sjögren's syndrome, and scleroderma.

blocking a. any antibody that by combining with an antigen blocks another immunologic reaction with the antigen. Immunotherapy (hypersensitization) for allergic disorders induces in most treated patients IgG blocking antibodies that can bind the allergen and prevent it from binding to cell-fixed IgE and trigger immediate hypersensitivity; thus it can induce partial immunologic tolerance. Blocking antibodies can prevent agglutination in serologic tests.

complement-fixing a. antibody (primarily IgM and the IgG subclasses 1, 2, and 3) that activates complement when reacted with antigen.

complete a. antibody capable of agglutinating cells in physiologic saline solution.

cross-reacting a. one that combines with an antigen other than the one that induced its production.

cytophilic a. cytotropic antibody.

cytotoxic a. any specific antibody directed against cellular antigens, which when bound to the antigen, activates the complement pathway or activates killer cells, resulting in cell lysis.

cytotropic a. any of a class of antibodies that attach to tissue cells (such as mast cells and basophils) through their Fc segments to induce the release of histamine and other vasoconstrictive amines important in immediate hypersensitivity reactions.

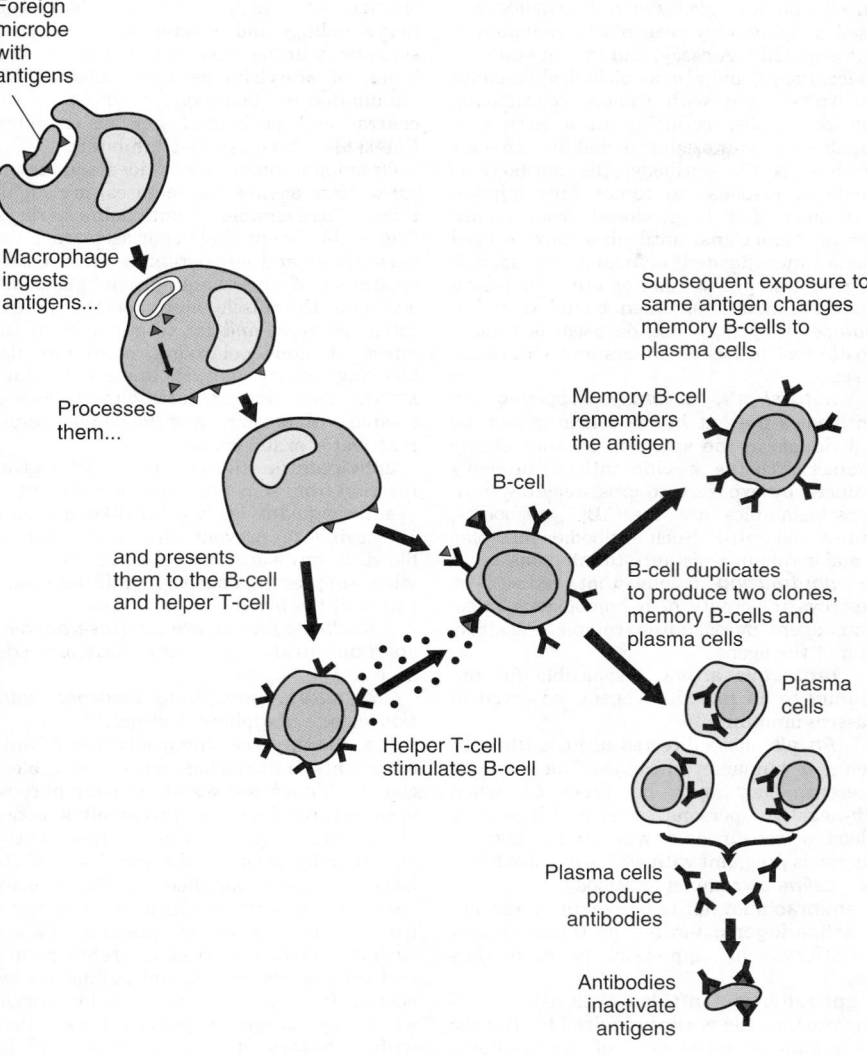

Foreign microbe with antigens

Macrophage ingests antigens...

Processes them...

and presents them to the B-cell and helper T-cell

Helper T-cell stimulates B-cell

B-cell

Subsequent exposure to same antigen changes memory B-cells to plasma cells

Memory B-cell remembers the antigen

B-cell duplicates to produce two clones, memory B-cells and plasma cells

Plasma cells

Plasma cells produce antibodies

Antibodies inactivate antigens

Antibody-mediated immunity. From Applegate, 2000.

In humans this antibody, also known as REAGIN, is of the immunoglobulin class known as IgE. Called also cytophilic antibody.

heterophil a. a characteristic antibody found with many cases of infectious mononucleosis; see also HETEROPHIL ANTIBODY.

immune a. a type of isoantibody induced by immunization, either by pregnancy or by transfusion, in contrast to natural antibodies.

incomplete a. 1. antibody that binds to erythrocytes or bacteria but does not produce agglutination; in blood banking, the nonagglutinating antibody is detectable in serum by using the antiglobulin (Coombs') test. For example, IgG anti-Rh antibodies do not agglutinate erythrocytes in physiologic saline whereas IgM antibodies do. 2. a univalent antibody fragment.

monoclonal a's (MOAB) proteins produced from a single CLONE of B LYMPHOCYTES; used as laboratory reagents in radioimmunoassays, ELISA assay, and immunofluorescence assays, and also as biological response MODIFIERS fused with rapidly reproducing myeloma cells, resulting in a HYBRIDOMA capable of synthesizing a massive amount of one specific antibody; the antibody is made in response to tumor cells injected into mice and is produced from mouse serum. Monoclonal antibodies may be used alone (unconjugated) or bound (conjugated) to radioisotopes, toxins, or other biological response modifiers. When bound to radioisotopes they may also be used as a diagnostic tool to locate tumors and metastatic disease.

natural a's, naturally occurring a's antibodies present in the serum of normal individuals in the apparent absence of any contact with the specific antigen, probably induced by exposure to cross-reacting antigens; examples are the ABO antibodies, anti-A and anti-B. Such antibodies may play a major role in resistance to infection.

neutralizing a. one that reduces or destroys infectivity of a homologous infectious agent by partial or complete destruction of the agent.

protective a. one responsible for immunity to an infectious agent, observed in passive immunity.

Rh a's those directed against Rh antigen(s) of human erythrocytes. Not normally present, they may be produced when Rh-negative persons receive Rh-positive blood by transfusion or when an Rh-negative person is pregnant with an Rh-positive fetus.

saline a. complete antibody.

antibrachium (an″te-bra′ke-um) forearm.

anticariogenic (an″te-, an″ti-kar″e-o-jen′-ik) effective in suppressing caries production.

anticathexis (an″tĭ-kah-thek′sis) in PSYCHOANALYSIS, the energy required for the ego to maintain repression of unacceptable ideas and impulses.

anticholelithogenic (an″te-ko″le-lith″o-jen′ik) 1. preventing the formation of gallstones. 2. an agent that so acts.

anticholesteremic (an″te-ko-les″ter-e′mik) 1. promoting a reduction of CHOLESTEROL levels in the blood. 2. an agent that has this effect.

anticholinergic (an″te-, an″ti-ko″lin-er′jik) 1. blocking the passage of impulses through the parasympathetic nerves. 2. an agent that has this effect; called also parasympatholytic.

anticholinesterase (an″te-, an″ti-ko″lin-es′ter-ās) an agent that inhibits ACETYLCHOLINESTERASE, the enzyme that breaks down ACETYLCHOLINE at junctions of cholinergic nerve endings and effector organs or postsynaptic neurons; this permits the accumulation of acetylcholine and increases the stimulation of cholinergic RECEPTORS in the central and peripheral nervous systems. Called also cholinesterase inhibitor.

Organophosphate insecticides and chemical-warfare agents (nerve gases) are highly toxic "irreversible" anticholinesterases; "reversible" anticholinesterases such as NEOSTIGMINE and PHYSOSTIGMINE are used for treatment of myasthenia gravis, glaucoma, and smooth muscle atony of the gastrointestinal tract and for termination of the effect of nondepolarizing neuromuscular blocking AGENTS and cholinergic blocking AGENTS. Poisoning by anticholinesterases is treated with atropine and the cholinesterase reactivator pralidoxime.

anticipate (an-tis′ĭ-pāt) to expect a given reaction from someone, such as a patient.

anticoagulant (an″te-, an″ti-ko-ag′u-lant) 1. serving to prevent the coagulation of blood. 2. any substance that, in vivo or in vitro, suppresses, delays, or nullifies COAGULATION of the blood.

a. citrate phosphate dextrose adenine solution citrate phosphate dextrose adenine.

a. citrate phosphate dextrose solution citrate phosphate dextrose.

a. therapy the therapeutic use of anticoagulants to discourage formation of blood clots within a blood vessel. Its main purpose is preventive; however, thrombolytic action of an anticoagulant can destroy a clot and thereby improve the condition of the ischemic tissue supplied by the affected vessel. Conditions in which this therapy is used include occlusive vascular disease, such as CORONARY OCCLUSION, cerebrovascular and venous THROMBOSIS, and pulmonary EMBOLISM. It is administered prophylactically when major surgery is planned for a patient with a history of arterial stasis, and for patients who must be immobilized for a prolonged period of time.

Anticoagulant agents include those that interfere with the formation of clots (ANTITHROMBOTICS), such as HEPARIN and the COUMARIN compounds, and those that are capable of disintegrating thrombi that have already formed (THROMBOLYTICS), such as STREPTOKINASE and UROKINASE. A third group of anticoagulants, the antiplatelet agents, prevent the clumping together of PLATELETS, a primary step in the formation of thrombi, especially in the cerebrovascular system.

These agents are classified as ANTITHROMBO-CYTICS and are not to be confused with or used as a substitute for other types of anticoagulants.

Patient Care. The major difficulties that may arise during the course of anticoagulant therapy are hemorrhage and drug interaction. Observation of the patient for early signs of internal as well as external spontaneous bleeding is of primary importance. Health care personnel responsible for the care of these patients must be knowledgeable about the various laboratory tests and interpretation of their results in the administration of anticoagulant drugs and in assessment of the patient.

The effects of anticoagulants can be enhanced or inhibited by a variety of drugs and chemical compounds, especially the salicylates, barbiturates, and antibiotics. Ambulatory patients must be cautioned against taking any other drugs in combination with an anticoagulant agent without first consulting with the health care provider who prescribed the drug. This includes nonprescription or "over-the-counter" drugs as well as prescription drugs. Dietary restrictions such as fasting diets or those that limit the intake or utilization of the fat-soluble vitamin K can result in increased pharmacologic action of an anticoagulant.

The patient and family should be given adequate instruction in the purposes of anticoagulant therapy, the effects and side effects of other drugs and dietary intake on anticoagulant agents, and the need for regular contact with members of the health care team so that adequate monitoring of the patient's status can be continued as long as the patient is receiving an anticoagulant.

Instruction of the patient and significant others should include prevention of accidental injury, basic first aid measures to control bleeding should an accident occur, the danger signs that warrant immediate medical attention, and assurance that bleeding can be controlled. A Medic Alert bracelet should be worn to alert health care professionals in an emergency situation that the patient is taking anticoagulants.

Women of childbearing age need counseling about the effects of anticoagulants on contraceptive methods and reproduction. Those who are taking an anticoagulant for prevention of emboli cannot use oral contraceptives or an intrauterine device, which could cause endometrial bleeding. Should a patient think she is or desires to be pregnant, the primary care provider should be notified at once. Warfarin crosses the placental barrier and can cause fatal hemorrhage in the fetus. It can also enter the

mother's milk and have an anticoagulant effect in the nursing baby. Heparin does not have these properties and can be substituted for warfarin when necessary.

anticodon (an″te-, an″ti-ko′don) a triplet of nucleotides in transfer RNA that is complementary to the codon in messenger RNA that specifies the amino acid. (See accompanying illustration.)

anticomplement (an″te-, an″ti-kom′plě-ment) a substance that counteracts the action of a complement.

anticonvulsant (an″te, an″ti-kon-vul′sant) 1. inhibiting convulsions. 2. an agent that has this effect, such as DIPHENYLHYDANTOIN (Dilantin), MEPHENYTOIN (Mesantoin), and TRIMETHADIONE. They are used in the treatment of EPILEPSY and in psychomotor and myoclonic seizures.

anticus (an-ti′kus) anterior.

anti-D antibody against D antigen, the most immunogenic of the antigenic markers of the Rh BLOOD GROUP. Commercial preparations of anti-D, Rh$_0$ (D) immune globulin, are administered to Rh-negative women following the birth of Rh-positive infants in order to prevent incompatibility of maternal blood with the D-antigen, which may cause ERYTHROBLASTOSIS FETALIS in a subsequent pregnancy. Called also anti-Rh$_0$.

antidepressant (an″te-, an″ti-de-pres′ant) 1. preventing or relieving depression. 2. an agent used for relief of symptoms of DEPRESSION. One type is the *tricyclic antidepressants,* so called because of their chemical structure, which has three fused rings; they block reuptake of the neurotransmitters NOREPINEPHRINE and SEROTONIN at nerve endings. This group includes AMITRIPTYLINE (ELAVIL), DESIPRAMINE (NORPRAMIN), DOXEPIN

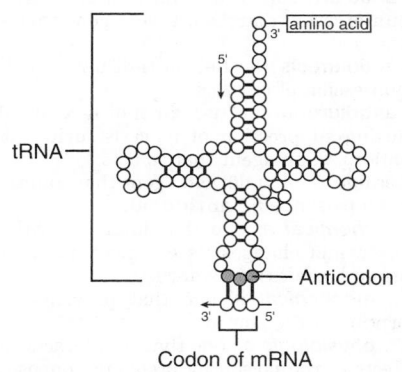

Anticodon. The three nucleotides (shaded) on a transfer RNA bind to a complementary messenger RNA codon. From Dorland's, 2000.

(SINEQUAN), IMIPRAMINE (TOFRANIL), NORTRIP-TYLINE (PAMELOR), and TRIMIPRAMINE (SURMON-TIL). Two drugs with different chemical structures but similar effects are AMOXAPINE (ASENDIN) and MAPROTILINE (LUDIOMIL). These drugs vary in the degree to which they affect reuptake of the two neurotransmitters. Also, some are sedating while others are alerting. The patient must take the drug for about 2 to 3 weeks before the full therapeutic effect is established.

An older group of antidepressants is the monoamine oxidase INHIBITORS ISOCARBOXAZID (MARPLAN), PHENELZINE (NARDIL), and TRANYLCY-PROMINE (PARNATE). These drugs inhibit MONO-AMINE OXIDASE, the enzyme that breaks down norepinephrine and serotonin released at nerve synapses. They are not as widely used as the tricyclic antidepressants because serious cardiovascular side effects (hypertension, headache, stroke syndrome) can occur when tyramine is ingested, and foods containing tyramine, such as cheese, certain beans, beer, and wine, must be avoided by patients taking monoamine oxidase inhibitors. A third class consists of the selective serotonin reuptake INHIBITORS, which inhibit reuptake of serotonin without affecting reuptake of norepinephrine. This group includes FLUOXETINE (PROZAC), PAROXETINE (PAXIL), and SERTRALINE (ZOLOFT). Drugs in this group are as effective as the tricyclic antidepressants but have fewer side effects. The most significant adverse reaction seen with this group is agitation, which can be lessened by decreasing the dose. Weight gain and sexual dysfunction may also occur.

antidiabetic (an″te-, an″ti-di″ah-bet′ik) 1. preventing or alleviating DIABETES. 2. antidiabetic AGENT.

antidiarrheal (an″te-, an″ti-di″ah-re′al) 1. counteracting diarrhea. 2. an agent that so acts.

antidiuresis (an″te-, an″ti-di″u-re′sis) the suppression of DIURESIS.

antidiuretic (an″te-, an″ti-di″u-ret′ik) 1. causing suppression of DIURESIS (urine formation). 2. an agent that so acts.

antidote (an′ti-dōt) an agent that counteracts a poison. adj., **antido′tal.**

   chemical a. one that interacts with a poison and changes its chemical nature to form a harmless substance.

   mechanical a. one that prevents absorption of the poison.

   physiologic a. one that counteracts the effects of the poison by producing opposing effects.

   universal a. a mixture formerly recommended as an antidote when the exact

poison is not known. There is, in fact, no known universal antidote. Activated CHAR-COAL is now being used for many poisons.

antidromic (an″te-drom′ik) conducting impulses in a direction opposite to the normal.

antidysenteric (an″te-, an″ti-dis″en-ter′ik) counteracting DYSENTERY.

antidyskinetic (an″te-, an″ti-dis″ki-net′ik) 1. relieving or preventing dyskinesia. 2. an agent that relieves or prevents dyskinesia.

antiemetic (an″te-e-met′ik) 1. useful in the treatment of vomiting. 2. an agent that relieves vomiting.

antiepileptic (an″te-ep″ĭ-lep′tik) 1. combating EPILEPSY. 2. a remedy for epilepsy.

antiestrogen (an″te-es′tro-jen) a substance capable of inhibiting the biological effects of estrogens.

antifebrile (an″te-, an″ti-feb′ril) antipyretic (def. 1).

antifibrinolysin (an″te-, an″ti-fi″bri-nol′ĭ-sin) antiplasmin.

antifibrinolytic (an″te-, an″ti-fi″bri-no-lit′-ik) 1. inhibiting fibrinolysis. 2. a substance that prevents FIBRINOLYSIS.

antifilarial 1. destructive to FILARIAE. 2. an agent having this effect.

antifolate (an″ti-fo′lāt) folic acid antagonist.

antifungal (an″te-, an″ti-fung′gal) 1. destructive to or checking the growth of fungi; called alsoantimycotic. 2. antifungal AGENT.

antigalactic (an″te-, an″ti-gah-lak′tik) 1. diminishing or stopping LACTATION. 2. an agent that so acts. Called also lactifuge.

antigen (an′ti-jen) any substance capable, under appropriate conditions, of inducing a specific IMMUNE RESPONSE and reacting with the products of that response; that is, with specific ANTIBODY or specifically sensitized T LYMPHOCYTES, or both. Antigens may be soluble substances, such as toxins and foreign proteins, or particulates, such as bacteria and tissue cells; however, only the portion of the protein or polysaccharide molecule known as the antigenic DETERMI-NANT combines with antibody or a specific receptor on a lymphocyte. Abbreviated Ag. See also IMMUNITY. adj., **antigen′ic.**

   allogeneic a. one occurring in some but not all individuals of the same species, e.g., histocompatibility antigens and human blood group antigens; called also isoantigen.

   a.-antibody reaction the reversible binding of antigen to homologous antibody by the formation of weak bonds between antigenic determinants on antigen molecules and antigen binding sites on immunoglobulin molecules.

   blood-group a's erythrocyte surface antigens whose antigenic differences determine BLOOD GROUPS.

cancer a. 125 (CA 125) a GLYCOPROTEIN antigen found in normal adult tissues such as the epithelium of the fallopian tubes, the endometrium, the endocervix, the pleura, and the peritoneum. Elevated levels are seen in association with epithelial ovarian carcinomas, particularly nonmucinous tumors, as well as with some other malignancies, various benign pelvic disorders, tuberculosis, and cirrhosis.

carcinoembryonic a. (CEA) an oncofetal glycoprotein antigen originally thought to be specific for adenocarcinoma of the colon, but now known to be found in many other cancers and some nonmalignant conditions. Its primary use is in monitoring the response of patients to cancer treatment.

CD a. any of a number of cell-surface MARKERS expressed by leukocytes and used to distinguish cell lineages, developmental stages, and functional subsets. Such markers can be identified by specific monoclonal ANTIBODIES and are numbered CD1, CD2, CD3, etc. (for cluster designation, according to how their specificity characteristics group together when analyzed by computer).

CD4 a. an antigen on the surface of helper T CELLS; the normal range of helper cells is 800 to 1200 per cubic mm of blood. The human immunodeficiency VIRUS binds to this antigen and infects and kills T CELLS bearing this antigen, thus gradually destroying the body's ability to resist infection. CD4 can be administered in a soluble form to increase the amount of it in the circulation and interfere with the ability of HIV to affect CD4 antigens on the cell.

class I a's major histocompatibility ANTIGENS found on virtually every cell, human erythrocytes being the only notable exception; they are the classic histocompatibility antigens recognized during graft REJECTION.

class II a's major histocompatibility ANTIGENS found only on immunocompetent cells, primarily B lymphocytes and macrophages.

conjugated a. antigen produced by coupling a hapten to a protein carrier molecule through covalent bonds; when it induces immunization, the resultant immune response is directed against both the hapten and the carrier.

cross-reacting a. 1. one that combines with antibody produced in response to a different but related antigen, owing to similarity of antigenic determinants. 2. identical antigens in two bacterial strains, so that antibody produced against one strain will react with the other.

extractable nuclear a's ENA; protein antigens, not containing DNA, that are extractable from cell nuclei in phosphate-buffered saline; anti-ENA antibodies are a component of the antinuclear antibodies occurring in systemic lupus erythematosus and other connective tissue diseases.

flagellar a. H antigen.

Forssman a. a heterogenetic ANTIGEN discovered in guinea pig tissues, capable of lysing sheep erythrocytes in the presence of complement. It is found usually in animal organs but occasionally in blood, and induces formation of an antibody (Forssman antibody, a type of heterophile antibody) only when combined with protein or hog serum. Davidsohn's Differential Test was historically used to differentiate between the heterophile sheep agglutinins in human serum that were due to Forssman antigen and those due to infectious mononucleosis; this is based upon the fact that boiled guinea pig kidney will absorb heterophile sheep cell agglutinins produced by Forssman antigen, but not those produced by infectious mononucleosis.

H a. (Ger. *Hauch,* film), the antigen that occurs in the FLAGELLA of motile bacteria.

hepatitis B core a. (HBcAg) a core protein antigen of the hepatitis B virus present inside complete virions (Dane particles) and in the nuclei of infected hepatic cells, indicating the presence of reproducing hepatitis B virus. The antigen is not present in the blood of infected individuals, but antibodies against it appear during the acute infection; they do not protect against reinfection.

hepatitis B e a. (HBeAg) an antigen of hepatitis B virus sometimes present in the blood during acute infection, usually disappearing afterward but sometimes persisting in chronic disease. Anti-HBe antibodies appear transiently during convalescence; they do not protect against reinfection.

hepatitis B surface a. (HBsAg) one present in the serum of those infected with HEPATITIS B, consisting of the surface coat lipoprotein of the hepatitis B virus. Tests for serum HbsAg are used in the diagnosis of hepatitis B and in testing blood products for infectivity.

heterogeneic a. xenogeneic antigen.

heterogenetic a., heterophil a., heterophile a. one capable of stimulating the production of antibodies that react with tissues from other animals or even plants.

histocompatibility a's genetically determined isoantigens present on the cell membranes of nucleated cells of most tissues, which incite an immune response when grafted onto a genetically disparate individual and thus determine the compatibility of tissues in transplantation. *Major histocompatibility antigens* are those that belong to the major histocompatibility COMPLEX, which in humans contains the HLA ANTIGENS. *Minor histocompatibility antigens* are those that can cause delayed tissue rejection.

HLA a's, human leukocyte a's see HLA ANTIGENS.

H-Y a. a minor histocompatibility ANTIGEN present in all tissues of normal males and coded for by a structural gene on the short arm of the Y chromosome; it is thought to promote the differentiation of indifferent gonads into testes, thus determining male sex.

isogeneic a. an antigen carried by an individual which is capable of eliciting an immune response in genetically different individuals of the same species, but not in an individual bearing it.

K a. a bacterial capsular antigen, a surface antigen external to the cell wall.

lymphogranuloma venereum a. a sterile suspension of *Chlamydia lymphogranulomatis;* used as a dermal reactivity indicator.

M a. a type-specific antigen that appears to be located primarily in the cell wall and is associated with virulence of *Streptococcus pyogenes.*

mumps skin test a. a sterile suspension of mumps virus; used as a dermal reactivity indicator.

nuclear a's the components of cell nuclei with which antinuclear antibodies react.

O a. (Ger. *ohne Hauch,* without film), the antigen that occurs in the bodies of bacteria.

oncofetal a. a gene product that is expressed during fetal development, but repressed in specialized tissues of the adult and that is also produced by certain cancers. In the neoplastic transformation, the cells dedifferentiate and these genes can be derepressed so that the embryonic antigens reappear. Examples are alpha-fetoprotein and carcinoembryonic antigen.

organ-specific a. any antigen that occurs exclusively in a particular organ and serves to distinguish it from other organs. Two types of organ specificity have been proposed: (1) first-order or tissue specificity is attributed to the presence of an antigen characteristic of a particular organ in a single species; (2) second-order organ specificity is attributed to an antigen characteristic of the same organ in many, even unrelated, species.

partial a. an antigen that does not produce antibody formation, but gives specific precipitation when mixed with the antibacterial immune serum.

pollen a. the essential polypeptides of the pollen of plants extracted with a suitable menstruum, used in diagnosis, prophylaxis, and desensitization in hay fever.

a. presentation the presentation of ingested antigens on the surface of macrophages in close proximity to histocompatibility ANTIGENS. Some populations of T LYMPHOCYTES can only be triggered by antigens that are presented in this way. Thus macrophages play a role in inducing cell-mediated immunity.

private a's antigens of the low-frequency blood groups, so called because they are found only in members of a single kindred.

prostate-specific a., prostatic specific a. an antigen that is elevated in all patients with prostatic cancer and in some with an inflamed prostate gland.

public a's antigens of the high-frequency blood groups, so called because they are found in many persons.

self a. an AUTOANTIGEN, a normal constituent of the body against which antibodies are formed in AUTOIMMUNE DISEASE.

sequestered a's the cellular constituents of tissue (e.g., the lens of the eye and the thyroid) sequestered anatomically from the lymphoreticular system during embryonic development and thus thought not to be recognized as "self." Should such tissue be exposed to the lymphoreticular system during adult life, an autoimmune response would be elicited.

somatic a's antigens, usually cell surface antigens, of the body of a bacterial cell, in contrast to flagellar or capsular antigens.

T a. 1. any of several antigens, coded for by the viral genome, associated with transformation of infected cells by certain DNA tumor viruses. Called also tumor antigen. 2. an antigen present on human ERYTHROCYTES that is exposed by treatment with NEURAMINIDASE or contact with certain bacteria. see *CD a.*

T-dependent a. one that requires the presence of helper T cells to stimulate antibody production by B cells; most antigens are T-dependent.

T-independent a. an antigen that can trigger B LYMPHOCYTES to produce antibodies without the participation of T LYMPHOCYTES. See also T-dependent antigen.

tumor a. 1. T antigen (def. 1). 2. tumor-specific antigen.

tumor-specific a. (TSA) any cell-surface antigen of a tumor that does not occur on normal cells of the same origin.

V a., Vi a. an antigen contained in the sheath of a bacterium, as *Salmonella typhosa* (the typhoid bacillus), and thought to contribute to its virulence.

xenogeneic a. an antigen common to members of one species but not to members of other species; called also heterogeneic antigen.

antigenemia (an″tĭ-jĕ-ne′me-ah) the presence of ANTIGEN, such as hepatitis B surface ANTIGEN, in the blood.

antigenicity (an″tĭ-jĕ-nis′ĭ-te) the property of being able to induce a specific IMMUNE RESPONSE or the degree to which a substance is able to stimulate an immune response; called also immunogenicity.

antigenuria (an″tĭ-jĕ-nu′re-ah) the presence of a specific ANTIGEN in the urine.

antiglaucoma (an″te-glaw-ko′mah, -glou-ko′mah) preventing or alleviating glaucoma.

antiglobulin (an″tĭ-glob′u-lin) an antibody directed against gamma globulin.

a. **test (AGT)** Coombs' test.

antihelix (an″te-he′liks) the semicircular ridge on the ear anterior and parallel to the HELIX; called also anthelix.

antihelmintic (an″te-, an″ti-hel-min′tik) anthelmintic.

antihemophilic (an″te-, an″ti-he″mo-fil′ik) 1. effective against the bleeding tendency in hemophilia. 2. an agent that has this effect.

antihemorrhagic (an″te-, an″ti-hem″o-raj′ik) 1. preventing or stopping HEMORRHAGE. 2. an agent that so acts.

antihistamine (an″te-, an″ti-his′tah-mēn) a drug that counteracts the effects of HISTAMINE, a normal body chemical that among its actions is believed to cause the symptoms of persons who are hypersensitive to various ALLERGENS. While the term antihistamine can broadly include any agent that blocks any histamine receptor, in practice it is usually used to denote those blocking the H_1 type of receptors (H_1 receptor ANTAGONISTS), those involved in allergic reactions. Agents blocking the H_2 type of receptors are usually called histamine H_2 receptor ANTAGONISTS, and include the agents used to inhibit gastric secretion in peptic ulcer. Antihistamines are used to relieve the symptoms of allergic reactions, especially HAY FEVER and other allergic disorders of the nasal passages. Some antihistamines have an antinauseant action that is useful in the relief of MOTION SICKNESS. Others have a sedative and hypnotic action and may be used as TRANQUILIZERS. Many are ingredients of compound preparations used to treat coughs or the common cold.

Patients for whom an antihistamine has been prescribed should be instructed

about the side effects of these drugs, including drowsiness, dizziness, and muscular weakness. These side effects present a special hazard in driving an automobile or operating heavy machinery. Other side effects include dryness of the mouth and throat and insomnia.

antihistaminic (an″te-, an″ti-his-tah-min′ik) 1. counteracting the effects of HISTAMINE. 2. ANTIHISTAMINE.

antihormone (an″te-hor′mōn) a substance that counteracts a hormone.

antihuman globulin (AHG) test direct COOMBS TEST.

antihypercholesterolemic (an″te-, an″ti-hi″per-ko-les″ter-ol-e′mik) 1. effective against elevated serum cholesterol levels. 2. an agent with this effect.

antihyperglycemic (an″te-, an″ti-hi″per-gli-se′mik) 1. counteracting high levels of glucose in the blood. 2. antihyperglycemic agent.

antihyperkalemic (an″te-, an″ti-hi″per-kah-le′mik) 1. effective in decreasing or preventing HYPERKALEMIA. 2. an agent with this effect.

antihyperlipidemic (an″te-, an″ti-hi″per-lip″ĭde′mik) 1. promoting a reduction of lipid levels in the blood. 2. an agent that promotes a reduction of lipid levels in the blood.

antihyperlipoproteinemic (an″te-, an″ti-hi″per-lip″o-pro″tēn-e′mik) 1. promoting a reduction of lipoprotein levels in the blood. 2. an agent that promotes a reduction of lipoprotein levels in the blood.

antihypertensive (an″te-, an″ti-hi″per-ten′siv) 1. effective against hypertension. 2. antihypertensive agent.

a. **agent** an agent that reduces high BLOOD PRESSURE; there are many different types of drugs that do this. DIURETICS inhibit the reabsorption of sodium in the renal tubules, causing an increase in urinary excretion of sodium and a decrease in the plasma volume and extracellular fluid volume. Drugs that act on adrenergic control of blood pressure include BETA-ADRENERGIC BLOCKING AGENTS such as PROPRANOLOL, which act at beta-adrenergic receptors in the heart and kidneys to reduce cardiac output and renin secretion, and others such as METHYLDOPA that act on alpha-adrenergic mechanisms in the central or sympathetic nervous system to reduce peripheral vascular resistance. VASODILATORS act directly on the arterioles to produce the same effect. Almost every case of hypertension can be controlled by one of these drugs or a combination of them. The proper combination is determined by the response of the individual patient. In some cases several drugs must be tried before the right combination is found.

Patient Education. Instruction of the patient and significant others is an essential part of antihypertensive therapy. Learning objectives are based on the patient's particular regimen of drug therapy, allowance of sodium intake, and other dietary restrictions, such as a low-calorie diet to combat obesity.

Some antihypertensive drugs can produce acute HYPOTENSIVE reactions. The patient will need to know how to prevent a hypotensive reaction and what measures to take should such a reaction occur.

Prevention of a hypotensive reaction includes avoiding hot baths and sudden immobility after exercise, both of which promote vasodilation and a lowering of arterial pressure. The patient also should be aware of the effect of sudden changes in position that can precipitate an attack of orthostatic HYPOTENSION. Pooling of blood in the lower limbs can divert it from the brain and other vital organs. This can sometimes be avoided by moving about frequently instead of standing motionless for long periods of time. Elastic stockings also help promote venous return from the legs and help prevent fainting from decreased cerebral blood supply.

Acute hypotension can be serious, but milder hypotensive reactions with faintness and weakness can be relieved at home if the patient lies down and elevates his lower extremities above the level of his head and flexes the thigh muscles to encourage the flow of blood from his feet and legs to his brain.

The patient on a diuretic that is not potassium-sparing will need instruction on the symptoms of potassium deficit, how to avoid potassium depletion, and when to notify the doctor should hypokalemia occur.

Limitation of SODIUM intake can be very confusing and emotionally stressful to the uninstructed patient. In order to comply with the prescribed restriction of sodium the patient will need to know about satisfying substitutes and alternative seasonings for food, to be aware of the necessity of reading labels carefully when buying prepared food and over-the-counter medications, and to recognize the relationship between sodium and high blood pressure and the reasons why high sodium intake is harmful to health and well-being.

antihypoglycemic (an″te-, an″ti-hi″po-gli-se′mik) 1. counteracting HYPOGLYCEMIA. 2. an agent that counteracts hypoglycemia.

antihypotensive (an″te-, an″ti-hi″po-ten′-siv) 1. counteracting low blood pressure. 2. an agent that counteracts low blood pressure.

antiinfective (an″te-in-fek′tiv) 1. capable of killing infectious agents or of preventing them from spreading. 2. a substance that counteracts infection; see also ANTIMICROBIAL AGENT.

antiinflammatory (an″te-in-flam′ah-tor-e) 1. counteracting or suppressing INFLAMMATION. 2. an agent that so acts.

antiketogenesis (an″te-, an″ti-ke″to-jen′ĕ-sis) inhibition of the formation of ketone bodies.

antiketogenic (an″te-, an″ti-ke″to-jen′ik) preventing or suppressing the development of ketones (ketone bodies) and thus preventing development of ketosis.

antilewisite (an″tĭ-loo′ĭ-sīt) dimercaprol.

antilipemic (an″te-, an″ti-lĭ-pe′mik) antihyperlipemic.

antilipidemic (an″te-, an″ti-lip″ĭ-de′mik) antihyperlipidemic.

antilithic (an″te-, an″ti-lith′ik) 1. preventing CALCULUS formation. 2. an agent that so acts.

antimalarial (an″te-, an″ti-mah-lar′e-al) 1. therapeutically effective against MALARIA. 2. antimalarial AGENT.

antimere (an′tĭ-mēr) one of the segments of the body bounded by planes at right angles to the long axis of the body. See PLANE (def. 2).

antimetabolite (an″te-, an″ti-mĕ-tab′o-līt) 1. a substance bearing a close structural resemblance to one required for normal physiological functioning, and exerting its effect by interfering with the utilization of the essential metabolite. 2. a class of antineoplastic AGENTS consisting of antimetabolites of substances required for cell growth and replication; the interference with cell function is phase specific, largely in the S phase of the cell cycle. The group includes CLADRIBINE, CYTARABINE, FLOXURIDINE, FLUDARABINE, FLUOROURACIL, MERCAPTOPURINE, METHOTREXATE, and THIOGUANINE. See also ANTINEOPLASTIC THERAPY.

antimethemoglobinemic (an″te-, an″ti-met″he-mo-glo″bĭ-ne′mik) 1. promoting reduction of methemoglobin levels in the blood. 2. an agent that has this effect.

antimetropia (an″te-, an″ti-mĕ-tro′pe-ah) difference in the refractive error of the two eyes, such as hyperopia in one eye with myopia in the other.

antimicrobial (an″te-, an″ti-mi-kro′be-al) 1. killing microorganisms, or suppressing their multiplication or growth. (See accompanying illustration.) 2. antimicrobial agent.

a. agent an agent that kills microorganisms or suppresses their multiplication or growth. Such agents are classified functionally according to the manner in which they adversely affect a microorganism.

One group interferes with the synthesis of the bacterial cell wall, resulting in cell lysis because the contents of the bacterial cell are hypertonic and therefore under high osmotic pressure. A weakening of the cell wall causes the cell to rupture, spill its contents, and be destroyed. The PENICILLINS, CEPHALOSPORINS, and BACITRACIN are examples of this group.

A second group interferes with the synthesis of nucleic acids. Without DNA and RNA synthesis a microorganism cannot replicate or translate genetic information. Such interference with reproduction of the cell produces a bacteriostatic effect. Examples of this group are GRISEOFULVIN and TETRACYCLINE.

A third group of antimicrobial agents changes the permeability of the cell membrane, causing a leakage of metabolic substrates essential to the life of the microorganism. Their action can be either bacteriostatic or bactericidal. Examples include AMPHOTERICIN B and POLYMYXIN B.

A fourth group of antimicrobial agents interferes with metabolic processes within the microorganism. They are structurally similar to natural metabolic substrates, but since they do not function normally, they interrupt metabolic processes. Most of these agents are bacteriostatic. Examples include the SULFONAMIDES, *p*-AMINOSALICYLIC ACID, and ISONIAZID.

The side effects of antimicrobials can be widespread and dangerous to the patient. Damage to the central nervous system, blood components, liver, kidney, and lung are possible. (See accompanying table.)

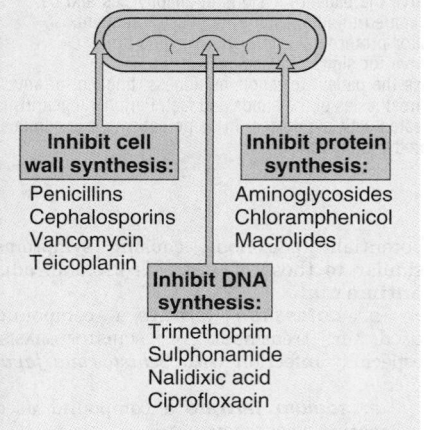

Mechanisms of antimicrobial action against bacteria. From Hart and Shears, 1997.

Inhibit cell wall synthesis:
Penicillins
Cephalosporins
Vancomycin
Teicoplanin

Inhibit protein synthesis:
Aminoglycosides
Chloramphenicol
Macrolides

Inhibit DNA synthesis:
Trimethoprim
Sulphonamide
Nalidixic acid
Ciprofloxacin

Additionally, debilitated and immunocompromised patients are susceptible to a superinfection by a second microorganism that is resistant to the antimicrobial that is being administered to them.

Local effects of antimicrobial therapy involving the gastrointestinal tract are the result of destruction of large numbers of microorganisms that normally inhabit the intestines. This produces alterations in the balance of microbial flora in the body. Broad-spectrum antibiotics are likely to inhibit the growth of some normal flora and allow yeasts and molds to flourish. An example of this is the occurrence of CANDIDIASIS when tetracycline is being taken. Other kinds of microorganisms that can replace normal gastrointestinal flora suppressed by antibiotic therapy are SALMONELLAE and *Clostridium difficile*. Large numbers of salmonellae in the stool of patients on antimicrobials greatly increases the possibility of cross-infection; hence, there is a need for enteric precautions in the care of these patients. *Clostridium difficile* produces a toxin that can cause severe pseudomembranous colitis (see antibiotic-associated COLITIS).

Special Considerations. Effective antimicrobial therapy depends on maintaining an optimum and stable level of the drug in the serum and body tissues. This demands meticulous care in the administration of the drug by the correct route and at the correct time. Patients who take antimicrobials at home need instruction in when and how to take the prescribed medication in order to obtain the desired effects. This includes knowledge of which foods to avoid because of food-drug interaction, whether to take the drug before or after meals, and the quantity of water or other liquid to take with the medication. Patients should be aware of the side effects of their specific medication, and which ones should be reported immediately. Laypersons may not be aware of the hazards of ignoring directions and discontinuing the drug when their symptoms subside, or of taking an antimicrobial prescribed for someone else. Failure to take only what is prescribed and in the full amount can contribute to the development of drug-resistant strains of microorganisms.

antimongolism (an″tĭ-mon′go-lizm) a term applied to syndromes associated with certain chromosomal abnormalities, in which some of the clinical signs, e.g., downward-slanting palpebral fissures, are the opposite of those seen in Down syndrome.

MAJOR ADVERSE EFFECTS ASSOCIATED WITH ANTIMICROBIAL THERAPY

Symptom	Drug or Class of Antimicrobial	Pertinent Observations and Interventions
Aplastic anemia, leukopenia, thrombocytopenia, gray syndrome	Chloramphenicol	Complete blood counts prior to therapy and every two days during treatment for leukopenia and thrombocytopenia. Aplastic anemia cannot be predicted by monitoring the blood. Adequate numbers of blood elements are not produced, resulting in symptoms associated with anemia. This reaction is usually fatal and may occur long after the drug is withdrawn. The risk of gray syndrome is reduced by careful monitoring of drug levels and discontinuation at the first signs of vomiting, gray discoloration of the skin, abdominal distention, or cyanosis.
Ototoxicity	Aminoglycosides, vancomycin, streptomycin	Audiometric testing; advise the patient to report tinnitus or fullness in the ears. Patients may experience vestibular changes, such as dizziness or vertigo. Frequent monitoring of serum drug levels.
Nephrotoxicity	Aminoglycosides, vancomycin, amphotericin B, polymyxins	Monitor the patient for dilute urine, elevated BUN, and creatinine. Proteinuria and casts are often noted.
Hepatotoxicity	Erythromycin, isoniazid	Erythromycin estolate should be avoided by patients with pre-existing hepatic disease.
	Rifampin, Tetracycline (especially in high doses or the presence of renal failure)	Observe the patient for signs of liver disease such as jaundice, abnormal liver function tests, dark urine, etc.
Colitis and diarrhea	Lincomycin, clindamycin	Colitis associated with the administration of clindamycin is characterized by profuse watery diarrhea, severe abdominal pain, and leukocytosis, Clindamycin is withdrawn and vancomycin treatment is begun.
	Tetracycline	Administer tetracycline with meals to reduce GI effects.
Damage to teeth, nails and bones	Tetracycline	Avoid use in children under eight. Avoid use during pregnancy.
Kernicterus	Sulfonamides	Sulfonamides are usually not administered to infants under two months, or late in pregnancy. They are not administered to nursing mothers.
Severe allergic reactions	Most common with penicillins	Observe the patient for signs of anaphylaxis and be prepared to administer emergency treatment.
Bleeding tendencies	Cephalosporins	Monitor prothrombin time and bleeding time. Observe for signs of bleeding.
Peripheral neuritis	Isoniazid	Advise the patient to report numbness, tingling, or any paresthesias of the hands and feet. Peripheral neuritis is treated with pyridoxine. In some patients it is administered prophylactically.

antimongoloid (an″tĭ-mon′go-loid) opposite to that characteristic of DOWN SYNDROME (formerly called *mongolism*), such as an antimongoloid slant of the palpebral fissures.

antimony (Sb) (an′tĭ-mo″ne) a chemical element, atomic number 51, atomic weight 121.75. (See Appendix 6.) Several of its salts are used in tropical medicine as treatments for SCHISTOSOMIASIS; however, they must be used with caution because they are potentially poisonous, causing symptoms similar to those of ARSENIC POISONING. adj., **antimo′nial.**

    a. potassium tartrate a compound used in treatment of SCHISTOSOMIASIS, especially infection with *Schistosoma japonicum.*

    a. sodium tartrate a compound used in treating SCHISTOSOMIASIS.

antimuscarinic (an″te-, an″tĭ-mus″kah-rin′ik) 1. effective against the toxic effects of MUSCARINE. 2. blocking the muscarinic RECEPTORS. 3. an agent that counteracts the effects of muscarine or blocks the muscarinic receptors.

antimyasthenic (an″te-, an″ti-mi′as-then′-ik) 1. counteracting or relieving muscular weakness in MYASTHENIA GRAVIS. 2. an agent that counteracts or relieves muscular weakness in myasthenia gravis.

antimycotic (an″ti-mi-kot′ik) 1. antifungal (def. 1). 2. antifungal AGENT.

antinarcotic (an″ti-nahr-kot′ik) relieving narcotic depression.

antinauseant (an″te-, an″ti-naw′ze-ant) 1. counteracting nausea. 2. an agent that so acts.

antineoplastic (an″te-, an″ti-ne″o-plas′tik) 1. inhibiting the maturation and proliferation of malignant cells. 2. antineoplastic AGENT.

a. therapy a regimen that includes CHEMOTHERAPY, aimed at destruction of malignant cells using a variety of agents that directly affect cellular growth and development. Chemotherapy is but one of a variety of methods available in the treatment of CANCER. Cancers particularly responsive to chemotherapy include CHORIOCARCINOMA, a highly malignant form of cancer that originates in the placenta; testicular carcinoma; and BURKITT'S LYMPHOMA, a malignancy most often found in African children. Combinations of drugs have successfully controlled acute leukemia in children and in persons with advanced stages of HODGKIN'S DISEASE.

Types of Antineoplastic Agents. The chemicals and drugs used in the treatment of cancer may be divided into several main groups. The first group, the ALKYLATING AGENTS, are capable of damaging the DNA of cells, thereby interfering with the process of replication; they are cell cycle phase nonspecific. Among these are BUSULFAN, CYCLOPHOSPHAMIDE, IFOSFAMIDE, and THIOTEPA; the NITROGEN MUSTARDS CHLORAMBUCIL, MECHLORETHAMINE, and MELPHALAN; and the NITROSOUREAS CARMUSTINE, LOMUSTINE, SEMUSTINE, and STREPTOZOCIN. The second group of drugs is the ANTIMETABOLITES; as the name suggests, they interfere with the cancer cell's metabolism. Some replace essential metabolites without performing their functions, while others compete with essential components by mimicking their functions and thereby inhibiting the manufacture of protein in the cell. Antimetabolites are cell cycle phase specific (S phase). Included in this group are CAPECITABINE, CLADRIBINE, CYTARABINE, FLOXURIDINE, FLUDARABINE, FLUOROURACIL, MERCAPTOPURINE, METHOTREXATE, and THIOGUANINE.

The third group is the ANTITUMOR ANTIBIOTICS. These agents have been isolated

from microorganisms and affect the function and/or synthesis of nucleic acids; they are cell cycle phase nonspecific. This group includes BLEOMYCIN SULFATE, DACTINOMYCIN, DAUNORUBICIN, DOXORUBICIN, EPIRUBICIN, IDARUBICIN, MITOMYCIN, MITOXANTRONE, PENTOSTATIN, PLICAMYCIN, and STREPTOZOCIN.

The fourth group is the *alkaloids;* the most important of which are the VINCA ALKALOIDS. They are cell cycle phase specific, exerting their effect during the M phase of cell mitosis and causing metaphase arrest. Included in this group are VINBLASTINE, VINCRISTINE, VINDESINE, and VINORELBINE TARTRATE.

The fifth group is the *hormones and antihormones,* which create an unfavorable environment for cancer cell growth. Hormones used in antineoplastic therapy include ESTROGENS, ANDROGENS, PROGESTINS, and CORTICOSTEROIDS. ANTIHORMONES include AMINOGLUTETHIMIDE, CHLOROTRIANISENE, FLUTAMIDE, GOSERELIN, LEUPROLIDE, and TAMOXIFEN.

There are a variety of other drugs, some whose mechanisms of action are known and others for whom the mechanism is unknown. Plant derivatives include the PODOPHYLLOTOXIN derivatives ETOPOSIDE and TENIPOSIDE, as well as PACLITAXEL, a derivative of the Pacific yew tree. Platinum coordination compounds include CARBOPLATIN and CISPLATIN. Other agents include ASPARAGINASE, DACARBAZINE, HYDROXYUREA, the INTERFERONS, LEVAMISOLE, MITOTANE, PROCARBAZINE, and TRETINOIN.

Patient Care. The drugs used in antineoplastic therapy are highly toxic and likely to produce troublesome or even extremely dangerous reactions; they should be administered only by qualified professionals. They may be given singly or in combination, depending on the type of malignancy and the stage of its development. The complexity of this type of therapy, particularly when used in conjunction with surgery or radiation therapy, demands a team of specialists, including medical oncologists, radiotherapists, nurse clinicians, and clinical pharmacologists, working cooperatively to accomplish the goals of the prescribed regimen.

It is especially important that members of the team be aware of and capable of dealing with the toxicity inherent in antineoplastic therapy. The management of drug toxicities requires a delicate balance between effective dosage to destroy malignant cells and the individual patient's tolerance of drug and dosage. Anorexia, nausea, and vomiting are among the milder but more troublesome effects of antibiotics, alkylating agents, and antimetabolites. It is necessary to work with each patient and help establish a routine that will incorporate administration of the drug, taking an antiemetic, and spacing meals so that adequate nutrition is provided and excessive weight loss is avoided. Stomatitis and diarrhea are also likely to appear as early signs of toxicity from antimetabolic and antibiotic drug therapy.

Drugs that suppress bone marrow function produce leukopenia, which in turn increases susceptibility to infection. If the patient is also receiving an IMMUNOSUP-PRESSANT such as PREDNISONE, resistance to infection is further compromised. The patient will need adequate rest, good nutrition, good habits of personal cleanliness, and avoidance of contact with those who have infectious diseases. If an infection does develop, it should receive prompt attention to minimize its effects and inhibit its progress. It may be necessary to alter the dosage of the antineoplastic drug until the infection subsides.

Bone marrow-suppressing drugs can also affect the platelet count, reducing it to a level at which bleeding can readily occur. Normal clotting is impaired by some cancer therapeutic agents and there is therefore the danger of internal bleeding anywhere in the body. Should the situation become severe, the drug dosage may need to be reduced or stopped altogether and platelet transfusions may be given.

Hormonal therapy frequently is accompanied by fluid retention. Measurement of intake and output, daily weight measurement, and observation for signs of surface edema or congestive heart failure are essential parts of patient care. Care of the patient with edema must include meticulous skin care. If DIURETICS are given, the patient must be watched for signs of potassium depletion. Another side effect of hormonal therapy may be changes in secondary sexual characteristics. These can be particularly embarrassing and emotionally disturbing to the patient.

Neurologic disorders may result from treatment with the plant alkaloids. These conditions may manifest themselves as impaired sensation, loss of coordination, and severe constipation. Although these neurological effects usually are reversible, especially if caught in the early stages, it may take months for the nerve cells to recover and resume normal function.

Many antineoplastic drugs cause alopecia (hair loss). This side effect can drastically alter the patient's body image and can be very disturbing psychologically. Wigs, hairpieces, and various head coverings can be used to mask the hair loss.

antinephritic (an″te-, an″ti-nĕ-frit′ik) effective against nephritis.

antineuralgic (an″te-, an″ti-noo-ral′jik) relieving neuralgia.

antineuritic (an″te-, an″ti-noo-rit′ik) relieving neuritis.

antinion (an-tin′e-on) the frontal pole of the head.

antioncogene (an″te-ong′ko-jēn″) tumor suppressor gene.

antiovulatory (an″te-ov′u-lah-to″re) suppressing ovulation.

antioxidant (an″te-ok′sĭ-dant) a substance that in small amounts will inhibit the oxidation of other compounds.

antiparasitic (an″te-, an″ti-par″ah-sit′ik) 1. destroying parasites. 2. an agent that destroys parasites.

antiparkinsonian (an″te-, an″ti-pahr″kin-so′ne-an) 1. effective in treatment of PARKIN-SONISM. 2. an agent that has this property.

antiparticle (an″tĭ-pahr′tĭ-k′l) either of a pair of elementary particles that have electric charges and magnetic moments of opposite sign and are the same in all other properties, such as mass, lifetime, and spin, e.g., the electron and positron. Every particle has an antiparticle. When antiparticles collide, they are annihilated, and their mass is converted to energy in the form of gamma rays.

antipediculotic (an″te-, an″ti-pĕ-dik″u-lo-t′ik) 1. effective against lice and in treatment of PEDICULOSIS. 2. an agent with this property.

antipepsin (an″te-pep′sin) an antienzyme that counteracts pepsin.

antiperistalsis (an″te-, an″ti-per″ĭ-stawl′-sis) upward waves of contraction sometimes occurring normally in the lower ileum, competing with the normal downward PERISTALSIS and retarding passage of intestinal contents into the cecum. adj., **antiperistal′tic.**

antiperistaltic (an″te-, an″ti-per′ĭ-stawl′-tik) 1. opposing the force of PERISTALSIS. 2. an agent with this effect. 3. pertaining to ANTIPERISTALSIS.

antiperspirant (an″te-, an″ti-per′spir-ant) 1. suppressing SWEATING. 2. an agent that so acts.

antiplasmin (an″te-, an″ti-plaz′min) a substance in the blood that inhibits plasmin. The most important is α_2-*antiplasmin*, which acts by forming stable complexes with free plasmin. It is also crosslinked to fibrin by coagulation factor XIII and inhibits the binding of plasminogen to fibrin. Inherited deficiency of α_2-antiplasmin results in tendency to severe bleeding, including extravasation into joints or their synovial cavities.

antiplastic (an″te-, an″ti-plas′tik) unfavorable to healing.

antipolycythemic (an″te-, an″ti-pol″e-si-the′mik) 1. effective against POLYCYTHEMIA. 2. an agent with this property.

antiport (an′ti-port) a cell MEMBRANE TRANSPORT mechanism that transports two molecules at once through the membrane in opposite directions. See also COUNTERTRANSPORT and SYMPORT.

antiprogestin (an″te-, an″ti-pro-jes′tin) a substance that inhibits the formation of progestational agents; the most common example is mifepristone.

antiprothrombin (an″te-, an″ti-pro-throm′bin) 1. directed against prothrombin. 2. a substance that retards the conversion of prothrombin into thrombin.

antiprotozoal (an″te-, an″ti-pro-to-zo′al) 1. destroying PROTOZOA or checking their growth or reproduction. 2. antiprotozoal AGENT.

antipruritic (an″te-, an″ti-proo-rit′ik) 1. preventing or relieving itching. 2. an agent that so acts.

antipsoriatic (an″te-, an″ti-sor″e-at′ik) 1. effective against psoriasis. 2. an agent effective against psoriasis.

antipsychotic (an″te-, an″ti-si-kot′ik) 1. modifying PSYCHOTIC behavior. 2. antipsychotic agent.

a. agent any drug that favorably modifies PSYCHOTIC symptoms; categories include the PHENOTHIAZINES, BUTYROPHENONES, THIOXANTHENES, DIBENZODIAZEPINES, DIPHENYL-BUTYLPIPERIDINES, DIHYDROINDOLONES, and DIBENZOXAZEPINES. They are chemically diverse but pharmacologically similar. Formerly called major tranquilizer.

Antipsychotics stabilize mood and reduce anxiety, tension, and hyperactivity. They are also effective in helping to control agitation and aggressiveness. Delusions and hallucinations are often modified and may

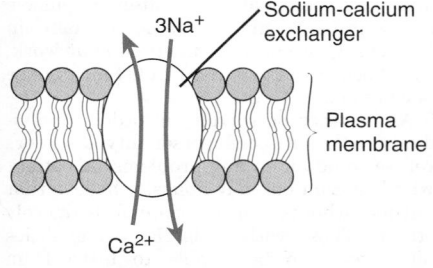

3Na⁺
Sodium-calcium exchanger

Plasma membrane

Ca²⁺

Cytosol

Antiport: sodium-calcium exchanger. The electrochemical gradient of Na⁺ is used to pump Ca²⁺ out of the cell and thereby regulate the cytosolic Ca²⁺ level.

be eliminated by such an agent, but once the drug is discontinued, the delusions and hallucinations often return within a short while. Different antipsychotic agents bind to dopamine, histamine, muscarinic, cholinergic, α-adrenergic, and serotonin receptors. Blockade of dopaminergic transmission in various areas is thought to be responsible for the major antipsychotic, antiemetic effects of these agents as well as neurologic side effects. The drugs are contraindicated in patients suffering from central nervous system depression, severe allergy, Parkinson's disease, or a blood dyscrasia. There also is the possibility of drug-drug interaction when neuroleptic drugs are given concurrently with barbiturates, alcohol, tricyclic antidepressants, antihypertensives, meperidine, anticonvulsants, or levodopa.

Many antipsychotics have alarming side effects (see extrapyramidal EFFECTS); thus there must be thorough patient education and individualized adjustments in dosage. The side effects can usually be minimized by gradually increasing the dosage until the optimum for the individual is reached. Side effects such as a discomforting restlessness and agitation (AKATHISIA), involuntary rhythmic movements of the trunk and limbs, PARKINSONISM, and tardive DYSKINESIA are often misinterpreted as symptoms of some unrelated disorder; these are often the reason for noncompliance or stopping of medication by patients. Approximately 20 per cent of the patients treated with neuroleptics for long periods develop tardive dyskinesia, a syndrome of choreoathetoid movements of the tongue, mouth, face, neck, limbs, and trunk, which may continue after the drug is stopped.

Antipsychotic agents are sometimes prescribed for conditions other than mental disorders. They can be beneficial in the control of nausea, in the treatment of intractable hiccups, in controlling the movement disorders associated with Huntington's chorea and Gilles de la Tourette's syndrome, and, in combination with other drugs, for the control of pain.

antipyretic (an″te-, an″ti-pi-ret′ik) 1. effective against FEVER; called also antifebrile. 2. something having this effect, such as a cold pack, aspirin, or quinine; antipyretic drugs dilate the blood vessels near the surface of the skin, thereby allowing more blood to flow through the skin, where it can be cooled by the air. An antipyretic can also increase perspiration, the evaporation of which cools the body. Called also febricide and febrifuge.

antipyrine (an″te-, an″ti-pi′rēn) a compound formerly used as an analgesic and antipyretic, now replaced by safer and more effective agents. Its current uses are as a component of multi-ingredient ear drop solutions and complexed with CHLORAL HYDRATE in DICHLORALPHENAZONE, a SEDATIVE and HYPNOTIC used for headaches. Called also phenazone.

antirachitic (an″te-, an″ti-rah-kit′ik) therapeutically effective against RICKETS.

antiretroviral (an″te-, an″ti-ret′ro-vi″ral) 1. effective against RETROVIRUSES. 2. an agent with this quality.

anti-Rh₀ anti-D.

antirheumatic (an″te-, an″ti-roo-mat′ik) counteracting RHEUMATISM and RHEUMATOID DISEASE.

antirickettsial (an″te-, an″ti-rī-ket′se-al) 1. effective against RICKETTSIAE. 2. an agent with this property.

antiscorbutic (an″te-, an″ti-skor-bu′tik) 1. preventing or relieving SCURVY. 2. an agent that so acts.

antisecretory (an″te-, an″ti-se-kre′to-re) 1. inhibiting or diminishing secretion; called also secretoinhibitory. 2. an agent that so acts, as certain drugs that inhibit or diminish gastric secretions.

antisense (an′te-, an′ti-sens) pertaining to the antisense STRAND of a nucleic acid.

antisepsis (an″tĭ-sep′sis) 1. the prevention of SEPSIS. 2. any procedure that reduces to a significant degree the microbial flora of skin or mucous membranes. See also ANTISEPTIC.

antiseptic (an″tĭ-sep′tik) 1. pertaining to ANTISEPSIS. 2. any substance that inhibits growth of microorganisms; this is contrasted to a GERMICIDE, which kills them outright. The category *antiseptics* is also not considered to include ANTIBIOTICS, which are usually taken internally, although it does include DISINFECTANTS. However, most disinfectants are too strong to be applied to body tissue and are generally used to clean inanimate objects such as floors and bathroom fixtures.

Antiseptics are divided into two types: *physical* and *chemical*. The most important physical antiseptic is heat, applied by boiling, autoclaving, flaming, or burning. These are among the oldest and most effective methods of disinfecting contaminated objects, water, and food. Chemical antiseptics have many applications: they are used in treating wounds and infections, in sterilizing (such as before an operation), and in general hygiene; they also have applications in the preservation of food and purification

of sewage. There are many different antiseptic substances to choose from; their strength and the speed at which they work are factors that influence the choice of which to use for a specific task.

urinary a. a drug that is excreted mainly by way of the urine and performs its antiseptic action in the bladder. These drugs may be given before examination of or operation on the urinary tract, and they are sometimes used to treat urinary tract infections.

antiserum (an′tĭ-se″rum) 1. a serum containing ANTIBODIES, such as one obtained from an animal that has been subjected to the action of antigen either by injection into the tissues or blood or by infection. See also IMMUNITY and IMMUNIZATION. Called also immune serum. 2. a reagent source of antibody, often sold commercially.

antisialagogue (an″te-, an″ti-si-al′ah-gog) an agent that inhibits the flow of SALIVA.

antisialic (an″te-, an″ti-si-al′ik) checking the flow of SALIVA.

antisocial (an″te-, an″ti-so′shal) 1. denoting behavior that violates the rights of others, societal mores, or the law. 2. denoting the specific personality traits seen in ANTISOCIAL PERSONALITY DISORDER.

a. personality disorder a PERSONALITY DISORDER characterized by a conspicuous disregard for the rights and needs of others. Antisocial behavior begins before the age of 15 and includes such behaviors as truancy, delinquency, theft, and vandalism. Adults with this disorder show a lack of maturity, unwillingness to take responsibility, and emotional instability. The chief characteristic of such persons is an apparent lack of conscience. Their behavior includes a variety of antisocial and criminal acts, such as theft, engaging in an illegal occupation (for example, selling drugs), repeated defaulting on debts, sexual promiscuity, and repeated lying. In addition, an antisocial personality is often impulsive and aggressive and is unable to maintain consistent, responsible functioning at work, at school, or as a parent. Substance abuse is common.

As in other personality disorders, individuals with antisocial personality disorders refuse to admit to any problems. A patient who is a criminal may honestly believe that anyone who is not a criminal is merely stupid. Those with antisocial personalities often seem to be unable to learn from experience. They also are seldom willing to accept psychiatric help and when they do agree to consult a mental health professional, it is often only to avoid the legal consequences of their activity.

antispasmodic (an″te-, an″ti-spaz-mod′ik) 1. preventing or relieving spasms. 2. an agent that prevents or relieves spasms. Called also spasmolytic.

antispastic (an″te-, an″ti-spas′tik) antispasmodic with specific reference to skeletal muscle.

antistreptococcic (an″te-, an″ti-strep″to-kok′sik) counteracting streptococcal infection.

antithenar (an″te-the′nar) placed opposite to the palm or sole.

antithrombin (an″te-throm′bin) any naturally occurring or therapeutically administered substance that neutralizes the action of thrombin and thus limits or restricts blood coagulation.

  a. I FIBRIN, referring to the capacity of fibrin to adsorb thrombin and thus neutralize it.

  a. III a naturally occurring inhibitor of blood coagulation; it is an α_2-globulin member of the SERPIN group, synthesized in the liver and found in the plasma and various extravascular sites. It inactivates THROMBIN as well as certain COAGULATION FACTORS and KALLIKREIN. Inherited deficiency of the protein, an autosomal dominant disorder, is associated with recurrent deep vein thrombosis and pulmonary emboli. Complications from the disorder are prevented and, in conjunction with heparin, treated with a preparation of antithrombin III from pooled human plasma, administered intravenously.

antithrombocytic (an″te-throm″bo-sit′ik) 1. preventing the aggregation of blood PLATELETS (THROMBOCYTES). 2. an agent that does this; see also ANTICOAGULANT.

antithromboplastin (an″te-throm″bo-plas′tin) any agent or substance that prevents or interferes with the interaction of blood COAGULATION FACTORS as they generate THROMBOPLASTIN.

antithrombotic (an″te-throm-bot′ik) 1. preventing or interfering with the formation of THROMBI. 2. an agent that has this effect, such as HEPARIN or COUMARIN. See also ANTICOAGULANT and THROMBOLYTIC.

antithyroid (an″te-thi′roid) suppressing or inhibiting thyroid activity.

antitoxin (an′tĭ-tok″sin) a particular kind of ANTIBODY produced in the body in response to the presence of a toxin; see also IMMUNITY. adj., **an′titoxic.**

  botulism a. an equine antitoxin against the toxins produced by the types A and B and/ or E strains of *Clostridium botulinum;* administered intravenously in the postexposure prophylaxis and treatment of botulism, other than infant botulism. Generally trivalent (ABE) antitoxin is used.

  diphtheria a. equine antitoxin from horses immunized against diphtheria toxin or the toxoid; administered intramuscularly or intravenously in the treatment of suspected cases of diphtheria.

  equine a. an antitoxin derived from the blood of healthy horses immunized against a specific bacterial toxin.

  tetanus a. equine antitoxin from horses that have been immunized against tetanus toxin or toxoid; used for the passive prevention and treatment of tetanus. It is rarely used, tetanus immune globulin being preferred.

antitragus (an″te-tra′gus) a projection on the ear opposite the TRAGUS.

antitrope (an′tĭ-trōp) one of two structures that are similar but oppositely oriented, like the right and the left hand.

α_1-antitrypsin alpha$_1$-antitrypsin.

antituberculotic (an″te-too-ber″ku-lot′ik) counteracting tuberculosis.

antitussive (an″te-, an″ti-tus′iv) 1. effective against cough. 2. an agent that suppresses coughing.

antiulcerative (an″te-ul′sah-ra″tiv, an″te-ul′ser-ah-tiv) 1. preventing the formation or promoting the healing of ulcers. 2. an agent that has these effects.

antiurolithic (an″te-u″ro-lith′ik) 1. preventing formation of urinary CALCULI. 2. an agent that so acts.

antivenin (an″te-, an″ti-ven′in) a material used to neutralize the VENOM of a poisonous animal; it is composed of concentrated purified antibodies from the serum of an immunized animal, frequently a horse.

  black widow spider a. antivenin (*Latrodectus mactans*).

  a. (Crotalidae) polyvalent a serum containing specific venom-neutralizing globulins, produced by immunizing horses with venoms of the fer-de-lance and the western, eastern, and tropical rattlesnakes, used for treatment of envenomation by most pit vipers throughout the world.

  a. (Latrodectus mactans) a serum containing specific venom-neutralizing globulins, prepared by immunizing horses against venom of the black widow spider (*L. mactans*).

  a. (Micrurus fulvius) a serum containing specific venom-neutralizing globulins, produced by immunization of horses with venom of the eastern coral snake (*M. fulvius*).

  North American coral snake a. antivenin (*Micrurus fulvius*).

  polyvalent crotaline a. antivenin (Crotalidae) polyvalent.

Antivert (an″tĭ-vert′) trademark for preparations of MECLIZINE hydrochloride, an antiemetic and antivertigo agent.

antiviral (an″te-, an″ti-vi′ral) 1. effective against viruses. 2. an agent effective against viruses.

antivitamin (an″te-, an″ti-vi′tah-min) a substance that inactivates or inhibits synthesis of a VITAMIN.

antixerotic (an″te-, an″ti-ze-rot′ik) preventing dryness.

antr(o)- word element [L.], *chamber; cavity;* often used with specific reference to the maxillary antrum or sinus.

antrectomy (an-trek′to-me) surgical excision of an antrum.

antritis (an-tri′tis) 1. inflammation of an antrum. 2. maxillary SINUSITIS.

antroatticotomy (an″tro-at″ĭ-kot′ah-me) atticoantrotomy.

antrocele (an′tro-sēl) accumulation of fluid in the maxillary antrum (sinus).

antronasal (an″tro-na′zal) pertaining to the maxillary antrum (sinus) and nasal fossa.

antroscope (an′tro-skōp) an instrument for inspecting the maxillary antrum (sinus).

antrostomy (an-tros′tah-me) incision of an ANTRUM with drainage.

antrotomy (an-trot′ah-me) incision of an antrum.

antrum (an′trum), pl. *an′tra, antrums* [L.] a cavity or chamber. adj., **an′tral.**

a. of Highmore maxillary sinus.

mastoid a. an air space in the mastoid portion of the temporal bone communicating with the middle ear and the mastoid cells.

a. maxilla′re, maxillary a. maxillary sinus.

pyloric a., a. pylo′ricum the proximal, expanded portion of the pyloric part of the stomach.

tympanic a., a. tympa′nicum mastoid antrum.

Anturane (an′tu-rān) trademark for a preparation of SULFINPYRAZONE, a uricosuric agent used in the management of GOUT.

anuclear (a-noo′kle-ar) having no nucleus.

anulus (an′u-lus), pl. *a′nuli* [L.] a small RING or encircling structure; also spelled annulus.

a. fibro′sus 1. fibrous ring of heart; any of four dense fibrous rings, one of which surrounds each of the major cardiac orifices. 2. fibrous ring of intervertebral disk; the circumferential ringlike portion of an intervertebral disk.

a. of spermatozoon a dark ringlike structure at the posterior end of the middle piece of a spermatozoon. Called also *ring centriole.*

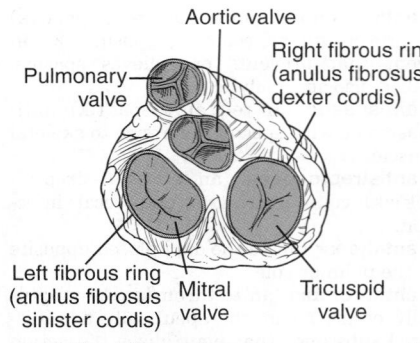

Anuli Fibrosi (Fibrous rings) of heart, one surrounding each of the two atrioventricular valves. From Dorland's, 2000.

anuresis (an″u-re′sis) 1. urinary retention. 2. anuria. adj., **anuret′ic.**

anuria (ah-nu′re-ah) 1. complete suppression of urine formation by the kidney. adj., **anu′ric.** 2. complete suppression of urine formation and excretion, as in acute RENAL FAILURE. Called also anuresis. adj., **anu′ric.**

anus (a′nus), pl. *a′nus* the opening of the rectum on the body surface. (See accompanying illustration.)

imperforate a. congenital absence of the normal opening of the rectum. Called also anal atresia and atresia ani.

anvil (an′vil) incus.

anxiety (ang-zi′ĭ-te) a multidimensional emotional state manifested as a somatic, experiential, and interpersonal phenomenon; a feeling of uneasiness, apprehension, or dread. These feelings may be accompanied by symptoms such as breathlessness, a choking sensation, palpitations, restlessness, muscular tension, tightness in the chest, giddiness, trembling, and flushing, which are produced by the action of the autonomic nervous system, especially the sympathetic part of it.

Anxiety may be rational, such as the anxiety about doing well in a new job, about one's own or someone else's illness, about passing an examination, or about moving to a new community. People also feel realistic anxiety about world dangers, such as the possibility of war, and about social and economic changes that may affect their livelihood or way of living. Most persons find healthy ways to deal with their normal quota of anxiety.

Nursing Diagnosis. Anxiety was accepted as a nursing diagnosis by the North America Nursing Diagnosis Association and defined as "a vague, uneasy feeling of discomfort or dread, accompanied by an autonomic response (the source often nonspecific or

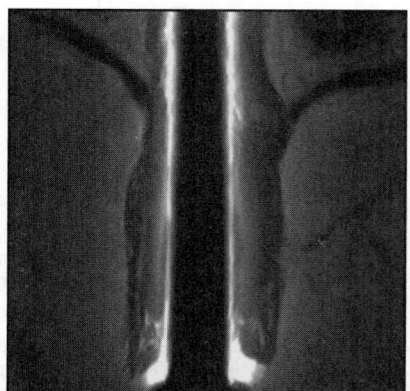 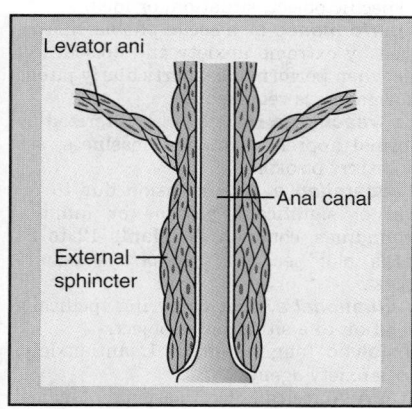

The anus. *Left,* Endoanal magnetic resonance image of the sphincter muscles. High-definition images can be obtained by using an endoanal MRI coil. *Right,* Explanatory diagram (coronal view in a normal patient). From Aspinall and Taylor Robinson, 2001.

unknown to the individual); a feeling of apprehension caused by anticipation of danger." It is an alerting signal that warns of apprehension caused by anticipation of danger and enables the individual to take measures to deal with the threat. It is differentiated from fear in that the anxious person cannot identify the threat, whereas the fearful person recognizes the source of fear.

Factors that can precipitate an attack of anxiety include any pathophysiological event that interferes with satisfaction of the basic human physiological needs. Situational factors include actual or perceived threat to self-concept, loss of significant others, threat to biological integrity, change in environment, change in socioeconomic status, and transmission of another person's anxiety to the individual. Other etiologic factors are associated with a threat to completion of developmental tasks at various life stages, for example, a threat to an adolescent in the completion of developmental tasks associated with sexual development, peer relationships, and independence.

Interventions. Measures to assist the individuals suffering from anxiety are aimed at helping them recognize their anxiety and their usual means of coping with it, and providing alternate, more healthful coping mechanisms that give a sense of physiological and psychological comfort.

a. disorders a group of mental disorders in which anxiety is the most prominent disturbance or in which anxiety is experienced if the patient attempts to control the symptoms. Everyone occasionally experiences anxiety as a normal response to a dangerous or unusual situation. In an anxiety disorder, the person feels the same emotion without any apparent reason and cannot identify the source of the threat that produces the anxiety, which actually has its origin in unconscious fears or conflicts.

People with anxiety disorders experience both the subjective emotion and various physical manifestations resulting from muscular tension and autonomic nervous system activity. This can produce a variety of symptoms, including sweating, dizziness, shortness of breath, insomnia, loss of appetite, and palpitations. The source of the anxiety lies in unconscious fears, unresolved conflicts, forbidden impulses, or threatening memories. Symptoms are often triggered by an apparently harmless stimulus that the patient unconsciously links with a deeply buried, anxiety-producing experience. Chronic anxiety can lead to various somatic alterations. The onset of anxiety may be gradual or sudden. Some persons experience incapacitating acute anxiety (as in panic disorder) while others manifest their anxiety through avoidant behavior patterns (phobias, obsessive-compulsive disorder). Anxiety disorders include: PANIC DISORDER, AGORAPHOBIA, SOCIAL PHOBIA, SPECIFIC PHOBIA, OBSESSIVE-COMPULSIVE DISORDER, POSTTRAUMATIC STRESS DISORDER, ACUTE STRESS DISORDER, GENERALIZED ANXIETY DISORDER, and SUBSTANCE-INDUCED ANXIETY DISORDER.

free-floating *a.* severe, generalized anxiety having no apparent connection to any specific object, situation, or idea.

performance *a.* a social phobia characterized by extreme anxiety and episodes of panic when performance, particularly public performance, is required.

a. reaction a reaction characterized by abnormal apprehension or uneasiness; see also ANXIETY DISORDERS.

separation *a.* apprehension due to removal of significant persons or familiar surroundings, common in infants 12 to 24 months old; see also SEPARATION ANXIETY DISORDER.

situational *a.* that occurring specifically in relation to a situation or object.

anxiolytic (ang″zĭ-o-lit′ik) 1. antianxiety. 2. antianxiety agent.

AOMA American Occupational Medical Association.

AONE American Organization of Nurse Executives.

AORN Association of Perioperative Registered Nurses (formerly called the Association of Operating Room Nurses).

aorta (a-or′tah), pl. *aor′tae, aortas* [L.] the great artery arising from the left ventricle, being the main trunk from which the systemic arterial system proceeds. It has four divisions: the ascending aorta, the aortic arch, the thoracic aorta, and the abdominal aorta. See Appendix of Arteries and see CIRCULATORY SYSTEM. (See accompanying illustration.)

overriding *a.* a congenital anomaly occurring in TETRALOGY OF FALLOT, in which the aorta is displaced to the right so that it appears to arise from both ventricles and straddles the ventricular septal defect.

aortalgia (a″or-tal′jah) pain in the region of the aorta.

aortic (a-or′tik) pertaining to the aorta.

a. arch syndrome any of a group of disorders adding to occlusion of the arteries arising from the aortic ARCH; such occlusion may be caused by atherosclerosis, arterial embolism, or other conditions. See also PULSELESS DISEASE.

a. septal defect a congenital anomaly in which there is abnormal communication between the ascending aorta and the pulmonary artery just above the semilunar valves.

aortitis (a″or-ti′tis) inflammation of the aorta.

aortocoronary (a-or″to-kor′ŏ-nar-e) pertaining to or communicating with the aorta and coronary arteries.

aortogram (a-or′to-gram) a radiograph that serves as a record of aortography.

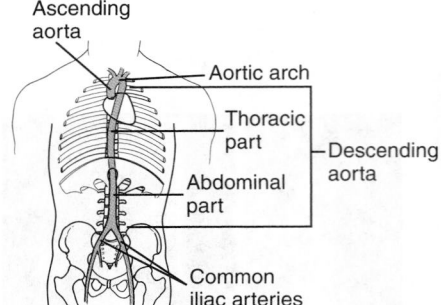

Aorta, arising from the left ventricle, ascending, arching, then descending through the thorax to the abdomen, where it divides into the common iliac arteries. From Dorland's, 2000.

aortography (a″or-tog′rah-fe) radiography of the aorta after introduction into it of a contrast material.

aortopathy (a″or-top′ah-the) any disease of the aorta.

aortoplasty (a-or′to-plas″te) surgical repair of the aorta; see also aortic RECONSTRUCTION.

aortorrhaphy (a″or-tor′ah-fe) suture of the aorta.

aortosclerosis (a-or″to-sklĕ-ro′sis) sclerosis of the aorta.

aortostenosis (a-or″ to-stĕ -no′ sis) narrowing of the aorta.

aortotomy (a″or-tot′ah-me) incision of the aorta.

AOTA American Occupational Therapy Association.

AP angina pectoris; anteroposterior; arterial pressure.

APA American Pharmaceutical Association; American Podiatric Association; American Psychiatric Association; American Psychological Association.

APA style a format for writing and documenting scholarly papers, developed by the American Psychological Association and frequently used in writings related to the health sciences.

APACHE [*A*cute *P*hysiology *a*nd *C*hronic *H*ealth *E*valuation] a patient classification system that predicts the risk of death in INTENSIVE CARE UNITS.

ap- see APO-.

ap(o)- word element [Gr.], *away from; separated.* Also *ap-*.

apancreatic (a-pan″kre-at′ik) due to absence of the pancreas.

aparalytic (a″par-ah-lit′ik) characterized by absence of paralysis.

apathy (ap′ah-the) lack of feeling or emotions; indifference.

APC abbreviation for the activated form of PROTEIN C.

APCC anti-inhibitor coagulant complex.

aperient (ah-pe′re-ent) 1. mildly CATHARTIC. 2. a substance that is mildly cathartic.

aperistalsis (ah″per-ĭ-stal′sis) absence of peristaltic action.

Apert's syndrome (ah-pārz′) an inherited disorder with autosomal dominant inheritance, characterized by conical deformity of the head, webbed FINGERS and TOES, and often other skeletal deformities, usually with mental retardation. Called also acrocephalosyndactyly, type I.

Apert-Crouzon disease (ah-pār′ kru-zaw′) a disorder formerly believed to combine hand and foot malformations associated with APERT'S SYNDROME with the facial characteristics of CROUZON'S DISEASE; it is now believed to be Apert's syndrome with unusually marked facial features.

apertura (ap″er-tu′rah), pl. *apertu′rae* [L.] aperture.

aperture (ap′er-chur) opening.

   inferior a. of minor pelvis, inferior a. of pelvis pelvic outlet.

   numerical a. an expression of the measure of efficiency of a microscope objective.

   superior a. of minor pelvis, superior a. of pelvis pelvic inlet.

apex (a′peks), pl. *apexes, a′pices* [L.] the pointed end of a cone-shaped part. adj., **ap′ical.**

   a. of lung the rounded upper extremity of either lung.

   root a. the terminal end of the root of the tooth.

apexogenesis (a″peks-o-jen′ĕ-sis) normal development of the root apex of a tooth.

APF acidulated phosphate fluoride, a preparation of sodium fluoride acidulated with phosphoric acid for topical application to the teeth in the prevention of dental caries; see SODIUM FLUORIDE.

aphagia (ah-fa′je-ah) refusal or loss of the ability to swallow. See also DYSPHAGIA.

aphakia (ah-fa′ke-ah) absence of the lens of an eye, occurring congenitally or as a result of trauma or surgery. adj., **apha′kic.**

aphalangia (a″fah-lan′jah) absence of fingers or toes.

aphasia (ah-fa′zhah) a type of SPEECH DISORDER consisting of a defect or loss of the power of expression by speech, writing, or signs, or of comprehension of spoken or written language, due to disease or injury of the brain centers, such as after STROKE SYNDROME on the left side.

Patient Care. Aphasia is a complex phenomenon manifested in numerous ways. The recovery period is often very long, even months or years. Because communication is such a vital part of everyday living, loss of the ability to communicate with words, whether in speaking or writing, can profoundly affect the personality and behavior of a patient. Although aphasic persons usually require extensive treatment by specially trained speech pathologists or therapists, all persons concerned with the care of the patient should practice techniques that will help minimize frustration and improve communication with such patients.

   amnestic a. anomic aphasia.

   anomic a. inability to name objects, qualities, or conditions. Called also amnestic or nominal aphasia.

   ataxic a. expressive aphasia.

   auditory a. loss of ability to comprehend spoken language. Called also word deafness.

   Broca's a. motor aphasia.

   conduction a. aphasia due to a lesion of the pathway between the sensory and motor speech centers.

   expressive a. motor aphasia.

   fluent a. that in which speech is well articulated (usually 200 or more words per minute) and grammatically correct but is lacking in content and meaning.

   global a. total aphasia involving all the functions that go to make up speech and communication.

   jargon a. that with utterance of meaningless phrases, either neologisms or incoherently arranged known words.

   mixed a. combined expressive and receptive aphasia.

   motor a. aphasia in which there is impairment of the ability to speak and write, owing to a lesion in the INSULA and surrounding OPERCULUM including Broca's motor speech area. The patient understands written and spoken words but has difficulty uttering the words. See also RECEPTIVE APHASIA. Called also logaphasia and Broca's, expressive, or nonfluent aphasia.

   nominal a. anomic aphasia.

   nonfluent a. motor aphasia.

   receptive a. inability to understand written, spoken, or tactile speech symbols, due to disease of the auditory and visual word centers, as in word blindness. See also motor aphasia. Called also logamnesia and sensory or Wernicke's aphasia.

   sensory a. receptive aphasia.

   visual a. alexia.

   Wernicke's a. receptive aphasia.

Apgar score (ap′gahr) a method for determining an infant's condition at birth by scoring the heart rate, respiratory effort, muscle tone, reflex irritability, and color.

The infant is rated from 0 to 2 on each of the five items, the highest possible score being 10. (See table.) Each of the factors is rated 60 seconds after birth and again five minutes later. The Apgar score is an objective way of assessing and describing an infant's adaptation to extrauterine life.

APHA American Public Health Association.

aphasic (ah-fa'zik) 1. pertaining to or affected with aphasia. 2. a person affected with aphasia.

aphasiologist (ah-fa″ze-ol'o-jist) a specialist in APHASIOLOGY.

aphasiology (ah-fa″ze-ol'o-je) the scientific study of APHASIA and specific neurologic lesions producing it.

aphemia (ah-fe'me-ah) a term formerly used to describe a type of motor APHASIA and more recently proposed as a synonym for APRAXIA OF SPEECH.

apheresis (af″ĕ-re'sis) any procedure in which blood is withdrawn from a donor, a portion (such as plasma, leukocytes, or platelets) is separated and retained, and the remainder is retransfused into the donor. Types include ERYTHROCYTAPHERESIS, LEUKAPHERESIS, LYMPHOCYTAPHERESIS, PLASMAPHERESIS, and PLATELETPHERESIS.. Called also hemapheresis and pheresis.

therapeutic a. separation of whole blood into its major components and removal of the abnormal, pathogenic component. Types include plasma exchange (PLASMAPHERESIS), removal of white blood cells (LEUKAPHERESIS), removal of platelets (THROMBOCYTAPHERESIS), and removal of red blood cells ERYTHROCYTAPHERESIS). The process is currently used as measure of last resort when conventional therapies are unsuccessful in controlling a chronic, debilitating, or potentially fatal disease. Its primary purpose is to modify the pathologic process so that other treatments can be more effective. It is not a cure. Plasmapheresis may be used in treatment of rheumatoid ARTHRITIS, MYASTHENIA GRAVIS, systemic LUPUS ERYTHEMATOSUS, and some malignancies, in which plasma constituents can interfere with the function of the immune system. Other diseases for which therapeutic apheresis might be used include certain blood DYSCRASIAS such as THROMBOCYTOSIS, POLYCYTHEMIA vera, and SICKLE CELL ANEMIA.

aphonia (a-fo'ne-ah) 1. loss of the voice; see also DYSPHONIA. 2. mutism.

aphonic (a-fon'ik) 1. pertaining to APHONIA. 2. without audible sound.

aphose (af'ōz) any subjective visual sensation due to absence or interruption of light sensation.

aphrasia (a-fra'zah) inability to speak or to understand phrases. See also APHASIA and MUTISM.

aphrodisiac (af″ro-diz'e-ak) 1. arousing sexual desire. 2. a drug that arouses sexual desire.

aphtha (af'thah), pl. *aph'thae* [L.] a small ulcer, such as the small oval or round ulcers covered with gray exudate and surrounded by a red halo characteristic of recurrent aphthous STOMATITIS.

aphthosis (af-tho'sis) a condition marked by presence of aphthae.

aphylaxis (af″ĭ-lak' sis) absence of phylaxis or immunity. adj., **aphylac'tic.**

apical (ap'ĭ-k'l) pertaining to an apex.

apicectomy (a″pĭ-sek'to-me) excision of the apex of the petrous portion of the temporal bone.

apicitis (a″pĭ-si'tis) inflammation of the apex of the lung or of the root of a tooth.

apicoectomy (a″pĭ-ko-ek'to-me) excision of the apical portion of the root of a tooth through an opening in overlying tissues of the jaw.

apicostomy (a″pĭ-kos'tah-me) dental trephination.

apiotherapy (a″pe-o-ther'ah-pe) the therapeutic use of products from bees, especially bee venom.

aplacental (a″plah-sen't'l) having no placenta.

aplanatic (ap″lah-nat'ik) correcting or not affected by spherical aberration.

aplasia (ah-pla'zhah) defective development or complete absence of an organ due to failure of development of the embryonic

APGAR SCORING CHART			
Sign	**0**	**1**	**2**
Heart rate	Absent	Below 100	Over 100
Respiratory effort	Absent	Slow, irregular	Good, crying
Muscle tone	Limp	Some flexion of extremities	Active motion
Response to catheter in nostril (tested after oropharynx is clear)	No response	Grimace	Cough or sneeze
Color	Blue, pale	Body pink, extremities blue	Completely pink

tissues or cells. 2. a hematologic disorder in which the normal progression of cell generation and development does not occur.

aplastic (a-plas′tik) pertaining to or characterized by aplasia; having no tendency to develop into new tissue.

a. anemia any form of anemia caused by bone marrow FAILURE or aplasia of the marrow. This may be due to chemical factors such as drugs, to physical factors such as radiation, to infection by a virus, or to idiopathic congenital defects of the stem cells of the bone marrow. It is characterized by a reduction or depletion of hemopoietic precursor cells with decreased production of leukocytes, erythrocytes, and platelets, resulting in peripheral blood PANCYTOPENIA.

apnea (ap′ne-ah) cessation of breathing, especially during sleep. The most common type is adult sleep APNEA. Central apnea in which there is failure of the central nervous system drive to respiration sometimes occurs in infants younger than 40 weeks after the date of conception.

adult sleep a. frequent and prolonged episodes in which breathing stops during sleep. Diagnosis is confirmed by monitoring the subject during sleep for periods of apnea and lowered blood oxygen levels. Sleep apnea is divided into three categories: (1) *obstructive,* resulting from obstruction of the upper airways; (2) *central,* caused by some pathology in the brain's respiratory control center; and (3) *mixed,* a combination of the two (see above).

Treatment. Obstructive and mixed types are amenable to therapy. Since many sleep apnea patients are overweight, weight loss improves the symptoms. Central sleep apnea is the most difficult to control. Medications to stimulate breathing have not proven beneficial. Mechanical ventilation or administration of oxygen during the night may help some patients.

The most common treatment for obstructive sleep apnea is nasal CONTINUOUS POSITIVE AIRWAY PRESSURE, which the patient uses during sleep; the positive pressure exerted prevents the airway from obstructing. Another method that may be tried is a dental appliance to move the jaw forward during sleep. In the most refractory cases, such as when an anatomical airway obstruction can be demonstrated, surgery to remove it may be performed after consultation with a surgeon experienced in evaluating and treating such obstructions. Another treatment that is occasionally used is insertion of a special type of tracheostomy TUBE that can be plugged during the day for normal use of the upper airway and opened at night to bypass upper airway obstruction

central a., central sleep a. see adult sleep APNEA.

deglutition a. a temporary arrest of the activity of the respiratory nerve center during an act of swallowing.

initial a. a condition in which a newborn fails to establish sustained respiration within two minutes of delivery.

late a. cessation of respiration in a newborn for more than 45 seconds after spontaneous breathing has been established and sustained.

mixed a. see adult sleep APNEA.

obstructive a., obstructive sleep a. see adult sleep APNEA.

primary a. cessation of breathing resulting when a fetus or newborn infant is deprived of oxygen; exposure to oxygen and stimulation usually restore respiration.

prolonged infantile a. sudden infant death syndrome.

secondary a. a period of time following primary apnea during which continued asphyxia of the fetus or newborn, with a fall in blood pressure and heart rate, necessitates artificial ventilation for resuscitation and reestablishment of ventilation.

sleep a. transient periods when breathing stops during sleep; see adult sleep APNEA.

apneumia (ap-noo′me-ah) congenital absence of the lungs.

apneusis (ap-noo′sis) sustained, gasping inhalation followed by short, inefficient exhalation, which can continue to the point of ASPHYXIA; it is often associated with lesions in a respiratory CENTER of the brain. adj., **apneu′stic.**

apochromatic (ap″o-kro-mat′ik) free from chromatic aberration.

apocrine (ap′o-krin) denoting that type of glandular secretion in which the secretory products become concentrated at the free end of the secreting cell and are thrown off, along with the portion of the cell where they have accumulated, as in the mammary gland. See also HOLOCRINE and MEROCRINE.

apodia (ah-po′de-ah) congenital absence of one or both feet.

apoenzyme (ap″o-en′zīm) the protein component of an enzyme that requires the presence of the prosthetic group (coenzyme) to form the functioning enzyme.

apoferritin (ap″o-fer′ĭ-tin) an apoprotein that can bind many atoms of iron per molecule to form FERRITIN, the form in which iron is stored in the liver and other tissues.

apolar (a-po′lar) having neither poles nor processes; without polarity.

apolipoprotein (ap″o-lip″o-pro′tēn) a non-lipid protein portion occurring in plasma LIPOPROTEINS; there are five families of apolipoproteins, grouped into four classes according to function, A, B, C, and E (the former apolipoprotein D has now been placed in class A). Apolipoproteins play a role in the transport of lipoproteins.

aponeurectomy (ap″o-noo-rek′to-me) excision of an aponeurosis.

aponeurorrhaphy (ap″o-noo-ror′ah-fe) suture of an aponeurosis.

aponeurosis (ap″o-noo-ro′sis), pl. *aponeuro′ses* a sheetlike tendinous expansion, mainly serving to connect a muscle with the parts it moves. adj., **aponeurot′ic.** (See accompanying illustration.)

aponeurositis (ap″o-noo-ro-si′tis) inflammation of an aponeurosis.

aponeurotomy (ap″o-noo-rot′ah-me) incision of an aponeurosis.

apophyseal (ap″o-fiz′e-al) pertaining to an apophysis.

apophysis (ah-pof′ĭ-sis), pl. *apoph′yses* [Gr.] any outgrowth or swelling, especially a bony outgrowth that has never been entirely separated from the bone of which it forms a part, such as a process, tubercle, or tuberosity.

apophysitis (ah-pof″ĭ-si′tis) inflammation of an apophysis.

apoplectiform (ap″o-plek′tĭ-form) resembling apoplexy.

apoplectoid (ap″o-plek′toid) resembling apoplexy.

apoplexy (ap′o-plek″se) old name for STROKE SYNDROME. adj., **apoplec′tic.**

apoprotein (ap″o-pro′tēn) the protein portion of a molecule or complex consisting of a protein molecule joined to a nonprotein protein molecule or molecules (such as a LIPOPROTEIN).

apoptosis (ap″op-to′sis) a morphologic pattern of cell death affecting single cells, marked by shrinkage of the cell, condensation of chromatin, formation of cytoplasmic blebs, and fragmentation of the cell into membrane-bound bodies that are eliminated by phagocytosis. It is a mechanism for cell deletion in the regulation of cell populations. Often used synonymously with programmed cell DEATH.

aporepressor (ap″o-re-pres′or) a repressor that is inactive until it combines with a corepressor.

aposthia (ah-pos′the-ah) congenital absence of the prepuce.

apothecaries' system a system used for measuring and weighing drugs and solutions, brought to the United States

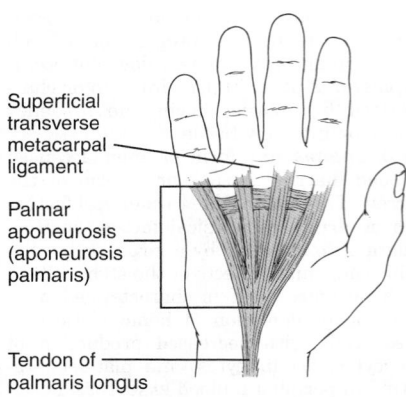

Superficial transverse metacarpal ligament

Palmar aponeurosis (aponeurosis palmaris)

Tendon of palmaris longus

Palmar aponeurosis. A fifth longitudinal band, radiating toward the base of the thumb, is sometimes present. From Dorland's, 2000.

from England during the colonial period; it has now been replaced by the METRIC SYSTEM. Its units are the GRAIN, SCRUPLE, DRAM, OUNCE, and POUND. Fractions are used to designate portions of a unit of measure: e.g., one-fourth grain is written gr. 1/4. The fraction 1/2 is written ss. There are two symbols in this system which are sometimes confused and always must be written clearly, those for drams and ounces. Lower case Roman numerals are used after the symbols: ʒiss reads drams one and one-half; ℥iii reads ounces three. See also Table of Weights and Measures in the Appendix.

apothecary (ah-poth′ĕ-kar″e) pharmacist.

apparatus (ap″ah-rat′tus), pl. *appara′tus, apparatuses* an arrangement of a number of parts acting together to perform a special function.

Golgi a. see GOLGI APPARATUS.

juxtaglomerular a. a collective term for the juxtaglomerular CELLS in a nephron.

lacrimal a. see LACRIMAL APPARATUS.

Wangensteen's a. a nasal suction apparatus connected with a duodenal tube for aspirating gas and fluid from stomach and intestine.

appendage (ah-pen′dij) a less important portion of an organ, or an outgrowth, such as a tail. Also, a limb or limblike structure.

appendectomy (ap″en-dek′to-me) excision of the vermiform appendix.

appendicectomy (ah-pen″dĭ-sek′to-me) appendectomy.

appendicitis (ah-pen″dĭ-si′tis) inflammation of the vermiform APPENDIX, a serious disease that usually requires surgical removal (APPENDECTOMY). When performed early the operation is comparatively simple and safe. When the appendix becomes inflamed and infected, rupture may occur within a matter of hours. Rupture of the appendix leads to PERITONITIS, one of the most serious of all diseases, although its danger has been reduced by antibacterial agents. (See accompanying illustration.)

Cause. If the tubelike appendix becomes plugged by a hard bit of fecal matter or by intestinal worms, or becomes inflamed from other causes, normal drainage cannot take place. Because the appendix is chiefly lymphatic tissue, an infection that produces enlarged lymph nodes elsewhere in the body also can increase the glandular tissue in the appendix and obstruct its lumen. Narrowing of the lumen makes the pouch-like organ more susceptible to bacterial infection. *Escherichia coli* and other types of bacteria multiply and cause inflammation and infection that spread to the peritoneal cavity unless the body's defenses are able to overcome the infection or the appendix is removed before it ruptures.

Symptoms. The classic symptoms of appendicitis are pain, nausea, vomiting, and low-grade fever in adults. Children tend to have higher fevers. The pain typically begins in the umbilical region and eventually localizes in the right lower quadrant of the abdomen over the site of the appendix. The pain is persistent and is aggravated by motion, causing the patient to bend over and tense the abdominal muscles (muscle guarding). Rebound pain occurs when the abdomen is deeply palpated and the hand is quickly removed from the abdomen. The patient also can feel pain in the area of the appendix when either a rectal or pelvic examination is done.

Other data that may support a diagnosis of appendicitis are obtained through a blood cell count. An elevated white cell count (leukocytosis) commonly accompanies appendicitis as it does other kinds of inflammation. Mild leukocytosis of 14,000 to 16,000 per mm^3 is common. A white cell count higher than 20,000 per mm^3 suggests a ruptured appendix and peritonitis.

Other diseases that can be mistaken for appendicitis are gallbladder attacks and kidney infection on the right side. The onset of pneumonia, rheumatic fever, or diabetic ketoacidosis can imitate appendicitis. In women, there is the possibility of a ruptured ectopic pregnancy, a twisted ovarian cyst, or a hemorrhaging ovarian follicle at the middle of the menstrual cycle.

Patient Care. When appendicitis is suspected because of symptoms exhibited by the patient, a health care provider should be notified immediately. The patient should lie down and remain as quiet as possible. It is best to give him nothing by mouth, and because of the danger of aggravating the condition and possibly causing rupture of the appendix, cathartics and laxatives are contraindicated. Applications of heat and the administration of laxatives or enemas are contraindicated for the same reasons. After the patient has been assessed and a diagnosis of appendicitis has been

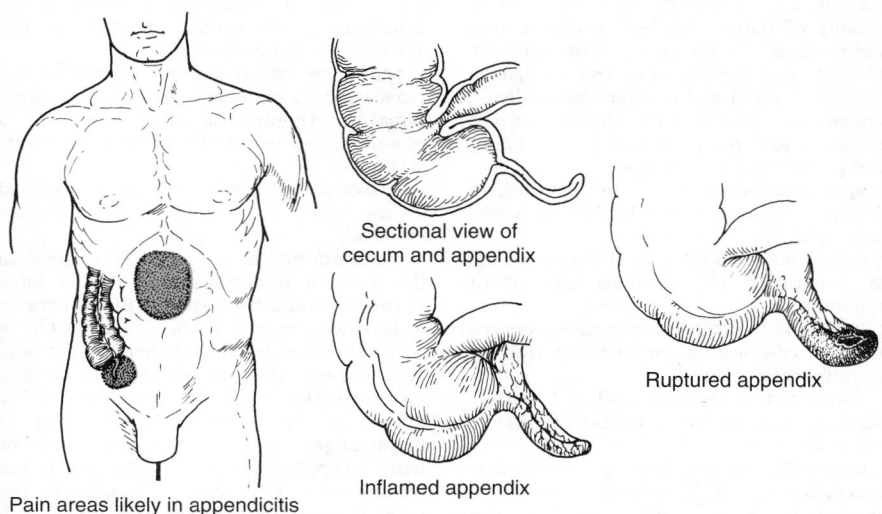

Sectional view of cecum and appendix

Ruptured appendix

Inflamed appendix

Pain areas likely in appendicitis

Appendicitis.

established, appendectomy will probably be performed as soon as possible.

During the preoperative phase it may be necessary to hydrate the patient with intravenous fluid therapy, especially when there has been prolonged nausea and vomiting. Decompression of the intestinal contents by suction via a nasogastric tube is also necessary in some cases.

Postoperative care is usually uneventful. The exception is when there has been a ruptured appendix; this serious condition warrants diligent and aggressive nursing care to overcome the effects of peritonitis with the resultant shifting of body fluids, hypovolemia (which can be life-threatening), and septic shock. Antibacterial drugs are administered to combat the infection. Gastric and intestinal decompression is maintained, and most surgeons advocate intraperitoneal draining by means of Penrose drains in order to prevent formation of abscesses and promote healing. The most common complications of appendectomy and peritonitis are (1) infection of the surgical wound, (2) paralytic ileus due to irritation of the small bowel, (3) abscesses, and (4) obstruction and adhesions.

Ongoing assessment of the patient includes observing the type and amount of drainage from the intestinal tract via the nasogastric tube and from the Penrose drain in the wound; appearance of the surgical incision; dressings applied and the frequency with which they are changed; evidence that bowel function is returning to normal, e.g., presence of bowel sounds, passing of flatus and fecal material; measurement of intake and output; tolerance of foods and liquids once the nasogastric tube is removed and decompression discontinued; and tolerance for physical activity, coughing and deep breathing, positioning, and postoperative exercises.

appendicolithiasis   (ah-pen″dĭ-ko-lĭ-thi′ah-sis) formation of calculi in the vermiform appendix.

appendicolysis (ah-pen″dĭ-kol′ĭ-sis) surgical separation of adhesions binding the appendix.

appendicostomy (ah-pen″dĭ-kos′tah-me) surgical creation of an opening into the vermiform appendix.

appendicular (ap″en-dik′u-lar) 1. pertaining to an appendix or appendage. 2. pertaining to the limbs.

appendix (ah-pen′diks), pl. *appen′dices, appendixes* [L.] 1. a slender outgrowth or appendage. 2. a small appendage near the juncture of the small intestine and the large intestine (ileocecal valve). An apparently useless structure, it can be the source of a serious illness, APPENDICITIS. Called also vermiform appendix. adj., **appendic′eal.**

  vermiform a. appendix (def. 2).

apperception (ap″er-sep′shun) conscious discernment of a sensory stimulus, understanding its significance as interpreted through one's own emotional outlook, experiences, and prior knowledge.

appersonation (ah-per″so-na′shun) appersonification.

appersonification (ap″er-son-ĭ-fĭ-ka′shun) unconscious identification with another person or delusional belief that one is another person.

appestat (ap′pĕ-stat) a brain center (probably in the hypothalamus) concerned in controlling the appetite.

appetite (ap′ĕ-tīt) the desire for food, stimulated by the sight, smell, or thought of food and accompanied by the flow of saliva in the mouth and gastric juice in the stomach. The stomach wall also receives an extra blood supply in preparation for its digestive activity. Appetite is psychological, dependent on MEMORY and associations, as compared with HUNGER, which is physiologically aroused by the body's need for food. Lack or loss of appetite, known as ANOREXIA, may be due to subjectively unpleasant food, surroundings, or company, or a symptom of either a physical disorder or an emotional disturbance. Excessive appetite may be an indication of either a metabolic disorder or an emotional disturbance.

applanometer (ap′lah-nom′ĕ-ter) a mechanical or electronic instrument for determining intraocular pressure in the detection of glaucoma.

appliance (ah-pli′ans) any of various devices used in dentistry to provide a functional or therapeutic effect, such as a PROSTHESIS, an OBTURATOR, or an orthodontic APPLIANCE.

  fixed a. an appliance that is attached to the teeth by cement or an adhesive material.

  orthodontic a. a device, either fixed to the teeth or removable, that applies force to the teeth and their supporting structures to produce changes in their relationship to each other and to control their growth and development. Used in orthodontic therapy to move the teeth into esthetically or physiologically better positions, such as better alignment within the dental arch or with the opposing dentition; also used in the treatment of fractures or injuries to the maxilla, to stabilize or immobilize the teeth and jaws. Called also braces.

application (ap″lĭ-ka′shun) the act of bringing something into contact or of starting an action.

heat/cold a. in the NURSING INTERVENTIONS CLASSIFICATION, a nursing INTERVENTION defined as stimulation of the skin and underlying tissues with heat or cold for the purpose of decreasing pain, muscle spasms, or inflammation.

appointment (ah-point′ment) 1. a meeting at a specific time and place, planned in advance. 2. designation of someone for an official position.

joint a. a formal agreement between a hospital or agency and an academic institution whereby a health care provider may hold a position divided between the hospital or agency and the academic faculty.

apposition (ap″o-zish′un) the placement or position of adjacent structures or parts so that they can come into contact.

appraisal (ah-prāz′al) the act of evaluating something.

health risk a. a systematic evaluation of factors in an individual, family, community, or other AGGREGATE that might lead to illness or other health problems.

performance a. the evaluation of an employee or student, comparing his or her job-related behavior with a standard of expectations for performance.

apprehension (ap″re-hen′shun) 1. perception and understanding. 2. anticipatory fear or anxiety.

approximal (ah-prok′sĭ-mal) close together.

approximation (ah-prok″sĭ-ma′shun) 1. the act or process of bringing into proximity or apposition. 2. a numerical value of limited accuracy.

successive a. shaping.

apraclonidine (ap″rah-klon′ĭ-dēn) an α₂-adrenergic RECEPTOR agonist used to reduce intraocular pressure in the treatment of open-angle GLAUCOMA and the treatment and prevention of ocular hypertension; administered topically to the conjunctiva as the hydrochloride salt.

apraxia (ah-prak′se-ah) loss of ability to carry out familiar purposeful movements in the absence of sensory or motor impairment, especially impairment of the ability to use objects correctly.

amnestic a. loss of ability to carry out a movement on command due to inability to remember the command.

a. of gait a common disorder of the elderly in which the patient walks with a broad-based gait, taking short steps and placing the feet flat on the ground.

motor a. impairment of skilled movements that is not explained by weakness of the affected parts; the patient appears clumsy rather than weak.

sensory a. loss of ability to make proper use of an object due to lack of perception of its purpose.

a. of speech a speech disorder similar to motor APHASIA, due to apraxia of mouth and neck muscles because of a lesion interfering with coordination of impulses from Broca's motor speech area. Called also aphemia.

aprobarbital (ap″ro-bahr′bĭ-tal) an intermediate-acting BARBITURATE, used as a SEDATIVE and HYPNOTIC; administered orally.

aproctia (ah-prok′she-ah) imperforate anus.

aprosopia (ap″ro-so′pe-ah) a developmental ANOMALY consisting of partial or complete absence of the face.

aprotinin (ap″ro-ti′nin) an inhibitor of proteolytic enzymes, used as an antihemorrhagic to reduce perioperative blood loss in patients undergoing cardiopulmonary BYPASS during coronary artery BYPASS graft; administered intravenously.

APTA American Physical Therapy Association.

APTT, aPTT activated partial thromboplastin time.

aptyalism (ap-ti′ah-lizm) absence or deficiency of saliva.

aptitude test (ap′tĭ-tōōd) one designed to measure the capacity for developing general or specific skills.

APUD cells [*a*mine *p*recursor *u*ptake and *d*ecarboxylation] a group of apparently unrelated cells that secrete most of the body's hormones, with the exception of steroids. Included are both specialized neurons and other endocrine cells that synthesize structurally related polypeptides and biogenic amines. The name comes from the fact that polypeptide production is linked to the uptake of a precursor amino acid and its decarboxylation in the cell to produce an amine. Examples of the peptide hormones are INSULIN, CORTICOTROPIN, GLUCAGON, and antidiuretic HORMONE. Examples of the amine hormones are DOPAMINE, NOREPINEPHRINE, SEROTONIN, and HISTAMINE.

apudoma (ah″pu-do′mah) a tumor derived from APUD CELLS, many of which secrete ectopic HORMONES.

apus (a′pus) a malformed fetus without feet; see also SYMMELIA.

apyretic (a″pi-ret′ik) afebrile.

apyrexia (a″pi-rek′se-ah) absence of fever. adj., **apyrexial, afebrile.**

apyrogenic (ah-pi″ro-jen′ik) not producing fever.

Aq. [L.] a′qua (water).

Aq. dest. a′qua destilla′ta (distilled water).

aqua (ak′wah) [L.] water.

aquaphobia (ak″wah-fo′be-ah) irrational fear of water.

aquaporin (ak″wah-po′rin) any of a family of proteins found in cell membranes and forming a functional component of water CHANNELS.

aqueduct (ak′wĕ-dukt″) any canal or passage.

cerebral a. a narrow channel in the midbrain connecting the third and fourth ventricles and containing cerebrospinal fluid.

a. of Fallopius the canal for the facial nerve in the temporal bone.

sylvian a., a. of Sylvius, ventricular a. cerebral aqueduct.

aqueous (a′kwe-us) watery; prepared with water.

Ar argon.

ara-A adenine arabinoside; see VIDARABINE.

ara-C cytarabine.

arachidonic acid (ah-rak″ĭ-don′ik) an essential FATTY ACID that cannot be synthesized by animal tissues and must be obtained in the diet.

arachnephobia (ah-rak″nĕ-fo′be-ah) arachnophobia.

arachnid (ah-rak′nid) any member of the class ARACHNIDA.

Arachnida (ah-rak′nĭ-dah) a class of animals of the phylum Arthropoda, including 12 orders, comprising such forms as spiders, scorpions, ticks, and mites.

arachnidism (ah-rak′nĭ-dizm) poisoning from a SPIDER BITE.

arachnitis (ar″ak-ni′tis) arachnoiditis.

arachnodactyly (ah-rak″no-dak′tĭ-le) extreme length and slenderness of the fingers or toes, as in MARFAN SYNDROME.

arachnoid (ah-rak′noid) 1. resembling a spider's web. 2. the delicate membrane interposed between the dura mater and the pia mater, and with them constituting the meninges.

arachnoiditis (ah-rak″noid-i′tis) inflammation of the ARACHNOID.

arachnophobia (ah-rak″no-fo′be-ah) irrational fear of spiders.

Aralen (ar′ah-len) trademark for a preparation of CHLOROQUINE, an antimalarial AGENT also used as a suppressant of LUPUS ERYTHEMATOSUS.

Aran-Duchenne disease (ah-rahn′ du-shen′) spinal muscular atrophy.

arbor (ahr′bor), pl. *ar′bores* [L.] a tree.

a. vi′tae treelike outlines seen on median section of the cerebellum.

arborescent (ahr″bo-res′ent) branching like a tree.

arborization (ahr″bor-ĭ-za′shun) a collection of branches, as the branching terminus of a nerve-cell process.

arbovirus (ahr′bo-vi′rus) a term used by epidemiologists to refer to any of numerous viruses that replicate in blood-feeding arthropods such as mosquitoes and ticks and are transmitted to humans by biting. adj., **arbovi′ral.**

arbutamine (ahr-bu′tah-mēn″) a synthetic CATECHOLAMINE used as a diagnostic aid in cardiac stress TESTING in patients unable to exercise sufficiently for the test; administered as the hydrochloride salt.

ARC AIDS-related complex; American Red Cross.

arc (ahrk) a part of the circumference of a circle, or a regularly curved line.

binauricular a. the arc across the top of the head from one auricular point to the other.

reflex a. the circuit traveled by impulses producing a reflex action: receptor organ, afferent nerve, nerve center, efferent nerve, effector organ in a muscle; see also REFLEX. (See accompanying illustration.)

arcate (ahr′kāt) arcuate.

arch (ahrch) a structure of bowlike or curved outline.

abdominothoracic a. the lower boundary of the front of the thorax.

a. of aorta, aortic a. the curving portion between the ascending aorta and the descending aorta, giving rise to the brachiocephalic trunk, the left common carotid artery, and the left subclavian artery.

aortic a's paired vessels arching from the ventral to the dorsal aorta through the branchial clefts of fishes and amniote embryos. In mammalian development, arch 1 largely disappears but may contribute to the maxillary and external carotid arteries; the dorsal portion of arch 2 persists and forms stems of the stapedial arteries; arch 3 joins the common to the internal carotid artery; arch 4 becomes the arch of the aorta and joins the aorta and subclavian artery; arch 5 disappears; and arch 6 forms the pulmonary arteries and, until birth, the ductus arteriosus.

branchial a's 1. four pairs of arched columns in the neck region of some aquatic vertebrates that bear the gills. (See accompanying illustration.) 2. pharyngeal arches.

dental a. either of the curving structures formed by the crowns of the upper and lower teeth in their normal positions (or by the residual ridge after loss of the

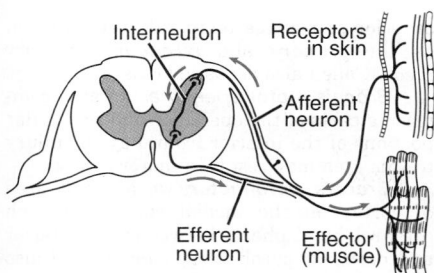

Three-neuron reflex arc. From Dorland's, 2000.

teeth); they are called the *inferior dental arch* (see mandibular arch) and the *superior dental arch* (see maxillary arch).

a's of foot the longitudinal and transverse arches of the foot. The longitudinal arch comprises the *medial arch* or *pars medialis,* formed by the calcaneus, talus, and the navicular, cuneiform, and the first three tarsal bones; and the *lateral arch* or *pars lateralis,* formed by the calcaneus, the cuboid bone, and the lateral two metatarsal bones. The transverse arch comprises the navicular, cuneiform, cuboid, and five metatarsal bones.

lingual a. a wire appliance that conforms to the lingual aspect of the dental arch, used to secure movement of the teeth in orthodontic work.

mandibular a. 1. the first branchial arch, being the rudiment of the maxillary and mandibular regions; it also gives rise to the malleus and incus. 2. the dental arch formed by the teeth of the mandible; called also inferior dental arch.

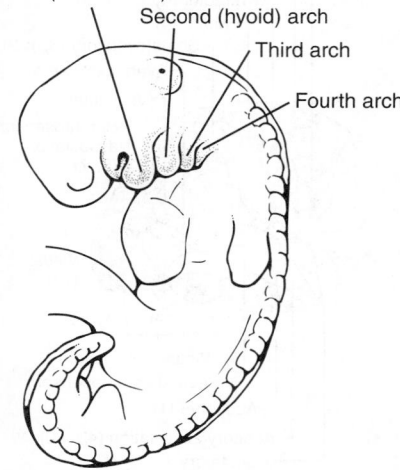

First (mandibular) arch
Second (hyoid) arch
Third arch
Fourth arch

Branchial arches. From Dorland's, 2000.

maxillary a. the dental arch formed by the teeth of the maxilla; called also superior dental arch.

neural a. vertebral arch.

palatal a. the arch formed by the roof of the mouth from the teeth on one side to those on the other.

pharyngeal a's structures in the neck region of the human embryo that are analagous to the branchial arches in lower vertebrates; the four pairs of pharyngeal arches are mesenchymal and later cartilaginous structures that develop during the first two months of embryonic life and are separated by clefts (the pharyngeal GROOVES). As the fetus develops, the arches grow to form structures within the head and neck. Two of them grow together and enclose the cervical sinus, a cavity in the neck. Called also branchial arches.

pubic a. the arch formed by the conjoined rami of the ischium and pubis of the two sides of the body.

pulmonary a's the most caudal of the aortic arches; it becomes the pulmonary artery.

tendinous a. a linear thickening of fascia over some part of a muscle.

vertebral a. the dorsal bony arch of a VERTEBRA, composed of the laminae and pedicles of a vertebra.

zygomatic a. the arch formed by the temporal PROCESS of the zygomatic bone and the zygomatic PROCESS of the temporal bone. See also anatomic Table of Bones in the Appendices.

arch- see ARCHI-.

archae(o)- see ARCHI-.

arche(o)- see ARCHI-.

archencephalon (ahrk″en-sef′ah-lon) the primordial brain from which the MIDBRAIN and FOREBRAIN develop.

archenteron (ahrk-en′ter-on) the central cavity that is the provisional gut in the GASTRULA; the primordial digestive cavity of the embryo.

archeocerebellum (ahr″ke-o-ser″ĕ-bel′um) the phylogenetically old part of the cerebellum.

archeocortex (ahr″ke-o-kor′teks) that portion of the cerebral CORTEX that, with the PALEOCORTEX, develops in association with the olfactory system, and which is phylogenetically older than the neocortex and lacks its layered structure.

archetype (ar′kĕ-tīp) in jungian psychology, a structural component of the collective unconcious, which is an inherited idea derived from the life experience of all of the members of the race and contained in the individual unconscious. The archetypes are the ideas, modes of thought, and patterns of reaction that are typical of all humanity and represent the wisdom of the ages. They appear in personified or symbolized form in dreams and visions and in mythology, legends, religion, fairy tales, and art. See also JUNG.

archi- word element [Gr.], *ancient; beginning; original; first; chief; leading.*

archinephron (ahr″kĭ-nef′ron) pronephros.

archipallium (ahr″kĭ-pal′e-um) that portion of the pallium, or cerebral cortex, which phylogenetically is the first to show the characteristic layering of the cellular elements.

arciform (ahr′sĭ-form) arcuate.

arctation (ahrk-ta′shun) stenosis.

arcuate (ahr′ku-āt) bent like a bow.

arcuation (ahr″ku-a′shun) a bending or curvature.

arcus (ahr′kus), pl. *ar′cus* [L.] arch; bow.

  a. adipo′sus arcus corneae.

  a. cor′neae, a. cornea′lis a white or gray opaque ring in the corneal margin; it may be present at birth or appear in childhood (see ARCUS JUVENILIS), but the condition is particularly common in those over 50 years old (see ARCUS SENILIS). It results from cholesterol deposits in or hyaline degeneration of the corneal stroma and may be associated with ocular defects or with familial HYPERLIPIDEMIA.

  a. juveni′lis ARCUS CORNEAE in young persons.

  a. seni′lis ARCUS CORNEAE in the elderly. (See Atlas 4, Part E).

ardeparin (ahr-de-par′in) a low molecular weight HEPARIN administered subcutaneously as the sodium salt as an anticoagulant and antithrombotic for prevention of deep venous THROMBOSIS and pulmonary THROMBOEMBOLISM after knee replacement surgery.

ARDS adult respiratory distress syndrome.

area (a′re-ah), pl. *a′reae, areas* [L.] a limited space or plane surface.

  acoustic a′s auditory areas.

  association a′s areas of the cerebral cortex (excluding primary areas) connected with each other and with the neothalamus; they are responsible for higher mental and emotional processes, including memory, learning, speech, and the interpretation of sensations. (See accompanying illustration.)

  auditory a′s two contiguous areas of the temporal lobe in the region of the anterior transverse temporal gyrus, known as the *primary* and *secondary auditory areas.* Called also acoustic areas.

  Broca's motor speech a. an area comprising parts of the opercular and triangular portions of the inferior frontal gyrus; injury to this area may result in motor APHASIA.

  Broca's parolfactory a. a small area of cortex on the medial surface of each cerebral hemisphere, between the anterior and posterior parolfactory sulci. Called also area subcallosa.

  Brodmann's a′s specific occipital and preoccipital areas of the cerebral CORTEX, distinguished by differences in the arrangement of their six cellular layers, and identified by numbering each area. They are considered to be the seat of specific functions of the brain.

  catchment a. 1. the geographical region drained by one body of water. 2. the area whose residents are served by a specialized health care agency. Called also catchment.

  contact a. proximal surface.

  embryonic a., germinal a., a. germinati′va embryonic DISK.

  Kiesselbach's a. an area on the anterior part of the nasal septum, richly supplied with capillaries, and a common site of epistaxis (nosebleed).

  language a. any nerve center of the cerebral cortex, usually in the dominant hemisphere, controlling the understanding or use of language.

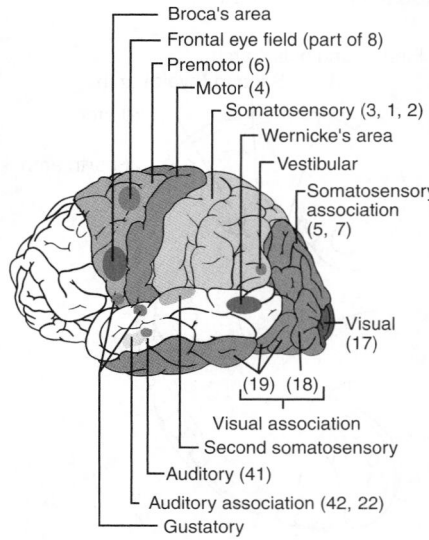

Broca's area
Frontal eye field (part of 8)
Premotor (6)
Motor (4)
Somatosensory (3, 1, 2)
Wernicke's area
Vestibular
Somatosensory association (5, 7)
Visual (17)
(19) (18)
Visual association
Second somatosensory
Auditory (41)
Auditory association (42, 22)
Gustatory

Area. Functional areas and lobes of the cerebrum.

motor a. any area of the cerebral cortex primarily involved in stimulating muscle contractions; most are in the precentral gyri. (See accompanying illustration.) See also premotor AREA, sensorimotor AREA, and Broca's motor speech AREA.

motor speech a. see Broca's motor speech AREA and Wernicke's AREA.

occupational performance a's categories of activities that make up an individual's occupational PERFORMANCE; they include ACTIVITIES OF DAILY LIVING, work activities, and play or leisure activities. A delay in any of these areas may be addressed by occupational therapy intervention.

olfactory a. 1. a general area of the brain, including the olfactory bulb, tract, and trigone, the anterior portion of the gyrus cinguli, and the uncus. 2. anterior perforated substance.

postcentral a., postrolandic a. an area just posterior to the central sulcus of the cerebral hemisphere that is the primary receiving area for general sensations.

precentral a. primary somatomotor area.

premotor a. an area of the motor cortex of the frontal lobe immediately in front of the precentral gyrus.

primary a. areas of the cerebral cortex comprising the motor and sensory regions.

primary receiving a's the areas of the cerebral cortex that receive the thalamic projections of the primary sensory modalities such as vision, hearing, and smell. (See accompanying illustration.) Called also sensory areas.

primary somatomotor a. an area in the posterior part of the frontal lobe just anterior to the central sulcus; different regions control motor activity of specific parts of the body. Called also precentral area and rolandic area.

projection a's those areas of the cerebral CORTEX that receive the most direct projection of the sensory systems of the body.

rolandic a. primary somatomotor area.

sensorimotor a. the cortex of the precentral and postcentral gyri, which are the motor area and the primary receiving area for general sensations, respectively.

sensory a's primary receiving areas.

sensory association a. an association area around the borders of a primary receiving area, where sensory stimuli are interpreted.

silent a. an area of the brain in which pathologic conditions may occur without producing symptoms.

somatic sensory a., somatosensory a. either of two cortical projection areas in or

near the postcentral gyrus where conscious perception of somatic sensations occurs, known as the *first* or *primary somatosensory area* and the *second* or *secondary somatosensory area.*

a. subcallo'sa, subcallosal a. Broca's parolfactory area.

a. under the curve (AUC) the area enclosed between the curve of a PROBABILITY with nonnegative values and the axis of the quality being measured; of the total area under a curve, the proportion that falls between two given points on the curve defines a probability density FUNCTION.

visual a's three areas *(first, second, and third visual areas)* of the visual CORTEX. The first visual area is better known as the striate cortex.

vocal a. rima glottidis.

Wernicke's a. originally a name for a speech center thought to be confined to the posterior part of the superior temporal gyrus next to the transverse temporal gyri; the term now refers to a wider zone that also includes the supramarginal and angular gyri.

areflexia (a″re-flek′se-ah) absence of the reflexes.

detrusor a. absence of contractions of the detrusor muscles of the urinary bladder.

arenavirus (ah-re′nah-vi″rus) any member of a family of spherical or pleomorphic RNA viruses containing host cell–derived RIBONUCLEOPROTEINS, including viruses that cause LASSA FEVER and lymphocytic CHORIOMENINGITIS; the natural hosts are rodents.

areola (ah-re′o-lah), pl. *are′olae* [L.] 1. a narrow zone surrounding a central area, e.g., the darkened area surrounding the NIPPLE of the mammary gland. 2. any minute space or interstice in a tissue.

Chaussier's a. the indurated area encircling a malignant pustule.

areolar (ah-re′o-lar) 1. containing minute spaces. 2. pertaining to an areola.

Argas (ahr′gas) a genus of ticks parasitic in poultry, other birds, and sometimes humans.

Argasidae (ahr-gas′ĭ-de) a family of arthropods, the soft TICKS.

argatroban (ahr-gat′ro-ban″) an ANTICOAGULANT that binds to the THROMBIN active site and inhibits various thrombin-catalyzed reactions; used in the prophylaxis and treatment of THROMBOCYTOPENIA resulting from treatment with HEPARIN, administered intravenously.

argentaffin (ahr-jen′tah-fin) staining readily with silver salts; see also argentaffin CELLS.

argentaffinoma (ahr″jen-taf″ĭ-no′mah) a carcinoid tumor of the gastrointestinal tract formed from argentaffin cells, usually in the terminal ileum or appendix; such tumors elaborate a variety of catecholamines that produce the symptom complex called CARCINOID SYNDROME. Called also carcinoid.

arginase (ahr′jĭ-nās) an enzyme of the liver that splits arginine into urea and ornithine.

arginine (Arg) (R) (ahr′jĭ-nēn) a nonessential AMINO ACID that occurs in proteins and is involved in the urea CYCLE and in the synthesis of CREATINE. Preparations of the base or the glutamate or hydrochloride salt are used in the treatment of hyperammonemia and in the assessment of pituitary function.

argininosuccinic acid (ahr″-jĭ-ne′no-suk-sin″ik) a compound normally formed in urea formation in the liver, but not normally present in urine.

argininosuccinicaciduria (ahr″jĭ-ne″no-suk-sin″ik-as″ĭ-du′re-ah) excretion in the urine of ARGININOSUCCINIC ACID, a feature of an inborn ERROR of metabolism marked also by mental retardation.

argipressin (ahr″gĭ-pres′in) arginine vasopressin.

argon (Ar) (ahr′gon) a chemical element, atomic number 18, atomic weight 39.948. (See Appendix 6.)

argyria (ahr-ji′re-ah) poisoning by silver or its salts; chronic argyria is marked by a permanent ashen-gray discoloration of the skin, conjunctivae, and internal organs, and there is usually a slate blue "silver line" on the gingival margin. Argyria can result from either industrial or medicinal exposure.

argyric (ahr-ji′rik) pertaining to silver.

argyrism (ahr′jĭ-rizm) argyria.

argyrophil (ahr-ji′ro-fil) easily impregnated with silver; said of cells or tissues that bind with silver salts, which can then be reduced to produce a brown or black stain.

argyrosis (ahr″jĭ-ro′sis) argyria.

arhinia (ah-rin′e-ah) congenital absence of the nose. Spelled also arrhinia.

Arias-Stella reaction (ah′ryahs stel′ah) nuclear and cellular hypertrophy of the endometrial epithelium associated with ectopic pregnancy.

ariboflavinosis (a-ri″bo-fla″vĭ-no′sis) deficiency of RIBOFLAVIN (vitamin B_2) in the diet, a condition marked by lesions in the corners of the mouth, on the lips, and around the nose and eyes, malaise, weakness, weight loss and, in severe cases, anemia, corneal or other eye changes, and seborrheic dermatitis. It is most common among people in regions such as Asia and the West Indies, where the diet contains large quantities of corn, potatoes, or rice, which lack riboflavin. A well-balanced diet will prevent riboflavin deficiency; it will also correct the disorder, with the help of supplementary doses of riboflavin and other vitamins.

Aristocort (ah-ris′to-cort) trademark for preparations of TRIAMCINOLONE, a PREDNISOLONE derivative that is a steroid ANTIINFLAMMATORY agent.

Arlidin (ahr′lĭ-din) trademark for a preparation of NYLIDRIN, a peripheral VASODILATOR.

arm (ahrm) 1. the part of the upper LIMB from the shoulder to the elbow; called also brachium. 2. in common usage, the entire upper LIMB. 3. a slender part or extension that projects from a main structure. 4. chromosome arm.

brawny a. a hard, swollen condition of the arm due to lymphedema following mastectomy.

chromosome a. either of the two segments of the chromosome separated by the centromere. The arms are equal in length when the centromere is in the median position and are unequal when the centromere is off center; the symbol p indicates the short arm and q the long arm. (See accompanying illustration.)

armamentarium (ahr″mah-men-tar′e-um) the entire equipment of a practitioner, such as medicines, instruments, and books.

armboard (ahrm′bord) a rigid flat piece of boardlike material, used to immobilize the arm when an intravenous device is placed close to an area of flexion.

ARMD age-related macular degeneration.

Arnold-Chiari syndrome (ahr′nold ke-ah′re) Arnold-Chiari DEFORMITY.

aromatase (ah-ro′mah-tās) an enzyme activity occurring in the endoplasmic reticulum and catalyzing the conversion of TESTOSTERONE to the aromatic compound ESTRADIOL.

aromatic (ar″o-mat′ik) 1. having a spicy fragrance. 2. denoting a compound containing a ring system stabilized by a closed circle of conjugated double bonds or nonbonding electron pairs, e.g., benzene or naphthalene.

ARPKD autosomal recessive POLYCYSTIC KIDNEY DISEASE.

arrector (ah-rek′tor), pl. *arrecto′res* [L.] raising, or that which raises; an erector muscle.

arrest (ah-rest′) sudden cessation or stoppage.

cardiac a. see CARDIAC ARREST.

epiphyseal a. premature arrest of the longitudinal growth of bone due to fusion of the epiphysis and diaphysis.

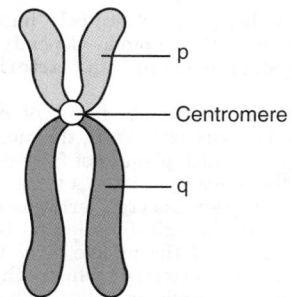

Chromosome arms. From Dorland's, 2000.

maturation a. interruption of the process of development, as of blood cells, before the final stage is reached.

arrhen(o)- word element [Gr.], *male; masculine.*

arrhenoblastoma (ah-re″no-blas-to′mah) a rare ovarian tumor that secretes male hormones and causes virilization.

arrhinia (ah-rin′e-ah) arhinia.

arrhythmia (ah-rith′me-ah) variation from the normal rhythm, especially of the heartbeat; see also DYSRHYTHMIA. adj., **arrhyth′mic.**

sinus a. the physiologic cyclic variation in heart rate, originating in the sinoatrial node and related to vagal impulses to the node; it occurs commonly in children (juvenile arrhythmia) and in the aged.

arrhythmogenic (ah-rith″mo-jen′ik) producing or promoting arrhythmia.

ARRT American Registry of Radiologic Technologists.

arseniasis (ahr″se-ni′ah-sis) chronic ARSENIC POISONING.

arsenic (As) (ahr′se-nik) a chemical element, atomic number 33, atomic weight 74.92. (See Appendix 6.) It is toxic by inhalation or ingestion, and CARCINOGENIC (see ARSENIC POISONING). In nature it occurs usually as one of its salts; in human environments it is often a pollutant in mining regions, and is used in dyes, household pesticides, and compounds used in agriculture. Arsenic compounds called ARSENICALS were formerly widely used in medicine.

a. poisoning poisoning due to systemic exposure to inorganic pentavalent arsenic. Arsenic is cumulative, storing permanently in hair, nails, and bone, and children are particularly susceptible. Arsenic is odorless and flavorless and has been found in elevated levels in the drinking water that flows through arsenic-rich rocks, leading to serious health problems in some countries. The antidote for arsenic poisoning is DIMERCAPROL. *Acute arsenic poisoning,*

which may result in shock and death, is marked by skin eruptions, swelling of eyelids and limbs, vomiting, diarrhea, and cramps. *Chronic arsenic poisoning* (called also arsenism), due to ingestion of small amounts over a long period of time, is marked by skin pigmentation with scaling, keratosis of the palms and soles, white lines on the fingernails, peripheral neuropathy, and confusion.

a. trioxide an oxidized form of arsenic, used in weed killers and rodenticides. It is also administered intravenously as an ANTINEOPLASTIC in the treatment of acute promyelocytic LEUKEMIA.

arsenical (ahr-sen′ĭ-k′l) 1. pertaining to arsenic. 2. a compound containing arsenic; arsenicals were once widely used in medicine, but have now mostly been replaced by ANTIBIOTICS. However, some are still used to treat infectious diseases, especially those caused by protozoa, as well as skin disorders and blood dyscrasias; they must be administered with caution because of their toxicity. All arsenicals are toxic to humans and some are CARCINOGENIC. See also ARSENIC POISONING.

arsenism (ahr′se-nizm) chronic ARSENIC POISONING.

arsine (ahr′sēn) any of several colorless, volatile ARSENICAL bases that are highly toxic and CARCINOGENIC; the most common one is AsH_3, arsenous hydride. Some of their compounds have been used in warfare, and a major industrial use is in the production of microelectronic components. Inhalation leads to massive red blood cell hemolysis with secondary renal failure and jaundice. A garliclike odor may be noted with high concentrations.

ART Accredited Record Technician; assisted reproductive technology; automated reagin test.

Artane (ahr′tān) trademark for preparations of TRIHEXYLPHENIDYL hydrochloride, an ANTIDYSKINETIC.

artefact (ahr′tĕ-fakt) artifact.

arteri(o)- word element [L., Gr.], *artery.*

arteria (ahr-te′re-ah), pl. *arte′riae* [L.] artery. See also anatomic Table of Arteries in the Appendices.

a. luso′ria an abnormally situated vessel behind the esophagus, usually the subclavian artery from the aortic arch; it may cause symptoms by compression of the esophagus, the trachea, or a nerve.

arterial (ahr-te′re-al) pertaining to an artery or to the arteries.

arteriectasis (ahr-tēr″e-ek′tah-sis) dilatation of an artery.

arteriectomy (ahr-tēr″e-ek′to-me) excision of an artery.

arteriogram (ahr-te′re-o-gram″) a radiograph of an artery.

arteriography (ahr-te″re-og′rah-fe) ANGIOGRAPHY of an artery or arterial system.

   catheter a. radiography of vessels after introduction of contrast material through a catheter inserted into an artery.

   coronary a. angiography of the coronary arteries, in which a cardiac CATHETER is inserted into an artery, usually the femoral or brachial artery, advanced under fluoroscopic guidance, and used to inject contrast medium directly into the coronary orifices. It is most often used in evaluations of patients with angina pectoris, prior to coronary artery surgery or percutaneous transluminal coronary ANGIOPLASTY.

   selective a. radiography of a specific vessel that is opacified by a medium introduced directly into it, usually via a catheter.

arteriol(o)- word element [L.], *arteriole.*

arteriola (ahr-te″re-o′lah), pl. *arterio′lae* [L.] arteriole.

   arterio′lae rec′tae re′nis vasa recta.

arteriole (ahr-te′re-ōl) a minute arterial branch. adj., **arterio′lar.**

arteriolith (ahr-te′re-o-lith″) hard, chalky mass (CONCRETION) in an artery.

arteriolitis (ahr-te″re-o-li′tis) inflammation of arterioles.

arteriology (ahr-te″re-ol′o-je) the anatomy or study of arteries and the arterial system.

arteriolonecrosis (ahr-te″re-o″lo-ně-kro′-sis) necrosis or destruction of arterioles.

arteriolosclerosis (ahr-te″re-o″lo-sklě-ro′-sis) sclerosis and thickening of the walls of arterioles. adj., **arteriolosclerot′ic.**

arteriomotor (ahr-te″re-o-mo′tor) involving or causing dilation or constriction of arteries.

arteriopathy (ahr-te″re-op′ah-the) any disease of an artery.

   hypertensive a. widespread involvement of the smaller arteries and arterioles, associated with hypertension and characterized primarily by hypertrophy of the tunica media.

arterioplasty (ahr-te′re-o-plas″te) surgical repair or reconstruction of an artery.

arteriopressor (ahr-te″re-o-pres′or) increasing arterial blood pressure.

arteriorrhaphy (ahr-te″re-or′ah-fe) suture of an artery.

arteriorrhexis (ahr-te″re-o-rek′sis) rupture of an artery.

arteriosclerosis (ahr-te″re-o-sklě-ro′sis) any of a group of diseases characterized by thickening and loss of elasticity of the arterial walls; popularly called "hardening of the arteries." Symptoms depend on the organ system involved. adj., **arteriosclerot′ic.**

There are three main forms of arteriosclerosis: (1) ATHEROSCLEROSIS, the most common type, in which plaques of fatty deposits form in the inner layer (TUNICA INTIMA) of the arteries; (2) Mönckeberg's arteriosclerosis, called also medial calcific sclerosis because of involvement of the middle layer (TUNICA MEDIA) of the arteries, where there is destruction of muscle and elastic fibers and formation of calcium deposits; and (3) arteriolar sclerosis or ARTERIOLOSCLEROSIS, which is marked by thickening of the walls of arterioles. All three forms may be present in the same patient, but in different blood vessels. When reference is made to hardening of the arteries, this usually refers to atherosclerosis; the terms *arteriosclerosis* and *atherosclerosis* are often used interchangeably.

It is the responsibility of the health care provider to help individuals modify or eliminate from their lives risk factors for the development of arteriosclerosis. These include cigarette smoking, obesity, elevated cholesterol levels, and sedentary life style.

   Mönckeberg's a. see ARTERIOSCLEROSIS.

   a. obli′terans arteriosclerosis in which proliferation of the intima has caused complete obliteration of the lumen of the artery. Cf. ENDARTERITIS OBLITERANS.

arteriospasm (ahr-te′re-o-spazm″) spasm of an artery, resulting in a decrease of its caliber.

arteriostenosis (ahr-te″re-o-stě-no′sis) constriction of an artery.

arteriotomy (ahr-te″re-ot′ah-me) incision of an artery.

arteriovenous (ahr-te″re-o-ve′nus) both arterial and venous; pertaining to both artery and vein.

arteritis (ahr″ter-i′tis), pl. *arteri′tides* inflammation of an artery.

   aortic arch a. pulseless disease.

   brachiocephalic a. pulseless disease.

   cranial a. temporal arteritis.

   giant cell a. temporal arteritis.

   hemolytic a., microangiopathic pulseless disease.

   a. obli′terans endarteritis obliterans.

   rheumatic a. generalized inflammation of arterioles and arterial capillaries occurring in rheumatic fever.

   Takayasu's a. pulseless disease.

   temporal a. a chronic vascular disease of unknown origin, occurring in the elderly, characterized by severe headache, fever, and accumulation of giant cells in the walls of medium-sized arteries, especially the

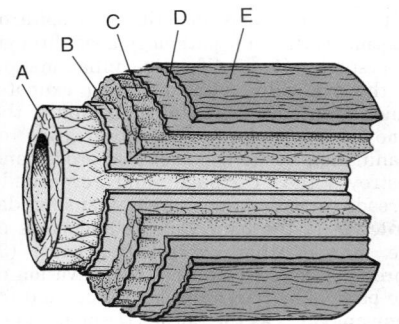

Representation of arterial coats: *A,* tunica intima; *B,* internal elastic lamina; *C,* tunica media; *D,* external elastic lamina; *E,* tunica externa. From Dorland's, 2000.

temporal arteries. Ocular involvement may cause visual impairment or blindness.

artery (ahr′ter-e) a vessel through which the blood passes away from the heart to various parts of the body. The wall of an artery consists typically of an outer coat (TUNICA ADVENTITIA), a middle coat (TUNICA MEDIA), and an inner coat (TUNICA INTIMA). (See accompanying illustration.) For names of specific arteries, see anatomic Table of Arteries in Appendices. See also Plate 8.

> **end a.** one that undergoes progressive branching without development of channels connecting with other arteries.

> **nutrient a.** any artery that supplies the marrow, or medulla, of a long bone.

arthr(o)- word element [Gr.], *joint; articulation.*

arthralgia (ahr-thral′jah) pain in a joint; called also arthrodynia.

arthrectomy (ahr-threk′to-me) excision of a joint.

arthritide (ahr′thrĭ-tīd) a skin eruption of gouty origin.

arthritis (ahr-thri′tis), pl. *arthri′tides* inflammation of a joint. adj., **arthrit′ic.** The term is often used by the public to indicate any disease involving pain or stiffness of the musculoskeletal system. Arthritis is not a single disease, but a group of over 100 diseases that cause pain and limit movement. The most common types are OSTEOARTHRITIS and rheumatoid ARTHRITIS.

> **acute a.** arthritis marked by pain, heat, redness, and swelling.

> **acute rheumatic a.** swelling, tenderness, and redness of many joints of the body, accompanying rheumatic fever.

> **hypertrophic a.** rheumatoid ARTHRITIS marked by hypertrophy of the cartilage at the edge of the joints; OSTEOARTHRITIS.

> **juvenile rheumatoid a.** rheumatoid ARTHRITIS in children under age 16, characterized by swelling, tenderness, and pain, involving one joint or several joints and lasting more than six weeks. It may lead to impaired growth and development, limitation of movement, and ANKYLOSIS and CONTRACTURES of joints. At times it is

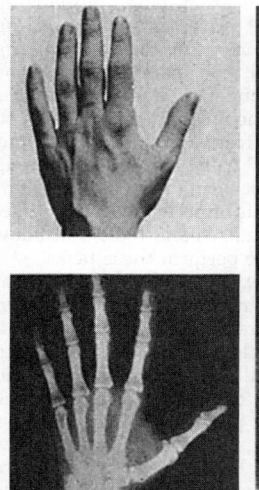
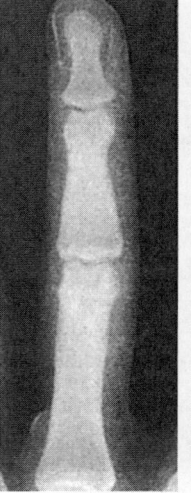
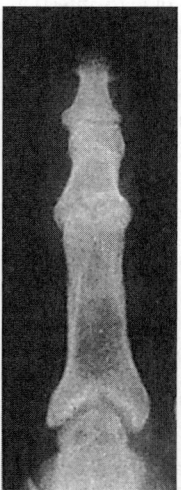
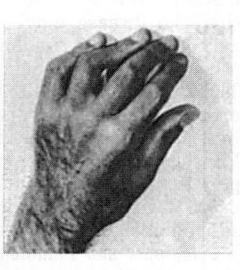
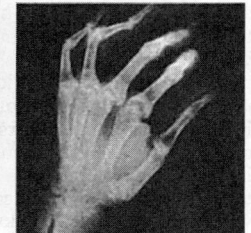

Arthritis of the fingers. *Left,* normal hand and finger. *Right,* arthritic hand and finger, with ankylosis, or "locking" of the joint by bone and scar tissue. Courtesy of Bergman Associates.

accompanied by systemic manifestations such as spiking fever, transient rash on the trunk and limbs, hepatosplenomegaly, generalized lymphadenopathy, and anemia, in which case it is known as STILL'S DISEASE or systemic onset juvenile rheumatoid arthritis.

Lyme a. Lyme disease.

psoriatic a. that associated with severe PSORIASIS, classically affecting the terminal interphalangeal joints.

rheumatoid a. a chronic systemic disease characterized by inflammatory changes occurring throughout the body's connective tissues. As such, it is classified as a COLLAGEN DISEASE. This form of arthritis strikes during the most productive years of adulthood, with onset in the majority of cases between the ages of 20 and 40. No age is spared, however, and the disease may affect infants as well as the very old. The disease affects men and women about equally in number, but three times as many women as men develop symptoms severe enough to require medical attention.

Etiology. The cause of rheumatoid arthritis is unknown and it is doubtful that there is one specific cause. It is regarded by some researchers as an AUTOIMMUNE DISEASE, in which the body produces abnormal antibodies against its own cells and tissues. Evidence to support this theory is found in the fact that there is an abnormally high level of certain types of IMMUNOGLOBULINS in the blood of patients suffering from rheumatoid arthritis. Other researchers contend that the disease may be due to infection, perhaps from an undefined virus or some other microorganism (e.g., *Mycoplasma*). There also is the possibility that rheumatoid arthritis is a genetic disorder in which one inherits a predisposition to the disease. Physical and emotional STRESS also play some part in the onset of acute attacks; however, psychological stress is implicated as a causative factor in the onset of many illnesses.

Symptoms and Pathology. In about 75 per cent of patients the onset of rheumatoid arthritis is gradual, with only mild symptoms at the beginning. Early symptoms include malaise, fever, weight loss, and morning stiffness of the joints. One or more joints may become swollen, painful, and inflamed. Some patients may experience only mild episodes of acute symptoms with lengthy remissions. The more typical patient, however, experiences increasingly severe and frequent attacks with subsequent joint damage and deformity. The pattern of remissions and exacerbations continues throughout the course of the disease.

If untreated, and sometimes in spite of treatment, the joint pathology goes through four stages: (1) proliferative inflammation of the synovium with increased exudate, which eventually leads to thickening of the synovium; (2) formation of a layer of granulation tissue (PANNUS) that erodes and destroys the cartilage and eventually spreads to contiguous areas, causing destruction of the bone capsule and parts of the muscles that control the joint; (3) fibrous ANKYLOSIS resulting from invasion of the pannus by tough fibrous tissue; and (4) bony ankylosis as the fibrous tissue becomes calcified.

In addition to the joint changes there is atrophy of muscles, bones, and skin adjacent to the affected joint. The most characteristic lesions of rheumatoid arthritis are subcutaneous nodules, which may be present for weeks or months and are most commonly found over bony prominences, especially near the elbow.

Because rheumatoid arthritis is a systemic disease, there is involvement of connective tissues other than those in the musculoskeletal system. Degenerative lesions may be found in the collagen in the lungs, heart, blood vessels, and pleura.

Patients with rheumatoid arthritis appear undernourished and chronically ill. Most are anemic because of the effect of the disease on blood-forming organs. The erythrocyte sedimentation rate is elevated and the WBC may be slightly elevated.

Treatment and Patient Care. Management of rheumatoid arthritis is aimed at providing rest and freedom from pain, minimizing emotional stress, preventing or correcting deformities, and maintaining or restoring function so that the patient can enjoy as much independence and mobility as possible. Occupational therapy is needed to teach patients effective ways to carry out such activities of daily living as grooming and self-care, preparing meals, and light housekeeping. This often involves using specially designed utensils and tools that allow deformed joints to perform these tasks.

Rest and Exercise. It is recommended that the patient with rheumatoid arthritis plan for 10 to 12 hours of sleep out of each 24. The patient should be careful to maintain good posture while lying in bed and avoid pillows or other devices that support the joints in a flexed position. A firm mattress is recommended, with only one pillow under the head. During periods of severe attacks, the patient may require continuous bed rest.

The purpose of rest is to allow the body's natural defenses against inflammation to work at optimal level. It is necessary, however, even in the acute phase to balance rest with prescribed exercises which take into account the severity of the case, the joints affected, and the patient's individual needs and tolerance.

Physical Therapy. The goals of physical therapy for the patient with rheumatoid arthritis are to prevent and correct deformities, control pain, strengthen weakened muscles, and improve function.

Therapeutic EXERCISE is of major importance in the physical therapy program established for the patient. It is necessary to enlist the patient's cooperation, and this can be done most effectively by explaining the purposes of the exercises and teaching ways to exercise that will not increase pain. In many instances proper exercise can actually diminish pain. The patient's tolerance for exercise must be carefully monitored. While it is expected that some discomfort may be present during exercise, there should not be persistent pain that continues for hours after the exercises have been done. If such pain and fatigue do occur, the exercise program should be reviewed and revised so that a good balance of rest and exercise is obtained. It should be remembered that overactivity can contribute to the inflammatory process.

Applications of heat or cold may be used in the management of rheumatoid arthritis. Heat applications improve circulation, promote relaxation, and relieve pain. When used in conjunction with exercise, heat can allow more freedom of joint movement. Various forms of heat therapy may be used, including dry heat, moist heat, DIATHERMY, and ULTRASOUND. For dry heat a therapeutic infrared heat lamp may be most convenient during home care. Hot water bottles or electric heating pads also may be used. For treatment of the hands, paraffin baths are effective. Wet heat can be applied by hot tub baths with the water temperature not exceeding 39°C (102°F) or by means of a towel dipped in hot water, wrung out, and applied to the joint. Whirlpool baths are effective, especially when prolonged treatment is indicated. Relief from pain and stiffness can be provided for some patients by applications of cold packs to the affected joints. This can be done by placing ice packs directly over the joint. When either heat or cold is used, care must be taken to protect the patient's skin. It should be remembered that rheumatoid arthritis affects the skin as well as other tissues.

Whenever it is necessary to handle the joints and limbs of a patient with rheumatoid arthritis, it is extremely important to move slowly and gently, avoiding sudden, jarring movements which stimulate muscle contraction and produce pain. The affected joints should be supported so that there is no excessive motion.

Medication. There is no drug that will cure arthritis. The health care provider does have a variety of medications that may be prescribed, depending on the needs and tolerance of the patient. It is important that the patient be advised of the expected results and possible undesirable side effects that may accompany ingestion of certain drugs. He or she should also be advised that therapeutic trials of several different drugs may be necessary. With this information at hand, he or she can work cooperatively with the physician in determining which drug or drugs can be most beneficial for treatment of the condition.

ASPIRIN was among the first drugs used to treat rheumatoid arthritis and remains a low-cost treatment option. It is a potent antiinflammatory agent when given at dosages that achieve a serum level of 20–30 mg/100 ml. For those prone to stomach upset or other gastrointestinal side effects from aspirin, enteric-coated tablets or antacid mixtures of aspirin are available.

Other nonaspirin, NONSTEROIDAL ANTI-INFLAMMATORY DRUGS (NSAIDs) include the indole derivatives INDOMETHACIN, SULINDAC, and TOLMETIN and the phenylalkanoic acid derivatives FENOPROFEN, IBUPROFEN, and NAPROXEN. Nowadays NSAIDs are the most used group of medications for treatment of arthritis. They may provide more relief than aspirin for certain patients, but they also may have side effects related to the gastrointestinal and nervous systems. COX-2 (cyclooxygenase-2) INHIBITORS are the latest class of NSAIDs. They have fewer gastrointestinal side effects than other NSAIDs.

CYTOTOXIC agents may also be used; these drugs act as IMMUNOSUPPRESSANTS and block the inflammatory process of the disease. METHOTREXATE is the most common of these. The dosage for the management of rheumatoid arthritis is much lower than the dosages for malignancies; thus the associated side effects are fewer. GOLD compounds or PENICILLAMINE may be prescribed for selected patients who cannot tolerate or are not responding well to more conservative methods of treatment.

The CORTICOSTEROIDS may be used in treating rheumatoid arthritis, but they are not a substitute for other forms of treatment. In some cases these drugs produce side effects that are more difficult to treat than arthritis. They also may worsen certain features of the disease rather than relieve them. Drugs included in this group are CORTISONE, HYDROCORTISONE, PREDNISONE, PREDNISOLONE, and DEXAMETHASONE.

Another group of medications that reduce inflammation are the biological response MODIFIERS. Members of this group used to treat arthritis include ETANERCEPT and IN-FLIXIMAB.

Surgical Intervention and Orthopedic Devices. In the past, surgical intervention was reserved for patients who had already suffered severe joint deformity. There is presently a trend toward the use of surgery in the early stages of the disease so that deformities and serious mechanical abnormalities can be prevented or at least modified.

One surgical procedure employed is SYNOVECTOMY (excision of the synovial membrane of a joint). The goal of this treatment is to interrupt the destructive inflammatory processes that eventually lead to ankylosis and invasion of surrounding cartilage and bone tissues.

Surgical repair of a hip joint (ARTHROPLASTY) may be performed when there is extensive damage and ambulation is not possible. The purpose of this procedure is to restore, improve, or maintain joint function. In cases in which it is not possible to restore the damaged hip joint there is a surgical procedure in which the diseased joint is completely replaced with a total hip prosthesis. The procedure is called a total hip REPLACEMENT. A similar procedure involving total replacement of the knee can be done when there is extensive damage to the knee joint.

Braces, casts, or splints are sometimes used to immobilize the affected part so that it can rest during an active stage of the disease. Devices that immobilize the affected joint also may allow for motion of adjacent muscle, thereby improving muscle strength and permitting more independence on the part of the patient. Braces also may be used to prevent deformities by maintaining good position of the joints.

Patient Education. Unfortunately, arthritis is so widespread and such a crippling disease that its victims may be easy prey for charlatans and promoters of "miraculous cures." The nature of the disease, with its unexplained remissions and relief of symptoms, makes it easy for unscrupulous individuals to convince the arthritic patient that some bizarre treatment they have used has indeed "cured" the arthritis. It is important that members of the health team recognize the need for patient education and work diligently with the patient and family so that they can cooperatively participate in a program of care that is most effective for the individual patient.

Home care is an essential part of the management of arthritis. To help in education of the public The Arthritis Foundation provides a number of pamphlets and other educational materials, supports a broad program of research and education, and helps finance improvement of local facilities for treatment of arthritis. The address of the foundation is The Arthritis Foundation, 1330 W. Peachtree St., Atlanta, GA 30309, telephone 404-872-7100.

suppurative a. inflammation of a joint with a purulent effusion into the joint, due chiefly to bacterial infection.

systemic onset juvenile rheumatoid a. Still's disease.

arthrocele (ahr'thro-sēl) a joint swelling.

arthrocentesis (ahr″thro-sen-te′sis) surgical puncture of a joint cavity for aspiration of fluid.

arthrochondritis (ahr″thro-kon-dri′tis) inflammation of the cartilage of a joint.

arthroclasia (ahr″thro-kla′zhah) surgical breaking down of an ankylosis to permit a joint to move freely.

arthrodesis (ahr″thro-de′sis) artificial ANKYLOSIS; surgical fusion of a joint.

arthrodia (ahr-thro′de-ah) gliding JOINT. adj., **arthro′dial.**

arthrodynia (ahr″thro-din′e-ah) arthralgia.

arthrodysplasia (ahr″thro-dis-pla′zhah) any abnormality of joint development.

arthroempyesis (ahr″thro-em″pi-e′sis) formation of pus within a joint.

arthroendoscopy (ahr″thro-en-dos′kah-pe) inspection of the interior of a joint with an endoscope.

arthrogram 1. a radiographic record after introduction of opaque contrast material into a joint. 2. a nuclear medicine study used to detect the loosening of a prosthetic device.

arthrography (ahr-throg′rah-fe) radiography of a joint.

air a. pneumoarthrography.

arthrogryposis (ahr″thro-grī-po′sis) 1. persistent flexion of a joint. 2. tetanoid spasm.

arthrolith (ahr'thro-lith) a hard mass (CONCRETION) within a joint.

arthrology (ahr-throl′o-je) the scientific study of the joints and ligaments; also applied to the body of knowledge relating thereto.

arthrolysis (ahr-throl′ĭ-sis) operative loosening of adhesions in an ankylosed joint.

arthrometer (ahr-throm′ĕ-ter) an instrument for measuring the angles of movements of joints.

arthro-ophthalmopathy (ahr″thro-of′-thal-mop′ah-the) an association of degenerative joint disease and eye disease.

arthropathy (ahr-throp′ah-the) any joint disease.

> ***Charcot's a.*** neuropathic arthropathy.

> ***chondrocalcific a.*** progressive polyarthritis with joint swelling and bony enlargement, most commonly in the small joints of the hand but also affecting other joints, characterized radiographically by narrowing of the joint space with subchondral erosions and sclerosis and frequently chondrocalcinosis.

> ***neuropathic a.*** chronic progressive degeneration of the stress-bearing portion of a joint, with hypertrophic changes at the periphery; it is associated with neurologic disorders involving loss of sensation in the joint. Called also Charcot's arthropathy.

> ***osteopulmonary a.*** clubbing of fingers and toes, and enlargement of ends of the long bones, in cardiac or pulmonary disease.

arthrophyma (ahr″thro-fi′mah) a joint swelling.

arthrophyte (ahr″thro-fīt) an abnormal growth in a joint cavity.

arthroplasty (ahr′thro-plas″te) plastic repair of a joint; called also joint replacement.

> ***total hip a.*** replacement of the femoral head and acetabulum with prostheses (*femoral* and *acetabular components*) that are anchored to the bone, done to replace a severely damaged hip joint. (See

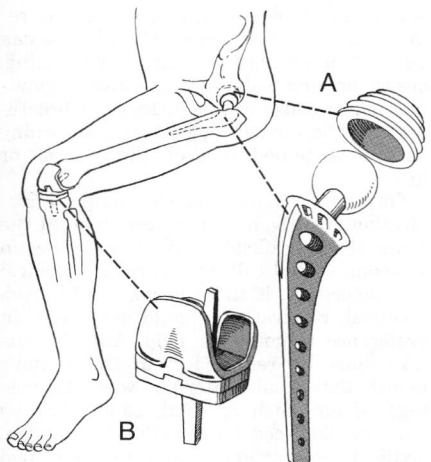

A, Total hip arthroplasty. A cementless prosthesis allows porous ingrowth of bone. *B,* Total knee arthroplasty using a tibial metal retainer and a femoral component. The femoral component is chosen individually for each person according to the amount of healthy bone present. From Polaski and Tatro, 1996.

accompanying illustration.) Called also total hip replacement.

Patient Care. The most frequent complications to guard against in these patients are infection and dislocation. An interdisciplinary team helps the patient with recovery and rehabilitation after surgery. Before surgery patients are given instruction to assure that they understand the nature of the surgery, its expected outcome, procedures and exercises that will be done postoperatively, and the correct use of aids to ambulation such as a walker, crutch, or cane.

In addition to routine postoperative care to avoid respiratory and circulatory complications, special care must be taken in positioning the patient. In order to prevent subluxation (dislocation) of the prosthesis, an abduction wedge is secured between the legs (usually in the operating room) and left in place until removed by the surgeon. The head of the patient's bed should not be raised more than 45 degrees.

Patients usually are allowed to stand at the bedside the first postoperative day, supported by a walker and two persons. Specific written permission for weight-bearing on the affected joint should be obtained from the surgeon before this is allowed. Patients often need additional instruction and help in transferring from bed to chair, wheelchair, and commode. Whenever a sitting position is assumed, the chair seat should be raised so that the hips are not flexed beyond a 90-degree angle.

Discharge planning should include instructions that will enable patients to care for themselves safely at home. These include: (1) It is safe to lie on your operated side. (2) For three months you should not cross your legs. (3) Place a pillow between your legs when you roll over on your abdomen or lie on your side in bed. (4) It is safe to bend your hip, but not beyond a right (90-degree) angle. (5) Faithfully continue the exercise program started in the hospital. Patients who need assistance in self-care are referred to a home health agency, social worker, or community health NURSE.

> ***total joint a.*** arthroplasty in which both sides of a joint are removed and replaced by artificial implants anchored to the bones; the most common joints treated are the hip, knee, elbow, and shoulder. Called also total joint replacement.

> ***total knee a.*** arthroplasty of both sides of the knee joint, with tibial, patellar, and femoral components.

arthropod (ahr″thro-pod) an individual of the phylum ARTHROPODA.

Arthropoda (ahr-throp'o-dah) a phylum of the animal kingdom that includes bilaterally symmetrical animals with hard, segmented bodies bearing jointed appendages; it embraces the largest number of known animals, with at least 740,000 species, divided into 12 classes. It includes the arachnids, crustaceans, and insects.

arthrosclerosis (ahr″thro-sklĕ-ro'sis) stiffening or hardening of the joints.

arthroscope (ahr'thro-skōp) an endoscope for examining the interior of a joint. The arthroscope is designed to allow passage of surgical instruments, thus permitting concurrent surgery within a joint. Arthroscopy is an alternative to surgical incision and creation of an open surgical wound. The procedure may be done under either local or general anesthesia. Postoperative complications rarely occur, but infection, bleeding into the joint, swelling, rupture of the synovium, thrombophlebitis, and joint injury are possible.

arthroscopy (ahr-thros'kah-pe) examination of the interior of a joint with an arthroscope.

arthrosis (ahr-thro'sis) 1. a joint or articulation. 2. disease of a joint.

arthrostomy (ahr-thros'tah-me) surgical creation of an opening in a joint, as for drainage.

arthrosynovitis (ahr″thro-sin″o-vi'tis) inflammation of the synovial membrane of a joint.

arthrotomy (ahr-throt'ah-me) incision of a joint.

arthroxesis (ahr-throk'sĕ-sis) scraping of diseased tissue from an articular surface.

articular (ahr-tik'u-lar) pertaining to a joint.

articulare (ahr-tik″u-la're) the point of intersection of the dorsal contours of the articular process of the mandible and the temporal bone.

articulate (ahr-tik'u-lāt) 1. to unite by joints; to join. 2. united by joints. 3. capable of expressing oneself orally.

articulatio (ahr-tik″u-la'she-o), pl. *articulatio'nes* [L.] synovial JOINT.

articulation (ahr-tik″u-la'shun) 1. any place of junction between two different parts or objects. 2. enunciation of words and sentences. 3. synovial JOINT.

articulator (ahr-tik'u-la″tor) a device for effecting a jointlike union.

dental a. a device that simulates movements of the temporomandibular joints or mandible, used in dentistry.

articulo mortis (ahr-tik'u-lo mor'tis) at the point or moment of death.

artifact (ahr'tĭ-fakt) 1. any artificial product; a structure or appearance that is not natural, but is due to manipulation. 2. distortion or fuzziness of an image caused by manipulation, such as during compression of a digital file.

film a. artificial images on x-ray films due to storage, handling, or processing.

phantom a. artificial images seen with conventional TOMOGRAPHY.

standardization a. an electrical stimulus of 1 mV deliberately introduced into the ELECTROCARDIOGRAM so that pulse amplitudes on the tracing can be adjusted to 10 mm. The amplitudes of the P, QRS, and T intervals can be accurately evaluated only on an electrocardiogram thus standardized.

artificial (ahr″tĭ-fish'al) made by art; not natural or pathologic.

a. respiration any method of forcing air into the lungs in a person who still has a pulse but whose breathing has stopped. Artificial respiration can be given with no equipment, so that it is an ideal emergency first aid procedure. Ideally, it should be given using a pocket face mask or a bag valve mask; in the absence of emergency resuscitation equipment, mouth-to-mouth RESUSCITATION may be done.

Indications. Artificial respiration can save a life whenever breathing has stopped but heartbeat has not, as in near-drowning, electric shock, choking, gas poisoning, drug poisoning, injury to the chest, or suffocation from other causes. It is also administered along with other procedures in cases of cardiac arrest. Usually one can tell that breathing has stopped by listening, observing, and feeling for respiratory movement. The cause of the stoppage of breathing may be obvious (as when a drowning person is pulled out of the water) or unknown.

Procedure. To be effective, artificial respiration must be begun immediately. At the same time artificial respiration is begun someone should call for emergency medical assistance, but if there is no one to send, artificial respiration should be given in preference to going for help. Any obstruction must be removed from the victim's mouth that would interfere with the passage of air, such as mud, sand, chewing gum, or displaced false teeth. Once begun, artificial respiration should be continued until the victim begins to breathe regularly by himself, until trained emergency personnel take charge, until the rescuer cannot continue because of fatigue, or until a physician determines that the patient is dead. Do not give up easily; victims have recovered as long as 4 hours after artificial respiration was started. If CARDIAC ARREST occurs, CARDIOPULMONARY RESUSCITATION should be started. If only one person is present, that person should provide both alternately.Once revived, the victim is kept quiet, covered to prevent chills, and given other first aid for SHOCK.

ARV AIDS-related virus.

aryl- a chemical prefix denoting a radical derived from an aromatic compound by removal of a hydrogen atom.

arytenoid (ar″ĭ-te′noid) shaped like a jug or pitcher, as the arytenoid cartilage or arytenoid muscle of the larynx.

arytenoidectomy (ar″ĭ-tĕ-noi-dek′to-me) excision of an arytenoid cartilage.

arytenoiditis (ar″ĭ-te-noi-di′tis) inflammation of the arytenoid muscle or cartilage.

arytenoidopexy (ar″ĭ-te-noi′do-pek″se) surgical fixation of arytenoid cartilage or muscle.

AS [L.] au′ris sinis′tra (left ear).

As arsenic.

ASA acetylsalicylic acid; American Society of Anesthesiologists; American Standards Association; American Surgical Association.

5-ASA 5-aminosalicylic acid; see MESALAMINE.

ASAHP American Society of Allied Health Professionals.

ASAS American Society of Abdominal Surgeons.

asbestiform (as-bes′tĭ-form) resembling asbestos.

asbestos (as-bes′tos) fibrous calcium and MAGNESIUM SILICATE, a nonburning compound used in roofing materials, insulation for electric circuits, brake linings, and many other products that must be fire resistant. Alternative materials are being developed to replace asbestos because fine asbestos fibers can be inhaled, causing ASBESTOSIS, pleural MESOTHELIOMA, and other types of lung cancer. In 1971, asbestos became the first material to be regulated by the Occupational Safety and Health Administration.

asbestosis (as″bes-to′sis) a form of PNEUMOCONIOSIS (SILICATOSIS) caused by inhalation of asbestos fibers, characterized by interstitial fibrosis, and associated with mesothelioma and bronchogenic carcinoma.

ascariasis (as″kah-ri′ah-sis) infection by the nematode Ascaris lumbricoides, seen in temperate and tropical regions of the world; it is common in the southern mountain region of the United States and is associated with poor sanitation such as when human feces is used as fertilizer. The Ascaris eggs develop into larvae in the soil and on growing plants on which feces have been deposited. When such vegetables are eaten without having been properly washed or cooked, live larvae are carried into the digestive system along with the food. Migrating from the intestines into the blood, then to the lungs and the esophagus, the larvae finally return to the intestines, where they grow to maturity, reaching a length ranging from 15 to 35 cm (6 to 14 in).

Ascaris infection may go unsuspected until a worm is passed in the stool. But there may be colic or other abdominal symptoms, and occasionally the worms are vomited during their passage through the esophagus. In children, "wandering worms" may emerge through the skin near the navel, and in adults, near the groin. Infected children usually are thin because the worms consume vital nutrients and inhibit the digestion of proteins. Loss of appetite and angioneurotic edema are common, and the face may be swollen.

Accurate diagnosis of the presence and extent of Ascaris infection usually depends on the detection of eggs in a stool sample examined microscopically. Treatment involves the use of medications such as MEBENDAZOLE or PYRANTEL. to destroy and expel the parasites, and is completely successful in nearly every case. Prevention of Ascaris infection depends primarily on the sanitary disposal of human feces and discontinuing their use as fertilizer. Also important are the thorough washing of hands before food is prepared, and the careful cleaning and cooking of possibly infected foods.

ascaricide (as-kar′ĭ-sīd) an agent destructive to ascarids. adj., **ascarici′dal.**

ascarid (as′kah-rid) any of the phasmid nematodes of the Ascaridoidea, which includes the genera Ascaridia, Ascaris, Toxocara, and Toxascaris.

Ascaris (as′kah-ris) a genus of NEMATODE (ROUNDWORM) PARASITES FOUND IN THE INTESTINES OF HUMANS AND OTHER VERTEBRATES. A. lumbricoi′des is the largest roundworm infecting humans, causing ASCARIASIS. (See accompanying illustration.)

ascaris a nematode of the genus Ascaris.

Aschelminthes (ash″el-min′thēz) a phylum of unsegmented, bilaterally symmetrical WORMS whose bodies are almost entirely covered with a cuticle; the class NEMATODA (roundworms) contains many important parasites.

ascites (ah-si′tēz) abnormal accumulation of serous fluid (EDEMA) within the peritoneal CAVITY. It may be associated with any of numerous disorders, including neoplastic

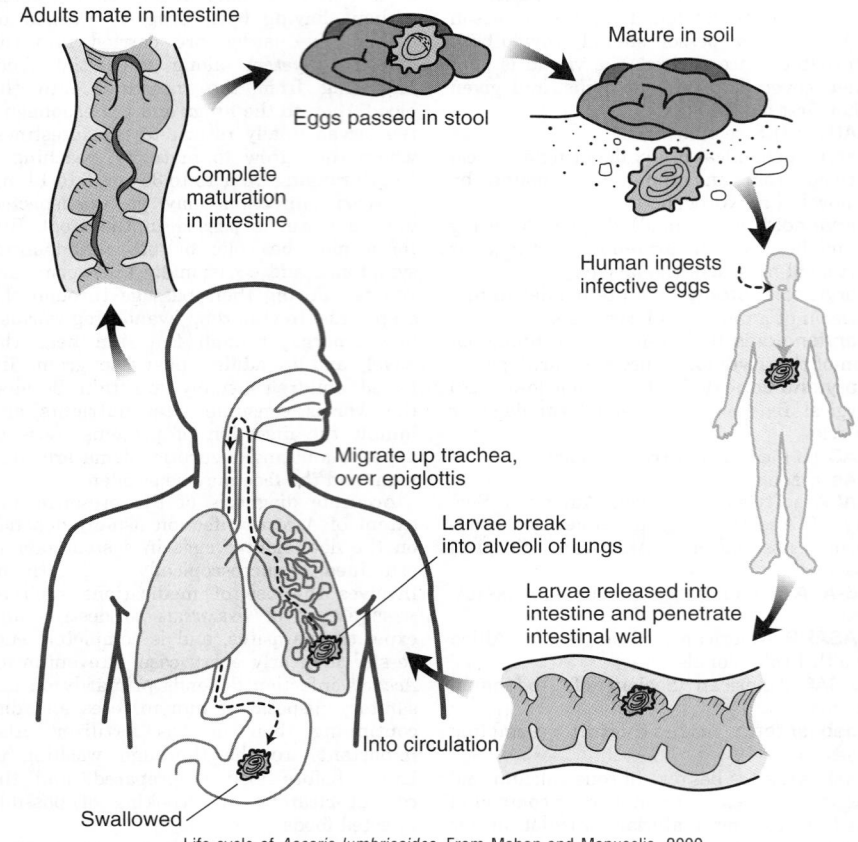

Adults mate in intestine

Eggs passed in stool

Mature in soil

Complete maturation in intestine

Human ingests infective eggs

Migrate up trachea, over epiglottis

Larvae break into alveoli of lungs

Larvae released into intestine and penetrate intestinal wall

Into circulation

Swallowed

Life cycle of *Ascaris lumbricoides.* From Mahon and Manuselis, 2000.

and inflammatory disorders of the peritoneum that produce increased permeability of the peritoneal capillaries; severe HYPOALBUMINEMIA from any cause; portal HYPERTENSION associated with CIRRHOSIS of the liver, advanced congestive HEART FAILURE, and constrictive PERICARDITIS; and HYPERALDOSTERONISM with increased retention of sodium and water. adj., **ascit′ic.**

In portal hypertension there is increased pressure within the sinusoids and hepatic veins. As the pressure increases there is movement of protein-rich plasma filtrate into the hepatic lymphatics. Some of the fluid enters the thoracic duct, but if the pressure is high enough, the excess fluid will ooze from the surface of the liver into the peritoneal cavity. Because the fluid has a high colloidal osmotic PRESSURE owing to its high protein content, it is not readily reabsorbed from the peritoneal cavity.

Treatment. Because ascites is symptomatic of an underlying disorder that can range from liver failure to endocrine disease, treatment of the primary disorder is a major goal. The problems of fluid and electrolyte imbalance that are associated with ascites, and the potential for mechanical trauma due to pressure against internal organs adjacent to the abdominal cavity necessitate some kind of symptomatic relief.

Medical treatment includes restriction of fluid and sodium intake and administration of DIURETICS. Supplementation of potassium and chloride may be necessary during diuretic therapy to avoid an imbalance of these electrolytes. Careful measurement of intake and output is essential,

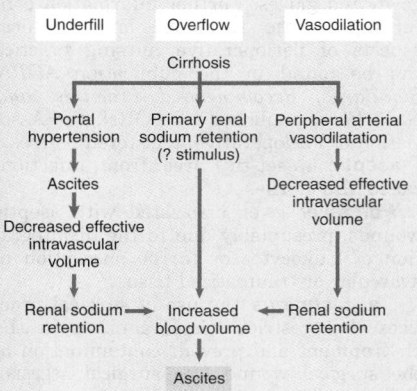

Pathogenesis of ascites: different theories. Three important factors in the production of ascites in cirrhosis are portal hypertension, hypoalbuminemia, and hepatic blockage of lymphatic flow with local overproduction. From Aspinall and Taylor-Robinson, 2002

and laboratory values for the electrolytes must be monitored frequently.

Surgical treatment was at one time almost entirely limited to abdominal PARACENTESIS for removal of large accumulations of ascitic fluid. It is, however, only a temporary measure that poses problems of rapid fluid shift, loss of protein, and the potential for introducing infectious agents into the peritoneum. A more effective procedure is the insertion of a peritoneovenous SHUNT (LeVeen SHUNT), which provides a means for continuous reinfusion of ascitic fluid into the venous system.

Patient Care. Assessment of the degree of fluid accumulation and the problems it presents to the patient can be done by measuring abdominal girth (see accompanying illustration), recording daily weight gain and loss, and determining the extent to which pressure from the fluid is interfering with respiration, circulation, and digestion. Most patients with ascites are more comfortable in high Fowler's position. When a change of position is necessary to maintain integrity of the skin and promote circulation, small pillows can be used to support the rib cage while the patient is lying on the side. Ascites is usually a chronic condition that is difficult to control. Management must include instruction to the patient and significant others, particularly the caregivers who will help with home care.

ascorbate (as-kor'bāt) a compound or derivative of ascorbic acid.

ascorbic acid (as-kor'bik) vitamin C, a substance found in many fruits (especially citrus fruits and tomatoes) and vegetables. It is an essential element of the diet; lack of it can lead to SCURVY or to less severe conditions, such as delayed healing of wounds. Solutions of ascorbic acid deteriorate rapidly, and it is not stored in the body to any extent. Large doses of commercial preparations may cause gastrointestinal irritation. Recommended dietary intakes are 60 mg daily for adults, an amount available from one to two oranges. See also VITAMIN.

Preparations of ascorbic acid are used as antiscorbutics and nutritional supplements, as as aids to improve absorption in the treatment of iron deficiency anemia and to improve chelation during deferoxamine therapy for chronic iron toxicity; administered orally or by intravenous or intramuscular injection. Ascorbic acid is also used as an aid in the radioactive labeling of red blood cells for various studies.

ascospore (as'ko-spor) a spore contained or produced in an ascus.

Ascriptin (ah-skrip'tin) trademark for a preparation of ASPIRIN with MAALOX (magnesium oxide and aluminum hydroxide), an analgesic, antipyretic, and antiinflammatory, and an inhibitor of platelet aggregation.

ascus (as'kus) the spore case of certain fungi.

ASD atrial septal defect.

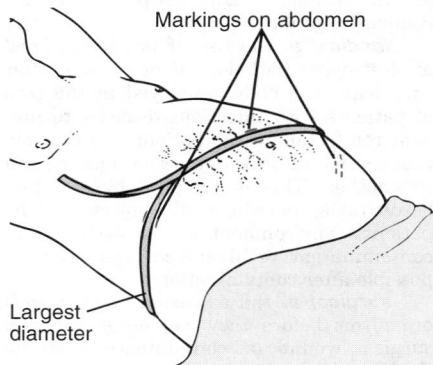

How to measure abdominal girth of a patient with ascites. With patient supine, the tape measure is brought around the largest diameter of the abdomen and a measurement is taken. Before the tape is removed, the abdomen is marked along the sides of the tape on the flanks (sides) and midline to ensure that later measurements are taken in a consistent manner. Redrawn from Ignatavicius and Workman, 2002.

PRINCIPLES OF SURGICAL ASEPSIS

1. All items used within a sterile field must be sterile.
2. Edges of sterile containers are not considered sterile once the package has been opened.
3. A sterile barrier that has been permeated must be considered contaminated.
4. Draped tables are sterile only at the top surface of the table.
5. Gowns are considered sterile in front from shoulder to table level; the sleeves are sterile between two inches above the elbow and the stockinette cuff.
6. Movement in and around a sterile field must not contaminate that field.
7. Sterile persons and items touch only sterile areas; unsterile persons or items touch only unsterile areas.
8. All items of doubtful sterility are considered contaminated.
9. The sterile field is created as close as possible to the time of use.
10. Sterile areas are continuously kept in view.

-ase suffix used in forming the name of ENZYMES, affixed to a stem indicating the substrate (luciferase), the general nature of the substrate (ENDOPEPTIDASE, PROTEINASE), or the type of reaction catalyzed (HYDROLASE).

asemasia (as″e-ma′zhah) asymbolia.

Asendin (ah-sen′din) trademark for a preparation of AMOXAPINE, a tricyclic ANTIDEPRESSANT.

asepsis (a-sep′sis) 1. freedom from infection or infectious material. 2. the absence of viable pathogenic organisms; see also ASEPTIC TECHNIQUE. adj., **asep′tic.** (See accompanying table.)

medical a. the use of practices aimed at destroying pathological organisms after they leave the body; employed in the care of patients with infectious diseases to prevent reinfection of the patient and to avoid the spread of infection from one person to another. This is achieved by ISOLATION PRECAUTIONS, in which the objects in the patient's environment are protected from contamination or disinfected as soon as possible after contamination.

surgical a. the exclusion of all microorganisms before they can enter an open surgical wound or contaminate a sterile field during surgery. See accompanying table. Measures taken include sterilization of all instruments, drapes, and all other inanimate objects that may come in contact with the surgical wound. All personnel coming in contact with the sterile field perform a surgical hand scrub with an antimicrobial agent and put on a surgical gown and gloves. Further information concerning ASEPTIC TECHNIQUE and technical aspects of perioperative nursing practice can be found in the publication *AORN Standards, Recommended Practices, and Guidelines,* published by AORN, the Association of Perioperative Registered Nurses.

aseptic (a-sep′tik) free from infection; called also sterile.

a. fever fever associated with aseptic wounds, presumably due to the disintegration of leukocytes or to the absorption of avascular or traumatized tissue.

a. technique the use of surgical practices that restrict microorganisms in the environment and prevent contamination of the surgical wound (see surgical ASEPSIS). Called also sterile technique.

asexual (a-sek′shoo-al) without sex; not pertaining to or involving sex.

ASGE American Society for Gastrointestinal Endoscopy.

ASH American Society of Hematology.

Ashman's phenomenon (ash′manz) a condition seen in atrial FIBRILLATION, in which a long cardiac cycle (R–R interval) is immediately followed by a short cycle with the next beat conducted aberrantly.

ASIA American Spinal Injury Association.

asialia (a″si-a′le-ah) aptyalism.

asiderosis (ah″sid-er-o′sis) deficiency of iron reserve of the body.

ASPAN American Society of Post Anesthesia Nurses.

asparaginase (as-par′ah-jin-ās″) an enzyme that catalyzes removal of the AMINE group that results in breakdown of ASPARAGINE; used as an antineoplastic AGENT against cancers such as acute lymphoblastic LEUKEMIA in which the malignant cells require exogenous asparagine for protein synthesis.

asparagine (ah-spar′ah-jēn) the β-amide of ASPARTIC ACID, a nonessential AMINO ACID that is also used as a culture medium for certain bacteria.

aspartame (ah-spar′tām) a synthetic compound of two amino acids, used as a low-calorie sweetener. It is 180 times as sweet as SUCROSE (table sugar); the amount equal in sweetness to a teaspoon of sugar contains 0.1 calorie. Aspartame does not promote the formation of dental caries. The amount of PHENYLALANINE it contains must be taken into account in the low-phenylalanine diet of patients with PHENYLKETONURIA.

aspartate (ah-spahr′tāt) any salt of aspartic acid; aspartic acid in dissociated form.

aspartate transaminase (AST) (ASAT) (ah-spahr′tāt trans-am′ĭ-nās) an enzyme that catalyzes the reversible transfer of an amino group from aspartate to α-ketoglutarate

ASPARTATE TRANSAMINASE (AST): NORMAL VALUES	
Newborn and infants:	16–72 UL
Child under five:	19–28 U/L
Adult under sixty:	8–20 U/L
Female adult over sixty:	10–20 U/L
Male adult over sixty:	11–26 U/L

to form glutamate and oxaloacetate, requiring the coenzyme pyridoxal phosphate; it is normally present in serum and in various body tissues, especially in the heart and liver. (See accompanying table.) It is released into the serum as the result of tissue injury, especially injury to the heart or liver, hence the concentration in the serum may be increased in myocardial infarction or acute damage to hepatic cells. Serum levels are also increased in some muscle diseases, such as progressive muscular dystrophy. Called also glutamic-oxaloacetic transaminase.

aspartic acid (ah-spahr′tik) a dibasic AMINO ACID, one of the nonessential amino acids, widely distributed in proteins and found as an excitatory neurotransmitter in the central nervous system.

aspecific (a″spĕ-sif′ik) not specific; not caused by a specific organism.

aspect (as′pekt) 1. that part of a surface viewed from a particular direction. 2. the look or appearance.

anterior a. that surface of the human body or a body part viewed from the front. Called also ventral aspect.

dorsal a. posterior aspect.

posterior a. that surface of the human body or a body part viewed from the back. Called also dorsal aspect.

ventral a. anterior aspect.

Asperger's syndrome (ahs′per-gerz) a PERVASIVE DEVELOPMENTAL DISORDER resembling AUTISTIC DISORDER, characterized by severe impairment of social interactions and restricted interests and behaviors, but lacking the delays in development of language, cognitive function, and self-help skills that additionally define autistic disorder; it may be equivalent to a high-functioning form of autistic disorder.

aspergilloma (as″per-jil-o′mah) the most common kind of fungus BALL formed by colonization of *Aspergillus* in a bronchus or lung cavity.

aspergillosis (as″per-jil-o′sis) a disease caused by species of *Aspergillus,* marked by inflammatory granulomatous lesions in the skin, ear, orbit, nasal sinuses, lungs, and sometimes bones and meninges.

bronchopulmonary a. infection of the lungs and bronchi by *Aspergillus;* see ASPERGILLOMA.

Aspergillus (as″per-jil′us) a genus of fungi (molds), several species of which are endoparasitic and opportunistic pathogens.

aspermatogenesis (a-sper″mah-to-jen′ĕ-sis) failure in a male of production of SPERMATOZOA.

aspermia (ah-sper′me-ah) 1. aspermatogenesis. 2. anejaculation.

asphyxia (as-fik′se-ah) pathological changes caused by lack of oxygen in respired air, resulting in a deficiency of oxygen in the blood (HYPOXIA) and an increase in carbon dioxide in the blood and tissues (HYPERCAPNIA). Symptoms include irregular and disturbed respirations, or a complete absence of breathing, and pallor or cyanosis. Asphyxia may occur whenever there is an interruption in the normal exchange of oxygen and carbon dioxide between the lungs and the outside air. Some common causes are drowning, electric shock, hanging, suffocation, lodging of a foreign body in the air passages, inhalation of smoke and poisonous gases, and trauma to or disease of the lungs or air passages. Treatment includes immediate remedy of the situation by ARTIFICIAL RESPIRATION and removal of the underlying cause whenever possible. See also SUFFOCATION. adj., **asphyx′ial, asphyx′iant.**

asphyxiant (as-fik′se-ant) any substance capable of producing asphyxia.

asphyxiate (as-fik′se-āt) to suffocate; to deprive of oxygen for utilization by the tissues.

asphyxiation (as-fix″e-a′shun) suffocation.

aspidium (as-pid′e-um) the dried products of a genus of plants known as male fern; it was formerly used to treat tapeworm infestations but was found to be highly toxic to the gastrointestinal tract.

aspirate (as′pĭ-rāt) 1. to withdraw fluid by negative pressure, or suction; see ASPIRATION (def. 3). 2. the fluid withdrawn this way.

aspiration (as″pĭ-ra′shun) 1. inhalation of some foreign material; aspiration of vomitus, blood, or mucus may occur when a person is unconscious or under the effects of a general anesthetic, and can be avoided by keeping the head turned to the side and removing all such foreign material from the air passages. (See accompanying illustration.) 2. withdrawal of fluid by an ASPIRATOR; the method is widely used in hospitals, especially during surgery, to drain the area of the body being operated on and keep it clear of excess blood and other fluids to

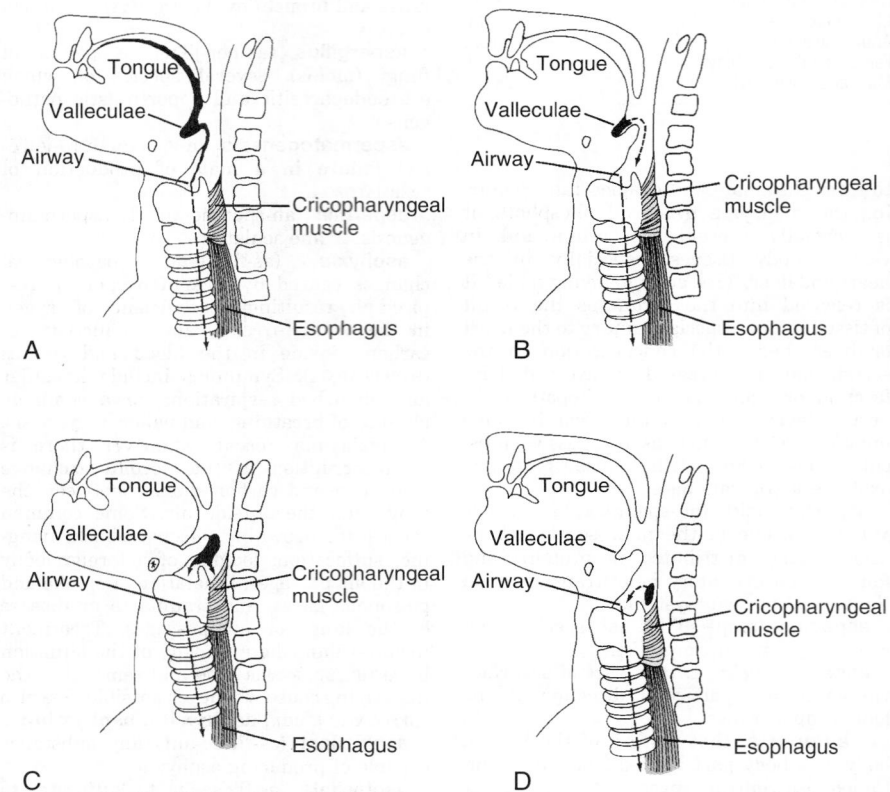

A, Types of aspiration. *A,* Aspiration before swallow caused by reduced tongue control. *B,* Aspiration before swallow caused by absent swallow response. *C,* Aspiration during swallow caused by reduced laryngeal closure. *D* Aspiration after swallow caused by pooled material in pyriform sinuses overflowing into airway. From Logemann J: *Evaluation and Treatment of Swallowing Disorders,* San Diego, College-Hill Press, 1983.

facilitate visualization of the surgical field. Sometimes after extensive surgery, suction drainage under the skin is used to speed the healing process.

meconium a. inhalation of MECONIUM by the fetus or newborn, which may result in atelectasis, emphysema, pneumothorax, or pneumonia.

risk for a. a NURSING DIAGNOSIS accepted by the North American Nursing Diagnosis Association, defined as a state in which an individual is at risk for entry of gastric secretions, oropharyngeal secretions, solids, or fluids into the tracheobronchial passage.

vacuum a. a form of induced ABORTION in which the uterine contents are removed by application of a vacuum through a hollow curet or a cannula introduced into the uterus.

aspirator (as′pĭ-ra″tor) an instrument for evacuating fluid by suction; see ASPIRATION (def. 3).

aspirin (as′pĭ-rin) ACETYLSALICYLIC ACID, a common NONSTEROIDAL ANTIINFLAMMATORY DRUG used to relieve pain and reduce fever, and specifically prescribed for rheumatic and arthritic disorders. See SALICYLATE for adverse reactions and poisoning. Aspirin should not be given to children who have viral infections, because this has been associated with the subsequent development of REYE'S SYNDROME. Because it interferes with platelet aggregation, aspirin has some value in the treatment of clotting disorders. It is given as a prophylactic measure to patients at risk for myocardial infarction or stroke syndrome and to those at risk of thromboembolism after certain surgical procedures. Administered orally or rectally.

asplenia (ah-sple′ne-ah) absence of the spleen.

asporogenic (as″po-ro-jen′ik) not producing spores; not reproduced by spores.

asporous (ah-spor′us) having no true spores.

ASRT American Society of Radiologic Technologists.

assay (as′a) determination of the purity of a substance or the amount of any particular constituent of a mixture.

biological a. bioassay; determination of the potency of a drug or other substance by comparing the effects it has on animals with those of a reference standard.

CH50 a. a test of total complement activity as the capacity of serum to lyse a standard preparation of sheep red blood cells coated with antisheep erythrocyte antibody. The reciprocal of the dilution of serum that lyses 50 per cent of the erythrocytes is the whole complement titer in CH50 units per milliliter of serum.

enzyme-linked immunosorbent a. **(ELISA)** any enzyme IMMUNOASSAY using an enzyme-labeled IMMUNOREACTANT (antigen or antibody) and an IMMUNOADSORBENT (antigen or antibody bound to a solid support). A variety of methods are used for measuring the unknown concentration, such as either competitive binding between the labeled reactant and unlabeled unknown or a sandwich technique in which the unknown antigen binds both the immunoadsorbent and labeled antibody. One of the uses of ELISA is to screen blood for antibody to the human immunodeficiency VIRUS; a positive result indicates probable exposure to the virus and possibly that the virus is in the blood. Since false-positives can occur, a back-up test is used to confirm positive findings. (See accompanying illustration.)

microhemagglutination a.–Treponema pallidum **(MHA-TP)** a *Treponema pallidum* hemagglutination assay using microtechniques; used in the detection of syphilis.

radioreceptor a. a radioligand assay in which a radiolabeled hormone is used to measure the concentration of specific cellular receptors for the hormone in tissue specimens, an example being radioassay of estrogen receptors in breast tissue.

thyroid-stimulating hormone a. thyroid-stimulating hormone test.

Treponema pallidum hemagglutination a. **(TPHA)** a treponemal antigen serologic test for SYPHILIS using tanned sheep red blood cells coated with antigen from the Nichol's strain of *Treponema pallidum* and treated patient serum; it is similar in sensitivity and specificity to the FTA-ABS test. This test is not useful for individuals who have had syphilis in the past.

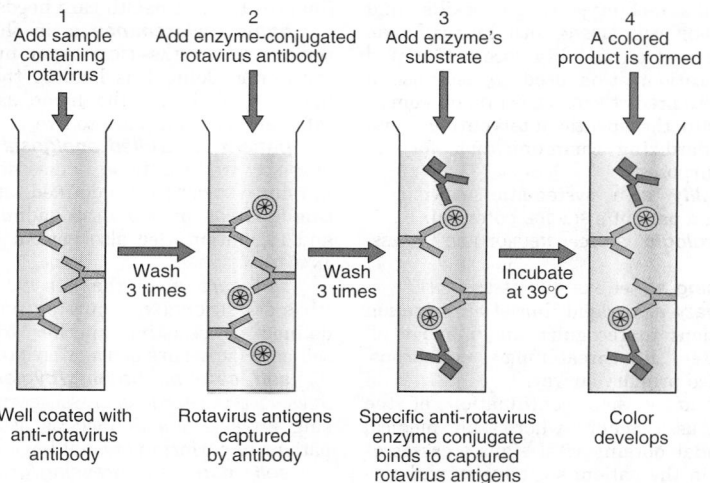

1 Add sample containing rotavirus

2 Add enzyme-conjugated rotavirus antibody

3 Add enzyme's substrate

4 A colored product is formed

Wash 3 times

Wash 3 times

Incubate at 39°C

Well coated with anti-rotavirus antibody

Rotavirus antigens captured by antibody

Specific anti-rotavirus enzyme conjugate binds to captured rotavirus antigens

Color develops

ELISA: With antigen capture ELISA, the wells are coated with antibody to the virus. The sample containing virus (1) is added and, after washing several times, enzyme conjugated to an antibody to the virus is added (2). Finally, after a further cycle of washing, the enzyme's substrate (3) is added. A colored product is formed if the viral antigen is present in the sample (4). From Hart and Shears, 1997.

TSH   a. thyroid-stimulating hormone test.

assertiveness (ah-ser′tiv-ness) a form of behavior characterized by a confident declaration or affirmation of a statement without need of proof. To assert oneself is to affirm one's rights or position withouteither aggressively transgressing the rights of another (assuming a position of dominance) or submissively permitting another to ignore or deny one's rights or rightful position.

a. training instruction and practice in techniques for dealing with interpersonal conflicts and threatening situations in an assertive manner, avoiding the extremes of aggressive and submissive behavior. Such training has as its goals enabling the learner to express personal feelings freely, speak up for his or her rights, communicate disagreement effectively, accept compliments comfortably, persist in expressing a legitimate complaint, and negotiate mutually satisfying solutions to interpersonal situations in which there is some type of conflict.

assessment (ah-ses′ment) an appraisal or evaluation.

fetal a. see FETAL ASSESSMENT.

focused a. a highly specific assessment performed on patients in the EMERGENCY DEPARTMENT, focusing on the system or systems involved in the patient's problem.

functional a. an objective review of an individual's mobility, transfer skills, and ACTIVITIES OF DAILY LIVING, including self care, sphincter control, mobility, locomotion, and communication. It is used to establish a baseline, to predict REHABILITATION outcomes, to evaluate therapeutic interventions, and for standardizing communication for RESEARCH purposes.

lethality a. a systematic method of assessing a patient's SUICIDE potential.

neurologic a. see NEUROLOGIC ASSESSMENT.

nursing a. see NURSING ASSESSMENT.

primary a. a rapid, initial examination of a patient to recognize and manage all immediate life-threatening conditions. Called also primary survey.

secondary a. a continuation of the primary assessment, where the medical professional obtains vital signs, reassesses changes in the patient's condition, and performs appropriate physical examinations.

assignment (ah-sīn′ment) the selection of something for a specific purpose.

random a. in a research study, the assignment of subjects to experimental (treatment) or control groups in such a way that each member of a sample has an equal chance of being assigned to a particular group. Random assignment ensures that the groups will be as alike as possible at the beginning of the study. Called also randomization.

assimilation (ah-sim″ĭ-la′shun) 1. conversion of nutritive material into living tissue; anabolism. 2. psychologically, absorption of new experiences into the existing psychologic makeup. 3. the process by which members of a culture change their lifeways in order to become totally integrated into another culture.

assistance (ah-sis′tans) help or aid.

anger control a. in the NURSING INTERVENTIONS CLASSIFICATION, a nursing INTERVENTION defined as the facilitation of expression of anger in an adaptive nonviolent manner.

breastfeeding a. in the NURSING INTERVENTIONS CLASSIFICATION, a nursing INTERVENTION defined as preparing a new mother to breastfeed her infant. See also BREASTFEEDING.

examination a. in the NURSING INTERVENTIONS CLASSIFICATION, a nursing INTERVENTION defined as providing assistance to the patient and another health care provider during a procedure or examination.

financial resource a. in the NURSING INTERVENTIONS CLASSIFICATION, a nursing INTERVENTION defined as assisting an individual/family to secure and manage finances to meet health care needs.

home maintenance a. in the NURSING INTERVENTIONS CLASSIFICATION, a nursing INTERVENTION defined as helping the patient/family to maintain the home as a clean, safe, and pleasant place to live.

patient controlled analgesia a. in the NURSING INTERVENTIONS CLASSIFICATION, a nursing INTERVENTION defined as facilitating control of ANALGESIA administration and regulation. See also patient controlled ANALGESIA.

self care a. in the NURSING INTERVENTIONS CLASSIFICATION, a nursing INTERVENTION defined as assisting another to perform self-care (ACTIVITIES OF DAILY LIVING).

self care a.: bathing/hygiene in the NURSING INTERVENTIONS CLASSIFICATION, a nursing INTERVENTION defined as assisting the patient to perform personal hygiene.

self care a.: dressing/grooming in the NURSING INTERVENTIONS CLASSIFICATION, a nursing INTERVENTION defined as assisting the patient with clothes and make-up.

self care a.: feeding in the NURSING INTERVENTIONS CLASSIFICATION, a nursing

self care a.: toileting in the NURSING INTERVENTIONS CLASSIFICATION, a nursing INTERVENTION defined as assisting another with ELIMINATION.

self-modification a. in the NURSING INTERVENTIONS CLASSIFICATION, a nursing INTERVENTION defined as reinforcement of a self-directed change initiated by the patient to achieve personally important goals.

smoking cessation a. in the NURSING INTERVENTIONS CLASSIFICATION, a nursing INTERVENTION defined as helping a patient to stop SMOKING.

surgical a. in the NURSING INTERVENTIONS CLASSIFICATION, a nursing INTERVENTION defined as assisting the surgeon/dentist with operative procedures and care of the surgical patient.

ventilation a. in the NURSING INTERVENTIONS CLASSIFICATION, a nursing INTERVENTION defined as promotion of an optimal spontaneous BREATHING pattern that maximizes oxygen and carbon dioxide exchange in the lungs.

weight gain a. in the NURSING INTERVENTIONS CLASSIFICATION, a nursing INTERVENTION defined as facilitating gain of body weight.

weight reduction a. in the NURSING INTERVENTIONS CLASSIFICATION, a nursing INTERVENTION defined as facilitating loss of weight and/or body fat.

assistant (ah-sis′tant) one who aids or helps another; an auxiliary.

dental a. see DENTAL ASSISTANT.

first a. a physician, physician's assistant, nurse practitioner, surgical technologist, or specially trained registered professional nurse who directly assists the surgeon by handling tissue, providing exposure, using surgical instruments and equipment, suturing, and providing hemostasis.

occupational therapy a. see OCCUPATIONAL THERAPY ASSISTANT.

personal digital a. (PDA) a small computer used to organize and easily access information; for example, clinical guidelines can be downloaded to this device.

physician a. see PHYSICIAN ASSISTANT.

second a. an individual who assists the surgeon or first assistant during an operative procedure by carrying out technical tasks such as holding retractors; this individual does not cut, clamp, or suture tissue. This role may be performed at the same time as the scrub role.

surgeon a. (SA) see SURGEON ASSISTANT.

association (ah-so″se-a′shun) 1. a state in which two attributes occur together either more or less often than expected by chance.

2. in neurology, a term applied to those regions of the brain (association AREAS) that link the primary motor and sensory AREAS. 3. in genetics, the occurrence together of two or more phenotypic characteristics more often than would be expected by chance. To be distinguished from linkage (q.v.). 4. in psychiatry, a connection between ideas or feelings, especially between conscious thoughts and elements of the unconscious, or the formation of such a connection.

clang a. see CLANGING.

free a. in PSYCHOANALYSIS, verbal expression by the patient of ideas as they arrive spontaneously, without censoring or withholding anything, no matter how distressing, embarrassing, trivial, or irrelevant it may seem. The analyst forms tentative explanations of the patient's associations and experiences but withholds them until they are validated by more material and until the patient is in a receptive frame of mind.

a. test one based on associative reaction, usually by mentioning words to a patient and noting what other words he or she gives as the ones called to mind; see ASSOCIATION (def. 4).

Association of Perioperative Registered Nurses (AORN) the professional organization of perioperative NURSES, which supports registered nurses in achieving optimal outcomes for patients undergoing operative or other invasive procedures. Formerly called the Association of Operating Room Nurses, which accounts for the abbreviation.

assumption (ah-sump′shun) a statement that is taken for granted or considered true, even though it may not have been scientifically tested.

AST Association of Surgical Technologists; aspartate transaminase.

astasia (as-ta′zhah) motor incoordination with inability to stand. adj., **astat′ic.**

a.-aba′sia motor incoordination with an inability to stand or walk despite normal ability to move the legs when sitting or lying down, a form of hysterical ataxia.

astatine (as′tah-tēn) a chemical element, atomic number 85, atomic weight 210, symbol At. (See Appendix 6.)

ASTDN Association of State and Territorial Directors of Nursing.

asteatosis (as″te-ah-to′sis) any disease in which persistent dry scaling of the skin suggests scantiness or absence of sebum.

aster (as′ter) a structure occurring in dividing cells, composed of microtubules radiating from a centrosome. The two asters

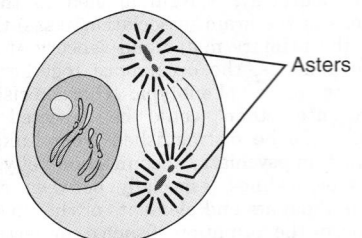

Asters

Asters separating in prophase of mitosis. From Dorland's, 2000.

are the poles of the spindle apparatus. (See accompanying illustration.)

astereognosis (ah-ster″e-og-no′sis) loss or lack of the ability to understand the form and nature of objects that are touched (STEREOGNOSIS), a form of tactile AGNOSIA.

asterion (as-te′re-on) the point on the surface of the skull where the lambdoid, parietomastoid, and occipitomastoid sutures meet. (See accompanying illustration.)

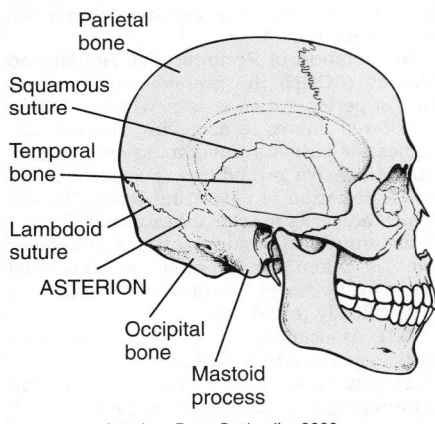

Parietal bone

Squamous suture

Temporal bone

Lambdoid suture

ASTERION

Occipital bone

Mastoid process

Asterion. From Dorland's, 2000.

asterixis (as″ter-ik′sis) a motor disturbance marked by intermittent lapses of an assumed posture as a result of intermittency of sustained contraction of groups of muscles; called liver flap because of its occurrence in coma associated with liver disease, but also observed in other conditions. (See accompanying illustration.)

asternal (a-ster′nal) 1. not joined to the sternum. 2. pertaining to asternia.

asternia (ah-ster′ne-ah) congenital absence of the sternum.

asteroid (as′ter-oid) star-shaped.

asthen(o)- word element [Gr.], *weak; weakness.*

asthenia (as-the′ne-ah) debility; loss of strength and energy; weakness. adj., **asthen′ic.**

neurocirculatory a. Da Costa syndrome.

tropical anhidrotic a. a rare condition occurring under conditions of heat stress, in which miliaria causes extensive occlusion of the sweat ducts producing anhidrosis and heat retention that may lead to weakness, dyspnea, tachycardia, elevation of body temperature, and collapse.

asthenocoria (as″thĕ-no-kor′e-ah) sluggishness of the pupillary light reflex.

asthenopia (as″thĕ-no′pe-ah) weakness or easy fatigue of the eye, with pain in the eyes, headache, and dimness of vision. adj., **asthenop′ic.**

accommodative a. asthenopia due to strain of the ciliary muscle.

muscular a. asthenopia due to weakness of the external ocular muscles.

asthenospermia (as″thĕ-no-sper′me-ah) reduced motility of spermatozoa in the semen.

asthma (az′mah) a condition marked by recurrent attacks of DYSPNEA, with airway inflammation and wheezing due to spasmodic constriction of the bronchi; it is also known as *bronchial asthma.* Attacks vary greatly from occasional periods of wheezing and slight dyspnea to severe attacks that almost cause suffocation. An acute attack that lasts for several days is called *status asthmaticus;* this is a medical emergency that can be fatal. adj., **asthmat′ic.**

Causes. Asthma can be classified into three types according to causative factors. *Allergic* or *atopic asthma* (sometimes called *extrinsic asthma*) is due to an ALLERGY to ANTIGENS; usually the offending allergens are suspended in the air in the form of pollen, dust, smoke, automobile exhaust, or animal dander. More than half of the cases of asthma in children and young adults are

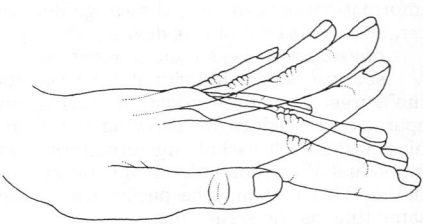

To elicit asterixis (flapping tremor) the patient extends the arm, dorsiflexes the wrist, and extends the fingers. The hand is observed for rapid, nonrhythmic extensions and flexions. From Ignatavicius and Workman, 2002.

of this type. *Intrinsic asthma* is usually secondary to chronic or recurrent infections of the bronchi, sinuses, or tonsils and adenoids. There is evidence that this type develops from a HYPERSENSITIVITY to the bacteria or, more commonly, viruses causing the infection. Attacks can be precipitated by infections, emotional factors, and exposure to nonspecific irritants. The third type of asthma, *mixed,* is due to a combination of extrinsic and intrinsic factors.

There is an inherited tendency toward the development of extrinsic asthma. It is related to a HYPERSENSITIVITY REACTION of the IMMUNE RESPONSE. The patient often gives a family medical history that includes allergies of one kind or another and a personal history of allergic disorders. Secondary factors affecting the severity of an attack or triggering its onset include events that produce emotional stress, environmental changes in humidity and temperature, and exposure to noxious fumes or other airborne allergens.

Symptoms. Typically, an attack of asthma is characterized by dyspnea and a wheezing type of respiration. The patient usually assumes a classic sitting position, leaning forward so as to use all the accessory muscles of respiration. The skin is usually pale and moist with perspiration, but in a severe attack there may be cyanosis of the lips and nailbeds. In the early stages of the attack coughing may be dry; but as the attack progresses the cough becomes more productive of a thick, tenacious, mucoid sputum. (See accompanying illustration.)

Treatment. The treatment of extrinsic asthma begins with attempts to determine the allergens causing the attacks. The cooperation of the patient is needed to relate onset of attacks with specific environmental substances and emotional factors that trigger or intensify symptoms. The patient with nonallergic asthma should avoid infections, nonspecific irritants, such as cigarette smoke, and other factors that provoke attacks.

Drugs given for the treatment of asthma are primarily used for the relief of symptoms. There is no cure for asthma but the disease can be controlled with an individualized regimen of drug therapy coupled with rest, relaxation, and avoidance of causative factors. Bronchodilators such as epinephrine and aminophylline may be used to enlarge the bronchioles, thus relieving respiratory embarrassment. Other drugs that thin the secretions and help in their ejection (expectorants) may also be prescribed.

The patient with status asthmaticus is very seriously ill and must receive special attention and medication to avoid excessive

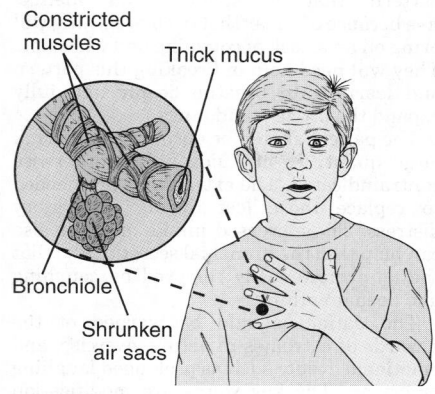

Symptoms	Physical findings
• Shortness of breath	• Rapid, shallow respirations
• Wheezing	• Rapid pulse
• Difficult breathing	• Pallor or cyanosis
• Cough	• Diminished breath sounds
• Anxiety	• Generalized retractions
	• Frequent pausing to catch the breath when talking
	• Hyperexpansion of the chest

An asthma attack with respiratory distress. From Frazier et al., 2000.

strain on the heart and severe respiratory difficulties that can be fatal.

Patient Care. Because asthma is a chronic condition with an irregular pattern of remissions and exacerbations, education of the patient is essential to successful treatment. The plan of care must be highly individualized to meet the needs of the patient and must be designed to encourage active participation in the prescribed program and in self care. Most patients welcome the opportunity to learn more about their disorder and ways in which they can exert some control over the environmental and emotional events that are likely to precipitate an attack.

Exercises that improve posture are helpful in maintaining good air exchange. Special deep breathing exercises can be taught to the patient so that elasticity and full expansion of lung and bronchial tissues are maintained. (See also LUNG and CHRONIC OBSTRUCTIVE PULMONARY DISEASE.) Some asthmatic patients have developed a protective breathing pattern that is shallow and ineffective because of a fear that deep breathing will bring on an attack of coughing and wheezing. They will need help in breaking this pattern and learning to breathe deeply and fully expand the bronchi and lungs.

The patient should be encouraged to drink large quantities of fluids unless otherwise contraindicated. The extra fluids are needed to replace those lost during respiratory distress. The increased intake of fluids also can help thin the bronchial secretions so that they are more easily removed by coughing and deep breathing.

The patient should be warned of the hazards of extremes in eating, exercise, and emotional events such as prolonged laughing or crying. The key words are modification and moderation to avoid overtaxing and overstimulating the body systems. Relaxation techniques can be very helpful, especially if the patient can find a method that effectively reduces tension.

Asthmatic patients fare better if they feel that they do have some control over their disease and are not necessarily helpless victims of a debilitating incurable illness. There is no cure for asthma but there are ways in which one can adjust to the illness and minimize its effects.

allergic a., atopic a. that due to an atopic ALLERGY; see ASTHMA.

bronchial a. asthma.

cardiac a. a term applied to breathing difficulties due to pulmonary edema in heart disease, such as left ventricular failure.

extrinsic a. 1. asthma caused by some factor in the environment, usually atopic in nature. 2. atopic asthma.

intrinsic a. that due to a chronic or recurrent infection; see ASTHMA.

occupational a. extrinsic asthma due to an allergen present in the workplace.

astigmatism (ah-stig′mah-tizm) an error of refraction in which a ray of light is not sharply focused on the retina, but is spread over a more or less diffuse area; it is due to differences in curvature in the refractive surfaces (CORNEA and LENS) of the eye. adj., **astigmat′ic.** Its exact cause is not known; some common types of astigmatism seem to run in families and may be inherited. Probably everyone has some astigmatism, since it is rare to find perfectly shaped curves in the cornea and lens, but the defect is rarely serious. If the refractive error is troublesome, corrective lenses may be needed.

compound a. that in which both principal meridians are either hyperopic (*compound hyperopic astigmatism*, with rays coming into focus behind the retina) or myopic (*compound myopic astigmatism*, with rays coming into focus in front of the retina).

corneal a. that due to the presence of abnormal curvatures on the anterior or posterior surface of the cornea.

hypermetropic a. hyperopic astigmatism.

hyperopic a. that in which the light rays are brought to a focus behind the retina.

irregular a. that in which the curvature varies in different parts of the same meridian or in which refraction in successive meridians differs irregularly.

lenticular a. astigmatism due to defect of the crystalline lens.

mixed a. that in which one principal meridian is hyperopic and the other myopic.

myopic a. that in which the light rays are brought to a focus in front of the retina.

regular a. that in which the refraction changes gradually in power from one principal meridian of the eye to the other, the two meridians always being at right angles; this condition is further classified as being *against the rule* when the meridian of greatest refractive power tends toward the horizontal, *with the rule* when it tends toward the vertical, and *oblique* when it lies 45 degrees from the horizontal and vertical.

astigmatometer (ah-stig″mah-tom′ĕ-ter) an apparatus used in measuring astigmatism.

astigmometer (as″tig-mom′ĕ-ter) astigmatometer.

astomia (ah-sto′me-ah) congenital atresia of the mouth. adj., **asto′matous.**

astragalectomy (ah-strag″ah-lek′to-me) excision of the astragalus.

astragalus (ah-strag′ah-lus) talus. adj., **astrag′alar.**

astraphobia (as″trah-fo′be-ah) irrational fear of thunder and lightning.

astringent (as-strin′jent) 1. causing contraction or arresting discharges. 2. an agent that causes contraction or arrests discharges, usually locally after topical application. Astringents act as protein precipitants and arrest discharge by causing shrinkage of tissue. Skin preparations such as shaving lotions often contain astringents such as aluminum acetate that help to reduce oiliness and excessive perspiration. Witch hazel is a common household astringent used to reduce swelling. Styptic pencils, used to stop bleeding from small cuts, contain astringents. Zinc oxide and calamine are astringents used in lotions, powders, and ointments to relieve itching and chafing in various forms of dermatitis. Some astringents, such as tannic acid, have been used in treating diarrhea; others, such as boric acid and sodium borate, help relieve the symptoms of inflammation of the mucous membranes of the throat or conjunctiva of the eye. Astringents have some bacteriostatic properties, though they are not generally used as antiseptics.

astroblast (as′tro-blast) a cell that develops into an ASTROCYTE.

astroblastoma (as″tro-blas-to′mah) an ASTROCYTOMA of Grade II, composed of cells with abundant cytoplasm and two or three nuclei.

astrocyte (as′tro-sīt) a neuroglial cell of ectodermal origin, characterized by fibrous or protoplasmic processes; collectively called ASTROGLIA or MACROGLIA. (See accompanying illustration.)

astrocytoma (as″tro-si-to′mah) a tumor composed of astrocytes; classified in order of malignancy as: *Grade I,* consisting of fibrillary or protoplasmic astrocytes; *Grade II* (astroblastoma); *Grades III* and *IV* (glioblastoma multiforme).

astroglia (ah-strog′le-ah) NEUROGLIA tissue made up of ASTROCYTES.

astrosphere (as′tro-sfēr) 1. the central mass of an aster, excluding the rays. 2. aster.

asymbolia (a″sim-bo′le-ah) loss of ability to understand symbols, such as words, figures, gestures, signs; called also asemasia.

asymmetry (a-sim′ĕ-tre) lack or absence of symmetry; dissimilarity in corresponding parts or organs on opposite sides of the body that are normally alike. In chemistry, lack of symmetry in the special arrangements of the atoms and radicals within the molecule or crystal. adj., **asymmet′rical.**

asymphytous (ah-sim′fī-tus) separate or distinct; not grown together.

asymptomatic (a″simp-to-mat′ik) showing no symptoms or signs of a disease or disorder.

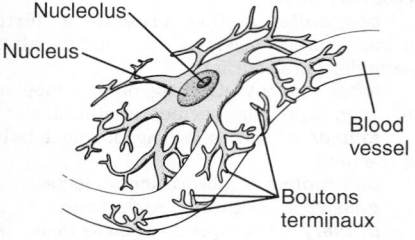

Nucleolus

Nucleus

Blood vessel

Boutons terminaux

Astrocyte in association with a blood vessel. From Dorland's, 2000.

asynchronism (a-sin′kro-nizm) occurrence at different times; disturbance of coordination.

asynchronous (a-sing′kro-nus) 1. pertaining to ASYNCHRONISM. 2. in cardiac PACING terminology, said of a PACEMAKER that cannot sense any spontaneous underlying cardiac electrical activity, so that pacing is done at a fixed, constant rate.

asynclitism (ah-sin′klī-tizm) 1. oblique presentation of the fetal head in labor, called anterior asynclitism when the anterior parietal bone is designated the point of presentation, and posterior asynclitism when the posterior parietal bone is so designated. 2. dyserythropoiesis.

asyndesis (ah-sin′dĕ-sis) a pattern of language in which words and phrases are juxtaposed without grammatical linkage; seen in schizophrenic and other mental disorders.

asynechia (a″sī-nek′e-ah) absence of continuity of structure.

asynergia (a″sin-er′je-ah) lack of coordination among parts or organs normally acting in unison. adj., **asyner′gic.**

asynovia (a″sī-no′ve-ah) absence or insufficiency of synovial secretion.

asyntaxia (a″sin-tak′se-ah) lack of proper and orderly embryonic development.

asystole (a-sis′to-le) cardiac standstill or arrest; absence of heartbeat. adj., **asystol′ic.**

At astatine.

Atabrine (at′ah-brin, at′ah-brēn) trademark for a preparation of QUINACRINE, an ANTHELMINTIC and antimalarial AGENT.

atactic (ah-tak′tik) pertaining to or characterized by ataxia; marked by incoordination or irregularity.

Atarax (at′ah-raks) trademark for preparations of HYDROXYZINE hydrochloride, an ANTIANXIETY AGENT, ANTIEMETIC, SEDATIVE, and ANTIPRURITIC.

ataraxia (at″ah-rak′se-ah) [Gr.] serenity, calmness, peace of mind.

atavism (at′ah-vizm) apparent inheritance of characters from remote ancestors. adj., **atavis′tic.**

ataxia (ah-tak′se-ah) failure of muscular coordination; irregularity of muscular action. adj., **atac′tic, atax′ic.**

　　cerebellar a. ataxia due to disease of the cerebellum.

　　Friedreich's a. see FRIEDREICH'S ATAXIA.

　　frontal a. disturbance of equilibrium associated with tumor of the frontal lobe.

　　hereditary a. Friedreich's ataxia.

　　hysterical a. ataxia recognizable as a conversion symptom; see also ASTASIA-ABASIA.

locomotor a. tabes dorsalis.

sensory a. ataxia due to loss of proprioception (joint position sense), resulting in poorly judged movements and becoming aggravated when the eyes are closed.

a.-telangiectasia a severe, autosomal recessive, progressive ataxia, associated with TELANGIECTASIAS (dilation of small blood vessels) in the skin and eyes; IMMUNODEFICIENCY with frequent infections of the respiratory tract from sinuses to lungs; and abnormal eye movements. Called also Louis-Bar's syndrome.

ataxiaphasia (ah-tak″se-ah-fa′zhah) inability to arrange words into sentences.

ataxophemia (ah-tak″so-fe′me-ah) dysarthria.

atel(o)- word element [Gr.], *incomplete; imperfectly developed.*

atelectasis (at″ĕ-lek′tah-sis) a collapsed or airless state of the lung, which may be acute or chronic, and may involve all or part of the lung. The primary cause is obstruction of the bronchus serving the affected area. adj., **atelectat′ic.**

In *congenital atelectasis* of the fetus or newborn, the lungs fail to expand normally at birth. This may be due to any of a variety of causes, including prematurity (often accompanying HYALINE MEMBRANE DISEASE); diminished nervous stimulus to breathing and crying; fetal hypoxia from any cause, including oversedation of the mother during labor and delivery; or obstruction of the bronchus by a mucous plug.

In older individuals atelectasis may be the result of airway obstruction, as by

Pneumothorax   Hydrothorax

Air   Tumor

A   B   C
COLLAPSE   COMPRESSION   OBSTRUCTION

Fluid

Mechanisms of atelectasis. *A,* Collapse of the lung in pneumothorax. *B,* Compression of the lung by pleural fluid. *C,* Resorption of the air from alveoli distal to an obstructed bronchus. Obstructive atelectasis is usually focal. Atelectasis of premature infants, which is caused by a deficiency of pulmonary surfactant, is not shown. From Damjanov, 2000.

secretions or a tumor (called *obstructive, absorption,* or *acquired atelectasis*); or it may be from a failure to deep breathe, such as postoperatively or because of neuromuscular disease. It occurs most commonly as a complication in the postoperative period, when deep breathing and incentive SPIROMETRY are often used to prevent or treat it. (See accompanying illustration.)

Symptoms. In acute atelectasis in which there is sudden obstruction of the bronchus, there may be dyspnea and cyanosis, elevation of temperature, a drop in blood pressure, or shock. In the chronic form, the patient may experience no symptoms other than gradually developing dyspnea and weakness.

X-ray examination may show a shadow in the area of collapse. If an entire lobe is collapsed, the x-ray will show the trachea, heart, and mediastinum deviated toward the collapsed area, with the diaphragm elevated on that side.

Treatment. Atelectasis in the newborn is treated by suctioning the trachea to establish an open airway, positive-pressure breathing, and administration of oxygen. High concentrations of oxygen given over a prolonged period tend to promote atelectasis and may lead to the development of retrolental fibroplasia in premature infants.

Acute atelectasis is treated by removing the cause whenever possible. To accomplish this, coughing, suctioning, and bronchoscopy may be employed. In atelectasis due to airway obstruction with secretions, chest physiotherapy is often useful. Chronic atelectasis usually requires surgical removal of the affected segment or lobe of lung. Antibiotics are given to combat the infection that almost always accompanies secondary atelectasis.

absorption a., acquired a. that produced by any factor, e.g., secretions, foreign body, tumor, or abnormal external pressure, that completely obstructs the airway, preventing intake of air into the alveolar sacs and permitting absorption of air into the bloodstream. Called also obstructive or secondary atelectasis.

congenital a. that present at birth (primary atelectasis) or immediately after (secondary atelectasis).

lobar a. that affecting only a lobe of the lung; called also segmental atelectasis.

lobular a. that affecting only a lobule of the lung.

obstructive a. absorption atelectasis.

passive a. relaxation atelectasis.

primary a. congenital atelectasis in which the alveoli have never been expanded with air.

relaxation a. atelectasis because of large amounts of air or fluid in the pleural cavity, as in pneumothorax or pleural effusion. Called also passive atelectasis.

round a., rounded a. a localized, reversible form in subjacent peripheral tissue, often following pleural effusion and characterized by focal pleural scarring.

secondary a. 1. congenital atelectasis in which resorption of the contained air has led to collapse of the alveoli. 2. acquired atelectasis.

segmental a. lobar atelectasis.

subsegmental a. that affecting only the part of a lung distal to an occluded segmental bronchus.

atelia (ah-te′le-ah) imperfect or incomplete development.

atelocardia (at″ĕ-lo-kahr′de-ah) imperfect development of the heart.

atelocephaly (at″ĕ-lo-sef′ah-le) imperfect development of the skull. adj., **atelocephal′ic, ateloceph′alous.**

atelomyelia (at″ĕ-lo-mi-e′le-ah) imperfect development of the spinal cord.

atenolol (ah-ten′o-lol) a cardioselective beta-adrenergic blocking agent used in the treatment of hypertension and chronic angina pectoris and the prevention and treatment of myocardial infarction and cardiac arrhythmias; administered orally or intravenously.

ATG antithymocyte globulin.

athelia (ah-the′le-ah) congenital absence of the nipples.

atherectomy (ath″er-ek′tŏ-me) the removal of atherosclerotic plaque from an artery using a rotary cutter inside a special catheter guided radiographically; it does not extend to the tunica intima as ENDARTERECTOMY does.

athermic (ah-ther′mik) without rise of temperature.

athermosystaltic (ah-ther″mo-sis-tal′tik) not contracting under the action of cold or heat; said of muscles.

atheroembolus (ath″er-o-em′bo-lus), pl. *atheroem′boli* an embolus composed of cholesterol or its esters, or of fragments of atheromatous plaques, typically lodging in small arteries.

atherogenesis (ath″er-o-jen′ĕ-sis) formation of abnormal fatty or lipid masses in arterial walls. adj., **atherogen′ic.**

atheroma (ath″er-o′mah) an abnormal mass of fatty or lipid material with a fibrous covering, existing as a discrete, raised plaque within the intima of an artery. adj., **atherom′atous.**

atheromatosis (ath″er-o″mah-to′sis) the presence of multiple atheromas.

atherosclerosis (ath″er-o″sklĕ-ro′sis) a common form of ARTERIOSCLEROSIS in which deposits of yellowing plaques (ATHEROMAS) containing cholesterol, other lipoid material,

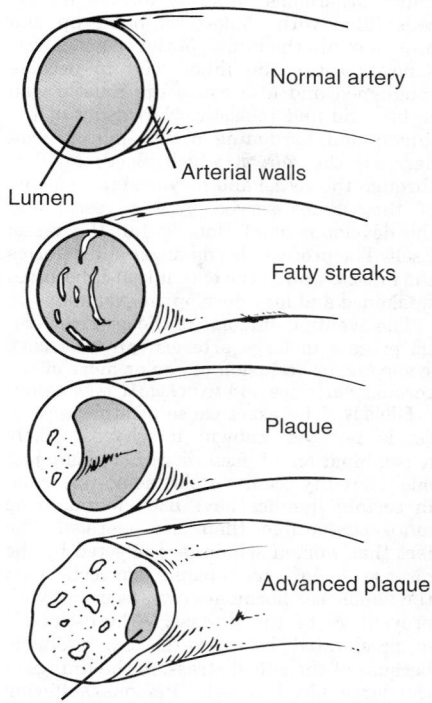

Cross-section of artery showing progressive narrowing of diameter due to atherosclerosis and plaque formation.

and lipophages are formed within the intima of large and medium-sized arteries. (See accompanying illustration.) adj., **atherosclerot′ic.**

The word *atherosclerosis* comes from the Greek, *athere,* meaning "soft, fatty, gruellike," and *scler-* meaning "hard." These terms are descriptive of the material deposited on the inner lining *(tunica intima)* of an artery and of the state of the arterial muscle walls once they have been affected by the disease.

In a normal artery the endothelial lining is tightly packed with cells that allow for the smooth passage of blood and act as a protective covering against harmful substances circulating in the bloodstream. The endothelial lining is surrounded by a sheath of muscle cells. In the earliest stage of atherosclerosis fatty streaks form along the intima. The lesions are widely scattered at first, but as the disease progresses they become more numerous and can eventually cover the entire intimal surface of an artery.

Later, atheromas of newly formed muscle cells filled with cholesterol build up and protrude into the lumen of the vessel. These deposits cause the inner wall to become roughened and also cause the muscle wall to be rigid and inelastic. Narrowing of the lumen and hardening of the muscle wall decrease the rate at which blood can flow through the vessel and may lead to ischemia of the tissues served by the vessel and the development of clots within the vessel itself. The process also damages and deforms the muscle wall to the extent that it becomes weakened and may develop an ANEURYSM.

The eventual outcome of the atherosclerotic process in large arteries can be STROKE SYNDROME, or occlusion of one or more of the coronary arteries and MYOCARDIAL INFARCTION.

Etiology. The exact cause of atherosclerosis is not yet known; it is most likely a combination of factors rather than just one. Heredity seems to play some role; men in certain families have been found to be more susceptible than the average. The fact that women seldom are affected by the disease before menopause suggests that the female sex hormones are associated with prevention of the disease. Atherosclerosis is accelerated by HYPERTENSION, probably because of the added stress on the linings of the large blood vessels. Persons suffering from disorders of metabolism, particularly DIABETES MELLITUS, are especially susceptible and tend to develop atherosclerosis earlier in life than persons who do not have these disorders. Another major factor is HYPERLIPID-EMIA, particularly high serum cholesterol, which is closely associated with the development of coronary heart disease (see HEART).

athetoid (ath′ĕ-toid) 1. resembling athetosis. 2. affected with athetosis.

athetosis (ath″ĕ-to′sis) repetitive involuntary, slow, sinuous, writhing movements. (See accompanying illustration.)

athlete's foot (ath′lēts) a fungal infection of the skin of the foot; called also TINEA

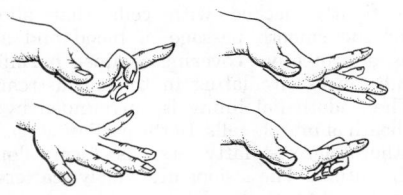

Positions of fingers in movements of athetosis. From Dorland's, 2000.

PEDIS. It causes itching and often blisters and cracks, usually between the toes. Causative agents are *Candida albicans, Epidermophyton floccosum,* and species of *Trichophyton,* which thrive in warmth and dampness. If not arrested, it can cause a rash and itching in other parts of the body as well. It is often recurrent, since the fungus survives under the toenails (see TINEA UNGUIUM) and reappears when conditions are favorable. Although athlete's foot is usually little more than an uncomfortable nuisance, its open sores provide excellent sites for more serious infections. Early treatment and health care supervision insure correct diagnosis and prevention of complications. Specific diagnosis is made by microscopic examination or culture of skin scrapings for the fungus.

Prevention includes keeping the feet dry and open to the air as much as possible, especially the areas between the toes. Small cotton pads may be used between the toes if this area is difficult to keep dry. Dusting powder may be used on the feet and sprinkled in the shoes to reduce accumulation of moisture. Topical fungicides may control cases in the early phases. For more severe cases, there are compounds such as GRISEOFULVIN taken by mouth, or topical preparations such as CLOTRIMAZOLE.

athrepsia (ah-threp′se-ah) extreme malnutrition and wasting of subcutaneous tissue and muscle; see also MARASMUS. adj., **athrep′tic.**

athymia (ah-thi′me-ah) 1. absence of functioning thymus tissue. 2. lack of feeling and emotion, as found in DEPRESSION and other mental disorders.

athyria (ah-thi′re-ah) 1. absence of functioning thyroid tissue. 2. hypothyroidism.

Ativan (at′ĭ-van) trademark for preparations of LORAZEPAM, an ANTIANXIETY AGENT, SEDATIVE, and ANTICONVULSANT.

atlantal (at-lan′t′l) pertaining to the atlas.

atlas (at′las) the first cervical VERTEBRA, the uppermost segment of the vertebral column, which supports the skull. (See accompanying illustration.)

atloaxoid (at″lo-ak′soid) pertaining to the atlas and axis.

atm atmosphere (def. 3).

atmosphere (at′mos-fēr) 1. the entire gaseous envelope surrounding the earth and subject to the earth's gravitational field. 2. the air or climate in a particular place. adj., **atmospher′ic.** 3. a unit of pressure, being that exerted by the earth's atmosphere at sea level; equal to 1.01325×10^5 pascals (approximately 760 mm Hg). Abbreviated atm.

at no atomic number.

atocia (ah-to′shah) sterility in the female.

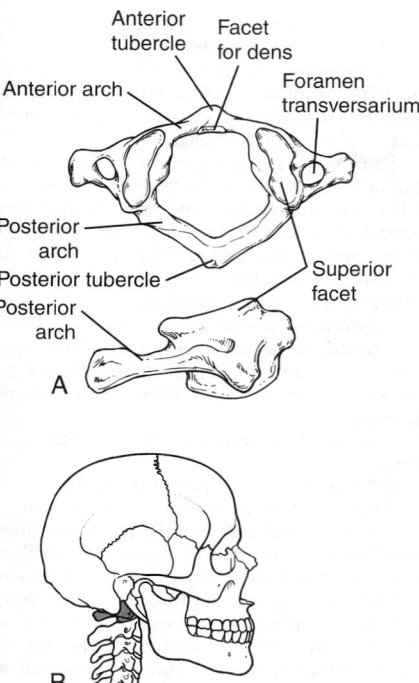

Anterior tubercle — Facet for dens

Anterior arch —

Foramen transversarium

Posterior arch —

Posterior tubercle —

Posterior arch —

Superior facet

A

B

Atlas. *(A), (top)* superior aspect; *(bottom)* transverse aspect. Note the absence of the body and spinous process. *(B),* position. From Dorland's, 2000.

atom (at′om) the smallest particle of an ELEMENT that has all the properties of the element. adj., **atom′ic.**

There are two main parts of an atom: the NUCLEUS and the electron cloud. The nucleus is made up of PROTONS, which carry a positive electrical charge, and (except in hydrogen) NEUTRONS, which contain one proton and one electron and carry no electrical charge. The electron cloud is made up of particles called ELECTRONS, which carry a negative electrical charge and move in orbits or "shells" around the nucleus. Different atoms have different numbers of protons, neutrons, and electrons in their makeup.

In a chemical change, atoms do not break up but act as individual units. The chemical behavior of an atom is controlled by the number and spatial arrangement of electrons in orbit around the nucleus. The atoms of radioactive elements are very unstable and are capable of emitting nuclear particles in a stream or "ray;" these particles are called RADIATIONS.

The atomic NUMBER of an element is the number of free protons (those not in neutrons) in the nucleus; it is equal to the net positive charge of the nucleus. The atomic WEIGHT is the weight of an atom of a substance as compared with the weight of an atom of carbon-12, which is taken as 12.

atomization (at″om-ĭ-za′shun) nebulization.

atomizer (at′om-i″zer) nebulizer.

atonia (ah-to′ne-ah) [L.] atony.

atony (at′ah-ne) lack of normal tone or strength; flaccidity. adj., **aton′ic.**

atopen (at′o-pen) the antigen responsible for atopy.

atopic (ah-top′ik) 1. displaced; ectopic. 2. pertaining to atopy.

atopy (at′o-pe) a clinical hypersensitivity state or allergy with a hereditary predisposition; the tendency to develop an allergy is inherited, although the specific clinical form (such as hay fever or asthma) is not. The antibody reagin is involved. Called also atopic, hereditary, or spontaneous allergy.

atorvastatin (ah-tor″vah-stat′in) an agent that inhibits cholesterol synthesis, used as the calcium salt in treatment of primary HYPERCHOLESTEROLEMIA and HYPERLIPIDEMIA; administered orally.

atovaquone (ah-to′vah-kwōn) an antibiotic used in treatment of mild to moderate *Pneumocystis carinii* PNEUMONIA and the prevention and treatment of falciparum MALARIA; administered orally.

atoxic (ah-tok′sik) not poisonous; not due to a poison.

ATP adenosine triphosphate.

ATPase adenosine triphosphatase.

Na⁺,K⁺-A. an enzyme that spans the plasma membrane and hydrolyzes adenosine triphosphate to provide the energy necessary to drive the cellular sodium PUMP.

ATPS ambient temperature and pressure, saturated; denoting a volume of gas saturated with water vapor at ambient temperature and barometric pressure.

atracurium (at″rah-cūr′e-um) a neuromuscular blocking AGENT of intermediate duration; used as the besylate salt for intravenous administration as an adjunct to anesthesia to induce skeletal muscle relaxation during surgery and facilitate mechanical ventilation.

atraumatic (a″traw-mat′ik) not producing injury or damage.

atresia (ah-tre′zhah) congenital absence or closure of a normal body opening or tubular structure; see also obstruction. adj., **atret′ic.**

anal a., a. a′ni imperforate anus.

aortic a. 1. congenital absence of the aortic ORIFICE. 2. absence or closure of the

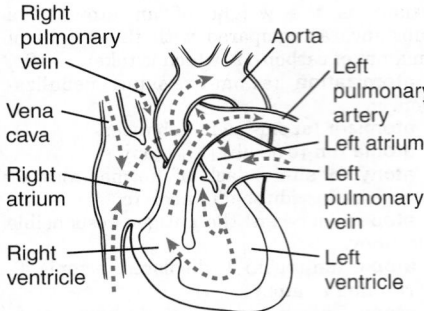

Right pulmonary vein
Aorta
Left pulmonary artery
Vena cava
Left atrium
Right atrium
Left pulmonary vein
Right ventricle
Left ventricle

Tricuspid atresia, here displaying a ventricular septal defect and normally related great arteries, the arrows showing the altered flow of blood through the heart. From Dorland's, 2000.

aortic ORIFICE, a rare congenital anomaly in which the left ventricle is hypoplastic, so that oxygenated blood passes from the left into the right atrium through a septal defect, and the mixed venous and arterial blood passes from the pulmonary artery to the aorta by way of a PATENT DUCTUS ARTERIOSUS.

aural a. absence of closure of the auditory canal.

biliary a. congenital obliteration or hypoplasia of one or more components of the bile ducts, resulting in persistent jaundice and liver damage.

choanal a. blockage of the posterior nares. When the blockage is bilateral in a newborn, it produces acute respiratory distress because neonates are nose-breathers. Diagnosis is confirmed if a catheter cannot be passed through the nares. Until surgery is done to relieve the obstruction, insertion of an airway may be necessary.

esophageal a. congenital lack of continuity of the esophagus, commonly accompanied by tracheoesophageal fistula, and characterized by accumulations of mucus in the nasopharynx, gagging, vomiting when fed, cyanosis, and dyspnea. Treatment should begin with suction of the upper esophageal pouch, followed by surgical repair by esophageal anastomosis and division of the fistula as soon as the infant's general condition permits.

follicular a., a. folli′culi the normal death of the ovarian follicle when unfertilized.

laryngeal a. congenital lack of the normal opening into the larynx.

mitral a. congenital obliteration of the mitral ORIFICE; it is associated with HYPOPLASTIC LEFT HEART SYNDROME and TRANSPOSITION OF GREAT VESSELS.

prepyloric a. congenital membranous obstruction of the gastric outlet, characterized by vomiting of gastric contents only. Called also pyloric atresia.

pulmonary a. congenital severe narrowing or obstruction of the pulmonary ORIFICE, with cardiomegaly, reduced pulmonary vascularity, and right ventricular atrophy. It is usually associated with TETRALOGY OF FALLOT, TRANSPOSITION OF GREAT VESSELS, or other cardiovascular anomalies.

pyloric a. prepyloric atresia.

tricuspid a. absence of the tricuspid ORIFICE, circulation being made possible by an ATRIAL SEPTAL DEFECT. (See accompanying illustration.)

urethral a. imperforation of the urethra.

atria (a′tre-ah) [L.] plural of ATRIUM.

atrial (a′tre-al) pertaining to an atrium.

a. natriuretic factor (ANF) a hormone produced in the cardiac atrium; it inhibits renin secretion and thus the production of ANGIOTENSIN, and stimulates ALDOSTERONE release. Its effect is increased excretion of water and sodium and a lowering of blood pressure, which reduces the workload of the heart.

a. septal defect a CONGENITAL HEART DEFECT in which the ostium primum or ostium secundum, openings in the septum primum of the embryonic heart, fail to close completely after birth. When an opening remains between the atria, some of the

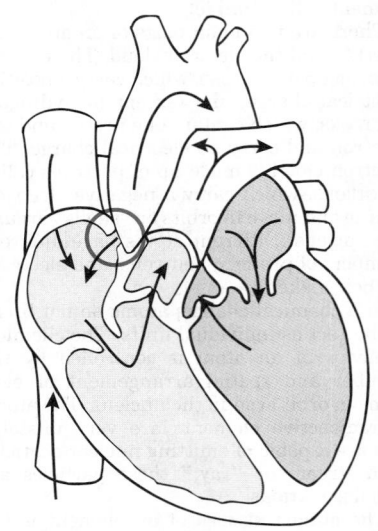

Atrial septal defect. The shunt is from left atrium to right atrium. From Betz et al., 1994.

oxygen-rich blood from the left atrium passes into the right atrium and travels back to the lungs without being first transported through the body. (See illustration.)

atrichous (ah-trik'us) 1. having no hair. 2. having no flagella.

atriomegaly (a″tre-o-meg'ah-le) abnormal enlargement of an atrium of the heart.

atriopeptin (a″tre-o-pep'tin) a peptide hormone that promotes the loss of fluid and electrolytes and the reduction of vascular tone.

atrioseptopexy (a″tre-o-sep'to-pek″se) surgical correction of a defect in the interatrial septum.

atrioseptoplasty (a″tre-o-sep'to-plas″te) repair of the interatrial septum.

atrioventricular (a″tre-o-ven-trik'u-ler) pertaining to or connecting an atrium and ventricle of the heart.

atrioventricularis communis (a″tre-o-ven-trik″u-lar'is kŏ-mu'nis) a congenital cardiac anomaly in which the endocardial cushions fail to fuse, the ostium primum persists, the atrioventricular canal is undivided, a single atrioventricular valve has anterior and posterior cusps, and there is a defect of the membranous interventricular septum.

atrium (a'tre-um), pl. *a'tria* [L.] a chamber affording entrance, especially the upper chamber (*a'trium cor'dis*) on either side of the heart, transmitting to the ventricle of the same side blood received from the pulmonary veins (left atrium) and from the venae cavae (right atrium).

Atromid-S (at'ro-mid) trademark for a preparation of CLOFIBRATE, used in treatment of HYPERLIPOPROTEINEMIA.

atrophia (ah-tro'fe-ah) [L.] atrophy.

atrophoderma (at″ro-fo-der'mah) atrophy of the skin.

atrophy (at'ro-fe) 1. decrease in size of a normally developed organ or tissue; see also WASTING. 2. to undergo or cause such a decrease. adj., **atroph'ic.**

acute yellow a. massive hepatic necrosis.

circumscribed cerebral a. PICK'S DISEASE.

disuse a. atrophy of a tissue or organ as a result of inactivity or diminished function.

gyrate a. of choroid and retina a rare hereditary, slowly progressive atrophy of the choroid and pigment epithelium of the retina; inherited as an autosomal recessive trait.

juvenile spinal muscular a. Kugelberg-Welander syndrome.

Leber's optic a. Leber's optic neuropathy.

lobar a. PICK'S DISEASE.

myelopathic muscular a. muscular atrophy due to lesion of the spinal cord, as in spinal muscular atrophy.

olivopontocerebellar a. any of a group of progressive hereditary disorders involving degeneration of the cerebellar cortex, middle peduncles, ventral pontine surface, and olivary nuclei. They occur in the young to middle-aged and are characterized by ataxia, dysarthria, and tremors similar to those of parkinsonism.

peroneal a., peroneal muscular a. progressive neuromuscular atrophy.

progressive neuromuscular a. hereditary muscular atrophy beginning in the muscles supplied by the fibular (peroneal) nerves, progressing slowly to involve the muscles of the hands and arms. Called also peroneal or peroneal muscular atrophy and Charcot-Marie-Tooth disease.

senile a. the natural atrophy of tissues and organs occurring with advancing age.

spinal muscular a. progressive degeneration of the motor cells of the spinal cord, beginning usually in the small muscles of the hands, but in some cases (scapulohumeral type) in the upper arm and shoulder muscles, and progressing slowly to the leg muscles. Called also Aran-Duchenne disease, Cruveilhier's disease, and Duchenne's disease.

subacute yellow a. submassive necrosis of the liver associated with broad zones of necrosis, due to viral, toxic, or drug-induced hepatitis; it may have an acute course with death from liver failure occurring after several weeks, or clinical recovery may be associated with regeneration of the parenchymal cells.

atropine (at'ro-pēn) an ANTICHOLINERGIC alkaloid found in BELLADONNA; it acts as a competitive antagonist of ACETYLCHOLINE at muscarinic RECEPTORS, blocking stimulation of muscles and glands by parasympathetic and cholinergic sympathetic nerves; used as the sulfate salt as a smooth muscle RELAXANT, as an ANTIARRHYTHMIC, as a PREANESTHETIC to reduce secretions, as an antidote to poisoning by organophosphorus compounds, cholinesterase inhibitors, or muscarine, and as a MYDRIATIC and CYCLOPLEGIC.

a. poisoning severe toxic reaction due to overdosage of atropine. Symptoms include dryness of mouth, thirst, difficulty in swallowing, dilated pupils, tachycardia, fever, delirium, stupor, and a rash on the face, neck, and upper trunk.

Treatment of atropine poisoning: This will depend on the patient, dose, and route of administration. A POISON CONTROL CENTER and emergency service should be contacted immediately if poisoning occurs in the home. Measures to be anticipated in the clinical setting include airway maintenance, monitoring, control of temperature, lavage, and sometimes administration of activated CHARCOAL.

atropinic (at″ro-pin'ik) having actions similar to those of ATROPINE; that is, antagonizing the MUSCARINIC effects of ACETYLCHOLINE.

ATS American Thoracic Society.

ATSDR Agency for Toxic Substances and Disease Registry, an agency of the United States Department of Health and Human Services.

attachment (ah-tach'ment) 1. the development of strong affectional ties between an infant and a significant other (mother, father, sibling, caretaker); this is a psychological, rather than a biological, process. 2. the initial stage of infection of a cell by a VIRUS, in which the viral ENVELOPE finds a suitable receptor on the cell surface, enabling the virus to enter. Called also adsorption.

risk for impaired parent/infant/child a. a NURSING DIAGNOSIS accepted by the North American Nursing Diagnosis Association, defined as disruption of the interactive process between parent/significant other and infant that fosters the development of a protective and nurturing reciprocal relationship. Possible causes include inadequacy of the parent or parent substitute (such as anxiety or substance abuse), illness in the child, physical separation, lack of privacy, and others.

attack (ah-tak') an episode or onset of illness.

anxiety a. panic attack.

heart a. 1. popular term for MYOCARDIAL INFARCTION. 2. any of various types of acute episodes of ISCHEMIC HEART DISEASE.

panic a. an episode of acute intense anxiety, with symptoms such as pounding or racing heart, sweating, trembling or shaking, feelings of choking or smothering, chest pain, nausea, dizziness, feelings of unreality, and chills or hot flashes. It is the essential feature of PANIC DISORDER and other ANXIETY DISORDERS as well as other psychiatric disorders such as schizophrenia and mood disorders.

transient ischemic a. see TRANSIENT ISCHEMIC ATTACK.

vagal a., vasovagal a. see VASOVAGAL ATTACK.

attapulgite (at″ah-pul'jit) a clay mineral that contains ALUMINUM SILICATE and is the main ingredient of FULLER'S EARTH; *activated attapulgite* is a heat-treated form that is administered orally in the treatment of diarrhea.

attempt (ah-tempt') a try or effort to achieve some goal.

suicide a. a serious effort to commit SUICIDE involving definite risk. The outcome frequently depends on circumstances alone and is not under the person's control.

attendant (ah-ten'dant) a person paid to perform personal services for those unable to care for themselves.

attention-deficit/hyperactivity disorder a childhood mental disorder characterized by inattention (such as distractibility, forgetfulness, not finishing tasks, and not appearing to listen), HYPERACTIVITY, and impulsivity (such as fidgeting and squirming, difficulty in remaining seated, excessive running or climbing, feelings of restlessness, difficulty awaiting one's turn, interrupting others, and excessive talking). Onset of the disorder is before age seven. Patterns of behavior vary in individual children and even in the same child from day to day, at times from hour to hour. The activity level improves during adolescence but attention problems often continue. Medications have been tried with varying degrees of success. Stimulants are often helpful as a palliative measure. Good results have also been obtained with clinical BEHAVIOR THERAPY, parent training, and contingency management.

The NATIONAL INSTITUTES OF HEALTH issued a consensus statement called *Diagnosis and Treatment of Attention Deficit Hyperactivity Disorder.* It makes note of the major controversy regarding use of psychostimulant medication for short and long term treatment of this condition. It also urges development of an integrated care model to provide services to individuals, families, and schools affected by the disorder.

attenuation (ah-ten″u-a'shun) 1. the act of thinning or weakening. 2. the change in the virulence of a pathogenic microorganism induced by passage through another host species, decreasing its virulence for the native host and increasing it for the new host. This is the basis for the development of live vaccines. 3. the change in a beam of radiation as it passes through matter. The intensity of the electromagnetic radiation decreases as its depth of penetration increases.

attic (at'ik) a small upper space of the middle ear, containing the head of the malleus and the body of the incus.

atticoantrotomy (at″ĭ-ko-an-trot'ah-me) surgical exposure of the epitympanic recess (attic) and mastoid antrum.

atticotomy (at″ĭ-kot′ah-me) incision into the epitympanic recess (attic).

attitude (at′ĭ-tood) 1. a posture or position of the body; in obstetrics, the relation of the various parts of the fetal body to one another. 2. a pattern of mental views established by cumulative prior experience.

atto- word element [Danish], *eighteen*; used in naming units of measurement to designate an amount one quintillionth (10^{-18}) the size of the unit to which it is joined; symbol a.

attraction (ah-trak′shun) the force or influence by which one object is drawn toward another.

    capillary a. the force that causes a liquid to rise in a fine-caliber tube.

attrition (ah-trĭ′shun) the wearing away of a substance or structure (such as the teeth) in the course of normal use.

at wt atomic weight.

atypia (a-tip′e-ah) deviation from the normal or typical state.

atypical (a-tip′ĭ-k'l) irregular; not conformable to the type.

Au gold (L. *au′rum*).

AUA American Urological Association.

AUC area under the curve.

audi(o)- word element [L.], *hearing.*

audioanalgesia (aw″de-o-an″al-je′ze-ah) reduction or abolition of the perception of pain by listening to recorded music to which has been added a background of "white noise."

audiogenic (aw″de-o-jen′ik) produced by sound.

audiogram (aw′de-o-gram″) 1. a graphic record of the findings by AUDIOMETRY. 2. the HEARING test done by AUDIOMETRY; it tests the ability to hear pure tones in each ear. A careful and complete audiogram will test both bone CONDUCTION and air CONDUCTION. A comparison between these two types of conduction can be useful in localizing which part of the hearing mechanism is responsible for any HEARING LOSS: if the loss is due to a problem with the portion of the middle ear that conducts sound from the ear canal to the inner ear, it is a *conductive hearing loss*; if it is due to the inner ear or the nerve that conducts sound signals to the brain, it is a *sensorineural hearing loss*. The results of audiograms are usually displayed in graph form; the amount of hearing is tested at different sound frequencies (measured in hertz). Most audiograms go from around 250 hertz to 4000 hertz. Lack of hearing at below 20 decibels on the graph is within the normal range; lack of hearing at above 20 decibels is considered abnormal. The American Speech-Language-Hearing Association has published guidelines for

audiologic screening, which are available at their web site: http://www.asha.com. In addition, the U.S. Preventive Services Task Force, part of the Agency for Healthcare Research and Quality, has recommendations on screening for hearing impairment and notes that there is good evidence that screening of newborns leads to earlier identification and treatment. The recommendations are available through the agency's web site: http://www.ahcpr.gov.

audiologist (aw″de-ol′o-jist) an allied health professional specializing in AUDIOLOGY, who provides services that include evaluation of HEARING function to detect hearing impairment and, if there is a hearing disorder, to determine the anatomical site involved and its cause; selection of appropriate hearing aids; and training in lip reading, hearing aid use, and maintenance of normal speech.

audiology (aw″de-ol′o-je) the science concerned with the sense of HEARING, especially in the evaluation and measurement of HEARING LOSS and the rehabilitation of those with impaired hearing. See also AUDIOLOGIST.

audiometer (aw″de-om′ĕ-ter) an apparatus used in AUDIOMETRY for testing the HEARING.

audiometry (aw″de-om′ĕ-tre) measurement of the acuity of HEARING through generation of tones of known frequencies and amplitudes. See also AUDIOGRAM (def. 2). adj., **audiomet′ric.**

    electrocochleographic a. measurement of electrical POTENTIALS from the middle ear or external auditory canal (cochlear MICROPHONICS and eighth nerve ACTION POTENTIALS) in response to acoustic stimuli.

    pure tone a. audiometry utilizing pure tones that are relatively free of noise and overtones.

    speech a. that in which the speech reception threshold in decibels and the ability to understand speech (speech discrimination) are measured.

audit (aw′dit) systematic review and evaluation of records and other data to determine the quality of the services or products provided in a given situation.

    nursing a. see NURSING AUDIT.

audition (aw-dish′un) hearing.

    chromatic a. chromesthesia.

auditory (aw′dĭ-tor″e) 1. pertaining to the EAR; called also aural and otic. 2. pertaining to the sense of hearing.

augmentation (awg-men-ta′shun) an adding on.

    bladder a. augmentation cystoplasty.

WINDOW ON AUDIOLOGY

The body's hearing mechanism is particularly complex but crucial Difficulty with hearing can be a life altering experience. Each individual and their particular hearing loss is different and requires individual and ongoing assistance. An audiologist is trained at the master's degree level to identify the nature of hearing difficulty and to work with individuals to improve the situation. Some programs award clinical doctorates (AuD.)

The British Columbia Association of Speech-Language Pathologists and Audiologists defines an audiologist as the hearing health-care professional who is educated and trained to evaluate and treat hearing, balance and related disorders.

The audiologist recommends the appropriate treatment, including aural rehabilitation, hearing aids, and other amplification devices. The services of audiologists include testing and diagnosing hearing and balance disorders in infants, children, and adults; selecting, fitting, and dispensing hearing aids and assistive listening, alerting, and captioning devices; working with adults and children who need aural rehabilitation such as auditory training and speechreading; educating consumers and professionals on the prevention of hearing loss; consulting and administering help through hearing conservation programs in industry to prevent hearing loss; consulting to federal, state or provincial, and local agencies on reducing community noise; and conducting research into environmental influences on hearing testing methods and new rehabilitative devices such as cochlear implants.

With the help of certified audiologists, people with hearing problems can receive assessment and treatment that can lead to better hearing. Audiologists are important members of the health care team and the treatment for hearing problems is the best it has ever been. Moreover, it keeps getting better.

BRENT McNEILL, DIP. T, M.A., AUD. (C)

---

breast a. popular name for augmentation MAMMAPLASTY.

augnathus (awg-nath′us) a malformed fetus with a double lower jaw.

aura (aw′rah), pl. *auras, au′rae* a peculiar sensation preceding the appearance of more definite symptoms. An *epileptic aura* precedes an epileptic SEIZURE and may involve visual disturbances, dizziness, numbness, or any of a number of sensations which the patient may find difficult to describe exactly. In epilepsy the aura serves a useful purpose in that it warns of an impending attack and gives the patient time to seek privacy and a safe place to lie down before the seizure actually begins.

A *migraine aura* precedes about 15 per cent of MIGRAINE headaches, warning the patient that an attack is imminent. When it occurs the patient should rest in a quiet, darkened room.

aural (aw′ral) 1. auditory (def. 1). 2. pertaining to an aura.

auranofin (aw-ran′o-fin) a gold-containing compound that is a disease-modifying antirheumatic DRUG used to treat active rheumatoid ARTHRITIS, usually that not adequately controlled by NONSTEROIDAL ANTIINFLAMMATORY DRUGS, or nondrug therapy such as physical therapy; administered orally.

aurantiasis (aw″ran-ti′ah-sis) yellowness of skin caused by intake of large amounts of food containing carotene.

auric (aw′rik) pertaining to gold.

auricle (aw′rĭ-k′l) 1. the projecting part of the ear lying outside the head; called also pinna. (See illustration.) 2. the ear-shaped appendage of either atrium of the heart; formerly used to designate the entire ATRIUM.

auricula (aw-rik′u-lah), pl. *auri′culae* [L.] auricle.

auricular (aw-rik′u-lar) pertaining to an auricle or ear.

auricularis (aw-rik″u-la′ris) [L.] pertaining to the ear.

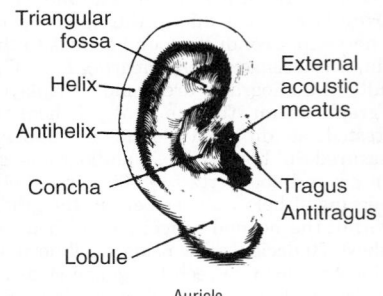

Triangular fossa

Helix

Antihelix

Concha

Lobule

External acoustic meatus

Tragus

Antitragus

Auricle.

auriculotemporal (aw-rik″u-lo-tem′po-ral) pertaining to the ear and the temporal region.

auris (aw′ris) [L.] ear.

auriscope (aw′rĭ-skōp) otoscope.

aurotherapy (aw″ro-ther′ah-pe) chrysotherapy.

aurothioglucose (aw″ro-thi″o-gloo′kōs) a gold preparation used in the treatment of early active rheumatoid ARTHRITIS (both adult and juvenile types) not controlled by nonsteroidal antiinflammatory drugs, rest, and physical therapy; administered intramuscularly.

auscultate (aw′skul-tāt) to examine by AUSCULTATION.

auscultation (aw″skul-ta′shun) listening for sounds produced within the body, chiefly to assess the condition of the thoracic or abdominal organs and vessels such as the heart, lungs, aorta, and intestines. Fetal heart tones can also be monitored during pregnancy by auscultation with a specialized stethoscope. It may be performed with the unaided ear *(direct* or *immediate auscultation)* or with a stethoscope *(mediate auscultation).* See also auscultatory SOUNDS.

auscultatory (aw-skul′tah-tor″e) pertaining to AUSCULTATION.

aut(o)- word element [Gr.], *self.*

autacoid (aw′tah-koid) local hormone.

authorization (aw″ther-ĭ-za′shun) permission.

insurance a. in the NURSING INTERVENTIONS CLASSIFICATION, a nursing INTERVENTION defined as assisting the patient and provider to secure payment for health services or equipment from a third party.

autism (aw′tizm) autistic disorder. adj., **autis′tic.**

infantile a. AUTISTIC DISORDER.

autistic (aw-tis′tik) pertaining to or exhibiting AUTISM.

a. disorder a PERVASIVE DEVELOPMENTAL DISORDER beginning before age three; called also autism and infantile autism. Characteristics include impairment in reciprocal social interaction (for example, lack of awareness of the existence of feelings in others), in verbal and nonverbal communication, and in capacity for symbolic play, as well as by a restricted repertoire of activities and interests. There may also be cognitive impairment, abnormally increased or decreased reactivity to certain stimuli, stereotypic behaviors, neurological abnormalities such as seizures or altered muscle tone, sleeping or eating pattern abnormalities, and severe behavioral problems. There are no delusions, hallucinations, or incoherence, and the facial expression is

intelligent and responsive. Often, children are self absorbed, inaccessible, and unable to relate to others, including parents; they may play happily alone for hours but have temper tantrums if interrupted. Language disturbances often include repetition of previously heard speech and reversal of the pronouns "I" and "you." Individuals with the disorder may show any of a wide spectrum of behaviors.

The cause of the syndrome is unknown. Early intervention programs have improved outcomes for affected children. Research studies have demonstrated that a highly structured, specialized educational program tailored to the child's individual needs can result in significant improvement in functional ability, although autism usually affects a person through life. Programs should incorporate the parents and other caregivers to maximize effectiveness. Appropriate support services often enable the child to remain in the community rather than being institutionalized.

autoagglutination (aw″to-ah-gloo″tĭ-na′shun) 1. clumping or agglutination of an individual's cells by his own serum (containing AUTOANTIBODY), as in autohemagglutination. Autoagglutination occurring at low temperatures is called *cold agglutination.* 2. nonspecific clumping or agglutination of particulate antigens that does not involve antibody.

autoagglutinin (aw″to-ah-gloo′tĭ-nin) a factor in serum capable of causing clumping together of the subject's own cellular elements.

autoamputation (aw″to-am″pu-ta′shun) 1. spontaneous detachment from the body and elimination of an appendage or an abnormal growth, such as a polyp. 2. ainhum.

autoantibody (aw″to-an′tĭ-bod″e) an antibody formed in response to, and reacting against, an antigenic constituent of the individual's own tissues.

autoantigen (aw″to-an′tĭ-jen) an ANTIGEN that, despite being a normal tissue constituent, is the target of a humoral or cell-mediated IMMUNE RESPONSE, such as in AUTOIMMUNE DISEASE.

autocatalysis (aw″to-kah-tal′ĭ-sis) an increase in the rate of a chemical reaction in which a product of the reaction itself hastens or intensifies the rate.

autochthonous (aw-tok′tho-nus) 1. originating in the same area in which it is found; said of pathological processes. 2. denoting a tissue graft to a new site on the same individual.

autoclasis (aw-tok′lah-sis) destruction of a part by influences within itself.

autoclave (aw′to-klāv) a self-locking apparatus for the sterilization of materials by steam under pressure. The autoclave allows steam to flow around each article placed in the chamber. The vapor penetrates cloth or paper used to package the articles being sterilized. Autoclaving is one of the most effective methods for destruction of all types of microorganisms, including spores. The amount of time and degree of temperature necessary for sterilization depend on the articles to be sterilized and whether they are wrapped or left directly exposed to the steam.

autocoid local hormone.

Autoclip (aw′to-klip″) trademark for a stainless steel surgical clip inserted by means of a mechanical applier that automatically feeds a series of clips for wound closing.

autocrine (aw′to-krin) denoting a mode of hormone action in which a hormone binds to receptors on and affects the function of the same cell that produced it.

autocytolysin (aw″to-si-tol′ĭ-sin) autolysin.

autocytolysis (aw″to-si-tol′ĭ-sis) autolysis.

autodigestion (aw″to-dĭ-jes′chun) dissolution of tissue by its own secretions.

autoecholalia (aw″to-ek″o-la′le-ah) parrotlike repetition of words and phrases initially uttered by the patient himself; seen in catatonic schizophrenia and in certain cerebral degenerative disorders.

autoeczematization (aw″to-ek-zem″ah-tĭ-za′shun) the spread, at first locally and later more generally, of lesions from an originally circumscribed focus of eczema.

autoeroticism (aw″to-ĕ-rot′ĭ-sizm) sexual self-gratification or arousal without the participation of another person, such as masturbation. See also ALLOEROTICISM. adj., **autoerot′ic.**

autoerotism (aw″to-er′o-tizm) autoeroticism.

autoerythrocyte sensitization syndrome (aw″to-e-rith′ro-sīt) painful bruising syndrome.

autogeneic (aw″to-jĕ-ne′ik) autologous.

autogenesis (aw″to-jen′ĕ-sis) self-generation; origination within the organism. adj., **autogenet′ic, autog′enous.**

autogenic training (aw″to-jen′ik) a method of self-induced deep relaxation, derived from hypnosis.

autograft (aw′to-graft) autologous GRAFT.

autohemagglutination (aw″to-he″mah-gloo″tĭ-na′shun) HEMAGGLUTINATION caused by an antibody produced in the subject's own body.

autohemagglutinin (aw″to-he″mah-gloo′-tĭ-nin) a HEMAGGLUTININ produced in the subject′ s own body.

autohemolysin (aw″to-he-mol′ĭ-sin) a HEMOLYSIN produced in the body of an animal which causes destruction of its own erythrocytes.

autohemolysis (aw″to-he-mol′ĭ-sis) HEMOLYSIS of the blood cells by the subject's own serum. adj., **autohemolyt′ic.**

a. test determination of spontaneous hemolysis in a blood specimen maintained under certain conditions, to detect the presence of certain hemolytic states.

autohemotherapy (aw″to-he″mo-ther′ah-pe) treatment with an AUTOTRANSFUSION.

autohypnosis (aw″to-hip-no′sis) self-induced hypnosis; the act or process of hypnotizing oneself.

autoimmune disease (aw″to-ĭ-mun′) disease associated with the production of antibodies directed against one's own tissues. The immunological mechanism of the body is dependent on two major factors: first, inactivation and rejection of foreign substances, and second, the ability to differentiate between the body's own material (SELF) and that which is foreign (NONSELF). It is not yet known exactly what causes the body to fail to recognize proteins as its own and to react to them as if they were foreign. Several possibilities have been identified as pertinent to the development of autoimmunity.

1. There may be a leakage of normally _inaccessible_ tissue antigen from its isolated location into an area where it comes into contact with the IMMUNOCOMPETENT cells of the RETICULOENDOTHELIAL SYSTEM. These reticuloendothelial cells do not recognize the formerly inaccessible antigen as "self" and react accordingly.

2. The antigens that are normally accessible to the RES cells may suddenly stimulate the production of autoantibodies. It is thought that this occurs as a result of the emergence of "forbidden clones" (colonies) of cells. Normally these cells are inactivated as a result of adaptive changes that occur during fetal life. For reasons not yet fully explained, these "forbidden clones" survive and emerge to produce an autoimmune reaction. It is believed that they may be activated by injury, disease, or a metabolic change in the body, or there may be a mutation of the forbidden clone cells and immunologically competent cells.

3. Certain body proteins may be so altered by viral infection, by combination with a drug or chemical, or by extensive trauma (as in a severe burn and myocardial infarction) that they are no longer recognized by the

Autoimmune disease can be viewed as a spectrum of disorders. At one end are *organ-specific* diseases, in which there is localized tissue damage resulting from the presence of specific auto-antibodies. An example is HASHIMOTO'S DISEASE of the thyroid, characterized by a specific lesion in the thyroid gland with infiltration by mononuclear cells, destruction of follicular cells, and production of antibodies with absolute specificity for certain thyroid constituents.

In the middle of the spectrum are disorders in which the lesion tends to be localized in one organ, but the antibodies are nonorgan specific. An example is primary biliary CIRRHOSIS, in which there is inflammatory cell infiltration of the small bile ductule, but the serum antibodies are not specific to liver cells.

At the other end of the spectrum are *non-organ specific* diseases, in which lesions and antibodies are widespread throughout the body and not limited to one target organ. Systemic LUPUS ERYTHEMATOSUS is an example of this type of autoimmune disease. Others include RHEUMATIC FEVER, rheumatoid ARTHRITIS, autoimmune hemolytic ANEMIA, idiopathic thrombocytopenic PURPURA, and postviral ENCEPHALOMYELITIS.

Treatment of autoimmune diseases varies with each specific disease, but in all cases the members of the health care team must strive to achieve a delicate balance between adequate suppression of the autoimmune reaction to avoid continued damage to the body tissues, and maintenance of sufficient functioning of the immune mechanism to protect the patient against foreign invaders.

autoimmunity (aw″to-ĭ-mu′nĭ-te) a condition characterized by a specific humoral or cell-mediated IMMUNE RESPONSE against the constituents of the body's own tissues (AUTOANTIGENS); it may result in HYPERSENSITIVITY REACTIONS or, if severe, in AUTOIMMUNE DISEASE.

autoimmunization (aw″to-im″u-nĭ-za′-shun) induction in an organism of an IMMUNE RESPONSE to its own tissue constituents.

autoinfusion (aw″to-in-fu′zhun) the forcing of blood toward the heart by measures such as bandaging of limbs or compressing of the abdominal aorta.

autoinoculation (aw″to-ĭ-nok″u-la′shun) inoculation with microorganisms from one's own body.

autoisolysin (aw″to-i-sol′ĭ-sin) autoantibody that causes complement-dependent lysis of cells (e.g., blood cells) of the individual in which it is formed and also those of other individuals of the same species.

autokeratoplasty (aw″to-ker′ah-to-plas″te) grafting of corneal tissue from one eye to the other.

autokinesis (aw″to-kĭ-ne′sis) voluntary motion. adj., **autokinet′ic.**

autolesion (aw″to-le′zhun) a self-inflicted injury.

autologous (aw-tol′o-gus) related to self; belonging to the same organism; called also autogeneic.

autolysate (aw-tol′ĭ-sāt) a substance produced by autolysis.

autolysin (aw-tol′ĭ-sin) a lysin originating in an organism and capable of destroying its own cells and tissues.

autolysis (aw-tol′ĭ-sis) the disintegration of cells or tissues by endogenous enzymes. adj., **autolyt′ic.**

automated reagin test (ART) a modification of the rapid plasma reagin (RPR) test for use with automated analyzers; used in clinical chemistry.

automatic (aw″to-mat′ik) spontaneous; done involuntarily; self-regulating.

automaticity (aw″to-mah-tis′ĭ-te) the ability of a cell to depolarize itself, reach threshold POTENTIAL, and produce a propagated ACTION POTENTIAL; cells with this capability are called AUTOMATIC CELLS.

abnormal a. a type of altered automaticity occurring in cells that do not normally possess that property, as in myocardial cells with severely depressed function that have lost their fast sodium channels.

altered a. ectopic automatic firing of myocardial cells; there are two types, enhanced normal automaticity and abnormal automaticity.

enhanced normal a. a type of altered automaticity seen in pacemaker CELLS, caused by a steepening of phase 4 such as occurs in the presence of excess catecholamines, which causes premature BEATS to occur.

automatism (aw-tom′ah-tizm) aimless and apparently undirected behavior that is not under conscious control and is performed without conscious knowledge; seen in psychomotor epilepsy, catatonic schizophrenia, dissociative fugue, and other conditions.

command a. the performance of suggested acts without exercise of critical judgment; seen in catatonic schizophrenia and in the hypnotic state.

autonomic (aw″to-nom′ik) not subject to voluntary control.

a. dysreflexia an uninhibited and exaggerated reflex of the AUTONOMIC NERVOUS SYSTEM to stimulation; called also hyperreflexia. The response occurs in 85 per cent of all patients who have spinal cord injury above the level of the sixth thoracic vertebra. It is potentially dangerous because of attendant vasoconstriction and immediate elevation of blood pressure, which in turn can bring about hemorrhagic retinal damage or STROKE SYNDROME. Less serious effects include severe headache; changes in heart rate; sweating, flushing, and "goose bumps" or piloerection above the level of the spinal cord injury; and pallor below that level.

Patient Care. Circumstances that can trigger autonomic dysreflexia are often related to stimulation of the bladder, bowel, and skin of the patient. Examples are a distended bowel or bladder, pressure on the skin, or any of a number of noxious stimuli.

Once the symptoms of autonomic dysreflexia are manifest, emergency care is indicated. Efforts are made to lower the blood pressure by placing the patient in a sitting position or elevating the head and upper body to a 45-degree angle. The stimulus must be identified and removed as gently and quickly as possible. If fecal impaction is the cause, the rectum should be coated with an anesthetic ointment prior to attempted removal of the impaction; this prevents increasing the stimulus to autonomic dysreflexia. The physician is notified so that appropriate medical intervention can be initiated. Antihypertensive drugs are a last resort. As soon as the cause is identified and removed, the dysreflexia will disappear. Patients who experience repeated attacks may require surgery to sever the nerves responsible for the exaggerated response to stimulation.

a. nervous system the branch of the NERVOUS SYSTEM that works without conscious control. The voluntary nervous system governs the striated or skeletal muscles, whereas the autonomic nervous system governs the glands, cardiac muscle, and smooth muscles such as those of the digestive system, respiratory system, and skin. The autonomic nervous system is divided into two subsidiary systems, the SYMPATHETIC NERVOUS SYSTEM and the PARASYMPATHETIC NERVOUS SYSTEM. See Plate 14.

autonomotropic (aw″to-no″mo-trop′ik) having an affinity for the autonomic nervous system.

autonomy (aw-ton′o-me) 1. the ability to function in an independent fashion. 2. in BIOETHICS, self-determination that is free from both controlling interferences by others and personal limitations preventing meaningful choice (such as inadequate understanding or faulty reasoning). Having the capacity to act with autonomy does not guarantee that a person will actually do so with full understanding and without external controlling influences. adj., **auton′omous.**

auto-PEEP (aw′to-pēp″) intrinsic positive end-expiratory pressure.

autophagia (aw″to-fa′ge-ah) 1. eating or biting of one's own flesh. 2. nutrition of the body by consumption of its own tissues. 3. autophagy.

autophagosome (aw″to-fa′go-sōm) a secondary lysosome in which elements of a cell's own cytoplasm are digested.

autophagy (aw-tof′ah-je) 1. lysosomal digestion of a cell's own cytoplasmic material. 2. autophagia.

autopharmacologic (aw″to-fahr″mah-ko-loj′ik) pertaining to substances (e.g., hormones) produced in the body that have pharmacologic activities.

autophony (aw-tof′ah-ne) abnormal hearing of one's own voice and respiratory sounds, usually as a result of a patulous eustachian tube.

autoplasty (aw′to-plas″te) 1. autotransplantation. 2. in psychoanalytic theory, adaptation by changing one's self rather than the external environment. adj., **autoplas′tic.**

autopsy (aw′top-se) examination of a body after death to determine the cause of death; it may be ordered by a coroner or medical examiner when the cause of death is unknown or the death has taken place under suspicious circumstances. Autopsies are also valuable sources of medical knowledge. Unless it is demanded by public authorities, an autopsy cannot be performed without permission of the next of kin of the deceased. Called also postmortem examination and necropsy.

autoradiograph (aw″to-ra′de-o-graf) the film produced by autoradiography.

autoradiography (aw″to-ra″de-og′rah-fe) the making of a radiograph of an object or tissue by recording on a photographic plate the radiation emitted by radioactive material within the object.

autoregulation (aw″to-reg″u-la′shun) control of certain phenomena by factors inherent in a situation; specifically, (1) maintenance by an organ or tissue of a constant blood flow despite changes in arterial pressure, and (2) adjustment of blood flow through an organ in accordance with its metabolic needs.

heterometric a. those intrinsic mechanisms controlling the strength of ventricular contractions that depend on the length of myocardial fibers at the end of diastole.

homeometric a. those intrinsic mechanisms controlling the strength of ventricular contractions that are independent of the length of myocardial fibers at the end of diastole.

autosensitization (aw″to-sen″sĭ-tĭ-za′-shun) development of sensitivity to one's own serum or tissues.

autoserum (aw″to-sēr′um) serum administered to the patient from whom it was derived.

autosite (aw′to-sīt) in unequal TWINS, the larger, more normal twin, to which the other (the parasitic FETUS) is attached.

autosome (aw′to-sōm) any of the 22 pairs of chromosomes in humans other than the pair concerned with determination of sex.

autosplenectomy (aw″to-sple-nek′to-me) almost complete disappearance of the spleen due to progressive fibrosis and shrinkage.

autosuggestion (aw″to-sug-jes′chun) self-suggestion; the process by which a person induces in himself an uncritical acceptance of an idea, belief, or opinion.

autotomography (aw″to-to-mog′rah-fe) a method of TOMOGRAPHY involving movement of the patient instead of the x-ray tube.

autotopagnosia (aw″to-top-ag-no′zhah) inability to orient correctly different parts of the body.

autotransfusion (aw″to-trans-fu′zhun) 1. reinfusion of a patient's own blood; see autologous TRANSFUSION. 2. in the NURSING INTERVENTIONS CLASSIFICATION, a nursing INTERVENTION defined as collecting and re-infusing blood which has been lost intra-operatively or postoperatively from clean wounds.

autotransplantation (aw″to-trans″planta′shun) transfer of tissue from one part of the body to another part. See also autologous GRAFT.

autotroph (aw′to-trōf) an autotrophic organism.

autotrophic (aw″to-trof′ik) capable of synthesizing necessary nutrients if water, carbon dioxide, inorganic salts, and a source of energy are available.

autovaccination (aw″to-vak″sĭ-na′shun) treatment with autovaccine.

autovaccine (aw″to-vak-sēn′) a vaccine prepared from cultures of organisms from the patient's own tissues or secretions.

autoxidation (aw″tok-sĭ-da′shun) the spontaneous reaction of a compound with molecular oxygen at room temperature.

autumn fever mud fever.

auxesis (awk-se′sis) increase in size of an organism, especially that due to growth

of its individual cells rather than increase in their number. adj., **auxet′ic.**

auxodrome (awk-so-drōm) the course of growth of a child as plotted on a specially devised graph called the Wetzel GRID.

auxotroph (awk′so-trōf) an auxotrophic organism.

auxotrophic (awk″so-trof′ik) 1. requiring a growth factor not required by the parental or prototype strain; said of microbial mutants. 2. requiring specific organic growth factors in addition to the carbon source present in a minimal medium.

AV, A-V atrioventricular; arteriovenous.

av avoirdupois.

avascular (a-vas′ku-ler) not vascular; bloodless.

avascularization (a-vas″ku-ler-ĭ-za′shun) diversion of blood from tissues, as by ligation or bandaging.

AVC trademark for preparations of SULFA-NILAMIDE, an ANTIMICROBIAL.

Avellis' syndrome (av-el′ēz) a syndrome in which a brain stem lesion limits innervation by the VAGUS NERVE unilaterally, causing paralysis of the vocal cord and soft palate on one side with loss of pain and temperature sensibility on the other side in the upper and lower limbs, neck, trunk, and skin over the scalp.

avidity (ah-vid′ĭ-te) 1. eagerness, or a strong attraction for something. 2. in immunology, an imprecise measure of the strength of antigen-antibody binding based on the rate at which the complex is formed.

avirulence (a-vir′u-lens) lack of virulence; lack of competence of an infectious agent to produce pathologic effects. adj., **avir′-ulent.**

avitaminosis (a-vi″tah-mĭ-no′sis) disease due to deficiency of VITAMINS in the diet. adj., **avitaminot′ic.**

avobenzone (av′o-ben′zōn) a SUNSCREEN that absorbs light in the UVA range.

avocational (av″o-ka′shun-al) pertaining to leisure time activities.

Avogadro's law (ah″vo-gah′drōz) equal volumes of perfect gases at the same temperature and pressure contain the same number of molecules.

avoidance (ah-void′ans) a conscious or unconscious DEFENSE MECHANISM consisting of refusal to encounter situations, activities, or objects that would produce conflict.

avoidant (ah-voi′dant) characterized by avoidance or moving away from something.

a. disorder of childhood and adolescence former name for a disorder now included under the diagnosis of social PHOBIA.

a. personality disorder a PERSONALITY DISORDER marked by extreme shyness and sensitivity to rejection. Because of this sensitivity, the person becomes socially withdrawn and forms relationships only with those willing to give uncritical acceptance. The self-esteem of such a person is naturally low. Fear of embarrassment prevents the patient from undertaking risks or new activities. In spite of the social withdrawal, the avoidant personality has a great desire for affection and companionship.

avoirdupois system (av′er-dŭ-poiz″) a system of weights based on POUNDS and OUNCES, widely used in English-speaking countries for commodities other than drugs, precious stones, and precious metals. See also Table of Weights and Measures in the Appendix.

avulsion (ah-vul′shun) the tearing away of a structure or part either accidentally or surgically.

awareness (ah-war′nes) consciousness.
sensory a. the ability to receive and differentiate sensory stimuli.

Axenfeld's anomaly (ak′sen-feldz) a developmental anomaly characterized by a circular opacity of the posterior peripheral cornea, and caused by an irregularly thickened, axially displaced Schwalbe's ring.

axenic (a-zen′ik) not contaminated by or associated with any foreign organisms; used in reference to pure cultures of microorganisms or to germ-free animals.

axi(o)- word element [L., Gr.], denoting relation to an axis; in dentistry, used in special reference to the long axis of a tooth.

Axid (ak′sid) trademark for preparations of NIZATIDINE, an antagonist of histamine H_2 RECEPTORS used to inhibit gastric acid secretion.

axilla (ak-sil′ah), pl. *axil′lae* [L.] the armpit.

axillary (ak′sĭ-lar″e) of or pertaining to the armpit.

axis (ak′sis), pl. *ax′es* 1. a line through a center of a body, or about which a structure revolves. the second cervical vertebra. adj., **ax′ial.** 2. the position of the cylindrical part of a LENS, used for correcting ASTIGMATISM; the range of values is from 0° to 180°.
celiac a. celiac trunk.
dorsoventral a. one passing from the posterior to the anterior surface of the body.
electrical a. of heart the preponderant direction of current flow through the heart, a consequence of the electromotive forces within the heart. It may be computed on either an *instantaneous* basis or a *mean* basis.

frontal a. an imaginary line running from right to left through the center of the eyeball.
a. of heart a line passing through the center of the base of the heart to the apex.
instantaneous electrical a. the electrical axis of the heart determined at a given point in time.
lead a. the imaginary direct line between the two electrodes of the bipolar leads or between the positive electrode and the reference point of the unipolar leads.
mean electrical a. the average direction of the activation or repolarization process during the cardiac cycle; it may be determined for any deflection (P, QRS, ST-T) and in the frontal, transverse, or sagittal plane.
optic a. 1. a line connecting the center of the anterior curvature of the cornea (anterior pole) with that of the posterior curvature of the sclera (posterior pole). 2. the hypothetical straight line passing through the centers of curvature of the front and back surfaces of a simple lens.
phlebostatic a. a point located by drawing an imaginary line from the fourth intercostal space at the sternum and finding its intersection with an imaginary line drawn down the center of the chest below the axillae. (See accompanying illustration.)
sagittal a. an imaginary line extending through the anterior and posterior poles of the eye.
visual a. an imaginary line passing from the midpoint of the visual field to the

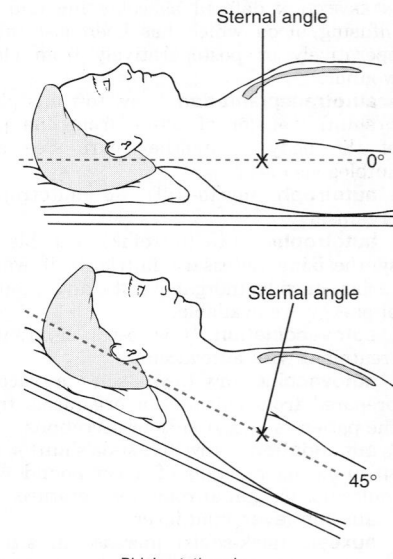

Phlebostatic axis.

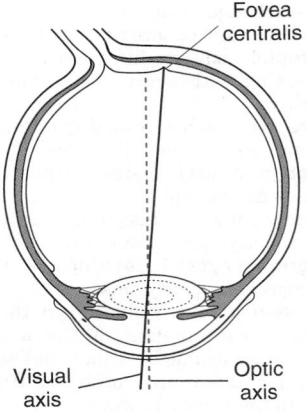

Fovea
centralis

Visual
axis

Optic
axis

Axes of the eye. From Dorland's , 2000.

fovea centralis. (See accompanying illustration.)

axoaxonic (ak″so-ak-son′ik) referring to a synapse between the axon of one neuron and the axon of another.

axodentritic (ak″ so-den-drit′ ik) referring to a synapse between the axon of one neuron and dentrites of another.

axolemma (ak″so-lem′ah) the surface membrane of an axon.

axolysis (ak-sol′ĭ-sis) degeneration of an axon.

axon (ak′son) the process of a nerve cell along which impulses travel away from the cell body. It branches at its termination, forming synapses at other nerve cells or effector organs. Many axons are covered by a myelin sheath formed from the cell membrane of a glial cell. adj., **ax′onal.**

axonapraxia (ak″son-ah-prak′se-ah) neurapraxia.

axoneme (ak′so-nēm) the central core of a cilium or flagellum, consisting of two central fibrils surrounded by nine peripheral fibrils.

axonopathy (ak″sŏ-nop′ah-the) a disorder disrupting the normal functioning of the axons.

axonotmesis (ak″son-ot-me′sis) nerve injury characterized by disruption of the axon and myelin sheath but with preservation of the connective tissue fragments, resulting in degeneration of the axon distal to the injury site; regeneration of the axon is spontaneous and of good quality.

axoplasm (ak′so-plasm) the cytoplasm of an AXON. adj., **axoplas′mic.**

axosomatic (ak″so-so-mat′ik) referring to a synapse between the axon of one neuron and the cell body of another.

Ayerza's disease (ah-yer′thaz) a form of polycythemia vera marked by chronic cyanosis, chronic dyspnea, chronic bronchitis, bronchiectasis, hepatosplenomegaly, and hyperplasia of bone marrow, and associated with sclerosis of the pulmonary artery.

azatadine (ah-zat′ah-dēn) an ANTIHISTAMINE with sedative and anticholinergic effects; used as the maleate salt in the treatment of nasal, eye, and skin manifestations of allergic reactions, including allergic rhinitis, conjunctivitis, and itching, and also as an ingredient in some cough and cold preparations, administered orally.

azathioprine (a″zah-thi′o-prēn) a MERCAPTOPURINE derivative used as an IMMUNOSUPPRESSIVE agent for prevention of transplant rejection in organ TRANSPLANTATION; as a disease-modifying antirheumatic DRUG for treatment of severe, progressive rheumatoid ARTHRITIS unresponsive to other agents; and for treatment of a number of AUTOIMMUNE DISEASES; administered orally as the base or intravenously as the sodium salt.

azelaic acid (az″ĕ-la′ik) a dicarboxylic acid occurring in whole grains and animal products; it has antibacterial effects on both aerobic and anaerobic organisms, particularly *Propionibacterium acnes* and *Staphylococcus epidermidis,* normalizes keratinization, and has a cytotoxic effect on malignant or hyperactive melanocytes; applied topically in the treatment of ACNE VULGARIS.

azelastine (ah-zel′as-tēn″) an ANTIHISTAMINE used intranasally as the hydrochloride salt in treatment of HAY FEVER and topically to the conjunctiva in treatment of allergic CONJUNCTIVITIS.

Azelex (az-ĕ-leks) trademark for a preparation of AZELAIC ACID, used for treating ACNE.

azeotrope (a′ze-o-trōp″) a mixture of two substances that has a constant boiling point and cannot be separated by fractional distillation. adj., **azeotrop′ic.**

azithromycin (az-ith″ro-mi′sin) a MACROLIDE antibiotic derived from ERYTHROMYCIN, effective against a wide range of gram-positive, gram-negative, and anaerobic bacteria; administered orally or intravenously.

azoospermia (a″zo-o-sper′me-ah) lack of live SPERMATOZOA in the semen; see also ASPERMATOGENESIS.

azote (a″zōt) nitrogen.

azotemia (az″o-te′me-ah) an excess of nitrogenous waste products in the blood. (This is the most precise name for the condition, although in the literature it is commonly referred to as *uremia.*) See also UREMIA. adj., **azote′mic.**

azotorrhea (az″o-to-re′ah) discharge of excessive quantities of nitrogenous matter in the stools.

azoturia (az″o-tu′re-ah) an excess of urea or other nitrogen compounds in the urine.

aztreonam (az′tre-o-nam″) a narrow-range ANTIBIOTIC effective against aerobic gram-negative bacteria; used for the treatment of infections caused by susceptible organisms. Administered intravenously or intramuscularly.

AZT zidovudine.

Azulfidine (ah-zul′fĭ-dēn) trademark for a preparation of SULFASALAZINE, used in the treatment of INFLAMMATORY BOWEL DISEASE and rheumatoid ARTHRITIS.

azure (azh′ūr) one of three metachromatic basic dyes (azures A, B, and C).

azuresin (azh″u-rez′in) a complex combination of azure A dye and carbacrylic cation–exchange resin used as a diagnostic aid in detection of gastric secretion.

azurophil (azh-u′ro-fil) a tissue constituent staining with azure or a similar blue aniline dye.

azurophilic (azh″u-ro-fil′ik) staining with azure or similar blue aniline dyes.

azygogram (az′ĭ-go-gram″) the film obtained by azygography.

azygography (az″ĭ-gog′rah-fe) radiography of the azygous venous system.

azygos (az′ĭ-gos) 1. any unpaired part, as the azygos vein. 2. azygous.

a. vein a vein beginning in the abdomen as a continuation of the ascending lumbar vein; it and its tributaries serve as vessels for the return of blood from the thorax to the superior VENA CAVA. The azygos vein also serves as a connecting link, through the ascending lumbar vein, between the venae cavae returning blood from above and below the heart. See anatomic Table of Veins in the Appendices.

azygous (az′ĭ-gus) having no fellow; unpaired. Called also azygos.

B bel; boron. See also POINT B.

β beta, the second letter of the Greek alphabet, often used to indicate the second member of a series, such as the β chain of HEMOGLOBIN. See also terms beginning BETA.

BA Bachelor of Arts.

Ba barium.

Babesia (bah-be′zhah) a genus of protozoa found as parasites in red blood cells and transmitted by ticks; its numerous species cause BABESIOSIS in both wild and domestic animals and a malarialike illness in humans.

babesiosis (bah-be″ze-o′sis) a group of tickborne diseases due to infection with protozoa of the genus *Babesia*, usually seen in wild or domestic animals as a type of anemia; it may spread to humans as a ZOONOSIS characterized by a malarialike fever with chills, sweats, myalgia, nausea and vomiting, hemolytic anemia, and splenomegaly.

Babinski reflex (sign) (bah-bin′ske) a reflex action of the toes, normal during infancy but abnormal after 12 to 18 months of age; after locomotion begins, it is indicative of abnormalities in the motor control pathways leading from the cerebral cortex and is widely used as a diagnostic aid in disorders of the central nervous system. It is elicited by a firm stimulus (usually scraping) on the sole of the foot, which results in dorsiflexion of the great toe and fanning of the smaller toes. Normally such a stimulus causes all the toes to bend downward. (See accompanying illustration.)

Babkin reflex (bab′kin) pressure by the examiner's thumbs on the palms of both hands of the infant results in opening of the infant's mouth; it is elicited in many newborn infants, normal and abnormal, except when lethargic or comatose.

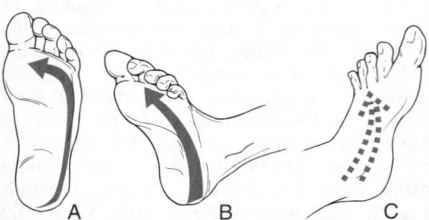

Normal and Babinski reflexes. *A,* Line of stimulation: Outer sole, heel to little toe. *B,* Plantar (normal) reflex. Toes curl inward. *C,* Positive Babinski reflex (always abnormal). Great toe bends upward; smaller toes fan outward.

baby (ba′be) infant.

blue b. an infant born with CYANOSIS, a bluish color due to abnormally low concentration of oxygen in the circulating blood, usually due to one or more defect(s) of the heart or great vessels. See also CONGENITAL HEART DEFECT.

collodion b. an infant affected with lamellar EXFOLIATION of the newborn.

B. Doe legislation a law that requires health care providers to provide treatment for severely handicapped newborns except when death appears inevitable, when treatment merely prolongs inevitable death, or when treatment is so futile as to be inhumane. The 1984 regulations give broader discretion to providers and parents than the original bill and carry out provisions of the Child Abuse Prevention Amendments of 1984.

bacampicillin (bah-kam″pĭ-sil′in) a semisynthetic penicillin of the AMPICILLIN class, administered orally as the hydrochloride salt; it is hydrolyzed to ampicillin in the body and has antibiotic activity and uses similar to those of the parent drug.

bacillary (bas′ĭ-lar″e) pertaining to bacilli or to rodlike structures.

b. dysentery the most common and violent form of dysentery, caused by bacteria of the genus *Shigella*. It is most common in the tropics, the subtropics, and East Asia and can be fatal, especially among children. It can erupt anyplace where sanitation is poor and large groups of people, including carriers of the disease, are crowded together.

The disease is spread through the feces of carriers who have the bacteria in their intestines; such individuals may have diarrhea or dysentery or may seem perfectly well in spite of carrying the disease. Infection may come after eating or drinking from anything contaminated with bacteria from the feces of these carriers. Even touching something contaminated and then touching the mouth can cause infection. Flies also spread the disease.

Attacks of bacillary dysentery are always acute after the incubation period of a few days. Temperature may rise as high as 40°C (104°F), sometimes with symptoms of dehydration, shock, and delirium. Bowel movements may be as many as 30 to 40 a day. Running its normal course, without special medicines, it is usually over within a few weeks from its outset, although an attack in a child may be more serious and last longer.

Ampicillin is the drug of choice for sensitive strains of *Shigella* in the United States and is usually effective in relieving the symptoms and controlling bacillary dysentery in a day or two.

The greatest threat of dysentery is from deficient fluid VOLUME and electrolyte imbalance, which must be corrected by the intravenous administration of fluids and electrolytes lost in the watery stools.

Although the usual dysenteric illness may last a few weeks if not treated with special medicines, symptoms of intestinal ulceration, diarrhea, and painful spasms in evacuating may in a few cases continue for a longer time.

bacillemia (bas″ĭ-le′me-ah) the presence of bacilli in the blood.

bacille (bah-sēl′) bacillus.

b. **Calmette-Guérin** (BCG) *Mycobacterium bovis* that has been rendered completely avirulent by cultivation over a long period on bile-glycerol-potato medium. See also BCG VACCINE and BCG SOLUTION.

bacilli (bah-sil′i) [L.] plural of BACILLUS.

bacilliform (bah-sil′ĭ-form) having the appearance of a bacillus; rod-shaped.

bacilluria (bas″il-u′re-ah) BACTERIURIA with BACILLI in the urine.

Bacillus (bah-sil′us) a genus of aerobic or facultatively anaerobic, spore-forming rods, most of which are gram-positive and motile. There are three pathogenic species: *B. an′thracis,* which causes anthrax; *B. ce′reus,* a common soil saprophyte that causes food poisoning by the formation of an enterotoxin in contaminated foods; and *B. sub′tilis,* a common soil and water saprophyte that often occurs as a laboratory contaminant and occasionally causes conjunctivitis. *B. subtilis* also produces the antibacterial agent BACITRACIN.

bacillus (bah-sil′us), pl. *bacil′li* [L.] 1. an organism of the genus *Bacillus.* 2. any rod-shaped bacterium.

anthrax b. *Bacillus anthracis.*

Calmette-Guérin b. BACILLE CALMETTE-GUÉRIN.

coliform bacilli gram-negative bacilli found in the intestinal tract that resemble *Escherichia coli,* particularly in the fermentation of lactose with gas.

colon b. *Escherichia coli.*

glanders b. *Pseudomonas mallei.*

Hansen's b. *Mycobacterium leprae.*

legionnaire's b. *Legionella pneumophila.*

tubercle b. *Mycobacterium tuberculosis.*

typhoid b. *Salmonella typhi.*

bacitracin (bas″ĭ-tra′sin) an ANTIBACTERIAL polypeptide elaborated by the licheniformis group of *Bacillus subtilis*; it is effective against a wide range of gram-positive and a few gram-negative bacteria; also used as the zinc salt. It is applied topically to the skin and eye.

backache (bak′āk″) any pain in the back, usually in the LUMBAR or CERVICAL region; it is often dull and continuous, but sometimes sharp and throbbing. This is the most common cause of disability and time lost from work for people 18 to 65 years old. Between 50 and 80 per cent of individuals will be disabled by back pain, even if only for a short period, at some time during their lives. About 60 per cent of all backache is related to non-sciatic muscle strain and ligament sprain. Approximately 30 per cent of backache can be attributed to the back component of SCIATICA, although leg pain is usually a more prominent feature. Roughly 10 per cent of backache can be attributed to other causes, such as urinary tract infection, kidney stones, multiple myeloma, metastatic carcinoma, osteoporosis, osteomalacia, abdominal aortic aneurysm, spondylosis, and spondylolisthesis.

A sudden action, using muscles that are already fatigued or out of condition, is particularly likely to cause acute strain. In such cases rest and time usually bring recovery. A very sharp, persistent pain following the use of unusual force against something (for example, trying to open a jammed window) could indicate a herniated intervertebral disk or sacroiliac strain. Night pain or pain that wakes the patient from sleep often points to a diagnosis of infection or tumor.

Treatment. The initial treatment for backache usually is nonoperative. NONSTEROIDAL ANTIINFLAMMATORY DRUGS and postural rest are the hallmarks of conservative therapy and are based on the principles of reducing inflammation about the spinal nerve or related structures such as the disk or posterior facet joints, and decreasing at least temporarily the tremendous loads borne by the spine. Epidural steroids are helpful in some cases. Surgical treatment is usually a last resort and involves excision of a herniated disk, LAMINECTOMY to allow the surgeon to visualize the area, with fusion to stabilize the spine or some other type of orthopedic surgery, depending on the cause of back pain. Minimally invasive surgical procedures may also be performed.

Chronic backache that does not respond to other modes of treatment sometimes can be relieved by TRANSCUTANEOUS

ELECTRICAL NERVE STIMULATION and other modalities such as back school, antidepressants, muscle-strengthening exercises, and weight-reduction programs.

backbone (bak′bōn″) SPINE (def. 2).

backcross (bak′cros″) in experimental genetics, union between a HETEROZYGOTE of the first generation and one of its parents or an organism genetically identical to one of its parents.

double b. the mating between a double heterozygote and a homozygote.

backflow (bak′flo) REFLUX or REGURGITATION (def. 1).

pyelovenous b. drainage from the renal PELVIS into the venous system occurring under certain conditions of back pressure.

backscatter (bak′skat″er) in radiology, radiation deflected by scattering processes at angles greater than 90 degrees to the original direction of the beam of radiation.

baclofen (bak′lo-fen) an analogue of γ-aminobutyric acid administered orally or intrathecally as a muscle RELAXANT and ANTISPASTIC in the treatment of spasticity of spinal origin, such as multiple sclerosis or spinal cord injury. It is also used intrathecally to treat spasticity of cerebral origin, such as trauma to the brain or cerebral palsy.

bacter(io)- word element [Gr.], *bacteria.*

bacteremia (bak″ter-e′me-ah) the presence of bacteria in the blood. (See accompanying table.)

bacteria (bak-te′re-ah) [L.] plural of BACTERIUM.

bactericidal (bak-tēr″ĭ-si′dal) destructive to bacteria.

bactericide (bak-tēr′ĭ-sīd) an agent that destroys bacteria.

bactericidin (bak″ter-ĭ-sīd′in) an antibody that causes complement-dependent lysis of bacteria.

bacterid (bak′ter-id) a skin eruption due to bacterial infection elsewhere in the body.

bacteriocidin (bak-te″-re-o-si′din) a bactericidal antibody.

bacteriologist (bak-te″re-ol′o-jist) an expert in the study of bacteria.

bacteriology (bak-te″re-ol′o-je) the scientific study of bacteria. adj., **bacteriolog′ic, bacteriolog′ical.**

bacteriolysin (bak-te″re-ol′ĭ-sin) an antibody that lyses bacterial cells.

bacteriolysis (bak-te″re-ol′ĭ-sis) destruction or dissolution of bacteria. adj., **bacteriolyt′ic.**

bacteriophage (bak-te′re-o-fāj″) a VIRUS that destroys bacteria by lysis; several varieties exist, and usually each attacks only one kind of bacteria. Certain types attach themselves to the cell membrane of the bacterium and instill a charge of DNA into the cytoplasm. DNA carries the genetic code of the virus, so that rapid multiplication of the virus takes place inside the bacterium. The growing viruses act as parasites, using the metabolism of the bacterial cell for growth and development. Eventually the bacterial cell bursts, releasing many more viruses capable of destroying similar bacteria. Called also bacterial virus. adj., **bacteriopha′gic.**

With some bacteria, notably those of the *Streptococcus* family, infection by certain phages can dramatically alter pathogenicity, converging previously innocuous microbes into deadly pathogenic strains. The so-called "flesh-eating" viruses are a striking example. They are relatively harmless bacteria until new geletic material is incorporated via a PHAGE or PLASMID.

temperate b. one whose genetic material (PROPHAGE) becomes an intimate part of the bacterial GENOME, persisting and being reproduced through many cell division cycles; the affected bacterial cell is known as a lysogenic BACTERIUM.

bacteriopsonin (bak-te″re-op′so-nin) an OPSONIN that acts on bacteria.

bacteriospermia (bak-te″re-o-sper′me-ah) the presence of bacteria in the semen.

bacteriostatic (bak-te″re-o-stat′ik) arresting the growth or multiplication of bacteria; also, an agent that so acts.

bacterium (bak-te′re-um), pl. *bacte′ria* [L.] any prokaryotic organism. adj., **bacte′rial.** Bacteria are single-celled microorganisms that differ from all other organisms (the eukaryotes) in lacking a true nucleus and organelles such as mitochondria, chloroplasts, and lysosomes. Their genetic material consists of a single loop of double-stranded DNA, whereas the genetic material of eukaryotes consists of multiple chromosomes, which are complex structures of DNA and protein.

MICROORGANISMS FREQUENTLY ASSOCIATED WITH BACTEREMIA

Acinetobacter
Citrobacter
Enterobacter
Escherichia coli
Klebsiella
Proteus
Pseudomonas
Salmonella
Serratia
Staphylococcus aureus

Bacteria reproduce by cell division about every 20 minutes, giving them a very high rate of population growth and evolution. Genetic material can be transferred between bacteria by three processes: TRANSFORMATION (absorption of naked DNA), TRANSDUCTION (transfer by a virus), and CONJUGATION (transfer by independently replicating DNA molecules, called PLASMIDS, which can be inserted into the bacterial DNA). Some bacteria can also form SPORES, dehydrated forms that are relatively resistant to heat, cold, lack of water, toxic chemicals, and radiation.

Most bacteria have a rigid cell wall outside of the cell membrane primarily composed of a dense layer of peptidoglycan, a network of polysaccharide chains with polypeptide crosslinks. Some antimicrobials, the PENICILLINS and CEPHALOSPORINS, act by interfering with peptidoglycan synthesis.

Bacteria can have any of three types of external structures: FLAGELLA (whiplike locomotor organelles), PILI (minute filamentous appendages), or a CAPSULE (a layer of gelatinous material around the cell). Various types of pili are involved in conjugation and in the adherence of bacteria to mucosal surfaces. The capsule protects the bacterium from phagocytosis. (See accompanying illustration.)

Classification of Bacteria. Bacteria are classified into two major groups, GRAM-POSITIVE and GRAM-NEGATIVE, based on their reaction to Gram STAIN. Other important classification characteristics are morphology and metabolic reactions. A spherical bacterium is called a COCCUS. Some species do not always completely separate when the cells divide and characteristically occur in pairs (see DIPLOCOCCUS), clusters (see STAPHYLOCOCCUS), or chains (see STREPTOCOCCUS). A rod-shaped bacterium is called a BACILLUS. Some species have tapered ends (*fusiform bacilli*) or are shaped like long threads (*filamentous bacilli*) or spirals (SPIROCHETES).

On the basis of their requirements for atmospheric oxygen, bacteria can be divided

GENERALIZED STRUCTURE OF BACTERIUM

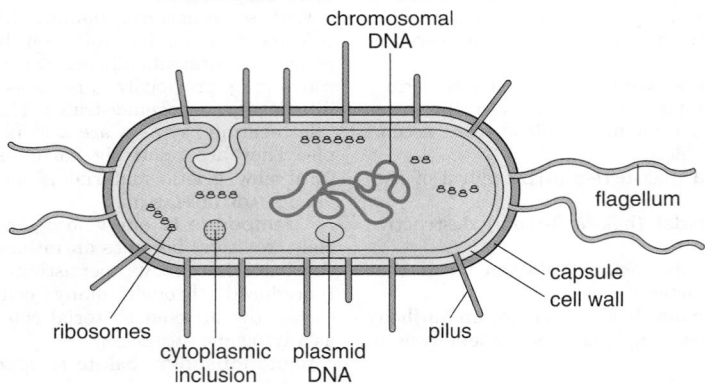

EXAMPLES OF BACTERIAL MORPHOLOGY

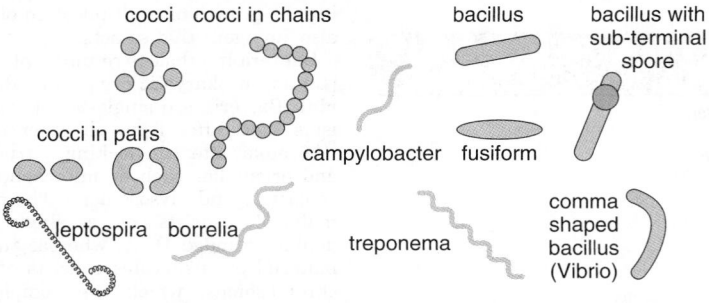

Bacterial structure and morphology. From Hart and Shears, 1997.

into *obligate aerobes,* which require oxygen; *obligate anaerobes,* which grow only in the absence of oxygen; and *facultative anaerobes,* which adapt to either environment. On the basis of their growth on a specific medium under aerobic and anaerobic conditions, certain groups are divided into *oxidizers,* those that use oxygen to metabolize sugars; *fermenters,* those that metabolize sugars in the absence of oxygen; and *nonutilizers,* which do not grow on the medium.

Two groups of prokaryotic organisms are sometimes not classified as bacteria. These are CYANOBACTERIA (the blue-green bacteria), which have aerobic photosynthesis like plants; and MYCOPLASMA, which lack cell walls.

Bacterial Infection. The skin, respiratory tract, and gastrointestinal tract are inhabited by a variety of bacteria. These normal flora are harmless or even helpful, protecting their host by interference with the growth of harmful bacteria. An opportunistic infection occurs when an organism indigenous to one part of the body invades another part where it is pathogenic. A commonly occurring example is infection of the urinary tract with *Escherichia coli* or other enteric bacilli.

There are many mechanisms by which pathogenic bacteria can be transmitted from person to person, including airborne infection, direct contact, contact with animals, transmission by insect vectors, or indirect transmission in drinking water, milk, or food or on inanimate objects. Although some diseases, such as CHOLERA and BOTULISM, are caused by toxins absorbed in the intestine, most diseases occur from bacteria that can attach to a mucosal surface, multiply, and invade tissue. To be pathogenic, bacteria must also be able to resist the host defenses: bactericidins, such as complement and lysozyme, in the blood, and phagocytosis and subsequent intracellular destruction by leukocytes.

Bacteria can cause disease by producing TOXINS, by causing INFLAMMATION or the formation of GRANULOMAS, or by inducing a HYPERSENSITIVITY REACTION. EXOTOXINS are extremely potent poisons produced by some gram-positive bacteria. These include NEUROTOXINS, such as tetanus toxin and botulinum toxin; ENTEROTOXINS, such as cholera toxin; and diphtheria TOXIN, which blocks protein synthesis, thereby causing tissue necrosis. ENDOTOXINS are lipopolysaccharides that are components of the outer membrane of gram-negative cell walls and are released on cell lysis. They can cause hypotension, fever, disseminated intravascular coagulation, and shock. Other toxins include HEMOLYSINS and LEUKOCIDINS, which destroy red and white blood cells; KINASES, which lyse blood clots; and enzymes that attack tissue.

Host resistance to infection is lowered in weak and debilitated patients and in those with a decreased ability to mount an effective immune response because of disease or the effects of drugs (such as corticosteroids, immunosuppressive agents, or cytotoxic agents).

A major problem in antimicrobial therapy is the evolution of antibiotic-resistant strains of bacteria, which are an important cause of serious NOSOCOMIAL INFECTIONS. Unnecessary overuse of ANTIMICROBIAL AGENTS speeds up the evolution of resistant strains. This problem is exacerbated by the transfer of resistance between different species by plasmids, producing multiple drug-resistant strains.

Diseases Caused by Bacteria. The different kinds of bacteria tend to affect different organs and systems of the body, producing infectious diseases, each with its own group of symptoms.

STAPHYLOCOCCI are generally found on the surface of the skin. When they invade the body tissue, for instance through a cut, they usually produce a local infection with inflammation and pus. Occasionally a strain of staphylococcus develops that can cause an infection affecting more than a local area of the body, but this is relatively rare.

The diseases produced by STREPTOCOCCI are often more serious. Streptococci tend to resist localization and may spread through the bloodstream. Among the diseases caused by streptococci are STREPTOCOCCAL SORE THROAT, RHEUMATIC FEVER, and SCARLET FEVER.

PNEUMONIA, MENINGITIS, and GONORRHEA are produced by different types of DIPLOCOCCI. The PNEUMOCOCCUS, which produces pneumonia, has its special effect on the lungs; the MENINGOCOCCUS has an affinity for the MENINGES of the brain and spinal cord. Both types of bacteria enter the body via the respiratory tract. GONORRHEA, spread by bacteria called GONOCOCCI, is usually spread by coitus.

CHOLERA, caused by a SPIRILLUM and spread by unsanitary water supplies, was formerly a dread epidemic disease. SYPHILIS, like gonorrhea, is spread most often by coitus. It also is caused by a spirillum.

BACILLI are responsible for many serious diseases, including PLAGUE, DIPHTHERIA, LEPROSY, TUBERCULOSIS, and TYPHOID FEVER. Prevention and control of the spread of many infectious diseases can be accomplished through IMMUNIZATION and proper sanitary conditions.

acid-fast b. one that is not readily decolorized by acids after staining, especially *Mycobacterium* and *Nocardia.*

blue-green bacteria see CYANOBACTERIA.

coliform b. one of the gram-negative rod-shaped bacteria that are normal inhabitants of the intestinal tract of humans and animals.

hemophilic bacteria bacteria that have a nutritional affinity for constituents of fresh blood or whose growth is significantly stimulated on blood-containing media.

lactic acid bacteria bacteria that, in suitable media, produce fermentation of carbohydrate materials to form lactic acid.

lysogenic b. any bacterial cell harboring in its GENOME the genetic material (PROPHAGE) of a temperate BACTERIOPHAGE and thus reproducing the bacteriophage in cell division; occasionally the prophage develops into the mature form, replicates, lyses the bacterial cell, and is free to infect other cells.

water b. a gram-negative bacterium capable of rapid growth in all types of water and producing pyrogenic infections, especially in immunocompromised hospital patients, occurring as contaminants in hemodialysis fluids and in flood waters. Genera of medical importance include *Aeromonas, Flavobacterium,* and *Pseudomonas.*

bacteriuria (bak-te″re-u′re-ah) bacteria in the urine. adj., **bacteriu′ric.**

bacteroid (bak′ter-oid) 1. resembling a bacterium. 2. a structurally modified bacterium.

Bacteroides (bak″tĕ-roi′dēz) a genus of gram-negative, anaerobic, rod-shaped bacteria. Organisms are part of the normal flora of the oral, respiratory, intestinal, and urogenital cavities of humans and animals; some species are potential pathogens, causing possibly fatal abscesses and bacteremias. Pathogenic species include *B. asaccharoly′ticus; B. fra′gilis,* the most common anaerobic bacterium causing human infection, most frequently implicated in intra-abdominal infections, but found in bacteremias, abscesses, and other lesions throughout the body; *B. fundibulifor′mis,* an animal pathogen also found in chronic ulcer of the colon in humans; *B. melaninoge′nicus,* which occurs in oral, lung, and brain abscesses and in mixed infections; and *B. thetaiotaomi′cron,* the second most common anaerobic bacterium causing human infection (after *B. fragilis*).

bacteroides (bak″tĕ-roi′dēz) 1. any rod-shaped bacteria that can take many different shapes. 2. an organism of the genus *Bacteroides.*

bacteruria (bak″ter-u′re-ah) bacteriuria.

Bactrim (bak-trim) trademark for combination preparations of TRIMETHOPRIM and SULFAMETHOXAZOLE, an ANTIMICROBIAL.

bag (bag) a flexible container; see also POCKET, POUCH and SAC.

colostomy b. a receptacle worn over the stoma by a COLOSTOMY patient, to receive the fecal discharge.

Douglas b. a receptacle for the collection of exhaled air, permitting measurement of respiratory gases; typically used to measure dead space to tidal volume ratio (V_D/V_T).

ileostomy b. any of various plastic or latex pouches attached to the stoma either for collection of fecal material as a continent ileal RESERVOIR or for collection of urine as a NEOBLADDER.

micturition b. a receptacle used for urine by ambulatory patients with urinary incontinence.

Politzer b. a soft bag of rubber for inflating the eustachian tube.

b. of waters popular name for the amniotic SAC.

bagassosis (bag″ah-so′sis) hypersensitivity PNEUMONITIS due to inhalation of dust from bagasse (the residue of cane after extraction of sugar).

BAL British antilewisite; see DIMERCAPROL.

balance (bal′ans) 1. an instrument for weighing. 2. equilibrium (def. 1). 3. postural control.

acid-base b. see ACID-BASE BALANCE.

analytical b. a balance used in the laboratory, sensitive to variations of the order of 0.05 to 0.1 mg.

fluid b. see FLUID BALANCE.

negative b. a state in which the amount of water or an electrolyte excreted from the body is greater than that ingested.

nitrogen b. see NITROGEN BALANCE.

positive b. a state in which the amount of water or an electrolyte excreted from the body is less than that ingested.

water b. fluid balance.

zero b. a state in which the amount of water or an electrolyte excreted from the body is exactly equal to that ingested; see EQUILIBRIUM (def. 1).

balanic (bah-lan′ik) pertaining to the glans penis or glans clitoridis.

balanitis (bal″ah-ni′tis) inflammation of the GLANS PENIS.

b. circumscrip′ta plasmacellula′ris a benign ERYTHROPLASIA characterized histologically by plasma cell infiltration of the dermis, and clinically by persistent inflammation usually involving the inner surface of the prepuce and glans associated with the development of a single erythematous, moist, shiny lesion.

erosive b. balanitis due to mixed microbial infection that progresses to gangrenous ulcerations of the penis similar to the lesions seen in noma of oral tissues.

gangrenous b. erosion of the glans penis leading to rapid destruction, believed to be due to continually unhygienic conditions together with secondary spirochetal infection.

balanoposthitis (bal″ah-no-pos-thi′tis) inflammation of glans penis and prepuce.

balanopreputial (bal″ah-no-pre-pu′she-al) pertaining to the glans penis and prepuce.

balanorrhagia (bal″ah-no-ra′je-ah) balanitis with free discharge of pus.

balantidiasis (bal″an-tī-di′ah-sis) infection by protozoa of the genus *Balantidium;* in man, *B. coli* may cause diarrhea and dysentery, with ulceration of the colon mucosa.

Balantidium (bal″an-tid′e-um) a genus of ciliated protozoa, including many species found in the intestine in vertebrates and invertebrates. *B. co′li* is a common parasite of swine and sometimes causes BALANTIDIASIS in humans.

baldness (bawld′nes) total or partial loss or absence of hair, especially absence of the hair from the scalp; called also ALOPECIA.

common b. androgenetic alopecia; in men called *common male baldness* and in women called *common female baldness.*

male pattern b. see androgenetic ALOPECIA.

ball (bawl) a more or less spherical mass. See also GLOBUS and SPHERE.

fungus b. a tumorlike granulomatous mass formed by colonization of a fungus in a body cavity, usually a bronchus or pulmonary cavity but occasionally a nasal cavity; the organism may disseminate through the bloodstream to the brain, heart, and kidneys. The most common type is the ASPERGILLOMA.

ballismus (bah-liz′mus) violent flinging movements of the limbs; called HEMIBALLISMUS when it affects only one side of the body.

balm (bahm) 1. balsam. 2. a soothing or healing medicine.

balneotherapy (bal″ne-o-ther′ah-pe) use of baths in the treatment of disease.

balsalazide (bal-sal′ah-zīd) a prodrug of the antiinflammatory mesalamine, to which it is converted in the colon; administered orally as the disodium salt in the treatment of ULCERATIVE COLITIS.

balsam (bawl′sam) a semifluid, fragrant, resinous, vegetable juice. Balsams are resins combined with oils, used in various preparations to treat irritated or denuded areas of the skin and mucous membranes. Stains from them may be difficult to remove. Balsam of Peru, or peruvian balsam, is used as a local

skin protectant and vasodilator. Tolu balsam is used as an ingredient in compound benzoin TINCTURE and as an expectorant.

Bamberger-Marie disease (bahm′berger mah-re′) hypertrophic pulmonary osteoarthropathy.

bancroftosis (ban″krof-to′sis) infection with *Wuchereria bancrofti.*

band (band) 1. a part, structure, or appliance that binds; for anatomical structures, see FRENULUM, TENIA, TRABECULA, or VINCULUM. 2. in dentistry, a thin metal strip fitted around a tooth or its roots. 3. in histology, a zone of a myofibril of striated muscle. 4. in cytogenetics, a segment of a chromosome stained brighter or darker than the adjacent bands; used in identifying the chromosomes and in determining the exact extent of chromosomal abnormalities. Called *Q-bands, G-bands, C-bands, T-bands,* etc., according to the staining method used. See also LAYER, STRIA, and STRIPE.

A b. the dark-staining zone of a SARCOMERE, whose center is traversed by the H band.

H b. a pale zone sometimes seen traversing the center of the A band of a striated MYOFIBRIL.

I b. the band within a striated myofibril, seen as a light region under the light microscope and as a dark region under polarized light.

M b. the narrow dark band in the center of the H band.

matrix b. a cylindrical metal band with a special clamp or holder (the matrix RETAINER); it is filled with softened impression compound and seated over a tooth so that the compound flows into the prepared cavity and an impression of the tooth can be obtained. It is also used for placement and contouring of certain restorative materials.

orthodontic b. a band fitted over a tooth to anchor an orthodontic fixed APPLIANCE.

Z b. a thin membrane in a MYOFIBRIL, seen on longitudinal section as a dark line in the center of the I band; the distance between Z bands delimits the SARCOMERES of striated muscle.

bandage (ban′dij) 1. a strip or roll of gauze or other material for wrapping or binding any part of the body. 2. to cover by wrapping with such material. Bandages may be used to stop the flow of blood, absorb drainage, cushion the injured area, provide a safeguard against contamination, hold a medicated dressing in place, hold a splint in position, or otherwise immobilize an injured part of the body to prevent further injury and to facilitate healing.

Application of Bandages. In applying a bandage: (1) If the skin is broken a sterile pad or several thicknesses of sterile gauze should be placed over the wound before tape or bandaging material is applied over the pad to hold it in place. Adhesive tape is never applied directly on a wound. (2) The bandage should not be made so tight that it interferes with circulation. A pressure bandage should be applied only for the purpose of arresting hemorrhage. (3) A bandage does not have to look good to be effective; in an emergency, that the bandage serves its purpose is more important than its appearance.

Ace b. trademark for a bandage of woven elastic material.

adhesive b. a sterile compress of layers of gauze or other material, affixed to a fabric or film coated with a pressure-sensitive adhesive.

cravat b. one made by bringing the point of a triangular bandage to the middle of the base and then folding lengthwise to the desired width.

demigauntlet b. one that covers the hand, but leaves the fingers uncovered.

Esmarch's b. a rubber bandage applied upward around a part (from the distal to the proximal part) to expel blood from it; the part is often elevated as the elastic pressure is applied. This is often used in conjunction with a pneumatic tourniquet. Called also Martin bandage.

figure-of-eight b. one in which the turns cross each other like the figure 8.

gauntlet b. one that covers the hands and fingers like a glove.

Martin b. Esmarch's bandage.

plaster b. a bandage stiffened with a paste of plaster of Paris.

pressure b. one for applying pressure, for the purpose of arresting hemorrhage; pressure is applied directly over the wound.

recurrent b. one used on a distal stump, such as that of a finger, toe, or limb, turned lengthwise to cover the end of the stump and secured in place by circular turns.

roller b. a tightly rolled, circular bandage of varying widths and materials, often prepared commercially. In an emergency, strips may be torn from a sheet or piece of yard goods and rolled. When more than a few inches of length is needed, rolling is essential for quick and clean bandaging.

Scultetus b. a large rectangular cloth bandage whose ends are split into many tails; the tails overlap each other and are tied or pinned across a compress covering the bandaged area, usually the abdomen.

spiral b. a roller bandage applied spirally around a limb.

tailed b. a square piece of cloth cut or torn into strips from the ends toward the center, with as large a center left as necessary. The bandage is centered over a compress on the wound and the ends are then tied separately. A four-tailed bandage is useful for wounds of the nose and chin.

triangular b. one made by folding or cutting a large square of cloth diagonally. It may form a sling for an injured arm, or can be folded several times into a cravat of any desired width.

banding (band'ing) 1. the act of encircling and binding with a thin strip of material. 2. in genetics, any of several techniques of staining chromosomes so that a characteristic pattern of transverse dark and light bands becomes visible, permitting identification of individual chromosome pairs.

Bandl's ring (bahn'd'lz) a pathologic retraction RING at the juncture of the upper and lower segments of the uterus occurring at any stage of dysfunctional or obstructed labor. Normally, as contractions progress during labor the upper segment of the uterus becomes thicker and more active while the lower segment becomes thin-walled, supple, and passive. The boundary between the two points is marked by a normal physiologic retraction RING. In difficult labor the ring can become hardened and more prominent. The pathologic ring is observed as an indentation in the abdomen as the ring rises against the abdominal wall. The uterine wall below the pathologic ring becomes thin and distended as labor continues. If obstruction to the passage of the fetus and placenta is not relieved, the lower segment of the uterus may rupture.

bank (bank) a stored supply of human material or tissues for future use by other individuals, such as a BLOOD BANK, bone bank, EYE BANK, or skin bank.

Banti's disease (ban'tēz) congestive splenomegaly.

Banting (ban'ting) Sir Frederick Grant (1891–1941). Canadian scientist. Born in Allison, Ontario, and educated at the University of Toronto, Banting undertook research on the internal secretion of the pancreas, and in 1921, with Charles Herbert Best, he discovered insulin. Banting and J. J. R. Macleod shared the Nobel prize for medicine in 1923. The Banting Research Foundation was established in 1924, and the Banting Institute was opened in Toronto in 1930. Banting was knighted in 1934.

bar (bahr) 1. a structure having greater length than width, and often some degree of rigidity. **2.** a heavy wire or a wrought or cast metal segment, longer than its width, used to connect parts of a removable partial denture. **3.** a long narrow rigid structure that a patient can grasp to assist in stabilization.

grab b. a fixed bar in the bathroom to assist a patient in preventing falls while bathing or toileting.

median b. a fibrotic formation across the neck of the prostate, producing obstruction of the urethra.

parallel b's a set of bars running parallel to each other; the patient holds them with the hands to ambulate safely.

tarsal b. tarsal coalition.

baragnosis (bar″ag-no′sis) impairment of the ability to perceive differences in weight or pressure.

barbiturate (bahr-bich′er-it) any of a class of SEDATIVE-HYPNOTIC agents derived from BARBITURIC ACID or THIOBARBITURIC ACID and classified into long-, intermediate-, short-, and ultrashort-acting classes. The ultra-short-acting barbiturates, such as THIOPENTAL, are used as intravenous ANESTHETICS. The long-acting barbiturate PHENOBARBITAL is an important ANTICONVULSANT used in treatment of EPILEPSY. Barbiturates should not be used as a routine medication for anxiety or insomnia. In addition to numerous side effects, the risk of DEPENDENCY is great. Barbiturates should be used only by the person for whom they have been prescribed. Abrupt WITHDRAWAL is associated with seizure activity.

Barbiturate poisoning was one of the most common methods of suicide in the industrialized world prior to the introduction of BENZODIAZEPINES. Barbiturate overdose is often fatal and should be treated with utmost promptness. If it occurs in the home, a POISON CONTROL CENTER should be contacted, as well as a health care provider and emergency services. The victim should be made to vomit *(only if awake)* and should be kept warm with breathing facilitated by proper positioning and removal of constricting clothing.

barbituric acid (bahr″bi-tu′rik) the parent substance of the BARBITURATES, not itself a central nervous system depressant.

barbotage (bahr″bo-tahzh′) [Fr.] repeated alternate injection and withdrawal of fluid with a syringe, as in gastric lavage or administration of an anesthetic agent into the subarachnoid space by alternate injection of part of the anesthetic and withdrawal of cerebrospinal fluid into the syringe.

baresthesia (bar″es-the′zhah) sensibility for weight or pressure.

baresthesiometer (bar″es-the″ze-om′ĕ-ter) an instrument for estimating the acuteness of the sense of weight or pressure.

bariatrics (bar″e-at′riks) a field of medicine encompassing the study of overweight, its causes, prevention, and treatment.

barium (Ba) (bar′e-um) a chemical element, atomic number 56, atomic weight 137.34. (See Appendix 6.) Ingestion of excessive amounts can be toxic, occasionally resulting in fatal hypokalemia and paralysis.

b. sulfate a water-insoluble salt used as an opaque contrast medium for x-ray examination of the digestive tract.

b. test x-ray examination using a barium mixture to help locate disorders in the esophagus, stomach, duodenum, and small and large intestines. Such conditions as peptic ulcer, benign or malignant tumors, colitis, or enlargement of organs that might be causing pressure on the stomach may be readily identified with the use of barium tests. If perforation exists or is suspected, the barium test should not be administered. It is important to evacuate the barium completely following the study; a mild laxative is usually prescribed for this purpose.

Barium sulfate is a harmless chalky, water-insoluble compound that does not permit x-rays to pass through it. Taken before or during an examination, it causes the intestinal tract to stand out in silhouette when viewed through a fluoroscope or seen on an x-ray film.

Two main types of tests are conducted with the use of barium: the barium meal or barium swallow, for radiologic examination of the upper gastrointestinal tract, and the barium enema for examination of the lower gastrointestinal tract. (See accompanying illustration.)

Barlow's syndrome (bar′lōz) MITRAL VALVE PROLAPSE.

baroceptor (bar′o-sep″ter) baroreceptor.

barognosis (bar″og-no′sis) conscious perception of weight; the faculty by which weight is recognized.

baro-otitis (bar″o-o-ti′tis) barotitis.

barophilic (bar″o-fil′ik) growing best under high atmospheric pressure; said of bacteria.

baroreceptor (bar″o-re-sep′ter) a sensory nerve terminal that is stimulated by changes in pressure, as those in blood vessel walls. Called also baroceptor and pressoreceptor.

barosinusitis (bar″o-si″nŭ-si′tis) a symptom complex due to differences in environmental atmospheric pressure and the air pressure in the paranasal sinuses.

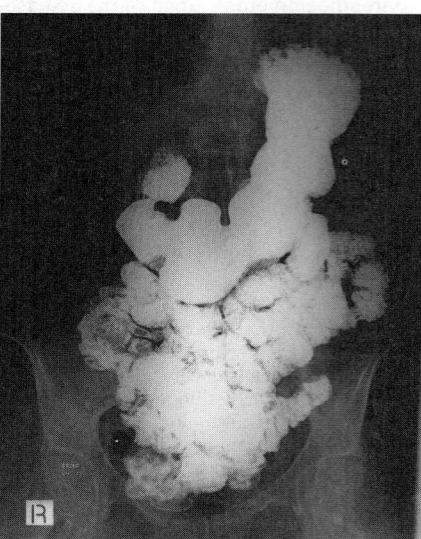

Barium test: Barium meal and follow-through. Normal stomach and small bowel. From Aspinall and Taylor-Robinson, 2001.

barotaxis (bar″o-tak′sis) stimulation of living matter by change of atmospheric pressure.

barotitis (bar″o-ti′tis) an inflammatory condition of the ear due to exposure to differing atmospheric pressures, such as those experienced when in an airplane.

b. **me′dia** a symptom complex consisting of ear pain, dizziness, and muffled hearing, caused by difference between the atmospheric pressure of the environment and air pressure in the middle ear.

barotrauma (bar″o-traw′mah) injury caused by pressure differences between the external environment and the inside of a bodily structure. Seen with structures of the ear, in high altitude flyers and others (see BAROTITIS MEDIA and BAROSINUSITIS). In the lung it is caused by excessive airway pressures, resulting in extra-alveolar air, as in PNEUMOTHORAX, PNEUMOMEDIASTINUM, or PNEUMOPERITONEUM.

barracuda any of various carnivorous marine fish of the genus *Sphaerena,* found in tropical waters; they are often eaten by humans but sometimes contain CIGUATOXIN and can cause CIGUATERA.

Barrett's syndrome (bar′ets) PEPTIC ULCER of the lower esophagus, often with stricture, due to the presence of columnar-lined epithelium in the esophagus, sometimes containing functional mucous cells, parietal cells, or chief cells, instead of the normal squamous cell epithelium. It is sometimes premalignant, followed by esophageal adenocarcinoma.

barrier (bar′e-er) 1. an obstruction. 2. a partition between two fluid compartments in the body. 3. a covering used to prevent contact with body fluids.

alveolar-capillary b., alveolocapillary b. see under MEMBRANE.

blood-air b. alveolocapillary membrane.

blood-aqueous b. the physiologic mechanism that prevents exchange of materials between the chambers of the eye and the blood.

blood-brain b. see BLOOD-BRAIN BARRIER.

blood-gas b. alveolocapillary membrane.

blood-testis b. a barrier separating the blood from the seminiferous tubules, consisting of special junctional complexes between adjacent Sertoli cells near the base of the seminiferous epithelium.

b. methods CONTRACEPTIVE methods such as CONDOMS and DIAPHRAGMS in which a plastic or rubber barrier blocks passage of SPERMATOZOA through the vagina or cervix. See discussion under CONTRACEPTION.

placental b. the tissue layers of the placenta which regulate the exchange of substances between the fetal and maternal circulation.

bartholinitis (bahr″to-lin-i′tis) inflammation of the Bartholin glands.

Barton (bahr′tun) Clara (1821–1912). Founder and first president of the American National Red Cross. Born in North Oxford, Massachusetts, she distributed supplies for the relief of wounded soldiers during the Civil War, and at its close organized a bureau of records in Washington to aid in the search of missing men. She assisted in organizing military hospitals when the Franco-Prussian War started in 1870, and began at once to establish an American Red Cross Society upon her return to the United States in 1873.

Barton (bahr′tun) George. An architect who in 1917 organized a group of individuals interested in the advancement of occupational therapy and served as the president of the group, The National Society for the Promotion of Occupational Therapy. Barton became interested in occupational therapy during a long convalescence when he recognized the importance of activity in assisting him to cope with his illness and deal with his disabilities. The National Society for the Promotion of Occupational Therapy became the American Occupational Therapy Association in 1921.

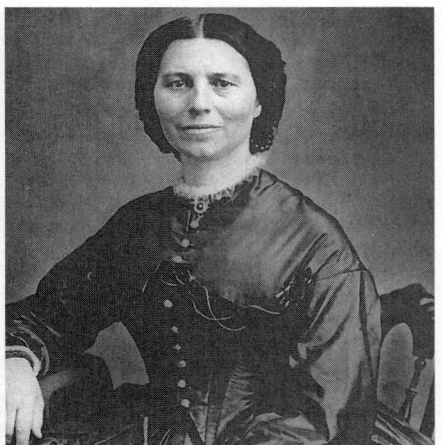

Clara Barton. Courtesy of American Red Cross.

Bartonella (bahr″to-nel′ah) a genus of bacteria of the family Bartonellaceae, made up of gram-negative cells in chains; it includes *B. bacillifor′mis,* the etiologic agent of BARTONELLOSIS (CARRIÓN'S DISEASE), and *B. hen′selae,* the etiologic agent of CAT-SCRATCH DISEASE.

Bartonellaceae (bahr″to-nel-la′se-e) a family of the order Rickettsiales, occurring as pathogenic parasites in the erythrocytes of humans and other animals.

bartonellosis (bahr″to-nel-o′sis) infection with *Bartonella bacilliformis,* transmitted by sandflies of the genus *Phlebotomus.* There are two distinct stages. The first stage (Oroya fever) is an acute, highly fatal, febrile illness associated with severe hemolytic anemia. The second stage (verruga peruana) is manifested by a chronic, benign skin eruption of hemangiomalike macules surrounded by hyperpigmentation borders. Called also Carrión's disease.

Bartter syndrome (bahr′ter) hypertrophy and hyperplasia of the juxtaglomerular CELLS of the kidney, producing hypokalemic ALKALOSIS and HYPERALDOSTERONISM, characterized by absence of hypertension in the presence of markedly increased plasma RENIN concentration and by insensitivity to the pressor effects of ANGIOTENSIN. It usually affects children and is perhaps hereditary.

baryesthesia (bar″e-es-the′zhah) baresthesia.

barylalia (bar″e-la′le-ah) indistinct, thick speech, resulting from a lesion of the central nervous system.

bas(o)- see BASI(O)-.

basal (ba′sal) pertaining to or situated near a base; in physiology, pertaining to the lowest possible level.

b. body temperature method a type of natural family PLANNING; see CONTRACEPTION.

Basaljel (ba′sil-jel″) trademark for basic aluminum carbonate gel.

base (bās) 1. the lowest part or foundation of anything. See also BASIS. 2. the main ingredient of a compound. 3. the nonacid part of a salt; a substance that combines with acids to form salts. In the chemical processes of the body, bases are essential to the maintenance of a normal ACID-BASE BALANCE. Excessive concentration of bases in the body fluids leads to ALKALOSIS. 4. a unit of a removable dental prosthesis. 5. in genetics, a nucleotide, particularly one in a nucleic acid sequence.

intermediary b. the layer of cement between a dental restoration and the tooth structure, acting as an insulator and protective barrier.

nitrogenous b. an aromatic, nitrogen-containing molecule that serves as a proton acceptor, e.g., purine or pyrimidine.

ointment b. a vehicle for the medicinal substances carried in an ointment.

purine b's a group of compounds of which purine is the base, including uric acid, adenine, xanthine, and theobromine. (See accompanying illustration.)

pyrimidine b's a group of chemical compounds of which pyrimidine is the base, including uracil, thymine, and cytosine, which are common constituents of nucleic acids.

Basedow's disease (bah′zĕ-dōz) Graves' disease.

baseline (bās′līn) an observation or value that represents the normal or beginning level of a measurable quality, used for comparison with values representing response to experimental intervention or an environmental stimulus, usually implying that the baseline and reponse values refer to the same individual or system.

basi(o)- word element [Gr.], *base or foundation; basion; chemical base.*

basic (ba′sik) 1. pertaining to or having properties of a base. 2. capable of neutralizing acids.

basicity (ba-sis′ĭ-te) 1. the quality of being a base, or basic. 2. the combining power of an acid.

Basidiobolus (bah-sid″e-ob′o-lus) a genus of perfect fungi of the group Phycomycetes, including *B. rana′rum,* the cause of entomophthoromycosis basidiobolae.

basidiobolomycosis entomophthoromycosis basidiobolae.

basidiospore (bah-sid′e-o-spor″) a type of sexual SPORE of certain higher fungi.

A

Purine

Adenine

Guanine

B

Pyrimidine

Thymine

Cytosine

Uracil

Bases. *A*, Purine and some substituted purine bases occurring in nucleic acids. *B*, Pyrimidine and some substituted pyrimidine bases occurring in nucleic acids. From Dorland's, 2000.

basidium (bah-sid′e-um), pl. *basi′dia* [L.] the clublike organ bearing basidiospores.

basihyoid (ba″sĭ-hi′oid) the body of the hyoid bone.

basilad (bas′ĭ-lad) toward the base.

basilar (bas′ĭ-ler) pertaining to a base or basal part.

basilateral (ba″sĭ-lat′er-al) both basilar and lateral.

basilemma (ba″sĭ-lem′ah) basement membrane.

basiliximab (bas″ĭ-lik′sĭ-mab) a monoclonal ANTIBODY that is an INTERLEUKIN-2 receptor antagonist; used in prophylaxis of acute organ rejection after renal transplantation.

basion (ba′se-on) the midpoint of the anterior border of the foramen magnum. (See accompanying illustration.)

basipetal (bah-sip′ĕ-t'l) descending toward the base; developing in the direction of the base.

basis (ba′sis), pl. *ba′ses* [Gr.] the lower, basic, or fundamental part of an object, organ, or substance. Anatomic nomenclature for the base of a structure or organ, or the part opposite to or distinguished from the APEX.

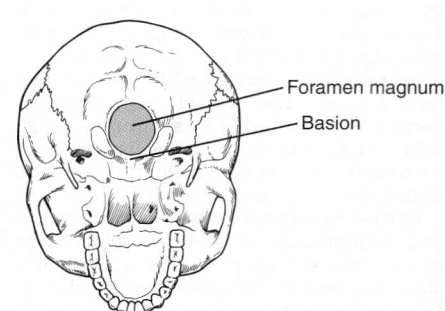

Basion, visible on the inferior view of the skull. From Dorland's, 2000.

b. pedun′culi ce′rebri the large bundle of nerve fiber tracts forming the ventral part of the cerebral peduncles, consisting of corticospinal, corticonuclear, corticopontine, parietotemporopontine, and frontopontine fibers descending from the cerebral cortex and terminating in the pons and spinal cord. Called also crus cerebri.

basisphenoid (ba″sĭ-sfe′noid) an embryonic bone that becomes the back part of the body of the sphenoid.

basket (bas·ket) a container made of material woven together, or something resembling such a container.

   Dormia b. a tiny apparatus consisting of four wires that can be advanced through an endoscope into a body cavity or tube, manipulated to trap a calculus or other object, and withdrawn.

basophil (ba′so-fil) 1. any structure, cell, or histologic element staining readily with basic dyes. 2. a granular LEUKOCYTE with an irregularly shaped, pale-staining nucleus that is partially constricted into two lobes, and with cytoplasm containing coarse bluish-black granules of variable size; about 1 per cent bring anticoagulants to inflamed tissues. Called also basophilic leukocyte. 3. one of the hormone-producing basophilic cells of the adenohypophysis; types include gonadotrophs and thyrotrophs. Called also beta cell. 4. basophilic.

basophilia (ba″so-fil′e-ah) 1. abnormal increase of basophils in the blood, seen in myxedema, hypothyroid conditions, ulcerative colitis, certain types of anemia, and other conditions. Called also basophilic leukocytosis. 2. the reaction of immature erythrocytes to basic dyes, so that they become blue or gray in color; stippling appears in lead poisoning. 3. basophilic leukocytosis.

basophilic (ba″so-fil′ik) 1. staining readily with basic dyes. 2. pertaining to basophils. 3. pertaining to or characterized by basophilia.

basophilism (ba-sof′ĭ-lizm) basophilia (def. 1).

basoplasm (ba′so-plazm) cytoplasm that stains with basic dyes.

Bassen-Kornzweig syndrome (bas′en korn′zwīg) abetalipoproteinemia.

bath (bath) 1. a medium, e.g., water, vapor, sand, or mud, with which the body is washed or in which the body is wholly or partially immersed for therapeutic or cleansing purposes; application of such a medium to the body. 2. the equipment or apparatus in which a body or object may be immersed.

   bed b. the cleansing of a patient in bed. A complete bed bath indicates that someone must totally wash a patient, as is done with an unconscious patient. A partial bed bath is one in which the patient is not totally dependent but is given a basin, soap, and water, as well as any assistance needed to maintain good hygiene.

   b. blanket a flannel covering used to prevent chilling when administering a bed bath.

   colloid b. a medicated bath prepared by adding soothing agents to the bath water such as gelatin, starch, or bran in order to relieve skin irritation and itching. The patient is dried by patting rather than rubbing the skin. Care must be taken to avoid chilling.

   contrast b. alternate immersion of a part in hot water and cold water.

   cool b. one in water from 18° to 24°C (65° to 75°F).

   emollient b. a bath in a soothing and softening liquid, used in various skin disorders.

   lukewarm b. warm bath.

   oatmeal b. a colloid bath containing oatmeal, used for treatment of dermatoses to soothe the skin and relieve itching.

   paraffin b. the dipping of a limb into a warm solution of PARAFFIN, or the brushing of paraffin onto the skin, to provide pain relief and increase mobility.

   sitz b. immersion of only the hips and buttocks, done to relieve pain and discomfort following rectal surgery, cystoscopy, or vaginal surgery; sitz baths also may be ordered for patients with cystitis or infections in the pelvic cavity. Temperature for a hot sitz bath is started at 35°C (95°F) and gradually increased to 40 to 43°C (104° to 110°F). The patient must be watched for fatigue and faintness, and an attendant must remain within calling distance. Cool compresses to the head or cool drinks during the bath promote comfort and relieve faintness. (See accompanying illustration.)

   sponge b. one in which the patient's body is not immersed but is wiped with a wet cloth or sponge; this is most often done for reduction of body temperature in presence of fever, in which case the water used is cool.

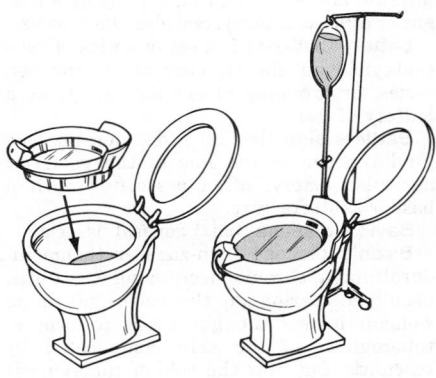

Disposable sitz bath. From Lammon et al., 1995.

tepid b. one in water 24° to 33°C (75° to 92°F).

warm b. one in water just under body temperature, 33° to 37°C (92° to 98°F).

whirlpool b. one in which the water is kept in constant motion by mechanical means and has a massaging action that can promote improved circulation and relaxation; often used in the treatment of soft tissue injuries and management of open wounds such as burns.

bath(o)- see BATHY-.

bathing (bāth'ing) in the NURSING INTERVENTIONS CLASSIFICATION, a nursing INTERVENTION defined as cleaning of the body for the purposes of relaxation, cleanliness, and healing.

bathmotropic (bath"mo-trop'ik) influencing the response of tissue to stimuli.

bathrocephaly (bath"ro-sef'ah-le) a developmental anomaly marked by a steplike posterior projection of the skull, caused by excessive growth of the lambdoid suture.

bathy- word element [Gr.], *deep.* Also BATH(O)-.

bathyanesthesia (bath"e-an"es-the'zhah) loss of deep sensibility.

bathyesthesia (bath"e-es-the'zhah) deep sensibility.

bathyhyperesthesia (bath"ĭ-hi"per-es-the'zhah) abnormally increased sensitiveness of deep body structures.

bathyhypesthesia (bath"ĭ-hi"pes-the'-zhah) abnormally diminished deep sensibility.

bathypnea (bath"ip-ne'ah) deep breathing.

Batten disease (bat'en) 1. Vogt-Spielmeyer disease. 2. more generally, any or all of the group of disorders constituting neuronal ceroid lipofuscinosis.

battered-child syndrome unexplained or inappropriately explained physical trauma and other manifestations of severe, repeated physical abuse of children, usually by a parent or other caretaker. See also CHILD ABUSE.

battery (bat'er-e) 1. a set or series of cells that yield an electric current. 2. any set, series, or grouping of similar things, as a battery of tests.

Battle's sign (bat"lz) a discoloration behind the ear in the line of the posterior auricular artery, often associated with a basilar skull fracture.

Bayle's disease (bālz) general paresis.

Bazin's disease (bah-zaz') erythema induratum; a chronic necrotizing vasculitis, usually occurring on the calves of young women; it was thought to be a form of tuberculosis of the skin complicated by vasculitis, but now the role of tuberculosis is in dispute.

BBT basal body temperature.

BCG bacille Calmette-Guérin.

BCG vaccine BACILLE CALMETTE-GUÉRIN vaccine, a TUBERCULOSIS vaccine containing living, avirulent, bovine-strain tubercle bacilli (*Mycobacterium bovis*). It may be administered percutaneously by a special technique using a multiple-puncture disk, intracutaneously, or intradermally, and it cannot be given when the patient is reactive to TUBERCULIN, when acute infectious disease is present, or when there is extensive skin disorder. It offers some protection against tuberculosis but cannot be relied on for total control of the disease. In a high percentage of cases the vaccine causes local ulcers at the site of administration. Public health officials in the United States recommend the use of BCG vaccine only for those persons living in communities having a high rate of tuberculosis cases. After vaccination with BCG, the patient will have a positive response to TUBERCULIN TESTS. See also BCG SOLUTION.

BCLS basic cardiac life support.

BCNU carmustine.

Bdellovibrio (del"o-vib're-o) a genus of small, gram-negative, rod-shaped or curved, actively motile bacteria that are obligate parasites of certain other gram-negative bacteria, including *Pseudomonas, Salmonella,* and coliform bacteria.

bdellovibrio (del"o-vib're-o) any microorganism of the genus *Bdellovibrio.*

B-E, BE, below-elbow; see under AMPUTATION.

Be chemical symbol, *beryllium.*

beaker (bēk'er) a round laboratory vessel of various materials, usually with parallel sides and often with a pouring spout.

BEAM *b*rain *e*lectric *a*ctivity *m*ap; trademark name for a map of brainwave activity derived from a computerized enhancement of electroencephalographic records.

beam (bēm) a unidirectional, or approximately unidirectional, emission of electromagnetic radiation or particles.

useful b. in radiology, that part of the primary radiation that is permitted to emerge from the tubehead assembly of an x-ray machine, as limited by the aperture or port and accessory collimating devices.

b. splitter a device that reflects light from the output phosphor of an image intensifier to a photographic recording. Called also image distributor.

beat (bēt) a throb or pulsation, as of the heart or of an artery.

apex b. the beat felt over the apex of the heart in the POINT OF MAXIMAL IMPULSE.

atrial b. an ectopic beat originating in an atrium.

capture b. 1. a heartbeat resulting from the production of a ventricular COM-PLEX by a supraventricular source following a period of atrioventricular DISSOCIATION. 2. in cardiac PACING terminology, the successful pacing of the heart by a pulse GENERATOR.

dropped b. absence of one ventricular contraction.

echo b. reciprocal beat.

ectopic b. a heartbeat originating at some point other than the sinus node.

escape b., escaped b. heartbeats that follow an abnormally long pause.

forced b. an extrasystole produced by artificial stimulation of the heart.

fusion b. in electrocardiography, a P or QRS complex that results from the concurrent activation of the atria or the ventricles by two stimuli in the same chambers. An *atrial fusion beat* results when the sinus beat coincides with an atrial ectopic beat, when two atrial ectopic beats coincide, or when an atrial or sinus beat coincides with retrograde conduction from a junctional focus. A *ventricular fusion beat* results when a ventricular beat coincides with a sinus beat, a ventricular ectopic beat, or a junctional beat.

junctional b. an ectopic beat originating at the atrioventricular JUNCTION; see also junctional RHYTHM.

premature b. a cardiac event resulting from discharge by an atrial, junctional, or ventricular focus before the next expected sinus beat and at an interval from the last sinus beat that is shorter than its own intrinsic rhythm.

reciprocal b. a heartbeat resulting from an atrial or ventricular COMPLEX caused by a return of an impulse to its chamber of origin; called also echo beat.

sinus b. a heartbeat with sinus RHYTHM.

ventricular b. an ectopic beat originating in a ventricle.

becaplermin (bĕ-kap'ler-min) a recombinant platelet-derived growth FACTOR used in treatment of chronic severe dermal ulcers of the lower limbs in DIABETES MELLITUS.

Beckwith-Wiedemann syndrome (bek'-with ve'dĕ-mahn) an autosomal dominant syndrome with variable expressivity, usually seen as a growth-related disorder in infants with risk of the development of hypoglycemia and tumors; other characteristics include UMBILICAL HERNIA, large protruding tongue, and GIGANTISM, often with VISCEROMEGALY, adrenocortical CYTOMEGALY, and dysplasia of the renal medulla. Information and peer support for families affected with this disorder can be obtained from the Beckwith-Wiedemann Support Network on the Internet at http://beckwith-wiedemann.org.

beclomethasone (bek"lo-meth'ah-sōn) a synthetic glucocorticoid administered, as the dipropionate salt, by inhalation for the chronic treatment of bronchial asthma and intranasally for seasonal and nonseasonal allergic rhinitis or other allergic or inflammatory nasal conditions, and to prevent recurrence of nasal polyps after surgical removal; also used topically for relief of inflammation and pruritus in certain dermatoses.

Beclovent (bek'lo-vent) trademark for a BECLOMETHASONE dipropionate metered dose INHALER used for bronchial asthma.

becquerel (Bq) (bek-ē-rel') the SI unit of radioactivity, defined as the quantity of a radionuclide that undergoes one decay per second; one CURIE equals 3.7×10^{10} becquerels.

bed (bed) 1. a supporting structure or tissue. 2. a couch or support for the body during sleep.

b. blocks square pieces of wood placed under the legs of a bed to change its incline; frequently used when a patient is in traction.

capillary b. the capillaries of a tissue, area, or organ considered collectively, and their volume capacity.

CircOlectric b. (ser"ko-lek'trik) an electrically operated frame similar in principle to the STRYKER FRAME. It can be rotated so that the patient is in a prone, supine, or erect position; this facilitates turning of patients with severe burns, those in some types of traction, or those with various types of spinal injuries.

Clinitron b. fluidized air bed.

b. cradle a frame placed over the body of a patient in bed for application of heat or cold or for protecting injured parts from coming into contact with the bed clothes. Cradles vary in size according to their intended purpose and can be used over the entire body or over one or more of the limbs.

flotation b. a waterbed or other fluid-filled mattress that distributes body weight evenly to minimize prolonged pressure in one area; used for immobilized or burned patients to prevent PRESSURE ULCERS.

fluidized air b. a bed that minimizes pressure and distributes weight evenly over the support surface. A gentle flow of temperature-controlled air is projected upward through numerous tiny openings called ceramic microspheres. Called also Clinitron bed. (See accompanying illustration.)

Gatch b. a bed fitted with jointed springs, which may be adjusted to various positions.

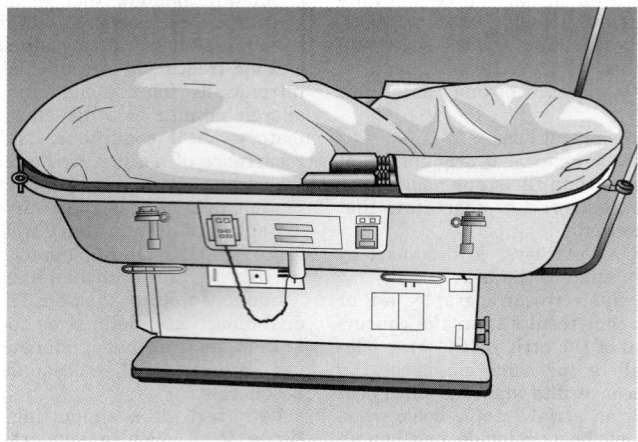

Clinitron bed or fluidized air bed. From Elkin et al., 2000.

nail b. the area of modified epidermis beneath the nail over which the nail plate slides as it grows.

Roto Rest b. trademark for an oscillating hospital bed used in the treatment of a variety of neurological conditions in which the patient must be kept still and in alignment. The bed can rock slowly back and forth, thereby preventing some HAZARDS OF IMMOBILITY. The patient is kept in place with a system of belts and specially designed pillows and packs. (See accompanying illustration.)

vascular b. the sum of the blood vessels supplying an organ or region.

bedbug (bed′bug″) a bug of the genus *Cimex,* a flattened, oval, reddish insect that inhabits houses, furniture, and neglected beds and feeds on man, usually at night.

bedpan (bed′pan″) a shallow vessel used for defecation or urination by patients confined to bed.

fracture b. a waste collection receptacle that is not as deep as a regular bedpan, utilized for patients in traction in order to disturb alignment as little as possible.

bed rest restriction of a patient's activities, either partially or completely. A person on *strict bed rest* must remain in bed at all times. Many patients are placed on *bed rest with bathroom privileges* and are permitted to ambulate to a toilet in the bathroom. Bed rest may be prescribed to maintain a pregnancy. It is associated with many HAZARDS OF IMMOBILITY and may be a greater stressor to the patient than a less restrictive activity prescription would be.

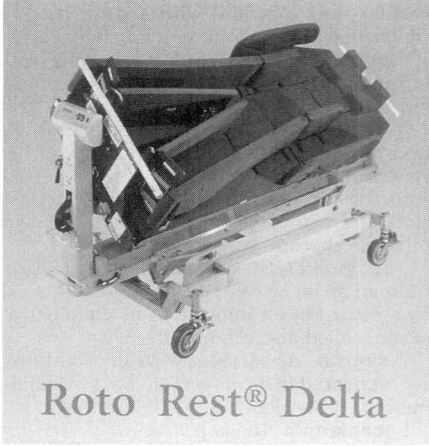

ROTO REST kinetic treatment table. ROTO REST is Kinetic Concepts' trademark for its oscillating bed. Courtesy of Kinetic Concepts, San Antonio, TX.

The cardiovascular, pulmonary, gastrointestinal, and musculoskeletal systems all suffer from inactivity and the recumbent position. Cardiac output and capacity, depth of respiration, and peristalsis decrease, while the risk of orthostatic hypotension, thromboembolism, and pulmonary disorders increases. Muscle tone, strength, and endurance decrease. Losses of muscle strength as much as 10 to 15 per cent have been demonstrated after only one week of bed rest. Over extended periods of immobility, collagen components of soft tissues begin to rearrange, resulting in joint capsule tightening and muscle contracture and atrophy. Osteoporotic changes with loss of bone density result from lack of weight bearing and reduction of muscular forces on the bones.

Measures to offset the deleterious effects of immobility are indicated for those confined to bed rest, specifically bed mobility and exercise. Such activities and exercises condition not only the musculoskeletal system, but also other body systems stressed by bed rest. Daily range of motion exercises prevent stiffness in muscles and joints and provide sensory and proprioceptive stimulation. Conditioning exercises enhance cardiac, pulmonary, and gastrointestinal function. Instruction and assistance with an appropriate exercise program can do much to promote the well-being of a patient immobilized by bed rest.

bedsore (bed'sor") pressure ulcer.

bed-wetting (bed'wet"ing) enuresis.

bee sting injury caused by the venom of a bee. The resulting pain can be relieved by SODIUM BICARBONATE, a few drops of AMMONIA, or calamine LOTION; a paste made from unseasoned meat tenderizer effectively breaks down the protein of the venom and diminishes its harmful effects. Cold compresses help prevent swelling. The skin should not be scratched as that may lead to infection. The insect's stinger should be removed as quickly as possible. A health care provider should be consulted promptly if the pain or swelling persists, if the sting is on the tongue or in the mouth, or if any systemic allergic reaction occurs, such as generalized URTICARIA (itching). Symptoms of a severe allergic reaction, such as collapse or swelling of the body, indicate ANAPHYLAXIS and require immediate medical treatment.

behavior (be-hāv'yer) the observable responses, actions, or activities of someone. adj., **behav'ioral.**

  adaptive b. behavior that fosters effective or successful individual interaction with the environment.

  contingent b. actions that are dependent upon a specific stimulus.

  b. disorder a general concept referring to any type of behavioral abnormality that is functional in origin.

  disorganized infant b. a NURSING DIAGNOSIS defined as alteration in integration and modulation of the physiological and behavioral systems of functioning (autonomic, motor, state-organizational, self-regulatory, and attentional-interactional systems) in an infant.

  health seeking b's see HEALTH SEEKING BEHAVIORS.

  b. modification 1. an approach to correction of undesirable conduct that focuses on changing observable actions. Modification of the behavior is accomplished through systematic manipulation of the environmental and behavioral variables related to the specific behavior to be changed. The principles and techniques of this method have been used in treatment of both physical and mental disorders, such as alcoholism, smoking, obesity, and stress. See also CONDITIONING. 2. in the NURSING INTERVENTIONS

WINDOW ON BED REST

Bed rest is one example of reduced activity. Other examples include immobilization of a limb in a cast, non-weight-bearing or limb unloading, the detraining of athletes in the off-season, or the effects of microgravity in space. The consequences of bed rest affect almost every system of the body.

The effects of reduced activity on muscle and bone have been studied to prepare astronauts for prolonged space travel. Muscle atrophy, decreased cross sectional area, and loss of muscle strength are characteristics of the muscle dysfunction that occurs. Thirty-day bed rest studies of healthy individuals reported breakdown of the contractile unit of the muscle. Muscle biopsy samples from astronauts indicated specific atrophy of one of the contractile proteins. This atrophy may render the muscle vulnerable to a reloading injury upon return to earth. This same process may occur in the muscles of patients on bed rest, and would explain the muscle soreness patients experience as they are remobilized. Joint contractures, or stiffness, may occur during bed rest because the tissues are vulnerable to decreased movement and loss of the usual joint stresses. In bone there is a loss of calcium and a resulting loss of bone mass, due to reduced skeletal loading. It appears that there is greater bone resorption than bone formation. The lower weight-bearing bones are more sensitive than the upper extremities to this reduced loading bone loss.

DONNA MAC INTYRE Dip (PT), BSR(PT), MPE, Ph.D.

CLASSIFICATION, a nursing INTERVENTION defined as promotion of a behavior change.

b. modification: social skills in the NURSING INTERVENTIONS CLASSIFICATION, a nursing INTERVENTION defined as assisting the patient to develop or improve interpersonal social skills.

readiness for enhanced organized infant b. a NURSING DIAGNOSIS defined as a pattern of modulation of the physiologic and behavioral systems of functioning (autonomic, motor, state-organizational, self-regulatory, and attentional-interactional systems) in an infant, which is satisfactory but can be improved, resulting in higher levels of integration in response to environmental stimuli.

risk for disorganized infant b. a NURSING DIAGNOSIS defined as the risk for alteration in integration and modulation of the physiological and behavioral systems of functioning in an infant; see also disorganized infant BEHAVIOR.

b. therapy a therapeutic approach in which the focus is on the patient's observable behavior, rather than on conflicts and unconscious processes presumed to underlie his maladaptive behavior. This is accomplished through systematic manipulation of the environmental and behavioral variables related to the specific behavior to be modified; operant conditioning, systematic desensitization, token economy, aversive control, flooding, and implosion are examples of techniques that may be used in behavior therapy. Studies of classical and operant CONDITIONING form the basis of behavior therapy, which has been used in treatment of both physical and mental disorders, such as alcoholism, smoking, obesity, and stress. See also BEHAVIOR MODIFICATION.

behavioral system model a CONCEPTUAL MODEL of nursing, formulated by Dorothy E. JOHNSON, concerned with structural or functional problems in the behavioral system and its subsystems.

behaviorism (be-hāv′yer-izm) a theory of psychology that takes into account primarily objectively observable, tangible, and measurable data, rather than subjective phenomena such as ideas and emotions, based on the hypothesis that all actions are conditioned reflexes responding to stimuli. See also BEHAVIOR THERAPY.

Behçet's syndrome (disease) (bĕ′chets) severe UVEITIS and retinal VASCULITIS, optic atrophy, and small, shallow, painful, white or gray lesions of the mouth and genitalia, often with other signs and symptoms suggestive of a diffuse VASCULITIS; it most often affects young males.

Bekhterev's (Bechterew's) disease (bek-ter′yefs) ankylosing spondylitis.

bel (bel) a unit of relative power intensity used for acoustic or electric power; a change of one bel is a tenfold power increase and approximately doubles loudness of most sounds. See also DECIBEL.

belching (belch′ing) eructation.

belemnoid (bĕ-lem′noid) 1. dart-shaped. 2. the styloid process.

belief (bĕ-lēf′) trust placed in a person or thing.

cultural b's shared statements that individuals in a cultural group hold as true. Cultural beliefs, which sometimes are expressed as proverbs, shape the values of a culture; these beliefs and values in turn affect that culture's practices. Cultural beliefs about health and illness influence health behavior and the significance of symptoms for an individual; for example, some people believe that cancer is sent by God while other people believe cancer is in part due to personal behavior and lifestyle.

Bell's palsy (belz) NEUROPATHY of the FACIAL NERVE, resulting in paralysis of the muscles on one side of the face. The person usually has sagging on one side of the mouth, with drooling and lack of ability to whistle. Care must be taken when eating to avoid inadvertent trauma. If the eye on the affected side cannot be closed, it may become tearful and inflamed. (See illustration.) Bell's palsy is often no more than a temporary condition lasting a few days or weeks. Occasionally it may be the result of a tumor pressing on the nerve or physical trauma to the nerve. In this event, recovery will depend on the success in treating the tumor or injury. More often, however, the cause is unknown. In many cases the deformity can be reduced by plastic surgery.

belladonna (bel″ah-don′ah) 1. Atropa belladonna (deadly nightshade), a plant that is the source of numerous alkaloids, such as ATROPINE and HYOSCYAMINE. 2. the dried leaves and fruiting tops of this plant, used in the pharmacologic preparation of ANTICHOLINERGIC medications for treatment of peptic ulcer and other gastrointestinal disorders. Also known as belladonna leaf.

b. poisoning a severe toxic condition due to accidental or purposeful overdosage of belladonna. (Some herbal remedies and over the counter medications have it as an ingredient, or the plant or parts of it may be ingested.) Symptoms include dryness of the mouth, thirst, dilated pupils,

B

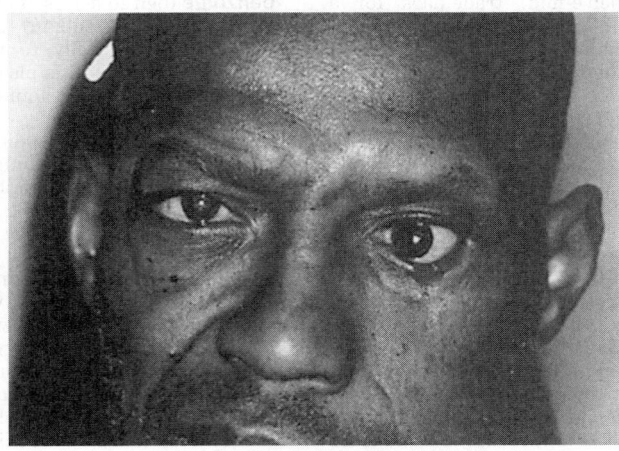

Bell's palsy. From McQuillan et al., 2002.

flushed skin or rash on the face, neck, and upper trunk, tachycardia, fever, delirium, and stupor. *Treatment* of belladonna poisoning will depend on the patient, dose, and route of administration. A POISON CONTROL CENTER or emergency services should be contacted immediately if poisoning occurs in the home. Airway maintenance, monitoring, administration of activated CHARCOAL, and control of temperature will be done in the clinical setting.

belly (bel′e) 1. abdomen. 2. venter (def. 1).

Belsey Mark IV operation (bel′ze) a procedure to correct gastroesophageal RE-FLUX, performed through a thoracic incision; the fundus of the stomach is wrapped 270 degrees around the circumference of the esophagus, leaving its posterior wall free.

belt (belt) 1. a strip of leather, canvas, or webbing that is worn around the waist. 2. to restrict by placing a circular binding around an area.

benactyzine (ben-ak′tĭ-zēn) an ANTICHOLIN-ERGIC and ANTIMUSCARINIC, used as the hydrochloride salt for its ANTIDEPRESSANT and ANTIANXIETY effects. It is contraindicated in patients with severe psychosis.

Benadryl (ben′ah-dril) trademark for preparations of DIPHENHYDRAMINE hydrochloride, an ANTIHISTAMINE.

benazepril (ben-a′zĕ-pril) an ANGIOTENSIN-CONVERTING ENZYME INHIBITOR administered orally as the hydrochloride salt in treatment of HYPERTENSION.

bendroflumethiazide (ben″dro-floo″mĕ-thi′ah-zīd) a thiazide DIURETIC and ANTI-HYPERTENSIVE AGENT; it enhances the excretion of sodium and chloride.

bends (bendz) decompression sickness.

Benedict's solution (ben′ĕ-dikts) a chemical solution used to determine the presence of glucose and other reducing substances in the urine.

Benedikt's syndrome (ben′ĕ-dikts) ipsilateral oculomotor paralysis, contralateral hyperkinesia, contralateral tremor and paralysis of the upper and lower limbs, with ipsilateral ataxia; due to damage to the third cranial nerve with involvement of the NUCLEUS RUBER and corticospinal TRACT.

beneficence (bĕ-nef′ĭ-sens) the doing of active goodness, kindness, or charity, including all actions intended to benefit others. It is contrasted to *benevolence,* which refers to the character trait or moral virtue of being disposed to act for the benefit of others. In BIOETHICS, the *principle of beneficence* refers to a moral obligation to act for the benefit of others. Not all acts of beneficence are obligatory, but a principle of beneficence asserts an obligation to help others further their interests. Obligations to confer benefits, to prevent and remove harms, and to weigh and balance the possible goods against the costs and possible harms of an action are central to bioethics.

Beneficence may be considered to include four components: (1) one ought not to inflict evil or harm (sometimes called the principle of NONMALEFICENCE); (2) one ought to prevent evil or harm; (3) one ought to remove evil or harm; and (4) one ought to do or promote good.

Benemid (ben′ĕ-mid) trademark for a preparation of PROBENECID, a uricosuric agent used mainly in the treatment of chronic GOUT and also for some forms of ARTHRITIS.

benign (be-nīn′) not recurrent; favorable for recovery with appropriate treatment. The opposite of MALIGNANT.

benoxinate (ben-ok′sĭ-nāt) a local ANESTHETIC applied to the conjunctiva for relatively short procedures; used as the hydrochloride salt.

benserazide (ben-ser′ah-zīd) an inhibitor of the decarboxylation of peripheral levodopa to dopamine, having actions similar to those of carbidopa. When given with levodopa, benserazide produces higher brain concentrations of dopamine with lower doses of levodopa, thus lessening the side effects seen with higher doses. It is used orally, in conjunction with levodopa, as an antiparkinsonian agent.

Benson's disease (ben′sunz) a unilateral condition of unknown origin, sometimes occurring with age, characterized by spherical and stellate opacities in the vitreous body, which appear to sparkle when illuminated by an examining light. Called also asteroid hyalitis.

bentoquatam (ben′to-kwah″tam) a topical skin protectant used to prevent or reduce allergic contact DERMATITIS from contact with POISON IVY, OAK, and SUMAC.

Bentyl (ben′til) trademark for preparations of DICYCLOMINE hydrochloride, an ANTICHOLINERGIC used as a gastrointestinal ANTISPASMODIC.

benzalkonium chloride (ben″zal-ko′ne-um) a quaternary ammonium compound used as a surface disinfectant and detergent, topical antiseptic, and antimicrobial preservative.

Benzedrex (ben′zĕ-dreks) trademark for a PROPYLHEXEDRINE inhaler, used as a vasoconstrictor to decongest the nasal mucosa.

benzene (ben′zēn) a liquid hydrocarbon, C_6H_6, obtained mainly as a byproduct of the destructive distillation of coal, used as a solvent. It is irritant, toxic, and CARCINOGENIC.

b. hexachloride (BHC) a chlorinated hydrocarbon; one isomer, gamma benzene hexachloride (LINDANE) is used as an insecticide, to kill lice.

benzethonium chloride (ben″zĕ-tho′ne-um) a quaternary ammonium compound used as a local antiseptic, pharmaceutical preservative, and detergent and disinfectant.

benzidine (ben′zĭ-dēn) a compound formed by the action of acids on hydrazobenzene, once widely used in testing for

occult blood; its use is now limited because it is toxic and carcinogenic.

benzoate (ben′zo-āt) a salt of BENZOIC ACID.

benzocaine (ben′zo-kān) a local anesthetic, applied topically to the skin and mucous membranes; it is also used to suppress the gag reflex in dental procedures, endoscopy, and intubation.

benzodiazepine (ben″zo-di-az′ĕ-pēn) any of a group of drugs having a common molecular structure and similar pharmacological activities, including antianxiety, muscle relaxing, and sedative and hypnotic effects. The group includes the sedative-hypnotics CHLORDIAZEPOXIDE (LIBRIUM), CLORAZEPATE (TRANXENE), DIAZEPAM (VALIUM), FLURAZEPAM (DALMANE), and OXAZEPAM (SERAX), which are used as ANTIANXIETY AGENTS; and CLONAZEPAM (KLONOPIN), an ANTICONVULSANT.

benzoic acid (ben-zo′ik) an antifungal AGENT used as a pharmaceutical and food preservative and, with salicylic acid, as a topical antifungal agent. The sodium salt, sodium benzoate, is also used as an antifungal agent and may be used as a test for liver function.

benzoin (ben′zo-in, ben-zo′in) 1. a balsamic resin from *Styrax benzoin* and other *Styrax* species, used primarily as a topical skin protectant and antiseptic. It also acts as an expectorant and thus is sometimes used in steam inhalations in treating respiratory disorders. 2. a highly toxic compound prepared from benzaldehyde and cyanide, used in organic synthesis.

benzol (ben′zol) benzene.

benzonatate (ben-zo′nah-tāt) an antitussive that depresses cough without affecting respiration, by anesthetizing stretch receptors in the respiratory passages, lungs, and pleura. It is administered orally in capsule or tablet form, but should not be chewed or dissolved in the mouth because the local anesthetic action may cause numbness of the oral mucosa.

benzothiadiazide (ben″zo-thi″ah-di′ah-zīd) thiazide.

benzothiadiazine (ben″zo-thi″ah-di′ah-zēn) thiazide.

benzoyl (ben′zo-il) the acyl radical formed from benzoic acid, $C_6H_5CO—$.

b. peroxide a topical antibacterial used in the treatment of acne vulgaris; it also has keratolytic, drying, and skin peeling actions which promote evacuation of comedones.

benzphetamine (benz-fet′ah-mēn) a sympathomimetic amine used as an oral anorectic in the form of the hydrochloride salt.

benzquinamide (benz-kwin′ah-mīd) an ANTIEMETIC compound with antihistaminic, mild anticholinergic, and sedative properties; used as the hydrochloride salt to prevent and treat nausea and vomiting associated with anesthesia and surgery. Administered intramuscularly or intravenously.

benzthiazide (benz-thi'ah-zīd) a thiazide DIURETIC used as an ANTIHYPERTENSIVE AGENT and for treatment of EDEMA.

benztropine (benz'tro-pēn) an ANTIDYSKINETIC used as the mesylate salt in the treatment of PARKINSONISM and for the control of drug-induced extrapyramidal reactions (except tardive dyskinesia); administered orally, intramuscularly, and intravenously.

benzyl (ben'zil) the hydrocarbon radical, C_7H_7 or $C_6H_5CH_2—$, found in benzyl alcohol and various other compounds.

b. benzoate one of the active substances in peruvian and tolu balsams, and produced synthetically; applied topically as a scabicide.

benzylpenicillin (ben'zil-pen-ĭ-sil'in) penicillin G.

benzylpenicilloyl polylysine a skin test ANTIGEN prepared from polylysine and a penicillic acid; intradermal reaction elicits a wheal and erythema response in those sensitive to PENICILLIN.

bepridil (bep'rĭ-dil) a CALCIUM CHANNEL BLOCKING AGENT used orally as the hydrochloride salt in treatment of chronic ANGINA PECTORIS.

beractant (ber-ak'tant) a substance obtained from bovine lungs, containing mostly phospholipids; it mimics the action of human pulmonary SURFACTANT and is used in prevention and treatment of RESPIRATORY DISTRESS SYNDROME OF THE NEWBORN. Administered by endotracheal intubation.

bereavement (be-rēv'ment) a deprivation causing grief and desolation, especially the death or loss of a loved one. The period of grief and mourning following a bereavement often resembles clinical depression. See also MOURNING and GRIEVING).

Berger's disease (ber'gerz) IgA nephropathy.

beriberi (ber"e-ber'e) an endemic form of polyneuritis due to an unbalanced diet, chiefly a lack of thiamine (vitamin B_1). It is more common in areas where refined rice is the main staple in the diet; however, improved refining processes, enrichment and fortification of grain and cereal products, and improved dietary habits have now decreased its incidence. In the United States, mild forms sometimes occur in persons on extremely restricted diets. Alcoholics, who tend to decrease food intake drastically during periods of drinking, may show signs of beriberi. See also ALCOHOLISM.

berkelium (Bk) (ber-ke'le-um) a chemical element, atomic number 97, atomic weight 247. (See Appendix 6.)

Berkow formula (ber'ko) a method for determining the percentage of total body surface affected by a BURN. The formula is derived from the RULE OF NINES; that is, certain body areas account for 9 per cent each and the total body area is given a value of 99. The remaining 1 per cent is allocated to the perineum. The age of the patient is taken into consideration when applying the Berkow formula. For example, the head of a 1-year-old child is proportionately larger than that of an adult; therefore, the 1-year-old's head would account for 19 per cent of total body surface, while the head of an adult would account for 7 per cent.

Bernstein test (bern'stīn) an acid perfusion test useful in differentiating esophageal pain from ANGINA PECTORIS. The test requires passage of a nasogastric tube and instillation of an acid solution into the esophageal area. A lack of discomfort from the presence of the acid rules out esophagitis.

berylliosis (bě-ril"e-o'sis) BERYLLIUM poisoning, usually involving the lungs and less often the skin, subcutaneous tissues, lymph nodes, liver, and other structures. The fumes, oxide, salts, and finely divided dust of beryllium all may cause a tissue reaction when inhaled or implanted in the skin. *Acute berylliosis* is basically a toxic or allergic PNEUMONITIS, sometimes with rhinitis, pharyngitis, and tracheobronchitis. *Chronic berylliosis,* which is more common, is characterized by development of granulomas and a diffuse interstitial inflammatory reaction with clinical and pathological findings often indistinguishable from those of SARCOIDOSIS.

beryllium (Be) (bě-ril'e-um) a chemical element, atomic number 4, atomic weight 9.012. (See Appendix 6.) Ingestion of excessive amounts can cause BERYLLIOSIS.

Besnier-Boeck disease (bez'ne-a bek') sarcoidosis.

Best's disease (bests) congenital MACULAR DEGENERATION.

bestiality (bes-te-al'ĭ-te) zoophilia (def. 2).

besylate (bes'ĭ-lāt) USAN contraction for benzenesulfonate.

beta (ba'tah) second letter of the Greek alphabet, β; used to denote the second position in a classification system. Often used in names of chemical compounds to distinguish one of two or more isomers or to indicate the position of substituent atoms or groups in certain compounds. Also used to distinguish types of radioactive decay; brain rhythms or waves; adrenergic receptors; secretory cells of the various organs of the body that stain with basic dyes, such as the beta cells of the pancreas; and the type of hemolytic streptococci that produce a zone of decolorization when grown on blood media.

b.-adrenergic blocking agent, b.-blocker any of a group of drugs that block the action of epinephrine at beta-adrenergic receptors on cells of effector organs. There are two types of these receptors: β_1-receptors in the myocardium and β_2-receptors in the bronchial and vascular smooth muscles. The principal effects of beta-adrenergic stimulation are increased heart rate and contractility, vasodilation of the arterioles that supply the skeletal muscles, and relaxation of bronchial muscles.

Because of their effects on the heart, these agents are used to treat ANGINA PECTORIS, HYPERTENSION, and cardiac ARRHYTHMIAS. And, because they decrease the workload of the heart, they are effective in reducing the long-term risk of mortality and reinfarction after recovery from the acute phase of a MYOCARDIAL INFARCTION. They are an important adjunct in treatment of HEART FAILURE and are also used for prophylaxis of MIGRAINE.

Nonselective beta-adrenergic blocking agents affect both types of receptors and can produce bronchospasm in patients with asthma or chronic obstructive pulmonary disease. If such patients need one of these drugs, they should be given a cardioselective one that preferentially blocks the β_1-receptors in the heart.

Nonselective agents include PROPRANOLOL (Inderal), used for treatment of angina, hypertension, arrhythmias, and migraine and for prophylaxis after the acute phase of a myocardial infarction; NADOLOL (Corgard), used for treatment of angina and hypertension; and TIMOLOL, used as an ophthalmic preparation (Timoptic) for treatment of glaucoma and as an oral preparation (Blocadren) for treatment of hypertension and for prophylaxis after the acute phase of a myocardial infarction. Cardioselective beta-adrenergic blocking agents are used for treatment of hypertension and include ATENOLOL (Tenormin) and METOPROLOL (Lopressor).

b. particles negatively charged particles emitted by radioactive elements, the result of disintegration of neutrons; their source is the unstable atoms of radioactive metals such as radium and uranium. There are three general types of emissions from radioactive substances: alpha and beta particles and gamma rays. Beta particles are less penetrating than gamma rays and may be used to treat certain conditions on or near the surface of the body. See also RADIATION and RADIATION THERAPY.

betacarotene (ba″tah-kar′o-tēn) beta-CAROTENE.

betacism (ba′tah-sizm) excessive use of the *b* sound in speaking.

Betadine (ba′tah-dēn) trademark for preparations of POVIDONE-IODINE, a topical antiinfective.

betahistine (ba″tah-his′tēn) a histamine analogue used as the hydrochloride salt as a vasodilator to reduce the frequency of attacks of vertigo in MENIERE'S DISEASE, especially in patients having a high frequency of such attacks; administered orally.

beta-hydroxybutyric acid (ba″tah-hi-drok″se-bu-tir′ik) one of the KETONE BODIES, occurring in abnormal amounts in diabetic ketoacidosis and in starvation due to fatty acid oxidation.

betaine (be′tah-ēn) the carboxylic acid derived by oxidation of choline; it acts as a transmethylating metabolic intermediate and is used in the treatment of homocystinuria. The hydrochloride salt is used as a gastric acidifier.

beta-ketobutyric acid (ba″tah-ke″to-bu-tir′ik) acetoacetic acid.

betamethasone (ba″tah-meth′ah-sōn) a synthetic GLUCOCORTICOID, the most active of the steroid ANTIINFLAMMATORY agents; used topically as the benzoate, dipropionate, or valerate salts as an antiinflammatory, topically or rectally as the sodium phosphate salt as an antiinflammatory, and systemically as the base or the combination of sodium phosphate and acetate salts as an antiinflammatory, as a replacement for adrenal insufficiency, and as an immunosuppressant.

betaxolol (ba-tak′so-lol) a cardioselective BETA-ADRENERGIC BLOCKING AGENT, used in the form of the hydrochloride salt; administered orally in treatment of hypertension and topically to the conjunctiva in treatment of GLAUCOMA and ocular hypertension.

bethanechol (bĕ-tha′nĕ-kol) a CHOLINERGIC agonist and PROKINETIC agent used in the form of the chloride salt as a smooth muscle RELAXANT in treatment of urinary retention. Hypotension and dyspnea may occur as side effects; if they do, the patient is placed in Fowler's position and ATROPINE is usually administered.

bevel (bev′el) 1. a slanting edge. 2. the slanted portion of a needle tip that facilitates nontraumatic entry into a vein. (See accompanying illustration.)

bexarotene (bek-sar′ah-tēn) a retinoid that modulates transcription and expression of genes involved in cellular differentiation and proliferation; used as an

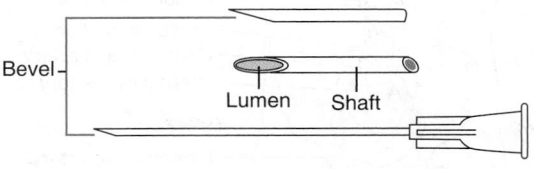

Beveled needle tip.

ANTINEOPLASTIC in the treatment of cutaneous T-cell LYMPHOMA, administered orally. It is also used topically in the treatment of cutaneous lesions of T-cell LYMPHOMAS and Kaposi's SARCOMA.

bezoar (be′zor) a mass formed in the stomach by compaction of ingested material that does not pass into the intestine.

BHC benzene hexachloride.

BHCDA Bureau of Health Care Delivery and Assistance, an agency of the Health Resources and Services Administration.

BHP blood hydrostatic pressure; the pressure exerted by the blood cells and plasma in the capillaries.

BHPR Bureau of Health Professions, an agency of the Health Resources and Services Administration.

BHRD Bureau of Health Resources Development, an agency of the Health Resources and Services Administration.

Bi bismuth.

bi- word element [L.], *two.*

biarticular (bi″ahr-tik′u-ler) diarthric.

biarticulate (bi″ahr-tik′u-lāt) pertaining to or having two joints.

bias (bi′as) 1. (in a measurement process) systematic error. 2. any influence or action at any stage of a study that systematically distorts the findings. 3. (of a statistical estimator) the difference between the expected value of the estimator and the true parameter value.

biauricular (bi-aw-rik′u-ler) pertaining to the auricles of the two ears; called also binauricular.

bibliotherapy (bib″le-o-ther′ah-pe) 1. the reading of selected books as part of the treatment of mental disorders or for mental health. 2. in the NURSING INTERVENTIONS CLASSIFICATION, a nursing INTERVENTION defined as the use of literature to enhance the expression of feelings and the gaining of insight.

bicalutamide (bi″kah-loo′tah-mīd) an ANDROGEN antagonist used as an adjunct, in combination with a luteinizing hormone–releasing HORMONE analogue, in treatment of prostatic carcinoma; administered orally.

bicameral (bi-kam′er-al) having two chambers or cavities.

bicapsular (bi-kap′su-ler) having two capsules.

bicarbonate (bi-kahr′bon-āt) any salt containing the HCO_3^- anion.

blood b., plasma b. the bicarbonate of the blood plasma, an important parameter of ACID-BASE BALANCE measured in BLOOD GAS ANALYSIS.

b. of soda sodium bicarbonate.

bicaudal (bi-kaw′dal) having two tails.

bicaudate (bi-kaw′dāt) bicaudal.

bicellular (bi-sel′u-ler) 1. made up of two cells. 2. having two chambers or compartments.

bicephalus (bi-sef′ah-lus) dicephalus.

biceps (bi′seps) a muscle having two heads. The biceps muscle of the upper limb flexes and supinates the forearm; the biceps muscle of the thigh flexes and rotates the lower limb laterally and extends the thigh. See anatomic Table of Muscles in the Appendices.

bichloride (bi-klor′īd) a chloride containing two equivalents of chlorine.

Bicillin C-R (bi-sil′in) trademark for combination preparations of the ANTIBIOTICS PENICILLIN G benzathine and PENICILLIN G procaine.

Bicillin L-A (bi-sil′in) trademark for preparations of PENICILLIN G benzathine, an ANTIBIOTIC.

bicipital (bi-sip′ĭ-t'l) having two heads; pertaining to a biceps muscle.

biconcave (bi-kon′kāv) having two concave surfaces.

biconvex (bi-kon′veks) having two convex surfaces.

bicornate (bi-kor′nāt) bicornuate.

bicornuate (bi-kor′nu-āt) having two horns or having horn-shaped branches (cornua).

bicorporate (bi-kor′po-rit) having two bodies.

bicuspid (bi-kus′pid) 1. having two CUSPS. 2. bicuspid valve (mitral valve). 3. premolar tooth; see TOOTH. 4. pertaining to a premolar tooth.

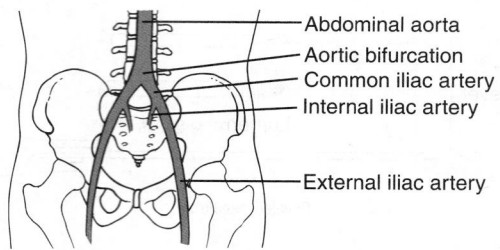

Bifurcatio aortae (aortic bifurcation), showing the branching of the abdominal aorta into the common iliac arteries, and from there to the internal and external iliac arteries. From Dorland's, 2000.

b.i.d. [L.] bis in di′e (twice a day).

Bielschowsky-Janský disease (byels-chov′ske yahn′ske) Janský-Bielschowsky disease.

bifid (bi′fid) cleft into two parts or branches.

Bifidobacterium (bi″fid-o-bak-tēr′e-um) a genus of obligate anaerobic lactobacilli commonly occurring in the feces.

bifocal (bi′fo-kal) of a lens, having two areas with different refractive powers.

b. glasses eyeglasses in which each lens is made up of two segments of different refractive powers, or strength. Generally, the upper part of the lens is used for ordinary or distant vision, and the smaller, lower section for near vision, for close work such as reading or sewing. Bifocal eyeglasses may be prescribed for PRESBYOPIA, which often occurs with aging.

biforate (bi-for′āt) having two perforations or foramina.

bifurcate (bi-fur′kāt) divided into two branches.

bifurcation (bi-fur-ka′shun) 1. a division into two branches, such as a blood vessel, or a tooth that has two roots. (See accompanying illustration.) 2. the site of such a division.

bigeminy (bi-jem′ĭ-ne) occurrence in pairs; especially, the occurrence of two beats of the pulse or two heartbeats in rapid succession.

bilateral (bi-lat′er-al) having two sides; pertaining to both sides.

bilayer (bi′la-er) a membrane consisting of two molecular layers, such as the cell membrane or the envelope of some viruses. (See accompanying illustration.)

bile (bīl) a clear yellow or orange fluid produced by the liver. It is concentrated and stored in the gallbladder, and is poured into the small intestine via the bile ducts when needed for digestion. Bile helps in alkalinizing the intestinal contents and plays a role in the emulsification, absorption, and digestion of fat; its chief constituents are conjugated bile salts, cholesterol, phospholipid, bilirubin, and electrolytes. The bile salts emulsify fats by breaking up large fat globules into smaller ones so that they can be acted on by the fat-splitting enzymes of the intestine and pancreas. A healthy liver produces bile according to the body's needs and does not require stimulation by drugs. Infection or disease of the liver, inflammation of the gallbladder, or the presence of gallstones can interfere with the flow of bile.

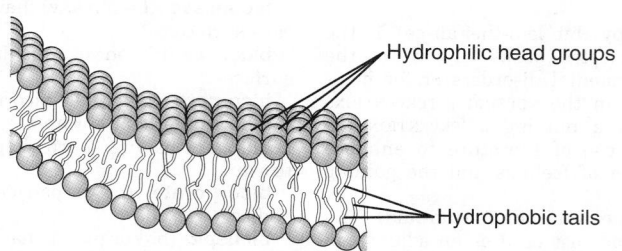

Lipid bilayer, a fluid barrier to permeability, with polar head groups exposed and hydrophobic tails sequestered. From Dorland's, 2000.

b. acids steroid acids derived from cholesterol; classified as primary, those synthesized in the liver, e.g., CHOLIC and CHENODEOXYCHOLIC ACIDS, or secondary, those produced from primary bile acids by intestinal bacteria and returned to the liver by enterohepatic circulation, e.g., DEOXYCHOLIC and LITHOCHOLIC ACIDS.

b. ducts the canals or passageways that conduct bile. There are three bile ducts: the hepatic duct drains bile from the liver; the cystic duct is an extension of the gallbladder and conveys bile from the gallbladder. These two ducts may be thought of as branches that drain into the "trunk," or common bile duct. The common bile duct passes through the wall of the small intestine at the duodenum and joins with the pancreatic duct to form the hepatopancreatic ampulla, or ampulla of Vater. At the opening into the small intestine there is a sphincter that automatically controls the flow of bile into the intestine.

The bile ducts may become obstructed by GALLSTONES, benign or malignant tumors, or a severe local infection. Various disorders of the GALLBLADDER or bile ducts are often diagnosed by ULTRASONOGRAPHY, radionuclide imaging, and x-ray examination of the gallbladder and bile ducts using a special contrast medium so that these hollow structures can be clearly outlined on the x-ray film.

bilharziasis (bil″har-zi′ah-sis) schistosomiasis.

bil(i)- word element [L.], *bile.*

biliary (bil′e-ar″e) pertaining to the bile, to the bile ducts, or to the gallbladder.

b. catheter, b. decompression catheter a catheter inserted via a skin incision through the liver and common BILE DUCT into the DUODENUM. Its purpose is to provide for drainage of bile past obstructed bile ducts and into the small intestine, where it aids digestion. Called also transhepatic biliary catheter.

Immediately after insertion, the proximal end of the catheter is attached to a drainage bag into which the bile temporarily flows. This permits observation of the catheter and amount of bile output. A three-way stopcock between catheter and drainage bag facilitates irrigation and maintains a closed drainage system to minimize contamination. After a few days the end of the catheter is capped with an adapter. The bile then flows interiorly through the catheter's ports above and below the obstruction.

Patient Care. While the catheter is attached to the drainage system the patient is monitored carefully for signs of obstruction and the drainage is observed. Bleeding

from the catheter can occur internally or externally. Hence the drainage is observed for excessive amounts of blood and the vital signs checked every 15 to 30 minutes for 2 hours, then every 4 hours for 8 to 16 hours or longer. The dressing and area around the insertion site are checked for bile leakage, which indicates that the catheter either is dislodged or is obstructed by debris. Fever and chills can indicate biliary sepsis.

After the drainage bag is removed and the catheter tip capped with an adapter, it is flushed once a day to ensure patency. The adjacent skin is observed for signs of irritation from bile leakage and the insertion site is assessed for signs of infection.

During the time observations, irrigations, and catheter care are being done, the patient and family are given instruction so that these procedures can be continued at home. They also are taught signs of complications that might arise if the catheter is not working as it should and the importance of getting help from a health care provider if the signs of complications appear.

Within about 2 weeks liver function improves and jaundice abates. Stool and urine color should return to normal, pruritus should be relieved, and the patient should be more comfortable. The biliary catheter does not cure the biliary obstruction. It is an alternative to surgical intervention when the patient is too ill to withstand surgery or has a terminal hepatic malignancy obstructing the flow of bile.

b. drainage test an examination of the contents of the duodenum at the site where the common bile duct empties into it. The test is used when other, more conventional diagnostic tests for gallbladder disease reveal no pathology but the patient's symptoms persist. Specimens are collected via the Rehfuss TUBE and examined for leukocytes, cholesterol crystals, and parasites.

biligenesis (bil″ĭ-jen′ĕ-sis) production of bile.

biligenic (bil″ĭ-jen′ik) producing bile.

biliousness (bil′yus-nes) a symptom complex comprising nausea, abdominal discomfort, headache, and constipation, formerly attributed to excessive bile secretion.

bilirachia (bil″ĭ-ra′ke-ah) the presence of bile pigments in the spinal fluid.

bilirubin (bil″ĭ-roo′bin) a yellow to orange bile PIGMENT produced by the breakdown of HEME and reduction of BILIVERDIN; it normally circulates in plasma and is taken up by liver cells and conjugated to form bilirubin diglucuronide, the water-soluble

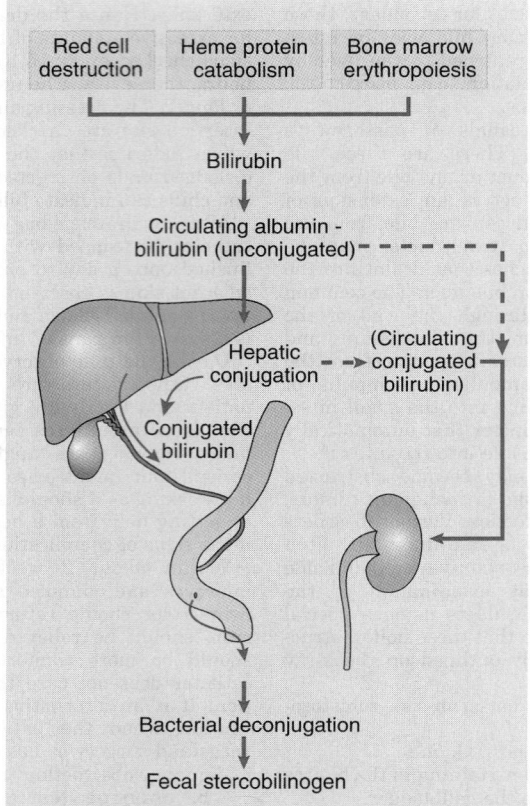

Bilirubin. The metabolism of bilirubin. Once bile is taken up and conjugated by the liver, some leakage of bilirubin mono- and diglucuronides does occur, but these normally account for less than 5% of circulating bilirubin. In bile, more than 80% is conjugated as the diglucuronide form. From Aspinall and Taylor-Robinson, 2001.

pigment excreted in the bile. (See accompanying illustration.) Failure of the liver cells to excrete BILE, or obstruction of the BILE DUCTS, can cause an increased amount of bilirubin in the body fluids and lead to obstructive JAUNDICE.

Another type of jaundice, HEMOLYTIC JAUNDICE, results from excessive destruction of erythrocytes. The more rapid the erythrocyte destruction and hemoglobin degradation, the greater the amount of bilirubin in body fluids.

Laboratory tests for the determination of bilirubin content in the blood are of value in diagnosing liver dysfunction and in evaluating HEMOLYTIC ANEMIAS.

Table (See accompanying table.) Bilirubin may be classified as indirect ("free" or unconjugated) while en route to the liver

BILIRUBIN: NORMAL VALUES

Total Bilirubin
Adult: 0.3–1.1 mg/dL or SI 5–17 µmol/L
Child: 0.2–0.8 mg/dL or SI 3.4–13.6 µmol/L
Full-term neonate: 6–10 mg/dL or SI up to 205 µmol/L

Direct Bilirubin
Adult: 0.1–0.4 mg/dL or SI < 5 µmol/L

Indirect Bilirubin
Adult: 0.2–0.8 mg/dL or SI 3.4–13.6 µmol/L

from its site of formation by reticuloendothelial cells, and direct (bilirubin diglucuronide) after its conjugation in the liver with glucuronic acid. Elevated indirect bilirubin levels indicate prehepatic jaundice, such as hemolytic jaundice, or certain types of hepatic jaundice involving inability to conjugate bilirubin. Elevated direct bilirubin levels indicate other types of hepatic jaundice, such as in viral or alcoholic hepatitis, or posthepatic jaundice, as in biliary obstruction.

Normally the body produces a total of about 260 mg of bilirubin per day. Almost 99 per cent of this is excreted in the feces; the remaining 1 per cent is excreted in the urine as UROBILINOGEN.

bilirubinemia (bil″ĭ-roo″bĭ-ne′me-ah) the presence of bilirubin in the blood.

bilirubinuria (bil″ĭ-roo″bĭ-nu′re-ah) the presence of bilirubin in the urine, a sign of liver disease or duct obstruction.

biliuria (bil″e-u′re-ah) the presence of bile PIGMENTS or bile SALTS in the urine.

biliverdin (bil″ĭ-ver′din) a green bile PIGMENT that is formed by catabolism of HEMOGLOBIN and converted to BILIRUBIN in the liver.

Billings method (bil′ingz) CERVICAL MUCUS METHOD; see discussion under CONTRACEPTION.

Billroth's operation (procedure) (bil′rōts) any of various partial or complete GASTRECTOMY operations; the *Billroth I* procedure is GASTRODUODENOSTOMY and the *Billroth II* procedure is GASTROJEJUNOSTOMY.

bilobate (bi-lo′bāt) having two lobes.

bilobular (bi-lob′u-ler) having two lobules.

bilocular (bi-lok′u-ler) having two compartments.

biloma (bi′lo-mah) an encapsulated collection of bile in the peritoneal cavity.

Biltricide (bil′trĭ-sīd) trademark for a preparation of PRAZIQUANTEL, an ANTHELMINTIC.

bimanual (bi-man′u-al) with both hands.

bimastoid (bi-mas′toid) pertaining to both mastoid PROCESSES.

bimatoprost (bĭ-mat′o-prost) a synthetic prostaglandin analogue that acts as an ocular hypotensive; applied topically to the conjunctiva in the treatment of open-angle GLAUCOMA and ocular HYPERTENSION.

binary (bi′nah-re) 1. made up of two elements or parts. 2. denoting a number system with a base of two.

binaural (bi-naw′ral, bin-aw′ral) pertaining to both EARS; called also binotic.

binauricular (bin″aw-rik′u-ler) biauricular.

bind (bīnd) 1. to wrap with a BINDER or bandage. 2. to form a weak, reversible chemical bond, such as antigen to antibody or hormone to receptor.

binder (bīnd′er) 1. a support bandage that wraps around the chest or abdomen and is secured with ties or Velcro. (See accompanying illustration.) 2. a substance that attaches to another, such as to facilitate its removal from the body; see BIND (def. 2).

phosphate b. a substance such as aluminum hydroxide, calcium acetate, or calcium carbonate that binds phosphate in the blood, removing it from circulation;

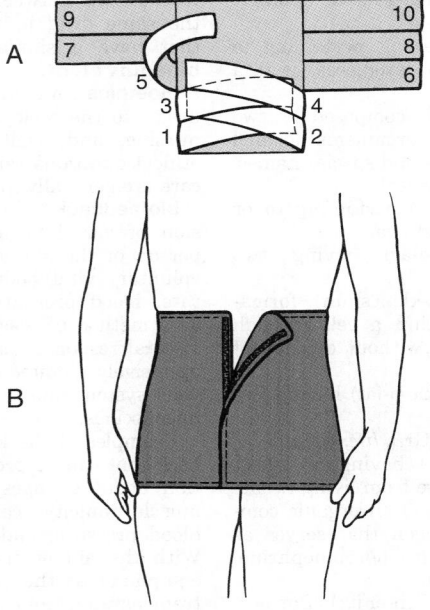

Abdominal binders. *A*, Scultetus. *B*, Straight. From Elkin et al., 2000.

used in treatment of hyperphosphatemia, such as in patients with end-stage renal disease or hypoparathyroidism.

binding-in (bīnd'ing-in″) bonding.

Binet's test (be-nāz′) a method of testing the mental capacity of children and youth by asking a series of questions adapted to and standardized upon the capacity of normal children of various ages. See also STANFORD-BINET TEST. Called also Binet-Simon test.

Binet-Simon test (be-na′ se-maw′) Binet's test.

Bing test (bing) a TUNING FORK TEST in which the vibrating fork is held against the mastoid PROCESS and the auditory meatus is alternately occluded and left open; an increase and decrease in loudness *(positive Bing)* is perceived by the normal ear and in sensorineural HEARING LOSS, whereas lack of a difference in loudness *(negative Bing)* is the perception in conductive HEARING LOSS.

binge (binj) 1. a period of uncontrolled or excessive self-indulgent activity, particularly of eating or drinking. 2. to engage in such activity; see also binge EATING.

binge-eating disorder an EATING DISORDER characterized by repeated episodes of binge EATING, as in BULIMIA NERVOSA, but not followed by inappropriate compensatory behavior such as purging, fasting, or excessive exercise.

bingeing (binj'ing) engaging in a binge, especially of eating.

binocular (bin-ok'u-ler) 1. pertaining to both eyes. 2. having two eyepieces, as in a microscope.

binomial (bi-no'me-al) composed of two terms, e.g., names of organisms formed by combination of genus and species names.

binotic (bin-ot'ik) binaural.

binovular (bin-ov'u-ler) pertaining to or derived from two distinct ova.

binuclear (bi-noo'kle-ar) having two nuclei.

binucleation (bi″noo-kle-a'shun) formation of two nuclei within a cell through division of the nucleus without division of the cytoplasm.

binucleolate (bi-noo'kle-o-lāt) having two nucleoli.

bi(o)- word element [Gr.], *life; living.*

bioactive (bi″o-ak'tiv) having an effect on or eliciting a response from living tissue.

bioamine (bi″o-ah-mēn′) an organic compound containing nitrogen that serves as a neurotransmitter, e.g., norepinephrine, serotonin, and dopamine.

bioaminergic (bi″o-am″in-er'jik) of or pertaining to neurons that secrete bioamines.

bioassay (bi″o-as′a) determination of the active power of a drug sample by comparing its effects on a live animal or an isolated organ preparation with those of a reference standard.

bioavailability (bi″o-ah-vāl″ah-bil′ĭ-te) the degree to which a drug or other substance becomes available to the target tissue after administration.

biochemistry (bi″o-kem'is-tre) the chemistry of living organisms and of their chemical constituents and vital processes.

biocidal (bi″o-si′d′l) destructive to living organisms; see also ANTIBIOTIC.

biocompatibility (bi″o-kom-pat″ĭ-bil′ĭ-te) the quality of not having toxic or injurious effects on biological systems. adj., **biocompat′ible.**

biodegradable (bi″o-de-grād'ah-b'l) susceptible of breakdown into simpler components by biological processes, as by bacterial or other enzymatic action.

biodegradation (bi″o-deg″rah-da'shun) the series of processes by which living systems render chemicals less noxious to the environment.

bioengineering (bi″o-en″jĭ-nēr'ing) the field of study that uses engineering techniques to improve the health and well-being of human beings; examples of its application are the design and manufacture of artificial limbs and body parts. Also called biomedical engineering.

bioequivalence (bi″o-e-kwiv'ah-lens) the relationship between two preparations of the same drug in the same dosage form that have a similar bioavailability. adj., **bioequiv′alent.**

bioethics (bi″o-eth′iks) the application of ETHICS to the biological sciences, medicine, nursing, and health care. The practical ethical questions raised in everyday health care are generally in the realm of bioethics.

biofeedback (bi″o-fēd′bak) 1. the provision of visual or auditory evidence to a person of the status of an autonomic (involuntary, vital) body function such as heart rate, blood pressure, or respiratory rate, as a method of teaching control of certain visceral responses previously thought to be exclusively dictated by the autonomic nervous system and therefore involuntary or unconscious.

Examples of the kinds of biological feedback that can be provided include information about changes in skin temperature, muscle tonicity, cardiovascular activities, blood pressure, and brain wave activities. With the aid of such sensitive electronic equipment as the electrocardiograph, electromyograph, and electroencephalograph, it is possible for the person to become consciously aware of the response being measured and to learn to control it. The feedback may be presented in the form of musical tones, lights, or direct visualization of scales or meters which indicate variance in the response.

In clinical biofeedback, the patient must practice the particular desired response many times under the supervision of professional persons who are skilled in the techniques of psychophysiology. An example in which biofeedback may be used clinically is in the treatment of RAYNAUD'S DISEASE, in which the patient learns to consciously raise skin temperature in the extremities and thus reduce vasoconstriction. 2. in the NURSING INTERVENTIONS CLASSIFICATION, a nursing INTERVENTION defined as assisting the patient to modify a body function using feedback from instrumentation.

alpha b. a procedure in which a person is presented with continuous information, usually auditory, on the state of his brainwave pattern, with the intent of increasing the percentage of alpha activity; this is done with the expectation that it will be associated with a state of relaxation and peaceful wakefulness. Called also alpha feedback.

biofilm (bi′o-film″) a thin layer of microorganisms adhering to the surface of a structure, which may be organic or inorganic, together with the polymers that they secrete.

biogenesis (bi″o-jen′ĕ-sis) the theory, opposed to spontaneous generation, that living matter always arises by the agency of preexisting living matter.

biogenic (bi″o-jen′ik) originating in a biological process.

bioimplant (bi″o-im′plant) denoting a prosthesis made of biosynthetic material.

bioincompatible (-in″kom-pat′ĭ-b′l) inharmonious with life; having toxic or injurious effects on life functions.

biokinetics (bi″o-ki-net′iks) the science of the movements of tissue and related phenomena that occur during the development of organisms.

biologic (bi″o-loj′ik) biological (def. 1).

biological (bi″o-loj′ĭ-k′l) 1. pertaining to biology. 2. a medicinal preparation made from living organisms and their products, such as a serum or vaccine.

b. clock the physiologic mechanism that governs the rhythmic occurrence of certain biochemical, physiologic, and behavioral phenomena in living organisms. See also biological RHYTHMS.

biologist (bi-ol′o-jist) a specialist in biology.

biology (bi-ol′o-je) scientific study of living organisms. adj., **biolog′ic, biolog′ical.**

molecular b. study of molecular structures and events underlying biological processes, including relation between genes and the functional characteristics they determine.

radiation b. scientific study of the effects of ionizing radiation on living organisms.

bioluminescence (bi″o-loo″mĭ-nes′ens) the production of light by chemicals (as in fireflies) occurring in living cells.

biomarker (bi′o-mahr″ker) tumor marker.

biomass (bi′o-mas) the entire assemblage of living organisms of a particular region, considered collectively.

biomaterial (bi″o-mah-tēr′e-al) any substance (other than a drug), synthetic or natural, that can be used as a system or part of a system that treats, augments, or replaces any tissue, organ, or function of the body; especially, material suitable for use in prostheses that will be in contact with living tissue.

biome (bi′ōm) a large, distinct, easily differentiated community of organisms arising as a result of complex interactions of climatic factors, flora, fauna, and substrate; usually designated according to kind of vegetation present, such as tundra, coniferous forest, deciduous forest, or grassland.

biomechanics (bi″o-mĕ-kan′iks) the application of mechanical laws to living structures. See also KINESIOLOGY.

biomedicine (bi″o-med′ĭ-sin) clinical medicine based on the principles of the natural sciences such as biology and biochemistry. adj., **biomed′ical.**

biomembrane (bi″o-mem′brān) any membrane, e.g., the cell membrane, of an organism. adj., **biomem′branous.**

biometrics (bi″o-met′riks) biometry.

biometry (bi-om′ĕ-tre) the application of statistical methods and measurement methods to biological phenomena.

biomicroscope (bi″o-mi′kro-skōp) a microscope for examining living tissue in the body.

biomicroscopy (bi″o-mi-kros′kah-pe) microscopic examination of living tissue in the body.

biomodulator (bi″o-mod′u-la-ter) biological response modifier.

biomolecule (bi″o-mol′ĕ-kūl) a molecule produced by living cells, e.g., a protein, carbohydrate, lipid, or nucleic acid.

bionecrosis (bi″o-nĕ-kro′sis) necrobiosis.

bionics (bi-on′iks) scientific study of how functions, characteristics, and phenomena observed in the living world can be applied to nonliving systems.

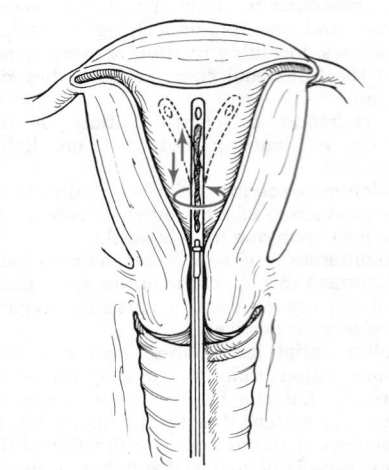

Technique for endometrial biopsy. Longitudinal strips of the endometrium are sampled using an in-and-out and rotational motion. From Rakel, 2000.

biophysics (bi″o-fiz′iks) the science dealing with the application of physical methods and theories to biological problems. adj., **biophys′ical.**

biophysiology (bi″o-fiz″e-ol′o-je) that portion of biology including organogenesis, morphology, and physiology.

bioprosthesis (bi″o-pros-the′sis) a prosthesis made of biological material.

biopsy (bi′op-se) removal and examination, usually microscopic, of tissue from the living body, often to determine whether a tumor is malignant or benign; biopsies are also done for diagnosis of disease processes such as infections. (See accompanying illustration.)

aspiration b. one in which tissue is obtained by application of suction through a needle attached to a syringe.

brush b. one in which the sample is obtained by a brush with stiff bristles introduced through an endoscope, such as for a tissue sample from an inaccessible place such as the renal pelvis or bronchus.

chorionic villus b. chorionic villus SAMPLING.

cone b. one in which an inverted cone of tissue is excised, as from the uterine cervix.

endoscopic b. removal of tissue by instruments inserted through an endoscope.

excisional b. removal of biopsy tissue by surgical cutting, such as a LUMPECTOMY.

fine-needle aspiration b. aspiration BIOPSY using a fine needle. For superficial

tissue such as the thyroid, breast, or prostate the needle is unguided, but for deep tissue it must be guided radiologically.

incisional b. biopsy of a selected portion of a lesion.

needle b., percutaneous b. one in which tissue is obtained by insertion through the skin of a special type of needle (see biopsy NEEDLE).

punch b. one in which tissue is obtained by a punch-type instrument.

sentinel node b. biopsy of a sentinel NODE (the first LYMPH NODE to receive lymphatic drainage from a malignant tumor). It is identified as follows: a dye and a radioactive substance are injected into the body, which causes certain nodes to "light up" like a sentinel, indicating that they are the most appropriate ones for examination. They are detected by both the light created by the dye and the radioactive substance that is monitored by a gamma CAMERA. If the sentinel NODES do not contain malignant cells, this usually eliminates the need for removal of more distal nodes. Called also intraoperative lymphatic mapping.

shave b. biopsy of a skin lesion by excising it with a cut parallel to the surface of the surrounding skin.

stereotactic b. biopsy of the brain using a STEREOTACTIC technique to locate the biopsy site. This can be done as a minimally invasive SURGERY technique. The patient's head is held in a special rigid frame so that a probe can be directed into the brain through a small hole in the skull.

sternal b. biopsy of bone marrow of the sternum removed by puncture or trephining; see also STERNAL PUNCTURE.

biopsychology (bi″o-si-kol′ah-je) psychobiology (def. 1).

bioreversible (bi″o-re-ver′sĭ-b'l) capable of being changed back to the original biologically active chemical form by processes within the organism; said of drugs.

biorhythm (bi′o-rith″m) a biological RHYTHM.

bioscience (bi″o-si′ens) the study of biology wherein all the applicable sciences (such as physics, chemistry, and others) are applied.

biosocial (bi″o-so′shul) pertaining to interrelationships between biological and social phenomena.

biosphere (bi′o-sfēr) 1. that part of the universe in which living organisms are known to exist; see also ATMOSPHERE. 2. the sphere of action between an organism and its environment.

biostatistics (bi″o-stah-tis′tiks) the application of statistics to biology, medicine, nursing, and other health-related professions.

biosynthesis (bi″o-sin′thĕ-sis) creation of a compound by physiologic processes in a living organism. adj., **biosynthet′ic.**

biota (bi-o′tah) all the living organisms of a particular area; the combined flora and fauna of a region.

biotelemetry (bi″o-tel-em′ĕ-tre) the use of TELEMETRY to record and measure certain vital phenomena occurring in living organisms.

bioterrorism the use, or threat of use, of biological agents to negatively affect the health of a population; the objective is to instill fear and disrupt the normal functioning of a society or culture.

biotherapy (bi″o-ther′ah-pe) the use of biological response MODIFIERS in treatment of cancer.

biotic (bi-ot′ik) 1. pertaining to all plant and animal life or living organisms. 2. pertaining to the biota.

biotin (bi′o-tin) a sulfur-containing member of the vitamin B complex that plays an essential role in GLUCONEOGENESIS and the synthesis of FATTY ACIDS. Food sources include liver, egg yolk, soy flour, cereals, and yeast. For recommended daily intake, see Section 4 of the appendices. See also VITAMIN.

biotoxicology (bi″o-tok″sĭ-kol′o-je) scientific study of poisons produced by living organisms, their cause, detection, and effects, and treatment of conditions produced by them.

biotoxin (bi′o-tok″sin) a poisonous substance produced by a living organism.

biotransformation (bi″o-trans″for-ma′-shun) the series of chemical alterations of a compound (e.g., a drug) occurring within the body, as by enzymatic activity.

biotype (bi′o-tīp) 1. a group of individuals having the same genotype. 2. any of a number of strains of a species of microorganisms having differentiable physiologic characteristics.

biovular (bi-ov′u-ler) binovular.

biparental (bi″pah-ren′t′l) derived from two parents, male and female.

biparous (bip′ah-rus) producing two ova or offspring at one time.

bipenniform (bi-pen′ĭ-form) doubly feather-shaped; said of muscles whose fibers are arranged on each side of a tendon like barbs on a feather shaft.

biperiden (bi-per′ĭ-den) a synthetic anticholinergic used as an ANTIDYSKINETIC to reduce the tremors of parkinsonism and for the treatment of drug-induced extrapyramidal reactions; administered orally as the hydrochloride salt and intramuscularly or intravenously as the lactate salt. Side effects are minor and include dryness of the mouth, blurring of vision, drowsiness, and nausea. Biperiden is contraindicated in patients with epilepsy and should be given with great care to patients with glaucoma.

biphenyl (bi-fen′il) diphenyl.

polybrominated b. (PBB) any of various brominated derivatives of biphenyl; uses and toxic hazards are similar to those of polychlorinated biphenyls. They typically are deposited in body fat stores and are rarely mobilized except through lactation.

polychlorinated b. (PCB) any of various chlorinated derivatives of biphenyl, toxic and carcinogenic nonbiodegradable compounds used as heat-transfer agents and electrical insulators; they are readily absorbed from the gastrointestinal tract, and those with a lower percentage of chlorine are associated with a higher toxicity but are more readily excreted.

bipolar (bi-po′lar) 1. having two poles or pertaining to both poles. 2. describing a neuron with processes at both ends. 3. pertaining to MOOD DISORDERS in which both manic or hypomanic episodes and depressive episodes occur.

b. disorders MOOD DISORDERS with a history of manic, mixed, or hypomanic EPISODES, usually with present or previous history of one or more major depressive EPISODES; included are *bipolar I disorder,* characterized by one or more manic or mixed episode(s); *bipolar II disorder,* characterized by one or more hypomanic episodes but no manic episodes, and CYCLOTHYMIC DISORDER. The term is sometimes used in the singular to refer to either bipolar I disorder, bipolar II disorder, or both.

bipotentiality (bi″po-ten″she-al′ĭ-te) ability to develop or act in either of two different ways.

biramous (bi-ra′mus) having two branches.

birefractive (bi″re-frak′tiv) doubly refractive.

birefringence (bi″re-frin′jens) the quality of transmitting light unequally in different directions.

birth (berth) a coming into being; the act or process of being born.

b. certificate a written, authenticated record of the birth of a child, required by state laws throughout the United States. After a birth is registered, a birth certificate is issued which represents legal proof of parentage, age, and citizenship, and is of great personal and legal importance. A birth certificate is required for many legal and business or personal transactions. Whether the child is born at home or at the hospital, the physician, midwife, or other attendant must report the birth to the local or state registrar. The report becomes a permanent record, and a certificate is issued to the parents. If a child dies during birth, an immediate report and certification of the birth and death are required, containing a statement of the cause of death.

b. control the concept of limiting the size of families by measures designed to prevent CONCEPTION. The movement of that name began in modern times as a humanitarian reform to conserve the health of mothers and the welfare of children, especially among the poor. More recently it has been superseded by the term *family planning*, which means planning the arrival of children to correspond with the desire and resources of the married couple. See also CONTRACEPTION.

multiple b. the birth of two or more offspring produced in the same GESTATION PERIOD.

premature b., preterm b. expulsion of the fetus from the uterus before termination of the normal GESTATION PERIOD, but after independent existence has become possible; defined as birth occurring before 37 completed weeks (295 days), counting from the first day of the last normal menstrual period. Approximately 6 to 8 per cent of all live births in the United States are premature, and premature births are the major cause of neonatal morbidity and mortality.

birthing (birth'ing) in the NURSING INTERVENTIONS CLASSIFICATION, a nursing INTERVENTION defined as the DELIVERING of a baby.

birthmark (berth'mahrk″) a congenital blemish or spot on the skin, of unknown cause, usually visible at birth or shortly after. Those appearing later occur at the location of a skin defect present at birth. See also NEVUS.

vascular b. hemangioma.

bisacodyl (bis-ak′o-dil) a contact LAXATIVE used before procedures involving the colon; administered orally or by rectal suppository, either as the base or as a complex with tannic acid (bisacodyl tannex).

bisacromial (bis″ah-kro′me-al) pertaining to the two acromial processes.

bisection (bi-sek′shun) division into two parts by cutting.

bisexual (bi-sek′shoo-al) 1. of or pertaining to BISEXUALITY; see also AMBISEXUAL and UNISEXUAL. 2. an individual exhibiting bisexuality.

bisexuality (bi-sek′shoo-al′ĭ-te) 1. true hermaphroditism; the condition of having gonads of both sexes. 2. sexual attraction to persons of both sexes; exhibition of both HOMOSEXUAL and HETEROSEXUAL behavior. 3. existence of the psychological qualities of both sexes, both masculinity and femininity, in the same person.

bisferious (bis-fēr′e-us) having two beats, as a bisferious PULSE.

bishydroxycoumarin (bis″hi-drok″se-koo′-mah-rin) former name for DICUMAROL.

bisiliac (bis-il′e-ak) pertaining to the two iliac bones or to any two corresponding points on them.

bis in die (bis in de′a) [L.] twice a day; abbreviated b.i.d.

bismuth (Bi) (biz′muth) a chemical element, atomic number 83, atomic weight 208.980. (See Appendix 6.) Its salts have been used for their antacid and mild astringent properties in relief of inflammatory diseases of the stomach and intestines, and as topical protectants in skin and anorectal disorders.

b. subsalicylate a bismuth salt of salicylic acid, administered orally in the treatment of diarrhea and gastric distress, including nausea, indigestion, and heartburn.

bismuthosis (biz″muth-o′sis) chronic bismuth poisoning, with anuria, stomatitis, dermatitis, and diarrhea.

bisoprolol (bis″o-pro′lol) a synthetic BETA-ADRENERGIC BLOCKING AGENT, used as the fumarate salt; administered orally as an ANTIHYPERTENSIVE AGENT.

bisphosphonate (bis-fos′fo-nāt) diphosphonate.

bisulfate (bi-sul′fāt) an acid sulfate combining a sulfate radical with a monovalent metal and a hydrogen ion.

bite (bīt) 1. seizure with the teeth. 2. a wound or puncture made by a living organism; see also at the name of the organism, such as INSECT BITES AND STINGS, SPIDER BITE, and SNAKEBITE. 3. an impression made by closure of the teeth upon some plastic material, such as wax. 4. occlusion (def. 2).

Animal Bite. Any animal bite that breaks the skin should be treated rapidly and with care. The wound should be washed at once with warm, soapy water and the victim taken to an emergency medical facility. Potential complications of an animal bite include tetanus, rabies, septicemia, and bone and muscle infections. Every effort should be made to catch an animal that has bitten someone, so that it may be confined and examined by the health department for signs of rabies. Whenever possible it should be caught alive because evidence of rabies disappears rapidly after death. If the animal is not caught, the bitten person is given antirabies treatment immediately.

Human Bite. Any human bite that penetrates the skin should be considered dangerous because a human bite can be contaminated with both aerobic and anaerobic organisms. The wound should be washed immediately with soap and water and a health care provider should be consulted. Antimicrobial therapy may be needed as there is a serious danger of infection, a danger that is more serious with human bites than with animal bites since many of the organisms carried by animals do not affect humans.

over-b. overbite.

stork b's see STORK BITES.

bitemporal (bi-tem′po-ral) pertaining to both temples or temporal bones.

biteplate (bīt′plāt″) an appliance, usually plastic or wire, worn in the palate as a diagnostic or therapeutic adjunct in orthodontics or prosthodontics.

bite-wing (bīt′wing″) a wing or fin attached along the center of the tooth side of a dental x-ray film and bitten on by the patient, permitting production of a bite-wing RADIOGRAPH.

bitolterol (bi-tol′ter-ol) a beta-adrenergic RECEPTOR agonist used as a BRONCHODILATOR; administered by inhalation as the mesylate salt in the treatment of bronchospasm associated with asthma and the treatment and prophylaxis of bronchospasm associated with chronic obstructive airway disease, including bronchitis and pulmonary emphysema.

bitrochanteric (bi-tro″kan-ter′ik) pertaining to both trochanters on one femur or to both greater trochanters.

bituminosis (bĭ-too″mĭ-no′sis) a form of coal workers' PNEUMOCONIOSIS due to dust from soft coal.

biuret (bi′u-ret) a urea derivative; its presence is detected after addition of sodium hydroxide and copper sulfate solutions by a pinkish-violet color (protein test) or a pink and finally a bluish color (urea test).

b. reaction the reaction in BIURET TESTS.

b. test either of the tests done with BIURET.

bivalent (bi-va′lent) 1. divalent. 2. the structure formed by a pair of homologous chromosomes joined by synapsis along their length during the ZYGOTENE and PACHYTENE stages of the first meiotic PROPHASE. After each homologous chromosome splits into two sister chromatids during the pachytene stage, this structure is called a TETRAD.

bivalirudin (bi-val′ĭroo-din) an inhibitor of the clot-promoting activity of thrombin, used in conjunction with aspirin as an ANTICOAGULANT in patients with unstable ANGINA PECTORIS who are undergoing percutaneous transluminal coronary ANGIOPLASTY; administered intravenously.

biventral (bi-ven′tral) 1. having two bellies. 2. digastric muscle.

biventricular (bi″ven-trik′u-ler) pertaining to or affecting both ventricles of the heart.

bizygomatic (bi-zi″go-mat′ik) pertaining to the two most prominent points of the two zygomatic ARCHES.

B-K, BK, below-knee; see transtibial AMPUTATION.

Bk berkelium.

Blackfan-Diamond syndrome (blak′fan di′ah-mond) congenital hypoplastic ANEMIA.

blackhead (blak′hed″) a plug of keratin and sebum within the dilated orifice of a hair follicle. The dark color is caused not by dirt but by the discoloring effect of air on the sebum in the clogged pore. Infection may cause it to develop into a pustule or boil. See also ACNE VULGARIS. Called also open comedo.

blackout (blak′owt″) temporary loss of vision and momentary unconsciousness due to diminished circulation to the brain and retina. Blackout refers specifically to a condition which sometimes occurs in aviators resulting from increased acceleration, which causes a decrease in blood supply to the brain cells. The term can also refer to other forms of temporary loss of consciousness and of FAINTING, as well as to temporary loss of memory and to certain forms of vertigo.

alcoholic b. anterograde amnesia experienced by alcoholics during episodes of drinking, even when not fully intoxicated; it is indicative of early but still reversible brain damage.

blackwater fever a severe complication of malaria characterized by intravascular hemolysis, hemoglobinuria, renal failure, and passage of dark brown or red urine, seen in association with intermittent quinine therapy, with *Plasmodium falciparum* infection in the nonimmune, or with interrupted exposure in the partially immune.

bladder (blad′er) 1. a membranous sac, such as one serving as a receptacle for secretion. Called also cyst and vesica. 2. urinary bladder.

atonic b. neurogenic bladder in which the bladder is dilated and poorly contracting and the lesion is not in the central nervous system.

atonic neurogenic b. neurogenic bladder due to destruction of sensory nerve fibers from the bladder to the spinal cord, marked by absence of control of bladder functions and of desire to urinate, bladder overdistention, and an abnormal amount of residual urine; it is usually associated with TABES DORSALIS or PERNICIOUS ANEMIA but may be seen with other conditions as well. Called also paralytic bladder.

automatic b. neurogenic bladder due to complete transection of the spinal cord above the sacral segments, marked by complete loss of micturition reflexes and bladder sensation, violent involuntary urination, and an abnormal amount of residual urine. Called also reflex neurogenic bladder.

autonomous b. neurogenic bladder due to a lesion in the sacral spinal cord that interrupts the reflex arc that controls the bladder. The lesion may be in the cauda equina, conus medullaris, sacral roots, or pelvic nerve. It is marked by loss of normal bladder sensation and contractility, inability to initiate urination normally, and stress INCONTINENCE.

b. cancer malignancy of the urinary bladder; this is the most common site of malignancy of the urinary system. It affects men more often than women, and it usually occurs in persons over age 50. Suspected contributing factors include exposure to industrial substances such as aniline dyes, and toxins in cigarette smoke. The artificial sweeteners saccharine and cyclamate have been shown to cause bladder tumors in other animals, but not in humans.

There are two commonly used staging systems, the ABCD system and the TNM system. The ABCD is an older system with broad descriptions. In 1997 the International Union Against Cancer (UICC) developed a new system using TNM STAGING (see Table).

The most common symptom of tumor of the bladder is painless HEMATURIA. It may come and go during the early stages of the disease, which gives the patient a false sense of security or causes him or her to be indifferent about seeking treatment. Later, there can be urinary frequency and dysuria.

Treatment. Treatment of bladder cancer depends on the type of tumor, its stage of development when first diagnosed, the patient's general state of health, and other factors. There are several chemotherapeutic agents that are applied locally by instillation and others that are given systemically; these have been shown to be of some usefulness, particularly when they are used in combinations. (See ANTINEOPLASTIC THERAPY.) Radiation therapy is often used in cases in which the disease is more advanced.

Surgery. Surgical treatment ranges from electric cauterization of the tumor mass to removal of the entire bladder (cystectomy) and diversion of the urinary flow through a surgically created opening to the skin or into an isolated segment of the ileum, called an ileal conduit. In some cases, only a portion of the bladder (*segmental resection*) is done. This is the procedure of choice when a tumor is located in the dome of the bladder or near the points at which the ureters empty into the bladder.

Patient Care. For patient care, see under urinary BLADDER.

gall b. gallbladder.

irritable b. a state of the bladder marked by increased frequency of contraction with associated desire to urinate.

motor paralytic b. neurogenic bladder due to impairment of the motor neurons or nerves controlling the bladder. The *acute* form is marked by painful distention and inability to initiate urination; the *chronic* form is marked by difficulty in initiating urination, straining, decreased size and force of the stream, interrupted stream, and recurrent infection of the urinary tract.

neurogenic b. any condition of dysfunction of the urinary bladder caused by a lesion of the central or peripheral nervous system.

paralytic b. atonic neurogenic bladder.

reflex neurogenic b. automatic bladder.

uninhibited neurogenic b. neurogenic bladder due to a lesion in the upper MOTONEURONS with subtotal interruption of corticospinal pathways, marked by urgency, frequent involuntary urination, and a small volume threshold of activity. It is associated with STROKE SYNDROME and MULTIPLE SCLEROSIS.

urinary b. a hollow container with muscular walls in the anterior part of the pelvic cavity; often called simply *the bladder*. It is joined to the kidneys by the URETERS and to the exterior of the body by the URETHRA. See illustration. Urine passes to the bladder from the kidneys every few seconds and remains there until the person URINATES (voids). Urination occurs when the sphincters (circular muscles) at the juncture of the bladder and urethra are relaxed and the muscular walls of the bladder contract, forcing the urine out. In the adult the sphincters can prevent urination even when the bladder is uncomfortably full, but in children full bladder control is slow to develop. BED-WETTING may normally continue to the age of 3 or 4 years.

Benign tumors of the bladder are relatively rare. Small, superficial ones can be treated by fulguration, using a cystoscope and an electric cautery. Normally, after fulguration there is minimal bleeding and the patient can be treated and sent home in 1 day. The bladder is the most common site of malignancy of the urinary system (see BLADDER CANCER).

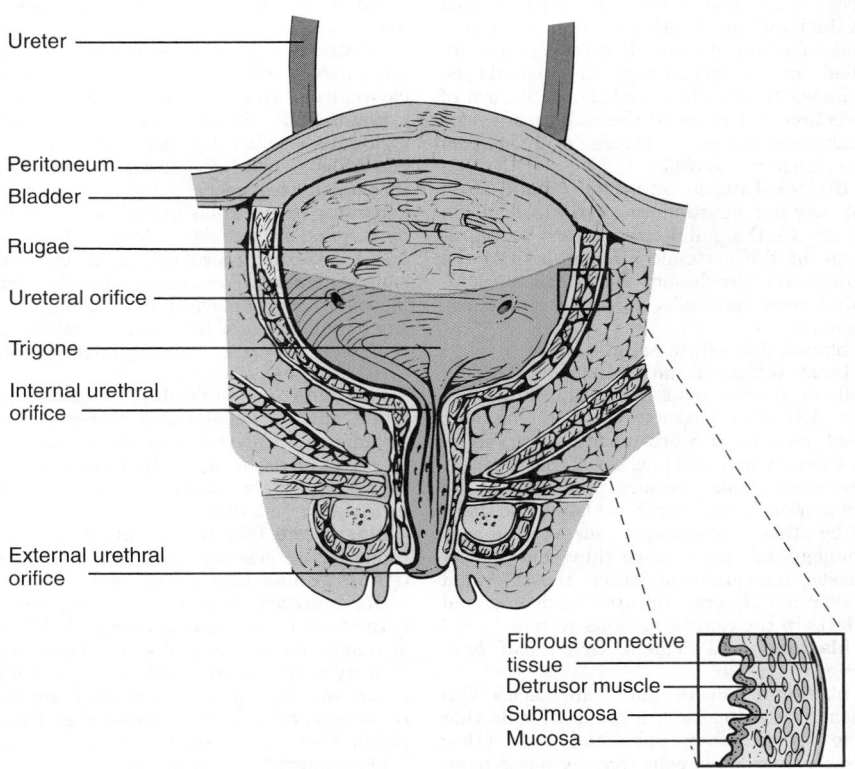

Ureter

Peritoneum
Bladder
Rugae
Ureteral orifice
Trigone
Internal urethral
orifice

External urethral
orifice

Fibrous connective
tissue
Detrusor muscle
Submucosa
Mucosa

Urinary bladder, with cross section of the bladder wall. From Applegate, 1995.

Diagnostic Procedures. One of the most common diagnostic procedures for bladder disorders of all kinds is CYSTOSCOPY, which allows direct visualization of the interior of the bladder. In CYSTOGRAPHY, a contrast medium or air is instilled into the bladder and x-rays are taken. CYSTOMETROGRAPHY is another procedure that is particularly useful in assessing the motor and sensory function of the bladder when the patient has a problem of incontinence or has difficulty voiding and emptying the bladder.

Surgery of the Bladder. For surgical treatment of bladder cancer, see BLADDER CANCER. CYSTOSTOMY is surgical incision into the bladder for removal of stones that cannot be passed through the urethra, for purposes of drainage, or for access to an enlarged prostate gland. Ultrasonic or mechanical dissolution of stones often can be done, thus avoiding the need for cystostomy; see also LITHOTRIPSY.

Patient Care. In all types of surgery involving the bladder the major concerns are

maintenance of the flow of urine and prevention of infection. The urinary system fulfills its primary function, i.e., the excretion of wastes, by continuously producing urine. If for any reason there is an obstruction to the flow of urine from the bladder, it will continue to fill, causing extreme discomfort and leading to possible rupture, or backflow of urine into the renal pelvis with resultant hydronephrosis. It is therefore essential that catheters and drainage tubes be monitored frequently and carefully.

The urine must be observed for signs of hemorrhage, the presence of clots or bits of tissue, and unusual color, odor, and concentration during both the preoperative and the postoperative periods. It is extremely important that intake and output be measured accurately. If an irrigation fluid is used either continuously or intermittently, the amount of fluid that is instilled into the bladder must be subtracted from the total amount of fluid collected in the drainage bag. In order to prevent infection extreme care must be used in the handling of catheters, drainage tubes, and collecting devices. If dressings are applied, as in cystostomy, they should be changed frequently to reduce the hazard of infection and to avoid the unpleasant odor that accompanies the leakage of urine from the incision.

Blalock-Taussig operation (shunt) (bla′-lok taw′sig) anastomosis of the subclavian artery to the pulmonary artery to shunt some of the systemic circulation into the pulmonary circulation; performed as palliative treatment of congenital pulmonary stenosis.

blanch (blanch) to become pale.

blast (blast) 1. an immature stage in cellular development before appearance of the definitive characteristics of the cell; used also as a word termination, as in AMELOBLAST and TROPHOBLAST. 2. blast cell. 3. the wave of air pressure produced by the detonation of high-explosive bombs or shells or by other explosions; it causes pulmonary damage and hemorrhage (lung blast, blast chest), laceration of other thoracic and abdominal viscera, ruptured eardrums, and effects in the central nervous system.

blast(o)- word element [Gr.], *a bud; budding.*

blastema (blas-te′mah) 1. in species with asexual REPRODUCTION, a group of cells that give rise to a new individual. 2. in other species, a group of cells that gives rise to an organ or part in either normal development or regeneration.

blastocoele (blas′to-sēl) the fluid-filled central segmentation cavity of the mass of the BLASTULA.

blastocyst (blas′to-sist) the mammalian conceptus in the post-morula stage, consisting of the trophoblast and an inner cell mass. (See accompanying illustration.)

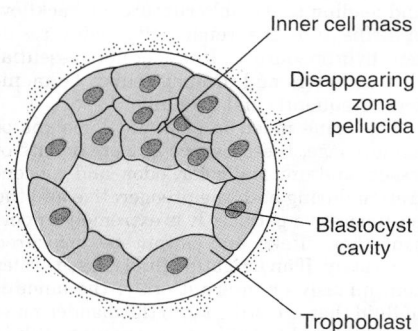

Early blastocyst. From Dorland's, 2000.

blastocyte (blas′to-sīt) an undifferentiated embryonic cell.

blastocytoma (blas″to-si-to′mah) blastoma.

blastoderm (blas′to-derm) a disk of cells lying betwen the yolk sac and the amniotic cavity, from which the embryo develops.

blastodisc (blas′to-disk) the convex structure formed by the BLASTOMERES at the animal pole of a ZYGOTE undergoing incomplete cleavage.

blastogenesis (blas″to-jen′ĕ-sis) 1. development of an individual from a blastema, i.e., by asexual reproduction. 2. transmission of inherited characters by the germ plasm. 3. morphological transformation of small lymphocytes into large lymphocytes (lymphoblasts) that accompanies lymphocyte ACTIVATION.

blastoma (blas-to′mah), pl. *blastomas, blasto′mata* A neoplasm composed of embryonic cells derived from the blastema of an organ or tissue. adj., **blasto′matous.**

blastomatosis (blas″to-mah-to′sis) the formation of BLASTOMAS.

blastomere (blas′to-mēr) one of the cells produced by cleavage of a fertilized ovum (ZYGOTE). Called also cleavage cell.

Blastomyces (blas″to-mi′sēz) a genus of pathogenic fungi growing as mycelial forms at room temperature and as yeastlike forms at body temperature; applied to the yeasts pathogenic for humans and other animals. *B. dermati′tidis* is the species that causes North American BLASTOMYCOSIS.

blastomycete (blas″to-mi′sēt) 1. any organism of the genus *Blastomyces.* 2. any yeastlike organism.

blastomycosis (blas″to-mi-ko′sis) 1. infection with any yeastlike organism. 2. an infection usually acquired through the pulmonary route, caused by *Blastomyces dermatitidis.* There may be suppurating tumors in the skin *(cutaneous b.)* or lesions in the lungs, bones, subcutaneous tissues, liver, spleen, and kidneys *(systemic b.).* It runs a fulminant, sometimes fatal, course in immunocompromised patients. Called also North American blastomycosis.

North American b. blastomycosis (def. 2).

South American b. paracoccidioidomycosis.

blastopore (blas′to-por) the opening of the archenteron to the exterior of the embryo at the gastrula stage.

blastospore (blas′to-spor) a spore formed by budding, as in yeast.

blastula (blas′tu-lah), pl. *blas′tulae* [L.] the usually spherical body produced by cleavage of a fertilized ovum (ZYGOTE), consisting of a single layer of cells (BLASTODERM) surrounding a fluid-filled cavity (BLASTO-COELE); it follows the MORULA stage.

blastulation (blas″tu-la′shun) conversion of the morula to the blastula by development of a blastocoele.

bleb (bleb) bulla (def. 1).

bleeder (blēd′er) 1. any blood vessel cut during surgery that requires clamping, cautery, or ligature. 2. slang term, now considered offensive, referring to a person who bleeds freely, especially one suffering from a condition in which the blood fails to clot properly, such as HEMOPHILIA.

bleeding (blēd′ing) 1. escape of blood from an injured vessel; see also HEMORRHAGE. 2. phlebotomy.

dysfunctional uterine b. bleeding from the nonmenstruating uterus when no organic lesions are present.

implantation b. that occurring at the time of implantation of the zygote in the decidua.

occult b. escape of blood in such small quantity that it can be detected only by chemical tests or by microscopic or spectroscopic examination.

b. time the time required for a standardized wound to stop bleeding. The *bleeding time test* is used as a screening procedure to detect both congenital and acquired platelet disorders; it measures the ability of platelets to arrest bleeding and hence gives an estimate of platelet number and level of functioning. There are several methods of performing the bleeding time. In *Ivy's test*, incisions are made on the forearm, a sphygmomanometer is inflated to a standard of 40 mm around the upper arm, and the time until cessation of bleeding is recorded. The *template method* is a variation in which a template with a slit in it is laid on the forearm, and the slit and the knife making the skin incision are both standardized. The most widely used template is the Simplate. Normally bleeding will cease in 2 to 9 minutes. Qualitative platelet disorders, thrombocytopenia (platelet count of less than $100,000/mm^3$), and the use of aspirin will prolong the bleeding time.

blenn(o)- word element [Gr.], *mucus.*

blennadenitis (blen″ad-ĕ-ni′tis) myxadenitis.

blennoid (blen′oid) mucoid.

blennorrhagia (blen″o-ra′jah) 1. blennorrhea. 2. old term for GONORRHEA.

blennorrhea (blen″o-re′ah) 1. any free discharge of mucus, especially a gonorrheal discharge from the urethra or vagina. 2. old term for GONORRHEA.

inclusion b. inclusion conjunctivitis.

blennothorax (blen″o-tho′raks) a PLEURAL EFFUSION containing mucus.

blennuria (blen-u′re-ah) mucus in the urine.

Blenoxane (blen′oks-ān) trademark for a preparation of BLEOMYCIN sulfate, an antineoplastic ANTIBIOTIC.

bleomycin (ble″o-mi′sin) an antitumor ANTIBIOTIC obtained from cultures of *Streptomyces verticellus.* It binds to DNA and causes single-strand breaks and double-strand scissions, impairing DNA synthesis and inhibiting RNA and protein synthesis. Administered by injection as the sulfate salt to treat lymphomas, soft tissue sarcomas, and cancers of the head and neck, cervix, skin, testes, lung, and other organs.

blephar(o)- word element [Gr.], *eyelid; eyelash.*

blepharadenitis (blef″ah-rad″ĕ-ni′tis) inflammation of the meibomian GLANDS; called also blepharoadenitis.

blepharal (blef′ar-al) palpebral.

blepharectomy (blef″ah-rek′to-me) partial or complete excision of an eyelid.

blepharism (blef′ah-rizm) spasm of the eyelid; continuous blinking.

blepharitis (blef″ah-ri′tis) inflammation of the glands and lash follicles along the margin of the EYELIDS; symptoms include itching, burning, photophobia, mucous discharge, crusted eyelids, and loss of eyelashes. Warm saline compresses may be used to soften secretions, and the eyelids are cleansed thoroughly. Exudate and scales should be removed by stroking downward and sideways. Antibiotic salve or eyedrops are administered as prescribed; in some cases systemic antibiotic therapy is indicated.

angular b. inflammation involving the outer angle of the eyelids.

nonulcerative b., squamous b. that in which the edge of the eyelid is covered with small white or gray scales.

ulcerative b. that marked by small ulcerated areas along the eyelid margin, multiple suppurative lesions, and loss of lashes.

blepharoadenitis (blef″ah-ro-ad″ĕ-ni′tis) blepharadenitis.

blepharoatheroma (blef″ah-ro-ath″er-o′mah) an encysted tumor or sebaceous cyst of an eyelid.

blepharochalasis (blef″ah-ro-kal′ah-sis) hypertrophy and loss of elasticity of the skin of the upper eyelid.

blepharoconjunctivitis (blef″ah-ro-konjunk″tĭ-vi′tis) inflammation of the eyelids and conjunctiva.

blepharoncus (blef″a-rong′kus) a tumor on the eyelid.

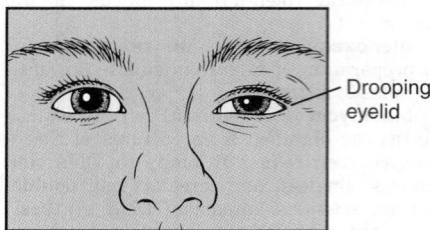

Drooping eyelid

Blepharoptosis. From Frazier et al., 2000.

blepharophimosis (blef″ah-ro-fi-mo′sis) abnormal narrowness of the palpebral FIS-SURES.

blepharoplasty (blef′ah-ro-plas″te) plastic surgery of an eyelid; called also tarsoplasty.

blepharoplegia (blef″ah-ro-ple′jah) paralysis of an eyelid.

blepharoptosis (blef″ah-rop-to′sis) ptosis (def. 2). (See accompanying illustration.)

blepharorrhaphy (blef″ah-ror′ah-fe) 1. suture of an eyelid. 2. tarsorrhaphy.

blepharospasm (blef′ah-ro-spaz″m) spasm of the orbicular muscle of the eyelid.

blepharostat (blef′ah-ro-stat″) an instrument for holding the eyelids apart.

blepharostenosis (blef″ah-ro-stě-no′sis) blepharophimosis.

blepharosynechia (blef″ah-ro-sī-nek′e-ah) growing together or adhesion of the eyelids.

blepharotomy (blef′ah-rot′ah-me) surgical incision of an eyelid; called also tarsotomy.

blind (blīnd) 1. not having the sense of sight. 2. pertaining to an experiment in which one or more of the groups receiving, administering, and evaluating treatment are unaware of which treatment any particular recipient is getting. See SINGLE BLIND, DOUBLE BLIND, and TRIPLE BLIND.

blindness (blīnd′nes) lack or loss of ability to see (see VISION). Legally, blindness is defined as less than 20/200 vision in the better eye with GLASSES (vision of 20/200 is the ability to see at 20 feet only what the normal eye can see at 200 feet). A person with 20° or less vision (*pinhole vision*) is also legally blind. In 2002, the number of people classified as legally blind in the United States was estimated at 10 million; millions more had severe visual impairments. The five leading causes of impaired vision and blindness in the United States are AGE-RELATED MACULAR DEGENERATION, CATA-RACT, GLAUCOMA, diabetic RETINOPATHY, and atrophy of the OPTIC NERVE. Besides health care problems, issues related to employment, independent living, and literacy should all be considered when caring for patients who are blind. The American Foundation for the Blind is a resource center for information related to visual problems. They can be contacted by calling 1-800-232-5463 or consulting their web site at http://www.afb.org.

blue b., blue-yellow b. popular names for imperfect perception of blue and yellow tints; see *tritanopia* and *tetartanopia*.

color b. COLOR VISION DEFICIENCY.

complete color b. monochromatic VISION.

day b. hemeralopia.

green b. imperfect perception of green tints; see DEUTERANOPIA and PROTANOPIA.

legal b. that defined by law, usually, maximal visual acuity in the better eye after correction of 20/200 with a total diameter of the visual field in that eye of 20°.

night b. see NIGHT BLINDNESS.

object b., psychic b. visual agnosia.

red b. popular name for PROTANOPIA.

red-green b., red-green color b. popular names for any imperfect perception of red and green tints, including all the most common types of COLOR VISION DEFI-CIENCY. See DEUTERANOMALY, DEUTERANOPIA, PROTANOMALY, and PROTANOPIA.

snow b. dimness of vision, usually temporary, due to the glare of the sun upon snow.

total color b. monochromatic VISION.

yellow b. popular name for TRITANOPIA.

blister (blis′ter) a vesicle, especially a BULLA.

blood b. a vesicle having bloody contents, as may be caused by a pinch or bruise.

fever b's herpes febrilis.

water b. one with clear watery contents.

Blocadren (blok′ah-dren) trademark for a preparation of TIMOLOL maleate, a BETA-ADRENERGIC BLOCKING AGENT used as an ANTIHYPERTENSIVE AGENT and in treatment of MYOCARDIAL INFARCTION and MIGRAINE.

block (blok) 1. obstruction. 2. to obstruct. 3. regional ANESTHESIA. 4. HEART BLOCK.

atrioventricular b. 1. any interruption of the conduction of electrical impulses from the atria to the ventricles; it can occur at the level of the atria, the atrioventricular node, the bundle of His, or the Purkinje system. See HEART BLOCK. 2. a type of HEART BLOCK in which the blocking is at the atrioventricular junction. It is *first degree* when atrioventricular conduction time is prolonged; it is called *second degree* or *partial* when some but not all atrial impulses reach the ventricle; and it is called *third degree* or *complete* when no atrial

ELECTROCARDIOGRAPHIC CRITERIA FOR BUNDLE BRANCH BLOCK

Left Bundle Branch Block
Complete
QRS interval ≥ 0.12 sec
Broad, notched, or slurred R wave — I, aVL, V5, V6
RS pattern — V5, V6 (occasional)
No Q waves — I, V5, V6
Intrinsicoid deflection > 0.06 sec — V1, V2
Intrinsicoid deflection normal — V1, V2
rS or QS — V1, V2
Shift to left of transitional zone
Incomplete
QRS internal > 0.10 sec, < 0.12 sec
Intrinsicoid deflection in left precordial lead 0.06 sec
No Q waves — I, V5, V6
Notching and/or slurring of ascending limb of R wave
    of left precordial lead (sometimes)

Right Bundle Branch Block
Complete
QRS interval ≥ 0.12 sec
rsr', rsR', or rSR' — V1, V2
Wide S in V6 (longer than R or > 40 msec, adults)
Intrinsicoid deflection may be > 0.05 sec — V1, normal
    — V5, V6
Incomplete
QRS interval < 0.12 sec
Other criteria as in complete r.b.b.b.

---

impulses at all reach the ventricle, so that the atria and ventricles act independently of each other.

atrioventricular b., complete see atrioventricular block.

atrioventricular b., first degree see atrioventricular block.

atrioventricular b., partial see atrioventricular block.

atrioventricular b., second degree see atrioventricular block.

atrioventricular b., third degree see atrioventricular block.

AV b. atrioventricular block.

Bier b. regional ANESTHESIA by intravenous injection, used for surgical procedures on the forearm or the lower leg; performed in a bloodless field maintained by a pneumatic tourniquet that also prevents anesthetic from entering the systemic circulation. Called also intravenous block and IV block.

bifascicular b. the combination of complete right bundle branch block with either left anterior fascicular block or left posterior fascicular block. This is an imprecise though commonly used term; specific terms defining the structures involved are preferred.

bundle branch b. (BBB) a form of HEART BLOCK involving delay or failure of conduction in one of the branches in the bundle of His, as determined by an electrocardiogram. It may be complete or incomplete, transient, permanent, or intermittent, and is also named according to involvement of the left or the right bundle branch. It is impossible to determine if bundle branch block is complete or not. When associated with acute anterior wall myocardial infarction, bundle branch block identifies a high-risk patient. See accompanying table.

bundle branch b., bilateral HEART BLOCK characterized by conduction disturbance in the right and left bundle branches; it may be alternate, intermittent, or permanent. Complete bilateral bundle branch block results in complete (third degree) atrioventricular block.

bundle branch b., complete HEART BLOCK characterized by absence of conduction in a bundle branch or conduction delay, causing ventricular activation to occur largely or exclusively through the contralateral bundle.

bundle branch b., incomplete HEART BLOCK characterized by delayed conduction within a bundle branch, resulting in a delay in activation of the ipsilateral ventricle.

bundle branch b., right HEART BLOCK characterized by a delay or failure of impulse propagation through the right BUNDLE BRANCH; it may be either complete or incomplete. See accompanying table.

caudal b. caudal anesthesia.

cervical plexus b. regional ANESTHESIA of the neck by injection of a local anesthetic into the cervical PLEXUS.

entrance b. a zone of depressed conduction surrounding a pacemaker focus, protecting it from discharge by an extraneous impulse but not necessarily from discharges by electrotonic influences.

epidural b. epidural anesthesia.

exit b. HEART BLOCK characterized by failure of an expected impulse to emerge from its focus of origin and propagate; this usually occurs with a parasystolic focus, but is also seen with sinus, junctional, and ventricular rhythms. In cardiac PACING it means that the pacemaker stimulus is not of sufficient amplitude to stimulate the heart, such as when there is a very high THRESHOLD.

fascicular b. HEART BLOCK characterized by certain abnormal QRS waveforms ascribed to conduction disturbance in the anterior and posterior divisions of the left bundle branch.

fascicular b., left anterior HEART BLOCK characterized by delay or interruption of impulse conduction in the anterior superior division of the left BUNDLE BRANCH, resulting in asynchronous activation of the left ventricle.

fascicular b., left posterior HEART BLOCK characterized by delay or interruption of impulse conduction in the posterior inferior division of the left BUNDLE BRANCH, resulting in asynchronous activation of the left ventricle.

femoral b. regional ANESTHESIA of the posterior thigh and the lower leg by injection of a local anesthetic around the femoral nerve just below the inguinal ligament at the lateral border of the fossa ovalis.

field b. regional ANESTHESIA by blocking conduction in nerves with chemical or physical agents.

heart b. see HEART BLOCK.

intravenous b. Bier block.

intraventricular b. impaired conduction within the ventricles due to absence of conduction within the bundle branches, their ramifications, or the ventricles.

intraventricular b., unspecified any HEART BLOCK characterized by an electrocardiographic pattern of intraventricular conduction disturbance and not qualifying as a bundle branch block or a fascicular block.

interventricular b. bundle branch block.

IV b. Bier block.

lumbar plexus b. regional ANESTHESIA of the anterior and medial aspects of the lower limb by injection of a local anesthetic into the lumbar PLEXUS.

mental b. blocking (def. 3).

metabolic b. the blocking of a biosynthetic pathway due to a genetic enzyme defect or to inhibition of an enzyme by a drug or other substance.

Mobitz type I b. a second degree atrioventricular block in which the P-R interval increases progressively until an atrial impulse is blocked. Called also Wenckebach's phenomenon or block.

Mobitz type II b. a second degree atrioventricular block in which the P-R interval is fixed, with periodic blocking of the atrial impulse to the ventricle.

nerve b. regional ANESTHESIA by injection of an anesthetic close to the appropriate nerve.

paracervical b. regional ANESTHESIA of the inferior hypogastric plexus and ganglia produced by injection of the local anesthetic into the lateral fornices of the vagina.

paraneural b. perineural block.

parasacral b. regional ANESTHESIA by injection of a local anesthetic around the sacral nerves as they emerge from the sacral foramina.

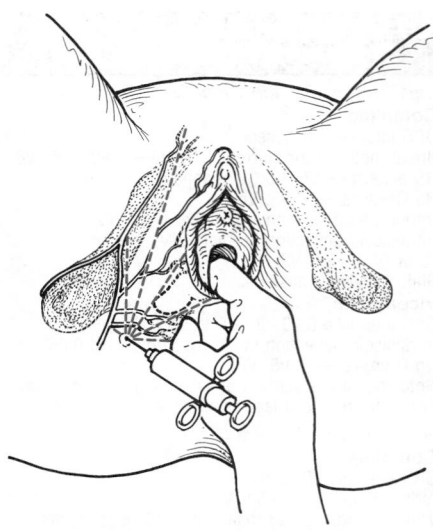

The pudendal block. The pudendal nerves can be effectively blocked by a local anesthetic, thereby anesthetizing the perineum. From Nichols and Zwelling, 1997.

paravertebral b. paravertebral anesthesia.

perineural b. regional ANESTHESIA produced by injection of the anesthetic agent close to the nerve. Called also paraneural anesthesia or block and perineural anesthesia.

presacral b. regional ANESTHESIA produced by injection of the local anesthetic into the sacral nerves on the anterior aspect of the sacrum.

pudendal b. regional ANESTHESIA produced by blocking the pudendal nerves, accomplished by injection of the local anesthetic into the tuberosity of the ischium. (See accompanying illustration.)

retrobulbar b. that performed by injection of a local anesthetic into the retrobulbar space to anesthetize and immobilize the eye.

sacral b. regional ANESTHESIA produced by injection of the local anesthetic into the extradural space of the spinal canal.

saddle b. regional ANESTHESIA in an area corresponding roughly with the areas of the buttocks, perineum, and inner aspects of the thighs, by introducing the anesthetic agent low in the dural sac. Called also saddle block anesthesia.

sinoatrial b. a type of HEART BLOCK characterized by partial or complete interference with the propagation of impulses from the sinoatrial node to the atria, resulting in delay or absence of the atrial response.

sinus b. 1. barosinusitis. 2. sinoatrial block.

spinal b. spinal anesthesia.

subarachnoid b. spinal anesthesia (def. 2).

trifascicular b. an imprecise term referring to HEART BLOCK characterized by failure of conduction, partial or complete, in all three of the fascicles of the intraventricular conduction system; i.e., there is simultaneous right bundle branch block, left anterior hemiblock, and left posterior hemiblock. In the setting of acute anterior wall myocardial infarction, this is an ominous sign. More precise terms referring to the specifically involved structures are preferred.

vagal b., vagus nerve b. regional ANESTHESIA produced by blocking of vagal impulses by injection of a solution of local anesthetic into the vagus nerve at its exit from the skull.

Wenckebach b. Mobitz type I block.

wrist b. regional ANESTHESIA of the hand by injection of a local anesthetic around the median, radial, and ulnar nerves at the wrist.

blockade (blok-ād′) 1. in pharmacology, the blocking of the effect of a neurotransmitter or hormone by a drug. 2. in histochemistry, a chemical reaction that modifies certain chemical groups and blocks a specific staining method. 3. regional anesthesia.

adrenergic b. selective inhibition of the response to sympathetic impulses transmitted by EPINEPHRINE or NOREPINEPHRINE at alpha or beta receptor sites of an effector organ or postganglionic adrenergic neuron. See also ADRENERGIC BLOCKING AGENT.

cholinergic b. selective inhibition of cholinergic nerve impulses at autonomic ganglionic synapses, postganglionic parasympathetic effectors, or neuromuscular junctions. See also cholinergic blocking AGENT.

ganglionic b. inhibition by drugs of nerve impulse transmission at autonomic ganglionic synapses; see also ganglionic blocking AGENT.

narcotic b. inhibition of the euphoric effects of narcotic drugs by the use of other drugs, such as methadone, in the treatment of addiction.

neuromuscular b. a failure in neuromuscular transmission that can be induced pharmacologically or result from any of various disturbances at the myoneural JUNCTION. See also neuromuscular blocking AGENT.

sympathetic b. block of nerve impulse transmission between a preganglionic sympathetic fiber and the ganglion cell.

blocker (blok′er) something that blocks or obstructs a passage or activity; see also ANTAGONIST and blocking AGENT.

α-**b.** alpha-adrenergic blocking agent.

β-**b., beta-b.** beta-adrenergic blocking agent.

calcium channel b. calcium channel blocking agent.

potassium channel b. potassium channel blocking agent.

sodium channel b. sodium channel blocking agent.

blocking (blok′ing) 1. interruption of an afferent nerve pathway (see BLOCK). 2. inhibition of an intracellular biosynthetic process; metabolic block. 3. thought blocking or thought deprivation; sudden cessation of the train of thought or speech, such as may occur in a period of extreme emotion or when a repressed painful thought is approached. 4. casting of tissue blocks in an embedding medium such as paraffin wax so that sections can be cut with a microtome.

blood (blud) the fluid that circulates through the heart, arteries, capillaries, and veins and is the chief means of transport within the body. It transports oxygen from the lungs to the body tissues, and carbon dioxide from the tissues to the lungs. It transports nutritive substances and metabolites to the tissues and removes waste products to the kidneys and other organs of excretion. It has an essential role in the maintenance of fluid balance.

In an emergency, blood cells and antibodies carried in the blood are brought to a point of infection, or blood-clotting substances are carried to a break in a blood vessel. The blood distributes hormones from the endocrine glands to the organs they influence. It also helps regulate body temperature by carrying excess heat from the interior of the body to the surface layers of the skin, where the heat is dissipated to the surrounding air.

Blood varies in color from a bright red in the arteries to a duller red in the veins. The total quantity of blood within an individual depends upon body weight; a person weighing 70 kg (154 lb) has about 4.5 liters of blood in the body.

Blood is composed of two parts: the fluid portion is called PLASMA, and the solid portion or *formed elements* (suspended in the fluid) consists of the blood cells (ERYTHROCYTES and LEUKOCYTES) and the PLATELETS. Plasma accounts for about 55 per cent of the volume and the formed elements account for about 45 per cent. (See accompanying illustration and table.)

Chemical analyses of various substances in the blood are invaluable aids in (1) the prevention of disease by alerting the patient and health care provider to potentially dangerous levels of blood constituents that could lead to more serious conditions, (2) diagnosis of pathologic conditions already present, (3) assessment of the patient's progress when a disturbance in blood chemistry exists, and (4) assessment of the patient's status by establishing baseline or "normal" levels for each individual patient.

In recent years, with the increasing attention to preventive health care and rapid progress in technology and automation, the use of a battery of screening tests performed by automated instruments has become quite common. These instruments are capable of performing simultaneously a variety of blood chemistry tests. Some of the more common screening tests performed on samples of blood include evaluation of ELECTROLYTE, ALBUMIN, and BILIRUBIN levels, BLOOD UREA NITROGEN (BUN), CHOLESTEROL, total protein, and such enzymes as LACTATE DEHYDROGENASE and ASPARTATE TRANSAMINASE. Other tests include ELECTROPHORESIS for serum proteins, BLOOD GAS ANALYSIS, GLUCOSE TOLERANCE TESTS, and measurement of IRON levels.

b. bank 1. a place of storage for blood. 2. an organization that collects, processes, stores, and transfuses blood. In most health agencies the blood bank is located in the pathology laboratory. It is operated by medical technologists under the direction of a pathologist.

b. bank technologist a CLINICAL LABORATORY SCIENTIST/MEDICAL TECHNOLOGIST who has postgraduate education in blood banking and is certified by the Board of Registry of the American Society of Clinical Pathologists; designated as MT(ASCP)SBB. Specialists in blood bank technology perform both routine and specialized tests in blood

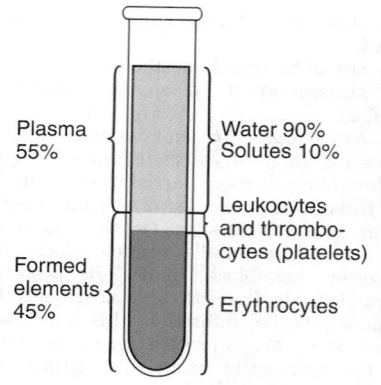

Plasma 55%

Water 90%
Solutes 10%

Leukocytes and thrombocytes (platelets)

Formed elements 45%

Erythrocytes

Composition of the blood, which constitutes 8% of total body weight. From Applegate, 2000.

FORMED ELEMENTS IN THE BLOOD			
Formed Element	Description	Number	Function
Erythrocytes	Biconcave disk; no nucleus; 7–8 μm in diameter	4.5–6.0 million/mm³	Transport oxygen and some carbon dioxide
Leukocytes	Nucleated cells	5000–9000/mm³	Part of the body's defense against disease
Neutrophils	Nucleus with 2 to 5 lobes; indistinct granules in the cytoplasm; 12–15 μm in diameter	60–70% or total WBCs	Phagocytosis
Eosinophils	Nucleus bilobed; red-staining granules in the cytoplasm; 10–12 μm in diameter	2–4% of total WBCs	Counteract histamine in allergic reactions; destroy parasitic worms
Basophils	Nucleus U-shaped or bilobed; granules in cytoplasm stain blue; 10–12 μm in diameter	Less than 1% of total WBCs	Release histamine and the anticoagulant heparin; called mast cells in the tissues
Lymphocytes	Agranulocyte; small cell with large round nucleus; 6–8 μm in diameter	20–25% of total WBCs	Produce antibodies; function in immunity
Monocytes	Large cells with bean-shaped nucleus; may be 20 μm in diameter	3–8% of total WBCs	Phagocytosis; engulf relatively large particles; called macrophages in the tissues
Thrombocytes	Cell fragments of megakaryocytes; 2–5 μm in diameter	250,000–500,000 mm³	Help control blood loss by forming platelet plug and releasing factors necessary for blood clotting

WBCs, white blood cells. Modified from Applegate, 2000.

bank immunohematology and perform transfusion services. The address of the American Association of Blood Banks is 8101 Glenbrook Road, Bethesda, MD 20814 (telephone 301-907-6582). The address of the Board of Registry of the American Society of Clinical Pathologists is P.O. Box 12270, Chicago, IL 60612. Their telephone number is 312-738-1336 and their web site is http://www.aabb.org.

b.-brain barrier BBB; the barrier separating the blood from the brain parenchyma everywhere except in the hypothalamus. It is permeable to water, oxygen, carbon dioxide, and nonionic solutes, such as glucose, alcohol, and general anesthetics, and is only slightly permeable to electrolytes and other ionic substances. Some small molecules, e.g., amino acids, are taken up across the barrier by specific transport mechanisms.

citrated b. blood treated with sodium citrate or citric acid to prevent its coagulation.

cord b. the blood contained in the umbilical vessels at the time of delivery of the infant. It is rich in stem cells that could be used in place of bone marrow for a transplant; thus, it is sometimes collected and stored for future use.

b. count determination of the number of blood cells in a given sample of blood, usually expressed as the number in a cubic millimeter; it may be either a complete blood COUNT or a count of just one of the elements such as an erythrocyte COUNT, leukocyte COUNT or a platelet COUNT. Methods include manual counts using a HEMACYTOMETER and automated counts using a flow cytometer, a Coulter counter, or other means. The blood count is useful in the diagnosis of various blood dyscrasias, infections, or other abnormal conditions and is one of the most common tests done on the blood. Called also blood cell count. (See accompanying table.)

defibrinated b. whole blood from which fibrin has been separated during the clotting process.

b. gas analysis laboratory studies of arterial and venous blood for the purpose of measuring oxygen and carbon dioxide levels and pressure or tension, and hydrogen ion concentration (pH). (See accompanying table.) Analyses of blood gases provide the following information:

Pa_{O_2}—partial pressure (P) of oxygen (O_2) in the arterial blood (a)

Sa_{O_2}—percentage of available hemoglobin that is saturated (Sa) with oxygen (O_2)

Pa_{CO_2}—partial pressure (P) of carbon dioxide (CO_2) in the arterial blood (a)

pH—an expression of the extent to which the blood is alkaline or acidic

COMPLETE BLOOD COUNT: NORMAL VALUES IN ADULTS

B

White Blood Cell Count (WBC):
$4.5-11 \times 10^3/\mu L$ or SI $4.5-11 \times 10^9/L$

Red Blood Cell Count (RBC):
Male: $4.6-6.2 \times 10^6/\mu L$ or SI $4.6-6.2 \times 10^{12}/L$
Female: $4.2-5.4 \times 10^6/\mu L$ or SI $4.2-5.4 \times 10^{12}/L$

Hemoglobin:
Male: 13.5–18 g/dL or SI 135–180 g/L
Female: 12–16 g/dL or SI 120–160 g/L

Hematocrit:
Male: 40–54% or 0.4–0.59 (volume fraction)
Female: 38–47% or SI 0.38–0.47 (volume fraction)

Red Cell Indices:
Mean Corpuscular Volume (MCV): 80–96 μm^3 or SI 80–96 fL
Mean Corpuscular Hemoglobin (MCH): 27–31 pg or SI 27–31 pg
Mean Corpuscular Hemoglobin Concentration (MCHC): 32–36% or 0.32–0.36 (concentration fraction)
Red Cell Distribution Width (RDW-CV): 13.1% (range: 11.6–14.6%) (Henry, 1990)

Platelet Count:
Adult: 150,000–450,000 cells/μL or SI 150–450 $\times 10^9/L$
Newborn: 84,000–478,000 cells/μL or SI 84–478 $\times 10^9/L$

HCO_3^-—the level of plasma bicarbonate; an indicator of the metabolic acid-base status

These parameters are important tools for assessment of a patient's ACID-BASE BALANCE. They reflect the ability of the lungs to exchange oxygen and carbon dioxide, the ability of the kidneys to control the retention or elimination of bicarbonate, and the effectiveness of the heart as a pump. Because the lungs and kidneys act as important regulators of the respiratory and metabolic acid-base balance, assessment of the status of a patient with any disorder of respiration and metabolism includes periodic blood gas measurements.

The partial pressure of a particular gas in a mixture of gases, as of oxygen in air, is the pressure exerted by that gas alone. It is proportional to the relative number of molecules of the gas, for example, the fraction of all the molecules in the air that are oxygen molecules. The partial pressure of a gas in a liquid is the partial pressure of a real or imaginary gas that is in equilibrium with the liquid.

Pa_{O_2} measures the oxygen content of the arterial blood, most of which is bound to

Examine the pH
Normal: 7.35–7.45
Acidemia: < 7.35
Alkalemia: > 7.45

Evaluate the Pa$_{O_2}$
Normal: 50–80 mm Hg for infants
            100 mm Hg young adults
            80 mm Hg elderly adults

Evaluate the Pa$_{CO_2}$
Normal: 32–45 mm Hg
Respiratory acidosis: > 45 mm Hg
Respiratory alkalosis: < 35 mm Hg
Assess the HCO$_3$
Normal: 22–26 mEq/L
Metabolic acidosis: < 22 mEq/L
Metabolic alkalosis: > 26 mEq/L

Evaluate the pH for Compensation
Compensated pH: Pa$_{CO_2}$ and HCO$_3$ are not normal in a
    fashion where one is acidotic and the other
    alkalotic.
Check for the presence of a mixed disorder.
Partial compensation: pH not within normal limits
Fully compensated: pH is normal

---

hemoglobin, forming oxyhemoglobin. The Sa$_{O_2}$ measures the oxygen in oxyhemoglobin as a percentage of the total hemoglobin oxygen-carrying capacity.

A Pa$_{O_2}$ of 60 mm Hg represents an Sa$_{O_2}$ of 90 per cent, which is sufficient to meet the needs of the body's cells. However, as the Pa$_{O_2}$ falls, the Sa$_{O_2}$ decreases rapidly. A Pa$_{O_2}$ below 55 indicates a state of hypoxemia that requires correction. Normal Pa$_{O_2}$ values at sea level are 80 mm Hg for elderly adults and 100 mm Hg for young adults.

However, some patients with CHRONIC OBSTRUCTIVE PULMONARY DISEASE can tolerate a Pa$_{O_2}$ as low as 70 mm Hg without becoming hypoxic. In caring for patients with this condition, it is important to know that attempts to elevate the Pa$_{O_2}$ level to the normal level can be dangerous and even fatal. It is best to establish a baseline for each individual patient before supplementary oxygen is given, and then to assess his condition and the effectiveness of his therapy according to this baseline.

The Pa$_{CO_2}$ gives information about the cellular production of carbon dioxide through metabolic processes, and the removal of it from the body via the lungs. The normal range is 32 to 45 mm Hg. Values outside this range indicate a primary respiratory problem associated with pulmonary function, or a metabolic problem for which there is respiratory compensation.

In the newborn the normal Pa$_{O_2}$ is 50 to 80 mm Hg. At 40 to 50 mm Hg cyanosis may become apparent. Respiratory distress in an infant who is unable to ventilate the lungs adequately will produce a drop in Pa$_{O_2}$ level. However, there is no marked increase in Pa$_{CO_2}$ level in some infants as in adults with respiratory distress because many infants can still eliminate carbon dioxide from the lungs even though weakness prevents inhaling an adequate oxygen supply. All infants being ventilated and receiving oxygen therapy require frequent blood gas analyses and also pH, base excess, and oxygen saturation levels to avoid oxygen toxicity and acid-base imbalance.

Blood pH gives information about the patient's metabolic state. A pH of 7.4 is considered normal; a value lower than 7.4 indicates acidemia and one higher than 7.4 alkalemia.

Because the amount of CO_2 in the blood affects its pH, abnormal Pa$_{CO_2}$ values are interpreted in relation to the pH. If the Pa$_{CO_2}$ value is elevated, and the pH is below normal, *respiratory acidosis* from either acute or chronic hyperventilation is suspected. Conversely, a Pa$_{CO_2}$ below normal and a pH above normal indicates *respiratory alkalosis*. When both the Pa$_{CO_2}$ and the pH are elevated, there is respiratory retention of CO_2 to compensate for *metabolic acidosis*. If both values are below normal, there is respiratory elimination of CO_2 (HYPERVENTILATION) to compensate for metabolic acidosis.

Abnormal levels of bicarbonate (HCO$_3^-$) in the plasma are also interpreted in relation to the pH in the diagnosis of disturbances in the *metabolic* component of the acid-base balance. The normal range for HCO$_3^-$ is 22 to 26 mEq per liter. Abnormally low levels of both HCO$_3^-$ and pH indicate acidosis of metabolic origin. Conversely, elevations of both of these values indicate metabolic alkalosis. The kidneys maintain bicarbonate levels by filtering bicarbonate and returning it to the blood; they also produce new bicarbonate to replace that which is used in buffering. Therefore, a decreased HCO$_3^-$ and an increased pH level indicate either retention of hydrogen ions by the kidneys or the elimination of HCO$_3^-$ in an effort to compensate for respiratory alkalosis. Conversely, if the HCO$_3^-$ level is increased and the pH is decreased, the kidneys have compensated for respiratory acidosis by retaining HCO$_3^-$ or by eliminating hydrogen ions.

    b. gas analysis, mixed venous blood gas analysis performed on a blood sample obtained from the pulmonary artery.

    b. gas analysis, transcutaneous the determination of PO$_2$ and PCO$_2$ by

ERYTHROCYTE ANTIGENS AND ANTIBODIES — ABO SYSTEM

Blood Group	Erythrocyte Antigens	Serum Antibodies
A	A	Anti-B
B	B	Anti-A
AB	AB	None
O	None	Anti-A, anti-B

placement of a heated electrode over the skin to get an inference of Pa_{O_2} and Pa_{CO_2}.

b. group the phenotype of ERYTHRO-CYTES defined by one or more cellular antigenic structural groupings under the control of allelic genes. In clinical practice there are four main blood groups or blood types: A, B, O, and AB (see table). In addition to this major grouping there is an Rh-hR system that is important in the prevention of ERYTHROBLASTOSIS FETALIS resulting from incompatibility of blood groups in mother and fetus.

The ABO blood group system was first introduced in 1900 by Karl Landsteiner; in 1920 group AB was discovered by van Descatello and Sturli. Identification of these four major blood groups represented a major step toward resolving the problem of blood transfusion reactions resulting from donor-recipient incompatibility. In 1938 Landsteiner and Weiner discovered another blood factor related to maternal-fetal incompatibility. The factor was named Rh because the researchers were using rhesus monkeys in their studies. Further research has uncovered additional factors in the Rh group.

Although more than 90 factors have been identified, many of these are not highly antigenic and are not, therefore, a cause for concern in the typing of blood for clinical purposes.

The term *factor,* in reference to blood groups, is synonymous with ANTIGEN, and the reaction occurring between incompatible blood types is an ANTIGEN-ANTIBODY REACTION. In cases of incompatibility, the antigen, located on the red blood cells, is an agglutinogen and the specific antibody, located in the serum, is an agglutinin. These are so named because whenever red blood cells with a certain factor come in contact with the agglutinin specific for it, there is agglutination or clumping of the erythrocytes.

In determining blood group, a sample of blood is taken and mixed with specially prepared sera. One serum, anti-A agglutinin, causes blood of group A to agglutinate; another serum, anti-B agglutinin, causes blood of group B to agglutinate. Thus, if anti-A serum alone causes clumping, the blood is group A; if anti-B serum alone causes clumping, it is group B. If both cause clumping, the blood group is AB, and if it is not clumped by either, it is identified as group O.

occult b. that present in such small amounts as to be detectable only by chemical tests or by spectroscopic or microscopic examination.

peripheral b. that obtained from acral areas, or from the circulation remote from the heart; the blood in the systemic circulation.

b. poisoning popular term for SEPTICE-MIA.

b. pressure 1. the pressure of the blood against the walls of any blood vessel. 2. the term usually refers to the pressure of the blood within the arteries, or arterial blood PRESSURE. This pressure is determined by several interrelated factors, including the pumping action of the heart, the resistance to the flow of blood in the arterioles, the elasticity of the walls of the main arteries, the blood volume and extracellular fluid volume, and the blood's viscosity, or thickness.

The pumping action of the heart refers to how hard the heart pumps the blood (force of heartbeat), how much blood it pumps (the cardiac output), and how efficiently it does the job. Contraction of the heart, which forces blood through the arteries, is the phase known as SYSTOLE. Relaxation of the heart between contractions is called DIASTOLE.

The main arteries leading from the heart have walls with strong elastic fibers capable of expanding and absorbing the pulsations generated by the heart. At each pulsation the arteries expand and absorb the momentary increase in blood pressure. As the heart relaxes in preparation for another beat, the aortic valves close to prevent blood from flowing back to the heart chambers, and the artery walls spring back, forcing the blood through the body between contractions. In this way the arteries act as dampers on the pulsations and thus provide a steady flow of blood through the blood vessels. Because of this, there are actually two blood pressures within the blood vessels during one complete beat of the heart: a higher blood pressure during systole (the *contraction phase*) and a lower blood pressure during diastole (the *relaxation phase*). These two blood pressures are known as the systolic pressure and the diastolic pressure, respectively.

It is generally agreed that a reading of 120 mm Hg systolic and 80 mm Hg diastolic are the norms for a blood pressure reading; that

CLASSIFICATION OF BLOOD PRESSURE FOR ADULTS AGE 18 AND OLDER*

Category	Systolic (mm Hg)	Diastolic (mm Hg)
Optimal	<120	<80
Normal	<130	<85
High Normal	130–139	85–89
Hypertension		
Stage 1 (Mild)	140–159	90–99
Stage 2 (Moderate)	160–179	100–109
Stage 3 (Severe)	≥ 180	≥ 110

Note: In addition to classifying stages of hypertension based on average blood pressure levels, the clinician should specify presence or absence of target-organ disease and additional risk factors. For example, a patient with diabetes and a blood pressure of 142/94 mm Hg plus left ventricular hypertrophy should be classified as "Stage 1 hypertension with target-organ disease (left ventricular hypertrophy) and with another major risk factor (diabetes)." This specificity is important for risk classification and management. From the Sixth Report of the Joint National Committee on Detection, Evaluation, and treatment of High Blood Pressure, Nov 1997.
*Not taking antihypertensive drugs and not acutely ill. When systolic and diastolic pressure fall into different categories, the higher category should be selected to classify the individual's blood pressure status. For instance, 160/92 should be classified as Stage 2, and 174/120 should be classified as Stage 3. Isolated systolic hypertension is defined as SBP 140 mm Hg or greater and DBP below 90 mm Hg and staged appropriately (e.g., 170/82 mm Hg is defined as Stage 2 isolated systolic hypertension.
Optimal blood pressure with respect to cardiovascular risk is below 128/80 mm Hg. However, unusually low readings should be evaluated for clinical significance.
Based on the average of two or more readings taken at each of two or more visits following an initial screening.

is, it represents the *average* blood pressure obtained from a large sampling of healthy adults. In general, a blood pressure of 95 mm Hg systolic and 60 mm Hg diastolic indicates HYPOTENSION. However, a reading equal to or below this level must be interpreted in the light of each patient's "normal" reading as determined by baseline data.

On the basis of validated research on the long-term effects of an elevated blood pressure, it is generally agreed that some degree of risk for major cardiovascular disease exists when the systolic pressure is greater than or equal to 140 mm Hg, and the diastolic pressure is greater than or equal to 90 mm Hg. Life expectancy is reduced at all ages and in both males and females when the diastolic pressure is above 90 mm Hg. (See accompanying table.)

Measurement of the Blood Pressure. The blood pressure is usually measured in the artery of the upper arm, with a

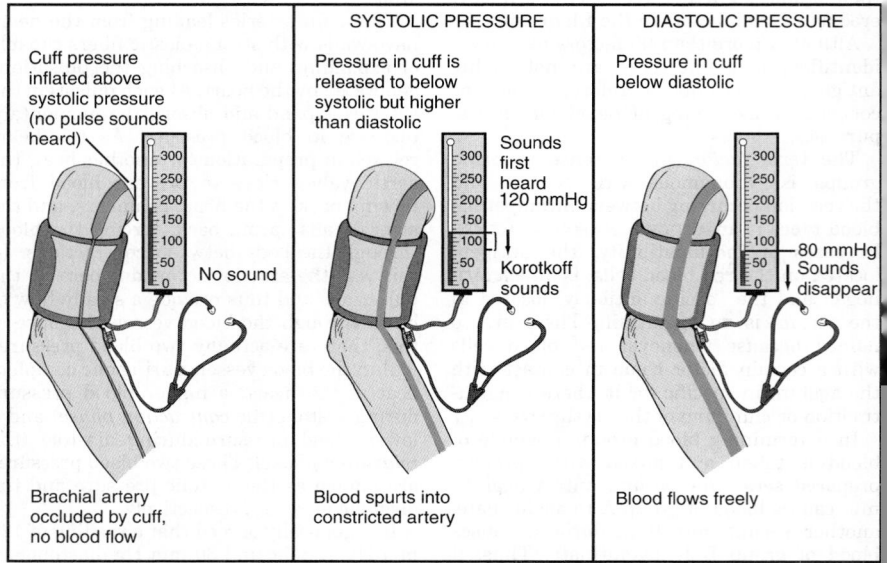

Measurement of blood pressure. From Applegate, 2000.

sphygmomanometer. (See accompanying illustration.) This consists of a rubber cuff and a gauge or column of mercury for measuring pressure. The rubber cuff is wrapped about the patient's arm, and then air is pumped into the cuff by means of a rubber bulb. As the pressure inside the rubber cuff increases, the flow of blood through the artery is momentarily checked.

A stethoscope is placed over the artery at the elbow and the air pressure within the cuff is slowly released. As soon as blood begins to flow through the artery again, Korotkoff SOUNDS are heard. The first sounds heard are tapping sounds that gradually increase in intensity. The initial tapping sound that is heard for at least two consecutive beats is recorded as the *systolic* blood pressure.

The first phase of the sounds may be followed by a momentary disappearance of sounds that can last from 30 to 40 mm Hg as the gauge needle (or mercury column) descends. It is important that this auscultatory GAP not be missed; otherwise, either an erroneously low systolic pressure or high diastolic pressure will be obtained.

During the second phase following the temporary absence of sound there are murmuring or swishing sounds. As deflation of the cuff continues, the sounds become sharper and louder. These sounds represent phase three. During phase four the sounds become muffled rather abruptly and then are followed by silence, which represents phase five.

Although there is disagreement as to which of the latter phases should represent the diastolic pressure, it is usually recommended that phase five, the point at which sounds disappear, be used as the diastolic pressure for adults, and phase four be used for children. The reason for this is that children, having a high cardiac output, often will continue to produce sounds when the gauge is at a very low reading or even at zero. In some adult patients whose arterioles have lost their elasticity, the fifth phase is also extremely low or nonexistent. In these cases, it is recommended that three readings be recorded: phase one and phases four and five. For example, the blood pressure would be written as 140/96/0. On most occasions, however, the blood pressure is written as a fraction. The systolic pressure is written as the top number, a line is drawn, and the diastolic pressure is written as the bottom number.

Errors in blood pressure measurement can result from failure of the cuff to reach and compress the artery. The cuff diameter should be 20 per cent greater than the diameter of the limb, the bladder of the cuff

must be centered over the artery, and the cuff must be wrapped smoothly and snugly to ensure proper inflation. When a mercury gauge is used, the meniscus should be at eye level to avoid a false reading.

Direct Measurement of Blood Pressure. Critically ill patients who require continuous monitoring of the blood pressure may have a catheter inserted into an artery and attached to a catheter-monitor-transducer system. The blood pressure is displayed on an oscilloscope at the bedside so that the patient's pressure can be determined at a glance. This intra-arterial technique of blood pressure monitoring provides accurate, objective, and continuous data on the patient's status.

b. pressure, mean arterial MAP; the average pressure within an artery over a complete cycle of one heartbeat; in the brachial artery, calculated to be the diastolic pressure plus 1/3 of the difference between the systolic and diastolic pressures.

b. stream bloodstream.

b. urea nitrogen see UREA NITROGEN.

b. volume 1. the total quantity of blood in the body; the plasma VOLUME added to the red cell VOLUME. 2. a laboratory test performed to determine this. The indicators used to determine these measurements are ^{125}I-labeled human serum albumin for plasma volume and ^{51}Cr-labeled erythrocytes for red cell volume. The regulation of blood volume in the circulatory system is affected by the intrinsic mechanism for fluid exchange at the capillary membranes and by hormonal influences and nervous reflexes that affect the excretion of fluids by the kidneys. A rapid decrease in the blood volume, as in hemorrhage, greatly reduces the cardiac output and creates a condition called SHOCK or circulatory shock. Conversely, an increase in blood volume, as when there is retention of water and salt in the body because of renal failure, results in an increase in cardiac output. The eventual outcome of this situation is increased arterial blood pressure.

The blood volume in the pulmonary circulation is approximately 12 per cent of the total blood volume. Such conditions as left-sided heart failure and mitral stenosis can greatly increase the pulmonary blood volume while decreasing the systemic volume. As would be expected, right-sided heart failure has the opposite effect. The latter condition has less serious effects because the volume of the systemic circulation is about seven times that of the pulmonary circulation and it is therefore better able to accommodate a change in fluid volume.

Tests. Clinical assessment of blood volume can be accomplished in a number of ways, for example, by measuring the patient's blood pressure while he is lying down, sitting, and standing. The quality and volume of peripheral pulses will give information about blood volume, as does determining the ease and speed with which a compressed vein will refill after pressure is released. Neck veins that are engorged indicate hypervolemia; the collapse of these veins indicates hypovolemia. A more accurate assessment can be done through the use of intravascular catheters such as the CENTRAL VENOUS PRESSURE catheter, which measures pressure in the right atrium, and the SWAN-GANZ CATHETER, which measures pressure on both sides of the heart.

Measurement of blood volume is accomplished by using substances that combine with red blood cells, for example, iron, chromium, and phosphate, or substances that combine with plasma proteins. In either case the measurement of the blood volume is based on the "dilution" principle. That is, the volume of any fluid compartment can be measured if a given amount of a substance is dispersed evenly in the fluid within the compartment, and then the extent of dilution of the substance is measured.

For example, a small amount of radioactive chromium (^{51}Cr), which is widely used to determine blood volume, is mixed with a sample of blood drawn from the patient. After about 30 minutes the ^{51}Cr will have entered the red blood cells. The sample with the tagged red blood cells is then returned by injection into the patient's bloodstream. About 10 minutes later a sample is removed from the patient's circulating blood and the radioactivity level of this sample is measured. The total blood volume is calculated according to this formula:

volume in mL =

$$\frac{\text{quantity of test substance instilled}}{\text{concentration per mL of dispersed fluid}}$$

When volume is used to arrive at the total blood volume, a dye (usually T-1824, also known as Evans blue) is injected into the circulating blood. The dye immediately combines with the blood proteins and within 10 minutes is dispersed throughout the circulatory system. A sample of blood is then drawn and the exact quantity of dye is measured. Using the information about plasma volume obtained by applying the above formula, the total blood volume can

be calculated, provided the hematocrit is also known. The formula for this calculation is:

$$\text{blood volume} = \text{plasma volume}$$
$$\times \frac{100}{100 - 0.87 \text{ hematocrit}}$$

whole b. that from which none of the elements has been removed, sometimes specifically that drawn from a selected donor under aseptic conditions, containing citrate ion or heparin, and used as a blood replenisher.

bloodstream (blud' strēm″) the blood flowing through the CIRCULATORY SYSTEM in the living body. Also written *blood stream.*

blooming (blōōm'ing) in radiology, a change in size of the focal spot, usually an increase.

Blount's disease (blunt) tibia vara.

blowpipe (blo'pīp) a tube through which a current of air is forced upon a flame to concentrate and intensify the heat.

blues (blōōz) popular term for a state of sadness; see DEPRESSION.

maternity b., postpartum b. popular terms for postpartum DEPRESSION.

Blumberg's sign (blum'bergz) pain on abrupt release of steady pressure (rebound tenderness) over the site of a suspected abdominal lesion, seen in peritonitis.

blur lack of sharpness in an x-ray image, usually due to patient motion.

blush (blush) sudden, brief erythema of the face and neck, resulting from vascular dilatation due to emotion or heat.

BMA British Medical Association.

BMI body mass index.

BMR basal metabolic rate.

BMT bone marrow transplantation.

BNA Basle Nomina Anatomica, a system of anatomic nomenclature adopted at the annual meeting of the German Anatomic Society in 1895; superseded by NOMINA ANATOMICA.

Bobath method (principles) (bo'baht) a neurophysiological rehabilitation approach based on a hierarchical nervous system; the principles focus on the inhibition of abnormal tone by using reflex inhibiting patterns and on the promotion of basic movement patterns that occur in an automatic fashion, such as equilibrium, righting reflexes, and other protective reactions. Called also neurodevelopmental treatment.

body (bod'e) 1. trunk (def. 1). 2. the largest and most important part of any organ. 3. any mass or collection of material.

acetone b's KETONE BODIES.

alkapton b's a class of substances with an affinity for alkali, found in the urine and causing the condition known as ALKAPTONUR-IA. The compound commonly found, and most commonly referred to by the term, is HOMOGENTISIC ACID.

amygdaloid b. a small mass of subcortical gray matter within the tip of the temporal lobe, anterior to the inferior horn of the lateral ventricle of the brain. It is part of the limbic system.

aortic b's small neurovascular structures on either side of the aorta in the region of the aortic arch, containing chemoreceptors that play a role in reflex regulation of respiration.

asbestos b's golden yellow bodies of various shapes, formed by the deposition of calcium salts, iron salts, and proteins on a spicule of ASBESTOS, found in the lungs, lung secretions, and feces of patients with ASBESTOSIS.

Aschoff b's submiliary collections of cells and leukocytes in the interstitial tissues of the heart in the myocarditis that accompanies RHEUMATIC FEVER; called also Aschoff's nodules.

asteroid b. an irregularly star-shaped inclusion body found in the giant cells in sarcoidosis and other diseases.

Babès-Ernst b. metachromatic granule.

Barr b. sex chromatin.

basal b. a modified centriole that occurs at the base of a flagellum or cilium.

carotid b's small neurovascular structures lying in the bifurcation of the right and left carotid arteries, containing chemoreceptors that monitor the oxygen content of the blood and help to regulate respiration.

ciliary b. see CILIARY BODY.

Donovan b's encapsulated bacteria (*Calymmatobacterium granulomatis*) found in lesions of GRANULOMA INGUINALE, visible when a Wright-stained smear of infected tissue is viewed under a microscope.

b. dysmorphic disorder a SOMATOFORM DISORDER in which a normal-appearing person is either preoccupied with an imagined defect in appearance or is overly concerned about a very slight physical anomaly. See also BODY IMAGE. Called also dysmorphophobia.

fimbriate b. corpus fimbriatum.

foreign b. a mass of material that is not normal to the place where it is found.

fruiting b. a specialized structure of certain fungi that produces the spores.

geniculate b., lateral either of the two metathalamus eminences, one on each side just lateral to the medial geniculate bodies, marking the termination of the optic tract.

geniculate b., medial either of the two metathalamus eminences, one on each side just lateral to the superior colliculi, concerned with hearing.

hematoxylin b. a dense, homogeneous particle, easily stainable with HEMATOXYLIN, consisting of nuclear material derived from an injured cell together with a small amount of cytoplasm. Hematoxylin bodies occur in SYSTEMIC LUPUS ERYTHEMATOSUS. Lymphocytes that ingest such particles are known as LE CELLS. Called also LE body.

Howell's b's, Howell-Jolly b's smooth, round remnants of nuclear chromatin seen in erythrocytes in megaloblastic and hemolytic anemia, in various leukemias and after splenectomy.

b. image the total concept, including conscious and unconscious feelings, thoughts, and perceptions, that a person has of his or her own body as an object in space independent and apart from other objects. The body image develops during infancy and childhood from exploration of the body surface and orifices, from development of physical abilities, and from play and comparison of the self with others. Changes in body image are particularly important in adolescence when attention is focused on appearance and attractiveness and relations with others. Body image is strongly influenced by parental attitudes that give the child a perception of certain body parts as good, clean, and attractive, or bad, dirty, and repulsive. The evolution of body image continues throughout life and incorporates such factors as a person's style of dress, hair style, and use of makeup, which symbolize social and professional status and other feelings about the self. Many clinical syndromes involve disturbances of body image. *Disturbed body image* is a NURSING DIAGNOSIS that was approved by the North American Nursing Diagnosis Association, defined as confusion in the mental picture of one's physical self. Surgery or trauma involving disfigurement or loss of a body part can be very threatening to a patient. Diseases involving a loss of body function, such as stroke syndrome, paraplegia, quadriplegia, coronary heart disease, and bowel or bladder incontinence, and diseases involving disfiguring skin lesions or the feeling of "rotting away" as in cancer or gangrene, can all cause changes in body image. Body image is frequently disturbed in schizophrenia, and patients may feel that their body or its parts are changing in size or shape or are ugly or threatening. Rape or violent physical assault can disturb the feeling of being secure in one's own body. Changes in body image involving sexual attractiveness or sexual identity, such as surgery or trauma involving the genitals or breasts and tubal ligation, hysterectomy, or vasectomy, can be especially difficult for the patient to deal with. Intrusive therapeutic or diagnostic procedures, such as insertion of a nasogastric tube, bladder catheterization, administration of intravenous fluids, endoscopy, and cardiac catheterization, can also threaten a patient's body image.

The reaction of a patient to an alteration in body image can include mourning the loss of the former body image, fear of rejection by significant others, hostility, and experiencing of "phantom" sensations from missing body parts. Patients with less ability to cope with their loss may respond with denial or depression. This can lead to a rejection of the altered body image and feelings of depersonalization that can involve avoidance of interpersonal contact and an unwillingness to discuss the deformity or to accept corrective medical treatment or vocational rehabilitation.

inclusion b's round, oval, or irregular-shaped bodies in the cytoplasm and nuclei of cells, as in disease caused by viral infection, such as rabies, smallpox, and herpes.

ketone b's see KETONE BODIES.

lamellar b. keratinosome.

Lafora's b's intracytoplasmic inclusions consisting of a complex of glycoprotein and acid mucopolysaccharide; widespread deposits are found in LAFORA'S DISEASE, a type of epilepsy.

LE b. hematoxylin body.

Leishman-Donovan b's round or oval bodies found in the reticuloendothelial cells, especially those of the spleen and liver, in KALA-AZAR; they are nonflagellate intracellular forms of *Leishmania donovani*. Also used to designate similar forms of *Leishmania tropica* found in macrophages in lesions of cutaneous LEISHMANIASIS.

mamillary b., mammillary b. either of the pair of small spherical masses in the interpeduncular fossa of the midbrain, forming part of the hypothalamus.

Masson b's cellular tissue that fills the pulmonary alveoli and alveolar ducts in rheumatic pneumonia; they may be modified Aschoff's bodies.

molluscum b's large homogeneous intracytoplasmic inclusions found in the stratum granulosum and stratum corneum in MOLLUSCUM CONTAGIOSUM, which contain replicating virus particles and cellular debris.

multilamellar b. any of the osmiophilic, lipid-rich, layered bodies found in the great alveolar cells of the lung.

Negri b's oval or round bodies in the nerve cells of animals dead of RABIES.

Nissl b's large granular bodies that stain with basic dyes, forming the reticular substance of the cytoplasm of neurons, composed of rough endoplasmic reticulum and free polyribosomes; ribonucleoprotein is one of their main constituents. Called also Nissl's granules.

olivary b. olive (def. 2).

paraaortic b's see PARA-AORTIC BODIES.

pineal b. see PINEAL BODY.

pituitary b. PITUITARY GLAND.

polar b's 1. the small cells consisting of a tiny bit of cytoplasm and a nucleus; they result from unequal division of the primary oocyte (*first polar body*) and, if fertilization occurs, of the secondary oocyte (*second polar body*). 2. metachromatic granules located at one or both ends of a bacterial cell.

psammoma b's usually microscopic, laminated masses of calcareous material, occurring in both benign and malignant epithelial and connective-tissue tumors, and sometimes associated with chronic inflammation.

quadrigeminal b's corpora quadrigemina.

b. of sternum the second or main part of the sternum, bounded by the manubrium above and the xiphoid process below. Called also gladiolus and corpus sterni.

striate b. corpus striatum.

trachoma b's inclusion bodies found in clusters in the cytoplasm of the epithelial cells of the conjunctiva in TRACHOMA.

vitreous b. the transparent gel filling the inner portion of the eyeball between the lens and retina. Called also vitreous and vitreous humor.

wolffian b. mesonephros.

boil (boil) a painful nodule formed in the skin by circumscribed inflammation of the dermis and subcutaneous tissue, enclosing a central slough or "core." Called also furuncle. Boils occur most frequently on the neck and buttocks, although they may develop wherever friction or irritation, or a scratch or break in the skin, allows the bacteria resident on the surface to penetrate the outer layer of the skin. A CARBUNCLE is a group of interconnected boils arising in a cluster of hair follicles.

Cause. Most boils and carbuncles are caused by *Staphylococcus aureus*. When these bacteria gain entrance to the skin, the infection settles in the hair follicles or the sebaceous glands. To combat the infection, large numbers of leukocytes travel to the site and attack the invading bacteria. Some bacteria and white cells are killed and they and their liquefied products form pus. The body's defenses may succeed in overcoming the invaders so that the boil subsides by itself, or the pus may build up pressure against the skin surface so that it ruptures, drains, and heals.

Boils most often afflict healthy persons but occasionally their appearance is a sign that the resistance is low, usually as the result of poor nutrition or illness. Patients with recurrent boils should be suspected of being chronic staphylococcal carriers. The nose is the most common carriage site.

Treatment. In most cases a single boil is not serious and will respond to incision and drainage. Systemic antibiotics are also sometimes indicated. Although complications are rare, a boil on or above the upper lip, on the nose or scalp, or in the outer ear can be serious because in these areas infection has easy access to the brain. Other danger zones are the armpit, the groin, and the breast of a woman who is nursing. If bacteria from a boil enter the bloodstream, septicemia may result (see BLOOD POISONING).

gum b. parulis.

bolometer (bo-lom′ĕ-ter) 1. an instrument for measuring the force of the HEARTBEAT. 2. an instrument for measuring minute degrees of radiant heat.

bolus (bo′lus) 1. a rounded mass of food or pharmaceutical preparation ready to be swallowed, or such a mass passing through the gastrointestinal tract. 2. a concentrated mass of pharmaceutical preparation, e.g., an opaque contrast medium, given intravenously or swallowed. 3. a mass of scattering material, such as wax or paraffin, placed between the radiation source and the skin to achieve a precalculated isodose pattern in the tissue irradiated.

alimentary b. the mass of food, made ready by mastication, that enters the esophagus at one swallow.

bombesin (bom′bĕ-sin) a tetradecapeptide neurotransmitter and hormone found in the brain and intestine; it is also found increased in cultures of small cell carcinoma of the lung.

bond (bond) the linkage between atoms or radicals of a chemical compound, or the symbol representing this linkage and indicating the number and attachment of the valencies of an atom in constitutional formulas, represented by a pair of dots or a line between atoms, e.g., H—O—H, H—C≡C—H or H:O:H, H:C:::C:H.

coordinate covalent b. a covalent bond in which one of the bonded atoms furnishes both of the shared electrons.

covalent b. a chemical bond between two atoms or radicals formed by the sharing of a pair (single bond), two pairs (double bond), or three pairs of electrons (triple bond).

disulfide b. a strong covalent bond, —S—S—, important in linking polypeptide chains in proteins, the linkage arising as a result of the oxidation of the sulfhydryl (SH) groups of two molecules of cysteine.

high-energy phosphate b. an energy-rich phosphate linkage present in adenosine triphosphate (ATP), phosphocreatine, and certain other biological molecules. On hydrolysis at pH 7 it yields about 8000 calories per mole, in contrast to the 3000 calories yielded by phosphate esters. The bond stores energy that is used to drive biochemical processes, such as the synthesis of MACROMOLECULES, contraction of muscles, and the production of the electrical POTENTIALS for nerve conduction.

high-energy sulfur b. an energy-rich sulfur linkage, the most important of which occurs in the acetyl-CoA molecule, the main source of energy in fatty acid biosynthesis.

hydrogen b. a weak, primarily electrostatic, bond between a hydrogen atom bound to a highly electronegative element (such as oxygen or nitrogen) in a given molecule, or part of a molecule, and a second highly electronegative atom in another molecule or in a different part of the same molecule.

ionic b. a chemical bond in which electrons are transferred from one atom to another so that one bears a positive and the other a negative charge, the attraction between these opposite charges forming the bond.

peptide b. the —CO—NH— linkage formed between the carboxyl group of one amino acid and the amino group of another; it is an amide linkage joining amino acids to form peptides.

bonding (bond′ing) 1. joining together securely with an adhesive substance. 2. the development of a close emotional tie to a mate or to a newborn; called also claiming and binding-in. It is thought that optimal bonding of the parents to a newborn requires a period of close contact in the first few hours after birth. The mother initiates bonding when she caresses her infant and exhibits certain behaviors typical of a mother tending her child. The infant's responses to this, such as body and eye movements, are a necessary part of the process. The length of time necessary for bonding depends on the health of the infant and mother, as well as on circumstances surrounding labor and delivery. The presence of the father during the birth increases his bonding to the infant.

dentin b. establishment of a micromechanical bond between cut dentin and the bonding agent.

    enamel b. tooth bonding.

    tooth b. the technique of fixing orthodontic brackets or other attachments directly to the enamel surface with orthodontic adhesives.

bone (bōn) 1. the hard, rigid form of connective tissue constituting most of the skeleton of vertebrates, composed chiefly of calcium salts. 2. any distinct piece of the skeleton of the body. See anatomic Table of Bones in the Appendices for regional and alphabetical listings of bones, and see color plates 1 and 2. Called also os. adj., **bo'ny.**

There are 206 separate bones in the human body. Collectively they form the SKELETAL SYSTEM, a structure bound together by ligaments at the joints and set in motion by the muscles, which are secured to the bones by means of tendons. Bones, ligaments, muscles, and tendons are the tissues of the body responsible for supporting and moving the body.

Some bones have a chiefly protective function. An example is the skull, which encloses the brain, the back of the eyeball, and the inner ear. Some, such as the pelvis, are mainly supporting structures. Other bones, such as the jaw and the bones of the fingers, are concerned chiefly with movement. The bone MARROW in the center manufactures blood CELLS. The bones themselves act as a storehouse of CALCIUM, which must be maintained at a certain level in the blood for the body's normal chemical functioning.

Structure and Composition. Bone is not uniform in structure but is composed of several layers of different materials. The outermost layer, the periosteum, is a thin, tough membrane of fibrous tissue. It gives support to the tendons that secure the muscle to the bone and also serves as a protective sheath. This membrane encloses all bones completely except at the joints where there is a layer of cartilage. Beneath the periosteum lie the dense, hard layers of bone tissue called compact bone. Its composition is fibrous rather than solid and it gives bone its resiliency. Encased within these layers is the tissue that makes up most of the volume of bone, called cancellous or spongy bone because it contains little hollows like those of a sponge. The innermost portion of the bone is a hollow cavity containing marrow. Blood vessels course through every layer of bone, carrying nutritive elements, oxygen, and other products. Bone tissue also contains a large number of nerves. The basic chemical in bone, which gives bone its hardness and strength, is calcium phosphate.

Development. Cartilage forms the major part of bone in the very young; this accounts for the great flexibility and resiliency of the infant skeleton. Gradually, calcium phosphate collects in the cartilage, and it becomes harder and more brittle. Some of the cartilage cells break loose, so that channels develop in the bone shaft. Blood vessels enter the channels, bearing with them small cells of connective tissue, some of which become osteoblasts, cells that form true bone. The osteoblasts enter the hardened cartilage, forming layers of hard, firm bone. Other cells, called osteoclasts, work to tear down old or excess bone structure, allowing the osteoblasts to rebuild with new bone. This renewal continues throughout life, although it slows down with age.

Cartilage formation and the subsequent replacement of cartilage by hard material is the mechanism by which bones grow in size. During the period of bone growth, cartilage grows over the hardened portion of bone. In time, this layer of cartilage hardens as calcium phosphate is added, and a fresh layer grows over it, and it too hardens. The process continues until the body reaches full growth. Long bones grow in length because of special cross-sectional layers of cartilage located near the flared ends of the bone. These harden and new cartilage is produced by the same process as previously described.

Bone Disorders. FRACTURE, a break in the bone, is the most common injury to the bone; it may be closed, with no break in the skin, or open, with penetration of the skin and exposure of portions of the broken bone. OSTEOPOROSIS is excessive brittleness and porosity of bone in the aged. OSTEOMYELITIS is a bone infection similar to a boil on the skin, but much more serious because blood supply to bone is less exquisite than that to other body organs and bone metabolizes more slowly, so that the infection can destroy the bone and invade other body tissues. OSTEOMALACIA is the term used for RICKETS when it occurs in adults. In these diseases there is softening of the bones, due to inadequate concentration of calcium or phosphorus in the body. The usual cause is deficiency of vitamin D, which is required for utilization of calcium and phosphorus by the body. In OSTEITIS FIBROSA CYSTICA, bone is replaced by fibrous tissue because of abnormal calcium metabolism. The condition usually is due to overactivity of the parathyroid glands. OSTEOMA refers to abnormal new growth, either benign or malignant, of the tissue of the bones. Although it is not common, it may occur in any of the bones of the body, and at any age.

alveolar b. the thin layer of bone making up the bony processes of the maxilla and mandible, surrounding and containing the teeth; it is pierced by many small blood vessels, lymphatic vessels, and nerves.

ankle b. talus.

brittle b's osteogenesis imperfecta.

bundle b. lamina dura.

cancellated b., cancellous b. bone composed of thin intersecting lamellae, usually found internal to compact bone.

cartilage b. bone developing within cartilage, ossification taking place within a cartilage model, as opposed to membranous bone.

cheek b. zygomatic bone.

collar b. clavicle.

compact b. bone substance that is dense and hard.

cortical b. the compact bone of the shaft of a bone that surrounds the marrow cavity.

cranial b's the bones that constitute the CRANIUM, including the occipital, sphenoid, temporal, parietal, frontal, ethmoid, lacrimal, and nasal bones, the inferior nasal concha, and the vomer. Some authorities also include the maxilla, zygomatic bone, and palatine bone. See anatomic Table of Bones in the Appendices.

ethmoid b. the sievelike bone that forms a roof for the nasal fossae and part of the floor of the anterior cranial fossa. See anatomic Table of Bones in the Appendices.

facial b's the bones that form the skeleton of the face, including the hyoid, palatine, and zygomatic bones, the mandible, and the maxilla. Some authorities include the lacrimal bones, nasal bones, inferior nasal concha, and vomer and exclude the hyoid bone. See anatomic Table of Bones in the Appendices.

flat b. one whose thickness is slight, sometimes consisting of only a thin layer of compact bone, or of two layers with intervening cancellous bone and marrow; usually curved rather than flat.

frontal b. the bone at the anterior part of the skull. See anatomic Table of Bones in the Appendices.

heel b. calcaneus.

hip b. the ilium, ischium, and pubis as a unit. See anatomic Table of Bones in the Appendices.

hyoid b. a horseshoe-shaped bone at the base of the tongue. See anatomic Table of Bones in the Appendices. Called also lingual bone.

incisive b. the portion of the maxilla bearing the incisors; developmentally, it is

the premaxilla, which in humans later fuses with the maxilla, but in most other vertebrates persists as a separate bone.

innominate b. hip bone.

jaw b. either the MANDIBLE (lower jaw) or the MAXILLA (upper jaw). See anatomic Table of Bones in the Appendices.

jugal b. zygomatic bone.

lingual b. hyoid bone.

long b. one whose length far exceeds its breadth and thickness.

malar b. zygomatic bone.

marble b's osteopetrosis.

mastoid b. mastoid PART of temporal bone.

membrane b., membranous b. bone that develops within a connective tissue membrane, in contrast to cartilage bone.

occipital b. the bone constituting the back and part of the base of the skull. See anatomic Table of Bones in the Appendices.

parietal b. one of two bones forming the sides and roof of the cranium. See anatomic Table of Bones in the Appendices.

pelvic b. hip bone.

petrous b. petrous PART of temporal bone.

pneumatic b. bone that contains air-filled spaces.

premaxillary b. premaxilla.

pterygoid b. pterygoid process.

rider's b. localized ossification sometimes seen on the inner aspect of the lower end of the tendon of the adductor muscle of the thigh in horseback riders.

shin b. tibia.

short b. one of approximately equal length, width, and thickness.

solid b. compact bone.

spongy b. cancellous bone.

squamous b. squamous PART of temporal bone.

sutural b. any of the variable and irregularly shaped bones in the sutures between the bones of the skull. Called also wormian bone.

temporal b. one of two bones forming part of the lateral and inferior surfaces of the skull and containing the organs of HEARING. See anatomic Table of Bones in the Appendices.

thigh b. femur.

turbinate b. a nasal CONCHA.

tympanic b. tympanic PART of temporal bone.

wormian b. sutural bone.

zygomatic b. the quadrilateral bone that forms a cheek. See anatomic Table of Bones in the Appendices.

bonelet (bōn′let) ossicle.

Bonine (bo'nēn) trademark for preparations of MECLIZINE, an antinauseant.

Boolean logic (boo'le-an) an algebra that permits operations on sets of elements; it is used in online literature searches. The principal Boolean operators are AND (intersection), OR (union), and NOT (difference).

booster phenomenon (boos'ter) on a TUBERCULIN TEST, an initial false negative result due to a diminished amnestic response that becomes positive on subsequent testing.

boot (boot) an encasement for the foot; a protective casing or sheath.

Gibney b. an adhesive tape support used in treatment of sprains and other painful conditions of the ankle, the tape being applied in a basket-weave fashion with strips placed alternately under the sole of the foot and around the back of the leg.

Unna's paste b. a dressing for varicose ulcers, consisting of a paste made from gelatin, zinc oxide, and glycerin, which is applied to the entire leg, then covered with a spiral bandage, this in turn being given a coat of the paste; the process is repeated until satisfactory rigidity is attained.

borate (bor'āt) any salt of boric acid.

borborygmus (bor''bor-ig'mus), pl. *borboryg'mi* a rumbling noise caused by propulsion of gas through the intestines; see also BOWEL SOUNDS.

border (bor'der) a bounding line, edge, or surface.

brush b. a specialization of the free surface of a cell, consisting of minute cylindrical processes (microvilli) that greatly increase the surface area. (See accompanying illustration.)

vermilion b. the exposed red portion of the upper and lower lips.

borderline (bor'der-līn'') 1. of a phenomenon, straddling the dividing line between two categories. 2. a term used in psychiatry for PERSONALITY DISORDERS originally viewed as being on the border between PSYCHOSIS and NEUROSIS. See BORDERLINE PERSONALITY DISORDER.

b. personality disorder a PERSONALITY DISORDER marked by various features of borderline personality organization, such as instability, impulsiveness, intense or poorly controlled anger, inability to tolerate being alone, and chronic feelings of emptiness. Affected individuals sometimes seem to be on the borderline of psychosis and are highly unstable in mood, behavior, self-image, and affect. None of the features of the condition are constant; behavior is highly unpredictable and such persons seldom achieve their full potential. Their interpersonal relationships are often stormy because of their shifts in attitude and their tendency to idealize, devalue, or manipulate others. Suicidal gestures and self-mutilation sometimes occur with this disorder. The American Psychiatric Association has published *Practice Guidelines for the Treatment of Patients with Borderline Personality Disorder*, which is printed on their web site at http://www.psych.org.

Bordet-Gengou phenomenon (bor-da'-zhaw-goo') complement fixation.

Bordetella (bor''dě-tel'ah) a genus of gram-negative aerobic cocci. *B. pertus'sis* is the etiologic agent of WHOOPING COUGH. *B. bronchisep'tica* and *B. parapertus'sis* are also found occasionally in whooping cough.

boric acid (bor'ik) a mild acid used as a buffer. It was formerly used as a household antiseptic for treating minor irritations of the skin and eyes. Because the powder is highly poisonous when taken internally, and since other antiseptics are more effective, boric acid is no longer recommended. Boric acid ointment (for external use only) occasionally helps in cases of mild skin irritations and keeps gauze dressing from sticking to a wound. It is also used as a pesticide to kill ants and cockroaches.

borism (bor'izm) BORON POISONING.

Bornholm disease (born'hōm) epidemic pleurodynia.

boron (B) (bōr'on) a chemical element, atomic number 5, atomic weight 10.811. (See Appendix 6.)

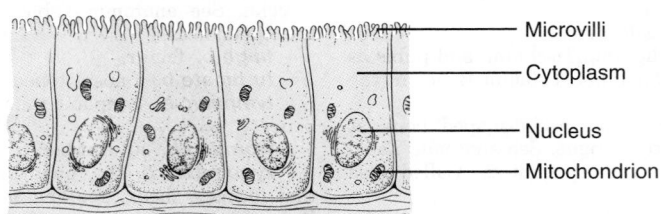

Brush border, characterized by closely packed microvilli. From Dorland's, 2000.

Microvilli

Cytoplasm

Nucleus

Mitochondrion

b. poisoning poisoning by BORON, BORIC ACID, or a borate salt. Symptoms include weakness, ataxia, tremors, convulsions, and often death. Called also borism.

Borrelia (bo-rel′e-ah) a genus of gram-negative, aerobic, spirochete bacteria that are parasites on mucous membranes and cause BORRELIOSIS and other conditions. *B. burgdor′feri,* transmitted by ixodid ticks, is the cause of ACRODERMATITIS CHRONICA ATROPHICANS, ERYTHEMA CHRONICUM MIGRANS, and LYME DISEASE. *B. recurren′tis* is transmitted by the human body louse *Pediculus humanus* and causes epidemic RELAPSING FEVER in various countries around the world. A number of other species are spread by tick bites and also cause RELAPSING FEVER.

borreliosis (bo-rel″e-o′sis) infection with spirochetes of the genus *Borrelia.*

Lyme b. a general term encompassing several different diseases that are caused by *Borrelia burgdorferi* and have similar manifestations, including LYME DISEASE, ACRODERMATITIS CHRONICA ATROPHICANS, and ERYTHEMA CHRONICUM MIGRANS.

boss (bos) a rounded eminence.

bosselated (bos′ĕ-lāt″ed) marked or covered with bosses.

botfly (bot′fli) an insect of the family Oestridae whose larvae (called *bots*) are parasitic, especially in horses and sheep. Genera include *Oestrus, Gasterophilus,* and *Dermatobia.*

botryoid (bot′re-oid) shaped like a bunch of grapes.

botryomycosis (bot″re-o-mi-ko′sis) a chronic purulent granulomatous bacterial infection usually caused by *Staphylococcus aureus.* Human infection is usually localized to the skin but may involve other organs such as the viscera and lymph nodes, especially in debilitated patients.

botuliform (bŏ-choo′lĭ-form) sausage-shaped.

botulin (boch′u-lin) botulinum toxin.

botulinal (boch″u-lĭ′nal) pertaining to *Clostridium botulinum* or to its toxin (botulinum toxin).

botulism (boch′u-lizm) 1. any poisoning caused by *Clostridium botulinum* in the body; it produces a NEUROTOXIN called botulinum TOXIN. 2. specifically, a rare but severe, often fatal, form of FOOD POISONING due to ingestion of improperly canned or preserved foods contaminated with *Clostridium botulinum.* Called also foodborne botulism. Symptoms include vomiting, abdominal pain, headache, weakness, constipation, and nerve paralysis (causing difficulty in seeing, breathing, and swallowing), with death from paralysis of the respiratory organs. To prevent botulism, home canning and preserving

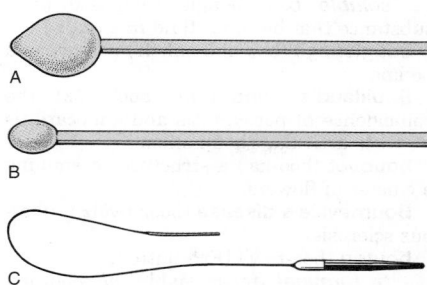

Bougies: *A,* Otis bougie à boule; *B,* olive-tipped bougie; *C,* filiform bougie. From Dorland's, 2000.

of all nonacid foods (that is, all foods other than fruits and tomatoes) must be done according to proper specific directions.

Treatment. Treatment is determined based on the type of botulism, but careful respiratory assessment and support are always required. An antitoxin to block the action of toxin circulating in the blood can be used for foodborne and wound botulism if the problem is diagnosed and treated early.

foodborne b. botulism (def. 2).

infant b. that affecting infants, typically 4 to 26 weeks of age, marked by constipation, lethargy, hypotonia, and feeding difficulty; it may lead to respiratory insufficiency. It results from toxin produced in the gut by ingested organisms, rather than from preformed toxins.

wound b. a form resulting from infection of a wound with *Clostridium botulinum.*

bougie (boo′zhe) a slender, flexible or rigid, hollow or solid, cylindrical instrument for introduction into the urethra or other tubular organ, usually for calibrating or dilating constricted areas. (See accompanying illustration.)

filiform b. a bougie of very slender caliber, generally used for exploration of small areas, such as sinus tracts, where false tracts could be easily created. The entering end is of smaller diameter, and the following end is threaded to allow for attachment of a following bougie.

following b. a flexible, tapered bougie attachable to a filiform bougie and allowing progressive dilatation without creation of false tracts.

Hurst b's a series of mercury-filled tubes of progressive diameter used for dilatation of the cardioesophageal region.

Maloney b's a series of mercury-filled tubes of progressive diameter, having cone-shaped tips.

soluble b. a bougie composed of a substance that becomes fluid *in situ.*

bougienage (boo″zhĕ-nahzh′) passage of a bougie.

Bouillaud's syndrome (boo′e-yōz) the coincidence of pericarditis and endocarditis in acute articular rheumatism.

bouquet (boo-ka′) a structure resembling a cluster of flowers.

Bourneville's disease (boorn-vēlz′) tuberous sclerosis.

bouton (boo-taw′) [Fr.] button.

b. terminal (ter-mĭ-nahl′), *pl.* boutons′ terminaux′ end-foot.

boutonneuse fever (boo-ton-ez′) a tick-borne disease endemic in the Mediterranean area, Crimea, Africa, and India, due to infection with *Rickettsia conorii,* with chills, fever, primary skin lesion (tache noire), and rash appearing on the second to fourth day.

bovine (bo′vīn) pertaining to, characteristic of, or derived from the ox (cattle).

bowel (bow′el) intestine.

b. bypass syndrome a syndrome that may occur one to six years after jejunoileal bypass, characterized by rash, malaise, myalgia, polyarthralgia, sterile skin pustules, and a flulike illness; it is probably caused by circulating immune complexes that include bacterial antigens resulting from bacterial overgrowth in the bypassed bowel.

b. sounds relatively high-pitched abdominal sounds caused by the propulsion of the intestinal contents through the lower alimentary tract. Auscultation of bowel sounds is best accomplished by using a diaphragm-type stethoscope rather than a bell-shaped one. Normal bowel sounds are characterized by bubbling and gurgling noises that vary in frequency, intensity, and pitch. In the presence of distention from flatus, the sounds are hyperresonant and can be heard over the entire abdomen.

The *absence* of bowel sounds is symptomatic of greatly decreased or totally absent peristaltic movement. This can occur in such conditions as paralytic ileus, advanced intestinal obstruction, gangrene of the bowel, enterocolic ulceration, myxedema, and spinal cord injury. In the early stages of bowel obstruction, high-pitched splashing sounds are heard in the intestine proximal to the obstruction. As the obstruction continues to constrict the lumen of the bowel, the sounds are of shorter duration and eventually cease altogether as the obstruction to the lumen of the bowel becomes complete.

Increased motility of the bowel usually results from some sort of irritating stimulus, such as gastroenteritis with diarrhea, bleeding in the intestine, and emotional disorders. Hyperactivity of the bowel produces a rush of sounds, with waves of loud, gurgling, and tinkling sounds called *borborygmi.*

b. training 1. a nursing INTERVENTION classification defined as assisting the patient to learn to evacuate the bowel at specific intervals. 2. a program designed to help the patient having difficulty with the regulation and control of DEFECATION. A program of this type may be indicated in cases ranging from chronic constipation to paralysis, as in PARAPLEGIA and HEMIPLEGIA. Patients who suffer from lesions or congenital anomalies of the intestinal tract also may benefit from such a program.

Before planning a program of bowel control it is necessary to determine the cause of the difficulty, the patient's former bowel habits, and specific symptoms. The plan devised will depend on the patient's needs and physical, mental, and emotional capacities for cooperation in the planning and implementation of the program. It is necessary to know whether the person can realistically be expected to achieve complete control, or if neural damage or anatomical and structural changes in the intestine prevent reaching this goal. For example, a COLOSTOMY patient cannot achieve complete control over bowel movements, but regulation of diet and fluid intake can affect the number and consistency of the stools, giving some sense of security. Diet also is important in all other types of bowel training in which the goal is regularity of defecation and stools of normal consistency.

It is important that patients participate as much as possible in planning the program. They will need to give an accurate history of bowel habits, former use of laxatives and enemas, usual time of day for bowel movements, and the frequency, and whether or not they are aware of the urge to defecate. As the program is carried out, revisions may be necessary as the patient learns which techniques are most helpful.

The major components of a bowel training program are choosing the location to ensure some degree of privacy, getting the patient into a sitting position, having him attempt defecation at a specific time that is most natural for him, regulating the food and fluid intake, and establishing some plan of regular exercise and physical activity.

In some cases of paralysis it may be necessary to stimulate bowel function through the use of suppositories and digital stimulation. Enemas, laxatives, and bulk-forming medications are used only if necessary, not on a regular basis if at all possible. These measures may be necessary, however, at the beginning of a bowel training program to remove constipated stool and FECAL IMPACTION.

Bowen's disease (bo′enz) intraepidermal squamous cell carcinoma, often occurring in multiple sites.

bowleg (bo′leg′) genu varum.

Boyle's law (boilz) at a constant temperature the volume of a perfect gas varies inversely with pressure; that is, as increasing pressure is applied, the volume decreases. Conversely, as pressure is reduced, volume is increased.

BP 1. blood pressure. 2. boiling point. 3. *British Pharmacopoeia*, a publication of the General Medical Council, describing and establishing standards for medicines, preparations, materials, and articles used in the practice of medicine, surgery, or midwifery.

bp boiling point.

bpm beats per minute.

Bq becquerel.

Br bromine.

brace (brās) 1. an orthopedic appliance or apparatus applied to the body, particularly the trunk and lower limbs, to support the weight of the body, to correct or prevent deformities, or to control involuntary movements. See also ORTHOSIS. 2. (in the plural) orthodontic APPLIANCE.

Milwaukee b. a brace consisting of a leather girdle and neck ring connected by metal struts; used to brace the spine in the treatment of SCOLIOSIS. (See accompanying illustration.)

neck b. cervical orthosis.

brachi(o)- word element [L., Gr.], *arm*.

brachial (bra′ke-al) pertaining to the upper LIMB.

b. plexus a nerve plexus partly in the neck and partly in the axilla, originating from the ventral branches of the last four cervical spinal nerves and most of the

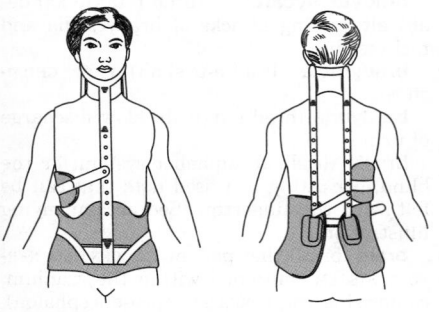

Milwaukee brace. From Bolander, 1994.

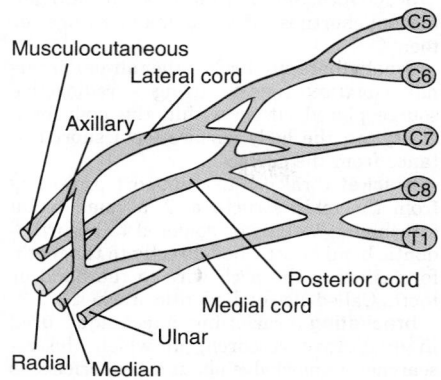

Brachial plexus.

ventral branch of the first thoracic spinal nerves. It has a *supraclavicular part* and an *infraclavicular part* that give off many of the principal nerves of the shoulder and upper limb. (See accompanying illustration.)

brachialgia (bra″ke-al′jah) pain in the arm.

brachiocephalic (bra″ke-o-sĕ-fal′ik) pertaining to the upper limb and the head.

brachiocrural (bra′ke-o-kroo′ral) pertaining to an upper and lower limb.

brachiocubital (bra″ke-o-ku′bĭ-t'l) pertaining to the arm and elbow or forearm, such as something extending from the upper arm to the forearm.

brachiocyrtosis (bra″ke-o-ser-to′sis) crookedness of the arm.

brachium (bra′ke-um), pl. *bra′chia* [L.] 1. arm (def. 1). 2. arm (def. 3).

brachy- word element [Gr.], *short.*

brachybasia (brak″e-ba′zhah) a slow, shuffling, short-stepped gait.

brachycardia (brak″e-kahr′de-ah) bradycardia.

brachycephalic (brak″e-sĕ-fal′ik) having a short wide head.

brachycephaly (brak″e-sef′ah-le) the state of being brachycephalic.

brachycheilia (brak″e-ki′le-ah) shortness of the lip.

brachydactyly (brak″e-dak′tĭ-le) abnormal shortness of the fingers and toes.

brachygnathia (brak″ig-na′the-ah) abnormal shortness of the mandible.

brachymetacarpia (brak″e-met″ah-kahr′pe-ah) abnormal shortness of the metacarpal bones.

brachymetatarsia (brak″e-met″ah-tahr′se-ah) abnormal shortness of the metatarsal bones.

brachyphalangia (brak″e-fah-lan′jah) abnormal shortness of a phalanx of a finger or toe.

brachytherapy (brak″e-ther′ah-pe) internal RADIATION THERAPY using a radioactive source placed either within the body or a cavity, on the body surface, or a short distance from the surface.

bracket (brak′et) 1. a support projecting from the main structure. 2. a small metal attachment welded or soldered to an orthodontic band or attached directly to the teeth, for fastening the arch wire to the band or tooth. Called also orthodontic bracket.

bracketing (brak′et-ing) a technique, used in qualitative research, in which the researcher's knowledge about an experience is suspended or set aside.

Braden Scale (bra′den) an assessment tool for predicting the risk of PRESSURE ULCERS, based on the total of scores given in the categories sensory perception, moisture, activity, mobility, nutrition, and friction and shear.

brady- word element [Gr.], *slow.*

bradyacusia (brad″e-ah-ku′ze-ah) dullness of hearing.

bradyarrhythmia (brad″e-ah-rith′me-ah) BRADYCARDIA associated with ARRHYTHMIA; the rate is 60 beats per minute or less. It is caused by conditions such as sinus bradycardia, sinoatrial block, and atrioventricular block.

bradycardia (brad″e-kahr′de-ah) slowness of the heartbeat, so that the pulse rate is less than 60 per minute. This can occur in normal persons, particularly during sleep; trained athletes also usually have slow pulse and heart rates. adj., **bradycar′diac.**

fetal b. a fetal heart rate of less than 120 beats per minute, generally associated with hypoxia; it is usually due to placental INSUFFICIENCY; it may also result from transfer of local anesthetics or beta-adrenergic blocking agents, and rarely to heart block associated with congenital heart disease or maternal collagen vascular disease.

nodal b. bradycardia in which the stimulus of the heart's contraction arises in the atrioventricular node or common bundle.

sinoatrial b., sinus b. a slow sinus rhythm, with a heart rate of less than 60 beats per minute in an adult; it is common in young adults and in athletes but is also a manifestation of some disorders.

b.-tachycardia syndrome any cardiac DYSRHYTHMIA characterized by alternating slow and fast heart rates, often resulting in hemodynamic compromise. See also SICK SINUS SYNDROME.

bradydysrhythmia an abnormal heart rhythm with rate less than 60 beats per minute in an adult; the term BRADYARRHYTHMIA is usually used instead.

bradyesthesia (brad″e-es-the′zhah) slowness or dullness of perception.

bradyglossia (brad″e-glos′e-ah) abnormal slowness of utterance.

bradykinesia (brad″e-kĭ-ne′zhah) abnormal slowness of movement. adj., **bradykinet′ic.**

bradykinin (brad″e-ki′nin) a nonapeptide KININ formed from a plasma protein, high-molecular-weight (HMW) kininogen by the action of kallikrein; it is a very powerful vasodilator that increases capillary permeability and, in addition, constricts smooth muscle and stimulates pain receptors.

bradylalia (brad″e-la′le-ah) abnormally slow utterance due to a central nervous system lesion; bradyphasia.

bradylexia (brad″e-lek′se-ah) abnormal slowness in reading, due neither to defect in intelligence or of vision, nor to ignorance of the alphabet.

bradylogia (brad″e-lo′jah) bradylalia.

bradyphagia (brad″e-fa′jah) abnormal slowness of eating.

bradyphasia (brad″e-fa′zhah) bradylalia.

bradyphemia (brad″e-fe′me-ah) slowness of speech.

bradyphrasia (brad″e-fra′zhah) bradylalia.

bradypnea (brad″e-ne′ah) respirations that are regular in rhythm but slower than normal in rate. This is normal during sleep; otherwise it is associated with disturbance in the brain's respiratory control center, as when the center is affected by opiate narcotics, alcohol, a tumor, a metabolic disorder, or a respiratory decompensation mechanism. See also HYPOPNEA and HYPOVENTILATION.

bradyspermatism (brad″e-sper′mah-tizm) abnormally slow EJACULATION of semen.

bradysphygmia (brad″e-sfig′me-ah) abnormal slowness of the pulse.

bradytachycardia (brad″e-tak″e-kar′de-ah) alternating attacks of bradycardia and tachycardia.

bradytocia (brad″e-to′shah) slow CHILDBIRTH.

bradyuria (brad″e-u′re-ah) slow discharge of urine.

braille (brāl) an alphabet system for the blind, consisting of raised dots that can be felt with the fingertip. (See accompanying illustration.)

brain (brān) that part of the CENTRAL NERVOUS SYSTEM contained within the cranium, comprising the FOREBRAIN (prosencephalon), MIDBRAIN (mesencephalon), and HINDBRAIN

A	B	C	D	E	F

G	H	I	J	K	L

M	N	O	P	Q	R

S	T	U	V	W	X

Y	Z

Braille alphabet based on six-dot system. From Stein et al., 2000.

(rhombencephalon); it develops from the embryonic neural tube. The brain is a mass of soft, spongy, pinkish gray nerve tissue that weighs about 1.2 kg in a human being. It is connected at its base with the SPINAL CORD, which is also part of the central nervous system. Called also encephalon. (See also color plates.)

The brain is made up of billions of nerve cells, intricately connected with each other. It contains nerve CENTERS (groups of NEURONS and their connections) which control many involuntary functions, such as circulation, temperature regulation, and respiration, and interpret sensory impressions received from the eyes, ears, and other sense organs. Consciousness, emotion, thought, and reasoning are functions of the brain. It also contains centers or areas for associative memory which allow for recording, recalling, and making use of past experiences.

Cerebrum. The largest and main portion of the brain, the cerebrum is made up of an outer coating, or cerebral CORTEX, consisting of gray MATTER, several cell layers deep, covering the cerebral HEMISPHERES. The cortex is the thinking and reasoning brain, the intellect, as well as the part of the brain that receives information from the senses and directs the conscious movements of the body. (See illustration.)

In appearance the cortex is rather like a relief map, with one very deep valley (longitudinal fissure) dividing it lengthwise into symmetrical halves, and each of the halves again divided by two major valleys and many shallower folds. The longitudinal fissure runs from the brow to the back of the head, and deep within it is a bed of matted white fibers, the CORPUS CALLOSUM, which connects the left and right cerebral HEMISPHERES.

The major folds of the cortex divide each hemisphere into four sections or lobes: the occipital LOBE at the back of the skull, the parietal LOBE at the side, the frontal LOBE at the forehead, and the temporal LOBE at the temple.

The Senses. The major senses of VISION and HEARING have been well mapped in the cortex; the center for vision is at the back, in the occipital lobe, and the center for hearing is at the side, in the temporal lobe. Two other areas have been carefully explored, the sensory and motor areas for the body, which parallel each other along the fissure of Rolando. In the sensory strip are the brain cells that register all sensations, and in the motor strip are the nerves that control the voluntary muscles. In both, the parts of the body are represented in an orderly way.

It is in the sensory areas of the brain that all perception takes place. Here sweet and sour, hot and cold, and the form of an object held in the hand are recognized. Here are sorted out the sizes, colors, depth, and space relationships of what the eye sees, and the timbre, pitch, intensity, and harmony of what the ear hears. The significance of these perceptions is interpreted in the cortex and other parts of the brain. A face is not merely seen; it is recognized as familiar or interesting or attractive. Remembering takes place at the same time as perception, so that other faces seen in the past, or experiences linked to that face are called up. Emotions may also be stirred. For this type of association the cortex draws on other parts of the brain by way of the communicating network of nerves.

Memory. In the temporal lobe, near the auditory area, is a center for MEMORY. This center appears to be a storehouse where memories are filed. When this area alone is stimulated, a particular event, a piece of music, or an experience long forgotten or deeply buried is brought to the individual's mind, complete in every detail. This is a very mechanical type of memory; when the stimulation is removed the memory ends. When it is applied again, the memory begins again, not where it left off, but from the beginning.

Brainstem. This is the stemlike portion of the brain connecting the cerebral hemispheres with the spinal cord, and comprising midbrain, pons, and medulla oblongata. Some consider it to include the diencephalon.

Thalamus. This organ lies beneath the cortex, deep within the cerebral hemispheres. It is a relay station for body sensations, and integrates these sensations on their way to the cortex. The thalamus is an organ of crude consciousness and of sensations of rough contact and extreme temperatures, either hot or cold. It is principally here that pain is felt. In the thalamus, responses are of the all-or-nothing sort; even mild stimuli would be felt as acutely painful if they were not graded and modified by the cortex.

Hypothalamus. This organ lies below the thalamus, at the base of the cerebrum. It is small (no larger than a lump of sugar), but takes part in such vital activities as the ebb and flow of the body's fluids and the regulation of metabolism, blood sugar levels, and body temperature. It directs the body's many rhythms, including those of activity and rest, appetite and digestion, sexual desire, and menstrual and reproductive cycles. The hypothalamus is also the body's emotional brain. It is the integrating center of the AUTONOMIC NERVOUS SYSTEM, with its sympathetic and parasympathetic branches, and is located close to the PITUITARY GLAND.

Midbrain. Just below the thalamus is the short narrow pillar of the midbrain. This contains a center for visual reflexes, such as moving the head and eyes, as well as a sound-activated center, obsolete in humans, for pricking up the ears.

Medulla Oblongata. Below the midbrain is the medulla oblongata, the continuation upward of the spinal cord. In the medulla, the great trunk nerves, both motor and sensory, cross over, left to right and right to left, producing the puzzling phenomenon by which the left cerebral hemisphere controls the right half of the body, while the right hemisphere controls the left half of the body. This portion of the brain also contains the centers that activate the heart, blood vessels, and respiratory system.

CEREBELLUM. The cerebellum (Latin for "little brain") is attached to the back of the brainstem, under the curve of the cerebrum. It is connected, by way of the midbrain, with the motor area of the cortex and with the spinal cord, as well as with the SEMICIRCULAR CANALS, the organs of balance. The function of the cerebellum is apparently to blend and coordinate motion of the various muscles involved in voluntary movements. It does not direct these movements; that is the function of the cortex. The cortex, however, operates in terms of movements, not of muscles. As a conscious function the cortex may, for example, direct the arm to pick up a glass of water; the cerebellum, which operates entirely below the level of consciousness, then translates this instruction into detailed actions by the 32 different muscles in the hand, plus several more in the arm and shoulder. When the cerebellum is injured, the patient's movements are jerky and uncoordinated.

Cranial Nerves. These are twelve nerves that arise within the skull. All but the OLFACTORY NERVE emerge from the brainstem. Most, with the important exception of the VAGUS NERVE, serve the head and neck. See also CRANIAL NERVES.

Protection of the Brain. The brain is protected by the bony SKULL and by three layers of membranes, the MENINGES. Between the middle and inner layer is a space filled with CEREBROSPINAL FLUID, which serves as a shock absorber. The same system of membranes and fluid protects the spinal cord. The brain is protected from harmful substances in the bloodstream by a barrier called the BLOOD-BRAIN BARRIER, which keeps some of the substances out of the brain entirely and delays the entry of others for hours or even days after they have penetrated the rest of the body.

b. abscess a localized suppurative lesion within the intracranial cavity; most cases are secondary to middle ear infections. Other causes include compound fracture of the skull with contamination of brain tissue, sinusitis, and infections of the face, lung or heart. Symptoms include fever, malaise, irritability, severe headache, convulsions, vomiting, and other signs of

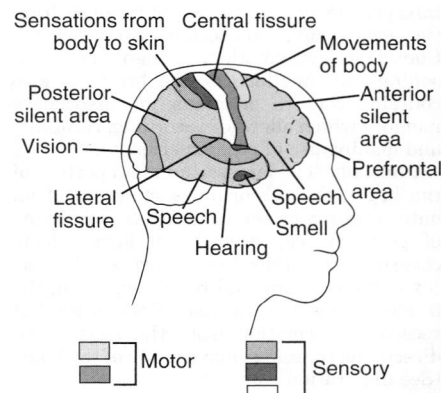

Projection areas of the brain.

intracranial hypertension. Treatment consists of surgical removal of the infected area and administration of antibiotics.

  b. death the irreversible cessation of all brain activity for an appropriate observation period, at least 24 hours, so that cardiopulmonary functions must be artificially maintained. A presidential commission in the USA accepted criteria for such a diagnosis, including cessation of all brain functions, including cerebral functions and brainstem (reflex) functions; irreversibility of the cessation; establishment of the cause of coma, sufficient to explain the loss of brain function; exclusion of possibility of recovery of brain function; and persistence of the cessation for an appropriate period of observation or trial of therapy. Complicating conditions must also be excluded. Called also irreversible coma.

  b. scanning a nuclear medicine procedure for the detection of brain tumors, areas of stroke syndrome, abscesses, hematomas, and other intracranial lesions. A radiopharmaceutical, such as ^{99m}Tc-pertechnetate, is injected intravenously and is carried to the brain, where it localizes around any lesion that alters the blood-brain barrier. A scintillation camera makes an image of the distribution of radioactivity in which a lesion appears as a region of increased activity. Computed TOMOGRAPHY brain scanning is an alternative procedure, which is more effective than radionuclide scans for the detection of some lesions.

  b. tumor a neoplasm of the intracranial portion of the central nervous system. Any abnormal growth within the skull creates a special problem because it is in a confined space and will press on normal brain tissue and interfere with the functions of the body controlled by the affected parts. This is true whether the tumor itself is benign or malignant. Fortunately, the functions of certain areas of the brain are well known, and a disturbance of some specific function guides the clinician to the affected area. If diagnosed early, a benign tumor often can be removed surgically with a good chance of recovery. Malignant tumors are more difficult to remove. The causes of brain tumors are not known. They are not common, but they can occur at any age and in any part of the brain. Some originate in the brain itself, while others metastasize from a tumor in another part of the body.

The symptoms of brain tumor vary and depend on the location and size of the tumor. Headache together with nausea is sometimes the first sign. The headache can be generalized or localized in one part of the head, and the pain is usually intense.

Vomiting can be significant if it is sudden and without nausea. Disturbances of vision, loss of coordination in movement, weakness, and stiffness on one side of the body are also possible symptoms. Loss of sight, hearing, taste, or smell may result from brain tumor. A tumor can also cause a distortion of any of these senses, such as seeing flashes at the sides of the field of vision, or smelling odors or hearing sounds that do not exist. It can affect the ability to speak clearly or to understand the speech of others. Varying degrees of weakness or paralysis in the arms or legs may appear. A tumor may cause convulsions. Changes in personality or mental ability are rare in cases of brain tumor. When such changes occur they may take the form of lapses of memory or absentmindedness, mental sluggishness, or loss of initiative.

  wet b. brain edema.

brainstem (brān′stem) the stemlike portion of the brain connecting the cerebral HEMISPHERES with the SPINAL CORD, and comprising the PONS, MEDULLA OBLONGATA, and MIDBRAIN; considered by some to include the DIENCEPHALON. Also written brain stem.

brainwashing (brān′wahsh-ing) any systematic effort aimed at instilling certain attitudes and beliefs in persons against their will, usually beliefs in conflict with their prior beliefs and knowledge. It initially referred to political indoctrination of prisoners of war and political prisoners.

branch (branch) a division or offshoot from a main stem, especially of blood vessels, nerves, or lymphatics. Called also ramus.

  bundle b. a branch of the bundle of His.

branchial (brang′ke-al) pertaining to, or resembling, gills of a fish or derivatives of homologous parts in higher animals.

  b. cyst a cyst formed deep within the neck from an incompletely closed pharyngeal GROOVE (branchial CLEFT), usually between the second and third pharyngeal ARCHES (branchial arches). These two arches grow together and enclose the cervical SINUS in the neck, which is a common site of a branchial cyst. Called also branchiogenic or branchiogenous cyst.

Branham's sign (bran′hamz) bradycardia produced by digital closure of an artery proximal to an arteriovenous fistula.

Branhamella (bran″hah-mel′ah) *Moraxella (Branhamella).*

brash (brash) heartburn.

  water b. heartburn with regurgitation of sour fluid or almost tasteless saliva into the mouth.

Braxton Hicks contractions (braks'ton hiks') light, usually painless, irregular contractions of the uterus throughout pregnancy, gradually increasing in intensity and frequency and becoming more rhythmic during the third trimester; they are often mistaken for true labor, and are sometimes referred to as "false labor." They may be stimulated by the descent of the head of the fetus into the pelvic inlet. Braxton Hicks contractions are not as regular and rhythmic as are true LABOR contractions.

breakdown (brāk'doun) 1. the act or process of ceasing to function, or the resulting condition. 2. an often sudden collapse in health, physical or mental. 3. loss of self-control.

nervous b. a nonspecific, popular name for any type of mental disorder that interferes with the affected individual's normal activities, often implying a severe episode of sudden onset.

breakthrough (brāk'throo") 1. a significant step forward in theory development or research. 2. in psychotherapy, a change in attitude or behavior following a period of little or no client insight.

breast (brest) the front of the chest, especially the modified cutaneous, glandular structure it bears, the mamma. In women the breasts are secondary sex organs with the function of producing milk after childbirth. The term breast is less commonly used to refer to the breasts of the human male, which neither function nor develop.

At the tip of each breast is an area called the areola, usually reddish in color; at the center of this area is the NIPPLE. About 20 separate lactiferous ducts empty into a depression at the top of the nipple. Each duct leads from alveoli within the breast called lobules, where the milk is secreted. Along their length, the ducts have widened areas that form reservoirs in which milk can be stored. The ducts and lobules form the glandular tissue of the breasts. Connective tissue covers the glandular tissue and is itself sheathed in a layer of fatty tissue. The fatty tissue gives the breast its smooth outline and contributes to its size and firmness. (See accompanying illustration.)

Surgery of the Breast. Surgical operations of the breast are done for a variety of reasons. MAMMOPLASTY refers to reconstructive surgery of the breast and includes procedures to enlarge the breasts (*augmentation mammoplasty*), reduce their size (*reduction mammoplasty*), or reconstruct one or both breasts so that they are equal in size and contour. With the advent of less radical surgery for breast malignancies, postmastectomy plastic surgery of the breast has become more commonplace. MASTECTOMY is surgical removal of breast tissue; it is most often done to treat breast cancer. Procedures can vary from a simple lumpectomy to a radical procedure in which the surgeon removes the internal mammary chain of lymph nodes, the entire breast, the underlying pectoral muscles, and the adjacent axillary lymph nodes.

b. cancer malignancy of the breast; it is second only to lung cancer as a cause of cancer deaths in North American women. It currently affects 1 in 9 women in the United States (11 per cent) and is called an epidemic by authorities. The incidence of breast cancer appears to be rising each year, even though when all age groups are considered its death rate has slightly declined in the past two decades. Risk factors include age over 40, close family member with breast cancer, onset of menses before age 13 or continuation beyond age 50, nulliparity, and first child after age 30.

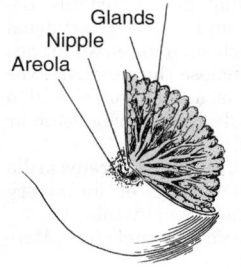

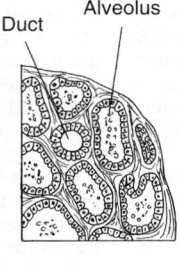

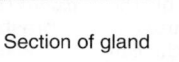

Section of gland

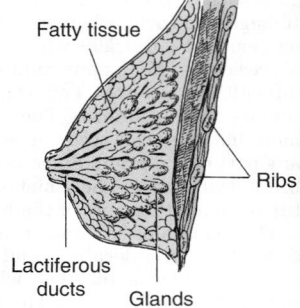

Breast, with detail and cross section.

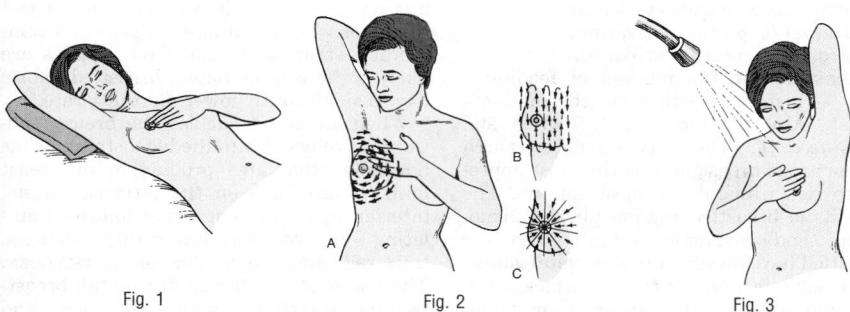

Fig. 1   Fig. 2   Fig. 3

Breast self-examination. From Lowdermilk et at., 2000. 1. The best time to do breast self-examination is after your period, when breasts are not tender or swollen. If you do not have regular periods or sometimes skip a month, do it on the same day every month. 2. Lie down and put a pillow under your right shoulder. Place your right arm behind your head (Fig. 1). 3. Use the finger pads of your three middle fingers on your left hand to feel for lumps or thickening. Your finger pads are the top third of each finger. 4. Press firmly enough to know how your breast feels. If you're not sure how hard to press, ask your health care provider, or try to copy the way your health care provider uses the finger pads during a breast examination. Learn what your breast feels like most of the time. A firm ridge in the lower curve of each breast is normal. 5. Move around the breast in a set way. You can choose either circles (Fig. 2, *A*), vertical lines (Fig. 2, *B*), or wedges (Fig. 2, *C*). Do it the same way every time. It will help you to make sure that you've gone over the entire breast area and to remember how your breast feels. 6. Gently compress the nipple between your thumb and forefinger and look for discharge. 7. Now examine your left breast using the finger pads of your right hand. 8. If you find any changes, see your health care provider right away. 9. You may want to check your breasts while standing in front of a mirror right after you do your breast self-examination each month. See if there are any changes in the way your breasts look: dimpling of the skin, changes in the nipple, or redness or swelling. 10. You may also want to do an extra breast self-examination while you're in the shower (Fig. 3). Your soapy hands will glide over the wet skin, making it easy to check how your breasts feel. 11. It is important to check the area between the breast and the underarm and the underarm itself. Also examine the area above the breast to the collarbone and to the shoulder.

Breast Self-Examination. Women should train themselves to perform a simple self-examination of the breasts (see illustration). The best time for this is just after menstruation when the breasts are normally soft. If any lump in the breast can be felt, a health care provider should be consulted immediately.

As with other forms of cancer, early detection and prompt treatment of malignancy of the breast are the keys to eradication of the disease. Studies have shown that breast self-examination has contributed to earlier detection and improved survival rates. It should be done monthly; more than 90 percent of breast cancers are discovered by the patients themselves either by chance or by routine self-examination. The American Cancer Society reports that only about 69 percent of women polled in the past had done self-examination at any time during the past year and less than 29 percent did it routinely each month.

Screening should begin by age 40 and should consist of a clinical examination every year and screening mammography every one or two years. Beginning at age 50, both the clinical examination and the mammography should be done once a year.

MAMMOGRAPHY is considered to be the best diagnostic method for early detection when tumors are small and not readily found by palpation. Other diagnostic techniques include thermography, ultrasonography, magnetic resonance imaging, and computerized tomography, but none of these is believed to be as accurate as mammography. The first symptom noted is usually a lump or nodule in the breast tissue; however, dimpling of the breast skin or changes in the nipple may be noted before a lump is found. Diagnosis of a malignant tumor is confirmed by biopsy.

Treatment. Options for treatment of breast cancer are based on the clinical stage of the disease when first diagnosed or when re-evaluated. Formerly, the most common procedure was radical mastectomy. However, improvements in irradiation equipment and procedures, alternative surgical techniques that are less mutilating, and more active participation of patients in making decisions about the mode of therapy have all resulted in significant changes in the treatment of breast cancer.

Additional information can be obtained by calling the National Cancer Institute's Cancer Information Service Hotline at 1-800-4-CANCER.

chicken b. pectus carinatum.
funnel b. pectus excavatum.
pigeon b. pectus carinatum.
breastfeeding the method of feeding a baby with milk directly from the mother's breast. Also written *breast feeding* and *breast-feeding*. There is strong research support that breast milk is the most appropriate nourishment for most infants. The benefits of breastfeeding are physical, emotional, and economic. Infants who are breastfed have lower rates of hospital admissions, ear infections, diarrhea, rashes, allergies, and other health problems than babies who receive infant formulas. Breastfeeding also benefits the mother by stimulating release of OXYTOCIN, which causes involution of the uterus following pregnancy. It can also be a very satisfying experience for the mother-baby pair and encourage bonding. Nevertheless, breastfeeding is a personal decision to be made by the mother with the support of health care providers. Mothers should be encouraged and supported to breastfeed, but they should not be made to feel guilty or inadequate if circumstances interfere with their ability to do so. Certain harmful agents and substances, such as the human immunodeficiency VIRUS, are transmitted through breast milk.

Breast milk is easily digested and of unique benefit to the baby, for whom it is perfectly formulated. It is sterile and contains nutrients needed by the infant in ideal proportions. It also contains IMMUNO-GLOBULINS. Breast milk is the standard against which all other infant formulas should be compared. The NATIONAL INSTITUTE OF ALLERGY AND INFECTIOUS DISEASES notes that there is no conclusive research evidence that breastfeeding helps prevent the development of food allergies as the child grows older. However, keeping an infant on exclusive breastfeeding does delay the onset of allergies by delaying the infant's exposure to foods that might prompt allergies. Based on research sponsored by the AGENCY FOR HEALTHCARE RESEARCH AND QUALITY, Vitamin D supplementation is recommended for dark-skinned infants and children who are fed only breast milk, beginning by two months of age.

The American Academy of Pediatrics, after an extensive review of the research, recommends that breast milk be almost the only food that a healthy infant receives for the first four to six months after birth. The Surgeon General of the United States and Healthy People 2010 Goals for the Nation have reviewed the research and set national goals related to increasing the number of mothers who breastfeed their infants. Moreover, in the underdeveloped countries where sanitation is poor and community water, milk, and food supplies are likely to be contaminated, breastfed babies have a significantly lower mortality rate.

When an infant suckles the breast, PRO-LACTIN is released into the bloodstream. This hormone stimulates production of breast milk. It also acts on the PITUITARY GLAND, interfering with the action of follicle-stimulating HORMONE and luteinizing HORMONE, thus reducing the production of ESTROGEN. The low level of estrogen during full breastfeeding interferes with OVULATION and MENSTRUATION, resulting in lactation AMENOR-RHEA.

As a rule, the baby nurses at both breasts during each feeding. The breast used to initiate the feeding should be alternated. Some babies nurse rapidly and others do it slowly. An infant should nurse 10 to 12 times a day initially. The intervals between the feedings will grow longer as the infant grows. Typically, a full-term infant will nurse every 2 to 3 hours.

Researchers and clinicians categorize breastfeeding as either *full* or *partial*. *Full breastfeeding* is either exclusive or almost exclusive (the latter allowing for water, juice, and infrequently given food). *Partial breastfeeding* is defined as either high (over 80 per cent breast milk), medium, or low (under 20 per cent breast milk). Occasional, irregular breastfeeding ("token" or "comfort feeding") is a category set apart from breastfeeding.

The LA LECHE LEAGUE is a voluntary organization that encourages breastfeeding and offers excellent support and guidance to nursing mothers. Local chapters may be listed in the telephone book, or their national office can be contacted by calling 1-800-LALECHE in the USA or 1-800-665-4324 in Canada. The web site for La Leche League International is http://www.la-lecheleague.org. Lactation CONSULTANTS can also offer assistance to mothers and health care providers.

effective b. a NURSING DIAGNOSIS accepted by the North American Nursing Diagnosis Association, defined as the state in which a mother-infant dyad/family exhibits adequate proficiency and satisfaction with the breastfeeding process.

ineffective b. a NURSING DIAGNOSIS accepted by the North American Nursing Diagnosis Association, defined as dissatisfaction or difficulty that a mother, infant, or child experiences with the breastfeeding process. Defining characteristics include lack of observable signs of oxytocin release, persistence of sore nipples beyond the first week of breastfeeding, insufficient emptying of each breast at each feeding, actual or perceived inadequate milk supply, nonsustained or insufficient opportunity for sucking at the breast, infant inability to attach correctly to the maternal breast, and infant arching of the back and crying at the breast. Related factors include prematurity, infant anomaly, and maternal anxiety or ambivalence.

interrupted b. a NURSING DIAGNOSIS accepted by the North American Nursing Diagnosis Association, defined as a break in the continuity of the breastfeeding process as a result of inability or inadvisability of putting the baby to the breast for feeding.

breath (breth) the air taken in and expelled during VENTILATION.

breathing (brēth'ing) VENTILATION (def. 2).

diaphragmatic b. 1. diaphragmatic RESPIRATION. 2. a type of breathing exercise that patients are taught to promote more effective aeration of the lungs, consisting of moving the diaphragm downward during inhalation and upward with exhalation.

frog b., glossopharyngeal b. respiration unaided by the primary or ordinary accessory muscles of respiration, the air being "swallowed" rapidly into the lungs by use of the tongue and the muscles of the pharynx; used by patients with chronic muscle paralysis to augment their vital capacity.

intermittent positive pressure b. (IPPB) see INTERMITTENT POSITIVE PRESSURE BREATHING.

mouth b. breathing through the mouth instead of the nose, usually because of some obstruction in the nasal passages.

b. pattern, ineffective a NURSING DIAGNOSIS approved by the North American Nursing Diagnosis Association, defined as INSPIRATION and/or EXPIRATION that does not provide adequate VENTILATION. Etiologic and contributing factors include disorders of the nervous system in which there is abnormal response to neural stimulation, as in spinal cord injury; impairment of musculoskeletal function, as in trauma to the chest; pain and discomfort associated with deep breathing, as after abdominal or thoracic surgery; fatigue and diminished energy level; inadequate lung expansion, as in poor body posture and positioning; inappropriate response to stress, as in hyperventilation; inflammation of respiratory structures; and tracheobronchial obstruction.

Subjective symptoms include reports of dyspnea, shortness of breath, pain

associated with breathing, complaints of dizziness, and previous episodes of emotional or physical stress or fear and anxiety. Objective symptoms include increased respiratory rate and changes in depth of respirations, fremitus, abnormal arterial blood gases, nasal flaring, orthopnea or assumption of the three-point position, in which the patient sits down and elevates the shoulders by stiffening each arm and pushing downward with the hands on the chair or bed, use of accessory muscles of respiration, increased anteroposterior diameter of chest (barrel CHEST), and altered chest excursion.

The goal of nursing intervention is to help the patient experience improved gas exchange by using a more effective breathing pattern. This might include teaching appropriate breathing exercises and proper use of accessory muscles of respiration, and encouraging body posture that maximizes expansion of the lungs. If postoperative pain is a contributing factor, providing support of the operative site to reduce strain during coughing or moving about could encourage deeper respirations and a more normal breathing pattern. If a causative factor is stress with resultant hyperventilation or some other ineffective breathing pattern, the patient may need help in developing more beneficial coping mechanisms such as relaxation techniques.

pursed-lip b. a breathing technique in which air is inhaled slowly through the nose and then exhaled slowly through pursed lips. This type of breathing is often used by patients with CHRONIC OBSTRUCTIVE PULMONARY DISEASE to prevent small airway collapse.

b.-related sleep disorder any of several disorders characterized by sleep disruption due to some sleep-related breathing problem, resulting in excessive sleepiness or insomnia. Included are central and obstructive sleep apnea syndromes (see adult sleep APNEA).

Breckinridge (brek'in-rij) Mary (1881–1965). American nurse, founder of the Frontier Nursing Service, a primarily midwifery service for women in remote areas of Kentucky. The Service, originally the Kentucky Committee for Mothers and Babies, was founded in 1925.

breech (brēch) buttocks.

bregma (breg'mah) the point on the surface of the skull at the junction of the coronal and sagittal sutures. adj., **bregmat'ic.** (See accompanying illustration.)

Brethine (breth'ēn) trademark for preparations sof TERBUTALINE sulfate, a bronchodilator.

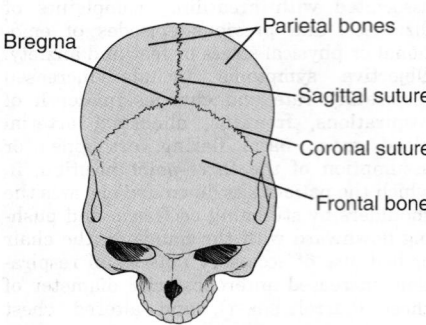

Bregma. From Dorland's, 2000.

bretylium (brĕ-til'e-um) an ADRENERGIC BLOCKING AGENT used in the form of the tosylate salt to control arrhythmias in certain cases of ventricular TACHYCARDIA or FIBRILLATION; administered by intravenous or intramuscular injection.

brevicollis (brev″ĭ-kol'is) shortness of the neck.

Brevital (brev'ĭ-tal) trademark for a preparation of METHOHEXITAL sodium, a BARBITURATE used as an anesthetic.

Bricker procedure (brik'er) ileal conduit.

bridge (brij) 1. a fixed partial DENTURE; see illustration.   2. pons. 3. a protoplasmic structure uniting adjacent elements of a cell, similar in plants and animals.

conjugative b. in bacterial CONJUGATION, a connection formed between two bacterial cells by the attachment of an F pilus from an F⁺ cell to an F⁻ cell.

disulfide b. disulfide bond.

bridgework (brij'werk) a partial denture retained by attachments other than clasps.

fixed b. one retained with crowns or inlays cemented to the natural teeth.

removable b. one retained by attachments which permit its removal.

brief psychotic disorder an episode of psychotic symptoms (incoherence, loosening of associations, delusions, hallucinations, disorganized or catatonic behavior) with sudden onset, lasting less than one month. If it occurs in response to a stressful life event, it may be called *brief reactive psychosis.*

Bright's disease (brīts) a broad descriptive term once used for kidney disease with proteinuria, usually glomerulonephritis; named for Richard Bright, an English physician who published a description of the diseases in 1827.

Brill's disease (brilz) recrudescent TYPHUS.

Brill-Symmers disease (bril' sim'erz) nodular lymphoma.

Brill-Zinsser disease (bril' zin'ser) recrudescent TYPHUS.

brim (brim) the upper edge of a bowllike structure.

pelvic b. pelvic inlet.

brimonidine (brĭ-mo'nĭ-dēn) an alpha-adrenergic RECEPTOR agonist used as the tartrate salt in treatment of open-angle GLAUCOMA and ocular hypertension; administered topically to the conjunctiva.

brinzolamide (brin-zo'lah-mīd) a carbonic anhydrase INHIBITOR used in treatment of open-angle GLAUCOMA and ocular hypertension.

Briquet's syndrome (bre-kāz') somatization disorder.

brisement (brēz-maw') [Fr.] a crushing, especially the breaking up of an ankylosis.

British antilewisite (BAL) dimercaprol.

BRM biological response modifier.

broach (brōch) 1. an elongated, tapered, and serrated cutting tool for shaping and enlarging holes. 2. barbed b.; root canal b.

barbed b. a thin, flexible, hand-operated or engine-driven endodontic instrument, usually tapered, with a series of sharply pointed barbs along the operative head; used for engaging and removing the

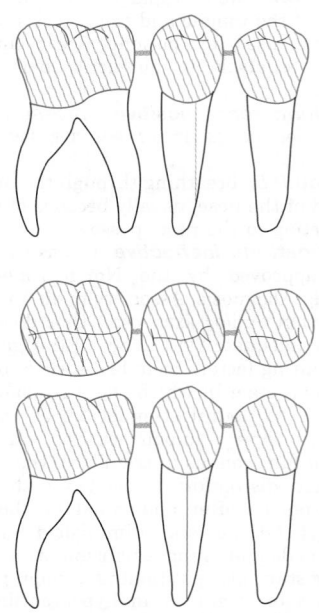

A bridge unit serves to restore a functional unit by replacing one or more missing teeth. A fixed bridge consists of abutment and pontic teeth splinted together. From Darby and Walsh, 1995.

dental pulp and other substances intact from the root canal or pulp chamber.

pathfinder b. root canal probe.

root canal b. a broach, usually barbed, used for removing the soft tissue contents of the root canal; see *barbed b.*

smooth b. root canal probe.

Brock syndrome (brok) middle lobe syndrome.

brokerage (bro´ker-aj) the process of acting as someone's representative, especially in negotiations.

culture b. in the NURSING INTERVENTIONS CLASSIFICATION, a nursing INTERVENTION defined as the deliberate use of culturally competent strategies to bridge or mediate between the patient's culture and the biomedical health care system.

bromelain (bro´mē-lān) any of a group of proteolytic enzymes that catalyze the cleavage of specific bonds in proteins. Different forms are derived from the fruit *(fruit b.)* and stem *(stem b.)* of the pineapple plant, *Ananas comosus.* As the concentrate *bromelains,* it is used as an ANTIINFLAMMATORY agent.

bromazepam (bro-maz´ĕ-pam) a BENZODIAZEPINE used as an ANTIANXIETY AGENT and as a SEDATIVE and HYPNOTIC; administered orally.

bromhidrosis (bro˝mĭ-dro´sis) the secretion of foul-smelling perspiration.

bromide (bro´mīd) any binary compound of BROMINE. Bromides produce depression of the central nervous system, and were once widely used for their sedative effect; because overdosage causes serious mental disturbances they are now seldom used, except occasionally in grand mal seizures. See also BROMISM.

bromidrosis (bro˝mĭ-dro´sis) bromhidrosis.

bromine (Br) (bro´mēn) a chemical element, atomic number 35, atomic weight 79.909. (See Appendix 6.)

bromism (bro´mizm) poisoning by excessive use of BROMINE or its compounds, seen when the bromine concentration in body fluids is high enough to have a toxic and depressant action on the central nervous system. The toxic level varies with the individual and is somewhat dependent on chloride intake because the bromide ion and the chloride ion are equally absorbed and distributed throughout the same fluid compartments. This means that in a person with a limited salt intake bromine accumulates more quickly and severe poisoning can occur after ingestion of an amount that would be relatively harmless for a person with a normal or high salt intake.

Bromism was much more common before the removal from the market of certain over-the-counter remedies high in bromide, advertised as "nerve tonics" or headache remedies. Symptoms include acne, coldness of arms and legs, fetid breath, sleeplessness, impotence, headache, irritability, emotional instability, malaise, and mental aberrations such as hallucinations, amnesia, and disorientation.

Treatment. Treatment consists of immediate curtailment of bromine ingestion and efforts to eliminate it from the body. Diuretics may be used, or enteric-coated tablets of ammonium and sodium chloride if they are not contraindicated by cardiac or renal disease. Removal of bromine from the system may take as long as several months. In severe, acute poisoning it may be removed by HEMODIALYSIS.

bromocriptine (bro˝mo-krip´tēn) an ergot alkaloid that acts as a DOPAMINE agonist; used as the mesylate salt to suppress prolactin secretion in the treatment of pituitary PROLACTINOMAS and of HYPERPROLACTINEMIA-associated amenorrhea, galactorrhea, infertility, or male hypogonadism. It is also used as an antidyskinetic, usually in conjunction with levodopa, in the treatment of PARKINSONISM, and is used as a growth hormone suppressant in the treatment of ACROMEGALY. Administered orally.

bromoderma (bro˝mo-der´mah) a skin eruption due to excessive use of BROMIDES.

bromodiphenhydramine (bro˝mo-di˝fenhi´drah-mēn) a sedating ANTIHISTAMINE used in the form of the hydrochloride salt in the treatment of nasal, eye, and skin manifestations of allergic reactions, including allergic rhinitis, conjunctivitis, and itching, and as an ingredient in some cough and cold preparations, administered orally.

bromomenorrhea (bro˝mo-men˝o-re´ah) menstruation characterized by an offensive odor.

brompheniramine (brōm˝fen-ir´ah-mēn) an ANTIHISTAMINE with sedative and anticholinergic effects; used as the maleate salt in the treatment of nasal, eye, and skin manifestations of allergic reactions, including allergic rhinitis, conjunctivitis, and itching, administered orally or by intramuscular, intravenous, or subcutaneous injection. The maleate salt is also an ingredient in some cold and cough preparations, administered orally.

Bromsulphalein (brōm-sul´fah-lēn) trademark for a preparation of SULFOBROMOPHTHALEIN sodium, a dye used in a liver function test called the SULFOBROMOPHTHALEIN TEST.

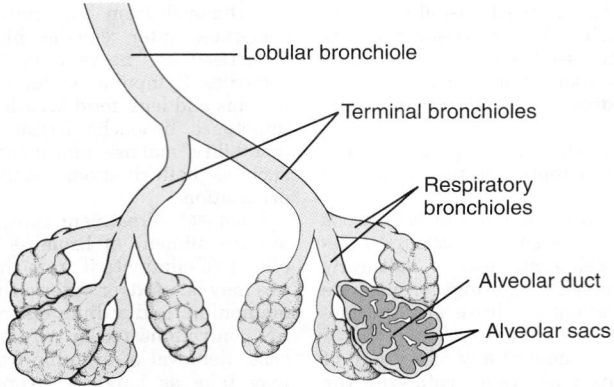

Lobular bronchiole

Terminal bronchioles

Respiratory bronchioles

Alveolar duct

Alveolar sacs

Respiratory bronchiole. From Dorland's 2000.

bronchadenitis (brong″kad-ĕ-ni′tis) inflammation of the bronchial glands.

bronchi (brong′ki) [L.] plural of BRONCHUS.

bronchial (brong′ke-al) pertaining to or affecting one or more bronchi.

b. challenge test a PULMONARY FUNCTION TEST in which an aerosol such as METHACHOLINE, HISTAMINE, or an ALLERGEN is administered to provoke BRONCHOSPASM; used in diagnosis of ASTHMA.

bronchiectasis (brong″ke-ek′tah-sis) chronic dilatation of the bronchi and bronchioles associated with secondary infection; types include *cylindrical, follicular, fusiform, saccular,* and *varicose,* named according to the nature of the dilatations. It is associated with chronic copious sputum production, and may be associated with an inherited ciliary dysfunction. The most immediate symptom is persistent coughing with sputum production. In advanced cases the sputum and breath may become foul-smelling, and the patient may suffer loss of appetite, anemia, fever, episodes of pneumonia, and a general lowering of resistance to infection. The principal treatment is chest physical therapy with antibiotics. Long-term care is essentially the same as for any patient with CHRONIC AIRFLOW LIMITATION.

bronchiloquy (brong-kil′o-kwe) bronchophony (def. 2).

bronchiocele (brong′ke-o-sēl″) bronchocele.

bronchiogenic (brong″ke-o-jen′ik) bronchogenic.

bronchiole (brong′ke-ōl) one of the successively smaller channels into which the segmental bronchi divide within the bronchopulmonary segments. adj., **bronchi′olar.**

respiratory b's the final branches of the bronchioles, communicating directly with the alveolar ducts; they are subdivisions of terminal bronchioles, have alveolar outcroppings, and themselves divide into several alveolar ducts. (See accompanying illustration and see color plates.)

terminal b. the last portion of a bronchiole that does not contain alveoli, i.e., one whose sole function is gas conduction; it subdivides into respiratory bronchioles.

bronchiolectasis (brong″ke-o-lek′tah-sis) dilatation of the bronchioles.

bronchiolitis (brong″ke-o-li′tis) inflammation of the bronchioles due to a viral infection; children are more often affected than adults. (See accompanying illustration.)

b. exudati′va, exudative b. inflammation of the bronchioles with exudation of Curschmann's spirals (coiled mucinous fibrils) and gray, tenacious sputum; often associated with asthma.

b. fibro′sa obli′terans chronic bronchiolitis with ingrowth of connective tissue from the wall of the terminal bronchi and occlusion of their lumina; it may be a complication of connective tissue disease or heart-lung transplant, and in children it may follow an acute attack of bronchiolitis or pneumonia.

b. obli′terans, obliterative b. bronchiolitis fibrosa obliterans.

bronchiolus (brong-ki′o-lus), pl. *bronchi′oli* [L.] bronchiole.

bronchiospasm (brong′ke-o-spaz″m) bronchospasm.

bronchiostenosis (brong″ke-o-stĕ-no′sis) bronchostenosis.

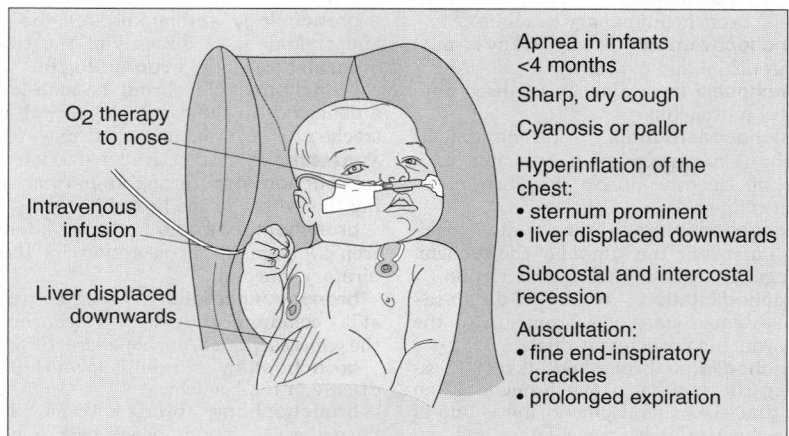

O₂ therapy to nose

Intravenous infusion

Liver displaced downwards

Apnea in infants
<4 months

Sharp, dry cough

Cyanosis or pallor

Hyperinflation of the chest:
• sternum prominent
• liver displaced downwards

Subcostal and intercostal recession

Auscultation:
• fine end-inspiratory crackles
• prolonged expiration

Clinical features of severe bronchiolitis in an infant. From Lissauer and Graham, 2002.

bronchitis (brong-ki′tis) inflammation of one or more bronchi. adj., **bronchit′ic.** Bronchitis may be either an acute or chronic disorder and frequently involves the trachea as well as the bronchi (TRACHEOBRONCHITIS). The acute stage of the disease often is an extension of an upper respiratory infection, which is usually viral in origin. Causes other than infectious agents are physical and chemical irritants that are inhaled in air polluted by dust, automobile exhaust, industrial fumes, and tobacco smoke.

Acute Bronchitis. This condition is most often seen in small children and in the elderly or the debilitated. It is particularly serious in small children because their bronchi are smaller and more easily obstructed. The elderly and debilitated are prime targets for complications of bronchitis because they are more susceptible to secondary infections. Symptoms include the early symptoms of an upper respiratory infection or common cold, which progress to chest pain, fever, and a dry, irritating cough. Later the cough becomes more productive of mucopurulent to purulent sputum. There may be moderate fever with accompanying chills, muscle soreness, and headache.

Clinical guidelines published by the American College of Physicians–American Society of Internal Medicine for treatment of acute bronchitis in otherwise healthy adults emphasize the importance of ruling out other serious illnesses such as PNEUMONIA when evaluating a patient with an acute cough illness. Use of routine antibiotic treatment for patients with acute bronchitis is not recommended, since there is no research support for it. The practitioner is urged to give a realistic prediction of the duration of the cough, typically 10 to 14 days. A determination is important of which symptoms are most troublesome to the patient. Most patients seek treatment because of the cough. Randomized controlled studies support the use of BRONCHODILATORS in selected patients. Cough preparations containing DEXTROMETHORPHAN or CODEINE may reduce the severity and duration of the cough. Nursing and respiratory therapy interventions are logical, including control of the environment and vaporized treatments, based on the pathophysiology of acute bronchitis.

Acute bronchitis and tracheobronchitis require a period of convalescence to avoid development of a chronic condition. Although the disease in its acute form occurs most often in the winter months, repeated bouts indicate a chronic bronchitis.

Chronic Bronchitis. This condition is characterized by increased secretion from the bronchial mucosa and obstruction of the respiratory passages. It interferes with the flow of air to and from the lungs and causes shortness of breath, persistent coughing with expectoration, and recurrent infection. There is no cure for the disorder and its management requires long-range rehabilitation involving patient education and cooperation in carrying out the prescribed regimen.

bronchoalveolar pertaining to a bronchus and alveoli; called also bronchovesicular.

bronchocandidiasis (brong″ko-kan″dĭ-di′ah-sis) bronchopulmonary candidiasis.

bronchocavernous (brong″ko-kav′er-nus) both bronchial and cavitary.

bronchocele (brong′ko-sēl) localized dilatation of a bronchus.

bronchoconstriction (brong″ko-kon-strik′shun) narrowing of a bronchus as a result of smooth muscle contraction, as in ASTHMA.

bronchoconstrictor (brong″ko-kon-strik′tor) 1. narrowing the lumina of the bronchi. 2. an agent that causes such constriction.

bronchodilatation (brong″ko-dil″ah-ta′-shun) a dilated state of a bronchus, or the site at which a bronchus is dilated.

bronchodilator (brong″ko-di-la′tor) 1. expanding the lumina of the bronchi. 2. an agent that does this. Epinephrine is one of the most powerful bronchodilators and can be administered by injection or by aerosol. Isoproterenol (Isuprel) affects the bronchi by relieving bronchospasm through its action on smooth muscle. It is one of the most widely used aerosol bronchodilators. Other drugs used to enlarge the lumen of the bronchi and thereby facilitate breathing and removal of secretions include isoetharine, atropine, and aminophylline.

bronchoesophageal (brong″ko-e-sof′ah-je′al) pertaining to or communicating with a bronchus and the esophagus.

bronchoesophagology (brong″ko-e-sof″-ah-gol′o-je) the branch of medicine concerned with the air passages (bronchi) and esophagus.

bronchoesophagoscopy (brong″ko-e-sof″ah-gos′kah-pe) instrumental examination of the bronchi and esophagus.

bronchofiberscope (brong″ko-fi′ber-skōp″) a flexible bronchoscope utilizing fiberoptics, often used for collection of sputum or tissue samples in the diagnosis of pneumonia or cancer. Called also fiberoptic bronchoscope.

bronchofibroscopy (brong″ko-fi-bros′-kah-pe) examination of the bronchi through a bronchofiberscope.

bronchogenic (brong″ko-jen′ik) originating in the bronchi.

bronchogram (brong′ko-gram) the film obtained by bronchography.

bronchography (brong-kog′rah-fe) radiography of the lungs after instillation of an opaque medium in the bronchi.

broncholith (brong′ko-lith) a hard mass or CONCRETION in a bronchus or bronchi, formed around an inorganic center or from calcified portions of lung tissue or adjacent lymph nodes. Called also bronchial calculus.

broncholithiasis (brong″ko-lĭ-thi′ah-sis) the presence of BRONCHOLITHS within the lumen of the tracheobronchial tree.

bronchology (brong-kol′o-je) the study and treatment of diseases of the tracheobronchial tree. adj., **broncholog′ic.**

bronchomalacia (brong″ko-mah-la′shah) a deficiency in the cartilaginous wall of the trachea or a bronchus that may lead to ATELECTASIS or obstructive EMPHYSEMA.

bronchomotor (brong″ko-mo′ter) affecting the caliber of the bronchi.

bronchomucotropic (brong″ko-mu″ko-trop′ik) augmenting secretion by the respiratory mucosa.

bronchopancreatic (brong″ko-pan″kre-at′ik) communicating with a bronchus and the pancreas, as a bronchopancreatic fistula.

bronchopathy (brong-kop′ah-the) any disease of the bronchi.

bronchophony (brong-kof′o-ne) 1. the normal voice SOUNDS heard over a healthy large bronchus. 2. abnormal voice SOUNDS heard over the lung, with the voice transmitted unusually clearly and with a high pitch; it is a type of PECTORILOQUY, indicating solidification of the lung tissue. Called also bronchiloquy.

whispered b. bronchophony heard through a stethoscope while the patient is whispering.

bronchoplasty (brong′ko-plas″te) plastic surgery of a bronchus to restore the integrity of the lumen.

bronchoplegia (brong″ko-ple′jah) paralysis of the muscles of the walls of the bronchial tubes.

bronchopleural (brong″ko-ploor′al) pertaining to a bronchus and the pleura, or communicating with a bronchus and the pleural cavity.

bronchopneumonia (brong″ko-noo-mo′-ne-ah) inflammation of the bronchi and lungs, usually beginning in the terminal bronchioles. See also PNEUMONIA.

bronchopneumopathy (brong″ko-noo-mop′ah-the) disease of the bronchi and lung tissue.

bronchopulmonary (brong″ko-pul′mo-nar″e) pertaining to the bronchi and lungs.

bronchorrhagia (brong″ko-ra′jah) hemorrhage from the bronchi.

bronchorrhaphy (brong-kor′ah-fe) suture of a bronchus.

bronchorrhea (brong″ko-re′ah) excessive discharge of mucus from the bronchi.

bronchoscope (brong′ko-skōp) an endoscope especially designed for passage through the trachea to permit inspection of the interior of the tracheobronchial tree and carrying out of endobronchial diagnostic and therapeutic maneuvers, such as taking

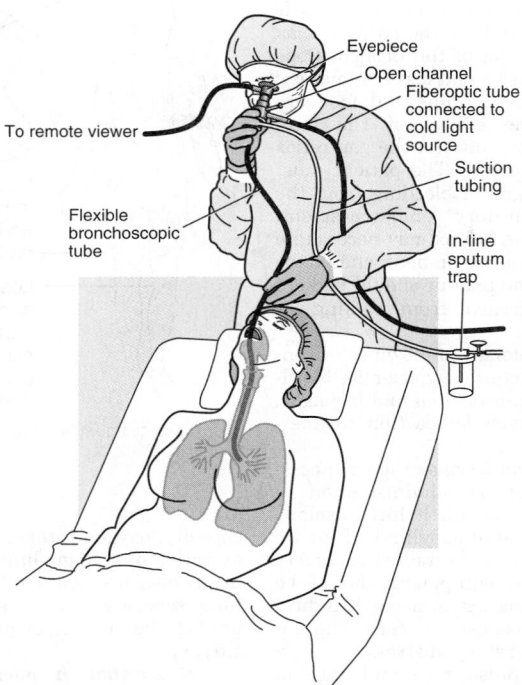

Flexible fiberoptic bronchoscopy. From Malarkey and McMorrow, 2000.

specimens for culture and biopsy and removing foreign bodies. adj., **bronchoscop'ic.**

fiberoptic b. bronchofiberscope.

bronchoscopy (brong-kos'kah-pe) inspection of the interior of the tracheobronchial tree through a bronchoscope, usually a fiberoptic one passed through the nose. (See accompanying illustration.) This is used as a diagnostic aid and for therapeutic purposes. As an aid to diagnosis the bronchoscope allows for visualization of the bronchial mucosa and removal of tissue for biopsy. Bronchial washings and collection of secretions are done at the time of bronchoscopy to obtain samples for culture and cytological examination. Therapeutically, the bronchoscope permits removal of foreign bodies that have been aspirated into the bronchial tree and also may be used to facilitate suctioning of the lower airway. The latter technique is done at the bedside and anesthesia is not considered necessary.

Patient Care. If the fiberoptic bronchoscope is used at the bedside as an adjunct to bronchial hygiene and removal of secretions, it should be used only by health care personnel who have been trained in the technique. It has the advantage of allowing for more precise suctioning with less trauma to the respiratory tract, because it is possible to visualize the areas needing suctioning and to reach lower segments not accessible to the larger suction catheter.

Bronchoscopy as a surgical diagnostic procedure requires preparation and instruction of patients in regard to the purpose of the procedure, what they can expect to be done, and how they may cooperate during the procedure. A topical anesthetic is used most often, but in some cases the patient may have general anesthesia.

Food and fluids are withheld for 8 hours before bronchoscopy is performed. The teeth should be brushed and the mouth rinsed thoroughly before the procedure to lessen the danger of introducing bacteria from the mouth into the bronchi. Dentures are removed and any loose teeth are brought to the attention of the physician. A mild sedative such as diazepam or midazolam may be given prior to the bronchoscopy. This medication plus instructions to the patient and a full explanation of what is going to be done will help the patient relax and make the passing of the bronchoscope into the bronchi easier and less traumatic.

After bronchoscopy, fluids and food are withheld until the effects of the local anesthetic have worn off and the gag reflex has returned completely. The patient must be observed for signs of bleeding from the throat and respiratory embarrassment. Since swelling of the larynx may necessitate a TRACHEOSTOMY, the equipment should be readily at hand. The patient should be kept quiet and discouraged from talking or coughing.

Potential problems following bronchoscopy include arterial hypoxemia, bleeding, pneumothorax, bronchial and laryngeal spasm, and anaphylactic reaction to anesthetic drugs.

Bronchospasm and laryngeal spasm necessitate the intravenous administration of medications such as methylprednisolone (Solu-Medrol) and aminophylline. If an intravenous line was not established before the procedure, the equipment should be at the bedside in case it is needed. Indications that bronchospasm is occurring include pallor, respiratory distress, and an elevation of the pulse rate and rate of respirations.

Supplemental oxygen is needed if arterial BLOOD GAS ANALYSIS or PULSE OXIMETRY indicates a drop in the Pa$_{O_2}$; hypoxemia can occur either before or after the procedure. Pulse oximetry and electrocardiographic readings are commonly monitored during the procedure. The amount and character of the sputum should be observed in case bleeding occurs, especially when a biopsy has been done during bronchoscopy. A foul-smelling, purulent sputum in the postoperative period probably indicates an infection. A sputum culture for bacteria and an antimicrobial sensitivity test are then commonly ordered.

Pneumothorax is not a common complication of bronchoscopy; should it occur, a thoracotomy tube must be inserted as soon as possible to allow for reexpansion of the lung. A trocar thoracic kit should be readily available.

fiberoptic b. bronchofibroscopy.

bronchospasm (brong′ko-spazm) bronchial spasm.

bronchospirography (brong″ko-spi-rog′-rah-fe) the recording of BRONCHOSPIROMETRY results.

bronchospirometry (brong″ko-spi-rom′ĕ-tre) use of a SPIROMETER to determine vital

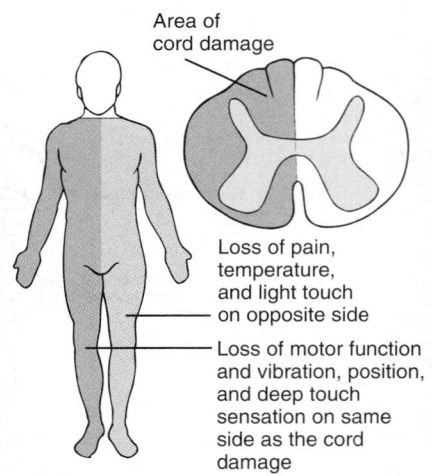

Area of cord damage

Loss of pain, temperature, and light touch on opposite side

Loss of motor function and vibration, position, and deep touch sensation on same side as the cord damage

Brown-Séquard syndrome. From Ignatavicius and Workman, 2002.

capacity, oxygen intake, and carbon dioxide excretion of a single lung, or to get simultaneous measurements of the function of each lung separately; it is sometimes used to predict the success of pulmonary resection surgery.

differential b. measurement of the function of each lung separately.

bronchostaxis (brong″ko-stak′sis) bronchorrhagia.

bronchostenosis (brong″ko-stĕ-no′sis) narrowing of a bronchial tube as a result of scarring or some other stricture; called also bronchiostenosis.

bronchostomy (brong-kos′tah-me) surgical creation of an opening through the chest wall into a bronchus.

bronchotomy (brong-kot′ah-me) incision of a bronchus.

bronchotracheal (brong″ko-tra′ke-al) tracheobronchial.

bronchovesicular (brong″ko-vĕ-sik′u-ler) bronchoalveolar.

bronchus (brong′kus), pl. *bron′chi* any of the larger passages conveying air to a lung (right or left principal bronchus) and within the lungs (lobar and segmental bronchi). See also RESPIRATION and see color plates.

Bronkometer (bron-kom′ĕ-ter) trademark for a preparation of ISOETHARINE mesylate inhalation aerosol, a bronchodilator.

Bronkosol (brong′ko-sol) trademark for a preparation of isoetharine hydrochloride inhalation, a bronchodilator.

brontophobia (bron″to-fo′be-ah) irrational fear of thunder.

brow (brow) the forehead, or either lateral half of it.

Brown-Séquard syndrome (brown-sa-kahr′) paralysis and loss of discriminatory and joint sensation on one side of the body and of pain and temperature sensation on the other, due to a lesion involving one side of the spinal cord. (See accompanying illustration.)

Brucella (broo-sel′ah) a genus of gram-negative, aerobic, nonmotile cocci or rod-shaped bacteria, the etiologic agent of BRU-CELLOSIS. *B. abor′tus,* which causes infectious abortion in cattle, is the most common cause of infection in humans; other species pathogenic for humans are *B. meliten′sis,* found in goats and sheep, and *B. su′is,* found in swine.

brucella (broo-sel′ah) any member of the genus *Brucella.* adj., **brucel′lar.**

Brucellergen (broo-sel′er-jen) trademark for a solution of nucleoproteins derived from *Brucella*; used in a skin test for brucella infection.

brucellosis (broo″sel-o′sis) a generalized infection involving primarily the reticulo-endothelial system, marked by remittent fluctuating fever, malaise, and headache. It is caused by various species of *Brucella* and is transmitted to humans from domestic animals such as pigs, goats, and cattle, especially through infected milk or contact with the carcass of an infected animal.

The disease is also called undulant fever because one of the major symptoms in humans is a fever that fluctuates widely at regular intervals. The symptoms in the beginning stages are difficult to notice and include loss of weight and increased irritability. As the illness advances, headaches, chills, diaphoresis, and muscle aches and pains appear. It is possible for these symptoms to persist for years, either intermittently or continuously, although most patients recover completely within 2 to 6 months. Diagnosis is confirmed by blood cultures or serologic agglutination tests.

Treatment consists of rest and supportive care with a prolonged antibiotic regimen. *Prevention* is best accomplished by the pasteurization of milk and a program of testing, vaccination, and elimination of infected animals.

Brudzinski's sign (broo-jin′skēz) 1. in meningitis, bending the patient's neck usually produces flexion of the knee and hip. 2. in meningitis, passive flexion of the lower limb on one side causes a similar movement in the opposite limb.

Brugia (broo′je-ah) a genus of filarial worms. *B. mala′yi* is a species similar to, and often found in association with,

bucc(o)- word element [L.], *cheek.*

bucca (buk′ah) [L.] cheek (def. 1).

buccal (buk′al) pertaining to or directed toward the cheek.

bucco-occlusal (buk″o-ŏ-kloo′zal) pertaining to or formed by the buccal and occlusal surfaces of a tooth.

buckling (buk′ling) the process or an instance of becoming crumpled or warped.

   scleral b. a technique for repair of detachment of the retina, in which indentations or infoldings of the sclera are made over the tears in the retina so as to promote adherence of the retina to the choroid.

buclizine (bu′klĭ-zēn) an ANTIHISTAMINE used mainly as an antinauseant in treatment of MOTION SICKNESS; administered orally as the hydrochloride salt.

bud (bud) 1. a structure on a plant, often round, that encloses an undeveloped flower or leaf. 2. something resembling the bud of a plant, especially a protuberance in the embryo from which an organ or part develops.

   end b. the remnant of the embryonic primitive knot, from which arises the caudal part of the trunk.

   limb b. one of the four lateral swellings appearing in vertebrate embryos, which develop into the two pairs of limbs.

   tail b. 1. the primordium of the caudal appendage. 2. end bud.

   taste b's end organs of the gustatory nerve containing the receptor surfaces for the sense of TASTE.

   ureteric b. a dorsal outgrowth of the mesonephric duct near its entry into the cloaca; it is the primordium of the ureter, renal pelvis, calices, and collecting tubules of the kidneys.

   b. of urethra bulb of urethra.

budding (bud′ing) 1. gemmation. 2. a method of release of VIRUS from a cell after REPLICATION has taken place: viral protein associates itself with an area of cell membrane, which forms a coat or ENVELOPE around the virus; some cellular proteins in the area of budding are replaced by virus-coded proteins.

budesonide (bu-des′o-nīd) a glucocorticoid ANTIINFLAMMATORY agent administered by inhalation to treat ASTHMA, intranasally to treat allergic RHINITIS and other inflammatory nasal conditions, rectally to treat ULCERATIVE COLITIS, and orally to treat Crohn's disease.

Buerger's disease (ber′gerz) thromboangiitis obliterans.

Buerger-Allen exercises (ber′ger al′en) specific exercises intended to improve

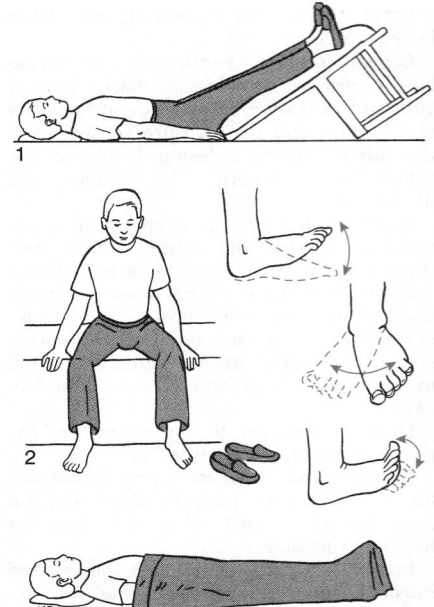

Buerger-Allen exercises. *1,* Elevate feet on padded chair or board for 1/2 to 3 minutes. *2,* Sit in relaxed position while each foot is flexed and extended then pronated and supinated for 3 minutes. The feet should become entirely pink. If the feet are blue or painful, elevate them and relax as necessary. *3,* Lie quietly for 5 minutes, keeping legs warm with a blanket. From Black and Matassarin-Jacobs, 1997.

circulation to the feet and legs. The lower extremities are elevated to a 45 to 90 degree angle and supported in this position until the skin blanches (appears dead white). The feet and legs are then lowered below the level of the rest of the body until redness appears (care should be taken that there is no pressure against the back of the knees); finally, the legs are placed flat on the bed for a few minutes. The length of time for each position varies with the patient's tolerance and the speed with which color change occurs. Usually the exercises are prescribed so that the legs are elevated for 2 to 3 minutes, down 5 to 10 minutes, and then flat on the bed for 10 minutes. (See accompanying illustration.)

buffalo hump a painless accumulation of fat on the upper back, seen in CUSHING'S SYNDROME.

buffer (buf′er) a substance that, by its presence in solution, increases the amount of acid or alkali necessary to produce a unit change in pH. The *bicarbonate buffer system* in the blood maintains a balance between bicarbonate and carbon dioxide ions and determimes the pH of the blood.

building (bil′ding) constructing; forming something by putting parts together.

   complex relationship b. in the NURSING INTERVENTIONS CLASSIFICATION, a nursing INTERVENTION defined as establishing a therapeutic relationship with a patient who has difficulty interacting with others.

bulb (bulb) a rounded mass or enlargement. adj., **bul′bar.**

   b. of aorta the enlargement of the aorta at its point of origin from the heart.

   auditory b. the membranous labyrinth and cochlea.

   b. of eye eyeball.

   gustatory b′s taste buds.

   hair b. the bulbous expansion at the proximal end of a hair, in which the hair shaft is generated.

   inferior b. of jugular vein a dilatation of the internal jugular vein just before it joins the brachiocephalic vein.

   Krause's b. end-bulb.

   olfactory b. the bulblike expansion of the olfactory tract on the under surface of the frontal lobe of each cerebral hemisphere.

   b. of penis bulb of urethra.

   superior b. of jugular vein a dilatation at the beginning of the internal jugular vein.

   taste b′s taste buds.

   b. of urethra the enlarged proximal part of the corpus spongiosum.

   b. of vestibule, vestibulovaginal b. a body consisting of paired masses of erectile tissue, situated one on either side of the vaginal orifice.

bulbar (bul′ber) 1. pertaining to a BULB. 2. pertaining to or involving the MEDULLA OBLONGATA, such as bulbar PARALYSIS.

bulbiform (bul′bĭ-form) bulb-shaped.

bulbitis (bul-bi′tis) inflammation of the bulb of the urethra.

bulbourethral (bul″bo-u-re′thral) pertaining to the bulb of the urethra.

bulbous (bul′bus) 1. bulbar. 2. bulbiform. 3. bearing or arising from a bulb.

bulbus (bul′bus), pl. *bul′bi* [L.] bulb.

   b. o′culi eyeball.

bulimia (bu-le′me-ah) [Gr.] episodic binge eating usually followed by behavior designed to negate the caloric intake of the ingested food, most commonly purging behaviors such as self-induced vomiting or laxative abuse but sometimes other methods such as excessive exercise or fasting. While most commonly associated with BULIMIA NERVOSA, it may also occur in other disorders, such as ANOREXIA NERVOSA. adj., **bulim′ic.**

   b. nervo′sa an EATING DISORDER characterized by episodic binge eating followed by behaviors designed to prevent weight gain, including purging, fasting, and excessive exercise. Episodes of binge eating involve intake of quantifiably excessive amounts of food within a short, discrete period as well as a sense of loss of control over food intake during these periods. The person with bulimia nervosa has a preoccupying pathological fear of becoming overweight, feels an unusually strong tie between self-worth and body shape and size, is aware that the eating pattern is abnormal, and frequently experiences feelings of self-recrimination. In contrast to persons with ANOREXIA NERVOSA, patients with bulimia nervosa tend to be somewhat older and more socially inclined, and to have fewer obsessive characteristics. Bulimia nervosa differs from anorexia nervosa in maintenance of a normal or near normal body weight; it is not diagnosed in the presence of anorexia nervosa.

bulla (bul′ah), pl. *bul′lae* [L.] 1. a circumscribed, fluid-containing, elevated lesion of the skin, usually more than 5 mm in diameter. Called also blister and bleb. 2. an anatomical structure with a blisterlike appearance. adj., **bul′late, bul′lous.**

bullosis (bŭ-lo′sis) the production of, or a condition characterized by, bullous lesions.

bumetanide (bu-met′ah-nīd) a loop DIURETIC used in treatment of edema, such as that associated with congestive HEART FAILURE or hepatic or renal disease, treatment of hypertension, usually in association with other drugs, and as an adjunct in treatment of acute pulmonary edema; administered orally, intramuscularly, or intravenously.

BUN blood urea nitrogen; see UREA NITROGEN.

bundle (bun′d′l) a collection of fibers or strands, as of muscle FIBERS or nerve FIBERS. See also TRACT and FASCICULUS.

   atrioventricular b. bundle of His.

   fundamental b., ground b. that part of the white matter of the spinal cord bordering the gray matter and containing fibers that travel for a distance of only a few segments of the cord.

   b. of His a band of cardiac muscle FIBERS connecting the atria with the ventricles of the heart; called also atrioventricular bundle. (See accompanying illustration.)

   medial forebrain b. a group of nerve FIBERS connecting the midbrain tegmentum and elements of the limbic system.

   Thorel's b. a bundle of muscle FIBERS in the human heart connecting the sinoatrial and atrioventricular nodes.

Bunge (bun′je) Helen L. (1906–1970). Nursing educator and researcher who

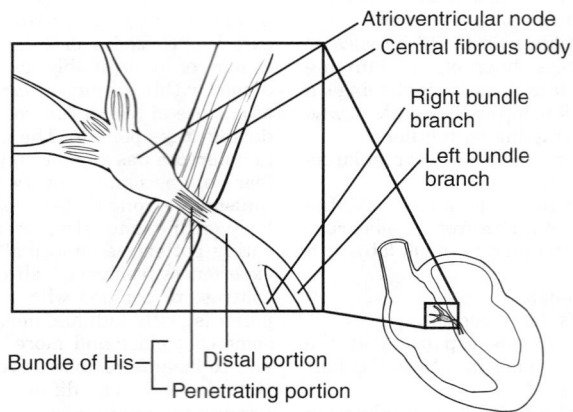

Bundle of His considered as the trunk of the bundle and excluding the bundle branches. From Dorland's, 2000.

served as Dean of the Frances Payne Bolton School of Nursing at Western Reserve University and later as executive officer of the Institute for Research and Services at Teachers College, Columbia University. As chairperson of the Committee on Research of the American Association of Collegiate Schools of Nursing, she helped to launch *Nursing Research,* of which she was editor and chairperson of the editorial board. She was a strong supporter of nursing research, believing that research is an integral part of nursing, not a field isolated from teaching and practice.

bunion (bun′yun) an abnormal prominence on the inner aspect of the first metatarsal head, with bursal formation, and resulting in lateral or valgus displacement of the great toe. Bunions can be caused by

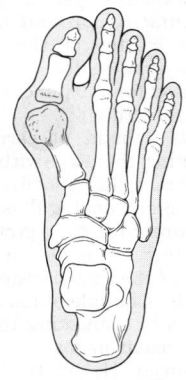

Bunion. From Dorland's, 2000.

congenital malformation of the bony structure of the foot or by joint disease such as rheumatoid arthritis, but they are most often caused by wearing shoes with pointed toes, especially ones that are high-heeled and too short. When the shoes do not fit properly they force the great toe toward the outer side of the foot. The result is continued pressure on the joint where the great toe articulates with the first metatarsal head. Chronic irritation causes a buildup of soft tissue and underlying bone in the area. Symptoms are swelling, redness, and pain. (See accompanying illustration.) Mild cases can be relieved by changing to properly fitting shoes. If there is severe pain making ambulation difficult or impossible, antiinflammatory agents may be effective. Surgical correction (*bunionectomy*) is indicated when all other measures fail.

bunionectomy (bun″yun-ek′to-me) excision of a bunion.

bunionette (bun″yun-et′) enlargement of the lateral aspect of the fifth metatarsal head.

bupivacaine (bu-piv′ah-kān) a local ANESTHETIC, used as the hydrochloride for local infiltration, peripheral nerve block, and retrobulbar, subarachnoid, sympathetic, caudal, or epidural block.

buprenorphine (bu″prĕ-nor′fĕn) a synthetic OPIOID agonist-antagonist derived from THEBAINE, used in the form of the hydrochloride salt as an analgesic for moderate to severe pain and as an anesthesia adjunct. Administered sublingually or by intramuscular or intravenous injection.

bupropion (bu-pro′pe-on) a compound structurally similar to AMPHETAMINE, used in the form of the hydrochloride salt as

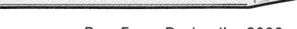

Bur. From Dorland's, 2000.

an ANTIDEPRESSANT and as an aid in smoking cessation to reduce the symptoms of nicotine WITHDRAWAL; administered orally.

bur (ber) a form of drill used for creating openings in bone or similar hard material. Also spelled burr. (See accompanying illustration.)

Burch procedure (berch) a type of bladder neck SUSPENSION for stress INCONTINENCE, consisting of fixation of the lateral vaginal fornices to the ileopectineal ligaments.

burden (ber'den) load.

   body b. chemicals stored in the body that may be detected by ANALYSIS.

buret (bu-ret') a glass tube with a capacity of the order of 25 to 100 mL and graduation intervals of 0.05 to 0.1 mL, with stopcock attachment, used to deliver an accurately measured quantity of liquid.

burette (bu-ret') buret.

Burkitt's lymphoma (berk'its) a form of undifferentiated LYMPHOMA, usually found in central Africa but also reported from other areas, and manifested most often as a large bone-destroying lesion in the jaw or as an abdominal mass. The EPSTEIN-BARR VIRUS (EB virus), a herpesvirus, has been isolated from Burkitt's lymphoma cells in culture, and has been implicated as a causative agent. Called also African lymphoma and Burkitt's tumor.

burn (bern) injury to tissues caused by contact with dry heat (fire), moist heat (steam or liquid), chemicals, electricity, lightning, or radiation. Safety measures in the home and on the job are extremely important in the prevention of burns. Burns have traditionally been classified according to degree: A *first-degree burn* involves a reddening of the skin area. In a *second-degree burn* the skin is blistered. A *third-degree burn* is the most serious type, involving damage to the deeper layers of the skin with necrosis through the entire skin. In some cases the growth cells of the tissues in the burned area may be destroyed. See accompanying table.

Another classification describes burns as *partial-thickness wounds* in which the epithelializing elements remain intact, and *full-thickness wounds* in which all of the epithelializing elements and those lining the sweat glands, hair follicles, and sebaceous glands are destroyed. A *deep thermal burn* is a deep partial-thickness wound that may have the white, waxy appearance of a full-thickness burn.

It is difficult to determine the depth of a wound at first glance, but any burn involving more than 15 per cent of the body surface is considered serious. Because surface area as well as depth is important in evaluating a burned patient's status, a method called the RULE OF NINES has been developed to determine surface area involvement. The head and each arm are figured at 9 per cent. The anterior and posterior trunk and the two legs comprise 18 or (2×9) per cent each, and the perineum is figured as 1 per cent. An improvement on the rule of nines, the BERKOW FORMULA, takes into account the age of the burn victim.

In a burn the *crust* is the dry, scablike covering that forms over a superficial burn. ESCHAR is a hard layer of tissue that results from full-thickness injury. It is considered to be a protective covering over the wound, serving as a barrier to bacterial invasion. Research indicates that eschar may be viable tissue that can contribute to healing and the prevention of scarring.

Immediate Treatment. The following steps should be taken for prompt and effective treatment of the various types of burns.

Major Burns. A burn is classified as major if it meets the following criteria: (1) in children, one that involves 10 to 15 per cent of total body surface and is a second- or third-degree burn; (2) in adults, one involving 25 to 30 per cent of total body surface, with deep partial-thickness or full-thickness destruction of epithelializing structures; (3) in children and adults, electrical burns, burns of the face and hands, or those that have traumatized the bronchi and lungs.

Emergency care at the scene of the injury includes application of cool water to neutralize the continued thermal effects of the burn agent and to dilute and wash away any chemicals that may be on the skin. In order to avoid SHOCK, no more than 10 to 20 per cent of the burned area should be cooled at one time. If there is evidence of a major burn, it is necessary to establish and maintain an airway. Respiratory problems are especially likely if the person was burned in an enclosed place or was burned on the face and neck. Singed nasal hairs, darkened oral and nasal membranes, hoarseness, and carbon particles in the sputum are indicative of thermal injury to the respiratory tract.

The victim should be wrapped in a clean, preferably sterile, sheet. A blanket is used to cover the unaffected areas and to maintain normal body temperature if possible. If available, an intravenous infusion of

BURN DEPTH CATEGORIES

Degree	Cause	Surface
First: minor except under the age of 18 months, over the age of 65 years, or if there is severe fluid loss	Flash flame, sunburn (ultraviolet)	Dry, no blisters, little or no edema
Second: (partial thickness):	Hot liquids or solids, flash flame, direct flame, chemical	Moist blebs and blisters
Minor: adults, less than 15%, children less than 10%		
Moderate: adult 15–30%, minor electrical or chemical, less than 15% but involving hands, feet, face, perineum children: 10–30%		
Severe: over 30%		
Third: (full thickness):	Hot liquids or solids, flame, chemical, electrical	Dry leathery eschar; charred vessels visible under eschar
Minor: less than 2%		
Moderate 2–10% or any involvement of hands, feet, face, perineum		
Severe: over 10% major chemical or electrical		

Ringer's lactate solution is begun. If intravenous therapy is not available and the victim is conscious and able to swallow, fluids can be given by mouth. Nausea, vomiting, and ileus *contraindicate* the administration of any food or liquids.

Clothing is removed from the burned area only if this does not further traumatize the skin. Burned clothing should be sent to the burn center, as it may help determine the chemicals and other substances that either caused or entered the wound. Absorbent cotton, oily salves, ointments, and creams should *not* be applied to moderate and severe burns. Blisters are not opened or disturbed in any way.

Minor Burns. For a small first-degree burn, the reddened area is immersed in clean cold water, or ice cubes are applied. This relieves the pain. Even first-degree burns are extremely serious if they involve a large area. They should receive prompt medical attention. Death may result if a first-degree burn covers as much as two thirds of the body area. On a child such burns are dangerous on a smaller area of the skin.

Chemical and Other Burns. For chemical burns, such as those caused by acids, the affected area should be bathed immediately with water, using plenty of water and continuing bathing the area until all of the chemical has been washed away. A health care worker should be called and first aid treatment should be given as for any similar heat burn. If the burned area is extensive, the victim should be given emergency CARE for a major burn.

If the area affected is the eye, it is held open and flushed gently but thoroughly with water. Then it is covered with a sterile dressing and medical aid is sought immediately.

In electrical burns, SHOCK is the main danger. It may be necessary to use ARTIFICIAL RESPIRATION. This should be begun as soon as contact with the current has been broken. A person stricken by lightning also requires artificial respiration if the shock has been severe enough to interfere with normal breathing.

Hospital Treatment. A major burn presents problems of respiratory impairment, disruption of fluid and electrolyte balance, disturbances of tissue perfusion and homeostasis, and the potential for infection, delayed healing, and unnecessary scarring. Long-term effects also include orthopedic deformities resulting from immobility.

In the United States, most severely burned patients are given emergency care in a local hospital and then transferred to a large burn center for intensive long-term care. Patients who show signs of trauma to the respiratory tract must be watched closely for signs of developing laryngeal edema and obstruction of the air passages.

BURN DEPTH CATEGORIES

Color	Pain Level	Depth	Healing Time
Erythematous	Painful	Epidermis only	2–5 days with no peeling or scarring; discoloration possible
Mottled white to pink, red	Very painful	Epidermis; papillary and reticular layers of dermis, possibly fat domes of subcutaneous layer	Superficial: 5–21 days without grafting; deep 21–35 days; with infection, becomes full thickness
Mixed white waxy, pearly; dark khaki, mahogany; charred	Little or no pain	Subcutaneous tissue; may include fascia, muscle, and bone	Smaller areas may heal from edges in several weeks; large areas require grafting, may take many months

This condition can develop any time from 4 to 48 hours after the accident. When wheezing on inhalation or other signs of respiratory distress occur, intubation, frequent suctioning, and VENTILATOR assistance may be needed.

Fluid loss by the evaporation of free water through the burned area causes disturbances in the extracellular and intracellular fluids. This can lead to burn shock, renal damage, and other life-threatening conditions. In addition to a loss of body water and changes in fluid composition, there are alterations in the composition of blood and the development of metabolic ACIDOSIS. If untreated, the changes in volume, concentration, and composition of extracellular fluid can be fatal. Information about the specific kinds of intravenous fluids that should be administered should be obtained from the burn center to which the patient will be transferred so that there is no break in the continuity of patient care.

In order to avoid nausea, vomiting, and the gastric and intestinal distention resulting from decreased peristaltic activity, a nasogastric tube is inserted and gentle suction applied. A retention catheter is inserted into the urinary bladder to obtain accurate measurement of output and periodic urine specimens for the determination of specific gravity and the presence of protein and blood.

In the EMERGENCY DEPARTMENT, the burn wounds are cleansed according to established protocol, using clean technique and avoiding excessive loss of body heat. The cleansed wounds are then usually covered with dry sterile dressings, or with saline-soaked dressings that are covered with dry bandages before the patient is transferred. Exposed bone and tendon *must be kept moist* at all times with sterile saline-soaked dressings.

The major cause of death in burn victims is infection. Immunization against tetanus by administration of tetanus toxoid is recommended. If the patient has not received basic immunization prior to injury, he is also given tetanus immune globulin (Hyper-Tet).

The kind of environment provided in special burn units in large medical centers varies, but all have the objectives of avoiding contamination of the wound. Some special units use complete reverse ISOLATION PRECAUTIONS and elaborate laminar air flow systems to maintain an environment that is as free of microorganisms as possible.

When the patient is cared for in a general hospital, it is recommended that some form of reverse isolation be used. Every effort should be made to protect the patient from autocontamination as well as from contamination from others and from the environment. It has been estimated that more than half of all burn wound infections can be traced to contamination by microorganisms such as *Staphylococcus* that originate in the patient. Physically isolating the patient from others should not be allowed to foster neglect and failure to attend to basic principles of cleanliness and good personal hygiene in day-to-day care.

Burn wounds can be treated in either of two ways: open or closed methods of therapy. In the open, exposed method of treatment no dressings are applied. Every effort is made to avoid disturbance of the eschar and the introduction of pathogenic microorganisms into the wound. If, however, the eschar causes a circumferential constriction of the trunk or an extremity, an escharotomy is indicated to prevent ischemic necrosis. ANTIMICROBIAL AGENTS are given systemically and, if the open method is used, they are applied topically. Examples of these topical medications include silver nitrate, silver sulfadiazine cream, and mafenide acetate.

The closed method of treatment may involve the application of dry occlusive dressings or wet dressings soaked in saline or some other solution preferred by the physician. The wet dressings require frequent changes when there is much exudate from the wound.

Immersion in water is especially helpful in cleansing the wound, removing debris and caked creams, and therapeutic EXERCISE is essential to avoid orthopedic deformities. See also HYDROTHERAPY.

Skin GRAFTING is done soon after the initial injury. The donor skin is best taken from the patient, but when this is not possible, the skin of a matched donor can be used. Prior to grafting, or in some cases as a substitute for it, the burn may be covered with either cadaver or porcine (pig) skin to keep it moist and free from exogenous bacterial infection.

Patient Care. The primary concerns in patient care are prevention of infection, avoidance of a fluid and electrolyte imbalance, and prevention of such orthopedic deformities as contractures and ankylosis. If the patient is confined to a bed or frame, all the hazards of immobility must be guarded against. In addition to these measures, it is especially important that good sanitation practices and sterile technique be carried out faithfully. Handwashing is of vital importance.

The patient must be protected from extremes of heat and cold whether dry or wet dressings are used. Dry dressings, which do not allow for circulation of air, can cause a buildup of body heat, especially in a febrile patient. The patient receiving wet dressings must be protected from drafts and other conditions that could produce chilling.

Careful and accurate taking and recording of vital signs is done periodically and any significant change reported immediately. An accurate record of intake and output is of primary importance. Because large amounts of body fluids and many essential minerals and salts can escape through burn wounds, it is imperative that a record be kept of fluids excreted through the kidneys or intestinal tract or by emesis. Observations should include not only the amount but also the color, concentration, unusual odor, or any other characteristic of the urine, emesis, or liquid stool.

A high-protein diet with supplemental vitamins and minerals is prescribed to aid in the repair of damaged tissue. Ingenuity and imagination may be needed to encourage the patient to eat meals as well as the between-meal feedings prescribed.

The patient who has suffered disfigurement from burns will have additional emotional problems in adjusting to a new body image. Burn therapy can be long and tedious for the patient and family. They will need emotional and psychological support as well as attention to their spiritual needs as they work their way through the many problems created by the physical and emotional trauma of a major burn.

acid b. injury to tissues caused by an acid, such as sulfuric acid or nitric acid. Emergency first aid for an acid burn of the skin includes immediate and thorough washing of the burn with water for 20 minutes and transportation of the victim with extensive burns to an emergency care facility. See also discussion of Chemical and Other Burns, under BURN.

burning mouth syndrome (bern′ing mouth) a burning sensation in the mouth that is often associated with MENOPAUSE.

burnout (bern′out) emotional and physical exhaustion resulting from a combination of exposure to environmental and internal stressors and inadequate coping and adaptive skills. In addition to signs of exhaustion, the person with burnout exhibits an increasingly negative attitude toward his or her job, low self-esteem, and personal devaluation.

Strategies for preventing and managing burnout include utilizing assertiveness techniques, improving problem-solving and decision-making skills, clarifying personal values and setting realistic personal goals, learning and using coping mechanisms to deal with emotions, ensuring oneself adequate relaxation and recreation, maintaining a healthy lifestyle, and minimizing stressors at work and at home.

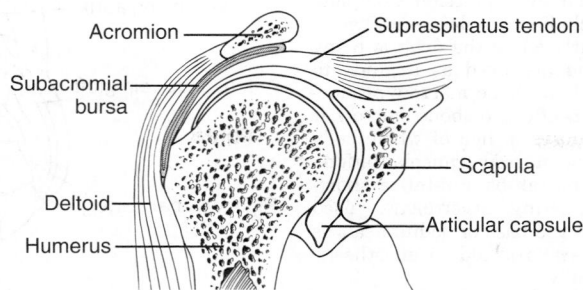

Subacromial bursa, lying between the acromion and supraspinatus tendon and extending between the deltoid and greater tubercle. From Dorland's, 2000.

Burow's solution (boor'ovz) a preparation of aluminum subacetate, glacial acetic acid, and water; used topically on the skin as an astringent and topical antiseptic and for relief of itching, and as an astringent gargle or mouthwash. Called also aluminum acetate solution.

burp (burp) 1. to expel gas from the stomach through the mouth; see ERUCTATION. 2. to assist an infant to expel gas from the stomach by upright positioning or gently rubbing or patting the back.

burr (ber) bur.

bursa (bur'sah), pl. *bur'sae* [L.] a small fluid-filled sac or saclike cavity situated in places in tissues where friction would otherwise occur. adj., **bur'sal**. Bursae function to facilitate the gliding of muscles or tendons over bony or ligamentous surfaces. They are numerous and are found throughout the body; the most important are located at the shoulder, elbow, knee, and hip. Inflammation of a bursa is known as BURSITIS.

b. of Fabricius an epithelial outgrowth of the cloaca in chick embryos, which develops in a manner similar to that of the THYMUS in mammals, atrophying after 5 or 6 months and persisting as a fibrous remnant in sexually mature birds. It contains lymphoid follicles, and before involution is a site of formation of B-LYMPHOCYTES associated with humoral IMMUNITY.

b. muco'sa, mucous b., synovial b. a closed synovial sac interposed between surfaces that glide upon each other; it may be subcutaneous, submuscular, subfascial, or subtendinous in location.

subacromial b. one between the ACROMION and the insertion of the supraspinatus muscle, extending between the deltoid and the greater tubercle of the HUMERUS. See illustration.

bursectomy (bur-sek'to-me) excision of a bursa.

bursitis (ber-si'tis) inflammation of a bursa; types are usually named for the bursa involved. The subdeltoid bursa in the shoulder is most commonly affected, but inflammation may develop in almost any bursa in the body. Excessive use of the joint is often the cause. *Acute bursitis* comes on suddenly; severe pain and limitation of motion of the affected joint are the principal symptoms. Resting the joint, moist heat, and the use of ANALGESICS or NONSTEROIDAL ANTIINFLAMMATORY DRUGS frequently are sufficient treatment. *Chronic bursitis* may follow the acute attacks. There is continued pain and limitation of motion around the joint. X-ray examination will usually reveal the deposit of calcium salts. If rest, heat, and medications do not relieve the condition, surgery may be required to remove the calcium deposits or free the area of chronic inflammation.

bursolith (bur'so-lith) a hard mass (CALCULUS) in a bursa.

bursopathy (bur-sop'ah-the) any disease of a bursa.

bursotomy (ber-sot'ah-me) incision of a bursa.

buspirone (bu-spi'rōn) an ANTIANXIETY AGENT not related chemically to others; administered orally as the hydrochloride salt.

Busse-Buschke disease (boos'ĕ boosh'kĕ) cryptococcosis.

busulfan (bu-sul'fan) an ALKYLATING AGENT that acts selectively on the bone marrow, depressing granulocyte formation, and is therefore used in the treatment of myelogenous LEUKEMIAS. It is also used for the treatment of MYELOPROLIFERATIVE DISORDERS, including POLYCYTHEMIA vera and myeloid METAPLASIA. Administered orally or intravenously. Side effects include nausea and vomiting, and heavy doses may lead to excessive bone marrow depression. Complete blood counts (including platelet counts) must be done frequently while the drug is being administered and are used as a guide to dosage and effects on bone marrow production. Because of its effects on bone marrow, it is used at high doses in lieu of whole body irradiation in bone marrow transplantation.

butabarbital (bu″tah-bahr′bĭ-tal) a short- to intermediate-acting BARBITURATE, used preoperatively as the base or sodium salt as a SEDATIVE and HYPNOTIC aid to anesthesia. Administered orally.

butacaine (bu′tah-kān) a local anesthetic; the sulfate salt is used as a topical anesthetic in the eye and on mucous membranes, in solution or ointment.

butalbital (bu-tal′bĭ-tal) an intermediate-acting BARBITURATE used as a SEDATIVE along with an analgesic in treatment of tension HEADACHE or MIGRAINE.

butamben (bu-tam′ben) 1. a local anesthetic used topically for the treatment of painful skin conditions. 2. a topical anesthetic, used as the base or as *b. picrate.*

butane (bu′tān) an aliphatic hydrocarbon, C_4H_{10}, from petroleum; used in pharmacy as an aerosol propellant.

butenafine (bu-ten′ah-fēn) a topical antifungal AGENT used as the hydrochloride salt in the treatment of ATHLETE'S FOOT, JOCK ITCH, and RINGWORM.

butethamine (bu-teth′ah-mēn) a local anesthetic; used in dentistry in the form of the hydrochloride salt.

Butisol (bu′tĭ-sol) trademark for preparations of BUTABARBITAL, a BARBITURATE.

butoconazole (bu″to-kon′ah-zōl) an IMIDAZOLE derivative used intravaginally in the form of the nitrate salt as a topical antifungal AGENT in treatment of vulvovaginal CANDIDIASIS.

butorphanol (bu-tor′fah-nol) a synthetic OPIOID used as an ANALGESIC and an adjunct to anesthesia in the form of the tartrate salt.

buttocks (but′oks) the two fleshy prominences formed by the gluteal muscles on the lower part of the back. Called also breech, clunes, and nates.

butyl (bu′til) a hydrocarbon radical, C_4H_9.

butyraceous (bu″tĭ-ra′shus) of a buttery consistency.

butyrate (bu′tĭ-rāt) a salt of butyric acid.

butyric acid (bu-tir′ik) a saturated fatty acid found in butter.

butyroid (bu′tĭ-roid) resembling butter.

butyrophenone (bu″tĭ-ro-fe′nōn) any of a class of structurally related ANTIPSYCHOTIC AGENTS; the prototype is HALOPERIDOL.

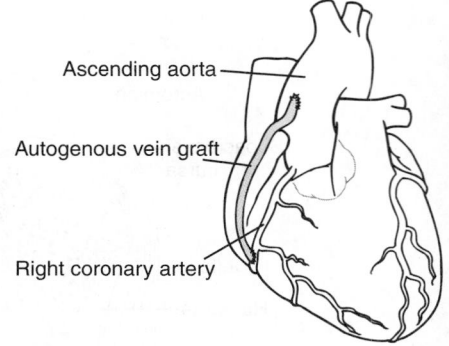

Bypass. Single artery bypass of an occluded right coronary artery. From Dorland's, 2000.

butyrous (bu′tĭ-rus) resembling butter.

bypass (bi′pas″) an auxiliary flow; a shunt; a surgically created pathway circumventing the normal anatomical pathway, such as in an artery or the intestine. (See accompanying illustration.)

aortocoronary b. coronary artery bypass.

aortofemoral b. insertion of a vascular prosthesis from the aorta to the femoral artery to bypass atherosclerotic occlusions in the aorta and the iliac artery.

aortoiliac b. insertion of a vascular prosthesis from the abdominal aorta to the femoral artery to bypass intervening atherosclerotic segments.

axillofemoral b. insertion of a vascular prosthesis or section of saphenous vein from the axillary artery to the ipsilateral femoral artery to relieve lower limb ischemia in patients in whom normal anatomic placement of a graft is contraindicated, as by abdominal infection or aortic aneurysm.

axillopopliteal b. insertion of a vascular prosthesis from the axillary artery to the popliteal artery to relieve lower limb ischemia in patients in whom the femoral artery is unsuitable for axillofemoral bypass.

cardiopulmonary b. diversion of the flow of blood from the entrance to the right atrium directly to the aorta, usually via a pump OXYGENATOR, avoiding both the heart and the lungs; a form of extracorporeal CIRCULATION used in HEART surgery.

coronary b., coronary artery b. a section of saphenous vein or other conduit grafted between the aorta and a coronary artery distal to an obstructive lesion in the latter; called also aortocoronary bypass.

extra-anatomic b. an arterial bypass that does not follow the normal anatomic pathway, such as an axillofemoral bypass.

extracranial/intracranial *b.* anastomosis of the superficial temporal artery to the middle cerebral artery to preserve function or prevent stroke or death in patients with stenosis of the internal carotid or middle cerebral artery.

femorofemoral *b.* insertion of a vascular prosthesis between the femoral arteries to bypass an occluded or injured iliac artery.

femoropopliteal *b.* insertion of a vascular prosthesis from the femoral to the popliteal artery to bypass occluded segments.

gastric *b.* see GASTRIC BYPASS.

hepatorenal *b.* insertion of a vascular prosthesis between the common hepatic artery and the renal artery, serving as a passage around an occluded segment of renal artery.

intestinal *b.*, jejunoileal *b.* see INTESTINAL BYPASS.

left heart *b.* diversion of the flow of blood from the pulmonary veins directly to the aorta, avoiding the left atrium and the left ventricle.

partial *b.* the deviation of only a portion of the blood flowing through an artery.

partial ileal *b.* anastomosis of the proximal end of the transected ileum to the cecum, the bypass of the portion of the small intestine resulting in decreased intestinal absorption of and increased fecal excretion of cholesterol; sometimes used in treatment of hyperlipidemia.

right heart *b.* diversion of the flow of blood from the entrance of the right atrium directly to the pulmonary arteries, avoiding the right atrium and right ventricles.

byssinosis (bis″ĭ-no′sis) a pulmonary disease seen in cotton textile workers and preparers of flax and soft hemp, due to inhalation of textile dust. Two forms are distinguished: *acute byssinosis,* seen in those who return to work after an absence and marked by tightness of the chest, wheezing, and coughing; and *chronic byssinosis,* seen in those with years of exposure and marked by permanent dyspnea. Called also brown lung. adj., **byssinot′ic.**

C

C canine (TOOTH); carbon (molecular carbon atoms are frequently designated C1, C2, C3, etc., or α-C, β-C, etc., beginning from one end or other standard reference point); large calorie; cathode; Celsius (SCALE); clonus; complement (C1 through C9); compliance (subscripts denote the structure, e.g., C_L lung compliance); contraction; coulomb; cytosine; cervical VERTEBRAE (C1 through C7).

C capacitance; clearance (subscripts denote the substance, e.g., C_I or C_{In} inulin clearance); heat capacity.

°C degree Celsius; see Celsius SCALE.

c small CALORIE; centi-.

χ² chi-square; see CHI-SQUARE TEST.

CA CARDIAC ARREST.

CA 125 cancer antigen 125.

Ca chemical symbol, *calcium;* cathode (cathodal); cancer.

cabergoline (cah-ber′go-lēn) a DOPAMINE receptor agonist used in treatment of HYPERPROLACTINEMIA; administered orally.

CABG coronary artery bypass graft; see under BYPASS.

cac(o)- word element [Gr.], *bad; ill.*

cache (kash) a memory mechanism used by a computer to accelerate access to information.

cachectin (kah-kek′tin) former name for tumor necrosis FACTOR α.

cachet (kah-sha′) [Fr.] a disk-shaped wafer or capsule enclosing a dose of medicine.

cachexia (kah-kek′se-ah) a profound and marked state of constitutional disorder; general ill health and malnutrition. adj. **cachec′tic.**

c. hypophysiopri′va symptoms resulting from total loss of pituitary function, including loss of sexual function, bradycardia, hypothermia, apathy, and coma.

malarial c. the physical signs resulting from antecedent attacks of severe malaria, including anemia, sallow skin, yellow sclera, splenomegaly, hepatomegaly, and, in children, retardation of growth and puberty.

pituitary c. SIMMONDS′ DISEASE.

cachinnation (kak″ĭ-na′shun) excessive, hysterical laughter.

cacogeusia (kak″o-ju′se-ah) a sensation of bad taste not related to the ingestion of specific substances.

cacomelia (kak″o-me′le-ah) dysmelia.

cacosmia (kak-oz′me-ah) a sensation of bad smell not related to a specific odor, or associated with olfactory stimuli usually considered to be pleasant.

CAD coronary artery disease.

cadaver (kah-dav′er) a dead body; generally applied to one preserved for anatomical study. adj., **cadav′eric, cadav′erous.**

cadaverine (kah-dav′er-in) a relatively nontoxic ptomaine, $C_5H_{14}N_2$, formed by decarboxylation of lysine; it is sometimes one of the products of *Vibrio proteus* and of *V. cholerae,* and occasionally found in the urine in cystinuria, where it causes an unpleasant odor.

cadmiosis (kad″me-o′sis) PNEUMOCONIOSIS due to inhalation of and tissue reaction to CADMIUM dust.

cadmium (Cd) (kad′me-um) a chemical element, atomic number 48. (See Appendix 6.) Inhalation of cadmium fumes causes pulmonary edema with proliferative interstitial pneumonia and various degrees of lung damage. Cadmium poisoning may occur due to occupational exposure, smoking, and ingestion of certain foods (kidneys and livers; seafoods such as mussels, oysters, and crabs; and some grains). Maternal cadmium exposure can cause abnormal embryonic development by interfering with normal zinc ion metabolic activities.

caduceus (kah-du′se-us) the wand of Hermes or Mercury; used as a symbol of the medical profession and as the emblem of the Medical Corps of the U.S. Army. Another symbol of medicine is the staff of Aesculapius, which is the official insignia of the American Medical Association.

cae- for words beginning thus, see also those beginning *ce-*.

caecum (se′kum) [L.] 1. the first part of the large intestine, forming a dilated pouch into which open the ILEUM, COLON, and vermiform APPENDIX. Spelled also *cecum.* 2. cul-de-sac.

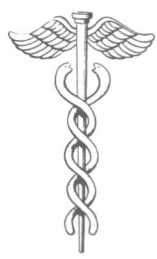

Caduceus.

caelotherapy (se″lo-ther′ah-pe) the therapeutic use of religion and religious symbols.

caffeine (kaf-ēn′) a xanthine compound found in coffee, tea, chocolate, and colas; it is a central nervous system stimulant, diuretic, striated muscle stimulant, and acts on the cardiovascular system. As the base or the citrate salt, it is used as a central nervous system stimulant and as an adjunct in the treatment of neonatal apnea; as the base it is also used in the treatment of vascular headaches and as an adjunct to analgesics.

caffeinism (kaf′ēn-izm) 1. physical dependence on CAFFEINE. 2. a disorder associated with excessive intake of CAFFEINE, defined as the presence of five or more of the following symptoms: restlessness, nervousness, excitement, insomnia, flushed face, diuresis, gastrointestinal disturbance, muscle twitching, rambling flow of thought and speech, tachycardia or cardiac arrhythmia, and periods of inexhaustibility. Called also caffeine intoxication.

Caffey's disease (kaf′fēz) infantile cortical hyperostosis.

cage (kāj) a box or enclosure.

rib c., thoracic c. the bony structure enclosing the THORAX, consisting of the ribs, vertebral column, and sternum.

CAI computer-assisted instruction.

caisson disease (ka′son) see DECOMPRESSION SICKNESS.

cal calorie.

calamine (kal′ah-mīn) a preparation of ZINC OXIDE and the coloring agent ferric oxide, used topically as a skin protectant and astringent. See also calamine LOTION.

Calan (kal′an) trademark for preparations of VERAPAMIL hydrochloride, a CALCIUM CHANNEL BLOCKING AGENT used to treat ANGINA PECTORIS, HYPERTENSION, and TACHYARRHYTHMIAS.

calcaneoapophysitis (kal-ka″ne-o-ah-pof″ĭ-si′tis) inflammation of the posterior part of the calcaneus, marked by pain and swelling.

calcaneoastragaloid (kal-ka″ne-o-ah-strag′ah-loid) pertaining to the calcaneus and astragalus.

calcaneodynia (kal-ka″ne-o-din′e-ah) pain in the heel.

calcaneus (kal-ka′ne-us) the irregular quadrangular bone at the back of the tarsus; called also heel bone. See anatomic Table of Bones in the Appendices.

calcar (kal′kar) 1. spur. 2. a spur-shaped structure.

c. a′vis an eminence on the medial wall of the occipital horn of the lateral ventricle, below the bulb of the occipital horn, produced by lateral extension of the calcarine sulcus.

calcareous (kal-kar′e-us) pertaining to or containing lime; chalky.

calcarine (kal′kar-in) 1. spur-shaped. 2. pertaining to the calcar avis.

calcariuria (kal-kar″e-u′re-ah) the presence of lime (calcium) salts in the urine; see HYPERCALCIURIA.

calcemia (kal-se′me-ah) hypercalcemia.

calcibilia (kal″sĭ-bil′yah) the presence of calcium in the bile.

calcic (kal′sik) of or pertaining to lime or calcium.

calcicosis (kal″sĭ-ko′sis) a form of PNEUMOCONIOSIS disease due to inhalation of marble dust.

calcifediol (kal″sĭ-fē-di′ol) 25-hydroxycholecalciferol (a form of VITAMIN D), used in the treatment of hypocalcemia, hypophosphatemia, rickets, and osteodystrophy associated with various medical conditions including chronic RENAL FAILURE and HYPOPARATHYROIDISM, administered orally.

calciferol (kal-sif′er-ol) 1. see VITAMIN D. 2. ergocalciferol.

calcific (kal-sif′ik) forming lime.

calcification (kal″sĭ-fĭ-ka′shun) the deposit of calcium salts, mostly calcium phosphate, in body tissues. The normal absorption of calcium is facilitated by parathyroid hormone and by vitamin D. When there are increased amounts of parathyroid hormone in the blood (as in HYPERPARATHYROIDISM), there is deposition of calcium in the alveoli of the lungs, the renal tubules, the thyroid gland, the gastric mucosa, and the arterial walls. Normally calcium is deposited in the bone matrix to insure stability and strength of the bone and in growing teeth.

dystrophic c. the deposition of calcium in abnormal tissue, such as scar tissue or atherosclerotic plaques, without abnormalities of blood calcium.

eggshell c. deposition of a thin layer of calcium around a thoracic lymph node, often seen in SILICOSIS.

calcinosis (kal″sĭ-no′sis) 1. a condition characterized by abnormal deposition of calcium salts in the tissues.

c. circumscrip′ta localized deposition of calcium in small nodules in subcutaneous tissues or muscle.

c. universa′lis widespread deposition of calcium in nodules or plaques in the dermis, panniculus, and muscles.

calcipenia (kal″sĭ-pe′ne-ah) deficiency of CALCIUM in the system; see also *hypocalcemia*.

calcipexis (kal″sĭ-pek′sis) **calcipexy** (kal′-sĭ-pek″se) fixation of calcium in the tissues. adj., **calcipec′tic, calcipex′ic.**

calciphilia (kal″sĭ-fil′e-ah) a tendency to calcification.

calciphylaxis (kal″sĭ-fĭ-lak′sis) a condition of induced HYPERSENSITIVITY characterized by formation of calcified tissue in response to administration of a challenging agent.

calcipotriene (kal″sĭ-po-tri′ēn) a synthetic derivative of CHOLECALCIFEROL (vitamin D₃), applied to the skin to treat psoriasis.

calciprivia (kal″sĭ-priv′e-ah) deprivation or loss of calcium; see also *hypocalcemia*. adj., **calcipriv′ic.**

calcitonin (kal″sĭ-to′nin) a polypeptide hormone secreted by the parafollicular or C cells of the THYROID GLAND; it is involved in plasma CALCIUM homeostasis and acts to decrease the rate of bone resorption. Preparations of calcitonin are called either calcitonin-human or calcitonin-salmon; the former is a synthetic polypeptide with the same sequence as that occurring naturally in humans, and the latter is either derived from salmon or is a synthetic polypeptide of the same sequence as that found in salmon. They are used in the treatment of severe HYPERCALCEMIA, PAGET'S DISEASE of bone, and postmenopausal OSTEOPOROSIS. Called also thyrocalcitonin.

calcitriol (kal′sĭ-tri′ol) 1,25-DIHYDROXYCHO-LECALCIFEROL; a form of VITAMIN D used as a calcium regulator in the management of HYPOCALCEMIA in conditions such as RICKETS, OSTEODYSTROPHY, HYPOPARATHYROIDISM, and complications of renal DIALYSIS; administered orally or intravenously.

calcium (Ca) (kal′se-um) a chemical element, atomic number 20, atomic weight 40.08. (See Appendix 6.) Calcium is the most abundant mineral in the body. In combination with phosphorus it forms calcium phosphate, the dense, hard material of the bones and teeth. It is an important cation in intracellular and extracellular fluid and is essential to the normal clotting of blood, the maintenance of a normal heartbeat, and the initiation of neuromuscular and metabolic activities.

Within the body fluids calcium exists in three forms. Protein-bound calcium accounts for about 47 per cent of the calcium in plasma; most of it in this form is bound to albumin. Another 47 per cent of plasma calcium is ionized. About 6 per cent is complexed with phosphate, citrate, and other anions.

Ionized calcium is physiologically active. One of its most important physiological functions is control of the permeability of cell membranes. Parathyroid hormone, which causes transfer of exchangeable calcium from bone into the blood stream, maintains calcium homeostasis by preventing either calcium deficit or excess.

Hypercalcemia: This is when the level of serum calcium rises above normal; neuromuscular activity begins to diminish. Symptoms include lethargy, muscle weakness (which, as the level of calcium increases, can progress to depressed reflexes and hypotonic muscles), constipation, mental confusion, and coma. The heartbeat also slows, which potentiates the effects of digitalis.

Hypocalcemia: This is a serum level of calcium that is below normal; it is manifested by increased neuromuscular irritability. When there is a deficit of ionized calcium, the nerve cells become more permeable, allowing leakage of sodium and potassium from the cells. This produces excitation of the nerve fibers and triggers uncontrollable activity of the skeletal muscles. Hence, as the calcium level continues to drop, the patient begins to experience muscle twitching and cramping, grimacing, and carpopedal spasm, which can quickly progress to tetany, laryngospasm, convulsions, cardiac arrhythmias, and eventually to respiratory and cardiac arrest. Relatively early signs of hypocalcemia are a positive TROUSSEAU'S SIGN and a positive CHVOSTEK'S SIGN.

Dietary sources of calcium include dairy products (such as milk and cheese), soybeans, fortified orange juice, dark green leafy vegetables (such as mustard greens and broccoli), sardines, clams, and oysters. The recommended dietary ALLOWANCE of calcium for children aged 4 to 8 is 800 mg, and that for women aged 50 to 70 is 1200 mg. (See tables in the Appendices for recommended dietary allowances across the life span.) It is difficult to meet these requirements without including milk or milk products in the daily diet. The most familiar calcium deficiency disease is RICKETS, in which the bones and teeth soften. However, it is believed that a large number of people suffer from subclinical calcium deficiency because of poor eating habits. Since calcium is essential to the formation and maintenance of strong bones, an adequate intake is important in the prevention of OSTEOPOROSIS.

c. acetate the calcium salt of acetic acid; administered orally as a source of calcium and as a phosphate BINDER, such as in patients with END-STAGE RENAL DISEASE. Also used as a pharmaceutical buffering agent.

c. carbonate an insoluble salt occurring naturally in bone, shells, and chalk; used as an ANTACID, calcium supplement, and phosphate BINDER, and for treatment of OSTEOPOROSIS.

c. channel blocker, c. channel blocking agent a drug such as NIFEDIPINE, DILTIAZEM, or VERAPAMIL that selectively blocks the influx of calcium ions through a calcium CHANNEL of cardiac muscle and smooth muscle cells; used in the treatment of Prinzmetal's ANGINA, chronic stable ANGINA, and cardiac ARRHYTHMIAS. Calcium channel blocking agents act to control arrhythmias by slowing the rate of sinoatrial node discharge and the conduction velocity through the atrioventricular node. They act in vasospastic angina to relax and prevent coronary artery spasm. The mechanism of action in classical angina is a lowering of myocardial oxygen utilization by dilating peripheral arteries and thereby reducing total peripheral resistance and the work of the heart. (See accompanying illustration.)

c. chloride a salt used in solution to restore electrolyte balance, treat hypocalcemia, and act as a treatment adjunct in cardiac arrest and in MAGNESIUM poisoning.

c. citrate a salt used as a calcium replenisher; also used in the treatment of hyperphosphatemia in renal OSTEODYSTROPHY.

c. glubionate a calcium replenisher, used as a nutritional supplement and for the treatment of hypocalcemia; administered orally.

c. gluceptate a calcium salt administered intramuscularly or intravenously in the prevention and treatment of HYPOCALCEMIA and as an electrolyte replenisher.

c. gluconate a calcium salt administered intravenously or orally in the treatment and prevention of hypercalcemia and as a nutritional supplement. It is also administered by injection as a treatment adjunct in cardiac arrest and in the treatment of hyperkalemia.

c. hydroxide an astringent compound used topically in solution or lotions.

c. lactate a calcium replenisher, administered orally in the treatment and prevention of hypocalcemia and as a nutritional supplement.

c. oxalate a salt of oxalic acid, which in excess in the urine may lead to formation of oxalate urinary CALCULI.

c. oxide lime (def. 1).

c. pantothenate a calcium salt of the dextrorotatory isomer of the B vitamin PANTOTHENIC ACID; used as a nutritional supplement. It is also available as *racemic calcium pantothenate,* which is a mixture of the dextrorotatory and levorotatory isomeric forms.

c. phosphate a salt containing calcium and the phosphate radical; *dibasic* and

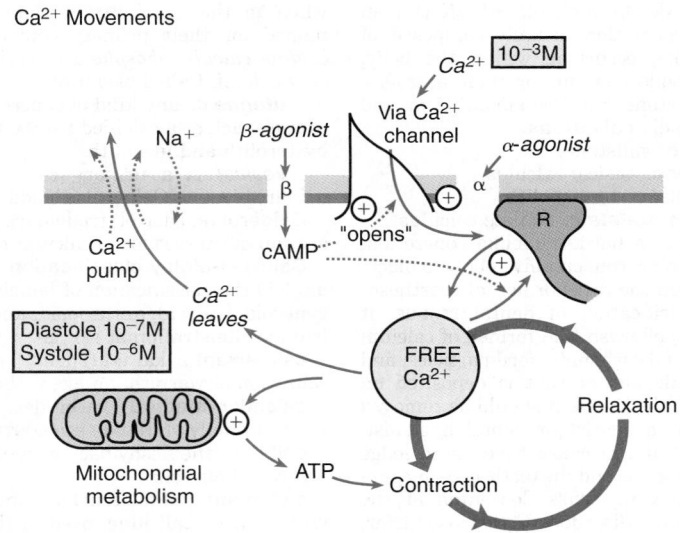

Physiologic activity of calcium channel blockers. (Data from Hardman J. and Limbird L., editors: Goodman and Gilman's The Pharmacologic Basis of Therapeutics, 9th ed., New York, McGraw-Hill, 1996; and the National Institutes of Health: The Sixth Report of the Joint National Committee on Prevention, Detection, Evaluation and Treatment of High Blood Pressure, NIH Pub. No. 98-4080, Washington, DC, GPO, 1998.) From Edmunds and Mayhew, 2000.

tribasic calcium phosphate are used as sources of calcium.

c. polycarbophil a hydrophilic agent used as a bulk LAXATIVE.

c. propionate a salt used as an ANTIFUNGAL preservative in foods and as a topical antifungal AGENT.

c. pyrophosphate the pyrophosphate salt of calcium, used as a polishing agent in dentifrices. Crystals of the dihydrate form occur in the joints in CALCIUM PYROPHOSPHATE DEPOSITION DISEASE.

c. pyrophosphate deposition disease an acute or chronic inflammatory ARTHROPATHY caused by deposition of crystals of CALCIUM PYROPHOSPHATE dihydrate in the joints and synovial fluid and CHONDROCALCINOSIS. Clinically, it may resemble numerous other connective tissue diseases such as ARTHRITIS and GOUT, or it may be asymptomatic. Acute attacks are sometimes called PSEUDOGOUT.

c. sulfate a compound of calcium and sulfate, occurring as GYPSUM or as PLASTER OF PARIS.

calciuria (kal″se-u′re-ah) hypercalciuria.

calcospherite (kal″ko-sfēr′ĭt) one of the minute globular bodies formed during calcification by chemical union of calcium particles and albuminous matter of cells.

calculogenesis (kal″ku-lo-jen′ĕ-sis) the formation of calculi.

calculosis (kal″ku-lo′sis) lithiasis.

calculus (kal′ku-lus), pl. *cal′culi* [L.] an abnormal concretion, usually composed of mineral salts, occurring within the body, chiefly in hollow organs or their passages. Called also stone. See also KIDNEY STONE and GALLSTONE. adj., **cal′culous.**

biliary c. gallstone.

bladder c. vesical calculus.

bronchial c. broncholith.

calcium oxalate c. oxalate calculus.

dental c. a hard, stonelike concretion, varying in color from creamy yellow to black, that forms on the teeth or dental prostheses through calcification of dental PLAQUE; it begins as a yellowish film formed of calcium phosphate and carbonate, food particles, and other organic matter that is deposited on the teeth by the saliva. It should be removed regularly by a dentist or dental hygienist; if neglected, it can cause bacteria to lodge between the gums and the teeth, causing gum infection, DENTAL CARIES, loosening of the teeth, and other disorders. Called also tartar.

gastric c. gastrolith.

intestinal c. enterolith.

lung c. a hard mass or CONCRETION formed in the bronchi around a small center of inorganic material, or from calcified portions of lung tissue or adjacent lymph nodes. Called also pneumolith.

mammary c. a concretion in one of the lactiferous ducts.

nasal c. rhinolith.

oxalate c. a hard urinary calculus of CALCIUM OXALATE; some are covered with minute sharp spines that may abrade the renal pelvic epithelium, and others are smooth. Called also calcium oxalate calculus.

phosphate c. a urinary calculus composed of a phosphate along with calcium oxalate and ammonium urate; it may be hard, soft, or friable, and so large that it may fill the renal pelvis and calices.

prostatic c. a concretion formed in the PROSTATE, chiefly of CALCIUM CARBONATE and phosphate. Called also prostatolith.

renal c. kidney stone.

staghorn c. a urinary calculus, usually a phosphate calculus, found in the renal PELVIS and shaped like the antlers of a stag because it extends into multiple CALICES.

urate c. uric acid calculus.

urethral c. a urinary calculus in the urethra; symptoms vary according to the patient's sex and the site of lodgment.

uric acid c. a hard, yellow or reddish-yellow urinary calculus formed from uric acid.

urinary c. a calculus in any part of the urinary TRACT; it is *vesical* when lodged in the bladder and *renal* (see KIDNEY STONE) when in the renal PELVIS. Common types named for their primary components are *oxalate calculi, phosphate calculi,* and *uric acid calculi.* Called also urolith.

uterine c. any kind of concretion in the uterus, such as a calcified MYOMA. Called also hysterolith and uterolith.

vesical c. a urinary calculus in the urinary bladder. Called also bladder calculus.

Calderol (kal′der-ol) trademark for a preparation of CALCIFEDIOL, a calcium regulator.

Caldwell-Moloy classification (kawld′wel mō-loi′) the classification of female pelves as gynecoid, android, anthropoid, and platypelloid (see illustration at PELVIS).

calefacient (kal″ĕ-fa′shent) causing a sensation of warmth; an agent that so acts.

calendar method (kal′en-der) a type of natural family PLANNING; see CONTRACEPTION.

calf (kaf) the fleshy back part of the lower leg; called also sura.

calfactant (kal-fak′tant) a pulmonary SURFACTANT from calf lung, used in the prophylaxis and treatment of neonatal RESPIRATORY DISTRESS SYNDROME; administered intratracheally by instillation via the ENDOTRACHEAL TUBE.

caliber (kal′ĭ-ber) the diameter of the lumen of a canal or tube.

calibration (kal″ĭ-bra′shun) determination of the accuracy of an instrument, usually by measurement of its variation from a standard, to ascertain necessary correction factors.

calicectasis (kal″ĭ-sek′tah-sis) dilatation of a calix of the kidney.

calicectomy (kal″ĭ-sek′to-me) excision of a calix of the kidney.

calices (kal′ĭ-sēz) [L.] plural of CALIX.

calicivirus (kah-lis′ĭ-vi″rus) any member of a family of RNA viruses that cause disease in humans and other animals; the species that most often causes human disease is Norwalk VIRUS.

caliculus (kah-lik′u-lus), pl. *cali′culi* a bud-shaped or cup-shaped structure.

California disease coccidioidomycosis.

californium (Cf) (kal″ĭ-for′ne-um) a chemical element, atomic number 98, atomic weight 249. (See Appendix 6.)

calipers (kal′ĭ-perz) an instrument with two bent or curved legs used for measuring thickness or diameter of a solid.

calisthenics (kal″is-then′iks) systematic exercise for attaining strength and gracefulness.

calix (ka′liks), pl. *ca′lices* [L.] a cuplike organ or cavity. adj., **calice′al.**

renal c. the subdivision of the renal PELVIS that encloses a renal PYRAMID.

Calliphora (kah-lif′o-rah) a genus of flies, the blowflies or bluebottle flies, which deposit their eggs in decaying matter, on wounds, or in body openings; the maggots are a cause of MYIASIS.

callosity (kah-los′ĭ-te) CALLUS (def. 1).

callosum (kah-lo′sum) corpus callosum.

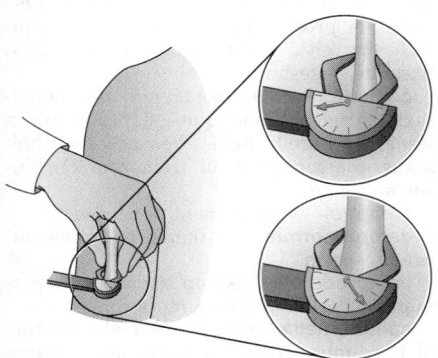

Skinfold calipers measure the thickness of subcutaneous fat tissue in millimeters. This gives a rough measurement of adiposity. (NOTE: Large caliper readings are read counterclockwise.) Courtesy of Dorice Czajka-Narins, in Mahan and Escott-Stump, 2000.

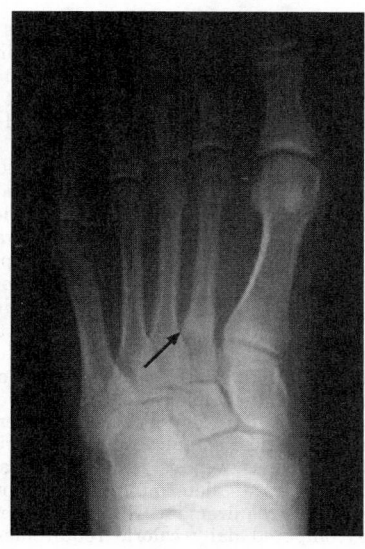

A fracture with callus formation (*arrow*) is demonstrated corresponding to the base of the second metatarsal. From Thrall and Ziessman, 2001.

callous (kal′us) of the nature of a callus; hard.

callus (kal′us) 1. localized hyperplasia of the horny layer of the epidermis due to pressure or friction. 2. an unorganized network of woven bone formed about the ends of a broken bone; it is absorbed as repair is completed (provisional callus), and ultimately replaced by true bone (definitive callus). (See accompanying illustration.)

calmative (kal′mah-tiv, kah′mah-tiv) sedative.

calming technique (kahl′ming) in the NURSING INTERVENTIONS CLASSIFICATION, a nursing INTERVENTION defined as reducing anxiety in a patient experiencing acute distress.

calmodulin (kal-mod′u-lin) a calcium-binding protein present in all nucleated cells, thought to be an essential mediator of most calcium-sensitive cellular processes.

calor (kal′er) [L.] heat; one of the cardinal signs of inflammation.

caloric (kah-lor′ik) pertaining to heat or to calories.

c. test a test of third, sixth, and eighth cranial nerves. Irrigation of the normal ear with warm water produces caloric NYSTAGMUS toward the irrigated side; irrigation with cold water produces similar nystagmus away from that side. Called also oculovestibular test.

calorie (kal'o-re) any of several units of heat defined as the amount of heat required to raise the temperature of 1 kilogram of water by 1 degree Celsius (1°C) at a specified temperature. The calorie used in chemistry and biochemistry is equal to 4.184 joules. Symbol cal. See also NUTRITION.

In referring to the energy content of foods it is customary to use the "large calorie," which is equal to 1 kilocalorie (kcal). Every bodily process, including the building up of cells, motion of the muscles, and the maintenance of body temperature, requires energy, which the body derives from the food it consumes. Digestive processes reduce food to usable "fuel," which the body "burns" in the complex chemical reactions that sustain life. The amount of energy required for these chemical processes varies. Factors such as weight, age, activity, and metabolic rate determine a person's daily calorie requirement. Nutrition experts have computed daily calorie requirements in terms of age and other factors. These tabulations serve only as guides; they cannot, of course, embrace all individual variations.

From its daily intake of energy foods, the body uses only the amount it needs for energy purposes. The remainder is stored as fat. If the average adult consumes more calories than the daily requirement, he or she will gain weight. However, if consumption is less than recommended daily requirements, the body will supplement its energy sources by drawing upon stores of fat and the person will lose weight.

calorimeter (kal″o-rim'ĕ-ter) an instrument for measuring the amount of heat produced in any system or organism.

calorimetry (kal″o-rim'ĕ-tre) measurement of the heat eliminated or stored in any system.

direct c. measurement of the amount of heat produced by a subject enclosed within a small chamber.

indirect c. measurement of the amount of heat produced by a subject by determination of the amount of oxygen consumed and the amount of carbon dioxide eliminated.

calvaria (kal-var'e-ah) the domelike superior portion of the cranium, comprising superior portions of the frontal, parietal, and occipital bones. Called also cranial vault. (See accompanying illustration.)

Calvé-Perthes disease (kal-va′-per′tēz) osteochondrosis of the epiphysis at the head of the femur.

calx (kalks) 1. lime or chalk. 2. heel.

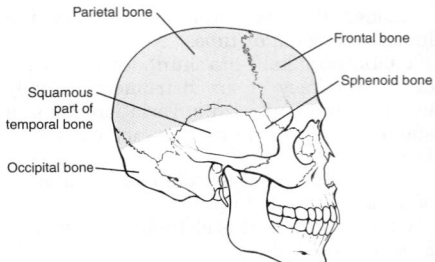

Calvaria. From Dorland's, 2000.

Calymmatobacterium (kah-lim″mah-to-bak-tēr′e-um) a genus of bacteria made up of gram-negative rods. *C. granulo'matis* causes GRANULOMA INGUINALE.

calyx (ka'liks) calix.

camera (kam'er-ah), pl. *ca'merae, cameras* [L.] a cavity or chamber.

Anger c. the original form of gamma camera. Because the Anger camera is by far the most frequently used type of gamma (or scintillation) camera today, the terms are often used interchangeably.

gamma c., scintillation c. an electronic instrument that produces photographs or cathode-ray tube images of the gamma ray emissions from organs containing tracer compounds. The original and most commonly used version is the ANGER C.

camisole (kam'ĭ-sōl) a device for restraining the limbs, especially the arms, of a violently disturbed person; it consists of a canvas jacket with long sleeves that can be fastened behind the back of the patient. Called also straitjacket and jacket restraint.

cAMP cyclic adenosine monophosphate.

camphor (kam'fer) a ketone derived from an Asian tree, *Cinnamomum camphora*, or produced synthetically; used topically for relief of itching and inhaled as a nasal decongestant.

campotomy (kam-pot'ah-me) the stereotaxic surgical technique of producing a lesion in Forel's fields, beneath the thalamus, for correction of tremor in Parkinson's disease.

campt(o)- word element [Gr.], *bent.*

camptocormia (kamp″to-kor′me-ah) camptospasm.

camptodactyly (kamp″to-dak′tĭ-le) permanent flexion of one or more fingers.

camptomelia (kamp″to-me′le-ah) bending of the limbs, producing permanent bowing or curving of the affected part. adj., **camptome'lic.**

camptospasm (kamp′to-spazm) a static deformity consisting of forward flexion of the trunk. Called also camptocormia.

Campylobacter (kam′pĭ-lo-bak″ter) a genus of gram-negative, microaerophilic to anaerobic, motile, curved or spiral rod-shaped bacteria, found in the oral cavity, intestinal tract, and reproductive organs of humans and animals. Certain subspecies of *C. fe′tus* are agents of acute gastroenteritis and can cause systemic infection in immunocompromised persons. *C. pylo′ri* is now known as *Helicobacter pylori.*

campylobacteriosis (kam″pĭ-lo-bak-tēr″e-o′sis) infection with organisms of the genus *Campylobacter.*

Canada-Cronkhite syndrome (kan′ah-dah-krong′-kīt) familial polyposis of the gastrointestinal tract associated with alopecia, nail dystrophy, and hyperpigmentation of the skin.

Canadian Nurses Association (CNA) the professional association for registered nurses in Canada. Its stated mission is "to foster excellence in nursing practice, education, research and management, to advocate high quality health care in Canada and internationally, and to speak on behalf of Canadian nurses on nursing and health related issues."

Canadian Nurses Association Testing Services a testing program administered by the Canadian Nurses Association for the purpose of licensure.

canal (kah-nal′) a relatively narrow tubular passage or channel.

adductor c. Hunter's canal.

Alcock's c. a tunnel formed by a splitting of the obturator fascia, which encloses the pudendal vessels and nerve.

alimentary c. see ALIMENTARY CANAL.

anal c. the terminal portion of the alimentary canal, from the rectum to the anus.

atrioventricular c. the common canal connecting the primordial atrium and ventricle; it sometimes persists as a congenital anomaly.

birth c. the canal through which the fetus passes in birth.

carotid c. one in the pars petrosa of the temporal bone, transmitting the internal carotid artery to the cranial cavity.

cervical c. the part of the uterine cavity lying within the cervix.

condylar c. an occasional opening in the condylar fossa for transmission of the transverse sinus; called also posterior condyloid foramen.

c. of Corti a space between the outer and inner rods of Corti.

femoral c. the cone-shaped medial part of the femoral sheath lateral to the base of Gimbernat's ligament.

haversian c. any of the anastomosing channels of the haversian system in compact bone, containing blood and lymph vessels, and nerves.

Hunter's c. a fascial tunnel in the middle third of the medial part of the thigh, containing the femoral vessels and saphenous nerve. Called also adductor canal.

hypoglossal c. an opening in the occipital bone, transmitting the hypoglossal nerve and a branch of the posterior meningeal artery; called also anterior condyloid foramen.

infraorbital c. a small canal running obliquely through the floor of the orbit, transmitting the infraorbital vessels and nerve.

inguinal c. the oblique passage in the lower anterior abdominal wall on either side, through which passes the round ligament of the uterus in the female, and the spermatic cord in the male.

medullary c. 1. spinal canal. 2. marrow cavity.

optic c. a passage for the optic nerve and ophthalmic artery at the apex of the orbit; called also optic foramen.

pulp c. root canal.

root c. that part of the pulp CAVITY extending from the pulp chamber to the apical foramen. Called also pulp canal.

sacral c. the continuation of the spinal canal through the sacrum.

Schlemm's c. venous SINUS of sclera.

semicircular c's see SEMICIRCULAR CANALS.

spinal c., vertebral c. the canal formed by the series of vertebral foramina together, enclosing the spinal cord and meninges.

Volkmann's c's canals communicating with the haversian canals, for passage of blood vessels through bone.

canaliculitis (kan″ah-lik″u-li′tis) inflammation of the lacrimal ducts.

canaliculus (kan″ah-lik′u-lus), pl. *canali′culi* [L.] an extremely narrow tubular passage or channel. adj., **canalic′ular.**

bile canaliculi fine tubular channels forming a three-dimensional network within the parenchyma of the liver. They join to form the bile ductules and eventually the hepatic duct.

bone canaliculi branching tubular passages radiating like wheel spokes from each bone lacuna to connect with the canaliculi of adjacent lacunae, and with the haversian canal.

lacrimal c. the short passage in an eyelid, beginning at the lacrimal point and draining tears from the lacrimal lake to the lacrimal sac; called also lacrimal duct. See also LACRIMAL APPARATUS.

mastoid c. a small channel in the temporal bone transmitting the auricular branch of the vagus nerve.

canalis (kah-na'lis), pl. *cana'les* [L.] a canal or channel.

canalization (kan"al-ī-za'shun) 1. formation of canals, natural or morbid. 2. surgical establishment of canals for drainage. 3. recanalization.

canaloplasty (kah-nal'o-plas"te) plastic reconstruction of a passage, as of the external acoustic meatus.

Canavan disease (kan'ah-van) a rare autosomal recessive form of LEUKODYSTROPHY, found especially in people of Ashkenazi Jewish descent, although it has also been seen in other ethnic groups. Characteristics include early onset, widespread DEMYELINATION and VACUOLATION of the cerebral white matter that gives it a spongy appearance, severe mental retardation, an enlarged head, atony of neck muscles, spasticity of arms and legs, and blindness. Death may occur as early as 18 months of age; in those who survive, there may be seizures, muscle weakness, stiffness, and feeding problems. Called also spongy degeneration of central nervous system.

cancellated (kan'sel-āt"ed) having a lattice-like structure.

cancellous (kan'sĕ-lus) of a reticular, spongy, or lattice-like structure; said mainly of bone tissue.

cancellus (kan-sel'us), pl. *cancel'li* [L.] the lattice-like structure in bone; any structure arranged like a lattice.

cancer (kan'ser) any malignant, cellular tumor. For specific types, see under the name, such as BREAST CANCER or LUNG CANCER. adj., **can'cerous.**

The term *cancer* encompasses a group of neoplastic diseases in which there is a transformation of normal body cells into malignant ones. This probably involves some change in the genetic material of the cells, deoxyribonucleic acid (DNA). ONCOGENES are the genes that organisms have evolved to regulate growth and repair of tissues. They are genetic codes for the proteins that function as signals that cells send and receive to regulate proliferation. These oncogenes are the targets of CARCINOGENS. MUTATION and TRANSFORMATION of oncogenes may permanently affect a cell's ability to control cell growth. Damage to the cell's genetic material may be caused by carcinogenic agents. Normal cell lines can be transformed into cancer cells by VIRUSES, chemical CARCINOGENS, and RADIATION. Transformed cell lines have the ability to develop into malignant neoplasms. Transformed cells may also be recognized by other characteristics which include altered antigenicity, diminished contact inhibition, reduced requirements for certain nutrients, and the ability to grow in suspension. The altered cells pass on inappropriate genetic information to their offspring and begin to proliferate in an abnormal and destructive way. Normally, cells reproduce regularly to replace worn-out tissues, repair injuries, and allow for growth during the developing years. After these processes have taken place, cellular reproduction stops. Clearly the body in its normal processes regulates cell growth in an orderly manner. In cancer, there is no regulation and cell reproduction and growth is disorderly. The dangers of cancer are related to this chaotic reproduction of malignant cells.

As the cancer cells continue to proliferate, the mass of abnormal tissue that they form enlarges, ulcerates, and begins to shed cells that spread the disease locally or to distant sites. This migration is called METASTASIS. Some cells penetrate neighboring tissues, destroying normal cells and taking their place. Others can enter the blood stream and lymphatic vessels and be carried along in the fluid to another part of the body. Another way malignancy can be spread is by entering a body cavity and coming in contact with a healthy organ; however, this is not common.

Causes. It is doubtful that one process is involved in the etiology of all cancers. The exact cause of conversion of normal cells into cancerous ones is still not completely understood. An important factor is permanent alteration in the DNA of the cell, which is passed on to subsequent generations, but we do not know what triggers the change in DNA structure and why some people succumb to a cancer and others do not. Cellular IMMUNITY undoubtedly plays some part in one's ability to stop the growth of cancer cells; it is believed by some that most persons develop many small cancers in their lifetime but do not develop clinical signs because their defense mechanisms destroy the malignant cells and prevent their replication.

Oncologists recognize that environmental, hereditary, and biological factors all play important roles in the development of cancer (see table). Environmental causes are believed to account for at least 50 per cent and perhaps, in some types, as much as 80 per cent of all cancers. For example, cigarette SMOKING is directly related to approximately 90 per cent of all cases of LUNG CANCER. Other environmental carcinogens include

WINDOW ON CANCER

Living with a chronic illness such as cancer is a complex process involving factors that influence a patient's responses and subsequent quality of life. Due to its focus on enhancing quality of life and providing symptom management, cancer nursing typifies the essence of professional nursing practice. This is also true in the area of cancer nursing research which, in many respects, has taken the lead in outlining important areas of inquiry, especially within the context of expanding chronic health problems. In the mid 1970s a program of research was initiated by McCorkle and her colleagues to develop standardized instruments so that the impact of illness and treatment could be documented. The Symptom Distress Scale and the Enforced Social Dependency Scale have been used in multiple clinical studies as dependent variables or outcome measures. These scales were designed respectively to describe patients' symptom profiles associated with various cancers and treatment efforts and to describe alterations in functional abilities and independence. In four home care nursing studies, the vital role professional nurses play in providing home care over time to patients with cancer and their family caregivers has been demonstrated. Patients receiving home care by professional nurses had less symptom distress, improved function, and better survival. Critical nursing behaviors demonstrated to be effective included: monitoring patient status, providing symptom management, executing complex care procedures, teaching patients and family caregivers, coordinating care, responding to the family, enhancing quality of living, and collaborating with other care providers. Results, to date, establish essential skills and knowledge associated with critical nursing behaviors. Additional work is needed to incorporate these behaviors into clinical practice as part of evidence-based practice.

RUTH MCCORKLE, PhD, FAAN

industrial pollutants and radiation. Among the chemical carcinogens are ARSENIC from mining and smelting industries; ASBESTOS from insulation, at construction sites and power plants; BENZENE from oil refineries, solvents, and insecticides; and products from coal combustion in steel and petrochemical industries. Each year new products that in all probability are carcinogenic are being produced by industrial operations. A major concern is the occupational and environmental hazards these chemicals present to those who work in or live near these plants.

RADIATION from prolonged exposure to the ultraviolet rays of the sun or from injudicious use of diagnostic and therapeutic procedures involving X-RAYS and RADIOACTIVE substances is also a significant factor in the incidence of cancer, particularly that of the skin, bone marrow, and thyroid.

HORMONES, especially the synthetic ESTROGENS given to prevent spontaneous ABORTION, are directly related to some cancers of the female reproductive organs.

VIRUSES as causal agents in the development of cancer have been subjected to intensive research efforts in recent years. The epidemiologic evidence is strongest for a relationship between hepatitis B VIRUS and hepatocellular CARCINOMA and between human T-lymphotropic VIRUS (HTLV)-1 and T-cell LYMPHOMA. Both have a geographic distribution of cancer prevalence and viral infection as well as case-by-case associations. The association between BURKITT'S LYMPHOMA and EPSTEIN-BARR VIRUS (EBV) is likewise strong, except that there seems to be a need for an associated IMMUNODEFICIENCY state, such as that induced by chronic MALARIA. Similarly, the association between EBV and high-grade lymphoma in Western countries seems to require that an immunodeficiency state be present, either congenital or induced by the HUMAN IMMUNODEFICIENCY VIRUS (HIV) or a drug such as CYCLOSPORINE.

The intriguing fact has been noted that viruses are capable of introducing new genetic material into a normal cell and transforming it into a malignant one, and that cell reproduction may be altered when viruses interact with such carcinogens as chemicals and radiation. Recent studies have shown that an extracellular enzyme, REVERSE TRANSCRIPTASE, plays an important role in the transmission of genetic information to the cell and thereby facilitates the reproduction of cancer cells.

The incidence of cancer in certain populations suggests that other factors are important in its development. It is known, for example, that some families show a high

CANCER RISK FACTORS

Breast
Nulliparity
Early menarche
Diet high in fat
First child after age 30
Family history of breast cancer
History of benign breast disease
History of ovarian cancer

Bladder
Cigarette smoking
Over age 65
Working in organic chemical, dye, rubber,
  or paint industry

Cervical
Low socioeconomic status
Adolescent sexual activity
Adolescent pregnancy
Multiple sexual partners
Multiparity
Maternal use of diethylstilbestrol during
  pregnancy

Colorectal
History of adenomatous polyps, ulcerative colitis,
  or Crohn's disease
Family history of colorectal cancer
Over age 40
Diet rich in animal fats and low in fiber

Endometrial
Obesity
Nulliparity
Diabetes mellitus
Hypertension
Late menopause

Esophageal
African American
Heavy use of alcohol with tobacco

Lung
Cigarette smoking
Exposure to second-hand smoke
Exposure to asbestos, high levels of indoor
  radon, heavy metals, or petroleum products

Oral
Heavy use of alcohol and tobacco
Poor oral hygiene
Vitamin A deficiency

Ovarian
Nulliparity
History of breast cancer
Living in a Western industrialized country

Prostate
African American
Family history
High-fat diet
Greater with increasing age

Skin
Fair complexion
Family history of melanoma
Personal history of dysplastic nevus
  syndrome
Ionizing radiation exposure
Work settings with sun exposure
Severe sunburn before age 20

Stomach
High intake of pickled, salted, or smoked foods
Poor vitamin A and C intake
Helicobacter pylori infection
Tobacco use

Testicular
Age 20–40
Caucasian
Cryptorchidism

incidence of malignancy among their members, but there is no definite hereditary pattern. There also is a high incidence of cancer in persons receiving drugs for immunosuppression, yet cancer itself is immunosuppressive. It is suggested that prolonged suppression of the body's immune RESPONSE may eventually impair its ability to distinguish between self and nonself and thus render it unable to destroy malignant cells. When cancer itself acts to suppress the immune response, it may be the result of an overwhelming demand on the body to destroy more foreign cells than it is prepared to cope with at any given time.

Aging is another factor to consider in development of malignancy. Although cancer can occur at any age, older persons are more susceptible, perhaps because their powers of adaptability are weakened and they have been exposed to carcinogens longer than have younger persons.

Classification. Cancers are classified on the basis of two factors: the type of tissue and the type of cell in which they arise. Using this classification system, it is possible to identify over 150 types of cancer in humans. In the classification of cancers according to the type of tissue from which they evolve, there are two main groups, SARCOMAS and CARCINOMAS. Sarcomas are of mesenchymal origin and affect such tissues as the bones and muscles; they tend to grow rapidly and to be very destructive. The carcinomas are of epithelial origin and make up the great majority of the glandular cancers and cancers of the breast, stomach, uterus, skin, and tongue. Cell type affects the appearance, rate of growth, and degree of malignancy. Thus, classification of tumors according to the type of cell from which they are derived is important in deciding the course of treatment for a specific malignancy.

TNM STAGING SYSTEM

T: Primary Tumor

TX	Primary tumor is not assessable
T0	No evidence of primary tumor
Tis	Carcinoma in situ
T1, T2, T3, T4	Progressive increase in tumor size and involvement locally

N: Regional Lymph Nodes

NX	Nodes are not assessable
N0	No metastasis to regional lymph nodes
N1, N2, N3	Increasing degrees of involvement of regional lymph nodes

Note: Extension of primary tumor directly into lymph nodes is considered metastasis to lymph nodes. Metastasis to a lymph node beyond the regional ones is considered to be a distant metastasis.

M: Distant Metastasis

MX	Presence of distant metastasis is not assessable
M0	No distant metastasis
MI	Presence of distant metastasis

Staging. An approach to describing and categorizing malignant tumors has been developed by the International Union Against Cancer (UICC) and the American Joint Committee on Cancer (AJCC). It is hoped that by standardizing the classification and staging of tumors, treatment protocols can be established and end results reporting can be utilized to determine the effectiveness of the suggested treatment. Whereas *classification* of tumors refers to the anatomical and histological descriptions of the tumor (see above), *staging* refers to the extent of the tumor. The three components of the staging system are the primary tumor (T), regional nodes (N), and metastasis (M). Subscripts may be used to describe the extent to which the malignancy has increased in size, its involvement of regional nodes, and its metastatic development (see table). For example, a tumor may be described as T1N2M0. DUKES' CLASSIFICATION is a system of staging colorectal tumors, based on the depth of invasion and degree of metastasis.

Precancers. Some potentially dangerous cancers appear first in the form of harmless changes in the body's tissues. The danger lies in the fact that such changes have a tendency to become malignant; hence they are known as PRECANCERS. Among them are sores that appear as thickened white patches (LEUKOPLAKIA) in the mouth and on the vulva, some MOLES, and any chronically irritated area on the skin or the mucous membranes of the mouth and tongue. POLYPS are also possible precancers.

Prevention. Because environmental conditions play an important role in the etiology of many cancers, prevention is aimed at identifying carcinogens, educating the general public about them, and encouraging their avoidance. Equally important, if not more so, is recognition of causative factors related to life style and personal habits. Perhaps the best example of this is the relationship between SMOKING and LUNG CANCER. When heavy consumption of ALCOHOL is combined with cigarette smoking, the risk for cancer of the larynx, esophagus, and mouth is greatly increased.

Nutritional balance is also important in the prevention of cancer. Certain foods and food additives contain specific carcinogenic agents. Nutritional deficiency can lower resistance and increase the risk of certain types of cancers. The decrease in incidence of stomach cancer in most Western countries may possibly be the result of an increase in consumption of fruits and vegetables, since vitamin B_{12} deficiency (PERNICIOUS ANEMIA) is known to be related to increased incidence of stomach cancer.

Studies have shown that a relationship exists between OBESITY and cancer, and between dietary excess, particularly consumption of large amounts of fats, and certain types of cancers. In general, overweight women are at increased risk for cancer of the endometrium, gallbladder, and kidney. Cancers associated with a high dietary intake of fat, with or without obesity, are those affecting the breast, ovary, endometrium, prostate, colon, and pancreas. Although neither saturated nor unsaturated fats are themselves carcinogenic, they act on the endocrine system and affect hormonal activity. The relationship of fat consumption to colon cancer is thought to be due to the effect of BILE ACIDS and their metabolites, which have been shown to act as tumor promoters in laboratory animals. In humans, patients with cancer of the colon typically have elevated levels of bile acid metabolites. Studies of various populations throughout the world have shown that bowel cancer is more prevalent among groups who eat large amounts of fat and very little food fiber. Hence the American Cancer Society recommends a low fat, high fiber diet for Americans.

The judicious use of hormones for therapeutic purposes also can reduce the incidence of some cancers. The widespread use of DIETHYLSTILBESTROL (DES) to prevent threatened or habitual abortion and premature labor, beginning in the 1940s, eventually resulted in development of vaginal and cervical cancer in a significant number of the female offspring of women who took the drug while pregnant. As was previously mentioned, estrogens prescribed for relief of menopausal symptoms have been implicated in cancer in women. It is recommended that the lowest possible therapeutic dose be given to relieve the symptoms of menopause and prevent osteoporosis.

Cancer of the skin and malignant MELANOMA are related to prolonged exposure to the ultraviolet radiation in sunlight. The incidence of cancer of the skin is increasing in those persons who value a deep suntan and spend a significant amount of time engaged in outdoor leisure activities. Also at risk are those whose work requires that they be exposed to sunlight for prolonged periods of time, such as farmers.

Since most occupational cancers are preventable, increased awareness on the part of industry and the provision of a safe workplace environment can decrease the incidence of many kinds of cancer. It is also necessary for workers to cooperate with management in reducing exposure to carcinogens by complying with rules for preventive measures.

Ultimately, the prevention of cancer depends upon knowledge of each person's risk factors for development of cancer, and that person's decision to avoid whenever possible those habits and practices that predispose to the disease. There also should be frequent examination and monitoring of those who are known to be at greater risk.

Detection. In addition to routine cancer-related checkups by a health care provider for early detection of cancer, self-examination and awareness of the early danger signs of cancer are suggested as means by which lay persons can participate in detecting it in its earliest stages.

Monthly self-examination of the BREAST is advocated for all adult women, including those who are postmenopausal. Monthly self-examination of the TESTES is recommended for all males, particularly those in the age group most at risk for testicular cancer, that is, between the ages of 15 and 34 years.

Another self-administered screening technique is the test for occult blood, a symptom of colorectal cancer. This requires only that a smear of fecal material be applied to a slide, which is sent to a clinical laboratory for examination. To avoid a false positive reading, the person participating in the test is given instructions regarding ingestion of

SEVEN EARLY DANGER SIGNS OF CANCER

Change in bowel or bladder habits
A sore that does not heal
Unusual bleeding or discharge
Thickening or lump in breast or elsewhere
Indigestion or difficulty swallowing
Obvious change in a wart or mole
Nagging cough or hoarseness

Note: These signs do not necessarily signify cancer, but if they occur, a physician should be consulted and an examination is advisable. There may be other symptoms, depending on location and type of malignancy.

meat and other foods that could interfere with accurate test findings.

Signs of Cancer. There are seven early warning signs of cancer (see table). *These signs do not necessarily signify cancer, but should they occur, a health care provider should be consulted and an examination is advisable.* Other signs and symptoms depend on location and type of malignancy present.

canceremia (kan″ser-e′me-ah) the presence of cancer cells in the blood.

cancericidal (kan″ser-ĭ-si′d′l) oncolytic; see ONCOLYSIS.

cancerigenic (kan″ser-ĭ-jen′ik) giving rise to a malignant tumor; see also CARCINOGENIC.

cancerophobia (kan″ser-o-fo′be-ah) cancerphobia.

cancerphobia (kan″ser-fo′be-ah) irrational fear of cancer or other tumors.

cancriform (kang′krĭ-form) resembling cancer.

cancroid (kang′kroid) 1. cancer-like. 2. a skin cancer of a low grade of malignancy.

cancrum (kang′krum) [L.] canker.

　　c. o′ris see NOMA.

　　c. puden′di see NOMA.

candela (cd) (kan-del′ah) the base SI UNIT of luminous intensity.

candesartan (kan″dĕ-sahr′tan) an angiotensin II receptor antagonist, used in the treatment of hypertension; administered orally as *candesartan cilexetil.*

candicidin (kan″dĭ-si′din) an antifungal AGENT derived from *Streptomyces griseus,* used principally to treat candidal VAGINITIS.

Candida (kan′dĭ-dah) a genus of yeastlike fungi that are commonly part of the normal flora of the mouth, skin, intestinal tract, and vagina, but can cause a variety of infections. *C. al′bicans* is the usual pathogen in humans. See also CANDIDIASIS.

candidemia (kan″dĭ-de′me-ah) the presence in the blood of fungi of the genus *Candida.*

candidiasis (kan″dĭ-di′ah-sis) infection by fungi of the genus *Candida,* generally

C. albicans, most commonly involving the skin, oral mucosa (THRUSH), respiratory tract, or vagina; occasionally there is a systemic infection or endocarditis. It is most often associated with pregnancy, glycosuria, diabetes mellitus, or use of antibiotics. The Centers for Disease Control and Prevention has found that in the United States this condition is the fourth most common cause of nosocomial infections of the blood stream. Called also candidosis and moniliasis.

The most prominent symptom of vaginitis due to *Candida* infection is severe itching. Sexual transmission is unlikely. Intravaginal cream containing MICONAZOLE or CLOTRIMAZOLE, applied each night for one week, usually clears up the infection. Difficulty or pain with swallowing, or retrosternal pain, may indicate candidiasis of the esophagus. Systemic antifungal therapy is indicated for esophagitis and other more severe forms of the disease. Therapeutic options include KETOCONAZOLE, FLUCONAZOLE, and AMPHOTERICIN B. Chronic suppressive therapy is sometimes required for severely IMMUNOCOMPROMISED patients. The Infectious Disease Society of America has published "Practice Guidelines for the Treatment of Candidiasis" on their web site, http://www.idsociety.org.

atrophic c. oral candidiasis marked by erythematous, pebbled patches on the hard or soft palate, buccal mucosa, and dorsal surface of the tongue, a complication of numerous different conditions such as vitamin deficiency, diabetes mellitus, or poorly fitting dentures. There are acute forms and a chronic form called DENTURE STOMATITIS.

bronchopulmonary c. candidiasis of the respiratory tree, occurring in a mild afebrile form manifested as chronic bronchitis, and in a usually fatal form resembling tuberculosis. Called also bronchocandidiasis.

chronic mucocutaneous c. a group comprising a number of varying forms of *Candida* infection, marked by chronic candidiasis of the skin and nails and the mucous membranes of the mouth and vagina that is resistant to treatment; it may be localized or diffuse, is sometimes familial, and may be associated with disorders of the immune and endocrine systems.

endocardial c. *Candida* endocarditis.

oral c. thrush.

pulmonary c. a type of fungal pneumonia caused by infection with *Candida* species, seen especially in IMMUNOCOMPROMISED patients or those with malignancies. Called also *Candida* pneumonia.

vaginal c., vulvovaginal c. candidal infection of the vagina, and usually also the vulva, commonly characterized by itching, creamy white discharge, vulvar redness and swelling, and dyspareunia. Called also Candida or candidal vaginitis and Candida or candidal vulvovaginitis.

candidid (kan′dĭ-did) a secondary skin eruption that is an expression of hypersensitivity to infection with *Candida* elsewhere on the body.

candidin (kan′dĭ-din) a skin test antigen derived from *Candida albicans,* used in testing for the development of delayed-type hypersensitivity to the microorganism.

candidosis (kan″dĭ-do′sis) candidiasis.

candiduria (kan″did-u′re-ah) the presence of *Candida* organisms in the urine.

cane (kān) an assistive DEVICE that provides partial support and balance for ambulation and standing.

adjustable c. a cane whose length can be easily altered.

quadripod c. a cane adapted for increased stability by providing a four-legged rectangular base of support.

tripod c. one similar to a quadripod cane except that its base is triangular with three legs.

white c. a cane used by the visually handicapped to increase awareness of the immediate environment; the white color is a sign to others that the user is blind.

canine (ka′nīn) 1. pertaining to or characteristic of dogs. 2. cuspid tooth; see TOOTH. 3. pertaining to a cuspid (canine) tooth.

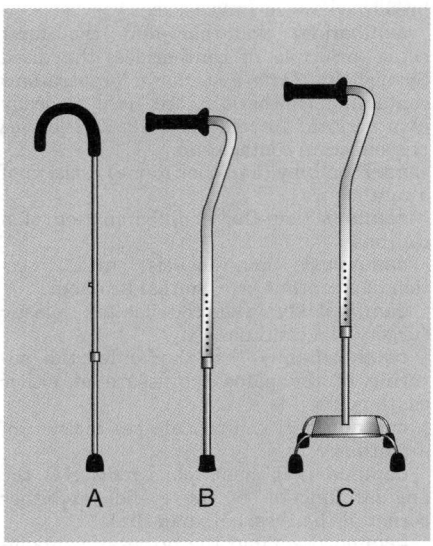

Cane. *A* and *B*, adjustable canes. *C*, quadripod (quad) cane.

canities grayness or whiteness of the scalp hair, especially as associated with aging. See also LEUKOTRICHIA and POLIOSIS.

canker (kang'ker) an ulceration, especially of the oral mucosa; see also recurrent aphthous STOMATITIS.

cannabinoid (kah-nab'ĭ-noid) any of the principles of *Cannabis,* including TETRAHYDROCANNABINOL and CANNABINOL.

cannabinol (kah-nab'ĭ-nol) a physiologically inactive principle from *Cannabis;* its tetrahydro derivative (TETRAHYDROCANNABINOL) is active.

cannabis (kan'ah-bis) the dried flowering tops of hemp plants *(Cannabis sativa),* which have euphoric principles; see MARIJUANA and HASHISH.

cannula (kan'u-lah) a tube for insertion into a vessel, duct, or cavity. During insertion its lumen is usually occupied by a trocar; following placement, the trocar is removed and the cannula remains patent as a channel for the flow of fluids.

nasal c. one that fits into the nostrils for delivery of OXYGEN THERAPY. Called also nasal prongs.

cannulate (kan'u-lāt) to introduce a cannula, which may be left in place.

cannulation (kan″u-la'shun) introduction of a cannula into a tubelike organ or body cavity.

canola oil (kah-no'lah) RAPESEED OIL that has been specifically prepared from plants bred to be low in ERUCIC ACID.

cantharidin (kan-thar'ĭ-din) the most active principle of cantharides, the dried Spanish fly, *Lytta vesicatoria;* preparations containing cantharidin are used topically as a vesicant to remove warts and lesions of molluscum contagiosum.

canthectomy (kan-thek'to-me) excision of a canthus.

canthitis (kan-thi'tis) inflammation of a canthus.

cantholysis (kan-thol'ĭ-sis) surgical section of a canthus or a canthal ligament.

canthoplasty (kan'tho-plas″te) plastic surgery of a canthus.

canthorrhaphy (kan-thor'ah-fe) the suturing of the palpebral fissure at either canthus.

canthotomy (kan-thot'ah-me) incision of a canthus.

canthus (kan'thus), pl. *can'thi* [L.] the angular junction of the eyelids at either corner of the eyes. adj., **can'thal.**

canting (kant'ing) the process for manufacturing x-ray grids, resulting in grid lines that are uniform and bilateral.

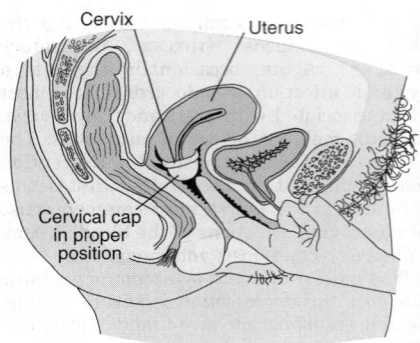

The cervical cap is inserted much like the diaphragm. The woman should check to be certain that it is placed over the cervix. From McKinney et al., 2000.

cap (kap) 1. a covering. 2. a maximum budgetary limit.

cervical c. a contraceptive device similar to the DIAPHRAGM but much smaller, consisting of a cup that fits directly over the cervix. It is only 60 per cent effective for women who have already given birth. (See accompanying illustration.)

cradle c. an oily yellowish crust that sometimes appears on the scalp of an infant, caused by excessive secretion by the sebaceous glands in the scalp. Treatment of mild cases consists of daily shampoo with mild soap. It can be loosened with an application of mineral oil or baby oil prior to shampooing. Called also milk crust and crusta lactea.

capacitance (C) (kah-pas″ĭ-tans) 1. the property of being able to store an electric charge. 2. the ratio of the charge stored by a capacitor to the voltage across the capacitor.

capacitation (kah-pas″ĭta'shun) the process by which the glycoprotein coat and the seminal proteins are removed from the surface of the sperm's ACROSOME by substances secreted by the uterus or fallopian tubes of the female genital tract, thereby permitting the acrosome REACTION to occur.

capacitor (kah-pas'ĭ-ter) a device for holding and storing charges of electricity, made of two conductors separated by insulating material. Called also condenser.

capacity (kah-pas'ĭ-te) the power to hold, retain, or contain, or the ability to absorb; usually expressed numerically as the measure of such ability.

closing c. (CC) the volume of gas in the lungs at the time of airway closure, the sum of the closing volume and the residual volume. See also CLOSING VOLUME.

decreased intracranial adaptive c. a NURSING DIAGNOSIS accepted by the North American Nursing Diagnosis Association, defined as the state in which intracranial fluid dynamic mechanisms that normally compensate for increases in intracranial volumes are compromised, resulting in repeated disproportionate increases in INTRACRANIAL PRESSURE in response to a variety of noxious and nonnoxious stimuli.

diffusing c. see DIFFUSING CAPACITY.

forced vital c. the maximal volume of gas that can be exhaled from full inhalation by exhaling as forcefully and rapidly as possible. See also PULMONARY FUNCTION TESTS.

functional residual c. the amount of gas remaining at the end of normal quiet respiration.

heat c. the amount of heat required to raise the temperature of a specific quantity of a substance by one degree Celsius.

inspiratory c. the volume of gas that can be taken into the lungs in a full inhalation, starting from the resting inspiratory position; equal to the tidal volume plus the inspiratory reserve volume.

maximal breathing c. maximum voluntary ventilation.

thermal c. heat capacity.

total lung c. the amount of gas contained in the lung at the end of a maximal inhalation. (See accompanying illustration.)

virus neutralizing c. the ability of a serum to inhibit the infectivity of a virus.

vital c. (VC) see VITAL CAPACITY.

capecitabine (kap″ĕ-si′tah-bēn) an oral ANTIMETABOLITE used in treatment of metastatic breast or colorectal carcinoma; administered orally.

CAPD continuous ambulatory peritoneal dialysis.

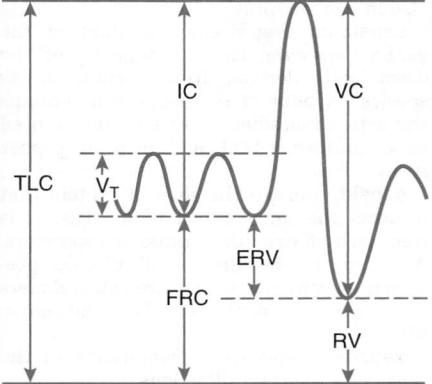

Subdivisions of total lung capacity: TLC, total lung capacity; V, tidal volume; IC, inspiratory capacity; FRC, functional residual capacity; ERV, expiratory reserve volume; VC, vital capacity; RV, residual volume. From Dorland's, 2000.

capillarectasia (kap″ĭ-lar″ek-ta′zhah) dilatation of capillaries.

Capillaria (kap″ĭ-lar′e-ah) a genus of parasitic nematodes. *C. hepa′tica* parasitizes the liver of various mammals, including humans. *C. philippinen′sis* is the most common cause of CAPILLARIASIS.

capillariasis (kap″ĭ-lah-ri′ah-sis) infection with nematodes of the genus *Capillaria*, especially *C. philippinensis*. Symptoms include severe diarrhea and malabsorption that can be fatal.

capillaritis (kap″ĭ-lar-i′tis) inflammation of the capillaries.

capillarity (kap″ĭ-lar′ĭ-te) the action by which the surface of a liquid where it is in contact with a solid, as in a capillary tube, is elevated or depressed.

capillary (kap′ĭ-lar″e) 1. pertaining to or resembling a hair. 2. in the CIRCULATORY SYSTEM, one of the minute vessels connecting arterioles and venules, the walls of which act as a semipermeable membrane for interchange of various substances between the blood and tissue fluid. Capillary walls consist of thin endothelial cells through which body fluids and dissolved substances can pass. At the arterial end, the blood pressure within the capillary is higher than the pressure in the surrounding tissues, and the blood fluid and some dissolved substances pass outward through the capillary wall. At the venous end, the pressure within the tissues is higher and waste material and fluids from the tissues pass into the capillary, to be carried away for disposal.

arterial c. a vessel lacking complete coats, intermediate between an arteriole and a capillary. Called also precapillary.

venous c. a type of minute vessel that lacks a muscular coat and is intermediate between a venule and a capillary. Called also postcapillary.

capillus (kah-pil′us), pl. *capil′li* [L.] a hair; used in the plural to designate the aggregate of hair on the scalp.

capitation (kap″ĭ-ta′shun) the annual fee paid to a health care practice by each participant in a health plan.

capitular (kah-pit′u-ler) pertaining to a capitulum or the head of a bone.

capitulum (kah-pit′u-lum), pl. *capi′tula* [L.] a small eminence on a bone, as on the distal end of the humerus, by which it articulates with another bone.

Capnocytophaga (kap″no-si-tof′ah-gah) a genus of anaerobic, gram-negative, rod-shaped bacteria that have been implicated in the pathogenesis of periodontal disease; they closely resemble *Bacteroides ochraceus*.

capnogram (kap′no-gram″) a graphic representation of inhaled and exhaled carbon dioxide concentrations in the form of continuous waves. (See accompanying illustration.)

capnography (kap-nog′grah-fe) the measurement of inhaled and exhaled carbon dioxide concentrations, as recorded on a capnogram.

capnometer (kap-nom′ĕ-ter) a device for measuring the end-tidal partial pressure of carbon dioxide.

capnometry (kap-nom′ĕ-tre) the determination of the end-tidal partial pressure of carbon dioxide.

capotement (kah-pōt-maw′) [Fr.] a splashing sound heard in dilatation of the stomach.

Capoten (kap′o-ten) trademark for a preparation of CAPTOPRIL, an ANTIHYPERTENSIVE AGENT.

capping (kap′ing) 1. the provision of a protective or obstructive covering. 2. the movement of cell surface antigens into a small region (cap) on the cell surface owing to the cross-linking of antigens by specific

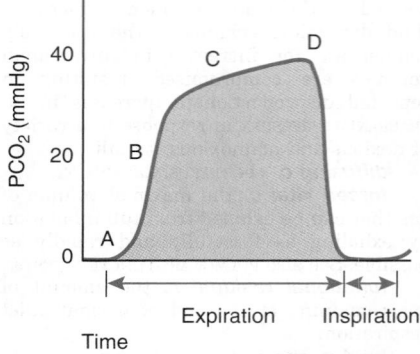

Normal capnogram. *A*, Carbon dioxide cleared from the anatomic dead space; *B*, dead space and alveolar carbon dioxide; *C*, alveolar plateau; *D*, end-tidal carbon dioxide tension ($P_{ET}CO_2$). From Dorland's, 2000.

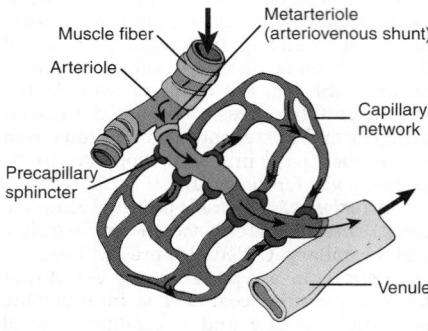

Precapillary sphincters open

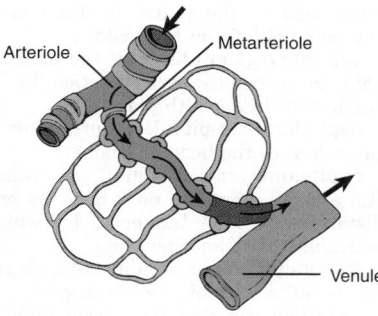

Sphincters closed–blood shunted to venule

Capillary. From Applegate, 2000.

antibody. 3. the covering of tooth cusps weakened by caries with a protective metal overlay. 4. colloquial term for replacement of the crown of a natural tooth with an artificial crown (cap).

pulp c. the covering of an exposed dental pulp with some material to provide protection against external influences and to encourage healing.

capreomycin (kap″re-o-mi′sin) a polypeptide antibiotic produced by *Streptomyces capreolus*, which is active against human strains of *Mycobacterium tuberculosis*; used as the disulfate salt.

capsaicin (cap-sa′ĭ-sin) a plant alkaloid irritating to the skin, the active ingredient of capsicum; used in a cream that is a counterirritant and topical analgesic, and also in pepper spray.

capsicum (kap′sĭ-kum) a plant of the genus *Capsicum*, the hot peppers, or the dried fruit derived from certain of its species (cayenne or red pepper); it contains the active ingredient CAPSAICIN and is used as a counterirritant and also in pepper spray.

capsid (kap′sid) the shell of protein that protects the nucleic acid of a virus; it is composed of structural units, or capsomers. According to the number of subunits possessed by capsomers, they are called dimers (2), trimers (3), pentamers (5), or hexamers (6).

capsitis (kap-si′tis) inflammation of the capsule of the crystalline lens.

capsomer (kap′so-mer) **capsomere** (kap′-so-mēr) a morphological unit of the capsid of a virus.

capsula (kap′su-lah), pl. *cap′sulae* [L.] capsule.

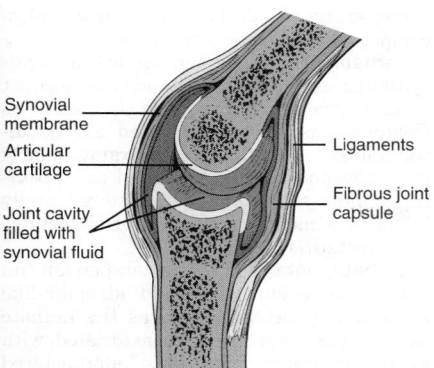

Capsule. Generalized structure of a synovial joint showing the joint or articular capsule. From Applegate, 2000.

capsulation (kap″su-la′shun) enclosure in a capsule.

capsule (kap′sul, kap′sūl) 1. an enclosing structure, as a soluble container enclosing a dose of medicine. 2. a cartilaginous, fatty, fibrous, or membranous structure enveloping another structure, organ, or part. adj., **cap′sular.**

articular c. the saclike envelope that encloses the cavity of a synovial joint by attaching to the circumference of the articular end of each involved bone. Called also joint capsule.

adipose renal c. the investment of fat surrounding the fibrous renal CAPSULE, continuous at the hilus with the fat in the renal sinus.

bacterial c. a gelatinous envelope surrounding a bacterial cell, usually polysaccharide but sometimes polypeptide in nature; it is associated with the virulence of pathogenic bacteria.

Bowman's c. the globular dilatation forming the beginning of a renal TUBULE and surrounding the GLOMERULUS. Called also glomerular capsule and malpighian capsule.

c's of the brain two layers of white matter in the substance of the brain; external capsule and internal capsule.

external c. the layer of white fibers between the putamen and claustrum.

fibrous renal c. the connective tissue investment of the kidney, which continues through the hilus to line the renal sinus.

Glisson's c. a sheath of connective tissue accompanying the hepatic ducts and vessels through the hepatic portal. In HEPATITIS it may become stretched, which is a common cause of pain.

glomerular c. Bowman's capsule.

c. of heart pericardium.

internal c. the fanlike mass of white fibers separating the lentiform nucleus laterally from the head of the caudate nucleus, the dorsal thalamus, and the tail of the caudate nucleus medially. The internal capsule carries both afferent and efferent fibers of the cerebral cortex.

joint c. articular capsule.

c. of lens the elastic sac enclosing the lens of the eye.

malpighian c. Bowman's capsule.

c. of pancreas a thin sheath of areolar tissue that invests the pancreas (but does not form a definite capsule), the septa of which extend into the gland and divide it into lobules.

renal c's the investing tissue around the kidney, divided into the fibrous renal CAPSULE and the adipose renal CAPSULE.

Tenon's c. the connective tissue enveloping the posterior eyeball.

capsulectomy (kap″su-lek′to-me) surgical excision of a capsule, such as a joint capsule or lens capsule; called also decapsulation.

capsulitis (kap″su-li′tis) inflammation of a capsule, such as that of the lens or joint.

adhesive c. adhesive inflammation between the joint capsule and the peripheral articular cartilage of the shoulder, with obliteration of the subdeltoid bursa; it is characterized by increasing pain, stiffness, and limitation of motion. There are three stages to the condition: the *painful stage* (3 to 8 months long); the *adhesive stage* (4 to 6 months long); and the *recovery stage* (1 to 3 months long). Sometimes popularly called by the misleading term frozen shoulder.

capsulolenticular (kap″su-lo-len-tik′u-ler) pertaining to the lens of the eye and its capsule.

capsuloplasty (kap′su-lo-plas″te) plastic repair of a joint capsule.

capsulorrhaphy (kap″su-lor′ah-fe) suture of a joint capsule.

capsulotomy (kap″su-lot′ah-me) incision of a capsule, as that of the lens, the kidney, or a joint.

captopril (kap′to-pril) an ANGIOTENSIN-CONVERTING ENZYME INHIBITOR used, usually with a diuretic, for treatment of HYPERTENSION or congestive HEART FAILURE in patients who have failed to respond to or developed unacceptable side effects with multiple drug regimens that usually include an ADRENERGIC BLOCKING AGENT, DIURETIC, and VASODILATOR. The most serious adverse reactions associated with its use include proteinuria, neutropenia, and agranulocytosis.

capture (kap′choor) 1. the production of a ventricular COMPLEX from a supraventricular source following a period of atrioventricular DISSOCIATION. 2. in cardiac PACING terminology, the successful pacing of the heart by a pulse GENERATOR.

caput (kap′ut), pl. *cap′ita* [L.] head. anatomical terminology for the expanded or chief extremity of an organ or part.

   c. medu′sae the dilated cutaneous veins around the umbilicus, seen mainly in the newborn and in patients suffering from cirrhosis of the liver.

   c. succeda′neum localized edema, congestion, and petechiae on the fetal and newborn scalp (presenting part), crossing the suture lines.

Carafate (kār′ah-fāt) trademark for preparations of SUCRALFATE, used as an ANTIULCERATIVE.

caramiphen (kah-ram′ĭ-fen) an anticholinergic AGENT with actions similar to but weaker than those of ATROPINE; the edisylate ester is administered orally as an ANTITUSSIVE and the hydrochloride ester is administered orally in treatment of PARKINSON'S DISEASE.

carbacephem (kahr″bah-sef′em) any of a class of ANTIBIOTICS closely related to the CEPHALOSPORINS in structure, antimicrobial activity, and use, but chemically more stable.

carbachol (kahr′bah-kol) a CHOLINERGIC agonist that is not hydrolyzed by acetylcholinesterase or pseudocholinesterase; it is used as a MIOTIC and to lower intraocular pressure in treatment of GLAUCOMA and after cataract surgery.

carbamazepine (kahr″bah-maz′ĕ-pēn) an ANTICONVULSANT and ANALGESIC used in the treatment of pain associated with trigeminal NEURALGIA and for control of complex partial SEIZURES or generalized tonic-clonic SEIZURES in patients who do not respond to PHENYTOIN, PHENOBARBITAL, or PRIMIDONE.

carbamide (kahr-bam′īd) urea.

   c. peroxide a compound of urea and hydrogen peroxide used as a cerumen-softening agent, dental cleanser, bleaching agent, and antiinflammatory.

carbaminohemoglobin (kahr-bam″ĭ-no-he′mo-glo″bin) a combination of carbon dioxide and hemoglobin, CO_2 HHb, being one of the forms in which carbon dioxide exists in the blood.

carbamoyl (kahr′bah-moil) the radical NH_2CO-.

carbamoyltransferase (kahr″bah-moil-trans′fer-ās) an enzyme that catalyzes the transfer of carbamoyl, as from carbamoyl-phosphate to L-ornithine to form orthophosphate and citrulline in the synthesis of UREA.

carbarsone (kahr′bahr-sōn) an arsenical compound used as an ANTIAMEBIC.

carbenicillin (kahr″ben-ĭ-sil′in) a semisynthetic PENICILLIN, with activity against certain gram-negative bacteria, such as *Pseudomonas aeruginosa;* used as the disodium salt, administered intramuscularly or intravenously. It is also used as *carbenicillin indanyl sodium,* administered orally in the treatment of urinary tract infections and prostatitis.

carbetapentane (kahr-ba″tah-pen′tān) an antitussive agent with mild atropine-like antisecretory activity; used as the tannate salt in treatment of cough associated with upper respiratory infections, administered orally.

carbidopa (kahr-bĭ-do′pah) an inhibitor of the decarboxylation of LEVODOPA in peripheral tissues; it does not cross the blood-brain barrier and is used in combination with levodopa to control the symptoms of PARKINSON'S DISEASE. In the presence of carbidopa, levodopa enters the brain in larger quantities, thus avoiding the need for excessively high doses of levodopa.

carbinoxamine (kahr″bĭ-nok′sah-mēn) an ANTIHISTAMINE with sedative and anticholinergic effects; used as the maleate salt in the treatment of nasal, eye, and skin manifestations of allergic reactions, including allergic rhinitis, conjunctivitis, and itching, and also as an ingredient in some cough and cold preparations, administered orally.

Carbocaine (kahr′bo-kān) trademark for preparations of MEPIVACAINE hydrochloride, a local ANESTHETIC.

carbohydrase (kahr″bo-hi′drās) any of a group of enzymes such as AMYLASE that catalyze the hydrolysis of higher carbohydrates to lower forms.

carbohydrate (kahr″bo-hi′drāt) a compound of carbon, hydrogen, and oxygen, the latter two usually in the proportions of water $(CH_2O)_n$. They are classified into mono-, di-, tri-, poly-, and heterosaccharides. Carbohydrates in food are an important and immediate source of energy for the body; 1 g of carbohydrate yields 4 calories. They are present, at least in small quantities, in most foods, but the chief sources are the SUGARS and STARCHES. Food substances that are almost pure sugar include granulated sugar, maple sugar, honey, and molasses. The MONOSACCHARIDES (simple sugars) include GLUCOSE and FRUCTOSE. GALACTOSE, another simple sugar, is produced by the digestion or hydrolysis of lactose. The DISACCHARIDES (double sugars) include SUCROSE (white sugar, found in sugar cane or sugar beets), MALTOSE, and LACTOSE. All ripe fruits and many vegetables contain natural sugars. The starches are present in such foods as rice, wheat, and potatoes. Carbohydrates may be stored in the body as glycogen for future use. If they are eaten in excessive amounts, however, the body changes them into fats and stores them in that form.

carbohydraturia (kahr″bo-hi″drah-tu′re-ah) excess of carbohydrates in the urine, such as in fructosuria, galactosuria, glycosuria, lactosuria, or pentosuria.

carbolic acid (kar-bol′ik) phenol (def. 1).

carbolism (kahr′bo-lizm) PHENOL (carbolic acid) poisoning.

carbon (C) (kahr′bon) a chemical element, atomic number 6, atomic weight 12.011. (See Appendix 6.)

c. 11 a radioactive isotope of carbon, atomic mass 11, having a half-life of 20.39 minutes; used as a TRACER in positron emission TOMOGRAPHY.

c. 14 a radioactive isotope of carbon, atomic mass 14, having a half-life of 5730 years; used as a TRACER in cancer and metabolic research.

carbonate (kahr′bon-āt) a salt of carbonic acid.

carbon dioxide an odorless, colorless gas, CO_2, resulting from oxidation of carbon, formed in the tissues and eliminated by the lungs; used in some pump oxygenators to maintain the carbon dioxide tension in the blood. It is also used in solid form; see carbon dioxide snow and carbon dioxide slush.

c. d. combining power the ability of blood plasma to combine with carbon dioxide; indicative of the alkali reserve and a measure of the acid-base balance of the blood.

c. d. content the amount of carbonic acid and bicarbonate in the blood; reported in millimoles per liter.

c. d.–oxygen therapy administration of a mixture of carbon dioxide and oxygen (commonly 5 per cent CO_2 and 95 per cent O_2 or 10 per cent CO_2 and 90 per cent O_2); used for improvement of cerebral blood flow, stimulation of deep breathing, and treatment of singultation (hiccupping). Carbon dioxide acts by stimulating the respiratory center; it also increases heart rate and blood pressure. Therapy is given for 6 minutes or less with a 5 per cent mixture and 2 minutes or less with a 10 per cent mixture. Potential adverse effects include headache, dizziness, dyspnea, nausea, tachycardia and high blood pressure, blurred vision, mental depression, coma, and convulsions.

c. d. slush solid carbon dioxide combined with a solvent such as acetone, and

sometimes also alcohol; used as an escharotic to treat skin lesions such as warts and moles and as a peeling agent in chemabrasion.

c. d. snow the solid formed by rapid evaporation of liquid CARBON DIOXIDE, giving a temperature of about $-79°C$ ($-110°F$). It has been used in cryotherapy to freeze the skin, thus producing local anesthesia and arrest of blood flow. See also carbon dioxide slush.

carbonic acid (kahr-bon′ik) aqueous solution of carbon dioxide, H_2CO_3.

c. a. anhydrase carbonic ANHYDRASE.

carbon monoxide a colorless, odorless, tasteless gas, CO, formed by burning carbon or organic fuels with a scanty supply of oxygen; it is the number one cause of unintentional poisoning around the world (see CARBON MONOXIDE POISONING). Inhalation causes central nervous system damage and asphyxiation. Carbon monoxide is present in the exhaust of gasoline engines, in the smoke of wood and coal fires, in manufactured gas such as that used in the household, and wherever carbon burns without a sufficient supply of oxygen.

c. m. poisoning poisoning by CARBON MONOXIDE, the most common type of gas poisoning around the world. When the gas is inhaled and comes in contact with the blood, it combines more readily with HEMOGLOBIN than OXYGEN does. Thus it takes the place of oxygen in the ERYTHROCYTES, and the tissues are deprived of their normal oxygen supply. The symptoms of carbon monoxide poisoning begin with dizziness, headache, weakness, shortness of breath, and sometimes nausea; the skin and mucous membranes become cherry red in color. Unconsciousness follows, with death from ASPHYXIA if a large enough quantity is inhaled.

Treatment. The victim of acute carbon monoxide poisoning should be moved immediately to an open area with fresh air. Administration of 100 per cent oxygen or hyperbaric OXYGEN via face mask may be indicated.

Prevention. Cases of carbon monoxide poisoning are usually accidental. It should be remembered that carbon monoxide has no odor and its presence may not be detected unless other gases, such as exhaust fumes from an automobile motor, are also escaping. Care should be taken to ensure proper ventilation of working and sleeping areas. It is extremely dangerous to leave an automobile motor running in a closed garage. Stoves and furnaces should be kept in good repair. Burners using gas, especially in a bedroom, should have a ventilator pipe to carry the exhaust to the outside.

carbon tetrachloride a clear, colorless, mobile liquid used as a solvent. The most common route of poisoning is by inhalation of its vapors; it can also be absorbed through the skin. Toxicity results from depression of central nervous system activity and degeneration of the liver and kidneys. Signs of acute poisoning include nausea, vomiting, diarrhea, headache, and in severe cases anuria that can be fatal. Since the toxic concentrations are below the odor threshold, carbon tetrachloride should always be used in a well-ventilated area.

carbonyl (kahr′bo-nil) the divalent organic radical, C=O, characteristic of aldehydes, ketones, carboxylic acid, and esters.

carboplatin (kahr″bo-plat′in) a PLATINUM coordination compound that interferes with functioning of cellular DNA; used as an antineoplastic AGENT to treat cancers of the ovary, lung, head and neck, testes, bladder, brain, and other organs.

carboprost a synthetic analogue of DINO-PROST, used as an OXYTOCIC for termination of pregnancy and missed abortion, administered intramuscularly.

carboxyhemoglobin (kahr-bok″se-he′mo-glo″bin) hemoglobin in which the sites usually bound to oxygen are bound to carbon monoxide molecules; carbon monoxide has an affinity for hemoglobin over 200 times that of oxygen. See CARBON MONOXIDE POISONING.

carboxyl (kahr-bok′sil) the monovalent radical, —COOH, found in those organic acids termed carboxylic acids.

carboxylase (kahr-bok′sĭ-lās) an enzyme that catalyzes the removal of carbon dioxide from the carboxyl group of alpha amino keto acids.

carboxylation (kahr-bok″sil-a′shun) the addition of a carboxyl group, as to pyruvate to form oxaloacetate.

carboxylesterase (kahr-bok″sil-es′ter-ās) an enzyme that catalyzes the hydrolysis of the esters of carboxylic acids.

carboxylic acid (kahr-bok-sil′ik) an organic compound containing the carboxy group (—COOH), which is weakly ionized in solution forming a carboxylate ion (—COO⁻).

carboxyltransferase (kahr-bok″sil-trans′-fer-ās) an enzyme that catalyzes carboxylation.

carboxy-lyase (kahr-bok′se-li′ās) any of a group of lyases that catalyze the removal of a carboxyl group; it includes the carboxy-lases and decarboxylases.

carboxymethylcellulose (kahr-bok″se-meth″il-sel′u-lōs) a substituted cellulose polymer of variable size, used as the sodium or calcium salt as a pharmaceutical suspending agent, tablet EXCIPIENT, and viscosity-increasing agent; the sodium salt is also used as a LAXATIVE.

carboxymyoglobin (kahr-bok″se-mi′o-glo″bin) a compound formed from myoglobin on exposure to carbon monoxide.

carboxypeptidase (kahr-bok″se-pep′tĭ-dās) an exopeptidase that acts only on the peptide linkage of a terminal amino acid containing a free carboxyl group.

carbuncle (kahr′bung-k′l) a necrotizing infection of skin and subcutaneous tissue composed of a cluster of BOILS (furuncles), usually due to *Staphylococcus aureus,* with multiple formed or incipient drainage sinuses. They are often a symptom of poor health. adj., **carbunc′ular.** Like boils, carbuncles are caused by pus-forming bacteria. These organisms are often present on the skin but are unable to do any damage unless resistance is lowered by such conditions as irritating friction, cuts, poor health, nutritional deficiency, or diabetes mellitus.

Treatment includes administration of antibiotics and incision and drainage when necessary to remove exudate. Efforts are made to determine the cause of the carbuncles so that it can be eliminated.

malignant c. anthrax.

carbunculoid (kahr-bung′ku-loid) resembling a carbuncle.

carbunculosis (kahr-bung″ku-lo′sis) a condition marked by the formation of numerous carbuncles.

carcinoembryonic (kahr″sī-no-em″bre-on′ik) occurring both in carcinoma and in embryonic tissue, such as carcinoembryonic ANTIGEN.

carcinogen (kahr-sin′o-jen) a substance that causes CANCER. The Environmental Protection Agency of the U.S. Government has three descriptors for classifying human carcinogenic potential: "known/likely," "cannot be determined," and "not likely."

carcinogenesis (kahr″sī-no-jen′ĕ-sis) production of cancer. (See accompanying illustration.)

carcinogenic (kahr″sin-o-jen′ik) 1. pertaining to a CARCINOGEN. 2. causing CANCER.

carcinogenicity (kahr″sī-no-jĕ-nis′ĭ-te) the ability or tendency to produce CANCER; see also CARCINOGEN.

carcinoid (kahr′sī-noid) 1. a yellow circumscribed tumor of the gastrointestinal tract or bronchus formed from chromaffin cells. See also CARCINOID SYNDROME. 2. argentaffinoma.

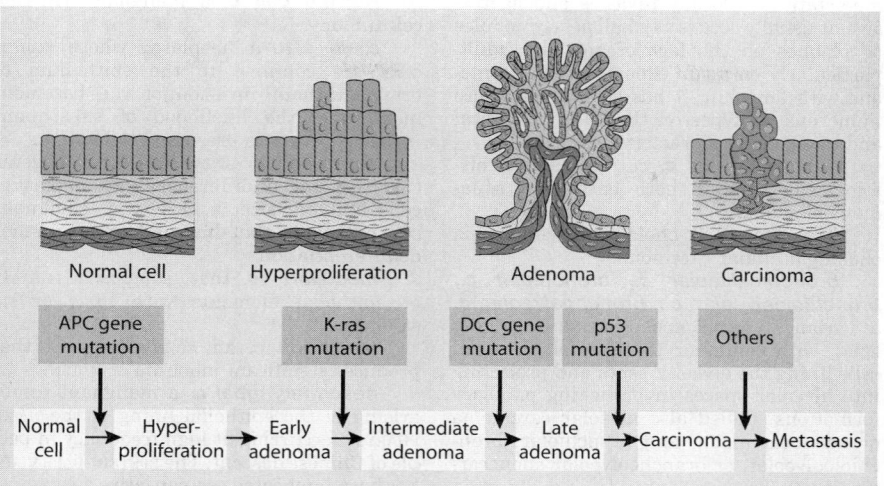

Normal cell	Hyperproliferation	Adenoma	Carcinoma
APC gene mutation	K-ras mutation	DCC gene mutation · p53 mutation	Others

Normal cell → Hyper-proliferation → Early adenoma → Intermediate adenoma → Late adenoma → Carcinoma → Metastasis

Multistep model of carcinogenesis. The stepwise genetic alterations that lead to colorectal cancer. From Aspinall and Taylor-Robinson, 2001.

c. syndrome a symptom complex associated with carcinoid tumors (ARGENTAFFINOMAS), marked by attacks of severe cyanotic flushing of the skin lasting from minutes to days and by watery diarrhea, bronchoconstrictive attacks, sudden drops in blood pressure, edema, and ascites. Symptoms are caused by SEROTONIN, PROSTAGLANDINS, and other biologically active substances secreted by the tumor.

The specific symptoms associated with this disorder depend upon the site of the primary tumor; tumors are found most commonly in the appendix and the terminal third of the ileum but can also be in the bronchi, ovaries, testes, and anywhere along the entire length of the alimentary tract. The full set of carcinoid symptoms are manifested only when the liver is involved.

Diagnosis of the condition is established by a 24-hour urine test for 5-HYDROXYINDOLE-ACETIC ACID (5-HIAA), the end product of the breakdown of TRYPTOPHAN to SEROTONIN. Patients with carcinoid syndrome may have very high levels of 5-HIAA, 100 to 500 mg in 24 hours.

Carcinoid tumors are not always benign and should be approached as if they were malignant growths. Surgical excision of the tumor and any associated mesenteric nodes is the treatment of choice. Chemotherapy can be used with metastatic disease, and other drugs are prescribed as indicated to manage the hypotension, diarrhea, flushing, and other symptoms. Efforts are made to improve nutrition and to avoid serotonin-containing foods, such as walnuts and bananas, which are known to precipitate an attack and make accurate diagnosis difficult.

carcinolysis (kahr″sĭ-nol-ĭ-sis) destruction of cancer cells. adj., **carcinolyt′ic.**

carcinoma (kahr″sĭ-no′mah), pl. *carcinomas, carcino′mata* a malignant new growth made up of epithelial cells tending to infiltrate surrounding tissues and to give rise to metastases. A form of CANCER, carcinoma makes up the majority of the cases of malignancy of the breast, uterus, intestinal tract, skin, and tongue.

adenocystic c., adenoid cystic c. carcinoma marked by cylinders or bands of hyaline or mucinous stroma separated or surrounded by nests or cords of small epithelial cells, occurring in the mammary and salivary glands, and mucous glands of the respiratory tract. Called also cylindroma.

alveolar c. bronchioloalveolar carcinoma.

basal cell c. the most common form of skin cancer, consisting of an epithelial tumor of the skin originating from neoplastic differentiation of basal CELLS, rarely metastatic but locally invasive and aggressive. It usually occurs as small pearly nodules or plaques on the face of an older adult, particularly on a sun-exposed area of someone with fair skin. It has been divided into numerous subtypes on the basis of clinical and histological characteristics.

basosquamous c. carcinoma that histologically exhibits both basal and squamous elements.

bile duct c. 1. cholangiocarcinoma. 2. cholangiocellular carcinoma.

bronchioalveolar c., bronchiolar c., bronchioloalveolar c., bronchoalveolar c. a variant type of ADENOCARCINOMA OF THE LUNG, with columnar to cuboidal epithelial cells lining the alveolar septa and projecting into alveolar spaces in branching papillary formations. Called also alveolar carcinoma or adenocarcinoma and bronchiolar, bronchioloalveolar, or bronchoalveolar adenocarcinoma.

bronchogenic c. any of a large group of carcinomas of the lung, so called because they arise from the epithelium of the bronchial tree. Four primary subtypes are distinguished: ADENOCARCINOMA OF THE LUNG, large cell CARCINOMA, small cell CARCINOMA, and squamous cell CARCINOMA.

cholangiocellular c. a rare type of hepatocellular CARCINOMA arising from the CHOLANGIOLES, consisting of two layers of cells surrounding a minute lumen. Called also bile duct carcinoma and cholangiocarcinoma.

chorionic c. choriocarcinoma.

clear cell c. 1. clear cell adenocarcinoma. 2. renal cell carcinoma.

colloid c. mucinous carcinoma.

cylindrical cell c. carcinoma in which the cells are cylindrical or nearly so.

embryonal c. a highly malignant germ cell TUMOR that is a primitive form of carcinoma, probably of primitive embryonal cell derivation; it usually arises in a GONAD and may be found either in pure form or as part of a mixed germ cell tumor.

epidermoid c. squamous cell carcinoma.

giant cell c. a poorly differentiated, highly malignant, epithelial neoplasm containing many large multinucleated tumor cells, such as occurs in the lungs.

hepatocellular c. primary carcinoma of the liver cells with hepatomegaly, jaundice, hemoperitoneum, and other symptoms of the presence of an abdominal mass. It is rare in North America and Western Europe but is one of the most common malignancies in parts of sub-Saharan Africa, Southeast Asia, East Asia, and elsewhere. A strong association seems to exist with chronic hepatitis B VIRUS infection.

Hürthle cell c. a malignant Hürthle cell tumor.

c. in si′tu a neoplasm whose tumor cells are confined to the epithelium of origin, without invasion of the basement membrane; the likelihood of subsequent invasive growth is presumed to be high.

large cell c. a type of bronchogenic CARCINOMA of undifferentiated (anaplastic) cells of large size, a variety of squamous cell CARCINOMA that has undergone further dedifferentiation.

medullary c. that composed mainly of epithelial elements with little or no stroma.

mucinous c. an ADENOCARCINOMA that produces significant amounts of MUCIN.

nasopharyngeal c. a malignant tumor arising in the epithelial lining of the NASOPHARYNX, occurring at high frequency in people of Chinese descent. The EPSTEIN-BARR VIRUS has been implicated as a causative agent.

non–small cell c. a general term comprising all lung carcinomas except small cell carcinoma, and including adenocarcinoma of the lung, large cell carcinoma, and squamous cell carcinoma.

oat cell c. a form of small cell CARCINOMA in which the cells are round or elongated and slightly larger than lymphocytes; they have scanty cytoplasm and clump poorly.

papillary c. carcinoma in which there are papillary growths that are irregular in nature arising from otherwise normal tissue; it can occur in the thyroid gland, the breast, or the bladder. Called also papillocarcinoma.

renal cell c. carcinoma of the renal PARENCHYMA, composed of tubular cells in varying arrangements; called also clear cell carcinoma.

scirrhous c. carcinoma with a hard structure owing to the formation of dense connective tissue in the stroma. Called also fibrocarcinoma.

c. sim′plex an undifferentiated carcinoma.

small cell c. a common, highly malignant form of bronchogenic CARCINOMA in the wall of a major bronchus, occurring mainly in middle-aged individuals with a history of tobacco smoking; it is radiosensitive and has small oval undifferentiated cells. Metastasis to the hilum and to mediastinal lymph nodes is common.

spindle cell c. squamous cell CARCINOMA marked by development of rapidly proliferating spindle CELLS.

squamous cell c. 1. carcinoma developed from squamous EPITHELIUM, having

TION. Initially local and superficial, the lesion may later invade and metastasize. 2. the form occurring in the skin, usually originating in sun-damaged areas or preexisting lesions. 3. in the lung, one of the most common types of bronchogenic CARCINOMA, generally forming polypoid or sessile masses that obstruct the airways of the bronchi. It usually occurs in middle-aged individuals with a history of smoking. There is frequent invasion of blood and lymphatic vessels with metastasis to regional lymph nodes and other sites. Called also epidermoid carcinoma.

transitional cell c. a malignant tumor arising from a transitional type of stratified epithelium, usually affecting the urinary bladder.

verrucous c. 1. a variety of squamous cell carcinoma that has a predilection for the buccal mucosa but also affects other oral soft tissue and the larynx. It is slow-growing and somewhat invasive. 2. Buschke-Löwenstein tumor, so called because it is histologically similar to the oral lesion.

carcinomatosis (kahr″sĭ-no″mah-to′sis) the condition of widespread dissemination of cancer throughout the body.

carcinomatous (kahr″sĭ-no′mah-tus) pertaining to or of the nature of cancer; malignant.

carcinophilia (kahr″sĭ-no-fil′e-ah) special affinity for cancerous tissue. adj., **carcinophil′ic.**

carcinophobia (kahr″sĭ-no-fo′be-ah) cancerphobia.

carcinosarcoma (kahr″sĭ-no-sahr-ko′-mah) a malignant tumor composed of carcinomatous and sarcomatous tissues.

embryonal c. Wilms' tumor.

carcinosis (kahr″sĭ-no′sis) carcinomatosis.

miliary c. that marked by development of numerous nodules resembling miliary tuberculosis.

Cardarelli's sign (kar-dar-el′ēz) transverse pulsation of the laryngotracheal tube in aneurysms and in dilatation of the arch of the aorta.

cardi(o)- word element [Gr.], *heart.*

cardia (kahr′de-ah) 1. the cardiac opening. 2. the cardiac part of the stomach; that part of the stomach surrounding the esophagogastric junction, distinguished by the presence of cardiac glands.

cardiac (kahr′de-ak) 1. pertaining to the HEART. 2. pertaining to the OSTIUM CARDIACUM.

c. arrest sudden and often unexpected stoppage of effective heart action. Either the periodic impulses that trigger the coordinated heart muscle contractions cease or ventricular FIBRILLATION or FLUTTER occurs in which the individual muscle fibers have

a rapid irregular twitching. The majority of victims of cardiac arrest suffer from ventricular fibrillation, and most have severe coronary artery disease. The only chance for survival for many who have unexpected cardiac arrest is successful implementation of emergency cardiac care and CARDIOPULMONARY RESUSCITATION (CPR). Reduction of the incidence of cardiac arrest and sudden death is a major concern of the American Heart Association and the American Red Cross.

Programs aimed at achieving the goal of reduced mortality from cardiac arrest include education of the general public in ways to avoid the development of coronary artery disease in the first place, and secondarily, training lay people and health care professionals and paraprofessionals in the techniques of CPR and emergency cardiac care.

Although cardiac arrest usually is related to preexisting coronary artery disease, there are other events in which the prompt delivery of CPR alone could mean survival for the victim. These include the cessation of heart and lung action as a result of drowning, suffocation, electrocution, drug overdose, and severe accidental trauma.

c. catheterization the insertion of a catheter into a vein or artery and guiding of it into the interior of the heart for purposes of measuring cardiac output, determining the oxygen content of blood in the heart chambers, and evaluating the structural components of the heart. It is indicated whenever it is necessary to establish a precise and definite diagnosis in order to determine whether heart surgery is necessary and to plan the surgical approach.

Patient Care. Patients scheduled for cardiac catheterization experience a high level of stress. They are fearful and anxious because the procedure involves the heart, has a potential for some rather serious complications, and could indicate a need for cardiac surgery. Prior to the catheterization the patient will need to know that it is not a surgical procedure, even though a consent form must be signed, food and fluids are restricted, and a surgical preparation of the catheter insertion site is done. The patient should be told of these and other preparations as well as the physical features of the laboratory in which the catheterization is to be done.

During the initial assessment it is important to find out whether the patient has any allergies. The contrast medium used contains iodide salts; if a patient is allergic to iodine or seafood, a contrast medium that

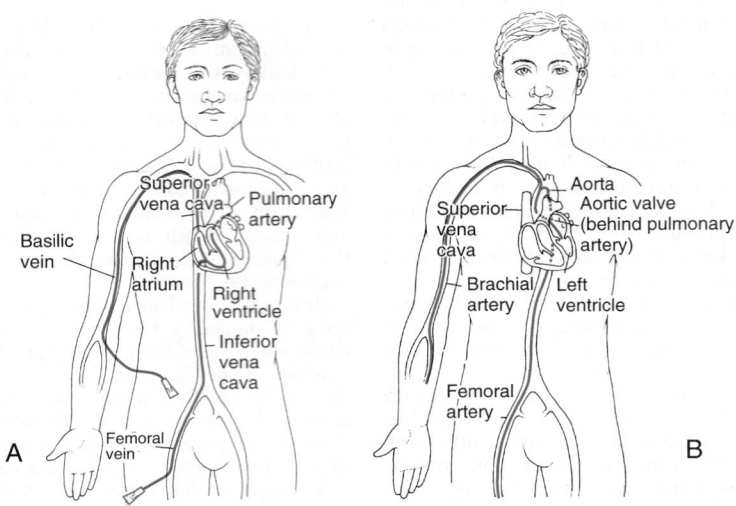

A, Right-sided heart catheterization. The catheter is inserted into the femoral vein and advanced through the inferior vena cava (or, if into an antecubital or basilic vein, through the superior vena cava), right atrium, and right ventricle and into the pulmonary artery. *B,* Left-sided heart catheterization. The catheter is inserted into the femoral artery or the antecubital artery. The catheter is passed through the ascending aorta, through the aortic valve, and into the left ventricle. From Ignatavicius and Workman, 2002.

does not contain iodine must be used, or antihistamines must be administered before the procedure. A mild tranquilizer or hypnotic may be given just before the procedure to help the patient relax, but a general anesthetic is not used. Patients need to know that they must be awake and cooperative during the procedure. They will be asked to stay in a certain position, cough, breathe deeply, and possibly exercise so that the heart's response to an increased workload can be evaluated. They should be reassured that the laboratory staff is ready and equipped to handle any emergency should the need arise.

Ideally, preprocedure visits by the physician and a member of the staff in the cardiac catheterization laboratory will provide patients with the information they need about the procedure, its purpose, and potential complications. However, because of anxiety the patient may not be able to assimilate the information and will have many questions not asked at the time of the visits. It is then the responsibility of the floor nurses to answer questions as honestly as they can and to provide emotional support and reassurance.

After the procedure the vital signs are checked periodically. It is especially important to check the pulses distal to the insertion site every half-hour for three hours, or as often as required by protocol, to be sure

there has been no clotting and obstruction of a blood vessel. The insertion site dressing is changed as needed and the site inspected for signs of infection. Thirst and diuresis are expected because of the effect of the dye used in the procedure. The patient should be encouraged to drink fluids to prevent hypotension and hasten excretion of the dye, which is potentially nephrotoxic. Mild discomfort also is expected and should respond to the prescribed analgesic. If the patient experiences severe pain the physician should be notified.

cardialgia (kahr″de-al′jah) pain in the heart.

cardioaccelerator (kahr″de-o-ak-sel′er-a″ter) quickening the heart action; an agent that so acts.

cardioactive (kahr″de-o-ak′tiv) having an effect on the heart.

cardioangiology (kahr″de-o-an″je-ol′o-je) the medical specialty dealing with the heart and blood vessels.

Cardiobacterium (kahr′de-o-bak-tēr′e-um) a genus of gram-negative, facultatively anaerobic, rod-shaped bacteria that are part of the normal flora of the nose and throat; *C. ho′minis* is a cause of ENDOCARDITIS.

cardiocele (kahr′de-o-sēl″) hernial protrusion of the heart through a fissure of the diaphragm or through a wound.

cardiocentesis (kahr″de-o-sen-te′sis) surgical puncture or incision of the heart.

cardiochalasia (kahr″de-o-kah-la′zhah) relaxation or incompetence of the sphincter action of the cardiac opening of the stomach.

cardiocirculatory (kar″de-o-ser′ku-lah-tor′e) pertaining to blood flow through the heart and vascular system.

cardiocirrhosis (kahr″de-o-sĭ-ro′sis) cardiac CIRRHOSIS.

cardiodiosis (kahr″de-o-di-o′sis) dilatation of the cardiac opening of the stomach.

cardiodynamics (kahr″de-o-di-nam′iks) study of the forces involved in the heart's action.

cardioesophageal (kahr″de-o-ĕ-sof′ah-je′al) pertaining to the cardia of the stomach and the esophagus, as the cardioesophageal junction or sphincter.

cardiogenesis (kahr″de-o-jen′ĕ-sis) development of the heart in the embryo.

cardiogenic (kahr″de-o-jen′ik) originating in the heart.

cardiogram (kahr′de-o-gram″) a tracing of a cardiac event produced by cardiography; see also ELECTROCARDIOGRAM.

cardiograph (kahr′de-o-graf″) an instrument for recording some element of the heart beat.

cardiography (kahr″de-og′rah-fe) the graphic recording of a physical or functional aspect of the heart, such as in ECHOCARDIOGRAPHY, ELECTROCARDIOGRAPHY, KINETO-CARDIOGRAPHY, PHONOCARDIOGRAPHY, and VIBROCARDIOGRAPHY.

   apex c. graphic recording of low-frequency pulsations at the anterior chest wall over the apex of the heart.

   ultrasonic c. echocardiography.

   vector c. vectorcardiography.

Cardio-Green (kahr′de-o-grēn″) trademark for a preparation of INDOCYANINE GREEN, a dye used as a diagnostic aid for determination of blood volume, cardiac output, and hepatic function.

cardiohepatic (kahr″de-o-hĕ-pat′ik) pertaining to the heart and liver.

cardioinhibitor (kahr″de-o-in-hib′ĭ-ter) an agent that restrains the heart's action.

cardioinhibitory (kahr″de-o-in-hib′ĭ-tor-e) restraining or inhibiting the heart movements.

cardiokinetic (kahr″de-o-kĭ-net′ik) 1. exciting or stimulating the heart. 2. an agent that so acts.

cardiokymography (kahr″de-o-ki-mog′-rah-fe) the recording of the motion of the heart by means of the electrokymograph. adj., **cardiokymograph′ic.**

cardiologist (kahr″de-ol′o-jist) a physician skilled in the diagnosis and treatment of heart disease.

cardiology (kar″de-ol′o-je) study of the heart and its functions.

cardiolysis (kahr″de-ol′ĭ-sis) the operation of freeing the heart from its adhesions to the sternal periosteum in adhesive mediastinopericarditis.

cardiomalacia (kahr″de-o-mah-la′shah) morbid softening of the muscular substance of the heart.

cardiomegaly (kahr″de-o-meg′ah-le) abnormal enlargement of the heart from either HYPERTROPHY or DILATATION.

cardiomelanosis (kahr″de-o-mel″ah-no′-sis) melanosis of the heart.

cardiomotility (kahr″de-o-mo-til′ĭ-te) the movement of the heart; motility of the heart.

cardiomyoliposis (kahr″de-o-mi″o-lĭ-po′-sis) fatty degeneration of the heart muscle.

cardiomyopathy (kahr″de-o-mi-op′ah-the) a general diagnostic term designating primary myocardial disease.

   alcoholic c. a congestive cardiomyopathy resulting in cardiac enlargement and low cardiac output occurring in chronic ALCOHOLICS; the heart disease in BERIBERI (thiamine deficiency) is also associated with alcoholism.

   congestive c. a syndrome characterized by cardiac enlargement, especially of the left ventricle, myocardial dysfunction, and congestive HEART FAILURE.

   hypertrophic c. an increase in heart muscle weight, particularly of the left ventricle and often involving the interventricular septum; it may affect the flow of blood from an atrium into the ventricle or out from the ventricle. This type of cardiomyopathy is frequently associated with IDIOPATHIC HYPERTROPHIC SUBAORTIC STENOSIS. Called also asymmetrical septal hypertrophy.

   hypertrophic obstructive c. a form of hypertrophic cardiomyopathy in which the location of the septal hypertrophy causes obstructive interference to left ventricular outflow. See also asymmetrical septal HYPERTROPHY.

   infiltrative c. myocardial disease resulting from deposition in the heart tissue of abnormal substances, as may occur in amyloidosis, hemochromatosis, and other disorders.

   primary c. that in which the basic pathologic process involves the myocardium itself and not other cardiac structures; the condition is of unknown etiology and not part of a disease affecting other organs.

   restrictive c. a form in which the ventricular walls are excessively rigid, impeding ventricular filling; it is marked by abnormal diastolic function but normal or nearly normal systolic function.

secondary c. any form that is due to another cardiovascular disorder or is a manifestation of a systemic disease such as sarcoidosis.

cardionephric (kahr″de-o-nef′rik) cardiorenal.

cardioneural (kahr″de-o-noor′al) pertaining to the heart and nervous system.

cardiopaludism (kahr″de-o-pal′u-dizm) heart disease due to malaria.

cardiopathy (kahr″de-op′ah-the) any disorder or disease of the heart.

cardiopericarditis (kahr″de-o-per″ĭ-kahr-di′tis) inflammation of the heart and pericardium.

cardiophobia (kahr″de-o-fo′be-ah) irrational dread of heart disease.

cardioplasty (kahr′de-o-plas″te) esophagogastroplasty.

cardioplegia (kahr″de-o-ple′jah) arrest of myocardial contraction, as by use of chemical compounds or cold in cardiac surgery. adj., **cardiopleg′ic.**

cardiopneumatic (kahr″de-o-noo-mat′ik) pertaining to the heart and respiration.

cardiopneumograph (kahr″de-o-noo′mo-graf) an apparatus for registering cardiopneumatic movements.

cardioprotectant (kahr″de-o-pro-tek′tant) 1. counteracting CARDIOTOXIC effects. 2. an agent that so acts.

cardioprotective (kahr″de-o-pro-tek′tiv) cardioprotectant.

cardioptosis (kahr″de-o-to′sis) downward displacement of the heart.

cardiopulmonary (kahr″de-o-pul′mo-nar″e) pertaining to the heart and lungs.

c. resuscitation (CPR) the manual application of chest compressions and ventilations to patients in CARDIAC ARREST, done in an effort to maintain viability until advanced help arrives. This procedure is an essential component of basic life support (BLS), basic cardiac life support (BCLS), and advanced cardiac life support (ACLS). The preliminary steps of CPR, as defined by the American Heart Association, are (1) calling for help; (2) establishing unresponsiveness in the victim by tapping or gently shaking and shouting at him or her; (3) positioning the victim in a supine position on a hard surface; (4) giving two breaths; and (5) checking the pulse. These are begun as quickly as possible; prompt action is essential for successful outcome. At the moment breathing and heart action stop, "clinical death" ensues. Within four to six minutes the cells of the brain, which are the most sensitive to lack of oxygen, begin to deteriorate. If breathing and circulation are not restored within this period of time, irreversible brain damage occurs and "biological death" takes place.

Although CPR is strongly recommended as a life-saving measure, it is not without danger; specific risks include rib fracture, damage to the liver or heart, and puncture of lungs or large blood vessels. All health care providers should receive instruction and practice in CPR under the direction of a qualified instructor. The public in general should also be encouraged to learn CPR for use in emergency situations.

Once it has been established that a person is in need of CPR, the rescuer immediately begins the "ABC's" of CPR: Airway, Breathing, and Circulation. Opening the airway and determining by look, sound, and feel is the first step for determining whether the person will be able to resume unassisted breathing. This is accomplished by lifting the chin up and back and bringing the mandible forward. If there is no evidence of spontaneous breathing, the rescuer corrects obstruction of the airway by a foreign body, when this is indicated. This is done by one or more of the following methods: back blows, manual chest thrusts, and finger sweeps. Once the airway is open, rescue breathing is started by means of mouth-to-mouth resuscitation (see ARTIFICIAL RESPIRATION).

The third element of CPR is circulation, which begins by establishing the presence or absence of a pulse. If there is no pulse, compression of the chest is begun. This consists of rhythmic applications of pressure on the lower half of the sternum (NOT on the xiphoid process, which may injure the liver). For a normal-sized adult, sufficient force is used to depress the sternum about 4 to 5 cm ($1\frac{1}{2}$ to 2 in). This raises intrathoracic pressure and produces the output of blood from the heart. When the pressure is released, blood is allowed to flow into the heart. Compressions should be maintained for one-half second; the same length of time is allowed for the relaxation period.

Chest compression is always accompanied by rescue breathing. The two must be coordinated so that there is regular and uninterrupted circulation of blood and aeration of the lungs.

CPR is a psychomotor skill and all health care providers should keep their certification current in order to be proficient in this procedure in case of emergency. The techniques of CPR provide basic life support (BLS) in all cases of respiratory and cardiac arrest. Standards and guidelines for CPR

C

Airway

Breathing

Circulation

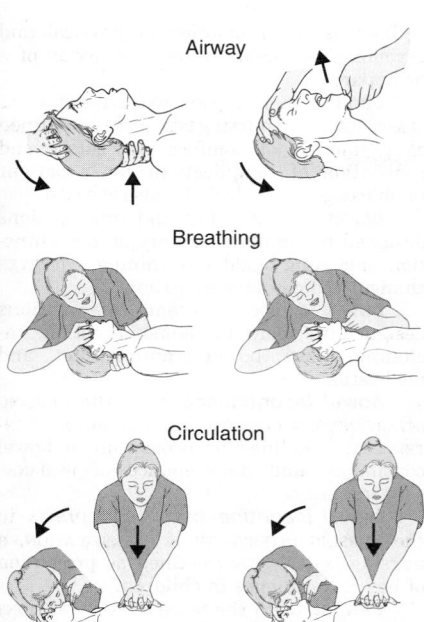

Cardiopulmonary resuscitation. *Airway:* One hand is placed under the neck to extend it. With the other hand the chin is lifted so that it points upward. Sometimes this maneuver clears the airway and is all that is necessary to reinstate spontaneous breathing. *Breathing:* The nostrils are pinched and the chin held in position so that the rescuer's mouth can make a tight seal over the victim's mouth. *Circulation:* Compression of the chest with a downward thrust is alternated with breathing. If one person is performing CPR, he or she first blows into the victim's lungs, applies pressure to the sternum 15 times, and then continues a cycle of 2 breaths to 15 compressions.

and emergency cardiac care (ECC), including BCLS and ACLS, have been developed cooperatively by the American Heart Association and the National Academy of Sciences–National Research Council. Reprints of these standards can be obtained from local chapters of the American Heart Association or from the American Heart Association, Distribution Department, 7272 Greenville Ave., Dallas, TX 75231-4596, telephone (800) 553-6321.

cardiopuncture (kahr″de-o-pungk′chur) cardiocentesis.

cardiopyloric (kahr″de-o-pi-lor′ik) pertaining to the cardiac opening of the stomach and the pylorus.

cardiorenal (kahr″de-o-re′nal) pertaining to the heart and kidneys; called also nephrocardiac.

cardiorespiratory (kahr″de-o-res′pĭ-rah-to″re) cardiopulmonary.

cardiorrhaphy (kahr″de-or′ah-fe) suture of the heart muscle.

cardiorrhexis (kahr″de-o-rek′sis) rupture of the heart.

cardiosclerosis (kahr″de-o-sklĕ-ro′sis) fibrous induration of the heart.

cardioselective (kahr″de-o-sĕ-lek′tiv) having greater activity on heart tissue than on other tissue.

cardiospasm (kahr″de-o-spazm) achalasia of the esophagus.

cardiotachometer (kahr″de-o-tah-kom′ĕ-ter) an instrument for continuously portraying or recording the heart rate.

cardiotachometry (kahr″de-o-tah-kom′ĕ-tre) continuous recording of the heart rate for long periods.

cardiotherapy (kahr″de-o-ther′ah-pe) the treatment of diseases of the heart.

cardiotocograph (kahr″de-o-to′ko-graf″) the instrument used in cardiotocography.

cardiotocography (kahr″de-o-to-kog′rah-fe) the monitoring of the fetal heart rate and uterine contractions, as during delivery.

cardiotomy (kahr″de-ot′ah-me) 1. surgical incision of the heart. 2. surgical incision into the cardia.

cardiotonic (kahr″de-o-ton′ik) 1. having a tonic effect on the heart. 2. an agent that so acts.

cardiotoxic (kahr′de-o-tok″sik) having a poisonous or deleterious effect upon the heart.

cardiovalvular (kahr″de-o-val′vu-ler) pertaining to the valves of the heart.

cardiovalvulotome (kahr″de-o-val′vu-lo-tōm″) an instrument for incising a heart valve.

cardiovascular (kahr″de-o-vas′ku-ler) pertaining to the heart and blood vessels.

cardioversion (kahr′de-o-ver″zhun) the delivery of a direct current COUNTERSHOCK synchronized with the QRS complex to the myocardium as an elective treatment to end TACHYDYSRHYTHMIAS. (For emergency treatment using a nonsynchronized current to terminate arrhythmia, see DEFIBRILLATION.) The goal of cardioversion is to restore sinoatrial control of the heart rhythm by depolarizing the entire myocardium at the moment of shock. The depolarization interrupts reentry CIRCUITS, thus ending myocardial FIBRILLATION and some other types of DYSRHYTHMIAS. The electric shock can be delivered directly to the myocardium in an open chest procedure, or through externally applied paddles placed on the chest.

Cardioversion is most effective in terminating arrhythmias due to continuous REENTRY, including atrial FLUTTER, atrial FIBRILLATION, paroxysmal supraventricular TACHYCARDIA, ventricular TACHYCARDIA, and ventricular FIBRILLATION. Patients who have had a recent myocardial infarction and resultant atrial, nodal, or ventricular tachycardia are the most frequent candidates for cardioversion. Those with severe, longstanding arrhythmias due to chronic extensive heart disease usually do not benefit from this procedure.

Cardioversion should be done only by trained physicians in a setting where resuscitation equipment and respiratory support are readily at hand. Serum POTASSIUM levels must be within normal limits at the time of procedure because HYPOKALEMIA increases the patient's chance of developing deadly post-conversion dysrhythmias. If necessary, potassium salts can be given prior to the procedure. DIGITALIS toxicity predisposes the patient to life-threatening dysrhythmias *during* cardioversion and the drug should be withheld several days prior to the anticipated procedure. HYPOXIA and ACIDOSIS may decrease the chances of successful cardioversion.

cardioverter (kahr′de-o-ver″ter) an energy-storage capacitor-discharge type of condenser that is discharged with an inductance; it delivers a direct-current shock which restores normal rhythm of the heart.

automatic implantable c.-defibrillator, *implantable c.-defibrillator* see under DEFIBRILLATOR.

carditis (kahr-di′tis) inflammation of the heart; MYOCARDITIS.

cardivalvulitis (kahr″di-val″vu-li′tis) inflammation of the heart valves.

care (kār) the services rendered by members of the health professions for the benefit of a patient. See also TREATMENT.

acute c. see ACUTE CARE.

admission c. in the NURSING INTERVENTIONS CLASSIFICATION, a nursing INTERVENTION defined as facilitating entry of a patient into a health care facility.

adult day c. a health care service provided for adults with a disability or illness who need partial or supplemental care and companionship during the day, when family members are working or otherwise unable to stay at home with a disabled relative. Among the services that may be offered at an adult day care center are nursing services (e.g., medication administration and health monitoring); nutritional and health education, health counseling; physical, speech, and occupational therapy; and socialization.

ambulatory c. health services or acute care services that are provided on an outpatient basis.

amputation c. in the NURSING INTERVENTIONS CLASSIFICATION, a nursing INTERVENTION defined as the promotion of physical and psychological healing after AMPUTATION of a body part.

bed rest c. in the NURSING INTERVENTIONS CLASSIFICATION, a nursing INTERVENTION defined as promotion of comfort and safety and prevention of complications for a patient unable to get out of bed. See also BED REST.

bladder c. activities and interventions designed to maintain urinary BLADDER function, including bladder retraining, CATHETER change, and catheter irrigation.

bowel c. activities and interventions designed to maintain BOWEL function, including ENEMA, bowel training, diet, and medication.

bowel incontinence c. in the NURSING INTERVENTIONS CLASSIFICATION, a nursing INTERVENTION defined as promotion of bowel continence and maintenance of PERIANAL skin integrity.

bowel incontinence c.: encopresis in the NURSING INTERVENTIONS CLASSIFICATION, a nursing INTERVENTION defined as promotion of bowel continence in children.

cardiac c. in the NURSING INTERVENTIONS CLASSIFICATION, a nursing INTERVENTION defined as the limitation of complications resulting from an imbalance between myocardial oxygen supply and demand for a patient with symptoms of impaired cardiac function.

cardiac c.: acute in the NURSING INTERVENTIONS CLASSIFICATION, a nursing INTERVENTION defined as the limitation of complications for a patient recently experiencing an episode of an imbalance between myocardial oxygen supply and demand resulting in impaired cardiac function.

cardiac c.: rehabilitative in the NURSING INTERVENTIONS CLASSIFICATION, a nursing INTERVENTION defined as the promotion of maximal functional activity level for a patient who has suffered an episode of impaired cardiac functon which resulted from an imbalance between myocardial oxygen supply and demand.

cast c. activities and interventions designed to protect and maintain an immobilized body part, including relief of pain, pressure or constriction of circulation. See also HAZARDS OF IMMOBILITY.

cast c.: maintenance in the NURSING INTERVENTIONS CLASSIFICATION, a nursing INTERVENTION defined as care of a cast after the drying period.

cast c.: wet in the NURSING INTERVENTIONS CLASSIFICATION, a nursing INTERVENTION defined as care of a new cast during the drying period.

cesarean section c. in the NURSING INTERVENTIONS CLASSIFICATION, a nursing INTERVENTION defined as the preparation and support of a patient delivering a baby by CESAREAN SECTION.

circulatory c.: arterial insuficiency in the NURSING INTERVENTIONS CLASSIFICATION, a nursing INTERVENTION defined as promotion of arterial circulation.

circulatory c.: mechanical assist device in the NURSING INTERVENTIONS CLASSIFICATION, a nursing INTERVENTION defined as temporary support of the circulation through the use of mechanical devices or pumps.

circulatory c.: venous insufficiency in the NURSING INTERVENTIONS CLASSIFICATION, a nursing INTERVENTION defined as promotion of venous circulation.

contact lens c. in the NURSING INTERVENTIONS CLASSIFICATION, a nursing INTERVENTION defined as the prevention of eye injury and lens damage by proper use of contact lenses.

continuing c. the level of care in the HEALTH CARE SYSTEM that consists of ongoing care of the physically handicapped, mentally retarded, emotionally retarded, and those suffering from chronic incapacitating illness.

cord c. specialized care of the remnants of a newborn's UMBILICAL CORD until it falls off, consisting of cleaning and precautions to prevent infection. Cleansing protocols continue until the site is completely healed.

critical c. intensive care.

culture-specific c. those assistive, supportive, or facilitative acts toward or for an individual or group with evident or anticipated needs that are congruent with the values and lifestyles of an individual, family, or group of a specific culture, as used in the CULTURAL CARE DIVERSITY AND UNIVERSALITY theory.

developmental c. in the NURSING INTERVENTIONS CLASSIFICATION, a nursing INTERVENTION defined as structuring the environment and providing care in response to the behavioral cues and states of the preterm infant.

direct c. the provision of services to a patient that require some degree of interaction between the patient and the health care provider. Examples include assessment, performing procedures, teaching, and implementation of a care plan.

dying c. in the NURSING INTERVENTIONS CLASSIFICATION, a nursing INTERVENTION defined as promotion of physical comfort and psychological peace in the final phase of life. See also DYING.

ear c. in the NURSING INTERVENTIONS CLASSIFICATION, a nursing INTERVENTION defined as prevention or minimization of threats to ear or hearing.

embolus c.: peripheral in the NURSING INTERVENTIONS CLASSIFICATION, a nursing INTERVENTION defined as limitation of complications for a patient experiencing, or at risk for, occlusion of peripheral circulation. See also EMBOLUS.

embolus c.: pulmonary in the NURSING INTERVENTIONS CLASSIFICATION, a nursing INTERVENTION defined as limitation of complications for a patient experiencing, or at risk for, occlusion of pulmonary circulation. See also EMBOLUS.

emergency c. in the NURSING INTERVENTIONS CLASSIFICATION, a nursing INTERVENTION defined as providing life-saving measures in life-threatening situations. See also EMERGENCY.

episodic c. interventions aimed at patient cure or restoration to previous level of functioning.

eye c. in the NURSING INTERVENTIONS CLASSIFICATION, a nursing INTERVENTION defined as the prevention or minimization of threats to eye or visual integrity.

family-centered maternity c. a pattern of caring for infants and their families used by Health and Welfare Canada. It is characterized by a great deal of flexibility and parental choice, and health care professionals are encouraged to individualize care. Breast feeding and rooming in are encouraged and grandparent and sibling visits are permitted.

foot c. see FOOT CARE.

hair c. in the NURSING INTERVENTIONS CLASSIFICATION, a nursing INTERVENTION defined as the promotion of neat, clean, and attractive hair.

health c. see HEALTH CARE SYSTEM.

high-risk pregnancy c. in the NURSING INTERVENTIONS CLASSIFICATION, a nursing INTERVENTION defined as identification and management of a high-risk pregnancy to promote healthy outcomes for mother and baby.

home health c. see HOME HEALTH CARE.

incision site c. in the NURSING INTERVENTIONS CLASSIFICATION, a nursing INTERVENTION defined as cleansing, monitoring, and promotion of healing in a wound that is closed with sutures, clips, or staples.

indirect c. services that are related to patient care but do not require interaction between the health care provider and the patient. Examples include charting and scheduling.

infant c. in the NURSING INTERVENTIONS CLASSIFICATION, a nursing INTERVENTION defined as the provision of developmentally appropriate family-centered care to the child under one year of age.

intensive c. the care of seriously ill patients in a special hospital unit; see INTENSIVE CARE UNIT. Called also critical care.

intrapartal c. in the NURSING INTERVENTIONS CLASSIFICATION, a nursing INTERVENTION defined as the monitoring and management of stages one and two of the birth process. See LABOR.

intrapartal c.: high-risk delivery in the NURSING INTERVENTIONS CLASSIFICATION, a nursing INTERVENTION defined as assisting vaginal birth of multiple or malpositioned fetuses.

kangaroo c. in the NURSING INTERVENTIONS CLASSIFICATION, a nursing INTERVENTION defined as promoting closeness between parent and physiologically stable preterm infant by preparing the parent and providing the environment for skin-to-skin contact.

kinlein c. kinlein.

long-term c. health care services required for an extended period of time by individuals unable to fully execute activities of daily living; it can be provided by a variety of agencies in outpatient settings as well as on an inpatient basis.

managed c. a method of health care delivery that focuses on collaboration among and coordination of all services to avoid overlap, duplication, and delays and to reduce costs. There is an emphasis on efficacy and timeliness of interventions to prevent unnecessary delays in discharge from the hospital or agency.

mouth c. see MOUTH CARE.

nail c. in the NURSING INTERVENTIONS CLASSIFICATION, a nursing INTERVENTION defined as promotion of clean, neat, attractive nails and prevention of skin lesions related to improper care of nails.

newborn c. in the NURSING INTERVENTIONS CLASSIFICATION, a nursing INTERVENTION defined as management of the NEONATE during the transition to extrauterine life and the subsequent period of stabilization.

ostomy c. in the NURSING INTERVENTIONS CLASSIFICATION, a nursing INTERVENTION defined as maintenance of elimination through a stoma and care of surrounding tissue. See also OSTOMY.

palliative c. supportive care.

perineal c. in the NURSING INTERVENTIONS CLASSIFICATION, a nursing INTERVENTION defined as maintenance of PERIANAL skin integrity and relief of perineal discomfort.

peripherally inserted central catheter c. in the NURSING INTERVENTIONS CLASSIFICATION, a nursing INTERVENTION defined as insertion and maintenance of a peripherally inserted central catheter.

personal c. the management of hygiene, including bathing, shampooing, shaving, nail trimming, dressing, and so on.

point of c. the location at which patient services are delivered.

postanesthesia c. in the NURSING INTERVENTIONS CLASSIFICATION, a nursing INTERVENTION defined as monitoring and management of the patient who has recently undergone general or regional anesthesia.

postmortem c. in the NURSING INTERVENTIONS CLASSIFICATION, a nursing INTERVENTION defined as providing physical care of the body of an expired patient and support for the family viewing the body.

postoperative c. see POSTOPERATIVE CARE.

postpartal c. in the NURSING INTERVENTIONS CLASSIFICATION, a nursing INTERVENTION defined as monitoring and management of the patient who has recently given birth.

pregnancy termination c. in the NURSING INTERVENTIONS CLASSIFICATION, a nursing INTERVENTION defined as the management of the physical and psychological needs of the woman undergoing a spontaneous or elective ABORTION.

prenatal c. 1. care of the pregnant woman before delivery of the infant. See also PREGNANCY. 2. in the NURSING INTERVENTIONS CLASSIFICATION, a nursing intervention defined as monitoring and management of the patient during pregnancy to prevent complications of pregnancy and promote a healthy outcome for both mother and infant.

preoperative c. see PREOPERATIVE CARE.

pressure ulcer c. in the NURSING INTERVENTIONS CLASSIFICATION, a nursing INTERVENTION defined as facilitation of healing in PRESSURE ULCERS.

preventive c. the level of care in the HEALTH CARE SYSTEM that consists of PUBLIC HEALTH services and related programs such as school health education.

primary c. the routine outpatient care that a patient receives at first contact with the HEALTH CARE SYSTEM.

prosthesis c. in the NURSING INTERVENTIONS CLASSIFICATION, a nursing INTERVENTION defined as the care of a removable appliance worn by a patient and the prevention of complications associated with its use. See also PROSTHESIS.

respiratory c. see RESPIRATORY CARE.

respite c. 1. services provided by a health care agency that permit a primary caregiver temporary relief from caring for an ill individual. 2. in the NURSING INTERVENTIONS CLASSIFICATION, a nursing INTERVENTION defined as the provision of short-term care to provide relief for a family CAREGIVER.

restorative c. the level of care in the HEALTH CARE SYSTEM that consists of follow-up care and rehabilitation to an optimal functional level.

secondary c. 1. treatment by specialists to whom a patient has been referred by primary care facilities; see also HEALTH CARE SYSTEM. 2. acute care.

self c. the performance of basic ACTIVITIES OF DAILY LIVING; see also under ASSISTANCE and DEFICIT.

skilled nursing c. the services provided by a registered nurse in a skilled nursing FACILITY. It currently includes observation during periods of acute or unstable illness; administration of intravenous fluids, enteral feedings, and intravenous or intramuscular medications; short-term bowel and bladder retraining; and changing of sterile dressings.

skin c. activities and interventions designed to maintain integrity of integument, including care of PRESSURE ULCERS and MASSAGE.

skin c.: topical treatments in the NURSING INTERVENTIONS CLASSIFICATION, a nursing INTERVENTION defined as the application of topical substances or manipulation of devices to promote skin integrity and minimize skin breakdown.

spiritual c. see SPIRITUAL CARE.

subacute c. comprehensive goal-oriented inpatient care designed for a patient who has had an acute illness, injury, or exacerbation of a disease process; it is rendered either immediately after or instead of acute care hospitalization, to treat specific active or complex medical conditions or to administer any necessary technically complex medical treatments in the context of the person's underlying long-term condition.

supportive c. interventions that help the patient achieve comfort but do not affect the course of a disease. Called also palliative care or treatment.

tertiary c. the level of care in the HEALTH CARE SYSTEM that consists of complex procedures given in a health care center that has highly trained specialists and often advanced technology.

total patient c. a method of organizing care of patients such that one practitioner carries out all care requirements.

traction/immobilization c. in the NURSING INTERVENTIONS CLASSIFICATION, a nursing INTERVENTION defined as management of a patient who has TRACTION and/or a stabilizing device to immobilize and stabilize a body part.

tube c. in the NURSING INTERVENTIONS CLASSIFICATION, a nursing INTERVENTION defined as management of a patient with an external drainage device exiting the body.

tube c.: chest in the NURSING INTERVENTIONS CLASSIFICATION, a nursing INTERVENTION defined as management of a patient with an external water-seal drainage device exiting the chest cavity.

tube c.: gastrointestinal in the NURSING INTERVENTIONS CLASSIFICATION, a nursing INTERVENTION defined as management of a patient with a gastrointestinal tube.

tube c.: umbilical line in the NURSING INTERVENTIONS CLASSIFICATION, a nursing INTERVENTION defined as management of a newborn with an umbilical catheter.

tube c.: urinary in the NURSING INTERVENTIONS CLASSIFICATION, a nursing INTERVENTION defined as management of a patient with urinary drainage equipment.

tube c.: ventriculostomy/lumbar drain in the NURSING INTERVENTIONS CLASSIFICATION, a nursing INTERVENTION defined as management of a patient with an external cerebrospinal fluid drainage system. See also VENTRICULOSTOMY and DRAIN.

urinary incontinence c. in the NURSING INTERVENTIONS CLASSIFICATION, a nursing INTERVENTION defined as assistance in promoting continence and maintaining perineal skin integrity. See also urinary INCONTINENCE.

urinary incontinence c.: enuresis in the NURSING INTERVENTIONS CLASSIFICATION, a nursing INTERVENTION defined as promotion of urinary continence in children.

urinary retention c. in the NURSING INTERVENTIONS CLASSIFICATION, a nursing INTERVENTION defined as assistance in relieving bladder distention. See also RETENTION OF URINE.

wound c. in the NURSING INTERVENTIONS CLASSIFICATION, a nursing INTERVENTION defined as prevention of wound complications and promotion of WOUND HEALING.

wound c.: closed drainage in the NURSING INTERVENTIONS CLASSIFICATION, a nursing INTERVENTION defined as maintenance of a pressure drainage system at the wound site.

career ladders the organization of education or experience for health care professionals so that they may increase their expertise and receive recognition for professional development.

caregiver (kār′giv″er) a lay individual who assumes responsibility for the physical and emotional needs of another who is incapable of self care. See also caregiver role FATIGUE and caregiver role STRAIN. Called also caretaker.

CareMaps trademark for a type of CRITICAL PATH.

caretaker (kār′tāk″er) caregiver.

caretaking (kār′tāk-ing) assuming responsibility for the physical or emotional needs of another who is incapable of self care. See also CAREGIVER.

CARF Commission on the Accreditation of Rehabilitation Facilities.

caries (kar′e-ēz, kar′ēz) decay, as of bone or teeth. adj., **ca′rious.**

> **bottle mouth c.** early childhood caries.

> **dental c.** see DENTAL CARIES.

> **dry c., c. sic′ca** a form of tuberculous caries of the joints and ends of bones.

> **early childhood c.** severe dental caries that are promoted by the sugars, acids, and sometimes *Streptococcus mutans* in a bottle of milk or juice left in contact with a child's primary teeth; this can also occur from contact with breast milk left in a sleeping child's mouth. The condition is preventable; no child should be permitted to fall asleep nursing on any liquid other than plain water. Called also bottle mouth caries.

> **recurrent c.** dental caries beneath the margin of an existing tooth restoration.

carina (kah-ri′nah), pl. *cari′nae* [L.] a ridgelike structure.

> **c. tra′cheae** a downward and backward projection of the lowest tracheal cartilage, forming a ridge between the openings of the right and left principal bronchi.

> **c. urethra′lis vagi′nae** the column of rugae in the lower anterior wall of the vagina, immediately below the urethra.

caring (kār′ing) an interpersonal process involving an emotional commitment to, and a willingness to act on behalf of, a person with whom one has a significant relationship. See also CARE. Caring is moral reflection but does not necessarily have a central moral principle. The BIOETHICS of caring may focus on relationship, responsibility, trust, fidelity, and sensitivity. Emphasis is on not only what the health care provider does but also on how the actions are performed, what motives underlie them, and whether they promote or thwart positive relationships.

cariogenesis (kar″e-o-jen′ē-sis) the development of caries.

cariogenic (kar″e-o-jen′ik) conducive to caries.

carious (kar′e-əs) [L. *cariosus*] affected with or of the nature of caries.

carisoprodol (kar″i-so′pro-dol) an ANALGESIC and skeletal muscle RELAXANT used to relieve symptoms of acute painful skeletomuscular disorders, administered orally.

Carmichael's law of anticipatory function (kahr′mi-k′lz) a law that helps establish a foundation for motor development, stating that a system will mature before it is needed.

carminative (kahr-min′ah-tiv) 1. relieving flatulence. 2. an agent that so acts.

carmustine (kahr-mus′tēn) a cytotoxic ALKYLATING AGENT of the nitrosourea group, used as an antineoplastic AGENT, primarily against brain tumors, multiple myeloma, colorectal carcinoma, Hodgkin's disease, and non-Hodgkin's lymphomas. Called also BCNU.

carnitine (kahr′nĭ-tēn) a derivative of betaine found in skeletal muscle and liver; it is necessary for the mitochondrial oxidation of fatty acids.

carnivore (kahr′nĭ-vor) any animal that eats primarily flesh, particularly mammals of the order Carnivora, which includes cats, dogs, bears, and others. adj., **carniv′orous.**

carnosinase (kahr′no-sĭ-nās) an enzyme that hydrolyzes carnosine (amino-acyl-L-histidine) and other dipeptides containing L-histidine into their constituent amino acids.

carnosine (kahr′no-sēn) a dipeptide composed of beta-alanine and histidine, found in skeletal muscle of vertebrates.

carnosinemia (kahr″no-sĭ-ne′me-ah) excessive amounts of carnosine in the blood; it has been associated with a progressive neurologic disease characterized by severe mental defect and myoclonic seizures, and is probably due to a genetic deficiency of carnosinase in the serum.

carnosinuria (kahr″no-sĭ-nu′re-ah) an AMINOACIDURIA characterized by an excess of CARNOSINE in the urine; it occurs in CARNOSINEMIA or may be dietary in origin, especially in young children.

carotenase (kar-ot′ĕ-nās) an enzyme that converts carotene into vitamin A.

carotene (kar′o-tēn) a yellow or red pigment found in many dark green, leafy, and yellow vegetables such as collards, turnips, carrots, sweet potatoes, and squash, as well as in yellow fruit, milk, egg yolk, and body fat; it is a chromolipoid hydrocarbon existing in four forms (α-, β-, γ-, and δ-carotene), which can be converted into VITAMIN A in the body.

> **beta c.** 1. the β isomer of carotene. 2. a preparation of this substance administered orally to prevent VITAMIN A deficiency and to

reduce PHOTOSENSITIVITY in patients with erythropoietic PROTOPORPHYRIA. Written also betacarotene and β-carotene.

carotenemia (kar″ah-te-ne′me-ah) hypercarotenemia.

carotenodermia (kar-ot″ĕ-no-der′me-ah) yellowness of the skin due to carotenemia.

carotenoid (kah-rot′ĕ-noid) 1. any member of a group of red, orange, or yellow pigmented lipids found in carrots, sweet potatoes, green leaves, and some animal tissues; examples are the carotenes, lycopene, and xanthophyll. 2. marked by yellow color. 3. lipochrome.

carotenosis (kar″o-tĕ-no′sis) deposition of CAROTENE in tissues, especially the skin.

caroticotympanic (kah-rot″ĭ-ko-tim-pan′-ik) pertaining to the carotid canal and tympanum.

carotid (kah-rot′id) pertaining to the principal artery of the neck (the carotid artery). See anatomic Table of Arteries in the Appendices.

c. endarterectomy surgical removal of atherosclerotic plaques within an extracranial carotid artery, usually the common carotid, done to prevent STROKE in patients with 70 per cent or greater carotid stenosis. Patients who have a stroke in evolution or have recently had a stroke are not good candidates for the procedure. Surgery at this time could cause an infarcted area of the brain to hemorrhage when its blood supply is suddenly increased. In addition, there is a low success rate for those patients who have total occlusion of the internal carotid arteries.

Patient Care. Immediately after surgery special monitoring is necessary to assess the patient's neurologic status, including level of consciousness, orientation, and motor activity, especially on the side opposite the surgery. Because of the location of the surgical incision, an enlarging hematoma can rapidly produce respiratory distress. Aspiration also is possible because a hematoma can obstruct the trachea and damage the laryngeal nerve, preventing closure of the glottis.

Crucial observations include evaluation of neck size, noting the patient's ability to swallow, close observation and measurement of drainage, and measurement of respiratory rate and character. A tracheostomy tray and suction apparatus should be available even after the patient is transferred from the recovery room or intensive care unit. Neurologic assessment is necessary to detect complications associated with postoperative cerebral ischemia and cranial nerve damage. Because ischemia of the myocardium is also a possibility, continuous electrocardiograph monitoring is required. Since blood pressure may be increased by surgery, postoperative hypertension is not uncommon. (See accompanying illustration.)

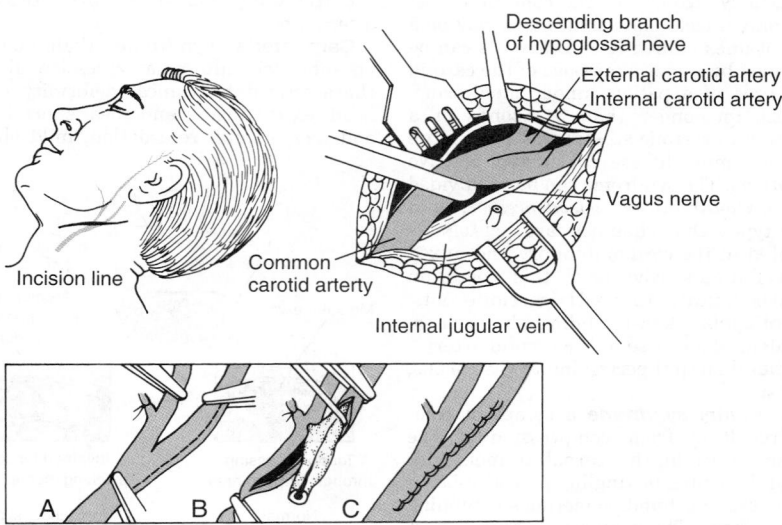

Descending branch of hypoglossal neve
External carotid artery
Internal carotid artery
Vagus nerve
Common carotid arterty
Internal jugular vein
Incision line
A   B   C

Carotid endarterectomy. Plaques are removed from the artery to improve blood flow. Modified from Black and Matassarin-Jacobs, 2001.

NATIONAL INSTITUTE FOR OCCUPATIONAL SAFETY AND HEALTH (NIOSH) CRITERIA FOR CARPAL TUNNEL SYNDROME

I. One or more of the following symptoms suggestive of carpal tunnel syndrome must be present:
Paresthesia
Hypoesthesia
Pain
Numbness affecting at least one part of the median nerve distribution of the hand

Symptoms should have lasted at least one week, or if intermittent have occurred on multiple occasions. Other causes of hand numbness should be excluded by clinical evaluation.

II. Objective findings consistent with carpal tunnel syndrome are present in the affected hand or wrist:
Either:
   Tinel's sign
   Positive Phalen's test
   Diminished or absent sensation to pin prick
Or:
   Electrodiagnostic findings indicative of median nerve dysfunction across the carpel tunnel

III. Evidence of work-relatedness is a history of a job involving one or more of the following activities before the development of symptoms:
Frequent, repetitive use of the same or similar movements of the hand or wrist on the affected side
Regular tasks requiring the generation of high force by the hand
Regular or sustained tasks requiring awkward hand positions of the affected side
Regular use of vibrating hand-held tools
Frequent or prolonged pressure over the wrist or base of the palm on the affected side

***

c. sinus syndrome syncope sometimes associated with convulsive seizures due to overactivity of the carotid sinus REFLEX. In certain susceptible persons the carotid SINUS is too easily stimulated and symptoms are produced by sudden turning of the head or the wearing of a tight collar. Transient attacks of numbness or weakness of the face, arm, or leg, headache, and in some cases APHASIA may also occur. The condition most commonly affects older males and may be a cause of unexplained falls. Diagnosis can be confirmed by a gentle massage of the carotid sinus area of a patient under monitoring. ASYSTOLE for longer than 3 seconds or a reduction in systolic BLOOD PRESSURE of more than 500 mm Hg are considered positive indications. The syndrome can be subdivided into *cardioinhibitory, vasodepressor,* and *mixed* types. Dual chamber cardiac PACING is indicated in the cardioinhibitory and mixed types. Patients who have this condition should be educated to avoid triggering events.

carotidynia (kah-rot″ĭ-din′e-ah) tenderness along the course of the carotid artery.

carpal (kahr′p'l) pertaining to the carpus, or wrist.

c. tunnel syndrome a symptom complex resulting from compression of the median nerve in the carpal tunnel, with pain and burning or tingling paresthesias in the fingers and hand, sometimes extending to the elbow. The disorder is found most often in middle-aged women. Excessive wrist movements, arthritis, hypertrophy of the bone and connective tissue in ACROMEGALY, and swelling of the wrist can produce the carpal tunnel syndrome. Treatment is usually conservative and consists of splinting the wrist to immobilize it for several weeks until the irritation of the median nerve has healed. In severe cases surgical resection of the carpal ligament is helpful.

carpectomy (kahr-pek′to-me) excision of a carpal bone.

Carpenter's syndrome (kahr′pen-terz) an inherited autosomal recessive disorder characterized by conical deformity of the head, extra fingers and toes, short fingers and toes, mental retardation, mild obesity,

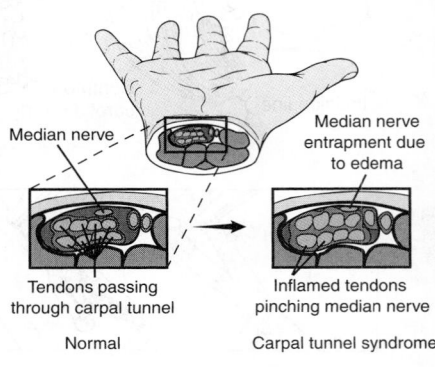

Median nerve
Median nerve entrapment due to edema

Tendons passing through carpal tunnel
Inflamed tendons pinching median nerve

Normal
Carpal tunnel syndrome

Carpal tunnel syndrome. Entrapment of the median nerve in the carpal tunnel space. From Frazier et al., 2000.

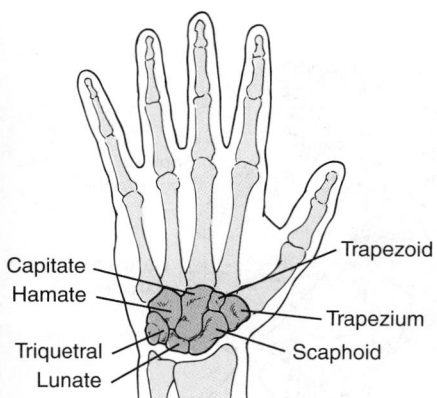

Capitate
Hamate
Triquetral
Lunate
Trapezoid
Trapezium
Scaphoid

Carpus, viewed from the dorsal aspect. The eighth bone, the pisiform, is palmar to the triquetral bone. From Dorland's, 2000.

HYPOGONADISM, and other anomalies. Called also acrocephalopolysyndactyly, type II.

carphenazine (kahr-fen′ah-zēn) a PHENO-THIAZINE ANTIPSYCHOTIC AGENT, used as the maleate salt.

carphology (kahr-fol′o-je) involuntary picking at the bedclothes, seen in states of great exhaustion and grave fevers.

carpometacarpal (kahr″po-met″ah-kahr′p′l) pertaining to the carpus and metacarpus.

carpopedal (kahr″po-pe′d′l) affecting the wrist and foot.

carpophalangeal (kahr″po-fah-lan′je-al) pertaining to the carpus and phalanges.

carpoptosis (kahr″po-to′sis) wristdrop.

carpus (kahr′pus) the joint between the arm and hand, made up of eight bones; the WRIST. (See accompanying illustration.) (See also table of BONES.)

carrier (kar′e-er) 1. an individual who harbors the specific organisms of a disease without manifest symptoms and is capable of transmitting the infection; the condition of such an individual is referred to as the carrier state. 2. in genetics, an individual who is heterozygous for a recessive gene and thus does not express the recessive phenotype but can transmit it to offspring. Only females can be carriers of X-linked recessive traits. 3. a substance that carries a radioisotopic or other label, as in a tracer study. A second isotope mixed with a particular isotope is also referred to as a carrier. See also CARRIER-FREE. 4. a transport protein that carries specific substances, e.g., in the blood or across cell membranes. 5. in immunology, a macromolecular substance to which a hapten is coupled in order to produce an immune response against the hapten. IMMUNE RESPONSES are usually produced only against large molecules capable of simultaneously binding both B CELLS and helper T CELLS.

carrier-free (kar′e-er-fre″) a term denoting a radioisotope of an element in pure form, i.e., essentially undiluted with a stable isotope carrier.

Carrión's disease (kah-re-ōnz′) bartonellosis.

carteolol (kahr′te-ah-lol) a BETA-ADRENERGIC BLOCKING AGENT with intrinsic sympathetic activity, administered orally as an antihypertensive and applied topically to the conjunctiva in the treatment of glaucoma and ocular hypertension.

cartilage (kahr′tĭ-lij) a specialized, fibrous connective tissue present in adults, and forming most of the temporary skeleton in the embryo, providing a model in which most of the bones develop, and constituting an important part of the organism's growth mechanism; the three most important types are hyaline cartilage, elastic cartilage, and fibrocartilage. Also, a general term for a mass of such tissue in a particular site in the body. (See accompanying illustration.)

alar c's the cartilages of the wings of the nose.

aortic c. the second costal cartilage on the right side.

arthrodial c., articular c. that lining the articular surfaces of synovial joints.

arytenoid c's two pyramid-shaped cartilages of the larynx.

connecting c. that connecting the surfaces of an immovable joint.

costal c. a bar of hyaline cartilage that attaches a rib to the sternum in the case of true ribs, or to the immediately above rib in the case of the upper false ribs.

cricoid c. a ringlike cartilage forming the lower and back part of the larynx.

diarthrodial c. articular cartilage.

elastic c. cartilage that is more opaque, flexible, and elastic than hyaline cartilage, and is further distinguished by its yellow color. The ground substance is penetrated in all directions by frequently branching fibers that give all of the reactions for elastin.

ensiform c. xiphoid process.

fibrous c. fibrocartilage.

floating c. a detached portion of semilunar cartilage in the knee joint.

hyaline c. flexible, somewhat elastic, semitransparent cartilage with an opalescent bluish tint, composed of a basophilic fibril-containing substance with cavities in which the chondrocytes occur. (See accompanying illustration.)

Meckel's c. the ventral cartilage of the first branchial arch.

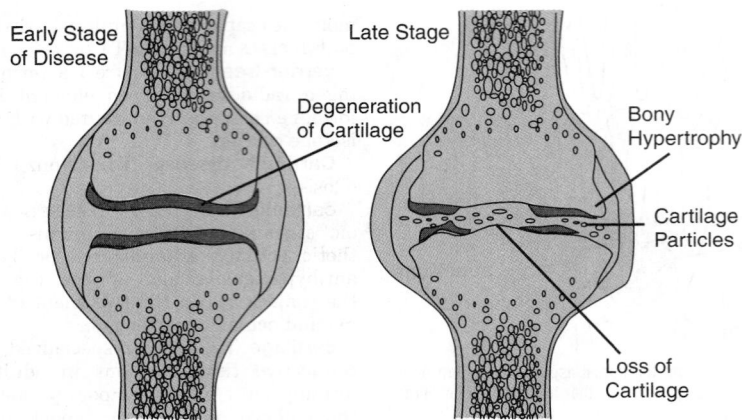

Early Stage of Disease

Late Stage

Degeneration of Cartilage

Bony Hypertrophy

Cartilage Particles

Loss of Cartilage

Involvement of joint and cartilage in osteoarthritis. From ARHP Arthritis Teaching Slide Collection, American College of Rheumatology.

permanent c. cartilage that does not normally become ossified.

Reichert's c. the dorsal cartilage of the second branchial arch.

reticular c. elastic cartilage.

semilunar c. one of the two interarticular cartilages of the knee joint.

temporary c. cartilage that is normally destined to be replaced by bone.

thyroid c. the shield-shaped cartilage of the larynx, underlying the laryngeal PROMINENCE on the surface of the neck.

vomeronasal c. either of the two narrow strips of cartilage, one on each side, of the nasal septum supporting the vomeronasal organ.

yellow c. elastic cartilage.

cartilaginiform (kahr″tĭ-lah-jin′ĭ-form) chondroid.

cartilaginous (kahr″tĭ-laj′ĭ-nus) consisting of or of the nature of cartilage.

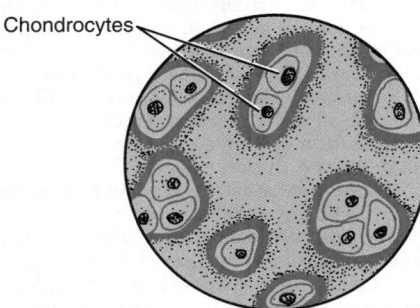

Chondrocytes

Hyaline cartilage. The matrix nearest the chondrocytes is intensely staining; although the matrix appears homogeneous, collagen fibrils may be visualized by polarized light or electron microscopy. From Dorland's, 2000.

cartilago (kahr″tĭ-lah′go), pl. *cartila′gines* [L.] cartilage.

Cartrol trademark for a preparation of CARTEOLOL hydrochloride, an ANTIHYPERTENSIVE AGENT.

caruncle (kar′ung-k'l) a small fleshy eminence, often abnormal.

hymenal c's small elevations of mucous membrane around the vaginal opening, being relics of the ruptured HYMEN; called also myrtiform caruncles.

lacrimal c. the red eminence at the medial angle of the eye.

myrtiform c's hymenal caruncles.

sublingual c. an eminence on either side of the frenulum of the tongue (frenulum linguae), on which the major duct of the sublingual gland and the duct of the submandibular gland open.

urethral c. a small, polyploid, red growth on the mucous membrane of the female urinary meatus, sometimes causing difficulty in urination.

caruncula (kah-rung′ku-lah), pl. *carun′culae* [L.] caruncle.

carvedilol (kahr′vĕ-dil″ol) a BETA-ADRENERGIC BLOCKING AGENT used in treatment of HYPERTENSION and as an adjunct in treatment of congestive HEART FAILURE; administered orally.

cary(o)- for words beginning thus, see those beginning *kary(o)-*.

casanthranol (kah-san′thrah-nol) a purified mixture of glycosides derived from CASCARA SAGRADA; a CATHARTIC.

cascade (kas-kād′) a series of steps or stages (as of a physiological process) that, once initiated, continues to the final step because each step is triggered by the preceding one, resulting in amplification of the signal, information, or effect at each stage. In electronics, the term is applied to multiple amplifiers. Examples in biochemistry include blood coagulation and the complement system.

coagulation c. the series of steps beginning with activation of the intrinsic or extrinsic PATHWAYS of coagulation, or of one of the related alternative pathways, and proceeding through the common PATHWAY of coagulation to the formation of the fibrin clot. (See illustration.)

cascara (kas-kar′ah) [Sp.] bark.

c. sagra′da dried bark of the shrub *Rhamnus purshiana*, used as a CATHARTIC.

case (kās) a particular instance of a disease or other problem; sometimes used incorrectly to designate the patient with the disease.

c. history the collected data concerning an individual, the family, and environment; it includes the medical history and any other information that may be useful in analyzing and diagnosing the case or for instructional or research purposes.

c. method a type of nursing care delivery system; see NURSING PRACTICE.

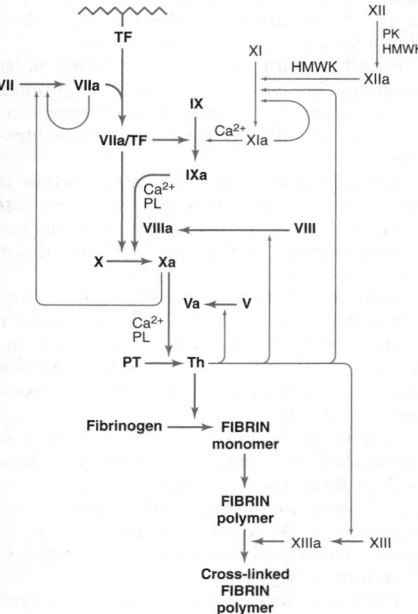

The coagulation cascade. This scheme emphasizes the understanding of 1, the importance of the tissue factor pathway in initiating clotting in vivo; 2, the interactions between pathways; and 3, the pivotal role of thrombin in sustaining the cascade by feedback activation of coagulation factors. HMWK = high-molecular-weight kininogen; PK = prekallikrein; PL = phospholipid; PT = prothrombin; TF = tissue factor; Th = thrombin. From Schafer, 1994.

c. mix the groups of patients requiring similar tests, procedures, and resources that are treated at a particular hospital. Case mix is a way to define a hospital's production and has been identified as a major factor in differing costs among hospitals and among individual patients.

caseation (ka″se-a′shun) 1. the precipitation of casein. 2. a form of necrosis in which tissue is changed into a dry, amorphous mass resembling cheese. Called also caseous degeneration or necrosis.

casein (ka′se-in) a phosphoprotein, the principal protein of milk, that is the basis of curd and of cheese. Casein, usually in the form of one of its salts, is added to the other ingredients of the diet to increase its protein content. NOTE: In British nomenclature casein is called caseinogen, and paracasein is called casein.

caseinogen (ka″se-in′o-jen) the British term for casein.

caseous (ka′se-us) resembling cheese or curd; cheesy.

Casoni's test (kah-so′nēz) intradermal injection of hydatid fluid followed by production of wheal-flare reaction denotes hydatid infection.

caspofungin (kas″po-fun′jin) an antifungal used as the acetate salt in the treatment of invasive aspergillosis, administered intravenously.

cassette (kah-set′) [Fr.] a light-proof housing for x-ray film and electrostatic imaging plates, containing front and back intensifying screens, between which the film is placed; a magazine for film or magnetic tape.

grid c. a cassette that has its front replaced by a built-in grid.

cast (kast) 1. a positive copy of an object. 2. to make such a copy. 3. a mold of a tube or hollow organ (such as a renal tubule or bronchiole), formed of effused matter and eliminated from the body. See also urinary CAST. 4. a positive copy or mold of the tissues of the jaws, made in an IMPRESSION, and over which denture bases or other restorations may be fabricated. 5. strabismus. 6. a stiff dressing or casing, usually made of plaster of Paris, used to immobilize body parts.

Patient Care. If the patient is confined to bed after a plaster of Paris cast is applied, it is necessary to provide a firm mattress protected by a waterproof material. Several small pillows should be available for placing under the curves of the cast to prevent remolding or cracking of the plaster and to provide adequate support of the patient. When handling a wet cast only the palm or flat of the hand is used so that the fingertips will not make indentations that might produce pressure against the patient's skin.

While the cast is drying it is left uncovered to allow circulation of air around it. Extreme heat should not be used to hasten drying of a plaster of Paris cast, as this may produce burns under the cast. Synthetic casts, however, may be set or cured with heat. To minimize crumbling of the edges and irritation of the skin around and under the cast, a strip of stockinette or adhesive tape is applied so that the rim of the cast is thoroughly covered. Observation of the patient for signs of impaired circulation, pressure against a nerve, or COMPARTMENTAL SYNDROME is extremely important. Any numbness, recurrent pain, or tingling should be reported at once. If a limb is enclosed in a cast it should be elevated to reduce swelling. Cyanosis or blanching of the fingers or toes extending from a cast usually indicates impaired blood flow, which may lead to serious complications if not corrected immediately.

renal c., urinary c. a cast formed from gelled protein precipitated in the renal tubules and molded to the tubular lumen; pieces of these casts break off and are washed out with the urine. Types named for their constituent material include epithelial, granular, hyaline, and waxy casts. In renal disease, casts may be seen containing red or white blood cells.

walking c. a lower extremity cast with an attached heel or other support so that the patient is able to ambulate while the cast is in place.

Castleman disease (kas'el-man) a benign or premalignant condition resembling lymphoma but without recognizable malignant cells; there are isolated masses of lymphoid tissue and lymph node hyperplasia, usually in the abdominal or mediastinal area.

castor oil (kas'ter) a fixed oil obtained from the seed of the castor bean plant *(Ricinus communis);* now used primarily as a topical EMOLLIENT. When taken internally it acts as a powerful CATHARTIC; because of its strength, other agents are now preferred for treatment of digestive disorders.

castrate (kas'trāt) 1. to deprive of the gonads, rendering the individual incapable of reproduction. 2. a castrated individual.

castration (kas-tra'shun) excision of the gonads (bilateral ORCHIECTOMY in a male or bilateral OOPHORECTOMY in a female), or destruction of the gonads, as by radiation or parasites. If this occurs before puberty, secondary sex CHARACTERS will fail to develop. See also EUNUCH.

female c. removal of the ovaries, or bilateral OOPHORECTOMY; called SPAYING in female animals.

male c. bilateral ORCHIECTOMY.

casualty (kazh'oo-al-te) 1. an accident; an accidental wound; death or disablement from an accident; also the person so injured. 2. in the armed forces, one missing from his unit as a result of death, injury, illness, or capture, because his whereabouts are unknown, or for other reasons.

casuistics (kaz"u-is'tiks) the recording and study of cases of disease.

CAT computerized axial TOMOGRAPHY.

cat(a)- word element [Gr.], *down; lower; under; against; along with; very.*

catabiosis (kat"ah-bi-o'sis) the natural aging of cells. adj., **catabiot'ic.**

catabolism (kah-tab'o-lizm) any destructive process by which complex substances are converted by living cells into simpler compounds, with release of energy; the opposite of ANABOLISM. See also METABOLISM. adj., **catabol'ic.**

catabolite (kah-tab'o-līt) a compound produced in catabolism.

catacrotism (kah-tak'rŏ-tizm) a pulse anomaly in which a small additional wave or notch appears in the descending limb of the pulse tracing. adj., **catacrot'ic.**

catadicrotism (kat"ah-di'krŏ-tizm) pulse anomaly in which two small additional waves or notches appear in the descending limb of the pulse tracing. adj., **catadicrot'ic.**

catagen (kat'ah-jen) the brief portion of the hair CYCLE in which growth of the HAIR (ANAGEN) stops and resting (TELOGEN) begins.

catagenesis (kat"ah-jen'ē-sis) involution or retrogression.

catalase (kat'ah-lās) a HEMOPROTEIN enzyme that specifically catalyzes the decomposition of hydrogen peroxide and is found in almost all cells except certain anaerobic bacteria. Deficiency results in ACATALASIA. adj., **catalat'ic.**

catalepsy (kat'ah-lep"se) a condition of diminished responsiveness usually characterized by a trancelike state and constantly maintained immobility, often with CEREA FLEXIBILITAS. Affected individuals may remain in one position for minutes, days, or even longer. adj., **catalep'tic.**

Catalepsy may accompany any of several different mental illnesses. It is common in catatonic schizophrenia and may also occur in epilepsy, hysteria, and cerebellar disorders; it may also be induced by hypnosis. The patient may sit with the hands flat on the knees and the head bowed or may remain in an awkward and uncomfortable position. The patient is not necessarily unaware of what is going on but does not respond. This apathetic condition may end as suddenly as it begins.

Patient Care. Regular skin care and exercise of the muscles and joints are necessary to prevent circulatory complications. Nutritional status requires attention and an adequate diet must be provided. Even though cataleptic patients may not be able to respond to spoken directions or conversation and are physically unable to move, they cannot be left in one position for long periods of time any more than can patients who are physically paralyzed. The mental state of these patients is such that they cannot recognize numbness or pain, nor can they communicate a need for attention.

Care must be used in conversations held within the patient's hearing. Total apathy does not indicate a loss of ability to hear or see what is going on. Sometimes it is of great help to these patients to have someone sit quietly beside them so that they are aware that someone cares and is genuinely interested in their welfare.

A sudden change in the patient's condition, with increased activity, may indicate progression from one state of extreme emotion to another. Restlessness or talkativeness usually do not indicate a dramatic improvement in mental condition. When the patient becomes more active the staff should be alert to the possibility of SUICIDE and attempts at self-mutilation. A person who has exhibited symptoms as severe as catalepsy is very ill and will need continued and long-term care to facilitate recovery from serious emotional problems.

cataleptiform (kat″ah-lep′tĭ-form) resembling CATALEPSY.

catalysis (kah-tal′ĭ-sis) increase in the velocity of a chemical reaction or process produced by the presence of a substance that is not consumed in the net chemical reaction or process; negative catalysis denotes the slowing down or inhibition of a reaction or process by the presence of such a substance. adj., **catalyt′ic.**

catalyst (kat′ah-list) any substance that brings about CATALYSIS.

catalyze (kat′ah-līz) to cause or produce catalysis.

catamnesis (kat″am-ne′sis) 1. the follow-up history of a patient after he is discharged from treatment or a hospital. 2. the history of a patient after the onset of a medical or psychiatric illness. adj., **catamnes′tic.**

cataphasia (kat″ah-fa′zhah) verbigeration.

cataphoria (kat″ah-fo′re-ah) a downward turning of the visual axes of both eyes after visual functional stimuli have been removed. adj., **cataphor′ic.**

cataphylaxis (kat″ah-fĭ-lak′sis) movement of leukocytes and antibodies to the site of an infection. adj., **cataphylac′tic.**

cataplasia (kat″ah-pla′zhah) atrophy with tissues reverting to earlier, or more embryonic conditions.

cataplexy (kat′ah-plek″se) a condition, often associated with NARCOLEPSY; marked by abrupt attacks of muscular weakness and hypotonia triggered by an emotional stimulus, such as mirth, anger, or fear. adj., **cataplec′tic.**

Catapres (kat′ah-pres) trademark for preparations of CLONIDINE hydrochloride, an ANTIHYPERTENSIVE AGENT and analgesic.

cataract (kat′ah-rakt) opacity of the LENS of the eye or its capsule. adj., **catarac′tous.**

Causes and Symptoms. Some cataracts result from injuries to the eye, exposure to great heat or radiation, or inherited factors. The great majority, however, are "senile" cataracts, which are apparently a part of the aging process of the human body.

Blurred and dimmed vision are often the first symptoms. The patient may find that a brighter reading light is needed, or objects must be held closer to the eyes for better vision. Continued clouding of the lens may cause double vision; eventually there may be a need for frequent changes of eyeglasses. These symptoms do not necessarily indicate cataract, but if any of them are present, an ophthalmologist should be consulted immediately.

Treatment. The only known effective treatment for cataract is surgical removal of the lens (lens extraction or cataract extraction). The procedure of choice was formerly intracapsular extraction, with total removal of the lens within its capsule. This may be done by forceps or by CRYOEXTRACTION using a supercooled metal probe that forms a bond with the lens capsule. The inner portion of the lens can be removed by emulsification and aspiration. More recently the removed cataract has been replaced with a plastic intraocular lens. In this procedure the inner portions of the lens (the nucleus and cortex) may be all that is removed; the capsule is retained and the intraocular lens is placed inside it.

The lens of the eye serves only to focus light rays upon the retina. After cataract extraction the loss of the natural lens is compensated for by either special eyeglasses or contact lenses. Implantation of a permanent artificial lens, either during cataract surgery or later, is an alternative to use of cataract spectacles and a removable contact lens.

Patient Care. Eye drops are administered to produce MYDRIASIS and VASOCONSTRICTION. Because these patients may have extremely poor eyesight, care should be taken that they do not injure themselves. (See also VISION.) Local anesthesia is usually preferred for the surgical procedure and preoperative medications are given to produce drowsiness. Ambulatory care surgery with same-day admission and discharge is becoming increasingly routine. Careful observation of the patient on follow-up visits is important. One needs to be on the alert for a complaint of pain in the eye followed by nausea and vomiting. These could be signs that the patient has increased intraocular pressure within the operative eye and measures need to be taken to reduce the pressure.

after-c. any membrane of the pupillary area after extraction or absorption of the lens. See also secondary cataract.

atopic c. cataract occurring, most often in the second to third decade, in those with longstanding atopic dermatitis.

brown c., brunescent c. senile cataract appearing as a brown opacity.

capsular c. one consisting of an opacity of the capsule of the lens.

complicated c. secondary cataract.

cortical c. an opacity in the cortex of the lens.

hypermature c. one in which the entire lens capsule is wrinkled and the contents have become solid and shrunken, or soft and liquid.

immature c., incipient c. an incomplete cataract; the lens is only slightly opaque and the cortex clear.

intumescent c. a mature cataract that progresses; the lens becomes swollen from the osmotic effect of degenerated lens protein, and this may lead to secondary angle closure (acute) glaucoma.

lenticular c. opacity of the lens not affecting the capsule.

mature c. a cataract that produces swelling and opacity of the entire lens; cataracts are removed before maturity.

presenile c. a subcapsular senile cataract in a person under 40 years of age.

secondary c. a cataract, usually posterior subcapsular, that arises from either disease (especially IRIDOCYCLITIS), degeneration (such as chronic GLAUCOMA or retinal DETACHMENT), or surgery (such as glaucoma filtering or retinal reattachment).

senile c. cataract with no obvious cause occurring in persons over 50 years old.

cataracta (kat″ah-rak′tah) [L.] cataract.

cataractogenic (kat″ah-rak″to-jen′ik) tending to induce the formation of cataracts.

catarrh (kah-tahr′) inflammation of a mucous membrane (particularly of the head and throat), with free discharge of mucus. adj., **catar′rhal.**

catathymia (kat″ah-thi′me-ah) the existence of unconscious material so emotionally charged or affect-laden that conscious effects are produced. adj., **catathy′mic.**

catatonia (kat″ah-to′ne-ah) a wide group of motor abnormalities, most involving extreme under- or overactivity, associated primarily with catatonic SCHIZOPHRENIA but also with other disorders. Included are motoric immobility, excessive motor activity, extreme negativism or mutism, unusual mannerisms, sterotypy, waxy flexibility, peculiarities of voluntary movement, echolalia, and echopraxia. adj., **cataton′ic.**

catatricrotism (kat″ah-tri′kro-tizm) a pulse anomaly in which three small additional waves or notches appear in the descending limb of the pulse tracing. adj., **catatricrot′ic.**

cat-bite fever an infectious disease of humans transmitted by the bite of a cat, caused by *Pasteurella multocida* and marked by formation of an abscess at the site of inoculation. NOTE: Not to be confused with CAT-SCRATCH DISEASE.

catchment (kach′ment) 1. the catching or collecting of water. 2. catchment area.

catecholamine (kat″ĕ-kol′ah-mēn″) any of a group of sympathomimetic amines (including dopamine, epinephrine, and norepinephrine), the aromatic portion of whose molecule is catechol.

The catecholamines play an important role in the body's physiological response to stress. Their release at sympathetic nerve endings increases the rate and force of muscular contraction of the heart, thereby increasing cardiac output; constricts peripheral blood vessels, resulting in elevated blood pressure; elevates blood glucose levels by hepatic and skeletal muscle glycogenolysis; and promotes an increase in blood lipids by increasing the catabolism of fats.

catecholaminergic (kat″ĕ-kol-am″in-er′jik) activated by or secreting catecholamines.

categorization (kat″ĕ-go-rī-za′shun) the identification of similarities and differences among pieces of received information.

category a unit in a classification system.

Major Diagnostic C. a group of similar DIAGNOSIS-RELATED GROUPS, such as all those affecting a given organ system of the body.

catgut (kat′gut) surgical GUT.

catharsis (kah-thahr′sis) 1. a cleansing of the bowels; called also evacuation and purgation. 2. the bringing into conscious-ness and the emotional reliving of a for-gotten (repressed) painful experience as a means of releasing anxiety and tension.

cathartic (kah-thahr′tik) 1. causing emptying of the bowels. 2. an agent that so acts; called also evacuant and purgative. 3. producing emotional catharsis.

   bulk c. one stimulating bowel evacua-tion by increasing fecal volume.

   lubricant c. one that acts by softening the feces and reducing friction between them and the intestinal wall.

   saline c. one that increases fluidity of intestinal contents by retention of water by osmotic forces, and indirectly increases motor activity.

   stimulant c. one that directly increases motor activity of the intestinal tract.

cathectic (kah-thek′tik) pertaining to cathexis.

cathepsin (kah-thep′sin) an endopeptidase found in most cells, which takes part in cell autolysis and self-digestion of tissues.

catheter (kath′ĕ-ter) a tubular, flexible instrument, passed through body channels for withdrawal of fluids from (or introduc-tion of fluids into) a body cavity.

   acorn-tipped c. one used in URETERO-PYELOGRAPHY to occlude the ureteral orifice and prevent backflow from the ureter dur-ing and following the injection of an opaque medium.

   Amplatz coronary c. a J-shaped angio-graphic catheter used as an alternative to a Judkins coronary catheter in coronary ar-teriography.

   angiographic c. one through which a contrast medium is injected for visualiza-tion of the vascular system of an organ. Such catheters may have preformed ends to facilitate selective locating (as in a renal or coronary vessel) from a remote entry site. They may be named according to the site of entry and destination, such as *femoral-renal* and *brachial-coronary.*

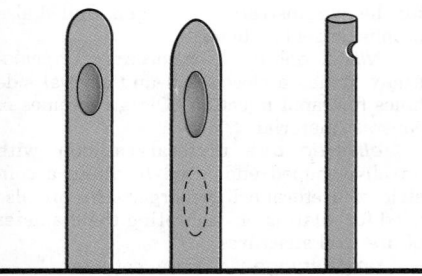

Straight catheters. May have one or two eyes, a round tip, or a "whistle" tip. These catheters are not self-retaining.

   arterial c. one inserted into an artery, used as part of a catheter-transducer-moni-tor system to continuously observe the BLOOD PRESSURE of critically ill patients. An arterial catheter also may be inserted for x-ray studies of the arterial system and for delivery of chemotherapeutic agents directly into the arterial supply of malignant tumors.

   atherectomy c. a catheter containing a rotating cutter and a collecting chamber for debris, used for ATHERECTOMY and ENDAR-TERECTOMY; it is inserted percutaneously under radiographic guidance.

   balloon c., balloon-tip c. a catheter with a balloon at the tip that may be inflated or deflated while the catheter is in place to create, enlarge, or occlude a pas-sageway; see also balloon ANGIOPLASTY. The pressure-sensitive balloon may be used to facilitate HEMODYNAMIC MONITORING.

   Braasch bulb c. a bulb-tipped ureteral catheter used for dilation and determination of the inner diameter of the ureter.

   Brockenbrough transseptal c. a spe-cialized cardiac catheter with a curved steel inner needle that can puncture the inter-atrial septum; used to catheterize the left ventricle when the aortic valve cannot be crossed in a retrograde approach.

   Broviac c. a central venous catheter similar to the Hickman catheter but with a smaller lumen.

   cardiac c. a long, fine catheter espe-cially designed for passage into the cham-bers of the heart, usually through a peripheral blood vessel under fluoroscopic control. See also CARDIAC CATHETERIZATION.

   Castillo c. a cardiac catheter similar to an Amplatz coronary catheter in shape and use, but shorter and introduced via the brachial artery.

   central venous c. a long, fine catheter inserted via a large vein into the superior vena cava or right atrium to administer parenteral fluids (as in PARENTERAL NUTRI-TION), antibiotics, or other therapeutic agents; it can also be used for measurement of CENTRAL VENOUS PRESSURE and for tempo-rary HEMODIALYSIS. See also CENTRAL VENOUS CATHETERIZATION.

   condom c. an external urinary collec-tion device that fits over the penis like a CONDOM; used in the management of urinary INCONTINENCE.

   conical c. a ureteral catheter that has a cone-shaped tip designed to dilate the lumen.

   Cournand c. a cardiac catheter with a single end hole; used for pressure measure-ment, usually in the right heart.

DeLee c. a catheter used to suction meconium and amniotic debris from the nasopharynx and oropharynx of neonates.

de Pezzer c. a self-retaining urethral catheter with a bulbous end.

directional atherectomy c. a type of atherectomy catheter whose direction can be shifted to shave off additional plaque.

double-channel c., double-lumen c., dual-lumen c. a catheter with two channels, one for injection and the other for removal of fluids; called also two-way catheter.

elbowed c. a catheter bent at an angle near the beak, used in cases of enlarged prostate. Called also prostatic catheter.

electrode c. a cardiac catheter containing one or more electrodes; it may be used to pace the heart or to deliver high-energy shocks.

end-hole c. a cardiac catheter with a hole in the tip, through which a guidewire may be passed or pressure monitored.

eustachian c. one for inflating the EUSTACHIAN TUBE.

female c. a short urethral catheter for passage through the female urethra.

femoral c. a central venous catheter inserted through the femoral vein.

fluid-filled c. an intravascular catheter connected by a saline-filled tube to an external pressure transducer; used to measure intravascular pressure.

Fogarty c. a type of balloon-tip catheter used to remove thrombi and emboli from blood vessels.

Foley c. an indwelling catheter retained in the bladder by a balloon inflated with air or liquid; see illustration.

Gensini coronary c. a catheter used for coronary arteriography, having an end-hole to accommodate a guidewire or monitor pressure as well as side holes for rapid injection of large volumes of contrast material.

Groshong c. a single or double lumen cardiac catheter inserted into the right atrium with an external port. Unlike the

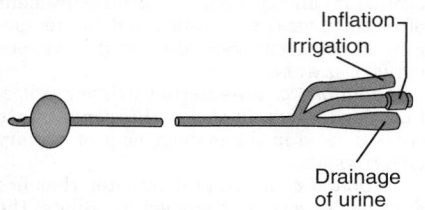

Inflation

Irrigation

Drainage of urine

Three-way Foley catheter. Three separate lumens are incorporated within the round shaft of the catheter for drainage of urine, inflation, and introduction of irrigating solutions into the bladder.

Hickman and Broviac catheters, this type has a valve at the distal end, eliminating the need for clamping and preventing blood from entering it when not in use.

Gruentzig balloon c. a flexible balloon catheter with a short guidewire fixed to the tip, used for dilation of arterial stenoses; the balloon is made of low-compliance plastic to reduce the risk of arterial rupture.

hemodialysis c. a catheter used on a temporary basis for vascular ACCESS for HEMODIALYSIS; usually some type of central venous catheter.

Hickman c. a type of central venous catheter used for long term administration of substances via the venous system, such as antibiotics, total PARENTERAL NUTRITION, or chemotherapeutic agents; it can be used for continuous or intermittent administration and may have either a single or a double lumen.

indwelling c. a urethral catheter designed to be held in place to drain urine from the bladder.

internal jugular c. a central venous catheter inserted through the internal jugular vein.

Judkins coronary c. a preformed J-shaped angiographic catheter used in coronary arteriography to cannulate and deliver contrast material to one of the coronary arteries via a percutaneous femoral route.

left coronary c. one designed for coronary arteriography of the left coronary artery.

Malecot c. 1. a two- or four-winged female catheter. 2. a tube with an expanded tip that is used for gastrostomy feedings.

manometer-tipped c. one with a small pressure transducer on its tip; used in measuring intravascular or intracardiac pressure.

multipurpose c. 1. a catheter with several functions or applications. 2. a catheter for coronary ANGIOGRAPHY that is shaped so that it can be used in either coronary artery.

nasal c. one made of flexible rubber or plastic with several holes near the end; used for the administration of oxygen. Called also oropharyngeal catheter.

NIH c. one used for coronary ARTERIOGRAPHY; it has a closed end and several side holes for rapid injection of large volumes of contrast material.

olive-tip c. a ureteral catheter with an olive-shaped end, used to dilate a constricted ureteral orifice; larger sizes are also used for dilating or calibrating the diameter of urethral strictures.

oropharyngeal c. nasal catheter.

pacing c. a cardiac catheter containing one or more electrodes on pacing wires; used as a temporary cardiac pacing lead.

Pezzer's c. de Pezzer catheter.

pigtail c. an angiographic catheter ending in a tightly curled tip that resembles the tail of a pig.

preformed c. a preshaped catheter designed to require less operator manipulation but usually restricted to a single function.

prostatic c. elbowed catheter.

right coronary c. one designed for coronary ARTERIOGRAPHY of the right coronary artery.

Robinson c. a straight urethral catheter with two to six openings to allow drainage, especially useful in the presence of blood clots which may occlude one or more openings.

self-retaining c. a urethral catheter constructed to be retained in the bladder and urethra; see *Foley catheter* and *indwelling catheter.*

snare c. one designed to remove intracardiac catheter fragments or pacing leads introduced iatrogenically.

Sones coronary c. a woven Dacron or polyurethane catheter used in coronary arteriography to cannulate and deliver contrast material to the coronary arteries via the brachial artery.

subclavian c. a central venous catheter inserted through the subclavian vein.

Swan-Ganz c. see SWAN-GANZ CATHETER.

Tenckhoff c. a cuffed silicone catheter that is permanently inserted into the abdominal cavity for infusion of dialyzing solution in patients undergoing PERITONEAL DIALYSIS.

Texas c. trademark for a commercially made condom catheter.

thermodilution c. a catheter used in THERMODILUTION for introduction of the cold liquid indicator into the cardiovascular system.

toposcopic c. a miniature catheter that can pass through narrow, tortuous vessels to convey chemotherapy directly to brain tumors.

tracheal c. one with small holes at the end, especially designed for removal of secretions during tracheal SUCTIONING.

transhepatic biliary c. biliary c.

transluminal endarterectomy c. a type of atherectomy catheter with a conical cutting window, inserted through the lumen of the vessel; debris is collected in a special vacuum bottle.

transtracheal c. a catheter inserted into the trachea through a tracheostomy for patients who cannot tolerate an oral or nasal cannula.

two-way c. double-lumen catheter.

ureteral c. a long, small gauge catheter designed for insertion directly into a ureter,

either through the urethra and bladder or posteriorly via the kidney.

urethral c. any of various types of catheters designed for insertion via the urethra into the urinary bladder. See also CATHETERIZATION.

whistle-tip c. a urethral catheter with a terminal opening as well as a lateral one.

winged c. a urethral catheter that has winglike projections on the end to retain it in the bladder.

catheterization (kath″ĕ-ter-ĭ-za′shun) 1. passage of a CATHETER into a body channel or cavity. See also CARDIAC CATHETERIZATION and CENTRAL VENOUS CATHETERIZATION. 2. introduction of a catheter via the urethra into the urinary bladder; called also urinary catheterization. This is often a nursing procedure, one that demands strict adherence to the principles of medical and surgical ASEPSIS so that pathogenic microorganisms are not introduced into the urinary system. Since the urinary tract is normally sterile, any break in technique during the insertion of a catheter, or in the care of an indwelling catheter that is left in the bladder for a period of time, may result in a serious infection.

Patient Care. About 40 per cent of all nosocomial infections are URINARY TRACT INFECTIONS, and of these, about 75 per cent are related to urologic instrumentation, usually an indwelling bladder catheter. Prevention of these infections is a challenge to the nursing staff and others concerned with care of the patient.

The smallest gauge catheter that will drain the bladder should always be chosen. It should be inserted gently to avoid trauma, and under sterile conditions to avoid introducing microorganisms into the urinary system. Once an indwelling catheter has been inserted an absolutely closed drainage system must be maintained. Special care must be taken to guard against tension on the catheter and kinking of the tubing, which can obstruct the flow of urine. Catheters should never be pinned to the bedclothing as this can result in accidental removal of the catheter or unnecessary pulling when the patient moves about in bed. The catheter is taped securely to the patient's body. Male, bedridden patients can have the catheter taped to the abdomen to avoid pressure at the junction of the penis and scrotum.

The tubing and collection bag should be arranged so that there is continuous gravity flow of urine. The bag must *always* be kept below the level of the bladder to avoid backflow of urine into the bladder. It also should never be inverted, for the same reason. This is especially important when the patient is being positioned, helped out of bed, or transported on a stretcher. The catheter should not be clamped nor should it be *routinely* irrigated and changed. Most authorities agree that catheters need changing only if they are obstructed, if contamination is suspected, or if there is a malfunction of the apparatus. When the collecting bag is being emptied, care must be taken to avoid contamination of the spout.

Patient care must also include attention to the area surrounding the urinary meatus. At least twice daily, or more often if necessary, the genital area should be washed gently with soap and water and dried thoroughly. Crusts and secretions around the catheter may be removed by gentle wiping with a gauze or cotton square saturated with a mild antiseptic. These measures will reduce the possibility of infection and ensure the comfort of the patient by eliminating unpleasant odors and irritation.

Because of the ever-present danger of urinary tract infection, routine orders for catheterization to relieve bladder distention should be avoided and alternatives to an indwelling catheter should be considered. One-time catheterization following surgery may not be necessary if other measures to induce voiding are tried. Patients who require continuous care because of incontinence or an inability to void normally may respond favorably to measures other than indwelling catheterization, such as condom drainage, suprapubic catheter drainage, and, for some carefully selected patients, self-catheterization.

cardiac c. see CARDIAC CATHETERIZATION.

central venous c. see CENTRAL VENOUS CATHETERIZATION.

urinary c. 1. catheterization (def. 2). 2. in the NURSING INTERVENTIONS CLASSIFICATION, a nursing INTERVENTION defined as insertion of a catheter into the bladder for temporary or permanent drainage of urine.

urinary c.: intermittent in the NURSING INTERVENTIONS CLASSIFICATION, a nursing INTERVENTION defined as regular periodic use of a catheter to empty the bladder.

catheterize (kath′ĕ-ter-īz″) to introduce a catheter into a body cavity; see CATHETERIZATION.

cathexis (kah-thek′sis) in psychiatry, conscious or unconscious investment of psychic energy in a person, idea, or any other object. adj., **cathec′tic.**

cathode (kath′ōd) the electrode at which reduction occurs and to which cations are attracted. adj., **cathod′ic.**

cation (kat′i-on) an ION with a positive charge. adj., **cation′ic.**

cat-scratch disease (fever) a benign, subacute, regional lymphadenitis resulting from a scratch or bite of a cat or a scratch from a surface contaminated by a cat. The causative agent is the bacterium *Bartonella henselae.* Cats thought to be associated with human infection show no signs of illness, and probably act only as vectors of the disease, conveying the causative agent on claws or teeth.

In half the cases, after several days there is a persistent sore at the site of the scratch, and fever and other symptoms of infection may develop. There is also swelling of the lymph nodes draining the infected part. In milder cases, the symptoms soon disappear, with no aftereffects. Sometimes the attack is more serious and the glands may require surgical incision and drainage. Occasionally meningoencephalitis is a serious complication. The disease is generally mild and lasts for about 2 weeks. In rare cases, it may persist for a period of up to 2 years.

No specific remedy exists for cat-scratch disease, although certain antibiotics appear to shorten its course. The main treatment consists simply of keeping the patient as comfortable as possible. The disease can, however, usually be prevented by avoiding cat scratches or bites or by thoroughly washing and disinfecting any wound that does occur.

NOTE: Not to be confused with CAT-BITE FEVER.

cauda (kaw′da), pl. *cau′dae* [L.] a tail or tail-like appendage.

c. equi′na the collection of spinal roots descending from the lower spinal cord and occupying the vertebral canal below the cord.

caudad (kaw′dad) directed toward the tail or distal end; opposite of cephalad.

caudal (kaw′d′l) 1. pertaining to a cauda. 2. situated more toward the cauda, or tail, than some specified reference point; away from the head.

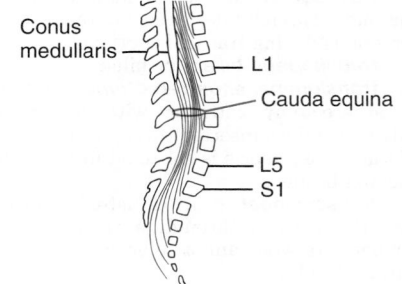

Cauda equina, descending from the conus medullaris of the spinal cord. From Dorland's, 2000.

caudate (kaw'dāt) having a tail.

caudatum (kaw-da'tum) the caudate nucleus.

caudoexternal (kaw''do-eks-ter'nal) situated on the outside of a dorsal aspect.

caudoinferior (kaw''do-in-fēr-e-or) situated behind and below.

caudolateral (kaw''do-lat''er-al) situated on the side and toward the dorsal aspect.

caudomedian (kaw''do-me'de-an) situated on the middle of a dorsal aspect.

caudosuperior (kaw''do-soo-pe'r-e-or) situated behind and above; used only when referring to ocular structures.

caul (kawl) a part of the amniotic sac that sometimes envelops the head of the fetus at birth.

caumesthesia (kaw''mes-the'zhah) a sensation of burning heat even though the body temperature is not elevated.

causalgia (kaw-zal'jah) a burning pain often associated with trophic skin changes in the hand or foot, caused by peripheral nerve injury. It may be aggravated by the slightest stimuli or it may be intensified by the emotions. It usually begins several weeks after the initial injury and the pain is described as intense, with patients sometimes taking elaborate precautions to avoid any stimulus that they know could cause a flare-up of symptoms. They often will go to great extremes to protect the affected limb and become preoccupied with such protection.

Any of a variety of injuries to the hand, foot, arm, or leg can lead to causalgia, but in most cases there has been some injury to the median nerve or sciatic nerve. Injections of a local anesthetic at the painful site may bring relief. Sympathectomy may be necessary to eliminate the severe pain, and in the majority of cases it is quite successful. Psychotherapy may be necessary when emotional instability is suspected. Emotional problems may result from the intense suffering characteristic of severe causalgia. Reflex sympathetic DYSTROPHY (also called chronic regional pain syndrome) is a variant of causalgia.

causality (kaw-zal'ĭ-te) the relationship between cause and effect.

CAUSN Canadian Association of University Schools of Nursing.

caustic (kaws'tik) 1. burning or corrosive; destructive to tissue. 2. having a burning taste. 3. a corrosive or escharotic agent.

cauterant (kaw'ter-ant) 1. any caustic material or application. 2. caustic.

cauterization (kaw''ter-ĭ-za'shun) destruction of tissue with a hot or cold instrument, electric current, caustic substance, or other agent. Called also cautery.

cauterize (kaw'ter-īz) to apply a CAUTERY; to perform CAUTERIZATION.

cautery (kaw'ter-e) 1. a caustic substance or hot or cold instrument used in cauterization. 2. cauterization.

   chemical c. chemocautery.

   cold c. cryocautery.

   electric c. electrocautery (def. 2).

cava (ka'vah) [L.] 1. plural of CAVUM. 2. VENA CAVA.

caveola (ka''ve-o'lah), pl. *caveo'lae* [L.] one of the minute pits or incuppings of the cell membrane formed during pinocytosis.

caverna (ka-ver'nah), pl. *caver'nae* [L.] cavity (def. 1).

cavernitis (kav''er-ni'tis) inflammation of the corpora cavernosa or corpus spongiosum of the penis.

cavernositis (kav''er-no-si'tis) cavernitis.

cavernosography (kav''er-no-sog'rah-fe) radiographic visualization of the corpus cavernosum of the penis.

   dynamic infusion c. radiographic imaging of the corporal bodies and associated vasculature following infusion of contrast medium or saline solution directly into the corpus cavernosum; used for detection of venous leaks.

cavernosometry (kav''er-no-som'ĕ-tre) measurement of the vascular pressure in the corpus cavernosum.

   dynamic infusion c. a graphic representation of intracorporal vascular pressure as a function of infused volume.

cavernostomy (kav''er-nos'tah-me) operative incision into a cavity to allow drainage, such as the drainage of a pulmonary abscess.

cavernous (kav'er-nus) 1. pertaining to a hollow. 2. cavitary.

cavitary (kav'ĭ-tar''e) characterized by the presence of a cavity or cavities.

cavitas (kav'ĭ-tas), pl. *cavita'tes* [L.] cavity (def. 1).

cavitation (kav''ĭ-ta'shun) 1. cavity. 2. the formation of cavities.

cavitis (ka-vi'tis) inflammation of a VENA CAVA.

cavity (kav'ĭ-te) 1. a hollow or space, or a potential space, within the body or one of its organs; called also caverna and cavum. 2. the lesion produced by DENTAL CARIES.

   abdominal c. the cavity of the body between the diaphragm above and the pelvis below, containing the abdominal organs.

   absorption c's cavities in developing compact bone due to osteoclastic erosion, usually occurring in the areas laid down first.

   amniotic c. the closed sac between the embryo and the amnion, containing amniotic fluid.

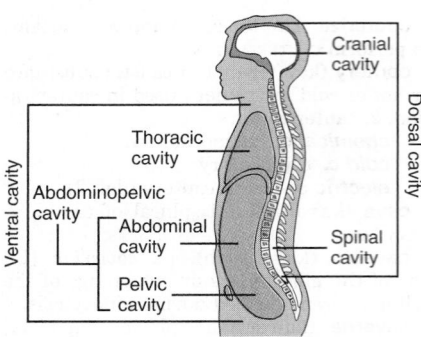

Cavities in the body. From Applegate, 2000.

cranial c. the space enclosed by the bones of the cranium.

glenoid c. a depression in the lateral angle of the scapula for articulation with the humerus.

marrow c., medullary c. the cavity that contains bone MARROW in the diaphysis of a long bone; called also medullary canal.

nasal c. the proximal portion of the passages of the respiratory system, extending from the nares to the pharynx; it is divided into left and right halves by the nasal septum and is separated from the oral cavity by the hard palate.

oral c. the cavity of the mouth, bounded by the jaw bones and associated structures (muscles and mucosa).

pelvic c. the space within the walls of the pelvis.

pericardial c. the potential space between the epicardium and the parietal layer of the serous pericardium.

peritoneal c. the potential space between the parietal and the visceral peritoneum.

pleural c. the potential space between the two layers of PLEURA.

pulp c. the pulp-filled central chamber in the crown of a tooth.

c. of septum pellucidum the median cleft between the two laminae of the septum pellucidum. Called also pseudocele, pseudocoele, and fifth ventricle.

serous c. a coelomic cavity, like that enclosed by the pericardium, peritoneum, or pleura, not communicating with the outside of the body and lined with a serous membrane, i.e., one which secretes a serous fluid.

tension c. cavities of the lung in which the air pressure is greater than that of the atmosphere.

thoracic c. the portion of the ventral body cavity situated between the neck and the diaphragm; it contains the pleural cavity.

tympanic c. the major portion of the middle ear, consisting of a narrow air-filled cavity in the temporal bone that contains the auditory ossicles and communicates with the mastoid air cells and the mastoid antrum by means of the aditus and the nasopharynx by means of the auditory tube. The middle ear and the tympanic cavity were formerly regarded as being synonymous.

uterine c. the flattened space within the uterus communicating proximally on either side with the fallopian tubes and below with the vagina.

cavography (ka-vog′rah-fe) radiography of the VENA CAVA.

cavum (ca′vum), pl. *ca′va* [L.] cavity (def. 1).

cavus (ka′vus) [L.] hollow.

CBC complete BLOOD COUNT.

cc cubic centimeter.

CCNE Commission on Collegiate Nursing Education.

CCNU lomustine.

CCU critical care unit; see INTENSIVE CARE UNIT.

CD curative DOSE; cadaveric DONOR.

CD$_{50}$ median curative DOSE.

Cd 1. cadmium. 2. caudal or coccygeal.

cd candela.

CD4 designation for an antigen found on helper T CELLS; see under ANTIGEN.

CDC Centers for Disease Control and Prevention.

cDNA complementary DNA.

Ce cerium.

CEA carcinoembryonic antigen.

cebocephaly (se″bo-sef′ah-le) a monkey-like deformity of the head, with the eyes close together and the nose defective.

cecal (se′k′l) pertaining to the cecum.

cecectomy (se-sek′to-me) excision of the cecum.

cecitis (se-si′tis) inflammation of the cecum.

Ceclor (se′klor) trademark for a preparation of CEFACLOR, a broad-spectrum CEPHALOSPORIN ANTIBIOTIC.

cec(o)- word element [L.], *cecum.*

cecocele (se′ko-sēl) a hernia containing part of the cecum.

cecocolopexy (se″ko-ko′lo-pek″se) an operation for fixation or suspension of the cecum and ascending colon.

cecocolostomy (se″ko-kah-los′tah-me) surgical anastomosis of the cecum and the colon.

cecoileostomy (se″ko-il″e-os′tah-me) ileocecostomy; surgical anastomosis of the ileum to the cecum.

cecopexy (se'ko-pek"se) fixation or suspension of the cecum to correct excessive mobility.

cecoplication (se"ko-plĭ-ka'shun) plication of the cecal wall to correct ptosis or dilatation.

cecorrhaphy (se-kor'ah-fe) suture or repair of the cecum.

cecosigmoidostomy (se"ko-sig"moi-dos'-tah-me) formation, usually by surgery, of an opening between the cecum and sigmoid.

cecostomy (se-kos'tah-me) surgical creation of an artificial opening or fistula into the cecum.

cecotomy (se-kot'ah-me) incision of the cecum.

cecum (se'kum) 1. caecum. 2. cul-de-sac.

cefaclor (sef'ah-klor) a semisynthetic broad-spectrum second-generation CEPHALOSPORIN ANTIBIOTIC administered orally in treatment of OTITIS MEDIA and infections of the respiratory tract, urinary tract, and skin and soft tissues.

cefadroxil (sef"ah-drok'sil) a semisynthetic first-generation CEPHALOSPORIN ANTIBIOTIC effective against a wide range of gram-positive and a very limited number of gram-negative bacteria.

Cefadyl (sef'ah-dil) trademark for a preparation of CEPHAPIRIN sodium, a CEPHALOSPORIN antibiotic.

cefamandole (sef"ah-man'dōl) a semisynthetic broad-spectrum second-generation CEPHALOSPORIN ANTIBIOTIC administered by injection in treatment of a wide variety of infections, usually as *cefamandole nafate,* a sodium salt.

cefazolin (sĕ-faz'o-lin) a semisynthetic first-generation CEPHALOSPORIN antibiotic effective against a wide range of gram-positive and a limited range of gram-negative bacteria; administered intramuscularly and intravenously as the sodium salt.

cefdinir (sef'dĭ-nir) a semisynthetic, third-generation CEPHALOSPORIN effective against a wide range of bacteria, used in the treatment of OTITIS MEDIA, BRONCHITIS, PHARYNGITIS, TONSILLITIS, SINUSITIS, bacterial PNEUMONIA, and skin and soft tissue infections; administered orally.

cefepime (sef'ĕpēm) a semisynthetic fourth-generation CEPHALOSPORIN ANTIBIOTIC; used in the treatment of infections of the skin and soft tissues and of the respiratory and urinary tracts. Administered intravenously or intramuscularly as the hydrochloride salt.

cefixime (sĕ-fik'sēm) a third-generation CEPHALOSPORIN antibiotic effective against a wide range of bacteria, used in the treatment of otitis media, bronchitis, pharyngitis, tonsillitis, gonorrhea, and urinary tract infections; administered orally.

cefonicid (sĕ-fon'ĭ-sid) a semisynthetic, second-generation, β-LACTAMASE–resistant CEPHALOSPORIN ANTIBIOTIC effective against a wide range of gram-positive and gram-negative bacteria; used as the sodium salt.

cefoperazone (sef"o-per'ah-zōn) a third-generation CEPHALOSPORIN antibiotic with a wide range of antimicrobial activity, especially effective against *Pseudomonas aeruginosa.*

cefotaxime (sef'o-tak"sēm) a third-generation CEPHALOSPORIN ANTIBIOTIC having a broad spectrum of activity, including against penicillinase-producing bacterial strains.

cefotetan (sef'o-te"tan) a β-LACTAMASE–resistant second-generation CEPHALOSPORIN antibiotic effective against a wide range of gram-positive and gram-negative bacteria, used as the disodium salt.

cefoxitin (sĕ-foks'ĭ-tin) a semisynthetic second-generation CEPHALOSPORIN antibiotic, especially effective against gram-negative organisms, with strong resistance to degradation by β-lactamase; administered intravenously as the sodium salt.

cefpodoxime (sef"po-dok'sēm) a broad-spectrum, β-LACTAMASE–resistant, third-generation CEPHALOSPORIN antibiotic effective against a wide range of gram-positive and gram-negative bacteria; used as cefpodoxime proxetil.

cefprozil (sef-pro'zil) a semisynthetic second-generation CEPHALOSPORIN antibiotic with a wide range of antimicrobial activity, used in the treatment of otitis media and infections of the respiratory and oropharyngeal tracts, skin, and soft tissues; administered orally.

ceftazidime (sef'ta-zĭ-dēm) a broad-spectrum third-generation CEPHALOSPORIN antibiotic effective against many different types of infections caused by susceptible organisms.

ceftibuten (sef-ti'bu-ten) a third-generation CEPHALOSPORIN antibiotic used in treatment of bronchitis, pharyngitis, tonsillitis, and acute otitis media; administered orally.

ceftizoxime (sef'tĭ-zoks'ēm) a third-generation CEPHALOSPORIN antibiotic; the sodium salt is used against a broad range of bacteria, administered intravenously or intramuscularly.

ceftriaxone (sef"tri-ak'sōn) a semisynthetic, β-lactamase–resistant, third-generation CEPHALOSPORIN effective against a wide range of gram-positive and gram-negative bacteria, used as the sodium salt.

cefuroxime (sef'u-rok'sēm) a semisynthetic, β-LACTAMASE–resistant, second-generation CEPHALOSPORIN ANTIBIOTIC effective against a wide range of gram-positive and gram-negative bacteria; used as the sodium salt and the axetil ester.

celecoxib (sel″ĕ-kok′sib) a NONSTEROIDAL ANTIINFLAMMATORY DRUG of the COX-2 INHIBITORS group, administered orally for symptomatic treatment of ARTHRITIS.

-cele word element [Gr.], *tumor; hernia; cavity.*

Celexa (sĕ-lek′sah) trademark for a preparation of CITALOPRAM hydrobromide, an antidepressant.

celi(o)- word element [Gr.], *abdomen; through the abdominal wall.*

celiac (se′le-ak) pertaining to the abdomen.

c. disease a MALABSORPTION SYNDROME characterized by marked atrophy and loss of function of the villi of the jejunum and occasionally the cecum. A distinction was formerly made between infantile, childhood, and adult forms, but they are now all considered to be the same entity. Called also celiac or nontropical sprue and gluten enteropathy.

The condition is related in some way to dietary gluten and is either a hypersensitive reaction to a protein in certain cereal grains or a local toxic inflammatory reaction to gluten. A hereditary factor has been implicated because the disease occurs in familial clusters. Diagnosis is usually made in young to middle-aged adults, but the onset of symptoms often is traced to early childhood.

The symptoms of celiac disease are fairly typical of all malabsorption syndromes. Manifestations include large, foul-smelling, bulky, frothy, and pale-colored stools containing much fat. There are recurrent attacks of diarrhea, with accompanying stomach cramps, alternating with constipation. There is some edema and abdominal distention as in severe malnutrition, extreme weight loss, asthenia, deficiency of vitamins B, D, and K, and electrolyte depletion.

Diagnosis is based on intestinal biopsy and demonstrated pathological changes in the structure of the absorbing cells of the small intestine. In many cases, elimination of gluten from the diet produces a dramatic improvement in symptoms and restoration of normal function of the small intestine. Some patients experience remission within a few days, while others continue to have symptoms for months.

Treatment consists of placing the patient on a gluten-free diet that excludes all cereal grains except corn and rice. Since many prepared foods contain wheat, barley, rye, or oats to provide bulk, the patient must be cautioned to read *all* labels on packaged foods, even ice cream, salad dressings, condiments, and foods one would not expect to contain cereal products. (See also GLUTEN.) Administration of corticosteroids may be necessary for some adults who do not respond to a gluten-free diet. There is evidence that celiac disease is associated with lymphoma and carcinoma of the small bowel; this is especially true of patients who have not been treated with a gluten-free diet.

celiectomy (se″le-ek′to-me) excision of an abdominal organ.

celiocolpotomy (se″le-o-kol-pot′ah-me) incision into the abdomen through the vagina.

celioenterotomy (se″le-o-en″ter-ot′ah-me) incision through the abdominal wall into the intestine.

celiogastrotomy (se″le-o-gas-trot′ah-me) incision through the abdominal wall into the stomach.

celioma (se″le-o′mah) a tumor of the abdomen.

celiomyomectomy (se″le-o-mi″o-mek′to-me) surgical removal of a uterine myoma (leiomyoma) performed through an abdominal incision.

celiomyositis (se″le-o-mi″o-si′tis) inflammation of the abdominal muscles.

celiopathy (se″le-op′ah-the) any abdominal disease.

celioscope (se′le-o-skōp″) laparoscope.

celioscopy (se″le-os′kah-pe) laparoscopy.

celiotomy (se″le-ot′ah-me) incision into the abdominal cavity.

vaginal c. incision into the abdominal cavity through the vagina.

cell (sel) 1. a small more or less enclosed space. 2. the intersection between a row and a column in a table where a specific numerical value is inserted. 3. a vessel that contains two metal electrodes (the ANODE and the CATHODE) and an electrolyte solution to produce an electric current; see also BATTERY. 4. the basic structural unit of living organisms. All living cells arise from other cells, either by division of one cell to make two, as in MITOSIS and MEIOSIS, or by fusion of two cells to make one, as in the union of the sperm and ovum to make the zygote in sexual reproduction. Cells are bounded by a structure called the *cell membrane* or *plasma membrane,* which is a *lipid bilayer* composed of two layers of phospholipids. Each layer is one molecule thick with the charged, hydrophilic end of the lipid molecules on the surface of the membrane and the uncharged hydrophobic fatty acid tails in the interior of the membrane.

Cells are divided into two classes, eukaryotic cells and prokaryotic cells. *Eukaryotic cells* have a true nucleus, which contains the genetic material, composed of the

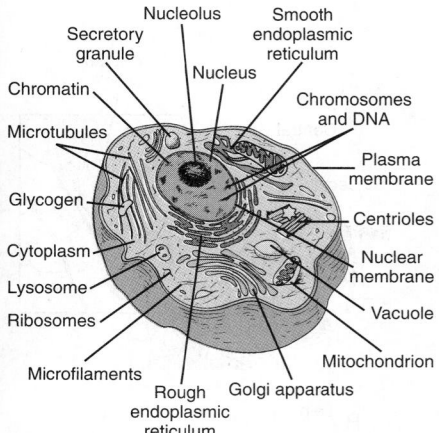

Generalized cell, showing the internal structures (organelles) in the cytoplasm and nucleus.

Labels for figure:
Secretory granule · Nucleolus · Smooth endoplasmic reticulum · Chromatin · Nucleus · Chromosomes and DNA · Microtubules · Plasma membrane · Glycogen · Centrioles · Cytoplasm · Nuclear membrane · Lysosome · Vacuole · Ribosomes · Mitochondrion · Microfilaments · Rough endoplasmic reticulum · Golgi apparatus

chromosomes, which are long linear structures composed of DEOXYRIBONUCLEIC ACID (DNA) and protein. The nucleus is bounded by a nuclear envelope, which is composed of two lipid bilayer membranes. *Prokaryotic cells,* the bacteria, have no nucleus, and their genetic material, consisting of a single loop of naked DNA, is not separated from the rest of the cell. Eukaryotic cells are larger and more complex than prokaryotic cells. They also have membrane-bounded structures, such as mitochondria, chloroplasts, the Golgi apparatus, the endoplasmic reticulum, and lysosomes, that prokaryotic cells lack.

The contents of a cell are referred to collectively as the *protoplasm.* In eukaryotic cells the contents of the nucleus are referred to as the *nucleoplasm* and the rest of the protoplasm as the *cytoplasm.*

The lipid bilayer of eukaryotic cells is impermeable to many substances, such as ions, sugars, and amino acids; however, membrane proteins move specific substances through the cell membrane by active or passive transport.

The cells of the body differentiate during development into many specialized types with specific tasks to perform. Cells are organized into TISSUES and tissues into ORGANS.

accessory c's cells, predominantly of the monocyte-macrophage lineage, that cooperate with B and T LYMPHOCYTES in the generation of the IMMUNE RESPONSE.

acinar c., acinic c., acinous c. any of the cells lining an ACINUS, especially applied to the zymogen-secreting cells of the pancreatic acini.

air c. 1. any minute bodily chamber filled with air, such as an alveolus of

the lung. 2. a cavity containing air and surrounded by a bodily structure, usually one of the bones of the head; see ethmoid air CELLS, mastoid air CELLS, and tubal air CELLS.

alpha c. 1. a type of cell in the ISLETS OF LANGERHANS that secretes GLUCAGON. 2. acidophil (def. 2).

alveolar c. any cell of the walls of the pulmonary alveoli; the term is often limited to alveolar epithelial cells (type I and type II alveolar cells) and alveolar macrophages. Called also pneumocyte and pneumonocyte.

Alzheimer c's 1. giant ASTROCYTES with large prominent nuclei found in the brain in hepatolenticular degeneration and hepatic comas. 2. degenerated astrocytes.

antigen-presenting c's any of several types of cells arising in the bone marrow and migrating to other body sites; their function seems to be the retention of ANTIGENS on their surfaces for presentation to the LYMPHOCYTES, thereby inducing an IMMUNE RESPONSE.

APUD c's see APUD CELLS.

argentaffin c's enterochromaffin cells containing cytoplasmic granules that stain with silver; they are located throughout the gastrointestinal tract (chiefly in the basilar portions of the gastric glands and the crypts of Lieberkühn) and secrete SEROTONIN.

argyrophilic c's enterochromaffin cells that require exposure to a reducing substance before their granules will react with silver; they are located in the fundic and pyloric glands between the basement lamina and zymogenic cells. See also *argentaffin cells.*

Askanazy c's large eosinophilic cells found in the thyroid gland in autoimmune THYROIDITIS and HÜRTHLE CELL TUMORS. Called also Hürthle cells.

automatic c's cells that show AUTOMATICITY; their activity arises spontaneously and does not have to be evoked.

B c's B lymphocytes.

band c. a neutrophil in which the nucleus is not yet multilobar like that of a polymorphonuclear leukocyte but is in the form of a continuous band or coil. Called also band neutrophil and stab cell or neutrophil.

basal c. an early KERATINOCYTE, present in the basal layer of the epidermis.

basal granular c's enteroendocrine cells.

beta c. 1. a type of basophilic cell in the pancreas that secretes INSULIN; beta cells make up most of the bulk of the ISLETS OF LANGERHANS and contain granules that are soluble in alcohol. 2. basophil (def. 3).

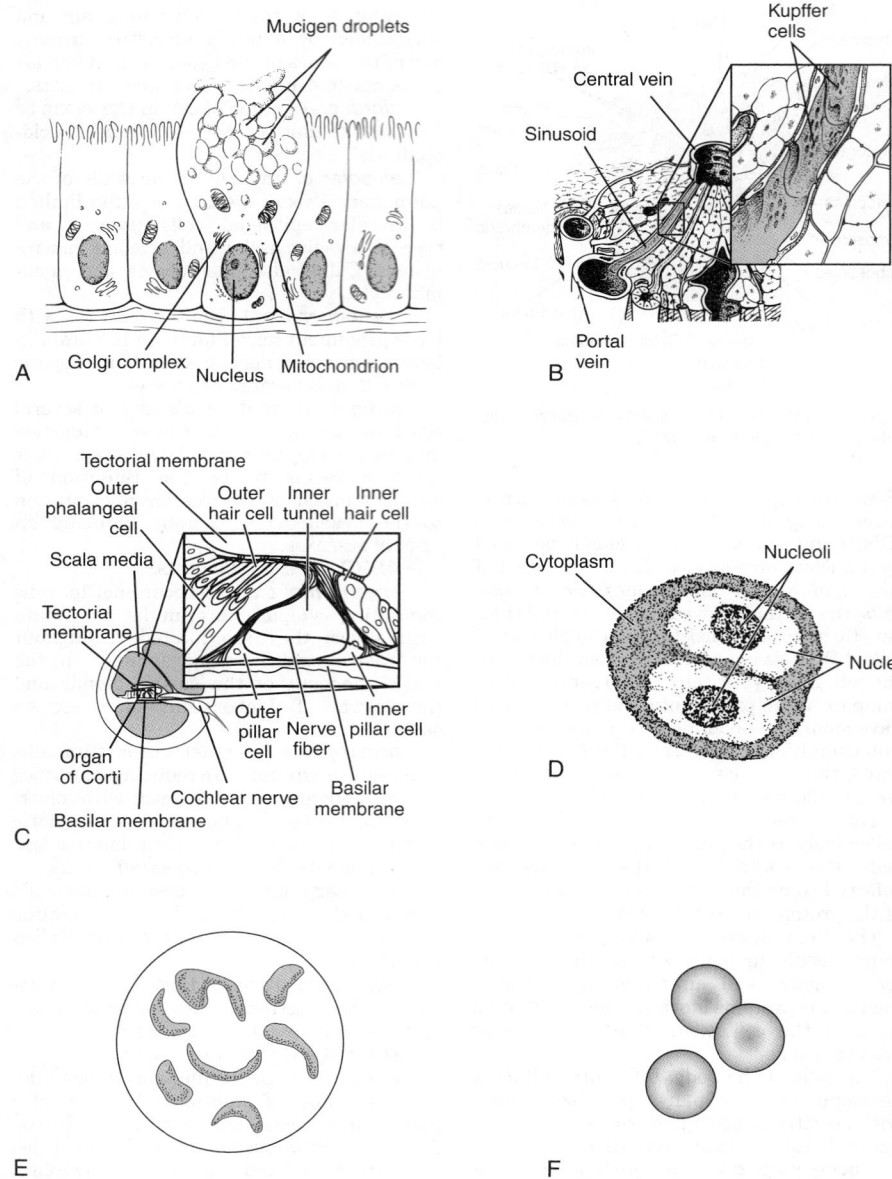

Types of cells. *A,* Goblet cell. *B,* Kupffer cells lining a hepatic sinusoid. *C,* Pilar cells forming the inner tunnel in the organ of Corti in the inner ear. *D,* Binucleate Reed-Sternberg cell. *E,* Sickle cells. *F,* Target cells. From Dorland's, 2000.

Betz c's large pyramidal ganglion cells forming a layer of the cerebral cortex.

blast c. in one theory of development, the least differentiated, totipotential blood cell without commitment as to its particular series, from which all blood cells are derived, preceding a stem cell. Called also blast, hematoblast, hemoblast, and hemocytoblast.

blood c. one of the formed elements of the blood; a LEUKOCYTE, ERYTHROCYTE, or

PLATELET. Called also blood corpuscle and hemocyte.

bone c. a type of nucleated cell found in the lacunae of bone; called also osteocyte.

burr c. a spiculed erythrocyte that has multiple small projections evenly spaced over the cell circumference; observed in azotemia, gastric carcinoma, and bleeding peptic ulcer. Called also crenocyte and echinocyte.

cartilage c. chondrocyte.

CD4 c's, CD4⁺ c's a major classification of T LYMPHOCYTES, referring to those that carry the CD4 ANTIGEN; most are helper CELLS. Called also CD4 T lymphocytes.

CD8 c's, CD8⁺ c's a major classification of T LYMPHOCYTES, referring to those that carry the CD8 ANTIGEN; the major subtypes are the cytotoxic T LYMPHOCYTES and the suppressor CELLS. Called also CD8 T lymphocytes.

chromaffin c's a type of APUD CELLS that stain readily with chromium salts, their cytoplasmic granules taking on a characteristic brown color; they are found in the adrenal medulla and in scattered groups in various organs along with epinephrine-containing cells.

chromophobe c's small faintly staining cells with scanty cytoplasm, found often in clusters in the center of the cell cords in the ADENOHYPOPHYSIS. They are increased in chromophobe or null-cell adenomas.

cleavage c. blastomere.

cytotoxic T c's cytotoxic T LYMPHOCYTES.

daughter c. a cell formed by division of a mother cell.

delta c. 1. a type of cell in the ISLETS OF LANGERHANS that secretes SOMATOSTATIN. 2. gonadotroph.

effector c. 1. a cell that becomes active in response to stimulation. 2. in immunology, a differentiated T LYMPHOCYTE that carries out some part of the IMMUNE RESPONSE.

enterochromaffin c's a group of enteroendocrine cells whose granules stain readily with silver and chromium salts, and which are sites of synthesis and storage of SEROTONIN. Based upon their staining reactions with silver, they have been divided between those that reduce silver without pretreatment (*argentaffin cells*) and those that require prior exposure to a reducing substance (*argyrophilic cells*).

enteroendocrine c's a group of APUD cells found scattered throughout the gastrointestinal epithelium, mainly at the base of the epithelium; their secretions affect gastrointestinal motility, pancreatic and biliary secretions, and gastrointestinal epithelial growth, as well as being regulators of other enteroendocrine products. Called also basal granular c's.

ethmoid c's, ethmoid air c's, ethmoidal c's, ethmoidal air c's paranasal sinuses occurring in groups within the ethmoid BONE and communicating with the ethmoidal infundibulum and bulla and the superior and highest meatuses. They are often subdivided into *anterior, middle,* and *posterior ethmoid cells,* groups of air CELLS named according to where they open into the nasal meatus. Called also ethmoid sinuses.

eukaryotic c. one with a true nucleus; see CELL.

excitable c. a cell that can generate an ACTION POTENTIAL at its membrane in response to DEPOLARIZATION and may transmit an impulse along the membrane; most are nerve cells or muscle cells, although other kinds of cells have also been shown to be excitable.

F c. in bacterial genetics, a cell with an inheritable mating type. The F⁺ cell (male donor) carries the F PLASMID (fertility plasmid), while the F⁻ cell (female recipient) lacks this factor.

foam c. a cell with a fluid-filled appearance due to the presence of complex lipoids; seen in XANTHOMA.

follicular center c. any of a series of B LYMPHOCYTES occurring normally in the germinal CENTER and pathologically in the neoplastic nodules of follicular center cell LYMPHOMA.

ganglion c. 1. a form of large nerve cell characteristic of ganglia. 2. any of those retinal cells that are the third and last neurons in the vertical linkage of the retina and are analogous to the relays in the spinal cord and brain stem.

Gaucher c. a large and distinctive cell characteristic of GAUCHER'S DISEASE, with one or more eccentrically placed nuclei and with fine wavy kerasin fibrils running parallel to the long axis of the cell, imparting a wrinkled, tissue-paper appearance to the gray or bluish opaque cytoplasm.

germ c. an OVUM or SPERMATOZOON or one of their immature stages; see also GAMETE. Called also sex cell.

giant c. a very large, multinucleate cell; applied to MEGAKARYOCYTES of bone marrow, to huge cells formed by coalescence and fusion of MACROPHAGES in the lesions of tuberculosis and other infectious granulomas and about foreign bodies, and to certain cancer cells.

glial c's neuroglia cells.

goblet c. a unicellular mucous gland found in the epithelium of various mucous membranes, especially that of the respiratory passages and intestines.

Golgi c's Golgi NEURONS.

granular c. one containing granules, such as a KERATINOCYTE in the STRATUM GRANULOSUM of the epidermis, when it contains a dense collection of darkly staining granules.

granulosa c's cells surrounding the GRAAFIAN FOLLICLE and forming the STRATUM GRANULOSUM and CUMULUS OOPHORUS; after ovulation they are transformed into lutein cells.

granulosa-lutein c's lutein CELLS of the CORPUS LUTEUM derived from granulosa cells.

hair c's neuroepithelial cells in the inner ear that have hairlike processes and participate in the sense of HEARING; they are found in the ORGAN OF CORTI, ampullar CREST, UTRICLE, and SACCULE and receive afferent and efferent fibers of either the cochlear nerve or the vestibular nerve.

hairy c. any of the abnormal cells with a flagellated or hairy appearance found in the blood in hairy cell LEUKEMIA.

heart failure c's, heart-lesion c's iron-containing, rust-colored MACROPHAGES found in the pulmonary alveoli and sputum in congestive HEART FAILURE.

HeLa c's cells of the first continuously cultured carcinoma strain, descended from a human cervical carcinoma; used in the study of life processes, including viruses, at the cell level.

helmet c. schistocyte.

helper c's, helper T c's T LYMPHOCYTES of the CD4 CELL group that cooperate with B LYMPHOCYTES for the synthesis of antibody to many antigens; they play an integral role in IMMUNOREGULATION.

Hürthle c's Askanazy cells.

immunologically competent c. immunocyte.

interstitial c's the cells of the connective tissue of the ovary or of the testis (Leydig's CELLS), which furnish the internal secretion of those structures.

islet c's the endocrine cells of the ISLETS OF LANGERHANS; see *alpha cell, beta cell,* and *delta cell.*

juxtaglomerular c's specialized cells, containing secretory granules, located in the tunica media of the afferent glomerular arterioles. They cause aldosterone production by secreting the enzyme renin and play a role in the regulation of blood pressure and fluid balance.

K c's 1. cells mediating antibody-dependent cell-mediated CYTOTOXICITY; they are small LYMPHOCYTES without T or B cell surface markers and recognize IgG antibody coating the target cell by means of Fc receptors. Lysis of the target cell is extracellular, requires direct cell-to-cell contact, and does not involve complement. Called also killer cells. 2. cells located predominantly in the midzone of the duodenal and jejunal mucosa that synthesize gastric inhibitory polypeptide.

killer c's 1. K cells (def. 1). 2. cytotoxic T LYMPHOCYTES.

killer T c's cytotoxic T LYMPHOCYTES.

Kupffer c's large, stellate or pyramidal, intensely phagocytic cells lining the walls of the hepatic sinusoids and forming part of the reticuloendothelial system.

LAK c's lymphokine-activated killer cells.

Langerhans c's star-shaped cells with long cytoplasmic processes, derived from precursor cells in the bone marrow, that appear clear on light microscopy and have a dark-staining, indented nucleus and characteristic rod- or tennis racquet–shaped inclusions (Birbeck GRANULES) in the cytoplasm. Langerhans cells are found principally in the epidermis, but they also occur in cells in other types of stratified epithelium and have been identified in the lung, lymph nodes, spleen, and thymus. They have surface markers characteristic of macrophages and are believed to induce contact allergic responses and other immune reactions in the skin by retaining antigen on the cell surface for presentation to lymphocytes.

LE c. see LE CELL.

Leydig c's interstitial cells of the testis, which secrete TESTOSTERONE.

luteal c's, lutein c's the plump, pale-staining, polyhedral cells of the CORPUS LUTEUM.

lymph c. lymphocyte.

lymphoid c's lymphocytes and plasma CELLS.

lymphokine-activated killer c's T LYMPHOCYTES that have been incubated with INTERLEUKIN-2; used as a BIOLOGICAL RESPONSE MODIFIER in the treatment of cancer. Called also LAK cells.

mast c. a connective tissue cell capable of elaborating basophilic, metachromatic cytoplasmic granules that contain histamine, heparin, hyaluronic acid, slow-reacting substance of anaphylaxis (SRS-A), and, in some species, serotonin.

mastoid c's, mastoid air c's air cells of various sizes and shapes in the mastoid PROCESS of the temporal bone.

memory c's T and B LYMPHOCYTES that mediate immunologic MEMORY; believed to retain information that permits a subsequent antigenic CHALLENGE to be followed by a more rapid efficient immunologic reaction than that seen with the first exposure.

Mexican hat c. target cell (def. 1).

mother c. a cell that divides to form new, or daughter, cells.

muscle c. any contractile cell peculiar to muscle. Smooth muscle cells are elongated spindle-shaped cells containing a single nucleus and longitudinally arranged myofibrils. For cardiac and skeletal muscle cells, see muscle FIBER. Called also myocyte.

natural killer c. NK cell.

NK c. a specialized type of lymphocyte capable of recognizing and destroying cancer cells and virus-infected cells. NK cells are important in natural resistance to tumors; when they are exposed to interleukin-2, they are activated and become more effective in killing tumor cells. Called also natural killer cell.

nerve c. neuron.

neuroglia c's, neuroglial c's the branching non-neural cells of the supporting tissue (the neuroglia) of the central nervous system; they are of three types: ASTROGLIA (MACROGLIA), OLIGODENDROGLIA, and MICROGLIA.

nonpacemaker c. a cardiac cell that is incapable of self-excitation and must wait in a state of equilibrium for an outside stimulus.

null c's LYMPHOCYTES that lack the surface antigens characteristic of B and T lymphocytes; such cells are seen in active systemic LUPUS ERYTHEMATOSUS and other disease states.

olfactory c's a set of specialized cells of the mucous membrane of the nose; the receptors for SMELL.

pacemaker c. a cardiac cell that exhibits the property of normal automaticity; examples are the cells of the sinus node and conduction system.

packed red blood c's red blood cells.

parafollicular c's ovoid epithelial cells in the thyroid follicles that secrete CALCITONIN.

pessary c. a markedly hypochromic ERYTHROCYTE in which the hemoglobin is present only as a circumferential rim.

pheochrome c's chromaffin cells.

Pick c's round, oval, or polyhedral cells with foamy, lipid-containing cytoplasm found in the bone marrow and spleen in NIEMANN-PICK DISEASE.

pillar c's rodlike cells in a double row in the inner ear, having their heads joined and their bases on the basilar membrane widely separated so as to form a spiral tunnel. Called also Corti's rods or fibers.

plasma c. a round or oval cell having a single, eccentrically placed nucleus containing coarsely clumped chromatin and abundant agranular, deep blue cytoplasm with a clear zone adjacent to the nucleus. Plasma cells are involved in the synthesis, storage, and release of immunoglobulin (humoral antibody). Pathological plasma cells are seen in MULTIPLE MYELOMA and Waldenström's MACROGLOBULINEMIA. Called also plasmacyte and plasmocyte.

prickle c. a dividing KERATINOCYTE of the prickle-cell layer of the epidermis, with delicate radiating processes connecting with other similar cells.

primordial germ c. the earliest type of germ CELL, originating elsewhere but migrating to the GONADS early in embryonic development. Called also gonocyte.

prokaryotic c. one without a true nucleus; see CELL.

Purkinje's c's large branching cells of the middle layer of the cerebellar cortex.

red c., red blood c. erythrocyte.

red blood c's the remaining red blood cells of whole blood from which plasma has been removed; used therapeutically in blood transfusions.

Reed-Sternberg c's giant histiocytic cells, typically multinucleate, which are the common histologic characteristic of HODGKIN'S DISEASE.

reticular c's the cells forming the reticular fibers of connective tissue; those forming the framework of lymph nodes, bone marrow, and spleen form part of the RETICULOENDOTHELIAL SYSTEM and may differentiate into MACROPHAGES.

reticuloendothelial c. a cell of the RETICULOENDOTHELIAL SYSTEM.

Rieder c. Rieder's lymphocyte.

Sala c's star-shaped cells of connective tissue in the fibers that form the sensory nerve endings situated in the pericardium.

Schwann c. any of the large nucleated cells whose cell membrane spirally enwraps the axons of myelinated peripheral neurons supplying the myelin SHEATH between two NODES OF RANVIER.

sensitized c. 1. a cell that has been immunologically activated by an antigen (primed). 2. an antibody-coated cell used in COMPLEMENT FIXATION TESTS.

Sertoli c's elongated cells in the tubules of the testes to which the spermatids become attached; they provide support, protection, and, apparently, nutrition until the spermatids are transformed into mature spermatozoa.

sex c., sexual c. germ cell.

sickle c. see SICKLE CELL.

signet-ring c. a cell in which the nucleus has been pressed to one side by an accumulation of intracytoplasmic mucin as occurs in KRUKENBERG'S TUMOR.

somatic c's the cells of the SOMATOPLASM; all the cells of the body except the germ cells.

spindle c. any of various cells that are shaped like SPINDLES, being more or less round in the middle with two ends that are pointed.

spur c. acanthocyte.

squamous c's flat, scalelike epithelial cells.

stab c. band cell

stellate c. any star-shaped cell, as a Kupffer cell or astrocyte, having many filaments extending in all directions.

stem c. 1. any precursor cell. 2. a blood cell progenitor, or mother cell, having the capacity for both replication and differentiation; it has PLURIPOTENTIALITY, giving rise to precursors of various different blood cell lines, such as the proerythrocyte and myeloblast, which cannot self-replicate and must differentiate into more mature daughter cells.

Sternberg giant c's, Sternberg-Reed c's Reed-Sternberg cells.

stippled c. an erythrocyte containing granules that take a basic or bluish stain with Wright's stain, seen in BASOPHILIA.

suppressor c's, suppressor T c's differentiated T LYMPHOCYTES of the CD8 CELLS group that inhibit humoral and cell-mediated IMMUNE RESPONSES; they play an integral role in IMMUNOREGULATION, and are believed to be operative in various autoimmune and other immunological disease states.

T c's T lymphocytes.

target c. 1. an abnormally thin erythrocyte that when stained has a dark center and a peripheral ring of hemoglobin, separated by a pale, unstained zone containing less hemoglobin; seen in various anemias and other disorders. Called also leptocyte and Mexican hat cell. 2. any cell selectively affected by a particular agent, such as a hormone or drug.

taste c's cells in the taste BUDS associated with the nerves of TASTE.

theca c's, theca-lutein c's lutein cells derived from the THECA interna.

totipotential c. an embryonic cell that is capable of developing into any variety of body cell.

tubal air c's air CELLS on the floor of the EUSTACHIAN TUBE close to the carotid canal.

tympanic c's, tympanic air c's spaces in the tympanic cavity between the bony projections of the floor or jugular wall; they sometimes communicate with the tubal air CELLS.

visual c's the neuroepithelial elements of the retina.

white c., white blood c. leukocyte.

cellobiase (sel″lo-bi′ăs) β-glucosidase.

cellular (sel′u-ler) pertaining to, or made up of, cells.

cellularity (sel″u-lar′ĭ-te) the state of a tissue or other mass as regards the number of its constituent cells.

cellulase (sel′u-lās) a concentrate of cellulose-splitting enzymes derived from *Aspergillus niger* and other sources; used as a digestive aid.

cellulitis (sel″u-li′tis) a diffuse inflammatory process within solid tissues, characterized by edema, redness, pain, and interference with function; it may be caused by infection with streptococci, staphylococci, or other organisms. It usually occurs in the loose tissues beneath the skin, but may also occur in tissues beneath mucous membranes or around muscle bundles or surrounding organs.

RYSIPELAS, a surface cellulitis of the skin, is characterized by patches of skin that are red, have sharply defined borders, and feel hot to the touch. Other types of skin cellulitis are also characterized by hot red patches, but the borders are less clearly defined. Red streaks extending from the patch indicate that lymph vessels have been infected.

Facial cellulitis is a type involving the face, especially the cheek or periorbital or orbital tissues, although other regions such as the neck may be affected. LUDWIG'S ANGINA is a cellulitis of the tissues of the floor of the mouth and neck, in the area around the submaxillary gland. *Orbital cellulitis* is an acute inflammation of the eye socket. (See accompanying illustration.)

Pelvic cellulitis involves the tissues surrounding the uterus and is better known as PARAMETRITIS.

Cellulitis is potentially dangerous but usually can be treated successfully with antimicrobials. Any cellulitis on the face

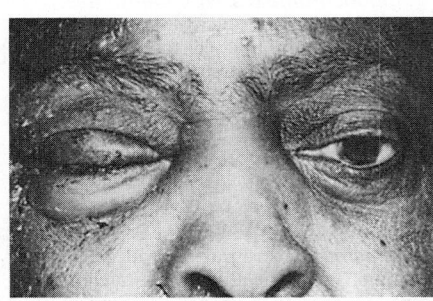

Orbital cellulitis. From McQuillan et al., 2002.

must be given special attention because the infection may extend directly to the cavernous sinuses of the brain.

eosinophilic c. WELLS SYNDROME.

cellulofibrous (sel″u-lo-fi′brus) partly cellular and partly fibrous.

celluloneuritis (sel″u-lo-noo-ri′tis) inflammation of neurons.

cellulose (sel′u-lōs) a carbohydrate forming the skeleton of most plant structures and plant cells. It is the most abundant polysaccharide in nature and is the source of dietary FIBER, preventing constipation by adding bulk to the stool. Good sources in the diet are vegetables, cereals, and fruits.

absorbable c., oxidized c. an absorbable oxidation product of cellulose, applied locally to stop bleeding.

c. sodium phosphate an insoluble, nonabsorbable cation exchange resin prepared from cellulose; it binds calcium and is used to prevent formation of calcium-containing KIDNEY STONES.

Celontin (se-lon′tin) trademark for a preparation of METHSUXIMIDE, an ANTICONVULSANT.

celoschisis (se-los′kĭ-sis) abdominal FISSURE.

celoscope (se′lo-skōp) celioscope.

celosomia (se″lo-so′me-ah) congenital fissure or absence of the sternum, with hernial protrusion of the viscera; see also THORACOCELOSCHISIS. Called also coelosomy.

celothelioma (se″lo-the″le-o′mah) mesothelioma.

celozoic (se″lo-zo′ik) inhabiting the intestinal canal of the body; said of parasites.

cement (se-ment′) 1. a substance that produces a solid union between two surfaces. 2. dental cement. 3. cementum.

dental c. any of various bonding substances that are placed in the mouth as a viscous liquid and set to a hard mass; used in restorative and orthodontic dental procedures as luting (cementing) agents, as protective, insulating, or sedative bases, and as restorative materials.

cementicle (se-men′tĭ-k'l) a small, discrete globular mass of cementum in the region of a tooth root.

cementoblast (se-men′to-blast) a large cuboidal cell, found between fibers on the surface of cementum, which is active in the formation of cementum.

cementoblastoma (se-men″to-blas-to′-mah) an odontogenic fibroma whose cells are developing into cementoblasts and in which there is only a small proportion of calcified tissue.

cementoclasia (se-men″to-kla′ze-ah) disintegration of the cementum of a tooth.

cementocyte (se-men′to-sīt) a cell found in lacunae of cellular cementum, frequently

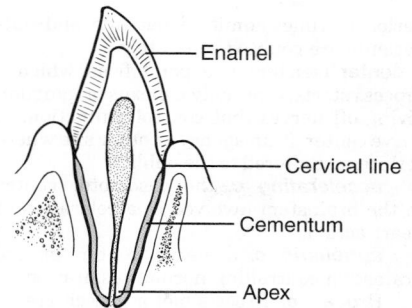

Cementum covering the anatomical root of an anterior tooth. Dorland's, 2000.

having long processes radiating from the cell body toward the periodontal surface of the cementum.

cementogenesis (se-men″to-jen′ĕ-sis) development of cementum on the root dentin of a tooth.

cementoma (se″men-to′mah) a mass of cementum lying free at the apex of a tooth, probably a reaction to injury.

cementosis (se″men-to′sis) proliferation of cementum.

cementum (se-men′tum) the bonelike connective tissue covering the root of a tooth and assisting in tooth support. (See accompanying illustration.)

CEN certified emergency nurse.

cen(o)- word element [Gr.], *new; empty;* or denoting relationship to a common feature.

cenesthesia (sen″es-the′zhah) the general sense of normal functioning of body organs. Called also somesthesia, somatesthesia, and somatognosis. adj., **cenesthe′sic, cenesthet′ic.**

cenosite (se′no-sīt) coinosite.

censor (sen′ser) a term used by Freud to refer to the mental faculty that guards the border between the UNCONSCIOUS and PRECONSCIOUS, preventing unconscious thoughts and wishes from coming into consciousness unless disguised, as in dreams. In Freud's later theory, the actions of the censor (displacement, condensation, symbolism, and repression) are considered DEFENSE MECHANISMS of the EGO and SUPEREGO.

censorship (sen′ser-ship) the action of the censor.

census an official count. In the hospital setting, the total number of patients admitted to the facility by midnight, or sometimes at another time of the day or evening.

average daily c. the average number of patients per day in a hospital over a given period of time; admitted patients and out-patients are counted separately.

center (sen'ter) 1. a point from which a process starts, especially a plexus or ganglion giving off nerves that control a function. 2. nerve center. 3. an agency or other site where services are offered to the public.

accelerating c. the vasomotor center in the brainstem involved in acceleration of heart action.

apneustic c. a nerve center in the brainstem controlling normal respiration.

Broca's c. Broca's motor speech area.

cardioinhibitory c. a vasomotor center in the medulla oblongata that exerts an inhibitory influence on the heart.

cardiovascular control c's vasomotor centers.

community mental health c. **(CMHC)** a mental health facility or group of affiliated agencies that provide services to a designated catchment area.

coughing c. a nerve center in the medulla oblongata, situated above the respiratory center, which controls the act of coughing.

deglutition c. a nerve center in the medulla oblongata that controls swallowing.

detente c. a residential care center of the KINLEIN type, using the ESCA theory of moving as the basis for the staff's actions to maintain the independence of residents who are experiencing lessened physical or mental capacity.

C's for Disease Control and Prevention **(CDC)** an agency of the United States Department of Health and Human Services whose headquarters is in Atlanta, Georgia. It is concerned with all phases of control of communicable, vector-borne, and occupational diseases, and with the prevention of disease, injury, and disability. Its responsibilities include epidemiology, surveillance, detection, laboratory science, ecological investigations, training, disease control methods, chronic disease prevention, health promotion, and injury prevention and control. Its major tasks include the licensing of qualified clinical laboratories for interstate commerce, maintenance of laboratories as reference centers for microorganisms and infectious diseases, and operation of extensive research programs in the prevention, detection and control of disease. The CDC's name has changed several times to reflect its expanding role; it has been called the Communicable Disease Center (1946), the Center for Disease Control (1970), and the Centers for Disease Control (1980). The latest name change, enacted by Congress in 1992, reflects the expansion of the scope of the CDC's mission to include health promotion and education. Because of the widespread recognition of the acronym CDC, that acronym continues to be used by the agency. The mailing address of the CDC is Centers for Disease Control and Prevention, 1600 Clifton Rd. NE, Atlanta, GA 30333, and the website is http://www.cdc.gov.

ejaculation c. a reflex center in the lumbar spinal cord that regulates ejaculation of semen during sexual stimulation.

erection c. a reflex center in the sacral spinal cord that regulates erection of the penis or clitoris. Called also genital center.

feeding c. a group of cells in the lateral hypothalamus that when stimulated cause a sensation of hunger; called also hunger center.

genital c. erection center.

germinal c. the area in the center of a lymph node containing aggregations of actively proliferating lymphocytes.

health c. 1. a community health organization providing ambulatory health care and referrals to appropriate service agencies, and coordinating the efforts of all health agencies. 2. an educational complex consisting of a medical college, nursing college, and various allied health professional schools.

heat-regulating c's thermoregulatory centers.

hunger c. feeding center.

medullary respiratory c. the nerve center in the MEDULLA OBLONGATA that coordinates respiratory movements.

micturition c's a nerve center controlling the bladder and inhibiting the tension of the vesical sphincter, situated in the lumbar enlargement.

nerve c. a collection of nerve cells in the CENTRAL NERVOUS SYSTEM that are associated together in the performance of some particular function, such as a primary AREA or an association AREA.

nursing c. a site where public health or primary care services, including patient education, assessment, and screening and preventive services are provided and managed by registered nurses.

c. of ossification any point in bones at which ossification begins.

pneumotaxic c. a nerve center in the upper pons that rhythmically inhibits inhalation.

poison c., poison control c. see POISON CONTROL CENTER.

rectovesical c. a reflex center in the spinal cord that regulates the rectum and bladder.

reflex c. any nerve center at which afferent sensory impressions are converted into efferent motor impulses.

respiratory c's a series of nerve centers (the apneustic, pneumotaxic, and medullary respiratory centers) in the medulla and pons that coordinate respiratory movements.

satiety c. a group of cells in the ventromedial hypothalamus that when stimulated suppress the desire for food.

senior c. a program supported by Title XX funding, providing recreational activities and lunch for a small fee for older adults in need of socialization. Health assessments and education may also be provided.

sudorific c. 1. a nerve center in the anterior hypothalamus controlling sweating. 2. any of several nerve centers in the medulla oblongata or spinal cord that exercise parasympathetic control over sweating. Called also sweat center.

> **swallowing c.** deglutition center.
> **sweat c.** sudorific center.
> **thermoregulatory c's** nerve centers in the hypothalamus that regulate the conservation and dissipation of heat.
> **thirst c.** a group of cells in the lateral hypothalamus that when stimulated cause a sensation of THIRST.
> **trauma c.** an institution officially designated as a site to which catastrophically injured patients can be brought quickly to receive specialized care. Trauma centers are classified as Level I, II, or III according to criteria developed by the Committee on Trauma of the American College of Surgeons, with Level I facilities having the equipment and personnel necessary to care for the most seriously injured patients.
> **vasoconstrictor c.** a nerve center in the medulla oblongata and lower pons that controls contraction of the blood vessels.
> **vasodilator c.** a nerve center in the medulla oblongata that causes dilation of blood vessels by repressing the activity of the vasoconstrictor center.
> **vasomotor c's** nerve centers in the medulla oblongata and the lower pons that regulate the caliber of the blood vessels and increase or decrease the heart rate and contractility. See also vasoconstrictor c. and vasodilator c. Called also cardiovascular control c's.
> **vomiting c.** a center in the lower central region of the medulla oblongata; its stimulation causes vomiting.
> **word c., auditory** Wernicke's area.

-centesis word element [Gr.], *puncture and aspiration of.*

centi- word element [L.], *hundred;* used *(a)* in naming units of measurement to indicate one hundredth (10^{-2}) of the unit designated by the root with which it is combined (symbol c), such as centimeter and *(b)* to denote one hundred, such as centipede.

centigrade (sen′tĭ-grād) having 100 gradations (steps or degrees); see also Celsius SCALE. (For equivalents of Celsius and Fahrenheit temperatures, see Appendix.)

centigray (cGy) (sen′tĭ-gra″) a unit of absorbed radiation dose equal to one hundredth (10^{-2}) of a gray, or 1 rad.

centimeter (cm) (sen′tĭ-me″ter) one hundredth (10^{-2}) of a meter.

> **cubic c.** (cm³) **(cc)** a unit of capacity, being that of a cube each side of which measures 1 cm; equal to 1 mL.

centr(o)- word element [L., Gr.], *center; central location.*

centrad (sen′trad) toward a center.

central (sen′tral) pertaining to a center; located at the midpoint.

> **c. cord syndrome** injury to the central portion of the cervical spinal cord resulting in disproportionately more weakness or paralysis in the upper extremities than in the lower; pathological change is caused by hemorrhage or edema.
> **c. fever** sustained fever resulting from damage to the thermoregulatory centers of the hypothalamus.
> **c. nervous system** the portion of the NERVOUS SYSTEM consisting of the BRAIN and SPINAL CORD. See also Plate 14.
> **c. venous catheterization** insertion of an indwelling catheter into a central vein

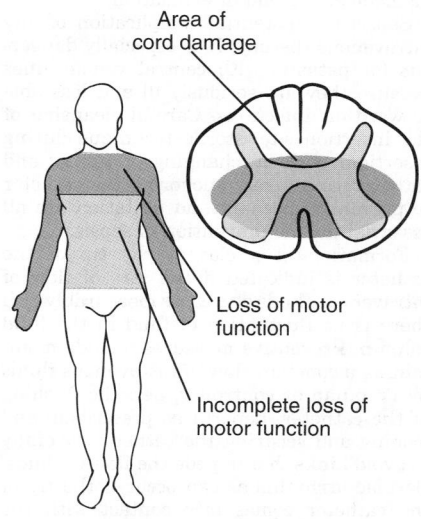

Central cord syndrome. From Ignatavicius and Workman, 2002.

for administering fluid and medications and for measuring CENTRAL VENOUS PRESSURE. The most common sites of insertion are the jugular and subclavian veins; however, such large peripheral veins as the saphenous and femoral veins can be used in an emergency even though they offer some disadvantages. The procedure is performed under sterile conditions and placement of the catheter is verified by x-rays before fluids are administered or central venous pressure measurements are made.

Selection of a large central vein in preference to a smaller peripheral vein for the administration of therapeutic agents is based on the nature and amount of fluid to be injected. Central veins are able to accommodate large amounts of fluid when shock or hemorrhage demands rapid replacement. The larger veins are less susceptible to irritation from caustic drugs and from hypertonic nutrient solutions administered during PARENTERAL NUTRITION.

Patient Care. Patients who have central venous lines are subject to a variety of complications. Air embolism is most likely to occur at the time a newly inserted catheter is connected to the intravenous tubing. Introduction of air into the system can be avoided by having the patient hold his breath and contract the abdominal muscles while the catheter and tubing are being connected. This maneuver increases intrathoracic pressure; if the patient is not able to cooperate, the connection should be made at the end of exhalation.

Sepsis is a potential complication of any intravenous therapy. It is especially dangerous for patients with central venous lines because they are seriously ill and less able to ward off infections. Careful cleansing of the insertion site, sterile technique during insertion, periodic changing of tubing and catheter, and firmly anchoring the catheter to prevent movement and irritation are all essential for the prevention of sepsis.

Formation of a clot at the tip of the catheter is indicated if the rate of flow of intravenous fluids decreases measurably or if there is no fluctuation of fluid in the fluid column. Preventive measures include maintaining a constant flow of intravenous fluids by IV pump or controller, periodic flushing of the catheter, heparin as prescribed, and looping and securing the catheter carefully to avoid kinks that impede the flow of fluids. Cardiac arrhythmias can occur if the tip of the catheter comes into contact with the atrial or ventricular wall. Changing the patient's position may eliminate the problem, but if ectopic rhythm persists, additional interventions are warranted.

c. venous pressure (CVP) the pressure of blood in the right atrium. Measurement of central venous pressure is made possible by the insertion of a catheter through the median cubital vein to the superior vena cava. The distal end of the catheter is attached to a manometer (or transducer and monitor) on which can be read the amount of pressure being exerted by the blood inside the right atrium or the vena cava. The manometer is positioned at the bedside so that the zero point is at the level of the right atrium. Each time the patient's position is changed the zero point on the manometer must be reset. For a multilumen catheter the distal port is used to measure central venous pressure; for a pulmonary artery catheter the proximal port is used.

An arterial line can also be used to monitor the central venous pressure. The waveform for a tracing of the pressure reflects contraction of the right atrium and the concurrent effect of the ventricles and surrounding major vessels. It consists of a, c, and v ascending (or positive) waves and x and y descending (or negative) waves. Since systolic atrial pressure (a) and diastolic (v) pressure are almost the same, the reading is taken as an average or mean of the two.

The normal range for CVP is 0 to 5 mm H_2O. A reading of 15 to 20 mm usually indicates inability of the right atrium to accommodate the current BLOOD VOLUME. However, the trend of response to rapid administration of fluid is more significant than the specific level of pressure. Normally the right heart can circulate additional fluids without an increase in central venous pressure. If the pressure is elevated in response to rapid administration of a small amount of fluid, there is indication that the patient is hypervolemic in relation to the pumping action of the right heart. Thus, CVP is used as a guide to the safe administration of replacement fluids intravenously, particularly in patients who are subject to pulmonary EDEMA. Central venous pressure indirectly indicates the efficiency of the heart's pumping action; however, pulmonary artery pressure is more accurate for this purpose.

A high venous pressure may indicate congestive HEART FAILURE, HYPERVOLEMIA, cardiac TAMPONADE in which the heart is unable to fill, or VASOCONSTRICTION, which affects the heart's ability to empty its chambers. Conversely, a low venous pressure indicates HYPOVOLEMIA and possibly a need to increase fluid intake.

centrencephalic (sen″tren-sĕ-fal′ik) pertaining to the center of the encephalon.

centric (sen′trik) pertaining to a center.

centriciput (sen-tris′ĭ-put) the central part of the upper surface of the head, located between the occiput and sinciput.

centrifugal (sen-trif′u-gal) 1. moving away from a center. 2. efferent (def. 1).

centrifugate (sen-trif′u-gāt) material subjected to centrifugation.

centrifugation (sen-trif″u-ga′shun) the process of separating lighter portions of a solution, mixture, or suspension from the heavier portions by centrifugal force.

centrifuge (cen′trĭ-fūj) 1. to rotate, in a suitable container, at extremely high speed, to cause the deposition of solids in solution. 2. a laboratory device for subjecting substances in solution to relative centrifugal force up to 25,000 times gravity.

centrilobular (sen″trĭ-lob′u-ler) pertaining to the central portion of a lobule.

centriole (sen′tre-ōl) either of the two cylindrical organelles located in the centrosome and containing nine triplets of microtubules arrayed around their edges; centrioles migrate to opposite poles of the cell during cell division and serve to organize the spindles. They are capable of independent replication and of migrating to form basal bodies.

ring c. a common misnomer for the ANULUS OF THE SPERMATOZOON, which is not actually a centriole.

centripetal (sen-trip′ĕ-t′l) 1. moving towards a center. 2. afferent (def. 1).

centrokinesia (sen″tro-kĭ-ne′zhah) movement originating from central stimulation. adj., **centrokinet′ic.**

centromere (sen′tro-mēr) the clear constricted portion of the chromosome at which the chromatids are joined and by which the chromosome is attached to the spindle during cell division. adj., **centromer′ic.**

centrosclerosis (sen″tro-sklĕ-ro′sis) osteosclerosis of the marrow cavity of a bone.

centrosome (sen′tro-sōm) a specialized area of condensed cytoplasm containing the centrioles and playing an important part in mitosis.

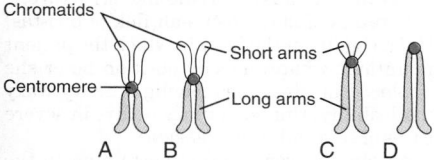

Position of the centromere in *A*, metacentric, *B*, submetacentric, *C*, acrocentric, and *D*, telocentric chromosomes. From Dorland's, 2000.

centrosphere (sen′tro-sfēr) centrosome.

centrostaltic (sen″tro-stal′tik) pertaining to a center of motion.

centrum (sen′trum), pl. *cen′tra* [L.] 1. a center. 2. the body of a vertebra.

CEP congenital erythropoietic porphyria.

cephal(o)- word element [Gr.], *head.*

cephalad (sef′ah-lad) toward the head; cranially.

cephaledema (sef″al-ĕ-de′mah) edema of the head.

cephalexin (sef″ah-lek′sin) a semisynthetic, first-generation CEPHALOSPORIN antibiotic, effective against a wide range of gram-positive and a limited number of gram-negative bacteria; administered orally as the base or the hydrochloride salt in the treatment of tonsillitis, otitis media, and infections of the genitourinary tract, of bones and joints, and of skin and soft tissues.

cephalhematocele (sef″al-he-mat′o-sēl) a hematocele under the pericranium, communicating with the sinuses of the dura mater.

cephalhematoma (sef″al-he″mah-to′mah) a localized effusion of blood beneath the periosteum of the skull of a newborn, due to disruption of the vessels during birth. Cephalhematoma, in contrast to CAPUT SUCCEDANEUM, does not cross cranial suture lines. It is firmer to the touch than an edematous area: it feels like a water-filled balloon. Cephalhematoma usually appears on the second or third day after birth and disappears within weeks or months.

cephalic (sĕ-fal′ik) pertaining to the head, or to the head end of the body.

cephalin (sef′ah-lin) a group of phospholipids found particularly in the brain and other nerve tissue.

cephalocaudal (sef″ah-lo-kau′d′l) pertaining to the long axis of the body, in a direction from head to tail; called also craniocaudal.

cephalocele (sĕ-fal″o-sēl) encephalocele.

cephalocentesis (sef″ah-lo-sen-te′sis) surgical puncture of the head.

cephalodactyly (sef″ah-lo-dak′tĭ-le) malformation of the head and digits.

Vogt's c. Apert-Crouzon disease.

cephalogram (sef″ah-lo-gram) cephalometric radiograph.

cephalogyric (sef″ah-lo-ji′rik) pertaining to turning motions of the head.

cephalohematoma (sef″ah-lo-he″mah-to′-mah) cephalhematoma.

cephalomelus (sef″ah-lom′ĕ-lus) a fetus with an accessory limb growing from the head.

cephalometer (sef″ah-lom′ĕ-ter) an instrument for measuring the head; an orienting device for positioning the head for radiographic examination and measurement.

cephalometry (sef″ah-lom′ĕ-tre) a branch of ANTHROPOMETRY, being the measurement of the dimensions of the head of a living person, taken either directly or by radiography. adj., **cephalomet′ric.**

cephalomotor (sef″ah-lo-mo′tor) moving the head; pertaining to motions of the head.

cephalonia (sef″ah-lo′ne-ah) a condition in which the head is abnormally enlarged, with sclerotic hyperplasia of the brain.

cephalopathy (sef″ah-lop′ah-the) any disease of the head.

cephalopelvic (sef″ah-lo-pel′vik) pertaining to the relationship of the fetal head to the maternal pelvis. Cephalopelvic disproportion is a major factor in delivery by cesarean section.

cephalosporin (sef″ah-lo-spor′in) any of ɩ large group of broad-spectrum ANTIBIOTICS from *Acremonium* (formerly *Cephalosporium*), a genus of soil-inhabiting fungi. Cephalosporins are similar in structure and antimicrobial action to PENICILLIN. The cephalosporins have been classified by "generations" according to general features of antimicrobial activity, with successive generations having increasing activity against gram-negative organisms and decreasing activity against gram-positive organisms.

cephalosporinase (sef″ah-lo-spor′in-ās) an enzyme that hydrolyzes the CO—NH bond in the lactam ring of cephalosporin, converting it to an inactive product.

Cephalosporium (sef″ah-lo-spo′re-um) former name for ACREMONIUM.

cephalostat (sef′ah-lo-stat″) a head-positioning device used in dental radiology, facial photography, cephalometry, and other procedures requiring exact positioning of the head.

cephalothin (sef′ah-lo-thin) a semisynthetic first-generation CEPHALOSPORIN antibiotic, effective against a wide range of gram-positive and a limited range of gram-negative bacteria.

cephalothoracic (sef″ah-lo-tho-ras′ik) pertaining to the head and thorax.

cephalothoracopagus (sef″ah-lo-thor″ah-kop′ah-gus) a twin fetus united at the head, neck, and thorax.

cephalotomy (sef″ah-lot′ah-me) 1. the cutting up of the fetal head to facilitate delivery. 2. dissection of the fetal head.

cephapirin (sef″ah-pi′rin) a semisynthetic first-generation CEPHALOSPORIN ANTIBIOTIC

effective against a wide variety of gram-positive and gram-negative bacteria; used as the sodium salt.

cephradine (sef′rah-dēn) a semisynthetic first-generation CEPHALOSPORIN antibiotic effective against a wide range of gram-positive and a limited range of gram-negative bacteria; administered orally or parenterally.

Cephulac (sef′u-lak) trademark for a preparation of LACTULOSE used to decrease blood ammonia levels in hepatic ENCEPHALOPATHY.

ceramic (sĕ-ram′ik) an object or material that is hard, brittle, and resistant to corrosion and heat, made by subjecting clay or a combination of minerals to high temperatures.

glass c. any of a number of forms of crystallized glass having a variety of properties and uses, including the manufacture of dental restorations; formed by heating to the point of crystallization an amorphous glass matrix to which impurities have been added to provide nuclei for crystal formation.

ceramidase (sĕ-ram′ĭ-dās) an enzyme occurring in most mammalian tissue that catalyzes the reversible acylation (incorporation of an acid radical) and deacylation (loss of an acid radical) in ceramides.

ceramide (ser′ah-mīd) the basic unit of the SPHINGOLIPIDS, consisting of sphingosine or a related base attached via its amino group to a long-chain fatty acid anion. Ceramides accumulate abnormally in FARBER'S DISEASE.

c. glucoside the major sphingolipid accumulated in Gaucher's disease.

c. lactosidosis a SPHINGOLIPIDOSIS in which ceramide lactoside accumulates in neural and visceral tissues owing to a deficiency of a β-galactosidase.

c. trihexoside the major sphingolipid accumulated in Fabry's disease.

cerat(o)- for words beginning thus, see those beginning KERAT(O)-.

cercaria (ser-kar′e-ah), pl. *cerca′riae* [L.] the final, free-swimming larval stage of a trematode parasite.

cerclage (ser-klahzh′) [Fr.] encircling of a part with a ring or loop, as for correction of an incompetent cervix uteri or fixation of the adjacent ends of a fractured bone.

cercus (ser′kus) a bristle-like structure.

cerea flexibilitas (sēr′e-ah flek″sī-bil′ĭ-tas) [L.] a rigidity of the body in which the patient maintains whatever body position he or she is placed in, the limbs having a heavy waxy malleability; this sometimes occurs in severe cases of catatonic SCHIZOPHRENIA.

cerebellar (ser″ĕ-bel′er) pertaining to the cerebellum.

cerebellitis (ser″ĕ-bel-i′tis) inflammation of the cerebellum.

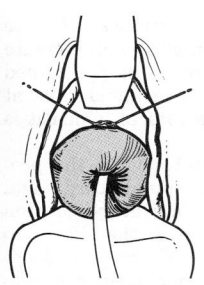

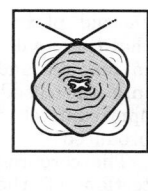

Cerclage of an incompetent cervix uteri, the inset showing the effect of the tightened suture.

cerebellum (ser″ĕ-bel′um) the part of the METENCEPHALON situated on the back of the BRAINSTEM, to which it is attached by three peduncles on each side (the cerebellar PEDUNCLES); it consists of a median lobe (VERMIS) and two lateral lobes (the cerebellar HEMISPHERES). See also BRAIN.

cerebral (ser′ĕ-bral, sĕ-re′bral) pertaining to the cerebrum.

   c. palsy a diagnostic term used to describe a type of nonprogressive neuromotor dysfunction; it is a disorder of movement and posture resulting from an insult to the immature brain. Cerebral dysfunction can occur because the central nervous system has not developed properly from the start (a developmental ANOMALY); or it can be the consequence of an injury to a previously normally developing nervous system. The insult of cerebral palsy is always static and nonprogressive; the lesion itself will not get worse. What often do change over time are the manifestations of the motor disorder and the emergence or recognition of associated deficits as the child grows and the nervous system matures. There is no universally accepted age-of-onset criterion for making the diagnosis. The upper age limit is often set at seven or eight years old for an acquired insult to be classified as cerebral palsy; this is the age when motor areas in the nervous system have largely reached maturation and therefore the potential for motor plasticity significantly diminishes. Prior to this age, function lost by damage to one area of the brain may be partially taken over by another area. However, there is not universal agreement on this age criterion.

   The child with cerebral palsy is at high risk for having associated deficits in neurological, cognitive, and perceptual abilities. Motor deficits are generally identified before delays in language or perceptual abilities are evident.

   Etiology. Cerebral palsy is relatively common, affecting 1 in 200 children. This number takes into account the full spectrum of the disorder, including milder cases, a broad definition of age of insult, and more complete case ascertainment. The exact cause cannot always be determined, but it usually develops before the age of three. The percentage due to prenatal anomalies and insults is usually considered to be 40 to 60 per cent. Damage to the fetal brain can occur as a result of maternal infections, drug or alcohol abuse, other teratogenic exposures, and genetic syndromes. Cerebral palsy is associated with preterm birth between 30 and 50 per cent of the time, but it is not clear whether or not this association is causal in nature. Thirty years ago, the belief was that most cerebral palsy was a consequence of birth-related injury to the brain, and obstetricians often took blame for "causing" the condition. More recently, there has been a shift in emphasis to unknown prenatal events as the causative factors, such as preterm birth, difficult deliveries, and prenatal or perinatal brain injuries. Any situation that interferes with the fetal oxygen supply can produce brain damage and cerebral palsy. These include premature separation of the placenta, prolapsed cord, and chronic placental insufficiency. Other potential causes during the perinatal and early postnatal period include HYPOGLYCEMIA, which can lead to cell death; HYPERNATREMIA, which results in cellular hyperosmolality, vascular lesions, and intracranial hemorrhage; and HYPERBILIRUBINEMIA. Postnatally acquired cerebral palsy is usually considered to be around 10 per cent of cases. Damage to the brain in childhood can result from infections of the meninges or brain cells; near-drowning or similar anoxic insults; cancers that although successfully treated leave permanent brain damage; head injury; or any of various STROKE SYNDROMES.

   Classification. The most common classification for cerebral palsy, based on the predominant clinical manifestations, distinguishes three major types: (1) *spastic*, in which there are exaggerated stretch reflexes, muscle spasticity, and a strong tendency to develop contractures; (2) *athetoid*, with purposeless, uncontrollable movements and muscle tension; and (3) *atactic*, in which the child has poor balance, poor coordination, and a staggering gait.

   Treatment. This varies according to the nature and extent of brain damage. Muscle relaxants and other medications may help reduce spasms. Orthopedic surgery, casts, braces, and traction can be used to correct or prevent associated deformities. Early muscle training and special exercises may also promote function, prevent deformity, and help the child lead a useful, productive life. If muscle training is not begun early, extensive rehabilitation may be necessary to correct faulty habits and poor muscle patterns the child has established. However, it is never too late for a complete evaluation of the condition of a patient with cerebral palsy. A rehabilitation program can produce good results later in life, not only in childhood. Anticonvulsant drugs are necessary when seizures are among the associated symptoms. Special education is important for children with cognitive impairments, as is attention to the other associated problems.

cerebration (ser″ĕ-bra′shun) normal and appropriate activity of the brain.

cerebritis (ser″ĕ-bri′tis) inflammation of the cerebrum.

cerebrocerebellar (ser″ĕ-bro-ser″ĕ-bel′er) pertaining to the cerebrum and the cerebellum.

cerebrohepatorenal syndrome (ser″ĕ-bro-hep″ah-to-re′nal) Zellweger syndrome.

cerebroid (ser′ĕ-broid) resembling cerebral substance.

cerebromacular (ser″ĕ-bro-mak′u-ler) pertaining to or affecting the brain and the macula retinae; called also maculocerebral.

cerebromalacia (ser″ĕ-bro-mah-la′shah) abnormal softening of the substance of the cerebrum.

cerebromeningitis (ser″ĕ-bro-men″in-ji′tis) meningoencephalitis.

cerebronic acid (ser″ĕ-bron′ik) a fatty acid derived from sphingomyelin, which is the principal hydroxy saturated acid from the brain.

cerebropathy (ser″ĕ-brop′ah-the) any disorder of the cerebrum; see also ENCEPHALOPATHY.

cerebrophysiology (ser″ĕ-bro-fiz″e-ol′o-je) the physiology of the brain.

cerebropontile (ser″ĕ-bro-pon′tīl) pertaining to the cerebrum and pons.

cerebrosclerosis (ser″ĕ-bro-sklĕ-ro′sis) morbid hardening of the substance of the cerebrum.

cerebroside (sĕ-re′bro-sīd) a general designation for sphingolipids in which sphingosine is combined with galactose or glucose; found chiefly in nervous tissue.

cerebrosis (ser″ĕ-bro′sis) cerebropathy.

cerebrospinal (ser″ĕ-bro-spi′nal) pertaining to the brain and spinal cord.

c. fluid the fluid within the subarachnoid space, the central canal of the spinal cord, and the four ventricles of the brain. The fluid is formed continuously by the choroid plexus in the ventricles, and, so that there will not be an abnormal increase in amount and pressure, it is reabsorbed into the blood by the arachnoid villi at approximately the same rate at which it is produced.

The cerebrospinal fluid aids in the protection of the brain, spinal cord, and meninges by acting as a watery cushion surrounding them to absorb the shocks to which they are exposed. There is a blood-cerebrospinal fluid barrier that prevents harmful substances, such as metal poisons, some pathogenic organisms, and certain drugs from passing from the capillaries into the cerebrospinal fluid.

The normal cerebrospinal fluid pressure is 5 mm Hg (100 mm H_2O) when the individual is lying in a horizontal position on his side. Fluid pressure may be increased by a brain tumor or by hemorrhage or infection in the cranium. HYDROCEPHALUS, or excess fluid in the cranial cavity, can result from either excessive formation or poor absorption of cerebrospinal fluid. Blockage of the flow of fluid in the spinal canal may result from a tumor, blood clot, or severance of the spinal cord. The pressure remains normal or decreases below the point of obstruction but increases above that point.

Cell counts, bacterial smears, and cultures of samples of cerebrospinal fluid are done when an inflammatory process or infection of the meninges is suspected. Since the cerebrospinal fluid contains nutrient substances such as glucose, proteins, and sodium chloride, and also some waste products such as urea, it is believed to play a role in metabolism. The major constituents of cerebrospinal fluid are water, glucose, sodium chloride, and protein. Information about changes in their concentrations is helpful in diagnosis of brain diseases.

Samples of cerebrospinal fluid may be obtained by LUMBAR PUNCTURE, in which a hollow needle is inserted between two lumbar vertebrae (below the lower end of the spinal cord), or into the cisterna cerebellomedullaris just below the occipital bone of the skull (cisternal puncture). Pressure of the cerebrospinal fluid is measured by a manometer attached to the end of the needle after it has been inserted.

cerebrotendinous (ser″ĕ-bro-ten′dī-nus) pertaining to the cerebrum and the tendons.

cerebrotomy (ser″ĕ-brot′ah-me) incision of the brain.

cerebrovascular (ser″ĕ-bro-vas′ku-ler) pertaining to the blood vessels of the cerebrum, or brain.

cerebrum (ser′ĕ-brum) the main portion of the BRAIN, occupying the upper part of

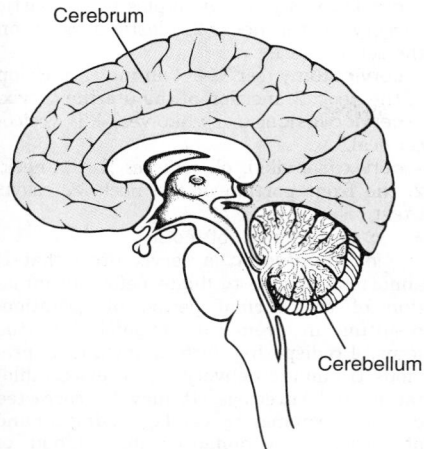

Cerebrum

Cerebellum

the cranial cavity; its two cerebral HEMISPHERES, united by the CORPUS CALLOSUM, form the largest part of the CENTRAL NERVOUS SYSTEM in humans. The term is sometimes extended to refer to the postembryonic FOREBRAIN and MIDBRAIN together or to the entire brain.

cerium (Ce) (sēr′e-um) a chemical element, atomic number 58, atomic weight 140.12. (See Appendix 6.)

cerivastatin (sĕ-riv′ah-stat″in) an inhibitor of an enzyme involved in the biosynthesis of CHOLESTEROL; used as an adjunct in the treatment of HYPERLIPIDEMIA. Withdrawn in the United States because it is associated with an increased risk for RHABDOMYOLYSIS.

certificate of need (CON) a document issued by a health systems agency or local health planning agency, giving formal permission for construction and modification of health agencies, major equipment expenditures, or new health services. An institution or individual health care provider can apply for such a certificate.

certification (ser″tĭ-fĭ-ka′shun) a process indicating that an individual or institution has met predetermined standards; many specialty areas have professional organizations that provide certification to individual practitioners. National associations may control the process and development of certification examinations conducted by their specialty interest groups.

Certified Postanesthesia Nurse (CPAN) see under NURSE.

Certified Respiratory Therapy Technician CRTT; a RESPIRATORY THERAPY TECHNICIAN who has been certified by the National Board for Respiratory Care.

Cerubidine (sĕ-roo′bĭ-dēn) trademark for a preparation of DAUNORUBICIN, an antitumor ANTIBIOTIC.

ceruloplasmin (sĕ-roo″lo-plaz′min) an alpha$_2$-globulin of the plasma, being the form in which most of the plasma copper is transported.

cerumen (sĕ-roo′men) a waxy secretion of the glands of the external acoustic meatus; ear wax. adj., **ceru′minal, ceru′minous.**

ceruminolysis (sĕ-roo″mĭ-nol′ĭ-sis) dissolution or disintegration of cerumen in the external acoustic meatus. adj., **ceruminolyt′ic.**

ceruminosis (sĕ-roo′mĭ-no′sis) excessive or disordered secretion of cerumen.

cervic(o)- word element [L.], *neck; cervix uteri.* See also terms beginning TRACHEL(O)-.

cervical (ser′vĭ-k′l) 1. pertaining to the NECK. 2. pertaining to the neck or cervix of any organ or structure.

c. cancer cancer of the cervix uteri, the third most common cause of cancer deaths in American women (after lung cancer and breast cancer). Its victims are usually women over 40. One of the first warning signs of cervical cancer is vaginal bleeding between menstrual periods, after coitus, or after menopause is established. There may also be increased vaginal discharge. The PAPANICOLAOU TEST should be done routinely every year in women over 40 to rule out the possibility of cervical malignancy. This test identifies cancer in its earliest stages while the malignancy can still be eradicated with relative ease.

Traditionally, a positive finding of abnormal cells from the cervix was an indication for cervical biopsy, which, if positive for malignancy, was an indication for total hysterectomy. Currently, this sequence is giving way to more selective methods of diagnosis and treatment. Special stains and colposcopy are used to define more clearly the nature and extent of abnormal changes in cervical cells. These techniques have permitted a greater use of localized excision of cervical tissues (conization) and CRYOSURGERY of early cancer zones, thereby avoiding total removal of the uterus.

c. mucus method a type of natural family PLANNING; see CONTRACEPTION.

c. rib syndrome pain over the shoulder, often extending down the upper limb or radiating up the back of the neck, due to compression of the nerves and vessels between a cervical rib and the anterior scalene muscle.

cervicectomy (ser′vĭ-sek′to-me) excision of the cervix uteri.

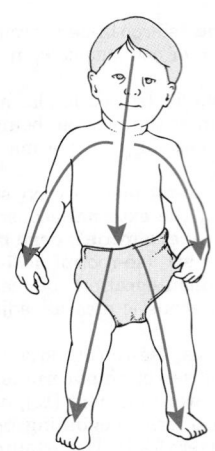

Cervicocephalocaudal development.

cervicitis (ser″vĭ-si′tis) inflammation of the cervix uteri.

cervicobrachialgia (ser″vĭ-ko-brak″e-al′-jah) pain in the neck radiating to the arm, due to compression of nerve roots of the cervical spinal cord.

cervicocephalocaudal (ser″vĭ-ko-sef″ah-lo-kaw′d'l) denoting a pattern of motor development that occurs in widening circles and proceeds ventrally and caudally.

cervicocolpitis (ser″vĭ-ko-kol-pi′tis) inflammation of the cervix uteri and vagina.

cervicodynia (ser″vĭ-ko-di′ne-ah) pain in the neck.

cervicofacial (ser″vĭ-ko-fa′shal) pertaining to the neck and face.

cervicoplasty (ser′vĭ-ko-plas″te) 1. plastic surgery on the neck. 2. plastic surgery on the cervix uteri.

cervicotomy (ser″vĭ-kot′ah-me) 1. incision of the neck. 2. incision of the uterine cervix.

cervicovesical (ser″vĭ-ko-ves′ĭ-k'l) vesicocervical.

cervix (ser′viks), pl. *cer′vices* [L.] 1. neck. 2. the front portion of the neck. 3. CERVIX UTERI.

c. den′tis neck of tooth.

incompetent c. a cervix uteri that is abnormally prone to dilate before termination of the normal period of gestation, resulting in premature expulsion of the fetus. Predisposing factors include a previous traumatic delivery and previous dilatation and curettage. It may be corrected during pregnancy by cerclage using a band of fascia or a nonabsorbable ribbon of Mersilene to constrict the cervical os.

c. u′teri, uterine c. the narrow lower end of the UTERUS between the isthmus and the opening of the uterus into the vagina.

CERVICAL CANCER is surpassed only by lung cancer and breast cancer as a cause of female cancer deaths in the United States. *Cervical erosion* refers to ulceration of the surface epithelium of the cervix resulting from trauma (as in childbirth) or infection. Cervical lacerations are likely to occur during childbirth. Most small lacerations heal by themselves, but more extensive tears in the cervix may require surgical repair. Cervical POLYPS are fleshy growths that form on the cervix, causing bleeding, and can be removed surgically.

c. vesi′cae urina′riae the lower, constricted part of the urinary bladder, near the opening of the urethra.

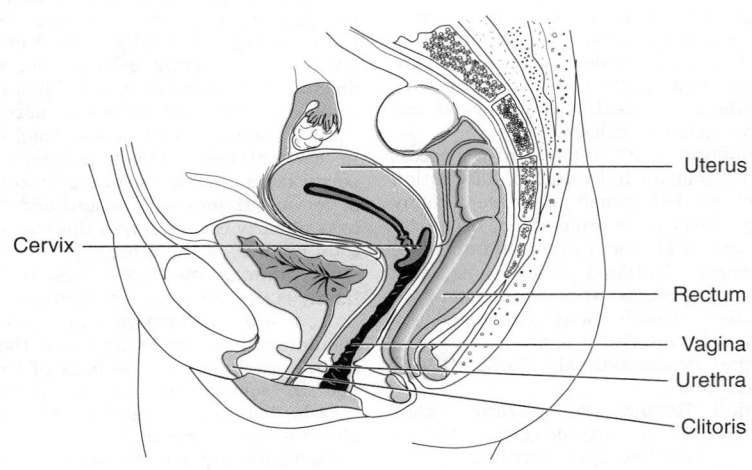

Organs of the female reproductive system. From Applegate, 2000.

cesarean section (sĕ-zar′e-an) delivery of a fetus by incision through the abdominal wall and uterus. The procedure takes its name from the Latin word *caedere,* to cut, and has no relation to the birth of Caesar as is sometimes believed. Indications for cesarean section include cephalopelvic DISPROPORTION, hemorrhage from ABRUPTIO PLACENTAE or PLACENTA PREVIA, fetal distress, and breech or shoulder PRESENTATION. (See illustration.) Called also abdominal delivery.

Between the 1970s and the 1990s the rate of cesarean sections in the United States rose from about 6 per cent of all deliveries to about 20 per cent. The increase was probably due to the development of safer surgical procedures and improved monitoring of the fetus, which can warn the obstetrician that the fetus is in distress during labor. Prolonged labor is now recognized as a serious threat to the fetus as well as the mother. Brain damage and other serious injuries can be avoided by performance of a cesarean section in such cases.

Another factor contributing to the increase in cesarean deliveries is adherence to the old dictum "once a cesarean, always a cesarean." Although the possibility of rupture of the uterus during a subsequent labor is greatly reduced when the incision is made in the lower uterine segment, many patients and their obstetricians are not willing to take the risk. This multiplies the statistical effect of the first cesarean section.

Normal vaginal delivery is preferred to a cesarean delivery, but when the mother or the fetus is in jeopardy, the surgical procedure provides a relatively safe alternative to prolonged labor and difficult application of forceps. Subsequent labors and deliveries can be accomplished by the vaginal route after a cesarean section with minimal risk, provided the patients are carefully selected and closely monitored during labor in a fully equipped obstetric unit that is staffed for any emergency.

cesium (Cs) (se′ze-um) a chemical element, atomic number 55, atomic weight 132.905. (See Appendix 6.)

Cestan-Chenais syndrome (ses-tan′-shen-āz′) a syndrome in which scattered lesions of the pyramid, sensory tracts, inferior cerebellar peduncle, nucleus ambiguus, and oculopupillary center cause HEMIPLEGIA and numbness on the opposite side from the lesions, ATAXIA with paralysis of the soft palate and vocal cords on the same side, and HORNER'S SYNDROME.

cesticidal (ses″tĭ-si′d′l) destructive to cestodes (TAPEWORMS).

Cestoda (ses-to′dah) a subclass of Cestoidea comprising the true TAPEWORMS,

which have a head (SCOLEX) and segments (PROGLOTTIDS). The adults are endoparasitic in the alimentary tract and associated ducts of various vertebrate hosts; their larvae may be found in various organs and tissues.

Cestodaria (ses″to-dar′e-ah) a subclass of Cestoidea, the unsegmented TAPEWORMS of that class, which are endoparasitic in the intestines and coelom of various primitive fishes and rarely in reptiles.

cestode (ses′tōd) 1. tapeworm. 2. resembling a TAPEWORM.

cestodology (ses″to-dol′o-je) the scientific study of TAPEWORMS.

cestoid (ses′toid) cestode.

Cestoidea (ses-toi′de-ah) a class of TAPEWORMS (phylum Platyhelminthes), characterized by a noncellular cuticular layer covering their bodies and by the absence of a mouth and digestive tract. Those most often infecting humans are in the subclass Cestoda.

cetalkonium (set″al-ko′ne-um) a cationic quaternary ammonium surfactant; the chloride salt is used as a topical antiinfective agent and disinfectant.

cetirizine (sĕ-tir′ĭ-zēn) a nonsedating ANTIHISTAMINE administered orally in the form of the hydrochloride salt for treatment of allergic RHINITIS and chronic hives, and as a treatment adjunct for ASTHMA.

cetrimonium (set″rĭ-mo′ne-um) a quaternary ammonium antiseptic and detergent; used as the bromide salt in topical applications to the skin for cleansing of wounds, preoperative disinfection, and treatment of seborrhea of the scalp; also used to cleanse utensils and to store surgical instruments.

cetrorelix (set″ro-rel′iks) a gonadotropin-releasing hormone antagonist, used to inhibit premature luteinizing hormone surges in women undergoing controlled ovarian stimulation during infertility treatment; administered subcutaneously.

cetylpyridinium (se″til-pi″rĭ-din′e-um) a cationic disinfectant used in the form of the chloride salt as a local antiinfective agent applied topically or sublingually to intact skin or mucous membrane.

cevimeline (sĕ-vim′ah-lēn) a cholinergic agonist used as the hydrochloride salt in the treatment of xerostomia associated with Sjögren's syndrome; administered orally.

CEU continuing education unit.

Cf californium.

cGMP cyclic guanosine monophosphate.

CGNA Canadian Gerontological Nursing Association.

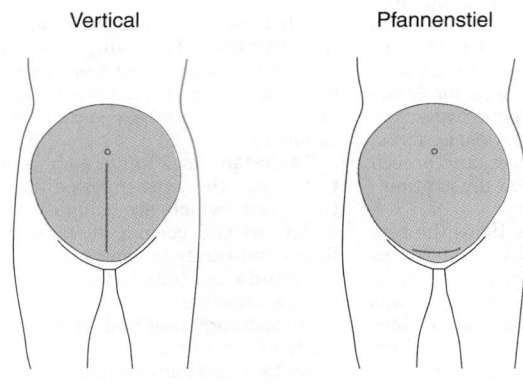

Vertical   Pfannenstiel

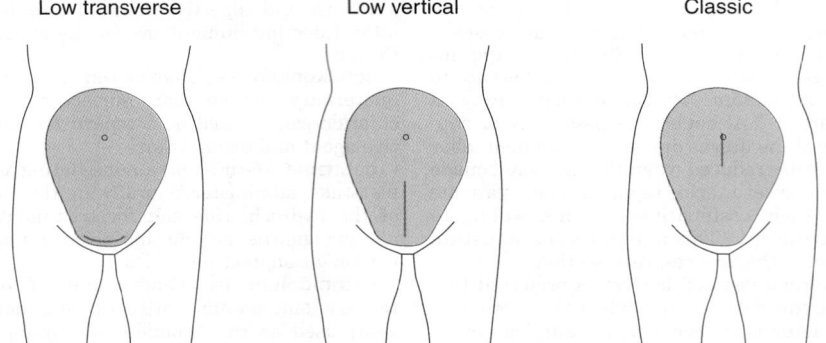

Low transverse   Low vertical   Classic

Uterine incisions for cesarean birth. The abdominal and uterine incisions do not always match. From McKinney et al., 2000.

CGS, cgs centimeter-gram-second system.

cGy centigray.

CH50 see CH50 ASSAY and CH50 UNIT.

Chaddock's sign (chad′oks) Chaddock's REFLEX.

Chadwick's sign (chad′wiks) a sign of PREGNANCY consisting of a dark bluish or purplish-red color of the VAGINAL or cervical mucosa as a result of increased blood supply to the area.

chafe (chāf) to irritate the skin by friction, usually from clothing, or the rubbing together of body surfaces, such as the thighs, when they are damp with perspiration, or the rubbing together of opposing skin folds. The skin folds of the obese are particularly subject to chafing. Tight shoes, badly fitting brassieres, and other clothing that binds, all cause chafing. Babies are particularly susceptible.

The irritation can usually be cleared up by keeping the parts dry, using a plain talcum powder, and, if necessary, substituting clothing that does not bind or rub. In some cases, a sterile dressing may be necessary to help relieve the rubbing. The best prevention is to keep the skin clean and dry and to wear clothing that fits properly.

Chagas' disease (shah′gahs) American trypanosomiasis.

chagasic (chah-gas′ik) pertaining to or due to Chagas' disease.

chain (chān) a collection of objects linked together in linear fashion, or end to end, as the assemblage of atoms or radicals in a chemical compound, or an assemblage of individual bacterial cells.

branched c. an open chain of atoms, usually carbon, with one or more side chains attached to it.

closed c. several atoms linked together so as to form a ring, which may be saturated, as in cyclopentane, or aromatic, as in benzene.

H c., heavy c. any of the large polypeptide chains of five classes that, paired with the L or light chains, make up the antibody molecule of an IMMUNOGLOBULIN; heavy chains bear the antigenic determinants that differentiate the classes of immunoglobulins. See also HEAVY CHAIN DISEASE.

J c. a polypeptide occurring in polymeric IgM and IgA molecules.

L c., light c. either of the two small polypeptide chains (molecular weight 22,000) that, when linked to H or heavy chains by disulfide bonds, make up the antibody molecule of an IMMUNOGLOBULIN monomer; they are of two types, kappa and lambda, which are unrelated to immunoglobulin class differences.

open c. a series of atoms united in a straight line; components of this series are related to methane.

c. reaction a chemical reaction that is self-propagating; each time a free radical is destroyed a new one is formed.

side c. a group of atoms attached to a larger chain or to a ring.

chalasia (kah-la′ze-ah) 1. relaxation of a bodily opening. 2. an incompetent or relaxed cardiac sphincter that permits REFLUX of the contents of the stomach into the esophagus. A cause of regurgitation in infants, it is considered a developmental event with no sequelae and gradual resolution.

chalazion (kah-la′ze-on), pl. *chala′zia, chalazions* [Gr.] a small eyelid mass resulting from chronic inflammation of a meibomian GLAND; it can sometimes be treated at home with the application of hot compresses, but while this method is usually successful with a STY, a similar infection that has not yet formed a cyst, chalazion often requires incision and drainage. Called also meibomian cyst.

chalcosis (kal-ko′sis) copper deposits in tissue.

chalicosis (kal″ĭ-ko′sis) PNEUMOCONIOSIS due to inhalation of particles of stone; called also flint disease.

challenge (chal′enj) 1. to administer a chemical substance to a patient for observation of whether the normal physiological response occurs. 2. in immunology, to administer antigen to evoke an immunologic response in a previously sensitized individual. 3. the administration of such a substance in order to assess for a response; called also provocation.

bronchial c., inhalational c. bronchial challenge test.

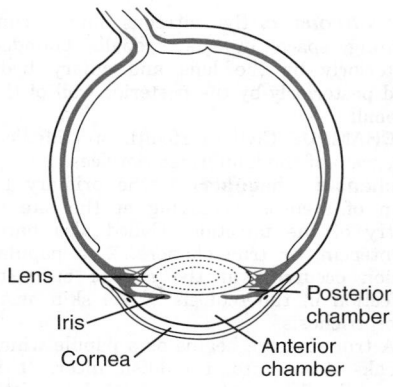

Chambers of the eye. From Dorland's, 2000.

chalone (kal′ōn) a group of tissue-specific, water-soluble substances that are produced within a tissue and that inhibit mitosis of the cells of that tissue and whose action is reversible.

chalybeate (kah-lib′e-āt) ferruginous.

chamaecephaly (kam″ě-sef′ah-le) the condition of having a low, flat head, i.e., a cephalic index of 70 or less. adj., **chamaecephal′ic.**

chamber (chām′ber) an enclosed space.

anterior c. the part of the aqueous humor-containing space of the eyeball between the cornea and iris.

counting c. the part of a hemacytometer consisting of a microscopic slide with a depression whose base is marked in grids, and into which a measured volume of a sample of blood or bacterial culture is placed and covered with a cover glass. The number of cells and formed blood elements in the squares is counted under a microscope and used as a representative sample for calculating the unit volume.

drip c. the expanded portion of intravenous tubing into which fluid falls, where the rate of flow can be monitored if necessary. See also INTRAVENOUS INFUSION.

hyperbaric c. an enclosed space in which gas (oxygen) can be raised to greater than atmospheric pressure; see also HYPERBARIC OXYGENATION.

ionization c. an enclosure containing two or more electrodes between which an electric current may be passed when the enclosed gas is ionized by radiation; used for determining the intensity of x-rays and other rays.

posterior c. that part of the aqueous humor–containing space of the eyeball between the iris and the lens.

vitreous c. the vitreous humor–containing space in the eyeball, bounded anteriorly by the lens and ciliary body and posteriorly by the posterior wall of the eyeball.

CHAMPUS Civilian Health and Medical Program of the Uniformed Services.

chancre (shang′ker) 1. the primary lesion of SYPHILIS, occurring at the site of entry of the infection. Called also hard, hunterian, or true chancre. 2. a papular lesion occurring at the site of entry of infection in tuberculosis of the skin or in sporotrichosis.

A true chancre begins as a papule which breaks down into a reddish ulcer. It is generally firm and accompanied by little or no pain. Although most frequently located on the external genitalia, it may be on the lips or fingers. In women, a chancre is sometimes concealed in the internal genitalia where it may not be seen or felt. Two or three may develop simultaneously. A chancre heals of its own accord without treatment, thus leading many persons infected with syphilis to believe they are cured. They are not, and if adequate medical treatment is not begun at this early and curable stage of syphilis, the disease will progress, doing irreparable damage.

chancroid (shang′kroid) a soft nonsyphilitic venereal sore caused by *Haemophilus ducreyi.* As in SYPHILIS, the first symptom of this disease may be the appearance of a sore, but the sore is soft, as opposed to the hard CHANCRE of syphilis. Chancroid is almost always spread by sexual contact, but in rare instances it may be transmitted indirectly from soiled dressings or towels. In the venereal infection, three to five days after exposure one or more small soft

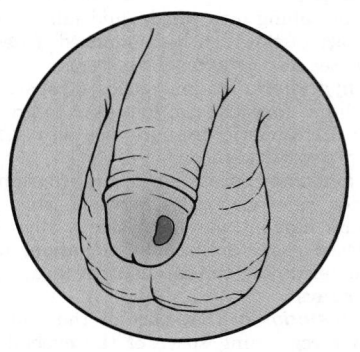

Chancre of primary syphilis. From Frazier et al., 2000.

sores appear on or near the external genitalia. These soon develop into ulcers with irregular edges, and the surrounding areas become red and swollen. In many cases, the infection spreads to the lymph nodes of the groin, causing swelling and tenderness. These masses usually require aspiration.

It is difficult to isolate *Haemophilus ducreyi.* The Centers for Disease Control and Prevention has therefore recommended the following criteria for diagnosis of chancroid: one or more painful genital ulcers, tender lymphadenopathy, suppurative adenopathy, and negative laboratory tests for *Treponema pallidum,* and HERPES SIMPLEX.

The recommended antibiotic therapy is any of four agents: AZITHROMYCIN, CEFTRIAXONE, ERYTHROMYCIN, and CIPROFLOXACIN. The patient should also be evaluated for syphilis, herpes simplex VIRUS, and the human immunodeficiency VIRUS. Patient education should focus on avoiding high-risk sexual activities; unprotected sexual intercourse during treatment places partners at risk.

chancrous (shang′krus) of the nature of chancre.

change (chānj) conversion of something to a different form.

culture c. the sum of the changes that occur in a culture over time in response to various circumstances; such changes result from contact between groups and forces within the culture.

reciprocal c′s the changes seen in leads facing the wall opposite to a myocardial infarction; they were formerly thought to be purely electrical but are now considered a sign of more extensive myocardial damage.

channel (chan′el) a passage, cut, or groove through which something can pass or flow across a solid structure.

calcium c., calcium-sodium c. a slow voltage-gated channel very permeable to calcium ions and slightly permeable to sodium ions, existing in three subtypes designated *L, M,* and *N* and located throughout the body; calcium channels are the main cause of ACTION POTENTIALS in certain smooth muscles, and the N channels regulate NEUROTRANSMITTER release.

fast c. a protein channel, such as a sodium channel, that becomes activated relatively quickly; a fast voltage-gated channel has a much lower activation potential than does the slow type. See also slow channel.

ligand-gated c. a protein channel that opens in response to the binding of a molecule (the ligand) to the protein, which causes a conformational change in the protein molecule. See also voltage-gated channel.

potassium c. a slow voltage-gated channel selective for the passage of potassium ions, found on the surface of a wide variety of cells, including nerve, muscle, and secretory cells; its functions include regulation of cell membrane excitability, regulation of repetitive low frequency firing in some neurons, and recovery of the nerve fiber membrane at the end of the ACTION POTENTIAL.

protein c. a watery pathway through the interstices of a protein molecule by which ions and small molecules can cross a membrane into or out of a cell by diffusion; protein channels play a vital role in DEPOLARIZATION and REPOLARIZATION of nerve and muscle fibers, and may have physical characteristics such as shape or diameter that particularly attract certain ions.

slow c. a protein channel such as the calcium channel that is slow to become activated; a slow voltage-gated channel has a much higher activation potential than does the fast type. See also fast channel.

sodium c. a type of fast channel selective for the passage of sodium ions. Voltage-gated sodium channels are the main causes of DEPOLARIZATION and REPOLARIZATION of nerve membranes during the ACTION POTENTIAL. In cardiac cells they produce phase 0 of the action potential.

voltage-gated c. a protein channel that can be opened or closed in response to changes in the electric POTENTIAL across a cell membrane. See also ligand-gated channel.

water c. a channel in a cell membrane that permits passage of water molecules; chemical substances such as VASOPRESSIN cause the opening of new channels and increase permeability.

character (kar'ak-ter) 1. a quality or attribute indicative of the nature of an object or organism. 2. in genetics, an observable property of an organism that is under genetic control; a trait. 3. in psychiatry, a term used, especially in the psychoanalytic literature, in much the same way as PERSONALITY, particularly for those personality traits shaped by life experiences and developmental processes. Compare TEMPERAMENT.

acquired c. a noninheritable modification produced in an animal as a result of its own activities or of environmental influences.

c. disorders personality disorders.

dominant c. a mendelian character that is expressed when it is transmitted by a single gene.

mendelian c's in genetics, the separate and distinct traits exhibited by an animal or plant and dependent on the genetic constitution of the organism.

primary sex c's those traits of the male and female directly concerned in reproduction.

recessive c. a mendelian character that is expressed only when transmitted by both genes (one from each parent) determining the trait.

secondary sex c's those traits specific to the male and female but not directly concerned in reproduction, such as facial hair, voice depth, and distribution of body fat.

sex-conditioned c., sex-influenced c. an autosomal trait whose full expression is conditioned by the sex of the individual, e.g., human baldness.

sex-linked c. one transmitted consistently to individuals of one sex only, being carried in the sex chromosome.

characteristic (kar″ak-ter-is'tik) 1. character. 2. typical of an individual or other entity.

demand c's cues regarding the purpose of the study or the behavior expected that an experimental subject perceives and responds to.

charcoal (chahr'kōl) carbon prepared by charring wood or other organic material.

activated c. the residue of destructive distillation of various organic materials, treated to increase its adsorptive power; used as a general purpose antidote.

Charcot's disease (shahr-kōz') neuropathic ARTHROPATHY.

Charcot-Marie-Tooth disease (shahr-ko'mah-re' tooth) progressive neuromuscular atrophy.

charlatan (shahr'lah-tan) a pretender to knowledge or skills not possessed; in medicine, a quack.

Charles' law (sharlz) at a constant pressure the volume of a given mass of perfect gas varies directly with the absolute temperature.

charleyhorse (chahr'le-hors) popular term for soreness and stiffness in a muscle, especially the quadriceps femoris muscles, due to overstrain or contusion. It usually occurs when muscles that have not been conditioned for hard use are put under a strain, with the result that some of the muscle fibers are strained or may actually tear. It is characterized by soreness, stiffness, and pain that often comes on very suddenly. Heat, such as from a warm bath, helps the condition, and aspirin is useful in relieving the pain. If the pain persists for several days, there may be some other muscle injury and a health care provider should be consulted.

chart (chart) a record of data in graphic or tabular form.

Amsler c's a set of charts used for the detection and measurement of visual field defects. The charts consist of various geometric patterns, such as grids or parallel lines, printed in white on a black background, with a dot in the center. The patient looks at the dot with one eye closed; defects in the visual field will cause the patient to see irregularities or blank spots in the pattern.

dental c. a record of a patient's dental history and treatment (see illustration).

genealogical c. a graph showing various descendants of a common ancestor, used to indicate those affected by genetically determined disease.

Ishihara c. the PSEUDOISOCHROMATIC chart used in the ISHIHARA TEST. (See Atlas 4, Part F.)

reading c. a chart with material printed in gradually increasing type sizes, used in testing acuity of near vision.

Reuss' c. a chart similar to the Ishihara CHART for testing color vision.

c. rounds review of a hospitalized patient's current records by a group of health care professionals. Chart rounds can be undertaken for a variety of reasons such as assessment of patient progress, planning of interventions, or education of staff.

Snellen's c. a chart printed with block letters in gradually decreasing sizes, used in testing visual acuity. (See accompanying illustration.)

charting (chahrt'ing) the keeping of a clinical record of the important facts about a patient and the progress of his or her illness. The patient's chart most often contains the history; laboratory reports; list of medications; results of physical examinations, consultations, and special diagnostic tests; treatments of the health care team; any problems; and the patient's response to interventions and treatment. See also PROBLEM-ORIENTED RECORD.

c. by exception a method of charting designed to minimize clerical activities; a notation is made only when there is a

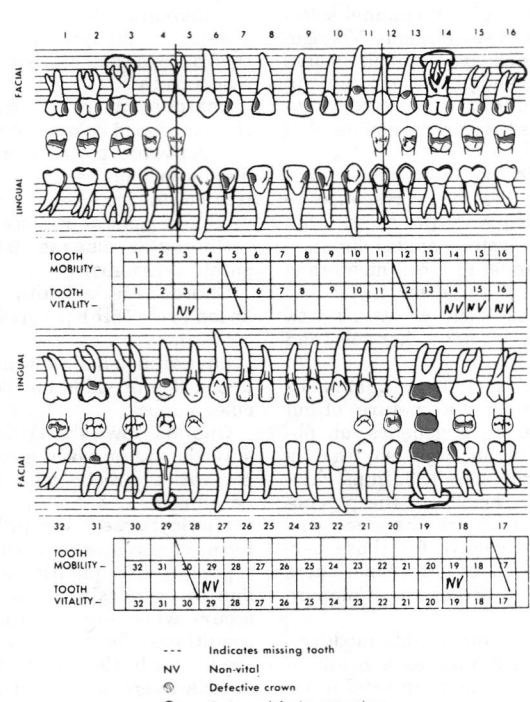

Dental chart showing caries and defective restorations. Adequate restorations are not charted. From Barsh, 1981.

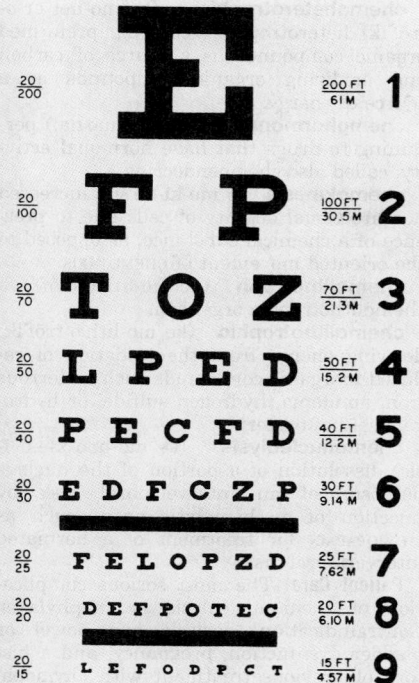

The Snellen chart is used to assess distant vision. From Malarkey and McMorrow, 2000.

deviation from the baseline or expected outcome, or when a procedure or expected activity is to be omitted.

ChB [L.] Chirur′giae Baccalau′reus (Bachelor of Surgery).

CHD coronary heart disease.

checking (chek′ing) inspecting, TESTING, or MONITORING.

controlled substance c. in the NURSING INTERVENTIONS CLASSIFICATION, a nursing INTERVENTION defined as promoting appropriate use and maintaining security of controlled SUBSTANCES.

emergency cart c. in the NURSING INTERVENTIONS CLASSIFICATION, a nursing INTERVENTION defined as systematic review of the contents of an emergency cart at established time intervals.

Chédiak-Higashi syndrome a lethal, progressive, autosomal recessive, systemic disorder associated with oculocutaneous albinism, massive leukocyte inclusions (giant lysosomes), histiocytic infiltration of multiple body organs, development of pancytopenia, hepatosplenomegaly, recurrent or persistent bacterial infections, and a possible predisposition to development of malignant lymphoma.

cheek (chēk) 1. the fleshy portion of either side of the face. Called also bucca and mala. 2. any fleshy protuberance resembling the cheek of the face.

cleft c. facial cleft caused by developmental failure of union between the maxillary and frontonasal prominences.

cheil(o)- word element [Gr.], *lip.*

cheilectropion (ki″lek-tro′pe-on) eversion of the lip.

cheilitis (ki-li′tis) inflammation of the lips.

actinic c., c. acti′nica involvement of the lips after exposure to actinic RAYS, with pain and swelling and development of a scaly crust on the vermilion border; it may be acute or chronic. Called also solar cheilitis. (See Atlas 3, Part E.)

angular c. single or multiple fissures and cracks at the corner of the mouth on one side or both sides, which in advanced stages may spread to the lips and cheeks. Causes include primary or superimposed infection with microorganisms such as *Candida albicans*, staphylococci, or streptococci; poor hygiene; drooling of saliva; overclosure of the jaws in patients without teeth or with ill-fitting dentures; riboflavin deficiency; or other causes. Called also perlèche.

solar c. actinic cheilitis.

cheilognathopalatoschisis (ki″lo-na″tho-pal″ah-tos′ki-sis) cleft of the lip, upper jaw, and hard and soft palates.

cheiloplasty (ki′lo-plas″te) plastic surgery of the lip.

cheilorrhaphy (ki-lor′ah-fe) suture of the lip; as in surgical repair of a congenital cleft lip.

cheilosis (ki-lo′sis) fissuring and dry scaling of the vermilion surface of the lips and angles of the mouth, a characteristic of riboflavin deficiency.

cheilotomy (ki-lot′ah-me) incision of the lip.

cheir(o)- word element [Gr.], *hand;* see also words beginning CHIR(O)-.

cheiralgia (ki-ral′jah) pain in the hand.

cheirarthritis (ki″rahr-thri′tis) inflammation of the joints of the hand and fingers.

cheirokinesthesia (ki″ro-kin″es-the′zhah) subjective perception of movements of the hand, especially in writing.

cheiropodalgia (ki″ro-po-dal′jah) pain in the hands and feet.

cheiropompholyx (ki″ro-pom′fo-liks) pompholyx.

cheirospasm (ki′ro-spazm) spasm of the muscles of the hand.

chelate (ke′lāt) 1. to combine with a metal in complexes in which the metal is part of a ring. 2. by extension, a chemical compound in which a metallic ion is sequestered and firmly bound into a ring within the chelating molecule. Chelates are used in chemotherapy of metal poisoning.

cheloid (ke'loid) keloid.

chem(o)- word element [Gr.], *chemical; chemistry.*

chemabrasion (kēm″ah-bra'zhun) superficial destruction of the epidermis and the upper layer of the dermis by application of a CAUTERANT to the skin; done to remove marks and lesions such as scars or tattoos. Called also chemical peel.

chemexfoliation (kēm″eks-fo″le-a'shun) chemabrasion.

chemical (kem'ĭ-k'l) 1. pertaining to chemistry. 2. a substance composed of chemical elements, or obtained by chemical processes.

chemiluminescence (kem″ĭ-loo″mĭ-nes'-ens) luminescence produced by direct transformation of chemical energy into light energy.

chemist (kem'ist) 1. an expert in chemistry. 2. (British) pharmacist.

chemistry (kem'is-tre) the science that treats of the elements and atomic relations of matter, and of the various compounds of the elements.

   colloid c. chemistry dealing with the nature and composition of colloids.

   inorganic c. the branch of chemistry dealing with compounds that do not contain carbon-carbon bonds (inorganic compounds).

   organic c. the branch of chemistry dealing with organic compounds, those characterized by carbon-carbon bonds, i.e., all compounds containing carbon except oxides of carbon, carbides, and carbonates.

chemoattractant (ke″mo-ah-trak'tant) a chemical (chemotactic) agent that induces an organism or a cell (e.g., a leukocyte) to migrate toward it.

chemoautotroph (ke″mo-aw'to-trōf) a chemoautotrophic organism.

chemoautotrophic (ke″mo-au″to-trof'ik) capable of synthesizing cell constituents from carbon dioxide by means of energy derived from inorganic reactions.

chemocautery (ke″mo-kaw'ter-e) CAUTERIZATION by application of a caustic substance.

chemodectoma (ke″mo-dek-to'mah) any benign, chromaffin-negative tumor of the chemoreceptor system, such as a tumor of the carotid, aortic, or tympanic body.

chemoendocrine (ke″mo-en'do-krīn) chemohormonal.

chemoheterotroph (ke″mo-het'er-o-trōf) a chemoheterotrophic organism.

chemoheterotrophic (ke″mo-het'er-o-trōf'ik) heterotrophic; requiring preformed organic compounds as a source of carbon and oxidizing organic compounds as a source of energy.

chemohormonal (ke″mo-hor-mo'nal) pertaining to drugs that have hormonal activity; called also chemoendocrine.

chemokinesis (ke″mo-kĭ-ne'sis) increased nondirectional activity of cells due to presence of a chemical substance, as opposed to the oriented movement of CHEMOTAXIS.

chemolithotroph (ke″mo-lith'o-trōf) a chemolithotrophic organism.

chemolithotrophic (ke″mo-lith'o-trōf'ik) deriving energy from the oxidation of reduced inorganic compounds such as ferrous iron, ammonia, hydrogen sulfide, or hydrogen; said of bacteria.

chemonucleolysis (ke″mo-noo″kle-ol'ĭ-sis) dissolution of a portion of the nucleus pulposus of an intervertebral disk by injection of a chemolytic agent such as CHYMOPAPAIN for treatment of a herniated intervertebral disk.

Patient Care. The most serious complication of chemonucleolysis is anaphylaxis. Contraindications include any bowel or bladder dysfunction, pregnancy, and a history of previous treatment with chymopapain, which could increase the possibility of an allergic reaction. Any of these conditions identified during preoperative assessment should be reported to the surgeon immediately.

Postoperatively the patient is monitored for signs of anaphylaxis, alteration in neurological status, and discomfort or pain due to muscle spasm.

chemo-organotroph (ke″mo-or'gah-no-trōf) a chemo-organotrophic organism.

chemo-organotrophic (ke″mo-or'gah-no-trōf'ik) deriving energy from the oxidation of organic compounds; said of bacteria.

chemopallidectomy (ke″mo-pal″ĭ-dek'to-me) destruction of tissue of the globus pallidus by a chemical agent.

chemoprophylaxis (ke″mo-pro″fĭ-lak'sis) prevention of disease by chemical means.

chemoprotectant 1. providing protection against the toxic effects of chemotherapy agents. 2. an agent that so acts.

chemopsychiatry (ke″mo-si-ki'ah-tre) the treatment of mental and emotional disorders by the use of drugs.

chemoradiotherapy combined modality THERAPY using CHEMOTHERAPY and RADIOTHERAPY, designed to reduce the need for surgery by maximizing the interaction between the radiation and the therapeutic agent or agents.

chemoreceptor (ke″mo-re-sep'ter) any of the special cells or organs adapted for excitation by chemical substances and located outside the central nervous system. The *carotid* and *aortic bodies* are chemoreceptors in the large arteries of the thorax and the neck; they are responsive to changes in the oxygen, carbon dioxide, and hydrogen ion concentrations in the blood. When oxygen concentration falls below normal in the arterial blood, they send impulses to stimulate the respiratory center so that there will be an increase in alveolar ventilation and thus an increase in the intake of oxygen by the lungs. Other chemoreceptors are the *taste buds,* which are sensitive to chemicals in the mouth, and the *olfactory cells* of the nose, which detect certain chemicals in the air.

chemosensitive (ke″mo-sen′sĭ-tiv) sensitive to changes in chemical composition.

chemosensory (ke″mo-sen′so-re) relating to the perception of chemical substances, as in odor detection.

chemosis (ke-mo′sis) edema of the conjunctiva of the eye.

chemosurgery (ke″mo-ser′jer-e) the removal of diseased tissue after first chemically treating it.

chemosynthesis (ke″mo-sin′thĕ-sis) the building up of chemical compounds under the influence of chemical stimulation, specifically the formation of carbohydrates from carbon dioxide and water as a result of energy derived from chemical reactions. adj., **chemosynthet′ic.**

chemotaxin (ke″mo-tak′sin) a substance, e.g., a complement component, that induces CHEMOTAXIS.

chemotaxis (ke″mo-tak′sis) list; movement (TAXIS) in response to the influence of chemical stimulation. adj., **chemotac′tic.**

   leukocyte c. the response of LEUKOCYTES to products formed in immunologic reactions, wherein leukocytes are attracted to and accumulate at the site of the reaction; a part of the inflammatory RESPONSE. See also INFLAMMATION.

chemotherapy (ke″mo-ther′ah-pe) the treatment of illness by chemical means; that is, by medication. adj., **chemotherapeu′tic.** The term was first applied to the treatment of infectious diseases, but it now is used to include treatment of mental illness and CANCER with drugs.

chemotic (ke-mot′ik) pertaining to or affected with CHEMOSIS.

chemotroph (ke′mo-trōf) a microorganism that derives energy from the oxidation of inorganic compounds.

chemotrophic (ke″mo-trōf′ik) deriving energy from the oxidation of organic (chemoorganotrophic) or inorganic (chemolithotrophic) compounds; said of bacteria.

chemotropism (ke-mot′ro-pizm) TROPISM elicited by chemical stimulation.

chenodeoxycholic acid (ke″no-de-ok″se-ko′lic) one of the primary BILE ACIDS in humans, usually found conjugated with GLYCINE or TAURINE; it facilitates fat absorption and cholesterol excretion. The pharmaceutical preparation, called CHENODIOL, is used in treatment of gallstones.

chenodiol (ke″no-di′ol) nonproprietary drug name for the bile acid CHENODEOXYCHOLIC ACID; administered orally to dissolve radiolucent cholesterol GALLSTONES; most are dissolved in one to two years of therapy.

cherubism (cher′ōo-bizm) hereditary and progressive bilateral swelling at the angle of the mandible, sometimes involving the entire jaw, imparting a cherubic look to the face, in some cases enhanced by upturning of the eyes.

chest (chest) thorax.

   barrel c. a rounded, bulging chest with abnormal increase in the anteroposterior diameter, showing little movement on respiration; seen in EMPHYSEMA, KYPHOSIS, and CHRONIC AIRFLOW LIMITATION.

   flail c. see FLAIL CHEST.

   funnel c. pectus excavatum.

   pigeon c. pectus carinatum.

   c. tube a tube inserted into the thoracic cavity for the purpose of removing air or fluid, or both. Chest tubes are attached to a closed drainage system (see illustration) so that normal pressures within the alveoli and the pleural cavity can be restored. These pressures are essential to adequate expansion and reinflation of the lung.

Chest tubes are indicated when the normally airtight pleural space has been penetrated through surgery or trauma, when a

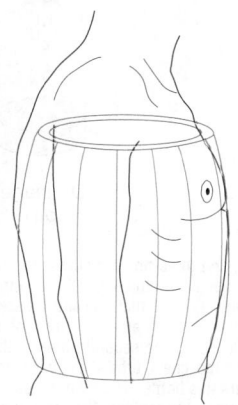

Barrel chest. From Herlihy et al., 2000.

defect in the alveoli allows air to enter the intrapleural space, and when there is an accumulation of fluid, as from PLEURAL EFFUSION. The effect of excessive amounts of air and fluid within the pleural space is collapse of the lung and the danger of MEDIASTINAL SHIFT.

Patient Care. It is important that those responsible for the personal care of a patient who has chest tubes inserted understand the basic mechanics of inflation and deflation of the LUNG, and the purpose of the

tubes and their location in each patient. In some cases one tube is inserted higher in the thorax (usually in the 2nd intercostal space) to remove air, and a second tube is placed lower (in the 8th or 9th intercostal space) to drain off fluids.

Chest tubes may be connected to a variety of closed drainage systems: a water-seal drainage system with one, two, or three bottles; and a self-contained system such as Pleur-evac. Whatever the type, the purpose of the system is to allow for drainage from the pleural cavity to the outside and at the same time prevent the

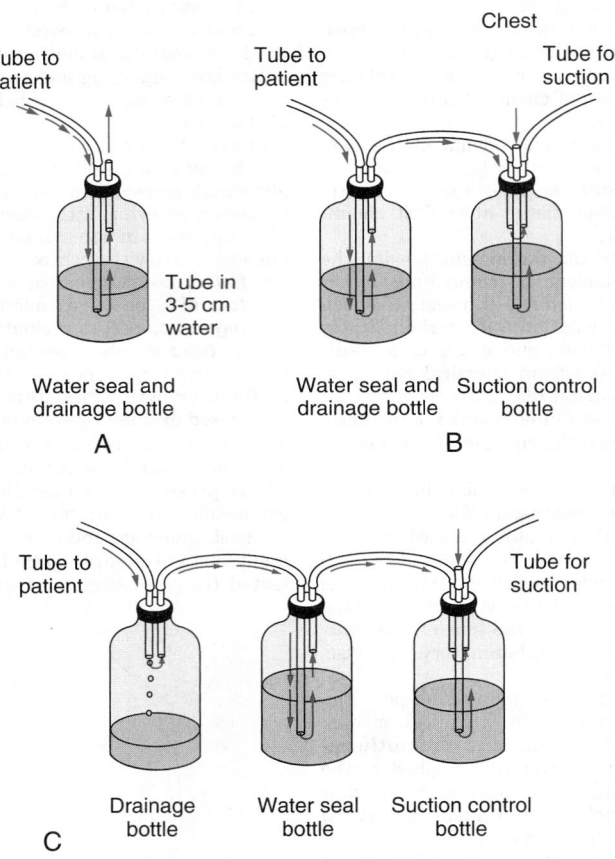

One-, two-, and three-bottle methods for providing a closed drainage system. *A*, In the one-bottle system the drainage via the chest tube enters the bottle through the glass tube which has one end submerged under water to form a seal. This provides a one-way valve that prevents a backflow of air into the pleural cavity, which could collapse the lung. As fluid and air from the pleural cavity enter the drainage bottle, the air that is displaced in the bottle is vented through the short tube above water level. *B*, The second bottle in the two-bottle system acts as a trap to control and decrease the amount of suction within the chest tube. Otherwise, the suction might be too forceful and damage the pleural membrane. No drainage enters this bottle. Its only purpose is to control the force of suction applied. *C*, The third bottle in the three-bottle system also is used to regulate the amount of suction. This can be done by adjusting the length of the glass tube that is under water.

entry of atmospheric air into the pleural cavity.

Precautions that must be taken in the maintenance of the drainage system are:

1. The bottles and collection apparatus of the system must be kept below the level of the chest to prevent backflow.

2. The lumens of the tubes must be kept open to allow for drainage. If they are obstructed there will be no fluctuation of the fluid level in the glass tube that is connected to the chest tube at one end and kept under water in the bottle at the other end. In the Pleur-evac, the liquid in the chamber should rise on the right side and fall on the left side. If there is evidence that the system is not working properly, this must be attended to immediately. Occlusion of the tubes can lead to a buildup of air and fluids in the pleural cavity and creation of a tension PNEUMOTHORAX.

3. The system must be a *closed* (airtight) system. There can be no leaks around connections, and the lower end of the glass tube must remain under water in the bottle.

The amount, color, and consistency of the fluid drainage should be checked at least once each hour for the first 24 hours after surgery. The chest tubes should be milked and stripped every one to two hours to assure patency and adequate drainage. The amount of air being removed is indicated by occasional bubbling in the water-seal chamber. Excessive bubbling may indicate air leaks in the tubing.

An important aspect of patient care is proper positioning to maintain adequate drainage. The positions allowed and the amount of mobility permitted will depend on the patient's surgical diagnosis, the placement of the tube(s), and preference of the attending physician. Frequent turning, coughing, and deep breathing are instituted on a regular basis to avoid serious pulmonary complications. An exception to the rule of turning is the pneumonectomy patient, who is placed in high Fowler's position and not turned for at least 24 hours after surgery. Chest PHYSICAL THERAPY and INTERMITTENT POSITIVE PRESSURE BREATHING (IPPB) treatments usually are ordered for all patients with chest tubes. Some patients may require a VENTILATOR during the immediate postoperative period.

The patient is observed for signs of respiratory distress and a buildup of air and fluid within the pleural cavity. Early correction of this condition can prevent mediastinal shift. Other signals that demand immediate attention are persistent bubbling in the underwater seal (fluid should fluctuate in the tube as the patient breathes), a

drainage through the tube that accumulates at a rate of more than 100 ml per hour, leakage of air at the junctions of the chest tube and tubing and bottles or self-contained unit, and a "putty" appearance caused by the leakage of air into subcutaneous tissues in the upper chest and neck. After a chest tube is removed, the wound is promptly sealed with a sterile petroleum jelly dressing to occlude the opening and prevent entry of air into the pleural space.

Cheyne-Stokes respiration (chān stōks) breathing characterized by rhythmic waxing and waning of the depth of respiration; the patient breathes deeply for a short time and then breathes very slightly or stops breathing altogether. The pattern occurs over and over, every 45 seconds to 3 minutes. Periodic breathing of this type is caused by disease affecting the respiratory centers, usually heart failure or brain damage.

chiasm (ki′azm) a decussation or X-shaped crossing.

optic c. a structure in the forebrain formed by the decussation of fibers of the optic nerve from each half of each retina. (See accompanying illustration.)

chiasma (ki-az′mah), pl. *chias′mata* [L.; Gr.] 1. chiasm. 2. in genetics, the points at which members of a chromosome pair are in contact during the prophase of meiosis and because of which recombination, or crossing over, occurs on separation. See also chiasma FORMATION.

chickenpox (chik′en-poks) an acute, highly contagious, viral disease, with mild constitutional symptoms and a maculopapular vesicular skin eruption; it is a common

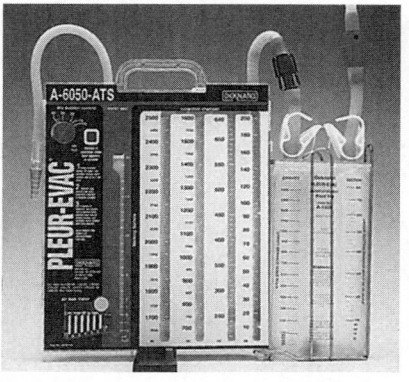

Pleur-evac Adult/Pediatric Chest Drainage Model A-6000. The Pleur-evac Chest Drainage Systems have been the world's most popular units since their inception in 1967. (Courtesy of Deknatel, Inc., Fall River, MA.)

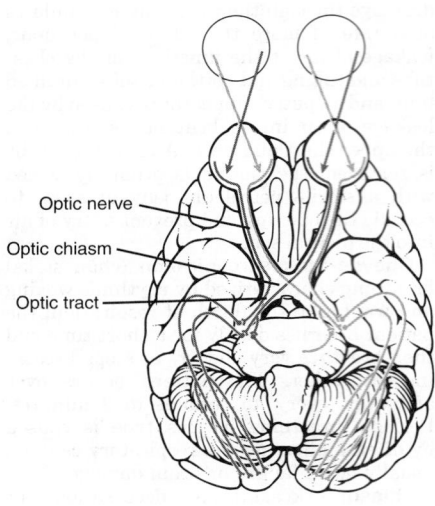

Optic nerve
Optic chiasm
Optic tract

childhood disease and is rarely severe, but it can be accompanied by severe symptoms in infants and adults. It is usually spread by either contact with blisters or droplet infection, and the average incubation period is 10 to 16 days. The period of contagion lasts about two weeks, beginning two days before the rash appears. The causative virus is human HERPESVIRUS 3 (formerly known as varicella-zoster virus). The same virus also causes HERPES ZOSTER (shingles), with the differences in the two diseases probably reflecting differences in the response to the virus. Called also varicella.

Symptoms. Chickenpox may begin with a slight fever, headache, backache, and loss of appetite. At the same time, or a day or two later, small red spots appear, usually on the back and chest first. Within a few hours the spots enlarge and a vesicle filled with a clear fluid appears in the center of each spot, surrounded by an area of reddened skin. After a day or two, the fluid turns yellow and a crust or scab forms. This crust peels off in from 5 to 20 days. During this period the patient experiences severe itching.

The vesicles do not appear all at once, but in crops, the number of crops depending on the severity of the case. Usually the eruptions are concentrated on the back and chest, with only a few appearing on the arms, legs, and face, but in severe cases they may cover almost all of the body. (See accompanying illustration.)

Prevention and Treatment. Children should receive one dose of chickenpox vaccine between 12 and 18 months of age, or at any age after that if they have not had chickenpox. Individuals over age 13 who have not had chickenpox or received the vaccine

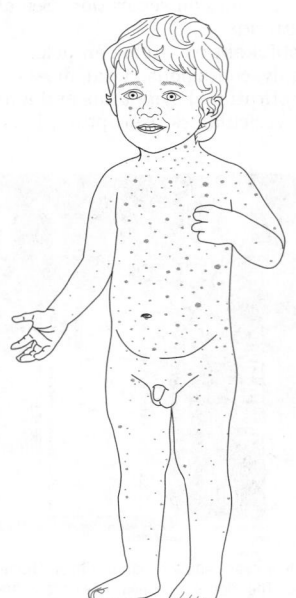

- Macular rash 24–48 hours following slight fever, malaise, anorexia

- Lesions appear in "crops," first on trunk and scalp, then moving sparsely to extremities. May appear in mucous membranes (mouth, genital area, rectum)

- Generally 3 successive eruptions over 3–4 days

- Lesions begin as a macular rash, develop into a red papular rash, then move quickly into teardrop vesicles with erythematous base. Vesicle becomes pustular and begins drying, and a crust develops.

- Rash varies from child to child

Chickenpox rash distribution. From McKinney et al., 2000.

should receive two doses, four to eight weeks apart. There are some contraindications to the use of the vaccine, such as women who are pregnant or are planning to conceive a child within a month.

Most cases of chickenpox are mild and require no special treatment except rest in bed and forcing fluids during the fever stage. For severe itching, emollient baths, calamine lotion, or other applications offer some relief. Since scratching the scabs may result in permanent scars and opens the way for other infections, the child's fingernails should be cut short and the hands washed often.

The Centers for Disease Control and Prevention recommends airborne and contact isolation. Other recommendations include after-exposure advisories. Varicella-zoster immune GLOBULIN (VZIG) should be used when appropriate, along with discharge of susceptible patients if possible. Exposed susceptible patients should be placed on airborne PRECAUTIONS beginning 10 days after exposure and continuing until 21 days after the last exposure (up to 28 days if VZIG has been given). Susceptible persons should not enter the room of patients on precautions if other immune caregivers are available. (See Atlas 2, part M.)

chigger (chig′er) the six-legged red larva of any of the mites of the family TROMBICULIDAE (see TROMBICULA and EUTROMBICULA); they attach to their host's skin and their bite produces a wheal, usually with severe itching and dermatitis. Some species are vectors of the rickettsiae of scrub TYPHUS. Called also harvest mite.

chigoe (chig′o) the sand flea, *Tunga penetrans,* of tropical and subtropical America and Africa. The pregnant female flea burrows into the skin of the feet, legs, or other part of the body, causing intense irritation and resulting in ulceration, sometimes leading to spontaneous amputation of a digit, if untreated.

chilblain (chil′blān) one of the mildest forms of cold injury, characterized by recurrent localized itching, swelling, painful erythema, and sometimes blistering and ulceration upon exposure to cold and dampness; it occurs chiefly on the fingers, toes, ears, and face, but may involve other areas of the body. (This condition should not be confused with FROSTBITE, another type of skin damage caused by exposure to cold.) The basic cause of chilblain is sensitivity to cold, sometimes due to circulatory disturbances that can be partially corrected by exercise and proper diet; severe cases require medical attention. Extreme heat or cold applications should not be applied directly to chilblains. Called also pernio.

child (chīld) the human young, from infancy to puberty.

c. abuse the nonaccidental use of physical force or the nonaccidental act of omission by a parent or other custodian responsible for the care of a child. Child abuse encompasses malnutrition and other kinds of neglect through ignorance as well as deliberate withholding from the child of the necessary and basic physical care, including the medical and dental care necessary for the child to grow up without threat to his or her physical and emotional survival. Examples of physical abuse range from burns and exposure to extreme cold to beating, poisoning, strangulation, and withholding of food and water. Members of the health care team should be alert for signs of child abuse and aware of the proper procedure for reporting suspected cases to local authorities.

Abusive parents come from all socioeconomic groups. Many have themselves been abused as children. They typically lack parenting skills and do not understand the normal developmental stages through which children progress and demand performance from their children that is clearly beyond a child's capability. Some engage in role reversal, looking to the child for protection and loving response, while at the same time denying the child satisfaction of his or her own needs. The majority of identified abusive parents are believed to want professional help in changing their behavior.

autistic c. a child suffering from AUTISTIC DISORDER.

exceptional c. a child with special learning needs; he or she may have learning disabilities, be handicapped, or be gifted.

childbed fever (chīld′bed) puerperal fever.

childbirth (chīld′berth) the process of giving birth to a child, including both LABOR and DELIVERY. Called also accouchement and parturition.

cooperative c., educated c. natural c. prepared childbirth.

prepared c. see PREPARED CHILDBIRTH.

chill (chil) a sensation of cold, with convulsive shaking of the body. A true chill, or rigor, results from an increase in chemical activity within the body and usually ushers in a considerable rise in body temperature. The pallor and coldness of a chill, and the PILOERECTION of the skin (goose flesh) that often accompanies it, are caused by constriction of the peripheral blood vessels. Chills are symptomatic of a wide variety of diseases. They usually do not accompany well-localized infections.

Patient Care. During a chill sufficient heat should be applied to maintain normal body temperature. Since the patient will most likely begin to have a sharp rise in body temperature immediately after or during the chill, it is best to use only a light blanket to alleviate the sensation of cold. In addition to this the patient's temperature should be taken every 30 minutes until it is stabilized.

Chilomastix (ki″lo-mas′tiks) a genus of pear- or lemon-shaped parasitic protozoa found in the intestines of various vertebrates, including humans. All species are considered nonpathogenic or only slightly pathogenic, but one species, *C. mesni′li,* has been associated with rare cases of watery diarrhea.

Chilopoda (ki-lop′o-dah) a class of ARTHROPODS that includes the centipedes.

chimera (ki-me′rah) an organism whose body contains different cell populations derived from different zygotes of the same or different species, occurring spontaneously or produced artificially.

chimerism (ki′mer-izm) the state of being a chimera; the presence in an individual of cells of different origin.

chin (chin) the anterior prominence of the lower jaw; called also mentum.

Chinese restaurant syndrome transient arterial dilatation due to ingestion of monosodium glutamate, which is sometimes used liberally in seasoning Chinese food, marked by throbbing head, lightheadedness, tightness of the jaw, neck, and shoulders, and backache.

chionablepsia (ki″o-nah-blep′se-ah) snow blindness.

chir(o)- word element [Gr.], *hand.* See also words beginning CHEIR(O)-.

chirality (ki-ral′ĭ-te) the property of handedness, of not being superimposable on a mirror image; the handedness of an asymmetric molecule, as specified by its optical rotation or absolute configuration.

chiropodist (ki-rop′ŏ-dist) former term for podiatrist.

chiropractic (ki″ro-prak′tik) a nonpharmaceutical, nonsurgical system of health care based on the self-healing capacity of the body and the primary importance of the proper function of the nervous system in the maintenance of health; therapy is aimed at removing irritants to the nervous system and restoring proper function. The most common method of treatment is by spinal manipulation and is primarily done for musculoskeletal complaints; other methods include lifestyle modification, nutritional therapy, and physiotherapy.

chiropractor (ki′ro-prak″ter) a practitioner in CHIROPRACTIC.

chi-square test a statistical procedure for determining significant differences between frequencies observed within the data and frequencies that were expected. There are two chi-squared tests: the chi-square test of *independence,* which tests whether two or more series of frequencies are independent of one another; and the chi-square test of *goodness of fit,* which tests whether an observed frequency distribution fits a specified theoretical model. Written also χ^2-test.

chitin (ki′tin) a horny polysaccharide, the principal constituent of shells of arthropods and shards of beetles, and found in certain fungi.

chlamydemia (klam″ĭ-de′me-ah) the presence of chlamydiae in the blood.

Chlamydia (klah-mid′e-ah) a widespread genus of gram-negative, nonmotile bacteria. They are obligate intracellular parasites that are totally dependent on the host cell for energy in the form of adenosine triphosphate (ATP), which they cannot synthesize. Outside a host they exist as elementary bodies that have a rigid cell wall and are unable to grow and divide. The elementary bodies attach to the host cells and are taken in by phagocytosis. Inside the phagosome they become reticulate bodies that have flexible cell walls and are able to grow and divide. Subsequent release of elementary bodies and lysis of the host cell permit infection of surrounding cells.

The genus *Chlamydia* contains two species, *C. tracho′matis* and *C. psit′taci. C. trachomatis* can cause TRACHOMA, inclusion CONJUNCTIVITIS, LYMPHOGRANULOMA VENEREUM, nongonococcal URETHRITIS, and a number of other genital infections. *C. psittaci* causes PSITTACOSIS.

The symptoms of sexually transmitted chlamydial infections may be mild; hence this is sometimes called "the silent STD." Victims may not be aware they have the disease and may not seek treatment until serious complications and unwitting transmission to other persons have occurred. Males who have symptoms usually have painful urination and a watery discharge from the penis. Women may suffer itching and burning in the genital area, an odorless, thick, yellow-white vaginal discharge, dull abdominal pain, and bleeding between menstrual periods. *C. trachomatis* causes about half of all PELVIC INFLAMMATORY DISEASE. Symptoms can appear from a week to five weeks after exposure to the bacteria, during which time almost all sexual contacts become infected.

Chlamydial infection during PREGNANCY can increase the risk of stillbirth or premature birth. The newborn is at risk for infection from its mother and may suffer from inclusion conjunctivitis. Chlamydial infection can also lead to pneumonia some weeks after birth, probably because of infectious material from the eye draining through the nasolacrimal ducts and being aspirated into the lungs.

Chlamydial infection is usually treated with an antibiotic; effective single antibiotic therapy is available. It is essential that condoms be used during sexual intercourse throughout the treatment period to prevent reinfection, and condom use is usually recommended for 3 to 6 months after treatment. As with all sexually transmitted diseases, both partners should be treated at the same time to prevent reinfection. If left untreated, chlamydial infection can cause scarring in the fallopian tubes and lead to infertility and tubal pregnancies. In the male, nongonococcal urethritis due to chlamydiae may lead to epididymitis and sterility.

The U.S. Preventive Services Task Force has drawn up guidelines that strongly recommend routine screening for *Chlamydia* infections for all sexually active women ages 25 and younger in order to insure detection. Printed copies of the Guidelines are available online through the National Guideline Clearinghouse at http://www.guideline.gov. They can also be obtained from the AHRQ Publications Clearinghouse by calling 1-800-358-9295.

chlamydia (klah-mid′e-ah) any member of the genus *Chlamydia.*

Chlamydiaceae (klah-mid″e-a′se-e) a family of bacteria containing a single genus, *Chlamydia.*

chlamydiosis (klah-mid″e-o′sis) any infection or disease caused by *Chlamydia.*

chlamydospore (klam′ĭ-do-spor″) a thick-walled terminal asexual spore formed by the rounding-up of a cell; it is not shed.

chloasma (klo-az′mah) hyperpigmentation in circumscribed areas of the skin; called also melasma.

c. gravida′rum melasma gravidarum.

chloracne (klor-ak′ne) an acneiform eruption, caused by exposure to chlorine compounds.

chloral (klor′al) 1. an oily liquid with a pungent, irritating odor; used in the manufacture of chloral hydrate and DDT. 2. chloral hydrate.

c. hydrate a SEDATIVE and HYPNOTIC used primarily as an adjunct to ANESTHESIA and for sedation of children before certain medical or dental procedures. It is now rarely used for management of INSOMNIA. The Health Care Financing Administration (HCFA) guidelines for long-term care facilities discourages the use of chloral hydrate. The National Institutes of Health Consensus Conference on the Treatment of Sleep Disorders of Older People noted that hypnotic medications such as this should not be the mainstay of management of most causes of disturbed sleep.

chlorambucil (klor-am′bu-sil) a NITROGEN MUSTARD ALKYLATING AGENT used as an antineoplastic AGENT.

chloramphenicol (klor″am-fen′ĭ-kol) a broad-spectrum ANTIBIOTIC with specific therapeutic activity against rickettsiae and many different bacteria. Side effects include serious, even fatal, blood dyscrasias in certain patients. Frequent blood tests are recommended during therapy.

chlorcyclizine (klor-si′klĭ-zēn) an ANTIHISTAMINE derived from PIPERAZINE, used as the hydrochloride salt; it has anticholinergic, antiemetic, local anesthetic, and mild sedative properties. Administered orally as a component of various cold and allergy preparations and topically to relieve itching.

chlordane (klor′dān) a poisonous chlorinated HYDROCARBON insecticide. Signs of acute poisoning include irritability, convulsions, and deep depression. Chronic exposure can result in liver degeneration.

chlordiazepoxide (klor″di-a″ze-pok′sīd) a BENZODIAZEPINE used as the base or hydrochloride salt in the treatment of ANXIETY DISORDERS and short-term or preoperative anxiety, for alcohol WITHDRAWAL, and as an antitremor agent; administered orally, intravenously, or intramuscularly.

chloremia (klo-re′me-ah) 1. chlorosis. 2. hyperchloremia.

chlorhexidine (klor-hek′sĭ-dēn) an antibacterial compound used in antimicrobial skin cleansers for surgical scrub, preoperative skin preparation, and cleansing skin wounds.

chlorhydria (klor-hi′dre-ah) hyperchlorhydria.

chloride (klor′īd) a salt of HYDROCHLORIC ACID; any binary compound of CHLORINE.

chloridorrhea (klor″īd-o-re′ah) diarrhea with an excess of chlorides in the stool.

chloriduria (klor″ĭ-du′re-ah) chloruresis.

chlorinated (klor'ĭ-nāt″ed) charged with chlorine.

chlorination (klor″ĭ-na'shun) the addition of chlorine to water or sewage to kill germs. Liquid chlorine has been found to be the most effective water disinfectant, and is almost invariably used in the United States for the purification of both public water supplies and swimming pools.

chlorine (Cl) (klor'ēn) a gaseous chemical element, atomic number 17, atomic weight 35.453. (See Appendix 6.) It is a disinfectant, decolorizer, and irritant poison. It is used for disinfecting, fumigating, and bleaching, either in an aqueous solution or in the form of chlorinated lime.

chlorite (klor'īt) a salt of chlorous acid; disinfectant and bleaching agent.

chloroacetophenone (CN) (klo″ro-as″ĕ-to-fe'nōn) a commonly used tear GAS.

o-chlorobenzylidenemalononitrile (klo″-ro-ben-zil″ĭ-dēn-mal″ah-no-ni'trīl) CS (def. 2).

chloroform (klor″o-form) a colorless, mobile liquid with an ethereal odor and sweet taste, used as a solvent; it is hepatotoxic and nephrotoxic when ingested. It was once used widely medicinally, such as for inhalation anesthesia and analgesia.

chlorolabe (klor'o-lāb) the pigment in retinal cones that is more sensitive to the green portion of the spectrum than are the other pigments (cyanolabe and erythrolabe).

chloroleukemia (klor″o-lu-ke'me-ah) 1. chloroma. 2. a tumor of rose or greenish color occurring in rats or mice with leukemia.

chloroma (klŏ-ro'mah) a malignant, green-colored tumor arising from MYELOID tissue, associated with myelogenous LEUKEMIA; it can occur anywhere in the body but has an affinity for the central nervous system, bone, and soft tissues of the head and neck. Called also granulocytic sarcoma.

Chloromycetin (klor″o-mi-se'tin) trademark for preparations of CHLORAMPHENICOL, a broad-spectrum ANTIBIOTIC.

chloromyeloma (klor″o-mi″ĕ-lo'mah) chloroma with multiple growths in bone marrow.

chlorophyll (klor'o-fil) any of a group of green pigments, containing a magnesium-porphyrin complex, that are involved in oxygen-producing photosynthesis. Preparations of water-soluble chlorophyll derivatives are sometimes applied topically for deodorization purposes. They may also be administered orally to deodorize ulcerative lesions as well as urine and feces in colostomy, ileostomy, or incontinence.

chlorophyllin (klor'o-fil-in) any of the water-soluble salts from CHLOROPHYLL, used topically and orally for deodorizing skin lesions and orally for deodorizing the urine and feces in colostomy, ileostomy, and incontinence; used particularly in the form of the copper complex.

chloroplast (klor'o-plast) the photosynthetic unit of a plant cell, containing all the chlorophyll.

chloroprivic (klor″o-pri'vik) deprived of chlorides; due to loss of chlorides.

chloroprocaine (klor″o-pro'kān) a local anesthetic, used as the hydrochloride salt.

chloropsia (klŏ-rop'se-ah) a defect of vision in which objects appear to have a greenish tinge.

chloroquine (klor'o-kwin) 1. an antimalarial and antiprotozoal AGENT, also used as a LUPUS ERYTHEMATOSUS suppressant. 2. an antiamebic and antiinflammatory agent used in treatment of MALARIA, GIARDIASIS, non-intestinal AMEBIASIS, LUPUS ERYTHEMATOSUS, and rheumatoid ARTHRITIS; used as the base, hydrochloride salt, or phosphate salt.

chlorothiazide (klor″o-thi'ah-zīd) a thiazide DIURETIC used in treatment of EDEMA, such as in congestive HEART FAILURE or liver disease, as well as of HYPERTENSION. Possible side effects include potassium depletion and other electrolyte imbalances; occasionally bone marrow depression with lowering of platelet and leukocyte counts, agranulocytosis, and aplastic anemia may occur.

chlorotrianisene (klor″o-tri-an'ĭ-sēn) a synthetic ESTROGEN used to suppress lactation in postpartum women, for palliative treatment in inoperable prostatic carcinoma, and for replacement therapy of estrogen deficiency; administered orally.

chloroxine (klo-rok'sēn) a synthetic antibacterial used in the topical treatment of dandruff and seborrheic dermatitis of the scalp.

chloroxylenol (klor″o-zi'lĕ-nol) a broad-spectrum antimicrobial used in the treatment of bacterial, fungal, and yeast infections of the skin and nails.

chlorphenesin (klor-fen'ĕ-sin) an ANTIBACTERIAL, antifungal, and antiprotozoal AGENT used in treatment of ATHLETE'S FOOT and other fungal and trichomonal infections of the skin and vagina; administered topically or intravaginally.

c. carbamate a centrally acting skeletal muscle RELAXANT used in treatment of musculoskeletal conditions characterized by skeletal muscle spasms; administered orally.

chlorpheniramine (klor″fen-ir'ah-mēn) an ANTIHISTAMINE with sedative and anticholinergic effects; used orally or by injection as the maleate salt in the treatment of nasal, eye, and skin manifestations of allergic reactions, including allergic rhinitis, conjunctivitis, and itching, and orally as the maleate or tannate salt or polistirex complex as an ingredient in various cough and cold preparations.

chlorphenoxamine (klor″fen-ok′sah-mēn) an agent used to reduce muscular rigidity in PARKINSONISM.

chlorpromazine (klor-pro′mah-zēn) a phenothiazine used in the form of the base or the hydrochloride salt as an ANTIPSYCHOTIC AGENT, ANTIEMETIC, and presurgical SEDATIVE, and in the treatment of intractable hiccups, acute intermittent porphyria, tetanus, and the manic phase of BIPOLAR DISORDER. It is also used to treat certain severe behavioral problems in children. Side effects include drowsiness and slight hypotension. In prolonged therapy the patient should be observed for jaundice. Some patients on long-term therapy develop persistent tardive dyskinesia.

chlorpropamide (klor-pro′pah-mīd) an oral SULFONYLUREA hypoglycemic AGENT useful in treatment of type 2 DIABETES MELLITUS in the adult whose condition is stabilized; it is contraindicated in patients with impairment of renal, thyroid, or hepatic function. Dosage is individually adjusted.

chlorprothixene (klor″pro-thik′sēn) a THIOXANTHENE drug having sedative, antiemetic, antihistaminic, anticholinergic, and alpha-adrenergic blocking activity; used to control symptoms of psychotic disorders.

chlortetracycline (klor″tet-rah-si′klēn) a broad-spectrum ANTIBIOTIC obtained from *Streptomyces aureofaciens,* used in the form of the hydrochloride salt as an ANTIBACTERIAL (effective against both gram-positive and gram-negative bacteria) and as an antiprotozoal AGENT. It is administered orally, intravenously, or topically to the skin or eye. Side effects include gastrointestinal disturbances, especially diarrhea.

chlorthalidone (klor-thal′ĭ-dōn) a diuretic with the same pharmacologic action as thiazide DIURETICS; used for treatment of hypertension and edema.

Chlor-Trimeton (klor-tri′mě-ton) trademark for preparations of CHLORPHENIRAMINE maleate, an ANTIHISTAMINE.

chloruresis (klor″u-re′sis) excretion of chlorides in the urine; called also chloriduria and chloruria. adj., **chloruret′ic.**

chloruria (klor-u′re-ah) chloruresis.

chlorzoxazone (klor-zok′sah-zōn) a skeletal muscle RELAXANT used to relieve discomfort of painful musculoskeletal disorders; administered orally.

ChM [L.] Chirur′giae Magis′ter (Master of Surgery).

CHO Comprehensive Health Organization.

choana (ko′ah-nah), pl. *cho′anae* [L.] 1. infundibulum. 2. [pl.] the paired openings between the nasal cavity and the nasopharynx.

choanoid (ko′ah-noid) infundibular (def. 2).

choke (chōk) 1. to interrupt respiration by obstruction or compression; called also strangle. 2. the condition resulting from such interruption; called also strangulation.

chokes (chōks) a burning sensation in the substernal region, with uncontrollable coughing, occurring during DECOMPRESSION.

chol(o)- word element [Gr.], *bile.*

cholagogue (ko′lah-gog) an agent that stimulates gallbladder contraction to promote bile flow. adj., **cholagog′ic.**

cholangi(o)- word element [Gr.], *bile duct.*

cholangiectasis (ko-lan″je-ek′tah-sis) dilatation of a bile duct.

cholangiocarcinoma (ko-lan″je-o-kahr″sĭ-no′mah) 1. an adenocarcinoma arising from the epithelium of the intrahepatic bile ducts, composed of eosinophilic cuboidal or columnar epithelial cells, with abundant fibrous stroma; mucus may be secreted but not bile. 2. cholangiocellular carcinoma.

cholangioenterostomy (ko-lan″je-o-en″-ter-os′tah-me) surgical anastomosis of a bile duct to the intestine.

cholangiogastrostomy (ko-lan″je-o-gas-tros′tah-me) surgical anastomosis of the bile duct to the stomach.

cholangiogram (ko-lan′je-o-gram″) the film obtained by cholangiography.

cholangiography (ko-lan″je-og′rah-fe) x-ray examination of the bile ducts, using a radiopaque dye as a contrast medium. In the intravenous method, the dye is administered intravenously and is excreted by the liver into the bile ducts. X-ray films are taken at 10-minute intervals as the dye is excreted via the cystic, hepatic, and common bile ducts into the intestinal tract. The excretion is usually completed within 4 hours. Preparation of the patient for the intravenous method requires restriction of fluids to concentrate the dye and may also include cleansing of the intestinal tract on the day prior to the examination with a laxative or enema so that fecal material and gas will not obscure the biliary tract.

Sometimes cholangiography is done after surgery of the gallbladder and biliary tract. In this method the radiopaque dye is injected directly into a tube that has been left in the biliary tract since the time of

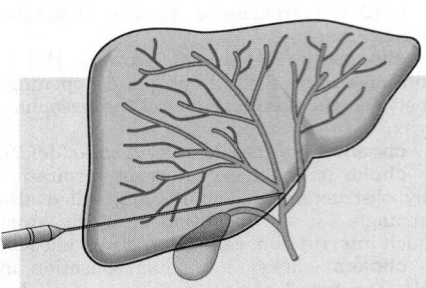

Percutaneous transhepatic cholangiography. The aspirating needle is passed through the patient's skin and liver tissue until the tip penetrates one of the hepatic ducts. Radiopaque medium is then instilled into the biliary tree to enhance radiographic visualization. From Malarkey and McMorrow, 2000.

surgery. Films are taken immediately after the dye is injected. If no obstruction is present, the biliary structures fill readily and rapidly empty into the intestinal tract.

When it is necessary for the surgeon to locate gallstones or other obstructive conditions at the time that surgery is being performed, the dye may be injected directly into the bile ducts. Films are taken in the operating room, and obstructions not otherwise discernible can be located and corrected while the patient is still anesthetized.

A patient who is jaundiced cannot undergo either intravenous cholangiography or oral CHOLECYSTOGRAPHY. An alternative route for the injection of the contrast dye and visualization of the biliary system is *percutaneous transhepatic cholangiography*. Under fluoroscopic control, a needle is introduced through the skin and into the liver where the contrast material is deposited. Obstructed and distended bile ducts can then be visualized. After visualization the ducts can be drained via the needle.

fine needle transhepatic c. (FNTC) transhepatic cholangiography performed by means of a very fine, highly flexible steel needle (skinny needle).

percutaneous transhepatic c. see CHO-LANGIOGRAPHY.

transhepatic c. cholangiography after introduction of radiopaque medium into the biliary system by percutaneous puncture of a bile duct.

transjugular c. cholangiography after catheterization of a hepatic vein via the internal jugular vein in the neck and entry into a bile duct by percutaneous puncture across the wall of the hepatic vein.

cholangiohepatoma (ko-lan″je-o-hep″ah-to′mah) primary carcinoma of the liver of mixed liver cell and bile duct cell origin.

cholangiole (ko-lan′je-ōl) one of the fine terminal elements of the bile duct system. adj., **cholangi′olar.**

cholangiolitis (ko-lan″je-o-li′tis) inflammation of the cholangioles. adj., **cholangiolit′ic.**

cholangioma (ko-lan″je-o′mah) cholangiocellular carcinoma.

cholangiopancreatography (ko-lan″je-o-pan″kre-ah-tog′rah-fe) radiographic examination of the bile ducts and pancreas after administration of a contrast medium.

endoscopic retrograde c. (ERCP) a procedure consisting of a combination of retrograde cholangiography and transhepatic cholangiography. The endoscope is advanced into the duodenum, the biliary tract is cannulated, and contrast medium is injected in order to demonstrate all portions of the biliary tree. See also GALLBLADDER.

cholangiostomy (ko″lan-je-os′tah-me) fistulization of a bile duct.

cholangiotomy (ko″lan-je-ot′ah-me) incision into a bile duct.

cholangitis (ko″lan-ji′tis) inflammation of a bile duct. adj., **cholangit′ic.**

cholanopoiesis (ko″lah-no-poi-e′sis) the synthesis of bile acids or of their conjugates and salts by the liver.

cholanopoietic (ko″lah-no-poi-et′ik) 1. promoting synthesis of bile acids. 2. an agent that so acts.

cholate (ko′lāt) a salt or ester of cholic acid.

chole- word element [Gr.], *bile.*

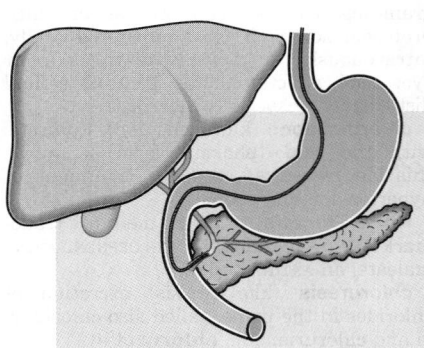

Endoscopic retrograde cholangiopancreatography. At the level of the duodenum, the papilla is located and the cannula is inserted through it. Once the cannula is in the ampulla of Vater, it is passed into the common bile duct. Once that phase of the examination is completed, the cannula is passed into the pancreatic duct. From Malarkey and McMorrow, 2000.

cholecalciferol (ko″le-kal-sif′er-ol) vitamin D_3, an oil-soluble vitamin used in the prevention of rickets. See also VITAMIN.

cholecyst(o)- word element [Gr.], *gallbladder.*

cholecystagogue (ko″le-sis′tah-gog) an agent that promotes evacuation of the gallbladder.

cholecystalgia (ko″le-sis-tal′jah) biliary colic.

cholecystectasia (ko″le-sis″tek-ta′zhah) distention of the gallbladder.

cholecystectomy (ko″le-sis-tek′to-me) excision of the GALLBLADDER, usually done to relieve the symptoms of CHOLECYSTITIS associated with GALLSTONES. During the operation a dye may be injected directly into the biliary ducts and a CHOLANGIOGRAM done to determine whether there are any stones within the ducts. If stones are known or suspected to be in the common bile duct, a T-tube is inserted to bypass the calculi and allow drainage of bile. The end of the tube is brought to the outside through a stab wound in the upper right quadrant and attached to a drainage bag. In spite of the intraoperative cholangiography, some patients will retain stones in the common bile duct after the surgery. LAPAROSCOPY is commonly used, which allows most patients to go home on the same day as surgery and return to full activity within a week.

Patient Care. During the preoperative period the patient will be given a thorough physical examination as well as specific tests for liver function and either radiologic or endoscopic studies of the gallbladder and biliary drainage system. Because nausea and flatulence are common problems in these patients, a nasogastric tube usually is inserted and attached to a decompression apparatus prior to surgery.

When the patient returns from surgery a careful check is made for drainage tubes inserted during the operation. Sometimes the drains are devised so that bile and serous fluid from the operative site drain directly onto the surgical dressings. Other drains or tubes such as a T-tube or Y-tube are attached to a drainage bag so that the amount of bile removed can be measured periodically. In either case, dressings over the wound are checked frequently for signs of bleeding or other abnormalities in the character and amount of drainage. When bile leakage is copious, as it sometimes is, the dressings will need to be reinforced and the outer layers changed as often as necessary to keep the patient dry and comfortable and to avoid irritation of the skin around the incision.

The nursing care plan of a patient with either a T-tube or a Y-tube should take into

C

account three major potential problems: infection, obstruction, and dislodgment of the tube. Monitoring for infection includes watching for elevation of body temperature above 100° F and inspection of the tube insertion site for redness, swelling, warmth, and purulent drainage. The patient also is watched for jaundice and complaints of pain in the right upper quadrant, drainage around the tube when it is clamped, nausea, vomiting, and very dark urine and clay-colored stools, all of which indicate obstruction of the common bile duct. The amount of drainage from the tube is measured and recorded at least once every eight hours. A marked decrease in amount could mean that the tube has become dislodged.

Biliary tract disease continues to occur in approximately 5 to 8 per cent of all post-cholecystectomy patients. The symptoms can appear within weeks after surgery or may occur years later and are the result of residual stones not removed at the time of surgery, newly formed gallstones, or stricture of the common bile duct. Infections and malignancies also can produce the symptoms of postcholecystectomy syndrome (PCS). Because of hormonal influences, women in the 40- to 49-year-old age group account for almost 80 per cent of patients with PCS. Treatment of the condition varies, but might entail more extensive surgery to provide a means by which bile can drain into the intestines.

cholecystenterostomy (ko″le-sis″ten-ter-os′tah-me) formation of a new communication between the gallbladder and the intestine.

cholecystic (ko″le-sis′tik) pertaining to the gallbladder.

cholecystitis (ko″le-sis-ti′tis) inflammation of the GALLBLADDER, acute or chronic.

Acute Cholecystitis. The most frequent cause of acute cholecystitis is GALLSTONES. Other causes include typhoid fever and a malignant tumor obstructing the biliary tract. The inflammation may be secondary to a systemic sepsis.

The symptoms of a mild inflammation may be very slight and include indigestion, moderate pain and tenderness in the upper right quadrant of the abdomen that is usually aggravated by deep breathing, malaise, and a low-grade fever. When gallstones or other disorders cause complete obstruction of the bile ducts, the symptoms are much more extreme. The pain becomes unbearable, the temperature may rise to 40°C (104°F), and there is nausea and vomiting.

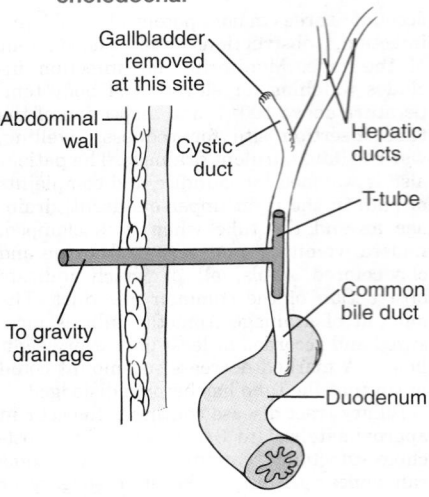

Gallbladder removed at this site

Abdominal wall

Cystic duct

Hepatic ducts

T-tube

Common bile duct

To gravity drainage

Duodenum

Placement of T-tube following cholecystectomy. From Monahan et al., 1994.

Treatment of acute cholecystitis may entail either cholecystectomy or cholecystostomy. In some cases the surgery may be postponed until the attack subsides.

Chronic Cholecystitis. Chronic cholecystitis progresses more slowly than acute cholecystitis, but it also is usually the result of gallstones or other conditions that lead to obstruction of the bile ducts and impaired gallbladder function. It is the most common disorder of the gallbladder.

The characteristic symptom of chronic cholecystitis is indigestion manifested by discomfort after eating, with flatulence and nausea. If the meal has been larger than usual, or high in fat content, the symptoms are more pronounced and there is eructation (belching) and regurgitation. There may also be vomiting and some pain in the upper right quadrant of the abdomen. It is not unusual for patients to suffer repeated episodes before seeking medical attention. Neglect of the situation may lead to permanent damage to the gallbladder and liver.

Diagnosis of cholecystitis is aided by the use of ULTRASONOGRAPHY to visualize an enlarged, inflamed gallbladder and detect the presence of gallstones. Radionuclide scanning is the most reliable diagnostic test for cholecystitis.

The preferred treatment of chronic cholecystitis with gallstones is cholecystectomy. If surgery is contraindicated for some reason, then the symptoms may be controlled to some extent by low-fat diet, restriction of alcohol intake, and spacing of meals so that large amounts of food are avoided and there is not a long interval between meals.

   emphysematous c. that due to gas-producing organisms, marked by gas in the gallbladder lumen, often infiltrating into the gallbladder wall and surrounding tissues.

   cholecystocolostomy (ko″le-sis″to-kah-los′tah-me) surgical anastomosis of the gallbladder and the colon.

   cholecystoduodenostomy (ko″le-sis″to-doo″o-dĕ-nos′tah-me) surgical anastomosis of the gallbladder and the duodenum.

   cholecystogastrostomy (ko″le-sis″to-gas-tros′tah-me) surgical anastomosis between the gallbladder and stomach.

   cholecystogram (ko″le-sis′to-gram) a radiograph of the gallbladder.

   cholecystography (ko″le-sis-tog′rah-fe) radiography of the gallbladder, using a radiopaque dye as contrast medium. adj., **cholecystograph′ic.** The purpose of the examination is to determine the ability of the gallbladder to fill, concentrate bile, and empty. The dye is administered in tablets the evening before the x-ray films are made. Other, more commonly used diagnostic tests are discussed at GALLBLADDER.

   cholecystojejunostomy (ko″le-sis″to-jĕ-joo-nos′tah-me) surgical anastomosis of the gallbladder and jejunum.

   cholecystokinin (ko″le-sis″to-ki′nin) a polypeptide hormone secreted in the small intestine, which stimulates gallbladder contraction and secretion of pancreatic enzymes.

   cholecystolithiasis (ko″le-sis″to-li-thi′ah-sis) the occurrence of gallstones (see CHOLE-LITHIASIS) within the gallbladder.

   cholecystolithotomy (ko″le-sis″to-li-thot′ah-me) incision of the GALLBLADDER for removal of GALLSTONES.

   cholecystopexy (ko″le-sis′to-pek″se) surgical suspension or fixation of the gallbladder.

   cholecystorrhaphy (ko″le-sis-tor′ah-fe) suture or repair of the gallbladder.

   cholecystostomy (ko″le-sis-tos′tah-me) the creation of an opening into the gallbladder for drainage.

   percutaneous c. the insertion of a catheter into the gallbladder under radiologic guidance for drainage or the removal of gallstones.

   cholecystotomy (ko″le-sis-tot′ah-me) incision of the gallbladder.

   choledoch(o)- word element [Gr.], *common bile duct.*

   choledochal (kol′ĕ-dok″al) pertaining to the common bile duct.

choledochectomy (kol″ĕ-do-kek′to-me) excision of part of the common bile duct.

choledochitis (kol″ĕ-do-ki′tis) inflammation of the common bile duct.

choledochoduodenostomy (ko-led″ah-ko-doo″o-dĕ-nos′-tah-me) surgical anastomosis of the common bile duct to the duodenum.

choledochoenterostomy (ko-led″ah-ko-en″ter-os′-tah-me) surgical anastomosis of the common bile duct to the intestine.

choledochogastrostomy (ko-led″ah-ko-gas-tros′tah-me) surgical anastomosis of the common bile duct to the stomach.

choledochojejunostomy (ko-led″ah-ko-je-joo-nos′tah-me) surgical anastomosis of the common bile duct to the jejunum.

choledocholithiasis (ko-led″ah-ko-lī-thi′ah-sis) the occurrence of calculi (see CHOLELITHIASIS) in the common bile duct.

choledocholithotomy (ko-led″ah-ko-lī-thot′ah-me) incision into the common bile duct for removal of GALLSTONES.

choledochoplasty (ko-led′ah-ko-plas″te) plastic repair of the common bile duct.

choledochorrhaphy (ko-led″ah-ko-kor′ah-fe) suture or repair of the common bile duct.

choledochoscopy (ko-led″ah-kos′kah-pe) the direct visualization of the biliary tract with an endoscope through a T-tube or incision into the common bile duct. Small calculi can be removed from the common bile duct during this procedure.

choledochostomy (ko″led-ah-kos′tah-me) creation of an opening into the common bile duct for drainage.

choledochotomy (ko″led-ah-kot′ah-me) incision into the common bile duct.

choledochus (ko-led′o-kus) the common bile duct.

Choledyl (ko′lĕ-dil) trademark for preparations of OXTRIPHYLLINE, a bronchodilator.

choleic (ko-le′ik) biliary.

cholelith (ko′lĕ-lith) gallstone.

cholelithiasis (ko″le-li-thi′ah-sis) the presence or formation of GALLSTONES; they may be either in the gallbladder (CHOLECYSTO-LITHIASIS) or in the common bile duct (CHOLEDOCHOLITHIASIS). adj., **cholelith′ic.**

cholelithotomy (ko″le-lī-thot′ah-me) incision of the biliary tract for removal of GALLSTONES; it may be either in the gallbladder (CHOLECYSTOLITHOTOMY) or in the common bile duct (CHOLEDOCHOLITHOTOMY).

cholelithotripsy (ko″le-lith′o-trip″se) **cholelithotrity** (ko″le-li-thot′ri-te) crushing of a gallstone.

cholemesis (ko-lem′ĕ-sis) vomiting of bile.

cholemia (ko-le′me-ah) bile or bile pigment in the blood. adj., **chole′mic.**

choleperitoneum (ko″le-per″i-to-ne′um) the presence of bile in the peritoneum.

cholepoiesis (ko″le-poi-e′sis) the formation of bile in the liver. adj., **cholepoiet′ic.**

cholera (kol′er-ah) an acute infectious enteritis endemic and epidemic in Asia, caused by *Vibrio cholerae,* marked by severe diarrhea and vomiting, with extreme fluid and electrolyte depletion, and by muscle cramps and prostration. Called also Asiatic cholera.

Immunization and modern methods of sanitation have all but eliminated cholera epidemics in the United States and Europe, but they are still a danger in many other parts of the world, such as in India and many tropical regions. Travelers to cholera-ridden areas should protect themselves by vaccination, but this does not provide complete immunity. The local drinking water should be boiled; uncooked foods should be avoided; food should be protected from flies; and fruits and vegetables should be peeled with their rinds discarded.

Transmission. *Vibrio cholerae* is carried in the cholera victim's feces, urine, and vomitus, and is transmitted to others in contaminated water or food. Once it has reached the intestines, the intestinal lining becomes inflamed and the passages distended with a thin, watery fluid.

Symptoms. Symptoms begin to appear at any time from a few hours to 5 days after contact; the usual incubation period is 3 days. When the disease is at its peak, diarrhea and vomiting occur with such frequency and abundance that dehydration results very rapidly. The skin is cyanotic and shriveled, the eyes are sunken and the voice is feeble. There may be painful muscular cramps throughout the body.

Treatment. Because alkaline substances are lost in the vomitus and feces, ACIDOSIS as well as dehydration must be combated. The fluids and electrolytes are replaced either orally or by administration of a water, glucose, and electrolyte solution. Acid intoxication may require intravenous administration of sodium bicarbonate. Guidelines for cholera control are available from the World Health Organization.

Asiatic c. see CHOLERA.

c. infan′tum a noncontagious diarrhea occurring in infants; formerly common in the summer months.

pancreatic c. a condition marked by profuse watery diarrhea, hypokalemia, and usually achlorhydria, and due to an islet-cell tumor (other than beta cell) of the pancreas.

choleragen (kol′er-ah-gen) the cholera enterotoxin; an extremely potent protein molecule elaborated by strains of *Vibrio* *cholerae* in the small intestine after ingestion of feces-contaminated water and food, where it acts on the epithelial cells to cause hypersecretion of chloride and bicarbonate and an outpouring of large quantities of isotonic fluid from the mucosal surface.

choleraic (kol″ĕ-ra′ik) of or pertaining to cholera, or of the nature of cholera.

choleresis (ko-ler′ĕ-sis) the secretion of bile by the liver.

choleretic (ko″ler-et′ik) 1. stimulating bile production by the liver. 2. an agent that so acts.

choleriform (ko-ler′ĭ-form) resembling cholera.

choleroid (kol′er-oid) resembling cholera.

cholestasis (ko″le-sta′sis) stoppage or suppression of bile flow, due to factors within (intrahepatic cholestasis) or outside the liver (extrahepatic cholestasis). adj., **cholestat′ic.**

cholesteatoma (ko″le-ste″ah-to′mah) a cystlike mass with a lining of stratified squamous epithelium, filled with desquamating debris frequently including cholesterol. Cholesteatomas are most common in the middle ear and mastoid region secondary to trauma or infection that undergoes faulty healing so that epithelium invaginates.

cholesteatosis (ko″le-ste″ah-to′sis) fatty degeneration due to cholesterol esters.

cholesterol (ko-les′ter-ol) a steroid alcohol found in animal fats and oils, bile, blood, brain tissue, milk, egg yolk, myelin sheaths of nerve fibers, liver, kidneys, and adrenal glands. It is a precursor of BILE ACIDS and STEROID hormones, and it occurs in the most common type of GALLSTONE, in ATHEROMA of the arteries, in various cysts, and in carcinomatous tissue. Most of the body's cholesterol is synthesized by the liver, but some is obtained in the diet from animal-derived foods. Plant-derived foods are cholesterol-free. Cholesterol is not transported free in the blood but is bound to certain proteins to form LIPOPROTEINS. Two important fractions of the serum lipoproteins are high-density lipoproteins (HDL) and low-density lipoproteins (LDL).

High levels of *total* serum cholesterol have been shown to be associated with a high risk for coronary artery disease and myocardial infarction. Research has drawn a distinction between HDL-C, the cholesterol carried on high-density lipoproteins and LDL-C, the cholesterol carried on low-density lipoproteins. The *balance* between HDL-C and LDL-C is more significant than the *total concentration* of cholesterol in the blood. The risk of coronary heart disease increases as LDL-C increases and HDL-C decreases.

Because HDL-C promotes the removal of excess cholesterol from the cells and its excretion from the body, it is thought to be beneficial rather than harmful. In contrast, LDL-C picks up cholesterol from ingested fats and from cells that synthesize it in the body and delivers it to blood vessels and muscles where it is deposited in the cells. The concentration of cholesterol in cells within the linings of the arteries contributes to the build-up of atherosclerotic plaques. (See also ATHEROSCLEROSIS.)

A third type of lipoprotein is known as very-low-density lipoprotein (VLDL). There is a preponderance of triglyceride and very little cholesterol in VLDL. Triglyceride is the basic type of lipid used for the storage of energy. The role of serum triglyceride in the formation of atherosclerotic plaques is not known. Those persons who are at high risk for heart disease, already have a heart condition, or are obese should limit the amount of fats and cholesterol in the foods they eat. LDL-C levels can be reduced by limiting dietary intake of saturated fat and cholesterol. Organ meats and egg yolks are high in cholesterol. HDL-C levels can be raised by exercise, stopping cigarette smoking, and losing excess body fat. (See accompanying illustration.)

Blood Cholesterol. Laboratory testing of cholesterol in the blood is often used as a preliminary test for a disorder of blood lipids. Although the normal values for total blood cholesterol vary according to age, diet, and nationality, levels above 200 mg/dl indicate a need for further testing and efforts to reduce the cholesterol level. In general, as the total cholesterol level rises above 150 mg/dl, the risk for coronary artery disease gradually increases. Persons with cholesterol levels above 260 mg/dl may require medication to lower their LDL-C levels and reduce the risk of heart disease.

Increased levels of cholesterol in the blood are found in cardiovascular disease and atherosclerosis, obstructive jaundice, hypothyroidism, nephrosis, and uncontrolled diabetes mellitus. Cholesterol exists in both a free and esterified form; the ratio of free to esterified cholesterol is significant in the diagnosis of certain diseases. For example, there is a markedly abnormal ratio of these two forms of cholesterol in hepatic biliary disease, infectious diseases, and extreme cholesterolemia.

Decreased levels of cholesterol in the blood are noted when there is malabsorption of cholesterol from the intestinal tract as in pernicious anemia, hemolytic

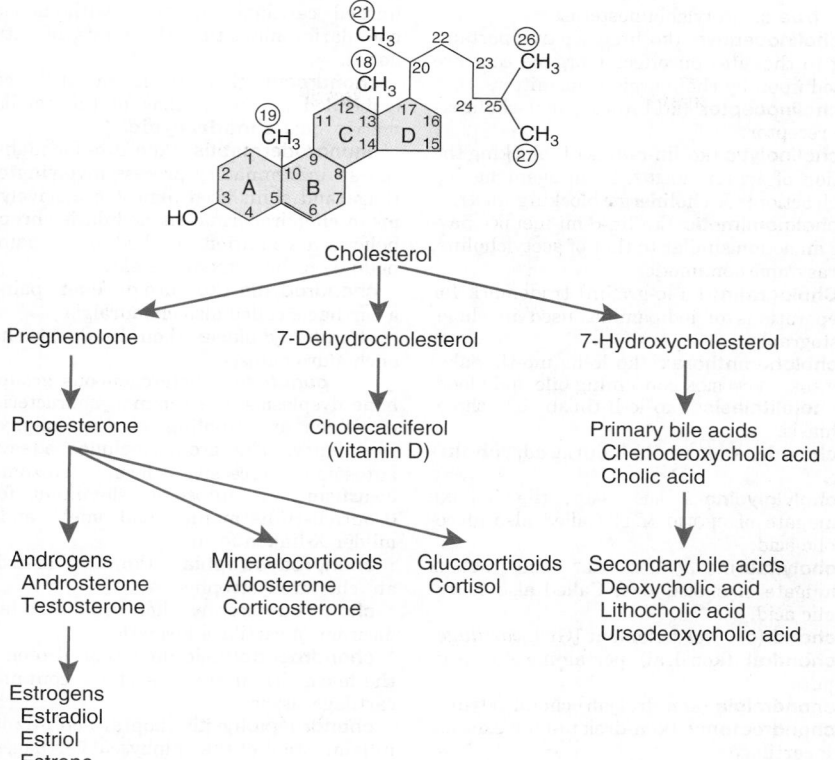

Structure and metabolism of cholesterol. From Dorland's, 2000.

jaundice, hyperthyroidism, and terminal cancer.

cholesterolemia (ko-les″ter-ol-e′me-ah) hypercholesterolemia.

cholesteroluria (ko-les″ter-ol-u′re-ah) the presence of cholesterol in the urine.

cholesterosis (ko-les″ter-o′sis) a condition in which cholesterol is deposited in tissues in abnormal amounts.

cholestyramine (ko-lĕ-stir′ah-mēn) see cholestyramine RESIN.

choletherapy (ko″le-ther′ah-pe) treatment by administration of bile salts.

cholic acid (ko′lik, kol′ik) one of the primary BILE ACIDS, usually found conjugated with GLYCINE or TAURINE; it facilitates fat absorption and cholesterol excretion.

choline (ko′lēn) an amine that occurs in PHOSPHATIDYLCHOLINE and ACETYLCHOLINE, and is an important methyl donor in intermediary metabolism. Choline is a lipotropic agent, a substance that decreases liver fat content by increasing phospholipid turnover. It was formerly considered to be a B VITAMIN and is now classified as a pseudovitamin, although it is still sometimes classified as part of the vitamin B complex. Vitamin B_{12} and folacin are involved in the synthesis of choline.

c. acetylase, c. acetyltransferase an enzyme that brings about the synthesis of acetylcholine.

c. magnesium trisalicylate see under TRISALICYLATE.

c. salicylate see SALICYLATE.

cholinergic (ko″lin-er′jik) 1. activated or transmitted by ACETYLCHOLINE; see also cholinergic FIBERS and cholinergic RECEPTORS. 2. an agent that resembles acetylcholine or simulates its action. Called also parasympathomimetic.

cholinesterase (ko″lin-es′ter-ās) an enzyme that splits acetylcholine into acetic acid and choline; it occurs primarily in the serum, liver, and pancreas. See also ACETYLCHOLINESTERASE.

true c. acetylcholinesterase.

cholinoceptive (ko″lin-o-sep′tiv) pertaining to the sites on effector organs that are acted upon by cholinergic transmitters.

cholinoceptor (ko″lin-o-sep′ter) cholinergic receptor.

cholinolytic (ko″lin-o-lit′ik) 1. blocking the action of ACETYLCHOLINE. 2. an agent having such action; see cholinergic blocking AGENT.

cholinomimetic (ko″lin-o-mi-met′ik) having an action similar to that of acetylcholine; parasympathomimetic.

Cholografin (ko″lo-gra′fin) trademark for preparations of iodipamide, used in cholecystography.

cholohemothorax (ko″lo-he″mo-thor′aks) a PLEURAL EFFUSION containing bile and blood.

chololithiasis (ko″lo-lĭ-thi′ah-sis) cholelithiasis.

choluria (ko-lu′re-ah) biliuria. adj., **choluˈric.**

cholylglycine a BILE SALT, the GLYCINE conjugate of CHOLIC ACID. Called also glycocholic acid.

cholyltaurine a BILE SALT, the TAURINE conjugate of CHOLIC ACID. Called also taurocholic acid.

chondr(o)- word element [Gr.], *cartilage.*

chondral (kon′dral) pertaining to cartilage.

chondralgia (kon-dral′jah) chondrodynia.

chondrectomy (kon-drek′to-me) excision of a cartilage.

chondri(o)- word element [Gr.], *cartilage; granule.*

chondrification (kon″drĭ-fĭ-ka′shun) conversion into cartilage.

chondritis (kon-dri′tis) inflammation of a cartilage.

chondroadenoma (kon″dro-ad″ĕ-no′mah) adenochondroma.

chondroangioma (kon″dro-an″je-o′mah) a benign MESENCHYMOMA containing cartilaginous and angiomatous elements.

chondroblast (kon′dro-blast) an immature cartilage-producing cell.

chondroblastoma (kon″dro-blas-to′mah) a benign tumor arising from young CHONDROBLASTS in the epiphysis of a bone.

chondrocalcinosis (kon″dro-kal″sĭ-no′sis) deposition of calcium salts in the cartilage of joints. When accompanied by attacks of goutlike symptoms, it is called pseudogout.

chondroclast (kon′dro-klast) a giant cell believed to be associated with absorption of cartilage.

chondrocostal (kon″dro-kos′t'l) pertaining to the ribs and costal cartilages.

chondrocranium (kon″dro-kra′ne-um) the cartilaginous cranial structure of the embryo from the seventh week to the middle of the third month, when it is a unified cartilaginous mass without clear boundaries indicating the limits of future bones.

chondrocyte (kon′dro-sīt) one of the cells embedded in the lacunae of the cartilage matrix. adj., **chondrocytˈic.**

chondrodermatitis (kon″dro-der″mah-ti′-tis) an inflammatory process involving cartilage and skin; used almost exclusively to mean chondrodermatitis nodularis chronica helicis, a condition marked by a painful nodule on the helix of the ear.

chondrodynia (kon″dro-din′e-ah) pain in a cartilage; called also chondralgia.

chondrodysplasia (kon″dro-dis-pla′zhah) enchondromatosis.

c. puncta′ta a heterogeneous group of bone dysplasias, the common characteristic of which is stippling of the epiphyses in infancy. The group includes a severe autosomal recessive form (rhizomelic dwarfism), an autosomal dominant form (Conradi-Hünermann syndrome), and a milder X-linked form.

chondrodystrophia (kon″dro-dis-tro′fe-ah) chondrodystrophy.

chondrodystrophy (kon″dro-dis′tro-fe) a disorder of cartilage formation.

chondroendothelioma (kon″dro-en″do-the″le-o′mah) an ENDOTHELIOMA containing cartilage tissue.

chondroepiphysitis (kon″dro-ep″ĭ-fiz-i′tis) inflammation of the epiphyseal cartilages.

chondrofibroma (kon″dro-fi-bro′mah) a FIBROMA with cartilaginous elements.

chondrogenesis (kon″dro-jen′ĕ-sis) formation of cartilage.

chondrogenic (kon″dro-jen′ik) giving rise to or forming cartilage.

chondroid (kon′droid) resembling CARTILAGE.

chondroitin sulfate (kon-dro′ĭ-tin) a glycosaminoglycan (mucopolysaccharide) which is widespread in connective tissue, particularly cartilage, and in the cornea.

chondrolipoma (kon″dro-lĭ-po′mah) a tumor containing cartilaginous and fatty tissue.

chondroma (kon-dro′mah), pl. *chondromas, chondro′mata* a tumor or tumorlike growth of cartilage cells. It may remain in the interior or substance of a cartilage or bone (true chondroma, or enchondroma), or may develop on the surface of a cartilage and project under the periosteum of a bone (ecchondroma, or ecchondrosis).

chondromalacia (kon″dro-mah-la′shah) abnormal softening of cartilage.

chondromatosis (kon″dro-mah-to′sis) formation of multiple chondromas.

synovial c. a rare condition in which cartilage is formed in the synovial membrane of joints, tendon sheaths, or bursae, sometimes becoming detached and producing a number of loose bodies.

chondromere (kon′dro-mēr) a cartilaginous vertebra of the fetal vertebral column.

chondrometaplasia (kon″dro-met″ah-pla′zhah) a condition characterized by metaplastic activity of the CHONDROBLASTS.

chondromyoma (kon″dro-mi-o′mah) a benign tumor with myomatous and cartilaginous elements.

chondromyxoma (kon″dro-mik-so′mah) MYXOMA with cartilaginous elements.

chondromyxosarcoma (kon″dro-mik″so-sahr-ko′mah) a SARCOMA containing cartilaginous and mucous tissue.

chondro-osseous (kon″dro-os′e-us) osteochondral.

chondropathy (kon-drop′ah-the) any disease of cartilage.

chondroplasia (kon″dro-pla′zhah) the formation of CARTILAGE by specialized cells (CHONDROCYTES).

chondroplast (kon′dro-plast) chondroblast.

chondroplasty (kon′dro-plas″te) plastic repair of cartilage.

chondroporosis (kon″dro-po-ro′sis) the formation of sinuses or spaces in cartilage.

chondrosarcoma (kon″dro-sahr-ko′ma) a malignant tumor derived from cartilage cells or their precursors.

chondrosis (kon-dro′sis) the formation of cartilage.

chondrosteoma (kon″dros-te-o′mah) osteochondroma.

chondrosternal (kon″dro-ster′nal) pertaining to the costal cartilages and sternum.

chondrosternoplasty (kon″dro-ster′no-plas″te) surgical correction of pectus excavatum.

chondrotomy (kon-drot′ah-me) the dissection or the surgical division of cartilage.

chondroxiphoid (kon″dro-zif′oid) pertaining to the xiphoid process.

chord (kord) chord.

chorda (kor′dah), pl. *chor′dae* [L.] a CORD or sinew. adj., **chor′dal.**

c. mag′na Achilles tendon.

chor′dae tendi′neae tendinous cords connecting the two atrioventricular valves to the appropriate papillary muscles in the heart ventricles. (See accompanying illustration.)

c. tym′pani a nerve originating from the facial nerve, distributed to the submandibular, sublingual, and lingual glands and the anterior two-thirds of the tongue; it is a parasympathetic and special sensory nerve.

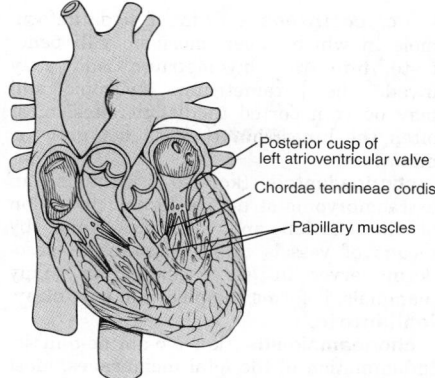

Posterior cusp of left atrioventricular valve

Chordae tendineae cordis

Papillary muscles

Chordae tendineae of the posterior cusps of atrioventricular valves in a cross-section of the heart. From Dorland's, 2000.

c. umbilica′lis umbilical cord.

c. voca′lis vocal cord.

Chordata (kor-da′tah) a phylum of the animal kingdom comprising all animals having a notochord during some developmental stage.

chordate (kor′dāt) 1. an animal of the CHORDATA. 2. having a NOTOCHORD.

chordee (kor′de) downward deflection of the penis, due to a congenital anomaly (hypospadias) or to urethral infection.

chorditis (kor-di′tis) inflammation of vocal or spermatic cords.

c. nodo′sa, c. tubero′sa the formation of small white nodules on one or both vocal cords in persons who use their voices excessively; see also vocal cord NODULES.

chordoma (kor-do′mah) a malignant tumor arising in the axial SKELETON from embryonic remains of the NOTOCHORD.

chordotomy (kor-dot′ah-me) cordotomy.

chorea (ko-re′ah) the ceaseless occurrence of rapid, jerky involuntary movements. adj., **chore′ic.**

acute c. Sydenham's chorea.

chronic c. HUNTINGTON'S CHOREA.

c. gravida′rum SYDENHAM'S CHOREA in early pregnancy, with or without a previous history of RHEUMATIC FEVER.

hereditary c., Huntington's c. see HUNTINGTON'S CHOREA.

Sydenham's c. see SYDENHAM'S CHOREA.

choreiform (ko-re′ĭ-form) resembling chorea.

choreoathetosis (ko″re-o-ath″ĕ-to′sis) a condition characterized by choreic and athetoid movements. adj., **choreoath′etoid.**

chorioadenoma (ko″re-o-ad″ĕ-no′mah) adenoma of the chorion.

c. destru′ens a form of hydatidiform mole in which molar chorionic villi penetrate into the myometrium and may invade the parametrium. Hydropic villi may be transported to distant sites, most often the lungs, but they do not grow as metastases.

chorioallantois (kor″e-o-ah-lan′to-is) an extraembryonic structure formed by union of the chorion and allantois, which by means of vessels in the associated mesoderm serves in gas exchange; in many mammals, it forms the placenta. adj., **chorioallanto′ic.**

chorioamnionitis (kor″e-o-am″ne-o-ni′tis) inflammation of the fetal membranes, most commonly due to bacterial or viral infection. It is usually the result of upward spread of vaginal organisms. Rupture of the amniotic membranes for over 24 hours before birth and prolonged labor are major predisposing factors. If the infection occurs when membranes are intact, it can result from ascending infections, from herpes, cytomegalovirus infection, or syphilis, or as a consequence of diagnostic amniocentesis.

chorioangioma (ko″re-o-an″je-o′mah) an angioma of the chorion.

choriocarcinoma (kor″e-o-kahr″sĭ-no′-mah) a malignant neoplasm of trophoblastic cells formed by abnormal proliferation of the placental epithelium, without production of chorionic villi. It is a malignant variant of gestational THROMBOPLASTIC disease and can occur following a full term pregnancy, pregnancy complicated by a MOLE, ectopic PREGNANCY, or ABORTION.

choriocele (kor′e-o-sēl″) protrusion of the chorion through an aperture.

chorioepithelioma (kor″e-o-ep″ĭ-the″le-o′mah) choriocarcinoma.

choriogenesis (kor″e-o-jen′ĕ-sis) the development of the chorion.

choriogonadotropin (ko″re-o-gon′ah-do-tro″pin) chorionic gonadotropin.

c. alfa human chorionic GONADOTROPIN produced by recombinant technology, used to induce ovulation and pregnancy in certain infertile, anovulatory women, and to increase the numbers of oocytes for patients attempting conception using assisted reproductive TECHNOLOGIES such as gamete intrafallopian TRANSFER (GIFT) or in vitro FERTILIZATION; administered subcutaneously.

chorioid (kor′e-oid) choroid.

chorioma (kor″e-o′mah) any trophoblastic proliferation, benign or malignant.

choriomeningitis (kor″e-o-men″in-ji′tis) cerebral meningitis with lymphocytic infiltration of the choroid plexus.

lymphocytic c. a form of viral MENINGITIS caused by an ARENAVIRUS; it usually occurs during the fall and winter months in adults between the ages of 20 and 40.

chorion (kor′e-on) an extraembryonic fetal membrane, composed of trophoblast lined with mesoderm; it develops villi, becomes vascularized, and forms the fetal part of the placenta.

c. frondo′sum the placental part of the chorion; it is covered by villi.

c. lae′ve the nonvillous, membranous part of the chorion.

chorionic (kor″e-on′ik) pertaining to the chorion.

c. villi numerous branching projections from the external surface of the CHORION that provide for exchange between the maternal and fetal circulation. Oxygen and nutrients in the maternal blood diffuse through the walls of the villi and enter the blood of the embryo or fetus. Carbon dioxide and waste products diffuse from blood in the fetal capillaries through the walls of the villi into the maternal blood. See also chorionic villus SAMPLING.

chorioretinal (kor″e-o-ret′ĭ-nal) pertaining to the choroid and retina.

chorioretinitis (kor″e-o-ret″ĭ-ni′tis) inflammation of the choroid and retina.

chorioretinopathy (kor″e-o-ret″ĭ-nop′ah-the) a noninflammatory process involving both the choroid and retina.

chorista (ko-ris′tah) defective development due to, or marked by, displacement of primordial tissue that is histologically normal.

choristoma (kor″is-to′mah) a mass of histologically normal tissue in an abnormal location.

choroid (kor′oid) the middle, vascular coat of the eye, between the sclera and the retina. adj., **choroid′al.** It contains an abundant supply of blood vessels and a large amount of brown pigment that serves to reduce reflection or diffusion of light when it falls on the retina. Adequate nutrition of the eye is dependent upon blood vessels in the choroid.

choroidea (ko-roi′de-ah) choroid.

choroideremia (ko-roi″der-e′me-ah) hereditary (X-linked) primary choroidal degeneration that, in males, eventually leads to blindness as degeneration of the retinal pigment epithelium progresses to complete atrophy; in females, it is nonprogressive and vision is usually normal.

choroiditis (kor″oi-di′tis) inflammation of the choroid.

choroidocyclitis (ko-roi″do-si-kli′tis) inflammation of the choroid and ciliary processes.

choroidoiritis (ko-roi″do-i-ri′tis) inflammation of the choroid and iris.

choroidoretinitis (ko-roi″do-ret″ĭ-ni'tis) inflammation of the choroid and retina.

Chotzen's syndrome (chot'senz) an autosomal dominant disorder characterized by conical deformity of the head, mildly webbed FINGERS and TOES, a wide space between the eyes, PTOSIS, and sometimes mental retardation. Called also acrocephalosyndactyly, type III.

Christian-Weber disease (kris'chan va'-ber) Weber-Christian disease.

Christmas disease (kris'mas) hemophilia B.

chrom(o)- word element [Gr.], *color.*

chromaffin (kro-maf'in) taking up and staining strongly with chromium salts, such as the chromaffin CELLS.

chromaffinoma (kro-maf″ĭ-no'mah) 1. any tumor containing chromaffin cells. 2. pheochromocytoma.

chromat(o)- word element [Gr.], *color; chromatin.*

chromate (kro'māt) any salt of chromic acid.

chromatic (kro-mat'ik) 1. pertaining to color; stainable with dyes. 2. pertaining to chromatin.

chromatid (kro'mah-tid) either of two parallel filaments joined at the centromere that make up a chromosome and that divide in cell division, each going to a different pole of the dividing cell and each becoming a chromosome of one of the two daughter cells.

chromatin (kro'mah-tin) the substance of the chromosomes, composed of DNA and basic proteins (histones), the material in the nucleus that stains with basic dyes.

   sex c. the persistent mass of the material of the inactivated X chromosome in cells of normal females; called also Barr body.

chromatin-negative lacking sex chromatin; characteristic of the nuclei of cells in a normal male.

chromatin-positive containing sex chromatin; characteristic of the nuclei of cells in a normal female.

chromatism (kro'mah-tizm) abnormal pigment deposits.

chromatogenous (kro″mah-toj'ē-nus) producing color or coloring matter.

chromatogram (kro-mat'o-gram) the record produced by chromatography.

chromatograph (kro-mat'o-graf) 1. to analyze by chromatography. 2. the apparatus used in chromatography.

chromatography (kro″mah-tog'rah-fe) a technique for analysis of chemical substances. The term *chromatography* literally means color writing, and denotes a method by which the substance to be analyzed is poured into a vertical glass tube containing an adsorbent, the various components of the substance moving through the adsorbent at different rates of speed, according to their degree of attraction to it, and producing bands of color at different levels of the adsorption column. The term has been extended to include other methods utilizing the same principle, although no colors are produced in the column. adj., **chromatograph'ic.**

The mobile phase of chromatography refers to the fluid that carries the mixture of substances in the sample through the adsorptive material. The stationary or adsorbent phase refers to the solid material that takes up the particles of the substance passing through it. Kaolin, alumina, silica, and activated charcoal have been used as adsorbing substances or stationary phases.

Classification of chromatographic techniques tends to be confusing because it may be based on the type of stationary phase, the nature of the adsorptive force, the nature of the mobile phase, or the method by which the mobile phase is introduced.

The technique is a valuable tool for the research biochemist and is readily adaptable to investigations conducted in the clinical laboratory. For example, chromatography is used to detect and identify in body fluids certain sugars and amino acids associated with inborn errors of metabolism.

   adsorption c. that in which the stationary phase is an adsorbent.

   affinity c. that based on a highly specific biologic interaction such as that between antigen and antibody, enzyme and substrate, or receptor and ligand. Any of these substances, covalently linked to an insoluble support or immobilized in a gel, may serve as the sorbent allowing the interacting substance to be isolated from relatively impure samples; often a 1000-fold purification can be achieved in one step.

   column c. the technique in which the various solutes of a solution are allowed to travel down a column, the individual components being adsorbed by the stationary phase. The most strongly adsorbed component will remain near the top of the column; the other components will pass to positions farther and farther down the column according to their affinity for the adsorbent. If the individual components are naturally colored, they will form a series of colored bands or zones.

Column chromatography has been employed to separate vitamins, steroids, hormones, and alkaloids and to determine the amounts of these substances in samples of body fluids.

exclusion c. that in which the stationary phase is a gel having a closely controlled pore size. Molecules are separated based on molecular size and shape, smaller molecules being temporarily retained in the pores.

gas c. a type of automated chromatography in which the mobile phase is an inert gas. Volatile components of the sample are separated in the column and measured by a detector. The method has been applied in the clinical laboratory to separate and quantify steroids, barbiturates, and lipids.

gas-liquid c. gas chromatography in which the substances to be separated are moved by an inert gas along a tube filled with a finely divided inert solid coated with a nonvolatile oil; each component migrates at a rate determined by its solubility in oil and its vapor pressure.

gel-filtration c., gel-permeation c. exclusion chromatography.

ion exchange c. that utilizing ion exchange RESINS, to which are coupled either cations or anions that will exchange with other cations or anions in the material passed through their meshwork.

molecular sieve c. exclusion chromatography.

paper c. a form of chromatography in which a sheet of blotting paper, usually filter paper, is substituted for the adsorption column. After separation of the components as a consequence of their differential migratory velocities, they are stained to make the chromatogram visible. In the clinical laboratory, paper chromatography is employed to detect and identify sugars and amino acids.

partition c. a process of separation of solutes utilizing the partition of the solutes between two liquid phases, namely the original solvent and the film of solvent on the adsorption column.

thin-layer c. that in which the stationary phase is a thin layer of an adsorbent such as silica gel coated on a flat plate. It is otherwise similar to paper chromatography.

chromatolysis (kro″mah-tol′ĭ-sis) 1. the solution and disintegration of the chromatin of cell nuclei. 2. disintegration of the Nissl bodies of a neuron as a result of injury, fatigue, or exhaustion.

chromatophil (kro-mat′o-fil) a cell or structure that stains easily. adj., **chromatophil′ic.**

chromatophore (kro-mat′o-for) any pigmentary cell or color-producing plastid.

chromatopsia (kro″mah-top′se-ah) a visual defect in which colored objects appear unnaturally colored and colorless objects appear tinged with color. The chromatopsias are named for the colors seen: cyanopsia, blue; chloropsia, green; erythropsia, red; xanthopsia, yellow. Chromatopsia may be caused by drugs, disturbance of the optic centers, cataract extraction, or dazzling light.

chromatoptometer (kro″mah-top-tom′ĕ-ter) a device for measuring color perception.

chromatoptometry (kro″mah-top-tom′ĕ-tre) measurement of color perception.

chromatoscope (kro-mat′to-skōp) an instrument used in CHROMATOSCOPY for testing color VISION.

chromatoscopy (kro″mah-tos′kah-pe) 1. the testing of color VISION using light beams to mix color stimuli. 2. the diagnosis of renal function by the color of urine following administration of dyes; called also chromoscopy.

chromaturia (kro″mah-tu′re-ah) abnormal coloration of the urine.

chromesthesia (kro″mes-the′zhah) association of imaginary color sensations with actual sensations of taste, hearing, or smell.

chromhidrosis (krōm″hĭ-dro′sis) secretion of colored sweat.

chromic acid (kro′mik) 1. a dibasic acid, H_2CrO_4; its salts are called chromates. 2. chromium trioxide.

chromidrosis (kro″mĭ-dro′sis) chromhidrosis.

chromium (Cr) (kro′me-um) a chemical element, atomic number 24, atomic weight 51.996. (See Appendix 6.) It is an essential dietary trace element, but hexavalent chromium is carcinogenic.

c. 51 a radioactive isotope of chromium having a half-life of 27.7 days and decaying by electron capture, emitting gamma rays. It is used to label red blood cells for measurement of red cell mass or volume, survival time, and sequestration studies, and for the diagnosis of gastrointestinal bleeding, and is used to label platelets to study their survival. Symbol ^{51}Cr.

Chromobacterium (kro″mo-bak-tēr′e-um) a genus of gram-negative, aerobic or facultatively anaerobic, usually nonpathogenic rod-shaped bacteria; *C. viola′ceum* may cause abscesses, diarrhea, and urinary tract and systemic infections.

chromoblast (kro′mo-blast) an embryonic cell that develops into a pigment cell.

chromoblastomycosis (kro″mo-blas″to-mi-ko′sis) a chronic fungal infection of the skin, usually beginning at the site of a puncture wound or other trauma on one leg or foot, but sometimes involving other areas of the body, with wartlike nodules or papillomas that may or may not ulcerate.

It is usually caused by *Phialophora verrucosa, Fonsecaea compactum, F. pedrosoi,* or *Cladosporium carrionii.* Called also chromomycosis and verrucose or verrucous dermatitis.

chromoclastogenic (kro″mo-klas″to-jen′-ik) giving rise to or inducing chromosomal disruption or damage.

chromocystoscopy (kro″mo-sis-tos′kah-pe) cystoscopy of the ureteral orifices after oral administration of a dye which is excreted in the urine.

chromocyte (kro′mo-sīt) any colored or pigmented cell.

chromodacryorrhea (kro″mo-dak″re-o-re′ah) the shedding of bloody tears.

chromogen (kro′mo-jen) any substance, itself without color, giving origin to a coloring matter.

chromogenesis (kro″mo-jen′ĕ-sis) the formation of color or pigment.

chromogenic (kro″mo-jen′ik) producing color or pigment.

chromomere (kro′mo-mēr) 1. any of the beadlike granules occurring in series along a chromonema. 2. granulomere.

chromomycosis (kro″mo-mi-ko′sis) chromoblastomycosis.

chromonema (kro″mo-ne′mah), pl. *chromone′mata* [Gr.] the coiled central thread of a chromatid along which lie the chromomeres. adj., **chromone′mal.**

chromophil (kro′mo-fil) any easily stainable structure. adj., **chromophil′ic.**

chromophobe (kro′mo-fōb) any cell, structure, or tissue that does not stain readily; applied especially to the chromophobe cells of the anterior lobe of the pituitary gland.

chromophobia (kro″mo-fo′be-ah) the quality of staining poorly with dyes. adj., **chromopho′bic.**

chromophore (kro′mo-for) any chemical group whose presence gives a decided color to a compound and that unites with certain other groups (auxochromes) to form dyes; called also color radical.

chromophoric (kro″mo-for′ik) 1. bearing color. 2. pertaining to a chromophore.

chromophose (kro′mo-fōz) a subjective sensation of a spot of color in the eye.

chromopsia (kro-mop′se-ah) chromatopsia.

chromoscopy (kro-mos′kah-pe) chromatoscopy (def. 2).

chromosome (kro′mo-sōm) in animal cells, a structure in the nucleus, containing a linear thread of DEOXYRIBONUCLEIC ACID (DNA), which transmits genetic information and is associated with RIBONUCLEIC ACID and HISTONES. In bacterial genetics, a closed circle of double-stranded DNA that contains

the genetic material of the cell and is attached to the cell membrane; the bulk of this material forms a compact bacterial nucleus. adj., **chromoso′mal.**

During cell division the material composing the chromosome is compactly coiled, making it visible with appropriate staining and permitting its movement in the cell with minimal entanglement. Each organism of a species is normally characterized by the same number of chromosomes in its somatic cells, 46 being the number normally present in humans, including 22 pairs of autosomes and the two sex chromosomes (XX or XY), which determine the sex of the organism. (See also HEREDITY.)

Chromosome Analysis. This can be done on fetal cells obtained by AMNIOCENTESIS or chorionic villus SAMPLING, on lymphocytes from a blood sample, on skin cells from a biopsy, or on cells from products of conception such as an aborted fetus. The cells are then cultured in the laboratory until they divide. Cell division is arrested in mid-metaphase by the drug Colcemid. The chromosomes can be stained by one of several techniques that produce a distinct pattern of light and dark bands along the chromosomes, and each chromosome can be recognized by its size and banding pattern. The chromosomal characteristics of an individual are referred to as the KARYOTYPE. It is also possible to make a PHOTOMICROGRAPH of a cell nucleus, cut it apart, and rearrange it so that the individual chromosomes are in order and labeled. The AUTOSOMES are numbered 1–22, roughly in order of decreasing length. The sex CHROMOSOMES are labeled X and Y. Karyotyping is useful in determining the presence of chromosome defects.

Before the chromosomes could be precisely identified they were placed in seven groups: A (chromosomes 1–3), B (4–5), C (6–12 and X), D (13–15), E (16–18), F (19–20), and G (21–22 and Y).

Chromosomal Abnormalities. The prevalence of chromosomal disorders cannot be fully and accurately determined because many of these disorders do not permit full embryonic and fetal development and therefore end in spontaneous abortion. About one in every 100 newborn infants do, however, have a gross demonstrable chromosomal abnormality. A large majority of cytogenetic abnormalities can be identified by cytogenetic analysis either before birth, by means of chorionic villus SAMPLING or AMNIOCENTESIS, or after birth.

Cytogenetic disorders with visible chromosomal abnormalities are evidenced by either an abnormal number of chromosomes or some alteration in the structure of one or more chromosomes. In the language of the geneticist, TRISOMY refers to the presence of an additional chromosome that is homologous with one of the existing pairs so that that particular chromosome is present in triplicate. An example of this type of disorder is a form of DOWN SYNDROME (*trisomy 21*). Another example is PATAU'S SYNDROME (*trisomy 13*), which produces severe anatomical malformations and profound mental retardation.

The term MONOSOMY refers to the absence of one of a pair of homologous chromosomes. Monosomy involving an autosome usually results in the loss of too much genetic information to permit sufficient fetal development for a live birth. Either trisomy or monosomy involving the sex chromosomes yields relatively mild abnormalities.

A condition known as MOSAICISM results from an error in the distribution of chromosomes between daughter cells during an early embryonic cell division, producing two and sometimes three populations of cells with different chromosome numbers in the same individual. Mosaicism involving the sex chromosomes is not uncommon.

Other abnormal structural changes in the chromosome are consequences of some kind of chromosomal breakage, with either the loss or rearrangement of genetic material. TRANSLOCATION involves the transfer of a segment of one chromosome to another. INVERSION refers to a change in the sequence of genes along the chromosome, which occurs when there are two breaks in a chromosome and the segment between the breaks is reversed and reattached to the wrong ends. DELETION occurs when a portion of a chromosome is lost. An example of this type of chromosomal abnormality is CRI DU CHAT SYNDROME, a deletion in the short arm of chromosome 5, marked by mental retardation and sometimes congenital heart defects. When deletion occurs at both ends of the chromosome, the two damaged ends can unite to form a circle and the rearrangement produces a ring CHROMOSOME. ISO-CHROMOSOMES form when the CENTROMERE divides along the transverse plane rather than the normal long axis of the chromosome so that both arms are identical. All of the previously described structural abnormalities can affect both autosomal and sex chromosomes.

The causes of chromosomal errors are not completely understood. In some conditions such as Down syndrome, late maternal age seems to be a factor. Other factors may include the predisposition of chromosomes to nondisjunction (failure to separate during meiosis), exposure to radiation, and viruses.

homologous c's the chromosomes of a matching pair in the diploid complement that contain alleles of specific genes.

c. painting fluorescent in situ hybridization.

Ph¹ c., Philadelphia c. an abnormality of chromosome 22, characterized by the translocation of genetic material from its long arm to chromosome 9, seen in the marrow cells of most patients with chronic myelogenous leukemia.

ring c. a chromosome in which both ends have been lost (deletion) and the two broken ends have reunited to form a ring-shaped figure.

sex c's the chromosomes responsible for determination of the sex of the individual that develops from a zygote; in mammals they are an unequal pair, the X and Y chromosomes.

somatic c. autosome.

X c. the female sex chromosome, being carried by half the male gametes and all female gametes; female diploid cells have two X chromosomes.

Y c. the male sex chromosome, being carried by half the male gametes and none of the female gametes; male diploid cells have an X and a Y chromosome.

chromotherapy (kro″mo-ther′ah-pe) the use of light of specific colors to treat health problems.

chron(o)- word element [Gr.], *time.*

chronaxie (kro′nak-se) the minimum time at which an electric current must flow at a voltage twice the RHEOBASE to cause a muscle to contract. In a strength-duration CURVE for muscle stimulation, it is the pulse WIDTH at a voltage twice that at the rheobase.

chronaxy (kro′nak-se) chronaxie.

chronic (kron′ik) persisting for a long time; applied to a morbid state, designating one showing little change or extremely slow progression over a long period.

c. airflow limitation (CAL) any pulmonary disorder occurring as a result of increased airway resistance or of decreased elastic recoil; the diseases most often associated are ASTHMA, chronic BRONCHITIS, and chronic pulmonary EMPHYSEMA. Called also chronic obstructive pulmonary disease.

Chronic airflow limitation has the highest morbidity rate of any significant chronic pulmonary disorder in the United States and is the second most common cause of hospital admissions. It is difficult to estimate its exact incidence because most diseases of the respiratory tract are not reportable and there is some confusion in definition of terms related to diseases of this type. However, the Social Security Administration reports that CAL ranked only second to heart disease as the cause of disability in men over the age of 40. The incidence of CAL is increasing and, although not all specific causes are known, factors contributing to its development and affecting its degree of severity have been identified. Heavy cigarette smoking is probably the most important factor, and others are industrial pollution, occupational exposure to irritating inhalants, allergy, autoimmunity, genetic predisposition, and chronic infections.

Prevention is best accomplished through education of the public about the hazards of cigarette smoking and air pollution and the need for early detection and prompt treatment of respiratory disorders that could become chronic in nature. The American Lung Association is particularly interested in education of lay persons in these matters and in the prevention of all types of respiratory disorders. This agency, which has local offices distributed throughout the country, is an excellent source of information about prevention and the latest developments in the treatment of respiratory diseases.

Symptoms. This is an insidious disease that can develop into advanced lung damage almost before its victim is aware that the condition is serious. The early symptoms are shortness of breath upon exertion, a mild cough (sometimes called "smoker's cough"), which occurs most often in the morning, and easy fatigability that follows even minimal physical effort. Prompt treatment of these symptoms can forestall the more serious effects of extensive lung damage; however, the destruction of lung tissue and bronchial mucosa damage that has already occurred by the time these symptoms appear is irreversible.

As the disease progresses, the symptoms of dyspnea, weakness, and cough become more severe. The patient has difficulty expelling air from the lungs and the cough becomes more productive of thick, tenacious sputum. The patient looks anxious and drawn and may speak in short, hesitant sentences. Symptoms related to disturbances of the respiratory and circulatory systems and ACID-BASE BALANCE may appear as these complications develop.

Complications. Destructive involvement of respiratory structures and the resultant impairment of circulatory function can produce serious life-threatening complications. Among these are acute respiratory failure, disturbance in the acid-base balance (which can occur either as uncompensated respiratory ACIDOSIS or metabolic ALKALOSIS), bronchopulmonary infections, COR PULMONALE (the result of increased resistance in pulmonary circulation), pulmonary EMBOLISM (especially if polycythemia is severe), and PEPTIC ULCER. BLOOD GAS ANALYSIS is helpful in evaluating effectiveness of blood gas exchange across alveolar walls. In severe chronic airflow limitation, the Pa_{CO_2} level is high while the Pa_{O_2} and the Sa_{O_2} levels are low.

Treatment and Patient Care. In general, treatment is concerned with restoring and maintaining existing lung function, relieving symptoms, and planning a program of rehabilitation tailored to accommodate the individual patient's physiologic needs, physical stamina, vocational needs, lifestyle, and personality. Specific measures of patient care are concerned with (1) initial and periodic evaluation of patient status, (2) maintenance of general health as much as possible, (3) prevention and control of infection, (4) improvement of ventilation, and (5) patient education.

Chronic airflow limitation is a disease that has no cure; its chronic nature requires an ongoing program of assessment and long-term care that is planned and revised as the patient's needs dictate. Whatever the patient care setting—acute care facility, outpatient clinic, long-term care facility, or home—the elements of care presented below are essential to the effective management of the condition.

Evaluation. Patient assessment begins with the taking of the patient's history and performing physical examination and lung function tests at the time the diagnosis is established. These measures, along with blood gas analysis at rest and after exercise, provide a baseline for periodic evaluation of the patient's status to determine the progress of the disease and the effectiveness of treatment.

When patients are informed about the purpose of the tests and therapy they are more likely to participate in the planned regimen of care and to become motivated to continue carrying out their responsibilities in the management of their illness. Those who work with the patient should clarify the goals and offer encouragement when they make progress toward those goals, no matter how slight the improvement might be. This implies, of course, that all members of the health care team have an understanding of the disease, the meaning of various test values, and the purpose of each aspect of care.

Maintenance of Health Status. It is important to communicate to these patients the concept of health status, particularly in regard to their position on the health-illness continuum. They cannot be completely disease-free or restored to their former state of health. They can, however, manage the disease symptoms for periods of time and some may even make progress toward a better state of health. For those patients who continue to deteriorate despite appropriate care, encouragement should be provided to maintain as much function as possible.

Poor appetite and the potential for dehydration are problems commonly associated with pulmonary disease. Purulent sputum, coughing, and fatigue can contribute to loss of interest in eating. Mouth breathing, increased respiratory rate, and frequent expectorating contribute to the loss of fluid.

Frequent oral hygiene and mouth care can help diminish mouth odor and unpleasant taste. A short period of rest just prior to each meal can help overcome the problem of fatigue. Meals should be spaced so that the stomach is not overloaded at any one time; five small meals, rather than three a day, can help avoid overfilling of the stomach and interference with breathing. Postural drainage and similar procedures should not be done on a full stomach, nor should they be scheduled just before a meal. Adequate hydration can be accomplished by an intake of at least 3000 ml of liquid each day. Unless contraindicated, this should include bouillon, fruit juices, and other liquids the patient finds enjoyable and refreshing.

Physical activity may be severely limited by CAL because of inadequate ventilation and decreased circulation. As with all other aspects of patient care, plans to increase exercise tolerance and promote physical activity should be designed according to the patient's cardiopulmonary status. Techniques to promote muscular relaxation and breathing control are the first step, followed by gradual increase in activity as the patient's progress and general physical condition permit.

Adequate rest is essential, but the HAZARDS OF IMMOBILITY must be avoided, especially in patients who are fearful that any physical activity may precipitate an exhausting episode of coughing and dyspnea. The goal is to provide sufficient rest so that the body's natural restorative processes can work, but to avoid long periods of sleeping and lying in bed during the day.

When the patient's cardiopulmonary condition is such that bed rest is prescribed, care is taken to avoid complete physical inactivity, which will only serve to increase problems of inadequate ventilation and muscle weakness. Proper positioning is essential and should be such that the neck is extended, with the chin well off the chest. Support under the thighs while the patient is supine will release tension on abdominal muscles, thereby facilitating movement of the diaphragm for deep breathing and effective coughing. The arms and hands should also be supported on pillows and positioned away from the sides to allow for maximum lung expansion without elevation of the upper chest. A foot board is placed so as to maintain good posture, promote comfort, and ensure good muscle tone in the legs and feet.

Prevention and Control of Infection. Acute respiratory infection can be fatal in patients with chronic airflow limitation. Chronic infections inflict further damage to the respiratory structures, lead to increased debilitation, and increase the likelihood of severe complications. Both acute and chronic infections produce increased secretions in the air passages, which further restrict the flow of air.

Contact with others who have an upper respiratory infection should be avoided, as should being in large crowds during the season when such infections are common. A high level of resistance should be maintained through good personal hygiene and adequate nutrition. Vaccines to guard against influenza are recommended. Patients should be taught to watch for changes in color and amount of sputum. If a change in sputum or any other symptoms of infection appear, this should be reported.

Improvement of Ventilation. It is obvious that measures to improve ventilation in the patient with CAL are of primary importance, and perhaps that is why so many ways have been devised to facilitate the flow of air to and from the lungs. Breathing is most difficult during the expiratory phase, making it difficult to remove trapped air and secretions. In addition, the bronchial walls are weakened in patients with emphysema and are subject to collapse. Health status and physical condition at the time the technique is used will affect the choice of method and its effectiveness.

Hydration is considered especially valuable in improvement of ventilation. Inhaled air should be moist so as to thin the secretions for removal and soothe the irritated mucous membranes. This can be accomplished through the use of vaporizers and humidifiers, either for environmental humidification in the patient's room or in conjunction with oxygen therapy and the administration of aerosols. Oral intake of fluids is also important. Bronchodilators, usually in the form of aerosols, sometimes as oral medications, are usually prescribed. The aerosol method of delivery depends on the ability of the patient to breathe deeply so that the medication reaches the lower segments of the respiratory tract.

Controlled deep breathing patterns are especially helpful in emptying the lungs and providing adequate ventilation. The patient with CAL is taught to expand the lower chest and to use the accessory muscles and diaphragm to improve the breathing pattern. Performance of these breathing patterns is important because patients probably are not in the habit of breathing in the most effective manner, making optimum use of remaining pulmonary function. The patient is taught slow, controlled, and steady breathing. Respiratory effort should be concentrated on slow expiratory flow through parted or pursed lips. Pushing the air out of the lungs too forcefully can bring on collapse of the airway structures. During instruction, the caregiver watches for signs of exhaustion and warns against overdoing the deep breathing until the patient has adjusted to it. A correct breathing pattern should be coordinated with all of the patient's daily activities so that it becomes habitual and is done without too much thought.

Effective coughing does not come easily to patients with this condition. They may have experienced too many episodes in which a dry hacking cough has caused exhaustion, increased dyspnea, and prevented removal of tenacious sputum from the air passages. They must be convinced that, when done correctly, coughing can remove mucous plugs and relieve rather than produce dyspnea. Patients should be warned that explosive coughing is not very effective, can damage the airways, and can lead to exhaustion. The objective of coughing is to move secretions upward gradually so that they can be expectorated.

POSTURAL DRAINAGE is also valuable in facilitating the removal of mucus from the air passages. The various maneuvers involved in this procedure are designed to take advantage of gravity flow as a means of clearing specified segments of the air passages when normal air flow is not sufficient to move secretions or stimulate the cough reflex. Chest percussion and vibration may be employed during postural drainage to loosen secretions. OXYGEN THERAPY is used as a supportive measure when there is decreased oxygenation of arterial blood. It can be administered to ambulatory patients being cared for at home. Blood gas analysis is an excellent guide in determining the need for initiating oxygen therapy and for monitoring dosage.

Patient Education. As with all chronic diseases that require long-term planning and management, patient education is of primary importance in successful execution of the plan. Each of the measures previously described involves instruction of the patient and family, particularly when care is carried out on an outpatient basis. The patient should be told *why* it is necessary to stop smoking, avoid other irritating inhalants, carry out good health practices, take medication only as prescribed, and faithfully perform techniques to improve ventilation. Those patients who follow the exercises prescribed for them often find they can lead more active lives than formerly. Exertional dyspnea becomes less severe and complications from infections caused by bacteria in secretions formerly trapped in the respiratory tract are less frequent. Active participation in a program of self-care gives these patients a sense of control and improves their self-esteem.

c. fatigue syndrome, c. fatigue and immunodeficiency syndrome persistent debilitating fatigue of recent onset, with reduction of physical activity to less than half of usual, accompanied by some combination of muscle weakness, sore throat, mild fever, tender lymph nodes, headaches, and depression, with the symptoms not attributable to any other known causes. Its nature is controversial; viral infection (including Epstein-Barr virus and human herpesvirus-6) may be associated with it, but no causal relationship has been demonstrated. A number of names have been used for this syndrome, including Iceland disease and benign myalgic encephalomyelitis.

c. granulomatous disease chronic suppurative lymphadenitis, eczematoid dermatitis, enlargement of the liver and spleen, and chronic pulmonary disease associated with a genetically determined defect in the intracellular bactericidal function of leukocytes.

c. obstructive lung disease (COLD), **c. obstructive pulmonary disease** (COPD) chronic airflow limitation.

c. regional pain syndrome reflex sympathetic dystrophy.

chronobiologist (kron″o-bi-ol′ah-jist) a specialist in CHRONOBIOLOGY.

chronobiology (kron″o-bi-ol′ah-je) the scientific study of the effect of time on living systems and of biological RHYTHMS. adj., **chronobiolog′ic, chronobiolog′ical.**

chronognosis (kron″og-no′sis) perception of the lapse of time.

chronograph (kron′o-graf) an instrument for recording small intervals of time.

chronophobia (kron″o-fo′be-ah) extreme, irrational fear of time; a type seen in prisoners is called prison NEUROSIS.

chronotropic (kron″o-trop′ik) affecting the time or rate.

chronotropism (kro-not′ro-pizm) interference with regularity of a periodical movement, such as the heart's action.

Chronulac (kron′u-lak) trademark for a preparation of LACTULOSE, a CATHARTIC.

chrys(o)- word element [Gr.], *gold.*

chrysiasis (kri-si′ah-sis) 1. deposition of gold particles in the tissues as a result of prolonged or excessive parenteral CHRYSO-THERAPY, which commonly causes adverse reactions consisting primarily of dermatitis, stomatitis, or transient mild proteinuria; more serious toxicity involves the hematopoietic system, liver, kidney, eye (cornea, lens), or other vital organs. 2. chrysoderma.

chrysoderma (kris″o-der′mah) a manifestation of CHRYSIASIS presenting as a permanent gray- to lilac-colored pigmentation on the face, eyelids, and other sun-exposed areas of the body.

Chrysops (kris′ops) a genus of small bloodsucking horse flies of warm regions, of the family Tabanidae. *C. disca′lis* is the deer fly, a host of TULAREMIA in the western United States, and *C. sila′cea* is an intermediate host of *Loa loa* in Africa.

chrysotherapy (kris″o-ther′ah-pe) treatment with GOLD salts, especially for rheumatoid ARTHRITIS; it is thought to work by affecting oxygen radicals or stabilizing lysosomes. The goals are to reverse, inhibit, or prevent damage to cartilage, bone, and other connective tissues. Use of this method has been declining as other treatments have become available. Called also gold therapy and aurotherapy.

Churg-Strauss syndrome (cherg strous) a form of systemic necrotizing vasculitis in which there is prominent lung involvement with severe asthma, eosinophilia, and granulomatous reactions. If present, skin lesions consist of tender subcutaneous nodules and bruiselike spots. Called also allergic granulomatosis, allergic granulomatous angiitis, and Churg-Strauss vasculitis.

Chvostek's sign (khvos′teks)) **Chvostek-Weiss sign** (khvos′tek-vīs′)) a spasm of the facial muscles elicited by tapping the facial nerve in the region of the parotid gland; seen in tetany.

chylangioma (ki-lan″je-o′mah) a tumor of intestinal lymph vessels filled with chyle.

chyle (kīl) the milky fluid taken up by the lacteals from the intestine during digestion, consisting of lymph and triglyceride fat (chylomicrons) in a stable emulsion, and conveyed by the thoracic duct to empty into the venous system.

chylemia (ki-le′me-ah) the presence of chyle in the blood.

chylifaction (ki″lĭ-fak′shun)) **chylification** (ki″lĭ-fĭ-ka′shun)) chylopoiesis.

chyliform (ki′lĭ-form) resembling chyle.

chylocele (ki′lo-sēl) elephantiasis scroti.

chyloderma (ki″lo-der′mah) elephantiasis.

chylomediastinum (ki″lo-me″de-ah-sti′-num) the presence of effused chyle in the mediastinum.

chylomicron (ki″lo-mi′kron) a particle of the class of LIPOPROTEINS responsible for the transport of exogenous CHOLESTEROL and TRIGLYCERIDES from the small intestine to tissues after meals. Chylomicrons are spherical particles with a core of triglycerides surrounded by a layer of phospholipids, cholesterol, and apolipoproteins.

chylomicronemia (ki″lo-mi″kro-ne′me-ah) an excess of chylomicrons in the blood.

chylopericardium (ki″lo-per″ĭ-kahr′de-um) the presence of effused chyle in the pericardium.

chyloperitoneum (ki″lo-per″ĭ-to-ne′um) the presence of effused chyle in the peritoneal cavity.

chylopneumothorax (ki″lo-noo″mo-thor′-aks) a PLEURAL EFFUSION containing effused chyle and air.

chylopoiesis (ki″lo-poi-e′sis) the formation of chyle. adj., **chylopoiet′ic.**

chylothorax (ki″lo-thor′aks) a PLEURAL EFFUSION consisting of chyle or a chylelike fluid; it may be either congenital (such as in babies) or acquired from trauma or disease states. There are two types: *chylous effusion,* due to leakage of chyle from the thoracic duct, and *chyliform* or *pseudochylous effusion,* consisting of chylelike fluid, the result of a chronic disease such as tuberculosis.

chylous (ki′lus) pertaining, mingled with, or of the nature of chyle.

chyluria (ki-lu′re-ah) the presence of chyle in the urine, giving it a milky appearance this follows obstruction of lymph flow which causes rupture of lymph vessels into the renal pelves, ureters, bladder, or urethra.

C

chyme (kīm) the semifluid, homogeneous, creamy or gruel-like material produced by action of the gastric juice on ingested food in the stomach and discharged through the pylorus into the duodenum.

chymification (ki″mĭ-fĭ-ka′shun) gastric DIGESTION.

chymopapain (ki″mo-pah-pān′) a proteolytic enzyme from the tropical tree *Carica papaya,* used in CHEMONUCLEOLYSIS of a HERNIATED DISK in the lumbar region.

chymotrypsin (ki″mo-trip′sin) 1. an enzyme with action similar to that of TRYPSIN, produced in the intestine by activation of CHYMOTRYPSINOGEN. 2. a preparation crystallized from an extract of the pancreas of the ox, used clinically for enzymatic dissolution of the zonular membrane of the eye.

chymotrypsinogen (ki″mo-trip-sin′o-jen) the inactive precursor of chymotrypsin, the form in which it is secreted by the pancreas.

Ci curie.

cib. ci′bus (food).

cicatrectomy (sik″ah-trek′to-me) surgical excision of a scar (cicatrix).

cicatricial (sik″ah-trish′al) pertaining to a cicatrix (scar).

cicatrix (sik′ah-triks, sĭ-ka′triks), pl. *cica′-trices* [L.] scar.

cicatrization (sik″ah-trī-za′shun) scarring; the formation of a cicatrix (scar).

ciclopirox (si″klo-pir′oks) a broad-spectrum antifungal AGENT with activity similar to that of the IMIDAZOLES, used topically as the olamine salt against skin infections.

cidofovir (si-dof′ah-vir) an antiviral nucleoside analogue used in treatment of cytomegalovirus RETINITIS in patients with acquired immunodeficiency syndrome; administered by intravenous infusion.

-cide word element [L.], *destruction or killing* (homicide); *an agent that kills or destroys* (germicide). adj., **-ci′dal.**

ciguatera (se″gwah-ta′rah) a form of FISH POISONING, marked by gastrointestinal and neurologic symptoms due to ingestion of tropical or subtropical marine fish such as the BARRACUDA, GROUPER, or SNAPPER that have CIGUATOXIN in their tissues.

ciguatoxin (se′gwah-tok″sin) a heat-stable toxin originating in a dinoflagellate as a pretoxin and concentrating in active form in the tissues of certain marine fish, causing CIGUATERA in humans who eat the fish.

cilastatin (si″lah-stat′in) an enzyme inhibitor used with IMIPENEM to decrease the metabolism of imipenem in the kidneys and increase its concentration in the urine; administered as the sodium salt.

cili(o)- word element [L.], *cilia; ciliary (body).*

cilia (sil′e-ah) sing. *cil′ium* [L.] 1. the eyelids or their outer edge. 2. the eyelashes. 3. minute hairlike processes that extend from a cell surface, composed of nine pairs of microtubules around a core of two microtubules. They beat rhythmically to move the cell or to move fluid or mucus over the surface.

ciliariscope (sil″e-ar′ĭ-skōp) an instrument for examining the ciliary region of the eye.

ciliarotomy (sil″e-ah-rot′ah-me) surgical division of the ciliary zone.

ciliary (sil′e-ar″e) pertaining to or resembling cilia; used particularly in reference to certain eye structures, as the ciliary body or muscle.

c. body the thickened part of the vascular tunic of the eye, connecting choroid and iris, made up of the ciliary muscle and the ciliary processes. These processes radiate from the ciliary muscle and give attachment to ligaments supporting the lens of the eye.

Ciliata (sil″e-a′tah) a class of protozoa (subphylum Ciliophora) whose members possess cilia throughout the life cycle; a few species are parasitic.

ciliate (sil′e-āt) 1. having cilia. 2. any individual of the Ciliata.

ciliated (sil′e-āt″ed) provided with cilia.

ciliectomy (sil″e-ek′to-me) 1. excision of a portion of the ciliary body. 2. excision of the portion of the eyelid containing the roots of the eyelashes.

Ciliophora (sil″e-of′o-rah) a subphylum of Protozoa, including two major groups, the ciliates and suctorians, and distinguished from the other subphyla by the presence of cilia at some stage in the existence of the member organisms.

cilium (sil′e-um) [L.] singular of CILIA.

cillosis (sil-o′sis) spasmodic quivering of the eyelid.

cilostazol (sī-lo′stah-zol) an agent that reversibly inhibits platelet aggregation and causes vasodilation, particularly in femoral vascular beds; administered orally to produce symptomatic relief in the treatment of intermittent claudication.

cimbia (sim′be-ah) a white band running across the ventral surface of the crus cerebri.

cimetidine (si-met′ĭ-dēn) an antagonist of histamine H_2 RECEPTORS, inhibiting the action of HISTAMINE at cell surface receptors of the gastric parietal cells and reducing basal gastric acid secretion and secretion stimulated by food, histamine, gastrin, caffeine, and insulin. It is used for the short-term (two months) treatment and, at reduced dosage, the long-term prevention of PEPTIC ULCERS, for the relief of symptoms associated with hyperacidity, such as heartburn and acid indigestion, and for the treatment of GASTROESOPHAGEAL REFLUX DISEASE, upper gastrointestinal bleeding, and pathological hypersecretory conditions such as ZOLLINGER-ELLISON SYNDROME. Treatment of peptic ulcer with cimetidine brings prompt relief and speeds ulcer healing. Antacids are also taken as needed for relief of pain. Cimetidine is used as the base or the hydrochloride salt, administered orally, intramuscularly, or intravenously.

Cimex (si'meks) a genus of blood-sucking insects (order Hemiptera), the bedbugs. *C. lectula'rius* is the common bedbug of temperate regions. Other species are limited to tropical and subtropical areas and feed on other animals as well as humans.

CINAHL Cumulative Index to Nursing and Allied Health Literature.

cinchona (sin-ko'nah) the dried bark of the stem or root of various South American trees of the genus *Cinchona;* it is the source of QUININE, CINCHONINE, and other alkaloids and was used as an antimalarial.

cinchonine an alkaloid of CINCHONA used as an antimalarial AGENT, chiefly in the form of the sulfate salt; administered orally.

cinchonism (sin'ko-nizm) toxicity due to overdosage of CINCHONA alkaloids; symptoms are tinnitus and slight deafness, photophobia and other visual disturbances, mental dullness, depression, confusion, headache, and nausea. Called also quininism.

cine- word element [Gr.], *movement.* See also words beginning KINE-.

cineangiocardiography (sin″e-an″je-o-kahr″de-og'rah-fe) the photographic recording of fluoroscopic images of the heart and great vessels by motion picture techniques.

cineangiography (sin″e-an″je-og'rah-fe) the photographic recording of fluoroscopic images of the blood vessels by motion picture techniques.

cinefluorography (sin″ĕ-floo'or-og'rah-fe) cineradiography.

cinemicrography (sin″ĕ-mi-krog'rah-fe) the making of motion pictures of a small object through the lens system of a microscope.

cinephlebography (sin″ĕ-flĕ-bog'rah-fe) cineradiography of the veins after administration of a contrast medium. In ascending functional cinephlebography, the contrast medium is introduced into a vein in a foot and its progress is observed as it courses through the tibial, popliteal, and iliac veins.

cineradiofluorography (sin″ĕ-ra″de-o-floo-rog'rah-fe) cineradiography.

cineradiography (sin″e-ra″de-og'rah-fe) the making of a motion picture record of successive images appearing on a fluoroscopic screen.

cinerea (sĭ-nēr'e-ah) the gray matter of the nervous system. adj., **cine'real.**

cinesi- for words beginning thus, see those beginning *kinesi-.*

cinet(o)- for words beginning thus, see those beginning *kinet(o)-.*

cingulectomy (sing″gu-lek'to-me) bilateral extirpation of the anterior half of the gyrus cinguli.

cingulotomy (sing″gu-lot'ah-me) the creation of lesions in the GYRUS CINGULI using STEREOTACTIC techniques; the primary psychiatric indication for this procedure is relief of intractable OBSESSIVE-COMPULSIVE DISORDER. It may also be done for relief of intractable pain. Research about it is ongoing.

cingulum (sing'gu-lum), pl. *cin'gula* [L.] 1. an encircling part or structure; a girdle. 2. a bundle of association fibers partly encircling the corpus callosum not far from the median plane, interrelating the cingulate and hippocampal gyri. 3. the lingual lobe of an anterior tooth. adj., **cing'ulate.**

cingulumotomy (sing″gu-lum-ot'ah-me) cingulotomy.

C1 INH C1 inhibitor.

Cinobac (sin'o-bak) trademark for a preparation of CINOXACIN, an antimicrobial agent used in the treatment of urinary tract infections.

cinoxacin (sin-ok'sah-sin) a QUINOLONE antimicrobial agent administered orally in the treatment of urinary tract infections due to *Escherichia coli, Proteus mirabilis, P. vulgaris, Klebsiella* species, including *K. pneumoniae,* and *Enterobacter* species.

ciprofloxacin (sip″ro-flok'sah-sin) a QUINOLONE antibacterial agent effective against many gram-positive and gram-negative bacteria, including some strains resistant to other agents such as penicillins.

circadian (ser″kah-de'an, ser-ka'de-an) denoting a period of one day, or repeating every day; see circadian RHYTHM.

c. rhythm sleep disorder a sleep disorder of the DYSSOMNIA group, consisting of a lack of SYNCHRONY between the schedule of sleeping and waking required by the external environment and that of the person's own circadian RHYTHM. The cause is usually environmental, such as rotating shift work or long-distance air travel, but some individuals simply have natural circadian rhythms sharply different from the predominant one of their society.

circinate (ser'sĭ-nāt) 1. circular. 2. annular.

circle (ser'k'l) a round figure, structure, or part.

  Berry's c's charts with circles on them for testing stereoscopic vision.

  cerebral arterial c. circle of Willis.

  Minsky's c. a device for the graphic recording of eye lesions.

  sensory c. a body area within which it is impossible to distinguish separately the impressions arising from two sites of stimulation.

  c. of Willis the anastomotic loop of blood vessels near the base of the brain. Called also cerebral arterial circle.

circulation (ser-ku-la'shun) 1. movement in a regular or circuitous course, returning to the point of origin. 2. the movement of blood through the heart and blood vessels by which food, oxygen, and internal secretions are carried to and wastes are carried from the body tissues; see also CIRCULATORY SYSTEM.

  collateral c. that carried on through secondary channels after obstruction of the principal channel supplying the part.

  coronary c. that within the coronary vessels, supplying the muscle of the heart.

  enterohepatic c. the cycle in which bile salts and other substances excreted by the liver are absorbed by the intestinal mucosa and returned to the liver via the portal circulation.

  extracorporeal c. circulation of blood outside the body, as through a HEMODIALYZER for removal of substances usually excreted in the urine, or a HEART-LUNG MACHINE for carbon dioxide–oxygen exchange.

  fetal c. see FETAL circulation.

  hepatic portal c. portal circulation (def. 2).

  persistent fetal c. a condition in newborns in which blood continues to flow through the FORAMEN OVALE and a PATENT DUCTUS ARTERIOSUS, bypassing the lungs and resulting in hypoxemia. Called also persistent pulmonary hypertension of the newborn.

  portal c. 1. the circulation of blood through larger vessels from the capillaries of one organ to those of another; see also portal SYSTEM. 2. specifically, the passage of blood from the gastrointestinal tract and spleen through the portal vein to the liver; called also hepatic portal circulation. (See illustration.)

  pulmonary c. see PULMONARY CIRCULATION.

  systemic c. the flow of blood from the left ventricle through the aorta, carrying oxygen and nutrient material to all the tissues of the body, and returning through

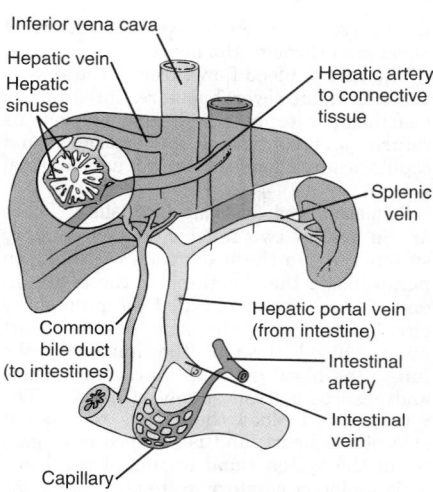

Portal and hepatic circulations.

the superior and inferior venae cavae to the right atrium.

  c. time the time required for blood to flow between two given points. It is determined by injecting a substance into a vein and then measuring the time required for it to reach a specific site, for example, arm-to-tongue time.

circuit (ser'kut) the round or course traversed by an electrical current. The circuit is said to be *closed* when it is continuous, so that the current may pass through it; it is *open, broken,* or *interrupted* when it is not continuous and the current cannot pass through it.

  reentrant c., reentry c. the circuit formed by the circulating impulse in REENTRY.

circulatory (ser'ku-lah-tor"e) pertaining to circulation.

  c. system the major system concerned with the movement of BLOOD and LYMPH, consisting of the HEART, blood VESSELS, and lymphatic VESSELS. (See also color plates.) The circulatory system transports to the tissues and organs of the body the oxygen, nutritive substances, immune substances, hormones, and chemicals necessary for normal function and activities of the organs; it also carries away waste products and carbon dioxide. It equalizes body temperature and helps maintain normal water and electrolyte balance.

  An adult has an average of 5 liters of blood in the body; the circulatory system carries this entire quantity on one complete circuit through the body every minute. In the course of 24 hours, over 6500 liters of blood pass through the heart.

The rate of blood flow through the vessels depends upon several factors: force of the heartbeat, rate of the heartbeat, venous return, and control of the arterioles and capillaries by chemical, neural, and thermal stimuli.

Pulmonary and Systemic Circulation. There are in reality two independent circulatory systems within the body, each with its own pump inside the sheathing of the heart. In one of these systems, called the pulmonary circulation, the right side of the heart pumps blood through the lungs. In the lungs, the blood gives up its carbon dioxide and absorbs a fresh supply of oxygen. The reoxygenated blood then flows to the left side of the heart, and is pumped out again to all the systems and organs of the body. This major circulatory system is called the systemic circulation.

The circulation of blood through the fetus bypasses the pulmonary circuit (see also FETAL CIRCULATION).

Arterial System. Blood pumped from the left side of the heart enters the aorta, the main arterial trunk of the systemic circulation. The aorta, which is about 1 inch in diameter, arches upward and toward the left side of the body. Just above the heart two coronary arteries branch off from the aorta. These arteries supply the muscles of the heart with blood.

Branching from the top of the aortic arch are three large arteries which supply the upper part of the body, the brachiocephalic trunk (which divides into the right carotid and right subclavian arteries) and the left carotid and left subclavian arteries. The carotid arteries supply the head and neck; the subclavian arteries supply the arms. The aorta then turns downward and passes through the trunk of the body, close to the vertebral column. Smaller arteries branch off from the aorta to supply the lungs, stomach, spleen, pancreas, kidneys, intestines, and other organs of the body. At about the level of the umbilicus, the aorta divides into two branches, the two iliac arteries, which supply the vessels of the pelvic organs and the legs.

The arteries so far named are the main conducting arteries. They consist of a smooth inner lining covered largely by elastic fibers that absorb the pulsations of the heart. As the heart beats, the elastic arterial walls damp the strong pulsations into a more nearly constant blood pressure.

Distributing arteries branch out from the conducting arteries. These arteries are composed largely of muscle fibers that encircle the smooth inner lining of the blood vessels and have the ability to contract and relax. The distributing arteries in turn branch out into arterioles, or little arteries, which are barely visible to the eye. The elastic walls of the arterioles and distributing arteries are under the control of the autonomic NERVOUS SYSTEM. The arterioles lead directly to the capillaries.

Blood passes through the aorta at the speed of about 40 cm per second when the body is at rest, and at a faster rate when it is active. As the blood spreads through the distributing arteries and arterioles, its speed gradually diminishes. By the time the blood has reached the capillaries, it has slowed to a speed about one-eightieth of that in the arteries.

Capillaries. The complex network of innumerable and microscopically small capillaries distributed throughout the tissues supplies blood to all cells in the body. Each capillary is about 10 microns in diameter, about the size of a single blood cell; thus the blood cells must make their way through the capillaries in single file.

Despite their minute size, the capillaries have a vast total area. The capillary "lake" can be called the climax of the circulatory system, for it is here that the vital work of the circulatory system is carried out. Nutrients leaving the blood capillaries enter the capillary lake, a collection of tissue fluid which bathes each cell. From there the nutrients permeate the walls of the cells. Waste products of cell metabolism enter the capillary lake and eventually pass through the capillary wall and into the blood circulation. The capillary walls are selective; i.e., they permit the exchange of special nutrients and chemicals and bar the passage of unwanted substances. For example, the cells making up the walls of the capillaries in the brain bar the passage of many substances that might injure the brain cells, and the capillaries in the placenta also act as a barrier against substances that might be harmful to the developing fetus.

Venous System. From the capillaries the blood returns to the heart via the veins, which together make up the venous system. The blood flows from the capillaries to minute venules, and then to the veins, in a network of blood vessels of ever-increasing size that parallels in reverse the branching of the arterial system. The walls of the veins, however, are thinner, less elastic, and less muscular than those of the arteries. And whereas the arteries are for the most part buried deep within the body for protection, the venous system has many superficial veins that run close to the surface of the skin. If an arterial blood vessel is cut, the blood flows from the cut in spurts, whereas blood from a cut vein flows steadily.

The blood returning to the heart collects into two main veins. Blood returning from the arms, head and upper chest flows into the superior vena cava; blood returning from the rest of the body flows into the inferior vena cava. Both these veins return the blood to the right side of the heart.

The blood from the lower part of the body must return to the heart against the force of gravity, since all the pressure built up by the heart has been dissipated in the capillaries. This is accomplished in several ways. The veins themselves contain one-way venous valves which work in pairs. When the blood is flowing in the correct direction, the venous valves are pressed against the walls of the veins, permitting unobstructed flow. If the blood should tend to flow backward, however, the venous valves fall inward and press against each other, effectively stopping the backward flow of blood. The blood is "milked" upward toward the heart principally by the massaging action of the abdominal and leg muscles as they press against the veins. Inspirations of air also force the blood through the venous system, as do the movements of the intestines. If the leg muscles do not move for long periods of time, the blood collects in the lower part of the body and the amount available for the brain is decreased.

Systemic Circuits. The circulatory system has been discussed so far as if the blood flowed through the body in a simple circular path. In fact, the blood can take one of several circuits through the body. Among these circuits are the coronary circuit through the arteries and veins of the heart; a circuit through the neck, head, and brain; a circuit through the digestive organs; and the renal circuit through the kidneys. The importance of the renal circulation lies in the fact that the kidneys act as the cleansing filter of the circulatory system, removing a variety of products that have been cast off from the cells and body tissues. At any given time, about one-quarter of all the blood pumped through the body is passing through the renal circuit.

The most complex circuit (portal circulation) is that which flows through the digestive system, picking up proteins, carbohydrates, fats, and chemicals from the intestines and delivering them to the tissues. Separate distributing arteries conduct the blood to the lower intestine, upper intestine, stomach, spleen, and pancreas. The veins leading from these organs combine to form the portal vein, which leads to the liver. Within the liver, the artery leading to the liver (the hepatic artery) and the portal vein subdivide themselves into a complex network of capillary-like vessels called sinusoids which bring the blood into closer contact with the cells of the liver. The liver cells withdraw glucose from the blood for storage as glycogen or release it as needed, and remove from the blood many harmful substances that might be toxic to body tissues. The blood leaving the liver flows to the inferior vena cava.

Lymphatic System. The cells, chemicals, and other components of the blood are suspended within the blood vessels in plasma. Similar fluid also fills the spaces between the tissue cells. Nutrients reaching the cells are carried there by this tissue fluid, and it also carries waste products from the cells to the capillaries. One function of the lymphatic system is to collect and return this fluid via the lymphatic vessels to the circulatory system. When this tissue fluid is within the lymphatic system, it is called lymph. In addition to draining off excess tissue fluid, the lymphatic capillaries also transport some waste products as well as dead blood cells, pathogenic organisms in case of infection, and malignant cells from cancerous growths. From the lymphatic capillaries the lymph is carried into larger lymphatic vessels which contain one-way valves similar to those in the veins. Lymph nodes are interspersed among the lymph vessels and filter their fluids. Eventually large lymph ducts (the thoracic duct and right lymphatic duct) empty into the right and left subclavian veins. The lymph is propelled by the same massaging action that causes the blood to circulate through the venous system. There are larger masses of lymphatic tissue called lymphatic organs, and among them are the SPLEEN, TONSILS, and THYMUS. These organs produce specialized leukocytes (lymphocytes) that help protect the body against infections (see also IMMUNITY).

circum- word element [L.], *around* or *encircling.*

circumcise (ser′kum-sīz) to perform circumcision.

circumcision (ser″kum-sizh′un) 1. in males, surgical removal of all or part of the foreskin (prepuce) of the penis; see discussion below. 2. **Female Circumcision** is any of various operations to remove part or all of the female external genitalia. It is a widespread practice in some parts of the world, especially in Africa, the Middle East, Indonesia, and Malaysia. In 1979 the WORLD HEALTH ORGANIZATION sponsored a conference in The Sudan that unanimously condemned this practice as indefensible on medical as well as humane grounds.

Female circumcision is classified according to the extent of what is removed. *Sunna circumcision* involves removal of the prepuce or excision of the tip of the clitoris or both. *Excision circumcision* usually includes removal of the clitoris, the labia majora, and the labia minora. *Infibulation* is the most extreme form, involving excision of all or part of the clitoris, labia minora, and medial aspect of the labia majora. The raw edges of the wound are sutured or otherwise held together until healing and scarring form a wall over the upper part of the vestibule. A small opening is left for the flow of urine and menstrual discharge. When a woman marries who has had this latter procedure done as an infant or child, she must be forcibly penetrated or the opening made larger. In these women such complications as painful intercourse, possible perineal lacerations, infections, and hemorrhage are common. At the time of childbirth the scar tissue must be cut and the opening enlarged to allow passage of the infant. Otherwise, both mother and child are at risk for serious complications.

Male Circumcision. This has been traditionally done for hygienic and medical reasons and is the oldest known religious rite. In the Jewish faith the circumcision is a ritual that is performed by a *mohel* (ordained circumciser) on the eighth day after birth if possible. The circumcision is followed by a religious ceremony during which the baby also receives his name.

Circumcision in the hospital usually is done very shortly after birth, provided the newborn is full-term and in good health. The procedure is not without risk from complications, the most common being infection, hemorrhage, and surgical trauma to the penis. Although there is some evidence of a relationship between lack of circumcision and penile cancer, which is relatively rare, poor hygiene seems equally important as an etiologic factor. Cancer of the prostate cannot be linked to lack of circumcision, nor are there good data to support a cause-effect relationship between cervical cancer in females and coitus with an uncircumcised spouse.

The American Academy of Pediatrics and the American College of Obstetricians have found no medically valid reasons for routine circumcision of newborns. While the practice is declining in the United States and is not routinely done in Canada, Great Britain, or Western European countries, almost two thirds of North American newborns are circumcised. For parents who are undecided about circumcision for their newborn sons, the American Academy of Pediatrics provides a brochure that can be obtained from AAP, Dept. C, 141 Northwest Point Blvd., Elk Grove Village, IL 60007. A stamped, self-addressed business envelope should accompany the request.

Patient Care. Preoperative care for the older male child or adult undergoing circumcision includes laboratory tests to determine coagulation or clotting time and a general checkup to assure that the patient is in good health. A mild sedative may be given, though newborns usually do not receive any special preoperative care or sedation.

The patient is watched closely after the operation for signs of bleeding; however, excessive bleeding is extremely rare. Other observations include watching for signs of infection, difficulty in urination, and jaundice. A sterile gauze dressing with ointment is usually placed over the penis when surgery is completed. The dressing is changed each time the diaper is changed, or, in young children and adults, after each urination. When the Plastibell method of circumcision is used, the penis and attached ring is cleansed with sterile water each time the diaper is changed. Healing usually takes place in five to seven days. (See accompanying illustration.)

circumduction (ser″kum-duk′shun) circular movement of a limb or of the eye.

circumflex (ser′kum-fleks) curved like a bow.

circumscribed (ser′kum-skrībd) bounded or limited; confined to a limited space.

circumstantiality (ser″kum-stan″she-al′ĭ-te) a disturbed pattern of speech or writing characterized by delay in getting to the point because of the interpolation of unnecessary details and irrelevant remarks; seen in persons with schizophrenia and obsessive-compulsive disorders. See also TANGENTIALITY.

circumvallate (ser″kum-val′āt) surrounded by a ridge or trench, as the circumvallate papillae.

circumventricular (ser″kum-ven-trik′u-ler) located around a ventricle, particularly in the brain.

cirrhosis (sĭ-ro′sis) a liver disease (actually a group of chronic diseases) characterized by loss of the normal microscopic lobular architecture and regenerative replacement of necrotic parenchymal tissue with fibrous bands of connective tissue

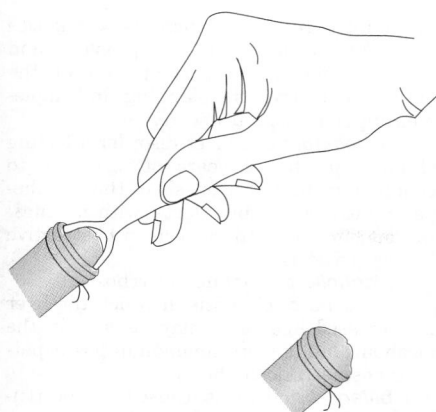

Circumcision using the Plastibell. The specialist places the Plastibell, a plastic ring, over the glans, draws the prepuce over it, and ties a suture around the prepuce and Plastibell. This procedure prevents bleeding when the excess prepuce is removed. The handle is removed, leaving only the ring in place over the glans. The Plastibell falls off in 5 to 8 days. From McKinney et al., 2000.

that eventually constrict and partition the organ into irregular nodules. It has a lengthy latent period, usually followed by the sudden appearance of abdominal pain and swelling, hematemesis, dependent edema, or jaundice. In advanced stages, ascites, pronounced jaundice, portal hypertension, and central nervous system disorders, which may end in hepatic COMA, become prominent. adj., **cirrhot′ic.**

Clinical Manifestations. The signs and symptoms are manifestations of interference with the major functions of the liver: (1) the storage and release of blood to maintain adequate circulating volume, (2) the metabolism of nutrients and the detoxification of poisons absorbed from the intestines, (3) the regulation of fluid and electrolyte balance, and (4) production of clotting factors.

The patient with alcoholic cirrhosis (Laënnec's CIRRHOSIS) may be admitted to the hospital with acute alcoholic hepatitis, marked by fever and dehydration. Prominent spider angiomas and redness of the palms of the hands (palmar erythema) are usually present. DELIRIUM TREMENS may be a difficult problem during the early phase of hospitalization. Data from liver function tests usually show elevated transaminase levels, elevated bilirubin levels, and decreased values for albumin and clotting factors. (See also ALCOHOLISM.)

Continued fluid and electrolyte imbalances and inefficient metabolism of nutrients produce ascites, hypoglycemia, and hypoproteinemia. Obstruction to the return of blood from the portal system causes increased pressure within the veins of the esophagus and stomach. These engorged vessels are subject to rupture with subsequent hemorrhage that is abetted by clotting disorders. JAUNDICE develops as a result of biliary obstruction.

Neurological symptoms begin with subtle changes in mental acuity, mild memory loss, poor reasoning ability, and irritability. Tremor of the outstretched hands (asterixis) is common. These symptoms become more severe and may eventually progress to delirium, suicidal tendencies, and coma.

Treatment. The major goals of treatment for the patient with cirrhosis are: (1) to maintain liver function at its current level and prevent further deterioration of the organ, (2) to maintain electrolytes within normal limits, (3) to maintain sufficient respiratory function, (4) to prevent or resolve gastrointestinal bleeding, and (5) to provide adequate nutritional intake and a positive nitrogen balance.

Since there is no cure for cirrhosis, supportive measures are instituted to help the liver rebuild and repair its damaged cells. Prevention of further deterioration of the cells is accomplished by removing the primary cause; for example, restriction of the intake of alcohol or other toxic agent, treatment of infection, and providing an adequate nutritional intake; supplemental vitamins are often prescribed.

Severe blood loss is compensated for by transfusions of whole blood. Excessive bleeding from esophageal varices may necessitate insertion of a Sengstaken-Blakemore tube. This device has three channels: one for inflation of the esophageal balloon, one for inflation of the gastric balloon, and a third for aspiration of stomach contents.

Relief of portal hypertension sometimes is accomplished by a surgical procedure called a portacaval shunt. The portal vein is surgically connected to the inferior vena cava to allow drainage of excessive amounts of blood from the portal system to the general circulation. A similar procedure called the splenorenal shunt involves connecting the splenic vein to the renal vein.

Removal of fluid from the abdominal cavity (abdominal PARACENTESIS) may be necessary to relieve respiratory embarrassment or pressure on the abdominal organs caused by ascites. A more permanent resolution of the problem of chronic ascites is surgical creation of a peritoneovenous SHUNT.

Hepatic ENCEPHALOPATHY and coma can be precipitated by any of a number of factors, including gastrointestinal bleeding, fluid and electrolyte and acid-base imbalances, intercurrent infection and fever, administration of analgesics and sedatives that are central nervous system depressants, and increased dietary protein intake.

Patients with chronic hepatic encephalopathy are placed on a protein-restricted diet. An antibiotic may be prescribed to reduce bacterial flora in the intestine. Surgical removal of all or part of the bacteria-laden colon is an alternative treatment, but the surgical risk is high in these chronically ill patients.

Patient Care. In view of the many functions of the liver, it is essential that a thorough assessment of the patient be done to identify specific problems before a plan of care is developed. Among the problems likely to be associated with cirrhosis are self-care deficit related to low energy level due to inadequate metabolism of carbohydrates; fluid volume excess, especially ascites; potential for impairment of skin integrity related to edema, jaundice, and itching; electrolyte imbalance related to poor storage of minerals; alteration in comfort; tendency to bleed excessively related to deficits of vitamin K and prothrombin and the presence of esophageal varices; potential for infection related to decreased levels of gamma globulins and dysfunction of phagocytic Kupffer cells; impaired gas exchange related to pressure against the lungs by ascitic fluid; potential for injury related to altered levels of consciousness; alteration in nutrition related to indigestion, nausea, inability of liver cells to metabolize food elements, or confusion and depression; and diarrhea related to diminished bile production and decreased tolerance to fatty acids.

Patients in the advanced stages of cirrhosis require periodic and thorough monitoring to detect blood loss in the form of hematemesis, tarry stools, bleeding gums, frequent and heavy nosebleeds, and bruising. In order to evaluate fluid status the fluid intake and output and daily weight are measured and recorded.

Dietary restrictions and prohibition of alcohol may result in noncompliance in some patients. Education must include the purpose of these restrictions, the expected effect and dosage of medications that have been prescribed, and the importance of adequate nutrition, rest, and preservation of independence within the patient's capabilities. Compliance may be improved by enhancing the patient's self-esteem, emphasizing personal strengths, encouraging the use of available community resources such as ALCOHOLICS ANONYMOUS if alcoholism is a problem, and providing for active participation of the patient and family in planning and implementing some aspects of care.

acholangic c. a liver disorder affecting children up to 12 years of age, due to complete or partial agenesis of the intrahepatic, intralobular bile ducts, with manifestations similar to those seen in obstructive biliary cirrhosis.

alcoholic c. Laënnec's cirrhosis.

atrophic c. cirrhosis in which the liver is decreased in size; it may be seen in the alcoholic, but is more common in posthepatic or postnecrotic cirrhosis.

biliary c. cirrhosis caused by obstruction or infection of the major extra- or intrahepatic bile ducts (except in *primary biliary cirrhosis*). It is marked by jaundice, abdominal pain, steatorrhea, and enlargement of the liver and spleen.

cardiac c. cirrhosis complicating heart disease, with recurrent intractable congestive HEART FAILURE. Called also cardiocirrhosis.

congestive c. cirrhosis resulting from increased hepatic venous pressure or thrombosis; commonly due to congestive HEART FAILURE (see cardiac CIRRHOSIS) or to obstruction of the hepatic vein.

fatty c. cirrhosis in which liver cells are infiltrated with fat (triglyceride), the infiltration usually being due to alcohol ingestion; see LAËNNEC'S CIRRHOSIS.

Laënnec's c. cirrhosis associated with chronic ALCOHOLISM. In the early stages, liver enlargement may reflect fatty infiltration of liver cells (fatty cirrhosis) with necrosis and inflammation due to acute alcohol injury; progressive fibrosis extending from portal areas separates uniform small regeneration nodules. Some attribute the condition to a nutritional deficiency associated with alcoholism and others to chronic exposure to alcohol as a hepatotoxin. Called also alcoholic cirrhosis.

macronodular c. morphological changes that cause the liver to become small and shrunken.

metabolic c. cirrhosis associated with metabolic diseases such as HEMOCHROMATOSIS, WILSON'S DISEASE, GLYCOGEN STORAGE DISEASE, GALACTOSEMIA, and disorders of AMINO ACID metabolism.

micronodular c. morphological changes in the liver resulting in an enlarged liver.

mixed c. morphological changes in the diseased liver that represent both the micronodular and macronodular patterns.

portal c. Laënnec's cirrhosis.

posthepatic c. cirrhosis (usually macronodular) resulting as a sequel to acute hepatitis.

postnecrotic c. cirrhosis following submassive necrosis of the liver (subacute yellow atrophy) due to toxic or viral hepatitis.

primary biliary c. a rare form of biliary CIRRHOSIS of unknown etiology, occurring without obstruction or infection of the major bile ducts, sometimes developing after the administration of such drugs as chlorpromazine and arsenicals. Affecting chiefly middle-aged women, it is characterized by chronic cholestasis with pruritus, jaundice, and hypercholesterolemia with xanthomas, and malabsorption.

secondary biliary c. cirrhosis resulting from chronic bile obstruction due to congenital atresia or stricture.

cirsectomy (ser-sek′to-me) excision of a portion of a varicose vein.

cirsoid (ser′soid) resembling a varix.

cirsomphalos (ser-som′fah-los) caput medusae.

cis (sis) [L.] 1. in organic chemistry, having certain atoms or radicals on the same side. 2. in genetics, denoting two or more loci, especially pseudoalleles, occurring on the same chromosome of a homologous pair. See also *trans*.

cisatracurium (sis″at-rah-kūr′e-um) a nondepolarizing neuromuscular blocking AGENT administered intravenously as the besylate salt administered intravenously to facilitate endotracheal intubation and to induce skeletal muscle relaxation, either as an adjunct to general anesthesia during surgery or during mechanical ventilation.

cisplatin (sis′plah-tin) a PLATINUM coordination compound whose main mode of action resembles that of ALKYLATING AGENTS with production of cross links between the two strands of DNA in the double helix so that DNA cannot be replicated and the cells cannot divide. It is used as an antineoplastic AGENT in the treatment of metastatic tumors of the testis, ovary, bladder, and head and neck. It can cause serious damage to the kidney, eighth cranial nerve, gastrointestinal tract, and bone marrow, can upset metabolic processes, and can produce hypocalcemia and hypomagnesemia. Called also DDP or *cis*-DDP.

cistern (sis′tern) a closed space serving as a reservoir for lymph or other body fluids, especially one of the enlarged subarachnoid spaces containing cerebrospinal fluid.

cisterna (sis-ter′nah), pl. *cister′nae* [L.] cistern.

c. cerebellomedulla′ris poste′rior the enlarged subarachnoid space between the undersurface of the cerebellum and the posterior surface of the medulla oblongata; called also cisterna magna.

c. chy′li the dilated portion of the thoracic duct at its origin in the lumbar region; called also receptaculum chyli.

c. mag′na c. cerebellomedullaris posterior.

cisternal (sis-ter′nal) pertaining to a cistern, especially the cisterna cerebellomedullaris.

c. puncture puncture of the cisterna cerebellomedullaris with a hollow needle inserted just between the occipital bone, to obtain a specimen of cerebrospinal fluid. See also LUMBAR PUNCTURE.

Patient Care. Preparation of the patient for this procedure should include a detailed explanation, because insertion of a needle so close to the brain may cause apprehension. The physician may request that the back of the neck be shaved. The patient is positioned on either side with the head bent forward and held firmly by an attendant. Complications seldom occur, but the patient should be observed for signs of dyspnea or cyanosis during and immediately after the procedure. A cisternal puncture is often done in the outpatient clinic, and the patient is allowed to go home soon after it is completed.

cisternography (sis″ter-nog′rah-fe) radiography of the basal cistern of the brain after subarachnoid injection of a contrast medium.

cis-trans test (sis trans) a test in microbial genetics to determine whether two mutations that have the phenotypic effects,

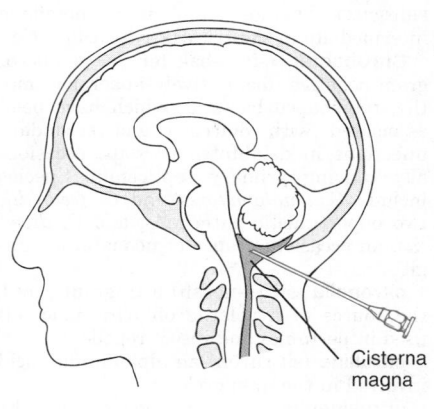

Cisterna magna

Cisternal puncture.

in a haploid cell or a cell with single phage infection, are located in the same gene or different genes; the test depends on the independent behavior of two alleles of a gene in a diploid cell or in a cell infected with two phages carrying different alleles.

cistron (sis'tron) the smallest unit of genetic material that must be intact to function as a transmitter of genetic information; as traditionally construed, approximately synonymous with gene.

citalopram (si-tal'o-pram) an ANTIDEPRESSANT used in the treatment of DEPRESSIVE DISORDERS, administered orally as citalopram hydrobromide.

citrate (sit'rāt, si'trāt) any anionic form, salt, or ester of citric acid.

c. phosphate dextrose (CPD) a solution containing citric acid, sodium citrate, monobasic sodium phosphate, and dextrose that is the primary ANTICOAGULANT used for preservation of whole blood or red blood cells for up to 21 days. The official USP name is anticoagulant citrate phosphate dextrose solution.

c. phosphate dextrose adenine (CPDA-1) an ANTICOAGULANT solution, containing citric acid, sodium citrate, monobasic sodium phosphate, dextrose, and adenine, used for the preservation of whole blood and red blood cells for up to 35 days; it extends red cell survival by providing adenine needed for the maintenance of red cell ATP levels. The official USP name is anticoagulant citrate phosphate dextrose adenine solution.

citric acid (sit'rik) a compound found in citrus fruits and acting as an antiscorbutic and diuretic. It functions as an ANTICOAGULANT in blood preservatives such as CITRATE PHOSPHATE DEXTROSE, and is a metabolic intermediate in the tricarboxylic acid cycle.

Citrobacter (sit'ro-bak"ter) a genus of gram-negative, facultatively anaerobic, motile, rod-shaped bacteria, which have been associated with diarrhea and secondary infections in debilitated persons, occasionally causing primary septicemia. Species include *C. amalona'ticus* and *C. freun'dii*, two opportunistic pathogens; and *C. diver'sus*, an occasional cause of neonatal meningitis.

citronella (sit'ro-nel'ah) a fragrant grass, the source of a volatile oil (citronella oil) used in perfumes and insect repellents.

citrulline (sit-rul'ēn) an alpha amino acid involved in the urea cycle.

citrullinemia (sit-rul"ĭ-ne'me-ah) the presence in the blood of excessive CITRULLINE, resulting from an inborn ERROR of

metabolism, marked by absence or deficiency of the enzyme argininosuccinate synthetase. The disorder, transmitted as an autosomal recessive trait, is manifested by hyperammonemia, vomiting, convulsions, and mental retardation.

citrullinuria (sit-rul"ĭ-nu're-ah) the presence in the urine of large amounts of citrulline, with increased levels also in both plasma and cerebrospinal fluid.

CK creatine kinase.

Cl chlorine.

cladosporiosis (klad"o-spor"e-o'sis) any infection with *Cladosporium*.

clade (klād) a grouping of genetic variants within a single species.

Cladosporium (klad"o-spor'e-um) a genus of imperfect fungi. *C. herba'rum* produces "black spot" on meat in cold storage at a temperature of $-8°$ C. *C. carrio'ni* is an agent of CHROMOBLASTOMYCOSIS.

cladribine (kla'drĭ-bēn) a purine ANTIMETABOLITE antineoplastic AGENT administered intravenously in the treatment of hairy cell LEUKEMIA.

Claforan (klaf'or-an) trademark for a preparation of CEFOTAXIME sodium, a broad-spectrum CEPHALOSPORIN ANTIBIOTIC.

claiming (klām'ing) bonding.

clairvoyance (klar-voi'ans) [Fr.] a form of extrasensory perception in which knowledge of objective events is acquired without the use of the senses.

clamp (klamp) a surgical device for compressing a part or structure.

clamping (klamp'ing) in the measurement of insulin secretion and action, the infusion of a glucose solution at a rate adjusted periodically to maintain a predetermined blood glucose concentration.

euglycemic c. a clamp technique in which the blood glucose is maintained at normal levels.

clanging (klang'ing) a pattern of speech in which words are selected because of sound rather than meaning, resulting in rhyming and punning (*clang association*) instead of logic; normal in young children but a sign of mental disturbance in older persons.

clap (klap) a slang term used by patients to refer to GONORRHEA.

clapotement (klah-pōt-maw') [Fr.] a splashing sound, as in succussion.

clarification (klar"ĭ-fĭ-ka'shun) 1. the clearing of a liquid from turbidity. 2. the making of a concept or statement easier to understand.

values c. in the NURSING INTERVENTIONS CLASSIFICATION, a nursing INTERVENTION defined as assisting another to clarify her or his own values in order to facilitate decision making.

clarificant (klah-rif′ĭ-kant) a substance that clears a liquid of turbidity.

clarithromycin (klah-rith″ro-mi′sin) a MACROLIDE antibiotic effective against a wide spectrum of gram-positive and gram-negative bacteria; used in the treatment of respiratory tract, skin, and soft tissue infections and of *Helicobacter pylori*–associated duodenal ulcer.

Clarke-Hadfield syndrome (klark had′-fēld) congenital pancreatic infantilism, with hepatomegaly, bulky stools, and extensive atrophy of the pancreas in an undersized and underweight child.

class (klas) 1. a taxonomic category subordinate to a phylum or subphylum and superior to an order. 2. in statistics, a subgroup of a population for which certain variables measured for individuals in the population fall within specific limits.

classification (klas″ĭ-fĭ-ka′shun) a systematic arrangement of similar entities on the basis of certain differing characteristics. For names of specific classifications, see under the names.

clastic (klas′tik) 1. undergoing or causing division. 2. separable into parts.

clastogenic (klas″to-jen′ik) giving rise to or inducing disruption or breakages, as of chromosomes.

clastothrix (klas′to-thriks) trichorrhexis nodosa.

clathrate (klath′rāt) 1. having the shape or appearance of a lattice. 2. a clathrate COMPOUND.

Claude's syndrome (klawdz) paralysis of the third (oculomotor) nerve on one side and asynergia on the other side, together with dysarthria.

claudication (klaw″dĭ-ka′shun) limping or lameness.

intermittent c. see INTERMITTENT CLAUDICATION.

jaw c. a complex of symptoms like those of intermittent claudication but seen in the muscles of mastication, occurring in giant cell arteritis.

venous c. intermittent claudication caused by venous stasis.

claustrophobia (klaws″tro-fo′be-ah) irrational fear of being shut in; fear of enclosed spaces, such as elevators and tunnels.

claustrum (klaws′trum), pl. *claus′tra* [L.] the thin layer of gray matter lateral to the external capsule of the lentiform nucleus, separating it from the white matter of the insula.

Claviceps (klav′ĭ-seps) a genus of parasitic fungi that infest various seed plants. *C. purpu′rea* is the source of ERGOT.

clavicle (klav′ĭ-k′l) an elongated, slender, curved bone lying horizontally at the root of the neck, in the upper part of the thorax; called also collar bone. See anatomic Table of Bones in the Appendices. adj., **clavic′ular.**

clavicotomy (klav″ĭ-kot′ah-me) surgical division of the clavicle.

clavicula (klah-vik′u-lah) [L.] the clavicle.

clavulanate (klav′u-lah-nāt) a β-LACTAMASE inhibitor used as the potassium salt in combination with penicillins in treating infections caused by β-lactamase–producing organisms.

clavus (kla′vus), pl. *cla′vi* [L.] corn.

c. hyste′ricus a sharp, painful sensation as if a nail were being driven into the head. It is usually regarded as a conversion symptom.

clawfoot (klaw′foot) a high-arched foot with the toes hyperextended at the metatarsophalangeal joint and flexed at the distal joints.

clawhand (klaw′hand) flexion and atrophy of the hand and fingers.

clearance (klēr′ans) the act of clearing; specifically, complete removal of a solute or substance from a specific volume of blood per unit time by processes such as hepatic clearance, renal clearance, or hemodialysis.

aerosol c. see AEROSOL CLEARANCE.

blood-urea c. urea clearance.

creatinine c. the volume of plasma cleared of CREATININE in a unit of time by the kidney system. Since creatinine is normally produced in fairly constant amounts as a result of the breakdown of PHOSPHOCREATINE and is excreted in the urine, an elevation in levels of it in the blood indicates a disturbance in kidney function.

hepatic c. the removal of a substance from the blood via the liver.

ineffective airway c. see AIRWAY CLEARANCE, INEFFECTIVE.

inulin c. an expression of the renal efficiency in eliminating INULIN from the blood, a measure of the glomerular filtration RATE.

mucociliary c. the clearance of mucus and other material from the AIRWAYS by the CILIA of the epithelial cells, which move mucus cephalad with every beat.

renal c. the rate at which a substance is removed from the blood via the kidneys; types commonly measured are creatinine CLEARANCE, inulin CLEARANCE, and urea CLEARANCE.

urea c. the volume of the blood cleared of urea per minute by either renal CLEARANCE or HEMODIALYSIS. Called also blood-urea clearance.

cleavage (klēv′ij) 1. division into distinct parts. 2. the early successive splitting of a fertilized ovum (ZYGOTE) into smaller cells (BLASTOMERES) by mitosis.

cleft (kleft) 1. a fissure or longitudinal opening, especially one occurring during embryonic development. 2. having such a fissure.

branchial c. 1. one of the slitlike openings in the gills of fish between the branchial ARCHES. 2. pharyngeal groove.

facial c. 1. any of the clefts between the embryonic prominences that normally unite to form the face. 2. failure of union of one of these embryonic clefts; depending on the site, this causes such developmental defects as cleft cheek, cleft mandible, or CLEFT LIP. Called also prosoposchisis.

c. lip, c. palate congenital fissure, or split, of the lip (cleft lip) or of the roof of the mouth (cleft palate); one or the other occurs in about one birth per thousand. Sometimes they are associated with clubfoot (talipes) or other anatomic defects. They have no connection with mental retardation. Although poor health of the mother during pregnancy may have some effect on the development of her child, the old superstition that psychologic experiences of the pregnant mother can cause cleft palate and cleft lip has no scientific basis. However, it is true that parents who were born with cleft palate or cleft lip are somewhat more likely than other parents to have children with these defects.

Cleft palate and cleft lip result from failure of the two sides of the face to unite properly at an early stage of prenatal development. The defect may be limited to the outer flesh of the upper lip (the term harelip, suggesting the lip of a rabbit, is both inaccurate and unkind), or it may extend back through the midline of the upper jaw through the roof of the palate. Sometimes only the soft palate, located at the rear of the mouth, is involved.

The infant with a cleft palate is unable to suckle properly, because the opening between mouth and nose through the palate prevents suction. Feeding must be done by other means, with a dropper, a cup, a spoon, or an obturator, a device inserted in the mouth to close the cleft while the baby is sucking. Cleft palate allows food to get into the nose, and it causes difficulty in chewing and swallowing. Later it will hinder speech, because consonants such as *g, b, d,* and *f,* which are normally formed by pressure against the roof of the mouth, are distorted by resonance in the nasal cavity.

The cleft may also prevent movements of the soft palate essential in clear speech.

Treatment. Treatment of cleft palate and cleft lip is by surgery, followed by measures to improve speech. A cleft palate should be reconstructed by plastic surgery when the child is about 18 months old, before he learns to talk. The corrective work usually requires only one operation. After surgery, the child often needs special training in speech to facilitate communication and maintain self-esteem. Cleft lip usually can be corrected by surgery when the child reaches a weight of 12 to 15 lb (5.4 to 7 kg), generally at the age of 2 to 3 months. Successful surgery often leaves only a thin scar and a greatly improved ability to form the *p, b,* and *m* sounds. A child born with a moderate degree of cleft palate or cleft lip can look forward to a life normal in appearance, speech, and manner if proper action is taken early. This means consulting and carefully following the advice of competent specialists in medicine, surgery, dentistry, and speech.

Patient Care. The main concerns during the preoperative period are maintenance of adequate nutrition, prevention of respiratory infections, and speech therapy to prevent development of bad habits of speech. Postoperative care must be aimed at prevention of trauma to or infection of the operative site. The child is not allowed to lie prone until the incision is completely healed. Elbow restraints are used to keep the fingers and hands away from the mouth. The patient is usually fed with a special syringe with a rubber tip as long as only liquids are allowed. When a soft diet is prescribed, care must be taken that the spoon or other eating utensils do not damage the suture line. Mouth care is given frequently to keep the mouth clean and reduce the danger of infection. Dental caries often occurs in patients with cleft palate and regular visits to the dentist are needed. Tender loving care, always a part of pediatric care, is even more necessary when caring for these children. They must be reassured and kept quiet so that crying and restlessness do not undo the work done by the surgeon. (See Atlas 1, Part A.) (See accompanying illustration.)

cleid(o)- word element [Gr.], *clavicle.*

cleidocranial (kli″do-kra′ne-al) pertaining to the clavicles and head.

cleidotomy (kli-dot′ah-me) surgical division of the clavicle of the fetus in difficult labor to facilitate delivery.

clemastine (klem′as-tēn) an ANTIHISTAMINE with sedative and anticholinergic effects; used as the fumarate salt in the treatment

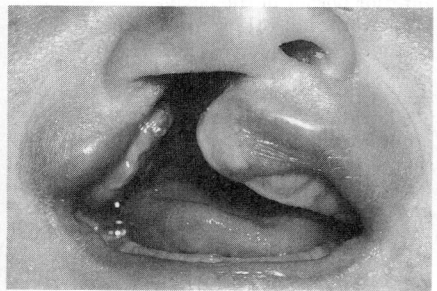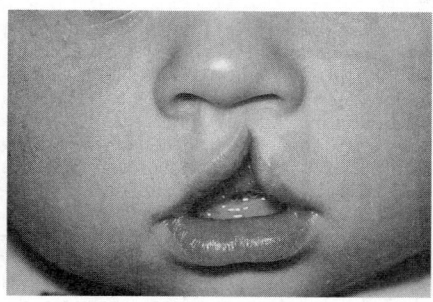

A, Severe and *B,* mild form of cleft lip/palate. From Mueller et al., 2001.

of nasal, eye, and skin manifestations of allergic reactions, including allergic rhinitis, conjunctivitis, and itching, and also as an ingredient in cough and cold preparations, administered orally.

Cleocin (kle´o-sin) trademark for preparations of CLINDAMYCIN, an ANTIBIOTIC.

clerk (klerk) an employee who keeps records and does other general office work.

unit c., ward c. a worker on a nursing unit who schedules patients for prescribed studies, prepares charts for patients, answers the phone on the unit, and handles other general clerical tasks. In some provinces of Canada, ward clerks of certain types of facilities are also trained to transcribe orders. Called also *unit secretary.*

click (klik) a brief, sharp sound, especially any of the short, dry clicking heart sounds during systole, indicative of various heart conditions.

click-murmur syndrome mitral valve prolapse.

clidinium (kli-din´e-um) an ANTICHOLINERGIC and ANTIMUSCARINIC with ANTISPASMODIC and ANTISECRETORY effects on the gastrointestinal tract; as *clindium bromide* it has been administered orally as adjunctive therapy in treatment of peptic ulcer and other gastrointestinal disorders.

client (kli´ent) the term most often used as a synonym for a PATIENT who receives health care in an ambulatory CARE setting, especially when health maintenance rather than illness care is the primary service provided. Sometimes this term is preferred to denote a collaborative relationship rather than a hierarchical one.

climacteric (kli-mak´ter-ik, kli″mak-ter´-ik) the complex of endocrine, somatic, and psychic changes occurring at the end of the female reproductive period (menopause); it may also accompany normal diminution of sexual activity in the male.

climax (kli´maks) the period of greatest intensity, as in the course of a disease.

clindamycin (klin″dah-mi´sin) 1. a semisynthetic ANTIBIOTIC that is a derivative of LINCOMYCIN; used to treat gram-positive penicillin-resistant infections. 2. a semisynthetic derivative of LINCOMYCIN used systemically, topically, and vaginally as an ANTIBACTERIAL, primarily against gram-positive bacteria; used also as the hydrochloride and phosphate salts and as the hydrochloride salt of the ester of clindamycin and palmitic acid (clindamycin palmitate hydrochloride).

clinic (klin´ik) 1. an establishment where patients are admitted for special study and treatment by a group of health care professionals practicing together. 2. a clinical lecture; examination of patients before a class of students; instruction at the bedside.

satellite c. a facility owned by a hospital but operated at a distant site.

walk-in c. a facility that offers health care services without an appointment.

clinical (klin´i-k'l) pertaining to a clinic or to the bedside; pertaining to or founded on actual observation and treatment of patients, as distinguished from theoretical or experimental.

c. laboratory scientist/medical technologist (CLS/MT) a laboratory professional who has all the skills possessed by a CLINICAL LABORATORY TECHNICIAN as well as the ability to perform complex analyses, fine line discrimination, and correction of errors. This technologist assumes responsibility and is held accountable for accurate results and establishes and monitors quality control and quality assurance programs, designing or modifying procedures as necessary. Academic programs are accredited by the National Accrediting Agency for Clinical Laboratory Sciences. Certification as MT is through the Board of Registry of the

American Society of Clinical Pathologists, whose address is P.O. Box 12270, Chicago, IL 60612 (telephone 312-738-1336). Certification as CLT is through the National Credentialing Agency for Medical Laboratory Personnel. The address of the American Society for Clinical Laboratory Sciences is 7910 Woodmont Ave., Suite 1301, Bethesda, MD 20814 (telephone 301-657-2768).

c. laboratory technician/medical laboratory technician (CLT/MLT) a laboratory professional skilled in the performance of clinical laboratory analyses. Associate degree or certificate programs are accredited by the National Accrediting Agency for Clinical Laboratory Sciences, whose address is 8410 W. Bryn Mawr Ave., Suite 670, Chicago, IL 60631 (telephone 773-714-8880). Certification as MLT(ASCP) is through the Board of Registry of the American Society of Clinical Pathologists, whose address is P.O. Box 12270, Chicago, IL 60612 (telephone 312-738-1336). Certification as CLT is through the National Credentialing Agency for Medical Laboratory Personnel, whose address is P.O. Box 15945-289, Lenexa, KS 66285 (telephone 913-438-5110).

clinician (klĭ-nish'an) an expert clinical practitioner and teacher.

   nurse c. see NURSE CLINICIAN.

clinicopathologic (klin″ĭ-ko-path″o-loj'ik) pertaining to both symptoms of disease and to its pathology.

Clinistix (klin'ĭ-stiks) trademark for glucose oxidase reagent strips used to test for glucose in urine. The strip is dipped into the urine and positive or negative results are indicated by the color of the strip.

Clinitest (klin'ĭ-test) trademark for alkaline copper sulfate reagent tablets used to test for reducing substances, such as sugars, in urine. The practice of periodic testing of urine for sugar in diabetic patients has been supplanted by blood GLUCOSE monitoring, which is far more accurate.

clinocephaly (kli″no-sef'ah-le) congenital flatness or concavity of the vertex of the head.

clinodactyly (kli″no-dak'til-e) permanent deviation or deflection of one or more fingers, as seen in TRISOMY 18 SYNDROME.

Clinoril (klin'o-ril) trademark for a preparation of SULINDAC, a NONSTEROIDAL ANTIINFLAMMATORY DRUG.

clip (klip) a metallic device for approximating the edges of a wound or for the prevention of bleeding from small individual blood vessels.

clition (klit'e-on) the midpoint of the anterior border of the clivus.

clitorectomy (klit″o-rek'to-me) clitoridectomy.

clitoridectomy (klit″o-rĭ-dek'to-me) excision of the clitoris.

clitoriditis (klit″o-rĭ-di'tis) clitoritis.

clitoridotomy (klit″ah-rĭ-dot'ah-me) incision of the clitoris.

clitorimegaly (kli″to-rĭ-meg'ah-le) enlargement of the clitoris.

clitoris (klit'o-ris) the small, elongated, erectile body in the female, situated at the anterior angle of the rima pudendi. See also VULVA.

clitorism (klit'o-rizm) 1. hypertrophy of the clitoris. 2. persistent erection of the clitoris.

clitoritis (klit″o-ri'tis) inflammation of the clitoris.

clitoromegaly (kli″to-ro-meg'ah-le) clitorimegaly.

clitoroplasty (kli'to-ro-plas″te) plastic surgery of the clitoris.

clivography (kli-vog'rah-fe) radiographic visualization of the clivus, or posterior cranial fossa.

clivus (kli'vus) [L.] a bony surface in the surface of the posterior cranial fossa sloping upward from the foramen magnum to the dorsum sellae.

cloaca (klo-a'kah), pl. *cloa′cae* [L.] 1. a common passage for fecal, urinary, and reproductive discharge in most lower vertebrates. 2. in mammalian embryos, the terminal end of the HINDGUT before division into rectum, bladder, and the PRIMORDIA of the reproductive ORGANS. 3. an opening in the covering or sheath of a necrosed bone. adj., **cloa′cal.**

cloacogenic (klo″ah-ko-jen'ik) originating from the CLOACA or from persisting cloacal remnants; said of a group of rare transitional-cell nonkeratinizing epidermoid anal cancers.

clobetasol (klo-ba'tah-sol) a synthetic CORTICOSTEROID used topically as the salt for the relief of inflammation and pruritus in corticosteroid-responsive dermatoses.

clocortolone (klo-cor'to-lōn) a synthetic CORTICOSTEROID used topically as the pivalate ester in the treatment of the inflammatory manifestations of corticosteroid-responsive dermatoses.

Cloderm (klo'derm) trademark for a preparation of CLOCORTOLONE pivalate, a synthetic glucocorticoid used in topical treatment of dermatoses.

clofazimine (klo-fa'zĭ-mēn) an antibacterial effective against *Mycobacterium* species, including *Mycobacterium leprae*.

clofibrate (klo-fi′brāt) an agent used to reduce elevated serum lipids in treatment of HYPERLIPOPROTEINEMIA, administered orally.

clomiphene (klo′mĭ-fēn) a nonsteroid ESTROGEN analogue used as the citrate salt to stimulate ovulation.

clomipramine (klo-mip′rah-mēn) 1. a tricyclic ANTIDEPRESSANT of the DIBENZAZEPINE class, used in the form of the hydrochloride salt. Also used as an ANTIANXIETY AGENT and investigationally to relieve symptoms of OBSESSIVE-COMPULSIVE DISORDER. 2. a tricyclic ANTIDEPRESSANT with anxiolytic activity, also used in treatment of obsessive-compulsive disorder, panic disorder, bulimia nervosa, cataplexy associated with narcolepsy, and chronic, severe pain; used as the hydrochloride salt.

clonality (klo-nal′ĭ-te) the ability to be CLONED.

clonazepam (klo-naz′ĕ-pam) a BENZODIAZEPINE used as an oral ANTICONVULSANT; also used as an antipanic agent in the treatment of panic disorders.

clone (klōn) 1. the genetically identical progeny produced by the natural or artificial asexual reproduction of a single organism, cell, or gene, such as plant cuttings, a cell culture descended from a single cell, or genes reproduced by recombinant DNA technology. 2. to establish or produce such a line of progeny. adj., **clo′nal.**
In 1997 a lamb was cloned in the United Kingdom, and in 2001 a cat was cloned in Texas. The idea of cloning animals remains a controversial subject that is being discussed by ethicists.

clonic (klon′ik) pertaining to or characterized by CLONUS.

clonicity (klo-nis′ĭ-te) the condition of being clonic.

clonicotonic (klon″ĭ-ko-ton′ik) both clonic and tonic.

clonidine (klo′nĭ-dēn) a centrally acting ANTIHYPERTENSIVE AGENT, administered orally as the hydrochloride salt; also used to treat migraine, dysmenorrhea, opioid withdrawal, vasomotor symptoms of menopause, and cancer-associated pain.

clonism (klon′izm) a succession of clonic spasms.

clonogenic (klo″no-jen′ik) giving rise to a clone of cells.

clonograph (klon′o-graf) an instrument for recording spasmodic movements of parts and tendon reflexes.

clonorchiasis (klo″nor-ki′ah-sis) infection of the biliary passages with the liver fluke *Clonorchis sinensis,* which may lead to inflammation of the biliary tree, proliferation of the biliary epithelium, and progressive portal fibrosis; extension into the liver

parenchyma may lead to fatty changes and cirrhosis.

Clonorchis (klo-nor′kis) a genus of liver flukes. *C. sinen′sis* is the cause of CLONORCHIASIS throughout eastern Asia from Vietnam to Korea.

clonospasm (klon′o-spazm) clonic spasm; see SPASM.

clonus (klo′nus) 1. alternate involuntary muscular contraction and relaxation in rapid succession. 2. a continuous rhythmic reflex tremor initiated by the spinal cord below an area of spinal cord injury, set in motion by reflex testing.
   ankle c., foot c. a series of abnormal reflex movements of the foot, induced by sudden dorsiflexion, causing alternate contraction and relaxation of the triceps surae muscle.
   toe c. abnormal rhythmic contraction of the great toe, induced by sudden passive extension of its first phalanx.
   wrist c. spasmodic contraction of the hand muscles, induced by forcibly extending the hand at the wrist.

clopidogrel (klo-pid′ah-grel) an inhibitor of platelet aggregation, used in the form of the bisulfate salt to prevent formation of THROMBI and prevent MYOCARDIAL INFARCTION, stroke, and vascular death in patients with atherosclerosis; administered orally.

clorazepate (klo-raz′ĕ-pāt) a BENZODIAZEPINE compound used as the dipotassium salt as an ANTIANXIETY AGENT, ANTICONVULSANT, and for the treatment of acute alcohol WITHDRAWAL symptoms; administered orally.

closing volume (CV) the difference between the closing CAPACITY and the residual VOLUME; the volume of gas in the lungs in excess of the residual volume at the time when small airways in the dependent portions of the lungs close during maximal exhalation, as measured by the single breath NITROGEN WASHOUT TEST. Closing volume normally increases with age, is also increased in obstructive airways disease, and can be used to detect small airways disease before symptoms appear. From residual volume, the patient inhales pure oxygen to total lung capacity, and then exhales slowly and evenly while the nitrogen concentration of the exhaled gas is recorded. Because the lower portions of the lung expand more during inspiration, the nitrogen remaining in the alveoli is mixed with more oxygen in the lower portions than in the upper portions. Thus, when the closing volume is reached there is a sharp rise in the nitrogen concentration, because most of the gas is coming from upper air spaces. The closing capacity is equal to closing volume plus residual volume.

Clostridium (klo-strid′e-um) a genus of gram-positive, obligate anaerobic or micro-aerophilic, spore-forming, rod-shaped bacteria. Several species cause gas GANGRENE, including *C. bifermen′tans, C. histioly′ticum, C. no′vyi, C. perfrin′gens* (the most common cause), and *C. sep′ticum.* Other species are *C. botuli′num,* the cause of BOTULISM; *C. diffi′cile,* the cause of antibiotic-associated COLITIS; and *C. te′tani,* the cause of TETANUS.

clostridium (klo-strid′e-um), pl. *clostri′dia* [L.] any individual of the genus *Clostridium.*

closure (klo′zher) 1. occlusion. 2. obstruction.

    delayed primary c. the surgical closing of a wound several days after the injury because the wound was initially too contaminated to close; called also healing by third intention.

    Vacuum Assisted C. **(VAC)** trademark for a system that uses the controlled negative pressure of a vacuum to promote healing of certain types of wound. The edges of the wound are made airtight with foam and a dressing, and a tube is placed in the wound, connecting to a canister that creates a vacuum. Infectious materials and other fluids are then sucked out of the wound.

    velopharyngeal c. closure of nasal air escape by the elevation of the soft palate and contraction of the posterior pharyngeal wall; see also velopharyngeal INSUFFICIENCY.

    visual c. identification of complete forms or objects from incomplete visual presentations.

clot (klot) 1. a semisolidified mass, as of blood or lymph; called also coagulum. 2. coagulate. See also CLOTTING.

    blood c. a coagulum in the blood stream formed of an aggregation of blood factors, primarily platelets, and fibrin with entrapment of cellular elements; see also THROMBUS. Some authorities differentiate thrombus formation from simple COAGULATION or clot formation. Called also cruor.

clotrimazole (klo-trim′ah-zōl) a synthetic broad-spectrum antifungal AGENT applied topically to the skin in the treatment of candidiasis and various forms of tinea, and administered intravaginally in the treatment of vulvovaginal candidiasis and orally in the prevention and treatment of candidiasis of the mouth and throat.

clotting (klot′ing) the formation of a jelly-like substance over the ends or within the walls of a blood vessel, with resultant stoppage of the blood flow; called also coagulation.

Clotting is one of the natural defense mechanisms of the body when injury occurs. A clot will usually form within 5 minutes after a blood vessel wall has been damaged. The exact process of clotting is not known; however, it is believed that the mechanism is initiated by the platelets, which adhere and aggregate as they come in contact with the injured surface. As they aggregate they release serotonin and other substances from their dense granules. Serotonin causes constriction of the blood vessels and reduction of blood flow. Thromboplastin unites with calcium ions and other substances that promote the formation of fibrin. When examined under a microscope, a clot consists of a mesh of fine threads of fibrin in which are embedded erythrocytes and leukocytes and small amounts of fluid (serum).

Twelve factors essential to normal blood clotting have been described; see COAGULATION FACTORS. At least four PLATELET FACTORS also exist that have a part in clotting.

It is possible for a clot to form within a blood vessel if the inner wall of the vessel has been roughened by injury or disease. Clots may form in conditions such as arteriosclerosis, varicose veins, and thrombophlebitis. An internal clot that remains at the place where it forms is called a thrombus; the general condition is called THROMBOSIS. If the clot (or pieces of it) breaks loose and flows through the blood vessels, it is called an embolus, and the condition is called EMBOLISM.

Clotting of the blood can be hastened by contact with injured tissue, by warming, by adding such coagulants as calcium, or by combination with thromboplastin and thrombin. The process can be retarded by cooling, by dilution, by adding oxalates and citrates, or by administration of substances such as heparin and dicumarol, called ANTICOAGULANTS.

clouding of consciousness a disturbance of consciousness in which a patient cannot think clearly and has difficulty paying attention to what is happening or what is being said. Clouding of consciousness may occur in organic disease that affects the oxygenation and metabolism of the brain, as well as in psychogenic disorders.

clove oil (klōv) a volatile oil from cloves (dried flowerbuds of *Syzygium aromaticum*); used as a flavoring agent and as a topical germicide and analgesic in dentistry.

cloxacillin (kloks″ah-sil′in) a semisynthetic PENICILLIN; its sodium salt is used in treating staphylococcal infections due to penicillinase-positive organisms.

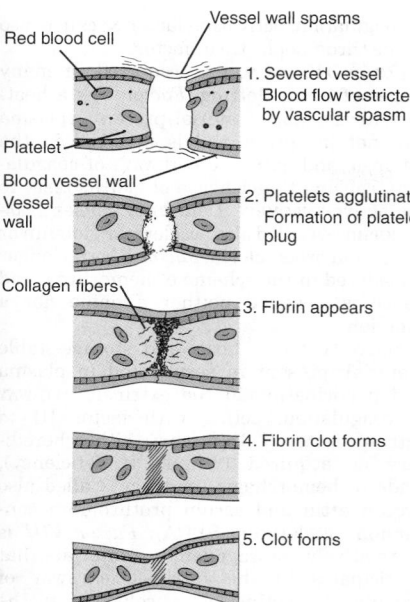

Red blood cell

Vessel wall spasms

Platelet

Blood vessel wall

Vessel wall

Collagen fibers

1. Severed vessel
Blood flow restricted by vascular spasm

2. Platelets agglutinate
Formation of platelet plug

3. Fibrin appears

4. Fibrin clot forms

5. Clot forms

The clotting process.

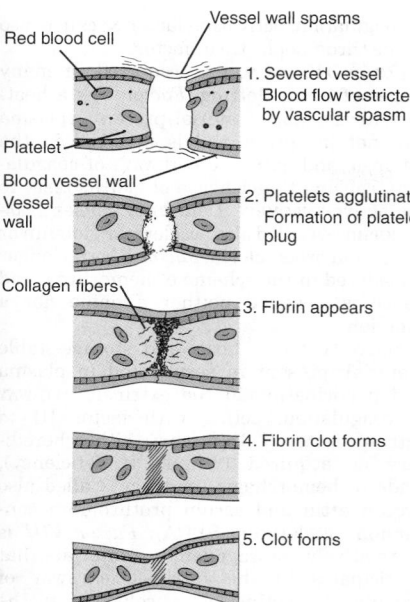

C3 NeF C3 nephritic factor.

cnemial (ne′me-al) tibial.

Cnidaria (ni-dar′e-ah) a phylum of marine invertebrates that includes sea anemones, hydras, jellyfish, and corals. See also COELENTERATA.

CNM certified nurse-midwife.

CNS central nervous system.

CO conscientious objection.

C/O complaint of.

Co cobalt.

CoA coenzyme A.

coadaptation (ko″ad-ap-ta′shun) the mutual, correlated, adaptive changes in two interdependent organs.

coagglutination (ko″ah-gloo″tĭ-na′shun) the aggregation of particulate antigens combined with agglutinins of more than one specificity.

coagulability (ko-ag″u-lah-bil′ĭ-te) capability of forming or of being formed into clots.

coagulant (ko-ag′u-lant) 1. promoting, accelerating, or making possible COAGULATION of blood. 2. an agent that promotes coagulation of blood.

coagulase (ko-ag′u-lās) a bacterial enzyme that reacts with a cofactor found in blood plasma to catalyze the formation of fibrin from fibrinogen. It is produced by most of the virulent strains of staphylococci, and by *Yersinia pestis*.

coagulate (ko-ag′u-lāt) 1. to cause CLOTTING. 2. to become clotted.

coagulation (ko-ag″u-la′shun) clotting. 1. in surgery, the disruption of tissue by physical means to form an amorphous residuum, as in ELECTROCOAGULATION or HOTOCOAGULATION. 2. in colloid chemistry, solidification of a sol into a gelatinous mass.

    blood c. clotting.

    diffuse intravascular c., disseminated intravascular c. (DIC) see DISSEMINATED INTRAVASCULAR COAGULATION.

    c. factors factors essential to normal blood CLOTTING, whose absence, diminution, or excess may lead to abnormality of the clotting. Twelve factors, commonly designated by Roman numerals, have been described (I–V and VII–XIII; VI is no longer considered to have a clotting function). (See table 6.)

Factor I is a high-molecular-weight plasma protein that is converted to fibrin through the action of thrombin; deficiency conditions are called AFIBRINOGENEMIA and HYPOFIBRINOGENEMIA. Called also fibrinogen. *Factor II* is a glycoprotein present in the plasma that is converted into THROMBIN in the common PATHWAY of coagulation; deficiency is called HYPOPROTHROMBINEMIA. Called also prothrombin. *Factor III* is involved in the extrinsic PATHWAY of coagulation, activating factor X; called also tissue thromboplastin or factor.

Factor IV is CALCIUM, required in many stages of blood clotting. *Factor V* is a heat- and storage-labile material, present in plasma and not in serum and is involved in the intrinsic and extrinsic PATHWAYS of coagulation, causing the cleavage of PROTHROMBIN to the active THROMBIN. Deficiency causes PARAHEMOPHILIA. Called also accelerator globulin or factor and proaccelerin. *Factor VI* is no longer considered in the scheme of hemostasis, and hence is assigned neither a name nor a function.

Factor VII is a heat- and storage-stable material, present in serum and in plasma and participating in the extrinsic PATHWAY of coagulation, acting with factor III to activate factor X. Deficiency, either hereditary or acquired (VITAMIN K deficiency), leads to hemorrhagic tendency. Called also proconvertin and serum prothrombin conversion accelerator (SPCA). *Factor VIII* is a relatively storage-labile material that participates in the intrinsic PATHWAY of coagulation, acting as a cofactor in the activation of factor X. Deficiency, an X-linked recessive trait, results in HEMOPHILIA A (classical hemophilia). Called also antihemophilic factor (AHF) and antihemophilic globulin (AHG). *Factor IX* is a relatively storage-stable substance involved in the intrinsic PATHWAY of coagulation, acting to activate factor X. Deficiency of this factor results in a hemorrhagic syndrome called HEMOPHILIA B (or Christmas disease), which is similar to classical hemophilia A. It is treated with purified preparations of the factor, derived from human plasma or recombinant, or with factor IX COMPLEX.

COAGULATION FACTORS	
Factor	**Other Name(s)**
Factor I	Fibrinogen
Factor II	Prothrombin
Factor III	Tissue thromboplastin
Factor IV	Calcium
Factor V	Proaccelerin
Factor VII	Proconvertin
Factor VIII	Antihemophilic factor
Factor IX	Christmas factor, plasma thromboplastin component
Factor X	Stuart-Prower factor
Factor XI	Plasma thromboplastin antecedent (PTA)
Factor XII	Hageman factor
Factor XIII	Fibrin-stabilizing factor
Prekallikrein	—
High-molecular-weight kininogen	HMWK

Called also plasma thromboplastin component (PTC) and antihemophilic factor B.

Factor X is a heat-labile material with some storage stability, which is involved in both intrinsic and extrinsic PATHWAYS of coagulation, uniting them to begin the common PATHWAY. Once activated, it complexes with calcium, phospholipid, and activated factor V to form PROTHROMBINASE, which cleaves and activates PROTHROMBIN to THROMBIN. Called also Stuart or Stuart-Prower factor. *Factor XI* is a stable factor involved in the intrinsic PATHWAY of coagulation, activating factor IX. Deficiency results in HEMOPHILIA C. Called also plasma thromboplastin antecedent (PTA) and antihemophilic factor C. *Factor XII* is a stable factor activated by contact with glass or other foreign substances, which initiates coagulation through the intrinsic PATHWAY by activating factor XI; called also Hageman factor. *Factor XIII* is a factor that polymerizes FIBRIN monomers, enabling fibrin to form a firm blood clot. Deficiency causes a clinical hemorrhagic diathesis. Called also fibrin-stabilizing factor.

coagulator (ko-ag′u-la″ter) a surgical device that utilizes electrical current or light to stop bleeding.

> ***argon beam c.* (ABC)** a device consisting of an electrode recessed inside a probe through which argon gas is passed; the energy from the electrode is carried by the jet of argon, which is directed at bleeding tissue to effect hemostasis.

coagulopathy (ko-ag″u-lop′ah-the) any disorder of blood coagulation.

> ***consumption c.*** disseminated intravascular coagulation.

coagulum (ko-ag′u-lum), pl. *coa′gula* [L.] clot.

coalescence (ko″ah-les′ens) a fusion or blending of parts.

coalition (co″ah-li′shun) the fusion of parts that are normally separate.

> ***tarsal c.*** the fibrous, cartilaginous, or bony fusion of two or more of the tarsal bones, often resulting in TALIPES planovalgus, although other deformities occur and some patients are asymptomatic; it may be congenital or acquired as a response to trauma, infection, or joint disease. Called also tarsal bar.

coarctate (ko-ahrk′tāt) 1. to press close together; contract. 2. pressed close together; restrained.

coarctation (ko″ahrk-ta′shun) stenosis.

> ***c. of aorta*** a CONGENITAL HEART DEFECT consisting of localized deformity of the TUNICA MEDIA of the aorta, causing narrowing (usually severe) of the lumen of the vessel (See illustration).

C

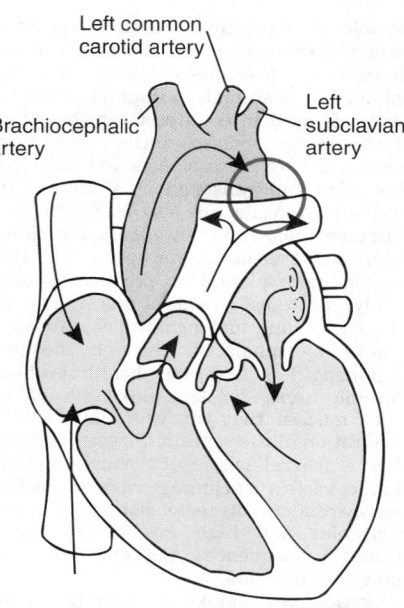

Coarctation of the aorta. Flow patterns are normal but are diminished distal to the coarctation. Blood pressure is increased in vessels leaving the aorta proximal to the coarctation. From Betz et al., 1994.

> ***reversed c.*** pulseless disease.

coat (kōt) 1. a membrane or other structure covering or lining a part or organ; in anatomic nomenclature called TUNICA. 2. the layer or layers of protective protein surrounding the nucleic acid in a virus. See also CAPSID.

> ***buffy c.*** the thin yellowish layer of leukocytes overlying the packed erythrocytes in centrifuged blood.

Coats' disease (kōts) exudative retinopathy.

cobalamin (ko-bal′ah-min) a cobalt-containing complex common to all members of the vitamin B_{12} group; see also VITAMIN.

cobalt (Co) (ko′bawlt) a chemical element, atomic number 27, atomic weight 58.933. (See Appendix 6.)

> ***c. 57*** a radioisotope of cobalt, atomic mass 57, having a half-life of 270 days; used as a label for cyanocobalamin. Symbol ^{57}Co.

> ***c. 60*** a radioisotope of cobalt, atomic mass 60, having a half-life of 5.27 years and a principal gamma ray energy of 1.33 MeV; used as a radiation therapy source. Symbol ^{60}Co.

cobra (ko′brah) any of numerous extremely poisonous ELAPID snakes commonly found in Africa, Asia, and India. They are capable of expanding the neck region to form a hood, and have two comparatively short, erect, deep grooved fangs. A serum obtained from animals inoculated with cobra venom is used in counteracting the effects of the venom. Species include the *Asian cobra* and *king cobra* of Asia and the *Egyptian cobra* found throughout Africa and the Arabian peninsula. See also SNAKEBITE.

cocaine (ko-kān') an alkaloid obtained from the leaves of various species of *Erythroxylon* (coca plants) or produced synthetically; used as a topical ANESTHETIC for surgery of mucous membranes. Abuse of cocaine by inhalation through the nose ("snorting") is a serious health problem. Chronic users develop ulceration of the nasal mucosa that can eventually lead to perforation of the septum. Its systemic toxic effects are related to its SYMPATHOMIMETIC characteristics, including vasoconstriction, tachycardia, and hypertension. Cardiac dysrhythmias and high fever have caused serious consequences and even death in some cocaine users.

crack c. a smokable form of cocaine prepared for illicit use, characterized by rapid absorption and onset of euphoric effects.

cocarcinogen (ko"kahr-sin'o-jen) an agent that increases the effect of a CARCINO-GEN by direct concurrent local effect on the tissue.

cocarcinogenesis (ko-kahr"sī-no-jen'ē-sis) the development, according to one theory, of cancer only in preconditioned cells as a result of conditions favorable to its growth.

cocci (kok'si) [L.] a plural of COCCUS.

Coccidia (kok-sid'e-ah) a subclass of sporozoa commonly parasitic in epithelial cells of the intestinal tract, but also found in the liver and other organs; it includes two genera, *Eimeria* and *Isospora*.

coccidia (kok-sid'e-ah) [L.] plural of COC-CIDIUM.

coccidial (kok-sid'e-al) of, pertaining to, or caused by Coccidia.

coccidian (kok-sid'e-an) 1. pertaining to Coccidia. 2. coccidium.

Coccidioides (kok-sid"ē-oi'dēz) a genus of pathogenic fungi. *C. im'mitis* is the etiologic agent of COCCIDIOIDOMYCOSIS.

coccidioidin (kok-sid"e-oi'din) a sterile preparation containing by-products of growth products of *Coccidioides immitis,* injected intracutaneously as a test for coccidioidomycosis.

coccidioidoma (kok-sid"e-oi-do'mah) residual pulmonary granulomatous nodules seen radiographically as solid round foci in COCCIDIOIDOMYCOSIS.

coccidioidomycosis (kok-sid"e-oi"do-mi-ko'sis) a fungal disease caused by infection with *Coccidioides immitis.* The fungus grows in hot, dry areas, especially in the southwestern United States, Mexico, and parts of Central and South America. Called also coccidioidosis and California disease. The disease occurs in a primary and in a secondary form. *Primary coccidioidomycosis* (called also VALLEY FEVER and SAN JOAQUIN VALLEY FEVER) is due to inhalation of windborne spores and varies in severity from symptoms like those of the common cold to influenzalike symptoms. *Secondary coccidioidomycosis* is a virulent, chronic, progressive, granulomatous disease resulting in involvement of cutaneous and subcutaneous tissues, viscera, central nervous system, and lungs. Treatment consists primarily of rest. Antibiotics may be given to prevent secondary bacterial infection. Amphotericin B or ketoconazole may be used to reduce risk of extrapulmonary dissemination or in the hope of having a remission after dissemination occurs.

coccidioidosis (kok-sid"e-oi-do'sis) coccidioidomycosis.

coccidiosis (kok-sid"e-o'sis) protozoal infection by coccidia. In humans it takes the form of *Isospora belli* in the stools; such infection is usually asymptomatic but occasionally causes a severe watery mucous diarrhea.

coccidium (kok-sid'e-um), pl. *cocci'dia* [L.] any member of the Coccidia; coccidian.

coccobacillus (kok"o-bah-sil'us), pl. *coccobacil'li* an oval bacterial cell intermediate between the coccus and bacillus forms. adj., **coccobac'illary.**

coccobacteria (kok"o-bak-tēr'e-ah) a common name for spheroid bacteria, or for various bacterial cocci.

coccoid (kok'oid) resembling a coccus.

coccus (kok'us), pl. *coc'ci* [L.] a spherical bacterium, usually slightly less than 1 μ in diameter, belonging to the Micrococcaceae family. It is one of the three basic forms of bacteria, the other two being BACILLUS (rod-shaped) and SPIRILLUM (spiral-shaped). A pathogenic coccus can almost always be classified as either a STAPHYLOCOCCUS (occurring in clusters), or a STREPTOCOCCUS (occurring in short or long chains). Both staphylococci and streptococci are gram-positive and do not form spores.

The staphylococci are responsible for many serious infections, especially *Staphylococcus aureus,* which is the causative agent in boils, abscesses, osteomyelitis, and a large variety of other infections. Staphylococci have received much attention in recent years because of the ability of most strains to develop a resistance to antibiotics.

The most dangerous streptococci are those of the beta-hemolytic type. Various species of streptococci cause SORE THROAT, SCARLET FEVER, MASTOIDITIS, and SEPTICEMIA.

coccyalgia (kok″se-al′je-ah) coccygodynia.

coccydynia (kok″si-din′e-ah) coccygodynia.

coccygeal (kok-sij′e-al) pertaining to or located in the region of the coccyx.

coccygectomy (kok″si-jek′to-me) excision of the coccyx.

coccygeus (kok-sij′e-us) pertaining to the coccyx.

coccygodynia (kok″si-go-din′e-ah) pain in the coccyx and neighboring region. Called also coccyalgia and coccydynia.

coccygotomy (kok″si-got′ah-me) freeing of the coccyx from its attachments.

coccyx (kok′siks) the small bone caudad to the sacrum in humans, formed by the union of four (sometimes five or three) rudimentary vertebrae, and forming the caudal end of the vertebral column.

cochlea (kok′le-ah) a spiral tube shaped like a snail shell, forming part of the inner ear; it is the essential organ of HEARING. adj., **coch′lear.**

The cochlea is filled with fluid and is connected with the middle ear by two membrane-covered openings, the oval WINDOW (fenestra vestibuli) and the round WINDOW (fenestra cochleae). Inside it is the ORGAN OF CORTI, a structure of highly specialized cells that translate sound vibrations into nerve impulses. The cells of this organ have tiny hairlike strands (cilia) that protrude into the fluid of the cochlea.

Sound vibrations are relayed from the TYMPANIC MEMBRANE (eardrum) by the bones of hearing in the middle ear to the oval window, where they set up corresponding vibrations in the fluid of the cochlea. These vibrations move the cilia of the organ of Corti, which then sends nerve impulses to the brain.

cochleariform (kok″le-ar′i-form) spoon-shaped.

cochlear implant a device consisting of a microphone, signal processor, external transmitter, and implanted receiver; the receiver is surgically implanted under the skin near the mastoid PROCESS above and behind the ear. It is an alternative to total DEAFNESS, although it does not actually restore HEARING. Deaf persons using the implant do not hear sounds in the same way hearing persons do, but they can be taught to interpret sounds transmitted by the device.

cochleitis (kok″le-i′tis) inflammation of the cochlea.

cochleotopic (kok″le-o-top′ik) relating to the organization of the auditory pathways and auditory area of the brain.

cochleovestibular (kok″le-o-ves-tib′u-ler) pertaining to the cochlea and vestibule of the ear.

coconsciousness (ko-kon′shus-nes) 1. a secondary CONSCIOUSNESS coexisting with the main stream of consciousness. 2. the edge of CONSCIOUSNESS.

code (kōd) 1. a set of rules governing one's conduct. 2. a system by which information can be communicated.

genetic c. see GENETIC CODE.

mode c., pacemaker c. a five-letter code used to describe the function of an artificial PACEMAKER.

C. for Nurses an ethical code adopted by the American Nurses' Association in 1950 and revised periodically, seeking to provide definite standards of practice and conduct for nurses. See nursing ETHICS.

V c. a numbered list of personal problems not attributable to specific mental disorders but nevertheless deserving of

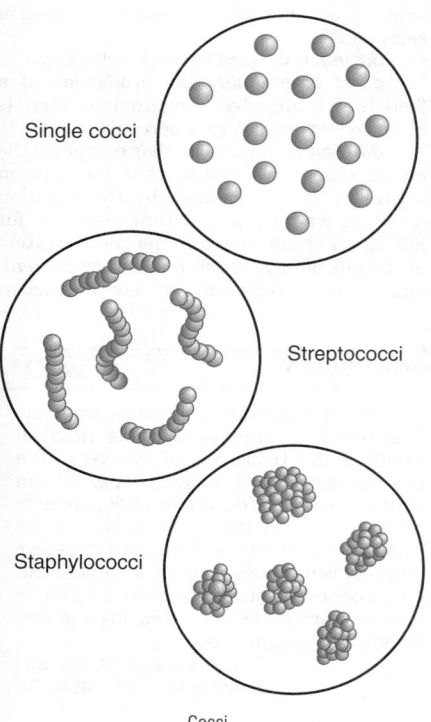

Single cocci

Streptococci

Staphylococci

Cocci.

attention or treatment by health care workers; it was drawn up by the World Health Organization and appears in a modified form in DSM-IV. It includes behaviors and conditions such as antisocial behavior, malingering, noncompliance with medical treatment, and bereavement.

codebook (kōd'book) a plan for data input that documents the location, or column number(s), and value for each variable and other information entered into a computer file.

codeine (ko'dēn) an alkaloid obtained from OPIUM or MORPHINE, used as the base or as the phosphate or sulfate salt as an opioid ANALGESIC, ANTITUSSIVE, and ANTIDIARRHEAL.

codependence (ko''de-pen'dens) a relationship in which the individual fears intimacy and establishes patterns of relating to another that are other-directed and entrapping. Codependent people tend to be highly organized, competent, energetic, strongly moral overachievers; they are devoted caretakers but are out of touch with their own needs and feelings.

codependency (ko''dĕ-pen'den-se) a condition in which one person supports, either overtly or inadvertently, the addictive behavior of another.

coding (kōd'ing) 1. the assigning of symbols or abbreviations to classify field notes into categories. 2. the process of transforming qualitative data into numerical data that can be entered into a computer file.

cod liver oil partially destearinated, fixed oil from fresh livers of *Gadus morrhua* and other fish of the family Gadidae; used as a source of vitamins A and D.

codon (ko'don) a series of three adjacent bases in one polynucleotide chain of a DNA or RNA molecule, which codes for a specific amino acid.

coe- for words beginning thus, see also those beginning *ce-*.

coefficient (ko''ĕ-fish'ent) 1. an expression of the change or effect produced by the variation in certain variables, or of the ratio between two different quantities. 2. in chemistry, a number or figure put before a chemical formula to indicate how many times the formula is to be multiplied.

   absorption c. absorptivity. 1. linear absorption coefficient. 2. mass absorption coefficient.

   Bunsen c. the number of milliliters of gas dissolved in a milliliter of liquid at atmospheric pressure (760 mm Hg) and a specified temperature. Symbol, α.

   confidence c. the probability that a confidence INTERVAL will contain the true value of the population parameter. For example, if the confidence coefficient is 0.95, 95 per cent of the confidence intervals so calculated for a large number of random samples would contain the parameter.

   correlation c. a numerical value that indicates the degree and direction of relationship between two variables; the coefficients range in value from +1.00 (perfect positive relationship) to 0.00 (no relationship) to −1.00 (perfect negative or inverse relationship).

   diffusion c. see DIFFUSION COEFFICIENT.

   c. of digestibility the proportion of a food that is digested compared to what is absorbed, expressed as a percentage.

   dilution c. a number that expresses the effectiveness of a disinfectant for a given organism. It is calculated by the equation $tc^n = k$, where t is the time required for killing all organisms, c is the concentration of disinfectant, n is the dilution coefficient, and k is a constant. A low coefficient

---

WINDOW ON CODEPENDENCY

Until recently, the term "codependency" described a person emotionally involved with a chemically dependent person. The codependent was someone who developed an unhealthy pattern of coping, as a reaction to another's alcohol or drug problem. Many definitions have been proposed to describe codependency; however, among the opinions of most experts is the notion that it is a disease entity with a definable onset, a set of physical and psychological symptoms, and a predictable medical course.

Recovery is possible from codependency. The simple awareness that the problem exists is the beginning of recovery. The process is slow and sometimes painful, but very worthwhile. Too often, codependents are aware of only the sorrow in life and the vicarious joy of others. Through awareness and recovery, those who are characteristically codependent can discover a full life of their own and experience great joy and love without strings attached.

Jo Ann Zerwekh, EdD, RN, and
Barbara Michaels, MSN, RN

indicates the disinfectant is effective at a low concentration.

linear absorption c. the fraction of a beam of radiation absorbed per unit thickness of absorber.

mass absorption c. the linear absorption coefficient divided by the density of the absorber.

phenol c. see PHENOL COEFFICIENT.

sedimentation c. the velocity at which a particle sediments in a centrifuge divided by the applied centrifugal field, the result having units of time (velocity divided by acceleration), usually expressed in Svedberg units (S), which equal 10^{-13} second. Sedimentation coefficients are used to characterize the size of macromolecules; they increase with increasing mass and density and are higher for globular than for fibrous particles.

-coele word element [Gr.], *cavity; space.*

Coelenterata (se-len″ter-a′tah) former name for a phylum of marine invertebrates now assigned to the phylum CNIDARIA.

coelenterate (se-len′ter-āt) 1. pertaining or belonging to the phylum CNIDARIA (Coelenterata). 2. an individual member of the phylum Cnidaria.

coeloblastula (se″lo-blas′tu-lah) the common type of blastula, consisting of a hollow sphere composed of blastomeres.

coelom (se′lom) body cavity, especially the cavity in the mammalian embryo between the somatopleure and splanchnopleure, which is both intra- and extraembryonic; it develops into the pleural, peritoneal, and pericardial cavities. adj., **coelom′ic.**

coelosomy (se″lo-so′me) celosomia.

coenzyme (ko-en′zīm) an organic molecule, usually containing phosphorus and some vitamins, sometimes separable from the enzyme protein; a coenzyme and an apoenzyme must unite in order to function (as a holoenzyme).

c. A a coenzyme essential for carbohydrate and fat metabolism; among its constituents are pantothenic acid and a terminal SH group, which forms linkages with various acids, e.g., acetic acid (acetyl CoA) and fatty acids (acyl CoA); abbreviated CoA.

c. Q any of a group of related quinones occurring in the lipid fraction of mitochondria and serving, along with the cytochromes, as an intermediate in electron transport; they are similar in structure and function to vitamin K_1.

coeur (ker) [Fr.] heart.

c. en sabot (on să-bo′), a heart whose shape on a radiograph vaguely resembles that of a wooden shoe; noted in tetralogy of Fallot.

cofactor (ko′fak-ter) an element or principle, e.g., a coenzyme, with which another must unite in order to function.

heparin c. II a member of the SERPIN group that inhibits THROMBIN.

cogener (ko′jĕ-ner) congener.

Cogentin (ko-jen′tin) trademark for preparations of BENZTROPINE mesylate, an ANTIDYSKINETIC.

cognator (cog′na-ter) in the ADAPTATION MODEL of nursing, one of two major internal processor subsystems (the other is the REGULATOR subsystem) by which an individual adapts to or copes with internal and external environmental stimuli. The cognator subsystem encompasses psychosocial pathways and apparatus for perceptual and information processing, learning, judgment, and emotion. It is related primarily to the four adaptive modes of the adaptation model: physiologic needs, self-concept, role function, and interdependence.

cognition (kog-nish′un) the act or process of knowing, perceiving, or remembering. adj., **cog′nitive.**

cohesion (ko-he′zhun) the intermolecular attractive force causing various particles of a single material to unite. adj., **cohe′sive.**

cohort (ko′hort) in research and statistics, a group of individuals who share a characteristic at some specific time and who are then followed forward in time, with data being collected at one or more suitable intervals. The most common use of the term is to describe a *birth cohort,* in which all the group members are born in a specified time period, but other common characteristics could define the cohort, such as marriage date, exposure to an infectious agent, or date of diagnosis or of treatment for a disease.

coil (koil) a winding structure. See also HELIX and SPIRAL.

coinfection (ko′in-fek″shun) simultaneous infection by separate pathogens, as by hepatitis B and hepatitis D viruses.

coinosite (koi′no-sīt) a free commensal organism.

coition (ko-ish′un) coitus.

coitophobia (ko″ĭ-to-fo′be-ah) irrational fear of coitus.

coitus (ko′ĭ-tus) sexual union by vagina between male and female; usually applied to the mating process in human beings. adj., **co′ital.**

c. incomple′tus, c. interrup′tus coitus in which the penis is withdrawn from the vagina before ejaculation, a widely used but unreliable method of contraception.

c. reserva′tus coitus in which ejaculation of semen is intentionally suppressed.

col(o)- word element [Gr.], *colon.*

colation (ko-la'shun) 1. the separation of solid particles from a liquid, by filtration or straining. 2. the product of such a process.

Colcemid (kol'sĕ-mid) trademark for a preparation of DEMECOLCINE, a cytotoxic alkaloid used in CHROMOSOME analysis.

colchicine (kol'chĭ-sēn) an alkaloid from *Colchicum autumnale* (meadow saffron), used in treatment of GOUT, including for termination of an attack of acute gout. Side effects include gastrointestinal symptoms and hypotension.

cold (kold) 1. COMMON COLD. 2. a relatively low temperature; the lack of heat. A total absence of heat is absolute ZERO, at which all molecular motion ceases. See also HYPOTHERMIA and FROSTBITE. 3. low in physiological activity. 4. low in radioactivity.

  common c. see COMMON COLD.

colectomy (ko-lek'to-me) excision of the colon or of a portion of it.

colesevelam (ko″lĕ-sev'ĕ-lam) a polymer that binds BILE ACIDS in the intestine and prevents them from being reabsorbed, resulting in decreased serum levels of total cholesterol, LDL CHOLESTEROL (LDL-C), and apolipoprotein B and increased levels of HDL CHOLESTEROL (HDL-C); administered orally as the hydrochloride salt as adjunctive therapy to reduce elevated LDL-C levels in patients with primary hypercholesterolemia.

Colestid (ko-les'tid) trademark for a preparation of COLESTIPOL, used in treatment of primary HYPERCHOLESTEROLEMIA.

colestipol (ko-les'tĭ-pol) an anion exchange RESIN used as adjunctive therapy to diet for the reduction of elevated serum cholesterol in patients with primary HYPERCHOLESTEROLEMIA.

colfosceril (kol-fos'ĕ-ril) a synthetic pulmonary SURFACTANT used as the palmitate ester in combination with TYLOXAPOL and an alcohol in prophylaxis and treatment of neonatal RESPIRATORY DISTRESS SYNDROME; instilled into the endotracheal tube for intratracheal administration.

colibacillemia (ko″lĭ-bas″ĭ-le'me-ah) the presence of *Escherichia coli* in the blood.

colibacillosis (ko″lĭ-bas″ĭ-lo'sis) infection with *Escherichia coli.*

colibacilluria (ko″lĭ-bas″ĭ-lu're-ah) BACTERIURIA with *Escherichia coli* in the urine; called also coliuria.

colibacillus (ko″le-bah-sil'us) *Escherichia coli.*

colic (kol'ik) acute paroxysmal abdominal pain. It is particularly common during the first three months of life; the infant has paroxysmal, unexplained crying and may pull up arms and legs, turn red-faced, and expel gas from the anus or belch it up from the stomach. The exact cause of infantile colic is not known but several factors may contribute to it, including excessive swallowing of air, too rapid feeding or overfeeding, parental anxiety, allergy to milk, or other feeding problems. It generally occurs at the same time of day, usually at the busiest period. The parents need sympathetic support and assurance that the condition is not serious and most infants gain weight and are healthy in spite of the colic.

  biliary c. colic due to passage of gallstones along the bile duct.

  gastric c. gastrodynia.

  lead c. colic due to lead poisoning.

  menstrual c. dysmenorrhea.

  renal c. intermittent, acute pain beginning in the kidney region and radiating forward and down to the abdomen, genitalia, and legs; the usual cause is calculi in a kidney or ureter. Symptoms include nausea, vomiting, diaphoresis, and a desire to urinate frequently.

colicky (kol'ik-e) pertaining to or affected by colic.

colicoplegia (kol″ĭ-ko-ple'jah) combined colic and paralysis produced by LEAD POISONING.

coliform (kol'ĭ-form) pertaining to fermentative gram-negative enteric bacilli, sometimes restricted to those fermenting lactose, i.e., *Escherichia, Klebsiella, Enterobacter,* and *Citrobacter.*

coliplication (ko″lĭ-plĭ-ka'shun) coloplication.

colipuncture (ko'lĭ-pungk″chur) colocentesis.

colistimethate (ko-lis″tĭ-meth'āt) an ANTIBIOTIC that is a COLISTIN derivative; the sodium salt is used in treatment of infections.

colistin (ko-lis'tin) an antibiotic produced by *Bacillus polymyxa* var. *colistinus,* or the same substance produced by other means; it is related chemically to POLYMYXIN, and used in treatment of infections.

colitides (ko-lit'ĭ-dēz) plural of COLITIS; inflammatory disorders of the colon considered collectively.

colitis (ko-li'tis) inflammation of the colon. There are many types of colitis, each with different etiologies; the differential diagnosis involves the clinical history, stool examinations, sigmoidoscopy, and radiologic studies such as a lower gastrointestinal series. One of the most common types is *idiopathic ulcerative colitis,* which is characterized by extensive ulcerations along the mucosa and submucosa of the bowel. Other types often can be traced to such etiologic factors as bacteria and viruses, drugs such as antibiotics, and radiation from x-rays or radioactive materials. Strong emotions can cause hypermotility of the gut and thereby produce symptoms typical of colitis. True colitis should be distinguished from IRRITABLE BOWEL SYNDROME (formerly referred to by other names such as *mucous colitis, irritable colon,* and *spastic colon*); in the latter condition there is no actual inflammation of the gastrointestinal mucosa. Almost all forms of colitis cause lower abdominal pain, bleeding from the bowel, and diarrhea. The patient may have as many as 20 bowel movements a day, resulting in serious depletion of body fluids and electrolytes. Treatment is aimed at eliminating or mitigating the underlying cause of the inflammatory process, resting and soothing the inflamed bowel, and restoring the nutritional status and fluid and electrolyte balance to normal.

antibiotic-associated c. colitis associated with antimicrobial therapy, most commonly with LINCOMYCIN or CLINDAMYCIN, but also with other broad-spectrum antibiotics, such as AMPICILLIN and TETRACYCLINE. It can range from mild nonspecific colitis and diarrhea to severe fulminant pseudomembranous COLITIS with profuse watery diarrhea, abdominal cramps, and fever. The inflammation may be caused by a toxin produced by *Clostridium difficile,* a microorganism that is normally present in the resident bowel flora of infants, but is rarely found in adults. Presumably, the disruption of the normal flora allows the growth of *C. difficile.*

collagenous c. a type of colitis of unknown etiology characterized by deposits of collagenous material beneath the epithelium of the colon, with crampy abdominal pain and watery diarrhea.

Crohn's c. Crohn's disease.

diversion c. inflammation in a non-functioning colonic pouch created by corrective surgery; it resolves following restoration of intestinal continuity.

ischemic c. acute vascular insufficiency of the colon, usually involving the portion supplied by the inferior mesenteric artery; symptoms include pain at the left iliac fossa, bloody diarrhea, low-grade fever, abdominal distention, and abdominal tenderness. The classic radiologic sign is thumbprinting, due to localized elevation of the mucosa by submucosal hemorrhage or edema. Ulceration may follow.

pseudomembranous c. a severe acute inflammation of the bowel mucosa, with the formation of pseudomembranous plaques; it is usually associated with antimicrobial therapy (antibiotic-associated COLITIS). The common symptoms are watery diarrhea, abdominal cramps, and fever. The pathologic lesions are yellow-green pseudomembranous plaques of mucinous inflammatory exudate distributed in patches over the colonic mucosa and sometimes also in the small intestine. Called also pseudomembranous enterocolitis.

radiation c. colitis resulting from radiation therapy to the abdominal region; it is manifested clinically by tenesmus, pain, rectal bleeding, diarrhea, and telangiectases. Malabsorption, ulceration, and partial or complete obstruction may follow.

ulcerative c. see ULCERATIVE COLITIS.

colitoxicosis (ko″lĭ-tok″sĭ-ko′sis) toxemia caused by *Escherichia coli.*

colitoxin (ko′lĭ-tok″sin) a toxin from *Escherichia coli.*

coliuria (ko″le-u′re-ah) colibacilluria.

collagen (kol′ah-jen) any of a family of extracellular, closely related proteins occurring as a major component of connective tissue, giving it strength and flexibility. Numerous types exist, each composed of TROPOCOLLAGEN units that share a common triple-helical shape but that vary somewhat in composition between types, with the types being localized to different tissues. adj., **collag′enous.**

c. diseases a group of diseases having in common certain clinical and histological features that are manifestations of involvement of CONNECTIVE TISSUE, i.e., those tissues that provide the supportive framework (musculoskeletal structures) and protective covering (skin and mucous membranes and vessel linings) for the body.

The basic components of connective tissue are cells and extracellular protein fibers embedded in a matrix or ground substance of large carbohydrate molecules and carbohydrate-protein complexes called mucopolysaccharides.

For the sake of clarity and organization, collagen diseases may be divided into two major groups: (1) those that are genetically determined and are a result of structural and biochemical defects, and (2) those that are acquired and in which immunological and inflammatory reactions are taking place within the tissues. Among the first group are those diseases caused by a lack of a specific enzyme necessary for proper storage and excretion of one or more mucopolysaccharides. Also included in this group are osteogenesis imperfecta, Ehlers-Danlos syndrome, and Marfan's syndrome. These disorders are distinguished by structural defects affecting the formation of the extracellular fibers called collagen.

Acquired connective tissue diseases are believed to develop as a result of at least two causative factors: a genetic factor and an abnormal immunological response. The exact role of these factors in the development of connective tissue diseases has not been firmly established, but there is strong evidence that immunological mechanisms are involved. Examples of collagen diseases that are most probably the result of an aberration of the immunological reactions that mitigate injury and inflammation of connective tissues are systemic lupus erythematosus, scleroderma, rheumatoid arthritis, rheumatic fever, polymyositis, and dermatomyositis.

collagenase (kŏ-laj′ĕ-nās) an enzyme that catalyzes the degradation of collagen.

collagenation (kŏ-laj″ĕ-na′shun) the appearance of collagen in developing cartilage.

collagenic (kol″ah-jen′ik) 1. producing collagen. 2. pertaining to collagen.

collagenitis (kŏ-laj″ĕ-ni′tis) inflammatory involvement of collagen fibers in the fibrous component of connective tissue, characterized by pain, swelling, and low-grade fever, and by increased erythrocyte sedimentation rate.

collagenoblast (kŏ-laj′ĕ-no-blast″) a cell arising from a FIBROBLAST and which, as it matures, is associated with COLLAGEN production; it may also form cartilage and bone by METAPLASIA.

collagenocyte (kŏ-laj′ĕ-no-sīt″) a mature collagen-producing cell.

collagenogenic (kŏ-laj″ĕ-no-jen′ik) pertaining to or characterized by collagen production; forming collagen or collagen fibers.

collagenolysis (kol″ah-jĕ-nol′ĭ-sis) dissolution or digestion of collagen. adj., **collagenolyt′ic.**

collagenosis (kol″ah-jĕ-no′sis) collagen disease.

collapse (kŏ-laps′) 1. a state of extreme prostration and depression, with failure of circulation. 2. abnormal falling in of the walls of a part or organ.

circulatory c. shock (def. 2).

collar (kol′er) a type of orthosis worn around the neck for support and stabilization. See also cervical ORTHOSIS.

cervical c. cervical ORTHOSIS.

Chandler c. a neck brace made of soft felt.

four poster c. a rigid brace with four upright rods to support the neck and reduce motion; it has chin and occipital supports.

Philadelphia c. a rigid, adjustable neck brace. (See accompanying illustration.)

collarette (kol′er-et′) 1. a narrow rim of loosened KERATIN overhanging the periphery

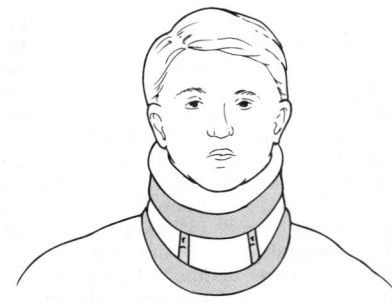

Philadelphia collar. From Dorland's, 2000.

of a circumscribed skin lesion, attached to the normal surrounding skin. 2. an irregular jagged line dividing the anterior surface of the iris into two regions, the pupillary ZONE and the ciliary ZONE. (See accompanying illustration.)

Biett's c. a type of papular SYPHILID in which the central papule is surrounded by a ring of scales.

collateral (kŏ-lat′er-al) 1. secondary or accessory; not direct or immediate. 2. a small side branch, as of a blood vessel or nerve.

collection (kŏ-lek′shun) a gathering together.

data c. the process of acquiring subjects and gathering information needed for a study; methods of collection will vary depending on the study design.

research data c. in the NURSING INTERVENTIONS CLASSIFICATION, a nursing INTERVENTION defined as collecting research data.

colliculectomy (kŏ-lik″u-lek′to-me) excision of the seminal colliculus.

colliculitis (kŏ-lik″u-li′tis) inflammation around the seminal colliculus.

colliculus (kŏ-lik′u-lus), pl. *colli′culi* [L.] 1. a small elevation. 2. either of the two pairs of rounded eminences in the midbrain concerned with visual and auditory reflexes.

seminal c. a prominent portion of the male urethral crest, on which are the

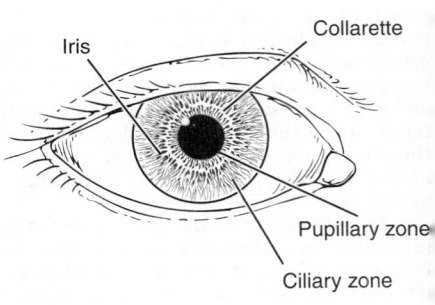

From Dorland's, 2000.

opening of the prostatic utricle and, on either side of it, the orifices of the ejaculatory ducts; called also verumontanum.

collimation (kol″ĭ-ma′shun) 1. in microscopy, the process of making light rays parallel; the adjustment or alignment of optical axes. 2. in radiology, the elimination of the more divergent portion of an x-ray beam. 3. in nuclear medicine, the use of a perforated absorber to restrict the field of view of a detector and reduce scatter.

collimator (kol′ĭ-ma″ter) a diaphragm or system of diaphragms made of an absorbing material, designed to define and restrict the dimensions and direction of a beam of radiation.

colliquative (kŏ-lik′wah-tiv) characterized by excessive liquid discharge, or by liquefaction of tissue.

collodiaphyseal (kol″o-di″ah-fiz′e-al) pertaining to the neck and shaft of a long bone, especially the femur.

collodion (kŏ-lo′de-on) a clear or slightly opalescent, highly flammable, syrupy liquid compounded of pyroxylin, ether, and alcohol, which dries to a transparent, tenacious film; used as a topical protectant, applied to the skin to close small wounds, abrasions, and cuts, to hold surgical dressings in place, and to keep medications in contact with the skin.

flexible c. a preparation of camphor, castor oil, and collodion, used as a topical protectant.

salicylic acid c. flexible collodion containing SALICYLIC ACID, used topically as a keratolytic.

colloid (kol′oid) 1. gluelike. 2. the translucent, yellowish, gelatinous substance resulting from colloid degeneration. 3. a chemical system composed of a continuous medium (the *continuous phase*) throughout which are distributed small particles, 1 to 1000 nm in size (the *disperse phase*), which do not settle out under the influence of gravity. Colloidal particles are not capable of passing through a semipermeable membrane, as in DIALYSIS. Solutes that can pass through a semipermeable membrane are sometimes called CRYSTALLOIDS. adj., **colloid′al.**

dispersion c. COLLOID (def. 3), particularly an unstable colloid system.

emulsion c. 1. lyophilic colloid 2. rarely, emulsion.

lyophilic c. a stable colloid system in which the disperse phase is relatively liquid, usually comprising highly complex organic substances, such as glue or starch, which readily absorb solvent, swell, and distribute uniformly through the continuous phase.

lyophobic c. an unstable colloid system in which the disperse phase particles tend to repel liquids, are easily precipitated, and cannot be redispersed with additional solvent.

stannous sulfur c. a sulfur colloid containing stannous ions; complexed with technetium 99m it is used as a diagnostic aid (bone, liver, and spleen imaging).

suspension c. lyophobic colloid.

colloidal (kŏ-loi′d′l) of the nature of a gel or gluelike substance in which particles are held in suspension.

c. gold test a test of cerebrospinal fluid based on alterations in the albumin-globulin ratios that occur in certain disorders of the central nervous system. Normal spinal fluid, when diluted and added to a colloidal gold suspension, will not precipitate the colloidal gold. The extent of precipitation is indicative of various diseases such as multiple sclerosis, poliomyelitis, and encephalitis. A positive reaction also occurs in the presence of neurosyphilis. The sample of spinal fluid must not contain blood because this will cause a false-positive reaction.

colloidin (kŏ-loi′din) a jelly-like principle produced in colloid degeneration.

collum (kol′um), pl. *col′la* [L.] the neck, or a necklike part.

c. den′tis neck of tooth.

c. distor′tum torticollis.

c. val′gum coxa valga.

collutory (kol′u-tor″e) a mouthwash or gargle.

collyrium (kŏ-lir′e-um), pl. *colly′ria* [L.] a lotion for the eyes; an eye wash.

coloboma (kol″o-bo′mah), pl. *colobomas, colobo′mata* [L.] 1. a defect of tissue. 2. particularly, a defect of some ocular tissue, usually due to failure of part of the fetal fissure to close; it may affect the choroid, ciliary body, eyelid (palpebral coloboma, colobo′ma palpebra′le), iris (colobo′ma i′ridis), lens (colobo′ma len′tis), optic nerve, or retina (colobo′ma re′tinae). A scotoma is usually present, corresponding to the area of the coloboma. (See accompanying illustration.)

colocecostomy (ko″lo-se-kos′tah-me) cecocolostomy.

colocentesis (ko″lo-sen-te′sis) surgical puncture of the colon.

coloclysis (ko-lok′lĭ-sis) irrigation of the colon.

coloclyster (ko″lo-klis′ter) an enema introduced into the colon through the rectum.

colocolostomy (ko″lo-kah-los′tah-me) surgical formation of an anastomosis between two portions of the colon.

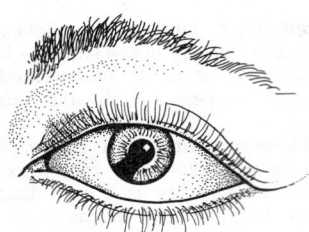

Coloboma of the iris. From Dorland's, 2000.

colocutaneous (ko″lo-ku-ta′ne-us) pertaining to the colon and skin, or communicating with the colon and the cutaneous surface of the body.

coloenteritis (ko″lo-en″ter-i′tis) enterocolitis.

colofixation (ko″lo-fik-sa′shun) fixation of the colon.

Cologel (kol′o-jel) trademark for a preparation of METHYLCELLULOSE, which acts as a mild LAXATIVE by increasing intestinal bulk.

coloileal (ko″lo-il′e-al) ileocolic.

colon (ko′lon) the part of the large intestine extending from the cecum to the rectum; it is divided as follows: the *ascending colon* passes upward from the cecum to the lower edge of the liver, where it bends and becomes the transverse colon; the *transverse colon* crosses the abdominal cavity from right to left below the stomach and then bends downward to become the descending colon; the *descending colon* then extends downward along the left side of the abdomen, and at the brim of the pelvis it becomes the *sigmoid colon,* an S-shaped curve leading down to the sacrum where it becomes the RECTUM. See also DIGESTIVE SYSTEM and see color plates. adj., **colon′ic.**

irritable c., nervous c., spastic c. terms formerly used for IRRITABLE BOWEL SYNDROME.

colonization (kol″ŏ-nĭ-za′shun) the development of a bacterial infection on an individual, as demonstrated by a positive culture. The infected person may have no signs or symptoms of infection while still having the potential to infect others.

colonography (ko″lon-og′rah-fe) imaging of the colon, as by computed tomography or magnetic resonance imaging.

colonopathy (ko″lon-op′ah-the) any disease or disorder of the colon.

colonorrhagia (ko″lon-o-ra′jah) hemorrhage from the colon.

colonoscope (ko-lon′o-skōp) an elongated flexible fiberoptic endoscope which permits visual examination of the entire colon.

colonoscopy (ko″lon-os′kah-pe) endoscopic examination of the colon, either transabdominally during laparotomy, or transanally by means of a colonoscope.

colony (kol′o-ne) a discrete group of organisms, as a collection of bacteria in a culture.

colopexy (kol′o-pek″se) surgical fixation or suspension of the colon.

coloplication (ko″lo-plĭ-ka′shun) the operation of taking a reef in the colon.

coloproctectomy (ko″lo-prok-tek′to-me) surgical removal of the colon and rectum.

coloproctitis (ko″lo-prok-ti′tis) inflammation of the colon and rectum; colorectitis.

coloproctostomy (ko″lo-prok-tos′tah-me) anastomosis of the colon to the rectum.

colopuncture (ko′lo-pungk″cher) colocentesis.

color (kul′er) 1. a property of a surface or substance due to absorption of certain light rays and reflection of others within the range of wavelengths (roughly 370 to 760 nm) adequate to excite the retinal receptors. 2. radiant energy within the range of adequate chromatic stimuli of the retina, i.e., between the INFRARED and the ULTRAVIOLET. 3. a sensory impression of one of the rainbow hues.

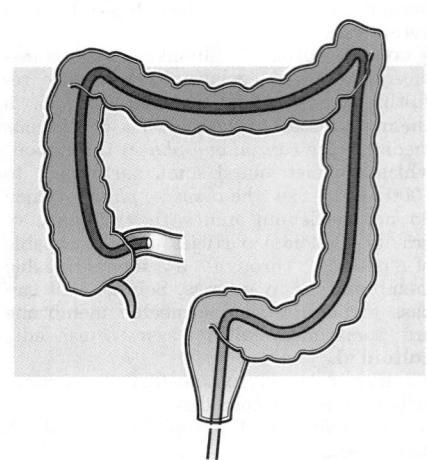

Colonoscopy. The endoscopic instrument is passed through the entire colon and into the distal segment of the ileum. The combination of the flexible tube, fiberoptics, and the light enables the examiner to visualize the entire mucosal surface, identifying sites of bleeding, inflammation, tissue irregularity, or abnormal tissue. From Malarkey and McMorrow, 2000.

primary c's a small number of fundamental colors. In visual science this refers to red, green, and blue, the colors specifically picked up by the retinal cones; mixtures of varying proportions of the primary colors will yield the 150 discriminable hues of normal human vision. In painting and printing, the primary colors are red, blue, and yellow.

c. vision deficiency inability to distinguish between certain colors, popularly called "color blindness." A complete deficiency (monochromatic VISION), the total inability to see colors, is rare, affecting only one person in 300,000. Much more common are the various types of partial deficiency. The most common is red-green confusion (see DEUTERANOPIA and PROTANOPIA), which affects approximately 8 million people in the United States.

Color vision is a function of the CONES in the retina of the eye, which are stimulated by light and transmit impulses to the brain. It is now thought that there are three types of cones, each type stimulated by one of the primary colors in light (red, green, and blue or violet). In red-green color vision deficiency, there is a deficiency of either red or green receptors, so that the two colors do not appear distinct from each other.

Color vision is usually tested by the ISHIHARA TEST with a series of PSEUDOISOCHROMATIC charts or plates. (See Atlas 4, Part F.) These have a letter, number, or symbol printed in dots of one color in the midst of dots of gray or other colors. The normal person can see the symbol with no difficulty, but the person with color vision deficiency cannot distinguish it from the background.

Although color vision deficiency may occasionally result from injuries, diseases, or certain drugs, most cases are hereditary. It is usually inherited by males through the mother, who carries the trait from her father although she is not color deficient herself. In some cases, if the grandfather is color deficient and the mother carries the trait, a daughter may inherit color vision deficiency, but the ratio of men to women with inherited forms is about 20 to 1. There is no known cure for color vision deficiency.

Colorado tick fever (kol″ŏ-rah′do) a febrile disease occurring in the Rocky Mountain and Pacific slope regions of the United States and Canada; it is caused by a virus and the vector is a tick, *Dermacentor andersoni*. The accompanying fever and flulike symptoms occur in two phases with a period of remission in between.

colorectitis (ko″lo-rek-ti′tis) inflammation of the colon and rectum; coloproctitis.

colorectostomy (ko″lo-rek-tos′tah-me) coloproctostomy.

colorectum (ko″lo-rek′tum) the distal 10 inches (25 cm.) of the bowel, including the distal portion of the colon and the rectum, regarded as a unit. adj., **colorec′tal.**

colorimeter (kul″er-im′ĕ-ter) an instrument for measuring the color or color intensity of a solution. See also SPECTROPHOTOMETER.

colorrhaphy (ko-lor′ah-fe) suture of the colon.

coloscope (kol′o-skōp) colonoscope.

coloscopy (ko-los′kah-pe) colonoscopy.

colosigmoidostomy (ko″lo-sig″moi-dos′-tah-me) the surgical anastomosis of a formerly remote portion of the colon to the sigmoid.

colostomy (kah-los′tah-me) an artificial opening (STOMA) created in the large intestine and brought to the surface of the abdomen for evacuating the bowels. It may be necessary in INTESTINAL OBSTRUCTION, perforation of the bowel, cancer, birth defects, and occasionally ULCERATIVE COLITIS. The altered patterns of discharge created by colostomy may be permanent or temporary, depending on the primary condition being treated. The most common types of colostomy are transverse, descending, and sigmoid, the name being derived from the site of the disorder and the location of the stoma.

A *transverse colostomy* may be located on the right, left, or midline of the abdomen. This type of colostomy usually is done as a temporary measure, allowing for discharge of feces while the diseased portion of the intestine returns to normal. Later, the two ends are anastomosed to restore continuity of the bowel. In most transverse colostomies a loop of the colon is brought out through an abdominal incision and an opening made through the intestine. Observation of the stoma as it functions can determine which side of the colostomy leads from the functioning colon and which side leads to the lower, nonfunctioning segment.

A *double-barreled colostomy* is one in which there are two separate stomas. The proximal or right-sided stoma provides an opening for the active segment of the colon; the distal or left-sided stoma opens into the inactive segment. The double-barreled colostomy may later be joined by anastomosis and returned to the abdominal cavity.

Permanent colostomies are usually made at the level of the descending and sigmoid colon. The colostomy is formed and the diseased portion of the colon and anus are removed (abdominoperineal resection) in a single operation. The stoma created in the descending colon and in the sigmoid colon is usually located on the left side of the abdomen. Hernias may occur around colostomies if there is a weakness of the fascia around the stoma. These can be troublesome and should be repaired surgically, but the success of such repairs is limited.

Patient Care. Unless otherwise prohibited by physical weakness or mental incompetence, colostomy care is directed toward helping the patient become totally self-sufficient in the care of the colostomy. Patients are taught to care for the physical aspects of a colostomy and are assisted in adjusting psychologically to a new method of handling solid body waste. This is accomplished in stages, doing for patients those things they cannot do, showing them the way they can be done, and encouraging them to accept responsibility for their own care. Once having overcome initial shock and apprehension at the prospect of colostomy care, most patients welcome the opportunity to care for themselves in privacy.

Prior to surgery the operative procedure is explained and the patient is encouraged at this time to ask questions that are of concern to him. The idea of an artificial anus in the abdominal wall may well be overwhelming to someone who has never heard of the operation. It is best to be open and matter-of-fact in discussing this with patients, remembering that they cannot be expected to absorb too much information at one time. They should be assured that their questions will be answered as they occur to them, that there will be someone to listen to them when they want to talk, and that there are many sources of information available to help with adjustment.

When the patient is ready to learn about caring for his own colostomy, printed information and teaching aids can be obtained through local offices of national health agencies. For example, the Rehabilitation Program of the American Cancer Society publishes a pamphlet entitled *Colostomies: A Guide,* and the United Ostomy Association provides pamphlets, audiovisual material, a quarterly bulletin, and a monthly newsletter. Many times it is helpful to have the patient talk with someone who has a colostomy and is living a normal active life. Certified Enterostomal Therapists are specially trained to work with colostomy patients and others who have permanent stomas.

Devices for collection of waste passing through the stoma vary in design according to the patient's progress. An open-ended bag is needed until bowel control is developed and then a closed pouch is used. Eventually some patients may need nothing more than a simple dressing over the stoma. Selection of a drainage pouch should be based on the size of the stoma. As the stoma shrinks following surgery, the pouch size is changed so that it fits correctly, not so small as to constrict the stoma, and not so large as to permit leakage around the stoma.

Skin care around the stoma is planned so that the area is kept clean and protected from the enzymes and acid in the digestive fluid. The area is washed with soap and water, dried thoroughly, and then a medicated skin barrier such as Stomahesive is applied. (See also STOMA.)

Irrigation of a colostomy is prescribed on an individual basis. Not all patients require irrigation to regulate fecal discharge. When irrigation is needed, the cone-shaped device is less hazardous and easier for most patients to use. Catheters sometimes cause difficulties in that the patients do not know how far to insert them, they may perforate the intestine, and there often is leakage of the irrigating fluid around the catheter during irrigation.

The diet of patients with a colostomy need not be severely restricted. They will need to notice which foods produce gas, diarrhea, and constipation and then adjust their diet to reduce difficulties arising from individual problems with certain foods. Food must be chewed well. Odors may be a source of worry for the patient until they are controlled with cleanliness, avoidance of gas-producing foods, and proper application of the pouch. Commercially produced deodorants are available.

Patients with temporary colostomies may undergo barium studies of the intestines. Preparation of the bowel for these radiologic studies should be carried out with care as the fluid and electrolyte balance of an ostomate can be easily upset. When the studies are completed, the barium must be removed in order to avoid intestinal obstruction.

Suppositories can be inserted into a colostomy stoma. If the patient has had a double-barreled colostomy, the choice of stoma for insertion of the suppository will depend on the desired action of the drug. A glycerine suppository to facilitate passage of fecal material through the stoma would be inserted into the *proximal* limb to achieve the desired action. Conversely, a drug that is to be absorbed from the intestine, for example for the relief of pain, is inserted into the *distal* limb, from which it will not be expelled through the stoma. Before inserting any kind of medication or a catheter for irrigation, the stoma should be digitally examined. The gloved finger is gently inserted into the stoma to determine the direction of the lumen of the intestine.

colostrum (ko-los′trum) the thin, yellow, milky fluid secreted by the mammary gland a few days before or after CHILDBIRTH.

colotomy (ko-lot′ah-me) incision of the colon.

colovaginal (ko″lo-vaj′ĭ-nal) pertaining to or communicating with the colon and vagina.

colovesical (ko″lo-ves′ĭ-k′l) pertaining to or communicating with the colon and urinary bladder.

colp(o)- word element [Gr.], *vagina.*

colpalgia (kol-pal′jah) vaginodynia.

colpatresia (kol″pah-tre′zhah) atresia, or occlusion of the vagina.

colpectasia (kol″pek-ta′zhah) distention or dilation of the vagina.

colpectomy (kol-pek′to-me) vaginectomy (def. 1).

colpeurysis (kol-pu′rĭ-sis) operative dilatation of the vagina.

colpitis (kol-pi′tis) vaginitis.

colpocele (kol′po-sēl) vaginocele (def. 1).

colpocleisis (kol″po-kli′sis) surgical closure of the vaginal canal.

colpocystitis (kol″po-sis-ti′tis) inflammation of the vagina and bladder.

colpocystocele (kol″po-sis′to-sēl) prolapse of the bladder into the vagina.

colpocytogram (kol″po-si′to-gram) a differential listing of the cells observed in smears from the vaginal mucosa.

colpocytology (kol″po-si-tol′o-je) the quantitative and differential study of cells exfoliated from the epithelium of the vagina.

colpomicroscope (kol″po-mi′kro-skōp) an instrument for examining stained tissues of the cervix *in situ.*

colpomicroscopy (kol″po-mi-kros′kah-pe) examination by means of a colpomicroscope.

colpoperineoplasty (kol″po-per″ĭ-ne′o-plas″te) plastic repair of the vagina and perineum.

colpoperineorrhaphy (kol″po-per″ĭ-ne-or′ah-fe) surgical repair of a tear of the vagina and perineum.

colpopexy (kol″po-pek″se) suture of a relaxed vagina to the abdominal wall.

colpoplasty (kol′po-plas″te) plastic surgery involving the vagina.

colpoptosis (kol″pop-to′sis) vaginocele (def. 2).

colporrhaphy (kol-por′ah-fe) 1. suture of the vagina. 2. the operation of denuding and suturing the vaginal wall to narrow the vagina.

colporrhexis (kol″po-rek′sis) laceration of the vagina.

colposcope (kol′po-skōp) 1. an instrument for examining the vulva, vagina, and cervix by means of a magnifying lens and a bright light, used to identify abnormal epithelium that warrants biopsy and to evaluate the cervix following a Pap smear. 2. vaginoscope. adj., **colposcop′ic.**

colpospasm (kol′po-spazm) vaginal spasm.

colpostenosis (kol″po-stĕ-no′sis) contraction or narrowing of the vagina.

colpostenotomy (kol″po-stĕ-not′ah-me) a cutting operation for stricture of the vagina.

colposuspension (kol″po-sus-pen′shun) bladder neck suspension.

colpotomy (kol-pot′ah-me) incision of the vagina with entry into the cul-de-sac; called also vaginotomy.

colpoxerosis (kol″po-ze-ro′sis) abnormal dryness of the vulva and vagina.

columella (kol″u-mel′ah), pl. *columel′lae* [L.] a little column.

c. na′si the fleshy external termination of the septum of the nose.

column (kol′um) an anatomical part or other structure that resembles a PILLAR.

anal c's vertical folds of mucous membrane at the upper half of the anal canal; called also rectal columns.

anterior c. the anterior portion of the gray substance of the spinal cord, in transverse section seen as a horn.

gray c. the longitudinally oriented parts of the spinal cord in which the nerve cell bodies are found, comprising the gray matter of the spinal cord.

lateral c. the lateral portion of the gray substance of the spinal cord, in transverse section seen as a horn; present only in the thoracic and upper lumbar regions.

posterior c. the posterior portion of the gray substance of the spinal cord, in transverse section seen as a horn.

rectal c's anal columns.

spinal c., vertebral c. SPINE (def. 2).

columna (ko-lum′nah), pl. *colum′nae* [L.] column.

Coly-Mycin M (kol′e-mi″sin) trademark for a preparation of COLISTIMETHATE sodium, an ANTIBIOTIC.

coma (ko′mah) a state of unconsciousness from which the patient cannot be aroused, even by powerful stimuli. Traumatic brain injuries are the most frequent cause; other causes include severe uncontrolled DIABETES MELLITUS, liver disease, kidney disease, and neurologic conditions. Evaluation of a patient in a coma is comprehensive. The underlying cause should be identified so that appropriate treatment can be initiated. MAGNETIC RESONANCE IMAGING, ELECTROENCEPHALOGRAPHY, and brainstem auditory evoked POTENTIALS give information about electrical activity of the brain in a patient who is comatose, although the results are not predictive of recovery. Some patients are able to emerge from a coma. In others, the coma may progress to a persistent vegetative STATE in which the functions of the brainstem and CIRCULATION remain relatively intact or may be supported with assistive technologies. Patients in irreversible coma may meet the criteria of BRAIN DEATH. (See accompanying illustration.)

Patient Care. Assessment of the patient in a coma includes an evaluation of vital signs, determination of LEVEL OF CONSCIOUSNESS, neuromuscular responses, and reaction of the pupils to light. In most hospitals a standard form is used to measure and record the patient's responses to stimuli in objective terms. The GLASGOW COMA SCALE is a standardized tool that aids in assessing a comatose patient and eliminates the use of ambiguous and easily misinterpreted terms such as unconscious and semicomatose. Additional assessment data are gathered relating to the underlying cause and the patient's immobility; these include evaluation of the gag and corneal reflexes. In the absence of gag reflex, regurgitation and aspiration are potential problems. Abnormal rigidity and posturing in response to noxious stimuli are motor responses to coma. DECORTICATE RIGIDITY is abnormal flexor posturing, with the arms, wrists, and fingers drawn up. The legs may be extended with plantar flexion. This type of rigidity usually indicates a lesion in the cerebral hemispheres or a disruption of the corticospinal tracts. DECEREBRATE RIGIDITY is abnormal extensor posturing: in response to painful stimuli the extremities extend rigidly and the palms turn outward. This type of rigidity is indicative of damage to the brainstem and as a rule is a sign of greater cerebral impairment than is decorticate rigidity.

Comatose patients are predisposed to all the HAZARDS OF IMMOBILITY, including impairment of skin integrity and development of PRESSURE ULCERS and CONTRACTURES. A multidisciplinary, coordinated plan of care is essential. Families should be encouraged to be actively involved in care of the patient. The health care team should also recognize the family's need for support; the emotional and financial impacts of coma are usually significant.

alcoholic c. coma accompanying severe alcoholic intoxication.

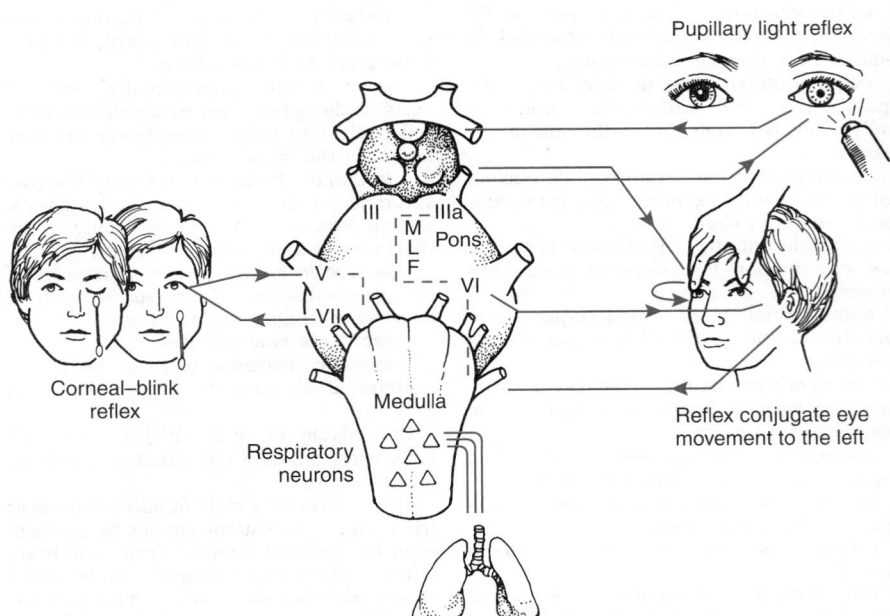

Schematic representation of major brain stem reflexes used in coma examination. From Marx et al., 2002.

alpha c. coma in which there are electroencephalographic findings of dominant alpha-wave activity.

diabetic c. the coma of severe diabetic ACIDOSIS; see also DIABETES MELLITUS.

hepatic c. coma accompanying cerebral damage resulting from degeneration of liver cells, especially that associated with CIRRHOSIS of the liver.

hyperglycemic hyperosmolar nonketotic c., hyperosmolar nonketotic c. see HYPERGLYCEMIC HYPEROSMOLAR NONKETOTIC COMA.

irreversible c. brain death.

Kussmaul's c. the coma and air hunger of diabetic ACIDOSIS.

myxedema c. an often fatal complication of long-term HYPOTHYROIDISM in which the patient is comatose with HYPOTHERMIA, depression of respiration, bradycardia, and hypotension; usually seen in elderly patients during cold weather.

c. vigil locked-in syndrome.

comatose (ko'mah-tōs) pertaining to or affected with coma.

Combivir (kom'bĭ-vir) trademark for a combination preparation of the nucleoside ANALOGUES ZIDOVUDINE and LAMIVUDINE, used in treatment of HIV infection and AIDS.

combustion (kom-bus'chun) rapid oxidation with emission of heat.

comedo (kom'ĕ-do), pl. *comedo'nes* [L.] 1. a plug of keratin and sebum within the dilated orifice of a hair follicle frequently containing the bacteria *Corynebacterium acnes, Staphylococcus albus,* and *Pityrosporum ovale;* see also ACNE VULGARIS.

closed c. whitehead (def. 1).

open c. blackhead.

comedogenic (kom''ĕ-do-jen'ik) producing a COMEDO or comedones.

comedomastitis mammary duct ectasia.

comes (ko'mēz), pl. *comi'tes* [L.] an artery or vein accompanying a nerve trunk.

commensal (kŏ-men'sal) 1. living on or within another organism, and deriving benefit without harming or benefiting the host individual. 2. a parasitic organism that causes no harm to the host.

commensalism (kŏ-men'sal-izm) symbiosis in which one population (or individual) is benefited and the other is neither benefited nor harmed.

comminuted (kom'ĭ-nūt''ed) broken or crushed into small pieces, as a comminuted fracture.

comminution (kom''ĭ-nu'shun) the act of breaking, or condition of being broken, into small fragments.

Commission on Collegiate Nursing Education (CCNE) an autonomous accrediting agency whose mission includes the

assessment and identification of nursing programs that engage in effective educational practices, having a scope of the institutions of higher education in the United States. Its mailing address is One Dupont Circle NW, Washington, DC 20036, and its phone number is 202-887-6791.

commissura (kom''ĭ-su'rah), pl. *commissu'rae* [L.] commissure.

commissure (kom'ĭ-shūr) 1. a site of union of corresponding parts, such as the angle of the lips or eyelids. 2. the site of junction between adjacent cusps of a cardiac VALVE.

anterior c. the band of fibers connecting the parts of the two cerebral HEMISPHERES.

c. of epithalamus a large fiber bundle that crosses the midline of the EPITHALAMUS just dorsal to the point where the cerebral aqueduct opens into the third ventricle.

middle c. a band of gray matter joining the optic thalami; it develops as a secondary adhesion and may be absent.

posterior c. commissure of epithalamus.

commissurorrhaphy (kom''ĭ-shūr-or'ah-fe) suture of the components of a COMMISSURE, to lessen the size of the orifice.

commissurotomy (kom''ĭ-sher-ot'ah-me) surgical incision or digital disruption of the components of a COMMISSURE to increase the size of the opening.

mitral c. the breaking apart of the adherent leaflets (COMMISSURE) of the mitral VALVE, a formerly common treatment for mitral STENOSIS.

commitment (kŏ-mit'ment) 1. a sense of responsibility and dedication. 2. the legal proceeding by which a person is confined to a psychiatric treatment center, usually involuntarily.

committee (kŏ-mit'e) a body of people delegated to perform some function.

ethics c. a group of individuals formed to protect the interests of patients and address moral issues. It normally includes a board member of the institution, a lay person, and an administrator. A member of the clergy may also be included, as well as an ethicist if one is available. Most ethics committees work in an advisory capacity; they can help patients and families make informed decisions and work with health care providers in order to make complex and difficult decisions. The ethics committee often reviews hospital policies and procedures for potential problems and may also reduce the potential for litigation against the institution.

commode (kŏ-mōd') TOILET (def. 2).

c. chair a portable toilet that can be placed at the bedside of a patient whose activity is limited; these are often used in the home when the patient is too debilitated to reach the bathroom. The receptacle for waste can be removed and emptied.

common cold an acute and highly contagious virus infection of the upper respiratory tract. Cold viruses are resistant to present antibiotics, and there is currently no really effective preventive vaccine that will work against them in all situations for all people. Having had a cold confers only a brief immunity. Called also acute rhinitis.

Symptoms. All colds are not identical, because of different causative agents and individual reactions. Usually the common cold starts with a runny nose, sneezing, a stuffy feeling in the head, slight headache, watering of the eyes, general aching and listlessness, inability to concentrate, and perhaps a slight fever. The affected membranes swell until the nasal passages are blocked. Often the inflammation spreads to the throat, causing sore throat and cough.

A cold usually begins to subside after several days. The nasal discharge lessens, the membranous swelling decreases and the patient is able to breathe through the nose again. The average cold lasts from 7 to 14 days. If at any stage the cold shows signs of getting worse—for example, if there are prolonged chills, fever above 39.5° C (103° F), aches in the chest, ears, or face, shortness of breath, coughing up of blood-streaked or rust-colored mucus, or persistent hoarseness—then a health care provider should be consulted.

Treatment. To help avoid complications of all kinds, it is best to take a cold seriously from the beginning. Rest and isolation at the first signs will speed recovery and prevent the passing on of the cold to others. Extra hours of rest or sleep at night are important. It is important to keep warm and avoid changing temperatures as much as possible and to drink plenty of liquids and eat in moderation. The nose should be blown gently, to avoid forcing the infection into the sinuses and ears. Aspirin brings the quickest and safest relief for adults. Antibiotics are *not* helpful for colds. They may be prescribed if complications occur.

SINUSITIS may occur when the infection spreads and causes inflammation of the membranes of the paranasal sinuses. The infection may also affect the membranes of the middle ear. Other complications may occur if the infection enters the lower respiratory system; these include LARYNGITIS, BRONCHITIS, and PNEUMONIA.

communicable disease (kŏ-mu′nĭ-kah-b′l) a disease whose causative agents may pass or be carried from one person to another directly or indirectly. Modes of transmission include (1) direct contact with body excreta or discharges from an ulcer, open sore, or respiratory tract; (2) indirect contact with inanimate objects such as drinking glasses, toys, or bed-clothing; and (3) vectors such as flies, mosquitoes, or other insects capable of spreading the disease. For special precautions to prevent the spread of communicable disease, see ISOLATION. Called also contagious disease.

communication (kŏ-mu′nĭ-ka′shun) the sending of information from one place or individual to another.

c. disorders MENTAL DISORDERS characterized by difficulties in speech or language severe enough to be a problem academically, occupationally, or socially; one such is STUTTERING.

impaired verbal c. a NURSING DIAGNOSIS approved by the North American Nursing Diagnosis Association, defined as decreased, delayed, or absent ability of an individual to receive, process, transmit, or use a system of symbols.

nonverbal c. the transmission of a message without the use of words.

communitarianism (cŏ-mu″nĭ-tar′e-an-izm) community-based theory.

community (kŏ-mu′nĭ-te) a group of persons residing together in face-to-face association; a group of persons with whom an individual identifies as a source of identity and potential support.

continuing care c. life care community.

life care c. a living arrangement for older adults that provides several levels of care within one facility or complex. As the resident requires more health supervision, he or she moves from areas that are more independent to those where care is provided under the supervision of a registered nurse. Life care communities usually require an entry fee as well as a monthly fee. Called also continuing care community.

therapeutic c. a specially structured mental treatment center, employing group and milieu therapy and encouraging the patient to function within social norms.

comorbid (ko-mor′bid) pertaining to a disease or other pathological process that occurs simultaneously with another.

comorbidity (ko″mor-bid′ĭ-te) 1. a COMORBID disease or condition. 2. the state of being

comorbid. 3. the extent to which two pathological conditions occur together in a given
population.

compaction (kom-pak′shun) a complication of labor in twin births in which there is
simultaneous full engagement of the leading
fetal poles of both twins, so that the true
pelvic cavity is filled and further descent is
prevented.

compartmental syndrome (kum-pahrt-
men′tal) a condition in which increased
tissue pressure in a confined anatomical
space causes decreased blood flow leading
to ischemia and dysfunction of contained
myoneural elements, marked by pain,
muscle weakness, sensory loss, and palpable
tenseness in the involved compartment.
Ischemia can lead to necrosis resulting in
permanent impairment of function.

compassion (kom-pă′shun) in bioethics, a
virtue combining concepts such as sympathy, empathy, fellow feeling, benevolence,
care, love, and sometimes pity and mercy.
These are character traits that enable
professionals to use their cognitive and
psychomotor skills of healing to meet the
needs of a particular patient. The need
for particularity in the healing relationship
makes compassion a moral virtue.

compatibility (kom-pat″ĭ-bil′ĭ-te) the quality of being COMPATIBLE; see also HISTOCOM-
PATIBILITY.

compatible 1. capable of harmonious coexistence; said of two or more medications
that are suitable for simultaneous administration without nullification or aggravation of
their effects. 2. denoting a donor and recipient
of a blood transfusion in which there is no
transfusion REACTION. 3. histocompatible.

Compazine (kom′pah-zēn) trademark for
preparations of PROCHLORPERAZINE, an ANTI-
PSYCHOTIC AGENT and ANTIEMETIC.

**Compendium of Pharmaceuticals and
Specialties (CPS)** a publication for Canadian health care providers, published by
the Canadian Pharmaceutical Association.
It contains drug monographs and has a
section of color illustrations of medications
for identification purposes.

compensation (kom″pen-sa′shun) 1. the
counterbalancing of any defect of structure
or function. 2. a mental process that may be
either conscious or, more frequently, an
unconscious DEFENSE MECHANISM by which a
person attempts to make up for real or
imagined physical or psychological deficiencies. 3. in cardiology, the maintenance of
an adequate blood flow without distressing
symptoms, accomplished by such cardiac
and circulatory adjustments as tachycardia,
cardiac hypertrophy, and increase of blood
volume by sodium and water retention.

competence (kom′pĕ-tens) 1. a principle
of professional practice, identifying the
ability of the provider to administer safe
and reliable care on a consistent basis. 2.
the ability of a patient to manage activities
of daily living.

complement (kom′plĕ-ment) a term originally used to refer to the heat-labile factor
in serum that causes immune CYTOLYSIS
(lysis of antibody-coated cells). It is now
used to refer to the entire functionally
related system comprising at least 20
distinct serum proteins, their cellular receptors, and related regulatory proteins; this
system is the effector not only of immune
cytolysis but also of other biologic functions
including ANAPHYLAXIS, PHAGOCYTOSIS, OPSONI-
ZATION, and HEMOLYSIS.
Complement activation occurs by two
different sequences, the *classical pathway*
and the *alternative pathway*. All of the
"components of complement," designated
C1 through C9 (C1 being composed of three
distinct proteins, C1q, C1r, and C1s), participate in the classical pathway; the alternative pathway lacks components C1, C2,
and C4 but adds FACTOR B, FACTOR D, and
PROPERDIN. Regulatory proteins include FAC-
TOR H, FACTOR I, CLUSTERIN, C3 nephritic
FACTOR, decay accelerating FACTOR, homologous restriction FACTOR, C1 INHIBITOR, C4
binding PROTEIN, membrane cofactor PROTEIN,
PROTECTIN, and VITRONECTIN.
The classical pathway is primarily
activated by the binding of C1 to antigen-
antibody complexes containing the IMMUNO-
GLOBULINS IgM or IgG. The alternative
pathway can be activated by IgA immune
complexes and also by nonimmunologic
materials including bacterial endotoxins,
microbial polysaccharides, and cell walls.
Activation of the classical pathway triggers
an enzymatic cascade involving C1, C4,
C2, and C3; activation of the alternative
pathway triggers a cascade involving C3
and factors B and D and properdin. Both
pathways result in cleavage of C5 and
formation of the membrane attack COMPLEX,
which in its final state creates a pore in the
cell wall and causes cell lysis. Complement
activation also results in the formation
of many biologically active complement
fragments that act as anaphylatoxins,
opsonins, or chemotactic factors. Fragments
resulting from proteolytic cleavage of
complement proteins are designated with
lower-case-letter suffixes, e.g., C3a.

c. fixation the combining of COMPLE-
MENT with the antigen-antibody complex,
rendering the complement inactive, or

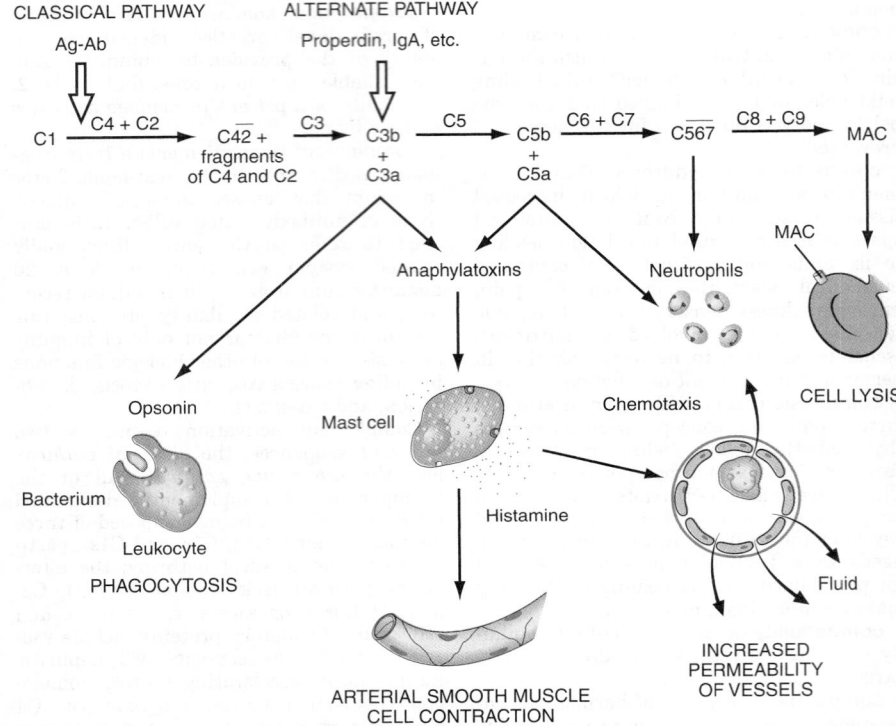

CLASSICAL PATHWAY

ALTERNATE PATHWAY

Complement activation. Activation of the classical and alternative pathways leads to a common terminal pathway from C5 to C9. These complement components form the final membrane attack complex (MAC). Other intermediate complexes and fragments are also biologically active: opsonins facilitate phagocytosis, anaphylatoxins act on mast cells and mediate a release of histamine which acts on blood vessels, and chemotactic fragments and intermediate complexes attract leukocytes to the site of inflammation. Redrawn from Damjanov, 2000.

fixed. Its presence or absence as free, active complement can be shown by adding sensitized blood cells to the mixture. If free complement is present, hemolysis occurs; if not, no hemolysis is observed. This reaction is the basis of many serologic tests for infection, including the WASSERMANN TEST for syphilis, and reactions for gonococcus infection, glanders, typhoid fever, tuberculosis, and amebiasis. Called also Bordet-Gengou phenomenon. See also IMMUNITY.

   c. fixation tests tests that use antigen-antibody reaction and result in hemolysis to determine the presence of various organisms in the blood; see also COMPLEMENT FIXATION.

complex (kom′pleks) 1. the sum, combination, or collection of various things or related factors, like or unlike; e.g., a complex of symptoms (see SYNDROME). 2. a group of interrelated ideas, mainly unconscious, that have a common emotional tone and

strongly influence a person's attitudes and behavior. 3. that portion of an electrocardiographic tracing which represents the systole of an atrium or ventricle.

   AIDS-related c. **(ARC)** a complex of signs and symptoms occurring in HIV infection including fever, weight loss, prolonged diarrhea, minor opportunistic infections, lymphadenopathy, and changes in cells of the immune system.

   antigen-antibody c. here the complex formed by the noncovalent binding of an antibody and antigen. Complexes of antibodies belonging to certain immunoglobulin classes may activate complement. Called also immune complex.

   anti-inhibitor coagulant c. **(AICC)** a concentrated fraction from pooled human plasma, which includes various coagulation factors. It is administered intravenously as an antihemorrhagic in hemophilic patients with inhibitors to COAGULATION FACTOR VIII.

atrial c. the P wave of the ELECTROCARDIOGRAM, representing electrical activity of the atria. See also ventricular COMPLEX.

castration c. in psychoanalytic theory, unconscious thoughts and motives stemming from fear of loss of the genitals as punishment for forbidden sexual desires.

Electra c. libidinous fixation of a daughter toward her father. This term is rarely used, since OEDIPUS COMPLEX is generally applied to both sexes.

factor IX c. a sterile, freeze-dried powder consisting of partially purified COAGULATION FACTOR IX fraction, as well as concentrated factor II, VII, and X fractions, of venous plasma from healthy human donors. It is used in the prophylaxis and treatment of bleeding in patients with HEMOPHILIA B, replacement of factor VII in patients deficient in that factor, and treatment of anticoagulant-induced hemorrhage. Administered intravenously.

Ghon c. primary complex (def. 1).

Golgi c. GOLGI APPARATUS.

HLA c. the human major histocompatibility complex, which contains the HLA ANTIGENS.

immune c. antigen-antibody complex.

inclusion c. one in which molecules of one type are enclosed within cavities in the crystalline lattice of another substance.

inferiority c. unconscious feelings of inadequacy, producing shyness or timidity or, as a compensation, exaggerated aggressiveness and expression of superiority; based on Alfred Adler's concept that everyone is born with a feeling of inferiority stemming from real or imagined physical or psychological deficiency, with the manner in which the inferiority is handled determining behavior.

interpolated premature ventricular c. a premature ventricular complex that does not interfere with the conduction of the next sinus beat, i.e., it lacks the usual following compensatory pause.

major histocompatibility c. (MHC) the chromosomal region containing genes that control the histocompatibility ANTIGENS; in humans it controls the HLA ANTIGENS.

membrane attack c. (MAC) C5b,6,7,8,9, the five-molecule complex that is the cytolytic agent of the COMPLEMENT system.

Oedipus c. see OEDIPUS COMPLEX.

primary c. 1. the combination of a parenchymal pulmonary lesion (*Ghon focus*) and a corresponding lymph node focus, occurring in primary tuberculosis, usually in children. Similar lesions may also be associated with other mycobacterial infections

and with fungal infections. 2. the primary cutaneous lesion at the site of infection in the skin, e.g., chancre in syphilis and tuberculous chancre.

QRS c. a group of waves seen on an ELECTROCARDIOGRAM, representing ventricular depolarization. Called also QRS wave. It actually consists of three distinct waves created by the passage of the cardiac electrical impulse through the ventricles and occurs at the beginning of each ventricular contraction. In a normal surface electrocardiogram the R wave is the upward deflection; the first downward deflection represents a Q wave and the final downward deflection is the S wave. The Q and S waves may be extremely weak and sometimes are absent.One abnormality of the QRS complex is increased voltage resulting from enlargement of heart muscle, which produces increased quantities of electric current. A low-voltage QRS complex may result from toxic conditions of the heart, most commonly from fluid in the pericardium. Pleural effusion and emphysema also can cause a decrease in the voltage of the QRS complex.

VATER c. an association of congenital anomalies consisting of *v*ertebral defects, imperforate *a*nus, *t*racheo*e*sophageal fistula, and *r*adial and *r*enal dysplasia.

ventricular c. the Q, R, S, and T waves of the ELECTROCARDIOGRAM, representing ventricular electrical activity. See also atrial COMPLEX.

complexion (kom-plek′shun) the color and appearance of the skin of the face.

complex regional pain syndrome reflex sympathetic dystrophy.

compliance (kom-pli′ans) 1. implementation by the patient of the therapeutic plan that has been established. 2. the quality of yielding to pressure or force without disruption, or an expression of the measure of ability to do so, as an expression of the distensibility of an air- or fluid-filled organ, such as the lung or urinary bladder, in terms of unit of volume per unit of pressure.

Lung compliance. This is a measure of the ability of the lung to distend in response to pressure without disruption; it expresses the unit volume of change in the lung per unit of pressure (ml/cm H_2O). Compliance or distensibility of the lung is increased in conditions such as EMPHYSEMA, in which the lung distends more readily, and is decreased in fibrotic conditions in which the lung distends with difficulty.The compliance of the lungs (C_L) and thorax (C_T)

determine the elastic resistance to VENTILA-TION. The total compliance of the lungs and thorax (C_{LT}) is given by the formula $1/C_{LT} = 1/C_L + 1/C_T$. C_L is measured by determining the intrapleural pressure at different end-inspiratory volumes. A balloon-tipped catheter is used to determine the intrapleural pressure, which is transmitted through the soft wall of the esophagus. C_L is usually divided by the functional residual capacity to give the specific compliance. Lung compliance is decreased in congestive heart failure and interstitial lung disease and increased in emphysema. C_{LT} can be measured by determining the change in lung volume for various amounts of pressure difference between the mouth and chest surface using a body PLETHYSMOGRAPH.

Bladder compliance. The compliance of the bladder is expressed in cubic centimeters per centimeter of water calculated as change in volume divided by change in pressure during cystometrography. The normal bladder has a compliance of no more than 2 cm increase in water pressure per 100 ml of fluid. Calculated as dV/dP, where dV is change in volume from 0 cc to bladder capacity and dP is change in pressure from 0 cc to bladder capacity, the normal value is greater than or equal to 50. Compromised bladder compliance causes decreased bladder capacity and predisposes the individual to urinary infection and upper urinary tract distress including pyelonephritis and compromised renal function.

dynamic c. compliance measured while an organ is expanding or contracting; in the lung it is measured at the moment between inhalation and exhalation (when flow rate is zero) and is calculated by dividing the tidal volume by the change in pressure during an exhalation. See also static COMPLIANCE.

effective static c. **(ESC)** an estimate of lung compliance calculated by dividing the exhaled tidal volume by the difference in inspiratory plateau PRESSURE and positive end-expiratory PRESSURE; used to reflect gross changes in lung compliance when chest wall compliance is controlled and remains relatively constant.

lung c. a measure of the ability of the lung to distend without disruption in response to pressure; see COMPLIANCE.

specific c. lung compliance in relation to the actual lung volume.

static c. compliance measured in the absence of any motion; see also dynamic COMPLIANCE.

complicating disease (kom′plĭ-kāt″ing) one that occurs in the course of some other disease as a complication.

complication (kom″plĭ-ka′shun) 1. one or more disease(s) concurrent with another disease. 2. the occurrence of two or more diseases in the same patient. 3. an injury or disorder occurring in a patient with a pre-existing condition.

component (com-po′nent) 1. a constituent element or part. 2. one part of a prosthesis system.

clinical c's the three classification schemes that make up the OMAHA SYSTEM: the PROBLEM CLASSIFICATION SCHEME arranges 40 NURSING DIAGNOSES (called client PROBLEMS) into four different domains; the INTERVENTION SCHEME assigns nursing INTERVENTIONS to the client problems; and the PROBLEM RATING SCALE FOR OUTCOMES assigns RATINGS to describe the client's problem-specific knowledge, behavior, and status at various points in the treatment process. See Appendix on the Omaha System.

M c. [*M*yeloma or *M*acroglobulinemia] structurally homogeneous protein in serum or urine appearing as a sharp spike in the beta or gamma globulin region on protein electrophoresis. The protein is in most cases a monoclonal IMMUNOGLOBULIN or heavy chain fragment, or a monoclonal immunoglobulin light chain or light chain fragment, either alone or with monoclonal immunoglobulin containing the same light chain. M components are characteristic of plasma cell DYSCRASIAS.

performance c's see PERFORMANCE COMPONENTS.

plasma thromboplastin c. **(PTC)** factor IX, one of the COAGULATION FACTORS.

composite (kom-poz′it) 1. made up of unlike parts. 2. composite RESIN.

compos mentis (kom′pos men′tis) [L.] sound of mind; sane.

compound (kom′pownd) 1. made up of diverse elements or ingredients. 2. a substance made up of two or more materials. 3. in chemistry, a substance made up of two or more elements in union. The elements are united chemically, which means that each of the original elements loses its individual characteristics once it has combined with the other element(s). When elements combine they do so in definite proportions by weight; this is why the union of hydrogen and oxygen always produces water. Sugar, salt, and vinegar are examples of compounds.

Organic compounds are those containing carbon atoms; inorganic compounds are those that do not contain carbon atoms.

clathrate c's inclusion complexes in which molecules of one type are trapped within cavities of another substance, such as within a crystalline lattice structure or large molecule.

quaternary ammonium c. an organic compound containing a quaternary ammonium group, a nitrogen atom carrying a single positive charge bonded to four carbon atoms, e.g., choline.

Comprehensive Health Organization (CHO) in Canada, a joint venture formed by community and provider interests operating a nonprofit corporation. Comprehensive health organizations combine the existing elements of the health care system into a unified whole and provide a range of health promotion and treatment services to a defined roster population.

compress (kom′pres) a pad of gauze or similar dressing, for application of pressure or medication to a restricted area, or for local applications of heat or cold.

compression (kom-presh′un) 1. the act of pressing upon or together; the state of being pressed together. 2. in embryology, the shortening or omission of certain developmental stages. 3. the flattening of soft tissue to improve optical density in radiographic procedures such as MAMMOGRAPHY.

compressor (kom-pres′er) something that causes compression.

air c. a device used to pressurize room air, which can then be used to power other devices, such as respiratory devices.

compromise (kom′pro-mīz) 1. to make a decision by mutual consent in which neither party has all demands met but both agree that it is acceptable. 2. to take an action or place a patient in a position that endangers health and well-being.

compulsion (kom-pul′shun) 1. a recurrent, unwanted, and distressing (ego-dystonic) urge to perform an act. 2. a compulsive act or ritual; a repetitive and stereotyped action that is performed to ward off some untoward event, although the patient recognizes that it does not do so in any realistic way. It serves as a defensive substitute for unacceptable unconscious ideas or impulses. Failure to perform the compulsive act gives rise to anxiety and tension. Common compulsions involve hand-washing, touching, counting, and checking. adj., **compul′sive.** See also OBSESSIVE-COMPULSIVE.

repetition c. in psychoanalytic theory, the impulse to reenact earlier emotional experiences.

compulsive personality disorder obsessive-compulsive personality disorder.

CON certificate of need.

conation (ko-na′shun) in psychology, the power that motivates effort of any kind; the conscious tendency to act.

conative (kon′ah-tiv) pertaining to the basic strivings of a person, as expressed in his behavior and actions.

concanavalin (kon″kah-nav′ah-lin) a lectin isolated from the jack bean (*Canavalia ensiformis*) that agglutinates mammalian erythrocytes and is a mitogen that stimulates predominantly T lymphocytes. Abbreviated ConA.

Concato's disease (kon-ka′tōz) progressive malignant polyserositis with large effusions into the pericardium, pleura, and peritoneum.

concave (kon′kāv) rounded and somewhat depressed or hollowed out.

concavity (kon-kav′ĭ-te) a depression or hollowed surface.

conceive (kon-sēv′) 1. to become pregnant. 2. take in, grasp, or form in the mind.

concentrate (kon′sen-trāt) 1. to bring to a common center; to gather at one point. 2. to increase the strength by diminishing the bulk of, as of a liquid; to condense. 3. a drug or other preparation that has been strengthened by evaporation of its nonactive parts.

***activated prothrombin complex c.* (APCC)** anti-inhibitor coagulant complex.

***prothrombin complex c.* (PCC)** factor IX complex.

concentration (kon″sen-tra′shun) 1. increase in strength by evaporation. 2. the ratio of the mass or volume of a solute to the mass or volume of the solution or solvent. 3. intense mental focus.

hydrogen ion c. see HYDROGEN ION CONCENTRATION.

mass c. the mass of a constituent substance divided by the volume of the mixture, as milligrams per liter (mg/l).

***mean corpuscular hemoglobin c.* (MCHC)** the average HEMOGLOBIN concentration in erythrocytes, conventionally expressed in "per cent," meaning grams per deciliter of red blood cells, obtained by dividing the blood hemoglobin concentration (in g/dl) by the hematocrit (in l/l): MCHC = Hb/Hct.

***minimal alveolar c.* (MAC)** the concentration of anesthetic that at a pressure of 1 atmosphere produces immobility in 50 per cent of subjects exposed to a noxious stimulus.

***minimal bactericidal c.* (MBC)** the lowest concentration of a given antibiotic required to kill a specific organism.

***minimal inhibitory c.* (MIC)** the lowest concentration of a given antibiotic that inhibits the growth of a specific organism.

molar c. the concentration of a substance expressed in terms of MOLARITY.

c. test a test of renal function based on the patient's ability to concentrate urine; see also FISHBERG CONCENTRATION TEST.

concept (kon'sept) the image of a thing held in the mind; an abstract notion. A concept is an element used in the development of a THEORY. It is generally agreed that the central concepts of the discipline of NURSING are ENVIRONMENT, HEALTH, NURSING, and *person.*

conception (kon-sep'shun) 1. the onset of PREGNANCY, marked by implantation of the BLASTOCYST; the formation of a viable ZYGOTE. 2. concept.

conceptualization (kon-sep″choo-al-ĭ-za′-shun) the process of thinking or imaging, resulting in the formation of a CONCEPT.

conceptual model a set of CONCEPTS, with propositions that describe them, express the relationship between them, or set forth the basic assumptions of the model. Both the concepts and the propositions of a conceptual model are abstract and very general and are often expressed in a vocabulary that is distinctive for each model; however, the concepts and propositions of a conceptual model are less abstract than those of a METAPARADIGM, from which a conceptual model is derived. A conceptual model provides a framework for the organization of the knowledge of a discipline, determining the focus of the discipline and serving as a guide for observation and interpretation.

For conceptual models developed by nursing theorists for the discipline of NURSING, see ADAPTATION MODEL; BEHAVIORAL SYSTEM MODEL; CONSERVATION MODEL; GENERAL SYSTEMS FRAMEWORK AND THEORY OF GOAL ATTAINMENT; HEALTH AS EXPANDING CONSCIOUSNESS; NEUMAN'S SYSTEMS MODEL; SCIENCE OF UNITARY HUMAN BEINGS; SELF-CARE MODEL; THEORY OF HUMAN BECOMING; and THEORY OF HUMAN CARING.

conceptus (kon-sep′tus) the whole product of CONCEPTION at any stage of development, from FERTILIZATION of the ovum to BIRTH, including extraembryonic membranes as well as the EMBRYO or FETUS.

concha (kong′kah), pl. *con′chae* [L.] a shell-shaped structure.

c. of auricle the hollow of the auricle of the external ear, bounded anteriorly by the tragus and posteriorly by the antihelix.

inferior nasal c. a bone forming the lower part of the lateral wall of the nasal cavity.

middle nasal c. the lower of two bony plates projecting from the inner wall of the ethmoidal labyrinth and separating the superior from the middle meatus of the nose.

sphenoidal c. a thin curved plate of bone at the anterior and lower part of the body of the sphenoid bone, on either side, forming part of the roof of the nasal cavity.

superior nasal c. the upper of two bony plates projecting from the inner wall of the ethmoidal labyrinth and forming the upper boundary of the superior meatus of the nose.

supreme nasal c. a third thin bony plate occasionally found projecting from the inner wall of the ethmoidal labyrinth, above the two usually found.

conchitis (kong-ki′tis) inflammation of a nasal CONCHA.

conchotomy (kong-kot′ah-me) turbinotomy.

conclination (kon″kli-na′shun) inward rotation of the upper pole of the vertical meridian of each eye.

concordance (kon-kor′dans) in genetics, the occurrence of a given trait in both members of a twin pair. adj., **concor′dant.**

concrescence (kon-kres′ens) a growing together of parts originally separate.

concretio (kon-kre′she-o) [L.] concretion.

c. cor′dis adhesive PERICARDITIS in which the pericardial cavity is obliterated, often with calcification of the pericardium.

concretion (kon-kre′shun) 1. a CALCULUS or hard inorganic mass in a natural cavity or in tissue. 2. abnormal union of adjacent parts. 3. the process of becoming harder or more solid.

concurrent (kon-ker′ent) happening at the same time; simultaneous.

concussion (kon-kush′un) a violent jar or shock, or the condition that results from such an injury.

c. of the brain alteration of CONSCIOUSNESS, transient or prolonged, due to a blow to the head; it may be followed by transient amnesia, vertigo, nausea, and weak pulse. Breathing often is unusually rapid or slow. Outward evidence of the injury may include bleeding and contusions (bruises). When consciousness is regained, the victim is likely to have severe headache and, possibly, blurred vision. If severely injured, the victim may lapse into a COMA.

Concussion is a type of traumatic brain injury (see also HEAD INJURY). In addition to the primary injury, concussion can precipitate an increase in INTRACRANIAL PRESSURE or other neurological sequelae such as bleeding that can emerge several hours or days after the trauma. It is critical for health care providers to monitor these secondary tissue damages. Education of the patient and family is important regarding signs and symptoms of an increase in intracranial pressure and when to seek emergency care. Most people, however, recover from a concussion with no permanent neurological deficits. Rest is the usual treatment. ACET-AMINOPHEN is usually prescribed for the associated headache.

condensation (kon″den-sa′shun) 1. the act of rendering or process of becoming more compact; compression. 2. the packing of dental filling material into a prepared tooth cavity. 3. a mental process in which one symbol stands for a number of components and contains all the emotions associated with them. 4. conversion from the gaseous state to the liquid or solid state; gas liquefaction.

condenser (kon-den′ser) 1. a vessel or apparatus for condensing gases or vapors. 2. a device for illuminating microscopic objects. 3. capacitor. 4. a dental tool used to pack filling material in a cavity.

condition (kon-dish′un) 1. to train; to subject to CONDITIONING. 2. the state in which an object or person exists.

conditioned response (kun-dish′und) a response that does not occur naturally in the animal but that may be developed by regular association of some physiologic function with an unrelated outside event, such as ringing of a bell or flashing of a light. Soon the physiologic function starts whenever the outside event occurs. Called also conditioned reflex. See also CONDITION-ING.

conditioning (kon-dish′un-ing) 1. in physical medicine, improvement of physical health by a program of exercises; called also physical conditioning. 2. in psychology, a form of learning in which a response is elicited by a neutral stimulus which previously had been repeatedly presented in conjunction with the stimulus that originally elicited the response. Called also classical or respondent conditioning.

The concept had its beginnings in experimental techniques for the study of reflexes. The traditional procedure is based on the work of Ivan P. Pavlov, a Russian physiologist. In this technique the experimental subject is a dog that is harnessed in a sound-shielded room. The neutral stimulus is the sound of a metronome or bell which occurs each time the dog is presented with food, and the response is the production of saliva by the dog. Eventually the sound of the bell or metronome produces salivation, even though the stimulus that originally elicited the response (the food) is no longer presented.

C

In the technique just described, the conditioned stimulus is the sound of the bell or metronome, and the conditioned response is the salivation that occurs when the sound is heard. The food, which was the original stimulus to salivation, is the unconditioned stimulus and the salivation that occurred when food was presented is the unconditioned response.

Reinforcement is said to take place when the conditioned stimulus is appropriately followed by the unconditioned stimulus. If the unconditioned stimulus is withheld during a series of trials, the procedure is called extinction because the frequency of the conditioned response will gradually decrease when the stimulus producing the response is no longer present. The process of extinction eventually results in a return of the preconditioning level of behavior.

aversive c. learning in which punishment or other unpleasant stimulation is used to associate negative feelings with an undesirable response.

classical c. conditioning (def. 2).

instrumental c., operant c. learning in which a particular response is elicited by a stimulus because that response produces desirable consequences (reward). It differs from classical conditioning in that the reinforcement takes place only after the subject performs a specific act that has been previously designated. If no unconditioned stimulus is used to bring about this act, the desired behavior is known as an operant. Once the behavior occurs with regularity the behavior may be called a conditioned response. The traditional example of instrumental conditioning uses the Skinner BOX, named after B. F. Skinner, an American behavioral psychologist. The subject, a rat, is kept in the box and becomes conditioned to press a bar by being rewarded with food pellets each time its early random movements caused it to press against the bar.

The principles and techniques related to instrumental conditioning are used clinically in BEHAVIOR THERAPY to help patients eliminate undesirable behavior and substitute for it newly learned behavior that is more appropriate and acceptable.

physical c. conditioning (def. 1).

respondent c. conditioning (def. 2).

work c. a physical exercise program designed to restore specific strength, flexibility, and endurance for return to work following injury, disease, or medically imposed rest; it may be part of a complete WORK HARDENING program when other aspects of functional restoration are required.

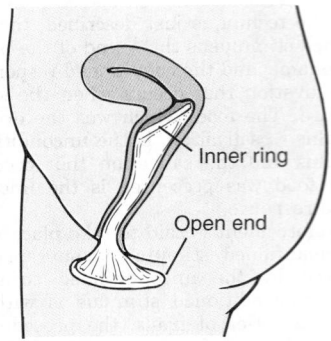

Female condom. When correctly in place, the female condom covers the cervix and lines the vaginal canal with the open end outside the vagina. From Nichols and Zwelling, 1997.

condom (kon′dum) a sheath or cover worn over the penis during sexual intercourse for CONTRACEPTION and prevention of SEXUALLY TRANSMITTED DISEASES.

female c. a long polyurethane sheath that is inserted into the vagina as a CONTRACEPTIVE; it has a flexible ring that fits over the cervix like a diaphragm and another ring that extends outside the vagina. See also CONTRACEPTION.

conduct (kon′dukt) behavior.

c. disorder a form of disruptive behavior disorder of childhood and adolescence characterized by a persistent pattern of antisocial conduct, in which rights of others or age-appropriate societal norms or rules are violated. Misconduct may include aggression to people or animals, destruction of property, deceitfulness or theft, and serious violations of rules.

conductance (kon-duk′tans) ability to conduct or transmit, as electricity or other energy or material.

airway c. in studies of respiration, an expression of the amount of air reaching the alveoli per unit of time per unit of pressure, the reciprocal of airway RESISTANCE.

social c. interaction appropriate to one's environment, making use of manners, respect for personal space, eye contact, gestures, active listening, and self expression; a PERFORMANCE COMPONENT of occupational therapy.

conduction (kon-duk′shun) conveyance of energy, as of heat, sound, or electricity.

aberrant ventricular c. the temporary abnormal intraventricular conduction of supraventricular impulses; called also ventricular aberration.

aerial c., air c. conduction of sound waves to the organ of HEARING in the inner ear through the air.

anterograde c. 1. forward conduction of impulses through a nerve. 2. in the heart, conduction of impulses from atria to ventricles.

atrioventricular c., AV c. the conduction of atrial impulses through the atrioventricular node and the His-Purkinje system to the ventricles.

bone c. conduction of sound waves to the inner ear through the bones of the skull.

concealed c. conduction that is not seen on the surface electrocardiogram but may be detected by its effect on subsequent impulses; common examples are the incomplete penetration of the AV junction during atrial FIBRILLATION, the Wenckebach type penetration during atrial FLUTTER, and the retrograde incomplete penetration following ventricular ectopic BEATS.

decremental c. a gradual decrease in the stimuli and response along a pathway of conduction; it occurs in nerve FIBERS with reduced membrane POTENTIALS.

retrograde c. transmission of a cardiac impulse backward in the ventricular to atrial direction; particularly, conduction from the atrioventricular node into the atria.

saltatory c. the rapid passage of an electric POTENTIAL between the NODES OF RANVIER in myelinated nerve fibers, rather than along the full length of the membrane.

conductivity (kon″duk-tiv′ĭ-te) capacity for conduction.

conductor (kon-duk′ter) any material capable of CONDUCTION.

electrical c. a substance that can conduct electricity because it has mobile electrons.

conduit (kon′doo-it) a channel for the passage of fluids.

ileal c. see ILEAL CONDUIT.

condylarthrosis (kon″dil-ahr-thro′sis) a modification of the spheroidal form of synovial joint, in which the articular surfaces are ellipsoidal rather than spheroid.

condyle (kon′dīl) a rounded projection on a bone, usually for articulation with another bone.

condylectomy (kon″dil-ek′to-me) excision of a condyle.

condylion (kon-dil′e-on) the most lateral point on the surface of the head of the mandible.

condyloid (kon′dĭ-loid) resembling a condyle.

condyloma (kon″dĭ-lo′mah), pl. *condylomata* [L.] an elevated wartlike lesion of the skin. adj., **condylo′matous.**

c.′ta acumina′ta sing. *condylo′ma acumina′tum.* Sexually transmitted venereal papillomatous lesions caused by the human PAPILLOMAVIRUS. The incubation period is one to three months. The growths are usually pinkish and occur around the cervix, vulva, perineum, anus and anal canal, urethra, and glans penis. They are often treated with weekly applications of podophyllum resin, 10 to 25 per cent in tincture of benzoin or by application of trichloroacetic acid. Especially resistant warts or extensive involvement may require electrocautery, cryosurgery, or recombinant interferon alfa-2b or alfa-n3. Called also genital or venereal warts. (See Atlas 2, Part H.)

flat c. condyloma latum.

giant c. Buschke-Löwenstein tumor.

c. la'tum a wide, flat, syphilitic condyloma occurring on moist skin, especially around the genitals or anus.

condylotomy (kon″dĭ-lot′ah-me) transection of a condyle.

condylus (kon′dĭ-lus), pl. *con'dyli* [L.] condyle.

cone (kōn) 1. a solid figure or body having a circular base and tapering to a point. 2. one of the conelike structures which, with the RODS, form the light-sensitive elements of the RETINA; the cones make possible the perception of color. See also EYE and VISION. Called also retinal cone. 3. in radiology, a conical or open-ended cylindrical structure formerly used as an aid in centering the radiation beam and as a guide to source-to-film distance. Cones were commonly attached to the x-ray tube prior to the use of the COLLIMATOR. 4. in root canal THERAPY, a solid substance with a tapered form, usually made of gutta-percha or silver, fashioned to conform to the shape of a root canal.

ether c. a cone-shaped device used over the face in administration of ether for anesthesia.

gutta-percha c. in root canal THERAPY, a plastic radiopaque cone made from gutta-percha and other ingredients, available in standard sizes according to the dimensions of root canal reamers and files; used to fill and seal the canal along with sealer cements. Called also gutta-percha point.

c. of light the triangular reflection of light seen on the tympanic membrane.

pressure c. the area of compression exerted by a mass in the brain, as in transtentorial herniation.

retinal c. cone (def. 2).

silver c. silver point.

conexus (kŏ-nek′sus), pl. *conex'us* [L.] a connecting structure; also spelled connexus.

confabulation (kon″fab-u-la′shun) unconscious filling in of gaps in memory with fabricated facts and experiences, commonly associated with organic pathology. It differs from lying in that the patient has no intention to deceive and believes the fabricated memories to be real.

conference (kon′fer-ens) a gathering for discussion or deliberation.

multidisciplinary care c. in the NURSING INTERVENTIONS CLASSIFICATION, a nursing INTERVENTION defined as planning and evaluating patient care with health professionals from other disciplines.

confidentiality (kon-fĭ-den-she-al′ĭ-te) a substantive rule in BIOETHICS saying that the information a patient reveals to a health care provider is private and has limits on how and when it can be disclosed to a third party; usually the provider must obtain permission from the patient to make such a disclosure.

configuration (kon-fig′u-ra′shun) 1. the general form, shape, or appearance of an object. 2. in chemistry, the arrangement in space of the atoms of a molecule.

conflict (kon′flikt) a mental struggle arising from the clash of incompatible or opposing impulses, wishes, drives, or external demands.

decisional c. (specify) a NURSING DIAGNOSIS accepted by the North American Nursing Diagnosis Association, defined as a state of uncertainty about the course of action to be taken when choice among competing actions involves risk, loss, or challenge to personal values.

extrapsychic c. that between the self and the external environment.

intrapsychic c. conflict between incompatible or opposing wishes, impulses, needs, thoughts, or demands within one's own mind.

parental role c. a NURSING DIAGNOSIS accepted by the North American Nursing Diagnosis Association, defined as experience by a parent of role confusion and conflict in response to crisis. See also PARENTING.

confluence (kon′floo-ens) a running together; a meeting of streams.

c. of sinuses the dilated point of confluence of the superior sagittal, straight, occipital, and two transverse sinuses of the dura mater.

confounding (kon-foun′ding) interference by a third variable so as to distort the association being studied between two other variables, because of a strong relationship with both of the other variables; a relationship between two causal factors such that their individual contributions can not be separated.

confrontation the act of facing or being made to face one's own attitudes and shortcomings, the way one is perceived, and the consequences of one's behavior, or of causing another to face these things. It is a therapeutic technique which demonstrates where change must begin, but which also has destructive potential.

confusion (kon-fu′zhun) disturbed orientation in regard to time, place, or person, sometimes accompanied by disordered CONSCIOUSNESS.

congener (kon′jĕ-ner) something closely related to another thing, or derived from the same source or stock, such as a member of the same genus, a muscle having the same function as another, or a chemical compound closely related to another in composition and exerting similar or antagonistic effects. adj., **congener′ic, congen′erous.**

congenital (kon-jen′ĭ-t′l) existing at, and usually before, birth; referring to conditions that are present at birth, regardless of their causation. Cf. HEREDITARY.

   c. heart defect a structural defect of the heart or great vessels or both, present at birth. Any number of defects may occur, singly or in combination. They result from improper development of the heart and blood vessels during the prenatal period. Congenital heart defects occur in about 8 to 10 of every 1000 live-born children in the United States. The most common types are TETRALOGY OF FALLOT, PATENT DUCTUS ARTERIOSUS, VENTRICULAR SEPTAL DEFECT, ATRIAL SEPTAL DEFECT, TRANSPOSITION OF GREAT VESSELS, and COARCTATION OF THE AORTA.

In many cases, depending on the severity of the defect and the physical condition of the patient, these congenital conditions can be treated by surgery. However, some are so minor that they do not significantly affect the action of the heart and do not require surgery. The cause of most of these conditions is unknown. Gene abnormalities account for about 5 per cent, and in a small number of other cases they may be seen in a child whose pregnant mother had rubella (German measles) during the first 2 or 3 months of pregnancy.

congestion (kon-jes′chun) abnormal accumulation of fluid, usually blood, in a body part, organ, or area.

congestive (kon-jes′tiv) pertaining to or associated with congestion.

conglobation (kon″glo-ba′shun) the act of forming, or the state of being formed, into a rounded mass.

conglutinant (kon-gloo′tĭ-nant) 1. promoting union, such as of the edges of a wound. 2. an adhesive used for this purpose.

conglutinating complement absorption test (CCAT) (kon-gloo′tĭ-nāt-ing kom′plĕ-ment ab-sorp′shun) a test resembling the COMPLEMENT FIXATION TEST, using the disappearance of CONGLUTININ activity as the indicator of antigen-antibody reaction.

conglutination (kon-gloo″tĭ-na′shun) 1. ADHESION (def. 2). 2. agglutination of bacteria or erythrocytes that is dependent upon both complement and antibodies.

conglutinin (kən-gloo′tĭ-nin) a nonimmunoglobulin bovine serum protein that aggregates immune complexes with conglutinogen activity (inactivated C3b) in the presence of divalent cations. It has been used as an indicator system, replacing COMPLEMENT FIXATION, in serologic tests, and in the detection of immune complexes. Not to be confused with IMMUNOCONGLUTININ.

   immune c. immunoconglutinin.

Conidiobolus (ko-nid″e-ob′o-lus) a genus of perfect fungi; *C. corona′tus* is usually a saprobe but sometimes causes ENTOMOPHTHOROMYCOSIS in humans and horses.

coniofibrosis (ko″ne-o-fi-bro′sis) PNEUMOCONIOSIS marked by an exuberant growth of connective tissue caused by a specific irritant, as in ASBESTOSIS, SILICOSIS, and SILICOTUBERCULOSIS.

coniosis (ko″ne-o′sis) a disease state caused by the inhalation of dust, such as BYSSINOSIS or PNEUMOCONIOSIS.

coniosporosis (ko″ne-o-spo-ro′sis) a condition characterized by asthmatic symptoms and acute pneumonitis, caused by inhalation of spores of *Coniosporium corticale,* a fungus growing under the bark of certain trees; observed in workers engaged in peeling logs.

coniotoxicosis (ko″ne-o-tok″sĭ-ko′sis) pneumoconiosis in which the irritant affects the tissues directly.

conization (ko″nĭ-za′shun) the removal of a cone of tissue, as in partial excision of the cervix uteri.

   cold c. that done with a cold knife, as opposed to electrocautery, to better preserve the histologic elements.

conjugata (kon″joo-ga′tah) the conjugate diameter of the pelvis; see PELVIC DIAMETER.

conjugate (kon′joo-gāt) 1. paired, or equally coupled; working in union. 2. a conjugate diameter of the pelvic inlet, especially the true conjugate diameter; see PELVIC DIAMETER.

conjugation (kon″joo-ga′shun) a joining. In unicellular organisms, a form of sexual reproduction in which two individuals join in temporary union to transfer genetic material. In biochemistry, the joining of a toxic substance with some natural substance of the body to form a detoxified product for elimination from the body.

conjunctiva (kon″junk-ti′vah), pl. *conjunc′tivae* [L.] the delicate membrane lining the eyelids (*palpebral conjunctiva*) and covering the eyeball (*ocular conjunctiva*). adj., **conjuncti'val.**

conjunctivitis (kon-junk″tĭ-vi′tis) inflammation of the CONJUNCTIVA; it may be caused by bacteria or a virus, or by allergic, chemical, or physical factors. Its infectious form (of bacterial or viral origin) is highly contagious. See also PINKEYE.

acute contagious c. a contagious inflammation of the CONJUNCTIVA caused by *Haemophilus aegypticus;* secretions must be handled with extreme care to prevent its spread. Popularly known as pinkeye.

acute hemorrhagic c. a highly contagious form due to infection with enteroviruses.

gonococcal c., gonorrheal c., a severe form caused by infection with gonococci, marked by greatly swollen conjunctivae and eyelids with a profuse purulent discharge. In newborns it is bilateral, acquired from an infected maternal vaginal passage. In adults it is usually unilateral and is acquired by autoinoculation into the eye of other gonococcal infections, such as URETHRITIS, either in oneself or in another person. Called also gonorrheal ophthalmia.

inclusion c. a type of conjunctivitis primarily affecting newborn infants, caused by a strain of *Chlamydia trachomatis,* beginning as an acute purulent form and leading to papillary hypertrophy of the palpebral conjunctiva.

neonatal c. ophthalmia neonatorum.

conjunctivoma (kon-junk″tĭ-vo′mah) a tumor of the eyelid composed of conjunctival tissue.

conjunctivoplasty (kon″junk-ti′vo-plas″te) plastic repair of the conjunctiva.

Conn's syndrome (konz) primary aldosteronism.

connective (kŏ-nek′tiv) serving as a link or binding.

connective tissue (kŏ-nek′tiv) a fibrous type of body tissue with varied functions; it supports and connects internal organs, forms bones and the walls of blood vessels, attaches muscles to bones, and replaces tissues of other types following injury. Connective tissue consists mainly of long fibers embedded in noncellular matter, the ground substance. The density of these fibers and the presence or absence of certain chemicals make some connective tissues soft and rubbery and others hard and rigid. Compared with most other kinds of tissue, connective tissue has few cells. The fibers contain a protein called COLLAGEN. Connective tissue can develop in any part of the body, and the body uses this ability to help repair or replace damaged areas.

Scar tissue is the most common form of this substitute. See also COLLAGEN DISEASES.

connector (kŏ-nek′ter) 1. anything serving as a link between two separate objects or units. 2. in electrocardiography, an insulated connection between the lead WIRES and the pulse GENERATOR, usually of the pin-and-socket type.

neutral c. in electrocardiography, one of the flat blades of the standard three-pin wall receptacle that provides a return path for the electrical current.

Y-c. see Y-CONNECTOR.

connexus (cŏ-nek′sus), pl. *connex′us* [L.] a connecting structure; also spelled conexus.

Conradi-Hünermann syndrome (kon-rah′de hu′ner-mahn) the autosomal dominant form of CHONDRODYSPLASIA PUNCTATA.

consanguinity (kon″sang-gwin′ĭ-te) blood relationship; kinship. adj., **consanguin′eous.**

conscience (kon′shens) 1. an inner moral sense that distinguishes right acts from wrong. Difficulties arise in how the conscience decides between good and bad. Conscience is not always an adequate justification for action. 2. the internalization of parental and social norms, related to the Freudian concept of SUPEREGO; this conception of conscience has no role in ethical deliberation. 3. in bioethics, the exercise and expression of a reflective sense of integrity, constitutive of reflection about the relationship between a specific course of action and a particular idea of the self and one's integrity. Appeals to conscience presume a prior decision about the rightness or wrongness of an act. Justification is adequate if it is based on universalizable principles; if justification is founded on religious beliefs, personal ideas, or a particular way of life, others cannot be held to them.

conscientiousness (kon″she-en′shus-nes) a principled commitment to do something, such as to provide health care.

conscientious objection (kon″she-en′shus) an appeal to CONSCIENCE in refusing to do, or seeking exemption from, acts that threaten a person's sense of integrity. Patients as well as physicians and nurses may appeal to conscience in refusing treatment or procedures. Called also conscientious refusal.

conscious (kon′shus) 1. having awareness of oneself and of one's acts and surroundings. 2. a state of alertness or awareness characterized by response to external stimuli. 3. the part of the mind that is constantly within awareness, one of the systems of Freud's topographic model of the mind.

consciousness (kon'shus-nes) 1. the state of being conscious; fully alert, aware, oriented, and responsive to the environment. 2. subjective awareness of the aspects of cognitive processing and the content of the mind. 3. the current totality of experience of which an individual or group is aware at any time. 4. in psychoanalysis, the conscious. 5. in Newman's conceptual model, HEALTH AS EXPANDING CONSCIOUSNESS, the informational capacity of the human system, or its capacity for interacting with the environment; consciousness is considered to be coextensive with the universe, residing in all matter.

clouding of c. see CLOUDING OF CONSCIOUSNESS.

levels of c. 1. an early FREUDIAN concept referring to the CONSCIOUS, PRECONSCIOUS, and UNCONSCIOUS. 2. the somewhat loosely defined states of awareness of and response to stimuli, generally considered an integral component of the assessment of an individual's neurologic status. Levels of consciousness range from full consciousness (behavioral wakefulness, orientation as to time, place, and person, and a capacity to respond appropriately to stimuli) to deep COMA (complete absence of response).

Consciousness depends upon close interaction between the intact cerebral hemispheres and the central gray matter of the upper brainstem. Although the hemispheres contribute most of the specific components of consciousness (memory, intellect, and learned responses to stimuli), there must be arousal or activation of the cerebral cells before they can function. For this reason, it is suggested that a detailed description of the patient's response to specific auditory, visual, and tactile stimuli will be more meaningful to those concerned with neurologic assessment than would the use of such terms as *alert, drowsy, stuporous, semiconscious,* or other equally subjective labels. Standardized systems, such as the GLASGOW COMA SCALE, aid in objective and less ambiguous evaluation of levels of consciousness.

Examples of the kinds of stimuli that may be used to determine a patient's responsiveness as a measure of consciousness include calling him by name, producing a sharp noise, giving simple commands, gentle shaking, pinching the biceps, and application of a blood pressure cuff. Responses to stimuli should be reported in specific terms relative to how the patient responded, whether the response was appropriate, and what occurred immediately after the response.

consensus statement a document developed by an independent panel of experts, usually multidisciplinary, convened to review the research literature for the purpose of advancing the understanding of an issue, procedure, or method.

consent (kon-sent') in law, voluntary agreement with an action proposed by another. Consent is an act of reason; the person giving consent must be of sufficient mental capacity and be in possession of all essential information in order to give valid consent. A person who is an infant, is mentally incompetent, or is under the influence of drugs is incapable of giving consent. Consent must also be free of coercion or fraud.

informed c. consent of a patient or other recipient of services based on the principles of autonomy and privacy; this has become the requirement at the center of morally valid decision making in health care and research. Seven criteria define informed consent: (1) competence to understand and to decide, (2) voluntary decision making, (3) disclosure of material information, (4) recommendation of a plan, (5) comprehension of terms (3) and (4), (6) decision in favor of a plan, and (7) authorization of the plan. A person gives informed consent only if all of these criteria are met. If all of the criteria are met except that the person rejects the plan, that person makes an informed refusal.

In nonemergency situations, written informed consent is generally required before many medical procedures, such as surgery, including biopsies, endoscopy, and radiographic procedures involving catheterization. The physician must explain to the patient the diagnosis, the nature of the procedure, including the risks involved and the chances of success, and the alternative methods of treatment that are available. Nurses or other members of the health care team may be involved in filling out the consent form and witnessing the signature of the patient or the parent or guardian, if the patient is a minor. In medical research, the patient must be informed that the procedure is experimental and that consent can be withdrawn at any time. In addition, the person signing the consent form must be informed of the risks and benefits of the experimental procedure and of alternative treatments.

conservation model a CONCEPTUAL MODEL of nursing, formulated by Myra E. LEVINE, concerned with the maintenance of the person's wholeness. The *person* is a holistic being, an organism that is a system of systems, and changes through adaptation. Adaptation is facilitated by the fight-or-flight mechanism, inflammatory processes, nonspecific bodily responses to stress, and perceptual awareness as experienced through the basic orienting, visual, auditory, taste-smell, and haptic systems. The *environment* includes internal and external components: the internal environment manifests HOMEORHESIS, a stabilized flow, in the face of continuous change; the external environment is further divided into perceptual, operational, and conceptual components. The perceptual environment encompasses stimuli that can be perceived by the sense organs. The operational environment encompasses environmental factors that cannot be perceived by the sense organs. The conceptual environment encompasses exchange of language, ability to think, and ability to experience emotions, as well as value systems, religious beliefs, and ethnic and cultural traditions.

Health is characterized as patterns of adaptive change. Adaptation is viewed as a matter of degree; some adaptations are successful, and some are not. Wellness in this model apparently refers to successful adaptation and wholeness. Illness is adaptation to noxious environmental forces, and disease is viewed as undisciplined and unregulated change.

Nursing is a human interaction whose goal is to promote wholeness. The recipient of nursing care is a patient, or a person who is temporarily dependent on the nurse. The patient is viewed as a partner or participant in nursing care. Nursing process is conservation, or keeping together, and is based on both the scientific method and messages given by the patient. Thus the nursing care plan is viewed as a testable hypothesis based on facts that provoke the nurse's attention. Although a specific nursing process is not explicit in Levine's writings, some components can be extracted from her publications. Assessment focuses on the patient's nursing requirements. The primary question is: To what extent is the person adapting successfully or effectively?

TROPHICOGNOSIS, an alternative to nursing diagnosis, is a nursing care judgment. One element of trophicognosis is the establishment of an objective and scientific rationale for nursing care; this includes identifying a basis for implementation of the prescribed medical or paramedical regimens, determining nursing processes demanded by medical treatment, and identifying the basis for implementation of the unique nursing needs of the patient. The second element is the implementation of nursing care. Nursing intervention is structured according to four conservation principles, including conservation of the patient's energy, conservation of the patient's structural integrity, conservation of the patient's personal integrity, and conservation of the patient's social integrity. Nursing interventions based on the conservation principles may be therapeutic, as when nursing intervention has a favorable influence on adaptation, or supportive, as when intervention can only maintain the status quo or fails to halt a downward course.

consolidation (kon-sol′ĭ-da′shun) 1. solidification; the process of becoming solidified or the condition of being solid; said especially of the lung as it fills with exudate in pneumonia. 2. the combination of parts into a whole.

constancy (kon′stan-se) the quality of remaining stable or unaltered.

> ***form c.*** the ability to recognize forms and objects as the same in spite of variation in environment, position, and size.

> ***object c.*** the capacity to understand that an absent person or object exists and will return.

constant (kon′stant) a fact or principle that is not subject to change.

> ***Avogadro's c.*** Avogadro's number.

constipation (kon″stĭ-pa′shun) 1. a change in normal bowel habits with decreased frequency of DEFECATION or passage of hard dry FECES. 2. a NURSING DIAGNOSIS accepted by the North American Nursing Diagnosis Association, defined as a decrease in frequency of defecation or passage of hard, dry feces.

Although many persons may experience a sense of incomplete evacuation of the colon and become concerned when daily bowel movements do not occur, the frequency of defecation can vary according to individual characteristics such as body build, level of physical activity, dietary habits, and custom. Constipation can be said to exist when a person reports a frequency of bowel elimination that is less than his or her usual pattern or when defecation occurs less than three times a week, stools are hard and well-formed and possibly less than the usual amount, straining at stool occurs regularly, and the person experiences headache, abdominal pain, a feeling of fullness in the abdomen or rectum, and either diminished appetite or nausea. Objective signs of constipation include discovery of a palpable mass in the abdomen and decreased bowel sounds.

Etiology. Constipation can result from a variety of causes. Such habits of daily living as lack of exercise, insufficient intake of water and dietary bulk, and chronic use of laxatives and enemas can contribute to the development of constipation. Other etiologic factors include neurologic, metabolic, and endocrine disorders such as stroke, spinal cord injury, and hypothyroidism; pain on defecation; decreased peristalsis related to aging or cardiopulmonary hypoxia; and the side-effects of some drugs.

Patient Care. Unless there is a demonstrable organic disorder causing constipation, regular bowel elimination is largely a matter of habit. Stress, tension, failure to take the time to defecate when the urge is felt, and insufficient fluid intake can all contribute to the problem. Among the goals of intervention are encouraging regular bowel function by adhering to healthful habits of diet and exercise, and developing an awareness of the need to establish a regular routine of elimination. For some people this may mean a change in lifestyle that entails addition of dietary fiber and regular physical exercise. For others it may be necessary to develop a more rational approach to the problem. Excessive concern over constipation and frequent use of laxatives can be as harmful as deliberately ignoring the need for regular elimination.

For those patients who have constipation related to an organic disease, a BOWEL TRAINING program may be appropriate.

perceived c. a NURSING DIAGNOSIS accepted by the North American Nursing Diagnosis Association, defined as the making by an individual of a self-diagnosis of constipation, and abuse of laxatives, enemas, and suppositories to ensure a daily bowel movement.

constitution (kon″stĭ-too′shun) 1. the make-up or functional habit of the body, determined by the genetic, biochemical, and physiologic endowment of the individual, and modified in great measure by environmental factors. 2. in chemistry, the atoms making up a molecule and the way they are linked, the property that distinguishes a compound from its structural isomers.

constitutional (kon″stĭ-too′shun-al) 1. pertaining to the constitution. 2. affecting the whole constitution of the body; not local.

c. disease one involving a system of organs or one with widespread symptoms.

constriction (kon-strik′shun) a narrowing or compression of a part; a stricture.

constrictor (kon-strik′ter) that which causes constriction.

consultant (kon-sul′tant) an individual with specialized expertise in an area who offers to share this unique knowledge with others.

lactation c. a health care professional, often with advanced certification, who provides education and management related to BREASTFEEDING.

consultation (kon″sul-ta′shun) 1. a deliberation of two or more health care professionals about diagnosis or treatment in a particular case. 2. the provision of expert advice and counseling by an individual with specialized knowledge, as a statistician consulting with health care team members regarding study design. 3. in the NURSING INTERVENTIONS CLASSIFICATION, a nursing INTERVENTION defined as using expert knowledge to work with those who seek help in problem-solving to enable individuals, families, groups, or agencies to achieve identified goals.

c.-liaison provision of psychiatric services at the request of another health professional, often for physically ill patients in a nonpsychiatric hospital.

telephone c. in the NURSING INTERVENTIONS CLASSIFICATION, a nursing INTERVENTION defined as eliciting patient's concerns, listening, and providing support, information, or teaching in response to the patient's stated concerns over the telephone.

consumption (kon-sump′shun) 1. the act of consuming, or the process of being consumed. 2. a wasting away of the body. 3. old name for pulmonary TUBERCULOSIS.

oxygen c. see OXYGEN CONSUMPTION.

prothrombin c. see PROTHROMBIN CONSUMPTION.

contact (kon′takt) 1. a mutual touching of two bodies or persons. 2. an individual known to have been sufficiently near an infected person to have been exposed to the transfer of infectious material.

c. dermatitis a skin rash marked by itching, swelling, blistering, oozing, and scaling, caused by direct contact between the skin and a substance to which the person is allergic or sensitive. The rash usually occurs only on that area of the body that has come into contact with the irritating substance. The most common form is that caused by POISON IVY, OAK, AND SUMAC. Other plants, too, sometimes cause an allergic reaction. Contact dermatitis may also be caused by industrial oils, medicines, cosmetics, perfumes, mouthwashes, deodorants, rubber, plastics, metals, and clothing made of various materials and treated with certain preservatives and dyes. A nonallergic form, primary-irritant dermatitis, may be induced by a substance acting as an irritant rather than as a sensitizer or allergen. Some soaps, detergents, and other cleansing products can cause a condition of the hands often referred to as "housewives' dermatitis" (or, popularly, "dishpan hands"). Called also contact allergy.

direct c., immediate c. transmission of infection from an infected host or reservoir to a susceptible individual by physical contact.

indirect c. transmission of infection to a susceptible host by means of inanimate objects (fomites) or a vector or through the air by dust or droplets.

c. lenses corrective lenses that fit directly over the cornea of the eye, for correction of refractive errors. They do not actually touch the surface of the eye, but float on a thin layer of the fluid that naturally moistens the eyeball. There are two main types of contact lenses, *hard* and *soft*. The hard lenses were the first to be developed and are still used because they are durable, easy to care for, and relatively inexpensive. They also provide good vision, especially in the correction of ASTIGMATISM. Their chief disadvantage is their inflexibility, which makes them difficult to fit to the shape of the eyeball. Soft lenses are more comfortable because of their flexibility, but they do not provide as sharp vision as that with conventional eyeglasses and hard lenses. Moreover, the surface of soft lenses can harbor bacteria; therefore there is a higher risk of infection. Gas-permeable lenses have the same advantages as hard lenses; that is, they are durable, easy to care for, and have a high optical quality. In addition, they allow passage of oxygen and carbon dioxide to and from the cornea, and tears flow more easily across the eye when these lenses are worn.

Contact lenses correct vision problems through the entire visual field and are more desirable than eyeglasses for certain kinds of eye disorders. For example, contact lenses eliminate the difficulties associated with the thick lenses of the cataract eyeglasses previously required for all patients following CATARACT extraction. Irregular scarring of the cornea cannot be helped by glasses, but contact lenses can improve vision when the cornea has been injured.

There are relatively few serious problems caused by wearing contact lenses. If they are properly fitted and the patient gets regular eye examinations, there should be no great difficulty. Signs of continued irritation and infection should be reported to the ophthalmologist promptly in order to avoid scarring and permanent loss of vision.

Patient Care. Patients wearing contact lenses who are hospitalized will need assistance in daily contact lens CARE regimens. The fact that a patient is wearing contact lenses is noted on the chart and the regimen of care included in the nursing care plan.

The manner in which the lenses have been cleaned at home by the patient should be determined. Some patients disinfect their lenses with a thermal disinfecting unit, but most use a chemical solution in which the lenses are soaked for a period of time, rinsed, and then reinserted. Removal and reinsertion of contact lenses is not difficult, but patients in a hospital or long-term care facility may not be able to do this for themselves. The usual routine for wearing lenses may need to be changed while patients are hospitalized. Medications such as sedatives, muscle relaxants, and hypnotics reduce the frequency of blinking, and certain other drugs such as anticholinergics and antihistamines can reduce tear production. Diminished blinking and a decrease in tearing can lead to dryness and irritation. This may be relieved by administering contact lens wetting agents to provide lubrication.

Contact lenses should not be left in the eyes of patients going to surgery. In addition, it is better to remove contact lenses before sedating patients, lest they accidentally rub their eyes or in some way remove the lenses in their sleep. Contact lenses that have been removed are stored in a solution to prevent their drying out or being lost.

Symptoms of overwearing or irritation include excessive tearing, redness, pain, and photophobia. When these symptoms appear the lenses should be removed and the ophthalmologist notified. If an infection is suspected, antibiotic eyedrops or ointment may be prescribed.

mediate c. indirect contact.

social c. communication or interactions between an individual or family and people outside the immediate household.

contactant (kon-tak′tant) an allergen capable of inducing delayed contact-type hypersensitivity of the epidermis after one or more episodes of contact.

contagion (kon-ta′jun) 1. the spread of disease from one individual to another. 2. a contagious disease.

contagious (kon-ta′jus) capable of being transmitted from one individual to another.

c. disease communicable disease.

containment the keeping of something within limits.

cost c. in the NURSING INTERVENTIONS CLASSIFICATION, a nursing INTERVENTION defined as management and facilitation of efficient and effective use of resources.

contaminant (kon-tam′ĭ-nant) something that causes CONTAMINATION.

contamination (kon-tam″ĭ-na′shun) 1. the soiling or making inferior by contact or mixture, as by introduction of organisms into a wound. 2. the deposition of radioactive material in any place where it is not desired, especially where its presence may be harmful or constitute a radiation hazard.

content (kon′tent) that which is contained within a thing.

latent c. in FREUDIAN theory, the hidden and unconscious true meaning of a symbolic representation, such as a DREAM or fantasy, as opposed to the manifest CONTENT.

manifest c. in FREUDIAN theory, the content of a DREAM or fantasy as it is experienced and remembered, and in which the latent CONTENT is disguised and distorted by displacement, condensation, symbolization, projection, and secondary elaboration.

context (kon′tekst) the setting, in time or space, surrounding the occurrence of a given event.

cultural c. the environment or situation that is relevant to the beliefs, values, and practices of the culture under study.

continence (kon′tĭ-nens) the ability to exercise voluntary control over natural impulses, such as the urge to defecate or urinate. adj., **con′tinent.**

continuous positive airway pressure (CPAP) a method of positive pressure VENTILATION used with patients who are breathing spontaneously, done to keep the alveoli open at the end of exhalation and thus increase oxygenation and reduce the work of breathing. When the same principle is used in mechanical ventilation, it is called positive end-expiratory PRESSURE.

contra- word element [L.], *against; opposed.*

contra-aperture (kon″trah-ap′er-cher) a second opening, such as one made in an abscess to facilitate the discharge of its contents or one made to facilitate arthroscopic repair of a joint. Called also counteropening.

contraception (kon″trah-sep′shun) prevention of CONCEPTION or IMPREGNATION; it may be achieved by several methods. (See also BIRTH CONTROL.)

Natural Family Planning (Fertility Awareness Methods). In these methods no artificial means are used; they are also known as *periodic abstinence,* and the older popular name for them was "the rhythm method." With these methods a woman seeks to plan or prevent pregnancy by avoiding intercourse on the fertile days of her MENSTRUAL CYCLE. This is safe and inexpensive and offers the advantage of being acceptable to religious groups who object to other contraceptive methods. Methods include the *calendar method, basal body temperature method,* and *cervical mucus method.*

Calendar and Body Temperature Methods. The *calendar method* depends on the fact that the period of possible conception lasts from about 2 days before ovulation through about 1 day after it, and during these days if conception is to be prevented the woman must abstain from intercourse. The other days of the cycle constitute the so-called "safe period." In practice, however, the safe period is considered to be shorter, since ovulation can occur anytime between the twelfth and sixteenth days of the cycle and any of these days must be counted as days of possible conception. (The first day of the cycle is the first day of MENSTRUATION.) To calculate the fertile period, it is necessary to keep an accurate record of menstrual cycles for 8 to 12 months. The length of the longest and shortest cycles must be carefully noted over this time. To find the first day she is likely to be fertile, subtract 20 days from her shortest cycle. To find the last day she is likely to be fertile, subtract 10 days from her longest cycle. The *body temperature method* attemps to determine when ovulation is taking place by daily readings of body temperature. The temperature becomes elevated after ovulation.

Cervical Mucus Method (Ovulation Method, Billings Method). Alterations in the amount and consistency of cervical MUCUS occur during the days around ovulation. This method is based on awareness of days of "dryness" and days of "wetness" during the menstrual cycle, and recognition of the significance of a unique "fertile mucus" that appears in the vaginal area at the time of ovulation. According to proponents of this method, appearance of the mucus signals the onset of the time during which impregnation can occur.

Success of the mucus method depends on the woman's ability to observe and recognize the characteristics of cervical discharge as indicated by a change in vaginal discharge, which gives warning of the period of ovulation. After the menstruation that begins the cycle, there are "early dry days" during which the cervical mucus is thick and gelatinous and is not seen or felt in the vaginal area. With the ripening of the ovum just prior to ovulation, the cervical mucus becomes abundant, clear, and stretchy. This is considered "fertile mucus," and it usually appears three days prior to ovulation, though the time may vary with individuals. It is clear, similar in appearance and consistency to the white of an uncooked egg. The vaginal area has a sensation of wetness or lubrication. The egg is released from the GRAAFIAN FOLLICLE within 24 to 48 hours of the peak of wetness.

It is recommended that those persons using the cervical mucus method of contraception refrain from sexual intercourse from the first appearance of the fertile mucus through the height of the sensation of wetness and then for an additional four days. The reason for this precaution is that the fertile mucus produced by the glands at the time of ovulation helps keep the SPERM alive and active and facilitates its penetration of the ovum. Should there be spermatozoa present before ovulation occurs, the mucus can help maintain their vitality until the egg is released from the follicle and is available for impregnation. The life span of the sperm is in part determined by presence of fertile mucus, so that waiting 96 hours after the period of wetness assures that the ovum has been released and expelled through the vaginal tract without becoming impregnated. A major advantage of this method over other natural contraceptive methods is that it can be used by women with irregular menstrual cycles and does not rely on extensive keeping of records of lengths of cycles.

Oral Contraceptives. Popularly called "the pill," these methods are considered safe, reliable, and effective. The oldest type are the *combined oral contraceptives*, which involve having a woman take, for a set number of days each month, oral forms of hormones or hormonelike products that duplicate the action of ESTROGEN and PROGESTERONE in different phases of each MENSTRUAL CYCLE.

Oral contraceptives can be obtained by prescription only, because they may produce serious cardiovascular side effects, especially in women who smoke. In women between the ages of 30 and 39, users of the pill who smoke are 5 times as likely to have a heart attack as users who do not smoke and 10 times as likely as nonusers who are nonsmokers. Positive effects of oral contraceptives include their protective effect against ovarian and endometrial cancer. They also have a protective effect against PELVIC INFLAMMATORY DISEASE, which is a major cause of female infertility. In addition, they tend to decrease menstrual cramps and pain, shorten the time of menstrual bleeding, and lessen the amount of blood loss. Contraindications to use of oral contraceptives include any history of thromboembolic disorders, cerebrovascular disease, or coronary artery disease; breast cancer, estrogen-dependent tumors, abnormal vaginal bleeding; and suspected pregnancy.

C

Progestin-Only Contraceptives. These differ from the combined oral contraceptives in that they contain no estrogen. The most common method is the injectable Norplant system, a long-lasting and effective method of contraception. A steroid, LEVONORGESTREL, is slowly diffused into the body from six capsules that are usually placed under the skin in a fanlike configuration on the inside of a woman's upper arm. The hormone is released at 34 mcg per day. Contraceptive action is due to ANOVULATION, an inadequate luteal phase in the menstrual CYCLE, changes in cervical mucus, and interference with OOCYTE maturation. The medication must be replaced every 5 years. Its noncontraceptive benefits include decreased anemia, decreased menstrual cramps, and reduced risk of endometrial cancer. Its disadvantages include high initial expense, the minor surgery required for discontinuation, alterations in bleeding patterns, acne, and hair loss. Contraindications for use include known or suspected pregnancy, unexplained vaginal bleeding, active thrombophlebitis, or known or suspected breast cancer. Research is currently being conducted on a two-rod system.

There is also a *progestin-only pill* (also called *minipill*). This is a hormonally active pill to be taken every day; its mechanism of action is the same as for other PROGESTINS. It is less effective than combined oral contraceptives, but estrogen-related side effects are avoided. Non-contraceptive benefits include decreased risk of PELVIC INFLAMMATORY DISEASE. Contraindications include unexplained vaginal bleeding and a history of ectopic pregnancy.

A common medication in this group is *Depo-Provera (medroxyprogesterone acetate),* which is given as an intramuscular injection every 3 months. The high levels of progestogen block the luteinizing hormone surge and thus suppress ovulation. The cervical mucus is thickened. Advantages include lack of estrogen-related side effects, freedom from compliance concerns, prolonged absence of menses, and the fact that this method is both highly effective and long-acting. Non-contraceptive benefits include decreased risk for endometrial cancer, pelvic inflammatory disease, and ectopic PREGNANCY. Disadvantages include the need to get an injection every 3 months, cyclic irregularities, delay in return of fertility, and possibly decreased bone density. Contraindications are the same as for other progestin-only methods.

Hormonal contraceptives for men. Research on hormonal contraceptives for the male is currently being conducted.

Emergency Contraception. Oral contraceptives that contain ETHINYL ESTRADIOL and NORGESTREL can be used for POSTCOITAL contraception. Two treatment doses are required, 12 hours apart, with the first as soon as possible following unprotected intercourse.

Permanent Sterilization. Irreversible contraceptive techniques involving surgical procedures include SALPINGECTOMY, tubal LIGATION, and VASECTOMY. Newer techniques utilizing endoscopy include hysteroscopic, culdoscopic, and laparoscopic STERILIZATION. There is a small rate of failure with most of these procedures.

Barrier Methods

Condom. This is a thin flexible sheath worn over the penis to prevent entry of spermatozoa into the vagina during sexual intercourse. It has many advantages as a contraceptive. Its effectiveness rate is reported to be 80 to 90 per cent, and use of this method encourages participation of the male in pregnancy prevention. Condoms are readily available, are relatively inexpensive, and can protect against SEXUALLY TRANSMITTED DISEASES. The addition of a SPERMICIDAL lubricant offers greater protection from unwanted pregnancies and sexually transmitted diseases.

Cervical Diaphragm. This is a cup-shaped device of molded rubber or other soft plastic material, with a flexible spring forming the circular outer edge. It is inserted in the vagina in such a position that it covers the uterine CERVIX and prevents entry of spermatozoa. It is used in conjunction with a spermicidal cream or jelly. (See *Jellies, Creams, Vaginal Film, Suppositories, and Foams,* below.) Although the diaphragm is 80 per cent effective when used with a spermicide, many women find it awkward to use, messy, or inconvenient because of the need for inserting it prior to sexual intercourse and using a spermicide.

Cervical Cap. This device is custom-fitted and has some advantages over the diaphragm. It fits more snugly, is more comfortable, and, because of a small one-way valve in its center, it permits the flow of menstrual blood and mucus, yet prohibits the travel of sperm from the vagina to the uterus. Because of the possible risk of TOXIC SHOCK SYNDROME, however, it should not be worn for more than 48 hours at a time.

Spermicidal Jellies, Creams, Vaginal Film, Suppositories, and Foams. NONOXYNOL 9 is the active agent in most SPERMICIDAL products in the United States. Consistent use is the most important factor in minimizing failure rates with spermicides. Nonoxynol 9 may decrease the risk of sexually transmitted diseases, but

it can cause vaginal irritation in some women. There are a number of contraceptive jellies, creams, and aerosol foams that are more powerful than those used with diaphragms and can be used without any mechanical device.

Female Condom. This is a thin polyurethane sheath containing two flexible rings. One ring lies inside at the closed end of the sheath and serves as an insertion mechanism and internal anchor. The other ring forms the external open edge and remains outside of the vagina. The external portion covers part of the perineum and provides protection to the labia and base of the penis during intercourse. Polyurethane is less susceptible than latex to deterioration during storage.

Intrauterine Devices (IUD's). Two of these are currently available in the United States. The CUT380A (ParaGard) is approved for 10 years of use. The ProgesteroneT (Progestasert System) is approved for 1 year of contraceptive protection. The IUD is a highly effective, safe, long-acting, single-decision method. It is a good method for women who have medical contraindications to oral contraceptives, want a long-acting reversible method, are lactating, or are post partum. However, screening is critical for identifying women at risk for IUD complications. Risks include pelvic inflammatory disease, heavy menses, and increased menstrual cramping. See also INTRAUTERINE DEVICE.

The Population Information Program at Johns Hopkins University publishes *Population Reports,* which provides current information on contraceptives.

contraceptive (kon″trah-sep′tiv) 1. diminishing the likelihood of or preventing CONCEPTION. 2. an agent that does this; see also CONTRACEPTION.

 oral c. a compound, usually hormonal, taken orally in order to block ovulation and prevent the occurrence of pregnancy. See also CONTRACEPTION.

contractile (kon-trak′til) having the power or tendency to contract in response to a suitable stimulus.

contractility (kon″trak-til′ĭ-te) a capacity for shortening in response to suitable stimulus.

contracting (kon′trakt-ing) negotiating and establishing an agreement.

 patient c. in the NURSING INTERVENTIONS CLASSIFICATION, a nursing INTERVENTION defined as negotiating an agreement with a patient to reinforce a specific behavior change.

contraction (kon-trak′shun) a drawing together; a shortening or shrinkage.

 Braxton Hicks c's see BRAXTON HICKS CONTRACTIONS.

carpopedal c. the condition resulting from chronic shortening of the muscles of the upper and lower limbs including the fingers and toes, seen in TETANY.

concentric c. contraction resulting in shortening of a muscle, used to perform positive work or to accelerate a body part. It is metabolically more demanding than an eccentric CONTRACTION. Called also shortening contraction.

Dupuytren's c. Dupuytren's contracture.

eccentric c. contraction in the presence of a resistive force that results in elongation of a muscle, used to perform negative work or to decelerate a body part. It is less metabolically demanding than a concentric contraction but may cause disruption of associated connective tissue with delayed soreness or frank injury if it occurs in an unaccustomed manner. Called also lengthening contraction.

end-diastolic premature ventricular c. a ventricular ectopic BEAT falling at the end of DIASTOLE; it may or may not be slightly premature and may or may not be a fusion beat.

haustral c's muscular contractions of the wall of the large intestine during which the haustra can be seen more easily; called also haustrations.

isometric c. muscle contraction without appreciable shortening or change in distance between its origin and insertion.

isotonic c. muscle contraction without appreciable change in the force of contraction; the distance between the origin and insertion becomes lessened.

lengthening c. eccentric contraction.

postural c. the state of muscular tension and contraction that just suffices to maintain the posture of the body.

segmental c's muscular contractions of the small intestine that serve to mix and transport chyme.

shortening c. concentric contraction.

c. stress test observation of the fetal heart rate in response to uterine contractions; see also FETAL MONITORING.

tetanic c., tonic c. physiological TETANUS.

Volkmann's c. Volkmann's contracture.

contracture (kon-trak′cher) abnormal shortening of muscle tissue, rendering the muscle highly resistant to stretching; this can lead to permanent disability. It can be caused by fibrosis of the tissues supporting the muscle or the joint, or by disorders of the muscle fibers themselves.Improper support and positioning of joints affected by arthritis or injury, and inadequate exercising of joints in patients with paralysis can result in contractures. For example, a patient with arthritis or severe burns may assume the most comfortable position and will resist changing position because motion is painful. If the joints are allowed to remain in this position, the muscle fibers that normally provide motion will stretch or shorten to accommodate the position and eventually will lose their ability to contract and relax.

In many cases contractures can be prevented by range of motion EXERCISES (active or passive), and by adequate support of the joints to eliminate constant shortening or stretching of the muscles and surrounding tissues.

Dupuytren's c. a flexion deformity of the fingers or toes, due to shortening, thickening, and fibrosis of the palmar or plantar fascia.

ischemic c. muscular contracture and degeneration due to interference with the circulation due to pressure or to injury or cold.

Volkmann's c. contraction of the fingers and sometimes of the wrist, or of analogous parts of the foot, with loss of power, after severe injury or improper use of a tourniquet or cast in the region of the elbow.

contrafissure (kon″trah-fish′er) a fracture in a part opposite the site of the blow.

contraindication (kon″trah-in″dĭ-ka′shun) any condition that renders a particular line of treatment improper or undesirable.

contralateral (kon″trah-lat′er-al) pertaining to, situated on, or affecting the opposite side.

contrasexual (kon-trah-sek′shoo-al) 1. in psychiatry, said of the personality traits that most people repress because they are characteristic of the opposite sex. 2. having SECONDARY SEX CHARACTERS appropriate to the opposite sex. Called also heterosexual.

contrecoup (kon″truh-koo′) [Fr.] denoting an injury, as to the brain, occurring at a site opposite to the point of impact.

control (kon-trōl′) 1. the governing or limitation of certain objects, events, or physical responses. 2. a standard against which experimental observations may be evaluated, as a procedure identical to the experimental procedure except for the absence of the one factor being studied. 3. conscious restraint and regulation of impulses and suppression of instincts and affects. 4. a patient or group differing from the case or treated group under study by lacking the disease or by having a different or absent treatment or regimen.

The controls and subjects usually otherwise have certain similarities to allow or enhance comparison between them.

automatic brightness c. an automated exposure device used in radiology; it senses light and adjusts itself to produce a predetermined fluoroscopic density.

automatic exposure c. a timer by which the exposure of x-ray film is determined by the radiographer but the length of exposure is determined by the equipment.

aversive c. in BEHAVIOR THERAPY, the use of unpleasant stimuli to change undesirable behavior.

birth c. see BIRTH CONTROL.

hemorrhage c. in the NURSING INTERVENTIONS CLASSIFICATION, a nursing INTERVENTION defined as reduction or elimination of rapid and excessive blood loss.

infection c. see INFECTION CONTROL.

infection c.: intraoperative in the NURSING INTERVENTIONS CLASSIFICATION, a nursing INTERVENTION defined as preventing NOSOCOMIAL infection in the operating room.

motor c. the generation and coordination of movement patterns to produce function; it may either control movements of the body in space or stabilize the body in space. See also *postural control.*

postural c. motor control that stabilizes the body in space by integrating sensory input about body position (somatosensory, visual, and vestibular input) with motor output to coordinate the action of muscles and keep the body's center of mass within its base of support. An important aspect of postural control is the RIGHTING REACTIONS. Called also BALANCE.

stimulus c. any influence exerted by the environment on behavior.

Controlled Substances Act a federal law that regulates the prescribing and dispensing of psychoactive DRUGS, including NARCOTICS, HALLUCINOGENS, DEPRESSANTS, and STIMULANTS. See table at DRUG DEPENDENCE.

contuse (kon-tōōz´) to bruise; to injure without breaking the skin.

contusion (kon-too´zhun) injury to tissues with skin discoloration and without breakage of skin; called also bruise. Blood from the broken vessels accumulates in surrounding tissues, producing pain, swelling, and tenderness, and the discoloration is the result of blood seepage just under the skin. Most heal without special treatment, but cold compresses may reduce bleeding if applied immediately after the injury, and thus may reduce swelling, discoloration, and pain.If a contusion is unusually severe, the injured part should be rested and slightly elevated; later application of heat may hasten absorption of blood. Serious complications may develop in some cases. Normally blood is drawn off from the bruised area in a few days, but occasionally blood clotted in the area may form a cyst or may calcify and require surgical treatment. Contusions may also be complicated by infection.

cerebral c. contusion of the brain following a HEAD INJURY. It may occur with extradural or subdural collections of blood, in which case the patient may be left with neurologic defects or EPILEPSY. (See also cranial HEMATOMA.)

conus (ko´nus), pl. *co´ni* [L.] 1. cone. 2. a cone-shaped structure. 3. posterior staphyloma of the myopic eye.

c. arterio´sus the anterosuperior portion of the right ventricle of the heart, at the entrance to the pulmonary trunk. Called also infundibulum.

c. medulla´ris the cone-shaped lower end of the spinal cord, at the level of the upper lumbar vertebrae.

convalescence (kon″vah-les´ens) the stage of recovery from an illness, operation, or injury.

convalescent (kon″vah-les´ent) 1. pertaining to or characterized by convalescence. 2. a patient who is recovering from a disease, operation, or injury.

convection (kon-vek´shun) the act of conveying or transmission; specifically, transmission of heat in a liquid or gas by the bulk movement of heated particles to a cooler area. See also convection CURRENT.

convergence (kon-ver´jens) the coordinated inclination of the two lines of sight towards their common point of fixation, or the point itself.

conversion (kon-ver´zhun) 1. the act of changing into something of different form or properties. 2. an unconscious DEFENSE MECHANISM by which the anxiety that stems from intrapsychic conflict is altered and expressed in a symbolic physical symptom such as pain, paralysis, loss of sight, or some other manifestation that has no organic or physiological basis. 3. manipulative correction of malposition of a fetal part during labor.

c. disorder a SOMATOFORM DISORDER characterized by symptoms or deficits affecting voluntary motor or sensory functioning and suggesting physical illness but produced by CONVERSION. Called also conversion reaction. Patients' anxiety is ''converted'' into any of a variety of somatic symptoms such as blindness, deafness, or paralysis, none of which have any organic basis. The anxiety may be the result of an inner conflict too difficult to face, and symptoms are aggravated in times of psychological stress. Patients often exhibit remarkable lack of concern, called *la belle indifférence*, about their symptoms, no matter how serious.

From their symptoms, patients achieve both the *primary gain* of relief from their anxiety and a number of *secondary gains* such as support and attention from others and the chance to avoid unpleasant responsibilities. Symptoms are often increased at times of psychological stress. The symptoms often have an important symbolic relationship to the patient's unconscious conflict, such as incapacitating illness in those who cannot acknowledge dependency needs. Symptoms are neither intentionally produced nor feigned, are not limited to pain or sexual dysfunction, and may affect a part of the body the patient considers weak. One of the first observed examples of conversion disorder was combat fatigue, in which soldiers became paralyzed and could not participate in battle.

Treatment of conversion disorder aims at helping the patient resolve the underlying conflict. Under former classifications, this disorder was called a neurosis (hysterical neurosis, conversion type).

convertase (kon-ver′tās) an enzyme of the complement system that activates specific components of the system.

convex (kon′veks) having a rounded, somewhat elevated surface.

convolution (kon″vo-lu′shun) a tortuous irregularity or elevation caused by the infolding of a structure upon itself.

convulsion (kon-vul′shun) a type of SEIZURE consisting of a series of involuntary contractions of the voluntary muscles. Such seizures are symptomatic of some neurologic disorder; they are not in themselves a disease entity. Convulsions can be produced by any of a number of chemical disorders, such as HYPOGLYCEMIA and HYPOCALCEMIA; metabolic disturbances and hormonal imbalances; brain cell injury from head trauma, tumors, degenerative neural disease, and stroke; anoxia and hemorrhage which deprive brain cells of vital substances; acute cerebral edema which interferes with normal brain cell function; and infection and high fever (*febrile convulsions*). Finally, EPILEPSY is one of the most common of all disorders associated with convulsions.

Patient Care. The plan for patient care should take into account the potential for injury to the patient during a seizure.

This includes observing the patient before, during, and after each convulsion, and when possible, preventing or minimizing environmental factors and events in the patient's daily life that are believed to precipitate a seizure.

Protection of the patient from injury is of primary concern. Once a seizure has begun, the person with the patient should remain calm, summon help, and try to help prevent injury to the patient, using mild restraint in order to avoid allowing the extremities to strike nearby hard objects. Vigorous restraint can cause orthopedic injuries, as the muscles contract strongly against resistance. Whatever the location, the patient should not be moved until after the seizure is over. If the patient has some warning and there is time before the seizure actually begins, a soft oral airway or folded towel can be placed between the teeth to prevent tongue biting. Hard objects should never be used to force open the mouth. It is not only useless to attempt this once the jaws are firmly fixed, but teeth can be broken and soft tissues severely injured by trying to force something into the mouth and between the teeth.

It is especially important to observe and report what happened before, during, and immediately after a seizure. This is a critical source of information in the diagnosis of the disorder leading to the convulsion. Observations should include: (1) the time the convulsion began, whether the patient had any warning or specific symptoms just before it, and the length of time it lasted; (2) where the seizure began and what parts of the body were involved; (3) whether the eyes deviated, and a description of the patient's level of consciousness before and during the seizure; (4) whether there was incontinence of urine or stool, vomiting, bleeding, or foaming or frothing at the mouth; (5) the effects of the seizure on the patient's pulse and respirations, and any other objective signs, such as change in skin color or profuse perspiration; and (6) the condition of the patient after the seizure was over (*postictal* symptoms and signs), such as lethargy, mental confusion, or speech impairment.

Careful attention to environmental factors such as noise or bright light, pain, exhaustion, and other seizure triggers can help identify conditions that might have precipitated seizure activity. Emotional events also should be considered as possible stimulants that can elicit uncontrollable activity.

If the seizures are recurring, as in epilepsy, the patient and the significant others will need instruction in the nature of the illness, an explanation of the prescribed regimen for medications, a list of potential seizure triggers that could precipitate an attack, how to prevent injury during a seizure, and when notification of the health care provider is indicated.

central c. a convulsion not triggered by any external cause but due to a lesion of the central nervous system; called also essential convulsion.

clonic c. a convulsion marked by alternating contracting and relaxing of the muscles. See also generalized tonic-clonic SEIZURE.

epileptiform c. any convulsion attended by loss of consciousness.

essential c. central convulsion.

febrile c. a seizure occurring in children age 3 months to 5 years in association with a fever at or above 39.5° C (103.2° F), often associated with a family history of febrile seizures. Treatment of children with febrile seizures with no evidence of neurologic dysfunction is usually limited to diagnosis and treatment of the underlying cause of the fever. Phenobarbital may be used to treat the seizure or used prophylactically when the child is ill or is receiving childhood immunizations. Called also febrile seizure.

tetanic c. a tonic SPASM without loss of consciousness and often associated with HYPOCALCEMIA. See also TETANY.

tonic c. prolonged contraction of the muscles, as a result of an epileptic discharge. See also generalized tonic-clonic SEIZURE.

uremic c. one due to uremia, or retention in the blood of material that should have been expelled by the kidneys.

convulsive (kon-vul′siv) pertaining to, characterized by, or of the nature of a convulsion.

Coombs' test (kōōmz) any of a number of tests to ascertain the presence or absence of IMMUNOGLOBULIN and COMPLEMENT in the coating of ERYTHROCYTES. Rabbit antihuman serum is used to act as a bridge between sensitized cells, yielding agglutination (a positive result). The tests can be used to differentiate between various types of HEMOLYTIC ANEMIAS, to determine minor blood types including the RH FACTOR, and to test for anticipated ERYTHROBLASTOSIS FETALIS.

direct C. t. the test used to detect in vivo sensitization of red blood cells and formation of cell-bound antibodies that may damage erythrocytes but will not cause visible agglutination. The erythrocytes are washed free of serum and unbound antibody, and antiglobulin (antiserum directed against human antibodies and complement components) is added. Agglutination indicates the presence of antibody. Clinically its most important use is in early diagnosis of erythroblastosis fetalis and autoimmune HEMOLYTIC ANEMIAS. It is used also in crossmatching blood for transfusions. Venous blood or blood from the umbilical cord may be used.

indirect C. t. a test for detecting antigen-antibody reactions that occur in vitro; used to determine incompatibility in transfusions when the recipient has a greater than normal risk of TRANSFUSION REACTION. It uses antiglobulin serum to detect the in vitro sensitization of red blood cells by serum. The test also can reveal the presence of anti-Rh antibodies in maternal blood during pregnancy. Either clotted blood or blood with an anticoagulant may be used. The patient's serum is incubated with donor red blood cells, the cells are washed, and antiglobulin added. Agglutination indicates the presence of incomplete sensitizing antibodies in the serum.

coordination (ko-or″dĭ-na′shun) 1. the harmonious functioning of interrelated organs and parts. 2. the putting of a group of things or individuals into harmonious working order. 3. the process of the motor apparatus of the brain that provides for the coworking of particular groups of muscles for the performance of definite adaptive useful responses. 4. a nursing INTERVENTION in the NURSING MINIMUM DATA SET; action geared to the integration of multidisciplinary treatment plans with the goal of smooth, continuous patient or client care.

preoperative c. in the NURSING INTERVENTIONS CLASSIFICATION, a nursing INTERVENTION defined as facilitating preadmission diagnostic testing and preparation of the surgical patient.

c. of services the management of health care resources so that the recipient of care has access to all needed services with no duplication.

COPD chronic obstructive pulmonary disease.

coping (ko′ping) the process of contending with life difficulties in an effort to overcome or work through them. National Conferences on the Classification of Nursing Diagnoses have accepted several NURSING DIAGNOSES associated with individual and family coping with the challenge of a client's changing or changed health status, including *Ineffective Individual Coping; Defensive Coping; Ineffective Family Coping: Disabling; Ineffective Family Coping: Compromised;* and *Family Coping: Potential for Growth.* See also COPING mechanisms.

compromised family c. a NURSING DIAGNOSIS accepted by the North American Nursing Diagnosis Association, defined as a situation in which a usually supportive primary person (family member or close friend) is providing insufficient, ineffective, or compromised support, comfort, assistance, or encouragement that may be needed by the client to manage or master adaptive tasks related to his/her health challenge. Compromised ineffective family coping may arise from inadequate or incorrect information; inadequate or incorrect understanding by the family member or close friend; temporary preoccupation by the significant person, who is trying to manage emotional conflicts and personal suffering and so is unable to perceive the client's needs or act effectively to fulfill them; temporary family disorganization and role changes; other crises or situations that the significant person may be facing; failure of the client to provide reciprocal support for the significant person; or prolonged disease or progression of the disability that exhausts the supportive capacity of significant people. Subjective data that could indicate compromised ineffective family coping might include an expression by the significant person of a lack of understanding or knowledge that interferes with effective assistance or support; a description by the significant person of preoccupation with such personal reactions to the client's illness or disability as fear, anticipatory grief, guilt, or anxiety; or expression of a preoccupation with similar reactions to other situational or developmental crises.

defensive c. a NURSING DIAGNOSIS accepted by the North American Nursing Diagnosis Association, defined as the state in which an individual has a repeated projection of falsely positive self-evaluation based on a self-protective pattern that defends against underlying perceived threats to positive self-regard. See also ineffective individual COPING.

disabled family c. a NURSING DIAGNOSIS accepted by the North American Nursing Diagnosis Association, defined as the behavior of a significant person (family member or other primary person) who disables his or her own capacities *and* the client's capacities to address tasks effectively that are essential to either person's adaptation to the health challenge. The significant person's coping response is disabling if it

involves short-term behaviors that are highly detrimental to the welfare of either the client or the significant person. Chronically disabling patterns by a primary person are described as continued use of selected coping skills that have interrupted the person's longer-term capacity to receive, store, or organize information or to react to it. Defining characteristics of this diagnostic category include neglectful care of the client in meeting basic human needs and in the treatment of illness, extreme denial of the existence of the client's health problem, intolerance, rejection, abandonment or desertion of the client, taking on the illness signs of the client, decisions and actions by the family which are detrimental to its economic or social well-being, impaired restructuring of a meaningful life for oneself and prolonged overconcern for the client, neglectful relationships with other family members, and development by the client of helplessness and inactive dependence.

ineffective individual c. a NURSING DIAGNOSIS accepted by the North American Nursing Diagnosis Association, defined as the inability to form a valid appraisal of the stressors, inadequate choices of practical responses, and/or inability to use available resources. Many stressors in everyday life can create tension and tax one's ability to cope with them; these include situational crises, crises associated with advancing through the stages of life (childhood to old age), personal vulnerability, multiple life changes, and poor or unhealthy habits of living (which might include inadequate relaxation, failure to take vacations, poor nutrition and lack of exercise, inadequate support systems, unmet expectations, work overload, unrealistic perceptions, and inadequate methods of coping).

Ineffective individual coping may be manifest when a person verbalizes an inability to cope or to ask for help, is unable to meet basic needs or role expectations, cannot use problem-solving techniques, has a high rate of illness or accidents, exhibits destructive behavior toward self or others (including excessive eating, drinking, or smoking), has high blood pressure, ulcers, irritable bowel, or other illnesses related to emotional tension, is a chronic worrier, or exhibits chronic depression.

Nursing interventions are aimed at determining the etiologic factors responsible for ineffective coping, assessing the effectiveness of the coping strategies being used by the person, facilitating an understanding of possible sources and consequences of prolonged challenge to one's ability to cope, supporting the person's strengths and effective coping mechanisms, and offering alternative strategies to ineffective and dysfunctional coping.

readiness for enhanced family c. a NURSING DIAGNOSIS accepted by the North American Nursing Diagnosis Association, defined as effective management of adaptive tasks by a family member involved with the client's health challenge, who now exhibits desire and readiness for enhanced health and growth in regard to self and in relation to the client. The family member is willing and ready for enhanced health and personal growth in regard to self and in relation to the client. Evidence that the family member's basic human needs are sufficiently gratified and that his or her adaptive tasks are effectively addressed so that goals related to self-actualization can emerge indicates potential for personal growth. Defining characteristics include an attempt to describe how the client's health crisis has influenced the family member's own values, priorities, goals, or relationships; evidence that the family member is moving toward a lifestyle that supports and optimizes wellness; and expression of interest in contacting another person or group of persons who have experienced a similar situation.

copiopia (ko″pe-o′pe-ah) eyestrain.

copolymer (ko-pol′ĭ-mer) a POLYMER containing monomers of more than one kind.

copper (Cu) (kop′er) a chemical element, atomic number 29, atomic weight 63.54. (See Appendix 6.) It is necessary for bone formation and for the formation of blood because it occurs in several oxidative enzymes including one involved in the transformation of inorganic iron into hemoglobin. There is little danger of deficiency in ordinary diets because of relatively abundant supply and minute daily requirements. Excessive copper in the body can be toxic, with vomiting, jaundice, hypotension, and sometimes coma; this may occur with excessive intake of medicinal copper salts or in metabolic conditions such as MENKES' SYNDROME or WILSON'S DISEASE.

c. 67 a radioisotope of copper, atomic mass 67, with a half-life of 2.58 days; used in radiotherapy as well as for imaging, tracer kinetic studies, and dosimetry.

copperhead (kop′er-hed) *Agkistrodon contortrix*, a venomous pit VIPER of the United States that has a brown to copper-colored body with dark bands. Called also highland moccasin. See also SNAKEBITE.

copr(o)- word element [Gr.], *feces.* See also words beginning STERC(O)-.

copremesis (kop-rem′ĕ-sis) the vomiting of fecal matter.

coproantibody (kop″ro-an′tĭ-bod-e) antibody found in the feces, chiefly secretory IgA.

coprolalia (kop″ro-la′le-ah) compulsive, stereotyped use of obscene language, particularly of words relating to feces; seen in some cases of schizophrenia and Gilles de la Tourette's syndrome.

coprolith (kop′ro-lith) fecalith.

coprology (kop-rol′o-je) scatology (def 1).

coprophagia (kop″ro-fa′jah) coprophagy.

coprophagy (kop-rof′ah-je) the ingestion of feces.

coprophilia (kop″ro-fil′e-ah) an absorbing interest in feces or filth, particularly a paraphilia in which sexual arousal or activity is linked to feces.

coprophilic (kop″ro-fil′ik) 1. pertaining to or characterized by coprophilia. 2. inhabiting feces or fecal-polluted water; said of microorganisms.

coprophobia (kop″ro-fo′be-ah) abnormal repugnance to defecation and to feces.

coprophrasia (kop″ro-fra′zhah) coprolalia.

coproporphyria (kop″ro-por-fir′e-ah) any of various types of porphyria characterized by elevated levels of coproporphyrin in the body.

hereditary c. a hepatic porphyria transmitted as an autosomal dominant trait, characterized biochemically by constant excretion of coproporphyrin III in the feces and intermittent urinary excretion of coproporphyrin, α-aminolevulinic acid (ALA), and porphobilinogen (PBG). The condition is usually asymptomatic, but acute attacks resembling those of acute intermittent PORPHYRIA can occur.

coproporphyrin (kop″ro-por′fi-rin) a PORPHYRIN occurring as several isomers; the III isomer, an intermediate in heme biosynthesis, is excreted in the feces and urine in hereditary coproporphyria and variegate porphyria; the I isomer, a side product, is excreted in the feces and urine in congenital erythropoietic porphyria.

coproporphyrinogen (kop″ro-por″fi-rin′o-jen) a PORPHYRINOGEN formed from UROPORPHYRINOGEN. Two isomers exist naturally, types I and III; the latter is a functional intermediate in heme biosynthesis while the former is produced in an abortive side reaction.

coproporphyrinuria (kop″ro-por″fi-rĭ-nu′re-ah) the presence of COPROPORPHYRIN in the urine; see COPROPORPHYRIA.

coprostasis (kop-ros′tah-sis) FECAL IMPACTION.

coprozoic (kop″ro-zo′ik) living in fecal matter.

copula (kop′u-lah) any connecting part or structure.

copulation (kop″u-la′shun) sexual union or coitus; the transfer of the sperm from male to female; usually applied to animals other than humans.

cor (kor) [L.] heart.

  c. adipo′sum a heart that has undergone fatty degeneration or that has an accumulation of fat around it.

  c. bovi′num a greatly enlarged heart resulting from a hypertrophied left ventricle.

  c. pulmona′le a serious cardiac condition in which there is right ventricular HEART FAILURE due to pulmonary hypertension secondary to disease of the blood vessels of the lungs. Acute cor pulmonale is an emergency situation arising from a sudden dilatation of the right ventricle as a result of pulmonary EMBOLISM. Chronic cor pulmonale develops gradually and is associated with such chronic obstructive pulmonary diseases as EMPHYSEMA, SILICOSIS, and pulmonary FIBROSIS following an infection. These conditions impair pulmonary circulation and thus create a "damming" effect on the blood flowing through the pulmonary artery. This in turn slows down the flow of blood from the right ventricle, and the ventricle becomes hypertrophied and dilated.

Signs and symptoms are similar to those of congestive HEART FAILURE from other causes: DYSPNEA, EDEMA of the lower extremities, enlargement of the liver, and distention of neck veins. The HEMATOCRIT is increased as the body attempts to compensate for impaired circulation by producing more erythrocytes.

Treatment. Treatment may involve use of drugs to decrease pulmonary vascular resistance, pulmonary EMBOLECTOMY, or even lung transplantation. More traditional treatments have included administration of bronchodilators and use of a mechanical ventilator to reduce hypoxia and dyspnea. For treatment of the heart failure, see HEART FAILURE.

coracoid (kor′ah-koid) 1. like a crow's beak. 2. the coracoid process, a projection from the upper part of the neck of the scapula, overhanging the shoulder joint.

cord (kord) any long, cylindrical, flexible structure; called also chord, chorda, and funiculus.

  spermatic c. the structure extending from the abdominal inguinal ring to the testis, comprising the pampiniform plexus, nerves, ductus deferens, testicular artery, and other vessels.

  spinal c. see SPINAL CORD.

  tethered c. a congenital anomaly resulting from defective closure of the neural tube; the conus medullaris is abnormally low and tethered by a short, thickened filum terminale, fibrous bands, intradural lipoma, or some other intradural abnormality. Surgical correction in infancy or early childhood is necessary to prevent progressive neurological deficit in the lower limb and bladder dysfunction.

  umbilical c. see UMBILICAL CORD.

  vocal c's see VOCAL CORDS.

cordal (kor′dal) pertaining to a cord; used specifically in referring to the vocal cords.

cordate (kor′dāt) cordiform.

cordectomy (kor-dek′to-me) excision of a cord, as of a vocal cord.

cordiform (kor′dĭ-form) heart-shaped.

cordising (kor′dis-ing) [L. *cordis* of the heart] a concept used in the ESCA philosophy of KINLEIN: caring from the heart, integrating truth, justice, and charity into one's actions.

corditis (kor-di′tis) inflammation of the spermatic cord.

cordocentesis (kor″do-sen-te′sis) percutaneous umbilical blood SAMPLING.

cordopexy (kor′do-pek″se) surgical fixation of a vocal cord.

cordotomy (kor-dot′ah-me) 1. section of a vocal cord. 2. surgical division of the anterolateral tracts of the spinal cord. Spelled also chordotomy.

Cordran (kor′dran) trademark for preparations of FLURANDRENOLIDE, a topical GLUCOCORTICOID used to treat dermatosis.

core(o)- word element [Gr.], *pupil of the eye.*

corectasis (kor-ek′tah-sis) morbid dilatation of the pupil of the eye.

corectome (ko-rek′tōm) a cutting instrument for iridectomy.

corectomy (ko-rek′to-me) iridectomy.

corectopia (kor″ek-to′pe-ah) abnormal location of the pupil of the eye.

core curriculum an organized program or course of study in a specialty area of practice.

coredialysis (ko″re-di-al′ĭ-sis) surgical separation of the external margin of the iris from the ciliary body.

corediastasis (ko″re-di-as′tah-sis) dilatation of the pupil.

corelysis (ko-rel′ĭ-sis) operative destruction of the pupil; especially detachment of adhesions of the pupillary margin of the iris from the lens.

coremorphosis (kor″e-mor-fo′sis) surgical formation of an artificial pupil.

corenclisis (kor″en-kli′sis) iridencleisis.

coreometer (ko″re-om′ĕ-ter) pupillometer.

coreoplasty (kor′re-o-plas″te) any plastic operation on the pupil.

corepressor (ko″re-pres′ser) a small molecule that combines with a protein aporepressor molecule to form an active substance, which then binds to an operator gene and inhibits the synthesis of an enzyme.

coretomy (ko-ret′o-me) iridectomy.

Corgard (kor′gard) trademark for a preparation of NADOLOL, a BETA-ADRENERGIC BLOCKING AGENT used as an antianginal and ANTIHYPERTENSIVE AGENT.

Cori's disease (ko′rēz) Forbes' disease.

corium (kor′e-um) dermis.

corn (korn) 1. *Zea mays,* a tall cereal plant that produces kernels on large ears and is the source of CORN OIL. 2. a circumscribed, conical, horny induration and thickening of the stratum corneum that causes severe pain by pressure on nerve endings in the corium. Corns are always caused by friction or pressure from poorly fitting shoes or hose. There are two kinds: the *hard corn,* usually located on the outside of the little toe or on the upper surfaces of the other toes; and the *soft corn,* found between the toes, usually the fourth and fifth toes, kept softened by moisture. Called also heloma.

c. oil a refined fixed oil obtained from the corn plant, *Zea mays;* used as a solvent and vehicle for medicinal agents and as a vehicle for injections. It has also been promoted as a source of polyunsaturated FATTY ACIDS in special diets.

cornea (kor′ne-ah) the clear, transparent anterior covering of the EYE (see also color plates). The cornea is subject to injury by foreign bodies in the eye, bacterial infection, and viral infection, especially by the herpesvirus that causes HERPES SIMPLEX. The herpesvirus that causes HERPES ZOSTER (shingles) can also infect the cornea. Prompt treatment of any corneal injury or infection is essential to avoid ulceration and loss of vision.

corneal (kor′ne-al) pertaining to the cornea.

c. reflex a reflex action of the eye resulting in automatic closing of the eyelid when the cornea is stimulated. The corneal reflex can be elicited in a normal person by gently touching the cornea with a wisp of cotton. Absence of the corneal reflex indicates deep coma or injury of one of the nerves carrying the reflex arc.

c. transplantation transplantation of a donor cornea into the eye of a recipient,

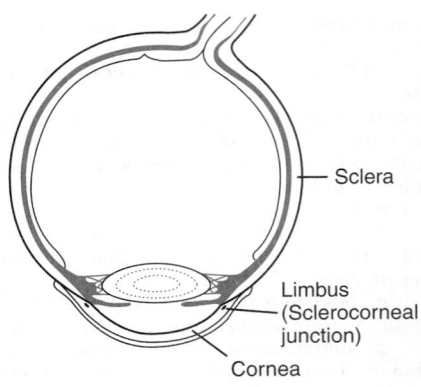

Cornea. From Dorland's, 2000.

done to improve the vision of patients with distorted curvature of the cornea (KERATOCONUS) or corneal edema, infection, trauma, or intractable pain. Vision should improve beginning the day after surgery with optimal vision 6 to 12 months later. Because the cornea does not have a blood supply, corneal transplants were one of the earliest successful types of organ transplants. Called also KERATOPLASTY.

corneitis (kor″ne-i′tis) keratitis.

corneoiritis (kor″ne-o-i-ri′tis) keratoiritis.

corneosclera (kor″ne-o-skle′rah) the cornea and sclera regarded as one organ.

corneous (kor′ne-us) 1. horny. 2. keratinous.

cornification (kor″nĭ-fĭ-ka′shun) 1. keratinization. 2. conversion of epithelium to the stratified squamous type.

cornified (kor″nĭ-fīd) converted into KERATIN; see also KERATINIZATION.

cornstarch (korn′stahrch) see STARCH (def. 2).

cornu (kor′noo), pl. cor′nua [L.] HORN.

c. ammo′nis hippocampus.

c. sacra′le either of two hook-shaped processes extending downward from the arch of the last sacral vertebra.

cornual [kor′noo-al] pertaining to a horn or cornu.

cornuate (kor′noo-āt) cornual.

corona (kŏ-ro′nah), pl. coro′nae, coronas [L.] crown; in anatomic nomenclature, an eminence or encircling structure that resembles a crown. adj., **cor′onal.**

c. radia′ta 1. the radiating crown of projection fibers passing from the internal capsule to every part of the cerebral cortex. 2. an investing layer of radially elongated follicle cells surrounding the zona pellucida of the ovum; it accompanies the oocyte during ovulation.

coronary (kor'ah-nar-e) encircling in the manner of a crown; said of anatomical structures such as vessels, ligaments, or nerves.

c. arteries two large arteries that branch from the ascending aorta and supply all of the heart muscle with blood (see also table of ARTERIES).

c. artery disease (CAD) atherosclerosis of the coronary arteries, which may cause angina pectoris, myocardial infarction, and sudden death. Both genetically determined and avoidable risk factors contribute to the disease; they include hypercholesterolemia, hypertension, smoking, diabetes mellitus, and low levels of high density lipoproteins (HDL).

c. heart disease (CHD) ischemic heart disease.

c. occlusion the occlusion, or closing off, of a coronary artery, usually caused by a narrowing of the lumen of the blood vessels by the plaques of ATHEROSCLEROSIS. Sometimes a plaque may rupture and release vasoactive or thrombogenic substances that lead to clot formation. If there is adequate collateral circulation to the heart muscle at the time of the occlusion, there may be little or no damage to the myocardial cells. When occlusion is complete, however, with no blood being supplied to an area of the myocardium, MYOCARDIAL INFARCTION results.

coronavirus (ko-ro'nah-vi"rus) any of a group of morphologically similar, ether-sensitive viruses, probably RNA, causing infectious bronchitis in birds, hepatitis in mice, gastroenteritis in swine, and respiratory infections in humans.

coroner (kor'ah-ner) an official of a local community who holds inquests concerning sudden, violent, or unexplained deaths.

coronoid (kor'ah-noid) shaped like a crow's beak, as the coronoid process.

coronoidectomy (kor"ah-noi-dek'tah-me) surgical removal of the coronoid PROCESS of the mandible.

corotomy (kah-rot'ah-me) iridotomy.

corpulency (kor'pu-len"se) obesity.

corpus (kor'pus), pl. *cor'pora* [L.] body.

c. al'bicans white fibrous tissue that replaces the regressing corpus luteum in the human ovary in the latter half of pregnancy, or soon after ovulation when pregnancy does not supervene.

c. amygdaloi'deum amygdaloid BODY.

cor'pora amyla'cea small hyaline masses of degenerate cells found in the prostate, neuroglia, and other sites.

c. callo'sum an arched mass of white MATTER in the depths of the longitudinal FISSURE, made up of transverse fibers connecting the cerebral HEMISPHERES.

c. caverno'sum either of the two columns of erectile tissue forming the body of the penis or clitoris.

c. fimbria'tum a band of white matter bordering the lateral edge of the lower cornu of the lateral ventricle of the brain.

c. genicula'tum see geniculate BODIES, lateral, and geniculate BODIES, medial.

c. hemorrha'gicum 1. an ovarian follicle containing blood. 2. a corpus luteum containing a blood clot. 3. a blood clot

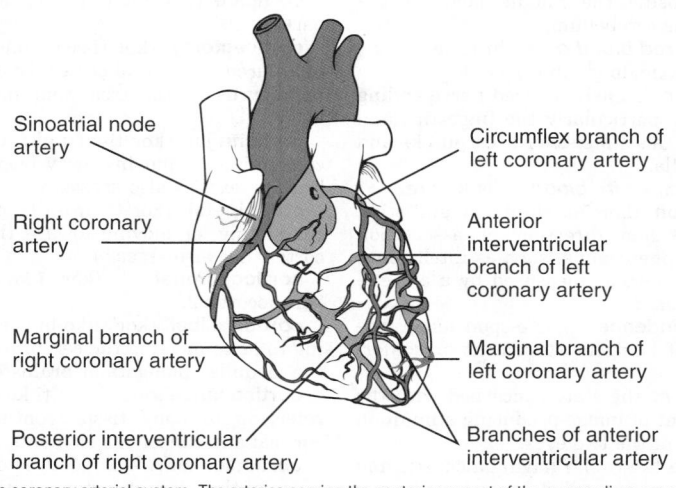

Sinoatrial node artery

Right coronary artery

Marginal branch of right coronary artery

Posterior interventricular branch of right coronary artery

Circumflex branch of left coronary artery

Anterior interventricular branch of left coronary artery

Marginal branch of left coronary artery

Branches of anterior interventricular artery

A view of the coronary arterial system. The arteries serving the posterior aspect of the myocardium are shown here in a lighter shade.

formed in the cavity left by rupture of a graafian follicle.

c. lu'teum a yellow glandular mass in the ovary formed by an ovarian follicle that has matured and discharged its ovum; see also OVULATION.

c. mammilla're mamillary BODY.

cor'pora quadrige'mina four rounded eminences on the posterior surface of the mesencephalon.

c. spongio'sum pe'nis a column of erectile tissue forming the urethral surface of the penis, in which the urethra is found.

c. ster'ni body of sternum.

c. stria'tum a subcortical mass of gray MATTER and white MATTER in front of and lateral to the THALAMUS in each cerebral HEMISPHERE.

c. u'teri that part of the uterus above the isthmus and below the orifices of the FALLOPIAN TUBES.

corpuscle (kor'pus'l) any small mass or body. adj., **corpus'cular.**

blood c. blood cell.

colostrum c's large rounded bodies in colostrum, containing droplets of fat and sometimes a nucleus.

Krause's c. end-bulb.

malpighian c. the funnel-like structure constituting the beginning of the structural unit of the kidney (nephron) and comprising the malpighian capsule and its partially enclosed glomerulus. Called also renal corpuscle.

Meissner's c. tactile corpuscle.

Purkinje's c's large, branched nerve cells composing the middle layer of the cortex of the cerebellum.

red c., red blood c. erythrocyte.

renal c. malpighian corpuscle.

tactile c. a medium-sized nerve ending in the skin, particularly the fingertips and lips; called also Meissner's corpuscle and tactile papilla.

white c., white blood c. leukocyte.

correlation (kor″ĕ-la'shun) in statistics, the degree and direction of association of variable phenomena, such as intelligence and birth order, as measured by a correlation COEFFICIENT.

correspondence (kor″ĕ-spon'dens) the condition of being in agreement or conformity.

retinal c. the state concerned with the impingement of image-producing stimuli on the retinas of the two eyes.

corrosive (kŏ-ro'siv) having a caustic and locally destructive effect; an agent having such effects.

Cort-Dome (kort'dōm) trademark for preparations of HYDROCORTISONE, a GLUCO-CORTICOID used topically and rectally as an antiinflammatory agent.

Cortef (kor'tef) trademark for preparations of HYDROCORTISONE, a GLUCOCORTICOID used as an antiinflammatory and immunosuppressant agent.

Cortenema (kort″en'ĕ-mah) trademark for a preparation of hydrocortisone ENEMA, used in treatment of ULCERATIVE COLITIS.

cortex (kor'teks), pl. *cor'tices* [L.] the outer layer of an organ or other structure, as distinguished from its inner substance or MEDULLA. adj., **cor'tical.**

adrenal c., c. of adrenal gland the outer, firm layer comprising the larger part of the ADRENAL GLAND; it secretes MINERALO-CORTICOIDS, ANDROGENS, and GLUCOCORTICOIDS.

cerebellar c. the superficial gray MATTER of the CEREBELLUM.

cerebral c., c. cerebra'lis the convoluted layer of gray MATTER covering each cerebral HEMISPHERE. See also BRAIN.

renal c. the granular outer layer of the kidney, composed mainly of glomeruli and convoluted tubules, extending in columns between the pyramids that constitute the renal medulla.

striate c. part of the occipital lobe that receives the fibers of the optic RADIATION and serves as the primary receiving area for VISION. Called also first visual area.

visual c. the area of the occipital lobe of the cerebral cortex concerned with VISION; the striate cortex is also called the *first visual area,* and the adjacent *second* and *third visual areas* serve as its association areas.

corticate (kor'tĭ-kāt) having a cortex or bark.

corticectomy (kor″tĭ-sek'to-me) excision of an area of cerebral cortex, as of a scar or microgyrus in the treatment of focal epilepsy.

corticifugal (kor″tĭ-sif'u-g'l) proceeding, conducting, or moving away from the cerebral cortex. See also EFFERENT.

corticipetal (kor″tĭ-sip'ĕ-t'l) proceeding, conducting, or moving toward the cerebral cortex. See also AFFERENT.

corticoadrenal (kor″tĭ-ko-ah-dre'nal) adrenocortical.

corticobulbar (kor″tĭ-ko-bul'ber) pertaining to or connecting the cerebral cortex and the medulla oblongata or brainstem.

corticocancellous (kor″tĭ-ko-kan'sĕ-lus) referring to bony tissue containing both cortical and cancellous elements.

corticoid (kor'tĭ-koid) corticosteroid, a hormone of the adrenal cortex, or other natural or synthetic compound with similar activity.

corticopontine (kor″tĭ-ko-pon′tīn) pertaining to or connecting the cerebral cortex and the pons.

corticospinal (kor″tĭ-ko-spi′nal) pertaining to or connecting the cerebral cortex and spinal cord.

corticosteroid (kor″tĭ-ko-ster′oid) any of the hormones produced by the ADRENAL CORTEX; also, their synthetic equivalents. Called also adrenocortical hormone and adrenocorticoid. All the hormones are steroids having similar chemical structures, but quite different physiologic effects. Generally they are divided into GLUCOCORTICOIDS (CORTISOL, CORTISONE, and CORTICOSTERONE), MINERALOCORTICOIDS (ALDOSTERONE and DESOXY-CORTICOSTERONE, and also CORTICOSTERONE) and ANDROGENS. Patients who must take exogenous adrenal corticosteroids to supplement a deficit in endogenous cortisol or as a treatment for metastatic breast cancer should be thoroughly instructed in self-medication. Their needs are somewhat similar to those of the insulin-dependent diabetic patient. They should know the prescribed dosage and basic therapeutic action of the oral corticosteroid preparation they are taking and should be aware of the importance of taking the medication at the same time every day. The medication should never be discontinued abruptly for any reason. It is advisable that the patient carry an extra prescription when traveling, in case the supply is used up before returning home. These patients also need to wear some form of medical identification so that all health care professionals with whom they come in contact will know that they are receiving hormones of this kind. This includes dentists, oral surgeons, EMERGENCY DEPARTMENT personnel, and others who might not be familiar with the patient's medical history.

corticosterone (kor″tĭ-kos′tĕ-rōn) a steroid hormone of the adrenal cortex; it affects carbohydrate, potassium, and sodium metabolism. It is usually classified as a GLUCOCORTICOID, but it also has slight MINERALOCORTICOID activity.

corticotrope (kor′tĭ-ko-trōp) corticotroph.

corticotroph (kor′tĭ-ko-trōf) a type of ACIDOPHIL found in the anterior lobe of the pituitary gland that secretes CORTICOTROPIN; it is synthesized as a large prohormone containing both corticotropin and β-lipotropin.

corticotrophic (kor″tĭ-ko-trof′ik) adrenocorticotropic.

corticotrophin (kor′tĭ-ko-tro″fin) corticotropin.

corticotropic (kor″tĭ-ko-trop′ik) 1. having a stimulating effect on the adrenal cortex. 2. adrenocorticotropic.

corticotropin (kor″tĭ-ko-tro′pin) 1. a hormone secreted by the anterior lobe of the PITUITARY GLAND that stimulates the cortex of the ADRENAL GLAND to secrete its hormones, including CORTICOSTERONE. If production of corticotropin falls below normal, the adrenal cortex decreases in size, and production of the cortical hormones declines. 2. a pharmaceutical preparation of animal-derived corticotropin, administered intravenously for diagnostic testing of adrenocortical function and subcutaneously or intramuscularly, in a slowly absorbed gel form (repository corticotropin), as an ANTICONVULSANT for treating infantile spasms. Called also adrenocorticotropic hormone (ACTH), adrenocorticotropin, and corticotrophin.

corticotropinoma (kor″tĭ-ko-tro″pin-o′mah) corticotroph adenoma.

Cortifoam (kor′tĭ-fōm) trademark for an aerosol foam containing 10 per cent HYDROCORTISONE acetate; used as an intrarectal ANTIINFLAMMATORY.

cortilymph (kor′tĭ-limf″) the fluid filling the intercellular spaces of the organ of Corti, similar in composition to PERILYMPH.

cortisol (kor′tĭ-sol) a hormone from the adrenal cortex, the principal GLUCOCORTICOID; called also 17-hydroxycorticosterone and, pharmaceutically, hydrocortisone. A synthetic preparation is used for its ANTIINFLAMMATORY actions.

cortisone (kor′tĭ-sōn) a GLUCOCORTICOID with significant MINERALOCORTICOID activity, isolated from the adrenal cortex, largely inactive in humans until it is converted to HYDROCORTISONE (CORTISOL). Cortisone, as the acetate ester, is used as an antiinflammatory and immunosuppressant and for replacement therapy in adrenocortical INSUFFICIENCY; administered orally or by intramuscular injection.

Cortisporin (kor″tĭ-spor′in) trademark for combination preparations of POLYMYXIN B, NEOMYCIN SULFATE, HYDROCORTISONE, and (in some preparations) BACITRACIN zinc. Uses include topical preparations for dermatoses and ophthalmic and otic preparations for inflammatory conditions where there is actual or potential risk of bacterial infection.

coruscation (kor″us-ka′shun) the sensation as of a flash of light before the eyes.

corybantism (kor″e-ban′tizm) wild, frenzied, and sleepless delirium.

corymbiform (ko-rim′bi-form) clustered; said of lesions grouped around a single, usually larger, lesion.

Corynebacteriaceae (ko-ri″ne-bak-tēr″e-a′se-e) a family of bacteria, made up of usually nonmotile rods, sometimes showing marked variation in form and sometimes beaded or banded with metachromatic granules.

Corynebacterium (ko-ri″ne-bak-tēr′e-um) a genus of gram-positive, nonmotile, straight to slightly curved rod-shaped bacteria. It includes both pathogenic and nonpathogenic organisms, which are widely distributed in nature. Species include *C. ac′nes,* found in ACNE lesions; *C. diphthe′riae,* the etiologic agent of DIPHTHERIA; *C. haemoly′ticum,* found in PHARYNGITIS and skin ulcers; *C. minutis′simum,* the causative agent of ERYTHRASMA; *C. pseudodiphtheri′-ticum,* a nonpathogenic inhabitant of the upper respiratory tract; *C. te′nuis,* the causative agent of TRICHOMYCOSIS AXILLARIS; *C. ul′cerans,* which causes nasopharyngeal infections; and *C. xero′sis,* an opportunistic pathogen found on the skin and mucous membranes and in the conjunctival sac.

coryneform (ko-ri′nĕ-form) club-shaped; denoting or resembling organisms of the family Corynebacteriaceae.

coryza (ko-ri′zah) acute rhinitis.

Cosmegen (kos′mĕ-jen) trademark for a preparation of DACTINOMYCIN, an antitumor ANTIBIOTIC.

cosmesis (koz-me′sis) 1. the preservation, restoration, or bestowing of bodily beauty. 2. the surgical correction of a disfiguring physical defect.

cosmetic (koz-met′ik) 1. beautifying; tending to preserve, restore, or confer comeliness. 2. a beautifying substance or preparation. 3. pertaining to surgical correction of a physical defect.

cost(o)- word element [L.], *rib.*

costa (kos′tah) [L.] a rib. adj., **cos′tal.**

costalgia (kos-tal′jah) 1. pain in the ribs. 2. pain in the costal muscles; called also pleurodynia.

costectomy (kos-tek′to-me) excision of a rib.

cost effective in the health sciences, pertaining to a situation in which funds spent to improve the health and well-being of a client or group reduces the overall cost of care. Increased productivity produces more output for the same input or produces the same output for less input. A change in practice that results in the same patient outcomes but uses fewer resources is cost effective. Health prevention and promotion strategies save potential costs in the long run. Nurse researchers have been able to demonstrate that the care of clinical nurse specialists can save significant health

care costs without reducing the quality of care.

costive (kos′tiv) 1. pertaining to, characterized by, or producing constipation. 2. an agent that so acts.

costiveness (kos′tiv-nes) constipation.

costocervical (kos″to-ser′vĭ-k'l) pertaining to the ribs and neck.

costochondral (kos″to-kon′dral) pertaining to a rib and its cartilage.

costoclavicular (kos″to-klah-vik′u-ler) pertaining to the ribs and clavicle.

costocoracoid (kos″to-kor′ah-koid) pertaining to the ribs and coracoid process.

costosternal (kos″to-ster′nal) pertaining to the ribs and sternum.

costosternoplasty (kos″to-ster′no-plas″te) surgical repair of funnel chest, a segment of rib being used to support the sternum.

costotomy (kos-tot′ah-me) incision or division of a rib or costal cartilage.

costotransverse (kos″to-trans-vers′) lying between the ribs and the transverse processes of the vertebrae.

costovertebral (kos″to-ver′tĕ-bral) pertaining to a rib and a vertebra.

costoxiphoid (kos″to-zi′foid) connecting the ribs and xiphoid cartilage.

cosyntropin (ko″sin-tro′pin) a synthetic CORTICOTROPIN used in the screening of adrenal INSUFFICIENCY on the basis of plasma cortisol response after intramuscular or intravenous injection.

COTA Certified Occupational Therapy Assistant.

cotransport (ko-trans′port) linking of the TRANSPORT of one substance across a membrane with the simultaneous transport of a different substance in the same direction. See also COUNTERTRANSPORT.

co-trimoxazole (ko″tri-moks′ah-zōl) a combination of trimethoprim and sulfamethoxazole, an antibacterial used primarily in the treatment of urinary tract infections and *Pneumocystis carinii* pneumonia; administered orally or intravenously..

cotton (kot′'n) 1. a plant of the genus *Gossypium.* 2. a textile material derived from the seeds of this plant.

   absorbable c. oxidized cellulose.

   absorbent c., purified c. cotton freed from impurities, bleached, and sterilized; used as a surgical dressing.

cottonmouth (kot′on-mouth) water moccasin.

cottonseed oil a fixed oil from seeds of cultivated varieties of the cotton plant, *(Gossypium)*; used as a solvent and vehicle for drugs.

cotyledon (kot″ĭ-le′don) 1. any subdivision of the uterine surface of the placenta. 2. irregular convex areas on the chorionic surface of the placenta, consisting of two or more stem villi and their many branch villi; by the end of the fourth month the DECIDUA BASALIS is almost entirely replaced by the cotyledons.

cough (kof) 1. a sudden noisy expulsion of air from the lungs; called also tussis. 2. to produce such an expulsion of air.

dry c. cough without expectoration.

productive c. cough attended with expectoration of material from the bronchi.

reflex c. a cough due to the irritation of some remote organ.

wet c. productive cough.

whooping c. see WHOOPING COUGH.

coughing (kof'ing) the production of COUGHS.

assisted c. a technique used to enhance the effectiveness of coughing for individuals such as quadriplegics who have ineffective diaphragmatic movement. The hands of the person assisting are placed on either side of the rib cage or on the upper abdomen under the diaphragm; the patient is instructed to exhale as the assistant pushes upward and inward.

coulomb (C) (koo'lom) the SI unit of electric charge, defined as the quantity of electrical charge transferred across a surface by 1 ampere in 1 second.

Coumadin (koo'mah-din) trademark for preparations of WARFARIN sodium, an ANTICOAGULANT.

coumarin (koo'mah-rin) 1. a principle extracted from the tonka bean, from which several ANTICOAGULANTS are derived that inhibit hepatic synthesis of vitamin K–dependent COAGULATION FACTORS. 2. any of these derivatives.

counseling (kown'sel-ing) in the NURSING INTERVENTIONS CLASSIFICATION, a nursing INTERVENTION defined as use of an interactive helping process focusing on the needs, problems, or feelings of the patient and significant others to enhance or support coping, problem solving, and interpersonal relationships.

genetic c. in the NURSING INTERVENTIONS CLASSIFICATION, a nursing INTERVENTION defined as use of an interactive helping process focusing on assisting an individual, family, or group, manifesting or at risk for developing or transmitting a birth defect or genetic condition, to cope.

lactation c. in the NURSING INTERVENTIONS CLASSIFICATION, a nursing INTERVENTION defined as the use of an interactive helping process to assist in maintenance of successful BREASTFEEDING.

nutritional c. in the NURSING INTERVENTIONS CLASSIFICATION, a nursing INTERVENTION defined as the use of an interactive helping process focusing on the need for diet modification.

preconception c. in the NURSING INTERVENTIONS CLASSIFICATION, a nursing INTERVENTION defined as providing information and support to individuals of childbearing age before pregnancy to promote health and reduce risk.

sexual c. in the NURSING INTERVENTIONS CLASSIFICATION, a nursing INTERVENTION defined as the use of an interactive helping process focusing on the need to make adjustments in sexual practice or to enhance coping with a sexual event or disorder.

counselor (kown'sel-er) one who gives advice or instruction.

vocational c. a professional who assists disabled individuals in assessing their strengths and weaknesses and selecting jobs or careers that maximize their potential to become contributing members of the workforce. The vocational counselor works as a member of the rehabilitation team to formulate a plan designed to achieve vocational goals.

count (kownt) a numerical computation or indication.

Addis c. the determination of the number of erythrocytes, leukocytes, epithelial cells, and casts, and the protein content in an aliquot of a 12-hour urine specimen; used in the diagnosis and management of kidney disease.

blood c., blood cell c. see BLOOD COUNT.

blood c., complete a series of tests of the peripheral blood, including the erythrocyte count, erythrocyte indices, leukocyte counts, and sometimes platelet count.

blood c., differential differential leukocyte count.

erythrocyte c. determination of the number of erythrocytes in a unit volume of blood that has been diluted in an isotonic solution, done with an automatic counter such as a flow cytometer. Called also red blood cell or red cell count.

leukocyte c. determination of the number of leukocytes in a unit volume of blood, usually after the erythrocytes have been lysed and the blood has been diluted; it may be done either manually with a hemacytometer or electronically. See *total leukocyte c.* and *differential leukocyte c.* Called also white blood cell or white cell count.

leukocyte c., differential a leukocyte count that calculates the percentages of different types. See also total leukocyte COUNT.

leukocyte c., total a leukocyte count measuring the total number of all the types in a given volume of blood. See also differential leukocyte count.

platelet c. determination of the total number of platelets per cubic millimeter of blood; the *direct platelet count* simply counts the cells using a microscope, and the *indirect platelet count* determines the ratio of platelets to erythrocytes on a peripheral blood smear and computes the number of platelets from the erythrocyte count.

red blood cell c., red cell c. erythrocyte count.

reticulocyte c. a calculation of the number of reticulocytes in 1 cu mm of peripheral blood, recorded either as an absolute number or as the percentage of the erythrocyte count. It provides a means of assessing the erythropoietic activity of the bone marrow.

white blood cell c., white cell c. leukocyte count.

counter (kown′ter) an instrument or apparatus by which numerical value is computed; in radiology, a device for enumerating ionizing events.

Coulter c. an automated instrument for performing blood counts, based on the principle that cells are poor electrical conductors compared with saline solution.

Geiger c., Geiger-Müller c. a radiation counter using a gas-filled tube that indicates the presence of ionizing particles. It is very sensitive to β particles but relatively insensitive to γ and x-rays.

scintillation c. a device for detecting ionization events, permitting determination of the concentration of radioisotopes in the body or other substance.

countercurrent (kown′ter-ker″ent) flowing in an opposite direction.

counterelectrophoresis (kown″ter-e-lek′-tro-fo-re′sis) counterimmunoelectrophoresis.

counterextension (kown″ter-ek-sten′-shun) traction in a proximal direction coincident with traction in opposition to it.

counterimmunoelectrophoresis (CIE) (kown″ter-im″u-no-e-lek″tro-fo-re′sis) a laboratory technique in which an electric current is used to accelerate the migration of antibody and antigen through a buffered diffusion medium. Antigens in a gel medium in which the pH is controlled are strongly negatively charged and will migrate rapidly across the electric field toward the anode. The antibody in such a medium is less negatively charged and will migrate in an opposite or "counter" direction toward the cathode. If the antigen and antibody are specific for each other, they combine and form a distinct precipitin line.

The technique of CIE was first applied clinically in 1970 to detect hepatitis B antigen. With modification and refinement it is becoming increasingly useful as a means of detecting antigens or antibodies specific for a variety of infectious diseases. It can be especially valuable as an aid to accurate diagnosis of clinical bacterial infections and the selection of specific therapeutic agents for control of infections once the causative organisms are identified.

counterincision (kown″ter-in-sizh′un) a second incision made to promote drainage or to relieve tension on the edges of a wound.

counterirritant (kown″ter-ir′ĭ-tant) producing counterirritation. an agent that so acts.

counterirritation (kown″ter-ir″ĭ-ta′shun) an irritation produced in one part of the body that is intended to relieve an irritation in some other part.

counteropening (kown″ter-o′pen-ing) contra-aperture.

counterpulsation (kown″ter-pul-sa′shun) a technique for assisting the circulation and decreasing the work of the heart by synchronizing the force of an external pumping device with cardiac systole and diastole. *External* counterpulsation is a noninvasive procedure in which the legs are encased in rigid tubular bags filled with air or water and connected to a pumping unit. *Internal* counterpulsation requires insertion of an intra-aortic balloon-tipped catheter, the distal end of which is attached to a pump that inflates the balloon. (See also INTRA-AORTIC BALLOON PUMP.)

External counterpulsation is less effective than internal counterpulsation, but it is easier to use and less hazardous to the patient. It employs the same general principles as internal counterpulsation by applying pressure against the blood vessels of the legs during diastole and release of pressure during systole. This has the effect of increasing venous return and enhancing systolic unloading of the left ventricle. The end result of external counterpulsation is that of augmenting coronary circulation and improving blood flow to the myocardium, improving systemic circulation, and reducing the workload of the heart, thereby lessening myocardial demand for and consumption of oxygen. Indications for external counterpulsation include cardiogenic shock and severe heart failure in acute situations such as myocardial infarction and open-heart surgery. It is a temporary measure that does not benefit patients with chronic heart failure.

counterpuncture (kown′ter-punk″chur) counteropening.

countershock (koun′tər-shok″) a high-intensity direct current shock delivered to the heart to interrupt ventricular FIBRILLA-TION and restore synchronous electrical activity.

counterstain (kown′ter-stān) a stain applied to render the effects of another stain more discernible.

countertraction (kown′ter-trak″shun) traction opposed to traction; used in reduction of fractures.

countertransference (kown″ter-trans-fe-r′ens) a TRANSFERENCE reaction of a psychoanalyst or other psychotherapist to a patient; that is, an emotional reaction that is generally a reflection of the therapist's own inner needs and conflicts but also may be a reaction to the client's behavior.

countertransport (kown″ter-trans′port) the simultaneous TRANSPORT of two substances across a membrane in opposite directions, either by the same CARRIER or by different carriers that are biochemically linked to each other. See also COTRANSPORT.

coup (koo) [Fr.] stroke.

   c. de sabre (koo-duh-sahb′) linear SCLERODERMA on the forehead or scalp, so-called because of its resemblance to the scar of a saber wound.

coupling (kup′ling) in electrocardiography, precise linkage of an ectopic complex to the preceding beat each time it occurs.

covalence (ko-va′lens) 1. the number of electron pairs an atom can share with other atoms. 2. one or more chemical bonds formed by sharing of electron pairs between atoms. adj., **cova′lent.**

covariance (ko-va′re-ans) a measure of the tendency of two random variables to vary together. It is the expected value of the product of the deviations of corresponding values of two random variables from their respective means.

coverglass (kuv′er-glas) a thin glass that covers a mounted microscopic object or a culture; called also coverslip.

coverslip (kuv′er-slip) coverglass.

cowperitis (kow″per-i′tis) inflammation of the bulbourethral (Cowper's) glands, located in the urethral sphincter.

cowpox (kow′poks) a mild pustular eruption affecting milk cows, usually confined to the udder and teats, caused by the VACCINIA virus, and transmissible to humans. Edward Jenner, in the 18th century, discovered that cowpox could be transmitted to humans who milked or tended cattle, and also noted that persons who contracted it in this way seldom contracted smallpox. This discovery led to VACCINATION against SMALLPOX.

coxa (kok′sah) [L.] 1. hip. 2. hip joint.

   c. pla′na flattening of the head of the femur resulting from osteochondrosis of its epiphysis.

   c. val′ga deformity of the hip joint with increase in the angle of inclination between the neck and shaft of the femur.

   c. va′ra deformity of the hip joint with decrease in the angle of inclination between the neck and shaft of the femur.

coxalgia (kok-sal′jah) 1. hip-joint disease. 2. pain in the hip; called also coxodynia.

Coxiella (kok″se-el′ah) a genus of bacteria of the family Rickettsiaceae, occurring as short rods; *C. burnet′ii*, is the causative agent of Q FEVER.

coxitis (kok-si′tis) inflammation of the hip joint.

coxodynia (kok″so-din′e-ah) coxalgia (def. 2).

coxofemoral (kok″so-fem′o-ral) pertaining to the hip and thigh.

coxotuberculosis (kok″so-too-ber″ku-lo′-sis) tuberculosis of the hip joint; hip-joint disease.

coxsackievirus (kok-sak′e-vi″rus) any member of a heterogeneous group of EN-TEROVIRUSES; in humans one species causes a disease resembling POLIOMYELITIS but without paralysis. Called also Coxsackie virus.

CPAN Certified Post Anesthesia Nurse.

CPAP continuous positive airway pressure.

CPD citrate phosphate dextrose.

CPDA-1 citrate phosphate dextrose adenine.

C Ped Certified Pedorthist.

cpm counts per minute.

CPR cardiopulmonary resuscitation; computerized patient record.

CPS Compendium of Pharmaceuticals and Specialties.

CPU central processing unit (on a computer).

cps cycles per second; see HERTZ.

CR 1. conditioned reflex (response). 2. dibenz(b,f)-1,4-oxazepine, a common tear GAS.

   Cr chromium.

crabs (krabz) popular name for PEDICULO-SIS PUBIS.

crackle (krak′l) rale.

cradle (kra′d′l) a frame placed over the body of a bed patient for application of heat or cold or for protecting injured parts from coming in contact with the bed clothes. Cradles vary in size according to their intended purpose and can be used over the entire body or over one or more extremities.

   bed c. see BED CRADLE.

electric c., heat c. a tunnel- or hood-shaped cradle equipped with light bulbs, for applications of heat to the patient's body.

cramp (kramp) a painful spasmodic muscular contraction.

heat c. spasm accompanied by pain, weak pulse, and dilated pupils; seen in workers in intense heat.

recumbency c's cramping in the muscles of the lower limbs and feet occurring while resting or during light sleep.

writers' c. a muscle cramp in the hand caused by excessive use in writing.

crani(o)- word element [L.] *skull.*

craniad (kra'ne-ad) in a cranial direction; toward the head end of the body; in humans, a synonym of superiorly.

cranial (kra'ne-al) pertaining to the cranium or to the head end of the body; in humans, a synonym of superior.

c. nerves nerves that are attached to the brain and pass through the openings of the skull; see anatomic Table of Nerves in the Appendices. There are 12 pairs of cranial nerves, symmetrically arranged so that they are distributed mainly to the structures of the head and neck. The one exception is the VAGUS NERVE, which extends down to serve structures in the chest and abdomen. Some of the cranial nerves are both sensory and motor (controlling motion as well as conducting sensory impulses), while others are either only sensory or only motor.

craniectomy (kra"ne-ek'to-me) excision of a segment of the skull.

craniocaudal (kra"ne-o-kaw'dal) cephalocaudal.

CRANIAL NERVES*	
I Olfactory	Sensory
II Optic	Sensory
III Oculomotor	Mixed
IV Trochlear	Mixed
V Trigeminal	
Ophthalmic	Sensory
Maxillary	Sensory
Mandibular	Mixed
VI Abducens	Motor
VII Facial	Mixed
VIII Vestibulocochlear	
Cochlear	Sensory
Vestibular	Sensory
IX Glossopharyngeal	Mixed
X Vagus	Mixed
XI Accessory	Motor
XII Hypoglossal	Motor

*See also anatomic table of nerves in the Appendices.

craniocele (kra'ne-o-sēl") encephalocele.

craniocerebral (kra"ne-o-ser'ĕ-bral) pertaining to the skull and cerebrum.

craniocleidodysostosis (kra"ne-o-kli"do-dis"os-to'sis) cleidocranial dysostosis.

craniodidymus (kra"ne-o-did'ĭ-mus) bicephalus.

craniofacial (kra"ne-o-fa'shal) of or pertaining to the cranium and face.

craniomalacia (kra"ne-o-mah-la'shah) abnormal softness of the bones of the skull.

craniometer (kra"ne-om'ĕ-ter) an instrument for measuring the skull in craniometry. adj., **craniomet'ric.**

craniometry (kra"ne-om'ĕ-tre) a branch of anthropometry, being the measurement of the dimensions and angles of a bony skull.

craniopagus (kra"ne-op'ah-gus) conjoined twins that are joined at the skull.

craniopharyngeal (kra"ne-o-fah-rin'je-al) pertaining to the cranium and pharynx.

craniopharyngioma (kra"ne-o-fah-rin"je-o'mah) a tumor arising from cell RESTS derived from Rathke's POUCH or some other part of the PITUITARY GLAND, often destroying the gland and causing deficits of the pituitary hormones.

cranioplasty (kra'ne-o-plas"te) any plastic operation on the skull.

craniopuncture (kra'ne-o-pungk"cher) puncture of the skull.

craniorachischisis (kra"ne-o-rah-kis'kĭ-sis) congenital fissure of the skull and vertebral column.

craniosacral (kra"ne-o-sa'kral) pertaining to the skull and sacrum.

cranioschisis (kra"ne-os'kĭ-sis) cranium bifidum.

craniosclerosis (kra"ne-o-sklĕ-ro'sis) abnormal calcification and thickening of the cranial bones.

craniospinal (kra"ne-o-spi'nal) pertaining to the skull and spine.

craniostenosis (kra"ne-o-stĕ-no'sis) deformity of the skull due to premature closure of the cranial sutures.

craniostosis (kra"ne-os-to'sis) congenital ossification of the cranial sutures.

craniosynostosis (kra"ne-o-sin"os-to'sis) premature closure of the cranial sutures, resulting in skull deformities such as OXYCEPHALY, PLAGIOCEPHALY, SCAPHOCEPHALY, or TRIGONOCEPHALY. See illustration.

craniotabes (kra"ne-o-ta'bēz) reduction in mineralization of the skull, with abnormal softness of the bone, usually affecting the occipital and parietal bones along the lambdoidal sutures.

craniotome (kra'ne-o-tōm") a cutting instrument used in craniotomy.

craniotomy (kra"ne-ot'ah-me) 1. any operation on the cranium. 2. puncture of the

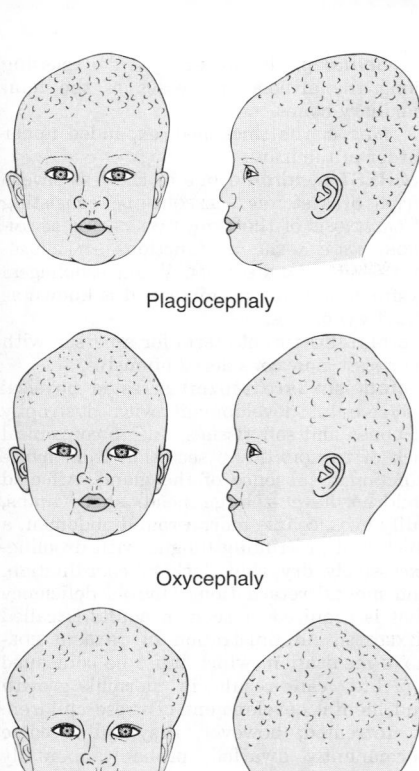

Plagiocephaly

Oxycephaly

Trigonocephaly

Examples of craniosynostosis.

skull and removal of its contents to decrease the size of the head of a dead fetus and facilitate delivery.

craniotympanic   (kra″ne-o-tim-pan′ik) pertaining to the skull and tympanum.

cranium (kra′ne-um), pl. *cra′nia* [L.] the large round superior part of the SKULL, enclosing the brain and made up of the cranial BONES.

c. bi′fidum incomplete formation of the skull, with defective formation of the brain and often an encephalocele or meningocele. Called also cranioschisis.

crater (kra′ter) an excavated area surrounded by an elevated margin, such as is caused by ulceration.

craterization (kra″ter-ĭ-za′shun) excision of bone tissue to create a crater-like depression.

crawl (krawl) to move the body along the ground through a synchronized action of the hands and knees.

cream (krēm) 1. the fatty part of milk from which butter is prepared, or a fluid mixture of similar consistency. 2. in pharmaceutical preparations, a semisolid dosage form being either an emulsion of oil and water or an aqueous microcrystalline dispersion of a long-chain fatty acid or alcohol.

creatinase (kre-at′ĭ-nās) an enzyme that catalyzes the decomposition of creatine into urea and ammonia.

creatine (kre′ah-tin) a nonprotein substance synthesized in the body from three amino acids: arginine, glycine (aminoacetic acid), and methionine. Creatine readily combines with phosphate to form phosphocreatine, or creatine phosphate, which is present in muscle, where it serves as the storage form of high-energy phosphate necessary for muscle contraction.

c. kinase an enzyme catalyzing the transfer of a phosphate group from phosphocreatine to ATP. It has three isoenzymes: CK_1, found primarily in the brain; CK_2, found in the myocardium; and CK_3, found in both skeletal muscle and the myocardium. The presence of CK_2 in the blood is strongly indicative of a recent myocardial infarction; it is present until about 72 hours after the attack.

creatinemia (kre″ah-tĭ-ne′me-ah) excessive creatine in the blood.

creatinine (kre-at′ĭ-nin) a nitrogenous compound formed as the end product of CREATINE metabolism. It is formed in the muscle in relatively small amounts, passes into the blood and is excreted in the urine. A laboratory test for the creatinine level in the blood may be used as a measurement of kidney function (see creatinine CLEARANCE).

c. clearance test a test of renal function based on the rate of creatinine CLEARANCE.

creatinuria (kre″ah-tĭ-nu′re-ah) increased concentration of CREATINE in the urine, as seen in MUSCULAR DYSTROPHY, POLIOMYELITIS, and various other conditions.

Credé's method (maneuver) (krĕ-dāz′) a technique for manual expression of urine from the bladder used in BLADDER TRAINING for paralyzed patients: the hands are held flat against the abdomen, just below the umbilicus. A firm downward stroke toward the bladder is repeated six or seven times, followed by pressure from both hands placed directly over the bladder to manually remove all urine.

creep (krēp) 1. a physical property of materials that results in progressive deformation when a constant load is applied over time; it allows soft tissues to tolerate applied loads by lengthening. 2. to move along the ground using the arms and legs for propulsion. The trunk does not touch the ground.

cremasteric (kre″mas-ter′ik) pertaining to the cremaster muscle.

crenated (kre′nāt-ed) scalloped or notched.

crenation (kre-na′shun) 1. the formation of abnormal notching around the edge of an erythrocyte (burr CELL). 2. the notched appearance of an erythrocyte due to its shrinkage after suspension in a hypertonic solution.

crenocyte (kre′no-sīt) burr cell.

creosol (kre′o-sol) one of the active constituents of CREOSOTE.

creosote (kre′o-sōt) a mixture of phenols from wood tar, formerly used as an expectorant and external antiseptic and now mainly used as a wood preservative. A mixture of the carbonates of various constituents of creosote (creosote carbonate) is used as an expectorant and antiseptic.

crepitant (krep′ĭ-tant) having a dry, crackling sound.

crepitation (krep″ĭ-ta′shun) 1. a dry, crackling sound or sensation; see crepitant RALE. 2. a sound like that produced by the grating of the ends of a fractured bone.

crepitus (krep′ĭ-tus) 1. the discharge of flatus from the bowels. 2. crepitation. 3. crepitant RALE.

crescent (kres′ent) 1. shaped like a new moon. 2. something with this shape. adj., **crescen′tic.**

Giannuzzi's c's crescent-shaped patches of serous cells surrounding the mucous tubercles in mixed glands.

sublingual c. the crescent-shaped area on the floor of the mouth, bounded by the lingual wall of the mandible and the base of the tongue.

cresol (kre′sol) a phenol from coal or wood tar; a mixture of isomeric cresol from coal tar or petroleum is used as a disinfectant and in making synthetic resins. Acute poisoning may result in rapid circulatory collapse; chronic poisoning may produce gastrointestinal symptoms, vertigo, skin rashes, jaundice, and uremia.

crest (krest) a projection, or projecting structure or ridge, especially one surmounting a bone or its border.

alveolar c. alveolar RIDGE.

ampullar c., ampullary c. the most prominent part of a localized thickening of the membrane that lines the ampullae of the semicircular DUCTS, covered with NEUROEPITHELIUM containing endings of the vestibular nerve.

dental c. the maxillary ridge passing along the alveolar processes of the fetal maxillary bones.

iliac c. the thickened, expanded upper border of the ILIUM.

CREST syndrome one of the less severe forms of systemic SCLERODERMA, consisting of CALCINOSIS of the skin, RAYNAUD'S PHENOMENON, ESOPHAGEAL dysfunction, SCLERODACTYLY, and TELANGIECTASIA. When esophageal dysfunction is not prominent, it is known as CRST syndrome.

cretin (kre′tin) old term for a person with CRETINISM; now considered offensive.

cretinism (kre′tĭ-nizm) arrested physical and mental development with dystrophy of bones and soft tissues, due to congenital lack of THYROID GLAND secretion from hypofunction or absence of the gland. Affected children have a large head, short limbs, puffy eyes, coarse hair, a round abdomen, a thick and protruding tongue with drooling, excessively dry skin, lack of coordination, and mental retardation. Thyroid deficiency that is acquired or seen in adults is called MYXEDEMA. Administration of THYROID HORMONE medication, which must be continued for life, can result in normal growth and mental development of these children. If untreated, however, they will become permanently dwarfed, probably mentally retarded, and sterile.

cretinoid (kre′tĭ-noid) resembling or suggestive of CRETINISM.

cretinous (kre′tĭ-nus) affected with CRETINISM.

Creutzfeldt-Jakob disease (kroits′felt-yah′kōp) a rare PRION DISEASE, associated with a number of different mutations of the prion PROTEIN gene. There are sporadic, infectious, and familial forms, the last inherited as an autosomal dominant trait, with onset usually in middle life, and a wide variety of clinical and pathological features. The most commonly seen are varying degrees of spongiform degeneration of neurons, neuronal loss, GLIOSIS, and amyloid plaque formation, with rapidly progressive dementia. Death may come soon or after several years. Most cases are sporadic, although infectious cases may occur after surgical procedures or injection of hormone from infected pituitary glands. *New variant Creutzfeld-Jakob disease* is a variant seen almost exclusively in the United Kingdom, caused by the same agent that causes bovine spongiform ENCEPHALOPATHY ("mad cow disease") in cattle.

crevice (krev′is) a fissure.

gingival c. the space between the cervical enamel of a tooth and the overlying unattached gingiva.

cribriform (krib'rĭ-form) perforated like a sieve.

cricoarytenoid (kri″ko-ar″ĭ-te'noid) pertaining to the cricoid and arytenoid cartilages.

cricoid (kri'koid) 1. ring-shaped. 2. the cricoid cartilage.

cricoidectomy (kri″koi-dek'to-me) excision of the cricoid cartilage.

cricopharyngeal (kri″ko-fah-rin'je-al) pertaining to the cricoid cartilage and pharynx.

cricothyroid (kri″ko-thi'roid) pertaining to the cricoid and thyroid cartilages.

cricothyrotomy (kri″ko-thi-rot'ah-me) incision through the skin and cricothyroid membrane to secure a patent airway for emergency relief of upper airway obstruction. Called also intercricothyrotomy. (See illustration.)

cricotomy (kri-kot'ah-me) incision of the cricoid cartilage.

cricotracheotomy (kri″ko-tra″ke-ot'ah-me) incision of the trachea through the cricoid cartilage.

cri du chat syndrome (kre-du-shah) [Fr.] a hereditary congenital syndrome characterized by a wide space between the eyes, microcephaly, severe mental deficiency, and a plaintive catlike cry caused by laryngeal abnormalities, due to deletion of part of the short arm of chromosome 5. (See illustration.)

Crigler-Najjar disease (syndrome) (krig'ler naj'er) a congenital hereditary non-hemolytic jaundice due to absence of the hepatic enzyme glucuronide transferase, marked by excessive amounts of unconjugated bilirubin in the blood, kernicterus, and severe central nervous system disorders.

crisis (kri'sis), pl. *cri'ses* [L.] 1. the turning point of a disease for better or worse;

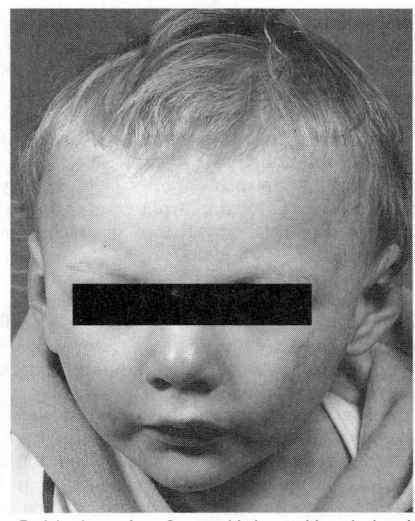

Facial view of a 2-year-old boy with cri du chat syndrome. From Mueller and Young, 2001.

especially a sudden change, usually for the better, in the course of an acute disease. 2. a sudden paroxysmal intensification of symptoms in the course of a disease. 3. life CRISIS.

addisonian c., adrenal c. the symptoms accompanying an acute onset or worsening of ADDISON'S DISEASE: anorexia, vomiting, abdominal pain, apathy, confusion, extreme weakness, and hypotension; if untreated these progress to shock and then death.

aplastic c. a SICKLE CELL CRISIS in which there is temporary bone marrow aplasia.

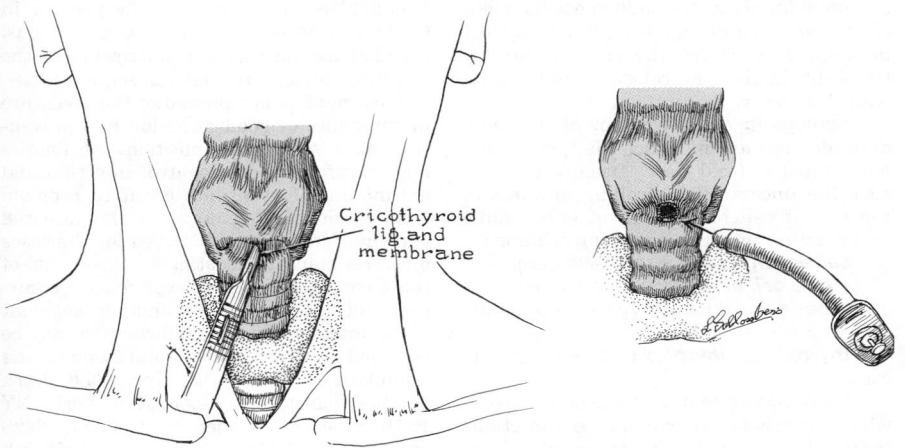

Cricothyrotomy. From Zuidema et al., 1985.

blast c. a sudden, severe change in the course of chronic granulocytic LEUKEMIA, characterized by an increased number of blasts, i.e., MYELOBLASTS or LYMPHOBLASTS.

catathymic c. an isolated, nonrepetitive act of violence that develops as a result of intolerable tension.

celiac c. an attack of severe watery diarrhea and vomiting producing dehydration and acidosis, sometimes occurring in infants with CELIAC DISEASE.

developmental c. maturational crisis.

hemolytic c. an uncommon SICKLE CELL CRISIS in which there is acute red blood cell destruction with jaundice.

hypertensive c. dangerously high BLOOD PRESSURE of acute onset.

identity c. a period in the psychosocial development of an individual, usually occurring during adolescence, manifested by a loss of the sense of the sameness and historical continuity of one's self, confusion over values, or an inability to accept the role the individual perceives as being expected by society.

life c. a period of disorganization that occurs when a person meets an obstacle to an important life goal, such as the sudden death of a family member, a difficult family conflict, an incident of domestic violence (spouse or child abuse), a serious accident, loss of a limb, loss of a job, or rape or attempted rape.

maturational c. a life CRISIS in which usual coping mechanisms are inadequate in dealing with a stress common to a particular stage in the life cycle or with stress caused by a transition from one stage to another. Called also developmental crisis.

myasthenic c. the sudden development of DYSPNEA requiring respiratory support in MYASTHENIA GRAVIS; the crisis is usually transient, lasting several days, and accompanied by fever.

oculogyric c. a symptom of an acute dystonic reaction in which the person demonstrates a fixed gaze, usually upward; also, the uncontrollable rolling upwards of the eye. It can be a result of encephalitis or a reaction to antipsychotic medications.

salt-losing c. see SALT-LOSING CRISIS.

sickle cell c. see SICKLE CELL CRISIS.

tabetic c. a painful paroxysm occurring in TABES DORSALIS.

thyroid c., thyrotoxic c. see THYROID CRISIS.

vaso-occlusive c. a SICKLE CELL CRISIS in which there is severe pain due to infarctions in the bones, joints, lungs, liver, spleen, kidney, eye, or central nervous system.

crista (kris'tah), pl. *cris'tae* [L.] crest.

cris'tae cu'tis dermal ridges.

c. gal'li a thick, triangular process projecting upward from the cribriform plate of the ethmoid bone.

critical path a concise document describing the common practices of all health care disciplines in relation to a specific type of case; it is a tool used in managed CARE and CASE MANAGEMENT representing specific practice patterns, patient populations, and limits on the length of stay. A critical path is a set of concurrent or sequential actions to achieve a goal or complete a project. The start and completion dates are the critical organizing factor. See also critical path DEVELOPMENT.

CRNA Certified Registered Nurse Anesthetist.

Crohn's disease (krōnz) inflammation of the gastrointestinal tract, usually the terminal portion of the ileum; called also Crohn's colitis, regional enteritis, and regional ileitis. The synonym "regional ileitis" is, however, misleading because Crohn's disease is not limited to the ileum.

Because it bears many similarities to ULCERATIVE COLITIS, Crohn's disease is sometimes considered as one manifestation of a disease entity called INFLAMMATORY BOWEL DISEASE. Like ulcerative colitis, Crohn's disease is a chronic, relapsing inflammatory disease that produces bouts of diarrhea, cramping of the abdomen, and fever. It is believed to be a genetic disorder, and is related in some way to an abnormal IMMUNE RESPONSE to an unidentified etiologic agent.

In contrast to ulcerative colitis, Crohn's disease only rarely is complicated by toxic megacolon and carcinoma of the colon. Rectal bleeding is not typically present in Crohn's disease, but abscesses, fistulas, perianal ulcerations, and narrowing of the intestinal lumen are common sequelae.

Treatment is symptomatic; the goals are maintenance of good nutrition and prevention of a secondary infection. Antibiotics may be prescribed to control infection and antiinflammatory agents given to promote healing. Surgical removal of the diseased portion of intestine is reserved for the cases most resistant to treatment, since half of those treated by surgery experience a recurrence of the disease in another segment of the intestine.Further information may be obtained by writing The Crohn's and Colitis Foundation of America Inc., 386 Park Avenue South, 17th floor, New York, NY 10016-8804, calling them at: 1-800-932-2423 or 1-212- 685-3440, or consulting their web site at http://www.ccfa.org.

cromolyn (kro′mō-lin) a drug that inhibits the release of chemical mediators of immediate sensitivity from basophils and mast cells, administered by inhalation or intranasally for prophylaxis and treatment of bronchial ASTHMA and allergic RHINITIS, orally for treatment of MASTOCYTOSIS, and topically to the conjunctiva for prevention and treatment of allergen-induced inflammation of the conjunctiva or cornea. It has the advantage of reducing or eliminating the need for steroids and sympathomimetics. Used in the form of its disodium salt, *cromolyn sodium*.

cross (kros) 1. a cross-shaped figure or structure. 2. any organism produced by CROSSBREEDING. 3. a method of crossbreeding.

crossbite (kros′bīt″) malocclusion in which the mandibular teeth are in buccal version (or completely lingual version in posterior segments) to the maxillary teeth.

crossbreeding (kros′brēd-ing) hybridization; the mating of organisms of different strains or species.

cross-cultural (kros″kul′cher-al) pertaining to the identification and analysis of distinct features of human behavior in different cultural, geographic, and social settings; intercultural and transcultural are sometimes substituted for this term.

cross-dressing (kros′dres-ing) the wearing of clothing specific to or characteristic of the opposite sex.

cross-eye esotropia.

crossing over the exchanging of material between homologous chromosomes, during the first meiotic division, resulting in new combinations of genes.

cross-link (kros′link″) a bond formed between polymer chains, either between different chains or between different parts of the same chain.

crossmatching (kros′mach′ing) a procedure vital in blood transfusions and organ transplantation. The recipient's erythrocytes or leukocytes are incubated with the donor's serum and vice versa. Various testing procedures are then performed to ensure that the donor and recipient have blood group COMPATIBILITY or HISTOCOMPATIBILITY. Also written *cross matching* and *cross-matching*.

cross-reaction (kros′re-ak-shun) an interaction between an antibody and an antigen closely related to the antigen that specifically stimulated synthesis of the antibody.

cross-reactivity (kros″re-ak-tiv′ĭ-te) the degree to which an antibody or antigen participates in CROSS-REACTIONS.

cross-resistance (kros-re-zis′tans) multidrug resistance.

crosstalk (kros′tawk) in cardiology, inappropriate detection of the atrial stimulus by the ventricular sensing mechanism, usually seen with dual chamber pacemakers; it can lead to ASYSTOLE. Pacemakers are now able to respond to crosstalk with an obligatory ventricular pacing stimulus at a shorter than average A-V interval.

cross-tolerance (kros′tol-er-ans) extension of the tolerance for a substance to others of the same class, even those to which the body has not been exposed previously.

crotalid (krot′ah-lid) pit viper.

Crotalus (krot′ah-lus) a large genus of venomous RATTLESNAKES with numerous species in North America and others in Central and South America. See also SNAKEBITE.

crotamiton (kro″tah-mi′ton) an ANTIPARASITIC used in the treatment of SCABIES; also used to relieve itching.

croup (krōōp) a condition resulting from acute partial obstruction of the upper airway, seen mainly in infants and young children; characteristics include resonant barking cough, hoarseness, and persistent stridor. It may be caused by a viral infection (usually a parainfluenzavirus), a bacterial infection (usually *Staphylococcus aureus, Streptococcus pneumoniae,* or *Streptococcus pyogenes,*) an allergy, a foreign body, or a tumor.

bacterial c., membranous c., pseudomembranous c. bacterial tracheitis.

Crouzon's disease (kroo-zonz′) craniofacial DYSOSTOSIS.

crown (krown) 1. the topmost part of an organ or structure, e.g., the top of the head. 2. artificial crown.

anatomical c. the upper, enamel-covered part of a tooth. (See illustration.)

artificial c. a metal, porcelain, or plastic reproduction of a crown affixed to the remaining natural structure of a tooth.

clinical c. that portion of a tooth visible above the gingiva.

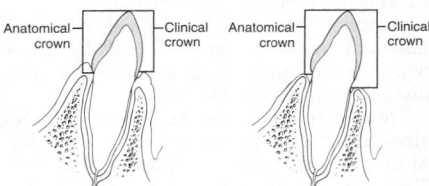

Anatomical and clinical crowns, demonstrating that the former are independent of the state of surrounding tissues while the latter depend on the height of the surrounding gingiva. From Dorland's, 2000.

crowning (krown'ing) the appearance of the fetal scalp at the vaginal orifice in childbirth.

CRP C-reactive protein.

CRST syndrome see CREST SYNDROME.

CRTT Certified Respiratory Therapy Technician.

crucial (kroo'shal) severe and decisive.

cruciate (kroo'she-āt) cruciform.

crucible (kroo'sĭ-b'l) a vessel for melting, burning, or dehydrating substances at high temperatures.

cruciform (kroo'sĭ-form) shaped like a cross; called also cruciate.

cruor (kroo'or) blood clot.

crurotomy (kroo-rot'ah-me) the cutting of a crus of the stapes, usually the anterior one.

crus (krus), pl. *cru'ra* [L.] 1. leg (def. 1). 2. a leglike part.

   c. ce'rebri basis pedunculi cerebri.

   c. of clitoris the continuation of the corpus cavernosum of the clitoris, diverging posteriorly to be attached to the pubic arch.

   crura of diaphragm two fibroelastic bands that arise from the lumbar vertebrae and insert into the central tendon of the diaphragm.

   crura of fornix two flattened bands of white matter that unite to form the body of the fornix of the cerebrum.

   c. of penis the continuation of each corpus cavernosum of the penis, diverging posteriorly to be attached to the pubic arch.

crush syndrome (krush) the edema, oliguria, and other symptoms of renal failure that follow crushing of a part, especially a large muscle mass, causing the release of myoglobin. See also RHABDOMYOLYSIS.

crust (krust) a formed outer layer, especially an outer layer of solid matter formed by drying of a bodily exudate or secretion.

   milk c. CRADLE CAP.

crusta (krus'tah), pl. *crus'tae* [L.] a crust.

   c. lac'tea CRADLE CAP.

Crustacea (krus-ta'shah) a class of ARTHROPODS including the lobsters, crabs, shrimps, wood lice, water fleas, and barnacles.

crutches (kruch'ez) artificial supports, made of wood or metal, used by those who need aid in walking because of injury, disease, or birth defect.

Types. Crutches are made in different sizes suitable for persons of various heights. Most are made of wood or tubular aluminum. The standard type is the tall crutch that fits under the armpit with double uprights and a small horizontal hand bar between them. The lower part may be adjustable to allow for extensions. There always should

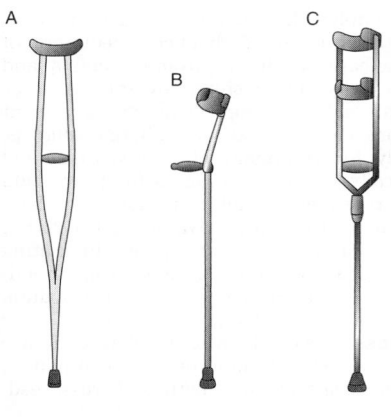

Axillary crutch   Lofstrand crutch   Elbow extension (Canadian) crutch

Types of crutches.

be a rubber tip at the base, preferably a suction tip, to prevent slipping.

Gaining in popularity is the Lofstrand crutch, which consists of a single tube of aluminum surmounted by a metal cuff that fits around the forearm. The user supports his weight on a handbar. He can release his hold on the handbar, as in grasping a handrail to climb stairs, without dropping the crutch. A variation of the Lofstrand crutch is the Canadian elbow extensor crutch, which goes farther up the arm.

In walking with crutches, the means of locomotion is transferred from the legs to the arms. The muscles of the arms, shoulders, back, and chest work together to manipulate the crutches. The kind of crutches used depends largely on the nature of the disability. In some cases, the legs may be partially able to function and bear some of the body's weight, so that there is less dependence on the crutches. In other cases, leg braces may be needed to supplement the crutches.

Gaits. The user is taught one of several standard methods or gaits, depending on the underlying condition. Eventually he or she should be able to master at least two gaits: a fast one for making speed in the open, and a slow one for crowded places, where the primary need is to maintain balance. A variety of gaits also helps to relieve fatigue because one set of muscles can rest while another works.In describing a gait each foot and crutch is called a point, so that a two-point gait, for example, means that two points of the total of four are in contact with the ground during the performance of one step. A three-point gait may be used when one leg is stronger than the other, meaning that two crutches and the weaker leg hit the ground simultaneously while the next step is made by the stronger leg alone. There is also the so-called tripod gait, swinging gait, and variations of them. (See accompanying illustration and see also GAIT ANALYSIS.)

Cruveilhier's disease (kroo-vāl-yāz′) 1. simple ulcer of the stomach. 2. spinal muscular atrophy.

Cruveilhier-Baumgarten syndrome (kroo-vāl-ya′ bowm′gahr-ten) cirrhosis of the liver with portal hypertension associated with congenital patency of the umbilical and paraumbilical veins.

cry(o)- word element [Gr.], *cold.*

cryalgesia (kri″al-je′ze-ah) pain on application of cold.

cryanesthesia (kri″an-es-the′zhah) loss of power of perceiving cold.

cryesthesia (kri″es-the′zhah) abnormal sensitiveness to cold.

cryoanalgesia (kri″o-an″al-je′ze-ah) the relief of pain by application of cold by cryoprobe to peripheral nerves.

cryoanesthesia (kri″o-an″es-the′zhah) local ANESTHESIA produced by applying a tourniquet and chilling the part to near freezing temperature; see also HYPOTHERMIA. Called also refrigeration anesthesia.

cryobank (kri′o-bank″) a facility for freezing and preserving semen at low temperatures (usually −196.5°C) for future use.

cryobiology (kri″o-bi-ol′o-je) the science dealing with the effect of low temperatures on biological systems.

cryocautery (kri′o-kaw″ter-e) CAUTERIZATION by freezing, using a substance such as liquid nitrogen or carbon dioxide snow, or a very cold instrument. Called also cold cautery.

cryoextraction (kri″o-eks-trak′shun) application of extremely low temperature for the removal of a lens that has a CATARACT.

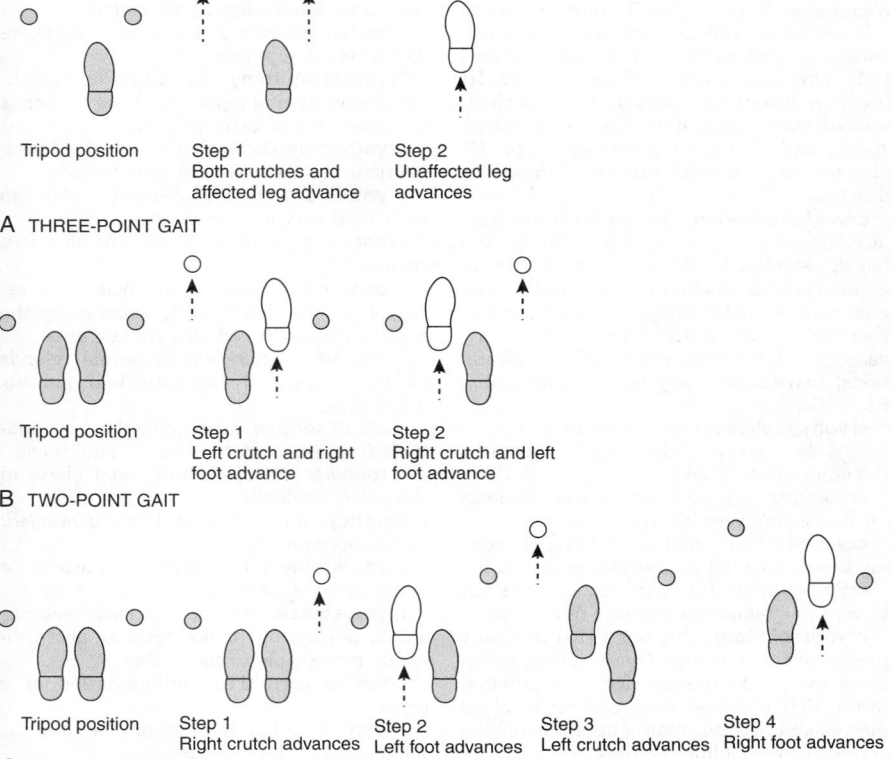

A THREE-POINT GAIT

Tripod position | Step 1 Both crutches and affected leg advance | Step 2 Unaffected leg advances

B TWO-POINT GAIT

Tripod position | Step 1 Left crutch and right foot advance | Step 2 Right crutch and left foot advance

C FOUR-POINT GAIT

Tripod position | Step 1 Right crutch advances | Step 2 Left foot advances | Step 3 Left crutch advances | Step 4 Right foot advances

Crutch-walking gaits. Note that all gaits begin from the tripod position.

cryoextractor (kri″o-eks-trak′ter) a cryoprobe used in cryoextraction.

cryofibrinogen (kri″o-fi-brin′o-jen) an abnormal fibrinogen that precipitates at low temperatures and redissolves at 37° C.

cryofibrinogenemia (kri″o-fi-brin″o-jĕne′me-ah) the presence of cryofibrinogen in the blood.

Cryogel (kri′o-jel) trademark name for a unit that can be used for therapeutic application of cold.

cryogenic (kri″o-jen′ik) producing low temperatures.

cryoglobulin (kri″o-glob′u-lin) a serum globulin (invariably an IMMUNOGLOBULIN) that precipitates at low temperature (e.g., 4°C) and redissolves at 37°C. Cryoglobulins are classified as *Type I,* monoclonal immunoglobulins; *Type II,* immune complexes involving monoclonal immunoglobulins with antibody activity against polyclonal immunoglobulins; or *Type III,* immune complexes involving polyclonal immunoglobulins (in most cases, these are globulin-antiglobulin immune complexes like Type II complexes). Types I and II occur in plasma cell DYSCRASIAS and LYMPHOPROLIFERATIVE DISORDERS as well as in asymptomatic "essential" CRYOGLOBULINEMIA. Types II and III occur in AUTOIMMUNE DISEASES such as rheumatoid ARTHRITIS, systemic LUPUS ERYTHEMATOSUS, and SJÖGREN'S SYNDROME. Type III also occurs in a wide variety of infectious diseases.

cryoglobulinemia (kri″o-glob″u-lin-e′me-ah) the presence of cryoglobulin in the blood, associated with a variety of clinical manifestations including Raynaud's phenomenon, vascular purpura, cold urticaria, necrosis of extremities, bleeding disorders, vasculitis, arthralgia, neurologic manifestations, hepatosplenomegaly, and glomerulonephritis.

cryohypophysectomy (kri-o-hi″po-fiz-ek′-to-me) destruction of the pituitary gland by the application of cold.

cryometer (kri-om′ĕ-ter) a thermometer for measuring very low temperature.

cryophilic (kri″o-fil′ik) preferring or growing best at low temperatures; psychrophilic.

cryophylactic (kri″o-fi-lak′tik) resistant to very low temperatures; said of bacteria.

cryoprecipitate (kri″o-pre-sip′ĭ-tāt) any precipitate that results from cooling, sometimes specifically the one rich in coagulation factor VIII obtained from cooling of blood plasma and used in treatment of hemophilia A (see antihemophilic FACTOR).

cryopreservation (kri″o-prez″er-va′shun) maintenance of the viability of excised tissue or organs by storing at very low temperatures.

cryoprobe (kri′o-prōb″) an instrument for applying extreme cold to tissue.

cryoprotective (kri″o-pro-tek′tiv) capable of protecting against injury due to freezing, as glycerol protects frozen red blood cells.

cryoprotein (kri″o-pro′tēn) a blood protein that precipitates on cooling.

cryoscopy (kri-os′kah-pe) examination of fluids based on the principle that the freezing point of a solution varies according to the amount and nature of the solute. adj., **cryoscop′ic.**

cryostat (kri′o-stat″) 1. a device by which temperature can be maintained at a very low level. 2. in pathology and histology, a chamber containing a microtome for sectioning frozen tissue.

cryosurgery (kri″o-ser′jer-e) destruction of tissue by application of extreme cold; SILVER NITRATE and solid CARBON DIOXIDE are commonly used. Uses include treatment of certain malignant lesions of the skin and mucous membranes, early removal of malignant lesions of the uterine cervix, and treatment of tumors that cannot be handled with traditional surgical techniques.

cryothalamectomy (kri″o-thal″ah-mek′to-me) cryothalamotomy.

cryothalamotomy (kri″o-thal″ah-mot′ah-me) destruction of a portion of the thalamus by application of extreme cold.

cryotherapy (kri″o-ther′ah-pe) the therapeutic use of cold; see also HYPOTHERMIA.

cryotolerant (kri″o-tol′er-ant) able to withstand very low temperatures.

crypt (kript) a blind pit or tube on a free surface.

 anal c's furrows, with pouchlike recesses at the lower end, separating the rectal columns; called also anal sinuses.

 c's of Lieberkühn intestinal glands on the surface of the intestinal mucous membrane.

 c's of tongue deep, irregular invaginations from the surface of the lingual tonsil.

 tonsillar c's epithelium-lined clefts in the palatine tonsils.

crypt(o)- word element [Gr.], *concealed; pertaining to a crypt.*

cryptectomy (krip-tek′to-me) excision or obliteration of a CRYPT.

cryptesthesia (krip″tes-the′zhah) subconscious perception of occurrences not ordinarily perceptible to the senses.

cryptitis (krip-ti′tis) inflammation of a crypt.

 anal c. inflammation of the mucous membrane of the anal CRYPTS.

cryptocephalus (krip″to-sef′ah-lus) 1. a developmental ANOMALY in which the head is inconspicuous. 2. a malformed fetus with this deformity.

cryptococcosis (krip″to-kok-o′sis) infection by *Cryptococcus neoformans,* which has a predilection for the brain and meninges but also invades the skin, lungs, and other parts. It is the most frequent fungal infection of the central nervous system, and the incidence is much higher in IMMUNOCOMPROMISED persons. Presenting symptoms of cryptococcosis of the central nervous system are often vague and include headache, subtle mental changes, and fever. Diagnosis is made by LUMBAR PUNCTURE. Treatment consists of intravenous amphotericin B or oral fluconazole. Supportive care will depend on the patient's symptoms.

Cryptococcus (krip″to-kok′us) a genus of yeastlike fungi. *C. neofor′mans* is a species of worldwide distribution that causes CRYPTOCOCCOSIS in humans.

cryptodeterminant (krip″to-de-ter′min-ant) hidden determinant.

cryptodidymus (krip″to-did′ĭ-mus) a developmental ANOMALY in which one fetus is enclosed within the body of the other.

cryptogenic (krip″to-jen′ik) of obscure or doubtful origin.

cryptoglioma (krip″to-gli-o′mah) a stage of retinal glioma in which the eyeball shrinks, masking the presence of the growth.

cryptolith (krip′to-lith) a concretion or STONE in a pit or blind tube of the body.

cryptomenorrhea (krip″to-men″o-re′ah) the occurrence of menstrual symptoms without external bleeding, as in imperforate hymen.

cryptomerorachischisis (krip″to-me″ro-rah-kis′kĭ-sis) spina bifida occulta.

cryptomnesia (krip″tom-ne′zhah) the recall of memories not recognized as such but thought to be original creations. adj., **cryptomne′sic.**

cryptophthalmia (krip″tof-thal′me-ah) cryptophthalmos.

cryptophthalmos (krip″tof-thal′mos) congenital absence of the palpebral fissure, the skin extending from the forehead to the cheek, with the eyeball malformed or rudimentary. Called also cryptophthalmia and cryptophthalmus.

cryptophthalmus (krip″tof-thal′mus) cryptophthalmos.

cryptopodia (krip″to-po′de-ah) swelling of the lower leg and foot, covering all but the sole of the foot.

cryptorchid (krip-tor′kid) 1. having undescended testes. 2. a male with undescended testes; see also CRYPTORCHIDISM.

cryptorchidectomy (krip″tor-kĭ-dek′to-me) excision of an undescended testis.

cryptorchidism (krip-tor′kid-izm) failure of one or both of the testes to descend into the scrotum. As the unborn male child develops, the testes first appear in the abdomen at about the level of the kidneys. They develop at this site, and in approximately the seventh month of fetal life start to descend to the upper part of the groin. From there they move into the inguinal canal and then, normally, into the scrotum. In its descent, a testis may sometimes be halted in the abdomen or within the canal, becoming an undescended testis. An improperly developed testis may never leave the abdomen, and it may not produce the hormones that induce secondary sex characters. A testis lodged in the canal may well produce these secondary sex characters, but cannot produce spermatozoa. Cases in which both testes fail to descend are uncommon; usually only one is involved and the other produces sufficient numbers of spermatozoa.

Treatment. Often the undescended testis can be brought down into the scrotum by medical treatment with the gonadotropic hormone, and for physical and psychologic reasons this method is preferred. Frequently, however, surgery (called ORCHIOPEXY) is required. This operation is not particularly serious and is usually successful. It is best performed before the patient is 5 to 7 years old, since operating at a later age may involve more risk to the cells that produce spermatozoa.

cryptorchism (krip-tor′kizm) cryptorchidism.

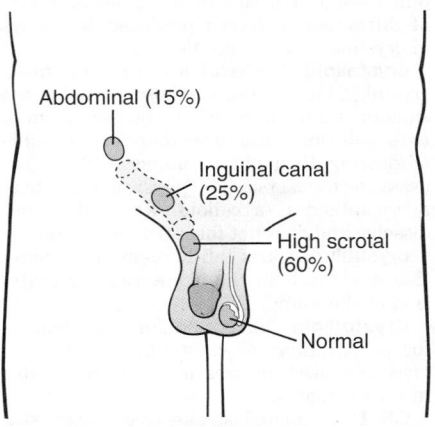

In cryptorchidism, the testis is not in the scrotum, but may be found in the inguinal canal or in the abdominal cavity. From Damjanov, 2000.

cryptosporidiosis (krip″to-spo-rid″e-o′sis) infection with protozoa of the genus *Cryptosporidium,* which may be associated with or contribute to enteric disease in calves, lambs, foals, and piglets. Human infection occurs both in immunocompetent persons, in whom it causes a self-limited diarrhea syndrome, and in immunocompromised patients, in whom it is much more serious, being manifested clinically as prolonged debilitating diarrhea, weight loss, fever, and abdominal pain, with occasional spread to the trachea and bronchial tree.

Cryptosporidium (krip″to-spo-rid′e-um) a genus of minute coccidian protozoa; they are parasitic in the intestinal tracts of many different vertebrates, including reptiles, birds, and mammals. See also CRYPTOSPORIDIOSIS.

cryptozygous (krip″to-zi′gus) having the calvaria wider than the face, so that the zygomatic ARCHES are concealed when the head is viewed from above.

crystal (kris′t'l) a homogeneous angular solid of definite form, with systematically arranged elemental units.

hydroxyapatite c. microscopic crystals of hydroxyapatite occurring in joints or bursae in a variety of connective tissue disorders.

crystallin (kris′tah-lin) a globulin in the crystalline lens of the eye.

crystalline (kris′tah-lin) 1. resembling a crystal in nature or clearness. 2. pertaining to crystals.

crystallography (kris″tah-log′rah-fe) the science dealing with the study of crystals.

x-ray c. the determination of the three-dimensional structure of molecules by means of diffraction patterns produced by x-rays of crystals of the molecules.

crystalloid (kris′tah-loid) 1. resembling a crystal. 2. a substance whose particles are smaller than those of a COLLOID, form a true solution, and are therefore capable of passing through a semipermeable MEMBRANE, as in DIALYSIS. The physical opposite of a crystalloid is a colloid, which does not dissolve and does not form true solutions.

crystalluria (kris″tah-lu′re-ah) the excretion of crystals in the urine, causing irritation of the kidney.

Crystodigin (kris″to-dij′in) trademark for preparations of crystalline DIGITOXIN, a glycoside used in treatment of congestive HEART FAILURE.

CS 1. completed stroke (see STROKE SYNDROME); *o*-chlorobenzylidenemalononitrile. 2. *o*-chlorobenzylidenemalononitrile, a commonly used tear GAS.

Cs cesium.

CSF cerebrospinal fluid.

CSM cerebrospinal meningitis.

C-spine cervical spine.

CT computed tomography.

C-terminal (ter′min-al) the end of the peptide chain carrying the free alpha carboxyl group of the last amino acid, conventionally written to the right. See also N-TERMINAL.

CTN Certified Transcultural Nurse.

Cu copper (L. *cu′prum*).

cu cubic.

cubital (ku′bĭ-tal) pertaining to the ELBOW; called also anconal and anconeal.

cubitus (ku′bĭ-tus) 1. elbow. 2. the entire upper limb distal to the humerus, including elbow, forearm, and hand. 3. ulna. adj., **cu′bital.**

c. val′gus deformity of the elbow in which it deviates away from the midline of the body when extended.

c. va′rus deformity of the elbow in which it deviates toward the midline of the body when extended.

cuboid (ku′boid) resembling a cube; applied particularly to a bone of the foot. See anatomic Table of Bones in the Appendices.

cueing (ku′ing) assisting an individual in the completion of a task by offering prompts.

cuffing (kuf′ing) formation of a cufflike surrounding border, as of leukocytes about a blood vessel observed in certain infections.

cuirass (kwe-ras′) a covering for the chest.

cul-de-sac (kul-dah-sak′) [Fr.] a pouch or tubular cavity closed at one end; called also caecum.

conjunctival c. the fold formed by the junction of the palpebral and the ocular conjunctiva; called also fornix of conjunctiva.

Douglas' c. a sac or recess formed by a fold of the peritoneum dipping down between the rectum and the uterus; called also rectouterine excavation or pouch.

culdocentesis (kul″do-sen-te′sis) transvaginal puncture of Douglas' cul-de-sac for aspiration of fluid.

culdoscope (kul′do-skōp) an endoscope used in culdoscopy.

culdoscopy (kul-dos′kah-pe) direct visual examination of the female viscera through an endoscope introduced into the pelvic cavity through the posterior vaginal fornix.

Culex (ku′leks) a genus of mosquitoes found throughout the world; many species transmit various disease-producing agents, e.g., microfilariae, sporozoa, and viruses.

culicide (ku′lĭ-sīd) an agent that destroys mosquitoes.

culicifuge (ku-lis'ĭ-fūj) an agent that repels culicine mosquitoes.

culicine (ku'lĭ-sin, ku'lĭ-sīn) 1. any member of the genus *Culex* or related genera. 2. pertaining to, involving, or affecting mosquitoes of the genus *Culex* or related species.

Cullen's sign (kul'enz) bluish discoloration around the umbilicus sometimes occurring in intraperitoneal hemorrhage, especially following rupture of the fallopian tube in ectopic pregnancy. A similar discoloration is seen in acute hemorrhagic pancreatitis.

culmen (kul'men), pl. *cul'mina* 1. acme or summit. 2. culmen cerebelli.

c. cerebel'li, c. of cerebellum the portion of the rostral lobe of the cerebellum that lies medially between the central lobule and the primary fissure.

cultivation (kul"tĭ-va'shun) the propagation of living organisms, applied especially to the growth of microorganisms or other cells in artificial media.

Cultural Care Diversity and Universality a theory of nursing formulated by Madeleine M. LEININGER, which evolved from

her study of nursing and anthropology and her clinical experiences; it recognizes culture as a missing link in nursing knowledge and practice. The concept of culture is derived from ANTHROPOLOGY, and the concept of care is identified as the essence of nursing. The ultimate goal of the theory is to provide culture-congruent nursing care practices. The SUNRISE MODEL was developed to depict the components of the theory, which posits that culture care has a WORLD VIEW and cultural and social structure learned through language and environment, which influence care and health patterns and expressions of individuals, families, groups, and institutions, all of which participate in diverse health systems, including both folk and professional systems. To provide culture congruent care, nurses use knowledge gained through analysis of the components of the model to make nursing care decisions based on cultural care preservation/maintenance, cultural care accommodation/negotiation, or cultural care repatterning/restructuring.

WINDOW ON CULTURAL CARE DIVERSITY AND UNIVERSALITY

The theory of Cultural Care Diversity and Universality holds that there are diverse and similar forms, expressions, values, patterns, and practices of care in Western and non-Western cultures. The theorist seeks to discover what is universal and diverse about human care worldwide. I predict that discovering, understanding, and using culturally based patterns of culture care with appropriate professional nursing care practices are essential to provide culturally congruent nursing care that is beneficial and satisfying to clients. The theorist contends that: 1) Culture care is essential for human growth, development, and survival, and to face death, 2) Culture care is essential to caring, for there can be no curing without caring, 3) Every culture has generic (lay, folk, or naturalistic) care and usually professional (learned and practiced) care, 4) Culture care values, beliefs, and practices tend to be embedded in world view and social structure features, i.e., religion, kinship, culture values, education, politics, technology, and economics, 5) Culture care differences between care-giver(s) and care-receivers may be quite striking and lead to different care outcomes or consequences, 6) The use of culture-specific care leads to indicators of health and well-being,

7) Nursing is a transcultural profession requiring exquisite transcultural nursing knowledge and skills. The Sunrise Model depicts the components of the theory, positing that culture care is influenced by and can explain health or well-being through in-depth and systematic study of the world view, cultural, and social features, and through the language, ethnohistory, and environmental context of individuals, families, groups, institutions, and communities who participate in generic and/or professional nursing in health care systems. Research findings explicated from these areas are essential to guide nurses to provide culturally congruent care through three modes of decisions or action: culture care preservation or maintenance, culture care accommodation, and negotiation or culture care repatterning and restructuring. Most importantly, this theory can be used to research and assess in all cultures and subcultures in the world and with either qualitative or quantitative paradigms. The construct of culturally competent care was coined by me in the 1960s as the goal of the Theory of Culture Care.

Madeleine Leininger, PhD, RN,
CTN, LHD, DS, FAAN

culture (kul′cher) 1. the propagation of microorganisms or of living tissue cells in special media conducive to their growth. 2. to induce such propagation. 3. the product of such propagation. 4. the shared values, beliefs, and practices of a particular group of people, which are transmitted from one generation to the next and are identified as patterns that guide the thinking and action of the group members. adj., **cul′tural.**

cell c. the maintenance or growth of animal cells in vitro, or a culture of such cells.

blood c. microbiologic examination of a blood sample to check for presence of microorganisms.

continuous flow c. the cultivation of bacteria in a continuous flow of fresh medium to maintain bacterial growth in logarithmic phase.

enrichment c. one grown on a medium, usually liquid, that has been supplemented to encourage the growth of a given type of organism.

hanging-drop c. a culture in which the material to be cultivated is inoculated into a drop of fluid attached to a coverglass inverted over a hollow slide.

primary c. a cell or tissue culture made by direct transfer from a natural source to an artificial medium.

selective c. one grown on a medium, usually solid, that has been supplemented to encourage the growth of a single species of microorganism. It may also include substances that inhibit the growth of other species.

shake c. a culture made by inoculating warm liquid agar culture medium in a tube and shaking to distribute contents evenly. Incubation of the resolidified culture allows the development of separated colonies; especially adaptable to obligate anaerobes.

slant c. one made on the surface of solidified medium in a tube which has been tilted to provide a greater surface area for growth.

c.-specific syndrome folk illnesses that are unique to a particular culture or geographical area. Each illness has a cluster of symptoms, signs, and behavioral changes that are recognized by members of the culture; usually, they also have a range of symbolic meanings and culturally agreed-upon treatments. Anorexia nervosa and Type A behavior pattern are examples of syndromes specific to industrialized cultures.

stab c. a culture into which the organisms are introduced by thrusting a needle deep into the medium.

streak c. a culture in which the surface of a solid medium is inoculated by drawing across it, in a zig-zag fashion, a wire inoculating loop carrying the inoculum.

suspension c. a culture in which cells multiply while suspended in a suitable medium.

tissue c. the maintaining or growing of tissue, organ primordia, or the whole or part of an organ in vitro so as to preserve its architecture and function.

type c. a culture of a species of microorganism usually maintained in a central collection of type cultures.

cumulus (ku′mu-lus), pl. *cu′muli* [L.] a small elevation.

c. oo′phorus a mass of follicular cells surrounding the ovum in the vesicular ovarian follicle.

cuneate (ku′ne-āt) wedge-shaped.

cuneiform (ku-ne′ĭ-form) wedge-shaped; applied particularly to three of the tarsal bones of the foot. See anatomic Table of Bones in the Appendices.

cuneus (ku′ne-us), pl. *cu′nei* [L.] a wedge-shaped lobule on the medial aspect of the occipital lobe of the cerebrum.

cuniculus (ku-nik′u-lus), pl. *cuni′culi* [L.] 1. a tunnel. 2. a burrow in the skin made by the itch mite, *Sarcoptes scabiei.*

cunnilingus (kun″ĭ-lin′gus) oral stimulation of the female genitals.

cup (kup) a depression or hollow.

eye c. 1. eyecup (def. 1). 2. excavation of optic disk.

glaucomatous c. a depression of the optic disk due to persistently increased intraocular pressure, broader and deeper than a physiologic cup, and occurring first at the temporal side of the disk.

physiologic c. excavation of optic disk.

cupola (ku′pŏ-lah) cupula.

cupping (kup′ing) 1. the formation of a cup-shaped depression. 2. percussion (def. 2). 3. the application of heated cups to the skin, creating suction. It is used in some cultures to treat headache, fever, chills, back pain, and similar complaints.

cupric (ku′prik) pertaining to or containing divalent copper.

c. sulfate a crystalline salt of copper used as an emetic, astringent, and fungicide, as an oral antidote to phosphorus poisoning, as a topical treatment of cutaneous phosphorus burns, and as a catalyst in iron deficiency anemia.

cupriuria (koo″pre-u′re-ah) hypercupriuria.

cuprous (ku′prus) pertaining to or containing monovalent copper.

cupruresis (ku″proo-re′sis) hypercupriuria.

cupula (ku′pu-lah), pl. *cu′pulae* [L.] a small, inverted cup or dome-shaped cap over a structure.

cupulolithiasis (ku″pu-lo-lĭ-thi′ah-sis) the presence of calculi in the cupula of the posterior semicircular duct.

curare (koo-rah′re) any of a wide variety of highly toxic extracts from various botanical sources, including various species of *Strychnos,* a genus of tropical trees; used originally as arrow poisons in South America. A form extracted from the shrub *Chondodendron tomentosum* has been used as a skeletal muscle RELAXANT.

curarization (koo″rar-ĭ-za′shun) administration of CURARE (usually in the form of TUBOCURARINE) to induce muscle relaxation.

curb cut (kerb kut) a portion of the curb that is removed so that the sidewalk gently slopes to the street, thus increasing access to the environment for individuals in wheelchairs.

cure (kūr) 1. the course of treatment of any disease, or of a special case. 2. the successful treatment of a disease or wound. 3. a system of treating diseases. 4. a medicine effective in treating a disease.

curet (ku-ret′) curette.

curettage (ku″rĕ-tahzh′) [Fr.] removal of material from the wall of a cavity or other surface by scraping with a CURETTE.

  suction c., vacuum c., a method of induced ABORTION, consisting of removal of the uterine contents, after dilatation, by means of a hollow curette introduced into the uterus, through which suction is applied.

curette (ku-ret′) 1. a loop, ring, or spoon-shaped instrument, attached to a handle and having sharp or blunt edges; used to scrape tissue from a surface. 2. to remove growths or other material from the wall of a cavity or other surface, using a curette.

curettement (ku-ret′ment) curettage.

curie (Ci) (ku′re) a unit of radioactivity, defined as the quantity of any radioactive nuclide in which the number of disintegrations per second is 3.700×10^{10}.

curie-hour (ku′re-owr″) a unit of dose equivalent to that obtained by exposure for one hour to radioactive material disintegrating at the rate of 3.7×10^{10} atoms per second.

curium (Cm) (ku′re-um) a chemical element, atomic number 96, atomic weight 247. (See Appendix 6.)

current (kur′ent) 1. something that flows. 2. specifically, electricity transmitted through a CIRCUIT.

  alternating c. a current that periodically flows in opposite directions; its AMPLITUDE fluctuates as a sine wave.

  convection c. a current caused by movement by CONVECTION of warmer fluid into an area of cooler fluid.

  direct c. a current that flows in one direction only; when modeled as a wave, its AMPLITUDE is constant. When used medically it is called *galvanic current.* This current has distinct and important polarity and marked secondary chemical effects.

  galvanic c. a steady direct CURRENT.

  c. of injury an electric current that flows between injured myocardium and normal myocardium, because such cells have a reduced membrane POTENTIAL; it may be either *diastolic* or *systolic.*

  c. of injury, diastolic the current that flows from injured to noninjured tissue during electrical DIASTOLE.

  c. of injury, systolic the current that flows from healthy tissue to injured tissue during electrical systole.

  inwardly rectifying c. current that RECTIFIES so that it passes more easily towards the interior of a cell.

  leakage c. the electrical current that exists in the parts or metal case of electrical equipment.

  outwardly rectifying c. current that RECTIFIES so that it passes more easily towards the exterior of a cell.

  potassium rectifying c's transmembrane currents that RECTIFY inwardly or outwardly to make adjustments in cellular functions; they are mainly responsible for the REPOLARIZATION phase of the ACTION POTENTIAL. There are at least six mechanisms by which potassium ions move across cardiac cell membranes in the role of rectifier.

curvature (ker′vah-chur) a nonangular deviation from a normally straight course.

  greater c. of stomach the left or lateral and inferior border of the stomach, marking the inferior junction of the anterior and posterior surfaces.

  lesser c. of stomach the right or medial border of the stomach, marking the superior junction of the anterior and posterior surfaces.

  penile c. curvature of the penis to one side when erect; called also clubbed penis.

  Pott's c. abnormal posterior curvature of the spine occurring as a result of POTT'S DISEASE.

  spinal c. abnormal deviation of the vertebral column, as in KYPHOSIS, LORDOSIS, and SCOLIOSIS.

curve (kerv) a line that is not straight, or that describes part of a circle, especially a line representing varying values in a graph.

  dose-effect c., dose-response c., a graphic representation of the effect caused by an agent (such as a drug or radiation) plotted against the dose, showing the relationship of the effect to changes in the dose.

growth c. the curve obtained by plotting increase in size or numbers against the elapsed time.

oxyhemoglobin dissociation c. a graphic curve representing the normal variation in the amount of oxygen that combines with hemoglobin as a function of the partial pressures of oxygen and carbon dioxide. The curve is said to shift to the right when less than a normal amount of oxygen is taken up by the blood at a given Po_2, and to shift to the left when more than a normal amount is taken up. Factors influencing the shape of the curve include changes in the blood pH, Pco_2, and temperature; the presence of carbon monoxide; alterations in the constituents of the erythrocytes; and certain disease states.

pulse c. sphygmogram.

Spee c., c. of Spee the anatomic curvature of the occlusal alignment of teeth, beginning at the tip of the lower canine, following the buccal cusps of the premolars and molars, and continuing to the anterior border of the ramus.

strength-duration c. a graphic representation of the relationship between the intensity of an electric stimulus at the motor point of a muscle and the length of time it must flow to elicit a minimal contraction; see also CHRONAXIE and RHEOBASE. In cardiac pacing it is useful in determining characteristics of a particular pacing electrode and determining the most efficient selection of pacing parameters for an appropriate safety margin.

survival c. a graph of the probability of survival versus time, commonly used to present the results of clinical trials, e.g., a graph of the fraction of patients surviving (until death, relapse, or some other defined endpoint) at each time after a certain therapeutic procedure.

Curvularia (ker″vu-lar′e-ah) a genus of imperfect fungi commonly found in soil and elsewhere; *C. luna′ta* is found in human MYCETOMAS.

Cushing's disease (koosh′ingz) Cushing's syndrome in which the hyperadrenocorticism is secondary to excessive pituitary excretion of adrenocorticotropic hormone.

Cushing's syndrome (koosh′ingz) a group of symptoms produced by an excess of free circulating cortisol from the ADRENAL CORTEX. This may be the result of: (1) excessive secretion of adrenocorticotropic hormone (ACTH) from the pituitary gland, which

may actually result from faulty release of corticotropin-releasing factor from the hypothalamus; (2) tumor of the adrenal cortex, causing hypersecretion of the glucocorticoids; (3) ectopic production of ACTH by extrapituitary tumors, most commonly lung carcinoma, medullary thyroid carcinoma, and thymoma; and (4) *iatrogenic* Cushing's syndrome resulting from overzealous administration of exogenous glucocorticoids.

Diagnosis of the disorder is established by laboratory findings of a continuous elevation of plasma CORTISOL. The symptoms and signs are a result of the action of this hormone and include fatty swellings in the interscapular area (buffalo hump) and in the facial area (moon face), distention of the abdomen, ecchymoses following even minor trauma, impotence, amenorrhea, high blood pressure, osteoporosis, and general weakness due to excessive protein catabolism and loss of muscle mass. There also can be hirsutism in females and streaked purple markings (atrophic striae) in the abdominal area as a result of collections of body fat. Patients who have a familial predisposition to diabetes mellitus frequently develop insulin-dependent diabetes mellitus as a result of the anti-insulin, diabetogenic properties of cortisol.

Treatment of Cushing's syndrome is becoming more effective as new modes of therapy become available. Pituitary Cushing's syndrome can be treated by surgical excision of the neoplasm using microsurgical techniques. Radiation with cobalt also is helpful in some cases. Drug therapy using adrenocorticolytic agents may be used as an adjunct to surgery and radiation or as an alternative when these modes of therapy are not feasible.

cushingoid (koosh′ing-oid) resembling the features, symptoms, and signs associated with CUSHING'S SYNDROME.

cushion (koosh′un) a fleshy, padlike anatomical structure.

endocardial c's swellings that form on the dorsal and ventral walls of the atrioventricular canal of the embryonic heart during the fourth week of gestation. As they are invaded by mesenchymal cells during the fifth week, they approach each other and fuse, dividing the atrioventricular canal into right and left canals.

cusp (kusp) a pointed or rounded projection, such as on the crown of a tooth, or a segment of a cardiac VALVE. See also VALVULA.

Carabelli c. an accessory fifth cusp on the lingual surface of many maxillary first molars; it may be unilateral or bilateral and varies in size from person to person.

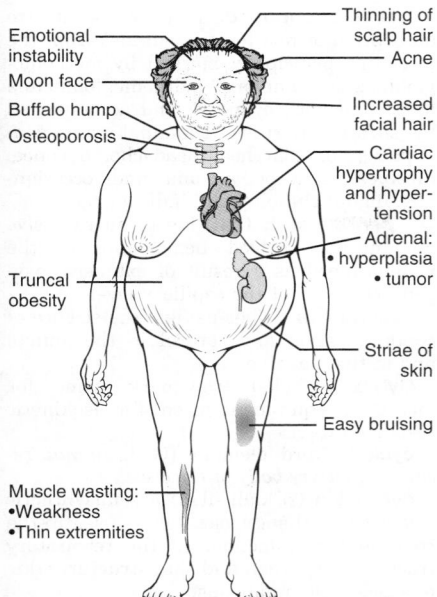

Emotional instability
Moon face
Buffalo hump
Osteoporosis
Truncal obesity
Muscle wasting:
•Weakness
•Thin extremities

Thinning of scalp hair
Acne
Increased facial hair
Cardiac hypertrophy and hypertension
Adrenal:
• hyperplasia
• tumor
Striae of skin
Easy bruising

Cushing's syndrome. From Damjanov, 1996.

semilunar c. any of the semilunar segments of the aortic VALVE (having posterior, right, and left cusps) or the pulmonary VALVE (having anterior, right, and left cusps).

cuspid (kus′pid) 1. having a CUSP. 2. cuspid tooth; see TOOTH. 3. pertaining to a cuspid tooth.

cuspis (kus′pis), pl. *cus′pides* [L.] cusp.

cutaneous (ku-ta′ne-us) pertaining to skin.

cutdown (kut′down) creation of a small incised opening, especially in a vein (venous cutdown) for venipuncture and venous access.

cuticle (ku′tĭ-k'l) 1. a layer of more or less solid substance covering the free surface of an epithelial cell. 2. the narrow band of epidermis extending from the nail wall onto the nail surface; called also eponychium and perionychium.

enamel c. primary cuticle.

primary c. a film on the enamel of unerupted teeth, considered to be the final product of degenerating ameloblasts after completion of enamel formation. Called also enamel cuticle and Nasmyth's membrane.

cutireaction (ku″tĭ-re-ak′shun) an inflammatory or irritative reaction of the skin, occurring in certain infectious diseases, or on application or injection of a preparation of the organism causing the disease.

cutis (ku′tis) skin.

c. anseri′na goose flesh.

c. hyperelas′tica Ehlers-Danlos syndrome.

c. lax′a a group of connective tissue disorders in which the skin hangs in loose pendulous folds, believed to be associated with decreased elastic tissue formation as well as an abnormality in elastin formation, and usually occurring as a hereditary disorder and occasionally in an acquired form.

cuvette (ku-vet′) [Fr.] a glass container generally having well-defined characteristics (dimensions, optical properties), used to contain solutions or suspensions for study.

CVA cerebral vascular accident; costovertebral angle.

CVID common variable immunodeficiency.

CVP central venous pressure.

cwt hundredweight.

Cx complaints.

cyan(o)- word element [Gr.], *blue.*

cyanhemoglobin (si″an-he′mo-glo″bin) a compound formed by the combination of hydrogen cyanide with hemoglobin; it gives the bright red color to the blood that is seen in cyanide poisoning.

cyanide (si′ah-nīd) a binary compound containing the radical CN— (cyanogen); since cyanide prevents tissue use of oxygen, most of its compounds are deadly poisons. Some inorganic compounds, such as cyanide salts, potassium cyanide, and sodium cyanide, are important in industry for extracting gold and silver from their ores or in electroplating, and other cyanide compounds are used in manufacture of synthetic rubber and textiles or as pesticides.

c. poisoning poisoning by cyanide or one of its compounds; most cyanide compounds are deadly poisons. Characteristics include nausea without vomiting, dizziness, convulsions, opisthotonos, and death from respiratory paralysis.

Treatment varies according to the nature of the poison. In the case of swallowed poison like hydrocyanic acid, the poison itself will cause vomiting. If the victim is able to swallow, milk or water may be given. A large dose of hydrocyanic acid will cause almost instant death. If a gas such as hydrogen cyanide has been inhaled, the victim should be taken into open air and given artificial respiration. Sodium thiosulfate and sodium nitrate are used as antidotes to cyanide poisoning.

While poisoning may occur following exposure to any substance that releases cyanide ions, it can also occur concurrently if another toxic ion is present (for example, with mercuric cyanide). In such a situation, ironically the symptoms of toxicity may change to those of the second ion when the antidote to cyanide is used.

cyanmethemoglobin (si″an-met-he′mo-glo″bin) a tightly bound complex of methemoglobin with the cyanide ion. The standard method of HEMOGLOBINOMETRY (measuring hemoglobin content) is determination of the amount of this compound after it is produced quantitatively from oxyhemoglobin, deoxyhemoglobin, carboxyhemoglobin, or methemoglobin (it cannot be produced from sulfhemoglobin).

cyanmetmyoglobin (si″an-met-mi′o-glo″-bin) a compound formed from metmyoglobin by addition of the cyanide ion.

Cyanobacteria the blue-green bacteria (formerly called blue-green algae), a subgroup of the kingdom Procaryotae, unicellular or filamentous phototrophic organisms that use water as an electron donor and produce oxygen in the presence of light. They are the only organisms that fix both carbon dioxide (in the presence of light) and nitrogen. Most species are photosynthetic and many are strong nitrogen fixers. Several species are common causes of water pollution and are often used as indicators of EUTROPHICATION of lakes and streams.

cyanocobalamin (si″ah-no-ko-bal′ah-min) 1. vitamin B_{12}, a substance having hematopoietic activity found in liver, fish meal, eggs, and other natural sources, or produced from cultures of *Streptomyces griseus;* it combines with intrinsic factor for absorption and is needed for erythrocyte maturation. Absence of intrinsic factor leads to malabsorption of cyanocobalamin and results in pernicious anemia. Called also extrinsic factor. See also VITAMIN.

c. Co-57 a radiopharmaceutical used in the SCHILLING TEST for the diagnosis of PERNICIOUS ANEMIA.

cyanolabe (si′ah-no-lāb″) the pigment in retinal cones that is more sensitive to the blue range of the spectrum than are chlorolabe and erythrolabe.

cyanopsia (si-ah-nop′se-ah) a chromatopsia in which objects appear tinged with blue.

cyanosed (si′ah-nōsd) cyanotic.

cyanosis (si″ah-no′sis) a bluish discoloration of the skin and mucous membranes due to excessive concentration of reduced hemoglobin in the blood. adj., **cyanot′ic.**

central c. that due to arterial unsaturation, the aortic blood carrying reduced hemoglobin.

enterogenous c. a syndrome due to absorption of nitrites and sulfides from the intestine, principally marked by methemoglobinemia and/or sulfhemoglobinemia associated with cyanosis, and accompanied by severe enteritis, abdominal pain, constipation or diarrhea, headache, dyspnea, dizziness, syncope, anemia, and, occasionally, digital clubbing and indicanuria.

peripheral c. that due to an excessive amount of reduced hemoglobin in the venous blood as a result of extensive oxygen extraction at the capillary level.

cybernetics (si″ber-net′iks) the science of communication and control in the animal and in the machine.

Cybex (si′beks) trademark name for pieces of equipment used for isokinetic resistive exercises.

cycl(o)- word element [Gr.], *round; recurring; ciliary body of the eye.*

cyclacillin (si″klah-sil′in) a semisynthetic PENICILLIN of the AMPICILLIN class used in the treatment of infections of the respiratory tract, urinary tract, and skin structures due to susceptible organisms.

cyclamate (si′klah-māt) a non-nutritive sweetener; nonprescription use of this substance in the United States was banned when animal testing showed that it may be carcinogenic.

cyclandelate (si-klan′dĕ-lāt) an antispasmodic acting on smooth muscle; used as a VASODILATOR for peripheral vascular disease.

cyclarthrosis (si″klahr-thro′sis) a pivot joint.

cyclase (si′klās) an enzyme that catalyzes the formation of a cyclic phosphodiester.

cycle (si′k'l) a succession or recurring series of events.

cardiac c. a complete cardiac movement, or heart beat, including systole, diastole, and the intervening pause. (See accompanying illustration.)

cell c. the cycle of biochemical and morphological events occurring in a reproducing cell population; it consists of the S phase, occurring toward the end of interphase, in which DNA is synthesized; the G_2 phase, a relatively quiescent period; the M phase, consisting of the four phases of mitosis; and the G_1 phase of interphase, which lasts until the S phase of the next cycle.

citric acid c. tricarboxylic acid cycle.

estrous c. the recurring periods of ESTRUS in adult females of most mammalian species and the correlated changes in the reproductive tract from one period to another.

hair c. the successive phases of the production and then loss of HAIR, consisting of ANAGEN, CATAGEN, and TELOGEN.

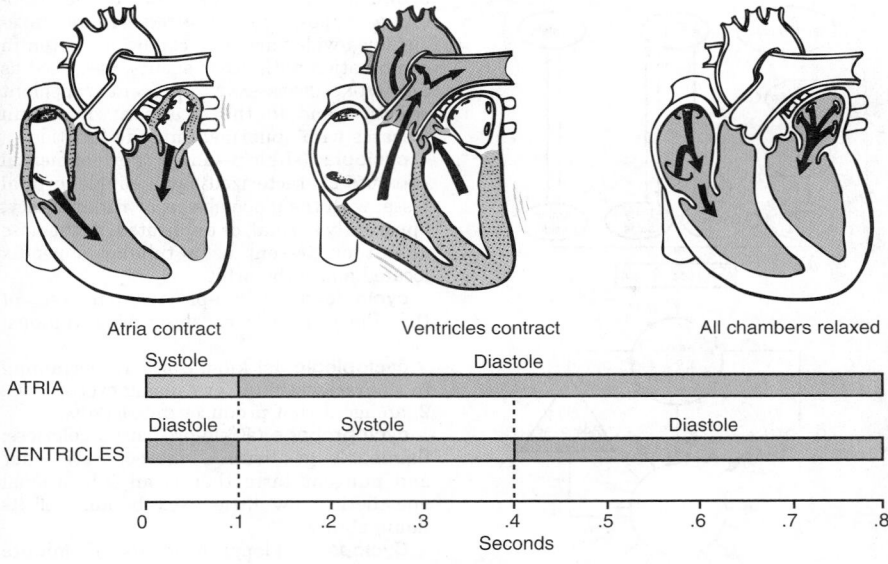

Cardiac cycle. From Applegate, 2000.

Krebs c. tricarboxylic acid cycle.

menstrual c. see MENSTRUAL CYCLE.

ovarian c. the sequence of physiologic changes in the ovary involved in ovulation; see also OVULATION and REPRODUCTION.

reproductive c. the cycle of physiologic changes in the reproductive organs, from the time of fertilization of the ovum through gestation and childbirth; see also REPRODUCTION.

sex c., sexual c. 1. the physiologic changes that recur regularly in the reproductive organs of nonpregnant female mammals. 2. the period of sexual reproduction in an organism that also reproduces asexually.

TCA c. tricarboxylic acid cycle.

tricarboxylic acid c. the cyclic metabolic mechanism by which the complete oxidation of the acetyl portion of acetyl-coenzyme A is effected; the process is the chief source of mammalian energy, during which carbon chains of sugars, fatty acids, and amino acids are metabolized to yield carbon dioxide, water, and high-energy phosphate bonds. (See illustration.) Called also citric acid cycle, Krebs cycle, and TCA cycle.

urea c. a cyclic series of reactions that produce UREA; it is a major route for removal of the ammonia produced in the metabolism of amino acids in the liver and kidney.

cyclectomy (si-klek'to-me) 1. excision of a piece of the ciliary body. 2. excision of a portion of the ciliary border of the eyelid.

cyclic (sik'lik) pertaining to or occurring in a cycle or cycles. The term is applied to chemical compounds that contain a ring of atoms in the nucleus.

cyclic AMP cyclic adenosine monophosphate.

cyclic GMP cyclic guanosine monophosphate.

cyclicotomy (si″klĭ-kot'ah-me) cyclotomy.

cycling (si'kling) the ending of an inspiratory phase of mechanical ventilation.

flow c. the delivery of gas under positive PRESSURE during inspiration until flow drops to a specified terminal level.

pressure c. the delivery of gas under positive PRESSURE during inspiration until an adjustable, preselected pressure has been reached.

timed c. the delivery of gas under positive PRESSURE during inspiration until an adjustable, preselected time interval has elapsed.

volume c. the delivery of gas under positive PRESSURE during inspiration until an adjustable, preselected volume has been delivered.

cyclitis (si-kli'tis) inflammation of the ciliary body.

cyclizine (si'klĭ-zēn) an ANTIHISTAMINE used in the form of the hydrochloride salt to treat nausea in MOTION SICKNESS.

cyclobenzaprine (si″klo-ben'zah-prēn) a skeletal muscle RELAXANT used to relieve

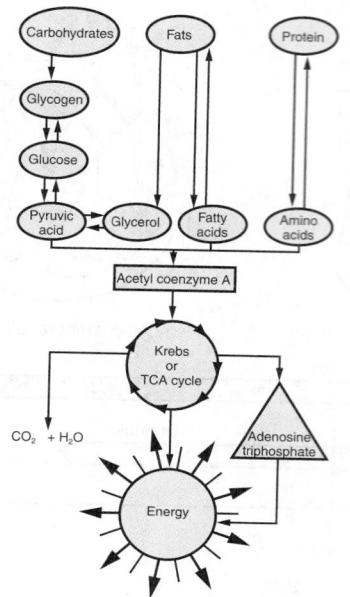

Central pathways of metabolism: How the body produces energy from the energy-containing nutrients using the tricarboxylic acid cycle. From Davis and Sherer, 1994.

painful muscle spasms, administered orally.

cyclochoroiditis (si″klo-ko″roi-di′tis) inflammation of the ciliary body and choroid.

cyclocryotherapy (si″klo-kri′o-ther′ah-pe) freezing of the ciliary body; done in the treatment of glaucoma.

cyclodialysis (si″klo-di-al′ĭ-sis) creation of a communication between the anterior chamber of the eye and the suprachoroidal space, in glaucoma.

cyclodiathermy (si″klo-di″ah-ther′me) destruction of a portion of the ciliary body by diathermy.

cyclokeratitis (si″klo-ker″ah-ti′tis) inflammation of the cornea and ciliary body.

cyclomethycaine (si″klo-meth′ĭ-kān) a local anesthetic.

cyclooxygenase (si″klo-ok′sĭ-jĕ-nās) an activity of the enzyme PROSTAGLANDIN ENDOPEROXIDE SYNTHASE.

cyclopentamine (si″klo-pen′tah-mēn) a sympathomimetic used as a nasal decongestant in the form of the hydrochloride salt.

cyclophoria (si″klo-for′e-ah) heterophoria in which there is deviation of the visual axis of one eye from the anteroposterior axis in the absence of visual fusional stimuli.

cyclophosphamide (si″klo-fos′fah-mīd) a cytotoxic ALKYLATING AGENT, one of the NITROGEN MUSTARDS, used in ANTINEOPLASTIC THERAPY for a wide variety of conditions, often in combination with other agents; also used as an IMMUNOSUPPRESSANT to prevent transplant rejection and in the treatment of certain diseases with abnormal immune function.

cyclopia (si-klo′pe-ah) a developmental ANOMALY characterized by a single orbital fossa, with the globe absent or rudimentary, apparently normal, or duplicated, or the nose absent or present as a tubular appendix located above the orbit.

cycloplegia (si″klo-ple′jah) paralysis of the ciliary muscle; paralysis of ACCOMMODATION.

cycloplegic (si″klo-ple′jik) 1. pertaining to, characterized by, or causing CYCLOPLEGIA. 2. an agent that produces CYCLOPLEGIA.

cyclopropane (si″klo-pro′pān) a colorless, flammable gas with a characteristic odor and pungent taste that is an inhalational anesthetic; now little used because of its flammability.

Cyclops (si′klops) a genus of minute crustaceans, species of which act as hosts of *Diphyllobothrium* and *Dracunculus*.

cyclops (si′klops) a malformed fetus exhibiting CYCLOPIA. Called also monops and monophthalmus.

cycloserine (si″klo-ser′ēn) an ANTIBIOTIC elaborated by *Streptomyces orchidaceus* or produced synthetically, used as a tuberculostatic and in the treatment of urinary tract infections.

cyclosis (si-klo′sis) movement of the cytoplasm within a cell, without external deformation of the cell wall.

Cyclospasmol (si″klo-spaz′mol) trademark for preparations of CYCLANDELATE, a peripheral VASODILATOR.

cyclosporin A (si″klo-spor′in) cyclosporine.

cyclosporine (si″klo-spōr′in) a cyclic peptide from an extract of soil fungi, an inhibitor of T CELL function; used as an IMMUNOSUPPRESSANT to prevent and treat rejection in organ transplant recipients and to treat severe PSORIASIS and as a disease-modifying antirheumatic DRUG.

cyclothymia (si″klo-thi′me-ah) cyclothymic disorder.

cyclothymic (si″klo-thi′mik) pertaining to or characterized by cyclothymia.

c. disorder a MOOD DISORDER characterized by numerous alternating short cycles of hypomanic and depressive periods with symptoms like those of manic and major depressive episodes but of lesser severity.

cyclotomy (si-klot′ah-me) incision of the ciliary muscle; cyclicotomy.

cyclotropia (si″klo-tro′pe-ah) STRABISMUS in which there is permanent deviation of the eye around the anteroposterior axis in the presence of visual fusional stimuli, resulting in diplopia.

cycrimine (si′krĭ-mēn) an ANTICHOLINERGIC used as the hydrochloride salt in the treatment of parkinsonism.

cyesis (si-e′sis) pregnancy. adj., **cyet′ic.**

cylindroid (sil′in-droid) 1. shaped like a cylinder. 2. a type of urinary CAST that tapers to a slender, sometimes twisted or curled, tail.

cylindroma (sil″in-dro′mah) 1. adenocystic carcinoma. 2. a benign skin tumor, usually on the face and scalp consisting of cylindrical masses of epithelial cells surrounded by a thick band of hyaline material. adj., **cylindrom′atous.**

cylindruria (sil″in-droo′re-ah) the presence of casts in the urine; see urinary CAST.

cymbocephaly (sim″bo-sef′ah-le) scaphocephaly.

cynophobia (sin″o-fo′be-ah) irrational fear of dogs.

cyotrophy (si-ot′ro-fe) nutrition of the fetus.

cyproheptadine (si″pro-hep′tah-dēn) an ANTIHISTAMINE with sedative, anticholinergic, and serotonin-blocking effects; used as the hydrochloride salt in the treatment of nasal, eye, and skin manifestations of allergic reactions, including allergic rhinitis, conjunctivitis, and itching, and also used in the prevention of MIGRAINE, administered orally.

cyrtometer (sir-tom′ĕ-ter) a device for measuring the curved surfaces of the body.

cyst (sist) 1. bladder. 2. an abnormal closed epithelium-lined sac in the body that contains a liquid or semisolid substance. Most are harmless, but they should be removed when possible because they occasionally may change into malignant growths, become infected, or obstruct a gland. There are four main types of cysts: retention cysts, exudation cysts, embryonic cysts, and parasitic cysts. 3. a stage in the life cycle of certain parasites, during which they are enveloped in a protective wall.

adventitious c. pseudocyst (def. 1).

alveolar c's dilatations of pulmonary alveoli, which may fuse by breakdown of their septa to form large air cysts (pneumatoceles).

arachnoid c. a fluid-filled cyst between the layers of the LEPTOMENINGES, lined with arachnoid membrane, usually in the sylvian fissure.

Baker c. a swelling on the back of the knee, due to escape of synovial fluid that has become enclosed in a sac of membrane.

Bartholin c. a mucus-filled cyst of a Bartholin gland, usually developing as a consequence of an obstruction of the duct by trauma, infection, epithelial hyperplasia, or congenital atresia or narrowing.

Blessig c's cystic spaces formed at the periphery of the retina.

blue dome c. 1. a benign retention cyst of the breast that shows a pale blue color. See also CYSTIC DISEASE OF BREAST. 2. a cyst due to ENDOMETRIOSIS, found in healed wounds such as those of an episiotomy or an incision for a cesarean section; it is usually found in the vaginal fornix or on the cervix.

Boyer c. an enlargement of the subhyoid bursa.

branchial c., branchiogenic c., branchiogenous c. see BRANCHIAL CYST.

bronchogenic c. a congenital cyst, usually in the mediastinum or lung, arising from anomalous budding during formation of the tracheobronchial tree, lined with bronchial epithelium that may contain secretory elements.

chocolate c. one filled with hemosiderin, causing a dark color, following local hemorrhage, such as may occur in the ovary in ovarian endometriosis.

choledochal c. a congenital cystic dilatation of the common bile duct, which may cause pain in the right upper quadrant, jaundice, fever, or vomiting, or be asymptomatic.

daughter c. a small parasitic cyst developed from the walls of a larger cyst.

dentigerous c. an odontogenic CYST surrounding the crown of a tooth, originating after the crown is completely formed.

dermoid c. see DERMOID CYST.

duplication c. a congenital cystic malformation of the alimentary tract, consisting of a duplication of the segment to which it is adjacent, occurring anywhere from the mouth to the anus but most frequently affecting the ileum and esophagus.

echinococcus c. hydatid cyst.

embryonic c. one developing from bits of embryonic tissue that have been overgrown by other tissues, or from developing organs that normally disappear before birth. An example is a BRANCHIAL CYST.

enteric c., enterogenous c. a cyst of the intestine arising or developing from some fold or pouch along the intestinal tract. Called also enterocyst and enterocystoma.

epidermal c., epidermoid c. an intradermal or subcutaneous cyst containing keratinizing squamous epithelium; it arises from occluded hair follicles. Called also wen.

epidermal inclusion c. a type of epidermal CYST occurring on the head, neck, or trunk, formed by keratinizing squamous epithelium with a granular layer.

epithelial c. 1. any cyst lined by keratinizing stratified squamous epithelium, found most often in the skin. 2. epidermal cyst.

exudation c. a cyst formed by the slow seepage of an exudate into a closed cavity.

false c. pseudocyst (def. 1).

follicular c. one due to occlusion of the duct of a follicle or small gland, especially one formed by enlargement of a graafian follicle as a result of accumulated transudate.

hydatid c. the larval stage of the tapeworms *Echinococcus granulosis* and *E. multilocularis*; each one contains daughter cysts that have many scoleces (mouths). See also HYDATID DISEASE. Called also echinococcus cyst and hydatid.

inclusion c. one formed by the inclusion of a small portion of epithelium or mesothelium within connective tissue along a line of fusion of embryonic processes; several types are found in the oral and nasal regions.

keratinizing c. one arising in the pilosebaceous apparatus, lined by stratified squamous epithelium and containing largely macerated keratin and often sufficient sebum to render the contents greasy or rancid.

meibomian c. chalazion.

mucus retention c. a mucus-containing retention CYST caused by blockage of a salivary gland duct.

multilocular c. 1. a cyst containing several loculi or spaces. 2. a hydatid CYST with many small irregular cavities that may contain scoleces but generally little fluid. 3. a thick-walled cyst in the kidney, found in clusters and usually unilaterally. In children it contains blastema and may develop into a Wilms tumor.

myxoid c. a nodular lesion usually overlying a distal interphalangeal finger joint in the dorsolateral or dorsomesial position, consisting of focal mucinous degeneration of the collagen of the dermis; not a true cyst, lacking an epithelial wall, it does not communicate with the underlying synovial space.

Naboth's c's, nabothian c's cysts that occur when mucus-producing glands in the columnar epithelium of the uterine cervix become covered over by squamous epithelium resulting from metaplasia; they are usually found in the transformation zone of the cervix. Called also Naboth's or nabothian follicles.

nasoalveolar c., nasolabial c. a fissural cyst arising outside the bones at the junction of the globular portion of the medial nasal process, lateral nasal process, and maxillary process.

odontogenic c. one derived from epithelium, usually containing fluid or semisolid material, which develops during various stages of ODONTOGENESIS; nearly always enclosed within bone.

parasitic c. one forming around larval parasites (tapeworms, amebas, trichinae), such as a hydatid CYST.

periapical c. a periodontal cyst involving the apex of an erupted tooth.

perineurial c. an outpouching of the perineurial space on the extradural portion of the posterior sacral or coccygeal nerve roots at the junction of the root and ganglion; it may cause low back pain and sciatica.

periodontal c. one in the periodontal ligament and adjacent structures, usually at the apex of the tooth (periapical CYST).

pilar c. a type of epidermal CYST, almost always found on the scalp, arising from the outer root sheath of the hair follicle.

pilonidal c. see PILONIDAL CYST.

radicular c. an epithelium-lined sac at the apex of a tooth.

Rathke's c's, Rathke's cleft c's groups of epithelial cells forming small colloid-filled cysts in the pars intermedia of the pituitary gland; they are vestiges of Rathke's POUCH and are closely related to CRANIOPHARYNGIOMAS.

retention c. a tumorlike accumulation of a secretion formed when the outlet of a secreting gland is obstructed. These cysts may develop in any of the secretory glands, such as the breast, pancreas, kidney, salivary or sebaceous glands, or mucous membranes.

sarcosporidian c. sarcocyst (def. 2).

sebaceous c. see SEBACEOUS CYST.

solitary bone c. a pathologic bone space in the metaphyses of long bones of growing children; it may be either empty or filled with fluid and have a delicate connective tissue lining.

subchondral c. a bone cyst within the fused epiphysis beneath the articular plate.

tarry c. 1. one resulting from hemorrhage into a corpus luteum. 2. a bloody cyst resulting from endometriosis.

theca-lutein c. a cyst of the ovary in which the cystic cavity is lined with theca CELLS.

traumatic bone c. a cavity (not a true cyst) formed in bone, particularly the mandible, in response to trauma. The hematoma precipitated by trauma is resorbed but bone is not replaced; the space formed is usually empty and lacks an epithelial lining.

unicameral bone c. solitary bone cyst.

wolffian c. a cyst of the broad ligament developed from vestiges of the mesonephros.

cyst(o)- word element [Gr.], *cyst; bladder.*

cystadenoma (sis-tad″ĕ-no′mah) cystoma blended with adenoma.

mucinous c. a multilocular, usually benign, tumor produced by ovarian epithelial cells and having mucin-filled cavities.

papillary c. any tumor producing patterns that are both papillary and cystic; called also papilloadenocystoma.

serous c. a cystic tumor of the ovary containing thin, clear yellow serum and some solid tissue.

Cystagon (sis′tah-gon) trademark for a preparation of CYSTEAMINE, used in treatment of nephropathic CYSTINOSIS.

cystalgia (sis-tal′jah) cystodynia.

cystathionine (sis″tah-thi′o-nēn) a thioester of HOMOCYSTEINE and SERINE; it serves as an intermediate in the transfer of a sulfur atom from METHIONINE to CYSTEINE.

cystathioninuria (sis″tah-thi″o-nin-u′re-ah) a hereditary disorder of CYSTATHIONINE metabolism, marked by increased concentrations in the urine, and due to deficiency of γ-cystathionase; mental retardation may be associated.

cysteamine (sis-te′ah-mēn″) a sulfhydryl amine that is part of COENZYME A; it reduces intracellular CYSTINE levels and is used in treatment of nephropathic CYSTINOSIS; administered orally.

cystectasia (sis″tek-ta′zhah) dilatation of the bladder.

cystectomy (sis-tek′to-me) 1. excision of a cyst. 2. excision or resection of the urinary bladder.

cysteine (sis-te′ēn) a sulfur-containing AMINO ACID, one of the nonessential amino acids, produced by enzymatic or acid hydrolysis of proteins; it is readily oxidized to CYSTINE and is sometimes found in urine.

cystencephalus (sis″ten-sef′ah-lus) a malformed fetus with a membranous sac in place of a brain.

cystic (sis′tik) 1. pertaining to or containing cysts. 2. pertaining to the urinary bladder or to the gallbladder.

c. disease of breast fibrocystic disease of breast.

c. fibrosis a hereditary disorder associated with widespread dysfunction of the exocrine glands, with accumulation of excessively thick and tenacious mucus and abnormal secretion of sweat and saliva; it is inherited as a recessive trait; both parents must be carriers. The cause is thought to be absence, insufficiency, or abnormality of some essential hormone or enzyme. Called

also cystic fibrosis of the pancreas and mucoviscidosis.

Effects. The symptoms and severity vary widely. Although cystic fibrosis is congenital, it may not manifest itself significantly during the early weeks or months of life, or it may cause intestinal obstruction and perforation in the newborn. The chief cause of complications is the extremely thick mucus produced. Normal mucus bathes and protects internal surfaces, transports chemicals produced in one organ through intricate small ducts to another organ, and carries bacteria, dirt, and wastes to be eliminated from the body; thus it needs to flow easily. The mucus of cystic fibrosis, in contrast, is highly adhesive. Bacteria and other matter stick to it, and it in turn clogs the lungs and usually interferes with the flow of digestive enzymes from the pancreas to the small intestine.

In the lungs, the mucus blocks the bronchioles, creating breathing difficulties. Infection develops, thereby increasing obstruction of the air passages. Air becomes trapped in the lungs (EMPHYSEMA), and scattered small areas eventually collapse (patchy ATELECTASIS). Repeated infections follow, inflaming and damaging lung tissue and leading to chronic lung disease. The organism that produces infection in cystic fibrosis is almost always a staphylococcus, but other organisms may be present in more severe cases. About half of children with cystic fibrosis have lung-related symptoms.

When mucus prevents the pancreatic enzymes from reaching the duodenum (as in about 80 per cent of cystic fibrosis patients), digestion is hindered. Fats especially are poorly digested and absorbed. The child may have a voracious appetite, yet fail to grow normally or gain weight. There may be marked signs of malnutrition. The outstanding symptom associated with pancreatic enzyme deficiency is frequent bulky, fatty, and foul-smelling feces.

Between 5 and 10 per cent of cystic fibrosis babies are born with intestines obstructed by puttylike intestinal secretions (meconium ILEUS) and die unless the condition is diagnosed promptly and relieved by surgery within the first few days of life. Such relief does not protect the child against the other manifestations of cystic fibrosis, although these may not appear until later.

Because cysts and scar tissue on the pancreas were observed during autopsy when the disease was first being differentiated from other conditions, it was given the name cystic fibrosis of the pancreas. Although this term describes a secondary rather than primary characteristic, it has been retained.

Diagnosis. Sweat in cystic fibrosis is excessively salty. Collapse of cystic fibrosis patients from salt loss during a heat wave led to recognition of the sweat abnormality. The sweat chloride test remains the cornerstone of diagnosis of cystic fibrosis. In children, a sweat chloride level above 60 mEq/l indicates cystic fibrosis. Newborn infants do not produce sufficient sweat for the test, but it has been noted that older babies "taste salty" when kissed. Supporting evidence can confirm the sweat test finding.

Treatment. Under careful supervision by the health care team, parents are taught the principles of home treatment of cystic fibrosis. The child may be required to sleep regularly in a plastic mist tent, into which a dense fog is pumped to help liquefy mucus and check infection. Aerosol therapy is generally prescribed. Extracts of animal pancreas taken with meals, which should be high in protein and low in fat, compensate for pancreatic deficiency. Physical therapy involving POSTURAL DRAINAGE together with "clapping" and "vibrating" aids in loosening the mucus so that it can be coughed up and expectorated.

It is estimated that in the United States cystic fibrosis occurs once in every few thousand births. Caucasians appear more subject to it than blacks, and among those of Asian descent it seems to be rare.

Patient Care. Maintenance of the child's nutritional status may be difficult because of his tendency to cough and vomit frequently during feedings, and also because of difficulty in breathing. Small amounts of food, given slowly and at frequent intervals, are best for infants as well as for small children with cystic fibrosis.

Skin care is important, especially for infants and toddlers who are not yet toilet trained. The stools are likely to be copious and extremely irritating to the skin. Frequent turning of the infant or bedridden child helps to prevent decubitus ulcers and lessens the danger of pneumonia, a constant threat to these children. Prevention of infection is a most important aspect of the care of these children because of their extreme vulnerability to disorders of the respiratory tract.

Education of the parents must include the dietary regimen; how to use the Croupette, a machine for AEROSOL THERAPY in the home; hygienic measures to prevent infections; and the importance of continuous medical follow-up and administration of medications prescribed for the child.

c. kidney disease, c. disease of kidney see ACQUIRED CYSTIC KIDNEY DISEASE and POLYCYSTIC KIDNEY DISEASE.

cysticercosis (sis″tĭ-ser-ko′sis) infection with cysticerci. In man, infection with the larval forms (Cysticercus cellulosae) of Taenia solium.

cysticercus (sis″tĭ-ser′kus), pl. cysticer′ci [Gr.] a larval form of tapeworm.

cystiform (sis′tĭ-form) resembling a cyst.

cystigerous (sis-tij′er-us) containing cysts.

cystine (sis′tēn, sis′tin) 1. a naturally occurring amino acid, the chief sulfur-containing component of the protein molecule. It is sometimes found in the urine and in the kidneys in the form of minute hexagonal crystals, frequently forming cystine calculus in the bladder.

c. storage disease Fanconi's syndrome (def. 2).

cystinemia (sis″tĭ-ne′me-ah) the presence of cystine in the blood.

cystinosis (sis″tĭ-no′sis) a hereditary inborn ERROR of metabolism, appearing in various forms. The early onset or infantile form may appear as early as 6 months of age and is marked by osteomalacia, aminoaciduria, phosphaturia, and deposition of CYSTINE throughout the tissues of the body, including the liver, bone marrow, kidney, spleen, and cornea, ending with chronic RENAL FAILURE. It is the most common cause of FANCONI SYNDROME (def. 2). The prognosis for children with the disease has improved greatly in recent decades. CYSTEAMINE (Cystagon) is administered to lower cystine levels within cells and may delay or prevent renal failure The benign or adult form of cystinosis does not affect the kidneys or shorten life span; deposition of cystine crystals occurs in the bone marrow, leukocytes, and corneas. The condition is usually diagnosed by ophthalmic examination. The late onset juvenile or adolescent type falls in between the other two, with ocular and renal manifestations but often no resultant renal failure.

cystinuria (sis″tĭ-nu′re-ah) a hereditary AMINOACIDURIA with persistent excessive urinary excretion of CYSTINE, LYSINE, ORNITHINE, and ARGININE, due to impairment of renal tubular reabsorption of these amino acids. The predominant clinical manifestation is formation of urinary cystine calculi (see KIDNEY STONE).

cystistaxis (sis″tĭ-stak′sis) oozing of blood from the mucous membrane into the bladder.

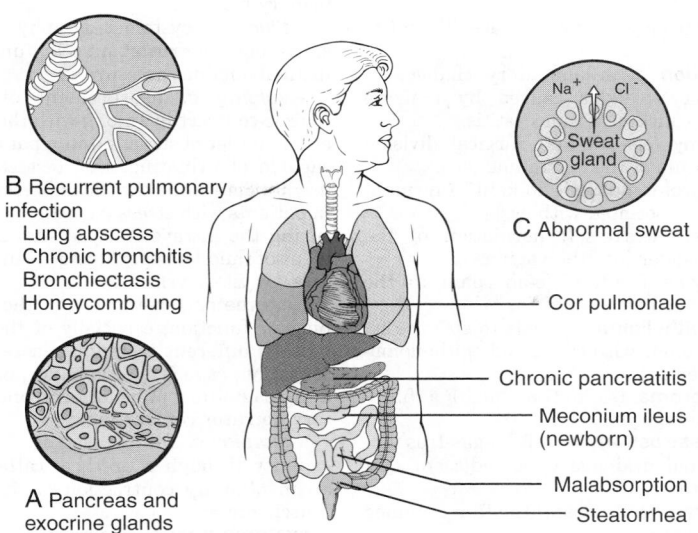

B Recurrent pulmonary
infection
   Lung abscess
   Chronic bronchitis
   Bronchiectasis
   Honeycomb lung

C Abnormal sweat

Cor pulmonale

Chronic pancreatitis

Meconium ileus
(newborn)

Malabsorption

Steatorrhea

A Pancreas and
exocrine glands

Cystic fibrosis. The abnormal chloride transport associated with cystic fibrosis in a lack of sodium chloride in the secretions of all exocrine glands, especially the pancreas, intestine, and bronchi. Redrawn from Damjanov, 2000.

cystitis (sis-ti′tis) inflammation of the urinary bladder; it may result from an *ascending* infection coming from the exterior of the body by way of the urethra, or from an infection *descending* from the kidney. A simple cystitis that does not involve the rest of the urinary tract is not as serious as the descending type in which the kidneys and ureters as well as the bladder are involved. Often cystitis is not an isolated infection but is a result of some other physical condition, such as urinary retention, calculi in the bladder, tumors, or neurologic diseases that impair normal bladder function.

Prevention of recurrent cystitis in females that is not attributable to abnormal structures or other factors mentioned previously may be achieved by good personal hygiene and the following measures: (1) always wipe the anal region from front to back after a bowel movement; (2) avoid wearing nylon pantyhose, tight slacks, or any clothing that traps perineal moisture and prevents evaporation; (3) do not wash underclothing in strong soap, and rinse underclothing well; (4) do not use bubble bath, perfumed soap, feminine hygiene sprays, or products containing hexachlorophene; (5) avoid prolonged bicycling, motorcycling, horseback riding, and traveling involving prolonged sitting, which can contribute to irritation of the urethral meatus and to development of an ascending cystitis;

and (6) do not ignore vaginal discharge or other signs of vaginal infection.

Symptoms and Treatment. The most common symptoms of cystitis are dysuria, frequency and urgency of urination, and in some cases hematuria. Chills and fever indicate involvement of the entire urinary tract and are not symptomatic of uncomplicated cystitis. Treatment of acute cystitis consists of antimicrobials, forcing of fluids, and bed rest. Hot sitz baths give some relief of the discomfort, and spasms of the bladder wall may respond to an antispasmodic drug such as hyoscyamine. Chronic cystitis is more difficult to cure and may require surgical dilatation of the urethra to facilitate drainage of urine. In many cases removal of the underlying cause, such as chronic vaginal infection, relieves the cystitis.

c. col′li inflammation of the bladder and bladder NECK.

hemorrhagic c. cystitis with severe hemorrhage, a dose-limiting toxic condition with administration of IFOSFAMIDE or CYCLOPHOSPHAMIDE, or a complication of bone marrow TRANSPLANTATION.

interstitial c. a type seen mainly in women, with the inflammatory lesion a small patch of red to brown mucosa surrounded by a network of radiating vessels, usually in the vertex and involving the entire thickness of the wall. The lesions are known as Hunner's ULCERS and often heal superficially so that they are difficult to detect.

radiation c. inflammatory changes in the urinary bladder caused by ionizing radiation; called also radiocystitis.

cystitomy (sis-tit′o-me) surgical division of the capsule of the crystalline lens.

cystocarcinoma (sis″to-kahr″sĭ-no′mah) carcinoma associated with cysts.

cystocele (sis′to-sēl) herniation of the urinary bladder into the vagina.

cystodynia (sis″to-din′e-ah) pain in the bladder; called also cystalgia.

cystoepithelioma (sis″to-ep′ĭ-the″le-o′mah) a tumor with cystic and epitheliomatous elements.

cystofibroma (sis″to-fi-bro′mah) a fibroma containing cysts.

cystogastrostomy (sis″to-gas-tros′tah-me) internal drainage of an adjacent cyst into the stomach.

cystogram (sis′to-gram) the film obtained by cystography.

voiding c. a radiogram of the urinary tract made while the patient is urinating.

cystography (sis-tog′rah-fe) radiography of the urinary BLADDER using a contrast medium, so that its outline can be seen clearly. This type of examination frequently is part of a complete x-ray study of the kidneys, urethra, and ureters as well as the bladder. (See also PYELOGRAPHY.) It is useful in diagnosing tumors or other defects in the bladder wall, vesicoureteral REFLUX, and calculi or other pathologic conditions of the bladder.

cystoid (sis′toid) 1. resembling a cyst. 2. a cystlike, circumscribed collection of softened material, having no enclosing capsule.

cystojejunostomy (sis″to-jě-joo-nos′tah-me) surgical anastomosis of a pancreatic cyst to the jejunum.

cystolith (sis′to-lith) vesical CALCULUS.

cystolithectomy (sis″to-lĭ-thek′to-me) cystolithotomy.

cystolithiasis (sis″to-lĭ-thi′ah-sis) the presence of calculi (vesical CALCULI) in the urinary bladder.

cystolithic (sis″to-lith′ik) pertaining to a vesical CALCULUS.

cystolithotomy (sis″to-lĭ-thot′ah-me) incision of the bladder for removal of a CALCULUS; called also cystolithectomy.

cystoma (sis-to′mah) a tumor containing cysts of neoplastic origin; a cystic tumor.

cystometer (sis-tom′ě-ter) an instrument for studying the neuromuscular mechanism of the bladder by means of measurements of pressure and capacity.

cystometrography (sis″to-met-rog′rah-fe) the graphic recording of the pressure exerted at varying degrees of filling of the urinary bladder.

filling c. cystometrography that measures both detrusor muscle function and intra-abdominal pressure.

voiding c. measurement of detrusor muscle contractility along with the detection of any outlet obstruction in a patient who is capable of urinating; this test can also be used to determine the "leak pressure point" in patients with stress INCONTINENCE, by measuring the intravesical pressure at the moment of fluid leakage during straining or the VALSALVA MANEUVER.

cystometry (sis-tom′ě-tre) the study of bladder function, especially of the detrusor muscle; different techniques assess bladder sensation, capacity, compliance, or presence and magnitude of voluntary and involuntary detrusor contractions.

simple c. filling of the bladder to capacity through a urethral catheter, until an involuntary contraction of the detrusor muscle occurs.

cystomorphous (sis″to-mor′fus) resembling a cyst or bladder.

cystoparesis (sis″to-pah-re′sis) paralysis of the urinary bladder; called also cystoplegia.

cystopexy (sis′to-pek″se) fixation of the bladder to the abdominal wall.

cystoplasty (sis′to-plas″te) plastic surgery of the bladder, usually referring to some type of augmentation cystoplasty.

augmentation c. enlargement of the bladder by grafting to it a detached segment of intestine (ENTEROCYSTOPLASTY) or stomach (GASTROCYSTOPLASTY). Called also bladder augmentation.

sigmoid c. augmentation CYSTOPLASTY using an isolated segment of the sigmoid colon for the graft.

cystoplegia (sis″to-ple′jah) cystoparesis.

cystoprostatectomy (sis″to-pros″tah-tek′tah-me) surgical removal of the urinary bladder and prostate.

cystoptosis (sis″top-to′sis) prolapse of part of the inner coat of the bladder into the urethra.

cystopyelitis (sis″to-pi″ě-li′tis) pyelocystitis.

cystopyelonephritis (sis″to-pi″ě-lo-ně-fri′tis) combined CYSTITIS and PYELONEPHRITIS.

cystorrhaphy (sis-tor′ah-fe) suture of the bladder.

cystorrhea (sis″to-re′ah) mucous discharge from the bladder.

cystosarcoma (sis″to-sahr-ko′mah) an unusually large fibroadenoma of the mammary gland, with a cellular, sarcoma-like stoma; it is locally aggressive and sometimes metastasizes.

cystoscope (sis′to-skōp) a hollow metal ENDOSCOPE especially designed for passing through the urethra into the bladder to permit visual inspection of the bladder interior. See also CYSTOSCOPY.

cystoscopy (sis-tos′kah-pe) examination of the BLADDER by means of a cystoscope, a hollow metal tube that is introduced into the urinary meatus and passed through the urethra and into the bladder. At the end of the cystoscope is an electric bulb that illuminates the bladder interior. By means of special lenses and mirrors the bladder mucosa is examined for inflammation, calculi, or tumors.

A catheter can be passed through the cystoscope into the bladder or, if necessary, beyond, into the ureters and kidneys. In this way samples of urine can be obtained for diagnostic purposes. Also, radiopaque fluids can be injected into the bladder or ureters for x-rays of the urinary tract (see also PYELOGRAPHY). (See illustration.)

Patient Care. Prior to the procedure the patient should be given an adequate explanation of its purpose and expected outcome, and of the need for proper preparation. Because the full cooperation of the patient is of crucial importance to a successful test, it is essential that the patient be told what is expected of him or her when the procedure is done under local anesthesia. During the procedure, if the patient is awake, the

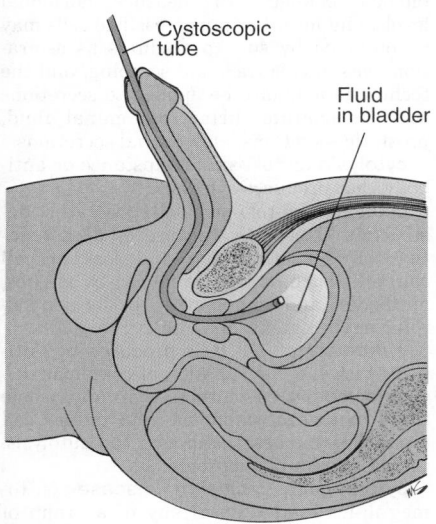

Cystoscopy: examination of the male bladder. The cystoscope is passed through the urethra into the bladder. Although shown here as a flexible scope, usually the scope is rigid. Through the scope fluid is instilled to maintain bladder distention. From Beare and Myers, 1998.

C

nurse or other attendant should be alert for indications of sudden pain, which could signify perforation of the urethra or other structures. Another complication that can occur in patients with a history of heart disease is cardiac arrhythmia.

The plan of care following cystoscopy should include observation of the amount and character of the urine. Some slight coloration from blood should be expected, but any frank bleeding and passing of clots should be reported to the surgeon. Other problems likely to require nursing intervention are discomfort from bladder spasms, back pain, a feeling of fullness and burning in the bladder region, and possible urinary retention. Nursing measures would include warm sitz baths, relaxation techniques to promote rest and provide relief from pain, and administration of prescribed medications.

If chilling and fever occur and do not respond to attempts to provide warmth and to increased fluid intake, there could be an infection in the urinary tract requiring antibacterial therapy.

cystostomy (sis-tos′tah-me) vesicostomy.

cystotomy (sis-tot′ah-me) vesicotomy.

cystoureteritis (sis″to-u-re″ter-i′tis) inflammation involving the urinary bladder and ureters.

cystoureterography (sis″to-u-re″ter-og′-rah-fe) radiography of the bladder and ureter.

cystourethrography (sis″to-u″re-throg′-rah-fe) radiography of the urinary bladder and urethra.

chain c. that in which a sterile beaded metal chain is introduced via a modified catheter into the bladder and urethra; used in evaluating anatomical relationships of the bladder and urethra.

cystourethroscope (sis″to-u-re′thro-skōp″) an ENDOSCOPE for examining the posterior urethra and bladder.

cystourethroscopy (sis″to-u″re-thros′kah-pe) use of a CYSTOURETHROSCOPE to evaluate lesions or foreign bodies in the bladder, urethral diverticula, fistulas, strictures, and other conditions. Called also urethrocystoscopy.

cyt(o)- word element [Gr.], *a cell.*

Cytadren (si′tah-dren) trademark for a preparation of AMINOGLUTETHIMIDE, an ANTIHORMONE used in treatment of CUSHING'S SYNDROME and investigationally for advanced breast carcinoma.

cytapheresis (sīt″ah-fĕ-re′sis) APHERESIS of blood cells; see *erythrocytapheresis, leukapheresis,* and *thrombocytapheresis.*

cytarabine (si-tar′ah-bēn) an ANTIMETABO-LITE antineoplastic AGENT that inhibits DNA polymerase and thus inhibits DNA synthesis during a specific phase of the cell cycle. Administered intravenously to treat acute myelogenous and other types of LEUKEMIA. It is also injected intrathecally to treat MENINGITIS associated with leukemia or lymphoma. Called also cytosine arabinoside.

-cyte word element [Gr.], *a cell.*

cytoanalyzer (si″to-an″ah-li′zer) an electronic optical apparatus for the detection of malignant cells in smears.

cytochalasin (si″to-kal′ah-sin) any of a group of fungal metabolites that affect the motility of polymorphonuclear leukocytes.

cytochemistry (si″to-kem′is-tre) the identification and localization of the different chemical compounds and their activities within the cell.

cytochrome (si′to-krōm) any of a class of HEMOPROTEINS, widely distributed in animal and plant tissue, whose main function is electron transport; distinguished according to their non–amino acid components as *a, b, c, d,* etc.

cytoclasis (si-tok′lah-sis) the destruction of cells. adj., **cytoclas′tic.**

cytodiagnosis (si″to-di″ag-no′sis) diagnosis based on examination of cells. adj., **cytodiagnos′tic.**

cytodifferentiation (si″to-dif′er-en″she-a′shun) the development of specialized structures and functions in embryonic cells.

cytodistal (si″to-dis′tal) denoting that part of an axon remote from the cell body.

cytogenesis (si″to-jen′ĕ-sis) the origin and development of the cell.

cytogenetic (si″to-jĕ-net′ik) 1. chromosomal. 2. pertaining to CYTOGENETICS.

    c. **technologist** a CLINICAL LABORATORY SCIENTIST who carries out diagnostic testing, including culturing, harvesting, staining, photomicroscopy, and chromosome analysis. Academic programs preparing practitioners are approved by the National Accrediting Agency for Clinical Laboratory Sciences; certification is through the National Credentialing Agency for Medical Laboratory Personnel. The address of the Association of Cytogenetic Technologists is P.O. Box 15945-288, Lenexa, KS 66285 (telephone 913-541-9077). The address of the National Credentialing Agency for Medical Laboratory Personnel is P.O. Box 15945-289, Lenexa, KS 66285 (telephone 913-438-5110).

cytogenetics (si″to-jĕ-net′iks) that branch of GENETICS devoted to the cellular constituents concerned in heredity, i.e., the CHROMOSOMES.

    clinical c. the branch of cytogenetics concerned with relations between chromosomal abnormalities and pathologic conditions.

cytogenic (si″to-jen′ik) 1. pertaining to cytogenesis. 2. forming or producing cells.

cytoglycopenia (si″to-gli″ko-pe′ne-ah) deficient glucose content of the body or blood cells.

cytohistogenesis (si″to-his″to-jen′ĕ-sis) development of the structure of cells.

cytohistology (si″to-his-tol′o-je) the combination of cytologic and histologic methods. adj., **cytohistolog′ic.**

cytokine a generic term for nonantibody proteins released by one cell population on contact with specific antigen, which act as intercellular mediators, as in the generation of an IMMUNE RESPONSE.

cytokinesis (si″to-kĭ-ne′sis) the division of the cytoplasm between daughter cells in MITOSIS or MEIOSIS.

cytologist (si-tol′o-jist) a specialist in cytology.

cytology (si-tol′o-je) the study of cells, their origin, structure, function, and pathology. adj., **cytolog′ic.**

    aspiration biopsy c. **(ABC)** the microscopic study of cells from superficial or internal lesions obtained by aspiration BIOPSY.

    exfoliative c. microscopic examination of cells desquamated from a body surface or lesion, done to detect malignancy or microbiologic changes, to measure hormonal levels, and for other purposes. The cells may be obtained by such procedures as aspiration, washing, smear, and scraping, and the technique may also be applied to secretions such as sputum, urine, abdominal fluid, prostatic secretions, and vaginal secretions.

cytolysin (si-tol′ĭ-sin) a substance or antibody that produces cytolysis.

cytolysis (si-tol′ĭ-sis) cell lysis; the destruction of cells by rupture or disintegration of the membrane and loss of cell contents, such as that produced by viruses, antibodies and complement, or by a hypotonic environment. See also CYTOTOXICITY.

    immune c. cell lysis produced by antibody with the participation of complement.

cytolysosome (si″to-li′so-sōm) a lysosome fused with mitochondria and other cell organelles and associated with cell autolysis. Called also autophagosome.

cytomegalic inclusion disease (si″to-meg′ah-lik in-kloo′zhun) any of a group of diseases caused by CYTOMEGALOVIRUS infection, marked by characteristic inclusion bodies in enlarged infected cells. In the fetus and infant, infection can be acquired in utero from the mother, transmitted from mother to infant in passage through the birth canal, or transmitted in the mother's milk. Most infected infants are asymptomatic, but in some there may be hepatosplenomegaly, jaundice, chorioretinitis, purpura, microcephaly, cerebral calcifications, and severe central nervous system sequelae with blindness, deafness, quadriplegia, and mental retardation. Acquired disease is transmitted via respiratory droplets, tissue or blood donation, or sexual transmission. Another acquired infection is cytomegalovirus MONONUCLEOSIS. In IMMUNOCOMPROMISED patients there may be a disseminated, sometimes fatal, infection as well as specific syndromes such as cytomegalovirus PNEUMONIA or cytomegalovirus RETINITIS.

Cytomegalovirus (si″to-meg′ah-lo-vi″rus) a genus of HERPESVIRUSES closely related to genus *Roseolovirus*, containing the single species human herpesvirus 5. It is transmitted by multiple routes and causes infection that is usually mild or subclinical but may be symptomatic (CYTOMEGALIC INCLUSION DISEASE).

cytomegalovirus (CMV) (si″to-meg′ah-lo-vi″rus) any of a subfamily of host-specific HERPESVIRUSES infecting humans, monkeys, and rodents, producing unique large cells with inclusion bodies. Opportunistic infection with this virus is common in IMMUNOCOMPROMISED individuals, causing clinical illnesses such as cytomegalovirus RETINITIS, pneumonia, esophagitis, colitis, adrenalitis, and hepatitis. It can also cause CYTOMEGALIC INCLUSION DISEASE, a variety of gastrointestinal infections, and ENCEPHALITIS. Most infections are mild in immunocompetent persons, but it has been associated with a syndrome called cytomegalovirus MONONUCLEOSIS.

c. disease cytomegalic inclusion disease.

cytomegaly (si″to-meg′ah-le) abnormal enlargement of a cell or group of cells.

adrenocortical c. abnormal enlargement of cells in the outer layer of the adrenal CORTEX.

Cytomel (si′to-mel) trademark for a preparation of LIOTHYRONINE sodium, a THYROID HORMONE preparation.

cytometaplasia (si″to-met″ah-pla′zhah) change in function or form of cells.

cytometer (si-tom′ĕ-ter) a device for counting cells.

flow c. an instrument used to perform flow CYTOMETRY.

cytometry (si-tom′ĕ-tre) the counting of cells, especially blood cells.

flow c. a cytometric technique in which cells suspended in a fluid flow one at a time through a focus of exciting light, which is scattered in patterns characteristic to the cells and their components; cells are frequently labeled with fluorescent markers so that light is first absorbed and then emitted at altered frequencies. A sensor detecting the scattered or emitted light measures the size and molecular characteristics of individual cells; tens of thousands of cells can be examined per minute and the data gathered is processed by computer.

cytomorphology (si″to-mor-fol′o-je) the morphology of body cells.

cytomorphosis (si″to-mor-fo′sis) the changes through which cells pass in development.

cytopathic (si″to-path′ik) pertaining to or characterized by pathologic changes in cells.

cytopathogenesis (si″to-path″o-jen′ĕ-sis) production of pathologic changes in cells. adj., **cytopathogenet′ic.**

cytopathologic (si″to-path″o-loj′ik) relating to cytopathology; denoting the changes in cells in disease.

cytopathological (si″to-path″o-loj′ĭ-k′l) cytopathologic.

cytopathologist (si″to-pah-thol′o-jist) an expert in the study of cells in disease; a cellular pathologist.

cytopathology (si″to-pah-thol′o-je) the study of cells in disease; cellular pathology.

cytopenia (si″to-pe′ne-ah) deficiency in numbers of any of the blood cell elements.

cytophagy (si-tof′ah-je) the ingestion of cells by phagocytes.

cytophilic (si″to-fil′ik) having an affinity for cells.

cytophylaxis (si″to-fi-lak′sis) 1. the protection of cells against cytolysis. 2. increase in cellular activity.

cytopipette (si″to-pi-pet′) a PIPETTE for taking cytological smears.

cytoplasm (si′to-plazm) the protoplasm of a cell surrounding the nucleus (nucleoplasm). adj., **cytoplas′mic.**

cytoprotectant (si″to-pro-tek′tant) cytoprotective.

cytoprotective (si″to-pro-tek′tiv) 1. protecting cells from noxious chemicals or other stimuli. 2. an agent that so protects; called also cytoprotectant.

cytoreduction (si″to-re-duk′shun) 1. decrease in the number of cells, such as in a tumor. 2. debulking.

cytoreductive (si″to-re-duk′tiv) reducing the number of cells, as in surgery for a tumor; see also DEBULKING.

cytosine (si′to-sēn) a pyrimidine base found in NUCLEIC ACIDS.

c. arabinoside cytarabine.

cytoskeleton (si″to-skel′ĕ-ton) a conspicuous internal reinforcement in the cytoplasm of a cell, consisting of tonofibrils, filaments of the terminal web, and other microfilaments. adj., **cytoskel′etal.**

cytosol (si′to-sol) the liquid medium of the cytoplasm, e.g., cytoplasm minus organelles and nonmembranous insoluble components. adj., **cytosol′ic.**

cytosome (si′to-sōm) the body of a cell apart from its nucleus.

cytostatic (si″to-stat′ik) 1. suppressing the growth and multiplication of cells. 2. an agent that so acts.

cytotaxis (si″to-tak′sis) the movement and arrangement of cells with respect to a specific source of stimulation. adj., **cytotac′tic.**

cytotechnologist (si″to-tek-nol′o-jist), a CLINICAL LABORATORY SCIENTIST specializing in CYTOLOGY. Certification is through the Board of Registry of the American Society of Clinical Pathologists, whose address is P.O. Box 12270, Chicago, IL 60612 (telephone 312-738-1336). The address of the American Society of Cytopathology is 400 W. 9th St., Wilmington, DE 19801 (telephone 302-429-8802).

cytothesis (si-toth′ĕ-sis) restitution of cells to their normal condition.

cytotoxic having destructive action on cells, usually only certain types of cells; see CYTOTOXICITY.

cytotoxicity (si″to-tok-sis′ĭ-te) 1. the degree to which an agent has specific destructive action on certain cells. 2. the possession of such destructive action, particularly in reference to lysis of cells by immune phenomena and to antineoplastic AGENTS that selectively kill dividing cells. adj., **cytotox′ic.**

antibody-dependent cell-mediated c. **(ADCC),** *antibody-dependent cellular c.* lysis of target cells coated with antibody by effector cells with cytolytic activity and specific immunoglobulin receptors called Fc receptors, including K cells, macrophages, and granulocytes. Lysis of the target cell is extracellular, requires direct cell-to-cell contact, and does not involve complement.

cell-mediated c. destruction of a target cell by specific lymphocytes, such as cytotoxic T lymphocytes or NK cells; it may be antibody-dependent (see ANTIBODY-DEPENDENT CELL-MEDIATED C.) or independent, as in certain cell-mediated HYPERSENSITIVITY REACTIONS.

cytotoxin (si′to-tok″sin) a toxin having a specific toxic action on cells of special organs.

cytotrophoblast (si″to-trof′o-blast) the cellular (inner) layer of the trophoblast.

cytotropism (si-tot′ro-pizm) 1. cell movement in response to external stimulation. 2. the tendency of viruses, bacteria, drugs, and other substances to exert their effect upon certain cells of the body.

Cytoxan (si-tok′san) trademark for preparations of CYCLOPHOSPHAMIDE, an antineoplastic AGENT.

cyturia (sī-tu′re-ah) the presence of cells of any sort in the urine.

D

D deuterium.

2,4-D 2,4-dichlorophenoxyacetic acid, a toxic chlorphenoxy HERBICIDE; it is a component of AGENT ORANGE.

d- abbreviation for *dextro-* (right or clockwise); a chemical prefix indicating an ENANTIOMER that rotates the plane of polarization of a beam of light in the clockwise direction, the other enantiomer being specified as *l-* (for *levo-*). The prefixes *d-* and *l-* are now being replaced by (+)- and (−)-, respectively, especially when the prefixes D- and L- are also used; for example, *l*-fructose is D-(−)-fructose.

D- chemical prefix specifying the relative configuration of an enantiomer, the mirror image configuration being specified L-. Carbohydrates are designated as D- or L- depending on their configuration at the asymmetric carbon atom most distant from the carbonyl functional group, being compared in chemical configuration to the standard substance D-GLYCERALDEHYDE. Amino acids are designated according to their configuration at the asymmetric carbon atom closest to the carbonyl group, with D-SERINE being the standard.

d day; deci-; deoxyribose (in specifying nucleosides and nucleotides, e.g., A is adenosine, dA is deoxyadenosine).

DA dietetic assistant.

Da symbol for *dalton.*

dacarbazine (dah-kahr′-bah-zēn) a cytotoxic ALKYLATING AGENT, used in ANTINEOPLASTIC THERAPY primarily for treatment of malignant melanoma and in combination chemotherapy for Hodgkin's disease and sarcomas. Unlike other alkylating agents, its primary target is not DNA; its major effect is inhibition of RNA and protein synthesis. Called also DTIC.

daclizumab (dah-kliz′u-mab) an IMMUNOSUPPRESSANT used to prevent acute organ rejection in renal transplant patients; administered intravenously.

Da Costa syndrome (dah′kos′tah) a syndrome characterized by palpitation, dyspnea, a sense of fatigue, fear of effort, and discomfort brought on by exercise or sometimes even slight effort; it is considered to be a manifestation of an ANXIETY DISORDER, with the physical symptoms being a reaction to something perceived to be dangerous or otherwise a threat to the person, causing autonomic responses or HYPERVENTILATION. Called also neurocirculatory asthenia.

dacry(o)- word element [Gr.], *tears* or *the lacrimal apparatus of the eye.*

dacryoadenalgia (dak″re-o-ad″ĕ-nal′jah) pain in a lacrimal gland.

dacryoadenectomy (dak″re-o-ad″ĕ-nek′to-me) excision of a lacrimal gland.

dacryoadenitis (dak″re-o-ad″ĕ-ni′tis) inflammation of a lacrimal gland.

dacryoblennorrhea (dak″re-o-blen″o-re′ah) mucous flow from the lacrimal apparatus.

dacryocele (dak′re-o-sēl″) dacryocystocele.

dacryocyst (dak′re-o-sist″) the lacrimal sac.

dacryocystalgia (dak″re-o-sis-tal′jah) pain in the lacrimal sac.

dacryocystectomy (dak″re-o-sis-tek′to-me) excision of the wall of the lacrimal sac.

dacryocystitis (dak″re-o-sis-ti′tis) inflammation of the lacrimal sac.

dacryocystoblennorrhea (dak″re-o-sis″to-blen″o-re′ah) chronic catarrhal inflammation of the lacrimal sac, with constriction of the lacrimal gland.

dacryocystocele (dak″re-o-sis′to-sēl) hernial protrusion of the lacrimal sac; called also dacryocele. (See illustration.)

dacryocystoptosis (dak″re-o-sis″top-to′-sis) prolapse of the lacrimal sac.

dacryocystorhinostenosis (dak″re-o-sis″-to-ri″no-stĕ-no′sis) narrowing of the duct leading from the lacrimal sac to the nasal cavity.

dacryocystorhinostomy (dak″re-o-sis″to-ri-nos′tah-me) surgical creation of an opening between the lacrimal sac and nasal cavity.

dacryocystorhinotomy (dak″re-o-sis″to-ri-not′ah-me) passage of a probe through the lacrimal sac into the nasal cavity.

dacryocystostenosis (dak″re-o-sis″to-stĕ-no′sis) narrowing of the lacrimal sac.

dacryocystostomy (dak″re-o-sis-tos′tah-me) surgical creation of a new opening into the lacrimal sac with drainage.

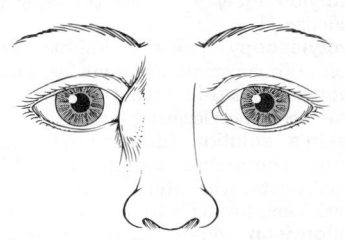

Dacryocystocele. From Dorland's, 2000.

dacryocystotomy (dak″re-o-sis-tot′ah-me) incision of the lacrimal sac and duct.

dacryohemorrhea (dak″re-o-he″mo-re′ah) the discharge of tears mixed with blood.

dacryolith (dak′re-o-lith″) a CALCULUS in a tear duct.

dacryolithiasis (dak″re-o-lĭ-thi′ah-sis) the presence of dacryoliths.

dacryoma (dak″re-o′mah) a tumorlike swelling due to obstruction of the lacrimal duct.

dacryon (dak′re-on) the point where the lacrimal, frontal, and upper maxillary bones meet.

dacryopyorrhea (dak″re-o-pi″o-re′ah) the discharge of tears mixed with pus.

dacryorrhea (dak″re-o-re′ah) excessive flow of tears.

dacryoscintigraphy (dak″re-o-sin-tig′rah-fe) scintigraphy of the lacrimal ducts.

dacryosolenitis (dak″re-o-so″lĕ-ni′tis) inflammation of a lacrimal duct.

dacryostenosis (dak″re-o-stĕ-no′sis) stricture or narrowing of a lacrimal duct.

dacryosyrinx (dak″re-o-sir′inks) 1. lacrimal duct. 2. a lacrimal fistula. 3. a syringe for irrigating the lacrimal ducts.

dactinomycin (dak″tĭ-no-mi′sin) an antitumor ANTIBIOTIC of the ACTINOMYCIN complex (actinomycin D), produced by *Streptomyces parvulus*. Used to treat RHABDOMYOSARCOMA and Wilms' TUMOR in children, as well as Ewing's SARCOMA, Kaposi's SARCOMA, osteogenic SARCOMA, soft tissue sarcomas, testicular carcinoma, and choriocarcinoma.

dactyl (dak′til) digit.

dactyl(o)- word element [Gr.], *a digit; a finger or toe.*

dactylitis (dak″tĭ-li′tis) inflammation of a FINGER or TOE.

dactylography (dak″tĭ-log′rah-fe) the study of fingerprints.

dactylogryposis (dak″tĭ-lo-grĭ-po′sis) permanent flexion of the fingers.

dactylology (dak″tĭ-lol′o-je) signing.

dactylolysis (dak″tĭ-lol′ĭ-sis) 1. surgical correction of syndactyly. 2. loss or amputation of a FINGER or TOE.

dactylomegaly (dak″tĭ-lo-meg′ah-le) megalodactyly.

dactyloscopy (dak″tĭ-los′kah-pe) examination of fingerprints for identification.

dactylus (dak′tĭ-lus) [Gr.] digit.

DAF decay accelerating factor.

Dakin's solution (da′kinz) an aqueous solution containing sodium hypochlorite and sodium bicarbonate; used as a local antibacterial and formerly to irrigate wounds.

dalfopristin (dal-fo′pris-tin) a semisynthetic ANTIBACTERIAL effective against a variety of gram-positive organisms. It is used in conjunction with QUINUPRISTIN in the treatment of serious BACTEREMIA caused by VANCOMYCIN-resistant ENTEROCOCCUS FAECIUM and complicated skin and skin structure infections caused by STREPTOCOCCUS PYOGENES or METHICILLIN-sensitive STAPHYLOCOCCUS AUREUS; administered intravenously.

Dalmane (dal′mān) trademark for a preparation of FLURAZEPAM hydrochloride, a SEDATIVE and HYPNOTIC.

dalteparin (dal-tep′ah-rin) an agent used as the sodium salt for prevention of pulmonary THROMBOEMBOLISM and deep venous thrombosis in at-risk abdominal surgery patients.

dalton (D) (Da) (dawl′ton) an arbitrary unit of mass, being $\frac{1}{12}$ the mass of the nuclide of carbon-12, equivalent to 1.657×10^{-24} g. Called also atomic mass unit.

Dalton's law (dawl′tonz) the pressure exerted by a mixture of nonreacting gases is equal to the sum of the partial pressures of the separate components; it holds true only at very low pressures.

daltonism (dawl′ton-izm) red-green color blindness.

dam (dam) 1. a barrier to obstruct the flow of water or other fluid. 2. rubber dam.

  dental d. rubber dam.

  rubber d. a sheet of thin latex rubber used by dentists to isolate a tooth or teeth from the fluids of the mouth during dental treatment, held in place by a clamp and frame. Occasionally these are used in surgical procedures to isolate tissues or structures. Called also dam.

damping (damp′ing) steady diminution of the amplitude of successive vibrations of a specific form of energy, as of electricity.

danaparoid (dah-nap′ah-roid) an agent used as the sodium salt in prophylaxis of pulmonary THROMBOEMBOLISM and deep venous THROMBOSIS.

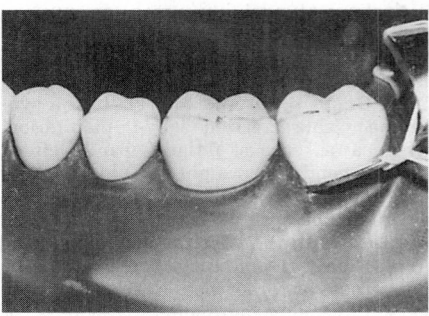

A well-sealed properly inverted rubber dam. From Darby and Walsh, 1994.

danazol (dan'ah-zol) a synthetic ANDROGEN that suppresses the ovarian-pituitary axis by inhibiting the release of GONADOTROPINS from the pituitary gland; administered orally for treatment of endometriosis, fibrocystic disease of the breast, hereditary angioedema, and gynecomastia.

D and C dilation and curettage.

dander (dan'der) small scales from the hair or feathers of animals, which may be a cause of allergy in sensitive persons.

dandruff (dan'druf) 1. a scaly material shed from the scalp; applied to that normally shed from the scalp epidermis as well as to the excessive scaly material associated with disease. The condition may spread unless checked and in rare cases may extend to the eyebrows, ears, nose, and neck, causing a reddening of the skin in those areas. 2. SEBORRHEIC DERMATITIS of the scalp.

Dandy-Walker syndrome (dan'de-wawk'-er) congenital hydrocephalus due to obstruction of the foramina of Magendie and Luschka.

Danocrine (dan'o-krin) trademark for a preparation of DANAZOL, an anterior pituitary suppressant used for treatment of endometriosis, fibrocystic disease of the breast, hereditary angioedema, and gynecomastia.

dantrolene (dan'tro-lēn) a skeletal muscle RELAXANT producing its effect primarily on the myoneural junction and the muscle tissue, and only secondarily on the central nervous system. It is used as the sodium salt, administered orally as an antispasmodic in conditions such as stroke, multiple sclerosis, and cerebral palsy; it is also used orally or intravenously in the prophylaxis and treatment of malignant hyperthermia.

dapiprazole (dah-pip'rah-zōl) an alpha-adrenergic blocking agent used topically to the conjunctiva as the hydrochloride salt to reverse pharmacologically-induced mydriasis.

dapsone (dap'sōn) an antibacterial used in treatment of LEPROSY and DERMATITIS HERPETIFORMIS and for prophylaxis of MALARIA caused by *Plasmodium falciparum*. Called also DDS.

Daranide (dar'ah-nīd) trademark for a preparation of DICHLORPHENAMIDE, a carbonic anhydrase INHIBITOR used in treatment of GLAUCOMA.

Darier's disease (dar'e-āz) keratosis follicularis.

Darling's disease (dahr'lingz) histoplasmosis.

dartoid (dar'toid) resembling the dartos.

dartos (dar'tos) the contractile tissue under the skin of the scrotum; called also tunica dartos.

Darvocet-N (dahr'vo-set) trademark for a preparation of PROPOXYPHENE napsylate and ACETAMINOPHEN, an ANALGESIC.

Darvon (dahr'von) trademark for preparations containing PROPOXYPHENE, an opioid ANALGESIC.

darwinism (dar'wĭ-nizm) the theory of EVOLUTION stating that change in a species over time is partly the result of a process of natural selection, which enables the species to continually adapt to its changing environment.

data (dat'ah, da'tah) pieces of information, such as those collected during a study; see data COLLECTION and data ANALYSIS.

   subjective d. information provided by the patient that focuses on perceptions and feelings.

database (da'tah-bās'') a collection of data or information. In online information retrieval, a collection of index records in machine readable form.

   bibliographic d. a database containing bibliographic records.

   full text d. a database containing the complete text of a source document such as a legal decision, news story, journal article, or other primary source.

daughter (daw'ter) 1. decay product. 2. arising from cell division, as a daughter cell.

daunorubicin (daw''no-roo'bĭ-sin) an antitumor ANTIBIOTIC of the ANTHRACYCLINE family, produced by a strain of *Streptomyces coeruleorubidus* and having antimitotic, cytotoxic, and immunosuppressive effects. As the hydrochloride salt it is administered intravenously in the treatment of acute lymphoblastic LEUKEMIA and acute myelogenous LEUKEMIA. As a liposome-encapsulated preparation of the citrate salt, it is administered intravenously in the treatment of advanced Kaposi's SARCOMA associated with ACQUIRED IMMUNODEFICIENCY SYNDROME (AIDS).

Davis (da'vis) Mary E. P. (1858–1924). Nursing educator and organizer and one of the founders of the *American Journal of Nursing*. She helped found the American Society of Superintendents of Training Schools for Nurses (later the League of Nursing Education), which became part of the National League for Nursing. She was a strong advocate of the development of nursing education, with its own theory and curriculum.

dB, db, decibel.

DBS deep brain stimulation.

D & C dilation of cervix and curettage (of uterus).

DDAVP trademark for preparations of DESMOPRESSIN acetate, a synthetic analogue of VASOPRESSIN used to treat central DIABETES INSIPIDUS, increased urination caused by trauma or surgery in the pituitary region, primary nocturnal ENURESIS, HEMOPHILIA A, and VON WILLEBRAND'S DISEASE.

DDP, *cis*-DDP, cisplatin.

DDS 1. Doctor of Dental Surgery. 2. dapsone.

DDT (dichlorodiphenyltrichloroethane) a moderately toxic chlorinated hydrocarbon pesticide, formerly widely used but now banned in the United States except for a few specialized purposes because its extremely long half-life causes ecological damage.

de- word element [L.], *down; from;* sometimes negative or privative, and often intensive.

deactivation (de-ak″tĭ-va′shun) the process of making or becoming inactive.

dead space 1. a space remaining in the tissues as a result of failure of proper closure of surgical or other wounds, permitting the accumulation of blood or serum. 2. the portions of the respiratory tract that are ventilated but not perfused by pulmonary circulation.

alveolar d. s. the difference between anatomical dead space and physiologic dead space, representing the space in alveoli occupied by air that does not participate in oxygen–carbon dioxide exchange (alveolar VENTILATION). It varies in different parts of the lungs and under different conditions.

anatomical d. s. the airways of the mouth, nose, pharynx, larynx, trachea, bronchi, and bronchioles.

equipment d. s. the volume of equipment that results in rebreathing of gases.

physiologic d. s. the sum of the anatomic and alveolar dead spaces; its volume (V_D) is determined by measuring the partial pressure of carbon dioxide in a sample of exhaled gas (PE_{CO_2}) and in the arterial blood (Pa_{CO_2}) and (with tidal volume of V_T) using the formula $V_D/V_T = (Pa_{CO_2}-PE_{CO_2})/Pa_{CO_2}$.

deaf (def) lacking the sense of HEARING or not having the full power of hearing; see HEARING LOSS.

deaf-mute (def′mūt″) old term for a person unable to hear or speak; now considered offensive.

deafness (def′nes) HEARING LOSS; lack or loss of all or a major part of the sense of HEARING. For types, see under hearing loss.

Alexander's d. congenital deafness due to cochlear aplasia involving chiefly the organ of Corti and adjacent ganglion cells of the basal coil of the cochlea; high-frequency hearing loss results.

central d. that due to causes in the auditory pathways or in the brain; see HEARING LOSS.

conduction d., conductive d. conductive HEARING LOSS.

functional d. functional HEARING LOSS.

hysterical d. functional hearing loss.

pagetoid d. that occurring in osteitis deformans of the bones of the skull (PAGET'S DISEASE).

sensorineural d. 1. that due to a defect in the inner ear or the acoustic nerve. See HEARING LOSS. 2. sensorineural HEARING LOSS.

word d. auditory aphasia.

deamidase (de-am′ĭ-dās) an enzyme that splits amides to form a carboxylic acid and ammonia.

deamidization (de-am″ĭ-dĭ-za′shun) the removal of an amido group from a molecule.

deaminase (de-am′ĭ-nās) an enzyme causing DEAMINATION (removal of the AMINE group from a compound); enzymes are named according to substrate, such as adenosine deaminase, cytidine deaminase, guanine deaminase, etc.

deamination (de-am″ĭ-na′shun) removal of the amino group, —NH_2, from a compound.

death (deth) the cessation of all physical and chemical processes that invariably occurs in all living organisms. (See also DYING.) There is at present no standardized diagnosis of clinical death or precise definition of human death. The most widely known and commonly accepted means of determining death evolved from several medical conferences held in the late 1960s for the purpose of defining irreversible COMA or nonfunctioning brain as a new criterion for death. The indications of deep irreversible coma (or brain DEATH) are (1) absolute unresponsiveness to externally applied stimuli; (2) cessation of movement and breathing, including no spontaneous breathing for three minutes after an artificial respirator has been turned off; and (3) complete absence of cephalic reflexes. The pupils of the eyes must be dilated and unresponsive to direct light. Use of the electroencephalogram is also recommended as being of value in confirmation of irreversible coma or death. If there is a flat electroencephalographic reading at the time of apparent death and a second flat reading 24 hours later, then the patient may be declared dead.

There are two exceptions to the above criteria. These are in regard to patients exhibiting marked hypothermia (body temperature below 32.2°C), and those suffering from severe central nervous system depression as a result of drug overdose.

It is recognized that the above criteria are limited in that the notion of irreversibility is not readily agreed upon and may take on new meaning as medical technology advances. The criteria are especially helpful as complements to the traditional criteria of absence of heart beat and lack of spontaneous respiration as indications of death.

In 1981, a Presidential Commission for the Study of Ethical Problems in Medicine and Biomedical and Behavioral Research strongly recommended that all of the United States recognize the cessation of brain function as a definition of death, even in cases in which life-support systems could maintain respiratory and circulatory functions by artificial means.

activation-induced cell d. (AICD) recognition and deletion of T lymphocytes that have been activated and so induced to proliferate. T lymphocytes are activated when a foreign agent is perceived, and AICD thereby prevents them from overgrowth. It is particularly important for regulation of lymphocytes that recognize self antigens.

black d. bubonic plague; see PLAGUE.

brain d., cerebral d. see BRAIN DEATH.

clinical d. the absence of heart beat (no pulse can be felt) and cessation of breathing.

cot d., crib d. sudden infant death syndrome (SIDS).

programmed cell d. the theory that particular cells are programmed to die at specific sites and at specific stages of development.

debility (de-bil′ĭ-te) asthenia.

débride (da-brēd′) [Fr.] to remove by débridement.

débridement (da-brēd-maw′) [Fr.] the removal of all foreign material and all contaminated and devitalized tissues from or adjacent to a traumatic or infected area until surrounding healthy tissue is exposed.

debriefing (de-brēf′ing) in health care research, informing the subjects of a study of the purpose of the study and the results that were obtained after the study is completed.

critical d. a conference or discussion held after an intense event or catastrophe; all aspects of the event are discussed and analyzed.

debris (dĕ-bre′) devitalized tissue or foreign matter.

debt (det) something owed.

oxygen d. the extra oxygen that must be used in the oxidative energy processes

after a period of strenuous exercise to reconvert lactic acid to glucose and decomposed ATP and creatine phosphate to their original states.

debulking (de-bulk′ing) removal of a major portion of the material that composes a lesion, such as the surgical removal of most of a tumor so that there is less tumor load for subsequent treatment by chemotherapy or radiation. Called also cytoreduction.

deca- word element [Gr.], 1. *ten;* also spelled deka-. 2. used in naming units of measurement to indicate a quantity 10 times the unit designated by the root with which it is combined.

Decadron (dek′ah-dron) trademark for preparations of DEXAMETHASONE, a steroid ANTIINFLAMMATORY agent.

decalcification (de-kal″sĭ-fĭ-ka′shun) 1. the process of removing calcareous matter. 2. the loss of calcium salts from bones or teeth.

decalcify (de-kal′sĭ-fĭ) to undergo DECALCIFICATION.

decannulation (de-kan″nu-la′shun) EXTUBATION of a cannula.

decantation (de-kan-ta′shun) the pouring of a clear supernatant liquid from a sediment.

decapitation (de-kap″ĭ-ta′shun) removal of the head, as of an animal, fetus, or bone.

decapsulation (de-kap″su-la′shun) capsulectomy.

decarboxylase (de″kahr-bok′sĭ-lās) any of the lyase class of enzymes that catalyze the removal of a carbon dioxide molecule from a compound.

decarboxylation (de″kahr-bok″sĭ-la′shun) removal of the carboxyl group from a compound.

decay (de-ka′) 1. the gradual decomposition of dead organic matter. 2. the process or stage of decline, as in old age.

tooth d. dental caries.

deceleration (de-sel″ĕ-ra′shun) the sudden stopping of movement, a frequent mechanism of motion injury. Common causes of deceleration INJURY are motor vehicle accidents and falls.

early d. in fetal heart rate monitoring, a transient decrease in heart rate that coincides with the onset of a uterine contraction.

late d. in fetal heart rate monitoring, a transient decrease in heart rate occurring at or after the peak of a uterine contraction and resulting from fetal hypoxia.

variable d's in fetal heart rate monitoring, a transient series of decelerations in heart rate that vary in duration, intensity, and relation to uterine contractions; they are abrupt in onset and cessation and result from vagus nerve firing in response to stimuli such as umbilical cord compression in the first stage of labor.

decerebrate (de-ser′ĕ-brāt) 1. to eliminate cerebral function by transection of the BRAINSTEM or ligation of the common carotid arteries and basilar artery at the center of the PONS. 2. a laboratory animal so prepared.

   d. rigidity a posture found in those with lesions of the upper part of the BRAINSTEM or severe bilateral lesions of the cerebrum; the patient lies in rigid extension with the arms internally rotated at the shoulders, elbows, knees, and hips extended, and fingers, ankles, and toes flexed. The jaw may be clenched with the neck hyperextended. (See illustration.) Called also decerebrate posturing.

decerebration (de-ser″ĕ-bra′shun) the act of decerebrating.

decholesterolization (de-ko-les″ter-ol-ĭ-za′shun) reduction of cholesterol levels in the blood.

deci- word element [L.], *one tenth;* used in naming units of measurement to indicate one tenth of the unit designated by the root with which it is combined (10^{-1}); symbol d.

decibel (des′ĭ-bel) a unit of relative power intensity equal to one tenth of a bel, used for electric or acoustic power measurements; one decibel equals approximately the smallest difference in acoustic power the human ear can detect and an increase of 10 decibels approximately doubles the loudness of a sound. Abbreviated dB or db.

decidua (de-sid′u-ah) a name applied to the endometrium during pregnancy, all of which except for the deepest layer is shed after childbirth; called also decidual or deciduous membranes. adj., **decid′ual.**

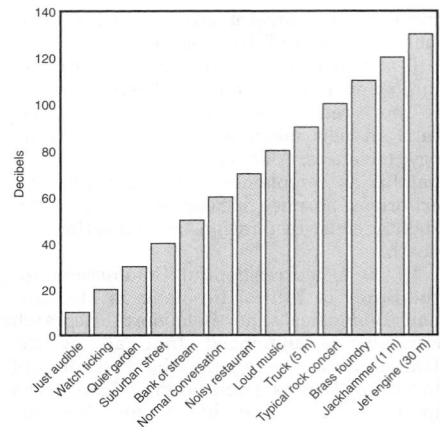

Examples of decibel levels in everyday situations. From Frazier et al., 1996.

   basal d., d. basa′lis that portion lying under the implanted ovum and chorion.

   capsular d., d. capsula′ris that portion directly overlying the implanted ovum and chorion, facing the uterine cavity.

   menstrual d., d. menstrua′lis the hyperemic uterine mucosa shed during menstruation.

   parietal d., d. parieta′lis true d., d. ve′ra the decidua exclusive of the area occupied by the implanted ovum and chorion.

deciduate (de-sid′u-āt) characterized by shedding.

deciduitis (de-sid″u-i′tis) a bacterial disease leading to changes in the decidua.

deciduoma (de-sid″u-o′mah) an intrauterine mass containing decidual cells.

deciduosis (de-sid″u-o′sis) the presence of decidual tissue or of tissue resembling the endometrium of pregnancy in an ectopic site.

deciduous (de-sid′u-us) falling off; subject to being shed, such as deciduous (primary) teeth. See TOOTH.

decile (des′īl) any of the nine values that divide the RANGE of a probability DISTRIBUTION into ten equal parts of equal probability; deciles are the 10th, 20th, 30th, etc. PERCENTILES.

deciliter (dL) (des′ĭ-le″ter) one tenth (10^{-1}) of a liter; 100 milliliters.

decitabine (DAC) (de-si′tah-bēn″) a cytotoxic compound used as an antineoplastic AGENT in treatment of acute leukemia.

declination (dek″lĭ-na′shun) cyclophoria.

declive (de-kliv′) a slope or a slanting surface. In anatomy, the part of the vermis of the cerebellum just caudal to the primary fissure. (See illustration.)

Arms extended
with wrists rotated

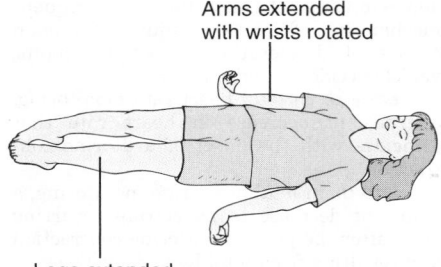

Legs extended
with feet internally rotated

Decerebrate rigidity (or posturing).

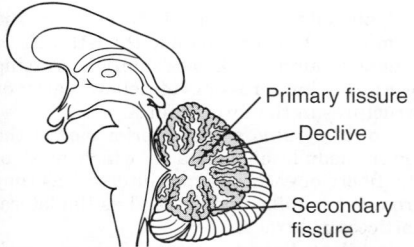

Median section of cerebellum, showing declive. From Dorland's, 2000.

- Primary fissure
- Declive
- Secondary fissure

D

declivis (de-kli′vis) [L.] declive.

decoloration (de-kul″er-a′shun) 1. removal of color; bleaching. 2. lack or loss of color.

decolorizer (de-kul′er-īz″er) an agent that removes color or bleaches.

decompensation (de″kom-pen-sa′shun) 1. any failure of homeostatic mechanisms. 2. inability of the heart to maintain adequate circulation; it is marked by dyspnea, venous engorgement, cyanosis, and edema. 3. in psychiatry, the failure of DEFENSE MECHANISMS, which results in progressive personality disintegration.

decomposition (de-kom″po-zish′un) 1. the separation of compound bodies into their constituent principles. 2. deterioration or decay of a substance.

decompression (de″kom-presh′un) return to normal environmental pressure after exposure to greatly increased pressure.

cerebral d. removal of a flap of the skull and incision of the dura mater for relief of intracranial pressure.

d. sickness a condition resulting from a too-rapid decrease in atmospheric pressure, as when a deep-sea diver is brought too hastily to the surface. The popular term *bends* is derived from the bodily contortions its victims undergo when atmospheric pressure is abruptly changed from a high pressure to a relatively lower one. Called also caisson disease and divers' paralysis. A similar condition, ALTITUDE SICKNESS, is suffered by aviators who ascend too rapidly to high altitudes. Decompression sickness may also be a complication in a type of oxygen therapy called HYPERBARIC OXYGENATION, in which the patient is placed in a high-pressure chamber to increase the oxygen content of the blood. Personnel and the patient within the chamber must be protected from decompression sickness when they emerge from the high-pressure chamber.

Cause. The phenomenon of decompression sickness is explained in terms of a law of physics: The greater the atmospheric pressure, the greater the amount of gas that can be dissolved in a liquid. The gas involved in this condition is the air we breathe, composed chiefly of nitrogen and oxygen. Under normal atmospheric pressure, nitrogen is present in the blood in dissolved form. If the atmospheric pressure is substantially increased, a proportionately greater amount of nitrogen will be dissolved in the blood. The same is true of oxygen, and this is the basis for hyperbaric oxygenation in the treatment of oxygen deficiency. The increase in pressure causes no ill effects. Nor will there be any ill effects if the pressure is gradually brought back to normal. When the decrease in pressure is slow, the nitrogen escapes safely from the blood as it passes through the lungs to be exhaled. If the pressure drops abruptly back to normal, the nitrogen is suddenly released from its state of solution in the blood and forms bubbles. Although the body is now under normal air pressure, expanding bubbles of nitrogen are present in the circulation and force their way into the capillaries, blocking the normal passage of the blood. This blockage (or air embolus) starves cells dependent on a constant supply of oxygen and other blood nutrients. Some of these cells may be nerve cells located in the limbs or in the spinal cord. When they are deprived of blood, an attack of decompression sickness occurs.

The oxygen in the blood reacts similarly when abnormal pressure is abruptly relieved. But because oxygen is dissolved more easily than nitrogen, and because some of the oxygen combines chemically with hemoglobin, the oxygen released in decompression forms fewer bubbles, and is therefore less troublesome.

Symptoms and Treatment. Symptoms include joint pain, dizziness, staggering, visual disturbances, dyspnea, and itching of the skin. Partial paralysis occurs in severe cases; collapse and insensibility are also possible. Only rarely is decompression sickness itself fatal, although a diver while in this condition may suffer a fatal accident unless he or she is rescued. Treatment consists of placing the victim in a decompression chamber where the air pressure is at the original higher level of pressure. If the victim is a diver, this is the pressure at the depth where he or she was working. Pressure in the chamber is then reduced to normal at a safe rate.

deconditioning (de-kon-dish′un-ing) the loss of muscle tone and endurance due to chronic disease, immobility, or loss of function.

decongestant (de″kon-jes′tant) 1. tending to reduce CONGESTION or swelling, usually of the nasal membranes. Called also decongestive. 2. an agent that has this effect; it may be inhaled, taken as spray or nose drops, or used orally in liquid or tablet form. Nasal decongestants act by reducing swelling of the membranes and thus opening up the nasal passages. Among the leading ones are EPINEPHRINE, EPHEDRINE, and PHENYLEPHRINE. ANTIHISTAMINES may also be effective either alone or in combination with decongestants. A decongestant must be used several times a day to be helpful; but excessive use may cause headaches, dizziness, or other disorders and sometimes the medicine itself may cause reactive nasal swelling.

decongestive (de″kon-jes′tiv) decongestant (def. 1).

decontamination (de″kon-tam-ĭ-na′shun) the freeing of a person or object from some contaminating substance such as war gas, radioactive material, or bacteria.

decorticate rigidity (de-kor′tĭ-kāt) abnormal flexor posturing of the limbs, indicative of a lesion in the cerebral HEMISPHERES or disruption of the corticospinal TRACTS. The patient exhibits bilateral adduction of the shoulders, pronation and flexion of the elbows and wrists, and extension, internal rotation, and plantar flexion of the lower extremities.

decortication (de-kor″tĭ-ka′shun) 1. removal of the outer covering from a plant, seed, or root. 2. removal of portions of the CORTEX of a structure or organ, as of the brain, kidney, or lung. 3. a surgical procedure to remove a residual clot or new scar tissue following a HEMOTHORAX or untreated EMPYEMA.

decrudescence (de″kroo-des′ens) diminution or abatement of the intensity of symptoms.

decubitus (de-ku′bĭ-tus), pl. *decu′bitus* [L.] 1. the act of lying down. 2. the position assumed in lying down. 3. obsolete term for PRESSURE ULCER. adj., **decu′bital.**

Andral's d. decubitus on the affected side, a position assumed in the early stages of pleurisy.

dorsal d. lying on the back.

lateral d. lying on one side, designated right lateral decubitus when the subject lies on the right side and left lateral decubitus when on the left side.

ventral d. lying on the stomach.

decussate (de-kus′āt) 1. to cross in the form of an X. 2. crossed like the letter X.

decussation (de″kus-sa′shun) a crossing over; the intercrossing of fellow parts or structures in the form of an X.

d. of pyramids the anterior part of the lower medulla oblongata in which most of the fibers of each pyramid intersect as they cross the midline and descend as the lateral corticospinal tracts.

dedifferentiation (de-dif″er-en″she-a′-shun) anaplasia.

deductible (de-duk′tĭ-b′l) the amount that the patient must pay before a third party payer will assume responsibility for health care charges; see also third party PAYMENT.

deduction (de-duk′shun) reasoning in which the conclusion follows necessarily from the premises; reasoning from the general to the particular.

deerfly fever (dēr′fli″) tularemia.

deet (dēt) diethyltoluamide.

DEF decayed/extraction/filled; see DEF RATE.

defatted (de-fat′ed) deprived of fat.

defecation (def″ĕ-ka′shun) elimination of wastes and undigested food, as feces, from the rectum.

defect (de′fekt) an imperfection, failure, or absence.

congenital heart d. see CONGENITAL HEART DEFECT.

aortic septal d. see AORTIC SEPTAL DEFECT.

atrial septal d. see ATRIAL SEPTAL DEFECT.

filling d. an interruption in the contour of the inner surface of stomach or intestine revealed by radiography, indicating excess tissue or substance on or in the wall of the organ.

neural tube d. see NEURAL TUBE DEFECT.

septal d. a defect in the cardiac septum resulting in an abnormal communication between opposite chambers of the heart. Common types are AORTIC SEPTAL DEFECT, ATRIAL SEPTAL DEFECT, and VENTRICULAR SEPTAL DEFECT. See also CONGENITAL HEART DEFECT.

defective (de-fek′tiv) 1. imperfect. 2. a person lacking in some physical, mental, or moral quality.

defeminization (de-fem″ĭ-nĭ-za′shun) loss of female sexual characteristics.

defense (de-fens′) behavior directed to protection of the individual from injury.

character d. any character trait, e.g., a mannerism, attitude, or affectation, which serves as a DEFENSE MECHANISM.

insanity d. a legal concept that a person cannot be convicted of a crime if he lacked criminal responsibility by reason of insanity at the time of commission of the crime.

d. mechanism in psychology, an unconscious mental process or coping pattern that lessens the anxiety associated with a situation or internal conflict and protects the person from mental discomfort. In the theory of PSYCHOANALYSIS, the EGO, following the reality principle, conforms to the demands of the outside world, but the ID (repressed unconscious), following the pleasure principle, pursues immediate gratification of desires and reduction of psychic tension. The SUPEREGO (conscience or morality) may take either side. Defense mechanisms develop in order to control impulses or feelings that lead to inner conflicts, to reach compromises between conflicting impulses, and to reduce inner tensions. They help to manage or avoid anxiety, aggression, hostility, resentment, and frustration. Defense mechanisms are not pathological in themselves; they can be a means of dealing with unbearable situations. Among the most common defense mechanisms are DENIAL, DISPLACEMENT, IDENTIFICATION, PROJECTION, RATIONALIZATION, REACTION-FORMATION, REPRESSION, and SUBLIMATION.

d. reaction a mental reaction that shuts out from consciousness ideas not acceptable to the ego. See also DEFENSE MECHANISM.

deferens (def'er-ens) [L.] deferent.

deferent (def'er-ent) conducting or progressing away, as from a center or specific site of reference.

deferential (def''er-en'shal) pertaining to the ductus deferens.

deferentitis (def''er-en-ti'tis) inflammation of the ductus deferens.

deferoxamine (de''fer-oks'ah-mēn) an iron-chelating agent isolated from *Streptomyces pilosus,* used as an antidote in IRON POISONING.

defervescence (def''er-ves'ens) the period of abatement of fever.

defibrillation (de-fib''rĭ-la'shun) termination of atrial or ventricular FIBRILLATION, usually by electric shock. Defibrillation by precordial shock is accomplished by delivering a nonsynchronized direct current to the myocardium. It is an emergency procedure, used to terminate a life-threatening ventricular arrhythmia. The electric shock is delivered either by placing metal paddles on the chest (*closed defibrillation*) or by applying paddles directly to the heart muscle, as in cardiac surgery. The high-voltage electrical current delivered during precordial shock causes complete depolarization of the heart muscle, disrupting all of the electrical circuits that are activating the heart muscle and causing ventricular

fibrillation. This allows the heart's natural pacemaker to regain control and regulation of the heart rate and rhythm.

The procedure carries some risk and should be done only by specially trained physicians, nurses, and paramedics. Cardiopulmonary resuscitation and the administration of intravenous fluids and drugs are essential components of defibrillation. Sodium bicarbonate is given to combat acidosis; lidocaine or amiodarone is given to forestall arrhythmias that may develop during and after defibrillation.

Electrocardiographic readings and assessment of ECG patterns are done prior to the procedure to verify the presence of a lethal arrhythmia, and afterwards to evaluate the effectiveness of the treatment. Some ECG machines and cardiac monitors can continue to function during defibrillation because they have been designed to withstand the electrical shock when it is delivered to the patient.

Burns of the skin may occur under the paddles at the time of defibrillation; steroid or lanolin-based ointments or creams are usually prescribed as treatment. The use of conduction gel and close contact of paddles to skin may prevent burns. More serious complications of defibrillation include cardiac arrest, respiratory arrest, neurologic impairment, pulmonary edema, and pulmonary and systemic emboli. The patient must be monitored carefully after the procedure for return of ventricular fibrillation. Additional observations include changes in blood pressure; pulse rate,

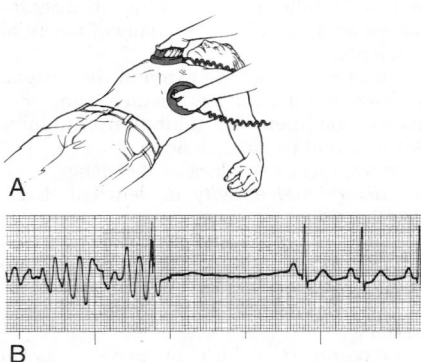

Defibrillation: *A,* Anterolateral paddle placement for external countershock. External paddles are placed at the second right intercostal space and at the anterior axillary line in the fifth left intercostal space. *B,* Ventricular fibrillation converted to normal sinus rhythm with external countershock. From Polaski and Tatro, 1996.

rhythm, and character; state of consciousness; and adequacy of ventilation.

defibrillator (de-fib′rĭ-la″ter) an apparatus used to produce defibrillation by application of brief electroshock to the heart, directly or through electrodes placed on the chest wall.

automatic external d. **(AED)** a portable defibrillator designed to be automated such that it can be used by persons without substantial medical training who are responding to a cardiac emergency.

automatic implantable cardioverter-d. **(AICD),** *implantable cardioverter-d.* **(ICD)** an implantable device that detects sustained ventricular TACHYCARDIA or FIBRILLATION and terminates it by a shock or shocks delivered directly to the myocardium, thus preventing sudden cardiac death. Three different types of electrodes may be used: a superior vena cava spring lead, a transvenous bipolar ELECTRODE, and a ventricular patch lead. One third of the patients who have had this device implanted have received spontaneous device COUNTERSHOCKS. Other reported side effects are similar to those of PACEMAKERS.

defibrination (de-fi″brĭ-na′shun) the destruction or removal of fibrin, as from the blood.

d. syndrome disseminated intravascular coagulation.

deficiency (de-fish′en-se) a lack or shortage; a condition characterized by the presence of less than the normal or necessary supply or competence.

color vision d. see COLOR VISION DEFICIENCY.

d. disease a condition due to dietary or metabolic deficiency, including all diseases caused by an insufficient supply of essential nutrients.

iron d. deficiency of iron in the system, as from blood loss, low dietary iron, or a disease condition that inhibits iron uptake. See IRON and iron deficiency ANEMIA.

deficit (def′ĭ-sit) a lack or deficiency.

diversional activity d. deficient diversional activity.

fluid volume d. deficient fluid volume.

hearing d. HEARING LOSS; see also communication ENHANCEMENT: hearing deficit.

knowledge d. see KNOWLEDGE DEFICIT (SPECIFY).

oxygen d. a lack of oxygen, as in HYPOXIA, ANOXIA, or insufficient oxygen delivery in comparison to oxygen consumption.

pulse d. the difference between the apical pulse and the radial pulse, obtained by having one person count the apical pulse as heard through a stethoscope over the

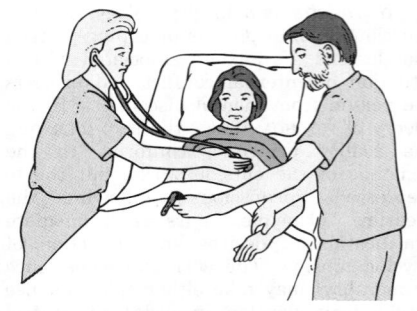

Assessing the apical-radial pulse to identify a pulse deficit. From Lammon et al., 1995.

heart and a second person count the radial pulse at the same time.

reversible ischemic neurologic d. a type of cerebral INFARCTION whose clinical course lasts longer than 24 hours but less than 72 hours; brain imaging usually reveals an infarct. See also STROKE SYNDROME.

self care d. any of a group of NURSING DIAGNOSES approved by the North American Nursing Diagnosis Association, defined as impaired ability to perform basic self care (ACTIVITIES OF DAILY LIVING) in the areas of feeding, bathing/hygiene, dressing/grooming, and toileting. Related factors include diminished strength and endurance, pain or discomfort, impaired mentation, neuromuscular disorder, depression, and anxiety. The defining characteristics for each functional level are readily observed and graded on a scale of 0 to 4. The suggested code for functional level classification is as follows: *0,* Completely independent; *1,* Requires use of equipment or device; *2,* Requires help from another person for assistance, supervision, or teaching; *3,* Requires help from another person and equipment or device; *4,* Dependent; does not participate in activity.

self care d., bathing/hygiene a NURSING DIAGNOSIS defined as impaired ability to perform or complete bathing/hygiene activities for oneself; see self care DEFICIT.

self care d., dressing/grooming a NURSING DIAGNOSIS defined as impaired ability to perform or complete dressing and grooming activities for oneself; see self care DEFICIT.

self care d., feeding a NURSING DIAGNOSIS defined as impaired ability to perform or complete feeding activities; see self care DEFICIT.

self care d., toileting a NURSING DIAGNOSIS defined as impaired ability to perform or complete one's own toileting activities; see self care DEFICIT.

speech d. SPEECH DISORDER; see also communication ENHANCEMENT: speech deficit.

visual d. partial or complete BLINDNESS; see communication ENHANCEMENT: visual deficit.

definition (def″ĭ-ni′shun) a statement of the meaning of a word or phrase.

conceptual d. an identification of the personal knowledge or connotative meaning of a word. These meanings are often difficult to express; the meaning is "known" but not easily put into words.

operational d. a definition, method, or procedure used to measure or represent a concept or variable in a specific situation.

deflection (de-flek′shun) a turning aside. In the electrocardiogram, a deviation of the curve from the isoelectric baseline; that is, any wave or complex.

H d. the segment on an electrocardiogram that represents activation of the bundle of His.

intrinsicoid d. measured on unipolar precordial leads, the interval from the earliest onset of the QRS complex to the peak of the last R wave, representing the arrival of the impulse under the electrode. Called also R peak time.

defluvium (de-floo′ve-um) [L.] a falling out, as of hair.

defluxion (de-fluk′shun) 1. a sudden disappearance. 2. a copious discharge, as of catarrh. 3. a falling out, as of hair.

deformability (de-form″ah-bil′ĭ-te) the ability of cells to change shape as they pass through narrow spaces, such as erythrocytes passing through the microvasculature.

deformation (de″for-ma′shun) 1. DEFORMITY, especially an alteration in shape or structure. 2. the process of adapting in shape or form.

elastic d. temporary elongation of tissue when a prolonged force has been applied. See also CREEP.

plastic d. permanent elongation of tissue when a prolonged nondisruptive mechanical force has been applied. See also CREEP.

deformity (de-for′mĭ-te) distortion of any part or of the body in general; called also malformation.

Arnold-Chiari d. a congenital anomaly in which the cerebellum and medulla oblongata protrude down into the cervical spinal canal through the foramen magnum; it is almost always associated with meningomyelocele and hydrocephalus.

Madelung's d. radial deviation of the hand secondary to overgrowth of the distal ulna or shortening of the radius.

degenerate 1. (de-jen′er-āt) to change from a higher to a lower form. 2. (de-jen′er-it) characterized by degeneration.

degeneration (de-gen″ĕ-ra′shun) deterioration; change from a higher to a lower form, especially change of tissue to a lower or less functionally active form. When there is chemical change of the tissue itself, it is true degeneration; when the change consists in the deposit of abnormal matter in the tissues, it is infiltration. adj., **degen′erative.**

caseous d. caseation (def. 2).

cerebromacular d., cerebroretinal d. 1. degeneration of brain cells and of the macula retinae, as occurs in TAY-SACHS DISEASE. 2. any lipidosis with cerebral lesions and degeneration of the retinal macula. 3. any form of neuronal ceroid-lipofuscinosis.

colloid d. degeneration with conversion of the tissues into a gelatinous or gumlike material.

cystic d. degeneration with formation of cysts.

fatty d. deposit of fat globules in a tissue.

fibroid d. degeneration of a LEIOMYOMA with subsequent FIBROSIS.

hepatolenticular d. Wilson's disease.

hyaline d. a regressive change in cells in which the cytoplasm takes on a homogeneous, glassy appearance; also used loosely to describe the histologic appearance of tissues.

hydropic d. a form in which the epithelial cells absorb much water.

lattice d. of retina a frequently bilateral, usually benign asymptomatic condition, characterized by patches of fine gray or white lines that intersect at irregular intervals in the peripheral retina, usually associated with numerous, round, punched-out areas of retinal thinning or retinal holes.

macular d. see MACULAR DEGENERATION.

macular d., congenital see STARGARDT'S DISEASE.

macular d., Stargardt's STARGARDT'S DISEASE.

mucoid d. degeneration with deposit of myelin and lecithin in the cells.

mucous d. degeneration with accumulation of mucus in epithelial tissues.

myofibrillar d. damage to selective cardiac cells when surrounding interstitial cells, nerves, and capillaries remain viable.

myxomatous d. mucous degeneration.

spongy d. of central nervous system, spongy d. of white matter Canavan disease.

subacute combined d. of spinal cord degeneration of both the posterior

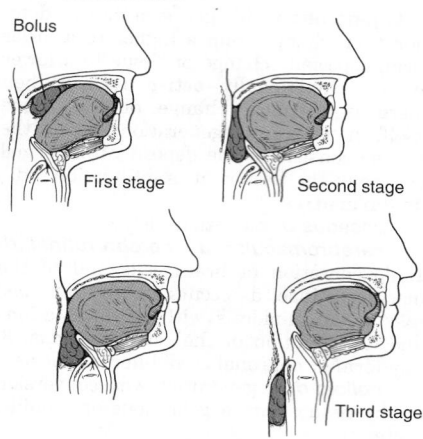

Bolus

First stage

Second stage

Third stage

The three stages of deglutition: *First stage*, voluntary lip closure and tooth approximation. *Second stage*, involuntary peristalsis carries the bolus of food down the esophagus; the nasal passage and pharyngeal airway is blocked. *Third stage*, the bolus of food passes the length of the esophagus and into the stomach via peristaltic waves. From Myers, 1995.

and lateral columns of the spinal cord, producing various motor and sensory disturbances; it is due to vitamin B_{12} deficiency and is usually associated with pernicious anemia. Called also Lichtheim's or Putnam-Dana syndrome.

wallerian d. fatty degeneration of a nerve fiber that has been severed from its nutritive source.

Zenker's d. Zenker's necrosis.

degenerative joint disease osteoarthritis.

degloving (de-gluv'ing) intra-oral surgical exposure of the bony mandibular chin; it can be performed in the posterior region if necessary.

deglutition (deg″loo-tish'un) swallowing.

deglicerolize (de-glis'er-ol-īz) to remove the glycerol cryopreservative medium from frozen red blood cells and replace it with an isotonic solution for transfusion.

degradation (deg″rah-da'shun) conversion of a chemical compound to one less complex, as by splitting off one or more groups of atoms. See also LYSIS.

degree (dĕ-gre') 1. a grade or rank within a series, especially a rank awarded to scholars by a college or university. 2. a unit of measure of temperature. 3. a unit of measure of arcs and angles, one degree being 1/360 of a circle. 4. one of the ranks or stages in a progressive series.

d's of freedom (df) the number of ways that the members of a sample can vary independently. For example, if a sample contains n scores and the sum of those scores is known, $n − 1$ scores are free to vary; the nth score, however, is not free to vary but is determined by the values of the other scores and the established sum of the scores. In this example, the degrees of freedom equal the sample size minus 1 ($df = n − 1$).

degustation (de″gus-ta'shun) the act or function of tasting.

dehiscence (de-his'ens) 1. a splitting open. 2. wound dehiscence.

d. of uterus rupture of the uterus following cesarean section, especially separation of the uterine scar prior to or during a subsequent labor.

wound d. separation of the layers of a surgical wound; it may be partial or only superficial, or complete with separation of all layers and total disruption. Complete dehiscence of an abdominal wound usually leads to EVISCERATION.

PATIENT CARE. Patients most at risk for wound dehiscence are those who are obese, malnourished, or dehydrated or have abdominal distention, a malignancy, or multiple trauma to the abdomen. Infected wounds are also prone to dehiscence. Those patients who smoke or have a chronic cough are also at risk. Careful monitoring of patients with a predisposition to delayed healing is essential for prevention or mitigation of wound separation, especially between the fifth and twelfth postoperative days, when dehiscence most often occurs. In about half the cases of dehiscence there is a noticeable increase in serosanguineous drainage on the wound dressing before separation of the outer layers becomes apparent. Patients also may report the feeling that something has "given way" in the wound. If evisceration has not occurred, the wound may be splinted with reinforced dressings, sterile towels, or a binder. This could prevent further separation and allow time to notify the surgeon. The patient should be instructed to lie quietly and, if it is an abdominal wound, to try to avoid increasing intra-abdominal pressure by coughing or straining in any way.

Should splinting an abdominal wound fail to prevent further separation and a spilling of the viscera through the opening, emergency surgery is imperative. Until the patient goes to surgery, the protruding intestines should be covered to prevent drying. Some authorities recommend that only dry sterile towels be used while others prefer covering the entire wound with a sterile towel moistened with povidone-iodine

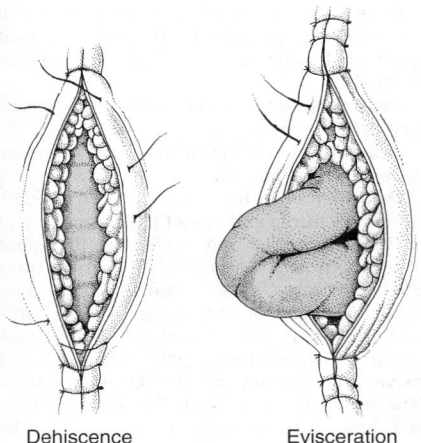

Dehiscence   Evisceration

The sutures are unable to keep the wound closed and the edges are no longer approximated. Dehiscence can lead to wound evisceration. From Ignatavicius and Workman, 2002.

(Betadine). Warming the solution to body temperature can help avoid shock to the intestines, but is not necessary if there is not time to do this.

   dehumidifier (de″hu-mid′ĭ-fi″er) an apparatus for reducing the content of moisture in the atmosphere.

   dehydratase (de-hi′drah-tās) any enzyme of the lyase class that catalyzes the removal of H_2O, leaving double bonds (or adding groups to double bonds).

   dehydration (de″hi-dra′shun) removal of water from the body or a tissue; or the condition that results from undue loss of water. DIARRHEA in infants is a common cause of this. Severe dehydration is a serious condition that may lead to SHOCK, ACIDOSIS, and accumulation of waste products in the body (as in UREMIA), sometimes resulting in death. Water accounts for more than half the body weight. Under normal conditions, the total 24-hour output of fluid in urine and feces and through the lungs and skin is about 2500 ml in adults. To make up for this loss, the same amount must be taken in to maintain FLUID BALANCE. When the fluid intake is insufficient or the output is excessive, deficient fluid VOLUME occurs. (See accompanying illustration.)

   dehydrocholesterol (de-hi″dro-ko-les′terol) a sterol found in the skin which, when properly irradiated by ultraviolet rays, forms vitamin D.

   activated 7-d. cholecalciferol.

   dehydrocholic acid (de-hi″dro-ko′lik) a synthetic BILE ACID used to increase output of bile by the liver and the filling of the gallbladder. Preparations of this acid are used to aid the digestion of fats and increase absorption of fat-soluble vitamins. Drugs containing dehydrocholic acid are contraindicated in cases of biliary obstruction. Because of the bitter taste on the tongue after it is injected into a vein, it is used to provide an end point for the measurement of arm-tongue circulation time.

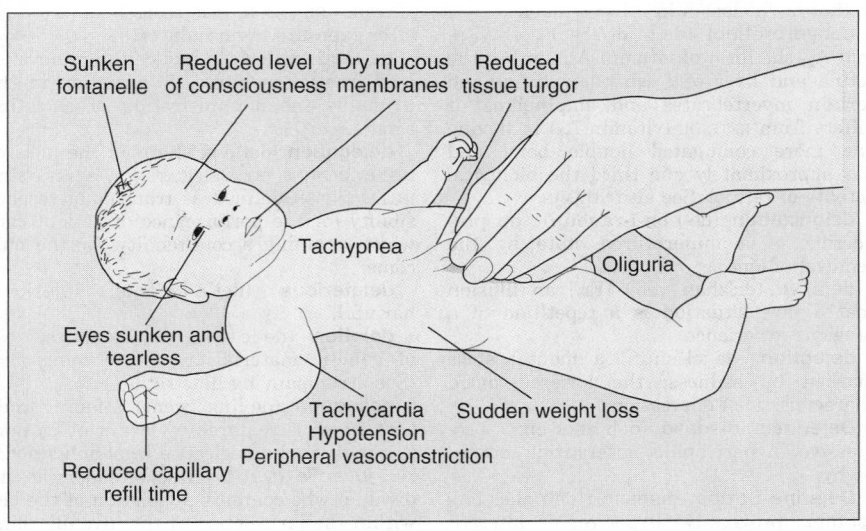

Clinical features of dehydration in an infant. From Lissauer and Graham, 2002.

11-dehydrocorticosterone (de-hi″dro-kor″tĭ-ko-stēr′ōn) one of the least active of the GLUCOCORTICOSTEROIDS produced by the adrenal cortex; it affects water and salt metabolism.

dehydroepiandrosterone (de-hi″dro-ep″ē-an-dros′ter-ōn) an androgen occurring in normal human urine and synthesized from cholesterol; its level decreases with age.

dehydrogenase (de-hi′dro-jen-ās″) an enzyme that mobilizes the hydrogen of a substrate so that it can pass to a hydrogen acceptor.

glucose-6-phosphate d. an enzyme necessary for the oxidation of glucose-6-phosphate, an intermediate in carbohydrate metabolism. Hereditary deficiency of this enzyme in the erythrocytes is associated with a tendency toward hemolysis upon ingestion of certain antimalarial AGENTS and SULFONAMIDE drugs and fava beans (see FAVISM.

lactate d. **(LDH)** an enzyme that catalyzes the interconversion of lactate and pyruvate. It is widespread in tissues and is particularly abundant in kidney, skeletal muscle, liver, and myocardium. It appears in elevated concentrations when these tissues are injured.

dehydrogenate (de-hi′dro-jen-āt″) to remove hydrogen from a molecule.

dehydroretinal (de-hi″dro-ret′ĭ-nal) the aldehyde of dehydroretinol, derived from the visual pigment porphyropsin, found in freshwater fishes and certain vertebrates and amphibians; its metabolic role is analogous to that of rhodopsin in other animals.

dehydroretinol (de-hi″dro-ret′ĭ-nol) vitamin A_2, the form of vitamin A found in the retina and liver of fresh-water fishes and certain invertebrates and amphibians; it differs from RETINOL (vitamin A_1) in having one more conjugated double bond and has approximately one third the biological activity of retinol. See also VITAMIN.

deionization (de-i″on-ī-za′shun) the production of a mineral-free state by the removal of ions.

déjà vu (da′zhah voo′) [Fr.] an illusion that a new situation is a repetition of a previous experience.

dejection (de-jek′shun) a mental state marked by sadness; the lowered mood characteristic of depression.

Dejerine's disease (deh″zher-ēnz′) progressive hypertrophic interstitial neuropathy.

Dejerine-Sottas disease (deh″zher-ēn′-sot′tahz) progressive hypertrophic interstitial neuropathy.

deka- a prefix used in naming units of measurement to indicate 10 times the unit specified by the root to which it is joined. Symbol dk.

delacrimation (de-lak″rĭ-ma′shun) excessive flow of tears.

delactation (de″lak-ta′shun) 1. weaning. 2. cessation of lactation.

Delano (del′ah-no) Jane A. (1862–1919). American nurse and one of the organizers of military nursing. She served as president of the Nurses' Associated Alumnae (now the American Nurses' Association) and as superintendent of the Army Nurse Corps and founded the American Red Cross Nursing Service. From 1909 until 1919, she served as director of the Department of Nursing of the American Red Cross, where she helped to develop a reserve for the Army Nurse Corps, with the result that a large number of well-trained nurses were available for duty in World War I.

Delatestryl (del″ah-tes′tril) trademark for a preparation of TESTOSTERONE, used for treatment of male HYPOGONADISM and delayed male puberty, and palliation of metastatic breast cancer in women.

delavirdine (del″ah-vir′dēn) an ANTIRETROVIRAL agent, that acts as a non-nucleoside reverse transcriptase INHIBITOR; administered orally as the mesylate salt in treatment of human immunodeficiency VIRUS infection.

delay (de-la′) a postponement to a later time.

atrioventricular d., AV d. atrioventricular INTERVAL (def. 2).

delayed reaction a reaction, such as an ALLERGIC REACTION, occurring hours to days after exposure to an inducer.

de-lead (de-led′) to induce the removal of lead from tissues and its excretion in the urine by the administration of chelating agents.

delegation (del″e-ga′shun) in the NURSING INTERVENTIONS CLASSIFICATION, a nursing INTERVENTION defined as transfer of responsibility for the performance of patient care while retaining accountability for the outcome.

deleterious (del″e-tēr′e-us) injurious; harmful.

deletion (de-le′shun) in genetics, loss of genetic material from a chromosome. (See accompanying illustration.)

delinquent (de-ling′kwent) 1. failing to do that which is required by law or obligation. 2. a person who neglects a legal obligation.

juvenile d. a juvenile offender; an individual who commits a violation of the law within the jurisdiction of the juvenile court system.

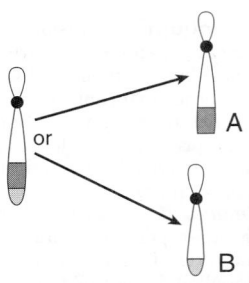
Examples of large-scale chromosomal deletions: *A*, terminal; *B*, interstitial. From Dorland's, 2000.

deliquescence (del″ĭ-kwes′ens) the condition of becoming moist or liquefied as a result of absorption of water from the air.

delirium (dĕ-lēr′e-um), pl. *deli'ria* An acute, transient disturbance of CONSCIOUS-NESS accompanied by a change in cognition and having a fluctuating course. Characteristics include reduced ability to maintain attention to external stimuli and disorganized thinking as manifested by rambling, irrelevant, or incoherent speech; there may also be a reduced level of CONSCIOUSNESS, sensory misperceptions, disturbance of the sleep-wakefulness cycle and level of psychomotor activity, disorientation to time, place, or person, and memory impairment. Delirium may be caused by a number of conditions that result in derangement of cerebral metabolism, including systemic infection, cerebral tumor, poisoning, drug intoxication or withdrawal, seizures or head trauma, and metabolic disturbances such as fluid, electrolyte, or acid-base imbalance, hypoxia, hypoglycemia, or hepatic or renal failure.

 alcohol withdrawal d., d. tre'mens an acute alcohol WITHDRAWAL syndrome that can occur in any person who has a history of drinking heavily and suddenly stops. It can occur with any form of alcoholic beverage, including beer and wine, and is most commonly seen in chronic alcoholics. The severity of the symptoms usually depends on the length of time the patient has had a problem of alcohol abuse and the amount of alcohol that had been drunk before the abstinence that precipitated the delirium. See also ALCOHOLISM.

Clinical Course. Generally, this syndrome begins a few days after drinking has ceased and ends within 1–5 days. It can be heralded by a variety of signs and symptoms. Some patients exhibit only mild tremulousness, irritability, difficulty in sleeping, an elevated pulse rate and hypertension, and increased temperature. Others

have generalized convulsions as the first sign of difficulty. Most persons exhibit severe memory disturbance, agitation, anorexia, and hallucinations. Hallucinations are likely to follow the early signs and usually, but not always, are unpleasant and threatening to the patient. These hallucinations can be of three types: auditory, visual, or tactile. Delusions often follow or accompany the hallucinations. These patients are unable to think clearly and sometimes become paranoid and greatly agitated. At this point they can become dangerous to themselves and others.

Generalized grand mal seizures can occur in delirium tremens. The hallucinations and delusions may continue, contributing to the state of agitation and precipitating seizures.

Treatment and Patient Care. Persons with delirium tremens are very ill and have multiple short-term and long-term problems. They should be kept in a quiet, nonstimulating environment and approached in a calm, reassuring manner. They must be watched closely and protected from self-injury during the period of delirium and also when they are convalescing from their illness and are likely to feel great remorse and depression. They should be observed for signs of extreme fatigue, pneumonia, or heart failure. Respiratory infections are quite common in these patients because of their weakened condition and inattention to personal hygiene. The diet should be high in fluid intake and carbohydrate content and low in fats. If the patient has cirrhosis, protein intake may be limited. Dietary supplements usually include vitamin preparations, especially the B complex vitamins. If the patient is unable to cooperate by taking fluids and food by mouth, tube feeding and intravenous fluids may be necessary. Tranquilizing agents and sedatives are useful for therapy.

deliver (de-liv′er) 1. to aid in childbirth. 2. to remove, as a fetus, placenta, or lens of the eye.

delivery (de-liv′er-e) 1. the bringing of something to a place. 2. expulsion or extraction of the child and fetal membranes at birth; see also LABOR. Called also accouchement.

 abdominal d. cesarean section.

 breech d. delivery of a fetus in breech presentation; see also BREECH EXTRACTION.

 controlled drug d. a system used in dentistry that delivers an ANTIMICROBIAL AGENT to the target site and maintains the desired concentration for enough time without development of resistant bacteria.

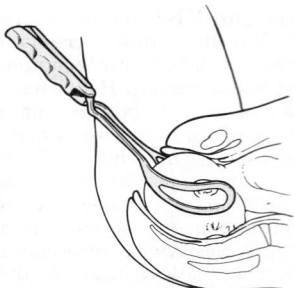

Forceps delivery. From Dorland's, 2000.

forceps d. extraction of a fetus from the maternal passages by application of forceps to the child's head. See illustration.

dellen (del′en) saucer-shaped excavations at the periphery of the cornea, usually on the temporal side.

delomorphous (del″o-mor′fus) having definitely formed and well-defined limits, as a cell or tissue.

Delphi technique (del′fi) a method of measuring the judgments of a group of experts, assessing priorities, or making forecasts. A questionnaire is sent to a panel of experts and the responses are summarized and subjected to statistical analysis. The outcome of the analysis is returned to the panel along with a second questionnaire. This procedure is repeated until a consensus is reached by the panel.

delta (del′tah) 1. the fourth letter of the Greek alphabet, Δ or δ; used in chemical names to denote the fourth of a series of isomeric compounds or the carbon atom fourth from the carboxyl group, or to denote the fourth of any series. 2. a triangular area.

Deltasone (del′tah-sōn) trademark for a preparation of PREDNISONE, a GLUCOCORTICOID used as an antiinflammatory and immunosuppressant.

Deltavirus (del′tah-vi″rus) a genus of satellite VIRUSES that require helper hepatitis B viruses for their replication. It contains a single species, hepatitis D virus.

deltoid (del′toid) 1. triangular. 2. the deltoid muscle (see anatomic Table of Muscles in the Appendices).

delusion (dĕ-loo′zhun) a false belief that is firmly maintained in spite of incontrovertible and obvious proof to the contrary and in spite of the fact that other members of the culture do not share the belief. adj., **delu′sional.**

bizarre d. one that is patently absurd, with no possible basis in fact.

d. of control the delusion that one's thoughts, feelings, and actions are not one's own but are being imposed by someone else or some other external force.

depressive d. a delusion that is congruent with a predominant depressed mood, such as a delusion of serious illness, poverty, or spousal infidelity.

erotomanic d. a delusional conviction that some other person, usually of higher status and often famous, is in love with the individual; it is one of the subtypes of DELUSIONAL DISORDER.

fragmentary d's unconnected delusions not organized around a coherent theme.

d. of grandeur, grandiose d. delusional conviction of one's own importance, power, or knowledge, or that one is, or has a special relationship with, a deity or a famous person. It is one of the subtypes of DELUSIONAL DISORDER.

d. of jealousy a delusional belief that one's spouse or lover is unfaithful, based on erroneous inferences drawn from innocent events imagined to be evidence and often resulting in confrontation with the accused. It is one of the subtypes of DELUSIONAL DISORDER.

mixed d. one in which no central theme predominates. It is one of the subtypes of DELUSIONAL DISORDER.

d. of negation, nihilistic d. a depressive delusion that the self, part of the self, part of the body, other persons, or the whole world has ceased to exist.

paranoid d's an older term for delusion of grandeur and delusion of persecution; its use is discouraged.

d. of persecution a delusion that one is being attacked, harassed, cheated, persecuted, or conspired against. It is one of the subtypes of DELUSIONAL DISORDER.

d. of reference a delusional conviction that ordinary events, objects, or behaviors of others have particular and unusual meanings specifically for oneself.

somatic d. a delusion that there is some alteration in a bodily organ or its function. It is one of the subtypes of DELUSIONAL DISORDER.

systematized d's a group of delusions organized around a common theme; typical of delusional disorders or paranoid schizophrenia.

delusional disorder a MENTAL DISORDER marked by well-systematized, logically consistent delusions with no other psychotic feature. There are six subtypes on the basis of the predominant delusional theme: persecutory, jealous, erotomanic, somatic, grandiose, and mixed. See also individual subtypes under DELUSION.

demand (de-mand′) activated only by the absence of an intrinsic cardiac event, used of an artificial PACEMAKER. See also demand PACEMAKER.

demecarium (dem″ĕ-kar′e-um) an ANTICHOLINESTERASE agent used topically as the bromide salt to produce miosis, reduce intraocular pressure, and potentiate accommodation in the treatment of open-angle GLAUCOMA and of closed-angle glaucoma after iridectomy, and in the management of accommodative ESOTROPIA.

demecolcine (dem″e-kol′sēn) a cytotoxic alkaloid derived from *Colchicum autumnale.* It is used in CHROMOSOME analysis to arrest cell division in mid-metaphase so that the chromosomes can be stained by one of several techniques that produce a distinct pattern of light and dark bands along the chromosomes, and each chromosome can be recognized by its size and banding pattern.

demeclocycline (dem″ĕ-klo-si′klēn) a broad-spectrum TETRACYCLINE antibiotic produced by a mutant strain of *Streptomyces aureofaciens;* administered orally as the hydrochloride salt.

dementia (dĕ-men′shah) a general loss of cognitive abilities, including impairment of memory as well as one or more of the following: aphasia, apraxia, agnosia, or disturbed planning, organizing, and abstract thinking abilities. It does not include loss of intellectual functioning caused by CLOUDING OF CONSCIOUSNESS (as in DELIRIUM), DEPRESSION, or other functional mental disorder (PSEUDODEMENTIA). Causes include a large number of conditions, some reversible and some progressive, that result in widespread cerebral damage or dysfunction. The most common cause is Alzheimer's disease; others include cerebrovascular disease, central nervous system infection, brain trauma or tumors, vitamin deficiencies, anoxia, metabolic conditions, endocrine conditions, immune disorders, prion diseases, Wernicke-Korsakoff syndrome, normal-pressure hydrocephalus, Huntington's chorea, multiple sclerosis, and Parkinson's disease.

d. of the Alzheimer type official name for ALZHEIMER'S DISEASE.

Binswanger's d. a progressive dementia of presenile onset due to demyelination of the subcortical white matter of the brain, with sclerotic changes in the blood vessels supplying it.

boxer's d. a syndrome more serious than boxer's traumatic encephalopathy, the result of cumulative injuries to the brain in boxers; characterized by forgetfulness, slowness in thinking, dysarthric speech, and slow, uncertain movements, especially of the legs.

epileptic d. a progressive mental and intellectual deterioration that occurs in a small fraction of cases of epilepsy; it is thought by some to be caused by degeneration of neurons resulting from circulatory disturbances during seizures.

multi-infarct d. vascular d.

paralytic d., d. paraly′tica general paresis.

d. prae′cox (*obs.*) schizophrenia.

presenile d. name given to dementia of the Alzheimer type when it occurs in persons younger than age 65.

senile d. name given to dementia of the Alzheimer type when it occurs in persons aged 65 or older.

substance-induced persisting d. that resulting from exposure to or use or abuse of a substance, such as alcohol, sedatives, anxiolytics, anticonvulsants, lead, mercury, carbon monoxide, or organophosphate insecticides, but persisting long after exposure to the substance ends, usually with permanent and worsening deficits. Individual cases are named for the specific substance involved.

vascular d. patchy deterioration of intellectual function resulting from damage by a significant cerebrovascular disorder.

Demerol (dem′er-ol) trademark for preparations of MEPERIDINE hydrochloride, an opioid ANALGESIC.

demilune (dem′e-lo̅o̅n) crescent (def. 2).

demineralization (de-min″er-al-ĭ-za′shun) excessive elimination of mineral or organic salts from the tissues of the body.

demodectic (dem″o-dek′tik) pertaining to or caused by *Demodex.*

Demodex (dem′o-deks) a genus of mites parasitic within the hair follicles of the host, including the species *D. folliculo′rum* in man, and several other species in domestic and other animals.

demography (de-mog′rah-fe) the science dealing with populations, including matters of health, disease, births, and mortality.

demucosation (de″mu-ko-za′shun) removal of the mucous membrane from a part.

demulcent (de-mul′sent) 1. soothing; bland. 2. a soothing mucilaginous or oily medicine or application.

Demulen (dem′u-len) trademark for preparations of ETHYNODIOL DIACETATE with ETHINYL ESTRADIOL; used as an oral CONTRACEPTIVE.

de Musset's sign (dĕ-mu-sāz′) rhythmic jerky movements of the head; seen in cases of aortic aneurysm and aortic insufficiency. Called also Musset's sign.

demyelinating disease (de-mi'ĕ-lin-āt"-ing) any condition characterized by destruction of myelin.

demyelination (de-mi'ĕ-lin-a'shun) destruction, removal, or loss of the myelin sheath of a nerve or nerves. Called also demyelinization and myelinolysis.

demyelinization (de-mi"ĕ-lin-ĭ-za'shun) demyelination.

denarcotize (de-nahr'ko-tīz) 1. to deprive of narcotics in the process of addiction treatment. 2. to remove the narcotic element from an opiate.

denasality (de"na-zal'ĭ-te) hyponasality.

denaturant (de-na'chur-ant) a denaturing agent.

denaturation (de-na"chur-a'shun) a change in the usual nature of a substance, as by the addition of methanol or acetone to alcohol to render it unfit for drinking, or the change in the physical properties of a substance, such as a protein or nucleic acid, caused by heat or certain chemicals that alter tertiary structure.

protein d. any nonproteolytic change in the chemistry, composition, or structure of a native protein that causes it to lose some or all of its unique or specific characteristics.

dendr(o)- word element [Gr.], *tree; treelike.*

dendraxon (den-drak'son) a nerve cell whose axon splits up into terminal filaments immediately after leaving the cell.

dendric (den'drik) pertaining to a dendrite.

dendriform (den'drĭ-form) tree-shaped.

dendrite (den'drīt) any of the threadlike extensions of the cytoplasm of a neuron; they typically branch into treelike processes, and compose most of the receptive surface of a neuron. (See accompanying illustration.)

dendritic (den-drit'ik) 1. branched like a tree. 2. pertaining to or possessing dendrites.

dendrodendritic (den"dro-den-drit'ik) referring to a synapse between dendrites of two neurons.

dendroid (den'droid) branched like a tree.

dendron (den'dron) dendrite.

denervation (de"ner-va'shun) interruption of the nerve connection to an organ or part.

dengue (deng'e; Spanish, dān'ga) a painful viral disease that flourishes in tropical climates throughout the world; the virus that causes it is carried by *Aedes* mosquitoes. Because of the intense pain in the bones, dengue is also known as "breakbone fever" and by other names based on the necessity of keeping the neck rigid, such as "dandy" and "giraffe." People who have had dengue are generally immunized against further attacks for 5 years, but epidemics tend to recur at five-year intervals. Occasional epidemics occur in the Gulf states of the United States.

Symptoms. The symptoms begin within a week after the bite of the infected mosquito and begin with a severe headache and pain behind the eyes. Within hours the characteristic pain in the back and joints begins. Movement is difficult, and the temperature may rise as high as 41°C (106°F). A pink rash, congested eyeballs, and a flushed face are outward signs. The disease usually has two stages of about 3 days and 2 days, separated by a period of 24 hours in which symptoms disappear and there may be hope that the attack is over. The second stage is marked by the earlier symptoms, and in addition a red rash appears on the trunk and lower extremities, often leading to peeling skin. The total course of the disease is rarely more than 6 or 7 days. Although the sufferer is exhausted and less resistant to other diseases, dengue by itself is rarely fatal. Convalescence is slow.

Treatment and Prevention. As there is no known remedy for dengue, the treatment is mainly palliative; analgesics to relieve the pain and a large intake of liquid are the basic essentials, along with maintenance of an environment conducive to rest. Aspirin should be avoided to prevent problems associated with thrombocytopenia that often occurs with the disease. The best method of preventing dengue is by controlling the mosquito, and in some areas this has been successful. In areas lacking mosquito control, protective clothing should be worn outside and mosquito netting used indoors to reduce the risk of infection.

denial (dĕ-ni'al) in psychiatry, a DEFENSE MECHANISM in which the existence of unpleasant internal or external realities is denied and kept out of conscious awareness. By keeping the stressors out of consciousness, they are prevented from causing anxiety.

ineffective d. a NURSING DIAGNOSIS accepted by the North American Nursing Diagnosis Association, defined as denial that is detrimental to health when a person makes a conscious or unconscious attempt to disavow the meaning or even the knowledge of an event in order to reduce anxiety or fear.

denidation (de"nĭ-da'shun) the degeneration and expulsion, during menstruation, of certain epithelial elements, potentially the nidus of an embryo.

denileukin diftitox (den"ĭ-loo'kin dif'tĭ-toks) a genetically engineered construct

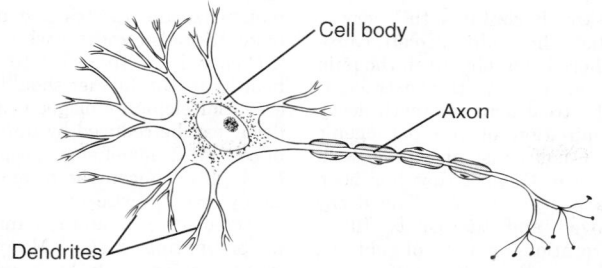

Dendrites in a multipolar neuron. From Dorland's, 2000.

containing amino acid sequences for specific diphtheria TOXIN fragments linked to sequences for INTERLEUKIN-2 (IL-2), so that the cytotoxic action of the diphtheria toxin is targeted to cells expressing a specific form of the IL-2 receptor, as in certain leukemias and lymphomas. It is used as an ANTINEOPLASTIC in the treatment of cutaneous T-cell LYMPHOMAS, administered intravenously.

Denny-Brown's syndrome (den'e-brownz) hereditary sensory radicular neuropathy.

dens (dens), pl. *den'tes* [L.] 1. TOOTH. 2. a toothlike structure such as the odontoid PROCESS.

densimeter (den-sim'ĕ-ter) densitometer (def. 1).

densitometer (den″-sĭ-tom'ĕ-ter) 1. an instrument for determining density or specific gravity of a liquid. 2. an instrument used to measure the degree of exposure (darkening) on photographic or x-ray film.

densitometry (den″sĭ-tom'ĕ-tre) determination of variations in density by comparison with that of another material or with a certain standard.

density (den'sĭ-te) 1. the ratio of the mass of a substance to its volume. 2. the quality of being compact. 3. the quantity of matter in a given space. 4. the quantity of electricity in a given area, volume, or time. 5. the degree of film blackening in an area of a photograph or radiograph.

dent(o)- word element [L.], *tooth; toothlike.*

dental (den't'l) pertaining to the teeth.

d. ***assistant*** a specially trained health care worker who provides direct support to the dentist. An educationally qualified dental assistant may be delegated to do intraoral procedures that do not require the professional skill and judgment of a dentist. Although not all states require formal education for dental assistants, minimum educational standards include a

program of approximately one academic year. Dental assistants may take the Certification Examination administered by the Dental Assisting National Board and earn the title of a Certified Dental Assistant (CDA). Some state boards of dentistry register dental assistants (RDA) after completion of a state-administered examination. Dental assistants may be members of their professional organization, the American Dental Assistants Association (ADAA), whose address is American Dental Assistants Association, 203 N. LaSalle St., Chicago, IL 60601.

d. ***caries*** a process of demineralization of tooth enamel, leading to destruction of ENAMEL and DENTIN, with cavitation of the tooth. Decayed and infected teeth can be the source of other infections throughout the body, and decayed or missing teeth can interfere with proper chewing of food, leading to nutritional deficiencies or disorders of digestion. Called also tooth decay.

Causes. The causes are not completely understood, but certain facts are known. Tooth decay seems to be a disease of civilization, possibly associated with refined foods. Lack of dental cleanliness is also closely associated. Decay occurs where food and bacteria such as *Lactobacillus* species and *Streptococcus mutans* adhere to the surface of the teeth, especially in pits or crevices, and form dental PLAQUE. It is believed that the action of the bacteria on sugars and starches creates LACTIC ACID, which can quickly and permanently dissolve tooth enamel. The acid produced in just 20 minutes after sugar comes into contact with plaque is enough to begin this process. In most people this occurs whenever sweet foods are eaten; thus, eating of sweet or starchy foods between meals or at bedtime can be harmful to the teeth unless they are thoroughly brushed and rinsed immediately afterward. Decay that is not treated will progress through the enamel and dentin into the PULP, which contains the nerves. When it reaches the pulp, it can cause intense pain. There is no relief until the pulp dies or is removed or the tooth is extracted.

Treatment. The treatment for tooth decay consists of elimination of the pathogenic microorganisms that cause it, along with regular dental care. Enamel that has been destroyed does not grow back. The decay must be removed and the cavity filled. FILLINGS (or restorations) may be of gold foil, baked porcelain, synthetic cements, silver amalgam, or cast gold inlays. When decay has reached the pulp, formerly extraction was usually necessary. Whenever possible, however, the exposed pulp is re-covered, or capped, and the tooth is then filled. New techniques of root canal THERAPY are saving many teeth that would formerly have been lost.

Prevention. *Flossing and Brushing the Teeth.* Cleanliness is the best weapon against caries and PERIODONTITIS. Bacteria and food particles must be removed before the enamel is penetrated. This means thorough brushing regularly each day, preferably after every meal. If it is impossible to brush after every meal, it is helpful to rinse the mouth by swishing water vigorously back and forth between and around the teeth. When the teeth are brushed, food particles that lodge between the teeth should also be removed with dental floss.

The dental floss should be strung tightly between the two index fingers or between the bows of a floss holder. Flossing and brushing should be done in an orderly sequence so that no area is neglected. The usual pattern is beginning at the upper right, progressing to the upper left, and then from the lower left to the lower right. The floss is gently inserted between the teeth and pulled against the surface of one tooth to a point slightly under the tissue of the gum. It is then moved up and down for several strokes. The adjacent tooth is cleaned in the same manner.

The "sulcular" technique for brushing the teeth is so called because the bristles of the brush are worked beneath the free gingival margin and into the space between the tooth and the gum (the *sulcus*). To accomplish this the bristles are placed at a 45 degree angle to the gum line. Pressure is then used to move the brush back and forth in a circular motion. The brushing is continued around the mouth in the same pattern as the flossing.

A disclosing dye may be used to determine the presence of plaque on the teeth.

Flavored mouthwash does not reduce plaque formation and is useful only to moisturize the tissues and improve mouth taste. (See also MOUTH CARE.)

Proper Diet. In order to help maintain healthy teeth, the diet should include all the essential elements of good nutrition. Tooth decay can be reduced by limiting the intake of certain forms of sugar, especially the rich or highly concentrated ones such as in candy or rich desserts.

FLUORIDATION is another important means of preventing caries. Many communities whose water is lacking in an adequate natural supply of fluoride add the chemical to their water supply. In communities that do not have fluoridation, dental professionals may add a fluoride solution directly to the teeth or may suggest other means of obtaining fluoride protection.

Correction of Malocclusion. Another factor leading to tooth decay is MALOCCLUSION (poor position of the teeth), which results in faulty closure of the jaws and uneven meeting of the teeth. This should be corrected early because it also can lead to inadequate nutrition because of difficulty in chewing, and if it is severe enough to distort the face, it may have psychologic effects.

dentate (den′tāt) notched; tooth-shaped.

dentia (den′she-ah) a condition relating to development or eruption of the teeth.

d. prae′cox premature eruption of the teeth; presence of teeth in the mouth at birth.

d. tar′da delayed eruption of the teeth, beyond the usual time for their appearance.

dentibuccal (den″tĭ-buk′al) pertaining to the cheek and teeth.

denticle (den′tĭ-k′l) 1. a small toothlike process. 2. a distinct calcified mass within the pulp chamber or in the dentin of a tooth.

dentification (den″tĭ-fĭ-ka′shun) formation of tooth substance.

dentifrice (den″tĭ-fris) a preparation for cleansing and polishing the teeth; some contain agents for whitening. Those containing FLUORIDE inhibit formation of DENTAL CARIES; those containing TRICLOSAN help inhibit formation of GINGIVITIS and PLAQUE.

dentigerous (den-tij′er-us) bearing teeth.

dentilabial (den′tĭ-la′be-al) pertaining to the teeth and lips.

dentilingual (den″tĭ-ling′gwal) pertaining to the teeth and tongue.

dentin (den′tin) the chief substance of the teeth, surrounding the tooth pulp and covered by the enamel on the crown and by cementum on the roots. adj., **den′tinal.**

dentinoblastoma (den″tĭ-no-blas-to′mah) dentinoma.

dentinogenesis (den″tĭ-no-jen′ĕ-sis) the formation of dentin.

d. imperfec′ta a hereditary disorder of tooth development, transmitted as an autosomal dominant trait, and characterized by discoloration of the teeth, ranging from dusky blue to brownish, poorly formed dentin with an abnormally low mineral content, obliteration of the root canal, and normal enamel. The teeth usually wear down rapidly, leaving short, brown stumps.

dentinoma (den″tĭ-no′mah) tumor of odontogenic origin, consisting mainly of dentin; called also dentinoblastoma.

dentinosteoid (den″tin-os′te-oid) a tumor composed of or containing dentin and bone.

dentinum (den-ti′num) dentin.

dentist (den′tist) a person who has received a degree from an accredited school of dentistry and is licensed to practice dentistry by a state board of dental examiners.

pediatric d. a dentist specializing in pediatric DENTISTRY.

dentistry (den′tis-tre) 1. that branch of the healing arts concerned with the teeth and associated structures of the oral cavity, including prevention, diagnosis, and treatment of disease and restoration of defective or missing teeth. 2. the work done by dentists, e.g., the creation of restoration, crowns, and bridges, and surgical procedures performed in and about the oral cavity. 3. the practice of the dental profession collectively.

operative d. dentistry concerned with restoration of parts of the teeth that are defective as a result of disease, trauma, or abnormal development to a state of normal function, health, and esthetics.

pediatric d. the branch of dentistry that deals with teeth and mouth conditions of children.

WINDOW ON DENTIST

Dentists are responsible for the oral health of their patients. The oral cavity contains both hard and soft tissues that, if diseased, can cause profound effects on the other systems of the human body. The muscles of mastication and the temporomandibular joint complete the stomatognathic system. The goal of the dentist is to maintain or reacquire optimal oral health for each patient.

General Dentists treat most of the patients. They provide primary dental care, preventive services, and restorative care. If necessary, general dentists can extract teeth or provide endodontic therapy. They may choose to refer patients to the various dental specialties.

Oral and Maxillofacial Surgeons provide the dental surgical services. Treated are extractions of erupted, embedded, and impacted teeth. Also, these dentists treat fractures of the jaws, and perform biopsies and removal of cysts and tumors. Through surgery they help to correct facial deformities and problems of the temporomandibular joint.

Endodontists are specialists in the treatment of the dental pulp. If that area is exposed, either by trauma or by caries, these dentists can relieve severe pain and save teeth. Because loose teeth cause effects on the other oral structures and the body, this is an important area of dental care.

Periodontists treat the supporting structures of the teeth. They are involved in the disease prevention or treatment of the gingiva, mucosa, intraoral muscles, alveolar bone, and supporting ligaments of the teeth. From initial hygiene to sophisticated periodontal surgery, a need is met to prevent tooth loss.

Orthodontists utilize different types of appliances to correct deformities of the jaws, teeth, or both. Some of them are either removable or bonded and cemented to the teeth. Sometimes, the problems are so severe that treatment is in conjunction with an oral surgeon.

Pediatric Dentists limit their practices by age. They perform restorative, preventive, and growth and developmental treatment. Most children in these offices receive primary care, but because of the extra training Pediatric Dentists treat difficult patients. Seen are children with complex treatment needs or behavioral issues, and medically compromised children.

In medicine, dentists provide the oral health care. Teeth allow a person to chew and enjoy a wide variety of foods, or teeth can be a source of pain and trouble. A healthy smile gives self esteem and is appealing for others. The mouth is the pathway of the digestive system and can be an entrance to the bloodstream. Dentists prevent dental disease that has the potential of becoming systemic, and restore its effects. Dentistry is an integral part of the health care network.

BURTON L. NUSSBAUM, DDS

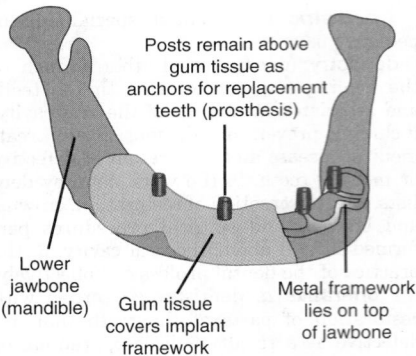

Posts remain above gum tissue as anchors for replacement teeth (prosthesis)

Lower jawbone (mandible)

Gum tissue covers implant framework

Metal framework lies on top of jawbone

A subperiosteal implant. From Darby and Walsh, 1995.

preventive d. dentistry concerned with maintenance of a normal masticating mechanism by fortifying the structures of the oral cavity against damage and disease.

prosthetic d. prosthodontics.

dentition (den-tish′un) the TEETH in the dental arch, usually referring to the natural teeth in position in the alveoli.

deciduous d. primary teeth; see TOOTH.

mixed d. the complement of teeth in the jaws after eruption of some of the permanent teeth, but before all the deciduous teeth are shed.

permanent d. permanent teeth; see TOOTH.

primary d. primary teeth; see TOOTH.

dentoalveolar (den″to-al-ve′o-lar) pertaining to a tooth and its alveolus.

dentofacial (den″to-fa′shal) of or pertaining to the teeth and alveolar process and the face.

dentulous (den′tu-lus) having natural teeth.

denture (den′cher) a complement of teeth, either natural or artificial; ordinarily used to designate an artificial replacement for the natural teeth and adjacent tissues.

complete d. an appliance replacing all the teeth of one jaw, as well as associated structures of the jaw.

fixed partial d. a partial DENTURE held in position by attachments to adjacent prepared natural teeth, roots, or implants; called also bridge.

implant d. an artificial denture or single tooth retained and stabilized by a framework or post implanted in the bone.

overlay d. a complete denture supported both by soft tissue (mucosa) and by a few remaining natural teeth that have been altered, as by insertion of a long or short coping, to permit the denture to fit over them.

partial d. a dental appliance that replaces one or more missing teeth, receiving support and retention from underlying tissues and some or all of the remaining teeth; it may be either permanently attached or removable. See fixed partial DENTURE and removable partial DENTURE.

removable partial d. a partial DENTURE made so that it can readily be removed from the mouth.

denucleated (de-noo′kle-āt″ed) deprived of the nucleus.

denudation (de″nu-da′shun) the stripping or laying bare of any part.

Denver classification (den′ver) the classification of human CHROMOSOMES on the basis of size and centromere position; the 23 pairs of chromosomes are classified in seven groups (A to G), in order of decreasing length. Used before it was possible to distinguish among the chromosomes of the groups.

Denver Developmental Screening test a test for identification of infants and preschool children with developmental delay.

deodorant (de-o′dor-ant) 1. destroying or masking offensive odors. 2. an agent that so acts.

deodorize (de-o′dor-īz) to neutralize or absorb odor.

deodorizer (de-o′dor-īz″er) a deodorizing agent.

deorsumversion (de-or″sum-ver′zhun) the turning downward of a part, especially of the eyes. (See accompanying illustration.)

deossification (de-os″ĭ-fĭ-ka′shun) loss or removal of the mineral elements of bone.

deoxidation (de-ok″sĭ-da′shun) the removal of oxygen from a chemical compound.

deoxy- a chemical prefix designating a compound containing one less atom of oxygen than the reference substance. See also DESOXY-.

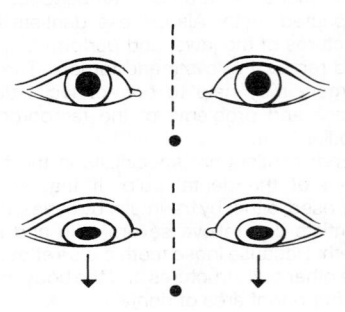

Deorsumversion. From Stein et al., 2000.

deoxycholic acid (de-ok″sĭ-ko′lik) a secondary BILE ACID, capable of forming soluble, diffusible complexes with fatty acids, and thereby allowing for their absorption in the small intestine.

deoxycorticosterone (de-ok″sĭ-kor′tĭ-kostēr′ōn) desoxycorticosterone.

deoxygenation (de-ok″sĭ-jĕ-na′shun) the act of depriving of oxygen.

2-deoxy-D-glucose (de-ok′sĭ-gloo′kōs) an ANTIMETABOLITE of glucose with ANTIVIRAL activity; it acts by inhibiting the glycosylation of glycoproteins and glycolipids; it has been investigated for treatment of herpesvirus infections.

deoxyhemoglobin (de-ok″sĭ-he′mo-glo″-bin) hemoglobin not combined with oxygen, formed when oxyhemoglobin releases its oxygen to the tissues.

deoxyribonuclease (DNase) (de-ok″sĭ-ri″bo-nu′kle-ās) an enzyme that catalyzes the hydrolysis (depolymerization) of deoxyribonucleic acid (DNA).

deoxyribonucleic acid (DNA) (de-ok″sĭ-ri″bo-nu-kle′ik) a NUCLEIC ACID of complex molecular structure occurring in cell nuclei as the basic structure of the GENES. DNA is present in all body cells of every species, including unicellular organisms and DNA viruses. The structure of DNA was first described in 1953 by J. D. Watson and F. H. C. Crick. DNA molecules are linear polymers of small molecules called *nucleotides,* each of which consists of one molecule of the five-carbon sugar *deoxyribose* bonded to a *phosphate* group and to one of four heterocyclic nitrogenous compounds referred to as *bases.* A single strand of DNA is made by linking the nucleotides together in a chain with bonds between the sugar and phosphate groups of adjacent nucleotides. It thus consists of a backbone of alternating sugar and phosphate groups with a base attached to each sugar as a side chain. The four bases are two purines, *adenine* (A) and *guanine* (G), and two pyrimidines, *cytosine* (C) and *thymine* (T). Single-stranded DNA can be synthesized with any specified sequence of bases, but in living cells the base sequence has a meaning: it specifies the amino acid sequence of all of the polypeptides and proteins made by the cell. And since all of the enzymes that catalyze biochemical reactions are proteins, the DNA contains the specifications for all of the biochemistry and structure of the cell.

The chemical basis of the genetic code lies in the ability of the bases to form hydrogen bonds with each other. Unlike the covalent bonds holding together the atoms of a single strand of DNA, hydrogen bonds are weak

and easily broken and reformed. Hydrogen bonding is governed by the base pairing rule: A always bonds with T, and C always bonds with G. A and T (or C and G) are called *complementary bases.* The genetic information is read and preserved by the matching up of complementary bases.

In cells, the DNA is double-stranded. The configuration of the DNA molecule resembles a ladder in which the sides are the sugar-phosphate backbones, which are antiparallel (they run in opposite directions), and the rungs are hydrogen-bonded complementary bases; thus, the entire sequence along the two strands is complementary. This whole structure is twisted so that the two strands form a double helix. Once before each cell division, a group of proteins splits the two strands apart, and as complementary nucleotides bond to the bases of each strand they are joined to form a new strand. This process is called *replication.* It results in the exact duplication of the DNA molecule, because each strand serves as a *template* (pattern) for the synthesis of its complementary strand. When the cell divides, one copy goes to each daughter cell. Thus, the genetic information is passed on from generation to generation without change except for rare mutations, which result from copying errors or incorrectly repaired breaks in the DNA molecule that change the base sequence.

The reading of the genetic code involves two processes: *transcription* and *translation.* In transcription, a length of DNA is used as a template to make a complementary strand of *messenger RNA* (mRNA). RNA (ribonucleic acid) is a nucleic acid like DNA. The only differences are that the sugar, ribose, has an extra oxygen atom, and the pyrimidine base, *uracil* (U), which also pairs with adenine, replaces thymine. In translation, the mRNA molecule is read by a structure called a ribosome, which produces the polypeptide specified by the mRNA message.

The genetic code is a triplet code. Every triplet of bases along the strand specifies a single amino acid. There are 64 possible triplets (codons) that can be formed from the four bases. Each one specifies that one of 20 different amino acids be inserted in a growing polypeptide chain or marks either the start or the end of a chain.

Two other types of RNA are involved in translation. *Ribosomal RNA* (rRNA) forms a large part of the ribosome. *Transfer RNA* (tRNA) is the means by which codons are matched with amino acids. tRNAs are small molecules with several self-complementary sections so that they fold up into a compact structure owing to bonding between complementary bases. One end of the molecule is a three-base anticodon, which bonds to its complementary codon on mRNA molecules. The other end is recognized by a specific enzyme that attaches the correct amino acid to it. During translation, the ribosome proceeds along the mRNA molecule and, as each codon is matched by a specific tRNA, the amino acid it carries is transferred to the growing polypeptide chain, and the process is repeated until the "stop" codon is reached. Like the mRNA molecules, rRNA and tRNA molecules are formed on DNA templates; the genetic material contains the information not only for polypeptide sequences but also for rRNA and tRNA sequences.

There is an enormous amount of information stored in the DNA of a cell. The 48 chromosomes of a human cell contain a total length of about 6 billion base pairs of DNA. This is enough to code for the thousands of enzymes and structural proteins in the cell. DNA is the molecule that directs all of the activities of living cells, including its own reproduction and perpetuation in generation after generation.

deoxyribonucleoprotein (de-ok″sĭ-ri″bo-noo″kle-o-pro′tēn) a nucleoprotein in which the sugar is D-2-deoxyribose.

deoxyribonucleoside (de-ok″sĭ-ri″bo-noo′-kle-o-sīd) a nucleoside having a purine or pyrimidine base bonded to deoxyribose.

deoxyribonucleotide (de-ok″sĭ-ri″bo-noo′-kle-o-tīd) a nucleotide having a purine or pyrimidine base bonded to deoxyribose,

The basic building blocks of DNA.

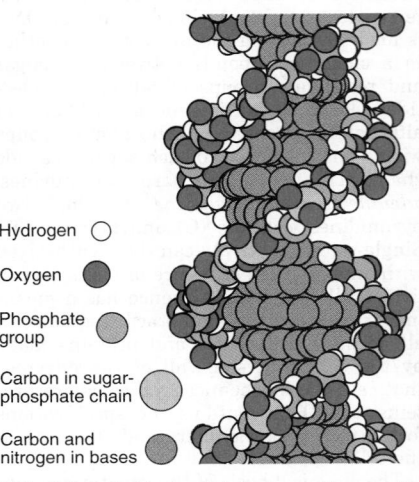

Hydrogen ○

Oxygen ●

Phosphate group ●

Carbon in sugar-phosphate chain ○

Carbon and nitrogen in bases ●

The helical, double-stranded structure of the gene. The outside strands are composed of phosphoric acid and the sugar deoxyribose. The internal molecules that connect the two strands of the helix are purine and pyrimidine bases; these determine the code of the gene.

deoxyribose (de-ok″sĭ-ri′bōs) an ALDOPEN-TOSE found in deoxyribonucleic acid, deoxy-ribonucleotides, and deoxyribonucleosides.

dependence (de-pen′dens) a need for something; sometimes used as a synonym for DRUG DEPENDENCE.

   chemical d., drug d. see DRUG DEPEN-DENCE.

   emotional d. psychological dependence.

   physical d., physiological d. DRUG DE-PENDENCE in which the drug is used to prevent WITHDRAWAL SYMPTOMS or in which it is associated with TOLERANCE, or both.

   psychoactive substance d. drug de-pendence.

   psychological d. DRUG DEPENDENCE in which the drug is used to obtain relief from tension or emotional discomfort; called also emotional dependence.

   substance d. drug dependence.

dependency (de-pen′den-se) a state of relying on another for love, affection, mothering, comfort, security, food, warmth, shelter, protection, and the like.

dependent (de-pen′dent) 1. pertaining to dependence or to dependency. 2. hanging down.

   d. personality disorder a PERSONALITY DISORDER marked by excessive need to be taken care of, with submissiveness and clinging and preoccupation with fears of abandonment, so that others are allowed to assume responsibility for major areas of one's life. Persons with the disorder need advice and reassurance in decision making, yield responsibility, initiative, and inde-pendence, avoid disagreement, voluntarily undertake unpleasant tasks to ensure fur-ther care, subordinate their own desires to those of the people they depend on to avoid jeopardizing those relationships, and feel discomfort or helplessness when alone, in-discriminately rushing to new relationships.

depersonalization (de-per″sun-al-ĭ-za′-shun) alteration in the perception of the self so that the usual sense of one's own reality is lost, manifested in a sense of unreality or self-estrangement, in changes of body image, or in a feeling that one does not control one's own actions and speech; seen in disorders such as depersonalization disorder (see also DISSOCIATIVE DISORDERS), depression, hypochondriasis, temporal lobe epilepsy, schizophrenia, and schizotypal personality disorder. Some authorities do not draw a distinction between this concept and DEREALIZATION, and use the term deper-sonalization to include both.

   d. disorder a DISSOCIATIVE DISORDER in which there are feelings of unreality and

strangeness in one's perception of self or of one's body image. Individuals with this disorder may feel as though they are in a dream or are not totally in control of their actions. Episodes of depersonalization are usually accompanied by dizziness, anxiety, fears of going insane, and derealization. Depersonalization as an isolated event oc-curs in many people without significantly affecting their functioning; it is considered a disorder only when it impairs the patient's daily activities, when it is not associated with some other mental disorder, and when the patient's perception of reality remains intact.

dephosphorylation (de-fos″for-ĭ-la′shun) removal of a phosphate group from an organic molecule.

depilate (dep′ĭ-lāt) to remove hair.

depilation (dep″ĭ-la′shun) removal of hair by the roots; called also epilation.

depilatory (de-pil′ah-tor″e) 1. removing or destroying hair. 2. an agent that does this. Called also epilatory.

depolarization (de-po″lar-ĭ-za″shun) the reduction of a membrane's resting POTENTIAL so that it becomes less negative. In cardiac physiology there are several forms: the normal slow diastolic depolarization of pacemaker CELLS; the slow but normal depolarization of cells of the atrioventricu-lar and sinoatrial nodes; the rapid phase 0 depolarization of normal atrial, His-Pur-kinje, and ventricular cells; and abnormal depolarization resulting from disease.

   phase 4 d. the slow reduction of the membrane POTENTIAL during phase 4 (elec-trical diastole); normal in pacemaker CELLS but sometimes abnormally accelerated.

   rapid d. the sudden reversal in electri-cal potential from negative to positive; it is represented by phase 0 of the ACTION POTENTIAL.

depolymerization (de″po-lim″er-ĭ-za′-shun) the conversion of a polymer into its component monomers.

Depo-Provera (de″po-pro-ver′ah) trade-mark for a preparation of MEDROXYPROGES-TERONE acetate for intramuscular injection, a progestational AGENT used in treatment of DYSMENORRHEA, metastatic cancer, and other conditions, as hormone replacement THER-APY, and as a long-acting CONTRACEPTIVE.

deposit (de-poz′it) 1. sediment or dregs. 2. extraneous inorganic matter collected in the tissues or in an organ of the body.

depot (de′po, dep′o) a body area in which a substance, e.g., a drug, can be accumu-lated, deposited, or stored and from which it can be distributed.

fat d. a site in the body in which large quantities of fat are stored, as in adipose tissue.

Depo-Testosterone (de″po-tes-tos′ter-ōn) trademark for a sustained-action preparation of TESTOSTERONE cypionate, used in treatment of HYPOGONADISM or delayed puberty in males and certain forms of metastatic breast cancer in females.

L-**deprenyl** (dep′rĕ-nil) selegiline.

depressant (de-pres′ant) 1. diminishing any function or activity; see also DEPRESSOR. 2. an agent that retards any function, especially a drug that acts on the central nervous system to depress activity at all levels by stabilizing neuronal membranes. Central nervous system depressants such as BARBITURATES and inhalational ANESTHETICS are used as sedatives, hypnotics, and anesthetics. ALCOHOL is also a depressant, although its first effect is sometimes stimulating.

cardiac d. an agent that depresses the rate or force of contractions of the heart.

depressed (de-prest′) carried below the normal level; associated with depression.

depression (de-presh′un) 1. a hollow or depressed area. 2. a lowering or decrease of functional activity. 3. in psychiatry, a mental state of altered mood characterized by feelings of sadness, despair, and discouragement; distinguished from grief, which is realistic and proportionate to a personal loss. Profound depression may be an illness itself, such as MAJOR DEPRESSIVE DISORDER (see also MOOD DISORDERS), or it may be symptomatic of another psychiatric disorder, such as SCHIZOPHRENIA. adj., **depres′-sive.** Depression is closely associated with a lack of confidence and self-esteem and with an inability to express strong feelings. Repressed anger is thought to be a powerful contributor to depression. The person feels inadequate to cope with the situations that arise in everyday life and so feels insecure.

Treatment of profound and chronic depression is often very difficult, requiring in most cases intensive psychotherapy to help the patient understand the underlying cause of the depression. ANTIDEPRESSANT drugs such as IMIPRAMINE hydrochloride (TOFRANIL) and AMITRIPTYLINE (ELAVIL) are often used in the treatment of profound depression. They are not true stimulants of the central nervous system, but they do block the reuptake of neurotransmitter substances, which may potentiate the action of norepinephrine and serotonin. MONOAMINE OXIDASE (MAO) INHIBITORS are also used. When antidepressants fail, a different technique such as ELECTROCONVULSIVE THERAPY may be used in conjunction with the psychotherapy.

Patient Care. Mild, sporadic depression is a relatively common phenomenon experienced by almost everyone at some time, but hospitalized patients are particularly susceptible to feelings of depression and a sense of loss and despair. Early signs of depression of this kind include pessimistic statements about one's illness and its prognosis, refusal to eat, diminished concern about personal appearance, and reluctance to make decisions. When depression is noted in a patient, it should be listed on the treatment plan along with suggestions for resolving it. When patients are depressed, they are likely to isolate themselves and avoid social contact even with those who are trying to help them. Since loss of contact with others contributes to depression, members of the health care team should persist in attempts to talk with these patients, by asking them questions, and actively listening when they attempt to express their feelings. One should be especially careful to avoid being judgmental when the patient does express despair, anger, hostility, or some negative feeling. Above all, it is important not to be condescending or to respond to statements with a meaningless cliché such as "Don't worry," or "I'm sure everything will turn out okay." These responses convey a lack of empathy with the patient's suffering and are an unrealistic approach to a problem that is very real.

Physical contact and touching may be misunderstood by depressed patients. Sometimes, it is better just to sit with them and calmly observe them without making them feel uncomfortable. Honest dialogue and expressions of support and concern can often improve their mood and sense of self worth.

Severely depressed patients usually express three basic feelings associated with their mental state. These are a lack of desire for socializing or physical activity, feelings of worthlessness and loss of self esteem, and thoughts of self-injury or destruction. In planning the care of the depressed patient, one must always consider these feelings and strive for some understanding of the reasons for the patient's behavior. Only by gradually gaining their attention and pointing out encouraging signs of progress can they be helped in their early attempts to return to reality and socialize with others.

Physical inactivity will require attention to adequate nutrition, a normal balance of fluid intake and output, proper elimination, and good skin care. Patients will need help in maintaining good personal hygiene. Severely depressed patients may be totally out of touch with reality and completely unresponsive to anyone else's presence. In such instances the health care provider may be able to do little more than demonstrate caring and empathy by remaining with the patient.

Consistency of care is helpful to depressed patients. They know what to expect, and thus are not repeatedly disappointed when their expectations are not met. An example is consistency in scheduling and carrying out treatments and routine care at the same time each day. A supportive family and interested friends should be involved in choosing and planning activities that are helpful.

Constant vigilance must be maintained to prevent the profoundly depressed patient from injuring himself or committing SUICIDE. Self-destructive behavior is a manifestation of the patient's feeling of worthlessness and loss of self esteem. An awareness of the potential dangers in such a situation should help the provider plan and provide a safe and congenial atmosphere, remaining alert to the early signs of a patient's intention to harm or destroy himself. In most cases suicide is most likely to occur when the patient is recovering from severe depression.

agitated d. major depressive disorder characterized by signs and symptoms of agitation, such as restlessness, racing thoughts, pacing, hand-wringing, sighing, or moaning.

congenital chondrosternal d. a congenital, deep, funnel-shaped depression in the anterior chest wall.

endogenous d. a type of depression caused by somatic or biological factors rather than environmental influences, in contrast to a REACTIVE DEPRESSION. It is often identified with a specific symptom complex—psychomotor retardation, early morning awakening, weight loss, excessive guilt, and lack of reactivity to the environment—that is roughly equivalent to the symptoms of major depressive disorder.

major d. major depressive disorder.

neurotic d. one that is not a PSYCHOTIC DEPRESSION. The term is now little used but has been used sometimes broadly to indicate any depression without psychotic features and sometimes more narrowly to denote only milder forms of depression (DYSTHYMIC DISORDER).

postpartum d. moderate to severe depression beginning slowly and sometimes undetectably during the second to third week post partum, increasing steadily for weeks to months and usually resolving

spontaneously within a year. Somatic complaints such as fatigue are common. It is intermediate in severity between the mood fluctuations experienced by the majority of new mothers and frank postpartum PSYCHOSIS.

psychotic d. strictly, MAJOR DEPRESSIVE DISORDER with psychotic features, such as hallucinations, delusions, mutism, or stupor. The term is often used more broadly to cover all severe depressions causing gross impairment of social or occupational functioning.

reactive d. a usually transient depression that is precipitated by a stressful life event or other environmental factor, in contrast to an ENDOGENOUS DEPRESSION.

retarded d. major depressive disorder characterized by signs and symptoms of psychomotor retardation, such as burdened movements and slowed, toneless speech.

situational d. reactive depression.

unipolar d. a type that is not accompanied by episodes of MANIA or HYPOMANIA, such as MAJOR DEPRESSIVE DISORDER or DYSTHYMIC DISORDER. The term is sometimes used more specifically as a synonym of major depressive disorder.

depressive (de-pres´iv) 1. tending to lower. 2. of or pertaining to depression.

d. disorders MOOD DISORDERS in which DEPRESSION is unaccompanied by episodes of mania or hypomania, including MAJOR DEPRESSIVE DISORDER and DYSTHYMIC DISORDER. See also BIPOLAR DISORDERS.

d. personality disorder a PERSONALITY DISORDER characterized by a persistent and pervasive pattern of depressive cognitions and behaviors, such as chronic unhappiness, low self-esteem, pessimism, critical and derogatory attitudes toward oneself and others, feelings of guilt or remorse, and an inability to relax or feel enjoyment.

depressomotor (de-pres″o-mo´ter) 1. retarding or abating motor activity. 2. an agent that so acts.

depressor (de-pres´or) 1. anything that depresses, such as a muscle, agent, or instrument. See also DEPRESSANT. 2. depressor nerve.

tongue d. an instrument for pressing down the tongue, allowing better visualization of the OROPHARYNX.

deprivation (dep-rĭ-va´shun) loss or absence of parts, organs, powers, or things that are needed.

emotional d. deprivation of adequate and appropriate interpersonal or environmental experience, usually in the early developmental years.

maternal d. the result of premature loss or absence of the mother or of lack of proper mothering; see also MATERNAL DEPRIVATION SYNDROME.

sensory d. a condition in which an individual receives less than normal sensory input. It can be caused by physiological, motor, or environmental disruptions. Effects include boredom, irritability, difficulty in concentrating, confusion, and inaccurate perception of sensory stimuli. Auditory and visual hallucinations and disorientation in time and place indicate perceptual distortions due to sensory deprivation. Symptoms can be produced by solitary confinement, loss of sight or hearing, paralysis, and even by ordinary hospital bed rest.

sleep d. a NURSING DIAGNOSIS accepted by the North American Nursing Diagnosis Association, defined as prolonged periods of time without SLEEP (sustained, natural, periodic suspension of relative consciousness).

thought d. blocking (def. 2).

de Quervain's disease (dĕ kār-vaz′) QUERVAIN'S DISEASE.

deradelphus (der″ah-del′fus) malformed twins fused at or near the navel and having one head.

derailment (de-rāl′ment) disordered thought or speech characteristic of schizophrenia and marked by constant jumping around from one topic to another before the first is fully realized, the topics often being clearly but indirectly related or unrelated.

derangement (de-rānj′ment) 1. older term for a MENTAL DISORDER. 2. disarrangement of a part or organ.

Dercum's disease (der′kumz) adiposis dolorosa.

derealization (de-re″al-ĭ-za′shun) loss of sensation of the reality of one's surroundings; the feeling that something has happened, that the world has been changed and altered, that one is detached from one's environment. It is seen most frequently in schizophrenia. See also DEPERSONALIZATION.

dereism (de′re-izm) dereistic THINKING. **derei′stic.**

derencephalus (der″en-sef′ah-lus) a fetus with a rudimentary skull and bifid cervical vertebrae, the brain resting in the bifurcation.

derepression (de″re-presh′un) 1. elevation of the level of an enzyme above the normal, either by lowering the corepressor concentration or by a mutation that decreases the formation of aporepressor or the response to the complete repressor. 2. the

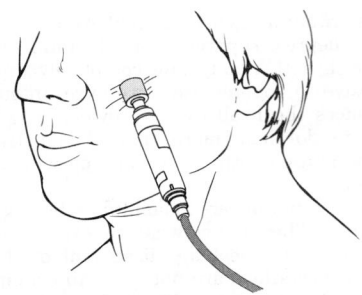

Dermabrader. From Dorland's, 2000.

inhibition of the repressor substance produced by the regulator genes with the result that the operator gene is free to initiate the process of polypeptide formation.

derma (der′mah) the skin, usually with special reference to the dermis.

dermabrader (derm″ah-brād′er) a surgical instrument used for removal or rounding out of scars and for other plastic surgery procedures. (See illustration.)

dermabrasion (derm″ah-bra′zhun) PLANING of the skin done by mechanical means such as sandpaper or wire brushes.

Dermacentor (der″mah-sen′ter) a genus of ticks parasitic on various animals, and vectors of disease-producing microorganisms.

D. anderso′ni a species of tick common in the western United States, parasitic on numerous wild mammals, most domestic animals, and humans. It is a vector of Rocky Mountain spotted fever, tularemia, Colorado tick fever, and Q fever in the United States, and is the cause of tick paralysis.

D. varia′bilis the chief vector of Rocky Mountain spotted fever in the central and eastern United States, the dog being the principal host of the adult forms, but also parasitic on cattle, horses, rabbits, and humans.

dermal (der′mal) 1. pertaining to the dermis. 2. pertaining to the skin; cutaneous; dermic.

dermat(o)- word element [Gr.], *skin.*

dermatitides (der″mah-tit′ĭ-dēz) plural of DERMATITIS; inflammatory conditions of the skin considered collectively.

dermatitis (der″mah-ti′tis), pl. *dermatitides* Inflammation of the skin. Dermatitis can result from various animal, vegetable, and chemical substances, from heat or cold, from mechanical irritation, from certain forms of malnutrition, or from infectious disease. In some cases, dermatitis may have a psychologic rather than a physical cause. The symptoms may include itching, redness, crustiness, blisters, watery discharges, fissures, or other changes in the normal condition of the skin. The treatment of dermatitis varies greatly and is determined by the cause. Cortisone-containing creams, lotions, and ointments are frequently prescribed as a palliative measure.

actinic d. that produced by exposure to actinic RAYS, such as that from the sun, ULTRAVIOLET RAYS X-RAYS, or GAMMA RAYS.

allergic contact d. CONTACT DERMATITIS due to allergic sensitization to various substances that produce inflammatory reactions in the skin of those who have acquired hypersensitivity to the allergen as a result of previous exposure to it.

atopic d. a chronic inflammatory skin disorder seen in individuals with a hereditary predisposition to a lowered cutaneous threshold to pruritus, often accompanied by allergic rhinitis, hay fever, and asthma, and principally characterized by extreme itching, leading to scratching and rubbing that in turn results in the typical lesions of eczema.

contact d. see CONTACT DERMATITIS.

diaper d. diaper RASH.

d. exfoliati′va neonato′rum exfoliative dermatitis supervening in bullous impetigo of the newborn; called also Ritter's disease.

exfoliative d. virtually universal erythema, desquamation, scaling, and itching of the skin and loss of hair; it may result from internal medication with such drugs as penicillin, quinine, sulfonamides, gold salts, and iodides.

factitial d. various types of self-inflicted lesions, usually produced by mechanical means, burning, or application of chemical irritants or caustics.

d. herpetifor′mis a chronic, relapsing multisystem disease with mainly cutaneous symptoms, presenting as a pruritic eruption with various combinations of grouped, erythematous, symmetrical, papular, papulovesicular, vesicular, eczematous, and bullous lesions, that usually heal with hyperpigmentation or occasionally hypopigmentation and sometimes scarring. It usually occurs in association with an asymptomatic type of CELIAC DISEASE. The cause is unknown, but immunogenic factors may play a role.

irritant d. a nonallergic type of CONTACT DERMATITIS due to exposure to a substance that damages the skin rather than acting as a sensitizer or allergen.

d. medicamento′sa drug eruption.

nickel d. a type of CONTACT DERMATITIS from prolonged exposure to NICKEL, such as in jewelry.

photocontact d. allergic contact dermatitis caused by the action of sunlight

on skin sensitized by a substance capable of causing this reaction, such as sandalwood oil, hexachlorophene, or a halogenated salicylanilide.

phototoxic d. an exaggerated sunburn-like reaction, sometimes with vesiculation, resulting in hyperpigmentation and desquamation, which occurs on the light-exposed areas of the skin as the cutaneous manifestation of phototoxicity.

poison ivy d., poison oak d. poison sumac d. *Rhus* dermatitis.

primary irritant d. irritant dermatitis.

rhus d., Rhus d. allergic contact dermatitis due to exposure to plants of the genus *Rhus;* see POISON IVY OAK AND SUMAC. Called also poison ivy dermatitis.

schistosome d. dermatitis caused by penetration of the skin by larvae (cercariae) of organisms of the genus *Schistosoma.*

seborrheic d., d. seborrhe′ica see SEBORRHEIC DERMATITIS.

stasis d. an eczematous eruption of the lower legs, usually due to impeded circulation, with edema, pigmentation, and often chronic ulceration.

d. venena′ta severe allergic contact dermatitis.

verrucose d., verrucous d. chromoblastomycosis.

x-ray d. radiodermatitis.

Dermatobia (der″mah-to′be-ah) a genus of botflies. The larvae of *D. ho′minis* are parasitic in the skin of humans, mammals, and birds.

dermatofibroma (der″mah-to-fi-bro′mah) a fibrous tumorlike nodule of the skin, usually on the extremities and especially the legs. Its etiology is not known, but it is most likely a neoplastic disorder. Although it is benign, itching and pain can be a source of severe discomfort.

dermatofibrosarcoma (der″mah-to-fi′-bro-sar-ko′mah) a FIBROSARCOMA of the skin, arising from the dermis and invading deeper subcutaneous tissue such as fat, fascia, and muscle.

dermatoglyphics (der″mah-to-glif′iks) the study of the patterns of ridges of the skin of the fingers, palms, toes, and soles; of interest in anthropology and law enforcement as a means of establishing identity and in medicine, both clinically and as a genetic indicator, particularly of chromosomal abnormalities such as trisomy 21 syndrome.

dermatographism (der″mah-tog′rah-fizm) urticaria due to physical allergy in which a pale, raised welt or wheal with a red flare on each side is elicited by stroking or scratching the skin with a dull instrument. adj., **dermatograph'ic.**

dermatoheteroplasty (der″mah-to-het′er-o-plas″te) the grafting of skin derived from an individual of another species.

dermatologic (der″mah-to-loj′ik) pertaining to dermatology; of or affecting the skin.

dermatological (der″mah-to-loj′ĭ-k'l) dermatologic.

dermatologist (der″mah-tol′o-jist) a physician who specializes in dermatology.

dermatology (der″mah-tol′o-je) the medical specialty concerned with the diagnosis and treatment of skin diseases.

dermatome (der′mah-tōm) 1. the area of skin supplied with afferent nerve fibers by a single posterior spinal root. 2. the lateral part of an embryonic somite. 3. an instrument for removing split-thickness skin grafts from donor sites; there are many different kinds, divided into three major types: knife, drum, and motor-driven.

drum d. a dermatome consisting of a cylindrical drumlike apparatus coated with adhesive that rolls over the skin while a blade moves across the surface and cuts the graft free.

knife d. the simplest type of dermatome, which is used to remove grafts by a freehand technique.

motor-driven d. a dermatome driven by a power source; motor-driven dermatomes cut with a back-and-forth blade action.

dermatomegaly (der″mah-to-meg′ah-le) cutis laxa.

dermatomere (der′mah-to-mēr″) any segment of the embryonic integument.

dermatomycosis (der″mah-to-mi-ko′sis) a superficial fungal infection of the skin or of its appendages.

dermatomyoma (der″mah-to-mi-o′mah) leiomyoma cutis.

dermatomyositis (der″mah-to-mi″o-si′tis) an acute, subacute, or chronic disease marked by nonsuppurative inflammation of the skin, subcutaneous tissue, and muscles, with necrosis of muscle fibers. It is in the group of illnesses known as COLLAGEN DISEASES. Among a variety of symptoms that point to the onset of the disease are fever, loss of weight, skin lesions, and aching muscles. As the disease progresses there

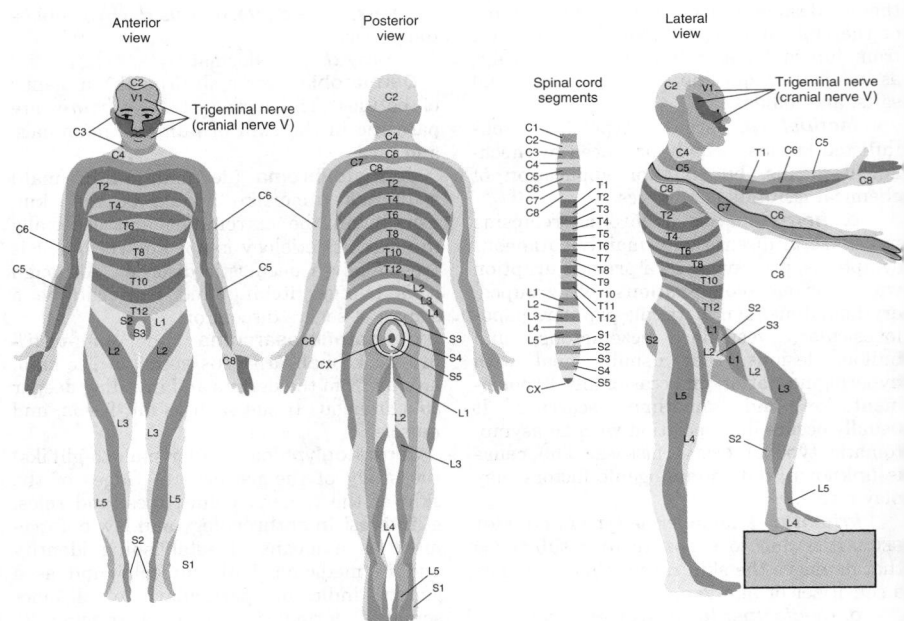

Dermatomes. Segmental dermatome distribution of spinal nerves to the front, back, and side of the body. *C,* Cervical segments; *T,* thoracic segments; *L,* lumbar segments; *S,* sacral segments; *CX,* coccygeal segment. Dermatomes are specific skin surface areas innervated by a single spinal nerve or group of spinal nerves. Dermatome assessment is done to determine the level of spinal anesthesia for surgical procedures and postoperative analgesia when epidural local anesthetics are used. From Thibodeau and Patton, 1999.

may be loss of the use of the arms and legs. Complications such as hardening may occur, similar to the changes seen in scleroderma. Occasionally steroids prove helpful in relieving symptoms, but the most beneficial treatment is physical therapy to maintain maximal use of the muscles.

dermatopathic (der″mah-to-path′ik) pertaining to or attributable to disease of the skin.

dermatopathology (der″mah-to-pah-thol′-o-je) pathology that is especially concerned with lesions of the skin.

dermatopathy (der″mah-top′ah-the) any disease of the skin; dermopathy.

Dermatophagoides pteronyssimus (der″-mah-tof′ah-goi′dēz ter″ŏ-nĭ-si′mus) the house dust mite, which is antigenic and can produce allergic ASTHMA in atopic persons.

dermatophilosis (der″mah-to-fi-lo′sis) an actinomycotic disease caused by *Dermatophilus congolensis*, affecting cattle, sheep, horses, goats, deer, and sometimes human beings. In humans it is marked by nonpainful pustules on the hands and arms; the lesions break down and form shallow red ulcers which regress spontaneously, leaving some scarring.

Dermatophilus (der″mah-tof′ĭ-lus) a genus of gram-positive, aerobic or facultatively anaerobic actinomycetes; *D. congolen′sis* is the etiologic agent of DERMATOPHILOSIS.

dermatophyte (der′mah-to-fīt″) a fungus parasitic upon the skin, usually a species of *Microsporum, Epidermophyton,* or *Trichophyton.* Called also cutaneous fungus.

dermatophytid (der″mah-tof′ĭ-tid) a secondary skin eruption which is an expression of hypersensitivity to a dermatophyte, especially *Epidermophyton,* infection, occurring on an area remote from the site of infection, most commonly on the hands, wrists, and sides of the fingers in association with tinea pedis.

dermatophytosis (der″mah-to-fi-to′sis) 1. any superficial fungal infection caused by a dermatophyte and involving the stratum corneum of the skin, hair, and nails, including ONYCHOMYCOSIS and the various forms of TINEA. Called also epidermomycosis and epidermophytosis. 2. tinea pedis.

dermatoplasty (der′mah-to-plas″te) a plastic operation on the skin; operative replacement of lost skin. adj., **dermatoplas′tic.**

dermatosclerosis (der″mah-to-sklĕ-ro′sis) scleroderma.

dermatosis (der″mah-to′sis), pl. *dermato′ses* Any noninflammatory disorder of the skin.

lichenoid d. any skin disorder characterized by thickening and hardening of the skin.

precancerous d. any skin condition in which the lesions, such as warts, nevi, or other excrescences, are likely to undergo malignant degeneration.

dermatotherapy (der″mah-to-ther′ah-pe) treatment of skin diseases.

dermatotropic (der″mah-to-trop′ik) having a specific affinity for the skin.

dermatozoon (der″mah-to-zo′on) any animal parasite on the skin; an ectoparasite.

dermis (der′mis) the true skin; the fibrous inner layer of the skin just beneath the epidermis, derived from the embryonic mesoderm, varying from 0.05 cm to 0.3 cm in thickness, well supplied with nerves and blood vessels and containing hair roots, sebaceous glands, and sweat glands; on the palms and soles the dermis bears ridges whose arrangement in whorls and loops is unique to the individual. Called also corium. adj., **der′mal, der′mic.**

dermoblast (der′mo-blast) the part of the mesoderm that develops into the true skin.

dermoid (der′moid) 1. skinlike. 2. a dermoid cyst.

d. cyst 1. a tumor of developmental origin consisting of a fibrous wall lined with stratified epithelium and containing hair follicles, sweat glands, sebaceous glands, nerve elements, and teeth; a teratoma. When these cysts occur in the ovary they may present no symptoms, but their long pedicles may cause twisting, resulting in acute abdominal pain. Treatment is surgical removal. 2. a benign teratoma of the ovary, found usually in young women, typically filled with sebaceous material and hair.

dermoidectomy (der″moi-dek′to-me) excision of a dermoid cyst.

dermolipectomy (der″mo-lĭ-pek′to-me) resection of excess skin and fat, usually from the abdomen.

dermopathy (der-mop′ah-the) any skin disease; dermatopathy. adj., **dermopath′ic.**

diabetic d. any of several cutaneous manifestations of DIABETES MELLITUS.

thyroid d. pretibial myxedema.

dermosynovitis (der″mo-sin″o-vi′tis) inflammation of the skin overlying an inflamed bursa or tendon sheath.

dermotropic (der″mo-trop′ik) dermatotropic.

dermovascular (der″mo-vas′ku-ler) pertaining to the skin and blood vessels of the skin.

derodidymus (der″o-did′ĭ-mus) dicephalus.

DES diethylstilbestrol.

descensus (de-sen′sus), pl. *descen′sus* [L.] downward displacement or prolapse.

d. tes′tis normal migration of the testis from its fetal position in the abdominal cavity to its location within the scrotum, usually during the last 3 months of gestation.

d. u′teri prolapse of uterus.

desensitization (de-sen″sĭ-tĭ-za′shun) 1. the prevention or reduction of immediate HYPERSENSITIVITY by administration of graded doses of allergen; see also IMMUNOTHERAPY. Called also hyposensitization. 2. in behavior therapy, the treatment of PHOBIAS and related disorders by intentionally exposing the patient, in imagination or in real life, to a hierarchy of emotionally distressing stimuli.

desensitize (de-sen′sĭ-tīz) 1. to deprive of sensation. 2. to subject to desensitization.

deserpidine (de-ser′pĭ-dēn) a RAUWOLFIA alkaloid, administered orally as an ANTIHYPERTENSIVE AGENT.

desert fever the primary form of COCCIDIOIDOMYCOSIS.

desflurane (des-floo′rān) an inhalational anesthetic used for induction and maintenance of general ANESTHESIA.

desiccant (des′ĭ-kant) 1. promoting dryness. 2. an agent that promotes dryness.

desiccate (des′ĭ-kāt) to render thoroughly dry.

desiccation (des″ĭ-ka′shun) the act of drying.

design (de-zīn′) a strategy that directs a researcher in planning and implementing a study in a way that is most likely to achieve the intended goal.

case study d. an investigation strategy involving extensive exploration of a single unit of study, which may be a person, family, group, community, or institution, or a very small number of subjects who are examined intensively. The number of variables is usually very large.

cohort d. longitudinal design.

cross-sectional d. a research strategy in which one or more group(s) of subjects are studied at one given point in time.

experimental d. a research design that eliminates all factors that influence outcome except for the cause being studied (independent variable). All other factors are controlled by randomization, investigator-controlled manipulation of the independent variable, and control of the study situation by the investigator, including the use of control groups.

longitudinal d. a research strategy in which one or more group(s) of subjects in various stages of development are examined simultaneously with the intent of inferring trends over time. The assumption is that the phenomenon under study progresses with time. Called also cohort design.

methodological d. a process used to develop the validity and reliability of instruments to measure constructs used as variables in research.

nonequivalent control group d. a study design in which the control group is not selected by random means.

partial correlation d. a design developed to eliminate the influence of a third variable on a relational pattern by holding it constant mathematically, so that the magnitude of the relationship between the two remaining variables can be determined.

path analysis d. a design to determine the accuracy of a theoretical model: a hypothesized causal model is developed from the theoretical model and the major variables within it are measured and relationships among them determined; regression analysis is used to determine whether the data are consistent with the model.

survey d. a design in which data are collected with questionnaires or through personal interviews with members of an identified population.

time dimensional d. an investigation strategy for the examination of sequence and patterns of change, growth, or trends across time; see also prospective STUDY and retrospective STUDY.

trend d. a research strategy to examine changes in the general population in relation to a particular phenomenon by means of data collected at predetermined intervals of time from different samples selected from the general population.

desipramine (des-ip′rah-mēn) a tricyclic ANTIDEPRESSANT of the DIBENZAZEPINE group, administered orally as the hydrochloride salt.

deslanoside (des-lan′o-sīd) a cardiotonic GLYCOSIDE obtained from lanatoside C, having the same actions and uses as DIGITALIS.

desloratadine (des″lah-rat′ah-dēn) a nonsedating antihistamine (H_1 receptor ANTAGONIST) used for treatment of allergic RHINITIS and chronic idiopathic urticaria; administered orally.

desm(o)- word element [Gr.], *ligament.*

desmitis (dez-mi′tis) inflammation of a ligament.

desmocranium (dez″mo-kra′ne-um) the mass of mesoderm at the cranial end of the notochord in the early embryo, forming the earliest stage of the skull.

desmography (dez-mog′rah-fe) a description of ligaments.

desmoid (dez'moid) 1. an unencapsulated, locally invasive, and rarely metastasizing fibromatous tumor arising in the muscle sheath, usually of the abdominal wall, which closely resembles FIBROSARCOMA. Called also desmoid tumor. 2. fibroid (def. 1).

desmology (dez-mol'o-je) the science of ligaments.

desmoma (dez-mo'mah) desmoid (def. 1).

desmopathy (dez-mop'ah-the) any disease of the ligaments.

desmoplasia (dez″mo-pla'zhah) the formation and development of fibrous tissue. adj., **desmoplas'tic.**

desmopressin (des″mo-pres'in) a synthetic analogue of VASOPRESSIN, used as an antidiuretic in central DIABETES INSIPIDUS and in primary nocturnal ENURESIS, and as an antihemorrhagic in HEMOPHILIA A and VON WILLEBRAND'S DISEASE.

desogestrel (des″o-jes'trel) a progestational AGENT having little androgenic activity; used in combination with an estrogen component as an oral CONTRACEPTIVE.

desonide (des'o-nīd) a synthetic CORTICOSTEROID used as a topical ANTIINFLAMMATORY agent in the treatment of steroid-responsive dermatoses.

desorb (de-sorb') to remove a substance from the state of absorption or adsorption.

desorption (de-sorp'shun) the process of being desorbed.

desoximetasone (des-ok″se-met'a-sōn) 1. a steroid used topically to relieve inflammation and itching in corticosteroid-responsive dermatoses. 2. a synthetic corticosteroid used topically for the relief of inflammation and pruritus in corticosteroid-responsive dermatoses.

desoxy- older form for DEOXY-.

desoxycorticosterone (des-ok″sĭ-kor″tĭ-ko-stēr'ōn) a MINERALOCORTICOID with no GLUCOCORTICOID activity, secreted in small amounts by the human adrenal cortex. It is used with a glucocorticoid for replacement therapy in adrenocortical INSUFFICIENCY and ADDISON'S DISEASE and for treatment of salt-losing ADRENOGENITAL SYNDROME.

Desoxyn (des-ok'sin) trademark for preparations of METHAMPHETAMINE hydrochloride, a central nervous system STIMULANT and PRESSOR drug.

desquamation (des″kwah-ma'shun) the shedding of epithelial elements, chiefly of the skin, in scales or sheets. adj., **desquam'-ative.**

desulfhydrase (de″sulf-hi'drās) an enzyme that splits cysteine into hydrogen sulfide, ammonia, and pyruvic acid.

desynchrony a condition in which the envronmental cues and patterns, such as sleeping and eating, conflict with an individual's existing pattern; one type is JET LAG.

detachment (de-tach'ment) the condition of being separated or disconnected.

d. of retina, retinal d. separation of the inner layers of the RETINA from the pigment epithelium, which remains attached to the choroid; it occurs most often as a result of degenerative changes in the peripheral retina and vitreous body, which produce holes or tears in the retina ranging from tiny breaks of less than 0.1 mm to extensive holes extending over the entire fundus. It is most common in persons over 40, and about two thirds of affected patients are myopic (nearsighted). Trauma to the eyeball, severe contusions, inflammatory lesions, and sometimes ocular surgery such as for a cataract can also lead to retinal detachment.

Symptoms. The onset of symptoms may be gradual or sudden, depending on the cause, size, number, and location of retinal holes. The patient usually sees flashes of light and then notices cloudy vision or loss of a portion of the visual field. Another common manifestation is the sensation of spots or moving particles in the field of vision. Treatment should be sought immediately when any of these occur. In severe retinal detachment there can be complete loss of vision.

Treatment. Retinal detachment is corrected surgically. Two outpatient modes of therapy currently in use are PHOTOCOAGULATION, using the light source of an argon laser; and CRYOSURGERY, in which a freezing probe is used to penetrate the tissues of the eye and encircle the hole or tear in the retina. Scar tissue eventually forms and seals the opening. Scleral BUCKLING is another treatment, which places the retinal breaks in contact with the pigment epithelium and choroid. Adhesions form and bind the sensory retinal layers to these structures. In some cases, such as vitreous

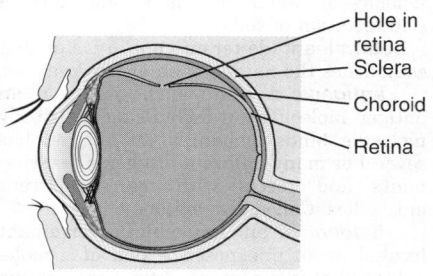

Retinal detachment. From Frazier et al., 2000.

hemorrhage, the surgeon performs a combined vitrectomy and humoral retinal repair. The purpose of the surgery is to remove vitreous that is opaque because of accumulated blood, and to stabilize the retina in apposition to the choroid. Aqueous humor eventually fills the space.

Pneumatic RETROPEXY, the most recently developed treatment, consists of injection of air or gas into the posterior vitreous cavity, followed by positioning of the patient so that the bubble rises, presses against the area of torn retina, and pushes it back into its normal position against the choroid. Laser photocoagulation and/or cryopexy is then done to create inflammation within the tissues, resulting in scarring and permanent reattachment of the area(s) of torn retina. This procedure is appropriate for only certain types and locations of retinal detachment.

Preoperative and postoperative care of the patient requires a thorough knowledge of the type of detachment afflicting the patient and the surgical procedure performed. Positioning of the patient and the level of physical activity allowed after surgery are determined by the surgeon. Before discharge from the hospital the patient will need instruction in follow-up care, especially the correct procedure for instilling eye drops.

detail (de'tāl) in radiology, the precise definition of structures.

detector (de-tek'ter) a device by which an object or condition can be discovered.

image d. any recording medium used in radiology, such as film or a cathode ray tube.

lie d. polygraph.

detergent (de-ter'jent) 1. purifying or cleansing. 2. an agent that purifies or cleanses. 3. in biochemistry, any of a class of agents structurally consisting of a nonpolar hydrocarbon chain and a hydrophilic polar head group, which reduce the surface tension of water, emulsify, and aid in solubilization of soil.

determinant (de-ter'mĭ-nant) a factor that establishes the nature of an entity or event.

antigenic d. a site on the surface of an antigen molecule to which a single antibody molecule binds; generally an antigen has several or many different antigenic determinants and reacts with many different antibodies. Called also epitope.

hidden d. an antigenic determinant located in an unexposed region of a molecule so that it is prevented from interacting with receptors on lymphocytes, or with

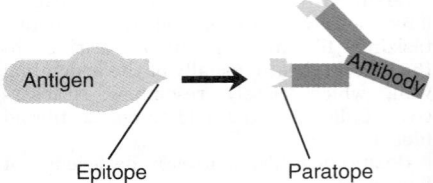

Antigens contain antigenic determinants (epitopes) and antibodies contain antibody combining sites (paratopes). From Copstead and Banasik, 2000.

antibody molecules, and is unable to induce an IMMUNE RESPONSE; it may appear following stereochemical alterations of molecular structure.

immunogenic d. the part of an immunogenic molecule that interacts with a helper T CELL in triggering antibody production as opposed to the antigenic determinant or hapten, which interacts with B CELLS.

determination (de-ter″mĭ-na'shun) the establishment of the exact nature of an entity or event.

embryonic d. the loss of pluripotentiality in any embryonic part and its start on the way to an unalterable fate.

sex d. the process by which the sex of an organism is fixed; associated, in man, with the presence or absence of the Y chromosome.

determinism (de-ter'mĭ-nizm) the theory that all phenomena are the result of antecedent conditions, nothing occurs by chance, and there is no free will.

detoxicate (de-tok'sĭ-kāt) detoxify.

detoxication (de-tok″sĭ-ka'shun) detoxification.

detoxification (de-tok″sĭ-fĭ-ka'shun) 1. reduction of the toxic properties of a substance. 2. treatment designed to assist in recovery from the toxic effects of a drug.

metabolic d. reduction of the toxic properties of a substance by chemical changes induced in the body, producing a compound which is less poisonous or more readily eliminated.

detoxify (de-tok'sĭ-fī) to subject to detoxification.

detrition (de-trish'un) the wearing away, as of teeth, by friction.

detritus (de-tri'tus) particulate matter produced by or remaining after the wearing away or disintegration of a substance or tissue.

detrusor (de-troo'ser) 1. a body part that pushes down, such as a muscle. 2. pertaining to the detrusor muscle of the bladder; see anatomic Table of Muscles in the Appendices.

detumescence (de″too-mes′ens) the subsidence of congestion and swelling.

deutan (doo′tan) a person exhibiting deuteranomaly or deuteranopia.

deuteranomaly (doo″ter-ah-nom′ah-le) a type of anomalous trichromatic VISION in which the second, green-sensitive, cones have decreased sensitivity. It is an X-linked trait, affecting about 5 per cent of white males in the U.S.A. and 0.25 per cent of females, and is the most common COLOR VISION DEFICIENCY.

deuteranope (doo′ter-ah-nōp″) a person exhibiting DEUTERANOPIA.

deuteranopia (doo″ter-ah-no′pe-ah) defective color vision, with confusion of greens and reds, and retention of the sensory mechanism for only the hues of blue and yellow. adj., **deuteranop′ic.**

deuteranopsia (doo″ter-ah-nop′se-ah) deuteranopia.

deuterium (D) (doo-tēr′e-um) the mass 2 isotope of hydrogen; it is available as a gas or heavy water and has been used as a tracer or indicator in metabolic studies.

deuteropathy (doo″ter-op′ah-the) a disease that is secondary to another disease.

devascularization (de-vas″ku-ler-ĭ-za′-shun) interruption of circulation of blood to a part due to obstruction or destruction of blood vessels supplying it. See also ISCHEMIA.

development (de-vel′up-ment) 1. growth and differentiation. 2. BUILDING or ENHANCEMENT.

cognitive d. the development of intelligence, conscious thought, and problem-solving ability that begins in infancy.

community health d. in the NURSING INTERVENTIONS CLASSIFICATION, a nursing INTERVENTION defined as facilitating members of a community to identify the community's health concerns, mobilize resources, and implement solutions.

critical path d. in the NURSING INTERVENTIONS CLASSIFICATION, a nursing INTERVENTION defined as constructing and using a timed sequence of patient care activities to enhance desired patient outcomes in a cost-efficient manner. See also CRITICAL PATH.

program d. in the NURSING INTERVENTIONS CLASSIFICATION, a nursing INTERVENTION defined as planning, implementing, and evaluating a coordinated set of activities designed to enhance wellness or to prevent, reduce, or eliminate one or more health problems of a group or community.

psychosexual d. 1. generally, the development of the psychological aspects of sexuality from birth to maturity. 2. In psychoanalytic theory, the development of object relations has five stages: the *oral stage* from birth to 2 years, the *anal stage* from 2 to 4 years, the *phallic stage* from 4 to 6 years, the *latency stage* from 6 years until puberty, and the *genital stage* from puberty onward; see also SEXUAL DEVELOPMENT.

psychosocial d. the development of the personality, including the acquisition of social attitudes and skills, from infancy through maturity.

risk for delayed d. a NURSING DIAGNOSIS accepted by the North American Nursing Diagnosis Association, defined as being at risk for delay of 25 per cent or more in one or more of the areas of social or self-regulatory behavior, or in cognitive, language, gross motor, or fine motor skills.

sexual d. see SEXUAL DEVELOPMENT.

staff d. 1. an educational program for health care providers conducted by a hospital or other institution; it includes orientation, in-service training, and continuing education. 2. in the NURSING INTERVENTIONS CLASSIFICATION, a nursing INTERVENTION defined as developing, maintaining, and monitoring competence of staff.

developmental (de-vel″up-men′t'l) 1. pertaining to development.

d. disorder 1. developmental disability. 2. a former classification of chronic disorders of mental development with onset in childhood. Such disorders are now classifed as MENTAL RETARDATION, LEARNING DISORDERS, MOTOR SKILLS DISORDER, COMMUNICATION DISORDERS, or PERVASIVE DEVELOPMENTAL DISORDERS.

d. tasks fundamental achievements that must be accomplished at each stage of life, arising at or near critical stages in the maturation of an individual; successful attainment leads to a healthy self-image and success with later tasks. Failure to achieve developmental tasks at one stage leads to unhappiness in the individual, disapproval of society, and difficulty in accomplishing later developmental tasks. Two major primary origins of developmental tasks are physical maturation and cultural pressures and privileges. Secondary origins are derived from the first two and are found in the aspirations and values of the individual.

Family developmental tasks are those that must be attained to assure survival of the family and its continuance as a unit. Examples include (1) providing shelter, food, clothing, health care, and other essentials needed by its members, (2) establishing ways of interacting, communicating, and expressing affection, (3) maintaining morale and motivation, (4) rewarding achievement, (5) meeting personal and family crises,

(6) setting attainable goals for family members, and (7) developing family loyalties and values.

deviant (de′ve-ant) 1. varying from a determinable standard. 2. a person with characteristics varying from what is considered standard or normal.

   sexual d. a person exhibiting sexual deviation.

deviation (de″ve-a′shun) 1. a turning away from the regular standard or course. 2. in ophthalmology, strabismus. 3. in statistics, the difference between a sample value and the mean.

   axis d. an axis shift in the frontal plane, as seen on an electrocardiogram. There are three types: *Left,* from −30° to −90°; *Right,* from +90° to +180°; and *Undetermined,* which may be either extreme left or extreme right, from −90° to +180°.

   conjugate d. dysfunction of the ocular muscles causing the two eyes to diverge to the same side when at rest.

   sexual d. sexual behavior or fantasy outside that which is morally, biologically, or legally sanctioned, often specifically one of the PARAPHILIAS.

   standard d. **(SD)** the dispersion of a random variable; a measure of the amount by which each value deviates from the mean. It is equal to the square root of the variance. For data that have a normal distribution, about 68 per cent of the data points fall within (plus or minus) one standard deviation from the mean and about 95 per cent fall within (plus or minus) two standard deviations. Symbol σ.

   ulnar d. a hand deformity, seen in chronic rheumatoid ARTHRITIS and LUPUS ERYTHEMATOSUS, in which swelling of the metacarpophalangeal joints causes the fingers to become displaced to the ulnar side. Called also ulnar drift. See illustration.

device (de-vīs′) something contrived for a specific purpose; usually a simple mechanical apparatus.

   assisting d′s, assistive d′s tools and implements that aid a person with a disability in carrying out mobility or ACTIVITIES OF DAILY LIVING.

   intrauterine d. see INTRAUTERINE DEVICE.

   left ventricular assist d. a circulatory support device consisting of a pump connected to an external pneumatic power source and control circuit; it has afferent and efferent conduits attached respectively to the left atrium or ventricle and the ascending aorta. Each conduit contains a porcine valve to ensure unidirectional blood flow and maintain systemic circulation

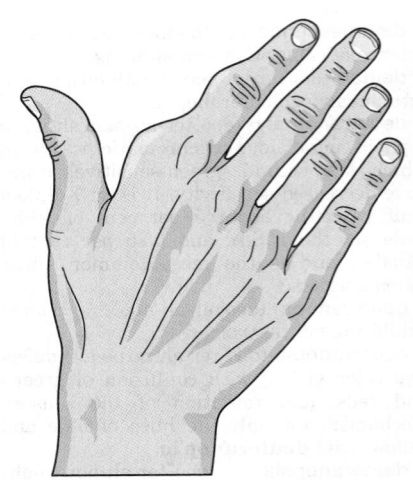

Ulnar deviation (ulnar drift) of the metacarpophalangeal joint, a characteristic sign of rheumatoid arthritis. From Pedretti and Early, 2001.

when the heart is unable to do so. The device is used as a bridge to transplantation.

   mobility d. a device such as a wheelchair, motorized scooter, cart, or stroller that permits the disabled individual to move about and have greater access to the environment.

   terminal d. the end piece of a prosthesis for the upper limb; it may be a hook or a mechanical or cosmetic hand.

devitalized (de-vi′tal-īzd) 1. devoid of vitality or life; dead. 2. of an organ or body part, having a blood supply so reduced that the oxygen supply will not support life.

DEXA dual energy x-ray absorptiometry.

dexamethasone (dek″sah-meth′ah-sōn) a synthetic steroid ANTIINFLAMMATORY agent used for various conditions, including collagen diseases and allergic states; it is also used for replacement therapy in adrenal insufficiency and in a screening test for the diagnosis of CUSHING′S SYNDROME.

dexbrompheniramine (deks″brōm-fen-ir′-ah-mēn) the dextrorotatory isomer of BROMPHENIRAMINE, having similar actions and uses as an ANTIHISTAMINE, but having approximately twice the activity by weight; used in the form of the maleate salt.

dexchlorpheniramine (deks″klor-fen-ir′ah-mēn) the dextrorotatory isomer of CHLORPHENIRAMINE, having similar actions and uses as an ANTIHISTAMINE, but having approximately twice the activity by weight; used in the form of the maleate salt.

Dexedrine (dek′sĕ-drēn) trademark for preparations of DEXTROAMPHETAMINE, a central nervous system STIMULANT.

dexmedetomidine (deks″med-ĕ-to′mĭ-dēn) a selective α₂-adrenergic RECEPTOR agonist, used as the hydrochloride salt as a SEDATIVE for patients in intensive care units; administered intravenously.

Dexon (dek′son) trademark for POLYGLYCOLIC ACID, a synthetic suture material that is absorbable and nonirritating.

dexpanthenol (deks-pan′thĕ-nol) the D-isomer of PANTHENOL, a coenzyme A precursor with cholinergic activity. Used to increase peristalsis in atony and paralysis of the lower intestine and as an antiflatulent; also used topically to stimulate skin healing in various eczemas and dermatoses.

dexrazoxane (deks″ra-zok′sān) a derivative of ETHYLENEDIAMINETETRAACETIC ACID (EDTA) used as a CARDIOPROTECTANT in ANTINEOPLASTIC THERAPY to counteract CARDIOMYOPATHY induced by DOXORUBICIN; administered intravenously.

dexter [L.] right; on the right side.

dextr(o)- word element [L.], *right*.

dextrality (dek-stral′ĭ-te) the preferential use, in voluntary motor acts, of the right member of the major paired organs of the body, such as the right eye, ear, hand, or leg. See also LATERALITY and HANDEDNESS

dextran (dek′stran) a water-soluble polysaccharide of GLUCOSE produced by the action of *Leuconostoc mesenteroides* on sucrose; used as an artificial plasma EXTENDER.

dextranomer (dek-stran′o-mer) small beads of highly hydrophilic dextran polymers used in débridement of secreting wounds, such as venous stasis ulcers; the sterilized beads are poured over secreting wounds to absorb wound exudates and prevent crust formation.

dextraural (dek-straw′ral) hearing better with the right ear.

dextrin (dek′strin) any of a range of glucose polymers of varying sizes formed during the hydrolysis of starch.

dextrin-1,6-glucosidase (deks″trin-glu-ko′sĭ-dās) dextrin 6-glucanohydrolase: an enzyme that catalyzes the hydrolysis of α-1-6-glucan links in dextrins containing short 1,6-linked side chains.

dextrinosis (dek″strĭ-no′sis) a condition characterized by accumulation in the tissues of an abnormal polysaccharide.

limit d. Forbes' disease.

dextrinuria (dek″strin-u′re-ah) presence of dextrin in the urine.

dextroamphetamine (dek″stro-am-fet′ah-mēn) the dextrorotatory isomer of AMPHETAMINE, having a more conspicuous STIMULANT effect on the central nervous system than the racemic form of amphetamine; used as the sulfate salt in the treatment of narcolepsy and attention-deficit/hyper-

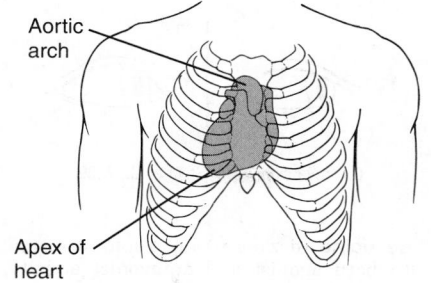

Aortic arch

Apex of heart

Dextrocardia. From Dorland's, 2000.

activity disorder. Abuse of this drug may lead to dependence.

dextrocardia (dek″stro-kahr′de-ah) location of the heart in the right side of the thorax, the apex pointing to the right. See illustration.

mirror-image d. location of the heart in the right side of the chest, the atria being transposed and the right ventricle lying anteriorly and to the left of the left ventricle.

dextrocularity (dek″strok-u-lar′ĭ-te) having greater visual power in the right eye, therefore using it more than the left.

dextromanual (dek″stro-man′u-al) right-handed.

dextromethorphan (dek″stro-meth′or-fan) a synthetic MORPHINE derivative used as an antitussive in the form of the hydrobromide salt.

dextropedal (dek-strop′ĕ-d'l) right-footed.

dextroposition (dek″stro-po-zish′un) displacement to the right.

dextropropoxyphene (dek″stro-pro-pok′-sĭ-fēn) propoxyphene.

dextrorotatory (dek″stro-ro′tah-tor″e) turning the plane of polarization, or rays of light, to the right.

dextrose (dek′strōs) older chemical name for D-glucose (see GLUCOSE); the term *dextrose* continues to be used to refer to glucose solutions administered intravenously for fluid or nutrient replacement.

dextrosinistral (dek″stro-sin′is-tral) extending from right to left; also applied to a left-handed person trained to use the right hand in certain performances.

dextrosuria (dek″stro-su′re-ah) glycosuria.

dextroversion (dek″stro-ver′zhun) 1. version to the right, especially movement of the eyes to the right. 2. location of the heart in the right chest, the left ventricle remaining in the normal position on the left, but lying anterior to the right ventricle. See illustration.

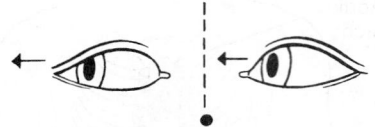

Dextroversion. From Stein et al., 2000.

dezocine (dez′o-sēn) an OPIOID ANALGESIC with both agonist and antagonist activity, used for short-term relief of pain; administered intramuscularly or intravenously.

df degrees of freedom.

DFA-TP test direct fluorescent antibody–*Treponema pallidum* test.

DHT dihydrotestosterone.

di- word element [Gr., L.], *two.*

dia- word element [Gr.], *through; between; apart; across; completely.*

diabetes (di″ah-be′tēz) a general term referring to any of various disorders characterized by excessive urination (POLYURIA); when used alone, the term refers to DIABETES MELLITUS. (See Atlas 4, Part D).

brittle d. diabetes that is difficult to control, characterized by unexplained oscillation between HYPOGLYCEMIA and diabetic KETOACIDOSIS. (This term was formerly much used, but it is not a classification used by the World Health Organization or the American Diabetes Association.)

bronze d. hemochromatosis.

central d. insipidus a metabolic disorder due to injury of the neurohypophyseal system, which results in a deficient quantity of antidiuretic hormone (ADH or vasopressin) being released or produced, resulting in failure of tubular reabsorption of water in the kidney. As a consequence, there is the passage of a large amount of urine having a low specific gravity, and great thirst; it is often attended by voracious appetite, loss of strength, and emaciation. Diabetes insipidus may be acquired through infection, neoplasm, trauma, or radiation injuries to the posterior lobe of the pituitary gland or it may be inherited or idiopathic. Treatment of pituitary diabetes insipidus consists of administration of vasopressin. A synthetic analogue of vasopressin (DDAVP) can be administered as a nasal spray, providing antidiuretic activity for 8 to 20 hours, and is currently the drug of choice. Patient care includes instruction in self-administration of the drug, its expected action, symptoms that indicate a need to adjust the dosage, and the importance of follow-up visits.

Patients with this condition should wear some form of medical identification at all times.

gestational d. DIABETES MELLITUS with onset or first recognition during pregnancy, usually during the second or third trimester. In some cases mild, undetected glucose intolerance was present before pregnancy. It often disappears after the end of the pregnancy, but many women with this condition develop permanent diabetes mellitus in later life. Although the disordered carbohydrate metabolism is usually mild, prompt detection and treatment are necessary to avoid fetal and neonatal morbidity and mortality.

maturity-onset d. of youth (MODY) an autosomal dominant variety of type 2 DIABETES MELLITUS characterized by onset in late adolescence or early adulthood.

d. mel′litus a broadly applied term used to denote a complex group of syndromes that have in common a disturbance in the oxidation and utilization of GLUCOSE, which may be secondary to a malfunction of the beta CELLS of the pancreas, whose function is the production and release of INSULIN. Because insulin is involved in the metabolism of carbohydrates, proteins, and fats, diabetes is not limited to a disturbance of glucose homeostasis alone. Insulin RESISTANCE may also sometimes play a role in the etiology of diabetes. The American Diabetes Association sponsored an international panel in 1995 to review the literature and recommend updates of the classification of diabetes mellitus. The definitions and descriptions that follow are drawn from the Report of the Expert Committee on the Diagnosis and Classification of Diabetes Mellitus. The report was first approved in 1997 and modified in 1999. Although other terms are found in older literature and remain in use, their use in current clinical practice is inappropriate. Epidemiologic and research studies are facilitated by use of a common language.

The Expert Committee notes that most cases of diabetes fall into two broad categories, which are called *Type 1* and *Type 2.* There are also other specific types, such as gestational DIABETES and impaired glucose homeostasis. See table for definitions of types of diabetes mellitus.

Incidence and Prevalence. It has been estimated that slightly over 6 per cent of the population is affected by some form of diabetes, or 17 million people in the USA and 1.2 to 1.4 million in Canada; many of these individuals are not diagnosed. Diabetes is ranked third as a cause of death, although the life span of patients with diabetes has increased due to improved methods of detection and better management. There is no cure for diabetes at the present time, but enormous strides have been made in the control of the disease. The patient must understand the importance of compliance with the entire treatment plan, including diet, exercise, and in some cases medication. The patient with diabetes is at increased risk for cardiovascular disease, renal failure, neuropathies, and diabetic RETINOPATHY. Research studies such as the Diabetes Control and Complications Trial have indicated that tight control of blood glucose levels resulted in the delay or prevention of retinopathy, nephropathy, and neuropathy.

Diagnosis. The most common diagnostic tests for diabetes are chemical analyses of the blood such as the fasting plasma GLUCOSE. Capillary blood glucose monitoring can be used for screening large segments of the population. Portable equipment is available and only one drop of blood from the fingertip or earlobe is necessary. Capillary blood glucose levels have largely replaced analysis of the urine for glucose. Testing for urinary glucose can be problematic as the patient may have a high renal threshold, which would lead to a negative reading for urinary glucose when in fact the blood glucose level was high.

Clinical Manifestations. Diabetes mellitus can present a wide variety of symptoms, from none at all to profound ketosis and coma. If the disease manifests itself late in life, patients may not know they have it until it is discovered during a routine examination, or when the symptoms of chronic vascular disease, insidious renal failure, or impaired vision cause them to seek medical help. The typical symptoms of diabetes mellitus are the three "polys:" POLYURIA, POLYDIPSIA, and POLYPHAGIA. Because of insulin deficiency, the assimilation and storage of glucose in muscle adipose tissues, and the liver is greatly diminished. This produces an accumulation of glucose in the blood and creates an increase in its osmolarity. In response to this increased osmotic pressure there is depletion of intracellular water and osmotic diuresis. The water loss creates intense thirst and

ETIOLOGIC CLASSIFICATION OF DIABETES MELLITUS

Type 1	Characterized by beta cell destruction, usually leading to absolute insulin deficiency. It has two forms: *Immune-Mediated Diabetes Mellitus*: Results from a cellular mediated autoimmune destruction of the beta cells of the pancreas. *Idiopathic Diabetes Mellitus*: Refers to forms of the disease that have no known etiologies.
Type 2	Diseases of insulin resistance that usually have relative (rather than absolute) insulin deficiency: Can range from predominant insulin resistance with relative insulin deficiency to predominant insulin deficiency with some insulin resistance.
Impaired Glucose Homeostasis	A metabolic stage intermediate between normal glucose homeostasis and diabetes. A risk factor for diabetes and cardiovascular disease. *Impaired Fasting Glucose*: Fasting plasma glucose higher than normal, and less than diagnostic. *Impaired Glucose Tolerance*: Plasma glucose higher than normal and less than diagnostic, following administration of a glucose load of 75 grams.
Gestational Diabetes Mellitus	Glucose intolerance in pregnancy: any degree of glucose intolerance with onset or first recognition during pregnancy. The definition applies whether insulin or only diet modification is used for treatment and whether or not the condition persists after pregnancy. It does not exclude the possibility that unrecognized glucose intolerance may have antedated or begun concomitantly with the pregnancy.
Other Specific Types	Diabetes caused by other identifiable etiologies: 1. Genetic defects of beta cell function (e.g., MODY 1,2,3) 2. Genetic defects in insulin action 3. Diseases of the exocrine pancreas (e.g., cancer of the pancreas, cystic fibrosis, pancreatitis) 4. Endocrinopathies (e.g., Cushing's) 5. Drug or chemical induced (e.g., steroids) 6. Infection (e.g., rubella, Coxsackie, CMV) 7. Uncommon forms of immune-related diabetes 8. Other genetic syndromes

increased urination. The increased appetite (POLYPHAGIA) is not as clearly understood. It may be the result of the body's effort to increase its supply of energy foods even though eating more carbohydrates in the absence of sufficient insulin does not meet the energy needs of the cells.

Fatigue and muscle weakness occur because the glucose needed for energy simply is not metabolized properly. Weight loss in type 1 diabetes patients occurs partly because of the loss of body fluid and partly because in the absence of sufficient insulin the body begins to metabolize its own proteins and stored fat. The oxidation of fats is incomplete, however, and the fatty acids are converted into ketone bodies. When the kidney is no longer able to handle the excess ketones the patient develops ketosis. The overwhelming presence of the strong organic acids in the blood lowers the pH and leads to severe and potentially fatal ketoacidosis.

The metabolism of body protein when sufficient amounts of insulin are not available causes an elevated BLOOD UREA NITROGEN. This first occurs because the nitrogen component of protein is discarded in the blood when the body metabolizes its own proteins to obtain the glucose it needs.

Persons with diabetes are prone to infection, delayed healing, and vascular disease. The ease with which poorly controlled diabetic persons develop an infection is thought to be due in part to decreased chemotaxis of leukocytes, abnormal phagocyte function, and diminished blood supply because of atherosclerotic changes in the blood vessels. An impaired blood supply means a deficit in the protective defensive cells transported in the blood. Excessive glucose allows organisms to grow out of control.

Another manifestation of diabetes mellitus is visual disturbance due to increased osmolarity of the blood and accumulation of fluid in the eyeball, which changes its shape. Once the diabetes is under control, visual problems should abate. Persistent vaginitis and urinary tract infection also may be symptoms of diabetes in females.

Sequelae. The long-term consequences of diabetes mellitus can involve both large and small blood vessels throughout the body. That in large vessels is usually seen in the coronary arteries, cerebral arteries, and arteries of the lower extremities and can eventually lead to MYOCARDIAL INFARCTION, STROKE, or GANGRENE of the feet and legs. ATHEROSCLEROSIS is far more likely to occur in

persons of any age who have diabetes than it is in other people. This predisposition is not clearly understood. Some believe that diabetics inherit the tendency to develop severe atherosclerosis as well as an aberration in glucose metabolism, and that the two are not necessarily related. There is strong evidence to substantiate the claim that optimal control will mitigate the effects of diabetes on the MICROVASCULATURE, particularly in the young and middle-aged who are at greatest risk for developing complications involving the arterioles. Pathologic changes in the small blood vessels serving the kidney lead to nephrosclerosis, pyelonephritis, and other disorders that eventually result in renal failure. Many of the deaths of persons with type 1 diabetes are caused by renal failure.

Visual impairment and blindness are common sequelae of uncontrolled diabetes. The three most frequently occurring problems involving the eye are diabetic RETINOPATHY, CATARACTS, and GLAUCOMA. PHOTOCOAGULATION of destructive lesions of the retina with laser beams can be used to delay further progress of pathologic changes and thereby preserve sight in the affected eye.

Another area of pathologic changes associated with diabetes mellitus is the nervous system (diabetic NEUROPATHY), particularly in the peripheral nerves of the lower extremities. The patient typically experiences a "stocking-type" anesthesia beginning about 10 years after the onset of the disease. There may eventually be almost total anesthesia of the affected part with the potential for serious injury to the part without the patient being aware of it. In contrast, some patients experience debilitating pain and HYPERESTHESIA, with loss of deep tendon reflexes.

Other problems related to the destruction of nerve tissue are the result of autonomic nervous system involvement. These include impotence, orthostatic hypotension, delayed gastric emptying, diarrhea or constipation, and asymptomatic retention of urine in the bladder.

Although age of onset and length of the disease process are related to the frequency with which vascular, renal, and neurologic complications develop, there are some patients who remain relatively free of sequelae even into the later years of their lives. Because diabetes mellitus is not a single disease but rather a complex constellation of syndromes, each patient has a unique response to the disease process.

Management. There is no cure for diabetes; the goal of treatment is to maintain blood glucose and lipid levels within normal limits and to prevent complications. In general, good control is achieved when the following occur: fasting plasma glucose is within a specific range (set by health care providers and the individual), glycosylated hemoglobin tests show that blood sugar levels have stayed within normal limits from one testing period to the next, the patient's weight is normal, blood lipids remain within normal limits, and the patient has a sense of health and well-being. The protocol for therapy is determined by the type of diabetes; patients with either type 1 or type 2 must pay attention to their diet and exercise regimens. Insulin therapy may be prescribed for patients with type 2 diabetes as well as any who are dependent on insulin. In most cases, the type 2 diabetes patient can be treated effectively by reducing caloric intake, maintaining target weight, and promoting physical exercise.

Diet. In general, the diabetic diet is geared toward providing adequate nutrition with sufficient calories to maintain normal body weight; the intake of food is adjusted so that blood sugar and serum cholesterol levels are kept within acceptable limits. Overweight diabetic patients should limit caloric intake until target weight is achieved. In persons with type 2 diabetes this usually results in marked improvement and may eliminate the need for drugs such as oral hypoglycemic AGENTS.

The patient, physician, nurse, and dietician must carefully evaluate the patient's life style, nutritional needs, and ability to comply with the proposed dietary prescription. There are a variety of meal planning systems that can be used by the patient with diabetes; each has benefits and drawbacks that need to be evaluated in order to maximize compliance. Two of the most frequently used ones are the *exchange system* (see accompanying table) and the *carbohydrate counting system*.

In the exchange system, foods are divided into six food groups (starch, meat, vegetable, fruit, milk, and fat) and the patient is taught to select items from each food group as

ordered. Items in each group may be exchanged for each other in specified portions. The patient should avoid concentrated sweets and should increase fiber in the diet. Special dietetic foods are not necessary. Patient teaching should emphasize that a diabetic diet is a healthy diet that all members of the family can follow.

The carbohydrate counting system focuses on matching the unit of insulin to the total number of grams of carbohydrate in food eaten. This system is the most accurate method for calculating insulin to food intake.

It is especially important that persons with diabetes who are taking insulin not skip meals; they must also be sure to eat the prescribed amounts at the prescribed times during the day. Since the insulin-dependent diabetic needs to match food consumption to the available insulin, it is advantageous to increase the number of daily feedings by adding snacks between meals and at bedtime.

Exercise. A program of regular exercise gives anyone a sense of good health and well-being; for persons with diabetes it gives added benefits by helping to control blood glucose levels, promoting circulation to peripheral tissues, and strengthening the heart beat. In addition, there is evidence that exercise increases the number of insulin receptor sites on the surface of cells and thus facilitates the metabolism of glucose. Many specialists in diabetes consider exercise so important in the management of diabetes that they prescribe rather than suggest exercise.

Persons with diabetes who take insulin must be careful about indulging in unplanned exercise. Strenuous physical activity can rapidly lower their blood sugar and precipitate a hypoglycemic reaction. For a person whose blood glucose level is over 250 mg/dl, the advice would be not to exercise at all. At this range, the levels of insulin are too low and the body would have

DIABETES: THE SIX FOOD EXCHANGE LISTS	
List 1: Milk Exchanges	Low fat, fortified, or whole milk
List 2: Vegetable Exchanges	½ cup of nonstarchy vegetables, excluding some vegetables like lettuce which can be used as desired by the patient
List 3: Fruit Exchanges	Fruits and fruit juices
List 4: Bread, Cereal, and Starchy Vegetables	Breads, cereal, starchy vegetables such as corn and potatoes, dried beans, peas, and lentils
List 5: Meat and Protein-Rich Exchanges	Meats, eggs, cheeses, and other high-protein foods
List 6: Fat Exchanges	Margarine, nuts, oils, cream cheese, and dressings

difficulty transporting glucose into exercising muscles. The result of exercise would be a rise in blood glucose levels.

Insulin Therapy. Exogenous INSULIN is given to patients with diabetes mellitus as a supplement to the insufficient amount of endogenous insulin that they produce. In some cases, this must make up for an absolute lack of insulin from the pancreas. Exogenous insulin is available in various types. It must be given by injection, usually subcutaneously, and because it is a potent drug, the dosage must be measured meticulously. Commonly, regular insulin, which is a fast-acting insulin with a short span of action, is mixed with one of the longer-acting insulins and both types are administered in one injection.

Human insulin (Humulin) is produced by recombinant DNA technology. This highly purified biosynthetic insulin reduces the incidence of allergic reactions and the changes in subcutaneous tissues (LIPODYSTROPHY) at sites of injection.

Recently, battery-operated insulin PUMPS have been developed that can be programmed to mimic normal insulin secretion more closely. A person wearing an insulin pump still must monitor blood sugar several times a day and adjust the dosage, and not all diabetic patients are motivated or suited to such vigilance. It is hoped that in the future an implantable or external pump system may be perfected, containing a glucose sensor. In response to data from the sensor the pump will automatically deliver insulin according to changing levels of blood glucose.

Oral Agents. Oral antidiabetic drugs (see hypoglycemic AGENTS) are sometimes prescribed for patients with type 2 diabetes who cannot control their blood glucose with diet and exercise. These are *not* oral forms of insulin; they are SULFONYLUREAS, chemically related to the sulfonamide antibiotics. Patients receiving them should be taught that the drug they are taking does not eliminate the need for a diet and exercise program. Only the prescribed dosage should be taken; it should never be increased to make up for dietary indiscretions or discontinued unless authorized by the physician.

Patient Education. Successful management of diabetes requires that the patient actively participate in and be committed to the regimen of care. The problem of poor control can cause serious or even deadly short-term and long-term complications, with devastating effects on the patient's longevity and sense of well being. There are many teaching aids available to help persons with diabetes understand their disease and comply with prescribed therapy. In general, a patient education program should include the following components:

1. *Monitoring of blood glucose status.* In the past, urine testing was an integral part of the management of diabetes, but it has largely been replaced in recent years by self monitoring of blood glucose. Reasons for this are that blood testing is more accurate, glucose in the urine shows up only after the blood sugar level is high, and individual renal thresholds vary greatly and can change when certain medications are taken. As a person grows older and the kidney is less able to eliminate sugar in the urine, the renal threshold rises and less sugar is spilled into the urine. The position statement of the American Diabetes Association on Tests of Glycemia in Diabetes notes that urine testing still plays a role in monitoring in type 1 and gestational diabetes, and in pregnancy with pre-existing diabetes, as a way to test for KETONES. All people with diabetes should test for ketones during times of acute illness or stress and when blood glucose levels are consistently elevated.

2. *Home glucose monitoring* using either a visually read test or a digital readout of the glucose concentration in a drop of blood. Patients can usually learn to use the necessary equipment and perform finger sticks. They keep a daily record of findings and are taught to adjust insulin dosage accordingly. More recent glucose monitoring devices can draw blood from other locations on the body, such as the forearm.

3. *Pathophysiology of diabetes mellitus,* including functions of the pancreas and the long-term effects of uncontrolled diabetes.

4. *Insulin administration* (if appropriate), including types of insulin and syringes, rotation of sites of injection, injection techniques, and pump therapy instructions.

5. *Signs and symptoms of* HYPERGLYCEMIA *and* HYPOGLYCEMIA, and measures to take when they occur. (See accompanying table.) It is important for patients to become familiar with specific signs that are unique to themselves. Each person responds differently and may exhibit symptoms different from those experienced by others. It should be noted that the signs and symptoms may vary even within one individual. Thus it is vital that the person understand all reactions that could occur. When there is doubt, a simple blood glucose reading will determine the actions that should be taken.

6. *Oral antidiabetic agents,* including information about drug-drug interactions, proper administration, and potential side effects.

7. *Personal hygiene and activities of daily living,* including general skin care, foot care, treatment of minor injuries to avoid infection, a formal exercise program as well as exercise at school or at work, recreational activity, and travel.

8. *Identification tag and card* and needed medical information.

9. *Information on what to do on "sick days"* when nausea, vomiting, or respiratory infection can interfere with the usual meals and exercise.

10. *Importance of keeping appointments* and staying in touch with a health care provider for consultation and assessment. Periodic evaluation of the binding of glucose to hemoglobin (glycosylated HEMOGLOBIN or HEMOGLOBIN A1C testing) can give information about the effectiveness of the prescribed regimen and whether any changes need to be made. The ADA position statement on tests of glycemia in diabetes recommends routine testing for all patients with diabetes. It should be a part of the initial assessment of the patient, with subsequent measurements every three months to determine if the patient's metabolic control has been reached and maintained. See illustration.

 nephrogenic d. insipidus a rare form caused by failure of the renal tubules to reabsorb water; there is excessive production of antidiuretic hormone but the tubules fail to respond to it. Characteristics include polyuria, extreme thirst, growth retardation, and developmental delay. The condition does not respond to exogenous vasopressin. It may be inherited as an X-linked trait or be acquired as a result of drug therapy or systemic disease.

 pituitary d. insipidus central diabetes insipidus.

DiaBeta (di″ah-ba′tah) trademark for a preparation of GLYBURIDE, an oral HYPOGLYCE-MIC used for type 2 DIABETES MELLITUS.

diabetic (di″ah-bet′ik) 1. pertaining to or characterized by diabetes. 2. a person with diabetes.

diabetogenic (di″ah-bet″o-jen′ik) producing diabetes.

diabetogenous (di″ah-be-toj′ĕ-nus) caused by diabetes.

Diabinese (di-ab′ĭ-nēs) trademark for a preparation of CHLORPROPAMIDE, an oral hypoglycemic AGENT.

diabrotic (di″ah-brot′ik) 1. ulcerative; caustic. 2. a corrosive or escharotic substance.

diacetylmorphine (di″ah-se″til-mor′fēn) heroin.

diacrisis (di-ak′rĭ-sis) 1. diagnosis. 2. a change in the character of secretions during an illness. 3. a disease characterized by a morbid state of the secretions.

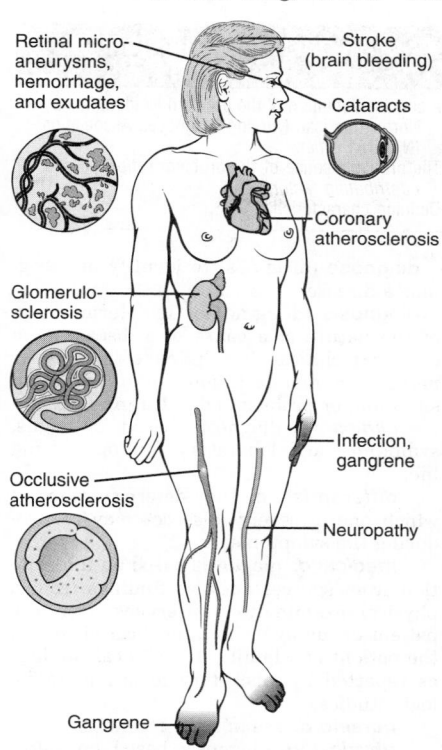

Complications of diabetes mellitus. From Damjanov, 2000.

diacritic (di″ah-krit′-ik) diagnostic; distinguishing.

diadochokinesia (di″ah-do″ko-kĭ-ne′zhah) the function of arresting one motor impulse and substituting one that is diametrically opposite, to permit sequential alternating movements, as pronation and supination of the arm.

Diagnex blue (di′ag-neks) trademark for a diagnostic agent for ACHLORHYDRIA; it is a means of GASTRIC ANALYSIS based on the fact that free HYDROCHLORIC ACID releases a dye (Azure A) from a resin base. Once the dye is released it is absorbed from the intestinal tract and excreted in the urine. If no hydrochloric acid is present in the stomach the dye will not appear in the urine. The test is valuable as a screening device to rule out achlorhydria and is much less disturbing than other methods of gastric analysis, which require the passage of a stomach tube. It does not, however, give conclusive evidence sufficient for diagnosis of cases in which there is no secretion of hydrochloric acid.

COMPONENTS OF THE NURSING DIAGNOSIS

A concise definition of the problem as identified by the North American Nursing Diagnoses Association (NANDA) (*title*)

The probable cause of the problem (*etiologic and contributing factors*)

Defining characteristics

---

diagnose (di'ag-nōs) to identify or recognize a disease.

diagnosis (di"ag-no'sis) 1. determination of the nature of a cause of a disease. 2. a concise technical description of the cause, nature, or manifestations of a condition, situation, or problem. adj., **diagnos'tic.**

   clinical d. diagnosis based on signs, symptoms, and laboratory findings during life.

   differential d. the determination of which one of several diseases may be producing the symptoms.

   medical d. diagnosis based on information from sources such as findings from a physical examination, interview with the patient or family or both, medical history of the patient and family, and clinical findings as reported by laboratory tests and radiologic studies.

   nursing d. see NURSING DIAGNOSIS.

   physical d. diagnosis based on information obtained by inspection, palpation, percussion, and auscultation.

   D.-Related Groups (DRG) a system of classification or grouping of patients according to medical diagnosis for purposes of paying hospitalization costs. In 1983, amendments to Social Security contained a prospective payment plan for most Medicare inpatient services in the United States. The payment plan was intended to control rising health care costs by paying a fixed amount per patient. The program of DRG reimbursement was based on the premise that similar medical diagnoses would generate similar costs for hospitalization. Therefore, all patients admitted for a surgical procedure such as hernia repair would be charged the same amount regardless of actual cost to the hospital. If a patient's hospital bill should total less than the amount paid by Medicare, the hospital is allowed to keep the difference. If, however, a patient's bill is more than that reimbursed by Medicare for a specific diagnosis, the hospital must absorb the difference in cost. See also appendix of Diagnosis-Related Groups.

diagnostician (di"ag-nos-tish'an) an expert in diagnosis.

Venn diagram. This depiction of the interactions of host, parasite, and environment provides a framework for understanding infectious processes. From Copstead, 1995.

diagnostics (di"ag-nos'tiks) the science and practice of diagnosis of disease.

diagram (di'ah-gram) a graphic representation, in simplest form, of an object or concept, made up of lines and lacking any pictorial content.

   Venn d. a diagram representing logical relationships using circles.

diakinesis (di"ah-kĭ-ne'sis) the stage of first meiotic prophase, in which the nucleolus and nuclear envelope disappear and the spindle fibers form.

dialysance (di-a'ĭ-sans) the minute rate of solute clearance through a membrane in dialysis.

dialysate (di-al'ĭ-sāt) 1. the fluid and solutes in a dialysis process that simply flow through the dialyzer and do not pass through the semipermeable membrane, being discarded along with removed toxic substances after they flow back out of the dialyzer. 2. diffusate (def. 2).

dialysis (di-al'ĭ-sis) [Gr.] 1. the diffusion of solute molecules through a semipermeable MEMBRANE, normally passing from the side of higher concentration to that of lower. A SEMIPERMEABLE membrane is one that allows the passage of certain smaller molecules of such crystalloids as GLUCOSE and UREA, but prevents passage of larger molecules such as the colloidal plasma PROTEINS and PROTOPLASM. adj., **dialyt'ic.** 2. hemodialysis.

   continuous ambulatory peritoneal d. (CAPD) peritoneal dialysis involving the continuous presence of dialysis solution in the peritoneal cavity; see discussion at PERITONEAL DIALYSIS.

   continuous cycling peritoneal d. (CCPD) a procedure similar to continuous ambulatory peritoneal dialysis but taking place at night, using a machine to make several fluid exchanges automatically. See discussion at PERITONEAL DIALYSIS.

d. dysequilibrium syndrome a condition occasionally seen following overly rapid HEMODIALYSIS, characterized by increased intracranial pressure that causes nausea, headache, vomiting, restlessness, and a decreased level of consciousness. The neurological complications may lead to coma and death if not treated. The cause of this syndrome is thought to be the rapid decrease in the blood UREA NITROGEN that accompanies dialysis. Called also dialysis dysequilibrium.

extracorporeal d. dialysis by a HEMODIALYZER; see also HEMODIALYSIS.

intermittent peritoneal d. (IPD) an older form of peritoneal dialysis in which dialysis solution is infused into the peritoneal cavity, allowed to equilibrate for 10 to 20 minutes, and then drained out. See discussion at PERITONEAL DIALYSIS.

kidney d. hemodialysis.

peritoneal d. see PERITONEAL DIALYSIS.

renal d. hemodialysis.

dialyzer (di′ah-līz″er) 1. an apparatus for performing DIALYSIS. 2. hemodialyzer.

diameter (di-am′ĕ-ter) the length of a straight line passing through the center of a circle and connecting opposite points on its circumference; hence the distance between the two specified opposite points on the periphery of a structure such as the cranium or pelvis.

cranial d's, craniometric d's imaginary lines connecting points on opposite surfaces of the cranium; the most important are biparietal, that joining the parietal eminences; bitemporal, that joining the extremities of the coronal suture; cervicobregmatic, that joining the center of the anterior fontanel and the junction of the neck with the floor of the mouth; frontomental, that joining the forehead and chin; occipitofrontal, that joining the external occipital protuberance and the most prominent midpoint of the frontal bone; occipitomental, that joining the external occipital protuberance and the most prominent midpoint of the chin; suboccipitobregmatic, that joining the lowest posterior point of the occiput and the center of the anterior fontanel.

pelvic d. see PELVIC DIAMETER.

diamniotic (di″am-ne-ot′ik) having or developing within separate amniotic cavities, as diamniotic twins.

Diamond-Blackfan syndrome (di′ah-mond blak′fan) congenital hypoplastic ANEMIA.

Diamox (di′ah-moks) trademark for preparations of ACETAZOLAMIDE, a carbonic anhydrase INHIBITOR used in treatment of

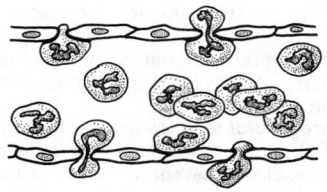

Diapedesis of leukocytes. From Dorland's, 2000.

glaucoma, epilepsy, mountain sickness, and other conditions.

diapedesis (di″ah-pĕ-de′sis) the outward passage of blood cells through intact vessel walls. See illustration.

diaphanography (di-af″ah-nog′rah-fe) TRANSILLUMINATION of the breast, with photography of the transilluminated light on infrared-sensitive film.

diaphanoscope (di″af′ah-nah-skōp) an instrument for TRANSILLUMINATION of a body cavity.

diaphanoscopy (di-af″ah-nos′kah-pe) transillumination.

diaphemetric (di″ah-fĕ-met′rik) pertaining to measurement of the sense of TOUCH.

diaphoresis (di″ah-fo-re′sis) SWEATING, especially of a profuse type.

diaphoretic (di″ah-fo-ret′ik) 1. pertaining to, characterized by, or promoting SWEATING. 2. an agent that promotes SWEATING; called also sudorific.

diaphragm (di′ah-fram) 1. the musculomembranous partition separating the thoracic and abdominal cavities. On its sides it is attached to the six lower ribs, at its front to the sternum, and at its back to the spine. The esophagus, aorta, vena cava, and numerous nerves pass through the diaphragm. When relaxed it is convex, but it flattens as it contracts during inhalation, thereby enlarging the chest cavity and allowing for expansion of the lungs. See also RESPIRATION. 2. any separating membrane or structure. 3. a disk with one or more openings or with an adjustable opening, mounted in relation to a lens or source of radiation, by which part of the light or radiation may be excluded from the area. 4. contraceptive diaphragm.

contraceptive d. a shallow dome-shaped disk used as a CONTRACEPTIVE, made of a soft plastic material such as latex. Its anterior lip fits behind the symphysis pubis and its posterior lip rests in the posterior fornix. It is used with a SPERMICIDE to prevent entrance of SPERMATOZOA into the cervical os. See also CONTRACEPTION.

pelvic d. the portion of the floor of the pelvis formed by the coccygeus muscles and the levator ani muscles, and their fascia.

polyarcuate d. one showing abnormal scalloping of margins on radiographic visualization.

urogenital d. a traditional but no longer valid concept that superior and inferior layers enclose the sphincter urethrae and deep transverse perineal muscles and together form a musculomembranous sheet that extends between the ischiopubic rami.

vaginal d. contraceptive diaphragm.

diaphragmatic (di″ah-frag-mat′ik) pertaining to a diaphragm.

d. hernia protrusion of some of the contents of the abdomen through an opening in the DIAPHRAGM and into the chest cavity. The condition may be congenital or acquired. *Congenital diaphragmatic hernia* in newborns is due to failure of the embryonic diaphragm to fuse. The opening in the diaphragm can be large enough to permit filling of the thoracic cavity with abdominal contents, thus interfering with normal expansion of the lungs. This produces respiratory distress, which is the outstanding feature of neonatal diaphragmatic hernia. HYPOXIA results from persistent fetal circulation that produces a right-to-left shunting via the foramen ovale and PATENT DUCTUS ARTERIOSUS. The severity of symptoms and age of onset depend on the extent of hypoplasia of the lungs and the degree of interference with ventilation. The condition constitutes a surgical emergency. Without immediate and successful intervention the neonate is likely to succumb to rapid and progressive respiratory failure.

At the moment of birth the neonate with this condition will show some degree of respiratory distress. The abdomen may appear sunken and the anterior-posterior chest diameter enlarged. Because the position of the heart can be shifted by the herniating organs, heart sounds are often heard on the side opposite the hernia, and bowel sounds may be heard in the chest cavity. A simple x-ray of the chest and abdomen will demonstrate loops of bowel in the chest, with the mediastinum shifted toward the contralateral side.

Surgical repair of the hernia and restoration of internal organs to their rightful place should be done as soon as possible. Before surgery the neonate is stabilized without delay. Nasogastric decompression is begun; intubation and assisted ventilation with supplemental oxygen may be necessary.

Postoperatively, the infant may remain extremely critical; at times extracorporeal membrane OXYGENATION will be necessary until the persistent fetal circulation resolves. It has been found that the survival rate for these neonates is greatly improved if they are cared for in an environment that is quiet, soothing, and as nonstressful as possible considering the intensive monitoring and care they must have.

Diaphragmatic hernia in the adult usually is a sliding type of hiatal HERNIA; that is, a part of the stomach slides upward into the thoracic cavity, following the normal path of the esophagus through an enlarged hiatal opening in the diaphragm. Causes include congenital weakness of the structures, trauma, relaxation of ligaments and skeletal muscles, or increased upward pressure from the abdomen. It is most often found in persons of middle age or older.

Small sliding hiatal hernias are found in the majority of persons undergoing an upper gastrointestinal series. Most are asymptomatic and do not require treatment. Those causing symptoms do so because of inflammation of the esophageal lining resulting from gastroesophageal REFLUX. Typically, the symptoms occur after a full meal and include HEARTBURN and indigestion. Large sliding hernias can cause intermittent abdominal and chest pain, difficult breathing, and cardiovascular symptoms. If the herniated portion of the stomach becomes incarcerated or is perforated, there is sudden sharp pain under the sternum and symptoms of obstruction. Although this rarely occurs, it is a surgical emergency.

The preferred treatment consists of small meals of bland, easily digested food, moderate exercise, and sleeping with the upper part of the body in a raised position. Surgical repair involves invasion of the abdominal and thoracic cavities and is reserved for severe cases that cannot be managed medically.

diaphragmatocele (di″ah-frag-mat′o-sēl) diaphragmatic hernia.

diaphragmitis (di″ah-frag-mi′tis) phrenitis.

diaphyseal (di″ah-fiz′e-al) pertaining to or affecting the shaft of a long bone (diaphysis).

diaphysectomy (di″ah-fī-zek′to-me) excision of part of a diaphysis.

diaphysial (di″ah-fiz′e-al) diaphyseal.

diaphysis (di-af′ĭ-sis), pl. *diaph′yses* [Gr.] 1. the portion of a long bone between the ends or extremities, which is usually articular, and wider than the shaft; it consists of a tube of compact bone, enclosing the medullary cavity. Called also shaft. 2. the portion of a bone formed from a primary center of ossification. See illustration.

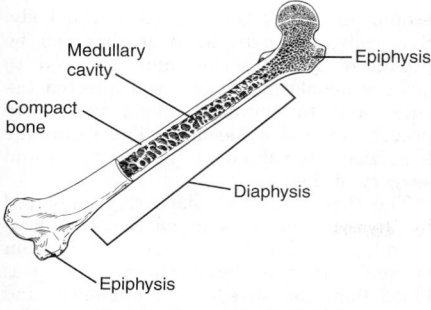

Diaphysis. From Dorland's, 2000.

Medullary cavity
Epiphysis
Compact bone
Diaphysis
Epiphysis

diapophysis (di″ah-pof′ĭ-sis) an upper transverse process of a vertebra.

diapyesis (di″ah-pi-e′sis) suppuration. adj., **diapyet′ic.**

diarrhea (di″ah-re′ah) rapid movement of fecal matter through the intestines resulting in poor absorption of water, nutritive elements, and electrolytes and producing abnormally frequent evacuation of watery stools. adj., **diarrhe′ic, diarrhe′al.**

Diarrhea is a NURSING DIAGNOSIS accepted by the North American Nursing Diagnosis Association, who defined it as "the state in which an individual experiences a change in normal bowel habits characterized by the frequent passage of loose, unformed stools." It can be caused by intestinal mucosal defects produced by infectious or chemical agents, toxins, which cause hypersecretion with no mucosal damage, osmotic agents, functional loss of intestinal segments, or emotional disorders which bring about increased peristalsis and increased secretion of mucus in the colon (psychogenic diarrhea or irritable colon); chronic recurrent diarrhea is a major symptom of CROHN'S DISEASE and of ULCERATIVE COLITIS. Concentrated tube feedings can cause diarrhea if adequate water is not given after each feeding.

In all types of diarrhea there is rapid evacuation of water and electrolytes resulting in a loss of these essential substances. Potassium supply especially is depleted by diarrhea, thus producing ACIDOSIS as well as deficient fluid VOLUME.

Symptoms. Diarrhea is accompanied by frequent and liquid bowel movements, abdominal cramps, and general weakness. The stools often contain mucus and may be blood streaked. In chronic diarrhea the patient is likely to be anemic and suffering from malnutrition.

Treatment. Mild cases of diarrhea of short duration can be treated conservatively with a bland diet, increased intake of liquids, and the administration of kaolin-pectin compounds to relieve the symptoms. Medicines are sometimes used to decrease peristalsis and relieve cramps. More severe and chronic cases can be symptomatic of a wide variety of disorders including glandular disturbances, deficiency diseases, allergies, and tumors of the intestinal tract. Since diarrhea is a symptom rather than a disease, extensive diagnostic procedures and laboratory tests may be necessary to determine the underlying cause. In the meantime symptomatic treatment must be instituted to relieve the dehydration, nutritional deficiencies, and disturbances of acid-base balance produced by the loss of water, food elements, and electrolytes in the stools. Liquids and semisolids may be given orally at frequent intervals if they can be tolerated. In cases in which vomiting accompanies the diarrhea or the stools occur with serious frequency, fluids may be given intravenously.

weanling d. a collection of diseases in the infant, described as a syndrome, associated with weaning from the breast. It is attributed to the introduction of other food and loss of the protective properties of breast milk.

diarrheogenic (di″ah-re″o-jen′ik) giving rise to diarrhea.

diarthric (di-ahr′thrik) pertaining to or affecting two different JOINTS; called also biarticular and diarticular.

diarthrodial (di″ahr-thro′de-al) of the nature of a diarthrosis.

diarthrosis (di″ahr-thro′sis), pl. *diarthro′-ses* [Gr.] synovial JOINT.

d. rotato′ria a joint characterized by mobility in a rotary direction.

diarticular (di″ahr-tik′u-lar) diarthric.

diascope (di′ah-skōp) a glass plate pressed against the skin to permit observation of changes produced in the underlying areas after the blood vessels are emptied and the skin is blanched.

diascopy (di-as′ko-pe) 1. examination by means of a diascope. 2. transillumination.

diastase (di′ah-stās) a combination of enzymes produced during germination of seeds, and contained in malt; it converts starch into maltose and then into glucose.

diastasis (di-as′tah-sis) 1. dislocation or separation of two normally attached bones between which there is no true joint. See illustration. 2. an abnormally large separation between associated bones, as between the ribs. 3. the rest period of the cardiac cycle, occurring just before systole. Called also diastasis cordis.

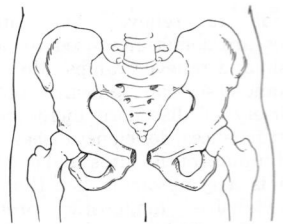

Diastasis of the pubic symphysis. From Dorland's, 2000.

d. rec'ti abdo'minis separation of the rectus muscles of the abdominal wall, sometimes occurring during pregnancy.

diastema (di″ah-ste′mah), pl. *diaste′mata* [Gr.] a space or cleft.

diastematocrania (di″ah-stem″ah-to-kra′ne-ah) congenital longitudinal fissure of the cranium.

diastematomyelia (di″ah-stem″ah-to-mi-e′le-ah) abnormal congenital division of the spinal cord by a bony spicule or fibrous band protruding from a vertebra or two, each of the halves being surrounded by a dural sac.

diastematopyelia (di″ah-stem″ah-to-pi-e′le-ah) congenital median fissure of the pelvis.

diastereoisomerism (di″ah-ster″e-o″i-som′er-izm) the relationship between two or more stereoisomers whose molecules are not mirror images of each other, for example, glucose and galactose or *cis* and *trans* isomers.

Diastix (di′ah-stiks) trademark for a reagent strip used for the semiquantitative determination of glucose in urine.

diastole (di-as′to-le) the phase of the cardiac CYCLE in which the heart relaxes between contractions; specifically, the period when the two ventricles are dilated by the blood flowing into them. See also BLOOD PRESSURE and HEART. adj., **diastol′ic.**

    electrical d. that time during which the cell rests; it is represented by phase 4 of the ACTION POTENTIAL.

diastrophic (di″ah-strahf″ik) bent or curved; said of structures, such as bones, deformed in such manner.

diataxia (di″ah-tak′se-ah) ataxia affecting both sides of the body.

diathermy (di′ah-ther″me) the use of high-frequency electromagnetic currents as a form of PHYSICAL THERAPY and in surgical procedures. The term diathermy is derived from the Greek words *dia* and *therma,* and literally means "heating through." adj., **diather′mal, diather′mic.**

Diathermy is used in physical therapy to deliver moderate heat directly to pathologic lesions in the deeper tissues of the body. Surgically, the extreme heat that can be produced by diathermy may be used to destroy neoplasms, warts, and infected tissues, and to cauterize blood vessels to prevent excessive bleeding. The technique is particularly valuable in neurosurgery and surgery of the eye.

The three forms of diathermy employed by physical therapists are short wave, ultrasound, and microwave. The application of moderate heat by diathermy increases blood flow and speeds up metabolism and the rate of ion diffusion across cellular membranes. The fibrous tissues in tendons, joint capsules, and scars are more easily stretched when subjected to heat, thus facilitating the relief of stiffness of joints and promoting relaxation of the muscles and decrease of muscle spasms.

Short wave diathermy machines utilize two condenser plates that are placed on either side of the body part to be treated. Another mode of application is by induction coils that are pliable and can be molded to fit the part of the body under treatment. As the high-frequency waves travel through the body tissues between the condensers or the coils, they are converted into heat. The degree of heat and depth of penetration depend in part on the absorptive and resistance properties of the tissues that the waves encounter.

The frequency allowed for short wave diathermy operations is under the control of the Federal Communications Commission. The frequencies assigned for short wave diathermy operations are 13.66, 27.33, and 40.98 megahertz. Most commercial machines operate at a frequency of 27.33 megahertz and a wavelength of 11 meters.

Short wave diathermy usually is prescribed for treatment of deep muscles and joints that are covered with a heavy soft-tissue mass, for example, the hip. In some instances short wave diathermy may be applied to localize deep inflammatory processes, as in pelvic inflammatory disease.

Ultrasound diathermy employs high-frequency acoustic vibrations which, when propelled through the tissues, are converted into heat. This type of diathermy is especially useful in the delivery of heat to selected musculatures and structures because there is a difference in the sensitivity of various fibers to the acoustic vibrations; some are more absorptive and some are more reflective. For example, in subcutaneous fat, relatively little energy is converted into heat, but in muscle tissues there is a much higher rate of conversion to heat.

The therapeutic ultrasound apparatus generates a high-frequency alternating current, which is then converted into acoustic vibrations. The apparatus is moved slowly across the surface of the part being treated. Ultrasound is a very effective agent for the application of heat, but it should be used only by a therapist who is fully aware of its potential hazards and the contraindications for its use.

Microwave diathermy uses radar waves, which are of higher frequency and shorter wavelength than radio waves. Most, if not all, of the therapeutic effects of microwave therapy are related to the conversion of energy into heat and its distribution throughout the body tissues. This mode of diathermy is considered to be the easiest to use, but the microwaves have a relatively poor depth of penetration.

Microwaves cannot be used in high dosage on edematous tissue, over wet dressings, or near metallic implants in the body because of the danger of local burns. Microwaves and short waves cannot be used on or near persons with implanted electronic cardiac pacemakers.

As with all forms of heat applications, care must be taken to avoid burns during diathermy treatments, especially to patients with decreased sensitivity to heat and cold.

surgical d. ELECTROCOAGULATION with an electrocautery of high frequency; often used for sealing blood vessels or stopping the bleeding of incised vessels.

diathesis (di-ath′ĕ-sis) an unusual constitutional susceptibility or predisposition to a particular disease. adj., **diathet′ic.**

diatomic (di″ah-tom′ik) 1. containing two atoms. 2. dibasic.

diatrizoate (di″ah-tri-zo′āt) the most commonly used water-soluble, iodinated, radiopaque x-ray contrast medium.

diaz(o)- the group —N═N—.

diazepam (di-az′ĕ-pam) a BENZODIAZEPINE used primarily as an ANTIANXIETY AGENT, and also used as a skeletal muscle RELAXANT, ANTICONVULSANT, antitremor agent, antipanic agent, as preoperative or preprocedural medication to relieve anxiety and tension, and in the management of alcohol withdrawal symptoms; administered orally, rectally, intravenously, or intramuscularly.

diaziquone (AZQ) (di-a′zĭ-kwŏn″) an ALKYLATING AGENT that acts by cross-linking DNA; used as an antineoplastic AGENT in treatment of primary brain tumors.

diazotize (di-az′o-tīz) to introduce the diazo group into a compound.

diazoxide (di″az-ok′sīd) a rapid-acting ANTIHYPERTENSIVE AGENT without diuretic activity; it has a longer duration of action than other rapid-acting antihypertensives, and is administered intravenously in treatment of malignant HYPERTENSION. It also inhibits INSULIN release and is therefore administered orally to treat HYPOGLYCEMIA due to HYPERINSULINISM.

dibasic (di-ba′sik) containing two replaceable hydrogen atoms, or furnishing two hydrogen ions.

dibenzazepine (di″ben-zaz′ĕ-pēn) any of a group of structurally related drugs including the tricyclic ANTIDEPRESSANTS CLOMIPRAMINE, DESIPRAMINE, IMIPRAMINE, and TRIMIPRAMINE.

dibenzodiazepine any of a class of structurally related heterocyclic drugs including the ANTIPSYCHOTIC AGENT clozapine.

dibenzoxazepine (di-benz″oks-az′ĕ-pēn) any of a class of structurally related heterocyclic drugs, including the ANTIPSYCHOTIC AGENT LOXAPINE and the ANTIDEPRESSANT AMOXAPINE.

dibenz(b,f)-1,4-oxazepine (di-benz″oks-az′ĕ-pēn) CR (def. 2).

Dibothriocephalus (di-both″re-o-sef′ah-lus) *Diphyllobothrium.*

dibucaine (di′bu-kān) a potent local ANESTHETIC applied rectally or topically to the anorectal region for treatment of hemorrhoids and other anorectal disorders, and topically to the skin in the treatment of minor skin disorders.

dicarboxylic acid (di-kahr-bok-sil′ik) any of various organic acids that contain two CARBOXYL groups, such as OXALIC ACID and TARTARIC ACID.

dicephalous (di-sef′ah-lus) having two heads.

dicephalus (di-sef′ah-lus) a malformed fetus with two heads; called also bicephalus and derodidymus.

dichloralphenazone (di-klor″al-fen′ah-zōn) a complex of CHLORAL HYDRATE and ANTIPYRINE (PHENAZONE), a SEDATIVE and HYPNOTIC used in combination with other agents for migraine and tension headache.

dichlorphenamide (di″klor-fen′ah-mīd) a carbonic anhydrase INHIBITOR used in the treatment of GLAUCOMA.

dichorial (di-kor′e-al) **dichorionic** (di-kor″e-on′ik) having two distinct chorions; said of dizygotic twins.

dichroism (di′kro-izm) the quality or condition of showing one color in reflected and another in transmitted light. adj., **dichro′ic.**

dichromacy (di-kro′mah-se) dichromatic VISION.

dichromate (di-kro′māt) a salt containing the bivalent Cr_2O_7 radical.

dichromatic (di″kro-mat′ik) 1. dichromic. 2. having dichromatic VISION.

dichromatism (di-kro′mah-tizm) 1. the quality of existing in or exhibiting two different colors. 2. dichromatic vision.

dichromic (di-kro′mik) having, or pertaining to, two colors.

diclofenac (di-klo′fen-ak) a NONSTEROIDAL ANTI-INFLAMMATORY DRUG used systemically as the potassium or sodium salt in the treatment of rheumatic and nonrheumatic inflammatory conditions, and as the potassium salt to relieve pain and dysmenorrhea; also applied topically to the conjunctiva as the sodium salt to reduce ocular inflammation or photophobia after certain kinds of surgery and to the skin to treat actinic KERATOSES.

dicloxacillin (di-kloks″ah-sil″in) a semisynthetic penicillinase-resistant PENICILLIN used as the sodium salt, primarily in the treatment of infections due to penicillinase-resistant staphylococci.

dicoelous (di-se′lus) 1. hollowed on each of two sides. 2. having two cavities.

Dicrocoelium (dik″ro-se′le-um) a genus of flukes. *D. dendri′ticum* is a liver fluke parasitic in domestic animals and occasionally humans.

dicrotism (di′kro-tizm) the occurrence of two sphygmographic waves or elevations to one beat of the pulse. adj., **dicrot′ic.**

dictyoma (dik″te-o′mah) diktyoma.

dicumarol (di-koo′mah-rol) a COUMARIN ANTICOAGULANT that acts by inhibiting the synthesis of vitamin K–dependent COAGULATION FACTORS (prothrombin and factors VII, IX, and X) and proteins C and S in the liver; used in the prevention and treatment of thromboembolic disorders.

dicyclomine (di-si′klo-mēn) an ANTICHOLINERGIC and ANTIMUSCARINIC with effects similar to those of ATROPINE; the hydrochloride salt is used as a gastrointestinal ANTISPASMODIC.

didactylism (di-dak′til-izm) the presence of only two digits on a hand or foot.

didanosine (di-dan′o-sēn) a nucleoside ANALOGUE ANTIRETROVIRAL agent used for the treatment of advanced human immunodeficiency VIRUS infection and ACQUIRED IMMUNODEFICIENCY SYNDROME; administered orally.

didelphia (di-del′fe-ah) uterus didelphys.

2′,3′-dideoxyadenosine (di″de-ok″se-ah-den′o-sēn) an ANTIRETROVIRAL agent whose base is adenine, used in treatment of human immunodeficiency VIRUS infection and AIDS.

dideoxycytidine (-si″ti-dēn) an ANTIRETROVIRAL agent whose base is cytosine; it acts by inhibiting reverse transcriptase and is used in treating human immunodeficiency VIRUS infection and AIDS.

dideoxyinosine (-in′o-sēn) didanosine.

dideoxynucleoside (-noo″kle-o-sīd) any of a group of synthetic nucleoside analogues, several of which are used as ANTIRETROVIRAL agents.

Didronel (di-dro′nel) trademark for preparations of ETIDRONATE disodium, a bone CALCIUM regulator.

didymitis (did″ĭ-mi′tis) inflammation of a testis.

didymous (did′ĭ-mus) occurring in pairs.

didymus (did′ĭ-mus) testis.

-didymus word element [Gr.], *fetus with duplication of parts; conjoined symmetrical twins.*

diecious (di-e′shus) sexually distinct; denoting species in which male and female genitals do not occur in the same individual. In botany, having staminate and pistillate flowers on separate plants.

dieldrin (di-el′drin) an effective, stable, but toxic chlorinated HYDROCARBON insecticide; it is prohibited in many states in the United States but is still used in some other countries.

dielectric (di″ə-lek′trik) 1. transmitting electric effects by INDUCTION, but not by CONDUCTION. The term is applied to an insulating substance through or across which electric force is acting or may act, by induction without conduction. 2. an insulating substance that transmits in this way, i.e., through or across which electric force is acting or may act, by induction without conduction.

diembryony (di-em′bre-on″e) the production of two embryos from a single zygote.

diencephalon (di″en-sef′ah-lon) 1. the posterior part of the PROSENCEPHALON, consisting of the hypothalamus, thalamus, metathalamus, and epithalamus; the subthalamus is often considered to be a distinct division. See also BRAINSTEM. 2. the posterior of the two brain vesicles formed by specialization of the prosencephalon in the developing embryo. See illustration.

dienestrol (di″en-es′trol) a synthetic ESTROGEN used in treatment of atrophic VAGINITIS and KRAUROSIS VULVAE.

Dientamoeba (di″ent-tah-me′bah) a genus of small highly active, usually nonpathogenic or mildly pathogenic ameboid protozoa parasitic in the large intestine of humans and certain monkeys. *D. fragilis* has been associated with human infection, which is manifested chiefly by diarrhea; abdominal pain; bloody, mucoid, or loose stools; and flatulence.

diet (di′et) 1. the customary amount and kind of food and drink taken by a

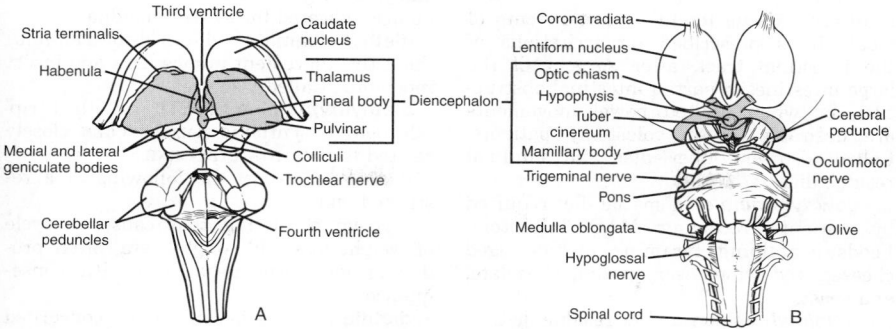

Diencephalon. Posterior (dorsal) *A* and anterior (inferior) *B* views of the base of the brain, showing the diencephalon in relation to the mesencephalon (midbrain) and rhombencephalon (hindbrain). From Dorland's, 2000.

person from day to day. 2. more narrowly, a regimen of food intake planned to meet specific requirements of the individual, including or excluding certain foods. See also NUTRITION.

acid-ash d. a special diet prescribed to increase the acidity of the urine so that alkaline salts will remain in solution. The diet may be given to aid in the elimination of fluid in certain kinds of edema, in the treatment of some types of urinary tract infection, and to inhibit the formation of alkaline urinary calculi. Meat, fish, eggs, and cereals are emphasized, with little fruit and vegetables and no milk or cheese.

alkali-ash d. a therapeutic diet prescribed to increase the alkalinity of the urine and dissolve uric acid and cystine urinary calculi. This type of diet changes the urinary pH so that certain salts are kept in solution and excreted in the urine. Emphasis is placed on fruits, vegetables, and milk. Meat, eggs, bread, and cereals are restricted.

bland d. one that is free from any irritating or stimulating foods.

DASH d. (Dietary Approach to Stop Hypertension) a diet high in fruits, vegetables, and low-fat dairy products; low in saturated and total fats; low in cholesterol; and high in fiber. Research studies support the hypothesis that this diet reduces BLOOD PRESSURE and may play a role in prevention of high blood pressure.

elemental d. one consisting of a well-balanced, residue-free mixture of all essential and nonessential amino acids combined with simple sugars, electrolytes, trace elements, and vitamins.

elimination d. one for diagnosis of food allergy, based on omission of foods that might cause symptoms in the patient.

Feingold d. a controversial diet for children with ATTENTION-DEFICIT/HYPERACTIVITY DISORDER, which excludes artificial colorings and flavorings, preservatives, and salicylates. The NATIONAL INSTITUTES OF HEALTH consensus statement, *Diagnosis and Treatment of Attention Deficit Hyperactivity Disorder,* notes that exclusion diets like this are an area warranting additional research.

gluten-free d. see GLUTEN-FREE DIET.

high calorie d. one that furnishes more calories than needed to maintain weight, often more than 3500–4000 calories per day.

high fat d. one that furnishes more than 35 per cent of its total calories from FATS; see also ketogenic diet.

high fiber d. one high in dietary fiber (typically more than 24 g daily), which decreases bowel transit time and relieves constipation.

high protein d. one containing large amounts of protein, consisting largely of meats, fish, milk, legumes, and nuts.

ketogenic d. one that produces ketones or acetones, or mild acidosis, such as one that is low in calories with insufficient carbohydrate and protein; it is occasionally used in the treatment of epilepsy. See also low fat diet.

liquid d. see LIQUID DIET.

low calorie d. one containing fewer calories than needed to maintain weight, e.g., less than 1200 calories per day for an adult.

low fat d. one containing limited amounts of fat.

low fiber d. low residue diet.

low purine d. one for mitigation of gout, omitting meat, fowl, and fish and substituting milk, eggs, cheese, and vegetable protein.

low residue d. one with a minimum of cellulose and fiber and restriction of connective tissue found in certain cuts of meat. It is prescribed for irritations of the intestinal tract, after surgery of the large intestine, in partial intestinal obstruction, or when limited bowel movements are desirable, as in colostomy patients. Called also low fiber diet and minimal residue diet.

low tyramine d. a special diet required by patients receiving MAO inhibitors. Foods containing tyramine include aged cheeses, red wine, beer, cream, chocolate, and yeast.

minimal residue d. low residue diet.

protein-sparing d. one consisting only of liquid protein or liquid mixtures of proteins, vitamins, and minerals, containing no more than 600 calories; it is designed to maintain a favorable nitrogen balance. Such diets have been used in weight loss programs, but are used only rarely now, usually only in inpatient settings.

purine-free d. low purine diet.

vegan d. the diet of a VEGAN; see also VEGANISM.

vegetarian d. see VEGETARIAN DIET.

dietary (di″ĕ-tar″e) 1. pertaining to diet. 2. a course or system of diet.

dietetic (di″ĕ-tet′ik) pertaining to diet or proper food.

dietetics (di″ĕ-tet′iks) the science of diet and nutrition.

diethylcarbamazine (di-eth″il-kahr-bam′-ah-zēn) an ANTIFILARIAL used as the citrate salt.

diethylenetriamine pentaacetic acid (DTPA) (di-eth″il-ēn-tri′ah-mēn pen″tah-ah-se′tik) pentetic acid.

diethylpropion (di-eth″il-pro′pe-on) a sympathomimetic amine used as an oral anorectic in the form of the hydrochloride salt.

diethylstilbestrol (DES) (di-eth″il-stil-bes′-trol) a synthetic nonsteroidal ESTROGEN used for palliative treatment of prostatic carcinoma and sometimes advanced breast carcinoma. It was formerly used to relieve vasomotor symptoms associated with menopause, and in primary ovarian failure, female HYPOGONADISM, atrophic VAGINITIS, KRAUROSIS VULVAE, and female CASTRATION. Most significantly, however, it was formerly widely used to prevent threatened abortion and premature labor. The female children who were thus exposed to the drug as fetuses have tended to have a variety of cervical abnormalities and an increased risk of clear cell ADENOCARCINOMA of the reproductive tract. Male offspring have sometimes had abnormal genitalia,

epididymal cysts, and abnormal semen analyses. Regular examinations and follow-up are indicated for these individuals.

diethyltoluamide (di-eth″il-tol-u′ah-mīd) the active ingredient in most tick and insect repellents. Called also deet.

diethyltryptamine (DET) (di-eth″il-trip′tah-mēn) a synthetic HALLUCINOGEN closely related to DIMETHYLTRYPTAMINE.

dieting (di′et-ing) the following of a restricted DIET.

_yo-yo d._ dieting that causes a cycle of weight loss and weight gain, often producing long-term negative health consequences.

dietitian (di″ĕ-tish′an) one concerned with the promotion of good health through proper diet and with the therapeutic use of diet in the treatment of disease. The dietitian may work in a variety of settings, including hospitals and other health care agencies, schools, hotels, and other commercial institutions where duties include both food service administration and therapeutic nutrition services, or may choose to enter the fields of education and research. Some dietitians practice independently either as consultants or private practitioners in the area of therapeutic dietetics. A bachelor's degree with a major in foods and nutrition or institutional management is the minimal educational requirement for a dietitian. Registration in the American Dietetic Association (ADA) requires satisfactory completion of either a one-year dietetic internship in a program approved by the Association, or three years' experience, two of which must have been served under the supervision of a member of the ADA. Additional education on the graduate level is necessary to qualify for positions in teaching, public health nutrition, and other specialty areas. The address of the American Dietetic Association is 216 W. Jackson Blvd., Chicago, IL 60606-6995.

Registered D. (RD) one meeting qualifications of the Commission on Dietetic Registration of the American Dietetic Association.

difenoxin (di″fĕ-nok′sin) an agent used as the hydrochloride salt for its ANTIPERISTALTIC action in treatment of DIARRHEA.

differential (dif″er-en′shal) 1. something that makes a distinction between two differing items. 2. the additional financial reward given to health care providers for working on a particular shift or in a particular unit. 3. in Canadian hospitals, the extra charge for a semiprivate or private room over the basic room rate subsidized by the provincial health plan.

differentiation (dif″er-en″she-a′shun) 1. the distinguishing of one thing from another. 2. the act or process of acquiring completely individual characteristics, such as occurs in the progressive diversification of cells and tissues in the embryo. 3. increase in morphological or chemical heterogeneity.

diffraction (dĭ-frak′shun) the bending or breaking up of a ray of light into its component parts.

diffusate (dĭ-fu′zāt) 1. material that has passed through a membrane. 2. specifically, the solutes that pass out of the blood into the dialysate fluid in a dialyzer; sometimes also referred to as the *dialysate.*

diffuse 1. (dĭ-fūs′) not definitely limited or localized. 2. (dĭ-fūz′) to pass through or to spread widely through a tissue or substance.

diffusing capacity (dĭ-fuz′ing) the rate at which a gas diffuses across the alveolocapillary MEMBRANE per unit difference in the partial pressure of the gas across the membrane, expressed in ml/min/mm Hg. Because of their high affinity for hemoglobin, both oxygen and carbon monoxide are limited in their rate of diffusion by their diffusing capacity. The diffusing capacity of the lung for these gases is symbolized by D_{LO_2} and D_{LCO}. The parameter usually measured is D_{LCO}. The normal value for the diffusing capacity of oxygen is 20 ml/min/mm Hg. If, during quiet breathing, the pressure difference of oxygen averages 11 mm Hg, a total of approximately 220 ml of oxygen diffuses through the respiratory membrane each minute. During strenuous exercise or other conditions that increase pulmonary activity, the diffusing capacity may increase to three times as much as that during rest. Pulmonary diseases that damage the respiratory membrane greatly interfere with the capacity of the oxygen to pass through the membrane and oxygenate the blood.

diffusion (dĭ-fu′zhun) 1. the state or process of being widely spread. 2. the spontaneous mixing of the molecules or ions of two or more substances resulting from random thermal motion; its rate is proportional to the concentrations of the substances and it increases with the temperature. In the body fluids the molecules of water, gases, and the ions of substances in solution are in constant motion. As each molecule moves about, it bounces off other molecules and loses some of its energy to each molecule it hits, but at the same time it gains energy from the molecules that collide with it.

The rate of diffusion is influenced by the size of the molecules; larger molecules move less rapidly, because they require more energy to move about. Molecules of a solution of higher concentration move more rapidly toward those of a solution of lesser concentration; in other words, *the rate of movement from higher to lower concentration is greater than the movement in the opposite direction.*

Other factors influencing the rate of diffusion from one substance to another are the size of the chamber in which the diffusion is taking place and the temperature within the chamber. *The rate of diffusion increases as the size of the chamber increases.* Molecular motion never ceases except at absolute zero; as the temperature increases so does the rate of motion of molecules. Thus, *the higher the temperature, the greater the molecular activity and, consequently, the greater the rate of diffusion.*

Many of the substances passing through the cell membrane are transported actively or passively by the process of diffusion. For certain hormones and other substances, there are TRANSPORT PROTEINS in the plasma membrane that bind to substances and transport them across the membrane; this type of transport is called *facilitated diffusion.* Without this constant motion of molecules there would be no exchange of nutrients and end products of cellular metabolism between the intracellular and extracellular fluid and the cell could not survive. The diffusion of water across cell membranes is called OSMOSIS.

The diffusion of gases through the respiratory membrane is essential to normal respiration. The rapidity and ease with which oxygen and carbon dioxide are diffused through the membrane are affected by the thickness of the membrane and its surface area, the diffusion coefficient of the gas in the water within the membrane, and the difference between the partial pressures of the gases in the alveoli and the blood.

The respiratory membrane is normally less than 1 micron in thickness, yet it is composed of three layers within the alveolus (surfactant and fluid layers and alveolar epithelium), an interstitial space between the alveolar epithelium and capillary membrane, and two layers in the capillary membrane. The thickness of the respiratory membrane can be affected by the presence of edematous fluid and by fibrotic changes in the membrane resulting from certain pulmonary diseases. An increase of fluid within the respiratory membrane and alveoli reduces the rate of diffusion because the gases must pass through the additional fluid as well as the other layers of the membrane. Thickening of the epithelial layers of the membrane, as in fibrosis, imposes additional restriction on the passage of gases.

The difference in the partial pressure of a gas in the alveoli and that same gas in the blood is a measure of the net tendency of that gas to pass through the respiratory membrane. The term partial pressure refers to the amount of pressure being exerted by a particular gas in a mixture of gases, the word *partial* referring to the part that is a particular gas in relation to the whole mixture. The partial pressure of oxygen, for example, reflects the number of oxygen molecules striking the surface of the membrane at any given point. The difference in the partial pressure refers to the difference in the amount of pressure being exerted by the oxygen molecules on the alveolar side of the membrane and the amount of pressure being exerted by the oxygen striking the same point from the opposite side. When the partial pressure of oxygen in the alveoli is greater than that of the oxygen in the blood, the oxygen molecules move across the membrane in the direction of the blood. The same is true in regard to carbon dioxide, which moves in the opposite direction when its partial pressure in the blood is greater than that in the alveoli. Partial pressures of oxygen and carbon dioxide are discussed in more detail under BLOOD GAS ANALYSIS. See illustration.

d. coefficient the number of milliliters of a gas that will diffuse at a distance of 0.001 mm over a square centimeter surface per minute, at 1 atm of pressure. The diffusion coefficient for any given gas is proportional to the solubility and molecular weight of the gas. The diffusion coefficient for oxygen is 1.0, for carbon dioxide it is 20.3, and for nitrogen it is 0.53. The diffusion capacity of a gas varies directly with the diffusion coefficient.

diflorasone (di-flor′ah-sōn) a synthetic CORTICOSTEROID used topically as the diacetate salt in the treatment of inflammation and pruritus in certain dermatoses.

diflucortolone (di-floo-kor′tah-lōn) a synthetic CORTICOSTEROID used as the valerate salt and applied topically in treatment of inflammation and pruritus of dermatoses.

diflunisal (di-floo′nĭ-sal) a SALICYLIC ACID derivative that, like ASPIRIN, has analgesic and antiinflammatory properties, although no antipyretic effects, but has fewer side effects than aspirin, does not affect bleeding time or function, and has a long half-life that permits twice daily dosage. It is used in the treatment of rheumatic and nonrheumatic inflammatory disorders, GOUT and CALCIUM PYROPHOSPHATE DEPOSITION DISEASE, dysmenorrhea, and vascular HEADACHES.

digastric (di-gas′trik) 1. having two bellies. 2. digastric muscle; see anatomic Table of Muscles in the Appendices.

digenetic (di-jĕ-net′ik) having two stages of multiplication, one sexual in the mature forms, the other asexual in the larval stages.

DiGeorge's syndrome (dĭ-jor′jez) a condition in which a child is born without a thymus gland, resulting in a complete absence of functional T cells. Normal B cell function is present.

digestant (di-jes′tant) 1. aiding or stimulating DIGESTION. 2. an agent that so acts.

digestion (dĭ-jes′chun) 1. the subjection of a substance to prolonged heat and moisture, so as to soften and disintegrate it. 2. the act or process of converting food into chemical substances that can be absorbed into the blood and utilized by the body tissue. See illustration. Digestion is accomplished by physically breaking down, churning, diluting, and dissolving the food substances, and also by splitting them chemically into simpler compounds. Carbohydrates are eventually broken down to monosaccharides

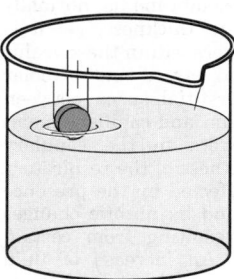 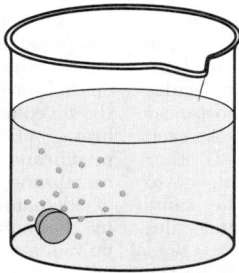 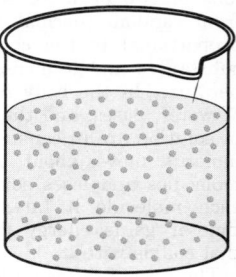

Simple diffusion. From Applegate, 2000.

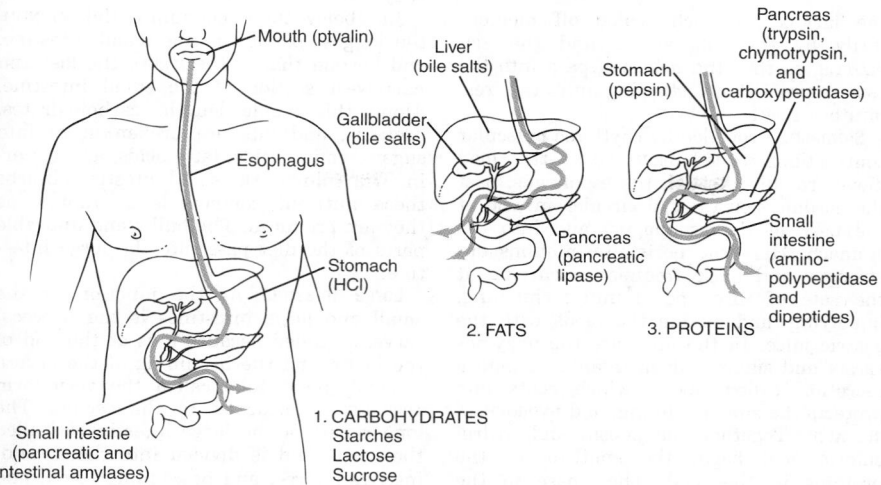

Digestion. 1. *Carbohydrates:* principally starches, lactose, and sucrose. Starches are acted on by the enzyme ptyalin (alpha-amylase) secreted in saliva, by hydrochloric acid (HCl) in the stomach, and by pancreatic amylase and intestinal amylase in the small intestine, which split the starches into maltose and isomaltose. These, in turn, are acted on by maltase and isomaltase and split into two molecules of glucose. Lactose is split by the enzyme lactase into a molecule of galactose and a molecule of glucose. The monosaccharides glucose, galactose, and fructose are absorbed from the small intestine into the blood. 2. *Fats:* emulsified by bile salts and agitation. The emulsified fats are acted upon by pancreatic and enteric lipase to form fatty acids, glycerol, and monoglycerides, which are absorbed through the intestinal walls. Small quantities of diglycerides and triglycerides are also absorbed. 3. *Proteins:* acted on chiefly in the stomach by pepsin, which splits proteins into proteoses, peptones, and polypeptides. In the small intestine they are acted on by the pancreatic enzymes trypsin, chymotrypsin, and carboxypeptidase to form polypeptides and amino acids. In the small intestine the peptidases complete the breakdown of the peptides into dipeptides and amino acids. Almost all proteins are eventually digested and absorbed either as amino acids or as dipeptides or tripeptides.

(simple sugars); proteins are broken down into amino acids; and fats are absorbed as fatty acids and glycerol (glycerin). The digestive process takes place in the alimentary canal or DIGESTIVE SYSTEM. The salivary glands, liver, gallbladder, and pancreas are located outside the alimentary canal, but they are considered accessory organs of digestion because their secretions provide essential enzymes.

 gastric d. digestion by the action of gastric juice.

 intestinal d. digestion by the action of intestinal juices.

 pancreatic d. digestion by the action of pancreatic juice.

 peptic d. gastric digestion.

 primary d. digestion occurring in the gastrointestinal tract.

 salivary d. the change of starch into maltose by the saliva.

 digestive (dĭ-jes′tiv) pertaining to digestion.

 d. system the organs that have as their particular function the ingestion, digestion, and absorption of food or nutritive elements. They include the MOUTH, TEETH, TONGUE, PHARYNX, ESOPHAGUS, STOMACH, and INTESTINES. The accessory organs of digestion, which contribute secretions important to digestion, include the SALIVARY GLANDS, PANCREAS, LIVER, and GALLBLADDER. (See also color plates.)

 Mouth. The mouth is the entrance to the alimentary canal; in it the teeth, tongue, and jaws begin the process of digestion by MASTICATION. SALIVA is secreted into the mouth by three separate pairs of glands (the SALIVARY GLANDS) located under the tongue, inside the lower jaw, and in the cheek. Saliva softens and lubricates the food, and dissolves some of it; it also contains an enzyme called PTYALIN that begins the conversion of starches into sugar. Saliva also moistens the inside of the mouth, the tongue, and the teeth, and rinses them after the food has departed on the next stage of its journey. Four passageways meet at the back of the throat: the oral and nasal passages, the LARYNX, and the ESOPHAGUS. In the act of SWALLOWING, the entrances to the nasal passages and the larynx are each sealed off momentarily by the soft PALATE and the EPIGLOTTIS, so that the food can pass into the ESOPHAGUS without straying into the respiratory TRACT.

Stomach. Propelled by rhythmic muscular contractions called PERISTALSIS, the food moves rapidly through the esophagus, past the cardiac SPHINCTER (a circular muscle at the base of the esophagus) and into the stomach. Here the peristaltic motions are stronger and more frequent, occurring at the rate of three per minute, churning, liquefying, and mixing the foods with the gastric juice. In the juice are the enzymes PEPSIN and LIPASE and, in infants, RENNIN; a secretion called MUCIN, which coats and protects the stomach lining; and HYDROCHLORIC ACID. Together the pepsin and hydrochloric acid begin the splitting of the proteins in the food. The lipase in the stomach is a rather weak fat-splitting enzyme, able to act only on fats that are already emulsified, such as those in cream and the yolk of egg; the intestine has a stronger lipase, and it is there that most fats are digested. The average adult stomach holds about 1.5 liters. The stomach reaches its peak of digestive activity nearly 2 hours after a meal and may empty in 3 to $4\frac{1}{2}$ hours; a heavy meal may take as long as 6 hours to pass into the small intestine.

Small Intestine. The food leaves the stomach in the form of CHYME, a thick, liquid mixture. It passes through the PYLORUS, a sphincter muscle opening from the lower part of the stomach into the duodenum. This sphincter is closed most of the time, opening each time a peristaltic wave passes over it. The stomach is much wider than the rest of the canal and also has a J-shaped curve at its bottom, so that the passage of food through the pylorus is automatically slowed until the food is of the right consistency to flow through the narrow opening into the intestine. The small intestine is about 6 meters (20 feet) long. The lining of the small intestine has deep folds and fingerlike projections called VILLI that give it a surface of about 9 square meters (100 square feet) through which absorption of food can take place.

The DUODENUM, a C-shaped curve with a length of about 25 cm (10 in), is the first and widest part of the small intestine. Into it flows the pancreatic juice, with enzymes that break down starch, protein, and fats. The common bile duct also empties into the duodenum. The bile emulsifies fats for the action of the fat-splitting enzymes.

Just below the duodenum is the JEJUNUM, the longest portion of the small intestine, and beyond that is the ILEUM, the last and narrowest section of the small intestine. Along this whole length, carbohydrates, proteins, and fats are broken down into sugars, amino acids, fatty acids, and glycerin. The lining of the small intestine absorbs these nutrient compounds as rapidly as they are produced. The bulky and unusable parts of the diet pass into the large intestine.

Large Intestine. At the junction of the small and large intestines is the ileocecal VALVE, so called because it is at the end of the ileum and the beginning of the CECUM. A small blind tube called the vermiform APPENDIX is attached to the cecum. The longer part of the large intestine is called the COLON and is divided into the ascending, transverse, and descending colon, and the sigmoid flexure, an S-shaped bend at the distal end of the colon. The sigmoid colon empties into the RECTUM. Along the 1.7 meters (5.5 feet) or so of the large intestine, the liquid in the waste is gradually reabsorbed through the intestinal walls. Thus the waste is formed into fairly solid feces and pushed down into the rectum for eventual evacuation. This takes from 10 to 20 hours. The evacuation consists of bacteria, cells cast off from the intestines, some mucus, and such indigestible substances as cellulose. The normal dark brown color of the FECES is caused by bile pigments.

Digibind (dij′ĭ-bīnd) trademark for a preparation of digoxin immune FAB (ovine), an antidote for DIGOXIN or DIGITOXIN overdose.

digit (dij′it) a FINGER or TOE.

digital (dij′ĭ-t′l) 1. pertaining to a finger or toe. 2. pertaining to an electronic system in which information is carried by a discontinuous signal that changes in frequency, amplitude, or polarity and has a finite number of levels, rather than a continuous range as in an ANALOG device.

Digitalis (dij″ĭ-tal′is) a genus of herbs. *D. lana′ta* yields digoxin and lanatoside and *D. purpu′rea,* the purple foxglove, has leaves that are a source of digitalis.

digitalis (dij″ĭ-tal′is) dried leaf of *Digitalis purpurea;* a cardiac GLYCOSIDE. All drugs prepared from this digitalis leaf are members of the same group and principles of administration are the same, although they vary according to speed of action and potency. Digitalis in its many forms is one of the most frequently prescribed drugs in the United States. It can be very effective in treatment of cardiac conditions, but its therapeutic range is narrow; a therapeutic dose is only about one third less than the dose that will induce toxicity. Moreover, physiologic changes due to age, electrolyte disturbances, renal impairment, metabolic disorders, and certain heart conditions can predispose a patient to digitalis toxicity. Other drugs can also alter the effects of digitalis and lead to toxicity.

Signs of Toxicity. Traditionally, nurses have been taught to count the patient's pulse or monitor the apical heartbeat for rate and rhythm before administering a digitalis preparation. A decreased pulse rate of 60 per minute or less is an indication that the drug should be temporarily discontinued. While this is the most typical sign of digitalis intoxication, there frequently are earlier symptoms that deserve attention. Some of the more common complaints expressed by patients who are in the early stages of toxicity are nausea, blurred vision, mental depression, disorientation, and malaise. Objective signs include vomiting, diarrhea, and confusion.

Drug Interactions. Unfortunately, most patients who take digitalis also have other drugs prescribed for the management of their illness. The risk of drug interactions and digitalis toxicity increases in proportion to the number of drugs being taken concurrently. One of the most common interactions is with a thiazide DIURETIC, which can enhance the effect of digitalis and can also lower potassium levels in the blood. Potassium decreases the likelihood of digitalis toxicity and so it is essential that hypokalemia be avoided. Since many patients who take digitalis are on restricted caloric and fluid intake, they cannot adequately replace lost potassium by eating enough potassium-rich foods and need a potassium supplement.

Patient Education. There is a danger of complacency about this drug because it is so familiar and so frequently prescribed for self-medication. Without unduly alarming the patient, it is imperative that the action of the drug and its potential for harm if it is not taken as prescribed and with caution are explained. The patient must be informed about the interactions of digitalis with over-the-counter drugs such as antacids and cold remedies that contain ephedrine. The patient should know the signs and symptoms of digitalis toxicity and appreciate the importance of notifying the primary health care provider should any of these signs appear. If the patient does not know how to check the pulse for rate

and rhythm, he or she will need to learn how and to learn why it is important to stop taking the drug and notify the physician should the pulse rate fall outside the normal range. There is so much that needs to be known in order to avoid the problems of toxicity inherent in the particular digitalis preparation that it is probably unrealistic to expect patients to remember all that they are told about taking the medication safely. Therefore it is best to give the patient the information in written form and go over the instructions with the patient and a member of the family in order to be sure that the instructions are understood.

digitalization (dij″ĭ-tal-ĭ-za′shun) the administration of digitalis in a dosage schedule designed to produce and then maintain optimal therapeutic concentrations of its cardiotonic glycosides.

digitation (dij″ĭ-ta′shun) 1. a fingerlike process. 2. surgical creation of a functioning digit by making a cleft between two adjacent metacarpal bones, after amputation of some or all of the fingers.

digitiform (dij′ĭ-tĭ-form″) fingerlike.

digitoxin (dij′ĭ-tok′sin) a cardiotonic GLYCOSIDE obtained from *Digitalis purpurea* and other species of the same genus; used in the treatment of congestive HEART FAILURE. It has a slowly developing action and slow elimination. Parenteral solutions should be diluted when given intravenously.

digitus (dij′ĭ-tus), pl. *di′giti* [L.] digit.

diglossia (di-glos′e-ah) bifid tongue.

diglyceride (di-glis′er-īd) a glyceride containing two fatty acid molecules in ester linkage.

dignathus (dig-na′thus) a malformed fetus with two lower jaws.

digoxin (dĭ-jok′sin) a cardiotonic GLYCOSIDE obtained from the leaves of *Digitalis lanata;* used in the treatment of congestive HEART FAILURE. It has a relatively rapid action and rapid elimination.

d. immune Fab (ovine) see under *Fab.*

dihydrocodeine (di-hi″dro-ko′dēn) a synthetic opioid ANALGESIC and ANTITUSSIVE.

dihydroergotamine (di-hi″dro-er-got′ah-mēn) hydrogenated ERGOTAMINE, an ALPHA-ADRENERGIC BLOCKING AGENT and VASOCONSTRICTOR used as ERGOTAMINE mesylate in treatment of MIGRAINE; administered intramuscularly, subcutaneously, intravenously, or intranasally.

dihydroindolone (di-hi″dro-in′do-lōn) any of a class of structurally related ANTIPSYCHOTIC AGENTS; the prototype is MOLINDONE.

dihydrotachysterol (di-hi″dro-tah-kis′ter-ol) an analogue of ERGOSTEROL, used as a calcium regulator in the management of HYPOCALCEMIA in conditions such as RICKETS, OSTEODYSTROPHY, HYPOPARATHYROIDISM, hypocalcemic TETANY, and complications of renal DIALYSIS; administered orally.

dihydrotestosterone (DHT) (di-hi″dro-testos′tē-rōn) an androgenic hormone formed in peripheral tissue from testosterone; thought to be the androgen responsible for development of the male primary sex CHARACTERS during embryogenesis and of male secondary sex CHARACTERS at puberty, and for adult male sexual function.

dihydroxyaluminum (di″hi-drok″se-ah-loo′mĭ-num) an aluminum compound having two hydroxyl groups in a molecule; available as dihydroxyaluminum aminoacetate and dihydroxyaluminum sodium carbonate, which are used as antacids.

dihydroxycholecalciferol (di″hi-drok″se-ko″le-kal-sif′er-ol) a group of active metabolites of CHOLECALCIFEROL (vitamin D₃), numbered according to the carbon atom(s) on which a hydroxyl group is substituted. 1,25-Dihydroxycholecalciferol (CALCITRIOL) is the most active derivative; it increases intestinal absorption of calcium and phosphate, enhances bone resorption, and prevents rickets, and, because of these activities at sites distant from the site of its synthesis, is considered to be a hormone.

diktyoma (dik″te-o′mah) a tumor of the ciliary epithelium resembling embryonic retinal tissue in structure.

dilaceration (di-las″er-a′shun) a tearing apart, as of a cataract. In dentistry, an abnormal angulation or curve in the root or crown of a formed tooth.

Dilantin (di-lan″tin) trademark for preparations of PHENYTOIN, an ANTICONVULSANT used in the treatment of EPILEPSY.

dilatation (dil″ah-ta′shun) 1. the condition, as of an orifice or tubular structure, of being dilated or stretched beyond normal dimensions by medications or instrumentation. 2. the act of dilating or stretching.

 d. of the heart compensatory enlargement of the cavities of the heart, with thinning of the walls.

dilate (di′lāt) to stretch an opening or hollow structure beyond its normal dimensions.

dilation (di-la′shun) 1. the act of dilating or stretching. 2. dilatation. 3. an increase in the diameter of a circular structure, such as the pupil.

 d. and curettage D and C; expanding of the ostium uteri to permit scraping of the walls of the uterus. See also ABORTION.

dilator (di-la′ter) a structure (muscle) that dilates, or an instrument used to dilate.

Dilaudid (di-law″did) trademark for preparations of HYDROMORPHONE, a opioid ANALGESIC.

dilemma (dĭ-lem′ah) any difficult or perplexing situation or problem; in bioethics, a situation requiring a choice between equally undesirable alternatives.

diltiazem (dil-ti′ah-zem) a CALCIUM CHANNEL BLOCKING AGENT that acts as a vasodilator; used as the hydrochloride salt in treatment of ANGINA PECTORIS, HYPERTENSION, and supraventricular TACHYCARDIA

diluent (dil′u-ent) 1. diluting or rendering less potent or irritant. 2. an agent that so acts.

dilute (di-loot′) to make a mixture or solution less concentrated by adding a fluid.

dilution (di-loo′shun) 1. reduction of concentration of an active substance by admixture of a neutral agent. 2. a substance that has undergone such a process.

 serial d. a set of dilutions in a mathematical sequence. In microbiological technique, serial dilutions are used to obtain a culture plate that yields a countable number of separate colonies. From this, a calculation of viable cells in the original suspension can be made, as a colony picked for pure culture.

dimenhydrinate (di″men-hi′drĭ-nāt) an antihistamine used as an antinauseant, antiemetic, and antivertigo agent, especially in prevention and treatment of MOTION SICKNESS, but also in other conditions in which nausea or vertigo may be a feature, administered orally, rectally, or by intramuscular or intravenous injection.

dimensionless (dĭ-men′shun-les) denoting a numerical constant or variable that has no units of measurement.

dimer 1. a compound formed by combination of two identical simpler molecules. 2. a capsomer having two structural subunits.

 D-d. a fragment of FIBRIN that is formed as a result of fibrin degradation. A positive test for its presence in the blood is suggestive of conditions such as thrombotic disease, sickle cell crisis, malignancy, disseminated intravascular coagulation, or recent surgery.

dimercaprol (di″mer-kap′rol) a colorless, liquid chelating agent used in the treatment of heavy METAL POISONING; it forms a relatively stable compound with arsenic, mercury, gold, and certain other metals, thus protecting the vital enzyme systems of the cells against the effects of the metals. It is sometimes diluted with water and used to wash the stomach, with some of the solution being left in the stomach. Side effects include tachycardia, hypertension, nausea and vomiting, severe headaches, and a sense of constriction of the chest; barbiturates are usually ordered to relieve the symptoms, which should subside within an hour. Dimercaprol has a disagreeable skunklike odor and should be handled carefully to avoid spilling. Called also British antilewisite.

Dimetane (di'mĕ-tān) trademark for preparations containing BROMPHENIRAMINE, an ANTIHISTAMINE.

dimethicone (di-meth'ĭ-kōn) a silicone oil used as a skin protectant; available as an ointment, spray, and cream. See also SIMETHICONE.

dimethisoquin (di″mĕ-thi'so-kwin) a local anesthetic; used topically to relieve pain, itching, and burning of the skin.

dimethyl sulfoxide (di-meth'il sul-fok'sīd) DMSO.

dimethyltryptamine (DMT) (di-meth″il-trip'tah-mēn) a hallucinogenic substance derived from the plant *Prestonia amazonica*.

dimorphism (di-mor'fizm) 1. the quality of existing in two distinct forms. adj., **dimor'phic, dimor'phous.**

sexual d. physical or behavioral differences associated with sex. 1. having some properties of both sexes, as in the early embryo and in some hermaphrodites.

Dinoflagellida (di″no-flah-jel'ĭ-dah) an order of minute, plantlike, chiefly marine protozoa. They may be present in sea water in vast numbers, causing a discoloration known as red tide or red water, which may result in the death of various marine animals and fish by exhaustion of their oxygen supply. Some species secrete a powerful neurotoxin that can cause a severe toxic reaction in humans who ingest shellfish that feed on the toxin-producing organisms.

dinoprost (di'no-prost) name given to PROSTAGLANDIN $F_{2\alpha}$ when used as a pharmaceutical; used as an OXYTOCIC for induction of abortion, to evacuate the uterus in the management of missed abortion, and in the treatment of hydatidiform mole. Available as the tromethamine salt.

dinoprostone (di″no-prōst'ōn) name given to PROSTAGLANDIN E_2 when used pharmaceutically; used as an OXYTOCIC for induction of ABORTION or of LABOR, to evacuate the uterus in the management of missed abortion, to aid ripening of the cervix prior to the induction of labor, and in the treatment of hydatidiform MOLE; administered intravaginally or intracervically.

dioctyl calcium sulfosuccinate (di-ok'til kal'se-um sul″fo-suk'sī-nāt) docusate calcium.

dioctyl sodium sulfosuccinate (di-ok'til so-de-um sul″fo-suk'sī-nāt) docusate sodium.

diopter (di-op'ter) a unit of refractive power of lenses: the reciprocal of the focal length in meters is the refractive power in diopters. Symbol D.

dioptometry (di″op-tom'ĕ-tre) the measurement of ocular accommodation and refraction.

dioptric (di-op'trik) pertaining to refraction or to transmitted and refracted light; refracting.

dioptrics (di-op'triks) the science of refracted light.

dioxin (di-ok'sin) a highly toxic and teratogenic chlorinated HYDROCARBON that is a trace contaminant in the HERBICIDES 2,4,5-T and AGENT ORANGE.

dioxybenzone (di-oks″ĭ-ben'zōn) a topical SUNSCREEN.

diperodon (di-per'o-don) a local ANESTHETIC used as the hydrochloride salt; applied to the skin for abrasions, irritations, and pruritus and intrarectally for relief of pain from HEMORRHOIDS.

Dipetalonema (di-pet″ah-lo-ne'mah) a genus of nematode parasites of the superfamily Filarioidea, including *D. per'stans* and *D. streptocer'ca*, species primarily parasitic in man, other primates serving as reservoir hosts.

diphallus (di-fal'us) a developmental anomaly characterized by partial or complete duplication of the penis; called also double penis.

diphemanil (di-fe'mah-nil) an ANTICHOLINERGIC and ANTIMUSCARINIC with effects similar to those of ATROPINE; used in the form of the methylsulfate salt to inhibit gastric mobility and secretion, relieve pylorospasm, control sweating, and relieve pruritus. Toxic symptoms are rare and include dry mouth, mydriasis, and fever. The drug is contraindicated in patients with glaucoma.

diphenhydramine (di″fen-hi'drah-mēn) an ANTIHISTAMINE with ANTICHOLINERGIC effects; the hydrochloride salt is used for relief of allergic symptoms, for treatment of ANAPHYLAXIS, PARKINSONISM, and MOTION SICKNESS or other causes of nausea, vomiting, or vertigo, and as an ANTITUSSIVE; administered orally, intramuscularly, or intravenously. The hydrochloride and citrate salts are used as SEDATIVES and HYPNOTICS and as ingredients in cough and cold preparations; administered orally.

diphenidol (di-fen'ĭ-dol) an ANTIEMETIC, used as the base or as the hydrochloride or pamoate salt in treatment of vertigo and to control nausea and vomiting.

diphenoxylate (di″fen-ok′sĭ-lāt) an agent derived from MEPERIDINE, used as the hydrochloride salt for its ANTIPERISTALTIC action in management of diarrhea.

diphenyl (di-fen′il) a colorless toxic compound used as a fungistat in containers for shipping citrus fruits; called also biphenyl.

diphenylbutylpiperidine (di-fen″il-bu″til-pi-per′ĭ-dēn) any of a class of structurally related, heterocyclic ANTIPSYCHOTIC AGENTS that includes PIMOZIDES.

diphenylhydantoin (di-fen″il-hi-dan′to-in) phenytoin.

diphonia (di-fo′ne-ah) the production of two different voice tones in speaking.

diphosphonate (di-fos′fo-nāt) any of a group of related phosphorus-containing compounds that are structurally similar to PYROPHOSPHATE but have enhanced stability to enzymatic and chemical hydrolysis and have affinity for sites of osteoid mineralization. They are used as sodium salts to inhibit bone resorption as well as complexed with technetium Tc 99m for bone imaging. The group includes ALENDRONATE, ETIDRONATE, and PAMIDRONATE. Called also bisphosphonate.

diphtheria (dif-thēr′e-ah) an acute, highly contagious childhood disease that generally affects the membranes of the throat and, less frequently, the nose; in rare instances it can affect other parts of the body, notably the skin, following an open wound. Caused by the bacillus *Corynebacterium diphtheriae,* it can be fatal if not treated promptly. However, repeated exposure to the causative organisms may provide a natural immunity. adj., **diphthe′rial, diphther′ic, diphtherit′ic.**

Diphtheria spreads in droplets of moisture from the mouth, nose, or throat of an infected person. It may also be spread by handkerchiefs, towels, eating utensils, or any other object used by an infected person or sprayed by his coughing or sneezing. It may also be transmitted by a healthy person who is nevertheless a carrier of the disease or by someone who is convalescing from diphtheria. The incubation period of the disease is generally between 2 and 5 days, sometimes longer. An infected person may continue to have the bacilli in his throat from 2 to 4 weeks after he has recovered from its effects.

Symptoms. The first symptoms of diphtheria usually include sore throat, fever, headache, and nausea. Patches of grayish or dirty-yellowish membrane form in the throat, and gradually grow into one membrane. This membrane, combined with swelling of the throat, may interfere with swallowing or breathing. In severe cases, when other measures fail, a tracheostomy may be necessary to restore breathing. The diphtheria bacillus also produces a toxin that spreads throughout the body and may damage the heart and nerves permanently. Diagnosis of the disease can be verified by identifying the causative organisms from throat cultures. Susceptibility to diphtheria is determined by the Schick test. A positive skin test indicates the absence of circulating antibodies to the diphtheria toxin, but a pseudoreaction can also occur.

Treatment. Diphtheria antitoxin is administered to counteract the toxic reaction from the bacillus. Prognosis depends on the severity of the infection and especially on how soon the antitoxin is given. Rest, antibiotics, and general hygienic measures are used to combat the infection. Oxygen is administered as necessary to relieve dyspnea and cyanosis. Cardiac complications are usually more severe in adults; thus the convalescent period is extended for these patients.

Prevention. Immunization should be begun between the sixth and eighth weeks of an infant's life. Diphtheria and tetanus toxoids and pertussis VACCINE (DTaP) is the preferred vaccine for all doses in the vaccination series. Booster doses are also needed later in life. (See also table under IMMUNIZATION.)

Once one of the most fatal diseases of childhood, cases of diphtheria and death from the disease have become almost nonexistent in countries where mass immunization has been practiced.

diphtheroid (dif′thĕ-roid) 1. resembling diphtheria or the diphtheria bacillus. 2. pseudodiphtheria.

diphthongia (dif-thon′je-ah) the production of double vocal sounds.

diphyllobothriasis (di-fil″o-both-ri′ah-sis) infection with *Diphyllobothrium.*

Diphyllobothrium (di-fil″o-both′re-um) a genus of large tapeworms. *D. la′tum* is the broad or fish tapeworm, an intestinal parasite of humans, dogs, cats, and other fish-eating mammals.

diphyodont (dif′e-o-dont″) having two dentitions, a primary and a permanent one.

dipivefrin (di-piv′ah-frin) an ester converted in the eye to EPINEPHRINE, lowering intraocular pressure by decreasing the production and increasing the outflow of aqueous humor; the hydrochloride salt is applied topically to the conjunctiva in treatment of open-angle or secondary GLAUCOMA.

diplacusis (dip″lah-koo′sis) the perception of a single auditory stimulus differently in one ear from in the other, so that two different sounds are heard.

diplegia (di-ple′jah) paralysis of like parts on either side of the body. adj., **diple′gic.**

diplobacillus (dip″lo-bah-sil′us), pl. *diplobacil′li* A short, rod-shaped organism occurring in pairs, joined end-to-end; diplobacterium.

diplobacterium (dip″lo-bak-tĕr′e-um) diplobacillus.

diploblastic (dip″lo-blas′tik) having two germ layers.

Diplococcus (dip″lo-kok′us) former name for a genus of bacteria of the tribe Streptococceae. *D. pneumo′niae* is now called *Streptococcus pneumoniae.*

diplococcus (dip″lo-kok′us), pl. *diplococ′ci* 1. any of the spherical, lance-shaped, or coffee bean–shaped bacteria occurring usually in pairs as a result of incomplete separation after cell division in a single plane. 2. any organism of the genus *Diplococcus.*

diploë (dip′lo-e) the spongy layer between the inner and outer compact layers of the flat bones of the skull. adj., **diploet′ic, diplo′ic.**

diplogenesis (dip″lo-jen′ĕ-sis) the production of a fetus that is double in part or almost completely.

diploid (dip′loid) 1. having a pair of each chromosome characteristic of a species (2n or, in man, 46). 2. a diploid individual or cell.

diploidy (dip′loi-de) the state of being diploid.

diplomyelia (dip″lo-mi-e′le-ah) lengthwise fissure and seeming doubleness of the spinal cord.

diplopia (dĭ-plo′pe-ah) the perception of two images of a single object; called also double vision.

> **binocular d.** double vision in which the images of an object are formed on noncorresponding points of the retinas.

> **crossed d.** horizontal diplopia in which the image belonging to the right eye is displaced to the left of the image belonging to the left eye (divergent strabismus).

> **direct d.** horizontal diplopia in which the image belonging to the right eye appears to the right of the image belonging to the left eye (convergent strabismus).

> **horizontal d.** diplopia in which the two images lie in the same horizontal plane, being either direct or crossed.

> **vertical d.** diplopia in which one image appears above the other in the same vertical plane.

diplosomatia (dip″lo-so-ma′shah) a condition in which complete twins are joined at some of their body parts.

diplosomia (dip″lo-so′me-ah) diplosomatia.

diplotene (dip′lo-tēn) the stage of the first meiotic prophase, following the pachytene, in which the two chromosomes in each bivalent begin to repel one another and a split occurs between the chromosomes.

dipole (di′pōl) 1. a molecule having separated charges of equal and opposite sign. 2. a pair of electric charges or magnetic poles separated by a short distance.

diprosopus (di-pros′o-pus) a malformed fetus with any degree of duplication of the face.

dipsogen (dip′sah-jen) an agent or measure that induces thirst and promotes ingestion of fluids. adj., **dipsogen′ic.**

dipsotherapy (dip″so-ther′ah-pe) the therapeutic limitation of the amounts of fluids ingested.

-dipsia word element [Gr.], thirst.

Diptera (dip′ter-ah) an order of insects, including flies, gnats, and mosquitoes.

dipterous (dip′ter-us) 1. having two wings. 2. pertaining to insects of the order Diptera.

dipygus (di-pi′gus) a malformed fetus with a double pelvis.

dipylidiasis (dip″ĭ-lĭ-di′ah-sis) infection with *Dipylidium caninum.*

Dipylidium (dip″ĭ-lid′e-um) a genus of tapeworms. *D. cani′num* is parasitic in dogs, cats, and occasionally humans.

dipyridamole (di″pi-rid′ah-mōl) a platelet INHIBITOR and coronary VASODILATOR, used to prevent clotting associated with mechanical heart valves and to treat transient ischemic attacks. It is also used as an adjunct in the prevention of myocardial reinfarction and as an adjunct in radionuclide myocardial perfusion imaging.

direct fluorescent antibody–*Treponema pallidum* test a treponemal antibody test for SYPHILIS using direct immunofluorescence to detect antibodies against *Treponema pallidum* in the serum. Called also DFA-TP test.

directive (dĭ-rek′tiv) a stated instruction or order. See also WILL.

> **advance d's** see ADVANCE DIRECTIVES.

director (dĭ-rek′ter) a grooved instrument for guiding a knife or other surgical instrument.

dirithromycin (di-rith″ro-mi′sin) a MACROLIDE ANTIBIOTIC used in treatment of bacterial infections of the respiratory tract, streptococcal pharyngitis, and skin and soft tissue infections; administered orally.

Dirofilaria (di″ro-fĭ-lar′e-ah) a genus of nematode parasites of the superfamily Filarioidea. *D. im′mitis* is common in dogs.

dirofilariasis (di″ro-fil″ah-ri′ah-sis) infection with nematodes of the genus *Dirofilaria;* it is common in dogs and occasionally seen in humans, causing symptoms such as coughing, chest pain, and sometimes hemoptysis.

dis- word element [L.], *reversal* or *separation.*

dis- word element [Gr.], *duplication.*

disability (dis″ah-bil′ĭ-te) **1.** impairment of function to below the maximal level, either physically or mentally. **2.** anything that causes such impairment. **3.** the United States Government defines a disability as "a physical or mental impairment that substantially limits one or more of an individual's major life activities:" this includes both those individuals with a record of an impairment and those regarded as having such an impairment. **4.** the World Health Organization defines disability as loss of function at the level of the whole person, which may include inability to communicate or to perform mobility, ACTIVITIES OF DAILY LIVING, or necessary vocational or avocational activities; rehabilitation is aimed at teaching patients to remediate or compensate and thus maximize functional independence. See also HANDICAP and IMPAIRMENT.

developmental d. a substantial handicap in mental or physical functioning, with onset before the age of 18 and of indefinite duration. Examples are autism, cerebral palsy, uncontrolled epilepsy, certain other neuropathies, and mental retardation.

disaccharidase (di-sak′ah-ri-dās″) an enzyme that hydrolyzes DISACCHARIDES; in humans the disaccharidases are located in the brush border membrane of the small intestine and hydrolyze the oligosaccharides and disaccharides produced after luminal digestion of starches and other carbohydrates. See also disaccharide INTOLERANCE.

disaccharide (di-sak′ah-rid, di-sak′ah-rīd) any of a class of sugars each molecule of which yields two molecules of monosaccharide on hydrolysis.

disarticulation (dis″ahr-tik″u-la′shun) amputation or separation at a joint; called also exarticulation.

disaster (dĭ-zas′ter) a situation that produces damage and varying amounts of destruction; there is a three-tiered classification for disasters, based on the number of casualties. See also EMERGENCY.

disc (disk) disk.

discectomy (dis-kek′to-me) diskectomy.

discernment insight related to a patient problem or dilemma; the ability to analyze and understand a patient situation.

discharge¹ (dis-charj′) **1.** to set free or liberate. **2.** to release from a health care setting.

discharge² (dis′charj) **1.** material or force set free. **2.** an EXCRETION or EVACUATION. **3.** release from a health care setting.

discission (dĭ-sizh″un) incision, or cutting into, as of a soft cataract.

discitis (dis-ki′tis) diskitis.

discogenic (dis″ko-jen′ik) caused by derangement of an intervertebral disk.

discography (dis-kog′rah-fe) diskography.

discoid (dis′koid) **1.** disk-shaped. **2.** a disklike medicated tablet. **3.** a disk-shaped dental EXCAVATOR designed to remove the carious dentin of a decayed tooth. See illustration.

discoplacenta (dis″ko-plah-sen′tah) a disk-shaped placenta.

discordance (dis-kor′dans) the occurrence of a given trait in only one member of a twin pair. adj., **discor′dant.**

discrete (dis-krēt′) made up of separated parts; characterized by lesions that do not become blended.

discrimination (dis-krim″ĭ-na′shun) **1.** the making of fine distinctions. **2.** actions based

TYPES OF DISABILITIES WITH EXAMPLES	

Communication Disorders
  Aphasia
  Apraxia
  Dysarthria
Cognitive Impairments
  Anorexia and Bulimia
  Alzheimer's Disease
  Dementia
  Mental Illness
Developmental Disabilities
  Autism
  Cerebral Palsy
  Epilepsy
  Mental Retardation
	Degenerative Nervous System Disorders
	  Huntington's Disease
	  Multiple Sclerosis
	  Myasthenia Gravis
	Medical Disabilities
	  Arthritis
	  Cardiovascular Diseases
	  Cancer
	  Respiratory Diseases
	Orthopedic Disorders
	  Congenital Anomalies
	  Paralysis
	  Spinal Cord Injury
	Sensory Impairments
	  Hearing Loss, Deafness
	  Diminished Visual Acuity, Blindness

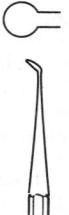
Discoid. From Dorland's, 2000.

on preconceived opinions without consideration of facts.

right-left d. the ability to differentiate one side of the body from the other.

discus (dis'kus), pl. *dis'ci* [L.] disk.

d. oo'phorus, d. ovi'gerus d. proli'gerus cumulus oophorus.

disease (dĭ-zēz') a definite pathological process having a characteristic set of signs and symptoms. It may affect the whole body or any of its parts, and its etiology, pathology, and prognosis may be known or unknown. For specific diseases, see under the specific name, as ADDISON'S DISEASE. See also ILLNESS, MAL, SICKNESS, and SYNDROME.

disengagement (dis"en-gāj'ment) emergence of the fetus, or part thereof, from the vaginal canal.

disequilibrium (dis"e-kwĭ-lib're-um) dysequilibrium.

dialysis d. dialysis dysequilibrium syndrome.

disinfect (dis"in-fekt') to free from pathogenic organisms, or to render them inert.

disinfectant (dis"in-fek'tant) 1. freeing from infection or infection-producing organisms. 2. an agent that does this. Heat and certain other physical agents such as live steam can be disinfectants, but in common usage the term is reserved for chemical substances such as MERCURY BICHLORIDE or PHENOL. Disinfectants are usually applied to inanimate objects since they are too strong to be used on living tissues. Chemical disinfectants are not always effective against spore-forming bacteria.

disinfection (dis"in-fek'shun) the act of disinfecting, using specialized cleansing techniques that destroy or prevent growth of organisms capable of infection.

terminal d. disinfection of a sick room and its contents at the termination of a disease.

disinfestation (dis"in-fes-ta'shun) destruction of insects, rodents, or other animal forms present on the person or his clothes or in his surroundings, and which may transmit disease.

disintegrant (dis-in'tĕ-grant) an agent used in pharmaceutical preparation of tablets, which causes them to disintegrate and release their medicinal substances on contact with moisture.

disintegration (dis"in-tĕ-gra'shun) 1. the process of breaking up or decomposing. 2. disruption of the integration functions of the personality in mental illness.

disintegrative disorder a PERVASIVE DEVELOPMENTAL DISORDER characterized by marked regression in a variety of skills, including language, social skills or adaptive behavior, play, bowel or bladder control, and motor skills, after at least two, but less than ten, years of apparently normal development.

disjunction (dis-junk'shun) the act or state of being disjoined. In genetics, the moving apart of bivalent chromosomes at the first anaphase of meiosis.

disk (disk) a circular or rounded flat plate; often spelled disc in names of anatomic structures.

articular d. a pad of fibrocartilage or dense fibrous tissue present in some synovial joints.

Bowman's d. one of the flat plates making up a striated muscle fiber.

choked d. papilledema.

ciliary d. pars plana.

embryonic d., germ d. germinal d. a flattened round bilaminar plate of cells in the BLASTOCYST of a mammal, where the first traces of the embryo are seen; called also embryonic or germinal area.

herniated d. see HERNIATED DISK.

intervertebral d. the layer of fibrocartilage between the bodies of adjoining VERTEBRAE; see also HERNIATED DISK.

intra-articular d's articular disk.

Merkel's d's small cup-shaped tactile receptors in the skin that are particularly sensitive to continuous pressure.

optic d. the intraocular part of the optic nerve formed by fibers converging from the retina and appearing as a pink to white disk in the retina; there are no sensory receptors in the region and hence no response to stimuli. Called also blind spot.

ruptured d. herniated disk.

slipped d. popular term for HERNIATED DISK.

diskectomy (dis-kek'to-me) excision of an intervertebral disk.

diskiform (dis'kĭ-form) in the shape of a disk.

diskitis (dis-ki'tis) inflammation of a disk, especially of an intervertebral disk.

diskography (dis-kog'rah-fe) radiography of the vertebral column after injection of radiopaque material into an intervertebral disk.

dislocation (dis″lo-ka′shun) displacement of a bone from a joint; called also luxation. The most common ones involve a finger, thumb, shoulder, or hip; less common are those of the mandible, elbow, or knee. Symptoms include loss of motion, temporary paralysis of the joint, pain, swelling, and sometimes shock. Dislocations are usually caused by a blow or fall, although unusual physical effort may also cause one. A few dislocations, especially of the hip, are congenital, usually from a faulty construction of the joint, and are best treated in infancy with a cast and possibly surgery. A dislocation should be treated as a fracture when first aid is administered. First aid includes checking for a pulse distal to the location and keeping the patient as still as possible. The patient is moved as a whole unit on a long board or a stretcher. As soon as possible the dislocation must be reduced by a surgeon.

   complete d. one in which the surfaces are entirely separated.

   compound d. one in which the joint communicates with the outside air through a wound.

   congenital d. of the hip a former name for developmental DYSPLASIA of the hip.

   pathologic d. one due to disease of the joint or to paralysis of the muscles.

   simple d. one in which there is no communication with the air through a wound.

dismemberment (dis-mem′ber-ment) amputation of a limb or a portion of it.

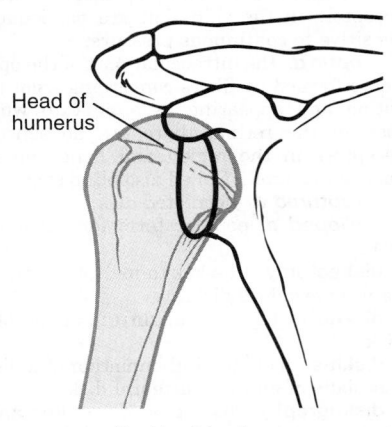

Shoulder dislocation.

dismutase (dis-mu′tās) any of a group of enzymes that have the ability to catalyze the reaction of two molecules of the same compound to yield two molecules in different oxidation states.

disomus (di-so′mus) a malformed fetus with a double trunk.

disopyramide (di″-so-pēr′ah-mīd) an agent used to control cardiac ARRHYTHMIAS; it suppresses and prevents recurrence of both unifocal premature ventricular contractions and those of multifocal origin, paired premature ventricular contractions, and episodes of ventricular tachycardia that are not persistent.

disorder (dis-or′der) a derangement or abnormality of function; a morbid physical or mental state. For specific disorders, such as the psychiatric disorders, see under the name, such as ANXIETY DISORDERS and PERSONALITY DISORDERS.

disorganization (dis-or″gan-ĭ-za′shun) the process of destruction of any organic tissue; any profound change in the tissues of an organ or structure that causes the loss of most or all of its proper characteristics.

disorientation (dis-o″re-en-ta′shun) the loss of proper bearings, or a state of mental confusion as to time, place, or identity.

dispensary (dis-pen′ser-e) 1. a place for dispensation of free or low-cost medical treatment. 2. any place where drugs or medicines are actually dispensed.

dispensatory (dis-pen′sah-tor″e) a book that describes medicines and their preparation and uses.

   D. of the United States of America a collection of monographs on unofficial drugs and drugs recognized by the Pharmacopeia of the United States, the Pharmacopoeia of Great Britain, and the National Formulary, also on general tests, processes, reagents, and solutions of the U.S.P. and N.F., as well as drugs used in veterinary medicine.

dispense (dis-pens′) to count, label, and disburse multiple doses of medications to a patient.

disperse (dis-pers′) to scatter the component parts, as of a tumor or the fine particles in a colloid system; also, the particles so dispersed.

dispersion (dis-per′zhun) 1. the act of scattering or separating; the condition of being scattered. 2. the incorporation of the particles of one substance into the body of another, comprising solutions, suspensions, and colloid systems. 3. a colloid system, particularly an unstable one.

displacement (dis-plās′ment) 1. malposition. 2. percolation. 3. a DEFENSE MECHANISM in which emotions, ideas, wishes, or impulses are unconsciously shifted from their original object to a more acceptable, usually less threatening, substitute. 4. in a chemical reaction, the replacement of one atom or group in a molecule by another.

display (dis-plaʹ) something presented for viewing, such as on a computer screen.

liquid crystal d. a thin membrane containing liquid crystals, used for displays in computers and monitoring equipment.

disposition (disʺpo-zĭʹshun) 1. a tendency, either physical or mental, toward a given disease. 2. the prevailing temperament or character, giving a degree of predictability to the response to a situation or other stimulus. 3. the plan for continuing health care of a patient following discharge from a given health care facility.

disproportion (disʺpro-porʹshun) a lack of the proper relationship between two elements or factors.

cephalopelvic d. abnormally large size of the fetal skull in relation to the maternal pelvis, leading to difficulties in delivery.

disruptive behavior disorders a group of mental disorders of children and adolescents consisting of behavior that violates social norms and is disruptive, often distressing others more than it does the person with the disorder. It includes CONDUCT DISORDER and OPPOSITIONAL DEFIANT DISORDER and is classified with ATTENTION-DEFICIT/HYPERACTIVITY DISORDER.

dissect (dĭ-sektʹ, di-sektʹ) to cut apart, or separate; especially, the exposure of structures of a cadaver for anatomical study.

dissection (dĭ-sekʹshun) 1. the act of dissecting. 2. a part or whole of an organism prepared by dissecting.

aortic d. a dissecting ANEURYSM of the aorta; the usual site is the thoracic aorta. There are two types, classified according to anatomical location: *Type A* involves the ascending aorta; *Type B* originates in the descending aorta. Acute aortic dissection is often fatal within one month of onset. Surgical treatment may be delayed in aneurysms involving the descending aorta until the blood pressure has been controlled and edema and friability of the aorta are diminished. The usual course of treatment for an aneurysm of the ascending aorta is immediate surgery. The surgical procedure for either type is aimed at either repairing the intimal tear or removing the affected portion of the aorta. This may be done by suturing the separated aortic layers back together or by removing the damaged section of the aorta and replacing it with a synthetic graft.

axillary d., axillary lymph node d. surgical removal of axillary LYMPH NODES, done as part of radical MASTECTOMY.

blunt d. separation of tissues along natural lines of cleavage, by means of a blunt instrument or finger.

lymph node d. lymphadenectomy.

lymph node d., retroperitoneal **(RPLND)** retroperitoneal LYMPHADENECTOMY.

sharp d. separation of tissues by means of the sharp edge of a knife or scalpel, or with scissors.

disseminated (dĭ-semʹĭ-nātʺed) scattered; distributed over a considerable area.

d. intravascular coagulation **(DIC)** a bleeding disorder characterized by abnormal reduction in the elements involved in blood clotting due to their use in widespread intravascular clotting. It may be a secondary complication of any of numerous obstetrical, surgical, infectious, hemolytic, and neoplastic disorders, all of which activate in some way the intrinsic coagulation sequence. Paradoxically, the intravascular clotting ultimately produces hemorrhage because of rapid consumption of fibrinogen, platelets, prothrombin, and COAGULATION FACTORS V, VIII, and X. Because of this pathology, the condition is sometimes called *defibrination syndrome* or *consumption coagulopathy.*

There may be signs and symptoms related to tissue hypoxia and infarction caused by the many microthrombi, but DIC is more often seen as an acute or chronic hemorrhagic disorder related to excessive and diffuse depletion of the elements needed for hemostasis. DIC should be suspected in any patient who has an unexplained tendency toward bleeding, and is suffering from one of the following types of clinical conditions: (1) those that introduce coagulation-promoting factors into the circulation, as in abruptio placentae, retained dead fetus, amniotic fluid embolism, metastatic carcinoma of the pancreas, lung, stomach, or prostate, and acute promyelocytic leukemia; (2) those that lead to stagnant blood flow, as in hypotension and polycythemia; (3) those accompanied by widespread endothelial injury, as in severe burns, trauma, heat stroke, and surgery, particularly surgery involving extracorporeal CIRCULATION; (4) various types of infections and bacteremias; and (5) snake bite and fat embolism.

The tendency toward excessive bleeding can appear suddenly and, with little warning, rapidly progress to severe or even fatal hemorrhage. Signs of DIC include continued bleeding from a venipuncture site, occult and internal bleeding, and, in some cases, profuse bleeding from all orifices. Other less obvious and more easily missed signs are generalized sweating, cold and mottled fingers and toes (due to capillary thrombi and hypoxia), and petechiae.

The diagnosis of DIC is confirmed by laboratory tests that show prolonged thrombin time, prothrombin time, and partial thromboplastin time; depressed platelet count and fibrinogen count; elevated fibrin split products (FSP); and a strongly positive protamine sulfate test. Assays for coagulation factors are commonly done to diagnose DIC; if the condition is present, the levels of these factors are reduced.

Extreme care must be taken to prevent complications related to bleeding. Injections should be avoided. Venipunctures should be limited whenever possible.

Treatment of DIC consists of replacement of the inadequate blood products and correction, when possible, of the underlying cause. When the primary disease cannot be treated, intravenous injections of heparin may inhibit the clotting process and raise the level of the depleted clotting factors. However, heparin therapy remains controversial as it can itself cause bleeding.

dissociation (dis-so″she-a′shun) 1. the act of separating or state of being separated. 2. the separation of a molecule into fragments produced by the absorption of light or thermal energy or by solvation. 3. segregation of a group of mental processes from the rest of a person's usually integrated functions of consciousness, memory, perception, and sensory and motor behavior, as in the separation of personality and aspects of memory or subpersonalities in the DISSOCIATIVE DISORDERS or in the segregation of an idea or object from its emotional significance, as is sometimes seen in schizophrenia.

atrial d. independent beating of the left and right atria, each with normal rhythm or with various combinations of normal rhythm, atrial FLUTTER, or atrial FIBRILLATION.

atrioventricular d. a condition in which the atria and the ventricles contract independently of each other, without synchronization of their rhythms.

electromechanical d. pulseless electrical activity.

isorhythmic atrioventricular d. a cardiac rhythm in which the atria and the ventricles beat independently and at approximately the same rate.

dissociative disorders (dĭ-so′se-ah-tive) a group of MENTAL DISORDERS characterized by a sudden, temporary change in consciousness, identity, memory, or motor behavior so that some part or more of these functions is lost. The DEFENSE MECHANISM of DISSOCIATION underlies these disorders and any organic basis for the changes must be ruled out. Dissociative disorders are uncommon and often bizarre defensive reactions to stress. They are complex and difficult to distinguish from each other. The commonality is a cluster of related mental events that are beyond the patient's recall but can spontaneously return to conscious awareness. The category includes: dissociative AMNESIA, dissociative FUGUE, DISSOCIATIVE IDENTITY DISORDER, and DEPERSONALIZATION DISORDER.

dissociative identity disorder a type of DISSOCIATIVE DISORDER in which more than one personality exists in the same individual. Each personality has unique memories, characteristic behaviors, and social relationships that determine the individual's actions when that personality is dominant; the various personalities are usually very different from one another and may even seem to be opposites. At least two of the personalities control the patient's behavior in turns, with the transition from one personality to another often being abrupt. The host personality is usually totally unaware of the alternate personalities and experiences only gaps of time when the others are in control as well as inability to recall important personal information. Called also MULTIPLE PERSONALITY DISORDER

dissolution (dis″o-loo′shun) 1. the process in which one substance is dissolved in another. 2. separation of a compound into its components by chemical action. 3. liquefaction. 4. death.

dissolve (dĭ-zolv′) 1. to cause a substance to pass into solution. 2. to pass into solution.

dissonance (dis′o-nans) discord or disagreement.

cognitive d. anxiety or similar unpleasant feelings resulting from a lack of agreement between a person's established ideas, beliefs, and attitudes and some more recently acquired information or experience.

distad (dis′tad) in a distal direction.

distal (dis′tal) remote; farther from any point of reference.

distance (dis′tans) the measure of space intervening between two objects or two points of reference.

interocclusal d. the distance between the occluding surfaces of the maxillary and mandibular teeth with the mandible in physiologic rest position.

interocular d. the distance between the eyes, usually used in reference to the interpupillary distance (the distance between the two pupils when the visual axes are parallel).

distemper (dis-tem′per) a name for several infectious diseases of animals, especially canine distemper, a highly fatal viral disease of dogs, marked by fever, loss of appetite, and a discharge from the nose and eyes.

distend (dis-tend′) to expand outward owing to pressure from within.

distention (dis-ten′shun) 1. the state of being distended, stretched out, or enlarged. 2. the act of distending.

distichia (dis-tik′e-ah) **distichiasis** (dis″tĭ-ki′ah-sis) the presence of a double row of eyelashes, one or both of which are turned against the eyeball.

distillate (dis′tĭ-lāt) a product of distillation.

distillation (dis″tĭ-la′shun) the process of vaporizing and condensing a substance to purify it or to separate a volatile substance from less volatile substances. Called also vaporization.

    fractional d. separation of volatilizable substances into a number of fractions, based on their different boiling points.

distobuccal (dis″to-buk′′l) pertaining to or formed by the distal and buccal surfaces of a tooth, or by the distal and buccal walls of a tooth cavity.

distobucco-occlusal (dis″to-buk″o-ŏ-kloo′zal) pertaining to or formed by the distal, buccal, and occlusal surfaces of a tooth.

distoclusion (dis-to-kloo′zhun) malrelation of the dental arches, with the lower jaw in a distal or posterior position in relation to the upper.

distolabial (dis″to-la′be-al) pertaining to or formed by the distal and labial surfaces of a tooth or the distal and labial walls of a tooth cavity preparation.

distolabioincisal (dis″to-la″be-o-in-si′zal) pertaining to or formed by the distal, labial, and incisal surfaces of a tooth.

distolingual (dis″to-ling′gwal) pertaining to or formed by the distal and lingual surfaces of a tooth, or the distal and lingual walls of a tooth cavity preparation.

distolinguoincisal (dis″to-ling″gwo-in-si′-zal) pertaining to or formed by the distal, lingual, and incisal surfaces of a tooth.

distolinguo-occlusal (dis″to-ling″gwo-ŏ-kloo′zal) pertaining to or formed by the distal, lingual, and occlusal surfaces of a tooth.

distomiasis (dis″to-mi′ah-sis) trematodiasis.

disto-occlusal (dis″to-ŏ-kloo′zal) pertaining to or formed by the distal and occlusal surfaces of a tooth, or the distal

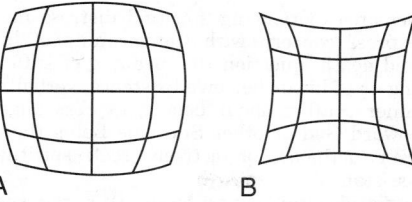

A, Barrel distortion; *B,* pincushion distortion. From Dorland's, 2000.

and occlusal walls of a tooth cavity preparation.

distortion (dis-tor′shun) 1. the state of being twisted out of a natural or normal shape or position. 2. in psychology, the process of altering or disguising unconscious ideas or impulses so that they become acceptable to the conscious mind. 3. in optics or radiology, deviation of an image from the true outline or shape of an object or structure; it may be a change in size or shape, an elongation, a foreshortening, or a magnification. See illustration.

distractibility (dis-trak″tĭ-bil′ĭ-te) inability to focus one's attention on the task at hand so that the attention is too frequently drawn to irrelevant and unimportant environmental stimuli.

distraction (dĭ-strak′shun) 1. diversion of attention. 2. separation of joint surfaces without rupture of their binding ligaments and without displacement. 3. surgical separation of the two parts of a bone after it is transected. 4. in the NURSING INTERVENTIONS CLASSIFICATION, a nursing INTERVENTION defined as purposeful focusing of attention away from undesirable sensations.

distress (dĭ-stres′) physical or mental anguish or suffering.

    respiratory d. see ADULT RESPIRATORY DISTRESS SYNDROME and RESPIRATORY DISTRESS SYNDROME OF NEWBORN.

    risk for spiritual d. a NURSING DIAGNOSIS accepted by the North American Nursing Diagnosis Association, defined as being at risk for an altered state of harmonious connectedness with all of life and the universe in which dimensions that transcend and empower the self may be disrupted.

    spiritual d. 1. discomfort related to religious, intellectual, or cultural concerns. 2. a NURSING DIAGNOSIS approved by the North American Nursing Diagnosis Association, defined as disruption in the life principle that pervades a person's entire being and that integrates and transcends his or her biological and psychosocial nature. The person experiencing spiritual distress may express concern with the meaning of life and death, question the meaning of suffering or of his or her own existence, verbalize inner conflict about beliefs, express anger toward God or other Supreme Being (however defined), or actively seek spiritual assistance.

distribution (dis″tri-bu′shun) 1. the specific location or arrangement of continuing or successive objects or events in space or time. 2. the extent of a ramifying structure such as an artery or nerve and its branches. 3. the geographical range of an organism or disease.

   frequency d. in statistics, a mathematical function that describes the distribution of measurements on a scale for a specific population.

   normal d. a symmetrical distribution of scores with the majority concentrated around the MEAN; for example, that representing a large number of independent random events. It is in the shape of a bell-shaped curve. Called also gaussian distribution. See illustration.

   probability d. a mathematical function that assigns to each measurable event in a sample group the probability that the event will occur.

disturbance (dis-tur′bans) a departure or divergence from that which is considered normal.

   body image d. former name for disturbed body IMAGE.

   sleep pattern d. former name for disturbed sleep PATTERN.

disulfiram (di-sul′fi-ram) ANTABUSE; a compound that, when used in the presence of ALCOHOL, produces distressing symptoms such as severe nausea and vomiting. It is a dangerous drug, should always be given under the supervision of a physician and is never given to a patient who is in a state of intoxication or does not have full knowledge of its effects. Disulfiram inhibits the oxidation of acetaldehyde produced by the metabolism of alcohol; the resultant accumulation of acetaldehyde in the body is what causes nausea, vomiting, palpitation, dyspnea, and lowered blood pressure. Occasionally this may lead to profound collapse.

disuse syndrome (dis-ūs′) deterioration of body systems as a result of prescribed or unavoidable inactivity. See also HAZARDS OF IMMOBILITY.

   risk for d. s. a NURSING DIAGNOSIS accepted by the North American Nursing Diagnosis Association, defined as a state in which an individual is at risk for deterioration of body systems owing to prescribed or unavoidable musculoskeletal inactivity.

Diucardin (di″u-kahr′din) trademark for preparations of HYDROFLUMETHIAZIDE, an ANTIHYPERTENSIVE agent.

diurese (di″u-rēs′) to cause DIURESIS; see also DIURETIC.

diuresis (di″u-re′sis) increased excretion of URINE; see also DIURETIC.

diuretic (di″u-ret′ik) 1. increasing DIURESIS (urine excretion). 2. an agent that does this, such as common substances like tea, coffee, and water, as well as medications. Types include loop diuretics, osmotic diuretics, potassium-sparing diuretics, and thiazide diuretics, with the most frequently prescribed being the THIAZIDES. Diuretics are used chiefly in treatment of edema resulting from conditions other than kidney disease; the abnormal kidney rarely responds to them. They are most useful in relieving edema accompanying congestive heart failure. Many, especially the thiazides, are used in the management of hypertension, particularly when used in conjunction with other kinds of antihypertensive agents.

   loop d's a group of diuretics that block active transport of chloride in the ascending limb of the loop of Henle, which stops coupled passive reabsorption of sodium. Some may cause OTOTOXICITY with reversible impaired hearing, and kidney damage from NEPHROTOXICITY; therefore these are contraindicated in renal disease. FUROSEMIDE, which belongs to this group, is a sulfonamide; hence, HYPERSENSITIVITY REACTION can develop in persons with a specific allergy.

   osmotic d's a group of diuretics that produce a rapid loss of sodium and water by inhibiting their reabsorption in the kidney tubules and loop of Henle; they also increase the osmolality of plasma, thus increasing diffusion of water from the intraocular and cerebrospinal fluids, and are used for reducing the pressure of these fluids. MANNITOL is clinically the most useful of this group, but it has significant

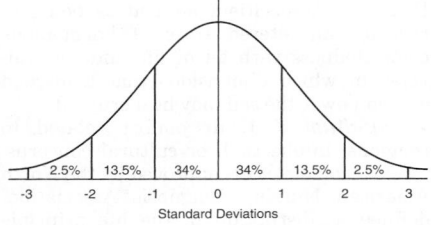

Normal distribution. The approximate percentage of the area (or frequency) lying under the curve between standard deviations is indicated. From Dorland's, 2000.

side effects such as pulmonary EDEMA and congestive HEART FAILURE.

potassium-sparing d's a group of diuretics that block the exchange of sodium for POTASSIUM and hydrogen ions in the distal tubule, causing an increase in excretion of sodium and chloride with a negligible increase in potassium excretion. They do not carry the threat of potassium loss, but they do present a potential problem of HYPERKALEMIA. TRIAMTERENE, one of the diuretics in this group, also can lead to HYPERGLYCEMIA in diabetic patients.

thiazide d's a group of diuretics in the THIAZIDE family; they decrease reabsorption of sodium by the kidney and thereby increase loss of water and sodium. They also increase urinary secretion of chloride, potassium, and, to some extent, bicarbonate ions. These are the most frequently prescribed diuretics, because they are moderately potent and have relatively few side effects. Most act within 1 hour after being taken and are excreted in 3 to 6 hours. Patients who are taking a thiazide diuretic should be monitored for electrolyte imbalances, metabolic acidosis, and, in the case of diabetic patients, hyperglycemia, which may necessitate an increase in their insulin dosage. Because gastrointestinal irritation can occur, it is advisable to take these diuretics at mealtime.

Diuril (di'u-ril) trademark for preparations of CHLOROTHIAZIDE, a diuretic.

diurnal (di-er'nal) pertaining to or occurring during the daytime, or period of light.

divagation (di"vah-ga'shun) incoherent or wandering speech and thought.

divalent (di-va'lent) bivalent; having a valence of two.

divalproex (di-val'pro-eks) an ANTICONVULSANT, used as *divalproex sodium,* a 1:1 compound of VALPROATE sodium and VALPROIC ACID in treatment of MIGRAINE, manic episodes of BIPOLAR DISORDER, and epileptic seizures, particularly absence seizures.

divergence (di-ver'jens) a moving apart, or inclination away from a common point. adj., **divergent.**

diverticular (di"ver-tik'u-ler) pertaining to or resembling a diverticulum.

d. disease a general term including the prediverticular state, diverticulosis, and diverticulitis.

diverticulectomy (di"ver-tik"u-lek'to-me) surgical excision of a diverticulum.

diverticulitis (di"ver-tik"u-li'tis) inflammation of a diverticulum, especially inflammation involving diverticula of the colon. Weakness of the muscles of the colon, sometimes produced by chronic constipation, leads to the formation of diverticula,

small blind pouches that form in the lining and wall of the colon. Inflammation may occur as a result of collections of bacteria or other irritating agents trapped in the pouches. Symptoms of diverticulitis include muscle spasms and cramplike pains in the abdomen, especially in the lower left quadrant. Diagnosis is confirmed by barium enema (see BARIUM TEST), in which the diverticula are clearly shown.

Treatment consists of bed rest, cleansing enemas, a bland or low-residue diet, and drugs to reduce infection. In severe cases portions of the affected bowel may require surgical removal and a temporary *colostomy.*

diverticulogram (di"ver-tik'u-lo-gram") a radiograph of a diverticulum.

diverticulosis (di"ver-tik"u-lo'sis) the presence of diverticula in the absence of inflammation. (See DIVERTICULITIS.)

diverticulum (di"ver-tik'u-lum), pl. *diverti'cula* [L.] a circumscribed pouch or sac occurring normally or created by herniation of the lining mucous membrane through a defect in the muscular coat of a tubular organ. See illustration.

ileal d. Meckel's diverticulum.

intestinal d. a pouch or sac formed by hernial protrusion of the mucous membrane through a defect in the muscular coat of the intestine.

Meckel's d. an occasional sacculation or appendage of the ileum, derived from an unobliterated yolk stalk.

pressure d., pulsion d. a sac or pouch formed by hernial protrusion of the mucous membrane through the muscular coat of the esophagus or colon as a result of pressure from within.

traction d. a localized distortion, angulation, or funnel-shaped bulging of the esophageal wall, due to adhesions resulting from an external lesion.

division (di-vizh'un) the act of separating into parts.

cell d. fission of a cell, the process by which cells reproduce.

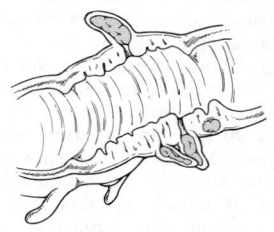

Intestinal diverticula. From Dorland's, 2000.

divulsion (dĭ-vul'shun) separation or pulling apart by force.

divulsor (dĭ-vul'ser) an instrument for dilating the urethra.

Dix (diks) Dorothea Lynde (1802–1887). American humanitarian. Born in Hampden, Maine, Miss Dix contributed to the establishment and improvement of many insane asylums and prisons in the United States, Europe, and Japan, beginning with the establishment of the Boston Lunatic Asylum in 1839. During the Civil War she was appointed Superintendent of Female Nurses and organized the first nurse corps of the United States Army.

dizygotic (di''zi-got'ik) pertaining to or derived from two separate ZYGOTES (fertilized ova; said of TWINS. See also MONOZYGOTIC.

dizygous (di-zi'gus) dizygotic.

dizziness (diz'e-nes) a disturbed sense of relationship to space; a sensation of unsteadiness and a feeling of movement within the head. VERTIGO is sometimes used erroneously as a synonym. See also DYSEQUI-LIBRIUM.

dL deciliter.

DL- chemical prefix (small capitals D and L) used with the D- and L- convention to indicate a racemic mixture of ENANTIOMERS.

dl- chemical prefix used with the *d* and *l* convention to indicate a racemic mixture of enantiomers; the prefix (±)- is used with the same meaning.

D$_{LCO}$ diffusing capacity of the lung for carbon monoxide.

D$_{LO_2}$ diffusing capacity of the lung for oxygen.

DLE discoid lupus erythematosus.

DMARD disease-modifying antirheumatic drug.

DMD Doctor of Dental Medicine.

DMF decayed, missing, filled; see DMF RATE.

DMSO dimethyl sulfoxide, an industrial solvent that has the ability to penetrate plant and animal tissues and to preserve living cells during freezing. It has been used investigationally as an agent to increase the penetrability of other substances and as a topical ANALGESIC and ANTIINFLAMMATORY. It has been approved by the U.S. Food and Drug Administration in a 50 per cent solution for direct instillation into the bladder for the treatment of interstitial cystitis. A 90 per cent solution, which has been approved only for veterinary use, is believed by some to be beneficial in the treatment of muscle sprains and strains, arthritis, spinal cord injuries, and the aftereffects of stroke when it is applied

externally and absorbed by the skin. Claims that it is effective for treating these disorders in humans have not been validated by research studies. It has been shown to produce some short-term side effects.

DMT dimethyltryptamine.

DNA deoxyribonucleic acid.

complementary DNA **(cDNA),** *copy DNA* **(cDNA)** synthetic DNA transcribed from a specific RNA through the reaction of the enzyme REVERSE TRANSCRIPTASE.

DNAR do not attempt resuscitation.

DNase deoxyribonuclease.

DNR do not resuscitate.

DNS, DNSc Doctor of Nursing Science.

DO Doctor of Osteopathy.

DOA dead on arrival; dead on admission.

dobutamine (do-bu'tah-mēn) a synthetic CATECHOLAMINE administered parenterally as the hydrochloride salt for inotropic support in short-term treatment of adults with cardiac decompensation due to depressed contractility resulting either from organic heart disease or from cardiac surgical procedures.

Dobutrex (do'bu-treks) trademark for a preparation of DOBUTAMINE hydrochloride, a synthetic CATECHOLAMINE used as a cardiotonic.

docetaxel (do''sĕ-tak's'l) an antineoplastic AGENT used in chemotherapy, particularly to treat carcinoma of the breast and non–small cell lung carcinoma; administered by intravenous infusion.

Dock (dok) Lavinia Lloyd (1858–1956). American pioneer in public health nursing. Beginning with her work with the United Workers of Norwich, Connecticut, she made valuable contributions to public health nursing, including work with Lillian WALD at the Henry Street Settlement in New York. In addition, she was active in the women's suffrage movement and an advocate of legislative control of nursing practice. She was also a prolific author; her works include *Materia Medica for Nurses,* one of the earliest nursing textbooks, and a four-volume *History of Nursing,* written with Adelaide NUTTING.

docosanol (do-ko'sah-nol) an antiviral agent effective against activity viruses with a lipid envelope, including herpes simplex virus; used topically in the treatment of recurrent herpes labialis.

doctor (dok'ter) 1. a holder of a diploma of the highest degree from a university, qualified as a specialist in a particular field of knowledge. 2. a practitioner of the healing arts, as one graduated from a college of medicine, osteopathy, chiropractic, optometry, podiatry, dentistry, or veterinary medicine, and licensed to practice.

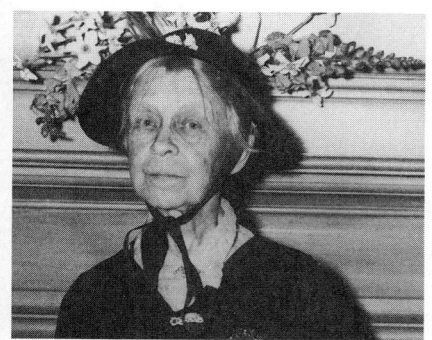

Lavinia Lloyd Dock. Special collections, Milbank Memorial Library, Teachers College, Columbia University.

documentation (dok″u-men-ta′shun) 1. written notations in a patient's record. 2. in the NURSING INTERVENTIONS CLASSIFICATION, a nursing INTERVENTION defined as recording of pertinent patient data in a clinical record.

docusate (dok′u-sāt) any of a group of anionic SURFACTANTS widely used as emulsifying, wetting, and dispersing agents.

   d. calcium an ionic surfactant used as a stool softener.

   d. potassium an anionic surfactant used as a stool softener; administered orally.

   d. sodium an ionic surfactant used as a stool softener.

DOE dyspnea on exertion.

dofetilide (do-fet′i-līd) an ANTIARRHYTHMIC that prolongs the duration of the cardiac action potential and the effective refractory period without affecting conduction velocity; used in the treatment of atrial arrhythmias, administered orally.

dol (dōl) a unit of pain intensity.

Dolan (do′lan) Margaret B. (1914–1974). Served as president of the American Nurses' Association, the American Public Health Association, and the National Health Council. She was active in public health nursing, serving on government advisory bodies, and urged community involvement by nurses. She was involved internationally in health care, serving as a consultant to the governments of Ghana and Thailand and as ANA representative at congresses of the International Council of Nurses.

dolasetron (do-las′ĕ-tron) a selective SEROTONIN receptor antagonist, used as the mesylate salt for the prevention of nausea and vomiting associated with chemotherapy or occurring after surgery; administered orally and intravenously.

dolich(o)- word element [Gr.], *long.*

dolichocephalic (dol″ĭ-ko-sĕ-fal′ik) having a narrow, long head.

dolichofacial (dol″ĭ-ko-fa′shal) having a long face.

dolichomorphic (dol″ĭ-ko-mor′fik) having a long, thin, asthenic body type.

dolichopellic (dol″ĭ-ko-pel′ik) having a long pelvis from front to back, with a pelvic index of 95 or above.

doll's eye phenomenon (reflex) (dolz i) the movement of the eyes as a unit in the opposite direction when the head is moved; it occurs in an individual with a depressed level of CONSCIOUSNESS when cranial nerves three and six are intact. Called also oculocephalic reflex.

Dolobid (dol′o-bid) trademark for a preparation of DIFLUNISAL, a NONSTEROIDAL ANTIINFLAMMATORY DRUG.

dolor (do′lor), pl. *dolo′res* [L.] PAIN; one of the cardinal signs of inflammation.

dolorific (do″lor-if′ik) producing pain.

dolorimeter (do″lor-im′ĕ-ter) an instrument for measuring pain in dols; see also ALGESIMETER.

dominance (dom′ĭ-nans) 1. the supremacy, or superior manifestation, in a specific situation of one of two or more competitive or mutually antagonistic factors. 2. the appearance, in the PHENOTYPE of a HETEROZYGOTE, of one of two mutually antagonistic parental characters.

dominant (dom′ĭ-nant) 1. exerting a ruling or controlling influence. 2. in genetics, capable of expression when carried by only one of a pair of homologous chromosomes; see dominant GENE. 3. an allele or trait that has this characteristic.

   d. side the half of the body in which a person is stronger; writing and eating are usually done with the hand on the dominant side. See also HANDEDNESS.

Donath-Landsteiner test (do′nath land′sti-ner) a test for paroxysmal hemoglobinuria based on the fact that the blood of patients with this disease contains isohemolysin and autohemolysin that unites with erythrocytes only at low temperatures (2° to 10°C), hemolysis occurring only after warming with the complement to 37°C.

donation (do-na′shun) 1. a gift. 2. the act of giving.

   oocyte d. a method of assisted reproductive TECHNOLOGY in which an OOCYTE from a fertile woman is aspirated for incubation in the uterus of a woman who has female factor INFERTILITY, such as after OOPHORECTOMY or premature MENOPAUSE. FERTILIZATION may be either in vitro or in utero.

donepezil (do-nep′ĕ-zil) a reversible ACETYLCHOLINESTERASE inhibitor, used as the

CLASSIFICATION OF HUMAN DONORS

Allogeneic	Tissue obtained from a blood relative (living related donor) or an unrelated individual (living unrelated donor) with an identical HLA type.
Autologous	Tissue that was previously removed from the recipient for later use.
Syngeneic	Tissue donated from an identical twin.

hydrochloride salt for treatment of mild to moderate symptoms of DEMENTIA OF THE ALZHEIMER TYPE; administered orally.

Donnatal (don'ah-tal) trademark for combination preparations of PHENOBARBITAL HYOSCYAMINE sulfate, ATROPINE sulfate, and SCOPOLAMINE hydrobromide, used for treatment of IRRITABLE BOWEL SYNDROME or PEPTIC ULCER.

donor (do'ner) 1. a person or organism that supplies an organ or tissue to be used in another body, usually either a cadaveric, living related, or living unrelated donor; see TRANSPLANTATION. 2. a substance or compound that contributes part of itself to another substance (acceptor).

cadaveric d. an organ or tissue donor who has already died; see cadaveric donor TRANSPLANTATION.

living nonrelated d. living unrelated donor.

living related d. one who is a close blood relative of the recipient; see living related donor TRANSPLANTATION.

living unrelated d. one who is not a close blood relative of the recipient; see living unrelated donor TRANSPLANTATION.

non–heart beating cadaveric d. a donor who has been pronounced dead according to the traditional criteria of lack of any pulse or detectable cardiac activity, but is not yet brain dead (see BRAIN DEATH). There are two types: The *controlled donor* is a person in a vegetative state who has signed a consent form or otherwise stated his or her wishes before becoming ill. Based on the patient's stated wishes and at the request of the next-of-kin, cannulas are placed into blood vessels for postmortem cooling of organs and the person is removed from life support. Once death has been declared, the organs are rapidly perfused with cold preservative solution and surgically removed. The *uncontrolled donor* is a person declared dead because of catastrophic injury to the heart, such as a gunshot wound to the heart. Cannulas are placed into blood vessels after death

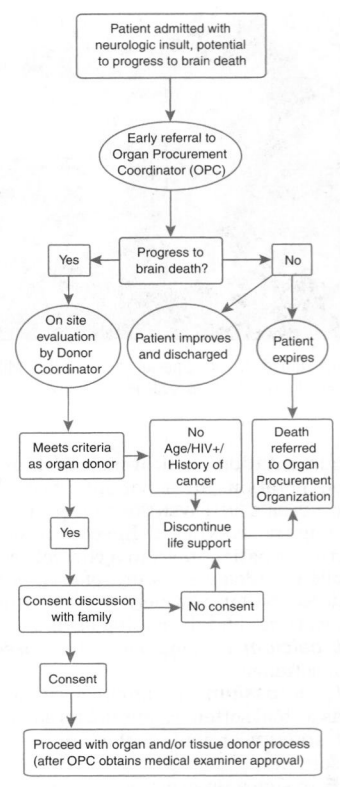

Algorithm for organ donation. From McQuillan, 2002.

and the organs are perfused and removed. This also requires consent of next-of-kin.

universal d. a person whose blood is type O in the ABO blood group system; such blood is sometimes used in emergency transfusion. Transfusion of blood cells rather than whole blood is preferred.

Donovania granulomatis (don-o-va'ne-ah gran-u-lo'mah-tis) *Calymmatobacterium granulomatis.*

dopa (do'pah) a compound produced by oxidation of tyrosine by tyrosinase; it is the precursor of DOPAMINE and an intermediate product in the biosynthesis of norepinephrine, epinephrine, and melanin. The naturally occurring form is L-dopa (see LEVODOPA), and is used to treat PARKINSON'S DISEASE and other forms of parkinsonism.

dopamine (do'pah-mēn) a compound produced by the decarboxylation of DOPA; it is the direct precursor in the synthesis of NOREPINEPHRINE and is also a NEUROTRANSMITTER in the central nervous system. It is administered intravenously to correct hemodynamic imbalance in persons with

SHOCK because it increases blood pressure, especially systolic pressure, as well as urinary output; it is also used as a cardiac stimulant.

dopaminergic (do'pah-mēn-er'jik) activated or transmitted by dopamine; pertaining to tissues or organs affected by dopamine.

dopant (do'pant) an impurity purposely added, as to a laser crystal or a semiconductor, during manufacturing in order to create a desired characteristic.

dopa-oxidase (do'pah-ok'sī-dās) an enzyme that oxidizes dopa to melanin in the skin, producing pigmentation.

doped (dōpt) having impurities (dopants) added purposely during manufacturing.

Doppler effect (dop'ler) the relationship of the apparent frequency of waves, as of sound, light, and radio waves, to the relative motion of the source of the waves and the observer, the frequency increasing as the two approach each other and decreasing as they move apart. The Doppler effect can be experienced when a train whistle or automobile horn produces a continuous sound as it approaches and passes a listener. The pitch of the sound suddenly falls as the source passes the listener.

Doppler ultrasonic flowmeter (dop'ler) a device for measuring blood flow that transmits sound at a frequency of several megahertz downstream along the flowing blood. Some of the sound waves are reflected by the moving red blood cells back toward the transducer. The difference in pitch between the transmitted and reflected sounds is produced as an audible tone and is proportional to the velocity of blood flow. Called also Doppler ultrasound flowmeter. A flowmeter can be incorporated into a stethoscope so that qualitative and quantitative measurements of the flow of blood through arteries and veins can be obtained. The Doppler flowmeter is capable of recording very rapid pulsatile changes in flow as well as steady flow; hence, it is helpful in assessing intermittent claudication, thrombus obstruction of deep veins, and other abnormalities of blood flow in the major arteries and veins.

There are various different types: a *laser Doppler flowmeter* is one in which blood flow is examined by a laser beam; the light is shifted by moving objects, mostly red blood cells, in accordance with the Doppler effect and the scattered light detected with a photodetector. A *transcranial Doppler flowmeter* is one that evaluates cerebral blood flow in the six intracranial arteries to assist in diagnosis of brain injury. One important use is for the detection of

vasospasm. It can also be used for the assessment of patients who are suspected to be brain dead or have suffered head trauma, and for monitoring of patients during surgery. The results of a TCD test are displayed on a color monitor and may be printed out.

D

   transcranial D. u. f., TCD ultrasound flowmeter an apparatus that evaluates cerebral blood flow in the six intracranial arteries to assist in diagnosis of brain injury. One important use is for the detection of vasospasm. It can also be used for the assessment of patients who are suspected to be brain dead or have suffered head trauma, and for monitoring of patients during surgery. The results of a TCD test are displayed on a color monitor and may be printed out.

Doriden (dor'ī-den) trademark for preparations of GLUTETHIMIDE, a SEDATIVE and HYPNOTIC.

dornase alfa (dor'nāz al'fah) recombinant human DEOXYRIBONUCLEASE I (DNase I) used to reduce the viscosity of sputum in CYSTIC FIBROSIS patients; administered by inhalation.

dors(o)- word element [L.], *the back; the dorsal aspect.*

dorsad (dor'sad) toward the back.

dorsal (dor'sal) directed toward or situated on the back surface, as opposed to ventral. See also POSTERIOR.

dorsalgia (dor-sal'jah) pain in the back.

dorsalis (dor-sa'lis) [L.] dorsal.

dorsiflexion (dor″sī-flek'shun) backward flexion or bending, as of the hand or foot.

dorsocephalad (dor″so-sef'ah-lad) toward the back of the head.

dorsolateral (dor″so-lat'er-al) pertaining to the back and side. See also POSTEROLATERAL.

dorsoventral (dor″so-ven'tral) 1. pertaining to the dorsal and ventral surfaces of a body. 2. directed from the back to the front; posteroanterior.

dorsum (dor'sum), pl. *dor′sa* [L.] 1. the back; the posterior surface of the human body in the anatomical POSITION. 2. the aspect of an anatomical structure or part corresponding in position to the back.

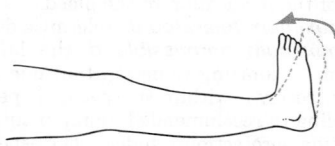

Dorsiflexion. From Lammon et al., 1995.

dorzolamide (dor-zo'lah-mīd) a CARBONIC ACID ANHYDRASE inhibitor, used in treatment of open-angle GLAUCOMA and ocular hypertension; administered topically to the conjunctiva as the hydrochloride salt.

dosage (do'sij) the determination and regulation of the size, frequency, and number of doses.

dose (dōs) the quantity to be administered at one time, as a specified amount of medication or a given quantity of radiation.

absorbed d. that amount of energy from ionizing radiations absorbed per unit mass of matter, expressed in rads.

air d. the intensity of an x-ray or gamma-ray beam in air, expressed in roentgens.

booster d. an amount of immunogen (vaccine, toxoid, or other antigen preparation), usually smaller than the original amount, injected at an appropriate interval after primary immunization to sustain the immune response to that immunogen.

curative d. (CD) a dose that is sufficient to restore normal health. See also median curative dose.

divided d. fractionated dose.

effective d. (ED) that quantity of a drug that will produce the effects for which it is administered. See also median effective dose.

erythema d. that amount of RADIATION that, when applied to the skin, causes ERYTHEMA (temporary reddening).

fatal d. lethal dose.

fractionated d. a fraction of the total dose prescribed, as of chemotherapy or radiation therapy, to be given at intervals, usually during a 24-hour period.

infective d. (ID) that amount of a pathogenic agent that will cause infection in susceptible subjects. See also median infective dose and tissue culture infective dose.

lethal d. (LD) that quantity of an agent that will or may be sufficient to cause death. See also median lethal dose and minimum lethal dose.

loading d. a dose of medication, often larger than subsequent doses, administered for the purpose of establishing a therapeutic level of the medication.

maintenance d. the amount of a medication administered to maintain a desired level of the medication in the blood.

maximum tolerated d. tolerance dose.

maximum permissible d. the largest amount of ionizing radiation that one may safely receive within a specified period according to recommended limits in current radiation protection guides. The specific amounts vary with age and circumstance.

median curative d. (CD$_{50}$) a dose that abolishes symptoms in 50 per cent of test subjects.

median effective d. (ED$_{50}$) a dose that produces the desired effect in 50 per cent of a population.

median infective d. (ID$_{50}$) that amount of pathogenic microorganisms that will produce demonstrable infection in 50 per cent of the test subjects.

median lethal d. (LD$_{50}$) the quantity of an agent that will kill 50 per cent of the test subjects; in radiology, the amount of radiation that will kill, within a specified period, 50 per cent of individuals in a large group or population.

median tissue culture infective d. (TCID$_{50}$) that amount of a pathogenic agent that will produce infection in 50 per cent of cell cultures inoculated.

minimum lethal d. 1. the amount of toxin that will just kill an experimental animal. 2. the smallest quantity of diphtheria toxin that will kill a guinea pig of 250-gm weight in 4 to 5 days when injected subcutaneously.

reference d. an estimate of the daily exposure to a substance for humans that is assumed to be without appreciable risk; it is calculated using the no observed adverse effect LEVEL and is more conservative than the older MARGIN OF SAFETY.

skin d. (SD) 1. the air dose of radiation at the skin surface, comprising the primary radiation plus backscatter. 2. the absorbed dose in the skin.

threshold d. the minimum dose of ionizing radiation, a chemical, or a drug that will produce a detectable degree of any given effect.

threshold erythema d. (TED) the single skin dose that will produce, in 80 per cent of those tested, a faint but definite erythema within 30 days, and in the other 20 per cent, no visible reaction.

tissue culture infective d. (TCID) that amount of a pathogenic agent that will produce infection when inoculated on tissue cultures; used with a numeric qualifier.

tolerance d. the largest quantity of an agent that may be administered without harm. Called also maximum tolerated dose.

dosimeter (do-sim'ĕ-ter) an instrument used to detect and measure exposure to radiation.

dosimetry (do-sim'ĕ-tre) scientific determination of amount, rate, and distribution of radiation emitted from a source of ionizing radiation.

dot (dot) a small spot or speck.

Gunn's d's white dots seen around the macula lutea on oblique illumination.

Maurer's d's irregular dots that stain red with Leishman's stain, seen in erythrocytes infected with *Plasmodium falciparum*.

Mittendorf's d. a congenital anomaly of the eye manifested as a small gray or white opacity just inferior and nasal to the posterior pole of the lens, representing the remains of the lenticular attachment of the hyaloid artery; it does not affect vision.

Schüffner's d's small granules seen in erythrocytes infected with the malarial parasite *Plasmodium vivax* when stained by certain methods. Called also Schüffner's granules.

Trantas' d's small white calcareous looking dots in the limbs of the conjunctiva in VERNAL CONJUNCTIVITIS.

double bind (dŭ′b′l bīnd′) a type of paradoxical communication or interaction in which one person demands a response to a message that contains mutually contradictory signals (verbal or nonverbal). The other person is unable to comment on the incongruity or to escape the situation.

double blind (dŭ′b′l-blīnd′) denoting a clinical TRIAL or other experiment in which neither the administrator nor the recipient, at the time of administration, knows which treatment a particular subject is receiving.

douche (dōōsh) a stream of water or air directed against a part of the body or into a cavity.

air d. a current of air blown into a cavity, particularly into the tympanum to open the eustachian tube.

vaginal d. irrigation of the vagina to cleanse the area, to apply medicated solutions to the vaginal mucosa and the cervix, or to apply heat in order to relieve pain, inflammation, and congestion. For the treatment to be effective the patient must be in the dorsal recumbent position with the hips level with the chest. Excessive pressure in administering the douche should be avoided so that solution is not forced through the cervix into the endometrial cavity.

Down syndrome (down) a congenital condition characterized by physical malformations and some degree of mental retardation; it was formerly known as mongolism because the patient's facial characteristics resemble those of persons of the Mongolian race. It is also called TRISOMY 21 SYNDROME because the disorder is concerned with a defect in CHROMOSOME 21. Causes are not known. There is a relatively high incidence in children of mothers in the older childbearing age, especially older than age 40. A particular type of the syndrome, seen in children of younger mothers, seems to have

a tendency to occur in certain families. The term TRISOMY refers to the presence of three representative chromosomes in a cell instead of the usual pair. In Down syndrome the twenty-first chromosome pair fails to separate when the germ cell (usually the ovum) is being formed. Thus the ovum contains 24 chromosomes, and when it is fertilized by a normal sperm carrying 23 chromosomes, the child is born with an extra chromosome (or total of 47) per cell.

Although not all of the physical characteristics of Down syndrome are always found in a child experiencing this disorder, there usually is a combination of several of them so that diagnosis at birth can be made without difficulty. These characteristics include a small, flattened skull, a short, flat-bridged nose, wide-set eyes, epicanthus, a protruding tongue that is furrowed and lacks a central fissure, short, broad hands and feet with a wide gap between the first and second toes, and a little finger that curves inward. The muscles are hypotonic and there is excessive mobility of the joints. The genitalia are often underdeveloped and congenital heart defects sometimes occur.

The National Down Syndrome Society maintains an informative web site at http://www.ndss.org. Their mailing address is National Down Syndrome Society, 666 Broadway, New York NY 10012. (See Atlas 1, Part D).

downloading (down′lōd-ing) a process by which an intelligent terminal is used to capture output from an information retrieval system in machine readable form for later processing and use by the searcher or end user.

down-regulation (down-reg-u-la′shun) a decrease in the number of RECEPTORS for a chemical or drug on cell surfaces in a given area, usually due to long-term exposure to the agent. See also UP-REGULATION.

doxacurium (dok″sah-ku′re-um) a long-acting neuromuscular blocking AGENT used as the chloride salt as a skeletal muscle RELAXANT during surgery and endotracheal intubation.

doxapram (dok′sah-pram) a respiratory stimulant, used as the hydrochloride salt for postanesthesia respiratory depression or for acute respiratory insufficiency associated with chronic obstructive pulmonary disease; administered intravenously.

doxazosin (dok-sa′zo-sin) a selective ALPHA-ADRENERGIC BLOCKING AGENT used as the mesylate derivative as an ANTIHYPERTENSIVE and in treatment of benign prostatic HYPERPLASIA; administered orally.

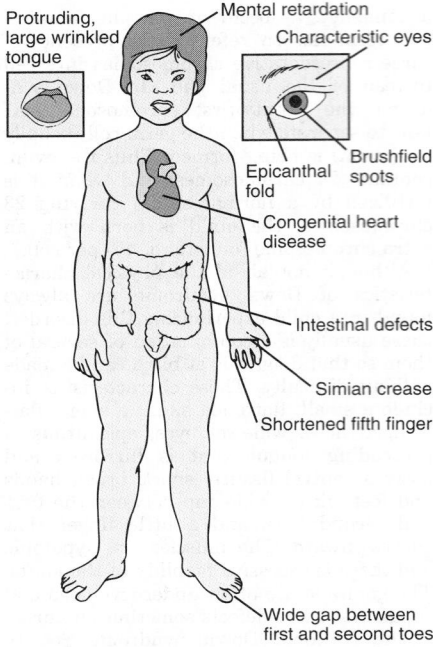

Typical features of Down syndrome. From Damjanov, 1996.

doxepin (dok′sĕ-pin) a tricyclic ANTIDE-PRESSANT, administered orally as the hydrochloride salt to treat depression, anxiety, chronic pain, peptic ulcer, pruritus, and other conditions.

doxercalciferol (dok″ser-kal-sif′er-ol) a synthetic analogue of VITAMIN D₂, used to reduce levels of circulating parathyroid HORMONE in treatment of secondary HYPER-PARATHYROIDISM associated with chronic RENAL FAILURE; administered orally or intravenously.

doxorubicin (dok″so-roo′bĭ-sin) an antitumor ANTIBIOTIC that binds to DNA, inhibits synthesis of nucleic acids, and inhibits cell division. It has one of the widest spectrums of antitumor activity of any antineoplastic AGENT and is administered intravenously as the hydrochloride salt. Side effects include bone marrow depression, alopecia, and cardiac toxicity; electroencephalogram monitoring is required during its administration. A liposome-encapsulated preparation of the hydrochloride salt is used in the treatment of Kaposi's SARCOMA associated with ACQUIRED IMMUNODEFICIENCY SYNDROME (AIDS).

doxycycline (dok″sĕ-si′klēn) a broad-spectrum semisynthetic ANTIBIOTIC, used as the hyclate and calcium salts against a wide range of gram-positive and gram-negative organisms; administered orally or intravenously.

doxylamine (dok″sil-am′ēn) an ANTIHISTA-MINE with sedative and anticholinergic effects; used as the succinate salt in the treatment of nasal, eye, and skin manifestations of allergic reactions, including allergic rhinitis, conjunctivitis, and itching, as an ingredient in cough and cold preparations, and in the short-term treatment of insomnia, administered orally.

DP Doctor of Pharmacy; Doctor of Podiatry.

DPH Department of Public Health; Diplomate in Public Health; Doctor of Public Health.

DPM Doctor of Podiatric Medicine.

DPT diphtheria, pertussis, and tetanus; used in reference to triple-antigen IMMUNIZA-TION against these diseases.

Dr Doctor.

dr dram.

dracunculiasis (drah-kung″ku-li′ah-sis) infection by nematodes of the genus *Dracunculus.*

dracunculosis (drah-kung′ku-lo′sis) dracunculiasis.

Dracunculus (drah-kung′ku-lus) a genus of parasitic NEMATODES. *D. medinen′sis* is a threadlike worm widely distributed in North America, Africa, the Middle East, Indonesia, and India; frequently found in the subcutaneous and intermuscular tissues of humans and certain other animals. See illustration.

draft (draft) a potion or dose.

drain (drān) 1. to withdraw liquid gradually. 2. any device by which a channel or open area may be established for exit of fluids or purulent material from a cavity, wound, or infected area. See also WOUND HEALING.

cigarette d. a drain made by drawing a small strip of gauze or surgical sponge into a rubber tube; called also Penrose drain.

Jackson-Pratt d. a closed wound drainage system comprising a drainage tube and collection vessel.

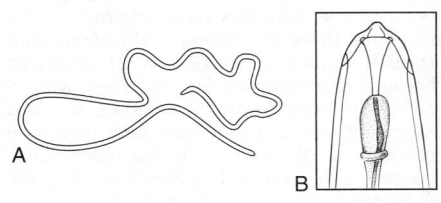

Dracunculus medinensis. From Dorland's, 2000.

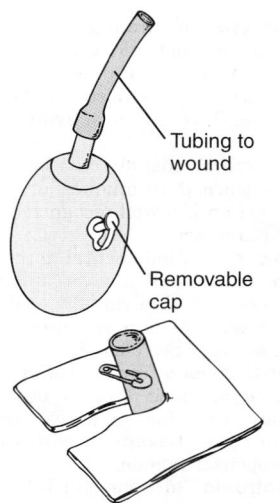

Top, Jackson-Pratt drain. *Bottom,* Penrose drain. From Lammon et al., 1995.

Penrose d. 1. cigarette drain. 2. a thin rubber tube that facilitates drainage from a closed or partially closed area.

sump d. a double-lumen drain that allows air entering the drained area through the smaller lumen to displace fluid into the larger lumen.

sump-Penrose d. a triple-lumen drain formed by placing a double-lumen tube within a Penrose drain.

wound d. see WOUND DRAIN.

drainage (drān'ij) systematic withdrawal of fluids and discharges from a wound, sore, or cavity.

capillary d. that effected by strands of hair, surgical gut, spun glass, or other material of small caliber which acts by capillary attraction.

closed d. airtight or water-tight drainage of a cavity so that air or contaminants cannot enter; for example, drainage of an empyema cavity carried out by means of an intercostal drainage tube passing into an airtight receiving vessel.

open d. drainage of a cavity through an opening in the chest wall into which one or more drainage tubes are inserted, the opening not being sealed against the entrance of outside air.

percutaneous d. drainage of an abscess or collection of fluid by means of a catheter inserted through the skin and positioned under the guidance of computed tomography or ultrasonography.

postural d. see POSTURAL DRAINAGE.

tidal d. drainage of the urinary bladder by an apparatus that alternately fills the bladder to a predetermined pressure and empties it by a combination of siphonage and gravity flow.

dram ($\mathfrak{z}$) **(dr)** (dram) a unit of weight which, in the APOTHECARIES' SYSTEM, equals 60 GRAINS, or $\frac{1}{8}$ OUNCE; in the AVOIRDUPOIS SYSTEM it equals 27.34 grains, or $\frac{1}{16}$ ounce.

fluid d. (fl dr) a unit of capacity (liquid measure) of the APOTHECARIES' SYSTEM, being 60 MINIMS, or the equivalent of 3.697 mL. In Great Britain, it is the *imperial fluid dram* and is equivalent to 3.55 mL. See also Table of Weights and Measures in the Appendix.

Dramamine (dram'ah-mēn) trademark for preparations of DIMENHYDRINATE or MECLIZINE hydrochloride, antihistamines effective against nausea and vomiting, especially in MOTION SICKNESS, and VERTIGO.

drawer tests (signs) (draw'er) either of two tests for integrity of the cruciate ligament of the knee: the knee is flexed to a 90° angle; at the femorotibial junction, if the tibia can be drawn too far forward *(anterior drawer test)* there is rupture of the anterior ligaments and if it can be drawn too far back *(posterior drawer test)* there is rupture of the posterior ligaments.

dream (drēm) 1. a mental phenomenon occurring during SLEEP in which images, emotions, and thoughts are experienced with a sense of reality. The interpretation of dream material is an important part of PSYCHOANALYSIS. According to psychoanalytic theory, dreams have both manifest CONTENT and latent CONTENT (see under *content*). The patient's free ASSOCIATIONS are used to discover the latent content and to discover how that affects waking life. 2. to experience such a phenomenon. Dreaming occurs during REM sleep; typically there are four or five such periods a night, with a total duration of about 90 minutes. The psychological interpretation of dreams was originated by Freud, who theorized that dreams enable the conscious expression of repressed unconscious impulses and wishes. Such wishes and impulses (*latent dream content*) are distorted and disguised so as to be acceptable to the conscious mind by the defensive processes of condensation, displacement, and symbolization and are then worked into a coherent story by secondary elaboration; this entire process (*dream work*) results in the dream as remembered by the dreamer (*manifest dream content*).

drepanocyte (drep'ah-no-sīt″) sickle cell. adj., **drepanocyt′ic.**

dressing (dres'ing) 1. any of various materials used for covering and protecting a WOUND. 2. in the NURSING INTERVENTIONS CLASSIFICATION, a nursing INTERVENTION defined as choosing, putting on, and removing clothes for a person who cannot do this for himself or herself.

    biologic d. one used in treatment of a burn or other large denuded area of skin to prevent infection and fluid loss; it may consist of synthetic material or a XENOGRAFT, ALLOGRAFT, or AUTOGRAFT

    hydrocolloid d. wafers or granules containing particles that interact with wound exudate to absorb the exudate by forming a gel.

    pressure d. one by which pressure is exerted on the covered area to prevent collection of fluids in underlying tissues; most commonly used after skin grafting and in treatment of burns.

    protective d. a light dressing to prevent exposure to injury or infection.

Dreves (drēvz) Katharine Densford (1890–1978). Nursing educator and organizer. As director of the Minnesota School of Nursing in Minneapolis, she was instrumental in development of a curriculum leading to a bachelor's degree in nursing and in establishing a continuing education program. She served as president of the American Nurses' Association and was active in the international organization of nursing, serving as vice-president of the International Council of Nurses.

DRG Diagnosis-Related Groups.

drift (drift) 1. slow movement away from the normal or original position. 2. a chance variation, as in gene frequency from one generation to another; the smaller the population, the greater are the random variations.

    antigenic d. relatively minor changes in the antigenic structure of a VIRUS strain, probably resulting from natural selection of variants circulating among an immune or partially immune population. See also antigenic SHIFT.

    ulnar d. ulnar deviation.

drill (dril) 1. instruction by repetition. 2. a device for cutting a hole or shaping something.

    bladder d. a technique of bladder TRAINING in which the patient is instructed to postpone voiding for an hour and a half, regardless of urgency or interim incontinence. The time interval between voiding episodes is increased in half-hour increments to a goal of two and a half to three hours.

drip (drip) the slow, drop-by-drop infusion of a liquid.

    postnasal d. drainage of excessive mucous or mucopurulent discharge from the postnasal region into the pharynx.

drive (drīv) 1. the force that activates human impulses. 2. to activate or cause to move.

    acquired d. goal-directed behavior satisfied by learned techniques or satisfiers. Drug addiction is a well-recognized example of an acquired drive.

    basic d. a fundamental force that is vital to survival of the organism. Such drives motivate individual, goal-directed activity related to hunger, thirst, sex, and physical activity. See also NEED.

dromostanolone (dro″mo-stan′o-lōn) an androgenic anabolic STEROID used as the propionate salt for palliative treatment of advanced metastatic breast cancer in postmenopausal women.

dromotropic (dro″mo-trop′ik) affecting conductivity of a nerve fiber.

dronabinol (dro-nab′in-ol) one of the major active substances in CANNABIS, used to treat nausea and vomiting in ANTINEOPLASTIC THERAPY and to treat anorexia associated with weight loss in ACQUIRED IMMUNODEFICIENCY SYNDROME; it is subject to abuse because of its psychotomimetic activity.

drop (drop) 1. a minute sphere of liquid as it hangs or falls. 2. to descend or cause to descend. 3. a descent or falling below the usual position.

droperidol (dro-per′ĭ-dol) a drug of the BUTYROPHENONE series, used for its ANTIANXIETY SEDATIVE, and ANTIEMETIC effects as a premedication prior to surgery and during induction and maintenance of anesthesia, as a postanesthesia antiemetic, and to produce conscious sedation; administered intravenously or intramuscularly. A combination of droperidol and FENTANYL citrate is administered intramuscularly to produce NEUROLEPTANALGESIA.

dropper (drop′er) a pipet or tube for dispensing liquids in drops.

dropsy (drop′se) old term for *edema.* adj., **drop′sical.**

drospirenone (dros-pi′rĕ-nōn) a spironolactone analogue that acts as a progestational agent; used in combination with an estrogen component as an oral contraceptive.

drowning (drown′ing) death from suffocation resulting from aspiration of water or other substance or fluid. Drowning occurs because the liquid prevents breathing. The lungs of a drowned person may contain very little water or other liquid. First aid measures are begun as soon as the individual is rescued from the water. Blankets and other coverings are used only to prevent loss of body heat. ARTIFICIAL RESPIRATION or other appropriate respiratory support should be administered at once to anyone who has stopped breathing. A victim who is unconscious but still breathing should be placed in a reclining position, preferably on the side. If the victim is not breathing and there is no evidence of a heart beat, CARDIOPULMONARY RESUSCITATION is begun immediately.

DrPH Doctor of Public Health.

drug (drug) 1. a chemical substance that affects the processes of the mind or body. 2. any chemical compound used in the diagnosis, treatment, or prevention of disease or other abnormal condition. 3. a substance used recreationally for its effects on the central nervous system, such as a NARCOTIC. DRUG ABUSE involving these substances may lead to DRUG DEPENDENCE or ADDICTION. 4. to administer such a substance to someone.

d. abuse the use of a drug or drugs for purposes other than those for which they are prescribed or recommended, involving a pathologic pattern of behavior (for example, difficulties with family or friends, aggressive behavior while intoxicated, absence from work, or legal problems). Drug abuse in conjunction with drug TOLERANCE or WITHDRAWAL constitutes drug DEPENDENCE. Specific SUBSTANCE USE DISORDERS include the following: abuse of AMPHETAMINES or similarly acting SYMPATHOMIMETICS CANNABIS COCAINE HALLUCINOGENS INHALANTS NICOTINE OPIOIDS, PCP, and SEDATIVES HYPNOTICS, and ANTIANXIETY AGENTS. Called also substance abuse and psychoactive substance abuse.

STIMULANTS affect the central nervous system, producing increased physical and mental activity, excitability, and prevention of sleep. Among the more popular stimulants are the AMPHETAMINES; these are dangerous because they alter judgment and obscure feelings. Prolonged use of these drugs can lead to acute toxic psychosis accompanied by hallucinations and delusions.

DEPRESSANTS favored by drug abusers include the BARBITURATES, the TRANQUILIZERS, and ALCOHOL. Their effect is opposite to that of stimulants and they often are taken as a means of "coming down from a high" produced by a stimulant. Sudden withdrawal from depressants can cause SEIZURE activity and even death. Combinations of barbiturates and alcohol, which compound the effect of each other, frequently lead to death.

Probably the best known of the HALLUCINOGENS is LSD; its use has declined in recent years because of public awareness of its long-term, if not permanent, effects on the psyche, producing "flashbacks" of an acute psychotic state, and its implication in chromosomal damage. Another popular hallucinogen is MESCALINE, which is derived from the peyote cactus.

The most popular addictive drugs are HEROIN (a NARCOTIC) and COCAINE and its derivative crack cocaine (central nervous system stimulants). These drugs are extremely potent and highly addictive; the complication of overdose is frequent. Crack is more insidious, addictive, and toxic than cocaine. Cardiac arrhythmias caused by its use may lead to sudden death.

d. dependence a state in which there is a compulsion to take a drug, either continuously or periodically, in order to experience its psychic effects or to avoid the discomfort of its absence. It is often subdivided into *psychological dependence* and *physiological dependence*. Some use the term more narrowly to refer only to physiological dependence, and in this sense it may be considered to be distinct from drug TOLERANCE, or it may be considered to be a state characterized by either tolerance or WITHDRAWAL. The last interpretation is the currently accepted official one. Called also substance dependence and psychoactive substance dependence. Drug dependence is characterized by a variable combination of several criteria, including (1) an overwhelming desire or need (compulsion) to continue use of the drug and to obtain it by any means, (2) a tendency to increase the dosage, (3) a psychological and usually a physical dependence on its effects, and (4) a detrimental effect on the individual and on society.

Treatment. The Center for Substance Abuse Treatment (CSAT) of the United States Department of Health and Human Services notes that "the challenge before us is to promote the most effective substance abuse treatment models to serve a multitude of needs among a very diverse population..." They released a consensus report with recommendations for improving the way in which alcohol and drug treatment services are delivered and paid for; it is part of the National Treatment Plan Initiative. The five major elements of the plan are that there must be an investment for results; that "there is no wrong door for treatment" (meaning that individuals with substance abuse problems should be able to access care from anywhere within the system); that there be a commitment to quality at all levels; that changes in attitude are needed to convince the public that recovery is possible; and that partnerships are needed, especially between the research and treatment communities, to ensure the use of evidence-based treatments. The National Treatment Plan Initiative is available online at http://www.natxplan.org or by writing to the Substance Abuse and Mental Health Services Administration, U.S. Department of Health and Human Services, 5600 Fishers Lane, Rockville MD 20857.

designer d. a recreational drug analogue similar in action to an existing recreational drug, most often created by making a slight alteration in the chemical structure of the older drug so that it is no longer a controlled substance; such drugs are developed and manufactured in illegal laboratories.

disease-modifying antirheumatic d. (DMARD) a classification of ANTIRHEUMATIC agents referring to their ability to modify the course of disease, as opposed to simply treating symptoms such as inflammation and pain. Agents in this group include AURANOFIN AZATHIOPRINE CYCLOSPORINE GOLD salts, HYDROXYCHLOROQUINE LEFLUNOMIDE METNOTREXATE D-PENICILLAMINE, and SULFASALAZINE.

d. interaction modification of the potency of one drug by another (or others) taken concurrently or sequentially. Some drug interactions are harmful and some may have therapeutic benefits. Present knowledge of drug interactions is limited and no single chart of drug interactions can be completely accurate in predicting the effects of a drug combination on an individual patient. For this reason any person responsible for administration of medications must be ever alert to the possibility of dangerous drug interaction any time drugs are given in combination. It is recommended that a clinical pharmacologist be consulted whenever the possibility of incompatibility is suspected in a multiple-drug regimen. Additives, for example, in an intravenous infusion may produce an adverse chemical interaction. Factors influencing these interactions include pH and chemical composition, especially the various buffering, stabilizing, and preserving chemicals present in commercially prepared intravenous solutions. Due to the variety and volume of drugs and chemicals available and the high potential of incompatibility, it is recommended that admixtures be restricted to a single additive in each intravenous solution administered.

Drugs may also interact with various foods. In general, these interactions fall into three categories: (1) food malabsorption; (2) nutritional status; and (3) alteration of drug response by nutrients. In teaching patients self-care in the taking of prescribed medications, one should explain the need for meticulously following directions related to the intake of food and drink while the medication regimen is being followed.

nonprescription d's see NONPRESCRIPTION DRUGS.

nonsteroidal antiinflammatory d. see NONSTEROIDAL ANTIINFLAMMATORY DRUG.

over the counter d's OVER THE COUNTER MEDICATIONS.

psychedelic d's chemical substances that produce hallucinations, distortions of perception, and sometimes psychotic-like behavior; see also PSYCHEDELIC.

psychoactive d., psychotropic d. psychoactive SUBSTANCE.

recreational d. a legal or illegal PSYCHOACTIVE SUBSTANCE that is used voluntarily for the satisfaction to be derived from it. It may also be used in the belief that some personal or social value will be achieved.

street d's drugs illegally obtained for use in DRUG ABUSE.

sulfa d. sulfonamide (def. 2).

druggist (drug'ist) pharmacist.

drunkenness inebriation.

sleep d. a condition of prolonged transition from sleep to waking, with partial alertness, disorientation, drowsiness, poor coordination, and sometimes excited or violent behavior.

drusen (droo'sen) 1. abnormal growths of hyaline in Bruch's membrane, the inner layer of the choroid of the eye, usually due to aging. 2. rosettes of granules occurring in the lesions of actinomycosis.

dry ice (dri is) carbon dioxide snow.

DSM-IV abbreviation for the *Diagnostic and Statistical Manual of Mental Disorders* (Fourth Edition), prepared by the Task Force on Nomenclature and Statistics of the American Psychiatric Association. It is the Association's official manual of mental disorders and provides detailed descriptions of categories of disorders as well as diagnostic criteria. Disorders are placed on one of five axes: *axis I* includes all the clinical syndromes and V codes except for personality disorders and mental retardation; *axis II* includes the personality disorders and mental retardation; *axis III* lists any coexisting physical disorders or conditions; *axis IV* assesses the severity of psychosocial and environmental stressors; and *axis V* consists of a global assessment of functioning, using a 100 point scale assessing the highest level of functioning during the past year and the current level of functioning.

DSM-IV-TR a text revision of the DSM-IV published in 2000, incorporating changes in diagnostic criteria for TOURETTE'S SYNDROME dementia of the alzheimer type dementia due to other medical conditions personality change due to a general medical condition, EXHIBITIONISM, FROTTEURISM, PEDOPHILIA, sexual SADISM, and VOYEURISM.

DT diphtheria and tetanus toxoids, pediatric use; see diphtheria TOXOID.

DTaP diphtheria and tetanus toxoids and pertussis vaccine in which the pertussis vaccine component is in the acellular rather than whole-cell form.

DTIC dacarbazine.

DTP diphtheria and tetanus toxoids and pertussis vaccine.

DTPA pentetic acid (diethylenetriamine pentaacetic acid).

DTR registered dietetic technician.

Dubin-Johnson syndrome (doo′bin jon′-son) hyperbilirubinemia II.

Duchenne's disease (du-shenz′) 1. spinal muscular atrophy. 2. bulbar paralysis. 3. tabes dorsalis.

Duchenne-Aran disease (du-shen′ar-ahn′) spinal muscular atrophy.

duct (dukt) a passage with well-defined walls, especially a tubular structure for the passage of excretions or secretions. adj., **ductal.**

   accessory d. of Santorini a tubular structure that drains the lower part of the head of the pancreas.

   alveolar d's small passages connecting the respiratory bronchioles and the alveolar sacs.

   Bartholin's d., d. of Bartholin the larger and longer of the sublingual ducts.

   bile d's, biliary d's see BILE DUCTS.

   cochlear d. a spiral membranous tube in the bony canal of the cochlea between Reissner's membrane and the basilar membrane; it is divided into the scala tympani, scala vestibuli, and spiral lamina. Called also scala media.

   common bile d. a duct formed by the union of the cystic and hepatic ducts; see also BILE DUCTS.

   cystic d. the passage connecting the gallbladder neck and the common bile duct.

   efferent d. any duct that gives outlet to a glandular secretion.

   ejaculatory d. the duct formed by union of the ductus deferens and the duct of the seminal vesicles, opening into the prostatic urethra on the colliculus seminalis.

   endolymphatic d. a canal connecting the membranous labyrinth of the ear with the endolymphatic sac.

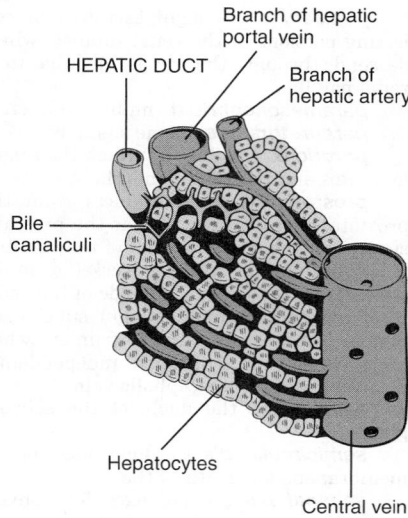

Hepatic duct. From Applegate, 2000.

   excretory d. one through which the secretion is conveyed from a gland.

   hepatic d. the excretory duct of the liver, or one of its branches in the lobes of the liver; see also BILE DUCTS.

   lacrimal d. the excretory duct of the lacrimal gland; see also LACRIMAL APPARATUS. Called also lacrimal canaliculus.

   lacrimonasal d. nasal duct.

   lactiferous d's ducts conveying the milk secreted by the lobes of the breast to and through the nipples.

   lymphatic d., left thoracic duct.

   lymphatic d's see LYMPHATIC DUCTS.

   mammary d. lactiferous ducts.

   mesonephric d. an embryonic duct of the mesonephros, which in the male becomes the epididymis, ductus deferens and its ampulla, seminal vesicles, and ejaculatory duct, and in the female is largely obliterated.

   müllerian d. either of the two paired embryonic ducts developing into the vagina, uterus, and fallopian tubes, and becoming largely obliterated in the male.

   nasal d., nasolacrimal d. the downward continuation of the lacrimal sac, opening on the lateral wall of the inferior meatus of the nose; see also LACRIMAL APPARATUS.

   pancreatic d. the main excretory duct of the pancreas, which usually unites with the common bile duct before entering the duodenum at the major duodenal papilla; see also BILE DUCTS.

papillary d's straight excretory or collecting portions of the renal tubules, which descend through the renal medulla to a renal papilla.

paramesonephric d. müllerian duct.

paraurethral d's Skene's glands.

parotid d. the duct by which the PAROTID GLANDS empty into the mouth.

prostatic d's minute ducts from the prostate, opening into or near the prostatic sinuses on the posterior wall of the urethra.

lymphatic d., right a vessel draining lymph from the upper right side of the body, receiving lymph from the right subclavian, jugular, and mediastinal trunks when those vessels do not open independently into the right brachiocephalic vein.

salivary d's the ducts of the salivary glands.

semicircular d's the long ducts of the membranous labyrinth of the ear.

seminal d's the passages for conveyance of spermatozoa and semen.

sublingual d's the excretory ducts of the sublingual salivary glands.

submandibular d., submaxillary d. the duct that drains the submandibular gland and opens at the sublingual caruncle.

tear d. lacrimal duct.

thoracic d. a duct beginning in the cisterna chyli and emptying into the venous system at the junction of the left subclavian and left internal jugular veins. It acts as a channel for the collection of lymph from the portions of the body below the diaphragm and from the left side of the body above the diaphragm.

ductile (duk′til) susceptible of being drawn out without breaking.

ductless (dukt′les) having no excretory duct.

ductopenia (duk″to-pe′ne-ah) deficiency in the number of ducts, particularly bile ducts; it may be focal or generalized.

ductule (duk′tūl) a minute duct.

ductulus (duk′tu-lus), pl. *duc′tuli* [L.] ductule.

ductus (duk′tus), pl. *duc′tus* [L.] duct.

d. arterio′sus a fetal blood vessel that joins the aorta and pulmonary artery.

d. de′ferens the excretory duct of the testis, which joins the excretory duct of the seminal vesicle to form the ejaculatory duct; called also vas deferens.

patent d. arteriosus see PATENT DUCTUS ARTERIOSUS.

d. veno′sus a major blood channel that develops through the embryonic liver from the left umbilical vein to the inferior vena cava.

Dukes' classification (dooks) a system of staging colorectal tumors based on evaluation of the depth of invasion of the carcinoma and the presence or absence of metastasis. The four stages are: *A,* confined to the mucosa and submucosa; *B,* invasion through the muscularis without lymph node involvement; *C,* invasion through the muscularis with regional node metastasis; and *D,* tumor metastasis to distant sites. See illustration.

Dukes' disease (dooks) a febrile disease of childhood marked by a characteristic skin rash; it is probably a mild form of scarlet fever.

dullness (dul′nes) a quality of sound elicited by percussion, being short and high-pitched with little resonance.

dumping syndrome nausea, weakness, sweating, palpitation, syncope, often a sensation of warmth, and sometimes diarrhea, occurring after ingestion of food in patients who have had partial GASTRECTOMY (see surgery of the stomach at STOMACH).

Patient Care. The symptoms experienced during dumping syndrome often are greater after ingestion of highly concentrated and refined carbohydrate foods. Hence the patient is instructed to avoid eating concentrated carbohydrates such as those in desserts and cereals sweetened with granulated sugar. To minimize the effects of the sudden entrance of large amounts of food into the jejunum, small, frequent meals are better than three large ones. Since fluids add to the volume of food ingested in a meal, the patient is encouraged to drink a limited amount of liquid during the meal and to avoid drinking fluids for an hour or two afterward. It also may be helpful for the patient to lie down and relax for about 30 minutes after eating.

duodenal (doo″o-de′nal) of or pertaining to the duodenum.

duodenectomy (doo″o-dě-nek′tah-me) excision of the duodenum, total or partial.

duodenitis (doo-od″ě-ni′tis) inflammation of the duodenum.

duodenocholedochotomy (doo″o-de″no-ko-led″ah-kot′ah-me) incision of the duodenum and common bile duct.

duodenoenterostomy (doo″o-de″no-en″ter-os′tah-me) anastomosis of the duodenum to some other part of the small intestine.

duodenography (doo″o-dě-nog′rah-fe) radiography of the duodenum.

duodenohepatic (doo″o-de″no-hě-pat′ik) pertaining to the duodenum and liver.

duodenoileostomy (doo″o-de″no-il′e-os′tah-me) anastomosis of the duodenum to the ileum.

Stage	Features	5-year survival
A	Tumor confined to the mucosa	90–95%
B1	Tumor growth into muscularis propria	75–80%
B2	Tumor growth through muscularis propria and serosa (full thickness)	60%
C1	Tumor spread to 1–4 regional lymph nodes	25–30%
C2	Tumor spread to more than 4 regional lymph nodes	
D	Distant metastases (liver, lung, bones)	<1%

Modified Dukes' staging system for colorectal cancer. From Aspinall and Taylor-Robinson, 2001.

duodenojejunostomy (doo″o-de″no-je″joo-nos′tah-me) anastomosis of the duodenum to the jejunum.

duodenorrhaphy (doo″o-dĕ-nor′ah-fe) suture of the duodenum.

duodenoscopy (doo″o-dĕ-nos′kah-pe) examination of the duodenum by an endoscope.

duodenostomy (doo″o-dĕ-nos′tah-me) surgical formation of a permanent opening into the duodenum.

duodenotomy (doo″o-dĕ-not′ah-me) incision of the duodenum.

duodenum (doo″o-de′num) the first or proximal portion of the small intestine, about 25 cm (10 inches) long, extending from the pylorus to the jejunum. It plays an important role in digestion of food because both the common bile duct and the pancreatic duct empty into it. It is subject to various disorders, the most common of which are PEPTIC ULCERS and obstruction due to dilatation of the intestine and stasis of the duodenal contents. The duodenum also may be the site of diverticula, fistulas, and occasionally tumors. See also DIGESTIVE SYSTEM.

duplication (doo-pli-ka′shun) 1. a doubling; in genetics, the presence of an extra segment of chromosome. See also REPEAT. 2. the process of copying a radiograph. 3. abnormal doubling of a body part.

dupp (dup) a syllable used to represent, or mimic, the second HEART SOUND.

durable power of attorney for health care advance directives.

dural (du′ral) pertaining to the dura mater.

dura mater (du′rah ma′ter) [L.] the outermost, toughest, and most fibrous of the three membranes (meninges) covering the brain and spinal cord.

Durand-Nicolas-Favre disease (du-ran′-ne-ko-lah′fav′r) lymphogranuloma venereum.

duroarachnitis (du″ro-ar″ak-ni′tis) inflammation of the dura mater and arachnoid.

Duroziez's disease (du-ro″ze-āz′) congenital mitral stenosis.

Duroziez's sign (du-ro″ze-āz′) Duroziez's MURMUR.

dust (dust) fine, dry particles of earth or any other substance small enough to be blown by the wind. See also CONIOSIS and PNEUMOCONIOSIS.

blood d. hemoconia.

Duvoid (doo′void) trademark for preparations of BETHANECHOL chloride, a smooth muscle RELAXANT used to treat urinary retention.

(dV/dt)max the most rapid rate of voltage change; in cellular electrophysiology it applies to phase 0 of the ACTION POTENTIAL.

DVM Doctor of Veterinary Medicine.

dwarf (dworf) an abnormally undersized person; see also *dwarfism.* adj., **dwar′fish.**

hypophysial d. pituitary dwarf.

hypothyroid d. a dwarf with HYPOTHYROIDISM or CRETINISM. See DWARFISM.

infantile d. a dwarf with INFANTILISM.

normal d. an individual who is undersized but perfectly formed.

pituitary d. a person with pituitary DWARFISM; called also hypophyseal dwarf.

renal d. a person with renal DWARFISM.

dwarfism (dwor′fizm) underdevelopment of the body; the state of being a DWARF. It may be the result of a developmental ANOMALY, of nutritional or hormone deficiencies, or of other diseases. The size of pygmies found in some parts of the world, such as the Philippines and equatorial Africa, is not the result of dwarfism; their small stature is a hereditary trait. Called also nanism and nanosomia. A dwarf in adulthood may be as small as 75 cm (30 inches) tall. The proportions of body to head and limbs may be normal or abnormal. In certain conditions the body may be deformed or the person may suffer from mental retardation.

ACHONDROPLASIA is a developmental anomaly that affects the growth of the bones.

The person's trunk is usually normal, but the head is unusually large and the limbs unusually small. Most fetuses with achondroplastic dwarfism are stillborn. Those who reach adulthood do not suffer lessening of their mental or sexual abilities, and may have unusual muscular strength. The condition does not significantly shorten the life span.

An infant who suffers from an insufficiency of THYROXINE, a hormone secreted by the thyroid gland, may develop the symptoms of CRETINISM, including an enlarged head, short limbs, puffy eyes, a thick and protruding tongue, dry skin, and lack of coordination. This can be treated by giving the patient an extract of thyroxine; early treatment can result in normal growth and development. If the condition is not treated, however, the child will grow up dwarfed, mentally retarded, and sexually sterile.

Pituitary dwarfism occurs when the pituitary gland does not produce enough growth HORMONE. This hormone plays a major role in growth of the skeleton and viscera; if it is not produced in large enough quantities, growth of the trunk will be curtailed, and the head and limbs will be in normal proportion to the small torso. Administration of purified human growth hormone has been shown to induce skeletal growth in these patients.

achondroplastic d. dwarfism due to ACHONDROPLASIA; see *dwarfism.*

pituitary d. dwarfism due to inadequate secretion of growth HORMONE by the PITUITARY GLAND; see DWARFISM.

renal d. dwarfism caused by RENAL FAILURE.

rhizomelic d. the autosomal recessive form of CHONDRODYSPLASIA PUNCTATA.

Dx diagnosis.

Dy dysprosium.

Dyazide (di'ah-zīd) trademark for a preparation of TRIAMTERENE and HYDROCHLOROTHIAZIDE, an ANTIHYPERTENSIVE AGENT.

dyclonine (di'klo-nēn) a bactericidal and fungicidal local anesthetic, used topically as the hydrochloride salt.

dydrogesterone (di''dro-jes'ter-ōn) an orally effective, synthetic PROGESTIN used mainly in the diagnosis and treatment of primary amenorrhea and severe dysmenorrhea, and in combination with ESTROGEN in dysfunctional menorrhagia.

dye (di) any of various colored substances containing auxochromes and thus capable of coloring substances to which they are applied; used for staining and coloring, as test reagents, and as therapeutic agents.

dying (di'ing) the last stage of life; a process that from a medical point of view begins when a person has a disorder that is untreatable and inevitably ends in DEATH, or the final stages of a fatal disease. Dying is a process, whereas death is an event. The essential task of the dying person is to work through psychologic responses toward the reality of approaching death to a final and peaceful acceptance of that reality.

Stages of Dying. Dr. Elisabeth Kübler-Ross, a psychiatrist, formulated a stage theory of dying. These stages represent the adaptive strategies of a dying person who is trying to come to grips with the finality of his or her terminal illness. Not every dying person proceeds through these stages in accordance with the proposed sequence; many alternate between one stage and another. Sometimes a patient will appear to have moved toward acceptance only to regress toward denial in response to some event. Dying is unique to the individual; no two people have the same life experiences or the same inner resources to deal with the vagaries of life and its inevitable end. However, being aware of what people who confront death have in common can be of benefit to those who care for them throughout the dying process.

The stages proposed by Kübler-Ross are not limited to adaptation to dying; they may also apply to anyone who has to deal with profound, unwanted change. Every change involves some loss, the end of something familiar and the beginning of something new. Unhappiness with the change can trigger denial and other psychologic responses that delay acceptance. The stages are *denial and disbelief, anger, bargaining, depression,* and *acceptance.*

Dr. George Engel proposed the theory that grief over the loss of a loved one brings about psychologic responses not too different from those exhibited by persons who are themselves dying. Moreover, it has been noted that severely handicapped and disabled persons who must change their lifestyle to accommodate the effects of illness or injury might also go through a process in which they move toward acceptance of a new self and a new way of life.

John Bowlby and C. Murray Parkes also described stages of grief, outlining four dimensions: (1) shock and numbness, (2) yearning and searching, (3) disorientation and disorganization, and (4) resolution and reorganization. These do not follow any particular order, and the stages may overlap.

Partnership for Caring is an educational council that provides programs tailored to meet the needs of laypersons and professional caregivers coping with the problems of terminal care. It also is the source of the Living Will and addresses legal and medical issues related to death and dying. Their mailing address is Partnership for Caring, 1620 Eye Street NW, Suite 202, Washington DC 20006, and their Internet web site is http://www.partnershipforcaring. org. Their telephone numbers are 202-296-8071 and 800-989-9455.

Dymelor (di′mĕ-lor) trademark for a preparation of ACETOHEXAMIDE, an oral hypoglycemic AGENT.

dynamic (di-nam′ik) pertaining to or manifesting force.

dynamics (di-nam′iks) 1. the scientific study of forces in action; a phase of mechanics. 2. the motivating or driving forces, physical or moral, in any field.

group d. the forces that underlie group interaction; the interactions among group members.

dynamograph (di-nam′o-graf) a self-registering dynamometer.

dynamometer (di″nah-mom′ĕ-ter) an instrument for measuring the force of muscular contraction.

dyne (dīn) a unit of force, being the amount that when acting continuously upon a mass of 1 g will impart to it an acceleration of 1 cm per second per second. It is equal to 10^{-5} newton.

dynein (di′ne-in) a protein from the microtubules of cilia and flagella, which functions as an ATP-splitting enzyme and is essential to the motility of cilia and flagella.

dyphilline (di-fil′in) a THEOPHYLLINE derivative used as a BRONCHODILATOR in the treatment of bronchial asthma or bronchospasm associated with chronic bronchitis or emphysema.

dys- word element [Gr.], *bad; difficult; disordered.*

dysacousia (dis″ah-koo′se-ah) **dysacousis** (dis″ah-koo′sis) dysacusis.

dysacusis (dis″ah-koo′sis) 1. a hearing impairment in which the loss is not measurable in decibels, as in disturbances in discrimination of speech or tone quality, pitch, or loudness. 2. a condition in which certain sounds produce discomfort.

dysaphia (dis-a′fe-ah) impairment of the sense of touch.

dysarthria (dis-ahr′thre-ah) imperfect articulation of speech due to disturbances of muscular control resulting from central or peripheral nervous system damage.

dysarthrosis (dis″ahr-thro′sis) 1. deformity or malformation of a joint. 2. dysarthria.

dysautonomia (dis″aw-to-no′me-ah) malfunction of the AUTONOMIC NERVOUS SYSTEM.

familial d. Riley-Day syndrome.

dysbarism (dis′bar-izm) any clinical syndrome caused by difference between the surrounding atmospheric pressure and the total gas pressure in the various tissues, fluids, and cavities of the body, including such conditions as barosinusitis, barotitis media, or expansion of gases in the hollow viscera.

dysbasia (dis-ba′ze-ah) difficulty in walking, especially that due to a nervous lesion.

dysbetalipoproteinemia (dis-ba″tah-lip″o-pro″tēn-e′me-ah) the accumulation of abnormal low-density LIPOPROTEINS (β-lipoproteins) in the blood.

familial d. familial HYPERLIPOPROTEINEMIA, type III.

dyscephaly (dis-sef′ah-le) malformation of the cranium and bones of the face. adj., **dyscephal′ic.**

dyschiria (dis-ki′re-ah) loss of power to tell which side of the body has been touched.

dyscholia (dis-ko′le-ah) a disordered condition of the bile.

dyschondroplasia (dis″kon-dro-pla′zhah) enchondromatosis.

dyschromatopsia (dis″kro-mah-top′se-ah) disorder of color vision.

dyschromia (dis-kro′me-ah) any disorder of pigmentation of the skin or hair.

dyschronism (dis-kro′nizm) separate in time; disturbance of any time relation.

dyscontrol syndrome (dis″kon-trōl′) a pattern of episodic, abnormal, and often violent and uncontrollable social behavior with little or no provocation; it may result from diseases of the limbic system or the temporal lobe or may accompany abuse of alcohol or other psychoactive substance.

dyscoria (dis-ko′re-ah) abnormality in shape or form of the pupil or in the reaction of the two pupils.

dyscorticism (dis-kor′tĭ-sizm) disordered functioning of the adrenal cortex.

dyscrasia (dis-kra′zhah) a condition related to a disease or pathologic state, usually referring to an imbalance of component elements. adj., **dyscrat′ic.**

blood d. a pathologic condition of the blood, usually referring to a disorder of the cellular elements of the blood.

plasma cell d′s a diverse group of neoplastic diseases involving proliferation of a single clone of cells producing a serum M component (a monoclonal IMMUNOGLOBULIN or immunoglobulin fragment); the cells usually have plasma CELL morphology, but may have lymphocytic or lymphoplasmacytic morphology. The group includes

MULTIPLE MYELOMA, Waldenström's MACROGLOB-ULINEMIA, the HEAVY CHAIN DISEASES, benign monoclonal GAMMOPATHY, and immunocytic AMYLOIDOSIS. Called also paraproteinemias and monoclonal gammopathies.

dyseidetic (dis″i-det′ik) DYSLEXIC regarding the sight or recognition of whole words.

dysembryoma (dis″em-bre-o′mah) teratoma.

dysencephalia splanchnocystica (disen″sĕ-fa′lyah splank″no-sis′tĭ-kah) Meckel-Gruber syndrome.

dysentery (dis′en-ter″e) any of a number of disorders marked by inflammation of the intestine, especially of the colon, with abdominal pain, tenesmus, and frequent stools often containing blood and mucus. The causative agent may be chemical irritants, bacteria, protozoa, viruses, or parasitic worms. adj., **dysenter′ic.** Dysentery is less prevalent today than in years past because of improved sanitary facilities throughout the world; it was formerly a common occurrence in crowded parts of the world and it particularly plagued army camps. It can be dangerous to infants, children, the elderly, and others who are in a weakened condition. In dysentery, there is an unusually fluid discharge of stool from the bowels, as well as fever, stomach cramps, and spasms of involuntary straining to evacuate, with the passage of little feces. The stool is often mixed with pus and mucus and may be streaked with blood.

 amebic d. see AMEBIC DYSENTERY.

 bacillary d. see BACILLARY DYSENTERY.

 viral d. a form caused by a virus, occurring in epidemics and marked by acute watery diarrhea. It is common in travelers who have eaten raw salads or fruit, or used contaminated tableware. With proper care, it should subside in 12 to 72 hours.

dysequilibrium (dis-e″kwĭ-lib′re-um) 1. any derangement of the SENSE OF EQUILIBRIUM; see also DIZZINESS and VERTIGO. 2. disturbance of a state of EQUILIBRIUM. Spelled also disequilibrium.

 dialysis d. DIALYSIS DYSEQUILIBRIUM SYNDROME.

dyserethesia (dis″er-ĕ-the′zhah) 1. impairment of sensibility. 2. an unpleasant abnormal sensation produced by a stimulus.

dysergia (dis-er′jah) motor incoordination due to defect of efferent nerve impulse.

dyserythropoiesis defective development of erythrocytes, such as ANISOCYTOSIS and POIKILOCYTOSIS.

dysesthesia (dis″es-the′zhah) 1. impairment of any sense, especially of the sense of touch. 2. a painful, persistent sensation induced by a gentle touch of the skin.

dysfibrogenemia (dis-fi″bro-jě-ne′me-ah) the presence in the blood of abnormal fibrinogen; both autosomal dominant and recessive forms are known.

dysfluency (dis-floo′enāse) the quality of being DYSFLUENT.

dysfluent (dis-floo′ent) proceeding with difficulty; said of SPEECH DISORDERS such as STUTTERING.

dysfunction (dis-fungk′shun) disturbance, impairment, or abnormality of functioning of an organ. adj., **dysfunc′tional.**

 erectile d. impotence.

 minimal brain d. former name for ATTENTION-DEFICIT/HYPERACTIVITY DISORDER.

 risk for peripheral neurovascular d. a NURSING DIAGNOSIS accepted by the North American Nursing Diagnosis Association, defined as being at risk for disruption in circulation, sensation, or motion of an extremity or limb.

 sexual d. see SEXUAL DYSFUNCTION.

dysgammaglobulinemia (dis-gam″mah-glob″u-lin-e′me-ah) an immunological deficiency state marked by selective deficiencies of one or more, but not all, classes of IMMUNOGLOBULINS, resulting in heightened susceptibility to those infectious diseases vulnerable to immunoglobulin-associated defense mechanisms. adj., **dysgammaglobuline′mic.**

dysgenesis (dis-jen′ě-sis) 1. defective development; see also DYSPLASIA and MALFORMATION.

 gonadal d. 1. defective development of the GONADS. 2. TURNER'S SYNDROME and its variants.

dysgerminoma (dis-jer″mĭ-no′mah) a solid, often radiosensitive, malignant ovarian neoplasm derived from undifferentiated germinal cells; the counterpart of SEMINOMA of the testis.

dysgeusia (dis-gu′ze-ah) distortion of the sense of taste.

dysglycemia (dis″gli-se′me-ah) any disorder of blood sugar metabolism.

dysgonic (dis-gon′ik) seeding badly; said of bacterial cultures that grow poorly.

dysgraphia (dis-gra′fe-ah) inability to write properly; it may be part of a language disorder due to disturbance of the parietal lobe or of the motor system.

dyshematopoiesis (dis-hem″ah-to-poi-e′sis) defective blood formation. adj., **dyshematopoiet′ic.**

dyshesion (dis-he′zhun) 1. disordered cell adherence. 2. loss of intercellular cohesion; a characteristic of malignancy.

dyshidrosis (dis-hĭ-dro′sis) 1. any disorder of the eccrine SWEAT GLANDS. 2. former name for pompholyx.

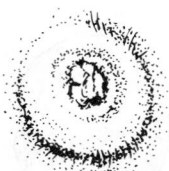

Warty dyskeratoma. From Dorland's, 2000.

dyskaryosis (dis″kar-e-o′sis) abnormality of the nucleus of a cell. adj., **dyskaryot′ic.**

dyskeratoma (dis″ker-ah-to′mah) a tumor from the KERATINOCYTES, characterized by abnormal, imperfect, or premature keratin development. See illustration.

warty d. a solitary brownish red nodule with a soft, yellowish, central keratotic plug, most commonly occurring on the face, neck, scalp, or axilla, or in the mouth; histologically it resembles an individual lesion of KERATOSIS FOLLICULARIS.

dyskeratosis (dis″ker-ah-to′sis) abnormal, premature, or imperfect development of the KERATINOCYTES. adj., **dyskeratot′ic.**

dyskinesia (dis-ki-ne′zhah) impairment of the power of voluntary movement.

primary ciliary d. any of a group of hereditary syndromes characterized by delayed or absent mucociliary clearance from the airways; often there is also lack of motion of sperm. One variety is KARTAGENER'S SYNDROME.

tardive d. an iatrogenic disorder produced by long-term administration of ANTIPSYCHOTIC AGENTS; it is characterized by oral-lingual-buccal dyskinesias that usually resemble continual chewing motions with intermittent darting movements of the tongue; there may also be choreoathetoid movements of the extremities. The disorder is more common in women than in men and in the elderly than in the young, and incidence is related to drug dosage and duration of treatment. In some patients symptoms disappear within several months after antipsychotic drugs are withdrawn; in others symptoms may persist indefinitely.

dyslalia (dis-la′le-ah) impairment of ability to speak associated with abnormality of external speech organs.

dyslexia (dis-lek′se-ah) inability to read, spell, and write words, despite the ability to see and recognize letters; a familial disorder with autosomal dominant inheritance that occurs more frequently in males. adj., **dyslex′ic.**

dyslipidemia (dis-lip″id-e′me-ah) abnormality in, or abnormal amounts of, lipids and lipoproteins in the blood; see HYPERLIPIDEMIA and HYPOLIPIDEMIA.

dyslipoproteinemia (dis-lip″o-pro″tēn-e′me-ah) the presence of abnormal concentrations of LIPOPROTEINS, or of abnormal lipoproteins, in the blood. See also HYPERLIPOPROTEINEMIA and HYPOLIPOPROTEINEMIA.

dyslogia (dis-lo′jah) impairment of speech due to a mental disorder.

dysmaturity (dis″mah-choor′ĭ-te) the condition in a fetus of being small or immature for gestational age with malnourishment and evidence of chronic stress in utero; usually seen in a postterm pregnancy.

pulmonary d. Wilson-Mikity syndrome.

dysmelia (dis-me′le-ah) malformation of a limb or limbs due to disturbance in embryonic development.

dysmenorrhea (dis″men-ŏ-re′ah) painful MENSTRUATION with cramps in the lower abdomen. adj., **dysmenorrhe′al.** *Primary dysmenorrhea* is painful menstruation with no detectable organic disease. *Secondary dysmenorrhea* is painful menstruation due to some pelvic pathology, such as ENDOMETRIOSIS PELVIC INFLAMMATORY DISEASE, or PROLAPSE OF THE UTERUS. Relief can often be obtained by simple hygienic measures such as adequate rest, avoidance of constipation, moderate exercise, applications of moderate heat to the abdomen, and removal of restricting clothing. See also PREMENSTRUAL SYNDROME.

Treatment. Severe primary dysmenorrhea requires more aggressive therapy. Drugs that may be helpful include ibuprofen (Motrin and Rufen), mefenamic acid (Ponstel), and naproxen sodium (Anaprox). Use of these drugs is not recommended for nursing mothers or in pregnancy. They also often have side effects related to irritation of the gastrointestinal tract. Taking the drug with meals or a glass of milk can mitigate the irritation. If the patient is not trying to conceive, preventive therapy, rather than symptomatic relief with analgesics, is the preferred mode of treatment. Because prostaglandins are known to produce increased uterine contractions and the cramping typical of dysmenorrhea, inhibition of ovulation can decrease endometrial production of prostaglandins and the concurrent increase in uterine activity. Therefore, oral contraceptives often prove to be effective. Similarly, prostaglandin synthetase inhibitors can provide relief in about 90 per cent of the cases if administration of medication is supplemented with patient education and reassurance. Therapy with these drugs can begin with the onset of bleeding, thus avoiding inadvertent intake of prostaglandin synthetase inhibitors in early pregnancy.

congestive d. that accompanied by great congestion of the uterus.

essential d. painful menstruation for which there is no demonstrable cause.

inflammatory d. that due to inflammation.

obstructive d. that due to mechanical obstruction to the discharge of menstrual fluid.

dysmetria (dis-me′tre-ah) inability to properly direct or limit motions.

dysmnesia (dis-ne′zhah) disordered memory; as in the AMNESTIC SYNDROME. adj. **dysmnes′tic.**

dysmorphism (dis-mor′fizm) 1. an abnormality in the development of form or structure. 2. ability to appear under different morphological forms. adj., **dysmor′phic.**

dysmorphophobia (dis-mor″fo-fo′be-ah) body dysmorphic disorder.

dysmyelination (dis-mi′ĕ-lin-a′shun) breakdown or defective formation of a myelin SHEATH, usually involving biochemical abnormalities.

dysmyotonia (dis″mi-o-to′ne-ah) muscular dystonia; abnormal tonicity.

dysontogenesis (dis″on-to-jen′ĕ-sis) defective embryonic development. adj., **dysontogenet′ic.**

dysopia (dis-o′pe-ah) defective vision.

dysorexia (dis″o-rek′se-ah) impaired or deranged appetite.

dysosmia (dis-oz′me-ah) distortion of the sense of smell.

dysostosis (dis″os-to′sis) defective ossification; a defect in the normal ossification of fetal cartilages.

cleidocranial d. an autosomal dominant condition in which there is defective ossification of the cranial bones, complete or partial absence of the clavicles, so that the shoulders may be brought together, or nearly together, in front, and dental and vertebral anomalies. See illustration.

craniofacial d. an autosomal dominant condition marked by a pointed or conical skull, protruding wide-set eyes, strabismus, parrot-beaked nose, and hypoplastic maxilla with relative mandibular prognathism. Called also Crouzon's disease.

mandibulofacial d. a hereditary disorder occurring in two different forms: the complete form is FRANCESCHETTI SYNDROME and the incomplete form is TREACHER COLLINS SYNDROME. Persons with the condition have downslanting eyes (ANTIMONGOLOID palpebral fissures); absence of all or part of the lower lid; underdeveloped cheekbones that appear depressed; a prominent nose, wide mouth, and small receding chin; underdeveloped,

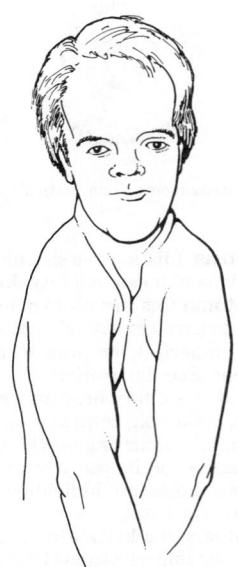

Cleidocranial dysostosis. From Dorland's, 2000.

malformed, or prominent ears; and small tufts of hair in front of the ears. There is often, but not always, some degree of HEARING LOSS, usually conductive.

metaphyseal d. a skeletal abnormality in which the epiphyses are normal or nearly so, and the metaphyseal tissues are replaced by masses of cartilage, producing interference with endochondral bone formation and expansion and thinning of the metaphyseal cortices.

orodigitofacial d. orofaciodigital syndrome.

dyspareunia (dis″pah-roo′ne-ah) difficult or painful sexual INTERCOURSE.

dyspepsia (dis-pep′se-ah) impairment of the power or function of digestion; usually applied to epigastric discomfort after meals. adj., **dyspep′tic.**

acid d. dyspepsia associated with excessive acidity of the stomach.

nonulcer d. dyspepsia in which the symptoms resemble those of peptic ulcer, although no ulcer can be detected. Because many patients with nonulcer dyspepsia have a *Helicobacter pylori* infection, *H. pylori* has been suggested as a cause. This has not been proven, however, and many patients still have dyspepsia after antibiotic treatment.

dysphagia (dis-fa′jah) difficulty in SWALLOWING; see also APHAGIA. There are numerous underlying causes, including stroke and other neurologic conditions, local trauma and muscle damage, and a tumor or swelling that partially obstructs the passage of food. The condition can range from mild discomfort, such as a feeling that there is a lump in the throat, to a severe inability to control the muscles needed for chewing and swallowing. Dysphagia can seriously compromise the nutritional status of a patient. Temporary measures such as TUBE FEEDING and PARENTERAL NUTRITION can remedy the immediate problem, but long-term goals for rehabilitation must focus on helping the patient recover the ability to swallow sufficient amounts of food and drink to assure adequate nutrition.

Measures intended to accomplish the goal of oral feeding are implemented only after determining the particular techniques that are most helpful for the individual patient. In general, placing the patient in an upright position, providing a pleasant and calm environment, being sure the lips are closed as the patient begins to swallow, and preparing and serving foods of the proper consistency are all helpful techniques. Stroke victims who have difficulty swallowing should be turned, or should turn their heads, to the unaffected side to facilitate swallowing. If dry mouth is a problem, there are artificial salivas available to moisten and lubricate the mouth. When drinking fluids, dysphagic patients should sip the liquid in small amounts.

esophageal d. dysphagia caused by an abnormality in the esophagus, such as a smooth muscle disorder that interferes with peristalsis or an obstruction from external compression or a stricture.

oropharyngeal d. dysphagia caused by difficulty in initiating the swallowing process, so that solids and liquids cannot move out of the mouth properly.

dysphasia (dis-fa′zhah) impairment of speech consisting in lack of coordination and failure to arrange words in their proper order; due to a central lesion; see also APHASIA. Called also dysphrasia.

dysphonia (dis-fo′ne-ah) any voice impairment; difficulty in speaking. adj., **dysphon′ic.**

d. clerico′rum clergyman's SORE THROAT.

dysphoria (dis-for′e-ah) [Gr.] disquiet; restlessness; malaise. adj. **dysphoret′ic, dysphor′ic.**

gender d. unhappiness with one's biological sex or its usual gender role, with the desire for the body and role of the opposite sex.

dysphrasia (dis-fra′zhah) dysphasia.

dyspigmentation (dis″pig-men-ta′shun) any abnormality of pigmentation of the skin or hair.

dysplasia (dis-pla′zhah) an abnormality of development; in pathology, alteration in size, shape, and organization of adult cells. See also DYSGENESIS. adj., **dysplas′tic.**

bronchopulmonary d. chronic lung disease of premature infants with hyaline membrane disease who have needed high concentrations of oxygen and assisted ventilation. Factors related to its development include alveolar damage due to hyaline membrane disease, oxygen toxicity, positive pressure ventilation, and endotracheal intubation. Treatment includes supportive measures and oxygen therapy. Recovery and normal pulmonary function usually occur by the age of 6 months to 1 year; however, some infants may exhibit limited tolerance to exercise.

craniometaphyseal d. metaphyseal dysplasia associated with overgrowth of the head bones, leonine FACIES, and increased distance between the eyes. (See illustration.)

cretinoid d. a developmental abnormality characteristic of cretinism, consisting of retarded ossification and smallness of the internal and reproductive organs.

cystic renal d. renal DYSPLASIA in which there are cysts.

developmental d. of the hip (DDH) instability of the hip joint leading to dislocation in the neonatal period. Although it may be associated with various neuromuscular disorders, such as myelodysplasia, or occur in utero, it most commonly occurs in neurologically normal infants and is multifactorial in origin. Usually there is laxity of the hip ligaments. Most affected infants are first-born children and 30 to 50 per cent present in the breech position. About 90 per cent of those affected are girls. The condition was formerly called congenital dislocation of the hip, but because the dislocation is not normally present at birth

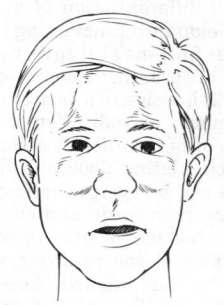

Craniometaphyseal dysplasia. From Dorland's, 2000.

but develops later, the term developmental dysplasia of the hip is preferred.

ectodermal d. any of a group of hereditary disorders involving absence or deficiency of tissues and structures derived from the embryonic ECTODERM, such as teeth, hair, nails, and certain glands.

fibromuscular d. dysplasia with fibrosis of the muscular layer of an artery wall, with collagen deposition and hyperplasia of smooth muscle, causing stenosis and hypertension. It most commonly occurs in the renal arteries and is a major cause of renovascular HYPERTENSION.

fibrous d. of bone thinning of the cortex of bone and replacement of bone marrow by gritty fibrous tissue containing bony spicules, causing pain, disability, and gradually increasing deformity; it may affect a single bone (monostotic fibrous dysplasia) or several or many bones (polyostotic fibrous dysplasia). When associated with melanotic pigmentation of the skin and endocrine disorders, it is known as ALBRIGHT'S SYNDROME.

metaphyseal d. a disturbance in enchondral bone growth, failure of modeling causing the ends of the shafts to remain larger than normal in circumference.

oculodentodigital d. a rare hereditary condition, characterized by bilateral microphthalmos, abnormally small nose with anteverted nostrils, hypotrichosis, dental anomalies, camptodactyly, syndactyly, and missing phalanges of the toes.

renal d. a congenital disorder of the kidney, with persistence of cartilage, undifferentiated mensenchyme, and immature collecting tubules, as well as with abnormal lobar organization and nearly always cysts; it may be unilateral or bilateral and total or subtotal. Total bilateral dysplasia is rapidly fatal in the neonatal period, while milder disease may be asymptomatic.

retinal d. a general term for a congenital defect resulting from the abnormal growth and differentiation of a retina that fails to develop into functioning tissue.

dyspnea (disp-ne'ah) breathlessness or shortness of breath; labored or difficult BREATHING. It is a sign of a variety of disorders and is primarily an indication of inadequate ventilation or of insufficient amounts of oxygen in the circulating blood. adj., **dyspne'ic.**

Dyspnea can be symptomatic of a variety of disorders, both acute and chronic. Acute conditions include acute infections and inflammations of the respiratory tract, obstruction by an inhaled foreign object, anaphylactic swelling of the tracheal and bronchial mucosa, and traumatic injury to the chest. Chronic disorders usually fall into the category of CHRONIC AIRFLOW LIMITATION, or are associated with pulmonary EDEMA and congestive HEART FAILURE. A fat embolism resulting from the release of fat particles from bone marrow at the time of a fracture of a long bone also can cause dyspnea.

PATIENT CARE. The dyspneic patient has some degree of difficulty in meeting the basic physiologic need for adequate levels of oxygen in the blood and the transportation of that oxygen to all cells of the body. Whatever the cause of dyspnea, the plan of care begins with treating the patient and providing adequate oxygenation.

A thorough assessment of the patient's condition is necessary in order to ascertain the extent of the problem and the urgency of the need. A current and past history are obtained and a physical examination completed as soon as possible. If the patient is acutely short of breath, corrective measures should be instituted promptly. In cases of acute respiratory distress, it may be necessary to intubate the patient, begin oxygen therapy, and obtain laboratory arterial blood gas data. If there is airway obstruction, clearing the airway is necessary, or a tracheotomy may be performed.

If the patient is suffering from an acute attack of dyspnea and has a history of chronic airflow limitation, certain nursing measures can help relieve anxiety and improve ventilation. The patient should respond favorably to a calm, reassuring manner and an explanation of what is being done to relieve the shortness of breath. High Fowler's POSITION or orthopneic POSITION with the arms resting on pillows on an overbed table will help improve chest expansion. Helping the patient relax muscles not needed for breathing conserves oxygen and promotes rest. If abdominal distention, ascites, or a massive tumor interferes with chest expansion and produces dyspnea, having the patient lie on one side and supporting the abdomen with pillows may provide some relief.

Once dyspneic patients are comfortable and less apprehensive, they may need instruction in prolonged, controlled exhalation. If they already know how to do pursed-lip breathing (inhaling slowly through the nose and exhaling slowly through pursed lips), they may need to be reminded of it and encouraged to use it to improve breathing.

Special observations and methods of assessment of a patient who has dyspnea include: auscultation of the chest for abnormal breath and voice SOUNDS, lung aeration,

RALES, and RHONCHI; inspection of the chest for respiratory rate and rhythm and for symmetrical expansion; inspection of the skin, lips, and nail beds for CYANOSIS; and percussion of the chest for abnormal RESONANCE. Results of arterial BLOOD GAS ANALYSES should be monitored and the patient observed for fatigability when engaged in various levels of activity.

exertional d. dyspnea provoked by physical effort or exertion.

functional d. respiratory distress not associated with organic disease and unrelated to exertion; often associated with anxiety states.

paroxysmal nocturnal d. respiratory distress related to posture (especially reclining at night), usually attributed to congestive HEART FAILURE with pulmonary EDEMA.

dyspragia (dis-pra′jah) painful performance of any function.

dyspraxia (dis-prak′se-ah) partial loss of ability to perform coordinated movements.

dysprosium (Dy) (dis-pro′ze-um) a chemical element, atomic number 66, atomic weight 162.50. (See Appendix 6.)

dysproteinemia (dis-pro″tēn-e′me-ah) 1. disorder of the protein content of the blood. 2. a plasma cell DYSCRASIA.

dysraphia (dis-ra′fe-ah) dysraphism.

dysraphism (dis-rāf′iz′m) incomplete closure of a RAPHE; defective fusion, particularly of the neural TUBE; see also NEURAL TUBE DEFECT.

dysreflexia (dis″re-flek′se-ah) 1. a condition of disordered response to stimuli.

autonomic d. 1. an uninhibited and exaggerated response of the autonomic nervous system to stimulation, as seen in many patients with high spinal cord injuries; see also AUTONOMIC DYSREFLEXIA. 2. a NURSING DIAGNOSIS accepted by the North American Nursing Diagnosis Association, defined as a life-threatening uninhibited sympathetic response of the nervous system to a noxious stimulus after a SPINAL CORD injury at T7 or above.

dysrhythmia (dis-rith′me-ah) disturbance of rhythm, such as of brain waves or the heartbeat.

cerebral d., electroencephalographic d. disturbance or irregularity in the rhythm of the brain waves as recorded by electroencephalography.

dyssebacia (dis″sē-ba′shah) a condition clinically indistinguishable from seborrheic dermatitis, due to alteration of the pattern of sebaceous gland retention, usually occurring as a manifestation of ARIBOFLAVINOSIS, and characterized by greasy scaling lesions involving the alae nasi, malar areas, canthi

of the eyes, and earlobes and sometimes the scrotum or vulva.

dyssomnia (dis-som′ne-ah) any of a group of primary SLEEP DISORDERS characterized by disturbances in the quality, amount, or timing of sleep, including primary INSOMNIA, primary HYPERSOMNIA, BREATHING-RELATED SLEEP DISORDER, CIRCADIAN RHYTHM SLEEP DISORDER, and NARCOLEPSY. See also PARASOMNIA.

dysspermia (dis-sper′me-ah) 1. an abnormality of the spermatozoa or of the semen. 2. difficult or painful emission of sperm or semen.

dysstasia (dis-sta′zhah) difficulty in standing. adj., **dysstat′ic.**

dyssynergia (dis″sin-er′jah) muscular incoordination.

d. cerebella′ris myoclo′nica dyssynergia cerebellaris progressiva associated with myoclonus epilepsy.

d. cerebella′ris progressi′va a condition marked by generalized intention tremors associated with disturbance of muscle tone and of muscular coordination; due to disorder of cerebellar function.

detrusor-sphincter d. contraction of the urethral sphincter muscle at the same time the detrusor muscle of the bladder is contracting, resulting in obstruction of normal urinary outflow; it may accompany detrusor hyperreflexia or instability.

dystectia (dis-tek′she-ah) defective closure of the neural tube.

dysthymia (dis-thi′me-ah) dysthymic disorder.

dysthymic disorder a chronic mood disorder characterized by depressed feeling (sad, blue, low), loss of interest or pleasure in one's usual activities, and other symptoms typical of depression but tending to be longer in duration and less severe than in major depressive disorder.

dysthyroid (dis-thi′roid) denoting defective functioning or development of the THYROID GLAND.

dystocia (dis-to′she-ah) abnormal labor or childbirth.

fetal d. that due to shape, size, or position of the fetus.

maternal d. that due to some condition inherent in the mother.

placental d. difficult delivery of the placenta.

dystonia (dis-to′ne-ah) impairment of muscular tonus. adj., **dyston′ic.**

tardive d. a variant of TARDIVE DYSKINESIA characterized by unusual posturing and movements.

dystopia (dis-to′pe-ah) malposition; displacement. adj., **dystop′ic.**

dystrophia (dis-tro'fe-ah) [Gr.] dystrophy.

d. adiposogenita'lis adiposogenital dystrophy.

d. epithelia'lis cor'neae dystrophy of the corneal epithelium, with erosions.

d. myoto'nica myotonic DYSTROPHY.

d. un'guium changes in the texture, structure, and/or color of the nails due to no demonstrable cause, but presumed by some to be attributable to some disturbance of nutrition.

dystrophoneurosis (dis-trof″o-noo-ro'sis) 1. any nervous disorder due to poor nutrition. 2. impairment of nutrition due to a nervous disorder.

dystrophy (dis'trah-fe) any disorder due to defective or faulty nutrition, especially MUSCULAR DYSTROPHY. adj., **dystroph'ic.**

adiposogenital d. adiposity of the feminine type, genital hypoplasia, changes in secondary sex characters, and metabolic disturbances; seen with lesions of the hypothalamus; see also ADIPOSOGENITAL DYSTROPHY.

Becker's muscular d., Becker type muscular d. a form closely resembling Duchenne's MUSCULAR DYSTROPHY, but having a later onset and milder course; transmitted as an X-linked recessive trait.

distal muscular d. distal myopathy.

Duchenne's muscular d., Duchenne type muscular d. The childhood type of MUSCULAR DYSTROPHY.

facioscapulohumeral muscular d. MUSCULAR DYSTROPHY affecting the face, shoulder, and upper arm muscles; called also Landouzy-Dejerine muscular dystrophy.

Landouzy-Dejerine d., Landouzy-Dejerine muscular d. facioscapulohumeral muscular dystrophy.

muscular d. see MUSCULAR DYSTROPHY.

myotonic d. a rare, slowly progressive, hereditary disease, marked by myotonia followed by muscular atrophy (especially of the face and neck), cataracts, hypogonadism, frontal balding, and cardiac disorders. Called also dystrophia myotonica, myotonia atrophica, and myotonia dystrophica.

progressive muscular d. MUSCULAR DYSTROPHY.

pseudohypertrophic muscular d. MUSCULAR DYSTROPHY affecting the shoulder and pelvic girdles, beginning in childhood and marked by increasing weakness, pseudohypertrophy of the muscles, followed by atrophy, and a peculiar swaying gait with the legs kept wide apart. Called also pseudohypertrophic muscular paralysis.

reflex sympathetic d. a syndrome of chronic pain that usually develops after a trauma or noxious stimulus, although the nerve injury cannot be immediately identified. The pain is not limited to the distribution of a single nerve and is often out of proportion to the precipitating event. It is most often described as a burning pain, and is accompanied by swelling, sweating, sensitivity to touch, and sometimes changes in tissue growth. Called also chronic or complex regional pain syndrome. Clinical practice guidelines have been published by the Reflex Sympathetic Dystrophy Syndrome Association of America and are available on their web site at http://www.rsds.org or by writing to Reflex Sympathetic Dystrophy Syndrome Association of America, P.O. Box 502, Milford CT 06460.

dysuria (dis-u're-ah) painful or difficult urination. adj., **dysu'ric.**

E

E emmetropia; enzyme; exa-.

E elastance; energy; expectancy; electromotive force; illumination.

ear (ēr) the organ of HEARING and EQUILIBRIUM. (See Plates.) It is made up of the outer (external) ear, the middle ear, and the inner (internal) ear.

The outer ear consists of the AURICLE or PINNA and the external acoustic MEATUS. The auricle collects sound waves and directs them to the external acoustic meatus; from there the waves travel through the external auditory canal to the EARDRUM (TYMPANIC MEMBRANE).

The middle ear is separated from the outer ear by the eardrum. It contains the three OSSICLES, the MALLEUS (hammer), INCUS (anvil), and STAPES (stirrup), so called because of their resemblance to these objects. These three small bones form a chain across the middle ear from the eardrum to the oval window. The stapes causes a membrane in the oval window to vibrate, and the vibrations are transmitted to the inner ear. The middle ear is connected to the nasopharynx by the EUSTACHIAN TUBE, through which the air pressure in the middle ear is equalized with the air pressure in the nose and throat. The middle ear is also connected with the cells in the mastoid bone just behind the outer ear. Two muscles attached to the ossicles contract when loud noises strike the tympanic membrane, limiting its vibration and thus protecting it and the inner ear from damage.

The inner ear (or LABYRINTH) contains the COCHLEA, as well as the nerves that transmit sound to the brain. It also contains the SEMICIRCULAR CANALS, which are essential to the SENSE OF EQUILIBRIUM.

When a sound strikes the ear it causes the tympanic membrane to vibrate. The ossicles function as levers, amplifying the motion of the tympanic membrane, and passing the vibrations on to the cochlea. From there the vestibulocochlear (eighth cranial) nerve transmits the vibrations, translated into nerve impulses, to the auditory center in the brain.

Diseases of the Ear. Infections and inflammations of the ear include OTOMYCOSIS, a fungal infection of the outer ear; OTITIS MEDIA, infection of the middle ear; and MASTOIDITIS, an infection of the mastoid cells. DEAFNESS may result from infection or from other causes such as old age, injury to the ear, hereditary factors, or conditions such as

OTOSCLEROSIS. Disorders of equilibrium may be caused by imperfect functioning of the semicircular canals or from LABYRINTHITIS, an inflammation of the inner ear. MÉNIÈRE'S DISEASE, believed to result from dilatation of the lymphatic channels in the cochlea, may also cause disturbances in balance.

Surgery of the Ear. Surgical procedures on the ear usually are indicated for chronic infection or hearing loss. An exception is MYRINGOTOMY, incision of the tympanic membrane, which is sometimes necessary to relieve pressure behind the eardrum and allow for drainage from an inflammatory process in the middle ear. Surgical procedures involving plastic reconstruction of the small bones of the middle ear are extremely delicate and have been made possible by the development of special instruments and technical equipment. STAPEDECTOMY and TYMPANOPLASTY are examples of this type of surgery, which has done much to preserve hearing that would otherwise be lost as a result of infectious destruction or sclerosis. Inner ear implants are now being performed to improve hearing in patients who have severe sensorineural hearing loss. Other surgical techniques for sensorineural hearing loss are in the developmental stage.

Patient Care. Care following surgery of the ear is aimed at preventing infection and promoting the comfort of the patient. Since the ear is so close to the brain, it is extremely important to avoid introducing pathogenic organisms into the operative site. The external ear and surrounding skin must be kept scrupulously clean. If the patient's hair is long it should be braided or arranged so that it does not come in contact with the patient's ear and side of the face. Aseptic technique must be used in all procedures carried out immediately before and after surgery.

The patient should be instructed to avoid nose blowing, especially after surgery, when there is a possibility that such an action can alter pressure within the ear. Observation of the patient after surgery of the ear includes assessing function of the facial nerve; evidence of dysfunction could include inability to wrinkle the forehead, close the eyes, pucker the lips, or bare the teeth. Any sign of facial nerve damage should be reported to the surgeon. VERTIGO is another common occurrence after surgery of the ear; it is usually only temporary and will subside as the operative site heals. The patient with

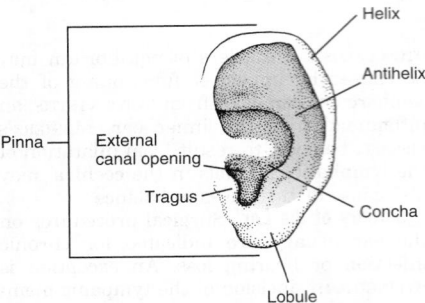

Anatomical features of the external ear. From Ignatavicius and Workman, 2002.

vertigo requires special protective measures such as side rails and support when out of bed, so as to avoid falls or other accidental injuries.

Most surgeons prefer that the dressings around the ear not be changed during the immediate postoperative period. Should excessive drainage require more dressings, these can be applied over the basic dressing. Any drainage should be noted and recorded, with excessive drainage reported immediately to the surgeon. (See also care of the patient with HEARING LOSS.)

beach e. OTITIS EXTERNA caused by irritation from ocean water and other beach conditions.

cauliflower e. a thickened and deformed ear caused by accumulation of fluid and blood clots in the tissue after repeated

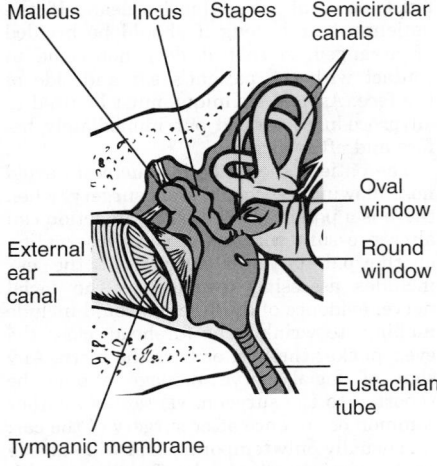

Structures of the middle ear.

injury; it is most often seen in boxers, for whom it is almost an occupational hazard. The ear will not recover its normal shape but can be restored to normal by plastic surgery.

swimmer's e., tank e. otitis externa.

earache (ēr'āk) pain in the ear; called also otalgia and otodynia.

eardrum (ēr'drum) TYMPANIC MEMBRANE.

early pregnancy test a do-it-yourself immunological PREGNANCY TEST, performed as early as 9 days after menstruation (missed period) was expected. Test materials consist of a mixture of human chorionic gonadotropin (HCG) antiserum and HCG-coated red blood cells in a glass test tube, a vial of water, and a medicine dropper.

earwax (ēr'waks) cerumen.

earwick (ēr'wik) a strip of gauze inserted into the external ear canal so that medicated drops applied to the outside pass along it and into the canal; used when the canal is obstructed by edema so that ear drops cannot be instilled.

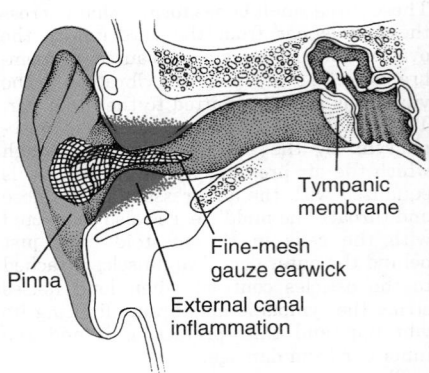

Earwick for instillation of antibiotics into the edematous external canal. From Ignatavicius and Workman, 2002.

eating (ēt'ing) the act of ingestion.

binge e. uncontrolled ingestion of large quantities of food in a given amount of time, often with a sense of lack of control over the activity. It is sometimes followed by purging.

e. disorder any in a group of disorders in which abnormal feeding habits are associated with psychological factors. Characteristics may include a distorted attitude toward eating, handling and hoarding food in unusual ways, loss of body weight, nutritional deficiencies, dental erosion, electrolyte imbalances, and denial of extreme thinness. More common conditions include ANOREXIA NERVOSA and BULIMIA NERVOSA. Persons with eating disorders of this kind characteristically misperceive themselves as either overweight or of normal weight. Eating disorders have reached epidemic proportions throughout the world, especially among women under the age of 25. The condition is seen only in countries in which food is readily available; it is not found in parts of the world where famine and starvation threaten.

Patient Care. Treatment of eating disorders usually is on an outpatient basis unless severe malnutrition and electrolyte imbalances demand aggressive therapy, severe depression and suicidal tendencies endanger the patient, or there is evidence that the patient cannot cope with daily living without resorting to abnormal eating patterns and purging. Additionally, the family and home environment may be creating unbearable tension because of a power struggle over the patient's abnormal eating pattern.

Although there are various modes of therapy for eating disorders, the goals of care are to help the patient (1) normalize eating behaviors, (2) develop a more realistic perception of his or her body and its need for food, (3) learn more healthful and effective adaptive coping mechanisms, (4) learn more about the issues and conflicts underlying the eating disorder, (5) utilize support systems more effectively, and (6) improve his or her sense of self-worth and self-esteem.

Nursing diagnostic categories that are commonly associated with eating disorders include alteration in nutrition, alteration in bowel elimination (constipation), ineffective family coping, self-care deficit (feeding), disturbance in self-concept, sexual dysfunction, spiritual distress, and role disturbance.

A holistic approach to correction of abnormal eating patterns requires an interdisciplinary approach and the cooperative and coordinated efforts of physicians, nurses, social workers, physical therapists, dieticians, and mental health workers.

Eaton-Lambert syndrome (e'ton lam'-bert) a myasthenia-like syndrome in which the weakness usually affects the limbs but ocular and bulbar muscles are spared; often associated with oat-cell carcinoma of the lung.

EBAA Eye Bank Association of America.

Ebstein's anomaly (eb'shtīnz) a malformation of the tricuspid valve, the septal and posterior leaflets being adherent to the wall of the right ventricle to a varying degree, producing tricuspid deficiency, and the anterior leaflet being normally attached to the annulus fibrosus; usually associated with an ATRIAL SEPTAL DEFECT.

eburnation (e"ber-na'shun) conversion of bone into a hard, ivory-like mass.

EBV Epstein-Barr virus.

ecaudate (e-kaw'dāt) tailless.

ecbolic (ek-bol'ik) oxytocic.

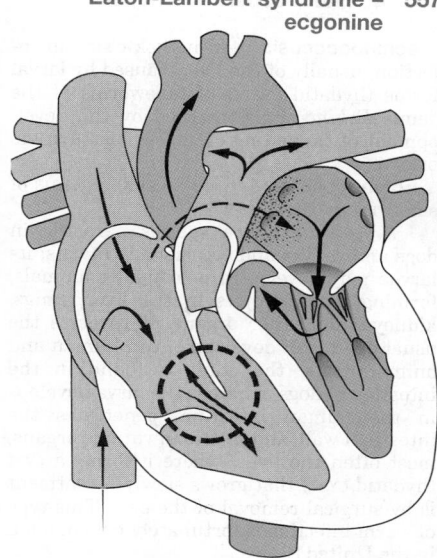

Ebstein's anomaly with tricuspid valve significantly displaced downward in the right ventricle; leakage occurs through the tricuspid valve back to the right atrium, and unoxygenated blood is shunted across the atrial-septal defect into the left atrium. From Betz et al., 1994.

ecchondroma (ek"on-dro'mah) a hyperplastic growth of cartilaginous tissue on the surface of a cartilage or projecting under the periosteum of a bone. Called also ecchondrosis.

ecchondrosis (ek"on-dro'sis) ecchondroma.

ecchymoma (ek"ĭ-mo'mah) swelling due to blood extravasation.

ecchymosis (ek"ĭ-mo'sis), pl. *ecchymo'ses* [Gr.] a hemorrhagic spot, larger than a petechia, in the skin or mucous membrane, forming a flat, rounded or irregular, blue or purplish patch. (See Atlas 2, Part R.) adj., **ecchymot'ic.**

eccrine (ek'rin) exocrine, with special reference to ordinary sweat glands.

eccritic (ek-krit'ik) 1. promoting excretion. 2. an agent that so acts.

eccyesis (ek"si-e'sis) ectopic pregnancy.

ECF extracellular fluid.

ECF-A eosinophil chemotactic factor of anaphylaxis; a primary mediator of Type I anaphylactic hypersensitivity. It is an acidic peptide (molecular weight 500) released by mast cells, which attracts eosinophils to areas where it is present.

ECG electrocardiogram.

ecgonine (ek'go-nin) the final basic product obtained by hydrolysis of COCAINE and several related alkaloids.

echinococcosis (e-ki″no-kok-o′sis) an infection, usually of the liver, caused by larval forms (hydatid CYSTS) of tapeworms of the genus *Echinococcus,* marked by the development of expanding cysts; see also HYDATID DISEASE.

Echinococcus (e-ki″no-kok′us) a genus of small TAPEWORMS.

E. granulo′sus a species parasitic in dogs and wolves and occasionally in cats; its larvae may develop in nearly all mammals, forming hydatid cysts in the liver, lungs, kidneys, and other organs. It reverses the usual process of development in human and animal hosts: the adult is found in the intestine of dogs, whereas the larva develops in the human intestine, penetrates the intestinal wall, and settles in various organs, most often the liver, where it forms a cyst (hydatid CYST) that grows slowly. Treatment is by surgical removal of the cyst. This type of worm infection is fortunately not common in the United States.

E. multilocula′ris a species whose adult forms usually parasitize the fox and wild rodents, although humans are sporadically infected. It resembles *E. granulosus,* but the larvae form alveolar or multilocular rather than unilocular cysts.

echinocyte (e-ki′no-sīt) burr cell.

echoacousia (ek″o-ah-koo′ze-ah) the subjective experience of hearing echoes after normally heard sounds.

echocardiogram (ek″o-kahr′de-o-gram″) the record produced by echocardiography.

echocardiography (ek″o-kahr″de-og′rah-fe) recording of the position and motion of the heart walls or internal structures of the heart and neighboring tissue by the echo obtained from beams of ultrasonic waves directed through the chest wall. It is based on the same principle as the oceanographic technique of depth-sounding; that is, it utilizes ULTRASOUND to delineate anatomical structures by recording on a graph the echoes from the heart structures. It is particularly useful in demonstrating, without danger to the patient, valvular and other structural deformities of the heart which formerly required CARDIAC CATHETERIZATION or some other elaborate procedure for accurate diagnosis. See also ULTRASONOGRAPHY.

Doppler e. an echocardiographic technique that records the flow of red blood cells through the cardiovascular system by means of Doppler ULTRASONOGRAPHY.

transesophageal e. (TEE) the introduction of a transducer attached to a fiberoptic endoscope into the esophagus to provide

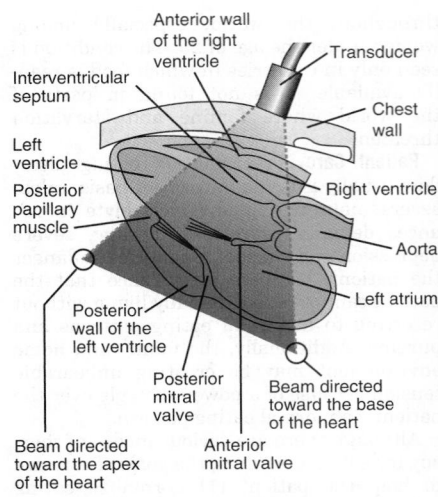

Echocardiographic imaging of the heart. From Ignatavicius and Workman, 2002.

two-dimensional cardiographic images or Doppler information. It is especially helpful in detecting enlargement of the cardiac chambers, septal defects, and pericardial effusion, and in assessing valvular function.

M-mode e. a technique in which a narrow stationary ultrasound beam is aimed through the heart and reflects back from each fluid-filled interface. The time the echo takes to return indicates the distance of the interface from the transducer. The M-mode scan thus provides a one-dimensional view that shows the motion of the heart valves and chamber walls over a period of time.

echogenic (ek″o-jen′ik) in ULTRASONOGRAPHY, giving rise to reflections (echoes) of ultrasound waves.

echography (ĕ-kog′rah-fe) ultrasonography.

echokinesis (ek″o-kĭ-ne′sis) echopraxia.

echolalia (ek″o-la′le-ah) stereotyped repetition of another person's words or phrases, seen in some cases of schizophrenia, particularly in catatonic schizophrenia, in Gilles de la Tourette's syndrome, and in neurological disorders such as transcortical aphasia.

echolucent (ek″o-loo′sent) permitting the passage of ultrasonic waves without giving rise to echoes, the representative areas appearing black on the sonogram.

echomatism (ĕ-ko′mah-tizm) echopraxia.

echomimia (ek″o-mim′e-ah) echopraxia.

echomotism (ek″o-mo′tizm) echopraxia.

echopathy (ĕ-kop′ah-the) stereotyped repetition of the words or actions of others, echolalia or echopraxia.

echophonocardiography (ek″o-fo″no-kahr″de-og′rah-fe) the combined use of echocardiography and phonocardiography.

echopraxia (ek″o-prak′se-ah) stereotyped imitation of the movements of another person; seen sometimes in catatonic schizophrenia and Gilles de la Tourette's syndrome.

echo-ranging (ek″o-rānj′ing) in ultrasonography, determination of the position or depth of a body structure on the basis of the time interval between the moment an ultrasonic pulse is transmitted and the moment its echo is received.

echothiophate (ek″o-thi″o-fāt) an ANTICHOLINESTERASE, used as the iodide salt for topical application to produce miosis, decrease intraocular pressure, and potentiate accommodation in treatment of open-angle GLAUCOMA, closed-angle glaucoma after iridectomy, and certain secondary types of glaucoma, and in the management of accommodative ESOTROPIA.

echovirus (ek′o-vi″rus) a species of viruses of the genus ENTEROVIRUS; the name was derived from the first letters of the description "enteric cytopathogenic human orphan." At the time of the isolation of the viruses the diseases they caused were not known, hence the term "orphan," but it is now known that they cause many different types of human disease, especially viral MENINGITIS, diarrhea, and various respiratory diseases.

eclampsia (e-klamp′se-ah) in pregnant women, the convulsive stage of PREECLAMPSIA-ECLAMPSIA SYNDROME; the convulsions are not attributable to other cerebral conditions such as epilepsy. It is a potentially life-threatening disorder characterized by hypertension, generalized edema, and proteinuria. Preeclampsia is a less severe, nonconvulsive form of the disorder. adj., **eclamp′tic.**

puerperal e. that occurring after or during childbirth.

uremic e. eclampsia due to uremia.

eclamptogenic (e-klamp″to-jen′ik) causing eclampsia.

ECMO extracorporeal membrane oxygenation.

ecologist (e-kol′o-jist) a specialist in ECOLOGY.

ecology (e-kol′o-je) the science of the relationship between organisms and their environments; the study of the effect of environment on the life history of organisms. adj., **ecolog′ic, ecolog′ical.**

ecomap (ek′o-map″) a family assessment tool consisting of a graphic representation of a family relationship with its environment. (See illustration.)

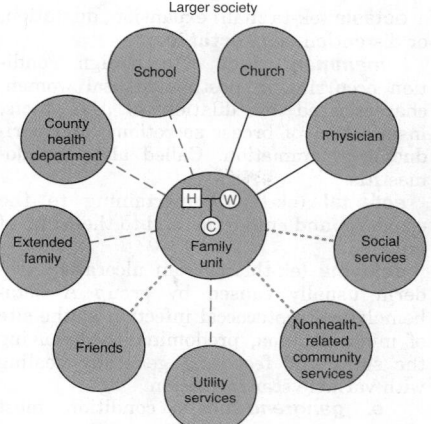

Larger society

Family ecomap of external relationships. Pictured here are but a few of the many that could be considered. Key: _____ Strong, supportive positive relationship; - - - - - Erratic, conflicted relationship, sometimes supportive and sometimes disruptive; •••• Negative, disruptive, or nonexistent relationship. From Betz et al., 1994.

econazole (ĕ-kon′ah-zōl) an IMIDAZOLE derivative used as the nitrate salt as a broad-spectrum antifungal AGENT, applied topically in the treatment of cutaneous candidiasis and various forms of TINEA.

economy (e-kon′o-me) the management of money or domestic affairs.

token e. a program of treatment in BEHAVIOR THERAPY, usually conducted in a hospital setting, in which the patient may earn tokens by engaging in appropriate personal and social behavior, or lose tokens by inappropriate or antisocial behavior; tokens may be exchanged for tangible rewards (such as food snacks or clothing) or for special privileges (such as watching television or passes to leave the hospital).

ecosystem (e″ko-sis′tem) the fundamental unit in ecology, comprising the living organisms and the nonliving elements interacting in a certain defined area.

ecotaxis (ek′o-tak″sis) the "homing" of recirculating lymphocytes to specific compartments of peripheral lymphoid tissues— B cells to B-dependent areas and T cells to T-dependent areas.

Ecstasy (ek′stah-se) popular name for 3,4-METHYLENEDIOXYMETHAMPHETAMINE, a hallucinogenic drug of abuse. See DRUG ABUSE.

ECT electroconvulsive therapy.

ect(o)- word element [Gr.], *external; outside.*

ectasia (ek-ta′zhah) expansion, dilatation, or distention. adj., **ectat′ic.**

mammary duct e. a benign condition occurring in postmenopausal women, characterized by dilation of the ducts, inspissation of breast secretions, and periductal inflammation. Called also comedomastitis.

ectental (ek-ten′t′l) pertaining to the ectoderm and entoderm, and to their line of junction.

ecthyma (ek-thi′mah) an ulcerative pyoderm usually caused by group A betahemolytic streptococcal infection at the site of minor trauma, predominantly involving the shins and feet, and generally healing with variable scar formation.

e. gangreno′sum a condition most often seen in debilitated patients in association with septicemia caused by gramnegative organisms, characterized by lesions that begin as vesicles that rapidly progress to pustulation and gangrenous ulcers with undermined purpuric edges.

ectoantigen (ek″to-an′tĭ-jen) 1. an antigen that seems to be loosely attached to the outside of bacteria. 2. an antigen formed in the ectoplasm (cell membrane) of a bacterium.

ectoblast (ek′to-blast) the ectoderm.

ectocardia (ek″to-kahr′de-ah) congenital displacement of the heart; exocardia.

ectocervix (ek″to-ser′viks) the part of the uterine cervix whose visible surface is covered with squamous epithelium. adj., **ectocer′vical.**

ectoderm (ek′to-derm) the outermost of the three primary germ layers of the embryo; from it are derived the epidermis and epidermic tissues such as nails, hair, and glands of the skin; the nervous system; external sense organs such as the eye and ear; and the mucous membranes of the mouth and anus. adj., **ectoder′mal, ectoder′mic.**

ectodermosis (ek″to-der-mo′sis) a disorder based on congenital maldevelopment of organs derived from the ectoderm.

ectoentad (ek″to-en′tad) from without inward.

ectoenzyme (ek″to-en′zīm) an extracellular enzyme.

ectogenous (ek-toj′ĕ-nus) originating outside the organism.

ectomere (ek′to-mēr) one of the blastomeres taking part in formation of the ectoderm.

ectomorph (ek′to-morf) an individual having a type of body build in which ectodermal tissues predominate: there is relatively slight development of both the visceral and body structures, the body being linear and delicate.

ectomorphy (ek′to-mor″fe) the condition of being an ectomorph. adj., **ectomor′phic.**

-ectomy word element [Gr.], *excision; surgical removal.*

ectoparasite (ek″to-par′ah-sīt) a parasite living on the surface of the host's body. adj., **ectoparasit′ic.**

ectophyte (ek′to-fīt) a vegetable parasite living on the surface of the host's body.

ectopia (ek-to′pe-ah) [L.] MALPOSITION, especially if congenital.

e. cor′dis congenital displacement of the heart outside the thoracic cavity.

e. len′tis displacement of the crystalline lens of the eye.

ectopic (ek-top′ik) 1. pertaining to or characterized by ECTOPIA. 2. located away from normal position. 3. arising or produced at an abnormal site or in a tissue where it is not normally found.

ectopy (ek′to-pe) ectopia.

ectosteal (ek-tos′te-al) pertaining to or situated outside a bone.

ectotherm (ek′to-therm″) 1. an animal that exhibits ectothermy. 2. poikilotherm.

ectothermic (ek″to-ther′mik) 1. pertaining to or characterized by ectothermy. 2. poikilothermic.

ectothermy (ek′to-ther″me) 1. the regulation of body temperature by the external environment, with thermoregulation being accomplished by the behavior of the

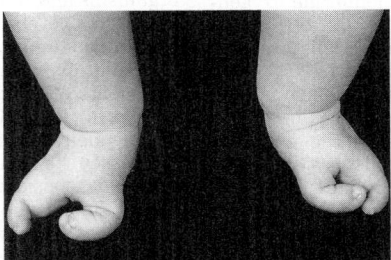

Appearance of the feet in a child with ectrodactyly. From Muller and Young, 2001.

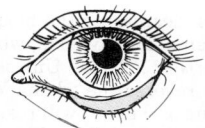
Ectropion. From Dorland's, 2000.

organism, such as seeking a different environment. 2. poikilothermy.

ectothrix (ek′to-thriks) a fungus that grows inside the shaft of a hair, but produces a conspicuous external sheath of spores.

ectozoon (ek″to-zo′on) ectoparasite.

ectr(o)- word element [Gr.], *miscarriage; congenital absence.*

ectrodactyly (ek″tro-dak′tĭ-le) congenital absence of all or part of a digit.

ectrogeny (ek-troj′ĕ-ne) congenital absence or defect of a part. adj., **ectrogen′ic.**

ectromelia (ek″tro-me′le-ah) gross hypoplasia or aplasia of one or more long bones of one or more limbs. adj., **ectromel′ic.**

ectromelus (ek-trom′ĕ-lus) an individual with rudimentary upper and lower limbs.

ectropion (ek-tro′pe-on) eversion or turning outward, as of the margin of an eyelid.

ectrosyndactyly (ek″tro-sin-dak′tĭ-le) a condition in which some digits are absent and those that remain are webbed; see also SYNDACTYLY.

eczema (ek′zĕ-mah) 1. any superficial inflammatory process involving primarily the epidermis, marked early by redness, itching, minute papules and vesicles, weeping, oozing, and crusting, and later by scaling, lichenification, and often pigmentation. 2. atopic DERMATITIS.

Eczema is a common allergic reaction in children but it also occurs in adults, usually in a more severe form. Childhood eczema often begins in infancy, the rash appearing on the face, neck, and folds of elbows and knees. It may disappear by itself when an offending food is removed from the diet, or it may become more extensive and in some instances cover the entire surface of the body. Severe eczema can be complicated by skin infections.

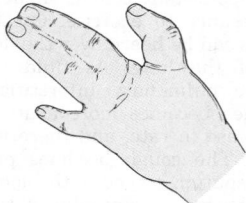
Ectrosyndactyly. From Dorland's, 2000.

Childhood eczema may persist for several years or return after the child is older. Persons suffering from childhood eczema may develop another allergic condition later, most often hay fever or asthma.

Cause and Treatment. Eczema is sometimes caused by an allergic sensitivity to foods such as milk, fish, or eggs. Inhalant allergens such as dust and pollens rarely cause eczema. Treatment involves the use of soothing baths, moisturizing creams, topical steroids, and oral antihistamines to alleviate itching. See also ALLERGY.

e. herpe′ticum disseminated herpes simplex (see KAPOSI'S VARICELLIFORM ERUPTION).

e. margina′tum tinea cruris.

e. vaccina′tum disseminated vaccinia (see KAPOSI'S VARICELLIFORM ERUPTION).

eczematoid (ek-zem′ah-toid) resembling eczema.

eczematous (ek-zem′ah-tus) characterized by or of the nature of eczema.

ED effective dose.

ED50 median effective dose.

ED90 the dose of a therapeutic agent that eradicates 90 per cent of the target pathogen.

EDC estimated (or expected) date of confinement; see NÄGELE'S RULE.

EDD estimated (or expected) date of delivery; see NÄGELE'S RULE.

edema (ĕde′mah) the accumulation of excess fluid in a fluid compartment. Formerly called dropsy and hydrops. adj., **edem′atous.** This accumulation can occur in the cells (*cellular edema*), in the intercellular spaces within tissues (*interstitial edema*), or in potential spaces within the body. Edema may also be classified by location, such as pulmonary edema or brain edema; types found in certain locations have specific names, such as ASCITES (peritoneal cavity), HYDROTHORAX (pleural cavity), or HYDROPERICARDIUM (pericardial sac). Massive generalized edema is called ANASARCA. Classification by location does not indicate whether the edema is cellular or interstitial or occupies a potential space (for example, brain edema may be either cellular or interstitial). Edema can be caused by a variety of factors, including conditions that affect osmotic pressure, such as hypotonic fluid overload, which allows the movement of water into the intracellular space, or hypoproteinemia, which decreases the concentration of plasma proteins and permits the passage of fluid out of the blood vessels into the tissue spaces. Other factors include poor lymphatic drainage; conditions that cause increased capillary pressure, such as

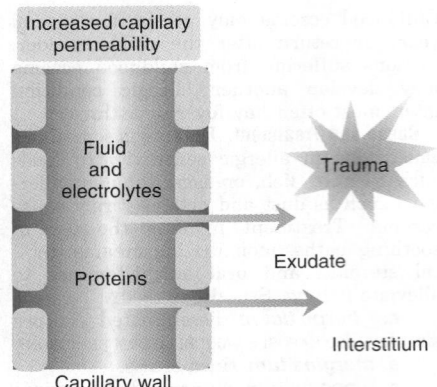

Increased capillary permeability

Fluid and electrolytes

Trauma

Proteins

Exudate

Interstitium

Capillary wall

Edema formation. With trauma, increased capillary permeability and dilation cause leaking into tissue space. Initially clear, exudate in the tissue space becomes more viscous with an increase in plasma protein. From Copstead and Banasik, 2000.

excessive retention of salt and water and heart failure; and conditions that increase capillary permeability, such as inflammation.

alveolar e. pulmonary edema in the alveoli, usually with hypoxemia and dyspnea.

brain e. cerebral edema.

cardiac e. a manifestation of congestive HEART FAILURE, due to increased venous and capillary pressures and often associated with renal sodium retention.

cellular e. edema caused by the entry of water into the cells, causing them to swell. This may occur because of decreased osmolality of the fluid surrounding the cells, as in hypotonic fluid overload, or increased osmolality of the intracellular fluid, as in conditions that decrease the activity of the sodium pump of the cell membrane, allowing the concentration of sodium ions within the cell to increase.

cerebral e. swelling of the brain caused by the accumulation of fluid in the brain substance. It may result from head injury, stroke, infection, hypoxia, brain tumors, obstructive hydrocephalus, and lead encephalopathy; it may also be caused by disturbances in fluid and electrolyte balance that accompany hemodialysis and diabetic ketoacidosis. The most common type is *vasogenic edema,* which may result from increased capillary pressure or from increased capillary permeability caused by trauma to the capillary walls. *Cellular edema* may occur in ischemia or hypoxia of the brain. Because the brain is enclosed in the solid vault of the skull, edema compresses the

blood vessels, decreasing the blood flow and causing ischemia and hypoxia, which in turn result in further edema. Unless measures are taken to reverse the edema, destruction of brain tissue and death will result.

dependent e. edema of the lowermost parts of the body relative to the heart; it is affected by gravity and position, so that the lower limbs are affected if the individual is standing, but the buttocks are affected if the individual is supine.

generalized e. edema that is caused by poor venous return; it is not localized by the effects of gravity, in contrast to dependent edema.

interstitial e. 1. edema caused by the accumulation of fluid in the extracellular spaces of a tissue. 2. pulmonary edema in the interstitial tissues; there is dyspnea but no hypoxemia.

e. neonato'rum sclerema neonatorum.

nonpitting e. edema in which pressure does not leave a depression in the tissues, such as in cellular EDEMA. See also pitting EDEMA.

pedal e. swelling of the feet and ankles.

peripheral e. edema affecting the extremities; seen in heart disease, Crohn's disease, and amyloidosis.

pitting e. edema in which external pressure leaves a persistent depression in the tissues (see PITTING); it occurs because the pressure pushes the excess fluid out of the intercellular spaces in the tissue. See also nonpitting EDEMA.

pulmonary e. diffuse extravascular accumulation of fluid in the tissues and air spaces of the LUNG due to changes in hydrostatic forces in the capillaries or to increased capillary permeability. It is most often symptomatic of left ventricular HEART FAILURE, but can also be a complication of mitral STENOSIS, aortic STENOSIS, ALTITUDE SICKNESS, acute HYPERTENSION, volume overload during intravenous therapy, or reduced serum oncotic pressure, as in patients who have NEPHROSIS, CIRRHOSIS, or HYPOALBUMINEMIA.

During the initial stage of pulmonary edema, patients may complain of restlessness and anxiety and the feeling that they are getting a COMMON COLD. Other signs include a persistent cough, slight DYSPNEA, and intolerance to exercise. On AUSCULTATION, RALES can be heard over the dependent portion of the lung. As fluid continues to fill the pulmonary interstitial spaces the dyspnea becomes more acute, respirations increase in rate, and there is audible wheezing. The cough becomes productive of frothy sputum tinged with blood, giving it a pinkish hue. Eventually, if the condition persists, the patient becomes less responsive to stimuli as levels of conscious-ness decrease. Ventricular arrhythmias develop and breath SOUNDS diminish. In some patients these phases are telescoped as the pulmonary edema develops rapidly and the final stages of respiratory insufficiency are evident in a very short period of time.

Treatment is aimed at enhancing gas exchange, reducing fluid overload, and strengthening and slowing the heart beat. To accomplish these goals the patient is often given oxygen by mask or through mechanically assisted ventilation. Drug therapy includes DIURETICS to remove excess alveolar fluid and MORPHINE to relieve anxi-ety and reduce the effort of breathing. Administration of other medications de-pends on the cause of the edema, as well as what other problems the patient may be having.

vasogenic e. that characterized by in-creased permeability of capillary endothelial cells; the most common form of cerebral EDEMA.

edemagen (ĕ-de′mah-jen) an irritant that elicits edema by causing capillary damage but not the cellular response of true inflam-mation.

edematogenic (ĕ-dem″ah-to-jen′ik) pro-ducing or causing edema.

edentia (e-den′shah) anodontia.

edentulism (e-den′tu-liz-em) the condi-tion of being without teeth.

edentulous (e-den′tu-lus) without teeth.

edetate (ed′ētāt) USAN contraction for ethylenediaminetetraacetate, a salt of ETH-YLENEDIAMINETETRAACETIC ACID (EDTA); the salts include *edetate disodium calcium,* used in the diagnosis and treatment of LEAD POISONING, and *edetate disodium,* used in the treatment HYPERCALCEMIA because of its affinity for calcium.

edetic acid (ĕ-det′ik) ethylenediamine-tetraacetic acid.

edisylate (ĕ-dis′ĭ-lāt) USAN contraction for 1,2-ethanedisulfonate.

edrophonium (ed″ro-fo′ne-um) a CHOLIN-ERGIC used in the form of the chloride salt as a CURARE antagonist and diagnostic agent in MYASTHENIA GRAVIS.

EDTA ethylenediaminetetraacetic acid.

educable (ej′u-kah-b′l) capable of being educated; formerly used to describe persons with mild MENTAL RETARDATION (IQ 50–70).

education (ed-u-ka′shun) 1. the process of sharing KNOWLEDGE. 2. the gaining of KNOWL-EDGE.

health e. see HEALTH EDUCATION.

parent e.: adolescent in the NURSING INTERVENTIONS CLASSIFICATION, a nursing INTER-VENTION defined as assisting parents to un-derstand and help their adolescent children.

parent e.: childrearing family in the NURSING INTERVENTIONS CLASSIFICATION, a nursing INTERVENTION defined as assisting parents to understand and promote the physical, psychological, and social growth and development of their toddler, preschool, or school-aged children.

parent e.: infant in the NURSING INTER-VENTIONS CLASSIFICATION, a nursing INTERVEN-TION defined as instruction on nurturing and physical care needed during the first year of life.

Edwards′ syndrome (ed′werdz) trisomy 18 syndrome.

Edwardsiella (ed-ward′se-el″ah) a genus of gram-negative, facultatively anaerobic, rod-shaped bacteria, which are pathogenic for aquatic animals and are occasional opportunistic pathogens for humans; *E. tar′da* can cause acute gastroenteritis and septic infections.

EEG electroencephalogram.

eelworm (ēl′werm) roundworm.

EENT eye, ear, nose, and throat.

E.E.S. trademark for a preparation of erythromycin ethylsuccinate, a broad-spec-trum antibacterial.

efavirenz (ef′ah-vi″renz) a non-nucleoside reverse transcriptase INHIBITOR, used as an ANTIRETROVIRAL in treatment of human im-munodeficiency VIRUS infection; adminis-tered orally.

effacement (ĕ-fās′ment) the obliteration of form or features; said of the cervix uteri during labor when it shortens from 1 or 2 cm in length to paper thin and there is no longer a cervical canal but only an external cervical os.

effect (ĕ-fekt′) a result produced by an action.

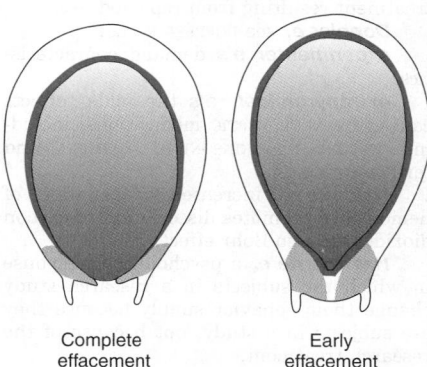

Complete effacement   Early effacement

Cervical dilation and effacement. During labor, the multigravida's cervix remains thicker than that of the nullipara. From McKinney et al., 2000.

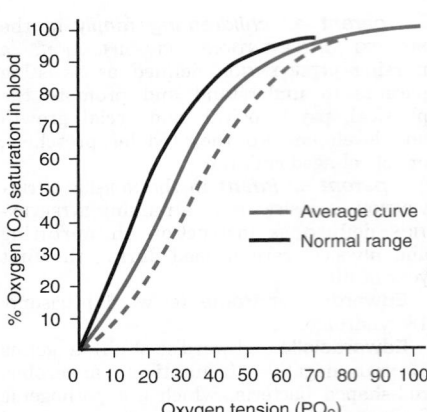

The Bohr effect causing a shift to the right in the oxyhemoglobin dissociation curve.

additive e. the combined effect produced by the action of two or more agents, being equal to the sum of their separate effects.

adverse e. a symptom produced by a drug or therapy that is injurious to the patient.

Bainbridge e. Bainbridge reflex.

Bohr e. decreased affinity of hemoglobin for oxygen caused by an increase of carbon dioxide; the oxyhemoglobin dissociation curve is displaced to the right because of higher partial pressure of carbon dioxide and lower pH. See also Haldane effect.

Crabtree e. the inhibition of oxygen consumption on the addition of glucose to tissues or microorganisms having a high rate of aerobic glycolysis; the converse of the Pasteur effect.

cumulative e. the action of a drug or treatment resulting from repeated use.

Doppler e. see DOPPLER EFFECT.

experimenter e's demand characteristics.

extrapyramidal e's the side effects caused by NEUROLEPTIC medications, including DYSTONIAS, PARKINSONISM, AKATHISIA, and tardive DYSKINESIA.

Haldane e. increased oxygenation of hemoglobin promotes dissociation of carbon dioxide; see also Bohr effect.

Hawthorne e. a psychological response in which the subjects in a research study change their behavior simply because they are subjects in a study, not because of the research treatment.

heel e. variation in x-ray beam intensity and projected focal spot size along the long axis of the x-ray tube from cathode to anode.

parallax e. the position of the image on each emulsion of dual emulsion film; it is accentuated by tube-angled x-ray techniques.

Pasteur e. the decrease in the rate of glycolysis and the suppression of lactate accumulation by tissues or microorganisms in the presence of oxygen.

photoelectric e. ejection of electrons from matter as a result of interaction with photons from high frequency electromagnetic radiation, such as x-rays; the ejected electrons may be energetic enough to ionize multiple additional atoms.

placebo e. the total of all nonspecific effects, both good and adverse, of treatment; it refers primarily to psychological and psychophysiological effects associated with the caregiver-patient relationship and the patient's expectations and apprehensions concerning the treatment. See also PLACEBO.

position e. in genetics, the changed effect produced by alteration of the relative positions of various genes on the chromosomes.

pressure e. the sum of the changes that are due to obstruction of tissue drainage by pressure.

proarrhythmic e. any new, more advanced form of ARRHYTHMIA caused by an ANTIARRHYTHMIC agent, especially those that produce hemodynamically important symptoms. These arrhythmias occur less than 30 days after initiation of treatment and are not due to a new event such as acute myocardial infarction or hypokalemia.

side e. a consequence other than that for which an agent is used, especially an adverse effect on another organ system.

Somogyi e. see SOMOGYI EFFECT.

effectiveness (ĕ-fek′tiv-nes) the ability to produce a specific result or to exert a specific measurable influence.

relative biological e. an expression of the effectiveness of other types of radiation in comparison with that of gamma or x-rays. Abbreviated RBE.

effector (ef-fek′ter) 1. an agent that mediates a specific effect, as an allosteric effector or an effector cell. 2. an organ that produces an effect, such as contraction or secretion, in response to nerve stimulation; see also RECEPTOR.

allosteric e. one that binds to an enzyme at a site other than the active site.

effemination (ĕ-fem″ĭ-na′shun) feminization (def. 2).

efferent (ef′er-ent) 1. conducting or progressing away from a center or specific site of reference, such as an efferent NERVE; called also centrifugal. See also AFFERENT and CORTICIFUGAL. 2. a fiber or nerve that so conducts.

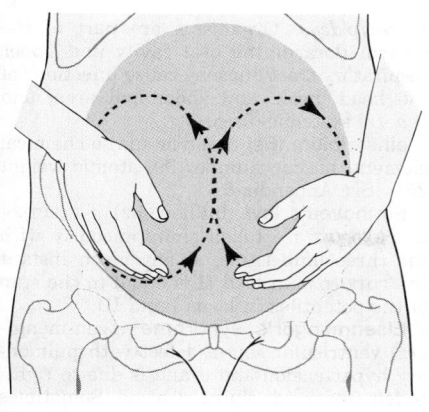

Effleurage.

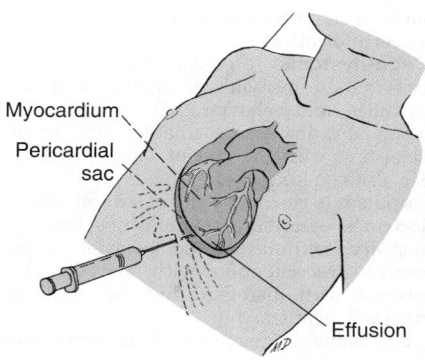

Accumulated fluid from a pericardial effusion evacuated by the subxiphoid approach to pericardiocentesis. From Polaski and Tatro, 1996.

effervescent (ef″er-ves′ent) bubbling; sparkling; giving off gas bubbles.

efficacy (ef′ĭ-kah″se) 1. the ability of a drug to achieve the desired effect. 2. the degree to which an intervention accomplishes the desired or projected outcomes.

effleurage (ef″loo-rahzh′) [Fr.] stroking movement in massage. During childbirth, a light circular stroke of the lower abdomen, done in rhythm to control breathing, to aid in relaxation of the abdominal muscles, and to increase concentration during a uterine contraction. The stroking is accomplished by moving the wrist only. Concentrating on the coordination of stroking and breathing is believed to block out some of the sensations created by the contracting uterus.

efflorescence (ef″lo-res′ens) 1. the quality of being EFFLORESCENT. 2. a rash or eruption.

efflorescent (ef″lo-res′ent) becoming powdery by losing the water of crystallization.

effluent (ef′floo-ent) something that flows out, especially a DISCHARGE that carries waste products.

effusion (ĕ-fu′zhun) 1. escape of a fluid into a part; exudation or transudation. 2. an exudate or transudate.

   chyliform e. see CHYLOTHORAX.
   chylous e. see CHYLOTHORAX.
   pericardial e. the accumulation of an abnormally large amount of pericardial fluid in the pericardium.
   pleural e. see PLEURAL EFFUSION.
   pseudochylous e. see CHYLOTHORAX.

eflornithine (ef-lor′nĭ-thēn″) an inhibitor of the enzyme catalyzing the decarboxylation of ORNITHINE; used topically as the hydrochloride salt to reduce unwanted facial hair in females. It has also been administered intravenously in treatment of African TRYPANOSOMIASIS.

Efudex (ef′u-deks) trademark for a preparation of FLUOROURACIL, an antineoplastic AGENT.

EGD esophagogastroduodenoscopy.

egesta (e-jes′tah) undigested material discharged from the body.

egestion (e-jes′chun) the casting out of undigested material.

egg (eg) 1. ovum. 2. oocyte. 3. a female reproductive cell at any stage before fertilization; after fertilization and fusion of the pronuclei it is called a ZYGOTE.

ego (e′go) in psychoanalytic theory, one of the three major parts of the personality, the others being the ID and the SUPEREGO. The word ego is Latin for "I," that is, self or individual as distinguished from other persons. The ego is represented by certain mental mechanisms, such as perception and memory, and specific DEFENSE MECHANISMS that are used to adjust to the demands of primitive instinctual drives (the id) and the demands of the external world (superego). The ego may be considered the psychologic aspect of one's personality, the id comprising the physiologic aspects and the superego the social aspects. The ego controls and directs an individual's actions and seeks compromises between the id impulses, social and parental prohibitions, and the pressures of reality.
   The word ego also is commonly used to express conceit or self-centeredness. This should not be confused with the psychiatric meaning described above.

egobronchophony (e″go-bron-kof′o-ne) egophony.

egocentric (e″go-sen′trik) self-centered, conceited, egotistical; preoccupied with one's own interests and needs; lacking concern for others.

ego-dystonic (e″go-dis-ton′ik) denoting aspects of a person's thoughts, impulses, attitudes, and behavior that are felt to be repugnant, distressing, unacceptable, or inconsistent with the rest of the personality. See also EGO-SYNTONIC.

egoism (e′go-izm) 1. any of several ethical doctrines describing relationships between morality, self-interest and behavior. 2. excessive preoccupation with oneself, self-interest with disregard for the needs of others. 3. egotism.

egomania (e″go-ma′ne-ah) extreme self-centeredness; extreme egotism.

egophony (e-gof′o-ne) increased resonance of voice SOUNDS, with a high-pitched bleating quality, heard especially over lung tissue compressed by PLEURAL EFFUSION; called also egobronchophony.

ego-syntonic (e″go-sin-ton′ik) denoting aspects of a person's thoughts, impulses, attitudes, and behavior that are felt to be acceptable and consistent with the rest of the personality. See also EGO-DYSTONIC.

egotism (e′go-tizm) 1. conceit, selfishness, self-centeredness, with an inflated sense of one's importance. 2. egoism (def. 2).

Ehlers-Danlos syndrome (a′lerz dan′los) a congenital hereditary syndrome of joint hyperextensibility, hyperelasticity and fragility of the skin, poor wound healing leaving parchment-like scars, capillary fragility, and subcutaneous nodules after trauma. Called also cutis hyperelastica.

Ehrlich (ār′lik) Paul (1854–1915). German bacteriologist. He studied medicine and was early drawn to research on aniline dyes. He did vast work on the problems of serology and immunity and is known preeminently for his discovery of salvarsan or "606," an arsenical compound later called arsphenamine, which was a cure for syphilis and the first effective chemotherapeutic agent against a microbial disease. He differentiated the leukemias, classified the leukocytes, described polychromatophilia, and is generally regarded as the founder of hematology. In 1908 Ehrlich shared with Metchnikoff the Nobel prize for medicine or physiology for his work in immunology.

eidetic (i-det′ik) denoting exact visualization of events or objects previously seen; a person having such an ability.

eidoptometry (i″dop-tom′ĕ-tre) measurement of the acuteness of visual perception.

Eikenella (i″kĕ-nel′ah) a genus of gram-negative, facultatively anaerobic, rod-shaped bacteria with a single species,

E. corro′dens. Organisms are part of the normal flora of the oral cavity and upper respiratory tract but may cause infections of the head, neck, and abdominal area, and general systemic disease.

einsteinium (Es) (īn-sti′ne-um) a chemical element, atomic number 99, atomic weight 254. (See Appendix 6.)

Einthoven's law (int′ho-venz) if ELECTRO-CARDIOGRAMS are taken simultaneously with the three limb LEADS, at any given instant the POTENTIAL in lead II is equal to the sum of the potentials in leads I and III.

Eisenmenger's syndrome (i′zen-meng′-erz) ventricular septal defect with pulmonary hypertension and cyanosis due to right-to-left (reversed) shunt of blood. Sometimes defined as pulmonary hypertension (pulmonary vascular disease) and cyanosis, with the shunt being at the atrial, ventricular, or great vessel area.

ejaculatio (e-jak″u-la′she-o) [L.] ejaculation.

    e. prae′cox premature ejaculation.

ejaculation (e-jak″u-la′shun) forcible, sudden expulsion of semen; especially expulsion of semen from the male urethra, a reflex action that occurs as a result of sexual stimulation. adj., **ejac′ulatory.** The three components of semen are expelled in quick succession. First to emerge is a lubricating fluid produced by the bulbourethral glands in the penis; next comes a fluid released into the urethral channel by the prostate, providing a neutral medium within which the sperm cells can swim; and lastly, the spermatic fluid, which has been stored in the seminal vesicles, is likewise injected into the urethral channel and ejaculated. See also REPRODUCTION.

    premature e. ejaculation consistently occurring either prior to, upon, or immediately after penetration and before desired, taking into account factors such as age, novelty of the specific situation and recent frequency of sexual activity.

    retarded e. male orgasmic disorder.

    retrograde e. ejaculation with discharge of the semen into the bladder rather than through the urethra to the outside. It often occurs after prostatectomy or spinal cord injury.

EKC epidemic keratoconjunctivitis.

EKG electrocardiogram.

EKY electrokymogram.

elaborate (e-lab′o-rāt) to produce complex substances out of simpler materials.

elaboration (e-lab″o-ra′shun) 1. the process of producing complex substances out of simpler materials. 2. in psychiatry, an unconscious mental process of expansion and embellishment of detail, especially of a symbol or representation in a dream.

elapid (el′ah-pid) 1. pertaining to the members of a family of pit VIPERS that includes the genera *Micruroides* and *Micrurus*. 2. any of the members of this group.

elastance (e-las′tans) the quality of recoiling on removal of pressure without disruption, or an expression of the measure of the ability to do so in terms of unit of volume change per unit of pressure change; it is the reciprocal of compliance.

elastase (e-las′tās) an enzyme capable of catalyzing the digestion of elastic tissue.

elastic (e-las′tik) capable of resuming normal shape after distortion.

elasticity (e″las-tis′ĭ-te) the quality of being elastic.

elastin (e-las′tin) a yellow scleroprotein, the essential constituent of elastic connective tissue; it is brittle when dry, but flexible and elastic when moist.

elastofibroma (e-las″to-fi-bro′mah) a tumor consisting of both elastin and fibrous elements.

elastoidosis (e-las″toi-do′sis) changes in the skin resembling ELASTOSIS.

nodular e. nodular ELASTOSIS of Favre and Racouchot.

elastolysis (e″las-tol′ĭ-sis) a defect in the elastic tissue, resulting in atrophy and laxity of the skin.

elastoma (e″las-to′mah) a tumor or focal excess of elastic tissue fibers or abnormal collagen fibers of the skin.

elastometer (e″las-tom′ĕ-ter) an instrument for measuring the elasticity of tissues.

elastorrhexis (e-las″to-rek′sis) a rupture of fibers composing elastic tissue.

elastosis (e″las-to′sis) 1. degeneration of elastic tissue. 2. degenerative changes in the dermal connective tissue with increased amounts of elastotic material. 3. any disturbance of the dermal connective tissue.

actinic e. premature aging of the skin due to prolonged exposure to sunlight, seen especially in light-skinned persons, characterized by inelasticity, thinning or sometimes thickening, wrinkling, dryness with fine scaling, and variable hyperpigmentation, often with development of cherry angiomas, telangiectasis, senile lentigines, ecchymosis, milia, and senile keratosis. Called also senile or solar elastosis.

nodular e. of Favre and Racouchot a type of actinic elastosis seen chiefly in elderly men, in which giant comedones, pilosebaceous cysts, and large folds of furrowed and yellowish skin are seen in the periorbital region; called also nodular elastoidosis.

e. perfo′rans serpigino′sa, perforating e. an elastic tissue defect, occurring alone or in association with other disorders, including DOWN'S SYNDROME and EHLERS-DANLOS SYNDROME, in which elastomas are extruded through small keratotic papules in the epidermis; the lesions are usually arranged in arc-shaped, continuous clusters on the sides of the nape, face, or arms.

senile e., solar e. actinic elastosis.

elastotic (e″las-tot′ik) 1. pertaining to or characterized by elastosis. 2. resembling elastic tissue; having the staining properties of elastin.

elation (e-la′shun) emotional excitement marked by acceleration of mental and bodily activity, with extreme joy and an overly optimistic attitude even in the face of negative circumstances.

Elavil (el′ah-vil) trademark for preparations of AMITRIPTYLINE hydrochloride, a tricyclic ANTIDEPRESSANT.

elbow (el′bo) 1. the bend of the upper LIMB; the area around the joint connecting the arm and forearm; see also elbow JOINT. Called also cubitus. 2. any angular bend.

The elbow joint connects the large bone of the upper arm, the humerus, with the two smaller bones of the lower arm, the radius and ulna. It is one of the body's more versatile joints, with a combined hinge and rotating action allowing the arm to bend and the hand to make a half turn. The flexibility of the elbow and shoulder joints together permits a nearly infinite variety of hand movements.

The action of the elbow is controlled primarily by the biceps and the triceps muscles. When the biceps contracts, the arm bends at the elbow. When the triceps contracts, the arm straightens. In each action, the opposite muscle exerts a degree of opposing tension, moderating the movement so that it is smooth and even instead of sudden and jerky.

As in other joints, the ends of the bones meeting at the elbow have a smooth covering of cartilage that minimizes friction when the joint is moved. The elbow joint is lubricated with synovia, and its movement is eased by the bursa, a small sac of connective tissue. The bones forming the joint are held together by tough, fibrous ligaments. The "funny bone" is not a bone but the ulnar nerve, a vulnerable and sensitive nerve lying close to the surface near the point of the elbow. Hitting it causes a tingling pain or sensation that may be felt all the way to the fingers.

Disorders of the Elbow. The elbows, like the knees, are continually exposed to bumps, twists, and wrenches. Elbow injuries include fracture of a bone near the joint, DISLOCATION, and tearing of tendons and ligaments.

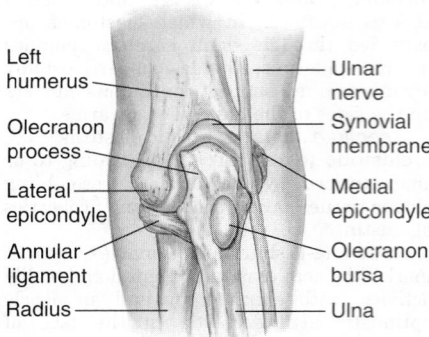

Left
humerus

Ulnar
nerve

Olecranon
process

Synovial
membrane

Lateral
epicondyle

Medial
epicondyle

Annular
ligament

Olecranon
bursa

Radius

Ulna

ELBOW—POSTERIOR VIEW

Elbow. From Jarvis, 2000.

Dislocation and fracture may occur together. ARTHRITIS may affect the elbow and make it stiff or impossible to move. Special exercises, manipulation, and heat therapy may be prescribed to help restore flexibility. BURSITIS can also cause pain in the elbow, often as a result of excessive use of the joint.

tennis e. a term often used for bursitis of the elbow but more accurately referring to tendinitis felt in the outer aspect of the elbow due to inflammation of the extensor tendon attached to the lateral humeral condyle. Rest and heat therapy usually relieve it. It affects both tennis players and others who put stress on the elbow.

elderly (el′der-le) aged.

frail e. 1. individuals over 65 years old who have functional impairments. 2. sometimes used to describe any adult over 75 years old.

ele(o)- word element [Gr.], *oil.*

electric shock shock caused by electric current passing through the body. (See illustration.) The longer the contact with electricity, the smaller the chance of survival. The victim's breathing may stop, and the body may appear stiff. In giving first aid, first the electric contact is broken as quickly as possible; this must be done with care so that the rescuer does not have exposure to the current. The rescuer, keeping in mind that water and metals are conductors of electricity, stands on a *dry* surface and does not touch the victim or electric wire with the bare hands. If the victim has stopped breathing and has no pulse, CARDIOPULMONARY RESUSCITATION is begun immediately.

electro- word element [Gr.], *electricity.*

electroaffinity (e-lek″tro-ah-fin′ĭ-te) electronegativity.

electroanalgesia (e-lek″tro-an″al-je′ze-ah) the reduction of pain by electrical stimulation of a peripheral nerve or the dorsal column of the spinal cord.

electrocardiogram (ECG, EKG) (e-lek″tro-kahr′de-o-gram″) the record produced by ELECTROCARDIOGRAPHY; a tracing representing the heart's electrical action derived by amplification of the minutely small electrical impulses normally generated by the heart.

electrocardiograph (e-lek″tro-kahr′de-o-graf″) the apparatus used in electrocardiography.

electrocardiography (e-lek″tro-kahr″de-og′rah-fe) the graphic recording from the body surface of the electric POTENTIAL of currents generated by the heart, as a means of studying the action of the heart muscle. adj., **electrocardiograph′ic.** With the modern electrocardiograph, the current that accompanies the action of the heart is amplified 3000 times or more, and it moves a small, sensitively balanced lever in contact with moving paper. The pattern of heart waves that is traced on the paper indicates the heart's rhythm and other actions.

The normal electrocardiogram is composed of a P wave, Q, R, and S waves known as the QRS COMPLEX, or QRS wave, and a T

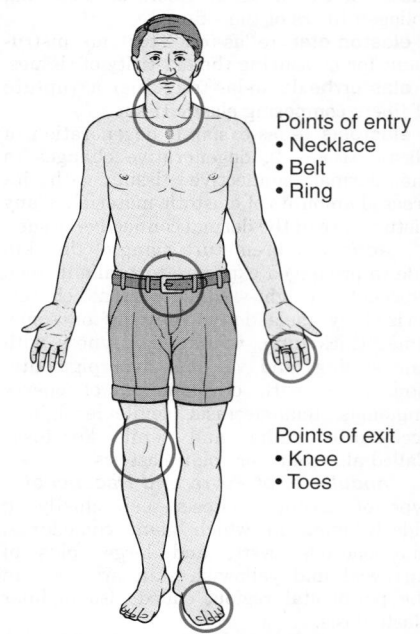

Points of entry
• Necklace
• Belt
• Ring

Points of exit
• Knee
• Toes

Common points of entry and exit for electrical burns. Severe internal damage can occur between these points. From Frazier et al., 2000.

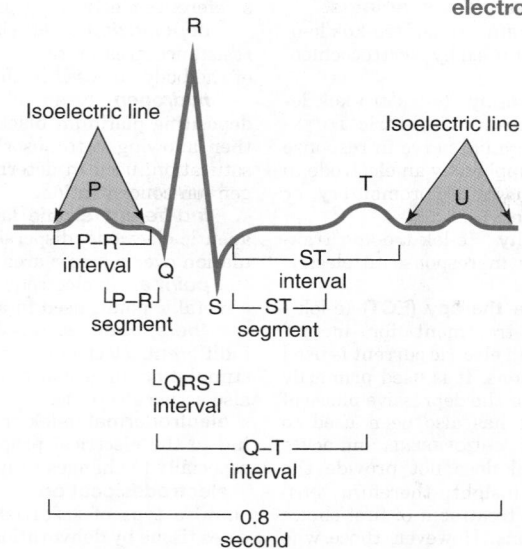

Normal electrocardiogram. *Heart action during P-R interval:* (1) Atrial contraction begins at peak of P wave. (2) P-R interval—atrial contraction. (3) Ventricles relaxed. *Heart action during QRS complex:* (1) Ventricular contraction begins at peak of R. (2) A-V (mitral and tricuspid) valves close, causing S₁ sound. (3) Ventricles contract. (4) Atrial relaxation begins. *Heart action during S-T segment:* (1) Semilunar valves open (aortic and pulmonic). (2) Ejection of blood from ventricles—systole. *Heart action during T wave:* (1) Slowing of ejection from ventricles. (2) Closure of semilunar valves (aortic and pulmonic) causing S₂ sound. *Heart action during T-P interval:* (1) Relaxation of ventricles. (2) A-V valves open. (3) Filling of ventricles, causing S₃ sound.

wave. The P wave occurs at the beginning of each contraction of the atria. The QRS wave occurs at the beginning of each contraction of the ventricles. The T wave seen in a normal electrocardiogram occurs as the ventricles recover electrically and prepare for the next contraction. There is a refractory period between these waves during which the muscle is inexcitable; this period is usually about 0.30 second.

The electric impulses in the heart muscle are picked up and conducted to the electrocardiograph by electrodes or LEADS connected to the body by small metal plates or other methods. The metal plates are moistened with a conductive paste and attached to the arms, legs, and chest (cardiac area) of the patient.

Electrocardiography is a valuable diagnostic tool, used in some routine physical examinations and when a heart disorder occurs or is suspected. It helps diagnose the damage that may have been inflicted on the heart muscle by a coronary occlusion, the progress of rheumatic fever, the presence of abnormal rhythms, or the effect of digitalis or other drugs. An electrocardiogram cannot always detect impending heart disease or all cardiovascular disorders. The readings are interpreted together with the results of other diagnostic tests.

electrocautery (e-lek″tro-kaw′ter-e) 1. an apparatus for surgical dissection and hemostasis, using heat generated by a high-voltage, high-frequency alternating current passed through an electrode. 2. the cauterization of tissue using such an instrument.

bipolar e. an electrocautery in which both active and return electrodes are incorporated into a single handheld instrument, so that the current passes between the tips of the two electrodes and affects only a small amount of tissue.

monopolar e., unipolar e. an electrocautery in which current is applied through a handheld active electrode and travels back to the generator through an inactive electrode attached to the patient (the grounding pad), so that the patient is part of the electrical circuit.

electrochemistry (e-lek″tro-kem′is-tre) the study of the relationships and transformations between chemical and electrical energy.

electrocoagulation (e-lek″tro-ko-ag″u-la′-shun) a type of ELECTROSURGERY by which tissue is coagulated using a modulated alternating current.

electrocochleogram (e-lek″tro-kok′le-o-gram) the record obtained by electrocochleography.

electrocochleography (e-lek″tro-kok″le-og′rah-fe) measurement of electric POTENTIALS of the eighth cranial nerve in response to acoustic stimuli applied by an electrode to the external acoustic canal, promontory, or tympanic membrane.

electrocontractility (e-lek″tro-kon″traktil′ĭ-te) contractility in response to electric stimulation.

electroconvulsive therapy (ECT) (e-lek″-tro-kon-vul′siv) a treatment for mental disorders in which an electric current is used to produce convulsions. It is used primarily to treat DEPRESSION or the depressive phase of BIPOLAR DISORDER; it has also been used to treat some forms of SCHIZOPHRENIA and acute MANIA. This method does not provide the patient with any insight; therefore ANTIDEPRESSANTS are the treatment of first choice for depressed persons. However, those who do not respond to medication or are unable to take it often experience dramatic improvement after electroconvulsive therapy. Formerly called electroshock therapy.

The procedure begins with administration of an intravenous anesthetic such as METHOHEXITAL or THIOPENTAL to induce general anesthesia and a muscle relaxant such as SUCCINYLCHOLINE to prevent a peripheral seizure that could carry the risk of bodily injury. Electric current is then applied unilaterally to the brain through an electrode placed on the skull. The goal is to produce a seizure in the central nervous system without causing any of the frightening manifestations of a grand mal SEIZURE; modern techniques using EEG recordings while administering ECT make this possible. Side effects occasionally include acute confusional state upon recovery from general anesthesia, which may last up to an hour. There may be a loss of memory, particularly of recent events. Basic principles of preoperative and postoperative nursing care apply.

electrocorticography (e-lek″tro-kor″tĭ-kog′rah-fe) electroencephalography with the electrodes applied directly to the cerebral cortex.

electrode (e-lek′trōd) either of two terminals of an electrically conducting system or cell; specifically, the uninsulated portion of a LEAD that is in direct contact with the body.

   active e. therapeutic electrode.

   calomel e. one capable of both collecting and giving up chloride ions in neutral or acidic aqueous media, consisting of mercury in contact with mercurous chloride; used as a reference electrode in pH measurements.

   depolarizing e. an electrode that has a resistance greater than that of the portion of the body enclosed in the circuit.

   hydrogen e. an electrode made by depositing platinum black on platinum and then allowing it to absorb hydrogen gas to saturation; used in determination of hydrogen ion concentration.

   indifferent e. one larger than a therapeutic electrode, dispersing electrical stimulation over a larger area.

   point e. an electrode having on one end a metallic point; used in applying current.

   therapeutic e. one smaller than an indifferent electrode, producing electrical stimulation in a concentrated area; called also active electrode.

electrodermal (e-lek″tro-der′mal) pertaining to the electrical properties of the skin, especially to changes in its resistance.

electrodesiccation (e-lek″tro-des″ĭ-ka′-shun) a type of ELECTROSURGERY that desiccates tissue by dehydration, which employs a spark gap type of generator to produce a highly or moderately damped alternating electrical current. It is usually used to remove small superficial growths on the skin.

electrodialyzer (e-lek″tro-di″ah-li′zer) a blood dialyzer utilizing an applied electric field and semipermeable membranes for separating the colloids from the solution.

electroejaculation (e-lek″tro-e-jak″u-la′-shun) electrical stimulation via the rectum to produce an EJACULATION of semen; this is commonly used for spinal cord injury or testicular cancer patients who cannot ejaculate and are attempting artificial INSEMINATION. It may also be used for those with abdominal injuries, multiple sclerosis, diabetic neuropathy, and ANEJACULATION from other causes, both physical and psychogenic.

electroencephalogram (EEG) (e-lek″tro-en-sef′ah-lo-gram″) the record produced by ELECTROENCEPHALOGRAPHY; a tracing of the electric impulses of the brain.

electroencephalograph (e-lek″tro-en-sef′-ah-lo-graf) the instrument used in electroencephalography.

electroencephalographic technologist EEG technologist; an allied health professional trained to obtain interpretable electroencephalographic recordings and who is able to apply electrodes in specified locations, conduct routine and special tests, and prepare the tracing for interpretation by the neurologist. Those having 1 year of training and 1 year of clinical experience and passing the certification examination of the American Board of Registration of Electroencephalograph Technologists are designated

Frontal-motor

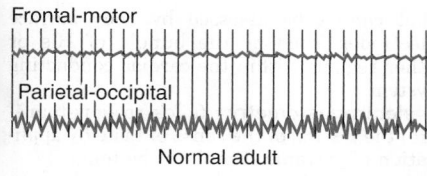

Parietal-occipital

Normal adult

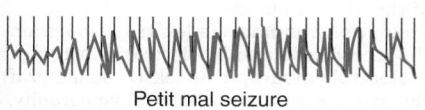

Petit mal seizure

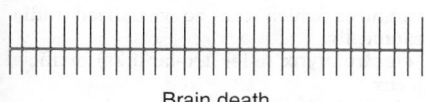

Brain death

Sample of electroencephalogram tracings showing normal activity, seizure activity, and brain death.

R EEG T, Registered Electroencephalographic Technologist.

electroencephalography (e-lek″tro-en-sef″ah-log′-rah-fe) the recording of changes in electric POTENTIALS in various areas of the brain by means of electrodes placed on the scalp, on the brain surface, or within the brain itself, and connected to a vacuum tube radio amplifier, which amplifies the impulses more than a million times. The impulses are of sufficient magnitude to move an electromagnetic pen that records the brain WAVES. adj., **electroencephalograph′ic.**

The rate, height, and length of the waves vary in different parts of the brain, and each individual has a unique and characteristic pattern. Age and degree of consciousness also cause the wave patterns to differ. Most of the recorded waves in a normal adult's EEG are the occipital alpha waves, which are best obtained from the back of the head (occipital region) when the subject is resting quietly, but not asleep, with the eyes closed. These waves are blocked by excitement or by opening the eyes.

The beta waves, obtained from the central and front parts of the head, are more closely related to the sensory-motor parts of the brain. These waves are blocked in the same way as are alpha waves, by opening the eyes. In a normal EEG the frequencies are predominantly within the range of alpha and beta rhythms at the rate of 8 to 30 hertz (cycles per second). During sleep the brain

cells generate higher voltage electrical waves, but the rhythm is slowed down to 2 or 3 hertz, sometimes with short "sleep" spindles of about 15 hertz. One should use the word "normal" with caution when speaking of EEG readings. Some persons with mild deviations from normal may have no evidence of cerebral disease, while others with readings within normal ranges may be suffering from a serious disorder.

Irregular slow waves of 2 to 3 hertz, called delta waves or the delta pattern, are normally found in deep sleep and in infants and young children, but they indicate an abnormality in the awake adult. Rhythmic slow waves of 4 to 7 hertz are called theta waves. "Electrical silence," or no evidence of brain activity, when demonstrated once and then again in 24 hours, has been taken as one of the criteria of DEATH.

Electroencephalography is widely used in studying brain function and in tracing the connections between the parts of the central nervous system. It is particularly valuable in diagnosing EPILEPSY, brain tumor, and other diseases of and injury to the brain.

Patient Care. The electroencephalograph is an extremely sensitive instrument, and readings can be greatly influenced by the actions and physiologic status of the subject. It is apparent, then, that the cooperation of the patient is needed, and that the patient should be properly prepared physically and psychologically in order to obtain an accurate and useful record of brain activity. Patients are more likely to be cooperative if they have had adequate preparation in the purpose of the test, how the procedure will be carried out, and what will be expected of them during the testing. Their fears about electricity and how it will be used must be allayed. They should know that the electrodes lead minute amounts of electrical charge *from* the body and that there is no danger of electric shock and no relationship of this procedure to electroshock therapy. In most instances the test is painless because the electrodes are attached to the scalp with collodion. If needle electrodes are to be used, however, patients should be told there will be mild discomfort because the needles are extremely small.

A sleep recording usually is taken when a seizure disorder is suspected. The patient will be expected to go to sleep during the test. Some EEG technicians encourage the patient to stay up later than usual the evening before the test and to awaken early in order to be more likely to fall asleep during testing. Medications to produce sleep are given only as a last resort because these drugs alter brain wave patterns. Infants and small children are not allowed to nap before the test.

Other aspects of physical preparation include withholding all anticonvulsants, tranquilizers, and stimulants for at least 24 to 48 hours prior to testing. This includes coffee, tea, cola drinks, and alcohol. Hypoglycemia affects the brain wave patterns and so the patient is told not to skip any meals.

At the beginning of the test a baseline EEG reading is obtained by having the patient lie quietly with the eyes closed in a dimly lit room. The patient is cautioned to avoid movement of the eyelids, mouth, or tongue because these activities can be particularly disruptive. Provocative or "stressing" techniques are sometimes used during the EEG testing. These are particularly useful in the diagnosis of epilepsy because they can evoke seizure potentials on the EEG. The two techniques most often used are HYPERVENTILATION and "photic" stimulation, which employs flickering lights to stimulate the brain. When these or any other techniques are anticipated, patients should be informed so they will not become unduly apprehensive before and during the testing.

electrofulguration (e-lek″tro-ful″gur-ra′-shun) a type of ELECTROSURGERY used to produce superficial desiccation of tissue.

electrogastrograph (e-lek″tro-gas′tro-graf) an instrument for recording the electrical activity of the stomach by means of swallowed gastric electrodes.

electrogastrography (e-lek″tro-gas-trog′-rah-fe) the recording of the electrical activity of the stomach as measured between its lumen and the body surface. adj., **electro-gastrograph′ic.**

electrogenic (e-lek″tro-jen′ik) pertaining to a physiological process that generates a significant current that directly contributes to the cell membrane POTENTIAL.

electrogram (e-lek′tro-gram) 1. any record produced by changes in electric POTENTIAL. 2. specifically, a CARDIOGRAM taken from the chambers of the heart or from a specific position within the chambers.

His bundle e. an intracardiac electrogram of potentials in the lower right atrium, atrioventricular node, and His-Purkinje system, obtained by positioning intracardiac electrodes near the tricuspid valve; it is used to pinpoint the site, extent, and mechanisms of arrhythmias and conduction defects.

intracardiac e. a record of changes in the electric potentials of specific cardiac loci as measured by electrodes placed within the heart via cardiac catheters; it is used for loci that cannot be assessed by body surface electrodes, such as the bundle of His or other regions within the cardiac conducting system.

electrogustometry (e-lek″tro-gus-tom′ĕ-tre) the testing of the sense of taste by application of galvanic stimuli to the tongue.

electrohysterography (e-lek″tro-his″ter-og′rah-fe) the recording of changes in electric POTENTIAL associated with contractions of the uterine muscle.

electrokymogram (e-lek″tro-ki′mo-gram) the record produced by electrokymography.

electrokymograph (e-lek″tro-ki′mo-graf) the instrument used in electrokymography.

electrokymography (e-lek″tro-ki-mog′-rah-fe) the photography on x-ray film of the motion of the heart or of other moving structures which can be visualized radiographically.

electrolarynx (e-lek″tro-lar′inks) artificial larynx.

electrolysis (e″lek-trol′ĭ-sis) destruction by passage of a galvanic current, as in disintegration of a chemical compound in solution or removal of excessive hair from the body.

electrolyte (e-lek′tro-līt) a chemical substance that, when dissolved in water or melted, dissociates into electrically charged particles (IONS) and thus is capable of conducting an electric current. The principal positively charged ions in the body fluids (CATIONS) are SODIUM (Na^+), POTASSIUM (K^+), CALCIUM (Ca^{2+}), and MAGNESIUM (Mg^{2+}). The most important negatively charged ions (ANIONS) are CHLORIDE (Cl^-), BICARBONATE (HCO_3^-), and PHOSPHATE (PO_4^{3-}). These electrolytes are involved in metabolic activities and are essential to the normal function of all cells. Concentration gradients of sodium and potassium across the cell membrane produce the membrane POTENTIAL and provide the means by which electrochemical impulses are transmitted in nerve and muscle fibers.

The concentration of the various electrolytes in body fluids is maintained within a

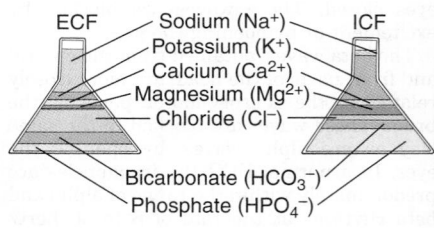

Electrolyte composition of body fluid.

COMMON ELECTROLYTE IMBALANCES

Calcium	Normal value: 4.5–5.5 mEq/liter or 9–11 mg/100 ml	
Hypercalcemia	> 11 mg/100 ml	Excess intake of calcium, as in taking antacids indiscriminately. Excess intake of vitamin D. Conditions that cause movement of calcium out of bones and into extracellular fluid, e.g., bone tumor, multiple fractures. Tumors of the lung, stomach, and kidney. Immobility and osteoporosis.
Hypocalcemia	< 8.5 mg/100 ml	Inadequate dietary intake of calcium and vitamin D. Impaired absorption of calcium from intestinal tract, as in diarrhea, sprue, overuse of laxatives and enemas containing phosphates (phosphorus tends to be more readily absorbed from the intestinal tract than calcium and suppresses calcium retention in the body). The parathyroid regulates calcium and phosphorus levels. Hyposecretion of parathyroid hormone can result in hypocalcemia.
Magnesium	Normal value: 1.5–2.5 mEq/liter	
Hypermagnesemia	> 2.5 mEq/liter	Overuse of antacids and cathartics containing magnesia; aspiration of sea water, as in near-drowning. Chronic kidney failure and adrenal insufficiency.
Hypomagnesemia	< 1.5 mEq/liter	Chronic malnutrition, chronic diarrhea. Bowel resection with ileostomy or colostomy, chronic alcoholism, prolonged gastric suction, acute pancreatitis, biliary or intestinal fistula, diuretic therapy, diabetic ketoacidosis.
Potassium	Normal value: 3.5–5.0 mEq/liter	
Hyperkalemia	> 5.5 mEq/liter	Conditions that alter kidney function or decrease its ability to excrete potassium. Intestinal obstruction that prevents elimination of potassium in the feces. Addison's disease, chronic heparin therapy, lead poisoning, insulin deficit, crushing injuries, and burns.
Hypokalemia	< 3.5 mEq/liter	Inadequate intake of potassium-rich foods. Loss of potassium in urine when kidneys do not reabsorb the mineral. Loss of potassium from intestinal tract as a result of diarrhea or vomiting, drainage from fistulas, overuse of gastric suction. Improper use of diuretics.
Sodium	Normal value: 135–145 mEq/liter	
Hypernatremia	> 147 mEq/liter	Insufficient water intake, as in comatose, mentally confused, or debilitated patients. Excessive sweating, diarrhea, failure of kidney to reabsorb water from urine. Administration of high-protein, hyperosmotic tube feedings and osmotic diuretics.
Hyponatremia	< 135 mEq/liter	Inadequate sodium intake, as in patients on low-sodium diets. Excessive intake or retention of water (kidney failure and heart failure). Loss of bile, which is rich in sodium, as a result of fistulas, drainage, gastrointestinal surgery, and suction. Loss of sodium through burn wounds. Administration of IV fluids that do not contain electrolytes.

narrow range. However, the optimal concentrations differ in the extracellular fluid and intracellular fluid. For example, the concentration of sodium in extracellular fluid (serum) is about 15 times higher than in the intracellular fluid. Conversely, the concentration of potassium is about 30 times higher within the cell than in the serum or extracellular fluid.

electrolyte imbalance. This exists when the serum concentration of an electrolyte is either too high or too low. (See accompanying table.) The terms for excessive and deficient blood levels of electrolytes are derived from the Greek prefixes *hyper-* (over) and *hypo-* (under), the English or Latin name of the electrolyte, and the Latin suffix *-emia.* For example, an excess of sodium (Latin, *natrium*) cations in the serum is called *hypernatremia,* and a deficit of these ions is called *hyponatremia.*

Stability of the electrolyte balance depends on adequate intake of water and the electrolytes, and on homeostatic mechanisms within the body that regulate the absorption, distribution, and excretion of water and its dissolved particles. Many conditions can interfere with these processes and result in an imbalance. For example, renal disease, in which the kidney nephron is unable to function normally, causes a retention of water, sodium, chloride, bicarbonate, and calcium as the glomerular filtration RATE falls. Even when the kidney structures are intact, electrolyte imbalances can result from an inadequate supply of blood to the nephrons or from imbalances of regulatory hormones such as ALDOSTERONE and antidiuretic HORMONE.

The effects of an electrolyte imbalance are not isolated to a particular organ or system. In general, however, imbalances in calcium concentrations affect the bones, kidney, and gastrointestinal tract. Calcium also influences the permeability of cell membranes and thereby regulates neuromuscular activity. Sodium affects the osmolality of blood and therefore influences blood volume and pressure and the retention or loss of interstitial fluid. Potassium affects muscular activities, notably those of the heart, intestines, and respiratory tract, and also affects neural stimulation of the skeletal muscles.

Assessment and nursing interventions related to electrolyte imbalance are shown in the accompanying table.

electrolytic (e-lek″tro-lit′ik) pertaining to electrolysis or to an electrolyte.

electromagnet (e-lek″tro-mag′net) a temporary MAGNET made by passing an electric current through a coil of wire surrounding a core of soft iron or steel.

electromagnetism (e-lek″tro-mag′nĕ-tizm) magnetism developed by an electric current.

electromyogram (e-lek″tro-mi′o-gram) the record obtained by electromyography.

electromyograph (e-lek″tro-mi′o-graf) the instrument used in electromyography.

electromyography (e-lek″tro-mi-og′rah-fe) the recording and study of the intrinsic electrical properties of skeletal muscle. adj., **electromyograph′ic.** When it is at rest, normal muscle is electrically silent, but when the muscle is active, an electrical current is generated. In electromyography the electrical impulses are picked up by needle electrodes inserted into the muscle and amplified on an oscilloscope screen in the form of wavelike tracings. The visual recording may be accompanied by auditory monitoring in which the sounds are amplified.

Electromyography is useful in diagnosing disorders of the nerves supplying the muscle (as in AMYOTROPHIC LATERAL SCLEROSIS and POLIOMYELITIS) and in disorders affecting the muscle tissues. Recordings usually are obtained while the muscle is relaxed, during voluntary contraction, and during muscle activity that is produced by nerve stimulation. In this way it is possible to determine the presence of a disorder, localize the site, and identify the specific disease producing muscle weakness.

electron (e-lek′tron) any of the negatively charged particles arranged in orbitals around the nucleus of an atom and determining all of the atom's physical and chemical properties except mass and radioactivity. Electrons flowing in a conductor constitute an electric current; when ejected from a radioactive substance, they are beta particles.

The number of electrons revolving around the nucleus of an atom is equal to its atomic number. An atom of oxygen, for instance, which has an atomic number of 8, has eight electrons in orbit around the nucleus in a manner similar to the planets revolving around the sun in our solar system.

Electrons greatly influence the behavior of an atom toward other atoms. The combination of various ELEMENTS to form compounds is brought about by the losing or gaining of electrons; the process is sometimes called "sharing" of electrons. For example, the combination of the elements sodium and chlorine produce the compound sodium chloride (table salt). This is accomplished by the transfer of one electron from the outer electron shell of the sodium atom to the outer electron shell of the chlorine atom. This combining of elements by the loss or gain of electrons is called electrovalence.

electronarcosis (e-lek″tro-nahr-ko′sis) 1. a treatment sometimes used to render an animal unconscious. 2. in humans, a rare treatment for psychiatric disorders using passage of an electric current through the brain via electrodes on the scalp; it is both less effective and more likely to cause side effects than is ELECTROCONVULSIVE THERAPY.

electron-dense (e-lek′tron-dens″) in electron microscopy, having a density that prevents electrons from penetrating.

electronegative (e-lek″tro-neg′ah-tiv) bearing a negative electric charge.

electronegativity (e-lek″tro-neg″ah-tiv′ĭ-te) the relative power of an atom or molecule to attract electrons.

electroneurography (e-lek″tro-nŏŏ-rog′rah-fe) the measurement of the conduction velocity and latency of peripheral nerves.

electroneuromyography (e-lek″tro-noor″-o-mi-og′rah-fe) electromyography in which the nerve of the muscle under study is stimulated by application of an electric current.

electronic (e″lek-tron′ik) pertaining to or carrying electrons.

electronystagmogram (e-lek″tro-nis-tag′-mo-gram) 1. the record obtained by ELECTRO-NYSTAGMOGRAPHY. 2. a test done using electronystagmography, assessing the balance mechanism of the inner ear. It involves running a cool liquid and then a warm liquid through a tube within the ear canal; the change in temperature stimulates the inner ear, which in turn causes rapid reflex eye movements. The movements are recorded, yielding information about the functioning of the balance mechanism.

electronystagmograph (e-lek″tro-nis-tag′mo-graf) the instrument used in electronystagmography; abbreviated ENG.

electronystagmography (e-lek″tro-nis″-tag-mog′rah-fe) graphic recordings of eye movements that provide objective documentation of induced and spontaneous NYSTAGMUS; see also ELECTRONYSTAGMOGRAM.

electro-oculogram (e″lek″tro-ok′u-lo-gram″) the electroencephalographic tracings made while moving the eyes a constant distance between two fixation points, inducing a deflection of fairly constant amplitude. Abbreviated EOG.

electro-olfactogram (EOG) (e-lek″tro-ol-fak′to-gram) a recording of changes in electric POTENTIAL detected by an electrode placed on the surface of the olfactory mucosa as the mucosa is subjected to an odorous stimulus.

electropherogram (e-lek″tro-fer′o-gram) electrophoretogram.

electrophile (e-lek′tro-fīl) a chemical compound that serves as an electron acceptor in a chemical reaction. adj., **electrophil′ic.**

electrophoresis (e-lek″tro-fo-re′sis) the movement of charged particles suspended in a liquid on various media (e.g., paper, gel, liquid) under the influence of an applied electric field. adj., **electrophoret′ic.** The various charged particles of a particular substance migrate in a definite and characteristic direction—toward either the anode or the cathode—and at a characteristic speed. This principle has been widely used in the separation of proteins and is therefore valuable in the study of diseases in which the serum and plasma proteins are altered. The principle also has been applied in the separation and identification of various types of human hemoglobin.

electrophoretogram (e-lek″tro-fo-ret′o-gram) the record produced on or in a supporting medium by bands of material which have been separated by the process of electrophoresis.

electrophrenic (e-lek″tro-fren′ik) pertaining to electrical stimulation of the phrenic nerve or diaphragm; see also electrophrenic RESPIRATION.

electropositive (e-lek″tro-poz′ĭ-tiv) bearing a positive electric charge.

electroresection (e-lek″tro-re-sek′shun) excision by electrosurgical means; see also ELECTROSECTION.

electroretinograph (e-lek″tro-ret′in-o-graf) ERG; an instrument for measuring the electrical response of the retina to light stimulation. The basic component of the ERG is a contact lens containing an electrode, which is placed on the surface of the eye. Electrical activity of the retina is magnified and recorded as waves similar to those seen on an electrocardiograph. Signals from a diseased retina are reduced in size and slower than normal. ERG is especially useful in confirming a diagnosis of RETINITIS PIGMENTOSA before visible signs can be detected with an ophthalmoscope.

electroscope (e-lek′tro-skōp) an instrument for measuring radiation intensity.

electrosection (ĕ-lek″tro-sek′shun) a type of ELECTROSURGERY used to incise or excise tissue.

electrosleep (e-lek′tro-slēp) the use of low-intensity electricity, below the threshold for inducing convulsions, in the treatment of insomnia, anxiety, or depression.

electrostimulation (e-lek″tro-stim″u-la′-shun) electric stimulation of tissues.

electrostriatogram (e-lek″tro-stri-a′to-gram) an ELECTROENCEPHALOGRAM showing differences in electric POTENTIAL recorded at various levels of the CORPUS STRIATUM.

electrosurgery (e-lek″tro-ser′jer-e) the use of high-frequency alternating current to remove, incise, or destroy tissue. This is accomplished by converting the electrical energy into heat through tissue resistance to the passage of the electrical current. Called also surgical diathermy. adj., **electrosur′gical.** Two types of current are used: damped and undamped; a *damped current* destroys and coagulates tissue and stops bleeding, and an *undamped current* destroys minimal tissue and incises tissue. Local anesthesia is required with electrosurgery except when very low current is used to remove small superficial lesions. Laser technology is now being used to perform some of the surgery previously done with electrosurgery. Lasers offer greater precision and application within organs such as the eye or the bronchus, which were once inaccessible to electrosurgery, and appear to destroy tumors more effectively.

Types. There are four basic types of electrosurgical technique: electrodesiccation, electrofulguration, electrocoagulation, and electrosection.

E

Electrodesiccation is desiccation of tissue by dehydration, using a spark gap type of generator to produce a highly or moderately damped current. The current is radiated through a monoterminal active electrode (usually a ball or needle), which is inserted into or applied directly to the lesion, and produces mass coagulation of the tissue surrounding the site of application or insertion of the electrode.

Electrofulguration is commonly considered to be a type of electrodesiccation, but the terms are not synonymous. Both techniques use the same kind of current and means of conduction, but in electrofulguration the electrode is held 1 or 2 mm from the operative area and is moved over the tissue so that a spray of sparks dries out the tissue, producing superficial desiccation and eschar formation.

Electrocoagulation is a biterminal technique that uses moderately damped or modulated undamped current and employs both an active concentrating electrode and an inactive dispersing electrode. The concentrating electrode, which may be a needle, disk, knife blade, bar, or ball, may contact or be inserted into the lesion to be destroyed; an adhesive dispersive pad, which may be placed in contact with or close to the operative site, is used as the dispersing electrode. Electrocoagulation produces various degrees of tissue coagulation or hemorrhage control, depending on the current used and the technique employed.

Another biterminal electrosurgical technique is *electrosection,* which uses slightly damped, modulated undamped, or undamped currents. The active electrode may be a knife blade, various types of wire loops, or a needle; an adhesive dispersive pad is used as the passive electrode. This technique is used in incising, excising, and planing procedures.

electrotaxis (e-lek″tro-tak′sis) TAXIS in response to electric stimuli.

electrotherapeutics (e-lek″tro-ther″ah-pu′tiks) electrotherapy.

electrotherapy (e-lek″tro-ther′ah-pe) treatment of disease by means of electricity; see also DIATHERMY.

  cerebral e. electrosleep.

electrotonic (e-lek″tro-ton′ik) 1. pertaining to electrotonus. 2. denoting the direct spread of CURRENT in tissues by electrical conduction, without the generation of new current by ACTION POTENTIALS.

electrotonus (e-lek-trot′o-nus) the altered electrical state of an excitable CELL when a constant electric current is passed through

it; for example, the changes in membrane POTENTIAL of excitable cells that cause a passive change in potential at every other point on the cell membrane.

electroureterography (e-lek″tro-u-re″ter-og′rah-fe) ELECTROMYOGRAPHY in which the ACTION POTENTIALS produced by peristalsis of the URETER are recorded.

electrovalence (e-lek″tro-va′lens) 1. the number of charges an atom acquires in a chemical reaction by gain or loss of electrons. 2. the bonding resulting from such transfer of electrons. adj., **electrova′lent.**

electroversion (e-lek″tro-ver′zhun) the act of electrically terminating a cardiac dysrhythmia.

electrovert (e-lek′tro-vert) to apply electricity to the heart or precordium to depolarize the heart and terminate a cardiac dysrhythmia.

electuary (e-lek′choo-ar″e) a medicinal preparation consisting of a powdered drug made into a paste with honey or syrup.

eledoisin (el′ĕ-doi′sin) a decapeptide from the posterior salivary gland of a species of small octopus, *Eledone;* it is a precursor of a large group of biologically active peptides. It has vasodilator, hypotensive, and extravascular smooth muscle stimulant properties.

eleidin (el-e′ĭ-din) a substance, allied to keratin, found in the cells of the stratum lucidum of the skin.

element (el′ĕ-ment) 1. any of the primary parts or constituents of a thing. 2. in chemistry, a simple substance that cannot be decomposed by ordinary chemical means; elements are the basic components of which all matter is composed.

Chemical elements are made up of ATOMS, each of which consists of a NUCLEUS with a cloud of negatively charged ELECTRONS revolving around it. The two major components of the nucleus are PROTONS and NEUTRONS. The number of protons in the atoms of a particular element is always the same, and therefore the physical and chemical properties of the element are always the same. It is possible, however, for a chemical element to exist in several different forms, the difference depending on the number of neutrons in the nucleus of its atoms. Different forms of the same element are called ISOTOPES.

There are at least 105 different chemical elements known. (See Appendix 6 for a list of the elements, and the symbol, atomic weight, and atomic number of each.) The atomic NUMBER of an element is determined by the number of protons in the nucleus of one of its atoms. The mass number of an isotope is determined by the total number of neutrons and protons in the nucleus.

Stable Chemical Elements. A stable chemical element is one that contains an optimal ratio or range of ratios between the number of protons and neutrons in the nucleus. A stable element does not spontaneously transmute into another element and therefore does not give off radiation. The stable elements are those that have an atomic number below 84, except for a few, such as potassium and rubidium, which are weakly radioactive.

Radioactive Chemical Elements. A RADIOACTIVE chemical element does not contain an optimal proton-to-neutron ratio in its atomic nuclei and therefore readily gives off nuclear particles until all nuclei have attained the optimal combination of protons and neutrons. The spontaneous releasing of its nuclear particles changes the radioactive atom into a new atom (transmutation).

As radioactive elements disintegrate and form new chemical elements, a tremendous amount of energy is released. This emission of energy and nuclear particles is called RADIATION. The radiations may be electrically charged particles having size and mass, such as ALPHA PARTICLES and BETA PARTICLES, or they may be nonparticulate and contain no electrical charges, such as GAMMA RAYS. Most radioactive elements give off either alpha or beta particles and at the same time emit gamma radiation.

formed e's of the blood the blood CELLS.

trace e. a chemical element present or needed in extremely small amounts by plants and animals; such elements include manganese, copper, cobalt, zinc, and iron.

eleoma (el″e-o′mah) a tumor or swelling caused by injection of oil into the tissues.

elephantiasis (el″ĕ-fan-ti′ah-sis) a chronic type of FILARIASIS marked by inflammation and obstruction of the lymphatics and hypertrophy of the skin and subcutaneous tissues, chiefly affecting the lower limbs and external genitals. The disease derives its name from the symptoms, particularly limb swelling, which makes the legs look like those of an elephant. The term is often applied to hypertrophy and thickening of the tissues that result from any cause.

True elephantiasis, or *elephantiasis filariensis*, is most often caused by a slender threadlike filarial parasite, *Wuchereria bancrofti,* which enters the lymphatic system, causing an obstruction to drainage. The filaria larvae are transmitted by mosquitoes or flies that carry blood infected with them. Elephantiasis is most often encountered in tropical or subtropical areas such as Central Africa and certain Pacific islands; it is rare or nonexistent in the temperate zone.

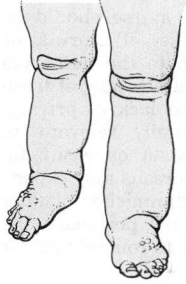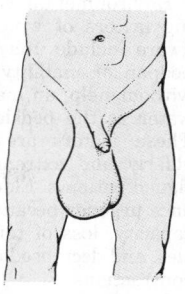

Elephantiasis of the legs and of the scrotum. From Dorland's, 2000.

The first visible signs are inflammation of the lymph nodes, with temporary swelling in the affected area, red streaks along the leg or arm, pain, and tenderness, attended by chills and fever (ELEPHANTOID FEVER), followed by formation of ulcers and tubercles, with thickening, discoloration, and fissuring of the skin. Specific drugs are administered for destruction of the parasites; bandages and elevation of the affected area help relieve the swelling. Sanitary control to eliminate the carrier insects is the most effective approach to elimination of this disease. (See accompanying illustration)

e. scro′ti that in which the scrotum is the main seat of the disease. Called also chylocele.

elephantoid fever a recurrent acute febrile condition occurring with filariasis; it may be associated with elephantiasis or lymphangitis.

elimination (e-lim″ĭ-na′shun) discharge from the body of indigestible materials and of waste products of body metabolism; see DEFECATION, URINATION, and CLEARANCE.

altered bowel e. a former NURSING DIAGNOSIS referring to change in normal DEFECATION patterns. See CONSTIPATION, DIARRHEA, and bowel INCONTINENCE.

bowel e. defecation.

impaired urinary e. a NURSING DIAGNOSIS accepted by the North American Nursing Diagnosis Association, defined as a disturbance in an individual's pattern of urine elimination (see URINATION). These changes are not to be confused with symptoms of pathologic conditions related to renal formation of urine, such as SUPPRESSION, ANURIA, and POLYURIA. Examples of changes that might be amenable to nursing interventions include those associated with DYSURIA, FREQUENCY, NOCTURIA, and urinary INCONTINENCE.

Environmental causative and contributing factors of which the nurse should be aware include unavailability of a urinal or bedpan or inability to go to the bathroom without help, an inadequate supply of fresh water at the bedside, and lack of privacy. These factors are especially relevant to elderly and extremely weak or easily fatigued patients. Elderly persons may experience urgency because of diminished bladder capacity, loss of tone in the perineal muscles, and decreased ability to control bladder contractions.

In some cases alteration in patterns of urination may be related to decreased attention to bladder cues because of the effects of certain drugs, such as tranquilizers and sedatives, or to psychologic factors, such as depression, anxiety, and confusion. See also BLADDER TRAINING.

urinary e. urination.

ELISA (e-li′sah) enzyme-linked immunosorbent ASSAY.

elixir (e-lik′ser) a clear, sweetened, alcohol-containing, usually hydroalcoholic liquid containing flavoring substances and sometimes active medicinal ingredients.

Elixophyllin (e-lik-so-fil′in) trademark for preparations of THEOPHYLLINE, a BRONCHODILATOR.

elliptocyte (e-lip′to-sīt) an abnormal oval or elliptical erythrocyte, as seen in ELLIPTOCYTOSIS. Called also ovalocyte.

elliptocytosis (e-lip″to-si-to′sis) any of several hereditary disorders in which most of the erythrocytes are ELLIPTOCYTES; it is characterized by increased erythrocyte destruction and anemia.

elongation (e-long-ga′shun) 1. the act or process of increasing in length. 2. a radiographic distortion in which the image is longer than what is being x-rayed.

Elspar (el′spahr) trademark for a preparation of ASPARAGINASE, an antineoplastic AGENT.

eluate (el′u-āt) the substance separated out by, or the product of, elution or elutriation.

eluent (e-lu′ent) the solution used in elution.

elution (e-loo′shun) in chemistry, separation of material by washing; the process of pulverizing substances and mixing them with water in order to separate the heavier constituents, which settle out in solution, from the lighter.

elutriation (e-loo″tre-a′shun) purification of a substance by dissolving it in a solvent and pouring off the solution, thus separating it from the undissolved foreign material.

Em. emmetropia.

emaciation (e-ma″se-a′shun) a wasted condition of the body; see WASTING.

emasculate (e-mas′ku-lāt) to CASTRATE a male.

emasculation (e-mas″ku-la′shun) bilateral ORCHIECTOMY.

embalming (em-bahm′ing) treatment of a dead body to retard decomposition.

embarrass (em-bar′as) to impede the function of; to obstruct.

embedding (em-bed′ing) fixation of tissue in a firm medium, in order to keep it intact during cutting of thin sections.

embole (em′bo-le) the reducing of a dislocated limb.

embolectomy (em″bo-lek′to-me) surgical removal of an embolus.

emboli (em′bo-li) [Gr.] plural of EMBOLUS.

embolic (em-bol′ik) pertaining to embolism or an embolus.

embolism (em′bo-lizm) the sudden blocking of an artery by a clot of foreign material (EMBOLUS) that has been brought to its site of lodgment by the blood current. The obstructing material is most often a blood clot, but it may be a fat globule, air bubble, piece of tissue, or clump of bacteria.

Symptoms. The symptoms of an embolism usually do not appear until the embolus lodges within a blood vessel and suddenly obstructs the blood flow; this usually occurs at divisions of an artery, where the vessel narrows. The signs of obstruction appear almost immediately with severe pain at the site. If the embolus lodges in a limb, the area becomes pale, numb, and cold to the touch, and normal arterial pulse below the site is absent. Fainting, nausea, vomiting, and eventually severe shock may occur if a large vessel is occluded. Unless the obstruction is relieved, gangrene of the adjacent tissues served by the affected vessel develops.

Prevention. Venous THROMBOSIS is the most common predisposing cause of embolism, particularly when a thrombus lodges in a limb. In order to prevent the development of emboli it is necessary to avoid venous STASIS in patients confined to bed because of surgery, illness, or injury. In addition to physical inactivity, heart failure and pressure on the veins of the legs and pelvis can inhibit blood flow and thus set the stage for inflammation, clot formation, and the possibility of embolism. Although frequent changing of position, exercise, and early ambulation are necessary to the prevention of thrombosis and embolism, sudden and extreme movements should be avoided. Under no circumstances should the legs be massaged to relieve "muscle cramps," especially when the pain is located in the calf and the patient has not been up and about; pain in the calf may be symptomatic of a thrombosis. The occurrence of an air embolism can be avoided by careful handling of equipment used for intravenous therapy, correct technique in administering intramuscular injections, and intra-arterial monitoring.

cerebral e. embolism of a cerebral artery, one of the three main causes of STROKE SYNDROME.

pulmonary e. (PE) obstruction of the pulmonary artery or one of its branches by an embolus. The embolus usually is a blood clot swept into circulation from a large peripheral vein, particularly a vein in the leg or pelvis. Factors that predispose a patient to this condition include: (1) *stasis of blood flow,* as in a patient who is on prolonged bed rest, is immobilized for some reason, or is aged, obese, or suffering from a burn; (2) *venous injury,* as from surgical procedures or trauma and fractures of the legs or pelvis; (3) *predisposition to clot formation* because of malignancy or use of oral contraceptives; (4) *cardiovascular disease;* (5) *chronic lung disease;* and (6) *diabetes mellitus.*The effects of pulmonary embolism will depend on the size of the embolus and the amount of lung tissue involved. When an embolus becomes lodged in a pulmonary blood vessel, it prevents adequate blood supply to the lung, interferes with the exchange of oxygen and carbon dioxide, and results in arterial hypoxemia. As pressure within the obstructed pulmonary artery increases there is strain on the right ventricle and it may eventually fail. Two other complications are pulmonary infarct and pulmonary hemorrhage.

Signs and symptoms of pulmonary embolism vary greatly, depending on the extent to which the lung is involved, the size of the clot, and the general condition of the patient. Simple, uncomplicated embolism produces such cardiopulmonary symptoms as dyspnea, tachypnea, persistent cough, pleuritic pain, and hemoptysis. Apprehension is a common symptom. On rare occasions the cardiopulmonary symptoms may be acute, occurring suddenly and quickly producing cyanosis and shock.

FIBRINOLYTIC therapy should be initiated as soon as possible for patients with massive or unstable pulmonary embolism. HEPARIN will not dissolve existing clots but is a drug often used in treatment of the condition; it prolongs clotting time and allows the body time to resolve the existing clot. The drug most often used in the treatment of PE is heparin, which prolongs clotting time and

allows the body time to resolve the existing clot.

Patient Care. Major goals in the care of patients at risk for pulmonary embolism are prevention and early detection. Those who are at risk and require diligent preventive measures and periodic monitoring are patients who have had surgery or cardiovascular disease associated with clot formation (such as after myocardial infarction or stroke), patients with multiple trauma, and those who are therapeutically immobilized.

Preventive measures include passive or active dorsiflexion of each foot at least ten times each hour; turning, coughing, and deep breathing after surgery; early ambulation whenever possible; and avoidance of pressure, such as propping pillows under the knees or bending the bed at the knees, that could produce venous stasis. Since patients receiving continuous intravenous therapy also are at risk for formation of clots and emboli, intravenous sites should be changed at frequent intervals.

Detection of pulmonary embolism in its earlier and more treatable stages demands constant vigilance for signs that a clot is forming or an embolus is in the blood stream. The more common signs of simple, uncomplicated embolism are listed above. Additionally, the patient is watched for increased jugular pressure, elevated pulse and heart rate, and friction rub. Eliciting Homans' sign (discomfort behind the knee on forced dorsiflexion of the foot), noting skin and temperature changes in the area of the calf, and assessing edema of the extremities are important monitoring activities in the care of patients at risk for pulmonary embolism.

embolization (em″bo-lĭ-za′shun) 1. the process or condition of becoming an embolus. 2. therapeutic introduction of a substance into a vessel in order to occlude it.

embololalia (em″bo-lo-la′le-ah) the interpolation of meaningless words or phrases in a spoken sentence.

embolophrasia (em″bo-lo-fra′zhah) embololalia.

embolus (em′bo-lus), pl. *em′boli* [Gr.] a clot or other plug, usually part or all of a THROMBUS, brought by the blood from another vessel and forced into a smaller one, thus obstructing circulation; see also EMBOLISM. (See accompanying illustration)

saddle e. one situated at the bifurcation of a large artery, sometimes blocking both branches.

embrasure (em-bra′zher) a space continuous with an interproximal space, produced by curvatures of teeth in contact in the

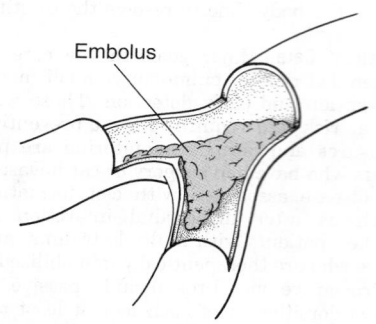

Embolus

Embolus impacted at the site of branching of an artery. From Dorland's, 2000.

same arch; it provides a passage through which food escapes from the occlusal surfaces during mastication.

embryectomy (em″bre-ek′to-me) excision of an extrauterine embryo or fetus.

embryo (em′bre-o) a new organism in the earliest stage of development. In humans this is defined as the developing organism from the fourth day after FERTILIZATION to the end of the eighth week. After that the unborn baby is usually referred to as the FETUS. adj., **em′bryonal, embryon′ic.**
Immediately after fertilization takes place, cell division begins and progresses at a rapid rate. At approximately 4 weeks the cell mass becomes a recognizable embryo from 7 to 10 mm long with rudimentary organs. The beginnings of the eyes, ears, and extremities can be seen. By the end of the second month the embryo has grown to a length of 2 to 2.5 cm, and the head is the most prominent part because of the rapid development of the brain; the sex can be distinguished at this stage.
At the time of fertilization the ovum contains the potential beginnings of a human being. As cell division takes place the cells of the BLASTODERM (embryonic disk) gradually form three layers from which all the body structures develop. The ECTODERM (outer layer) gives rise to the epidermis of the skin and its appendages, and to the nervous system. The MESODERM (middle layer) develops into muscle, connective tissue, the circulatory organs, circulating lymph and blood cells, endothelial tissues within the closed vessels and cavities, and the epithelium portion of the urogenital system. From the ENDODERM (internal layer) are derived those portions not arising from the ectoderm, the liver, the pancreas, and the lungs.

embryocardia (em″bre-o-kahr′de-ah) a symptom in which the heart sounds resemble those of the fetus, there being very little difference in the quality of the first and second sounds.

embryoctony (em″bre-ok′to-ne) destruction of the living embryo or fetus.

embryolethality (em″bre-o-le-thal′ĭ-te) embryotoxicity that causes death of the embryo. adj., **embryole′thal.**

embryologist (em″bre-ol′o-jist) an expert in embryology.

embryology (em″bre-ol′o-je) the science of the development of the individual during the embryonic stage and, by extension, in several or even all preceding and subsequent stages of the life cycle. adj., **embryolog′ic.**

embryoma (em″bre-o′mah) any of various neoplasms thought to be derived from embryonic cells or tissues, such as dermoid cysts, teratomas, and embryonal carcinomas.

embryonization (em-bre″o-nī-za′shun) reversion of a tissue or cell to the embryonic form.

embryonoid (em′bre-ŏ-noid″) resembling an embryo.

embryopathy (em″bre-op′ah-the) a morbid condition of the embryo or a disorder resulting from abnormal embryonic development, with consequent congenital anomalies. See also FETOPATHY.
  rubella e. rubella syndrome.

embryoplastic (em′bre-o-plas″tik) pertaining to or concerned in formation of an embryo.

embryotomy (em″bre-ot′ah-me) dismemberment of the fetus in difficult labor in which a normal delivery is impossible.

embryotoxicity (em″bre-o-tok-sis′ĭ-te) toxic effects on the embryo of a substance that crosses the placental barrier; see also EMBRYOLETHALITY and TERATOGENESIS. adj. **embryotox′ic.**

embryotoxon (em″bre-o-tok′son) arcus corneae.
  anterior e. arcus corneae.
  posterior e. Axenfeld's anomaly.

embryotroph (em′bre-o-trōf″) the total nutriment (histotroph and hemotroph) made available to the embryo.

embryotrophy (em″bre-ot′ro-fe) the nutrition of the early embryo.

emedastine (em″ĕ-das′tēn) an ANTIHISTAMINE applied topically to the conjunctiva as *emedastine difumarate* in treatment of allergic CONJUNCTIVITIS.

emedullate (e-med′u-lāt) to extract bone marrow.

emergency (e-mer′jen-se) an unlooked for or sudden occurrence, often dangerous, such as an accident or an urgent or pressing need.

E

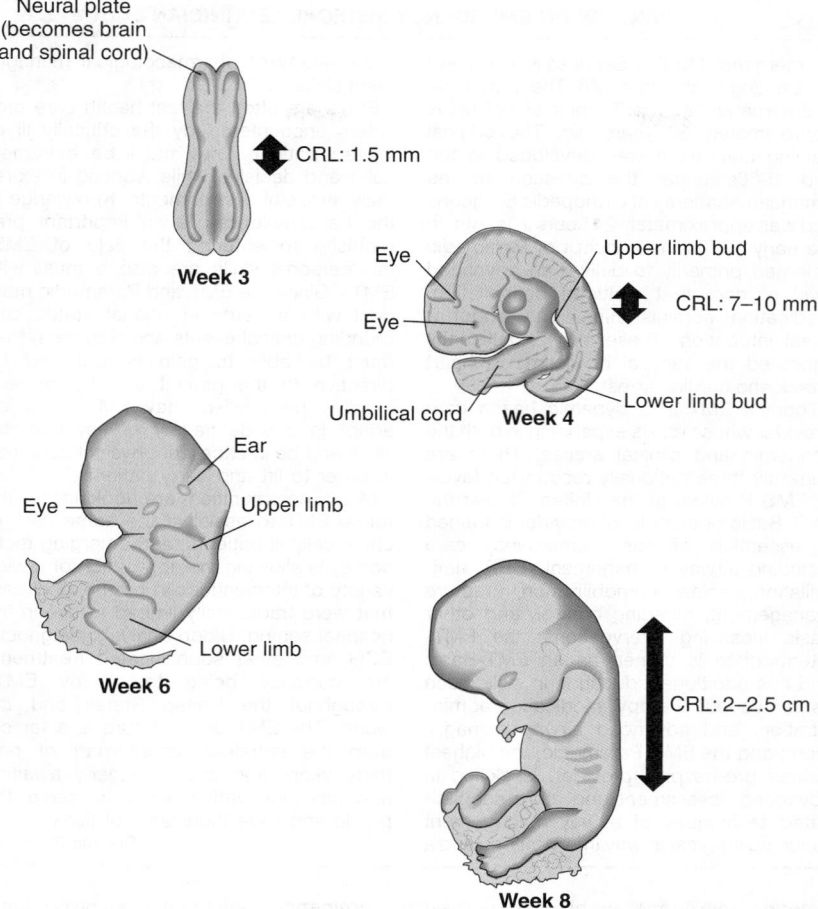

Neural plate (becomes brain and spinal cord)

CRL: 1.5 mm

Week 3

Eye

Upper limb bud

Eye

CRL: 7–10 mm

Umbilical cord **Week 4**

Lower limb bud

Ear

Eye

Upper limb

Lower limb

Week 6

CRL: 2–2.5 cm

Week 8

Embryonic development from 3 weeks through the eighth week after fertilization. CRL is crown-to-rump length. From McKinney et al., 2000.

e. department an area of a hospital especially equipped and staffed for emergency CARE. Popularly called emergency room.

e. medical technician (EMT) a provider of emergency CARE (health care at the basic life support level); this may include spinal immobilization, administration of oxygen, and control of bleeding. In some states there are modular training programs where an EMT can add skills to the basic level.

emergent (e-mer′jent) 1. coming out from a cavity or other part. 2. coming on suddenly.

emesis (em′ĕ-sis) VOMITING. Also used as a word termination, as in HEMATEMESIS.

emetic (e-met′ik) 1. causing VOMITING. 2. an agent that does this; examples are a strong solution of salt, MUSTARD water, powdered IPECAC, and ipecac syrup. Emetics should not be used when lye or other strong alkalis or acids have been swallowed, since vomiting may rupture the already weakened walls of the esophagus. Examples of such acids and alkalis are sodium hydroxide (caustic soda), potassium hydroxide (caustic potash), and carbolic acid. Emetics should also be avoided when kerosene, gasoline, nail polish remover, or lacquer thinner has been swallowed, since vomiting of these substances may draw them into the lungs.

WINDOW ON EMERGENCY MEDICAL TECHNICIAN

Emergency Medical Services is a new and exciting health care field. The formal title of Emergency Medical Technician or EMT is approximately 30 years old. The original training curriculum was developed in the mid 1960s under the direction of the American Academy of Orthopedic Surgeons and was approximately 24 hours in length. In the early 1970s the concept of Paramedic emerged primarily to deliver an advanced level of care that included defibrillation, medication administration, and endotracheal intubation. These skills significantly improved the survival of victims of heart attack and cardiac arrest.

Today's EMT is a dynamic health care provider whose role is expanding in both the academic and clinical arenas. There are currently three nationally recognized levels of EMS Provider in the United States: the EMT-Basic or entry level provider is trained in essentials of basic emergency care including airway management, CPR, defibrillation, spinal immobilization, fracture management, bleeding control, and other basic lifesaving interventions; the EMT-Intermediate is trained as an EMT-Basic and has additional education in skills such as intravenous therapy, medication administration, and advanced airway management; and the EMT-Paramedic, the highest trained pre-hospital provider, is skilled in advanced assessment and more sophisticated techniques of airway management including surgical airway interventions and a wide variety of pharmacological management skills.

EMTs are often the first health care providers encountered by the critically ill or injured patient. They must be extremely calm and decisive while working in extremely stressful environments. Knowledge in the basic sciences is an important prerequisite to entering the field of EMS. Interpersonal skills are also a must with EMTs. Since the EMT and Paramedic must deal with extreme emotional states surrounding critical events and disasters, they must be able to gain control and be directive to the patient and bystanders. Finally, the modern day EMT must be adept in a wide variety of psychomotor skills and be in excellent physical condition in order to lift and carry patients.

Many communities are looking to the future EMT to assist in the home care of chronically ill patients, and emerging technology is allowing the application of a wide variety of interventions in pre-hospital care that were traditionally limited to use in the hospital setting. Blood analysis, diagnostic ECG, and other sophisticated treatments are currently being tested by EMTs throughout the United States and the world. The EMT of the future is a far cry from the untrained counterpart of only thirty years ago and is eagerly awaiting new and innovative ways to serve the public and save thousands of lives.

EDWARD STAPLETON

---

emetine (em′ĕ-tēn) an alkaloid derived from ipecac or produced synthetically; its hydrochloride salt is used as an ANTIAMEBIC.

emetocathartic (em″ĕ-to-kah-thahr′tik) 1. both emetic and cathartic. 2. an agent with these effects.

emetogenic (em″ĕ-to-jen′ik)   EMETIC (def. 1).

EMF electromotive force.

-emia word element [Gr.], *condition of the blood.*

emic (e′mik) pertaining to expressions, perceptions, beliefs, and practices that are specific to a given cultural system; an emic view of a cultural system is a description from the perspective of the participant in the system, rather than that of the observer. See also ETIC.

emigration (em″ĭ-gra′shun) the escape of leukocytes through the walls of small blood vessels; diapedesis.

eminence (em′ĭ-nens) a projection or boss.

eminentia (em″ĭ-nen′shah), pl. *eminen′tiae* [L.] eminence.

emissary (em′ĭ-sar″e) 1. affording an outlet, as an emissary vein (see anatomic Table of Veins in the Appendices). 2. emissary vein.

emission (e-mish′un) 1. a discharge. 2. an involuntary discharge of semen.

nocturnal e. reflex emission of semen during sleep.

thermionic e. the application of heat, such as to a filament, resulting in the emission of electrons and ions.

emmetrope (em′ĕ-trōp) a person who has no refractive error of vision.

emmetropia (em″ĕ-tro′pe-ah) the ideal optical condition, parallel rays coming to a focus on the retina. adj., **emmetrop′ic.**

emollient (e-mol′yent) 1. soothing and softening, as an emollient bath given for skin disorders. 2. an agent having this effect on the skin or an irritated internal surface.

emotion (e-mo′shun) a state of arousal characterized by alteration of feeling tone and by physiologic behavioral changes. The external manifestation of emotion is called AFFECT; a pervasive and sustained emotional state, MOOD. adj., **emo′tional.** The physical form of emotion may be outward and evident to others, as in crying, laughing, blushing, or a variety of facial expressions. However, emotion is not always reflected in one's appearance and actions even though psychic changes are taking place. Joy, grief, fear, and anger are examples of emotions.

empathize (em′pah-thīz) to experience or feel empathy.

empathy (em′pah-the) intellectual and emotional awareness and understanding of another person's thoughts, feelings, and behavior, even those that are distressing and disturbing. Empathy emphasizes understanding; sympathy emphasizes sharing of another person's feelings and experiences.

emphysema (em″fĭ-se′mah, em″fi-ze′mah) 1. any pathologic accumulation of air in tissues or organs. 2. chronic pulmonary emphysema.

bullous e. emphysema in which bullae form in areas of lung tissue so that these areas do not contribute to respiration.

chronic pulmonary e. a type of CHRONIC AIRFLOW LIMITATION in the lungs that develops slowly over a period of years and in some persons may gradually lead to serious

disability. It is found most often in heavy smokers and in more men than women; however, this may simply reflect past differences in smoking habits. It becomes disabling between the ages of 50 and 80. Some authorities suggest that a defect in the elastic tissue of the lungs may make certain persons more susceptible. The condition is found with some frequency in aged persons whose lungs have lost their natural elasticity.

This condition is one of the major causes of death in industrialized countries. As with other respiratory ailments, one factor may be the increasing air pollution that accompanies urbanization, industrialization, and the growing number of automobiles. Another factor may be the increase in tobacco smoking. Continuance of smoking seriously aggravates the disease.

As the lungs become less efficient, breathing becomes more difficult for these patients. There is often a persistent cough that is moist and wheezing in nature. Patients often develop a barrel CHEST and have an anxious facial expression. Cardiac complications, especially enlargement and dilatation of the right ventricle with resultant right heart failure (COR PULMONALE), may develop.

A worldwide strategy for the diagnosis, management, and prevention of all forms of chronic airflow limitation has been developed by the WORLD HEALTH ORGANIZATION and the NATIONAL HEART, LUNG, AND BLOOD INSTITUTE. It is known as the GOLD initiative.

distal acinar e. interlobular emphysema.

hypoplastic e. pulmonary emphysema due to a developmental abnormality, resulting in a reduced number of alveoli, which are abnormally large.

interlobular e. accumulation of air in the septa between lobules of the lungs; called also distal acinar emphysema.

interstitial e. the escape of air into the connective tissue of the lung, mediastinum (see PNEUMOMEDIASTINUM), or subcutaneous tissue (see *subcutaneous emphysema*); it results from a tear or rupture of the respiratory passages or alveoli, which may be associated with bronchiolar obstruction or be caused by a penetrating wound of the chest wall or lung.

intestinal e. pneumatosis cystoides intestinalis.

lobar e. emphysema involving less than all the lobes of the affected lung, such as unilateral emphysema.

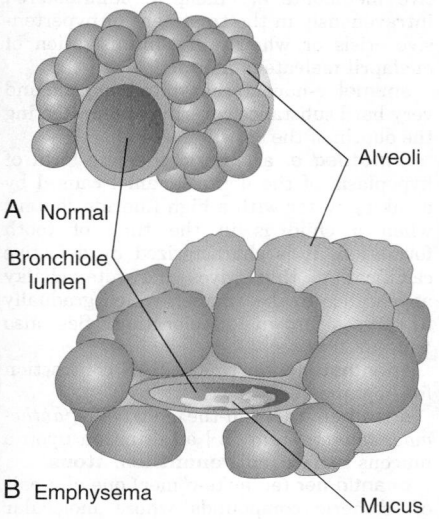

A, Terminal bronchiole in cross-section. B, Terminal bronchiole with narrowed lumen resulting from a loss of surrounding alveoli. From Copstead and Banasik, 2000.

A Normal

Bronchiole lumen

Alveoli

B Emphysema

Mucus

lobar e., congenital, lobar e., infantile a condition characterized by overinflation, commonly affecting one of the upper lobes and causing respiratory distress in early life.

panacinar e., panlobular e. generalized obstructive emphysema affecting all lung segments, with atrophy and dilatation of the alveoli and destruction of the vascular bed.

pulmonary e. see chronic pulmonary EMPHYSEMA.

pulmonary interstitial e. (PIE) a form of BAROTRAUMA that occurs mainly in premature infants, in which air leaks from the alveoli of the lungs into the interstitial space; it is often associated with underlying lung disease or the use of mechanical ventilation.

subcutaneous e. interstitial emphysema characterized by the presence of air in the subcutaneous tissue, usually caused by intrathoracic injury, and in most instances associated with PNEUMOTHORAX and PNEUMOMEDIASTINUM.

surgical e. subcutaneous emphysema following surgery.

unilateral e. emphysema affecting only one lung; it may be either congenital (such as from defects in circulation) or acquired (SWYER-JAMES SYNDROME).

vesicular e. panacinar emphysema.

emphysematous (em″fĭ-sem′ah-tus) of the nature of or affected with emphysema.

empirical (em-pir′ĭ-k′l) based on experience; determined from experimental data, as opposed to theoretical.

empowerment (em-pow′er-ment) the gaining by individuals or groups of the capability to fully participate in decision-making processes in an equitable and fair fashion.

emprosthotonos (em″pros-thot′o-nos) tetanic forward flexure of the body.

empty sella syndrome a syndrome diagnosed radiologically in which the diaphragm of the sella turcica is vestigial, the sella turcica forms an extension of the subarachnoid space and is filled with cerebrospinal fluid, and the pituitary fossa appears to be empty, although the pituitary gland is present in a flattened form.

empyema (em″pi-e′mah) 1. abscess. 2. a PLEURAL EFFUSION containing pus; it occurs as an occasional complication of pleurisy or some other respiratory disease. Symptoms include dyspnea, coughing, chest pain on one side, malaise, and fever. THORACENTESIS may be done to confirm the diagnosis and determine the specific causative organism. Called also pyothorax and purulent or suppurative pleurisy (see PLEURISY).

empyesis (em″pi-e′sis) a pustular eruption.

EMT emergency medical technician.

emulgent (e-mul′jent) 1. causing a straining or purifying process. 2. old term for an agent that stimulates flow of bile or urine.

emulsifier (emul′sĭ-fi″er) a substance used to make an emulsion.

emulsion (e-mul′shun) a mixture of two immiscible liquids, one being dispersed throughout the other in small droplets; a colloid system in which both the dispersed phase and the dispersion medium are liquids. Margarine, cold cream, and various medicated ointments are emulsions. In some emulsions the suspended particles tend to join together and settle out; hence the container must be shaken each time the emulsion is used.

film e. a dehydrated gel emulsion of light- or radiation-sensitive silver halide that is applied to a suitable base.

emulsoid (e-mul′soid) 1. lyophilic colloid. 2. rarely, emulsion.

emunctory (e-mungk′to-re) 1. excretory or cleansing. 2. an excretory organ or duct.

E-Mycin (e-mi′sin) trademark for a preparation of ERYTHROMYCIN, a broad-spectrum ANTIBIOTIC.

enalapril (e-nal′ah-pril) an ANGIOTENSIN-CONVERTING ENZYME INHIBITOR, used as *enalapril maleate* in the treatment of hypertension, congestive heart failure, and asymptomatic left ventricular dysfunction.

enalaprilat (ĕ-nal′-ah-pril-at″) an angiotensin-converting enzyme inhibitor, the active metabolite of enalapril, administered intravenously in the treatment of hypertensive crisis or when oral administration of enalapril maleate is impractical.

enamel (e-nam′el) the white, compact, and very hard substance covering and protecting the dentin of the crown of a tooth.

mottled e. a chronic endemic form of hypoplasia of the dental enamel caused by drinking water with a high fluoride content when a child is in the time of tooth formation. It is characterized by defective calcification that gives a white chalky appearance to the enamel, which gradually undergoes brown discoloration. See also dental FLUOROSIS.

enanthate (en-an′thāt) USAN contraction for heptanoate.

enanthema (en″an-the′mah), pl. *enanthemas, enanthe′mata* [L.] an eruption upon a mucous surface. adj., **enanthem′atous.**

enantiomer (en-an′te-o″mer) one of a pair of isomeric compounds whose molecular structures are mirror images of each other.

enantiomerism (en-an″te-om′er-izm) the relationship between two stereoisomers

Enantiomerism. From Dorland's, 2000.

having molecules that are mirror images of each other; enantiomers have identical chemical and physical properties in an achiral environment but form different products when reacted with other chiral molecules and exhibit optical activity. The enantiomer that rotates a beam of polarized light in the clockwise direction is indicated by the prefix (+)-, formerly *d*- or dextro-; the other enantiomer rotates light in a counterclockwise direction and is indicated by the prefix (−)-, formerly *l*- or levo-. See also DL-. (See accompanying illustration)

enantiomorph (en-an′te-o-morf″) 1. enantiomer. 2. either of two crystals exhibiting enantiomerism. adj., **enantiomor′phic.**

enarthrosis (en″ahr-thro′sis) a joint in which the rounded head of one bone is received into a socket in another, permitting motion in any direction; called also ball-and-socket joint.

encainide (en-ka′nīd) a sodium channel blocking AGENT that acts on the Purkinje FIBERS and MYOCARDIUM; used as the hydrochloride salt in treatment of life-threatening ARRHYTHMIAS.

encapsulation (en-kap″su-la′shun) enclosure within a capsule.

encephal(o)- word element [Gr.], *brain.*

encephalatrophy (en″sef-ah-lat′ro-fe) atrophy of the brain.

encephalic (en″sĕ-fal′ik)) 1. within the skull. 2. pertaining to the brain.

encephalitis (en-sef″ah-li′tis), pl. *encephali′tides* Inflammation of the brain. adj., **encephalit′ic.**

There are many types, depending on the causative agent and the structures involved. A large percentage are caused by viruses; some are transmitted from animals to humans, as in equine encephalitis, and some between humans, as in herpes encephalitis. The symptoms may be mild, with headache and a general malaise and muscle ache similar to that associated with influenza. The more acute and serious symptoms may include fever, delirium, convulsions, coma, and, in a significant number of patients, death.

Treatment is essentially symptomatic and is aimed at control of high fever, maintenance of fluid and electrolyte balance, and constant maintenance of respiratory and urinary function as required. Except for encephalitis caused by HERPESVIRUSES, drug therapy is mainly supportive, such as anticonvulsants, glucocorticoids to reduce cerebral edema, sedatives to minimize restlessness, and aspirin or some other mild analgesic to relieve headache and control fever. Herpes viral encephalitis is treated with VIDARABINE, which is effective only against herpesviruses.

Convalescence from acute cases with serious damage to the central nervous system usually is prolonged, and efforts at physical rehabilitation are needed to overcome the neurological and musculoskeletal complications that may develop. In some cases personality changes and emotional disturbances may require extensive treatment.

Patient Care. During the acute phase of the disease the patient is monitored for alterations in neurologic function. Assessment of level of consciousness, neuromuscular response, and pupil size, as well as evaluation of cranial nerve function and other aspects of a neurologic assessment, are an integral part of care. Increased intracranial pressure is likely; therefore fluid balance is watched closely to avoid aggravating this condition by administering too many fluids.

The patient will need frequent position changes and range of motion exercises to maintain skin integrity and joint motion. During position changes, bathing, and other procedures involving movement of the patient, care should be taken to avoid overstimulating the patient, increasing intracranial pressure, or aggravating neck and head pain. A mild laxative or stool softener should be given to avoid constipation, which can lead to straining at the stool, which in turn can increase intracranial pressure.

A quiet and nonstimulating environment, including a darkened room, is necessary to avoid triggering convulsions and to relieve headache and promote rest. If the patient is comatose, special care will be required as for any patient in COMA. Since DELIRIUM often is symptomatic of encephalitis, the patient will need reassurance and support while suffering from confusion and disorientation. Family members also will need reassurance that behavior changes and other symptoms associated with irritated nerve tissues are not necessarily permanent and usually abate as the patient's condition improves. If severe neurologic deficits do remain after the acute phase, the family will need assistance in obtaining and utilizing long-term rehabilitation services.

acute disseminated e. acute disseminated ENCEPHALOMYELITIS.

Central European e. the milder form of tick-borne ENCEPHALITIS, first noted in Central Europe.

Economo's e. a form of epidemic encephalitis, the original type described by von Economo, marked by increasing languor, apathy, and drowsiness, passing into lethargy; it was observed in various parts of the world between 1915 and 1926. Called also lethargic encephalitis.

epidemic e. any viral encephalitis that occurs in epidemics; common types are Japanese B encephalitis, St. Louis encephalitis, and tick-borne encephalitis.

equine e. equine encephalomyelitis.

granulomatous amebic e. a chronic, usually fatal opportunistic infection caused by *Acanthamoeba* species in debilitated, immunocompromised, diabetic, or alcoholic patients.

herpes e. that caused by a herpesvirus, resembling equine ENCEPHALOMYELITIS.

e. hyperplas'tica an acute nonsuppurating form of encephalitis.

Japanese B e. a form of epidemic ENCEPHALITIS of varying severity occurring in Japan and other Pacific islands, China, eastern Russia, and elsewhere in eastern and northeastern Asia.

La Crosse e. encephalitis caused by the La Crosse VIRUS, transmitted by *Aedes triseriatus,* seen primarily in children, chiefly in the midwestern United States.

lead e. encephalitis with cerebral edema due to LEAD POISONING.

lethargic e. Economo's encephalitis.

e. periaxia'lis diffu'sa Schilder's disease.

postinfection e., postvaccinal e. acute disseminated encephalomyelitis.

Russian spring-summer e. the severe form of epidemic ENCEPHALITIS acquired in forests from infected ticks, but also transmitted in other ways, as by ingestion of the flesh or milk of infected animals. It ranges in severity from mild to fatal, with degenerative changes in organs other than those of the nervous system.

St. Louis e. a viral disease first observed in 1932 in Illinois; it occurs in the late summer and early fall and is clinically similar to western equine ENCEPHALOMYELITIS.

It is usually transmitted by *Culex* mosquitoes.

tick-borne e. a form of epidemic ENCEPHALITIS usually spread by the bites of ticks of the genus *Ixodes* that are infected with FLAVIVIRUSES. It ranges in severity from mild to fatal and there may be degenerative changes in organs other than those of the nervous system. The more common, severe form is Russian spring-summer ENCEPHALITIS, and a milder form is called Central European ENCEPHALITIS.

West Nile e. a mild, febrile, sporadic disease caused by the West Nile VIRUS, transmitted by *Culex* mosquitoes, occurring chiefly in the summer; frequently, infection does not lead to encephalitis. It may be of sudden onset, and symptoms may include drowsiness, severe frontal headache, maculopapular rash, abdominal pain, loss of appetite, nausea, and generalized lymphadenopathy. It is widespread in Africa and also occurs in southern Europe, the Middle East, southern Asia, and more recently North America. Called also West Nile fever.

encephalocele (en-sef'ah-lo-sēl″) hernial protrusion of brain substance and meninges through a congenital or traumatic opening of the skull.

occipital e. an encephalocele in the occipital region, the most common kind seen in the Western Hemisphere. (See accompanying illustration.)

encephalocystocele (en-sef″ah-lo-sis'to-sēl) hydroencephalocele.

encephalography (en-sef″ah-log'rah-fe) radiography demonstrating the intracranial fluid-containing spaces after the withdrawal of cerebrospinal fluid and introduction of air or other gas; it includes pneumoencephalography and ventriculography.

encephaloid (en-sef'ah-loid) 1. resembling the brain or brain substance. 2. medullary carcinoma.

encephalolith (en-sef'ah-lo-lith″) a CALCULUS in the brain.

encephalology (en-sef″ah-lol'o-je) the sum of knowledge regarding the brain, its functions, and its diseases.

encephaloma (en-sef″ah-lo'mah) 1. any swelling or tumor of the brain. 2. medullary carcinoma.

encephalomalacia (en-sef″ah-lo-mah-la'-shah) softening of the brain.

encephalomeningitis (en-sef″ah-lo-men″-in-ji'-tis) meningoencephalitis.

encephalomeningocele (en-sef″ah-lo-mĕ-ning'go-sēl) encephalocele.

encephalomere (en-sef'ah-lo-mēr″) one of the segments making up the embryonic brain.

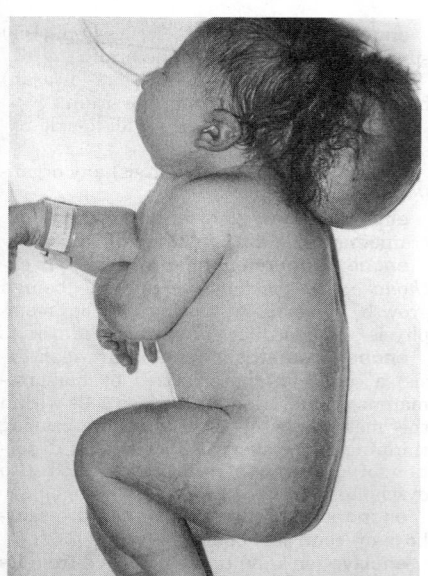

A baby with a large occipital encephalocele. From Mueller and Young, 2001.

encephalometer (en-sef″ah-lom′ĕ-ter) an instrument used in locating certain of the brain regions.

encephalomyelitis (en-sef″ah-lo-mi″ĕ-li′-tis) inflammation of the brain and spinal cord.

   acute disseminated e. an acute or subacute encephalomyelitis or myelitis occurring most commonly following an acute viral infection, especially measles, but sometimes occurring without a recognizable antecedent. Clinical manifestations include fever, headache, vomiting, and drowsiness progressing to lethargy and coma; tremor, seizures, and paralysis may also occur. Mortality ranges from 5 to 20 per cent, and many survivors have residual neurologic deficits.

   benign myalgic e. chronic fatigue syndrome.

   equine e. a type of encephalomyelitis in horses and mules, caused by an alphavirus and spread to humans by mosquitoes; it occurs in summer epizootics in the Western Hemisphere. Three forms are recognized: eastern, western, and Venezuelan. Called also equine encephalitis.

   equine e., eastern a viral disease similar to western equine encephalomyelitis, but occurring in a region extending from New Hampshire to Texas and as far west as Wisconsin, and in Canada, Mexico, the Caribbean, and parts of Central and South America.

   equine e., Venezuelan a viral disease of horses and mules, transmissible to humans; the causative agent was first isolated in Venezuela. The infection in humans resembles influenza, with little or no indication of nervous system involvement.

   equine e., western a viral disease of horses and mules, communicable to humans, occurring chiefly as a meningoencephalitis with little involvement of the medulla oblongata or spinal cord; observed in the United States chiefly west of the Mississippi River.

   granulomatous e. a disease marked by granulomas and necrosis of the walls of the cerebral and spinal ventricles.

   postinfectious e., postvaccinal e. acute disseminated encephalomyelitis.

encephalomyeloneuropathy (en-sef″ah-lo-mi″-ĕ-lo-noō-rop′ah-the) a disease involving the brain, spinal cord, and nerves.

encephalomyelopathy (en-sef″ah-lo-mi″ĕ-lop′ah-the) a disease involving the brain and spinal cord.

encephalomyeloradiculitis (en-sef″ah-lo-mi″ĕ-lo-rah-dik″u-li′tis) inflammation of the brain, spinal cord, and spinal nerve roots.

encephalomyeloradiculopathy (en-sef″-ah-lo-mi″ĕ-lo-rah-dik″u-lop′ah-the) a disease involving the brain, spinal cord, and spinal nerve roots.

encephalomyocarditis (en-sef″ah-lo-mi″o-kahr-di′tis) a viral disease characterized by degenerative and inflammatory changes in skeletal and cardiac muscle and by lesions of the central nervous system resembling those of poliomyelitis.

encephalon (en-sef′ah-lon) brain.

encephalopathy (en-sef″ah-lop′ah-the) any degenerative disease of the brain.

   AIDS e. HIV encephalopathy.

   anoxic e. hypoxic encephalopathy.

   biliary e., bilirubin e. kernicterus.

   bovine spongiform e. a PRION DISEASE of adult cattle in the British Isles with neurologic symptoms. It is transmitted by feed containing protein in the form of meat and bone meal derived from infected animals. The etiologic agent is also the cause of new variant CREUTZFELDT-JAKOB DISEASE. Called also mad cow disease.

   boxer's e., boxer's traumatic e. a syndrome due to cumulative head blows absorbed in the boxing ring, characterized by slowing of mental function, occasional bouts of confusion, and scattered memory loss. It may progress to the more serious BOXER'S DEMENTIA. See also POSTCONCUSSIONAL SYNDROME.

dialysis e. a degenerative disease of the brain associated with longterm use of HEMODIALYSIS, marked by speech disorders and constant myoclonic jerks, progressing to global dementia.

hepatic e. a condition, usually occurring secondary to advanced liver disease, marked by disturbances of consciousness that may progress to deep coma (hepatic coma), psychiatric changes of varying degree, flapping tremor, and fetor hepaticus.

HIV e., HIV-related e. a progressive primary encephalopathy caused by infection with human immunodeficiency VIRUS type I, manifested by a variety of cognitive, motor, and behavioral abnormalities. Called also AIDS encephalopathy.

hypernatremic e. a severe hemorrhagic encephalopathy induced by the hyperosmolarity accompanying hypernatremia and dehydration.

hypertensive e. a complex of cerebral phenomena such as headache, convulsions, and coma that occur in the course of malignant HYPERTENSION.

hypoxic e. encephalopathy caused by hypoxia from either decreased rate of blood flow or decreased oxygen content of arterial blood; mild cases cause temporary intellectual, visual, and motor disturbances, and severe cases can cause permanent brain damage within five minutes. Called also anoxic encephalopathy.

lead e. brain disease caused by LEAD POISONING.

mitochondrial e. encephalopathy associated with mitochondrial abnormalities, such as MELAS SYNDROME and MERRF SYNDROME.

portal-systemic e., portasystemic e. hepatic encephalopathy.

progressive subcortical e. Schilder's disease.

subacute spongiform e., transmissible spongiform e. prion disease.

traumatic e. 1. boxer's encephalopathy. 2. postconcussional syndrome.

Wernicke's e. a neurological disorder characterized by confusion, apathy, drowsiness, ataxia of gait, nystagmus, and ophthalmoplegia; it is due to thiamine deficiency, usually from chronic alcohol abuse. It is almost invariably accompanied by or followed by KORSAKOFF'S SYNDROME and frequently accompanied by other nutritional polyneuropathies. See also WERNICKE-KORSAKOFF SYNDROME.

encephalopuncture (en-sef'ah-lo-pungk"-chur) surgical puncture of the brain.

encephalopyosis (en-sef"ah-lo-pi-o'sis) suppuration or abscess of the brain.

encephalorrhagia (en-sef"ah-lo-ra'jah) hemorrhage within or from the brain.

encephalosclerosis (en-sef"ah-lo-sklě-ro'sis) hardening of the brain.

encephalosis (en"sef-ah-lo'sis) any organic brain disease.

encephalotomy (en"sef-ah-lot'ah-me) 1. craniotomy (def. 2). 2. incision of the brain.

enchondroma (en"kon-dro'mah), pl. *enchondromas, enchondro'mata* A benign growth of cartilage arising in the metaphysis of a bone. adj., **enchondro'matous.**

enchondromatosis (en-kon"dro-mah-to'sis) a condition characterized by hamartomatous proliferation of cartilage cells within the metaphysis of several bones, causing thinning of the overlying cortex and distortion of the growth in length. Called also dyschondroplasia.

enchondrosarcoma (en-kon"dro-sahr-ko'mah) central chondrosarcoma.

enclave (en'klāv) tissue detached from its normal connection and enclosed within another organ.

encopresis (en"ko-pre'sis) fecal incontinence.

encysted (en-sist'ed) enclosed in a sac, bladder, or cyst.

end(o)- word element [Gr.], *within; inward.*

endadelphos (end"ah-del'fos) a fetus in which a parasitic twin is enclosed within the body of the other twin (the autosite).

endaortitis (en"da-or-ti'tis) inflammation of the TUNICA INTIMA of the aorta.

endarterectomy (en"dahr-ter-ek'to-me) excision of thickened atheromatous areas of the innermost coat of an artery; see also ATHERECTOMY.

carotid e. see CAROTID ENDARTERECTOMY.

endarterial (end"ar-tēr'e-al) intra-arterial.

endarteritis (en"dahr-ter-i'tis) inflammation of the TUNICA INTIMA of an artery; called also endoarteritis.

e. obli'terans a form in which the lumina of the smaller vessels become narrowed or obliterated as a result of proliferation of the tissue of the intimal layer. See also ARTERIOSCLEROSIS OBLITERANS.

endaural (end-aw'ral) within the ear.

endbrain (end'brān) telencephalon.

end-bulb (end'bulb) one of the small encapsulated bodies at the end of sensory nerve fibers in skin, mucous membranes, muscles, and other areas. Called also Krause's bulb or corpuscle.

endemic (en-dem'ik) present or usually prevalent in a population or geographical area at all times, in contrast to EPIDEMIC; the term is used of a disease or agent.

endemoepidemic (en″de-mo-ep″ĭ-dem′ik) endemic, but occasionally becoming epidemic.

endergonic (en″der-gon′ik) characterized or accompanied by the absorption of energy; requiring the input of free energy.

end feel a characteristic sensation perceived by the examiner when the end of joint RANGE OF MOTION is reached. The six types of joint end feel most often used are bone to bone, soft tissue approximation, spasm end feel, empty end feel, capsular end feel, and springy block.

end-foot (end′foot) a buttonlike or knoblike terminal enlargement on a naked nerve fiber that ends in a synapse with dendrites of another cell. Called also bouton terminal.

ending (end′ing) a finishing or final part of something, especially the peripheral termination of a nerve or nerve fiber. Called also terminatio and terminus.

free nerve e. the type of neural receptor with the simplest form, in which the peripheral nerve fiber divides into fine branches that terminate freely in connective tissue or epithelium.

endoangiitis (en″do-an″je-i′tis) endangiitis.

endoappendicitis (en″do-ah-pen″dĭ-si′tis) inflammation of the mucous membrane of the vermiform appendix.

endoarteritis (en″do-ar″ter-i′tis) endarteritis.

endoblast (en′do-blast) endoderm.

endobronchitis (en″do-brong-ki′tis) inflammation of the epithelial lining of the bronchi.

endocardial (en″do-kahr′de-al) 1. situated or occurring within the heart. 2. pertaining to the endocardium.

e. cushions elevations on the atrioventricular canal of the embryonic heart that later help form the interatrial septum.

endocarditis (en″do-kahr-di′tis) exudative and proliferative inflammatory alterations of the endocardium, characterized by the presence of vegetations on the surface of the endocardium or in the endocardium itself, and most commonly involving a heart valve, but also affecting the inner lining of the cardiac chambers or the endocardium elsewhere. adj., **endocardit′ic**.

Patient Care. Treatment for bacterial or infectious endocarditis by intravenous antibiotic therapy usually lasts for about four weeks. During that time the patient usually is hospitalized and placed on therapeutic bed rest to reduce the workload of the heart. Throughout the course of treatment the patient must be protected from the hazards of immobility and possible complications from intravenous therapy. Because the potential for embolization is rather high during and for a few weeks after treatment, the patient is watched closely for such symptoms as hematuria, pleuritic chest pain, paresis, and pain in the upper left quadrant of the abdomen, which could indicate vascular occlusion or infarction of the kidney, pulmonary vessels, cerebral vessels, or spleen.

Urinary output is measured and laboratory test data on renal status such as BUN and creatinine are monitored for signs of renal infarction or drug toxicity. Since congestive HEART FAILURE is sometimes a complication of endocarditis, the patient is watched for edema, dyspnea, neck vein distention, and other signs of disturbance in the heart's pumping action.

Before discharge the patient and family are taught the symptoms of fever, fatigue, and other signs of relapse that could occur up to two or more weeks after therapy. During this time the patient is warned against excessive physical exertion, but normal activities of daily living can be resumed safely if approved by the health care provider. Patients who are susceptible to bacterial endocarditis are cautioned to notify their physicians before having dental work and invasive diagnostic procedures that might introduce microorganisms into the body. It may be recommended that prophylactic antibiotics be given before, during, and immediately after procedures of this kind.

atypical verrucous e. nonbacterial endocarditis found in association with systemic lupus erythematosus; called also Libman-Sacks disease or endocarditis.

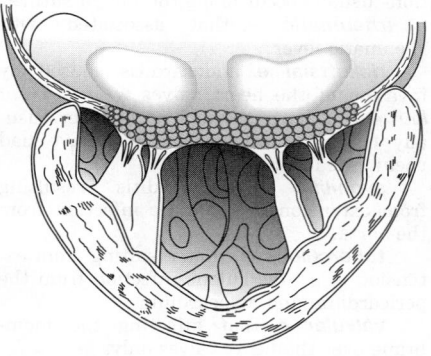

Endocarditis is characterized by the presence of vegetations (called Aschoff bodies) on the surface of the endocardium, most commonly the mitral valve. From Betz et al., 1994.

bacterial e. infectious endocarditis, acute or subacute, caused by various bacteria, including streptococci, staphylococci, enterococci, gonococci, and gram-negative bacilli. Bacterial endocarditis can be treated effectively in about 70 per cent of cases by intravenous antibiotic therapy.

Candida e. mycotic endocarditis caused by a species of *Candida;* called also endocardial candidiasis.

infectious e., infective e. that due to infection with microorganisms, especially bacteria and fungi: the *acute* form may be due to staphylococci, pneumococci, gonococci, streptococci, and other bacteria or to other microorganisms; the *subacute* form may be caused by viridans streptococci, fungi, or other microorganisms.

Libman-Sacks e. atypical verrucous endocarditis.

Löffler's e., Löffler's fibroplastic parietal e. endocarditis associated with EOSINO-PHILIA, marked by fibroplastic thickening of the endocardium, resulting in congestive HEART FAILURE, persistent TACHYCARDIA, HEPATOMEGALY, SPLENOMEGALY, serous effusions into the pleural cavity, and EDEMA of the limbs.

mural e. that affecting the lining of the walls of the heart chambers only.

mycotic e. infectious endocarditis, usually subacute, due to various fungi, most commonly species of *Candida, Aspergillus,* and *Histoplasma.*

nonbacterial thrombotic e. that in which the vegetations, single or multiple, consist of fibrin and other blood elements.

parietal e. mural endocarditis.

prosthetic valve e. infectious endocarditis as a complication of implantation of a prosthetic valve in the heart; the vegetations usually occur along the line of suture.

rheumatic e. that associated with rheumatic fever.

rickettsial e. endocarditis caused by invasion of the heart valves with *Coxiella burnetii;* it is a sequela of Q fever, usually occurring in persons who have had rheumatic fever.

syphilitic e. endocarditis resulting from extension of syphilitic infection from the aorta.

tuberculous e. that resulting from extension of a tuberculous infection from the pericardium and myocardium.

valvular e. that affecting the membrane over the heart valves only.

vegetative e., verrucous e. endocarditis, infectious or noninfectious, the characteristic lesions of which are vegetations or verrucae on the endocardium.

endocardium (en″do-kahr′de-um) the endothelial lining membrane of the cavities of the heart and the connective tissue bed on which it lies.

endocervicitis (en″do-ser″vĭ-si′tis) inflammation of the endocervix.

endocervix (en″do-ser′viks) 1. the glandular cells lining the canal of the cervix uteri. 2. the region of the opening of the cervix uteri into the uterine cavity. adj., **endocer′vical.**

endochondral (en″do-kon′dral) situated, formed, or occurring within cartilage.

endocolitis (en″do-ko-li′tis) inflammation of the mucous membrane of the colon.

endocranial (en″do-kra′ne-al) intracranial.

endocranitis (en″do-kra-ni′tis) inflammation of endocranium.

endocranium (en″do-kra′ne-um) the endosteal layer of the dura mater of the brain.

endocrine (en′do-krin) 1. secreting internally. 2. pertaining to internal secretions; hormonal.

e. glands ductless organs or groups of cells that secrete regulatory substances (HORMONES) and release them directly into the circulation. The endocrine SYSTEM and the nervous SYSTEM are the two major control systems of the body, and their functions are interrelated. Hormonal activity is mostly concerned with regulating metabolic activities by controlling the rates at which chemical reactions take place within cells, the transport of substances across the cell membrane, and activities related to growth and reproduction. The word *hormones* is applied to substances released by the endocrine glands that have physiologic effects on target organs (which can be other endocrine glands) and tissues distant from the gland. There are, however, local hormones (AUTACOIDS) secreted at the site of the tissue being affected, such as ACETYLCHOLINE and SEROTONIN.

The interactions between hormones and metabolic activities throughout the body are controlled by negative feedback. The system is a closed loop in which either an excess or a deficit of some hormone initiates a response that results in its return to a level within normal range. For example, the level of THYROXINE in the serum is responsive to the level of THYROTROPIN released by the anterior PITUITARY GLAND, which in turn responds to the level of thyrotropin-releasing HORMONE released by the hypothalamus; the release of these hormones responds to the level of thyroxine. Excessive amounts of thyroxine eventually result in reduction in the amount of it released from the thyroid gland.

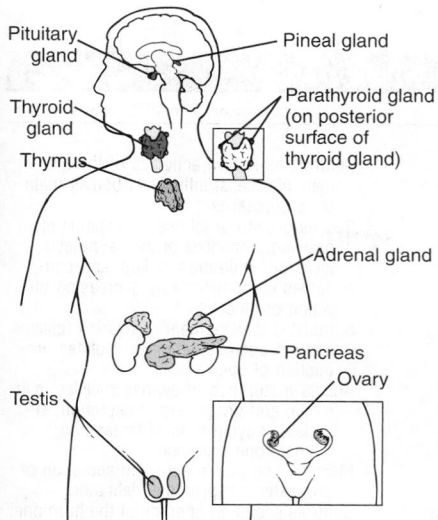

Pituitary gland

Pineal gland

Thyroid gland

Parathyroid gland (on posterior surface of thyroid gland)

Thymus

Adrenal gland

Pancreas

Ovary

Testis

The endocrine glands. From Applegate, 2000.

Similarly, a lower than normal concentration of it in the serum will initiate changes that eventually raise its levels by stimulating its release from the thyroid gland.

The major endocrine glands are the HY-POTHALAMUS; the PITUITARY, THYROID, PARA-THYROID, and ADRENAL GLANDS; the alpha and beta cells of the PANCREAS; and the gonads (OVARIES and TESTES).

Disorders of the endocrine glands are not simply a matter of overproduction or underproduction of a particular hormone. Hyperfunction and hypofunction of these glands can be classified according to the source of the dysfunction.

A *primary* disorder is one in which the gland responsible for synthesis and production of specific hormones is not functioning normally and is releasing too much or too little of one or more hormones. An example is HYPOTHYROIDISM resulting from surgical or radiotherapeutic destruction of the thyroid gland.

A *secondary* endocrine disorder is one in which dysfunction of one gland (usually the PITUITARY GLAND) causes dysfunction of another gland. An example is hyposecretion of CORTICOTROPIN from the anterior lobe of the pituitary gland. This results in secondary adrenocortical insufficiency and a deficit of GLUCOCORTICOIDS and MINERALOCORTICOIDS.

In a *tertiary* endocrine disorder, two control steps are involved, as when a disorder of the HYPOTHALAMUS causes improper inhibition or release of a releasing hormone

that influences the pituitary gland. Dysfunction of the pituitary then affects some other endocrine gland that is normally stimulated by a pituitary hormone.

endocrinologist (en″do-krĭ-nol′o-jist) a specialist in ENDOCRINOLOGY.

endocrinology (en″do-krĭ-nol′o-je) 1. the study of HORMONES, the endocrine SYSTEM, and their role in the physiology of the body. 2. a medical specialty concerned with the diagnosis and treatment of disorders of the endocrine SYSTEM.

endocrinopathy (en″do-krĭ-nop′ah-the) any disease due to disorder of the endocrine system. adj., **endocrinopath′ic.**

endocrinotherapy (en″do-kri″no-ther′ah-pe) treatment of disease by the administration of endocrine preparations; hormonotherapy.

endocytosis (en″do-si-to′sis) the uptake by a cell of material from the environment by invagination of the plasma membrane; it includes both PHAGOCYTOSIS and PINOCYTOSIS.

endoderm (en′do-derm) the innermost of the three primary germ layers of the embryo; from it are derived the epithelium of the pharynx, respiratory tract (except the nose), digestive tract, bladder, and urethra. Called also endoblast, entoderm, entoblast, and hypoblast.

endodontics (en″do-don′tiks) the branch of dentistry concerned with the etiology, prevention, diagnosis, and treatment of conditions that affect the tooth pulp, root, and periapical tissues.

endodontist (en″do-don′tist) a dentist who specializes in endodontics.

endodontitis (en″do-don-ti′tis) pulpitis.

endodontium (en″do-don′she-um) dental pulp.

endoenteritis (en″do-en″tĕ-ri′tis) inflammation of the intestinal mucosa.

endogamy (en-dog′ah-me) 1. fertilization by union of separate cells having the same chromatin ancestry. 2. restriction of marriage to persons within the same community. adj., **endog′amous.**

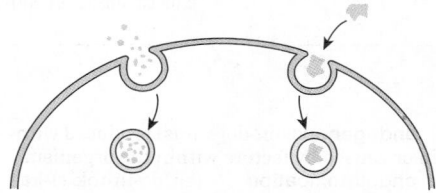

Endocytosis. Shown are pinocytosis of small fluid droplets *(left)* and phagocytosis of a large particle *(right)*. From Dorland's, 2000.

FUNCTIONS OF ENDOCRINE GLANDS

Gland	Hormone	Action on Target Tissues
Pituitary		
Anterior lobe	Thyroid-stimulating hormone (TSH); also called thyrotropin	Controls all known activities of thyroid glandular cells; influences body's metabolic processes
	Growth hormone (GH); also called somatotropic hormone (SH) and somatotropin	Causes growth of all tissues capable of growing; enhances protein synthesis, increases utilization of fats, and conserves carbohydrate by decreasing utilization of glucose.
	Follicle-stimulating hormone (FSH)	Stimulates development of ovarian follicles and estrogen secretion; stimulates production of sperm
	Luteinzing hormone (LH)	Affects maturation of ovarian follicles, ovulation, and progesterone secretion; stimulates Leydig cells of testes and testosterone secretion
	Prolactin (PRL)	Maintains corpus luteum and secretion of progesterone; promotes lactation
	Adrenocorticotrophic hormone (ACTH); also called adrenocorticotropin and corticotropin	Controls secretion of some of the hormones of the adrenal cortex, e.g., the glucocorticoids (chiefly cortisol and, to some extent, aldosterone and adrenal sex hormones)
Posterior lobe	Vasopressin (VP); also called antidiuretic hormone (ADH)	Elevates blood pressure in relatively high doses; conserves water by decreasing urinary output
	Oxytocin (OT)	Activates uterine contraction and, in response to sexual stimulation, transports sperm during coitus; increases secretion of milk
Intermediate part	Melanocyte-stimulating hormone (MSH)	Increases pigmentation of skin
Thyroid	Thyroxine (T_4); also called tetraiodothyronine and levothyroxine	Stimulate metabolism (catabolic phase), e.g., increase respiratory rate and utilization of oxygen, production of body heat, gluconeogenesis, strength and force of heart rate, and enhance muscle tone
	Calcitonin	Decreases serum calcium
Parathyroid	Parathyroid hormone (PTH); also called parathormone	Maintains constant serum level of calcium
Adrenal		
Cortex	Glucocorticoids (chiefly cortisol)	Increase protein breakdown, impair utilization of glucose, and increase hepatic output of glucose, hence are called diabetogenic hormones; essential for survival under stress
	Mineralocorticoids (chiefly aldosterone)	Promote retention of sodium and loss of potassium and hydrogen in urine
	Androgens and estrogens	(See under Testes and Ovaries)
Medulla	Epinephrine, norepinephrine (to a much smaller extent)	Increase cardiac output, elevate blood glucose and blood lipids, raise blood pressure

(continued)

endogenous (en-doj′ĕ-nus) produced within or caused by factors within the organism.

endointoxication (en″do-in-tok″sĭ-ka′-shun) poisoning by an endogenous toxin.

endolaryngeal (en″do-lah-rin′je-al) situated on or occurring within the larynx.

endolymph (en′do-limf) the fluid contained in the membranous labyrinth of the ear; it is entirely separate from the PERILYMPH.

endolysin (en-dol′ĭ-sin) a bactericidal substance in cells; acting directly on bacteria.

FUNCTIONS OF ENDOCRINE GLANDS—*cont'd"*

Gland	Hormone	Action on Target Tissues
Ovaries	Estrogens: beta-estradiol, estrone, and estriol	Cause proliferation and growth of sexual organs and other reproductive tissues; induce proliferative phase of the menstrual cycle
	Progesterone	Prepares endometrium for implantation of the fertilized ovum, decreases frequency of uterine contractions, promotes secretory changes in mucosal lining of uterine tubes for nutrition of fertilized ovum, prepares mammary tissue for lactation
Placenta	Human chorionic gonadotropin (hCG)	Maintains the corpus luteum and stimulates progesterone secretion
	Human placental lactogen (hPL)	Acts in combination with prolactin to induce lactation; also promotes growth and acts as an insulin antagonist
Testes	Androgens: testosterone, dihydrotestosterone, androstenedione	Promote development of male sex characteristics in fetus, stimulate descent of testes into scrotum, stimulate protein production, responsible for masculinization
Islets of Langerhans of Pancreas		
Beta cells	Insulin	Promotes uptake, storage, and use of glucose, particularly by liver, muscles, and fat tissue, increases transport of glucose into cells and their usage of glucose, causes active transport of many amino acids into cells, promotes protein synthesis and inhibits catabolism of proteins, depresses rate of gluconeogenesis, and has synergistic effect with GH
Alpha cells	Glucagon	Causes glycogenolysis in liver and release of glucose, which raises blood glucose level; increases rate of gluconeogenesis, which causes continued hyperglycemia
Delta cells	Somatostatin	Inhibits secretion of both insulin and glucagon; also secreted by hypothalamus as growth hormone-inhibiting hormone
Thymus	Thymosin	Induces differentiation of T-lymphocytes involved in cell-mediated immunity

endometriosis (en″do-me″tre-o′sis) a condition in which tissue more or less perfectly resembling the endometrium occurs outside the uterine cavity, usually in the pelvic cavity. adj., **endometriot′ic.**

Cause. Currently the cause of endometriosis is unknown. Researchers propose three possible causes: (1) the expulsion of endometrial tissue during menstruation upward through the fallopian tubes and into the pelvic cavity, where it is implanted on the ovaries or peritoneum, (2) a hormonal change or other event that triggers transformation of coelomic epithelium to endometrial endothelium, and (3) a combination of these two in which transported endometrium chemically induces undifferentiated mesenchymal cells to form endometrial tissue. Women may be asymptomatic, and symptoms vary among women and in one woman over time.

Symptoms may include secondary dysmenorrhea, dyspareunia, abnormal bleeding, and impaired fertility due to adhesions.

Treatment. Therapy is based on the age of the patient, her desire for pregnancy, and the extent of the endometrial growth. In young women with mild disease, combination oral contraceptives are often used. In more advanced cases, hormonally induced menopause may be indicated, because endometriosis regresses with menopause. In older women and in cases of extensive growth, surgical treatment is indicated. Conservative surgical treatment includes laparoscopy for lysis of adhesions and laser vaporization of endometrial lesions.

endometritis (en″do-me-tri′tis) inflammation of the endometrium.

puerperal e. endometritis following childbirth.

syncytial e. a benign tumorlike lesion with infiltration of the uterine wall by large syncytial trophoblastic cells.

tuberculous e. inflammation of the endometrium, usually also involving the fallopian tubes, due to infection by *Mycobacterium tuberculosis,* with the presence of tubercles.

endometrium (en″do-me′tre-um), pl. *endome′tria* [Gr.] the mucous membrane lining the uterus. adj., **endome′trial.**

endomitosis (en″do-mi-to′sis) mitosis taking place without dissolution of the nuclear membrane, and not followed by cytoplasmic division, resulting in doubling of the number of chromosomes within the nucleus. adj., **endomitot′ic.**

endomorph (en′do-morf) an individual having a type of body build in which endodermal tissues predominate: there is relative preponderance of soft roundness throughout the body, with large digestive viscera and fat accumulations, and with large trunk and tapering extremities.

endomorphy (en′do-mor″fe) the condition of being an endomorph. adj., **endomor′phic.**

endomyocarditis (en″do-mi″o-kahr-di′tis) inflammation of the endocardium and myocardium.

endomysium (en″do-mis′e-um) the sheath of delicate reticular fibrils that surrounds each muscle fiber.

endoneuritis (en″do-noo-ri′tis) inflammation of the endoneurium.

endoneurium (en″do-noor′e-um) the interstitial connective tissue in a peripheral nerve, separating individual nerve fibers. Called also Henle's sheath and connective tissue sheath of Key and Retzius. adj., **endoneu′rial.**

endonuclease (en″do-noo′kle-ās) an enzyme that cleaves internal bonds of polynucleotides.

restriction e's enzymes that cleave large DNA molecules at specific sequences of four to six nucleotides. See also RECOMBINANT DNA TECHNOLOGY.

endoparasite (en″do-par′ah-sīt) a parasite that lives within the body of the host. adj., **endoparasit′ic.**

endopelvic (en″do-pel′vik) within the pelvis.

endopeptidase (en″do-pep′tĭ-dās) any PEPTIDASE that catalyzes the cleavage of

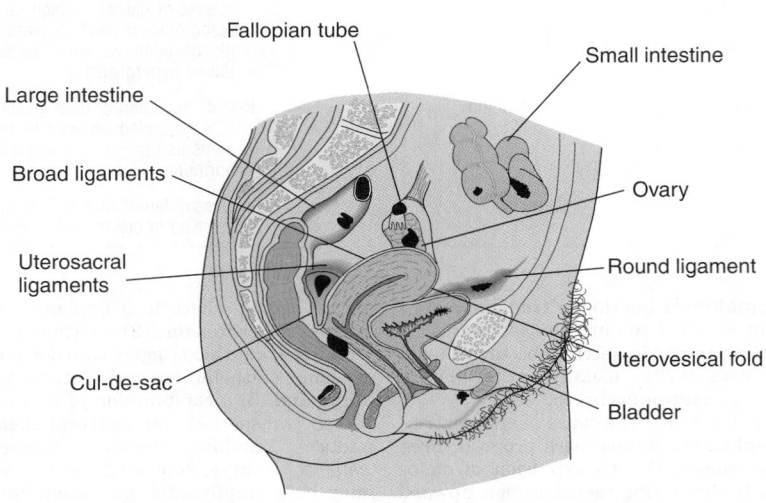

Common sites of endometriosis. From McKinney et al., 2000.

internal bonds in a polypeptide or protein. Inhibition of the action of endopeptidases (proteases) in viruses causes formation of noninfectious particles; certain antiviral drugs work in this way (see protease INHIBITORS). Called also protease and proteinase.

endopericarditis (en″do-per″ĭ-kahr-di′tis) inflammation of the endocardium and pericardium.

endoperimyocarditis (en″do-per″ĭ-mi″o-kahr-di′-tis) inflammation of the endocardium, pericardium, and myocardium.

endoperitonitis (en″do-per″ĭ-to-ni′tis) inflammation of the serous lining of the peritoneal cavity.

endophlebitis (en″do-flĕ-bi′tis) inflammation of the TUNICA INTIMA of a vein.

endophthalmitis (en″dof-thal-mi′tis) inflammation of the ocular cavities and their adjacent structures.

endophyte (en′do-fīt) a parasitic plant organism living within its host's body.

endophytic (en″do-fit′ik) 1. pertaining to an endophyte. 2. growing inward; proliferating on the interior of an organ or structure.

endoprosthesis (en″do-pros-the′sis) a hollow stent inserted into a bile duct to allow internal biliary drainage across an obstruction.

endopyelotomy (en″do-pi″ĕ-lot′ah-me) an incision procedure to correct a stenosed ureteropelvic JUNCTION by cutting from within using an instrument inserted through an endoscope.

endoreduplication (en″do-re-du″plĭ-ka′-shun) replication of chromosomes without subsequent cell division.

end-organ (end or′gan) one of the larger, encapsulated endings of sensory nerves. Written also end organ.

endorphin (en-dor′fin) one of a group of opiate-like peptides produced naturally by the body at neural synapses at various points in the central nervous system pathways, where they modulate the transmission of pain perceptions. The term *endorphin* was coined by combining the words *endogenous* and *morphine*. Like morphine, endorphins raise the pain threshold and produce sedation and euphoria; the effects are blocked by naloxone, a narcotic antagonist.

endorsement (en-dors′ment) the examination by a State Board of Nursing of the credentials of a nurse licensed in a different state, and the determination that the nurse is eligible to receive a nursing license in the second state.

endosalpingitis (en″do-sal″pin-ji′tis) inflammation of the endosalpinx.

endosalpingoma (en″do-sal″ping-go′mah) adenomyoma of the fallopian tube.

endosalpingiosis (en″do-sal-pin″-je-o′sis) 1. endometriosis involving the fallopian tube. 2. ovarian endometriosis in which the abnormal mucosa resembles tubal mucosa rather than endometrium.

endosalpinx (en″do-sal′pinks) the mucous membrane lining the FALLOPIAN TUBE.

endoscope (en′do-skōp) an instrument used for direct visual inspection of hollow organs or body cavities. Specially designed endoscopes are used for such examinations as BRONCHOSCOPY, CYSTOSCOPY, GASTROSCOPY, and PROCTOSCOPY. Although the design may vary according to the specific use, all endoscopes have similar working elements. The viewing part (scope) may be a hollow metal or fiber tube fitted with a lens system that permits viewing in a variety of directions. There is also a light source, power cord, and power source. Accessories that might be used for diagnostic or therapeutic purposes include suction tip, tubes, and suction pump; forceps for removal of biopsy tissue or a foreign body; biopsy brushes; an electrode tip for cauterization; as well as a video camera, video monitors, and image recorder.

endoscopy (en-dos′kah-pe) visual examination of interior structures of the body with an endoscope. adj., **endoscop′ic**.

endosepsis (en″do-sep′sis) septicemia originating from causes inside the body.

endoskeleton (en′do-skel″ĕ-ton) the cartilaginous and bony skeleton of the body, exclusive of that part of the skeleton of dermal origin.

endosmosis (en″dos-mo′sis) inward osmosis; inward passage of liquid through a membrane of a cell or cavity, by which one fluid passes through a septum into a cavity that contains fluid of a different density. adj., **endosmot′ic**.

endospore (en′do-spor) 1. a thick-walled body formed within the vegetative cells of certain bacteria (e.g., *Bacillus, Clostridium, Sarcina*) that can withstand adverse environmental conditions for prolonged periods; under favorable conditions it will germinate

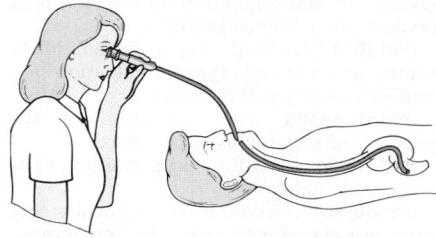

Upper GI endoscopy. From Lammon et al., 1995.

to form a vegetative bacterium. 2. an asexual fungal SPORE produced within the hyphae or cell, as in a spherule of *Coccidioides immitis* or in a SPORANGIUM.

endosteal (en-dos'te-al) 1. pertaining to the endosteum. 2. occurring or located within a bone.

endosteitis (en-dos″te-i′tis) inflammation of the endosteum.

endosteoma (en-dos″te-o′mah) a tumor in the medullary cavity of a bone.

endosteum (en-dos′te-um) the tissue lining the medullary cavity of a bone.

endostoma (en″dos-to′mah) endosteoma.

endotendineum (en″do-ten-din′e-um) the delicate connective tissue separating the secondary bundles (fascicles) of a tendon.

endothelia (en″do-the′le-ah) [L.] plural of ENDOTHELIUM.

endothelial (en″do-the′le-al) pertaining to or made up of endothelium.

endothelioid (en″do-the′le-oid) resembling endothelium.

endothelioma (en″do-the″le-o′mah) a tumor arising from the endothelial lining of blood vessels.

endotheliosis (en″do-the″le-o′sis) proliferation of endothelial elements.

  glomerular capillary e. a renal lesion typical of ECLAMPSIA; it is characterized by deposition of fibrous material in and beneath the cells of the grossly swollen glomerular capillary endothelium, resulting in near total or total occlusion of the capillaries.

endothelium (en″do-the′le-um), pl. *endothe′lia* [Gr.] the layer of epithelial cells that lines the cavities of the heart and of the blood and lymph vessels, and the serous cavities of the body.

endotherm (en′do-therm″) 1. an animal that exhibits endothermy. 2. homeotherm.

endothermal (en″do-ther′m'l) endothermic.

endothermic (en″do-ther′mik) 1. characterized or accompanied by the absorption of heat. 2. pertaining to or characterized by ENDOTHERMY. 3. homeothermic.

endothermy (en′do-ther″me) 1. diathermy. 2. thermal regulation by internal heat production. 3. homeothermy.

endothrix (en′do-thriks) a dermatophyte whose growth and spore production are confined chiefly within the shaft of a hair.

endotoxemia (en″do-tok-se′me-ah) the presence of endotoxins in the blood.

endotoxic (en′do-tok″sik) pertaining to or possessing endotoxin.

endotoxin (en′do-tok″sin) a heat-stable toxin associated with the outer membranes of certain gram-negative bacteria, including

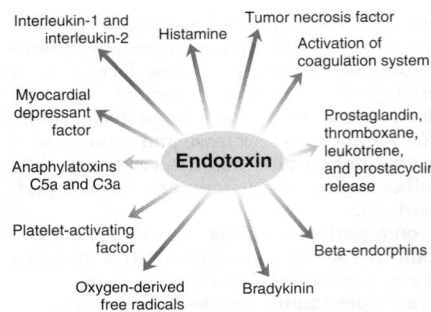

Results of endotoxin release. From Copstead, 1995.

Brucella, Neisseria, and *Vibrio* species. Endotoxins are not secreted but are released only when the cells are disrupted; they are less potent and less specific than the EXOTOXINS; and they do not form TOXOIDS. In large quantities they produce hemorrhagic shock and severe diarrhea; smaller amounts cause fever, altered resistance to bacterial infection, leukopenia followed by leukocytosis, and numerous other biologic effects.

endotracheal (en″do-tra′ke-al) within the trachea.

  e. tube an AIRWAY catheter inserted in the trachea during endotracheal INTUBATION to assure patency of the upper airway by allowing for removal of secretions and maintenance of an adequate air passage. Endotracheal intubation may be accomplished through the mouth using an orotracheal tube, or through the nose using a nasotracheal tube. Numerous different endotracheal tubes are available. Tubes for adults are almost always "cuffed" to prevent air and aspiration leakage and allow for their use with a mechanical ventilator. (Pediatric tubes are not cuffed, since the airway is narrower at the distal end.) The cuff is a balloonlike device that fits over the lower end of the tube and is attached to a narrow tube that extends outside the body and allows for inflation of the cuff. Once the cuff is inflated there is no flow of air through the trachea other than that going through the endotracheal tube. Care should be taken not to overinflate the cuff.

  Passage of an endotracheal tube during surgery is a well-established and long-used technique. In recent years the procedure has become a part of medical management of ventilatory failure as an alternative to TRACHEOTOMY. Tube placement is verified by watching the tube pass through the vocal cords, listening to the lungs and stomach, and checking it radiographically within one hour of placement. Adjunct techniques such as CAPNOMETRY and pulse OXIMETRY can also be

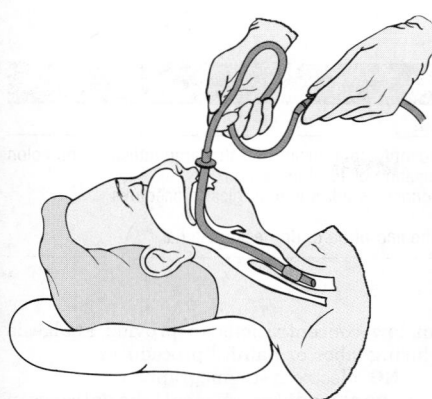

Suctioning an endotracheal tube. From Lammon et al., 1995.

used to verify placement. Endotracheal intubation has the advantages of not requiring a surgical procedure as does tracheotomy, of removal of the tube (extubation) being less involved, and of the procedure being able to be repeated as necessary.

The endotracheal tube cannot be used for long-term relief of ventilatory failure. A TRACHEOSTOMY is required for long-term VENTILATOR-dependent patients.

Complications of endotracheal intubation include damage to the vocal cords, erosion, and eventual stricture of the larynx. Pulmonary infections may result from interference with the normal protective mechanisms of the glottis and from the introduction of pathogenic organisms into the respiratory tract and difficulty in their removal by coughing.

Patient Care. The respiratory apparatus for assisted ventilation must be stabilized. Secure anchoring of the tube and apparatus is necessary to prevent tension on or misplacement of the tube. Its position is checked periodically by AUSCULTATION, chest X-RAY, or CAPNOGRAPHY.

The inhaled air must be adequately humidified; the normal humidifying function of the upper respiratory tract is not present because the tube bypasses that area. Inhaled air must also be protected from contamination as much as possible. SUCTIONING of secretions via the tube is done with gentleness and according to the basic guidelines established for this procedure. The patient will require mouth care and frequent observation for signs of pressure against the lips and nose. An emergency tracheotomy tray and an extra endotracheal tube are kept at the bedside. Since a patient with an endotracheal tube in place cannot talk,

means must be arranged to assist with communication. During an emergency, medications that can be administered through the endotracheal tube include EPINEPHRINE, ATROPINE, and LIDOCAINE.

endovasculitis (en″do-vas″ku-li′tis) endangiitis.

end plate a flat termination.

motor e. p. the discoid expansion of a terminal branch of the axon of a motor nerve fiber, which apposes the sole plate of a skeletal muscle fiber, forming the neuromuscular JUNCTION.

endrin (en′drin) a highly toxic chlorinated HYDROCARBON insecticide; it is a stereoisomer of DIELDRIN.

end-stage renal disease chronic RENAL FAILURE that is irreversible; at this stage serum CREATININE and BLOOD UREA NITROGEN (BUN) levels continue to rise and there is UREMIA with impairment of all body systems.

endurance (en-doo′rens) the ability to sustain an activity over a period of time.

Enduron (en′du-ron) trademark for a preparation of METHYCLOTHIAZIDE, a diuretic.

end user a person with need for information who employs an information retrieval system, either directly or through a search specialist.

enema (en′ĕ-mah) [Gr.] 1. introduction of fluid into the rectum. 2. a solution introduced into the rectum to promote evacuation of feces or as a means of administering nutrient substances, medicinal substances, or opaque material for radiologic examination of the lower intestinal tract; see also BARIUM TEST. Unless otherwise prescribed, the solution is warmed to 40.5°C (105°F), the patient is placed in Sims' POSITION or knee-chest POSITION, and the rectal tube is inserted. The container of fluid is usually held about 45 cm (18 in) above the buttocks for a cleansing enema. Various types of enema are shown in the accompanying table.

Fleet e. trademark for an enema containing, in each 100 ml, 16 g sodium biphosphate and 6 g sodium phosphate, packaged in a plastic squeeze bottle fitted with a 5-cm prelubricated rectal tube.

hydrocortisone e. an aqueous solution of HYDROCORTISONE administered rectally as an antiinflammatory in treatment of ULCERATIVE COLITIS.

energy (en′er-je) power that may be translated into motion, overcoming resistance or causing a physical change; the ability to do work. Energy assumes several forms; it may be thermal (in the form of heat), electrical, mechanical, chemical, radiant, or kinetic. In doing work, the energy is

ENEMAS	
Type	**Purpose**
Barium enema	Diagnostic test to identify abnormalities in the large intestine and colon
Cleansing enema	Treatment of constipation or fecal impaction
(Tap water, normal saline	Preparation for diagnostic studies and surgical procedures
or soapsuds)	
Retention enema	Lubrication and softening of hard, dry fecal material

changed from one form to one or more other form(s). In these changes some of the energy is "lost" in the sense that it cannot be recaptured and used again. Usually there is loss in the form of heat, which escapes or is dissipated unused; all energy changes give off a certain amount of heat.

All activities of the body require energy, and all needs are met by the consumption of food containing energy in chemical form. The human diet comprises three main sources of energy: CARBOHYDRATES, PROTEINS, and FATS. Of these three, carbohydrates most readily provide the kind of energy needed to activate muscles. Proteins work to build and restore body tissues. The body transforms chemical energy derived from food by the process of METABOLISM, an activity that takes place in the individual cell. Molecules of the food substances providing energy pass through the cell wall. Inside the cell, chemical reactions occur that produce the new forms of energy and yield by-products such as water and waste materials; see also ADENOSINE TRIPHOSPHATE.

free e., Gibbs free e. **(G)** the energy equal to the maximum amount of work that can be obtained from a process occurring under conditions of fixed temperature and pressure.

nuclear e. energy that can be liberated by changes in the nucleus of an atom (as by fission of a heavy nucleus or by fusion of light nuclei into heavier ones with accompanying loss of mass).

enervation (en″er-va′shun) 1. lack of nervous energy. 2. removal of a nerve or a section of a nerve.

enflagellation (en-flaj″ĕ-la′shun) the formation of FLAGELLA; called also flagellation.

enflurane (en′floo-rān) a potent inhalational ANESTHETIC, widely used for induction and maintenance of general ANESTHESIA. It is nonflammable, induction and recovery are smooth and rapid, and the depth of anesthesia is rapidly altered. The incidence of arrhythmias and postoperative nausea and vomiting are somewhat less than with HALOTHANE or METHOXYFLURANE. It is also used

in low concentrations to provide analgesia during labor or painful procedures.

ENG electronystagmograph.

engagement (en-gāj′ment) the entrance of the largest diameter of the fetal head into the smallest diameter of the maternal pelvis.

engastrius (en-gas′tre-us) a double fetus in which one fetus is contained within the abdomen of the other.

engineering (en″jĭ-nēr′ing) the application of scientific and mathematical principles to useful ends, such as in the development of mechanical devices, systems, or processes.

biomedical e. bioengineering.

engorgement (en-gorj′ment) 1. distention of a body part or organ with blood or other fluids. 2. hyperemia.

breast e. swelling of the breast due to an increase in blood and lymph supply as a precursor to lactation.

engraftment (en-graft′ment) incorporation of grafted tissue into the body of the host.

engram (en′gram) a lasting mark or trace. In psychology, it is the lasting trace left in the psyche by anything that has been experienced psychically; a latent memory picture.

enhancement (en-hans′ment) the process of making something greater; see also PROMOTION.

body image e. in the NURSING INTERVENTIONS CLASSIFICATION, a nursing INTERVENTION defined as improving a patient's BODY IMAGE (conscious and unconscious perceptions and attitudes toward his/her body).

communication e.: hearing deficit in the NURSING INTERVENTIONS CLASSIFICATION, a nursing INTERVENTION defined as assistance in accepting and learning alternate methods for living with diminished HEARING.

communication e.: speech deficit in the NURSING INTERVENTIONS CLASSIFICATION, a nursing INTERVENTION defined as assistance in accepting and learning alternate methods for living with impaired SPEECH.

communication e.: visual deficit in the NURSING INTERVENTIONS CLASSIFICATION, a nursing INTERVENTION defined as assistance in accepting and learning alternate methods for living with diminished VISION.

coping e. in the NURSING INTERVENTIONS CLASSIFICATION, a nursing INTERVENTION defined as assisting a patient in COPING with perceived STRESSORS, changes, or threats that interfere with meeting life demands and roles.

cough e. in the NURSING INTERVENTIONS CLASSIFICATION, a nursing INTERVENTION defined as promotion of patient COUGHING by deep inhalation with subsequent generation of high intrathoracic pressures and compression of underlying lung parenchyma for the forceful expulsion of air.

developmental e.: adolescent in the NURSING INTERVENTIONS CLASSIFICATION, a nursing INTERVENTION defined as facilitating optimal physical, cognitive, social, and emotional growth of individuals during the transition from childhood to adulthood.

developmental e.: child in the NURSING INTERVENTIONS CLASSIFICATION, a nursing INTERVENTION defined as facilitating or teaching parents/caregivers to facilitate the optimal gross motor, fine motor, language, cognitive, social, and emotional growth of preschool and school-aged children.

edge e. a sharp increase in contrast on a xeroradiograph where there is an abrupt difference in the tissue densities of adjacent structures.

learning readiness e. in the NURSING INTERVENTIONS CLASSIFICATION, a nursing INTERVENTION defined as improving the ability and willingness to receive information.

religious ritual e. in the NURSING INTERVENTIONS CLASSIFICATION, a nursing INTERVENTION defined as facilitating participation in religious practices.

role e. in the NURSING INTERVENTIONS CLASSIFICATION, a nursing INTERVENTION defined as assisting a patient, significant other, or family to improve relationships by clarifying and supplementing specific role behaviors.

security e. in the NURSING INTERVENTIONS CLASSIFICATION, a nursing INTERVENTION defined as intensifying a patient's sense of physical and psychological safety.

self-awareness e. in the NURSING INTERVENTIONS CLASSIFICATION, a nursing INTERVENTION defined as assisting a patient to explore and understand his/her thoughts, feelings, motivations, and behaviors.

self-esteem e. in the NURSING INTERVENTIONS CLASSIFICATION, a nursing INTERVENTION defined as assisting a patient to increase his or her personal judgment of self-worth.

sleep e. in the NURSING INTERVENTIONS CLASSIFICATION, a nursing INTERVENTION defined as facilitation of regular SLEEP/wake cycles.

socialization e. in the NURSING INTERVENTIONS CLASSIFICATION, a nursing INTERVENTION defined as facilitation of another person's ability to interact with others.

support system e. in the NURSING INTERVENTIONS CLASSIFICATION, a nursing INTERVENTION defined as the facilitation of a support SYSTEM for the patient by family, friends, and/or community.

enkephalin (en-kef'ah-lin) either of two pentapeptides, composed of four identical amino acids and either leucine or methionine, referred to as leu-enkephalin and met-enkephalin. The enkephalins function as neurotransmitters or neuromodulators at many locations in the brain and spinal cord and are involved with pain perception, movement, mood, behavior, and neuroendocrine regulation; they are also found in nerve plexuses and exocrine glands of the gastrointestinal tract.

enlargement (en-larj'ment) an increase in size; see also *hypertrophy*.

image e. an increase in the size of an x-ray image that is affected by the focal film distance as well as the object film distance.

enol (e'nol) an organic compound in which one carbon of a double-bonded pair is also attached to a hydroxyl group, thus a TAUTOMER of the ketone form. The term is also used as a prefix or infix, often italicized.

enolase (e'no-lās) an enzyme in glycolytic systems that changes phosphoglyceric acid into phosphopyruvic acid.

enophthalmos (en″of-thal'mos) a backward displacement of the eyeball into the orbit.

enostosis (en″os-to'sis) a bony growth within a bone cavity or on the internal surface of the bone cortex.

enoxacin (ĕ-nok'sah-sin) an antibacterial effective against many gram-positive and gram-negative bacteria; administered orally in the treatment of gonorrhea and urinary tract infections.

enoxaparin (e-nok″sah-par'in) a low molecular weight HEPARIN, used as the sodium salt to prevent pulmonary EMBOLISM and deep venous THROMBOSIS following hip or knee replacement or high-risk abdominal surgery; administered subcutaneously as the sodium salt. It is also used together with WARFARIN in the treatment of deep venous thrombosis and together with ASPIRIN in the prevention of coronary THROMBOSIS associated with unstable ANGINA or certain kinds of MYOCARDIAL INFARCTION.

enoximone (en-ok'sĭ-mōn) a VASODILATOR similar to INAMRINONE; used as a cardiotonic in the short-term management of congestive HEART FAILURE, administered intravenously.

ensiform (en′sĭ-form) xiphoid (def. 1).

ensomphalus (en-som′fah-lus) a double fetus with blended bodies, two separate navels, and two umbilical cords.

enstrophe (en′stro-fe) entropion.

ensulizole (en-sul′-ĭ-zōl) a water-soluble absorber of ultraviolet B radiation, used topically as a SUNSCREEN.

ENT ears, nose, and throat; see *otorhinolaryngology.*

entacapone (en-tak′ah-pōn) an ANTIDYSKINETIC agent used in conjunction with LEVODOPA and CARBIDOPA to enhance dopaminergic stimulation of the brain and the antiparkinsonian activity of levodopa in the treatment of idiopathic PARKINSON′S DISEASE, administered orally.

entad (en′tad) toward a center; inwardly.

ental (en′tal) inner; central.

entamebiasis (en″tah-me-bi′ah-sis) infection by *Entamoeba;* see AMEBIC DYSENTERY.

Entamoeba (en″tah-me′bah) a genus of amebas parasitic in invertebrates and vertebrates, including humans. *E. co′li* and *E. gingiva′lis* are nonpathogenic forms found in the human intestine and mouth. *E. histoly′tica* causes AMEBIC DYSENTERY and liver abscesses.

entasia (en-ta′zhah) a constrictive spasm; tonic spasm.

enter(o)- word element [Gr.], *intestine.*

enteral (en′ter-al) enteric.

enterectomy (en″ter-ek′to-me) excision of a portion of the intestine.

enteric (en-ter′ik) pertaining to the small intestine; called also enteral.

  e.-coated of tablets, having a special coating that prevents release and absorption of their contents until they reach the intestine.

enteritis (en″tĕ-ri′tis) inflammation of the intestine, especially the small intestine, a general condition that can be produced by a variety of causes. Bacteria and certain viruses may infect the intestinal tract and produce symptoms of abdominal pain, nausea, vomiting, and diarrhea. Similar effects may result from poisonous foods such as mushrooms and berries, or from a harmful chemical present in food or drink. Enteritis may also be the consequence of overeating or alcoholic excesses.

Rest and bland diet are generally prescribed. In cases of bacterial infection antibiotics may be helpful. Severe dehydration, which may accompany enteritis, is treated with replacement of lost fluids and ELECTROLYTES. See also DIARRHEA; bowel ELIMINATION, altered; and deficient fluid VOLUME.

  membranous e., mucomembranous e., mucous e. mucous colitis.

  e. necro′ticans an inflammation of the intestines due to *Clostridium perfringens* type F, characterized by necrosis.

  phlegmonous e. a condition with symptoms resembling those of peritonitis, which may be secondary to other intestinal diseases, e.g., chronic obstruction, strangulated hernia, carcinoma.

  e. polypo′sa enteritis marked by polypoid growths in the intestine, due to proliferation of the connective tissue.

  regional e. Crohn's disease.

enteroanastomosis (en″ter-o-ah-nas″to-mo′sis) enteroenterostomy.

Enterobacter (en″ter-o-bak′ter) a genus of gram-negative, facultatively anaerobic, motile, rod-shaped bacteria. Organisms are widely distributed in nature and occur in the intestinal tracts of humans and animals. They are frequently a cause of nosocomial infections.

Enterobacteriaceae (en″ter-o-bak-tēr″e-a′se-e) a family of gram-negative, facultatively anaerobic, rod-shaped bacteria, usually motile, made up of saprophytes and plant and animal parasites of worldwide distribution, found in soil, water, and plants and in animals from insects to humans. In humans, disease is produced by both invasive action and production of toxin. Species not normally associated with disease are often opportunistic pathogens. Enterobacteriaceae have been responsible for as many as half of the nosocomial infections reported annually in the United States, most frequently by species of *Escherichia, Klebsiella, Enterobacter, Proteus, Providencia,* and *Serratia.*

enterobiasis (en″ter-o-bi′ah-sis) infection with nematodes of the genus *Enterobius,* especially *E. vermicularis* (the PINWORM); called also oxyuriasis.

Pinworm infection does not produce the fatigue and loss of weight that characterize *Ascaris* infection; adult pinworms migrate to the anal region, usually at night, and deposit eggs, which cause irritation of the skin around the anus, leading to painful scratching and restless sleep. This irritation is the usual sign of the infection, although there may also be vague intestinal discomfort. Adult worms may appear in the feces, but the infection is transmitted by the eggs, which may be transferred to clothing, bedclothes, and toilet seats from the skin around the anus. A common method of detection is to apply clean adhesive tape to the rectal area immediately upon awakening. The tape can then be placed sticky side down on a glass slide. The health care provider will examine the slide under a microscope for evidence of infestation.

In scratching, the infected person is likely to collect the minute eggs on the hands and under the fingernails, and, until washing thoroughly, will shed the eggs on anything touched. The infection spreads to other persons when the eggs are carried to their mouths either by inhalation or on contaminated food, in beverages, or on hands. Widespread pinworm infection is explained by the fact that the eggs, which develop into mature worms only in a human body, can remain dormant but alive and infective for a considerable time in dust or air; they are not killed by most household disinfectants.

Enterobius vermicularis infection is treated by an anthelmintic such as MEBENDA-ZOLE, PIPERAZINE, or PYRVINIUM. Equally important, instructions for disinfecting bedclothes and other material that may harbor eggs must be followed carefully to avoid reinfection and spread of pinworms to other members of the family.

Enterobius (en″ter-o′be-us) a genus of ROUNDWORMS. *E. vermicula′ris* is the SEAT-WORM or PINWORM, a small white spindle-shaped worm about 1 cm long, parasitic in the upper part of the large intestine, and occasionally in the female genitals and bladder. Infection is frequent in children, sometimes causing itching.

enterocele (en′ter-o-sēl″) 1. any intestinal hernia; see terms under HERNIA. 2. posterior vaginal hernia.

enterocentesis (en″ter-o-sen-te′sis) surgical puncture of the intestine.

enteroclysis (en″ter-ok′lĭ-sis) the injection of liquids into the intestine.

enterococcemia (en″ter-o-kok-se′me-ah) the presence of enterococci in the blood.

Enterococcus (en″ter-o-kok′us) a genus of gram-positive, facultatively anaerobic bacteria of the family Streptococcaceae, formerly classified in the genus *Streptococcus*. *E. faeca′lis* and *E. fae′cium* are normal inhabitants of the human intestinal tract that occasionally cause urinary tract infections, infective endocarditis, and bacteremia; *E. a′vium* is found primarily in the feces of chickens and may be associated with appendicitis, otitis, and brain abscesses in humans.

enterococcus (en″ter-o-kok′us), pl. *enterococ′ci* [Gr.] an organism belonging to the genus *Enterococcus*.

enterocoele (en′ter-o-sēl″) the body cavity formed by outpouchings from the archenteron.

enterocolectomy (en″ter-o-ko-lek′to-me) resection of part of the intestine, including the ileum, cecum, and colon.

enterocolitis (en″ter-o-ko-li′tis) inflammation of the small intestine and colon.

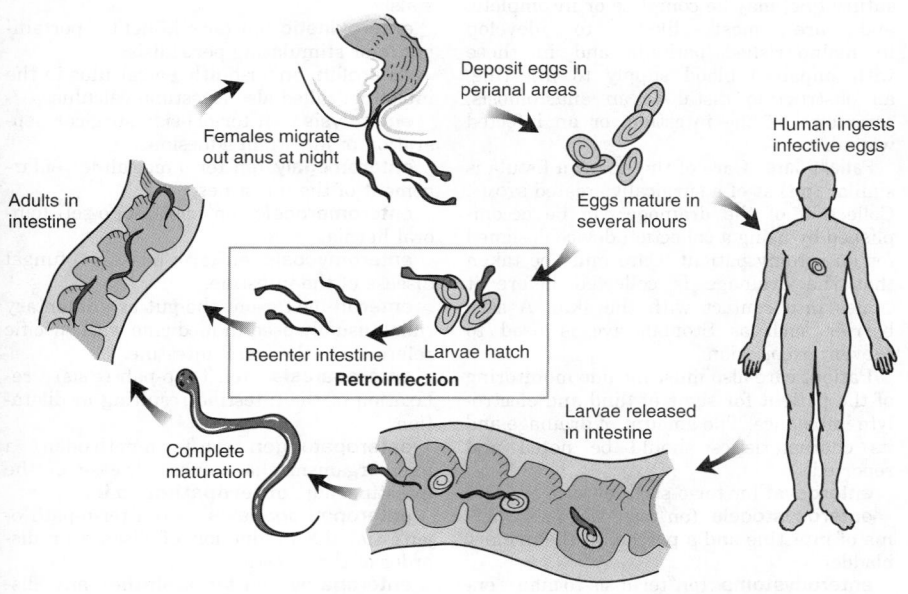

Life cycle of *Enterobius vermicularis*. From Mahon and Mansuelis, 2000.

Deposit eggs in perianal areas

Human ingests infective eggs

Females migrate out anus at night

Eggs mature in several hours

Adults in intestine

Reenter intestine   Larvae hatch
Retroinfection

Larvae released in intestine

Complete maturation

antibiotic-associated e. that in which treatment with antibiotics alters the bowel flora and results in diarrhea or pseudomembranous ENTEROCOLITIS. See also antibiotic-associated COLITIS.

hemorrhagic e. enterocolitis characterized by hemorrhagic breakdown of the intestinal mucosa, with inflammatory cell infiltration.

necrotizing e. the development of necrotic patches in the intestine that interfere with digestion and absorption; see also NECROTIZING ENTEROCOLITIS.

pseudomembranous e. an acute inflammation of the bowel mucosa, with the formation of pseudomembranous plaques, usually associated with antimicrobial therapy. See also pseudomembranous COLITIS.

enterocolostomy (en″ter-o-kah-los′tah-me) surgical anastomosis of the small intestine to the colon.

enterocutaneous (en″ter-o-ku-ta′ne-us) pertaining to or communicating with the intestine and the skin, or surface of the body.

e. fistula one in which there is communication between the intestinal tract and the skin. Some fistulas are created surgically, with gastrostomy, esophagostomy, or colostomy. Others may result from surgical trauma, breakdown of an intestinal anastomosis, or erosions around a surgical drain or tube. Fistulas frequently occur at a suture line, may be complete or incomplete, and are most likely to develop in malnourished patients and in those with impaired blood supply to intestine, an obstruction distal to an anastomosis, carcinoma of the intestine, or an infected wound.

Patient Care. Care of the site of a fistula is similar to that of a surgically created STOMA. Collection of the drainage can be accomplished by using a collection device designed for an ostomy patient. Care must be taken that the drainage is collected before it comes into contact with the skin. A skin barrier such as Stomahesive is used to prevent excoriation.

Patient care also must include monitoring of the patient for signs of fluid and electrolyte imbalance. The amount of drainage and its characteristics should be noted and reported.

enterocyst (en′ter-o-sist″) enteric cyst.

enterocystocele (en″ter-o-sis′to-sēl) hernia of intestine and a portion of the urinary bladder.

enterocystoma (en″ter-o-sis-to′mah) enteric cyst.

enterocystoplasty (en″ter-o-sis′to-plas″te) the most common type of augmentation CYSTOPLASTY, using a portion of intestine for the graft. Common types include ILEOCYSTOPLASTY, ILEOCECOCYSTOPLASTY, and sigmoid CYSTOPLASTY.

enterodynia (en″ter-o-din′e-ah) pain in the intestine.

enteroenterostomy (en″ter-o-en″ter-os′-tah-me) surgical anastomosis between two segments of the intestine.

enteroepiplocele (en″ter-o-e-pip′lo-sēl) hernia of the intestine and omentum.

enterogastritis (en″ter-o-gas-tri′tis) gastroenteritis.

enterogastrone (en″ter-o-gas′trōn) any of various hormones that mediate the humoral inhibition of gastric secretion and motility.

enterogenous (en″ter-oj′ĕ-nus) 1. arising from the FOREGUT. 2. originating within the small intestine.

enterogram (en′ter-o-gram″) an instrumental tracing of the movements of the intestine.

enterohepatitis (en″ter-o-hep″ah-ti′tis) inflammation of the intestine and liver.

enterohepatocele (en″ter-o-hep′ah-to-sēl″) an umbilical hernia containing intestine and liver.

enterohydrocele (en″ter-o-hi′dro-sēl) hernia with hydrocele.

enterokinase (en″ter-o-ki′nās) enteropeptidase.

enterokinesia (en″ter-o-ki″ne′zhah) peristalsis.

enterokinetic (en″ter-o-kĭ-net′ik) pertaining to or stimulating peristalsis.

enterolith (en′ter-o-lith″) a calculus in the intestine; called also intestinal calculus.

enterolysis (en″ter-ol′ĭ-sis) surgical separation of intestinal adhesions.

enteromegaly (en″ter-o-meg′ah-le) enlargement of the intestines.

enteromerocele (en″ter-o-mĕr′o-sēl) femoral hernia.

enteromycosis (en″ter-o-mi-ko′sis) fungal disease of the intestine.

enteron (en′ter-on) the gut or alimentary canal; usually used in medicine with specific reference to the small intestine.

enteroparesis (en″ter-o-pah-re′sis) relaxation of the intestine resulting in dilatation.

enteropathogen (en″ter-o-path′o-jen) a microorganism that causes disease of the intestine. adj., **enteropathogen′ic.**

enteropathogenesis (en″ter-o-path″o-jen′ĕ-sis) the production of disease or disorder of the intestine.

enteropathy (en″ter-op′ah-the) any disease of the intestine.

gluten e., gluten sensitive e. celiac disease.

protein-losing e. a nonspecific term referring to conditions, e.g., adult CELIAC DISEASE, associated with excessive loss of enteric plasma proteins.

enteropeptidase (en″ter-o-pep′tĭ-dās) an enzyme of the intestinal juice secreted by the duodenal mucosa; it activates the proteolytic enzyme of the pancreatic juice by converting trypsinogen into trypsin.

enteropexy (en′ter-o-pek″se) surgical fixation of the intestine to the abdominal wall.

enteroplasty (en′ter-o-plas″te) plastic repair of the intestine.

enteroplegia (en″ter-o-ple′jah) adynamic ileus.

enteroptosis (en″ter-op-to′sis) abnormal downward displacement of the intestine. adj., **enteroptot′ic.**

enterorrhagia (en″ter-o-ra′je-ah) intestinal hemorrhage.

enterorrhaphy (en″ter-or′ah-fe) suture of the intestine.

enterorrhexis (en″ter-o-rek′sis) rupture of the intestine.

enteroscope (en′ter-o-skōp″) an instrument for inspecting the inside of the intestine.

enterosepsis (en″ter-o-sep′sis) sepsis developing from the intestinal contents.

enterospasm (en′ter-o-spazm″) intestinal colic.

enterostasis (en″ter-o-sta′sis) intestinal stasis.

enterostenosis (en″ter-o-stĕ-no′sis) narrowing or stricture of the intestine.

enterostomal (en″ter-o-sto′mal) relating to or having undergone an ENTEROSTOMY.

e. therapist one who is certified to assist in the specialized care of patients who have undergone ENTEROSTOMY or who require special skin or wound care; see also STOMA. Information about local therapists available for consultation can be obtained by writing to Wound Ostomy and Continence Nurses Society, 4700 W. Lake, Glenview, IL 60025.

enterostomy (en″ter-os′tah-me) the artificial formation of a STOMA, a permanent opening into the intestine through the abdominal wall. See also COLOSTOMY and ILEOSTOMY.

enterotomy (en″ter-ot′ah-me) incision of the intestine.

enterotoxemia (en″ter-o-tok-se′me-ah) a condition characterized by the presence in the blood of toxins produced in the intestines.

enterotoxigenic (en″ter-o-tok″sĭ-jen′ik) producing, produced by, or pertaining to production of enterotoxin.

enterotoxin (en′ter-o-tok″sin) a toxin specifically affecting cells of the intestinal mucosa, causing vomiting and diarrhea, such as those elaborated by species of *Bacillus, Clostridium, Escherichia, Staphylococcus,* and *Vibrio.*

enterotoxism (en″ter-o-tok′sizm) autointoxication of enteric origin.

enterotropic (en″ter-o-trop′ik) affecting the intestines.

enterovaginal (en″ter-o-vaj′ĭ-nal) pertaining to or communicating with the intestine and the vagina, as an enterovaginal fistula.

enterovenous (en″ter-o-ve′nus) communicating between the intestinal lumen and the lumen of a vein.

enterovesical (en″ter-o-ves′ĭ-k′l) pertaining to or communicating with the urinary bladder and intestine; called also vesicoenteric and vesicointestinal.

enterovirus (en′ter-o-vi″rus) any member of a genus of PICORNAVIRUSES, usually infecting the gastrointestinal tract and being discharged in the feces; included are the POLIOVIRUSES, COXSACKIEVIRUSES, ENTEROVIRUSES, and others. adj., **enterovi′ral.**

enterozoon (en″ter-o-zo′on), pl. *enterozo′a* An animal parasite in the intestines. adj., **enterozo′ic.**

enthesis (en′thĕ-sis) the site of attachment of a muscle or ligament to bone.

enthesopathy (en-thĕ-sop′ah-the) disorder of the muscular or tendinous attachment to bone.

enthetobiosis (en-thet″o-bi-o′sis) dependency of an organism on a mechanical device implanted within the body, such as an electronic cardiac pacemaker.

ent(o)- word element [Gr.], *within; inner.*

entoblast (en′to-blast) endoderm.

entochoroidea (en″to-ko-roi′de-ah) the inner layer of the choroid of the eye.

entoderm (en′to-derm) endoderm.

entoectad (en″to-ek′tad) from within outward.

entomere (en′to-mēr) a blastomere normally destined to become endoderm.

entomion (en-to′me-on) the tip of the posteroinferior, or mastoid, angle of the parietal bone.

entomology (en″to-mol′o-je) that branch of biology concerned with the study of insects.

medical e. that concerned with insects that cause disease or serve as vectors of pathogens.

Entomophthorales (en″to-mof″tho-ra′lēz) an order of fungi that are usually parasitic in insects but sometimes infect humans, causing ENTOMOPHTHOROMYCOSIS.

E

entomophthoromycosis any disease in humans or other animals caused by fungi of the order ENTOMOPHTHORALES; human infections usually occur in apparently physiologically and immunologically normal individuals, although opportunistic infections also occur.

 e. basidio'bolae a chronic infection caused by *Basidiobolus ranarum*, in which gradually enlarging granulomas form in the subcutaneous tissues of the arms, chest, and trunk. Multiple purulent ulcers may develop; seen in children and adolescents in tropical areas of Indonesia, India, and Africa. Called also basidiobolomycosis.

 e. conidio'bolae infection by *Conidiobolus coronatus,* a form of ZYGOMYCOSIS usually involving the nose and paranasal sinuses (RHINOENTOMOPHTHOROMYCOSIS). Sometimes, especially in weak or immunocompromised patients, it can spread to the central nervous system and cause fatal rhinocerebral zygomycosis.

entopic (en-top'ik) occurring in the proper place.

entoptic (en-top'tik) originating within the eye.

entoptoscopy (en″top-tos'kah-pe) inspection of the interior of the eye.

entoretina (en″to-ret'ĭ-nah) the nervous or inner layer of the retina.

entotic (en-tot'ik) situated in or originating within the ear.

entozoon (en″to-zo'on), pl. *entozo'a* An internal animal parasite. adj., **entozo'ic.**

entropion (en-tro'pe-on) inversion, or the turning inward, as of the margin of an eyelid.

 e. u'veae inversion of the margin of the pupil.

entropy (en'trŏ-pe) 1. in thermodynamics, a measure of the part of the internal energy of a system that is unavailable to do work. In any spontaneous process, such as the flow of heat from a hot region to a cold region, entropy always increases. 2. the tendency of a system to move toward randomness. 3. in information theory, the negative of information, a measure of the disorder or randomness in a physical system. The theory of statistical mechanics proves that this concept is equivalent to entropy as defined in thermodynamics. 4. diminished capacity for spontaneous change, as occurs in the psyche in aging.

enucleate (e-noo'kle-āt) to remove whole and clean, as the eye from its socket.

enucleation (e-noo″kle-a'shun) removal of an organ or other mass intact from its supporting tissues, as of the eyeball from the orbit.

enuresis (en″u-re'sis) a type of urinary INCONTINENCE, usually referring to involuntary discharge of urine during sleep at night (*nocturnal enuresis* or bed-wetting), such as in a child beyond the age when bladder control should have been achieved. adj., **enuret'ic.** It can occur as a result of such organic conditions as structural defects or infections of the urinary tract, neurologic deficit and resultant loss of control, nocturnal epilepsy, diabetes mellitus and diabetes insipidus, which increase urine flow, and renal disorders that impair the kidney's ability to concentrate urine. If no organic basis can be found for bed-wetting, psychogenic factors are considered.

Patient Care. Efforts to manage enuresis require patience on the part of parents and understanding that the child may be embarrassed by the condition and its effects. Reprimands and punishment are not appropriate and only make matters worse. The child also needs to be encouraged to participate in planning and implementing the program of care and to have hope and confidence that the problem can be overcome.

Among the techniques used to manage nocturnal enuresis are restricting fluids after the evening meal, bladder TRAINING to help enlarge the capacity of the bladder, and fully awakening the child once or twice during the night to walk to the bathroom and urinate. Electronic devices that establish a conditioned reflex response to waken the child the moment urination starts are successful in some cases. An ANTICHOLINERGIC drug may be prescribed as an adjunct to any of these techniques. DESMOPRESSIN acetate nasal spray (DDAVP) may also be used.

envelope (en've-lŏp) 1. an encompassing structure or membrane. 2. in virology, the outer LIPOPROTEIN coat of a large virus, surrounding the CAPSID and usually furnished, at least partially, by the host cell. Called also peplos. 3. in bacteriology, the cell wall and the plasma membrane considered together.

 nuclear e. the condensed double layer of lipids and proteins enclosing the cell nucleus and separating it from the cytoplasm; its two concentric membranes, inner and outer, are separated by a perinuclear space.

envenomation (en-ven″o-ma'shun) POISONING by VENOM.

environment (en-vi'ron-ment) the aggregate of surrounding conditions or influences on an individual.

envy a desire to have another's possessions or qualities for oneself.

penis e. in psychoanalysis, the concept that the female envies the male his possession of a penis, first described by Freud as occurring during the phallic stage in little girls as they become aware of anatomical differences between the sexes. It is often used more broadly for the women's generalized envy of men or their characteristics.

enzacamene (en″zah-kam′ēn) an absorber of ultraviolet radiation, used topically as a SUNSCREEN.

enzygotic (en″zi-got′ik) developed from one zygote.

enzymatic (en″zi-mat′ik) of, relating to, caused by, or of the nature of an ENZYME.

enzyme (en′zīm) any protein that acts as a catalyst, increasing the rate at which a chemical reaction occurs. The human body probably contains about 10,000 different enzymes. At body temperature, very few biochemical reactions proceed at a significant rate without the presence of an enzyme. Like all catalysts, an enzyme does not control the direction of the reaction; it increases the rates of the forward and reverse reactions proportionally.

Enzymes work by binding molecules so that they are held in a particular geometric configuration that allows the reaction to occur. Enzymes are very specific; few molecules closely fit the binding site. Each enzyme catalyzes a specific type of chemical reaction between a few closely related compounds, which are called *substrates* of the enzyme.

Enzymes are given names ending in *-ase*. In older names, the suffix is added to the name of the substrate, as in amylase, an enzyme that breaks down the polysaccharide amylose. In newer names, the suffix is added to the type of reaction, as in lactate dehydrogenase, an enzyme that converts lactate to pyruvate by transferring a hydrogen atom to nicotinamide-adenine dinucleotide (NAD).

Regulation of Enzymes. The reaction rate of an enzyme-catalyzed reaction varies with the pH, temperature, and substrate concentration. Under physiologic conditions the rates of many reactions are controlled by substrate concentrations. Certain key reactions are controlled by one of three different mechanisms.

In *allosteric regulation,* the enzyme can bind molecules, which are referred to as *effectors,* at a site other than the active site, which is referred to as an *allosteric site.* In many biochemical pathways the enzyme that catalyzes the first reaction in the pathway is inhibited by the final product of the last reaction, so that when sufficient product is present the whole pathway is shut down. This is an example of negative FEEDBACK.

Many enzymes are regulated by *phosphorylation.* A phosphate group is attached to the enzyme by another enzyme, called a *protein kinase.* When the enzyme is phosphorylated it changes its shape and thus its activity. Phosphorylation activates some enzymes and inactivates others; by this means one protein kinase can control several enzymes.

All enzymes are controlled by their rate of synthesis. Like all proteins, enzymes are synthesized by ribosomes, which translate the genetic information coded in the DEOXY-RIBONUCLEIC ACID (DNA) of the CHROMOSOMES into the specific amino acid sequence of the enzyme. The expression of many genes is controlled by the processes of *genetic regulation.* Thus, although each cell contains the information to make all of the body's enzymes, it actually makes only those appropriate for its specific type of cell. The synthesis of some enzymes can be induced or repressed by the action of specific hormones, substrates, or products so that the enzyme is produced only when metabolic conditions require its presence.

Inborn Errors of Metabolism. Hundreds of genetic diseases that result from deficiency of a single enzyme are now known. Many of these diseases fall into two large classes. The *aminoacidopathies* result from deficiency of an enzyme in the major pathway for the metabolism of a specific amino acid. The amino acid accumulates in the blood, and it or its metabolites are excreted in the urine. The *lysosomal storage diseases* result from deficiency of a lysosomal enzyme and the accumulation of the substance degraded by that enzyme in lysosomes of cells throughout the body. The stored material is usually a complex substance, such as glycogen, a sphingolipid, or a mucopolysaccharide.

An example of an aminoacidopathy is PHENYLKETONURIA (PKU), which results from a deficiency of the enzyme phenylalanine hydroxylase, which converts the amino acid phenylalanine to tyrosine. Phenylalanine accumulates in the blood and phenylpyruvic acid is excreted in the urine. The phenylalaninemia eventually results in mental retardation due to defective formulation of myelin. However, PKU can be detected at birth by a screening test for phenylalanine in the blood, and clinical symptoms can be avoided by strict adherence to a low-phenylalanine diet.

An example of a lysosomal storage disease is TAY-SACHS DISEASE, which results from a deficiency of the enzyme hexosaminidase A.

The stored substance is a sphingolipid, GM_2-ganglioside, which accumulates in nerve tissue, causing blindness and mental deterioration. No cure is possible, but antenatal diagnosis can be made by determining hexosaminidase A activity in fetal fibroblasts from an amniotic fluid specimen drawn by AMNIOCENTESIS. It is also possible to identify carriers (heterozygotes) who are at risk for having children with the disease.

Enzyme Assays. Several enzymes are important in clinical pathology. Enzymes characteristic of a tissue are released into the blood when the tissue is damaged; hence assays of serum enzyme levels can aid in the diagnosis or monitoring of specific diseases. Lipase and amylase levels are useful in pancreatic diseases; alkaline phosphatase (ALP), lactate dehydrogenase (LD), aspartate transaminase (AST or GOT), and alanine transaminase (ALT or GPT) in liver diseases; and LD and creatine kinase (CK) in myocardial infarction. ALP is also released in bone diseases. Many enzymes have different forms (*isoenzymes*) in different organs. The isoenzymes can be separated by electrophoresis in order to determine the origin of the enzyme. Isoenzymes of LD, CK, and ALP have the most clinical utility. See accompanying table.

> **activating e.** one that activates a given amino acid by attaching it to the corresponding transfer ribonucleic acid.

> **brancher e., branching e.** α-glucan-branching glycosyltransferase: an enzyme involved in conversion of amylose to amylopectin; deficiency of this enzyme causes amylopectinosis.

> **constitutive e.** one produced by a microorganism regardless of the presence or absence of the specific substrate acted upon.

> **debrancher e., debranching e.** dextrin-1,6-glucosidase: an enzyme that acts on glucose residues of the glycogen molecule and is important in glycogenolysis; deficiency of this enzyme causes Forbes' disease.

> **induced e., inducible e.** one whose production requires or is stimulated by a specific small molecule, the inducer, which is the substrate of the enzyme or a compound structurally related to it.

> **proteolytic e.** one that catalyzes the hydrolysis of proteins and various split products of proteins, the final product being small peptides and amino acids.

> **repressible e.** one whose rate of production is decreased as the concentration of certain metabolites is increased.

> **respiratory e's** enzymes of the mitochondria, e.g., cytochrome oxidase, which serve as catalysts for cellular oxidations.

enzymic (en-zi′mik) enzymatic.

enzymology (en″zi-mol′o-je) the study of enzymes and enzymatic action.

enzymopathy (en″zi-mop′ah-the) an inborn ERROR of metabolism consisting of defective or absent enzymes, as in GLYCOGENOSIS or MUCOPOLYSACCHARIDOSIS.

ENZYMES: NORMAL VALUES	
Aspartate amino-transferase (AST) or serum glutamic oxaloacetic transaminase	**Adult:** 8–20 U/L **Older Adult:** Male: 11–26 U/L Female: 10–20 U/L **Child (< 5 years):** 19–28 U/L **Infant:** 15–60 U/L **Newborn:** 16–72 U/L
Creatine phosphokinase (CPK) or creatine kinase (CK)	**Adult Male:** 5–35 µg/ml 20–170 U/L < 90 U/L 5–55 mU/ml **Adult Female:** 5–25 µg/ml 10–135 U/L < 80 U/L 5–35 mU/ml **Male Child:** 0–70 U/L **Female Child:** 0–50 U/L **Newborn:** 10–200 U/L
CPK isoenzymes CPK-MM (skeletal muscles)	90–97% of total CPK or SI 0.90–0.97 (fraction of total CPK)
CPK-MB (heart)	0–6% of total CPK or SI 0.00–0.06% (fraction of total CPK)
Lactic acid dehydrogenase (LDH)	60–120 U/ml (Wacker scale) 150–450 U/ml (Wroblewski-La Due scale)
LDH isoenzymes LDH1 Heart, red blood cells	70–200 U/L 14–26% or SI 0.14–0.26 (fraction of total LDH)
LDH2 Reticuloendothelial cells and kidney	29–39% or SI 0.29–0.39 (fraction of total LDH)
LDH3 Lungs, lymphatics, spleen, and others	20–26% or SI 0.20–0.26 (fraction of total LDH)
LDH4 Kidney, placenta, and liver	8–16% or SI 0.08–0.16 (fraction of total LDH)
LDH5 Kidney, liver, and skeletal muscle	6–16% or SI 0.06–0.16 (fraction of total LDH)
Serum alphahydroxy-butyrate dehydrogenase	50–250 U/L

EOG electro-oculogram; electro-olfactogram.

eosin (e′o-sin) any of a class of rose-colored stains or dyes, all being bromine derivatives of fluorescein; eosin Y, the sodium salt of tetrabromofluorescein, is much used in histologic and laboratory procedures.

eosinopenia (e″o-sin″o-pe′ne-ah) abnormal deficiency of eosinophils in the blood.

eosinophil (e″o-sin′o-fil″) 1. a cell or other element readily stainable by EOSIN. 2. a granular LEUKOCYTE with a nucleus that usually has two lobes connected by a thread of chromatin, and cytoplasm containing coarse, round granules of uniform size. Called also eosinophilic leukocyte.

eosinophilia (e″o-sin″o-fil′e-ah) 1. the formation and accumulation of an abnormally large number of eosinophils in the blood; see also HYPEREOSINOPHILIA. Called also eosinophilic leukocytosis. 2. the condition of being readily stained with EOSIN. adj., **eosinophil′ic.**

tropical e., tropical pulmonary e. a subacute or chronic form of occult filariasis, usually involving *Brugia malayi* or *Wuchereria bancrofti* , occurring in the tropics. It is characterized by episodic nocturnal wheezing and coughing, strikingly elevated eosinophilia, and diffuse reticulonodular infiltrations of the lung. Sometimes the lymph nodes and spleen are greatly enlarged.

eosinophilia-myalgia syndrome a sometimes fatal syndrome of severe myalgia associated with marked peripheral eosinophilia, associated with the ingestion of oral preparations of L-TRYPTOPHAN; long-term sequelae include scleroderma and progressive neuropathy.

eosinophilic (e″o-sin″o-fil′ik) staining readily with eosin; pertaining to eosinophils or to eosinophilia.

eosinophiluria (e″o-sin″o-fil-u′re-ah) the presence of eosinophils in the urine, as in certain drug sensitivity conditions or disorders of the genitourinary tract.

EPA Environmental Protection Agency.

epallobiosis (ep-al″lo-bi-o′sis) dependency on an external life-support system, as on a HEART-LUNG MACHINE or HEMODIALYZER.

epaxial (ep-ak′se-al) situated above or upon an axis.

epencephalon (ep″en-sef′ah-lon) 1. cerebellum. 2. metencephalon.

ependyma (ĕ-pen′dĭ-mah) the membrane lining the cerebral ventricles and the central canal of the spine. adj., **epen′dymal.**

ependymoma (ĕ-pen″dĭ-mo′mah) a tumor composed of differentiated ependymal cells; most are slow growing and benign, but occasionally one is malignant.

ephapse (e-faps′) a point of lateral contact (other than a synapse) between nerve fibers across which impulses are conducted directly through the nerve membranes. adj., **ephap′tic.**

ephebiatrics (e-fe″be-at′riks) the branch of medicine that deals especially with the diagnosis and treatment of diseases and problems peculiar to youth.

ephedrine (ĕ-fed′rin, ef′ĕ-drin) an ADRENERGIC alkaloid obtained from several species of the shrub *Ephedra* or produced synthetically; used as a BRONCHODILATOR, ANTIASTHMATIC, central nervous system STIMULANT, and PRESSOR agent. Administered orally, parenterally, or intranasally as the hydrochloride, sulfate, or tannate salt. Besides its prescribed uses, it is also an ingredient in numerous supplements, with claimed benefits including weight loss, increased energy, and enhanced athletic performance.

ephelis (ĕ-fe′lis), pl. *ephe′lides* [Gr.] a freckle.

epi- word element [Gr.], *upon.*

epiandrosterone (ep″e-an-dros′ter-ōn) an androgenic steroid less active than androsterone and excreted in small amounts in normal human urine.

epiblepharon (ep″ĭ-blef′ah-ron) a developmental anomaly in which a horizontal fold of skin stretches across the border of the eyelid, pressing the lashes against the eyeball.

epibulbar (ep″ĭ-bul′ber) situated upon the eyeball.

epicanthus (ep″ĭ-kan′thus) a vertical fold of skin on either side of the nose, sometimes covering the inner canthus; a normal characteristic in persons of certain races, but anomalous in others. adj., **epican′thal, epican′thic.**

epicardia (ep″ĭ-kahr′de-ah) the lower portion of the esophagus, extending from the esophageal hiatus to the cardia, the upper orifice of the stomach.

epicardial (ep″ĭ-kahr′de-al) pertaining to the visceral pericardium (epicardium) or to the epicardia.

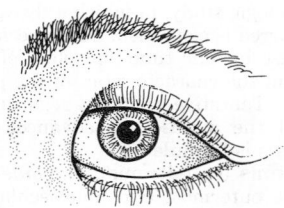

Epicanthus. From Dorland's, 2000.

epicardium (ep″ĭ-kahr′de-um) the inner layer of the serous pericardium, which is in contact with the heart.

epichorion (ep″ĭ-kor′e-on) the portion of the uterine mucosa enclosing the implanted conceptus.

epicondyle (ep″ĭ-kon′dīl) an eminence upon a bone, above its condyle.

epicondylitis (ep″ĭ-kon″dī-li′tis) inflammation of an epicondyle or of tissues adjoining the humeral epicondyle. Called also tennis elbow.

epicranium (ep″ĭ-kra′ne-um) the structures collectively that cover the skull.

epicritic (ep″ĭ-krit′ik) determining accurately; said of cutaneous nerve fibers sensitive to fine variations of touch or temperature.

epicystotomy (ep″ĭ-sis-tot′ah-me) suprapubic cystotomy.

epidemic (ep″ĭ-dem′ik) occuring suddenly in numbers clearly in excess of normal expectancy, in contrast to ENDEMIC or SPORADIC. The term is used especially of infectious diseases but is also applied to any disease, injury, or other health-related event occurring in such outbreaks.

   e. hemorrhagic fever an acute infectious disease thought to be transmitted to humans by mites or chiggers; characteristics include fever, purpura, peripheral vascular collapse, and acute renal failure.

epidemicity (ep″ĭ-dĕ-mis′ĭ-te) the state or quality of being epidemic.

epidemiologist (ep″ĭ-de″me-ol′o-jist) one who specializes in epidemiology.

epidemiology (ep″ĭ-de″me-ol′o-je) the science concerned with the study of the factors determining and influencing the frequency and distribution of disease, injury, and other health-related events and their causes in a defined human population for the purpose of establishing programs to prevent and control their development and spread. Also, the sum of knowledge gained in such a study.

   analytic e. the second stage in an epidemiologic study, in which hypotheses generated in the descriptive phase are tested.

   descriptive e. the first stage in an epidemiologic study, in which a disease that has occurred is examined. Data necessary in this phase include time and place of occurrence and the characteristics of the persons affected. Tentative theories regarding the cause of the disease are advanced and a hypothesis is formulated.

epidermis (ep″ĭ-der′mis), pl. *epider′mides* [Gr.] the outermost and nonvascular layer of the skin, derived from the embryonic ectoderm, varying in thickness from 0.07 to 1.4 mm. On the palmar and plantar surfaces it comprises, from within outward, five layers: (1) *basal layer* (stratum basale), composed of columnar cells arranged perpendicularly; (2) *prickle-cell* or *spinous layer* (stratum spinosum), composed of flattened polyhedral cells with short processes or spines; (3) *granular layer* (stratum granulosum), composed of flattened granular cells; (4) *clear layer* (stratum lucidum), composed of several layers of clear, transparent cells in which the nuclei are indistinct or absent; and (5) *horny layer* (stratum corneum), composed of flattened, cornified, non-nucleated cells. In the epidermis of the general body surface, the clear layer is usually absent. adj., **epider′mal, epider′mic.**

epidermitis (ep″ĭ-der-mi′tis) inflammation of the epidermis.

epidermodysplasia (ep″ĭ-der″mo-dis-pla′-zhah) faulty development of the EPIDERMIS.

   e. verrucifor′mis the widespread and persistent (sometimes lasting decades) dissemination of VERRUCA PLANA associated with a tendency to malignant degeneration. It typically begins in early childhood with the development of flat-topped papules that increase in number and coalesce to form large plaques, especially on the knees, elbows, and trunk. Familial occurrence and mental retardation are often associated with the disorder.

epidermoid (ep″ĭ-der′moid) 1. resembling the epidermis. 2. any tumor occurring at a noncutaneous site and formed by inclusion of epidermal cells.

epidermoidoma (ep″ĭ-der″moi-do′mah) a cerebral or meningeal tumor formed by inclusion of ectodermal elements at the time of closure of the neural groove.

epidermolysin (ep″ĭ-der-mol′ĭ-sin) exfoliatin.

epidermolysis (ep″ĭ-der-mol′ĭ-sis) a loosened state of the epidermis with formation of blebs and bullae either spontaneously or at the site of trauma.

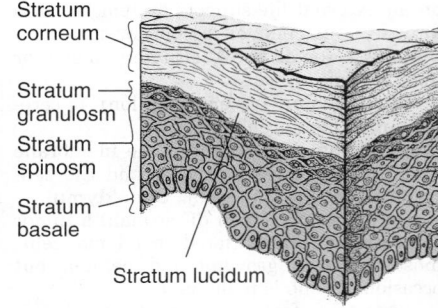

Stratum corneum

Stratum granulosm

Stratum spinosm

Stratum basale

Stratum lucidum

Section of epidermis. From Dorland's, 2000.

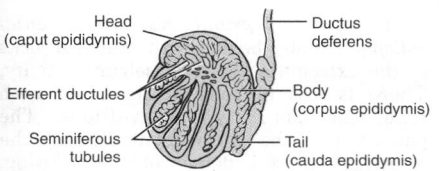

Head (caput epididymis)
Ductus deferens
Efferent ductules
Body (corpus epididymis)
Seminiferous tubules
Tail (cauda epididymis)

Vertical section of testis showing the head, body, and tail of the epididymis. From Dorland's, 2000.

e. bullo′sa a variety with development of bullae and vesicles, often at the site of trauma; in the hereditary forms, there may be severe scarring after healing, or extensive denuded areas after rupture of the lesions.

epidermomycosis (ep″ĭ-der″mo-mi-ko′sis) dermatophytosis.

epidermophytid (ep″ĭ-der-mof′ĭ-tid) dermatophytid.

Epidermophyton (ep″ĭ-der-mof′ĭ-ton) a genus of fungi. *E. flocco′sum* attacks both skin and nails but not hair, and is one of the causative organisms of TINEA CRURIS, TINEA PEDIS, and ONYCHOMYCOSIS.

epidermophytosis (ep″ĭ-der″mo-fi-to′sis) 1. a fungal skin infection due to *Epidermophyton*. 2. dermatophytosis.

e. cru′ris tinea cruris.

epididymectomy (ep″ĭ-did″ĭ-mek′to-me) excision of the epididymis.

epididymis (ep″ĭ-did′ĭ-mis), pl. *epididy′mides* [Gr.] an elongated, cordlike structure along the posterior border of the testis, whose coiled duct provides for the storage, transport, and maturation of spermatozoa. adj., **epidi′dymal.**

epididymitis (ep″ĭ-did″ĭ-mi′tis) inflammation of the epididymis. Nonspecific epididymitis may result from an infection in the urinary tract, especially in the prostate. Rarely it may be traced to an infection elsewhere in the body. Tuberculosis, mumps, and gonorrhea may be complicated by epididymitis. Symptoms include sudden severe pain in the testes followed by scrotal swelling and tenderness. Treatment is usually with antibiotics, rest in bed, and avoidance of alcoholic beverages, sexual excitement, and strenuous physical exercise until all symptoms have disappeared.

epididymo-orchitis (ep″ĭ-did″ĭ-mo-or-ki′-tis) inflammation of an epididymis and testis; called also orchiepididymitis.

epididymotomy (ep″ĭ-did″ĭ-mot′ah-me) incision of the epididymis.

epididymovasostomy (ep″ĭ-did″ĭ-mo-vas-os′tah-me) surgical anastomosis of the epididymis to the ductus deferens.

epidural (ep″ĭ-du′ral) situated upon or outside the dura mater.

epidurography (ep″ĭ-du-rog′rah-fe) radiography of the spine after a radiopaque medium has been injected into the epidural space.

epiestriol (ep″e-es′tre-ol) an estrogenic steroid found in pregnant women.

epigastralgia (ep″ĭ-gas-tral′jah) pain in the epigastrium.

epigastrium (ep″ĭ-gas′tre-um) the upper and middle region of the abdomen, located within the sternal angle. adj., **epigas′tric.**

epigenesis (ep″ĭ-jen′ĕ-sis) the development of an organism from an undifferentiated cell, consisting in the successive formation and development of organs and parts that do not preexist in the zygote. adj., **epigenet′ic.**

epiglottis (ep″ĭ-glot′is) the lidlike cartilaginous structure overhanging the entrance to the larynx. adj., **epiglot′tic.** The muscular action of swallowing closes the opening to the trachea by placing the larynx against the epiglottis. This prevents food and drink from entering the larynx and trachea, directing it instead into the esophagus. (See Plates.)

epiglottitis (ep″ĭ-glŏ-ti′tis) supraglottitis.

epilate (ep′ĭ-lāt) depilate.

epilation (ep″ĭ-la′shun) depilation.

epilatory (e-pil′ah-tor″e) depilatory.

epilemma (ep″ĭ-lem′ah) endoneurium.

epilepsy (ep′ĭ-lep″se) paroxysmal transient disturbances of nervous system function resulting from abnormal electrical activity of the brain. Epilepsy is not one specific disease, but rather a group of symptoms that are manifestations of any of a number of conditions involving overstimulation of nerve cells of the brain. The estimated incidence is 0.5 per cent of the population, making this a relatively

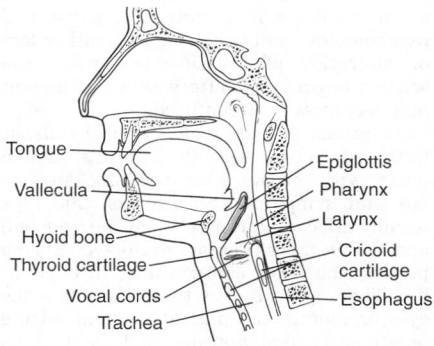

Tongue
Vallecula
Hyoid bone
Thyroid cartilage
Vocal cords
Trachea
Epiglottis
Pharynx
Larynx
Cricoid cartilage
Esophagus

Epiglottis in a sagittal section of the head and neck. From Dorland's, 2000.

common disease. Over 70 per cent of patients have their first attack (or SEIZURE) either during childhood or after age 50. The type of seizure varies with age of onset.

Types. There are several methods for classifying types of epilepsy. On the basis of origin, it may be either *idiopathic (cryptogenic, essential, genetic)* or *symptomatic (acquired, organic)*. Symptomatic epilepsy has a physical cause, such as a brain tumor, injury to the brain at birth, a wound or blow to the head, or an endocrine disorder.

One classification of epileptic seizures, called the Clinical and Electroencephalographical Classification of Epileptics of the International League Against Epilepsy, identifies four main types: (1) *partial seizures,* including those that begin locally, which are subdivided into (A) partial seizures with elementary symptomatology, (B) partial seizures with complex symptomatology (those with impairment of consciousness only, psychomotor symptomatology, and psychosensory symptomatology), and (C) partial seizures that are secondarily generalized; (2) *generalized seizures that are bilaterally symmetrical and without local onset;* (3) *unilateral seizures* (those involving only one hemisphere); and (4) *other unclassified epileptic seizures.*

Types According to Symptoms. The manifestations of epilepsy depend on the area of the brain where the abnormal discharge occurs. *Simple partial seizures,* called also *focal seizures,* result from a localized cortical discharge. The symptoms may be either motor, sensory, autonomic, or any combination of the three. *Complex partial seizures,* as in *psychomotor (temporal lobe) epilepsy,* usually, but not always, originate in the temporal lobe of the brain, often with a preceding aura. As the name implies, there are many different cognitive, affective, and psychomotor symptoms. There is either loss or alteration of consciousness when the seizure begins, and afterwards the patient may feel drowsy or confused.

An attack of *petit mal (absence) epilepsy* lasts only a few seconds and has sudden onset with no aura or warning and no postictal symptoms. Seizures of this type usually affect children between the ages of 5 and 12 years and may disappear during puberty, but they can continue throughout life. There typically is a twitching about the eyes or mouth, the patient remains sitting or standing, and appears to have had no more than a lapse of attention or a moment of absent-mindedness.

An attack of *grand mal (tonic-clonic) epilepsy* usually begins with bilateral jerks of the extremities or focal seizure activity. There is loss of consciousness and both tonic and clonic type convulsions. The patient may be incontinent during the attack and there is danger of tongue biting. In the postictal phase the patient is confused and drowsy.

Atonic or *akinetic seizures* are characterized by loss of body tone that can produce nodding of the head, weakness of the knees, or total collapse and falling. The patient usually remains conscious during the attack.

Diagnosis. A complete assessment of the patient's status is necessary, including a medical history, physical and neurological examination, and laboratory studies of the blood and spinal fluid. The latter are especially useful in determining whether an infection is the cause of the seizures. A CT scan may demonstrate a causative lesion. The diagnosis is confirmed by an electroencephalogram, which is helpful in locating the site and possibly the cause of the seizures.

Treatment. Medical management with anticonvulsant drugs is the preferred therapy for about 95 per cent of patients with epilepsy. Surgical intervention for the remaining 5 per cent involves removal of the portion of brain tissue believed to be responsible for the seizures. Because of the dangers inherent in the surgery, this mode of therapy is reserved for those patients who do not respond to medical management and in whom the focus of seizure activity is accessible.

The major antiepileptic drugs are phenytoin (Dilantin), which is usually the drug of choice, phenobarbital, primidone (Mysoline), carbamazepine (Tegretol) for complex partial tonic-clonic seizures, and ethosuximide (Zarontin) and clonazepam (Klonopin) for absence seizures. Valproic acid (Depakene) is also used in the treatment of absence seizures. The choice of drug and calculation of optimal dosage is very difficult and highly individualized.

All of the anticonvulsant drugs can produce unpleasant side effects. They include gingival hyperplasia, rash, and, in the case of Dilantin, fever and leukopenia. Physical dependence can become a problem in patients taking phenobarbital or primidone, which is largely converted to phenobarbital in the blood stream. Toxic side effects are also common and include drowsiness, ataxia, nausea, sedation, and dizziness. The untoward effects of anticonvulsant drug therapy require close monitoring of the patient's response to therapy and regulation of dosage as indicated.

Patient Care. Emergency care of the patient having a seizure includes clearing the immediate area to protect the patient and others, administering 100 per cent oxygen by face mask, and intravenous administration of antiepileptic medication. No one should force an object into the patient's mouth to hold it open (such as a comb, bite block, or wallet), as such objects might obstruct the airway. Do not attempt to restrain the patient, as that may cause harm to both the rescuer and the patient.

Until a diagnosis of epilepsy is confirmed, observations made before, during, and after each of the seizures can provide important information to the diagnostician. Such data also can help prepare an effective plan of care for managing the seizures once a definitive diagnosis is made.

Just before a seizure (the *preictal* stage) the patient may experience an abnormal somatic, visceral, or psychic sensation called an aura. The presence or absence of the aura and its nature (if it is present) should be noted and recorded. If a patient does experience a particular kind of aura just before each seizure, this information can be useful when planning care for prevention of injury. It also is helpful to note what the patient was doing just before the seizure began. If a particular emotional event or environmental or physiologic condition is found to trigger the seizures, the patient might be able to use this information to avoid or minimize the recurrence of seizures.

During the *interictal* stage (while the seizure is occurring) significant data include the time the seizure begins and its duration; where in the body the seizure begins and what parts of the body are involved; whether the head or eyes turn to one side and, if so, to which side; whether there is incontinence of urine or stool, bleeding, or foaming or frothing at the mouth; effects of the seizure on the vital signs; and changes in skin color or profuse perspiration.

During the *postictal* period the patient is assessed for lethargy, confusion, impaired speech, and reports of headache or muscle soreness.

The successful long-term management of epilepsy requires coordinated effort on the part of the patient, family, and health care professionals. Patient and family education and support are essential components of any plan of care. Epileptic patients must take their prescribed medications on their own and actively participate in the management of their illness. They and those upon whom they are dependent (as in the case of children) must know the nature of the illness, the purpose and expected effects of treatment, the side effects of the drug they are taking and its potential for interaction with other drugs that could inhibit or enhance its anticonvulsant action, and the signs and symptoms of drug intolerance that should be reported to the physician or nurse.

Education should also include information about possible seizure triggers and ways in which they might be avoided. Alcohol is especially dangerous for epileptic persons because most antiepileptic drugs are sedatives and cardiopulmonary depressants. The combination of drug and alcohol could cause loss of consciousness or even death. Moreover, alcohol acts as a seizure trigger in some persons.

It is important that patients with epilepsy wear some form of medical identification. In spite of efforts to educate the general public about the nature of epilepsy and its effects on those who have it, there remains some social stigma attached to epilepsy. Therefore, many patients do not want their friends, classmates, or employers to know they have the disease. Efforts must be made to improve the self-esteem of these people. Local chapters of the Epilepsy Association of America offer programs and opportunities for social interaction and group support to help persons with epilepsy and their families deal with the psychosocial effects of the disease. Information and guidance to a local chapter can be obtained by contacting the Epilepsy Association of America, 111 W. 55th St., New York, NY 10019.

The Epilepsy Foundation of America, 4351 Garden City Dr., Suite 406, Landover, MD 20785, supplies information on all aspects of epilepsy and can refer patients and their families to specialists and clinics in their locality.

One of the major challenges to persons working in the health field and concerned with the care of patients with epilepsy is the dispelling of myths and superstitions about the disease and the propagation of accurate information. Most persons with epilepsy can lead normal lives with few restrictions, but many are subjected to unfair employment practices and social stigma because of prejudices resulting from the general public's ignorance of the effects of epilepsy.

absence e. petit mal epilepsy.

audiogenic e. reflex epilepsy brought on by sound.

grand mal e. a form attended by loss of consciousness and convulsive movements, as distinguished from petit mal epilepsy. See EPILEPSY.

jacksonian e. a form of epilepsy characterized by unilateral clonic movements that start in one group of muscles and spread systematically to adjacent groups, reflecting the march of the epileptic activity through the motor cortex.

myoclonus e. any form of epilepsy accompanied by MYOCLONUS; one type is LAFORA'S DISEASE.

petit mal e. a relatively mild type of epilepsy in which the person loses consciousness only momentarily, in contrast to *grand mal epilepsy*; called also absence epilepsy. See EPILEPSY.

photogenic e. reflex epilepsy brought on by flickering light.

psychomotor e. temporal lobe epilepsy.

reflex e. epileptic seizures occurring in response to sensory stimuli (tactile, visual, auditory, or musical).

temporal lobe e. a type manifested by impaired consciousness of variable degree, with the patient carrying out bizarre but coordinated movements; called also psychomotor epilepsy. See EPILEPSY.

epileptic (ep″ĭ-lep′tik) pertaining to or affected with epilepsy.

epileptiform (ep″ĭ-lep′tĭ-form) 1. resembling epilepsy or its manifestations. 2. occurring in severe or sudden paroxysms.

epileptogenic (ep″ĭ-lep″to-jen′ik) causing an epileptic seizure.

epileptoid (ep″ĭ-lep′toid) epileptiform (def. 1).

epimenorrhagia (ep″ĭ-men″o-ra′jah) too frequent and excessive menstruation.

epimenorrhea (ep″ĭ-men″o-re′ah) abnormally frequent menstruation.

epimer (ep″ĭ-mer) one of two or more optical isomers that differ only in the configuration around one asymmetric carbon atom. adj., **epimer′ic.**

epimerase (ĕ-pim′er-āse) an ISOMERASE enzyme that catalyzes a change in asymmetric groups in substrates (EPIMERS) that have more than one center of asymmetry.

epimere (ep′ĭ-mēr) the dorsal portion of a somite, from which are formed muscles innervated by the dorsal ramus of a spinal nerve.

epimerization (ĕ-pim″er-ĭ-za′shun) the changing of one epimeric form of a compound into another, as by enzymatic action.

epimorphosis (ep″ĭ-mor-fo′sis) the regeneration of a piece of an organism by proliferation at the cut surface. adj., **epimor′phic.**

epimysium (ep″ĭ-mis′e-um) the fibrous sheath around an entire skeletal muscle.

epinephrine (ep″ĭ-nef′rin) a hormone produced by the adrenal MEDULLA; called also adrenaline (British). Its function is to aid in the regulation of the sympathetic branch of the AUTONOMIC NERVOUS SYSTEM. At times when a person is highly stimulated, as by fear, anger, or some challenging situation, extra amounts of epinephrine are released into the bloodstream, preparing the body for energetic action. Epinephrine is a powerful VASOPRESSOR that increases blood pressure and increases the heart rate and cardiac output. It also increases GLYCOGENOLYSIS and the release of glucose from the liver, so that a person has a suddenly increased feeling of muscular strength and aggressiveness.

Some disorders of the adrenal glands, such as ADDISON'S DISEASE, reduce the output of epinephrine below normal. By contrast, excessive activity of those glands, as sometimes seen in highly emotional persons, tends to produce tenseness, palpitation, high blood pressure, perhaps diarrhea, and overaggressiveness. Certain adrenal tumors also result in the production of too much epinephrine. Removal of the tumor relieves symptoms.

Epinephrine is also produced synthetically and can be administered parenterally, topically, or by inhalation. It acts as a VASOCONSTRICTOR, ANTISPASMODIC, and SYMPATHOMIMETIC, and it is used as an emergency heart stimulant as well as to relieve symptoms in allergic conditions such as urticaria (hives), asthma, and other conditions requiring bronchodilation and as an adjunct to local and regional anesthesia. It is the most effective drug for counteracting the lethal effects of anaphylactic shock. It is also used topically in the eye in the treatment of GLAUCOMA.

epinephryl borate (ep″ĭ-nef′ril) a compound containing EPINEPHRINE as a borate complex; used in treatment of GLAUCOMA.

epineural (ep″ĭ-noor′al) situated upon a neural arch.

epineurium (ep″ĭ-noor′e-um) the sheath of a peripheral nerve. adj., **epineu′rial.**

epiphysiolysis (ep″ĭ-fiz″e-ol′ĭ-sis) separation of the epiphysis from the diaphysis of a bone.

epiphysis (e-pif′ĭ-sis), pl. *epi′physes* [Gr.] 1. the end of a long bone, usually wider than the shaft, and either entirely cartilaginous or separated from the shaft by a cartilaginous disk. 2. part of a bone formed from a secondary center of ossification, commonly found at the ends of long bones, on the margins of flat bones, and at tubercles and processes; during the period of longitudinal growth, epiphyses are separated from the main portion of the bone by cartilage. adj., **epiphys′eal.**

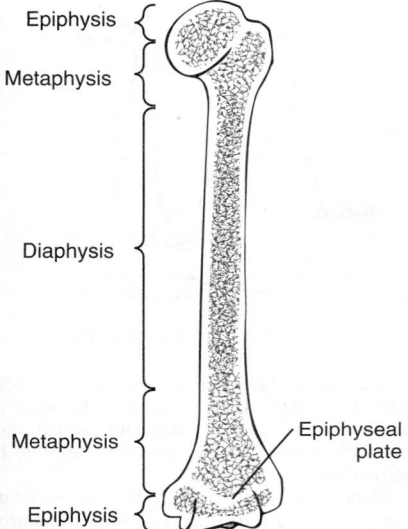

Epiphysis

Metaphysis

Diaphysis

Metaphysis — Epiphyseal plate

Epiphysis

Structure and composition of a typical long bone showing the epiphysis. From Copstead, 1995.

e. ce′rebri PINEAL BODY.

epiphysitis (e-pif″ĭ-si′tis) inflammation of an epiphysis or of the cartilage joining the epiphysis to a bone shaft.

epipial (ep″ĭ-pi′al) situated upon the PIA MATER.

epiplocele (e-pip′lo-sēl) omental hernia.

epiploon (e-pip′lo-on) [Gr.] the greater omentum. adj., **epiplo′ic.**

epiretinal (ep″ĭ-ret′ĭ-nal) overlying the retina.

epirubicin (ep″e-roo′bĭ-sin) an antitumor ANTIBIOTIC of the ANTHRACYCLINE group, having the same actions as DOXORUBICIN but a lower toxicity; administered intravenously in the treatment of carcinoma of the breast, ovary, stomach, colon, and rectum, as well as leukemia, lymphoma, and multiple myeloma.

episclera (ep″ĭ-skle′rah) the loose connective tissue forming the sclera and the conjunctiva.

episcleral (ep″ĭ-skle′ral) 1. overlying the sclera. 2. pertaining to the episclera.

episcleritis (ep″ĭ-skle-ri′tis) inflammation of the episclera and adjacent tissues.

episioperineoplasty (ě-piz″e-o-per″ĭ-ne′o-plas″te) plastic repair of the vulva and perineum.

episioperineorrhaphy (ě-piz″e-o-per″ĭ-ne-or′ah-fe) suture of the vulva and perineum.

episioplasty (ě-piz′e-o-plas″te) plastic repair of the vulva.

episiorrhaphy (ě-piz″e-or′ah-fe) 1. suture of the labia majora. 2. suture repair of an episiotomy.

episiostenosis (ě-piz″e-o-stě-no′sis) narrowing of the vulvar orifice.

episiotomy (ě-piz″e-ot′ah-me) surgical incision into the perineum and vagina for obstetrical purposes. The incision is repaired by PERINEORRHAPHY.

episode (ep′ĭ-sōd) a single noteworthy happening in the course of a longer series of events, such as one critical period of several during a prolonged illness.

hypomanic e. a period of elevated, expansive, or irritable mood similar to a

Median or midline

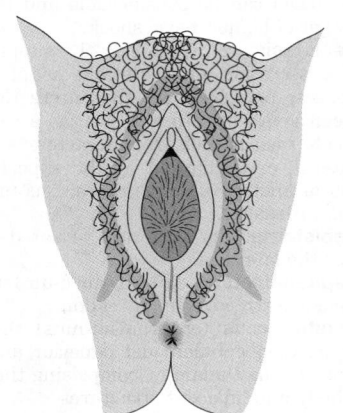

Mediolateral

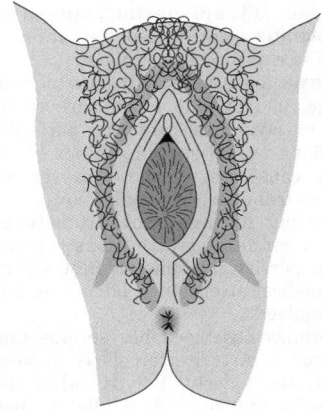

Types of episiotomy. From McKinney et al., 2000.

MANIC EPISODE but not as severe; see also BIPOLAR DISORDERS and MOOD DISORDERS.

major depressive e. a period of daily and day-long depressed mood or loss of interest or pleasure in virtually all activities. Also present is some combination of altered appetite, weight, or sleep patterns, psychomotor agitation or retardation, difficulty thinking or concentrating, lack of energy and fatigue, feelings of worthlessness, self-reproach, or inappropriate guilt, recurrent thoughts of death or suicide, and plans or attempts to commit suicide. See also BIPOLAR DISORDERS and MOOD DISORDERS.

manic e. a period of predominantly elevated, expansive, or irritable mood accompanied by some of the following symptoms: inflated self-esteem, decreased need for sleep, talkativeness, flight of ideas, distractibility, hyperactivity, hypersexuality, and recklessness. See also BIPOLAR DISORDERS and MOOD DISORDERS.

mixed e. a period during which the criteria are met both for a major depressive episode and for a manic episode nearly every day, with rapidly alternating moods and with symptoms characteristic of each type of episode. See also BIPOLAR DISORDERS and MOOD DISORDERS.

episodic (ep″ĭ-sod′ik) having symptom-free periods that alternate with the presence of symptoms.

episome (ep′ĭ-sōm″) in bacterial genetics, any accessory extrachromosomal replicating genetic element that can exist either autonomously or integrated with the chromosome.

epispadias (ep″ĭ-spa′de-as) a congenital malformation with absence of the upper wall of the urethra; it occurs in both sexes, but more commonly in the male, with the urethral opening somewhere on the dorsum of the penis. adj., **epispa′diac, epispa′dial.**

episplenitis (ep″ĭ-sple-ni′tis) inflammation of the capsule of the spleen.

epistaxis (ep″ĭ-stak′sis) hemorrhage from the nose, usually due to rupture of small vessels overlying the anterior part of the cartilaginous nasal septum. Minor bleeding may be caused by a blow on the nose, irritation from foreign bodies, or vigorous nose-blowing during a cold; sometimes it occurs in connection with menstruation. If bleeding persists in spite of first aid measures, medical attention is advisable. Called also nosebleed.

Sometimes nosebleed has serious underlying causes. Arteriosclerosis is a possible cause in the elderly. Polyps, other fleshy growths in the nose, food allergy, hypertension, vitamin deficiencies, or a disease

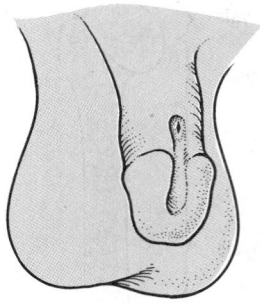

Epispadias. From Dorland's, 2000.

producing a bleeding tendency may produce nosebleed. If the nose bleeds often or profusely, or if the bleeding is difficult to stop, a health care provider should be consulted.

Bleeding from the nose that does not originate in the nose itself is a serious indication that some damage has been done internally, either by injury or disease. Medical attention is necessary to trace the bleeding to its source. The blood probably originates in the stomach, the lungs, within the skull, or in passages related to these parts.

First Aid Measures: The victim should sit up with the head tilted forward to avoid aspiration of blood. The soft portion of the nose is grasped firmly between the thumb and forefinger, for 5 to 15 minutes. Once bleeding stops the patient should rest for an hour or so and for several hours should avoid stooping, lifting, or vigorously blowing the nose. If bleeding continues, a health care provider may have to pack the nose. Sometimes cauterization of the bleeding vessel is necessary. In some cases surgery to clip the vessels may be done. Blood loss from a nosebleed can be considerable and there is danger of hemorrhagic shock.

epistasis (ĕ-pis′tah-sis) 1. suppression of a secretion or excretion, as of blood, menses, or lochia. 2. the interaction between genes at different loci, as a result of which one hereditary character is unexpressed, or is masked by the superimposition of another upon it. See also DOMINANCE. adj., **epistat′ic.**

episternal (ep″ĭ-ster′nal) situated on or over the sternum.

epitendineum (ep″ĭ-ten-din′e-um) the fibrous sheath covering a tendon.

epithalamus (ep″ĭ-thal′ah-mus) the part of the diencephalon just superior and posterior to the thalamus, comprising the pineal body and adjacent structures.

epithelial (ep″ĭ-the′le-al) pertaining to or composed of epithelium.

epithelialization (ep″ĭ-the″le-al-ĭ-za′shun) healing by the growth of epithelium over a denuded surface.

epithelialize (ep″ĭ-the′le-al-īz) to cover with epithelium.

epitheliitis (ep″ĭ-the″le-i′tis) inflammation of the epithelium.

epithelioid (ep″ĭ-the′le-oid) resembling epithelium.

epitheliolysis (ep″ĭ-the″le-ol′ĭ-sis) destruction of epithelial tissue. adj., **epitheliolyt′ic.**

epithelioma (ep″ĭ-the″le-o′mah) 1. a neoplasm of epithelial origin, ranging from benign (adenoma and papilloma) to malignant (carcinoma). 2. the term is sometimes used loosely and incorrectly as a synonym for CARCINOMA. adj., **epithelio′matous.**

   e. adenoi′des cys′ticum trichoepithelioma.

epithelium (ep″ĭ-the′le-um), pl. *epithe′lia* [Gr.] the cellular covering of internal and external surfaces of the body, including the lining of vessels and other small cavities. It consists of cells joined by small amounts of cementing substances. Epithelium is classified into types on the basis of the number of layers deep and the shape of the superficial cells.

   ciliated e. epithelium bearing vibratile, hairlike processes (cilia) on its free surface.

   columnar e. epithelium whose cells are of much greater height than width.

   cuboidal e. epithelium whose cells are of approximately the same height and width, and appear square in transverse section.

   germinal e. thickened peritoneal epithelium covering the gonad from earliest development; formerly thought to give rise to germ cells.

   glandular e. that composed of secreting cells.

   pigmentary e., pigmented e. that made of cells containing granules of pigment.

   sense e., sensory e. neuroepithelium (def. 1).

   simple e. that composed of a single layer of cells.

   squamous e. that composed of flattened platelike cells.

   stratified e. epithelium made up of cells arranged in layers.

   transitional e. a type characteristically found lining hollow organs, such as the urinary bladder, that are subject to great mechanical change due to contraction and distention; originally thought to represent a transition between stratified squamous and columnar epithelium.

epithelization (ep″ĭ-the″lĭ-za′shun) epithelialization.

epitonic (ep″ĭ-ton′ik) abnormally tense or tonic.

epitope (ep′ĭ-tōp) antigenic determinant.

epitrichium (ep″ĭ-trik′e-um) periderm.

epitrochlea (ep″ĭ-trok′le-ah) the inner condyle of the humerus.

epitympanum (ep″ĭ-tim′pah-num) epitympanic RECESS. adj., **epitympan′ic.**

epizoic (ep″ĭ-zo′ik) pertaining to or caused by an epizoon.

epizoon (ep″ĭ-zo′on), pl. *epizo′a* [Gr.] an external animal parasite.

epizootic (ep″ĭ-zo-ot′ik) attacking many animals in any region at the same time; widely diffused and rapidly spreading.

   e. disease 1. a disease that affects a large number of animals in some particular region within a short period of time. 2. a disease of high morbidity that is only occasionally present in an animal community.

epoetin (e-po′ĕ-tin) a form of human ERYTHROPOIETIN produced by recombinant technology and having the same amino acid sequence and mechanism of action as endogenous erythropoietin. Used in treatment of ANEMIA from various causes, including chronic RENAL FAILURE, ZIDOVUDINE therapy, and cancer CHEMOTHERAPY; also used prior to surgery in anemic patients to reduce the need for blood transfusion. Administered intravenously or subcutaneously. It is available in two forms, designated *epoetin alfa* (the form used in the United States) and *epoetin beta* (used in various other countries). Called also recombinant human erythropoietin.

eponychium (ep″o-nik′e-um) 1. cuticle. 2. the horny fetal epidermis at the site of the future nail.

eponym (ep′o-nim) a name or phrase formed from or including a person's name, such as HODGKIN'S DISEASE, Cowper's GLANDS, or SCHICK TEST. adj., **eponym′ic, epon′-ymous.**

epoöphoron (ep″o-of′o-ron) a vestigial structure associated with the ovary.

epoprostenol (e″po-pros′tĕ-nol) name for PROSTACYCLIN when used pharmaceutically; it is used in the form of the sodium salt as an inhibitor of platelet aggregation for blood contacting nonbiological systems, as in renal dialysis, as a pulmonary ANTIHYPERTENSIVE, and as a VASODILATOR.

epoxide (ĕ-pok′sīd) an organic compound resulting from the union of an oxygen atom with two other atoms, usually carbon, that are themselves joined together. Commonly referred to as epoxy. See also epoxy RESIN.

epoxy (ĕ-pok′se) 1. epoxide. 2. epoxy RESIN.

EPP erythropoietic protoporphyria.

eprosartan (ep″ro-sar′tan) an ANGIOTENSIN II antagonist that causes vasodilation and decreases the effects of aldosterone; used as an ANTIHYPERTENSIVE, administered orally.

EPS electrophysiological studies.

Epstein-Barr virus (ep′stīn bahr′) a HER-PESVIRUS of the genus *Lymphocryptovirus*, one of the etiologic agents of infectious MONONUCLEOSIS. It has been isolated from cells cultured from Burkitt's lymphoma and has been found in certain cases of nasopharyngeal carcinoma. There may be an association between EBV and CHRONIC FATIGUE SYNDROME. High titers of EBV are present in some tumors, but a causative role has not been proven. Called also EB virus.

EP test erythrocyte protoporphyrin test.

eptifibatide (ep″tĭ-fib′ah-tīd) an inhibitor of platelet aggregation used for prevention of THROMBOSIS in patients with ACUTE CORONARY SYNDROME or undergoing certain percutaneous coronary procedures; administered intravenously.

epulis (ep-u′lis), pl. *epu′lides* [Gr.] any tumor of the gingiva.

giant cell e., e. gigantocellula′ris a sessile or pedunculated lesion of the gingiva, or less often the mucous membrane covering edentulous ridges; it is an inflammatory reaction to injury or hemorrhage.

Eq equivalent.

Equagesic (ek″wah-je′sik) trademark for a combination preparation of the ANALGESIC ASPIRIN and the muscle RELAXANT MEPROBAMATE; used as an ANTISPASMODIC.

Equanil (ek′wah-nil) trademark for preparations of MEPROBAMATE, an ANTIANXIETY AGENT.

equation (e-kwa′zhun) an expression of equality between two parts.

Henderson-Hasselbalch e. a formula for calculating the pH of a buffer solution such as blood plasma, $pH = pK_a + \log [BA/HA]$; [HA] is the concentration of a free weak acid; [BA] the concentration of the ionized form of this acid; pK_a the acid dissociation constant, a measure of the ionization equilibrium of the acid.

equianalgesic (e-kwe-an″al-je′zik) approximately equal in ability to relieve pain; said of drugs, doses, or routes of administration. (See accompanying table.)

equifinality (e″kwĭ-fi-nal′ĭ-te) a principle of general SYSTEMS theory stating that an open system can attain a time-independent state not dependent on initial conditions and determined only by the system parameters.

equilibration (e″kwĭ-lĭ-bra′shun) the achievement of a balance between opposing elements or forces.

mandibular e. 1. the act or acts done to put the mandible into equilibrium with the maxilla. 2. a condition in which all the forces acting upon the mandible are neutralized.

equilibrium (e″kwĭ-lib′re-um) 1. harmonious adjustment of different elements or parts; called also balance. 2. a state of chemical balance in the body, reached when the tissues contain the proper proportions of various salts and water. See also ACID-BASE BALANCE and FLUID BALANCE. 3. SENSE OF EQUILIBRIUM.

dynamic e. the condition of balance between varying, shifting, and opposing forces that is characteristic of living processes.

equilin (ek′wĭ-lin) an ESTROGEN isolated from the urine of pregnant horses; see also conjugated ESTROGENS.

equine (e′kwīn) pertaining to, characteristic of, or derived from the horse.

equinovalgus (e-kwi″no-val′gus) TALIPES equinovalgus.

equinovarus (e-kwi″no-var′us) TALIPES equinovarus.

equipment (e-kwip′ment) necessary tools or provisions.

durable medical e. nonexpendable articles primarily used for medical purposes in cases of illness or injury; this includes hospital beds, respirators, walkers, and apnea monitors.

equipotential (e″kwĭ-po-ten′shal) having similar and equal power or capability.

equipotentiality (e″kwĭ-po-ten″she-al′ĭ-te) the quality or state of having similar and equal power; the capacity for developing in the same way and to the same extent.

equivalent (e-kwiv′ah-lent) 1. of equal value or force. 2. in chemistry, having the same valence. 3. see equivalent WEIGHT.

anxiety-e. translation of anxiety into a kind of emotional activity, e.g., the experiencing or expression of angry feelings.

full time e. (FTE) the equivalent of one full time staff member; a total number of full time equivalents is planned for in making budget allocations. A combination of part time staff members can be used to equal one full time equivalent.

Er erbium.

Erb-Goldflam disease (erb′ gōlt′flahm) myasthenia gravis.

erbium (Er) (er′be-um) a chemical element, atomic number 68, atomic weight 167.26. (See Appendix 6.)

ERCP endoscopic retrograde CHOLANGIO-PANCREATOGRAPHY.

erectile (e-rek′tīl) capable of erection.

erection (e-rek′shun) 1. the condition of becoming rigid and elevated, as erectile tissue when filled with blood. 2. especially the swelling and rigidity that occur in the penis as a result of sexual or other types of stimulation. Impulses received by the nervous system stimulate a flow of blood from the arteries leading to the penis, where the erectile tissue fills with blood, and the penis becomes firm and erect. Erection makes possible the transmission of semen into the body of the female (see REPRODUCTION). Erection can also occur to some extent in the clitoris and the nipples of the female. Dysfunction of the process of erection in a male is called IMPOTENCE.

erector (e-rek′tor) a structure that erects, as a muscle that holds up or raises a part.

erg (erg) a unit of work or energy, being the work performed when a force of 1 dyne moves its point of operation through a distance of 1 cm; equal to 10^{-7} joule.

ergasia (er-ga′zhah) term coined by Adolf MEYER to describe the total activity or functioning of a person, encompassing both behavior and mental activity. He defined a group of "ergasias," conceived of as behavioral patterns that are reactions or adaptations to genetic, developmental, and environmental factors, as alternatives to psychiatric diagnoses. For example, *merergasia,* partial impairment of functioning, included most behaviors now classified as ANXIETY DISORDERS.

ergocalciferol (er″go-kal-sif′er-ol) vitamin D_2; a sterol occurring naturally in fungi and some fish oils or synthesized from ERGOSTEROL, and similar to CHOLECALCIFEROL in activity and metabolism; it is administered orally or added to food (e.g., milk) as a dietary source of VITAMIN D. It is also used in treatment of hypocalcemia, hypophosphatemia, rickets, and osteodystrophy associated with various medical conditions including chronic RENAL FAILURE and HYPOPARATHYROIDISM, administered orally, intramuscularly, or intravenously.

ergograph (er′go-graf) an instrument for measuring work done in muscular action.

ergoloid mesylates (er′go-loid) hydrogenated ERGOT alkaloids used for relief of signs and symptoms of idiopathic decline in mental capacity (including impairment of recent memory, confusion, and disorientation) in persons over sixty.

ergometer (er-gom′ĕ-ter) an instrument that measures the amount of work performed during muscular activity; see also DYNAMOMETER.

ergonovine (er″go-no′vin) an alkaloid obtained from ERGOT or produced synthetically, used as the maleate salt as an OXYTOCIC and as a provocative test in detection of Prinzmetal's ANGINA due to coronary artery spasm.

ergosterol (er-gos′ter-ol) a sterol occurring in animal and plant tissues which on irradiation by ULTRAVIOLET RAYS converts to VITAMIN D_2, a potent agent for the prevention of RICKETS, ERGOCALCIFEROL.

ergot (er′got) the dried sclerotium of the fungus *Claviceps purpurea,* which attacks rye plants. Ergot alkaloids are used as OXYTOCICS and in treatment of MIGRAINE. Consumption of excessive amounts of ergot can cause the toxicity known as ERGOTISM.

ergotamine (er-got′ah-min) an alkaloid derived from ERGOT, used as the tartrate salt in treatment of MIGRAINE and cluster HEADACHES; administered orally, sublingually, rectally, or by oral inhalation.

ergotherapy (er″go-ther′ah-pe) treatment of disease by physical effort.

ergotism (er′go-tizm) chronic poisoning produced by ingestion of ERGOT, marked by cerebrospinal symptoms, spasm, cramps, a kind of dry gangrene of the extremities, and burning pain related to intense peripheral vasoconstriction.

erogenous (ĕ-roj′ĕ-nus) arousing erotic feelings.

erosion (e-ro′zhun) an eating or gnawing away; a shallow or superficial ulceration; in dentistry, the wasting away or loss of substance of a tooth by a chemical process that does not involve known bacterial action. adj., **ero′sive.**

cervical e. destruction of the squamous epithelium of the vaginal portion of the cervix, due to irritation and later ulceration.

erotic (ĕ-rot′ik) 1. charged with sexual feeling. 2. pertaining to sexual desire.

eroticism (ĕ-rot′ĭ-sizm) erotism.

erotism (er′o-tizm) a sexual instinct or desire; the expression of one's instinctual energy or drive, especially the sex drive.

E

anal e. in psychoanalytic theory, fixation of libido at (or regression to) the anal phase of infantile development, producing egotistic, dogmatic, stubborn, miserly character.

genital e. in psychoanalytic theory, achievement and maintenance of libido at the genital phase of psychosexual development, permitting acceptance of normal adult relationships and responsibilities.

oral e. in psychoanalytic theory, fixation of libido at (or regression to) the oral phase of infantile development, producing passive, insecure, sensitive character.

erotize (er′o-tīz) to endow with erotic meaning or significance.

erotogenic (ĕ-rot″o-jen′ik) producing erotic feeling.

erotomania (ĕ-rot″o-ma′ne-ah) 1. a disorder in which the subject believes that a person, usually older and of higher social status, is deeply in love with him or her; failure of the object of the delusion to respond to the subject's advances are rationalized, and pursuit and harassment of the object of the delusion may occur. 2. occasionally, hypersexuality.

erotophobia (ĕ-rot″o-fo′be-ah) fear of love, especially of sexual feelings and activity.

errhine (er′īn) 1. promoting a nasal discharge. 2. an agent that has this effect.

error (er′or) a defect or mistake in structure or function.

inborn e. of metabolism a genetically determined biochemical disorder in which a specific enzyme defect produces a metabolic block that may have pathologic consequences at birth, as in phenylketonuria, or in later life.

measurement e. the difference between what exists in reality and what is measured by a measurement method.

Type I e. the rejection of a null HYPOTHESIS that is true.

Type II e. acceptance of a null HYPOTHESIS that is false.

erucic acid (ĕ-roo′sik as′id) a monounsaturated FATTY ACID that is a major constituent of certain oils, such as RAPESEED OIL. Because it has been linked to cardiac muscle damage, oils such as CANOLA OIL were developed that are low in erucic acid.

eructation (e″ruk-ta′shun) the oral ejection of gas or air from the stomach; belching.

eruption (e-rup′shun) 1. the act of breaking out, appearing, or becoming visible, as eruption of the teeth. 2. visible efflorescent lesions of the skin due to disease, with redness, prominence, or both; a rash. adj., **erup′tive.**

creeping e. 1. a peculiar eruption that appears to migrate, due to burrowing beneath the skin by certain larvae; it has the appearance of subcutaneous tunnels that are red and vesicular at the advancing end and dry and encrusted at older portions. 2. LARVA MIGRANS.

drug e. an adverse cutaneous reaction produced by ingestion, parenteral use, or local application of a drug, which may produce various morphologic patterns and types of lesions; called also dermatitis medicamentosa.

Kaposi's varicelliform e. a generalized and serious vesiculopustular eruption of viral origin, superimposed on preexisting atopic dermatitis; it may be due to the herpes simplex virus (eczema herpeticum) or vaccinia (eczema vaccinatum).

ERV expiratory reserve volume.

Erwinia (er-win′e-ah) a genus of gram-negative, facultatively anaerobic, motile, rod-shaped bacteria. *E. herbi′cola* has been associated with nosocomial septicemia.

erysipelas (er″ĭ-sip′ĕ-las) a febrile disease characterized by inflammation and redness of the skin and subcutaneous tissues, and due to Group A hemolytic streptococci; it is a form of CELLULITIS. The visible symptoms are round or oval patches on the skin that promptly enlarge and spread, becoming swollen, tender, and red. The affected skin is hot to the touch, and, occasionally, the adjacent skin blisters. Headache, vomiting, fever, and sometimes complete prostration can occur. Penicillin is the treatment of choice. Care must be taken to avoid spreading the disease to other areas of the body. Adj., **erysipel′atous.**

coast e. a cutaneous manifestation of onchocerciasis seen in Central America, so called because of its resemblance to streptococcal erysipelas.

swine e. a contagious and highly fatal disease of pigs, caused by *Erysipelothrix rhusiopathiae.*

erysipeloid (er″ĭ-sip′ĕ-loid) 1. bacterial cellulitis due to infection with *Erysipelothrix rhusiopathiae,* usually occurring as an occupational disease associated with the handling of infected fish, shellfish, meat, or poultry. There are three forms: a usually self-limited, mild localized form manifested by an erythematous and painful swelling at the site of inoculation, which spreads peripherally with central clearing; a generalized or diffuse form, which may be accompanied by fever and arthritis symptoms and resolves spontaneously; and a rare and sometimes fatal systemic form associated with endocarditis. **2.** loosely, erysipelas like.

Erysipelothrix (er″i-sip′ĕ-lo-thriks″) a genus of gram-positive, rod-shaped bacteria. It contains one species, *E. rhusiopa′thiae,* the causative agent of swine erysipelas, which also infects sheep, turkeys, and rats. In humans the usual type of infection is an erythematous, edematous lesion, commonly on the hand, resulting from contact with infected meat, hide, or bones. See also ERYSIPELOID.

erythema (er″ĭ-the′mah) redness of the skin caused by congestion of the capillaries in the lower layers of the skin. It occurs with any skin injury, infection, or inflammation.

e. chro′nicum mi′grans a ring-shaped erythema due to the bite of a tick of the genus *Ixodes;* it begins as an erythematous plaque several weeks after the bite and spreads peripherally with central clearing. Often there are also systemic symptoms, including chills, fever, headache, vomiting, backache, and stiff neck. See also LYME DISEASE.

gyrate e., e. gyra′tum erythema multiforme characterized by the development of lesions that tend to migrate and spread peripherally with central clearing.

e. ab ig′ne permanent erythema produced by prolonged exposure to excessive nonburning heat. It is seen most often on the legs of women, but under appropriate environmental circumstances, it can occur anywhere on the body in either sex.

e. indura′tum a chronic necrotizing vasculitis, usually occurring on the calves of young women; see also BAZIN'S DISEASE.

e. infectio′sum a mild, self-limiting disease of childhood characterized by a lace-like skin rash symmetrically distributed on the hands, arms, and legs, with few or no other symptoms; occasionally there is a low grade fever, and the condition often clears up without specific treatment. The incubation period is six days to two weeks. This disease is contagious and originally was believed to be a form of rubella; because the rash can resemble that of scarlet fever and German measles, it is important to differentiate this mild condition from those more serious ones. Called also fifth disease.

e. margina′tum a type of erythema multiforme in which the reddened areas are disk-shaped, with elevated edges.

e. margina′tum rheuma′ticum a superficial, often asymptomatic, form of gyrate erythema associated with some cases of rheumatic fever, which is characterized by the presence on the trunk and extensor

surfaces of the extremities of a transient eruption of flat to slightly indurated, nonscaling, and usually multiple lesions.

e. mi′grans geographic tongue.

e. multifor′me a symptom complex representing a reaction of the skin and mucous membranes secondary to various known, suspected, and unknown factors, including infections, ingestants, physical agents, malignancy, and pregnancy. The conditions in the complex are characterized by the sudden onset of a reddened macular, bullous, papular, or vesicular eruption, the characteristic lesion being the iris, bull's eye, or target lesion, which consists of a central papule with two or more concentric rings. The complex includes a mild self-limited mucocutaneous form (erythema multiforme minor) and a severe, sometimes fatal, multisystem form (STEVENS-JOHNSON SYNDROME).

e. nodo′sum a type of PANNICULITIS occurring usually as a HYPERSENSITIVITY REACTION to multiple provoking agents, including various infections, drugs, sarcoidosis, and certain enteropathies. It may also be of idiopathic origin. It most often affects young women and is characterized by the development of crops of transient, inflammatory, nonulcerating nodules that are usually tender, multiple, and bilateral, and most commonly located on the shins; the lesions involute slowly, leaving bruiselike patches without scarring. The acute disease is often associated with fever, malaise, and arthralgias. A chronic variant sometimes occurs without any serious associated systemic disease.

toxic e., e. tox′icum a generalized erythematous or erythematomacular eruption due to administration of a drug or to bacterial or other toxins or associated with various systemic diseases.

e. tox′icum neonato′rum a benign, idiopathic, very common, generalized, transient eruption occurring in infants during the first week of life, usually consisting of small papules or pustules that become sterile, yellow-white, firm vesicles surrounded by an erythematous halo and some edema.

erythematous (er″ĭ-them′ah-tus) characterized by ERYTHEMA.

erythemogenic (er″ĭ-the″mo-jen′ik) producing or causing erythema.

erythr(o)- word element [Gr.], *red; erythrocyte.*

erythrasma (er″ĭ-thraz′mah) a chronic bacterial infection of the major skin folds due to *Corynebacterium minutissimum,* marked by red or brownish patches on the skin.

erythrism (ĕ-rith'rizm) redness of the hair and beard with a ruddy complexion. adj., **erythris'tic.**

erythrityl (ĕ-rith'rĭ-til) the univalent radical from erythritol.

e. tetranitrate a VASODILATOR used in ANGINA PECTORIS and coronary insufficiency; because of its explosiveness it must be diluted, as with lactose.

erythroblast (ĕ-rith'ro-blast) a term originally used for any type of nucleated ERYTHROCYTE, but now usually limited to one of the nucleated precursors of an erythrocyte, i.e. one of the developmental stages in the erythrocytic SERIES, in contrast to a MEGALOBLAST. In this usage, it is called also normoblast.

basophilic e. a nucleated precursor in the erythrocytic SERIES, preceding the polychromatophilic erythroblast and following the proerythroblast; the cytoplasm is basophilic, the nucleus is large with clumped chromatin, and the nucleoli have disappeared. Called also basophilic normoblast.

orthochromatic e. see NORMOBLAST.

polychromatic e., polychromatophilic e. see NORMOBLAST.

erythroblastemia (ĕ-rith″ro-blas-te'me-ah) erythroblastosis.

erythroblastoma (ĕ-rith″ro-blas-to'mah) a tumor composed of cells that resemble MEGALOBLASTS.

erythroblastosis (ĕ-rith″ro-blas-to'sis) the presence of erythroblasts in the circulating blood; called also erythroblastemia. adj., **erythroblastot'ic.**

e. feta'lis, e. neonato'rum a blood DYSCRASIA of the newborn characterized by agglutination and hemolysis of erythrocytes and usually due to incompatibility between the infant's blood and that of the mother. In most cases the fetus or infant has Rh-positive blood and its mother has Rh-negative blood (see RH FACTOR). Another form is seen when the fetus or infant has blood of type A or B and the mother has blood of type O; it is much milder than the Rh type because anti-A and anti-B antibodies only occasionally cross the placenta. Called also hemolytic disease of the newborn.

In Rh incompatibility the mother builds up ANTIBODIES against the red blood cells of the fetus; these pass through the placenta, enter the fetal circulation., and proceed to rapidly destroy the fetal red blood cells. In order to compensate for this, there is an ever-increasing effort on the part of the fetus to avoid anemia. This results in the release of very immature red blood cells (ERYTHROBLASTS). Thus an extremely high percentage of fetal erythrocytes are erythroblasts, giving the condition its name of erythroblastosis.

Symptoms. If it survives under these circumstances, at birth the baby is jaundiced and usually anemic. The immune bodies from the mother's blood usually circulate in the baby's blood for 1 to 2 months after birth, continuing the destruction of red blood cells unless an exchange TRANSFUSION is done. Other symptoms depend on the number of red cells destroyed and the amount of damage done to other tissues of the body, such as the brain and central nervous system.

Treatment. The usual treatment for erythroblastosis fetalis is exchange TRANSFUSION in which the infant's blood is replaced with Rh-negative blood. This measure stops the destruction of the infant's red blood cells, and gradually the Rh-negative blood is replaced with the baby's own blood. In about 6 weeks the immune bodies left over from the mother's blood have been destroyed and are no longer a menace to the baby. Exposure to ultraviolet light (PHOTOTHERAPY) breaks down the bilirubin causing the jaundice and reduces the number of transfusions that are required.

Developments in the management of erythroblastosis include AMNIOCENTESIS and intrauterine fetal transfusion. The former is puncture of the amniotic sac through the maternal abdomen and is done for the purpose of obtaining a sample of AMNIOTIC FLUID for analysis. This allows for determination of concentration of bilirubin pigments and protein in the amniotic fluid; a high concentration indicates excessive destruction of fetal erythrocytes. If there is a mild hemolysis the mother is watched closely and allowed to deliver at term. In more severe cases, induced labor and premature delivery are usually advised so that further destruction of erythrocytes will not take place and an exchange transfusion can be performed as soon as possible. For cases of very severe hemolysis it has been recommended that an intrauterine transfusion be administered to the fetus. This is a delicate procedure that involves certain risks, and is advised only if the mother's past history and the present evidence indicate that the infant would not survive or would suffer damage from erythroblastosis.

erythrochromia (ĕ-rith″ro-kro'me-ah) hemorrhagic, red pigmentation of the cerebrospinal fluid.

Erythrocin (ĕ-rith'ro-sin) trademark for preparations of ERYTHROMYCIN, a broad-spectrum ANTIBIOTIC.

erythroclasis (er″i′-throk′lah-sis) fragmentation of the red blood cells. adj., **erythroclas′tic.**

erythrocyanosis (ĕ-rith″ro-si″ah-no′sis) coarsely mottled bluish or red discoloration on the lower limbs, especially of girls; thought to be a circulatory reaction to exposure to cold.

erythrocytapheresis (ĕ-rith″ro-si″tah-fer′ĕ-sis) the withdrawal of blood, separation and retention of red blood cells, and retransfusion of the remainder into the donor.

erythrocyte (ĕ-rith′ro-sīt) one of the formed elements in the peripheral BLOOD, constituting the great majority of the cells in the blood. (For immature forms see erythrocytic SERIES.) In humans the normal mature erythrocyte is a biconcave disk without a nucleus, about 7.7 micrometers in diameter, consisting mainly of HEMOGLOBIN and a supporting framework called the STROMA. Erythrocyte formation (ERYTHROPOIESIS) takes place in the red bone marrow in the adult, and in the liver, spleen, and bone marrow of the fetus. It requires an ample supply of dietary elements such as iron, cobalt, copper, amino acids, and certain vitamins. Called also red cell or corpuscle and red blood cell or corpuscle.

The functions of erythrocytes include transportation of oxygen and carbon dioxide. They owe their oxygen-carrying ability to HEMOGLOBIN, a combination of an iron-containing prosthetic group *(heme)* with a protein *(globin)*. Hemoglobin attracts and forms a loose connection with free oxygen, and its presence enables blood to absorb some 60 times the amount of oxygen that the plasma by itself absorbs. Oxyhemoglobin is red, which gives oxygenated blood its red color. Erythrocytes are stored in the spleen, which acts as a reservoir for the blood system and discharges the cells into the blood as required. The spleen may discharge extra erythrocytes into the blood during emergencies such as hemorrhage or shock.

Erythrocytes also are important in the maintenance of a normal ACID-BASE BALANCE, and, since they help determine the viscosity of the blood, they also influence its specific gravity. Their average life span is 120 days. They are subjected to much wear and tear in circulation and eventually are removed by cells of the RETICULOENDOTHELIAL SYSTEM, particularly in the liver, bone marrow, and spleen. In spite of this constant destruction and production of erythrocytes, the body maintains a fairly constant number, between 4 and 5 million per mm^3 of blood in women and 5 to 6 million per mm^3 in men. A decreased number constitutes one form of ANEMIA.

The events in the life of erythrocytes. Nucleated red blood cell (RBC) precursors stimulated by erythropoietin form erythrocytes in the bone marrow. Normal synthesis of hemoglobin occurs only in the presence of nutrients, iron, vitamin B$_{12}$, and folic acid. Mature RBCs are released into circulation. The old or defective RBCs are degraded in the spleen. Iron and globin are reutilized immediately. Bilirubin is released in bile into the intestine. From Damjanov, 1996.

Erythrocytes are destroyed whenever they are exposed to solutions that are not isotonic to blood plasma. If they are placed in a solution that is more dilute than plasma (distilled water for example) the cells will swell until osmotic pressure bursts the cell membrane. If they are placed in a solution more concentrated than plasma, the cells will lose water and shrivel or crenate. It is for this reason that solutions to be given intravenously must be isotonic to plasma.

Aged red cells are ingested by macrophages in the spleen and liver. The iron is transported by the plasma protein TRANSFERRIN to the bone marrow, where it is incorporated into new red cells. The heme group is converted to bilirubin, a bile pigment secreted by the liver. About 180 million red blood cells are destroyed every minute. Since the number of cells in the blood remains more or less constant, this means that about 180 million red blood cells are manufactured every minute.

Determination of the red blood cell volume is usually done as a preliminary step in determination of the total BLOOD VOLUME. A radioactive substance, usually chromium, is used to "tag" cells of a sample of blood drawn from the patient. The sample is then reintroduced into the circulating blood and subsequent samples are taken to be evaluated for degree of radioactivity. The degree of dilution is used to calculate total blood volume.

e. protoporphyrin test EP test; a screening test for lead toxicity; erythrocyte protoporphyrin levels are determined by direct fluorometry of whole blood or fluorescence analysis of whole blood extracts. Levels will be increased in either lead poisoning or iron deficiency.

e. sedimentation rate the rate at which erythrocytes settle out of unclotted blood in one hour. The test is based on the fact that inflammatory processes cause an alteration in blood proteins, resulting in aggregation of the red cells, which makes them heavier and more likely to fall rapidly when placed in a special vertical test tube. Normal ranges vary according to the type of tube used, each type being of a different size. The most common methods and the normal range for each are: *Wintrobe method,* 0 to 6.5 mm per hour for men, 0 to 15 mm per hour for women; and *Westergren method,* 0 to 15 mm per hour for men, 0 to 20 mm per hour for women.

The erythrocyte sedimentation rate is often inconclusive and is not considered specific for any particular disorder. It is most often used as a gauge for determining the progress of an inflammatory disease such as rheumatic fever, rheumatoid arthritis, or a respiratory infection. The information provided by this test must be used in conjunction with results from other tests and clinical evaluations.

erythrocythemia (ĕ-rith″ro-si-the′me-ah) polycythemia.

erythrocytic (ĕ-rith″ro-sit′ik) 1. pertaining to, characterized by, or of the nature of erythrocytes. 2. pertaining to the erythrocytic series.

erythrocytorrhexis (ĕ-rith″ro-si″to-rek′sis) a morphologic change in erythrocytes, consisting in the escape from the cells of round,

shiny granules and splitting off of particles; called also plasmorrhexis.

erythrocytosis (ĕ-rith″ro-si-to′sis) increase in the total red blood cell mass secondary to any of a number of nonhematogenic systemic disorders in response to a known stimulus (secondary POLYCYTHEMIA), in contrast to primary POLYCYTHEMIA (polycythemia vera).

stress e. an apparent POLYCYTHEMIA seen in active, anxiety-prone persons, resulting from diminished plasma volume.

erythroderma (ĕ-rith″ro-der′mah) abnormal redness of the skin over widespread areas of the body.

congenital ichthyosiform e. a generalized hereditary dermatitis with scaling, occurring in a bullous form (epidermolytic HYPERKERATOSIS) and a nonbullous form (lamellar ICHTHYOSIS).

e. desquamati′vum Leiner's disease.

psoriatic e. a generalized psoriasis vulgaris, showing the chemical characteristics of exfoliative dermatitis.

erythrodontia (ĕ-rith″ro-don′she-ah) reddish brown pigmentation of the teeth.

erythrogenesis (ĕ-rith″ro-jen′ĕ-sis) erythropoiesis.

e. imperfec′ta congenital hypoplastic anemia (def. 1).

erythrogenic (ĕ-rith″ro-jen′ik) 1. producing a sensation of red. 2. erythemogenic. 3. erythropoietic.

erythroid (er′ĭ-throid) 1. of a red color; reddish. 2. pertaining to any of the cells in the erythrocytic SERIES.

erythrokeratodermia (ĕ-rith″ro-ker″ah-to-der′-me-ah) reddening and HYPERKERATOSIS of the skin.

e. varia′bilis a rare, dominantly inherited ichthyosis characterized by circumscribed areas of erythema that undergo changes in size, shape, and distribution over a period of days, with plaques of yellow-brown scales that occur in the areas of erythema. The usual onset is at birth or in the first year of life, and the disease runs a chronic course with remissions and exacerbations.

erythrokinetics (ĕ-rith″ro-ki-net′iks) the kinetics of erythrocytes, described by laboratory measurements of total red cell volume, rate of red cell production, and red cell life-span (rate of destruction).

erythrolabe (ĕ-rith′ro-lāb) the pigment in retinal cones that is more sensitive to the red range of the spectrum than are the other pigments (chlorolabe and cyanolabe).

erythroleukemia (ĕ-rith″ro-loo-ke′me-ah) a malignant blood DYSCRASIA, one of the MYELOPROLIFERATIVE DISORDERS, with atypical

ERYTHROBLASTS and MYELOBLASTS in the peripheral blood.

acute e. a form of acute myelogenous LEUKEMIA representing erythroleukemia in which malignant leukocyte precursors have proliferated and become predominant.

erythromelalgia (ĕ-rith″ro-mel-al′jah) acromelalgia.

erythromycin (ĕ-rith″ro-mi′sin) a broad-spectrum ANTIBIOTIC produced by a strain of *Streptomyces erythreus,* administered orally, parenterally, and topically to the skin or to the eye, and effective against a wide variety of organisms, including gram-negative and gram-positive bacteria. Available forms include the estrolate ester and the ethylsuccinate, gluceptate, lactobionate, and stearate salts.

erythron (er′ĭ-thron) the circulating erythrocytes in the blood, their precursors, and all the body elements concerned in their production.

erythroneocytosis (ĕ-rith″ro-ne″o-si-to′-sis) the presence of immature erythrocytes in the blood.

erythropenia (ĕ-rith″ro-pe′ne-ah) deficiency in the number of erythrocytes.

erythrophage (ĕ-rith′ro-fāj) a phagocyte that ingests erythrocytes.

erythrophagia (ĕ-rith″ro-fa′jah) erythrophagocytosis.

erythrophagocytosis phagocytosis of erythrocytes; called also erythrophagia.

erythrophil (ĕ-rith′ro-fil) 1. a cell or other element that stains easily with red. 2. erythrophilous.

erythrophilous (er″ĭ-throf′ĭ-lus) easily staining red.

erythrophobia (ĕ-rith″ro-fo′be-ah) 1. irrational fear of the color red, often accompanied by fear of blood (hematophobia). 2. fear of blushing; a distressing tendency to blush frequently.

erythroplakia (ĕ-rith″ro-pla′ke-ah) a red patch in the mouth with a velvet appearance, often a sign of oral cancer.

erythroplasia (ĕ-rith″ro-pla′zhah) a condition of the mucous membranes characterized by red papular lesions.

e. of Queyrat a form of epithelial dysplasia, which may range in severity from mild disorientation of epithelial cells with variable cellular pleomorphism to changes of carcinoma in situ and even invasive carcinoma, usually found on the glans penis and prepuce of uncircumcised middle-aged and older men; occasionally it may involve the lips, oral mucosa, tongue, vulva, or glabrous skin. It is typically characterized by the development of a slowly growing, circumscribed, erythematous, usually moist, velvety, and shiny patch.

erythropoiesis (ĕ-rith″ro-poi-e′sis) the formation of erythrocytes; called also erythrogenesis. adj., **erythropoiet′ic.**

erythropoietin (ĕ-rith″ro-poi′ĕ-tin) a glycoprotein hormone secreted by the kidney in the adult and by the liver in the fetus, which acts on stem cells of the bone marrow to stimulate red blood cell production (erythropoiesis).

recombinant human e. epoetin.

erythroprosopalgia (ĕ-rith″ro-pros″o-pal′-jah) a disorder similar to ERYTHROMELALGIA, but with the redness and pain in the face.

erythropsia (er″ĭ-throp′se-ah) a chromatopsia in which objects appear tinged with red.

erythrosine (ĕ-rith′ro-sēn) a coloring agent used to disclose plaque on teeth.

erythrosis (er″ĭ-thro′sis) 1. reddish or purplish discoloration of the skin and mucous membranes, as in polycythemia vera. 2. hyperplasia of the hematopoietic tissue.

erythrostasis (ĕ-rith″ro-sta′sis) the stoppage of erythrocytes in the capillaries, as in sickle cell anemia.

Erythrovirus (e-rith′ro-vi″rus) a genus of PARVOVIRUSES containing viruses that infect ERYTHROCYTE progenitor cells; it includes the species B19 VIRUS.

erythruria (er″ĭ-throo′re-ah) CHROMATURIA in which the urine is red.

Es einsteinium.

esca (es′kah) [exercise of *self care agency*] a philosophical concept guiding the practice of KINLEIN; the moving or dynamic power within each person that is integral to any action taken in thought, word, or deed.

escape (es-kāp′) the act of becoming free.

vagal e. the exhaustion of or adaptation to neural chemical mediators in the regulation of systemic arterial pressure.

ventricular e. extrasystole in which a ventricular pacemaker becomes effective before the sinoatrial pacemaker; it usually occurs with slow sinus rates and often, but not necessarily, with increased vagal tone.

eschar (es′kahr) 1. a slough produced by a thermal burn or a corrosive application, or by gangrene. 2. tache noire.

escharotic (es-kah-rot′ik) 1. capable of producing an eschar; corrosive. 2. a corrosive or caustic agent.

escharotomy (es″kah-rot′ah-me) surgical incision of the eschar and superficial fascia of the chest or a circumferentially burned limb in order to permit the cut edges to separate and restore blood flow to unburned tissue. Edema may form beneath the inelastic eschar of a full-thickness burn and compress arteries, thus impairing blood flow and necessitating an escharotomy. The incision is protected from infection with the same antimicrobial agent being used on the burn wound.

Escherichia (esh″ĕ-rik′e-ah) a genus of gram-negative, facultatively anaerobic, rod-shaped bacteria found in the large intestine of humans and other warm-blooded animals; most species are either nonpathogenic or opportunistic pathogens. *E. co′li* is the principal species and forms the greater part of the normal intestinal flora. Some strains of it may cause urinary tract infections, abscesses, conjunctivitis, and sometimes septicemia, as well as diarrheal diseases, especially in children.

Escherichieae (esh″er-ĭ-ki′e-e) a tribe of bacteria (family Enterobacteriaceae), comprising the coliform bacteria.

escutcheon (es-kuch′un) 1. a shield or something shaped like a shield. 2. the shieldlike pattern of distribution of the pubic hair.

Esidrix (es′ĭ-driks) trademark for a preparation of HYDROCHLOROTHIAZIDE, a diuretic.

-esis word element [Gr.], *state; condition.*

eso- word element [Gr.], *within.*

esmolol (es′mo-lol) a cardioselective BETA-ADRENERGIC BLOCKING AGENT used as the hydrochloride salt in treatment of ARRHYTHMIAS for short-term control of atrial FIBRILLATION, atrial FLUTTER, and noncompensatory sinus TACHYCARDIA.

esogastritis (es″o-gas-tri′tis) inflammation of the gastric mucosa.

esomeprazole (es″o-mep′rah-zōl) a proton pump INHIBITOR administered orally as the magnesium salt in treatment of GASTROESOPHAGEAL REFLUX DISEASE and in the treatment of duodenal ULCER associated with *Helicobacter pylori* infection.

esophageal (ĕ-sof″ah-je′al) of or pertaining to the esophagus.

esophagectasia (ĕ-sof″ah-jek-ta′zhah) dilatation of the esophagus.

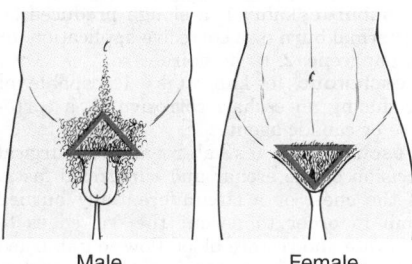

Male   Female

Normal escutcheon distribution of male and female pubic hair.

esophagectomy (ĕ-sof″ah-jek′to-me) excision of a portion of the esophagus.

esophagism (ĕ-sof′ah-jizm) spasm of the esophagus.

esophagitis (ĕ-sof″ah-ji′tis) inflammation of the esophagus.

peptic e., reflux e. a chronic, potentially life-threatening disease manifested by the various sequelae associated with reflux of the stomach and duodenal contents into the esophagus (gastroesophageal REFLUX); it is often accompanied by HEARTBURN and REGURGITATION, although not all patients with those symptoms have pathologic changes. It may occur as a primary condition or be associated with other diseases such as hiatal HERNIA.

esophagobronchial (ĕ-sof″ah-go-brong′-ke-al) bronchoesophageal.

esophagocele (ĕ-sof′ah-go-sēl″) abnormal distention of the esophagus; protrusion of the esophageal mucosa through a rupture in the muscular coat.

esophagocoloplasty (ĕ-sof″ah-go-ko′lo-plas″te) excision of a portion of the esophagus and its replacement by a segment of the colon.

esophagodynia (ĕ-sof″ah-go-din′e-ah) pain in the esophagus.

esophagoenterostomy (ĕ-sof″ah-go-en″-ter-os′tah-me) surgical formation of an anastomosis between the esophagus and the small intestine.

esophagoesophagostomy (ĕ-sof″ah-go-ĕ-sof″ah-gos′tah-me) anastomosis between two formerly remote parts of the esophagus.

esophagogastrectomy (ĕ-sof″ah-go-gas-trek′to-me) excision of the esophagus and stomach.

esophagogastric (ĕ-sof″ah-go-gas′trik) gastroesophageal.

esophagogastroanastomosis (ĕ-sof″ah-go-gas″tro-ah-nas″to-mo′sis) esophagogastrostomy.

esophagogastroduodenoscopy (ĕ-sof″-ah-go-gas″tro-doo″od-ĕ-nos′kah-pe) EGD; endoscopic examination of the interior of the esophagus, stomach, and initial portion of the duodenum. The procedure usually is done for diagnostic purposes and permits removal of samples of tissue for further study. In some cases the procedure is done to locate and remove a foreign object that has become lodged in the esophagus.

Patient Care. Prior to the procedure, foods and liquids are withheld to facilitate inspection of the mucosa and prevent vomiting and aspiration. A local anesthetic may be used to ease discomfort. Although there should be no severe pain associated with the examination, it can be uncomfortable and sometimes exhausting for the patient.

Since there may be some allergic reaction to the anesthetic, the patient is observed for dyspnea, excitement, dizziness, or headache. An emergency tray containing epinephrine and other drugs for treatment of anaphylaxis should be readily available.

Following any endoscopic examination of the upper gastrointestinal tract the patient is watched for signs of excessive bleeding and perforation. If a local anesthetic has been used, foods and liquids are withheld until normal reflex action returns and there is no danger of aspiration. Hoarseness and a mild sore throat may persist for a few days after the examination.

esophagogastroplasty (ĕ-sof″ah-go-gas′-tro-plas″te) plastic repair of the esophagus and stomach.

esophagogastroscopy (ĕ-sof″ah-go-gas-tros′kah-pe) endoscopic inspection of the esophagus and stomach.

esophagogastrostomy (ĕ-sof″ah-go-gas-tros′tah-me) anastomosis of the esophagus to the stomach.

esophagography (ĕ-sof″ah-gog′rah-fe) radiography of the esophagus.

esophagojejunostomy (ĕ-sof″ah-go-je″-joo-nos′tah-me) anastomosis of the esophagus to the jejunum.

esophagomalacia (ĕ-sof″ah-go-mah-la′-she-ah) softening of the walls of the esophagus.

esophagomyotomy (ĕ-sof″ah-go-mi-ot′ah-me) incision through the muscular coat of the esophagus.

esophagoplasty (ĕ-sof′ah-go-plas″te) plastic repair of the esophagus.

esophagoplication (ĕ-sof″ah-go-pli-ka′-shun) infolding of the wall of an esophageal pouch.

esophagoptosis (ĕ-sof″ah-gop-to′sis) prolapse of the esophagus.

esophagorespiratory (ĕ-sof″ah-go-re-spi′-rah-tor″e) pertaining to or communicating with the esophagus and respiratory tract (trachea or a bronchus).

esophagoscope (ĕ-sof′ah-go-skōp″) an endoscope for examination of the esophagus.

esophagoscopy (ĕ-sof′ah-gos′kah-pe) direct visual examination of the esophagus with an esophagoscope.

esophagostenosis (ĕ-sof″ah-go-stĕ-no′sis) stricture of the esophagus.

esophagostomy (ĕ-sof″ah-gos′tah-me) the creation of an artificial opening into the esophagus.

esophagotomy (ĕ-sof″ah-got′ah-me) incision of the esophagus.

esophagotracheal (ĕ-sof″ah-go-tra′ke-al) tracheoesophageal.

esophagus (ĕ-sof′ah-gus) the musculomembranous passage extending from the pharynx to the stomach, 25 to 30 cm (10 to 12 in) long in an adult, consisting of an outer fibrous coat, a muscular layer, a submucous layer, and an inner mucous membrane. The junction between the stomach and esophagus is closed by a muscular ring known as the cardiac sphincter, which opens to allow the passage of food into the stomach. See also DIGESTIVE SYSTEM and Plates.

Disorders of the Esophagus. The most common disorders of the esophagus often involve either an obstruction or a backward flow of food and gastric juice (gastroesophageal REFLUX). Foreign bodies, accidentally swallowed and lodged in the esophageal passage, can obstruct the flow of foods and fluids, as can malignant or benign tumors. The term ACHALASIA is used to describe a particular disturbance in motility which leads to obstruction at the level of the cardiac sphincter.

ESOPHAGITIS, inflammation of the mucous membrane lining the esophagus, may occur in conjunction with GASTROENTERITIS or as a result of reflux of gastric contents into the esophagus. The symptoms of hiatal HERNIA are due in large part to this type of reflux. Hiatal hernia is a protrusion of the stomach, colon, or other intestinal organs through the esophageal hiatus, a narrow opening in the diaphragm through which the esophagus normally passes. When the herniation occurs the normal downward passage of food is interrupted.

Esophageal VARICES are varicose veins of the esophagus and occur most often as a result of obstruction in the portal circulation, especially in portal hypertension. They are potentially dangerous since they tend to rupture easily and may result in serious hemorrhage. Visual examination of the interior lining of the esophagus is accomplished by ESOPHAGOSCOPY.

esophoria (es″o-for′e-ah) heterophoria in which there is deviation of the visual axis of one eye toward that of the other eye in the absence of visual fusional stimuli.

esosphenoiditis (es″o-sfe″noi-di′tis) osteomyelitis of the sphenoid bone.

esotropia (es″o-tro′pe-ah) STRABISMUS in which there is manifest deviation of the visual axis of one eye toward that of the other eye, resulting in DIPLOPIA; called also cross-eye and convergent strabismus. adj., **esotrop′ic.**

ESP extrasensory perception.

ESR erythrocyte sedimentation rate.

essence (es′ens) 1. that which is or necessarily exists as the cause of the properties of a body. 2. a solution of a volatile OIL in alcohol.

essential (ĕ-sen'shal) 1. constituting the necessary or inherent part of a thing; giving a substance its peculiar and necessary qualities. 2. indispensable; required in the diet, as essential fatty acids. 3. idiopathic; self-existing; having no obvious external cause.

EST electroshock therapy.

estazolam (es-taz'o-lam) a BENZODIAZEPINE used as a SEDATIVE and HYPNOTIC in treatment of insomnia; administered orally.

ester (es'ter) a compound formed from an alcohol and an acid by removal of water.

esterase (es'ter-ās) any enzyme that catalyzes the hydrolysis of an ester into its alcohol and acid.

esterification (es-ter″ĭ-fĭ-ka'shun) conversion of an acid into an ester by combination with an alcohol and removal of a molecule of water.

esterify (es-ter'ĭ-fi) to combine with an alcohol with elimination of a molecule of water, forming an ester.

esterolysis (es″ter-ol'ĭ-sis) the hydrolysis of an ester into its alcohol and acid. adj., **esterolyt'ic.**

esthematology (es″them-ah-tol'o-je) esthesiology.

esthesiogenic (es-the″ze-o-jen'ik) producing sensation.

esthesiology (es-the″ ze-ol' o-je) the scientific study or description of the sense organs and sensations.

esthesiometer (es-the″ze-om'ĕ-ter) an instrument for measuring tactile sensibility; tactometer.

esthesiophysiology (es-the″ze-o-fiz″e-ol'o-je) the physiology of sensation and sense organs.

esthesodic (es″thĕ-zod'ik) conducting or pertaining to conduction of sensory impulses.

esthetics (es-thet'iks) the branch of philosophy dealing with beauty; in dentistry, a philosophy concerned especially with the appearance of a dental restoration, as achieved through its color or form.

estimate (es'tĭ-ma) 1. a rough calculation or one based on incomplete data. 2. a statistic used to characterize the value of a population parameter. Called also estimator. 3. (es'tĭ-māt) to produce or use such a calculation or statistic.

estimator (es'tĭ-ma″ter) estimate (def. 2).

estival (es'tĭ-val, ĕ-sti'val) pertaining to or occurring in summer.

estivation (es″tĭ-va'shun) a dormant state in which certain animals pass the summer; see also HIBERNATION.

estivoautumnal (es″tĭ-vo-aw-tum'nal) occurring in summer and autumn.

estolate (es'to-lāt) USAN contraction for propionate lauryl sulfate.

estradiol (es″trah-di'ol, es-tra'de-ol) 1. the most potent naturally occurring ovarian and placental ESTROGEN in mammals; it prepares the uterus for implantation of the fertilized ovum and promotes the maturation of and maintenance of the female accessory reproductive organs and secondary sex CHARACTERS. 2. a preparation of this hormone used in estrogen replacement THERAPY for conditions such as female HYPOGONADISM, OVARIECTOMY, or primary ovarian failure, and in treatment of abnormal uterine bleeding, vasomotor menopausal symptoms, postmenopausal OSTEOPOROSIS, atrophic VAGINITIS, and certain advanced breast or prostatic carcinomas. Used most often in the form of estradiol cypionate, estradiol valerate, or ethinyl estradiol.

estramustine (es″trah-mus'tēn) an antineoplastic AGENT containing ESTRADIOL joined to MECHLORETHAMINE; administered orally for palliative treatment of metastatic or progressive carcinoma of the prostate; used as *estramustine phosphate sodium.*

estrin (es'trin) estrogen.

estrinization (es″trin-ĭ-za'shun) production of the cellular changes in the vaginal epithelium characteristic of ESTRUS.

estriol (es'tre-ol) a relatively weak human ESTROGEN that is a metabolic product of estradiol and estrone found in high concentration in the urine of females.

estrogen (es'tro-jen) a generic term for any of the estrus-producing compounds (female sex hormones), including ESTRADIOL, ESTRIOL, and ESTRONE. Called also estrogenic hormone. In humans, the estrogens are formed in the ovary, adrenal cortex, testis, and fetoplacental unit, and are responsible for female secondary sex characteristic development, and during the menstrual cycle, act on the female genitalia to produce an environment suitable for fertilization, implantation, and nutrition of the early embryo. Uses for estrogens include oral CONTRACEPTIVES, hormone replacement THERAPY, advanced prostate or postmenopausal breast carcinoma treatment, and osteoporosis prophylaxis.

conjugated e's a mixture of the sodium salts of the sulfate esters of ESTRONE and EQUILIN; therapeutic uses are similar to those of other estrogens; administered orally, intravenously, intramuscularly, or intravaginally.

esterified e's a mixture of esters of estrogenic substances, principally ESTRONE, having therapeutic uses similar to those of other estrogens.

estrogenic (es″tro-jen′ik) estrus-producing; having the properties of, or properties similar to, an estrogen.

estrone (es′trōn) an ESTROGEN isolated from pregnancy urine, the human placenta, and palm kernel oil, and also prepared synthetically; used in estrogen replacement THERAPY for hypogonadism, ovariectomy, primary ovarian failure, atrophic vaginitis, vasomotor menopausal symptoms such as hot flashes, and vulvar atrophy, and in the treatment of dysfunctional uterine bleeding and advanced prostate cancer. Administered intramuscularly or intravaginally. See also conjugated ESTROGENS and esterified ESTROGENS.

estrophilin (es″tro-fil′in) a cell protein that acts as a receptor for estrogen, found in estrogenic target tissue and in estrogen-dependent tumors and metastases.

estropipate (es″tro-pi′pāt) a preparation of PIPERAZINE and ESTRONE sulfate, having actions and uses similar to those of other estrogen preparations for treatment of estrogen deficiency states and for prevention of osteoporosis. Administered orally or intravaginally.

estruation (es″troo-a′shun) estrus.

estrum (es′trum) estrus.

estrus (es′trus) the recurrent, restricted period of sexual receptivity in female mammals other than human females, marked by intense sexual urge. See also estrous CYCLE. Called also estruation, estrum, and heat. adj., **es′trual, es′trous.**

esu electrostatic units.

etanercept (e-tan′er-sept) a soluble tumor necrosis FACTOR receptor that inactivates tumor necrosis factor, used in treatment of rheumatoid ARTHRITIS; administered subcutaneously.

etching (ech′ing) the cutting of a hard surface such as metal or glass by a corrosive chemical, usually an acid, in order to create a design.

    acid e. etching of dental enamel with an acid in order to roughen the surface, increase retention of resin sealant, and promote mechanical retention.

ethacrynate (eth-ah-krin′āt) a salt, ester, or the conjugate base of ETHACRYNIC ACID; the sodium salt has the same loop DIURETIC actions as the acid; administered parenterally.

ethacrynic acid (eth″ah-krin′ik) a loop DIURETIC used orally in the treatment of edema, including that associated with congestive heart failure or hepatic or renal disease, ascites, and hypertension.

ethambutol (ĕ-tham′bu-tol) an ANTIBACTERIAL agent specifically effective against *Mycobacterium tuberculosis*; it is administered orally as the hydrochloride salt, in

conjunction with one or more other antituberculous drugs, in the treatment of pulmonary TUBERCULOSIS.

ethanol (eth′ah-nol) a transparent, colorless, volatile, flammable liquid that is the major ingredient of alcoholic beverages. Excessive ingestion results in acute intoxication, with psychological, gastrointestinal, neurological, and motor abnormalities; ingestion during pregnancy can harm the fetus. See also ALCOHOLISM. The pharmaceutical preparation is called ALCOHOL. Called also ethyl or grain alcohol.

ethanolamine (eth″ah-nol′ah-mēn) monoethanolamine.

    e. oleate the oleate salt of monoethanolamine, used as a sclerosing agent in treatment of varicose veins and esophageal varices.

ethchlorvynol (eth-klor′vī-nol) a nonbarbiturate SEDATIVE and HYPNOTIC used for the short-term treatment of insomnia; administered orally.

ether (e′ther) 1. an organic compound containing an oxygen atom bonded to two carbon atoms. 2. diethyl or ethyl ether: a colorless, transparent, mobile, very volatile, highly flammable liquid with a characteristic odor; it was the first inhalational anesthetic used for surgical ANESTHESIA, but is now rarely used in the United States or Canada because of its flammability.

ethereal (e-the′re-al) 1. pertaining to, prepared with, containing, or resembling ether. 2. evanescent; delicate.

etherization (e″ther-ī-za′shun) induction of anesthesia by means of ether.

ethicist (eth′ī-sist) in health care, a person with graduate education, preferably doctoral, who is expert in BIOETHICS and has broad knowledge in philosophy and medicine or nursing, and whose job it is to help sort through difficult clinical situations to find ethical solutions.

ethics (eth′iks) 1. a branch of philosophy dealing with values pertaining to human conduct, considering the rightness and wrongness of actions and the goodness or badness of the motives and ends of such actions. 2. systematic rules or principles governing right conduct. Each practitioner, upon entering a profession, is invested with the responsibility to adhere to the standards of ethical practice and conduct set by the profession. adj., **eth′ical.**

    applied e. practical ethics.

    descriptive e. a type of nonnormative ethics that simply reports what people believe, how they reason, and how they act.

WINDOW ON ETHICIST

Management and resolution of ethical dilemmas is facilitated by careful, informed deliberation. This is a complex process; the particularity of each dilemma must be looked at in context of this situation or this patient. To analyze the conflict, it can be useful to refer to five basic types of moral conflict. These types, with examples, are: (1) conflict between ethical principles. A patient is competent to give informed consent for a potentially life-saving procedure, but refuses. The patient's condition is becoming worse. Here the conflict may be between respect for autonomy and beneficence. (2) Conflict of evidence. A family makes a decision for an incompetent patient without an advance directive, and the family stands to gain or lose when the patient dies. Conflict of evidence was a problem in the early years of AIDS when the risk to health care professionals was unclear. (3) Conflict between unsatisfactory alternatives. Using limited funds to treat one child with a rare condition or provide immunization for a whole community of children. Using limited funds for the cheapest single-chamber pacemaker for all pacemaker patients, or treating only some of the patients by implanting those who need them with the more expensive, appropriate pacemaker. (4) Conflict between role obligations and personal ethics or conflict between different roles. A nurse who because of personal beliefs objects to working in an operating room where abortions are done. A first line manager who must decide between using limited funds for emergency equipment or for overtime to provide adequate staff. (5) Conflict between law and ethics. What is legal may not be ethical and what is ethical may not be legal. Slavery, separate but equal racial policies, and involuntary sterilization have been legal; they are unethical practices. Abortion and euthanasia may or may not be ethical depending on individual philosophy. Likewise, they may or may not be legal, depending on the society and its philosophy.

To resolve an ethical dilemma it is essential to gather all of the facts relevant to the particular problem. Use people and other resources to get necessary information. Call for a consultation with an ethicist or refer the problem to the ethics committee. Reach agreement on definition of terms and on a common framework of moral principles, concepts, and ideas. It helps to know exactly what it is you are talking about. Explore the problem using examples and counterexamples. Expose the inconsistencies inherent in a line of reasoning. Make a decision after thorough discussion and contemplation. Evaluate the decision and its consequences.

CAROLINE CAMUNAS, RN, EdD

medical e. the values and guidelines governing decisions in medical practice.

nonnormative e. ethics whose objective is to establish what factually or conceptually is the case, not what ethically ought to be the case. Two types are *descriptive ethics* and *metaethics*.

normative e. an approach to ethics that works from standards of right or good action. There are three types of normative theories: *virtue theories, deontological theories,* and *teleological theories.*

nursing e. the values and ethical principles governing nursing practice, conduct, and relationships. The Code for Nurses, adopted by the American Nurses' Association (ANA) in 1950 and revised periodically, is intended to provide definite standards of practice and conduct that are essential to the ethical discharge of the nurse's responsibility. Further information on the Code, interpretative statements that clarify it, and guidance in implementing it in specific situations can be obtained from committees and councils on nursing practice of State Nurses' Associations or from the ANA Nursing Practice Department.

practical e. the attempt to work out the implications of general theories for specific forms of conduct and moral judgment; formerly called applied ethics.

professional e. the ethical norms, values, and principles that guide a profession and the ethics of decisions made within the profession.

ethinamate (ĕ-thin′ah-māt) a short-acting, nonbarbiturate SEDATIVE.

ethinyl (eth′ĭ-nil) the radical HC≡C—, derived from acetylene.

e. estradiol an estrogen derived from estradiol, used together with a progestational agent as a component of many oral contraceptives, in hormone replacement therapy, and as an antineoplastic in the treatment of advanced breast and prostate cancers; administered orally.

ethiodized oil an iodinated oil used as a radiopaque x-ray contrast medium in various diagnostic procedures.

ethionamide (ĕ-thi″on-am´īd) an ANTIBACTERIAL effective against *Mycobacterium tuberculosis;* used in the treatment of pulmonary TUBERCULOSIS, administered orally.

ethmocarditis (eth″mo-kahr-di´tis) inflammation of the connective tissue of the heart.

ethmoid (eth´moid) 1. sievelike; cribriform. 2. ethmoid BONE.

ethmoidal (eth-moi´dal) pertaining to the ethmoid bone.

ethmoidectomy (eth″moi-dek´to-me) excision of the ethmoid cells or of a portion of the ethmoid bone.

ethmoiditis (eth″moi-di´tis) 1. inflammation of the ethmoid bone. 2. ethmoid sinusitis.

ethmoidotomy (eth″moi-dot´ah-me) incision into the ethmoid sinus.

ethnic (eth´nik) pertaining to a social group whose members share cultural bonds or physical (racial) characteristics.

ethnicity (eth-nis´ĭ-te) affiliation due to shared linguistic, racial, or cultural background; intrinsic elements of one's heritage acquired from one's socially defined forebears that are based on perceptions of cultural differences among groups living in close proximity.

ethnocare (eth´no-kar″) care patterns that are known and preferred within a specific culture.

ethnography (eth-nog´rah-fe) 1. a description of the activities of a group and the beliefs held by group members. 2. study of the lifestyles, beliefs, and norms of a selected group through observation, participation, and analysis. Ethnographic research includes studies of patterns of behavior, known as culture traits, and the relationships between patterns of behavior. Ethnographic inquiry may be on selected topics, such as health and illness, and may ask questions such as "Do fathers in this culture attend the birth of a child?" or "What does a family member do immediately after the birth of a child?"

ethnology (eth-nol´o-je) 1. the branch of anthropology that deals with the study of the origin and descent of human races and ethnic groups and their distribution and relationships. 2. the science of comparing and analyzing transcultural differences and similarities and developing theoretical postulations and generalizations from the findings.

ethnonursing (eth″no-ners´ing) a research method for describing, documenting, and explaining nursing care phenomena by the study of the beliefs, values, and practices concerning nursing care that belong to a specific culture, as reflected by the language, beliefs, and values of the members of that culture.

ethoheptazine (eth″o-hep´tah-zēn) an ANALGESIC, used as the citrate salt to control mild to moderate pain; administered orally.

ethologist (ĕ-thol´o-jist) a person skilled in ethology.

ethology (ĕ-thol´o-je) the scientific study of animal behavior, particularly in the natural state. adj., **etholog´ical.**

ethopropazine (eth″o-pro´pah-zēn) an ANTIDYSKINETIC used as the hydrochloride salt in the treatment of PARKINSONISM and for the control of drug-induced extrapyramidal reactions (except tardive dyskinesia); administered orally.

ethosuximide (eth″o-suk´sĭ-mīd) an ANTICONVULSANT used in the treatment of petit mal EPILEPSY; administered orally.

ethotoin (eth´o-toin) an ANTICONVULSANT used in the treatment of grand mal EPILEPSY and temporal lobe EPILEPSY, administered orally

ethoxzolamide (eth″ok-zol´ah-mīd) a carbonic anhydrase INHIBITOR used in treatment of glaucoma and edema.

ethyl (eth´il) the monovalent radical, C_2H_5.

e. chloride a local anesthetic sprayed on intact skin to produce anesthesia by superficial freezing caused by its rapid evaporation.

ethylene (eth´ĭ-lēn) a colorless, highly flammable gas with a slightly sweet taste and odor, used as an inhalation anesthetic to induce general ANESTHESIA.

e. glycol a solvent with a sweet, acrid taste, used as an antifreeze. Acute poisoning by ingestion can result in central nervous system depression, vomiting, hypotension, coma, convulsions, renal damage, and death. While damage is thought to be due to the formed oxalic acid, ethanol is a good treatment because it competitively inhibits alcohol dehydrogenase. The unaltered ethylene glycol is then excreted in the urine.

e. oxide a gaseous, flammable ALKYLATING AGENT with a broad spectrum of activity, capable of killing both spores and viruses; it must be mixed with CO_2 or fluorocarbons because it is explosive above 3 per cent. It is used in hospitals, surgery, dentistry, and the pharmaceutical and other industries for disinfecting and sterilizing instruments and equipment that would be destroyed by heat or would be adversely affected by immersion in water or other media. Its optimal germicidal effect occurs after a 3-hour exposure at 30°C.

Ethylene oxide is toxic because it alkylates tissue constituents; it is carcinogenic and may produce adverse reproductive effects. Inhalation may cause nausea, vomiting, and neurological disorders, and severe exposure may be fatal. Before items exposed to ethylene oxide can be used they must be aired for 5 days at room temperature or for 8 hours at 120° C to remove any trace of the gas. This is also true for articles of clothing, such as gloves and shoes, that have been exposed, because chemical burns can occur when the contaminated clothing comes in contact with the skin.

ethylenediamine (eth″ĭ-lēn-di″ah-mēn) a clear liquid with an ammonia like odor and a strong alkaline reaction; complexed with theophylline, it forms AMINOPHYLLINE.

ethylenediaminetetraacetic acid (EDTA) (eth″ĭ-lēn-di″ah-mēn-tet″rah-ah-se′tik) a chelating agent that binds calcium and other metals; used as an anticoagulant for preserving blood specimens. Also used medicinally; see EDETATE. Called also edetic acid.

ethylnorepinephrine (eth″ĭl-nor-ep″ĭ-nef′-rin) a synthetic ADRENERGIC, used as the hydrochloride salt in treatment of ASTHMA.

ethynodiol (ĕ-thi″no-di′ol) a progestational AGENT used, as the diacetate salt, in combination with an ESTROGEN component as an oral CONTRACEPTIVE.

etic (et′ik) pertaining to expressions, perceptions, beliefs, and practices that are universal, or at least shared by several cultural groups; an etic view of a cultural system is one from the perspective of an outsider, based on universal and generalized explanations of behavior, rather than the perspective of the members of the system under study. See also EMIC.

etidocaine (ĕ-te′do-kān) 1. a local anesthetic of the amide type, used as the hydrochloride salt for percutaneous infiltration anesthesia, peripheral nerve block, and caudal and epidural block. 2. a local anesthetic used as the hydrochloride salt for infiltration anesthesia, peripheral nerve block, retrobulbar block, and epidural block.

etidronate (e″tĭ-dro′nāt) a bone CALCIUM regulator used as the disodium salt in the treatment of symptomatic OSTEITIS DEFORMANS, for the prevention of heterotopic ossification due to spinal cord injury or following total hip REPLACEMENT, and for the treatment of hypercalcemia associated with malignancy. It is also used in bone scanning, complexed with TECHNETIUM 99M.

etiolation (e″te-o-la′shun) 1. blanching or paleness of a plant grown in the dark due to lack of chlorophyll. 2. the process by which the skin becomes pale when deprived of sunlight.

etiology (e″te-ol′ah-je) the science dealing with causes of disease. adj., **etiolog′ic, etiolog′ical.**

ET-NANB enterically transmitted non-A, non-B (hepatitis); see HEPATITIS E.

etodolac (e-to-do′lak) a NONSTEROIDAL ANTIINFLAMMATORY DRUG used as an analgesic and antiinflammatory, especially to treat ARTHRITIS; administered orally.

etomidate (ĕ-tom′ĭ-dāt) a SEDATIVE and HYPNOTIC, administered intravenously for induction and maintenance of general anesthesia and as a supplement to low-potency anesthetics for maintenance of anesthesia during short operative procedures.

etoposide (e-to-po′sīd) a semisynthetic derivative of PODOPHYLLOTOXIN used as the base or the phosphate salt as an antineoplastic AGENT in treatment of carcinoma of the testes, lung, or bladder, lymphoma, acute myelocytic LEUKEMIA, Ewing's SARCOMA, and Kaposi's SARCOMA; administered orally or intravenously.

Eu europium.

eu- word element [Gr.], *normal; good; well; easy.*

Eubacterium (u″bak-tē′re-um) a genus of gram-positive, anaerobic, rod-shaped organisms occurring as saprophytes in soil and water. They are normal flora of the skin and body cavities and occasionally cause soft tissue infection. Species include *E. alactoly′ticum, E. len′tum,* and *E. limo′sum.*

eucalyptol (u″kah-lip′tol) a colorless liquid obtained from EUCALYPTUS OIL and other sources; used as an expectorant, flavoring agent, and local anesthetic.

eucalyptus oil (u″kah-lip′tus) a volatile oil from fresh leaf of species of *Eucalyptus,* the chief constituent of which is EUCALYPTOL; it is used as a pharmaceutical flavoring agent and as an expectorant and local antiseptic.

Eucaryotae (u-kar″e-o′te) a kingdom of organisms that includes higher plants and animals, fungi, protozoa, and most algae (except blue-green algae), all of which are made up of eukaryotic CELLS; see also EUKARYOTE.

eucaryote (u-kar′e-ōt) eukaryote.

euchlorhydria (u″klor-hi′dre-ah) the presence of the normal amount of HYDROCHLORIC ACID in the gastric juice.

eucholia (u-ko′le-ah) normal condition of the bile.

euchromatin (u-kro′mah-tin) that state of chromatin in which it stains lightly, is

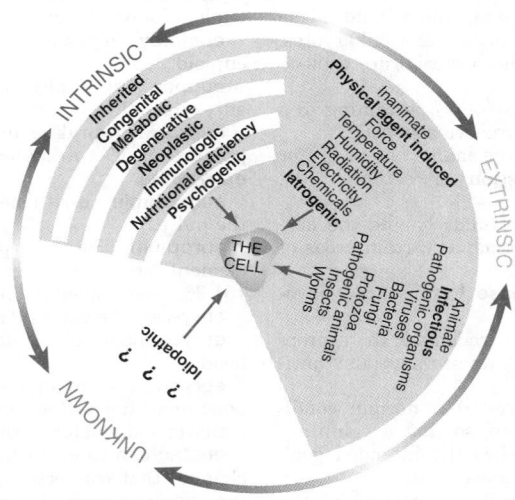

Etiology classification of disease. Illustrated here are the contributions of intrinsic, extrinsic, and unknown factors to disease causation. From Copstead and Banasik, 2000.

genetically active, and is considered to be partially or fully uncoiled.

euchromatopsy (u-kro′mah-top″se) normal color vision.

eucrasia (u-kra′zhah) 1. a state of health; proper balance of different factors constituting a healthy state. 2. a state in which the body reacts normally to ingested or injected drugs, proteins, or other substances.

eudiemorrhysis (u″di-ĕ-mor′ĭ-sis) the normal flow of blood through the capillaries.

eudipsia (u-dip′se-ah) ordinary, normal thirst.

euesthesia (u″es-the′zhah) a normal state of the senses.

eugenics (u-jen′iks) the study and control of procreation as a means of improving hereditary characteristics of future generations. The concept has sometimes been used in a pseudoscientific way as an excuse for unethical, racist, or even genocidal practices such as involuntary sterilization or certain other practices in Nazi Germany and elsewhere.

 macro e. eugenics policies that affect whole populations or groups. This has sometimes led to racism and genocide, such as the Nazi policies of sterilization and extermination of ethnic groups.

 micro e. eugenics policies affecting only families or kinship groups; such policies are directed mainly at women and thus raise special ethical issues.

 negative e. that concerned with prevention of reproduction by individuals considered to have inferior or undesirable traits.

 positive e. that concerned with promotion of optimal mating and reproduction by individuals considered to have desirable or superior traits.

eugenol (u′jĕ-nol) a dental topical ANALGESIC and protective obtained from clove oil or other sources.

euglobulin (u-glob′u-lin) one of a class of globulins characterized by being insoluble in water but soluble in saline solutions.

euglycemia (u″gli-se′me-ah) a normal level of glucose in the blood. adj., **euglyce′mic.**

eugonic (u-gon′ik) growing luxuriantly; said of bacterial cultures.

eukaryon (u-kar′e-on) 1. a highly organized nucleus bounded by a nuclear membrane, a characteristic of cells of higher organisms. 2. eukaryote.

eukaryosis (u″kar-e-o′sis) the state of having a true nucleus.

Eukaryotae (u-kar″e-o′te) Eucaryotae.

eukaryote (u-kar′e-ōt) an organism of the Eucaryotae, whose cells (eukaryotic CELLS) have a true nucleus that is bounded by a nuclear membrane, contains the CHROMOSOMES, and divides by MITOSIS. Eukaryotic cells also contain membrane-bound organelles, such as mitochondria, chloroplasts, lysosomes, and the Golgi apparatus. Plants and animals, protozoa, fungi, and algae (except blue-green algae) are eukaryotes. Other organisms (the bacteria) are PROKARYOTES.

eukaryotic (u″kar-e-ot′ik) pertaining to a EUKARYON or EUKARYOTE; see also CELL.

eukinesia (u″kĭ-ne′zhah) normal or proper motor function or activity. adj., **eukinet′ic.**

eulaminate (u-lam′ĭ-nāt) having the normal number of laminae, as certain areas of the cerebral cortex.

Eulenburg's disease (oil′en-burgz) myotonia congenita.

Eulexin (u-lek′sin) trademark for a preparation of FLUTAMIDE, an ANTIANDROGEN antineoplastic AGENT.

eumetria (u-me′tre-ah) a normal condition of nerve impulse, so that a voluntary movement just reaches the intended goal; the proper range of movement.

eunuch (u′nuk) a male deprived of the testes or external genitals, especially one castrated before puberty so that male secondary sex CHARACTERS fail to develop. See also CASTRATION.

eunuchoid (u′nŭ-koid) 1. resembling a eunuch. 2. a person who resembles a eunuch.

eunuchoidism (u′nŭ-koi-dizm) HYPOGONADISM in a male; deficiency of the testes or of their secretion, with deficient SECONDARY SEX CHARACTERS.

female e. hypogonadism in which the ovaries fail to function at puberty, resulting in infertility, absence of development of secondary sex characteristics, infantile sexual organs, and excessive growth of the long bones.

hypergonadotropic e. hypergonadotropic HYPOGONADISM.

hypogonadotropic e. hypogonadotropic HYPOGONADISM.

eupancreatism (u-pan′kre-ah-tizm) normal functioning of the pancreas.

eupepsia (u-pep′se-ah) good digestion; the presence of a normal amount of pepsin in the gastric juice. adj., **eupep′tic.**

euphoretic (u″fo-ret′ik) 1. producing EUPHORIA. 2. an agent that so acts.

euphoria (u-for′e-ah) an exaggerated feeling of physical and mental well-being, especially when not justified by external reality. Euphoria may be induced by drugs such as opioids, amphetamines, and alcohol and is also a feature of MANIA. adj., **euphor′ic.**

euphoriant (u-for′e-ant) euphoretic.

euplastic (u-plas′tik) readily becoming organized or healed; adapted to tissue formation.

euploid (u′ploid) 1. having a balanced set or sets of chromosomes, in any number. 2. a euploid individual or cell.

euploidy (u′ploi-de) the state of being euploid.

eupnea (ūp-ne′ah) normal respiration. adj., **eupne′ic.**

eupraxia (u-prak′se-ah) intactness of reproduction of coordinated movements. adj., **euprac′tic.**

eurhythmia (u-rith′me-ah) regularity of the pulse.

europium (Eu) (u-ro′pe-um) a chemical element, atomic number 63, atomic weight 151.96. (See Appendix 6.)

eury- word element [Gr.], *wide; broad.*

eurycephalic (u″rĭ-sĕ-fal′ik) having a wide head.

euryon (u′re-on) a point on either parietal bone marking either end of the greatest transverse diameter of the skull.

eustachian tube (u-sta′ke-an) the narrow channel that connects the middle ear with the nasopharynx; it serves to equalize pressure on either side of the tympanic membrane (eardrum). In children this tube is wider and shorter than in adults, and thus children are especially prone to OTITIS MEDIA, infection of the middle ear that originates in the pharynx and travels through the tube. Called also auditory tube. (See also Plates.)

euthanasia (u″thah-na′zhah) 1. an easy or painless death. 2. the deliberate ending of life of a person suffering from an incurable disease. In recent years the concept has been broadened to include the practice of withholding extraordinary means or "heroic measures," and thus allowing the patient to die (see extraordinary TREATMENT). A distinction was traditionally made between *positive* or *active euthanasia,* in which there is a deliberate ending of life and an action is taken to cause death in a person, and *negative* or *passive euthanasia,* which is the withholding of life-preserving procedures and treatments that would prolong the life of one who is incurably and terminally ill and could not survive without them. However, now all euthanasia is generally understood to be active, and so the more accurate term *forgoing life-sustaining treatment* is replacing *passive euthanasia.* See also ADVANCE DIRECTIVES.

voluntary e. see assisted SUICIDE.

euthermic (u-ther′mik) characterized by the proper temperatures; promoting warmth.

euthyroid (u-thi′roid) having a normally functioning thyroid gland.

eutocia (u-to′she-ah) normal labor or childbirth.

Eutrombicula (u″trom-bik′u-lah) a sub-genus of the mite genus *Trombicula*. *E. alfreddugè′si* (called also *Trombicula alfreddugèsi*) is the common CHIGGER of the United States.

eutrophication (u″tro-fi-ka′shun) the accidental or deliberate promotion of excessive growth (multiplication) of one kind of organism to the disadvantage of other organisms in the same ecosystem.

eV electron volt.

evacuant (e-vak′u-ant) 1. emptying. 2. CATHARTIC (defs. 1 and 2). 3. a remedy that empties any organ, such as a CATHARTIC, EMETIC, or DIURETIC.

evacuation (e-vak″u-a′shun) 1. an emptying. 2. catharsis (def. 1). 3. feces.

evagination (e-vaj″ĭ-na′shun) an outpouching of a layer or part.

evaluation (e-val″u-a′shun) a critical appraisal or assessment; a judgment of the value, worth, character, or effectiveness of something; measurement of progress. A broad view of evaluation in health care includes three approaches, directed toward STRUCTURE, PROCESS, and OUTCOME, depending on the focus of evaluation and the criteria or standards being used.

Structure evaluations are concerned with physical facilities, equipment, staffing, and other characteristics of the facility or agency that have an effect on the quality of care being provided. *Process evaluations* center on the activities of the provider and what the provider has done to assess, plan, and implement nursing care. The criteria used in process evaluations in nursing are the Standards of Nursing Practice developed by the American Nurses' Association. Structure and process evaluations are primarily concerned with QUALITY ASSURANCE and NURSING AUDITS. *Outcome evaluations* focus on the patient and goals set forth in the care plan and therefore are patient- and goal-oriented. Thus, outcome evaluation is the measurement of a patient's progress or lack of progress toward achievement of specified goals.

The purpose of the evaluation is to determine whether outcome criteria have been met and how care for the patient might be improved. Evaluation is *not* done to find fault or lay blame for inefficiency, incompetence, or carelessness. It is done for the purpose of improvement, by identifying specific areas that need change for the better. Some weaknesses that could be found during evaluation are vague or inaccurate statement of the problem because of poor assessment or faulty analysis and interpretation of data, unrealistic goal-setting due to over-estimating capabilities of the patient or

available resources, and well-intentioned but inappropriate nursing interventions that do not effectively meet the hoped-for outcome criteria.

Evaluation of direct care and the effectiveness of care plans and interventions is an ongoing activity. It serves to direct reassessment of patient status, the reordering of priorities, new goal-setting, and revision of nursing care as indicated.

The basic components of evaluation are (1) identifying the parameters of the subject of appraisal, (2) developing criteria specific to the topic within the parameters, (3) data gathering, (4) measuring the data against the criteria, and (5) employing the results of assessment for improvement of the process, status, behavior, or activity evaluated.

Parameters are the exact dimensions or fixed limits that clearly define the area of evaluation. They establish the frame of reference within which the process will take place and are essential to accurate interpretation and meaningful use of the results of the evaluation. Parameters to be considered might include the framework of time within which the data gathering will take place, description of the kinds of data to be obtained, and specification of the patient population selected for evaluation of patient care. In a NURSING AUDIT, for example, the medical records chosen for audit might be those of patients whose admission and discharge dates were within a specific period of time, and whose age range and diagnoses were similar. Since it is a *nursing* audit, the kind of data collected should be limited to information related to the area of nursing activities and the resulting patient care outcomes recorded on the patient's chart.

In the assessment of a patient's status on the health/illness continuum, the parameters might limit the appraisal to respiratory function, neuromuscular function, emotional status, or any of a number of areas that are important to accomplishing the overall goals and objectives of health care for that specific patient.

Data gathering involves the collection of information that gives factual and objective evidence about the subject being evaluated. The evidence may be obtained through observation, interview, the review of patient records, and, as in the case of assessment of a patient's health/illness status, through such procedures as laboratory analysis and testing, radiologic studies, and other diagnostic techniques, as well as a physical assessment or examination and history taking.

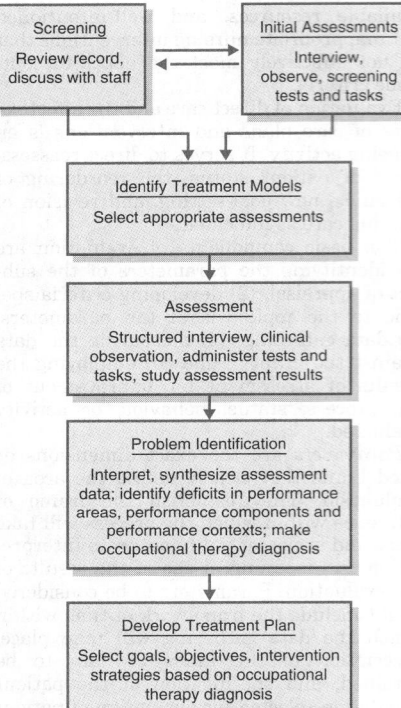

The evaluation process using occupational therapy as an exemplar. From Pedretti and Early, 2001.

The data collected become documented evidence, which is then measured against the established criteria. If the evidence indicates that all of the criteria are being met, there is no indication of a problem in the area of evaluation. If the evidence shows that certain criteria are not met, these deficiencies are identified as the ones needing attention so that there can be progress toward the stated goals.

criterion-referenced e. evaluation of performance by judging an individual's behavior, performance, or knowledge against specific criteria or standards. See also criterion-referenced TESTING.

formative e. evaluation that involves feedback regarding progress being made; it involves the continuous gathering of evaluative data throughout a learning experience.

normative-referenced e. evaluation in which the scores of an individual are interpreted in light of the norm or distribution of scores of others taking the same test; progress is determined by how well the individual compares with peers.

outcome e. see EVALUATION.

process e. see EVALUATION.

product e. in the NURSING INTERVENTIONS CLASSIFICATION, a nursing INTERVENTION defined as determining the effectiveness of new products or equipment.

structure e. see EVALUATION.

summative e. evaluation that involves one statement of the extent of achievement of objectives or goals; it involves the gathering of evaluative data at the end of a learning experience.

Evans blue (ev′anz) an odorless green, bluish green, or brown powder dye, used as a diagnostic acid in estimation of blood volume. The dye is injected into the bloodstream and after a sufficient period of time samples of the blood are taken to determine the degree of dilution of the dye.

evasion (e-va′zhun) in psychiatry, suppression of an idea that comes next in a thought sequence and substitution of a closely related idea. It is a form of paralogia.

eventration (e″ven-tra′shun) 1. herniation of the intestines; see HERNIA. 2. removal of the abdominal viscera.

    e. of the diaphragm, diaphragmatic e. elevation of the dome of the diaphragm into the thoracic cavity, usually due to phrenic nerve paralysis.

eversion (e-ver′zhun) a turning inside out; a turning outward.

    cervical e. the columnar glandular epithelium on the surface of the cervix surrounding the cervical os.

evert (e-vert′) to turn inside out; to turn outward.

evisceration (e-vis″er-a′shun) 1. extrusion of viscera outside the body, especially through a surgical incision (see illustration). 2. removal of abdominal viscera; called also eventration. 3. in ophthalmology, the

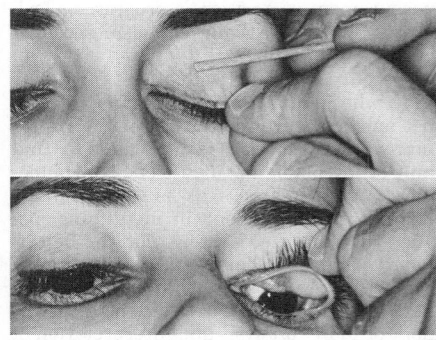

Eversion of the upper eyelid over an applicator. From Stein et al., 2000.

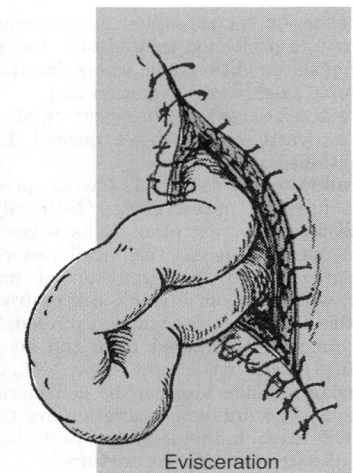

Evisceration

Wound evisceration requires immediate attention. The surgeon must be notified. Using sterile technique, cover the wound site with gauze or a sterile towel moistened in sterile saline. Take measures to prevent shock. Do not leave the person's side. From Polaski and Tatro, 1996.

removal of the contents of the eyeball, with the sclera being left intact.

evolution (ev″o-lu′shun) the process of development in which an organ or organism becomes more and more complex by the differentiation of its parts; a continuous and progressive change according to certain laws and by means of resident forces.

convergent e. the development, in animals that are only distantly related, of similar structures or functions in adaptation to similar environments.

evulsion (e-vul′shun) forcible extraction.

ex- word element [L.], *away from; without; outside;* sometimes used to denote *completely.*

ex(o)- word element [Gr.], *outside of; outward.*

exa- word element used in naming units of measurement to designate a quantity 10^{18} (a quintillion, or million million million) times the unit to which it is joined. Symbol E.

exacerbation (eg-zas″er-ba′shun) increase in severity of a disease or any of its symptoms.

examination (eg-zam″ĭ-na′shun) inspection or investigation, especially as a means of diagnosing disease.

breast e. in the NURSING INTERVENTIONS CLASSIFICATION, a nursing INTERVENTION defined as inspection and palpation of the breasts and related areas.

mental status e. a standardized procedure to gather data to determine etiology,

diagnosis, prognosis, and treatment for patients with mental disorders.

pelvic e. physical assessment of the internal pelvic organs. It includes inspection with a speculum, a PAPANICOLAOU SMEAR, bimanual palpation, and a rectovaginal examination.

physical e. examination of the bodily state of a patient by ordinary physical means, as inspection, palpation, percussion, and auscultation.

postmortem e. autopsy.

exanthem (eg-zan′them) 1. a skin eruption or rash. 2. a disease in which skin eruptions or rashes are a prominent manifestation.

e. su′bitum roseola infantum.

exanthema (eg″zan-the′mah), pl. *exanthemas, exanthem′ata* [Gr.] exanthem.

exanthematous (eg″zan-them′ah-tus) characterized by or of the nature of an eruption or rash.

exarticulation (eks″ar-tik″u-la′shun) disarticulation.

excavation (eks″kah-va′shun) 1. the act of hollowing out. 2. a hollowed-out space, or pouchlike cavity.

atrophic e. cupping of the optic disk, due to atrophy of the optic nerve fibers.

e. of optic disk, physiologic e. a normally occurring depression in the center of the optic disk.

rectouterine e. Douglas' cul-de-sac.

rectovesical e. the space between the rectum and bladder in the peritoneal cavity of the male.

vesicouterine e. the space between the bladder and uterus in the peritoneal cavity of the female.

excavator (eks′kah-va″ter) a scoop or gouge for surgical use.

excerebration (ek″ser-ĕ-bra′shun) removal of the brain.

excess (ek′ses) an amount more than is normal or necessary.

fluid volume e. excess fluid volume.

exchange (eks-chānj′) 1. the substitution of one thing for another. 2. to substitute one thing for another.

gas e. the passage of oxygen and carbon dioxide in opposite directions across the alveolocapillary MEMBRANE.

health care information e. in the NURSING INTERVENTIONS CLASSIFICATION, a nursing INTERVENTION defined as providing patient care information to health professionals in other agencies.

impaired gas e. a NURSING DIAGNOSIS approved by the North American Nursing Diagnosis Association, defined as excess or deficit in oxygenation and/or carbon dioxide elimination at the alveolocapillary MEMBRANE (see gas EXCHANGE). Etiological and contributing factors include an altered oxygen supply, changes in the alveolar-capillary membrane, altered blood flow, and altered oxygen-carrying capacity of the blood. Defining characteristics include changes in mental status such as confusion, somnolence, restlessness, and irritability; ineffective coughing and inability to move secretions from the air passages; hypercapnia; and hypoxia. For specific medical treatments and nursing interventions, see AIRWAY CLEARANCE, INEFFECTIVE; breathing PATTERNS, ineffective; CHRONIC AIRFLOW LIMITATION; and ANEMIA.

plasma e. see PLASMA EXCHANGE.

excipient (ek-sip′e-ent) any more or less inert substance added to a drug to give it suitable consistency or form; called also vehicle.

excise (ek-sīz′) to remove by cutting.

excision (ek-sizh′un) removal, as of an organ, by cutting; called also resection.

excitability (ek-sīt″ah-bil′ĭ-te) irritability.

excitant (ek-sīt′ant) stimulant.

excitation (ek″si-ta′shun) an act of irritation or stimulation; a condition of being excited or of responding to a stimulus; the addition of energy, as the excitation of a molecule by absorption of photons.

anomalous atrioventricular e. Wolff-Parkinson-White syndrome.

indirect e. electrostimulation of a muscle by placing the electrode on its nerve.

excitement (ek-sīt′ment) response to stimuli, often used specifically to denote excessive responsiveness to stimuli, particularly of an emotional nature, and often leading to impulsive activity.

psychomotor e. psychomotor acceleration.

excitomotor (ek-si″to-mo′tor) tending to produce motion or motor function; an agent that so acts.

excitosecretory (ek-si″to-se-kre′to-re) producing increased secretion.

excitovascular (ek-si″to-vas′ku-ler) stimulating the circulatory system.

exclave (eks′klāv) a detached part of an organ.

exclusion (ek-skloo′zhun) a shutting out or elimination; surgical isolation of a part, as of a segment of intestine, without removal from the body.

excoriation (ek″sko-re-a′shun) a scratch or abrasion of the skin.

excrement (ek′skrĕ-ment) 1. feces. 2. excretion (def. 2).

excrementitious (ek″skrĕ-men-tish′us) 1. pertaining to excrement. 2. fecal.

excrescence (ek-skres′ens) an abnormal outgrowth; a projection related to a disease or pathologic condition. adj., **excres′cent.**

excreta (ek-skre′tah) excretion (def. 2).

excrete (ek-skrēt′) to throw off or eliminate, as waste matter, by a normal discharge. Called also void.

excretion (ek-skre′shun) 1. the act, process, or function of excreting. Ordinarily, what is meant by excretion is DEFECATION, the evacuation of feces. Technically, excretion can refer to the expulsion of any matter, whether from a single cell or from the entire body, or to the matter excreted. 2. waste material eliminated from the body, including FECES, URINE, and SWEAT. Mucus and carbon dioxide also can be considered excretions. The organs of excretion are the intestinal tract, kidneys, lungs, and skin. Called also excreta. adj., **ex′cretory.**

excursion (ek-skur′zhun) a range of movement regularly repeated in performance of a function, e.g., excursion of the jaws in mastication. adj., **excur′sive.**

lateral e. sideward movement of the mandible between the position of closure and the position in which cusps of opposing teeth are in vertical proximity.

excystation (ek″sis-ta′shun) escape from a cyst or envelope, as in that stage in the life cycle of parasites occurring after the cystic form has been swallowed by the host.

exemestane (ek″sĕ-mes′tān) an AROMATASE inactivator structurally related to ANDROSTENEDIONE; used as an ANTINEOPLASTIC in the treatment of advanced breast carcinoma in postmenpausal women, administered orally.

exenteration (ek-sen″ter-a′shun) 1. surgical removal of the inner organs; evisceration. 2. in ophthalmology, removal of the entire contents of the orbit.

pelvic e. excision of the organs and adjacent structures of the pelvis.

exercise (ek′ser-sīz) performance of physical exertion for improvement of health or correction of physical deformity.

active e. motion imparted to a part by voluntary contraction and relaxation of its controlling muscles.

active assistive e. voluntary contraction of muscles controlling a part, assisted by a therapist or by some other means.

aerobic e. a type of physical activity that increases the heart rate and promotes increased use of oxygen in order to improve the overall body condition.

ballistic stretching e's rapid, jerky movements employed in exercises to stretch muscles and connective tissue.

Buerger-Allen e's see BUERGER-ALLEN EXERCISES.

cardiovascular e. exercises to promote improved capacity of the cardiovascular system. They must be administered at least twice weekly, with most programs conducted three to five or more times weekly. The contraction of major muscle groups must be repeated often enough to elevate the heart rate to a target level determined during testing. Used in the treatment of compromised cardiovascular systems, as in cardiac rehabilitation, or as a preventive measure.

corrective e. therapeutic exercise.

endurance e. any exercise that involves the use of several large groups of muscles and is thus dependent on the delivery of oxygen to the muscles by the cardiovascular system; used in both physical fitness programs and testing of cardiovascular and pulmonary function.

isokinetic e. dynamic muscle activity performed at a constant angular velocity.

isometric e. active exercise performed against stable resistance, without change in the length of the muscle.

isotonic e. active exercise without appreciable change in the force of muscular contraction, with shortening of the muscle.

Kegel e's see KEGEL EXERCISES.

McKenzie e. an exercise regimen used in the treatment of low back pain and sciatica, prescribed according to findings during mechanical examination of the lumbar spine and using a combination of lumbar motions, including flexion, rotation, side gliding, and extension. It is sometimes referred to as *McKenzie extension exercises,* but this is a misnomer because the regimen involves movements other than extension.

muscle-setting e. voluntary contraction and relaxation of skeletal muscles without changing the muscle length or moving the associated part of the body. Called also static exercise.

passive e. motion imparted to a segment of the body by another individual, machine, or other outside force, or produced by voluntary effort of another segment of the patient's own body.

pelvic floor e's 1. a combination of endurance and strength exercises of the pelvic floor (circumvaginal or perianal) muscles, used in the management of stress urinary incontinence; the patient is taught to isolate and contract muscles once or twice a day. 2. in the NURSING INTERVENTIONS CLASSIFICATION, a nursing INTERVENTION defined as pelvic muscle exercise strengthening and training of the levator ani and urogenital muscles through voluntary,

repetitive contraction to decrease stress, urge, or mixed types of urinary INCONTINENCE.

quadriceps setting e. an isometric exercise to strengthen muscles needed for ambulation. The patient is instructed to contract the quadriceps muscle while at the same time elevating the heel and pushing the knee toward the mat.

range of motion (ROM) e's exercises that move each joint through its full RANGE OF MOTION, that is, to the highest degree of motion of which each joint normally is capable; they may be either active or passive. See accompanying figure.

resistance e's, resistive e's activities designed to increase muscle strength, performed against an opposing force; the resistance may be either isometric, isotonic, or isokinetic.

static e. muscle-setting exercise.

static stretching e's the placement of muscles and connective tissues at their greatest length by steady force in the direction of lengthening. Short duration forces can be obtained manually, but special traction devices, splints, and casts are generally used to apply low-intensity forces for prolonged periods (30 minutes or longer). Warming the soft tissue before or during stretching will generally facilitate lengthening.

e. stress tests tests used in EXERCISE TESTING.

e. testing a technique for evaluating circulatory response to physical stress; it involves continuous electrocardiographic monitoring during physical exercise, the objective being to increase the intensity of physical exertion until a target heart rate is reached or signs and symptoms of cardiac ischemia appear. Called also stress testing.

Clinical exercise testing has become an important tool in screening for and diagnosing early ischemic heart disease that cannot be detected by a standard resting EKG, and in predicting the probability of the development of the condition in later years. The technique cannot determine the location of the lesion causing cardiac ischemia and therefore must be supplemented with angiocardiography when coronary occlusion is detected.

Common forms of exercise used include the treadmill and the bicycle ERGOMETER. These procedures must be performed in a clinical setting where health care personnel are available in the event symptoms develop during exercise, such as dyspnea,

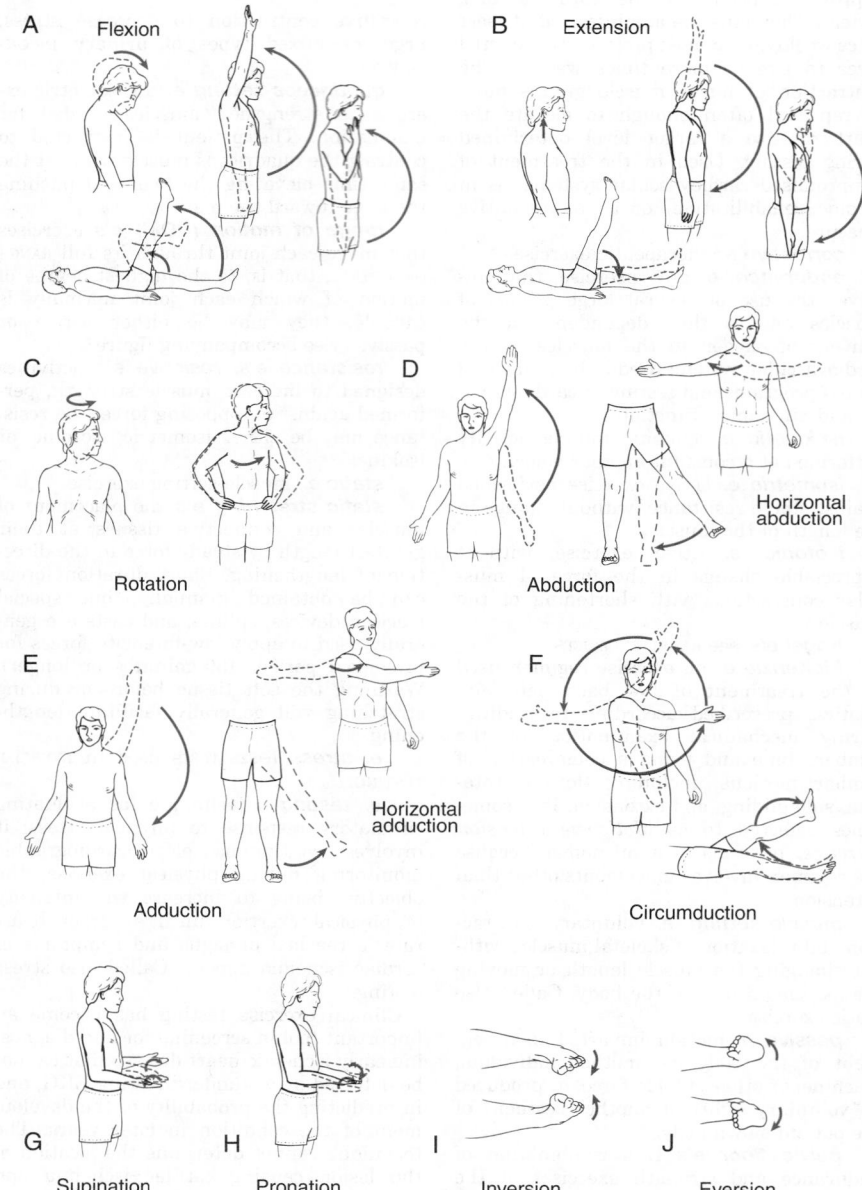

A, Flexion B, Extension C, Rotation D, Abduction, Horizontal abduction E, Adduction, Horizontal adduction F, Circumduction G, Supination H, Pronation I, Inversion J, Eversion

Examples of range of motion exercises. *A*, Flexion: The bending of a joint. *B*, Extension: A movement opposite to flexion in which a joint is in a straight position. *C*, Rotation: Pivoting a body part around its axis, as in shaking the head. *D*, Abduction: A movement of a limb away from the median plane of the body; the fingers are abducted by spreading them apart. *E*, Adduction: Moving toward the midline of the body or to the central axis of a limb. *F*, Circumduction: A combination of movements that cause a body part to move in a circular fashion. *G*, Supination: Extension of the forearm to bring the palm of the hand upward. *H*, Pronation: Movement of the forearm in the extended position that brings the palm of the hand to a downward position. *I*, Inversion: Movement of the ankle to turn the sole of the foot medially. *J*, Eversion: Movement of the sole of the foot laterally. From Lammon et al., 1995.

vertigo, extreme fatigue, severe arrhythmias, or other abnormal EKG readings.

Exercise testing also may be used to assess the pulmonary status of a patient with a respiratory disease. As the patient performs specific exercises, blood samples are drawn for BLOOD GAS ANALYSIS, and ventilatory function tests such as tidal volume, total lung capacity, and vital capacity are conducted.

therapeutic e. the scientific use of bodily movement to restore normal function in diseased or injured tissues or to maintain a state of well-being; called also corrective exercise. As with any type of therapy, a therapeutic exercise program is designed to correct specific disabilities of the individual patient. The program is evaluated periodically and modified as indicated by the patient's progress and response to the prescribed regimen. Exercises affect the body locally and systemically and bring about changes in the nervous, circulatory, and endocrine systems as well as the musculoskeletal system.

Among the types of therapeutic exercise are those that (1) increase or maintain mobility of the joints and surrounding soft tissues, (2) develop coordination through control of individual muscles, (3) increase muscular strength and endurance, and (4) promote relaxation and relief of tension.

Joint Mobility. In the absence of a disability that prohibits mobility, the regular day-to-day activities of living maintain the normal movements of the joints. If, however, motion is restricted for any reason, the soft tissues become dense and hard and adaptive shortening of the connective tissues takes place. These changes begin to develop within four days after a joint has been immobilized and are evident even in a normal joint that has been rendered immobile. It is for this reason that therapeutic exercises to prevent loss of joint motion are so important and should be begun as soon as possible after an injury has occurred or a disease process has begun.

Prevention of the loss of joint motion is much less costly and time-consuming than correction of tissue changes that seriously impair joint mobility. It is recommended that each joint should be put through its full range of motion three times at least twice daily. If the patient is not able to carry out these exercises, he is assisted by a therapist or member of the family who has been instructed in the exercises. Inflammation of the joint, as in arthritis, may cause some pain on motion, and so passive exercises are done slowly and gently with the joint as relaxed as possible. Procedures that stretch tight muscles to increase joint motion should be done only by a skilled therapist who understands the hazards of fracture and bleeding within the joint, which can occur if the exercises are done improperly or too strenuously.

Muscle Training. Exercises of this type are taught to the patient who has lost some control over a major skeletal muscle. By learning precise and conscious control over a specific muscle, the patient is able to strengthen and coordinate its movement with normal motor patterns and thus enhance mobility. Muscle training or neuromuscular re-education demands full cooperation of the patient, who must be capable of understanding the purpose of the exercises, following directions, and giving full attention to the muscle isolated for retraining. The sessions are held in a quiet, comfortable atmosphere to facilitate concentration by the patient.

The development of conscious control over individual muscles is useful in the rehabilitation of patients with a variety of disorders, including physical trauma, diseases such as poliomyelitis that affect the motor neurons, and congenital disorders such as cerebral palsy. It involves a systematic program of sequential activities under the direction of a therapist knowledgeable in the technique. Although it requires much effort on the part of the patient and the therapist, the attainment of muscle control and coordination is a satisfying reward.

Muscle Strength and Endurance. Improvement of muscle strength and endurance is particularly important in the rehabilitation of patients whose goal is to return to an active and productive life after a debilitating illness or disabling injury. The exercises are prescribed according to the individual needs of the patient and usually involve more than one group of muscles.

Strengthening (force increasing) exercises are prescribed after an examination has shown weakness in individual muscles or muscle groups. These exercises are usually administered with relatively high resistance and few (3 to 10) repetitions. A group of exercises, called a *set,* is followed by a few minutes of rest. Three to 5 sets for a muscle or group constitute one bout of exercises. Strengthening exercises are often performed daily in early stages of rehabilitation, but less often later in treatment.

Endurance exercises stimulate changes in the involved muscle or muscles, resulting in improved capacity for repeated contraction (e.g., increased ability to use metabolites). When conducted over a sufficient length of time and with several muscle groups, they may also produce central effects of the cardiovascular system (see cardiovascular exercise). Endurance exercises employ relatively low resistance and numerous (15 or more) repetitions. Endurance exercises are generally administered daily.

Relief of Tension. Exercises that promote relaxation of the muscles and provide relief from the effects of tension are useful in a wide variety of disorders ranging from mild tension headache to insomnia. Patients who are especially tense may require several sessions of instruction in relaxation before they can learn the technique.

Williams' e's, Williams' flexion e's a therapeutic exercise regimen used in the treatment of low back pain; it seeks to reduce lumbar lordosis through flexion of the lumbar spine and strengthening of the abdominal musculature.

exergonic (ek″ser-gon′ik) accompanied by the release of free energy.

exflagellation (eks-flaj″ĕ-la′shun) the protrusion or formation of flagelliform MICRO-GAMETES from a MICROGAMETOCYTE in malarial parasites and some related sporozoa.

exfoliatin (eks-fo″le-a′tin) an erythrogenic epidermolytic, heat-stable, acid-labile EXO-TOXIN produced by certain strains of *Staphylococcus aureus* (phage group II), which causes intraepidermal separation by disturbing the adhesive forces between cells in the stratum granulosum to give rise to the clinical manifestations of STAPHYLOCOCCAL SCALDED SKIN SYNDROME. Called also epidermolysin.

exfoliation (eks-fo″le-a′shun) 1. a falling off in scales or layers. 2. the normal loss of primary teeth after loss of their root structure. adj., **exfo′liative.**

lamellar e. of newborn a congenital hereditary disorder in which the infant is born covered with a collodionlike or parchmentlike membrane that peels off within 24 hours, after which there may be complete healing, or the scales may reform and the process may be repeated. In the more severe form, the infant (harlequin FETUS) is covered with thick, horny, armorlike scales and usually either is stillborn or dies shortly after birth. Called also ichthyosis congenita and lamellar ichthyosis of newborn.

exhalation (eks″hah-la′shun) 1. the giving off of watery or other vapor, or of an effluvium. 2. a vapor or other substance exhaled or given off. 3. the act of breathing out; called also expiration and halitus.

exhaustion (eg-zaws′chun) 1. a state of extreme mental or physical fatigue. 2. the state of being drained, emptied, consumed, or used up.

heat e. see HEAT EXHAUSTION.

exhibitionism (ek″sī-bish′un-izm) a paraphilia characterized by repeated acts of exposing the genitals to an unsuspecting stranger to achieve sexual excitement, with no attempt at further sexual activity with the stranger. It occurs almost exclusively in males, and in adults it is difficult to correct. It may be resorted to by an individual who is unable for physical or psychologic reasons to gain sexual gratification by normal means. A common cause is a feeling of sexual inadequacy; for this the exposure is a compensation. Exhibitionism may also be a form of masochism in which a feeling of guilt drives the person to behavior for which he knows he will be punished. Psychotherapy is necessary to deal with this type of sexual deviation.

exhibitionist (ek″sī-bish′un-ist) a person who indulges in exhibitionism.

Exna (eks′nah) trademark for a preparation of BENZTHIAZIDE, an ANTIHYPERTENSIVE.

exocardia (ek″so-kahr′de-ah) congenital displacement of the heart; ectocardia.

exocolitis (ek″so-ko-li′tis) inflammation of the outer coat of the colon.

exocrine (ek′so-krin) 1. secreting externally via a duct. 2. denoting such a gland or its secretion.

exocytosis (ek″so-si-to′sis) 1. the discharge from a cell of particles that are too large to diffuse through the wall; the opposite of endocytosis. 2. the aggregation of migrating LEUKOCYTES in the epidermis as part of the inflammatory RESPONSE.

exodeviation (ek″so-de″ve-a′shun) a turning outward; in ophthalmology, exotropia.

exoenzyme (ek″so-en′zīm) an enzyme that acts outside the cell that secretes it.

exoerythrocytic (ek″so-ĕ-rith″ro-sit′ik) occurring or situated outside the red blood cells (erythrocytes), a term applied to a stage in the development of malarial parasites that takes place in cells other than erythrocytes.

exogamy (ek-sog′ah-me) 1. protozoan fertilization by union of elements that are not derived from the same cell. 2. marriage outside a particular group.

exogenous (eks-oj′ĕ-nus) 1. developed or originating outside the organism, as exogenous disease. 2. growing by additions to the outside.

exomphalos (eks-om'fah-los) 1. hernia of the abdominal viscera into the umbilical cord. 2. UMBILICAL HERNIA.

exonuclease (ek″so-noo'kle-ās) an enzyme that cleaves single mononucleotides from the end of a polynucleotide chain.

exopeptidase (ek″so-pep'tĭ-dās) a proteolytic enzyme whose action is limited to terminal peptide linkages.

exophoria (ek″so-for'e-ah) heterophoria in which there is deviation of the visual axis of an eye away from that of the other eye in the absence of visual fusional stimuli. adj., **exopho′ric.**

exophthalmos (ek″sof-thal′mos) abnormal protrusion of the eye. adj., **exophthal′-mic.** It results in a marked stare and is usually due to HYPERTHYROIDISM. Occasionally the condition is caused by an infection of the eye or a tumor behind the eye.

exophthalmometry (ek″sof-thal-mom′ĕ-tre) measurement of the extent of protrusion of the eyeball in exophthalmos. adj., **exophthalmomet′ric.**

exophytic (ek″so-fit′ik) growing outward; in oncology, proliferating externally or on the surface epithelium of an organ or other structure in which the growth originated.

exorbitism (ek-sor′bĭ-tizm) protrusion of the eyeball.

exoserosis (ek″so-se-ro′sis) an oozing of serum or exudate.

exoskeleton (ek″so-skel′ĕ-ton) an external hard framework to the bodies of certain animals, derived from the ECTODERM, such as a crustacean's shell; it supports and protects the soft tissues. In vertebrates the term is sometimes applied to structures produced by the epidermis, such as hair, nails, hoofs, and teeth.

exosmosis (ek″sos-mo′sis) osmosis or diffusion from within outward.

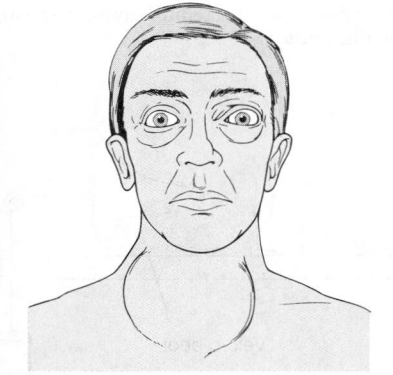

Exophthalmos and goiter in Graves' disease. From Frazier et al., 2000.

exostosis (ek″sos-to′sis) [Gr.] a benign new growth projecting from a bone surface and characteristically capped by cartilage. adj., **exostot′ic.**

    e. cartilagi′nea a variety of osteoma consisting of a layer of cartilage developing beneath the periosteum of a bone.

    hereditary multiple e. a generally benign, hereditary disorder of enchondral growth of bone, marked by exostoses near the extremities of the diaphysis of long bones.

Exosurf (ek′so-surf″) a commercially available synthetic surfactant preparation, which is used in the treatment of RESPIRATORY DISTRESS SYNDROME OF THE NEWBORN.

exothermal (ek″so-ther′m′l) exothermic.

exothermic (ek″so-ther′mik) marked or accompanied by the evolution of heat; liberating heat or energy.

exotoxin (ek′so-tok″sin) a potent toxin formed and excreted by the bacterial cell and found free in the surrounding medium; exotoxins are the most poisonous substances known. They are protein in nature and heat labile, and are detoxified with retention of antigenicity by treatment with formaldehyde. Bacteria of the genus *Clostridium* are the most frequent producers of exotoxins; DIPHTHERIA, BOTULISM, and TETANUS are all caused by such toxins. adj., **ex′otoxic.**

exotropia (ek″so-tro′pe-ah) STRABISMUS in which there is permanent deviation of the visual axis of one eye away from that of the other, resulting in DIPLOPIA; called also walleye and divergent strabismus. adj., **exotro′pic.**

expander (ek-span′der) extender.

    plasma volume e. artificial plasma extender.

expectancy (ek-spek′tan-se) the expected value or probability of occurrence for a specific event.

    life e. the number of years, based on statistical averages, that a given person of a specific age, class, or other demographic variable may be expected to continue living.

expectorant (ek-spek′to-rant) 1. promoting EXPECTORATION. 2. an agent that so acts.

    liquefying e. an expectorant that promotes the ejection of mucus from the respiratory tract by decreasing its viscosity.

expectoration (ek-spek″to-ra′shun) 1. the coughing up and spitting out of material from the lungs, bronchi, and trachea. 2. sputum.

experiment (ek-sper′ĭ-ment) a procedure done in order to discover or demonstrate some fact or general truth. adj., **experimen′tal.**

E

control e. one made under standard conditions, to test the correctness of other observations.

expirate (eks'pĭ-rāt) exhaled air or gas.

single e. the gas exhaled at a single breath.

expiration (ek″spĭ-ra'shun) 1. exhalation (def. 3). 2. termination, or death. 3. a time after which a medication or agent has lost its potency. adj., **expi'ratory.**

expire (ek-spīr') 1. to exhale. 2. to die. 3. to be no longer useful because of deterioration, such as a medication.

explant 1. (eks-plant') to take from the body and place in an artificial medium for growth. 2. (eks'plant) tissue taken from the body and grown in an artificial medium.

explantation (ex-plan-ta'shun) the removal of an IMPLANT.

exploration (eks″plo-ra'shun) investigation or examination for diagnostic purposes. adj., **explo'ratory.**

exposure (eks-po'zhur) 1. the act of laying open, as surgical exposure. 2. the condition of being subjected to something, as to infectious agents or extremes of weather or radiation, which may have a harmful effect. 3. in radiology, a measure of the amount of ionizing radiation at the surface of the irradiated object, such as a person's body; calculated by multiplying milliamperage times exposure time in seconds, expressed in units of milliampere seconds (mAs). See also X-RAYS.

x-ray e. see EXPOSURE (def. 3).

expression (eks-presh'un) 1. the aspect or appearance of the face as determined by the physical or emotional state. 2. the act of squeezing out or evacuating by pressure. 3. gene expression.

gene e. 1. the flow of genetic information from gene to protein. 2. the process, or the regulation of the process, by which the effects of a gene are manifested. 3. the manifestation of a heritable trait in an individual carrying the gene or genes that determine it.

expressivity (eks″pres-iv'ĭ-te) the extent to which a heritable trait is manifested by an individual carrying the principal gene or genes that determine it.

expulsive (eks-pul'siv) driving or forcing out; tending to expel.

exsanguination (eks-sang″gwĭ-na'shun) extensive blood loss due to internal or external hemorrhage.

exsiccation (ek″sĭ-ka'shun) the act of drying out; in chemistry, the deprival of a crystalline substance of its water of crystallization.

exstrophy (ek'stro-fe) the turning inside out of an organ, such as the urinary BLADDER.

e. of the bladder congenital absence of a portion of the abdominal wall and bladder wall, the bladder appearing to be turned inside out, with the internal surface of its posterior wall showing through the opening in the anterior wall.

e. of cloaca, cloacal e. a developmental anomaly in which two segments of bladder (HEMIBLADDERS) are separated by an area of intestine with a mucosal surface, resembling a large red tumor in the midline of the lower abdomen.

ext. external; extract.

extended endocardial resection procedure (EERP) surgical removal of all visible endocardial fibrosis around the base of a left ventricular aneurysm; done to relieve ventricular tachycardia in patients with ischemic heart disease in whom intraoperative cardiac mapping is not possible.

extended-release (ek-stend'ed-re-lēs') allowing a twofold or greater reduction in frequency of administration of a drug in comparison with the frequency required by a conventional dosage form.

extender (ek-sten'der) something that enlarges or prolongs; called also expander.

artificial plasma e., plasma volume e. a substance that can be transfused to maintain fluid volume of the blood in event of great necessity, supplemental to the use of whole blood and plasma. Called also plasma volume expander.

extension (ek-sten'shun) 1. the movement by which the two ends of any jointed part are drawn away from each other. 2. a movement bringing the members of a limb into or toward a straight condition.

Buck's e. a temporary type of lightweight traction applied to the distal end of a fractured lower limb; the foot of the bed is raised so that the body makes counterextension; often used to reduce muscle spasm. (See illustration.)

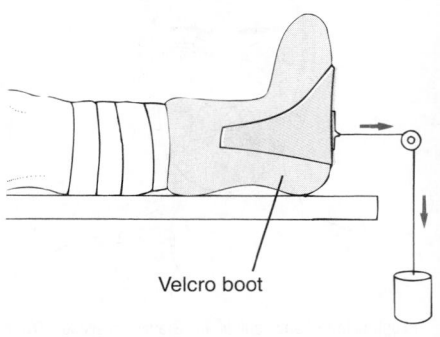

Velcro boot

Buck's extension.

nail e. extension exerted on the distal fragment of a fractured bone by means of a nail or pin driven into the fragment.

extensor (ek-sten′ser) [L.] 1. causing EXTENSION. 2. a muscle that extends a joint; see MUSCLE.

exteriorize (eks-te′re-er-īz) 1. to form a correct mental reference of the image of an object seen. 2. in psychiatry, to turn one's interest outward. 3. to transpose an internal organ to the exterior of the body.

extern (eks′tern) 1. a medical student or graduate in medicine who assists in patient care in the hospital but does not reside there. 2. a student nurse employed by an institution to provide care and develop clinical skills outside of the hours spent in school.

external (eks-ter′nal) situated or occurring on the outside. In anatomy, situated toward or near the outside. See also LATERAL.

externalization (eks-ter″nal-ĭ-za′shun) 1. the tendency to perceive in the external world and in external objects components of one's own personality, including instinctual impulses, conflicts, moods, attitudes, and ways of thinking. 2. the process of learning the difference between self and non-self in childhood. 3. the process by which external rather than internal stimuli become capable of arousing a drive, such as hunger.

externus (ek-ster′nus) external; in anatomy, denoting a structure farther from the center of an organ or cavity.

exteroception (ek″ster-o-sep′shun) the perception of stimuli originating outside or at a distance from the body.

exteroceptor (ek″ster-o-sep′tor) a sensory nerve ending stimulated by the immediate external environment, such as those in the skin and mucous membranes. adj., **exteroceptive.**

exterofective (ek″ster-o-fek′tiv) responding to external stimuli; a term applied to the cerebrospinal nervous system.

extima (ek′stĭ-mah) outermost; the outermost coat of a blood vessel; the adventitia.

extinction (eks-ting′shun) in psychology, the disappearance of a CONDITIONED RESPONSE as a result of its not being reinforced; also, the process by which the disappearance is accomplished. See also CONDITIONING.

extirpation (ek″ster-pa′shun) complete removal or eradication of an organ or tissue.

extorsion (eks-tor′shun) tilting of the upper part of the vertical meridian of the eye away from the midline of the face.

extortor (eks-tor′ter) an extraocular muscle that produces EXTORSION, such as the inferior oblique or the inferior rectus muscle.

extra- word element [L.], *outside; beyond the scope of; in addition.*

extra-anatomic (eks″trah-an″ah-tom′ik) not following the normal anatomic path; said of certain arterial bypass procedures.

extra-articular (ek″strah-ahr-tik′u-ler) situated or occurring outside a joint.

extracapsular (ek″strah-kap′su-ler) situated or occurring outside a capsule.

extracellular (ek″strah-sel′u-ler) situated or occurring outside a cell or cells.

extracorporeal (ek″strah-kor-por′e-al) located or occurring outside the body.

extracorticospinal (ek″strah-kor″tĭ-ko-spi′nal) outside the corticospinal tract.

extract (ek′strakt) a concentrated preparation of a vegetable or animal drug.

    allergenic e. an extract of allergenic components from a crude preparation of an allergen, such as weed, grass, or tree pollen, molds, house dust, or animal dander, used for diagnostic skin testing or for IMMUNOTHERAPY for allergy.

    cell-free e. the solution obtained by rupturing cells and removing all particulate matter.

extraction (ek-strak′shun) 1. the process or act of pulling or drawing out. 2. the preparation of an EXTRACT.

    breech e. extraction of an infant from the uterus in cases of breech presentation.

    flap e. removal of a cataract by making a flap in the cornea.

    menstrual e. a form of induced ABORTION in which a flexible cannula is inserted through an undilated cervix for the purpose of removing the fertilized embryo and endometrium. The cannula is attached to a syringe, which is used to aspirate the uterine contents and induce the onset of the "missed period." This technique is not always effective, and sometimes a second procedure is required. It should be done within two weeks of a missed menstrual period.

    serial e. the selective extraction of primary teeth during an extended period of time to allow autonomous adjustment.

    tooth e. forcible removal of a tooth; called also odontectomy.

    vacuum e. removal of the uterine contents by application of a vacuum, done either for delivery of a viable fetus or for an ABORTION.

extractive (ek-strak′tiv) any substance present in an organized tissue, or in a mixture in a small quantity, and requiring extraction by a special method.

extractor (ek-strak′ter) an instrument for pulling out a body part, foreign body, or calculus.

    basket e. a device for removal of calculi from the upper urinary tract, consisting of a network of filaments on a catheter that is passed into the ureter through a ureteroscope; the filaments surround the calculus and snare it so that it is withdrawn when the catheter is withdrawn.

vacuum e. a device to assist delivery consisting of a metal traction cup that is attached to the fetus' head; negative pressure is applied and traction is made on a chain passed through the suction tube.

extradural (ek″strah-du′ral) situated or occurring outside the dura mater.

extraembryonic (ek″strah-em″bre-on′ik) external to the embryo proper, as the extraembryonic coelom or the extraembryonic membranes.

extramastoiditis (ek″strah-mas″toi-di′tis) inflammation of tissues adjoining the mastoid PROCESS.

extramural (eks″trah-mu′ral) situated or occurring outside the wall of an organ or structure.

extraosseous (eks″trah-os′e-us) occurring outside a bone or bones.

extraplacental (eks″trah-plah-sen′t'l) independent of the placenta.

extrapolation (ek-strap″o-la′shun) inference of one or more unknown values on the basis of that which is known or has been observed; usually applied to estimation beyond the upper and lower ranges of observed data as opposed to INTERPOLATION between data points.

extrapsychic (eks″trah-si′kik) occurring outside the mind; taking place between the mind and the external environment.

extrapulmonary (eks″trah-pul′mo-nar″e) not connected with the lungs.

extrapyramidal (eks″trah-pī-ram′ĭ-d'l) outside the pyramidal tracts.

e. disease, e. syndrome any of a group of clinical disorders marked by abnormal involuntary movements, alterations in muscle tone, and postural disturbances; the group includes PARKINSONISM, CHOREA, ATHETOSIS, and others.

e. system a functional, rather than anatomical, unit comprising the nuclei and fibers (excluding those of the pyramidal tract) involved in motor activities; they control and coordinate especially the postural, static, supporting, and locomotor mechanisms. It includes the corpus striatum, subthalamic nucleus, substantia nigra, and red nucleus, along with their interconnections with the reticular formation, cerebellum, and cerebrum; some authorities include the cerebellum and vestibular nuclei. Called also extrapyramidal tract.

extrasystole (ek″strah-sis′to-le) a premature cardiac contraction that is independent of the normal rhythm and arises in response to an impulse outside the sinoatrial node.

atrial e. one in which the stimulus is thought to arise in the atrium elsewhere than at the sinoatrial node.

atrioventricular e. one in which the stimulus is thought to arise in the atrioventricular node.

interpolated e. a contraction taking place between two normal heartbeats.

nodal e. atrioventricular extrasystole.

retrograde e. a premature ventricular contraction followed by a premature atrial contraction, due to transmission of the stimulus backward, usually over the bundle of His.

ventricular e. one in which either a pacemaker or a re-entry site is in the ventricular structure.

extratubal (ek″strah-too′b'l) outside a tube.

extrauterine (ek″strah-u′ter-in) situated or occurring outside the uterus.

extravasation (eks-trav″ah-za′shun) 1. a discharge or escape, as of blood, from a vessel into the tissues. 2. the inadvertent administration of a vesicant into the tissues; the intensity of the irritating action is so severe that plasma escapes from the extracellular space and blisters are formed. Large extravasations of some medications may lead to contractures, with the need for débridement and grafting and in severe cases amputation. This term must be distinguished from intravenous INFILTRATION and FLARE. 3. blood or another substance so discharged.

extravascular (ek″strah-vas′ku-ler) situated or occurring outside a vessel or the vessels.

extraversion (ek″strah-ver′zhun) extroversion.

extravert (ek′strah-vert) extrovert.

extremitas (ek-strem′ĭ-tas), pl. *extremita′tes* [L.] extremity.

extremity (ek-strem′ĭ-te) 1. the distal or terminal portion of elongated or pointed structures. 2. limb.

extrinsic (ek-strin′sik) of external origin.

extroversion (eks″tro-ver′zhun) extraversion; 1. a turning inside out. 2. direction of one's energies and attention outward from the self.

extrovert (ek′stro-vert) 1. a person whose interest is turned outward. 2. to turn one's interest outward to the external world.

extrude (ek-strood′) 1. to force out, or to occupy a position distal to that normally occupied. 2. in dentistry, to occupy a position occlusal to that normally occupied.

extrusion (ek-stroo'zhun) 1. a pushing out. 2. in dentistry, the condition of a tooth pushed too far forward from the line of occlusion as a result of injury or of lack of opposing occlusal force.

extubation (eks"too-ba'shun) removal of a previously inserted tube, such as an endotracheal tube, catheter, drain, or feeding tube, from an organ, orifice, or other body structure. See also INTUBATION.

endotracheal e. in the NURSING INTERVENTIONS CLASSIFICATION, a nursing INTERVENTION defined as purposeful removal of the ENDOTRACHEAL TUBE from the nasopharynx or oropharyngeal airway.

exuberant (eg-zu'ber-ant) copious or excessive in production; showing excessive proliferation.

exudate (eks'u-dāt) a fluid with a high content of protein and cellular debris that has escaped from blood vessels and has been deposited in tissues or on tissue surfaces, usually as a result of inflammation.

exudation (eks"u-da'shun) 1. the escape of fluid, cells, or cellular debris from blood vessels and deposition in or on the tissue. 2. exudate.

exudative (eks-oo'dah-tiv) of or pertaining to a process of exudation.

exumbilication (eks"um-bil"ĭ-ka'shun) 1. marked protrusion of the navel. 2. umbilical hernia.

ex vivo (eks" ve'vo) outside the living body; denoting removal of an organ (e.g., the kidney) for reparative surgery, after which it is returned to the original site.

eye (i) the organ of VISION; see also Plates. In the embryo the eye develops as a direct extension of the brain, and thus is a very delicate organ. To protect the eye the bones of the skull are shaped so that an orbital cavity protects the dorsal aspect of each eyeball. In addition, the conjunctival sac covers the front of the eyeball and lines the upper and lower eyelids. Tears from the lacrimal duct constantly wash the eye to remove foreign objects, and the lids and eyelashes help protect the front of the eye.

Structure. The eyeball has three coats. The CORNEA is the clear transparent layer on the front of the eyeball; it is a continuation of the SCLERA (the white of the eye), the tough outer coat that helps protect the delicate mechanism of the eye. The CHOROID is the middle layer and contains blood vessels. The third layer, the RETINA, contains rods and cones, which are specialized cells that are sensitive to light. Behind the cornea and in front of the lens is the iris, the circular pigmented band around the pupil. The iris works much like the diaphragm in a camera, widening or narrowing the pupil to adjust to different light conditions.

Function. (See also VISION.) The refraction or bending of light rays so that they focus on the retina and can thus be transmitted to the optic nerve is accomplished by three structures: the aqueous humor, a watery substance between the cornea and lens; the lens, a crystalline structure just behind the iris; and the vitreous humor, a jelly-like substance filling the space between the lens and the retina. Unlike the lens of a camera, the lens of the eye focuses by a process called accommodation. This means that when the eye sees something in the distance, muscles pull the lens, stretching it until it is thin and almost flat, so that the light rays are only slightly bent as they pass through it. When the object is close, the muscles relax and the elastic lens becomes thicker, bending the light rays and focusing them on the retina.

Because the eye must function under many different circumstances, there are two types of nerve cells in the retina, with different shapes: the CONES and the RODS. They cover the full range of adaptation to light, the cones being sensitive in bright light, and the rods in dim light. The cones are responsible for color vision. There are three types of cones, each containing a substance that reacts to light of a different color, one set for red, one for green, and one for violet. These are the primary colors in light, which, when mixed together, give white. White light stimulates all three sets of color cells; any other color stimulates one or two.

The optic nerve, which transmits the nerve impulses from the retina to the visual center of the brain, contains nerve fibers from the many nerve cells in the retina. The small spot where it leaves the retina does not have any light-sensitive cells, and is called the blind spot.

The eyes are situated in the front of the head in such a way that human beings have stereoscopic vision, the ability to judge distances. Because the eyes are set apart, each eye sees farther around an object on its own side than does the other. The brain superimposes the two slightly different images and judges distances from the composite image.

Disorders of the Eye. If the eyeball is too short or too long, the lens focuses the image not on the retina but behind or in front of it. The former condition is called HYPEROPIA (or farsightedness) and the latter MYOPIA (or nearsightedness). An irregularity in the curvature of the cornea or lens can cause the impaired vision of ASTIGMATISM. STRABISMUS (or squint or crossed eyes) is usually caused by weakness in muscles that control movement of the eyeball. CONJUNCTIVITIS is an inflammation of the membrane that covers the front of the eyeball and lines the eyelids. When small pieces of the retina become detached from the underlying layers, the result is a retinal DETACHMENT; surgery may be necessary to prevent blindness. PRESBYOPIA (usually taking the form of hyperopia) occurs in older persons and develops as the lens loses its elasticity with the passing years. Correction is easily made with properly prescribed eyeglasses.

Foreign bodies in the eyes are common occurrences. Protective eyewear should be worn by individuals at risk. Cinders, grit, or other foreign bodies are best removed by lifting the eyelid by the lashes. The foreign body will usually remain on the surface of the lid, and can easily be removed. Particles embedded in the eyeball must be removed by a qualified health care professional.

Eyestrain is fatigue of the eyes caused by improper use, uncorrected defects in the vision, or an eye disorder. Symptoms may include aching or pains in the eyes, or a hot, scratchy feeling in the eyelids. Headache, blurring or dimness of vision, and sometimes dizziness or nausea may also occur.

artificial e. a glass or plastic prosthesis inserted in the eye socket to replace the eyeball; most are designed to be worn day and night. When patients become debilitated and unable to care for such a prosthesis, they must depend on members of the health care team to give proper care according to the chosen preferred routine.

Cleaning of a prosthetic eye is similar in principle to care of dentures; both are handled with care to avoid damage and are cleansed according to good hygienic principles. The prosthesis is removed while the patient is lying down so that it falls into the hand and is not likely to be dropped and broken. It is removed by depressing the lower eyelid, allowing the prosthesis to slide out and down. Mild soap and water are most often used for cleansing the prosthesis. Alcohol or other chemicals can damage prostheses made of plastic. If it is not replaced in the socket immediately after cleansing, it is stored in water or contact lens soaking solution. Insertion of the prosthesis is done by lifting the upper eyelid with the thumb or forefinger and placing its notched edge toward the nose. It is placed as far as possible under the upper lid and then the lower lid is depressed to allow it to slip into place. The process can be made easier by first moistening the prosthesis with

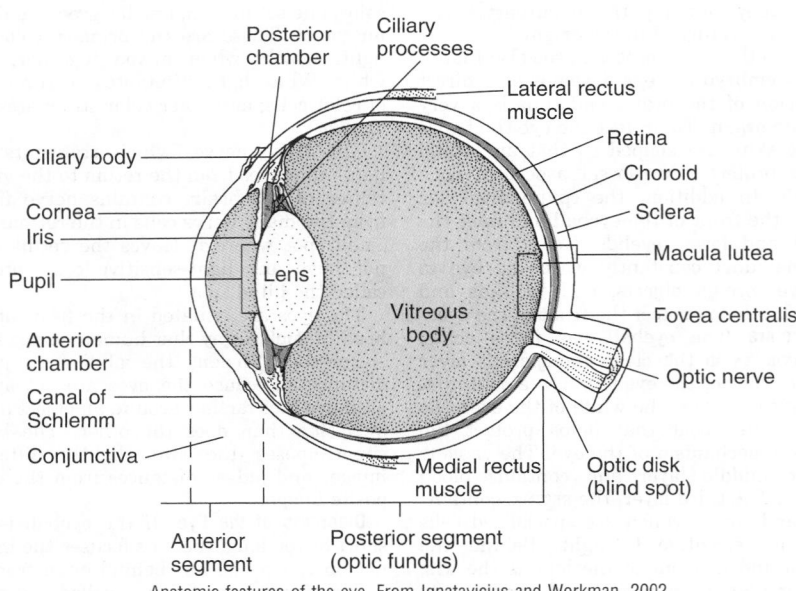

Anatomic features of the eye. From Ignatavicius and Workman, 2002.

water. If it is necessary to wipe the eye area of a patient wearing a prosthesis, one should gently wipe toward the nose in order not to dislodge the prosthesis.

cross e. esotropia.

dry e. keratoconjunctivitis sicca.

pink e. popular term for acute contagious conjunctivitis.

raccoon e's ecchymotic areas surrounding both eyes, suggestive of a basilar skull fracture.

wall e. exotropia.

eyeball (i'bawl) the ball or globe of the eye; called also bulbus oculi, bulb of eye, and globus.

eye bank an institution or agency whose primary purpose is to collect, prepare, and supply to ophthalmologists eye tissue for transplantation. Those institutions equipped with special laboratory facilities also conduct research and store eye tissue. The Eye Bank Association of America (EBAA) coordinates eye banks in the United States and establishes medical ethical standards for the various collecting and distributing agencies throughout the country. Individuals wishing to donate their eyes may make arrangements to do so prior to their death, or the legal next-of-kin may give permission for the donation at the time of death. At the present time, the demand for

usable eyes is far greater than the available supply. The address of a nearby eye bank, as well as other information about this service, can be obtained by writing to Eye Bank Association of America, 1015 18th St. NW, Suite 1010, Washington, DC 20036, or by consulting their website at http://www.restoresight.org.

eyebrow (i'brow) 1. supercilium; the transverse elevation at the junction of the forehead and the upper eyelid. 2. supercilia; the hairs growing on this elevation.

eyecup (i'kup) 1. a small vessel formerly used for application of cleansing or medicated solution to the exposed area of the eyeball. 2. excavation of optic disk.

eyeglasses (i'glasez) glasses.

eyeground (i'grownd) the fundus of the eye as seen with an ophthalmoscope.

eyelash (i'lash) cilium; one of the hairs growing on the edge of an eyelid.

eyelid (i'lid) either of two movable folds (upper and lower) protecting the anterior surface of the eyeball.

eyepiece (i'pēs) the lens or system of lenses of a MICROSCOPE (or telescope) nearest the user's eye, serving to further magnify the image produced by the objective. Called also ocular.

E

F

F Fahrenheit (SCALE); farad; fertility (PLASMID); visual field; fluorine; formula; French (SCALE).

F₁ first filial generation.

F₂ second filial generation.

°F degree Fahrenheit; see Fahrenheit SCALE.

f femto-.

FAAN Fellow, American Academy of Nursing.

FAB classification *(French-American-British)* a classification of acute LEUKEMIA produced by a three-nation joint collaboration; acute lymphoblastic LEUKEMIA is subdivided into three types and acute myelogenous LEUKEMIA is subdivided into eight types.

Fab [*f*ragment, *a*ntigen-*b*inding] originally, either of two identical fragments, each containing an antigen combining site, obtained by papain cleavage of the IgG molecule; now generally used as an adjective in terms such as Fab *fragment* or *region,* referring to an "arm" of any IMMUNOGLOBULIN monomer, i.e., one light CHAIN and the adjoining heavy CHAIN V_H and C_H1 domains.

   digoxin immune F. (ovine) a preparation of antigen-binding fragments derived

---

Acute leukemia: morphological classification
Acute Myeloid (AML)
M_0: minimally differentiated M_1: without maturation M_2: with maturation M_3: hypergranular promyelocytic M_4: myelomonocytic M_5: (a) monoblastic, (b) monocytic M_6: erythroleukemia M_7: megakaryoblastic Rare types (e.g. eosinophilic, natural killer)
Acute Lymphoblastic (ALL)
L_1: small, monomorphic L_2: large, heterogeneous L_3: Burkitt-cell type

French-American-British (FAB) classification of acute leukemias: the myeloid leukemias are divided into eight types (M_{0-7}) and the lymphoblastic leukemias into three (L_{1-3}). From Hoffbrand and Pettit, 2000.

---

from specific antidigoxin antibodies produced in sheep that have been immunized with digoxin coupled as a hapten to human serum albumin, used as an antidote to life-threatening DIGOXIN and DIGITOXIN overdose; administered intravenously.

fabella (fah-bel′ah), pl. *fabel′lae* [L.] a sesamoid fibrocartilage in the gastrocnemius muscle; see anatomic Table of Bones in the Appendices.

fabere sign (fah-bēr′) (from the movements necessary to elicit it: *f*lexion, *ab*duction, *e*xternal *r*otation, and *e*xtension) Patrick's test.

fabism (fa′bizm) favism.

Fabry's disease (syndrome) (fah′brēz) a SPHINGOLIPIDOSIS transmitted as an X-linked recessive trait, in which the glycolipid trihexosyl ceramide is deposited in various tissues, especially the kidneys; the deficient enzyme is α-galactosidase A. It is marked by purpuric skin lesions (angiokeratomas), central nervous system symptoms, and death due to progressive renal failure. Called also angiokeratoma corporis diffusum.

FAB test fluorescent antibody test.

face (fās) 1. the anterior, or ventral, aspect of the head from the forehead to the chin, inclusive. 2. any presenting aspect or surface. adj., **fa′cial.**

   f. lift popular name for RHYTIDECTOMY.

   moon f. the peculiar rounded face seen in various conditions, such as in Cushing's syndrome, or after administration of adrenal corticoids.

face-lift popular name for RHYTIDECTOMY.

facet (fas′et) a small, plane surface on a hard body, such as a bone.

facetectomy (fas″ĕ-tek′to-me) excision of the articular facet of a vertebra.

faci(o)- word element [L.], *face.*

facial (fa′shal) pertaining to or directed toward the face.

   f. nerve the seventh CRANIAL NERVE; its motor fibers supply the muscles of facial expression, a complex group of cutaneous muscles that move the eyebrows, skin of the forehead, corners of the mouth, and other parts of the face concerned with frowning, smiling, or any of the many other expressions of emotion. The sensory fibers of the facial nerve provide a sense of taste in the anterior two thirds of the tongue, and also supply the submaxillary, sublingual, and lacrimal glands for secretion. Irritation of the facial nerve can produce a paralysis known as BELL'S PALSY, which usually involves only one side of the face with a resulting distortion of facial expression such as inability to close the eye or part of the mouth on the affected side. See anatomic Table of Nerves in the Appendices.

facies (fa′she-ēz), pl. *fa′cies* [L.] 1. face. 2. a specific SURFACE of a body structure, part, or organ. 3. the EXPRESSION or appearance of the face.

   adenoid f. the dull expression with open mouth, in children with hypertrophy of the pharyngeal tonsils (ADENOIDS).

   f. hepa′tica a thin face with sunken eyeballs, sallow complexion, and yellow conjunctivae, characteristic of certain chronic liver disorders.

   f. hippocra′tica a drawn, pinched, and livid appearance indicative of approaching death.

   leonine f. a peculiar, deeply furrowed, lionlike appearance of the face seen in certain cases of advanced lepromatous leprosy and in other diseases associated with facial edema.

   Parkinson's f., parkinsonian f. a stolid masklike expression of the face, with infrequent blinking, which is pathognomonic of PARKINSON'S DISEASE.

facilitation (fah-sil″ĭ-ta′shun) 1. PROMOTION or ASSISTANCE. 2. the enabling of a process or leading of a group. 3. the increased excitability of a neuron after stimulation by a subthreshold presynaptic impulse; the resistance is diminished so that a second application of the stimulus evokes the reaction more easily.

   forgiveness f. in the NURSING INTERVENTIONS CLASSIFICATION, a nursing INTERVENTION defined as assisting an individual to forgive and/or experience forgiveness in relationship with self, others, and higher power.

   grief work f. in the NURSING INTERVENTIONS CLASSIFICATION, a nursing INTERVENTION defined as assistance with the resolution of a significant loss. See also GRIEF.

   grief work f., perinatal in the NURSING INTERVENTIONS CLASSIFICATION, a nursing INTERVENTION defined as assistance with the resolution of a perinatal loss.

   guilt work f. in the NURSING INTERVENTIONS CLASSIFICATION, a nursing INTERVENTION defined as helping another to cope with painful feelings of responsibility; actual or perceived.

   learning f. in the NURSING INTERVENTIONS CLASSIFICATION, a nursing INTERVENTION defined as promoting the ability to process and comprehend information.

   meditation f. in the NURSING INTERVENTIONS CLASSIFICATION, a nursing INTERVENTION defined as facilitating a person to alter his/her level of awareness by focusing specifically on an image or thought.

   pass f. in the NURSING INTERVENTIONS CLASSIFICATION, a nursing INTERVENTION defined as arranging a leave for a patient from a health care facility.

   proprioceptive neuromuscular f. **(PNF)** a neuromuscular treatment method for restoring movement and mobility using sensory inputs to direct motions in diagonal patterns; it emphasizes that movements must be specific and directed toward a goal.

   self-responsibility f. in the NURSING INTERVENTIONS CLASSIFICATION, a nursing INTERVENTION defined as encouraging a patient to assume more responsibility for his or her own behavior.

   spiritual growth f. in the NURSING INTERVENTIONS CLASSIFICATION, a nursing INTERVENTION defined as facilitation of growth in a patient's capacity to identify, connect with, and call upon the source of meaning, purpose, comfort, strength, and hope in his/her life.

   visitation f. in the NURSING INTERVENTIONS CLASSIFICATION, a nursing INTERVENTION defined as promoting beneficial visits by family and friends.

facilitative (fah-sil′ĭ-ta″tiv) in pharmacology, denoting a reaction arising as an indirect result of drug action, as development of an infection after the normal microflora has been altered by an antibiotic.

facility (fah-sil′ĭ-te) an agency or other site where an activity or process is carried out.

   independent living f's congregate housing.

   intermediate care f. **(ICF)** a health related facility designed to provide custodial care for individuals unable to care for themselves because of mental or physical infirmity; not considered by the government to be a medical facility, it can receive no reimbursement under Medicare, generally receiving the bulk of its financing under Medicaid. Federal regulations require that an ICF have a registered nurse as director of nursing and a licensed nurse on duty at least 8 hours a day; other staffing requirements vary from state to state.

   skilled nursing f. **(SNF)** a type of NURSING HOME recognized by the Medicare and Medicaid systems as meeting long term health care needs for individuals who have the potential to function independently after a limited period of care. A multidisciplinary team guides health care and rehabilitative services, including skilled nursing CARE.

faciobrachial (fa″she-o-bra′ke-al) pertaining to the face and arm.

faciocervical (fa″she-o-ser′vĭ-k'l) pertaining to the face and neck.

faciolingual (fa″she-o-ling′gwal) pertaining to the face and tongue.

facioplegia (fa″she-o-ple′jah) facial PARALYSIS. adj., **faciople′gic.**

facioscapulohumeral (fa″she-o-skap″u-lo-hu′mer-al) pertaining to the face, scapula, and arm.

FACNM Fellow of the American College of Nuclear Medicine.

FACOG Fellow of the American College of Obstetricians and Gynecologists.

FACP Fellow of the American College of Physicians.

FACS Fellow of the American College of Surgeons.

FACSM Fellow of the American College of Sports Medicine.

factitial (fak-tish′al) artificially produced; produced unintentionally.

factitious (fak-tish′us) artificial; not natural.

f. disorder a MENTAL DISORDER characterized by repeated, knowing simulation of physical or psychological symptoms for no apparent purpose other than obtaining treatment. Unlike MALINGERING there is no recognizable motive for feigning illness. It is subtyped on the basis of whether the predominant signs and symptoms are physical (MUNCHAUSEN SYNDROME), psychological, or both. See also GANSER SYNDROME.

f. disorder by proxy a form of FACTITIOUS DISORDER in which one person (usually a mother) intentionally fabricates or induces signs and symptoms of one or more physical (MUNCHAUSEN SYNDROME BY PROXY) or psychological disorders in another person under their care (usually a child) and subjects that person to needless and sometimes dangerous or disfiguring diagnostic procedures or treatment, without any external incentives for the behavior existing.

factor (fak′ter) an agent or element that contributes to the production of a result.

accelerator f. factor V, one of the COAGULATION FACTORS.

f. I see COAGULATION FACTORS.

f. II see COAGULATION FACTORS.

f. III see COAGULATION FACTORS.

f. IV see COAGULATION FACTORS.

f. V see COAGULATION FACTORS.

f. VI see COAGULATION FACTORS.

f. VII see COAGULATION FACTORS.

f. VIII see COAGULATION FACTORS.

f. IX see COAGULATION FACTORS.

f. X see COAGULATION FACTORS.

f. XI see COAGULATION FACTORS.

f. XII see COAGULATION FACTORS.

f. XIII see COAGULATION FACTORS.

angiogenesis f. a substance that causes the growth of new blood vessels, found in tissues with high metabolic requirements such as cancers and the retina. It is also released by hypoxic macrophages at the edges or outer surface of a wound and initiates revascularization in wound healing.

antihemophilic f. (AHF) 1. factor VIII, one of the COAGULATION FACTORS. 2. a preparation of factor VIII administered intravenously for the prevention or treatment of hemorrhage in patients with HEMOPHILIA A and the treatment of von Willebrand disease, hypofibrinogenemia, and coagulation factor XIII deficiency. Included are preparations derived from human plasma (antihemophilic factor, cryoprecipitated antihemophilic factor) or porcine plasma (antihemophilic factor [porcine]) and those produced by recombinant technology antihemophilic factor [recombinant]).

antihemophilic f. A factor VIII, one of the COAGULATION FACTORS.

antihemophilic f. B factor IX, one of the COAGULATION FACTORS.

antihemophilic f. C factor XI, one of the COAGULATION FACTORS.

antihemorrhagic f. vitamin K.

antinuclear f. (ANF) antinuclear antibody.

antirachitic f. vitamin D.

atrial natriuretic f. (ANF) a hormone produced in the cardiac atrium; an inhibitor of renin secretion and thus of the production of angiotensin, and a stimulator of aldosterone release. Its effect is increased excretion of water and sodium and a lowering of blood pressure.

f. B a COMPLEMENT component that participates in the alternative complement pathway.

blastogenic f. lymphocyte-transforming factor.

carative f's in the THEORY OF HUMAN CARING, a set of ten factors that offer a descriptive topology of interventions including (1) a humanistic-altruistic system of values; (2) faith-hope; (3) sensitivity to self and others; (4) a helping-trusting, human care relationship; (5) the expression of positive and negative feelings; (6) a creative problem-solving caring process; (7) transpersonal teaching and learning; (8) a supportive, protective, and/or corrective mental, physical, societal, and spiritual environment; (9) human needs assistance; and (10) existential-phenomenological-spiritual forces.

Christmas f. factor IX, one of the COAGULATION FACTORS.

citrovorum f. folinic acid.

clotting f's COAGULATION FACTORS.

C3 nephritic f. (C3 NeF) an autoantibody that stabilizes the alternative COMPLEMENT pathway C3 convertase, preventing its inactivation by FACTOR H, resulting in complete consumption of plasma C3; it is found in the serum of many patients with type II membranoproliferative GLOMERULONEPHRITIS.

coagulation f's see COAGULATION FACTORS.

colony-stimulating f. (CSF) any of a number of glycoproteins responsible for the proliferation, differentiation, and functional activation of hematopoietic progenitor cells; specific factors are named for the cell lines that they stimulate. Used to promote bone marrow proliferation in aplastic anemia, following cytotoxic chemotherapy, or following bone marrow TRANSPLANTATION. Types include granulocyte, granulocyte-macrophage, and macrophage colony-stimulating factors.

f. D a factor that when activated serves as a SERINE esterase in the alternative COMPLEMENT pathway.

decay accelerating f. (DAF) a protein of most blood as well as endothelial and epithelial cells, CD55 (see CD ANTIGEN); it protects the cell membranes from attack by autologous COMPLEMENT.

endothelial-derived relaxant f., endothelial-derived relaxing f. endothelium-derived relaxing f. (EDRF) nitric oxide.

extrinsic f. cyanocobalamin.

F f., fertility f. F plasmid.

fibrin-stabilizing f. (FSF) factor XIII, one of the COAGULATION FACTORS.

Fitzgerald f. high-molecular-weight kininogen.

Fletcher f. prekallikrein.

granulocyte colony-stimulating f. (G-CSF) a colony-stimulating FACTOR that stimulates production of NEUTROPHILS from precursor cells.

granulocyte-macrophage colony-stimulating f. (GM-CSF) a colony-stimulating FACTOR that binds to stem CELLS and most MYELOCYTES and stimulates their differentiation into GRANULOCYTES and MACROPHAGES.

growth f. any substance that promotes skeletal or somatic growth; usually a mineral, hormone, or vitamin.

f. H a COMPLEMENT system regulatory protein that inhibits the alternative pathway of complement activation.

Hageman f. (HF) factor XII, one of the COAGULATION FACTORS. See illustration.

hematopoietic growth f's a group of substances with the ability to support hematopoietic colony formation in vitro, including erythropoietin, interleukin-3, and

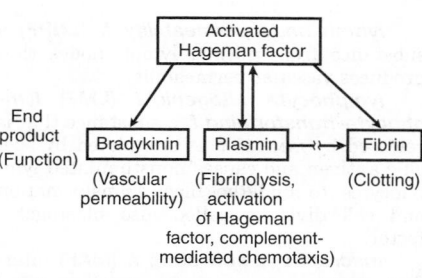

Activation of Hageman factor (factor XII) leads to increased vascular permeability, clotting, and thrombolysis. From Damjanov, 2000.

colony-stimulating factors. All except erythropoietin stimulate mature cells, have overlapping capabilities to affect progenitor cells of several blood cell lines, and also affect cells outside the hematopoietic system.

histamine-releasing f. (HRF) a LYMPHOKINE, believed to be produced by macrophages and B lymphocytes, that induces the release of histamine by IgE-bound basophils. It occurs in late phase allergic reaction, six or more hours after contact with the antigen, in sensitive individuals.

homologous restriction f. (HRF) a regulatory protein that binds to the membrane attack COMPLEX in autologous cells, inhibiting the final stages of COMPLEMENT activation.

f. I a plasma enzyme that regulates both classical and alternative pathways of COMPLEMENT activation by inactivating their C3 convertases.

immunoglobulin-binding f. (IBF) a lymphokine having the ability to bind IgG complexed with antigen and prevent complement activation.

insulinlike growth f's (IGF) insulinlike substances in serum that do not react with insulin antibodies; they are growth hormone–dependent and possess all the growth-promoting properties of the somatomedins.

intensification f. in radiology, the comparative increase in light transmission when films are exposed in the presence of intensifying screens compared to that in the absence of screens.

intrinsic f. a glycoprotein secreted by the parietal cells of the gastric glands, necessary for the absorption of CYANOCOBALAMIN (vitamin B_{12}). Its absence results in PERNICIOUS ANEMIA.

LE f. an immunoglobulin that reacts with leukocyte nuclei, found in the serum in systemic lupus erythematosus.

lymph node permeability f. (LNPF) a substance from normal lymph nodes that produces vascular permeability.

lymphocyte mitogenic f. (LMF), lymphocyte-transforming f. a substance that is released by LYMPHOCYTES stimulated by specific antigen and causes nonstimulated lymphocytes to undergo blast transformation and cell division; called also blastogenic factor.

macrophage-activating f. (MAF) interferon-α.

macrophage colony-stimulating f. (M-CSF) a colony-stimulating FACTOR secreted by MACROPHAGES, stimulated endothelial cells, and most tissues, that stimulates the production of macrophages from precursor cells and maintains the viability of mature macrophages in vitro.

macrophage chemotactic f. (MCF) a lymphokine that attracts macrophages to the invasion site.

macrophage-derived growth f. a substance released by macrophages below the surface of a wound that induces the proliferation of fibroblasts.

macrophage inhibition f., macrophage inhibitory f. migration inhibitory factor.

migration inhibition f., migration inhibitory f. a LYMPHOKINE that inhibits MACROPHAGE migration.

minification f. in radiology, the gain in light achieved by a reduction in size of the output phosphor from the input phosphor size.

osteoclast-activating f. (OAF) a lymphokine that stimulates bone resorption; it may be involved in the bone resorption associated with multiple myeloma and other hematologic neoplasms or inflammatory disorders such as rheumatoid arthritis and periodontal disease.

f. P properdin.

platelet f's see PLATELET FACTORS.

platelet-activating f. (PAF) a substance released by basophils and mast cells in immediate HYPERSENSITIVITY reactions, and by macrophages and neutrophils in other inflammatory reactions; it leads to bronchoconstriction, platelet aggregation, and release of vasoactive substances from platelets.

platelet-derived growth f. a substance contained in platelets and capable of inducing proliferation of vascular endothelial cells, vascular smooth muscle cells, fibroblasts, and glial cells; its action contributes to the repair of damaged vascular walls.

R f. R plasmid.

releasing f's factors elaborated in one structure (as in the hypothalamus) that effect the release of hormones from another structure (as from the anterior pituitary gland), including corticotropin-releasing factor, melanocyte-stimulating hormone–releasing factor, and prolactin-releasing factor. Applied to substances of unknown chemical structure, while substances of established chemical identity are called *releasing hormones.*

resistance f. R f.

Rh f. a type of agglutinogen found on some erythrocytes; see also RH FACTOR.

rheumatoid f. (RF) antibodies directed against antigenic determinants on IgG molecules, found in the serum of about 80 per cent of patients with classic or definite rheumatoid arthritis; but in only about 20 per cent of patients with juvenile rheumatoid arthritis; rheumatoid factors may be IgM, IgG, or IgA antibodies, although serologic tests measure only IgM. Rheumatoid factors also occur in other connective tissue diseases and infectious diseases.

risk f. an agent or situation that is known to make an individual or population more susceptible to the development of a specific negative condition.

stable f. factor VII, one of the COAGULATION FACTORS.

Stuart f., Stuart-Prower f. factor X, one of the COAGULATION FACTORS.

sun protection f. (SPF) a numerical rating of the amount of protection afforded by a SUNSCREEN; the higher the number, the more protection is provided.

tissue f. factor III, one of the COAGULATION FACTORS.

transfer f. (TF) a factor occurring in sensitized lymphocytes that can transfer delayed hypersensitivity to a formerly nonreactive individual; see also TRANSFER FACTOR.

tumor necrosis f. (TNF) either of two LYMPHOKINES produced primarily by cells of the IMMUNE SYSTEM, capable of causing in vivo hemorrhagic necrosis of certain tumor cells but not normal cells. They also destroy cells associated with the inflammatory RESPONSE. They have been used as experimental anticancer agents but can also induce SHOCK when bacterial endotoxins cause their release. *Tumor necrosis factor α,* formerly called *cachectin,* contains 157 amino acids and is produced by macrophages, eosinophils, and NK cells. *Tumor necrosis factor β* is lymphotoxic and contains 171 amino acids.

vascular endothelial growth f. (VEGF), vascular permeability f. (VPF) a peptide factor that stimulates the proliferation of cells of the endothelium of blood vessels;

it promotes tissue vascularization and is important in blood vessel formation in tumors.

von Willebrand's f. (vWF) a glycoprotein synthesized in endothelial cells and megakaryocytes that circulates complexed to COAGULATION FACTOR VIII. It is involved in adhesion of platelets to damaged epithelial surfaces and may participate in platelet aggregation. Deficiency results in the prolonged bleeding time seen in VON WILLEBRAND'S DISEASE.

facultative (fak'ul-ta"tiv) not obligatory; pertaining to or characterized by the ability to adjust to particular circumstances or to assume a particular role.

faculty (fak'ul-te) 1. a normal power or function, especially of the mind. 2. the teaching staff of an institute of learning.

FAD flavin adenine dinucleotide.

fae- for words beginning thus, see those beginning *fe-*.

Fahr-Volhard disease (fahr fōl'hahrt) the malignant form of arteriolar nephrosclerosis.

failure (fāl'yer) inability to perform or to function properly.

adult f. to thrive a NURSING DIAGNOSIS accepted by the North American Nursing Diagnosis Association, defined as a progressive functional deterioration of a physical and cognitive nature. The individual's ability to live with multisystem diseases, cope with ensuing problems, and manage his/her care are remarkably diminished.

bone marrow f. failure of the hematopoietic function of the bone marrow; see also bone marrow SUPPRESSION.

congestive heart f. see congestive HEART FAILURE.

heart f. see HEART FAILURE.

kidney f. renal failure.

multiple organ f. failure of two or more organ systems in a critically ill patient; see also MULTIPLE ORGAN FAILURE.

renal f. see RENAL FAILURE.

respiratory f. see RESPIRATORY FAILURE.

f. to thrive, f. to thrive syndrome physical and developmental retardation in infants and small children. The syndrome can be seen in children with a physical illness, but the term is most often taken to mean failure to thrive due to psychosocial effects such as maternal deprivation. The syndrome was first noticed when European psychiatrists studied the development of babies who had spent the first five years of their lives in institutions where they were deprived of the emotional warmth of a mother, father, or other primary caregiver.

Characteristics of the failure to thrive syndrome include lack of physical growth (for example, weight and height below the third percentile for age) and below normal achievement in fine and gross motor, social-adaptive, and language skills as assessed by psychometric testing using a tool such as the Denver Developmental Screening Test. Additionally, the child with this syndrome displays withdrawing behavior, avoidance of eye contact, and stiffness or flaccid posture when held. These children often have a history of irritability, feeding problems, and disturbed sleep patterns.

Parents of infants with failure to thrive syndrome typically display feelings of concern and inadequacy. The infant who is feeding poorly and is irritable may elicit a response in the caregiver that reflects tension and frustration. The need for comfort and nurturing by the infant may not met, and this may lead to a cycle that exacerbates feeding problems.

Intervention encompasses identification of infants and mothers at risk for the syndrome and care of both mother or primary caregiver and infant. The major goals are to encourage the mother to express her feelings without fear of rejection, to model the role of mother and teach her nurturing behaviors, and to promote her self-esteem and confidence. Important nursing goals in the care of the infant include providing optimal nutrition, comfort, and rest; meeting the infant's psychosocial needs; and supplying emotional nurturance and sensory stimulation appropriate to the assessed developmental level.

ventilatory f. respiratory failure.

faint (fānt) a temporary loss of CONSCIOUSNESS that is self-correcting, caused by generalized cerebral ischemia; called also syncope. It may be due to a nervous reaction stemming from such causes as fear, hunger, pain, or an emotional or physical shock. Although this may be considered a mild form of SHOCK, it is not as serious as true shock and usually is not accompanied by the rapid, weak pulse and cold, clammy skin characteristic of that condition. The person who is about to faint should be made to lie down with the legs elevated and collar and clothing loosened. If this is not feasible, the head is lowered between the knees for about five minutes. Prolonged loss of consciousness indicates a condition more serious than fainting and calls for medical attention.

fair treatment see RIGHT TO FAIR TREATMENT.

falcial (fal′shal) pertaining to a falx.

falciform (fal′sĭ-form) sickle-shaped.

falcular (fal′ku-ler) falciform.

fall (fawl) a coming down freely, usually under the influence of gravity.

risk for f's a NURSING DIAGNOSIS accepted by the North American Nursing Diagnosis Association, defined as increased susceptibility to falling that may cause physical harm.

fallopian tube (fah-lo′pe-an) a slender tube extending laterally from the UTERUS toward the OVARY, one on each side, allowing passage of OVA to the cavity of the uterus and of SPERMATOZOA in the opposite direction. Called also uterine tube and oviduct.

When the mature OVUM leaves the ovary it enters the fringed opening of the fallopian tube, through which it travels slowly to the uterus. When conception takes place, the tube is usually the site of FERTILIZATION. Obstruction or infection within the fallopian tubes is a major cause of INFERTILITY. The removal of one tube by surgery, or the failure of a tube to function, ordinarily leaves the other tube intact and able to perform its function in reproduction. Occasionally the fertilized ovum implants in the wall of the fallopian tube, resulting in an ectopic, or tubal PREGNANCY.

false-negative (fawls′ neg′ah-tiv) 1. denoting a test result that wrongly excludes an individual from a diagnostic or other category. 2. an individual so excluded. 3. an instance of such a result; called also false-negative reaction.

false-positive (fawls′ poz′ĭ-tiv) 1. denoting a test result that wrongly assigns an individual to a diagnostic or other category. 2. an individual so categorized. 3. an instance of such a result; called also false-positive reaction.

falsification (fawl″sĭ-fĭ-ka′shun) a deliberate misstatement or misrepresentation.

retrospective f. unconscious distortion of memories of past experiences to conform to present emotional needs.

falx (falks), pl. *fal′ces* [L.] a sickle-shaped structure.

f. cerebel′li the fold of DURA MATER separating the cerebellar HEMISPHERES.

f. ce′rebri a sickle-shaped fold of DURA MATER in the longitudinal fissure, which separates the two cerebral HEMISPHERES.

famciclovir (fam-si′klo-vir) a prodrug of penciclovir that is converted to the active drug following administration, used in the treatment of herpes zoster, of genital herpes, and of mucocutaneous herpes simplex in immunocompromised patients; administered orally.

familial (fah-mil′e-al) occurring in or affecting members of a family more than would be expected by chance.

f. Mediterranean fever a hereditary disease usually occurring in Armenians and Sephardic Jews, and marked by short recurrent attacks of fever with pain in the abdomen, chest, or joints, and erythema

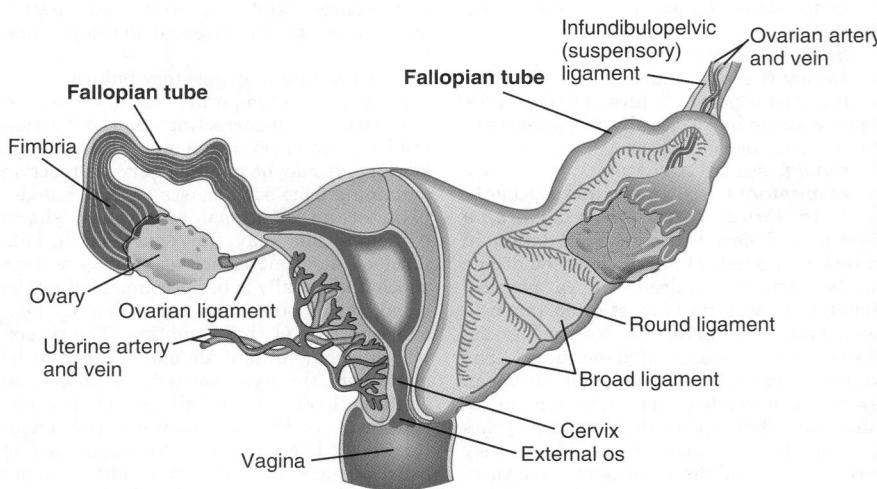

Fallopian tube. From McKinney et al., 2000.

resembling that seen in erysipelas; it is sometimes complicated by amyloidosis.

f. *periodic fever* a rare autosomal dominant syndrome that includes an abnormality on the cell receptor for tumor necrosis FACTOR; characteristics include periodic fever with any of various skin disorders lasting for four days to three weeks, as well as mild systemic manifestations such as abdominal pain, headache, and chest pain. Called also tumor necrosis factor receptor–associated periodic syndrome.

family (fam′ĭ-le) 1. a group of people related by blood or marriage or a strong common bond, such as those descended from a common ancestor, or a husband, wife, and their children. 2. a taxonomic category below an order and above a genus.

blended f. a family unit composed of a married couple and their offspring including some from previous marriages.

dysfunctional f. one in which adult caregivers are unable to consistently fulfill their family responsibilities.

extended f. a nuclear family and their close relatives, such as the children's grandparents, aunts, and uncles.

nuclear f. a family consisting of a two-generation relationship of parents and children, living together and more or less isolated from their extended family.

nuclear dyad f. a husband and wife with no children.

f. of origin the family in which a person grew up.

f. processes the psychosocial, physiological, and spiritual functions and relationships within the family unit; for NURSING DIAGNOSES, see under PROCESS.

single-parent f. a lone parent and offspring living together as a family unit.

skewed f. a family in which one spouse is severely dysfunctional and the other spouse assumes an acquiescent, peacemaking stance to maintain equilibrium.

famotidine (fam-o′tĭ-dēn) an antagonist of histamine H$_2$ RECEPTORS, inhibiting the action of HISTAMINE at cell surface receptors of the gastric parietal cells and reducing basal gastric acid secretion and secretion stimulated by food, histamine, gastrin, caffeine, and insulin. It is administered orally for the short-term (two months) treatment and, at reduced dosage, the long term prevention, of PEPTIC ULCERS, for the relief of symptoms associated with hyperacidity, such as heartburn and acid indigestion, and for the treatment of GASTROESOPHAGEAL REFLUX DISEASE, upper gastrointestinal bleeding, and pathological hypersecretory conditions such as ZOLLINGER-ELLISON SYNDROME.

Fanconi syndrome (fan-ko′nē) 1. a rare hereditary disorder, transmitted as an autosomal recessive trait, characterized by pancytopenia, hypoplasia of the bone marrow, and patchy brown discoloration of the skin due to the deposition of melanin, and associated with multiple congenital anomalies of the musculoskeletal and genitourinary systems. Called also Fanconi anemia. 2. any of a group of diseases marked by dysfunction of the proximal renal tubules, with generalized hyperaminoaciduria, renal glycosuria, hyperphosphaturia, and bicarbonate and water loss; the most common cause is cystinosis, but it is also associated with other genetic diseases and occurs in idiopathic and acquired forms.

F and R (of pulse) force and rhythm.

Fannia (fan′e-ah) a genus of flies whose larvae have caused both intestinal and urinary infestation in humans.

fantasy (fan′tah-se) a daydream; an imagined situation or sequence of events. Fantasy can serve as a realistic rehearsal of future events; it may also serve as an unconscious DEFENSE MECHANISM providing wish-fulfillment, gratification of repressed impulses, and resolution of unconscious conflicts.

FAOTA Fellow, American Occupational Therapy Association.

FAP familial adenomatous polyposis.

farad (F) (far′ad) the SI UNIT of electric CAPACITANCE; the capacitance of a condenser that charged with 1 coulomb gives a difference of potential of 1 volt.

Farber's disease (fahr′berz) a LYSOSOMAL STORAGE DISEASE and SPHINGOLIPIDOSIS, transmitted as an autosomal recessive trait, due to deficiency of the enzyme CERAMIDASE.

farcy (fahr′se) the more chronic and constitutional form of GLANDERS.

farsightedness (fahr-sīt′ed-nes) hyperopia.

fascia (fash′e-ah), pl. *fas′ciae* [L.] a sheet or band of fibrous tissue such as lies deep to the skin or invests muscles and various body organs. adj., **fas′cial.**

aponeurotic f. a dense, firm, fibrous membrane investing the trunk and limbs and giving off sheaths to the various muscles.

f. cribro′sa the superficial fascia of the thigh covering the saphenous opening (fossa ovalis femoris).

crural f. the investing fascia of the lower limb.

deep f. aponeurotic fascia.

endothoracic f. that beneath the serous lining of the thoracic cavity.

F

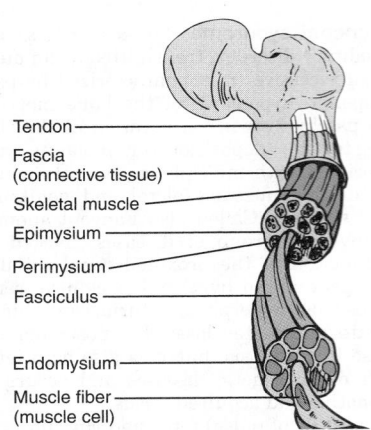

Tendon
Fascia (connective tissue)
Skeletal muscle
Epimysium
Perimysium
Fasciculus
Endomysium
Muscle fiber (muscle cell)

Organization and connective tissue components of skeletal muscle. From Applegate, 2000.

f. la′ta the external investing fascia of the thigh.

Scarpa's f. the deep, membranous layer of the subcutaneous abdominal fascia.

superficial f. 1. a fascial sheet lying directly beneath the skin. 2. subcutaneous tissue.

thyrolaryngeal f. the fascia covering the thyroid gland and attached to the cricoid cartilage.

transverse f. that between the transversalis muscle and the peritoneum.

fascicle (fas′ĭ-k′l) fasciculus.

fascicular (fah-sik′u-ler) clustered together; pertaining to or arranged in bundles or clusters; pertaining to a fascicle.

fasciculated (fah-sik′u-lāt-ed) clustered together or occurring in bundles, or fasciculi.

fasciculation (fah-sik″u-la′shun) 1. the formation of fascicles. 2. a small local involuntary muscular contraction visible under the skin, representing spontaneous discharge of a number of fibers innervated by a single motor nerve filament.

fasciculus (fah-sik′u-lus), pl. *fasci′culi* [L.] a small BUNDLE or TRACT, especially of nerve or muscle fibers. Called also fascicle.

cuneate f. of medulla oblongata the continuation into the medulla oblongata of the cuneate fasciculus of spinal cord.

cuneate f. of spinal cord the lateral portion of the dorsal funiculus of the spinal cord, composed of ascending fibers that end in the nucleus cuneatus.

gracile f. of medulla oblongata the continuation into the medulla oblongata of the gracile fasciculus of spinal cord.

gracile f. of spinal cord the median portion of the dorsal funiculus of the spinal cord, composed of ascending fibers that end in the nucleus gracilis.

fasciectomy (fas″e-ek′to-me) excision of fascia.

fasciitis (fas″e-i′tis) inflammation of a fascia.

necrotizing f. a fulminating group A streptococcal infection beginning with severe or extensive cellulitis that spreads to involve the superficial and deep fascia, producing thrombosis of the subcutaneous vessels and gangrene of the underlying tissues. A cutaneous lesion usually serves as a portal of entry for the infection, but sometimes no such lesion is found.

nodular f., proliferative f. a benign, reactive proliferation of fibroblasts in the subcutaneous tissues and commonly associated with the deep fascia.

pseudosarcomatous f. a benign soft tissue tumor occurring subcutaneously and sometimes arising from deep muscle and fascia.

fasciodesis (fas″e-od′ĕ-sis) suture of a fascia to skeletal attachment.

Fasciola (fah-si′o-lah) a genus of trematodes. *F. hepa′tica* is a common liver fluke of herbivores and is occasionally found in humans.

fasciola (fah-si′o-lah), pl. *fasci′olae* [L.] 1. a small band or striplike structure. 2. a small bandage. adj., **fasci′olar.**

fascioliasis (fas″e-o-li′ah-sis) infection with *Fasciola.*

fasciolopsiasis (fas″e-o-lop-si″ah-sis) infection with *Fasciolopsis.*

Fasciolopsis (fas″e-o-lop′sis) a genus of trematodes. *F. bus′ki* is a large intestinal fluke found in humans and a few other animals throughout Asia.

fascioplasty (fas′e-o-plas″te) plastic repair of a fascia.

fasciorrhaphy (fas″e-or′ah-fe) suture of a lacerated fascia.

fasciotomy (fas″e-ot′ah-me) incision of a fascia.

fast (fast) 1. immovable, or unchangeable; resistant to the action of a specific drug, stain, or destaining agent. 2. abstention from food.

fastigium (fas-tij′e-um) [L.] 1. the highest point in the roof of the fourth ventricle of the brain. 2. the acme, or highest point. adj., **fastig′ial.**

Fastin (fas′tin) trademark for a preparation of PHENTERMINE hydrochloride, an appetite suppressant.

fat (fat) 1. the adipose TISSUE of the body. 2. a TRIGLYCERIDE (or triacylglycerol) that is an ester of FATTY ACIDS and GLYCEROL. Each fat molecule contains one glycerol residue connected by ester linkages to three fatty acid residues, which may be the same or different. The fatty acids may have no double bonds in the carbon chain (saturated fatty acids), one double bond (monounsaturated), or two or more double bonds (polyunsaturated). Essential fatty acids cannot be synthesized by the body but must be obtained from the diet or from intravenous infusion of lipids.

Saturated and Unsaturated Fats. All of the common unsaturated fatty acids are liquid (oils) at room temperature. Through the process of hydrogenation, hydrogen can be incorporated into certain unsaturated fatty acids so that they are converted into solid fats for cooking purposes. Margarine is an example of the hydrogenation of unsaturated fatty acids into a solid substance.

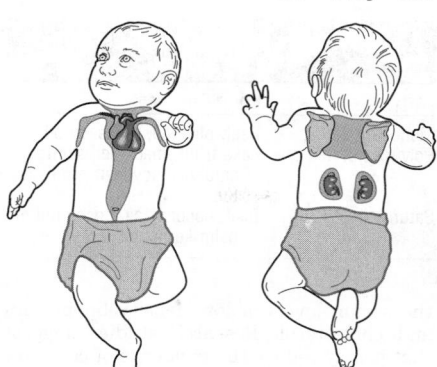

Sites of brown fat in the neonate. From McKinney et al., 2000.

brown f. a thermogenic type of adipose tissue containing a dark pigment, and arising during embryonic life in certain specific areas in many mammals, including humans (see illustration); it is prominent in the newborn. Called also brown adipose tissue.

neutral f. fat (def. 2).

polyunsaturated f. a fat containing polyunsaturated FATTY ACIDS; see also FAT.

saturated f. a fat containing saturated FATTY ACIDS; see also FAT.

unsaturated f. a fat containing unsaturated FATTY ACIDS; see also FAT.

fatal (fa′tal) pertaining to or resulting in death; called also lethal.

fatigability (fat″ĭ-gah-bil′ĭ-te) easy susceptibility to fatigue.

fatigue (fah-tēg′) 1. loss of the ability of a muscle to respond to stimuli. 2. a NURSING DIAGNOSIS accepted by the North American Nursing Diagnosis Association, defined as an overwhelming sustained exhaustion and decreased capacity for physical and mental work at the usual level. Fatigue is a normal reaction to intense physical exertion, emotional strain, or lack of rest. When it is not relieved by rest, it may have a more serious origin; it may be a symptom of poor physical condition, a specific disease or oncoming disease, or severe emotional stress. Sometimes fatigue is psychological in origin. Tiredness and a loss of interest in one's work may actually result from boredom with the daily routine. If one is certain that there is nothing wrong physically, steps should be taken to vary the daily round, to seek new and more active ways to spend leisure time, perhaps to revive old interests that have been neglected. See also ACTIVITY INTOLERANCE.

caregiver role f. excessive fatigue of a CAREGIVER caused by the neglect of his or her personal needs due to the demands of physical and emotional care of someone else.

vocal f. phonasthenia.

fatty (fat′e) pertaining to or characterized by fat.

f. acid an organic compound of carbon, hydrogen, and oxygen that combines with GLYCEROL to form FAT. All fats are esters of fatty acids and glycerol, the fatty acids usually accounting for 90 per cent of the fat molecule. A fatty acid consists of a long chain of carbon atoms with a carboxylic acid group at one end. Saturated fatty acids have no double bonds in the carbon chain. They are solid at room temperature and are the components of the common animal fats, such as butter and lard. Unsaturated fatty acids contain one or more double bonds. The unsaturated fatty acids are liquid at room temperature and are found in oils such as olive oil and linseed oil. Polyunsaturated fatty acids have two or more double bonds.

Fatty acids that cannot be synthesized by the human body and must be obtained from dietary sources are called *essential fatty acids*; these include linoleic acid, linolenic acid, and arachidonic acid. A deficiency of an essential fatty acid can lead to eczema or other skin disorders. Such deficiencies are rare, however, because the fatty acids occur in abundance in many foods, such as butter, whole milk, egg yolk, nuts, and vegetables. Consumption of less saturated fat and more polyunsaturated fat lowers

F

COMMON FOOD SOURCES OF FATTY ACIDS	
Fatty Acids	**Food Sources**
Monosaturated	Beef, olive oil, rapeseed oil
Polyunsaturated	Lake trout, mackerel, salmon, sardines, soybean products, tuna
Saturated	Beef, coconut oil, cocoa butter, palm kernel oil

the serum levels of low density lipoprotein and cholesterol. Research studies suggest that it may reduce the incidence of coronary artery disease.

fauces (faw′sēz) THROAT. adj., **fau′cial.**

faucitis (faw-si′tis) SORE THROAT (def. 1).

faveolate (fah-ve′o-lāt) honeycombed; alveolate.

faveolus (fah-ve′o-lus) [L.] foveola.

favism (fa′vizm) an acute hemolytic anemia caused by ingestion of fava beans or inhalation of the pollen of the plant, usually occurring in certain individuals as a result of a genetic abnormality with a deficiency of an enzyme, glucose-6-phosphate dehydrogenase, in the erythrocytes. Called also fabism.

favus (fa′vus) a type of RINGWORM, most often involving the scalp but sometimes affecting glabrous (smooth) skin, with formation of prominent honeycomblike masses, usually due to *Trichophyton schoenleini.*

FDA Food and Drug Administration.

F-duction (ef-duk′shun) in bacterial genetics, the process whereby part of the bacterial chromosome is attached to the autonomous F factor (fertility factor) and thus is transferred with high frequency from the donor (male) bacterium to the recipient (female) bacterium. Called also sexduction.

Fe iron (L. *fer′rum*).

fear (fēr) the unpleasant emotional state consisting of psychological and psychophysiological responses to a real external threat or danger. See also ANXIETY. Fear is a NURSING DIAGNOSIS accepted by the North American Nursing Diagnosis Association, who defined it as a response to a perceived threat that is consciously recognized as a danger. Causative factors may include separation from one's support system in a potentially threatening situation such as hospitalization, diagnostic test, or treatment; knowledge deficit or unfamiliarity; language barrier; sensory impairment; and phobic stimulus or phobia.

Persons experiencing fear may verbalize increased tension, apprehension, diminished self-assurance, panic, or a jittery feeling. Objective signs include increased alertness; concentration on the source of fear; attack and fight-or-flight behaviors; and evidence of sympathetic nerve stimulation such as cardiovascular excitation, superficial vasoconstriction, and dilation of the pupils. Interventions are aimed at helping the individual to identify effective and ineffective coping behaviors, promote effective coping strategies, and maintain psychological equilibrium.

febricide (feb′ri-sīd) ANTIPYRETIC (def. 2).

febrifacient (feb″ri-fa′shent) pyrogenic.

febrifuge (feb′ri-fūj″) ANTIPYRETIC (def. 2).

febrile (feb′ril) 1. pertaining to FEVER. 2. characterized by fever; called also feverish, pyrectic, and pyretic.

fecal (fe′k'l) pertaining to or of the nature of feces.

   f. impaction accumulation of putty-like or hardened feces in the rectum or sigmoid. The condition often occurs in patients with long-standing bowel problems and chronic constipation. It also may develop when barium is introduced into the intestinal tract and not completely removed.

Symptoms include painful defecation, feeling of fullness in the rectum, and constipation or a diarrheic stool. Rectal examination reveals a hard or putty-like mass. The condition can be prevented in most cases by adequate removal of barium after radiologic studies, and by careful monitoring of the bowel movements of patients with problems of bowel elimination.

Fecal impaction usually requires digital removal with a gloved finger to break up the mass. Prior to removal the patient may be given an oil retention ENEMA to help soften the mass.

fecalith (fe′kah-lith) an intestinal concretion formed around a center of fecal material. Called also coprolith.

fecaloid (fe′kah-loid) resembling feces.

fecaloma (fe″kah-lo′mah) a tumorlike accumulation of feces in the rectum; called also stercoroma.

fecaluria (fe″kal-u′re-ah) the presence of fecal matter in the urine.

feces (fe′sēz) [L.] body waste discharged from the intestine; called also stool, excrement, and excreta. The feces are formed in the colon and pass down into the rectum by the process of peristalsis. When the rectum is sufficiently distended, nerve endings in its wall signal a need for evacuation, which is made possible by a voluntary relaxation of the sphincter muscles around the outer part of the anus.

The frequency of bowel movements varies according to the individual body make-up, type of intestine, eating habits, physical activity, and custom. Although one bowel movement a day is the average, a movement every 2 or 3 days may be considered normal. A balanced diet and an established routine can promote regular bowel movements.

Characteristics. Normally feces are soft and formed and brownish in color. An abnormality in color, odor, or consistency usually indicates a disorder of the intestinal tract or of the accessory organs of the digestive system. Black, tarry feces may indicate intestinal bleeding, especially in the upper portion of the tract. Some drugs, such as those containing iron or bismuth, can produce tarry feces. Bright red blood in the feces can indicate a wide variety of disorders ranging from HEMORRHOIDS to a malignancy of the rectum. Clay-colored feces result from an absence or deficiency of BILE in the intestinal tract, indicating obstruction of the biliary tract or decreased production of bile by the liver. Greenish-colored feces often accompany diarrhea, especially in infants, and may be caused by growth of certain bacteria.

Bulky, fatty feces with a foul odor are characteristic of CYSTIC FIBROSIS. Other causes of fatty feces include gallbladder disease, pancreatic disorders, SPRUE, and excessive intake of fat in the diet. Feces containing large amounts of mucus often occur in COLITIS and IRRITABLE BOWEL SYNDROME.

The feces of a newborn, full-term infant is called MECONIUM. It is a dark greenish brown color, smooth and semisolid in consistency.

Disinfection. In many types of communicable diseases it is necessary to decontaminate the feces before they are flushed into the sewage system. Chlorinated lime, Lysol, or formalin may be used for this purpose. The contents of the bedpan used by the patient should be thoroughly covered with the disinfectant and allowed to stand for several hours. The contents are then disposed of in a hopper or commode, and the bedpan is rinsed and sterilized, preferably with live steam or by autoclave.

Observations. Because the characteristics of the feces can be of help in the diagnosis of various diseases, it is important to inspect the stool for color, consistency, odor, and number of stools per day. Abnormalities should be noted on the patient's chart or reported to the physician.

Specimens. A sample of feces (stool specimen) may be required as a diagnostic aid.

The specimen should be collected in a bedpan and transferred into a sterile container, using a wooden spatula or tongue blade for this purpose. In order for certain types of intestinal parasites to be discovered in the feces, the specimen must be fresh and kept warm until examined in the laboratory. Microorganisms that may be detected include the typhoid and paratyphoid bacilli, the anthrax bacilli, and *Entamoeba histolytica,* which causes AMEBIC DYSENTERY. Specimens of the feces may be examined for occult (hidden) blood. This test is indicated when intestinal bleeding is suspected but the stools do not appear to contain blood when examined by gross inspection.

feculent (fek′u-lent) 1. having dregs or sediment. 2. excrementitious. 3. fecal.

fecundation (fe″kun-da′shun) fertilization.

fecundity (fe-kun′dĭ-te) the ability to produce offspring frequently and in large numbers. In demography, the physiological ability to reproduce, as opposed to fertility.

feeblemindedness (fe″b′l-mīnd′ed-nes) former name for MENTAL RETARDATION, now considered offensive.

feedback (fēd′bak) the return of some of the output of a system as input so as to exert some control in the process. Feedback controls are a type of self-regulating mechanism by which certain activities are sustained within prescribed ranges. For example, the serum concentration of oxygen is affected in part by the rate and depth of respirations and is, therefore, an output of the respiratory system. If the concentration of oxygen drops below normal, this information is transmitted as *input* to the respiratory control center. The control center is thereby stimulated to increase the rate of respirations in order to return the oxygen concentration in the blood to within normal range.

This series of events is an example of *negative feedback,* which always causes the controller to respond in a manner that opposes a deviation from the normal level (setpoint). It is, therefore, a corrective action that returns a factor within the system to a normal range. *Positive feedback* tends to increase a deviation from the setpoint. In other words, positive feedback reinforces and accelerates either an excess or deficit of a factor within the system. See also HOMEOSTASIS.

alpha f. alpha biofeedback.

feedforward (fēd-for′werd) the anticipatory effect that one intermediate in a

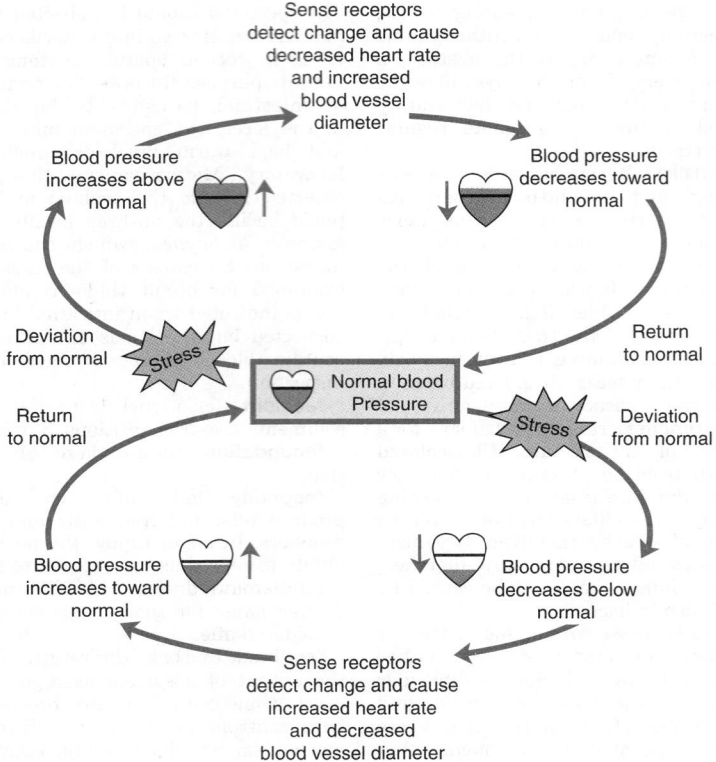

Physiologic example of negative feedback. From Applegate, 2000.

metabolic or endocrine control system exerts on another intermediate further along in the pathway; such effect may be positive or negative.

feeding (fēd′ing) 1. the taking of food. 2. the giving of food. 3. in the NURSING INTERVENTIONS CLASSIFICATION, a nursing INTERVENTION defined as providing nutritional intake for a patient who is unable to feed self.

artificial f. feeding of a baby with food other than mother's milk.

bottle f. in the NURSING INTERVENTIONS CLASSIFICATION, a nursing INTERVENTION defined as preparation and administration of fluids to an infant via a bottle.

breast f. breastfeeding.

enteral tube f. in the NURSING INTERVENTIONS CLASSIFICATION, a nursing INTERVENTION defined as delivering nutrients and water through a gastrointestinal tube.

forced f. administration of food by force to those who cannot or will not receive it.

intravenous f. administration of nutrient fluids through a vein; see also INTRAVENOUS INFUSION and PARENTERAL NUTRITION.

supplemental f. a planned additional food or nutrient that is added to the usual diet, often as a powder, formula, or tablet.

tube f. see TUBE FEEDING.

Feer disease (fār) erythredema polyneuropathy.

FEF forced expiratory flow.

Fehling's solution (fa′lingz) an alkaline cupric sulfate solution used to test for glucose.

felbamate (fel′bah-māt″) an ANTICONVULSANT used in treatment of EPILEPSY; administered orally.

Feldene (fel′dēn) trademark for preparations of PIROXICAM, a NONSTEROIDAL ANTIINFLAMMATORY DRUG used in treatment of ARTHRITIS.

fellatio (fĕ-la′she-o) oral stimulation or manipulation of the penis.

felodipine (fĕ-lo′dĭ-pēn) a CALCIUM CHANNEL BLOCKING AGENT used as a vasodilator in treatment of HYPERTENSION.

felon (fel′on) an extremely painful abscess involving the pulp of the distal phalanx of a finger; called also whitlow.

feltwork (felt′werk) a complex of closely interwoven fibers, as of nerve fibers.

Felty's syndrome (fel′tēz) a syndrome of splenomegaly with chronic rheumatoid arthritis and leukopenia; there are usually pigmented spots on the skin of the lower extremities, and sometimes there is other evidence of hypersplenism such as anemia or thrombocytopenia.

female (fe′māl) 1. an individual of the sex that produces ova or bears young. 2. feminine.

    f. orgasmic disorder persistently delayed or absent orgasm in a female after a normal sexual excitement phase of adequate focus, intensity, and duration. See also MALE ORGASMIC DISORDER.

    f. sexual arousal disorder a SEXUAL DYSFUNCTION involving failure by a female either to attain or maintain the lubrication and swelling response of sexual excitement during sexual activity, after adequate stimulation, causing significant distress or interpersonal difficulty. Both physiological (such as endocrine) and psychological factors may be involved. Formerly called frigidity. See also MALE ERECTILE DISORDER.

feminine (fem′ĭ-nin) pertaining to the female sex, or having qualities normally characteristic of the female.

feminism (fem′ĭ-nizm) old term for FEMINIZATION (def. 2).

feminization (fem″ĭ-nī-za′shun) 1. the normal induction or development of female secondary sex CHARACTERS. 2. the induction or development of female secondary sex CHARACTERS in the male.

    testicular f. complete androgen RESISTANCE.

femoral (fem′o-ral) pertaining to the femur or to the thigh.

femorocele (fem′o-ro-sēl″) femoral hernia.

femorotibial (fem″o-ro″tib′e-al) tibiofemoral.

femto- word element [Danish], *fifteen;* used in naming units of measurement to indicate one quadrillionth (10^{-15}) of the unit designated by the root with which it is combined; symbol f.

femur (fe′mur), pl. *fem′ora, femurs* [L.] 1. the thigh bone, extending from the pelvis to the knee; the longest and strongest bone in the body. Its proximal end articulates with the acetabulum, a cup-like cavity in the pelvic girdle. The greater and lesser

trochanters are the two processes (prominences) at the proximal end of the femur. See anatomic Table of Bones in the Appendices. 2. thigh.

fenestra (fĕ-nes′trah), pl. *fenes′trae* [L.] window.

    f. coch′leae round window.

    f. vesti′buli oval window.

fenestrate (fen′es-trāt) to pierce with one or more openings.

fenestration (fen″es-tra′shun) 1. the presence of openings in a body part. 2. the creation of openings to allow for viewing of parts. 3. the surgical creation of a new opening in the labyrinth of the ear for the restoration of hearing in otosclerosis. 4. loss or lack of supporting bone around the root of a tooth.

    alveolar plate f. apical fenestration.

    aorticopulmonary f. aortic septal defect.

    apical f. a condition sometimes seen in children, consisting of round or oval openings perforating the plate of bone that overlies a pulpless primary tooth. Called also alveolar plate fenestration.

fenfluramine (fen-floor′ah-mēn) an appetite suppressant used as the hydrochloride salt; unlike the AMPHETAMINES, it seems to depress rather than stimulate the central nervous system.

fenofibrate (fen″o-fi′brāt) an agent chemically related to CLOFIBRATE, used to treat HYPERLIPIDEMIA; administered orally.

fenoldopam (fe-nol′do-pam) a VASODILATOR used for short-term, inpatient management of severe HYPERTENSION, administered intravenously as the mesylate salt.

fenoprofen (fen″o-pro′fen) a NONSTEROIDAL ANTIINFLAMMATORY DRUG used in the treatment of rheumatoid arthritis, osteoarthritis, and other rheumatic and nonrheumatic inflammatory disorders, pain, dysmenorrhea, and vascular headaches; administered orally as the calcium salt.

fenoterol (fen″o-ter′ol) a beta$_2$-adrenergic RECEPTOR agonist used as a BRONCHODILATOR for the treatment and prophylaxis of reversible bronchospasm; administered by inhalation as the hydrobromide salt.

fentanyl (fen′tah-nil) an opioid ANALGESIC used as the citrate salt in the induction and maintenance of anesthesia, as an adjunct to anesthesia, in combination with DROPERIDOL (or similar agent) to induce NEUROLEPTANALGESIA, and in the management of chronic severe pain.

ferment (fer′ment) 1. to undergo fermentation. 2. any substance that causes fermentation.

fermentation (fer″men-ta′shun) the anaerobic enzymatic conversion of organic compounds, especially carbohydrates, to simpler compounds, especially to lactic acid or ethyl alcohol, producing energy in the form of ATP.

fermium (Fm) (fer′me-um) a chemical element, atomic number 100, atomic weight 253. (See Appendix 6.)

ferning (fern′ing) the appearance of a fernlike pattern in a dried specimen of cervical mucus, an indication of the presence of estrogen, usually seen at the midpoint of the MENSTRUAL CYCLE; it can be helpful in the determination of OVULATION. The same phenomenon occurs with premature rupture of the fetal MEMBRANES.

-ferous word element [L.], *bearing; producing.*

ferredoxin (fer″ē-dok′sin) a nonheme iron-containing protein having a very low oxidation-reduction potential; the ferredoxins participate in electron transport in photosynthesis, nitrogen fixation, and various other biological processes.

ferric (fer′ik) containing iron in its plus-three oxidation state, Fe(III) (sometimes designated Fe^{3+}).

f. chloride $FeCl_3$, used as a reagent and as a diagnostic aid in PHENYLKETONURIA.

ferritin (fer′ĭ-tin) the complex of IRON and APOFERRITIN, a major form in which iron is stored in the body.

ferrokinetics (fer″o-kĭ-net′iks) the turnover or rate of movement of iron in the body from plasma transferrin to erythrocyte precursors in the bone marrow to circulating erythrocytes to macrophages in the reticuloendothelial system and back to plasma transferrin. Ferrokinetic studies, using the radioisotope iron-59 as a tracer, measure kinetic parameters *(plasma iron clearance half-time, plasma iron turnover, red cell utilization,* and *erythrocyte iron turnover)* helpful in evaluating certain anemias and in detecting abnormal iron storage or extramedullary hematopoiesis by external counting over the liver, spleen, and bone marrow.

ferroprotein (fer″o-pro′tēn) a protein combined with an iron-containing radical; ferroproteins are respiratory carriers.

ferrotherapy (fer″o-ther′ah-pe) therapeutic use of iron and iron compounds.

ferrous (fer′us) containing iron in its plus-two oxidation state, Fe(II) (sometimes designated Fe^{2+}).

f. fumarate an oral iron preparation used in the treatment of iron deficiency.

f. gluconate a hematinic that is less irritating to the gastrointestinal tract than

other hematinics, and generally used as a substitute when ferrous sulfate cannot be tolerated.

f. sulfate the most widely used hematinic for the treatment of iron deficiency anemia. It is believed to be less irritating than equivalent amounts of ferric salts and is more effective.

All iron preparations should be administered after meals, never on an empty stomach. The patient should be warned that the drugs cause stools to turn dark green or black. Overdosage may cause severe systemic reactions.

ferruginous (fĕ-roo′jĭ-nus) containing IRON or iron rust; called also chalybeate.

fertility (fer-til′ĭ-te) 1. the capacity to conceive or to induce conception. adj., **fer′tile.** INFERTILITY is the inability to conceive after one year of sexual relations without contraception, or the inability to carry pregnancy to a live birth. It affects about one in six couples of childbearing age. STERILITY is complete inability to conceive children, and is relatively rare. 2. fertility rate.

assisted f. technologies that have developed to deal with INFERTILITY. Methods include: artificial INSEMINATION; in vitro FERTILIZATION; CRYOPRESERVATION of preembryos, ova, sperm, and embryos; MICROMANIPULATION of oocytes and embryos in vitro; gamete intrafallopian TRANSFER; surrogate gestational mothers; oocyte and sperm donation; and uses of embryos, fetuses, and cadavers. All such methods involve the separation of REPRODUCTION from COITUS and can raise ethical or legal questions such as: (1) the high value placed on genetic parenthood, (2) equitable access to techniques for those of different economic levels or racial groups, especially in times when access to ordinary health care is problematic for many, (3) women's control over their bodies and reproduction, and (4) the expending of considerable resources for producing children biologically related to their parents when the world's population continues to grow and there are many children without parents who could be adopted.

f. awareness methods natural family planning.

fertilization (fer″tĭ-lĭ-za′shun) in human REPRODUCTION, the process by which the male's SPERM unites with the female's OOCYTE, creating a new life. The sex and other biologic traits of the new individual are determined by the combined genes and chromosomes that exist in the sperm and oocyte. See also *conception* and *reproduction.* Called also fecundation and impregnation. After injection into the vagina, millions of sperm cells (SPERMATOZOA) make use of their whiplike tails to swim through the cervix toward the uterus. Most are destroyed along the way by secretions in the vagina, but some reach the uterus and a few may enter the FALLOPIAN TUBES. A very small number may survive as long as 48 hours. If during this period only one sperm succeeds in entering a fallopian tube and meeting there an oocyte ready to be fertilized, conception can occur. This event is possible only during a period of about 4 days of the month. After the sperm lodges in the oocyte, the tail disappears, but the head unites with the oocyte to form the ZYGOTE.

in vitro f. the process by which conception takes place in a laboratory medium; the term literally means fertilization "in glass." A lay term for the product of in vitro fertilization is "test tube baby."

The treatment cycle involves the following steps: (1) Induction of ovulation with fertility drugs, such as clomiphene citrate, injectable follicle-stimulating hormone/luteinizing hormone, or both, to produce multiple ovarian follicles. When the largest follicle reaches 20 mm in diameter the patient is given an injection of human chorionic gonadotropin to induce expulsion of the oocyte from the follicle. (2) Laparoscopy and follicular aspiration for the harvesting of oocytes. (3) Maturation of retrieved oocytes and inoculation with the husband's or donor's sperm. (4) Incubation of the resulting embryos until they reach the two- to six-cell stage. (5) Transfer of an embryo via catheter into the patient's uterus; at this point intensive intervention ceases, the pregnancy is considered normal, and no further manipulation is required.

in vivo f. union of the sperm and ovum within the reproductive tract of the female; usually taken to mean artificial INSEMINATION in which the sperm is artificially introduced into the vagina, cervix, or uterine cavity to overcome the problem of INFERTILITY.

fervescence (fer-ves′ens) increase of fever or body temperature.

fester (fes′ter) to SUPPURATE superficially.

festinant (fes′tĭ-nant) accelerating.

festination (fes″tĭ-na′shun) festinating gait.

festoon (fes-tōōn′) a carving in the base material of a denture that simulates the contours of the natural tissues it is replacing.

fetal (fe′t'l) of or pertaining to a fetus or to the period of its development.

f. acoustic stimulation test a test used to assess fetal health in compromised pregnancies; a vibroacoustic stimulus such as an electronic artificial larynx is applied either externally or directly to the fetus and resultant fetal movements, cardioacceleration, and alterations in respiration are compared to those of normal fetuses.

f. alcohol syndrome a group of symptoms characterized by mental and physical abnormalities of the infant and linked to the maternal intake of alcohol during pregnancy. Clinical manifestations, which can be present in varying degrees, include prenatal and postnatal growth deficiency, mental retardation, irritability in infancy, hyperactivity in childhood, microcephaly, short palpebral fissures, smooth philtrum, thin vermilion border of upper lip, small distal phalanges, and ventricular septal defects. Although the exact amount of alcohol consumption that will produce fetal damage is unknown, the risk and extent of abnormalities are most likely to be increased when the daily intake of pure alcohol exceeds 2 ounces. The periods of gestation during which the alcohol is most likely to result in fetal damage are three to four and a half months after conception and during the last trimester. Abstinence from alcohol during pregnancy is recommended.

f. assessment determination of the well-being of the fetus; techniques and procedures include: (1) medical and nursing histories and physical examination of the mother, (2) assays of amniotic fluid obtained by AMNIOCENTESIS, (3) ULTRASONOGRAPHY, (4) chemical assessment of placental function, (5) electronic and ultrasonic fetal heart rate monitoring, and (6) chorionic villus SAMPLING. Extensive and thorough assessment of the health status of the fetus is indicated when maternal characteristics, obstetrical complications, and familial and genetic factors place the fetus at risk.

AMNIOTIC FLUID assay is most often done to establish the diagnosis of a genetic disorder, to monitor the fetus sensitized against the mother's RH FACTOR, or to determine fetal lung maturity. Cells floating in the amniotic fluid sample can be examined to detect genetic disorders caused by chromosomal abnormalities and to detect certain metabolic aberrations. NEURAL TUBE DEFECTS such as SPINA BIFIDA and ANENCEPHALY are detected by analyzing the amniotic fluid for ALPHA-FETOPROTEIN (AFP). When an open neural tube defect is present, the amount of alpha-fetoprotein can be increased as much as eight times the normal value.

The amniotic fluid also can be assayed for BILIRUBIN, an indicator of the severity of Rh incompatibility between maternal and fetal blood. Fetal lung maturity can be assessed by evaluating the presence of pulmonary

SURFACTANT, a phospholipid protein, in the amniotic fluid. In normal fetal development the production of surfactant, a substance essential to lung expansion and adequate ventilation after birth, begins at about the 22nd week of gestation; however, surfactant is not present in sufficient quantities until 35 to 36 weeks. Two of its principal constituents, LECITHIN and SPHINGOMYELIN, can be evaluated by measuring the LECITHIN-SPHINGOMYELIN RATIO (L/S ratio) in a sample of amniotic fluid. In general, a ratio greater than 2:1 indicates that the fetal lungs are mature and the newborn infant is not likely to develop RESPIRATORY DISTRESS SYNDROME of the newborn.

ULTRASONOGRAPHY is a noninvasive technique helpful in diagnosing unusual fetal presentations, placenta previa, multiple pregnancy, and fetal abnormalities such as hydrocephalus and hydronephrosis. It also can be used to trace fetal growth by periodic measurement of the biparietal diameter of the head of the fetus, femur length, or head:abdominal circumference ratio.

Chorionic villus SAMPLING is a technique by which a small sample is obtained from the fetal portion of the placenta by aspiration through the cervical canal. It can be used for diagnosis of genetic abnormalities as early as the first trimester.

Chemical assessment of the nutritive and respiratory functions of the placenta can be accomplished by determining the amount of the hormone ESTRIOL in the maternal blood or urine. Throughout gestation a normally functioning placenta produces increasing amounts of estriol, the precursors for the production of which are provided by the fetal adrenal glands. Thus, a normal estriol value in maternal blood or urine indicates that both the placenta and the fetus are healthy.

Fetal monitoring using either ultrasound or direct electronic monitoring equipment to measure fetal heart rate and uterine contractions and the NONSTRESS TEST to evaluate fetal heart rate changes in response to uterine contractions and fetal movements are discussed under FETAL MONITORING.

f. circulation the circulation of blood from the placenta to and through the fetus and back to the placenta. Fetal circulation can be traced as follows: The oxygenated blood is carried from the placenta to the fetus via the umbilical vein. About half of this blood passes through the hepatic capillaries and the rest flows through the ductus venosus into the inferior vena cava. Blood from the vena cava is mostly deflected through the foramen ovale into the left atrium, then to the left ventricle, into the ascending aorta and on to the head and upper body. The arterial oxygenation of this blood is approximately 25 to 28 mm Hg; thus the fetal coronary circulation and brain receive the blood with the highest level of oxygenation.

Deoxygenated blood from the superior vena cava flows into the right atrium, right ventricle, and then into the pulmonary artery. Because of high pulmonary vascular resistance, only about 5 to 10 per cent of the blood in the pulmonary artery flows to the lungs, the majority of it being shunted through the patent ductus arteriosus and then down the descending aorta. The Pa_{O_2} of the blood in the descending aorta is about 22 mm Hg.

Postnatal Changes. After birth the changes in circulation involve closure of three fetal channels, the ductus venosus, the foramen ovale, and the ductus arteriosus. The ductus venosus closes with the clamping of the umbilical cord and inhibition of blood flow through the umbilical vein. The foramen ovale functionally closes after the first few breaths as pressure within the left atrium rises above that in the right atrium. The ductus arteriosus constricts partly in response to higher arterial oxygen levels that occur after the first few breaths. Other postnatal changes include a decrease in pulmonary vascular resistance and a decrease in pulmonary artery pressure. These changes result in the transport of 100 per cent of the cardiac output from the right heart to the lungs for oxygenation and then to the left heart and thence to the aorta.

f. monitoring continuous intrapartal monitoring of the fetal heart rate and uterine contractions for the purpose of reducing preventable fetal and neonatal death by more accurate diagnosis and correction of

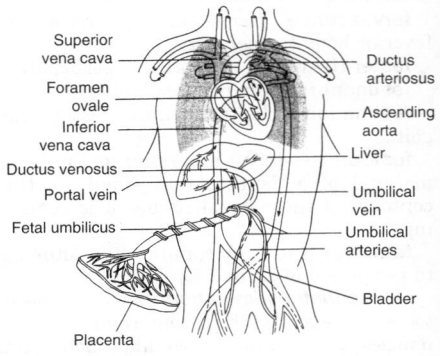

A simplified scheme of the fetal circulation. From Betz et al., 1994.

problems related to fetal distress during labor, such as compression of the umbilical cord or placental insufficiency.

Noninvasive (Indirect) Monitoring. The fetal heart rate is measured using the techniques of ULTRASONOGRAPHY or PHONOCARDIOGRAPHY. Evaluations of this kind provide good data on the fetal heart rate and, unlike direct fetal monitoring, can be used while the amniotic membranes are still intact and the cervix has not yet dilated. These techniques are easier to use than invasive techniques but do not provide information as accurate and precise as that obtained by direct monitoring.

The duration and relative strength of uterine contractions and the length of intervals between them can be measured externally by placing a tokodynamometer on the mother's abdomen at the site of greatest uterine activity. The force of contractions is displayed on a screen. Layers of fat in obese patients and restlessness of the mother interfere with precise external monitoring of uterine contractions. Therefore high-risk patients can be more effectively monitored by internal techniques. (See accompanying illustration.)

Invasive (Direct) Monitoring. Invasive techniques of fetal and maternal monitoring require direct access to the fetus and amniotic sac via the vagina and dilated cervix. Direct electrocardiography of the fetal heart is accomplished by attaching an electrode to the fetal presenting part. Proper placement of the electrode makes the risk to the mother and fetus negligible, and the data obtained are extremely accurate. Direct monitoring of uterine contractions uses an intrauterine amniotic fluid catheter to measure intrauterine pressure changes.

Simultaneous monitoring of the fetal heart rate and uterine contractions is essential to accurate interpretation of events taking place within the uterus during labor. Patterns of a slowing heart rate (deceleration) or increase in rate (acceleration) are examined in the context of the phase of the contraction in which the change in rate occurs. For example, decelerations that take place early during uterine contractions may indicate compression of the fetal head, a normal and expected event. However, a deceleration occurring late in the contraction may indicate placental pathology and uteroplacental insufficiency, a very serious and life-threatening condition. However, maternal hypotension and uterine hypotonus, both of which can be alleviated or corrected, may also cause late deceleration.

Contraction Stress Tests: Oxytocin Challenge Test. The purpose of this test, which is usually not done before the 28th week of gestation, is to assess the respiratory function of the placenta; that is, to determine whether the placenta and fetus will be able to withstand the stress of repetitive contractions during labor, and if they cannot, when and how delivery of the infant should be carried out. It is indicated for high-risk mothers, such as those with diabetes, hypertensive disease of pregnancy, history of a previous stillbirth, or anything else affecting the health status of the fetus. The oxytocin challenge test should not be attempted if placenta previa is present or if the mother has had a previous delivery by midline-incision cesarean section.

OXYTOCIN is given to stimulate enough uterine contractions to provide a sample of fetal response and determine whether there is adequate placental respiratory reserve to maintain the fetus for the remainder of the pregnancy and through labor. Data from the recorded fetal heart rate patterns during contractions are used to assess the status of the fetus and to make decisions about either allowing the pregnancy to continue until the fetus is more mature, or intervening promptly to avoid severe and perhaps fatal stress on the fetus.

Prior to the administration of the oxytocin, the fetal heart rate is monitored for 30 minutes or more to determine baseline variability and fetal movement. Spontaneous movement of the fetus without oxytocin may mean it is not necessary. However, if there is no spontaneous movement, oxytocin is given in quantities sufficient to trigger three or four contractions.

Nipple Stimulation. This involves the application of warm, moist washcloths to the breasts, followed by 10 minutes of massaging and rolling of the nipples. If it is successful in inducing uterine contractions, it obviates the need for an oxytocin challenge test.

Nonstress Test. This test relies on spontaneous fetal activity rather than on oxytocin-induced fetal movement to assess fetal response to uterine contractions. If there is no spontaneous fetal activity, it may be elicited by external rubbing or gentle pressure on the mother's abdomen. Fetal heart rate is monitored externally and correlated with fetal activity. Acceleration of the heart rate can also be induced by vibroacoustic stimulation using an external source of sound such as an artificial larynx applied to the maternal abdomen over the fetal head. Increased confidence in the validity and accuracy of the nonstress test has led to its widespread use and, in many cases, its preference over the more time-consuming and often contraindicated oxytocin challenge test.

Accelerations and Decelerations. Periodic heart rate changes are evaluated in reference to a fetal "baseline" that is determined when there is no stress present. Deviations from the baseline occur in response to uterine contractions and fetal activity that affect fetal oxygenation and transfer of carbon dioxide.

Accelerations are transient increases of the fetal heart rate, occurring at the same time as uterine contractions and coming at anytime during labor. They may be the earliest indicators of fetal distress; however, without other abnormalities of fetal heart rate pattern, they are thought to be reassuring when in response to manipulation, stimulation, or fetal movement.

Decelerations are decreases in the fetal heart rate. The three types are early, late, and variable. *Early deceleration* is believed to be caused by fetal head compression. The fetal heart rate returns to the baseline at or before the end of the uterine contraction and is not associated with an abnormality. *Late deceleration* occurs after the uterus has begun to contract and may not cease with the contraction. It is an ominous sign of fetal distress, is believed to be caused by uteroplacental insufficiency, and is frequently associated with high-risk pregnancy and with maternal hypotension or uterine hyperactivity. *Variable deceleration* occurs at various times in relation to uterine contractions. It could be associated with umbilical cord compression and may be relieved by changing the mother's position.

Early signs that suggest fetal distress include irregularity and mild variable decelerations. Early signs of fetal compromise that are more ominous include further decreased variability, heart rate increased over baseline, and variable or late decelerations. Late signs of fetal distress include no variability, severe variable or late decelerations with minimal variability, bradycardia in relation to baseline heart rate, and a sinusoid pattern to the fetal heart rate.

fetalization (fe″tal-ĭ-za′shun) retention in the adult of structures or other characteristics that at an earlier stage of evolution were only infantile and were lost as the organism matured.

fetation (fe-ta′shun) 1. development of the fetus. 2. pregnancy.

feticide (fēt′ĭ-sīd) destruction of the fetus.

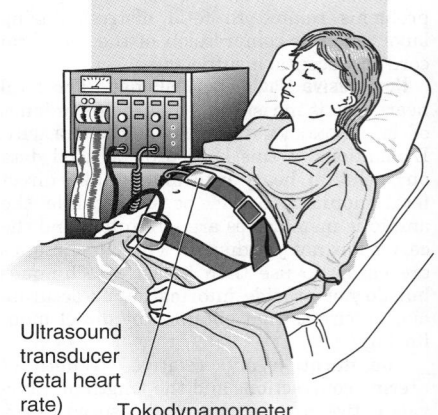

Ultrasound transducer (fetal heart rate) Tokodynamometer (uterine activity)

External fetal monitoring. The heart rate of the fetus is evaluated, particularly in response to uterine activity or contractions. From Malarkey and McMorrow, 2000.

fetid (fet′id) having a rank, disagreeable smell.

fetish (fet′ish, fe′tish) 1. a material object, such as an idol, charm, or talisman, believed by primitive people to have supernatural powers. 2. an inanimate object used to obtain sexual gratification.

fetishism (fet′ish-izm) 1. the worship of fetishes. 2. use of FETISHES as a preferred or necessary adjunct to sexual arousal.

> **transvestic f.** a PARAPHILIA of heterosexual males, characterized by recurrent, intense sexual urges, arousal, or orgasm associated with fantasized or actual CROSS-DRESSING, to the extent that this causes significant distress or impairment in the person's life. Called also transvestism.

fetography (fe-tog′rah-fe) radiography of the fetus in utero.

fetology (fe-tol′o-je) the branch of medicine dealing with the fetus in utero.

fetometry (fe-tom′ĕ-tre) measurement of the fetus, especially of its head.

fetopathy (fe-top′ah-the) a disease or disorder seen in a fetus; see also EMBRYOPATHY.

fetoplacental (fe″to-plah-sen′t′l) pertaining to the fetus and placenta.

α-fetoprotein (fe″to-pro′tēn) alpha-fetoprotein.

fetor (fe′tor) stench or offensive odor.

> **hepatic f., f. hepa′ticus** the peculiar odor of the breath characteristic of hepatic disease.

> **f. o′ris** halitosis.

fetoscope (fe′to-skōp) 1. a specially designed stethoscope for listening to the fetal heart beat. 2. an endoscope for viewing the fetus in utero.

fetoscopy (fe-tos'kah-pe) viewing of the fetus in utero by means of the fetoscope; this is now only rarely done, having been replaced by percutaneous umbilical blood SAMPLING. adj., **fetoscop'ic.**

fetotoxicity (fe"to-tok-sis'ĭ-te) toxic effects on a fetus of a substance that crosses the placental barrier; see also EMBRYOTOXICITY. adj., **fetotox'ic.**

fetus (fe'tus) [L.] the developing young in the uterus, specifically the unborn offspring in the postembryonic period, which in humans is from the third month after fertilization until birth. See also EMBRYO.

The stages of growth of the fetus are fairly well defined. At the end of the first month it has grown beyond microscopic size. After 2 months it is a little over 2.5 cm long, its face is formed, and its limbs are partly formed. By the end of the third month it is 8 cm long and weighs about 30 g; its limbs, fingers, toes, and ears are fully formed, and its sex can be distinguished.

After 4 months the fetus is about 20 cm long and weighs over 200 g. The mother can feel its movements, and usually the health care provider can hear its heartbeat. The eyebrows and eyelashes are formed, and the skin is pink and covered with fine hair called LANUGO. By the fifth month the fetus's body is covered with a cheeselike substance (VERNIX CASEOSA), which serves to protect it in its watery environment. By the end of the fifth month it is 30 cm long, weighs 450 g, and has hair on its head. At the end of the sixth month it is 35 cm long and weighs 900 g, and its skin is very wrinkled.

After 7 months the fetus is 40 cm long and weighs over 1.3 kg, with more fat under its skin. In the male, the testes have descended into the scrotum. By the end of the eighth month it is 45 cm long, may weigh 2.3 kg, and has a good chance of survival if it is born at that time. At the end of 9 months, the average length of a fetus is 50 cm and the average weight is 3.2 kg. adj., **fe'tal.**

   calcified f. a dead fetus that has become calcified *in utero;* called also lithopedion.

   f. in fe'tu a small, imperfect fetus, incapable of independent life, contained within the body of another fetus.

   harlequin f. an infant with a severe and dramatic form of congenital ICHTHYOSIS, manifested by HYPERKERATOSIS with rigid skin; death usually occurs in the first six weeks of life.

   mummified f. a dead fetus that is dried up and shriveled.

   f. papyra'ceus a dead fetus flattened by being pressed against the uterine wall by a living twin.

   parasitic f. in unequal TWINS, an incomplete minor fetus attached to a larger, more completely developed fetus (the AUTOSITE).

FEV forced expiratory volume.

fever (fe'ver) 1. an abnormally high body temperature; called also pyrexia. adj., **fe'brile, fe'verish.** 2. any disease characterized by marked increase of body temperature. For specific diseases, see the eponymic or descriptive name, such as ROCKY MOUNTAIN SPOTTED FEVER or TYPHOID FEVER. Other conditions involving elevated body temperature include HEAT EXHAUSTION and HEAT STROKE.

Normal body temperature when the body is at rest is 37°C (98.6°F). This is an average or mean body temperature that varies from person to person and from hour to hour in an individual. The route by which a body temperature is measured affects the reading. The normal *oral* temperature ranges from 36° to 37.5°C (96.8° to 99.5°F). If the temperature is measured *rectally,* the norm would be 0.5°C (1°F) higher. An *axillary* temperature would be 0.5°C (1°F) lower. Because of these differences, the number should always be followed by the route by which the temperature was taken when the reading is recorded.

Factors that can cause a temporary elevation in body temperature include age, physical activity, emotional stress, and ovulation. If a person has a consistently elevated temperature, fever is said to exist. A *low-grade* fever is marked by temperatures between 37.5° and 38.2°C (99.5° and 101°F) when taken orally. A *high-grade* fever is present when the oral temperature is above 38.2°C (101°F).

Types of fever include *continued* or *continuous fever,* one lasting more than 24 hours without significant variation or any return to normal body temperature; *intermittent fever,* in which at least once during a 24-hour period the fever spikes are separated by a return to normal body temperature; *remittent fever,* in which elevated body temperature shows fluctuations each day but never returns to normal; and *recurrent* (or *relapsing*) *fever,* in which periods of fever and normal body temperature alternate and last about 5 to 7 days each.

The regulation of body temperature is under the control of the HYPOTHALAMUS. *Thermolysis,* or dissipation of body heat, is regulated by the anterior hypothalamus in conjunction with the parasympathetic nervous system. The overall effect of heat loss is accomplished by vasodilation of the peripheral blood vessels, increased sweating, and decreased metabolic and muscular

F

activities. The production and conservation of body heat, or *thermogenesis,* is regulated by the posterior hypothalamus in conjunction with the sympathetic nervous system. The mechanisms by which body heat is produced and conserved are in opposition to those that increase heat loss; that is, by constriction of cutaneous blood vessels, decreased sweat gland activity, and increased metabolic and muscular activities.

Fever develops when there is some disturbance in the homeostatic mechanisms by which the hypothalamus maintains a balance between heat production and peripheral heat loss. Although dehydration, cerebral hemorrhage, heat stroke, thyroxine, and certain other drugs can cause an elevated body temperature or hyperthermia, fever, in the precise sense of the term, occurs as a result of inflammation or infection, or both. During the infectious and inflammatory processes certain substances called *pyrogens* are produced within the body. These *endogenous* pyrogens are the result of inflammatory reactions, such as those that occur in tissue damage, cell necrosis, rejection of transplanted tissues, malignancy, and antigen-antibody reactions. *Exogenous* pyrogens are introduced into the body when it is invaded by bacteria, viruses, fungi, and other kinds of infectious organisms.

Endogenous pyrogens act directly on the hypothalamus, affecting its thermostatic functions by "resetting" it to a higher temperature. When this happens, all of the physiologic activities concerned with heat production and conservation operate to maintain body temperature at a higher setpoint. The symptoms of chill and shivering are the result of increased muscular activity, which is an attempt by the body to raise its temperature to the higher setting. This increased muscular activity is accompanied by an elevation of the metabolic rate, which in turn increases the demand for nutrients and oxygen. Outward signs of these internal activities include a higher pulse rate, increased respirations, and thirst caused by the loss of extracellular water via the lungs. The pulse rate increases at the rate of about eight to ten beats per minute for each degree of temperature rise.

Once the body temperature reaches the setpoint of the hypothalamic thermostat, the mechanisms of heat production and heat loss keep it at a fairly constant level and the fever persists. This is sometimes called the *second stage of fever.* If it continues, fluid and electrolyte losses become more severe and there is evidence of cellular dehydration. During this stage DELIRIUM in older persons and CONVULSIONS in infants and children can occur. Febrile convulsions in children are believed to be closely related to cerebral damage that becomes evident as afebrile convulsions later in life.

Prolonged fever eventually brings about tissue destruction owing to the catabolism of body proteins. Because of this the patient experiences muscle aches and weakness, malaise, and the excretion of albumin in the urine. Anorexia also is present. If the body does not receive a sufficient supply of energy from dietary intake to meet its metabolic needs, it catabolizes its own fat and protein. The patient then rapidly loses weight and can develop KETOSIS and metabolic ACIDOSIS.

The period during which a fever abates is called the period of *defervescence.* It may occur rapidly and dramatically, as the temperature falls from peak to normal in a matter of hours. This is called the *crisis,* that is, the critical point at which the fever is broken. A more gradual resetting of the thermostat and slow decline of the fever is called *resolution* of the fever by *lysis.*

Treatment. It is not always necessary to reduce fever and in many cases it may be best not to treat it, at least until its cause is determined. The fever pattern can provide diagnostic information and is not necessarily harmful unless it is extremely high or the patient has cardiac or respiratory disease and cannot tolerate the additional tachycardia and dyspnea that may accompany fever. An elevated body temperature can inhibit bacterial replication and the action of viruses, spirochetes, and other pathogenic microorganisms.

If it is decided that treatment is necessary, there are two major goals: to identify the cause and to provide symptomatic relief. Antipyretic drugs such as aspirin and acetaminophen (Tylenol) are generally safe and effective. However, acetaminophen is preferred in children and when the patient has gastrointestinal sensitivity, allergy to aspirin, or a clotting disorder or is suspected of having Reye's syndrome.

Fluids and electrolytes are replaced orally or intravenously as indicated by laboratory tests and signs of dehydration. Frequent, small feedings of high-calorie, high-protein foods are recommended to combat fatigue and debility caused by the increased metabolic rate. The selection of oral liquids and foods should be based on the patient's preferences. Vitamin supplements may be prescribed in prolonged, low-grade fevers.

Patient Care. The patient with acute hyperpyrexia or hyperthermia will require extreme measures to lower the body temperature as quickly and safely as possible in order to prevent brain damage. Victims of heat stroke should be cooled rapidly. In order to keep the temperature at a tolerable level until the thermostat is reset, a cooling blanket or hypothermia mattress may be used. Care must be taken to maintain the integrity of the skin and avoid sudden and extreme hypothermia when such a device is used. Other measures include sponging parts of the body with cool water to increase heat loss through evaporation of moisture. The part being sponged should be left exposed to the air until it is almost dry, and then should be lightly covered while another part is being sponged. A cold compress on the forehead helps to reduce the fever and relieve headache and delirium. An alternative to sponging and a cool bath is the application of ice packs to specific parts of the body, such as the abdomen, groin, axillae, and spine. Fanning can also be effective, especially if the patient's torso is covered with a sheet saturated with water.

Chills are uncomfortable and sometimes frightening to the patient. When the patient complains of feeling chilled or cold, some form of external warmth should be provided. An extra blanket is helpful as is a hot water bottle filled with warm, *not hot,* water. As the body temperature declines the difference between body temperature and environmental temperature will decrease and the patient will begin to feel warmer. During the second stage of fever the patient may complain of feeling hot; the skin feels warm to the touch and the face is flushed. These symptoms are the result of vasodilation of surface blood vessels, an attempt by the body to prevent further escalation of the body temperature.

f. of unknown origin (FUO) a febrile illness of at least three weeks' duration with a temperature of at least 38.3°C on at least three occasions and failure to establish a diagnosis in spite of intensive inpatient or outpatient evaluation (three outpatient visits or three days' hospitalization). The duration of febrile illness needed to establish a diagnosis of FUO varies among authorities and is sometimes given as shorter than three weeks. Classic fever of unknown origin, as defined by the preceding criteria, is distinguished from neutropenic and nosocomial FUO, as well as that associated with human immunodeficiency virus infection. In the neutropenic form, fever is accompanied by a neutrophil level that is lower than 500/mm^3 or is expected to fall below that level within one or two days. The nosocomial form is a fever that occurs on several occasions in a hospitalized patient in whom neither fever nor infection was present on admission. In HIV-associated FUO, fever occurs in a person with human immunodeficiency virus infection on several occasions over a period of four weeks of outpatient care or three days of hospitalization. In all three of these forms of FUO, the cause of the fever cannot be determined after three days of investigation, including two days of incubation of cultures.

feverfew (fe′ver-fu″) the dried leaves of the herb *Tanacetum parthenium,* used for migraine, arthritis, rheumatic diseases, and allergy.

feverish (fe′ver-ish) febrile.

fexofenadine (fek″so-fen′ah-dēn) an H$_1$-receptor antagonist used as an ANTIHISTAMINE in the treatment of HAY FEVER and of chronic idiopathic URTICARIA; administered orally as the hydrochloride salt.

fiber (fi′ber) 1. an elongated threadlike structure. 2. dietary fiber. 3. nerve f.

A f's myelinated fibers of the somatic nervous system having a diameter of 1 to 22 μm and a conduction velocity of 5 to 120 meters per second.

accelerating f's, accelerator f's adrenergic fibers that transmit the impulses that accelerate the heart beat.

adrenergic f's nerve fibers of the sympathetic nervous system that liberate NOREPINEPHRINE (and possibly small amounts of EPINEPHRINE) at a synapse when a nerve impulse passes.

alpha f's motor and proprioceptive fibers of the A type having conduction velocities of 70 to 120 meters per second and ranging from 13 to 22 micrometers in diameter.

arcuate f's any of the bow-shaped fibers in the brain, such as those connecting adjacent gyri in the cerebral cortex, or the external or internal arcuate fibers of the medulla oblongata.

association f's nerve fibers that interconnect portions of the cerebral CORTEX within a HEMISPHERE. Short association fibers interconnect neighboring gyri; long fibers interconnect more widely separated gyri and are arranged into BUNDLES or FASCICULI.

B f's myelinated preganglionic autonomic axons having a fiber diameter less than 3 μm and a conduction velocity of 3 to 15 meters per second.

beta f's touch and temperature fibers of the A type having conduction velocities of 30 to 70 meters per second and ranging from 8 to 13 micrometers in diameter.

C f's postganglionic unmyelinated fibers of the autonomic nervous system; also, the unmyelinated fibers at the dorsal roots and at free nerve endings having a diameter of 0.3 to 1.3 μm and a conduction velocity of 0.6 to 2.3 meters per second.

cholinergic f's nerve fibers such as the parasympathetic fibers that liberate ACETYLCHOLINE at a synapse when a nerve impulse passes.

collagen f's, collagenous f's the soft, flexible, white fibers that are the most characteristic constituent of all types of connective tissue, consisting of the protein collagen, and composed of bundles of fibrils that are in turn made up of smaller units (MICROFIBRILS) that show a characteristic crossbanding with a major periodicity of 65 nm.

Corti's f's pillar cells.

crude f. the fiber that remains after food is digested with alkali and acid, which destroys all soluble and some insoluble fiber. It is mainly lignin and cellulose.

depressor f's afferent nerve fibers that when stimulated reflexly cause diminished vasomotor tone and thus decreased arterial pressure.

dietary f. that portion of ingested foodstuffs that cannot be broken down by intestinal enzymes and juices and, therefore, passes through the small intestine and colon undigested. It is composed of CELLULOSE (which is the "skeleton" of plants), HEMICELLULOSE, GUMS, LIGNIN, PECTIN, and other carbohydrates indigestible by humans. Dietary fiber is not to be confused with *crude fiber,* which is the term used in the USDA Handbook and other tables listing the composition of foods. Crude fiber is mainly lignin and cellulose and is the residue remaining after a food has been subjected to a standardized treatment with dilute acid and alkali. Crude fiber measurements usually underestimate actual total dietary fiber by at least 50 per cent.

Vegetables, cereals, and fruits are the main sources of dietary fiber. Although bran is advertised as an excellent source of fiber, it is not unique nor is it as nutritious as fruits and vegetables and some other whole unprocessed cereals. The typical diet in Western countries contains 10 to 30 grams of dietary fiber.

The primary effects of dietary fiber are to increase the bulk of the stool and make it softer by taking up water as it passes through the colon, and to absorb organic wastes and toxins and carry them out of the intestinal tract. The increase in stool bulk hastens the passage of feces and may reduce the length of time the intestinal wall is exposed to toxic substances.

Benefits of a High Fiber Diet. Dietary fiber is helpful in the treatment and prevention of uncomplicated constipation. Unlike strong LAXATIVES, it presents no problems when taken on a long-term basis. METAMUCIL, a medicinal fecal softener, is made from seed husks and is often prescribed for persons having problems with normal bowel activity. Hemorrhoids are aggravated by straining on defecation, and so there is some basis for recommending a high fiber diet for persons who have this condition.

The symptoms of diverticular disease, which is an outpouching of the wall of the colon with subsequent inflammation, are relieved by a high fiber diet. There is evidence to support the theory that the more rapid passage of softer stools through the colon decreases the pressure exerted against its walls and thereby prevents formation of diverticula.

The symptoms of IRRITABLE BOWEL SYNDROME often can be mitigated by fiber. The bulk of fiber keeps the colon mildly distended, thus preventing the development of pockets of high pressure that cause spasm. However, INFLAMMATORY BOWEL DISEASE in which there is a narrowing of the bowel, as in some cases of CROHN'S DISEASE, can be worsened by more roughage in the intestinal tract.

Fiber does have the capacity to unite with intestinal bile salts and dietary cholesterol, preventing their absorption from the gut and hastening their elimination via the intestinal tract. Because of these properties, fiber has been advocated as a preventive measure against the formation of gallstones and the production of atherosclerotic plaques in the blood vessels.

In diabetes mellitus, fiber, when eaten with other foods, somewhat reduces the rise in blood glucose that occurs after eating. Fiber slows the rate of carbohydrate breakdown and absorption from the intestinal tract. The American Cancer Society suggests a diet rich in fiber as a way to lower the incidence of certain kinds of cancer, particularly colorectal cancer.

Some people may have difficulties with a high fiber diet. It can produce abdominal pain, bloating, flatus, and diarrhea. These side effects can be controlled if the fiber is introduced to the diet in small amounts and with an increase in fluid intake. Excessive amounts of fiber can also impair absorption of essential minerals.

elastic f's yellowish fibers of elastic quality traversing the intercellular substance of connective tissue.

gamma f's fibers that conduct touch and pressure impulses and innervate the intrafusal fibers of the muscle spindle; they conduct at velocities of 15 to 40 meters per second and range from 3 to 7 μm in diameter.

gray f's unmyelinated fibers found largely in the sympathetic nerves.

insoluble f. that not soluble in water, composed mainly of lignin, cellulose, and hemicelluloses and primarily found in the bran layers of cereal grains. Its actions include increasing fecal bulk and decreasing free radicals in the gastrointestinal tract.

intrafusal f's modified muscle fibers which, surrounded by fluid and enclosed in a connective tissue envelope, compose the muscle spindle.

light f's muscle fibers poor in sarcoplasm and more transparent than dark fibers.

Mahaim f's short direct connections between the lower atrioventricular node or bundle of His and the ventricular septum, resulting in preexcitation of the ventricular septum and a delta wave. Only right sided connections have been described.

medullated f's, medullated nerve f's myelinated fibers.

motor f's nerve fibers transmitting motor impulses to a muscle fiber.

muscle f. any of the cells of skeletal or cardiac MUSCLE tissue. Skeletal muscle fibers are cylindrical multinucleate cells containing contracting MYOFIBRILS, across which run transverse striations. Cardiac muscle fibers have one or sometimes two nuclei, contain myofibrils, and are separated from one another by an intercalated disk; although striated, cardiac muscle fibers branch to form an interlacing network.

muscle f's, fast twitch paler-colored muscle fibers of larger diameter than slow twitch fibers, and having less sarcoplasm and more prominent cross-striping; used for forceful and rapid contractions over short periods of time.

muscle f's, slow twitch small dark muscle fibers rich in mitochondria, myoglobin, and sarcoplasm and with only faint cross-striping; designed for slow but repetitive contractions over long periods of time.

myelinated f's grayish white nerve fibers encased in a myelin SHEATH; see MYELIN.

nerve f. a slender process of a NEURON, especially the prolonged AXON that conducts nerve impulses away from the cell; classified as either myelinated FIBERS or unmyelinated

FIBERS according to whether they have or do not have a myelin SHEATH.

nonmedullated f's unmyelinated fibers.

osteogenetic f's, osteogenic f's precollagenous fibers formed by osteoclasts and becoming the fibrous component of bone matrix.

postganglionic f's nerve fibers passing to involuntary muscle and gland cells, the cell bodies of which lie in the autonomic ganglia.

preganglionic f's nerve fibers passing to the autonomic ganglia, the cell bodies of which lie in the brain or spinal cord.

pressor f's afferent nerve fibers that when stimulated reflexly cause or increase vasomotor tone and thus increase arterial pressure.

projection f's bundles of axons that connect the cerebral cortex with the subcortical centers, brain stem, and spinal cord.

Purkinje f's modified cardiac fibers in the subendocardial tissue that constitute the terminal ramifications of the conducting system of the heart. The term is sometimes used loosely to denote the entire system of conducting fibers.

radicular f's fibers in the roots of the spinal nerves.

ragged red f's muscle fibers characterized by large collections of structurally abnormal MITOCHONDRIA below the sarcolemmal surface and within the fiber itself that stain red; seen in mitochondrial MYOPATHY and certain other myopathic disorders.

reticular f's immature connective tissue fibers, staining with silver, forming the reticular framework of lymphoid and myeloid tissue, and occurring in interstitial tissue of glandular organs, the papillary layer of the skin, and elsewhere.

Sharpey's f's 1. collagenous fibers that pass from the periosteum and are embedded in the outer circumferential and interstitial lamellae of bone. 2. terminal portions of principal fibers that insert into the cementum of a tooth.

soluble f. that with an affinity for water, either dissolving or swelling to form a gel; it includes gums, pectins, mucilages, and some hemicelluloses, and is primarily found in fruits, vegetables, oats, barley, legumes, and seaweed. It acts to decrease the rate of stomach emptying and increase transit time through the intestine, and also binds bile acids, increasing their excretion. Soluble fiber appears to specifically lower levels of low-density LIPOPROTEIN CHOLESTEROL.

somatic f's, somatic nerve f's nerve fibers, afferent or efferent, that stimulate or activate skeletal muscle and somatic tissues.

spindle f's the microtubules radiating from the centrioles during mitosis and forming a spindle-shaped configuration.

unmyelinated f's nerve fibers that lack a myelin SHEATH; see MYELIN.

visceral f's, visceral nerve f's nerve fibers, afferent or efferent, that stimulate or activate smooth muscle and glandular tissues.

fibercolonoscope (fi″ber-ko-lon′o-skōp) a fiberscope for viewing the colon.

fibergastroscope (fi″ber-gas′tro-skōp) a fiberscope for viewing the stomach.

fiber-illuminated (fi′ber-ĭ-loo″min-a′ted) transmitting light by means of bundles of glass or plastic fibers, utilizing a lens system to transmit the image; said of endoscopes of such design.

fiberoptic (fi″ber-op′tik) pertaining to fiberoptics; coated with flexible glass or plastic fibers having special optical properties and orientation.

fiberoptics (fi″ber-op′tiks) the transmission of an image along flexible bundles of glass or plastic fibers each of which carries an element of the image.

fiberscope (fi′ber-skōp″) a flexible endoscope whose lumen is coated with fiberoptic glass or plastic fibers that have the optical property of transmitting images.

fibr(o)- word element [L.], *fiber; fibrous.*

fibra (fi′brah), pl. *fi′brae* [L.] fiber.

fibrates (fi′brāts) a general term for FIBRIC ACID derivatives, such as GEMFIBROZIL.

fibric acid (fi′brik) any of a group of compounds structurally related to CLOFIBRATE used to reduce plasma levels of TRIGLYCERIDES and CHOLESTEROL.

fibril (fi′bril) a minute fiber or filament. adj., **fi′brillar, fi′brillary**.

collagen f's delicate fibrils of collagen in connective tissue, composed of molecules of tropocollagen in linear array. In Type I collagen, the most common type, the tropocollagen molecules are associated in periodic, staggered arrays that give the appearance of cross-banding, forming unit fibrils; these unit fibrils are aggregated in bundles to form larger fibrils, with longitudinal striations, which may themselves be aggregated into fibers.

muscle f. MYOFIBRIL.

fibrillation (fi″brĭ-la′shun) 1. a small, local, involuntary, muscular contraction, due to spontaneous activation of single muscle cells or muscle fibers. 2. the quality of being made up of fibrils. 3. the initial degenerative

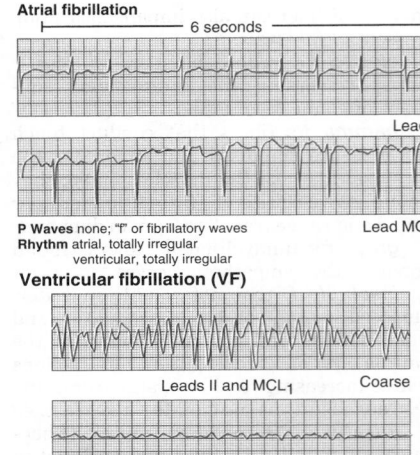

Atrial fibrillation

|← 6 seconds →|

Lead II

Lead MCL₁

P Waves none; "f" or fibrillatory waves
Rhythm atrial, totally irregular
ventricular, totally irregular

Ventricular fibrillation (VF)

Leads II and MCL₁   Coarse

Fine

Fibrillation on an electrocardiographic tracing. From Fenstermacher and Hudson, 1995.

changes in osteoarthritis, marked by softening of the articular cartilage and development of vertical clefts between groups of cartilage cells.

atrial f. a reentrant cardiac ARRHYTHMIA marked by rapid randomized contractions of the atrial myocardium, causing a totally irregular rapid atrial rate. It is recognizable on an ELECTROCARDIOGRAM by the absence of P waves and an irregular ventricular response. It may be controlled by drug therapy or CARDIOVERSION.

ventricular f. a cardiac ARRHYTHMIA marked by fibrillary contractions of the ventricular muscle due to rapid repetitive excitation of myocardial fibers with ineffectual ventricular contraction; on the surface electrocardiogram it is characterized by lack of identifiable QRS complexes. This is a frequent cause of CARDIAC ARREST. An apparatus called a DEFIBRILLATOR is used to alleviate it by delivering an electric shock to the heart muscle; this depolarizes the myocardium and ends the irregular contractions so that the heart can resume normal, regular contractions.

fibrillogenesis (fi-bril″o-jen′ĕ-sis) the formation and development of fibrils.

fibrin (fi′brin) an insoluble protein that is essential to CLOTTING of blood, formed from fibrinogen by action of thrombin.

fibrinocellular (fi″brĭ-no-sel′u-ler) made up of fibrin and cells.

fibrinogen (fi-brin′o-jen) a high-molecular-weight protein in the blood plasma that by the action of THROMBIN is converted into

FIBRIN; called also FACTOR I. In the CLOTTING mechanism, fibrin threads form a meshwork for the basis of a blood clot. Most of the fibrinogen in the circulating blood is formed in the liver. Normal quantities of fibrinogen in the plasma vary from 100 to 700 mg per 100 ml of plasma.

Commercial preparations of human fibrinogen are used to restore blood fibrinogen levels to normal after extensive surgery, or to treat diseases and hemorrhagic conditions that are complicated by AFIBRINOGENEMIA.

f. degradation products fragments of fibrinogen or fibrin degraded by plasmin, which are found in the serum and urine of patients with disseminated intravascular coagulation (DIC) and in the urine of patients who have had renal transplants.

fibrinogenemia (fi-brin″o-jĕ-ne′me-ah) hyperfibrinogenemia.

fibrinogenolysis (fi-brin″o-jĕ-nol′ĭ-sis) the proteolytic destruction of fibrinogen in the circulating blood. adj., **fibrinogenolyt′ic.**

fibrinogenopenia (fi-brin″o-jen″o-pe′ne-ah) hypofibrinogenemia.

fibrinoid (fi′brĭ-noid) 1. resembling fibrin. 2. a homogeneous, eosinophilic, relatively acellular refractile substance with some of the staining properties of fibrin.

fibrinolysin (fi″brĭ-nol′ĭ-sin) 1. plasmin. 2. a preparation of proteolytic enzyme formed from profibrinolysin (plasminogen) by action of physical agents or by specific bacterial kinases; used to promote dissolution of thrombi.

fibrinolysis (fi″brĭ-nol′ĭ-sis) the dissolution of fibrin by enzymatic action. adj. **fibrinolyt′ic.**

fibrinopeptide (fi″brĭ-no-pep′tīd) either of two peptides (A and B) split off from fibrinogen during blood CLOTTING by the action of thrombin.

fibrinoscopy (fi″brin-os′kah-pe) inoscopy.

fibrinous (fi′brĭ-nus) pertaining to or of the nature of fibrin.

fibrinuria (fi″brĭ-nu′re-ah) discharge of fibrin in the urine.

fibroadenoma (fi″bro-ad″ĕ-no′mah) ADENOMA containing fibrous elements.

fibroadipose (fi″bro-ad′ĭ-pōs) both fibrous and fatty.

fibroangioma (fi″bro-an″je-o′mah) an ANGIOMA containing much fibrous tissue.

fibroareolar (fi″bro-ah-re′o-ler) both fibrous and areolar.

fibroblast (fi′bro-blast) an immature fiber-producing cell of connective tissue capable of differentiating into a chondroblast, collagenoblast, or osteoblast. Called also fibrocyte. adj., **fibroblas′tic.**

Fibrinolysis. From Copstead, 1995.

fibroblastoma (fi″bro-blas-to′mah) any tumor arising from FIBROBLASTS, now classified as either FIBROMAS or FIBROSARCOMAS.

fibrocalcific (fi″bro-kal-sif′ik) pertaining to or characterized by partially calcified fibrous tissue.

fibrocarcinoma (fi″bro-kahr″sĭ-no′mah) scirrhous carcinoma.

fibrocartilage (fi″bro-kahr′tĭ-lij) cartilage made up of parallel, thick, compact collagenous bundles, separated by narrow clefts containing the typical cartilage cells (chondrocytes).

fibrochondritis (fi″bro-kon-dri′tis) inflammation of FIBROCARTILAGE.

fibrochondroma (fi″bro-kon-dro′mah) CHONDROMA (cartilaginous tumor) containing areas of FIBROSIS.

fibrocollagenous (fi″bro-ko-laj′ĕ-nus) both fibrous and collagenous; pertaining to or composed of fibrous tissue mainly composed of collagen.

fibrocyst (fi′bro-sist) cystic fibroma.

fibrocystic (fi″bro-sis′tik) characterized by an overgrowth of fibrous tissue and the development of cystic spaces, especially in a gland.

f. disease of breast a disorder characterized by single or multiple benign tumors in the breast; it is the most common disorder of premenopausal women between the ages of 30 and 55, has a familial tendency, and usually abates after menopause. It is due to abnormal hyperplasia of the ductal epithelium and dilatation of the ducts of the mammary gland. Called also chronic cystic mastitis, cystic disease of the breast, and Schimmelbusch's disease.

The tumors of true fibrocystic breast disease can be fluid-filled cysts that arise from glandular elements (blue dome CYSTS), or solid fibrous growths containing connective tissue elements (FIBROADENOMAS). It was once believed that women with this disorder had a two to three times greater than average risk of developing breast cancer; however, recent studies have shown the risk to be only about 1.6 times greater. Since this disorder does predispose a woman to a breast malignancy, it is recommended that it be carefully monitored by periodic examinations, radiologic studies, and biopsies to identify malignant changes in their earliest stages. Baseline mammography is done for the young patient, and routine regular mammograms are done for the older patient.

Since many cases subside on their own after menopause, it is believed that the cyclic appearance of symptoms is linked to estrogen levels.

Symptoms. The most outstanding symptom of fibrocystic disease of the breast is the presence of one or more lumps in the breast. There also is a feeling of breast fullness and tenderness that is more noticeable each month during the premenstrual period. The presence of cysts and lumps in the breast can produce anxiety for the patient and make self-examination more difficult. Additionally, the frequent examinations needed to rule out malignant changes add to physical discomfort and psychologic stress.

Treatment and Patient Care. Medical treatment usually consists of hormonal therapy with synthetic androgen; a commonly used agent is DANAZOL. Synthetic androgens depress ovarian functions, causing a lessening of symptoms. However, common side effects such as menstrual irregularities, weight gain, edema, and acne do occur. Hormonal therapy is usually reserved for those women who cannot find relief through more conservative therapy.

Among the self-help methods that have been successful are reduction of stressors in their lives and dietary restriction of all forms of methylxanthines, particularly caffeine. If the patient is able to eliminate her intake of caffeine, it usually takes at least two months for the effects of the restriction to become apparent. Other measures that have had varying degrees of success include limiting salt and taking a mild diuretic during the week before menstruation begins, applying warm compresses to the breast, wearing a brassiere that gives good support, and taking a mild nonprescription analgesic for discomfort.

Patient education includes instruction in self-examination of the breast with emphasis on the importance of doing this each month. Once the woman becomes accustomed to the location and size of her breast lumps she is better able to detect any change that might occur. The ideal time for breast self-examination is five to seven days after menstruation when swelling and tenderness are usually at a minimum.

f. disease of the pancreas cystic fibrosis.

fibrocystoma (fi″bro-sis-to′mah) cystic fibroma.

fibrodysplasia (fi″bro-dis-pla′zhah) abnormality in development of fibrous connective tissue.

fibrodysplasia ossificans progressiva (FOP) A rare genetic disease characterized by acute soft-tissue swelling after minor trauma, such as dental work or intramuscular injections, that leads to heterotopic bone formation.

fibroelastic (fi″bro-e-las′tik) both fibrous and elastic.

fibroelastosis (fi″bro-e″las-to′sis) overgrowth of fibroelastic elements.

endocardial f. a condition characterized by left ventricular hypertrophy and conversion of the endocardium into a thick fibroelastic coat, with ventricular capacity sometimes reduced, but often increased, leading to HEART FAILURE.

fibroenchondroma (fi″bro-en″kon-dro′-mah) ENCHONDROMA (benign growth of cartilage) containing fibrous elements.

fibroepithelioma (fi″bro-ep″ĭ-the″le-o′mah) a tumor composed of both fibrous and epithelial elements.

fibroglia (fi-brog′le-ah) border fibrils in close relation to the surface of fibroblasts.

fibroglioma (fi″bro-gli-o′mah) a GLIOMA containing excessive fibrous tissue.

fibrohistiocytic (fi″bro-his″te-o-sit′ik) having both FIBROUS and HISTIOCYTIC elements.

fibroid (fi′broid) 1. having a FIBROUS structure; resembling a FIBROMA. 2. fibroma. 3. LEIOMYOMA; *fibroids* is a colloquial term for LEIOMYOMA UTERI.

fibroidectomy (fi″broi-dek′to-me) uterine MYOMECTOMY.

fibrolipoma (fi″bro-lĭ-po′mah) a LIPOMA containing excessive fibrous tissue.

fibroma (fi-bro′mah), pl. *fibromas, fibro′ mata* a tumor composed mainly of fibrous or fully developed connective tissue. Called also fibroid and fibroid tumor.

ameloblastic f. an odontogenic fibroma, marked by simultaneous proliferation of both epithelial and mesenchymal tissue, without formation of enamel or dentin.

cementifying f. cementoblastoma; a tumor usually occurring in the mandible of older persons and consisting of fibroblastic tissue containing masses of cementum-like tissue.

chondromyxoid f. of bone a benign slowly growing tumor of chondroblastic origin, usually affecting the long bones of the lower limb.

cystic f. one that has undergone cystic degeneration.

f. myxomato'des myxofibroma.

nonosteogenic f. a degenerative and proliferative lesion of the medullary and cortical tissues of bone.

odontogenic f. a rare benign tumor of the jaw arising from the embryonic portion of the tooth germ, the dental papilla, or dental follicle.

ossifying f., ossifying f. of bone a benign, relatively slow-growing, central bone tumor, usually of the jaws, especially the mandible, which is composed of fibrous connective tissue within which bone is formed.

fibromatoid (fi-bro'mah-toid) resembling FIBROMA.

fibromatosis (fi″bro-mah-to'sis) 1. the presence of multiple FIBROMAS. 2. the formation of a fibrous tumorlike nodule arising from the deep fascia, with a tendency to local recurrence.

f. gingi'vae, gingival f. a noninflammatory fibrous hyperplasia of the gingivae and palate, manifested as a dense, smooth, or nodular overgrowth of the tissues. It is usually inherited as an autosomal dominant trait, but some cases are idiopathic and others are produced by drugs.

palmar f. fibromatosis involving the palmar fascia, and resulting in Dupuytren's contracture.

plantar f. fibromatosis involving the plantar fascia manifested as single or multiple nodular swellings, sometimes accompanied by pain but usually unassociated with contractures.

fibromatous (fi-bro'mah-tus) pertaining to or of the nature of fibroma.

fibromuscular (fi″bro-mus'ku-ler) both fibrous and muscular.

fibromyalgia (fi″bro-mi-al'jah) diffuse aching pain and stiffness in the muscles and joints.

fibromyitis (fi″bro-mi-i'tis) inflammation of muscle with fibrous degeneration.

fibromyoma (fi″bro-mi-o'mah) leiomyoma.

fibromyomectomy (fi″bro-mi″o-mek'to-me) uterine MYOMECTOMY.

fibromyositis (fi″bro-mi″o-si'tis) inflammation of fibromuscular tissue.

fibromyxoma (fi″bro-mik-so'mah) myxofibroma.

fibromyxosarcoma (fi″bro-mik″so-sahr-ko'mah) a SARCOMA containing fibrous and mucous elements.

fibronectin (fi″bro-nek'tin) an adhesive glycoprotein: one form circulates in plasma and acts as an opsonin, and another is a cell-surface protein that mediates cellular adhesive interactions.

fibroneuroma (fi″bro-noo-ro'mah) neurofibroma.

fibropapilloma (fi″bro-pap″ĭ-lo'mah) a PAPILLOMA containing much fibrous tissue.

fibroplasia (fi″bro-pla'zhah) the formation of fibrous tissue, as occurs normally in the healing of a wound or abnormally in certain tissues. adj., **fibroplas'tic.**

retrolental f. retinopathy of prematurity.

fibrosarcoma (fi″bro-sahr-ko'mah) a SARCOMA arising from collagen-producing FIBROBLASTS.

odontogenic f. a malignant tumor of the jaws, originating from one of the mesenchymal components of the tooth or tooth germ.

fibroserous (fi″bro-sēr'us) composed of both fibrous and serous elements.

fibrosis (fi-bro'sis) formation of fibrous tissue; see also fibroid DEGENERATION. adj., **fibrot'ic.**

congenital hepatic f. a developmental disorder of the liver, marked by formation of irregular broad bands of fibrous tissue containing multiple cysts formed by disordered terminal bile ducts, resulting in vascular constriction and portal hypertension.

cystic f., cystic f. of pancreas see CYSTIC FIBROSIS.

diffuse idiopathic interstitial f., diffuse interstitial pulmonary f. idiopathic pulmonary fibrosis.

endomyocardial f. an idiopathic type of MYOCARDIOPATHY that is endemic in various parts of Africa and rarely in other areas, characterized by CARDIOMEGALY, marked thickening of the endocardium with dense white fibrous tissue that may extend to involve the inner myocardium, and by congestive HEART FAILURE.

idiopathic pulmonary f. chronic inflammatory progressive fibrosis of the pulmonary alveolar walls, with steadily progressive dyspnea, resulting in death from oxygen lack or right heart failure. Most cases are of unknown origin, although some are thought to result from pneumoconiosis, hypersensitivity pneumonitis, scleroderma, and other diseases.

mediastinal f. development of hard white fibrous tissue in the upper portion of the mediastinum, sometimes obstructing the air passages and large blood vessels; called also fibrosing or fibrous mediastinitis.

periureteral f. retroperitoneal fibrosis.

pleural f. fibrosis of the visceral pleura so that part or all of a lung becomes covered with a plaque or a thick layer of nonexpansible fibrous tissue. The more extensive form is called FIBROTHORAX.

postfibrinous f. that occurring in tissues in which fibrin has been deposited.

proliferative f. that in which the fibrous elements continue to proliferate after the original causative factor has ceased to operate.

pulmonary f. idiopathic pulmonary fibrosis.

retroperitoneal f. deposition of fibrous tissue in the retroperitoneal space, producing vague abdominal discomfort, and often causing blockage of the ureters, with resultant hydronephrosis and impaired renal function, which may result in renal failure. Called also Ormond disease.

f. u'teri a morbid condition characterized by overgrowth of the smooth muscle and increase in the collagenous fibrous tissue of the uterus, producing a thickened, coarse, tough myometrium.

fibrositis (fi″bro-si'tis) inflammatory hyperplasia of the white fibrous tissue, especially of the muscle sheaths and fascial layers of the locomotor system, causing pain and stiffness; called also muscular rheumatism.

fibrothorax (fi″bro-thor'aks) adhesion of the two layers of pleura, so that the lung is covered by a thick layer of nonexpansible fibrous tissue (called *dry pleurisy;* see PLEURISY). It is often a consequence of traumatic HEMOTHORAX or of pleural EFFUSION.

fibrous (fi'brus) composed of or containing fibers.

fibrovascular (fi″bro-vas'ku-ler) both fibrous and vascular.

fibula (fib'u-lah) the lateral and smaller of the two bones of the lower leg. See anatomic Table of Bones in the Appendices.

fibular (fib'u-ler) pertaining to the FIBULA; called also peroneal.

ficin (fi'sin) a highly active, crystallizable endopeptidase from the sap of fig trees, which catalyzes the hydrolysis of many proteins at acid (4.1) pH.

FICS Fellow of the International College of Surgeons.

field (fēld) 1. an area or open space, as an operative field or visual field. 2. a range of specialization in knowledge, study, or occupation. 3. in embryology, the developing region within a range of modifying factors.

auditory f. the space or range within which stimuli will be perceived as sound.

disturbed energy f. a NURSING DIAGNOSIS defined as a disruption of the flow of energy surrounding a person's being that results in disharmony of the body, mind, and/or spirit.

energy f. the flow of energy surrounding a person.

extended f. in RADIATION THERAPY, such as for malignant LYMPHOMA, an area of irradiation beyond the involved FIELD. See also under IRRADIATION.

high-power f. the area of a slide visible under the high magnification system of a microscope.

individuation f. a region in which an organizer influences adjacent tissue to become a part of a total embryo.

inverted Y f. in RADIATION THERAPY, such as for malignant LYMPHOMA, a circumscribed area of irradiation below the diaphragm, covering the spleen, extending down the midline, and branching inferiorly to form tails across the inguinal areas.

involved f. in RADIATION THERAPY, such as for malignant LYMPHOMA, the irradiated area when irradiation has been limited to sites of detectable macroscopic disease. See also under IRRADIATION.

low-power f. the area of a slide visible under the low magnification system of a microscope.

magnetic f. that portion of space about a MAGNET in which its action is perceptible.

mantle f. in RADIATION THERAPY, such as for malignant LYMPHOMA, a circumscribed area of irradiation around the shoulders and chest, including the neck, clavicular regions, axillae, and mediastinum. See also under IRRADIATION.

morphogenetic f. an embryonic region out of which definite structures normally develop.

operating f., operative f. an isolated area where surgery is performed; it must be kept sterile by aseptic techniques (see surgical ASEPSIS). Called also surgical field.

sterile f. an operative FIELD that is properly sterile according to surgical ASEPSIS. It includes having all furniture and equipment covered with sterile drapes and all personnel being properly attired.

surgical f. operative field.

visual f. (F) (vf) the area within which stimuli will produce the sensation of sight with the eye in a straight-ahead position.

fifth disease (fifth) erythema infectiosum. In 1905 a French physician assigned numbers to the common childhood diseases characterized by rashes; German measles was "first disease," scarlet fever was "third disease," and so on. Although the numerical nomenclature in general has disappeared, the name fifth disease has persisted.

fight-or-flight reaction alarm reaction.

figure (fig′ūr) an object of a particular form or shape.

hexaxial f. a figure consisting of the axes of the six limb leads drawn through a central point.

triaxial f. a figure formed by the axes of the three bipolar limb leads drawn through a central point.

fila (fi′lah) [L.] plural of FILUM.

filaceous (fi-la′shus) composed of filaments.

filament (fil′ah-ment) 1. a delicate fiber or thread. 2. in an x-ray tube, the wire (cathode) that makes electrons available for interaction with the anode when it is heated to incandescence to form an electron cloud.

actin f. one of the thin contractile filaments in a myofibril, composed mainly of actin; each actin filament is surrounded by three myosin filaments.

myosin f. one of the thick contractile filaments in a myofibril, composed mainly of myosin; each myosin filament is surrounded by six actin filaments.

filamentous (fil″ah-men′tus) composed of long, threadlike structures.

filaria (fĭlar′e-ah), pl. *fila′riae* [L.] a NEMATODE of the superfamily FILARIOIDEA. adj., **fila′rial.**

filariasis (fil″ah-ri′ah-sis) any infection with FILARIAE; the organism causing the most common form is *Wuchereria bancrofti.* Most often encountered in central Africa, the southwest Pacific, and eastern Asia, the disease also occurs in the West Indies and in tropical South and Central America. It is transmitted by the *Culex* mosquito or by mites or flies. The larvae invade lymphoid tissues and then grow to adult worms 2 to 5 cm long. The resulting obstruction of the lymphatic circulation causes swelling, inflammation, and pain. Repeated infections over many years, with impaired circulation and formation of excess connective tissue, may cause enlargement of the affected part, usually a limb or the scrotum. In cases of extreme enlargement, known as ELEPHANTIASIS, the part may swell to many times its normal size. The larvae can be killed by treatment with diethylcarbamazine. Edema of the legs can be reduced by rest and by the use of pressure bandages. The prognosis is favorable for all but the most severe cases.

filaricide (fĭ-lar′ĭ-sīd) an agent that destroys FILARIAE. adj., **filaricid′al.**

filariform (fĭ-lār′ĭ-form) resembling filariae; threadlike.

Filarioidea (fĭ-lar″e-oi′de-ah) a superfamily of parasitic NEMATODES (FILARIAE), the adults of which are threadlike worms that invade the tissues and body cavities, where the female deposits microfilariae (prelarvae). These microfilariae are ingested by bloodsucking insects in whom they pass their developmental stage and are returned to humans by the bites of such insects. See also FILARIASIS.

file (fīl) a collection of records, which may constitute a DATABASE or be a component of one.

digital f. a patient record or part of a record that has been converted to a format that can be transmitted or viewed on a computer.

filgrastim (fil-gras′tim) a human granulocyte colony-stimulating factor produced by recombinant technology; used to enhance neutrophil function, stimulating hematopoiesis and decreasing neutropenia; administered intravenously or subcutaneously.

filiform (fil′ĭ-form, fi′lĭ-form) 1. threadlike. 2. an extremely slender bougie.

fillet (fil′et) 1. a loop, as of cord or tape, for making traction during surgery. 2. in the nervous system, a long band of nerve fibers.

filling (fil′ing) 1. the material inserted into a prepared tooth cavity, usually gold, amalgam, cement, or a synthetic resin. 2. the process of inserting, condensing, shaping, and finishing a filling in a prepared tooth cavity or root canal. Called also *restoration.*

film (film) 1. a thin layer or coating. 2. a thin sheet of material (e.g., gelatin, cellulose acetate) specially treated for use in photography or radiography; used also to designate the sheet after exposure to the energy to which it is sensitive.

bite-wing f. an x-ray film with a protruding tab to be held between the upper and lower teeth, used for a bite-wing RADIOGRAPH of oral structures.

gelatin f., absorbable a sterile, nonantigenic, absorbable, water-insoluble coating used as an aid in surgical closure and repair of defects in the dura mater and pleura and as a local hemostatic.

spot f. a radiograph of a small anatomic area obtained either by rapid exposure during fluoroscopy to provide a permanent record of a transiently observed abnormality, or by limitation of radiation passing through the area to improve definition and detail of the image produced. See also spot-film RADIOGRAPHY.

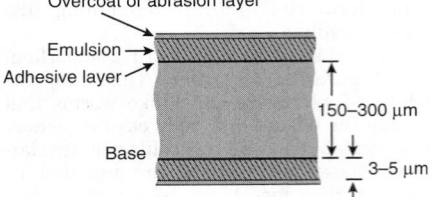

Overcoat or abrasion layer
Emulsion →
Adhesive layer
Base
150–300 μm
3–5 μm

Cross-sectional view of radiographic film. The bulk of the film is the base. The emulsion contains the diagnostic information. From Bushong, 2001.

x-ray f. film sensitized to x-rays, either before or after exposure.

film badge (film baj) a pack of radiographic film or films worn as a badge, used for the detection and approximate measurement of radiation exposure of personnel.

filopressure (fi′lo-presh″er) compression of a blood vessel by a thread.

filter (fil′ter) 1. a device for eliminating or separating certain elements, as (*a*) particles of certain size from a solution, or (*b*) rays of certain wavelength from a stream of radiant energy. 2. to cause such separation or elimination.

membrane f. a filter made up of a thin film of collodion, cellulose acetate, or other material, available in a wide range of defined pore sizes, the smaller ones being capable of retaining all the known viruses.

Millipore f. trademark for a device used to filter nutrient solutions as they are administered intravenously.

vena cava f., vena caval f. a filter used in the inferior VENA CAVA to prevent pulmonary EMBOLISM.

Wood's f. a nickel-oxide filter that holds back all but a few violet rays and passes ULTRAVIOLET RAYS of about 365 nm; see also Wood's LIGHT.

filterable (fil′ter-ah-b′l, fil′trah-b′l) capable of passing through the pores of a FILTER; usually referring to living infectious agents such as VIRUSES that can pass through a filter that retains the usual pathogenic BACTERIA. This attribute was key in the initial discovery of viruses.

filtrable filterable.

filtrate (fil′trāt) a liquid or gas that has passed through a filter.

filtration (fil-tra′shun) passage through a filter or other material that prevents passage of certain molecules, particles, or substances.

filum (fi′lum), pl. *fi′la* [L.] a threadlike structure or part.

f. termina′le a slender, threadlike prolongation of connective tissue from the conus medullaris to the back of the coccyx.

fimbria (fim′bre-ah), pl. *fim′briae* [L.] 1. a fringe, border, or edge; a fringelike structure. 2. pilus (def. 2).

fimbriae of fallopian tube the numerous divergent fringelike processes on the distal part of the infundibulum of the FALLOPIAN TUBE; called also fimbriae of uterine tube.

f. hippocam′pi the band of white matter along the median edge of the ventricular surface of the hippocampus.

fimbriae of uterine tube fimbriae of fallopian tube.

fimbriate (fim′bre-āt) fringed.

finasteride (fi-nas′ter-īd) an inhibitor of 5α-REDUCTASE, used in the treatment of benign prostatic hyperplasia and as a hair growth stimulant in the treatment of androgenetic alopecia; administered orally.

finger (fing′ger) one of the five digits of the hand.

baseball f. mallet finger.

clubbed f. one affected by CLUBBING.

hammer f. mallet f.

index f. forefinger.

mallet f. partial permanent flexion of the terminal phalanx of a finger caused by a ball or other object striking the end or back of the finger, resulting in rupture of the attachment of the extensor tendon. Called also baseball or hammer finger.

webbed f's SYNDACTYLY of the fingers.

finger-nose test (fing′ger nōz) a test for coordinated movements of the extremities; the patient is directed to close the eyes, and, with arm extended to one side, slowly try to touch the end of the nose with the tip of the index finger.

fingerprint (fing′ger-print) 1. an impression of the cutaneous ridges of the fleshy distal portion of a finger. 2. in biochemistry, the characteristic pattern of a peptide after subjection to an analytical technique.

DNA f., genetic f. the highly specific HYBRIDIZATION pattern generated by tandem REPEATS and other patterns of the DNA in an individual's GENOME.

first aid (ferst′ ād′) 1. emergency care and treatment of an injured or ill person before complete medical and surgical treatment can be secured. 2. in the NURSING INTERVENTIONS CLASSIFICATION, a nursing INTERVENTION defined as providing initial care of a minor injury.

FISH fluorescent in situ hybridization.

fish poisoning poisoning due to ingestion of poisonous fish; some have the poison in their muscles, skin, or other organs, while others secrete poisons. It is marked by various gastrointestinal and neurological disturbances that sometimes can be fatal. The most common kinds are CIGUATERA and TETRODOTOXISM. Called also ichthyosarcotoxism.

Fishberg concentration test (fish′berg) a test for renal function; the patient is given supper with not more than 200 mL of fluid and nothing thereafter. Urine voided during the night is discarded. The morning urine is saved, the patient kept in bed, and the urine of 1 hour later and of 2 hours later is saved. If the specific gravity of any of these 3 specimens is less than 1.024 there is impairment of renal concentration.

Fisher syndrome (fish′er) a variant of acute idiopathic POLYNEURITIS characterized by areflexia, ataxia, and ophthalmoplegia.

fission (fish′un) 1. the act of splitting. 2. asexual reproduction in which the cell divides into two (binary fission) or more (multiple fission) daughter parts, each of which becomes an individual organism. 3. nuclear fission; the splitting of the atomic nucleus, with release of energy.

binary f. the halving of the nucleus and then of the cytoplasm of the cell, as occurs in protozoa.

fissiparous (fĭ-sip′ah-rus) propagated by fission.

fissula (fis′u-lah) [L.] a small cleft.

fissura (fĭsu′rah), pl. *fissu′rae* [L.] fissure.

fissure (fish′er) 1. a narrow slit or cleft, especially one of the deeper or more constant furrows separating the gyri of the brain. 2. a deep cleft in the surface of a tooth, usually due to imperfect fusion of the enamel of the adjoining dental lobes. It can be treated with a dental SEALANT to decrease risk of CARIES.

abdominal f. a congenital cleft in the abdominal wall; see also GASTROSCHISIS and THORACOCELOSCHISIS. Called also celoschisis.

anal f., f. in ano a painful lineal ulcer at the margin of the anus.

anterior median f. a longitudinal furrow along the midline of the ventral surface of the spinal cord and medulla oblongata.

f. of Bichat transverse fissure (def. 2).

branchial f. pharyngeal groove.

central f. fissure of Rolando.

collateral f. a longitudinal fissure on the inferior surface of the cerebral hemisphere between the fusiform gyrus and the hippocampal gyrus.

Henle's f's spaces filled with connective tissue between the muscular fibers of the heart.

hippocampal f. one extending from the splenium of the corpus callosum almost to the tip of the temporal lobe; called also hippocampal sulcus.

longitudinal f. the deep fissure between the two cerebral HEMISPHERES.

palpebral f. the longitudinal opening between the eyelids.

portal f. porta hepatis.

posterior median f. 1. a shallow vertical groove in the closed part of the medulla oblongata, continuous with the posterior median fissure of the spinal cord. 2. a shallow vertical groove dividing the spinal cord throughout its length in the midline posteriorly; called also posterior median sulcus.

presylvian f. the anterior branch of the fissure of Sylvius.

pudendal f. rima pudendi.

Rolando's f., f. of Rolando a groove running obliquely across the superolateral surface of a cerebral HEMISPHERE, separating the frontal LOBE from the parietal LOBE. Called also central fissure and central sulcus.

f. of round ligament one on the visceral surface of the liver, lodging the round ligament in the adult.

sylvian f., f. of Sylvius one extending laterally between the temporal and frontal lobes, and turning posteriorly between the temporal and parietal lobes.

transverse f. 1. porta hepatis. 2. the transverse cerebral fissure between the diencephalon and the cerebral hemispheres; called also fissure of Bichat.

zygal f. any of the fissures on the cerebral cortex that consist of two branches connected by a stem.

fistula (fis′tu-lah), pl. *fistulas, fis′tulae* [L.] any abnormal tubelike passage within body tissue, usually between two internal organs or leading from an internal organ to the body surface. Some fistulas are created surgically for diagnostic or therapeutic purposes; others occur as result of injury or as congenital abnormalities. Among the many kinds of fistulas, the anal type (FISTULA IN ANO) is one of the most common. It generally develops as a result of a break or fissure in the wall of the anal canal or rectum, or an abscess there. Treatment is by surgery.

In women, difficult labor in childbirth may result in formation of a vesicovaginal FISTULA between the bladder and the vagina with resulting leakage of urine into the vagina. In a vesicointestinal FISTULA, there is leakage of urine from the bladder into the intestine. In a rectovaginal FISTULA, feces escape through the wall of the anal canal or rectum into the vagina. This condition, formerly a serious hazard of childbirth, is now rare; like other kinds of fistula, it can be corrected by surgery.

With the types of fistulas described here, typical symptoms are pain in the affected region and an abnormal discharge through the skin near the anus or through the vagina. Fistulas at different places of the body may be caused by TUBERCULOSIS, ACTINOMYCOSIS (a fungus infection), the presence of DIVERTICULA, or certain other serious diseases, and the fistula itself may be a site of infection and discomfort.

abdominal f. one between a hollow abdominal organ and the surface of the abdomen.

anal f., f. in a′no one opening on the cutaneous surface near the anus, which may or may not communicate with the rectum.

arteriovenous f. one between an artery and a vein, either pathologic (such as a varicose ANEURYSM) or surgically created to ensure an access site for HEMODIALYSIS. The site must be allowed 6 to 8 weeks to mature before it can be cannulated. Such a fistula may be the anastomosis of a natural artery and vein, a bovine graft, or a synthetic polytetrafluoroethylene (PTFE) graft. The bovine graft is taken from the bovine carotid artery and anastomosed to the vein and artery of the patient. In a PTFE graft, fibers are woven into a mesh called Gore-Tex and made into a sleeve and flange; this is available in a variety of sizes.

Precautions necessary to insure patient safety when caring for an individual with an arteriovenous fistula include frequent assessments for adequate circulation in the fistula and the distal extremity. A bruit or thrill can be heard over the access site. Blood pressure measurements, withdrawal of blood, injections, and administration of intravenous fluids should not be done on the extremity with such a fistula.

blind f. one open at one end only, opening on the skin (external blind fistula) or on an internal surface (internal blind fistula).

branchial f. a persistent pharyngeal GROOVE (branchial CLEFT).

Brescia-Cimino f. an arteriovenous fistula for HEMODIALYSIS access, connecting the cephalic vein and radial artery.

bronchopleural f. one between a bronchus and the pleural cavity, causing an air leak into the pleural cavity; sometimes seen as a complication of empyema, fibrosis, or pneumonia.

cerebrospinal fluid f. one between the subarachnoid space and a body cavity, such as from head trauma or bone erosion, with leakage of cerebrospinal fluid, usually in the form of RHINORRHEA or OTORRHEA.

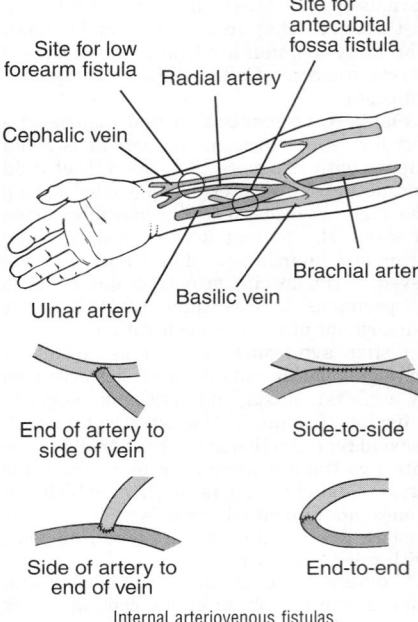

Internal arteriovenous fistulas.

complete f. one extending from the skin to an internal body cavity.

craniosinus f. one between the cerebral space and a paranasal sinus, permitting escape of cerebrospinal fluid into the nose.

Eck's f. an artificial communication made between the portal vein and the vena cava.

enterocutaneous f. see ENTEROCUTANEOUS FISTULA.

enterovesical f. one connecting some part of the intestine with the urinary bladder; called also *vesicoenteric f.*

fecal f. one between the colon and the external surface of the body, discharging feces.

gastric f. 1. one communicating between the stomach and some other body part. 2. a passage created artificially through the abdominal wall into the stomach.

horseshoe f. one near the anus, having a semicircular tract with both openings on the skin.

incomplete f. blind fistula.

perilymph f. rupture of the round WINDOW with leakage of PERILYMPH into the inner ear, so that changes in middle ear pressure directly affect the inner ear, causing sensorineural DEAFNESS as well as dizziness, vertigo, nausea, and vomiting. Head trauma and dramatic changes in atmospheric pressure are the most common causes. The usual treatment is restriction in activity (sometimes with complete bed rest), so that the fistula can heal. Surgical repair may be necessary, consisting of placement of a graft over the defect.

pilonidal f. PILONIDAL SINUS.

pulmonary arteriovenous f. a congenital fistula between the pulmonary arterial and venous systems, allowing unoxygenated blood to enter the systemic circulation.

rectovaginal f. one between the rectum and vagina.

rectovesical f. one between the rectum and urinary bladder.

salivary f. one between a salivary duct or gland and the cutaneous surface, or into the mouth through an abnormal pathway.

thoracic f. one communicating with the thoracic cavity.

umbilical f. one communicating with the intestine or urachus at the umbilicus.

urinary f. any fistula communicating between the urinary tract and another organ or the surface of the body.

vesicoenteric f., vesicointestinal f. enterovesical fistula.

vesicovaginal f. one from the bladder to the vagina.

fistulectomy (fis″tu-lek′to-me) excision of a fistula.

fistulization (fis″tu-lĭ-za′shun) 1. the process of becoming fistulous. 2. surgical creation of a fistula.

fistulotomy (fis″tu-lot′ah-me) incision of a fistula.

fistulous (fis′tu-lus) pertaining to or of the nature of a fistula.

fixation (fik-sa′shun) 1. the act or operation of holding, suturing, or fastening in a fixed position. 2. the condition of being held in a fixed position. 3. in psychiatry, a term with two related but distinct meanings: (*a*) arrest of development at a particular stage (if this is temporary it is a normal reaction to difficulties, but if continued it is a cause of emotional problems); and (*b*) a close and suffocating attachment to some person, especially a childhood figure such as a parent. 4. in microscopy, the treatment of material so that its structure can be examined in greater detail with minimal alteration of the normal state, and also to provide information concerning the chemical properties (as of cell constituents) by interpretation of fixation reactions. 5. in chemistry, the process whereby a substance is removed from the gaseous or solution phase and localized, as in carbon dioxide or nitrogen fixation. 6. in ophthalmology, direction of the gaze so that the visual image of the object falls on the fovea centralis. 7. in film processing, the chemical removal of all

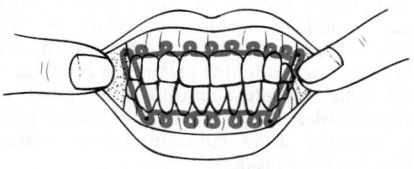

Teeth wired in intermaxillary fixation. From Ignatavicius et al., 1995.

unexposed and undeveloped silver compounds of the film emulsion, as on x-ray films.

complement f. see COMPLEMENT FIXATION.

intermaxillary f. (IMF) a technique used to stabilize a fractured jaw; the teeth are wired or banded together. Extreme caution must be exercised to insure that oral secretions and vomitus are not aspirated as the patient is unable to expectorate any fluids. Antiemetics are often administered to prevent vomiting. Wire cutters should be kept with the patient at all times.

fixative (fik′sah-tiv) an agent used in preserving a histologic or pathologic specimen so as to maintain the normal structure of its constituent elements.

fixer (fik′ser) the chemical used to remove unexposed, underdeveloped silver compounds and to harden gelatin or emulsion on film.

flaccid (flak′sid) 1. weak, lax, or soft; applied especially to muscles. 2. atonic.

flagella (flah-jel′ah) plural of FLAGELLUM.

flagellar (flah-jel′er) of or pertaining to a flagellum.

flagellate (flaj′ĕ-lāt) 1. having flagella. 2. any microorganism having flagella. 3. mastigote. 4. to practice FLAGELLATION.

flagellation (flaj″ĕ-la′shun) 1. whipping or being whipped to achieve erotic pleasure. 2. exflagellation. 3. the formation or arrangement of flagella on an organism or surface.

flagelliform (flah-jel′ĭ-form) shaped like a flagellum or lash.

flagellin (flaj′ĕ-lin) a protein (mol. wt. approximately 40,000) occurring in the flagella of bacteria, which is composed of subunits arranged in several-stranded helix formation somewhat resembling myosin in structure, and sometimes containing ε-N-methyl lysine. Its composition varies with the species; thus flagellin antibodies are species specific.

flagellosis (flaj″ĕ-lo′sis) infection with MASTIGOTES (flagellates).

F

flagellum (flah-jel'um), pl. *flagel'la* [L.] a long, mobile, whiplike appendage arising from a basal body at the surface of a cell, serving as a locomotor organelle; in eukaryotic cells, flagella contain nine pairs of microtubules arrayed around a central pair; in bacteria, they contain tightly wound strands of flagellin.

Flagyl (flag'l) trademark for preparations of METRONIDAZOLE, an ANTIBACTERIAL and antiprotozoal AGENT.

flail (flāl) exhibiting abnormal or pathologic mobility, such as a FLAIL CHEST or a flail JOINT.

   f. chest a loss of stability of the chest wall due to three or more ribs that are broken in two or more places as a result of a crushing chest injury. The loose chest segment moves in a direction in the reverse of normal; that is, the segment moves inward during inhalation and outward during exhalation (PARADOXICAL RESPIRATION). Other manifestations include shortness of breath, cyanosis, and extreme pain in the area of trauma.

   Emergency treatment is aimed at stabilizing the loose chest segment to reduce ineffective and exhausting chest movement and provide for adequate ventilation of the lungs. The patient is transported lying on the affected side to further stabilize the chest wall and enable the use of the unaffected side for respiration.

flame (flām) 1. the luminous, irregular appearance usually accompanying combustion, or an appearance resembling it. 2. to render sterile by exposure to a flame.

flank (flangk) lateral region.

flap (flap) 1. a mass of tissue for GRAFTING, usually including skin, only partially removed from one part of the body so that it retains its own blood supply during transfer to another site. 2. an uncontrolled movement.

   advancement f. sliding flap.

   axial pattern f. a myocutaneous flap containing an artery in its long axis.

   free f. an island flap detached from the body and reattached at the distant recipient site by microvascular anastomosis.

   island f. a flap consisting of skin and subcutaneous tissue, with a pedicle made up of only the nutrient vessels.

   jump f. one cut from the abdomen and attached to a flap of the same size on the forearm. The forearm flap is transferred later to some other part of the body to fill a defect there.

   myocutaneous f. a compound flap of skin and muscle with adequate vascularity to permit sufficient tissue to be transferred to the recipient site. See also axial pattern flap and random pattern flap.

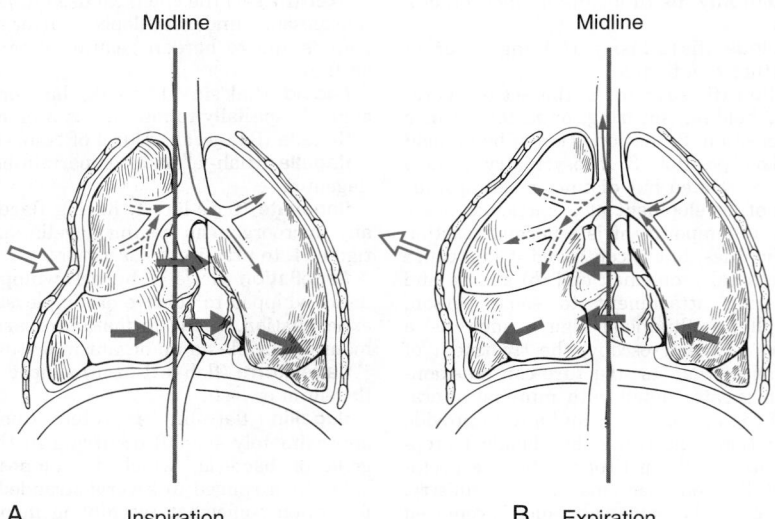

Flail chest. *A,* Inspiration. As intrapleural pressure becomes increasingly negative, the flail segment and its underlying lung tissue are sucked inward, collapsing the lung on the affected side and shifting the mediastinum toward the unaffected side. *B,* Expiration. As intrapleural pressure becomes less negative, the flail segment and underlying tissue are pushed outward, and the mediastinum shifts to the affected side. Some air moves between the lungs instead of passing through the upper airways. Large arrows indicate structural movement; dashed arrows indicate abnormal air movement; small arrows indicate normal air movement; open arrows indicate flail segment movement. From Kitt et al., 1995.

pedicle f. a flap consisting of the full thickness of the skin and the subcutaneous tissue, attached by tissue through which it receives its blood supply. Called also pedicle graft.

random pattern f. a myocutaneous flap with a random pattern of arteries, as opposed to an axial pattern flap.

rope f. tube flap.

rotation f. a local pedicle flap whose width is increased by having the edge distal to the defect form a curved line; the flap is then rotated and a counterincision is made at the base of the curved line, which increases the mobility of the flap.

skin f. a full-thickness mass or flap of tissue containing epidermis, dermis, and subcutaneous tissue.

sliding f. a flap carried to its new position by a sliding technique; called also advancement flap.

tube f., tubed pedicle f. a bipedicle flap made by elevating a long strip of tissue from its bed except at the two extremities, the cut edges then being sutured together to form a tube.

flare (flār) 1. a diffuse area of redness on the skin around the point of application of an irritant, due to vasomotor reaction. 2. a red streak or patchy urticaria along a vein, usually associated with the intravenous infusion of a hypotonic solution or of certain medications. It normally disappears within one to two hours, and almost never lasts longer than 12 to 24 hours.

flask (flask) a laboratory vessel, usually of glass and with a constricted neck.

flatfoot (flat´foot) a condition in which one or more arches of the foot have flattened out; called also pes planus, pes valgus, platypodia, and tarsoptosis.

flatness (flat´nes) a peculiar sound lacking resonance, heard on percussing an abnormally solid part.

flatulence (flat´u-lens) excessive formation of gases in the stomach or intestine.

flatulent (flat´u-lent) characterized by flatulence; distended with gas.

flatus (fla´tus) 1. gas or air in the gastrointestinal tract. 2. gas or air expelled through the anus.

flatworm (flat´werm) an individual organism of the phylum PLATYHELMINTHES; those parasitic in humans include TAPEWORMS and FLUKES. Called also platyhelminth.

flav(o)- word element [L.], *yellow.*

flavin (fla´vin) any of a group of water-soluble yellow pigments widely distributed in animals and plants, including riboflavin and yellow enzymes.

f. adenine dinucleotide (FAD) a coenzyme that is a condensation product of

riboflavin phosphate and adenylic acid; it forms the prosthetic group (non–amino acid component) of certain enzymes, including D-amino acid oxidase and xanthine oxidase, and is important in electron transport in mitochondria.

f. mononucleotide (FMN) a derivative of riboflavin consisting of a three-ring system (isoalloxazine) attached to an alcohol (ribitol); it acts as a coenzyme for a number of oxidative enzymes, including L-amino acid oxidase and cytochrome C reductase.

Flavivirus a genus of FLAVIVIRUSES of worldwide distribution, containing about 75 species in 9 serogroups. It includes the viruses that cause YELLOW FEVER, DENGUE, Japanese B ENCEPHALITIS, KYASANUR FOREST DISEASE, St. Louis ENCEPHALITIS, tick-borne ENCEPHALITIS, and West Nile ENCEPHALITIS. Mosquitoes are the most common vector, with some species being tick-borne and some having no known vector.

flavivirus (fla´vī-vi″rus) any in a family of RNA viruses that includes significant causes of human disease. See *Flavivirus* and *Hepacivirus.*

Flavobacterium (fla″vo-bak-tēr´e-um) a genus of gram-negative, aerobic or facultatively anaerobic, rod-shaped bacteria, characteristically producing a yellow pigment. Organisms occur widely in soil and water and are opportunistic pathogens in humans. *F. meningosep´ticum* causes a highly fatal meningitis with septicemia in premature and newborn infants and a milder bacteremia in adults; *F. odora´tum* occurs in wound infections and urinary tract infections.

flavoenzyme (fla´vo-en´zīm) any enzyme containing a flavin nucleotide (FMN or FAD) as a prosthetic group (non–amino acid component).

flavoprotein (fla″vo-pro´tēn) a conjugated protein containing a flavin nucleotide.

flavoxate (fla-voks´āt) a smooth muscle RELAXANT administered orally as the hydrochloride salt as a urinary tract ANTISPASMODIC for relief of symptoms associated with various urologic disorders.

fl dr fluid dram.

flea (fle) a small, wingless, bloodsucking insect. Many fleas are ectoparasites and may act as disease carriers; they act as vectors of such diseases as plague, tularemia, and brucellosis.

flecainide (flĕ-ka´nīd) a sodium channel blocking AGENT that decreases the rate of cardiac conduction and increases the ventricular refractory period; used as the acetate salt in treatment of life-threatening ARRHYTHMIAS.

Fleming (flem'ing) Sir Alexander (1881–1955). Scottish bacteriologist and discoverer of PENICILLIN. He was born at Lochfield in Scotland and served as a captain in the army medical corps during World War I. The first result of his search for an antibacterial substance that would not be toxic to human tissue was the discovery of lysozyme, but his epochal discovery was of penicillin in 1938. In 1943 he was made fellow of the Royal Society, was knighted and given the John Scott medal in 1944, and was awarded the Nobel prize in 1945.

flesh (flesh) the soft muscular tissue of the body.

goose f. transitory erection of the hair follicles due to contraction of the arrectores muscles, a reflection of sympathetic nerve discharge such as occurs with cold or shock; called also cutis anserina.

proud f. exuberant amounts of soft, edematous, unhealthy-looking granulation tissue developing during healing of large surface wounds.

flex (fleks) to bend or put in a state of FLEXION.

Flexeril (flek'sah-ril) trademark for a preparation of CYCLOBENZAPRINE hydrochloride, a skeletal muscle RELAXANT.

flexibilitas (flek″sĭ-bil'ĭ-tas) [L.] flexibility.

ce'rea f. CEREA FLEXIBILITAS.

flexibility (flek″sĭ-bil'ĭ-te) the state of being unusually pliant.

waxy f. cerea flexibilitas.

flexion (flek'shun) 1. the act of bending or the condition of being bent. 2. in obstetrics, the normal bending forward of the head of the fetus in the uterus or birth canal so that the chin rests on the chest, thereby presenting the smallest diameter of the vertex.

plantar f. bending of the toes or foot downwards toward the sole.

flexor (flek'ser) 1. causing FLEXION. 2. a muscle that FLEXES a joint; see MUSCLE.

flexorplasty (flek'ser-plas″te) plastic surgery of flexor muscles.

flexura (flek-shoo'rah), pl. *flexu'rae* [L.] flexure.

flexure (flek'sher) a bend or fold.

caudal f. the bend at the aboral end of the embryo.

cephalic f. the curve in the mid-brain of the embryo.

cervical f. a bend in the neural tube of the embryo at the junction of the brain and spinal cord.

colic f., left the angular junction of the transverse and descending colon.

colic f., right the angular junction of the ascending and transverse colon.

dorsal f. one of the flexures in the mid-dorsal region of the embryo.

duodenojejunal f. the bend at the junction of the duodenum and jejunum.

hepatic f. right colic flexure.

lumbar f. the ventral curvature in the lumbar region of the back.

mesencephalic f. a bend in the neural tube of the embryo at the level of the mesencephalon, or mid-brain.

pontine f. a flexure of the hindbrain in the embryo.

sacral f. caudal flexure.

sigmoid f. sigmoid colon.

splenic f. left colic flexure.

flight of ideas a nearly continuous flow of rapid speech that jumps from topic to topic, usually based on discernible associations, distractions, or plays on words, but in severe cases so rapid as to be disorganized and incoherent. It is most commonly seen in manic episodes but may also occur in other mental disorders, such as in manic phases of schizophrenia.

flint disease (flint) chalicosis.

floaters (flo'ters) "spots before the eyes"; deposits in the vitreous of the eye, usually moving about and probably representing fine aggregates of vitreous protein occurring as a benign degenerative change.

floating (flōt'ing) the temporary assignment of a nurse to a different patient care unit from the usual assignment.

floccillation (flok″sĭ-la'shun) carphology; involuntary picking at the bedclothes, seen in grave fevers and in conditions of great exhaustion.

floccose (flok'ōs) wooly; said of bacterial growth composed of short, curved chains variously oriented.

flocculation (flok″u-la'shun) the formation of a precipitate or agglomerate in the form of downy tufts or floccules.

f. test any serologic test in which FLOCCULATION takes place; usually applied to a variant form of the PRECIPITIN REACTION.

flocculent (flok'u-lent) containing downy or flaky shreds.

flocculus (flok'u-lus), pl. *floc'culi* [L.] 1. a small tuft, as of wool or similar material, or small mass of other fibrous material such as one of the flakes of a flocculent solution. 2. one of the small paired, partially detached lateral lobules continuous with the nodule of the CEREBELLUM, separated from each cerebellar HEMISPHERE by a fissure; they form part of the flocculonodular LOBE.

flooding (flud'ing) in behavior therapy, a form of DESENSITIZATION for the treatment of phobias and related disorders in which the patient is repeatedly exposed to highly distressing stimuli without being able to escape but without danger, until the lack of reinforcement of the anxiety response causes its extinction. In general, the term is used for actual exposure to the stimuli, with IMPLOSION used for imagined exposure, but the two terms are sometimes used synonymously to describe either or both types of exposure. Compare systematic DESENSITIZATION.

flora (flor′ah) the collective plant organisms of a given locality.

intestinal f. the bacteria normally residing within the lumen of the intestine; some are aids in digestion and food breakdown.

flow (flo) 1. the movement of a liquid or gas. 2. the amount of a fluid that passes through an organ or part in a specified time; called also flow rate.

forced expiratory f. **(FEF)** the rate of airflow recorded in measurements of forced vital CAPACITY, usually calculated as an average flow over a given portion of the expiratory curve; the portion between 25 and 75 per cent of forced vital capacity is called the maximal midexpiratory FLOW. Called also forced expiratory flow rate.

laminar f. smooth, uninterrupted flow as of a gas through a tube.

maximal expiratory f. $FEF_{200-1200}$; the rate of airflow at forced vital CAPACITY, represented graphically as the slope of the line connecting the points 200 mL and 1200 mL on the forced expiratory volume curve. See also PULMONARY FUNCTION TESTS. Called also maximal expiratory flow rate.

maximal midexpiratory f. FEF_{25-75}; the maximum rate of airflow measured between expired volumes of 25 and 75 per cent of the VITAL CAPACITY during a forced expiration; represented graphically as the slope of the line connecting the points on the forced expiratory volume curve at 25 and 75 per cent of the forced vital capacity. See also PULMONARY FUNCTION TESTS. Called also maximal midexpiratory flow rate.

renal plasma f. **(RPF)** the amount of plasma that perfuses the kidneys per unit time, approximately 90 per cent of the total constitutes the *effective renal plasma flow,* the portion that perfuses functional renal tissue such as the glomeruli.

turbulent f. flow that is agitated or haphazard.

flowmeter (flo′me-ter) an apparatus for measuring the rate of flow of liquids or gases.

Doppler ultrasonic f., Doppler ultrasound f. see DOPPLER ULTRASONIC FLOWMETER.

ultrasonic f. ultrasound flowmeter.

ultrasonic Doppler f. Doppler ultrasonic flowmeter.

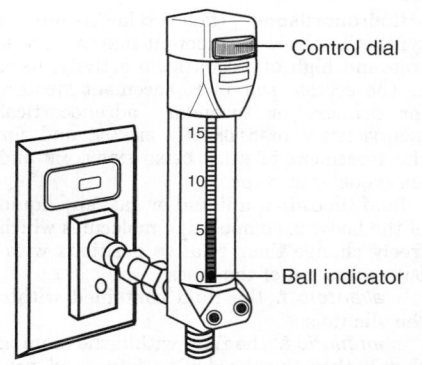

An oxygen flowmeter. From Lammon et al., 1995.

ultrasound f. any of various types of flowmeters that use ULTRASOUND techniques to measure blood flow, such as the DOPPLER ULTRASONIC FLOWMETER.

ultrasound Doppler f. Doppler ultrasonic flowmeter.

flow sheet a patient care record that documents interventions through the use of check marks and brief notations.

floxuridine (floks-ūr′ĭ-dēn) an ANTIMETABOLITE, derived from FLUOROURACIL and used as an antineoplastic AGENT by intra-arterial administration for treatment of liver metastases from gastrointestinal malignancies.

fl oz fluid ounce.

flu (floo) popular name for INFLUENZA.

intestinal f. see INTESTINAL FLU.

fluconazole (floo-kon′ah-zōl) a triazole antifungal AGENT used in the systemic treatment of CANDIDIASIS and cryptococcal MENINGITIS.

fluctuation (fluk″choo-a′shun) a variation, as about a fixed variation or mass; a wave-like motion.

flucytosine (floo-si′to-sēn″) an antifungal AGENT used in the treatment of severe candidal and cryptococcal infections.

Fludara (floo-dar′ah) trademark for a preparation of FLUDARABINE phosphate, an antineoplastic AGENT.

fludarabine (floo-dar′ah-bēn) an ADENINE analogue and PURINE ANTIMETABOLITE that inhibits DNA synthesis; administered intravenously as the phosphate salt as an antineoplastic AGENT in the treatment of chronic lymphocytic LEUKEMIA.

fludeoxyglucose F 18 (floo″de-ok″se-gloo′-kōs) radiolabeled 2-deoxy-D-glucose; used in positron emission tomography in the diagnosis of brain disorders, cardiac disease, and tumors of various organs.

fludrocortisone (floo″dro-kor′tĭ-sōn) a synthetic steroid with potent MINERALOCORTI-COID and high GLUCOCORTICOID activity, used as the acetate salt in replacement THERAPY for primary or secondary adrenocortical INSUFFICIENCY in ADDISON'S DISEASE and for the treatment of SALT-LOSING SYNDROME and ADRENOGENITAL SYNDROME.

fluid (floo′id) 1. a liquid or gas; any liquid of the body. 2. composed of molecules which freely change their relative positions without separation of the mass.

allantoic f. the fluid contained within the allantois.

amniotic f. the fluid within the amnion that bathes the developing fetus and protects it from mechanical injury; see also AMNIOTIC FLUID.

f. balance a state in which the volume of body water and its solutes is within normal limits and there is normal distribution of fluids within the intracellular and extracellular compartments. The total weight of body fluids should be about 60 per cent of the body weight, and it should be distributed so that one third is extracellular fluid and two thirds intracellular fluid. Although this distribution remains constant in a healthy individual, there is continuous movement of fluid into and out of the various compartments.

Most organs are concerned in some way with the maintenance of fluid balance within the body; however, the KIDNEYS play a major role in regulating most of the constituents of the fluids. It is in the renal tubules that water is reabsorbed into the blood stream or allowed to enter the urine for excretion. The antidiuretic hormone controls this process. It is also in the distal tubules of the kidneys that some sodium reabsorption takes place and this process is influenced by the hormone aldosterone.

Water and sodium are particularly important in fluid balance because they are the components directly affecting the concentration (OSMOLALITY) of the fluids and, therefore, their distribution. The body does not tolerate differences in osmotic pressure. Thus, whenever there is an imbalance in the concentration of fluids, there is shifting of the fluids, with water moving from the less concentrated fluid to the more concentrated until an equilibrium is established. In addition to these osmotic factors, the movement of fluids in and out of compartments is affected by capillary permeability, arterial and venous blood pressure, and the rate of flow of blood through the capillaries.

The adaptive mechanisms for maintaining normal volume and distribution of fluids inside and outside the cells function only as long as there is adequate and _equal_ intake and output of water and electrolytes. When either gains or losses of these components of body fluids are excessive and prolonged, a fluid imbalance exists.

An accurate measuring and recording of fluid intake and output can be a valuable aid in detecting imbalances and in determining the amount needed for fluid replacement when a fluid volume deficit is found. In addition to measurement and recording of intake and output and evaluation of the clinical signs of fluid imbalance, certain laboratory tests are helpful in the accurate assessment of a patient's hydration status. Among these are OSMOLALITY, SODIUM, and blood UREA NITROGEN.

body f's the fluids within the body, composed of water, electrolytes, and non-electrolytes. The volume and distribution of body fluids vary with age, sex, and amount of adipose tissue. Throughout life there is a slow decline in the volume of body fluids; obesity decreases the relative amount of water in the body. It has two components: the intracellular FLUID and the extracellular FLUID.

cerebrospinal f. the fluid contained within the ventricles of the brain, the subarachnoid space, and the central canal of the spinal cord; see also CEREBROSPINAL FLUID.

crevicular f. gingival fluid.

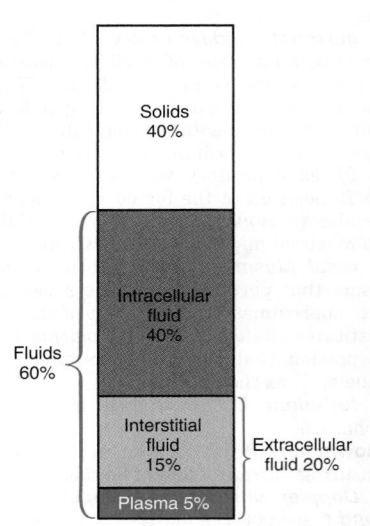

The body fluids diagrammed, showing extracellular fluid volume, intracellular fluid volume, blood volume, and total body fluids.

extracellular f. a general term for all the body FLUIDS outside the cells, comprising about one third of the body fluids. It can be further subdivided into interstitial FLUID and intravascular FLUID (PLASMA). Extracellular fluid consists of ultrafiltrates of the blood plasma and transcellular fluid (that produced by active cellular secretion). It circulates in the spaces between the cells and brings to the cells the nutrients and other substances needed for their functioning. See also FLUID BALANCE.

gingival f. tissue fluid that seeps in minute amounts into the gingival sulcus through its well; called also crevicular fluid and sulcular fluid.

interstitial f. the extracellular FLUID bathing most tissues, constituting the environment of body cells, excluding the fluid within the lymph and blood vessels. It is low in protein, is formed by filtration through the capillaries, and drains away as lymph.

intracellular f. any fluid that is within the membranes of the cells of the body; this comprises about two thirds of the total body FLUIDS. It serves as a medium for the basic materials needed by cells for growth, repair, and performance of other functions. Intracellular fluid contains relatively large amounts of positively charged potassium ions and smaller amounts of sodium ions, in contrast to extracellular FLUID. See also FLUID BALANCE.

intravascular f. a term sometimes used to refer to that part of the extracellular FLUID that is within the blood vessels, in other words, the PLASMA.

meconium-stained f. amniotic fluid that is stained green, a symptom of fetal hypoxia; caused by relaxation of the fetus' anal sphincter and escape of meconium.

seminal f. semen.

spinal f. the fluid within the spinal canal.

sulcular f. gingival fluid.

synovial f. the transparent viscid fluid secreted by the synovial membrane and found in joint cavities, bursae, and tendon sheaths; called also synovia. Analysis of synovial fluid aspirated from a joint can reveal any of various joint diseases: these include noninflammatory diseases such as traumatic arthritis and osteoarthritis; inflammatory joint diseases such as systemic lupus erythematosus, gout, and rheumatoid arthritis; and septic diseases such as tuberculous, gonorrheal, and septic arthritis.

The fluid is withdrawn under strict aseptic technique and sent to a laboratory, where it is evaluated for color, quantity,

viscosity, pH, and microscopically examined for a white blood cell count and differential. Special testing includes microscopic examination for formed elements such as crystals and bacteria and chemical analysis for glucose, protein, and enzymes. Special care must be used in handling samples of aspirated synovial fluid and dressings soiled with the fluid. This is especially true if septic arthritis is suspected.

After aspiration of fluid, ice packs are applied to the joint for 24 to 36 hours as necessary to minimize pain and swelling. Pillows may be used to support a painful joint. A pressure bandage is applied to stabilize the joint if a large amount of fluid has been withdrawn. Although patients may resume usual activities after the procedure, excessive use of the joint should be avoided for a few days. Patients are taught to assess the joint for signs of infection and to report them if they occur.

tissue f. interstitial fluid.

fluidextract (floo″id-ek′strakt) a liquid preparation of a vegetable drug, containing alcohol as a solvent or preservative, or both, of such strength that each milliliter contains the therapeutic constituents of 1 g of the standard drug it represents.

fluidram (floo′ĭ-dram) fluid dram.

fluke (flook) an organism of the class TREMATODA, characterized by a body that is usually flat and often leaflike; flukes can infect the blood, liver, intestines, and lungs. Called also trematode.

Flukes are not common in the United States but are a serious problem in many Asian, tropical, and subtropical countries. The Chinese liver fluke, *Clonorchis sinensis,* enters the body in raw or improperly cooked fish and may cause enlargement of the liver, jaundice, anemia, and weakness. Another liver fluke, *Fasciola hepatica,* is occasionally found in humans; it causes obstruction of the bile ducts and enlargement of the liver. Blood flukes such as *Schistosoma* penetrate the skin, make their way to the blood and travel to various parts of the body (see also SCHISTOSOMIASIS).

Treatment varies according to the type of fluke involved and requires careful medical supervision. Proper cooking of fish provides protection against liver fluke infection. Since snails are carriers of flukes, their destruction, usually by poison, is an effective preventive measure in areas where fluke infection is a problem.

flumazenil (floo-ma′zĕ-nil″) a BENZODIAZE-PINE agonist that competitively binds to receptor sites in the central nervous system;

used to reverse the effects of benzodiazepines after sedation, general ANESTHESIA, or overdose.

flumen (floo'men), pl. *flu'mina* [L.] a stream.

flu'mina pilo'rum the lines along which the hairs of the body are arranged.

flunisolide (floo-nis'o-līd) a steroid ANTI-INFLAMMATORY agent administered as an aerosol spray for treatment of bronchial ASTHMA and seasonal or perennial allergic RHINITIS when conventional treatment is unsatisfactory.

fluocinolone (floo″o-sin'o-lōn) a synthetic CORTICOSTEROID used topically as *f. acetonide* for the relief of inflammation and pruritus in certain dermatoses.

fluocinonide (floo″o-sin'o-nīd) a synthetic CORTICOSTEROID used topically for the relief of inflammation and pruritus in certain dermatoses.

fluorescein (floo-res'ēn) a fluorescing dye; the sodium salt is used as a contrast medium in retinal angiography and as a diagnostic aid for revealing corneal lesions and fitting contact lenses.

fluorescence (floo-res'ens) the property of emitting light while exposed to light, the wavelength of the emitted light being longer than that of the absorbed light.

f. microscopy the use of a fluorescence MICROSCOPE to identify microorganisms or specific tissue constituents that have been stained with a FLUOROCHROME or a fluorochrome-labeled substance (such as an antibody to a tissue antigen). A FLUORESCENT ANTIBODY TEST can be used in place of time-consuming culture methods for identifying bacteria. See also IMMUNOFLUORESCENCE.

fluorescent (floo-res'ent) pertaining to or characterized by FLUORESCENCE.

f. antibody test a test for the distribution of cells expressing a specific protein by binding ANTIBODY specific for the protein and detecting complexes by fluorescent labeling of the antibody. Called also FAB test.

f. treponemal antibody absorption test the standard treponemal antigen test for SYPHILIS: Nonspecific antibodies are removed from patient serum, which is then reacted with *Treponema pallidum* fixed to a glass slide. Specific antibodies adhering to the treponemes are demonstrated with fluorescein-labeled antihuman globulin. Positive tests are seen in about 85 per cent of cases of primary syphilis, 100 per cent in secondary syphilis, and 98 per cent in late syphilis. The test remains positive for life even after syphilis has been successfully treated. Called also FTA-ABS test.

fluoridation (floor″-ĭ-da'shun) treatment with FLUORIDES; the addition of fluorides to community drinking water as a measure to reduce the incidence of DENTAL CARIES. Minute traces of fluoride are found in almost all food, but the quantity apparently is too small to meet the requirements of the body in building tooth enamel that resists cavities. Drinking water containing one part fluoride to one million parts of water does meet this need and has been found to reduce tooth decay in children by as much as 40 per cent. Since few natural water supplies contain the necessary amount of fluoride, it usually must be added if protection against tooth decay is desired. Statistics indicate that 20 per cent of the teenagers who drank fluoridated water from birth have teeth totally free of caries. The practice of fluoridating water is rated among the most cost-effective preventive programs in public health.

There also is evidence that topically applied fluoride solutions help alleviate periodontal disease by removing bacteria from the site and rebuilding supporting bone tissue around the teeth. Dental professionals may apply fluoride solutions directly to a child's teeth, beginning at age 5 or 6 and repeating the treatment each year throughout life. This has been found to reduce caries by about 40 per cent.

The dentist or other health care provider may prescribe chewable fluoride tablets if fluoride is not available in drinking water. However, use of these tablets must be carefully supervised, since an excess of fluoride causes dental FLUOROSIS. Like most medicines, fluoride in large amounts is a poison. A dentifrice containing fluoride, or fluoride in gel form, may also prove effective. A dentist or dental hygienist should be consulted before any fluoride preparation is used.

fluoride (floor'īd) any binary compound of fluorine.

f. poisoning a toxic condition that sometimes occurs with ingestion of excessive fluoride. *Acute fluoride poisoning* involves an immediate physiological reaction, with nausea, vomiting, hypersalivation, abdominal pain, and diarrhea. *Chronic fluoride poisoning* is a physiological reaction to long term exposure to high levels of fluoride and is characterized by dental FLUOROSIS, skeletal FLUOROSIS, and kidney damage. Called also fluorosis.

systemic f. a fluoride ingested in water, supplements, or some other form. See also FLUORIDATION.

topical f. a fluoride applied directly to the teeth, especially of children, in a DENTAL CARIES prevention program.

fluorimeter (floo-rim′ĕ-ter) fluorometer.

fluorimetry (floo-rim′ĕ-tre) fluorometry.

fluorine (F) (floor′ēn) a chemical element, atomic number 9, atomic weight 18.998. (See Appendix 6.)

   f. 18 a radioactive isotope of fluorine, atomic mass 18, having a half-life of 1.8925 hours; it has been used as a TRACER in positron emission TOMOGRAPHY.

fluorochrome (floor′-o-krōm) a fluorescent compound, as a dye, used to mark protein with a fluorescent label.

fluorodopa F 18 (floor″o-do′pah) a radiolabeled compound of FLUORINE and LEVODOPA, used for positron emission TOMOGRAPHY of the cerebrum.

fluorography (floo-rog′rah-fe) photofluorography.

fluorometer (floo-rom′ĕ-ter) the instrument used in fluorometry, consisting of an energy source (e.g., a mercury arc lamp or xenon lamp) to induce fluorescence, filters or monochromators for selection of the wavelength, and a detector.

fluorometholone (floor″o-meth′o-lōn) a synthetic GLUCOCORTICOID used topically for treatment of allergic and inflammatory conditions of the eye.

fluorometry (floo-rom′ĕ-tre) an analytical technique for identifying and characterizing minute amounts of a substance by excitation of the substance with a beam of ultraviolet light and detection and measurement of the characteristic wavelength of the fluorescent light emitted.

fluorophotometry (floor″o-fo-tom′ĕ-tre) fluorometry.

   vitreous f. the measurement of light given off by intravenously injected fluorescein that has leaked through the retinal vessels into the vitreous; done to detect the breakdown of the blood-retinal barrier, an early ocular change in diabetes mellitus.

fluoroquinolone (floor″o-kwin′o-lōn) any of a subgroup of QUINOLONES that have a broader spectrum of activity than quinolones such as NALIDIXIC ACID.

fluororadiography (floor″o-ra″de-og′rah-fe) photofluorography.

fluoroscope (floor′o-skōp″) an instrument for visual observation of the body by means of X-RAY. The patient is put into position so that the part to be viewed is placed between an x-ray tube and a fluorescent screen. X-rays from the tube pass through the body and project the bones and organs as images on the screen. Examination by this method is called fluoroscopy.

   The advantage of the fluoroscope is that the action of joints, organs, and entire systems of the body can be observed

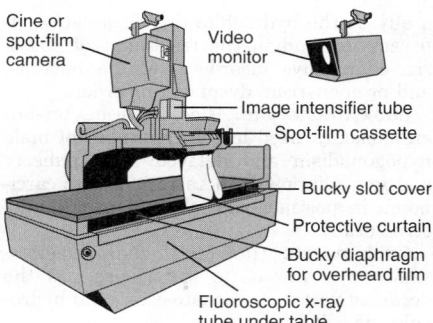

Fluoroscope and associated parts. From Bushong, 2001.

directly. The use of radiopaque media and radiolucent agents aids in this process.

fluoroscopy (floo″ros′kah-pe) examination by means of the fluoroscope.

fluorosis (floo″ro′sis) a condition due to ingestion of excessive amounts of fluorine or its compounds; see FLUORIDE POISONING.

   chronic endemic f. that due to unusually high concentrations of fluoride, usually in the natural drinking water supply, typically causing dental fluorosis characterized by a mottled appearance of the teeth. Combined osteosclerosis and osteomalacia can also occur in occupational exposures to vapors and dust.

   dental f. hypoplasia of the dental enamel resulting from prolonged ingestion of drinking water containing high levels of fluoride, manifested by the condition called mottled ENAMEL.

   skeletal f. skeletal changes due to long term ingestion of excessive fluoride; they may include HYPEROSTOSIS, OSTEOPETROSIS, and OSTEOPOROSIS.

fluorouracil (floor″o-u′rah-sil) a URACIL analogue that interferes with DNA synthesis; used intravenously as an ANTIMETABOLITE antineoplastic AGENT for palliative treatment of carcinomas of the breast and gastrointestinal tract; also used topically for treatment of actinic keratoses and superficial basal cell carcinomas. Called also 5-fluorouracil (5-FU).

Fluosol-DC (floo′o-sol) trademark for a type of inert substance with a high oxygen-carrying capacity that can be transfused for the temporary carrying of oxygen in the blood.

Fluothane (floo′o-thān) trademark for a preparation of HALOTHANE, a general anesthetic.

fluoxetine (floo-ok′sĕ-tēn) a selective serotonin reuptake inhibitor administered orally as the hydrochloride salt as an ANTI-DEPRESSANT and in the treatment of obsessive-compulsive disorder, bulimia nervosa, and premenstrual dysphoric disorder.

fluoxymesterone (floo-ok″se-mes′ter-ōn) an ANDROGEN used in the treatment of male hypogonadism and delayed male puberty and in palliation of metastatic breast carcinoma in postmenopausal women; administered orally.

fluphenazine (floo-fen′ah-zēn) a PHENO-THIAZINE ANTIPSYCHOTIC AGENT, used as the decanoate ester, enanthate ester, and hydrochloride salt.

fluprednisolone (floo″pred-nis′o-lōn) a glucocorticoid ANTIINFLAMMATORY agent used in the treatment of joint diseases and allergic disorders.

flurandrenolide (floor″an-dren′o-līd) a synthetic CORTICOSTEROID used topically for relief of inflammation and pruritus in dermatoses.

flurazepam (floor-az′ĕ-pam) a BENZODIAZE-PINE used as a SEDATIVE and HYPNOTIC for treatment of insomnia; administered orally as the hydrochloride salt.

flurbiprofen (floor-bi′pro-fen) a NONSTEROI-DAL ANTIINFLAMMATORY DRUG, administered orally in the treatment of ARTHRITIS, ankylosing SPONDYLITIS, BURSITIS, TENDINITIS, soft tissue injuries, and DYSMENORRHEA. The sodium salt is applied topically to the conjunctiva to inhibit MIOSIS during and inflammation following ophthalmic surgery.

flush (flush) 1. transient episodic redness of the face and neck caused by certain diseases, ingestion of certain drugs or other substances, heat, emotional factors, or physical exertion. 2. the rapid delivery of a bolus of solution through an intravenous line or catheter for the purpose of maintaining patency or insuring the complete delivery of all fluids in the lumen.

hectic f. a persistent or chronic flush associated with chronic debilitating disease, usually febrile.

heparin f. a dilute solution of heparin that is used to flush an intravenous line or arterial catheter.

malar f. a redness of the cheeks caused by excitement.

flutamide (floo′tah-mīd) a nonsteroidal ANTIANDROGEN administered orally in the treatment of advanced or metastatic prostatic carcinoma.

fluticasone (floo-tik′ah-sōn″) a steroid ANTIINFLAMMATORY agent, used as the propionate salt topically in treatment of itching or inflammation, intranasally for allergic RHINITIS and other inflammatory nasal conditions, and nasal POLYPS, and by inhalation in treatment of ASTHMA.

flutter (flut′er) a rapid vibration or pulsation.

atrial f. a cardiac arrhythmia in which the atrial contractions are rapid (230–380 per minute), but regular. Two types, I and II, are distinguished according to rate; Type I is also more amenable to CARDIOVERSION. In *Type I* the atrial rate is usually 290 to 310 per minute but can range from 230 to 350. In *Type II* the atrial rate is usually 360 to 380 per minute but can range from 340 to 430.

diaphragmatic f. peculiar wavelike fibrillations of the diaphragm of unknown cause.

impure f. atrial flutter in which the atrial rhythm is irregular.

mediastinal f. see MEDIASTINAL FLUTTER.

pure f. atrial flutter in which the atrial rhythm is regular.

ventricular f. a possible transition stage between ventricular tachycardia and ventricular fibrillation, the electrocardiogram showing rapid, uniform, and virtually regular oscillations, 250 or more per minute.

flutter-fibrillation (flut′er-fi-bri-la′shun) a supraventricular arrhythmia whose pattern on the electrocardiogram resembles both atrial FLUTTER and atrial FIBRILLATION.

fluvastatin (floo′vah-stat″in) an inhibitor of CHOLESTEROL biosynthesis used as the sodium salt in the treatment of HYPERLIPID-EMIA and to slow the progression of ATHERO-SCLEROSIS associated with CORONARY HEART DISEASE.

fluvoxamine (floo-vok′sah-mēn) a selective serotonin reuptake INHIBITOR, used as the maleate salt to relieve the symptoms of OBSESSIVE-COMPULSIVE DISORDER; administered orally.

flux (fluks) 1. an excessive flow or discharge. 2. the rate of the flow of some quantity (or magnetic field) per unit area.

magnetic f. (Φ) a quantitative measure of a magnetic field.

fly (fli) a dipterous, or two-winged insect, which is often the vector of organisms causing disease.

Fm fermium.

FMN flavin mononucleotide.

foam (fōm) 1. a dispersion of a gas in a liquid or solid, e.g., whipped cream or foam rubber. 2. frothy saliva, produced particularly on exertion or pathologically. 3. to produce, or cause to produce, froth.

focal (fo′kal) pertaining to or having a FOCUS.

f. disease a localized disease.

focus (fo′kus), pl. *fo′ci* [L.] 1. the point of convergence of light rays or sound waves. 2. the chief center of a morbid process.

Ghon f. the primary parenchymal lesion of primary pulmonary TUBERCULOSIS in children; when associated with a corresponding lymph node focus, it is known as the primary or Ghon COMPLEX. Called also Ghon tubercle.

grid f. in radiology, a determination made by drawing an imaginary line from the outside of the width of the grid to where it intersects with a centering point. Called also grid radius.

focusing (fo'kus-ing) the act of converging at a point.

isoelectric f. electrophoresis in which the protein mixture is subjected to an electric field in a gel medium in which a pH gradient has been established; each protein then migrates until it reaches the site at which the pH is equal to its isoelectric point.

foe- for words beginning thus, see those beginning *fe-*.

fog (fog) 1. a colloid system in which the dispersion medium is a gas and the dispersed particles are liquid. 2. an artifact seen on a radiograph caused by unintentional exposure to reducing contrast.

fogging (fog'ing) in ophthalmology, a method of determining refractive error in astigmatism, the patient being first made artificially myopic by means of plus spheres, in order to relax all accommodation before using cylinders.

fold (fōld) plica; a thin margin curved back on itself, or doubling.

amniotic f. the folded edge of the amnion where it rises over and finally encloses the embryo.

aryepiglottic f. a fold of mucous membrane extending on each side between the lateral border of the epiglottis and the summit of the arytenoid cartilage.

circular f's the permanent transverse folds of the luminal surface of the small intestine.

costocolic f. a fold of peritoneum passing from the left colic flexure to the adjacent part of the diaphragm; called also phrenicocolic ligament.

gastric f's the series of folds in the mucous membrane of the stomach.

gluteal f. the crease separating the buttocks from the thigh.

head f. a fold of blastoderm at the cephalic end of the developing embryo.

interdigital f. the free border of the web connecting the bases of adjoining digits.

lacrimal f. a fold of mucous membrane at the lower opening of the nasolacrimal duct.

mucosal f., mucous f. a fold of mucous membrane.

nail f. the fold of palmar skin around the base and sides of the nail of a finger or toe.

neural f. one of the paired folds lying on either side of the neural plate that form the neural tube.

semilunar f. of conjunctiva a mucous fold at the medial angle of the eye.

serosal f., serous f. a fold of serous membrane.

spiral f. a spirally arranged elevation in the mucosa of the first part of the cystic duct.

tail f. a fold of the blastoderm at the caudal end of the developing embryo.

transverse f's three permanent transverse folds in the rectum.

ventricular f., vestibular f. a false vocal cord.

vestigial f. a pericardial fold enclosing the remnant of the embryonic left anterior cardinal vein.

vocal f's true VOCAL CORDS.

folate (fo'lāt) the anionic form of FOLIC ACID.

folic acid (fo'lik) a vitamin of the B complex; it is involved in the synthesis of amino acids and DNA. Green vegetables, liver, and yeast are major food sources; folic acid can also be produced synthetically. Folic acid deficiency (leading to megaloblastic ANEMIA) may result from the inability of the body to use the vitamin. Because of the important role of folate in prevention of neural tube defects, it is now recommended that 400 μg of folate be taken daily before conception occurs. See also VITAMIN.

f. a. antagonist an antimetabolite of folic acid; some are used as antineoplastic AGENTS because they interfere with DNA replication and cell division by inhibiting the enzyme dihydrofolate reductase. Examples include TRIMETHOPRIM, an ANTIBACTERIAL; PYRIMETHAMINE, an antimalarial AGENT; and METHOTREXATE, an antineoplastic AGENT.

folie (fo-le') [Fr.] psychosis; insanity.

f. à deux mental disorder affecting two persons who share the same delusions; formally classified as SHARED PSYCHOTIC DISORDER.

f. du pourquoi (doo-poor-kwah') psychopathologic constant questioning.

f. gémellaire (zha″mĕ-lār') psychosis occurring simultaneously in twins.

folinic acid (fo-lin'ik) the 5-formyl derivative of tetrahydrofolic acid, a metabolically active derivative of FOLIC ACID used to treat folic acid deficiencies and as an antidote to FOLIC ACID ANTAGONISTS. Called also citrovorum factor and leucovorin.

folium (fo′le-um), pl. *fo′lia* [L.] a leaflike structure, especially one of the leaflike subdivisions of the cerebellar cortex.

follicle (fol′ĭ-k'l) a sac or pouchlike depression or cavity. adj., **follic′ular**.

   atretic ovarian f. an involuted ovarian follicle.

   dental f. the structure within the substance of the jaws enclosing a tooth before its eruption; the dental sac and its contents.

   gastric f's lymphoid masses in the gastric mucosa.

   graafian f. see GRAAFIAN FOLLICLE.

   hair f. one of the tubular invaginations of the epidermis enclosing the hairs, and from which the hairs grow.

   lymph f., lymphatic f. 1. lymph node. 2. lymphatic nodule (def. 2).

   Naboth's f's, nabothian f's Naboth's cysts.

   ovarian f. the ovum and its encasing cells, at any stage of its development.

   primary ovarian f. an immature ovarian follicle consisting of an immature ovum and the few specialized epithelial cells surrounding it.

   primordial ovarian f. an ovarian follicle consisting of an ovum enclosed by a single layer of cells.

   sebaceous f. a hair follicle with a relatively large sebaceous gland, producing a relatively insignificant hair.

   solitary f's 1. areas of concentrated lymphatic tissue in the mucosa of the colon. 2. small lymph follicles scattered throughout the mucosa and submucosa of the small intestine. Called also solitary glands.

   thyroid f's discrete cystlike units filled with a colloid substance rich in iodine; they constitute the lobules of the THYROID GLAND.

   vesicular ovarian f. GRAAFIAN FOLLICLE.

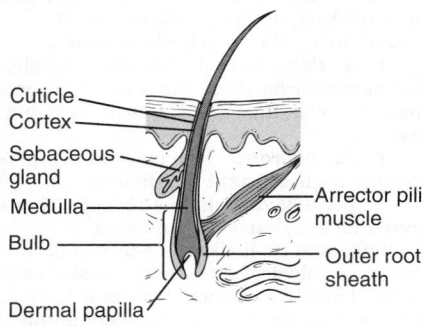

Cuticle
Cortex
Sebaceous gland
Medulla
Bulb
Arrector pili muscle
Outer root sheath
Dermal papilla

Diagram of a hair follicle showing layers of hair schematically. From Copstead, 1995.

folliculitis (fŏ-lik″u-li′tis) inflammation of a follicle(s); used ordinarily in reference to hair follicles, but sometimes in relation to follicles of other kinds.

   f. bar′bae sycosis barbae.

   gram-negative f. a superinfection complicating long-term systemic antibiotic treatment of acne vulgaris, particularly tetracyclines, usually caused by species of *Enterobacter, Klebsiella,* or *Proteus.*

   keloid f. infection of hair follicles of the back of the neck and scalp, occurring chiefly in men, producing large, irregular keloid plaques and scarring.

folliculoma (fŏ-lik″u-lo′mah) granulosa-theca cell tumor.

folliculus (fŏ-lik′u-lus), pl. *folli′culi* [L.] follicle.

follitropin (fol′ĭ-tro″pin) follicle-stimulating HORMONE; *follitropin alfa* and *follitropin beta* are forms produced by genetically modified hamster cells and used in the treatment of INFERTILITY.

follow-up (fol′o up) some further action taken after a procedure is finished, such as contact by a health care agency days or weeks after a patient has undergone treatment.

   telephone f.-u. in the NURSING INTERVENTIONS CLASSIFICATION, a nursing INTERVENTION defined as providing results of testing or evaluating patient's response and determining potential for problems as a result of previous treatment, examination, or testing, over the telephone.

fomentation (fo″men-ta′shun) treatment by warm, moist applications; also, the substance thus applied.

fomes (fo′mēz), pl. *fo′mites* [L.] an inanimate object or material on which disease-producing agents may be conveyed.

fomivirsen (fo-miv′er-sin) an ANTIVIRAL agent administered by intravitreal injection in the treatment of cytomegalovirus RETINITIS associated with ACQUIRED IMMUNODEFICIENCY SYNDROME (AIDS); used as the sodium salt.

Fonsecaea (fon″se-se′ah) a genus of imperfect fungi. *F. compac′tum* and *F. pedro′soi* are etiologic agents of CHROMOBLASTOMYCOSIS.

Fontan procedure (faw-tah′) functional correction of a tricuspid atresia by anastomosis of, or insertion of a nonvalved prosthesis between, the right atrium and the pulmonary artery with closure of the interatrial communication.

fontanel (fon″tah-nel′) fontanelle.

fontanelle (fon″tah-nel′) one of the membrane-covered spaces remaining at the junction of the sutures in the incompletely ossified skull of the fetus or infant. Actually

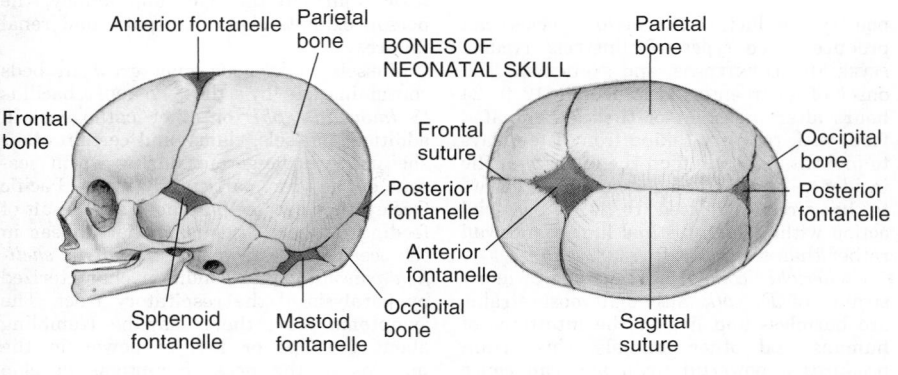

Fontanelles. From Jarvis, 2000.

there are two soft spots close together, representing gaps in the bone structure which will be filled in by bone during the normal process of growth. The anterior fontanelle is diamond shaped and lies at the junction of the frontal and parietal bones. This fontanelle usually fills in and closes between the eighth and fifteenth months of life. The posterior fontanelle lies at the junction of the occipital and parietal bones, is triangular in shape, and usually closes by the third or fourth month of life. Though these "soft spots" may appear very vulnerable, they may be touched gently without harm. Care should be exercised that they be protected from strong pressure or direct injury.

food (fo͞od) a nourishing substance that is eaten or otherwise taken into the body to sustain life, provide energy, or promote growth.

accessory f's foods high in calories and low in nutritive value, often used to increase palatability of foods with higher nutritive value, for example, gravy that is added to mashed potatoes.

functional f's foods and food supplements marketed for presumed health benefits, such as vitamin supplements and certain herbs; called also nutraceuticals.

f. poisoning any of a group of acute illnesses due to ingestion of contaminated food. It may result from allergy; toxemia from foods, such as those inherently poisonous or those contaminated by poisons; or foods containing poisons formed by bacteria or foodborne infections. Food poisoning usually causes inflammation of the gastrointestinal tract (GASTROENTERITIS); this may occur suddenly, soon after the poisonous

food has been eaten. The symptoms are acute, and include tenderness; pain or cramps in the abdomen; nausea, vomiting, or diarrhea; weakness; and dizziness.

The Division of Bacterial and Mycotic Diseases of the Centers for Disease Control and Prevention reports that the most commonly recognized foodborne infections are those caused by the bacteria *Campylobacter, Salmonella,* and *Escherichia coli* O157:H7. Some CALICIVIRUSES, especially the Norwalk VIRUS, are also common causes of food poisoning. There are more than 250 known foodborne diseases.

Bacterial Food Poisoning. Bacterial food poisoning may be from any of a number of different microorganisms, and includes (among other types) BOTULISM, CAMPYLO-BACTERIOSIS, *Escherichia coli* infection, SAL-MONELLOSIS, and SHIGELLOSIS.

Campylobacteriosis (*Campylobacter* infection) is the most common foodborne illness. Contaminated or undercooked poultry or meat, unpasteurized (raw) milk, and contaminated water may cause the disease, even though this organism is commonly found in the intestinal tracts of humans and other animals without causing symptoms of illness. Symptoms of campylobacteriosis usually occur within two to ten days of ingesting the bacteria and include mild to severe diarrhea, fever, nausea, vomiting, and abdominal pain. Children, the elderly, and IMMUNOCOMPROMISED persons are particularly at risk. The bacteria is now recognized as a major contributing factor in the development of GUILLAIN-BARRÉ SYNDROME.

SALMONELLOSIS (poisoning with *Salmonella*) is the second most common type of food poisoning. The source is usually a poultry product. *Salmonella* species can produce three types of illnesses: TYPHOID FEVER, GASTROENTERITIS, and SEPTICEMIA. The onset of gastroenteritis is usually 12 to 24 hours after ingestion of the contaminated food, with recovery taking from a few days to months, depending on the severity of the incident. The pathologic activity appears to be directly related to local bacterial action within the intestinal lumen and wall rather than from a toxin.

Escherichia coli O157:H7 is one of many strains of *E. coli;* although most strains are harmless and live in the intestines of humans and other animals, this strain produces a powerful toxin and can cause severe illness. It is most frequently associated with ingestion of undercooked ground beef. Other sources of infection include contaminated sprouts, lettuce, salami, unpasteurized (raw) milk, and juice. Swimming in or drinking water contaminated with sewage can also cause infection. The most common symptoms are abdominal cramps and bloody diarrhea. It is also possible to experience nonbloody diarrhea or no symptoms. Usually there is little or no fever, and the illness may resolve in five to ten days. HEMOLYTIC UREMIC SYNDROME occurs in 2 to 7 per cent of patients.

Norwalk VIRUS is another cause of food poisoning, usually associated with GASTROENTERITIS. Symptoms are often mild, consisting of nausea, vomiting, diarrhea, and abdominal pain. Headache and low-grade fever may occur. The fecal-oral route via contaminated water or food is the usual method of transmission. Shellfish and salad ingredients are the foods most often implicated. Norwalk viruses are responsible for about one third of the cases of viral GASTROENTERITIS in persons over the age of two years.

Other Poisonous Plants, Berries, and Shellfish. There are a number of poisonous berries and over 80 kinds of poisonous mushrooms. Children are frequently tempted by poisonous holly berries or the berries that grow on privet (the shrub often used for hedges). Adults often place their faith in misinformation about differences between poisonous and edible mushrooms. Although it is possible to learn to identify poisonous mushrooms and berries, it is much wiser to play safe. Children should be taught not to eat things they find in the woods or fields.

Mushroom poisoning can produce seizures, severe abdominal pain, intense thirst, nausea, vomiting, diarrhea, dimness of vision, and symptoms resembling those of alcoholic intoxication. Symptoms appear six to 15 hours after eating. Later, because of toxic injury to the liver and kidney, the person exhibits signs of hepatic and renal failure.

Mussels and clams may grow in beds contaminated by the TYPHOID bacillus *(Salmonella typhi)* or other pathogens. In addition, mussels, clams, and certain other shellfish are dangerous during warm seasons of the year, particularly in the Pacific Ocean; they become poisonous as a result of feeding on microorganisms that appear in the ocean in warm weather. *Paralytic shellfish poisoning* is a condition characterized by paralysis of the respiratory tract. The symptoms vary; there may be trembling about the lips or loss of power in the muscles of the neck. Symptoms develop quickly, within five to 30 minutes after eating.

BOTULISM is the most dangerous, but fortunately the rarest, type of food poisoning. Botulism-causing *Clostridium botulinum* bacteria and their spores are often present in the environment. The spores can be found on the surfaces of fruits and vegetables, as well as in seafood. Home-canned, low-acidic foods were once a common source for this type of poisoning. The bacteria and spores themselves are harmless; the dangerous substance is the botulinum TOXIN produced by the bacteria when they grow. Botulism results in a descending pattern of weakness and paralysis. When it is suspected, serum, feces, and any remaining food should be tested for botulinum toxin; food and fecal samples can also be cultured for *Clostridium botulinum*. In infant botulism, the toxin is produced when *C. botulinum* spores germinate in the intestines. Most cases in infants are caused by inhalation of airborne spores, but infants under one year old should not be given honey, which can contain *C. botulinum* spores.

Treatment. For most bacterial food poisoning, treatment is largely supportive and consists of rest, nothing by mouth until vomiting stops, medication for the diarrhea, and intravenous replacement of fluids and electrolytes as needed. While most bacterial poisonings are self-limiting, botulism must be treated promptly with ANTITOXIN and respiratory support; the greatest threat to life is respiratory failure. A large proportion of persons with botulism whose cases are misdiagnosed or treated improperly have a fatal outcome.

In general, antibiotics are not effective in treating bacterial food poisoning. However, care will be individualized to the patient dependent upon the organism causing the infection and the condition of the patient.

Prevention of food poisoning by proper handwashing techniques and appropriate food handling should be emphasized.

In the United States, the Center for Food Safety and Applied Nutrition of the Food and Drug Administration has published the *Foodborne Pathogenic Microorganisms and Natural Toxins Handbook,* a valuable source for basic facts on this subject.

Food and Drug Administration (FDA) an agency of the United States Department of Health and Human Services whose principal purpose is to enforce the Federal Food, Drug and Cosmetic Act. The agency insures that foods for sale in the United States are safe, pure, and wholesome; that drugs and therapeutic devices are safe and effective; that cosmetics are harmless; and that all these products are correctly labeled and packaged. The FDA is also responsible for enforcing the federal act that requires informative labels on any household product that is toxic, corrosive, irritant, or inflammable or generates pressure through decomposition or heat.

If a product in interstate commerce is proved to be faulty, the FDA is authorized to bring court action or seize the adulterated or incorrectly labeled merchandise and to prosecute the responsible person or company.

foot (foot) 1. the distal part of the lower limb of a primate, upon which the individual stands and walks. 2. something resembling this structure. 3. a unit of linear measure, 12 inches, equal to 0.3048 meter.

athlete's f. see ATHLETE'S FOOT.

Bock-Greissinger f. a prosthetic foot that allows ankle motion.

f. care 1. preventive and therapeutic measures to avoid complications and possibly amputation in patients with diabetes, peripheral arterial occlusive disease, and other disorders associated with circulatory stasis. 2. in the NURSING INTERVENTIONS CLASSIFICATION, a nursing INTERVENTION defined as cleansing and inspecting the feet for the purposes of relaxation, cleanliness, and healthy skin.

Assessment. Evaluation of the circulatory status of the feet includes noting the amplitude and other characteristics of the popliteal, posterior tibial, and dorsalis pedis pulses. Temperature changes can be assessed by comparing one foot and leg with the other, using the back of the hand and noting areas of coolness and heat. "Hot spots" on the foot could indicate a localized inflammation.

COMPARISONS AND CONTRASTS OF COMMON CAUSES OF FOOD POISONING

Causative Organism	Onset (incubation)	Causative Agent	Source	Recovery
Staphylococcus aureus	1–6 hours	Heat-resistant enterotoxin	Many food sources: custards, cream sauces, and processed meats most frequently involved	1–3 days
Clostridium perfringens	8–24 hours	Heat-labile enterotoxin	Animal products: frequently beed	12–24 hours
Salmonella (gastroenteritis)	12–24 hours	Local bacterial action in intestinal lumen and wall	Mainly meat, especially poultry products	Several days to months, mortality < 1%
			Nonfood sources: human-human or human-pet route; poor sanitation	
Shellfish poisoning: 1. *Salmonella typhi*	7–14 days	Bacteria in an organ		
2. **Paralytic shellfish poisoning (PSP)**	5–30 minutes	Saxitoxin (neurotoxin with curarelike action)	Accumulated toxin in shellfish, e.g., mussels and clams; from their food; often associated with "Red Tide" blooms of organisms	If victim survives the first 10–12 hours, prognosis is good Respiratory support may be needed

Abnormal skin color is significant. A bluish, mottled, pale, or ashen color indicates poor circulation if the feet have been exposed to a warm room temperature for five minutes or more. Irritation from poorly fitting shoes can cause localized areas of redness.

Vascular filling capacity is tested by applying pressure to superficial veins on the top of the foot and then releasing the pressure and noting refilling. There should be evidence of blood returning to the vessels within 15 seconds. Refilling that is prolonged beyond 20 seconds is indicative of insufficient circulation.

Another technique for evaluating circulatory status in the feet and legs is related to changes in position. While the patient is lying flat, the feet are elevated above the level of the heart for two full minutes. If the soles, heels, and toes turn pale after 30 seconds, there probably is vascular insufficiency. The patient then dangles the legs and the examiner notes whether color returns to the toes within the normal time of 10 seconds. Delayed return of color indicates poor circulation.

Excessive pressure or a rubbing action on the foot by poorly fitting shoes can produce overgrowth of the corneous layer of the skin, predisposing it to cracking, formation of calluses, and eventually ulceration.

Preventive Measures. All patients with peripheral vascular disease should be taught proper care of their feet. This includes avoiding injury by wearing well-fitting shoes that protect the feet whenever the patient is up and about. Circular garters should not be worn and the legs should not be crossed while sitting. Cleanliness is essential. Since nails should be filed when they are soft and pliable, the ideal time for nail care is immediately after a soaking. The nails should be filed straight across; no sharp instruments such as a razor or knife should ever be used to trim either the nails or corns. Calluses and corns should be treated by a podiatrist. Feet that are dry and scaly can be softened by using a lanolin-based lotion or cream.

dangle f., drop f. 1. a condition in which the foot hangs in a plantar-flexed position, due to lesion of the fibular nerve. 2. plantar FLEXION of the foot associated with IMMOBILITY and weakness of the lower limbs. Proper positioning and range of motion EXERCISES may help prevent this complication of immobility.

flat f. flatfoot.

immersion f. a condition resembling trench foot occurring in persons who have spent long periods in water.

Madura f. MYCETOMA of the foot.

march f. painful swelling of the foot, usually with fracture of a metatarsal bone, after excessive foot strain.

Morton's f. Morton's NEURALGIA.

SACH f. a prosthetic foot with a solid ankle and a cushion heel.

SAFE f. a prosthetic foot with a stationary attachment and a flexible endoskeleton.

f. slap a gait pattern often seen with a foot prosthesis; the prosthesis lands flatly on the ground, making a loud noise.

trench f. a condition of the feet resembling FROSTBITE, due to the prolonged action of water on the skin combined with circulatory disturbance due to cold and inaction.

footboard (foot′bord) a device placed at the foot of the bed in such a way that the feet rest firmly against it and are at right angles to the legs. It is used to relieve the weight of the bedclothes and to maintain proper positioning of the feet while a patient is confined to bed. Its purpose is to prevent development of FOOTDROP. It also helps maintain good posture by preventing the patient from slipping down in bed.

A footboard can be an adjustable metal device attached to the bed, a wooden apparatus, or an improvised structure made for a patient in the home from a cardboard box. Many patients, of all ages, wear high top sneakers in connection with the use of a footboard; these help the patient maintain proper alignment of the feet, and the rubber soles keep the feet from slipping away from the footboard. Specialized orthotic devices to keep the foot in good alignment may also be used.

footdrop (foot′drop) 1. a contracture deformity associated with bed rest and immobility, resulting in the inability to place the heel on the ground. 2. dropping of the foot

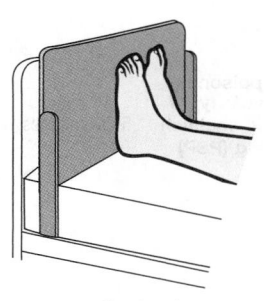

Footboard.

from paralysis of anterior muscles of the lower limb.

footplate (foot′plāt) the flat portion of the stapes, which is set into the oval window on the medial wall of the middle ear.

foramen (fo-ra′men), pl. *fora′mina* [L.] a natural opening or passage, especially one into or through a bone.

    aortic f. aortic hiatus.

    apical f. an opening at or near the apex of the root of a tooth.

    auditory f., external the external acoustic meatus.

    auditory f., internal the passage for the auditory (vestibulocochlear) and facial nerves in the petrous part of the temporal bone.

    cecal f., f. cae′cum 1. a blind opening between the frontal crest and the crista galli. 2. a depression on the dorsum of the tongue at the median sulcus.

    condyloid f., anterior hypoglossal canal.

    condyloid f., posterior condylar canal.

    epiploic f. omental foramen.

    ethmoidal foramina, fora′mina eth-moida′lia small openings in the ethmoid bone at the junction of the medial wall with the roof of the orbit, the anterior transmitting the nasal branch of the ophthalmic nerve and the anterior ethmoid vessels, the posterior transmitting the posterior ethmoid vessels.

    incisive f. one of the openings of the incisive canals into the incisive fossa of the hard palate.

    interventricular f. a passage from the third to the lateral ventricle of the brain.

    intervertebral f. a passage for a spinal nerve and vessels formed by notches on the pedicles of adjacent vertebrae.

    jugular f. an opening formed by the jugular notches of the temporal and occipital bones.

    f. mag′num a large opening in the anterior inferior part of the occipital bone, between the cranial cavity and spinal canal.

    mastoid f. an opening in the temporal bone behind the mastoid PROCESS.

    f. of Monro interventricular foramen.

    obturator f. the large opening between the pubic bone and the ischium.

    omental f. the opening connecting the greater and the lesser peritoneal sacs, situated below and behind the porta hepatis; called also epiploic foramen.

    optic f. optic canal.

    f. ova′le 1. the septal opening in the fetal heart that provides a communication between the atria; it normally closes at

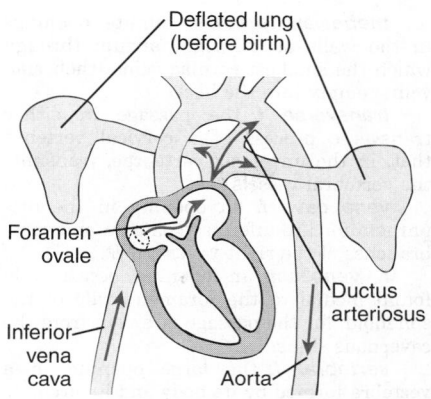

The fully developed embryonic heart showing the foramen ovale and ductus arteriosus. From Copstead and Banasik, 2000.

birth. Failure to close results in an ATRIAL SEPTAL DEFECT. 2. an aperture in the great wing of the sphenoid for vessels and nerves.

    petrosal f., f. petro′sum a small opening sometimes present behind the foramen ovale for transmission of the lesser petrosal nerve.

    f. rotun′dum a round opening in the great wing of the sphenoid for the maxillary branch of the trigeminal nerve.

    sacral foramina, anterior eight passages (four on each side) on the pelvic surface of the sacrum for the anterior branches of the sacral nerves.

    sacral foramina, posterior eight passages (four on each side) on the dorsal surface of the sacrum for the posterior branches of the sacral nerves.

    Scarpa's f. an opening behind the upper medial incisor, for the nasopalatine nerve.

    sciatic f. either of two openings (the greater and smaller sciatic foramina), formed by the sacrotuberal and sacrospinal ligaments in the sciatic notch of the hip bone.

    sphenopalatine f. a space between the orbital and sphenoidal processes of the palatine bone, opening into the nasal cavity and transmitting the sphenopalatine artery and the nasal nerves.

    spinous f. a hole in the great wing of the sphenoid for the middle meningeal artery.

    supraorbital f. passage in the frontal bone for the supraorbital vessels and nerve; often present as a notch bridged only by fibrous tissue.

thebesian foramina minute openings in the walls of the right atrium through which the smallest cardiac veins (thebesian veins) empty into the heart.

transverse f. the passage in either transverse process of a cervical vertebra that, in the upper six vertebrae, transmits the vertebral vessels.

vena cava f. an opening in the diaphragm for the inferior VENA CAVA and some branches of the right VAGUS NERVE.

f. veno'sum an opening occasionally found medial to the foramen ovale of the sphenoid, for the passage of a vein from the cavernous sinus.

vertebral f. the large opening in a vertebra formed by its body and its arch.

f. of Vesalius foramen venosum.

Weitbrecht's f. a foramen in the capsule of the shoulder joint.

f. of Winslow epiploic foramen.

Forbes' disease (forbz) GLYCOGEN STORAGE DISEASE (type III), a condition in which deficiency of the debrancher enzyme dextrin-1,6-glucosidase affects the heart and liver, with hepatomegaly, hypoglycemia, acidosis, stunted growth, and a doll-like face. Called also Cori's disease and limit dextrinosis.

force (fors) energy or power; that which originates or arrests motion or other activity.

electromotive f. the force that, by reason of differences in POTENTIAL, causes a flow of electricity from one place to another, giving rise to an electric CURRENT.

reserve f. energy above that required for normal functioning. In the heart it is the power that will take care of the additional circulatory burden imposed by bodily exertion.

shearing f's see SHEAR.

van der Waals f's the relatively weak, short-range forces of attraction existing between atoms and molecules, which results in the attraction of nonpolar organic compounds to each other (hydrophobic bonding).

forceps (for'seps) [L.] a two-bladed instrument with a handle, used for compressing or grasping tissues in surgical operations, handling sterile dressings, and other purposes.

alligator f. a grasping forceps with a scissorlike handle and blades opening in a vertical plane similar to the jaws of an alligator.

bayonet f. a forceps whose blades are offset from the axis of the handle.

capsule f. a forceps for removing the lens capsule in cataract.

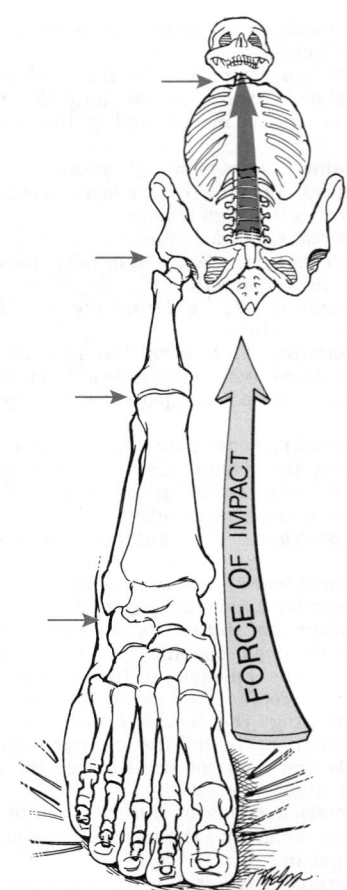

Forces resulting from a fall are transmitted up to the spine through the long leg bones and pelvis. From McQuillan et al., 2002.

Chamberlen f. the original form of obstetric forceps, invented in the sixteenth century.

clamp f. a forceps-like clamp with an automatic lock, for compressing arteries or other structures.

dressing f. forceps with scissor-like handles for grasping lint, drainage tubes, etc., in dressing wounds.

Magill f. forceps used to introduce an endotracheal tube into the trachea during nasotracheal intubation.

obstetric f. forceps for extracting the fetal head from the maternal passages.

rongeur f. a forceps designed for use in cutting bone.

thumb f. a forceps with serrated blades and with or without teeth.

tissue f. a forceps without teeth or with one or more small teeth at the end of

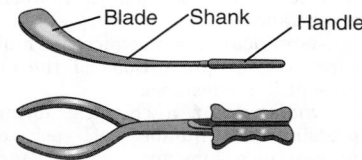

Solid blade Tucker-McLean forceps

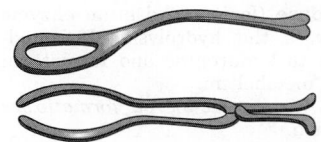

Piper forceps, used to deliver the head when the fetus is in a breech presentation

Obstetric forceps and their application. From McKinney et al., 2000.

each blade, designed for handling tissues with minimal trauma during surgery.

Fordyce's disease (for′dīs-ez) a developmental anomaly marked by enlarged and ectopic sebaceous glands that appear as minute yellowish papules on the oral mucosa.

forearm (for′ahrm) the part of the upper LIMB between the elbow and wrist; called also antebrachium.

forebag (for′bag) forewaters.

forebrain (for′brān) prosencephalon.

foreconscious (for′kon-shus) preconscious.

forefinger (for′fing-ger) the second finger, counting the thumb as first; called also index finger.

forefoot (for′foot) the front part of the foot.

foregut (for′gut) the endodermal canal of the embryo cephalic to the junction of the yolk stalk, giving rise to the pharynx, lung, esophagus, stomach, liver, and most of the small intestine.

forehead (for′hed) the part of the face above the eyes; the anterior portion of the cranium. Called also frons.

foreign (for′en) 1. not normal or usual to a place. 2. in immunology, pertaining to substances not recognized as "self" and capable of inducing an IMMUNE RESPONSE.

f. body reaction a granulomatous INFLAMMATORY RESPONSE evoked by the presence of a foreign BODY in the tissues; a characteristic feature of this is the formation of foreign body giant cells (see giant CELL).

foremilk (for′milk) 1. the first milk to be drawn out during BREASTFEEDING. 2. colostrum.

forensic (fo-ren′zik) pertaining to or applied in legal proceedings.

foreplay (for′pla) the sexually stimulating, usually pleasurable, play preceding intercourse.

foreshortening (for-shor′ten-ing) a distortion that gives the appearance of decreased depth in an image that is being studied radiographically.

foreskin (for′skin) a loose fold of skin that covers the glans penis; it is a continuation of the loose skin that covers the entire penis and scrotum. Its removal is called CIRCUMCISION. Called also prepuce.

Patient Care. In the uncircumcised male the foreskin is retracted at least daily and the glans penis washed with soap and water. In the newborn, assessment includes inspecting the foreskin and underlying penis for evidence of adhesions, interference with urination or other abnormalities. Before discharge the parents are taught how to clean the genitals of an uncircumcised male infant.

forewaters (for′wah-terz) the part of the amniotic sac that pouches into the uterine cervix in front of the presenting part of the fetus. Called also forebag.

fork (fork) a pronged instrument.

tuning f. a device that produces harmonic vibration when its two prongs are struck; used to test hearing and bone conduction. See TUNING FORK TESTS.

formaldehyde (for-mal′dĕ-hīd) a gaseous compound with strongly disinfectant properties. It is used in a 37 per cent solution (formaldehyde solution; also called formol or formalin) as a disinfectant and as a preservative and fixative for pathological specimens. The gas is toxic and carcinogenic.

formalin (for′mah-lin) formaldehyde solution; see FORMALDEHYDE.

Foreskin (prepuce)

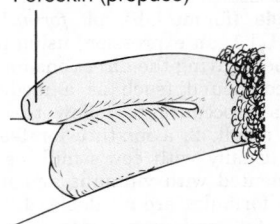

Uncircumcised penis

Foreskin. From Lammon et al., 1995.

formamidase (form-am′ĭ-dās) an enzyme that catalyzes the hydrolysis of formyl-kynurenine to kynurenine and formate in tryptophan metabolism.

formatio (for-ma′she-o), pl. *formatio′nes* [L.] formation.

formation (for-ma′shun) 1. the process of giving shape or form; the creation of an entity, or of a structure of definite shape. 2. a structure of definite shape.

   chiasma f. the process by which a chiasma is formed; it is the cytologic basis of genetic recombination, or crossing over.

   compromise f. in psychoanalysis a substituted idea or act representing and permitting partial expression of a repressed conflict.

   concept f. the ability to organize a variety of information to form thoughts and ideas, a cognitive PERFORMANCE COMPONENT in occupational therapy.

   reaction f. a DEFENSE MECHANISM in which a person adopts conscious attitudes, interests, or feelings that are the opposites of unconscious feelings, impulses, or wishes. For example, a person may use revulsion or repugnance to defend against an unconscious desire or attraction.

formic acid (for′mik) a colorless, pungent liquid with vesicant properties, from nettles and ants and other insects; derivable from oxalic acid and from glycerin and from the oxidation of formaldehyde.

formication (for″mĭ-ka′shun) a tactile hallucination in which there is a sensation of tiny insects crawling over the skin; most commonly seen in cocaine or amphetamine intoxication.

formiciasis (for″mĭ-si′ah-sis) a morbid condition caused by ant bites.

formiminoglutamic acid (FIGLU) (form-ĭ-me″no-gloo-tam′ik) a product of histidine metabolism. The urine FIGLU concentration is elevated in some individuals with folic acid deficiency.

formol (for′mol) formaldehyde solution; see FORMALDEHYDE.

formula (for′mu-lah), pl. *formulas, for′-mulae* [L.] 1. an expression, using numbers or symbols, giving the directions for preparing a compound (such as a medicine) or giving a procedure to follow to obtain a desired result. 2. a mixture for feeding an infant, usually with cow's milk as a base, supplemented with vitamins and minerals. Various formulas are available, differing in protein, fat, and carbohydrate content in order to meet the nutritional requirements or restrictions of individual infants.

   chemical f. a combination of symbols used to express the chemical components of a substance.

   empirical f. a chemical formula that expresses the proportions of the elements present in a substance.

   molecular f. a chemical formula expressing the number of each element present in a substance, without indicating how they are linked.

   spatial f., stereochemical f. a chemical formula giving the numbers of atoms of each element present in a molecule of a substance, which atom is linked to which, the types of linkages involved, and the relative positions of the atoms in space.

   structural f. a chemical formula showing the spatial arrangement of the atoms and the linkage of every atom.

formulary (for′mu-lar″e) a collection of formulae.

   National F. a book of standards for certain pharmaceuticals and preparations not included in the U.S.P; revised every 5 years, and recognized as a book of official standards by the Pure Food and Drug Act of 1906. Abbreviated N.F.

formyl (for′mil) the radical, HCO or H·C:O——, of formic acid.

fornix (for′niks), pl. *for′nices* [L.] an anatomical archlike structure.

   f. of conjunctiva conjunctival cul-de-sac.

Fortaz (for′taz) trademark for a preparation of CEFTAZIDIME, a CEPHALOSPORIN antibiotic.

Fort Bragg fever pretibial fever.

fortified (for′tĭ-fīd) containing nutrients that have been artificially added to foods that do not naturally contain them, such as milk fortified with vitamin D.

fortitude (for′tĭ-tood) in bioethics, a virtue consisting of a firm, sustained, moral courage or patient endurance of misfortune, pain, or other difficulties. As in all the virtues, the emphasis is on sustainability, not on individual acts.

forward-bending maneuver a method of detecting retraction signs in neoplastic changes in the breasts; the patient bends forward from the waist with chin held up and arms extended toward the examiner. If retraction is present, an asymmetry in the breast is seen.

foscarnet (fos-kahr′net) an agent that inhibits replication of viruses, used as the sodium salt in treatment of cytomegalovirus RETINITIS and HERPES SIMPLEX in immunocompromised patients.

fosfomycin (fos-fo-mi′sin) an antibacterial agent active against a wide range of gram-positive and gram-negative bacteria, used in the treatment of urinary tract infection; administered orally as the tromethamine salt.

fosinopril (fo-sin′o-pril) an angiotensin-converting enzyme INHIBITOR administered orally as the sodium salt to treat hypertension and congestive HEART FAILURE.

fosphenytoin (fos′fen-ĭ-toin″) a PRODRUG of PHENYTOIN used as the sodium salt in treatment of EPILEPSY, excluding the petit mal type; administered intravenously or intramuscularly.

fossa (fos′ah), pl. *fos′sae* [L.] a trench or channel; in anatomy, a hollow or depressed area.

amygdaloid f. the depression in which the tonsil is lodged.

cerebral f. any of the depressions on the floor of the cranial cavity.

condylar f., condyloid f. either of two pits on the lateral portion of the occipital bone.

coronoid f. a depression in the humerus for the coronoid process of the ulna.

cranial f. any one of the three hollows (anterior, middle, and posterior) in the base of the cranium for the lobes of the brain.

digastric f. a depression on the inner surface of the mandible, giving attachment to the anterior belly of the digastric muscle.

epigastric f. 1. one in the epigastric region. 2. urachal fossa.

ethmoid f. the groove in the cribriform plate of the ethmoid bones, for the olfactory bulb.

glenoid f. mandibular fossa.

hyaloid f. a depression in the front of the vitreous body, lodging the lens.

hypophyseal f. a depression in the sphenoid lodging the pituitary gland; called also pituitary fossa.

iliac f. a concave area occupying much of the inner surface of the ala of the ilium, especially anteriorly; from it arises the iliac muscle.

incisive f. a slight depression on the anterior surface of the maxilla above the incisor teeth.

infraclavicular f. the triangular region of the chest just below the clavicle, between the deltoid and pectoralis major muscles.

infratemporal f. an irregularly shaped cavity medial or deep to the zygomatic arch.

interpeduncular f. a depression on the inferior surface of the midbrain, between the two cerebral peduncles, the floor of which is the posterior perforated substance.

ischiorectal f. a potential space between the pelvic diaphragm and the skin below it; an anterior recess extends a variable distance.

mandibular f. a depression in the inferior surface of the pars squamosa of the temporal bone at the base of the zygomatic process, in which the condyle of the mandible rests; called also glenoid fossa.

mastoid f. a small triangular area between the posterior wall of the external acoustic meatus and the posterior root of the zygomatic process of the temporal bone.

nasal f. the portion of the nasal cavity anterior to the middle meatus.

navicular f. 1. the lateral expansion of the urethra of the glans penis. 2. a depression on the internal pterygoid process of the sphenoid, giving attachment to the tensor veli palatini muscle. 3. vestibular fossa.

f. ova′lis cor′dis a fossa in the right atrium of the heart; the remains of the fetal foramen ovale.

f. ova′lis fe′moris the depression in the fascia lata that is bridged by the cribriform fascia and perforated by the great saphenous vein.

ovarian f. a shallow pouch on the posterior surface of the broad ligament of the uterus in which the ovary is located.

paravesical f. the fossa formed by the peritoneum on each side of the urinary bladder.

pituitary f. hypophyseal fossa.

popliteal f. the hollow at the posterior part of the knee.

subarcuate f. a depression in the posterior inner surface of the pars petrosa of the temporal bone.

subpyramidal f. a depression on the internal wall of the middle ear.

subsigmoid f. a fossa between the mesentery of the sigmoid flexure and that of the descending colon.

supraspinous f. a depression above the spine of the scapula.

temporal f. an area on the side of the cranium bounded posteriorly and superiorly by the temporal lines, anteriorly by the frontal and zygomatic bones, and laterally by the zygomatic arch, lodging the temporal muscle.

tibiofemoral f. a space between the articular surfaces of the tibia and femur mesial or lateral to the inferior pole of the patella.

urachal f. one on the inner abdominal wall, between the urachus and the hypogastric artery.

vestibular f., f. of vestibule of vagina the vaginal vestibule between the vaginal orifice and the fourchette (frenulum of pudendal labia). Called also navicular fossa.

fossette (fŏ-set′) 1. a small depression. 2. a small, deep corneal ulcer.

fossula (fos′u-lah), pl. *fos′sulae* [L.] a small fossa.

Fothergill's disease (foth′er-gilz) 1. scarlatina anginosa. 2. tic douloureux.

foulage (foo-lahzh′) [Fr.] kneading and pressing of the muscles in massage; called also pétrissage.

fourchette (foor-shet′) [Fr.] frenulum of pudendal labia.

Fournier's disease (foor-nyāz′) Fournier's GANGRENE.

fovea (fo′ve-ah), pl. *fo′veae* [L.] a small pit or depression often used alone to indicate the central fovea of the retina.

central f. of retina, f. centra′lis re′tinae a small pit in the center of the MACULA LUTEA, composed of slim elongated CONES; it is the area of clearest vision, because here the layers of the retina are spread aside, permitting light to fall directly on the cones.

foveate (fo′ve-āt) pitted.

foveation (fo″ve-a′shun) formation of pits on a surface, as on the skin; a pitted condition.

foveola (fo-ve′o-lah), pl. *fove′olae* [L.] a minute pit or depression.

Fox-Fordyce disease (foks for′dīs) a chronic, usually pruritic disease chiefly seen in women, characterized by the development of small follicular papular eruptions of apocrine gland–bearing areas, especially the axillae and pubes, caused by obstruction and rupture of the intraepidermal portion of the ducts of affected apocrine glands.

FPG fasting plasma GLUCOSE.

Fr francium.

fractionation (frak″shun-a′shun) 1. in radiology, division of the total dose of radiation into small doses given at intervals. 2. in chemistry, separation of a substance into components, as by distillation or crystallization. 3. in histology, isolation of components of living cells by differential centrifugation.

fracture (frak′chur) 1. the breaking of a part, especially a bone. 2. a break in continuity of bone; it may be caused by trauma, twisting due to muscle spasm or indirect loss of leverage, or by disease that results in OSTEOPENIA. See illustration.

Treatment. Immediate first aid consists of SPLINTING the bone with no attempt to reduce the fracture; it should be splinted "as it lies," which means supporting it in such a way that the injured part will remain steady and will resist jarring if the victim is moved. Later it will be treated by REDUCTION, which means that the broken ends are

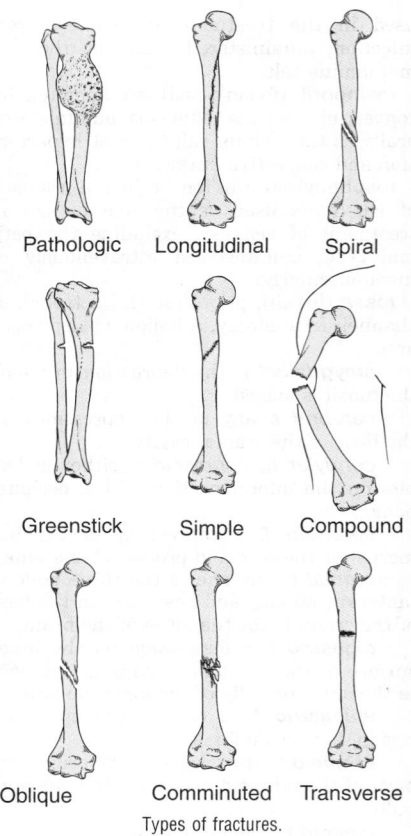

Pathologic   Longitudinal   Spiral

Greenstick   Simple   Compound

Oblique   Comminuted   Transverse

Types of fractures.

pulled into alignment and the continuity of the bone is established so that healing can take place. Fracture healing is truly a process of regeneration. Fractures heal with normal bone, not with scar tissue. Closed reduction is performed by manual manipulation of the fractured bone so that the fragments are brought into proper alignment; no surgical incision is made. Open fractures are highly contaminated and must be débrided and copiously irrigated in the operating room. A fracture may also require internal fixation with pins, nails, metal plates, or screws to stabilize the alignment. Once closed reduction is accomplished, the bone is immobilized by application of a CAST or by an apparatus exerting TRACTION on the distal end of the bone.

avulsion f. separation of a small fragment of bone cortex at the site of attachment of a ligament or tendon.

Barton's f. fracture of the distal end of the radius into the wrist joint.

COMPLICATIONS OF FRACTURES

Complication	Cause	Findings
Compartment Syndrome	Circulation is compromised due to an increase within the muscle compartments of an extremity. Histamine is released from the ischemic muscle tissue causing edema and more pressure. A cycle of ischemia and edema is established which can lead to tissue necrosis if not interrupted.	Initially the character of the pulse will weaken and the skin in the extremity will pale. Symptoms then progress to cyanosis, paresis and severe pain. If left untreated, irreversible neuromuscular damage will occur within 4 to 6 hours.
Fat Emboli	The release of fat globules from the fractured bone into the blood stream. This complication is more likely to be related to fractures of long bones.	Restlessness and apprehension, respiratory distress, tachycardia, hypertension, fever, and petechiae over neck and upper thoracic area. Laboratory findings that accompany this disorder include an increased erythrocyte sedimentation rate and serum lipase level as well as a decreased serum albumin, decreased red blood cells, and decreased platelet counts.
Infection	Interruption in the integrity of the integument. Instrumentation in the area of fracture.	Typical of those associated with either a local or systemic infection; these include fever, pain, tachycardia, elevated white blood cell counts and, in the case of a local infection, erythema in the area surrounding the fracture. Gas gangrene may also cause confusion on the part of the patient.
Avascular Necrosis	An interruption in the blood supply to the bony tissue, which results in death of the bone.	Pathological fractures.
Pulmonary Emboli	Immobility precipitated by the fracture.	Restlessness and apprehension, dyspnea, blood gas changes.

Bennett's f. fracture of the base of the first metacarpal bone, running into the carpometacarpal joint, complicated by subluxation.

blow-out f. fracture of the orbital floor caused by a sudden increase of intraorbital pressure due to traumatic force; the orbital contents herniate into the maxillary sinus so that the inferior rectus or inferior oblique muscle may become incarcerated in the fracture site, producing diplopia on looking up.

closed f. one that does not produce an open wound, as opposed to an open fracture. See illustration. Called also simple fracture.

Colles' f. fracture of the lower end of the radius, the distal fragment being displaced backward.

comminuted f. one in which the bone is splintered or crushed, with three or more fragments. See illustration.

complete f. one involving the entire cross section of the bone.

compound f. open fracture.

compression f. one produced by compression.

depressed f., depressed skull f. fracture of the skull in which a fragment is depressed.

direct f. one at the site of injury.

dislocation f. fracture of a bone near an articulation with concomitant dislocation of that joint.

double f. fracture of a bone in two places.

Dupuytren's f. Pott's fracture.

Duverney's f. fracture of the ilium just below the anterior inferior spine.

fissure f. a crack extending from a surface into, but not through, a long bone.

greenstick f. one in which one side of a bone is broken and the other is bent, most commonly seen in children. See illustration.

impacted f. fracture in which one fragment is firmly driven into the other.

incomplete f. one that does not involve the complete cross section of the bone.

indirect f. one distant from the site of injury.

interperiosteal f. greenstick fracture.

intrauterine f. fracture of a fetal bone incurred in utero.

Jefferson's f. fracture of the atlas (first cervical vertebra).

lead pipe f. one in which the bone cortex is slightly compressed and bulged on one side with a slight crack on the other side of the bone.

Le Fort f. bilateral horizontal fracture of the maxilla. Le Fort fractures are classified as follows: *Le Fort I fracture,* a horizontal segmented fracture of the alveolar process of the maxilla, in which the teeth are usually contained in the detached portion of the bone. *Le Fort II fracture,* unilateral or bilateral fracture of the maxilla, in which the body of the maxilla is separated from the facial skeleton and the separated portion is pyramidal in shape; the fracture may extend through the body of the maxilla down the midline of the hard palate, through the floor of the orbit, and into the nasal cavity. *Le Fort III fracture,* a fracture in which the entire maxilla and one or more facial bones are completely separated from the craniofacial skeleton; such fractures are almost always accompanied by multiple fractures of the facial bones.

longitudinal f. one extending along the length of the bone. See illustration.

Monteggia's f. one in the proximal half of the shaft of the ulna, with dislocation of the head of the radius.

oblique f. one in which the break extends in an oblique direction. See illustration.

open f. one in which a wound through the adjacent or overlying soft tissue communicates with the outside of the body; this must be considered a surgical emergency. The compounding may come from within (by a bone protruding through the skin) or from without (e.g., by a bullet wound communicating with the bone). See illustration. Called also compound fracture.

pathologic f. one due to weakening of the bone structure by pathologic processes such as neoplasia or osteomalacia; see illustration. Called also spontaneous fracture.

pertrochanteric f. fracture of the femur passing through the greater trochanter.

ping-pong f. an indented fracture of the skull, resembling the indentation that can be produced with the finger in a ping-pong ball; when elevated it resumes and retains its normal position.

Pott's f. fracture of lower part of the fibula with serious injury of the lower tibial articulation.

simple f. closed fracture.

Smith's f. reversed Colles' fracture.

spiral f. one in which the bone has been twisted and the fracture line resembles a spiral. See illustration.

spontaneous f. pathologic fracture.

sprain f. the separation of a tendon from its insertion, taking with it a piece of bone.

stellate f. one with a central point of injury, from which radiate numerous fissures.

Stieda's f. a fracture of the internal condyle of the femur.

transcervical f. one through the neck of the femur.

transverse f. one at right angles to the axis of the bone. See illustration.

trophic f. one due to a nutritional (trophic) disturbance.

fracture-dislocation (frak′chur-dis″lo-ka′-shun) a fracture of a bone near a joint, also involving dislocation.

frae- for words beginning thus, see those beginning *fre-*.

fragilitas (frah-jil′ĭ-tas) [L.] fragility.

f. cri′nium a brittleness of the hair.

f. os′sium conge′nita osteogenesis imperfecta.

fragility (frah-jil′ĭ-te) susceptibility, or lack of resistance, to influences capable of causing disruption of continuity or integrity.

f. of blood erythrocyte fragility.

capillary f. abnormal susceptibility of capillary walls to rupture with EXTRAVASATION.

erythrocyte f. unusual susceptibility of erythrocytes to hemolysis under certain conditions; see *mechanical fragility* and *osmotic fragility.*

mechanical f. unusual susceptibility of certain erythrocytes to hemolysis under mechanical stress.

osmotic f. susceptibility of certain erythrocytes to hemolysis when exposed to increasingly hypotonic solutions; seen in some forms of HEMOLYTIC ANEMIA and SPHEROCYTOSIS. A test of osmotic fragility is used in diagnosis of some types of hemolytic anemia.

fragmentation (frag″men-ta′shun) division into small pieces.

frambesia (fram-be′ze-ah) yaws.

frambesioma (fram-be″ze-o′mah) mother yaw; the initial cutaneous lesion of YAWS.

frame (frām) a rigid supporting structure or a structure for immobilizing a part.

Balkan f. an apparatus for continuous extension in treatment of fractures of the femur, consisting of an overhead bar, with pulleys attached, by which the leg is supported in a sling.

Bradford f. a rectangular structure of gas pipe across which are stretched two strips of canvas, once used as a bed frame for patients with fractures or disease of the hip or spine.

quadriplegic standing f. a device for supporting in the upright position a patient whose four limbs are paralyzed.

Stryker f. see STRYKER FRAME.

framework (frām′werk) the basic structure about which something is formulated or built.

conceptual f., theoretical f. an organization or matrix of concepts that provides a focus for inquiry.

Framingham Heart Study a longitudinal study begun in 1948 in which there is and has been continuous gathering of data on the health and habits of the adult inhabitants of Framingham, Massachusetts. Data from this study have shown relationships between cardiovascular disease and such variables as smoking, diet, lack of exercise, and other facets of a person's lifestyle.

Franceschetti syndrome (frahn″chĕ-sket′e) the complete form of mandibulofacial DYSOSTOSIS.

Francisella (fran″sĭ-sel′ah) a genus of gram-negative, aerobic, coccoid or rod-shaped bacteria; *F. tularen′sis* (formerly called *Pasteurella tularensis*) is the etiologic agent of TULAREMIA.

francium (Fr) (fran′se-um) a chemical element, atomic number 87, atomic weight 223. (See Appendix 6.)

Frankel classification (frank′l) ASIA scale.

Franklin (frank′lin) Martha M. (1870–1968). Founder of the National Association of Colored Graduate Nurses and activist for racial equality in nursing. Her concern for improved professional status for black nurses led to the foundation of the NACGN in 1908. The goals of the NACGN were to promote the standards and welfare of all nurses and to eliminate racial discrimination in the nursing profession. The organization was merged with the American Nurses' Association in 1951.

FRC functional residual capacity.

FRCP Fellow of the Royal College of Physicians.

FRCS Fellow of the Royal College of Surgeons.

freckle (frek′l) a benign, small, tan to brown macule occurring on sun-exposed skin, especially in children and tending to fade in adult life. Freckles resemble lentigines, but they darken after exposure to sunlight, whereas lentigines do not, and in freckles, the number of melanocytes is not increased. Called also ephelis.

melanotic f. of Hutchinson see lentigo maligna MELANOMA.

Freeman (fre′man) Ruth B. (1906–1982). American educator and author in the field of public health nursing; she served on the faculty at New York University, the School of Public Health at the University of Minnesota, and The Johns Hopkins University. She was the author of many works on public health nursing and administration, including *Techniques of Supervision in Public Health Nursing* and *Community Health Nursing Practice*. In addition, she was a member of many professional organizations in the field of PUBLIC HEALTH NURSING.

freeze-drying (frēz′-dri″ing) a method of tissue preparation in which the tissue specimen is frozen and then dehydrated at low temperature in a high vacuum. See also LYOPHILIZATION.

freeze-etching (frēz′-ech″ing) a method used to study unfixed cells by electron microscopy, in which the object to be studied is placed in 20 per cent glycerol, frozen at $-100°$C, and then mounted on a chilled holder.

freeze-fracturing (frēz′-frak″chur-ing) a method of preparing cells for electron-microscopical examination: a tissue specimen is frozen at $-150°$C, inserted into a vacuum chamber, and fractured by a microtome; a platinum carbon replica of the exposed surfaces is made, freed of the underlying specimen, and then examined.

freeze-substitution (frēz′-sub″-stĭ-too″-shun) a modification of freeze-drying in which the ice within the frozen tissue is replaced by alcohol or other solvents at a very low temperature.

freezing point the temperature at which a liquid begins to freeze; for water, the freezing point is $0°$ C, or $32°$ F.

Frei's disease (frīz) lymphogranuloma venereum.

Freiberg's disease (fri′bergz) osteochondrosis of the head of the second metatarsal bone.

Frejka pillow (frej′kah) a small pillow or splint used with infants to maintain hip abduction in cases of dislocation. Straps over the shoulder help keep the pillow in place.

fremitus (frem′ĭ-tus) a vibration perceptible on palpation or auscultation; see also THRILL.

tactile f. a type of vocal fremitus found over an area of secretions.

tussive f. one felt on the chest while the patient coughs.

vocal f. (VF) transmission of the spoken voice to the chest wall, detectable by auscultation or palpation; it is increased with lung consolidation and decreased with pleural effusion, pneumothorax, and airway obstruction.

frenectomy (fre-nek'to-me) excision of a frenum or frenulum.

frenoplasty (fre'no-plas"te) the correction of an abnormally attached frenum or frenulum, by surgically repositioning it.

frenotomy (fre-not'ah-me) the cutting of a frenum or frenulum.

frenulectomy (fren"u-lek'tŏ-me) frenectomy.

frenuloplasty (fren'u-lo-plas"te) frenoplasty.

frenulum (fren'u-lum), pl. *fren'ula* [L.] a small fold of integument or mucous membrane that limits the movements of an organ or part.

f. of clitoris a fold formed by union of the labia minora on the undersurface of the clitoris.

f. of ileocecal valve a fold formed by the joined extremities of the ileocecal valve, partially encircling the lumen of the colon.

f. labio'rum puden'di fourchette.

f. lin'guae frenulum of tongue.

f. of lip a median fold of mucous membrane connecting the inside of each lip to the corresponding gum.

f. of prepuce of penis a fold under the penis connecting it with the prepuce.

f. of pudendal labia the posterior junction of the labia minora; called also fourchette.

f. of superior medullary velum a band lying in the superior medullary velum at its attachment to the inferior colliculi.

f. of tongue the vertical fold of mucous membrane under the tongue, attaching it to the floor of the mouth; called also frenulum linguae.

frenum (fre'num), pl. *fre'na* [L.] a restraining structure or part; see also FRENULUM.

frequency (fre'kwen-se) 1. the number of occurrences of a periodic or recurrent process in a unit of time, such as the number of electrical cycles per second measured in HERTZ. In cardiac PACING terminology, frequency is expressed by the formula: frequency $= 12 \times$ pulse width. 2. the number of occurrences of a particular event or the number of members of a population or statistical sample falling in a particular class. 3. relative frequency.

radio f. the range of frequencies of electromagnetic RADIATION between 10 kilohertz and 100 gigahertz, used for radio communication.

relative f. the ratio of the number of occurrences of a specified phenomenon in a population to the total size of the population.

urinary f. URINATION at short intervals without increase in daily volume of urinary output, due to reduced bladder capacity or CYSTITIS.

Freud (froid) Sigmund (1856–1939). Clinical neurologist and founder of PSYCHOANALYSIS. Born in Freiberg in Moravia, and educated at the University of Vienna, he studied in Paris in 1885 under the neurologist J. M. Charcot, who encouraged him to investigate hysteria from a psychologic point of view. Freud stressed the existence of an unconscious that exerts a dynamic influence on consciousness, and was led to develop his method of "free association" in order to discover these buried memories. He emphasized the role of sexuality in the development of neurotic conditions, and published *Interpretation of Dreams* (1900), *Psychopathology of Everyday Life* (1901), and many more works. He was also director of the *International Journal of Psychology*. After fleeing the Nazi regime in Vienna in 1938, he died in London.

freudian (froi'de-an) 1. pertaining to Sigmund Freud, the founder of PSYCHOANALYSIS or his psychological theories and method of psychotherapy (psychoanalytic theory and technique). 2. an adherent or user of freudian theory or methods.

friable (fri'ah-b'l) easily pulverized or crumbled.

friction (frik'shun) the act of rubbing.

Fried's rule (frēds) the dose of a drug for an infant less than 2 years old is obtained by multiplying the child's age in months by the adult dose and dividing the result by 150.

Friedländer's disease (frēd'len-derz) endarteritis obliterans.

Friedreich's ataxia (frēd'rīks) hereditary sclerosis of the dorsal and lateral columns of the spinal cord, usually beginning in childhood or youth. It is attended by ataxia, speech impairment, scoliosis, and peculiar swaying and irregular movements, with paralysis of the muscles, especially of the lower extremities.

Friedreich's disease (frēd'rīks) 1. paramyoclonus multiplex. 2. Friedreich's ataxia.

frigidity (frĭ-jid'ĭ-te) 1. coldness. 2. former name for FEMALE SEXUAL AROUSAL DISORDER.

frigorific (frig'o-rif'ik) producing coldness.

Fröhlich's syndrome (fra'liks) adiposogenital dystrophy.

frolement (frōl-maw') [Fr.] 1. a rustling sound heard on auscultation in pericardial disease. 2. a brushing movement in massage.

frons (fronz) [L.] forehead.

frontad (frun'tad) toward a front, or frontal aspect.

frontal (frun't'l) 1. pertaining to the FORE-HEAD. 2. denoting a longitudinal plane passing through the body from side to side, and dividing it into front and back parts.

frontalis (fron-ta'lis) [L.] frontal.

frost (frost) a deposit resembling frozen dew or vapor.

    urea f. the appearance on the skin of salt crystals left by evaporation of the sweat in URHIDROSIS.

frostbite (frost'bīt) injury to tissues due to exposure to cold. Usually the first areas of the body to freeze are the nose, ears, fingers, and toes. The flesh feels cold to the touch, and frozen parts become pale and feel numb. There may also be some prickly or itchy sensation. A person suffering from frostbite may feel no warning pain. In mild cases, proper treatment can rather quickly restore normal circulation of blood. In more serious cases the area may become painfully inflamed, and blistering may follow. Especially severe frostbite can cause death of the injured tissues and GANGRENE.

Mild frostbite usually appears as a shallow, blanched wheal on the nose, ears, fingers, or toes. After rewarming, the area is slightly reddened for several hours and then resumes a normal appearance. If the frostbite is more severe, deeper tissues are affected and the area appears waxy and feels doughlike to the touch. With rewarming, the area becomes edematous and the patient feels itching, burning, and deep pain. Later on, mild edema may remain and the skin becomes mottled, cyanotic, or red without blistering. Over the following weeks the pain and edema should subside, but the skin may peel and the patient may experience increased sensitivity to cold in that area until healing is complete.

Blistering occurs in deeper frostbite. The vesicles may contain pink or clear fluid that has leaked from damaged cells and tissues. Eventually the vesicles contract and dry out, leaving an eschar that sloughs off and exposes new skin underneath if there has been adequate circulation to the part.

Severe frostbite damages all layers of soft tissue down to connective tissue and bone. The frostbitten area is hard and wooden and appears lifeless. There is no sensation of pain and the patient cannot voluntarily move the frozen part. With rewarming there are aching pain, burning, and blistering. If there is no pain or other sensation after rewarming, the tissue may be dead and amputation may be indicated.

Treatment. Rewarming is best done in an emergency care facility where assessment of the extent of frostbite can be done and appropriate measures taken to rewarm the frostbitten part without further damaging tissue. In the field, it is best to keep the part as warm as possible to prevent further freezing. Blankets and warm clothing are appropriate and, if possible, the frozen area can be placed in contact with any other part of the body that is warm. Rubbing and massaging the area is not recommended because it can only serve to further damage frozen tissue. The victim should not smoke and should avoid caffeine and alcohol because any of these can further restrict blood circulation.

Emergency medical care, if the patient cannot be brought to the hospital and rewarming must be done in the field, includes rapid rewarming in water baths not exceeding 40.6°C (105°F). Hot water can cause further tissue destruction. Tetanus prophylaxis is administered as necessary. If severely frostbitten tissue swells to the point of totally restricting circulation, a fasciotomy may be required to allow adequate blood supply. Vesicles are left intact but frostbitten fingers and toes should be separated with cotton balls and a loose dressing applied. If the patient will be taken outside for transport to a medical facility, rewarming should be started at the hospital.

frottage (frŏ-tazh') 1. a rubbing movement in massage. 2. frotteurism.

frotteur (frŏ-tur') one who practices frotteurism.

frotteurism (frŏ-tu'rizm) a PARAPHILIA in which there are repetitive sexual urges to gain gratification by rubbing against another person, often acted out in a public place. Called also frottage.

frozen section a specimen of tissue that has been quick-frozen, cut by microtome, and stained immediately for rapid diagnosis of possible malignant lesions. A specimen processed in this manner is not satisfactory for detailed study of the cells, but it is valuable because it is quick and gives the surgeon immediate information regarding the malignancy of a piece of tissue.

fructofuranose (fruk″to-fu'rah-nōs) the combining and more reactive form of fructose.

β-fructofuranosidase (fruk″to-fu″rah-no'sĭ-dās) an enzyme occurring in yeasts and other organisms that catalyzes the hydrolysis of sugars with a terminal unsubstituted β-D-fructofuranosyl residue.

fructokinase (fruk″to-ki′nās) an enzyme that catalyzes the transfer of a high-energy phosphate group to D-FRUCTOSE.

fructose (fruk′tōs) a monosaccharide found in honey and many sweet fruits; it is used in solution as a fluid and nutrient replenisher. Called also levulose and fruit sugar.

fructosemia (fruk″to-se′me-ah) the presence of fructose in the blood, as in fructose intolerance.

fructoside (fruk′to-sīd) a compound that bears the same relation to fructose as a glucoside does to glucose.

fructosuria (fruk″to-su′re-ah) the presence of fructose in the urine.

essential f. a benign, autosomal recessive disorder of carbohydrate metabolism due to a defect in fructokinase and manifested only by fructose in the blood and urine.

fructosyl (fruk′to-sil) a radical of fructose.

fruit (froot) the matured ovary of a plant, including the seed and its envelopes.

frustration (frus-tra′shun) 1. the blocking or thwarting of purposes, desires, actions, or impulses. 2. a feeling of tension arising when such thwarting occurs.

FSF fibrin-stabilizing factor (factor XIII, one of the COAGULATION FACTORS).

FSH follicle-stimulating hormone.

FSH/LH-RH follicle-stimulating hormone and luteinizing hormone releasing hormone.

FSH-RH follicle-stimulating hormone releasing hormone.

FTA-ABS test fluorescent treponemal antibody absorption test.

5-FU 5-fluorouracil; see *fluorouracil.*

fuchsin (fūk′sin) any of several red to purple dyes, sometimes specifically basic fuchsin.

acid f. a mixture of sulfonated fuchsins; used in various complex stains.

basic f. a histologic stain, containing predominantly pararosaniline and rosaniline.

fucose (fu′kōs) a monosaccharide occurring as L-fucose in a number of mucopolysaccharides and mucoproteins.

fucosidase (fu-ko′sĭ-dās) an enzyme occurring in two forms that catalyzes the hydrolysis of fucoside to an alcohol and fucose.

fucoside (fu′ko-sīd) an acetal derivative of fucose.

fucosidosis (fu″ko-sĭ-do′sis) a hereditary disease due to deficient enzymatic activity of fucosidase and resulting in accumulation of fucose in all tissues; marked by progressive cerebral degeneration, muscle weakness with eventual spasticity, emaciation, cardiomegaly, thick skin, and excessive sweating.

FUDR 1. abbreviation for FLOXURIDINE. 2. trademark for a preparation of floxuridine, an ANTINEOPLASTIC.

FUdR floxuridine.

-fugal word element [L.], *driving away; fleeing from; repelling.*

fugue (fūg) a pathological state of altered CONSCIOUSNESS in which an individual may act and wander around as though conscious but his behavior is not directed by his complete normal personality and is not remembered after the fugue ends.

dissociative f., psychogenic f. a DISSOCIATIVE DISORDER characterized by an episode in which an individual forgets his past, assumes a partial or complete new identity, and travels away from home or work, in some cases taking up a new name, occupation, and lifestyle. During the fugue, patients are unaware that they have forgotten anything and seem to other people to be behaving normally; following recovery, they recall nothing that happened during the fugue. The disorder is usually related to emotional conflicts due to some traumatic, stressful, or overwhelming event, remits spontaneously, and rarely recurs.

fulgurate (ful′gu-rāt) 1. to come and go like a flash of lightning. 2. to destroy by contact with electric sparks generated by a high-frequency current.

fulguration (ful″gu-ra′shun) destruction of living tissue by electric sparks generated by a high-frequency current.

direct f. that in which an insulated electrode with a metal point is connected to the uniterminal and an electric spark is allowed to impinge on the area being treated.

indirect f. that in which the patient is connected directly by a metal handle to the uniterminal and the operator uses an active electrode to complete an arc from the patient.

fuller's earth (ful′erz erth) an impure aluminum silicate that has decolorizing and purifying properties. It is an absorbent used in the management of PARAQUAT poisoning; the mode of action is by tightly binding paraquat to the clay in the formulation, which takes place in the gastrointestinal tract and facilitates elimination in the feces.

fulminate (ful′mĭ-nāt) to occur suddenly with great intensity. adj., **ful′minant.**

Fulvicin (ful′vĭ-sin) trademark for preparations of GRISEOFULVIN, an antifungal AGENT.

fumarase (fu′mah-rās) an enzyme that catalyzes the interconversion of fumarate and malate.

fumarate (fu'mar-āt) a salt of fumaric acid.

fumaric acid (fu'mar-ik) an unsaturated dibasic acid, the *trans* isomer of maleic acid and an intermediate in the tricarboxylic acid CYCLE.

fumigation (fu''mĭ-ga'shun) exposure to disinfecting fumes.

function (fungk'shun) the special, normal, or proper action of any part or organ.

   probability density f. in statistics, a mathematical function that describes the DISTRIBUTION of measurements for a population. It is a curve that describes the population.

functional (fungk'shun-al) 1. pertaining to or fulfilling a FUNCTION. 2. affecting the function but not the structure.

   f. disease, f. disorder a disease or disorder of physiological function having no known organic basis. Although not strictly correct, the term is often used in psychiatry for disorders that are PSYCHOGENIC and in other branches of medicine to refer to any that are IDIOPATHIC.

   f. method a type of nursing care delivery system; see NURSING PRACTICE.

fundectomy (fun-dek'to-me) fundusectomy.

fundiform (fun'dĭ-form) shaped like a loop or sling.

fundoplication (fun''do-pli-ka'shun) mobilization of the lower end of the ESOPHAGUS and plication of the FUNDUS of the stomach up around it, in the treatment of reflux ESOPHAGITIS that may be associated with disorders such as hiatal HERNIA.

fundus (fun'dus), pl. *fun'di* [L.] the bottom or base of anything; anatomic nomenclature for the bottom or base of an organ, or the part of a hollow organ farthest from its MOUTH. adj., **fun'dal, fun'dic.**

   f. of bladder the base or posterior surface of the urinary BLADDER, which contains the TRIGONE OF THE BLADDER and the outlet where urine empties through the internal urethral ORIFICE.

   f. of eye the back portion of the interior of the eyeball, visible through the pupil by use of the ophthalmoscope. (See Atlas 4, Part A).

   f. of gallbladder the inferior, dilated portion of the gallbladder.

   f. of stomach the part of the stomach to the left and above the level of the opening between the stomach and esophagus.

   f. tym'pani the floor of the tympanic cavity.

   f. u'teri, f. of uterus the part of the uterus above the orifices of the fallopian tubes.

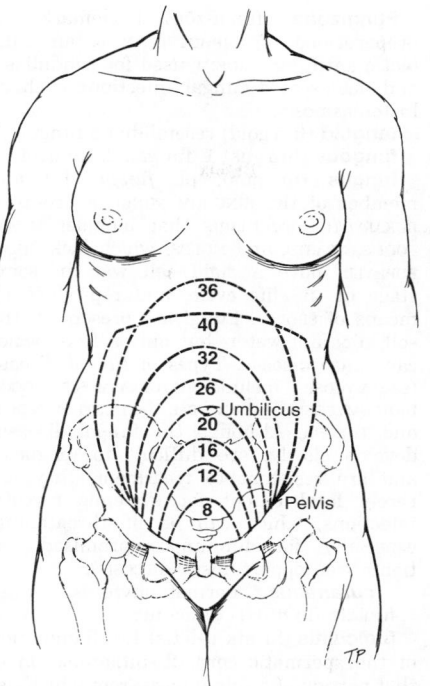

The fundus of the uterus grows in a predictable pattern during the weeks of pregnancy. From McQuillan et al., 2002.

funduscope (fun'dŭ-skōp) ophthalmoscope. adj., **funduscop'ic.**

fundusectomy (fun''dŭ-sek'to-me) excision of the fundus of an organ, as of the fundus of the stomach or uterus.

fungal (fun'g'l) pertaining to a fungus; called also fungous.

fungate (fun'gāt) to produce fungus-like growths; to grow rapidly, like a fungus.

fungemia (fun-je'me-ah) the presence of fungi in the blood stream.

Fungi (fun'ji) in the classification of living organisms, one of the kingdoms of eukaryotic organisms; see FUNGUS.

fungi (fun'ji) [L.] plural of FUNGUS.

fungicide (fun'jĭ-sīd) an agent that destroys fungi. adj., **fungici'dal.**

fungiform (fun'jĭ-form) shaped like a fungus, or mushroom.

fungistasis (fun''jĭ-sta'sis) inhibition of the growth of fungi. adj., **fungistat'ic.**

fungistat (fun'jĭ-stat) a substance that checks the growth of fungi.

fungitoxic (fun'jĭ-tok''sik) exerting a toxic effect on fungi.

Fungizone (fun'jĭ-zōn) trademark for preparations of AMPHOTERICIN B, an antibiotic antifungal AGENT used for candidiasis and deep-seated fungal infections such as histoplasmosis.

fungoid (fun'goid) resembling a fungus.

fungous (fun'gus) 1. fungal. 2. fungoid.

fungus (fun'gus), pl. *fun'gi* [L.] any member of the KINGDOM FUNGI, a group of EUKARYOTIC organisms that includes MUSHROOMS, YEASTS, and MOLDS, which lack CHLOROPHYLL, have a rigid cell wall in some stage of the life cycle, and reproduce by means of SPORES. Fungi are present in the soil, air, and water, but only a few species can cause disease. Types of fungal disease (see MYCOSIS) include HISTOPLASMOSIS, COCCIDIOIDOMYCOSIS, RINGWORM, ATHLETE'S FOOT, and THRUSH. Although the fungal diseases develop slowly, are difficult to diagnose, and are resistant to treatment, they are rarely fatal except for systemic mycotic infections, which can be life-threatening, especially for immunocompromised patients (see opportunistic MYCOSIS).

cutaneous f. dermatophyte.

funicle (fu'nĭ-k'l) funiculus.

funiculitis (fu-nik″u-li'tis) 1. inflammation of the spermatic cord. 2. inflammation of that portion of a spinal nerve root which lies within the intervertebral canal.

funiculoepididymitis (fu-nik″u-lo-ep″ĭ-did″i-mi'tis) inflammation of the spermatic cord and the epididymis.

funiculus (fu-nik'u-lus), pl. *funic'uli* [L.] CORD: anatomical nomenclature for a cordlike structure or part, especially one of the large bundle of nerve tracts that make up the white matter of the spinal cord. adj. **funic'ular.**

anterior f. ventral funiculus.

dorsal f. the white substance of the spinal cord lying on either side between the posterior median sulcus and the dorsal root.

lateral f., f. latera'lis the lateral mass of fibers on either side of the spinal cord, between the anterolateral and posterolateral sulci.

posterior f. dorsal funiculus.

f. sperma'ticus the spermatic cord.

ventral f. the white substance of the spinal cord lying on either side between the ventral median fissure and the ventral roots of the spinal nerves.

funiform (fu'nĭ-form) resembling a rope or cord.

FUO fever of unknown origin.

Furadantin (fūr″ah-dan'tin) trademark for preparations of NITROFURANTOIN, an antibacterial used in urinary tract infections.

furazolidone (fu″rah-zol'ĭ-dōn) a NITROFURAN antibacterial and antiprotozoal used against many gram-negative intestinal bacteria in control of diarrhea and enteritis.

furcal (fur'kal) forked.

furcation (fur-ka'shun) the anatomical area where the roots divide on a multirooted tooth.

furfuraceous (fur″fu-ra'shus) scaly or branny; called also pityroid.

furosemide (fur-o'sĕ-mīd) a loop DIURETIC used for treatment of edema and hypertension.

furrow (fur'o) a groove or trench.

atrioventricular f. the transverse groove marking off the atria of the heart from the ventricles.

digital f. any one of the transverse folds across the joints on the palmar surface of a finger.

gluteal f. the furrow that separates the buttocks.

furuncle (fu'rung-k'l) boil.

furunculoid (fu-rung'ku-loid) resembling a furuncle or boil.

furunculosis (fu-rung″ku-lo'sis) 1. the persistent sequential occurrence of furuncles (BOILS) over a period of weeks or months. 2. the simultaneous occurrence of a number of furuncles.

Fusarium (fu-sa're-um) a genus of fungi; some species are plant pathogens and some are opportunistic infectious agents of humans and other animals.

fuscin (fus'in) a brown pigment of the retinal epithelium.

fusible (fu'zĭ-b'l) capable of being melted.

fusiform (fu'zĭ-form) shaped like a SPINDLE; long and thin with tapering ends.

fusimotor (fu″sĭ-mo'ter) denoting motor nerve fibers (of gamma motoneurons) that innervate intrafusal fibers of the muscle spindle.

fusion (fu'zhun) 1. the act or process of melting. 2. the merging or coherence of adjacent parts or bodies. 3. the coordination of separate images of the same object in the two eyes into one. 4. the operative formation of an ankylosis or arthrosis.

diaphyseal-epiphyseal f. operative establishment of bony union between the epiphysis and diaphysis of a bone.

spinal f. surgical creation of ankylosis between contiguous vertebrae; used in treatment of spondylosis and ruptured intervertebral disk. Called also spondylosyndesis.

fusional (fu'zhun-al) marked by fusion.

Fusobacterium (fu″so-bak-tē're-um) a genus of gram-negative, anaerobic, rod-shaped bacteria found as normal flora in the mouth and large bowel and often in necrotic tissue, probably as secondary invaders. Species include *F. gonidiafor'-mans* and *F. morti'ferum (occurring in respiratory, urogenital, and gastrointestinal infections); F. necro'phorum* (occurring in disseminated infections involving necrotic lesions, abscesses, and bacteremia); and *F. navifor'me, F. nuclea'tum, F. rus'sii,* and *F. va'rium* (occurring in abscesses and other infections).

fusocellular (fu″zo-sel′u-ler) having spindle-shaped cells.

fusospirillosis (fu″zo-spi″ri-lo′sis) necrotizing ulcerative gingivitis.

fusospirochetal (fu″zo-spi″ro-ke′t'l) of or caused by fusiform bacilli and spirochetes.

fusospirochetosis (fu″zo-spi″ro-ke-to′sis) infection with fusobacteria and streptococci.

futility (fu-til′i-te) the quality of not leading to a desired result.

medical f. the judged futility of medical care, used as a reason to limit care. Two reasons for making this judgment are (1) to conserve resources and (2) to protect clinician integrity. The types are physiologic futility and normative futility.

normative f. a judgment of medical futility made for a treatment that is seen to have a physiologic effect but is believed to have no benefit.

physiologic f. a judgment of medical futility based on the observation of no physiologic effect of the treatment.

FVC forced vital capacity.

G

G gram (or grams); gingival; glucose; gonidial.

g gram.

g standard gravity.

γ gamma, the third letter of the Greek alphabet, often used to indicate the third member of a series, such as the γ chain of HEMOGLOBIN. See also terms beginning GAMMA.

Ga gallium.

gabapentin (gab″ah-pen′tin) an anticonvulsant chemically related to γ-aminobutyric acid, used in treatment of partial SEIZURES; administered orally.

GAD generalized anxiety disorder.

gadolinium (Gd) (gad″o-lin′e-um) a chemical element, atomic number 64, atomic weight 157.25. (See Appendix 6.)

gadopentetate dimeglumine (gad″o-pen′-tĕ-tāt di-meg′loo-mēn) a PARAMAGNETIC agent used as a contrast agent in MAGNETIC RESONANCE IMAGING of intracranial, spinal, and associated lesions.

GAF Global Assessment of Functioning; see under SCALE.

gag (gag) 1. a surgical device fitting between the upper and lower jaws to prevent the mouth from closing during operative procedures of the mouth or throat. 2. to retch, or strive to vomit; see also gag REFLEX.

gain (gān) the increase achieved by amplification of a signal.

brightness g. a factor in intensification of radiographs; minification factor multiplied by flux gain.

flux g. in radiology, acceleration of electrons that strike the output phosphor in radiology; it serves as a factor in the intensification of IMAGES.

gait (gāt) the manner or style of walking.

g. analysis evaluation of the manner or style of walking, usually done by observing the individual walking naturally in a straight line. The normal forward step consists of two phases: the *stance phase,* during which one leg and foot are bearing most or all of the body weight, and the *swing phase,* during which the foot is not touching the walking surface and the body weight is borne by the other leg and foot. In a complete two-step cycle both feet are in contact with the floor at the same time for about 25 per cent of the time. This part of the cycle is called the *double-support phase.*

An analysis of each component of the three phases of ambulation is an essential part of the diagnosis of various neurologic disorders and the assessment of patient progress during rehabilitation and recovery from the effects of a neurologic disease, a musculoskeletal injury or disease process, or amputation of a lower limb.

antalgic g. a limp adopted so as to avoid pain on weight-bearing structures, characterized by a very short stance phase.

ataxic g. an unsteady, uncoordinated walk, with a wide base and the feet thrown out, coming down first on the heel and then on the toes with a double tap.

double-step g. a gait in which there is a noticeable difference in the length or timing of alternate steps.

drag-to g. a gait in which the feet are dragged (rather than lifted) toward the CRUTCHES.

equine g. a walk accomplished mainly by flexing the hip joint; seen in crossed leg PALSY.

festinating g. one in which the patient involuntarily moves with short, accelerating steps, often on tiptoe, with the trunk flexed forward and the legs flexed stiffly at the hips and knees. It is seen in PARKINSON'S DISEASE and other neurologic conditions that affect the basal GANGLIA. Called also festination.

four-point g. a gait in forward motion using crutches: first one crutch is advanced, then the opposite leg, then the second crutch, then the second leg, and so on. See accompanying illustration.

gluteal g. the gait characteristic of paralysis of the gluteus medius muscle, marked by a listing of the trunk toward the affected side at each step.

helicopod g. a gait in which the feet describe half circles, as in some conversion disorders.

hemiplegic g. a gait involving flexion of the hip because of footdrop and circumduction of the leg.

intermittent double-step g. a hemiplegic gait in which there is a pause after the short step of the normal foot, or in some cases after the step of the affected foot.

Oppenheim's g. a gait marked by irregular oscillation of the head, limbs, and body; seen in some cases of multiple sclerosis.

scissors g. a crossing of the legs while advancing with slow, small steps.

spastic g. a walk in which the legs are held together and move in a stiff manner, the toes seeming to drag and catch.

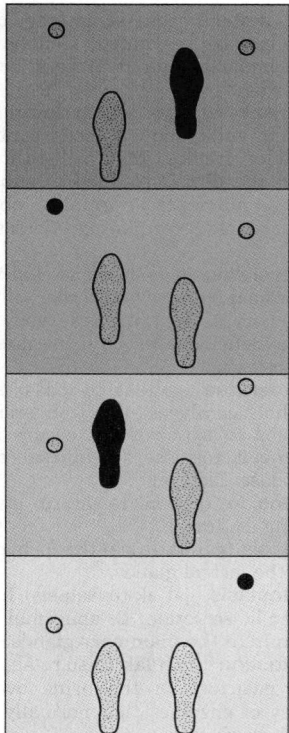

Four-point gait. From Elkin et al., 2000.

steppage g. the gait in FOOTDROP in which the advancing leg is lifted high in order that the toes may clear the ground. It is due to paralysis of the anterior tibial and fibular muscles, and is seen in lesions of the lower motor neuron, such as multiple neuritis, lesions of the anterior motor horn cells, and lesions of the cauda equina.

stuttering g. a walking disorder characterized by hesitancy that resembles stuttering; seen in some hysterical or schizophrenic patients as well as in patients with neurologic damage.

swing-through g. that in which the CRUTCHES are advanced and then the legs are swung past them.

swing-to g. that in which the CRUTCHES are advanced and the legs are swung to the same point.

tabetic g. an ataxic gait in which the feet slap the ground; in daylight the patient can avoid some unsteadiness by watching his feet.

three-point g. that in which both crutches and the affected leg are advanced

together and then the normal leg is moved forward. See illustration at CRUTCHES.

two-point g. that in which the right foot and left crutch or cane are advanced together, and then the left foot and right crutch. See illustration at CRUTCHES.

waddling g. exaggerated alternation of lateral trunk movements with an exaggerated elevation of the hip, suggesting the gait of a duck; characteristic of MUSCULAR DYSTROPHY.

galact(o)- word element [Gr.], *milk.*

galactacrasia (gah-lak″tah-kra′zhah) an abnormal state of the breast milk.

galactagogue (gah-lak′tah-gog) 1. promoting the flow of milk. 2. an agent that promotes the flow of milk.

galactemia (gal″ak-te′me-ah) the presence of galactose in the blood.

galactic (gah-lak′tik) 1. pertaining to milk. 2. galactagogue.

galactischia (gal″ak-tisk′e-ah) suppression of milk secretion.

galactobolic (gah-lak″to-bol′ik) of or relating to the action of neurohypophyseal peptides which contract the mammary myoepithelium and cause ejection of milk.

galactocele (gah-lak′to-sēl) a milk-containing, cystic enlargement of the mammary gland; called also lactocele.

galactography (gal″ak-tog′rah-fe) radiography of the mammary ducts after injection of a radiopaque substance into the duct system.

galactokinase (gah-lak″to-ki′nās) an enzyme that catalyzes the first step in the metabolism of galactose, the transfer of a phosphate group from ATP to galactose, producing galactose-1-phosphate.

g. deficiency a rare type of galactosemia transmitted as an autosomal recessive trait, caused by a deficiency of galactokinase. The only clinical manifestation is the development of cataracts during the first year of life, which can be prevented by a low-galactose diet.

galactophore (gah-lak′to-for) 1. galactophorous. 2. a milk duct.

galactophoritis (gah-lak″to-fo-ri′tis) inflammation of the milk ducts.

galactophorous (gal″ak-tof′o-rus) conveying milk.

galactophygous (gal″ak-tof′ĭ-gus) antigalactic (def. 1).

galactoplania (gah-lak″to-pla′ne-ah) secretion of milk in some abnormal part.

galactopoiesis (gah-lak″to-poi-e′sis) production of milk by the mammary glands; called also lactogenesis.

galactopoietic (gah-lak″to-poi-et′ik) pertaining to, marked by, or promoting milk production; called also lactogenic.

galactorrhea (gah-lak″to-re′ah) excessive or spontaneous milk flow; persistent secretion of milk irrespective of nursing. Called also lactorrhea. See also HYPERLACTATION.

g.-amenorrhea syndrome galactorrhea occurring with amenorrhea, sometimes associated with increased levels of PROLACTIN; several different types are known.

galactosamine (gah-lak″to-sam′in) an amino derivative of galactose.

galactose (gah-lak′tōs) a monosaccharide sugar of the ALDOSE group, derived from LACTOSE. D-galactose is found in lactose, in cerebrosides of the brain, in the sugar beet, and in many gums and seaweeds; L-galactose is found in flaxseed mucilage.

g. tolerance test a laboratory test done to determine the liver's ability to convert the sugar galactose into glycogen. Two methods may be used. The oral method requires about 5 hours to complete, and the intravenous method, which is more accurate, requires about 2 hours. With the oral method, elimination of more than 3 g of galactose in the urine during a 5-hour period indicates liver damage. With the intravenous method, all galactose should have been eliminated from the blood 45 minutes after its injection.

galactosemia (gah-lak″to-se′me-ah) a genetically determined biochemical disorder in which there is a lack of an enzyme necessary for proper metabolism of galactose. Normally the lactose in milk is initially broken down into its glucose and galactose components. The galactose is then changed by enzymatic action into glucose. When the conversion of galactose to glucose does not take place, the galactose accumulates in the tissues and blood. There are two types: classic galactosemia and GALACTOKINASE DEFICIENCY.

Classic galactosemia is due to a deficiency of the enzyme galactose-1-phosphate uridyl transferase, and is transmitted as an autosomal recessive trait. The disorder becomes manifest soon after birth and is characterized by feeding problems, vomiting and diarrhea, abdominal distention, enlargement of the liver, mental retardation, and elevated blood and urine levels of both galactose and galactose-1-phosphate.

Galactosemia is diagnosed by demonstrating that the activity of the enzyme galactose-1-phosphate uridyltransferase is absent. If the disease is detected early, before there is damage to the central nervous system, the symptoms of the disorder can be prevented. Genetic counseling is important for families affected by this disorder.

Treatment consists of exclusion from the diet of milk and all foods containing galactose or lactose. Milk substitutes are used and the diet is planned to substitute necessary nutrients normally obtained from products containing lactose or galactose.

galactosialidosis (gah-lak″to-si-al″ĭdo′sis) an autosomal recessive disorder clinically almost identical to SIALIDOSIS type II but due to a deficiency of both SIALIDASE and β-GALACTOSIDASE.

galactosidase (gah-lak″to-si′dās) an enzyme that catalyzes the conversion of GALACTOSIDE to GALACTOSE; it occurs in two forms: α-galactosidase (melibiase) and β-galactosidase (lactase).

galactoside (gah-lak′to-sīd) a glycoside containing GALACTOSE.

galactosis (gal″ak-to′sis) the formation of milk by the lacteal glands.

galactostasis (gal″ak-tos′tah-sis) 1. cessation of milk secretion. 2. abnormal collection of milk in the mammary glands.

galactosuria (gah-lak″to-su′re-ah) presence of galactose in the urine owing to deficiency of enzymes that normally would convert it to glucose.

galantamine (gah-lan′tah-mēn) a reversible competitive inhibitor of ACETYLCHOLINESTERASE used as the hydrobromide salt in the treatment of mild to moderate ALZHEIMER'S DISEASE, administered orally.

galea (ga′le-ah) [L.] a helmet-shaped structure.

g. aponeuro′tica aponeurosis connecting the frontal and occipital bellies of the occipitofrontal muscle.

Galen (ga′len) Claudius Galenus (A.D. 130–200). Celebrated Greek physician to Roman Emperor Marcus Aurelius. Although he did not dissect the human cadaver, he made many valuable anatomic and physiologic observations on animals (applying many of them inaccurately to humans). His writings on these and other subjects were extensive, and his influence on medicine was profound for many centuries. His teleology "nature does nothing in vain" was particularly attractive to the medieval mind, although it was stultifying for advances in medical thought and practice.

galenicals (gah-len′ĭ-kals) **galenics** (gah-len′iks) medicines prepared according to the formulas of GALEN. The term is now used to denote standard preparations containing one or several organic ingredients, as contrasted with pure chemical substances.

galeophobia (ga″le-o-fo′be-ah) ailurophobia.

gall (gawl) bile.

gallamine triethiodide (gal′ah-mēn tri″ē-thi′o-dīd) a quaternary ammonium compound used as the triethiodide salt as a skeletal muscle RELAXANT during surgery and other procedures, such as endoscopy or intubation, administered intravenously.

gallbladder (gawl′blad-er) the pear-shaped organ located below the liver. It serves as a storage place for BILE.

Diagnostic Studies. Laboratory tests helpful in the diagnosis of gallbladder and biliary tract diseases include evaluation of direct bilirubin and alkaline phosphatase, both of which are elevated in biliary tract disease. The presence of bile in the urine is indicative of biliary obstruction.

One of the most common radiologic techniques for diagnosis of gallbladder disease is *ultrasonography.* It is a noninvasive procedure that can help differentiate between biliary obstruction and liver disease. Abnormal patterns on the graph can show an enlarged gallbladder, obstruction of the common bile duct, dilatation in the biliary tree, and the presence of stones in the gallbladder and common bile duct. Ultrasonography has the advantages of being quick, requiring no special preparation of the patient, and avoiding the risks of exposure to radiation from x-rays.

Another commonly used radiologic study is *radionuclide imaging,* using an intravenous injection of ^{99}Tc iminodiacetic acid (HIDA) or some other radioisotope that has an affinity for the biliary tree and concentrates at that site.

Oral *cholecystography,* in which an iodinated radiopaque contrast medium is ingested, absorbed by the intestines, and excreted by the liver in the bile, is useful in opacification of the gallbladder. However, this method can be used only in patients without acute symptoms.

Percutaneous transhepatic cholangiography can be used to visualize the biliary ducts in jaundiced patients. A needle is inserted through the skin into the liver. The contrast medium is then injected into the liver and subsequently excreted in the biliary system. Obstructions and distention of the bile ducts can thus be observed, after which the ducts are drained of bile that has accumulated behind the obstruction.

When a suspected disorder of the gallbladder cannot be identified by any of the above procedures, the physician may choose to perform *endoscopic retrograde cholangiopancreatography* (ERCP). Under fluoroscopic control the endoscope is inserted into the mouth and guided through the esophagus and down to the descending duodenum. Cannulas are then directed through the endoscope and placed in the common bile duct; through them a contrast medium is injected into the ducts so that they can be inspected by fluoroscopy.

Unfortunately, none of the diagnostic tests is completely reliable, and between 5 and 10 per cent of patients with biliary disease have repeated normal test values. Many such patients eventually have exploratory surgery because of persistence of symptoms. In such cases the gallbladder is often inflamed but without stones, or it may contain grains of sand too small to be visualized by the testing procedures.

Surgery of the Gallbladder and the Biliary Tree. The most common operation on the biliary system is CHOLECYSTECTOMY, the removal of the gallbladder. CHOLECYSTOSTOMY, or drainage of the gallbladder, is rarely done today. CHOLEDOCHOTOMY, exploration of the common bile duct, is indicated if there are stones or a tumor obstructing the major drainage system. The duct is generally explored directly, but in difficult cases it may be approached through the wall of the duodenum.

Biliary surgery is usually followed by leakage of bile from the repaired common

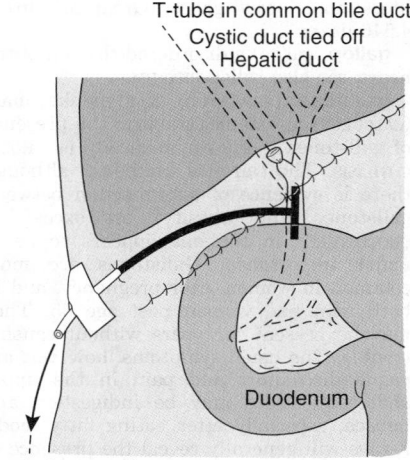

T-tube in common bile duct
Cystic duct tied off
Hepatic duct

Duodenum

To drainage collection

T-tube placement in gallbladder surgery. The surgeon ties off the cystic duct and sutures the T-tube into the common bile duct, with the short arms of the T-tube toward the hepatic duct and duodenum. The long arm of the T-tube exits the body near the incision site. Skin suture and tape secure placement. From Polaski and Tatro, 1996.

duct or from the gallbladder bed. Accordingly, many surgeons drain the gallbladder bed with a soft drain for several days. If the common duct is opened, drainage of bile can be accomplished by the insertion of a T-tube, which decompresses the common duct until it is healed. T-tubes are generally left in place for 10 days or more in order to develop a tract through which bile can drain after the T-tube is removed. A T-tube cholangiogram is usually performed prior to the removal of the tube in order to determine that the common bile duct is patent and free of stones. If stones are found, they can be removed through the tube tract by instruments inserted under x-ray control.

Minimally invasive techniques of surgery are dramatically changing cholecystectomy. Laser and endoscopic procedures to remove the gallbladder do not require insertion of a T-tube.

gallium (Ga) (gal′e-um) a chemical element, atomic number 31, atomic weight 69.72. (See Appendix 6.)

    g. 67 a radioisotope of gallium, atomic mass 67, having a half-life of 3.26 days; used in the imaging of tumors, especially of soft tissue, and sites of inflammation and abscess.

gallon (gal′on) 1. a unit of liquid measure (4 quarts, or 3.785 liters, or 3785 ml). 2. a measure of liquid volume, 4 quarts. A standard gallon (United States) is 3.785 liters; an imperial gallon (Great Britain) is 4.546 liters.

gallop (gal′op) a disordered rhythm of the heart; see also gallop RHYTHM.

gallstone (gawl′stōn) a stonelike mass (CALCULUS) in the GALLBLADDER; the presence of gallstones is known medically as CHOLELITHIASIS. The cause is unknown, although there is evidence of a connection between gallstones and obesity; an excess of CHOLESTEROL in the bile appears to be of major importance. Gallstones are most common in women after pregnancy, and in both men and women past age 35. They may be present for years without causing trouble. The usual symptoms, however, are vague discomfort and pain in the upper abdomen. There may be indigestion and nausea, especially after eating fatty foods. X-rays will generally reveal the presence of gallstones, either directly or by use of a dye introduced into the gallbladder (CHOLECYSTOGRAPHY).

The most common complication of gallstones occurs when one of the stones escapes from the gallbladder and travels along the common bile duct, where it may lodge, blocking the flow of bile to the intestine and causing obstructive jaundice. This condition should be corrected by surgery before the liver is damaged or problems with infection ensue.

When a gallstone travels through or obstructs a bile duct it can cause biliary COLIC, with severe pain. The pain is located in the upper right quadrant of the abdomen and radiates as far as the SCAPULA. MORPHINE is usually not given to relieve the pain because it increases spasm of the biliary sphincters. MEPERIDINE, which does not have this side effect, is the preferred medication for pain. Treatment may also include insertion of a nasogastric tube for the purpose of gastric suction to relieve distention in the upper gastrointestinal tract. URSODIOL is a drug that can dissolve gallstones and reduce the need for surgery.

Laparoscopic surgery is the usual method of treatment and is performed as soon as the patient is able to withstand it. In most cases the gallbladder is removed and a tube is inserted to establish drainage of bile that has been dammed up by the stone. (See also discussion of surgery at GALLBLADDER.) For those patients unable to withstand CHOLECYSTECTOMY (gallbladder removal) but who still require drainage, CHOLECYSTOSTOMY is indicated.

galvanism (gal′van-izm) 1. a unidirectional electric current derived from a chemical battery. 2. the therapeutic use of such a current.

    dental g. the production of galvanic current in the oral cavity due to the presence of two or more dissimilar metals in dental restorations that are bathed in saliva, or a single metal and two electrolytes (such as saliva and pulp tissue fluid); sometimes the current may be high enough to irritate the dental pulp and cause pain.

galvanocontractility (gal″vah-no-kon″-trak-til′ĭ-te) contractility in response to stimulation by galvanic current.

galvanometer (gal″vah-nom′ĕ-ter) an instrument for measuring current by electromagnetic action.

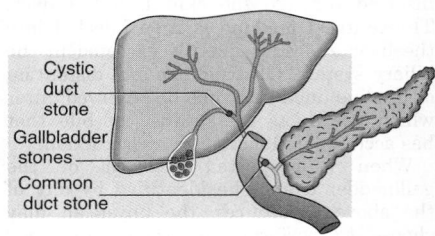

Cystic duct stone

Gallbladder stones

Common duct stone

Common anatomic locations of gallstones. From Malarkey and McMorrow, 2000.

galvanopalpation (gal″vah-no-pal-pa′-shun) testing of nerves of the skin by means of galvanic current.

gambling (gamb′ling) betting money or other valuables on the outcome of a game or other event.

pathological g. an IMPULSE CONTROL DISORDER consisting of persistent failure to resist the urge to gamble, to such an extent that personal, family, and vocational life are seriously disrupted.

gamete (gam′ēt) 1. one of two haploid reproductive cells, male (SPERMATOZOON) and female (OOCYTE), whose union is necessary in sexual reproduction to initiate the development of a new individual. 2. the malarial parasite in its sexual form in a mosquito's stomach, either male (MICROGAMETE) or female (MACROGAMETE); the latter is fertilized by the former to develop into an OOKINETE. adj., **gamet′ic.**

gametocide (gam′ē-to-sīd′) an agent that destroys gametes or gametocytes. adj., **gametoci′dal.**

gametocyte (gah-met′o-sīt) 1. an OOCYTE or SPERMATOCYTE; a cell that produces GAMETES. 2. the sexual stage of the malarial parasite in the blood which may produce gametes when taken into the mosquito host; it may be male (microgametocyte) or female (macrogametocyte).

gametogenesis (gam″ē-to-jen′ē-sis) the development of the male and female sex cells (gametes). adj., **gametogen′ic.**

gametogony (gam″ē-tog′o-ne) 1. the development of MEROZOITES into male and female gametes, which later fuse to form a zygote. 2. reproduction by means of gametes.

gamma (gam′ah) the third letter of the Greek alphabet, γ, used in names of chemical compounds to distinguish one of three or more isomers or to indicate the position of substituting atoms or groups.

g. chain disease a type of HEAVY CHAIN DISEASE that resembles a malignant lymphoma, with symptoms of lymphadenopathy, hepatosplenomegaly, and recurrent infections.

g. globulin 1. a class of plasma proteins composed almost entirely of IMMUNOGLOBULINS, the proteins that function as ANTIBODIES. Production of gamma globulin may be increased in the body when there is invasion by harmful microorganisms. An abnormal amount in the blood, a condition known as HYPERGAMMAGLOBULINEMIA, may be indicative of a chronic infection or certain malignant blood diseases. There is also a rare condition, AGAMMAGLOBULINEMIA, in which the body is unable to produce gamma globulin; patients suffering from this are extremely

susceptible to infection and must be given frequent injections of gamma globulin serum. 2. immune globulin.

g. rays, γ-rays electromagnetic emissions from radioactive substances; they are similar to and have the same general properties as x-rays but are produced through the disintegration of certain radioactive elements. They consist of high energy photons, have short wavelengths, and have no mass and no electric charge. Gamma rays are sometimes used in the treatment of deep-seated malignancies (see RADIATION THERAPY).

gamma-aminobutyric acid (gam″ah-ah-me″no-bu-tir′ik) γ-aminobutyric acid; see under *A.*

gamma benzene hexachloride (gam′ah ben′zēn hek″sah-klor′īd) lindane.

gammacism (gam′ah-sizm) imperfect utterance of velar consonants, especially *g* and *k* sounds.

gammaglobulinopathy (gam″ah-glob″u-lin-op′-ah-the) gammopathy.

gammopathy (gam-mop′ah-the) abnormal proliferation of the lymphoid cells producing IMMUNOGLOBULINS; the gammopathies include MULTIPLE MYELOMA, MACROGLOBULINEMIA, and Hodgkin's disease. Called also gammaglobulinopathy.

monoclonal g's plasma cell dyscrasias.

Gamna's disease (gam′nahz) splenomegaly with thickening of the splenic capsule and the presence of small brownish areas (Gamna's nodules), iron-containing pigment being deposited in the splenic pulp.

gamogenesis (gam″o-jen′ē-sis) sexual reproduction.

ganciclovir (gan-si′klo-vir) a derivative of ACYCLOVIR used in the form of the base or the sodium salt in treatment of CYTOMEGALOVIRUS infections of the retina; administered orally, intravenously, or by intravitreous injection or implantation.

gangli(o)- word element [Gr.], *ganglion.*

ganglial (gang′gle-al) pertaining to a ganglion.

gangliated (gang′gle-āt″ed) ganglionated.

gangliectomy (gang″gle-ek′to-me) ganglionectomy.

gangliform (gang′glī-form) having the form of a ganglion.

gangliitis (gang″gle-i′tis) ganglionitis.

ganglioblast (gang′gle-o-blast″) an embryonic cell of the cerebrospinal ganglia.

gangliocyte (gang′gle-o-sīt) a ganglion cell.

gangliocytoma (gang″gle-o-si-to′mah) ganglioneuroma.

ganglioform (gang′gle-o-form″) gangliform.

ganglioglioma (gang″gle-o-gli-o′mah) a glioma rich in mature neurons or ganglion cells.

ganglioglioneuroma (gang″gle-o-gli″o-noŏ-ro′mah) ganglioneuroma.

ganglioma (gang″gle-o′mah) ganglioneuroma.

ganglion (gang′gle-on), pl. *gan′glia, ganglions* [Gr.] 1. a knot or knotlike mass; in anatomic nomenclature, a group of nerve cell bodies located outside the central nervous system. The term is occasionally applied to certain nuclear groups within the brain or spinal cord, such as the basal ganglia. 2. a form of cystic tumor occurring on an aponeurosis or tendon, as in the wrist. adj., **gan′glial, ganglion′ic.**

autonomic ganglia aggregations of cell bodies of neurons of the autonomic nervous system; the parasympathetic and the sympathetic ganglia combined.

basal ganglia basal nuclei.

cardiac ganglia ganglia of the superficial cardiac plexus under the arch of the aorta.

carotid g. an occasional small enlargement in the internal carotid plexus.

celiac ganglia two irregularly shaped ganglia, one on each crus of the diaphragm within the celiac plexus.

cerebrospinal ganglia those associated with the cranial and spinal nerves.

cervical g. 1. any of the three ganglia (inferior, middle, and superior) of the sympathetic trunk in the neck region. 2. one near the cervix uteri.

cervicothoracic g. a ganglion on the sympathetic trunk anterior to the lowest cervical or first thoracic vertebra. It is formed by a union of the seventh and eighth cervical and first thoracic ganglia. Called also stellate ganglion.

cervicouterine g. one near the cervix uteri.

ciliary g. a parasympathetic ganglion in the posterior part of the orbit.

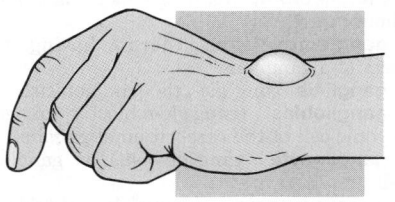

Ganglion. From Frazier et al., 2000.

cochlear g. the sensory ganglion located within the spiral canal of the MODIOLUS. It consists of bipolar cells that send fibers peripherally to the organ of Corti and centrally to the cochlear nuclei of the brainstem. Called also spiral ganglion and Corti's ganglion.

Corti's g. cochlear ganglion.

craniospinal ganglia collections of sensory neurons that form nodular enlargements on the dorsal roots of the spinal nerves and on the sensory roots of cranial nerves.

dorsal root g. spinal ganglion.

false g. an enlargement of a nerve that does not have a true ganglionic structure.

Frankenhäuser's g. cervical ganglion (def. 2).

gasserian g. trigeminal ganglion.

geniculate g. the sensory ganglion of the facial nerve, on the geniculum of the facial nerve.

g. im′par a ganglion commonly found on the front of the coccyx, where the sympathetic trunks of the two sides unite.

inferior g. 1. the lower of two ganglia of the glossopharyngeal nerve as it passes through the jugular foramen. 2. the lower of two ganglia of the vagus nerve as it passes through the jugular foramen.

jugular g. superior ganglion (defs. 1 and 2).

Ludwig's g. a ganglion near the right atrium of the heart, connected with the cardiac plexus.

lumbar ganglia the ganglia on the sympathetic trunk, usually four or five on either side.

lymphatic g. LYMPH NODE.

otic g. a parasympathetic ganglion next to the medial surface of the mandibular division of the trigeminal nerve, just inferior to the foramen ovale. Its postganglionic fibers supply the parotid gland.

parasympathetic ganglia aggregations of cell bodies of cholinergic neurons of the parasympathetic nervous system; these ganglia are located near to or within the wall of the organs being innervated. See also Plates.

petrous g. inferior ganglion (def. 1).

pterygopalatine g. a parasympathetic ganglion in a fossa in the sphenoid bone, formed by postganglionic cell bodies that synapse with preganglionic fibers from the fascial nerve via the nerve of the pterygopalatine canal. Called also sphenopalatine ganglion.

sacral ganglia those of the sacral part of the sympathetic trunk, usually three or four on either side.

Scarpa's g. vestibular ganglion.

sensory g. any of the ganglia of the peripheral nervous system that transmit sensory impulses; also, the collective masses of nerve cell bodies in the brain subserving sensory functions.

simple g. a cystic tumor in a tendon sheath.

sphenopalatine g. pterygopalatine ganglion.

spinal g. the cerebrospinal ganglion on the dorsal root of each spinal nerve; called also dorsal root ganglion.

spiral g. cochlear ganglion.

stellate g. cervicothoracic ganglion.

submandibular g. a parasympathetic ganglion located superior to the deep part of the submandibular gland, on the lateral surface of the hyoglossal muscle; its postganglionic fibers supply the sublingual and submandibular glands.

superior g. 1. the upper of two ganglia on the glossopharyngeal nerve as it passes through the jugular foramen. 2. the upper of two ganglia of the vagus nerve just as it passes through the jugular foramen. Called also jugular ganglion.

sympathetic ganglia aggregations of cell bodies of adrenergic neurons of the sympathetic nervous system; these ganglia are arranged in chainlike fashion on either side of the spinal cord. See also Plates.

thoracic ganglia the ganglia on the thoracic portion of the sympathetic trunk, 11 or 12 on either side.

trigeminal g. a ganglion on the sensory root of the fifth cranial nerve, situated in a cleft within the dura mater on the anterior surface of the pars petrosa of the temporal bone, and giving off the ophthalmic and maxillary and part of the mandibular nerve. Called also gasserian or semilunar ganglion.

tympanic g. an enlargement on the tympanic branch of the glossopharyngeal nerve.

vestibular g. the sensory ganglion of the vestibular part of the eighth cranial nerve, located in the upper part of the lateral end of the internal acoustic meatus. Called also Scarpa's ganglion.

Walther's g. glomus coccygeum.

Wrisberg's ganglia cardiac ganglia.

wrist g. cystic enlargement of a tendon sheath on the back of the wrist.

ganglionated (gang′gle-o-nāt″ed) provided with ganglia; called also gangliated.

ganglionectomy (gang″gle-o-nek′to-me) excision of a ganglion; called also gangliectomy.

ganglioneuroma (gang″gle-o-nu-ro′mah) a benign neoplasm composed of nerve fibers

and mature ganglion cells; called also gangliocytoma, ganglioglioneuroma, and ganglioma.

ganglionic (gang″gle-on′ik) pertaining to a ganglion.

ganglionitis (gang″gle-o-ni′tis) inflammation of a ganglion; called also gangliitis.

ganglionostomy (gang″gle-o-nos′tah-me) surgical creation of an opening into a cystic tumor on a tendon sheath or aponeurosis.

ganglioplegic (gang″gle-o-ple′jik) 1. blocking transmission of impulses through the sympathetic and parasympathetic ganglia. 2. an agent that so acts.

ganglioside (gang′gle-o-sīd) a class of galactose-containing cerebrosides found in central nervous system tissues; they are glycolipids of the basic composition ceramide-glucose-galactose-N-acetyl neuraminic acid. The form GM_1 accumulates in tissues in generalized gangliosidosis, the form GM_2 in Tay-Sachs disease.

gangliosidosis (gang″gle-o-si-do′sis), pl. *gangliosido′ses* a lipid storage disorder marked by accumulation of GANGLIOSIDES in tissues due to an enzyme defect. In generalized gangliosidosis, a hereditary defect in β-galactosidase causes accumulation of ganglioside GM_1, resulting in mental retardation, hepatomegaly, skeletal deformities, and, often, a cherry-red spot. In TAY-SACHS DISEASE, a defect of hexosaminidase A results in accumulation of ganglioside GM_2.

gangrene (gang′grēn) the death of body tissue, generally in considerable mass, usually associated with loss of vascular (nutritive) supply, and followed by bacterial invasion and putrefaction. Although it usually affects the extremities, gangrene sometimes may involve the internal organs. Symptoms depend on the site and include fever, pain, darkening of the skin, and an unpleasant odor. If the condition involves an internal organ, it is generally attended by pain and collapse. Treatment includes correcting the causes and is frequently successful with modern medications and surgery.

Types of Gangrene. The three major types are moist, dry, and gas gangrene. Moist and dry gangrene result from loss of blood circulation due to various causes; gas gangrene occurs in wounds infected by anaerobic bacteria, among which are various species of *Clostridium*, which break down tissue by gas production and by toxins.

Moist gangrene is caused by sudden stoppage of blood, resulting from burning by heat or acid, severe freezing, physical accident that destroys the tissue, a tourniquet

G

that has been left on too long, or a clot or other embolism. At first, tissue affected by moist gangrene has the color of a bad bruise, is swollen, and often blistered. The gangrene is likely to spread with great speed. Toxins are formed in the affected tissues and absorbed.

Dry gangrene occurs gradually and results from slow reduction of the blood flow in the arteries. There is no subsequent bacterial decomposition; the tissues become dry and shriveled. It occurs only in the extremities, and can occur with arteriosclerosis, in old age, or in advanced stages of DIABETES MELLITUS. BUERGER'S DISEASE can also sometimes cause dry gangrene. Symptoms include gradual shrinking of the tissue, which becomes cold and lacking in pulse, and turns first brown and then black. Usually a line of demarcation is formed where the gangrene stops, owing to the fact that the tissue above this line continues to receive an adequate supply of blood.

Gas gangrene results from dirty lacerated wounds infected by anaerobic bacteria, especially species of *Clostridium*. It is an acute, severe, painful condition in which muscles and subcutaneous tissues become filled with gas and a serosanguineous exudate.

Internal Gangrene. In strangulated HERNIA, a loop of intestine is caught in the bulge and its blood supply is cut off; gangrene may occur in that section of tissue. In acute APPENDICITIS, areas of gangrene may occur in the walls of the appendix with consequent rupture through a gangrenous area. In severe cases of CHOLECYSTITIS, which is usually associated with GALLSTONES, gangrene may develop where the stones compress the mucous membrane. Thrombosis of the mesenteric artery may result in gangrene. Gangrene can be a rare complication of lung abscess in pneumonia; a symptom is brown sputum with a foul smell.

Prevention. To prevent gangrene in an open wound, the wound should be kept as clean as possible. Special wound care is particularly important in patients with diabetes mellitus, malnutrition, and immunodeficiency. FROSTBITE is especially dangerous, for the freezing impedes circulation, skin becomes tender and easily broken, and underlying cells are destroyed.

Fournier's g. an acute gangrenous infection of the scrotum, penis, or perineum following local trauma, operative procedures, an underlying urinary tract disease,

or a distant acute inflammatory process. Called also Fournier's disease.

gas g. a condition often resulting from dirty, lacerated wounds in which the muscles and subcutaneous tissue become filled with gas and a serosanguineous exudate. It is due to species of *Clostridium* that break down tissue by gas production and by toxins.

gangrenous (gang′grĕ-nus) pertaining to, marked by, or of the nature of gangrene.

ganirelix (gan″ĭ-rel′iks) a synthetic compound derived from, and an antagonist to, gonadotropin-releasing HORMONE; used as the acetate salt to inhibit premature luteinizing HORMONE (LH) surges in women undergoing ovarian hyperstimulation in the treatment of female INFERTILITY, administered subcutaneously.

Ganser syndrome (gan′ser) the giving of inappropriate, ridiculous, or approximate answers to questions, sometimes associated with amnesia, disorientation, perceptual disturbances, and conversion symptoms; it is most commonly seen in malingering prisoners feigning psychosis.

Gantrisin (gan′trĭ-sin) trademark for preparations of SULFISOXAZOLE, a SULFONAMIDE antibiotic.

gap (gap) an opening or hiatus.

anion g. the concentration of plasma anions not routinely measured by laboratory screening, accounting for the difference between the routinely measured anions and cations and equal to the plasma sodium − (chloride + bicarbonate); used in the evaluation of acid-base disorders.

auscultatory g. a period in which Korotkoff SOUNDS disappear during auscultation of a patient's BLOOD PRESSURE.

Garamycin (gar″ah-mi′sin) trademark for preparations of GENTAMICIN, an ANTIBIOTIC.

Gardner's syndrome (gahrd′nerz) familial polyposis of the colon associated with osseous and soft tissue tumors.

Gardnerella (gahrd″ner-el′ah) a genus of gram-negative, rod-shaped bacteria having one species, *G. vagina′lis* (formerly called *Haemophilus vaginalis*). It is found in the normal female genital tract and is the causative organism for nonspecific VAGINITIS. *Gardnerella* infection is one of the most common and most contagious of the SEXUALLY TRANSMITTED DISEASES and is thought to be in association with infections by anaerobic organisms. The major symptom is increased vaginal discharge that is thin and gray, has a fishy odor, and has a pH between 5 and 5.5. There usually is no itching or sign of mucosal irritation since the organism does not invade the vaginal mucosa; if such symptoms do occur, it suggests that a concomitant infection is present. Treatment is with METRONIDAZOLE (Flagyl). The sexual partner should be treated concurrently if reinfection is to be avoided.

gargle (gahr′g'l) 1. a solution for rinsing the mouth and throat. 2. to rinse the mouth and throat by holding a solution in the open mouth and agitating it by expulsion of air from the lungs.

gargoylism (gahr′goil-izm) Hurler's syndrome.

garment (gahr′ment) an article of clothing.

   pneumatic antishock g. an inflatable garment used to combat shock, stabilize fractures, promote hemostasis and increase peripheral vascular resistance. Called also MAST suit.

   pressure g. a garment that applies continual pressure over large areas of healing skin after burns, trauma, and surgical intervention; worn continually for several months to a year, it limits hypertrophy and contraction of scar tissue.

gas (gas) any elastic aeriform fluid in which the molecules are widely separated from each other and so have free paths.

   alveolar g. the gas in the alveoli of the lungs, where gas EXCHANGE with the capillary blood takes place.

   blood g's the partial pressures of oxygen and carbon dioxide in blood; see BLOOD GAS ANALYSIS.

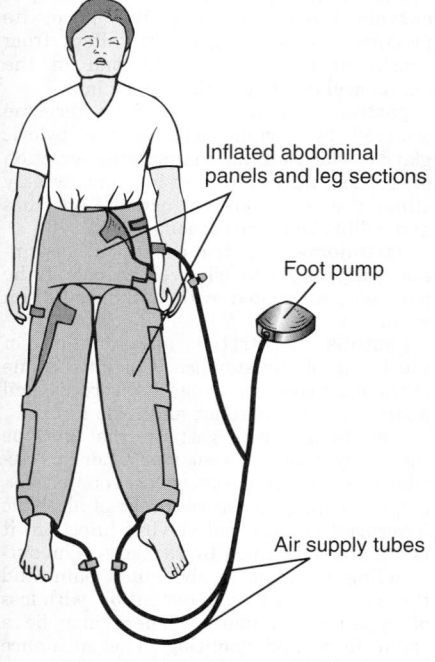

Pneumatic antishock garment (MAST suit).

Inflated abdominal panels and leg sections

Foot pump

Air supply tubes

   laughing g. nitrous oxide.

   g. pains pains caused by distention of the stomach or intestines by accumulation of air or other gases. The presence of gas is indicated by distention of the abdomen, belching, or discharge of gas through the rectum. Gas-forming foods include highly flavored vegetables such as onions, cabbage, and turnips; members of the bean family; and fruits such as melons and raw apples. Some seasonings and other chemical irritants also produce gas.

   tear g. any of various irritant vapors dispensed by AEROSOL and causing pain and severe LACRIMATION in humans; some also cause irritation of exposed mucous membranes as well as vomiting. Common ones include CHLOROACETOPHENONE (CN), o-chlorobenzylidenemalononitrile (see CS), and dibenz(b,f)-1,4-oxazepine (see CR); the most common of the three is CS (also known as MACE).

gas bloat syndrome a condition in which voluntary eructation is impossible; it is a common complication following fundoplication procedures.

gaster (gas′ter) [Gr.] stomach.

Gasterophilus (gas″ter-of′ĭ-lus) a genus of flies, the horse botflies, the larvae of which develop in the gastrointestinal tract of horses and may sometimes infect humans.

gastr(o)- word element [Gr.], *stomach.*

gastradenitis (gas″trad-ĕ-ni′tis) inflammation of the gastric glands.

gastralgia (gas-tral′jah) gastrodynia.

gastrectomy (gas-trek′to-me) excision of the entire STOMACH (total gastrectomy) or part of it (partial or subtotal gastrectomy); this may be indicated in cases of malignant tumors or gastric ULCERS not responsive to medical management or those complicated by perforation or hemorrhage. See accompanying illustrations.

gastric (gas′trik) pertaining to, affecting, or originating in the stomach.

   g. analysis analysis of the stomach contents by microscopy and tests to determine the amount of HYDROCHLORIC ACID present. The tests performed are of value in diagnosing PEPTIC ULCER, cancer of the stomach, and PERNICIOUS ANEMIA. Gastric secretions are collected by continuous or intermittent aspiration via nasogastric tube. There is a wide overlap of the ranges of normal and abnormal values; hence intermediate values are not indicative of pathology. A total absence of acid (pH above 6.0) occurs in almost all cases of pernicious anemia and in some patients with advanced gastric carcinoma. Hypersecretion

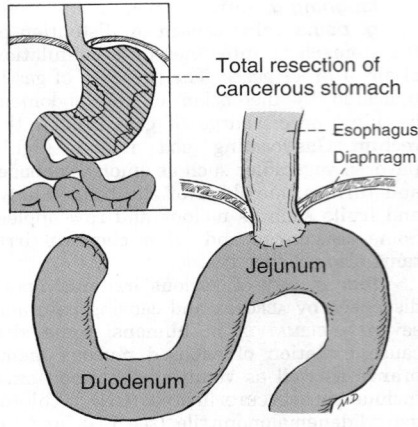

Total resection of cancerous stomach

Esophagus
Diaphragm

Jejunum

Duodenum

Total gastrectomy (inset) with anastomosis of esophagus to the jejunum (esophagojejunostomy) is the principal intervention for extensive gastric cancer. From Polaski and Tatro, 1996.

of hydrochloric acid is characteristic of ZOL-LINGER-ELLISON SYNDROME, which is marked by intractable, sometimes fulminating peptic ulcer, gastric hyperacidity, and gastrin-secreting pancreatic tumors.

g. bypass surgical creation of a small gastric pouch that empties directly into the jejunum through a gastrojejunostomy, thereby causing food to bypass the duodenum; done for the treatment of gross OBESITY.

g. juice the secretion of glands in the walls of the stomach for use in digestion. Its

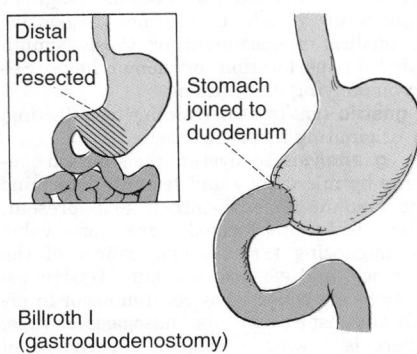

Distal portion resected

Stomach joined to duodenum

Billroth I
(gastroduodenostomy)

Subtotal gastrectomy removes acid-secreting portions of the stomach. After removing the distal stomach (inset) a surgeon sutures the remaining portion of the stomach to the duodenum (Billroth I procedure) or to the proximal jejunum (Billroth II procedure). From Polaski and Tatro, 1996.

essential ingredients are PEPSIN, an enzyme that breaks down proteins in food, and HYDROCHLORIC ACID, which destroys bacteria and helps in the digestive process.

At the sight and smell of food, the stomach increases its output of gastric juice. When the food reaches the stomach, it is thoroughly mixed with the juice, the breakdown of the proteins is begun and the food then passes on to the duodenum for the next stage of digestion.

Normally the hydrochloric acid in gastric juice does not irritate or injure the delicate stomach tissues. However, in certain persons the stomach produces too much gastric juice, especially between meals when it is not needed, and the gastric secretions presumably erode the stomach lining, producing a PEPTIC ULCER, and also hinder its healing once an ulcer has formed.

g. partitioning a procedure of the treatment of morbid obesity consisting of the creation of a small pouch in the proximal stomach by two rows of staples, which are deliberately interrupted at one point to allow passage of food from the pouch to the rest of the stomach. This procedure is rarely done today because of its high failure rate. The two favored operations are the gastric bypass and the vertical banded GASTROPLASTY.

gastricism (gas′trĭ-sizm) gastric disorder.

gastricsin (gas-trik′sin) a proteolytic enzyme isolated from gastric juice; its precursor is pepsinogen but differs from pepsin in molecular weight and in the amino acid content at the N terminal.

gastrin (gas′trin) a polypeptide hormone secreted by certain cells of the pyloric glands, which strongly stimulates secretion of gastric acid and pepsin, and weakly stimulates secretion of pancreatic enzymes and gallbladder contraction.

gastrinoma (gas″trin-o′mah) a gastrin-secreting, non-beta islet cell tumor of the pancreas, associated with Zollinger-Ellison syndrome.

gastritis (gas-tri′tis) inflammation of the lining of the stomach. Gastritis is one of the most common stomach disorders, and occurs in acute, chronic, and toxic forms.

acute g. severe gastritis that may be caused by intake of ASPIRIN or other NONSTEROIDAL ANTIINFLAMMATORY DRUGS, FOOD POISONING, overeating, excessive intake of alcoholic beverages, or bacterial or viral infection; it is often accompanied by ENTERITIS. The outstanding symptom is abdominal pain, and there is also a feeling of distention, with loss of appetite and nausea. There may be a slight fever and vomiting. The substance causing the irritation can often be identified, in which case it should be avoided. Treatment may include the use of ANTACIDS. A bland diet of liquids and easily digested food should be followed for 2 or 3 days. Simply prepared solid foods in small quantities can then be added.

atrophic g. chronic gastritis with atrophy of the mucous membranes and glands.

chronic g. gastritis that occurs repeatedly or continues over a period of time. Although pain, especially after eating, and symptoms associated with indigestion may occur in chronic gastritis, most patients are asymptomatic; however, the condition may lead to hemorrhage and ulcer formation. Among its possible causes are *Helicobacter pylori*, vitamin deficiencies, abnormalities of the gastric juice, ulcers, hiatus hernia, excessive use of alcohol, or a combination of any of these.

Chronic gastritis is treated with a bland diet; food should be taken frequently and in small amounts. Antacids or anticholinergics may also be used in moderation to minimize stomach acidity. If bleeding is a problem that cannot be controlled by conservative measures, partial gastrectomy, pyloroplasty, vagotomy, or total gastrectomy may be indicated.

giant hypertrophic g. Ménétrier's disease.

toxic g. gastritis resulting from ingestion of a corrosive substance such as a strong acid or POISON. There is an acute burning sensation and cramping stomach pain, accompanied by diarrhea and vomiting; the vomit may be bloody. The victim may collapse. This condition is an emergency and immediate measures must be taken to prevent serious damage to the tissues of the stomach. First aid measures are begun at once to flush out and neutralize the poison.

gastroanastomosis (gas″tro-ah-nas″to-mo′sis) gastrogastrostomy.

gastrocamera (gas″tro-kam′er-ah) a small camera which can be passed down the esophagus to photograph the inside of the stomach.

gastrocardiac (gas″tro-kahr′de-ak) pertaining to the stomach and the heart.

gastrocele (gas′tro-sēl) hernial protrusion of the stomach or of a gastric pouch.

gastrocolic (gas″tro-kol′ik) pertaining to or communicating with the stomach and colon.

gastrocolitis (gas″tro-ko-li′tis) inflammation of the stomach and colon.

gastrocolostomy (gas″tro-kah-los′tah-me) surgical anastomosis of the stomach to the colon.

gastrocolotomy (gas″tro-ko-lot′ah-me) incision into the stomach and colon.

gastrocutaneous (gas″tro-ku-ta′ne-us) pertaining to the stomach and skin, or communicating with the stomach and the cutaneous surface of the body, as a gastrocutaneous fistula.

gastrocystoplasty (gas″tro-sis′to-plas″te) augmentation CYSTOPLASTY using a portion of the stomach for the graft.

gastrodiaphany (gas″tro-di-af′ah-ne) examination of the stomach by transillumination of its walls with a small electric lamp passed down the esophagus.

gastrodidymus (gas″tro-did′ĭ-mus) symmetrical conjoined twins joined in the abdominal region.

gastroduodenal (gas″tro-doo″o-de′nal) pertaining to the stomach and duodenum.

gastroduodenitis (gas″tro-doo″o-dĕ-ni′tis) inflammation of the stomach and duodenum.

gastroduodenoscopy (gas″tro-doo″o-dĕ-nos′kah-pe) endoscopic examination of the stomach and duodenum.

gastroduodenostomy (gas″tro-doo″o-dĕ-nos′tah-me) anastomosis between the stomach and the duodenum; called also Billroth I procedure.

gastrodynia (gas″tro-din′e-ah) pain in the stomach; called also gastralgia and stomachalgia.

gastroenteralgia (gas″tro-en″ter-al′jah) pain in the stomach and intestines.

gastroenteric (gas″tro-en-ter′ik) gastrointestinal.

gastroenteritis (gas″tro-en″tĕ-ri′tis) inflammation of the lining of the stomach and intestine. Psychologic causes may include fear, anger, and other forms of emotional upset. Allergic reactions to certain foods can cause the condition, as can irritation by excessive use of alcohol. Severe gastroenteritis, with such symptoms as headache, nausea, vomiting, weakness, diarrhea, and gas pains, may result from various infectious and contagious diseases, such as TYPHOID FEVER, INFLUENZA, and FOOD POISONING.

eosinophilic g. a disorder, commonly associated with intolerance to specific foods, marked by infiltration of the mucosa of the small intestine and frequently the stomach by eosinophils, with edema but without vasculitis and by eosinophilia of the peripheral blood. Symptoms depend on the site and extent of the disorder.

gastroenteroanastomosis (gas″tro-en″-ter-o-ah-nas″to-mo′sis) surgical anastomosis of the stomach to the small intestine.

gastroenterocolitis (gas″tro-en″ter-o-ko-li′tis) inflammation of the stomach, small intestine, and colon.

gastroenterologist (gas″tro-en″ter-ol′o-jist) a physician specializing in gastroenterology.

gastroenterology (gas″tro-en″ter-ol′o-je) the study of the stomach and intestine and their diseases.

gastroenteropathy (gas″tro-en″ter-op′ah-the) any disease of the stomach and intestine.

gastroenteroptosis (gas″tro-en″ter-op-to′sis) downward displacement or prolapse of the stomach and intestine.

gastroenterostomy (gas″tro-en″ter-os′-tah-me) surgical anastomosis of the stomach to the intestine; see GASTRODUODENOSTOMY, GASTROJEJUNOSTOMY, and GASTROILEOSTOMY.

gastroenterotomy (gas″tro-en″ter-ot′ah-me) incision into the stomach and intestine.

gastroesophageal (gas″tro-ĕ-sof′ah-je′al) pertaining to the stomach and esophagus.

g. reflux disease (GERD) any of various conditions resulting from gastroesophageal REFLUX, ranging in seriousness from mild to life-threatening; principal characteristics are heartburn and regurgitation. When there is damage to the esophageal epithelium, it is known as reflux ESOPHAGITIS.

gastroesophagitis (gas″tro-e-sof′ah-ji′tis) inflammation of the stomach and esophagus.

gastroesophagostomy (gas″tro-e-sof″ah-gos′tah-me) surgical anastomosis between the stomach and esophagus.

gastrofiberscope (gas″tro-fi′ber-skōp) a fiberscope for viewing the stomach.

gastrogastrostomy (gas″tro-gas-tros′tah-me) surgical creation of an anastomosis of two previously remote portions of the stomach, such as anastomosis between the pyloric and cardiac ends of the stomach, performed for hourglass contraction of the stomach, a condition in which the organ contracts at the middle.

gastrogavage (gas″tro-gah-vahzh′) artificial feeding through a tube passed into the stomach.

gastrogenic (gas″tro-jen′ik) originating in the stomach.

Gastrografin (gas″tro-gra′fin) trademark for a preparation of meglumine diatrizoate, a diagnostic radiopaque medium.

gastrograph (gas′tro-graf) an instrument for registering motions of the stomach.

gastrohepatic (gas″tro-hĕ-pat′ik) pertaining to the stomach and liver.

gastrohepatitis (gas″tro-hep″ah-ti′tis) inflammation of the stomach and liver.

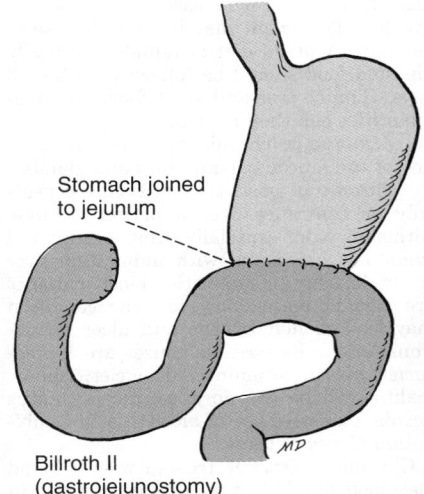

Stomach joined to jejunum

Billroth II
(gastrojejunostomy)

Gastrojejunostomy (Billroth II procedure). From Polaski and Tatro, 1996.

gastroileac (gas″tro-il′e-ak) pertaining to the stomach and ileum.

gastroileitis (gas″tro-il″e-i′tis) inflammation of the stomach and ileum.

gastroileostomy (gas″tro-il″e-os′tah-me) surgical anastomosis of the stomach to the ileum.

gastrointestinal (gas″tro-in-tes′tĭ-nal) pertaining to the stomach and intestine.

g. protein loss test administration of a radioisotope-labeled protein intravenously to determine the loss of plasma proteins in the gastrointestinal tract.

gastrojejunocolic (gas″tro-je-joo″no-kol′-ik) pertaining to the stomach, jejunum, and colon.

gastrojejunostomy (gas″tro-je-joo-nos′-tah-me) surgical anastomosis of the stomach to the jejunum; called also Billroth II procedure.

gastrolienal (gas″tro-li-e′nal) gastrosplenic.

gastrolith (gas′tro-lith) a calculus in the stomach; called also gastric calculus.

gastrolithiasis (gas″tro-lĭ-thi′ah-sis) the presence or formation of gastroliths.

gastrology (gas-trol′o-je) study of the stomach and its diseases.

gastrolysis (gas-trol′ĭ-sis) surgical division of perigastric adhesions to mobilize the stomach.

gastromalacia (gas″tro-mah-la′shah) softening of the wall of the stomach.

gastromegaly (gas″tro-meg′ah-le) enlargement of the stomach.

gastromycosis (gas″tro-mi-ko′sis) fungal infection of the stomach.

gastromyxorrhea (gas″tro-mik″so-re′ah) excessive secretion of mucus by the stomach.

gastroparalysis (gas″tro-pah-ral′ĭ-sis) gastroparesis.

gastroparesis (gas″tro-pah-re′sis) paralysis of the STOMACH; called also gastroparalysis and gastroplegia.

gastropathy (gas-trop′ah-the) any disease of the stomach.

gastropexy (gas′tro-pek″se) surgical fixation of the stomach.

Hill posterior g. a surgical procedure to correct gastroesophageal REFLUX. An abdominal approach is used to perform a 180 degree FUNDOPLICATION around the esophagus. The reduced gastroesophageal junction is anchored by sutures between the proximal lesser curvature and the preaortic fascia and sutures are placed in the crura to narrow the hiatus.

Gastrophilus (gas-trof′ĭ-lus) *Gasterophilus.*

gastrophrenic (gas″tro-fren′ik) pertaining to the stomach and diaphragm.

gastroplasty (gas′tro-plas″te) plastic repair of the stomach.

vertical banded g. a form of gastric partitioning in which a vertical pouch is created in the upper stomach, banded with nonabsorbable mesh to prevent dilatation of the stoma.

gastroplegia (gas″tro-ple′jah) gastroparesis.

gastroplication (gas″tro-plĭ-ka′shun) treatment of gastric dilatation by stitching a fold in the stomach wall.

gastroptosis (gas″trop-to′sis) downward displacement of the stomach.

gastropulmonary (gas″tro-pul′mo-nar″e) pertaining to the stomach and lungs.

gastropylorectomy (gas″tro-pi″lo-rek′to-me) excision of the pyloric part of the stomach.

gastropyloric (gas″tro-pi-lor′ik) pertaining to the stomach and pylorus.

gastrorrhagia (gas″tro-ra′jah) hemorrhage from the stomach.

gastrorrhaphy (gas-tror′ah-fe) suture of the stomach.

gastrorrhea (gas″tro-re′ah) excessive secretion by the glands of the stomach.

gastroschisis (gas-tros′kĭ-sis) a congenital fissure of the abdominal wall with protrusion of viscera.

gastroscope (gas′tro-skōp) an endoscope especially designed for passage into the stomach to permit examination of its interior. The gastroscope is a hollow, cylindrical tube fitted with special lenses and lights. The newer types of gastroscope are made of glass fiber (fiberscope) which is more flexible. Each glass fiber reflects light and creates a mirror effect, making it possible to "go around corners," and facilitating visualization of the curvature of the stomach.

gastroscopy (gas-tros′kah-pe) inspection of the interior of the stomach with a gastroscope.

Patient Care. For 6 to 8 hours prior to the examination the patient is not allowed to take any food or liquids by mouth. The stomach should be empty during the procedure to facilitate inspection of its lining and to avoid vomiting and aspiration of liquids into the lungs.

A SEDATIVE is given 30 minutes to 1 hour before the examination. The patient is awake during the procedure, which is not painful but is uncomfortable and exhausting. The sedatives help relieve apprehension and fear so that the patient can be more cooperative during the examination.

A local anesthetic such as cocaine or tetracaine (Pontocaine) is sprayed on the posterior pharynx to depress the gag reflex and reduce local reaction to the passage of the gastroscope. The patient is watched for toxic reaction to these drugs, and an emergency tray containing an airway, barbiturates, and epinephrine must be readily available.

After the procedure is completed the patient should be provided with rest and an opportunity to sleep. Foods and liquids are withheld until the gag reflex returns (usually about 4 hours). During the first two hours after gastroscopy the patient's vital signs should be checked periodically, especially if biopsies have been taken during the procedure and there is danger of bleeding.

gastrospasm (gas′tro-spazm) spasm of the stomach.

gastrosplenic (gas″tro-splen′ik) pertaining to the stomach and spleen; gastrolienal.

gastrostaxis (gas″tro-stak′sis) the oozing of blood from the stomach mucosa.

gastrostenosis (gas″tro-stĕ-no′sis) contraction or shrinkage of the stomach.

gastrostogavage (gas-tros″to-gah-vahzh′) feeding through a gastric fistula.

gastrostolavage (gas-tros″to-lah-vahzh′) irrigation of the stomach through a gastric fistula.

gastrostomy (gas-tros′tah-me) the creation of an opening into the stomach. This procedure is done to provide for the administration of food and liquids when stricture of the esophagus or other conditions make swallowing impossible. In the past gastrostomies were carried out in the operating room through an abdominal incision and formal laparotomy. Advances in endoscopic technology have led to techniques of introduction of the tube in a minimally percutaneous manner. Tubes placed in this fashion need special placement and a health care provider should be consulted before the tube is manipulated.

Patient Care. A patient who is to undergo this type of surgery usually has been ill for some time and often has nutritional deficiencies brought on by a steadily increasing difficulty in swallowing. Sometimes the patient is a small child who has accidentally swallowed lye or some other caustic substance, or it may be an adult who has taken a corrosive poison in an attempted suicide. Some elderly patients with obstructive carcinoma of the esophagus or throat may also require gastrostomy.

A primary consideration in the care of these patients is their acceptance of the gastrostomy as a substitute for eating. There are many social and emotional factors associated with eating and sharing a meal with others. Health care providers must be sensitive to the problems these patients will encounter in their adjustment to the changes a gastrostomy may bring to their lives. Whenever possible patients are taught self care in preparation of food, the feeding procedure, and peristomal skin care. It is important that they have privacy while doing this and that they be encouraged to ask questions and seek assistance from the members of the health care team.

The skin around the opening must be protected from irritation by the gastric juices, which may leak from the opening and act as a corrosive on the skin. In some cases the gastrostomy tube can be removed after each feeding. A device called the Barnes-Redo prosthesis is available for use by patients with a permanent gastrostomy; it is designed so that a cap can be fitted over a nylon tube permanently installed in the opening. When food or liquids are to be given the cap is unscrewed and a catheter is passed into the nylon tube. After feeding is completed the catheter is removed and the cap is screwed tightly over the nylon tube.

Feedings for a gastrostomy patient are gradually increased according to tolerance. At first, water and glucose are given at regular intervals. If there is no leakage and the patient has no difficulty with these liquids, other liquids and puréed foods are gradually added until a full meal can be tolerated.

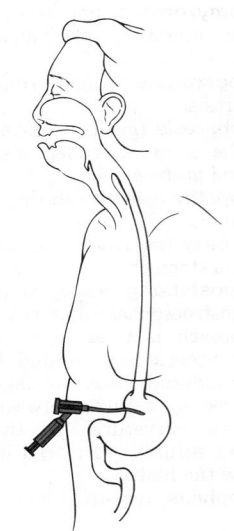

Gastrostomy. From Lammon et al., 1995.

In order to stimulate gastric secretions and aid digestion, these patients should see, smell, and taste small amounts of food before each feeding. It is recommended that they be allowed to chew small bits of food even though they cannot swallow them. This allows for proper stimulation of the gums and teeth and helps promote the health of the mouth and teeth.

Feedings should be warmed before they are given through the tube. Although commercially prepared liquid feedings are more convenient, they often cause diarrhea and are not as nutritionally adequate as regular meals. The foods to be given through the tube should be cooked until they are soft and then puréed in an electric blender. They can be diluted with the water in which they have been cooked, so that no vitamins are lost. A clinic dietitian usually must work very closely with the patient and family, instructing them in the planning and preparation of the patient's meals and offering suggestions for a variety of foods that will provide a well-balanced diet.

gastrothoracopagus (gas″tro-thor″ah-kop′ah-gus) symmetrical conjoined twins joined at the abdomen and thorax.

gastrotomy (gas-trot′ah-me) incision into the stomach.

gastrotropic (gas″tro-trop′ik) having affinity for or exerting a special effect on the stomach.

gastrotympanites (gas″tro-tim″pah-ni′-tēz) tympanitic distention of the stomach.

gastrula (gas′troo-lah) an embryo in the stage following the blastula stage; the simplest type consists of two layers of cells, the ectoderm and entoderm, which have invaginated to form the archenteron and an opening, the blastopore.

gastrulation (gas″troo-la′shun) the process by which a blastula becomes a gastrula or, in forms without a true blastula, the process by which three germ cell layers are acquired.

gatch (gach) to adjust mechanisms on a bed to achieve angulation of the mattress, especially elevation of the knee area.

gate (gāt) 1. an electronic circuit that passes a pulse only when a signal (the gate pulse) is present at a second input. 2. a mechanism for opening or closing a protein CHANNEL in a cell membrane, regulated by a signal such as increased concentration of a NEUROTRANSMITTER, change in electrical potential, or physical binding of a ligand molecule to the protein to cause a conformational change in the protein molecule. 3. to open and close selectively and function as a gate.

gatifloxacin (gat″ĭ-flok′sah-sin) a broad-spectrum ANTIBIOTIC effective against many gram-positive and gram-negative bacteria; administered orally and intravenously in the treatment of bacterial complication of chronic BRONCHITIS, acute SINUSITIS, community-acquired PNEUMONIA, GONORRHEA, PYELONEPHRITIS, and URINARY TRACT INFECTIONS due to susceptible organisms.

gating (gāt′ing) 1. controlling access or passage through GATES or CHANNELS. 2. selection of electrical signals by a GATE, which passes signals only when a control signal, the gate pulse, is present, or which passes only signals with certain characteristics, such as a pulse height. 3. substrate-binding– or ligand-binding–induced opening and closing of a biologic membrane channel, believed to be due to conformational changes in proteins lining the channels.

cardiac g. selective acquisition of cardiac function information at specific points in the cardiac cycle by using information from the electrocardiographic signal to time the cardiac cycle and control image sampling. It has been used in digital subtraction angiography, computed tomography, nuclear cardiology, and magnetic resonance imaging.

gatophobia (gat″o-fo′be-ah) ailurophobia.

Gaucher's disease (go-shāz′) a hereditary disorder of glucocerebroside metabolism, marked by the presence of Gaucher's CELLS in the bone marrow, and by hepatosplenomegaly and erosion of the cortices of long bones and pelvis. *Type 1,* the adult form, is associated with moderate anemia and thrombocytopenia, and yellowish pigmentation of the skin. *Type 2,* the infantile form, also has marked central nervous system impairment. In *type 3,* the juvenile form, there are rapidly progressive systemic manifestations but moderate central nervous system involvement.

Gault (gawlt) Alma E. (1891–1981). American nursing educator and activist for racial equality in nursing. As dean of Meharry Medical College School of Nursing in Nashville, Tennessee, she developed diploma and baccalaureate programs; Meharry also became the first predominantly African American school to become a member of the American Association of Collegiate Schools of Nursing. She was also active in promoting membership of African American students in nursing organizations, as well as being a campaigner for social reform. In addition, she helped organize the Southern Regional Conference of State Leagues of Nursing Education to promote regional planning for nursing education.

gauntlet (gawnt′let) a bandage covering the hand and fingers like a glove.

gauze (gawz) a light, open-meshed fabric of muslin or similar material used in bandages, dressings, and surgical sponges.

absorbent g. white cotton cloth of various thread counts and weights, supplied in various lengths and widths and in different forms (rolls or folds).

petrolatum g. sterile absorbent gauze saturated with white petrolatum; used as a non-adherent protective covering for wounds.

zinc gelatin impregnated g. absorbent gauze impregnated with zinc GELATIN for use as a skin protectant.

gavage (gah-vahzh′) [Fr.] 1. forced feeding, especially through a tube passed into the stomach; see also TUBE FEEDING. 2. superalimentation.

gaze (gāz) 1. to look in one direction for a period of time. 2. the act or state of looking steadily in one direction.

Gd gadolinium.

Ge germanium.

Gee's disease (gēz) **Gee-Herter disease** (ge′ her′ter) **Gee-Herter-Heubner disease** (ge′ her′ter hoib′ner) the infantile form of CELIAC DISEASE.

Gee-Thaysen disease (ge′ ti′sen) the adult form of CELIAC DISEASE.

gegenhalten (ga″gen-hahlt′en) [Ger.] an involuntary resistance to passive movement as may occur in cerebral cortical disorders.

Geister (gīs′ter) Janet M. (1885–1964). American nursing writer, editor, researcher, and consultant. As a field worker for the U.S. Children's Bureau, she conducted surveys of infant and maternal mortality in Chicago, Montana, and Kentucky. During World War I she made one of the first studies of children's day care centers and helped develop a mobile clinic to bring health care to isolated rural areas. She also conducted studies of nursing education, visiting nursing, and hospitals for the National Organization for Public Health Nursing and was active in a number of professional organizations.

gel (jel) 1. a colloid in which the solid disperse phase forms a network in combination with that of the fluid continuous phase, resulting in a viscous semirigid sol. 2. to form such a compound or any similar semisolid material.

gelatin (jel′ah-tin) a substance obtained by partial hydrolysis of collagen derived from skin, white connective tissue, and bones of animals; used as a suspending agent, in manufacture of capsules and suppositories, sometimes as an adjuvant protein food, and suggested for use as a plasma substitute. In absorbable film and sponge, it is used in surgical procedures.

　　zinc g. a preparation of zinc oxide, gelatin, glycerin, and purified water, used as a topical skin protectant. See also Unna's paste BOOT.

gelatinize (jĕ-lat′ĭ-nīz) 1. to convert into gelatin. 2. to become converted into gelatin.

gelatinoid (jĕ-lat′ĭ-noid) resembling gelatin.

gelatinous (jĕ-lat′ĭ-nus) like jelly or softened gelatin.

gelation (jĕ-la′shun) conversion of a sol into a gel.

Gelfilm (jel′film) trademark for absorbable gelatin film, used as an aid in surgical closure and repair of defects in the dura mater and pleura.

Gelfoam (jel′fōm) trademark for preparations of absorbable gelatin sponge, used as a local hemostatic.

Gell and Coombs classification (jel; kōōmz) a classification of immune mechanisms of tissue injury, comprising four types of HYPERSENSITIVITY REACTIONS: *type I,* immediate HYPERSENSITIVITY reactions, mediated by interaction of IgE antibody and antigen and release of histamine and other mediators; *type II,* antibody-mediated hypersensitivity reactions, due to antibody-antigen interactions on cell surfaces; *type III,* immune complex–mediated hypersensitivity reactions, local or general inflammatory RESPONSES due to formation of circulating immune complexes and their deposition in tissues; and *type IV* cell-mediated hypersensitivity reactions, delayed HYPERSENSITIVITY reactions initiated by sensitized T lymphocytes either by release of lymphokines or by T-cell–mediated cytotoxicity.

gelosis (jĕ-lo′sis) a hard, swollen lump in a tissue, especially in muscle.

gemcitabine (jem-sit′ah-bēn) an antineoplastic AGENT used in chemotherapy for pancreatic ADENOCARCINOMA and non–small cell lung CARCINOMA; administered by intravenous infusion as the hydrochloride salt.

gemellology (jem″el-ol′o-je) the scientific study of twins and twinning.

gemfibrozil (jem-fib′ro-zil) an ANTILIPIDEMIC agent used for treatment of patients with very high serum TRIGLYCERIDE levels (type IV HYPERLIPOPROTEINEMIA) who do not respond to dietary management.

geminate (jem′ĭ-nāt) paired; occurring in twos.

gemmation (jĕ-ma′shun) development of a new organism from a protuberance on the cell body of the parent, a form of asexual REPRODUCTION; called also budding.

gemmule (jem′ūl) 1. a reproductive bud, the immediate product of GEMMATION. 2. any of the little spinelike processes on the dendrites of a nerve cell.

gemtuzumab ozogamicin (gem-too′zoo-mab″ o″zo-gah-mi′sin) a recombinant DNA-derived monoclonal antibody conjugated with a cytotoxic antitumor antibiotic, used as an ANTINEOPLASTIC in the treatment of relapsed acute myelogenous LEUKEMIA, administered intravenously.

-gen word element [Gr.], *an agent that produces.*

genal (je′nal) pertaining to the cheek; buccal.

gender (jen′der) sex (def. 1); see also gender IDENTITY and gender ROLE.

　　g. identity disorder a disturbance of gender identification in which the affected person has an overwhelming desire to change their anatomic sex or insists that they are of the opposite sex, with persistent discomfort about their assigned sex or about filling its usual gender role; the disorder may become apparent in childhood or not appear until adolescence or adulthood. Individuals may attempt to live as members of the opposite sex and may seek hormonal and surgical treatment to bring their anatomy into conformity with their belief (see TRANSSEXUALISM). It is not the same as TRANSVESTISM.

gene (jēn) one of the biologic units of heredity, self-reproducing, and located at a definite position (locus) on a particular chromosome. Genes make up segments of the complex DEOXYRIBONUCLEIC ACID (DNA) molecule that controls cellular reproduction and function. There are thousands of genes in the chromosomes of each cell nucleus; they play an important role in heredity because they control the individual physical, biochemical, and physiologic traits inherited by offspring from their parents. Through the genetic code of DNA they also control the day-to-day functions and reproduction of all cells in the body. For example, the genes control the synthesis of structural proteins and also the enzymes that regulate various chemical reactions that take place in a cell.

The gene is capable of replication. When a cell multiplies by mitosis each daughter cell carries a set of genes that is an exact replica of that of the parent cell. This characteristic of replication explains how genes can carry hereditary traits through successive generations without change.

allelic g. allele.

complementary g's two independent pairs of nonallelic genes, neither of which will produce its effect in the absence of the other.

DCC g. (deleted in colorectal carcinoma) a gene normally expressed in the mucosa of the colon but reduced or absent in a small proportion of patients with colorectal cancer.

dominant g. one that produces an effect (the phenotype) in the organism regardless of the state of the corresponding allele. An example of a trait determined by a dominant gene is brown eye color. See also HEREDITY.

histocompatibility g. one that determines the specificity of tissue antigenicity (HLA ANTIGENS) and thus the compatibility of donor and recipient in tissue transplantation and blood transfusion.

holandric g's genes located on the Y chromosome and appearing only in male offspring.

immune response (Ir) g's genes of the major histocompatibility COMPLEX that govern the IMMUNE RESPONSE to individual immunogens.

immune suppressor (Is) g's genes that govern the formation of suppressor T LYMPHOCYTES.

immunoglobulin g's the genes coding for immunoglobulin heavy and light chains, which are organized in three loci coding for κ light chains, λ light chains, and heavy chains.

K-ras g. a type of ONCOGENE.

lethal g. one whose presence brings about the death of the organism or permits survival only under certain conditions.

major g. a gene whose effect on the phenotype is always evident, regardless of how this effect is modified by other genes.

mutant g. one that has undergone a detectable MUTATION.

operator g. one serving as a starting point for reading the genetic code, and which, through interaction with a repressor, controls the activity of structural genes associated with it in the operon.

g. pool all of the genes possessed by all of the members of a population that will reproduce.

recessive g. one that produces an effect in the organism only when it is transmitted by both parents, i.e., only when the individual is homozygous. See also HEREDITY.

regulator g., repressor g. one that synthesizes repressor, a substance which, through interaction with the operator gene, switches off the activity of the structural genes associated with it in the operon.

sex-linked g. a gene carried on a sex chromosome (X or Y); only X linkage has clinical significance. See X-linked GENE.

g. splicing RECOMBINANT DNA TECHNOLOGY.

structural g. one that forms templates for messenger RNA and is thereby responsible for the amino acid sequence of specific polypeptides.

tumor suppressor g. a gene whose function is to limit cell proliferation and loss of whose function leads to cell transformation and tumor growth; called also anti-oncogene.

X-linked g. a gene carried on the X chromosome; the corresponding trait, whether dominant or recessive, is always expressed in males, who have only one X chromosome. the term "X-linked" is sometimes used synonymously with "sex-linked," since no genetic disorders have as yet been associated with genes on the Y chromosome.

genera (jen'er-ah) [L.] plural of GENUS.

general adaptation syndrome all nonspecific systemic reactions of the body to prolonged systemic stress, including the ALARM REACTION, resistance, and exhaustion.

generalization (jen″er-al-ĭ-za′shun) the formation of a general principle or idea; inductive reasoning.

g. of learning the application of previously learned concepts and behaviors to similar situations, a cognitive PERFORMANCE COMPONENT of occupational therapy.

generalized anxiety disorder GAD; an ANXIETY DISORDER characterized by the presence of excessive, uncontrollable anxiety and worry about two or more life circumstances for six months or longer, accompanied by some combination of restlessness, fatigue, muscle tension, irritability, disturbed concentration or sleep, and somatic symptoms.

general systems framework and theory of goal attainment a conceptual model system for nursing, formulated by Imogene M. KING, comprising three dynamic, interacting systems (the personal, interpersonal and social systems), with specific concepts related to each system.

generation (jen″er-a′shun) 1. the process of reproduction. 2. a class composed of all individuals removed by the same number of successive ancestors from a common predecessor, or occupying positions on the same level in a genealogical (pedigree) chart.

alternate g. reproduction by alternate asexual and sexual means in an animal or plant species.

asexual g., direct g. production of a new organism not originating from union of gametes.

first filial g. the first-generation offspring of two parents; symbol F_1.

parental g. the generation with which a particular genetic study is begun; symbol P_1.

second filial g. all of the offspring produced by two individuals of the first filial generation; symbol F_2.

sexual g. production of a new organism from the cell formed by the union of a male gamete (SPERMATOZOON) and a female gamete (OOCYTE).

spontaneous g. the discredited concept of continuous generation of living organisms from nonliving matter.

generative (jen′er-ah-tiv″) pertaining to reproduction.

generator (jen′ĕ-ra″tor) 1. something that produces or causes to exist. 2. a machine that converts mechanical to electrical energy.

pulse g. the power source for an artificial PACEMAKER, usually powered by a long-lasting lithium battery and a microprocessor chip with appropriate electronic components to regulate the output of the battery; it supplies impulses to the implanted electrodes, either at a fixed rate or in a programmed pattern.

generic (jĕ-ner′ik) 1. pertaining to a genus. 2. nonproprietary; denoting a drug name not protected by a trademark, usually descriptive of the drug's chemical structure.

genesiology (jĕ-ne″ze-ol′o-je) the scientific study of REPRODUCTION.

genesis (jen′ĕ-sis) creation; origination; used as a word termination joined to an element indicating the thing created, e.g., carcinogenesis.

genetic (jĕ-net′ik) 1. pertaining to reproduction or to birth or origin. 2. inherited.

g. code the arrangement of nucleotides in the polynucleotide chain of a chromosome; it governs the transmission of genetic information to proteins, i.e., determines the sequence of amino acids in the polypeptide chain making up each protein synthesized by the cell. Genetic information is coded in DNA by means of four bases: two purines (adenine and guanine) and two pyrimidines (thymine and cystosine). Each adjacent sequence of three bases (a codon) determines the insertion of a specific amino acid. In RNA, uracil replaces thymine.

g. map 1. the location of mutations along the length of a chromosome, as determined by recombination experiments. The unit of length is the centimorgan (cM), one crossover per meiosis. 2. the sequence of base pairs along the DNA of a chromosome, a technique being applied to humans.

g. marker a gene having alleles that are all expressed in the phenotype, that is, they are codominant, and which can be used to study inheritance. The various blood group systems and serum or red blood cell proteins easily detected by electrophoresis or immunodiffusion are commonly used markers.

geneticist (jĕ-net′ĭ-sist) a specialist in genetics.

genetics (jĕ-net′iks) the branch of biology dealing with the phenomena of heredity and the laws governing it.

biochemical g. the study of the fundamental relationships between genes, protein, and metabolism. This involves the study of the cause of many specific heritable diseases. These include those resulting from the improper synthesis of hemoglobins and protein, such as SICKLE CELL DISEASE and THALASSEMIA, both of which are hereditary anemias; some 200 inborn errors of metabolism, such as PHENYLKETONURIA and GALACTOSEMIA, in which lack or alteration of a specific enzyme prohibits proper metabolism of carbohydrates, proteins, or fats and thus produces pathologic symptoms; and genetically determined variations in response to certain drugs, for example, isoniazid.

clinical g. the study of the causes and inheritance of genetic disorders. In addition to the diseases mentioned under biochemical genetics, other aspects of clinical genetics include the study of chromosomal aberrations, such as those that cause mental retardation and DOWN SYNDROME, and immunogenetics, or the genetic aspects of the IMMUNE RESPONSE and the transmission of genetic factors from generation to generation.

Many pediatric hospital admissions involve genetic disorders. In obstetrics and neonatal medicine, prenatal diagnosis of genetic defects and improvement of pre- and perinatal conditions are a major concern. In adults, such diseases as breast cancer, coronary artery disease, hypertension, and diabetes mellitus have all been found to have predisposing genetic components that are relevant to identification of risk factors and early diagnosis.

Geneva Convention an international agreement of 1864, whereby, among other pledges, the signatory nations pledged themselves to treat the wounded and the army medical and nursing staff as neutrals on the field of battle.

genic (jen′ik) pertaining to or caused by the genes.

-genic word element [Gr.], *giving rise to; causing.*

genicular (jĕ-nik′u-lar) pertaining to the knee.

geniculate (jĕ-nik′u-lāt) bent, like a knee.

geniculum (jĕ-nik′u-lum), pl. *geni′cula* [L.] a little knee; used in anatomic nomenclature to designate a sharp kneelike bend in a small structure or organ.

genit(o)- word element [L.], *genital organs.*

genital (jen′ĭ-tal) 1. pertaining to REPRODUCTION or to the reproductive organs. 2. (in the plural) reproductive organs; see REPRODUCTIVE ORGANS, FEMALE and REPRODUCTIVE ORGANS, MALE.

g. ulcer syndrome any of the group of diseases causing ulcerations of the genitalia, most commonly syphilis or herpes simplex, but also chancroid, lymphogranuloma venereum, granuloma inguinale, or trauma.

genitalia (jen″ĭ-ta′le-ah) reproductive organs; see REPRODUCTIVE ORGANS, FEMALE and REPRODUCTIVE ORGANS, MALE.

ambiguous g. genital organs with characteristics typical of both male and female, as seen in HERMAPHRODITISM and some types of PSEUDOHERMAPHRODITISM.

genitocrural (jen″ĭ-to-kroor′al) pertaining to the genitalia and the thigh.

genitofemoral (jen″ĭ-to-fem′o-ral) genitocrural.

genitography (jen″ĭ-tog′rah-fe) radiography of the urogenital sinus and internal duct structures after injection of a contrast medium through the sinus opening.

genitoplasty (jen′ĭ-to-plas″te) plastic surgery on the genital organs.

genitourinary (jen′ĭ-to-u′rĭ-ner″e) pertaining to the urinary system and genitalia; called also urinogenital and urogenital.

genocopy (jen′o-kop″e) an individual whose PHENOTYPE mimics that of another genotype but whose character is determined by a distinct assortment of genes.

genodermatosis (je″no-der″mah-to′sis) a genetic disorder of the skin, usually generalized.

G

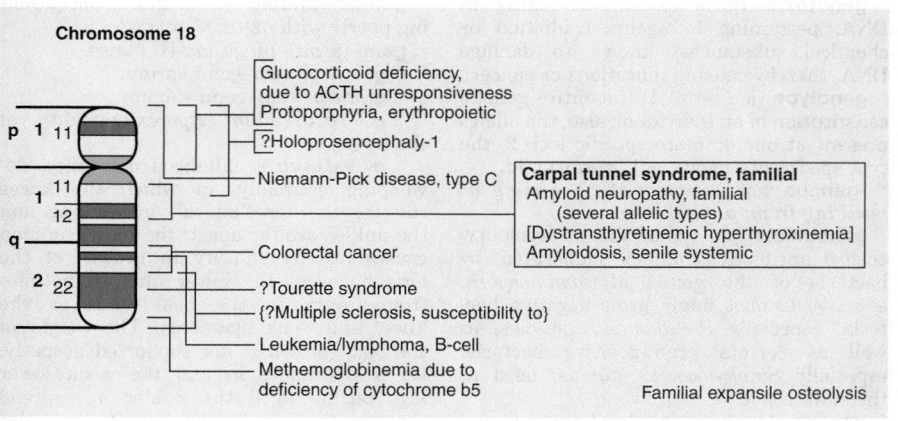

A gene map of Chromosome 18. From Copstead, 1996.

Chromosome 18

Glucocorticoid deficiency, due to ACTH unresponsiveness
Protoporphyria, erythropoietic
?Holoprosencephaly-1
Niemann-Pick disease, type C
Colorectal cancer
?Tourette syndrome
{?Multiple sclerosis, susceptibility to}
Leukemia/lymphoma, B-cell
Methemoglobinemia due to deficiency of cytochrome b5

Carpal tunnel syndrome, familial
Amyloid neuropathy, familial
   (several allelic types)
[Dystransthyretinemic hyperthyroxinemia]
Amyloidosis, senile systemic

Familial expansile osteolysis

p 1 11
1 11
12
q
2 22

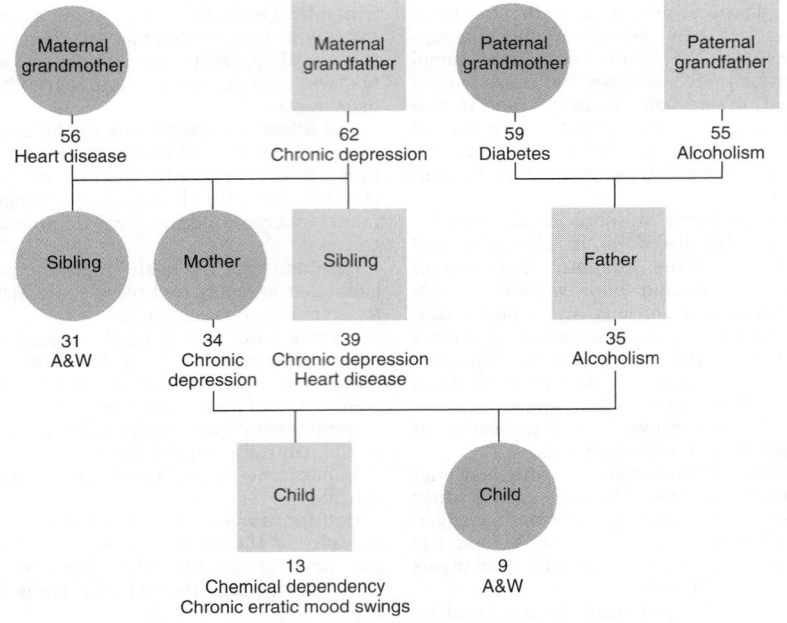

A family genogram of disease patterns. (A&W = alive and well) From Betz et al., 1994.

genogram (je′no-gram) a family assessment tool consisting of a family tree diagram depicting family dispersals, losses, roles, and organizational patterns over three or more generations.

genome (je′nōm) the complete set of GENES, hereditary factors contained in the haploid set of CHROMOSOMES; the human genome has an estimated 30,000 to 40,000 genes. adj., **genom′ic**.

genotoxic (je′no-tok″sik) damaging to DNA; pertaining to agents (radiation or chemical substances) known to damage DNA, thereby causing mutations or cancer.

genotype (jen″o-tīp) 1. the entire genetic constitution of an individual; also, the alleles present at one or more specific loci. 2. the type species of a genus. adj., **genotyp′ic**.

-genous word element [Gr.], *arising or resulting from; produced by*.

gentamicin (jen″tah-mi′sin) an AMINOGLYCOSIDE antibiotic complex elaborated by bacteria of the genus *Micromonospora*, effective against many gram-negative bacteria, especially *Pseudomonas* species, as well as certain gram-positive bacteria, especially *Staphylococcus aureus;* used as the sulfate salt.

gentian (jen′shan) the dried rhizome and roots of *Gentiana lutea.*

g. violet an antibacterial, antifungal, and anthelmintic dye, applied topically in the treatment of infections of the skin and mucous membranes associated with gram-positive bacteria and molds and also used to treat banked blood drawn from patients in areas endemic for CHAGAS' DISEASE, to kill trypanosomes in the blood.

gentianophilic (jen″shan-o-fil′ik) staining readily with GENTIAN VIOLET.

gentianophobic (jen″shan-o-fo′bik) staining poorly with GENTIAN VIOLET.

genu (je′nu), pl. *ge′nua* [L.] knee.

g. extror′sum genu varum.

g. intror′sum genu valgum.

g. recurva′tum hyperextensibility of the knee joint.

g. val′gum a childhood deformity, developing gradually, in which the knees rub together or "knock" in walking and the ankles are far apart; the most common causes are irregularity in growth of the long bones of the lower limb (sometimes from injury to the bone ends at the knee) and weak ligaments. The weight of the body, which is not supported properly, turns the knees in and the weak lower legs buckle until the ankles are spread far apart. See illustration. Called also knock-knee.

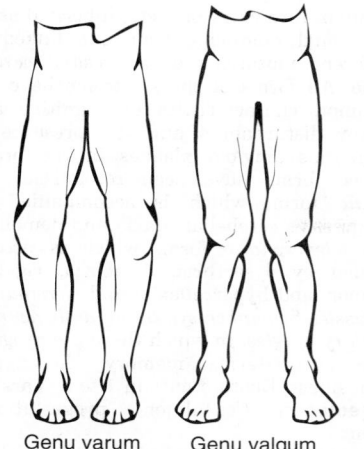

Genu varum   Genu valgum

Genu varum and genu valgum. From Copstead and Banasik, 2000.

Genu valgum in young children varies in seriousness. Milder cases may disappear after early childhood as bones, ligaments, and muscles strengthen and coordination improves. More serious cases can often be corrected by strengthening exercises and by proper manipulation of the joints. Sometimes braces are used to ensure the proper alignment of growing legs. In a very young child, genu valgum involves only the soft bone ends where the bone grows. If allowed to continue for a number of years, the condition can lead to abnormal developments in body structure. The sooner corrective measures are taken, the more effective the treatment is likely to be.

g. va′rum an outward curvature of one or both lower limbs near the knee; see illustration. Called also bowleg.

genus (je′nus), pl. *gen′era* [L.] a taxonomic category (taxon) subordinate to a tribe (or subtribe) and superior to a species (or subgenus).

geo- word element [Gr.], *the earth; soil.*

geode (je′ōd) a dilated lymph space.

geomedicine (je″o-med′ĭ-sin) the branch of medicine dealing with the influence of climatic and environmental conditions on health.

geophagia (je″o-fa′jah) the habit of eating clay or earth, a form of PICA.

geophagy (je-of′ah-je) geophagia.

geotaxis (je″o-tak′sis) TAXIS in response to gravity; movement influenced by gravity.

geotrichosis (je″o-trĭ-ko′sis) a candidiasis-like infection due to *Geotrichum candidum,* which may attack the bronchi, lungs, mouth, or intestinal tract.

Geotrichum (je-ot′rĭ-kum) a genus of yeastlike fungi. *G. can′didum* is found in dairy products and feces.

G. can′didum a species found in the feces and dairy products.

geotropism (je-ot′ro-pizm) TROPISM in response to gravity, i.e., either toward or away from the earth; growth influenced by gravity.

ger(o)- word element [Gr.], *old age; the aged.*

geratology (jer″ah-tol′o-je) gerontology.

GERD gastroesophageal reflux disease.

geriatric (jer″e-at′rik) 1. pertaining to elderly persons or to the aging process. 2. pertaining to geriatrics.

geriatrician (jer″e-ah-trish′an) a physician specializing in geriatrics.

geriatrics (jer″e-at′riks) the branch of health care dealing with the problems of AGING and diseases of the AGED; it is related to the science of GERONTOLOGY, which is the study of the aging process in all its aspects, social as well as biologic. Geriatrics grows increasingly important as modern medicine and a rising standard of living lengthen life expectancy and increase the proportion of aged persons in society.

An important part of geriatrics is helping older persons live happy and satisfying lives. Geriatric specialists encourage their patients to follow useful and interesting pursuits and to adopt a sound mental attitude toward aging itself. The prevention of disease is also important in geriatrics, and stress is placed on suitable exercise, rest, and nutrition, and on maintenance of proper body weight. Regular and thorough medical examinations are another essential factor in the control of illness.

In geriatrics, there is also concern for the older person's psychological welfare, such as social contacts, economic security, interest in living, work opportunities after retirement, and continuing sense of belonging to society. Geriatrics recognizes that health of mind is essential to the health of the body.

germ (jerm) 1. a pathogenic microorganism. 2. living substance capable of developing into an organ, part, or organism as a whole; a primordium.

wheat g. the embryo of wheat, which contains tocopherol, thiamine, riboflavin, and other vitamins.

germanium (Ge) (jer-ma′ne-um) a chemical element, atomic number 32, atomic weight 72.59. (See Appendix 6.)

germicidal (jer″mĭ-si′dal) destructive to pathogenic microorganisms.

germicide (jer′mĭ-sīd) an agent that destroys pathogenic microorganisms; see ANTIBIOTIC and ANTIMICROBIAL.

germinal (jer′mĭ-nal) pertaining to or of the nature of a germ CELL or the primordial stage of development.

germination (jer″mĭ-na′shun) the sprouting of a seed, spore, or plant embryo.

germinative (jer′mĭ-na″tiv) pertaining to germination or to a germ cell.

germinoma (jer″mĭ-no′mah) a type of germ cell TUMOR consisting of large round cells with vesicular nuclei, usually found in the ovary, undescended testis, anterior mediastinum, or pineal gland; in males these are called SEMINOMAS and in females DYSGERMINOMAS.

germline (jerm′lĭn) the sequence of cells in the line of direct descent from zygote to gametes, as opposed to somatic cells (all other body cells). Mutations in germline cells are transmitted to offspring; those in somatic cells are not.

geroderma (jer″o-der′mah) dystrophy of the skin and genitals, giving the appearance of old age.

gerodermia (jer″o-der′me-ah) geroderma.

gerodontics (jer″o-don′tiks) dentistry dealing with the dental problems of the AGED. adj., **gerodon′tic**.

gerodontist (jer″o-don′tist) a dentist specializing in gerodontics.

gerodontology (jer″o-don-tol′o-je) study of the dentition and dental problems in the AGED.

geromarasmus (jer″o-mah-raz′mus) the emaciation sometimes characteristic of old age.

geromorphism (jer″o-mor′fizm) premature senility.

geront(o)- word element [Gr.], *old age; the aged.*

gerontal (jĕ-ron′tal) senile.

gerontic (jĕ-ron′tik) senile.

gerontologist (jer″on-tol′o-jist) a health care provider specializing in gerontology.

gerontology (jer″on-tol′o-je) the scientific study of AGING.

gerontopia (jer″on-to′pe-ah) senopia.

gerontotherapeutics (je-ron″to-ther″ah-pu′tiks) the science of retarding and preventing the development of many of the aspects of AGING.

gerontotoxon (jer-on″to-tok′son) arcus corneae.

geropsychiatry (jer″o-si-ki′ah-tre) a subspecialty of psychiatry dealing with mental health and illness in the elderly.

Gerstmann-Sträussler-Scheinker syndrome (gerst′mahn-shtrois′ler-shĭn′ker) a group of rare PRION DISEASES, inherited as an autosomal dominant trait but linked to different mutations of the PRION PROTEIN gene. All forms of the syndrome have the common characteristics of cognitive and motor disturbances and the presence of numerous amyloid plaques in the brain. Three forms have been recognized: the *ataxic* form, which is accompanied by progressive cerebellar ataxia and dementia; the *telencephalic* form, which is accompanied by dysarthria, dementia, rigidity, tremor, and hyperreflexia; and *Gerstmann-Strässler-Scheinker syndrome with neurofibrillary tangles,* in which there are progressive short-term memory loss and clumsiness. Death occurs in 1 to 5 years.

gestagen (jes′tah-jen) progestational agent.

gestalt (gĕ-stawlt′, gĕ-shtawlt′) [Ger.] form, shape; a whole perceptual configuration.

gestaltism (gĕ-stawl′tizm) the theory in psychology that the objects of mind, as immediately presented to direct experience, come as complete unanalyzable wholes or forms (Gestalten) that cannot be split up into parts.

gestation (jes-ta′shun) the period of development of the young in viviparous animals, from the time of fertilization of the oocyte (ovum) to birth; see also PREGNANCY.

g. period the duration of PREGNANCY; in the human female, the average length, calculated from the first day of the last normal menstrual period, is 280 days, or 6 lunar months. The normal limits of the human gestation period are from 37 weeks (259 days) to 42 weeks (293 days); days and weeks are counted as completed days and weeks. If one counts from the moment of conception, the length of time is 266 days (280−14 days).

gestational (jes-ta′shun-al) pertaining to gestation.

g. age the estimated age or stage of maturity of a CONCEPTUS. Gestational age of the newborn INFANT can be estimated by noting various physical characteristics that normally appear at each stage of fetal development. *Gestational age assessment* of the newborn is facilitated by using a scoring system such as the one developed by Dubowitz and Dubowitz, or a modification of it by Ballard.

As the preterm newborn emerges from the birth canal it will be covered with a rather heavy coating of vernix caseosa; the full-term newborn has only a small amount of this cheeselike substance in body creases and the hair. By the 40th to 42nd week of gestation the skin of the newborn is pale and opaque, whereas the skin of the baby born before this period of gestation may be thin and transparent; venules can be seen under the skin on the abdomen.

At about 20 weeks the body is covered with fine hair called *lanugo*, which begins to disappear as maturation continues, first from the face, then the trunk, and finally from the extremities. At nine months gestation lanugo is usually seen only over the shoulders. Wrinkling of the soles of the feet is another indication of the newborn's gestational age. It occurs first near the toes and progresses toward the heels so that by the 40th week the entire sole is covered with creases. The preterm newborn will have smooth soles with only a few creases. "Cotton wool" hair that tends to stick together in small bunches so that it is difficult to distinguish one strand from another is common until the 38th week of gestation. This sign is of less significance in black infants. Cartilage of the ear can also be used to assess gestational age. Until about 32 or 33 weeks the pinnae stay folded when bent inward; by 36 weeks they spring back when released. At term they are firm enough to stand erect from the sides of the head.

gestosis (jes-to'sis), pl. *gesto'ses* any disorder of pregnancy, such as PREECLAMP-SIA-ECLAMPSIA SYNDROME.

Gestuno (ges-too'no) old name for International Sign Language.

gesture (jes'cher) an act made or something said to signify intention or attitude.

suicidal g. a more serious warning than a suicide THREAT; it may be followed by a planned suicidal act that attracts attention without seriously injuring the subject.

GeV gigaelectron volt.

GFR glomerular filtration rate.

GH-RH growth hormone–releasing hormone.

GI gastrointestinal; globin (zinc) insulin.

giantism (ji'an-tizm) 1. gigantism. 2. excessive size or numbers of cells or nuclei.

Giardia (je-ahr'de-ah) a genus of flagellate protozoa parasitic in the intestines of humans and other animals, which may cause protracted, intermittent diarrhea with symptoms suggesting malabsorption. *G. lamb'lia* (called also *G. intestina'lis*) causes GIARDIASIS.

giardiasis (je″ahr-di'ah-sis) a common infection of the lumen of the small intestine with *Giardia lamblia,* and spread via contaminated food and water and by direct person-to-person contact. Most of those infected are asymptomatic, but a small percentage of cases present a wide range of symptoms, including nonspecific

gastrointestinal discomfort, mild to profuse diarrhea, nausea, lassitude, anorexia, and weight loss.

gibbosity (gĭ-bos'ĭ-te) kyphosis.

gibbous (gib'us) humped; protuberant.

gibbus (gib'us) hump.

GIFT gamete intrafallopian transfer.

Gierke's disease (gēr'kez) GLYCOGEN STOR-AGE DISEASE (type I), a condition in which deficiency of the hepatic enzyme glucose-6-phosphatase results in liver and kidney involvement, with hepatomegaly, hypoglycemia, hyperuricemia, and gout. Called also von Gierke's disease and hepatorenal glycogenosis.

giga- word element [Gr.], *huge;* used in naming units of measurement to designate an amount one billion (10^9) times the size of the unit to which it is joined; symbol G.

gigantism (ji-gan'tizm, ji'gan-tizm) abnormal overgrowth of the body or a part; excessive size and stature. Generally applied to a rare abnormality of the PITUITARY GLAND, which secretes excessive GROWTH HORMONE before the growing ends of the bones have closed. This causes a child to become an unusually tall adult; if the abnormality is extreme, the individual may reach a height of 2.4 meters (8 feet) or more, although the body proportions usually are normal.

The opposite condition, DWARFISM, is caused by underproduction of the same hormone. (Overproduction of growth hormone in adults causes ACROMEGALY.) Gigantism can be corrected only by early diagnosis in childhood and removal by surgery of part of the pituitary gland or by x-ray treatment.

cerebral g. gigantism in the absence of increased levels of growth hormone, attributed to a cerebral defect; infants are large, and accelerated growth continues for the first 4 or 5 years, the rate being normal thereafter. The hands and feet are large, the head is large, narrow and long, and the eyes have an antimongoloid slant with an abnormally wide space between them. The child is clumsy, and mental retardation of varying degree is usually present. Called also Sotos syndrome.

pituitary g. that caused by oversecretion of growth hormone by the pituitary gland; see *gigantism.* Called also Launois syndrome.

gigantomastia (ji-gan″to-mas'te-ah) extreme MACROMASTIA.

Gilbert disease (zhēl-bār') 1. hyperbilirubinemia I. 2. a relatively common, hereditary, benign or subclinical form of

G

HYPERBILIRUBINEMIA caused by reduced rates of hepatic uptake and conjugation of BILIRUBIN. Patients may have mild, intermittent JAUNDICE, fatigue, and weakness. Although the disease is present from birth, it usually presents clinically in the second or third decade of life. No treatment is necessary and the prognosis is excellent. Called also Gilbert syndrome and hyperbilirubinemia I.

Gilles de la Tourette's syndrome (disease) (zhĕl′ dĕ lah too-rets′) a syndrome comprising both multiple motor and one or more vocal tics that occur for at least one year, either intermittently or sometimes numerous times in one day. Obsessions, compulsions, hyperactivity, distractibility, and impulsivity are often associated. Onset is in childhood, and tics often lessen in severity and frequency and may even remit during adolescence and adulthood. Called also Tourette's syndrome.

gingiv(o)- word element [L.], *gingiva.*

gingiva (jin-ji′vah, jin′ji-vah), pl. *gin′givae* [L.] the part of the oral mucosa covering the tooth-bearing border of the jaw; called also gum.

   alveolar g. attached gingiva.

   areolar g. the portion attached to the alveolar process by loose areolar connective tissue.

   attached g. that portion of the gingiva which is firm and resilient and is bound to the underlying cementum and the alveolar bone, thus being immovable. Called also alveolar gingiva.

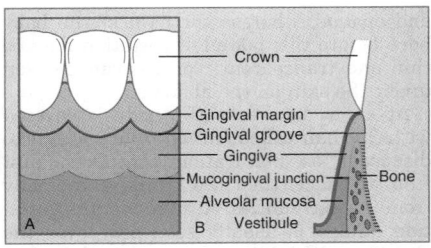

Anatomical relationship of normal gingiva in facial view (A) and in cross-section (B). From Darby and Walsh, 1994.

   free g. the portion that surrounds the tooth and is not directly attached to the tooth surface.

gingival (jin′ji-val) pertaining to the gingivae.

   g. disease any disease of the gingivae, such as GINGIVITIS. The American Academy of Periodontology classifies gingival disease as a major group of periodontal diseases and distinguishes two main subgroups, those gingival diseases induced by dental plaque and those attributed to other causes. The plaque-induced diseases may be associated with endocrine changes, medications, systemic disease, or malnutrition. The other causes of gingival lesions include viral infections, fungal infections, genetic predispositions, systemic conditions, allergic reactions, traumatic lesions, and a variety of others. See table at PERIODONTAL DISEASE.

gingivalgia (jin″ji-val′jah) pain in the gingiva.

gingivectomy (jin″ji-vek′to-me) surgical excision of all loose infected and diseased

TERMINOLOGY USED TO DESCRIBE OBSERVATIONS ASSOCIATED WITH CLINICAL ASSESSMENT OF THE GINGIVA			
Characteristic	**Terminology**	**Description**	**Example**
Gingival Color	Location: Distribution: Severity: Quality:	Generalized or localized Diffuse, marginal, or papillary Slight, moderate, severe Red, bright red, pink, cyanotic	Localized slight marginal redness linguals of #18, 19, 30, 31, all other areas coral pink, uniform in color
Gingival Contour	Location: Distribution: Severity: Quality:	Generalized or localized Diffuse, marginal, or papillary Slight, moderate, severe Bulbous, flattened, punched out, cratered	Localized moderately cratered papilla #6–11, #22–27, all other areas within normal limits
Consistency of Gingiva	Location: Distribution: Severity: Quality:	Generalized or localized Diffuse, marginal, or papillary Slight, moderate, severe Firm (fibrotic), spongy (edematous)	Generalized moderate marginal sponginess more severe on facial #8, #9, all other areas coral pink with moderate, generalized melanin pigmentation
Surface Texture of Gingiva	Location: Distribution: Quality:	Generalized or localized Diffuse, marginal, or papillary Smooth, shiny, eroded, stippling	Localized smooth gingiva on facial #7, #8, all other areas with generalized stippling

From Darby and Walsh, 1994.

gingival tissue to eradicate periodontal infection and reduce the depth of the gingival sulcus.

gingivitis (jin″jĭ-vi′tis) inflammation of the GUMS. Bleeding is a primary symptom, and other symptoms include swelling, redness, pain, and difficulty in chewing. Gingivitis can lead to the more serious disorder known as PERIODONTITIS. There are numerous causes, of which the primary one is pathogenic microorganisms in the crevices between the gums and the teeth. Other contributing factors are general poor health, host response to inflammation, hormonal imbalances, malnutrition, reactions to certain medications, irregular teeth, badly fitting fillings or dentures that irritate the gums, systemic disease, and infections such as herpetic GINGIVOSTO-MATITIS. Gingivitis is best prevented by correct brushing and flossing of the teeth and proper oral HYGIENE. A good diet containing the necessary minerals and vitamins is also important. Vitamin deficiencies and anemia and other blood dyscrasias are often accompanied by gingivitis.

acute necrotizing ulcerative g. **(ANUG),** *acute ulcerative g.* necrotizing ulcerative gingivitis.

Dilantin g. generalized hyperplasia of the gingiva, which may also rarely involve other areas of the oral mucosa, resulting in overgrowth of the fibrous tissue from the interaction of plaque accumulation with the anticonvulsive agent Dilantin (phenytoin).

necrotizing ulcerative g. **(NUG)** an inflammatory destructive disease of the gingivae that has a sudden onset with periods of remission and exacerbation. It is marked by ulcers of the gingival papillae that become covered with sloughed tissue and circumscribed by linear erythema. Fetid breath, increased salivation, and spontaneous gingival hemorrhage are additional features. It may extend to other parts of the oral mucosa, with lesions involving the palate or pharynx (see also VINCENT'S ANGINA). The etiology is uncertain, but many authorities believe it is caused by a bacterial complex in the presence of predisposing factors such as preexisting gingival disease, smoking, severe stress, radical changes in

CLINICAL FEATURES OF GINGIVITIS

Acute inflammation
Bleeding upon probing
Exudate may be present
Gingival margin greater than 1–2 mm above the cementoenamel junction

eating or sleeping patterns, or nutritional deficiency. It has also been associated with IMMUNODEFICIENCY conditions such as infection with the human immunodeficiency VIRUS (HIV). Although the disease often occurs in an epidemic pattern, it has not been shown to be contagious. Called also acute necrotizing ulcerative or acute ulcerative gingivitis.

pregnancy g. any of various gingival changes ranging from gingivitis to the so-called pregnancy tumor.

Vincent's g. necrotizing ulcerative gingivitis.

gingivoglossitis (jin″jĭ-vo-glŏ-si′tis) inflammation of the gingiva and tongue.

gingivolabial (jin″jĭ-vo-la′be-al) pertaining to the gingivae and lips.

gingivoplasty (jin′jĭ-vo-plas″te) surgical remodeling of the gingiva.

gingivosis (jin″jĭ-vo′sis) a chronic, diffuse inflammation of the gums, with desquamation of the papillary epithelium and mucous membrane.

gingivostomatitis (jin″jĭ-vo-sto″mah-ti′tis) inflammation of the gingiva and oral mucosa.

herpetic g. that due to infection with herpes simplex VIRUS, with redness of the oral tissues, formation of multiple vesicles and painful ulcers, and fever.

necrotizing ulcerative g. that due to extension to the oral mucosa of necrotizing ulcerative GINGIVITIS; see also VINCENT'S ANGINA. Called also Plaut's or pseudomembranous angina.

ginglymus (jing′glĭ-mus) hinge joint.

ginkgo (ging′ko) the dried leaves of the deciduous tree *Ginkgo biloba,* used for symptomatic relief of brain dysfunction, for intermittent claudication, and for tinnitus and vertigo of vascular origin.

girdle (ger′d'l) an encircling or confining structure.

pectoral g. shoulder girdle.

pelvic g. the encircling bony structure supporting the lower limbs.

shoulder g., thoracic g. the encircling bony structure supporting the upper limbs.

gitalin (jit′ah-lin) a mixture of DIGITALIS glycosides used as a CARDIOTONIC in congestive HEART FAILURE and cardiac ARRHYTHMIAS. Called also amorphous gitalin.

glabella (glah-bel′ah) the area on the frontal bone above the nasion and between the eyebrows.

glabrous (gla′brus) smooth and bare.

glacial (gla′sh'l) designating a highly pure state of certain acids, such as acetic acid, so called because the freezing point is only slightly below room temperature.

gladiolus (glah-di′o-lus) body of sternum.

glairy (glār′e) resembling white of an egg.

gland (gland) an aggregation of cells specialized to secrete or excrete materials not related to their ordinary metabolic needs. Glands are divided into two main groups, endocrine and exocrine. adj., **glan′-dular.** The ENDOCRINE GLANDS, or ductless glands, discharge their secretions (hormones) directly into the blood; they include the adrenal, pituitary, thyroid, and parathyroid glands, the islands of Langerhans in the pancreas, the gonads, the thymus, and the pineal body. The exocrine GLANDS discharge through ducts opening on an external or internal surface of the body; they include the salivary, sebaceous, and sweat glands, the liver, the gastric glands, the pancreas, the intestinal, mammary, and lacrimal glands, and the prostate. The LYMPH NODES are sometimes called lymph glands but are not glands in the usual sense.

acinous g. one made up of one or more ACINI (oval or spherical sacs).

adrenal g. see ADRENAL GLAND.

apocrine g. one whose discharged secretion contains part of the secreting cells.

areolar g′s Montgomery's glands.

axillary g′s lymph nodes in the axilla.

Bartholin g′s two small mucus-secreting glands, one on each side in the lower pole of the labium majus and connected to the surface by a duct lined with transitional cells, which opens just external to the hymenal ring. Their exact function is not clear but they are believed to secrete mucus to moisten the vestibule during sexual excitement. Called also major vestibular glands.

Bowman's g′s olfactory glands.

bronchial g′s seromucous glands in the mucosa and submucosa of the bronchial walls.

Brunner's g′s glands in the submucosa of the duodenum that secrete intestinal juice; called also duodenal glands.

buccal g′s seromucous glands on the inner surface of the cheeks; called also genal glands.

bulbocavernous g′s, bulbourethral g′s two glands embedded in the substance of the sphincter of the male urethra, posterior to the membranous part of the urethra; their secretion lubricates the urethra; called also Cowper's glands.

cardiac g′s mucus-secreting glands of the cardiac part (cardia) of the stomach.

celiac g′s lymph nodes anterior to the abdominal aorta.

ceruminous g′s cerumin-secreting glands in the skin of the external auditory canal.

cervical g′s 1. the lymph nodes of the neck. 2. compound clefts in the wall of the uterine cervix.

ciliary g′s sweat glands that have become arrested in their development, situated at the edges of the eyelids; called also Moll's glands.

circumanal g′s specialized sweat and sebaceous glands around the anus; called also Gay's glands.

Cobelli's g′s mucous glands in the esophageal mucosa just above the cardia.

coccygeal g. glomus coccygeum.

compound g. one made up of a number of smaller units whose excretory ducts combine to form ducts of progressively higher order.

Cowper's g′s bulbourethral glands.

ductless g′s ENDOCRINE GLANDS.

duodenal g′s Brunner's glands.

Ebner's g′s serous glands at the back of the tongue near the taste buds.

eccrine g. one of the ordinary or simple SWEAT GLANDS, which are of the MEROCRINE type.

endocrine g′s see ENDOCRINE GLANDS.

exocrine g′s glands that discharge their secretions through ducts opening on

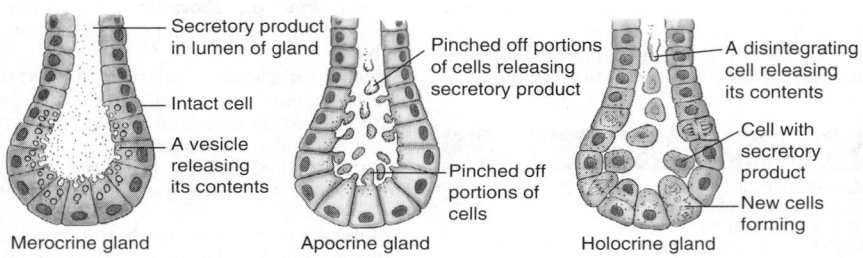

Merocrine gland — Secretory product in lumen of gland; Intact cell; A vesicle releasing its contents

Apocrine gland — Pinched off portions of cells releasing secretory product; Pinched off portions of cells

Holocrine gland — A disintegrating cell releasing its contents; Cell with secretory product; New cells forming

Classification of glands according to mode of secretion. From Applegate, 2000.

internal or external surfaces of the body; see GLAND.

fundic g's, fundus g's numerous tubular glands in the mucosa of the fundus and body of the stomach that contain the cells that produce acid and pepsin.

gastric g's the secreting glands of the stomach, including the fundic, cardiac, and pyloric glands.

Gay's g's circumanal glands.

genal g's buccal glands.

glossopalatine g's mucous glands at the posterior end of the smaller sublingual glands.

haversian g's synovial villi.

holocrine g. one whose discharged secretion contains the entire secreting cells.

intestinal g's straight tubular glands in the mucous membrane of the intestines, in the small intestine opening between the bases of the villi, and containing argentaffin cells. Called also crypts or glands of Lieberkühn.

jugular g. a lymph node behind the clavicular insertion of the sternocleidomastoid muscle.

Krause's g. an accessory lacrimal gland deep in the conjunctival connective tissue, mainly near the upper fornix.

lacrimal g's the glands that secrete tears; see also LACRIMAL APPARATUS.

g's of Lieberkühn intestinal glands.

lingual g's the seromucous glands on the surface of the tongue.

lingual g's, anterior seromucous glands near the apex of the tongue.

Littre's g's 1. preputial glands. 2. the male urethral glands.

lymph g. lymph node.

major vestibular g's Bartholin glands.

mammary g. a specialized gland of the skin of female mammals, which secretes milk for the nourishment of their young; it exists in a rudimentary state in the male. See also BREAST.

meibomian g's sebaceous follicles between the cartilage and conjunctiva of the eyelids. Called also tarsal glands.

merocrine g. one whose discharged secretion contains no part of the secreting cells.

mixed g's 1. seromucous glands. 2. glands that have both exocrine and endocrine portions.

Moll's g's ciliary glands.

Montgomery's g's sebaceous glands in the mammary areola; called also areolar glands.

mucous g's glands that secrete mucus.

olfactory g's small mucous glands in the olfactory mucosa; called also Bowman's glands.

parathyroid g's see PARATHYROID GLANDS.

parotid g's see PAROTID GLANDS.

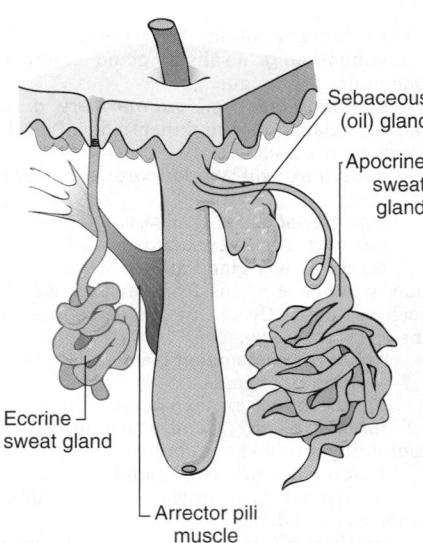

Glands: The relationship of the hair follicle, eccrine and apocrine sweat glands and sebaceous glands. From Copstead, 1995.

peptic g's gastric glands that secrete pepsin.

pineal g. PINEAL BODY.

pituitary g. see PITUITARY GLAND.

preputial g's small sebaceous glands of the corona of the penis and the inner surface of the prepuce, which secrete smegma; called also Littre's glands and Tyson's glands.

prostate g. prostate.

pyloric g's the mucin-secreting glands of the pyloric part of the stomach.

salivary g's see SALIVARY GLANDS.

sebaceous g. a type of holocrine gland of the corium that secretes an oily material (SEBUM) into the hair follicles.

sentinel g. an enlarged lymph node, considered to be pathognomonic of some pathologic condition elsewhere.

seromucous g's glands that are both serous and mucous.

serous g. a gland that secretes a watery albuminous material, commonly but not always containing enzymes.

sex g., sexual g. gonad.

simple g. one with a nonbranching duct.

Skene's g's the largest of the female urethral glands, which open into the urethral orifice; they are regarded as homologous with the prostate. Called also paraurethral ducts.

solitary g's solitary FOLLICLES.

sublingual g. a salivary gland on either side under the tongue.

submandibular g., submaxillary g. a salivary gland on the inner side of each RAMUS OF THE MANDIBLE.

sudoriferous g., sudoriparous g. SWEAT GLAND.

suprarenal g. ADRENAL GLAND.

sweat g. see SWEAT GLAND.

target g. any gland affected by a secretion or other stimulus from another gland, such as those affected by the secretions of the PITUITARY GLAND.

tarsal g's meibomian glands.

thymus g. thymus.

thyroid g. see THYROID GLAND.

tubular g. any gland made up of or containing a tubule or tubules.

Tyson's g's preputial glands.

unicellular g. a single cell that functions as a gland, e.g., a goblet cell.

urethral g's mucous glands in the wall of the urethra; in the male, called also Littre's glands.

uterine g's simple tubular glands found throughout the thickness and extent of the ENDOMETRIUM; they become enlarged during the premenstrual period.

vesical g's mucous glands sometimes found in the wall of the urinary bladder, especially in the area of the trigone.

vulvovaginal g's Bartholin's glands.

Waldeyer's g's glands in the attached edge of the eyelid.

Weber's g's the tubular mucous glands of the tongue.

glanders (glan′derz) a disease of horses that is communicable to humans, caused by *Pseudomonas mallei;* it is marked by a purulent inflammation of the mucous membranes and an eruption of nodules on the skin that coalesce and break down, forming deep ulcers, which may end in necrosis of cartilage and bones. The more chronic and constitutional form is known as FARCY.

glandilemma (glan″dī-lem′ah) the capsule or outer envelope of a gland.

glandula (glan′du-lah), pl. *glan′dulae* [L.] gland.

glandular (glan′du-lar) 1. pertaining to or of the nature of a gland. 2. balanic.

g. fever infectious MONONUCLEOSIS.

glandule (glan′dūl) a small gland.

glans (glanz), pl. *glan′des* [L.] a small, rounded mass or glandlike body.

g. clito′ridis the erectile tissue on the free end of the clitoris.

g. pe′nis the cap-shaped expansion of the corpus spongiosum at the end of the penis.

glanular (glan′u-lar) pertaining to the glans penis or to the glans clitoris.

Glanzmann disease (glahnz′-man) Glanzmann THROMBASTHENIA.

glass (glas) 1. a hard, brittle, often transparent material, usually consisting of the fused amorphous silicates of potassium or sodium, and of calcium, with silica in excess. 2. a container, usually cylindrical, made from this material.

glasses (glas′ez) LENSES arranged in a frame holding them in the proper position in front of the eyes, as an aid to VISION. Called also eyeglasses and spectacles.

bifocal g. glasses with bifocal LENSES; see also BIFOCAL GLASSES.

trifocal g. glasses with trifocal LENSES.

glatiramer (glah-tir′ah-mer) an IMMUNOMODULATOR used as the acetate ester to reduce relapses in MULTIPLE SCLEROSIS; administered by subcutaneous injection.

glaucoma (glaw-, glou-ko′mah) a group of diseases of the eye characterized by increased intraocular pressure, resulting in pathological changes in the optic DISK and typical visual field defects, and eventually BLINDNESS if it is not treated successfully. adj., **glauco′matous.** Glaucoma strikes more than 2 per cent of all those over 40 years of age in the United States. It rarely occurs in anyone under 40. The cause is unknown, but there is a hereditary tendency toward the development of most common forms of glaucoma. Early detection and treatment are essential to prevention of permanent loss of vision. Any person over 40 with a family history of glaucoma should have his intraocular pressure checked once a year.

The normal eye is filled with aqueous humor in an amount carefully regulated to maintain the shape of the eyeball. In glaucoma, the balance of this fluid is disturbed; fluid is formed more rapidly than it leaves the eye, and pressure builds up. The increased pressure damages the retina and disturbs the vision, such as by loss of side vision. If not relieved by proper treatment, the pressure will eventually damage the optic nerve, interrupting the flow of impulses and causing blindness.

Classification. Glaucoma can be divided into three major types: *adult primary glaucoma, secondary glaucoma,* and *congenital glaucoma.* The most common type of adult primary glaucoma is *open-angle glaucoma,* in which there are "open" chamber angles but there is resistance to the outward flow of aqueous humor. This type of glaucoma, also called chronic simple glaucoma, is

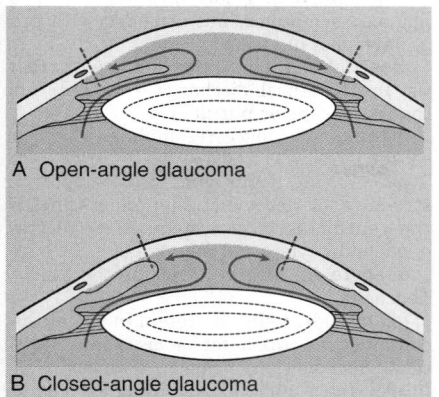

A Open-angle glaucoma

B Closed-angle glaucoma

Glaucoma. *A,* in open-angle glaucoma, the obstruction occurs in the trabecular meshwork. *B,* in closed-angle glaucoma, the trabecular meshwork is covered by the root of the iris or adhesions between the iris and cornea. From Damjanov, 1996.

characterized by very few symptoms in the early stages; thus, many people have the disease without knowing it. There may be some hazy vision and mild discomfort in the eye and later there is a barely noticed loss of peripheral vision. As the disease progresses there is reduced visual acuity and greatly increased intraocular pressure that can cause the appearance of colored rings or halos around bright objects.

Another form of adult primary glaucoma is *angle-closure glaucoma (narrow angle glaucoma),* which can be either acute or chronic. In this type of glaucoma the chamber angle is narrowed or completely closed because of forward displacement of the final roll and root of the iris against the cornea. This closure obstructs the flow of aqueous humor from the eyeball and permits a buildup of pressure.

Secondary glaucoma occurs as a result of a variety of disorders, such as uveitis, neoplastic disease, trauma, and degenerative changes in the eye.

Congenital glaucoma is due to the defective development of the structures in and around the anterior chamber of the eye and results in impairment of the aqueous humor.

Treatment. Open-angle glaucoma is treated medically through the use of BETA-ADRENERGIC BLOCKING AGENTS such as TIMOLOL, MIOTICS to facilitate aqueous outflow, and carbonic anhydrase INHIBITORS to reduce the rate at which aqueous humor is produced. Patients must be informed about this problem and made to understand that they must continue

the prescribed medications for the rest of their lives. An alternative treatment is laser PHOTOCOAGULATION of the angle.

Angle-closure glaucoma is usually treated surgically. If it becomes acute, it is a medical and surgical emergency. If the excessive intraocular pressure is not relieved promptly by medical and surgical means, nerve fibers in the optic disk are destroyed and vision is irretrievably lost. Laser surgical techniques for relief of intraocular pressure include IRIDOTOMY and TRABECULOPLASTY.

Iridotomy involves perforation of the root of the iris, which provides an additional route for the escape of excess aqueous from the posterior to the anterior chambers and the trabecular meshwork.

In trabeculoplasty the spaces of the trabecular meshwork are enlarged by a series of microscopic lesions. Eventually scars form and contract, thus widening the spaces and allowing better aqueous flow.

Laser surgery can be done on an outpatient basis. A local anesthetic is used and patients feel only mild pricking sensations as the laser pulses strike and coagulate tissue. A retrobulbar anesthetic may be used to immobilize the eye during laser surgery.

Patient Care. Early diagnosis and prompt treatment in order to prevent the serious consequences of increased intraocular pressure are a major concern of health care professionals. Screening techniques for early detecting include measurement of intraocular pressure in populations most at risk. Verification of the diagnosis of glaucoma is necessary once suspected cases are found. The general public should be aware of the danger signals of glaucoma and the importance of prompt and diligent treatment. All persons over 40 should have regular testing for glaucoma.

Those most at risk for glaucoma are (1) diabetics, (2) persons with recently controlled hypertension, (3) African Americans (who have an incidence rate of glaucoma-related blindness that is eight times that seen in other ethnic groups), (4) those with a family history of glaucoma, (5) persons with facial hemangiomas or other nevi, and (6) victims of eye injury.

Patients who already have symptoms of glaucoma and are being treated with drugs must be informed about the nature of their eye disorder, the expected effects of each medication, and the importance of faithfully following the regimen of care. Since some patients experience undesirable side effects from these medications, they are told to report them promptly so that the medications can be evaluated by the ophthalmologist.

The combinations of drugs used to treat glaucoma in individual patients can vary considerably. In some cases patients may take as many as four or five drugs. They will need to know about each drug and may need help in devising a schedule for taking them.

Drugs are prescribed either to enhance the outflow of aqueous or to decrease its production, or both. Miotic drugs such as PILOCARPINE facilitate aqueous outflow by stretching the iris away from the trabecular meshwork. Pilocarpine also constricts the pupil, which reduces visual acuity. EPINEPHRINE, ACETAZOLAMIDE, METHAZOLAMIDE, and the beta-adrenergic blocking agent TIMOLOL decrease production of aqueous.

Prescribed eyedrops and oral medications must be taken on an uninterrupted basis. Patients in acute care and long-term care facilities are sometimes allowed to keep their glaucoma medications at their bedsides if they are able to administer the eyedrops and medications themselves. If they are not able to do so, it is imperative that treatment for glaucoma not be neglected while caregivers are focusing their attention on more immediate medical needs of patients.

Care of the patient after laser surgery is relatively simple compared with treatment after more traditional surgery. The patient may experience mild headache and blurred vision for the first 24 hours after surgery and there will be transient distortion of the pupil and a mild iritis. Topical steroids and a cycloplegic to prevent movement of the ciliary muscle may be prescribed. The patient should be told to report any sudden severe eye pain immediately and to keep all appointments for follow-up care.

An elevated intraocular pressure may persist for a week or longer postoperatively and so glaucoma medications are continued until the follow-up visit and perhaps longer if intraocular pressure remains high. (See Atlas 4, Part B).

congenital g., infantile g. a congenital type that may be fully developed at birth with enlarged eyes and hazy corneas, or may develop at any time up to two or three years of age.

juvenile g. congenital glaucoma differing from the infantile form in that it occurs in older children and young adults, and there is no gross enlargement of the eyeball.

g. sim′plex glaucoma without pronounced symptoms, but attended with progressive loss of vision.

gleet (glēt) 1. chronic gonorrheal urethritis. 2. a urethral discharge, especially one that is mucous or purulent.

glenoid (gle′noid) resembling a pit or socket.

glia (gli′ah) neuroglia; the supporting structure of nervous tissue, consisting, in the central nervous system, of astrocytes, oligodendrocytes, and microglia.

gliacyte (gli′ah-sīt) a cell of the glia or neuroglia.

gliadin (gli′ah-din) a protein in wheat that contains the toxic factor associated with celiac disease.

glial (gli′al) of or pertaining to glia or neuroglia.

gliclazide (glik′lah-zīd) a SULFONYLUREA compound used as a hypoglycemic AGENT in treatment of type 2 DIABETES MELLITUS.

glimepiride (gli-mep′ĭ-rīd) a SULFONYLUREA compound used as a HYPOGLYCEMIC in treatment of type 2 DIABETES MELLITUS; administered orally.

glioblastoma (gli″o-blas-to′mah) any malignant ASTROCYTOMA.

g. multifor′me ASTROCYTOMA grade III or IV; a rapidly growing tumor, usually of the cerebral hemispheres, composed of SPONGIOBLASTS, ASTROBLASTS, and ASTROCYTES.

glioma (gli-o′mah) a tumor composed of NEUROGLIA in any of its states of development; sometimes extended to include all intrinsic neoplasms of the brain and spinal cord, such as ASTROCYTOMAS, EPENDYMOMAS, and so on. Called also neuroglioma and neurospongioma. adj., **glio′matous.**

g. re′tinae retinoblastoma.

gliomatosis (gli″o-mah-to′sis) excessive development of the NEUROGLIA, especially of the spinal cord, in certain cases of SYRINGOMYELIA.

glioneuroma (gli″o-noo-ro′mah) GLIOMA combined with NEUROMA.

gliosarcoma (gli″o-sahr-ko′mah) GLIOMA combined with SARCOMA.

gliosis (gli-o′sis) an excess of ASTROGLIA in damaged areas of the central nervous system.

glipizide (glip′ĭ-zīd) a SULFONYLUREA used as a hypoglycemic in patients with type 2 DIABETES MELLITUS whose blood glucose cannot be controlled by diet and exercise alone; administered orally.

glissade (glĭ-sād′) [Fr.] a gliding involuntary movement of the eye in changing the point of fixation; it is a slower, smoother movement than is a saccade. adj., **glissad′ic.**

glissonitis (glis″o-ni′tis) inflammation of Glisson's capsule.

globi (glo'bi) [L.] 1. plural of GLOBUS. 2. encapsulated globular masses containing bacilli; seen in smears of lepromatous leprosy lesions.

globin (glo'bin) 1. the protein constituent of HEMOGLOBIN. 2. any of a group of proteins similar to the typical globin.

globoid (glo'boid) globe-shaped; spheroid.

globoside (glob'o-sīd) a sphingoglycolipid containing acetylated amino sugars and simple hexoses, occurring in human serum, spleen, liver, and erythrocytes, and accumulating in tissues in Sandhoff's disease.

globule (glob'ūl) a small spherical mass; a little globe or pellet, as of medicine. adj., **glob'ular.**

globulin (glob'u-lin) any of numerous proteins that are insoluble in water or highly concentrated salt solutions but soluble in moderately concentrated salt solutions. All plasma proteins except albumin and prealbumin are globulins. The plasma globulins are separated into five fractions by serum protein electrophoresis (SPE). In order of decreasing electrophoretic mobility these fractions are the alpha$_1$-, alpha$_2$-, beta$_1$-, and beta$_2$-globulins, and the gamma globulins.

The globulins include carrier proteins, which transport specific substances; acute phase reactants, which are involved in the inflammatory process; coagulation factors; complement components; and immunoglobulins. Examples are transferrin, a beta$_1$-globulin that transports iron, and alpha$_1$-antitrypsin, an acute phase reactant that inhibits serum proteases. The GAMMA GLOBULIN fraction is almost entirely composed of IMMUNOGLOBULINS.

accelerator g. factor V, one of the COAGULATION FACTORS.

antihemophilic g. (AHG) factor VIII, one of the COAGULATION FACTORS.

antilymphocyte g. (ALG) the gamma globulin fraction of antilymphocyte SERUM; used as an IMMUNOSUPPRESSANT in organ transplantation. The term is sometimes used interchangeably with *antithymocyte globulin.*

antithymocyte g. (ATG) the gamma globulin fraction of antiserum derived from animals (such as rabbits) that have been immunized against human thymocytes; an immunosuppressive agent that causes specific destruction of T lymphocytes, used in treatment of allograft REJECTION. The term is sometimes used interchangeably with *antilymphocyte globulin.*

bacterial polysaccharide immune g. (BPIG) a human immune GLOBULIN derived from the blood plasma of adult human donors immunized with *Haemophilus*

influenzae type b, pneumococcal, and meningococcal polysaccharide vaccines; used for passive immunization of infants under 18 months of age.

cytomegalovirus immune g. a purified immunoglobulin derived from pooled adult human plasma selected for high titers of antibody against CYTOMEGALOVIRUS; administered intravenously for treatment and prophylaxis of CYTOMEGALOVIRUS DISEASE in transplant recipients.

gamma g. 1. see GAMMA GLOBULIN. 2. immune globulin.

hepatitis B immune g. (HBIG) a specific immune GLOBULIN derived from plasma of human donors with high titers of antibodies against hepatitis B surface antigen (HBsAg); used for postexposure prophylaxis following contact with HBsAg-positive materials, also administered to infants of HBsAg-positive mothers.

hyperimmune g. any of various immune GLOBULIN preparations especially high in antibodies against certain specific diseases.

immune g. 1. immunoglobulin. 2. a concentrated preparation containing mostly GAMMA GLOBULINS, predominantly IgG, from a large pool of human donors; used for passive immunization against measles, hepatitis A, and varicella and for treatment of hypogammaglobulinemia or agammaglobulinemia in immunodeficient patients, administered intramuscularly. See also IMMUNE G. INTRAVENOUS (HUMAN).

immune g. intravenous (human) a preparation of immune GLOBULIN suitable for intravenous administration; used in the treatment of primary immunodeficiency disorders and idiopathic thrombocytopenic purpura, and as an adjunct in the treatment of Kawasaki disease and the prevention of infections associated with chronic lymphocytic leukemia, bone marrow transplantation, and pediatric human immunodeficiency virus infection.

immune human serum g. immune globulin (def. 2).

immune serum g. immune g. (def. 2).

pertussis immune g. a specific immune GLOBULIN derived from the blood plasma of human donors immunized with pertussis vaccine; used for the prophylaxis and treatment of PERTUSSIS.

rabies immune g. a specific immune GLOBULIN derived from plasma of human donors hyperimmunized with rabies VACCINE; administered in conjunction with rabies vaccine in cases of bite or scratch exposure to known or suspected rabid animals.

respiratory syncytial virus immune g. intravenous a preparation of IMMUNOGLOBU-LIN G from pooled adult human plasma selected for high titers of antibodies against respiratory syncytial VIRUS; used for passive immunization of infants and young children.

Rh₀(D) immune g. a specific immune GLOBULIN derived from human blood plasma containing antibody to the erythrocyte factor $Rh_0(D)$; used to prevent Rh-sensitization of Rh-negative females and thus prevent erythroblastosis fetalis in subsequent pregnancies; administered within 72 hours after exposure to Rh-positive blood resulting from delivery of an Rh-positive child, abortion or miscarriage of an Rh-positive fetus, or transfusion of Rh-positive blood. It is also used as a platelet count stimulator in the treatment of idiopathic thrombocytopenic PURPURA.

serum g's all plasma proteins except albumin, which is not a globulin, and fibrinogen, which is not in the serum. The serum globulins are subdivided into alpha-, beta-, and gamma-globulins on the basis of their relative electrophoretic mobilities.

specific immune g. a preparation of immune GLOBULIN derived from a donor pool preselected for high antibody titer against a specific antigen, such as hepatitis B immune GLOBULIN.

tetanus immune g. a specific immune GLOBULIN derived from the blood plasma of human donors who have been immunized with tetanus TOXOID; used in the prophylaxis and treatment of TETANUS.

thyronine-binding g. (TBG), thyroxine-binding g. an acidic glycoprotein that is the main binding PROTEIN in the blood for THY-ROXINE, and less firmly for TRIIODOTHYRONINE.

vaccinia immune g. a specific immune GLOBULIN derived from the blood plasma of human donors who have been immunized with vaccinia virus smallpox vaccine; used as a passive immunizing agent.

varicella-zoster immune g. (VZIG) a specific immune GLOBULIN derived from plasma of human donors with high titers of varicella-zoster antibodies; used for prevention or amelioration of VARICELLA in immunocompromised patients exposed to the disease and in neonates whose mothers develop varicella in the perinatal period.

globulinuria (glob″u-lin-u′re-ah) PROTEIN-URIA in which GLOBULIN is excreted in the urine.

globus (glo′bus), pl. *glo′bi* [L.] 1. sphere. 2. a spherical structure. 3. eyeball.

g. hyste′ricus the subjective sensation of a lump in the throat.

g. pal′lidus the smaller and more medial part of the lentiform nucleus of the brain; it is divided into two parts, lateral and medial, by the medial medullary lamina.

glomangioma (glo-man″je-o′mah) glomus tumor.

glomectomy (glo-mek′to-me) excision of a glomus.

glomera (glom′er-ah) [L.] plural of GLOMUS.

glomerular (glo-mer′u-lar) pertaining to or of the nature of a glomerulus, especially a renal glomerulus.

glomeruli (glo-mer′u-li) [L.] plural of GLOMERULUS.

glomerulitis (glo-mer″u-li′tis) inflammation of the glomeruli of the kidney.

glomerulonephritis (glo-mer″u-lo-nĕ-fri′-tis) a variety of NEPHRITIS characterized by inflammation of the capillary loops in the glomeruli of the kidney. It occurs in acute, subacute, and chronic forms and may be secondary to an infection, especially with the hemolytic streptococcus.

diffuse g. a severe form of glomerulonephritis with proliferative changes in more than half the glomeruli, frequently with epithelial crescent formation and necrosis; it is often seen in cases of advanced systemic lupus erythematosus.

IgA g. IgA nephropathy.

lobular g., membranoproliferative g. a chronic glomerulonephritis characterized by mesangial cell proliferation and irregular thickening of the glomerular capillary wall. There are two subtypes: *Type I* is marked by subendothelial deposits and activation of the classic COMPLEMENT pathway. *Type II* is marked by heavy deposits in the glomerular basement membrane and activation of the alternative COMPLEMENT pathway. Both types occur in older children and young adults and follow a slowly progressing course with irregular remissions ultimately resulting in RENAL FAILURE.

membranous g. a form characterized by proteinaceous deposits on the glomerular capillary basement MEMBRANE or by thickening of the membrane, with circulating antigen-antibody COMPLEXES indicating immune complex disease; it may be secondary to any of numerous other conditions. In some cases it may develop into the nephrotic syndrome. Called also membranous nephropathy.

mesangiocapillary g. membranoproliferative glomerulonephritis.

rapidly progressive g. acute glomerulonephritis marked by a rapid progression to END-STAGE RENAL DISEASE and histologically by profuse epithelial proliferation, often with epithelial crescents; principal signs are

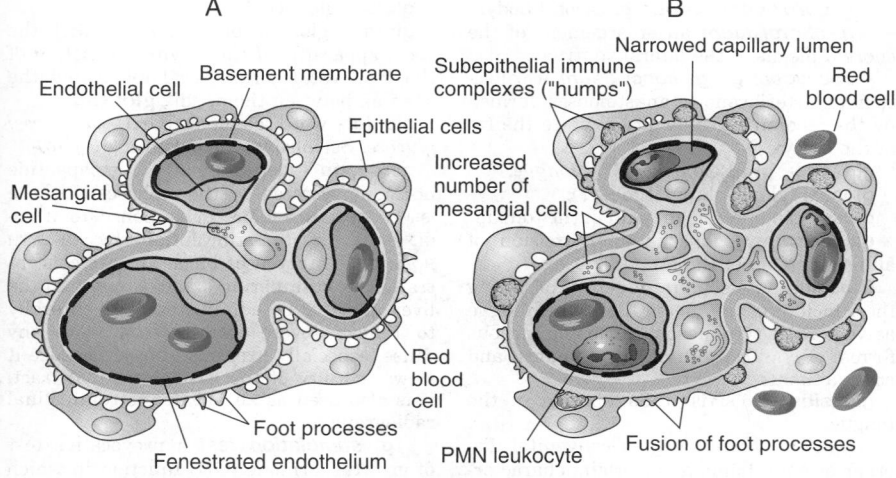

A

Endothelial cell
Basement membrane
Epithelial cells
Mesangial cell
Red blood cell
Foot processes
Fenestrated endothelium

B

Narrowed capillary lumen
Subepithelial immune complexes ("humps")
Red blood cell
Increased number of mesangial cells
PMN leukocyte
Fusion of foot processes

Histologic appearance of acute glomerulonephritis. *A*, Normal glomerulus. *B*, Glomerulonephritis. The glomerulus appears hypercellular and the capillaries are narrowed or occluded. From Damjanov, 2000.

anuria, proteinuria, hematuria, and anemia. Plasmapheresis or high doses of corticosteroids may lead to recovery of renal function.

glomerulonephropathy (glo-mer″u-lo-nĕ-frop′ah-the) any noninflammatory disease of the renal glomeruli.

glomerulopathy (glo-mer″u-lop′ah-the) any disease, especially any noninflammatory disease, of the renal glomeruli.

   diabetic g. intercapillary glomerulosclerosis.

glomerulosclerosis (glo-mer″u-lo-sklĕ-ro′sis) arteriolar nephrosclerosis.

   diabetic g., intercapillary g. a degenerative complication of DIABETES MELLITUS in which there is glomerular mesangial expansion with either diffuse lesions or nodular (Kimmelstiel-Wilson) LESIONS; symptoms include albuminuria, nephrotic edema, hypertension, renal insufficiency, and retinopathy. The type with nodular lesions is also called Kimmelstiel-Wilson syndrome.

   focal segmental g. focal sclerosing lesions of the renal glomeruli, with proteinuria, hematuria, hypertension, and the NEPHROTIC SYNDROME; it may be idiopathic or secondary to another condition. Called also focal glomerular sclerosis.

glomerulus (glo-mer′u-lus), pl. *glomer′uli* [L.] 1. a small tuft or cluster, such as a small convoluted mass of capillaries. 2. a network of vascular tufts encased in the malpighian capsule of the kidney. adj., **glomer′ular.**

The glomerulus is an integral part of the NEPHRON, the basic unit of the KIDNEY. Each nephron is capable of forming urine by itself, and each kidney has approximately a million nephrons. The specific function of each glomerulus is to bring blood (and the waste products it carries) to the nephron. As the blood flows through the glomerulus, about one fifth of the plasma passes through the glomerular membrane, collects in the malpighian capsule, and then flows through the renal tubules. Much of this fluid passes back into the blood via the small capillaries around the tubules (peritubular capillaries). The continuous filtration of fluid from the glomeruli and its reabsorption into the peritubular capillaries are made possible by a high pressure in the glomerular capillary bed and a low pressure in the peritubular bed.

Any disease of the glomerulus, such as acute or chronic glomerulonephritis, must be considered serious because it interferes with the basic functions of the kidneys, that is, filtration of liquids and excretion of certain end products of metabolism and excess sodium, potassium, and chloride ions that may accumulate in the blood.

glomoid (glo′moid) resembling a glomus.

glomus (glo′mus), pl. *glom′era* [L.] a small histologically recognizable body composed primarily of fine arterioles connecting directly with veins, and having a rich nerve supply.

   aortic g., g. aor′ticum aortic body.

g. caro'ticum, carotid g. carotid body.

g. choroi'deum an enlargement of the choroid plexus of the lateral ventricle.

coccygeal g., g. coccy'geum a collection of arteriovenous anastomoses formed by the median sacral artery close to the tip of the coccyx.

gloss(o)- word element [Gr.], *tongue.*

glossal (glos'al) lingual (def. 1).

glossalgia (glŏ-sal'jah) pain in the tongue.

glossectomy (glŏ-sek'to-me) excision of all or a portion of the tongue.

Glossina (glŏ-si'nah) a genus of biting flies, including the tsetse flies, which serve as vectors of trypanosomes causing various forms of TRYPANOSOMIASIS in humans and other animals.

glossitis (glŏ-si'tis) inflammation of the tongue.

median rhomboid g. a congenital disorder of noninflammatory origin, characterized by a somewhat rhomboid reddish, smooth, and shiny lesion with some opalescent spots, occurring at about the middle third of the dorsal surface of the tongue.

glossocele (glos'o-sēl) swelling and protrusion of the tongue.

glossodynia (glos"o-din'e-ah) pain in the tongue.

glossograph (glos'o-graf) an apparatus for registering tongue movements in speech.

glossolalia (glos"o-la'le-ah) gibberish that simulates coherent speech.

glossology (glŏ-sol'o-je) the sum of knowledge regarding the tongue.

glossopathy (glŏ-sop'ah-the) any disease of the tongue.

glossopharyngeal (glos"o-fah-rin'je-al) pertaining to the tongue and pharynx.

g. nerve the ninth CRANIAL NERVE; it supplies the carotid sinus, mucous membrane, and muscles of the pharynx, soft palate, and posterior third of the tongue, and the taste buds in the posterior third of the tongue. By serving the carotid sinus, the glossopharyngeal nerve provides for reflex control of the heart. It is also responsible for the swallowing reflex, for stimulating secretions of the parotid glands, and for the sense of taste in the posterior third of the tongue. See also anatomic Table of Nerves in the Appendices.

glossoplasty (glos'o-plas"te) plastic surgery of the tongue.

glossorrhaphy (glŏ-sōr'ah-fe) suture of the tongue.

glossospasm (glos'o-spazm) spasm of the tongue.

glossotomy (glŏ-sot'ah-me) incision of the tongue.

glossotrichia (glos"o-trik'e-ah) hairy tongue.

glottic (glot'ik) glottal.

glottis (glot'is), pl. *glot'tides* [Gr.] the vocal apparatus of the larynx, consisting of the true vocal cords (vocal folds) and the opening between them. adj., **glot'tal.**

gluc(o)- word element [Gr.], *sweetness; glucose.* See also words beginning *glyc(o)-.*

glucagon (gloo'kah-gon) a polypeptide hormone secreted by the alpha cells of the ISLETS OF LANGERHANS in response to HYPOGLYCEMIA or to stimulation by GROWTH HORMONE. It increases blood glucose concentration by stimulating GLYCOGENOLYSIS in the liver and can be administered parenterally to relieve severe HYPOGLYCEMIA from any cause, especially HYPERINSULINISM. Because it slows motility of the gastrointestinal tract, it is also used as an aid in gastrointestinal radiography.

g. stimulation test a provocative test of growth hormone (GH) function in which the fasting serum level of GH is measured after administration of glucagon.

glucagonoma (gloo"kah-gon-o'mah) a glucagon-secreting tumor of the alpha cells of the islets of Langerhans.

gluceptate (gloo-sep'tāt) USAN contraction for glucoheptonate.

glucocerebroside (gloo"ko-ser'ĕ-bro-sīd) a CEREBROSIDE containing a glucose sugar; it accumulates in the tissues in Gaucher's disease.

glucocorticoid (gloo"ko-kor'tĭ-koid) any corticoid substance that increases GLUCONEOGENESIS, raising the concentration of liver GLYCOGEN and blood GLUCOSE; the group includes CORTISOL, CORTISONE, and CORTICOSTERONE. The release of glucocorticoids from the adrenal cortex is initially triggered by corticotropin-releasing HORMONE (CRH) elaborated by the hypothalamus. The target organ for this factor is the anterior lobe of the pituitary gland, which reacts to the presence of CRH by releasing CORTICOTROPIN (ACTH). ACTH, in turn, stimulates the release of the glucocorticoids from the adrenal cortex. (See also ADRENAL GLAND.)

The principal glucocorticoid hormone is CORTISOL, which regulates the metabolism of proteins, carbohydrates, and lipids. Specifically, it increases the catabolism or breakdown of protein in bone, skin, muscle, and connective tissue. Cortisol also diminishes cellular utilization of glucose and increases the output of glucose from the liver.

Because of their effects on glucose levels and fat metabolism, all the glucocorticoids are referred to as anti-insulin diabetogenic hormones. They increase the blood sugar level, raise the concentration of plasma lipids, and, when insulin secretion is insufficient, promote formation of KETONE BODIES, thus contributing to KETOACIDOSIS.

Other physiologic processes within the body can occur only in the presence of or with the "permission of" the glucocorticoids. For example, the secretion of digestive enzymes by gastric cells and the normal excitability of myocardial and central nervous system neurons require a certain level of glucocorticoids.

Glucocorticoids also promote transport of amino acids into the extracellular compartment, making them more readily available for the production of energy. In times of stress the glucocorticoids influence the effectiveness of the CATECHOLAMINES DOPAMINE, EPINEPHRINE, and NOREPINEPHRINE. For example, the presence of cortisol is essential to norepinephrine-induced vasoconstriction and other physiologic phenomena necessary for survival under stress. This particular property of cortisol demonstrates the one identifiable relationship between hormones from the adrenal cortex and those from the adrenal medulla. One of the medullary hormones is NOREPINEPHRINE, which is secreted in large quantities when the gland is stimulated by the sympathetic nervous system in response to stress.

Another effect of cortisol is that of dampening the body's inflammatory RESPONSE to invasion by foreign agents. When present in large amounts, cortisol inhibits the release of HISTAMINE and counteracts potentially destructive reactions, such as increased capillary permeability and the migration of leukocytes. Since the IMMUNE RESPONSE can damage body cells as well as those of foreign agents, the antiinflammatory protective mechanisms of cortisol help preserve the integrity of body cells at the site of the inflammatory response.

glucofuranose (gloo″ko-fu′rah-nōs) a form of glucose in which carbon atoms 1 and 4 are bridged by an oxygen atom.

glucogenic (gloo″ko-jen′ik) giving rise to or producing sugar.

glucokinase (gloo″ko-ki′nās) an enzyme that in the presence of ATP catalyzes glucose to glucose-6-phosphate.

glucokinetic (gloo″ko-ki-net′ik) activating sugar so as to maintain the sugar level of the body.

gluconeogenesis (gloo″ko-ne″o-jen′ĕ-sis) the synthesis of glucose from noncarbohydrate sources, such as amino acids and glycerol. It occurs primarily in the liver and kidneys whenever the supply of carbohydrates is insufficient to meet the body's

energy needs. Gluconeogenesis is stimulated by cortisol and other GLUCOCORTICOIDS and by the thyroid hormone thyroxine. Formerly called glyconeogenesis.

glucophore (gloo′ko-fōr) the group of atoms in a molecule that gives the compound a sweet taste.

glucopyranose (gloo″ko-pir′ah-nōs) a form of glucose in which carbon atoms 1 and 5 are bridged by an oxygen atom.

glucosamine (gloo-ko′-sah-mēn) an amino derivative of glucose occurring in many glycoproteins and mucopolysaccharides.

glucose (gloo′kōs) 1. D-glucose, $C_6H_{12}O_6$, a MONOSACCHARIDE of the ALDOSE group, found in certain foodstuffs, especially fruit, and in normal blood; it is the chief source of energy for living organisms. In pharmaceuticals, called dextrose. 2. liquid glucose.

Glucose is the end product of carbohydrate digestion; soon after digestion other monosaccharides (FRUCTOSE and GALACTOSE) are converted into glucose. Because of this conversion, glucose is the only monosaccharide present in significant amounts in the body fluids. The metabolism of glucose produces energy for the body cells; the rate of metabolism is controlled by insulin. Glucose that is not needed for energy is stored in the form of glycogen as a source of potential energy, readily available when needed. Most of the glycogen is stored in the liver and muscle cells. When these and other body cells are saturated with glycogen, the excess glucose is converted into fat and stored as adipose tissue.

The normal fasting level for glucose in the blood is between 70 and 90 mg per 100 dl. Unusually high levels of glucose in the blood (HYPERGLYCEMIA) may indicate such diseases as DIABETES MELLITUS, HYPERTHYROIDISM, or hyperpituitarism. Levels of blood sugar below 40 mg per 100 dl (HYPOGLYCEMIA) may be caused by diseases of the kidneys or liver, hypopituitarism, and hyperinsulinism, an uncommon condition in which too much insulin is produced. A GLUCOSE TOLERANCE TEST is done to assess the ability of the body to metabolize glucose.

fasting plasma g. **(FPG)** a measurement of the concentration of glucose in the plasma after the patient has not eaten for at least 8 hours.

liquid g. a thick, sweet, syrupy liquid obtained by incomplete hydrolysis of starch and consisting chiefly of dextrose, with dextrins, maltose, and water; used as a pharmaceutic aid. Sometimes simply called glucose. It is not interchangeable with DEXTROSE for intravenous injection.

G

g.-1-phosphate an intermediate in carbohydrate metabolism.

g.-6-phosphate an intermediate in carbohydrate metabolism.

g. tolerance test a test of the body's ability to use glucose; it is often done to detect abnormalities of carbohydrate metabolism such as occur in DIABETES MELLITUS, HYPOGLYCEMIA, and liver and adrenocortical dysfunction.

In the standard *oral glucose tolerance test,* the patient is given a single dose of glucose in a fasting stomach and blood and urine specimens are collected periodically for up to 6 hours. A blood sample is taken for measurement of fasting glucose before the test dose is given. Then glucose is given; it may be dissolved in water and flavored with lemon juice, or as a commercial preparation such as a carbonated drink or gelatin; the latter are more palatable and provide a precise amount of glucose. One half hour after the glucose is ingested a blood sample and urine specimen are obtained. The specimens are collected at hourly intervals for the next 4 or 5 hours as indicated. Each specimen must be labeled with the exact time it was collected. The patient may be allowed to drink water during the testing period but may not drink anything else or eat or smoke until the test is completed. The patient is usually fed a high-carbohydrate diet for 3 days before the test.

glucosidase (gloo-ko'sĭ-dās) an enzyme of the hydrolase class that splits glucoside, occurring as α-, β-, and α-1,3-glucosidase; α-glucosidase (maltase) occurs in intestinal juice, and β-glucosidase (cellobiase) in the kidney, liver, and intestinal mucosa.

α-glucosidase (gloo-ko'sĭ-dās) any of a group of enzymes that catalyze the hydrolysis of certain α-D-glucose residues from oligosaccharides and polysaccharides and yield free α-D-glucose. Called also maltase.

β-glucosidase (gloo-ko'sĭ-dās) any of a group of enzymes that catalyze the hydrolysis of terminal, nonreducing, β-linked glucose residues from glycosides.

glucosuria (gloo″ko-su're-ah) glycosuria.

glucuronate (gloo-ku'ro-nāt) a salt, ester, or anionic form of glucuronic acid.

glucuronic acid (gloo″ku-ron'ik) a uronic acid formed by oxidation of C-6 of glucose to a carboxy group; it occurs in PROTEOGLYCANS (mucopolysaccharides), and is important in the conjugation of XENOBIOTICS; it is conjugated to many poisons and drugs by the liver, forming GLUCURONIDES, which markedly decreases their toxicity and enhances their excretion by the liver, intestine, and kidney.

β-glucuronidase (gloo″ku-ron'ĭ-dās) an enzyme that attacks glycosidic linkages in natural and synthetic glucuronides and has been implicated in estrogen metabolism and cell division; occurs in the spleen, liver, and endocrine glands.

glucuronide (gloo-ku'ron-īd) any glycosidic compound of glucuronic acid; glucuronides, which are generally inactive, constitute the major proportion of the metabolites of many phenols, alcohols, and carboxylic acids.

glutamate (gloo'tah-māt) a salt of glutamic acid; in biochemistry, the term is often used interchangeably with glutamic acid.

glutamic acid (gloo-tam'ik) a dibasic AMINO ACID, one of the nonessential amino acids; it is also an inhibitory neurotransmitter in the central nervous system. Its hydrochloride salt is used as a gastric acidifier. See also MONOSODIUM GLUTAMATE.

glutamic-oxaloacetic transaminase (GOT) (gloo-tam'ik oks″ah-lo-ah-se'tik trans-am'ĭ-nās) aspartate transaminase.

glutamic-pyruvic transaminase (GPT) (gloo-tam'ik pi-roo'vik trans-am'ĭ-nās) alanine transaminase.

glutaminase (gloo-tam'ĭ-nās) an enzyme that catalyzes the splitting of glutamine into glutamic acid and ammonia.

glutamine (gloo'tah-min) an amide of GLUTAMIC ACID, one of the nonessential AMINO ACIDS; it is an important carrier of urinary ammonia and is broken down in the kidney by the enzyme GLUTAMINASE.

glutaral (gloo'tah-ral) glutaraldehyde.

glutaraldehyde (gloo″tah-ral'dĕ-hīd) a disinfectant used in aqueous solution for sterilization of heat-sensitive equipment and instruments; it is a broad-spectrum microbicide effective against all vegetative bacteria, fungi, and viruses, is sporicidal, and may be used as a liquid sterilant with an extended exposure time. It is also used as a tissue fixative for light and electron microscopy.

glutathione (gloo″tah-thi'ōn) a tripeptide of glutamic acid, cysteine, and glycine; the reduced form (GSH) serves as a reducing agent in many biochemical reactions, being converted to oxidized glutathione (GSSG) in which the cysteine residues of two glutathione molecules are connected by a disulfide bridge. Reduced glutathione is important in protecting erythrocytes from oxidation and hemolysis; deficiency causes sensitivity to oxidant drugs.

glutathionuria (gloo″tah-thi″o-nu're-ah) the excretion of excessive amounts of GLUTATHIONE in the urine, sometimes due to a hereditary enzyme deficiency that can cause mental retardation.

gluteal (gloo′te-al) pertaining to the buttocks; called also natal and pygal.

gluten (gloo′ten) the protein derivative of wheat and other grains that gives dough its tough elastic character; avoidance of this substance will alleviate CELIAC DISEASE (nontropical sprue) in certain persons, as well as immunologic disturbances in which there is an allergy to gliadin, a component of gluten.

   g.-free diet a diet in which wheat must be avoided, as well as other grains such as barley, oats, and rye that contain analogues to wheat gluten. Exceptions to this essentially grain-free diet are corn, rice, and millet. Wheat starch, which has been washed free of GLIADIN, is not restricted nor are there restrictions on carbohydrates or fats.

   Patient Care. Following a gluten-free diet can relieve the problems associated with gluten allergy but preparing and enjoying gluten-free meals demands constant vigilance and motivation. Patients and family members who purchase and prepare patients' foods should read the labels on processed foods very carefully. Many contain hidden and unexpected wheat flour, for example, tomato catsup and ice cream. Processors also mix unacceptable and acceptable gluten-free soybeans and grains together in the same product. If there are any questions about the contents of a product, manufacturers will provide lists of their foods that are permissible on a gluten-free diet.

   Foods to be avoided are listed in the accompanying table, as well as possible sources of hidden gluten. Additional information and recipes for baking with nongluten flours can be obtained from a dietitian or from publications found in most large bookstores.

glutethimide (gloo-teth′ĭ-mīd) a nonbarbiturate SEDATIVE and HYPNOTIC.

glutinous (gloo′tĭ-nus) adhesive; sticky.

glutitis (gloo-ti′tis) inflammation of the gluteal muscles.

glyburide (gli′būr-īd) a SULFONYLUREA compound used as a HYPOGLYCEMIC in treatment of type 2 DIABETES MELLITUS; administered orally.

glyc(o)- word element [Gr.], *sweetness; glucose.* See also words beginning *gluc(o)-.*

glycan (gli′kan) polysaccharide.

glycemia (gli-se′me-ah) the presence of glucose in the blood.

glyceraldehyde (glis″er-al′dĕ-hīd) a compound, glyceric aldehyde, formed by the oxidation of glycerol.

glyceride (glis′er-īd) an organic acid ester of glycerin, designated, according to the number of ester linkages, as a mono-, di-, or triglyceride.

glycerin (glis′er-in) a clear, colorless, syrupy liquid, used as an osmotic DIURETIC to reduce intraocular pressure, a LAXATIVE, a soothing agent in cough preparations, and as a moistening agent and solvent for drugs; it is a trihydric sugar alcohol, being the alcoholic component of fats. See also GLYCEROL.

glycerol (glis′er-ol) a trihydric sugar alcohol, $CH_2OH \cdot CHOH \cdot CH_2OH$, which is a component of fats. It is an intermediate in the metabolism of fatty acids and serves as a phosphate acceptor. Pharmaceutical preparations are called glycerin.

glycerolize (glis′er-o-līz) to treat with or preserve in glycerol, as in the exposure of red blood cells to glycerol solution so that glycerol diffuses into the cells before they are frozen for preservation.

glycerose (glis′er-ōs) a sugar formed by oxidizing glycerin; there are two glyceroses, glyceraldehyde and dihydroxyacetone.

glyceryl (glis′er-il) the mono-, di-, or trivalent radical formed by the removal of

G

GLUTEN-FREE DIET	
Foods to be Avoided	**Hidden Sources**
Modified food starch	Meat and vegetable sauces
Hydrolyzed vegetable protein	Dressings
Emulsifiers (e.g., lecithin) or binders	Gravies
Flour (it is wheat unless otherwise stated)	Bread crumbs in cooked dishes
Buckwheat	Batters for fried meat and fish
Monosodium glutamate	Malt flavoring, as in some corn flakes
Starch (unless it is corn or potato starch)	and other cereals
Instant coffee, except Nescafé	
Malt	
Beer, rye, gin, Scotch, and bourbon whiskey	
Commercial chocolate milk	

hydrogen from one, two, or three of the hydroxy groups of glycerol.

g. triacetate triacetin.

g. trinitrate nitroglycerin.

glycine (gli′sēn) a nonessential AMINO ACID that functions as an inhibitory neurotransmitter in the central nervous system; used as a gastric antacid and dietary supplement, and as a bladder irrigation in transurethral prostatectomy. Called also aminoacetic acid.

glycinemia hyperglycinemia.

glycocalyx (gli″ko-kal′iks) the glycoprotein-polysaccharide covering that surrounds many cells.

glycocholate (gli″ko-ko′lāt) a salt of glycocholic acid.

glycocholic acid (gli″ko-ko′lik) cholylglycine.

glycogen (gli′ko-jen) a polysaccharide that is the chief carbohydrate storage material in animals, being converted to GLUCOSE by DEPOLYMERIZATION; it is formed by and largely stored in the liver, and to a lesser extent in muscles, and is liberated as needed.

g. disease glycogen storage disease.

g. storage disease any of a group of genetically determined disorders of glycogen metabolism, marked by abnormal storage of glycogen in the body tissues. *Type I* is called GIERKE'S DISEASE; *type II* is called POMPE'S DISEASE; *type III* is called FORBES' DISEASE; *type IV* is called AMYLOPECTINOSIS; *type V* is called MCARDLE DISEASE; and *type VI* is called HERS' DISEASE. In *type VII,* a deficiency in PHOSPHO-FRUCTOKINASE affects muscle and erythrocytes, with temporary weakness and cramping of skeletal muscle after exercise. In *type VIII,* the enzyme deficiency is unknown, but the liver and brain are affected, with hepatomegaly, truncal ataxia, and nystagmus; the neurologic deterioration progresses to hypertonia, spasticity, and death. In *type IX,* a deficiency in liver phosphorylase kinase results in marked hepatomegaly, which may disappear in early adulthood. In *type X,* a lack of activity of cyclic AMP–dependent kinase affects the liver and muscle, with mild clinical symptoms. Called also glycogen disease and glycogenosis.

glycogenase (gli′ko-jĕ-nās) an enzyme that splits glycogen into dextrin and maltose.

glycogenesis (gli″ko-jen′ĕ-sis) the conversion of glucose to glycogen for storage in the liver. adj., **glycogenet′ic.**

glycogenic (gli″ko-jen′ik) pertaining to, characterized by, or promoting glycogenesis; pertaining to glycogen.

glycogenolysis (gli″ko-jĕ-nol′ĭ-sis) the splitting up of glycogen in the liver, yielding glucose.

glycogenosis (gli″ko-jĕ-no′sis) glycogen storage disease.

generalized g. Pompe's disease.

hepatorenal g. Gierke's disease.

myophosphorylase deficiency g. McArdle disease.

glycogeusia (gli″ko-gu′se-ah) a sweet taste in the mouth.

glycohemoglobin (gli″ko-he″mo-glo′bin) glycosylated hemoglobin. (See HEMOGLOBIN A_{1C}.)

glycolipid (gli″ko-lip′id) a lipid containing carbohydrate groups, usually galactose but also glucose, inositol, or others; the glycolipids include the cerebrosides.

glycolysis (gli-kol′ĭ-sis) the anaerobic enzymatic conversion of glucose to lactate or pyruvate, resulting in energy stored in the form of ATP, as occurs in muscle. adj., **glycolyt′ic.**

glyconeogenesis (gli″ko-ne″o-jen′ĕ-sis) gluconeogenesis.

glyconucleoprotein (gli″ko-noo″kle-o-pro′tēn) nucleoprotein bearing carbohydrate groups.

glycopenia (gli″ko-pe′ne-ah) a deficiency of sugar in the tissues.

glycopeptide (gli″ko-pep′tīd) any of a class of peptides that contain carbohydrates, including those that contain amino sugars.

glycopexis (gli″ko-pek′sis) fixation or storing of sugar or glycogen. adj., **glycopec′tic.**

glycophilia (gli″ko-fil′e-ah) a condition in which a small amount of glucose produces hyperglycemia.

glycophorin (gli″ko-for′in) any of several related proteins that can project through the thickness of the cell membrane of erythrocytes; they attach to oligosaccharides at the outer cell membrane surface and to contractile proteins (spectrin and actin) at the cytoplasmic surface.

glycoprotein (gli″ko-pro′tēn) any of a class of conjugated proteins consisting of a compound of protein with a carbohydrate group.

α1-acid g. an acute phase PROTEIN found in blood plasma, an indicator of tissue necrosis and inflammation. Called also orosomucoid.

P-g. a cell-surface protein occurring normally in the colon, small intestine, adrenal glands, kidney, and liver, and also expressed by tumor cells. It is a modulator of multidrug RESISTANCE, mediating the transport of antineoplastic AGENTS out of tumor cells.

variable surface g. any of several glycoproteins that form the antigenic protein coating of *Trypanosoma brucei.* The organisms contain numerous genes encoding hundreds of such glycoproteins and, by expressing individual ones successively, evade the IMMUNE SYSTEM of the host.

glycoptyalism (gli″ko-ti′ah-lizm) glycosialia.

glycopyrrolate (gli″ko-pir′o-lāt) a synthetic ANTICHOLINERGIC used as an antispasmodic to help treat peptic ulcer and other gastrointestinal disorders, a preanesthetic antisialagogue to decrease salivation and respiratory secretions associated with anesthesia, and an antiarrhythmic to counteract arrhythmias associated with induction of anesthesia or surgery; administered orally, intramuscularly, or intravenously.

glycorrachia (gli″ko-ra′ke-ah) the presence of sugar in the cerebrospinal fluid.

glycorrhea (gli″ko-re′ah) any sugary discharge from the body.

glycosamine (gli-ko′sah-mēn) an amino sugar.

glycosaminoglycan (gli″kōs-ah-me″no-gli′kan) any of the carbohydrates containing amino sugars occurring in proteoglycans, e.g., hyaluronic acid or chondroitin sulfate.

glycosaminolipid (gli″kōs-ah-me″no-lip′-id) any of a class of lipids that contain amino sugars.

glycosecretory (gli″ko-se-kre′to-re) concerned in secretion of glycogen.

glycosialia (gli″ko-si-a′le-ah) glucose in the saliva; called also glycoptyalism.

glycosialorrhea (gli″ko-si″ah-lo-re′ah) excessive flow of saliva containing sugar.

glycosidase (gli-ko′sī-dās) any of a large group of hydrolytic enzymes acting on glycosyl compounds.

glycoside (gli″ko-sīd) any compound containing a carbohydrate molecule (sugar), particularly any such natural product in plants, convertible, by hydrolytic cleavage, into a sugar and a nonsugar component (aglycone), and named specifically for the sugar contained, such as fructoside (fructose), glucoside (glucose), or pentoside (pentose).

cardiac g. any of a group of glycosides occurring in certain plants (*Digitalis,* etc.), having a characteristic action on the contractile force of the heart muscle.

glycosphingolipid (gli″ko-sfing″o-lip′id) a fatty acid containing the carbohydrate sugar glucose or galactose.

glycostatic (gli″ko-stat′ik) tending to maintain a constant sugar level.

glycosuria (gli″ko-su′re-ah) the presence of GLUCOSE in the urine; called also dextrosuria and glucosuria.

renal g. glycosuria due to inability of the renal tubules to reabsorb glucose completely.

glycosyl (gli′ko-sil) a radical derived from a carbohydrate.

glycosylated hemoglobin test (gli-ko′sī-lāt″ed) measurement of the percentage of HEMOGLOBIN A molecules that have formed a stable ketoamine linkage between the hemoglobin and glucose; this can be used to assess the control of blood glucose levels. In persons with a normal blood glucose level it amounts to about 7 per cent of the total; in those with DIABETES MELLITUS it is about 14.5 per cent. The higher the blood glucose levels have been over the previous three months, the higher the glycosylated hemoglobin will be.

glycosylation (gli-ko″-sī-la′shun) the formation of linkages with glycosyl groups.

glycotropic (gli″ko-trop′ik) having an affinity for or attracting sugar; antagonizing the effects of insulin, causing hyperglycemia.

glycyrrhiza (glis″ĭ-ri′zah) licorice.

gm gram.

GMP guanosine monophosphate.

3′,5′-GMP, cyclic GMP cyclic guanosine monophosphate.

gnath(o)- word element [Gr.], *jaw.*

gnathic (nath′ik) pertaining to the jaw or cheeks.

gnathion (nath′e-on) the most outward and everted point on the profile curvature of the chin.

gnathitis (nath-i′tis) inflammation of the jaw.

gnathocephalus (nath″o-sef′ah-lus) a malformed fetus in which the head consists primarily of the jaws.

gnathodynamometer (nath″o-di″nah-mom′ĕ-ter) an instrument for measuring the force exerted in closing the jaws.

gnathology (nah-thol′o-je) the science dealing with the masticatory apparatus as a whole. adj., **gnatholog′ic.**

gnathoplasty (nath′o-plas″te) plastic repair of the jaw or cheek.

gnathoschisis (nah-thos′kĭ-sis) cleft JAW.

gnathostat (nath′o-stat) a jaw-positioning device used in dental radiology, facial photography, cephalometry, and other procedures requiring exact positioning of the jaws.

gnathostomiasis (nath″o-sto-mi′ah-sis) infection with the nematode *Gnathostoma spinigerum,* acquired from eating undercooked fish infected with the larvae.

gnosia (no′se-ah) the faculty of perceiving and recognizing. adj., **gnos′tic.**

gnotobiotics (no″to-bi-ot′iks) 1. the science of maintaining a microbiologically

G

controlled environment. 2. the science of raising laboratory animals whose microflora and microfauna are specifically known in their entirety.

Gn-RH gonadotropin-releasing hormone.

goals (gōlz) measurable milestones that are established to indicate the success of a plan.

   long term g. goals that are the ultimate results desired when a plan is established or revised.

   short term g. goals that can be achieved in a limited period of time and frequently lead to the achievement of a long term goal.

goiter (goi'ter) enlargement of the THYROID GLAND, causing a swelling in the front part of the neck; called also struma. adj., **goit'rous.**

   If there is evidence of pressure against the throat, or the possibility of a malignancy, the goiter may be removed surgically. Simple endemic goiter is usually caused by lack of iodine in the diet. In GRAVES' DISEASE, goiter is accompanied by excessive thyroid hormones in the blood and symptoms of hyperthyroidism.

   aberrant g. goiter of a supernumerary thyroid gland.

   adenomatous g. that caused by adenoma or multiple colloid nodules of the thyroid gland.

   Basedow g. a colloid GOITER that has become hyperfunctioning after administration of iodine.

   colloid g. one that is large and soft and has distended spaces filled with COLLOID.

   cystic g. one with cysts formed by mucoid or colloid degeneration.

   diffuse toxic g. exophthalmic goiter.

   endemic g. goiter occurring widely in a geographic region where the food or water is deficient in iodine. Treatment consists of iodine replacement; although this will not cure the condition, it can stop it from enlarging, and iodine administered in advance will prevent development of goiter.

   exophthalmic g. any type accompanied by EXOPHTHALMOS.

   fibrous g. goiter in which the thyroid capsule and stroma are hyperplastic.

   follicular g. parenchymatous goiter.

   intrathoracic g. one with part of the enlarged gland in the thoracic cavity.

   iodide g. that occurring in reaction to iodides at high concentrations, due to inhibition of iodide organification.

   multinodular g. one with circumscribed nodules within the gland.

   nontoxic g. that occurring sporadically and not associated with hyperthyroidism or hypothyroidism.

   parenchymatous g. one with increase in follicles and proliferation of epithelium.

   perivascular g. one that surrounds a large blood vessel.

   retrovascular g. one with processes behind a large blood vessel.

   substernal g. one whose lower part lies beneath the sternum.

   suffocative g. one that causes dyspnea due to pressure.

   toxic multinodular g. hyperthyroidism arising in a multinodular GOITER, usually of long standing.

   vascular g. one due chiefly to dilatation of the blood vessels of the thyroid gland.

goitrogen (goi'tro-jen) a goiter-producing agent.

goitrogenic (goi-tro-jen'ik) producing goiter.

goitrogenicity (goi″tro-jĕ-nis'ĭ-te) the tendency to produce goiter.

gold (Au) (gōld) chemical element, atomic number 79, atomic weight 196.967. (See Appendix 6.) Gold and many of its compounds are used in medicine, especially in treating rheumatoid arthritis. Gold salts are among the most toxic of therapeutic agents and must be given only under strict medical supervision. Toxic reactions may vary from mild to severe kidney or liver damage and blood dyscrasias.

   g. 198 a radioisotope of gold having a half-life of 2.7 days, used as either a solid (seed) or a colloidal solution. It has been used for intracavitary or interstitial RADIATION THERAPY and has also been used, in colloidal form, as a SCINTISCANNING agent. Symbol ^{198}Au.

   g. sodium thiomalate a gold preparation used as a disease-modifying antirheumatic DRUG in treatment of early active rheumatoid ARTHRITIS not controlled by NONSTEROIDAL ANTIINFLAMMATORY DRUGS, rest, and physical therapy; administered intramuscularly.

golden hour the first hour following a traumatic injury; patients who are in the operating room within one hour of injury have a much higher survival rate.

Goldflam's disease (gōlt'flahmz) myasthenia gravis.

Goldflam-Erb disease (gōlt'flahm erb') myasthenia gravis.

Golgi apparatus (gol'je) a complex cellular organelle consisting mainly of a number of flattened sacs (cisternae) and associated vesicles, which is involved in the synthesis of glycoproteins, lipoproteins, membrane-bound proteins, and lysosomal enzymes. The sacs form primary lysosomes and secretory vacuoles. Called also Golgi complex.

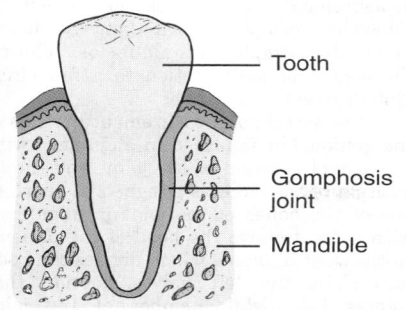

Tooth

Gomphosis joint

Mandible

The only joint in the human body that is a gomphosis joint is that between a tooth and the mandible or maxilla.

Goltz syndrome (gōlt′s) focal dermal hypoplasia.

GoLYTELY (go-līt′le) trademark for a preparation of POLYETHYLENE GLYCOL-3350 and the electrolytes sodium sulfate, sodium bicarbonate, sodium chloride, and potassium chloride; administered orally in an aqueous solution as a gentle CATHARTIC prior to studies that require bowel preparation.

gomitoli (go-mit′o-li) a network of capillaries in the upper infundibular stem (of the hypothalamus), which surround terminal arterioles of the superior hypophyseal arteries and that lead into the portal veins to the adenohypophysis.

gomphosis (gom-fo′sis) a type of fibrous joint in which a conical process is inserted into a socket-like portion.

gon(o)-¹ word element [Gr.], *seed; semen.*

gon(o)-² word element [Gr.], *knee.*

gonad (go′nad) a gamete-producing gland; the OVARY in the female or the TESTIS in the male. Called also sex gland. adj., **gonad′al, gonad′ial.** The ovary produces the OOCYTE (OVUM) and the testis produces the SPERMATOZOON. In addition, the gonads secrete hormones that influence the development of the reproductive organs at puberty, and they control other physical traits that differentiate men from women (secondary sex CHARACTERS), such as pitch of the voice and body form and size. The hormones produced by the ovary include ESTROGEN and PROGESTERONE. The principal hormone produced by the testis is TESTOS-TERONE.

gonadectomy (go″nah-dek′to-me) surgical removal of a gonad.

gonadopathy (go″nah-dop′ah-the) any disease of the gonads.

gonadorelin (go″nah-do-rel′in) synthetic luteinizing hormone–releasing HORMONE; used as the acetate or hydrochloride salt in

evaluation of HYPOGONADISM and as the acetate salt in the treatment of delayed puberty, infertility, and AMENORRHEA.

gonadotrope (go-nad′o-trōp) gonadotroph.

gonadotroph (go-nad′o-trōf) 1. a type of BASOPHIL in the adenohypophysis whose granules secrete follicle-stimulating hormone and luteinizing hormone. 2. a gonadotropic substance.

gonadotrophic (go″nah-do-trof′ik) gonadotropic.

gonadotrophin (go′nah-do-tro″fin) gonadotropin.

gonadotropic (go″nah-do-trop′ik) stimulating the GONADS; said of hormones of the anterior PITUITARY GLAND.

gonadotropin (go′nah-do-tro″pin) any hormone having a stimulating effect on the gonads. Two such hormones are secreted by the anterior PITUITARY GLAND: follicle-stimulating hormone and luteinizing hormone, both of which are active, but with differing effects, in the two sexes. Called also gonadotropic hormone.

chorionic g., human chorionic g. **(HCG) (hCG)** 1. a glycopeptide hormone that is produced by cells of the fetal placenta and maintains the function of the CORPUS LUTEUM during the first few weeks of pregnancy. It is thought to promote STEROIDOGENESIS in the fetoplacental unit and to stimulate fetal testicular secretion of TESTOSTERONE. It can be detected by IMMUNOASSAY in the maternal urine within days after FERTILIZATION; this provides the basis for the most commonly used PREGNANCY TEST. 2. the same principle obtained from the urine of pregnant women, used in treatment of certain cases of CRYPTORCHIDISM and male HYPOGONADISM, to induce ovulation and pregnancy in certain infertile, anovulatory women, and to increase the numbers of OOCYTES for patients attempting conception using assisted reproductive TECHNOLOGIES such as gamete intrafallopian TRANSFER or in vitro FERTILIZATION; administered intramuscularly. See also CHORIOGONADOTROPIN ALFA.

gonaduct (go′nah-dukt) the duct of a GONAD; a FALLOPIAN TUBE or seminal duct.

gonagra (go-nag′rah) gout in the knee.

gonalgia (go-nal′jah) pain in the knee.

gonarthritis (gon″ahr-thri′tis) inflammation of the knee joint.

gonarthrocace (gon″ahr-throk′ah-se) tuberculous arthritis of the knee joint.

gonarthrotomy (gon″ahr-throt′ah-me) incision into the knee joint.

gonecystolith (gon″ĕ-sis′to-lith) a concretion in a seminal vesicle.

G

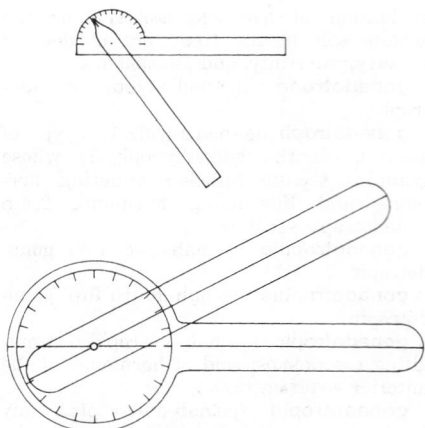

Two examples of universal goniometers commonly used by the clinician. From Kottke and Lehmann, 1990.

gonecystopyosis (gon″ĕ-sis″to-pi-o′sis) suppuration of a seminal vesicle.

gonidium (go-nid′e-um) [L.] 1. the algal component of the THALLUS of a lichen. 2. a motile reproductive unit of certain nitrogen-fixing bacteria. adj., **gonid′ial.**

goniometer (go″ne-om′ĕ-ter) an instrument for measuring angles; the instrument used in GONIOMETRY.

finger g. one for measuring the limits of flexion and extension of the joints between the phalanges of the fingers.

goniometry (go″ne-om′ĕ-tre) the measurement of range of motion in a joint. The technique may be used as a diagnostic or therapeutic measure to determine the functional status of a patient with a musculoskeletal or neurological disability. There are a variety of tools and techniques by which joint motion can be measured, but for most clinical purposes the simple universal goniometer is an adequate instrument. The system for recording measurements of range of motion may be somewhat complex or it may be based upon the simple technique of relating the degree of joint motion to a full circle (360 degrees).

In this system of measurement the axis of the goniometer is placed in alignment with the axis of rotation of the joint, and the 0° position of the circle is assigned in terms of one of the bones of the joint in alignment with a point above the head of the patient. In the sagittal plane, which divides the body into right and left halves, motion that rotates the distal member of the joint toward the 0° position is flexion, and motion which rotates it away from the 0° position is extension. In the frontal plane, which divides the body into ventral and dorsal portions, motion toward the 0° position is abduction (that is, toward the midline of the body), and motion away from the 0° position is adduction.

The 360° system for measurement of joint motion is relatively simple and easily understood by members of the health care team. For this reason it is frequently used. It is especially important, however, that all persons using this or any other system for joint measurement communicate with one another and come to a mutual understanding of the terms to be used and the purposes for which goniometry is being utilized.

gonion (go′ne-on), pl. *go′nia* [Gr.] the most inferior, posterior, and lateral point on the angle of the mandible. adj., **go′nial.**

goniopuncture (go″ne-o-pungk′cher) insertion of a knife blade through the clear cornea, just within the limbus, across the anterior chamber of the eye and through the opposite corneoscleral wall, in treatment of glaucoma.

gonioscope (go′ne-o-skōp″) an optical instrument for examining the angle of the anterior chamber of the eye and for demonstrating ocular motility and rotation.

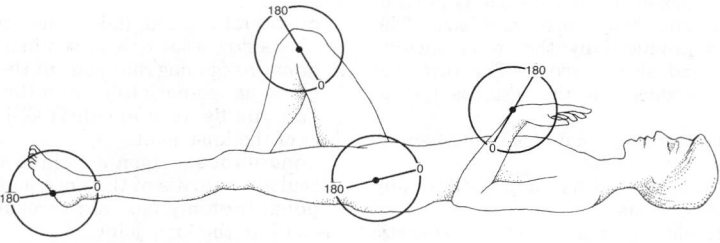

The full-circle or 360° system of goniometry applied to several joints of the body, illustrating the locations of the zero degree (0°) position. From Kottke and Lehmann, 1990.

gonioscopy (go″ne-os′kah-pe) examination of the angle of the anterior chamber of the eye with a gonioscope.

goniotomy (go″ne-ot′ah-me) an operation for glaucoma; it consists in opening Schlemm's canal under direct vision.

gonococcemia (gon″o-kok-se′me-ah) the presence of gonococci in the blood.

gonococcide (gon″o-kok′sīd) an agent destructive to gonococci.

gonococcus (gon″o-kok′us), pl. *gonococ′ci.* an individual of the species *Neisseria gonorrhoeae,* the etiologic agent of GONORRHEA. adj., **gonococ′cal.**

gonocyte (gon′o-sīt) primordial germ cell.

gonophore (gon′o-for) an accessory reproductive organ, such as a FALLOPIAN TUBE.

gonorrhea (gon″o-re′ah) a highly contagious bacterial infection of the genitourinary system, one of the most common sexually transmitted diseases in the United States. It is caused by the bacterial organism *Neisseria gonorrhoeae,* or GONOCOCCUS. Characteristically, the bacteria attacks the mucous membranes of the genital and urinary organs, producing inflammation and pus. In adults the disease is almost always contracted by coitus or intimate contact with an infected person. Gonococcal pharyngitis and proctitis occur in both males and females as a result of orogenital or anogenital contact with an infected partner. These infections frequently present no symptoms in the early stages. However, if left untreated, gonococcal proctitis can produce rectal abscesses, fistulas, or strictures. adj., **gonorrhe′al.**

Symptoms. The first symptoms of genital gonorrhea usually appear within a week after exposure to the gonococcus, but they may take as long as 3 weeks to develop; 10–40 per cent of males and 10–80 per cent of females with gonorrhea are asymptomatic. In men the inflammation generally causes a painful burning sensation during urination, and the infected penis discharges a whitish fluid, or pus. If the condition remains untreated, the discharge increases and continues for 2 or 3 months. As the infection spreads to other membranes, complications such as inflammation of the prostate and the testes may result and can cause sterility.

A woman infected with gonorrhea may feel no pain and notice no early symptoms. She may, however, experience pain in the lower abdomen, with or without a burning sensation during urination or a whitish discharge from the vagina. If the infection is allowed to reach other organs of her reproductive system, the ovaries and the fallopian tubes may become inflamed and sterility can result.

If uncontrolled, the gonococcal infection may spread to contiguous organs, or it can become blood borne, so that sites of infection may occur in multiple and varied locations, such as the valves of the heart, meninges, joints, peritoneum, and skin.

Occasionally the gonococci may attack the membranes of the eye, resulting in blindness if untreated. This is not common in adults, but the eyes of babies may be infected at birth during passage through the birth canal of an infected mother. The condition that results is called OPHTHALMIA NEONATORUM, and in the past it was a major cause of blindness in babies. Today it is usual (and required by law in some states) for all newborn infants to receive eye drops of penicillin or silver nitrate at birth as a protection against gonorrheal infection.

Diagnosis and Treatment. Diagnosis is confirmed by the presence of gonococci in the discharge from the penis or vagina or in fluid from any affected area. Gonorrhea is treated aggressively with antibiotics. Penicillin is no longer the treatment of choice because of the development of resistant organisms. CEFTRIAXONE, CIPROFLOXACIN, and OFLOXACIN are the current treatments of choice. The patient is usually treated for concurrent CHLAMYDIAL infection with doxycycline hyclate or tetracycline.

Education and social support are critical to eliminating the disease in at-risk populations. The possibility of reinfection or infection of sexual partners should be discussed with the patient, as well as the importance of identifying and treating all sexual partners. Sexual abstinence or the use of a condom should be stressed. Oral sexual activity should be avoided if there is a pharyngeal infection.

gonycampsis (gon″ĭ-kamp′sis) abnormal curvature of the knee.

gonyocele (gon′e-o-sēl″) synovitis or tuberculous arthritis of the knee.

gonyoncus (gon″e-ong′kus) tumor of the knee.

Goodell's sign (goo-delz′) softening of the cervix uteri and vagina, a probable sign of pregnancy.

Goodman's syndrome (good′manz) acrocephalopolysyndactyly, type IV.

Goodpasture's syndrome (good′paschurz) an AUTOIMMUNE DISEASE in which GLOMERULONEPHRITIS and pulmonary hemorrhage are produced by COMPLEMENT-mediated tissue damage caused by antibodies directed against the glomerular and alveolar basement MEMBRANES. It is characterized by PROTEINURIA, HEMATURIA, HEMOPTYSIS, and

G

DYSPNEA; the glomerulonephritis usually progresses to RENAL FAILURE.

Goodrich (good'rich) Annie W. (1866–1954). originator and dean of the Army School of Nursing and first dean of the Yale University School of Nursing, the first autonomous school of nursing in a university in the United States; she also developed the program for the Yale Graduate School of Nursing. The Yale curriculum aimed to produce well-educated nurses with a sound scientific background, able to care for the whole patient. She served as president of the International Council of Nurses, the American Nurses' Association, and the Association of Collegiate Schools of Nursing. For her contributions and her leadership, she received a number of awards, both in the United States and abroad.

good samaritan law a law that provides protection against claims of malpractice for medical practitioners who render emergency care at the scene of an accident except when gross negligence or willful misconduct can be proved. Most states have passed such laws; all the laws cover doctors, and about half the laws cover nurses.

Goostray (goos'tray) Stella (1886–1969). American nursing educator, author, and scholar. She graduated from Children's Hospital of Boston, and received a bachelor of science degree from Teachers College, Columbia University, and a master of education degree from Boston University. She served on the Board of Directors of the *American Journal of Nursing* and as secretary of the National League for Nursing, and wrote a number of books in the field of nursing.

goserelin (go'sĕ-rel''in) a synthetic gonadotropin-releasing HORMONE; upon administration it initially stimulates release of follicle-stimulating HORMONE and luteinizing HORMONE and on prolonged administration later suppresses them. It is used as the acetate salt to treat breast and prostate carcinomas and endometriosis and to thin the endometrium prior to endometrial ablation; administered by subcutaneous implant.

GOT glutamic-oxaloacetic transaminase; see ASPARTATE TRANSAMINASE.

gouge (gowj) a hollow chisel for cutting and removing bone.

goundou (goon-doo') a late sequel of YAWS and endemic SYPHILIS, manifested by massive PERIOSTITIS of the nasal processes of the maxillae with formation of bony hornlike growths at the sides of the nose, distortion of facial features, and eventual destruction of the nose and orbit.

gout (gowt) a form of ARTHRITIS in which URIC ACID appears in excessive quantities in the blood and may be deposited in the joints and other tissues. During an acute attack there is swelling, inflammation, and extreme pain in a joint, frequently that of the big toe. After several years of attacks, the chronic form of the disease may set in, permanently damaging and deforming joints and destroying cells of the kidney. Most cases occur in men and the first attack rarely occurs before the age of 30.

Causes. The causes of gout include excessive production of uric acid, as an inherited condition or as a side effect of chemotherapy for tumors, and impairment of clearance due to the ANTIHYPERTENSIVE AGENT HYDROCHLOROTHIAZIDE or to low-dose ASPIRIN.

Acute Gout. This form usually strikes without warning. The affected joint, which in 70 per cent of cases is that of the big toe, becomes swollen, inflamed, and very painful. The first attack may follow an operation, infection, or minor irritation such as tight shoes, or it may have no apparent cause. The patient may have a headache or fever, and often cannot walk because of the pain.

Without treatment, acute attacks of gout usually last a few days or weeks. The symptoms then disappear completely until the next attack. As the disease progresses, the attacks tend to last longer and the intervals between attacks become shorter.

A definite diagnosis of gout is made by identifying needle-shaped sodium urate crystals in the synovial fluid aspirated from an affected joint. The crystals may be seen inside polymorphonuclear leukocytes. Acute gouty arthritis is an example of an acute inflammatory process. Serial serum uric acid levels are also monitored; levels consistently above 8 mg/100 ml are an abnormal finding.

Treatment. An acute attack of gout can be treated successfully with any of several medicines. COLCHICINE has long been used; in most cases it relieves the pain and swelling in 72 hours or less, although it does not affect the high concentration of uric acid. INDOMETHACIN is a NONSTEROIDAL ANTIINFLAMMATORY DRUG that is particularly effective against acute gout and has become the treatment of choice. Aspirin should be avoided during acute attacks. The dietary management of gout is a subject of disagreement among researchers.

Chronic Gout. After a number of acute attacks of gout, the patient who goes without medical treatment may develop symptoms of chronic gout. This seldom occurs less than 10 years after the first acute attack. Joints affected by chronic gout degenerate in the same way as those affected by rheumatoid ARTHRITIS and may eventually lose their ability to move.

Treatment. Chronic gout is treated with PROBENECID, ALLOPURINOL, or other medicines that promote urinary excretion of uric acid. Other treatment may also be necessary if the kidney is involved. With appropriate treatment, gout should be well controlled.

Management Between Attacks. If acute gout is recognized at an early stage and treated correctly, the development of the chronic form can generally be prevented. Weight should be kept within normal limits, and increasing daily intake of liquids is beneficial because it encourages urine production.

GPT glutamic-pyruvic transaminase; see ALANINE TRANSAMINASE.

gr grain.

graafian follicle (grafʹe-an) a small sac, embedded in the OVARY, that encloses an OVUM. At puberty each ovary has a large number of immature follicles (primordial FOLLICLES), each of which contains an undeveloped egg cell.

About every 28 days between puberty and the onset of menopause, one of the follicles develops to maturity, or ripens, into a graafian follicle (or vesicular ovarian follicle). As it ripens, it increases in size. The ovum within becomes larger, the follicular wall becomes thicker, and fluid collects in the follicle and surrounds the ovum. The follicle also secretes estradiol, the hormone that prepares the endometrium to receive a fertilized egg. As the follicle matures, it moves to the surface of the ovary and forms a projection. When fully mature, the graafian follicle breaks open and releases the ovum, which passes into the FALLOPIAN TUBES. This release of the ovum is called OVULATION; it occurs midway in the menstrual cycle, generally about 14 days after the commencement of the menstrual flow.

The released ovum travels down the tube to the uterus, a process that takes about 3 days. Meanwhile, the empty graafian follicle in the ovary becomes filled with cells containing a yellow substance, the CORPUS LUTEUM. The corpus luteum secretes PROGESTERONE, a hormone that causes further change in the endometrium, allowing it to provide a good milieu in which a ZYGOTE (fertilized ovum) can grow through the stages of gestation to become a FETUS.

gracile (grasʹil) slender; delicate.

Gradenigo's syndrome (grah-dĕ-neʹgōz) paralysis of the abducens nerve and unilateral headache in chronic suppurative OTITIS MEDIA, caused by direct spread of the infection to involve the abducens and trigeminal nerves.

gradient (graʹde-ent) rate of increase or decrease of a variable value, or its representative curve.

edge g. in radiology, the penumbra or partial shadow on a radiograph caused by the three-dimensional shape of an object.

electrochemical g. the difference in ion CONCENTRATION and electrical POTENTIAL from one point to another, so that ions tend to move passively along it.

graduate (grajʹoo-at) 1. person who has received a degree from a university or college. 2. a measuring vessel marked by a series of lines.

graduated (grajʹu-āt″ed) marked by a succession of lines, steps, or degrees.

graft (graft) 1. any tissue or organ for IMPLANTATION or TRANSPLANTATION. 2. to

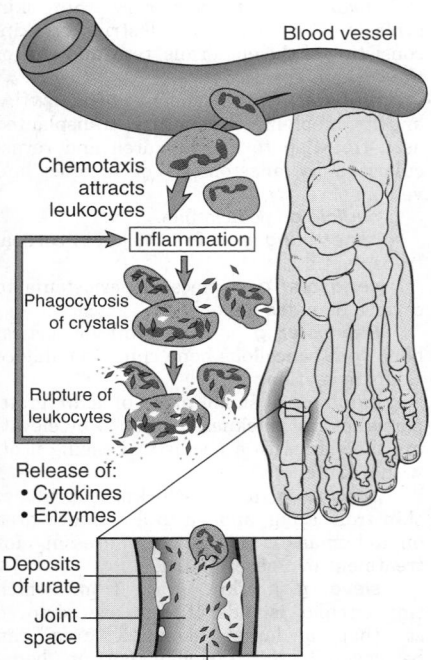

Blood vessel

Chemotaxis attracts leukocytes

Inflammation

Phagocytosis of crystals

Rupture of leukocytes

Release of:
• Cytokines
• Enzymes

Deposits of urate

Joint space

Uric acid crystals

Gouty arthritis. Deposits of uric acid crystals in the connective tissue have a chemotactic effect and cause exudation of leukocytes into the joint. The inflammation most often affects the metatarsophalangeal joint of the big toe. From Damjanov, 2000.

implant or transplant such tissues. This term is preferred over TRANSPLANT in the case of skin grafts. See also IMPLANT.

allogeneic g. allograft.

autodermic g., autoepidermic g. a skin graft taken from the patient's own body.

autologous g., autoplastic g. a graft taken from another area of the patient's own body; called also autograft.

avascular g. a graft of tissue in which not even transient vascularization is achieved.

bone g. bone transplanted from one site to another.

bypass g. an AUTOGRAFT consisting of a segment of vein or artery grafted into place in a BYPASS.

cable g. a nerve graft made up of several sections of nerve in the manner of a cable.

coronary artery bypass g. (CABG) see under BYPASS.

cutis g. dermal graft.

delayed g. a skin graft that is sutured back into its bed and subsequently used after several days.

dermal g., dermic g. a skin graft of DERMIS, used instead of fascia in various plastic procedures.

epidermic g. a skin graft in which a piece of EPIDERMIS is implanted on a raw surface.

fascia g. a graft of fibrous tissue, usually taken from the external investing fascia of the lower limb (FASCIA LATA).

fascicular g. a nerve graft in which bundles of nerve fibers are approximated and sutured separately.

filler g. one used for the filling of defects, as the filling of depressions with fatty tissue or of a bony cyst cavity with bone chips or dried cartilage.

free g. a graft of tissue completely freed from its bed, in contrast to a flap.

full-thickness g. a skin graft consisting of the full thickness of the skin, with little or none of the subcutaneous tissue. See accompanying illustration.

heterodermic g. a skin graft taken from a donor of another species.

heterologous g., heteroplastic g. xenograft.

homologous g. a graft of tissue obtained from the body of another animal of the same species but with a genotype differing from that of the recipient; called also allograft and homograft.

inlay g. a skin graft or mucosal graft applied by spreading the graft over a stent

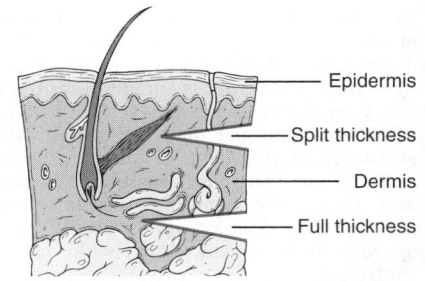

Diagram of a cross-section of the skin, demonstrating split thickness and full thickness skin grafts. From Roberts and Hedges, 1991.

and suturing the graft and mold into a prepared pocket.

isogeneic g., isologous g. isoplastic g. syngraft.

lamellar g. replacement of the superficial layers of an opaque cornea by a thin layer of clear cornea from a donor eye.

mesh g. a type of split-thickness graft in which many tiny splits have been made in the skin to allow it to be stretched to cover a larger area.

Ollier-Thiersch g. a very thin skin graft in which long, broad strips of skin, consisting of the epidermis, rete, and part of the corium, are used.

omental g. a segment of OMENTUM and its supplying vasculature, transplanted as a free flap to another area and revascularized by anastomosis of arteries and veins.

pedicle g. pedicle flap.

penetrating g. a full-thickness corneal transplant.

periosteal g. a piece of periosteum to cover a denuded bone.

Phemister g. a bone graft of cortical bone with cancellous bone chips to enhance callus formation.

pinch g. a small piece of skin graft, partial or full thickness, obtained by elevating the skin with a needle and slicing it off with a knife.

porcine g. a split-thickness graft of skin from a pig, applied to a denuded area on a human as a temporary dressing for treatment of a severe burn.

sieve g. a skin graft from which tiny circular islands of skin are removed so that a larger denuded area can be covered, the sievelike portion being placed over one area, and the individual islands over surrounding or other denuded areas.

skin g. a piece of skin transplanted to replace a lost portion of skin; see also skin GRAFTING.

G

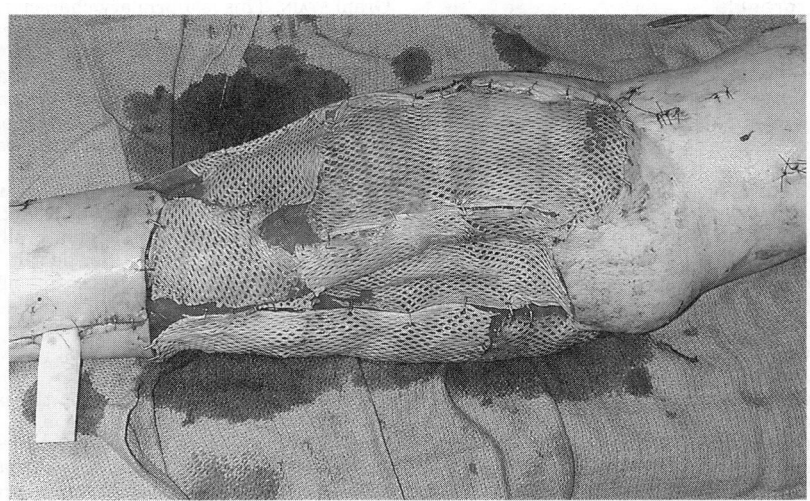

Mesh skin graft applied to the leg. From McQuillan et al., 2002.

split-skin g., split-thickness g. a skin graft consisting of the epidermis and a portion of dermis. See accompanying illustration.

syngeneic g. syngraft.

thick-split g. a skin graft consisting of the epidermis and about two thirds of the dermis.

Thiersch g. Ollier-Thiersch graft.

grafting (graft′ing) TRANSPLANTATION. The term *grafting* is preferred in the case of skin grafting and of synthetic grafts such as arteriovenous grafts.

skin g. implantation of patches of healthy skin on a denuded area to provide epithelial covering; the skin may come from another area with healthy skin from the patient's own body or from the body of a skin donor. The most important function of skin grafting is to promote healing of large surfaces that have been burned or wounded, or that have become ulcerous or cancerous. If burns or other injuries are extensive, grafting can prevent extensive scarring with unsightly tissue that cannot perform all the necessary functions of normal skin. Skin contractures can thus be avoided.

The skin to be grafted is cut usually from the chest, thigh, buttock, abdomen, lower part of the neck, or behind the ear. It may be removed in very thin strips or as a thin layer of superficial skin, and it must be placed in its new location without delay. If delay is unavoidable, it is placed in a saline solution or refrigerated. In this kind of free graft, the skin is cut entirely away from the body before transplantation and then is sewed into place; a pressure dressing is applied or a tissue glue is used. Afterwards the skin must depend for its nourishment on the surrounding tissue in the new location.

If a large thick area of skin containing much underlying tissue is to be moved, the traditional method has been to do this by means of a pedicle FLAP. For example, an injured hand that needs skin grafting would be strapped against the abdominal wall to receive a pedicle graft of skin from the abdomen. However, the introduction of MICROSURGERY has eliminated much of the need for this kind of graft.

A skin graft can sometimes be made by the simple procedure of cutting a piece of healthy skin from one part of the body, such as the back or the thigh, and stitching it to the injured area. Small arteries from the tissues surrounding the injured area then grow into the graft, nourish it with blood and promote normal growth. If the area to be covered is large, a number of separate patches may be stitched to it, forming islands of skin that will enlarge with healing until the entire area is covered. This is called "postage stamp" or pinch grafting.

With the advent of microsurgery, much of the inconvenience and lengthy waiting necessary for successful grafting of skin flaps have been eliminated. It is now possible for a surgeon to perform what are called *free-tissue transfers*. The skin flap is removed from the donor site and transferred directly to the distant recipient site where circulation to the free flap is reestablished by microvascular anastomoses.

There are many different types of skin GRAFTS, including DERMAL or DERMIC, EPIDERMIC, FULL-THICKNESS, SPLIT-THICKNESS, THICK-SPLIT, INLAY, MESH, PINCH, SIEVE, and OLLIER-THIERSCH GRAFTS. See also FLAP.

graft-versus-host disease (reaction) (GVH disease) a condition that occurs when immunologically competent cells or their precursors are transplanted into an immunocompromised recipient (host) that is not histocompatible with the donor. Because the host is immunocompromised, the graft is not rejected. Immunocompetent T LYMPHOCYTES derived from the donor tissue recognize the recipient's tissue as foreign or NONSELF and react with it, producing clinical manifestations including edema, erythema, ulceration, loss of hair, and heart and joint lesions similar to those of connective tissue disorders. This condition is a frequent complication of bone marrow TRANSPLANTATION. TISSUE TYPING and HLA ANTIGEN matching of the donor and recipient reduce the possibility of graft-versus-host disease.

Graham's law (gra′amz) the rate of diffusion of a gas through porous membranes varies inversely with the square root of its density.

grain (grān) 1. a seed, especially of a cereal plant. 2. the smallest unit in the APOTHECARIES′ and AVOIRDUPOIS SYSTEMS, equal to 0.065 of a GRAM; abbreviated gr.

gram (g) (gram) a unit of mass in the SI system; one thousandth of a kilogram. (See also Table of Weights and Measures in the Appendix and SI UNITS.)

-gram word element [Gr.], *written; recorded.*

gramicidin (gram″ĭ-si′din) an ANTIBIOTIC produced by *Bacillus brevis,* applied topically in pyodermic, ocular, and other localized infections due to susceptible gram-positive organisms. It is also one of the two major components of TYROTHRICIN, the other being TYROCIDINE.

gram-negative (gram-neg′ah-tiv) losing the stain or decolorized by alcohol in Gram's method of staining; see Gram STAIN. This is a primary characteristic of bacteria having a cell wall composed of a thin layer of PEPTIDOGLYCAN covered by an outer membrane of LIPOPROTEIN and LIPOPOLYSACCHARIDE.

gram-positive (gram-poz′ĭ-tiv) retaining the stain or resisting decolorization by alcohol in Gram's method of staining; see Gram STAIN. This is a primary characteristic of bacteria whose cell wall is composed of PEPTIDOGLYCAN and TEICHOIC ACIDS.

grandiose (gran′de-ōs″) in psychiatry, pertaining to exaggerated belief or claims of one's importance or identity, often manifested by delusions of great wealth, power, or fame.

granisetron (gră-nis′ĕ-tron) an ANTIEMETIC used in conjunction with cancer chemotherapy or radiotherapy; administered orally or intravenously as the hydrochloride salt.

granular (gran′u-lar) made up of or marked by the presence of granules or grains.

granulatio (gran″u-la′she-o), pl. *granulatio′nes* [L.] granulation.

granulation (gran″u-la′shun) 1. the process of forming granulation tissue. 2. the process of forming cytoplasmic granules. 3. granule (def. 1). 4. any granular material on the surface of a tissue, membrane, or organ. 5. the rendering of hard or metallic substances into granules or grains.

arachnoid g's enlarged arachnoid villi projecting into the venous sinuses and creating slight depressions on the inner surface of the cranium.

exuberant g's excessive proliferation of granulation tissue in the healing of a wound.

granule (gran′ūl) 1. a small particle or grain. 2. a small pill made of sucrose.

acidophil g's granules staining with acid dyes.

aleuronoid g's colorless myeloid colloidal bodies found in the base of pigment cells.

alpha g's 1. oval granules found in blood platelets; they are lysosomes containing acid phosphatase. 2. large granules in the alpha CELLS of the islets of Langerhans; they secrete GLUCAGON. 3. acidophilic granules in the ACIDOPHILS of the adenohypophysis.

amphophil g's granules that stain with both acid and basic dyes.

azurophil g's, azurophilic g's coarse reddish granules that contain myeloperoxidase and stain easily with azure dyes, found in mature neutrophils and their precursor cells.

Babès-Ernst g. metachromatic granule.

basophil g. 1. a granule that stains with basic dyes. 2. one of the coarse bluish-black granules found in BASOPHILS. 3. (in plural) beta granules (def. 2).

beta g's 1. granules in the beta CELLS of the islets of Langerhans; they secrete INSULIN. 2. basophilic granules in the BASOPHILS of the adenohypophysis.

Birbeck g's rod- or tennis racquet–shaped inclusions with a central linear, longitudinally striated nucleus, found in the cytoplasm of Langerhans' cells.

chromatic g's, chromophilic g's Nissl bodies.

cone g's the nuclei of the visual cells in the outer nuclear layer of the retina that are connected with the CONES.

eosinophil g. one of the coarse round granules that stain with eosin and are found in EOSINOPHILS.

iodophil g's granules staining brown with iodine, seen in polymorphonuclear leukocytes in various acute infectious diseases.

lamellar g. keratinosome.

metachromatic g. a granular cell inclusion that stains a color different from that of the dye used. In certain bacteria, yeasts, yeastlike fungi, and protozoa, metachromatic granules appear red when stained with a blue dye. They are composed of complex polyphosphate, lipid, and nucleoprotein molecules (volutin) and serve as an intracellular phosphate reserve. Called also Babès-Ernst body or granule.

Nissl's g's Nissl bodies.

oxyphil g's acidophil granules.

pigment g's small masses of coloring matter in pigment cells.

rod g's the nuclei of the visual cells in the outer nuclear layer of the retina; they are connected with the RODS.

Schüffner's g's Schüffner's DOTS.

seminal g's the small granular bodies in the semen.

granuloadipose (gran″u-lo-ad′ĭ-pōs) showing fatty degeneration containing granules of fat.

granuloblast (gran′u-lo-blast″) an immature granulocyte.

granulocyte (gran′u-lo-sīt″) granular LEUKOCYTE. adj., **granulocyt′ic.**

band-form g. band cell.

granulocytopathy (gran″u-lo-si-top′ah-the) any disorder of the granulocytes.

granulocytopenia (gran″u-lo-si″to-pe′ne-ah) a reduction in the number of granular leukocytes in the blood that is less severe than AGRANULOCYTOSIS; called also granulopenia.

granulocytopoiesis (gran″u-lo-si″to-poi-e′sis) granulopoiesis. adj., **granulocytopoiet′ic.**

granulocytosis (gran″u-lo-si-to′sis) an excess of granulocytes in the blood.

granuloma (gran″u-lo′mah), pl. *granulomas, granulo′mata* an imprecise term applied to (1) any small nodular, delimited aggregation of mononuclear inflammatory cells, or (2) a similar collection of modified macrophages resembling epithelial cells,

usually surrounded by a rim of lymphocytes, often with multinucleated giant cells. Some granulomas contain eosinophils and plasma cells, and fibrosis is commonly seen around the lesion. Granuloma formation represents a chronic inflammatory response initiated by various infectious and noninfectious agents.

apical g. modified granulation tissue containing elements of chronic inflammation located adjacent to the root apex of a tooth with infected necrotic pulp.

actinic g. an annular lesion seen on skin chronically exposed to the sun, with a raised border and a center that appears normal but is actually ELASTOTIC.

benign g. of thyroid chronic inflammation of the thyroid gland, converting it into a bulky tumor that later becomes extremely hard.

coccidioidal g. the secondary stage of COCCIDIOIDOMYCOSIS.

dental g. one usually surrounded by a fibrous sac continuous with the periodontal ligament and attached to the root apex of a tooth.

eosinophilic g. 1. Langerhans cell histiocytosis. 2. a disorder similar to eosinophilic gastroenteritis, characterized by localized nodular or pedunculated lesions of the submucosa and muscle walls, especially of the pyloric area of the stomach, caused by infiltration of eosinophils, but without peripheral eosinophilia and allergic symptoms.

g. fissura′tum a firm, whitish, fissured, fibrotic granuloma of the gum and buccal mucosa, occurring on an edentulous alveolar ridge and between the ridge and the cheek.

foreign-body g. a localized histiocytic reaction to a foreign body in the tissue.

giant cell reparative g., central a lesion of the jaws composed of a spindle cell stroma punctuated by multinucleate giant cells, considered by most to be a central lesion of the bone of the jaws, presenting an inflammatory reaction to injury or hemorrhage. Some, however, consider it to be a giant cell tumor occurring in both benign and malignant forms, and others consider it to be a form of osteogenic sarcoma, varying in degree of malignancy.

g. inguina′le a granulomatous disease that is associated with uncleanliness and is caused by the microorganism *Calymmatobacterium granulomatis* (sometimes called a Donovan BODY). Called also granuloma venereum. Although granuloma inguinale is often considered to be a venereal disease, research does not support the hypothesis that it is transmitted by sexual contact. It is possible that natural resistance to the disease is high, so that only a few of the persons exposed are affected. About 10 days to 3 months may elapse after exposure until appearance of the first symptoms, usually small painless ulcers that bleed easily. Swelling in the groin may then follow. A new ulcer or ulcers may appear as the old one heals, so that granuloma inguinale may eventually cover the reproductive organs, buttocks, and lower abdomen, with extensive sores and a foul odor. As persons who have the disease seem to develop little immunity to it, granuloma inguinale can be present for many years.

Treatment of the disease may be with streptomycin. tetracyclines, or lincomycin. There is no known preventive for granuloma inguinale, although it is rare where sanitary living conditions prevail. The drainage from lesions may be infectious and handwashing and basic cleanliness are required. The Centers for Disease Control and Prevention recommends standard PRECAUTIONS.

lipoid g. xanthoma.

lipophagic g. a granuloma attended by the loss of subcutaneous fat.

Majocchi's g. trichophytic granuloma.

midline g. a rare disease of unknown etiology, characterized by granulomatous lesions of the nasal mucosa, sinuses, palate, and pharynx. Massive, progressive, erosive lesions that destroy the involved soft tissue, cartilage, and bone and sometimes extend to the brain are typical. Untreated cases are fatal (lethal midline granuloma).

paracoccidioidal g. paracoccidioidomycosis.

peripheral giant cell reparative g. giant cell epulis.

pyogenic g. a benign, solitary nodule resembling granulation tissue, found anywhere on the body, commonly intraorally, usually at the site of trauma as a response of the tissues to a nonspecific infection.

sarcoid g. the granuloma seen with SARCOIDOSIS, consisting of multinucleated giant cells surrounded by macrophages and epithelioid cells derived from macrophages.

swimming pool g. a chronic granulomatous bacterial infection caused by contamination of an abrasion sustained in a swimming pool by *Mycobacterium marinum*, which histologically and clinically resembles tuberculosis. It tends to heal spontaneously within a few months to 2 years.

g. telangiecta'ticum a form characterized by numerous dilated blood vessels.

trichophytic g. a form of TINEA CORPORIS seen mainly on the lower legs, due to infection of hairs by the fungus *Trichophyton*; characteristics include raised, circumscribed, boggy granulomas that are disseminated or arranged in chains. Lesions are slowly absorbed or undergo necrosis, leaving depressed scars. Called also Majocchi's granuloma.

g. tro'picum yaws.

g. vene'reum granuloma inguinale.

granulomatosis (gran″u-lo″mah-to′sis) any condition involving the formation of multiple GRANULOMAS.

allergic g. CHURG-STRAUSS SYNDROME.

eosinophilic g. Langerhans cell histiocytosis.

Langerhans cell g. Langerhans cell HISTIOCYTOSIS.

lymphomatoid g. a multisystem disease involving predominantly the lungs, skin, central nervous system, and kidneys, caused by invasion and destruction of vessels by atypical lymphoreticular cells. Many affected patients develop frank lymphoma. It usually affects males, and the most frequent presenting symptoms are cough, shortness of breath, and chest pain. Extrapulmonary manifestations are common, with skin lesions being present in many cases.

g. sidero'tica a condition in which brownish nodules are seen in the enlarged spleen.

Wegener's g. a multisystem disease chiefly affecting males, characterized by necrotizing granulomatous vasculitis involving the upper and lower respiratory tracts, glomerulonephritis, and variable degrees of systemic, small vessel vasculitis, which is generally considered to represent an aberrant HYPERSENSITIVITY REACTION to an unknown antigen.

granulomatous (gran″u-lom′ah-tus) composed of granulomas.

granulopenia (gran″u-lo-pe′ne-ah) agranulocytosis.

granuloplastic (gran′u-lo-plas″tik) forming granules.

granulopoiesis (gran″u-lo-poi-e′sis) the formation and development of GRANULOCYTES; called also granulocytopoiesis. adj., **granulopoiet′ic.**

granulosa cell tumor (gran″u-lo′sah) an ovarian tumor originating in the granulosa CELLS, the solid mass of cells surrounding the GRAAFIAN FOLLICLE; it may be associated with excessive production of ESTROGEN, inducing endometrial hyperplasia with menorrhagia.

granulosa-theca cell tumor an ovarian tumor predominantly composed of either granulosa CELLS (follicular cells) or theca CELLS, and often associated with excessive production of ESTROGEN, with hyperplasia of the breast and ENDOMETRIUM and carcinoma of the endometrium. When luteinized, i.e., having cells resembling those of the corpus luteum, it is known as LUTEOMA.

granulosis (gran″u-lo′sis) the formation of granules.

g. ru′bra na′si redness and marked sweating confined to the nose and surrounding area of the face, with red papules and sometimes many small vesicles, seen most often in children, and usually subsiding at puberty.

graph (graf) a diagram or curve representing data and varying relationships between sets of data.

-graph word element [Gr.], *a writing recording instrument; the record made by such an instrument.*

graphospasm (graf′o-spazm) writer's cramp.

-graphy word element [Gr.], *writing or recording; a method of recording.* adj., **graph′ic.**

GRASP a patient classification system.

gravel (grav′el) calculus occurring in small particles.

Graves' disease (grāvz) a syndrome in which THYROTOXICOSIS is associated with diffuse GOITER, infiltrative EXOPHTHALMOS, and sometimes infiltrative DERMOPATHY, now known to be an AUTOIMMUNE DISEASE. As in the other autoimmune thyroid diseases, HASHIMOTO'S DISEASE and primary thyroid atrophy, 60 to 80 per cent of patients have autoantibodies against thyroglobulin or thyroid microsomes. About 80 per cent of patients with Graves' disease also have autoantibodies against some components of the thyroid cell membrane that alter or block the binding sites for THYROTROPIN. Other symptoms and signs include hand tremors, nausea, diarrhea, increased metabolism, profuse perspiration, nervous irritability, skin changes, hyperglycemia, anemia, and tachycardia. The first stage of treatment uses antithyroid drugs, such as PROPYLTHIOURACIL and METHIMAZOLE to suppress thyroid hormone secretion, and BETA-ADRENERGIC BLOCKING AGENTS to control the symptoms of HYPERTHYROIDISM. In severe cases, surgery or radioactive iodine therapy is used to ablate the gland permanently.

gravid (grav′id) pregnant.

gravida (grav′ĭ-dah) a pregnant woman; called gravida I (primigravida) during the first pregnancy, gravida II (secundigravida) during the second, and so on.

gravidic (grah-vid′ik) occurring in pregnancy.

gravidocardiac (grav″ĭ-do-kahr′de-ak) pertaining to heart disease in pregnancy.

gravimetric (grav″ĭ-met′rik) pertaining to measurement by weight; performed by weight, as the gravimetric method of drug assay.

gravity (grav′ĭ-te) 1. the phenomenon by which two bodies having mass are attracted to each other. 2. the gravitational attraction near a large body having mass, particularly near or on the surface of a planet or star.

specific g. see SPECIFIC GRAVITY.

standard g. (g) the acceleration due to gravity at mean sea level, 9.80616 meters per second squared.

Gravlee Jet Washer (grav′le) a diagnostic instrument consisting of a cannula, an adjustable rubber flange, a saline reservoir, and a 30 ml syringe, and employed to obtain endometrial cells for cytologic and histologic examination. The procedure of endometrial washing, for which the Gravlee Jet Washer is used, provides a relatively quick and easy means of screening for endometrial carcinoma in its early stages.

gray (gra) the SI unit of absorbed radiation dose, defined as the transfer of 1 joule of energy per kilogram of absorbing material (1 J/kg); 1 gray equals 100 rads.

gray baby syndrome gray syndrome.

gray syndrome (gra) a potentially fatal condition seen in neonates, particularly premature infants, due to a reaction to CHLORAMPHENICOL, characterized by an ashen gray cyanosis, listlessness, weakness, and hypotension. Called also gray baby syndrome.

green (grēn) 1. a color between yellow and blue, produced by energy with wavelengths between 490 and 570 nm. 2. a dye or stain with this color.

indocyanine g. a dye used intravenously in determination of blood volume and flow, cardiac output, and hepatic function.

Greenfield's disease (grēn′fēldz) the infantile form of metachromatic LEUKODYS-TROPHY.

GRH growth hormone–releasing hormone.

grid (grid) 1. a grating. 2. in radiology, a device consisting essentially of a series of narrow lead strips closely spaced on their edges and separated by spacers of low density material; used to reduce the amount of scattered radiation reaching the x-ray film. 3. a chart with horizontal and perpendicular lines for plotting curves.

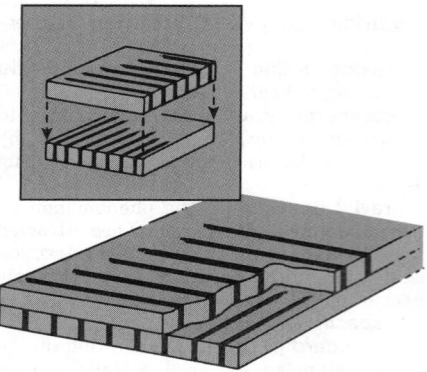

Cross-hatched grids are fabricated by sandwiching two linear grids together so that their grid strips are perpendicular. From Bushong, 2001.

Amsler g. see Amsler CHARTS.

baby g. a direct-reading chart on infant growth.

cross-hatched g. two linear grids that are superimposed at right angles to each other, used for maximal scatter cleanup.

g. cutoff differences in radiographic intensity that are caused by improper focusing of the lead lines of a grid.

focused g. a linear grid in which all of the lead strips are aligned in a tilted fashion toward a centering point.

linear g. a grid designed to permit the passage of the primary beam by having lead lines aligned in the same direction separated by radiolucent interspacing material. There are two types, *parallel* and *focused*.

Wetzel g. a direct-reading chart for evaluating physical fitness in terms of body build, developmental level, and basal metabolism.

grief (grēf) 1. keen mental suffering or distress over affliction or loss. 2. mental suffering or distress in response to a threatened or real loss, as loss of a body part or function, death of another person, or loss of one's possessions, job, status, or ideals; see also MOURNING. Various theorists have proposed stages of grieving; see descriptions under DYING.

grieving (grēv′ing) feeling or showing sorrow in reaction to an actual or perceived specific loss, or to one that is anticipated. See also GRIEF and DYING.

The North American Nursing Diagnosis Association recognizes two types of grieving as NURSING DIAGNOSES: In *anticipatory grieving* a person may deny the potential loss, or express feelings of sorrow, guilt, or anger over the threatened loss; physiological signs may include a choked feeling or changes in eating habits, sleep patterns, activity level, libido, or communication patterns. *Dysfunctional grieving* is characterized by the emotional and physiological signs listed above as well as expression of unresolved issues, difficulty expressing loss, interference with life functioning, developmental regression, and changes in concentration and pursuit of tasks.

grip (grip) 1. a grasping or clasping. 2. popular term for INFLUENZA.

devil's g. epidemic pleurodynia.

grippe (grip) popular term for INFLUENZA.

griseofulvin (gris″e-o-ful′vin) an antibiotic administered orally as an antifungal AGENT for infections of the skin, nails, and scalp. Treatment usually must be prolonged and the patient must be watched for signs of leukopenia, which often occurs when the drug is administered over a long period of time.

groin (groin) inguen.

grommet (grom′et) a tube inserted through the TYMPANIC MEMBRANE for drainage of the middle ear.

groove (groov) a narrow, linear hollow or depression.

branchial g. pharyngeal groove.

Harrison's g. a horizontal groove along the lower border of the thorax corresponding to the costal insertion of the diaphragm; seen in advanced rickets in childhood.

medullary g., neural g. that formed by the beginning invagination of the neural plate of the embryo to form the neural tube.

pharyngeal g. a groove between a pair of pharyngeal ARCHES in a mammalian embryo, homologous to the branchial CLEFT of a fish, formed by rupture of the membrane separating a corresponding entodermal pouch and ectodermal groove.

gross (grōs) coarse or large; visible to the naked eye.

ground (grownd) 1. a path of conduction from an electrical CIRCUIT to the earth. 2. to connect an electrical circuit or electrical equipment to the earth. 3. zero electrical POTENTIAL.

group (groop) 1. an assemblage of objects having certain things in common. 2. a number of atoms forming a recognizable and usually transferable portion of a molecule.

activity g's groups of individuals with similar needs for occupational therapy who are working on the correction of problems that they hold in common.

azo g. the bivalent radical, $-N{=}N-$.

blood g. see BLOOD GROUP.

control g. see CONTROL (def. 3).

encounter g. a sensitivity group in which the members strive to gain emotional rather than intellectual insight, with emphasis on the expression of interpersonal feelings in the group situation.

focus g's individuals with a common interest who meet to explore a problem in depth.

PLT g. [*p*sittacosis-*l*ymphogranuloma venereum-*t*rachoma] alternative name for genus *Chlamydia*.

prosthetic g. 1. an organic radical, nonprotein in nature, which together with a protein carrier forms an enzyme. 2. a cofactor tightly bound to an enzyme, i.e., it is an integral part of the enzyme and not readily dissociated from it. 3. a cofactor that may reversibly dissociate from the protein component of an enzyme; a coenzyme.

sensitivity g., sensitivity training g. a nonclinical group intended for persons without severe emotional problems, focusing on self-awareness, self-understanding, and interpersonal interactions and aiming to develop skills in leadership, management, counseling, or other roles. Called also T-group and training group.

support g. 1. a group made up of individuals with a common problem, usually meeting to express feelings, vent frustrations, and explore effective coping strategies. Education is a component of some support groups. 2. in the NURSING INTERVENTIONS CLASSIFICATION defined as the use of a group environment to provide emotional support and health-related information for members.

T-g. sensitivity group.

g. therapy a form of psychotherapy in which a group of patients meets regularly with a group leader, usually a therapist. The group may be balanced, having patients with diverse problems and attitudes, or it may be composed of patients who all have similar diagnoses or issues to resolve. In some groups, patients may be basically mentally healthy but trying to work through external stressors, such as job loss, natural disasters, or physical illness. Self-help groups are groups of people with a commonality of diagnosis (e.g., alcoholism, overeating, or a particular chronic physical illness) or of experience (e.g., rape, incest) and a leader who may be not a therapist but rather one who has experienced a similar problem or situation.

From hearing how the group leader or other members feel about this behavior, the patient may gain insight into his or her anxieties and conflicts. The group may provide emotional support for self-revelation and a structured environment for trying out new ways of relating to people. In contrast, there are other groups that focus on altering behavior, with less or minimal attention paid to gaining insight into the causes of the problems.

therapy g. in the NURSING INTERVENTIONS CLASSIFICATION, a nursing INTERVENTION defined as the application of psychotherapeutic techniques to a group, including the utilization of interactions between members of the group. See also GROUP THERAPY.

training g. sensitivity group.

grouper (grōōp′er) any of various usually large marine fish of the genera *Epinephelus* and *Mycteroperca*, found in tropical waters; they are often eaten by humans but sometimes contain CIGUATOXIN and can cause CIGUATERA.

group-transfer (grōōp″trans′fer) denoting a chemical reaction (excluding oxidation and reduction) in which molecules exchange functional groups, a process catalyzed by enzymes called transferases.

growth (grōth) 1. the progressive development of a living thing, especially the process by which the body reaches its point of complete physical development. 2. an abnormal formation of tissue, such as a tumor.

Human Growth. Human growth from infancy to maturity involves great changes in body size and appearance, including the development of the sexual characteristics. The growth process is not a steady one: at some times growth occurs rapidly, at others slowly. Individual patterns of growth vary widely because of differences in heredity and environment. Children tend to have physiques similar to those of their parents or of earlier forebears; however, environment may modify this tendency. Living conditions, including nutrition and hygiene, have considerable influence on growth.

Glands and Growth. The regulators of growth are the ENDOCRINE GLANDS, which are themselves subject to hereditary influence. The PITUITARY GLAND secretes growth hormone, which controls general body growth, particularly the growth of the skeleton, and also influences METABOLISM. In addition to influencing growth directly, the pituitary gland has a central role in regulating the other endocrine glands. These other glands in turn control many body functions, and they secrete the various hormones that directly regulate metabolism.

Variations in Growth Rates. The growth of different individuals varies a great deal. It should be remembered that the rate of growth we call "normal" is really only an average rate. There is a wide range of growth rates, almost all of them quite normal. Of the children of a given sex and age, only about two thirds will have physical measurements that fall close to the average.

Growth in height occurs as a result of maturation of the skeleton. When the long bones have reached maturity at about age 18, linear growth stops. In general, the birth weight of the average baby doubles in 5 to 6 months and triples by the end of the first year. At the end of the second year of life birth weight quadruples and then there is a steady increase of 2 to 2.75 kg (4.4 to 6 lb.) each year until the child reaches puberty, at which time there is a period of rapid growth in weight and height.

delayed g. and development a NURSING DIAGNOSIS accepted by the North American Nursing Diagnosis Association, defined as deviation from age group norms.

risk for disproportionate g. a NURSING DIAGNOSIS accepted by the North American Nursing Diagnosis Association, defined as being at risk for growth above the 97th percentile or below the 3rd percentile for age, crossing two percentile channels.

Gruber's syndrome (groo'berz) Meckel-Gruber syndrome.

grumous (groo'mus) lumpy or clotted.

gryposis (grĭ-po'sis) abnormal curvature, as of the nails.

GSH the reduced form of GLUTATHIONE.

GSSG the oxidized form of GLUTATHIONE.

GU genitourinary.

guaiac (gwi'ak) a resin from certain Caribbean trees, used as a reagent.

g. test one for occult blood; glacial acetic acid and guaiac are mixed with the specimen; on addition of hydrogen peroxide, the presence of blood is indicated by a blue tint.

guaifenesin (gwi-fen'ĕ-sin) an expectorant believed to act by reducing sputum viscosity.

guanabenz (gwah'nah-benz) an α_2-adrenergic agonist used in the form of the base or the acetate ester as an ANTIHYPERTENSIVE.

guanadrel (gwah'nah-drel) an adrenergic neuron blocking AGENT, used in the treatment of HYPERTENSION; used as the sulfate salt.

guanethidine (gwahn-eth'ĭ-dēn) an ADRENERGIC BLOCKING AGENT; the monosulfate salt is used as an ANTIHYPERTENSIVE AGENT.

guanfacine (gwahn'fah-sēn) an α_2-adrenergic agonist used in the form of the hydrochloride salt as an antihypertensive.

guanidoacetic acid (gwahn″ĭ-do-ah-se′-tik) an intermediate product in the synthesis of creatine.

guanine (gwah'nēn) a purine base, one of the fundamental components of NUCLEIC ACIDS (DNA and RNA).

guanosine (gwah'no-sēn) a nucleoside, guanine riboside, one of the major constituents of RNA.

cyclic g. monophosphate a cyclic nucleotide, guanosine 3′,5′-cyclic monophosphate, an intracellular "second messenger" similar in action to cyclic ADENOSINE monophosphate; the two cyclic nucleotides activate different protein kinases and usually produce opposite effects on cell function. Abbreviated 3′,5′-GMP, cGMP, and cyclic GMP.

g. monophosphate (GMP) a nucleotide important in metabolism and RNA synthesis.

g. triphosphate (GTP) a nucleotide required for RNA synthesis and involved in energy metabolism.

guard (gahrd) a protective device.

mouth g. any of various removable intraoral appliances that protect the teeth and sometimes the lips and cheeks during contact sports.

guarded (gahr'ded) of uncertain outcome; said of a patient condition.

guidance (gi'dans) 1. a guide. 2. an act of guiding.

anticipatory g. in the NURSING INTERVENTIONS CLASSIFICATION, a nursing INTERVENTION defined as the preparation of a patient for an anticipated development and/or situational crisis.

health system g. in the NURSING INTERVENTIONS CLASSIFICATION, a nursing INTERVENTION defined as facilitating a patient's location and use of appropriate health services.

Guillain-Barré syndrome (ge-yă′ bah-ra′) a relatively rare disease affecting the peripheral nervous system, especially the spinal nerves, as well as the cranial nerves. Pathologic changes include demyelination, inflammation, edema, and nerve root compression. The cause is unknown; however, it usually follows a febrile illness such as respiratory infection or gastroenteritis within 10 to 21 days and is believed by some to be related to an autoimmune mechanism. Because it is characterized by a flaccid paralysis, it is sometimes mistaken for POLIOMYELITIS. Called also acute idiopathic polyneuritis, acute postinfectious polyneuritis, and Landry's paralysis.

The early symptoms are fever, malaise, nausea, or prostration. Muscular weakness usually starts in the lower extremities and tends to go upward through the body, but it may affect the facial muscles and arms first and then move downward. The paralysis is not accompanied by loss of sensation, but rather by abnormal sensations of tingling and numbness. The classic cerebrospinal fluid findings are of an elevated protein level without an increase in the number of leukocytes. The cerebrospinal fluid pressure is within normal limits.

The progression of the paralysis may stop at any point. Once the weakness reaches its maximum, the paralysis remains unchanged for days or weeks. Improvement begins spontaneously and continues for weeks, or rarely, months. The prognosis for full recovery is good.

Guillain-Barré syndrome affects primarily the ventral roots of the spinal cord, hence the motor disturbances. The sensory counterpart of this syndrome affects the dorsal roots and is usually called *Guillain-Barré-Strohl syndrome*. The symptoms of this disease include severe stabbing pains at first, followed by abnormally exaggerated response to painful stimuli.

Patient Care. There is no specific treatment for the disease. It must run its course and for this reason skilled patient care is imperative, particularly in the acute phase, when respiratory failure requiring prolonged mechanical ventilation is a very real possibility. All measures needed to prevent complications in patients who cannot move about in bed are required. The experience of paralysis and sensory disturbances is an ordeal for them. They will need continued physical and psychological support throughout all stages of recovery, which may last for weeks or months, depending on the individual patient.

guillotine (ge′o-tēn) a surgical instrument with a sliding blade for excising a tonsil or the uvula.

Gull's disease (gulz) atrophy of the thyroid gland with myxedema.

gullet (gul′et) esophagus.

gum (gum) 1. a mucilaginous excretion of various plants. 2. gingiva.

 karaya g., sterculia g. see KARAYA GUM.

gumboil (gum′boyl) parulis.

gumma pl. *gummas, gum′mata* 1. a soft, gummy tumor occurring in tertiary syphilis. 2. late benign syphilis.

gummatous (gum′ah-tus) of the nature of gumma.

gummy (gum′e) 1. resembling a gum. 2. resembling a gumma.

Günther disease (gūn′ter) congenital erythropoietic porphyria.

gurney (ger′ne) a wheeled cot used in hospitals.

gustation (gus-ta′shun) the act of tasting or the sense of taste. adj., **gus′tatory**.

gut (gut) 1. intestine. 2. the primordial digestive tube, consisting of the FOREGUT, MIDGUT, and HINDGUT. 3. surgical gut.

 chromic g., chromicized g. surgical gut treated with a chromic salt to increase its resistance to absorption in tissues.

 surgical g. an absorbable sterile strand prepared from collagen derived from healthy mammals, used for absorbable SUTURES. It was originally prepared from the submucous layer of the intestines of sheep. Called also catgut.

Guthrie test (guth′re) a screening tool used with infants to determine the level of PHENYLALANINE in the blood. Blood from the head is placed on filter paper, which is then placed on agar plates with a strain of *Bacillus subtilis* that requires phenylalanine for growth. If there is excessive phenylalanine in the blood sample, a halo will form around the filter paper, and additional tests are required to determine the seriousness of the HYPERPHENYLALANINEMIA.

gutta (gut′ah), pl. *gut′tae* [L.] drop.

gutta-percha (gut″ah-per′chah) the coagulated, dried, purified latex of trees of the genera *Palaguium* and *Payena,* most commonly *Palaguium gutta;* used in orthopedics for fracture splints, in surgery for temporary sealing of cavities, and in dentistry in the form of cones for filling root canals or sticks for sealing cavities over treatment.

guttat. [L.] *gutta′tim* (drop by drop).

guttate (gut′āt) resembling a drop.

guttatim (gŭ-ta′tim) [L.] drop by drop.

guttural (gut′er-al) pertaining to the THROAT; see also PHARYNGEAL.

Gy gray.

gymnospore (jim′no-spor) a spore without a protective envelope.

gyn(o)- word element [Gr.], *woman.*

gynaec(o)- for words beginning thus, see those beginning *gynec(o)-*.

gynandrism (gi-, jĭ-nan′drizm) 1. female PSEUDOHERMAPHRODITISM. 2. hermaphroditism. 3. masculinization in a female.

gynandroblastoma (gi-, jĭ-nan″dro-blas-to′mah) an ovarian tumor containing elements of both ARRHENOBLASTOMA and GRANULOSA CELL TUMOR; it produces both ANDROGENIC and ESTROGENIC effects.

gynandroid (gi-, jĭ-nan′droid) 1. a hermaphrodite, a female pseudohermaphrodite, or a female exhibiting masculinization. 2. pertaining to or characterized by such a condition.

gynandromorph (gi-, ji-nan'dro-morf) an organism exhibiting gynandromorphism.

gynandromorphism (gi-, ji-nan"dro-mor'-fizm) the presence of chromosomes of both sexes in different tissues of the body, which produces a mosaic of male and female sex characteristics. adj., **gynandro-mor'phous**.

gyne- word element [Gr.], *woman.*

gynec(o)- word element [Gr.], *woman.*

gynecogenic (gi"ně-, jin"ě-ko-jen'ik) producing female characteristics.

gynecography (gi"ně-, jin"ě-kog'rah-fe) radiography of the female reproductive organs.

gynecoid (gi"ně-, jin'ě-koid,) woman-like.

gynecologist (gi"ně-, jin"ě-kol'ah-jist) a physician who specializes in the medical care of conditions unique to women.

gynecology (gi"ně-, jin"ě-kol'ah-je) the study of diseases unique to women, especially those of the genital tract and breasts.

gynecomastia (gi"ně-, jin"ě-ko-mas'te-ah) enlargement of one or both breasts in a male, usually seen in adolescents or elderly men due to excessive estrogen activity; occasionally there is even excretion of milk.

gynecopathy (gi"ně-, jin"ě-kop'ah-the) any disease unique to women.

Gyne-Lotrimin (gi"ně-lo'tri-min) trademark for a preparation of CLOTRIMAZOLE, an antifungal AGENT.

gynephobia (gi"ně-, jin"ě-fo'be-ah) irrational fear of or aversion to women.

gynogenesis (gi"no-, jin"o-jen'ě-sis) development of an egg that is stimulated by a sperm in the absence of any participation of the sperm nucleus.

gynopathic (gi"no-, jin"o-path'ik) pertaining to disease of women.

gynoplastics (gi"no-, jin'o-plas"tiks) plastic or reconstructive surgery of female reproductive organs. adj., **gynoplas'tic**.

gypsum (jip'sum) native CALCIUM SULFATE, which when calcined becomes PLASTER OF PARIS; used in making plaster casts for fractures and for taking dental impressions.

gyrate (ji'rāt) convoluted; ring- or spiral-shaped.

gyration (ji-ra'shun) revolution about a fixed center.

gyrectomy (ji-rek'to-me) excision or resection of a cerebral gyrus, or a portion of the cerebral cortex.

Gyrencephala (ji"ren-sef'ah-lah) a group of higher mammals, including humans and other primates, having cerebral hemispheres marked by convolutions.

gyrencephalic (ji"ren-sě-fal'ik) 1. pertaining to the Gyrencephala. 2. having cerebral hemispheres marked by convolutions.

gyrospasm (ji'ro-spazm) rotatory spasm of the head.

gyrus (ji'rus), pl. *gy'ri* [L.] one of the many CONVOLUTIONS of the surface of the cerebral HEMISPHERES caused by infolding of the cortex, separated by fissures or sulci; called also cerebral gyrus.

angular g. one continuous anteriorly with the supramarginal gyrus.

annectent gyri various small folds on the cerebral surface that are too inconstant to bear specific names; called also gyri transitivi.

Broca's g. inferior frontal gyrus.

central g., anterior precentral gyrus.

central g., posterior postcentral gyrus.

cerebral g. gyrus.

cingulate g., g. cin'guli an arch-shaped convolution situated just above the corpus callosum.

frontal g. any of the three (inferior, middle, and superior) gyri of the frontal lobe.

fusiform g. one on the inferior surface of the hemisphere between the inferior temporal and parahippocampal gyri, consisting of a lateral (lateral occipitotemporal gyrus) and a medial (medial occipitotemporal gyrus) part.

hippocampal g., g. hippocam'pi one on the inferior surface of each cerebral hemisphere, lying between the hippocampal and collateral fissures; called also parahippocampal gyrus.

infracalcarine g., lingual g. one on the occipital lobe that forms the inferior lip of the calcerine sulcus and, together with the cuneus, the visual cortex.

marginal g. the middle frontal gyrus.

occipital g. any of the three (superior, middle, and inferior) gyri of the occipital lobe.

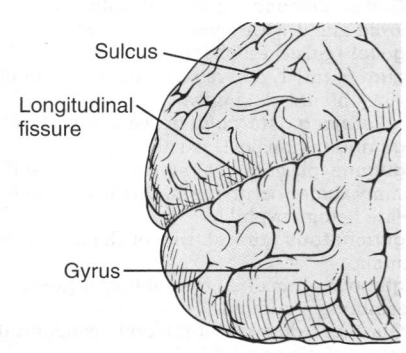

Cerebral gyri. From Applegate, 1996.

occipitotemporal g., lateral the lateral portion of the fusiform gyrus.

occipitotemporal g., medial the medial portion of the fusiform gyrus.

orbital gyri irregular gyri on the orbital surface of the frontal lobe.

parahippocampal g. hippocampal gyrus.

paraterminal g. a thin sheet of gray matter in front of and ventral to the genu of the corpus callosum.

postcentral g. the convolution of the frontal lobe immediately behind the central sulcus; the primary sensory area of the cerebral cortex; called also posterior central gyrus.

precentral g. the convolution of the frontal lobe immediately in front of the central sulcus; the primary motor area of

the cerebral cortex; called also anterior central gyrus.

g. rec′tus a cerebral convolution on the orbital aspect of the frontal lobe.

supramarginal g. that part of the inferior parietal convolution which curves around the upper end of the fissure of Sylvius.

temporal g. any of the gyri of the temporal lobe, including inferior, middle, superior, and transverse temporal gyri; the more prominent of the latter (anterior transverse temporal gyrus) represents the cortical center for hearing.

gy′ri transiti′vi annectent gyri.

uncinate g. the uncus.

G

H

H hydrogen; Hounsfield unit.

h. [L.] ho′ra (hour).

H⁺ symbol, *hydrogen ion.*

h hecto-; hour.

HA hepatitis A.

HAART highly active antiretroviral therapy.

habena (hah-be′nah), pl. *habe′nae* [L.] the peduncle of the pineal body.

habenula (hah-ben′u-lah), pl. *haben′ulae* [L.] 1. any frenulum, especially one of a series of structures in the cochlea. 2. a triangular area in the dorsomedial surface of the thalamus anterior to the pineal gland. adj., **haben′ular.**

habilitation (hah-bil″ĭ-ta′shun) the assisting of a child with achieving developmental skills when impairments have caused delaying or blocking of initial acquisition of the skills. Habilitation can include cognitive, social, fine motor, gross motor, or other skills that contribute to mobility, communication, and performance of ACTIVITIES OF DAILY LIVING and enhance quality of life.

habit (hab′it) 1. an action that has become automatic or characteristic by repetition. 2. predisposition; bodily temperament.

habituation (hah-bich″u-a′shun) 1. the gradual adaptation to a stimulus or to the environment. 2. the extinction of a conditioned reflex by repetition of the conditioned stimulus. 3. older term denoting sometimes tolerance and other times a psychological dependence resulting from the repeated consumption of a drug, with a desire to continue its use, but with little or no tendency to increase the dose.

habitus (hab′ĭ-tus) 1. posture or position of the body. 2. physique; body build and constitution. See also body TYPE.

hachement (ahsh-maw′) [Fr.] a hacking or chopping stroke in massage.

hae- for words beginning thus, see also those beginning *he-*.

haema (he′mah) [Gr.] blood.

Haemophilus (he-mof′ĭ-lus) a genus of hemophilic gram-negative bacteria. *H. aphro′-philus, H. parainfluen′zae,* and *H. paraphro′-philus* are part of the normal oral flora and are occasionally associated with endocarditis. Pathogenic species include *H. aegyp′tius,* the cause of PINKEYE (acute contagious conjunctivitis); *H. ducrey′i,* the cause of CHANCROID; and *H. influen′zae,* a species once thought to cause epidemic INFLUENZA. A species formerly called *H. vagina′lis* is now called *Gardnerella vaginalis. H. influenzae* type b, rather than causing INFLUENZA, can cause MENINGITIS, PNEUMONIA, and serious throat and ear infections, particularly in children under the age of five years; vaccination against it is recommended for all children.

hafnium (Hf) (haf′ne-um) a chemical element, atomic number 72, atomic weight 178.49. (See Appendix 6.)

Hailey-Hailey disease (ha′le ha′le) benign familial pemphigus.

hair (hār) 1. any thin, threadlike structure. 2. especially, the specialized epidermal structure produced only by mammals, developing from a papilla sunk in the CORIUM. The life cycle of a hair (hair CYCLE) consists of three phases, called ANAGEN, CATAGEN, and TELOGEN. Called also pilus. 3. the aggregate of such structures.

bamboo h. trichorrhexis nodosa.

beaded h. hair marked with alternate swellings and constrictions; seen in MONILETHRIX.

burrowing h. one that grows horizontally in the skin, causing a papule that may become infected; see also pili cuniculati, under PILUS.

club h. a hair whose root is surrounded by a bulbous enlargement composed of keratinized cells, preliminary to normal loss of the hair from the follicle.

Frey's h's stiff hairs mounted in a handle; used for testing the sensitiveness of pressure points of the skin.

ingrown h. one that has curved and reentered the skin, causing a papule that may become infected. See also pili incarnati, under PILUS.

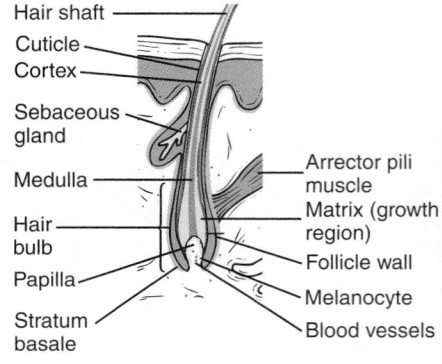

Hair shaft — Cuticle — Cortex — Sebaceous gland — Medulla — Hair bulb — Papilla — Stratum basale — Arrector pili muscle — Matrix (growth region) — Follicle wall — Melanocyte — Blood vessels

Structure of hair and hair follicles. From Applegate, 2000.

WINDOW ON HAEMOPHILUS INFLUENZAE, TYPE b

Haemophilus influenzae, type b (Hib) used to be the leading cause of invasive bacterial disease in children under the age of 5; it was manifested as meningitis, epiglottitis, pneumonia, septic arthritis, and cellulitis. Prior to the start of effective immunization in 1991, it affected more than 20,000 Americans each year, with a mortality rate of 4.5%, most of whom were children. Morbidity was high, especially from meningitis, where 38% of those affected developed blindness, deafness, paralysis, and/or mental retardation. Hib colonizes in the nasopharynx and is spread by respiratory droplets. While there are 6 types of Haemophilus influenzae (a–f), type b is the most dangerous. The first Hib vaccines were introduced in 1974 but were ineffective in children under the age of 2, the ages when most children were affected. Current vaccines are conjugated, connecting Hib to an immunogenic protein, such as diphtheria toxoid, Neisseria meningitidis, or tetanus toxoid; there is NO antibody response to these additional proteins.

It is recommended that all children be immunized against Hib, starting at 2 months of age. The initial series varies depending on the brand; some include doses at 2 and 4 months, others at 2, 4, and 6 months. All brands have a booster around 15 months of age. If a child is over 15 months and has not been immunized against Hib, only one dose is needed. No vaccine is recommended after 17 months of age. By 2000, there had been a 99% decrease in the incidence of Hib. Hib vaccines are very safe and can be given simultaneously with other vaccines if different sites are used.

JANICE SELEKMAN DNSc, RN

---

lanugo h. the fine hair on the body of the fetus.

moniliform h. beaded hair.

pubic h. the hair on the external genitalia; called also pubes.

sensory h's hairlike projections on the surface of sensory epithelial cells.

tactile h's hairs sensitive to touch.

taste h's short hairlike processes projecting freely into the lumen of the pit of a taste bud from the peripheral ends of the taste cells.

terminal h. the coarse hair on various areas of the body during adult years.

twisted h. a hair that is twisted through an axis of 180 degrees at spaced intervals, being abnormally flattened at the site of twisting. See also pili torti, under PILUS.

hairball (hār′bawl) trichobezoar; a concretion of hair sometimes found in the stomach or intestines of humans or other animals.

halation (hah-la′shun) indistinctness of the visual image caused by strong illumination coming from the same direction as the object being viewed.

halazepam (hal-az′e-pam) a benzodiazepine oral ANTIANXIETY AGENT.

halazone (hal′ah-zōn) a white, crystalline powder used as a disinfectant for water supplies.

halcinonide (hal-sin′o-nīd) a synthetic CORTICOSTEROID used topically as an anti-inflammatory and antipruritic in the treatment of certain dermatoses.

Haldol (hal′dol) trademark for a preparation of HALOPERIDOL, an ANTIPSYCHOTIC AGENT.

half-life (haf′līf′) the time required for the decay of half of a sample of particles of a radionuclide or elementary particle; see also RADIOACTIVITY. Symbol t_{12} or T_{12}.

half-time (haf′tīm′) the time required for one half of a quantity of a substance to be eliminated from a system when the substance is eliminated at a rate proportional to its concentration. Symbol t_{12} or T_{12}.

halfway house a residence for patients (e.g., mental patients, drug addicts, alcoholics) who do not require hospitalization but who need an intermediate degree of care until they can return to the community.

halide (hal′īd) a compound of a halogen with an element or radical.

halisteresis (hah-lis″ter-e′sis) deficiency of mineral salts (calcium) in a part, as in osteomalacia.

halitosis (hal″ĭ-to′sis) offensive odor of the breath.

halitus (hal′ĭ-tus) exhalation (def. 3).

Hall (hawl) Lydia E. (1906–1969) founder and first director of the Loeb Center for Nursing and Rehabilitation at Montefiore Hospital in the Bronx. Her work as a researcher and consultant at the New York Heart Association and as project director of nursing and long-term illnesses for the Division of Chronic Illnesses and Tuberculosis of the U.S. Public Health Service led her to believe that the nurse-patient relationship is therapeutic in itself and that the chief need of the chronically ill patient is professional nursing care. The establishment of the Loeb Center, providing professional nursing care in an institutional setting, enabled her to put her theories into practice.

Hallervorden-Spatz syndrome (hal′er-for″den-spatz′) a hereditary disorder involving marked reduction in the number of myelin sheaths of the globus pallidus and substantia nigra, with accumulations of iron pigment, progressive rigidity beginning in the legs, choreoathetoid movements, dysarthria, and progressive mental deterioration.

hallucination (hah-loo″sĭ-na′shun) a sensory impression (sight, touch, sound, smell, or taste) that has no basis in external stimulation. Hallucinations can have psychologic causes, as in mental illness, or they can result from drugs, alcohol, organic illnesses, such as brain tumor or senility, or exhaustion. When hallucinations have a psychologic origin, they usually represent a disguised form of a repressed conflict. adj. **hallu′cinative, hallu′cinatory.**

auditory h. a hallucination of hearing; the most common type.

gustatory h. a hallucination of taste.

haptic h. tactile hallucination.

hypnagogic h. a vivid, dreamlike hallucination occurring at sleep onset.

hypnopompic h. a vivid, dreamlike hallucination occurring on awakening.

kinesthetic h. a hallucination involving the sense of bodily movement.

olfactory h. a hallucination of smell.

somatic h. a hallucination involving the perception of a physical experience occurring within the body.

tactile h. a hallucination of touch.

visual h. a hallucination of sight.

hallucinogen (hah-loo′sĭ-no-jen″) a chemical agent capable of producing HALLUCINATIONS. adj., **hallucinogen′ic.** Drugs that have hallucinogenic properties include LSD, MESCALINE, and PSILOCYBIN. Certain mushrooms, seeds, and cactus buttons (such as PEYOTE) are also hallucinogenic. The experiences brought about by the use of hallucinogens involve a more acute "awareness" of one's environment and a distorted response to visual, auditory, and tactile stimuli. They

can also cause a person to exhibit behavior symptomatic of a psychotic state of mind. Indiscriminate use of these compounds can bring on PSYCHOSIS and may result in permanent brain damage. DRUG ABUSE with hallucinogens has led to the regulation of their distribution by the Food and Drug Administration.

hallucinogenesis (hah-loo″sĭ-no-jen′ĕ-sis) the production of hallucinations.

hallucinosis (hah-lu″sĭ-no′sis) a state characterized by HALLUCINATIONS without other impairment of consciousness. adj. **hallucinot′ic.**

organic h. a term used in a former system of classification, denoting an ORGANIC MENTAL SYNDROME characterized by HALLUCINATIONS caused by a specific organic factor and not associated with CLOUDING OF CONSCIOUSNESS (DELIRIUM), intellectual impairment (DEMENTIA), mood disturbance, or prominent delusions (ORGANIC DELUSIONAL SYNDROME). Such disorders are now mainly classified as substance-induced psychotic disorders and psychotic disorders due to a general medical condition. See also SUBSTANCE-INDUCED DISORDERS.

hallux (hal′uks), pl. *hal′luces* [L.] the great toe.

h. doloro′sus a painful disease of the great toe, usually associated with flatfoot.

h. flex′us hallux rigidus.

h. mal′leus hammer toe affecting the great toe.

h. ri′gidus painful flexion deformity of the great toe with limitation of motion at the metatarsophalangeal joint.

h. val′gus angulation of the great toe toward the other toes of the foot.

h. va′rus angulation of the great toe away from the other toes of the foot.

halo (ha′lo) a circular structure, such as a luminous circle seen surrounding an object or light.

Fick's h. a colored circle appearing around a light, experienced by wearers of contact lenses.

h. glaucomato′sus, glaucomatous h. a narrow light zone surrounding the optic disk in glaucoma.

senile h. a zone of variable width around the optic disk, due to exposure of various elements of the choroid as a result of senile atrophy of the pigmented epithelium.

halobetasol (hal″o-ba′tah-sol) a very high potency synthetic CORTICOSTEROID used topically in the form of the propionate as an ANTIINFLAMMATORY and ANTIPRURITIC agent.

halogen (hal′o-jen) an element of group VII of the periodic table, the members of which form similar (saltlike) compounds in combination with sodium. The halogens are bromine, chlorine, fluorine, iodine, and astatine.

halofantrine (-fan′trēn) an antimalarial agent used as the hydrochloride salt in treatment of acute MALARIA due to *Plasmodium falciparum* or *P. vivax*.

halometer (hah-lom′ĕ-ter) 1. an instrument for measuring ocular HALOS. 2. an instrument for estimating the size of ERYTHROCYTES by measuring the halos formed around them when a beam of light shines on them and is diffracted.

haloperidol (hal″o-per′ĭ-dol) an ANTIPSYCHOTIC AGENT of the butyrophenone group; used for the management of symptoms of psychoses and for control of the vocal utterances and tics of GILLES DE LA TOURETTE'S SYNDROME.

halophil (hal′o-fil) a microorganism that requires a high concentration of salt for optimal growth.

halophilic (hal″o-fil′ik) pertaining to or characterized by an affinity for salt; requiring a high concentration of salt for optimal growth.

haloprogin (hah″lo-pro′jin) a synthetic topical antifungal AGENT used in the treatment of TINEA.

Halotestin (hal″o-tes′tin) trademark for a preparation of FLUOXYMESTERONE, an androgen used in the palliative treatment of metastatic breast cancer and in replacement THERAPY for male HYPOGONADISM and delayed male puberty.

halothane (hal′o-thān) an inhalational anesthetic used for induction and maintenance of general ANESTHESIA.

Ham test one for paroxysmal nocturnal HEMOGLOBINURIA, performed by incubating red blood cells in an acid environment; a positive test may be obtained in other forms of anemia.

hamartia (ham-ahr′she-ah) a defect of tissue combination during development.

hamartoblastoma (ham-ahr″to-blas-to′mah) a tumor developing from a HAMARTOMA.

hamartoma (ham″ahr-to′mah) a benign tumorlike nodule composed of an overgrowth of mature cells and tissues normally present in the affected part, but often with one element predominating.

hamartomatous (ham″ahr-to′mah-tus) pertaining to a disturbance in growth of a tissue in which the cells of a circumscribed area outstrip those of the surrounding areas.

hamate (ham′āt) shaped like a hook, as the hamate bone (see anatomic Table of Bones in the Appendices). See also UNCINATE.

Hamman's disease (ham′anz) interstitial emphysema of the lungs due to spontaneous rupture of the alveoli.

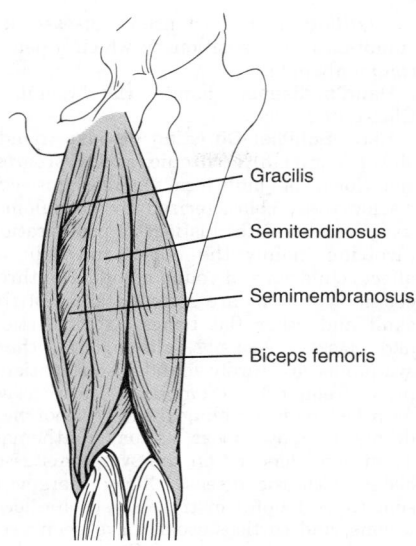

The inner and outer hamstrings.

Hamman-Rich syndrome (ham′an rich′) idiopathic pulmonary fibrosis.

hammer (ham′er) malleus.

hamstring (ham′string) one of the tendons that laterally and medially bound the depression in the popliteal FOSSA (posterior region of the knee).

inner h's the tendons of the gracilis, sartorius, and two other muscles of the lower limb (see anatomic Table of Muscles in the Appendices).

outer h. the tendon of the biceps muscle of the thigh (see anatomic Table of Muscles in the Appendices).

hamulus (ham′u-lus), pl. *ham′uli* [L.] any hook-shaped process.

hand (hand) the terminal part of the upper limb of a human or a nonhuman primate.

ape h. one with the thumb permanently extended.

cleft h. a malformation in which the division between the fingers extends into the metacarpus; also, a hand with the middle digits absent.

claw h. see CLAWHAND.

drop h. wristdrop.

lobster-claw h. cleft hand.

obstetrician's h. the contraction of the hand in tetany; the hand is flexed at the wrist, the fingers are flexed at the metacarpophalangeal joints but extended at the interphalangeal joints, and the thumb is strongly flexed into the palm.

writing h. in Parkinson's disease, assumption of the position by which a pen is commonly held.

Hand's disease (handz) Hand-Schüller-Christian disease.

Hand-Schüller-Christian disease (hand'-shil'er kris'chan) a chronic, slowly progressive form of multifocal Langerhans cell HISTIOCYTOSIS, characterized by granulomatous lesions with histiocyte proliferation involving mainly the bones and skin; it affects children and young adults. The three classic symptoms are softened areas of the skull and other flat bones, EXOPHTHALMOS, and DIABETES INSIPIDUS, although all three symptoms are rarely found in one patient. OTITIS frequently accompanies the disease. Skin lesions resembling those of seborrheic dermatitis may appear, as may xanthomas. Treatment depends on the symptoms associated with the disease. X-ray therapy is sometimes helpful in treating specific local lesions, and corticosteroids have been used with success in some cases. Complete recovery does occur, but about 40 per cent of the cases end fatally. Called also Hand's disease, Schüller's disease, Schüller-Christian disease, and chronic idiopathic xanthomatosis.

H and E hematoxylin and eosin (stain).

handedness (hand'ed-nes) the preferential use of the hand of one side in all voluntary motor acts; see also DEXTRALITY and SINISTRALITY.

hand-foot-and-mouth disease a mild, highly infectious viral disease of children, with vesicular lesions in the mouth and on the hands and feet.

handicap (han'de-kap) 1. a term that is considered offensive when used to denote a physical or mental IMPAIRMENT or characteristic that prevents a person from participating independently in any ACTIVITY OF DAILY LIVING. 2. according to the World Health Organization, a disadvantage that interferes with performance of life roles and is social, cultural, economic, or environmental in nature. For example, social stigma or environmental barriers may interfere with the employment of a person using a wheelchair even when the person is able to function independently (i.e., lacks a true DISABILITY).

hangnail (hang'nāl) a shred of CUTICLE at one side of a nail; it is prevented by gently pushing the cuticle instead of cutting it, and is treated by clipping off the shred of skin and applying antiseptic to prevent infection.

hangover (hang'o-ver) unpleasant symptoms that occur 4 to 6 hours after excessive ingestion of alcohol; see ALCOHOLISM.

Hanot's disease (ah-nōz') biliary cirrhosis.

Hansen's disease (han'sunz) leprosy.

Hantavirus (han'tah-vi''rus) a genus of viruses that cause epidemic hemorrhagic fever or pneumonia in humans, who are probably infected by contact with the waste products of rodents.

haphalgesia (haf''al-je'ze-ah) pain on touching objects.

haphephobia (haf''e-fo'be-ah) irrational fear of being touched.

haploid (hap'loid) having half the number of chromosomes characteristically found in the somatic (diploid) cells of an organism; typical of the gametes of a species whose union restores the diploid number.

haploidentity (hap''lo-i-den'tĭ-te) the condition of having the same antigenic phenotype at certain specified loci; said of donor-recipient combinations in transplantation studies.

haploidy (hap'loi-de) the state of being haploid.

haploscope (hap'lo-skōp) an instrument that presents two separate views to the two eyes so that the views may be seen as one integrated view; it is used to measure, test, or stimulate various binocular functions. adj., **haploscop'ic**.

haplotype (hap'lo-tīp) 1. a set of alleles of a group of closely linked genes, such as the HLA complex, which are usually inherited as a unit, an individual inheriting a complete haplotype from each parent. 2. the genetic constitution of an individual at a set of linked genes.

hapten (hap'ten) a small molecule, not antigenic by itself, that can react with specific antibodies and elicit the formation of such antibodies when conjugated to a larger antigenic molecule, usually a protein, called in this context the carrier. Antibody production involves activation of B LYMPHOCYTES by the hapten and helper T CELLS by the carrier.

haptic (hap'tik) tactile.

haptics (hap'tiks) the study of the sense of TOUCH.

haptoglobin (hap'to-glo''bin) a group of serum alpha$_2$-globulin glycoproteins that bind free hemoglobin; three phenotypes, with differing abilities to bind hemoglobin, are distinguished electrophoretically.

Harada syndrome (hah-rah'dah) Vogt-Koyanagi-Harada syndrome.

hardening (hahr'den-ing) 1. sclerosis. 2. the process of making more firm.

h. of arteries popular term for ARTERIOSCLEROSIS.

work h. see WORK HARDENING.

hardiness (hahr'dĭ-nes) a complex personality attribute that has been identified as a component in the maintenance of health and is the focus of intensive research activities. Generally, there are three elements that contribute to hardiness: control, commitment, and challenge. Control is the belief that an individual can influence events or occurrences, commitment is the deep feeling of involvement in daily activities, and challenge is viewed as an opportunity for development.

harelip (har'lip) cleft lip.

harmonic acceleration test (hahr-mon'ik-ak-sel″er-a'shun) rotation of a patient in a chair in the darkness, with monitoring of eye movements; with normal vestibulo-ocular reflexes the eyes should undergo similar rotatory NYSTAGMUS in both eyes in the direction opposite to that of the rotation.

harness (har'nes) a support device used to immobilize a body part or hold it in position.

   Pavlik h. a device used correct hip dislocations in infants with developmental dysplasia of the hip, consisting of a set of straps that hold the hips in flexion and abduction.

Hartmann's operation (hahrt'manz) resection of a diseased portion of the colon, with the proximal end of the colon brought out as a colostomy and the distal stump or rectum being closed by suture. Bowel continuity can later be restored.

Hartmannella (hahrt″mah-nel'ah) a genus of free-living protozoa found in fresh water and soil, species of which can cause a primary amebic meningoencephalitis, especially in immunocompromised hosts.

hartmannelliasis (hahrt″mah-nel-i'ah-sis) infection with *Hartmannella.*

Hartnup disease (hahrt'nup) a genetically determined disorder of intestinal and renal transport of neutral alpha-amino acids, with pellagra-like skin lesions, transient cerebellar ataxia, constant renal aminoaciduria and other biochemical abnormalities.

harvest (hahr'vest) to remove tissues or cells from a donor for transplantation.

harvest fever spirochetosis affecting harvest workers, due to *Leptospira interrogans* serogroup *grippotyphosa,* with fever, diarrhea, conjunctivitis, stupor, and vomiting.

Harvey (hahr've) William (1578–1657). English physician and physiologist. Born at Folkestone in Kent, he attended the universities of Cambridge and Padua, and announced in 1628 his discovery of the circulation of blood, which was a model of accurate experimentation and inductive proof and the first application of quantitative demonstration in any biologic investigation. His *De generatione animalium* is

important in the history of embryology, for in it Harvey rejected the doctrine of preformation of the fetus and stated that almost all animals, including humans, are produced from eggs.

Hashimoto's disease (hash″ĭ-mo'tō) a progressive type of autoimmune THYROIDITIS characterized by goiter and gradually developing hypothyroidism with lymphocytic infiltration of the gland and circulating antithyroid antibodies; women are most commonly affected, and there is a familial predisposition to the disease. Called also Hashimoto's thyroiditis or struma.

hashish (hash-ēsh') a preparation of resin scraped from the flowering tops of the plant *Cannabis sativa,* smoked or chewed for its intoxicating effects; it is far more potent than MARIJUANA.

hashitoxicosis (hash″ĭ-tok″sĭ-ko'sis) excessive functional activity of the thyroid gland in patients with HASHIMOTO'S DISEASE, in whom decreased thyroid function would ordinarily be expected.

hatchet (hach'et) a bibeveled or single beveled cutting dental instrument having its cutting edge in line with the axis of its blade; used for breaking down tooth structures undermined by caries, for smoothing cavity walls, and for sharpening line and point angles.

haustration (haws-tra'shun) 1. the formation of a haustrum. 2. a haustral CONTRACTION. 3. haustrum.

haustrum (haws'trum), pl. *haus'tra* [L.] one of the pouches of the colon, produced by adaptation of its length to the TAENIA COLI, or by collection of circular muscle fibers 1 or 2 cm apart; the haustra are responsible for the sacculated appearance of the colon. (See accompanying illustration.)

HAV hepatitis A virus.

Haverhill fever (ha'ver-il) an acute form of RAT-BITE FEVER caused by *Streptobacillus moniliformis* and transmitted by the bite of an infected rat. Characteristics include an erythematous eruption and more or less generalized arthritis, with adenitis, headache, and vomiting. It was first described in Haverhill, Massachusetts, in 1926.

haversian (ha-ver'shan) named for the English physician and anatomist Clopton Havers, 1650–1702.

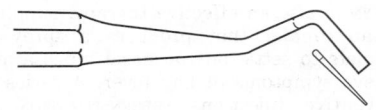

Hatchet. From Dorland's, 2000.

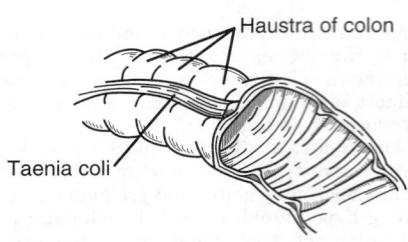

Haustra of colon

Taenia coli

Haustrum. From Dorland's, 2000.

hay fever an atopic ALLERGY characterized by sneezing, itching and watery eyes, nasal discharge, and a burning sensation of the palate and throat. It is a localized anaphylactic reaction to an extrinsic allergen, usually pollen or the spores of molds. When the allergen comes in contact with cell-bound IMMUNOGLOBULIN E in the tissues of the conjunctiva, nasal mucosa, and bronchial tree, the tissues release mediators of ANAPHYLAXIS and produce the characteristic symptoms of hay fever.

The amount of pollen in the air varies with the season and geographic area. East of the Rocky Mountains, the peak of the regional hay fever season occurs between mid-August and mid-September, when the air is heavy with the pollen of the ragweed plant. An appreciable number of hay fever sufferers are also reactive to the spring pollens from grasses and trees. Mold-bearing plants such as wheat, barley, and corn are prevalent in the agricultural areas of the Midwest, and attacks of hay fever caused by mold spores are common there as these crops ripen.

Hay fever should be recognized as more than a mere nuisance. By causing lack of sleep and loss of appetite, it can lower the body's resistance to disease. It can cause inflammation of the ears, sinuses, throat, and bronchi. Some hay fever sufferers develop ASTHMA.

Hay fever can be relieved, although not cured, by ANTIHISTAMINES and SYMPATHOMIMETIC drugs such as EPHEDRINE and PHENYLPROPANOLAMINE hydrochloride. LORATADINE and DESLORATADINE are newer antihistamines that do not cause the drowsiness, mental dullness, and sleepiness that were traditionally associated with antihistamines. CROMOLYN is also an effective therapy, supplied in an inhaler that produces a spray of droplets to settle on the nasal mucosa and relieve symptoms of hay fever. A series of preventive injections (DESENSITIZATION or HYPOSENSITIZATION) may be recommended in advance of the hay fever season. This consists of administering controlled and gradually increasing amounts of the offending substance in order to develop a certain amount of immunity. Air conditioning may help give relief by filtering much of the pollen from the air.

   nonseasonal h. f., perennial h. f. nonseasonal allergic rhinitis.

   hazards of immobility complications that are associated with a limited or absolute lack of movement by the patient; various members of the health care team may collaborate to assist the patient in avoiding these problems. See accompanying table, and see also DISUSE SYNDROME.

   HB hepatitis B.

   Hb hemoglobin.

   HBcAg hepatitis B core antigen.

   HBeAg hepatitis B e antigen.

   HBIG hepatitis B immune globulin.

   HBO hyperbaric oxygenation.

   HBsAg hepatitis B surface antigen.

   HBV hepatitis B virus.

   HCFA Health Care Financing Administration, former name for the Centers for Medicare and Medicade Services (CMS).

   HCG, hCG human chorionic gonadotropin.

   HCl hydrochloric acid.

   HD hemodialysis.

   H disease Hartnup disease.

   HDL high-density LIPOPROTEIN.

   HDL-C high-density-lipoprotein cholesterol; see CHOLESTEROL.

   H & E (stain) hematoxylin and eosin.

   He helium.

   head (hed) 1. the anterior or superior part of a structure or organism. 2. in vertebrates, the part of the body containing the brain and the organs of special sense. Called also caput.

   articular h. an eminence on a bone by which it articulates with another bone.

   h. injury traumatic injury to the head resulting from a fall or violent blow. Such an injury may be open or closed and may involve a brain CONCUSSION, skull fracture, or contusions of the brain. All head injuries are potentially dangerous because there can be a slow leakage of blood from damaged blood vessels into or around the brain. Such a process will gradually increase pressure within the skull and compress the surrounding brain (see HEMATOMA).

   One of the most common complications of head injury is *subdural hematoma,* resulting from the oozing of blood from the cortical veins and the small blood vessels that lie between the arachnoid and the dura mater. A less common but more serious complication that constitutes an extreme surgical

HAZARDS OF IMMOBILITY

System	Complication	Prevention Measures
Cardiovascular	Orthostatic hypotension	Active and passive range of motion exercises
	Increased venous stasis leading to thrombus formation and embolism	Antiembolic stockings
Gastrointestinal	Constipation	Increased activity level
	Decreased GI motility	High fiber diet
		Adequate fluid intake
Integumentary	Pressure ulcers	Frequent turning and repositioning
	Interruptions in skin integrity	Use of pressure relieving devices
		Adequate nutrition
		Frequent inspection of skin
Musculoskeletal	Contractures	Range of motion exercises
	Osteoporosis	Weight bearing when possible
	Muscle weakness and atrophy	Maintaining good body alignment
Neurologic	Disorientation	Control of sensory stimulation
		Frequent orientation to person, place and time
		Maintaining an appropriate sleep-wake schedule
Renal	Calculi	Increased fluid intake
	Urinary tract infection	Maintain an acidic urine
Respiratory	Pneumonia	Frequent repositioning
		Coughing and deep breathing exercises

emergency is *epidural hematoma,* a collection of blood in the space between the skull and the dura mater. The leaking of blood into the epidural space is the result of the rupture of a large meningeal artery. It progresses rapidly and therefore requires immediate treatment. A third complication that may occur following head injury is HERNIATION of either the brainstem or a part of the cerebellum through the tentorial hiatus (*transtentorial herniation*). This is an extreme emergency demanding immediate relief of pressure against the blood vessels serving the brain stem and cerebellum.

Long-term effects of head injury include chronic headache, disturbances in mental and motor function, diabetes insipidus, and a host of other symptoms that may or may not be psychogenic. Organic brain damage and posttraumatic epilepsy resulting from scar formation are possible sequels to head injury.

Treatment. The method of treatment will depend on the kind and amount of damage inflicted on the brain and surrounding membranes. Surgical procedures to relieve intracranial pressure include the drilling of burr holes in the skull to aspirate accumulated blood, and intracranial surgery to remove hematomas. Edema of brain tissue may be reduced by the intravenous administration of mannitol. DEXAMETHASONE (DECADRON), a STEROID ANTIINFLAMMATORY agent that has little salt-retaining action, is often used. If no immediate surgery is indicated, the physician may choose to treat the head injury conservatively, with rest and quiet and the careful monitoring of the patient for signs of change in the neurologic status.

Patient Care. Continuous monitoring of the vital signs and assessment of the patient's neurologic status are essential to the care of the patient with a head injury. Fluid intake and output are measured and recorded and are limited according to the degree of edema present. Intravenous fluids must be given with caution and oral liquids allowed as soon as the patient is able to swallow. An excessively large urinary output is reported immediately, as this may indicate damage to the hypothalamus and suppression of antidiuretic hormone.

Any one of the following symptoms should be reported to the physician: (1) changes in the patient's blood pressure, pulse, or respiratory rate, especially slowing of the pulse with a rising blood pressure; (2) extreme restlessness or excitability following a period of comparative calm; (3) changes in the level of consciousness; (4) headache that increases in intensity; (5) vomiting, especially persistent, projectile vomiting; (6) unequal size of pupils; (7) inability to move one of the extremities; (8) leakage of spinal fluid (clear yellow or pink-tinged) from the nose or ear.

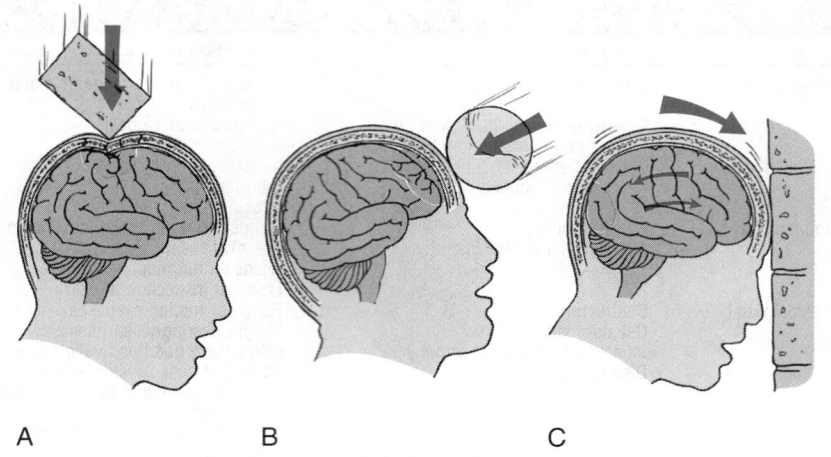

A　　　　　B　　　　　C

Some mechanisms of head injury. Head injury results from penetration or impact. *A,* A direct injury (blow to skull) may fracture the skull. Contusion and laceration of the brain may result from fractures. Depressed portions of the skull may compress or penetrate brain tissue. *B,* In the absence of skull fracture, a blow to the skull may cause the brain to move enough to tear some of the veins going from the cortical surface to the dura. Subsequently, subdural hematoma may develop. Note the areas of cerebral contusion (shaded in red). *C,* Rebound of the cranial contents may result in an area of injury opposite the point of impact. Such an injury is called a contrecoup injury. In addition to the three injuries depicted, secondary phenomena may result from the injury and cause additional brain dysfunction or damage. For example, ischemia, especially cerebral edema, may occur, elevating intracranial pressure. From Polaski and Tatro, 1996.

When leakage of spinal fluid is suspected, this can be verified by using a Clinistix test for sugar. If it is positive, the leaking fluid is spinal fluid rather than mucus. When there is leakage of spinal fluid through the nose, the patient must be warned not to blow the nose. Leakage of spinal fluid from the nose or the ear demands absolute bed rest with the head elevated 30 degrees to maintain neutral intracranial pressure and promote healing.

Patients who are unconscious must be watched closely for respiratory difficulty or inability to swallow. If the patient cannot swallow, the head must be turned to the side and the mouth and trachea suctioned as necessary to prevent aspiration of mucus into the lungs. A TRACHEOSTOMY set and VENTILATOR should be readily at hand in case severe respiratory embarrassment occurs.

Side rails are applied and the headboard of the bed is padded with pillows or a blanket if the patient is delirious or if convulsions are anticipated. An accurate record of the patient's intake and output is kept and the patient is observed for signs of retention of urine, incontinence, or abdominal distention.

sperm h., h. of spermatozoon the oval anterior end of a SPERMATOZOON, which contains the male pronucleus and is surrounded by the ACROSOME. See illustration at SPERMATOZOON.

headache (hed′āk) pain in the head; see also MIGRAINE. One of the most common ailments of humans, it is a symptom rather than a disorder in itself; it accompanies many diseases and conditions, including emotional distress. Although recurring headache may be an early sign of serious organic disease, relatively few headaches are caused by disease-induced structural changes. Most result from vasodilation of blood vessels in tissues surrounding the brain, or from tension in the neck and scalp muscles.

Immediate attention by a health care provider is indicated when (1) a severe headache comes on suddenly without apparent cause; (2) there are accompanying symptoms of neurological abnormality, for example, blurring of vision, mental confusion, loss of mental acuity or consciousness, motor dysfunction, or sensory loss; or (3) the headache is highly localized, as behind the eye or near the ear, or in one location in the head. Fever and stiffness of the neck accompanying the headache may indicate MENINGITIS.

cluster h. a migraine-like disorder marked by attacks of unilateral intense pain over the eye and forehead, with flushing and watering of the eyes and nose; attacks last about an hour and occur in clusters.

exertional h. one occurring after exercise.

histamine h. cluster headache.

lumbar puncture h. headache in the erect position, and relieved by recumbency, following lumbar puncture, due to lowering of intracranial pressure by leakage of cerebrospinal fluid through the needle tract.

migraine h. migraine.

organic h. headache due to intracranial disease or other organic disease.

tension h. a type due to prolonged overwork or emotional strain, or both, affecting especially the occipital region.

toxic h. headache due to systemic poisoning or associated with illness.

vascular h. a classification for certain types of headaches, based on a proposed etiology involving abnormal functioning of the blood vessels or vascular system of the brain; included are MIGRAINE, cluster headache, toxic headache, and headache caused by elevated blood pressure.

heading (hed′ing) a word or term found at the beginning of all or part of a piece of printed material.

Medical Subject h's (MeSH) see MeSH.

MeSH h's subject headings.

subject h's the terms chosen from medical subject headings (MeSH) to index the references appearing in MEDLINE and other NATIONAL LIBRARY OF MEDICINE databases. Called also MeSH terms and MeSH headings.

healing (hēl′ing) 1. the process of returning to health; the restoration of structure and function of injured or diseased tissues. The healing processes include blood clotting, tissue mending, scarring, and bone healing. See also WOUND HEALING. 2. the process of helping someone return to health; COMPASSION by a health care provider is part of this. Authentic perception of the experience of illness in the particular person is the essential basis.

h. by first intention, h. by primary intention WOUND HEALING in which restoration of continuity occurs directly by fibrous adhesion, without formation of granulation tissue; it results in a thin scar. (See illustration.)

h. by second intention WOUND HEALING by union by adhesion of granulating surfaces, when the edges of the wound are far apart and cannot be brought together. Granulations form from the base and sides of the wound toward the surface. (See illustration.)

h. by third intention 1. WOUND HEALING by the gradual filling of a wound cavity by

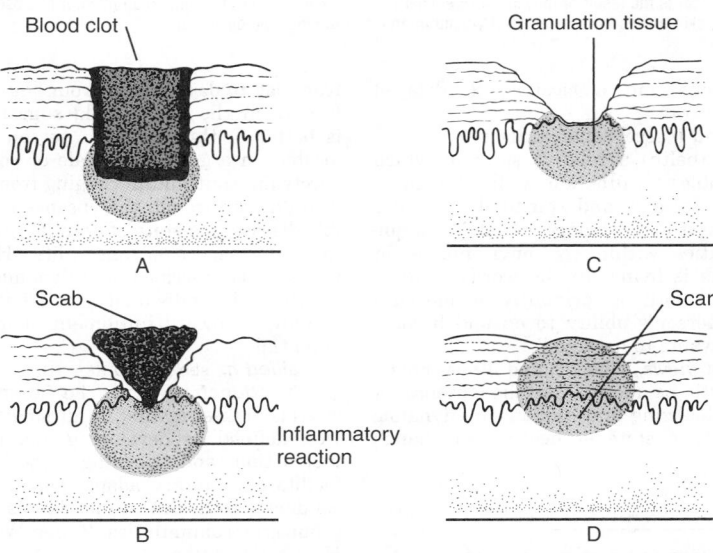

Healing by primary, or first intention. In primary wound healing there is no tissue loss. *A,* Incised wound is held together by a blood clot and possibly by sutures or surgical clamps. An inflammatory process begins in adjacent tissue at the moment of injury. *B,* After several days, granulation tissue forms as a result of migration of fibroblasts to the area of injury and formation of new capillaries. Epithelial cells at wound margin migrate to clot and seal the wound. Regenerating epithelium covers the wound. *C,* Scarring occurs as granulation tissue matures and injured tissue is replaced with connective tissue.

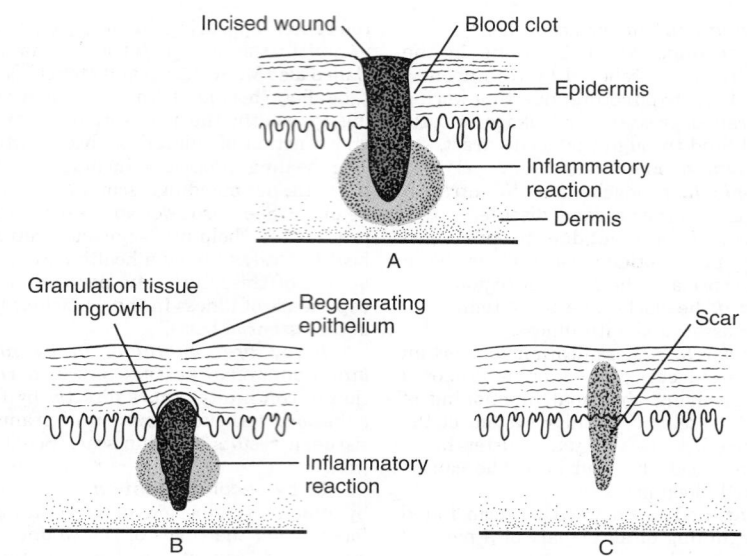

Healing by second intention occurs when there is tissue loss, as in extensive burns and deep ulcers. The healing process is more prolonged than in healing by primary intention because large amounts of dead tissue must be removed and replaced with viable cells. *A,* Open area is more extensive; inflammatory reaction is more widespread and tends to become chronic. *B,* Healing may occur under a scab formed of dried exudate, or dried plasma proteins and dead cells (eschar). *C,* Fibroblasts and capillary buds migrate toward center of would to form granulation tissue, which becomes a translucent red color as capillary network develops. Granulation tissue is fragile and bleeds easily. *D,* As granulation tissue matures, marginal epithelial cells migrate and proliferate over connective tissue base to form a scar. Contraction of skin around scar is the result of movement of epithelial cells toward center of wound in an attempt to close the defect. Surrounding skin moves toward center of wound in an effort to close the defect.

granulations and a cicatrix. 2. delayed primary CLOSURE.

wound h. see WOUND HEALING.

health (helth) a relative state in which one is able to function well physically, mentally, socially, and spiritually in order to express the full range of one's unique potentialities within the environment in which one is living. In the words of René Dubos, "health is primarily a measure of each person's ability to do and become what he wants to become."

Current views of health and illness recognize health as more than the absence of disease. Realizing that humans are dynamic beings whose state of health can change from day to day or even from hour to hour, leaders in the health field suggest that it is better to think of each person as being located on a graduated scale or continuous spectrum (continuum) ranging from obvious dire illness through the absence of discernible disease to a state of optimal functioning in every aspect of one's life. High-level WELLNESS is described as a dynamic process in which the individual is actively engaged in moving toward fulfillment of his or her potential.

allied h. see ALLIED HEALTH.

h. education. 1. in the NURSING INTERVENTIONS CLASSIFICATION, a nursing INTERVENTION defined as developing and providing instruction and learning experiences to facilitate voluntary adaptation of behavior conducive to health in individuals, families, groups, or communities. 2. See Window on Health Education.

h. as expanding consciousness a CONCEPTUAL MODEL of nursing formulated by Margaret A. NEWMAN which offers a paradigm based on the view of health as the undivided wholeness of the person in

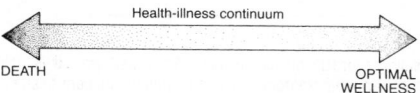

A common concept of health as a continuum ranging from optimal wellness at one end to illness culminating in death at the other end.

WINDOW ON HEALTH EDUCATION

Health education uses multidisciplinary theories and behavioral and organizational change principles that enable individuals, groups, and communities to achieve personal, environmental, and social health. In addition to individual behavior change, the field supports social and environmental policies that have the potential to promote health and prevent disease and disability. The work of professional health education specialists has expanded rapidly in the last two decades because of changes in national health policy that have placed emphasis on the underlying behavioral, social, and environmental determinants of disease and premature death, particularly risk factors that are potentially modifiable through individual behavior change. Thus, health education is an important strategy in the nation's effort to achieve the *Year 2010* goals and objectives for health promotion and disease prevention.

Certified health education specialists (CHES) are professionals who have met required health education training qualification, have successfully passed a competency-based examination, and satisfy the continuing education requirement to maintain the credential. Individuals who are certified by the National Commission for Health Education Credentialing, Inc., must demonstrate knowledge and skills in seven major areas. These responsibilities include assessing individual and community health education needs; planning, implementing, and evaluating effective health education programs; coordinating the provision of health education services; acting as resource persons in health education; and communicating health and health education needs, concerns, and resources. Those who have taken an advanced level of health education study are expected to have more specialized competencies in these seven areas as well

as to apply appropriate research principles and techniques in health education, and to manage and supervise health education programs in a variety of practice settings, including school, patient-care, workplace, and community settings. Health educators utilize a variety of intervention methods such as social marketing and mass communication to promote health among individuals, communities, and society. There are more than 300 professional preparation programs in community and school health education at the baccalaureate, master's, and doctoral levels to prepare health education researchers and practitioners.

An increasing body of cumulative research that has evaluated the impact and outcomes of health education indicates that educational intervention can be a cost-effective prevention strategy and promote appropriate utilization of health services. Planned health education programs not only positively influence health-related knowledge, attitudes, skills, and behaviors, but also can improve health status through changes in social norms, organizational practices, and public policies. Emerging research in health education is focusing on issues such as identifying combinations of intervention strategies that result in sustained changes of behavior and health status among people with infectious and chronic disease, multiple-behavior intervention and transbehavioral measures of outcome, determining the time and resources necessary to achieve "dose response" in health education programs, and adapting health education programs that have demonstrated effectiveness in dominant population groups for use in culturally, racially, and linguistically diverse groups.

JOHN P. ALLEGRANTE, PhD
M. ELAINE AULD, MPH, CHES

---

interaction with the environment. The four key concepts of her model are *consciousness, movement, space,* and *time.* Consciousness is defined as the informational capacity of the human system, or the capacity of the system to interact with the environment. Movement is the manifestation of consciousness, viewed as waves of energy and energy transformation in the space and time of a person's life.

Person and environment are defined as co-extensive, open energy fields. The two evolve together and move toward increasing complexity and diversity, manifested in patterns of interaction that occur along continua of time and space. Person is also defined as a specific pattern of consciousness.

Health is a process of expanding consciousness that synthesizes disease and non-disease and is recognized by patterns

WINDOW ON HEALTH AS EXPANDING CONSCIOUSNESS

This theory of health and nursing was stimulated by my concern for those for whom health as the absence of disease is not a reality. Nurses often relate to such people: people facing the uncertainty, debilitation, loss, and eventual death associated with chronic illness. The theory of health as expanding consciousness asserts that *every* person in *every* situation, no matter how disordered and hopeless it may seem, is part of the universal process of expanding consciousness—a process of becoming more of oneself, of finding greater meaning in life, and of reaching new heights of connectedness with other people and the world in which one lives. These characteristics of higher consciousness have been illustrated by research depicting persons facing life-threatening diseases and other crises. Nurses practicing within this perspective experience the joy of participating in the expanding process of others and find that their own lives are enhanced and expanded by the process.

MARGARET A. NEWMAN, PhD, RN, FAAN

of person-environment interaction. An understanding of *pattern* is basic to an understanding of health, and involves the movement from looking at parts to looking at the whole. Pattern is defined as information that depicts the whole, and gives an understanding of the meaning of relationships.

Nursing is an integrative force within the new paradigm of health seen as the undivided wholeness of the person in interaction and as a process of evolving consciousness. The *nursing process* is modified by Newman and encompasses nursing diagnosis/intervention based on the unique configuration of each person-environment interaction. Intervention is broadly intepreted as the recognition and augmentation of person-environment patterns, where the nurse and the client evolve together toward expanding consciousness.

h. care system an organized plan of health services. The term usually is used to refer to the system or program by which health care is made available to the population and financed by government, private enterprise, or both. In a larger sense, the elements of a health care system embrace the following: (1) personal health care services for individuals and families, available at hospitals, clinics, neighborhood centers, and similar agencies, in physicians' offices, and in the clients' own homes; (2) the public health services needed to maintain a healthy environment, such as control of water and food supplies, regulation of drugs, and safety regulations intended to protect a given population; (3) teaching and research activities related to the prevention, detection, and treatment of disease; and (4) third party (health insurance) coverage of system services.

In the United States, the spectrum of health care has been defined by the Department of Health and Human Services as encompassing six levels of health care. The first level of care is *preventive care,* which is primarily provided by school health education courses and community and public health services.

Primary care is the usual point at which an individual enters the health care system. Its major task is the early detection and prevention of disease and the maintenance of health. This level of care also encompasses the routine care of individuals with common health problems and chronic illnesses that can be managed in the home or through periodic visits to an outpatient facility. Providers of care at the primary level include family members as well as the professionals and paraprofessionals who staff community and neighborhood health centers, hospital outpatient departments, physicians' offices, industrial health units, and school and college health units.

Secondary or *acute care* is concerned with emergency treatment and critical care involving intense and elaborate measures for the diagnosis and treatment of a specified range of illness or pathology. Entry into the system at this level is either by direct admission to a health care facility or by referral. Provider groups for secondary care include both acute- and long-term care hospitals and their staffs.

Tertiary care includes highly technical services for the treatment of individuals and families with complex or complicated health needs. Providers of tertiary care are health professionals who are specialists in a particular clinical area and are competent to work in such specialty agencies as psychiatric hospitals and clinics, chronic disease centers, and the highly specialized units of general hospitals; for example, a coronary care unit. Entry into the health care system at this level is gained by referral from either the primary or secondary level.

Respite care is that provided by an agency or institution for long-term care patients on a short-term basis to give the primary caretaker(s) at home a period of relief.

Restorative care comprises routine follow-up care and rehabilitation in such facilities as nursing homes, halfway houses, inpatient facilities for alcohol and drug abusers, and in the homes of patients served by home health care units of hospitals or community-based agencies.

Continuing care is provided on an ongoing basis to support those persons who are physically or mentally handicapped, elderly and suffering from a chronic and incapacitating illness, mentally retarded, or otherwise unable to cope unassisted with daily living. Such care is available in personal care homes, domiciliary homes, inpatient health facilities, nursing homes, geriatric day care centers, and various other types of facilities. See also HOME HEALTH CARE.

holistic h. a system of preventive care that takes into account the whole individual, one's own responsibility for one's well-being, and the total influences—social, psychological, environmental—that affect health, including nutrition, exercise, and mental relaxation.

h. maintenance organization (HMO) any of a variety of health care delivery systems with structures ranging from group practice through independent practice models or independent practice associations (IPAs). They provide alternatives to the fee-for-service private practice of medicine and other allied health professions. Although the type of organizational pattern, membership, and ownership of the organization may vary among HMOs, all have the major goal of allowing for investment in and incentives to use a prepaid, organized, comprehensive health care system that serves a defined population. The enrolled population enters into a contract with the organization, agreeing to pay, or have paid on their behalf, a fixed sum, in return for which the HMO makes available the health care personnel, facilities, and services that the population may require. The services are available on a 24-hour-a-day, 7-day-a-week basis. Some HMOs may provide directly the entire range of health services, including rehabilitation, dental, and mental health care. Others may agree to provide directly or arrange to pay only for physicians' services, in-hospital care, and outpatient emergency and preventive medical services. The kinds of services available are stipulated in the contract between the organization and its enrolled population. The emphasis of a health maintenance organization is on preventive rather than crisis-oriented medical care.

public h. see PUBLIC HEALTH.

h. seeking behaviors a NURSING DIAGNOSIS accepted by the North American Nursing Diagnosis Association, defined as a state in which a person in stable health is actively seeking ways to alter his or her personal habits or environment in order to move toward a higher level of health. "Stable health" is defined as the achieving of age-appropriate illness prevention measures, with reporting of good or excellent health, and signs or symptoms of disease, when present, being controlled.

sexual h. see SEXUAL HEALTH.

healthy (helth'e) pertaining to, characterized by, or promoting health.

hearing (hēr'ing) the sense by which sounds are perceived, or the capacity to perceive sound; sound waves must be converted into nerve impulses that can be interpreted by the brain. The organ of hearing is the EAR, which is divided into three sections, the outer, middle, and inner ear, each with its own role in hearing. Connecting the middle ear with the nasopharynx is the eustachian tube, through which air enters to equalize the pressure on both sides of the tympanic membrane (eardrum). Called also audition. See accompanying illustration.

h. aid an instrument to amplify sounds for those with HEARING LOSS. There are two types of electronic hearing aids: the air-conduction type, which is worn in the external acoustic meatus, and the bone-conduction type, which is worn in back of the ear over the mastoid process.

Those who have conductive HEARING LOSS can often use any one of the better aids with good results. Patients with OTOSCLEROSIS will probably need the bone-conduction type of instrument. Those with sensorineural HEARING LOSS (caused by injury to the vestibulo-cochlear nerve), or a mixed type, may have more trouble selecting a suitable hearing aid and may get less satisfactory results.

Those wearing a hearing aid for the first time should have special training in its proper use. A hearing aid picks up and amplifies all sounds in the vicinity. Often a person whose hearing has declined gradually will have lost the facility to ignore background noises. When one first tries a hearing aid, one's ears will be assaulted by the

H

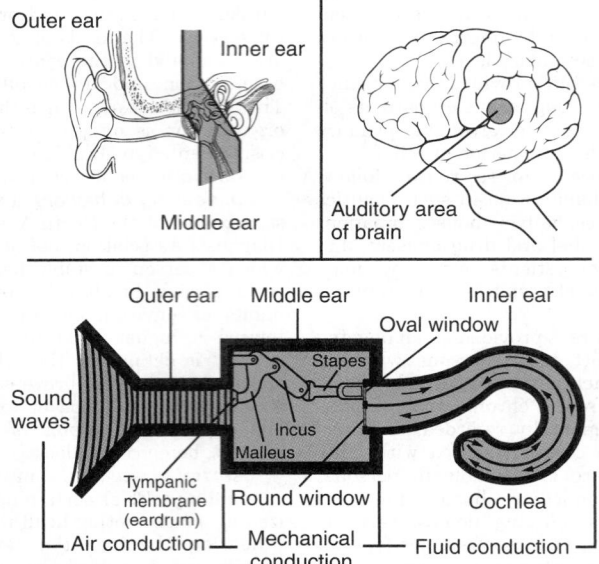

As sound is conducted from the external ear to the inner ear, the sound waves undergo considerable transformation. The tympanic membrane (eardrum), ossicles, and cochlea act as a mechanical transformer to concentrate the sound waves so that they can be picked up by nerve endings in the inner ear and transmitted to the brain.

sounds of passing cars, of doors slamming, of telephones ringing. Training in how to filter out these noises and concentrate on the essential is necessary if the person is to get good results from the hearing aid. For best results, this should be combined with lessons in lipreading.

A COCHLEAR IMPLANT can help profoundly deaf persons recognize and interpret various sounds. It does not restore hearing but can improve the quality of life for the deaf.

hearing loss partial or complete loss of the sense of HEARING; called also deafness. The number of hearing impaired individuals has steadily increased over the past few decades. While improved detection and reporting of impaired hearing can account for some of this increase, other contributing factors include an aging population and increased noise levels in the environment.

Types of Hearing Loss. There are three broad categories of hearing loss: conductive, sensorineural, and central. *Conductive hearing loss* is associated with impaired transmission of sound waves through the external ear canal to the bones of the middle ear. A blockage of the external ear or dysfunction of the middle ear will produce conductive loss of hearing.

Examples of common causes of conductive hearing loss are obstruction of the ear canal by cerumen or a foreign object, perforated eardrum, otitis media, otosclerosis, and congenital malformations of the outer or middle ear.

Sensorineural hearing loss is associated with some pathological change in structures within the inner ear or in the acoustic nerve. Normally, sound waves received by the external and middle ear are conveyed to the fluid in the cochlea of the inner ear. On the surface of its basilar membrane lies the organ of Corti, which contains mechanically sensitive cells. These minute structures act as end-organs that generate nerve impulses in response to sound vibrations. Thus the mechanical energy of sound vibrations is transformed into electrical energy that stimulates the nerve fibers of the acoustic (eighth cranial) nerve. The impulses are then transmitted to the brain, where the cerebral cortex decodes or interprets the sound. A sensorineural hearing loss results when there is dysfunction in either the perception or the interpretation of sound waves. Common causes of sensorineural hearing loss include hereditary disease, aging (presbycusis), noise damage, viral

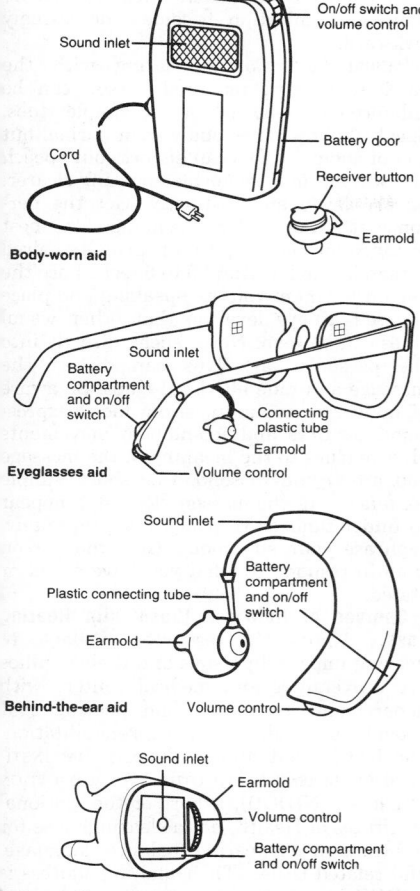

On/off switch and volume control

Sound inlet

Cord

Battery door

Receiver button

Earmold

Body-worn aid

Sound inlet

Battery compartment and on/off switch

Connecting plastic tube

Earmold

Eyeglasses aid

Volume control

Sound inlet

Battery compartment and on/off switch

Plastic connecting tube

Earmold

Behind-the-ear aid

Volume control

Sound inlet

Earmold

Volume control

Battery compartment and on/off switch

In-the-ear aid

Hearing aids. From Lammon et al., 1995.

childhood infections, skull fractures and intracranial tumors, oxytoxic drugs, and Rh incompatibility during fetal life.

Central hearing loss occurs when there is a pathologic condition above the junction of the acoustic nerve and the brainstem. Brain tumors, vascular changes that suddenly deprive the structures of the inner ear of their blood supply, stroke syndrome, and erythroblastosis fetalis are examples of pathologic conditions that can produce central hearing loss.

Preventing Hearing Loss. Not all cases of hearing loss can be prevented, but there are measures that are known to be effective in curtailing the incidence and severity of many types of hearing loss. For example, excessive environmental noise is a major contributing factor that is avoidable or at least manageable. Permanent damage to hearing can result when the structures of the inner ear and nerve cells are repeatedly bombarded with loud sound waves which reduce their blood supply. The cells thus lost are replaced by scar tissue that cannot transmit sound waves and impulses. If one's occupation requires continued exposure to loud noises, ear protection devices should be worn to mitigate the harmful effect.

Excessive noise in one's environment often can be greatly reduced by lowering the volume on radios and other music appliances, especially those with headphones. Authorities recommend that one should avoid continual exposure to music amplified to more than 104 to 111 decibels. It is believed that the loss of hearing associated with aging may not be an inevitable outcome of growing older, but rather a lasting effect of living in an increasingly noisy environment.

Efforts to reduce the risk of ATHEROSCLEROSIS can help prevent hearing loss by lowering the possibility of atherosclerotic plaque in the blood vessels supplying the delicate structures of the inner ear, and also by minimizing the risk of stroke.

There are some drugs that are particularly toxic to the ear. Examples are ASPIRIN, which can produce tinnitus and temporary deafness; the antibiotics ERYTHROMYCIN, KANAMYCIN, NEOMYCIN, and STREPTOMYCIN; the NONSTEROIDAL ANTIINFLAMMATORY DRUGS FENOPROFEN and INDOMETHACIN; the DIURETIC FUROSEMIDE (LASIX); and several drugs used in the chemotherapeutic treatment of malignancies. Any person taking a prescribed medication should be alert for hearing-related problems while taking the drug and report such problems as soon as they appear.

Prompt attention to and successful treatment of ear infections is another means by which hearing loss can be prevented. Symptoms such as ringing in the ears, a feeling of pressure in the ear, or increasing hearing difficulty call for medical consultation.

Great progress has been made in the treatment of conditions that once almost always resulted in impaired hearing. One example is the use of antibiotics to manage ear infections. Another is the development of microsurgery, which enables the surgeon to operate freely in the crowded inner chambers of the ear. Two such surgical procedures are STAPEDECTOMY and TYMPANOPLASTY. In a stapedectomy to correct otosclerosis the diseased stapes or stirrup is removed and replaced by a prosthesis that allows the chain of sound transmission to function again. Tympanoplasty is useful in correcting some types of conductive hearing loss. If chronic ear infection or injury has destroyed one or more of the ossicles, they can be rebuilt or replaced surgically.

Detecting Hearing Loss. In the infant and very young child hearing loss is evidenced by a lack of response to the sounds in the immediate environment. As the infant matures and begins to approach the age at which talking should begin, there may be either a failure to talk at all by age two or scarcely intelligible speech after age three.

Emotional and behavioral disorders can be signs of hearing loss in children and adults. The frustration they feel in trying to cope with their disability can be manifested by irritability, hyperactivity, hostility, and withdrawal. Other signs include speaking in either a very loud or very soft voice; habitually saying "What?" and failing to follow instructions; facial expressions indicating difficulty in understanding what is being said; and inappropriate responses to questions asked or statements made during a conversation.

Among the tests used to evaluate hearing are tuning fork tests such as the WEBER TEST and the RINNE TEST. A TYMPANOGRAM provides information about the movement of the eardrum. Evaluation of hearing acuity by AUDIOMETRY uses a special machine for testing sound perception.

Rehabilitation. For those cases of hearing loss that cannot be corrected, some form of rehabilitation is prescribed to make the best of whatever hearing remains and to improve the person's quality of life and socialization. The HEARING AID is helpful for persons with certain kinds of hearing loss. It should be selected with the help of an audiologist or an otologist because different types of hearing loss require different types of hearing aids. Careful training in the proper use of the hearing aid is also necessary to assure that the person wearing it will achieve maximum benefit.

An important tool in rehabilitation of the profoundly hearing impaired is training in SIGNING and lip READING. For lip reading, the patient is taught to use visual clues, such as facial expression and body movements, as well as movements of the lips and tongue.

A third component of rehabilitation of the hearing impaired is speech THERAPY. Profoundly deaf persons cannot hear their own voices, and those who have never heard spoken language have difficulty learning to speak coherently. Those who have lost their hearing over a period of time often suffer a gradual deterioration in their speech so that communication becomes increasingly awkward.

Patient Care. Communicating with the partially hearing impaired person can be enhanced by following a few simple rules. Speak slightly more loudly than normal but do not shout, as this can distort your speech and will not make your message any clearer. Speak slowly and distinctly. Get the person's attention before speaking. The best distance for speaking to a hearing-impaired person is 1 to 2 meters (3 to 6 feet). Face the person to whom you are speaking and place yourself at eye level so that other visual clues can be seen. Never speak directly into the person's ear. This can distort the message and hide all visual clues. Be aware of nonverbal communication; facial expressions, gestures, and lip and body movements all give clues to the meaning of the message you are trying to send. Use short, simple sentences. If the person does not appear to understand or responds inappropriately, rephrase your statement. Give the person time to respond to what you have asked or stated.

Sources of Help for Those with Hearing Loss. Among the resources available to hearing impaired persons and their families are universities and medical centers with departments of speech and hearing that provide lip-reading classes, rehabilitation and hearing aid clinics. The NATIONAL INSTITUTE ON DEAFNESS AND OTHER COMMUNICATION DISORDERS (NIDCD), a part of the National Institutes of Health, has a clearinghouse for information on hearing, balance, language, and related issues. Their mailing address is NIDCD Information Clearinghouse, 1 Communication Ave., Bethesda, MD 20892, and their web site is http://www.nidcd.nih.gov. They can be reached by telephone at (voice) 1-800-241-1044 or (TDD/TTY) 1-800-241-1055. Other societies and organizations devoted to helping the hearing impaired include The Better Hearing Institute, 515 King Street, Suite 420, Alexandria VA 22314, which operates a toll-free "Hearing Help line" at 1-800-327-9355; and The Alexander Graham Bell Association for the Deaf, 3417 Volta Pl. NW, Washington, DC 20007. Web site http://www.hear-it.org is a world wide hearing information web site.

central h. l. central deafness.

conductive h. l. that due to a defect of the sound-conducting apparatus, i.e., of the external auditory canal or middle ear. See HEARING LOSS.

functional h. l. hearing loss that lacks any organic lesion; called also hysterical deafness and nonorganic hearing loss.

mixed h. l. hearing loss that is both conductive and sensorineural in nature.

nonorganic h. l. functional hearing loss.

ototoxic h. l. deafness caused by ingestion of toxic substances or medications that affect the eighth CRANIAL NERVE.

paradoxic h. l. that in which the hearing is better during loud noise.

sensorineural h. l. that due to a defect in the inner ear or the acoustic nerve. See HEARING LOSS.

transmission h. l. conductive hearing loss.

heart (hahrt) the hollow muscular organ lying slightly to the left of the midline of the chest. The heart serves as a pump controlling the blood flow in two circuits, the pulmonary and the systemic. See also CIRCULATORY SYSTEM, and see Plates.

Divisions of the Heart. The SEPTUM, a thick muscular wall, divides the heart into right and left halves. Each half is again divided into upper and lower quarters or chambers. The lower chambers are called VENTRICLES and the upper chambers are called ATRIA. The right side of the heart, consisting of the right atrium and right ventricle, receives deoxygenated blood and sends it into the pulmonary circuit. The left side, consisting of the left atrium and left ventricle, receives oxygenated blood and sends it into the systemic circuit.

Valves of the Heart. The atrioventricular VALVES connect an atrium and a ventricle: between the right atrium and right ventricle is the tricuspid VALVE and between the left atrium and left ventricle is the mitral VALVE. The semilunar VALVES are valves at the blood's exit points from the heart: the pulmonary VALVE opens from the right ventricle into the pulmonary artery, and the aortic VALVE opens from the left ventricle into the aorta. These valves, both within the heart and leading out of it, open and shut in such a way as to keep the blood flowing in one direction through the heart's two separate pairs of chambers: fro atrium to ventricle and out through its appropriate artery.

Layers of the Heart. The heart wall is composed of three layers of tissues. Its chambers are lined by a delicate membrane, the ENDOCARDIUM. The thick muscular wall essential to normal pumping action of the heart is called the MYOCARDIUM. The thin but sturdy membranous sac surrounding the exterior of the heart is called the PERICARDIUM.

The Heart's Pacemaker. The heart is made up of special muscle tissue, capable of continuous rhythmic contraction without tiring. The impulse that starts the contraction of the heart has its origin in an area of

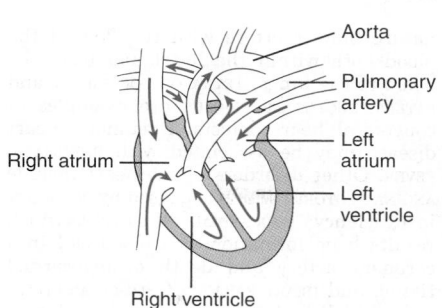

Blood enters the right atrium from the body and then passes into the right ventricle, where it is pumped into the lungs. It returns from the lungs into the right atrium. It enters the left ventricle and then is pumped to the body via the aorta.

H

the right atrium called the sinoatrial NODE; it is this special tissue that acts as the normal PACEMAKER for the heart. The impulse is transmitted in a fraction of a second through the atria to another group of similarly sensitive fibers called the atrioventricular NODE, through the BUNDLE OF HIS, down the bundle BRANCHES, and to the Purkinje FIBERS, resulting in contraction of the ventricles.

Pumping Action. Although the right and left sides of the heart serve two separate branches of the circulation, each with its distinct function, they are coordinated so that the heart efficiently serves both sides with a single pumping action. The valve action on both sides is also coordinated with the two phases of the pumping action. Thus during DIASTOLE, the relaxation phase, oxygen-poor blood returning from the systemic circulation and accumulated in the right atrium pours into the right ventricle. At the same time, the oxygen-rich blood that has accumulated in the left atrium returning from the pulmonary circulation pours into the left ventricle. The walls of both atria contract to press blood into the relaxed ventricles. In the next contraction phase (SYSTOLE), the valves between the atria and ventricles close and the ventricles contract, forcing the blood through the pulmonary artery and the aorta. At the end of the contraction the pulmonary and aortic valves snap shut, preventing any backward flow of the blood into the ventricles. Diastole follows, the ventricles again filling with the blood from their respective atria, and the cycle is repeated.

Disorders of the Heart. The heart is subject to a variety of disorders. Among them are CONGENITAL HEART DEFECTS, which begin or exist at the time of birth. Disorders of this nature may interfere with the flow of the blood both within the heart and from the heart to the lungs. TETRALOGY OF FALLOT and PATENT DUCTUS ARTERIOSUS are examples of congenital heart defects. Rheumatic heart disease may be associated with RHEUMATIC FEVER. Other disorders of the heart include ANGINA PECTORIS, which is caused by coronary insufficiency; MYOCARDIAL INFARCTION, which results from formation of a blood clot in a coronary artery and death of myocardial tissue; and HEART FAILURE. Cardiac ARRHYTHMIAS are disturbances in the normal rate and rhythm of the heartbeat.

Diagnostic Tests. Many different diagnostic procedures are available for the examination of the heart. Along with a history and physical examination, an ELECTROCARDIOGRAM (ECG) is routinely obtained. It shows a tracing of the electrical excitation that spreads through the heart during each beat. It is the definitive source of information about cardiac arrhythmias, and also gives diagnostic information about myocardial infarctions.

Exercise stress testing is a valuable tool for detecting persons who have some degree of coronary heart disease. The test subject performs maximal exercise while being monitored by ECG. A positive stress test occurs when the subject cannot sustain the exercise for the duration of the test, cannot attain a normal maximal heart rate, or shows ECG changes indicative of ischemia. When stress testing is used for screening purposes, it is not diagnostic. However, persons with a positive stress test are 13 times more likely to develop significant coronary artery or heart disease and should work to reduce their risk factors. Stress testing is also used to evaluate the severity of known coronary disease and to guide the rehabilitation of a patient with coronary disease.

PHONOCARDIOGRAPHY is the recording of heart sounds and murmurs. It is more precise than AUSCULTATION with a stethoscope because it provides a permanent visual record that can be used to obtain precise timing information and can be used as baseline data for comparison with later findings.

ECHOCARDIOGRAPHY is a type of diagnostic ULTRASONOGRAPHY that provides information about the structure and function of the heart. It is a comfortable technique for the patient and is capable of establishing a diagnosis for several types of heart disease, especially those involving the valves. Types include *M-mode, Doppler,* and *transesophageal echocardiography.*

Several types of RADIOISOTOPE examination are used to detect heart disease. A radioisotope imaging agent is injected into the patient, and a scintillation camera is then used to make an image of the distribution of radioactivity.

THALLIUM 201 has an affinity for heart tissue; when injected intravenously, it is carried to areas with adequate perfusion. Myocardial infarcts and areas of acute ischemia or scarring appear as "cold spots" (areas of no uptake of thallium) on the SCINTIGRAM. When the isotope is injected during maximal exercise in an exercise stress test, the scan shows areas of inadequate perfusion and is a better indicator of coronary disease than a stress test alone.

Radiopharmaceuticals that label the blood pool can be used with a computerized scintillation camera to evaluate ventricular performance. Images of the first pass of the radioisotope through the heart can be used to determine the cardiac output and ejection fraction, the size of the ventricles, and regional wall motion.

The imaging agents used for bone scans, such as TECHNETIUM 99M pyrophosphate or diphosphonate, also have an affinity for areas of acute ischemic tissue damage. "Hot spots" on the scintigram (areas of isotope uptake) show areas of acute infarction. The scan is usually negative by approximately 6 days after an infarction.

CARDIAC CATHETERIZATION is an invasive technique used when definitive data are required to decide whether heart disease should be treated medically, surgically, or through interventional cardiology techniques such as percutaneous transluminal ANGIOPLASTY, STENTS, or VALVULOPLASTY. A catheter is inserted into a vein or artery, usually the brachial artery or the femoral vein or artery, and guided into the heart. Tracings of the pressure pulses within the chambers during the heart cycle are obtained. Cardiac output, pulmonary artery pressures, the orifice area of valves, and the degree of left-to-right shunting can be determined.

ANGIOCARDIOGRAPHY is the x-ray examination of the heart after injection of a radiopaque contrast medium through a catheter at various locations in the heart. The films show the size and motion of the heart chambers and can demonstrate aortic or mitral REGURGITATION. In coronary ARTERIOGRAPHY the contrast medium is injected through a catheter into the orifice of each coronary artery. The films show atherosclerotic obstructions of the arteries and are useful in planning coronary bypass surgery, percutaneous transluminal angioplasty, or stents.

Prevention of Heart Disease. Although heart disease remains the leading cause of death in industrialized countries, its mortality rate has steadily declined since the early 1970s. A major factor in this decline is the development of more effective preventive measures and modes of treatment for ischemic heart disease. These advances include open heart surgery to repair congenital defects and replace malfunctioning valves; vascular surgery to repair or bypass obstructions in the coronary arteries and aorta; newer and more accurate diagnostic tests and procedures for detecting problems involving the heart and blood vessels; antimicrobial therapy for the treatment of rheumatic fever, syphilis, and other infectious diseases that are damaging to the heart; more sophisticated monitoring equipment and intensive care units; and aggressive medical treatment and management of heart disease and hypertension.

All these contributions to the control and correction of cardiovascular diseases are important in the reduction of mortality rates and improvement in patients' quality of life. Nevertheless, it is also important for prevention that there be an improvement of the general public's awareness of the causes and risk factors of cardiac disorders. Major risk factors that can be avoided, modified, or corrected include cigarette SMOKING, elevated blood lipids, OBESITY, habitual dietary excesses, lack of exercise, HYPERTENSION, and excessive STRESS. Health professionals can promote reduction in the incidence of heart disease by educating the public about these risk factors and by encouraging active participation in preventive measures, particularly in those that involve changes in lifestyle.

heartbeat (hahrt′bēt) the cycle of contraction of the heart muscle; it begins with an electrical impulse in the sinoatrial node, which serves as the normal PACEMAKER for the heart. (See accompanying illustration.)

heart block impairment of conduction in heart excitation; often applied specifically to atrioventricular BLOCK. See types listed at BLOCK.

When isolated impulses from the atria fail to reach the ventricles, heartbeats are missed and the block is called incomplete. When no impulses reach the ventricles from the atria the heart block is complete, with the result that the atria and the ventricles beat at separate rates. In this case the beats of the atria and ventricles remain regular but the rate of the ventricular beats is much slower.

Heart block can occur with various forms of heart disease and as a result of excessive

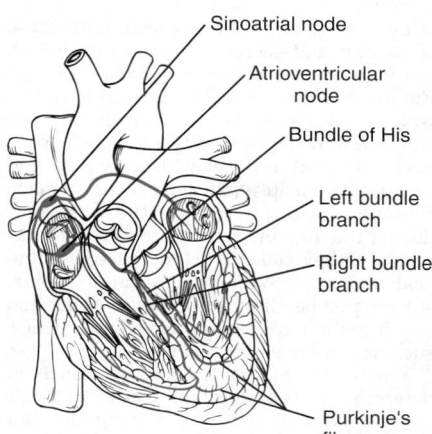

Heartbeat: The conduction system of the heart that is involved in the cycle of contraction. From Frazier et al., 2000.

dosages of certain medications such as digitalis. A particularly severe form of heart block is STOKES-ADAMS DISEASE, in which sudden unconsciousness results from the slowed heartbeat. It may be accompanied by convulsions.

The treatment for heart block caused by digitalis overdosage is to stop the medication. When there is hemodynamic instability, an antidote, digoxin immune F$_{AB}$ (ovine) (Digibind), can be administered intravenously for more rapid reduction of serum levels. If there is no response, temporary cardiac PACING is indicated.

heartburn (hahrt′burn) a burning sensation in the ESOPHAGUS, or below the sternum in the region of the heart, one of the common symptoms of INDIGESTION. Called also pyrosis.

Heartburn often occurs when there is distention of a part of the esophagus, particularly the lower part. This may happen with gastroesophageal REFLUX (regurgitation by the stomach of part of its contents upward into the esophagus). Since this matter is acidic, it acts as an irritant, producing discomfort or pain.

Excessive acidity (HYPERACIDITY) is thought to be a cause of heartburn, occurring when the stomach secretes an excessive amount of HYDROCHLORIC ACID. Recent evidence, however, indicates that hyperacidity in itself may not be the actual cause, and that heartburn results from excessive gastric secretions only when there is improper eating so that REFLUX takes place.

The functions of the stomach, both those of motion and secretion, are controlled by the VAGUS NERVE, one of the cranial nerves. Emotional stress can stimulate this nerve, which in turn starts the churning of the stomach and the flow of the various gastric juices; it can also cause contraction and spasm of the pylorus. If some of the stomach contents are displaced into the esophagus during this nervous activity, heartburn may result. Other causes include gastroesophageal reflux accompanying hiatal hernia, stooping or bending after a large meal, and the ingestion of certain foods and drugs, such as alcohol and aspirin.

Treatment of heartburn is aimed at determining its underlying cause. Antacids may be used to relieve the symptoms but they will not cure heartburn and should not be used indiscriminately. Antacid therapy is the key maneuver along with instituting small meal size and elevation of the head of the bed to prevent reflux.

heart failure inability of the heart to maintain cardiac output sufficient to meet the body's needs; it most often results from myocardial failure affecting the right or left ventricle.

    backward h. f. a concept of heart failure emphasizing the resultant passive engorgement of the systemic venous system that.

    congestive h. f. **(CHF)** that which occurs as a result of impaired pumping capability of the heart that is not keeping up with the metabolic needs of body tissues and organs; it is associated with abnormal retention of water and sodium. It ranges from mild congestion with few symptoms to life-threatening fluid overload and heart failure. Congestive heart failure results in an inadequate supply of blood and oxygen to the body's cells. The decreased cardiac output causes an increase in the blood volume within the vascular system. Congestion within the blood vessels interferes with the movement of body fluids in and out of the various fluid compartments, so that fluid accumulates in the tissue spaces, causing edema.

There are three general kinds of pathologic conditions that can bring about congestive heart failure: (1) *ventricular failure,* in which the contractions of the ventricles become weak and ineffective, as in myocardial ischemia from coronary artery disease; (2) *mechanical failure* of the ventricles to fill with blood during the diastole phase of the cardiac cycle, which can occur when the mitral valve is narrowed, as in rheumatic mitral stenosis, or when there is an accumulation of fluid within the pericardial sac (cardiac TAMPONADE) pressing against the ventricles, preventing them from accepting a full load of blood; and (3) an *overload* of

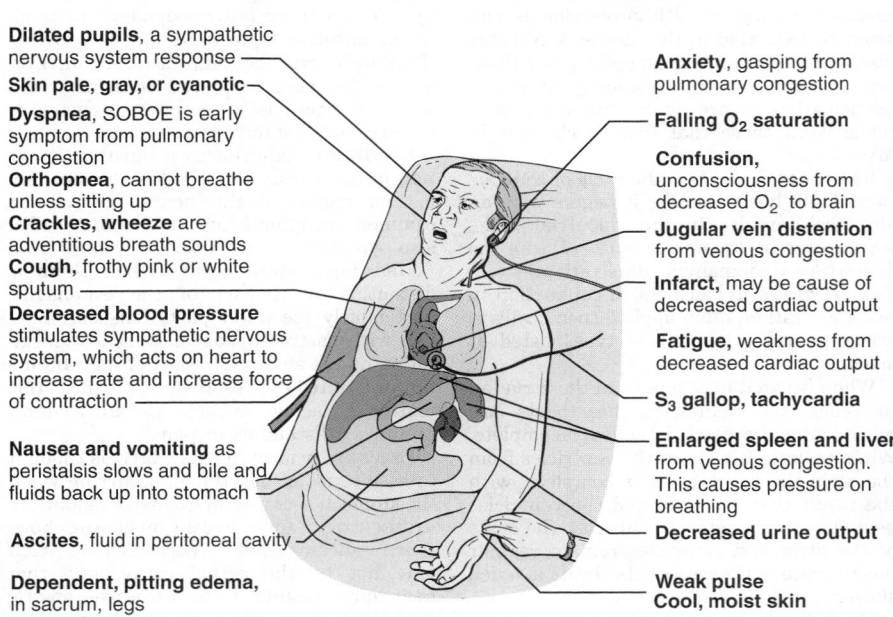

Dilated pupils, a sympathetic nervous system response

Skin pale, gray, or cyanotic

Dyspnea, SOBOE is early symptom from pulmonary congestion

Orthopnea, cannot breathe unless sitting up

Crackles, wheeze are adventitious breath sounds

Cough, frothy pink or white sputum

Decreased blood pressure stimulates sympathetic nervous system, which acts on heart to increase rate and increase force of contraction

Nausea and vomiting as peristalsis slows and bile and fluids back up into stomach

Ascites, fluid in peritoneal cavity

Dependent, pitting edema, in sacrum, legs

Anxiety, gasping from pulmonary congestion

Falling O$_2$ saturation

Confusion, unconsciousness from decreased O$_2$ to brain

Jugular vein distention from venous congestion

Infarct, may be cause of decreased cardiac output

Fatigue, weakness from decreased cardiac output

S$_3$ gallop, tachycardia

Enlarged spleen and liver from venous congestion. This causes pressure on breathing

Decreased urine output

Weak pulse
Cool, moist skin

Clinical portrait of congestive heart failure. (SOBOE = shortness of breath on exertion) From Jarvis, 1996.

blood in the ventricles during the systole phase of the cycle. High BLOOD PRESSURE, aortic STENOSIS, and aortic REGURGITATION are some of the conditions that can cause ventricular overload.

Compensatory Mechanisms. In an attempt to compensate for inadequate pumping of the heart, the body uses three basic adaptive mechanisms which, though they are effective for a brief period of time, will eventually become insufficient to meet the oxygen needs of the body. These mechanisms are also responsible for many of the symptoms experienced by the patient with congestive heart failure.

First, the failing heart attempts to maintain a normal output of blood by enlarging its pumping chambers so that they are capable of holding a greater volume of blood. This increases the amount of blood ejected from the heart, but it also leads to fluid overload within the blood vessels and excessive accumulation of body fluids in all of the fluid compartments.

Second, the heart begins to increase its muscle mass in order to strengthen the force of its contractions. This results in ventricular hypertrophy and a need for more oxygen. Eventually, the coronary arteries can no longer meet the oxygen demands of the enlarged myocardium and the patient experiences angina pectoris owing to ischemia.

Third, there is a response from the sympathetic nervous system. The involuntary muscle of the heart is regulated by autonomic, or involuntary, innervation. In response to failing contractility of the myocardial cells, the sympathetic nervous system activates adaptive processes that increase the heart rate, redistribute peripheral blood flow, and retain urine. These mechanisms are responsible for the symptoms of diaphoresis, cool skin, tachycardia, cardiac arrhythmias, and oliguria.

The combined efforts of these three compensatory mechanisms achieve a fairly normal level of cardiac output for a period of time. During this phase of congestive heart failure, the patient is said to have *compensated* CHF. When these mechanisms are no longer effective the disease progresses to the final stage of impaired heart function and the patient has *decompensated* CHF.

Clinical Symptoms. Left-sided heart failure produces dyspnea of varying intensity. In the early stages, shortness of breath occurs only when the patient is physically active. Later, as the heart action becomes more seriously impaired, the dyspnea is present even when the patient is resting. In

advanced cases, the patient must sit up in order to breathe (ORTHOPNEA). Attacks of breathlessness severe enough to wake the patient frequently occur during sleep (paroxysmal nocturnal DYSPNEA). These attacks usually are accompanied by coughing and wheezing, and the patient seeks relief by sitting upright. Orthopnea and paroxysmal nocturnal dyspnea are related to congestion of the pulmonary blood vessels and edema of the lung tissues. They are aggravated by lying down because in the prone position quantities of blood in the lower extremities move upward into the blood vessels of the lungs.

Fluid retention is another common symptom of congestive heart failure. In left-sided failure there is higher than normal pressure of blood in the pulmonary vessels. This increased pressure forces fluid out of the intravascular compartment and into the tissue spaces of the lungs, causing pulmonary edema. Right-sided failure causes congestion in the capillaries of the peripheral circulation and results in edema and congestion of the liver, stomach, legs, and feet, and in the sacral region in bedridden patients.

Decreased cardiac output also affects the kidneys by reducing their blood supply, which in turn causes a decrease in the rate of glomerular filtration of plasma from the renal blood vessels into the renal tubules. Sodium and water not excreted in the urine are retained in the vascular system, adding to the blood volume. The diminished blood supply to the kidney also causes it to secrete renin, which indirectly stimulates the secretion of aldosterone from the adrenal gland. Aldosterone in turn acts on the renal tubules, causing them to increase reabsorption of sodium and water, and thus to further increase the volume of body fluids.

Treatment. Medical management of congestive heart failure is aimed at improving contractility of the heart, reducing salt and water retention, and providing rest for the heart muscle. Drugs used to accomplish these goals include DIGITALIS glycosides to slow and strengthen the heartbeat, VASODILATORS such as nitroprusside and phentolamine to reduce resistance to the flow of blood being pumped from the heart, DIURETICS to assist in the elimination of water and sodium in the urine, and ANGIOTENSIN CONVERTING ENZYME INHIBITORS to reduce blood pressure, inhibit aldosterone release, and reduce peripheral arterial resistance. BETA-BLOCKERS are an important adjunct in

H

treatment of heart failure, helping to decrease the sympathetic response. Electroconversion of atrial FIBRILLATION enlists the help of the atria to fill the ventricles to maximum capacity. Biventricular PACING or restoration of cardiac SYNCHRONY is helpful for patients with interventricular conduction delay and a wide QRS COMPLEX.

Patient Care. Hospitalized patients with severe congestive heart failure present problems related to their needs for physical and mental rest, adequate aeration of the lungs and oxygenation of the tissues, prevention of circulatory stasis, maintenance of the integrity of the skin, restoration and maintenance of fluid and electrolyte balances, and adequate nutrition. The care plan should include frequent monitoring of the vital signs, intake and output, daily weight, serum electrolyte and blood gas levels, and nutritional intake. Patients are placed on sodium-restricted diets and limited fluid intake; they should have a good understanding of the reason for this before leaving the hospital. They should also have a plan for regular exercise as tolerated. Since it is likely that they will continue taking several kinds of medications after returning home, patients or family members should be taught about the pharmacologic action of each drug, the need for taking it exactly as prescribed, any precautions to be taken, and any untoward reactions that warrant notification of the physician, nurse practitioner, or physician's assistant.

forward h. f. a concept of heart failure emphasizing the inadequacy of cardiac output as the primary cause.

high-output h. f. that in which cardiac output remains high, associated with conditions such as hyperthyroidism, anemia, and emphysema.

left-sided h. f., left ventricular h. f. failure of the left ventricle to maintain a normal output of blood; it does not empty completely and thus cannot accept all the blood returning from the lungs via the pulmonary veins, which become engorged. Fluid seeps out of the veins through the pulmonary capillaries and collects in the interstitial tissue of the lung, causing pulmonary edema that eventually leads to right ventricular heart failure as well.

low-output h. f. that in which cardiac output is diminished, associated with cardiovascular diseases such as coronary artery disease, hypertension, and cardiomyopathy.

right-sided h. f., right ventricular h. f. failure of proper functioning of the right ventricle, with subsequent engorgement of the systemic veins, producing pitting edema, enlargement of the liver, and ascites.

heart-lung machine a mechanical device that temporarily takes over the functions of the heart and lungs; it is used as an aid in some surgeries, especially cardiovascular surgery. The "heart" of the machine is a pump that draws blood from the patient's vessels before it reaches the heart. The blood is routed through a "lung" chamber (usually made of plastic), where it receives oxygen. The oxygenated blood is then returned to the patient's vessels and pumped through the circulatory system. (This method of circulating the blood outside the patient's body is known as extracorporeal CIRCULATION.) Called also pump oxygenator.

heart murmur any sound in the heart region other than normal heart sounds; it may be caused by several different factors, including movement of blood through narrowed or stenotic heart valves and blood leaking through a valve that does not close properly. In many cases a murmur may be of the innocent or "functional" type, with no heart disease at all, so that it causes no trouble. The presence of such murmurs varies from time to time and they often go away completely.

heart sounds the sounds heard on the surface of the chest in the heart region; they are amplified by and heard more distinctly through a stethoscope. They are caused by the vibrations generated during the normal cardiac cycle and may be produced by muscular action, valvular actions, motion of the heart, or blood passing through the heart.

The *first heart sound* (S_1) is heard as a firm but dull "lubb" sound. It consists of four components: a low-frequency, indistinct vibration caused by ventricular contraction; a louder sound of higher frequency caused by closure of the mitral and tricuspid valves; a vibration caused by opening of the semilunar valves and early ejection of blood from the ventricles; and a low-pitched vibration produced by rapid ejection.

The *second heart sound* (S_2) is shorter and higher pitched than the first, is heard as a "dupp" and is produced by closure of the aortic and pulmonary valves.

The *third heart sound* (S_3) is very faint and is caused by blood rushing into the ventricles. It can be heard in most normal persons between the ages of 10 and 20 years.

The *fourth heart sound* (S_4) is rarely audible in a normal heart but can be

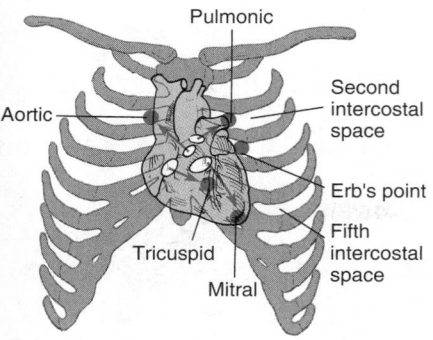

Precordial locations for cardiac palpation and auscultation of heart sounds. Closure of the mitral and tricuspid valves produces the S_1 heart sound; closure of the pulmonic and aortic (semilunar) valves produces the S_2 sound. From Polaski and Tatro, 1996.

demonstrated on graphic records. It is short and of low frequency and intensity, and is caused by atrial contraction. The vibrations arise from atrial muscle and from blood flow into, and distention of, the ventricles.

Abnormalities in Heart Sounds. Decreased compliance of a ventricle is characterized by a GALLOP or triple rhythm. Accentuation of the third heart sound (protodiastolic or ventricular gallop) is caused by the filling of a poorly compliant ventricle with blood under high venous pressure. A presystolic or atrial gallop is an accentuated fourth heart sound and is also caused by blood filling a poorly compliant ventricle. Merging of the third and fourth heart sounds is called a mesodiastolic or summation gallop. A very rare abnormality in which four heart sounds are heard distinctly is called a "locomotive" rhythm.

HEART MURMURS are sounds other than the normal heart sounds emanating from the heart region. They are often heard as blowing or hissing sounds as blood leaks back through diseased and malfunctioning valves or as blood is pushed through narrowed or stenotic valve orifices.

HEAT human erythrocyte agglutination test.

heat (hēt) 1. energy that raises the temperature of a body or substance. 2. estrus. 3. a rise in temperature. 4. to cause to increase in temperature.

Heat is associated with molecular motion, and is generated in various ways, including combustion, friction, chemical action, and radiation. The total absence of heat is absolute zero, at which all molecular activity ceases.

Body Heat. *Heat Production.* Body heat is the byproduct of the metabolic processes of the body. The hormones THYROXINE and EPINEPHRINE increase metabolism and consequently increase body heat. Muscular activity also produces body heat. At complete rest (basal metabolism) the amount of heat produced by muscular activity may be as low as 25 per cent of the total body heat. During exercise or shivering the percentage may rise to 60 per cent. Body temperature is regulated by the thermostatic center in the HYPOTHALAMUS. A body temperature above the normal range is called FEVER.

Heat Loss. Loss of body heat occurs in three ways: by radiation (heat waves), by conduction to air or objects in contact with the body, and by evaporation of perspiration. Some body heat is lost in exhalation of air and in elimination of urine and feces.

Applications of External Heat. *Purposes.* Local applications of heat may be used to provide warmth and promote comfort, rest, and relaxation. Heat is also applied locally to promote suppuration and drainage from an infected area by hastening the inflammatory process; to relieve congestion and swelling by dilating the blood vessels, thereby increasing circulation; and to improve repair of diseased or injured tissues by increasing local metabolism.

Effects. Factors that determine the physiologic action of heat include the type of heat used, length of time it is applied, age and general condition of the patient, and area of body surface to which the heat is applied. Moist heat is more penetrating than dry heat. Prolonged applications of heat produce an increase in skin secretions, resulting in a softening of the skin and a lowering of its resistance. Extreme heat produces constriction of the blood vessels; moderate heat produces vascular dilation. Repeated applications of heat will result in an increased tolerance to heat so that the individual may be burned without being aware of it. Elderly persons and infants are more susceptible to burns from high temperatures.

Heat applied to an infected area can localize the infection; for this reason, external heat should not be applied to the abdomen when appendicitis is suspected, because it may lead to rupture of the inflamed appendix.

h. exhaustion a disorder resulting from overexposure to heat or to the sun; long exposure to extreme heat or too much activity under a hot sun causes excessive sweating, which removes large amounts of salt and fluid from the body. When salt and fluid levels fall too far below normal, heat exhaustion may result. Called also heat prostration.

Symptoms. The early symptoms are headache and a feeling of weakness and dizziness, usually accompanied by nausea and vomiting. There may also be cramps in the muscles of the arms, legs, or abdomen. These first symptoms are similar to the early signs of SUNSTROKE, or heat stroke, but the disorders are not the same and should be treated differently. In heat exhaustion, the person turns pale and perspires profusely. The skin is cool and moist, pulse and breathing are rapid, and body temperature remains at a normal level or slightly below (in sunstroke the body temperature may be dangerously elevated). The patient may seem confused and may find it difficult to coordinate body movements; loss of consciousness seldom occurs.

Treatment. In cases of heat exhaustion, the victim should lie quietly in a cool place until transported to an emergency facility. The restoration of normal blood volume will be a priority. Stabilization of electrolytes is also important. If the person is able to safely swallow, sips of cool replacement fluid should be provided. Measures to reduce body temperature are employed.

If the condition is accompanied by cramps, the pain may be relieved by lightly stretching the affected muscles in addition to administering replenishing fluids. In cases of severe heat exhaustion and cramps, hospitalization may be necessary. Serum electrolyte levels are monitored to guide adequate replacement.

Prevention. Heat exhaustion and other heat disorders may be prevented by avoiding long exposure to sun or heat. The elderly, the very young, individuals with chronic diseases, and athletes exercising in the sun are at high risk. When the weather is very hot, or when working in an extremely hot place, it is essential to maintain adequate hydration. Regular rest periods are necessary. In the event of weakness or dizziness, persons should stop working at once and rest in a cool place.

It is possible for indoor temperatures to exceed the outdoor temperature. Poor ventilation can lead to an unhealthy situation that contributes to heat exhaustion. For this reason, adequate temperature control indoors is important in prevention of serious health problems.

latent h. the amount of heat absorbed or given off by a body without changing

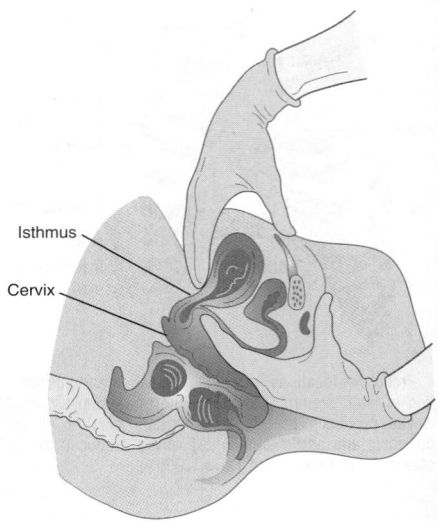

Hegar's sign—compressibility of the lower uterus—reflects softening of the isthmus of the cervix. From McKinney et al., 2000.

temperature, as when it undergoes a change of state.

prickly h., h. rash miliaria.

specific h. the ratio of the heat capacity of a substance to that of water; it is equivalent to the amount of heat required to raise the temperature of one gram of the substance by one degree Celsius, since the corresponding value for water is defined as 1.0.

heavy chain disease a rare monoclonal GAMMOPATHY characterized by neoplastic proliferation of plasma cells and precursors that secrete immunoglobulin heavy CHAINS. It is often accompanied by hepatosplenomegaly, lymphadenopathy, and soft tissue tumors. There are three varieties, each characterized by a specific heavy chain: ALPHA CHAIN DISEASE, GAMMA CHAIN DISEASE, and MU CHAIN DISEASE.

hebetic (hĕ-bet'ik) pubertal.

hebetude (heb'ĕ-tood) mental dullness; apathy.

hecatomeric (hek"ah-to-mer'ik) having processes that divide in two, one going to each side of the spinal cord; said of certain neurons.

hect(o)- word element [Fr.], *hundred;* used in naming units of measurements to designate an amount 100 times (10^2) the size of the unit to which it is joined; symbol h.

hedonism (he'don-izm) 1. pleasure-seeking behavior. 2. the ethical doctrine that regards pleasure and happiness as the highest good. 3. in psychology, the theory that the attainment of pleasure and the avoidance of pain are the prime motivators of human behavior. adj. **hedon′ic.**

heel (hēl) 1. the hindmost part of the foot; called also calx. 2. the hindmost portion of an elongated structure, or something else comparable to the heel of the foot.

    Thomas h. a shoe correction consisting of a heel one half inch longer and an eighth to a sixth of an inch higher on the inside; used to bring the heel of the foot into varus and to prevent depression in the region of the head of the talus.

Heerfordt's disease (hār′forts) uveoparotid fever.

Hegar's sign (ha′gahrz) compressibility and softening of the lower uterine segment, a probable sign of pregnancy; the lower uterine segment just above the cervix becomes so soft that when compressed between two fingers its wall cannot be felt or feels extremely thin.

height (hīt) the vertical measurement of something.

    h. of contour the measurement of a tooth from the lingual to the vestibular surface at its greatest bulge.

Heimlich maneuver (hīm′lik) a technique for removing foreign matter from the airway of a choking victim; the technique may be carried out with the victim in a standing position or lying down.

Standing Position. The rescuer stands behind the victim and wraps his arms around the victim's waist, allowing the victim's head, arms, and upper torso to hang forward. A fist is made with one hand and held with the other. The thumb side of the fist is then placed against the victim's abdomen at a point slightly above the umbilicus and below the rib cage. The rescuer's fist is then pressed into the victim's abdomen with a forceful upward thrust. The maneuver may be repeated if necessary to clear the air passages.

Supine Position. The victim is placed on the back with the head turned to one side. The rescuer kneels astride the victim's hips and places both hands on the abdomen, one hand upon the other. The heel of the lower hand is placed slightly above the umbilicus and below the rib cage. Pressure is applied to the victim's abdomen with a forceful upward thrust. The maneuver may be repeated if necessary to clear the air passages.

Heine-Medin disease (hi′nĕ ma′din) the major illness of POLIOMYELITIS.

helcoid (hel′koid) like an ulcer.

heli(o)- word element [Gr.], *sun.*

helical (hel′ĭ-k'l) spiral (def. 2).

helicine (hel′ĭ-sin) spiral (def. 2).

Helicobacter pylori (hel″ĭ-ko-bak′ter pi-lo′ri) a gram-negative spiral bacterium that causes gastritis and pyloric ulcers in humans; a history of *H. pylori* infection is

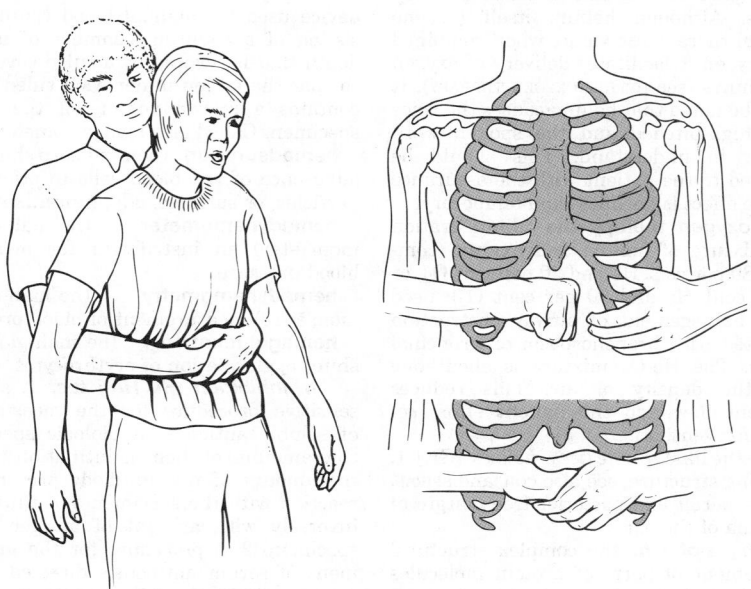

Heimlich maneuver.

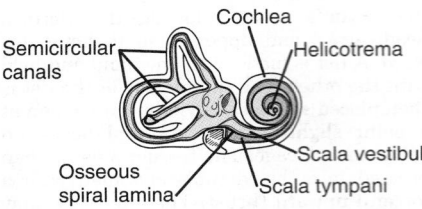

Helicotrema, shown in the interior of the right osseous labyrinth. From Dorland's, 2000.

associated with gastric carcinoma; Formerly called *Campylobacter pylori.*

helicoid (hel'ĭ-koid) spiral (def. 2).

helicotrema (hel''ĭ-ko-tre'mah) the passage that connects the scala tympani and the scala vestibuli at the apex of the cochlea.

helicy (he'lĭ-se) a principle of HOMEODY-NAMICS in the SCIENCE OF UNITARY HUMAN BEINGS; the continuous, innovative, and unpredictable increasing diversity of human and environmental field patterns.

helium (He) (he'le-um) a chemical element, atomic number 2, atomic weight 4.003. (See Appendix 6.) Helium is a chemically inert element that is odorless, tasteless, and noncombustible. Because of its low density it is easily moved through the air passages and therefore requires little effort in breathing on the part of the patient in respiratory distress. Although helium itself has no chemical therapeutic value, when combined with oxygen it facilitates delivery of oxygen to the lungs (see HELIUM-OXYGEN THERAPY). It should be noted that helium causes the voice to be high-pitched and the spoken word difficult to understand. This should be explained to the patient with the assurance that the effect is harmless and temporary.

h.-oxygen therapy the administration of a mixture of helium and oxygen (commonly 80 per cent He and 20 per cent O_2, or 70 per cent He and 30 per cent O_2); used in the management of airway obstruction associated with bronchospasm or bronchial asthma. The He-O_2 mixture is about one third the density of air. This reduces turbulent flow and the patient effort required for ventilation.

helix (he'liks), pl. *he'lices, helixes* [Gr.] 1. a winding structure; see also COIL and SPIRAL. 2. the superior and posterior free margin of the pinna of the ear.

α-h., alpha h. the complex structural arrangement of parts of protein molecules in which a single polypeptide chain forms a right-handed helix.

double h., Watson-Crick h. the structure of DEOXYRIBONUCLEIC ACID (DNA), consisting of two coiled chains, each of which contains information completely specifying the other chain.

Hellin's law (hel'inz) one in about 89 pregnancies ends in the birth of twins; one in 89^2, or 7921, of triplets; one in 89^3, or 704,969, of quadruplets.

helminth (hel'minth) a parasitic worm; see NEMATODE and TREMATODE.

helminthemesis (hel''min-them'ĕ-sis) the vomiting of worms.

helminthiasis (hel''min-thi'ah-sis) vermination (def. 1).

helminthology (hel''min-thol'o-je) the scientific study of parasitic worms.

helminthoma (hel''min-tho'mah) a tumor caused by a parasitic worm.

heloma (he-lo'mah) corn.

h. du'rum hard corn; see CORN.

h. mol'le soft corn; see CORN.

helotomy (he-lot'ah-me) excision or paring of a corn or callus.

helplessness (help'les-nes) a feeling that one's efforts as an individual will not influence the outcome of a situation. Patients may experience learned helplessness as a result of overly rigid institutional rules or behaviors of staff members. Individualized care fosters self-esteem and will assist in the prevention of helplessness.

hem(o)- word element [Gr.], *blood.* See also words beginning *hema-* and *hemat(o)-.*

hemacytometer (he''mah-si-tom'ĕ-ter) a device used for manual blood counts, consisting of a counting chamber of uniform depth that is covered by a ruled cover glass so that the region under each ruled square contains a known volume of the diluted specimen. Called also hemocytometer.

hemadsorption (hem''ad-sorp'shun) the adherence of red blood cells to other cells, particles, or surfaces. adj., **hemadsor'bent.**

hemadynamometer (he''mah-di''nah-mom'ĕ-ter) an instrument for measuring blood pressure.

hemadynamometry (he''mah-di''nah-mom'ĕ-tre) measurement of blood pressure.

hemagglutination (he''mah-gloo''tĭ-na'shun) agglutination of erythrocytes.

h. inhibition (HI, HAI) test 1. a highly sensitive procedure for the measurement of soluble antigens in biologic specimens; the amount of hemagglutination reflects the amount of free antibody present after reaction with the specimen and thus varies inversely with amount of antigen in the specimen. 2. a procedure for the measurement of serum antibodies directed against a hemagglutinating virus; the highest dilution of serum that completely inhibits hemagglutination by a standardized viral preparation is reported as the hemagglutination titer.

hemagglutinin (he″mah-gloo′tĭ-nin) an antibody that causes agglutination of erythrocytes.

    cold h. one that acts optimally at temperatures near 4°C.

    warm h. one that acts optimally at temperatures near 37°C.

hemal (he′mal) 1. ventral to the spinal axis, where the heart and great vessels are located, as, e.g., the hemal arches. 2. HEMIC. 3. pertaining to the blood vessels; see *vascular*.

hemanalysis (he″mah-nal′ĭ-sis) analysis of the blood.

hemangiectasis (he-man″je-ek′tah-sis) dilatation of blood vessels.

hemangioameloblastoma (he-man″je-o-ah-mel′o-blas-to′mah) a highly vascular AMELOBLASTOMA.

hemangioblast (he-man′je-o-blast″) a mesodermal cell that gives rise to both vascular endothelium and hemocytoblasts.

hemangioblastoma (he-man″je-o-blas-to′-mah) a benign blood vessel tumor of the cerebellum, spinal cord, or retina, consisting of proliferated blood vessel cells and ANGIO-BLASTS. Those arising in the cerebellum (cerebellar hemangioblastoma) may be cystic and associated with VON HIPPEL-LINDAU DISEASE. Called also *angioblastoma*.

    cerebellar h. hemangioblastoma of the CEREBELLUM, often cystic; an autosomal dominant form is associated with VON HIP-PEL-LINDAU DISEASE.

hemangioendothelioblastoma (he-man″-je-o-en″do-the″le-o-blas-to′mah) a tumor of mesenchymal origin of which the cells tend to form endothelial cells and line blood vessels.

hemangioendothelioma (he-man″je-o-en″do-the″le-o′mah) a rare, well-differentiated endothelial tumor with an appearance between that of a HEMANGIOMA and a SARCOMA; sometimes considered to be identical to a HEMANGIOSARCOMA.

hemangiofibroma (he-man″je-o-fi-bro′-mah) a HEMANGIOMA containing fibrous tissue.

hemangioma (he-man″je-o′mah) a congenital vascular malformation consisting of a benign tumor made up of newly formed blood vessels clustered together; it may be present at birth in various parts of the body, including the liver and bones. In the majority of cases it appears as a network of small blood-filled capillaries near the surface of the skin, forming a reddish or purplish birthmark.

    cavernous h. a congenital vascular malformation that has a soft, spongy consistency and may contain a large amount of blood. It usually appears during the first few postnatal weeks and disappears by the age of 9 years. The most common sites are head, neck, and viscera such as the liver, spleen, or pancreas. Treatment varies according to the size of the lesion.

    strawberry h. a circumscribed capillary hemangioma, which may be present at birth or may appear soon after birth. These are most common on the head, neck, and trunk and appear as small macules that develop into raised purplish-red lobulated tumors. Most involute by age 2 to 3.

hemangiomatosis (he-man″je-o-mah-to′-sis) the presence of multiple hemangiomas.

hemangiopericytoma (he-man″je-o-per″ĭ-si-to′-mah) a tumor composed of spindle CELLS with a rich vascular network, which apparently arises from PERICYTES.

hemangiosarcoma (he-man″je-o-sahr-ko′-mah) a malignant tumor of vascular tissue; called also angiosarcoma.

hemapheresis (hem″ah-fer′ĕ-sis) apheresis.

hemarthros (he-mahr′thrōs) hemarthrosis.

hemarthrosis (he″mahr-thro′sis) blood in a joint cavity; called also hemarthros.

hemat(o)- word element [Gr.], *blood.* See also words beginning *hema-* and *hem(o)-*.

hematemesis (he″mah-tem′ĕ-sis) the vomiting of blood. The appearance of the vomit depends on the amount and character of the gastric contents at the time blood is vomited and on the length of time the blood has been in the stomach. Gastric acids change bright red blood to a brownish color and the vomit is often described as "coffee-ground" in color. Bright red blood in the vomit indicates a fresh hemorrhage and little contact of the blood with gastric juices. The most common causes of hematemesis are PEPTIC ULCER, GASTRITIS, esophageal VARICES or lesions, and cancer of the stomach. Benign tumors, traumatic postoperative bleeding, and swallowed blood from points in the nose, mouth, and throat can also produce hematemesis.

hematencephalon (he″mah-ten-sef′ah-lon) effusion of blood into the brain.

hemathermous (he″mah-ther′mus) homeothermic.

hematic (he-mat′ik) 1. HEMIC. 2. HEMATINIC.

hematidrosis (he″mah-tĭ-dro′sis) excretion of bloody sweat.

hematin (he′mah-tin) 1. the hydroxide of HEME; it stimulates the synthesis of GLOBIN, inhibits the synthesis of PORPHYRIN, and is a component of CYTOCHROMES and

PEROXIDASES; it is also used as a reagent. 2. hemin (def. 1).

hematinemia (he″mah-tĭ-ne′me-ah) the presence of heme in the blood.

hematinic (he″mah-tin′ik) 1. improving the quality of the blood. 2. an agent that does this, increasing the HEMOGLOBIN level and the number of ERYTHROCYTES; examples are IRON preparations, liver extract, and the B complex VITAMINS.

hematinuria (he″mah-tin-u′re-ah) the presence of hematin in the urine, seen in hemoglobinuria.

hematobilia (he″mah-to-bil′e-ah) hemobilia.

hematoblast (he′mah-to-blast″) blast cell.

hematocele (he′mah-to-sēl″) an effusion of blood into a cavity, especially into the TUNICA VAGINALIS TESTIS.

hematochezia (he″mah-to-ke′ze-ah) blood in the feces.

hematochromatosis (he″mah-to-kro″-mah-to′sis) hemochromatosis.

hematochyluria (he″mah-to-ki-lu′re-ah) the discharge of blood and chyle in the urine, as seen in FILARIASIS.

hematocolpometra (he″mah-to-kol″po-me′trah) accumulation of menstrual blood in the vagina and uterus.

hematocolpos (he″mah-to-kol′pos) accumulation of menstrual blood in the vagina.

hematocrit (he-mat′o-krit) the volume percentage of erythrocytes (packed red blood CELLS) in whole blood; also, the procedure used in its determination. The hematocrit (which means literally, "to separate blood") is determined by centrifuging a blood sample to separate the cellular elements from the plasma; the results of the test indicate the ratio of cell volume to plasma volume and are expressed as milliliters of packed cells per 100 ml of blood, or in volumes per 100 ml. The normal range is 40 to 54 volumes per 100 ml for males, and 37 to 47 volumes per 100 ml for females. The hematocrit, in conjunction with other hematologic tests, provides information about the size, functioning capacity, and number of erythrocytes.

hematocyst (he′mah-to-sist″) effusion of blood into the bladder or in a cyst.

hematogenic (he″mah-to-jen′ik) 1. hematopoietic. 2. hematogenous.

hematogenesis (he″mah-to-jen′ĕ-sis) hematopoiesis.

hematogenous (he″mah-toj′ĕ-nus) produced by or derived from the blood; disseminated through the bloodstream or by the circulation.

hematoid (he′mah-toid) like blood.

hematoidin (he″mah-toi′din) a hematogenous pigment apparently identical to BILIRUBIN but formed in the tissues from hemoglobin, particularly under conditions of reduced oxygen tension.

hematologist (he″mah-tol′o-jist) a specialist in hematology.

hematology (he″mah-tol′o-je) the branch of medical science dealing with the blood and blood-forming tissues, including morphology, physiology, and pathology. adj., **hematolog′ic.**

hematolymphangioma (he″mah-to-lim-fan″je-o′mah) a tumor composed of blood and lymph vessels.

hematolysis (hem″ah-tol′ĭ-sis) hemolysis.

hematoma (he″mah-to′mah) A localized collection of extravasated blood, usually clotted, in an organ, space, or tissue; contusions (bruises) and black eyes are familiar forms that are seldom serious. Hematomas can occur almost anywhere on the body; they are almost always present with a fracture and are especially serious when they occur inside the skull, where they may produce local pressure on the brain. In minor injuries the blood is absorbed unless infection develops.

Cranial Hematoma. The two most common kinds of cranial hematomas are *epidural* and *subdural* (*dural* refers to the dura mater). Epidural hematoma occurs between the dura mater and the skull. It is most often caused by a heavy blow to the head that damages the upper surface of the dura mater. Blood seeps into the surrounding tissue, forming a tumorlike mass or hematoma. Since the skull is rigid, the hematoma presses inward against the brain; if the pressure continues, the brain can be affected. An epidural hematoma is the result of rupture of a relatively large meningeal artery, so that there is a rapid leakage of blood, causing increased intracranial pressure that can be fatal in a short period of time.

A subdural hematoma occurs beneath the dura mater, between the tough casing and the more delicate membranes covering the tissue of the brain, the pia-arachnoid. This kind of injury is more often caused by the head striking an immovable object, such as the floor, than by a blow from a moving object. There may be no severe head injury or fracture. A blow to the head can cause the brain to move violently, tearing blood vessels and forming a swelling that may include fluid from the brain tissue. A chronic subdural hematoma may remain and increase in size. (See also HEAD INJURY.)

Symptoms. The most common symptoms of epidural hematoma occur within a few hours after injury. There can be a sudden or gradual loss of consciousness, partial or full paralysis on the side opposite the injury, and dilation of the pupil of the eye on the same side as the injury.

The symptoms of chronic subdural hematoma are similar to those of a brain tumor, and may come and go. There may be subtle personality changes, or the patient may become confused, weak in various parts of the body, vague, and drowsy.

Subdural hematoma occasionally occurs in babies as a result of birth injury. Unless the injury is discovered and treated at an early stage, the child's mental and physical development may be retarded, and spastic paralysis can occur. Early surgery is usually successful in preventing permanent symptoms and disabilities.

Treatment. Prompt surgery is the only treatment for epidural hematoma. The clotted blood is removed by a combination of suction and irrigation methods through openings made in the skull, and the bleeding is controlled. The same surgery is used for subdural hematomas.

Septal Hematoma. Injury to the nose sometimes causes hematoma of the nasal septum. Its symptoms include nasal obstruction and headache. The condition may be treated by incision and drainage or may clear up spontaneously in a few weeks. If the hematoma becomes infected, an abscess may result, requiring drainage and treatment with antibiotics.

hematomediastinum (he″mah-to-me″de-ah-sti′num) effusion of blood into the mediastinum.

hematometra (he″mah-to-me′trah) an accumulation of menstrual blood in the uterus.

hematometry (he″mah-tom′ĕ-tre) measurement of various parameters of the blood, such as the complete blood COUNT.

hematomyelia (he″mah-to-mi-e′le-ah) hemorrhage into the substance of the spinal cord.

hematomyelitis (he″mah-to-mi″ĕ-li′tis) acute myelitis with bloody effusion into the spinal cord.

hematomyelopore (he″mah-to-mi″ĕ-lo-por″) formation of canals in the spinal cord due to hemorrhage.

hematonephrosis (he″mah-to-nĕ-fro′sis) the presence of blood in the renal pelvis; called also hemonephrosis.

hematopathology (he″mah-to-pah-thol′o-je) hemopathology.

hematophagous (he″mah-tof′ah-gus) subsisting on blood.

hematophilia (he″mah-to-fil′e-ah) hemophilia.

hematopoiesis (he″mah-to-poi-e′sis) the formation and development of blood cells.

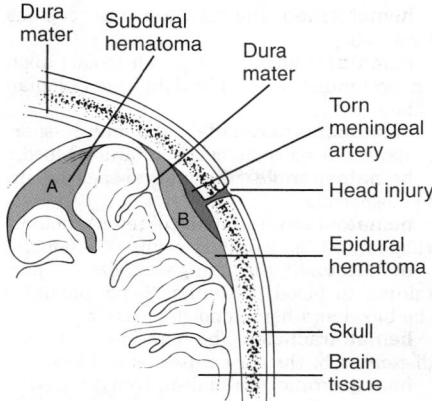

Subdural and epidural hematoma. *A,* Subdural hematoma. As a result of trauma to the head, small ruptured blood vessels leak blood into the space under the dura mater. The hematoma forms between the dura mater and the arachnoid membrane. *B,* Epidural hematoma. The result of a head injury that tears a large meningeal artery, causing the collection of a large amount of blood above the dura mater. The large epidural hematoma compresses brain tissue. If not relieved, subdural and epidural hematomas can be fatal.

In the embryo and fetus it takes place in a variety of sites including the liver, spleen, thymus, lymph nodes, and bone marrow; from birth throughout the rest of life it is mainly in the bone marrow with a small amount occurring in lymph nodes. Called also hematogenesis, hemogenesis, and hemopoiesis.

   extramedullary h. the formation and development of blood cells outside the bone marrow, as in the spleen, liver, and lymph nodes.

   hematopoietic (he″mah-to-poi-et′ik) 1. pertaining to HEMATOPOIESIS (formation of blood cells). 2. promoting hematopoiesis. 3. an agent that promotes HEMATOPOIESIS.

   hematoporphyria (he″mah-to-por-fēr′e-ah) a constitutional state marked by an abnormal quantity of porphyrin (uroporphyrin and coproporphyrin) in the tissues and secreted in the urine, pigmentation of the face (and later of the bones), sensitivity of the skin to light, vomiting, and intestinal disturbance; see PORPHYRIA.

   hematoporphyrin (he″mah-to-por′fi-rin) a hematogenous pigment that is an iron-free derivative of heme, a product of the decomposition of hemoglobin.

   hematorrhachis (he″mah-tor′ah-kis) hematomyelia; hemorrhage into the vertebral canal.

hematorrhea (he″mah-to-re′ah) copious hemorrhage.

hematosalpinx (hem″ah-to-sal′pinks) an accumulation of blood in the fallopian tube.

hematospermatocele (he″mah-to-sper-mat′o-sēl) a spermatocele containing blood.

hematospermia (he″mah-to-sper′me-ah) hemospermia.

hematosteon (he″mah-tos′te-on) hemorrhage into the medullary cavity of a bone.

hematotoxic (he′mah-to-tok″sik) 1. pertaining to blood poisoning. 2. poisonous to the blood and hematopoietic system.

hematotrachelos (he″mah-to-trah-ke′los) distention of the cervix uteri with blood.

hematotropic (he″mah-to-trop′ik) having a special affinity for or exerting a specific effect on the blood or blood cells.

hematotympanum (he″mah-to-tim′pah-num) hemorrhage into the middle ear.

hematoxylin (he″mah-tok′sī-lin) an acid coloring matter obtained from the wood of a tree (*Haematoxylon campechianum*); used as a stain for histologic specimens and as an indicator.

hematuria (he″mah-tu′re-ah) the discharge of blood in the urine, making the urine either slightly blood-tinged, grossly bloody, or a smoky brown color. Microscopic examination of a urine specimen can reveal red blood cells not evident to the naked eye; however, this *microscopic hematuria* is not always pathognomonic. *Gross hematuria* that is visible to the naked eye is symptomatic of disease or injury to a part of the urinary system. Bladder tumors, cystitis, urethritis, and small kidney stones passing along the ureter can cause blood in the urine. Vascular diseases, some types of kidney disorders, and (sometimes but not always) traumatic injury to the kidney can also produce hematuria.

Patient Care. Assessment activities include noting and recording the amount of urine and color and the presence or absence of clots and bits of tissue. Moreover, the patient should be asked at what point during urination the blood is noticed. This information can help locate the site of the source of bleeding. If bright red blood is noticed at the onset of urination, it is likely that the problem is somewhere in the urethra. If blood is noticed at the end of urination, the site probably is near the neck of the bladder. Bleeding throughout voiding indicates that blood is coming from a site above the bladder neck and has been well mixed with urine in the bladder before elimination. Blood that has remained in the urinary tract long enough to deteriorate will give the urine a smoky, brownish color.

Additional information includes any pain or burning associated with urination, as well as pain in the region of the bladder or over the kidney. Hematuria not associated with pain is characteristic of neoplasms of the kidney or bladder in the early stages.

False hematuria or *pseudohematuria* is a reddish color to the urine that is not associated with presence of blood. Patients taking PYRVINIUM pamoate (Povan) or PYRIDIUM should be told that their urine will have a red, red-brown, or red-orange color, so that they will not think this is hematuria.

heme (hēm) the nonprotein, insoluble, iron protoporphyrin constituent of hemoglobin, of various other respiratory pigments, and of many cells, both animal and vegetable. It is an iron compound and constitutes the pigment portion or protein-free part of the hemoglobin molecule, and is responsible for its oxygen-carrying properties.

hemeralopia (hem″er-al-o′pe-ah) defective vision in a bright light; called also day blindness and night sight.

hemi- word element [Gr.], *half.*

hemiacardius (hem″e-ah-kahr′de-us) an unequal twin in which the heart is rudimentary, its circulation being assisted by the other twin.

hemiachromatopsia (hem″e-ah-kro″mah-top′se-ah) loss of the normal perception of color in half, or in corresponding halves, of the visual field.

hemiamyosthenia (hem″e-ah-mi″os-the′-ne-ah) lack of muscular power on one side of the body.

hemianacusia (hem″e-an″ah-koo′ze-ah) HEARING LOSS in one ear.

hemianalgesia (hem″e-an″al-je′ze-ah) analgesia on one side of the body.

hemianencephaly (hem″e-an″en-sef′ah-le) congenital absence of one side of the brain.

hemianesthesia (hem″e-an″es-the′zhah) anesthesia of one side of the body.

   crossed h., h. crucia′ta loss of sensation on one side of the body and loss of pain and temperature sense on the opposite side.

hemianopia (hem″e-ah-no′pe-ah) defective vision or BLINDNESS in half of the visual field; usually applied to bilateral defects caused by a single lesion. adj., **hemianop′ic, hemianop′tic.**

Patient Care. Visual field deficit on one side often occurs as a result of STROKE SYNDROME. Patients with this problem are unable to perceive objects to the side of the visual midline. The visual loss is contralateral, i.e., it is on the side opposite the brain lesion. To facilitate self care, commonly

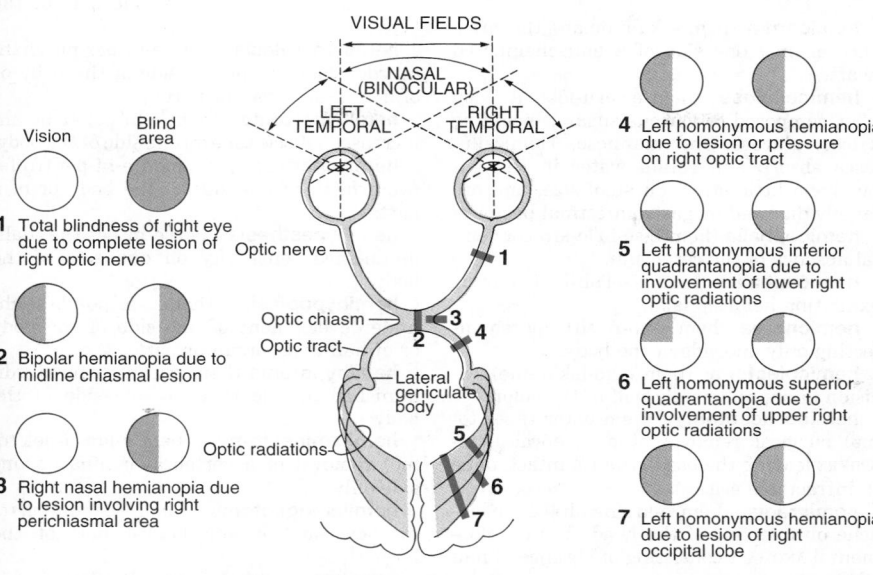

VISUAL FIELDS

NASAL (BINOCULAR)

LEFT TEMPORAL   RIGHT TEMPORAL

Vision   Blind area

1 Total blindness of right eye due to complete lesion of right optic nerve

Optic nerve

2 Bipolar hemianopia due to midline chiasmal lesion

Optic chiasm
Optic tract

3 Right nasal hemianopia due to lesion involving right perichiasmal area

Optic radiations

Lateral geniculate body

4 Left homonymous hemianopia due to lesion or pressure on right optic tract

5 Left homonymous inferior quadrantanopia due to involvement of lower right optic radiations

6 Left homonymous superior quadrantanopia due to involvement of upper right optic radiations

7 Left homonymous hemianopia due to lesion of right occipital lobe

Visual field defects associated with hemianopia. From Polaski and Tatro, 1996.

used articles such as the water pitcher, meal tray, and call bell are placed on the unaffected side. The patient should be approached from and communicated with while standing or sitting on the side in which vision is best. When in visual contact with the patient, caregivers should move slowly toward and past the visual boundary to stimulate scanning to the affected side. Auditory and visual stimulation on the affected side can help improve and maintain residual sight on that side.

homonymous h. hemianopia affecting the right halves or the left halves of the visual fields of both eyes. The patient must turn the head from side to side to compensate for the defect. Often it is due not to any pathology in the eye itself but to damage to the optic tract or occipital lobe.

hemianopic (hem″e-ah-nop′ik) pertaining to or characterized by HEMIANOPIA.

h. pupillary reaction in certain cases of hemianopia, light thrown upon one side of the retina causes the iris to contract, while light thrown upon the other side arouses no response.

hemianopsia (hem″e-ah-nop′se-ah) hemianopia.

hemianosmia (hem″e-an-oz′me-ah) absence of the sense of smell in one nostril.

hemiapraxia (hem″e-ah-prak′se-ah) inability to perform coordinated movements on one side of the body.

hemiataxia (hem″e-ah-tak′se-ah) ataxia on one side of the body.

hemiathetosis (hem″e-ath″ĕ-to′sis) athetosis of one side of the body.

hemiatrophy (hem″e-at′ro-fe) atrophy of one side of the body or one half of an organ or part.

hemiaxial (hem″e-ak′se-al) at any oblique angle to the long axis of the body or a part.

hemiballism (hem″e-bal′izm) hemiballismus.

hemiballismus (hem″e-bah-liz′mus) violent motor restlessness of half of the body, most marked in the upper limbs.

hemibladder (hem′e-blad″er) a half bladder, as seen in exstrophy of the cloaca; the urinary bladder is formed as two physically separated parts, each with its own ureter.

hemiblock (hem′e-blok″) failure in conduction of electrical impulse in either of the two main divisions of the left branch of the BUNDLE OF HIS; the interruption may occur in either the anterior (superior) or posterior (inferior) division. Hemiblock accompanied by an anterior wall MYOCARDIAL INFARCTION is a particularly serious finding.

left anterior h. a conduction block of the anterior superior division of the left bundle branch; left anterior hemiblock with acute anterior wall MYOCARDIAL INFARCTION is a particularly serious finding.

hemic (he′mik, hem′ik) pertaining to blood; called also hemal and hematic.

hemicardia (hem″e-kahr′de-ah) the presence of only one side of a four-chambered heart.

hemicellulose (hem″e-sel′u-lōs) a food fiber composed of various sugars, including xylose, glucose, and mannose. Hemicelluloses absorb and retain water in the gut but have little effect on stool size, and are largely digested by gastrointestinal bacteria.

hemicephalia (hem″e-sĕ-fa′le-ah) congenital absence of the cerebrum.

hemicephalus (hem″e-sef′ah-lus) a fetus exhibiting hemicephalia.

hemichorea (hem″e-ko-re′ah) chorea affecting only one side of the body.

hemicolectomy (hem″e-ko-lek′to-me) excision of approximately half of the colon.

hemicorticectomy (hem″e-kor″tĭ-sek′to-me) surgical removal of a cerebral HEMI-SPHERE leaving the basal GANGLIA intact; done in intractable EPILEPSY.

hemicrania (hem″e-kra′ne-ah) 1. headache on one side of the head. 2. a developmental ANOMALY consisting of absence of half of the cranium.

hemicraniosis (hem″e-kra″ne-o′sis) hyperostosis of one side of the cranium and face.

hemidiaphoresis (hem″e-di″ah-fo-re′sis) hemihyperhidrosis.

hemidysesthesia (hem″e-dis″es-the′zhah) a disorder of sensation affecting only one side of the body.

hemidystrophy (hem″e-dis′tro-fe) unequal development of the two sides of the body.

hemiectromelia (hem″e-ek″tro-me′le-ah) a developmental ANOMALY consisting of imperfect limbs on one side of the body.

hemiepilepsy (hem″e-ep′ĭ-lep″se) epilepsy affecting one side of the body.

hemifacial (hem″e-fa′sh′l) affecting one side of the face.

hemigastrectomy (hem″e-gas-trek′to-me) excision of half of the stomach.

hemigeusia (hem″e-goo′zhah) absence of the sense of taste on one side of the tongue.

hemiglossectomy (hem″e-glos-ek′to-me) excision of half of the tongue.

hemiglossitis (hem″e-glos-i′tis) inflammation of half of the tongue.

hemignathia (hem″e-na′the-ah) a developmental ANOMALY characterized by partial or complete lack of the lower jaw on one side.

hemihidrosis (hem″e-hi-dro′sis) sweating on one side of the body only.

hemihypalgesia (hem″e-hi″pal-je′ze-ah) diminished sensitivity to pain on one side of the body.

hemihyperesthesia (hem″e-hi″per-es-the′zhah) increased sensitivity of one side of the body.

hemihyperhidrosis (hem″e-hi″per-hi-dro′-sis) excessive sweating on one side of the body.

hemihyperplasia (hem″e-hi″per-pla′zhah) overdevelopment of one side of the body or of half of an organ or part.

hemihypertonia (hem″e-hi″per-to′ne-ah) increased muscle tone on one side of the body.

hemihypertrophy (hem″e-hi-per′tro-fe) overgrowth of one side of the body or of a part.

hemihypesthesia (hem″e-hi″pes-the′zhah) diminished sensitivity on one side of the body.

hemihypoplasia (hem″e-hi″po-pla′zhah) underdevelopment of one side of the body or of half of an organ or part.

hemihypotonia (hem″e-hi″po-to′ne-ah) diminished muscle tone on one side of the body.

hemilaminectomy (hem″e-lam″ĭ-nek′to-me) removal of a vertebral lamina on one side only.

hemilaryngectomy (hem″e-lar″in-jek′to-me) excision of one lateral half of the larynx.

hemilateral (hem″e-lat′er-al) affecting one side of the body only.

hemimelia (hem″e-me′le-ah) congenital absence of all or part of the distal half of a limb.

hemimelus (hem-im′ĕ-lus) an individual exhibiting hemimelia.

hemin (he′min) 1. a porphyrin chelate of iron, derived from red blood cells; the chloride of HEME. It is used to treat the symptoms of various PORPHYRIAS. 2. hematin (def. 1).

heminephrectomy (hem″e-nĕ-frek′to-me) excision of part (half) of a kidney.

hemiopia (hem″e-o′pe-ah) hemianopia.

hemipagus (hem-ip′ah-gus) twin fetuses joined laterally at the thorax.

hemiparalysis (hem″e-pah-ral′ĭ-sis) paralysis of one side of the body.

hemiparanesthesia (hem″e-par″an-es-the′zhah) anesthesia of the lower half of one side.

hemiparaplegia (hem″e-par″ah-ple′jah) paralysis of the lower half of one side.

hemiparesis (hem″e-pah-re′sis) paresis (paralysis) affecting one side of the body.

hemiparesthesia (hem″e-par″es-the′zhah) PARESTHESIA (abnormal sensations) on one side.

hemiparetic (hem″e-pah-ret′ik) 1. pertaining to hemiparesis. 2. one affected with hemiparesis.

hemipeptone (hem″e-pep′tōn) a form of peptone obtained from pepsin digestion.

hemiplegia (hem″e-ple′jah) paralysis of one side of the body; usually caused by a brain lesion, such as a tumor, or by STROKE SYNDROME. The paralysis occurs on the side opposite the brain disorder; this is explained by the fact that motor axons from the cerebral cortex enter the medulla oblongata and form two well-defined bands known as the pyramidal TRACTS. The majority of the fibers in these tracts cross to the opposite side; therefore damage to the right cerebral HEMISPHERE affects motor control of the left half of the body. See STROKE SYNDROME for symptoms and care of the patient with hemiplegia. adj., **hemiple′gic.**

Hemiptera (hem-ip′ter-ah) the true bugs, an order of arthropods (class Insecta) with over 30,000 species, usually characterized by the presence of two pairs of wings and mouth parts adapted for piercing or sucking.

hemirachischisis (hem″e-rah-kis′kĭ-sis) fissure of the vertebral column without prolapse of the spinal cord.

hemisacralization (hem″e-sa″kral-ĭ-za′-shun) fusion of the fifth lumbar vertebra to the first segment of the sacrum on only one side.

hemisection (hem″e-sek′shun) 1. division into two equal parts. 2. surgical removal of one root of a large mandibular molar along with the corresponding crown area.

hemisectomy (hem″e-sek′tah-me) amputation of one root of a two-rooted mandibular tooth. See also APICOECTOMY.

hemispasm (hem′e-spazm) spasm affecting only one side.

hemisphere (hem′ĭ-sfēr) half of a spherical or roughly spherical structure or organ.

cerebral h. one of the paired structures constituting the largest part of the brain, which together comprise the extensive cerebral cortex, centrum semiovale, basal ganglia, and rhinencephalon, and contain the lateral ventricle. See also BRAIN.

cerebellar h. either of the paired portions of the CEREBELLUM lateral to the VERMIS.

dominant h. the cerebral HEMISPHERE that is more concerned than the other in the integration of sensations and the control of many functions. See also LATERALITY.

hemispherectomy (hem″ĭ-sfēr-ek′to-me) surgical removal of a cerebral HEMISPHERE; done in intractable EPILEPSY.

hemispherium (hem″ĭ-sfēr′e-um), pl. *hemisphe′ria* [L.] hemisphere.

hemithorax (hem″e-thor′aks) one side of the chest; the cavity lateral to the mediastinum.

hemithyroidectomy (hem″e-thi″roi-dek′-to-me) excision of one lobe of the thyroid.

hemivertebra (hem″e-ver′tĕ-brah) a developmental ANOMALY in which one side of a vertebra is incompletely developed.

hemizygosity (hem″e-zi-gos′ĭ-te) the state of having only one of a pair of ALLELES transmitting a specific character. adj., **hemizy′gous.**

hemizygote (hem″e-zi′gōt) an individual exhibiting HEMIZYGOSITY, such as males with the X CHROMOSOME.

hemoaccess (he′mo-ak′ses) vascular access.

hemobilia (he″mo-bil′e-ah) bleeding into the biliary passages.

hemoblast (he′mo-blast″) blast cell.

hemocatheresis (he″mo-kah-ther′ĕ-sis) the destruction of erythrocytes.

Hemoccult (he′mo-kult) trademark for a guaiac reagent strip test for occult blood.

hemochorial (he″mo-ko′re-al) denoting a type of placenta in which maternal blood comes in direct contact with the chorion.

hemochromatosis (he″mo-kro″mah-to′-sis) a disorder of IRON metabolism with excess deposition of iron in the tissues, bronze skin pigmentation, cirrhosis of the liver, and diabetes mellitus; see also HEMOSIDEROSIS and SIDEROSIS. Called also bronze diabetes and iron storage disease. adj., **hemochromatot′ic.**

hemoclasis (he-mok′lah-sis) HEMOLYSIS.

hemoconcentration (he″mo-kon″sen-tra′-shun) increase in the proportion of formed elements in the blood, as a result of a decrease in its fluid content.

hemoconia (he″mo-ko′ne-ah), pl. *hemoco′-niae* [L.] minute colorless bodies found in blood, thought to be products of the disintegration of erythrocytes. Called also blood dust and hemokonia.

hemoconiosis (he″mo-ko″ne-o′sis) presence in blood of excessive amounts of hemoconia.

hemocyte (he′mo-sīt″) blood cell.

hemocytoblast (he″mo-si′to-blast) blast cell.

hemocytology (he″mo-si-tol′o-je) the study of blood cells.

hemocytolysis (he″mo-si-tol′ĭ-sis) hemolysis.

hemocytometer (he″mo-si-tom′ĕ-ter) a device used in manual blood cell counts consisting of a counting chamber of uniform depth that is covered by a ruled cover glass so that the region under each ruled square contains a known volume of the diluted blood specimen.

hemocytotripsis (he″mo-si′to-trip′sis) disintegration of blood cells by pressure.

hemodiafiltration (he″mo-di″ah-fil-tra′-shun) a technique of HEMODIALYSIS in which blood flow is accelerated to twice that of conventional dialysis; the speed of blood flow is 500 ml/min, so that this technique requires two dialyzers in series and replaces the rapid loss of volume with backfiltration from dialysate to blood. Patients who can benefit from this technique must have acceptable blood pressure levels, fully operative and stable fistulas to accommodate the rapid flow rate, and ability to comply with fluid restrictions. They must be monitored much more closely during this treatment than during more conventional hemodialysis, but they can be dialyzed for two rather than the standard four hours per session. Called also high flux hemodiafiltration.

hemodiagnosis (he″mo-di″ag-no′sis) diagnosis by examination of the blood.

hemodialysis (he″mo-di-al′ĭ-sis) the use of principles of DIALYSIS for removal of certain elements from the blood while it is being circulated outside the body in a HEMODIALYZER or through the peritoneal cavity (see PERITONEAL DIALYSIS). The procedure is used to remove toxic wastes from the blood of a patient with acute or chronic RENAL FAILURE. Called also dialysis, kidney dialysis, and renal dialysis. adj., **hemodialyt′ic.**

Either the membrane lining the peritoneal cavity (in peritoneal dialysis) or a synthetic membrane (in *extracorporeal hemodialysis*) may be used as the dialyzing membrane. In the latter, the patient's blood is pumped from the arterial circulation through the hemodialyzer to the venous circulation. In the dialyzer, it flows past a cellulosic or synthetic semipermeable membrane while DIALYSATE fluid flows past the other side of the membrane. Small molecules and ions diffuse through the membrane, passing from the side on which the concentration is higher to the side on which it is lower. The dialysate fluid contains no UREA or CREATININE, so that these constituents are removed at maximum rates. The concentrations of electrolytes are adjusted according to the needs of the patient. If the patient has HYPERKALEMIA or HYPERNATREMIA, the excess ions of potassium or sodium are also removed. Other electrolytes are adjusted so that serum pH and electrolyte levels are not changed by the dialysis. Large molecules and blood cells cannot pass through the membrane and, therefore, stay in the blood.

Two commonly used accesses to the patient's vascular system are the *external shunt* and the *internal arteriovenous (AV) fistula.* An external shunt is usually indicated when dialysis must begin immediately. It requires two lengths of specially prepared tubing; one for insertion in a vein and the other in an artery, usually in the forearm. Between dialysis treatments, the tubes are joined by a connector. Although the external shunt has the advantage of being immediately available for use in an emergency, it has the potential of becoming infected or obstructed with clots, and, if the integrity of the system is disrupted, rapid and copious blood loss may occur.

The internal AV fistula is surgically created by anastomosing an artery to a vein; that is, the vein is arterialized or made into a large superficial vessel that is easily accessible by venipuncture. The fistula must heal gradually and become mature before a cannula can be inserted. When END-STAGE RENAL DISEASE is inevitable, the fistula can be prepared months in advance for use when symptoms of UREMIA appear.

Patient Care. Hemodialysis treatments for chronic renal failure are usually done two to three times a week. The problems that a patient on hemodialysis may experience are fluid overload (HYPERVOLEMIA), electrolyte imbalance, and alterations in blood components, leading to anemia or platelet abnormalities resulting in a tendency to bleed excessively. Another problem is infection, either of the access site and the blood or in the urinary or respiratory tract because of urinary or pulmonary stasis. Infection with human immunodeficiency VIRUS is also a possibility since blood has not always been routinely screened for this virus and clients may have been infected. Precautions must be taken when handling any blood products or the dialysis equipment.

Patients who depend on hemodialysis to prolong their lives require extensive instruction in the care of their cannulae and access sites. Some individuals receive intensive training and are able to undergo hemodialysis at home. A partner must be trained in order to safely administer home hemodialysis. Follow up care, instruction, and evaluation by health care professionals are imperative to ensure patient safety.

Patients also must know about special precautions for avoiding the complications that accompany long-term hemodialysis. The purposes for prescribed medications should be explained, as well as side effects that should be reported. These drugs may include multivitamins, antacids, iron supplements, antihypertensives, digitalis, vasodilators, and antibiotics. Rigid dietary and fluid intake restrictions are particularly difficult for some patients and their families. Patient compliance can be a major

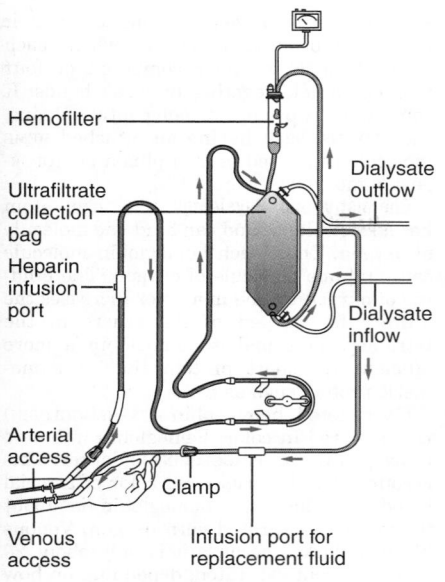

Hemofilter

Ultrafiltrate collection bag

Heparin infusion port

Dialysate outflow

Dialysate inflow

Arterial access

Clamp

Venous access

Infusion port for replacement fluid

A hemodialysis circuit.

monitoring of intra-arterial blood pressure, pulmonary artery pressure, left atrial pressure, and central venous pressure. Invasive pressure monitoring requires the insertion of a catheter into an artery (usually the radial, brachial, or femoral artery), vein (the antecubital, jugular, or subclavian vein), or a heart chamber. The SWAN-GANZ CATHETER is a pulmonary catheter that can permit measurement of pulmonary artery diastolic and systolic pressure, pulmonary-capillary wedge pressure (PCWP), left atrial filling pressure, central venous pressure, and cardiac output.

In all physiologic monitoring systems the catheter is connected to a pressure extension line attached to a transducer in an airtight, solution-filled system. The transducer converts pressure into an electrical signal that is displayed on an oscilloscope or recorder. The amplifier enlarges the signal being produced by the transducer; it contains a digital or analogue meter to indicate pressure, controls for setting alarms, audible and visual alarm systems, and a selector switch for systolic, diastolic, and mean pressures.

Invasive hemodynamic pressure monitoring permits continuous assessment of the status of critically ill patients and their response to ongoing therapy, thus providing information essential for more precise diagnosis and prompt correction of a problem. Measurement of intra-arterial blood pressure is especially helpful in the care of hemodynamically unstable patients, including those receiving potent drugs that affect the vascular system. Pulmonary artery pressure readings are indicated for patients in cardiogenic shock secondary to myocardial infarction, and for monitoring pulmonary congestion due to elevated pulmonary wedge pressure. Central venous pressure measures right-sided heart pressures (in the vena cava and right atrium) to determine the adequacy of central venous return.

The major risks of invasive hemodynamic pressure monitoring are sepsis, bleeding, cardiac arrhythmias, and the formation of thrombi and emboli.

hemodynamics (he″mo-di-nam′iks) the study of the movements of the blood and the forces concerned therein. adj., **hemodynam′ic.**

hemoendothelial (he″mo-en-do-the′le-al) denoting a type of placenta in which maternal blood comes in contact with the endothelium of chorionic vessels.

hemofiltration (he″mo-fil-tra′shun) the removal of waste products from the blood by

challenge to caregivers who also must work with family members to help them deal with changes in sexual activities, role reversal, financial burdens, and encouragement of self-care and independence for the patient, balanced with as much support as necessary.

Additionally, caregivers should take time to examine their personal feelings and clarify their values in regard to patients' rights to treatment or refusal of it, and allowing patients to die with dignity.

Heparin is given before treatment is begun to patients who are to be treated by extracorporeal hemodialysis in order to prevent clotting of the blood during the procedure.

hemodialyzer (he″mo-di′ah-liz″er) an apparatus by which hemodialysis may be performed; blood is brought in contact with a semipermeable membrane on whose other side is a dialysate solution of such composition as to secure diffusion of certain elements out of the blood. Popularly called *artificial kidney.*

hemodilution (he″mo-di-loo′shun) increase in the fluid content of blood, resulting in diminution of the concentration of formed elements.

hemodynamic monitoring continuous monitoring of the movement of blood and the pressures being exerted in the veins, arteries, and chambers of the heart. Current invasive techniques permit the

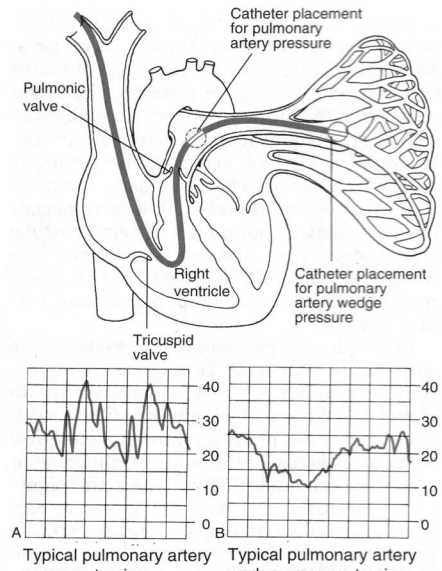

Cardiac pressure waveforms can be visualized on the oscilloscope in hemodynamic monitoring. *A,* Typical pulmonary artery pressure tracing. *B,* Typical pulmonary artery wedge pressure tracing. From Ignatavicius and Workman, 2002.

using large amounts of ULTRAFILTRATION with reinfusion of sterile replacement fluid. See also HEMOPERFUSION.

continuous arteriovenous h. a form of continuous renal replacement THERAPY consisting of hemofiltration with arteriovenous ACCESS using small-volume, low-resistance filters powered by the patient's arterial pressure, without need for a mechanical pump; used as an alternative to conventional HEMODIALYSIS in patients with acute RENAL FAILURE.

continuous venovenous h. a process similar to continuous arteriovenous hemofiltration but using venovenous ACCESS and a mechanical pump.

hemoflagellate (he″mo-flaj′ĕ-lāt) any flagellate protozoan parasitic in the blood.

hemofuscin (he″mo-fūs′in) a brownish-yellow pigment resulting from hemoglobin decomposition; it gives urine a deep ruddy color.

hemogenesis (he″mo-jen′ĕ-sis) HEMATOPOIESIS.

hemogenic (he″mo-jen′ik) HEMATOPOIETIC (def. 1).

hemoglobin (he′mo-glo″bin) the main functional constituent of the red blood cell,

serving as the oxygen-carrying protein; it is a type of HEMOPROTEIN in which each molecule is a tetramer composed of four monomers held together by weak bonds. It consists of two pairs of polypeptide chains, the GLOBINS, each having an attached HEME molecule composed of iron plus a PROTOPORPHYRIN molecule. Symbol Hb.

Chemistry and Physiology. The iron atom has a free valence and can bind one molecule of oxygen. Thus, each hemoglobin molecule can bind one molecule of oxygen. The binding of oxygen by one monomer increases the affinity for oxygen of the others in the tetramer. This makes hemoglobin a more efficient transport protein than a monomeric protein such as MYOGLOBIN.

Oxygenated hemoglobin (OXYHEMOGLOBIN) is bright red in color; hemoglobin unbound to oxygen (DEOXYHEMOGLOBIN) is darker. This accounts for the bright red color of arterial blood, in which the hemoglobin is about 97 per cent saturated with oxygen. Venous blood is darker because it is only about 20 to 70 per cent saturated, depending on how much oxygen is being used by the tissues. The affinity of hemoglobin for carbon monoxide is 210 times as strong as its affinity for oxygen. The complex formed (CARBOXYHEMOGLOBIN) cannot transport oxygen. Thus, carbon monoxide poisoning results in hypoxia and asphyxiation.

Another form of hemoglobin that cannot transport oxygen is METHEMOGLOBIN, in which the iron atom is oxidized to the +3 oxidation state. During the 120-day life span of a red blood cell, hemoglobin is slowly oxidized to methemoglobin. At least four different enzyme systems can convert methemoglobin back to hemoglobin. When these are defective or overloaded, METHEMOGLOBINEMIA can result, with high methemoglobin levels causing dyspnea and cyanosis.

A secondary function of hemoglobin is as part of the blood buffer system. The histidine residues in the globin chains act as weak bases to minimize the change in blood pH that occurs as oxygen is absorbed and carbon dioxide released in the lungs and as oxygen is delivered and carbon dioxide taken up from the tissues.

As erythrocytes wear out or are damaged, they are ingested by macrophages of the reticuloendothelial system. The porphyrin ring of heme is converted to the bile pigment BILIRUBIN, which is excreted by the liver. The iron is transported to the bone marrow to be incorporated in the hemoglobin of newly formed erythrocytes.

The hemoglobin concentration of blood varies with the hematocrit. The normal values for the blood hemoglobin concentration are

The normal value for hemoglobin with age, gender, race, and geographic location. Values are slightly higher for those who live at high attitudes.

Newborn	14–24 g/dl or SI 140–240 g/L
Infant	10–15 g/dl or SI 100–150 g/L
Child	11–16 g/dl or SI 110–160 g/L
Adult Female	12–16 g/dl or SI 120–160 g/L
Adult Male	13.5–18 g/dl or SI 135–180 g/L

13.5 to 18.0 g/100 ml in males and 12.0 to 16.0 g/100 ml in females. The normal mean corpuscular hemoglobin CONCENTRATION, which is the concentration within the red blood cells, is 32 to 36 g/100 ml.

Variant and Abnormal Hemoglobins. There are six different types of globin chains, designated by the Greek letters α, β, γ, δ, ε, and ζ. The composition of a hemoglobin is specified by a formula such as $\alpha_2\beta_2$, which indicates a tetramer containing two α chains and two β chains. The chains are coded by different genes, which are turned on and off during development in order to produce hemoglobins with the oxygen-carrying properties required at each developmental stage. In the first three months of embryonic development, when blood cells are produced in the yolk sac, embryonic hemoglobins such as Hb Gower ($\alpha_2{}^A\varepsilon_2$) or Hb Portland ($\zeta_2\gamma_2$) are produced. As erythropoiesis shifts to the liver and spleen, the fetal hemoglobin Hb F ($\alpha_2\gamma_2$) appears. When erythropoiesis shifts to the bone marrow during the first year of life, the adult hemoglobins Hb A ($\alpha_2\beta_2$) and Hb A_2 ($\alpha_2\delta_2$) begin to be produced.

Many abnormal hemoglobins arising from mutations have been discovered. Some have altered oxygen affinity, some are unstable, and in some the iron atom is oxidized, resulting in congenital METHEMOGLOBINEMIA. Some mutations result in a reduced rate of hemoglobin synthesis. All such conditions are known as HEMOGLOBINOPATHIES.

The most common hemoglobinopathy is SICKLE CELL DISEASE, caused by a mutation replacing the sixth amino acid in the β chain, normally glutamic acid, by valine. The variant hemoglobin $\alpha_2\beta^S{}_2$ is known as Hb S. Mutations resulting in reduced synthesis of one of the chains are called THALASSEMIAS. They can result from deletion of the gene for a chain or from a mutation in the regulatory gene that controls the synthesis of the chain.

h. A_{1c} hemoglobin A with a glucose group attached to the amino terminal of the beta chain; it is made at a slow constant rate during the 120-day life span of the erythrocyte. It accounts for 3 to 6 per cent of the total hemoglobin in a normal person and up to 12 per cent in persons with diabetes mellitus. Increased levels correlate with glucose intolerance in diabetics; with good diabetic control its level returns to normal range, so that periodic assays can be helpful in evaluating effective control of diabetes.

glycated h., glycosylated h. any of various hemoglobins with GLUCOSE attached nonenzymatically; the most common one is hemoglobin A_{1c}. The percentage of

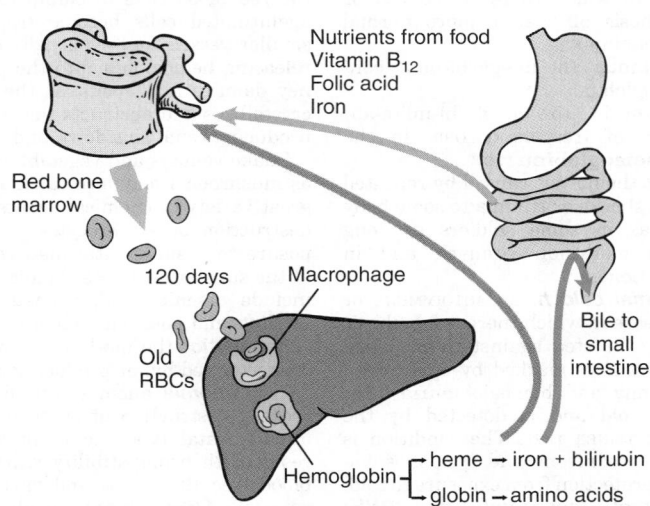

The life cycle of red blood cells and the breakdown of hemoglobin. From Polaski and Tatro, 1996.

hemoglobin that is glycosylated can be assessed over a long period of time as a gauge of blood sugar control; the normal range for a nondiabetic person is between 4 and 6 per cent.

mean corpuscular h. (MCH) the average hemoglobin content of an erythrocyte, conventionally expressed in picograms per red cell, obtained by multiplying the blood hemoglobin concentration (in g/dl) by 10 and dividing by the red cell count (in millions per ml): MCH = Hb/RBC.

hemoglobinemia (he″mo-glo″bĭ-ne′me-ah) presence of free hemoglobin in the blood plasma.

hemoglobinolysis (he″mo-glo″bĭ-nol′ĭ-sis) the splitting up of hemoglobin.

hemoglobinometer (he″mo-glo″bĭ-nom′ĕ-ter) a laboratory instrument for colorimetric determination of the hemoglobin content of the blood.

hemoglobinometry (he″mo-glo-bĭ-nom′ĕ-tre) measurement of the hemoglobin content of the blood, usually with a hemoglobinometer after the hemoglobin has been converted to cyanmethemoglobin.

hemoglobinopathy (he″mo-glo″bĭ-nop′ah-the) 1. any hematologic disorder due to alteration in the genetically determined molecular structure of HEMOGLOBIN, with characteristic clinical and laboratory abnormalities, resulting in conditions such as hemolytic ANEMIA, SICKLE CELL ANEMIA, or THALASSEMIA. 2. sometimes more specifically, a hemoglobin disorder in which the amino acid sequence is altered, as opposed to THALASSEMIA, in which there is reduced or absent synthesis of one or more normal polypeptide chain(s).

hemoglobinous (he″mo-glo′bĭ-nus) containing hemoglobin.

hemoglobinuria (he″mo-glo″bĭ-nu′re-ah) the presence of free HEMOGLOBIN in the urine. adj., **hemoglobinu′ric.**

march h. hemolysis caused by repeated uncushioned shocks or trauma to some body part, such as in some soldiers on long marches, in marathon runners, and in karate practitioners.

paroxysmal cold h. an AUTOIMMUNE or postviral disease in which there is a biphasic IgG antibody directed against the P blood group antigen. It is marked by episodes of hemoglobinemia and hemoglobinuria after exposure to cold and is detected by the DONATH-LANDSTEINER TEST. The condition is treated with prednisone and cyclophosphamide and by protection from exposure to cold.

paroxysmal nocturnal h. (PNH) an acquired blood cell abnormality with proliferation of abnormal red blood cells (PNH cells) that are readily hemolyzed by complement, and episodes of severe hemolysis and thrombosis, particularly of the hepatic veins. It is detected by the HAM TEST. Treatment is with androgens or prednisone and, during thrombotic episodes, with heparin.

hemogram (he′mo-gram) a graphic representation of a detailed blood assessment such as the complete blood COUNT or the differential leukocyte COUNT.

hemokinesis (he″mo-kĭ-ne′sis) CIRCULATION. adj., **hemokinet′ic.**

hemokonia (he″mo-ko′ne-ah) hemoconia.

hemolymph (he′mo-limf) 1. blood and lymph. 2. the bloodlike fluid of invertebrates having open blood-vascular systems.

hemolymphangioma (he″mo-lim-fan″je-o′mah) hematolymphangioma.

hemolysate (he-mol′ĭ-sāt) the product of HEMOLYSIS.

hemolysin (he-mol′ĭ-sin) a substance that liberates hemoglobin from erythrocytes by interrupting their structural integrity.

hemolysis (he-mol′ĭ-sis) rupture of ERYTHROCYTES with release of HEMOGLOBIN into the plasma. Some microbes form substances called HEMOLYSINS that have the specific action of destroying red blood cells; the beta-hemolytic streptococcus is an example. Intravenous administration of a hypotonic solution or plain distilled water will also destroy red blood cells by causing them to fill with fluid until their membranes rupture.

In a transfusion reaction or in ERYTHROBLASTOSIS FETALIS, incompatibility causes the red blood cells to clump together. The agglutinated cells become trapped in the smaller vessels and eventually disintegrate, releasing hemoglobin into the plasma. Kidney damage may result as the hemoglobin crystallizes and obstructs the renal tubules, producing renal shutdown and uremia.

Snake venoms and vegetable poisons such as mushrooms may also cause hemolysis. A great variety of chemical agents can lead to destruction of erythrocytes if there is exposure to a sufficiently high concentration of the substance. These chemical hemolytics include arsenic, lead, benzene, acetanilid, nitrites, and potassium chlorate.

hemolytic (he″mo-lit′ik) pertaining to, characterized by, or producing hemolysis.

h. anemia anemia caused by the increased destruction of ERYTHROCYTES. A frequently fatal type occurs in infants as a result of Rh incompatibility with the mother's blood (see RH FACTOR and ERYTHROBLASTOSIS FETALIS). Other types result from mismatched blood transfusions; from industrial poisons such as benzene, trinitrotoluene (TNT), or aniline; and from hypersensitivity to certain antibiotics and tranquilizers (drug-induced hemolytic ANEMIA). Another important cause is mechanical obstruction caused by microvascular or valvular abnormalities. In addition, it sometimes occurs as a result of a disorder of the IMMUNE RESPONSE in which B-cell–produced antibodies fail to recognize the body's own erythrocytes and directly attack and destroy them (autoimmune hemolytic ANEMIA). Finally, some types of hemolytic anemia appear in the course of other diseases such as LEUKEMIA, HODGKIN'S DISEASE, other types of cancer, acute ALCOHOLISM, and liver diseases. Along with the usual symptoms of anemia, the patient may exhibit jaundice. If the cause of the condition can be determined, and if it can be successfully treated, there is a good chance of recovery. STEROIDS and TRANSFUSION therapy are used to treat some types. In other cases, surgical removal of the spleen may bring about great improvement.

h. disease of newborn erythroblastosis fetalis.

h. jaundice a rare, chronic, and generally hereditary disease characterized by periods of excessive hemolysis due to abnormal fragility of the erythrocytes, which are small and spheroidal. It is accompanied by enlargement of the spleen and by jaundice. The hereditary form is also known as familial acholuric JAUNDICE; there is also a rare acquired form. See also HYPERBILIRUBINEMIA.

h. uremic syndrome a form of thrombotic MICROANGIOPATHY with RENAL FAILURE, HEMOLYTIC ANEMIA, and severe THROMBOCYTOPENIA and PURPURA, usually seen in children but occurring at any age. Some authorities consider it identical to thrombotic thrombocytopenic PURPURA.

hemolyze (he′mo-līz) 1. to subject to HEMOLYSIS. 2. to undergo hemolysis.

hemomediastinum (he″mo-me″de-ah-sti′-num) an effusion of blood into the mediastinum.

hemometra (he″mo-me′trah) hematometra.

hemonephrosis (he″mo-ně-fro′sis) hematonephrosis.

hemopathology (he″mo-pah-thol′o-je) the study of diseases of the blood; called also hematopathology.

hemopathy (he-mop′ah-the) any disease of the blood. adj., **hemopath′ic.**

hemoperfusion (he″mo-per-fu′zhun) the passing of large volumes of blood over an adsorbent substance outside the body in order to remove toxic substances. See also HEMOFILTRATION.

hemopericardium (he″mo-per″ĭ-kahr′de-um) an accumulation of blood in the pericardial cavity.

hemoperitoneum (he″mo-per″ĭ-to-ne′um) an effusion of blood in the peritoneal cavity.

hemopexin (he″mo-pek′sin) a heme-binding serum protein.

hemophagocyte (he″mo-fag′o-sīt) a cell that destroys blood CELLS.

hemophil (he′mo-fil) 1. thriving on blood. 2. a microorganism that grows best in media containing hemoglobin.

hemophilia (he″mo-fil′e-ah) a hereditary disorder characterized by a strong tendency to bleed. The most common types are carried as sex-linked genes with females carrying the trait and disease manifestations almost always in males. (Occasionally, women carrying the trait for hemophilia A or B have bleeding manifestations themselves, probably as a result of nonrandom inactivation of their X chromosomes and overexpression of the X chromosome coding for hemophilia; these women are referred to as *symptomatic carriers*.) All daughters of affected men will be carriers for the gene of hemophilia.

The two most common types are *hemophilia A* and *hemophilia B*. Over 80 per cent of patients have hemophilia A (*classical hemophilia*), which is characterized by a deficiency of COAGULATION FACTOR VIII. Hemophilia B (called also Christmas disease) affects about 15 per cent of hemophiliacs and is characterized by a deficiency of COAGULATION FACTOR IX. Other coagulation factor deficiencies are less common, with patients suffering either milder bleeding or thrombotic episodes.

Symptoms. Bleeding in hemophilic patients is variable, depending on the level of deficiency of the clotting factor. Approximately 60 per cent of persons with hemophilia A or B are severely affected and may have spontaneous bleeding without any recognized trauma. Soft tissue bleeding from the neck, lower face, and tongue may cause grave consequences if not treated. Hematuria and gastrointestinal bleeding are likely, and HEMARTHROSIS (bleeding into joints) can lead to painful stiffening and permanent disability. The leading cause of death, however, is intracranial bleeding. Hemorrhagic complications can be avoided or minimized with early and adequate factor replacement therapy.

Hemophilia A is characterized by a factor VIII level of from 0 to 30 per cent of normal. The partial thromboplastin time (PTT) is usually prolonged. The platelet count,

H

bleeding time, and prothrombin time (PT) are normal. In hemophilia B there is a low factor IX level and the prothrombin time is usually prolonged.

Treatment. The treatment of persons with hemophilia depends on the severity of their disease and the nature of a given bleeding episode. Several therapeutic materials are available for correction of the clotting defect in hemophilia A. Factor VIII is present in commercial lyophilized factor VIII concentrates, CRYOPRECIPITATE, fresh whole blood, and fresh frozen PLASMA. Purified factor VIII concentrate, however, is the treatment of choice. Successful treatment of those with mild hemophilia A can often be done with DESMOPRESSIN (DDAVP). While factor IX is present in fresh frozen plasma, it is not concentrated in cryoprecipitate, so that the latter is not useful for treatment of hemophilia B. Factor IX is present in two commercially prepared concentrates, known as *factor IX complex concentrates* and *coagulation factor IX concentrates.*

All persons with hemophilia should be immunized with hepatitis B vaccine. Suspected bleeding into the central nervous system must be promptly treated; when this happens, consultation with or transfer to a Hemophilia Treatment Center is mandatory. Early treatment of hemarthroses is essential for maintenance of joint health; infusions administered within 4 to 6 hours of onset of symptoms are sufficient to stop bleeding and restore joint function. Medically supervised home infusion therapy has become an integral part of the comprehensive care of patients with bleeding disorders and has facilitated the treatment of bleeding episodes outside the hospital setting.

Patient Care. Advances in therapy have greatly improved the prognosis and management of hemophilia, but new issues have emerged, including the impact on immune status of purer factor concentrates, escalating financial considerations, and therapeutics for infections with hepatitis B, hepatitis C, and the human immunodeficiency virus. Multidisciplinary comprehensive care that incorporates patient and family educational strategies continues to be an essential element of care. Surgery and dental care require a team approach by individuals with specialized knowledge and expertise, in order to ensure favorable outcomes. A diagnosis of hemophilia presents many challenges, not the least of which are psychosocial issues.

Excellent sources of information for both professionals and nonprofessionals are the National Hemophilia Foundation, 110 Greene St., Suite 303, New York, NY 10012 (telephone 212-219-8180) and the Hemophilia and AIDS/HIV Network for the Dissemination of Information ("HANDI") at the same address (telephone 800-42-HANDI).

h. A classical hemophilia, a sex-linked condition due to deficiency of COAGULATION FACTOR VIII; see HEMOPHILIA.

h. B a form similar to hemophilia A but due to a deficiency of COAGULATION FACTOR IX; called also Christmas disease. See HEMOPHILIA.

h. C an inherited disorder caused by a lack of COAGULATION FACTOR XI.. It has been observed mostly in persons of Ashkenazi Jewish ancestry and is characterized by recurring episodes of minor bleeding and mild bruising, severe prolonged bleeding after surgical procedures, and prolonged recalcification and partial thromboplastin times. Called also plasma thromboplastin antecedent deficiency, PTA deficiency, and Rosenthal syndrome.

hemophilic (he″mo-fil′ik) 1. pertaining to hemophilia. 2. in bacteriology, growing well on culture media containing blood or having a nutritional requirement for constituents of fresh blood.

Hemophilus (he-mof′ĭ-lus) *Haemophilus.*

hemophobia (he″mo-fo′be-ah) irrational fear of blood.

hemophthalmia (he″mof-thal′me-ah) extravasation of blood inside the eye.

hemopleura (he″mo-ploo′rah) hemothorax.

hemopneumopericardium (he″mo-noo″-mo-per″ĭ-kahr′de-um) accumulated blood and air in the pericardium; called also pneumohemopericardium.

hemopneumothorax (he″mo-noo″mo-thor′aks) PNEUMOTHORAX with an accumulation of blood in the pleural cavity; called also pneumohemothorax.

hemopoiesis (he″mo-poi-e′sis) hematopoiesis. adj., **hemopoiet′ic.**

hemoprecipitin (he″mo-pre-sip′ĭ-tin) a precipitin that precipitates erythrocytes.

hemoprotein (he″mo-pro′tēn) a conjugated protein whose nonprotein portion is HEME; examples include CATALASE, CYTOCHROME, HEMOGLOBIN, and MYOGLOBIN.

hemopsonin (he″mop-so′nin) an opsonin that renders erythrocytes more liable to phagocytosis.

hemoptysis (he-mop′tĭ-sis) coughing and spitting of blood as a result of bleeding from any part of the respiratory tract. In true hemoptysis the sputum is bright red and frothy with air bubbles; it must not be confused with the dark red or black color of HEMATEMESIS.

Although recent developments in drug therapy have reduced the incidence of serious bleeding in tuberculous patients, TUBERCULOSIS remains a common cause of hemoptysis. Other causes may be bronchitis, bronchiectasis, lung abscess, or malignancy. In acute pneumonia the sputum may be bright red or it may contain old blood which gives it a characteristic rusty appearance. Vascular disorders such as congestive HEART FAILURE and pulmonary infarction can also cause hemoptysis.

Patient care includes placing the affected lung in the dependent position and keeping the airway free of blood either by coughing or suctioning. Although violent coughing is not desirable, the patient can be instructed to cough with the glottis open and without straining. Selective bronchial intubation, bronchial embolization, or surgery may be required if bleeding persists.

parasitic h. a disease due to infection of the lungs with lung flukes of the genus *Paragonimus,* with cough and spitting of blood and gradual deterioration of health.

hemorrhage (hem′ŏ-rij) the escape of blood from a ruptured vessel; it can be either external or internal. Blood from an artery is bright red in color and comes in spurts; that from a vein is dark red and comes in a steady flow. Aside from the obvious flow of blood from a wound or body orifice, massive hemorrhage can be detected by other signs, such as restlessness, cold and clammy skin, thirst, increased and thready pulse, rapid and shallow respirations, and a drop in blood pressure. If the hemorrhage continues unchecked, the patient may complain of visual disturbances, ringing in the ears, or extreme weakness.

capillary h. oozing of blood from minute vessels.

cerebral h. a hemorrhage into the cerebrum; one of the three main causes of cerebral vascular accident (STROKE SYNDROME).

concealed h. internal hemorrhage.

fibrinolytic h. that due to abnormalities of FIBRINOLYSIS and not HYPOFIBRINOGENEMIA.

internal h. that in which the extravasated blood remains within the body.

intracranial h. bleeding within the cranium, which may be extradural, subdural, subarachnoid, or cerebral.

petechial h. subcutaneous hemorrhage occurring in minute spots.

postpartum h. that which follows soon after labor.

primary h. that which soon follows an injury.

secondary h. that which follows an injury after a considerable lapse of time.

hemorrhagenic (hem″o-rah-jen′ik) causing hemorrhage.

hemorrhagic (hem″o-raj′ik) pertaining to or characterized by hemorrhage.

h. disease of newborn a self-limited hemorrhagic disorder of the first days of life, caused by deficiency of vitamin K–dependent blood COAGULATION FACTORS II, VII, IX, and X.

h. fevers a group of viral diseases of diverse etiology but having many similar clinical characteristics: increased capillary permeability, leukopenia, and thrombocytopenia are common to all. The distribution of hemorrhagic fevers is worldwide but they occur mainly in the tropics; they are usually transmitted to humans by arthropod bites or contact with infected rodents. They are manifested by sudden onset, fever, headache, generalized myalgia, backache, conjunctivitis, and severe prostration, followed by various hemorrhagic symptoms, which result in focal inflammatory reaction and necrosis, with mild leukocytosis.

hemorrhea (he″mo-re′ah) hematorrhea.

hemorrheology (he″mo-re-ol′o-je) the scientific study of the deformation and flow properties of cellular and plasmatic components of blood in macroscopic, microscopic, and submicroscopic dimensions and the rheologic properties of vessel structure with which the blood comes in direct contact.

hemorrhoid (hem′ŏ-roid) an enlarged (varicose) vein in the mucous membrane inside or just outside the rectum; called also PILE.

Internal hemorrhoids usually are first noticed when minor bleeding occurs with defecation. Pain occurs rarely, unless there is an associated disorder such as an anal fissure, thrombosis, or strangulation of the affected vein. External hemorrhoids produce varying degrees of pain, feelings of pressure, itching, irritation, and a palpable mass. Bleeding occurs only if the external hemorrhoid is injured or ulcerated and begins to break down.

Hemorrhoids are caused by increased pressure on the veins of the anus. Prolonged sitting, constipation, and hard, dry stools that are difficult to pass can lead to straining and sitting at stool for long periods of time, all of which add pressure on the anal veins. Failure to follow through on the urge to defecate can also lead to hemorrhoids. In women, probably the single most common cause is pregnancy.

External hemorrhoids can be treated by local applications of cold and an astringent cream, by sitz baths, and by avoidance of constipation. Internal hemorrhoids may

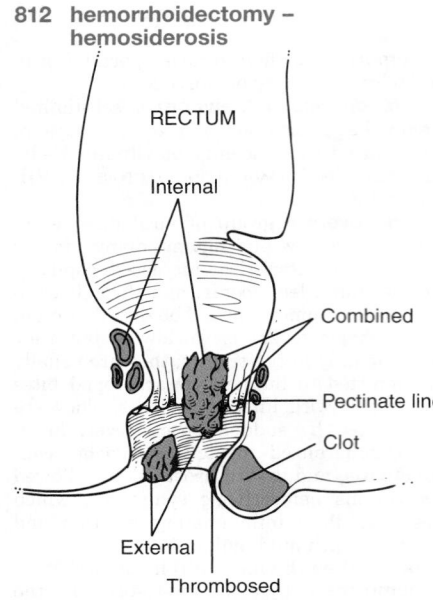

RECTUM

Internal

Combined

Pectinate line

Clot

External

Thrombosed

Types of hemorrhoids.

require sclerosing or cryosurgery to obliterate the affected tissue. More advanced, chronic hemorrhoids usually must be removed surgically by ligation and excision (HEMORRHOIDECTOMY) or by BARRON LIGATION.

external h. one distal to the pectinate line.

internal h. one originating above the pectinate line and covered by mucous membrane.

prolapsed h. an internal hemorrhoid that has descended below the pectinate line and protruded outside the anal sphincter.

strangulated h. an internal hemorrhoid that has prolapsed sufficiently and for a long enough time for its blood supply to become occluded by the constricting action of the anal sphincter.

hemorrhoidectomy (hem″ŏ-roi-dek′to-me) surgical excision of HEMORRHOIDS. *Barron ligation* (or *rubber band ligation*) is a conservative surgical technique in which the hemorrhoids are bound with rubber bands so that the ligated portion sloughs away after several days. Laser procedures are also used.

Patient Care. Postoperatively the patient must be monitored for signs of hemorrhage; this is an uncommon occurrence but one that can develop quickly. The patient may be kept in either a prone position to relieve pressure on the operative site or a supine position (for a short period) with a rubber air ring under the buttocks for support.

Warm sitz baths are usually begun the day after surgery, to relieve discomfort. Compresses of witch hazel or some other astringent agent may be applied to reduce swelling and promote healing. Difficulty in evacuating often occurs during the immediate postoperative period. The two most effective methods of relieving discomfort are keeping the area clean with multiple showers or sitz baths and maintaining a soft stool with a high-fiber diet and such agents as Metamucil.

hemosiderin (he″mo-sid′er-in) a pigment that is a product of HEMOLYSIS; it is an insoluble form of storage IRON that is visible microscopically both with and without the use of special stains.

hemosiderinuria (he″mo-sid″er-in-u′re-ah) the presence of HEMOSIDERIN in the urine, such as in HEMOCHROMATOSIS; called also urinary siderosis.

hemosiderosis (he″mo-sid″ĕ-ro′sis) a focal or general increase in tissue iron stores without associated tissue damage.

hepatic h. the deposit of an abnormal quantity of HEMOSIDERIN in the liver, when this is not associated with CIRRHOSIS, as HEMOCHROMATOSIS is.

pulmonary h. the deposition of abnormal amounts of HEMOSIDERIN in the lungs, due to bleeding into the lung interstitium.

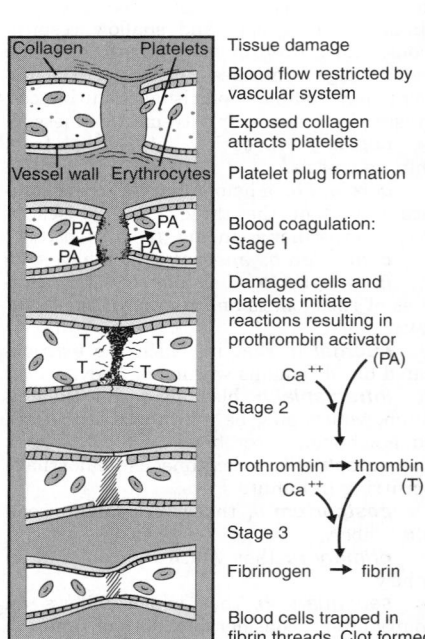

		Tissue damage
Collagen	Platelets	Blood flow restricted by vascular system
		Exposed collagen attracts platelets
Vessel wall	Erythrocytes	Platelet plug formation
		Blood coagulation: Stage 1
		Damaged cells and platelets initiate reactions resulting in prothrombin activator (PA)
		Ca^{++} Stage 2
		Prothrombin → thrombin Ca^{++} (T) Stage 3
		Fibrinogen → fibrin
		Blood cells trapped in fibrin threads. Clot formed

Hemostasis. From Polaski and Tatro, 1996.

hemospermia (he″mo-sper′me-ah) the presence of blood in the semen; called also hematospermia.

hemostasis (he″mo-sta′sis, he-mos′tah-sis) 1. arrest of the escape of blood by either natural means (clot formation or vessel spasm) or artificial means (compression or ligation). 2. interruption of blood flow to a part.

hemostat (he′mo-stat) 1. an instrument, such as a clamp, that stops HEMORRHAGE by compressing a bleeding vessel. 2. a chemical or mechanical agent that stops HEMORRHAGE from an open vessel.

hemostatic (he″mo-stat′ik) 1. checking blood flow. 2. hemostat (def. 2).

hemostyptic (he″mo-stip′tik) hemostatic.

hemotherapy (he″mo-ther′ah-pe) the use of blood in treating disease.

hemothorax (he″mo-thor′aks) a PLEURAL EFFUSION containing blood; called also hemopleura.

hemotoxic (he′mo-tok″sik) hematotoxic.

hemotoxin (he′mo-tok″sin) an EXOTOXIN characterized by hemolytic activity.

hemotroph (he′mo-trōf) the total of all the nutritive material from the circulating blood of the maternal body, utilized by the early embryo. adj., **hemotroph′ic.**

HemoVac (he′mo-vak) trademark for a portable wound suction device that is compressed to provide gentle suction; an internal spring slowly expands to create a negative suction pressure of approximately 45 mg Hg. (See accompanying illustration.)

Henoch-Schönlein syndrome (hen′ok shern′lĭn) Henoch-Schönlein purpura.

Henry's law (hen′rēz) the solubility of a gas in a liquid solution at constant temperature is proportional to the partial pressure of the gas above the solution.

Hepacivirus the hepatitis C VIRUSES, a genus of FLAVIVIRUSES that cause HEPATITIS C.

hepadnavirus (hĕ-pad′nah-vi″rus) any member of a family of DNA VIRUSES that cause HEPATITIS B in humans and other animals; the human pathogens are in genus *Orthohepadnavirus.*

hepar (he′pahr) [L.] liver.

heparan sulfate (hep′ah-ran) a sulfated mucopolysaccharide structurally related to heparin, which occurs normally in the liver, aorta, and lung; it is an accumulation product in several mucopolysaccharidoses.

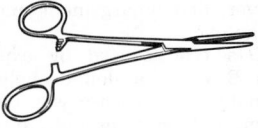

Hemostat. From Dorland's, 2000.

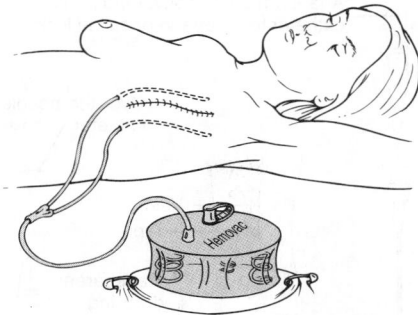

The HemoVac system. From Lammon et al., 1995.

H

heparin (hep′ah-rin) 1. an acid mucopolysaccharide present in many tissues, especially the liver and lungs, and having potent ANTICOAGULANT properties. It also has lipotrophic properties, promoting transfer of fat from blood to the fat depots by activation of the enzyme lipoprotein LIPASE. 2. a mixture of active principles capable of prolonging blood clotting time, obtained from domestic animals; used in the prophylaxis and treatment of clotting disorders, such as THROMBOPHLEBITIS, pulmonary EMBOLISM, disseminated intravascular COAGULATION, acute MYOCARDIAL INFARCTION, or STROKE SYNDROME, and to prevent clotting during extracorporeal CIRCULATION, blood TRANSFUSION, and blood sampling.

h. lock a type of intermittent intravenous device for the administration of heparin. It does not require a continuous flow of fluids; the intravenous fluid flow can be disconnected and the heparin lock filled with a heparin solution that maintains patency of the needle. (See accompanying illustration.)

heparinize (hep′ah-rĭ-nīz″) to treat with heparin.

hepat(o)- word element [Gr.], *liver.*

hepatalgia (hep″ah-tal′jah) pain in the liver.

hepatatrophia (hep″ah-tah-tro′fe-ah) atrophy of the liver.

hepatectomize (hep″ah-tek′to-mīz) to deprive of the liver by surgical removal.

hepatectomy (hep″ah-tek′to-me) surgical excision of all (total hepatectomy) or part (partial or subtotal hepatectomy) of the liver.

hepatic (hĕ-pat′ik) pertaining to the liver.

hepatic(o)- word element [Gr.], *hepatic duct.*

hepaticoduodenostomy (hĕ-pat″ĭ-ko-doo″o-dĕ-nos′tah-me) anastomosis of the hepatic duct to the duodenum.

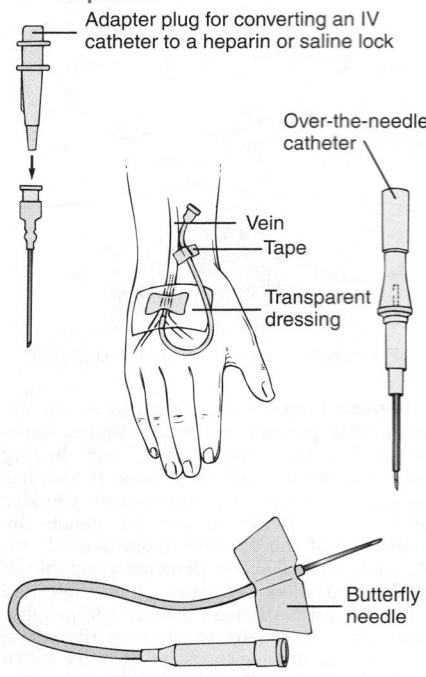

Adapter plug for converting an IV
catheter to a heparin or saline lock

Over-the-needle
catheter

Vein
Tape

Transparent
dressing

Butterfly
needle

Two types of heparin or saline lock sets. From Lammon
et al., 1995.

hepaticoenterostomy (hĕ-pat″ĭ-ko-en″ter-
os′tah-me) anastomosis of the hepatic duct to
the intestine (duodenum or jejunum).

hepaticogastrostomy (hĕ-pat″ĭ-ko-gas-
tros′tah-me) anastomosis of the hepatic
duct to the stomach.

hepaticojejunostomy (hĕ-pat″ĭ-ko-jĕ-joo-
nos′tah-me) anastomosis of the hepatic duct
to the jejunum.

hepaticolithotomy (hĕ-pat″ĭ-ko-lĭ-thot′ah-
me) incision of the hepatic duct with removal of calculi.

hepaticolithotripsy (hĕ-pat″ĭ-ko-lith′o-
trip″se) the crushing of a calculus in the
hepatic duct.

hepaticostomy (hĕ-pat″ĭ-kos′tah-me) fistulization of the hepatic duct.

hepaticotomy (hĕ-pat″ĭ-kot′ah-me) incision of the hepatic duct.

hepatitis (hep″ah-ti′tis), pl. *hepati′tides*
Inflammation of the liver.

h. A a type dependent on exposure to
hepatitis A VIRUS from an infected person;
the primary mode of transmission is the
oral-fecal route. Peak viral excretion occurs
during the two-week period before the onset
of jaundice, and before the infected person

becomes clinically ill. Thus, the greatest
danger of infection is during the incubation
period and early prodromal phase of the
disease, when the person is probably not
aware of being ill. As the disease progresses
and jaundice appears, the excretion of
viruses declines rapidly, the person becomes
less infectious, and there is less danger of
cross-infection. Called also infectious hepatitis.

Hepatitis A primarily affects children and
young adults, especially in environments
with poor sanitation and overcrowding. It is
often a mild disease with symptoms similar
to "flu," and therefore may be either
misdiagnosed or ignored completely. It does
not usually cause lasting damage to the
liver; it can, however, produce profound
fatigue, anorexia, fever, and generalized
aching for weeks. Other symptoms include
abdominal pain, clay-colored stools, dark
urine, and jaundice.

Treatment is primarily symptomatic and
supportive. Rest is recommended in order to
avoid complications from liver damage.
Patients need help dealing with the fatigue.
In 98 per cent of the cases there is total
recovery. Younger patients seem to have
less severe symptoms than do those who are
older. Education and good sanitation practices are an essential component of the
management of this disease. An inactivated
vaccine is available and is recommended for
persons in certain high-risk groups, such as
those traveling or living in areas where
hepatitis A is endemic.

Educational materials on the disease are
available online at the web site of the
Centers for Disease Control and Prevention:
http://www.cdc.gov. There are also guidelines from the Advisory Committee on
Immunization Practices. Printed materials
can be obtained from the Superintendent
of Documents, U.S. Government Printing
Office, Washington DC 20402-9371.

alcoholic h. liver inflammation resulting from ALCOHOLISM, often a precursor of
CIRRHOSIS of the liver.

amebic h. invasion of the liver parenchyma by trophozoites of *Entamoeba
histolytica,* leading to amebic abscess.

anicteric h. viral HEPATITIS without
JAUNDICE, tending to occur chiefly in infants
and young children; symptoms include mild
anorexia and gastrointestinal disturbances,
slight fever, and enlargement and tenderness of the liver.

h. B a type caused by exposure to
hepatitis B VIRUS, a double-shelled virus.
Traditionally, this disease was believed to
be transmitted only through contact with
blood and blood products, such as in blood

transfusions or contaminated needles. However, it is now known that the virus can be transmitted via such body fluids as tears, saliva, and semen, which makes it qualify as a SEXUALLY TRANSMITTED DISEASE. In addition to these parenteral and nonparenteral modes of transmission, there is "vertical TRANSMISSION," infection of an infant by its mother either during pregnancy or after birth. Called also serum hepatitis.

Whereas the hepatitis A VIRUS usually has been eliminated from the body by the time jaundice appears, the body is not always able to rid itself of the hepatitis B virus so easily. The virus can persist in body fluids for years or even a lifetime. Carriers of the disease not only are a threat to others, but also are at risk themselves for chronic hepatitis, CIRRHOSIS of the liver, and primary hepatocellular CARCINOMA. Because the symptoms of hepatitis B vary in intensity, some infected individuals are not aware that they have had the disease.

Symptoms can vary from undetectable to jaundice, joint pain, and a rash, with the potential for internal bleeding owing to an increased prothrombin TIME. The onset of hepatitis B is more insidious and less abrupt than that of hepatitis A. Patients at greatest risk for necrosis of liver cells as a result of hepatitis are the elderly and those who have diabetes mellitus, cancer, or some other severe illness, particularly a condition that requires surgery and transfusions. Hepatitis B has been successfully treated with INTERFERON, the nucleoside analog LAMIVUDINE, and combinations of the two. Hepatitis B VACCINE is prepared by isolating hepatitis B surface ANTIGEN from the plasma of asymptomatic carriers. Because it does not contain intact virus particles, it is noninfectious. The vaccine produces immunity in about 95 per cent of people. It is recommended for immunization of certain high-risk groups, such as physicians, dentists, nurses, aides, and laboratory technicians; staff and residents of institutions; and IMMUNOCOMPROMISED patients and those requiring HEMODIALYSIS or frequent transfusions.

h. C a viral disease caused by exposure to hepatitis C VIRUS, the most common form of post-transfusion hepatitis and also seen after parenteral drug abuse. Its epidemiology is idiosyncratic; although many infected patients have no known risk factors except sexual relations with an infected person, studies of serologically discordant couples reveal negligible rates of transmission. It is a common type of acute sporadic hepatitis, with approximately 50 per cent of acutely infected persons developing chronic hepatitis. Chronic infection is generally mild and asymptomatic, but CIRRHOSIS may occur. Approximately half of hepatitis C patients resopnd to treatment with INTERFERON-α and RIBAVIRIN.

cholangiolitic h., cholestatic h. inflammation of the bile ducts associated with obstructive jaundice, usually occurring as a form of viral hepatitis; symptoms include progressively deepening jaundice, pruritus, dark urine, acholic stools, and a protracted course.

chronic h. chronic inflammatory liver disease; it is defined as *chronic* when it has lasted longer than 3 to 6 months. It is divided by findings on liver biopsy into *chronic active hepatitis* and *chronic persistent hepatitis*.

In *chronic active hepatitis* the liver biopsy shows mononuclear and plasma cell infiltration of the portal areas and surrounding parenchyma in a "piecemeal" necrosis picture. Connective tissue fibrosis from portal area to parenchyma is also found. Untreated chronic active hepatitis has a high mortality rate. It is often a result of viral infection but can also be secondary to drug sensitivity, such as to METHYLDOPA (Aldomet) or ISONIAZID. In this case treatment involves stopping administration of the offending drug. STEROID therapy is sometimes recommended for those patients with evidence of aggressive inflammation and necrosis as identified by liver biopsy. AZATHIOPRINE and small doses of steroids may also be used in individuals who cannot tolerate large doses of steroids. Besides the pharmacologic intervention, bed rest is encouraged during the active phase. Home care is usually appropriate during convalescence.

In *chronic persistent hepatitis* the liver biopsy shows a mononuclear cell infiltrate around the portal area only and not extending into the parenchyma. Fibrosis of the portal area, even if present, is slight. This form of chronic hepatitis is most likely secondary to a viral infection. No treatment is needed, as the condition slowly resolves on its own.

Some authorities feel that the terms *chronic active hepatitis* and *chronic persistent hepatitis* are obsolete and represent different stages of the same viral diseases. However, the terms continue to be widely used.

h. D, delta h. infection with the hepatitis D VIRUS, requiring antecedent or simultaneous infection with hepatitis B VIRUS; manifestations are similar to those of HEPATITIS B, whose severity it may increase.

LABORATORY FINDINGS IN CHRONIC HEPATITIS

Chronic Active Hepatitis
AST (SGOT) > 10 times normal (or > 5 times normal with twice the normal amount of gamma globulin)
Bilirubin elevated
Possible serologic markers

Chronic Persistent Hepatitis
AST (SGOT) levels rarely > 2–10 times normal and the gamma globulin usually normal
Bilirubin usually normal
No characteristic serologic abnormalities

direct toxic h. toxic hepatitis.

h. E a type of viral hepatitis caused by exposure to hepatitis E VIRUS, transmitted by the fecal-oral route, usually via contaminated water. Chronic infection does not occur, but acute hepatitis may be fatal in pregnant women. Called also enterically transmitted non-A, non-B h.

enterically transmitted non-A, non-B h. (ET-NANB) hepatitis E.

fulminant h. an acute fulminating form of hepatitis with coma, resulting from massive hepatic NECROSIS. It may be due to (1) toxic liver injury, as in CARBON TETRACHLORIDE poisoning or ACETAMINOPHEN overdose; (2) a HYPERSENSITIVITY REACTION to a drug, such as HALOTHANE; or (3) viral HEPATITIS. Death is usually caused by acute yellow atrophy of the liver, in which the organ becomes smaller than normal, has a soft consistency, and is reddish brown in color. The disease is characterized by severe preicteric symptoms, an early appearance of jaundice, a sharp rise in temperature, and hemorrhages from the mucous membranes and into the skin because of prolongation of the prothrombin time. In the final stages, there is confusion, drowsiness, and stupor, followed by coma, which deepens until death occurs.

Unfortunately, no treatment is available for this type of hepatitis. With supportive care measures such as control of bleeding, infection, and electrolyte imbalances, the mortality rate is still 80 to 90 per cent.

h. G a posttransfusion disease caused by the hepatitis G VIRUS, ranging in severity from asymptomatic infection to fulminant hepatitis.

infectious h. hepatitis A.

non-A, non-B h. acute viral HEPATITIS occurring without the serologic markers of HEPATITIS A or B; it may be either HEPATITIS C or HEPATITIS E.

serum h. hepatitis B.

toxic h. hepatitis produced by a HEPATOTOXIN such as *Amanita phalloides* toxin, CARBON TETRACHLORIDE, or any of various drugs.

viral h. hepatitis caused by one of the hepatitis viruses; see HEPATITIS A, HEPATITIS B, HEPATITIS C, HEPATITIS D, and HEPATITIS E. There is no specific treatment or drug that kills the hepatitis viruses and can overcome an active infection. Supportive care is given to help the patient's natural defenses overcome the disease. It is important to maintain adequate hydration and nutrition and to get enough rest to lessen the likelihood of complications.

Patient Care. Vital signs and prothrombin time should be monitored regularly, as well as levels of AST, ALT, and serum bilirubin. Jaundice, urticaria, nausea, abdominal pain, arthralgia, and other symptoms should be noted and recorded when present. The care plan for the patient should include measures to provide rest and an adequate dietary intake to meet energy requirements. Fluid intake and output and the color and other characteristics of urine and stools should be noted and recorded.

The patient, family, and close contacts need instruction about isolation precautions and an explanation of why they are imposed as long as the patient can spread the infection. They also need guidance about being immunized when this is indicated. Although viral hepatitis can be a mild disease, it has the potential for becoming serious in some patients and presenting problems of silent gastrointestinal bleeding and neurologic dysfunction, including mental confusion and even profound coma.

hepatization (hep″ah-tĭ-za′shun) CONSOLIDATION of tissue into a liverlike mass, especially as occurs in the lung in lobar PNEUMONIA. The early stage, in which the pulmonary exudate is blood stained, is called *red hepatization*. The later stage, in which the red blood cells disintegrate and a fibrinosuppurative exudate persists, is called *gray hepatization*.

hepatoblastoma (hep″ah-to-blas-to′mah) a malignant intrahepatic tumor consisting chiefly of embryonic tissue, occurring in infants and young children.

hepatocarcinoma (hep″ah-to-kahr″sĭ-no′mah) hepatocellular carcinoma.

hepatocele (hep′ah-to-sēl″) hernia of the liver.

hepatocellular (hep″ah-to-sel′u-ler) pertaining to or affecting liver cells.

hepatocholangiocarcinoma (hep″ah-to-ko-lan″je-o-kahr″sĭ-no′mah) cholangiohepatoma.

hepatocholangitis (hep″ah-to-ko″lan-ji′tis) inflammation of the liver and bile ducts.

THE HEPATOTROPIC VIRUSES*				
Virus	Molecular Biology	Route of Transmission	Chronicity of Infection	Possibility of Causing Acute Liver Failure?
Hepatitis A	RNA virus; non-enveloped member of picornavirus family	Feco-oral	Acute only	Yes, but rare (< 0.3%); more likely in older patients (> 50 yrs) or if pre-existing chronic liver disease
Hepatitis B	Member of hepadnavirus family Double-stranded DNA genome; uses reverse transcriptase	Parenteral	5–10% of adults and 95% of neo- nates develop chronic infection	Yes, but < 1%
Hepatitis C	Enveloped single-strand RNA virus; related to flaviviridae	Parenteral	Acute infection usually subclini- cal; chronicity in 50–80%	Controversial; extremely rare in western nations; may occur in association with other viruses
Hepatitis D	Single-strand circular RNA virus; requires HBV in order to persist and be transmitted	Parenteral	Found in about 5% of HBV carriers; may cause acute or chronic hepa- titis	May cause fulminant hepatitis either as superadded infec- tion with HBV or as naïve coinfection
Hepatitis E	Non-enveloped single- strand RNA virus; mem- ber of flaviviridae family	Feco-oral	Acute only	Rare; most likely in third trimester of pregnancy
Hepatitis G	Single-strand RNA virus; member of flaviviridae family	Parenteral	Persists in about 20% of cases	Almost certainly not (but may be acquired from blood prod- ucts given during fulminant hepatitis)

*From Aspinall RJ and Taylor-Robinson SD: Mosby's Color Atlas and Text of Doctroenterology and Liver Disease. Edinburgh: Mosby International Ltd., 2002.

hepatocirrhosis (hep″ah-to-sǐ-ro′sis) cirrhosis of the liver.

hepatocystic (hep″ah-to-sis′tik) pertaining to the liver and gallbladder.

hepatocyte (hep′ah-to-sīt″) a hepatic cell.

hepatodynia (hep″ah-to-din′e-ah) pain in the liver.

hepatogastric (hep″ah-to-gas′trik) pertaining to the liver and stomach.

hepatogenic (hep″ah-to-jen′ik) 1. giving rise to or forming liver tissue. 2. hepatogenous.

hepatogenous (hep″ah-toj′ĕ-nus) 1. originating in or caused by the liver. 2. hepatogenic.

hepatogram (hep′ah-to-gram″) a radiograph of the liver.

hepatography (hep″ah-tog′rah-fe) radiography of the liver.

hepatojugular (hep″ah-to-jug′u-ler) pertaining to the liver and jugular vein.

hepatolienography (hep″ah-to-li″ĕ-nog′rah-fe) radiography of the liver and spleen.

hepatolith (hep′ah-to-lith″) a calculus in the liver.

hepatolithectomy (hep″ah-to-lǐ-thek′to-me) removal of a calculus from the liver.

hepatolithiasis (hep″ah-to-lǐ-thi′ah-sis) the presence of calculi in the biliary ducts of the liver.

hepatology (hep″ah-tol′o-je) the scientific study of the liver and its diseases.

hepatolysin (hep″ah-tol′ĭ-sin) a cytolysin destructive to liver cells.

hepatolysis (hep″ah-tol′ĭ-sis) destruction of the liver cells. adj., **hepatolyt′ic.**

hepatoma (hep″ah-to′mah) 1. a tumor of the liver. 2. hepatocellular carcinoma.

hepatomalacia (hep″ah-to-mah-la′she-ah) softening of the liver.

hepatomegaly (hep″ah-to-meg′ah-le) enlargement of the liver.

hepatomelanosis (hep″ah-to-mel′ah-no′-sis) melanosis of the liver.

hepatomphalocele (hep″ah-tom′fah-lo-sēl″) umbilical hernia with liver involvement in the hernial sac.

hepatonephric (hep″ah-to-nef′rik) pertaining to the liver and kidney.

hepatopathy (hep″ah-top′ah-the) any disease of the liver.

hepatopexy (hep′ah-to-pek″se) surgical fixation of a displaced liver to the abdominal wall.

H

hepatopleural (hep″ah-to-ploo′ral) pertaining to the liver and pleura or pleural cavity.

hepatopneumonic (hep″ah-to-noomon′ik) pertaining to, affecting, or communicating with the liver and lungs.

hepatoportal (hep″ah-to-por′t′l) pertaining to the portal system of the liver.

hepatopulmonary (hep″ah-to-pul′monar″e) hepatopneumonic.

hepatorenal (hep″ah-to-re′nal) pertaining to the liver and kidneys.

h. syndrome oliguria and renal failure in a patient with anatomically and morphologically normal kidneys in the presence of liver failure. Prognosis is poor.

hepatorrhaphy (hep″ah-tor′ah-fe) surgical repair of the liver.

hepatorrhexis (hep″ah-to-rek′sis) rupture of the liver.

hepatoscan (hep′ah-to-skan″) a surface scintiscan of the liver.

hepatoscopy (hep″ah-tos′kah-pe) examination of the liver.

hepatosis (hep″ah-to′sis) any functional disorder of the liver.

serous h. veno-occlusive disease of the liver.

hepatosplenitis (hep″ah-to-sple-ni′tis) inflammation of the liver and spleen.

hepatosplenography (hep″ah-to-splenog′rah-fe) radiography of the liver and spleen.

hepatosplenomegaly (hep″ah-to-sple″nomeg′ah-le) enlargement of the liver and spleen.

hepatotomy (hep″ah-tot′ah-me) incision of the liver.

hepatotoxin (hep′ah-to-tok″sin) a toxin that destroys liver cells. adj., **hep′atotoxic.**

hepatotropic (hep″ah-to-trop′ik) having a special affinity for or exerting a specific effect on the liver.

Hepatovirus (hep′ah-to-vi″rus) the hepatitis A VIRUSES, a genus of PICORNAVIRUSES.

hept(a)- (hep′tah) word element [Gr.], *seven.*

COMMON HEPATOTOXIC MEDICATIONS

Acetaminophen
Aspirin
Isoniazid
Phenytoin
Methotrexate
Tetracyclines
Quinidine
Many other medications can also be hepatotoxic. A current pharmacology reference should always be consulted.

heptachromic (hep″tah-kro′mik) 1. pertaining to or exhibiting seven colors. 2. having vision for all seven colors of the spectrum.

heptose (hep′tōs) a sugar whose molecule contains seven carbon atoms.

herbicide (her′bĭ-sīd) an agent that is destructive to weeds or causes an alteration in their normal growth.

hereditary (hĕ-red′ĭ-tar″e) transmissible or transmitted from parent to offspring; genetically determined.

heredity (hĕ-red′ĭ-te) the genetic transmission of traits from parents to offspring. The hereditary material is contained in the OVUM (oocyte) and SPERM, so that the child's heredity is determined at the moment of conception.

Chromosomes and Genes. Inside the nucleus of each germ cell are structures called CHROMOSOMES, composed of DEOXYRIBONUCLEIC ACID (DNA) on a framework of protein. GENES are segments of the DNA molecule; there are thousands of them in each cell, each carrying a specific hereditary trait, which may be physical, biochemical, or physiologic. Thus genes affect not only the physical appearance of an individual but also the physiologic makeup, the tendency to develop certain diseases, and the daily activities of all the cells of the body.

The human ovum and the human sperm each contain 23 chromosomes. Aside from the pair determining the sex, each chromosome in the sperm is similar in shape and size to one in the ovum. When the sperm penetrates the ovum, the fertilized ovum thus contains 23 pairs of chromosomes, or 46 chromosomes in all. The fertilized ovum (ZYGOTE) then begins to reproduce itself by dividing (MITOSIS). The original cell divides and forms two cells, each of these divides and forms a total of four cells, and so on until a many-celled embryo begins to take form. In the process of cell division, the chromosomes in the nucleus have the ability to make duplicates of themselves. They do not split in two, but instead each one produces another chromosome exactly like itself. When the two cells are formed from one, the chromosomes are divided so that each cell contains the same number and kind of chromosomes as the original. For this reason, all the cells in the developing embryo and in the human body, except the ovum and sperm, contain identical sets of 46 chromosomes.

The ovum and the sperm are formed by a special process of cell division (MEIOSIS) in which each sperm or ovum receives only one member of each chromosome pair. If this were not true, and sperm or ova contained the full complement of 46 chromosomes, the cells of the offspring would have 92 chromosomes, their offspring would have 184, and so on. As it is, the amount of hereditary material in the body cells remains constant from generation to generation.

In the formation of the germ cells, it is a matter of chance which member of each pair of chromosomes goes to a given ovum or sperm. It is also purely a matter of chance which sperm fertilizes an ovum. All in all,, there are about 70 trillion possible combinations of chromosomes that a child could inherit.

Inherited Traits. Although many details of human heredity are not known, we know that the child receives a set of genes from the parents. These genes (hereditary determinants) develop into characteristics reflecting those of the parents, grandparents, and other ancestors. Before birth these inherited traits are influenced by conditions within the mother's body; after birth they can be shaped by environmental influences such as diet, training, and education.

Some specific aspects of human heredity are well understood. One member of a chromosome pair is contributed by one parent and the other by the other parent. A gene in one chromosome acts on the same trait as a gene in the same position on the other chromosome. It has been found that one gene may be more powerful in its influence than the other gene that acts on the same trait. The more powerful gene is called a dominant GENE and the other is called a recessive GENE.

Sex-Linked Traits. Certain hereditary traits are known as sex-linked because they are carried on the X chromosome. Color blindness is an example. This condition, in which colors appear as varying shades of gray, is rare in females but appears in about 8 per cent of the male population. The genes for color vision are located on the X chromosomes, and the gene for normal vision is dominant to that for color blindness. A female having one gene for normal vision on one X chromosome and one for color blindness on the other will have normal vision, since the color blindness gene is recessive. A male, however, having only one X chromosome, will be color blind if that chromosome has the recessive gene, since there is no corresponding dominant gene to suppress it. It is possible for a female to be color blind, if she has two of the recessive genes, but it is quite rare that these two genes come together in one person.

Another characteristic associated with sex is baldness. The gene for baldness is

dominant in males and recessive in females. Thus a male need have only one gene for baldness for the trait to be expressed, but a female must have two.

Hereditary Diseases. These should be distinguished from congenital birth defects. A congenital defect is one that the infant is born with, such as a cleft lip, a birthmark, or congenital syphilis, but the defect can arise during conception or pregnancy and not be related to heredity. Hereditary diseases, on the other hand, are passed from generation to generation by genes. Some diseases, such as cystic fibrosis, are transmitted by recessive genes.

Role of Mutation. Mutation is the term used for a spontaneous change in a chromosome or gene. Normally chromosomes duplicate themselves exactly during cell division. Occasionally, however, the new cells contain an altered gene or chromosome. If the mutation occurs in an ovum or sperm involved in reproduction, the new trait will be expressed in the offspring.

Many mutations are so minor that they have no visible effect. A mutation that is very harmful will usually result in the death of the fetus and spontaneous abortion. Occasionally a mutation is beneficial. Favorable mutations gradually tend to spread through a population. The accumulation of mutations over millions of years has contributed to evolution.

heredofamilial (her″ē-do-fah-mil′e-al) occurring in certain families under circumstances that implicate a hereditary basis.

Herellea (hĕ-rel′e-ah) a genus of nonmotile, paired, gram-negative, enteric bacilli, including *H. vagini′cola*, a species causing various nosocomial infections.

Hering-Breuer reflexes (her′ing broy′er) inflation and deflation reflexes that help regulate the rhythmic ventilation of the lungs, thereby preventing overdistention and extreme deflation. These reflexes arise outside the respiratory CENTER in the brain; that is, the receptor sites are located in the respiratory tract, mainly in the bronchi and bronchioles. They are activated by either a stretching or a non-stretching and compression of the lung; the impulses are transmitted from the receptor sites through the vagus nerve to the brainstem and thence to the respiratory center.

The *inflation reflex* acts to inhibit inhalation and thereby prevent further inflation. When the lung tissue is stretched by inflation, the stretch receptors respond by sending impulses to the respiratory center, which in turn slows down the rate of inhalations. As the expiratory phase begins, the receptors are no longer stretched, impulses are no longer sent, and inhalation can begin again. This is called the Hering-Breuer *deflation reflex*. Besides cessation of impulses from stretch receptors, there may also be an activation of compression receptors that transmit impulses that inhibit exhalation, thus allowing inhalation to begin.

hermaphrodism (her-maf′ro-dizm) hermaphroditism.

hermaphrodite (her-maf′ro-dīt) an individual with HERMAPHRODITISM, presence of tissue of both male and female gonads; the ovaries and testes may be present as separate organs, or ovarian and testicular tissue may be combined in the same organ (OVOTESTIS).

hermaphroditism (her-maf′ro-di-tizm″) presence of both ovarian and testicular tissue and of ambiguous morphologic criteria of sex, a rare condition in human beings. Hermaphroditism is not to be confused with PSEUDOHERMAPHRODITISM, in which an individual has only one kind of gonad but has significant secondary sex CHARACTERS typical of the opposite sex.

bilateral h. that in which gonadal tissue typical of both sexes occurs on each side of the body.

false h. pseudohermaphroditism.

lateral h. presence of gonadal tissue typical of one sex on one side of the body and typical of the other sex on the opposite side.

transverse h. that in which the external genital organs are typical of one sex and the gonads typical of the other sex.

true h. coexistence in the same person of both ovarian and testicular tissue, with somatic characters typical of both sexes.

unilateral h. presence of gonadal tissue typical of both sexes on one side and of only an ovary or a testis on the other.

hermetic (her-met′ik) impervious to the air.

hernia (her′ne-ah) the abnormal protrusion of part of an organ or tissue through the structures normally containing it. adj., **her′-nial.** A weak spot or other abnormal opening in a body wall permits part of the organ to bulge through. A hernia may develop in various parts of the body, most commonly in the region of the abdomen *(abdominal hernia)*, and may be either acquired or congenital. An old popular term for hernia is *rupture*, but this term is misleading because it suggests tearing and nothing is torn in a hernia. Although various supports and trusses can be tried in an effort to contain

the hernia, the best treatment for this condition is HERNIORRHAPHY, surgical repair of the weakness in the muscle wall through which the hernia protrudes.

Bochdalek's h. congenital posterolateral DIAPHRAGMATIC HERNIA, with extrusion of bowel and other abdominal viscera into the thorax; due to failure of closure of the pleuroperitoneal hiatus.

cerebral h., h. ce′rebri protrusion of brain substance through a defect in the skull.

crural h. femoral hernia.

diaphragmatic h. see DIAPHRAGMATIC HERNIA.

fat h. hernial protrusion of peritoneal fat through the abdominal wall.

femoral h. protrusion of a loop of intestine into the femoral canal, a tubular passageway that carries nerves and blood vessels to the thigh; this type occurs more often in women than in men. Called also crural hernia and femorocele.

hiatal h., hiatus h. protrusion of a structure, often a portion of the stomach, through the esophageal hiatus of the diaphragm; see DIAPHRAGMATIC HERNIA.

Holthouse's h. an inguinal hernia that has turned outward into the groin.

incarcerated h. a hernia so occluded that it cannot be returned by manipulation; it may or may not become strangulated. Called also irreducible hernia.

incisional h. hernia after operation at the site of the surgical incision, owing to improper healing or to excessive strain on the healing tissue; such strain may be caused by excessive muscular effort, such as that involved in lifting or severe coughing, or by obesity, which creates additional pressure on the weakened area.

inguinal h. hernia occurring in the groin, or inguen, where the abdominal folds of flesh meet the thighs. It is often the result of increased pressure within the abdomen, whether due to lifting, coughing, straining, or accident. Inguinal hernia accounts for about 75 per cent of all hernias.

A sac formed from the peritoneum and containing a portion of the intestine or omentum, or both, pushes either directly outward through the weakest point in the abdominal wall (direct hernia) or downward at an angle into the inguinal canal (indirect hernia). *Indirect inguinal hernia* (the common form) occurs more often in males because it follows the tract that develops when the testes descend into the scrotum before birth, and the hernia itself may descend into the scrotum. In the female, the hernia follows the course of the round ligament of the uterus.

Inguinal hernia begins usually as a small breakthrough. It may be hardly noticeable, appearing as a soft lump under the skin, no larger than a marble, and there may be little pain. As time passes, the pressure of the contents of the abdomen against the weak abdominal wall may increase the size of the opening and, accordingly, the size of the lump formed by the hernia. In the early stages, an inguinal hernia is usually reducible—it can be pushed gently back into its normal place. Inguinal hernia usually requires HERNIORRHAPHY.

intra-abdominal h., intraperitoneal h. a congenital anomaly of intestinal positioning, occurring within the abdomen, in which a portion of bowel protrudes through a defect in the peritoneum or, as a result of abnormal rotation of the intestine during embryonic development, becomes trapped in a sac of peritoneum.

irreducible h. incarcerated hernia.

mesocolic h. an intra-abdominal hernia in which the small intestine rotates incompletely during development and becomes trapped within the mesentery of the colon.

Morgagni's h. congenital retrosternal DIAPHRAGMATIC HERNIA, with extrusion of tissue into the thorax through the foramen of Morgagni.

paraesophageal h. hiatal hernia in which part or almost all of the stomach protrudes through the hiatus into the thorax to the left of the esophagus, with the gastroesophageal junction remaining in place.

posterior vaginal h. downward protrusion of the pouch of Douglas, with its intestinal contents, between the posterior vaginal wall and the rectum; called also enterocele. See illustration.

reducible h. one that can be returned by manipulation.

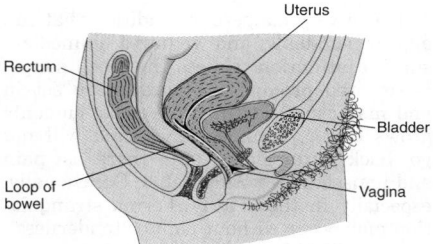
Posterior vaginal hernia. From McKinney et al., 2000.

Richter's h. incarcerated or strangulated hernia in which only a portion of the circumference of the bowel wall is involved.

rolling h. paraesophageal hernia.

scrotal h. an inguinal hernia that has passed into the scrotum.

sliding h. hernia of the cecum (on the right) or the sigmoid colon (on the left) in which the wall of the viscus forms a portion of the hernial sac, the remainder of the sac being formed by the parietal peritoneum.

sliding hiatal h. the most common type of DIAPHRAGMATIC HERNIA; a hiatal hernia in which the upper stomach and the cardioesophageal junction protrude upward into the posterior mediastinum. The protrusion, which may be fixed or intermittent, is partially covered by a peritoneal sac.

slip h., slipped h. sliding hernia.

strangulated h. one that is tightly constricted. As any hernia progresses and bulges out through the weak point in its containing wall, the opening in the wall tends to close behind it, forming a narrow neck. If the neck becomes pinched tight enough to cut off the blood supply, the hernia will quickly swell and become strangulated.

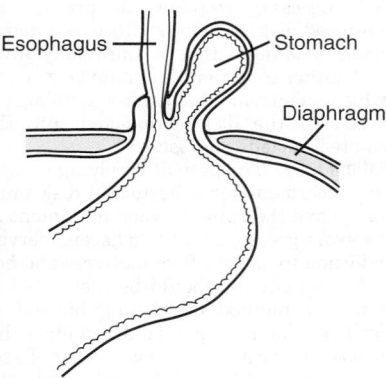
Paraesophageal hernia. From Dorland's, 2000.

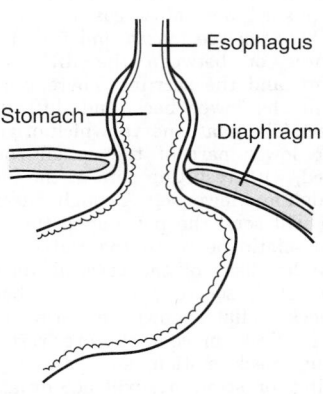
Sliding hiatal hernia. From Dorland's, 2000.

This is a very dangerous condition that can appear suddenly and requires immediate surgical attention. Unless the blood supply is restored promptly, gangrene can set in and may cause death. If a hernia suddenly grows larger, becomes tense, and will not go back into place, and there is pain and nausea, it is strangulated. Occasionally, especially in the elderly, hernia strangulation may occur without pain or tenderness.

umbilical h. see UMBILICAL HERNIA.

vaginal h. hernia into the vagina; called also colpocele.

herniated disk (her'ne-āt″ed) protrusion of all or part of the NUCLEUS PULPOSUS through the weakened or torn outer ring (anulus fibrosus) of an intervertebral DISK; it occurs most often in the lower back and occasionally in the neck or upper portion of the spinal column. Called also disk herniation, herniation of intervertebral disk or of nucleus pulposus, ruptured disk, and, popularly, "slipped disk."

Causes and Symptoms. Between each pair of vertebrae lies a pad of cartilage and fiber (the anulus fibrosus) that encloses a soft, mucoid central portion (the nucleus pulposus). The pads act as cushions between the vertebrae, absorbing ordinary shocks and strains, and shifting position to accommodate various movements of the spine. If the nucleus pulposus herniates through a weakened outer ring, it can impinge on spinal nerve roots as they exit from the spinal canal, or on the spinal cord itself, causing severe pain. Herniation may be caused by injury or by sudden straining with the spine in an unnatural position. It may also come on gradually as a result of a progressive deterioration of the disks.

Symptoms depend upon the location and the extent to which the disk material has been pushed out. Most cases involve the disks between the fourth and fifth lumbar vertebrae or between the fifth lumbar vertebra and the sacrum. There is severe pain in the lower back and difficulty in walking. The sciatic nerve, which originates in the lower part of the spinal cord, is affected, with resulting pain at the back of the thigh and lower leg. A cough, sneeze, or strain will send the pain along the course of the sciatic nerve to the calf or ankle. When the disks of the cervical vertebrae are affected, severe pain in the back of the neck radiates down the arms to the fingers. Neck movements are restricted, and any neck motion, such as coughing, sneezing, or straining, will accentuate the pain.

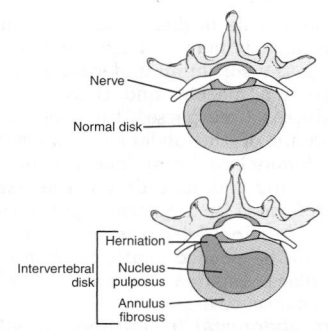

Transverse section showing normal intervertebral disk and ruptured intervertebral disk with herniation of the nucleus pulposus (herniated disk).

Diagnosis and Treatment. Careful examination is necessary to distinguish this condition from other disturbances of the spine. This may include laboratory tests, x-ray examinations, MYELOGRAPHY, MAGNETIC RESONANCE IMAGING (MRI), and CT scans. The x-rays or MRI may reveal pathologic changes in the spine and narrowing of the space between the vertebrae.

Treatment varies according to the seriousness of the condition. Conservative treatment for a herniated disk in the lower back consists of bed rest with leg- and back-strengthening exercises, as well as muscle relaxants and analgesics to relieve pain. Pelvic traction may be applied. In chronic cases the wearing of a surgical support may be helpful. Care must be taken to avoid aggravating the condition by excessive physical effort. Herniated disks in the neck are treated in a similar manner with bed rest, analgesics, anti-inflammatory agents, and traction. A collar may be worn to immobilize the neck when the patient is out of bed. If the response to these measures is inadequate or if the condition becomes disabling, surgery may be necessary to relieve the pressure on the injured disk. MICRODISKECTOMY is a newer surgical technique that is minimally invasive. Another treatment is CHEMONUCLEOLYSIS, in which an enzyme that causes shrinkage in the size of the disk is injected into the herniated nucleus pulposus.

Patient Care. The patient receiving conservative treatment for a herniated disk must always have the spine in good alignment so as to avoid pressure on the adjacent nerves. In addition to using a firm mattress and bed boards, the patient should be instructed in the proper method of turning himself or herself by "log-rolling." To accomplish this the patient crosses arms over chest, flexes the knee opposite the side being turned onto, and then rolls over "in one piece," being sure that the spine is not bent forward or twisted. Training in good posture and body mechanics, especially during lifting or stooping, are important in preventing recurrence of acute episodes.

herniation (her″ne-a′shun) abnormal protrusion of an organ or other body structure through a defect or natural opening in a covering membrane, muscle, or bone. (See also HERNIA.)

   caudal transtentorial h. transtentorial herniation.

   central h. a downward shift of the brainstem and the diencephalon due to a supratentorial lesion, causing Cheyne-Stokes respirations with pinpoint nonreactive pupils.

   cingulate h. a shift of the cingulate gyrus to below the falx cerebri.

   disk h., h. of intervertebral disk h. of nucleus pulposus herniated disk.

   tentorial h. transtentorial herniation.

   tonsillar h. protrusion of the cerebellar tonsils through the foramen magnum.

   transtentorial h. downward displacement of medial brain structures through the tentorial notch by a supratentorial mass, exerting pressure on the underlying structures, including the brainstem; this is a life-threatening situation because of pressure on the third cranial nerve, with symptoms including dilated, nonreactive pupils, ptosis, and a decreased level of consciousness. Called also caudal transtentorial herniation, tentorial herniation, and uncal herniation.

   uncal h. transtentorial herniation.

hernioid (her′ne-oid) resembling hernia.

hernioplasty (her′ne-o-plas″te) see HERNIORRHAPHY.

herniorrhaphy (her″ne-or′ah-fe) surgical repair of HERNIA, with suture of the abdominal wall. When the weakened area is very large, some type of strong synthetic material is sewn over the defect to reinforce the area; this type of repair is sometimes specifically called HERNIOPLASTY, although the two terms are often used interchangeably. Postoperative care is similar to that for any type of abdominal surgery. The patient is protected from respiratory infections, which may cause coughing and undue strain on the suture line. Ambulation is usually not restricted, and the physician instructs the patient in activities that can be resumed after discharge from the hospital.

heroin (her′o-in) a highly addictive NARCOTIC derived from MORPHINE. Because of its vulnerability to abuse, its medicinal use and sale are prohibited in the United States and many other countries. (See DRUG ABUSE.) Called also diacetylmorphine.

herpangina (herp″an-ji′nah) an infectious disease caused by either group A or B coxsackievirus or by echoviruses, chiefly affecting young children in the summer, and characterized by vesiculoulcerative lesions on the mucous membranes of the mouth and throat, dysphagia, fever, vomiting, and prostration.

herpes (her′pēz) any inflammatory skin disease caused by a HERPESVIRUS and characterized by formation of small vesicles in clusters. When used alone the term may refer to either HERPES SIMPLEX or HERPES ZOSTER.

   h. cor′neae herpetic inflammation involving the cornea.

   h. febri′lis a variety of HERPES SIMPLEX usually found on or around the lips and nostrils but occasionally on other mucoid tissues. It is generally caused by human

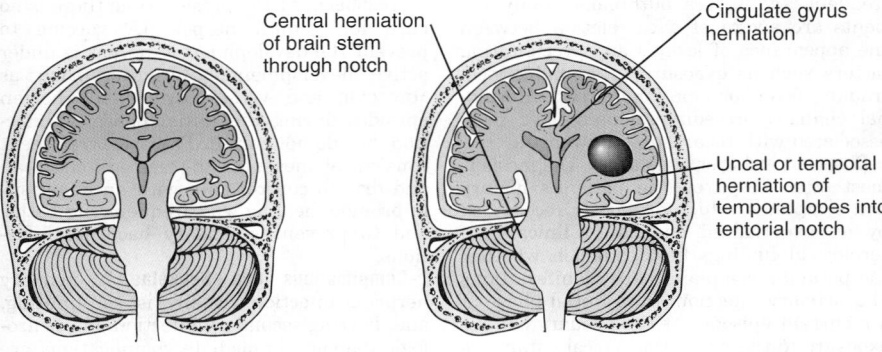

Central herniation of brain stem through notch

Cingulate gyrus herniation

Uncal or temporal herniation of temporal lobes into tentorial notch

Normal position of brain tissue

Position of brain tissue with herniation

Herniation syndromes. From Ignatavicius and Workman, 2002.

H

HERPESVIRUS 1, although occasionally it may be caused by human HERPESVIRUS 2. It is usually a concomitant of fever, but may also develop in situations of other stresses without fever or prior illness. The virus is carried by most people but usually lies quiescent. There is no cure for the condition, but some medications increase comfort. Antiviral medications used in this way include ACYCLOVIR and VALACYCLOVIR. Called also fever blisters and cold sores.

genital h., h. genita'lis HERPES SIMPLEX of the genitals, a common sexually transmitted disease, usually caused by human HERPESVIRUS 2 but occasionally by human HERPESVIRUS 1. If it is present at term in the pregnant female, it may lead to infection of the neonate (see maternal HERPES). The incidence of active genital herpes is difficult to determine precisely because many cases present mild symptoms, are self-limiting, and are not called to the attention of health care personnel. However, it is clear that the disease has reached epidemic proportions in the United States. It is highly contagious and is transmitted by direct person-to-person contact (not limited to sexual contact). Autoinoculation via the hands is possible; for example, from a lip ulcer to the genital area or from the lip or genitals to the eye. Once the virus gains access to the body it enters the nervous system and invades nerve cells located near the site of infection, such as in the sacral ganglia. The virus lies dormant in nerve cells and can remain there indefinitely, predisposing the person to recurrent outbreaks. Factors contributing to recurrent genital herpes are not well understood. Some infected persons experience no recurrences while others have frequent and severe outbreaks. Many patients are aware of a correlation between the appearance of lesions and precipitating factors such as exposure to sunlight, local trauma, fever, or emotional stress. Hormonal changes preceding menses have been associated with recurrences in women.

Diagnosis and Symptomatology. Diagnosis is most often based on the patient's history and symptoms, which are easily recognized by an experienced clinician. Clinical and serological findings help establish whether the patient's complaints are manifestations of a primary infection or an initial phase of a recurrent episode. At the primary or first exposure to the virus, the typical cutaneous lesions may or may not be present and no antibodies to the virus are found in the patient's serum. The presence of such antibodies at the time of an initial episode indicates a previous herpes infection. Since the virus dwells in the lesions and nerve cells and not in the blood, antibody titers, smears, and cultures taken from the lesions can be helpful in identifying the stage of the disease.

Typically, recurrent episodes become milder and less frequent; however, some patients may experience weekly or monthly outbreaks that are severe and painful. Those with recurrent herpes usually have high antibody titers. Paradoxically, it has been noted that the higher the antibody titer the more severe the symptoms and the more frequent the recurrences. Thus, it is apparent that the body's immune system is not effective in providing protection against herpes infection or in mitigating its effects.

A genital rash and mild itching usually are the earliest signs of infection. Eventually vesicles on the surface of the skin form, and then enlarge, break open, and ulcerate. The lesions are painful, especially during coitus, and can cause intense itching, and, if the urethra is involved, painful urination. The disease affects both sexes. In the male, vesicles are found principally on the glans penis, shaft of the penis, and prepuce, and may extend to the scrotum and inner thighs. In the female, vesicular eruptions usually involve the vulva, vagina, and cervix, and may extend to the perineum, inner thighs, and buttocks. Lesions of the cervix can vary from small superficial ulcers with diffuse inflammation to a single, large, necrotic ulcer. Other symptoms include malaise, fever, and anorexia. There also can be involvement of neural structures and the manifestation of neurologic symptoms. The characteristic lesions usually last from one to three weeks in either the initial stage or during periodic outbreaks.

Treatment. At the present time there is no cure for genital herpes. (A vaccine to prevent the development of herpes is under active development.) Antivirals such as ACYCLOVIR and VALACYCLOVIR help shorten episodes during the initial phase of infection, but do not cure it. Palliative treatment consists of measures to keep lesions clean and dry, to control pain with an analgesic, to promote healing with frequent sitz baths, and to prevent secondary bacterial infections.

Complications and Sequelae. A primary herpetic infection usually is self-limiting, and, barring secondary infection and neurologic damage, immediate complications are rare. In some instances the infection may be complicated by urethral stricture, MENINGOENCEPHALITIS, labial fusion, or lymphatic suppuration. Although there is no conclusive evidence that herpesvirus infection actually leads to cervical cancer, women with genital herpes are eight times more likely to develop carcinoma in situ than are those whose serum lacks antibodies to the virus.

Patient Care. Probably the greatest needs of patients with herpes are accurate information and support and counseling to help them cope with the emotional impact and fears about the disease and its effects. The palliative treatments presented above can provide symptomatic relief. In addition, the patient should be told to try to keep the lesions clean and dry. Loose cotton clothing avoids trapping moisture in the genital area. The person should not use perfumed soaps or sprays, and women should not use feminine deodorants or douches. Management of stress can be important in controlling symptoms; ineffective or harmful coping mechanisms can aggravate the condition and delay healing. The emotional impact of genital herpes often is overwhelming to persons who learn they have the disease. Since there currently is no cure, preventive medication, or vaccine and the infection can be transmitted by intimate contact, patients often feel anger, guilt, fear, or anxiety. Support groups can provide patients opportunities to ventilate their anger and talk about their guilt. In a group of persons with similar problems, they can learn that there are others who have had much the same feelings and have managed to work through them and develop a more positive attitude. The American Social Health Association (ASHA) sponsors self-help groups and provides educational materials; their address is P.O. Box 13827, Research Triangle Park, NC 27709.

Fear of cancer is very real in these patients; females are encouraged to have a Pap smear every six months. Early detection is almost guaranteed with such frequent examinations, and the cure rate in these cases is 100 per cent. Another source of anxiety for female patients is the effect of herpes on fertility and the welfare of infants born of mothers with herpes (see maternal HERPES).

h. labia′lis herpes febrilis affecting the vermilion boder of the lips.

maternal h. active genital HERPES during pregnancy and the perinatal period. Herpes infection during early pregnancy can result in a viral SEPTICEMIA and spontaneous ABORTION. Infants born of mothers with active herpes during which there is shedding of the virus at the time of delivery are likely to become infected during a vaginal delivery. Of those who contract herpes from their mothers, about 50 per cent will not survive. Of the ones who do survive, half will suffer from permanent neurological or visual damage.

Protective measures such as cesarean section for delivery improve the chances of avoiding infection in the newborn. During the last trimester it is best if the woman abstains from sexual intercourse if there is any history of either partner having herpes. When there is such a history, it is recommended that frequent cervical viral cultures be done to determine whether vaginal delivery is safe.

With early diagnosis and cesarean section many infants can be protected from infection, but only if the membranes are intact or have been ruptured no more than 4 to 6 hours before the operation. After that length of time it is assumed that an ascending infection has reached the fetus. Mothers who have no active lesions at the time of birth and two negative cervical smears for the virus within a week of delivery can safely deliver their newborns vaginally.

Wound and skin precautions are followed in the care of the mother if she has recurrent herpes (see above). An isolation nursery and wound/skin precautions are recommended for newborns delivered (whether vaginally or by cesarean section) to women with active genital herpes. Some authorities recommend isolation precautions the entire time the newborn is in the hospital and until the incubation period of 21 days has passed.

progenital h., h. progenita′lis herpes genitalis.

h. sim′plex an acute viral disease caused by a HERPESVIRUS and marked by groups of vesicles on the skin, each about 3 to 6 mm in diameter. *Type 1 herpes simplex,* or HERPES LABIALIS, is usually found on the borders of the lips or nostrils and has been nicknamed "kissing herpes." It may accompany fever (HERPES FEBRILIS or *fever blisters*), although there may also be other precipitating factors, such as the common cold, sunburn, skin abrasions, and emotional disturbances. *Type 2 herpes simplex,* or genital HERPES, is usually found on or around the genital area. Infection of the newborn from a mother with the condition (see maternal HERPES) has a fatality rate of 50 per cent and many survivors have significant neurological or ocular sequelae.

traumatic h., wrestler's h. a self-limiting cutaneous herpesvirus infection following trauma, the virus entering through burns or other wounds; the temperature

H

rises moderately, and vesicles appear around the wound.

h. zos′ter an acute viral disease caused by a herpesvirus (the same virus that causes CHICKENPOX); characteristics include inflammation of spinal ganglia and a vesicular eruption along the area of distribution of a sensory nerve. Called also shingles and zoster. It may appear in persons who have been exposed to chickenpox, and it sometimes accompanies other diseases such as pneumonia, tuberculosis, and lymphoma or is triggered by trauma or injection of certain drugs. In some cases it appears without any apparent reason for activation.

Treatment is symptomatic and is aimed at relieving the pain and itching of the blisters. Local applications of calamine lotion or other lotions to dry the blisters may help. Herpes zoster is a very exhausting disease, especially for elderly people, because the constant itching and pain are difficult to control, even with systemic analgesics in some cases.

Herpes zoster affecting the eye causes severe conjunctivitis and possible ulceration and scarring of the cornea if not treated successfully.

Herpes zoster is a communicable disease and therefore requires some type of isolation, the specific precautions depending on whether the disease is localized or disseminated and also on the condition of the patient. Localized lesions in immunocompromised patients often become disseminated. Persons susceptible to varicella-zoster (chickenpox) should stay out of the patient's room. This includes hospital personnel as well as other patients. If there is any question as to the proper procedures for prevention of the spread of herpes zoster, the CDC *Guidelines for Infection Control in Hospital Personnel* should be consulted.

h. zos′ter auricula′ris, h. zos′ter o′ticus Ramsay Hunt syndrome.

herpesvirus (her′pēz-vi′rus) any in a large family of DNA viruses that cause disease in humans and many other animal species. They mature in the nucleus of the infected cell, where they induce formation of a characteristic inclusion BODY and sometimes of a cytoplasmic inclusion body.

The strains affecting humans (*human herpesvirus*) cause the disease called HERPES as well as numerous other conditions. Some infections are primarily nongenital, such as HERPES LABIALIS, HERPES ZOSTER, and CHICKENPOX. Others are primarily genital (see genital HERPES), affecting the mucocutaneous border of the genitalia in either sex. In neonates, a cutaneous herpes infection can be contracted during birth, or possibly transplacentally, and renal transplant recipients sometimes contract a type of cutaneous herpes. Other herpesvirus infections include CYTOMEGALIC INCLUSION DISEASE and infectious MONONUCLEOSIS. Herpesviruses can also cause benign aseptic MENINGITIS and encephalitis. The most recently discovered human herpesvirus is HHV-8, which has also been called *Kaposi sarcoma virus* because it appears to be an etiologic agent of Kaposi SARCOMA.

Antibodies against CYTOMEGALOVIRUS have a low incidence in the general population but are much more common in certain groups, such as up to 50 per cent in urban gay men. Infection with human herpesvirus 1 is almost universal in North America and Europe. By early adulthood neutralizing antibodies to this species are estimated to be present in 40 to 100 per cent of the population. The majority of individuals with a *primary* infection present no symptoms and the disease goes undiagnosed. The primary infection is almost always self-limited, but recurrent reactivation can present severe clinical manifestations that are difficult to treat.

After the primary infection is healed, the virus remains in the body, a virus-host balance is established, and the disease enters a quiescent or latent stage during which no active lesions are apparent. However, some patients have postherpetic NEURALGIA for months, with tingling, burning, or other sensations along a dermatome.

Despite the presence of circulating antibody, the quiescent stage can be interrupted by reactivation of the disease. During the active phase the local lesions usually reappear at the site of the primary infection. The factors that precipitate recurrent episodes are not fully understood, but it is known that in institutions, other conditions of overcrowding, and other situations where people have unusual emotional stress, minor epidemics do occur, enhancing predisposition to overt disease. Excess exposure to sunlight and IMMUNOSUPPRESSION can trigger the re-emergence of overt manifestations in the form of SHINGLES.

The herpesviruses are among the few viruses that can be pharmacologically treated. Many respond well to ACYCLOVIR.

human h. 1 a virus of the genus *Simplexvirus* that is the etiologic agent of Type 1 HERPES SIMPLEX (HERPES LABIALIS). Primary infection usually occurs in early childhood and is often asymptomatic, although

HERPES GROUP OF VIRUSES

Virus Type	Infection
Cytomegalovirus	Congenital infection, cytomegalovirus infection, mononucleosis
Epstein-Barr Virus	Burkitt lymphoma, chronic Epstein-Barr infection, infectious mononucleosis, nasopharyngeal carcinoma
Herpes Simplex Virus	
Types I	"Cold sores," infection of the lips, mouth, eyes and skin, encephalitis in adults
Type II	Genital herpes, encephalitis in infants, and neonatal infection
Varicella Zoster Virus	Chickenpox (varicella), herpes zoster (shingles)

gingivostomatitis and pharyngitis may occur. Called also herpes simplex virus 1.

human h. 2 a virus of the genus *Simplexvirus* that is the etiologic agent of Type 2 HERPES SIMPLEX (genital HERPES). Called also herpes simplex VIRUS 2.

human h. 3 a virus of the genus *Varicellovirus* that is the etiologic agent of CHICKENPOX and HERPES ZOSTER.

human h. 4 Epstein-Barr virus.

human h. 5 the sole species of the genus *Cytomegalovirus,* the cause of CYTO-MEGALIC INCLUSION DISEASE.

human h. 6 a species of virus that is the etiologic agent of ROSEOLA INFANTUM; most healthy adults carry the virus without having any symptoms.

human h. 8 a species that has been implicated as a causative agent of Kaposi SARCOMA.

herpetic (her-pet′ik) 1. pertaining to or of the nature of herpes. 2. relating to or caused by herpesviruses.

herpetiform (her-pet′ĭ-form) resembling herpes.

Hers' disease (herz) GLYCOGEN STORAGE DISEASE (type VI), a condition in which deficiency of liver phosphorylase affects the liver and leukocytes, with hepatomegaly, mild hypoglycemia, mild acidosis, and growth retardation.

hersage (ār-sahzh′) [Fr.] surgical separation of the fibers of a peripheral nerve.

hertz (Hz) (herts) the SI unit of frequency, equal to one cycle per second.

HERV human endogenous retroviruses.

hetacillin (het″ah-sil′in) a semisynthetic PENICILLIN that is converted in the body to AMPICILLIN and has actions and uses similar to those of ampicillin.

hetastarch (het′ah-stahrch) an artificial colloid produced by addition of hydroxyethyl ether groups into amylopectin; used as an artificial plasma EXTENDER for treatment of shock.

heter(o)- word element [Gr.], *other; dissimilar.*

heteradelphus (het″er-ah-del′fus) conjoined twins with one fetus markedly more developed than the other.

heterecious (het″er-e′shus) requiring different hosts in different stages of development; a characteristic of certain parasites.

heterergic (het″er-er′jik) having different effects; said of two drugs, of which one produces a particular effect and the other does not.

heteresthesia (het″er-es-the′zhah) variation of cutaneous sensibility on adjoining areas.

heteroagglutination (het″er-o-ah-gloo″tĭ-na′-shun) agglutination of particulate antigens of one species by agglutinins derived from another species.

heteroagglutinin (het″er-o-ah-gloo′tin-in) an agglutinin that is capable of heteroagglutination.

heteroantibody (het″er-o-an″tĭ-bod′e) an antibody combining with antigens originating from a species foreign to the antibody producer.

heteroantigen (het″er-o-an′tĭ-jen) an antigen originating from a species foreign to the antibody producer.

heteroblastic (het″er-o-blas′tik) originating in a different kind of tissue.

heterocellular (het″er-o-sel′u-ler) composed of cells of different kinds.

heterocephalus (het″er-o-sef′ah-lus) a malformed fetus with two heads of unequal size.

heterochromatin (het″er-o-kro′mah-tin) that state of chromatin in which it is dark-staining, genetically inactive, and tightly coiled.

constitutive h. the chromatin in regions of the chromosomes that are invariably heterochromatic; it contains highly repetitive sequences of DNA that are genetically inactive and serves as a structural element of the chromosome.

facultative h. the chromatin in regions of the chromosomes that become heterochromatic in certain cells and tissues; for

H

example, it makes up the inactive X chromosome in female somatic cells.

heterochromia (het″er-o-kro′me-ah) diversity of color in a part normally of one color.

h. i′ridis difference in color of the iris in the two eyes, or in different areas in the same iris.

heterochronia (het″er-o-kro′ne-ah) irregularity in time; occurrence at abnormal times.

heterochronic (het″er-o-kron′ik) 1. pertaining to or characterized by heterochronia. 2. denoting different ages or stages of development, as between an excised organ and an implanted one in transplantation operations. 3. a difference in the rate or time of occurrence between two processes.

heterocyclic (het″er-o-sik′lik) having or pertaining to a closed chain or ring formation that includes atoms of different elements.

heterocytotropic (het″er-o-si″to-trop′ik) having an affinity for cells from different species.

heterodermic (het″er-o-der′mik) denoting skin for grafting taken from an animal of another species; see heterodermic GRAFT.

heterodont (het′er-o-dont″) having teeth of different shapes, such as the molars and incisors of humans.

heterodromous (het″er-od′ro-mus) moving or acting in other than the usual or forward direction.

heteroeroticism (het″er-o-ĕ-rot′ĭ-sizm) 1. sexual feeling directed toward another person, sometimes specifically one of the opposite sex. 2. alloeroticism (def. 1). 3. a stage in which the erotic energy is directed toward objects other than oneself, specifically to those of the opposite sex. adj. **heteroerot′ic.**

heteroerotism (het″er-o-er′o-tizm) heteroeroticism.

heterogamety (het″er-o-gam′ĕ-te) production of unlike GAMETES; said especially of the human male, who produces two types of sperm, one containing the x chromosome and the other containing the y chromosome. adj., **heterogamet′ic.**

heterogamy (het″er-og′ah-me) the conjugation of GAMETES differing in size and structure to form the ZYGOTE from which the new organism develops; this occurs in higher life forms.

heterogeneity (het″er-o-jĕ-ne′ĭ-te) the state or quality of being heterogeneous. In genetics, the production of identical or similar phenotypes by different genetic mechanisms. A phenotype resembling a known phenotype but determined by a different genetic mechanism is called a genocopy or genetic mimic.

heterogeneous (het″er-o-je′ne-us) 1. consisting of or composed of dissimilar elements or ingredients; not having a uniform quality throughout. 2. in genetics, said of a trait that can be produced by different genes or combinations of genes.

heterogenesis (het″er-o-jen′ĕ-sis) 1. metagenesis. 2. asexual generation.

heterogenote (het′er-o-je″nōt) a cell that has an additional genetic fragment, different from its intact genotype; usually resulting from transduction.

heterogenous (het″er-oj′ĕ-nus) xenogeneic.

heterogony (het″er-og′o-ne) metagenesis.

heterograft (het′er-o-graft″) xenograft.

heterohemagglutination (het″er-o-he″mah-gloo″tĭ-na′shun) agglutination of erythrocytes by a hemagglutinin derived from an individual of a different species.

heterohemagglutinin (het″er-o-he″mah-gloo′tĭ-nin) a hemagglutinin that agglutinates erythrocytes of organisms of other species.

heterohemolysin (het″er-o-he-mol′ĭ-sin) a hemolysin that destroys erythrocytes of animals of species other than that of the animal in which it is formed.

heterokeratoplasty (het″er-o-ker′ah-to-plas″te) grafting of corneal tissue taken from an individual of another species.

heterokinesis (het″er-o-kĭ-ne′sis) the differential distribution of the sex chromosomes in the developing gametes of a heterogametic organism.

heterolalia (het″er-o-la′le-ah) heterophasia.

heterolateral (het″er-o-lat′er-al) contralateral.

heterologous (het″er-ol′o-gus) 1. made up of tissue not normal to the part. 2. xenogeneic. 3. possessing different alleles in regard to a given characteristic.

heterolysin (het″er-ol′ĭ-sin) an antibody that lyzes cells of species other than the one in which it is formed.

heterolysis (het″er-ol′ĭ-sis) destruction of cells of one species by lysin from another species. adj., **heterolyt′ic.**

heteromeric (het″er-o-mer′ik) sending processes through one of the commissures to the white matter of the opposite side of the spinal cord.

heterometaplasia (het″er-o-met″ah-pla′-zhah) formation of tissue foreign to the part where it is formed.

heterometropia (het″er-o-mĕ-tro′pe-ah) the state in which the refraction in the two eyes differs.

heteromorphosis (het″er-o-mor-fo′sis) the development, in regeneration, of an organ or structure different from the one that was lost.

heteromorphous (het″er-o-mor′fus) of abnormal shape or structure.

heteronomous (het″er-on′ŏ-mus) subject to different laws; in biology, subject to different laws of growth or specialized along different lines.

hetero-osteoplasty (het″er-o-os′te-o-plas″-te) osteoplasty with bone taken from an individual of another species.

heteropagus (het″er-op′ah-gus) conjoined twins consisting of unequally developed components.

heteropathy (het″er-op′ah-the) abnormal or morbid sensibility to stimuli.

heterophagosome (het″er-o-fag′o-som) an intracytoplasmic vacuole formed by phagocytosis or pinocytosis, which becomes fused with a lysosome, subjecting its contents to enzymatic digestion.

heterophagy (het″er-of′ah-je) the taking into a cell of exogenous material by phagocytosis or pinocytosis and the digestion of the ingested material after fusion of the newly formed vacuole with a lysosome.

heterophasia (het″er-o-fa′ze-ah) the utterance of words other than those intended by the speaker.

heterophemia (het″er-o-fe′me-ah) heterophasia.

heterophil (het′er-o-fil″) 1. a finely granular polymorphonuclear leukocyte represented by neutrophils in human, but characterized in other mammals by granules that have variable sizes and staining characteristics. 2. heterophilic (def. 1).

  h. antibody a characteristic antibody found with INFECTIOUS MONONUCLEOSIS, demonstrated in 90 to 95 per cent of adolescents and adults and 50 per cent of children with the disease. It declines in titer after acute illness has resolved but may be detectable for up to 9 months after disease onset.

heterophile (het′er-o-fil) heterophil.

heterophilic (het″er-o-fil′ik) 1. having affinity for other antigens or antibodies besides the one for which it is specific. 2. staining with a type of stain other than the usual one.

heterophonia (het″er-o-fo′ne-ah) any abnormality of the voice.

heterophoria (het″er-o-for′e-ah) failure of the visual axes to remain parallel after the visual fusional stimuli have been eliminated. The various forms of heterophoria are spoken of as phorias, their direction being indicated by the appropriate prefix, as *cyclo*phoria, *eso*phoria, *exo*phoria, *hyper*phoria, and *hypo*phoria. adj., **heterophor′ic.**

heterophthalmia (het″er-of-thal′me-ah) difference in the direction of the axes, or in the color, of the two eyes.

Heterophyes (het″er-o-fi′ēz) a genus of minute TREMATODES found in the middle third of the small intestines of humans and certain other mammals; various species are found from Egypt and Turkey across Asia to Japan and the Philippines.

heteroplasia (het″er-o-pla′zhah) replacement of normal by abnormal tissues; malposition of normal cells. adj., **heteroplas′tic.**

  progressive osseous h. osteoma cutis.

heteroploid (het′er-o-ploid″) 1. characterized by heteroploidy. 2. an individual or cell with an abnormal number of chromosomes.

heteroploidy (het′er-o-ploi″de) the state of having an abnormal number of chromosomes.

heteropsia (het″er-op′se-ah) unequal vision in the two eyes.

heteropyknosis (het″er-o-pik-no′sis) 1. the quality of showing variations in density throughout. 2. a state of differential condensation observed in different chromosomes, or in different regions of the same chromosome; it may be attenuated (negative heteropyknosis) or accentuated (positive heteropyknosis). adj., **heteropyknot′ic.**

heterosexual (het″er-o-sek′shoo-al) 1. pertaining to, characteristic of, or directed toward the opposite sex. 2. a person with erotic interests directed toward the opposite sex. 3. contrasexual (def. 1).

heterosexuality (het″er-o-sek″shoo-al′ĭ-te) sexual attraction to or activity with persons of the opposite sex.

heterosis (het″er-o′sis) the existence, in the first generation hybrid, of greater vigor than is shown by either parent.

heterosuggestion (het″er-o-sug-jes′chun) suggestion received from another person, as opposed to autosuggestion.

heterotaxia (het″er-o-tak′se-ah) abnormal position of viscera.

heterotherm (het′er-o-therm″) an animal that exhibits heterothermy.

heterothermy (het′er-o-ther″me) the exhibition of widely different body temperatures at different times or under different conditions, as in species that hibernate. adj., **heterother′mic.**

heterotonia (het″er-o-to′ne-ah) a state characterized by variations in tension or tone. adj., **heteroton′ic.**

heterotopia (het″er-o-to′pe-ah) displacement or misplacement of parts. adj., **heterotop′ic.**

heterotransplant (het″er-o-trans′plant) 1. tissue taken from one animal and transplanted into one of a different species. 2. heterologous GRAFT.

heterotransplantation (het″er-o-transplan-ta′shun) xenogeneic transplantation.

heterotrichosis (het″er-o-trĭ-ko′sis) growth of hairs of different colors on the body.

heterotroph (het′er-o-trōf′) a heterotrophic organism.

heterotrophic (het″er-o-trof′ik) unable to synthesize metabolic products from inorganic materials; requiring complex organic substances (growth factors) for nutrition.

heterotropia (het″er-o-tro′pe-ah) failure of the visual axes to remain parallel when fusion is possible; see also STRABISMUS.

heterotypic (het″er-o-tip′ik) pertaining to, characteristic of, or belonging to a type different from the one being discussed or examined. adj., **heterotyp′ical.**

heteroxenous (het″er-ok′sĕ-nus) requiring more than one host to complete the life cycle; said of certain parasites.

heterozygosity (het″er-o-zi-gos′ĭ-te) the state of having different ALLELES in regard to a given character. adj., **heterozy′gous.**

heterozygote (het″er-o-zi′gōt) an individual exhibiting heterozygosity.

Heubner-Herter disease (hoib′ner her′ter) celiac disease of infants.

heuristic (hu-ris′tik) 1. encouraging or promoting investigation; conducive to discovery. 2. denoting a strategy for learning in which the student uses a tool or device for finding a way to achieve a goal or solve a problem.

HEW Department of Health, Education, and Welfare, a department of the United States government that was replaced by the Department of Health and Human Services (HHS).

hex(a)- word element [Gr.], *six.*

hexachlorophene (hek″sah-klor′ro-fēn) a detergent and germicidal compound commonly incorporated in soaps and dermatologic agents.

hexad (hek′sad) 1. a group or combination of six similar or related entities. 2. an element with a valence of six.

hexavalent (hek″sah-va′lent) having a valence of six.

hexokinase (hek″so-ki′nās) an enzyme that catalyzes the transfer of a high-energy phosphate group of a donor to D-glucose, producing D-glucose-6-phosphate.

hexosamine (hek′sōs-am″in) a nitrogenous sugar in which an amino group replaces a hydroxyl group.

hexose (hek′sōs) a monosaccharide containing six carbon atoms in a molecule.

hexosephosphate (hek″sōs-fos′fāt) an ester of glucose with phosphoric acid that aids in the absorption of sugars and is important in carbohydrate metabolism.

hexylcaine (hek′sil-kān) a local anesthetic, used as the hydrochloride salt.

hexylresorcinol (hek″sil-rĕ-zor′sī-nol) a phenol compound with bactericidal properties used as an antiseptic in mouthwashes and skin wound cleansers.

HF Hageman factor (factor XII, one of the COAGULATION FACTORS).

Hf hafnium.

Hg mercury (L. *hydrargy′rum*).

Hgb hemoglobin.

HGH, hGH human growth hormone.

HHCC Home Health Care Classification.

HHNK hyperglycemic hyperosmolar nonketotic (coma).

HHS Department of Health and Human Services, a department of the United States Government.

5-HIAA 5-hydroxyindoleacetic acid.

hiatus (hi-a′tus) [L.] an OPENING, gap, or cleft. adj., **hia′tal.**

   aortic h., h. aor′ticus the opening in the diaphragm through which the aorta and thoracic duct pass.

   esophageal h., h. esophage′us the opening in the diaphragm for the passage of the esophagus and the vagus nerves.

Hib *Haemophilus influenzae,* type b.

hibernation (hi″ber-na′shun) a dormant state in which certain animals pass the winter, marked by deep sleep and sharp reduction in body temperature and metabolism.

   artificial h. a state of reduced metabolism, muscle relaxation, and a twilight sleep resembling narcosis, produced by controlled inhibition of the sympathetic nervous system and causing attenuation of the homeostatic reactions of the organism.

hibernoma (hi″ber-no′mah) a rare benign tumor made up of large polyhedral cells with a coarsely granular cytoplasm, occurring on the back or around the hips.

hiccough (hik′up) hiccup.

hiccup (hik′up) spasmodic involuntary contraction of the diaphragm that results in uncontrolled breathing in of air; it is accompanied by a peculiar noise produced by a beginning inhalation that is suddenly checked by closure of the glottis. Hiccups have many different possible causes, such as rapid eating, irritation in the digestive or respiratory system, or irritation of the diaphragm muscle itself; they sometimes occur as a complication following some kinds of surgery or in serious diseases such as uremia and epidemic encephalitis; and they may have a purely emotional cause. The condition is serious only when it persists for a long time; hiccups usually stop after a few minutes. Called also hiccough and singultus.

Standard home remedies for hiccups include holding the breath, swallowing sugar or a bread crust, pulling the tongue forward, applications of cold to the back of the neck, simply sipping water slowly, and breathing into a paper bag. The bag has the effect of cutting off normal exchange of air with the surrounding atmosphere. The air in the bag, after a few breaths, will have an increasingly high carbon dioxide content, and so will the air in the lungs, and finally the blood. As a result, the automatic respiratory centers in the brain call for stronger and deeper breathing to get rid of the carbon dioxide. This frequently makes the contractions of the diaphragm more regular and eliminates the hiccups. (Patients should be cautioned not to use this paper bag method for longer than one minute at a time.) In extreme cases of prolonged hiccups, sedatives or antianxiety agents may be necessary.

Hicks contractions (hiks) Braxton Hicks contractions.

HICPAC Hospital Infection Control Practices Advisory Committee.

hidr(o)- word element [Gr.], *sweat.*

hidradenitis (hi″drad-ĕ-ni′tis) inflammation of the SWEAT GLANDS.

h. suppurati′va a severe, chronic, recurrent pus-producing infection of the apocrine sweat glands.

hidradenoid (hi-drad′ĕ-noid) resembling a SWEAT GLAND; having components resembling elements of a sweat gland.

hidradenoma (hi″drad-ĕ-no′mah) any of various tumors of the skin whose components resemble epithelial elements of SWEAT GLANDS; they may be nodular (solid) or papillary.

hidrocystoma (hid″ro-sis-to′mah) a retention cyst of a SWEAT GLAND.

hidropoiesis (hid″ro-poi-e′sis) the formation of SWEAT. adj., **hidropoiet′ic.**

hidroschesis (hi-dros′kĕ-sis) anhidrosis.

hidrotic (hi-drot′ik, hi-drot′ik) 1. sudoriparous. 2. diaphoretic.

hierarchy of needs see NEED.

high-altitude sickness ALTITUDE SICKNESS.

high-grade (hi′grād′) occurring near the high end of a range, as of a malignancy.

hillock (hil′ok) a small prominence or elevation.

hilum (hi′lum), pl. *hi′la* [L.] a depression or pit at the part of an organ where vessels and nerves enter.

hilus (hi′lus), pl. *hi′li* [L.] hilum.

hindbrain (hīnd′brān) rhombencephalon.

hindfoot (hīnd′foot) the posterior portion of the foot, comprising the region of the talus and calcaneus.

hindgut (hīnd′gut) a pocket formed beneath the caudal portion of the developing embryo, which develops into the distal portion of the small intestine, the colon, and the rectum.

hip (hip) the area around the articulation of the FEMUR and the ACETABULUM at the base of the lower trunk. (See also hip JOINT and see Appendices.) At each hip joint, the smooth round head of the femur fits into the acetabulum. The joint is covered by a tough, flexible protective capsule and is heavily reinforced by strong ligaments that stretch across the joint. As in most joints, where the ends of the bones meet they are covered with a layer of cartilage that reduces friction and absorbs shock. The synovial membrane lines the socket and lubricates the joint with synovial fluid. Cushioning is provided by small fluid-filled sacs, or bursae. Called also coxa. (See accompanying illustration.)

h.-joint disease tuberculosis of the hip joint; called also coxalgia.

Hippel's disease (hip′elz) angiomatosis confined chiefly to the retina.

hippocampus (hip″o-kam′pus) [L.] a curved elevation of gray matter on the floor of the inferior horn of the lateral ventricle; it is an important functional component of the limbic system.

Hippocrates (hĭ-pok′rah-tēz) (late 5th century B.C.). "Father of Medicine." Son of a priest-physician, he was born on the island of Cos. By stressing that there is a natural cause for disease he did much to dissociate the care of the sick from the influence of magic and superstition. His carefully kept records of treatment and solicitous observation of ill persons provided a foundation for clinical medicine in the case report; by also reporting unsuccessful methods of treatment, he anticipated the modern scientific attitude. See also HIPPOCRATIC OATH.

Hippocratic (hip″o-krat′ik) relating to HIPPOCRATES.

H. Oath a moral code for ethical conduct and practice in medicine, established according to the ideals of HIPPOCRATES. The text is as follows: "I swear by Apollo the physician, by Aesculapius, Hygeia, and Panacea, and I take to witness all the gods, all the goddesses, to keep according to my ability and my judgment the following oath: To consider dear to me as my parents

H

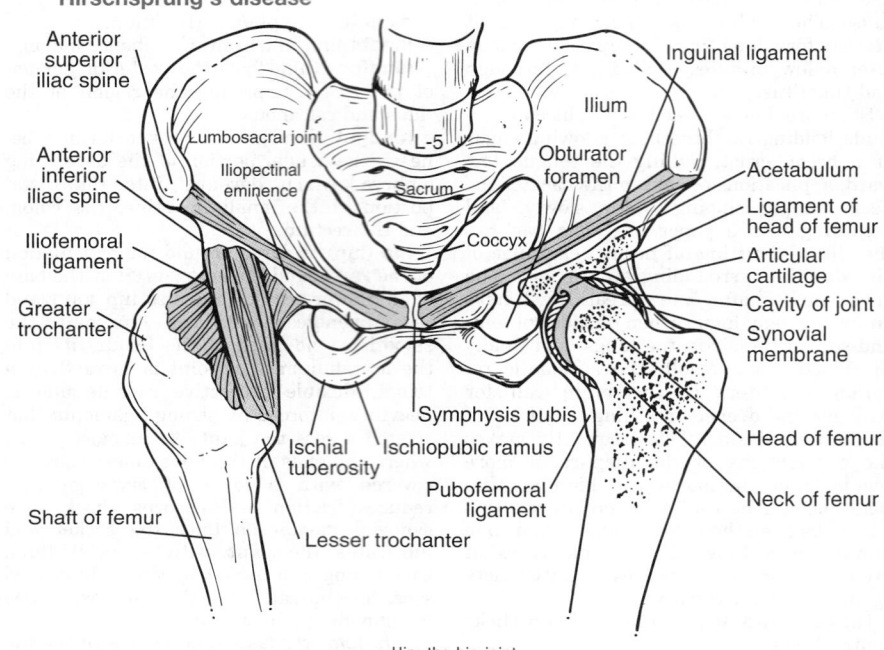

Hip: the hip joint.

him who taught me this art; to live in common with him and if necessary to share my goods with him; to look upon his children as my own brothers, to teach them this art if they so desire without fee or written promise; to impart to my sons and the sons of the master who taught me and the disciples who have enrolled themselves and have agreed to the rules of the profession, but to these alone, the precepts and the instruction. I will prescribe regimens for the good of my patients according to my ability and my judgment and never do harm to anyone. To please no one will I prescribe a deadly drug, nor give advice which may cause his death. Nor will I give a woman a pessary to procure abortion. But I will preserve the purity of my life and my art. I will not cut for stone, even for patients in whom the disease is manifest; I will leave this operation to be performed by practitioners (specialists in this art). In every house where I come I will enter only for the good of my patients, keeping myself far from all intentional ill-doing and all seduction, and especially from the pleasures of love with women or with men, be they free or slaves. All that may come to my knowledge in the exercise of my profession or outside of my profession or in daily commerce with men, which ought not to be spread abroad, I will keep secret and will never reveal. If I keep this oath faithfully, may I enjoy my life and practice my art, respected by all men and in all times; but if I swerve from it or violate it, may the reverse be my lot."

hippuric acid (hĭ-pu′rik) a compound formed by conjugation of benzoic acid and glycine; it occurs in the urine of herbivorous animals, rarely in human urine.

hippus (hip′us) abnormal exaggeration of the rhythmic contraction and dilation of the pupil, independent of changes in illumination or in fixation of the eyes.

hirci (her′si), sing. *hir′cus* [L.] the hairs growing in the axilla.

Hirschsprung's disease (hirsh′sproongz) congenital absence of the parasympathetic nerve ganglia in the anorectum or proximal rectum, or in some cases the entire colon, resulting in the absence of peristalsis in the affected portion of the colon and a consequent massive enlargement of the colon, constipation, and obstruction. Severe cases may require surgery in early infancy; less severe cases can be treated with enemas and laxatives but surgery often is required eventually. A temporary COLOSTOMY is

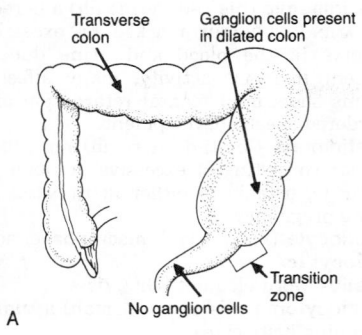

Transverse colon — Ganglion cells present in dilated colon

No ganglion cells — Transition zone

A

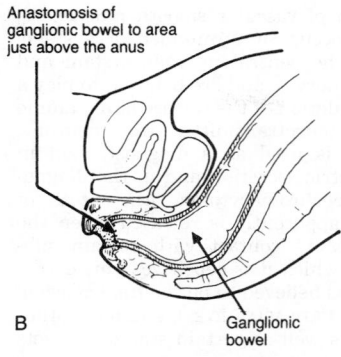

Anastomosis of ganglionic bowel to area just above the anus

Ganglionic bowel

B

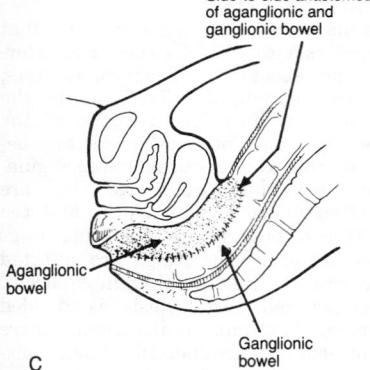

Side-to-side anastomosis of aganglionic and ganglionic bowel

Aganglionic bowel

Ganglionic bowel

C

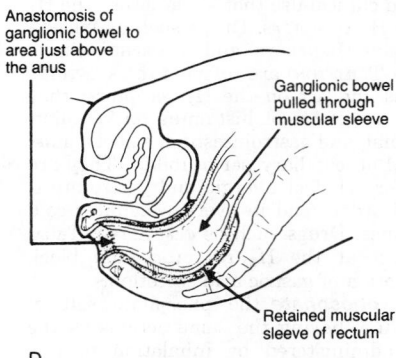

Anastomosis of ganglionic bowel to area just above the anus

Ganglionic bowel pulled through muscular sleeve

Retained muscular sleeve of rectum

D

Hirschsprung's disease and surgical procedures for repair. *A*, lack of ganglionic cells in a segment of the colon prevents the transmission of normal peristaltic waves and results in an intestinal obstruction. *B*, Swenson procedure: Aganglionic bowel is completely resected and ganglionic bowel is anastomosed to anus. *C*, Duhamel procedure: Ganglionic bowel is anastomosed side-to-side to aganglionic bowel and to the anus. *D*, Soave procedure: Ganglionic bowel is brought through a retained muscular sleeve of the rectum and anastomosed to the rectum. From Betz et al., 1994.

performed to relieve symptoms of bowel obstruction. Later, the aganglionic section of bowel is removed and the integrity of the intestine is restored. Called also aganglionic or congenital megacolon.

hirsute (her′sōōt) shaggy; hairy.

hirsuties (her-soo′she-ēz) hirsutism.

hirsutism (her′soo-tizm) abnormal hairiness, especially in women.

hirudicide (hĭ-roo′dĭ-sīd) an agent destructive to leeches.

hirudin (hĭ-roo′din) the active principle of the buccal secretion of leeches; it prevents clotting of the blood. A product made with recombinant technology is used as an ANTICO-AGULANT.

His's disease (his′ez) trench fever.

His-Werner disease (his ver′ner) trench fever.

hist(o)- word element [Gr.], *tissue.*

histaminase (his-tam′ĭ-nās) an enzyme that inactivates histamine.

histamine (his′tah-mēn) an amine, $C_5H_9N_3$, produced by decarboxylation of HISTIDINE, found in all body tissues. It induces capillary dilation (which increases capillary permeability and lowers blood pressure); contraction of most smooth muscle tissue; increased gastric acid secretion; and acceleration of the heart rate. It is also a mediator of immediate HYPERSENSITIVITY. adj., **histamin′ic.**

There are three types of cellular histamine RECEPTORS : H_1 *receptors* mediate contraction of smooth muscle and capillary dilation, and H_2 *receptors* mediate acceleration of heart rate and promotion of gastric acid secretion. Both types mediate contraction of vascular smooth muscle. H_3 receptors occur in a number of systems including the central nervous system and peripheral nerves, and are believed to play a role in regulation of the release of histamine and other neurotransmitters from neurons. Histamine is used as a diagnostic aid in testing gastric secretion and in the diagnosis of pheochromocytoma. An excess of histamine apparently is released when the body comes in contact with certain substances to which it is sensitive. This excess histamine is believed to be the final cause of HAY FEVER, URTICARIA (HIVES), and most other allergies, as well as certain stomach upsets and some headaches.

There are two types of histamine antagonists in clinical use that act at either the H_1 or the H_2 receptors. Drugs such as DIPHENHYDRAMINE (BENADRYL) and CHLORPHENIRAMINE (CHLOR-TRIMETON) are referred to as ANTIHISTAMINES and act on the H_1 receptors; they block the effects of histamine on vascular, bronchial, and gastrointestinal smooth muscle and on capillary permeability. They are used for relief of allergic and gastrointestinal disorders and in over-the-counter cold medicines. Drugs such as CIMETIDINE (TAGAMET) act at the H_2 receptors and block stimulation of gastric acid secretion.

h. phosphate the phosphate salt of histamine, having the same actions as the base; administered by inhalation to test airway hyperresponsiveness in diagnosis of ASTHMA, subcutaneously as a positive control in skin testing for allergy, and as a diagnostic aid to assess production of HYDROCHLORIC ACID in the stomach.

h. test 1. a formerly used test in which histamine was injected to stimulate gastric secretion and measure output of gastric acid. 2. a formerly used test for presence of a PHEOCHROMOCYTOMA; persons with such a tumor would show first a fall and then a marked rise in BLOOD PRESSURE. 3. a skin prick test used in evaluation of patients with ALLERGIES; skin responses to ALLERGENS are compared to the response to a histamine wheal.

histaminemia (his″tah-min-e′me-ah) histamine in the blood.

histaminergic (his″tah-min-er′jic) pertaining to the effects of HISTAMINE at histamine RECEPTORS of target tissues, which are blocked by ANTIHISTAMINES.

histidase (his′tĭ-dās) an enzyme of the liver that converts histidine to urocanic acid.

histidine (his′tĕ-dēn) a naturally occurring AMINO ACID, one of the essential amino acids, necessary for optimal growth of

infants; its decarboxylation results in formation of HISTAMINE.

histidinemia (his″tĭ-dĭ-ne′me-ah) a hereditary AMINOACIDOPATHY marked by excessive HISTIDINE in the blood and urine due to deficient HISTIDASE activity; many affected persons show mild mental retardation and disordered speech development.

histidinuria (his″tĭ-dĭ-nu′re-ah) an AMINOACIDURIA consisting of excessive HISTIDINE in the urine, usually in either HISTIDINEMIA or during pregnancy.

histiocyte (his′te-o-sīt″) macrophage. adj., **histiocyt′ic**.

histio- word element [Gr.], *tissue.*

histiocytoma (his″te-o-si-to′mah) a tumor containing histiocytes.

histiocytosis (his″te-o-si-to′sis) a condition marked by the abnormal appearance of histiocytes in the blood.

Langerhans cell h. a generic term that encompasses a group of disorders characterized by proliferation of Langerhans CELLS, which are specialized cells found in the epidermis that function as part of the immune system. These disorders are believed to arise from disturbances in regulation of the immune system. Children are more often affected than adults, and the bone marrow, endocrine system, and lungs may be involved (the lungs are affected more commonly in adults than in children). Langerhans cell histiocytosis is divided into unifocal and multifocal variants; there is also an acute, disseminated form (LETTERER-SIWE DISEASE). This group of disorders was formerly called histiocytosis X and was classified in three forms: Letterer-Siwe disease, Hand-Schüller-Christian disease, and eosinophilic granuloma. Called also eosinophilic granuloma, eosinophilic granulomatosis, and Langerhans cell granulomatosis.

Langerhans cell h., acute disseminated Letterer-Siwe disease.

Langerhans cell h., multifocal Langerhans cell histiocytosis occurring as erosive accumulations of proliferating Langerhans cells. It occurs most commonly in the marrow cavities of bones, but may also affect the skin, gingiva, lungs, and stomach. When the triad of involvement of the bones of the skull, exophthalmos, and diabetes insipidus is present, it is referred to as *Hand-Schüller-Christian disease.*

Langerhans cell h., unifocal Langerhans cell histiocytosis occurring as a single osteolytic lesion, usually in a long or flat bone; it may be asymptomatic or may produce bone pain, tenderness, and swelling and, sometimes, pathologic fracture.

h. X former name for Langerhans cell histiocytosis.

histiogenic (his″te-o-jen′ik) formed by the tissues.

histioid (his′te-oid) histoid.

histoblast (his′to-blast) a tissue-forming cell.

histochemistry (his″to-kem′is-tre) that branch of histology that deals with the identification of chemical components in cells and tissues.

histoclinical (his″to-klin′ĭ-k'l) combining histological and clinical evaluation.

histocompatibility (his″to-kom-pat″ĭ-bil′ĭ-te) 1. the quality of a cellular or tissue graft enabling it to be accepted and functional when transplanted to another organism. 2. the degree to which two individuals are histocompatible. adj., **histocompat′ible.**

histodialysis (his″to-di-al′ĭ-sis) disintegration or breaking down of tissue.

histodifferentiation (his″to-dif″er-en″she-a′shun) the acquisition of tissue characteristics by cell groups during development.

histogenesis (his″to-jen′ĕ-sis) differentiation of cells into the specialized tissues forming the various organs and parts of the body.

histogram (his′to-gram) a graph in which values found in a quantitative study are represented by lines or symbols placed horizontally or vertically, to indicate frequency distribution.

histoid (his′toid) 1. developed from one kind of tissue. 2. resembling one of the tissues of the body.

histoincompatibility (his″to-in″kom-pat″ĭ-bil′ĭ-te) the quality of a cellular or tissue graft preventing its acceptance or functioning when transplanted to another organism; said of the relationship between the genotypes (histocompatibility genes) of donor and host in which a graft generally will be rejected. adj., **histoincompat′ible.**

histokinesis (his″to-kĭ-ne′sis) movement in the tissues of the body.

histologic technician an allied health professional trained in tissue processing technique (fixation, dehydration, embedding, sectioning, routine and special staining, and mounting of tissue specimens) and also in histology and histochemistry. Graduates of accredited 1-year programs who pass the certification examination of the American Society of Clinical Pathologists are designated HT(ASCP), Histologic Technician.

histologist (his-tol′o-jist) one who specializes in histology.

histology (his-tol′o-je) that department of anatomy dealing with the minute structure, composition, and function of tissues. adj., **histolog′ic, histolog′ical.**

    pathologic h. the science of diseased tissues.

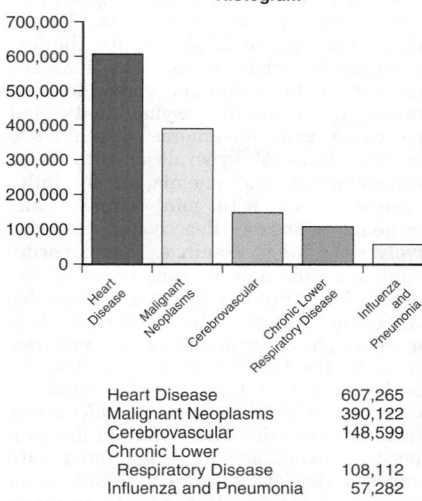

Histogram

Heart Disease	607,265
Malignant Neoplasms	390,122
Cerebrovascular	148,599
Chronic Lower Respiratory Disease	108,112
Influenza and Pneumonia	57,282

Leading causes of death in the United States, 1999.

histolysis (his-tol′ĭ-sis) breaking down of tissues. adj., **histolyt′ic.**

histoma (his-to′mah) any tissue tumor.

histone (his′tōn) a simple protein, soluble in water and insoluble in dilute ammonia, found combined as salts with acidic substances, such as nucleic acids or the globin of hemoglobin.

histopathology (his″to-pah-thol′o-je) pathologic histology.

histophysiology (his″to-fiz″e-ol′o-je) the correlation of function with the microscopic structures of cells and tissues.

Histoplasma (his″to-plaz′mah) a genus of fungi. *H. capsula′tum* causes HISTOPLASMOSIS in humans.

histoplasmin (his″to-plaz′min) a skin test antigen prepared from the fungus *Histoplasma capsulatum*. Because positive skin tests are common in endemic areas and indicate only previous exposure, not necessarily active disease, histoplasmin is not useful in diagnosis of HISTOPLASMOSIS. It is used primarily in epidemiologic surveys and in testing for cutaneous anergy in diagnosis of immunodeficiency.

histoplasmoma (his″to-plaz-mo′mah) a rounded granuloma of the lung due to infection with *Histoplasma capsulatum;* seen radiographically as a coin-shaped lesion.

histoplasmosis (his″to-plaz-mo′sis) a systemic fungal disease caused by inhalation of dust contaminated by *Histoplasma capsulatum;* it is not transmitted from one person to another. It is particularly common in rural areas of the midwestern United States, but is worldwide in distribution, including in urban areas. The infection begins in the lungs and may spread to other organs; it is usually asymptomatic but may cause acute pneumonia, disseminated reticuloendothelial hyperplasia with hepatosplenomegaly and anemia, or an influenzalike illness with joint effusion and erythema nodosum. Reactivated infection involves the lungs, meninges, heart, peritoneum, and adrenals in that order of frequency. On x-ray the lungs may resemble tuberculous lungs. The preferred drug for treatment of histoplasmosis is AMPHOTERICIN B. In the USPHS/IDSA *Guidelines for the Prevention of Opportunistic Infections in Persons with Human Immunodeficiency Virus,* persons with HIV infection are cautioned to avoid activities associated with increased risk of exposure to *Histoplasma capsulatum,* such as cleaning chicken coops, disturbing soil underneath bird roosting sites, or exploring caves.

   ocular h. disseminated choroiditis resulting in scars in the periphery of the fundus near the optic nerve, and characteristic disciform macular lesions; *Histoplasma capsulatum* is implicated strongly as the causative agent.

   historrhexis (his″to-rek′sis) the breaking up of tissue.

   history (his′to-re) a systematic account of events.

   case h. see CASE HISTORY.

   health h. a holistic assessment of all factors affecting a patient's health status, including information about social, cultural, familial, and economic aspects of the patient's life as well as any other component of the patient's life style that affects health and well-being. The health history is designed to assess the effects of health care deviations on the patient and the family, to evaluate teaching needs, and to serve as the basis of an individualized plan for addressing wellness.

   medical h. information obtained from the patient to aid in establishing a medical diagnosis and developing a treatment plan.

   nursing h. a written record providing data for assessing the nursing care needs of a patient.

   histotechnician/histotechnologist (his″-to-tek-nish′an his″to-tek-nol′ŏ-jist) HT/HTL; a CLINICAL LABORATORY TECHNICIAN specializing in the preparation of body tissue specimens for fixation, dehydration, embedding, sectioning, decalcification, microincineration, and routine and special staining. The histotechnologist performs all the functions of the histotechnician as well as identifying tissue structures, cell components, and their staining characteristics. Histotechnologists may serve as supervisors or educators. Academic programs are accredited by the National Accrediting Agency for Clinical Laboratory Sciences. Certification is through the Board of Registry of the American Society of Clinical Pathologists, whose address is P.O. Box 12270, Chicago, IL 60612 (telephone 312-738-1336). The address of the National Society for Histotechnology is 4201 Northview Drive, Suite 502, Bowie, MD 20716-1073 (telephone 301-262-6221).

   histotechnologist (his″to-tek-nol′o-jist) see HISTOTECHNICIAN/HISTOTECHNOLOGIST.

   histothrombin (his″to-throm′bin) thrombin derived from connective tissue.

   histotome (his′to-tōm) a cutting instrument used in microtomy; microtome.

   histotomy (his-tot′ah-me) dissection of tissues; microtomy.

   histotoxic (his′to-tok″sik) poisonous to tissue.

   histotroph (his′to-trōf) the sum total of nutritive material derived from maternal tissue other than the blood, utilized by the early embryo.

   histotrophic (his″to-trof′ik) 1. encouraging formation of tissue. 2. pertaining to histotroph.

   histotropic (his″to-trop′ik) having affinity for tissue cells.

   histrelin (his-trel′in) a synthetic preparation of gonadotropin-releasing HORMONE, used as the acetate ester in treatment of precocious PUBERTY.

   histrionic personality disorder a PERSONALITY DISORDER characterized by dramatic, attention-seeking, overly reactive, and intensely expressed behavior. Individuals with this disorder are prone to emotional display, such as angry outbursts and tantrums. They are often perceived by others as shallow and fickle; in their relationships they may be superficially charming but are frequently demanding and inconsiderate of others. Their behavior is often inappropriately sexually seductive or provocative, and they demand to be the center of attention, often using physical appearance to draw attention. Emotional expression is shallow and rapidly shifting. They may make manipulative suicide threats or attempts.

   hit 1. in library science, a retrieved document relevant to a search question that has been posed. 2. slang term for a single dose of a drug, used in reference to DRUG ABUSE.

HIV human immunodeficiency virus.

HIV-positive having a positive reaction on a test for the human immunodeficiency virus; used to indicate that an individual has been infected with the human immunodeficiency virus but does not yet have AIDS. Persons who are HIV-positive require sensitive counseling, information regarding transmission of the virus, and close supervision of their health status.

hives (hīvz) urticaria.

HI latent hyperopia.

HLA antigens the human major histocompatibility COMPLEX, located on the short arm of chromosome 6. Five loci have been identified, designated HLA-A, HLA-B, HLA-C, HLA-D, and HLA-DR (D related), each with multiple alleles, designated by numerals (e.g., HLA-B5). Provisionally identified alleles are designated by the letter *w* (e.g., HLA-Bw22). Called also human leukocyte antigens.

The HLA-A, -B, and -C loci gene products are cell surface antigens occurring on the surface of all nucleated cells. They are the most important antigens in transplant rejection, when donor and recipient HLA antigens do not match. The HLA-A, -B, and -C antigens are recognized by killer T cells that lyse the target cells. They are also involved in the cell-mediated lysis of virus-infected cells.

The HLA-D and -DR loci gene products are cell surface antigens of B lymphocytes and macrophages. They are involved in ANTIGEN PRESENTATION and other forms of cooperation between immunocompetent cells and also in the stimulation of transplant rejection.

A statistical association has been shown between certain HLA antigens and a number of diseases (e.g., HLA-B27 and ankylosing SPONDYLITIS). Such an association may be due to a genetic defect at a locus closely linked to the HLA locus, such as the immune response (Ir) genes or certain complement components (C2, C4, C8, factor B), or may be due to a defect in cell-mediated cytotoxicity or another mechanism that involves the HLA antigens.

Hm manifest hyperopia.

hMG human menopausal gonadotropin.

HMO health maintenance organization.

Ho holmium.

hoarseness (hors'nes) a rough quality of the voice.

Hodgkin's disease (hoj'kinz) a form of malignant LYMPHOMA characterized by painless, progressive enlargement of the LYMPH NODES, SPLEEN, and lymphoid tissues generally. It often begins in a cervical lymph node on the side of the neck and

HLA ANTIGEN–ASSOCIATED DISEASES

Specific HLA Antigens	Diseases
B8	Chronic autoimmune hepatitis
B27	Ankylosing spondylitis
B35	Subacute thyroiditis
B47	Congenital adrenal hyperplasia
Cw6	Psoriasis
D/DR3	Celiac disease
	Graves disease
	Idiopathic Addison disease
	Myesthenia gravis
	Systemic lupus erythematosus
D/DR4	Pemphigus
	Rheumatoid arthritis

spreads in a contiguous fashion through the body. It accounts for less than 1 per cent of all malignancies in the United States and is seen more in developed countries than in developing countries and more in males than in females. An unusual characteristic is that it has two peaks on its incidence curve, one between 15 and 35 years of age and the other between 55 and 75. CHEMOTHERAPY and RADIATION THERAPY have increased the survival rate. The rate of survival depends on the stage at which treatment is begun; in Stages I and II the five-year survival rate is 85 per cent. Called also Hodgkin's lymphoma

Signs and Symptoms. The first sign of the disease usually is an enlargement of lymph nodes in the cervical, axillary, or inguinal chains. Severe itching is often an early symptom of the disorder; signs may also include fever, night sweats, and weight loss of greater than 10 per cent.

As Hodgkin's disease progresses, it spreads through the lymphatic system, involving other lymph nodes elsewhere in the body as well as the spleen, liver, and bone marrow. The lymph nodes and the spleen and liver may swell, and by obstructing other organs may cause coughing, breathlessness, or enlargement of the abdomen. The patient often becomes NEUTROPENIC, THROMBOCYTOPENIC, or ANEMIC and because of blood changes the body becomes less able to combat infections.

There are several different staging systems, classifying the disease according to stages of development of malignancy; the stages are helpful in establishing the prognosis and prescribing treatment. The most commonly used is the Cotswold or Modified Ann Arbor Staging System. In Stage I only one localized lymph node region is involved.

Stage IE indicates involvement of a single extralymphatic organ. Stage II indicates two or more involved nodes on the same side of the diaphragm. Stage IIE indicates involvement of an extralymphatic organ and one or more nodes on the same side of the diaphragm. IIS designates splenic involvement with localization below the diaphragm. In Stage III there is disease on both sides of the diaphragm, sometimes with splenic involvement (IIIS) or extralymphatic organ involvement (IIIE), or both (IIISE). In Stage IV there is diffuse involvement of one or more extralymphatic organs or tissues with or without associated lymph node involvement. The presence or absence of systemic manifestations should be indicated by adding the letter A or B to the stage number, where A indicates asymptomatic and B indicates fever, night sweats, and weight loss of more than 10 per cent of body weight.

Diagnosis. The diagnosis of Hodgkin's disease requires the histologic identification of the characteristic malignant cell of the disease, the Reed-Sternberg CELL. The accepted histopathologic classification distinguishes four different disease patterns: LYMPHOCYTE predominance, mixed cellularity, lymphocyte depletion, and nodular sclerosis. The evaluation required for staging includes a history and physical examination; CT scans of the chest, abdomen, and pelvis; laboratory tests, including a complete BLOOD COUNT, serum ALKALINE PHOSPHATASE, and liver and kidney function tests; and sometimes GALLIUM scanning or LYMPHANGIOGRAPHY; and a surgical lymph node biopsy. Osseous involvement is evaluated with bone marrow biopsy and bone scans. The evaluation of abdominal involvement may require exploratory LAPAROTOMY or SPLENOTOMY.

Treatment and Care. If the disease is localized (Stages IA, IIA, or IIIA), the treatment of choice is RADIATION THERAPY capable of delivering a high dose of radiation deep into the tissues. CHEMOTHERAPY is recommended for patients with systemic involvement (Stages IB, IIB, and IIIB). The chemotherapeutic agents are administered in combination and intermittently so that there is a synergistic cytotoxic effect without overlapping toxicities. Drugs are chosen according to their effect on different phases of cell growth and proliferation. (See also ANTINEOPLASTIC THERAPY.) Often it is decided to employ both chemotherapy and radiation therapy, especially in treating bulky tumor involvement of nodes and spleen.

After recovery, follow-up care is extremely important. There is an increased risk of developing other cancers later in life.

Hodgson's disease (hoj′sunz) aneurysmal dilatation of the proximal part of the aorta; it is sometimes accompanied by dilatation of the heart.

hodoneuromere (ho″do-noor′o-mēr) a segment of the embryonic trunk with its pair of nerves and their branches.

Hoffmann's sign (hof′manz) 1. increased mechanical irritability of the sensory nerves in TETANY; the ulnar nerve is usually tested. 2. a sudden nipping of the nail of the index, middle, or ring finger produces flexion of

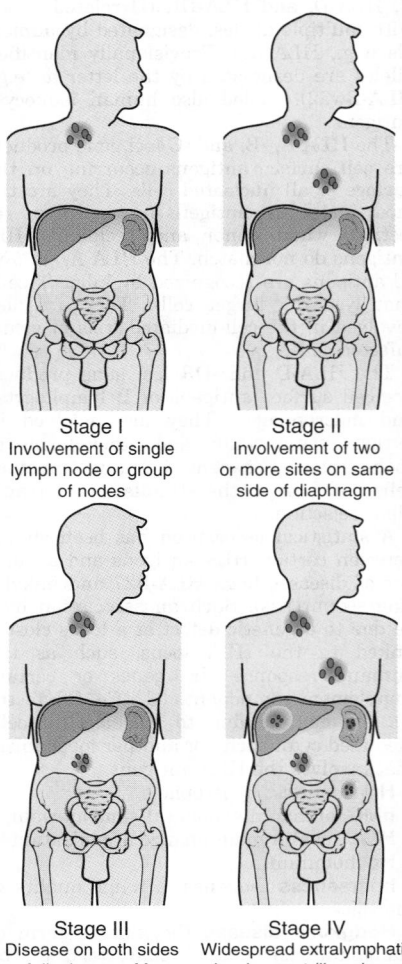

Stage I
Involvement of single lymph node or group of nodes

Stage II
Involvement of two or more sites on same side of diaphragm

Stage III
Disease on both sides of diaphragm. May include spleen or localized extranodal disease

Stage IV
Widespread extralymphatic involvement (liver, bone marrow, lung, skin)

Staging of Hodgkin's disease. From Damjanov, 1996.

the terminal phalanx of the thumb and of the second and third phalanx of some other finger; called also digital reflex.

hol(o)- word element [Gr.], *entire; whole.*

holandric (hol-an′drik) inherited exclusively through the male descent; transmitted through genes located on the Y chromosome.

holistic (ho-lis′tik) pertaining to totality, or to the whole. In recent years, there has been a growing interest in the concept of holistic health and the notion that the physical, mental, social, and spiritual aspects of a person's life must be viewed as an integrated whole. This leads to a broader concept of patient/client care in which emotional and social needs are dealt with as well as physical needs.

Hollander test (hol′an-der) a gastric function test that measures the response of gastric secretory cells to insulin-induced HYPOGLYCEMIA; used to evaluate the completeness of a VAGOTOMY.

Holmgren test (holm′gren) one for detection of imperfect perception of color, based on matching various strands of yarn.

holmium (Ho) (hol′me-um) a chemical element, atomic number 67, atomic weight 164.930. (See Appendix 6.)

holoacardius (hol″o-ah-kahr′de-us) a malformed monozygotic twin fetus in which the heart is entirely absent.

holoblastic (hol″o-blas′tik) undergoing cleavage in which the entire oocyte (ovum) participates; completely dividing.

holocrine (hol′o-krin) wholly secretory, denoting that type of glandular secretion in which the entire secreting cell, along with its accumulated secretion, forms the secreted matter of the gland, as in the sebaceous glands. See also APOCRINE and MEROCRINE.

holodiastolic (hol″o-di″ah-stol′ik) pertaining to the entire diastole.

holoendemic (hol″o-en-dem′ik) endemic at a high level in a population, affecting most of the children and so affecting the adults in the population less often; see also HYPERENDEMIC.

holoenzyme (hol″o-en′zīm) the active compound formed by combination of a coenzyme and an apoenzyme.

hologynic (hol″o-jin′ik) inherited exclusively through the female descent; transmitted through genes located on attached X chromosomes.

holoprosencephaly (hol″o-pros″en-sef′ah-le) a developmental ANOMALY consisting of failure of cleavage of the prechordal mesoderm with a deficit in the forebrain and midline facial development; in the severe form there may be CYCLOPIA. It is sometimes associated with TRISOMY 13 SYNDROME.

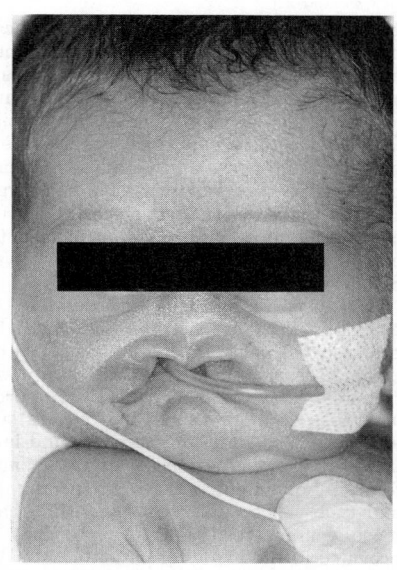

The facial features in holoprosencephaly. The eyes are close together and there is a midline cleft lip. From Mueller and Young, 2001.

holorachischisis (hol″o-rah-kis′ki-sis) fissure of the entire vertebral column with prolapse of the spinal cord.

holosystolic (hol″o-sis-tol′ik) pertaining to the entire systole.

hom(o)- word element [Gr.] 1. *same; similar.* 2. chemical prefix indicating addition of one CH_2 group to the main compound.

Homans' sign (ho′manz) discomfort behind the knee on forced dorsiflexion of the foot; a sign of thrombosis in the lower limb.

homatropine (ho-mat′ro-pēn) an ANTICHOLINERGIC and ANTIMUSCARINIC producing sympathetic blockade effects similar to but weaker than those of ATROPINE; the hydrobromide salt is used as a MYDRIATIC and CYCLOPLEGIC and the methylbromide salt is used as an inhibitor of gastric spasm and secretion.

home (hōm) a place where someone lives.

h. health care services provided by a certified agency using an interdisciplinary team to meet the needs of patients being cared for in out-of-hospital settings such as private homes, boarding homes, hospices, shelters, and so on. Caregivers include professional and practical nurses, nursing assistants, physical therapists, occupational therapists, speech therapists, and other professionals. The rising costs of hospitalization and the impact of diagnosis-related group (DRG) reimbursement for Medicare patients have contributed to the phenomenal increase in home health care agencies in the United States. Additionally, technological advances now make it possible for patients to receive many treatments at home that formerly were administered only in a hospital. Examples include oxygen therapy, intravenous drug perfusion (including administration of antineoplastics and antibiotics), and peritoneal dialysis. See also home health AGENCY.

A variety of agencies and services are available in many communities. Some are privately owned and operated for profit (proprietary), others are affiliated with hospitals, and some are private nonprofit agencies. As more third-party payers such as federal and state governments and large insurance companies certify these agencies for reimbursement, growth in the number and type can be expected to continue, and more complicated types of care may be provided in the homes of patients.

h. maintenance, impaired a NURSING DIAGNOSIS approved by the North American Nursing Diagnosis Association, defined as inability to independently maintain a safe and growth-promoting immediate environment. Related factors are any illness, injury, or knowledge deficit that can contribute to a person's inability to attend to cleaning, repairing, and maintaining the home and providing basic needs and comforts for the self and family members. Age-related factors might include special needs of an infant or of an elderly person with functional disabilities or sensory loss. In some cases impaired management of home maintenance could be related to insufficient family organization or planning, inadequate financial resources, or impaired cognitive or emotional functioning.

Nursing interventions are focused on determining the nature of the problem, assessing the family's ability to deal with it, and identifying available resources for assistance. Plans for utilizing available resources are developed with family members. These might include procuring a part-time homemaker, obtaining supportive assistance such as legal aid or nutritional care, or providing therapeutic care by nurses, speech therapists, physical therapists or other professionals who are involved in home health care.

nursing h. see NURSING HOME.

residential care h., rest h. a residence where room, board, and personal care are provided for individuals who need assistance and supervision. The focus is generally on dependent elderly persons who cannot live independently but do not require regular nursing care, and on younger individuals who have mental illness or mental retardation.

home(o)- word element [Gr.], *similar; same; unchanging.*

Home Health Care Classification (HHCC) a system developed by Dr. Virginia Saba to assess and classify patients receiving HOME HEALTH CARE.

Home Health Care Classification System a computerized classification system for HOME HEALTH CARE, assessing and classifying home health Medicare patients in order to predict their need for nursing and other home health care services, as well as their outcomes of care.

homeodynamics (ho″me-o-di-nam′iks) a way of viewing human beings, postulated by Martha E. ROGERS. Changes in the life process of human beings are irreversible, nonrepeatable, rhythmical in nature, and evidence growing complexity of pattern and organization. Change proceeds by continuous patterning of the human and environmental energy fields in the form of resonating waves and reflects the continuous interaction between the two at any given point in space-time.

homeomorphous (ho″me-o-mor′fus) of like form and structure.

homeopathy (ho″me-op′ah-the) a system of therapeutics founded by Samuel Hahnemann (1755–1843) in which diseases are treated by drugs that are capable of producing in healthy persons symptoms like those of the disease to be treated, the drug being administered in minute doses. adj., **homeopath′ic.**

homeoplasia (ho″me-o-pla′zhah) formation of new tissue like that normal to the part. adj., **homeoplas′tic.**

homeorhesis (ho″me-o-re′sis) a stabilized flow. The term has been proposed as a substitute for HOMEOSTASIS, which implies a static rather than a fluid state in the internal environment, while homeorhesis takes into account the fluidity of change within a space-time continuum and more accurately describes the adaptations and constant interactions necessary to one's well-being in a changing environment.

homeostasis (ho″me-o-sta′sis) the tendency of biological systems to maintain relatively constant conditions in the internal environment while continuously interacting with and adjusting to changes originating within or outside the system. See also BALANCE and EQUILIBRIUM. adj., **homeostat′ic.** The term is considered by some to be misleading in that the word element-STASIS

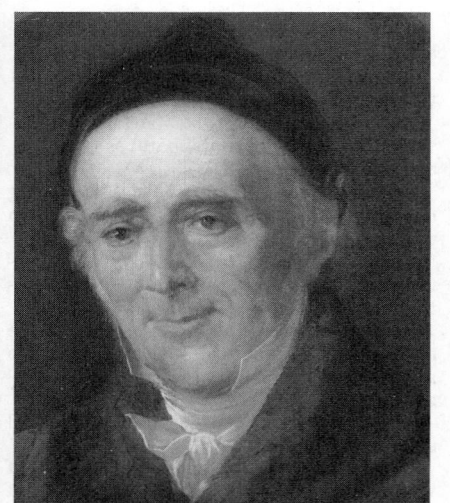

Samuel Hahnemann, founder of homeopathy. Courtesy of the Hahnemann University Archives, Medical College of Pennsylvania and Hahnemann University, Philadelphia, PA.

implies a static or fixed and unmoving state, whereas homeostasis actually involves continuous motion, adaptation, and change in response to environmental factors.

It is through homeostatic mechanisms that body temperature is kept within normal range, the osmotic pressure of the blood and its hydrogen ion concentration (pH) is kept within strict limits, nutrients are supplied to cells as needed, and waste products are removed before they accumulate and reach toxic levels of concentration. These are but a few examples of the thousands of homeostatic control systems within the body. Some of these systems operate within the cell and others operate within an aggregate of cells (organs) to control the complex interrelationships among the various organs.

homeotherapy (ho″me-o-ther′ah-pe) treatment with a substance similar to the causative agent of the disease.

homeotherm (ho′me-o-therm″) 1. an animal that exhibits homeothermy, a warm-blooded animal. 2. endotherm.

homeothermy (ho′me-o-ther″me) the maintenance of a constant body temperature despite changes in the environmental temperature. adj., **homeother′mal, homeother′mic.**

homeotypical (ho″me-o-tip′ĭ-k′l) resembling the normal or usual type.

homergic (hŏm-er′jik) having the same effect; said of two drugs each of which produces the same overt effect.

Homo (ho′mo) [L.] the genus of primates containing the single living species *H. sapiens* (human beings).

homocyclic (ho″mo-sik′lik) having or pertaining to a closed chain or ring formation that contains only atoms of the same element.

homocysteine (ho″mo-sis′te-ēn) a sulfur-containing amino acid homologous with CYSTEINE and produced by demethylation of METHIONINE; it can form CYSTINE or methionine.

homocystine (ho″mo-sis′tēn) a homologue of CYSTINE that results from demethylation of METHIONINE.

homocystinuria (ho″mo-sis″tin-u′re-ah) an inborn ERROR of metabolism of sulfur amino acids due to lack of the enzyme cystathionine synthase; it is characterized by HOMOCYSTINE in the urine and by mental retardation, hepatomegaly, ECTOPIA LENTIS (displacement of the lens), and cardiovascular and skeletal disorders.

homocytotropic (ho″mo-si′to-trop′ik) having an affinity for cells of individuals of the same species.

homodromous (ho-mod′ro-mus) moving or acting in the same or in the usual direction.

homoeroticism (ho″mo-ĕ-rot′ĭ-sizm) sexual feeling directed toward a person of the same sex. adj. **homoerot′ic.**

homoerotism (ho″mo-er′o-tizm) homoeroticism.

homogametic (ho″mo-gah-met′ik) having only one kind of GAMETE with respect to the sex chromosomes, as in the human female, all of whose ova contain only the X chromosome.

homogenate (ho-moj′ĕ-nāt) material obtained by homogenization.

homogeneity (ho″mo-jĕ-ne′ĭ-te) the state of being homogeneous.

homogeneous (ho″mo-je′ne-us) of uniform quality, composition, or structure.

homogenesis (ho″mo-jen′ĕ-sis) reproduction by the same process in each generation.

homogenic (ho″mo-jen′ik) homozygous (see HOMOZYGOSITY).

homogenicity (ho″mo-jĕ-nis′ĭ-te) homogeneity.

homogenize (ho-moj′ĕ-nīz) to convert into material that is of uniform quality or consistency throughout; to render homogeneous.

homogentisic acid (ho″mo-jen-tis′ik) 2,5-dihydroxyphenyl acetic acid, an intermediate product in the metabolism of TYROSINE and PHENYLALANINE, excreted in the urine in the inborn ERROR of metabolism known as PHENYLKETONURIA.

homograft (ho′mo-graft) ALLOGRAFT.

homolateral (ho″mo-lat′er-al) ipsilateral.

homologous (ho-mol′ŏ-gus) 1. corresponding in structure, position, origin, or other aspects. 2. allogeneic. 3. pertaining to an antibody and the antigen that elicited its production.

homologue (hom′ŏ-log) 1. any organ or part similar in origin or structure but not always in function, as the arms of a human and the wings of a bird or the hands and feet of a human and the paws of a dog. 2. in chemistry, one of a series of compounds distinguished by addition of a CH_2 group in successive members.

homology (ho-mol′ŏ-je) the state of being homologous.

homolysin (ho-mol′ĭ-sin) a lysin produced by injection into the body of an antigen derived from an individual of the same species.

homonomous (ho-mon′ŏ-mus) subject to the same laws; in biology, subject to the same laws of growth or developed along the same line.

homonymous (ho-mon′ĭ-mus) 1. having the same or corresponding sound or name. 2. standing in the same relation.

homophilic (ho″mo-fil′ik) reacting only with specific antigen.

homoplastic (ho″mo-plas′tik) 1. pertaining to homoplasty. 2. allogeneic. 3. denoting organs or parts, as the wings of birds and insects, that resemble one another in structure and function but not in origin or development.

homoplasty (ho′mo-plas″te) 1. allogeneic TRANSPLANTATION. 2. similarity between organs or their parts not due to common ancestry.

homorganic (hom″or-gan′ik) produced by the same or by homologous organs.

homosalate (ho″mo-sal′āt) a SUNSCREEN effective against ULTRAVIOLET B rays, applied topically to the skin.

homosexual (ho″mo-sek′shoo-al) 1. pertaining to the same sex; directed toward a person of the same sex; the opposite of heterosexual. 2. one who is sexually attracted to persons of the same sex.

h. panic an acute severe episode of anxiety, due to unconscious conflicts involving sexual identity, in which there is the fear or delusional conviction that the person is thought by others to be a homosexual or is in danger of sexual attack by a person of the same sex, often accompanied by agitation, guilt, hallucinations, or depression.

homosexuality (ho″mo-sek″shoo-al′ĭ-te) sexual orientation toward or activity with persons of the same sex.

homotherm (ho′mo-therm) homeotherm. adj. **homother′mal, homother′mic.**

homotopic (ho″mo-top′ik) occurring at the same place upon the body.

homotype (ho′mo-tīp) a part having reversed symmetry with its mate, as the hand. adj., **homotyp′ic.**

homoxenous (ho-mok′sĕ-nus) requiring only one host in the life cycle; said of certain parasites.

homozygosis (ho″mo-zi-go′sis) the formation of a zygote by the union of gametes that have one or more identical alleles.

homozygosity (ho″mo-zi-gos′ĭ-te) the state of having identical alleles in regard to a given character or characters. adj., **homozy′gous.**

homozygote (ho″mo-zi′gōt) an individual exhibiting homozygosity.

homunculus (ho-mung′ku-lus) a dwarf without deformity or disproportion of parts.

hookworm (hook′werm) a parasitic ROUNDWORM, found mostly in the southeastern United States, that enters the human body through the skin and migrates to the intestines, where it attaches itself to the intestinal wall and sucks blood for nourishment. The hookworm most common in the United States and Central America is *Necator americanus,* which literally means "American killer." It is about 1 cm (half an inch) long, with sharp hooklike teeth and a muscular gullet used in sucking blood. The female, slightly larger than the male, can lay more than 10,000 eggs a day, any one of which can hatch into a larva and invade the human body. Another common hookworm is *Ancylostoma duodenale.* (See illustration.)

h. disease NECATORIASIS, ANCYLOSTOMIASIS, or infection with some other type of hookworm. Once fairly common, it is now largely confined to rural or poor areas where modern sanitation is lacking.

Larval hookworms enter the body by burrowing through the skin, usually that of the sole of the foot. The first sign of the disease may appear on the skin as small eruptions that develop into pus-filled blisters; this condition is sometimes called "ground itch." The hookworms then enter blood vessels and are carried by the blood into the lungs. After they leave the lungs, they propel themselves up the trachea, are swallowed and washed through the stomach, and end up in the intestines. Here, if left alone, they will establish a parasitic relationship, using their host's body as a source of nourishment.

By the time they reach the intestines, about 6 weeks after they entered the body

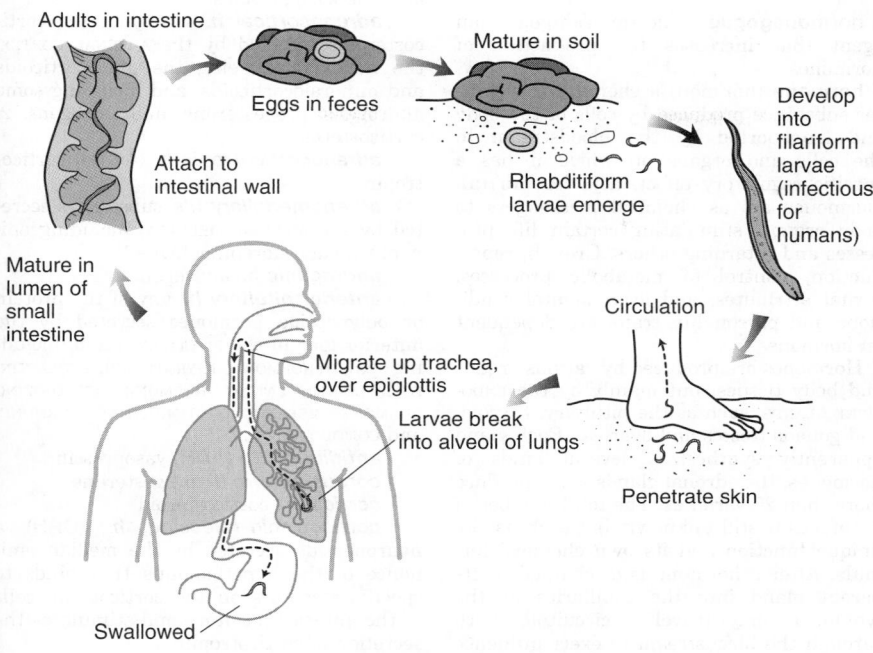

Life cycle of a hookworm. From Mahon and Manuselis, 2000.

as larvae, the worms are full-grown adults. Each worm now attaches itself by hooked teeth to the intestinal wall, where it sucks its host's blood by contraction and expansion of its gullet. If large numbers of worms are present, they can cause considerable loss of blood and severe anemia. The symptoms include pallor and loss of energy; the appetite may increase. The thousands of eggs laid every day by each female worm pass out of the body in the stool, in which they can easily be seen. If the stool is not properly disposed of, the larvae that hatch from the eggs may infect other persons.

Treatment and Prevention. A nutritious, high-protein diet supplemented by iron is given to relieve anemia and improve health. Drug treatment is with pyrantel pamoate or mebendazole. When left untreated, hookworms can cause not only anemia but also bronchial inflammation and occasionally stunting of growth, mental retardation, and even death. Hookworm infection can be prevented by installation of sanitary toilets or, if that is not possible, by disposal of human feces in deep holes so that the soil with which the human foot comes in contact is not contaminated. Shoes should be worn outdoors to protect the feet from infection.

hopelessness (hōp′les-nes) 1. a loss of confidence that future events or occurrences will be positive. 2. a NURSING DIAGNOSIS accepted by the North American Nursing Diagnosis Association, defined as the subjective state in which an individual sees limited or no alternatives or personal choices available and is unable to mobilize energy on his or her own behalf. Hopelessness is associated with poor health outcomes and may be counteracted for some patients by the maintenance of a positive environment that fosters independence and self-confidence.

hordeolum (hōr-de′o-lum) sty.

horizon (hŏ-ri′zon) a specific anatomic stage of embryonic development, of which 23 have been defined, beginning with the unicellular zygote (fertilized egg) and ending 7 to 9 weeks later with the beginning of the fetal stage.

horizontal (hor-ĭ-zon′tal) 1. parallel to the plane of the horizon. 2. spreading from one individual to another; see horizontal TRANSMISSION.

hormesis (hor-me′sis) stimulation by a subinhibitory concentration of a toxic substance.

hormonagogue (hor-mōn'ah-gog) an agent that increases the production of hormones.

hormone (hor'mōn) a chemical transmitter substance produced by cells of the body and transported by the bloodstream to the cells and organs on which it has a specific regulatory effect. adj., **hormo'nal.** Hormones act as chemical messengers to body organs, stimulating certain life processes and retarding others. Growth, reproduction, control of metabolic processes, sexual attributes, and even mental conditions and personality traits are dependent on hormones.

Hormones are produced by various organs and body tissues, but mainly by the ENDOCRINE GLANDS, such as the pituitary, thyroid, and gonads (testes and ovaries). Each gland apparently synthesizes several kinds of hormones; the adrenal glands alone produce more than 25 varieties. The total number of hormones is still unknown, but each has its unique function and its own chemical formula. After a hormone is discharged by its parent gland into the capillaries or the lymph, it may travel a circuitous path through the bloodstream to exert influence on cells, tissues, and organs (target organs) far removed from its site of origin.

One of the best-known endocrine hormones is INSULIN, a protein manufactured by the beta cells of the islands of Langerhans in the pancreas that is important in carbohydrate metabolism. Other important hormones are THYROXINE, an iodine-carrying amino acid produced by the thyroid gland; CORTISONE, a member of the steroid family from the adrenal glands; and the sex hormones, ESTROGEN from the ovaries and ANDROGEN from the testes. Certain hormone substances can be synthesized in the laboratory for treatment of human disease. Animal hormones can also be used, as endocrine hormones are to some extent interchangeable among species. Extracts from the pancreas of cattle, for example, enabled diabetes sufferers to live normal lives even before the chemistry of insulin was fully understood.

Endocrine hormone synthesis and secretion is controlled and regulated by a closed-loop system. Negative FEEDBACK loops maintain optimal levels of each hormone in the body. If there are abnormally high levels of a hormone in the blood, feedback to the gland responsible for its production inhibits secretion. If there are abnormally low levels, the gland is stimulated to step up production and secretion. In this way a homeostatic balance is maintained. (See also ENDOCRINE GLANDS.)

adrenocortical h. 1. any of the corticosteroids secreted by the ADRENAL CORTEX, the major ones being the glucocorticoids and mineralocorticoids, and including some androgens, progesterone, and estrogens. 2. corticosteroid.

adrenocorticotropic h. (ACTH) corticotropin.

adrenomedullary h's substances secreted by the ADRENAL MEDULLA, including epinephrine and norepinephrine.

androgenic h. androgen.

anterior pituitary h. any of the protein or polypeptide hormones secreted by the anterior lobe of the PITUITARY GLAND, including GROWTH HORMONE, THYROTROPIN, PROLACTIN, FOLLICLE-STIMULATING HORMONE, LUTEINIZING HORMONE, MELANOCYTE-STIMULATING HORMONE, and CORTICOTROPIN.

antidiuretic h. (ADH) vasopressin.

corpus luteum h. progesterone.

cortical h. corticosteroid.

corticotropin-releasing h. (CRH) a neuropeptide secreted by the median eminence of the hypothalamus that binds to specific receptors on the corticotroph cells of the anterior pituitary and stimulates the secretion of corticotropin.

ectopic h's those secreted by tumors of nonendocrine tissues but having the same physiologic effects as their normally produced counterparts. It is not known exactly how the synthesis and secretion of endocrine hormones from nonendocrine tissues occurs. Most of these tumors are derived from tissues that have a common embryonic origin with endocrine tissues. When the cells undergo neoplastic transformation, they can revert to a more primitive stage of development and begin to synthesize hormones.

Ectopic hormones present serious problems for patients and add to the complexity of caring for those with certain kinds of neoplastic diseases. These hormones do not respond to the feedback mechanisms that regulate normal hormonal production; hence, surgery and destruction of the tumorous tissue by radiation and chemotherapy are the treatments of choice.

estrogenic h. estrogen.

follicle-stimulating h. (FSH) one of the gonadotropins of the anterior pituitary, which stimulates the growth and maturity of graafian follicles in the ovary, and stimulates spermatogenesis in the male.

follicle-stimulating h. and luteinizing h.–releasing h. (FSH/LH-RH) luteinizing hormone–releasing hormone.

follicle-stimulating h.–releasing h. (FSH-RH) luteinizing hormone–releasing hormone.

gonadotropic h. gonadotropin.

gonadotropin-releasing h. (Gn-RH) luteinizing hormone–releasing hormone.

growth h. (GH) any of several related polypeptide hormones secreted by the anterior lobe of the PITUITARY GLAND that directly influence protein, carbohydrate, and lipid metabolism and control the rate of skeletal and visceral growth; their secretion is in part controlled by the hypothalamus. It is used pharmaceutically as SOMATREM and SOMATROPIN. Called also somatotrophin, somatotropin, and somatotrophic or somatotropic hormone.

growth h. release–inhibiting h. somatostatin.

growth h.–releasing h. (GH-RH) a neuropeptide elaborated by the median eminence of the hypothalamus that binds to specific receptors on the somatotroph cells of the anterior pituitary and stimulates the secretion of growth hormone.

interstitial cell–stimulating h. luteinizing hormone.

lactation h., lactogenic h. prolactin.

local h. a substance with hormone like properties that acts at an anatomically restricted site; most are rapidly degraded. Called also autacoid and autocoid.

luteinizing h. (LH) a GONADOTROPIN of the anterior pituitary gland, acting with follicle-stimulating hormone to cause ovulation of mature follicles and secretion of estrogen by thecal and granulosa cells of the ovary; it is also concerned with corpus luteum formation. In the male, it stimulates development of the interstitial cells of the testes and their secretion of testosterone. Called also interstitial cell–stimulating hormone.

luteinizing h.–releasing h. (LH-RH) a decapeptide hormone of the hypothalamus, which stimulates the release of follicle-stimulating hormone and luteinizing hormone from the pituitary gland; it can be used in the differential diagnosis of hypothalamic, pituitary, and gonadal dysfunction. Called also follicle-stimulating hormone–releasing hormone, follicle-stimulating hormone and luteinizing hormone–releasing hormone, and gonadotropin-releasing hormone.

melanocyte-stimulating h. (MSH) a substance from the anterior PITUITARY GLAND of certain other animals but not humans; it influences the formation or deposition of MELANIN in the body and pigmentation of the skin.

neurohypophyseal h's those stored and released by the neurohypophysis, i.e., oxytocin and vasopressin.

parathyroid h. (PTH) a polypeptide hormone secreted by the parathyroid glands that influences calcium and phosphorus metabolism and bone formation.

placental h's hormones secreted by the placenta, including chorionic gonadotropin, and other substances having estrogenic, progestational, or adrenocorticoid activity.

progestational h. 1. progesterone. 2. progestational agent.

prolactin-inhibiting h. a hormone released by the HYPOTHALAMUS that inhibits the secretion of PROLACTIN by the anterior PITUITARY GLAND.

prolactin-releasing h. any of various hormones elaborated by the HYPOTHALAMUS that stimulate the release of PROLACTIN by the anterior PITUITARY GLAND. Most such activity is exerted by VASOACTIVE INTESTINAL POLYPEPTIDE, although in humans thyrotropin-releasing HORMONE can also have this action.

sex h's see SEX HORMONES.

somatotrophic h., somatotropic h. growth hormone.

somatotropin release–inhibiting h. somatostatin.

somatotropin-releasing h. (SRH) growth hormone–releasing hormone.

steroid h's hormones that are biologically active STEROIDS; they are secreted by the adrenal CORTEX, TESTIS, OVARY, and PLACENTA and include the progestational AGENTS, GLUCOCORTICOIDS, MINERALOCORTICOIDS, ANDROGENS, and ESTROGENS. They act by binding to specific receptors to form complexes, which then enhance or inhibit the expression of specific genes.

thyroid h's see THYROID HORMONES.

thyroid-stimulating h. (TSH) thyrotropin.

thyrotropin-releasing h. (TRH) a tripeptide hormone of the hypothalamus, which stimulates release of thyrotropin from the pituitary gland. In humans, it also acts as a prolactin releasing factor. It is used in the diagnosis of mild hyperthyroidism and Graves disease, and in differentiating between primary, secondary, and tertiary hypothyroidism.

hormonogen (hor-mo'no-jen″) prohormone.

hormonopoiesis (hor-mo″no-poi-e'sis) the production of hormones. adj., **hormonopoiet'ic.**

hormonotherapy (hor-mo″no-ther'ah-pe) treatment by the use of hormones; endocrinotherapy.

horn (horn) 1. a pointed projection such as the paired processes on the head of various animals, or other structure resembling them in shape. **2.** an excrescence or projection shaped like the horn of an animal.

anterior h. of spinal cord the horn-shaped configuration presented by the anterior column of the spinal cord in transverse section; called also ventral horn of spinal cord.

cicatricial h. a hard, dry outgrowth from a scar, often scaly and occasionally osseous.

dorsal h. of spinal cord posterior horn of spinal cord.

lateral h. of spinal cord the horn-shaped configuration presented by the lateral column of the spinal cord in transverse section.

posterior h. of spinal cord the horn-shaped configuration presented by the posterior column of the spinal cord in transverse section; called also dorsal horn of spinal cord.

sebaceous h. a hard outgrowth of the contents of a sebaceous cyst.

ventral h. of spinal cord anterior horn of spinal cord.

warty h. a hard, pointed outgrowth of a wart.

horny (hor'ne) pertaining to or resembling a horn; called also corneous, keratic, and keratinous.

Horner syndrome (hor'ner) sinking in of the eyeball, ptosis of the upper eyelid, slight elevation of the lower lid, constriction of the pupil, narrowing of the palpebral fissure, and anhidrosis caused by paralysis of the cervical sympathetic nerve supply.

horopter (hor-op'ter) the sum of all points seen in binocular vision with the eyes fixed.

hospice (hos'pis) originally, a medieval guest house or way station for pilgrims and travelers. The term is currently used to designate either a place or a philosophy of care for persons in the last stages of life and their families. For decades there have been hospices in England, free-standing facilities unaffiliated with hospitals and autonomous in terms of professional procedures. These hospices were the predecessors of the hospices now found in the United States.

A hospice program provides palliative and supportive care for terminally ill patients and their families. The concept of hospice is that of a caring community of professional and nonprofessional people, supplemented by volunteer services. The emphasis is on dealing with emotional and spiritual problems as well as medical problems. Of primary concern is control of pain and other symptoms, on keeping the patient at home for as long as possible or desirable, and

on making his or her remaining days as comfortable and meaningful as possible. After the patient dies family members are given support throughout their period of bereavement.

hospital (hos'pit'l) an institution for the care and treatment of the acutely sick and injured.

day h. a facility that offers professional health care, such as psychiatric care or rehabilitation services, to individuals who require services but are able to return to their homes overnight.

H. Infection Control Practices Advisory Committee a committee established in 1991 by the United States Government with members appointed by the Secretary of Health and Human Services. It provides advice and guidance related to ISOLATION practices and serves as an advisory committee to the CENTERS FOR DISEASE CONTROL AND PREVENTION for updating guidelines and policy statements related to control of NOSOCOMIAL INFECTION.

open h. **1.** a mental hospital, or section of a hospital, without locked doors or other forms of physical restraint. **2.** a hospital to which health care providers who are not staff members may send their own patients and supervise their treatment.

hospitalization (hos''pit'l-ĭ-za'shun) **1.** the placing of a patient in a hospital. **2.** the period of confinement in a hospital.

partial h. a psychiatric treatment program for patients who do not need full-time hospitalization, involving a special facility or an arrangement within a hospital setting to which the patient may come for treatment during the day and return home at night (day hospital); or return at night after a day in the community (night hospital); or return for weekends only (weekend hospital).

host (hōst) **1.** an animal or plant that harbors and provides sustenance for another organism (the parasite). **2.** the recipient of an organ or other tissue derived from another organism (the donor).

accidental h. one that accidentally harbors an organism that is not ordinarily parasitic in the particular species.

definitive h., final h. a host in which a parasite attains sexual maturity.

intermediate h. a host in which a parasite passes one or more of its asexual stages; usually designated first and second, if there is more than one.

paratenic h. a potential or substitute intermediate host that serves until the appropriate definitive host is reached, and in which no development of the parasite occurs; it may or may not be necessary to the completion of the parasite's life cycle.

primary h. definitive host.

reservoir h. an animal (or species) that is infected by a parasite, and which serves as a source of infection for humans or another species.

secondary h. intermediate host.

transfer h. one that is used until the appropriate definitive host is reached, but is not necessary to completion of the life cycle of the parasite.

hot 1. characterized by high temperature. 2. radioactive; particularly used to denote the presence of significantly or dangerously high levels of radioactivity.

hot line (hot′ līn″) telephone assistance for those in need of crisis intervention (q.v.), as in suicide prevention, usually available 24 hours a day, seven days a week, and staffed by nonprofessionals with mental health professionals serving as advisors or in a back-up capacity.

hour (our) 1. the time something occurs. 2. a unit of time, being 60 minutes, or 3600 seconds. 3. a unit of educational credit.

contact h. a unit of credit for educational offerings, based on a mathematical formula. Continuing education programs that wish to award contact hours are carefully reviewed by the health care professionals for which the educational experience is designed.

golden h. the first hour following a traumatic injury. See GOLDEN HOUR.

housing (howz′ing) one or more buildings where people live.

congregate h. a living arrangement for healthy older adults in which residents live in their own apartments and may take their meals in a common dining room, with various opportunities for socialization with other residents. Housekeeping and maintenance services are provided, but health maintenance services are scheduled independently by the residents. Called also independent living facilities.

Hp haptoglobin.

HPL, hPL human placental lactogen.

hr hour.

HRF histamine-releasing factor; homologous restriction factor.

HRSA Health Resources and Services Administration, an agency of the United States Department of Health and Human Services.

HSA human serum albumin.

HSV herpes simplex virus.

5-HT serotonin (5-hydroxytryptamine).

ht. height.

HTLV human T-lymphotropic virus.

Hubbard tank (hub′erd) a tank designed for full immersion of the body, used for HYDROTHERAPY. A narrow section at the middle of the tank allows the therapist to reach the patient, and wider sections at each end permit full abduction of the patient's legs and arms. The tank is fitted with an aerator that agitates the water and provides gentle massage and débridement of wounds. An overhead crane facilitates transfer of the patient to and from the tank. The Hubbard tank is especially useful in the treatment of patients with extensive burns and those with chronic multiple joint disorders.

Huhner test (hoon′er) determination of the number and condition of spermatozoa in mucus aspirated from the canal of the cervix uteri within 2 hours after coitus.

hum (hum) a low, steady, prolonged sound.

venous h. a continuous blowing, singing, or humming murmur heard on auscultation over the right jugular vein in the sitting or erect position; it is an innocent sign that is obliterated on assumption of the recumbent position or on exerting pressure over the vein.

human erythrocyte agglutination test an adaptation of the sheep cell agglutination test; human Rh-positive cells coated with incomplete anti-Rh antibody are used instead of the sheep red blood cells sensitized with rabbit gamma globulin. The sera of some patients with rheumatoid arthritis will agglutinate these cells. The agglutination may be inhibited by some normal sera, and not others, and this test is the basis for the determination of the inherited gamma globulin groups (Gm system). Abbreviated HEAT.

Human Genome Project (hu′man je′nōm) an international effort, begun in the late 1980s, for mapping the sequence and analyzing the structure of all the DNA in the human GENOME. It is producing a very large amount of genetic information. Ethics has been a major concern in all aspects of the project, including development, design, and implementation. Ethical use of the information is concerned with the control, diffusion, and use within the context of a free market economy.

humectant (hu-mek′tant) 1. moistening. 2. a moistening or diluent medicine.

humeral (hu′mer-al) of or pertaining to the humerus.

humeroradial (hu″mer-o-ra′de-al) pertaining to the humerus and radius.

humeroscapular (hu″mer-o-skap′u-ler) pertaining to the humerus and scapula.

H

humeroulnar (hu″mer-o-ul′ner) pertaining to the humerus and ulna.

humerus (hu′mer-us), pl. *hu′meri* [L.] the bone of the upper arm, extending from shoulder to elbow, consisting of a shaft and two enlarged extremities. The proximal end has a smooth round head that articulates with the SCAPULA to form the shoulder joint. Just below the head are two rounded processes called the greater and lesser tubercles; the area just below the tubercles is called the "surgical neck," because of its liability to fracture. The distal end of the humerus has two articulating surfaces: the TROCHLEA, which articulates with the ULNA, and the CAPITULUM, which articulates with the RADIUS at the elbow. See accompanying illustration and see Appendices.

humidifier (hu-mid′ĭ-fi″er) an apparatus for controlling humidity by adding moisture to the air.

humidity (hu-mid′ĭ-te) the degree of moisture in the air.

absolute h. the actual amount of vapor in the atmosphere, expressed in milligrams per liter.

relative h. the percentage of moisture in the air as compared to the amount necessary to cause saturation, which is taken as 100.

h. therapy the therapeutic use of water to prevent or correct a moisture deficit in the respiratory tract. Under normal conditions the respiratory tract is kept moist by humidifying mechanisms that allow for evaporation of water from the respiratory mucosa. If these mechanisms fail to work,

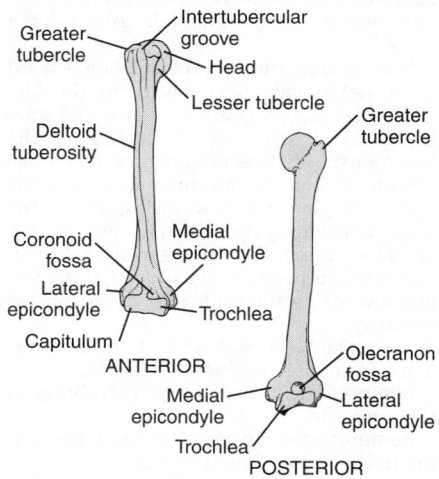

Humerus. From Applegate, 2000.

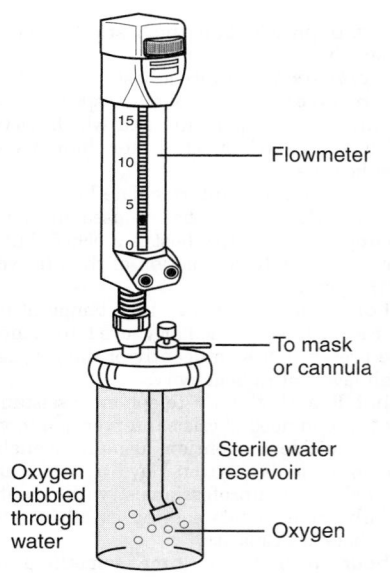

A bubble humidifier. From Lammon et al., 1995.

are bypassed (such as with an ENDOTRACHEAL TUBE), or are inadequate to overcome the drying and irritating effects of therapeutic gases and mucosal crusting, some form of humidification must be provided.

The principal reasons for employing humidity therapy are: (1) to prevent drying and irritation of the respiratory mucosa, (2) to facilitate ventilation and diffusion of oxygen and other therapeutic gases being administered, and (3) to aid in the removal of thick and viscous secretions that obstruct the air passages. Another important use of water aerosol therapy is to aid in obtaining an induced sputum specimen.

Humidity therapy may be delivered in a variety of ways. Humidifiers and vaporizers increase the water content of an environment and are limited to the treatment of upper respiratory disorders because they produce particles that are too large to penetrate deeply into the lungs. Nebulizers generate clouds or mists of particles that are extremely small and thus capable of penetrating more deeply into the bronchioles and small structures of the lower respiratory tract. Examples of these include jet instruments and ultrasonic nebulizers.

humor (hu′mor), pl. *humors, humo′res* [L.] 1. any fluid or semifluid in the body, adj., **hu′moral.** 2. in the NURSING INTERVENTIONS CLASSIFICATION, a nursing INTERVENTION defined as facilitating the patient to perceive, appreciate, and express what is funny, amusing, or ludicrous in order to establish relationships, relieve tension, release anger, facilitate learning, or cope with painful feelings.

aqueous h. the fluid produced in the eye and filling the spaces (anterior CHAMBER and posterior CHAMBER) in front of the LENS and its attachments. It diffuses out of the eye into the blood and is regarded as the lymph of the eye, although its composition is different from that of the lymph in the rest of the body.

ocular h. either of the humors of the eye—aqueous or vitreous.

vitreous h. the fluid portion of the vitreous BODY; often used to designate the entire vitreous body.

hump (hump) a rounded eminence; called also gibbus.

dowager's h. popular name for dorsal KYPHOSIS caused by multiple wedge fractures of the thoracic vertebrae seen in OSTEOPOROSIS.

hunchback (hunch'bak) old term for KYPHOSIS, now considered offensive.

hunger (hung'ger) a craving, as for food.

air h. Kussmaul's respiration.

husk (husk) an outer covering or shell, as of some fruits and seeds.

psyllium h. the cleaned, dried seed coat from the seeds of *Plantago* species; used as a bulk-forming LAXATIVE.

Hunter (hun'ter) John (1728–1793). "Founder of scientific surgery." Born in England, he learned dissection from his brother William and then acquired extensive knowledge of gunshot wounds in the army, of which he was later appointed surgeon-general. Upon retiring from the army, he practiced surgery and lectured on anatomy and surgery. His merit rests with the sound pathologic reasons upon which his surgical procedures were based. Hunter was also the first to study teeth scientifically. In 1783 he was elected a member of the Royal Society of Medicine and of the Royal Academy of Surgery at Paris.

Huntington's chorea (disease) (hunt'ingtunz) a rare hereditary disease characterized by quick involuntary movements, speech disturbances, and mental deterioration due to degenerative changes in the cerebral cortex and basal ganglia; it appears in adulthood, usually between the ages of 30 and 45, and the patient's condition deteriorates over a period of about 15 years to total incapacitation and death. There is not currently any treatment that can cure this disorder, although sedatives and anti-anxiety agents may relieve symptoms in the early stages. As the disease progresses, admission to a psychiatric facility is usually necessary. Called also chronic or hereditary chorea.

Hurler's syndrome (hoor'lerz) the prototypical form of MUCOPOLYSACCHARIDOSIS, with a gargoyle-like face, dwarfism, severe somatic and skeletal changes, severe mental retardation, cloudy corneas, deafness, cardiovascular defects, hepatosplenomegaly, and joint contractures. It is due to a deficiency of the enzyme α-L-iduronidase, and is transmitted as an autosomal recessive trait. Called also gargoylism.

Hürthle cell tumor (hĕrt'lĕ) a new growth of the thyroid gland composed wholly or predominantly of Askanazy CELLS (Hürthle CELLS) having abundant granular, eosinophilic cytoplasm. Such tumors are usually benign (Hürthle cell ADENOMA) but on occasion may be locally invasive or may rarely metastasize (Hürthle cell CARCINOMA).

Hutchinson-Gilford syndrome (huch'in-sun- gil'ford) progeria.

HVL half-value layer.

hyal(o)- word element [Gr.], *glassy.*

hyalin (hi'ah-lin) a translucent albuminoid substance obtainable from the products of amyloid degeneration.

hyaline (hi'ah-lĭn) glassy; pellucid.

h. membrane disease a disorder of newborns, typically preterm, characterized by the formation of a hyalinlike membrane lining the terminal respiratory passages. Newborns with this disease do not secrete adequate quantities of SURFACTANT, which is secreted by the epithelium of the alveoli and normally decreases the surface tension of the fluids lining the alveoli and bronchioles so that air can pass through the fluids and into the alveoli. If the surface tension is not kept low by adequate supplies of surfactant, the alveoli cannot fill with air and there is partial or complete collapse of the lung (ATELECTASIS). Thus the newborn with hyaline membrane disease suffers from respiratory insufficiency with severe DYSPNEA and CYANOSIS. The condition is treated with surfactant instillation, oxygen, and positive pressure. See also RESPIRATORY DISTRESS SYNDROME OF THE NEWBORN.

hyalinization (hi"ah-lin"ĭ-za'shun) conversion into a substance resembling glass.

hyalinosis (hi"ah-lĭ-no'sis) hyaline degeneration.

hyalinuria (hi"ah-lĭ-nu're-ah) hyalin in the urine.

hyalitis (hi"ah-li'tis) inflammation of the vitreous BODY; called also vitreitis and vitritis.

asteroid h. hyalitis marked by spherical or star-shaped bodies in the vitreous; see also BENSON'S DISEASE.

h. puncta′ta a form marked by small opacities.

h. suppurati′va purulent inflammation of the vitreous body.

hyalohyphomycosis (hi″ah-lo-hi″fo-mi-ko′sis) a HYPHOMYCOSIS caused by mycelial fungi with colorless walls; most are opportunistic.

hyaloid (hi′ah-loid) pellucid; like glass.

hyalomere (hi′ah-lo-mēr″) the pale, homogeneous portion of a blood platelet.

Hyalomma (hi″ah-lom′ah) a genus of ticks found on humans and other animals in Africa, Asia, and Europe; they may transmit disease and cause serious injury by their bite.

hyalonyxis (hi″ah-lo-nik′sis) surgical puncture of the vitreous body.

hyaloplasm (hi′ah-lo-plazm″) the more fluid, finely granular substance of the cytoplasm of cells.

hyaloserositis (hi″ah-lo-sēr″o-si′tis) inflammation of serous membranes marked by conversion of the serous exudate into a pearly coating of the affected organ.

hyalosis (hi″ah-lo′sis) degenerative changes in the vitreous humor.

asteroid h. the presence of spherical or star-shaped opacities in the vitreous humor.

hyaluronate (hi″ah-lōo′ro-nāt) a salt, anion, or ester of hyaluronic acid. The sodium salt and a derivative of it are used as analgesics in the treatment of osteoarthritis of the knee, administered by intra-articular injection.

hyaluronic acid (hi″ah-lōo-ron′ik) a glycosamino-glycan found in lubricating proteoglycans of synovial fluid, vitreous humor, cartilage, blood vessels, skin, and the umbilical cord.

hyaluronidase (hi″ah-lu-ron′ĭ-dās) 1. an enzyme that catalyzes the hydrolysis of HYALURONIC ACID, the "cement material" of connective tissues; it is found in human testes, as well as in leeches, snake venom, and spider venom, and is produced by various pathogenic bacteria, enabling them to spread through tissue. 2. a preparation derived from the secretion of mammalian testes, used to promote absorption and diffusion of solutions injected subcutaneously. When it is mixed with fluids administered subcutaneously, absorption is more rapid and less uncomfortable. This is especially valuable when large amounts of fluid must be given by hypodermoclysis instead of intravenously. The hyaluronidase should be dissolved just before it is used and usually is injected with the first portion of the fluid to be given. Hyaluronidase

should not be given in areas where there is infection. Since it hastens absorption, it must be given with caution when administered with toxic drugs, as a toxic reaction can occur rapidly.

hybrid (hi′brid) an offspring of parents of different strains, varieties, or species.

hybridization (hi″brid-ĭ-za′shun) 1. the production of HYBRIDS. 2. molecular hybridization.

fluorescent in situ h. (FISH) a genetic MAPPING technique using fluorescent tags for analysis of chromosomal aberrations and genetic abnormalities. Called also chromosome painting.

molecular h. in molecular biology, formation of a partially or wholly complementary nucleic acid duplex by association of single strands, usually between DNA and RNA strands or previously unassociated DNA strands, but also between RNA strands; used to detect and isolate specific sequences, measure homology, or define other characteristics of one or both strands.

hybridoma (hi″brī-do′mah) a somatic cell hybrid formed by fusion of normal lymphocytes and tumor (lymphoma) cells. B cell hybridomas are the most useful source of monoclonal antibodies; the hybridoma cells are able to produce antibody like the normal parent and to proliferate indefinitely in culture like the parent tumor cells.

hyclate (hi′klāt) USAN contraction for monohydrochloride hemiethanolate hemihydrate.

hydatid (hi′dah-tid) 1. hydatid CYST. 2. any cystlike structure.

h. disease an infection, usually of the liver, caused by larval forms (hydatid cysts) of TAPEWORMS of the genus *Echinococcus,* and characterized by the development of expanding cysts. In the infection caused by *E. granulosus,* single or multiple cysts that are unilocular in character are formed, and in that caused by *E. multilocularis,* the host's tissues are invaded and destroyed as the cysts enlarge by peripheral budding. Called also echinococcosis.

h. of Morgagni a cystlike remnant of the müllerian duct attached to a testis or fallopian tube.

sessile h. the HYDATID OF MORGAGNI connected with a testis.

stalked h. the HYDATID OF MORGAGNI connected with a FALLOPIAN TUBE.

hydatidiform (hi″dah-tid′ĭ-form) resembling a HYDATID; see also hydatidiform MOLE.

hydatidocele (hi″dah-tid′o-sēl) a tumor of the scrotum containing hydatids.

hydatidoma (hi″dah-tĭ-do′mah) a tumor containing hydatids.

hydatidosis (hi″dah-tǐ-do′sis) hydatid disease.

hydatidostomy (hi″dah-tǐ-dos′tah-me) incision and drainage of a hydatid cyst.

hydatiduria (hi″dah-tǐ-du′re-ah) excretion in the urine of material from hydatid CYSTS involving the urinary tract.

Hydergine (hi′der-jēn) trademark for preparations of ERGOLOID MESYLATES, ergot alkaloids used to combat mild to moderate DEMENTIA in the elderly.

hydr(o)- word element [Gr.], *hydrogen; water.*

hydraeroperitoneum (hi-dra″er-o-per″ĭ-to-ne′um) water and gas in the peritoneal cavity.

hydragogue (hi″drah-gog) 1. increasing the fluid content of the feces. 2. a CATHARTIC that causes evacuation of watery feces.

hydralazine (hi-dral′ah-zēn) an ANTIHYPERTENSIVE AGENT and VASODILATOR, administered orally, intramuscularly, or intravenously as the hydrochloride salt in treatment of peripheral vascular disease, essential and early malignant hypertension, thrombophlebitis, and other conditions in which dilation of blood vessels of the extremities is desired. Dosage is adjusted to the individual patient's response. BLOOD PRESSURE should be checked frequently, especially during parenteral administration. Side effects are rare with therapeutic doses, but the drug must be administered with caution to patients with coronary artery disease, advanced kidney damage, and existing or incipient stroke syndrome.

hydramnios (hi-dram′ne-os) excess of AMNIOTIC FLUID; i.e., more than 2000 ml. Amniotic fluid volume should increase gradually, reaching a peak of approximately 1000 ml between 34 and 36 weeks of pregnancy.

hydranencephaly (hi″dran-en-sef′ah-le) absence of the cerebral HEMISPHERES, their normal site being occupied by CEREBROSPINAL FLUID.

hydrargyrum (hi-drahr′jĕ-rum) [L.] mercury (symbol Hg).

hydrarthrosis (hi″drahr-thro′sis) an accumulation of watery fluid in the cavity of a joint. adj., **hydrarthro′dial.**

hydratase (hi′drah-tās) an enzyme that catalyzes the hydration-dehydration of C—O linkages.

hydrate (hi′drāt) 1. a compound of water with a radical. 2. a salt or other compound that contains water of crystallization.

hydration (hi-dra′shun) the absorption of or combination with water.

hydraulics (hi-draw′liks) the science dealing with the mechanics of liquids.

hydrazine (hi′drah-zēn) a gaseous diamine, H_4N_2, or any of its substitution derivatives.

Hydrea (hi-dre′ah) trademark for a preparation of HYDROXYUREA, an antineoplastic AGENT.

hydremia (hi-dre′me-ah) excess of water in the blood, so that it has a low osmolality; see also HYPO-OSMOLALITY.

hydrencephalocele (hi″dren-sef′ah-lo-sēl″) hydroencephalocele.

hydroa (hi-dro′ah) a vesicular or bullous eruption.

h. vaccinifor′me a vesicular and bullous eruption, which may be preceded by pruritus and burning sensation, having a tendency to recur each summer during childhood on sun-exposed areas of the skin.

hydroalcoholic (hi″dro-al″kah-hol′ik) pertaining to or containing both water and alcohol.

hydroappendix (hi″dro-ah-pen′diks) distention of the vermiform appendix with watery fluid.

hydrocalycosis (hi″dro-kal″ĭ-ko′sis) a usually asymptomatic cystic dilatation of a major renal calix, lined by transitional epithelium, and due to obstruction of the infundibulum.

hydrocarbon (hi″dro-kahr′bon) an organic compound that contains carbon and hydrogen only.

alicyclic h. one that has cyclic structure and aliphatic properties.

aliphatic h. one in which no carbon atoms are joined to form a ring.

aromatic h. one that has cyclic structure and a closed conjugated system of double bonds.

chlorinated h. any hydrocarbon compound with chlorine substitutions; many are toxic. They are used mainly as refrigerants, industrial solvents, dry cleaning fluids, and insecticides (such as DDT and DIELDRIN). Some have been used as anesthetics, such as CHLOROFORM.

hydrocele (hi′dro-sēl) a circumscribed collection of fluid; especially, a painless swelling of the scrotum caused by fluid in the TUNICA VAGINALIS TESTIS, the outermost covering of the testes. It can be removed by withdrawing the fluid by tapping through the outer layer of tissue, or by cutting away the outer layer of tissue. The latter operation makes it impossible for the hydrocele to recur. (See accompanying illustration.)

hydrocelectomy (hi″dro-se-lek′to-me) excision of a hydrocele.

hydrocephalocele (hi″dro-sef′ah-lo-sēl″) hydroencephalocele.

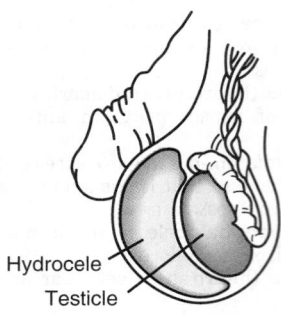

Hydrocele. From Dorland's, 2000.

hydrocephaloid (hi″dro-sef'ah-loid) resembling hydrocephalus.

h. disease a condition resembling hydrocephalus, but with depressed fontanels, following severe diarrhea.

hydrocephalus (hi″dro-sef'ah-lus) a condition caused by enlargement of the cranium caused by abnormal accumulation of CEREBROSPINAL FLUID within the cerebral ventricular system; popularly known as *water on the brain.* Although it occurs occasionally in adults, it is usually associated with a congenital defect, usually a NEURAL TUBE DEFECT. adj., **hydrocephal'ic.**

There are two types of hydrocephalus, distinguished according to whether there is abnormal absorption of the cerebrospinal fluid or an obstruction to its flow. In *communicating hydrocephalus* there is some abnormality in the capacity to absorb fluid from the arachnoid space. There is no obstruction to the flow of fluid between the ventricles. In *noncommunicating hydrocephalus* there is an obstruction at some point in the ventricular system. The cause of noncommunicating hydrocephalus usually is a congenital abnormality, such as stenosis of the aqueduct of Sylvius, congenital atresia of the foramina of the fourth ventricle, or spina bifida cystica. Infections, intraventricular hemorrhage (a frequent problem in premature infants), trauma, and tumors can produce acquired communicating hydrocephalus.

Medical treatment has had only limited success in controlling the secretion of cerebrospinal fluid and relieving hydrocephalus. The most effective treatment is surgical correction employing a shunting technique. The basic components of the shunt are a ventricular catheter, a valve, and a distal catheter. Multiple perforations along the ventricular catheter permit the drainage of fluid from the ventricle. The valve is constructed so that fluid will flow in one direction only, and some valves have a pumping chamber to facilitate drainage. The distal catheter may be positioned at any of a number of sites, the most common being the peritoneal cavity (ventriculoperitoneal shunt) and the right atrium (ventriculoatrial shunt).

Patient Care. The child with hydrocephalus requires frequent and careful changing of position of the head as well as of the body. Pressure sores on the head are a constant threat because of the weight and size of the head and the child's inability to move it. The child should be picked up and held frequently, especially during feeding periods. Care must be taken that the head is well supported while the child is being held. An important aspect of care is preparation of the patient and family for discharge and care at home.

hydrocephaly (hi″dro-sef'ah-le) hydrocephalus.

hydrochloric acid (hi″dro-klor'ik) HCl, a normal constituent of GASTRIC JUICE in humans and other animals. The absence of free hydrochloric acid in the stomach, called ACHLORHYDRIA or gastric anacidity, may be found with chronic GASTRITIS, gastric carcinoma, PERNICIOUS ANEMIA, PELLAGRA, and ALCOHOLISM.

hydrochloride (hi″dro-klor'id) an addition of HYDROCHLORIC ACID with an organic base.

hydrochlorothiazide (hi″dro-klor″o-thi'ah-zīd) a thiazide DIURETIC used as an ANTIHYPERTENSIVE AGENT and for treatment of EDEMA.

hydrocholecystis (hi″dro-ko″le-sis'tis) distention of gallbladder with watery fluid.

hydrocholeresis (hi″dro-ko″lĕ-re'sis) secretion of bile relatively low in specific gravity, viscosity, and total solid content.

hydrocholeretic (hi″dro-ko″ler-et'ik) 1 pertaining to or producing HYDROCHOLERESIS. 2. an agent that so acts.

hydrocodone (hi″dro-ko'dōn) a semisynthetic opioid ANALGESIC similar to but more active than CODEINE; used as the bitartrate salt or polistirex complex as an oral analgesic and antitussive. Continued use may cause addiction.

hydrocolloid (hi″dro-kol'oid) a colloid in which water is the dispersion medium; one type is used in dentistry as an impression material.

hydrocolpos (hi″dro-kol'pos) collection of watery fluid in the vagina.

hydrocortisone (hi″dro-kor'tĭ-sōn) the pharmaceutical term for CORTISOL, the principal GLUCOCORTICOID secreted by the adrenal gland; the base and its salts, including *h. acetate, h. butyrate, h. cypionate, h. pro-butate, h. sodium phosphate, h. sodium succinate,* and *h. valerate,* are used in replacement therapy for adrenocortical insufficiency and as antiinflammatory and immunosuppressant agents in the treatment of a wide variety of disorders.

Hydrocortone (hi″dro-kor′tōn) trademark for preparations of HYDROCORTISONE, a corticosteroid.

hydrocyanic acid (hi″dro-si-an′ik) hydrogen cyanide.

hydrocyst (hi′dro-sist) a cyst with watery contents.

hydrocytosis (hi″dro-si-to′sis) stomatocytosis.

HydroDIURIL (hi″dro-di′u-ril) trademark for a preparation of HYDROCHLOROTHIAZIDE, a DIURETIC and ANTIHYPERTENSIVE AGENT.

hydroencephalocele (hi″dro-en-sef′ah-lo-sēl″) hernial protrusion through a cleft in the skull of brain tissue containing fluid; called also hydrocephalocele and hydrencephalocele.

hydroflumethiazide (hi″dro-floo″mě-thi′-ah-zīd) a thiazide DIURETIC used as an ANTIHYPERTENSIVE AGENT and for treatment of EDEMA.

hydrogel (hi′dro-jel) a gel that contains water.

hydrogen (H) (hi′dro-jen) a chemical element, atomic number 1, atomic weight 1.00797. (See Appendix 6.) It exists as the mass 1 isotope (protium, or light or ordinary hydrogen), mass 2 isotope (deuterium, heavy hydrogen), and mass 3 isotope (tritium).

h. cyanide an extremely poisonous colorless liquid or gas, HCN, a decomposition product of various naturally occurring glycosides and a common cause of cyanide poisoning. Inhalation of the gas can cause death within a minute. Called also hydrocyanic acid.

heavy h. deuterium.

h. ion concentration the degree of concentration of hydrogen ions (the acid element) in a solution. Its symbol is pH, and it expresses the degree to which a solution is acidic or alkaline. The pH range extends from 0 to 14, pH 7 being neutral, a pH of less than 7 indicating acidity, and one above 7 indicating alkalinity. See also ACID-BASE BALANCE.

h. peroxide H_2O_2, an antiseptic with a mildly antibacterial action. A 3 per cent solution foams on touching skin or mucous membrane and appears to have a mechanical cleansing action.

h. sulfide H_2S, a poisonous gas with an offensive smell, released from decaying organic material, natural gas, petroleum, and sulfur deposits, and sometimes used as a chemical reagent.

hydrogenase (hi′dro-jen-ās″) an enzyme that catalyzes the reduction of various substances by combining them with molecular hydrogen.

hydrogenate (hi′dro-jen-āt″) to cause to combine with hydrogen; to reduce with hydrogen.

hydrogymnastics (hi″dro-jim-nas′tiks) therapeutic exercise performed in water.

hydrokinetic (hi″dro-kĭ-net′ik) relating to movement of water or other fluid, as in a whirlpool bath.

hydrokinetics (hi″dro-kĭ-net′iks) the science dealing with fluids in motion.

hydrolase (hi′dro-lās) one of the six main classes of enzymes, comprising those that catalyze the hydrolysis of a compound.

hydro-lyase (hi″dro-li′ās) an enzyme that catalyzes the removal of a hydrogen atom and a hydroxyl group from the substrate molecule as water and the formation of a double bond.

hydrolysate (hi-drol′ĭ-zāt) any compound produced by hydrolysis.

protein h. a mixture of amino acids prepared by splitting a protein with acid, alkali, or enzyme. Such preparations provide the nutritive equivalent of the original material in the form of its constituent amino acids and are used as nutrient and fluid replenishers in special diets or for patients unable to take ordinary food proteins.

hydrolysis (hi-drol′ĭsis), pl. *hydrol′yses* the cleavage of a compound by the addition of water, the hydroxyl group being incorporated in one fragment and the hydrogen atom in the other. adj., **hydrolyt′ic.**

hydroma (hi-dro′mah) hygroma.

hydromeningitis (hi″dro-men″in-ji′tis) meningitis with serous effusion.

hydromeningocele (hi″dro-mě-ning′go-sēl) protrusion of the meninges through a defect in the skull or vertebral column, forming a fluid-containing sac.

hydrometer (hi-drom′ě-ter) an instrument for determining the specific gravity of a fluid.

hydrometra (hi″dro-me′trah) collection of watery fluid in the uterus.

hydrometrocolpos (hi″dro-me″tro-kol′-pos) collection of watery fluid in the uterus and vagina.

hydrometry (hi-drom′ě-tre) measurement of specific gravity with a hydrometer. adj., **hydromet′ric.**

hydromicrocephaly (hi″dro-mi″kro-sef′-ah-le) smallness of the head with an abnormal amount of cerebrospinal fluid.

hydromorphone (hi″dro-mor′fōn) a MORPHINE alkaloid with effects similar to

Supratentorial

Tentorium
Infratentorial

1. Upward
2. Downward

Hydromyelia accompanying an Arnold-Chiari deformity. From Betz et al., 1994.

morphine but greater and of shorter duration; used as the hydrochloride salt as an ANALGESIC, ANTITUSSIVE, and anesthesia adjunct, administered orally, subcutaneously, intramuscularly, intravenously, or rectally.

hydromphalus (hi-drom′fah-lus) a cystic accumulation of watery fluid at the umbilicus.

hydromyelia (hi″dro-mi-e′le-ah) dilatation of the central canal of the spinal cord with an abnormal accumulation of fluid. (See accompanying illustration.)

hydromyelomeningocele (hi″dro-mi″ĕ-lo-mĕ-ning′go-sēl) a defect of the spine marked by protrusion of the membranes and tissue of the spinal cord, forming a fluid-filled sac.

hydromyoma (hi″dro-mi-o′mah) a leiomyoma with cystic degeneration.

hydronephrosis (hi″dro-nĕ-fro′sis) distention of the renal PELVIS and CALICES with urine; if it is allowed to progress, the functioning units of the kidney are destroyed. The collecting tubules dilate and the muscular walls of the pelvis and calices stretch, are replaced by fibrous tissue, and eventually form a large, fluid-filled, functionless sac. adj., **hydronephrot′ic.**

The cause of hydronephrosis is obstruction or atrophy of the urinary TRACT. Mechanical obstruction may result from ureteral tumors, calculi, benign or malignant hyperplasia of the prostate, or carcinoma of the bladder, urethra, or glans penis. Inflammatory obstruction is the outcome of a urinary tract infection that produces edema and narrowing of the ureters or urethra. Rarely there occurs during pregnancy a loss of muscle tone in the urinary tract. The atony is thought to be induced by placental hormones.

Symptoms. The patient usually complains of recurrent attacks of pain in the kidney region. The pain may be described as dull and nagging, or sharp. Examination of the urine often reveals the presence of pus and blood; there is fever if infection develops. If both kidneys are involved, uremia develops as the functional units of the kidneys are destroyed.

Diagnosis is established by extensive urologic examination with detailed PYELOGRAPHY, which usually reveals the cause of the obstruction and accumulation of fluid in the pelvis.

Treatment. The urinary tract must be drained by whatever means necessary; this may involve a simple dilatation of the ureter

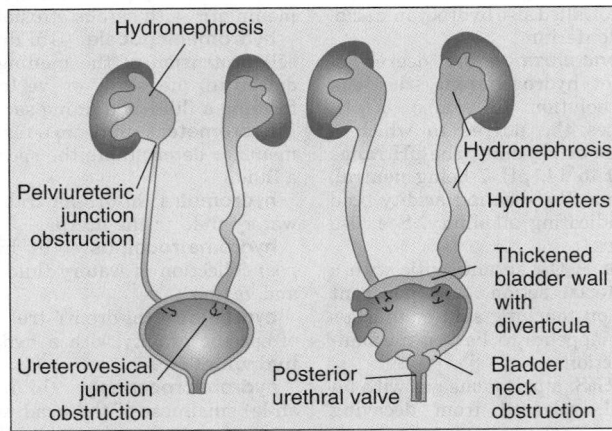

Obstruction to urine flow results in dilation of the urinary tract proximal to the site of obstruction. Obstruction may be at the pelviureteric or vesicoureteric junction (left), the bladder neck or urethra (right). From Lissauer and Young, 2002.

or urethra or it may require surgery of the affected kidney. When URINARY TRACT INFECTION is present as a cause or result of the hydronephrosis, urinary antiseptics and antibiotics are administered until the urine becomes sterile.

hydronium (hi-dro′ne-um) the hydrated proton H_3O^+; it is the form in which the proton (hydrogen ion, H^+) exists in aqueous solution, a combination of H^+ and H_2O.

hydropericarditis (hi″dro-per″ĭ-kahr-di′-tis) pericarditis with watery effusion.

hydropericardium (hi″dro-per″ĭ-kahr′de-um) an abnormal collection of fluid in the pericardial cavity.

hydroperitoneum (hi″dro-per″ĭ-to-ne′um) ASCITES.

hydrophilia (hi″dro-fil′e-ah) the property of absorbing water; having a strong affinity for water.

hydrophilic (hi″dro-fil′ik) readily absorbing moisture; hygroscopic; having strongly polar groups that readily interact with water.

hydrophilous (hi″drof′ĭ-lus) hydrophilic.

hydrophobia (hi″dro-fo′be-ah) 1. irrational fear of water. 2. choking, gagging, and fear on attempts to drink in the acute neurologic phase of rabies, caused by pain from spasms of the pharynx or larynx. 3. former term for RABIES.

hydrophobic (hi″dro-fo′bik) 1. repelling water; insoluble in water; not readily absorbing water. 2. rabid.

hydrophthalmos (hi″drof-thal′mos) 1. a type of glaucoma characterized by enlargement and distention of the fibrous coats of the eyeball. 2. congenital GLAUCOMA.

hydrophthalmus (hi″drof-thal′mus) 1. hydrophthalmos. 2. congenital glaucoma.

hydrophysometra (hi″dro-fi″so-me′trah) collection of fluid and gas in the uterus.

hydropneumatosis (hi″dro-noo″mah-to′-sis) collection of fluid and gas in the tissues.

hydropneumogony (hi″dro-noo-mo′go-ne) injection of air into a joint to detect the presence of effusion.

hydropneumopericardium (hi″dro-noo″-mo-per″ĭ-kahr′de-um) fluid and gas in the pericardium; called also pneumohydropericardium.

hydropneumoperitoneum (hi″dro-noo″-mo-per″ĭ-to-ne′um) fluid and gas in the peritoneal cavity.

hydropneumothorax (hi″dro-noo″mo-thor′aks) a collection of fluid and gas within the pleural cavity; called also pneumohydrothorax.

Hydropres (hi′dro-pres) trademark for a preparation of HYDROCHLOROTHIAZIDE and RESERPINE, an ANTIHYPERTENSIVE AGENT.

hydrops (hi′drops) [L.] old term for EDEMA. adj., **hydrop′ic**.

fetal h., h. feta′lis gross edema of the entire body of the newborn infant, in erythroblastosis fetalis.

hydropyonephrosis (hi″dro-pi″o-nĕ-fro′-sis) urine and pus in the renal pelvis.

hydroquinone (hi″dro-kwin′ōn) a topical agent used to bleach hyperpigmented skin.

hydrorrhea (hi″dro-re′ah) a copious watery discharge.

h. gravida′rum watery discharge from the gravid uterus.

hydrosalpinx (hi″dro-sal′pinks) accumulation of watery fluid in a fallopian tube.

hydroscheocele (hi-dros′ke-o-sēl″) a scrotal hernia containing fluid.

hydrosol (hi′dro-sol) a colloid in which the dispersion medium is a liquid.

hydrostatic (hi″dro-stat′ik) pertaining to a liquid in a state of equilibrium or the pressure exerted by a stationary fluid.

hydrostatics (hi″dro-stat′iks) the science of equilibrium of fluids.

hydrosulfuric acid (hi″dro-sul-fu′rik) hydrogen sulfide.

hydrosyringomyelia (hi″dro-sĭ-ring″go-mi-e′le-ah) syringomyelia.

hydrotaxis (hi″ro-tak′sis) TAXIS of motile organisms or cells in response to the influence of water or moisture.

hydrotherapy (hi″dro-ther′ah-pe) the external use of water in the treatment of disease and injury. adj., **hydrotherapeu′-tic**. Because of its physical properties related to the conduction of heat, buoyancy, and cleansing action, water is an ideal agent for applications of heat and cold to obtain desired physiological effects, débridement of wounds that are extensive and not easily cleansed by other methods, and the implementation of programs of therapeutic EXERCISE.

Applications of moist heat and warm water help relieve pain and improve circulation, promote relaxation and reduce muscle tightness, and serve to localize infections. Examples of hydrotherapeutic measures of this type include warm baths, hot packs, and compresses of toweling, wool, and other cloth materials. Special equipment such as the HUBBARD TANK and whirlpool baths are fitted with devices that mechanically agitate the water, thereby providing gentle massage and a cleansing action in addition to the therapeutic effects of heat.

Applications of cold water include cold packs, ice compresses, cold baths on all or part of the body, and cold showers. The cold water decreases body temperature, reduces swelling and constricts blood vessels, thereby reducing blood flow to the treated part. Brief applications of cold water increase the pulse and respiration rates and produce a rise in blood pressure. Removal from the cold water to a warmer environment induces relaxation and brings about a decrease in the vital signs.

The special properties of buoyancy, cohesion, and viscosity make water a particularly useful medium in which exercises may be carried out. For patients who cannot tolerate weight bearing on the joints, walking exercises underwater are of great value. The buoyant effect of the water in an exercise pool allows for a wider range of motion and permits fuller use of the muscles with less discomfort. This is especially important in exercising painful arthritic joints. The cohesion and viscosity of water account for its resistance to objects moving through it. This resistance can be used to good advantage in the progressive improvement of muscle strength and endurance by exercise. An additional benefit of underwater exercising is its psychological impact on the patient who has impaired mobility. In the water he has a feeling of movement accomplished with relatively more ease than outside the water and thus has a good "body image" of mobility.

Water under pressure may be applied in a spray or jet stream to all or a part of the body for the purpose of providing stimulation and massage, depending on the amount of pressure used. This procedure, called a douche, may also be used to provide a cleansing action to the part being treated.

hydrothermal (hi″dro-ther′mal) pertaining to the temperature effects of water, as in hot baths.

hydrothermic (hi″dro-ther′mik) hydrothermal.

hydrothionemia (hi″dro-thi″o-ne′me-ah) hydrogen sulfide in the blood.

hydrothionuria (hi″dro-thi″o-nu′re-ah) 1. hydrogen sulfide in the urine. 2. the presence of HYDROGEN SULFIDE in the urine after an individual has inhaled this toxic gas.

hydrothorax (hi″dro-thor′aks) a PLEURAL EFFUSION containing serous fluid.

hydrotropism (hi-drot′ro-pizm) TROPISM in response to the presence of water or moisture.

hydrotubation (hi″dro-too-ba′shun) introduction of saline solution into the fallopian tube; saline solution containing dye is used in determining patency of the tube, and saline solution containing hydrocortisone followed by chymotrypsin is used in maintaining patency after salpingostomy.

hydrotympanum (hi″dro-tim′pah-num) a collection of serous fluid in the middle ear.

hydroureter (hi″dro-u-re′ter) distention of the ureter with fluid, due to obstruction.

hydrous (hi′drus) containing water.

hydrovarium (hi″dro-var′e-um) a collection of serous fluid in an ovary.

hydroxide (hi-drok′sīd) the OH⁻ anion or a compound containing the OH⁻ ion.

hydroxocobalamin (hi-drok″so-ko-bal′ah-min) an analogue of CYANOCOBALAMIN (vitamin B_{12}) having exceptionally long-acting hematopoietic activity; used in the treatment of PERNICIOUS ANEMIA and other macrocytic anemias.

hydroxy- a chemical prefix indicating presence of the univalent radical OH.

hydroxyamphetamine (hi-drok″se-am-fet′-ah-mēn) an ADRENERGIC used as a nasal decongestant, pressor, and mydriatic.

hydroxyapatite (hi-drok″se-ap′ah-tīt) an inorganic constituent of bone matrix and teeth, imparting rigidity to these structures.

β-hydroxybutyric acid (hi-drok″sī-bu-tir′-ik) one of the KETONE BODIES that is excreted in diabetic ketoacidosis.

hydroxychloroquine (hi-drok″sī-klor′o-kwin) an ANTIINFLAMMATORY and antiprotozoal AGENT, used as the sulfate salt in treatment of malaria, lupus erythematosus, and rheumatoid arthritis.

25-hydroxycholecalciferol (hi-drok″sī-ko′le-kal-sif′er-ol) a metabolically activated form of CHOLECALCIFEROL (vitamin D_3) synthesized in the liver.

17β-hydroxycorticosterone cortisol.

5-hydroxyindoleacetic acid (hi-drok″se-in″dōl-ah-se′tic) a product of serotonin metabolism excreted in large amounts in patients with carcinoid tumors. Abbreviated 5-HIAA.

hydroxyl (hi-drok′sil) the univalent radical OH.

hydroxylase (hi-drok′sī-lās) any enzyme that brings about the coupled oxidation of two donors, with incorporation of oxygen into one of them.

hydroxylysine (hi-drok″sī-li′sēn) a naturally occurring amino acid.

hydroxyprogesterone (hi-drok″se-pro-jes′ter-ōn) 1. 17α-hydroxyprogesterone; an intermediate formed in the conversion of cholesterol to cortisol, androgens, and estrogens. 2. a synthetic preparation of the caproate ester, used in treatment of dysfunctional uterine BLEEDING and menstrual cycle abnormalities, and in the diagnosis of endogenous estrogen production; administered orally.

hydroxyproline (hi-drok″sī-pro′lēn) an amino acid produced in the digestion of hydrolytic decomposition of proteins, especially of collagens.

hydroxyprolinemia (hi-drok″se-pro″lēn-e′me-ah) an autosomal recessive AMINOACIDOPATHY characterized by an excess of free HYDROXYPROLINE in the plasma and urine, due to a defect in the enzyme hydroxyproline oxidase.

hydroxypropyl cellulose (hi-drok″se-pro′-pil sel′u-lōs) a water-soluble derivative of cellulose, used as an pharmaceutic aid and also applied topically to the conjunctiva to protect and lubricate the cornea in the treatment of dry eye.

hydroxypropyl methylcellulose (hi-drok″-se-pro′pil meth″il-sel′u-lōs) hypromellose.

5-hydroxytryptamine (5-HT) (hi-drok″sĭ-trip′tah-mēn) serotonin.

hydroxyurea (hi-drok″se-u-re′ah) an antineoplastic AGENT that blocks the conversion of ribonucleotides to deoxyribonucleotides, thus stopping DNA synthesis; used in the treatment of melanoma, resistant chronic myelocytic leukemia, and recurrent, metastatic, or inoperable ovarian carcinoma. It is also used in SICKLE CELL DISEASE to reduce the frequency of painful crises and to reduce the need for blood transfusions.

hydroxyzine (hi-drok′sĭ-zēn) a compound chemically related to PIPERAZINE, used as *hydroxyzine hydrochloride* or *hydroxyzine pamoate* as an ANTIANXIETY AGENT and ANTIEMETIC, in urticaria and other manifestations of allergic dermatoses, and as an adjunct to preoperative and postoperative medications. Administered orally or intramuscularly.

hydruria (hi-droo′re-ah) excessive dilution of the urine, so that it has a low osmolality or specific gravity. See also HYPO-OSMOLALITY.

hygiene (hi′jēn) 1. the science of health and its preservation. 2. personal hygiene. adj., **hygien′ic.**

bronchial h. in the OMAHA SYSTEM, activities directed toward maintenance of respiratory or pulmonary function, including inhalation therapy, percussion, and cannula insertion.

dental h. 1. oral hygiene. 2. the profession practiced by a dental HYGIENIST.

mouth h., oral h. the personal maintenance of cleanliness and hygiene of the teeth and oral structures by toothbrushing, tissue stimulation, gum massage, hydrotherapy, and other procedures recommended by the dentist or dental hygienist for the preservation of dental and oral health. Called also dental hygiene. (See table.)

hygienics (hi″jen′iks) a system of principles for promoting health.

hygienist (hi′jen-ist) a specialist in hygiene.

dental h. a dental health specialist whose primary concern is nonsurgical periodontal therapy, maintenance of dental health, and prevention of oral disease. Patient education in proper brushing and interdental cleaning (such as with floss or a water jet) is also a major responsibility of the dental hygienist. In most states the

H

WINDOW ON DENTAL HYGIENE

The dental hygienist is a licensed, professional member of the health care team who integrates the roles of educator, consumer advocate, practitioner, manager, change agent, and researcher to support total health through the promotion of oral health and wellness.

The purpose of dental hygiene is to promote and maintain oral wellness and, thereby, contribute to the quality of life. If the state of an individual's oral health changes, the dental hygienist, within the scope of dental hygiene practice, provides the highest quality of dental care to direct the person back to oral wellness. If oral wellness cannot be achieved, dental hygiene care helps to maximize the degree of oral health. In addition, the dental hygienist assists individuals in seeking other health care services as needed.

Dental hygiene is described as the study of preventive oral health care and the

management of behaviors required to prevent oral disease and promote health. The central concepts in dental hygiene include the client, the environment, health/oral health, dental hygiene actions, their relationship, and the factors that affect them. Dental hygiene involves assessment, diagnosis, planning of interventions, and evaluation, through oral disease prevention, treatment, oral health promotion, and collaboration.

Societal health needs continue to change. The predicted changes in the health care system require the dental hygiene profession to reflect on the way it views itself, its social responsibilities, its role in health care, and its clients. In this age of consumerism, wellness, and self-care, the role of the dental hygienist is assuming more value to the public than ever before.

MICHELE LEONARDI DARBY, BSDH, MS

TAXONOMY OF DENTAL HYGIENE DIAGNOSIS BASED ON THE HUMAN NEEDS CONCEPTUAL MODEL OF DENTAL HYGIENE WITH POSSIBLE ETIOLOGY, DEFINING CHARACTERISTICS, AND CLIENT GOALS			
Human Need Related to Oral Health	Dental Hygiene Diagnosis Based on Human Needs	Related to (Cause/Etiology)	As Evidenced by (Defining Characteristics)	Goal/Expected Behavior
Freedom from pain/stress	Deficit in the need for freedom from pain/stress	Immunosuppression Inadequate self-monitoring Anesthesia, paresthesia Oral surgery, dental procedure, dental hygiene procedure Untreated dental disease Lack of resources	Client-specific indicators: e.g., too much anxiety, fear, inability to experience pain relief, lack of appropriate pain signals, overresponse to painful stimuli	Client-specific
Self-determination and responsibility	Deficit in the need for self-determination and responsibility	Need for parental supervision of oral hygiene Partial self-care deficit Total self-care deficit Educational deficit Skill deficit Lack of motivation Impaired physical, mental ability Role conflicts	Client-specific indicators: e.g., various physical indicators of oral disease, client's health-seeking behavior	Client-specific
Nutrition	Deficit in the need for nutrition	Recent acquisition of implants, appliances Sugar in diet Fluoride deficit Knowledge deficit Lack of resources (time, money) Recent oral or maxillofacial surgery	Client-specific indicators: e.g., physical indicators of oral status; socioethnocultural indicators; lack of knowledge about diet and nutrition	Client-specific
Wholesome body image	Deficit in the need for a wholesome body image	Acquisition of oral prosthesis Visible dental disease or disorder Halitosis Malocclusion Acquisition of orthodontic appliances	Client-specific indicators: e.g., physical indicators of oral disease; client's subjective responses of dissatisfaction with his oral condition	Client-specific

Safety	Deficit in the need for safety	Participation in sports Improper use of oral healthcare product Educational deficit Paresthesia, anesthesia Oral habit Potential for oral infection Potential for oral injury Concern about infection control, radiation safety, fluoride safety, previous negative experience Inadequate oral health behaviors	Client-specific indicators: e.g., Physical indications of oral injury, or potential for oral injury, vital signs, client's subjective expectations that reveals threats to safety	Client-specific
Skin and mucous membrane integrity of the head and neck	Deficit in the need for skin and mucous membrane integrity of the head and neck		Client-specific indicators: e.g., various physical indicators of oral disease	Client-specific
Conceptualization and problem solving	Deficit in the need for conceptualization, problem solving	Educational deficit, lack of knowledge	Client-specific indicators: e.g., client inability to verbalize information about various oral disease processes	Client-specific
Territoriality	Deficit in the need for territoriality	Physical proximity of the healthcare provider as determined by psychosociocultural factors	Client-specific indicators: e.g., client's verbal and nonverbal indicators of discomfort and proximity, position, body mechanisms	Client-specific
Biologically sound dentition	Deficit in the need for a biologically sound dentition	Nutrition and diet Educational and diet Nonadherence Inadequate self-monitoring	Client-specific indicators: e.g., physical indicators of oral disease, defect, or disability; poorly fitting appliances; presence of calculus, plaque, stain, abrasion, attrition	Client-specific
Appreciation and respect	Deficit in the need for appreciation and respect	Lack of acceptance	Client-specific indicators: e.g., client's subjective expressions of dissatisfaction	Client-specific

(continued)

H

TAXONOMY OF DENTAL HYGIENE DIAGNOSIS BASED ON THE HUMAN NEEDS CONCEPTUAL MODEL OF DENTAL HYGIENE WITH POSSIBLE ETIOLOGY, DEFINING CHARACTERISTICS, AND CLIENT GOALS—cont'd

Human Need Related to Oral Health	Dental Hygiene Diagnosis Based on Human Needs	Related to (Cause/Etiology)	As Evidenced by (Defining Characteristics)	Goal/Expected Behavior
Value system	Deficit in the need for a value system regarding oral health	Client's belief system Client's culture Client's life pattern Nonadherence Lack of knowledge or educational deficit Inadequate self-monitoring Health-seeking behaviors of client	Client-specific indicators: e.g., client's verbalization about the importance of oral health, client's lifestyle, client's oral health behaviors	Client-specific

From Darby and Walsh, 1995

dental hygienist must work under the general supervision of a licensed dentist. The minimum education required for dental hygienist licensure is two academic years of college in an accredited dental hygiene program with an associate's degree and a certificate in dental hygiene. Dental hygiene is also offered in bachelor's and master's degree programs. The registered dental hygienist (RDH) must have successfully completed the written and practical examinations required by the state in which he or she wishes to practice.

Dental hygienists may be members of their professional organization, the American Dental Hygienists' Association (ADHA), whose address is 444 N. Michigan Ave., Suite 3400, Chicago, IL 60611.

hygr(o)- word element [Gr.], *moisture.*

hygroma (hi-gro'mah), pl. *hygromas, hygro'mata* an accumulation of fluid in a sac, cyst, or bursa. adj., **hygrom'atous.**

cystic h., h. cys'ticum an endothelium-lined, fluid-containing lesion of lymphatic origin, encountered most often in infants and children and occurring in various regions of the body, most commonly in the posterior triangle of the neck, behind the sternocleidomastoid muscle (hygroma colli cysticum).

Fleischmann's h. enlargement of a bursa in the floor of the mouth, to the outer side of the genioglossus muscle.

hygrometer (hi-grom'ĕ-ter) an instrument for measuring atmospheric moisture.

hygroscopic (hi″gro-skop'ik) readily absorbing moisture.

Hygroton (hi'gro-ton) trademark for a preparation of CHLORTHALIDONE, a diuretic.

hymen (hi'men) the membranous fold partly or completely closing the vaginal orifice. adj., **hy'menal.**

hymenectomy (hi″men-ek'to-me) excision of the hymen.

hymenitis (hi″men-i'tis) inflammation of the hymen.

hymenolepiasis (hi″men-o-lep-i'ah-sis) infection due to tapeworms of the genus *Hymenolepis.*

Hymenolepis (hi″men-ol'ĕ-pis) a genus of TAPEWORMS. *H. diminu'ta, H. lanceola'ta,* and *H. na'na* have been found in humans.

hymenotomy (hi″men-ot'ah-me) incision of the hymen.

hyoepiglottidean (hi″o-ep″ĭ-glŏ-tid'e-an) pertaining to the hyoid bone and epiglottis.

hyoglossal (hi″o-glos'al) pertaining to the hyoid bone and tongue or to the hyoglossal muscle.

hyoid (hi'oid) 1. shaped like a U. 2. pertaining to the hyoid bone; see Appendix 3-3.

hyoscine (hi'o-sēn) scopolamine.

hyoscyamine (hi′o-si′ah-mēn) an ANTICHOLINERGIC and ANTIMUSCARINIC alkaloid from plant species of the genus *Hyoscyamus* and others. It is the levorotatory component of ATROPINE with actions similar to those of atropine but with more potent effects. Used primarily as a gastrointestinal or urinary tract ANTISPASMODIC agent.

hyp(o)- word element [Gr.], *abnormally decreased; deficient; beneath; under.*

hypacusia (hi″pah-ku'ze-ah) slightly diminished acuteness of the sense of hearing.

hypalgesia (hi″pal-je'ze-ah) diminished sensibility to pain. adj., **hypalge'sic.**

hypamnios (hi-pam'ne-os) oligohydramnios.

hypanakinesia (hi″pan-ah-kĭ-ne'zhah) hypokinesia.

hypaxial (hi-pak'se-al) beneath an axis, as the axis of the vertebral column.

hyper- word element [Gr.], *abnormally increased; excessive.*

hyperabsorption (hi″per-ab-sorp'shun) increased intestinal absorption of a substance.

hyperacid (hi″per-as'id) abnormally or excessively acid.

hyperacidity (hi″per-ah-sid'ĭ-te) excessive acidity.

hyperactivity (hi″per-ak-tiv'ĭ-te) 1. abnormally increased muscular activity or function. 2. former name for, and now a principal sign of, ATTENTION-DEFICIT/HYPERACTIVITY DISORDER. adj. **hyperac'tive.**

hyperacusia (hi″per-ah-ku'zhah) hyperacusis.

hyperacusis (hi″per-ah-ku'sis) abnormal acuteness of the sense of hearing.

hyperacute (hi″per-ah-kūt') extremely acute.

hyperadenosis (hy″per-ad″ĕ-no'sis) enlargement of glands.

hyperadiposis (hi″per-ad″ĭ-po'sis) extreme fatness.

hyperadrenalemia (hi″per-ah-dre′nah-le'me-ah) increased amount of adrenal secretion in the blood.

hyperadrenalism (hi″per-ah-dre′nahl-iz-um) overactivity of the adrenal glands.

hyperadrenocorticalism (hi″per-ah-dre″no-kor'tĭ-kahl-iz-um) hypersecretion of hormones by the adrenal cortex; see CUSHING'S SYNDROME. Called also hyperadrenocorticism and hypercorticism.

hyperadrenocorticism (hi″per-ah-dre′no-kor'tĭ-siz-um) hyperadrenocorticalism.

hyperalbuminemia (hi″per-al-bu″mĭ-ne'me-ah) excessive albumin content of the blood.

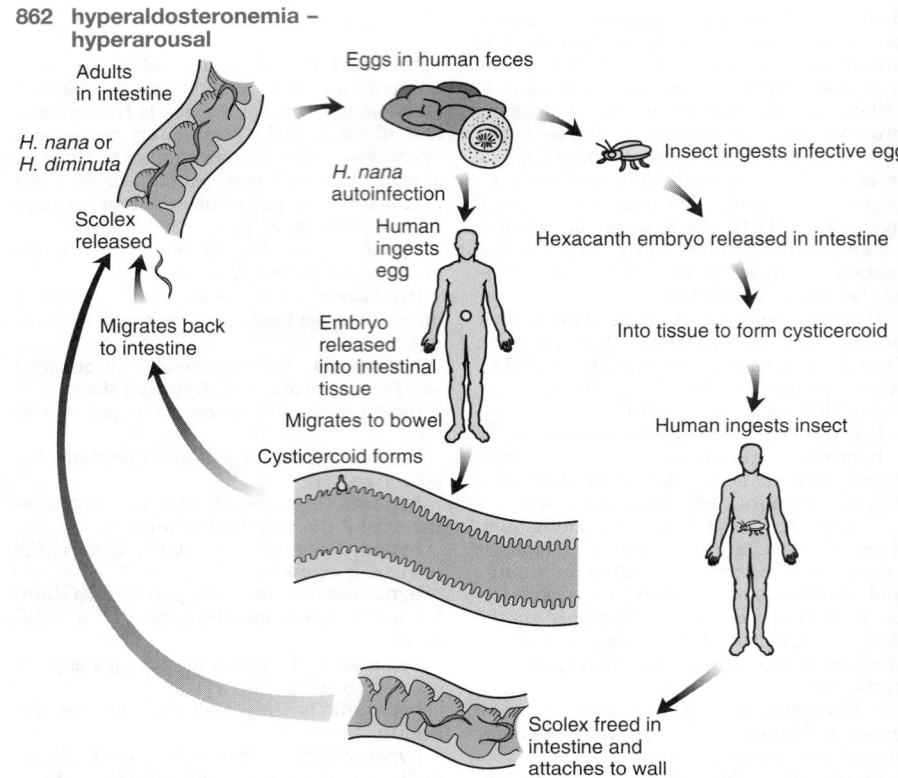

Life cycle of *Hymenolepis nana*. From Mahon and Manuselis, 2000.

hyperaldosteronemia (hi″per-al-dos″ter-o-ne′me-ah) excess of aldosterone in the blood.

hyperaldosteronism (hi″per-al-dos′ter-ōn-izm) aldosteronism.

hyperaldosteronuria (hi″per-al-dos″ter-o-nu′re-ah) excess of aldosterone in the urine.

hyperalgesia (hi″per-al-je′ze-ah) excessive sensitivity to pain. adj., **hyperalge′sic.**

hyperalimentation (hi″per-al″ĭ-men-ta′-shun) PARENTERAL NUTRITION. Although this term is commonly used, it is technically incorrect, since parenteral nutrition does not involve an abnormally increased or excessive amount of feeding.

hyperalkalinity (hi″per-al″kah-lin′ĭ-te) excessive alkalinity.

hyperalphalipoproteinemia (hi″per-al″-fah-lip″o-pro″tēn-e′me-ah) the presence of abnormally high levels of high-density LIPO-PROTEINS (α-lipoproteins) in the serum.

hyperammonemia (hi″per-am″mo-ne′me-ah) elevated levels of AMMONIA or its compounds in the blood. A congenital form occurs in two types: *Type 1,* due to deficiency of the enzyme ornithine carbamoyltransferase, is marked by vomiting, lethargy, coma, and hepatomegaly; symptoms are aggravated by protein ingestion. *Type 2,* due to deficiency of the enzyme carbamoyl phosphate synthetase (ammonia), is marked by vomiting, lethargy, and flaccidity and by elevated plasma and urinary levels of glycine. Hyperammonemia may also occur in nongenetic diseases such as severe liver disease.

hyperammonuria (hi″per-am″o-nu′re-ah) increased excretion of AMMONIA in the urine, as with HYPERAMMONEMIA; called also ammoniuria.

hyperamylasemia (hi″per-am″il-a-se′me-ah) abnormally high levels of amylase in the blood serum.

hyperanakinesia (hi″per-an″ah-kĭ-ne′zhah) excessive motor activity.

hyperaphia (hi″per-a′fe-ah) abnormal acuteness of the sense of touch. adj., **hyperaph′ic.**

hyperarousal (hi″per-ah-row′zal) a state of increased psychological and physiological tension marked by such effects as reduced pain tolerance, anxiety, exaggerated startle responses, insomnia, fatigue, and accentuation of personality traits.

hyperazotemia (hi″per-az″o-te′me-ah) excess of nitrogenous matter in the blood.

hyperazoturia (hi″per-az″o-tu′re-ah) azoturia.

hyperbaric (hi″per-bar′ik) characterized by greater than normal pressure or weight; applied to gases under greater than atmospheric pressure, or to a solution of greater specific gravity than another taken as a standard of reference.

h. oxygenation **(HBO)** exposure to OXYGEN under pressure greater than normal atmospheric pressure. This treatment is given to patients who, for various reasons, need more oxygen than they can take in by breathing in the normal atmosphere or using an oxygen mask. Called also high pressure oxygenation.

The patient is placed in a sealed enclosure called a hyperbaric chamber. Compressed air is introduced to raise the atmospheric pressure to several times normal. At the same time the patient is given pure oxygen through a face mask. The increase in atmospheric pressure forces enough air into the patient so that the pressure within the body equals that in the hyperbaric chamber. Thus all the tissues become flooded with more than the usual supply of oxygen. While the patient is in the chamber, pressure changes are controlled with extreme care to avoid injury to the lungs or other tissues.

Use of Hyperbaric Oxygenation. This treatment may be administered in many types of disorders in which oxygen supply is deficient. If, because of injury or disease, the heart or lungs are unable to maintain good circulation and oxygenation, the increase in oxygen can temporarily compensate for this reduction. If injury or disease has caused the breaking or blocking of arteries, an extra supply of oxygen in the vessels that are still functioning will help.

DECOMPRESSION SICKNESS related to diving is one of the most common uses for hyperbaric oxygen therapy. The effectiveness of this therapy has also been demonstrated for treatment of arterial gas emboli, treatment and prevention of bone damage caused by radiation therapy, and treatment of clostridial MYONECROSIS. It is also sometimes used to promote healing in skin grafts.

CARBON MONOXIDE POISONING can also be treated by hyperbaric oxygenation. Carbon monoxide, displacing the oxygen from hemoglobin, usually causes asphyxiation, but hyperbaric oxygenation can often keep patients alive until the carbon monoxide has been eliminated from the body.

Claims have been advanced about the effectiveness of hyperbaric oxygenation for a wide variety of disorders and diseases, including cancer, neurological disorders, and arthritis. To date, there have been no randomized clinical trials supporting such uses.

hyperbarism (hi″per-bar′izm) a condition due to exposure to ambient gas pressure or atmospheric pressures exceeding the pressure within the body.

hyperbetalipoproteinemia (hi″per-ba″tah-lip″o-pro″-tēn-e′me-ah) increased accumulation of low-density LIPOPROTEINS (β-lipoproteins) in the blood.

hyperbilirubinemia (hi″per-bil″ĭ-roo″bĭ-ne′me-ah) an excess of BILIRUBIN in the blood, occurring as a result of liver or biliary tract dysfunction or with excessive destruction of red blood cells. It is classified as *conjugated* or *unconjugated,* according to the type of bilirubin present. Jaundice is manifested when excess bilirubin is deposited in the skin and mucous membranes.

h. I Gilbert disease.

h. II a chronic idiopathic jaundice, transmitted as an autosomal recessive trait, that affects the excretory function of the liver. The resulting increase in serum conjugated bilirubin is caused by defective transport of conjugated bilirubin into the biliary tract. The condition is generally harmless. Called also Dubin-Johnson syndrome.

conjugated h., Type III a form of conjugated hyperbilirubinemia; probably the result of a primary defect in the storage or hepatic uptake of bilirubin.

h. in the newborn excess serum bilirubin in the newborn due either to overproduction of bilirubin, as in excessive destruction of erythrocytes, or to reduction in glucuronide conjugation in the liver. If a high level of bilirubinemia is left untreated, KERNICTERUS may occur as a result of free unconjugated bilirubin entering the brain tissue and causing neurotoxic damage. The exact level at which kernicterus will occur in individual newborns has not been established. There is evidence that bilirubin levels as low as 6 to 9 mg/dl in very-low-birth-weight and preterm infants puts them at risk for kernicterus and brain damage.

Treatment. The goal of therapy is to reduce serum bilirubin and prevent kernicterus, which virtually disappears when bilirubin levels are controlled. PHOTOTHERAPY is the standard treatment for nonhemolytic hyperbilirubinemia. It may be used prophylactically in newborns at high risk, for example, in preterm, low-birth-weight, and very-low-birth-weight newborns. Exchange TRANSFUSIONS are used for treatment of moderate to severe hemolytic disease, or when excessive bilirubinemia in preterm newborns is not controlled by phototherapy.

Patient Care. Newborns most at risk for hyperbilirubinemia are those who are preterm, who display bruising, or who have blood incompatibilities, an enclosed hemorrhage such as cephalhematoma, polycythemia, an intrauterine infection, congenital red blood cell abnormality, or congenital hypothyroidism or galactosemia.

Observation of the newborn for jaundice is of primary importance, especially those predisposed to hyperbilirubinemia. Yellowing of the skin is first apparent on the face, progressing downward as it increases in severity. The time at which jaundice is first noticed also is significant. Laboratory data can provide information on the levels of direct and indirect serum bilirubin, the hematocrit, variations in red cell morphology, reticulocyte count, Coombs' test and crossmatching of the infant's cells and maternal serum to detect abnormal antibodies when infant and mother are of the same blood type, and special tests for enzyme deficiencies and galactosemia.

Clinical jaundice is investigated when the jaundice appears in the first 12 hours of life and serum bilirubin levels rise at the rate of more than 3 mg per hour. These signs are indicative of hemolytic jaundice, which may require an exchange transfusion. Physiologic jaundice, which is due to immature liver function, rarely becomes apparent before the third day of life or persists beyond the first week and does not exceed 12 mg in term infants.

Other observations include noting any bruising, which causes hemolysis of erythrocytes and release of the bilirubin component, and assessment for cephalhematoma, which has the same effect as bruising because accumulated red blood cells are broken down. Intestinal obstruction also can lead to a buildup of serum bilirubin. The unevacuated stool contains bile which is broken down by intestinal flora into its basic components, thus allowing the release of bilirubin into the blood stream.

Care of the newborn receiving phototherapy includes protection of the skin and eyes from ultraviolet radiation. Care of the newborn receiving an exchange TRANSFUSION is discussed under that topic.

hyperbrachycephalic (hi″per-brak″e-sĕ-fal′ik) having a very short, wide head.

hyperbradykininemia (hi″per-brad″e-ki″-nin-e′me-ah) an excess of BRADYKININ in the blood.

hyperbradykininism (hi″per-brad″e-ki′-nin-izm) a syndrome in which elevated blood levels of BRADYKININ are associated with a fall in systolic blood pressure on standing, increased diastolic pressure and heart rate, and purplish discoloration and ecchymoses of the lower limbs.

hypercalcemia (hi″per-kal-se′me-ah) excess of calcium in the blood; called also calcemia. See CALCIUM, and see table of Electrolyte Imbalances at ELECTROLYTE.

idiopathic h. a condition of infants, associated with vitamin D intoxication, characterized by elevated serum calcium levels, increased skeletal density, mental deterioration, and nephrocalcinosis.

h. of malignancy abnormal elevation of serum calcium associated with malignant tumors, resulting from osteolysis caused by bone metastases or by the action of circulating osteoclast-activating factors released from distant tumor cells (known as *humoral hypercalcemia of malignancy*).

hypercalciuria (hi″per-kal″se-u′re-ah) excess of CALCIUM in the urine, such as in HYPERCALCEMIA or in defective renal tubular reabsorption of calcium.

hypercapnia (hi″per-kap′ne-ah) excess of CARBON DIOXIDE in the blood, indicated by an elevated PaCO₂ as determined by BLOOD GAS ANALYSIS, and resulting in respiratory ACIDOSIS. Called also hypercarbia. adj., **hypercap′nic.**

permissive h. VENTILATION that allows PaCO₂ to rise slowly over time as the pH becomes normalized; the goal is to reduce tidal volume and rate while preventing VOLUTRAUMA; patients may need to be sedated during this.

hypercarbia (hi″per-kahr′be-ah) hypercapnia.

hypercarotenemia (hi″per-kar″ah-tĕ-ne′me-ah) an elevated level of CAROTENE in the blood, resulting from excessive ingestion of CAROTENOIDS or from decreased ability to convert carotenoids to VITAMIN A; it is often characterized by yellowing of the skin (see CAROTENOSIS). Called also carotenemia.

hypercatharsis (hi″per-kah-thahr′sis) excessive purgation.

hypercellularity (hi″per-sel″u-lar′ĭ-te) abnormal increase in the number of cells present, as in bone marrow. adj., **hypercell′-ular.**

hyperchloremia (hi″per-klo-re′me-ah) excess of chlorides in the blood; this occurs as a result of fluid deficit for which the kidney seeks to compensate by reabsorbing large amounts of water and the chloride dissolved in it. The signs and symptoms of hyperchloremia are the same as those of ACIDOSIS. adj., **hyperchlore′mic.**

hyperchlorhydria (hi″per-klor-hi′dre-ah) excess of HYDROCHLORIC ACID in the gastric juice.

hypercholesteremia (hi″per-ko-les″ter-e′me-ah) hypercholesterolemia.

hypercholesterolemia (hi″per-ko-les″ter-ol-e′me-ah) excess of CHOLESTEROL in the blood.

    familial h. hyperlipoproteinemia (type II).

hypercholia (hi″per-ko′le-ah) excessive secretion of bile.

hyperchromatism (hi″per-kro′mah-tizm) 1. excessive pigmentation. 2. degeneration of cell nuclei, which become filled with particles of pigment, or chromatin. 3. increased staining capacity. adj., **hyperchromat′ic.**

hyperchromatosis (hi″per-kro″mah-to′-sis) hyperchromatism.

hyperchromia (hi″per-kro′me-ah) 1. hyperchromatism. 2. abnormal increase in the hemoglobin content of erythrocytes. adj., **hyperchro′mic.**

hyperchylia (hi″per-ki′le-ah) excessive secretion of gastric juice.

hyperchylomicronemia (hi″per-ki″lo-mi″-kro-ne′me-ah) the presence in the blood of an excessive number of particles of fat (chylomicrons).

hypercoagulability (hi″per-ko-ag″u-lah-bil′ĭ-te) abnormally increased coagulability of the blood.

hypercorticism (hi″per-kor′tĭ-sizm) HYPERADRENOCORTICALISM.

hypercryalgesia, hypercryesthesia (hi″-per-kri″al-je′ze-ah, hi″per-kri″es-the′zhah) particularly severe sensitivity to cold.

hypercupriuria (hi″per-ku-pre-u′re-ah) excretion of excessive copper in the urine, as seen in copper poisoning, Wilson's disease, and similar conditions. Called also cupriuria and cupruresis.

hypercyanotic (hi″per-si″ah-not′ik) extremely cyanotic.

hypercythemia (hi″per-si-the′me-ah) polycythemia.

hypercytosis (hi″per-si-to′sis) old term for LEUKOCYTOSIS.

hyperdactyly (hi″per-dak′tĭ-le) polydactyly.

hyperdicrotic (hi″per-di-krot′ik) markedly dicrotic.

hyperdipsia intense THIRST of relatively brief duration.

hyperdistention (hi″per-dis-ten′shun) excessive DISTENTION.

hyperdiuresis (hi″per-di″u-re′sis) excessive DIURESIS (secretion of urine).

hyperdontia (hi″per-don′she-ah) a condition characterized by the presence of supernumerary teeth.

hyperdynamia (hi″per-di-na′me-ah) hyperactivity (def. 1). adj., **hyperdynam′ic.**

hyperemesis (hi″per-em′ĕ-sis) excessive vomiting. adj., **hyperemet′ic.**

    h. gravida′rum excessive and pernicious VOMITING during pregnancy, usually in the first trimester, a more serious condition than the simple MORNING SICKNESS that is common during the first trimester. The exact cause is not known; however, it is thought to be related to trophoblastic activity and production of chorionic GONADOTROPIN and may be aggravated by psychologic factors. It is more common in association with hydatidiform mole and multiple gestation, both of which are associated with elevated levels of chorionic gonadotropin.

Symptoms. The patient complains of uncontrollable nausea, persistent retching and vomiting, inability to take any food by mouth, and exhaustion due to restlessness and lack of sleep. As the condition persists the patient becomes severely dehydrated, develops a fever, and may show signs of peripheral nerve involvement and jaundice. The urine may contain blood, bile, albumin, and ketone bodies as starvation develops. Although hyperemesis gravidarum is rarely fatal, these latter symptoms indicate a grave illness that demands prompt treatment.

Treatment. The physical symptoms of the patient are relieved by intravenous administration of fluids and nutrients and mild sedation to promote rest and relaxation. There is some controversy as to the value of psychotherapy; however, it is generally agreed that the patient will need help in overcoming emotional problems and situational tension if they contribute to the occurrence of the disorder. Dietary treatment may include limiting the intake of liquids, eating a snack of crackers or dry toast before arising, and avoiding excessive fat in the diet.

Patient Care. The hospitalized patient should be placed in a quiet, well-ventilated room that is free from odors or sights that may cause nausea. Fluid intake and output are monitored and mouth care is given frequently. Food and liquids are resumed on a prescribed schedule that gradually progresses to a regular diet. The patient should be encouraged to talk about her feelings if she indicates a desire to do so. The caregivers should be alert to signs of depression or fears of pregnancy, labor, or the responsibilities of motherhood. Recovery is much more likely if the patient is able to vocalize her fears and seek aid in solving any situational or emotional conflicts that may contribute to her illness. Those who care for her should be sympathetic, optimistic, and reassuring in discussing her condition with her.

h. lacten′tium vomiting by nursing babies.

hyperemia (hi″per-e′me-ah) an excess of blood in a part; called also engorgement. adj., **hypere′mic.**

active h., arterial h. that due to local or general relaxation of arterioles.

leptomeningeal h. congestion of the pia-arachnoid.

passive h. that due to obstruction of flow of blood from the area.

reactive h. that due to increase in blood flow after its temporary interruption.

venous h. passive hyperemia.

hyperencephalus (hi″per-en-sef′ah-lus) acranius.

hyperendemic (hi″per-en-dem′ik) equally endemic, at a high level, in all age groups of a population; see also HOLOENDEMIC.

hypereosinophilia (hi″per-e″o-sin″o-fil′e-ah) extreme EOSINOPHILIA. adj., **hypereosinophil′ic.**

hypereosinophilic syndrome (hi″per-e″o-sin″o-fil′ik) any of several diseases characterized a massive increase in the number of EOSINOPHILS in the blood and bone marrow, with eosinophilic infiltration of other organs. Symptoms vary, depending on the organ involved, and may include pruritic skin ulcers or erythroderma, endomyocarditis, lymph node or spleen enlargement, and ophthalmologic or gastrointestinal complications. EOSINOPHILIC LEUKEMIA is a potentially fatal member of the group.

hyperepinephrinemia (hi″per-ep″ĭ-nef′rĭ-ne′me-ah) excessive epinephrine in the blood.

hyperequilibrium (hi″per-e″kwĭ-lib′re-um) excessive tendency to vertigo.

hypererethism (hi″per-er′ĕ-thizm) extreme irritability.

hypererythrocythemia (hi″per-ĕ-rith″ro-si-the′me-ah) polycythemia.

hyperesophoria (hi″per-es″o-for′e-ah) deviation of the visual axes upward and inward.

hyperesthesia (hi″per-es-the′zhah) a state of abnormally increased sensitivity to stimuli. adj., **hyperesthet′ic.**

hyperexophoria (hi″per-ek″so-for′e-ah) deviation of the visual axes upward and outward.

hyperextension (hi″per-ek-sten′shun) extension of a limb or part beyond the normal limit.

hyperferremia (hi″per-fĕ-re′me-ah) excess of iron in the blood; called also siderosis. adj., **hyperferre′mic.**

hyperfibrinogenemia (hi″per-fi-brin″o-jĕ-ne′me-ah) excessive fibrinogen in the blood; fibrinogenemia.

hyperfiltration (hi″per-fil-tra′shun) an elevation in the filtration rate of the renal glomeruli, often a sign of early insulin-dependent diabetes mellitus.

hyperflexion (hi″per-flek′shun) flexion of a limb or part beyond the normal limit.

hyperfunction (hi″per-fungk′shun) excessive functioning of a part or organ.

hypergalactia, hypergalactosis (hi″per-gah-lak′she-ah, hi″per-gal″ak-to′sis) excessive secretion of milk.

hypergammaglobulinemia (hi″per-gam″-ah-glob″u-lin-e′me-ah) increased gamma globulins in the blood. adj., **hypergammaglobuline′mic.**

monoclonal h′s an excess of homogeneous immunoglobulin molecules of a single specificity in the blood following proliferation of a clone of immunoglobulin-producing cells.

hypergastrinemia (hi″per-gas″trin-e′me-ah) an excess of gastrin in the blood.

hypergenesis (hi″per-jen′ĕ-sis) excessive development.

hypergenitalism (hi″per-jen′ĭ-tal-izm) HYPERGONADISM.

hypergeusesthesia, hypergeusia (hi″per-gōōs″es-the′zhah, hi″per-goo′zhah) increased sensitivity of taste.

hyperglandular (hi″per-glan′du-ler) marked by excessive glandular activity.

hyperglobulia (hi″per-glo-bu′le-ah) excess of erythrocytes; erythrocytosis; polycythemia.

hyperglobulinemia (hi″per-glob″u-line′-me-ah) excess of globulin in the blood.

hyperglucagonemia (hi″per-gloo″kah-gon-e′me-ah) abnormally high levels of glucagon in the blood.

hyperglycemia (hi″per-gli-se′me-ah) excess of glucose in the blood; see also DIABETES MELLITUS.

hyperglycemic (hi″per-gli-se′mik) 1. characterized by or causing hyperglycemia. 2. an agent that has this effect.

h. hyperosmolar nonketotic (HHNK) coma a metabolic derangement in which there is an abnormally high serum GLUCOSE level without KETOACIDOSIS. It can occur as a complication of borderline and unrecognized DIABETES MELLITUS, in pancreatic disorders that interfere with the production of INSULIN, as a complication of extensive burns, and in conditions marked by an excess of steroids, as in steroid therapy, or acute stress conditions, such as infection. It also may develop during total PARENTERAL NUTRITION, HEMODIALYSIS, or PERITONEAL DIALYSIS. Called also hyperosmolar nonketotic coma.

Symptoms. The hyperglycemia of HHNK coma is usually extreme, with fasting blood sugar levels ranging from 600 to 3000 mg per 100 ml of blood. In contrast to typical diabetic coma, however, the serum acetone level is normal or only slightly elevated. This occurs because, although there is sufficient insulin available to avoid ketosis, there is not enough to metabolize the glucose and thereby relieve the hyperglycemia.

Hyperosmolality, resulting from the extremely high concentration of sugar in the blood, causes a shift of water from the intracellular fluid (the less concentrated solution) into the blood (the higher concentrated solution). This results in cellular dehydration. Another symptom of HHNK coma, polyuria, occurs because the high plasma osmolality prevents the normal osmotic return of water to the blood by the renal tubules, and it is excreted in the urine. This leads to a decreased blood volume, which severely hampers the kidney's excretion of glucose and a vicious cycle is begun.

Treatment. It is essential that HHNK coma be recognized early and treatment begun immediately to break the chain of metabolic aberrations that are occurring. It is estimated that the mortality rate of HHNK coma is 60 to 70 per cent; the probable reason for this is failure to recognize the condition and institute prompt corrective measures.

Insulin is administered in small doses, the amount and frequency depending on periodic assessment of blood glucose levels. The objective is to avoid the extremes of hyperglycemia and insulin shock. Intravenous fluids are administered cautiously, so that the sodium and water deficits can be corrected without producing extreme shifts of water from the blood into the intracellular compartment and thus failing to correct the hyperosmolar condition of the blood. Electrolytes other than the sodium lost through diuresis also must be replaced as indicated by laboratory findings.

Patient Care. Fluid volume deficit plays a major role in the development of severe HHNK coma; thus patient care is concerned with careful monitoring of those patients susceptible to its development, especially the elderly, the debilitated, and the mild or unsuspected diabetic. Maintenance of an adequate fluid balance can do much to prevent the hyperosmolar condition and the development of a chain of

events that can rapidly lead to coma and death.

hyperglyceridemia (hi″per-glis″er-ĭ-de′-me-ah) excess of glycerides in the blood.

hyperglycinemia (hi″per-gli″sĭ-ne′me-ah) a hereditary AMINOACIDOPATHY involving excessive GLYCINE in the blood and urine. One form is characterized by episodic vomiting, lethargy, dehydration, ketosis, and increased susceptibility to infection; a second form by generalized hypotonia, lethargy, absence of reflexes, and periodic myoclonic jerks. Called also glycinemia.

hyperglycinuria (hi″per-gli″sin-u′re-ah) an AMINOACIDURIA consisting of excessive GLYCINE in the urine; see HYPERGLYCINEMIA.

hyperglycogenolysis (hi″per-gli″ko-jĕ-nol′ĭ-sis) excessive splitting up of glycogen (glycogenolysis).

hyperglycorrhachia (hi″per-gli″ko-ra′ke-ah) excessive sugar in the cerebrospinal fluid.

hyperglycosuria (hi″per-gli″ko-su′re-ah) extreme GLYCOSURIA.

hypergnosis (hi″per-no′sis) an exaggerated perception, for example, expansion of an isolated idea into a complex philosophical system; seen in paranoia.

hypergonadism (hi″per-go′nad-izm) abnormally increased functional activity of the gonads, with excessive growth and precocious sexual development.

hypergonadotropic (hi″per-gon″ah-do-trop′ik) relating to or caused by excessive amounts of gonadotropins.

hyperhemoglobinemia (hi″per-he″mo-glo″bĭ-ne′me-ah) an excess of hemoglobin in the blood.

hyperhidrosis (hi″per-hi-dro′sis) excessive SWEATING. adj., **hyperhidrot′ic.**

emotional h. an autosomal dominant disorder of the eccrine sweat glands, most often of the palms, soles, and axillae, in which emotional stimuli (e.g., anxiety) and sometimes mental or sensory stimuli elicit volar or axillary sweating (usually not both in the same individual); eccrine sweat glands in other areas of the body are affected less often and are less sensitive to such stimuli.

hyperhydration (hi″per-hi-dra′shun) a state of excess fluids in the body; called also overhydration.

hyperidrosis (hi″per-i-dro′sis) hyperhidrosis.

hyperimmune (hi″per-im-mūn′) possessing very large quantities of specific antibodies in the serum.

hyperimmunoglobulinemia (hi″per-im″u-no-glob″u-lin-e′me-ah) abnormally high levels of immunoglobulins in the serum.

hyperinflation (hi″per-in-fla′shun) excessive inflation or expansion, as of the lungs; overinflation.

hyperinsulinism (hi″per-in′su-lin-izm″) 1. excessive secretion of insulin by the pancreas, resulting in hypoglycemia. 2. insulin shock from overdosage of insulin.

hyperinvolution (hi″per-in″vo-lu′shun) superinvolution.

hyperirritability (hi″per-ir″ĭ-tah-bil′ĭ-te) pathological responsiveness to slight stimuli.

hyperisotonic (hi″per-i″so-ton′ik) denoting a solution containing more than 0.45 per cent salt, in which exosmosis causes abnormal notching around the edges of erythrocytes (CRENATION).

hyperkalemia (hi″per-kah-le′me-ah) abnormally high POTASSIUM concentration in the blood, most often due to defective renal excretion, as in kidney disease, severe and extensive burns, intestinal obstruction, or ADDISON'S DISEASE. See table of Electrolyte Imbalances at ELECTROLYTE. adj., **hyperkale′mic.**

Potassium levels greater than 7 mEq per liter can produce electrocardiographic abnormalities, which are first evident as peaked T waves and depressed P waves; later there are widened QRS waves; and eventually there will be ASYSTOLE. Other signs and symptoms include muscular weakness, tingling of the hands, feet, and tongue, and a slow irregular pulse. As the amount of serum potassium continues to rise to above 8 mEq per liter, there is potential for respiratory paralysis, asystole or ventricular FIBRILLATION, and CARDIAC ARREST. Treatment consists of removing the excess potassium from the body with DIALYSIS, or giving intravenous sodium bicarbonate, calcium, or hypertonic glucose and insulin to shift potassium into the cells. Cation exchange resins may also be given orally or by enema to remove potassium.

hyperkeratinization (hi″per-ker″ah-tin-ĭ-za′shun) excessive development of KERATIN in the epidermis, usually on the palms of the hands or soles of the feet.

hyperkeratosis (hi″per-ker″ah-to′sis) 1. hypertrophy of the horny layer of the skin, or any disease characterized by it. 2. hypertrophy of the cornea. adj., **hyperkeratot′ic.**

epidermolytic h. a hereditary autosomal dominant form of ICHTHYOSIS, present at birth. Characteristics include generalized redness of the skin and severe hyperkeratosis with small, hard wartlike scales over the entire body, accentuated in areas that flex or bend and sometimes involving the palms and soles. In infancy and childhood, there are recurrent bullae, most often on the lower limbs.

follicular h. a skin condition characterized by excessive development of keratin in hair follicles, resulting in rough, cone-shaped, elevated papules, the openings of which are often closed with a white plug of encrusted sebum. Deficiencies of vitamins A and E, B complex vitamins, and essential fatty acids have all been implicated in the etiology. Called also phrynoderma.

h. lenticula′ris per′stans an autosomal dominant skin disorder, usually occurring in the third or fourth decade of life, characterized by pink, red, or yellow to brown scaly papules on the lower leg and back of the foot, and sometimes on the trunk, thigh, arm, back and palm of the hand, or sole of the foot.

hyperketonemia (hi″per-ke″to-ne′me-ah) abnormally increased concentration of ketone bodies in the blood.

hyperketonuria (hi″per-ke″to-nu′re-ah) ketonuria.

hyperketosis (hi″per-ke-to′sis) excessive formation of ketone.

hyperkinemia (hi″per-ki-ne′me-ah) abnormally high cardiac output.

hyperkinesia (hi″per-kĭ-ne′zhah) hyperactivity.

hyperkinesis (hi″per-kĭ-ne′sis) hyperactivity.

hyperkinetic (hi″per-kĭ-net′ik) pertaining to or marked by hyperactivity (hyperkinesis).

h. syndrome former name for ATTENTION-DEFICIT/HYPERACTIVITY DISORDER.

hyperlactation (hi″per-lak-ta′shun) LACTATION in greater than normal amount or for a longer than normal period; see also GALACTORRHEA. Called also superlactation.

hyperleukocytosis (hi″per-loo″ko-si-to′sis) extreme LEUKOCYTOSIS, as seen in certain forms of leukemia.

hyperlipemia (hi″per-lĭ-pe′me-ah) hyperlipidemia.

carbohydrate-induced h. hyperlipoproteinemia (type IV).

fat-induced h. hyperlipoproteinemia (type I).

hyperlipidemia (hi″per-lip″i-de′me-ah) elevated concentrations of any or all of the lipids in the blood. Called also hyperlipemia and lipemia.

hyperlipoproteinemia (hi″per-lip″o-pro″tēn-e′me-ah) an excess of LIPOPROTEINS in the blood, due to a disorder of lipoprotein metabolism; it may be acquired or hereditary. The *acquired* form occurs secondary to another disorder or as a result of environmental factors such as diet. The *hereditary* form is classified into five major phenotypes based on clinical features, enzymatic abnormalities, and serum lipoprotein electrophoretic patterns: *Type I* may be manifested clinically by repeated bouts of abdominal pain and vomiting, recurrent acute pancreatitis, eruptive xanthomas, hepatosplenomegaly, and lipemia retinalis. *Type II* (called also familial hypercholesterolemia) is an autosomal dominant condition characterized by tendinous and tuberous XANTHOMAS, XANTHELASMAS, early onset of corneal arcus, and accelerated atherosclerosis; children homozygous for the defect may have coronary artery disease and MYOCARDIAL INFARCTIONS in childhood. *Type III* is characterized chiefly by planar XANTHOMAS and is related to familial DYSBETALIPOPROTEINEMIA. *Type IV* is marked by mild HYPERTRIGLYCERIDEMIA and is related to TANGIER DISEASE and is marked by increased incidence of vascular disease, abnormal glucose tolerance, and family history of DIABETES MELLITUS. *Type V* is characterized by severe HYPERTRIGLYCERIDEMIA and may include diabetes mellitus, eruptive xanthomas, and recurrent acute PANCREATITIS.

hyperliposis (hi″per-lĭ-po′sis) excess of fat in the blood (HYPERLIPIDEMIA) or tissues.

hyperlysinemia (hi″per-li″sēn-e′me-ah) a congenital type of AMINOACIDOPATHY characterized by elevated levels of lysine in the blood, and marked by vomiting, spasticity, coma, and mental retardation; symptoms are related to protein intake.

hypermagnesemia (hi″per-mag″nĕ-se′me-ah) an abnormally high MAGNESIUM content of the blood plasma. See table of Electrolyte Imbalances at ELECTROLYTE.

hypermastia (hi″per-mas′te-ah) 1. polymastia. 2. macromastia.

hypermenorrhea (hi″per-men″o-re′ah) excessive MENSTRUATION; causes include uterine tumors, pelvic inflammatory disease, abnormal conditions of pregnancy, and endocrine disturbances. It may cause anemia. Called also menorrhagia.

hypermetabolism (hi″per-mĕ-tab′o-lizm) increased metabolism.

   extrathyroidal m. abnormally elevated basal metabolism unassociated with thyroid disease.

hypermetria (hi″per-me′tre-ah) ataxia in which movements overreach the intended goal.

hypermetrope (hi″per-met′rōp) hyperope.

hypermetropia (hi″per-mĕ-tro′pe-ah) farsightedness; hyperopia.

hypermnesia (hi″perm-ne′zhah) extreme retentiveness or unusual clarity of memory. adj. **hypermnes′ic.**

hypermorph (hi′per-morf) in genetics, a hypermorphic mutant gene, i.e., one exaggerating or increasing normal activity. adj., **hypermor′phic.**

hypermotility (hi″per-mo-til′ĭ-te) excessive or abnormally increased motility, as of the gastrointestinal tract.

hypermyotonia (hi″per-mi″o-to′ne-ah) excessive muscular tonicity.

hypermyotrophy (hi″per-mi-ot′ro-fe) excessive development of muscular tissue.

hypernasality (hi″per-na-zal′ĭ-te) a quality of voice in which the emission of air through the nose is excessive due to velopharyngeal INSUFFICIENCY, so that the voice is high-pitched and speech intelligibility deteriorates. Called also rhinolalia aperta.

hypernatremia (hi″per-na-tre′me-ah) an excess of SODIUM in the blood, indicative of water loss exceeding the sodium loss. See table of Electrolyte Imbalances at ELECTROLYTE. adj., **hypernatre′mic.**

hyperneocytosis (hi″per-ne″o-si-to′sis) HYPERLEUKOCYTOSIS with an excessive number of immature forms of leukocytes.

hypernephroma (hi″per-nĕ-fro′mah) renal cell carcinoma.

hypernutrition (hi″per-nu-trish′un) overfeeding and its ill effects.

hyperonychia (hi″per-o-nik′e-ah) hypertrophy of the nails.

hyperope (hi′per-ōp) a person with hyperopia.

hyperopia (hi″per-o′pe-ah) a defect of VISION in which parallel light rays reaching the eye come to focus behind the retina, vision being better for distant objects than for near. Called also farsightedness.

Most children are born with some degree of farsightedness. As the child grows this decreases and usually disappears by the age of 8 years. If the child is excessively farsighted, however, the constant effort to focus may cause headaches and fatigue. Eyeglasses used to correct hyperopia are convex; that is, they bend the light rays toward the center, helping the lens of the eye to focus them on the retina.

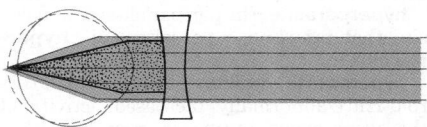

Refraction and correction in hyperopia. From Ignatavicius and Workman, 2002.

hyperorchidism (hi″per-or′kĭ-dizm) abnormally increased secretion by the testes.

hyperorexia (hi″per-o-rek′se-ah) excessive appetite.

hyperorthocytosis (hi″per-or″tho-si-to′sis) hyperleukocytosis with normal proportions of the various forms of leukocytes.

hyperosmia (hi″per-oz′me-ah) increased sensitivity of smell.

hyperosmolality (hi″per-oz″mo-lal′ĭ-te) an increase in the osmolality of the body fluids.

hyperosmolarity (hi″per-oz″mo-lar′ĭ-te) abnormally increased osmotic concentration of a solution.

hyperostosis (hi″per-os-to′sis) excessive growth of bony tissue. adj., **hyperostot′ic.**

frontal internal h., h. fronta′lis inter′na a new formation of bone tissue protruding in patches on the internal surface of the cranial bones in the frontal region, most commonly affecting women near menopause.

generalized cortical h. a hereditary disorder beginning during puberty, marked by osteosclerosis of the skull, mandible, clavicles, ribs, and diaphyses of long bones, associated with elevated blood alkaline phosphatase.

infantile cortical h. a syndrome seen in infants under six months of age, marked by fever, arthralgias, and swelling and cortical thickening of facial, trunk, and long bones. Called also Caffey's disease.

hyperoxaluria (hi″per-ok″sah-lu′re-ah) an excess of OXALATES in the urine, which can lead to formation of KIDNEY STONES. Called also oxaluria.

enteric h. formation of calcium oxalate CALCULI in the urinary tract, occurring after extensive resection or disease of the ileum, due to excessive absorption of oxalate from the colon.

primary h. an autosomal recessive disorder characterized by urinary excretion of oxalate, with nephrolithiasis, nephrocalcinosis, early onset of renal failure, and often a generalized deposit of calcium oxalate.

hyperoxemia (hi″per-ok-se′me-ah) excessive acidity of the blood.

hyperoxia (hi″per-ok′se-ah) an abnormally increased supply or concentration of oxygen.

hyperparasite (hi″per-par′ah-sīt) a parasite that preys on a parasite. adj., **hyperparasit′ic.**

hyperparathyroidism (hi″per-par″ah-thi′-roid-izm) abnormally increased activity of the PARATHYROID GLAND; it may be either primary or secondary. *Primary* hyperparathyroidism is associated with either neoplasia (chiefly adenomas) or hyperplasia; adenomas of the parathyroids account for about 85 per cent of all cases. Since hyperparathyroidism is a common cause of increased calcium levels, HYPERCALCEMIA discovered during routine serum chemistry profiles often leads to diagnosis of the condition.

An excess of parathyroid HORMONE leads to alteration in the function of cells of bone, renal tubules, and gastrointestinal mucosa. It may result in KIDNEY STONES and calcium deposits in the renal tubules; in generalized decalcification of bone (OSTEOMALACIA), resulting in pain and tenderness of bones and spontaneous fractures, and in HYPERCALCEMIA that could lead to muscular weakness and gastrointestinal symptoms such as anorexia, nausea, vomiting, and abdominal pains.

Secondary hyperparathyroidism develops as a compensatory mechanism when the serum calcium level is persistently below normal, as in chronic renal disease, VITAMIN D deficiency, or intestinal malabsorption syndromes, all of which can cause insufficient absorption of calcium and vitamin D.

The National Institutes of Health (NIH) Consensus Development Conference on Diagnosis and Management of Asymptomatic Primary Hyperparathyroidism addressed the diagnosis and management of the condition. Symptoms can be vague, and are most often related to elevated calcium levels; determinations of calcium and parathyroid hormone levels are required. The use of thiazide DIURETICS or LITHIUM can elevate levels of both parathyroid hormone and calcium, so that the levels should be evaluated after discontinuation of these medications before a diagnosis is made. Imaging studies may be helpful in diagnosis of a parathyroid adenoma or determination of its location.

Candidates for medical management of hyperparathyroidism can have a mildly elevated serum calcium level. There should be no history of life-threatening hypercalcemia, and renal and bone status should be normal. The patient should be monitored frequently for alterations in blood pressure, serum calcium and creatinine levels, creatinine CLEARANCE, urinary calcium, and bone density. Dehydration and immobilization should be avoided and diuretics should be used with caution. Dietary calcium should be neither liberalized nor restricted. Treatment of HYPERTENSION and replacement of ESTROGEN in post-menopausal women are also recommended.

Surgical treatment is indicated when parathyroid-related symptoms involve the skeletal, renal, or gastrointestinal systems.

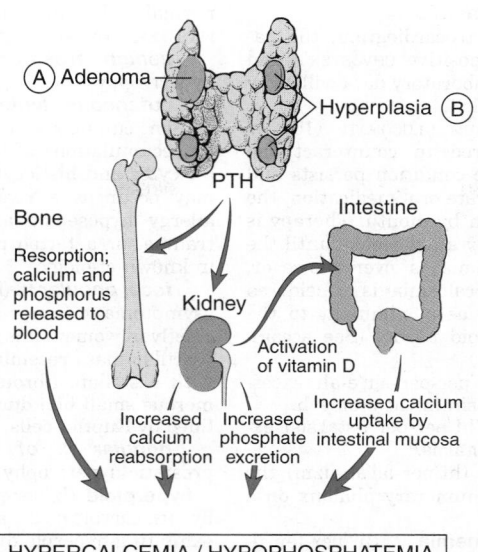

Metabolic consequences of hyperparathyroidism. PTH, parathyroid hormone. From Damjanov, 2000.

Other indications include markedly elevated serum calcium level (1 to 1.6 mg per dL [0.25 to 0.40 mmol per L] above accepted normal range); history of an episode of life-threatening hypercalcemia; reduced creatinine clearance (30% less than that expected); presence of kidney stones on radiograph with markedly elevated urinary calcium excretion (greater than 400 mg per 24 hours [10 mmol per day]); substantially reduced bone mass as determined by direct measurement (more than 2 standard deviations below that expected); significant neuromuscular or psychological symptoms without other obvious cause; request by the patient for surgery; anticipation of problems with follow-up; and coexistent illnesses that complicate management. The usual procedure is a subtotal PARATHYROIDECTOMY that leaves some parathyroid tissue to continue normal endocrine function.

Patient Care. Postoperative care includes careful monitoring of the patient for complications of hemorrhage, infection, HYPOPARATHYROIDISM and HYPOCALCEMIA, and damage to the laryngeal nerve.

When the patient returns from surgery, the operative site is assessed carefully. The side and back of the neck, as well as the anterior dressing, should be observed for any bleeding. The amount and other characteristics of drainage are noted and recorded, vital signs are monitored closely,

and the patient is observed for signs of respiratory difficulty. Accumulations of subcutaneous fluid must be watched carefully as they can contribute to infection and tissue necrosis. Unless otherwise indicated, the patient is placed in the semi-Fowler POSITION postoperatively. The rationale for this is that it makes breathing easier, promotes drainage from the operative site, and decreases pressure on the skin and suture line. At the time dressings are changed, wound drainage is noted. A milky drainage after feeding could indicate a chylous fistula, a rare complication resulting from injury to the thoracic duct during surgery or postoperative damage to and necrosis of adjacent tissues.

Mild, transient hypoparathyroidism and resultant hypocalcemia occur in about 70 per cent of patients after parathyroidectomy, probably because the removal of parathyroid tissue demands readjustment of the body to the decreased production of parathyroid hormone, to the interrupted blood supply to the gland, and to any trauma to the parathyroid tissue left after surgery. Patients with transient postoperative hypoparathyroidism will exhibit symptoms of hypocalcemia and neuromuscular irritability. The patient should be monitored carefully for any signs of TETANY. In addition to nervousness, hyperreflexia of tendons, convulsions, and prolonged Q-T interval on the electrocardiogram, the patient may present positive CHVOSTEK'S and TROUSSEAU'S SIGNS. Laboratory data will show a serum calcium deficit.

Intravenous CALCIUM GLUCONATE (10 per cent) is administered to counteract the hypocalcemia. If the condition persists and the patient can tolerate oral medication, the calcium can be given by mouth. Therapy is often needed for only a few weeks until the transient hypocalcemia is over; however, some level of hypocalcemia is considered desirable as it acts as a stimulant to the remaining parathyroid tissue. (See accompanying illustration.)

hyperpepsinia (hi″per-pep-sin′e-ah) excessive secretion of pepsin in the stomach.

hyperperistalsis (hi″per-per″ĭ-stal′sis) excessively active peristalsis.

hyperphalangism (hi″per-fal′an-jizm) the presence of a supernumerary phalanx on a finger or toe.

hyperphenylalaninemia (hi″per-fen″il-al″ah-nĭ-ne′me-ah) an excess of PHENYLALA-NINE in the blood, as in PHENYLKETONURIA.

hyperphonesis (hi″per-fo-ne′sis) intensification of the sound in auscultation or percussion.

hyperphoria (hi″per-fo′re-ah) HETERO-PHORIA in which there is permanent upward deviation of the visual axis of an eye in the absence of visual stimuli.

hyperphosphatasemia (hi″per-fos″fah-ta-se′me-ah) high levels of alkaline phosphatase in the blood; see HYPERPHOSPHATASIA.

hyperphosphatasia (hi″per-fos″fah-ta′-zhah) a hereditary condition transmitted as an autosomal recessive trait, marked by abnormally high alkaline phosphatase levels in the serum and by macrocranium, short neck and thorax, lateral bowing of the femurs, and anterior bowing of the tibias.

hyperphosphatemia (hi″per-fos″fah-te′me-ah) an excess of phosphates in the blood.

hyperphosphaturia (hi″per-fos″fah-tu′re-ah) an excessive amount of phosphates in the urine, such as in hyperparathyroidism, rickets, or inability of renal tubules to reabsorb phosphorus.

hyperpigmentation (hi″per-pig″men-ta′-shun) abnormally increased PIGMENTATION.

hyperpituitarism (hi″per-pĭ-too′ĭ-tah-rizm″) a condition due to pathologically increased activity of the PITUITARY GLAND, especially increased secretion of GROWTH HORMONE, resulting in ACROMEGALY or GIGAN-TISM.

hyperplasia (hi″per-pla′zhah) abnormal increase in volume of a tissue or organ caused by the formation and growth of new normal cells. See also HYPERTROPHY and PROLIFERATION. adj., **hyperplas′tic.**

benign prostatic h. benign prostatic hypertrophy.

cutaneous lymphoid h. a group of benign cutaneous disorders characterized by accumulations of large numbers of lymphocytes and histiocytes in the skin, which may occur as a reaction to insect bites, allergy hyposensitization injections, light, trauma, or a tattoo pigment or may be of unknown etiology.

focal nodular h. (FNH) a benign, usually asymptomatic tumor of the liver, occurring chiefly in women; it is a firm, nodular, highly vascular mass resembling cirrhosis, usually with a stellate fibrous core containing numerous small bile ducts, and having vessels lined by Kupffer cells.

nodular h. of the prostate benign prostatic hypertrophy.

hyperploid (hi′per-ploid) 1. characterized by HYPERPLOIDY. 2. an individual or cell exhibiting hyperploidy.

hyperploidy (hi′per-ploi″de) the state of having more than the typical number of chromosomes in unbalanced sets, as in DOWN SYNDROME.

hyperpnea (hi″perp-ne′ah) increase in depth of breathing, which may or may not be accompanied by an increase in the respiratory rate. Maximal hyperpnea occurs during strenuous exercise. See also HYPER-VENTILATION. adj., **hyperpne′ic.**

hyperpolarization (hi″per-po″ler-ĭz-a′shun) any increase in the amount of electrical charge separated by the cell membrane and hence in the strength of the membrane POTENTIAL. In cardiology this is the process by which an electrical fiber, at the end of phase 3 REPOLARIZATION, becomes more negative than usual.

hyperponesis (hi″per-po-ne′sis) excessive action-potential output from the motor and premotor areas of the cortex. adj., **hyperponet′ic.**

hyperposia (hi″per-po′ze-ah) abnormally increased ingestion of fluids for relatively brief periods.

hyperpotassemia (hi″per-pot″ah-se′me-ah) hyperkalemia.

hyperpragia (hi″per-pra′je-ah) excessive mental activity. adj. **hyperprag′ic.**

hyperpraxia (hi″per-prak′se-ah) abnormal activity; restlessness.

hyperprebetalipoproteinemia (hi″per-pre-ba″tah-lip″o-pro″tēn-e′me-ah) an excess of very-low-density LIPOPROTEINS (pre-beta lipoproteins) in the blood.

hyperprolactinemia (hi″per-pro-lak″tin-e′me-ah) increased levels of PROLACTIN in the blood; in women it is associated with amenorrhea and often galactorrhea, and it has been reported to cause impotence in men.

hyperprolinemia (hi″per-pro″li-ne′me-ah) a hereditary, usually benign AMINOACIDOPA-THY marked by excessive PROLINE in the blood.

hyperprosexia (hi″per-pro-sek′se-ah) pre-occupation with one idea to the exclusion of all others.

hyperproteinemia (hi″per-pro″te-ne′me-ah) an excess of protein in the blood.

hyperproteosis (hi″per-pro″te-o′sis) a condition due to excess of protein in the diet.

hyperpselaphesia (hi″perp-sel″ah-fe′-zhah) increased tactile sensitiveness.

hyperpyrexia (hi″per-pi-rek′se-ah) hyperthermia. adj., **hyperpyrex′ial, hyperpyrex′ic.**

   malignant h. malignant hyperthermia.

hyperreactive (hi″per-re-ak′tiv) showing a greater than normal response to stimuli.

hyperreactivity (hi″per-re-ak-tiv′ĭ-te) the quality of being HYPERREACTIVE; see also IRRITABILITY. Called also hyperresponsiveness.

hyperreflexia (hi″per-re-flek′se-ah) exaggeration of reflexes, sometimes due to excessive activity of the sympathetic NERVOUS SYSTEM; see also AUTONOMIC DYSREFLEXIA.

   detrusor h. the occurrence of unstable bladder contractions in the presence of known neurological disease; see also detrusor INSTABILITY.

hyperreninemia (hy″per-re″nin-e′me-ah) a condition of elevated levels of RENIN in the blood, which may lead to ALDOSTERONISM and HYPERTENSION.

hyperresonance (hi″per-rez′o-nans) exaggerated resonance on percussion.

hyperresponsive (hi″per-re-spon′siv) hyperreactive.

hyperresponsiveness (hi″per-re-spon′siv-nes) hyperreactivity.

hypersalemia (hi″per-sah-le′me-ah) abnormally increased content of salt in the blood.

hypersalivation (hi″per-sal″ĭ-va-shun) ptyalism.

hypersarcosinemia (hi″per-sahr″ko-sēn-e′me-ah) sarcosinemia.

hypersecretion (hi″per-se-kre′shun) excessive secretion.

hypersensitivity (hi″per-sen″sĭ-tiv′ĭ-te) a state of altered reactivity in which the body reacts with an exaggerated IMMUNE RESPONSE to a foreign agent; ANAPHYLAXIS and ALLERGY are forms of hypersensitivity. The hypersensitivity states and resulting hypersensitivity REACTIONS are usually subclassified by

the GELL AND COOMBS CLASSIFICATION. adj., **hypersen′sitive.**

   contact h. that produced by contact of the skin with a chemical substance having the properties of an antigen or hapten.

   delayed h. **(DH),** *delayed type h.* **(DTH)** the type of hypersensitivity exemplified by the tuberculin reaction, which (as opposed to immediate hypersensitivity) takes 12 to 48 hours to develop and which can be transferred by lymphocytes but not by serum. Delayed hypersensitivity can be induced by most viral infections, many bacterial infections, all mycotic infections, and a few protozoal infections (leishmaniasis and toxoplasmosis). The scope of the term is sometimes expanded to cover all aspects of cell-mediated immunity including contact dermatitis, granulomatous reactions, and allograft rejection.

   immediate h. antibody-mediated hypersensitivity occurring within minutes when a sensitized individual is exposed to antigen; clinical manifestations include systemic anaphylaxis and atopic allergy (allergic rhinitis, asthma, dermatitis, urticaria, and angioedema). The first exposure to the antigen induces the production of IgE antibodies (cytotropic antibodies, reagin) that bind to receptors on mast cells and basophils. Subsequent exposure to the antigen triggers production and release of a diverse array of mediators of hypersensitivity that act on other cells producing symptoms such as bronchospasm, edema, mucous secretion, and inflammation.

   h. reaction the exaggerated or inappropriate immune response occurring in HYPERSENSITIVITY, in response to a substance either foreign or perceived as foreign and resulting in local or general tissue damage. Such reactions are usually classified as types I–IV on the basis of the GELL AND COOMBS CLASSIFICATION.

hypersensitization (hi″per-sen″sĭ-ti-za′-shun) the induction of hypersensitivity.

hypersexuality (hi″per-sek″shoo-al′-ĭ-te) abnormally increased sexual desire or activity; nymphomania; satyriasis.

hypersomnia (hi″per-som′ne-ah) excessive sleeping or sleepiness, as in any of a group of sleep disorders.

   primary h. a dyssomnia consisting of persistent excessive sleepiness and sleeping, with prolonged sleep episodes or regularly occurring voluntary or involuntary napping, but not due to any other physical or psychological condition.

hypersomnolence (hi″per-som′no-lens) hypersomnia.

H

hypersplenism (hi″per-splen′izm) a condition characterized by exaggeration of the hemolytic function of the spleen, resulting in deficiency of peripheral blood elements, and by hypercellularity of the bone marrow and splenomegaly.

hypersthenia (hi″per-sthe′ne-ah) 1. increased strength or tonicity. 2. abnormal strength or excessive tension of the entire body or a part. adj., **hypersthen′ic.**

hypersthenuria (hi″per-sthĕ-nu′re-ah) increased osmolality of the urine.

hypertelorism (hi″per-te′lo-rizm) abnormally increased distance between two organs or parts.

  ocular h., orbital h. increase in the interocular distance, often associated with cleidocranial or craniofacial dysostosis and sometimes with mental deficiency.

hypertensinogen (hi″per-ten-sin′o-jen) angiotensinogen.

hypertension (hi″per-ten′shun) persistently high BLOOD PRESSURE. In adults, it is generally agreed that a blood pressure is abnormally high when the systolic pressure is equal to or greater than 140 mm Hg and the diastolic pressure is equal to or greater than 90 mm Hg.

A diagnosis of hypertension should be based on a series of readings rather than a single measurement that could be influenced by emotional state or physical activity. Hypertension is not a single disease entity in the usual sense, but rather a major indicator of the prognosis for future development of cardiovascular, cerebrovascular, and renal disease. Data from numerous studies indicate that a diastolic pressure above 90 mm Hg reduces life expectancy in persons of all ages and both sexes. Furthermore, studies have shown that an elevation in systolic pressure is as dangerous and likely to lead to cardiovascular disease as an elevated diastolic pressure.

Hypertension is a major threat to life and health. It is estimated that one in four Americans has high blood pressure. Although the disease primarily affects men over 35 and women over 45 years of age, it is not limited to older persons. Screening clinics have detected hypertension in increasing numbers of teenagers. Between 2 and 6 per cent of adolescents have persistent blood pressure elevations. Prevalence rates for prepubertal children have been reported to be as high as 1 per cent. Hypertension is more severe and more prevalent in blacks than in whites, by an overall ratio of two to one. Socioeconomic status does not seem to be a factor; the disease is distributed throughout all social, economic, and educational levels.

Statistical data on causes of death do not reflect the role of hypertension as a major contributing factor. Hypertensive individuals usually die from damage to the blood vessels in such vital organs as the heart, brain, and kidney. Hypertension increases the risk for heart disease and stroke, two of the leading causes of death in the United States.

Types and Causative Factors. There are two major types of hypertension: essential (primary or idiopathic) and secondary hypertension. *Essential hypertension* is by far the most common, accounting for about 95 per cent of all known cases. The cause of this form is not known; there are probably several different contributing factors, such as age (blood pressure tends to rise throughout life), obesity, smoking, heredity, and an aggressive, hyperactive personality. A stressful environment also can produce a tendency toward high blood pressure.

It is known that there is a direct relationship between hypertension and ATHEROSCLEROSIS. Elevated blood pressure levels

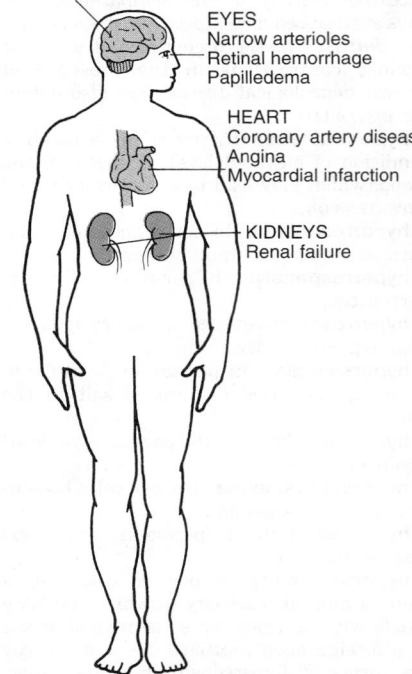

BRAIN
Transient ischemic attacks
Cerebrovascular accident

EYES
Narrow arterioles
Retinal hemorrhage
Papilledema

HEART
Coronary artery disease
Angina
Myocardial infarction

KIDNEYS
Renal failure

Long-term effects of hypertension on body organs. From Linton et al., 2000.

speed up the atherosclerotic process, and the complications of essential hypertension are directly related to this accelerated disease process. Essential hypertension is insidious and usually asymptomatic, although headache and flushing sometimes occur. As the disease progresses the patient may experience fatigue, dizziness, palpitations, tachycardia, and nosebleeds. Eventually, the effects of uncontrolled hypertension become manifest in the form of heart disease, stroke, or renal disease.

Examination of the retina can be a reliable index to the extent to which high blood pressure has damaged blood vessels throughout the body. By visualizing the retinal arterioles with an ophthalmoscope it is possible to estimate the effects of hypertension elsewhere in the body. If there is little or no sclerosis of the retinal arterioles but the patient has consistently high blood pressure readings, the hypertension probably is still labile or is in its earliest stages.

Malignant or *accelerated hypertension* is a particularly severe form of essential hypertension. Diastolic pressures of 130 to 170 mm Hg are not unusual in these patients. The most common symptoms are morning headache, blurred vision, dyspnea related to early pulmonary edema, and symptoms of uremia, including elevated blood urea nitrogen and serum creatinine levels. Malignant hypertension is treated as a medical emergency as soon as it is diagnosed because it can be fatal if not treated immediately. It causes progressive damage to blood vessels in the kidney and can cause cerebral hemorrhage. With proper care malignant hypertension can be kept under control for years. Without adequate treatment it is often fatal within two years.

Secondary hypertension is actually a symptom of a variety of underlying or primary diseases, such as renal vascular disease (e.g., atherosclerosis or stenosis of the renal artery), renal parenchymal disease, dysfunction of the adrenal cortex or medulla, atherosclerosis of the systemic arteries, and coarctation of the aorta. The most commonly contributing disorders are those that interfere with the supply of blood to the kidney. The resulting ischemia of renal tissue stimulates the secretion of RENIN, an enzyme that catalyzes the conversion of ANGIOTENSINOGEN to ANGIOTENSIN I. Other enzymes in the body then convert angiotensin I to angiotensin II, the most potent vasoconstrictor known.

Angiotensin II acts directly on the blood vessels and also acts as a physiologic stimulant to the adrenal gland and the production of aldosterone. Hence there is a twofold effect: (1) an increase in peripheral resistance due to vasoconstriction and a resulting elevation of blood pressure, and (2) a retention of sodium and water by the renal tubules in response to increased levels of serum ALDOSTERONE. The retained sodium and water increase blood volume, since they remain in the vascular system rather than being excreted by the kidney. The result is an increased cardiac output and an elevation of blood pressure.

Although the above mechanisms are responsible for elevation of blood pressure in many patients with renal hypertension, they do not completely explain the hypertension. Other factors being studied as possible causes include failure of the kidney either to secrete vasopressors or to inactivate pressor substances produced elsewhere in the body. Another possibility is that there are factors other than the renin-angiotensin-aldosterone axis responsible for the retention of water and sodium by the renal tubules.

Treatment. The regimen of therapy prescribed for a patient with essential hypertension is based on the level of blood pressure and the number of risk factors that are present. Patients who have extreme hypertension need immediate attention to bring the blood pressure down to safer levels and avoid catastrophic effects such as heart failure and cerebral hemorrhage. Those who have "mildly" or "moderately" high blood pressure associated with obesity, intolerance to glucose, high levels of serum lipids, or a smoking habit need additional help in reducing these risk factors.

Nonpharmacologic modes of therapy include weight loss, limiting SODIUM intake, stopping smoking, and limiting intake of fat. The DASH DIET ("Dietary Approaches to Stop Hypertension") has been reported to substantially lower blood pressure in studies by the NATIONAL HEART, LUNG, and BLOOD INSTITUTE. Other beneficial measures for reduction of stress and promotion of relaxation are through BIOFEEDBACK, relaxation techniques, and meditation.

Pharmacologic treatment will depend on the severity of the blood pressure elevation, presence of target organ damage, and presence of other risk factors. Considerations for individualizing drug treatment for hypertension can be found in the Sixth Report of the Joint National Committee on Prevention, Evaluation, and Treatment of High Blood Pressure. ANTIHYPERTENSIVE AGENTS may be prescribed either singly or in combination.

H

Patient Care. The greatest challenge in the continued control and management of essential hypertension is gaining the cooperation of the patient/client and compliance with the prescribed regimen of care. Hypertension is a chronic health problem that must be dealt with for the rest of the patient's life. Because the disease is often without severe symptoms, requires alterations in lifestyle and changes in lifelong habits, and demands continued surveillance by health care professionals, many patients become discouraged and fail to follow the advice and counsel offered to them. In order to keep patients participating in a program of control, they must be given a clear understanding of the pathology of the disease and the rationale for each aspect of therapy. Prevention of high blood pressure should be the priority.

There are many reasons why patients cannot or will not take an active part in managing their high blood pressure and avoiding its complications. Some discontinue their medications once they begin to feel better, and others stop taking them because they experience unpleasant side effects and do not realize that other medications can be substituted. It is difficult for some patients to accept the fact that their illness will persist throughout life and that, although there are means by which the disease can be managed, these modes of therapy are effective only insofar as each patient is willing and able to accept a part of the responsibility for carrying out the prescribed regimen.

Patient and family education should include information about the factors contributing to hypertension, the changes that uncontrolled hypertension can bring about within the body, the purpose of each prescribed medication, the importance of following the prescribed diet, the expected results of weight loss and other recommendations, and the need to consult with health care professionals on a regular basis for support and guidance. (See Atlas 4, Part C).

essential h., idiopathic h. hypertension without a discoverable organic cause.

malignant h. a severe hypertensive state with poor prognosis; it is characterized by papilledema of the ocular fundus, vascular hemorrhagic lesions, thickening of walls of small arteries and arterioles, and left ventricular hypertrophy.

ocular h. persistently elevated intraocular pressure in the absence of any other signs of GLAUCOMA; it may or may not progress to chronic simple glaucoma.

persistent pulmonary h. of the newborn persistent fetal CIRCULATION.

portal h. abnormally increased pressure in the portal circulation due to narrowing of the capillary branches of the portal vessels. The result is impairment of the liver's ability to detoxify wastes and transport nutrients, resulting in hepatic encephalopathy, anorexia, and metabolic acidosis. The increased pressure can lead to escape of fluids through the liver capsule and into the abdominal cavity (ASCITES). Resistance to blood flow in the hepatic sinusoids can cause esophageal varices and dilatation of abdominal and rectal veins.

pregnancy-induced h. (PIH) A potentially life-threatening hypertensive disorder that occurs after the 20th week of pregnancy. Formerly called *toxemia of pregnancy*, it is characterized by high blood pressure, proteinuria, generalized edema, and weight gain. Pregnancy-induced hypertension should be distinguished from other blood pressure disorders such as chronic hypertension. The American College of Obstetricians and Gynecologists classifies hypertensive disorders of pregnancy into six categories.

renovascular h. hypertension due to occlusive disease of the renal arteries such as renal artery stenosis or fibromuscular dysplasia.

systemic venous h. elevation of systemic venous pressure, usually detected by inspection of the jugular veins.

hypertensive (hi″per-ten′siv) 1. characterized by increased tension or pressure. 2. causing HYPERTENSION. 3. a person with hypertension.

hypertensor (hi″per-ten′ser) pressor.

hyperthecosis (hi″per-the-ko′sis) hyperplasia and excessive luteinization of the cells of the inner stromal layer of the ovary.

hyperthelia (hi″per-the′le-ah) the presence of supernumerary nipples.

hyperthermalgesia (hi″per-ther″mal-je′-zhah) abnormal sensitiveness to heat.

hyperthermesthesia (hi″per-therm″es-the′zhah) increased sensibility for heat.

hyperthermia (hi″per-ther′me-ah) 1. greatly increased temperature; see also FEVER. Called also hyperpyrexia. adj., **hyperther′mal, hyperther′mic.** 2. a NURSING DIAGNOSIS accepted by the North American Nursing Diagnosis Association, defined as the state in which an individual's body temperature is elevated above his or her normal range.

malignant h. a syndrome affecting patients undergoing general ANESTHESIA, marked by rapid rise in body temperature, signs of increased muscle metabolism, and usually rigidity. The sensitivity is inherited as an autosomal dominant trait.

hyperthrombinemia (hi″per-throm″bĭ-ne′me-ah) an excess of thrombin in the blood.

hyperthymia (hi″per-thi′me-ah) 1. excessive emotionalism. 2. excessive activity, verging on hypomania. adj., **hyperthy′mic.**

hyperthymism (hi″per-thi′mizm) excessive THYMUS activity.

hyperthyroidism (hi″per-thi′roi-dizm) excessive functional activity of the THYROID GLAND; see also THYROTOXICOSIS. It affects women far more frequently than men, with peak incidence between 30 and 50 years of age, and is commonly part of GRAVES′ DISEASE, a syndrome that may include GOITER and EXOPHTHALMOS. It is also seen in association with THYROIDITIS, thyroid cancer, molar PREGNANCY, HYPEREMESIS GRAVIDARUM, and toxic multinodular GOITER. Several different physiologic mechanisms may cause increased hyperthyroidism: increased synthesis and secretion of thyroid hormones, excessive release of the hormones, or ingestion of excessive amounts of the hormones. adj., **hyperthy′roid.**

Symptoms. Manifestations vary from mild symptoms of weakness, insomnia, weight loss, and tremulousness to extreme tachycardia, palpitations, exertional DYSPNEA, and ankle edema. The hyperthyroid patient's metabolic rate is greatly accelerated, speeding up bodily processes. Severity of symptoms is related to patient age, length of illness, and level of excess thyroid hormone in circulation.

The best screening test for hyperthyroidism is the THYROID-STIMULATING HORMONE (TSH) TEST (or assay). Other laboratory tests that may be performed include assessments of free TRIIODOTHYRONINE and free THYROXINE, the TRIIODOTHYRONINE RESIN UPTAKE TEST, and RADIOIMMUNOASSAY for triiodothyronine. Selected cases, such as hyperthyroidism during pregnancy, may warrant evaluation of thyroid antibodies. A RADIOACTIVE IODINE UPTAKE TEST or thyroid scan may also be useful evaluations.

Treatment. General measures of support for the patient suffering from hyperthyroidism include physical and emotional rest and a high caloric, nutritional diet supplemented with vitamins and calcium. The choice of additional medications and/or surgical intervention will depend on the age of the patient, the cause of the hyperthyroidism, and the patient's response to selected therapies.

Radioactive iodine (RADIOIODINE) is usually the drug of choice; either ^{125}I or ^{131}I may be used. Clinical Guidelines have been

developed by the American Association of Clinical Endocrinologists and the American College of Endocrinology. They note that some clinicians are hesitant to use radioactive iodine in treatment of any woman of childbearing age, but there is no evidence to back up such fears. However, treatment with radioactive iodine is contraindicated during pregnancy and on the nursing mother, and a waiting period of six months is advised after the end of treatment before initiation of pregnancy. Some patients may require treatment with antithyroid drugs before radioactive iodine. Careful monitoring of the patient is required as thyroid function diminishes. Many patients experience HYPOTHYROIDISM following treatment; it may occur immediately or may be delayed until a considerable time later.

The dosage depends on the size of the gland and its sensitivity to radiation. The radioactive iodine is administered orally, usually in one small dose. Some individuals receiving these small doses may require two or even three doses. Radioactive iodine takes several months to achieve the desired effect, and symptoms usually improve after about four weeks. Antithyroid medication and BETA-BLOCKERS may be necessary to control the symptoms associated with hyperthyroidism during this initial time period. All patients receiving radioactive iodine must be observed for signs of THYROID CRISIS resulting from radiation-induced thyroiditis.

Antithyroid Drugs. The antithyroid drugs, especially PROPYLTHIOURACIL, are prescribed in pregnancy and in cases where remission of the disease is a goal. The prime candidates for this therapy are patients with small goiters and mild symptoms. It is important that the patient take the medication in the prescribed time and strictly according to schedule. Propylthiouracil produces AGRANULOCYTOSIS, which can develop quickly. For this reason patients receiving this drug must be instructed to report to the physician any sore throat, fever, or rash, so that white blood cell counts can be done and the patient's condition evaluated.

Iodine preparations often are given routinely for 10 to 14 days prior to surgery to reduce the vascularity of the thyroid. Another important use of antithyroid drugs is in treatment of thyroid crisis. Iodine preparations such as a saturated solution of POTASSSIUM IODIDE have only a temporary effect.

Surgery. Subtotal THYROIDECTOMY is now rarely done as a treatment for hyperthyroidism. It is reserved for special circumstances,

H

such as a pregnant woman who cannot tolerate antithyroid medications or a patient with a large, nodular goiter. It may also be done on a patient who refuses treatment with radioactive iodine.

Patient Care. Patients with hyperthyroidism are subject to a variety of complex and long-term problems of physical and mental health. Among the nursing diagnoses commonly seen in these patients are agitation and irritability related to increased metabolic rate; anxiety and psychologic stress related to frequent diagnostic testing and its outcomes and to ongoing treatments; nutritional imbalance: less than body requirements, related to elevated metabolic rate; alteration in comfort related to heat intolerance and diaphoresis; potential for injury related to thyroid crisis; and disturbance in self-concept related to uncontrollable emotional outbursts, weight loss, and chronic nature of the illness.

Because of the increased irritability, it is helpful to keep environmental stimuli at a minimum. Patients should be approached in a calm and unhurried manner and their wishes regarding visitors during hospitalization respected. To assure as much rest and sleep as possible, meals and treatments are scheduled so that the patient has periods of uninterrupted rest. When at home or work, the patient is encouraged to take time for rest. Physical and mental rest are important because stress can act as a stimulus to and cause increased activity of the thyroid.

Information about tests and prescribed treatments should be provided to the patient and family. Caloric intake is increased to a daily intake of 3000 calories, and may require supplemental feeding to maintain desired body weight. Consultation with a dietitian can help improve the patient's understanding of and compliance with the prescribed diet. Patients and their families need to understand the nature of the illness, its effect on emotions, and the importance of complying with the regimen of care. They should report regularly to professional caregivers for support and guidance.

hyperthyroxinemia (hi″per-thi-rok″sin-e′me-ah) an excess of thyroxine in the blood.

hypertonia (hi″per-to′ne-ah) abnormally increased tonicity, as of skeletal muscles or the walls of arteries.

hypertonic (hi″per-ton′ik) 1. pertaining to or characterized by an increased tonicity or tension. 2. having an osmotic pressure greater than that of the solution with which it is compared.

hypertonicity (hi″per-to-nis′ĭ-te) the state or quality of being hypertonic.

hypertrichosis (hi″per-trĭ-ko′sis) hirsutism.

h. lanugino′sa persistent or acquired production of lanugo. It may be a congenital, autosomal dominant disorder in which there is excessive hair distributed over the entire body throughout life, usually in association with other congenital anomalies; or it may be acquired, with the degree of hairiness being variable, usually involving the face, and in most cases associated with internal carcinoma.

hypertriglyceridemia (hi″per-tri-glis″er-ĭ-de′me-ah) an excess of TRIGLYCERIDES in the blood; a familial form occurs in HYPERLIPOPROTEINEMIA types I and IV.

hypertrophy (hi-per′tro-fe) increase in volume of a tissue or organ produced entirely by enlargement of existing cells. See also HYPERPLASIA and PROLIFERATION. adj., **hypertro′phic.**

asymmetrical septal h. 1. hypertrophic cardiomyopathy. 2. the term is sometimes limited to cases of hypertrophic CARDIOMYOPATHY in which the hypertrophy is localized to the interventricular septum. See also hypertrophic obstructive CARDIOMYOPATHY.

benign prostatic h. **(BPH)** age-associated enlargement of the prostate resulting from proliferation of glandular and stromal elements, beginning generally in the fifth decade of life; it may cause urethral compression and obstruction. Called also benign prostatic hyperplasia and nodular hyperplasia of the prostate.

cardiac h. enlargement of myocardial cells and hyperplasia of nonmuscular cardiac components due to pressure and volume overload and sometimes to neurohumoral factors.

compensatory h. that which results from an increased workload due to some physical defect, such as in an organ where one part is defective, or in one kidney when the other is absent or nonfunctional.

functional h. hypertrophy of an organ or part caused by its increased activity.

ventricular h. hypertrophy of the myocardium of a ventricle, due to chronic pressure overload; it is manifest electrocardiographically by increased QRS complex voltage, frequently accompanied by repolarization changes.

hypertropia (hi″per-tro′pe-ah) vertical STRABISMUS in which there is permanent upward deviation of the visual axis of one eye.

hyperuricemia (hi″per-u″rĭ-se′me-ah) an excess of uric acid or urates in the blood. adj., **hyperurice′mic.**

hyperuricosuria (hi″per-u″rĭ-ko-su′re-ah) an excess of uric acid or urates in the urine; called also hyperuricuria and uricosuria.

hyperuricuria hyperuricosuria.

hypervalinemia (hi″per-val″ĭ-ne′me-ah) an inborn ERROR of metabolism characterized by elevated levels of VALINE in the blood and urine and by FAILURE TO THRIVE.

hypervascular (hi″per-vas′ku-ler) extremely vascular.

hyperventilation (hi″per-ven″tĭ-la′shun) abnormally fast and deep breathing, the result of either an emotional state or a physiological condition. Emotional causes include acute anxiety and emotional tension, such as in nervous, anxious patients who may have other functional disturbances related to emotional problems. Physiological causes include a rapid decrease in INTRACRANIAL PRESSURE, other neurologic problems, and metabolic, pulmonary, and cardiovascular conditions. More prolonged hyperventilation may be caused by certain disorders of the central nervous system, or by drugs that increase the sensitivity of the respiratory centers (such as high concentrations of SALICYLATES). Transient respiratory ALKALOSIS commonly occurs when a person is hyperventilating. Iatrogenic hyperventilation may be seen in critically ill patients receiving mechanical ventilation.

It was formerly considered standard practice to hyperventilate patients following severe head injuries. However, now practice guidelines published by the American Association of Critical Care Nurses note that current research does not conclusively support this practice, and they urge judiciousness in its use. The Cochrane review is another study that notes that more clinical trials are required to determine the efficacy of hyperventilation in treatment of head trauma.

Symptoms of hyperventilation in the anxious patient include "faintness" or impaired consciousness without actual loss of consciousness. At the outset the patient may feel a tightness of the chest, a sensation of smothering, and some degree of apprehension. Other symptoms may be related to the heart and digestive tract, such as palpitation or pounding of the heart, fullness in the throat, and pain over the stomach region. In prolonged attacks the patient may exhibit tetany with muscular spasm of the hands and feet, and perioral numbness.

Short-term immediate treatment consists of having the patient slow the rate of breathing. Determining the underlying physical or emotional cause is necessary; the type of treatment depends on the cause.

Medication, stress reduction measures, and controlled breathing exercises will control hyperventilation. Health care providers are no longer advised to use the technique of rebreathing into a paper bag, because of the danger of HYPOXIA.

h. syndrome a complex of symptoms that accompany hypocapnia caused by hyperventilation, including palpitation, a feeling of shortness of breath or air hunger, lightheadedness or giddiness, profuse perspiration, and tingling sensations in the fingertips, face, or toes. Prolonged overbreathing may result in vasomotor collapse and loss of consciousness. Hyperventilation that is unrecognized by the patient is a common cause of the symptoms associated with chronic anxiety or panic attacks.

hypervigilance (hi″per-vij′ĭ-lans) abnormally increased arousal, responsiveness to stimuli, and screening of the environment for threats; it is often associated with delusional or paranoid states.

hyperviscosity (hi″per-vis-kos′ĭ-te) excessive viscosity, as of the blood.

h. syndrome any of various syndromes associated with increased VISCOSITY of the blood. One type is due to serum HYPERVISCOSITY and is characterized by spontaneous bleeding with neurologic and ocular disorders. Another type is characterized by POLYCYTHEMIA with retarded blood flow, organ congestion, reduced capillary perfusion, and increased cardiac effort. A third group includes conditions in which the deformability of ERYTHROCYTES is impaired, such as SICKLE CELL ANEMIA.

hypervitaminosis (hi″per-vi″tah-mĭ-no′sis) a condition produced by ingestion of excessive amounts of VITAMINS; symptom complexes are associated with excessive intake of vitamins A and D (hypervitaminosis A and hypervitaminosis D).

hypervolemia (hi″per-vo-le′me-ah) abnormal increase in the volume of circulating blood plasma in the body; see also excess fluid VOLUME.

hypesthesia (hi″pes-the′hzah) hypoesthesia.

hypha (hi′fah), pl. *hy′phae* [L.] 1. one of the filaments or threads composing the mycelium of a fungus. 2. branching filamentous outgrowths produced by certain bacteria (e.g., *Actinomyces, Hyphomicrobium*), sometimes forming a mycelium.

hyphedonia (hīp″he-do′ne-ah) pathologic diminution of power of enjoyment.

hyphema (hi-fe′mah) hemorrhage into the anterior chamber of the eye. (See accompanying illustration.)

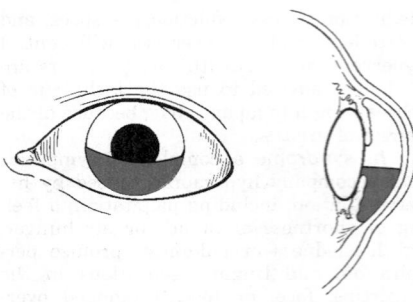

Hyphema, or hemorrhage in the anterior chamber. *A*, front view. *B*, side view. From Stein et al., 2000.

hyphemia (hi-fe′me-ah) 1. deficiency of blood to a part. 2. hyphema.

hyphidrosis (hīp″hi-dro′sis) HYPOHIDROSIS.

Hyphomycetes (hi″fo-mi-se′tēz) the mycelial (hyphal) fungi, i.e., the molds.

hyphomycosis (hi″fo-mi-ko′sis) any infection caused by an imperfect fungus of the form-class *Hyphomycetes*; the group has been divided into HYALOHYPHOMYCOSIS and PHAEOHYPHOMYCOSIS based on the color of the mycelium and wall of the fungus.

hypn(o)- word element [Gr.], *sleep; hypnosis.*

hypnagogic (hip″nah-goj′ik) 1. hypnotic (def. 1). 2. occurring just before sleep; applied to hallucinations occurring at sleep onset.

hypnagogue (hip′nah-gog) 1. hypnotic (def. 1). 2. hypnotic (def. 2).

hypnalgia (hip-nal′jah) pain during sleep.

hypnoanalysis (hip″no-ah-nal′ĭ-sis) psychoanalysis with use of hypnosis to help uncover unconscious material.

hypnoanesthesia (hip″no-an″es-the′zhah) reduction of sensitivity to pain by hypnosis.

hypnodontics (hip″no-don′tiks) the application of hypnosis and controlled suggestion in the practice of dentistry.

hypnogenic (hip″no-jen′ik) hypnotic (def. 1).

hypnoid (hip′noid) pertaining to or resembling hypnosis or sleep.

hypnology (hip-nol′o-je) the scientific study of sleep or hypnosis.

hypnopompic (hip″no-pom′pik) persisting after sleep; applied to hallucinations occurring on awakening.

hypnosis (hip-no′sis) 1. a state of altered CONSCIOUSNESS, usually artificially induced, in which there is a focusing of attention and heightened responsiveness to suggestions and commands. Contrary to popular belief, hypnosis is not sleep but rather intense concentration, something like the familiar experience of being engrossed in a book to the extent of shutting out the outside world.

State of Hypnosis. The nature of hypnosis and the way it works are still largely unknown. One widely accepted theory is that the person's ego—that is, the part of the mind that consciously restrains instincts—is temporarily weakened under hypnosis at the person's own wish. How deeply one responds depends on many psychologic and biologic factors. The ability to respond to hypnosis varies from person to person; it tends to increase after successive experiences.

Use of Hypnosis. A common medical use of hypnosis is in treating mental illness. Historically, Sigmund Freud developed his theory of the unconscious as a result of his experiments with a hypnotized patient. Out of this theory came some of the techniques of PSYCHOANALYSIS. By lessening the mind's unconscious defenses, hypnosis can make some patients able to recall and even reexperience important childhood events that have long been forgotten or repressed by the conscious mind.

In certain cases when the use of anesthetics is not advisable, hypnosis has been used successfully during dental treatment, setting of fractures, and childbirth, usually in addition to pain-killing medicines. 2. in the NURSING INTERVENTIONS CLASSIFICATION, a nursing INTERVENTION defined as assisting a patient to induce an altered state of consciousness to create an accurate awareness and a directed focus experience.

hypnotherapy (hip″no-ther′ah-pe) the therapeutic use of hypnotism.

hypnotic (hip-not′ik) 1. causing sleep; called also somniferous. 2. an agent that causes sleep; called also somnifacient. 3. pertaining to or of the nature of hypnosis or hypnotism.

hypnotism (hip′no-tizm) the study of or the method or practice of inducing hypnosis.

hypnotize (hip′no-tīz) to induce hypnosis.

hypo (hi′po) 1. a colloquial abbreviation of hypodermic. 2. sodium thiosulfate, used as a photographic fixing agent.

hypoacidity (hi″po-ah-sid′ĭ-te) decreased acidity.

hypoactive sexual desire disorder a SEXUAL DYSFUNCTION consisting of persistently or recurrently low level or absence of sexual fantasies and of desire for sexual activity, causing pronounced distress or interpersonal difficulties.

hypoacusis (hi″po-ah-ku′sis) slightly diminished HEARING.

hypoadrenalism (hi″po-ah-dren′al-izm) deficiency of adrenal activity, as in Addison's disease.

hypoadrenocorticism (hi″po-ah-dre″nokor′tĭ-sizm) adrenocortical insufficiency.

hypoalbuminemia (hi″po-al-bu″mĭ-ne′me-ah) abnormally low levels of albumin in the blood.

hypoalbuminosis (hi″po-al-bu-mĭ-no′sis) abnormally low level of albumin.

hypoaldosteronism (hi″po-al-dos′ter-ōn-izm) deficiency of aldosterone in the body.

hypoalimentation (hi″po-al″ĭ-men-ta′-shun) insufficient nourishment.

hypoazoturia (hi″po-az″o-tu′re-ah) diminished nitrogenous material in the urine.

hypobaric (hi″po-bār′ik) characterized by less than normal pressure or weight; applied to gases under less than atmospheric pressure, or to solutions of lower specific gravity than another taken as a standard of reference.

hypobarism (hi″po-bar′izm) the condition resulting from exposure to ambient gas pressure or atmospheric pressures that are below those within body tissues, fluids, cavities.

hypobaropathy (hi″po-bar-op′ah-the) 1. the disturbances experienced in high altitudes due to reduced air pressure; see HIGH ALTITUDE SICKNESS and MOUNTAIN SICKNESS. 2. hypobarism.

hypoblast (hi′po-blast) endoderm.

hypocalcemia (hi″po-kal-se′me-ah) diminished levels of CALCIUM in the blood; see table of Electrolyte Imbalances at ELECTROLYTE.

hypocalciuria (hi″po-kal″se-u′re-ah) an abnormally diminished amount of calcium in the urine.

hypocapnia (hi″po-kap′ne-ah) deficiency of CARBON DIOXIDE in the blood; it results from HYPERVENTILATION and eventually leads to ALKALOSIS. Called also hypocarbia. adj., **hypocap′nic.**

hypocarbia (hi″po-kahr′be-ah) hypocapnia.

hypocellularity (hi″po-sel″u-lar′ĭ-te) abnormal decrease in the number of cells present, as in bone marrow.

hypochloremia (hi″po-klo-re′me-ah) an abnormally low level of CHLORIDE in the blood; signs and symptoms are those of ALKALOSIS. adj., **hypochlore′mic.**

hypochlorhydria (hi″po-klor-hi′dre-ah) deficiency of HYDROCHLORIC ACID in the gastric juice.

hypochlorous acid (hi″po-klor′us) an unstable compound used as a disinfectant and bleaching agent.

hypochloruria (hi″po-klor-u′re-ah) diminished chloride content in the urine.

hypocholesteremia, hypocholesterolemia (hi″po-kah-les″tĕ-re′me-ah, hi″po-kah-les″ter-ol-e′me-ah) an abnormally low level of cholesterol in the blood.

hypochondria (hi″po-kon′dre-ah) 1. plural of HYPOCHONDRIUM. 2. hypochondriasis.

hypochondriac (hi″po-kon′dre-ak) 1. pertaining to the hypochondrium. 2. pertaining to hypochondriasis. 3. a person affected with hypochondriasis.

hypochondriasis (hi″po-kon-dri′ah-sis) a SOMATOFORM DISORDER marked by a preoccupation with one's health bodily functions and by exaggeration of normal sensations (such as heart beats, sweating, peristaltic action, and bowel movements) and minor complaints (such as a runny nose, minor aches and pains, or slightly swollen lymph nodes) into a strong belief of serious problems needing medical attention. Negative results of diagnostic evaluations and reassurance by health care providers only increase the patient's anxious concern about his health, although the concern is not of delusional intensity. adj., **hypochon′driac, hypochondri′acal.**

hypochondrium (hi″po-kon′dre-um), pl. *hypochon′dria* the upper abdominal region on either side, just below the thorax; called also hypochondriac region. adj., **hypochon′drial.**

hypochondroplasia (hi″po-kon″dro-pla′-zhah) a common disorder of CARTILAGE development transmitted as an autosomal dominant trait; clinical features resemble those of ACHONDROPLASIA but are milder, such as short stature with a long trunk and short limbs, broad and short fingers; the face is normal in appearance.

hypochromasia (hi″po-kro-ma′zhah) 1. staining less intensely than normal. 2. hypochromia (def. 1).

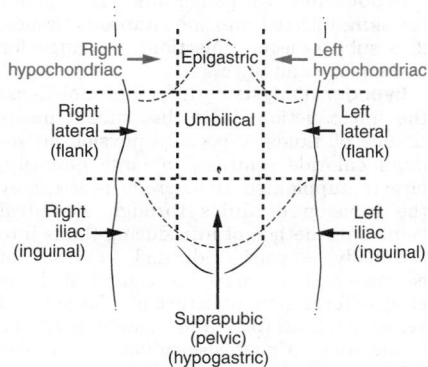

Left and right hypochondrium (hypochondriac region). From Lammon et al., 1995.

H

hypochromatism (hi″po-kro′mah-tizm) 1. abnormally deficient pigmentation, especially deficiency of chromatin in a cell nucleus. 2. HYPOCHROMIA (def. 1).

hypochromatosis (hi″po-kro″mah-to′sis) the gradual fading and disappearance of the nucleus (the chromatin) of a cell.

hypochromia (hi″po-kro′me-ah) 1. decrease of hemoglobin in the erythrocytes so that they are abnormally pale. Called also hypochromasia. adj., **hypochro′mic.** 2. hypochromatism (def. 1).

hypochylia (hi″po-ki′le-ah) deficiency of chyle.

hypocitraturia (hi″po-sī-tra-tu′re-ah) excretion of urine containing an abnormally small amount of citrate; an important cause of the formation of oxalate urinary CALCULI.

hypocomplementemia (hi″po-kom′plĕ-men-te′me-ah) abnormally low complement levels in the blood.

hypocorticism (hi″po-kor′tĭ-sizm) adrenocortical insufficiency.

hypocupremia (hi″po-ku-pre′me-ah) abnormally diminished concentration of copper in the blood.

hypocyclosis (hi″po-si-klo′sis) insufficient accommodation in the eye.

hypocythemia (hi″po-si-the′me-ah) deficiency in the number of erythrocytes in the blood.

hypodactyly (hi″po-dak′tĭ-le) oligodactyly.

Hypoderma (hi″po-der′mah) a genus of parasitic insects, the ox-warble or heel flies, whose larvae cause warbles in cattle and a form of larva migrans in humans.

hypodermiasis (hi″po-der-mi′ah-sis) a creeping ERUPTION of the skin in humans and cattle caused by the larvae of *Hypoderma*.

hypodermic (hi″po-der′mik) 1. beneath the skin; injected into subcutaneous tissues. 2. a subcutaneous, injection; a syringe for making such an injection.

hypodermoclysis (hi″po-der-mok′lĭ-sis) the introduction into the subcutaneous tissues of fluids, especially physiologic sodium chloride solution, in large quantity; largely supplanted in current practice by the infusion of fluids through a central vein. This method of introducing fluids into the body is contraindicated in cases of edema, and it may be complicated by abscess formation, puncture of a large blood vessel, and necrosis and sloughing of the tissues due to poor absorption. Called also subcutaneous infusion.

hypodipsia (hi″po-dip′se-ah) abnormally diminished thirst.

hypodynamia (hi″po-di-na′me-ah) abnormally diminished power. adj., **hypodynam′ic.**

hypoeccrisia (hi″po-e-kriz′e-ah) abnormally diminished excretion. adj., **hypoeccrit′ic.**

hypoechoic (hi″po-ĕ-ko′ik) in ultrasonography, giving off few echoes; said of tissues or structures that reflect relatively few of the ultrasound waves directed at them.

hypoergia (hi″po-er′je-ah) hyposensitivity to allergens.

hypoergic (hi″po-er′jik) 1. less energetic than normal. 2. pertaining to or characterized by hypoergy.

hypoergy (hi″po-er′je) abnormally diminished reactivity; hyposensitivity.

hypoesophoria (hi″po-es″o-for′e-ah) deviation of the visual axes downward and inward.

hypoesthesia (hi″po-es-the′zhah) abnormally decreased sensitivity to stimuli, particularly to TOUCH. Called also hypesthesia. adj., **hypoesthet′ic.**

hypoexophoria (hi″po-ek″so-for′e-ah) deviation of the visual axes downward and laterally.

hypoferremia (hi″po-fĕ-re′me-ah) deficiency of IRON in the blood.

hypofertility (hi″po-fer-til′ĭ-te) subfertility. adj., **hypofer′tile.**

hypofibrinogenemia (hi″po-fi-brin″o-jĕ-ne′me-ah) deficiency of FIBRINOGEN in the blood; called also fibrinogenopenia. See also AFIBRINOGENEMIA.

hypofunction (hi″po-fungk′shun) diminished functioning.

hypogalactia (hi″po-gah-lak′she-ah) deficiency of milk secretion. adj., **hypogalac′tous.**

hypogammaglobulinemia (hi″po-gam″ah-glob″u-lin-e′me-ah) abnormally low levels of all classes of immunoglobulins, associated with heightened susceptibility to infectious diseases; see also AGAMMAGLOBULINEMIA, DYSGLOBULINEMIA, and IMMUNODEFICIENCY.

common variable h. common variable IMMUNODEFICIENCY.

physiologic h. a normal period of hypogammaglobulinemia seen in all infants at about 5–6 months of age as the level of transplacentally acquired maternal immunoglobulins declines before endogenous immunoglobulin synthesis rises to normal levels.

transient h. of infancy prolongation of the normal physiologic hypogammaglobulinemia of infancy caused by delayed development of endogenous immunoglobulin production and associated with increased susceptibility to infections.

X-linked h. X-linked AGAMMAGLOBULINEMIA.

hypoganglionosis (hi″po-gang″gle-o-no′ sis) deficiency in the number of myenteric ganglion cells in the distal segment of the large bowel, resulting in constipation; a variant of congenital megacolon.

hypogastric (hi″po-gas′trik) pertaining to the hypogastrium.

hypogastrium (hi″po-gas′tre-um) the lowest middle abdominal region.

hypogenesis (hi″po-jen′ĕ-sis) defective development.

hypogenitalism (hi″po-jen′ĭ-tah-lizm) lack of sexual development because of deficient activity of the gonads; hypogonadism.

hypogeusesthesia (hi″po-goos-es-the′-zhah) hypogeusia.

hypogeusia (hi″po-goo′zhah) diminished sensitivity of TASTE; called also amblygeustia and hypogeusesthesia.

hypoglossal (hi″po-glos′al) sublingual.

h. nerve the twelfth CRANIAL NERVE; its modality is purely motor, serving the intrinsic muscles of the tongue and other muscles beneath the tongue. See Appendix 3-5.

hypoglucagonemia (hi″po-gloo″kah-gon-e′me-ah) abnormally reduced levels of glucagon in the blood.

hypoglycemia (hi″po-gli-se′me-ah) an abnormally low level of GLUCOSE in the blood, usually because glucose has been either removed at an excessive rate or secreted into the blood at a decreased rate. Overproduction of INSULIN by the islets of Langerhans or an overdose of exogenous insulin can lead to increased utilization of glucose, causing it to be removed from the blood at an accelerated rate. Some large tumors of the retroperitoneal area and tumors of the islets of Langerhans can increase the production of insulin and result in rapid removal of glucose from the blood. Because the liver is the source of most of the glucose entering the blood while a person is fasting, damage to the liver cells can result in impaired ability to convert glycogen to glucose. If secretion of the adrenocortical hormones, especially the GLUCOCORTICOIDS, is deficient, the protein precursors of glucose are not available and the blood glucose level drops as the liver's glycogen supply is depleted.

Symptoms. Hypoglycemia may be tolerated by normal persons for brief periods of time without symptoms; however, if the blood sugar level remains very low for a long time, symptoms of cerebral dysfunction develop. These include mental confusion, hallucinations, convulsions, and eventually deep coma as the nervous system is deprived of the glucose needed for its normal metabolic activities. Other symptoms are a

result of a greatly increased secretion of epinephrine, a normal response to hypoglycemia. The patient then experiences increased pulse rate, tachycardia, a rise in blood pressure, sweating, and anxiety.

Treatment. An acute episode requires careful assessment, with prompt measurement of capillary blood glucose levels. The American Diabetes Association notes than when symptoms occur, corrective action can often be taken by eating carbohydrates. The patient who is unconscious or who is experiencing seizures related to low blood sugar should receive an intravenous bolus of dextrose (50 per cent solution). A family member should be taught to administer glucagon to patients who may experience hypoglycemia and lose consciousness at home. Glucagon can also be administered to the hospitalized patient in an emergency situation when a vein cannot be located.

Specific treatment depends on the primary cause of hypoglycemia. If hyperinsulinism is due to a tumor or hyperplasia of the islands of Langerhans, surgical intervention is necessary to remove this cause of hypoglycemia. The large sarcomas of the retroperitoneal or mediastinal areas that cause hyperinsulinism also must be treated surgically.

Reactive or *postprandial hypoglycemia*, thought to be a precursor of diabetes mellitus, is a form of low blood sugar that develops rather suddenly several hours after ingestion of a high carbohydrate meal. It is characterized by a blood sugar level of 50 mg/100 ml or less, and symptoms of palpitations, sweating, anxiety, hunger, and tremulousness. The usual treatment for this form of chronic hypoglycemia involves dietary changes that are aimed at avoiding extremes in blood glucose level and maintaining an adequate level of glucose in the blood at all times. The diet is high in protein and fat and low in carbohydrate content and is given in frequent, small feedings during the day and before retiring. This regimen avoids extreme fluctuations in blood glucose concentration by restricting carbohydrate intake, and supplies adequate precursors of glycogen through the protein intake.

hypoglycemic (hi″po-gli-se′mik) 1. pertaining to or characterized by HYPOGLYCEMIA. 2. a hypoglycemic AGENT.

hypoglycogenolysis (hi″po-gli″ko-jĕ-nol′ĭ-sis) defective splitting up of glycogen in the body.

hypoglycorrhachia (hi″po-gli″ko-ra′ke-ah) abnormally low sugar content in the cerebrospinal fluid.

hypogonadism (hi″po-go′nad-izm) decreased functional activity of the GONADS, with retardation of growth, sexual development, and SECONDARY SEX CHARACTERS. The American Association of Clinical Endocrinologists has published "Clinical Practice Guidelines for the Evaluation and Treatment of Hypogonadism in Adult Male Patients." These are available online at their web site: http://www.aace.com.

hypergonadotropic h. that associated with secretion of high levels of gonadotropins, as in KLINEFELTER'S SYNDROME. Called also hypergonadotropic eunuchoidism.

hypogonadotropic h. that due to lack of gonads or of gonadotropin secretion. Called also hypogonadotropic eunuchoidism.

hypogonadotropic (hi″po-gon″ah-do-trōp′ik) relating to or caused by deficiency of gonadotropin.

hypohidrosis (hi″po-hī-dro′sis) abnormally diminished secretion of sweat. adj., **hypohidrot′ic.**

hypokalemia (hi″po-kah-le′me-ah) abnormally low POTASSIUM concentration in the blood; see table of Electrolyte Imbalances at ELECTROLYTE. It may result from potassium loss through the kidneys or gastrointestinal tract (vomiting or diarrhea), uncontrolled diabetes mellitus with polyuria, increased adrenocortical secretion, steroid therapy, diuretic therapy, excessive diaphoresis, or burns or other injuries. The earliest signs are weakness and muscle cramps and numbness and tingling that usually begin in the lower extremities. Other symptoms include nausea and vomiting, which can further contribute to potassium deficit. Paralysis of the muscles of respiration can produce respiratory arrest. Neurologic involvement can lead to confusion, irritability, and coma. The heart is particularly sensitive to potassium deficiency. The electrocardiographic abnormalities presented are depression of the T wave and elevation of the U wave. Susceptibility to digitalis toxicity is increased when a patient has hypokalemia. Replacement of potassium can be accomplished by administration of potassium chloride, either orally or intravenously.

hypokalemic (hi″po-kah-le′mik) 1. pertaining to or characterized by hypokalemia. 2. an agent that so acts.

hypokinesia (hi″po-kī-ne′zhah) abnormally diminished motor activity. adj., **hypokinet′ic.**

hypolactasia (hi″po-lak-ta′zhah) deficiency of lactase activity in the intestines.

hypoleydigism (hi″po-li′dig-izm) abnormally diminished secretion of androgens by Leydig's cells.

hypolipidemic (hi″po-lip″ĭ-de′mik) promoting the reduction of lipid concentrations in the serum.

hypolipoproteinemia (hi″po-lip″o-pro-te-ne′me-ah) the presence of abnormally low levels of LIPOPROTEINS in the serum, as in TANGIER DISEASE.

hypoliquorrhea (hi″po-li″kwo-re′ah) chronic deficiency of cerebrospinal fluid.

hypomagnesemia (hi″po-mag″nĕ-se′me-ah) abnormally low MAGNESIUM content of the blood, manifested chiefly by neuromuscular hyperirritability. See table of Electrolyte Imbalances at ELECTROLYTE.

hypomania (hi″po-ma′ne-ah) an abnormality of mood resembling MANIA (persistent elevated or expansive mood, hyperactivity, inflated self-esteem, and so on) but of lesser intensity. adj., **hypoman′ic.**

hypomastia (hi″po-mas′te-ah) micromastia.

hypomenorrhea (hi″po-men″o-re′ah) diminution of menstrual flow or duration.

hypomere (hi′po-mēr) 1. one of the ventrolateral portions of the fusing myotomes in embryonic development, forming muscles innervated by the ventral rami of the spinal nerves. 2. the lateral plate of mesoderm that develops into the walls of the body cavities.

hypometabolism (hi″po-mĕ-tab′o-lizm) decreased metabolism; low metabolic rate.

hypometria (hi″po-me′tre-ah) ataxia in which movements fall short of the intended goal.

hypomnesia (hi″pom-ne′zhah) defective memory.

hypomorph (hi′po-morf) in genetics, a hypomorphic mutant gene, i.e., showing only a slight reduction of the activity it influences. adj., **hypomor′phic.**

hypomotility (hi″po-mo-til′ĭ-te) deficient power of movement in any part.

hypomyotonia (hi″po-mi″o-to′ne-ah) deficient muscular tonicity.

hypomyxia (hi″po-mik′se-ah) decreased secretion of mucus.

hyponasality (hi″po-na-zal′ĭ-te) a quality of voice in which there is a complete lack of nasal emission of air and nasal resonance, so that the voice is low-pitched. Persons with this condition sound as if they have a cold. Called also rhinolalia clausa.

hyponatremia (hi″po-na-tre′me-ah) deficiency of SODIUM in the blood, considered to be present when the sodium concentration is less than 135 mEq per liter. See table of Electrolyte Imbalances at ELECTROLYTE. It can occur as a result of inadequate sodium intake, as in a sodium-restricted diet, excessive water ingestion or retention, or excessive wasting of salt. Symptoms include muscular weakness and twitching, progressing to convulsions if unrelieved; alterations in level of consciousness; mental confusion; and anxiety. When its cause is salt WASTING, there is an accompanying loss of body fluids. Treatment is based on correction of the underlying cause.

hyponeocytosis (hi″po-ne″o-si-to′sis) leukopenia with the presence of immature leukocytes in the blood.

hyponoia (hi″po-noi′ah) sluggish mental activity.

hyponychial (hi″po-nik′e-al) subungual.

hyponychium (hi″po-nik′e-um) the thickened epidermis beneath the free distal end of the nail of a digit. adj., **hyponych′ial.**

hypo-orthocytosis (hi″po-or″tho-si-to′sis) leukopenia with a normal proportion of the various forms of leukocytes.

hypo-osmolality (hi″po-oz″mo-lal′ĭ-te) a decrease in the osmolality of the body fluids; body fluid volume increases and solute volumes usually decrease. Symptoms are those of HYPONATREMIA such as cerebral edema with disorientation, focal neurologic deficits, and seizures.

hypopancreatism (hi″po-pan″kre-ah-tizm) diminished activity of the pancreas.

hypoparathyroidism (hi″po-par″ah-thi′roi-dizm) the condition produced by greatly reduced function of the parathyroid glands or by the removal of these bodies as a treatment for HYPERPARATHYROIDISM. The lack of parathyroid hormone leads to a fall in serum calcium level, which may result in increased neuromuscular excitability and, ultimately, in tetany. There is also a rise in the plasma phosphate level, which results in a decrease in bone resorption and an increased density of bone. There also may be dermatologic, ophthalmologic (cataracts), psychiatric, and dental symptoms.

Treatment consists of raising the lowered calcium content of the blood. There are various forms in which calcium can be administered, and calcium injections will bring immediate improvement. However, if there is complete absence of parathyroid function the patient will have to continue to take oral preparations of calcium indefinitely.

hypoperfusion (hi″po-per-fu′zhun) decreased blood flow through an organ, as in hypovolemic SHOCK; if prolonged, it may result in permanent cellular damage and death.

hypophalangism (hi″po-fal′an-jizm) absence of a phalanx on a finger or toe.

hypopharynx (hi″po-far′inks) laryngopharynx.

hypophonesis (hi″po-fo-ne′sis) diminution of the sound in auscultation or percussion.

hypophonia (hi″po-fo-ne′ah) a weak voice due to incoordination of the vocal muscles.

hypophoria (hi″po-for′e-ah) HETEROPHORIA in which there is permanent downward deviation of the visual axis of an eye in the absence of visual stimuli.

hypophosphatasia (hi″po-fos″fah-ta′zhah) an inborn ERROR of metabolism marked by abnormally low serum ALKALINE PHOSPHATASE activity; it is manifested by RICKETS in infants and children and by OSTEOMALACIA in adults. It is most severe in babies under six months of age.

hypophosphatemia (hi″po-fos″fah-te′me-ah) deficiency of phosphates in the blood; see also HYPOPHOSPHATASIA. adj., **hypophosphate′mic.**

hypophosphaturia (hi″po-fos″fah-tu′re-ah) abnormally decreased levels of urinary phosphate.

hypophrenic (hi″po-fren′ik) below the diaphragm.

hypophyseal (hi″po-fiz′e-al) pituitary (def. 1).

hypophysectomy (hi-pof′ĭ-sek′to-me) surgical removal of part or all of the PITUITARY GLAND (hypophysis), usually a surgical procedure but sometimes done chemically by injection of alcohol into the SELLA TURCICA. The primary indication is as treatment for a pituitary tumor. Because of its influence on the adrenal CORTEX and other endocrine glands, removal of a portion of the pituitary gland can reduce the hypoglycemic effects of CORTICOTROPIN, THYROTROPIN, and PROLACTIN. Similarly, malignancies of the BREAST or PROSTATE that are sensitive to hormones respond to removal of the pituitary hormones that stimulate the breast, ovaries, prostate, and adrenal glands. Elimination of these secondary hormones creates an environment hostile to the tumor cells. Hypophysectomy does not cure the malignancy but does help relieve the pain associated with growth of the tumor. The procedure is also under investigation as a treatment for diabetic RETINOPATHY. (See accompanying illustration.)

hypophyseoportal (hi″po-fiz″e-o-por′tal) hypophysioportal.

hypophysial (hi″po-fiz′e-al) pituitary (def. 1).

hypophysioportal (hi″po-fiz″e-o-por′tal) pertaining to the portal system of the PITUITARY GLAND, in which hypothalamic venules connect with capillaries of the anterior pituitary. Also spelled hypophyseoportal.

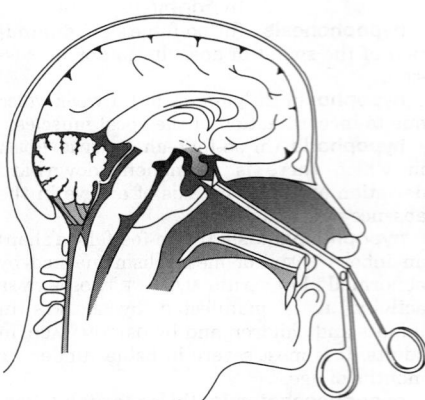

A transsphenoidal hypophysectomy. This approach leaves normal pituitary tissue undisturbed. From Ignatavicius and Workman, 2002.

hypophysioprivic (hi″po-fiz″e-o-priv′ik) due to deficiency of hormonal secretion of the pituitary gland.

hypophysis (hi-pof′ĭ-sis) [Gr.] pituitary gland.

hypopigmentation (hi″po-pig″men-ta′shun) abnormally decreased pigmentation resulting from decreased melanin production.

hypopituitarism (hi″po-pĭ-too′ĭ-tah-rizm) the condition resulting from diminution or cessation of hormonal secretion by the pituitary gland, especially the anterior pituitary. Symptoms vary with the degree of dysfunction.

hypoplasia (hi″po-pla′zhah) incomplete development or underdevelopment of an organ or tissue. adj., **hypoplas′tic.**

focal dermal h. a hereditary disorder found exclusively in females, transmitted as an X-linked dominant trait, characterized typically by linear areas of hypoplasia of the skin with herniation of underlying tissue through the defects; TELANGIECTASIAS; linear or reticular areas of skin discoloration; localized superficial fatty deposits in the skin; papillomas of mucous membranes or skin around various orifices; and anomalies of the extremities, including webbed FINGERS and TOES and absence of some or all of the digits (oligodactyly or adactyly). There may also be other defects affecting the eyes, teeth, or other body systems. Called also Goltz syndrome.

hypoplastic left heart syndrome congenital hypoplasia or atresia of the left VENTRICLE, the aortic or mitral VALVE, and the ascending AORTA, with respiratory distress, cardiac failure, and death in infancy.

hypoplasty (hi′po-plas″te) hypoplasia.

hypopnea (hi-pop′ne-ah) abnormal decrease in depth and rate of respiration; see also BRADYPNEA and HYPOVENTILATION. adj., **hypopne′ic.**

hypoporosis (hi″po-po-ro′sis) deficient callus formation after bone fracture.

hypoposia (hi″po-po′ze-ah) abnormally diminished ingestion of fluids.

hypopotassemia (hi″po-pot″ah-se′me-ah) hypokalemia.

hypopraxia (hi″po-prak′se-ah) abnormally diminished activity.

hypoprosody (hi″po-pros′o-de) diminution of the normal variation of stress, pitch, and rhythm of speech.

hypoproteinemia (hi″po-pro″te-ne′me-ah) deficiency of protein in the blood.

hypoprothrombinemia (hi″po-pro-throm″bĭ-ne′me-ah) deficiency of prothrombin in the blood.

hypopselaphesia (hi″pop-sel″ah-fe′zhah) dullness of tactile sensitiveness.

hypoptyalism (hi″po-ti′ah-lizm) abnormally decreased SALIVATION, as in XEROSTOMIA.

hypopyon (hi-po′pe-on) pus in the anterior chamber of the eye.

hyporeactive (hi″po-re-ak′tiv) showing less than normal response to stimuli.

hyporeflexia (hi″po-re-flek′se-ah) diminution or weakening of reflexes.

hyporeninemia (hi″po-re′nin-e′me-ah) low levels of RENIN in the blood.

hyposalemia (hi″po-sah-le′me-ah) diminution of salt levels in the blood.

hyposalivation (hi″po-sal′ĭ-va′shun) hypoptyalism.

hyposcleral (hi″po-skle′ral) beneath the sclera.

hyposecretion (hi″po-se-kre′shun) diminished secretion.

hyposensitivity (hi″po-sen″sĭ-tiv′ĭ-te) 1. abnormally decreased sensitivity. 2. the state of being less sensitive to a specific allergen after repeated and gradually increasing doses of the offending substance. adj., **hyposen′sitive.**

hyposensitization (hi″po-sen″sĭ-tĭ-za′shun) desensitization.

hyposexuality (hi″po-sek″shoo-al′ĭ-te) abnormally decreased sexual desire.

hyposmia (hi-poz′me-ah) diminished sensitivity of smell.

hyposmolarity (hi-poz″mo-lar′ĭ-te) abnormally decreased osmolar concentration of a solution.

hyposomatotropism (hi″po-so″mah-to-tro′pizm) deficient secretion of somatotropin (growth hormone) or secretion of inactive somatotropin, resulting in short stature.

hyposomnia (hi″po-som′ne-ah) reduced time of sleep.

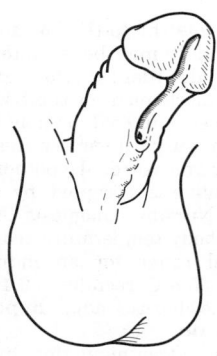

Hypospadias with chordee. From Dorland's, 2000.

hypospadiac (hi″po-spa′de-ak) 1. pertaining to hypospadias. 2. a person affected with hypospadias.

hypospadias (hi″po-spa′de-as) a developmental anomaly in which the urethra opens inferior to its normal position, usually in males with the opening on the underside of the penis or on the perineum. In *perineal hypospadias* the opening on the perineum is accompanied by severe deformity of the penis and testes so that the individual has male pseudohermaphroditism.

female h. a developmental anomaly in the female in which the urethra opens into the vagina.

hypospermatogenesis (hi″po-sper″mah-to-gen′ĕ-sis) abnormally decreased production of SPERMATOZOA; see also ASPERMATOGENESIS.

hyposplenism (hi″po-splen′izm) diminished functioning of the spleen.

hypostasis (hi-pos′tah-sis) poor or stagnant circulation, often with a deposit or sediment, in a dependent part of the body or an organ.

hypostatic (hi″po-stat′ik) 1. pertaining to, due to, or associated with HYPOSTASIS. 2. pertaining to certain inherited traits that are particularly liable to be suppressed by other traits; see EPISTASIS.

hyposthenia (hi″pos-the′ne-ah) diminished strength or tonicity. adj., **hyposthen′ic.**

hyposthenuria (hi″pos-thĕ-nu′re-ah) excretion of urine of low specific gravity.

hypostomia (hi″po-sto′me-ah) a developmental ANOMALY characterized by abnormal smallness of the mouth, the slit being vertical instead of horizontal.

hypostypsis (hi″po-stip′sis) moderate astringency. adj., **hypostyp′tic.**

hyposynergia (hi″po-sĭ-ner′je-ah) defective coordination.

hypotelorism (hi″po-te′lo-rizm) abnormally decreased distance between two organs or parts.

ocular h., orbital h. abnormal decrease in the intraocular distance.

hypotension (hi″po-ten′shun) diminished tension; lowered BLOOD PRESSURE. A consistently low blood pressure (systolic pressure less than 100 mm of mercury) usually is no cause for concern. In fact, low blood pressure often is associated with long life. However, extremely low blood pressure may be a sign of a serious condition such as SHOCK, massive HEMORRHAGE, HYPOVOLEMIA, or severe DEHYDRATION from nausea and vomiting. In shock there is a disproportion between the blood volume and the capacity of the CIRCULATORY SYSTEM, resulting in greatly reduced blood pressure. Hypotension may also be associated with ADDISON'S DISEASE or inadequate THYROID function, but in both cases the primary disease produces so many other symptoms that the hypotension is not a major focus for concern.

orthostatic h., postural h. a fall in blood pressure (usually defined as a 20 to 30 point change in pulse or blood pressure), associated with dizziness, syncope, and blurred vision, occurring when a person goes from lying down or sitting to standing; it can be acquired or idiopathic, transient or chronic, and may occur alone or secondary to a disorder of the central nervous system such as the SHY-DRAGER SYNDROME.

supine h. vena caval syndrome.

hypotensive (hi″po-ten′siv) 1. characterized by or causing diminished tension or pressure, as abnormally low blood pressure. 2. a person with abnormally low blood pressure.

hypotensor (hi″po-ten′ser) a substance that lowers the blood pressure.

hypothalamus (hi″po-thal′ah-mus) the portion of the diencephalon lying beneath the thalamus at the base of the cerebrum, and forming the floor and part of the lateral wall of the third ventricle. Anatomically, it includes the optic chiasm, mammillary bodies, tuber cinereum, infundibulum, and pituitary gland (hypophysis), but for physiologic purposes, the pituitary gland is considered a distinct structure. adj., **hypothalam′ic.**

The hypothalamus may be divided into four regions: the *dorsal region,* consisting of the nucleus of the lenticular ansa; the *anterior region,* consisting of the lateral and medial preoptic nuclei, the supraoptic and paraventricular nuclei, and the anterior hypothalamic nucleus; the *intermediate region,* consisting of the arcuate and tuberal nuclei, the lateral hypothalamic area, and the ventromedial, dorsomedial, and dorsal hypothalamic nuclei; and the *posterior region*, consisting of the lateral and medial nuclei of the mammillary body and the posterior hypothalamic nucleus. The hypothalamic nuclei activate, control, and integrate many of the involuntary functions necessary for living. The various hypothalamic centers influence peripheral autonomic mechanisms, endocrine activity, and many somatic functions, such as a general regulation of water balance, body temperature, sleep, thirst, and hunger, and the development of secondary sex characters.

Because of its influence on the release and inhibition of pituitary hormones, the hypothalamus indirectly plays an important role in the regulation of protein, fat, and carbohydrate metabolism, body fluid volume and electrolyte content, and internal secretion of endocrine hormones. The hormones synthesized and secreted by the special neurons of the hypothalamus are called *hypothalamic releasing hormones* or *factors* and *hypothalamic inhibiting hormones* or *factors* (see accompanying table); they act directly on the tissues of the pituitary gland. There are also stimulating and inhibiting factors that influence the release and retention of other anterior pituitary hormones.

The hypothalamic hormones or factors are secreted directly into the veins in the lower part of the hypothalamus and are transported directly to the tissues of the pituitary gland. This transportation network is called the *hypothalamo-hypophysial portal system*. The secretion of the hypothalamic hormones is a part of a regulatory negative FEEDBACK system that continuously operates to maintain homeostasis.

hypothenar (hi-poth'ĕ-ner) 1. the fleshy eminence on the palm along the ulnar margin. 2. relating to this eminence.

hypothermia (hi″po-ther′me-ah) low body temperature; it may be symptomatic of a disease or disorder of the temperature-regulating mechanism of the body, may be due to exposure to cold, or may be induced for certain surgical procedures or as a therapeutic measure. Hypothermia is a NURSING DIAGNOSIS accepted by the North American Nursing Diagnosis Association, defined as body temperature reduced below the normal range for an individual but not below 35.6°C rectally (36.4°C rectally for the newborn). adj., **hypother′mic.**

Emergency treatment for hypothermia includes administration of warm intravenous fluid and use of esophageal rewarming tubes and special rewarming blankets. Resuscitation efforts such as cardiopulmonary resuscitation should continue until the patient is warmed to a normal core temperature; if there is no other change, the patient may be pronounced dead.

accidental h. unintended lowering of body heat due to prolonged exposure to cold. Hypothermia is a chilling of the entire body, but the extremities can withstand temperatures as much as 10 to 15°C (20 to 30°F) lower than the torso, where vital organs are located. When the core temperature drops even a few degrees, physiologic changes can lead to fatal cardiac arrhythmias and respiratory failure. Persons most at risk for accidental hypothermia include the very young, the very thin, the very old, the mentally challenged or emotionally unstable, alcohol and drug abusers, and the homeless. Symptoms range from mild shivering and complaints of feeling chilled to loss of consciousness, absence of reflexes, and barely detectable pulse and respirations.

Prevention and Treatment. Accidental hypothermia can be avoided by eating high-energy foods, exercising when in the cold,

HYPOTHALAMIC HARMONES REGULATING PITUITARY FUNCTION	
TSH–releasing hormone (TRH)	Stimulates release of thyroid–stimulating hormone (TSH) and release of thyroxine (T_4)
Corticotropin–releasing hormone	Stimulates release of corticotropin (ACTH)
Gonadotropin–releasing hormone (GnRH)	Stimulates release of follicle–stimulating hormone (FSH) and luteinizing (LH)

Growth hormone–regulating hormones
  Growth hormone–releasing hormone (GHRH)
  Somatostatin
	Dual control system, one stimulating, the other inhibiting release of growth hormone (GH)

Prolactin–regulating hormones
  Prolactin–inhibiting hormone
  Prolactin–releasing hormone
	Predominant effect is inhibiting release of prolactin
	Stimulates release of prolactin after suckling and acute stress

wearing layers of clothing, and covering the head. From one half to two thirds of the body heat is lost through the head. For persons on a fixed or limited income, suggestions for avoiding hypothermia in a cold home must be realistic. Blankets and quilted covers that snap together to form a snug bag are alternatives to turning up the thermostat. A loose knitted cap worn day and night can help reduce loss of body heat. Persons who live alone may need help in finding another individual or agency that can check on them daily when the outside temperatures are very low.

The diagnosis of hypothermia may be missed if a clinical thermometer such as the kind used to measure fever is employed to determine the core temperature of a potential hypothermia victim. These thermometers rarely register temperatures below 34.5°C (94.1°F), while the patient's actual temperature can be as low as 30°C (86°F). Emergency departments should be equipped with special monitoring equipment that gives a true picture of the body temperature.

Once hypothermia is diagnosed, rewarming is indicated. Outside a medical facility the rewarming should be gradual so as to avoid respiratory and cardiac problems associated with rapidly sending cold blood back to the heart. The torso is warmed first by wrapping it in warm blankets or submersion in a tepid bath. Once the core temperature reaches 35°C (95°F), the extremities are warmed.

environmental h. accidental hyperthermia due to heat loss due to a combination of convection, conduction, and radiation to the surrounding ambient air.

induced h. deliberate reduction of the temperature of all or part of the body; sometimes used as an adjunct to anesthesia in surgical procedures involving a limb, and as a protective measure in cardiac and neurologic surgery. The hypothermia may be continued only for the duration of the operation or it may be prolonged for as long as 5 days, depending on the reason for its use. See also hypothermia TREATMENT.

Local Hypothermia. This is a type of refrigeration ANESTHESIA restricted to a part of the body, such as a limb. It usually is used to produce surgical anesthesia immediately before amputation. Advantages include minimal risk of shock, lowering of cell metabolism, and elimination of the need for inhalation anesthesia in patients who are poor surgical risks. The part to be anesthetized is packed in ice or wrapped in a special refrigeration unit consisting of coiled tubes. Tourniquets are applied to the limb to inhibit circulation and avoid general chilling of the patient. The limb is chilled for 3 to 5 hours before amputation.

General Hypothermia. Generalized lowering of the body temperature decreases the metabolism of tissues and thereby the need for oxygen; it is used in various surgical procedures, especially on the heart. The core temperature is maintained between 26°C and 32°C (78.8°F and 89.6°F).

To induce general hypothermia, the patient is wrapped in a cooling blanket containing coils through which cold water or an antifreeze, or both, are circulated. The fastest method for achieving hypothermia is extracorporeal cooling of the blood; the patient's blood is removed through a cannula inserted in a large vessel, circulated through refrigerated coils and returned via another cannulated vessel.

Rewarming of the patient is accomplished simply by removing cooling blankets and allowing the temperature to rise gradually and naturally. In most cases regular blankets are used to maintain body warmth. External heat in the form of hot water bottles or warm tub baths, if used at all, must be applied with extreme caution to avoid burning the patient.

Patient Care. During hypothermia and the rewarming process the patient's temperature, pulse, respiration, and blood pressure must be checked frequently. Special electronic thermometers are often used so that the body temperature can be monitored at all times. In prolonged hypothermia, cardiac irregularities or respiratory difficulties may develop quickly; the patient must be watched constantly for changes in the vital signs, and any changes must be reported immediately. The skin also should be observed for signs of developing pressure ulcers, edema, or marked discoloration.

The patient should be turned at least every 2 hours, with special attention to proper positioning and good body alignment. Decreased secretion of saliva and mouth-breathing demand frequent mouth care. The eyes may need to be irrigated frequently and covered with compresses moistened with physiologic saline solution or artificial tears if the corneal reflex is diminished and eye secretions are reduced.

Intake and output are measured and recorded. An indwelling catheter is inserted prior to induction of hypothermia and is left in place until normal body temperature is established. This is necessary because urinary output is diminished during hypothermia. Fluids are given intravenously and the oral intake of food and liquids is prohibited because of depression of the gag reflex.

Shivering during prolonged hypothermia must be avoided as it tends to elevate the body temperature and increase metabolic needs, thereby defeating the purpose of hypothermia.

During the rewarming process the patient must be observed for signs of increased tendency to bleed and of gastric distention; these are common complications. After the body temperature returns to normal and becomes stabilized, the patient is allowed to progress to a normal diet and physical activities.

moderate h. body temperature of 23° to 32°C, resulting from surface cooling.

profound h. body temperature of 12° to 20°C.

regional h. temperature reduction in a limb or organ resulting from application of external cold or perfusion with a cold solution.

symptomatic h. pathologic reduction of body temperature as a result of decreased heat production or increased heat loss. Hypothyroidism, severe blood loss with circulatory failure, and damage to the heat-producing cells of the hypothalamus can lead to decreased heat production. Prolonged exposure to cold, overdosage of antipyretic drugs, such as aspirin, and profuse sweating (diaphoresis) are some causes of increased heat loss and resultant hypothermia.

hypothesis (hi-poth′ĕ-sis) a supposition that appears to explain a group of phenomena and is advanced as a bases for further investigation.

alternative h. the hypothesis that is formulated as an opposite to the null hypothesis in a statistical test.

complex h. a prediction of the relationship between two or more independent variables and two or more dependent variables.

directional h. a statement of the specific nature (direction) of the relationship between two or more variables.

Lyon h. a hypothesis about development of X chromosomes in the embryo; see LYON HYPOTHESIS.

Monro-Kellie h. (mun-ro′ kel′e) an explanation of the maintenance of intracranial pressure: The skull is viewed as a closed container housing brain tissue, blood, and cerebrospinal fluid; a change in any of these three components will affect the other two. If the volume added to the cranial vault is equal to the volume displaced, the intracranial volume will not change.

nondirectional h. a statement that a relationship exists between two variables, without predicting the exact nature (direction) of the relationship.

null h. the hyothesis that the effect, relationship, or other manifestation of variables and data under investigation does not exist; an example would be the hypothesis that there is no difference between experimental and control groups in a clinical trial.

h. test the abstract procedure that is the theoretical basis of most statistical tests. A hypothesis test decides between two hypotheses, the *null hypothesis* (H_0) that the effect under investigation does not exist and the *alternative hypothesis* (H_1) that some specified effect does exist, based on the observed value of a *test statistic* whose sampling distribution is completely determined by H_0. The decision is made to reject H_0 and by implication to accept H_1 when the test statistic falls within a given set of values called the *critical region*. This region is so determined that the probability of rejecting H_0 when it is in fact true (a so-called *Type I error,* the reporting as significant results that are only the result of random variation and not a real effect), is set at a specified level (symbol α). When this level is set before the data are collected, usually at 0.05 or 0.01, it is called the *significance level* or α *level*. It is now more common to report the smallest α at which the null hypothesis can be rejected; this is called the *significance probability* or *P value.* The ability of the test to accept a true alternative (and thus to detect a real effect when it exists) is termed the *power* of the test. Note that no statistical test actually tests the H_1.

hypothrombinemia (hi″po-throm″bīne′-me-ah) deficiency of thrombin in the blood, resulting in a tendency to bleed.

hypothymia (hi″po-thi′me-ah) abnormally diminished emotional tone, as in depression. adj., **hypothy′mic.**

hypothymism (hi″po-thi′mizm) diminished thymus activity.

hypothyroid marked by deficiency of THYROID activity; called also thyroprival and thyroprivic.

hypothyroidism (hi″po-thi′roi-dizm) deficiency of THYROID GLAND activity, with underproduction of THYROXINE, or the condition resulting from it. In its severe form it is called MYXEDEMA and is characterized by physical and mental sluggishness, obesity, loss of hair, enlargement of the tongue, and thickening of the skin. In children the condition is known as CRETINISM. Called also athyria. adj., **hypothy′roid.**

pituitary h. secondary hypothyroidism caused by a defect or lesion of the PITUITARY GLAND that interferes with production of THYROTROPIN; the majority of cases are caused by tumors.

primary h. hypothyroidism due to disease of the thyroid gland itself, usually accompanied by increased levels of THYROTROPIN.

secondary h. that caused by THYROTROPIN deficiency.

hypotonia (hi″po-to′ne-ah) abnormally decreased tonicity or strength.

hypotonic (hi″po-ton′ik) 1. having an abnormally reduced tonicity or tension. 2. having an osmotic pressure lower than that of the solution with which it is compared.

hypotoxicity (hi″po-tok-sis′ĭte) abnormally reduced toxic quality.

hypotransferrinemia (hi″po-trans-fer″ĭ-ne′me-ah) deficiency of transferrin in the blood.

hypotrichosis (hi″po-trĭ-ko′sis) presence of less than the normal amount of hair.

hypotrophy (hi-pot′ro-fe) abiotrophy.

hypotropia (hi″po-tro′pe-ah) vertical STRABISMUS in which there is permanent downward deviation of the visual axis of one eye.

hypotympanotomy (hi″po-tim″pah-not′-ah-me) surgical opening of the hypotympanum.

hypotympanum (hi″po-tim′pah-num) the lower part of the cavity of the middle ear, in the temporal bone.

hypouricemia (hi″po-u″rĭ-se′me-ah) deficiency of uric acid in the blood, along with xanthinuria, due to deficiency of xanthine oxidase, the enzyme required for conversion of hypoxanthine to xanthine and of xanthine to uric acid.

hypoventilation (hi″po-ven″tĭ-la′shun) a state in which there is a reduced amount of air entering the pulmonary alveoli (decreased alveolar VENTILATION), which causes an increase in arterial CARBON DIOXIDE level. See also HYPOPNEA and BRADYPNEA.

hypovitaminosis (hi″po-vi″tah-mĭno′sis) a condition produced by lack of an essential VITAMIN.

hypovolemia (hi″po-vo-le′me-ah) abnormally decreased volume of circulating blood in the body; see also hypovolemic SHOCK. adj., **hypovole′mic.**

hypovolia (hi″po-vo′le-ah) diminished water content or volume, as of extracellular fluid.

hypoxanthine (hi″po-zan′thēn) an intermediate product of uric acid synthesis, formed from adenylic acid and itself a precursor of xanthine.

hypoxemia (hi″pok-se′me-ah) deficient oxygenation of the blood. The most reliable

method for measuring the degree of hypoxemia is BLOOD GAS ANALYSIS to determine the partial pressure of oxygen in the arterial blood. Insufficient oxygenation of the blood may lead to HYPOXIA.

hypoxia (hi-pok′se-ah) diminished availability of OXYGEN to the body tissues; its causes are many and varied and includes a deficiency of oxygen in the atmosphere, as in ALTITUDE SICKNESS; pulmonary disorders that interfere with adequate ventilation of the lungs; anemia or circulatory deficiencies, leading to inadequate transport and delivery of oxygen to the tissues; and finally, edema or other abnormal conditions of the tissues themselves that impair the exchange of oxygen and carbon dioxide between capillaries and tissues. adj., **hypox′ic.**

Signs and symptoms vary according to the cause. Generally they include dyspnea, rapid pulse, syncope, and mental disturbances such as delirium or euphoria. CYANOSIS is not always present and in some cases is not evident until the hypoxia is far advanced. The localized pain of ANGINA PECTORIS due to hypoxia occurs because of impaired oxygenation of the myocardium. Discoloration of the skin and eventual ulceration that sometimes accompany varicose veins are a result of hypoxia of the involved tissues.

The *treatment* of hypoxia depends on the primary cause but usually includes administration of oxygen by inhalation (see OXYGEN THERAPY). In some vascular diseases, administration of VASODILATORS may help increase circulation, hence oxygen supply, to the tissues.

affinity h. hypoxia resulting from failure of the hemoglobin to release oxygen to the tissues, as may occur with a left-shifted oxyhemoglobin dissociation curve.

anemic h. hypoxia due to reduction of the oxygen-carrying capacity of the blood as a result of a decrease in the total hemoglobin or an alteration of the hemoglobin constituents.

circulatory h. stagnant hypoxia.

histotoxic h. that due to impaired utilization of oxygen by tissues, as in cyanide poisoning.

hypoxemic h., hypoxic h. that due to insufficient oxygen reaching the blood, as at the decreased barometric pressures of high altitudes.

stagnant h. that due to failure to transport sufficient oxygen because of inadequate blood flow, as in heart failure.

hypromellose (hi-pro′mə-lōs) a PROPYLENE GLYCOL ether of METHYLCELLULOSE, supplied in differing degrees of viscosity; used as a suspending and viscosity-increasing agent and tablet binder, coating, and EXCIPIENT in pharmaceutical preparations, and applied topically to the conjunctiva to protect and lubricate the cornea. Called also *hydroxypropyl methylcellulose.*

   h. phthalate a phthalic acid ester of hydroxypropyl methylcellulose, used as a coating agent for tablets and granules.

hyps(o)- word element [Gr.], *height.*

hypsarhythmia (hip″sah-rith′me-ah) hypsarrhythmia.

hypsarrhythmia (hip″sah-rith′me-ah) a term for an electroencephalographic abnormality sometimes observed in infants, with random high-voltage slow waves and spikes arising from multiple foci and spreading to all cortical areas; the disorder is characterized by spasms or quivering spells, and is commonly associated with mental retardation.

hypsokinesis (hip″so-kĭ-ne′sis) a backward swaying or falling in erect posture, seen in PARKINSON'S DISEASE and other neurologic disorders.

hyster(o)- word element [Gr.], *uterus; hysteria.*

hysteralgia (his″tĕ-ral′jah) pain in the uterus; called also hysterodynia.

hysteratresia (his″ter-ah-tre′zhah) atresia of the uterus.

hysterectomy (his″tĕ-rek′to-me) surgical removal of the UTERUS. Within the past decade this has become a common major surgery in the United States. Controversy continues over whether many hysterectomies are really necessary. In making the decision for hysterectomy, patients often seek a second medical opinion and are encouraged to discuss options with health care givers and family members. Clinical indications for hysterectomy include pelvic relaxation; pain associated with congestion, endometriosis, or chronic pelvic inflammatory disease; fibroid tumors; recurrent ovarian cysts; excessive and debilitating bleeding; and cervical, ovarian, and uterine malignancies, premalignancy, and other high-risk conditions.

Potential Complications. Whether the surgery is vaginal or abdominal will affect the location of the surgical site and incidence of complications. In general, abdominal incisions are made horizontally and low in the abdomen just above the symphysis. The vaginal route usually is chosen when a patient is obese, when abdominal scarring from previous surgery is present, and for removal of a prolapsed uterus or one in which stage 0 cancer is localized in the cervix.

Incisions made above and around the cervix in vaginal hysterectomy heal more rapidly than do abdominal incisions, and intestinal complications such as ileus are less likely. However, vaginal hysterectomy patients have a higher incidence of postoperative bleeding and infections, especially of the urinary tract.

Patient Care. Two major areas of concern in the care of patients having a hysterectomy are psychosocial implications and physical care during the perioperative period.

Psychosocial Implications. The psychosocial impact of removal of the uterus is a major concern of professional caregivers. Patients may be misinformed about basic anatomical and physiological features of the female reproductive tract and the functions of the uterus, fallopian tubes, and ovaries, or they may not know the effects of the contemplated surgery and are anxious about how it might influence their roles as women.

There should be sufficient time to determine what the patient knows, to answer her questions, and to dispel any misinformation she might have. Preoperative teaching does not necessarily mean that it is done the night before surgery. In fact, at that time the patient may be preoccupied with anxieties about major surgery and fears about pain and perhaps death. In that state of mind she would probably be unable to assimilate most factual information presented to her. At this point relieving the patient's anxiety is a top priority.

A patient's ability to adjust to the loss of a reproductive organ will be influenced by her sense of self as a woman, her age and previous socialization in regard to the roles of women, and the attitudes and expectations of her spouse, family and friends. Negative or positive attitudes can arise from her beliefs about how the surgery will affect her sexual expression and function and her vocational and avocational involvement and enjoyment of life. If the woman has experienced long-term pain and discomfort or has no desire to have more children, she may be favorably disposed toward the surgery. However, she may feel a profound sense of loss and purpose in her life. Negative attitudes toward the hysterectomy can have serious and adverse psychologic effects months or even years after the surgery.

Physical Care After Surgery. Measures such as coughing, turning, deep breathing, and early ambulation to avoid circulatory and respiratory stasis are appropriate whether the hysterectomy is abdominal or vaginal.

Bleeding is a potential danger because of the abundant vascularity of the female pelvis. Dressings and perineal pads are checked regularly every two to four hours, or more often as indicated. The patient who has had vaginal surgery usually has a vaginal packing with a drain attached to the distal end. Some vaginal bleeding and oozing of serosanguineous fluid can be expected, but if there is frank bleeding of more than a light menstrual flow, or if the patient is passing clots around the pack, there is cause for concern. Heavy bleeding, a rapidly distended abdomen, referred shoulder pain, and change in vital signs are signs of an emergency that requires a return to the operating room to find and stop the source of blood loss.

Patients with an abdominal incision are monitored and dressings checked for excessive bleeding. If there is evidence of increasingly larger deposits of blood on the dressing, reinforcement of the dressing and notification of the surgeon are indicated.

The urinary output and characteristics of the urine are observed for signs of urinary tract infection. If the patient has an indwelling catheter, special catheter care is necessary. A poorly draining catheter or one that is totally blocked can lead to bladder distention and abdominal pressure. To avoid additional pressure on the abdomen and sutures, the patient is positioned on her side or back with her knees slightly flexed. High Fowler's position is contraindicated and there should be no pillows or break in the bed to produce pressure behind the knees.

Prior to discharge from the hospital the patient is given instructions in self-care; these should be written so that the patient can refer to them at home if necessary. They should include information about surgical menopause and estrogen therapy if the ovaries were removed; restrictions on douching and sexual intercourse; prevention of constipation; care of the incision; and reportable symptoms such as redness, swelling, pain, or drainage at the operative site and elevation of body temperature. Abdominal cramps and changes in bowel habits also should be reported to the professional caregiver.

The patient should also have opportunities to discuss personal contacts regarding sexual activity and her new body image. Although this may have been discussed during the preoperative period, she may be more receptive after the surgery is over and she is on the way to recovery. Some hospitals and clinics have support groups for women contemplating or recovering

from hysterectomy. These can be a great support to patients and provide them with additional information and a forum for expressing and dealing with their emotional reactions to hysterectomy.

abdominal h. that performed through the abdominal wall. Called also abdominohysterectomy and laparohysterectomy.

cesarean h. cesarean section followed by removal of the uterus.

radical h. hysterectomy with excision of the pelvic lymph nodes and wide lateral excision of parametrial and paravaginal supporting structures.

subtotal h. that in which the cervix is left in place.

total h. that in which the uterus and cervix are completely excised.

vaginal h. that performed through the vagina.

hysteresis (his-tĕ-re′sis) 1. the failure of coincidence of two associated phenomena, such as that exhibited in the differing temperatures of gelation and of liquefaction of a reversible colloid. 2. a phenomenon exhibited by a physical system in which the system's response to an outside influence depends not only on the instantaneous magnitude of the influence but also on the system's previous history, as when a material undergoing cyclical loading exhibits a loss of energy between cycles of loading and unloading. 3. in cardiac PACING terminology, the number of pulses per minute below the programmed pacing rate that the heart must drop in order to cause initiation of pacing; it can be programmed in by a pulse GENERATOR.

hystereurysis (his″ter-u′rĭ-sis) dilation of the ostium uteri.

hysteria (his-ter′e-ah) a now somewhat nebulous term formerly used widely in psychiatry. Its meanings included *classic hysteria* (now called SOMATIZATION DISORDER); *hysterical neurosis* (now divided into CONVERSION DISORDER and DISSOCIATIVE DISORDERS); and *hysterical personality* (now called HISTRIONIC PERSONALITY). adj. **hyster′ic, hyster′ical.**

hysterics (his-ter′iks) popular term for an uncontrollable emotional outburst.

hysterocele (his′ter-o-sēl″) hernia of the uterus.

hysterocleisis (his″ter-o-kli′sis) surgical closure of the ostium uteri.

hysterodynia (his″ter-o-din′e-ah) hysteralgia.

hysteroepilepsy (his″ter-o-ep′ĭ-lep″se) hysteria with attacks imitating epileptic seizures.

hysterography (his″tĕ-rog′rah-fe) 1. the graphic recording of the strength of uterine contractions in labor. 2. radiography of the uterus after instillation of a contrast medium.

hysteroid (his″ter-oid) resembling hysteria.

hysterolith (his′ter-o-lith″) uterine calculus.

hysterolysis (his″ter-ol′ĭ-sis) freeing of the uterus from adhesions.

hysterometry (his″tĕ-rom′ē-tre) measurement of the uterus.

hysteromyoma (his″ter-o-mi-o′mah) leiomyoma of the uterus.

hysteromyomectomy (his″ter-o-mi″o-mek′tah-me) local excision of a leiomyoma of the uterus.

hysteromyotomy (his″ter-o-mi-ot′ah-me) incision of the uterus.

hysteropathy (his″tĕ-rop′ah-the) any uterine disease; called also metropathy.

hysteropexy (his′ter-o-pek″se) fixation of a displaced uterus by surgery.

hysteroptosis (his″ter-op-to′sis) prolapse of the uterus.

hysterorrhaphy (his″ter-or′ah-fe) 1. suture of the uterus. 2. hysteropexy.

hysterorrhexis (his″ter-o-rek′sis) rupture of the uterus.

hysterosalpingectomy (his″ter-o-sal″pin-jek′tah-me) excision of the uterus and fallopian tubes.

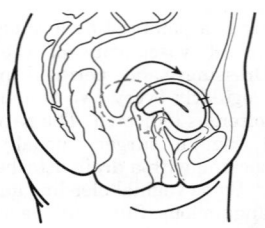

Hysteropexy, with fixation to the anterior abdominal wall. From Dorland's, 2000.

hysterosalpingography (his″ter-o-sal″-ping-gog′-rah-fe) radiography of the uterus and fallopian tubes.

hysterosalpingo-oophorectomy (his″ter-o-sal-ping″go-o″of-o-rek′tah-me) excision of the uterus, fallopian tubes, and ovaries.

hysterosalpingostomy (his″ter-o-sal″-ping-gos′tah-me) anastomosis of a fallopian tube and the uterus.

hysteroscope (his′ter-o-skōp″) an endoscope used in direct visual examination of the canal of the uterine cervix and the cavity of the uterus.

hysterospasm (his′ter-o-spazm) spasm of the uterus.

hysterotomy (his″ter-ot′ah-me) incision of the uterus.

abdominal h. incision of the uterus through the wall of the abdomen. Called also abdominohysterotomy and laparohysterotomy.

Hz hertz.

I

I incisor; iodine; inosine (in nucleotides).

-ia word element, *state; condition.*

IAET International Association for Enterostomal Therapy.

-iasis word element [Gr.], *condition; state.*

iatr(o)- word element [Gr.], *medicine; physician.*

iatric (i-at'rik) pertaining to medicine or to a physician.

iatrogenic (i-at″ro-jen'ik) resulting from the activity of a health care provider or institution; said of any adverse condition in a patient resulting from treatment by a physician, nurse, or allied health professional.

ibuprofen (i-bu'pro-fen) a NONSTEROIDAL ANTIINFLAMMATORY DRUG used as an ANALGESIC and ANTIPYRETIC and for symptomatic relief of dysmenorrhea, vascular headaches, rheumatoid ARTHRITIS, OSTEOARTHRITIS, and other rheumatic and nonrheumatic inflammatory disorders. It is similar in action to ASPIRIN but less apt to cause gastrointestinal side effects.

ibritumomab tiuxetan (i″brĭ-tu-mo'mab ti-uk'sĕ-tan) a RADIOPHARMACEUTICAL agent consisting of the monoclonal ANTIBODY RITUXIMAB conjugated with YTTRIUM 90C208; used in treatment of refractory LYMPHOMAS that are positive for CD20 antigen (see CD ANTIGEN).

ibutilide (ĭ-bu'tĭ-līd) a cardiac DEPRESSANT used in treatment of atrial ARRHYTHMIAS; administered by intravenous infusion as the fumarate salt.

IC inspiratory capacity.

ICD International Classification of Diseases (of the World Health Organization); intrauterine contraceptive device; implantable cardioverter-defibrillator.

Iceland disease chronic fatigue syndrome.

I-cell disease mucolipidosis II.

ICF intermediate care facility.

ichthammol (ik'tham-ol) an ammoniated coal tar product, used in ointment form for certain skin diseases.

ichthyoid (ik'the-oid) fishlike.

ichthyology (ik″the-ol'o-je) the study of fish.

ichthyophagous (ik″the-of'ah-gus) eating or subsisting on fish.

ichthyosarcotoxin (ik″the-o-sahr'ko-tok″-sin) a toxin found in the flesh of poisonous fishes.

ichthyosarcotoxism (ik″the-o-sahr″ko-tok'sizm) FISH POISONING.

ichthyosis (ik″the-o'sis) any in a group of skin disorders characterized by increased or aberrant KERATINIZATION, resulting in dryness, roughness, and scaliness of the skin. Many descriptive metaphors such as *alligator, collodion, crocodile, fish,* and *porcupine skin* have been used to describe the various types and stages of ichthyosis. Most ichthyoses are genetically determined, but some may be acquired and develop in association with systemic diseases or may be a prominent feature in certain genetic syndromes. The term is commonly used alone to refer to ichthyosis vulgaris. (See Atlas 2, Part L.) adj., **ichthyot'ic.**

i. **conge'nita, congenital *i.*** lamellar EXFOLIATION of newborn.

harlequin i. the ichthyosis affecting a harlequin FETUS.

i. **hys'trix** a rare form of epidermolytic hyperkeratosis marked by generalized, dark brown, linear, wartlike ridges somewhat like porcupine skin.

lamellar i. a congenital, chronic form of ichthyosis present at birth, inherited as an autosomal recessive trait, in which the affected infant is born encased in a collodion-like membrane (see collodion BABY) that is soon shed, the skin then becoming covered with large, coarse scales with involvement of all of the flexures as well as the palms and soles. Universal erythroderma and pruritus are characteristic, and ectropion of variable degree is usually present. Formerly called congenital ichthyosiform erythroderma (nonbullous type). (See Atlas 2, Part K.)

lamellar i. of newborn lamellar exfoliation of newborn.

i. linea'ris circumflex'a a congenital autosomal recessive disorder present at birth, characterized by the presence of generalized redness and scaling of the skin associated with migratory lesions and HYPERHIDROSIS of the palms and soles.

i. vulga'ris the most common form of ichthyosis, inherited as an autosomal dominant trait, having an onset sometime after the first year of life, especially near puberty. There is prominent fine scaling, principally on the extensor surfaces of the extremities and back (the flexures are spared and there is little scaling of the abdomen and face), together with accentuated markings and creases on the palms and soles; atopy is often present.

X-linked i. a chronic form of ichthyosis affecting only males, transmitted as an

X-linked recessive trait, that may be present at birth or appear in early infancy. It is characterized by the presence of prominent, very adherent scales, often brown, especially on the neck, extremities, trunk, and buttocks.

ichthyotoxin (ik'the-o-tok"sin) any toxic substance derived from fish. See also FISH POISONING.

ichthyotoxism (ik"the-o-tok'sizm) any intoxication due to an ICHTHYOTOXIN.

ICN International Council of Nurses.

ICS International College of Surgeons.

ICSH interstitial cell–stimulating hormone (luteinizing hormone).

ICSI intracytoplasmic sperm injection.

ictal (ik'tal) pertaining to, characterized by, or due to a stroke or an acute epileptic seizure.

icteric (ik-ter'ik) pertaining to or affected with jaundice.

icterogenic (ik"ter-o-jen'ik) causing jaundice.

icterohepatitis (ik"ter-o-hep"ah-ti'tis) inflammation of the liver with marked jaundice.

icteroid (ik'ter-oid) resembling jaundice.

icterus (ik'ter-us) jaundice.

   i. neonato'rum jaundice in newborn infants, as seen in ERYTHROBLASTOSIS FETALIS. Called also neonatal jaundice and jaundice of the newborn.

   i. prae'cox mild jaundice developing within the first 24 hours of life (before physiologic jaundice normally occurs), due to ABO blood group incompatibility between mother and infant; it usually clears rapidly and spontaneously, only occasionally resulting in hemolytic disease.

ictus (ik'tus), pl. *ic'tus* [L.] a SEIZURE, stroke, blow, or sudden attack. adj., **ic'tal.**

ICU intensive care unit.

ID infective DOSE.

ID$_{50}$ median infective DOSE.

id (id) a freudian term used to describe that part of the personality which harbors the unconscious, instinctive impulses that lead to immediate gratification of primitive needs such as hunger, the need for air, the need to move about and relieve body tension, and the need to eliminate. Id impulses are physiologic and body processes, as opposed to the EGO and SUPEREGO, which are psychologic and social processes. The id is dominated by the pleasure principle and some gratification of the id impulses is necessary for survival of a person's personality.

   i. reaction a localized or generalized, sterile secondary skin eruption occurring in sensitized patients as a result of circulation of allergenic products from a primary site of infection; the morphology and site of the lesion vary.

-id word element [Gr.], 1. *having the shape of, resembling.* 2. *an* ID REACTION *associated with the disorder specified by the root word.*

Idamycin (i"dah-mi'sin) trademark for a preparation of IDARUBICIN, an antitumor ANTIBIOTIC.

idarubicin (i"dah-roo'bĭ-sin) an antitumor ANTIBIOTIC of the ANTHRACYCLINE group, administered intravenously in the treatment of acute myelogenous LEUKEMIA.

IDDM insulin-dependent diabetes mellitus, former name for type 1 DIABETES MELLITUS.

-ide suffix indicating a binary compound.

idea (i-de'ah) a mental impression or conception.

   autochthonous i. a persistent idea, originating within the mind, usually from the unconscious, but seeming to have come from an outside source and often therefore felt to be of malevolent origin.

   dominant i. one that controls or colors every action and thought.

   fixed i. a persistent morbid impression or belief that cannot be changed by reason.

   overvalued i. a false or exaggerated belief sustained beyond logic or reason but with less rigidity than a delusion, also often being less patently unbelievable.

   i. of reference the incorrect idea that the words and actions of others refer to one's self, or the projection of the causes of one's own imaginary difficulties upon someone else.

ideal (i-de'al) a pattern or concept of perfection.

   ego i. the component of the superego containing the internalized image of what one desires to become, which the ego strives to attain. It is formed through conscious or unconscious identification with a person who plays a significant role or has a place of esteem in the life of the developing child, or through emulation of such a person.

idealization (i-de"al-ĭ-za'shun) a conscious or unconscious mental mechanism in which the individual overestimates an admired aspect or attribute of another person.

ideation (i"de-a'shun) the formation of ideas or images. adj., **idea'tional.**

   suicidal i. recurring thoughts of or preoccupation with SUICIDE.

idée fixe (e-da' fēks') fixed idea.

identification (i-den"tĭ-fī-ka'shun) 1. the defining or ascertaining of something. 2. a largely unconscious process, often a DEFENSE

MECHANISM, by which an individual takes as his or her own the characteristics, postures, achievements, or other identifying traits of other persons or groups. This plays a major role in development of the SUPEREGO and of awareness and acceptance of the standards and rules accepted by society. However, as individuals mature emotionally, their own self-identity should become clearer as they relate more to their own personal achievements and less to the accomplishments and successes of others with whom they identify. Overuse of identification as a defense mechanism denies one the opportunity of enjoying the benefits and self-satisfaction derived from one's own accomplishments. Identification is not to be confused with imitation, which is a conscious process.

risk i. in the NURSING INTERVENTIONS CLASSIFICATION, a nursing INTERVENTION defined as analysis of potential risk FACTORS, determination of health risks, and prioritization of risk reduction strategies for an individual or group.

risk i.: childbearing family in the NURSING INTERVENTIONS CLASSIFICATION, a nursing INTERVENTION defined as the identification of an individual or family likely to experience difficulties in parenting, and prioritization of strategies to prevent parenting problems.

risk i.: genetic in the NURSING INTERVENTIONS CLASSIFICATION, a nursing INTERVENTION defined as identification and analysis of potential genetic risk factors in an individual, family, or group.

identity (i-den′tĭ-te) the aggregate of characteristics by which an individual is recognized by himself and others.

disturbed personal i. a NURSING DIAGNOSIS accepted by the North American Nursing Diagnosis Association, defined as the inability to distinguish between the self and nonself.

gender i. a person's concept of himself or herself as being male and masculine or female and feminine, or ambivalent, usually based on physical characteristics, parental attitudes and expectations, and psychological and social pressures. It is the private experience of gender ROLE.

ideogenetic (i″de-o-jĕ-net′ik) related to mental processes in which images of sense impressions are used, rather than ideas that are ready for verbal expression.

ideology (i″de-ol′o-je, id″e-ol′o-je) 1. the science of the development of ideas. 2. the body of ideas characteristic of an individual or of a social unit.

ideomotion (i″de-o-mo′shun) motion or muscular action induced by a dominant idea rather than by reflex or volition.

idi(o)- word element [Gr.], *self; peculiar to a substance or organism.*

idiocy (id′e-ah-se) old term for profound MENTAL RETARDATION, now considered offensive.

amaurotic familial i. former name for neuronal ceroid-lipofuscinosis.

mongolian i. former name for DOWN SYNDROME or the marked mental retardation associated with it. The term is now considered offensive.

idioglossia (id″e-o-glos′e-ah) imperfect articulation, with utterance of meaningless vocal sounds. adj., **idioglot′tic.**

idiogram (id′e-o-gram) a drawing or photograph of the chromosomes of a particular cell.

idiopathic (id″e-o-path′ik) self-originated; occurring without known cause.

i. disease one that exists without any connection with any known cause.

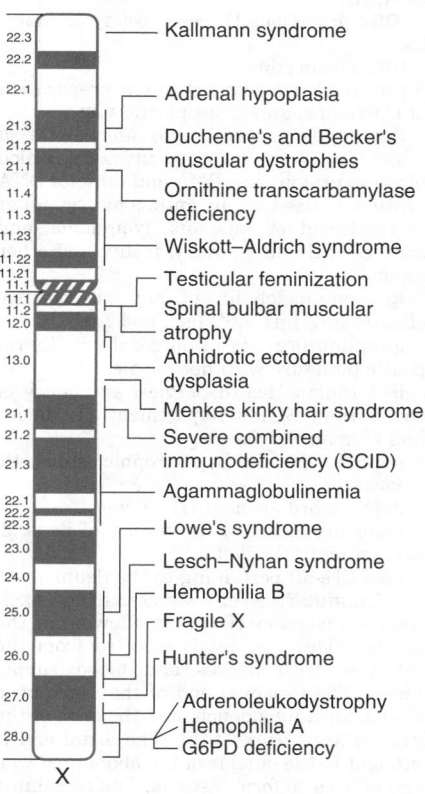

Idiogram of the X chromosome, showing some of the many disorders located on it. From Lissauer and Graham, 2002.

idiopathy (id″e-op′ah-the) a disease state or condition that arises without known cause.

idiosyncrasy (id″e-o-sing′krah-se) 1. a habit or quality of body or mind peculiar to any individual. 2. an abnormal susceptibility to an agent (e.g., a drug) that is peculiar to the individual. adj., **idiosyncrat′ic.**

idiot (id′e-ot) old term for profound MENTAL RETARDATION, now considered offensive.

i. savant a person who is generally mentally retarded, yet has a particular mental faculty developed to an unusually high degree, such as for mathematics or music.

idiotrophic (id″e-o-trof′ik) capable of obtaining its own nourishment.

idioventricular (id″e-o-ven-trik′u-lar) pertaining to the cardiac ventricle alone.

idoxuridine (i″doks-ūr′ĭ-dēn) a PYRIMIDINE analogue that prevents replication of DNA viruses; used topically in HERPES SIMPLEX keratitis.

IDSA Infectious Disease Society of America.

IDU idoxuridine.

Ifex (i′feks) trademark for a preparation of IFOSFAMIDE, an antineoplastic AGENT.

ifosfamide (i-fos′fah-mīd) an ALKYLATING AGENT, one of the NITROGEN MUSTARDS, which binds to protein and DNA and inhibits DNA synthesis. Used as an antineoplastic AGENT in treatment of leukemia, lymphoma, and cancers of the lung, ovary, testes, and other organs.

Ig immunoglobulin of any of the five classes: IgA, IgD, IgE, IgG, and IgM.

ignipuncture (ig″nĭ-pungk′chur) therapeutic puncture with hot needles.

IHS Indian Health Service, an agency of the United States Department of Health and Human Services.

IHSS idiopathic hypertrophic subaortic stenosis.

ile(o)- word element [L.], *ileum.*

ileac (il′e-ak) 1. of the nature of ileus. 2. pertaining to the ileum.

ileal (il′e-al) pertaining to the ileum.

i. conduit use of a segment of the ILEUM for the diversion of urinary flow from the ureters. The segment is resected from the intestine with nerves and blood supply intact. The proximal end of the segment is closed, forming a pouch, and the ends of the ureters are sutured to it. The distal end is brought to the outside of the abdominal wall and effaced to form a stoma. The remaining ends of the small intestine are anastomosed to reestablish bowel continuity, the ileal loop no longer being a part of the intestinal tract. Called also urinary ileostomy, ileal loop, and Bricker procedure.

Indications for an ileal conduit include surgical removal of the bladder for severe trauma or malignancy, congenital defect of the urinary tract, and neurogenic nonfunctioning bladder in which other devices to maintain urinary flow are unsatisfactory.

Prior to surgery, the placement of the stoma is determined by a thorough examination of the abdomen while the patient assumes various body positions. The site is selected so that old scar tissue, skin folds, bony prominences, and the umbilicus are avoided, thus providing a smooth surface for attachment of a drainage bag. Individuals wearing braces for ambulation must have the stoma placed so that there is no pressure on it from the appliance.

Patient Care. Physical care of the patient with urinary diversion via an ileal conduit and collection of the urine outside the body is essentially the same as for any patient with a stoma. The following information is specific to problems of urinary diversion. However, persons with a stoma of any kind share many of the same problems, especially those related to the psychosocial impact of this kind of surgery. These common problems are discussed under STOMA.

Major concerns related to the physical care of a patient with an ileal conduit are peristomal skin care, monitoring urinary flow, control of odor, and selection and care of the collection device.

Protection of the skin around the stoma requires attention to cleanliness and providing a protective barrier to prevent contact between the skin and the urine. Because there is continuous drainage of urine down the ureters from the kidney, there is always the threat of damage to the integrity of the skin from continued exposure to the caustic urine. It is not so much the flow of urine across the skin that is a cause for concern as it is the pooling of stagnant urine on the skin.

Additionally, moisture has a tendency to collect under the faceplate of the collection appliance, thus providing an ideal environment for yeast and mold infections. To avoid this the area is cleaned periodically with soap and water and thoroughly dried. A protective barrier of some type (there are several alternatives) is then applied. Topical medications such as Mycolog ointment, Kenalog spray, or Mycostatin powder may be used to prevent or treat infections.

The appliance usually must be emptied several times a day, depending on fluid intake and whether a leg bag is used to collect the urine. At the time urine is

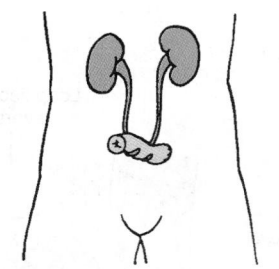

Ileal conduit. From Polaski and Tatro, 1996.

emptied its amount and characteristics are noted in much the same way one observes urine that has collected in the bladder and been voided normally.

The major causes of odor problems in urinary diversion are improper techniques in cleaning and storing appliances, inadequate use of deodorant acidifiers, urinary tract infections, a poor quality collection pouch that allows leakage, and poor basic hygiene. Dietary factors also must be considered as possible causes; for example, asparagus causes a peculiar odor in the urine.

The pouches used for collection of urine usually are cleaned with soap and water and rinsed in a white vinegar solution to help eliminate odor. Manufacturers of collection devices offer detailed instructions for the proper cleaning and storing of reusable appliances.

ileectomy (il″e-ek′to-me) excision of the ileum.

ileitis (il″e-i′tis) inflammation of the ILEUM; it may result from infection, obstruction, severe irritation, or faulty absorption of material through the intestinal walls. See also CROHN'S DISEASE. The advanced stage is marked by hardening, thickening, and ulceration of parts of the bowel lining. An obstruction may cause the development of a fistula. A common symptom of ileitis is pain in the lower right quadrant of the abdomen or around the umbilicus. Other symptoms include loss of appetite, loss of weight, anemia, and diarrhea, which may alternate with periods of constipation. Treatment may require medication to remove any source of infection, special diet, or surgery if there is obstruction.

  distal i. Crohn's disease.

  regional i., terminal i. Crohn's disease.

ileoanal (il″e-o-a′nal) pertaining to or connecting the ileum and the anus.

  i. reservoir a pouch for the collection of feces, created surgically in a two stage operation. The first stage involves removal of the rectal mucosa, an abdominal CO-LECTOMY, and construction of a fecal reservoir from loops of ileum; a temporary ILEOSTOMY is created at this time to allow the ileoanal reservoir to heal. Several months later the patient returns for closure of the ileostomy so that discharge of feces through the anus is possible.

ileocecal (il″e-o-se′kal) pertaining to the ileum and cecum.

ileocecocystoplasty (il″e-o-se″ko-sis′to-plas″te) augmentation CYSTOPLASTY using an isolated segment of the ileum and cecum for the graft.

ileocecostomy (il″e-o-se-kos′tah-me) surgical anastomosis of the ileum to the cecum.

ileocolic (il″e-o-kol′ik) pertaining to the ileum and colon.

ileocolitis (il″e-o-ko-li′tis) inflammation of the ileum and colon.

  i. ulcero′sa chro′nica chronic ileocolitis with fever, rapid pulse, anemia, diarrhea, and right iliac pain.

ileocolostomy (il″e-o-kah-los′tah-me) surgical anastomosis of the ileum to the colon.

ileocolotomy (il″e-o-ko-lot′ah-me) incision of the ileum and colon.

ileocystoplasty (il″e-o-sis′to-plas″te) augmentation CYSTOPLASTY using an isolated segment of the ileum for the graft.

ileocystostomy (il″e-o-sis-tos′tah-me) use of an isolated segment of ileum to create a passage from the urinary bladder to an opening in the abdominal wall.

ileoileostomy (il″e-o-il″e-os′tah-me) surgical anastomosis between two parts of the ileum.

ileorectal (il″e-o-rek′tal) pertaining to or communicating with the ileum and rectum.

ileorrhaphy (il″e-or′ah-fe) suture of the ileum.

ileosigmoidostomy (il″e-o-sig″moi-dos′-tah-me) surgical anastomosis of the ileum to the sigmoid colon.

ileostomy (il″e-os′tah-me) an artificial opening (STOMA) created in the ILEUM and brought to the surface of the abdomen for the purpose of evacuating feces. This may be done in the treatment of ULCERATIVE COLITIS, CROHN'S DISEASE, congenital defects of the bowel, cancer, trauma, and other conditions requiring bypass of the colon.

An ileostomy may be temporary or permanent. When the ileostomy is done in conjunction with partial or complete removal of the colon and anus, it is always permanent. The stoma created by ileostomy usually is located in the right lower quadrant of the abdomen.

Patient Care. Patients with an ileostomy require physical care similar to that given

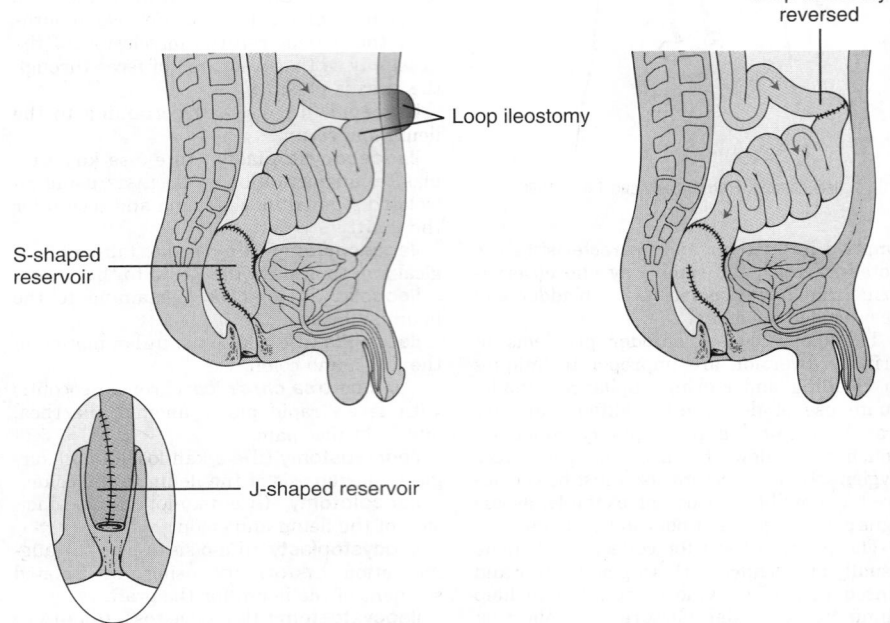

Stage 1.
After removal of the colon, a temporary loop ileostomy is created and an ileoanal reservoir is formed. The reservoir is created in an S-shaped reservoir (using three loops of ileum) or a J-shaped reservoir (suturing a portion of ileum to the rectal cuff, with an upward loop).

Stage 2.
After the reservoir has had time to heal–usually several months–the temporary loop ileostomy is reversed, and stool is allowed to drain into the reservoir.

Creation of an ileoanal reservoir. From Ignatavicius et al., 1995.

patients with a COLOSTOMY. The major difference is that the fecal material from an ileostomy will be more liquid and the passage of feces through the stoma less predictable than in a colostomy. The farther along the intestinal tract a stoma is located, the firmer the stool.

The psychosocial impact of surgery for either urinary or fecal diversion is a major concern of patients and their professional caregivers, families, and significant others. The problems related to this kind of surgery and the changes it brings in self-concept and fulfillment of roles are shared by all patients who must live with a stoma. Hence the emotional and psychological care of these patients is presented under STOMA.

The appliance for collection of feces is worn continuously and emptied every 4 to 5 hours. There is a continuous flow of liquid feces through an ileostomy. There should be no problem with persistent odor if the appliance is well made, worn correctly, and washed and rinsed frequently. Manufacturers of collection devices provide detailed information about cleaning and storage of their products.

Obstruction and diarrhea are common problems to be avoided. In regard to obstruction, the major offenders are foods that absorb water, for example, hard nuts, dried fruits, corn (including popcorn), and foods high in fiber. Particles from these foods are not small enough to pass through the ileostomy stoma; hence they inhibit the passage of feces and produce abdominal cramping and vomiting. Relief of blockage requires oral administration of enzymes to promote digestion, gentle lavage, and massage of the abdomen to encourage passage of the obstructing material. As a last resort, surgery may be necessary to remove the obstruction. Laxatives are *never* given; they will only aggravate the problem. Patients are taught the symptoms of obstruction and the necessity of consulting a health care professional should they occur and self-care measures not be effective.

Diarrhea is a more frequent problem in patients with an ileostomy than in patients with other types of fecal diversion and it is more likely to result in fluid and electrolyte imbalance than it would in a person who defecates normally. Although the fecal material passing through an ileostomy is already semi-liquid, patients can learn the difference between what is normal for them and what is indicative of diarrhea.

Dietary restrictions, other than the foods that could cause an obstruction, are not severe. The ostomate usually begins with a bland diet and gradually adds foods one at a time, noting whether a particular food causes problems of flatus, abdominal cramps, or diarrhea. Patients are warned that eating too quickly, not chewing food thoroughly, and swallowing air while eating can contribute to the problem of flatulence.

continent i. an ileostomy that maintains continence of feces, usually through construction of a continent ileal RESERVOIR; the ileostomy must be drained by the patient several times a day. See also KOCK POUCH.

urinary i. ileal conduit.

ileotomy (il″e-ot′ah-me) incision of the ileum.

Iletin (il′ĕ-tin) trademark for preparations of INSULIN for injection.

ileum (il′e-um) the distal portion of the small intestine, extending from the jejunum to the cecum.

duplex i. congenital duplication of the ileum.

ileus (il′e-us) failure of appropriate forward movement of bowel contents. It may be secondary to either mechanical obstruction of the bowel *(mechanical ileus)* or a disturbance in neural stimulation *(adynamic ileus).* Ileus is a surgical emergency that may or may not require surgical intervention; the cause needs to be established promptly.

Adynamic (or paralytic) ileus often accompanies peritonitis and is also found accompanying the colicky pains of gallstones or kidney stones; following spinal cord injury, pneumonia, or other generalized conditions; or being caused by peritoneal contamination by pus (from a perforated appendix) or acid (from a perforated ulcer). Mechanical ileus is that due to adhesions, ischemia, tumor, or stone and requires prompt decompression of the bowel to prevent perforation.

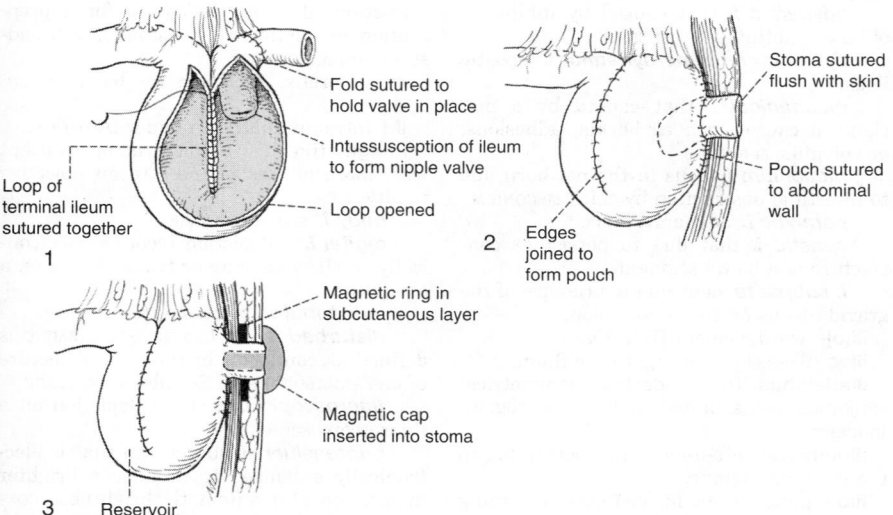

1, Fold sutured to hold valve in place
Intussusception of ileum to form nipple valve
Loop opened
Loop of terminal ileum sutured together

2, Stoma sutured flush with skin
Pouch sutured to abdominal wall
Edges joined to form pouch

3   Reservoir
Magnetic ring in subcutaneous layer
Magnetic cap inserted into stoma

Continent ileostomy (Kock pouch) with Maclet ring device. *1,* Loop of terminal ileum is sutured together and cut open. Using forceps, surgeon intussescepts distal ileum to form nipple valve. *2,* Free edges sutured together to form reservoir; stoma sutured flush with skin, and pouch sutured to abdominal wall. *3,* Magnetic ring is implanted in subcutaneous layer and stoma closed with magnetic cap. From Polaski and Tatro, 1996.

Symptoms. The principal symptoms of ileus are abdominal pain and distention, constipation, and vomiting in which the vomitus may contain fecal material. If the intestinal obstruction is not relieved, the circulation in the wall of the intestine is impaired and the patient appears extremely ill with symptoms of SHOCK and DEHYDRATION.

Treatment. Distention of the abdomen is relieved by decompression, which involves intubation with a long, balloon-tipped tube (e.g., MILLER-ABBOTT TUBE) that extends to the site of the obstruction, and use of constant suction. Because of the disruption in absorption of fluids and nutrients from the intestinal tract, fluids, electrolytes, and glucose are given intravenously. Surgical intervention to remove the cause of ileus is usually necessary when the obstruction is complete or the bowel is likely to become gangrenous. The type of surgical procedure will depend on the condition of the bowel and the cause of the obstruction. In some cases ileostomy or colostomy, either temporary or permanent, may be necessary. In cases of paralytic ileus due to causes other than contamination by pus or acid, tube decompression may be sufficient, but even in these patients, surgery may be needed to protect the bowel from overdistention and perforation. See also INTESTINAL OBSTRUCTION for patient care.

adynamic i. that caused by inhibition of bowel motility; see ILEUS.

dynamic i., hyperdynamic i. spastic ileus.

mechanical i. that caused by a mechanical cause, such as hernia, adhesions, or volvulus; see ILEUS.

meconium i. ileus in the newborn due to intestinal obstruction by thick MECONIUM.

paralytic i. adynamic ileus.

spastic i. that due to persistent contracture of a bowel segment.

i. subpar′ta ileus due to pressure of the gravid uterus on the pelvic colon.

ili(o)- word element [L.], *ilium.*

iliac (il′e-ak) pertaining to the ilium.

iliadelphus (il″e-ah-del′fus) symmetrical conjoined twins united in the iliac region; iliopagus.

iliofemoral (il″e-o-fem′o-ral) pertaining to the ilium and femur.

ilioinguinal (il″e-o-ing′gwĭ-nal) pertaining to the iliac and inguinal regions.

iliolumbar (il″e-o-lum′bar) pertaining to the iliac and lumbar regions.

iliopagus (il″e-op′ah-gus) symmetrical conjoined twins united in the iliac region.

iliopectineal (il″e-o-pek-tin′e-al) pertaining to the ilium and pubes.

iliotrochanteric (il″e-o-tro″kan-ter′ik) pertaining to the ilium and femoral trochanter.

ilium (il′e-um), pl. *i′lia* [L.] the lateral, flaring portion of the hip bone. adj., **il′iac.** (See also table of BONES.)

illness (il′nes) disease.

folk i. the experience of symptoms that are not identifiable with biomedical categories of disease; causes include natural forces, supernatural factors, interpersonal factors, and emotions. An example is *susto,* which is a Hispanic term for fright caused by a traumatic experience. Symptoms include listlessness, loss of appetite, and withdrawal. *Curanderos* (folk healers) treat the illness with prayers, rituals, and laying on of hands.

psychosomatic i. SOMATOFORM DISORDER.

illumination (ĭ-loo″mĭ-na′shun) 1. the lighting up of a part, cavity, organ, or object for inspection. 2. the luminous flux per unit area of a given surface; SI UNIT, lux. Symbol *E.*

darkfield i., dark-ground i. the casting of peripheral light rays upon a microscopical object from the side, the center rays being blocked out; the object appears bright on a dark background.

illuminator (ĭ-loo′mĭ-na″tor) the source of light for viewing an object.

illusion (ĭ-loo′zhun) a mental impression derived from misinterpretation of an actual sensory stimulus. adj., **illu′sional.**

Ilosone (il′o-sōn) trademark for a preparation of ERYTHROMYCIN estolate, a broad-spectrum ANTIBIOTIC.

im- a prefix, replacing *in-* before *b, m,* and *p.*

IM intramuscular; see under INJECTION.

image (im′ahj) a picture or concept with more or less likeness to an objective reality.

body i. see BODY IMAGE.

digital i. a depiction recorded electronically to allow viewing or transmission on a computer.

i. distributor beam splitter.

disturbed body i. a NURSING DIAGNOSIS defined as confusion in the mental picture of one's personal self. See also BODY IMAGE.

fluoroscopic i. a visual depiction on a fluoroscopy screen.

i. intensifier a fluoroscope that is electronically enhanced to produce a brighter image; see also automatic brightness CONTROL, brightness GAIN, and VIGNETTING.

latent i. the invisible change in radiographic film that is caused by x-radiation or light and is made visible by development of the film.

magnification i. direct radiographic enlargement requiring a fractional focus tube of 0.3 mm or less.

manifest i. the change on an x-ray film that becomes visible when the latent IMAGE undergoes appropriate chemical processing.

mirror i. 1. the image of light made visible by the reflecting surface of the cornea and lens when illuminated through the slit lamp. 2. an image with right and left relations reversed, as in the reflection of an object in a mirror.

motor i. the organized cerebral model of the possible movements of the body.

phantom i. an artifact seen in conventional linear TOMOGRAPHY.

imagery (im'ij-re) 1. a group of IMAGES or mental pictures. 2. the use of IMAGES to describe something.

simple guided i. in the NURSING INTERVENTIONS CLASSIFICATION, a nursing INTERVENTION defined as purposeful use of imagination to achieve relaxation and/or direct attention away from undesirable sensations.

imaging (im'ij-ing) the production of diagnostic images, e.g., radiography, ultrasonography, or scintigraphy.

digital subtraction i. a technique in radiography in which electronic subtraction allows the visualization of individual images; see also digital subtraction ANGIOGRAPHY.

electrostatic i. a method of visualizing deep structures of the body, in which an electron beam is passed through the patient and the emerging beam strikes an electrostatically charged plate, dissipating the charge according to the strength of the beam. A film is then made from the plate.

gated cardiac blood pool i. equilibrium radionuclide angiocardiography.

horizontal beam i. a grid positioning technique in radiology in which the grid cassette is positioned with its lead lines perpendicular to the floor.

hot spot i., infarct avid i. infarct avid scintigraphy.

magnetic resonance i. see MAGNETIC RESONANCE IMAGING.

myocardial perfusion i. myocardial perfusion SCINTIGRAPHY.

imago (ĭ-ma'go), pl. *imagoes, ima'gines* [L.] 1. the adult or definitive form of an insect. 2. in psychoanalysis, an idealized, unconscious mental image of a key person in one's early life.

imatinib (ĭ-mă'tĭ-nib″) an inhibitor acting specifically on an abnormal enzyme form that is created by the Philadelphia chromosome abnormality and present in chronic myeloid leukemia. It is used in the treatment of chronic myeloid leukemia during blast

crisis, accelerated phase, or chronic phase after failure of interferon-α therapy, administered orally as the mesylate salt.

imbalance (im-bal'ans) 1. dysequilibrium (def. 2). 2. lack of BALANCE; especially lack of balance between muscles, as in insufficiency of ocular muscles.

autonomic i. defective coordination between the sympathetic and parasympathetic nervous systems, especially with respect to vasomotor activities.

electrolyte i. serum concentrations of an electrolyte that are either higher or lower than normal; see discussion and table under ELECTROLYTE.

fluid volume i. abnormally decreased or increased fluid VOLUME or rapid shift from one compartment of body FLUID to another. See also deficient fluid VOLUME and excess fluid VOLUME.

risk for fluid volume i. a NURSING DIAGNOSIS accepted by the North American Nursing Diagnosis Association, defined as being at risk for a decrease, increase, or rapid shift from one to the other of intravascular, interstitial, and/or intracellular FLUID; this refers to body fluid loss, gain, or both. See also deficient fluid VOLUME and excess fluid VOLUME.

sympathetic i. vagotonia.

vasomotor i. autonomic imbalance.

imbecile (im'bĕ-sil) old term for a person with an intermediate grade of MENTAL RETARDATION, now considered offensive.

imbecility (im″bĕ-sil'ĭ-te) old term for intermediate forms of MENTAL RETARDATION, now considered offensive.

imbibition (im″bĭ-bish'un) absorption of a liquid.

imbricated (im'brĭ-kāt″ed) overlapping like shingles.

imidazole (im″id-az'ōl) 1. an organic compound in which two of the five atoms that make up the ring are nitrogen atoms. It is an antimetabolite and inhibitor of histamine and is used as an insecticide. 2. any of a class of antifungal AGENTS that contain this compound.

imide (im'īd) any compound containing the bivalent group =NH.

imiglucerase (im″ĭ-gloo'ser-ās) an analogue of the enzyme lacking in GAUCHER'S DISEASE, used for treating the adult form of the disease; administered by intravenous infusion.

imine (ĭ-mēn') an organic compound containing an imino group.

imino- a prefix used to denote the presence of the bivalent group =NH attached to nonacid radicals.

imino acid (ĭ-me′no) proline or hydroxyproline, the two amino acids in which the amino group is part of a closed ring.

iminoglycinuria (ĭ-me″no-gli″sin-u′re-ah) a benign hereditary disorder of renal tubular reabsorption of GLYCINE, PROLINE, and HYDROXYPROLINE, marked by excessive levels of all three substances in the urine.

imipenem (im″ĭ-pen′em) a β-lactam antibiotic with a broad spectrum of activity against gram-positive and gram-negative organisms. Because it is metabolized in the kidneys, it is administered with the enzyme inhibitor CILASTATIN in order to decrease the amount of it that is degraded by an enzyme in the kidneys.

imipramine (ĭ-mip′rah-mēn) a tricyclic ANTIDEPRESSANT of the DIBENZAZEPINE group, used also in the treatment of childhood enuresis, panic disorder, chronic pain, attention-deficit/hyperactivity disorder, cataplexy associated with narcolepsy, urinary incontinence, and bulimia nervosa. Administered orally or intramuscularly as the hydrochloride salt and orally as the pamoate salt.

imiquimod (im″ĭ-kwim′od) a biologic response MODIFIER used topically in the treatment of venereal warts of the external genitalia and perianal region.

immature (im″ah-chōōr′) unripe or not fully developed.

immersion (ĭ-mer′zhun) 1. the plunging of a body into a liquid. 2. the use of the microscope with the object and object glass both covered with a liquid. 3. a state of being deeply involved in something.

cultural i. the process of becoming familiar with a culture by extensive questioning and by active participation in the life of the culture, a technique used in ethnographic research for gaining increased familiarity with language, sociocultural norms, traditions, and other social dimensions in a culture.

i. foot a condition resembling trench foot occurring in persons who have spent long periods in water.

immiscible (ĭ-mis′ĭ-b′l) not susceptible to being mixed.

immobility (ĭ-mo-bil′ĭ-te) lack of movement; the state of not being movable; see also hazards of immobility.

immobilization (ĭ-mo″bil-ĭ-za′shun) the rendering of a part incapable of being moved.

immobilize (im-mo′bil-īz) to render incapable of being moved, as by a cast.

immobilizer (ĭ-mo′bĭ-li″zer) an object or apparatus that immobilizes.

sternal-occipital-mandibular i. (SOMI) any of a variety of cervical orthoses that have two or three posts running between head plates and a jacket or corset.

immune (ĭ-mūn′) 1. being highly resistant to a disease because of the formation of humoral antibodies or the development of immunologically competent cells, or both, or as a result of some other mechanism, as interferon activities in viral infections. 2. characterized by the development of humoral antibodies or cellular IMMUNITY, or both, following antigenic CHALLENGE. 3. produced in response to antigenic challenge, as immune serum globulin.

i. response the reaction to and interaction with substances interpreted by the body as NOT-SELF, the result being humoral and cellular IMMUNITY. Called also immune reaction. The immune response depends on a functioning THYMUS and the conversion of stem cells to B and T LYMPHOCYTES. These lymphocytes contribute to ANTIBODY production, cellular immunity, and immunologic memory.

Disorders of the Immune Response. Pathologic conditions associated with an abnormal immune response (immunopathy) may result from (1) immunodepression, that is, an absent or deficient supply of the components of either humoral or cellular immunity, or both; (2) excessive production of gamma globulins; (3) overreaction to antigens of extrinsic origin, that is, antigens from outside the body; and (4) abnormal response of the body to its own cells and tissues.

Those conditions arising from IMMUNOSUPPRESSION include AGAMMAGLOBULINEMIA (absence of GAMMA GLOBULINS) and HYPOGAMMAGLOBULINEMIA (a decrease of circulating antibodies). Factors that may cause or contribute to suppression of the immune response include (1) congenital absence of the thymus or of the stem cells that are precursors of B and T lymphocytes; (2) malnutrition, in which there is a deficiency of the specific nutrients essential to the life of antibody-synthesizing cells; (3) cancer, viral infections, and extensive burns, all of which overburden the immune response mechanisms and rapidly deplete the supply of antigen-specific antibody; (4) certain drugs, including alcohol and heroin, some antibiotics, antipsychotics, and the antineoplastics used in the treatment of cancer.

Overproduction of GAMMA GLOBULINS is manifested by an excessive proliferation of plasma cells (MULTIPLE MYELOMA). HYPERSENSITIVITY is the result of an overreaction to substances entering the body. Examples of this kind of inappropriate immune response include HAY FEVER, drug and food ALLERGIES,

AUTOIMMUNE DISEASES are manifestations of the body's abnormal response to and inability to tolerate its own cells and tissues. For reasons not yet fully understood, the body fails to interpret its own cells as SELF and, as it would with other foreign (NOT-SELF) substances, utilizes antibodies and immunologically competent cells to destroy and contain them.

i. system a complex system of cellular and molecular components whose primary function is distinguishing SELF from NONSELF and defense against foreign organisms or substances; see also IMMUNE RESPONSE. The primary cellular components are LYMPHOCYTES and MACROPHAGES, and the primary molecular components are ANTIBODIES and LYMPHOKINES; GRANULOCYTES and the COMPLEMENT system are also involved in immune responses but are not always considered part of the immune system per se.

i. complex disease local or systemic disease caused by the formation of circulating antibody-antigen immune complexes and their deposition in tissue, due to activation of complement and to recruitment and activation of leukocytes in type III HYPERSENSITIVITY REACTIONS.

immunifacient (ĭ-mu″nĭ-fa′shent) producing immunity; said of diseases, such as diphtheria and typhoid, that produce immunity against reinfection, which lasts for some time after an infection.

immunity (ĭ-mu′nĭ-te) the condition of being IMMUNE; the protection against infectious disease conferred either by the IMMUNE RESPONSE generated by immunization or previous infection or by other nonimmunologic factors. It encompasses the capacity to distinguish foreign material from SELF, and to neutralize, eliminate, or metabolize that which is foreign (NONSELF) by the physiologic mechanisms of the immune response.

The mechanisms of immunity are essentially concerned with the body's ability to recognize and dispose of substances which it interprets as foreign and harmful to its

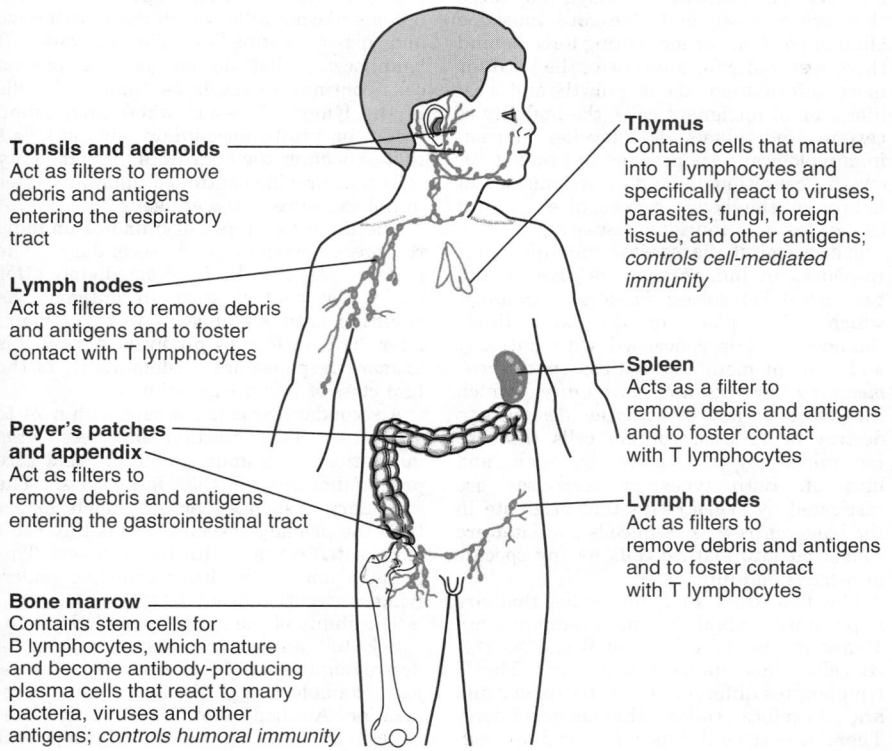

Tonsils and adenoids
Act as filters to remove debris and antigens entering the respiratory tract

Lymph nodes
Act as filters to remove debris and antigens and to foster contact with T lymphocytes

Peyer's patches and appendix
Act as filters to remove debris and antigens entering the gastrointestinal tract

Bone marrow
Contains stem cells for B lymphocytes, which mature and become antibody-producing plasma cells that react to many bacteria, viruses and other antigens; *controls humoral immunity*

Thymus
Contains cells that mature into T lymphocytes and specifically react to viruses, parasites, fungi, foreign tissue, and other antigens; *controls cell-mediated immunity*

Spleen
Acts as a filter to remove debris and antigens and to foster contact with T lymphocytes

Lymph nodes
Act as filters to remove debris and antigens and to foster contact with T lymphocytes

Major organs and tissues of the immune system in the child. From McKinney et al., 2000.

well-being. When such a substance enters the body, complex chemical and mechanical activities are set into motion to defend and protect the body's cells and tissues. The foreign substance, usually a protein, is called an ANTIGEN, that is, one that generates the production of an antagonist. The most common response to the antigen is the production of ANTIBODY. The antigen–antibody REACTION is an essential component of the overall immune response. A second type of activity, cellular response, is also an essential component.

The various and complex mechanisms of immunity are basic to the body's ability to protect itself against specific infectious agents and parasites, to accept or reject cells and tissues from other individuals, as in blood transfusions and organ transplants, and to protect against cancer, as when the immune system recognizes malignant cells as not-self and destroys them.

There has been extensive research into the body's ability to differentiate between cells, organisms, and other substances that are SELF (not alien to the body), and those that are NONSELF and therefore must be eliminated. A major motivating force behind these research efforts has been the need for more information about growth and proliferation of malignant cells, the inability of certain individuals to develop normal immunological responses (as in IMMUNODEFICIENCY conditions), and mechanisms of failure of the body to recognize its own tissues (as in AUTOIMMUNE DISEASES).

Immunological Responses. Immunological responses in humans can be divided into two broad categories: *humoral immunity,* which takes place in the body fluids (humors) and is concerned with antibody and complement activities; and *cell-mediated* or *cellular immunity,* which involves a variety of activities designed to destroy or at least contain cells that are recognized by the body as alien and harmful. Both types of responses are instigated by LYMPHOCYTES that originate in the bone marrow as stem cells and later are converted into mature cells having specific properties and functions.

The two kinds of lymphocytes that are important to establishment of immunity are T LYMPHOCYTES (T cells) and B LYMPHOCYTES (B cells). (See under LYMPHOCYTE.) The T lymphocytes differentiate in the THYMUS and are therefore called thymus-dependent. There are several types involved in cell-mediated immunity, delayed hypersensitivity, production of lymphokines, and the

regulation of the immune response of other T and B cells.

The B lymphocytes are so named because they were first identified during research studies involving the immunologic activity of the bursa of Fabricius, a lymphoid organ in the chicken. (Humans have no analogous organ.) They mature into plasma CELLS that are primarily responsible for forming antibodies, thereby providing humoral immunity.

Humoral Immunity. At the time a substance enters the body and is interpreted as foreign, antibodies are released from plasma cells and enter the body fluids where they can react with the specific antigens for which they were formed. This release of antibodies is stimulated by antigen-specific groups (clones) of B lymphocytes. Each B lymphocyte has IgM IMMUNOGLOBULIN receptors that play a major role in capturing its specific antigen and in launching production of the immunoglobulins (which are antibodies) that are capable of neutralizing and destroying that particular type of antigen.

Most of the B lymphocytes activated by the presence of their specific antigen become plasma cells, which then synthesize and export antibodies. The activated B lymphocytes that do not become plasma cells continue to reside as "memory" cells in the lymphoid tissue, where they stand ready for future encounters with antigens that may enter the body. It is these memory cells that provide continued immunity after initial exposure to the antigens.

There are two types of humoral immune response: primary and secondary. The primary response begins immediately after the initial contact with an antigen; the resulting antibody appears 48 to 72 hours later. The antibodies produced during this primary response are predominantly of the IgM class of immunoglobulins.

A secondary response occurs within 24 to 48 hours. This reaction produces large quantities of immunoglobulins that are predominantly of the IgG class. The secondary response persists much longer than the primary response and is the result of repeated contact with the antigens. This phenomenon is the basic principle underlying consecutive IMMUNIZATIONS.

The ability of the antibody to bind with or "stick to" antigen renders it capable of destroying the antigen in a number of ways; for example, agglutination and opsonization. Antibody also "fixes" or activates COMPLEMENT, which is the second component of the humoral immune system. Complement is the name given a complex series of enzymatic proteins which are present but inactive in normal serum. When complement fixation takes place, the antigen, antibody, and complement become bound together. The cell membrane of the antigen (which usually is a bacterial cell) then ruptures, resulting in dissolution of the antigen cell and a leakage of its substance into the body fluids. This destructive process is called lysis.

Cellular Immunity. This type of immune response is dependent upon T lymphocytes, which are primarily concerned with a delayed type of immune response. Examples of this include rejection of transplanted organs, defense against slowly developing bacterial diseases that result from intracellular infections, delayed hypersensitivity reactions, certain autoimmune diseases, some allergic reactions, and recognition and rejection of self cells undergoing alteration, for example, those infected with viruses, and cancer cells that have tumor-specific antigens on their surfaces. These responses are called *cell-mediated immune responses.*

The T lymphocyte becomes sensitized by its first contact with a specific antigen. Subsequent exposure to the antigen stimulates a host of chemical and mechanical activities, all designed to either destroy or inactivate the offending antigen. Some of the sensitized T lymphocytes combine with the antigen to deactivate it, while others set about to destroy the invading organism by direct invasion or the release of chemical factors. These chemical factors, through their influence on macrophages and unsensitized lymphocytes, enhance the effectiveness of the immune response.

Among the more active chemical factors are LYMPHOKINES, which are potent and biologically active proteins; their names are often descriptive of their functions: Ones that directly affect the macrophages are the macrophage chemotactic FACTOR, which attracts MACROPHAGES to the invasion site; migration inhibitory FACTOR, which causes macrophages to remain at the invasion site; and macrophage-activating FACTOR, which stimulates the metabolic activities of these large cells and thereby improves their ability to ingest the foreign invaders.

Another factor, a protein called INTERFERON, is produced by the body cells, especially T lymphocytes, following viral infection or in response to a wide variety of inducers, such as certain nonviral infectious agents and synthetic polymers.

A portion of the population of T lymphocytes is transformed into killer CELLS by the lymphocyte-transforming FACTOR (blastogenic factor). These activated lymphocytes produce a lymphotoxin or cytotoxin that damages the cell membranes of the antigens, causing them to rupture.

In order to ensure an ample supply of T lymphocytes, two factors are at work: lymphocyte-transforming FACTOR stimulates lymphocytes that have already undergone conversion to sensitized T lymphocytes, so that they increase their numbers by repeated cell division and clone formation; in the absence of antigens, transfer FACTOR takes over the task of sensitizing those lymphocytes that have not been exposed to antigen.

It is apparent that the immune response brings about intensive activity at the site of invasion; it is not only the pathogen that is destroyed, but invariably, there is death or damage to some normal tissues.

Interactions Between the Two Systems. There are several areas in which the cellular and humoral systems interact and thereby improve the efficiency of the overall immune response. For example, a by-product of the enzymatic activity of the complement system acts as a chemotactic factor, attracting T lymphocytes and macrophages to the invasion site. In another example, although T lymphocytes are not required for the production of antibody, there is optimal antibody production after interaction between T and B lymphocytes.

For a discussion of abnormalities of the immune response system, see IMMUNE RESPONSE.

Types of Immunity. An individual may be naturally immune to certain pathological conditions or may acquire immunity through either active or passive means.

Natural immunity is a genetic characteristic of an individual and is due to the particular species and race to which one belongs, to one's sex, and to one's individual ability to produce immune bodies. All humans are immune to certain diseases that affect animals of the lower species; males are more resistant to some disorders than are females, and vice versa. Persons of one race are more susceptible to some diseases than those of another race that has had exposure to the infectious agents through successive generations. One's individual ability to produce immune bodies, and thereby ward off pathogens, is influenced by one's state of physical health, one's nutritional status, and one's emotional response to stress.

In order for an individual to acquire immunity one's body must be stimulated to produce its own immune response components (active immunity) or these substances must be produced by other persons or animals and then passed on to the person (passive immunity). *Active immunity* can be established in two ways: by having the disease or by receiving modified pathogens and toxins. When an individual is exposed to a disease and the pathogenic organisms enter the body, the production of antibody is initiated. After recovery from the illness, memory cells remain in the body and stand ready as a defense against future invasion. It is possible, through the use of vaccines, bacterins, and modified toxins (toxoids), to stimulate the production of specific antibodies without having an attack of the disease. These are artificial means by which an individual can acquire active immunity.

Sometimes it is desirable to provide "ready-made" immune bodies, as in cases in which the patient has already been exposed to the antigen, is experiencing the symptoms of the disease, and needs reinforcements to help mitigate its harmful effects. Examples of conditions for which an individual may be given such *passive immunity* include tetanus, diphtheria, and a venomous snake bite. The patient is given immune serum, which contains GAMMA GLOBULIN, antibodies (including antitoxin) produced by the animal from which the serum was taken.

It is not always necessary that the patient actually suffer from the disease and exhibit its symptoms before passive immunity is provided. In some instances in which exposure to an infectious agent is suspected, immune bodies may be given to ward off a full-blown attack or at least to lessen its severity.

Another way in which immunity can be passively acquired is across the placental barrier from fetus to mother. The maternal antibody thus acquired serves as protection for the newborn until he can actively establish immunity on his own. Although humoral immunity can be acquired in this way, cellular immunity cannot.

acquired i. specific immunity attributable to the presence of antibody and to a heightened reactivity of antibody-forming cells, specifically immune lymphoid cells (responsible for cell-mediated immunity), and of phagocytic cells, following prior exposure to an infectious agent or its antigens, or passive transfer of antibody or immune lymphoid cells (adoptive immunity).

adoptive i. passive immunity of the cell-mediated type conferred by the administration of sensitized lymphocytes from an immune donor.

artificial i. acquired (active or passive) immunity produced by deliberate exposure to an antigen, such as a vaccine.

immunization (im″u-nĭ-za′shun) the process of rendering a subject immune, or of becoming immune. Called also INOCULATION and VACCINATION. The word VACCINE

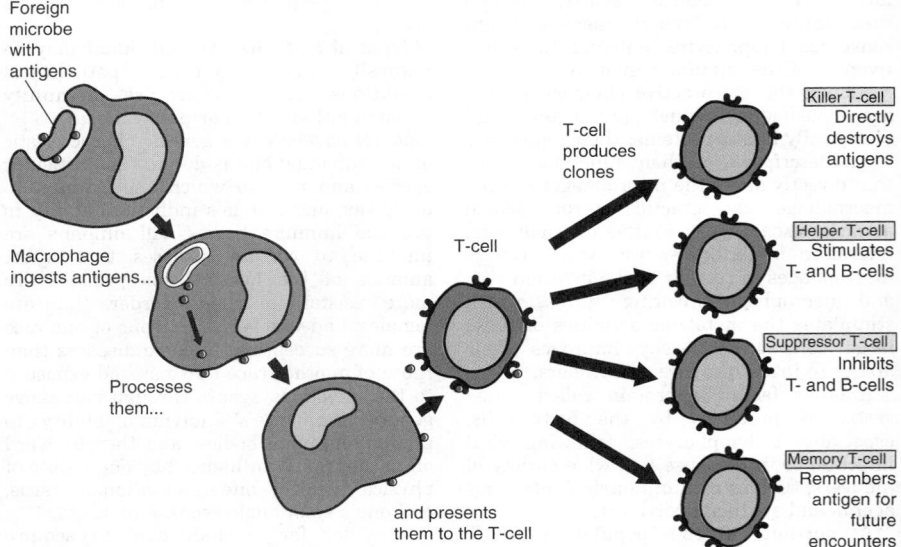

Foreign microbe with antigens

Macrophage ingests antigens...

Processes them...

and presents them to the T-cell

T-cell

T-cell produces clones

Killer T-cell
Directly destroys antigens

Helper T-cell
Stimulates T- and B-cells

Suppressor T-cell
Inhibits T- and B-cells

Memory T-cell
Remembers antigen for future encounters

Cell-mediated immunity. From Applegate, 2000.

originally referred to the substance used to immunize against SMALLPOX, the first immunization developed. Now, however, the term is used for any preparation used in active immunization.

The Centers for Disease Control and Prevention has an Advisory Committee on Immunization Practice that reviews childhood immunization schedules yearly. The recommended childhood immunization schedule is reprinted in Appendix 7-1. In Canada, the Health Protection Branch Laboratory Center for Disease Control, Health Canada, National Advisory Committee on Immunization publishes a recommended childhood vaccination schedule for Canada (reprinted in Appendix 7-3). Adult immunization schedules for the United States and Canada are found in Appendices 7-2 and 7-4.

active i. stimulation with a specific antigen to promote antibody formation in the body. The antigenic substance may be in one of four forms: (1) dead bacteria, as in TYPHOID FEVER immunization; (2) dead viruses, as in the Salk POLIOMYELITIS injection; (3) live attenuated virus, e.g., smallpox vaccine and Sabin polio vaccine (taken orally); and (4) toxoids, altered forms of toxins produced by bacteria, as in immunization against TETANUS and DIPHTHERIA.

Since active immunization induces the body to produce its own antibodies and to go on producing them, protection against disease will last several years, in some cases for life.

Active immunization is not without risks, although research supports the efficacy of immunization programs as a measure to reduce the incidence of infectious disease. Paradoxically, the more successful an immunization program and the higher the immunization rate, the more likely it becomes that a vaccine will cause more illness and injury than its target disease. Thus the risk of disease is less threatening than the risk of an adverse reaction to the vaccine that will prevent it.

In an effort to immunize larger numbers of children against preventable infectious diseases public health officials and health care professionals in the 50 states, the District of Columbia, Puerto Rico, the Virgin Islands, and Guam now enforce laws requiring children to be immunized before they enter school. Those children who come to school with incomplete or nonexistent records of immunizations are refused admittance until they are immunized.

Circumstances that require postponement of immunization include acute febrile illness, immunologic deficiency, pregnancy,

immunosuppressive therapy, and administration of gamma globulin, plasma, or whole blood transfusion 6 to 8 weeks prior to the scheduled immunization.

Because of their potential for triggering ANAPHYLAXIS in hypersensitive persons, all immunizing agents should be given with caution and only after a health history has been completed on the patient. Emergency equipment and drugs should be readily at hand in all clinics and other facilities where immunizing agents are administered.

passive i. transient immunization produced by the introduction into the system of pre-formed antibody or specifically sensitized lymphoid cells. The person immunized is protected only as long as these antibodies remain in his blood and are active—usually from 4 to 6 weeks.

immunize (im′u-nīz) to render immune.

immunoablative (im″mu-no-ab′lah-tiv) IMMUNOSUPPRESSANT with removal and destruction of a cell population, such as in the ablative step preceding bone marrow TRANSPLANTATION.

immunoadjuvant (im″u-no-aj′ah-vent, im″u-no-ad-joo′vent) a nonspecific stimulator of the IMMUNE RESPONSE, such as BCG VACCINE or Freund's complete and incomplete adjuvants.

immunoadsorbent (im″u-no-ad-sor′bent) a preparation of antigen attached to a solid support or antigen in an insoluble form, which adsorbs homologous antibodies from a mixture of immunoglobulins.

immunoassay (im″u-no-as′a) any of several methods for the quantitative determination of chemical substances, such as hormones, drugs, and specific proteins, that utilize the highly specific binding between an antigen or hapten and homologous antibodies, including radioimmunoassay, enzyme immunoassay, and fluoroimmunoassay.

immunobiological (im″u-no-bi″o-loj′ĭ-k′l) an antigenic or antibody-containing preparation derived from a pool of human or animal donors, including vaccines, toxoids, immune globulins, and antitoxins; used for immunization and immune therapy.

immunobiology (im″u-no-bi-ol′o-je) that branch of biology dealing with immunologic effects on such phenomena as infectious disease, growth and development, recognition phenomena, hypersensitivity, heredity, aging, cancer, and transplantation.

immunoblast (im′u-no-blast″) a mitotically active B or T LYMPHOCYTE.

immunoblastic (im″u-no-blas′tik) pertaining to or involving immunoblasts.

immunochemistry (im″u-no-kem′is-tre) 1. the study of the chemical basis of immunological phenomena. 2. the application of antibodies as chemical reagents.

immunochemotherapy (im″u-no-ke″mo-ther′ah-pe) a combination of immunotherapy and chemotherapy.

immunocompetence (im″u-no-kom′pĕtens) the capacity to develop an IMMUNE RESPONSE following exposure to antigen. Called also immunoresponsiveness. adj., **immunocom′petent.**

immunocomplex (im″u-no-kom′pleks) antigen-antibody complex.

immunocompromised (im″u-no-kom′promīzd) having the IMMUNE RESPONSE attenuated by administration of immunosuppressive drugs, by irradiation, by malnutrition, or by certain disease processes such as the viral infection that produces the acquired immunodeficiency syndrome (AIDS).

immunoconglutinin (im″u-no-kon-gloo′tin-in) an AUTOANTIBODY, usually of the IMMUNOGLOBULIN M class, that is specific for activated C3 and C4 components of COMPLEMENT. It is found in low titer in most normal sera and in increased levels in certain infectious diseases, in AUTOIMMUNE DISEASE, and after immunization with many antigens.

immunocyte (im′u-no-sīt) any cell of the lymphoid series that can react with antigen to produce antibody or to participate in cell-mediated immunity or delayed HYPERSENSITIVITY reactions; called also immunologically competent cell.

immunocytoadherence (im″u-no-si″to-ad-hēr′ens) the formation of ROSETTES by the binding of red blood cells bearing a homologous antigen to lymphocytes bearing surface immunoglobulin (B lymphocytes); used to identify B LYMPHOCYTES.

immunodeficiency (im″u-no-de-fish′ense) a deficiency of IMMUNE RESPONSE or a disorder characterized by deficient immune response; classified as antibody (B cell), cellular (T cell), or combined deficiency disorders. Antibody immunodeficiencies are marked by hypo- or DYSGAMMAGLOBULINEMIA, recurrent bacterial otitis media, and sinopulmonary infections. Cellular immunodeficiencies are characterized by recurrent low-grade or opportunistic INFECTIONS, by GRAFT-VERSUS-HOST DISEASE or reaction after blood transfusions, and by severe disease after immunization with live vaccines. See also ACQUIRED IMMUNODEFICIENCY SYNDROME.

common variable i. (CVID) a heterogeneous group of disorders characterized by HYPOGAMMAGLOBULINEMIA, decreased antibody production in response to antigenic challenge, and recurrent pyogenic infections, often associated with hematologic and autoimmune disorders. Most patients have normal numbers of circulating B CELLS but lack plasma CELLS and appear to have an intrinsic defect of B cell differentiation. However, two other forms are also recognized: that due to a disorder of T LYMPHOCYTE regulation and that due to production of autoantibodies against T and B lymphocytes.

severe combined i. (SCID) any of several rare congenital diseases, some of autosomal recessive and some of X-linked inheritance, in which both humoral and cell-mediated IMMUNITY fail to develop normally and T LYMPHOCYTES are absent or nearly so. In some forms, B LYMPHOCYTES are also absent. Early diagnosis is essential to prevent opportunistic INFECTIONS. Persistent DIARRHEA, chronic mucocutaneous CANDIDIASIS, and FAILURE TO THRIVE may occur in infancy. Blood transfusions can result in GRAFT-VERSUS-HOST DISEASE and routine vaccinations in fatal infection. Unless immune function is restored by a matched-donor bone marrow or fetal tissue transplantation or the patient is kept in complete isolation, the prognosis is poor.

immunodermatology (im″u-no-der″mahtol′o-je) the study of immunologic phenomena as they affect skin disorders and their treatment or prophylaxis.

immunodiffusion (im″u-no-dĭ-fu′zhun) the diffusion of antigen and antibody from separate reservoirs to form decreasing concentration gradients in hydrophilic gels.

immunoelectrophoresis (im″u-no-e-lek″tro-fo-re′sis) a method of distinguishing proteins and other materials on the basis of their electrophoretic mobility and antigenic specificities.

rocket i. electrophoresis in which antigen migrates from a well through agar gel containing antiserum, forming cone-shaped (rocket) precipitin bands.

immunofiltration (im″u-no-fil-tra′shun) the extraction of antigen or antibody in pure form using an IMMUNOADSORBENT.

immunofluorescence (im″u-no-floo″o-res′ens) a method of determining the location of antigen (or antibody) in a tissue section or smear using a specific antibody (or antigen) labeled with a FLUOROCHROME. There are two major types of immunofluorescence techniques, both based on the antigen–antibody REACTION, in which the antibody attaches itself to a specific antigen.

In the *direct fluorescent antibody* (DFA) method, the antibody coats the antigen, for example, a bacterial cell, and cannot be easily removed by elution (washing). The antibody remains attached to the cell after all nonantibody globulin has been washed away. Since the antibody has been rendered fluorescent by conjugation with fluorescein or another dye, the outline of the bacterial cell that it coats can readily be seen with a special microscope.

In the *indirect fluorescent antibody* (IFA) method, the specific antibody is allowed to react with the antigen. The nonantibody globulin is then washed off. This is then treated with a labeled antibody to the specific antibody. For example, if the specific antibody was raised in a rabbit, it is then treated with fluorescein-labeled anti-rabbit globulin, which results in a combination of this labeled antibody with the rabbit immunoglobulin already attached to the antigen.

Fluorescent antibody studies have been used in the detection of numerous bacterial, viral, fungal, and protozoan infections and in the identification of many microscopic tissue constituents.

immunogen (im'u-no-jen) any substance capable of eliciting an IMMUNE RESPONSE.

immunogenetics (im''u-no-jĕ-net'iks) the study of the genetics of the IMMUNE RESPONSE, such as the study of immune response genes or the association of HLA ANTIGENS with disease susceptibility, or the generation of antibody diversity. adj., **immunogenet'ic.**

immunogenic (im''u-no-jen'ik) producing immunity; evoking an IMMUNE RESPONSE.

immunogenicity (im''u-no-jĕ-nis'ĭ-te) the ability of a substance to provoke an IMMUNE RESPONSE or the degree to which it provokes a response. adj., **immunogen'ic.**

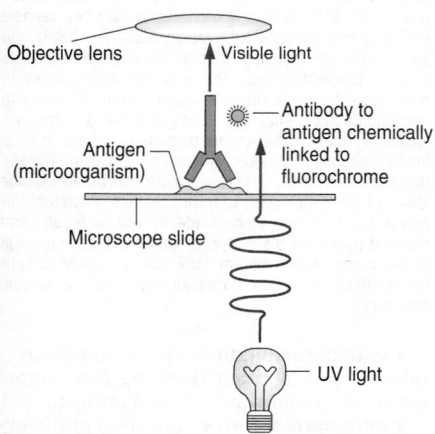

Objective lens — Visible light
Antibody to antigen chemically linked to fluorochrome
Antigen (microorganism)
Microscope slide
UV light

Direct immunofluorescence. In direct immunofluorescence the object is visualized using a fluorescein-tagged antibody. From Hart and Shears, 1997.

immunoglobulin (im''u-no-glob'u-lin) a protein of animal origin with known ANTIBODY activity. Immunoglobulins are major components of what is called the humoral IMMUNE RESPONSE system. They are synthesized by LYMPHOCYTES and plasma CELLS and found in the serum and in other body fluids and tissues, including the urine, spinal fluid, lymph nodes, and spleen. (See also IMMUNITY.) Each immunoglobulin molecule consists of four polypeptide chains: two heavy CHAINS (H chains) and two light CHAINS (L chains). There are five antigenically different kinds of H chains, and this difference is the basis for the classification of immunoglobulins. The five major classes of immunoglobulins (Ig) are IgA, IgD, IgE, IgG, and IgM. (See accompanying figure.) Each class varies in its chemical structure and in its number of antigen-binding sites and adheres to and reacts only with the specific antigen for which it was produced.

Two types of IgA have been identified. They are serum IgA and secretory IgA (sIgA). In sIgA two IgA molecules are linked by a polypeptide called the secretory piece and by a J CHAIN. Secretory IgA is present in nonvascular fluids, such as saliva, bile, synovial fluid, and intestinal and respiratory tract secretions. Both IgA types are known to have antiviral properties; their production is stimulated by oral vaccines and aerosol immunizations.

IgD is found in trace quantities in the serum (about 3 mg/dl). It serves as a B LYMPHOCYTE surface receptor.

IgE is called the reaginic antibody and is generally present in increased levels in persons with allergy. Its normal mean serum concentration is 0.03 mg/dl. When IgE attaches itself to cells within the body, such as those of the mucous membrane or skin, the cells become sensitized to allergens, causing them to release HISTAMINE and histamine-like substances when they come in contact with the allergen. Such allergic reactions as HIVES, HAY FEVER, ASTHMA, and ANAPHYLACTIC SHOCK are manifestations of IgE-mediated reactions.

IgG is the most abundant of the five classes of immunoglobulins. Its normal mean serum concentration is 1240 mg/dl. It is the major antibody in the secondary humoral response of immunity, serves to activate the complement system, and is frequently involved in OPSONIZATION. IgG is the only immunoglobulin that can cross the placental barrier.

IgM is principally concerned with the primary antibody response, appearing soon

after initial invasion by an antigen and
capable of destroying the antigen when it is
first introduced. Its normal mean serum
concentration is 120 mg/dl. Like IgG, IgM
activates the COMPLEMENT system and
together these two classes of immunoglobulins serve as specific ANTITOXINS against
the toxins of DIPHTHERIA, TETANUS, BOTULISM,
and ANTHRAX microorganisms, and snake
venoms.

immunohistochemical (im″u-no-his″to-
kem′ĭ-kal) denoting the application of
antigen–antibody interactions to histochem-
ical techniques, as in the use of immunofluorescence.

immunoincompetent (im″u-no-in-kom′-
pĕ-tent) immunocompromised.

immunologist (im″u-nol′o-jist) a specialist
in immunology.

immunology (im″u-nol′o-je) the branch of
biomedical science encompassing the study
of the structure and function of the immune
system (basic immunology); immunization,
organ transplantation, blood banking, and
immunopathology (clinical immunology);
laboratory testing of cellular and humoral
immune function (laboratory immunology);
and the use of antigen–antibody reactions in
other laboratory tests (serology and immunochemistry). adj., **immunolog′ic.**

immunomodulation (im″u-no-mod″u-la′-
shun) adjustment of the IMMUNE RESPONSE to
a desired level, as in IMMUNOPOTENTIATION,
IMMUNOSUPPRESSION, or induction of immunologic TOLERANCE.

immunomodulator (im″u-no-mod′u-lāt-
er) an agent that causes IMMUNOMODULATION.

immunopathogenesis (im″u-no-path″o-
jen′ĕ-sis) the process of development of a
disease in which an IMMUNE RESPONSE or its
products are involved.

immunopathology (im″u-no-pah-thol′o-je)
1. that branch of biomedical science
concerned with IMMUNE RESPONSES to disease,
with IMMUNODEFICIENCY diseases, and with
diseases caused by immune mechanisms. 2.
the structural and functional manifestations associated with IMMUNE RESPONSES to
disease or with diseases caused by immune
mechanisms. adj., **immunopatholog′ic.**

immunophysiology (im″u-no-fiz″e-ol′o-je)
the physiology of immunological processes.

immunopotency (im″u-no-po′ten-se) the
immunogenic capacity of an individual
antigenic determinant on an antigen
molecule to initiate antibody synthesis.

immunopotentiation (im″u-no-po-
ten″she-a′shun) accentuation of the response to an immunogen by administration
of another substance.

MOLECULAR STRUCTURE OF IMMUNOGLOBULINS

THE FIVE CLASSES

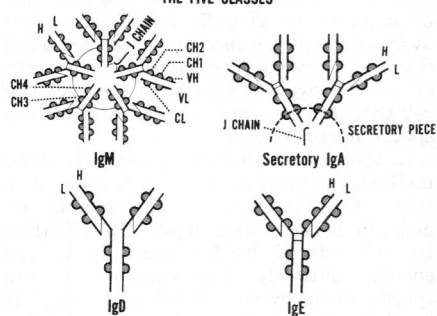

STRUCTURE OF IMMUNOGLOBULIN G & A SUBCLASSES

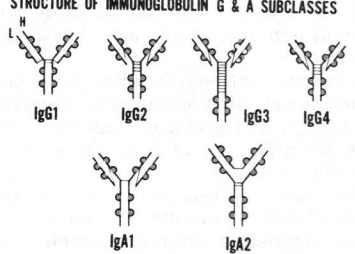

Schematic representation of the basic four-polypeptide
chain, monomeric unit structure of immunoglobulin
molecules. Heavy (H) chains determine *class.* Those in
IgG are gamma, in IgM are mu, in IgA are alpha, in IgD are
delta, and in IgE are epsilon. The two *types* of light (L)
chains (kappa and lambda) are shared in common by all
five immunoglobulin classes, although only one *type* is
present in any individual molecule. Both heavy and light
chains have looped structures referred to as domains or
regions. Heavy chains possess one variable (VH) (wherein
the antigen-binding site resides) and three constant (CH1,
CH2, CH3) regions, with the exception of IgM and IgE
which contain one variable (VH) and four constant regions
(CH1, CH2, CH3, CH4). Light chains contain one variable
(VL) and one constant (CL) region each. The heavy and
light chains are fastened together by disulfide bonds as
well as covalent forces. The disulfide bonds differ in
number at the *hinge* (inter H chain) region according to
immunoglobulin subclass. Antigen-binding sites are
located in the variable (aminoterminus) regions of each
immunoglobulin monomer. IgM and dimeric or multimeric
IgA molecules have J chains which are associated with the
ability of these molecules to form polymers. Secretory IgA
contains a secretory piece made by epithelial cells and
believed to protect the molecule from enzymatic cleavage
in the hinge region. Serum IgA2 has no heavy to light
chain disulfide bonds, whereas IgA1 has a classic
structure.

immunoprecipitation (im″u-no-pre-sip″ĭ-
ta′shun) precipitation resulting from interaction of specific antibody and antigen.

immunoproliferative (im″u-no-pro-lif′er-
ah-tiv) characterized by the proliferation of
the lymphoid cells producing IMMUNOGLOBU-
LINS, as in the GAMMOPATHIES.

i. small intestine disease the gastrointestinal form of alpha chain disease, characterized by diarrhea, malabsorption, abdominal pain, clubbing, plasma cell infiltration of the lamina propria of the small bowel, and presence of an abnormal alpha heavy chain fragment in the serum; it frequently evolves into primary malignant lymphoma.

immunoradiometry (im″u-no-ra″de-om′ĕ-tre) the use of radiolabeled antibody (in the place of radiolabeled antigen) in RADIO-IMMUNOASSAY techniques. adj., **immunoradiomet′ric.**

immunoreactant a substance that participates in an IMMUNE RESPONSE; an ANTIGEN or ANTIBODY.

immunoregulation (im″u-no-reg′u-la′-shun) the control of specific IMMUNE RESPONSES and interactions between B and T LYMPHOCYTES and MACROPHAGES.

immunoregulator (im″u-no-reg′u-la″ter) a substance such as INTERFERON that participates in IMMUNOREGULATION.

immunoresponsiveness (im″u-no-respon′siv-ness) immunocompetence.

immunoscintigraphy (im″u-no-sin-tig′rah-fe) scintigraphic imaging of a lesion using radiolabeled monoclonal antibodies or antibody fragments specific for antigen that is associated with the lesion.

immunosorbent (im″u-no-sor′bent) immunoadsorbent.

immunostimulant (im″u-no-stim′u-lant) an agent capable of stimulating an IMMUNE RESPONSE, usually used to refer to agents other than adjuvants.

immunostimulation (im″u-no-stim″u-la′-shun) stimulation of an IMMUNE RESPONSE, such as by BCG VACCINE.

immunosuppressant (im″u-no-sŭ-pres′-ant) an agent capable of suppressing IMMUNE RESPONSES.

immunosuppression (im″u-no-sŭ-presh′-un) inhibition of the IMMUNE RESPONSE to unfamiliar antigens that may be present; used in TRANSPLANTATION procedures to prevent rejection of the transplant or graft, and in AUTOIMMUNE DISEASE, ALLERGY, MULTIPLE MYELOMA, and other conditions.

immunosuppressive (im″u-no-sŭ-pres′iv) 1. pertaining to or inducing immunosuppression. 2. immunosuppressant.

immunosurveillance (im″u-no-ser-va′-lens) the monitoring function of the immune system whereby it recognizes and reacts against aberrant cells arising within the body.

immunotherapy (im″u-no-ther′ah-pe) passive IMMUNIZATION of an individual by administration of preformed ANTIBODIES (SERUM or GAMMA GLOBULIN) actively produced

in another individual. By extension, the term has come to include the use of immunopotentiators, replacement with immunocompetent lymphoid tissue (e.g., bone marrow or thymus), and infusion of specially treated white blood cells. Because the IMMUNE RESPONSE is a process of surveillance, recognition, and attack of foreign cells, immunotherapy has emerged as a promising mode of treatment for cancer. In general, there are three basic approaches to immunotherapy: active (specific and nonspecific), passive, and adoptive.

Nonspecific immunotherapy relies on general immune stimulants to activate the whole immune system. In the past decade, immunotherapy against cancer has involved the use of the bacille Calmette-Guérin vaccine (BCG VACCINE), which is evolved from strains of *Mycobacterium tuberculosis,* and is used to provide some immunity to tuberculosis. A growing body of knowledge allows scientists to devise mechanisms to utilize an individual's own defenses to attack foreign cells, such as cancer cells. One drawback to the use of general immune stimulants is that there is a limit to how much the immune system can be forced to respond. At some point there is an automatic dampening of the response which controls immunologic activities so as to protect the body from attack by its own destructive immune cells.

Specific immunotherapy is being actively investigated. Particularly promising is the technique that involves the use of specific antibodies for types of tumor cells, which have been "loaded" with either antineoplastic drugs or radioactive materials. When injected into the bloodstream of a patient with that particular kind of tumor, the "loaded" antibodies attach to the surface of the malignant cells. Thus, the antineoplastic drug or radiation does more damage to the malignant cells than to nonmalignant cells that the antibody does not bind to.

Adaptive immunotherapy is a technique in which a cancer patient's white blood cells are withdrawn and cultured in the laboratory with interleukin-2. The leukocytes thus treated are infused into the patient's bloodstream to stimulate the immune system.

Immunotherapy is also used in the DESENSITIZATION or HYPOSENSITIZATION of individuals allergic to specific ALLERGENS. Minute amounts of allergen to which the person is allergic are administered by injection in increasing doses over prolonged periods of time, in order to provoke production of large quantities of *blocking antibody* (predominantly IgG), which prevents an immediate HYPERSENSITIVITY REACTION from occurring. Presumably, the blocking antibody prevents the reaction by competing locally or in the circulation for the antigen.

immunotransfusion (im″u-no-trans-fu′-zhun) transfusion of blood from a donor previously rendered immune to the disease affecting the patient.

impacted (im-pak′ted) being wedged in firmly. In obstetrics, denoting twins so situated during delivery that the pressure of one against the other prevents complete engagement of either.

impaction (im-pak′shun) the condition of being wedged in firmly.

   bony i. a dental impaction in which the blockage consists of both bone and soft tissue.

   dental i. the blocking of a tooth by a physical barrier, such as a neighboring tooth, so that it cannot erupt; see also impacted TOOTH.

   fecal i. see FECAL IMPACTION.

   soft tissue i. a dental impaction in which the blockage consists of soft tissue only.

impaired environmental interpretation syndrome a NURSING DIAGNOSIS accepted by the North American Nursing Diagnosis Association, defined as a consistent lack of orientation to person, place, time, or circumstances over more than 3 to 6 months, necessitating a protective environment. See also DISORIENTATION.

impairment (im-pār′ment) 1. a decrease in strength or value. 2. any abnormality of, partial or complete loss of, or loss of the function of, a body part, organ, or system; this may be due directly or secondarily to pathology or injury and may be either temporary or permanent. Examples include muscle weakness, incontinence, pain, and loss of joint motion. See also DISABILITY and HANDICAP.

   functional aerobic i. **(FAI)** a ratio comparing the duration of a test performed by the patient with the duration of the test that would be expected for a healthy

Impaction of the third molar. From Dorland's, 2000.

individual of the same age, sex, and activity level, expressed as a percentage.

impalpable (im-pal′pah-b'l) not detectable by touch.

impar (im′pahr) not even; unequal; unpaired.

impatent (im-pa′tent) closed; not PATENT.

impedance (im-pe′dans) 1. obstruction or opposition to passage or flow, as of an electric current or other form of energy. 2. the resistance in alternating current circuits, represented by the letter Z in mathematical formulas. Medical equipment is often rated according to impedance to allow for optimum performance by matching impedance ratings. A TRANSFORMER can be used between components to cause the impedances of unequal systems to match.

   acoustic i. an expression of the opposition to passage of sound waves, being the product of the density of a substance and the velocity of sound in it.

imperforate (im-per′fo-rāt) not open; abnormally closed.

impermeable (im-per′me-ah-b'l) not permitting passage, as for fluid.

impetigo (im″pĕ-ti′go) a contagious skin disorder, caused by STREPTOCOCCI, STAPHYLOCOCCI, or a combination of organisms and marked by vesicles or bullae that become pustular, rupture, and form yellow crusts; called also impetigo contagiosa or impetigo vulgaris. Impetigo usually occurs in children, especially very young infants because of their low resistance, and is spread by direct contact with the moist discharges of the lesions. If not properly treated, it can be serious or even fatal to newborn infants. Isolation of the patient is recommended if patient hygiene is poor or the patient is a newborn in a hospital. Gowns and gloves are worn if soiling is likely. Impetigo is a particular problem for hospital patients, who may become infected by infected hospital staff. Treatment may consist of local applications of an antibiotic ointment, keeping the lesions and surrounding skin clean, and exposing the lesions to air to encourage drying. Systemic antibiotics are often recommended. (See Atlas 2, Part G).

   bullous i. a highly contagious type of impetigo, caused by *Staphylococcus aureus* and characterized by large pustules surrounded by reddened areas; transmission is by direct contact, by fomites, or by autoinoculation causing secondary infections in areas of the body not originally affected.

implant 1. (im-plant′) to insert or graft material, such as tissue or radioactive material, into intact tissues or a body cavity; see also TRANSPLANT. 2. (im′plant) any material inserted or grafted into the body.

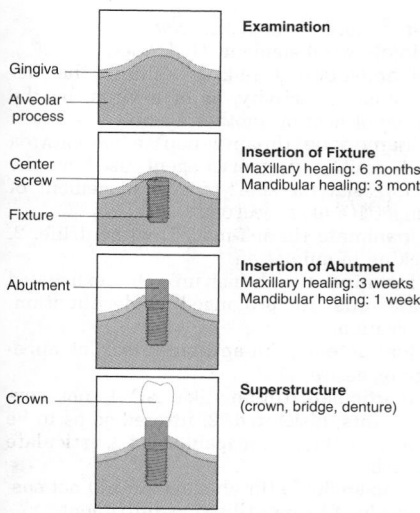

	Examination
Gingiva — Alveolar process —	
Center screw — Fixture —	**Insertion of Fixture** Maxillary healing: 6 months Mandibular healing: 3 months
Abutment —	**Insertion of Abutment** Maxillary healing: 3 weeks Mandibular healing: 1 week
Crown —	**Superstructure** (crown, bridge, denture)

Sequence of treatment with osseointegrated dental implants. From Darby and Walsh, 1995.

cochlear i. see COCHLEAR IMPLANT.

dental i. a prosthetic tooth with an anchoring structure surgically implanted beneath the mucosal or periosteal layer or in the bone.

penile i. penile prosthesis.

implantation (im″plan-ta′shun) 1. the insertion of an organ or tissue in a new site in the body. 2. the attachment and embedding of the ZYGOTE (fertilized ovum) in the ENDOMETRIUM in pregnancy; called also nidation. 3. the insertion or grafting into the body of biological, living, inert, or radioactive material.

implantology (im″plan-tol′o-je) the science dealing with implants.

implementation (im″ple-men-ta′shun) putting an instrument or plan into action. Implementation as a phase of the NURSING PROCESS involves putting the plan of care (nursing INTERVENTIONS) into effect. The nurse coordinates her activities with those of others responsible for contributing to patient care and delegates responsibility to other professional and technical care-givers as appropriate. During implementation the care PLAN is tested for effectiveness. Nursing interventions may not have had the desired effect, or a change in the patient's condition may present more critical problems that have a higher priority, thus requiring revision of the plan and different interventions.

implosion (im-plo′zhun) see FLOODING.

imposition (im″po-zi′shun) the forcing of something upon a person or group without consent.

cultural i. the tendency of a person or group to impose their values and patterns of behavior onto other persons.

impotence (im′po-tens) inability of the male to achieve or maintain an erection of sufficient rigidity to perform sexual intercourse successfully. An impotent man may produce sufficient numbers of normal spermatozoa; the condition is related to infertility only insofar as it prevents coitus with and impregnation of the female partner. Called also erectile dysfunction. adj., **im′potent.**

Etiology. Causes of impotence are usually classified as either physiological (*organic impotence*) or psychological (*psychogenic impotence,* officially called MALE ERECTILE DISORDER).

Organic Impotence. Diabetes mellitus, thyroid disease, and dysfunction of the pituitary gland or testes can cause impotence, as can certain medications. Other organic causes include arterial ischemia associated with atherosclerosis of the aorta and common iliac arteries, extensive pelvic surgery such as radical prostatectomy, spinal cord injury and other neurologic disorders, and a history of cigarette smoking. Because certain medications can cause impotence, it is recommended that in cases of recent impotence it be determined whether the patient has started on a new drug. The most common offenders are diuretics, antihypertensives, and vasodilators. Alcohol, which sometimes is ignored as a drug, is often a contributor to the problem of impotence.

Occasional successful sexual function and early morning erections do not preclude the possibility of endocrine dysfunction. Since abnormally low levels of testosterone frequently are the primary cause of impotence, it is recommended that determination of the blood level of testosterone be an integral part of the total evaluation of the impotent patient.

Psychogenic Impotence. In the past, psychological factors were frequently listed as the most common cause of impotence. However, research has now demonstrated that physical factors are actually more common than psychological ones.

Treatment. PROSTATITIS or another acute infection affecting the genitalia can cause temporary impotence that clears up in response to antibiotics. The smooth muscle relaxant SILDENAFIL (VIAGRA) was introduced in 1998 as a treatment for organic impotence. Administration of TESTOSTERONE may be indicated if low levels of this hormone are found in a blood sample. If impotence is organic and does not respond to other therapies, a penile prosthesis can be implanted; this is usually done surgically by a UROLOGIST. Other therapies include the use of vacuum tumescence devices and penile injection of pharmacologic agents that cause dilation.

organic i. impotence that has a physiological origin. See IMPOTENCE.

psychogenic i., psychological i. impotence that has an emotional or psychological cause; called also MALE ERECTILE DISORDER. See IMPOTENCE.

impregnation (im″preg-na′shun) 1. fertilization. 2. saturation.

impressio (im-pres′e-o), pl. *impressio′nes* [L.] impression (def. 1).

impression (im-presh′un) 1. a slight indentation or depression, as one produced in the surface of one organ by pressure exerted by another. 2. a negative imprint of an object made in some plastic material that later solidifies. 3. an effect produced upon the mind, body, or senses by some external stimulus or agent.

basilar i. 1. platybasia. 2. basilar invagination.

imprinting (im′print-ing) a rapid kind of learning of certain species-specific behavior patterns that occurs with exposure to the proper stimulus at a critical stage of early life.

impulse (im′puls) 1. a sudden pushing force. 2. a sudden uncontrollable determination to act. 3. nerve impulse.

cardiac i. a heartbeat palpated over the left side of the chest at the apex of the heart. See also POINT OF MAXIMAL IMPULSE.

i. control disorders a group of MENTAL DISORDERS characterized by repeated failure to resist an impulse to perform some act harmful to oneself or to others. In spite of the act's being socially unacceptable or inconsistent with the rest of the person's personality or lifestyle, he or she feels pleasure or emotional release upon doing it. Disorders in this category include INTERMITTENT EXPLOSIVE DISORDER, KLEPTOMANIA, pathological GAMBLING, PYROMANIA, and TRICHOTILLOMANIA.

nerve i. the electrochemical process propagated along nerve fibers.

impulsion (im-pul′shun) blind obedience to internal drives, without regard for acceptance by others or pressure from the superego; seen in children and in adults with weak defensive organization.

IMV intermittent mandatory ventilation.

In indium.

in-¹ word element [L.], *in, within,* or *into.*

in-² word element [L.], *not.*

in(o)- word element [Gr.], *fiber.*

inactivation (in-ak″tĭ-va′shun) the destruction of activity, as of a virus, by the action of heat or another agent.

inamrinone (in-am′rĭ-nōn) a VASODILATOR and positive INOTROPIC agent used as the lactate salt for short-term management of congestive HEART FAILURE.

inanimate (in-an′ĭ-mat) 1. without life. 2. lacking in animation.

inanition (in″ah-nish′un) the exhausted state due to prolonged undernutrition; starvation.

inappetence (in-ap′ĕ-tens) lack of appetite or desire.

inarticulate (in″ahr-tik′u-lat) 1. not having joints; disjointed. 2. uttered so as to be unintelligible; incapable of articulate speech.

inassimilable (in″ah-sim′ĭ-lah-b′l) not susceptible of being utilized as nutriment.

inattention (in″ah-ten′shun) lack of attention.

selective i. 1. unilateral neglect. 2. the ignoring or otherwise screening out of stimuli that are threatening, anxiety-producing, or felt to be unimportant.

inborn (in′born) 1. genetically determined, and present at birth; see also inborn ERROR of metabolism. 2. congenital.

inbreeding (in′brēd-ing) the mating of closely related individuals or of individuals having closely similar genetic constitutions.

incandescent in radiology, said of a heated filament that is emitting electrons; see also thermionic EMISSION.

incarceration (in-kahr″sĕ-ra′shun) unnatural retention or confinement of a part.

incest (in′sest) sexual activity between persons so closely related that marriage between them is legally or culturally prohibited.

incidence (in′sĭ-dens) the rate at which a certain event occurs, as the number of new cases of a specific disease occurring during a certain period in a population at risk, in contrast to PREVALENCE.

incident (in′sĭ-dent) 1. an unusual or noteworthy occurrence. 2. impinging upon, as incident radiation.

mass casualty i. a catastrophic event in which there are over 100 casualties; see table at DISASTER.

multiple casualty i. a catastrophic event that results in 10 to 100 casualties; see table at DISASTER.

multiple patient i. a catastrophic event that results in less than 10 casualties; see table at DISASTER.

incineration (in-sin″ĕ-ra′shun) the act of burning to ashes.

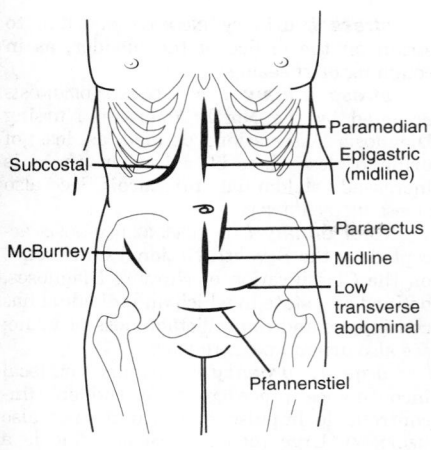

Various abdominal incisions. From Dorland's, 2000.

Labels on figure: Subcostal; McBurney; Paramedian; Epigastric (midline); Pararectus; Midline; Low transverse abdominal; Pfannenstiel

incipient (in-sip′e-ent) beginning to exist; coming into existence.

incisal (in-si′sal) pertaining to the cutting edge of an anterior tooth.

incision (in-sizh′un) 1. a cut or a wound made by a sharp instrument. 2. the act of cutting.

incisive (in-si′siv) 1. having the power of cutting; sharp. 2. pertaining to the incisor teeth.

incisor (I) (in-si′zor) 1. adapted for cutting. 2. incisor tooth; see TOOTH.

incisure (in-si′zher) notch.

Rivinus' i., tympanic i. tympanic NOTCH.

inclination (in″kli-na′shun) a sloping or leaning; the angle of deviation from a particular line or plane of reference.

i. of the pelvis the angle between the plane of the pelvic inlet and the horizontal plane.

inclusion (in-kloo′zhun) 1. the act of enclosing or the condition of being enclosed. 2. anything that is enclosed; a cell inclusion.

cell i. a usually lifeless, often temporary, constituent in the cytoplasm of a cell.

fetal i. a partially developed embryo enclosed within the body of its twin.

incoagulability (in″ko-ag″u-lah-bil′ĭ-te) the state of being incapable of coagulation. adj., **incoag′ulable.**

incompatible (in″kom-pat′ĭ-b'l) not suitable for combination, simultaneous administration, or transplantation; mutually repellent.

incompatibility (in″kom-pat″ĭ-bil′ĭ-te) the quality of being incompatible.

incompetence (in-kom′pě-tens) 1. inability to function properly. 2. the legal status of a person determined by the court to be unable to manage his own affairs. 3. insufficiency.

aortic i. aortic INSUFFICIENCY.

mitral i. mitral INSUFFICIENCY.

pulmonary i. pulmonary INSUFFICIENCY.

tricuspid i. tricuspid INSUFFICIENCY.

valvular i. valvular INSUFFICIENCY.

incompetent (in-kom′pě-tent) 1. not able to function properly. 2. a person who is unable to perform the required functions of everyday living. 3. a person determined by the courts to be unable to manage his own affairs.

incontinence (in-kon′tĭ-nens) 1. inability to control excretory functions. 2. immoderation or excess. adj., **incon′tinent.**

bowel i. 1. fecal incontinence. 2. a NURSING DIAGNOSIS accepted by the North American Nursing Diagnosis Association, defined as a state in which an individual has a change in normal bowel habits, with involuntary bowel movements.

continuous i. continuous urinary leakage from a source other than the urethra, such as a fistula.

fecal i., i. of the feces inability to control DEFECATION; both physiologic and psychological conditions can be contributing factors. Called also encopresis and bowel incontinence. See also bowel ELIMINATION, altered. Physiologic causes include neurologic sensory and motor defects such as those occurring in stroke and spinal cord injury; pathologic conditions that impair the integrity of the sphincters, such as tumors, lacerations, fistulas, and loss of sensory innervation; altered LEVELS OF CONSCIOUSNESS; and severe diarrhea. Psychological factors include anxiety, confusion, disorientation, depression, and despair.

There is potential for physical and psychological stress when a person is unable to control his or her bowel movements. Damage to the integrity of the skin and its breakdown into pressure ULCERS is always a possibility no matter how hard caregivers might try to keep the patient clean and dry. Psychologically the person is likely to suffer from loss of self-esteem and is certain to experience some alteration in self-image. From the time of toilet training a person is expected to be able to handle the tasks of bowel elimination. An adult who for some reason is no longer able to do this is often embarrassed by and ashamed of the inability to perform this most basic of self-care activities.

Patient Care. Assessment of the problem of fecal incontinence should be extensive and thorough so that a realistic and effective plan of care can be implemented. Sometimes all that is needed is a regularly scheduled time to offer the patient a bedpan or help using a bedside commode or going to the bathroom. If diarrhea is a problem it may be that dietary intake needs changing or tube feedings are not being administered correctly. Dietary changes may also help the patient who has a stoma leading from the intestine. In cases of neurologic or neuromuscular deficit, retraining for bowel elimination is a major part of rehabilitation of the patient. Frequently, it is possible to help a patient achieve control by means of a well-planned and executed BOWEL TRAINING program.

Biofeedback techniques can be helpful in many cases. The person learns to maintain higher tone in the anal sphincter through use of a balloon device that provides feedback information about pressures in the rectum. With practice the person can learn better control and develop a more acute awareness of the need to defecate.

functional i. incontinence due to impairment of physical or cognitive functioning.

functional urinary i. a NURSING DIAGNOSIS accepted by the North American Nursing Diagnosis Association, defined as an inability of a usually continent person to reach the toilet in time to avoid the unintentional loss of urine. See also urinary INCONTINENCE.

overflow i., paradoxical i. urinary INCONTINENCE due to pressure of retained urine in the bladder after the bladder has contracted to its limits; there may be a variety of presentations, including frequent or constant dribbling or symptoms similar to those of stress or urge INCONTINENCE.

reflex i. the urinary INCONTINENCE that accompanies detrusor HYPERREFLEXIA.

reflex urinary i. a NURSING DIAGNOSIS accepted by the North American Nursing Diagnosis Association, defined as an involuntary loss of urine at somewhat predictable intervals, whenever a specific bladder volume is reached. See also reflex INCONTINENCE.

risk for urge urinary i. a NURSING DIAGNOSIS accepted by the North American Nursing Diagnosis Association, defined as the state of being at risk for involuntary loss of urine associated with a sudden strong sensation of urinary urgency. See also urge urinary INCONTINENCE.

severe stress urinary i. severe stress incontinence as a result of incompetence of the sphincter mechanism.

stress i. urinary INCONTINENCE due to strain on the orifice of the bladder, as in coughing or sneezing.

stress urinary i. a NURSING DIAGNOSIS accepted by the North American Nursing Diagnosis Association, defined as loss of urine of less than 50 ml when there is increased abdominal pressure. See also stress INCONTINENCE.

total urinary i. a NURSING DIAGNOSIS accepted by the Seventh National Conference on the Classification of Nursing Diagnoses, defined as a state in which an individual has continuous and unpredictable loss of urine; see also urinary INCONTINENCE.

urge i., urgency i. urinary or fecal incontinence preceded by a sudden, uncontrollable impulse to evacuate (see also URGENCY). Urge incontinence of urine is a major complaint of patients with URINARY TRACT INFECTIONS and is also present in some women two or three days before onset of the menstrual period.

urge urinary i. a NURSING DIAGNOSIS accepted by the North American Nursing Diagnosis Association, defined as the involuntary passage of urine soon after feeling a strong sense of urgency to urinate; see also urge INCONTINENCE.

urinary i., i. of urine loss of control of the passage of urine from the bladder; see also ENURESIS. It can be caused by pathologic, anatomic, or physiologic factors affecting the urinary tract, as well as by factors entirely outside it. See also urinary ELIMINATION, altered.

Patient Care. The Agency for Health Care Policy and Research (AHCPR) convened an interdisciplinary, non-Federal panel of physicians, nurses, allied health care professionals, and health care consumers that has identified and published Clinical Practice Guidelines for Urinary Incontinence in Adults. Identification and documentation of urinary incontinence can be improved with more thorough medical history taking, physical examination, and record keeping. Routine tests of lower urinary tract function should be performed for initial identification of incontinence. There are also situations that require further evaluation by qualified specialists.

The guidelines provide an informed framework for selecting appropriate behavioral, pharmacologic, and surgical treatment and supportive services that can be used to treat urinary incontinence. The panel concluded that behavioral techniques such as bladder training and pelvic muscle exercises are effective, low cost interventions that can reduce incontinence significantly in varied populations. Surgery, except in very specific cases, should be considered only after behavioral and pharmacologic interventions have been tried. The panel found evidence in the literature that treatment can improve or cure urinary incontinence in most patients. The address of the AHCPR is Agency for Health Care Policy and Research, P.O. Box 8547, Silver Spring, MD 20907. They can also be called toll free at (800) 358-9295.

incoordination (in″ko-or″dĭ-na′shun) lack of normal adjustment of muscular motions; failure to work harmoniously.

incorporation (in-kor″po-ra′shun) 1. the union of one substance with another, or with others, in a composite mass. 2. an unconscious DEFENSE MECHANISM in which a person figuratively ingests the psychic representation of another person, or parts of another person.

increment (in′krĕ-ment) an increase or addition; the amount by which a value or quantity is increased. adj., **incremen′tal.**

incrustation (in″krus-ta′shun) 1. the formation of a crust. 2. a crust, scab, or scale.

incubate (in′ku-bāt) 1. to subject to or to undergo incubation. 2. material that has undergone incubation.

incubation (in″ku-ba′shun) 1. the provision of proper conditions for growth and development, as for bacterial or tissue cultures. 2. the development of an infectious disease from time of the entrance of the pathogen to the appearance of clinical symptoms. 3. the development of the embryo in the egg of oviparous animals. 4. the maintenance of an artificial environment for a newborn, especially a premature INFANT.

i. period the interval of time required for development; especially the time between invasion of the body by a pathogenic organism and appearance of the first symptoms of disease. Incubation periods vary from a few days to several months, depending on the causative organism and type of disease.

incubator (in′ku-ba″ter) an apparatus for maintaining optimal conditions for growth and development, such as temperature and humidity, especially one used in the early care of premature infants, or one used for cultures. The primary purpose of the incubator used for preterm newborns is to surround the infant with some of the environmental conditions normally provided in the uterus and necessary until he reaches approximately the level of development of a full-term infant.

The temperature within the incubator is regulated so that the infant's temperature is maintained between 35.5° and 36.6°C

(96° to 98°F). Humidity is kept at 50 to 60 per cent unless there is respiratory difficulty, in which case the humidity may be raised as high as 85 to 100 per cent. Oxygen is added in concentrations not exceeding 30 to 40 per cent only as long as the infant is cyanotic because of the danger of RETROLENTAL FIBROPLASIA with high concentrations of oxygen.

incudal (ing′ku-dal) pertaining to the incus.

incudectomy (ing″ku-dek′to-me) excision of the incus.

incudiform (ing-ku′dĭ-form) anvil-shaped.

incudomalleal (ing″ku-do-mal′e-al) pertaining to the incus and malleus.

incudomalleolar (ing″ku-do-mal″e-o′ler) incudomalleal.

incudostapedial (ing″ku-do-stah-pe′de-al) pertaining to the incus and stapes.

incurable (in-kūr′ah-b′l) 1. not susceptible of being cured. 2. a person with a disease that cannot be cured.

incus (ing′kus) the middle of the three ossicles of the EAR; called also anvil. See also color plates.

indanedione (in″dān-di′ōn) any of a group of synthetic ANTICOAGULANTS derived from 1,3-indanedione, such as ANISINDIONE. They act by impairing hepatic synthesis of the vitamin K-dependent COAGULATION FACTORS (prothrombin and factors VII, IX, and X).

indapamide (in-dap′ah-mīd) a thiazide DIURETIC used in treatment of EDEMA, such as in congestive HEART FAILURE or liver disease, as well as of HYPERTENSION.

independent 1. freestanding, capable of functioning in an autonomous fashion. 2. a process or activity that can be implemented without the assistance of another.

Inderal (in′der-al) trademark for preparations of PROPRANOLOL hydrochloride, a BETA-ADRENERGIC BLOCKING AGENT.

index pl. *indexes, in′dices* [L.] 1. the numerical ratio of measurement of any part in comparison with a fixed standard. 2. forefinger.

Barthel I. an objective, standardized tool for measuring functional status. The individual is scored in a number of areas depending upon independence of performance. Total scores range from 0 (complete dependence) to 100 (complete independence).

bleeding i. any of various methods of assessing bleeding in the gingival sulcus before or after treatment.

body mass i. (BMI) the weight in kilograms divided by the square of the height in meters, a measure of body fat that gives an indication of nutritional status.

cardiac i. cardiac output corrected for body size.

cephalic i. 100 times the maximum breadth of the skull divided by its maximum length.

citation i. an index listing all publications appearing in a set of source publications (e.g., articles in a defined group of journals) that cite a given publication in their bibliographies.

Colour I. a publication of the Society of Dyers and Colourists and the American Association of Textile Chemists and Colorists containing an extensive list of dyes and dye intermediates. Each chemically distinct compound is identified by a specific number, the C.I. number, avoiding the confusion of trivial names used for dyes in the dye industry.

erythrocyte indices the mean corpuscular VOLUME, mean corpuscular HEMOGLOBIN, and mean corpuscular hemoglobin CONCENTRATION. These are all useful for evaluating ANEMIAS because they provide information on the size of the ERYTHROCYTES and the concentration of HEMOGLOBIN. Called also red cell or red blood cell indices.

glycemic i. a ranking of foods based on the response of postprandial blood SUGAR levels as compared with a reference food, usually either white bread or GLUCOSE. See table.

left ventricular stroke work i. (LVSWI) an index of the amount of work performed by the heart.

leukopenic i. a fall of 1000 or more in the total leukocyte count within 1.5 hours after ingestion of a given food; it indicates allergic hypersensitivity to that food.

I. Medicus a monthly publication of the NATIONAL LIBRARY OF MEDICINE in which the world's leading biomedical literature is indexed by author and subject.

opsonic i. a measure of opsonic activity determined by the ratio of the number of microorganisms phagocytized by normal leukocytes in the presence of serum from an individual infected by the microorganism, to the number phagocytized in serum from a normal individual.

phagocytic i. any arbitrary measure of the ability of neutrophils to ingest native or opsonized particles determined by various assays; it reflects either the average number of particles ingested or the rate at which particles are cleared from the blood or culture medium.

red blood cell indices, red cell indices erythrocyte indices.

refractive i. the refractive power of a medium compared with that of air (assumed to be 1).

short increment sensitivity i. (SISI) a hearing test in which randomly spaced, 0.5-second tone bursts are superimposed at 1- to 5-decibel increments in intensity on a carrier tone having the same frequency and an intensity of 20 decibels above the speech recognition threshold.

therapeutic i. originally, the ratio of the maximum tolerated dose to the minimum curative dose; now defined as the ratio of the median lethal dose (LD_{50}) to the median effective dose (ED_{50}). It is used in assessing the safety of a drug.

indican (in'dĭ-kan) 1. a substance formed by decomposition of tryptophan in the intestines and excreted in the urine. 2. a yellow indoxyl glycoside from indigo plants.

indicanuria (in''dĭ-kan-u're-ah) an excess of indican in the urine.

GLYCEMIC INDEX FOR SELECTED FOODS AND BEVERAGES USING WHITE BREAD REFERENCE

	White Bread = 100
Low glycemic index (< 60)	
Apple	52
Barley, pearled	36
Butter Beans	44
Kellogg's All Bran Fruit and Nuts Cereal	55
Red Lentils	36
Rice Bran Cereal	27
Soy Milk	43
Spaghetti	59
Tomato Soup	54
Medium glycemic index (60–85)	
Baked Beans, canned	69
Kellogg's Special K Cereal	77
Instant Noodles	67
Pita Bread	82
Popcorn	79
Rice, brown	79
Snickers Bar	57
Sponge Cake	66
Yams	73
High glycemic index (> 85)	
Carrots	101
Cheerios	106
Couscous	93
French Baguette	136
Ice Cream	87
Pretzels	116
Pumpkin	107
Rice Cakes	117
Watermelon	103

indication (in″dĭ-ka′shun) a sign or circumstance that points to or shows the cause, treatment, or some other aspect of a disease.

indicator (in′dĭ-ka″ter) 1. the index finger, or the extensor muscle of the index finger. 2. any substance that indicates the appearance or disappearance of a chemical by a color change or attainment of a certain pH.

prognostic i's factors such as STAGING, tumor type, and laboratory studies that may indicate treatment effectiveness and outcomes.

indifférence (ă-de″fa-rahns′) [Fr.] indifference.

la belle i. an inappropriately complacent attitude towards their condition and physical symptoms, seen in patients with conversion disorder.

indigestion (in″dĭ-jes′chun) lack or failure of digestive function; commonly used to denote vague abdominal discomfort after meals. Among the symptoms of indigestion are heartburn, nausea, flatulence, cramps, a disagreeable taste in the mouth, belching, and sometimes vomiting or diarrhea. Ordinary indigestion can result from eating too much or too fast; from eating when tense, tired, or emotionally upset; from food that is too fatty or spicy; and from heavy food or food that has been badly cooked or processed.

Indigestion and its symptoms may also accompany other disorders such as allergy, migraine, influenza, typhoid fever, food poisoning, peptic ulcer, inflammation of the gallbladder (chronic cholecystitis), appendicitis, and coronary occlusion.

indigitation (in-dij″ĭ-ta′shun) intussusception (def. 1).

indigotindisulfonate sodium (in″di-go-tin″di-sul′fo-nāt) a bluish dye used as a diagnostic aid in cystoscopy.

indinavir (in-di′nah-vir) an HIV protease INHIBITOR that causes the virus to form noninfectious particles; used orally as the sulfate salt in the treatment of HIV infection and AIDS.

indium (In) (in′de-um) a chemical element, atomic number 49, atomic weight 114.82. (See Appendix 6.)

i. 111 an artificial isotope of indium, having a half-life of 2.81 days and emitting gamma rays; it is used as a radioactive tracer in nuclear medicine.

individuation (in″dĭ-vid″u-a′shun) 1. the process of developing individual characteristics. 2. differential regional activity in the embryo occurring in response to organizer influence. 3. in jungian psychology, the process of maturation and development and realization of the individual personality. In immature personalities, the process of

individuation and self-realization is delayed. See also JUNG.

Indocin (in′do-sin) trademark for preparations of INDOMETHACIN, a NONSTEROIDAL ANTIINFLAMMATORY DRUG.

indocyanine green (in″do-si′ah-nēn) a dye used intravenously as a diagnostic aid in the determination of blood volume, cardiac output, and hepatic function.

indole (in′dōl) a compound obtained from coal tar and indigo and produced by decomposition of tryptophan in the intestine, where it contributes to the peculiar odor of feces. It is excreted in the urine in the form of indican.

indolent (in′do-lent) 1. causing little pain. 2. slow growing.

indomethacin (in″do-meth′ah-sin) a NONSTEROIDAL ANTIINFLAMMATORY DRUG used in the treatment of rheumatoid ARTHRITIS, OSTEOARTHRITIS, ankylosing SPONDYLITIS, and various other rheumatic and nonrheumatic inflammatory conditions, dysmenorrhea, and vascular headache. The trihydrated sodium salt is used to induce closure in certain cases of patent ductus arteriosus.

indoxyl (in-dok′sil) an oxidation product of indole formed in tryptophan decomposition, and excreted in the urine as indican.

indoxyluria (in-dok″sil-u′re-ah) an excess of indoxyl in the urine.

induced psychotic disorder shared psychotic disorder.

inducer (in-do͞os′er) in biosynthesis, a compound that induces synthesis of a specific enzyme or sequence of enzymes, by antagonizing the corresponding repressor, or by some other mechanism.

induction (in-duk′shun) 1. the process or act of causing to occur. 2. the production of a specific morphogenetic effect in the embryo through evocators or organizers, or the production of anesthesia or unconsciousness by use of appropriate agents. 3. the generation of an electric current or magnetic properties in a body because of its proximity to an electrified or magnetized object. 4. reasoning from particular instances to general conclusions.

labor i. in the NURSING INTERVENTIONS CLASSIFICATION, a nursing INTERVENTION defined as initiation or augmentation of LABOR by mechanical or pharmacological methods.

ovulation i. treatment of INFERTILITY in the female by administration of hormones that stimulate the ovaries.

inductor (in-duk′tor) a tissue elaborating a chemical substance that acts to determine the growth and differentiation of embryonic parts.

indurated (in'du-rāt"ed) hardened; abnormally hard. Called also sclerous.

induration (in"du-ra'shun) 1. the quality of being hard. 2. the process of becoming hard; called also hardening and sclerosis. 3. an abnormally hard spot or place. adj., **indura'tive.**

black i. the hardening and pigmentation of the lung tissue seen in coal workers' PNEUMOCONIOSIS.

brown i. 1. a deposit of altered blood pigment in the lung in pneumonia. 2. increase of the pulmonary connective tissue and excessive pigmentation, due to chronic congestion from valvular heart disease, or to anthracosis. See also gray induration.

cyanotic i. hardening of an organ from chronic venous congestion.

granular i. cirrhosis.

gray i. induration of lung tissue in or after pneumonia, without the pigmentation seen in brown induration.

red i. red, congested lung tissue seen in idiopathic pulmonary FIBROSIS.

indusium griseum (in-doo'ze-um gris'e-um) [L.] a thin layer of gray matter on the dorsal surface of the corpus callosum.

indwelling (in'dwel-ing) pertaining to a catheter or other tube left within an organ or body passage for drainage, maintenance of patency, or administration of drugs or nutrients.

inebriant (ĭ-ne'bre-ant) 1. causing alcohol INTOXICATION. 2. an agent that has that effect.

inebriation (ĭ-ne"bre-a'shun) 1. INTOXICATION with ALCOHOL; see also ALCOHOLISM. 2. a state resembling alcoholic intoxication. Called also drunkenness.

inelastic (in"e-las'tik) lacking elasticity.

inert (in-ert') inactive.

inertia (in-er'shah) [L.] inactivity; inability to move spontaneously.

colonic i. weak muscular activity of the colon, leading to distention of the organ and constipation.

uterine i. sluggishness of uterine contractions in labor.

in extremis (in ek-stre'mis) [L.] at the point of death.

infancy (in'fan-se) the first 12 months of life.

infant (in'fant) a human child from birth (see newborn INFANT) to the end of the first year of life. Emotional and physical needs at this time include love and security, a sense of trust, warmth and comfort, feeding, and sucking pleasure.

Growth and Development. Development is a continuous process, and each child progresses at his own rate. There is a developmental sequence, which means that the changes leading to maturity are specific and orderly. The various types of growth and development and the accompanying changes in appearance and behavior are interrelated; that is, physical, emotional, social, and spiritual developments affect one another in the progress toward maturity.

Development of muscular control proceeds from the head downward (cephalocaudal development). The infant controls the head first and gradually acquires the ability to control the neck, then the arms, and finally the legs and feet. Movements are general and random at first, beginning with use of the larger muscles and progressing to specific smaller muscles, such as those needed to handle small objects. Factors that influence growth and development are hereditary traits, sex, environment, nationality and race, and physical makeup. See also GROWTH.

large-for-gestational-age i. a preterm, term, or postterm infant who is above the 90th percentile for GESTATIONAL AGE in head circumference, body weight, or length.

low-birth-weight i. one that weighs less than 2500 grams at birth. This standard is routinely used for infants in developed countries, but infants born in other countries typically weigh less at birth. In India the criterion for normal birth weight is 2150 grams and in Malaysia it is 2000 grams.

newborn i. a human infant from the time of birth through the 28th day of life. At birth, the GESTATIONAL AGE as well as birth weight is assessed and the newborn classified accordingly; for example, large for gestational age, preterm (premature), or low birth weight. Called also neonate and newborn.

premature i., preterm i. one born before a gestational age of 37 completed weeks (259 days). The duration of gestation is measured from the first day of the last menstrual period and is expressed in completed days or weeks.

postmature i., postterm i. one born any time after the beginning of the forty-second week (288 days) of gestation.

small-for-gestational-age i. a preterm, term, or postterm infant who is below the 10th percentile for GESTATIONAL AGE in head circumference, body weight, or length.

term i. one born at a gestational age of 37 to 42 completed weeks (259 to 293 completed days).

very-low-birth-weight i. one that weighs less than 1000 grams at birth.

Patient Care. Low-birth-weight and very-low-birth-weight infants require special care and support, preferably in a neonatal INTENSIVE CARE UNIT (NICU), until sufficient weight is gained and the infants have matured and are able to thrive without elaborate support systems.

At the time of delivery, whether cesarean or vaginal, a skilled neonatal team should be present to provide immediate care. After resuscitation measures under a radiant warmer are completed and the newborn is stabilized, transfer to the NICU is done without interruption of warming and oxygen therapies.

Among the problems associated with low birth weight are hypothermia, respiratory distress, hyperbilirubinemia, fluid and electrolyte imbalance, susceptibility to infection, and feeding problems.

Very-low-birth-weight newborns and infants are at significant risk for hypothermia because of their small body mass, large surface area, thin skin, minimal subcutaneous tissues, and posture. Thermoregulation is provided through the use of a standard incubator or a radiant warmer. Radiant warmers have the advantage of accessibility for caregivers and improved visibility of the infant. Their chief disadvantage is increased insensible water loss.

Neonatal RESPIRATORY DISTRESS SYNDROME is the major cause of death in newborns. Atelectasis can lead to hypoxemia and elevated serum carbon dioxide levels and all the problems related to inadequate gas exchange. Oxygen therapy must be administered with caution because of the danger of retinopathy.

The treatment of HYPERBILIRUBINEMIA remains a challenge because of lack of consensus on the level of serum bilirubin concentration at which therapy should begin, the uncertain diagnosis of kernicterus, and the currently limited knowledge of the blood–brain barrier. It is believed that these infants are at critical risk for bilirubin-related brain damage at serum concentrations as low as 6 to 9 mg/dl. Phototherapy is the treatment of choice and may be given prophylactically in some institutions to all infants weighing less than 1000 grams.

The management of fluid and electrolyte administration to maintain proper balance is highly complex. Factors taken into consideration are proportion of body, composition of water, renal function, and insensible water loss. Fluid and electrolyte status must be closely monitored. Overhydration is a hazard because it has been implicated in the development of such serious complications as pulmonary edema, patent ductus arteriosus, and necrotizing enterocolitis in these infants.

Low-birth-weight and very-low-birth-weight infants are particularly susceptible to infection because their immunologic system is deficient. Additionally, equipment and care related to long-term respiratory and nutritional support, together with frequent laboratory testing, increase exposure to infectious agents. Infection control measures must be adhered to faithfully. In some NICUs reverse isolation is required for all infants weighing less than 1000 grams.

Since the skin of these infants is highly permeable and easily traumatized, every effort must be made to preserve its integrity. Routine care to preserve the integrity of the skin, caution in the use of topical ointments and antiseptic preparations, and minimal handling also are essential.

At the beginning, nutritional support in the form of total PARENTERAL NUTRITION may be necessary until enteral feedings are feasible. Oral feedings usually are initiated by the end of the first week of life. Continuous gastric feedings via infusion pump have the advantage of preventing vomiting and aspiration and abdominal distention associated with intermittent feedings of larger amounts. The enteral feedings given in this manner include breast milk (donor or mother) and special formulas.

Discharge planning and follow-up care are begun upon admission to the NICU. Individual family needs should be assessed and available community resources identified. Parental education and support are provided throughout the time the infant is in the NICU. At the time of discharge parents should be confident of their ability to care for the infant, knowledgeable about sources available to them, and able to utilize those resources to the fullest.

infantile (in′fan-tīl) relating to infancy; having features or traits characteristic of early childhood.

infantilism (in-fan′tĭ-lizm, in′fan-tĭ-lizm) persistence of the characteristics of childhood into adult life, marked by mental retardation, underdevelopment of the reproductive organs, and often dwarfism.

infarct (in′fahrkt) a localized area of ischemic necrosis produced by anoxia following occlusion of the arterial supply or the venous drainage of the tissue, organ, or part.

   anemic i. one due to sudden interruption of arterial circulation to the area.

   hemorrhagic i. one that is red owing to oozing of erythrocytes into the injured area.

infarctectomy (in″fahrk-tek′to-me) surgical removal of an INFARCT.

infarction (in-fark′ shun) 1. infarct. 2. formation of an infarct.

    cardiac i. myocardial infarction.

    cerebral i. an ischemic condition of the brain, causing a persistent focal neurologic deficit in the area affected.

    myocardial i. see MYOCARDIAL INFARCTION.

    pulmonary i. localized necrosis of lung tissue caused by obstruction of the arterial blood supply, most often due to pulmonary embolism. Clinical manifestations range from the subclinical to pleuritic chest pain, dyspnea, hemoptysis, and tachycardia.

infection (in-fek′shun) invasion and multiplication of microorganisms in body tissues, as in an infectious disease. The infectious process is similar to a circular chain with each link representing one of the factors involved in the process. An infectious disease occurs only if each link is present and in proper sequence. These links are (1) the causative agent, which must be of sufficient number and virulence to destroy normal tissue; (2) reservoirs in which the organism can thrive and reproduce; for example, body tissues and the wastes of humans, animals, and insects, and contaminated food and water; (3) a portal through which the pathogen can leave the host, such as the respiratory tract or intestinal tract; (4) a mode of transfer, such as the hands, air currents, vectors, fomites, or other means by which the pathogens can be moved from one place or person to another; and (5) a portal of entry through which the pathogens can enter the body of (6) a susceptible host. Open wounds and the respiratory, intestinal, and reproductive tracts are examples of portals of entry. The host must be susceptible to the disease, not having any immunity to it, or lacking adequate resistance to overcome the invasion by the pathogens. The body responds to the invasion of causative organisms by the formation of ANTIBODIES and by a series of physiologic changes known as INFLAMMATION.

The spectrum of infectious agents changes with the passage of time and the introduction of drugs and chemicals designed to destroy them. The advent of antibiotics and the resultant development of resistant strains of bacteria have introduced new types of pathogens little known or not previously thought to be significantly dangerous to man. A few decades ago, gram-positive organisms were the most common infectious agents. Today the gram-negative microorganisms, and *Proteus, Pseudomonas,* and *Serratia* are particularly troublesome, especially in the development of hospital-acquired infections. It is predicted that in future decades other lesser known pathogens and new strains of bacteria and viruses will emerge as common causes of infections.

The development of resistant strains of pathogens can be limited by the judicious use of ANTIBIOTICS. This requires culturing and sensitivity testing for a specific antibiotic to which the identified causative organism has been found to be sensitive. If the patient has been receiving a broad-spectrum antibiotic prior to culture and sensitivity testing, this should be discontinued as soon as the specific antibiotic for the organism has been found. It would be helpful, too, if the general public understood that antibiotics are not cure-alls and that there is danger in using them indiscriminately. In some instances an antibiotic can upset the normal flora of the body, thus compromising the body's natural resistance and making it more susceptible to a second infection (SUPERINFECTION) by a microorganism resistant to the antibiotic.

Although antibacterials have greatly reduced mortality and morbidity rates for many infectious diseases, the ultimate outcome of an infectious process depends on the effectiveness of the host's IMMUNE

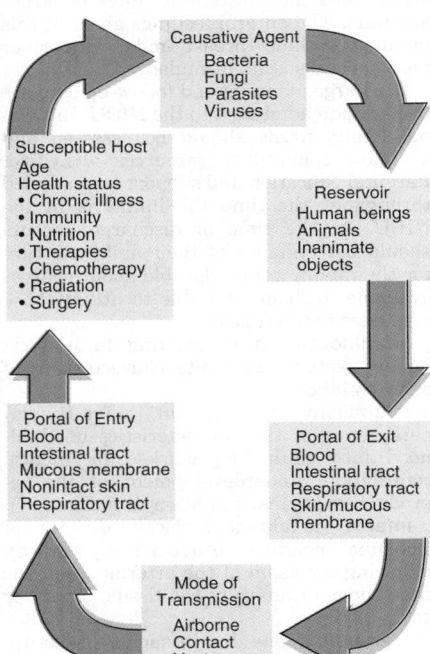

Chain of infection.

RESPONSES. The antibacterial drugs provide a holding action, keeping the growth and reproduction of the infectious agent in check until the interaction between the organism and the immune bodies of the host can subdue the invaders.

Intracellular infectious agents include viruses, mycobacteria, *Brucella, Salmonella,* and many others. Infections of this type are overcome primarily by T LYMPHOCYTES and their products, which are the components of cell-mediated IMMUNITY. Extracellular infectious agents live outside the cell; these include species of *Streptococcus* and *Haemophilus*. These microorganisms have a carbohydrate capsule that acts as an antigen to stimulate the production of antibody, an essential component of humoral IMMUNITY.

Infection may be transmitted by direct contact, indirect contact, or vectors. Direct contact may be with body excreta such as urine, feces, or mucus, or with drainage from an open sore, ulcer, or wound. Indirect contact refers to transmission via inanimate objects such as bed linens, bedpans, drinking glasses, or eating utensils. Vectors are flies, mosquitoes, or other insects capable of harboring and spreading the infectious agent.

Patient Care. Major goals in the care of patients with threatening, suspected, or diagnosed infectious disease include the following: (1) prevent the spread of infection, (2) provide physiologic support to enhance the patient's natural curative powers and resources for warding off or recovering from an infection, (3) provide psychologic support, and (4) prepare the patient for self-care if this is feasible.

Special precautions for prevention of the spread of infection can vary from strict ISOLATION of the patient and such measures as wearing gloves, mask, or gown to simply using care when handling infective material. No matter what the diagnosis or status of the patient, handwashing before and after each contact is imperative.

Unrecognized or subclinical infections pose a threat because many infectious agents can be transmitted when symptoms are either mild or totally absent.

In the care of patients for whom special precautions have not been assigned, gloves are indicated whenever there is direct contact with blood, wound or lesion drainage, urine, stool, or oral secretions. Gowns are worn over the clothing whenever there is copious drainage and the possibility that one's clothes could become soiled with infective material.

When a definitive diagnosis of an infectious disease has been made and special precautions are ordered, it is imperative that everyone having contact with the patient adhere to the rules. Family members and visitors will need instruction in the proper techniques and the reason they are necessary.

Physiologic support entails bolstering the patient's external and internal defense mechanisms. Integrity of the skin is preserved. Daily bathing is avoided if it dries the skin and predisposes it to irritation and cracking. Gentle washing and thorough drying are necessary in areas where two skin surfaces touch, for example, in the groin and genital area, under heavy breasts, and in the axillae. Lotions and emollients are used not only to keep the skin soft but also to stimulate circulation. Measures are taken to prevent pressure ulcers from prolonged pressure and ischemia. Mouth care is given on a systematic basis to assure a healthy oral mucosa.

The total fluid intake should not be less than 2000 ml every 24 hours. Cellular dehydration can work against adequate transport of nutrients and elimination of wastes. Maintenance of an acid urine is important when urinary tract infections are likely as when the patient is immobilized or has an indwelling urinary catheter. This can be accomplished by administering vitamin C daily. Nutritional needs are met by whatever means necessary, and may require supplemental oral feedings or total PARENTERAL NUTRITION. The patient will also need adequate rest and freedom from discomfort. This may necessitate teaching her or him relaxation techniques, planning for periods of uninterrupted rest, and proper use of noninvasive comfort measures, as well as judicious use of analgesic drugs.

Having an infectious disease can alter patients' self-image, making them feel self-conscious about the stigma of being infectious or "dirty," or making them feel guilty about the danger they could pose to others. Social isolation and loneliness are also potential problems for the patient with an infectious disease.

Patients also can become discouraged because some infections tend to recur or to involve other parts of the body if they are not effectively eradicated. It is important that they know about the nature of their illness, the purposes and results of diagnostic tests, and the expected effect of medications and treatments.

Patient education should also include information about the ways in which a particular infection can be transmitted, proper handwashing techniques, approved disinfectants to use at home, methods for handling and disposing of contaminated articles, and any other special precautions that are indicated. If patients are to continue taking antibacterials at home, they are cautioned not to stop taking any prescribed medication even if symptoms abate and they feel better.

airborne i. infection by inhalation of organisms suspended in air on water droplets or dust particles.

i. control 1. in the NURSING INTERVENTIONS CLASSIFICATION, a nursing INTERVENTION defined as minimizing the acquisition and transmission of infectious agents. 2. the use of surveillance, investigation, and compilation of statistical data in order to reduce the spread of infection, particularly nosocomial infections.

Practitioners in infection control are often nurses employed by hospitals. They have titles such as Infection Control Officer and Infection Control Nurse, and they function as liaisons between staff nurses, physicians, department heads, the infection control committee, and the local health department. Such practitioners also assume some responsibility for teaching patients and their families, as well as employees of the hospital.

The CENTERS FOR DISEASE CONTROL AND PREVENTION is an excellent source of information related to infection control; their web site is http://www.cdc.gov. Another source of help and support for infection control practitioners is the Association for Practitioners in Infection Control and Epidemiology, 1275 K St., NW, Suite 100, Washington, DC 20005-4006.

cross i. infection transmitted between patients infected with different pathogenic microorganisms.

droplet i. infection due to inhalation of respiratory pathogens suspended on liquid particles exhaled by someone already infected.

dustborne i. infection by inhalation of pathogens that have become affixed to particles of dust.

endogenous i. that due to reactivation of organisms present in a dormant focus, as occurs, for example, in tuberculosis.

exogenous i. that caused by organisms not normally present in the body but which have gained entrance from the environment.

mixed i. infection with more than one kind of organism at the same time.

nosocomial i. see NOSOCOMIAL INFECTION.

opportunistic i. infection by an organism that does not ordinarily cause disease but becomes pathogenic under certain circumstances, as when the patient is IMMUNOCOMPROMISED.

pyogenic i. infection by pus-producing organisms, most commonly species of *Staphylococcus* or *Streptococcus*.

risk for i. a NURSING DIAGNOSIS accepted by the North American Nursing Diagnosis Association, defined as a state in which an individual is at increased risk for being invaded by pathogenic organisms.

secondary i. infection by a pathogen following an infection by a pathogen of another kind.

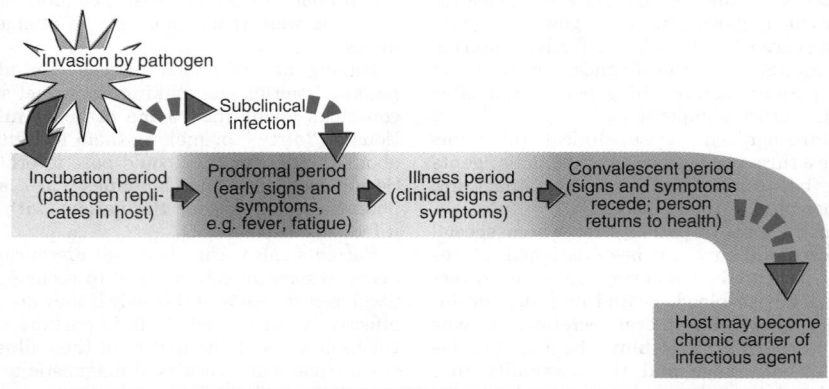

Period of communicability
Stages of infection. Each period varies with different pathogens and different diseases.

subclinical i. infection associated with no detectable symptoms but caused by microorganisms capable of producing easily recognizable diseases, such as poliomyelitis or mumps; this may occur in an early stage of the infection, with signs and symptoms appearing later during the course of the infection, or the symptoms and signs may never appear. It is detected by the production of antibody, or by delayed hypersensitivity exhibited in a skin test reaction to such antigens as tuberculoprotein.

terminal i. an acute infection occurring near the end of a disease and often causing death.

urinary tract i. see URINARY TRACT INFECTION.

vector-borne i. infection caused by microorganisms transmitted from one host to another by a carrier, such as a mosquito, louse, fly, or tick.

waterborne i. infection by microorganisms transmitted in water.

infectious (in-fek′shus) caused by or capable of being communicated by infection.

i. disease one due to organisms ranging in size from viruses to parasitic worms; it may be contagious in origin, result from nosocomial organisms, or be due to endogenous microflora from the nose and throat, skin, or bowel. See also COMMUNICABLE DISEASE.

An *emerging infectious disease* is one that is endemic in a given population but that has begun increasing in frequency or developing resistance to drug therapy or other treatments.

infective (in-fek′tiv) infectious, capable of producing infection; pertaining to or characterized by the presence of pathogens.

inferior (in-fēr′e-or) situated below, or directed downward; in anatomy, used in reference to the lower surface of a structure, or to the lower of two (or more) similar structures.

infertility (in″fer-til′ĭ-te) the inability to conceive and produce viable offspring. adj., **infer′tile.** The diagnosis of infertility is not usually considered valid until after one year of engaging in sexual relations with the same partner without contraception. Formerly, a couple's inability to have children was almost always ascribed to infertility in the female. It is now known that about 35 per cent of the cases of infertility are due to male factors, about 35 per cent to female factors, and the remaining 30 per cent to a combination of male and female factors. Most specialists subject both partners to an infertility study. More than half the couples who consult a specialist with a problem of infertility can achieve a live birth. About 5 per cent become fertile spontaneously without any treatment.

Diagnostic tests commonly used to identify female-related causes of infertility include a general pelvic examination, culdoscopy, and laparoscopy. In order to check ovulation, the health care provider may ask the patient to keep a basal temperature chart or, if indicated, an endometrial biopsy may be performed.

One cause of infertility is infection or obstruction within the fallopian tubes. The principal infections are gonorrhea and tuberculosis. A rare occurrence is the growth of a tumor in a tube. Tests to determine tubal patency include the Rubin test, which involves injecting carbon dioxide into the uterus under controlled pressure. The gas goes into the tubes and, if the tubes are open, escapes into the abdomen, from which it is harmlessly discharged. In some cases, it is thought that the gas may unblock obstructed fallopian tubes, as well as detect them. Similar information is obtained by HYSTEROSALPINGOGRAPHY, in which a radiopaque material is instilled into the uterus and fallopian tubes and x-rays of the structures are obtained.

Direct inspection of the cervix can be helpful in finding infections and chronic inflammations that could prevent conception. A postcoital test called the HUHNER TEST gives information about the ability of the sperm to survive in the cervical mucus.

Tests to identify male-related factors causing infertility include semen analysis to determine the number and motility of sperm. A low or absent sperm count could be caused by trauma to the sperm-producing cells, as in excessively high temperature of the scrotal sac resulting from inflammation, or radioactive damage to the cells. Certain drugs can also adversely affect the sperm-producing cells. Chronic prostatitis, prostatectomy, and hormonal factors can decrease motility of the sperm. A stricture in the vas deferens blocks the transporting of sperm. Strictures can result from infection, trauma, and congenital malformations. Deposition of the sperm in the vaginal tract can be hindered by premature ejaculation, impotence, and congenital malformations of the penis.

Both partners are usually given a general physical examination and a complete sexual history is taken. Painful intercourse (dyspareunia) can contribute to infertility by diminishing the frequency of intercourse. This condition can be due to malfunction of the glands that lubricate the vaginal wall. The difficulty can also be psychologic in origin, the result of sexual fears or inhibition.

The most serious condition of this type is VAGINISMUS, in which the muscles in the vagina contract, blocking the entry of the penis and making penetration impossible.

In addition to the sexual history, a medical history can raise a suspicion of an endocrine disorder, for example, hypothyroidism, or a genetic disorder, such as Turner's syndrome in women and Klinefelter's syndrome in men. If a chromosomal disorder is suspected, a buccal smear may be done for chromosomal studies.

Treatment. Treatment for relieving infertility is highly individualized. Detection of the cause and prescription of treatment should be conducted by a specialist in the area of fertility, who is better informed than general practitioners about current methods of diagnosis and treatment, and should be supportive of both partners. Feelings of anger, helplessness, grief, and other emotions can be very intense and may require great understanding and support. Either partner may feel that infertility is a threat to his or her sexuality and sexual self-image.

If the infertility cannot be corrected, as in women who fail to ovulate or men who have no sperm-producing cells, there are alternatives. Adoption is becoming more difficult because of the availability of birth control methods and the fact that more than 70 per cent of unwed mothers now choose to keep and raise their children themselves. Artificial INSEMINATION is an alternative for couples who have no moral or religious objection to the procedure. Since there is less social pressure to have children in modern Western cultures, some couples do not consider infertility a problem.

infestation (in″fes-ta′shun) parasitic attack or subsistence on the skin and/or its appendages, as by insects, mites, or ticks; sometimes used to denote parasitic invasion of the organs and tissues, as by helminths.

infiltrate (in-fil′trāt) 1. to penetrate the interstices of a tissue or substance. 2. material so deposited; called also infiltration.

infiltration (in″fil-tra′shun) 1. the pathological accumulation in tissue or cells of substances not normal to them or in amounts in excess of the normal. 2. infiltrate (def. 2). 3. the deposition of a solution directly into tissue; see infiltration ANESTHESIA.

adipose i. fatty infiltration.

calcareous i. deposit of lime and magnesium salts in the tissues.

cellular i. the migration and accumulation of cells within the tissues.

fatty i. 1. a deposit of fat in tissues, especially between cells. 2. the presence of fat vacuoles in the cell cytoplasm.

intravenous i. 1. the movement of a needle or cannula from within a vessel into the surrounding tissue. The typical symptoms are a slowed flow of fluids, swelling, pallor, coolness of the skin, and discomfort in the area; severity of the symptoms will depend on the amount and type of fluid infused. 2. inadvertent administration of parenteral fluid into the tissues.

infirm (in-ferm′) weak; feeble, as from disease or old age.

infirmary (in-fer′mah-re) a hospital or place where the sick or infirm are maintained or treated.

inflammagen (in-flam′ah-jen) an irritant that elicits both edema and the cellular response of inflammation.

inflammation (in″flah-ma′shun) a localized protective response elicited by injury or destruction of tissues, which serves to destroy, dilute, or wall off both the injurious agent and the injured tissue. adj., **inflam′matory.**

The inflammatory RESPONSE can be provoked by physical, chemical, and biologic agents, including mechanical trauma, exposure to excessive amounts of sunlight, x-rays and radioactive materials, corrosive chemicals, extremes of heat and cold, or by infectious agents such as bacteria, viruses, and other pathogenic microorganisms. Although these infectious agents can produce inflammation, infection and inflammation are not synonymous.

The classic signs of inflammation are *heat, redness, swelling, pain,* and *loss of function.* These are manifestations of the physiologic changes that occur during the inflammatory process. The three major components of this process are (1) changes in the caliber of blood vessels and the rate of blood flow through them (hemodynamic changes); (2) increased capillary permeability; and (3) leukocytic exudation.

Hemodynamic changes begin soon after injury and progress at varying rates, according to the extent of injury. They start with dilation of the arterioles and the opening of new capillaries and venular beds in the area. This causes an accelerated flow of blood, accounting for the signs of heat and redness. Next follows *increased permeability* of the microcirculation, which permits leakage of protein-rich fluid out of small blood vessels and into the extravascular fluid compartment, accounting for the inflammatory edema.

Leukocytic exudation occurs in the following sequence. First, the LEUKOCYTES move to the endothelial lining of the small blood vessels (*margination*) and line the endothelium in a tightly packed formation (*pavementing*). Eventually, these leukocytes move through the endothelial spaces and escape into the extravascular space (*emigration*). Once they are outside the blood vessels they are free to move and, by CHEMOTAXIS, are drawn to the site of injury. Accumulations of NEUTROPHILS and MACROPHAGES at the area of inflammation act to neutralize foreign particles by PHAGOCYTOSIS.

Chemical mediators of the inflammatory process include a variety of substances originating in the plasma and the cells of uninjured tissue, and possibly from the damaged tissue. The major kinds of mediators are (1) *vasoactive amines,* such as HISTAMINE and SEROTONIN; (2) *plasma endopeptidases* that comprise three interrelated systems, the kinin system that produces BRADYKININ, the complement system that produces proteins that interact with antigen–antibody complexes and mediate immunologic injury and inflammation, and the clotting system that increases vascular permeability and chemotactic activity for the leukocytes; (3) PROSTAGLANDINS, which can reproduce several aspects of the inflammatory process; (4) neutrophil products; (5) lymphocyte factors; and (6) other mediators, such as slow-reacting SUBSTANCE of anaphylaxis and endogenous PYROGEN.

Hormonal Response. Some hormones, such as CORTISOL, have an ANTIINFLAMMATORY action that limits inflammation to a local reaction while others are proinflammatory. Thus, the endocrine system has a regulatory effect on the process of inflammation so that it can be balanced and beneficial in the body's attempts to recover from injury.

acute i. inflammation, usually of sudden onset, marked by the classical signs of heat, redness, swelling, pain, and loss of function, and in which vascular and exudative processes predominate.

catarrhal i. a form affecting mainly a mucous surface, marked by a copious discharge of mucus and epithelial debris.

chronic i. prolonged and persistent inflammation marked chiefly by new connective tissue formation; it may be a continuation of an acute form or a prolonged low-grade form.

exudative i. one in which the prominent feature is an exudate.

fibrinous i. one marked by an exudate of coagulated fibrin.

granulomatous i. a form, usually chronic, attended by formation of granulomas.

interstitial i. inflammation affecting chiefly the stroma of an organ.

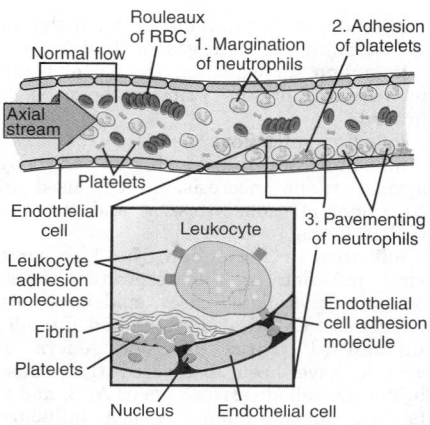

Cellular changes in inflammation. *1,* Margination of neutrophils brings these inflammatory cells in close contact with the endothelium. *2,* Adhesion of platelets results in the release of mediators of inflammation and coagulation. Fibrin strands are the first signs of clot formation. *3,* Pavementing of leukocytes is mediated by adhesion molecules activated by the mediators of inflammation released from platelets and leukocytes. RBC, red blood cells. From Damjanov, 2000.

parenchymatous i. inflammation affecting chiefly the essential tissue elements of an organ.

productive i., proliferative i. one leading to the production of new connective tissue fibers.

pseudomembranous i. an acute inflammatory RESPONSE to a powerful necrotizing toxin (such asdiphtheria TOXIN), characterized by formation on a mucosal surface of a false membrane composed of precipitated fibrin, necrotic epithelium, and inflammatory leukocytes.

purulent i. suppurative inflammation.

serous i. one producing a serous exudate.

subacute i. a condition intermediate between chronic and acute inflammation, exhibiting some of the characteristics of each.

suppurative i. one marked by pus formation.

toxic i. one due to a poison, e.g., a bacterial product.

traumatic i. one that follows a wound or injury.

ulcerative i. that in which necrosis on or near the surface leads to loss of tissue and creation of a local defect (ulcer).

inflammatory bowel disease any of various inflammatory diseases of the bowel whose etiology is unknown, including CROHN'S DISEASE and ULCERATIVE COLITIS.

inflation (in-fla′shun) distention or the act of distending, with air, gas, or fluid.

inflection (in′flek-shun) the act of bending inward, or the state of being bent inward.

inflexion inflection.

infliximab (in-flik′sĭ-mab) an antibody against tumor necrosis FACTOR, used in treatment of CROHN'S DISEASE and rheumatoid ARTHRITIS.

influenza (in″floo-en′zah) [Ital.] an acute viral infection of the respiratory tract, occurring in isolated cases, epidemics, and pandemics. Called also grippe and flu. adj., **influen′zal.** Three different genera of viruses have been discovered that cause influenza, called INFLUENZAVIRUS A, B, and C (species names influenza A VIRUS, influenza B VIRUS, and influenza C VIRUS). Influenza B and influenza C viruses are chiefly associated with sporadic epidemics among children and young adults. Most older adults carry antibodies against influenza because of repeated exposure to the viruses. Subtypes of influenza A virus are designated based on the antigens HEMAGGLUTININ and NEURAMINIDASE; because they can undergo antigenic SHIFT they are responsible for widespread epidemics.

Symptoms. Influenza has a short incubation period. Symptoms appear suddenly, and although the virus enters the respiratory tract it soon affects the entire body. The symptoms include fever, chills, headache, sore throat, cough, gastrointestinal disturbances, muscular pain, and neuralgia.

Treatment. There is no drug that will cure influenza, but over-the-counter medications may minimize discomfort. Rest, increased fluid intake, and aspirin to relieve aches and discomfort and help control fever are prescribed for adults. Children are also treated symptomatically, but without aspirin.

Prevention. A vaccine is available, although it does not always provide complete immunity against all forms of influenza viruses that may be present. In its *Guidelines for the Prevention and Treatment of Influenza and the Common Cold,* the American Lung Association recommends vaccination for people over 50, pregnant women who will be more than three months pregnant during flu season, residents of nursing homes or other chronic care facilities, and health care providers (the latter because they could transmit the virus to persons in high risk groups). Systemic reactions to the vaccine occasionally occur. Toxic reactions include fever, malaise, and muscle pain within 6 to 12 hours after injection. An immediate reaction can occur as a result of allergic HYPERSENSITIVITY. In about 10 cases per million vaccinations, GUILLAIN-BARRÉ SYNDROME occurs. Preventive measures other than vaccination include avoiding contact with persons who have influenza, avoiding crowded places when there is a local epidemic, and observing good personal hygiene to increase the body's resistance.

Influenzavirus (in″floo-en′zah-vi′rus) former genus name for the viruses that cause INFLUENZA, now found to be two different genera, which were named INFLUENZAVIRUS A and INFLUENZAVIRUS B.

I. A a genus of viruses containing the agent of INFLUENZA A. See also influenza VIRUS.

I. B a genus of viruses containing the agent of INFLUENZA B. See also influenza VIRUS.

I. C a genus of viruses containing the agent of INFLUENZA C. See also influenza VIRUS.

informatics (in″for-mat′iks) the management of information and knowledge by computers.

information (in″for-ma′shun) 1. knowledge obtained by learning. 2. knowledge that is exchanged through communication, either verbal, written or data.

preparatory sensory i. in the NURSING INTERVENTIONS CLASSIFICATION, a nursing INTERVENTION defined as describing in concrete and subjective terms the typical sensory experiences and events associated with an upcoming stressful health care procedure or treatment.

infra- word element [L.], *beneath.*

infra-axillary (in″frah-ak′sĭ-ler″e) below the axilla.

infraclavicular (in″frah-klah-vik′u-lar) subclavian.

infraclusion (in″frah-kloo′zhun) a condition in which the occluding surface of a tooth does not reach the normal occlusal plane and is out of contact with the opposing tooth.

infracostal (in″frah-kos′tal) subcostal.

infraction (in-frak′shun) incomplete bone fracture without displacement.

infradian (in″frah-de′an) pertaining to the rhythmic repetition of certain phenomena of living organisms in cycles of less frequency than one a day; see also infradian RHYTHM.

infrahyoid (in″frah-hi′oid) subhyoid.

inframaxillary (in″frah-mak′sĭ-ler″e) sub maxillary.

infranuclear (in″frah-noo′kle-ar) below nucleus.

WINDOW ON INFORMATICS

The term *informatics*, widely used in Europe, is used almost exclusively in health care in the United States. Today, the field is engaging some of the most original and creative minds in health care professions. The generic term *health care informatics* highlights the interdisciplinary nature of the field. The terms *medical informatics*, *nursing informatics*, and *dental informatics* underscore the relevance of informatics to the individual health care professions. Today we are seeing the development of informatics departments, informatics curricula, and even informatics degrees. As health care professionals strive to harness the power of technology, many look to the American Medical Informatics Association (AMIA) and the International Medical Informatics Association (IMIA).

Such power does not come without risk. Developments in health care informatics pose grave challenges. We must create organizations which can use the capabilities that informatics can provide. We must educate professionals to be able to develop new technologies as well as use them. We must evaluate the care we provide and assess the technologies we use to do so.

The power of informatics is to make "caring and technology meet." We can see its power in point of care terminals, health professional workstations, and networked environments, which give us access to information when, where, and how we need it. We will truly know the power of informatics when the patient record can go everywhere with the patient, from doctor's office to hospital, and can include whatever information there is on the patient and the patient's problems. We all stand to gain from realizing the World Health Organization's goal of "Informatics in Support of Global Health."

MARION J. BALL, EdD

infraorbital (in″frah-or′bĭ-tal) lying under or on the floor of the orbit; called also suborbital.

infrapatellar (in″frah-pah-tel′ar) below or beneath the PATELLA; called also subpatellar.

infrared (in″frah-red′) denoting electromagnetic RADIATION of wavelength greater than that of the red end of the spectrum, i.e., of 0.75–1000 μm. Infrared rays are sometimes subdivided into *long-wave* or *far infrared* (about 3.0–1000 μm) and *short-wave* or *near infrared* (about 0.75–3.0 μm). They are capable of penetrating body tissues to a depth of 1 cm. Sources of infrared rays include heat lamps, hot water bottles, steam radiators, and incandescent light bulbs. Infrared rays are used therapeutically to promote muscle relaxation, to speed up the inflammatory process, and to increase circulation to a part of the body. See also HEAT.

infrascapular (in″frah-skap′u-lar) subscapular.

infrasonic (in″frah-son′ik) below the frequency range of sound waves.

infraspinous (in″frah-spi′nus) beneath the spine of the scapula.

infrasternal (in″frah-ster′nal) substernal.

infratentorial (in″frah-ten-tor′e-al) beneath the tentorium of the cerebellum.

infratrochlear (in″frah-trok′le-ar) beneath the trochlea.

infraversion (in″frah-ver′zhun) 1. downward deviation of the eye. (See accompanying illustration.) 2. infraclusion.

infundibuliform (in″fun-dib′u-lĭ-form) infundibular (def. 2).

infundibular (in-fun-dib′u-ler) 1. pertaining to an INFUNDIBULUM. 2. funnel-shaped; called also choanoid.

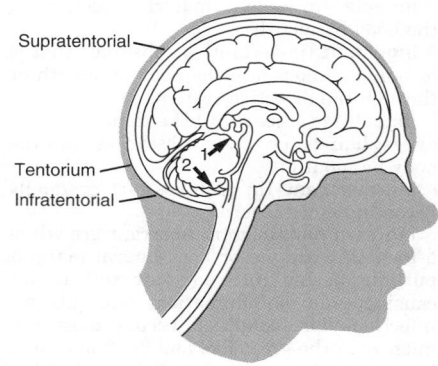

1. Upward
2. Downward

Infratentorial: infratentorial herniations. From Betz et al., 1994.

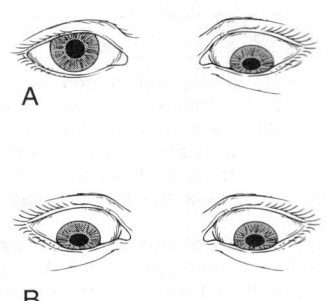

A

B

Infraversion of one *A* or both *B* eyes. From Dorland's, 2000.

infundibulum (in-fun-dib′u-lum), pl. *in-fundi′bula* [L.] 1. any funnel-shaped passage; called also choana. 2. conus arteriosus.

ethmoidal i. 1. a passage connecting the nasal cavity with the anterior ethmoidal CELLS and frontal SINUS. 2. a sinuous passage connecting the middle meatus of the nose with the anterior ethmoidal cells and often with the frontal sinus.

i. of hypothalamus a hollow, funnel-shaped mass in front of the tuber cinereum, extending to the posterior lobe of the pituitary gland.

i. of uterine tube the distal, funnel-shaped portion of the fallopian (uterine) tube.

infusion (in-fu′zhun) 1. the steeping of a substance in water to obtain its soluble principles. 2. the product obtained by this process. 3. the slow therapeutic introduction of fluid other than blood into a vein.

intravenous i. see INTRAVENOUS INFUSION.

subcutaneous i. hypodermoclysis.

ingesta (in-jes′tah) material taken into the body by mouth.

ingestant (in-jes′tant) a substance that is or may be taken into the body by mouth or through the digestive system.

ingestion (in-jes′chun) the taking of food, drugs, liquids, or other substances into the body by mouth.

ingravescent (in″grah-ves′ent) gradually becoming more severe.

ingrown nail (in′grōn) aberrant growth of a toenail, with one or both lateral margins pushing deeply into adjacent soft tissue, causing pain, inflammation, and possible infection. The condition occurs most frequently in the great toe, and is often caused by pressure from tight-fitting shoes. Another common cause is improper cutting of the toenails, which should be cut straight across or with a curved toenail scissors so that the sides are a little longer than the middle.

inguen (ing′gwen), pl. *in′guina* [L.] the junctional region betwen the abdomen and thigh; either of the abdominal REGIONS lateral to the suprapubic (hypogastric) region. Called also groin and iliac or inguinal REGION. adj., **in′guinal.**

inguinal (ing′gwĭ-nal) pertaining to the groin.

INH isoniazid.

inhalant (in-ha′lant) 1. a substance that is or may be taken into the body by way of the nose and trachea (through the respiratory system). 2. a class of psychoactive substances whose volatile vapors are subject to abuse; see SUBSTANCE ABUSE.

inhalation (in″hah-la′shun) 1. the drawing of air or other substances into the airways and lungs; see also ASPIRATION. Called also inspiration. 2. any drug or solution of drugs administered (as by means of nebulizers or aerosols) by the nasal or oral respiratory route.

inhaler (in-ha′ler) 1. an apparatus for administering vapor or volatilized medications by inhalation. 2. ventilator.

metered dose i. an inhaler used to deliver aerosolized medications in fixed doses to patients with respiratory disease.

inheritance (in-her′ĭ-tans) 1. the acquisition of characters or qualities by transmission from parent to offspring. 2. that which is transmitted from parent to offspring; see also GENE, DEOXYRIBONUCLEIC ACID, and HEREDITY.

intermediate i. inheritance in which the phenotype of the heterozygote falls between that of the two homozygotes.

maternal i. the transmission of characters that are dependent on peculiarities of the egg cytoplasm produced, in turn, by nuclear genes.

inhibition (in″hĭ-bish′un) 1. arrest or restraint of a process. 2. in psychoanalysis, the conscious or unconscious restraining of an impulse or desire. adj., **inhib′itory.**

competitive i. inhibition of enzyme activity by an inhibitor (a substrate analogue) that competes with the substrate for binding sites on the enzymes.

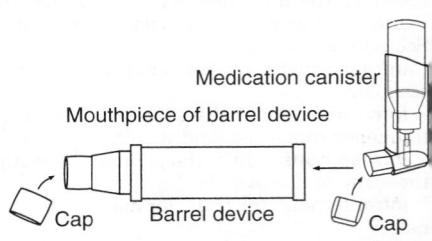

Medication canister

Mouthpiece of barrel device

Cap   Barrel device   Cap

Metered dose inhaler with a barrel device. From Lammon et al., 1995.

contact i. inhibition of cell division and cell motility in normal animal cells when in close contact with each other.

noncompetitive i. inhibition of enzyme activity by substances that combine with the enzyme at a site other than that utilized by the substrate.

inhibitor (in-hib´ĭ-tor) 1. any substance that interferes with a chemical reaction, growth, or other biologic activity. 2. a chemical substance that inhibits or checks the action of a tissue organizer or the growth of microorganisms. 3. an effector that reduces the catalytic activity of an enzyme.

ACE i's, angiotensin-converting enzyme i's see ANGIOTENSIN-CONVERTING ENZYME INHIBITORS.

angiogenesis i. a group of drugs that prevent growth of new blood vessels into a solid tumor.

aromatase i's a class of drugs that inhibit AROMATASE activity and thus block production of ESTROGENS; used to treat BREAST CANCER and ENDOMETRIOSIS.

C1 i. (C1 INH) a member of the SERPIN group, an inhibitor of C1, the initial component activated in the classical complement PATHWAY. Deficiency of or defect in the protein causes hereditary ANGIOEDEMA.

carbonic anhydrase i. an agent that inhibits the enzyme CARBONIC ANHYDRASE; used in treatment of GLAUCOMA and sometimes for EPILEPSY, familial periodic PARALYSIS, acute MOUNTAIN SICKNESS, and KIDNEY STONES of uric acid.

cholinesterase i. anticholinesterase.

COX-2 i's, cyclooxygenase-2 i's a group of NONSTEROIDAL ANTIINFLAMMATORY DRUGS that act by inhibiting CYCLOOXYGEN-ASE-1 activity; they have fewer gastrointestinal side effects than other NSAIDs. Two members of the group are CELECOXIB and ROFECOXIB.

gastric acid pump i. an agent that inhibits gastric acid secretion by blocking the action of H^+,K^+-ATPase at the secretory surface of gastric parietal cells; called also *proton pump i.*

HIV protease i. any of a group of antiretroviral drugs active against the human immunodeficiency virus; they prevent protease-mediated cleavage of viral polyproteins, causing production of immature viral particles that are noninfective. Examples include INDINAVIR sulfate, NELFINAVIR mesylate, RITONAVIR, and SAQUINAVIR.

HMG-CoA reductase i's a group of drugs that competitively inhibit the enzyme that catalyzes the rate-limiting step in CHOLESTEROL biosynthesis, and are used to lower plasma lipoprotein levels in the treatment of HYPERLIPOPROTEINEMIA. Called also statins.

MAO i. monoamine oxidase inhibitor.

membrane i. of reactive lysis (MIRL) protectin.

monoamine oxidase i. any of a group of drugs that inhibit the action of MONOAMINE OXIDASE, the enzyme that breaks down NOREPINEPHRINE and SEROTONIN, prescribed for their ANTIDEPRESSANT action; the most widely used ones are ISOCARBOXAZID, PHENELZINE, and TRANYLCYPROMINE. They are also used in the prevention of MIGRAINE.

α_2-plasmin i. α_2-antiplasmin.

plasminogen activator i. (PAI) any of several regulators of the fibrinolytic system that act by binding to and inhibiting free plasminogen ACTIVATOR. Their concentration in plasma is normally low, but is altered in some disturbances of bodily HEMOSTASIS. *PAI-1* is an important fast-reacting inhibitor of t-plasminogen ACTIVATOR and u-plasminogen ACTIVATOR. Its synthesis, activity, and release are highly regulated; elevated levels of it have been described in a number of disease states. *PAI-2* is a normally minor inhibitor that greatly increases in concentration during pregnancy and in certain disorders. *PAI-3* is protein C inhibitor.

platelet i. any of a group of agents that inhibit the clotting activity of platelets; the most common ones are ASPIRIN and DIPYRIDAMOLE. See also antiplatelet THERAPY.

protease i. 1. a substance that blocks activity of endopeptidase (protease), such as in a virus. 2. HIV protease inhibitor.

protein C i. the primary inhibitor of activated anticoagulant PROTEIN C; it is a glycoprotein of the serpin family of proteinase inhibitors and also inhibits several other proteins involved in coagulation (thrombin, kallikrein, and coagulation factors X and XI) and urokinase. Called also plasminogen activator inhibitor 3.

proton pump i. gastric acid pump i.

reverse transcriptase i. a substance that blocks activity of the REVERSE TRANSCRIPTASE of a RETROVIRUS and is used as an ANTIRETROVIRAL agent. Some are NUCLEOSIDES or nucleoside ANALOGUES, and those that are not are therefore often called *non-nucleoside reverse transcriptase inhibitors.*

selective serotonin reuptake i. (SSRI) any of a group of drugs that inhibit the inactivation of SEROTONIN by blocking its absorption in the central nervous system; used as ANTIDEPRESSANTS and in the treatment of OBSESSIVE-COMPULSIVE DISORDER and PANIC DISORDER.

serine protease i., serine proteinase i. serpin.

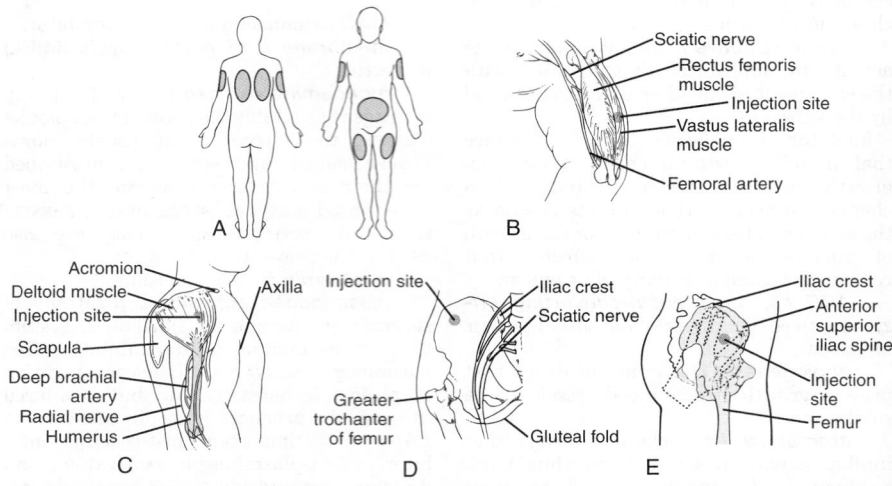

Sites for injections. *A*, subcutaneous injection sites. *B*, intramuscular injection site for children in the vastus lateralis muscle. *C*, *D*, and *E*, intramuscular injection sites for adults: *C*, deltoid muscle injection site. *D*, injection site in the buttock (dorsogluteal site). *E*, injection site in the anterolateral thigh (ventrogluteal site).

topoisomerase i's a class of antineo-plastic AGENTS that interfere with the ar-rangement of DNA in cells.

inion (in′e-on) the external occipital protuberance. adj., **in′ial.**

iniopagus (in″e-op′ah-gus) conjoined twins joined at the occiput.

initis (ĭ-ni′tis) myositis.

injected (in-jek′ted) 1. introduced by injection. 2. congested.

injection (in-jek′shun) 1. congestion. 2. the forcing of a liquid into a part, as into the subcutaneous tissues, the vascular tree, or an organ. 3. a substance so forced or administered; in pharmacy, a solution of a medicament suitable for injection.

Immunizing substances, or inoculations, are generally given by injection. Some medicines cannot be given by mouth because chemical action of the enzymes and digestive fluids would change or reduce their effectiveness, or because they would be removed from the body too quickly to have any effect. Occasionally a medication is injected so that it will act more quickly. In addition to the most common types of injections described below, injections are sometimes made into arteries, bone mar-row, the spine, the sternum, the pleural space of the chest region, the peritoneal cavity, and joint spaces. In sudden heart failure, heart-stimulating drugs may be injected directly into the heart (intracardiac injection).

hypodermic i. subcutaneous injection.

intracutaneous i. intradermal injec-tion.

intracytoplasmic sperm i. (ICSI) a MI-CROMANIPULATION technique used in male factor INFERTILITY; a single SPERMATOCYTE is inserted into an OOCYTE by MICROPUNCTURE.

intradermal i. injection of small amounts of material into the corium or substance of the skin, done in diagnostic procedures and in administration of regional anesthetics, as well as in treatment proce-dures. In certain allergy tests, the allergen is injected intracutaneously. These injections are given in an area where the skin and hair are sparse, usually on the inner part of the forearm. A 25-gauge needle, about 1 cm long, is usually used and is inserted at a 10- to 15-degree angle to the skin.

intramuscular i. injection into the sub-stance of a muscle, usually the muscle of the upper arm, thigh, or buttock. Intramuscular injections are given when the substance is to be absorbed quickly. They should be given with extreme care, especially in the buttock, because the sciatic nerve may be injured or a large blood vessel may be entered if the injection is not made correctly into the upper, outer quadrant of the buttock. The deltoid muscle at the shoulder is also used, but less commonly than the gluteus muscle of the buttock; care must be taken to insert the needle in the center, 2 cm below the acromion.

Injections into the anterolateral aspect of the thigh are considered the safest because there is less danger of damage to a major blood vessel or nerve. The area permits multiple injections, is more accessible, and is easier to stabilize, particularly in pediatric patients or others who are restless and uncooperative. The vastus lateralis muscle is located by identifying the trochanter and the side of the knee cap and then drawing a visual line between the two. The distance is then divided into thirds and the needle inserted into the area identified as the middle third.

The needle should be long enough to insure that the medication is injected deep into the muscle tissue. The gauge of the needle depends on the viscosity of the fluid being injected. As a general rule, not more than 5 ml is given in an intramuscular injection for an adult. The maximum for an infant is 0.5 ml, and the injection is made into the vastus lateralis muscle. The needle is inserted at a 90-degree angle to the skin. When the gluteus maximus muscle is the site chosen for the injection, the patient should be in a prone position with the toes turned in if possible. This position relaxes the muscle and makes the injection less painful.

intrathecal i. injection of a substance through the theca of the spinal cord into the subarachnoid space. Patients receiving intrathecal chemotherapy for metastatic malignancy of the central nervous system should maintain a flat or Trendelenburg position for one hour after treatment to achieve optimum distribution of the drug.

intravenous i. an injection made into a vein. Intravenous injections are used when rapid absorption is called for, when fluid cannot be taken by mouth, or when the substance to be administered is too irritating to be injected into the skin or muscles. In certain diagnostic tests and x-ray examinations a drug or dye may be administered intravenously. (See also INTRAVENOUS INFUSION.)

jet i. injection of a drug in solution through the intact skin by an extremely fine jet of the solution under high pressure.

subcutaneous i. injection made into the subcutaneous tissues. Although usually fluid medications are injected, occasionally solid materials such as steroid hormones may be injected in small, slowly absorbed pellets to prolong their effect. Subcutaneous injections may be given wherever there is subcutaneous tissue, usually in the upper outer arm or thigh. A 25-gauge needle about 2 cm long is usually used, held at a 45-degree angle to the skin, and the amount injected should not exceed 2 ml in an adult. Subcutaneous insulin injections may be given at a 90-degree angle

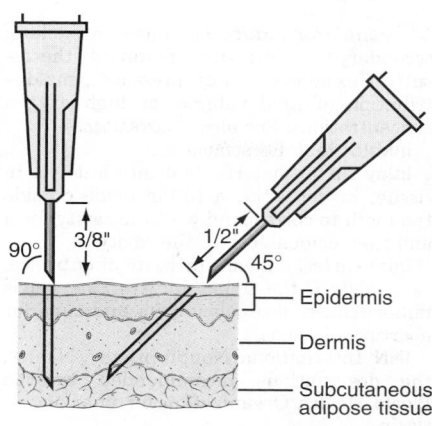

Angle of needle insertion for administering a subcutaneous injection. From Lammon et al., 1995.

with an insulin syringe. Called also hypodermic injection.

Z-track i. see Z-TRACK INJECTION.

injury (in′ju-re) harm or hurt; usually applied to damage inflicted on the body by an external force. Called also trauma and wound.

brain i. impairment of structure or function of the brain, usually as a result of a trauma.

deceleration i. a mechanism of motion injury in which the body is forcibly stopped but the contents of the body cavities remain in motion due to inertia; the brain is particularly vulnerable to such trauma.

head i. see HEAD INJURY.

risk for i. a NURSING DIAGNOSIS approved by the North American Nursing Diagnosis Association, defined as the state in which a person is at risk for injury as a result of environmental conditions interacting with the individual's adaptive and defensive resources. Any pathophysiological condition such as altered level of consciousness, impaired sensory perception, tissue hypoxia, and pain or fatigue can contribute to or be the cause of personal injury. Age-related factors include infancy and early childhood, advanced age, and the 20- to 29-year age group in which accidents and harmful lifestyles are major causes of illness and death.

risk for perioperative-positioning i. a NURSING DIAGNOSIS approved by the North American Nursing Diagnosis Association, defined as being at risk for injury as a result of the environmental conditions found in the PERIOPERATIVE setting.

ventilator-induced i. injury to the lung secondary to VENTILATOR treatment, the result of excessive airway pressures, maldistribution of tidal volume, or high oxygen concentrations. See also BAROTRAUMA.

inkblot test Rorschach test.

inlay (in'la) material laid into a defect in tissue; in dentistry, a filling made outside the tooth to correspond with the cavity form and then cemented into the cavity.

inlet (in'let) a means or route of entrance.

pelvic i. the upper limit of the pelvis minor; called also pelvic brim and superior aperture of pelvis.

INN International Nonproprietary Names, the designations recommended by the World Health Organization for pharmaceuticals.

innate (ĭ-nāt') inborn.

innervation (in″er-va'shun) 1. the distribution or supply of nerves to a part. 2. the supply of nervous energy or of nerve stimulation sent to a part.

innidiation (ĭ-nid″e-a'shun) development of cells in a part to which they have been carried by metastasis.

innocent (in'o-sent) benign.

innocuous (ĭ-nok'u-us) harmless.

innominate (ĭ-nom'ĭ-nāt) nameless, anonymous, such as the innominate artery or vein. See anatomic Tables of Arteries and Veins in the Appendices.

inochondritis (in″o-kon-dri'tis) fibrochondritis.

inoculability (ĭ-nok″u-lah-bil'ĭ-te) the state of being inoculable.

inoculable (ĭ-nok'u-lah-b'l) 1. susceptible of being inoculated; transmissible by inoculation. 2. not immune against a transmissible disease.

inoculation (ĭ-nok″u-la'shun) introduction of pathogenic microorganisms, injective material, serum, or other substances into tissues of living organisms or into culture media; introduction of a disease agent into a healthy individual to produce a mild form of the disease, followed by IMMUNITY.

inoculum (ĭ-nok'u-lum), pl. *inoc'ula* [L.] material used in inoculation.

inodilator (in″o-di-la'ter) an agent with both positive inotropic and vasodilator effects.

inogenous (in-oj'ĕ-nus) produced from or forming tissue.

inoperable (in-op'er-ah-b'l) not susceptible to treatment by surgery.

inorganic (in″or-gan'ik) 1. having no organs. 2. not of organic origin. 3. in chemistry, said of substances not derived from hydrocarbons.

inoscopy (in-os'kah-pe) diagnosis of disease by artificial digestion (as by enzymes outside the body) and examination of fibers or fibrinous matter from body products such as sputum, blood, or effusions. Called also fibrinoscopy.

inosemia (in″o-se'me-ah) 1. the presence of inositol in the blood. 2. an excess of fibrin in the blood.

inosine (I) (in'o-sēn) a purine nucleoside containing the base hypoxanthine and the sugar ribose, which occurs in transfer RNAs.

i. monophosphate **(IMP)** a nucleotide produced by removal of the AMINE group from ADENOSINE MONOPHOSPHATE in metabolism of PURINE nucleotides.

inosinic acid (in″o-sin'ik) a mononucleotide constituent of muscle, made up of hypoxanthine, ribose, and phosphoric acid.

inositol (ĭ-no'sĭ-tol) a cyclic sugar alcohol; usually referring to the most abundant isomer, *myo*-inositol, which is found in many plant and animal tissues and is often classified as part of the VITAMIN B complex.

inosituria (in″o-sĭ-tu're-ah) the presence of inositol in the urine.

inotropic (in″o-trop'ik) affecting the force of muscular contractions.

inpatient (in'pa-shent) a patient who comes to a hospital or other health care facility for diagnosis or treatment that requires an overnight stay.

inquest (in'kwest) a legal inquiry before a coroner or medical examiner, and usually a jury, into the manner of death.

insalubrious (in″sah-loo'bre-us) injurious to health.

insanity (in-san'ĭ-te) a medically obsolete term for mental derangement or disorder. Insanity is now a purely legal term, denoting a condition due to which a person lacks criminal responsibility for a crime and therefore cannot be convicted of it. adj., insane'.

inscriptio (in-skrip'she-o), pl. *inscriptio'nes* [L.] inscription.

i. tendi'nea intersectio tendinea.

inscription (in-skrip'shun) 1. a mark or line. 2. the second part of a PRESCRIPTION, the part containing names and amounts of the ingredients.

insect (in'sekt) any individual of the class Insecta.

i. bites and stings injuries caused by the mouth parts and venom of insects (see also BEE STING). Similar conditions are caused by members of the class ARACHNIDA, which includes the spiders, scorpions, ticks, and mites; see also SPIDER BITE. The most common biting insects are mosquitoes and ants. Bites and stings can be the cause of much discomfort, but there is usually no real danger, unless the individual experiences an allergic or ANAPHYLACTIC REACTION. More commonly, a local infection can develop from scratching the site of the bite. Some insects establish themselves on the skin as parasites, others inject poison, and still others transmit disease. A knowledge of first aid measures for bites and stings can do much to relieve discomfort, prevent infection, and sometimes even save a life.

Insecta (in-sek'tah) a class of arthropods whose members are characterized by division of the body into three distinct regions: head, thorax, and abdomen.

insecticide (in-sek'tĭ-sīd) an agent that kills insects. adj., **insecti'dal.**

insemination (in-sem″ĭ-na'shun) the deposit of seminal fluid within the vagina or cervix.

   artificial i. that done by artificial means. There are two primary types: *Artificial insemination by husband* (AIH) involves depositing the husband's or sexual partner's sperm from a specimen, obtained during masturbation, into the vagina, cervical canal, or uterine cavity of the recipient. *Donor insemination* or *Artificial insemination by donor* (AID) involves the same techniques but the sperm is from a donor other than the husband or partner.

insensible (in-sen'sĭ-b'l) 1. devoid of sensibility or CONSCIOUSNESS. 2. not perceptible to the senses.

insertion (in-ser'shun) 1. the act of implanting, or condition of being implanted. 2. the site of attachment, as of a muscle to the bone that it moves. 3. in genetics, a rare nonreciprocal type of TRANSLOCATION in which a segment is removed from one chromosome and then inserted into a broken region of a nonhomologous chromosome.

   airway i. and stabilization in the NURSING INTERVENTIONS CLASSIFICATION, a nursing INTERVENTION defined as insertion or assisting with insertion and stabilization of an artificial AIRWAY. See also artificial airway MANAGEMENT.

   intravenous (IV) i. in the NURSING INTERVENTIONS CLASSIFICATION, a nursing INTERVENTION defined as insertion of a needle into a peripheral vein for the purpose of INTRAVENOUS INFUSION of fluids, blood, or medications.

   thought i. the delusion that thoughts that are not one's own are being inserted into one's mind.

   velamentous i. attachment of the umbilical cord to the edge of the placenta.

insidious (in-sid'e-us) coming on stealthily; of gradual and subtle development.

insight (in'sīt) 1. in psychiatry, the patient's awareness and understanding of the origins and meaning of his attitudes, feelings, and behavior and of his disturbing symptoms; self-understanding. 2. in problem solving, the sudden perception of the appropriate relationships of things that results in a solution.

in situ (in si'tu) [L.] in its normal place; confined to the site of origin.

insoluble (in-sol'u-b'l) not susceptible of being dissolved.

insomnia (in-som'ne-ah) abnormal wakefulness; a SLEEP DISORDER consisting of an inability to fall asleep easily or to remain asleep throughout the night. The frequency of persistent insomnia is high; epidemiologic data indicate that it is the most common sleep disorder in the industrialized world. The causes may be physical, psychological, psychiatric, or presence of a specific sleep disorder. adj., **insom'niac.**

   The American Academy of Sleep Medicine recommends that health care practitioners should screen all patients for symptoms of insomnia during health examinations. Fatigue, irritability, reduction in memory, and loss of ability to concentrate are among the daytime manifestations of insomnia.

   The treatment of insomnia must be individualized, based on the underlying cause. Physical and mental health problems must be addressed, although they cannot always be successfully treated. Specific medications for sleep, such as SEDATIVES, HYPNOTICS, and other agents are frequently used but are often asociated with development of TOLERANCE, or with rebound insomnia when they are discontinued. Nonpharmacologic treatments that have strong research support include the following: stimulus control to retrain the person who is unable to sleep so that he or she reassociates the bed and bedroom with sleep; progressive muscle relaxation; paradoxical intention therapy where the patient stays awake to eliminate performance anxiety related to sleep; BIOFEEDBACK; and multicomponent (cognitive) therapy.

   Numerous papers and guidelines to support evidence-based practice in the management of insomnia are available by writing to the American Academy of Sleep Medicine, 6301 Bendel Road NW, Suite 101, Rochester, MN 55901 or looking at their web site at http://www.aasmnet.org/practiceparameters.htm.

   fatal familial i. an inherited PRION DISEASE, transmitted as an autosomal dominant trait. The cause is unknown, but it seems to affect primarily the THALAMUS with disruptions in the sleep-wake cycle. Onset is typically in midlife, characterized by progressive insomnia, hallucinations, and motor abnormalities followed by stupor and coma ending in death within 6 months to 3 years of onset. There may also be excessive sweating, elevated body temperature and blood pressure, and tachycardia.

primary i. a dyssomnia characterized by persistent difficulty initiating or maintaining sleep or by persistently nonrefreshing sleep, but not due to any other psychological or physical condition.

insonate (in-so′nāt) to expose to ultrasound waves.

insorption (in-sorp′shun) movement of a substance into the blood, especially from the gastrointestinal tract into the circulating blood.

inspection (in-spek′shun) visual examination for detection of features or qualities perceptible to the eye.

inspersion (in-sper′zhun) sprinkling, as with powder.

inspirate (in′spĭ-rāt) inhaled air or other gas.

inspiration (in″spĭ-ra′shun) inhalation (def. 1). adj., **inspi′ratory.**

inspissated (in-spis′āt-ed) being thickened, dried, or made less fluid by evaporation or absorption of liquid components.

instability (in-stah-bil′ĭ-te) lack of constancy; excessive likelihood of change.

detrusor i. the occurrence during bladder filling of contractions that compromise capacity or produce urinary leakage.

instep (in′step) the dorsal part of the arch of the foot.

instillation (in″stĭ-la′shun) 1. administration of a liquid drop by drop. 2. the putting of something into something else by a slow, persistent process.

hope i. in the NURSING INTERVENTIONS CLASSIFICATION, a nursing INTERVENTION defined as facilitation of the development of a positive outlook in a given situation.

instinct (in′stinkt) a complex of unlearned responses characteristic of a species. adj., **instinc′tive.**

death i. Freud's concept of an unconscious drive toward dissolution and death, in opposition to the life instinct.

herd i. the instinct or urge to be one of a group and to conform to its standards of conduct and opinion.

life i. Freud's concept of all the constructive tendencies of the organism aimed at maintenance and perpetuation of the individual and species, in opposition to the death instinct.

institutionalism (in-stĭ-too′shun-al-izm) social breakdown syndrome.

institutionalization (in″stĭ-too″shun-al′ĭ-za′shun) 1. commitment of a patient to a health care facility for treatment, often psychiatric. 2. in patients hospitalized for a long period, the development of excessive dependency on the institution and its routines, with diminishing of the will to function independently.

Institutional Review Board a group of peers in a clinical setting that examines a research proposal to insure patient safety and addresses the ethics of the proposed study.

instruction (in-struk′shun) teaching.

computer-assisted i. CAI; instructional activities that use a computer as the primary vehicle for teaching content or processes rather than one-to-one interaction with a student.

instrument (in′stroo-ment) 1. a tool or implement. 2. a device for accomplishing a desired activity.

OARS i. (Older Adult Resources and Services) a questionnaire used as a community assessment tool to determine the level of functioning of older adults in the five areas of mental health, physical health, social resources, economic resources, and activities of daily living. It must be administered by a trained individual and can be administered in separate segments if assessment of only one area is desired. The responses to the questionnaire can be used to determine choices of supportive services for the geriatric population.

instrumentarium (in″stroo-men-tar′e-um) the equipment or instruments required for any particular operation or purpose; the physical adjuncts with which a health care provider combats disease.

instrumentation (in″stroo-men-ta′shun) 1. the use of tools, appliances, or apparatus in the treatment of a patient. 2. the application of specific rules to develop a measurement device or instrument in a research study.

Harrington i. a system of metal hooks and rods inserted surgically into the posterior elements of the spine to provide distraction and compression in treatment of scoliosis and other deformities.

insudation (in″soo-da′shun) 1. the accumulation, as in the kidney, of a substance derived from the blood. 2. the substance so accumulated.

insufficiency (in″sŭ-fish′en-se) inability to perform properly an allotted function; called also incompetence.

adrenal i. abnormally diminished activity of the ADRENAL GLAND; called also hypoadrenalism.

adrenocortical i. abnormally diminished secretion of CORTICOSTEROIDS by the ADRENAL CORTEX; see also ADDISON'S DISEASE. Called also hypoadrenocorticism and hypocorticism.

aortic i. inadequate closure of the aortic VALVE, permitting aortic REGURGITATION.

coronary i. decreased supply of blood to the myocardium resulting from constriction or obstruction of the coronary arteries, but not accompanied by necrosis of the myocardial cells. Called also myocardial ischemia.

ileocecal i. inability of the ileocecal VALVE to prevent backflow of contents from the cecum into the ileum.

mitral i. inadequate closure of the mitral VALVE, permitting mitral REGURGITATION.

placental i. dysfunction of the PLACENTA, with reduction in the area of exchange of nutrients; it often leads to fetal growth retardation.

pulmonary i. 1. pulmonary valve insufficiency. 2. RESPIRATORY INSUFFICIENCY.

pulmonary valve i. inadequate closure of the pulmonary VALVE, permitting pulmonic REGURGITATION.

respiratory i. see RESPIRATORY INSUFFICIENCY.

thyroid i. hypothyroidism.

tricuspid i. incomplete closure of the tricuspid VALVE, resulting in tricuspid REGURGITATION.

valvular i. failure of a cardiac valve to close perfectly, causing valvular REGURGITATION; see also aortic, mitral, pulmonary, and tricuspid insufficiency.

velopharyngeal i. inadequate velopharyngeal CLOSURE, due to a condition such as CLEFT PALATE or muscular dysfunction, resulting in defective speech.

venous i. inadequacy of the venous VALVES and impairment of venous return from the lower limbs (venous STASIS), often with edema and sometimes with stasis ULCERS at the ankle.

insufflation (in″sŭ-fla′shun) 1. the blowing of a powder, vapor, or gas into a body cavity. 2. a drug administered by this method, especially a powder or aerosol carried into the respiratory passages.

perirenal i. injection of air around the kidney for radiologic examination of the adrenal glands.

tracheal gas i. continuous insufflation of a low flow of fresh gas to the distal endotracheal tube, believed capable of flushing out the anatomical dead space and thus reducing Paco$_2$.

tubal i. Rubin's test.

insufflator (in′sŭ-fla″tor) an instrument used in insufflation.

insula (in′su-lah), pl. *in′sulae* [L.] a triangular area of the cerebral cortex that forms the floor of the lateral cerebral fossa; called also island of Reil.

insular (in′su-lar) pertaining to the insula or to an island, as the islets of Langerhans.

insulation (in″sŭ-la′shun) 1. the surrounding of a space or body with material designed to prevent the entrance or escape of radiant energy. 2. the material so used.

insulin (in′su-lin) 1. the major fuel-regulating hormone of the body, a double-chain protein formed from proinsulin in the beta CELLS of the islets of Langerhans in the PANCREAS. Insulin promotes the storage of glucose and the uptake of amino acids, increases protein and lipid synthesis, and inhibits lipolysis and gluconeogenesis. Secretion of insulin is a response of the beta cells to a stimulus; the primary stimulus is GLUCOSE, and others are AMINO ACIDS and hormones such as SECRETIN, PANCREOZYMIN, and GASTRIN. These chemicals play an important role in maintaining normal blood glucose levels by triggering insulin release after a meal. After insulin is released from the beta cells, it enters the blood stream and is transported to cells throughout the body. The cell membranes have insulin receptors to which the hormone becomes bonded or "fixed." An interaction between the insulin and its receptors leads to biochemical processes that include (1) the transport of glucose, amino acids, and certain ions across the membrane and into the cell body; (2) the storage of glycogen in liver and muscle cells; (3) the synthesis of triglycerides and storage of fat; (4) the synthesis of protein, RNA, and DNA, and (5) inhibition of gluconeogenesis, degradation of glycogen and protein, and lipolysis. Although insulin increases the transport of glucose across the cell membrane of most cells, in the brain glucose enters the cells by simple diffusion through the blood–brain barrier. 2. a preparation of the hormone, first discovered in 1921, used in treatment of DIABETES MELLITUS; it may be bovine or porcine in origin (prepared from the pancreas of the animals) or a recombinant human type, although insulin of bovine origin is no longer available in the United States. Recombinant human types may duplicate exactly the human insulin protein sequence, or may be analogues with small differences in sequence. Commercially prepared insulin is available in various types

INSULIN PREPARATIONS			
Type	Onset	Peak	Duration (hours)
Short or very fast Acting Humalog Novalog	5–15 minutes	45–90 minutes	3–4
Short or Fast Acting Regular (Actrapid, Velosulin)	30 minutes	2–4 hours	4–8
Short or Fast Acting Humulin R Novolin R	30 minutes–1 hour	30 minutes–1 hour	5–8
Short or Fast Acting Iletin II Regular	30 minutes–2 hours	3–4 hours	4–6
Intermediate Acting Humulin L Humulin N Novolin L Novolin N	1–3 hours	6–12 hours	20
Intermediate Acting NPH (Insulatard)	2–4 hours	6–8 hours	12–15
Intermediate Acting Lente	1–2 hours	6–12 hours	18–24
Long Acting Ultralente	4–6 hours	8–15 hours	18–24
Long Acting or **Ultralong Acting** Lantus	4–6 hours	No peak	24 +

that differ in the speed with which they act and in the duration of their effectiveness. There are several different types of insulin, usually classified by their onset and duration of action. (See table.)

Patients with diabetes react differently in the rate at which they absorb and utilize exogenous insulin; therefore, the duration of action varies from person to person. Moreover, the site of injection, volume of injection, and the condition of the tissues into which the insulin is injected can alter its rate of absorption and peak action times, and exercising the limb which has been injected immediately after injection can increase the speed of absorption. Insulin is measured in units.

Problems of Insulin Therapy. The problem of either too much or too little insulin is always a potential hazard for the person on insulin therapy. The causes, symptoms, and treatment of hypoglycemic or insulin reaction and hyperglycemia are discussed under DIABETES MELLITUS. Other problems of insulin therapy include INSULIN ALLERGY, INSULIN RESISTANCE, INSULIN REBOUND due to the SOMOGYI EFFECT, and LIPODYSTROPHIES or other localized tissue changes at injection sites.

Lipodystrophies are localized manifestations of disordered fat metabolism at the sites of insulin injection. Tissue HYPERTROPHY can be seen as a mass of fibrous scar tissue and is sometimes called "insulin tumor." ATROPHY of the tissues at the injection site appears as dimpling and pitting of the skin and underlying tissues. These problems are more common in adult females and in children. Atrophy of the tissues is relatively harmless, but hypertrophy can cause malabsorption of the insulin and a possible misdiagnosis of insulin resistance. Measures that can help prevent lipodystrophies include (1) systematic rotation of injection sites, (2) warming insulin to room temperature before injection, (3) pinching the skin when injecting the insulin so that it is deposited between fat and muscle tissue, and (4) use of human insulin.

i. allergy a HYPERSENSITIVITY REACTION to insulin, usually a reaction to its protein components. More purified insulins have now been developed that are less likely to cause an allergic reaction and other complications. Human insulin, prepared by recombinant genetic engineering, eliminates many problems associated with repeated insulin injections, because of reduced antibody concentrations.

i. pump a device consisting of a syringe filled with a predetermined amount of short-acting insulin, a plastic cannula and a needle, and a pump that periodically

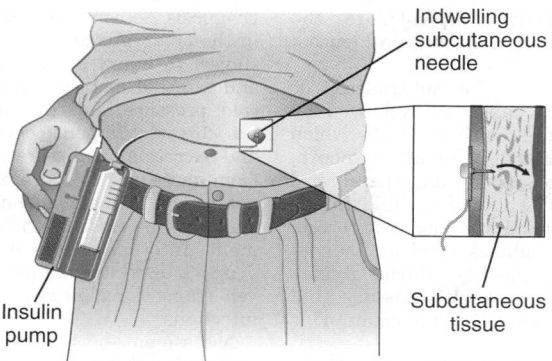

Indwelling
subcutaneous
needle

Insulin
pump

Subcutaneous
tissue

Insulin pumps are worn externally and connected to an indwelling subcutaneous needle, usually inserted in the abdomen. From Black and Matassarin-Jacobs, 2001.

delivers the desired amount of insulin. The basal rate of insulin delivery usually is one pulse every 8 minutes, but the pump can deliver as many as 60 pulses at a time. Before each meal or snack the patient manually administers a bolus of insulin by adjusting the pump setting to the desired one-time dose. Some insulin pumps will automatically reset themselves to the basal rate of infusion after each bolus. Research is ongoing regarding implantable pumps that release insulin in response to the pump's glucose sensor. This method could potentially administer insulin in a manner resembling the normal absorption from the pancreas.

i. rebound extreme fluctuations in blood sugar levels owing to overreaction of the body's homeostatic feedback mechanisms for control of glucose metabolism. When exogenous insulin is given, the HYPO-GLYCEMIA triggers an outpouring of GLUCAGON and EPINEPHRINE, both of which raise the blood sugar concentration markedly. Although the patient may actually have periods of hypoglycemia, urine and blood glucose tests will show HYPERGLYCEMIA. Treatment is aimed at modifying the extremes by gradually lowering the insulin dosage so as to reduce stimulation of the feedback system of glucose regulation. The patient may need to take smaller doses of insulin or take it at more frequent intervals and at different times during the day

i. resistance impairment of the normal biologic response to insulin, which may result from abnormalities in the B-cell products, binding of insulin to antagonists such as anti-insulin antibodies, defects in or reduced numbers of receptors, and defects in the insulin action cascade in the target cell.

Diabetic persons with this problem require more than 100 units daily, and some may need as much as 500 or 1000 units daily. Besides diabetes, the condition has also been associated with diseases such as OBESITY, ACROMEGALY, UREMIA, and certain rare, possibly genetic, AUTOIMMUNE DISEASES.

i. sensitivity test a test used to differentiate DIABETES MELLITUS from pituitary and adrenal diabetes. A test dose of exogenous insulin will produce a rapid and marked decrease in blood glucose if the pancreas is not secreting sufficient quantities of insulin. A much less dramatic response is produced if hyperglycemia is due to excessive secretion of either pituitary or adrenocortical hormones rather than insufficient insulin production.

insulinase (in′su-lin-ās) an enzymatic activity in body tissues that destroys or inactivates insulin; this effect is probably due to several nonspecific proteases.

insulinemia (in″su-lin-e′me-ah) the presence of insulin in the blood.

insulinogenesis (in″su-lin″o-jen′ĕ-sis) the formation and release of insulin by the islets of Langerhans.

insulinogenic (in″su-lin″o-jen′ik) relating to insulinogenesis.

insulinoma (in″su-lin-o′mah) a tumor of the beta cells of the islets of Langerhans; although usually benign, it is one of the chief causes of hypoglycemia.

insulitis (in″su-li′tis) cellular infiltration of the ISLETS OF LANGERHANS, a reaction similar to that observed in AUTOIMMUNE DISEASES.

insuloma (in″su-lo′mah) insulinoma.

insulopenic (in″su-lo-pe′nik) diminishing, or pertaining to a decrease in, the level of circulating insulin.

insusceptibility (in″sŭ-sep″tĭ-bil′ĭ-te) the state of being unaffected or uninfluenced; immunity.

intake (in′tāk) 1. the substances, or quantities thereof, taken in and used by the body; this refers to all routes by which fluids enter the body, including by mouth, rectum, irrigation tube, and parenteral administration. The record of fluid intake and output is called a FLUID BALANCE record. 2. the process of admission of an individual to a health facility, during which data regarding the health history and other pertinent personal information is gathered.

integrality (in″tě-gral′ĭ-te) a part of the principle of HOMEODYNAMICS in the SCIENCE OF UNITARY HUMAN BEINGS; the continuous mutual human field and environmental process.

integration (in″tě-gra′shun) 1. assimilation; anabolic action or activity. 2. the combining of different acts so that they cooperate toward a common end; coordination. 3. constructive assimilation of knowledge and experience into the personality. 4. in bacterial genetics, assimilation of genetic material from one bacterium (donor) into the chromosome of another (recipient).

bilateral i. the coordinated use of both sides of the body during activity.

i. of learning the incorporation of previously acquired concepts and behaviors into a variety of new situations, a cognitive PERFORMANCE COMPONENT of occupational therapy.

primary i. the recognition by a child that his or her body is a unit apart from the environment; it is probably not achieved before the second half of the first year of life.

secondary i. the sublimation of the separate elements of the early sexual instinct into the mature psychosexual personality.

vertical i. the structuring of hospital services in such a manner that a continuum of care is provided.

integrity (in-teg′rĭ-te) 1. soundness; freedom from serious flaws or impediments. 2. in bioethics, a virtue consisting of soundness of and adherence to moral principles and character and standing up in their defense when they are threatened or under attack. This involves consistent, habitual honesty and a coherent integration of reasonably stable, justifiable moral values, with consistent judgment and action over time. Some ethicists feel that integrity is the first or primary virtue.

impaired skin i. a NURSING DIAGNOSIS accepted by the North American Nursing Diagnosis Association, defined as alteration in the epidermis and/or dermis. The skin is subject to injury from a variety of external and internal factors. Extremes of heat and cold; pressure, shearing, and other mechanical forces; allergens; chemicals; radiation; and excretions and secretions such as those from an ostomy or a draining wound are all potentially damaging conditions and substances that exist in the external environment. Internal factors include emaciation, drugs, altered circulation and impaired oxygen transport, altered metabolic state, and infections.

Assessment of the skin should include such subjective data as reported itching or pain and a history of exposure to solar or other radiation or to an allergen, infectious agent, or parasite, or to extreme heat or cold. Objective data include any skin lesion and its distribution, size, and appearance; the appearance of the skin adjacent to lesions; localized or generalized edema; the characteristics of secretions; odor; the texture, elasticity, and thickness of the skin surface; and observation of scratching, rubbing of the skin, or restlessness.

impaired tissue i. a NURSING DIAGNOSIS accepted by the North American Nursing Diagnosis Association, defined as a state in which an individual has damage to a mucous membrane or to corneal, integumentary, or subcutaneous tissue.

risk for impaired skin i. a NURSING DIAGNOSIS accepted by the North American Nursing Diagnosis Association, defined as a state in which an individual's skin is at risk of being adversely altered.

integument (in-teg′u-ment) 1. a covering or investment. 2. the natural covering of the body; see SKIN.

integumentary (in-teg″u-men′tar-e) 1. pertaining to or composed of skin. 2. serving as a covering.

integumentum (in-teg″u-men′tum) [L.] integument.

in tela (in te′lah) [L.] in tissue; relating especially to stained histologic preparations.

intellect (in′tě-lekt) the mind, thinking faculty, or understanding.

intellectualization (in″tě-lek″choo-al-ĭ-za′-shun) an unconscious DEFENSE MECHANISM in which reasoning is used to avoid confronting an objectionable impulse and thus to defend against anxiety.

intelligence (in-tel′ĭ-jens) the ability to comprehend or understand. It is basically a combination of reasoning, MEMORY, imagination, and JUDGMENT; each of these faculties relies upon the others. Intelligence is not an entity within a person but a combination of cognitive skills and knowledge made evident by behaviors that are adaptive.

In speaking of general intelligence, authorities often distinguish between a number of different kinds of basic mental ability. One of these is verbal aptitude, the ability to understand the meaning of words and to use them effectively in writing or speaking. Another is skill with numbers, the ability to add, subtract, multiply, and divide and to use these skills in problems. The capacity to work with spatial relationships, that is, with visualizing how objects take up space, is still another (for example, how two triangles can fit together to make a square). Perception, memory, and reasoning may also be considered different basic abilities.

These abilities are the ones that are usually examined by intelligence tests. There are others, however, that may be as important or more important. Determination and perseverance make intelligence effective and useful. Artistic talent, such as proficiency in art or music, and creativity, the ability to use thought and imagination to produce original ideas, are difficult to measure but are certainly part of intelligence.

i. quotient **(I.Q.)** a numerical expression of intellectual capacity obtained by multiplying the mental age of the subject, ascertained by testing, by 100 and dividing by his or her chronologic age.

i. test a set of problems or tasks posed to assess an individual's innate ability to judge, comprehend, and reason.

intensionometer (in-ten″se-o-nom′ĕ-ter) an instrument for measuring the intensity of X-RAYS. Two series of plates, separated by an air gap that serves as the DIELECTRIC, are connected to opposite terminals in a closed chamber. An electric circuit is completed when the air becomes ionized by the roentgen rays, and the difference in electric POTENTIAL is registered by deflection of a GALVANOMETER needle.

intensity (in-ten′sĭ-te) strength, force, or concentration.

i. of nursing care a term in the NURSING MINIMUM DATA SET, defined as the total time and STAFF MIX of nursing personnel resources consumed by an individual patient or client during the episode of care under review.

intensive care unit (ICU) a hospital unit in which is concentrated special equipment and specially trained personnel for the care of seriously ill patients requiring immediate and continuous attention (intensive CARE). Called also critical care unit.

intensivist (in-ten′sĭ-vist) a physician who specializes in the provision of intensive CARE; see also INTENSIVE CARE UNIT.

intention (in-ten′shun) 1. a goal. 2. a manner of HEALING. 3. a surgical procedure or operation.

inter- word element [L.], *between.*

interacting systems framework former name for the GENERAL SYSTEMS FRAMEWORK AND THEORY OF GOAL ATTAINMENT.

interaction (in″ter-ak′shun) 1. the quality, state, or process of (two or more things) acting on each other. 2. reciprocal actions or influences among people, such as mother-child, husband-wife, client-nurse, or parent-teacher.

drug i. see DRUG INTERACTION.

impaired social i. a NURSING DIAGNOSIS accepted by the North American Nursing Diagnosis Association, defined as a state in which an individual participates in either an insufficient or an excessive quantity of social exchange, or with an ineffective quality of social exchange. See also SOCIAL ISOLATION.

interarticular (in″ter-ahr-tik′u-lar) between articulating surfaces.

interatrial (in″ter-a′tre-al) between the atria of the heart.

interbrain (in′ter-brān) diencephalon.

intercalary (in-ter′kah-ler″e) inserted between; interposed.

intercalated (in-ter′kah-la″ted) inserted between.

intercartilaginous (in″ter-kahr″tĭ-laj′ĭ-nus) between, or connecting, cartilages.

intercellular (in″ter-sel′u-lar) between the cells.

interchondral (in″ter-kon′dral) intercartilaginous.

intercilium (in″ter-sil′e-um) the space between the eyebrows.

interclavicular (in″ter-klah-vik′u-lar) between the clavicles.

intercondylar (in″ter-kon′dĭ-lar) between two condyles.

intercostal (in″ter-kos′tal) between two ribs.

intercourse (in′ter-kors) 1. mutual exchange. 2. sexual intercourse.

sexual i. 1. coitus. 2. any physical contact between two individuals involving stimulation of the genital organs of at least one.

intercricothyrotomy (in″ter-kri″ko-thi-rot′ah-me) cricothyrotomy.

intercritical (in″ter-krit′ĭ-kal) denoting the period between attacks, as of gout.

intercultural (in″ter-kul′cher-al) cross-cultural.

intercurrent (in″ter-kur′ent) pertaining to a process that occurs during the course of some other event.

i. disease a disease occurring during the course of another disease with which it has no connection.

interdependent (in″ter-dĕ-pen′dent) pertaining to actions or activities that require one individual to work with another. Interdependent nursing actions are those that are performed by the nurse after mutual determination by the nurse and the physician. They also include activities directed by the physician but requiring nursing judgment to perform.

interdigital (in″ter-dij′ĭ-tal) between two digits (fingers or toes).

interdigitation (in″ter-dij′ĭ-ta′shun) 1. an interlocking of parts by finger-like processes. 2. one of a set of finger-like processes.

interface (in′ter-fās″) 1. in chemistry, the boundary between two systems or phases. 2. a connection between two computer subsystems, or the hardware required to exchange data through such a connection, or an area of computer storage that can be accessed by more than one system.

interfascicular (in″ter-fah-sik′u-lar) between adjacent fascicles.

interfemoral (in″ter-fem′o-ral) between the thighs.

interference (in″ter-fēr′ens) 1. opposition to or hampering of some activity. 2. impairment of cardiac impulse conduction due to refractoriness of the tissue; the refractoriness is a physiological response to passage of a preceding impulse. 3. a premature contact point on the occlusal surface of the teeth.

electromagnetic i. electrical signals of nonphysiological origin that may affect PACEMAKER function; they can either inappropriately inhibit pacemaker output or trigger unnecessary pulses. Pacemakers with bipolar leads are less sensitive to this.

occlusal i's areas of interference on teeth that hamper proper occlusion and smooth, gliding, harmonious jaw movements.

interferon (in″ter-fēr′on) any of a family of glycoprotein biological response MODIFIERS used as antineoplastic AGENTS and IMMUNO-REGULATORS; they inhibit cellular growth, alter the state of cellular differentiation, have effects on the cell cycle, interfere with oncogene expression, alter cell surface antigen expression, have effects on antibody production, and regulate cytotoxic effector cells.

i.-α the major interferon produced by virus-induced leukocyte cultures; its primary producer cells are null CELLS, and its major activities are antiviral activity and activation of NK CELLS.

i. alfa-2a a synthetic form of interferon-α produced by recombinant technology that acts as a biologic response modifier, used as an antineoplastic in the treatment of hairy cell leukemia and AIDS-related Kaposi's sarcoma; administered intramuscularly or subcutaneously.

i. alfa-2b a synthetic form of interferon-α produced by recombinant technology that acts as a biologic response modifier, used in the treatment of veneral warts, hepatitis B, and chronic hepatitis C and as an antineoplastic in the treatment of hairy cell leukemia, malignant melanoma, non-Hodgkin's lymphomas, multiple myeloma, mycosis fungoides, and AIDS-related Kaposi's sarcoma; administered intramuscularly, subcutaneously, or intralesionally.

i. alfacon-1 a synthetic interferon related to both α and β interferons, produced by recombinant DNA technology; used in the treatment of chronic hepatitis C virus infection, administered subcutaneously.

i. alfa-n3 a highly purified mixture of natural human interferon proteins that acts as a biologic response modifier; used in the treatment of venereal warts, administered intralesionally.

i.-β the major interferon produced by double-stranded RNA-induced fibroblast cultures; the major producer cells are FIBRO-BLASTS, epithelial cells, and MACROPHAGES, and its major activity is antiviral.

i. beta-1a a synthetic form of interferon-β produced by recombinant DNA techniques that acts as a biologic response modifier; used in the treatment of relapsing forms of multiple sclerosis; administered intramuscularly.

i. beta-1b a synthetic modified form of interferon-β produced by recombinant DNA techniques; used as a biologic response modifier in the treatment of relapsing forms of multiple sclerosis; administered subcutaneously.

i.-γ the major interferon produced by lymphocyte cultures that have been immunologically stimulated by mitogens or antigens; the major producer cells are T LYMPHOCYTES, and its major activity is IMMUNOREGULATION.

i. gamma-1b a synthetic form of interferon-γ produced by recombinant technology that acts as a biologic response modifier and antineoplastic. It is used to reduce the frequency and severity of serious infections associated with chronic granulomatous disease, administered subcutaneously.

interfibrillar (in″ter-fi′bril-ar) between fibrils.

interfilar (in″ter-fi′lar) between or among the fibrils of a reticulum.

intergluteal (in″ter-gloo′te-al) between the buttocks; called also internatal.

interictal (in″ter-ik′tal) occurring between attacks or paroxysms.

interkinesis (in″ter-ki-ne′sis) the period between the first and second divisions in meiosis.

interleukin (in′ter-loo″kin) one of several proteins important for lymphocyte proliferation. *Interleukin-1* (IL-1) is produced by macrophages and induces the production of interleukin-2 by T cells that have been stimulated by antigen or mitogen. *Interleukin-2* (IL-2), produced by T cells, stimulates the proliferation of T cells bearing specific receptors for IL-2; these receptors are expressed in response to antigenic stimulation. IL-2 also seems to induce the production of interferon and is used as an anticancer drug in the treatment of a wide variety of solid malignant tumors. Another interleukin, *interleukin-3* (IL-3) is necessary for the differentiation of suppressor T cells.

interlobar (in″ter-lo′bar) between lobes.

interlobitis (in″ter-lo-bi′tis) interlobular PLEURISY.

interlobular (in″ter-lob′u-lar) between lobules.

intermaxillary (in″ter-mak′sĭ-ler″e) between the maxillae.

intermediate (in″ter-me′de-at) 1. placed between; see also MEDIAL and MEDIAN. 2. resembling, in part, each of two extremes. 3. a substance formed in a chemical process that is essential to formation of the end product of the process.

intermedin (in″ter-me′din) melanocyte-stimulating hormone.

intermedius (in″ter-me′de-us) [L.] intermediate; in anatomy, denoting a structure lying between a lateral and a medial structure.

intermeningeal (in″ter-mĕ-nin′je-al) between the meninges.

intermittent (in″ter-mit′ent) marked by alternating periods of activity and inactivity.

i. claudication a group of symptoms characterized by pain, cramping, and weakness in the calf muscles of one or both lower limbs, brought on by walking and relieved by resting for a few minutes. It is a form of arterial occlusive disease and is caused by atherosclerotic lesions of the limbs, which diminish blood supply to the muscles of the lower leg. Called also angina cruris. Treatment has traditionally involved vascular reconstructive surgery to bypass the diseased portion of the vessel. Modification of risk factors has also proved beneficial, such as smoking cessation, weight loss, and introduction of a graduated program of walking and exercise.

i. explosive disorder a rare IMPULSE CONTROL DISORDER in which a periodic loss of control of aggressive impulses results in serious assault or destruction of property; the outbursts are totally out of proportion to any apparent stress.

i. positive pressure breathing (IPPB) a form of RESPIRATORY THERAPY using a VENTILATOR for the treatment of selected patients with ATELECTASIS, those needing occasional assistance breathing, or those requiring some types of AEROSOL medications. As the name implies, this involves application of pressure only during the inspiratory phase, in order to help the patient breathe more deeply. It is used when other less expensive, less invasive forms of respiratory care have not been effective. Called also intermittent positive pressure ventilation.

Because of their compact size and capability of operating independently of an electrical current, IPPB machines are used widely. Similar treatment can also be delivered with a volume-, pressure-, or time-limited ventilator or manual resuscitation device. The American Association for Respiratory Care has published detailed and comprehensive clinical practice guidelines for the use of intermittent positive pressure breathing, which are available online at http://www.rcjournal.com/online_resources/cpgs/ippbcpg.hotmail.

intermural (in″ter-mu′ral) between the walls of an organ or organs.

intermuscular (in″ter-mus′ku-lar) between muscles.

intern (in′tern) 1. an allied health professional undertaking a learning experience supervised by a more experienced clinician. 2. a medical or dental graduate serving and residing in a hospital preparatory to being licensed to practice medicine or dentistry. 3. in some states, a physical therapy student enrolled in an educational program in a college or university whose school has a contractual agreement for clinical education with a physical therapy program in a hospital or clinic. In other states, a physical therapist who has completed the required academic coursework but is supervised by a licensed, practicing physical therapist. 4. a graduate professional nurse who is enrolled in a nursing internship program. Nursing internships are transitional programs for new graduates; they last longer (usually three months to a year) and are more comprehensive than traditional hospital orientation programs for new staff nurses. The goals of nursing internship are to ease the transition from the student role to the staff nurse role, and to guide new nurses in developing basic and specialized nursing skills.

The nurse intern works under the direction of a preceptor who serves as a role model as well as a support person and guide in clinical practice. The internship includes working a designated number of hours in the clinical setting and attending classes and seminars. Benefits to the facility offering an internship program include easier recruitment and retention of nurses and increased effectiveness of nursing care.

internal (in-ter′nal) situated or occurring within or on the inside, as in a hollow structure; in anatomy, many structures formerly called internal are now termed MEDIAL.

internalization (in-ter″nal-ĭ-za′shun) a mental mechanism whereby certain external attributes, attitudes, or standards are unconsciously taken as one's own.

internatal (in″ter-na′tal) intergluteal.

International Association for Enterostomal Therapy (IAET) a group comprising a wide variety of health care professions with the common goal of improving the care of patients with stomas or skin care problems. IAET publishes the *Journal of Enterostomal Therapy*, numerous newsletters, and *The Cost Benefits of ET Nursing in Modern Healthcare Delivery*.

International System of Units see SI UNITS.

International Union Against Cancer (UICC) [Fr. *Union Internationale Contre le Cancer*] an international, non-governmental organization founded in 1933 addressing all aspects of cancer control. See CANCER.

interneuron (in″ter-noo′ron) a neuron between the primary afferent neuron and the final motor neuron (motoneuron). Also any neuron whose processes lie entirely within a specific area, such as the olfactory lobe.

internist (in-ter′nist) a specialist in internal medicine.

internode (in′ter-nōd) a space between two nodes.

internship (in′tern-ship) 1. the position of an INTERN in a hospital. 2. the term of service of an intern.

internuclear (in″ter-noo′kle-ar) situated between nuclei or between nuclear layers of the retina.

internuncial (in″ter-nun′se-al) transmitting impulses between two different parts.

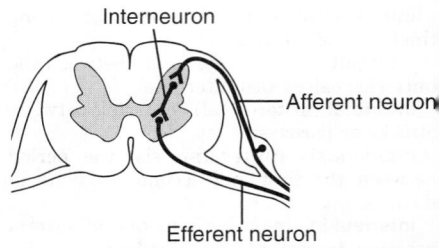

Interneuron

Afferent neuron

Efferent neuron

Interneuron as part of a three-neuron reflex arc in the spinal cord. From Dorland's, 2000.

internus (in-ter′nus) [L.] internal; in anatomy, denoting a structure nearer to the center of an organ or part.

interoceptor (in″ter-o-sep′tor) a sensory nerve terminal located in and transmitting impulses from the viscera. adj., **interoceptive.**

interofective (in″ter-o-fek′tiv) affecting the interior of the organism, usually with reference to the autonomic nervous system.

interolivary (in″ter-ol′ĭ-ver″e) between the olivary bodies.

interorbital (in″ter-or′bĭ-tal) between the orbits.

interosseous (in″ter-os′e-us) between two bones.

interpalpebral (in″ter-pal′pĕ-bral) between the eyelids.

interparietal (in″ter-pah-ri′ĕ-tal) 1. intermural. 2. between the parietal bones.

interparoxysmal (in″ter-par″ok-siz′mal) between paroxysms.

interphalangeal (in″ter-fah-lan′je-al) situated between two contiguous phalanges.

interphase (in′ter-fāz) the interval between two successive cell divisions, during which the chromosomes are not individually distinguishable.

interplant (in′ter-plant) an embryonic part isolated by transference to an indifferent environment provided by another embryo.

interpolation (in-ter″po-la′shun) the determination of intermediate values in a series on the basis of observed values.

interpretation (in-ter″prĕ-ta′shun) 1. an explanation. 2. in psychotherapy, the therapist's periodic explanation to the patient of the latent CONTENT or hidden meanings of the patient's mental phenomena as expressed through free ASSOCIATION, descriptions of DREAMS, and other aspects.

laboratory data i. in the NURSING INTERVENTIONS CLASSIFICATION, a nursing INTERVENTION defined as the critical analysis of patient laboratory data in order to assist with clinical decision making.

interproximal (in″ter-prok′sĭ-mal) between two adjoining surfaces, as between the proximal surfaces of adjacent teeth.

interpubic (in″ter-pu′bik) between the pubic bones.

interpupillary (in″ter-pu′pĭ-ler″e) between the pupils.

interscapular (in″ter-skap′u-lar) between the scapulae.

intersectio (in″ter-sek′she-o) [L.] intersection.

i. tendínea a fibrous band traversing the belly of a muscle, dividing it into two parts; called also inscriptio tendinea.

intersection (in″ter-sek′shun) a site at which one structure crosses another.

intersex (in′ter-seks) 1. hermaphrodite. 2. pseudohermaphrodite. 3. intersexuality.

female i. a female PSEUDOHERMAPHRODITE.

male i. a male PSEUDOHERMAPHRODITE.

true i. a true HERMAPHRODITE.

intersexuality (in″ter-sek″shoo-al′ĭ-te) 1. hermaphroditism. 2. pseudohermaphroditism.

interspace (in′ter-spās) a space between similar structures.

interspinal (in″ter-spi′nal) between two of the spinous PROCESSES of vertebrae.

interstice (in-ter′stis) an interval, space, or gap in a tissue or structure.

interstitial (in″ter-stish′al) pertaining to or situated between parts or in the interstices of a tissue.

interstitium (in″ter-stish′e-um) 1. interstice. 2. interstitial tissue.

intertransverse (in″ter-trans-vers′) situated between or connecting the transverse processes of the vertebrae.

intertrigo (in″ter-tri′go) an erythematous skin eruption occurring on apposed surfaces of the skin, as the creases of the neck, folds of the groin and armpit, and beneath pendulous breasts. It is caused by moisture, warmth, friction, sweat retention, and infectious agents. Fungal infections, such as with *Candida*, may complicate the condition. Symptoms include burning, itching, moistness, redness, maceration, and sometimes erosions, fissures, and exudations. It is most likely to occur in obese persons, and particularly in those with diabetes mellitus. Intertrigo is most prevalent in hot and humid regions.

In treatment of intertrigo, the apposing body surfaces should be thoroughly cleansed and dried, and then sprinkled with talcum powder containing zinc oxide. Cornstarch is not recommended as it can serve as a glucose-rich culture medium for the growth of bacteria. Sometimes gauze strips between the adjacent skin surfaces will help keep the area dry and exposed to air.

intertubular (in″ter-too′bu-lar) between tubules.

interureteral (in″ter-u-re′ter-al) interureteric.

interureteric (in″ter-u″rĕ-ter′ik) between the ureters.

intervaginal (in″ter-vaj′ĭ-nal) between sheaths.

interval (in′ter-val) the space between two objects or parts; the lapse of time between two events.

AA i. the interval between two consecutive atrial stimuli.

atrioventricular i., AV i. 1. P–R interval. 2. in dual chamber PACING, the length of time between the sensed or paced atrial event and the next sensed or paced ventricular event, measured in milliseconds; called also atrioventricular or AV delay.

cardioarterial i. the time between the apical beat and arterial pulsation.

confidence i. an estimated statistical interval for a parameter, giving a range of values that may contain the parameter and the degree of confidence that it is in fact there.

coupling i. the distance between two linked events in the CARDIAC CYCLE.

His-ventricular (H-V) i. an interval of the ELECTROGRAM of the BUNDLE OF HIS, measured from the earliest onset of the His potential to the onset of ventricular activation as recorded on eight of the intracardiac bipolar His bundle leads or any of the multiple surface ECG leads; it reflects conduction time through the His-Purkinje SYSTEM.

lucid i. 1. a brief period of remission of symptoms in a psychosis. 2. a brief return to CONSCIOUSNESS after loss of consciousness in HEAD INJURY.

PA i. the interval from the onset of the P wave on the standard ELECTROCARDIOGRAM (or from the atrial deflection on the high right atrial ECG) to the A wave on the His bundle ECG; it represents intra-atrial conduction time.

postsphygmic i. the short period (0.08 second) of ventricular DIASTOLE, after the sphygmic PERIOD, and lasting until the atrioventricular valves open.

P–R i. in electrocardiography, the time between the onset of the P wave (atrial activity) and the QRS complex (ventricular activity).

presphygmic i. the first phase of ventricular SYSTOLE, being the period (0.04–0.06 second) immediately after closure of the atrioventricular valves and lasting until the semilunar valves open.

QRST i., Q–T i. in the electrocardiogram, the length of time between ventricular DEPOLARIZATION (the Q wave) and REPOLARIZATION (the T wave); it begins with the onset of the QRS complex and ends with the end of the T wave.

VA i. [ventricular-atrial interval] the interval between a ventricular stimulus and the succeeding atrial stimulus; it is equal to the AA INTERVAL minus the atrioventricular INTERVAL.

intervalvular (in″ter-val′vu-lar) between valves.

intervascular (in″ter-vas′ku-lar) between blood vessels.

intervention (in″ter-ven′shun) interposition or interference in the affairs of another to accomplish a goal or end; see also IMPLEMENTATION.

crisis i. 1. counseling or psychotherapy for patients in a life crisis that is directed at supporting the patient through the crisis and helping the patient cope with the stressful event that precipitated it. 2. in the NURSING INTERVENTIONS CLASSIFICATION, a nursing INTERVENTION defined as use of short-term counseling to help the patient cope with a crisis and resume a state of functioning comparable to or better than the pre-crisis state.

nursing i. an action for which nurses are responsible that is intended to benefit a patient or client.

percutaneous coronary i. (PCI) the management of coronary artery occlusion by any of various catheter-based techniques, such as percutaneous transluminal coronary ANGIOPLASTY, ATHERECTOMY, angioplasty using the excimer laser, and implantation of coronary STENTS and related devices.

Intervention Scheme one of the three clinical components of the OMAHA SYSTEM; it is an organized framework of actions and activities used by nurses and other health care professionals to standardize care planning and interventions. It consists of four broad categories, 52 targets, and client-specific information. See Appendix on the Omaha System.

interventricular (in″ter-ven-trik′u-lar) between the ventricles of the heart.

intervertebral (in″ter-ver′tĕ-bral) between two vertebrae.

intervillous (in″ter-vil′us) between or among villi.

intestinal (in-tes′tĭ-nal) pertaining to the intestine.

i. bypass a surgical procedure in which all but a short section of the proximal jejunum and terminal ileum is bypassed in order to bring about malabsorption of digested food. The procedure is done for the purpose of correcting OBESITY. Patients having this type of surgery must be meticulously managed so that severe nutritional CIRRHOSIS and serious loss of water and electrolytes are avoided. Called also jejunoileal bypass and jejunoileal shunt.

i. flu a popular term for what may be any of several disorders of the stomach and intestinal tract. The symptoms are nausea, diarrhea, abdominal cramps, and fever. During the acute stage all foods should be avoided. Carbonated soft drinks such as ginger ale or cola can be taken in moderation to relieve the nausea. When the symptoms subside, the diet should at first be confined to liquids and soft, bland foods. Milk and dairy products, butter and fats generally, fruits, and greens should be avoided completely until the patient is free of all symptoms.

i. obstruction any hindrance to the passage of the intestinal contents. Causes may be mechanical or neural or both. Some of the more common mechanical causes are HERNIA, ADHESIONS of the peritoneum, VOLVULUS, INTUSSUSCEPTION, malignant or benign tumor, congenital defect, and local inflammation, as in DIVERTICULITIS. Failure of peristalsis (adynamic ILEUS) is frequently associated with PERITONITIS; it also may occur with GALLSTONES, UREMIA, heavy metal poisoning, infection, and spinal injury.

SYMPTOMS. The most characteristic symptoms are abdominal pain, vomiting, and distention. The symptoms may be mild at first and in its early stages the condition can be confused with less serious disorders of the intestinal tract. Under no circumstances should the patient be given a CATHARTIC or other LAXATIVE, because that will aggravate the situation. If the obstruction continues the patient suffers from dehydration and shock because of inadequate absorption of fluids, electrolytes, and nutrients from the intestinal tract. If the bowel becomes strangulated and circulation to the bowel wall is obstructed, the patient shows signs of peritonitis with extreme tenderness and rigidity of the abdomen.

Diagnosis. The diagnosis of obstruction can usually, but not always, be made from plain abdominal radiographs. If there is a question, a gastrointestinal series with barium will usually resolve the issue quickly.

Treatment. The basic steps of treatment are decompression of the intestine, replacement of fluids and electrolytes, and removal of the cause of the obstruction. Decompression is accomplished by intubation with a special tube (usually the MILLER-ABBOTT TUBE) designed to reach past the pyloric sphincter and into the intestine. Constant suction is then applied to remove accumulations of gas and liquids. Fluids, sodium chloride, and glucose are administered intravenously at a specific rate as prescribed. Transfusions of whole blood plasma may be given as necessary to restore normal blood values.

Surgical removal of the cause of obstruction is necessary in cases of complete obstruction. If there is no evidence of strangulation of the bowel, the surgeon may choose to postpone surgery until dehydration and shock have been overcome and a normal electrolyte balance is restored. The type of surgical procedure performed depends on the cause of the obstruction and whether or not the intestine is gangrenous. In some cases a colostomy may be necessary along with removal of the damaged portion of the bowel. A surgical incision into the cecum with insertion of a drainage tube (CECOSTOMY) may be done when intestinal intubation is not successful in relieving distention.

PATIENT CARE. Assessment of the patient with intestinal obstruction includes noting the location and character of abdominal pain, degree of distention, character of the bowel sounds, and occurrence or absence of bowel movements or passing of flatus. Should defecation occur, a specimen is saved for examination and laboratory analysis. If there is vomiting, the amount and special characteristics of the vomitus should be noted and recorded. In severe cases of obstruction of the small bowel the vomitus may contain fecal material because of the reversal of peristalsis and forcing of the intestinal contents backward into the stomach. Foods and fluids by mouth are restricted. Frequent mouth care is necessary to relieve the dryness and foul taste that accompanies intestinal obstruction and vomiting. Urinary output is measured and recorded because of the possibility of decreased urinary output related to dehydration.

Preoperative Care. If conservative measures fail to relieve the obstruction, or if the bowel has become strangulated, surgery is indicated. Suction siphonage, once initiated, is continued and the intestinal tube is left in place when the patient goes to the operating room.

Postoperative Care. Routine postoperative care of the patient with abdominal surgery is indicated. Specific measures depend on the type of surgical procedure done. Suction siphonage is usually continued until peristalsis resumes. Results of the assessment of bowel sounds and the passing of flatus or feces should be noted on the patient's chart because they indicate a return of normal peristaltic movements of the bowel. In some cases a cecostomy tube or rectal tube is inserted during surgery; the tube is attached to a drainage system and the amount and type of material collected in the system are recorded. If there is evidence that the tube has become obstructed the surgeon should be notified. The skin around the site of insertion of a cecostomy tube should be protected with a skin barrier. The area must be washed frequently to avoid erosion of the skin by intestinal contents leaking around the tube. (See COLOSTOMY for patient care after that procedure.)

i. tract the small and large intestines in continuity; this long, coiled tube is the part of the DIGESTIVE SYSTEM where most of the digestion of food takes place. (See color plates.) The *small intestine* has three parts: the DUODENUM (connected to the stomach), the JEJUNUM, and the ILEUM. The small intestine is small in diameter but very long (about 6.1 m). The *large intestine,* which starts just below the ileum, is about 1.5 m long. It is made up of the CECUM (to which the APPENDIX is attached), the COLON (comprising the ascending, transverse, and descending colon and the sigmoid), and the RECTUM.

The digestion of food is completed in the small intestine. The digested food is absorbed through the walls of the small intestine into the blood. Indigestible parts of the food pass into the large intestine. Here the liquid from the wastes is gradually absorbed back into the body through the intestinal walls. The waste itself is formed into fairly solid feces and pushed down into the rectum for evacuation.

Among the disorders of the intestinal tract are the disturbances of function, such as DIARRHEA, CONSTIPATION, and IRRITABLE BOWEL SYNDROME; the organic diseases, ULCERATIVE COLITIS, APPENDICITIS, and ILEITIS; and communicable diseases, such as DYSENTERY. Irritable bowel syndrome is characterized by constipation, sometimes alternating with diarrhea. Ulcerative colitis is a disorder in which ulcers may appear in the wall of the large intestine. Ileitis is a disorder of the ileum, or lower portion of the small intestine. A symptom of both is diarrhea. Dysentery, which is characterized by diarrhea, is the result of infection by bacteria, viruses, or various parasites.

intestine (in-tes'tin) the part of the ALIMENTARY CANAL extending from the pyloric opening of the stomach to the anus. It is a membranous tube, comprising the small intestine and large intestine; called also bowel and gut. See also INTESTINAL TRACT, and see color plates.

intestinum (in″tes-ti′num) [L.] intestine.

intima (in′ti-mah) 1. innermost. 2. tunica intima.

intimal (in′ti-mal) pertaining to the TUNICA INTIMA.

intimitis (in″ti-mi′tis) endangiitis.

intolerance (in-tol′er-ans) inability to withstand or consume; inability to absorb or metabolize nutrients.

activity i. a NURSING DIAGNOSIS accepted by the North American Nursing Diagnosis Association, defined as a state in which a person has insufficient physiological or psychological energy to endure or complete necessary or desired daily activities. Causes include generalized weakness, sedentary lifestyle, imbalance between oxygen supply and demand, and bed rest or immobility. Defining characteristics include verbal report of fatigue or weakness, abnormal heart rate or blood pressure response to activity, exertional discomfort, and dyspnea.

carbohydrate i. inability to properly metabolize one or more carbohydrate(s), such as GLUCOSE, FRUCTOSE, or one of the disaccharides.

disaccharide i. inability to properly metabolize one or more DISACCHARIDE(S), usually due to deficiency of the corresponding DISACCHARIDASE(S), although it may have other causes such as impaired absorption. After ingestion of the disaccharide there may be abdominal symptoms such as diarrhea, flatulence, borborygmus, distention, and pain. One common type is lactose INTOLERANCE.

drug i. the state of reacting to the normal pharmacologic doses of a drug with the symptoms of overdosage.

exercise i. limitation of ability to perform work or exercise at normally accepted levels, as measured in EXERCISE TESTING.

glucose i. inability to properly metabolize GLUCOSE, a type of carbohydrate intolerance; see DIABETES MELLITUS.

lactose i. a disaccharide intolerance specific for LACTOSE, usually due to an inherited deficiency of LACTASE activity in the intestinal mucosa.

risk for activity i. a NURSING DIAGNOSIS accepted by the North American Nursing

Diagnosis Association, defined as the state in which an individual is at risk of having insufficient physiological or psychological energy to endure or complete required daily activities. See also activity INTOLERANCE.

Patient Care. Nursing activities and interventions are aimed at identifying those factors that contribute to activity intolerance, providing evidence of the patient's progress to the higher level of activity possible for the patient, and reducing signs of physiologic intolerance to increased activity (blood pressure and respiratory and pulse rates). Once the contributing factors are identified, plans are made to avoid or minimize them. For example, if inadequate sleep or rest periods are a factor, the nurse plans with the patient scheduled periods of uninterrupted rest during the day. Inadequate sleep at night should be assessed and appropriate interventions planned and implemented. Making an objective record of the patient's progress toward increased activity tolerance can help alleviate depression or lack of incentive, both of which can be contributing factors. Such assessment data could include measurements of blood pressure, pulse, and respiratory rates before and after an activity, gradual increase in the distance walked, and gradual resumption of responsibility for ACTIVITIES OF DAILY LIVING.

intorsion (in-tor′shun) tilting of the upper part of the vertical meridian of the eye toward the midline of the face.

intoxication (in-tok″si-ka′shun) 1. stimulation, excitement, or impaired judgment caused by a chemical substance, or as if by one. 2. substance INTOXICATION, especially that due to ingestion of ALCOHOL (see discussion at ALCOHOLISM). Alcohol intoxication is defined legally according to a person's blood alcohol level; the definition is 0.10 per cent or more in most states in the U.S. and 0.8 per cent or more in Canada. 3. poisoning.

alcohol idiosyncratic i. a term previously used for marked behavioral change, usually belligerence, produced by ingestion of small amounts of alcohol that would not cause intoxication in most persons. It is now felt that there is no evidence for a distinction between this condition and any other form of alcohol intoxication.

caffeine i. caffeinism (def. 2).

cannabis i. physiological and psychological symptoms following the smoking of MARIJUANA or HASHISH, including euphoria, preoccupation with auditory and visual stimuli, and apathy. Intoxication occurs almost immediately after smoking and peaks within 30 minutes.

pathological i. alcohol idiosyncratic i.

substance i. a type of SUBSTANCE-INDUCED DISORDER, consisting of reversible, substance-specific, maladaptive behavioral or psychological changes directly resulting from the physiologic effects on the central nervous system of recent ingestion of or exposure to a drug of abuse, medication, or toxin. Specific cases are named on the basis of etiology, e.g., alcohol intoxication.

water i. a condition resulting from undue retention of water with decrease in sodium concentration, marked by lethargy, nausea, vomiting, and mild mental aberrations; in severe cases there may be convulsions and coma.

intra- word element [L.], *inside of; within.*

intra-abdominal (in″trah-ab-dom′ĭ-nal) within the abdomen.

intra-aortic balloon pump (IABP) a mechanical aid to the circulatory function of the heart that acts to provide internal COUNTERPULSATION. The basic components of the device are a catheter tipped with a balloon and a pump machine that inflates the balloon with either helium or carbon dioxide. The balloon is inserted via a femoral artery cutdown and guided under fluoroscopic control to a position in the descending thoracic aorta just distal to the left subclavian artery. In some models, the balloon is tri-segmented. When inflation begins in a tri-segmented balloon, the middle segment is inflated first, then the distal ends inflate simultaneously; there is no occlusion of the aorta. An alternative type of balloon catheter consists of only one segment with a second small balloon just distal to the main one; the smaller balloon partially occludes the aorta only during diastole, thus providing directional flow.

The pump console contains signal processing, drive, and timing and control mechanisms for appropriate inflation and deflation. The system also contains a display and diagnostic unit.

The physiologic effect of the IABP is to improve coronary blood flow and systemic circulation. It does this by (1) augmenting aortic root pressure during ventricular diastole at the time of maximum blood flow, and (2) reducing the workload of the heart by decreasing the amount of residual blood in the aortic arch, thereby decreasing resistance to the flow of blood from the ventricle. Inflation of the balloon during diastole just after aortic valve closure, and deflation just prior to ventricular systole reduces the pressure workload of the left ventricle and lessens oxygen demand and consumption by the myocardium. Timing of the inflation–deflation cycle is based on the

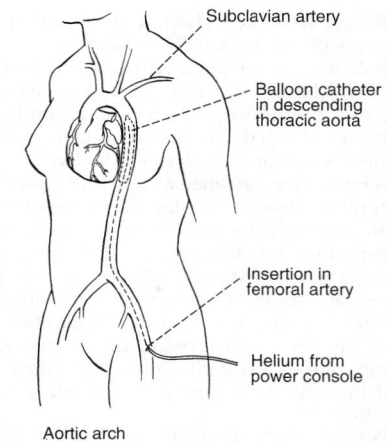

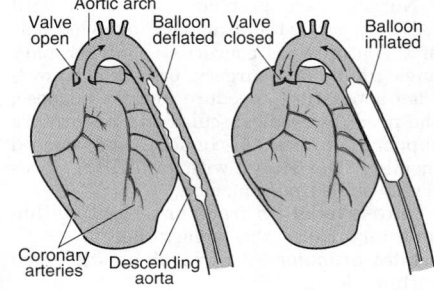

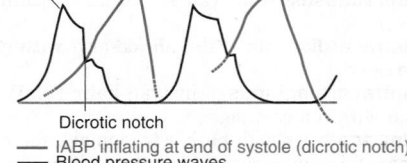

Intra-aortic balloon pump (IABP). From Polaski and Tatro, 1996.

arterial pulse wave configuration seen on the console's display screen. Adjustments to the cycle are made according to the site of arterial wave sampling, heart rate, and the depth of diastolic dip.

Indications for employment of the IABP include cardiogenic shock or severe pump failure secondary to acute myocardial infarction or following open-heart surgery, unstable angina resistant to drug therapy, and refractory ventricular irritability after myocardial infarction. The effect of improved oxygenation of the myocardium can result in reversal of ischemic damage resulting from infarction, and limitation of the size of the myocardial infarction.

Following insertion of the IABP catheter and initiation of the pumping action, nursing care is focused on proper administration of medications, monitoring the patient's response and the function of the equipment for evidence of safe and effective pumping, observation for ischemia of the limb in which the catheter is inserted, and observation for side effects and complications, such as excessive bleeding from the insertion site or formation of a hematoma, wound inflammation and infection, abdominal or back pain, reduction in platelet count and hematocrit and other signs of clotting abnormalities, and thrombus formation.

Nursing care problems associated with IABP include patient anxiety involving fear of the procedure, concerns about coronary angiography and surgery, or lack of knowledge about the procedure and its purpose; the need for cardiovascular and respiratory support; physical discomfort; and limited mobility. The patient with an IABP requires highly skilled nursing care.

intra-arterial (in″trah-ahr-tēr′e-al) within an artery; called also endarterial.

intra-articular (in″trah-ahr-tik′u-lar) within a joint.

intracanalicular (in″trah-kan″ah-lik′u-lar) within canaliculi.

intracapsular (in″trah-kap′su-lar) within a capsule.

intracardiac (in″trah-kahr′de-ak) within the heart.

intracartilaginous (in″trah-kahr″tĭ-laj′ĭ-nus) within a cartilage.

Intracath (in′trah-kath″) trademark for a type of intravenous cannulation device in which a rigid needle is surrounded by a plastic catheter and they are inserted as a unit; when the vein is successfully entered the rigid needle is removed and the catheter is advanced into the vein.

intracellular (in″trah-sel′u-lar) within a cell or cells.

intracervical (in″trah-ser′vĭ-kal) within the canal of the cervix uteri.

intracisternal (in″trah-sis-ter′nal) within a subarachnoid cistern.

intracranial (in″trah-kra′ne-al) within the cranium.

i. pressure (ICP) the pressure of the CEREBROSPINAL FLUID in the subarachnoid space, the space between the skull and the brain; the normal range is between 50 and 180 mm H_2O (approximately 4 to 13 mm Hg). A reading above 200 mm H_2O (about 15 mm Hg) is considered abnormally high; however, intracranial pressure, like arterial blood pressure, can fluctuate markedly and quickly during certain activities. For example, a transient elevation of pressure occurs during VALSALVA'S MANEUVER. Straining at stool, isometric exercises, and similar activities can momentarily raise the intracranial pressure to as high as 1360 mm H_2O. While signs of sustained increased intracranial pressure can be significant in the assessment of a patient with a neurologic disorder, momentary increases in intracranial pressure are not in themselves necessarily detrimental.

The level of intracranial pressure can be inferred by determining the pressure of lumbar spinal fluid during a spinal tap, but this is not the most accurate method and it can be dangerous. Removal of even a small amount of spinal fluid from a patient with a significantly high intracranial pressure can alter the pressure difference between the spinal column and the cranial cavity and cause herniation of the midbrain downward into the foramen magnum. A more accurate and continuous measurement of intracranial pressure can be obtained by monitoring pressure within the cerebral ventricles (cerebral ventricular pressure).

Causes of Increase in Pressure. The skull is a rigid container that holds the brain, blood vessels, and cerebrospinal fluid. There is room for some expansion within the skull, but not much, and any condition that causes an increase in volume in one or more of the structures within the cranium will cause an increase in pressure within the contained area. A tumor or swelling of brain tissue can increase the volume, as can extravascular leakage of blood and the formation of clots, dilatation of the cerebral vessels, and excess production, impeded outflow, or insufficient absorption of cerebrospinal fluid, as in HYDROCEPHALUS.

Increased fluid volume creates pressure against the structures inside the cranium, disrupting the blood and oxygen supply, and resulting in cellular hypoxia. As the pressure increases, the brain mass shifts or is distorted, causing compression of the neurons and nerve tracts or of the cerebral arteries. The effect of increased volume can be generalized, as in brain edema from lead poisoning, or focal. Cellular hypoxia resulting from direct pressure on the brain cells, distortion of the brain mass, or occlusion of cerebral blood vessels accounts for the signs and symptoms of increased intracranial pressure. A sustained increase in the pressure causes persistent hypoxia, irreversible damage to the brain cells, and eventually death.

Signs and Symptoms. The four classic groups of intracranial signs of increased intracranial pressure are (1) altered levels of consciousness; (2) changes in sensory and motor function; (3) changes in pupil size, equality, and reaction to light, and extraocular movements; and (4) changes in vital signs and patterns of respiration. However, only a few of these signs occur early in the process and then usually only at peak pressures.

Altered levels of consciousness occur as a result of compression of the ascending reticular activating system pathways and the resulting hypoxia of the cells of these tissues as well as the cells of the cortex. As compression increases the patient becomes more difficult to arouse. Assessment of the patient is based on the extent to which he is oriented and able to respond to stimuli. (See also levels of CONSCIOUSNESS.)

Motor and sensory dysfunction are the result of pressure on the cortex and the upper motor and sensory pyramidal pathways. The motor fibers descend through the brain stem where most of them cross over (decussate) in the medulla oblongata and then extend into the spinal cord. Sensory fibers ascend from the spinal cord to the brain stem and from there to the sensory areas in the parietal lobe of the brain. These fibers also decussate in either the spinal cord or the medulla. Assessment of the patient for motor and sensory dysfunction would include an evaluation of movement and strength of the extremities and a comparison of right side to left; perception of touch, pressure, and deep pain; and the presence or absence of the BABINSKI REFLEX.

Changes in pupil size, equality, and reaction to light, and extraocular movements are indicative of compression of the third, fourth, and sixth cranial nerves. Assessment of these changes should be as accurate and objective as possible. Unilateral and bilateral evaluations are important and usually are recorded by a drawing of the actual size of each pupil or by precise measurements using a small metric ruler.

Vital sign changes come very late in the process of cellular hypoxia and indicate that pressure is being exerted on the lower brain stem and medulla. If not relieved, these changes quickly accelerate and death ensues. Compression of the brain stem causes a rise in the systolic blood pressure and a widening of the pulse pressure followed by a sharp drop in blood pressure. The pulse rate slows and then rises sharply owing to blocking of the parasympathetic

impulses. As pressure on the respiratory center builds up there are changes in the rate, rhythm, and ratio of inspiration to expiration, and periods of apnea.

Earlier in the process, more subtle changes in the neurologic status of the patient can be detected by an experienced practitioner and are extremely important for prompt intervention and correction of the problem before irreversible damage is done. Signs and symptoms frequently noted early in the process and at peak pressure include increased restlessness, mental dullness, disorganized and unfocused behavior, such as plucking at the bedclothes, and increasingly severe headache. Another significant event is a *transient* worsening of the neurologic status as indicated by changes in the four classic signs and symptoms. These transient changes reflect a situation in which a critical volume of intracranial contents has been reached; small increases beyond that point are likely to lead to rapid and sustained increases in pressure. This situation demands immediate intervention for relief of compression of vital neuronal structures.

Patient Care. In addition to a thorough understanding of the pathophysiologic changes brought on by increased intracranial pressure and the signs and symptoms they produce, the nurse and other health professionals should be aware of factors that can precipitate increases in intracranial pressure. It is known, for example, that hypercapnia, profound hypoxia, and certain anesthetics can cause vasodilation of cerebral vessels and an increase in intracranial pressure. Patients who are known to be at risk for increases in pressure should not be given vasodilating drugs whenever such therapy can be avoided. The blood gases and chest sounds of these patients should be monitored periodically to determine whether there is adequate ventilation and oxygenation. Maintenance of a patent airway and adequate oxygenation by means of oxygen therapy, if necessary, are essential to the prevention of an escalating intracranial pressure.

Other protective measures for patients at risk for sudden increases in intracranial pressure include careful positioning to avoid flexion of the neck, extreme flexion of the hip, or the prone position. Elevating the head 15 to 30 degrees decreases baseline pressure. The patient also should avoid the Valsalva maneuver when moving about in bed and when defecating. Isometric exercises to avoid the hazards of immobility are contraindicated but passive range-of-motion exercises are not.

i. pressure monitoring 1. ICP monitoring; continuous monitoring of INTRACRANIAL PRESSURE. The three basic techniques used are intraventricular, subarachnoid (subdural), and epidural, with the intraventricular technique being the most common. 2. in the NURSING INTERVENTIONS CLASSIFICATION, a nursing INTERVENTION defined as the measurement and interpretation of patient data to regulate intracranial pressure.

In ICP monitoring, ventricular-fluid pressures are recorded from a zero baseline; the normal range is 0 to 15 mm Hg. Pressures usually are expressed in mm Hg rather than mm H_2O in order to facilitate comparison with mean systemic arterial pressures. The difference between mean ventricular pressure and mean arterial pressure indicates the pressure at which the brain is being perfused with blood.

ICP monitoring gives a far more accurate picture of forces at work within the closed cranial cavity than does clinical observation of the patient for signs of increased intracranial pressure. Most authorities agree that dangerously high levels of intracranial pressure exist well before clinical symptoms become evident. Invasive monitoring of pressure also provides access for cerebrospinal fluid drainage to relieve pressure, for procurement of samples of cerebrospinal fluid for laboratory evaluations, and for observation of volume–pressure responses to therapeutic intervention.

i. pressure screw a device for measuring the degree of pressure being exerted within the subarachnoid space. Monitoring can be done on a continuous or an intermittent basis. The screw is inserted through a burr hole in the frontal area of the skull just behind the hairline and a capped 3-way stop cock is attached to the pressure screw. High-pressure tubing joined to the screw leads to a manometer on which pressure changes can be directly visualized, or to equipment which displays the information on an oscilloscope or graph. Readings on changes in intracranial pressure can thus be obtained by watching the manometer or by monitoring the oscilloscope or graphic display. When the manometer is used, point zero is established after positioning the patient with the head of the bed elevated 30 degrees.

Through the use of the intracranial pressure screw, elevations in intracranial pressure can be detected before changes in the vital signs and other symptoms of increased pressure become apparent. In this way measures can be taken to reduce the pressure before irreversible damage is done to the brain tissue.

The major risks of the intracranial pressure screw are infection and leakage of cerebrospinal fluid, either of which necessitates removal of the screw.

intracutaneous (in″trah-ku-ta′ne-us) within the substance of the skin.

i. test one that involves introduction of an antigen between the layers of the skin and evaluation of the reaction elicited by it.

intracystic (in″trah-sis′tik) within the bladder or a cyst.

intradermal (in″trah-der′mal) within the dermis.

intraductal (in″trah-duk′tal) within a duct.

intradural (in″trah-doo′ral) within or beneath the dura mater.

intrafusal (in″trah-fu′zal) pertaining to the striated fibers within a muscle spindle.

intrahepatic (in″trah-hĕ-pat′ik) within the liver.

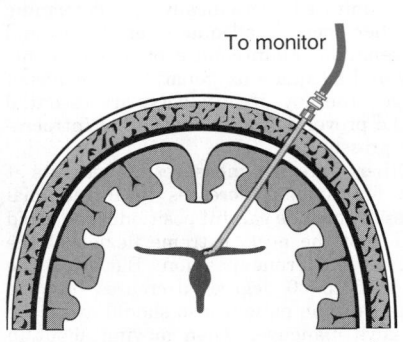

Ventricular Catheter (Ventriculostomy)

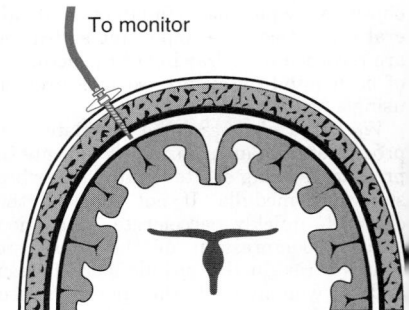

Subarachnoid Screw (bolt)

Intracranial pressure monitoring. From Polaski and Tatro, 1996.

intralesional (in″trah-le′zhun-al) occurring in or introduced directly into a localized lesion.

Intralipid (in″trah-lip′id) trademark for an intravenous fat emulsion used to prevent or correct deficiency of essential fatty acids and to provide calories in high density form during total PARENTERAL NUTRITION.

intralobar (in″trah-lo′bar) within a lobe.

intralocular (in″trah-lok′u-lar) within the loculi of a structure.

intraluminal (in″trah-loo′mĭ-nal) within the lumen of a tubular structure.

intramedullary (in″trah-med′u-lār″e) 1. within the spinal cord. 2. within the medulla oblongata. 3. within the marrow cavity of a bone.

intramural (in″trah-mu′ral) within the wall of an organ; called also intraparietal.

intramuscular (in″trah-mus′ku-lar) within the muscular substance.

intraocular (in″trah-ok′u-lar) within the eye.

intraoperative (in″trah-op′er-a″tiv) occurring during a surgical operation.

intraoral (in″trah-o′ral) within the mouth.

intraorbital (in″trah-or′bĭ-tal) within the orbit.

intraparietal (in″trah-pah-ri′ĕ-tal) 1. intramural. 2. within the parietal region of the brain.

intrapartum (in″trah-pahr′tum) occurring during labor or delivery.

intraperitoneal (in″trah-per″ĭ-to-ne′al) within the peritoneal cavity.

intrapleural (in″trah-ploor′al) within the pleura.

intrapsychic (in″trah-si′kik) arising, occurring, or situated within the mind.

intrapulmonary (in″trah-pul′mo-ner″e) within the substance of the lung.

intrasegmental (in″trah-seg-men′tal) within a single segment, such as a bronchopulmonary segment or spinal segment.

intraspinal (in″trah-spi′nal) within the substance of the spinal column.

intrasternal (in″trah-ster′nal) within the sternum.

intrathecal (in″trah-the′kal) 1. within a sheath. 2. through the theca of the spinal cord into the subarachnoid space.

intrathoracic (in″trah-tho-ras′ik) within the thorax.

intratracheal (in″trah-tra′ke-al) endotracheal.

intratubal (in″trah-too′bal) within a tube.

intratympanic (in″trah-tim-pan′ik) within the tympanic cavity.

intrauterine (in″trah-u′ter-in) within the uterus.

CORRECT POSITION
IUD inserted up to the top
wall of the uterus

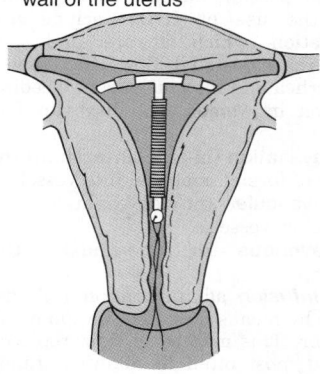

Intrauterine contraceptive device (IUD). From Nichols and Zwelling, 1997.

***i. device* (IUD),** *i. contraceptive device* a mechanical device inserted into the uterine cavity for the purpose of CONTRACEPTION. These devices are made of metal, plastic, or other substances and are manufactured in various sizes and shapes. Their effectiveness is based on their alteration of the endometrium and consequent disruption of implantation; there is generally no effect on the menstrual cycle.

After the IUD has been inserted, the patient is instructed to have yearly follow-up examinations. Contraindications to insertion include recent pelvic infection, suspected pregnancy, cervical stenosis, myoma of the uterus, and abnormal uterine bleeding. IUDs are not recommended for women who have never been pregnant because of the severe pain and bleeding that they produce in the majority of these patients.

The IUD is not 100 per cent effective and its use carries some risks. The device does not prevent ovulation or extrauterine implantation; therefore, ectopic pregnancy must be suspected when irregular bleeding or pelvic pain develops in a patient with an IUD. Four to five per cent of all pregnancies occurring in women with IUDs are likely to be outside the uterus. The increased risk for pelvic inflammatory disease is from three to five times that of women who do not use an IUD. Because pelvic inflammatory disease frequently leads to an inability to conceive as a result of scarring and narrowing of the fallopian tubes, the IUD also increases the chances for infertility. Many experts advise against the use of IUDs in women under 25 years of age and in those who hope to have children later in life.

Other possible adverse effects associated with the use of IUDs include uterine perforation, which is rare, and severely increased menstrual flow. Increased dysmenorrhea and intermenstrual bleeding are common in women who have an IUD in place.

intravasation (in-trav″ah-za′shun) the entrance of foreign material into vessels.

intravascular (in″trah-vas′ku-lar) within a vessel or vessels.

intravenous (in″trah-ve′nus) within a vein.

    i. infusion administration of fluids into a vein by means of a steel needle or plastic catheter. This method of fluid replacement is used most often to maintain fluid and electrolyte balance, or to correct fluid volume deficits after excessive loss of body fluids, in patients unable to take sufficient volumes orally. An additional use is for prolonged nutritional support of patients with gastrointestinal dysfunction (total PAR-ENTERAL NUTRITION).

Besides these uses, many medications are administered by intravenous infusion. A *piggyback intravenous infusion* is the intermittent delivery of an additional fluid or medication through the primary intravenous line from a second source of fluid with a secondary set of intravenous tubing. (See illustration.) A *push intravenous infusion* is the direct injection of medication into a vein through an intravenous line, needle, or catheter.

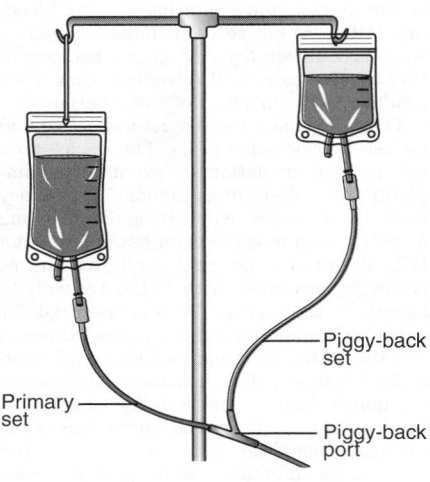

Primary set

Piggy-back set

Piggy-back port

Piggyback intravenous infusion set.

Manufacturers' instructions must be followed for preparation and administration of all such medications. The fluid to be infused and the flow rate are by prescription. With intravenous infusions of medication, the danger of drug incompatibility is very real. Incompatibility charts are not entirely reliable as sources of information about chemical interaction of drug additives combined in an intravenous infusion. For this reason admixing should be done by a clinical pharmacologist. Intravenous antibiotics should be mixed only with electrolytes. Because of their local irritating effects on the vein, doses of potassium chloride and dextrose solutions with a concentration higher than 10 per cent should not be given through a peripheral vein. Unless otherwise directed by the manufacturer, it is best to dilute all intravenous medications before administering them. When medications must be reconstituted with a solvent or removed from a glass ampule, a transfer filter should be used to filter out particulate matter. Once medications have been added to an intravenous solution the container should be checked every 30 minutes. A flowmeter is applied to the container of fluid and set to maintain the desired rate of flow. Infusion pumps are used and maintained according to hospital policy.

intraventricular (in″trah-ven-trik′u-lar) within a ventricle.

intravital (in″trah-vi′tal) occurring during life.

intra vitam (in′trah vi′tam) [L.] during life.

intrinsic (in-trin′sik) situated entirely within, or pertaining exclusively to, a part.

    i. PEEP intrinsic positive end-expiratory pressure.

introitus (in-tro′ĭ-tus) [L.] an entrance.

introjection (in″tro-jek′shun) an unconscious DEFENSE MECHANISM considered immature, in which loved or hated external objects are absorbed into the self as a means of diminishing anxiety by reducing the fear of loss (in the case of a loved object) or by internalizing the aggressive characteristic and putting it under control (in the case of a hated object).

intromission (in″tro-mish′un) the entrance of one part or object into another.

introspection (in″tro-spek′shun) contemplation or observation of one's thoughts and feelings; self-analysis. adj., **introspec′tive.**

introsusception (in″tro-sŭ-sep′shun) intussusception.

introversion (in″tro-ver′zhun) 1. the turning outside in, more or less completely, of an organ, or the resulting condition. 2. preoccupation with oneself, with reduction of interest in the outside world.

introvert (in'tro-vert) 1. a person whose interest is turned inward to the self. 2. to turn one's interest inward to the self. 3. a structure that can be turned or drawn inwards. 4. to turn a part or organ inward upon itself.

intubate (in'too-bāt) to perform intubation.

intubation (in"too-ba'shun) the insertion of a tube, as into the larynx; see also CANNULATION and CATHETERIZATION. The purpose of intubation varies with the location and type of tube inserted; generally it is done to allow drainage, to maintain an open airway, or to administer anesthetics or oxygen.

Intubation into the stomach or intestine is done to remove gastric or intestinal contents for the relief or prevention of distention, or to obtain a specimen for analysis. Another example of intubation is when a tube is inserted into the common bile duct to allow for drainage of bile from ducts draining the liver, done after surgery on the gallbladder or the common bile duct. Endotracheal intubation can be achieved by insertion of an ENDOTRACHEAL TUBE, sometimes containing a stylet, via the mouth or nose with the aid of a laryngoscope. It is done for the purpose of assuring patency of the upper airway. TRACHEOSTOMY is a form of endotracheal intubation.

gastrointestinal i. in the NURSING INTERVENTIONS CLASSIFICATION, a nursing INTERVENTION defined as insertion of a tube into the gastrointestinal tract.

intuiting (in-too'it-ing) a technique used in qualitative RESEARCH when the researcher focuses all awareness and energy on the subject of interest and gains insights by INTUITION.

intuition (in"too-ĭ'shun) an awareness or knowing that seems to come unbidden and usually cannot be logically explained.

intumescence (in"too-mes'ens) 1. a swelling, normal or abnormal. 2. the process of swelling. adj., **intumes'cent.**

intussusception (in"tŭ-sŭ-sep'shun) 1. prolapse of one part of the intestine into the lumen of an immediately adjacent part, causing INTESTINAL OBSTRUCTION. 2. the reception into an organism of matter, such as food, and its transformation into new protoplasm.

Intussusception is one of the most common causes of intestinal obstruction in infancy. Most cases occur in children during the first year of life, and some cases occur in the second year, but very few thereafter. The condition may be caused by a growth in the intestine or by any condition that causes the intestine to contract strongly. Usually, the cause is not known. The condition becomes apparent when a healthy, thriving infant suddenly experiences paroxysms of abdominal pain, with vomiting and restlessness. The infant usually cries out with pain and draws the knees up to the chest. The abdomen becomes tender and distended as the obstruction progresses and a sausage-shaped mass is felt in the upper right quadrant. Stools appear red and jellylike due to the presence of blood.

Diagnosis is confirmed by barium enema, which in about 75 per cent of uncomplicated cases has a therapeutic effect, reducing the invagination by hydrostatic force. Surgical intervention involves manual reduction and, if a portion of the intestine has been irreparably damaged, bowel resection. (See accompanying illustration.)

intussusceptum (in"tŭ-sŭ-sep'tum) the portion of intestine that has prolapsed in intussusception.

intussuscipiens (in"tŭ-sŭ-sip'e-ens) the portion of the intestine containing the intussusceptum.

inulin (in'u-lin) a starch occurring in the rhizome of certain plants, which on hydrolysis yields fructose. It is used as a measure of glomerular function in tests of renal function.

inunction (in-ungk'shun) the act of anointing or applying an ointment by rubbing.

in utero (in u'ter-o) [L.] inside the uterus.

invaginate (in-vaj'ĭ-nāt) to infold one portion of a structure within another portion.

invagination (in-vag"ĭ-na'shun) 1. the infolding of one part within another part of a structure, as of the blastula during gastrulation. 2. intussusception.

basilar i. a developmental deformity of the occipital bone and upper end of the cervical spine in which the latter appears to have pushed the floor of the occipital bone upward; see also *platybasia*. Called also basilar impression.

invasive (in-va'siv) 1. reaching or taking over surrounding tissues; see INVASIVENESS (def. 2). 2. involving puncture or incision of the skin or insertion of an instrument or injection of foreign material into the body; said of diagnostic techniques and procedures.

invasiveness (in-va'siv-nes) 1. the ability of microorganisms to enter the body and spread in the tissues. 2. the ability to infiltrate and actively destroy surrounding tissue, a property of malignant tumors. adj., **inva'sive.**

inventory (in'ven-tor"e) a comprehensive list of personality traits, aptitudes, and interests.

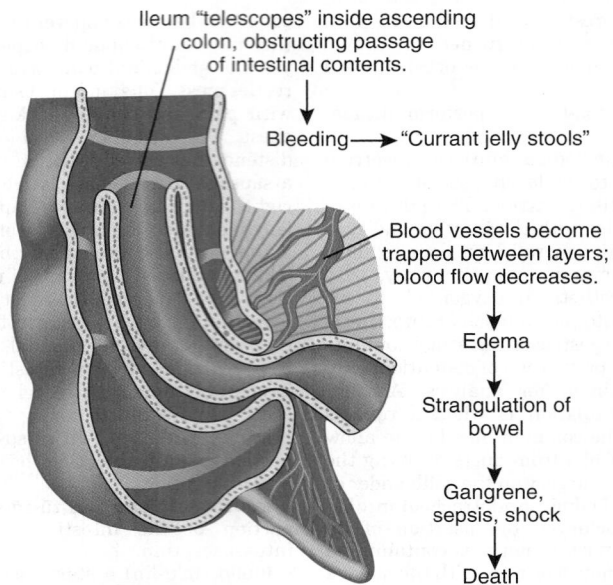

Ileum "telescopes" inside ascending colon, obstructing passage of intestinal contents.

↓

Bleeding ──→ "Currant jelly stools"

Blood vessels become trapped between layers; blood flow decreases.

↓

Edema

↓

Strangulation of bowel

↓

Gangrene, sepsis, shock

↓

Death

Intussusception. From McKinney et al., 2000.

California Personality I. CPI; a self-report, true-false questionnaire designed to measure aspects of personality style. It is generally used in counseling situations or for less than severe psychopathology.

Millon Clinical Multiaxial I. MCMI; a true-false, self-report questionnaire designed to produce a profile of the personality style and structure underlying mental disorders.

Minnesota Multiphasic Personality I. MMPI; a psychological test in questionnaire form in which the answers to true-false statements show dimensions of the subject's personality structure and provide comparison with responses made by persons in various diagnostic categories.

inversion (in-ver′zhun) 1. a turning inward, inside out, or other reversal of the normal relation of a part. 2. in psychiatry, a term used by Freud for homosexuality. 3. a chromosomal aberration due to the inverted reunion of the middle segment after breakage of a chromosome at two points, resulting in a change in sequence of genes or nucleotides.

invertebrate (in-ver′tĕ-brāt) 1. having no vertebral column. 2. any animal that has no vertebral column.

invest (in-vest′) 1. to envelop in or cover another tissue or part (as fascia). 2. to surround, envelop, or embed in an investment material.

investing (in-vest′ing) the covering or enveloping of a tissue or part by another tissue, such as a fascia.

investment (in-vest′ment) 1. any tissue, such as fascia, that envelops or covers other tissues or parts. 2. a material applied as a soft paste to a pattern that hardens to form a mold for casting.

inveterate (in-vet′er-it) confirmed and chronic; long-established and difficult to cure.

in vitro (in ve′tro) [L.] within a glass; observable in a test tube; in an artificial environment.

in vivo (in ve′vo) [L.] within the living body.

involucrum (in″vo-lu′krum) [L.] a covering or sheath, as of a sequestrum.

involuntary (in-vol′un-tar″e) performed independently of the will.

involution (in″vo-lu′shun) 1. a rolling or turning inward. 2. one of the movements involved in the gastrulation of many animals. 3. a retrograde change of the entire body or in a particular organ, as the retrograde changes in the female genital organs that result in normal size after delivery. 4. the progressive degeneration occurring naturally with advancing age,

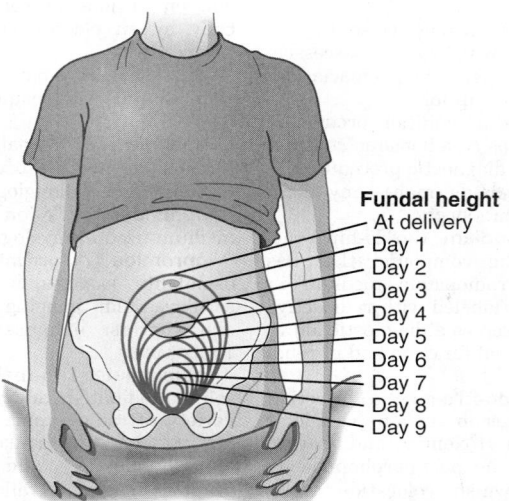

Fundal height
- At delivery
- Day 1
- Day 2
- Day 3
- Day 4
- Day 5
- Day 6
- Day 7
- Day 8
- Day 9

Involution of the uterus. Height of the uterine fundus decreases by approximately 1 cm/day. From McKinney et al., 2000.

resulting in shriveling of organs or tissues. adj., **involu′tional.**

iobenguane (i″o-ben′gwān) a NOREPI-NEPHRINE analogue that is taken up by the neuroendocrine cells and concentrated in the hormone storage vesicles; labeled with radioactive iodine, it is used for diagnostic imaging of neuroendocrine tumors and disorders of the adrenal MEDULLA.

iocetamic acid (i″o-sĕ-tam′ik) a water-soluble iodinated radiopaque x-ray contrast medium used in oral CHOLECYSTOGRAPHY.

iodamide (i-o′dah-mīd) a water-soluble, radiopaque, iodinated radiographic contrast medium; used for intravenous excretory urography.

Iodamoeba (i-o″dah-me′bah) a genus of amebas, including *I. buetsch′lii,* parasitic in man, and *I. su′is,* found in pigs.

iodide (i′o-dīd) a binary compound of IODINE, such as potassium iodide; it inhibits the release of THYROXINE from the THYROID GLAND.

iodination (i″o-dǐ-na′shun) the incorporation or addition of iodine in a compound.

iodine (I) (i′o-dīn) a chemical element, atomic number 53, atomic weight 126.904. (See Appendix 6.) Iodine is essential in nutrition, being especially prevalent in the colloid of the THYROID GLAND. It is used in the treatment of HYPOTHYROIDISM and as a topical antiseptic. Iodine is a frequent cause of poisoning (see IODISM). Deficiency of iodine causes GOITER. Since iodine salts are opaque

to x-rays, they can be combined with other compounds and used as contrast media in diagnostic x-ray examinations of the gallbladder and kidneys.

i. 123 a radioactive isotope of iodine having a half-life of 13.2 hours and emitting gamma rays and x-rays. It is used in diagnostic imaging and as radiation sources in radiation therapy. Symbol ^{123}I.

i. 125 a radioisotope of iodine having a half-life of 60.14 days and emitting gamma rays; used as a label in radioimmunoassays and other *in vitro* tests, and also for thyroid imaging. Symbol ^{125}I.

i. 131 a radioactive isotope of iodine having a half-life of 8.04 days and emitting beta particles and gamma rays. It is used as a tracer in diagnostic imaging and as a radiation source in radiation therapy. Symbol ^{131}I.

protein-bound i. a test of THYROID function; see also PROTEIN-BOUND IODINE TEST.

radioactive i. RADIOIODINE.

i. solution a transparent, reddish brown liquid, each 100 ml of which contains 1.8 to 2.2 g of iodine and 2.1 to 2.6 g of sodium iodide; a local antiinfective agent.

strong i. solution Lugol's solution.

iodinophilous (i″o-din-of′ĭ-lus) easily stainable with iodine.

iodipamide (i″o-dip′ah-mīd) a radiopaque medium used in the form of its meglumine and sodium salts in cholangiography and cholecystography.

iodism (i′o-dizm) chronic poisoning by IODINE or iodides, with coryza, excessive salivation, frontal headache, emaciation, weakness, and skin eruptions.

iodized oil an iodine addition product of vegetable oil; used as a radiopaque contrast medium in various diagnostic procedures.

iododerma (i″o-do-der′mah) any skin lesion resulting from IODISM.

iodohippurate sodium (i-o″do-hip′u-rāt) an iodine-containing compound that has been used as a radiopaque medium in pyelography. When labeled with radioactive iodine, it may be used as a diagnostic aid in determination of renal function and in renal imaging.

iodophilia (i″o-do-fil′e-ah) a reaction shown by leukocytes in certain pathologic conditions, as in toxemia and severe anemia, in which the polymorphonuclears show diffuse brownish coloration when treated with iodine or iodides.

iodophor (i-o′do-for) any of various compounds of iodine with carriers, used as surgical scrubs and surface disinfectants.

iodoquinol (i-o″do-kwin′ol) an amebicide used in the treatment of amebic dysentery; also used topically as an antibacterial and antifungal.

iodotherapy (i″o-do-ther′ah-pe) treatment with iodine or iodides.

ion (i′on) an atom or group of atoms having a positive (CATION) or negative (ANION) electric charge by virtue of having gained or lost an electron; substances forming ions are called ELECTROLYTES. adj., **ion′ic.**

dipolar i. an ion that has both positive and negative regions of charge.

hydrogen i. the positively charged HYDROGEN atom (H^+), which is the positive ion of all ACIDS. See also HYDROGEN ION CONCENTRATION.

hydroxyl i. the negatively charged group, OH^-, present to excess in alkaline solutions.

Ionamin (i-o′nah-min) trademark for a preparation of PHENTERMINE, an appetite suppressant.

ionization (i″on-ī-za′shun) 1. any process by which a neutral atom or molecule gains or loses electrons, thus acquiring a net charge, as the dissociation of a substance in solution into ions or ion production by the passage of radioactive particles. 2. iontophoresis.

ionophore (i′on-o-for″) any molecule, as of a drug, that increases the permeability of cell membranes to a specific ion.

ionophose (i′o-no-fōz″) a sensation of seeing the color violet.

iontophoresis (i-on″to-fo-re′sis) the introduction of ions of soluble salts into the body by an electric current. adj., **iontophoret′ic.**

iopamidol (i″o-pam′ĭ-dol) a nonionic, water-soluble radiopaque medium used in myelography.

iopanoic acid (i″o-pah-no′ik) an iodinated radiopaque medium used in oral cholecystography and cholangiography.

iophendylate (i″o-fen′dĭ-lāt) a radiopaque medium used in myelography.

iopromide (i″o-pro′mīd) a nonionic, low-osmolality RADIOPAQUE medium used for cardiovascular imaging, excretory urology, and contrast enhancement in computed TOMOGRAPHY.

iothalamate (i″o-thal′ah-māt) a water-soluble iodinated radiopaque medium for a variety of radiographic procedures, including ANGIOGRAPHY, ARTHROGRAPHY, UROGRAPHY, CHOLANGIOGRAPHY, and computed tomographic imaging. Available as *iothalamate meglumine, iothalamate sodium,* or a mixture of the two salts.

ioversol (i″o-ver′sol) a nonionic contrast medium used in ANGIOGRAPHY and UROGRAPHY and for contrast enhancement in computed TOMOGRAPHY.

ioxaglate (i″ok-sag′lāt) a low-osmolality radiopaque medium, used as the meglumine or sodium salt.

ioxilan (i-ok′sĭ-lan) a low-viscosity, low-osmolality, nonionic contrast agent used in ARTERIOGRAPHY, excretory UROGRAPHY, and computed TOMOGRAPHY.

ipecac (ip′ĕ-kak) the dried rhizome and roots of *Cephaelis ipecacuanha* or *Cephaelis acuminata;* used as an emetic or expectorant.

ipodate (i′po-dāt) a radiopaque contrast medium used in cholecystography.

IPPB intermittent positive pressure breathing.

ipratropium (ip-rah-tro′pe-um) an ANTICHOLINERGIC and ANTIMUSCARINIC, used in the form of the bromide salt as an aerosol BRONCHODILATOR in treatment of bronchospasm and as a nasal spray for the relief of RHINORRHEA.

iproplatin (i′pro-plat″in) an analogue of CISPLATIN, used as an antioneoplastic AGENT, administered intravenously; its actions are similar to those of cisplatin but its toxicities are different and usually milder.

irbesartan (ir″bĕ-sahr′tan) an ANGIOTENSIN II receptor antagonist used as an ANTIHYPERTENSIVE, administered orally.

ipsi- word element [L.], *same; self.*

ipsilateral (ip″sĭ-lat′er-al) situated on or affecting the same side.

IPV poliovirus vaccine inactivated.

IQ intelligence quotient.

Ir iridium.

irid(o)- word element [Gr.], *iris of the eye; a colored circle.*

iridal (i″rĭ-dal) pertaining to the iris.

iridalgia (i″rĭ-dal′jah) pain in the iris.

iridauxesis (ir″id-awk-se′sis) thickening of the iris.

iridectomesodialysis (ir″ĭ-dek″to-me″so-di-al′ĭ-sis) surgical formation of an artificial iris by excision and separation of adhesions around the inner edge of the iris.

iridectomy (ir″ĭ-dek′to-me) excision of a full-thickness piece of the iris.

iridectropium (ir″ĭ-dek-tro′pe-um) eversion of the iris.

iridemia (ir″ĭ-de′me-ah) hemorrhage from the iris.

iridencleisis (ir″ĭ-den-kli′sis) surgical incarceration of a slip of the iris within a corneal or limbal incision to act as a wick for aqueous drainage in glaucoma.

irideremia (ir″ĭ-der-e′me-ah) congenital absence of the iris.

irides (ir′ĭ-dēz) [Gr.] plural of IRIS.

iridescence (ir″ĭ-des′ens) the condition of gleaming with bright and changing colors. adj., **irides′cent.**

iridesis (i-rid′ĕ-sis) repositioning of the pupil by fixation of a sector of iris in a corneal or limbal incision.

iridic (i-rid′ik) pertaining to the iris.

iridium (Ir) (ĭ-rid′e-um, i-rid′e-um) a chemical element, atomic number 77, atomic weight 192.2. (See Appendix 6.)

iridoavulsion (ir″ĭ-do-ah-vul′shun) complete tearing away of the iris from its periphery.

iridocapsulitis (ir″ĭ-do-kap″su-li′tis) inflammation of the iris and lens capsule.

iridocele (i-rid′o-sēl) hernial protrusion of part of the iris through the cornea.

iridochoroiditis (ir″ĭ-do-ko″roi-di′tis) inflammation of the iris and choroid.

iridocoloboma (ir″ĭ-do-kol″o-bo′mah) congenital fissure or coloboma of the iris.

iridoconstrictor (ir″ĭ-do-kon-strik′tor) a muscle or agent that constricts the pupil of the eye.

iridocyclectomy (ir″ĭ-do-si-klek′to-me) excision of part of the iris and of the ciliary body.

iridocyclitis (ir″ĭ-do-si-kli′tis) inflammation of the iris and ciliary body.

heterochromic i. a unilateral lowgrade form leading to depigmentation of the iris of the affected eye; called also heterochromic uveitis.

iridocyclochoroiditis (ir″ĭ-do-si″klo-ko″roi-di′tis) inflammation of the iris, ciliary body, and choroid.

iridocystectomy (ir″ĭ-do-sis-tek′-to-me) excision of part of the iris to form an artificial pupil.

iridodesis (ir″ĭ-dod′ĕ-sis) iredesis.

iridodialysis (ir″ĭ-do-di-al′ĭ-sis) separation or loosening of the iris from its root at the ciliary body, either from trauma or from surgical accident.

iridodilator (ir″ĭ-do-di-la′tor) a muscle or agent that dilates the pupil of the eye.

iridodonesis (ir″ĭ-do-do-ne′sis) tremulousness of the iris on movement of the eye, occurring in subluxation of the lens.

iridokeratitis (ir″ĭ-do-ker″ah-ti′tis) inflammation of the iris and cornea.

iridokinesia (ir″ĭ-do-kĭ-ne′zhah) **iridokinesis** (ir″ĭ-do-kĭ-ne′sis) contraction and expansion of the iris. adj., **iridokinet′ic.**

iridoleptynsis (ir″ĭ-do-lep-tin′sis) thinning or atrophy of the iris.

iridology (ir″ĭ-dol′o-je) the study of the iris as associated with disease.

iridomalacia (ir″ĭ-do-mah-la′shah) softening of the iris.

iridomesodialysis (ir″ĭ-do-me″so-di-al′ĭ-sis) surgical loosening of adhesions around the inner edge of the iris.

iridomotor (ir″ĭ-do-mo′tor) pertaining to movements of the iris.

iridoncus (ir″ĭ-dong′kus) tumor or swelling of the iris.

iridoparalysis (ir″ĭ-do-pah-ral′ĭ-sis) iridoplegia.

iridoperiphakitis (ir″ĭ-do-per″ĭ-fah-ki′tis) inflammation of the lens capsule.

iridoplegia (ir″ĭ-do-ple′jah) paralysis of the sphincter of the iris, with lack of contraction or dilation of the pupil; called also iridoparalysis.

iridoptosis (ir″ĭ-dop-to′sis) prolapse of the iris.

iridopupillary (ir″ĭ-do-pu′pĭ-ler″e) pertaining to the iris and pupil.

iridorhexis (ir″ĭ-do-rek′sis) 1. rupture of the iris. 2. the tearing away of the iris.

iridoschisis (ir″ĭ-dos′kĭ-sis) splitting of the mesodermal stroma of the iris into two layers, with fibrils of the anterior layer floating in the aqueous.

iridosclerotomy (ir″ĭ-do-sklĕ-rot′ah-me) incision of the sclera and of the edge of the iris in glaucoma.

iridosteresis (ir″ĭ-do-stĕ-re′sis) removal of all or part of the iris.

iridotasis (ir″ĭ-dot′ah-sis) stretching of the iris in treatment of glaucoma.

iridotomy (ir″ĭ-dot′ah-me) incision of the iris.

irinotecan (i″rĭ-no-te′kan) an antineoplastic AGENT used as the hydrochloride salt in treatment of colorectal carcinoma.

iris (i′ris), pl. *i′rides* [Gr.] the circular pigmented membrane behind the cornea, perforated by the pupil. It is the most anterior portion of the vascular tunic of the EYE and is made up of a flat bar of circular muscular fibers surrounding the pupil, a thin layer of plain muscle fibers by which the pupil is dilated, and, posteriorly, two layers of pigmented epithelial cells. (See also color plates.)

iritis (i-ri′tis) inflammation of the IRIS; it may be acute, occurring suddenly with pronounced symptoms, or chronic, with less severe but longer-lasting symptoms. adj., **irit′ic.**

Cause. The cause is often obscure; iritis is frequently associated with rheumatic diseases (particularly rheumatoid arthritis), diabetes mellitus, syphilis, diseased teeth, tonsillitis, and other infections. It may also be caused by trauma.

Symptoms. Iritis is characterized by severe pain, usually radiating to the forehead and becoming worse at night. The eye is usually red and the pupil contracts and may be irregular in shape; there is extreme sensitivity to light, together with blurring of vision and tenderness of the eyeball. The iris becomes swollen and discolored. If not treated promptly, iritis can be dangerous because of scarring and adhesions that may cause impaired vision and possibly blindness.

Treatment. Caring for iritis calls for treatment of the underlying cause and then dilation of the pupil with atropine drops to prevent scarring or adhesions. Certain steroid drugs may be used to reduce the inflammation quickly. Warm compresses may also help to lessen the inflammation and pain. A protective covering allows the eye to rest.

With proper treatment, acute iritis usually clears up fairly quickly, although it may recur. For permanent relief, elimination or control of the underlying cause is necessary.

serous i. iritis with a serous exudate.

iritoectomy (ir″ĭ-to-ek′to-me) surgical excision of deposits of after-cataract on the iris, together with iridectomy, to form an artificial pupil.

iritomy (i-rit′o-me) iridotomy.

iron (Fe) (i′ern) a chemical element, atomic number 26, atomic weight 55.847. (See Appendix 6-1.) Iron is chiefly important to the human body because it is the main constituent of HEMOGLOBIN, CYTOCHROME, and other components of respiratory enzyme systems. A constant although small intake of iron in food is needed to replace ERYTHROCYTES that are destroyed in the body processes. Most iron reaches the body in food, where it occurs naturally in the form of iron compounds. These are converted for use in the body by the action of the hydrochloric acid produced in the stomach. This acid separates the iron from the food and combines with it in a form that is readily assimilable by the body. Vitamin C enhances absorption of iron, and alkalis hamper absorption.

IRON DEFICIENCIES. The amount of new iron needed every day by the adult body is about 18 mg. A child needs more in proportion to weight. Although these amounts are very small, iron deficiencies may cause serious disorders. Three stages of iron deficiency are distinguished: *iron depletion* or *prelatent iron deficiency,* in which bodily stores are mildly depleted but no change in hematocrit or serum iron levels is detectable; *latent iron deficiency,* in which the serum iron level has dropped but the hematocrit is unchanged and there is no anemia; and iron deficiency ANEMIA, a serious condition characterized by low to absent iron stores, low hematocrit, and other blood abnormalities. A great loss of blood, such as may result from bleeding ulcers, hemorrhoids, or injury, is the most common cause of a deficiency of iron. Women who lose much blood in menstruation may have to supplement their diet with iron-rich food. Iron deficiency sometimes occurs in pregnancy as a result of increased demands on the mother's blood. It may also occur in infants, since milk contains little iron. Although babies are born with an extra supply of hemoglobin, by the age of 2 or 3 months they need iron-rich food to supplement milk.

Iron preparations, such as ferrous sulfate, may be necessary in the treatment of iron deficiency anemia; they should be administered after meals, never on an empty stomach. The patient should be warned that the drugs cause stools to turn dark green or black. Overdosage may cause severe systemic reactions.

An acute iron deficiency may warrant parenteral administration of an iron supplement. Hypersensitivity to iron supplements often occurs in patients with other known allergies. In other patients the parenteral administration of iron can cause vomiting, chills, fever, headache, joint pain, and urticaria.

Food Sources of Iron. Liver is the richest source of iron; 200 g (6 ounces) of liver contains a whole day's supply for an adult. Other iron-rich foods include lean meat, oysters, kidney beans, whole wheat bread, kale, spinach, egg yolk, turnip greens, beet greens, carrots, apricots, and raisins.

i. 59 a radioisotope of iron having a half-life of 44.5 days; used in ferrokinetics tests to determine the rate at which iron is cleared from the plasma and incorporated in red blood cells. Symbol ^{59}Fe.

i. dextran a complex of iron and dextran of low molecular weight; administered intravenously or intramuscularly as a hematinic.

i. poisoning poisoning from ingestion of excessive iron or iron-containing compounds, such as in children who eat iron supplement tablets like candy; symptoms include ulceration of the gastrointestinal tract, vomiting, vasodilation with shock, metabolic acidosis, liver injury, and coagulation disturbances.

i. storage disease hemochromatosis.

i. sucrose a complex of ferric hydroxide, $Fe(OH)_3$, in sucrose; used intravenously to treat iron deficiency ANEMIA in hemodialysis patients receiving supplemental ERYTHROPOIETIN therapy.

irotomy (i-rot′ah-me) iridotomy.

irradiate (ĭ-ra′de-āt) to treat with radiant energy.

irradiation (ĭ-ra″de-a′shun) 1. RADIATION THERAPY. 2. the dispersion of nervous impulse beyond the normal path of conduction. 3. the exposure of a substance to RADIATION, which consists of any of numerous kinds of rays that travel at the speed of light. Every living thing is subject to some irradiation by cosmic rays, ULTRAVIOLET RAYS in sunlight, and other natural radiation in the environment, all of which is usually slight and harmless. In large amounts,

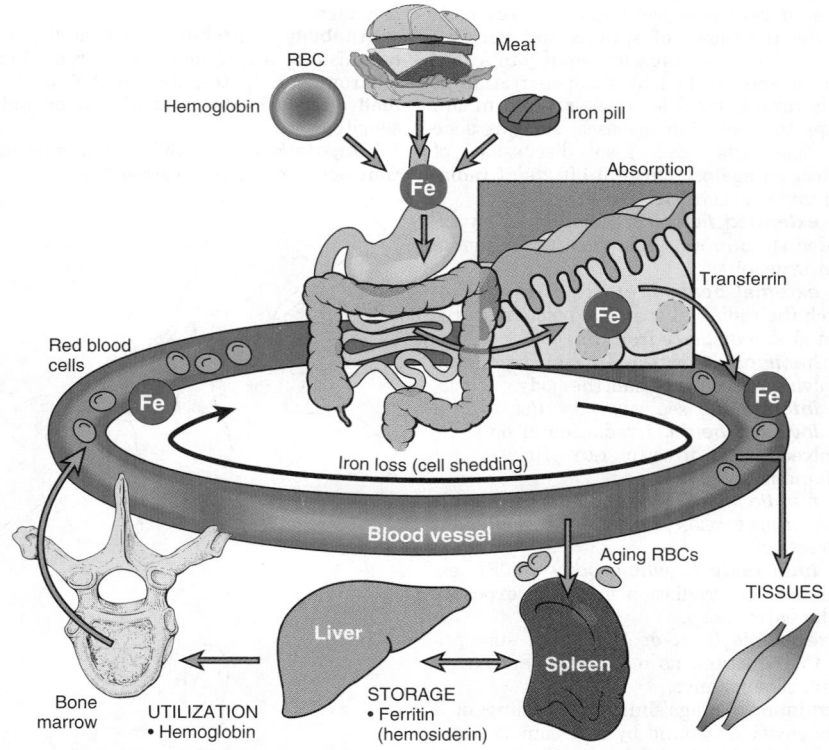

Iron metabolism. Uptake of heme iron or ferrous iron occurs in the intestine. From the intestine, iron is transported on transferrin to the liver or the bone marrow. Transferrin binds to red blood precursors in the bone marrow and delivers iron for incorporation into hemoglobin. Red blood cells in the circulation contain 60 percent to 80 percent of body iron. Old red blood cels are destroyed in the spleen. The iron is bound to transferrin for recirculation. Approximately 20 percent to 30 percent of iron is stored in the form of hemosiderin in the spleen, liver, and bone marrow. The remaining iron is in the respiratory enzymes of somatic cells. Iron is lost by desquamation of skin and intestinal cells. From Damjanov, 2000.

however, certain kinds of radiation cause direct harm to living cells, especially those rays that have a greater frequency and produce more energy. Irradiation of certain foods, including milk, kills harmful bacteria, prevents spoilage, and sometimes increases its vitamin efficiency. X-ray photography is used in industrial research and in diagnosis of disorders within the body.

RADIATION THERAPY usually refers to treatment by X-RAYS and GAMMA RAYS. X-rays are produced by bombarding a tungsten target with high-speed electrons in a vacuum tube; gamma rays are emitted during the decay of radioisotopes. X-rays may be employed to kill organisms causing skin diseases, for example, or to destroy the abnormal cells that form tumors. Gonads, blood cells, and cancer cells are especially sensitive to radiation, particularly to x-rays and gamma rays.

Other rays are also used medically. Infrared rays produce a radiant heat used for the treatment of sprains and bursitis; tissues such as muscles and joints are relaxed and soothed by the penetration of these rays. Ultraviolet rays are used in sun lamps to treat skin diseases, such as acne and psoriasis. See also discussion of protection against harmful effects of radiation under RADIATION.

extended field i. irradiation of an extended FIELD in RADIATION THERAPY for malignant LYMPHOMA.

external beam i. RADIATION THERAPY in which the radiation is emitted from a source located at a distance from the body.

hemibody i. external beam irradiation involving exposure of half the body.

interstitial i. see RADIATION THERAPY.

involved field i. irradiation of only the involved FIELD in RADIATION THERAPY for malignant LYMPHOMA.

mantle field i. irradiation of a mantle FIELD in RADIATION THERAPY for malignant LYMPHOMA.

total body i., whole-body i. TBI; external beam irradiation involving exposure of the entire body.

irreducible (ir″rē-doo′sĭ-b'l) not susceptible to reduction, as a fracture, hernia, or chemical substance.

irrigation (ir″ĭ-ga′shun) 1. washing of a body cavity or wound by a stream of water or other fluid. A steady, gentle stream is used; pressure should be sufficient to reach the desired area, but not enough to force the fluid beyond the area to be irrigated. Pressure may be applied manually, such as with a bulb syringe or mechanical device, or by gravity. The greater the height of the container of solution, the greater will be the pressure exerted by the stream of solution. There are also specially designed irrigating units that deliver a pulsed flow of fluid. Return flow of solution must always be allowed for. Directions about the type of solution to be used, the strength desired, and correct temperature should be followed carefully. Aseptic technique must be observed if sterile irrigation is ordered.   2. a liquid used for such washing.

bladder i. in the NURSING INTERVENTIONS CLASSIFICATION, a nursing INTERVENTION defined as instillation of a solution into the bladder to provide cleansing or medication.

bowel i. in the NURSING INTERVENTIONS CLASSIFICATION, a nursing INTERVENTION defined as instillation of a substance into the lower gastrointestinal tract.

wound i. in the NURSING INTERVENTIONS CLASSIFICATION, a nursing INTERVENTION defined as flushing of an open wound to cleanse and remove debris and excessive drainage.

irritability (ir″ĭ-tah-bil′ĭ-te) 1. ability of an organism or a specific tissue to react to the environment. 2. the state of being abnormally responsive to slight stimuli, or unduly sensitive.

myotatic i. the ability of a muscle to contract in response to stretching.

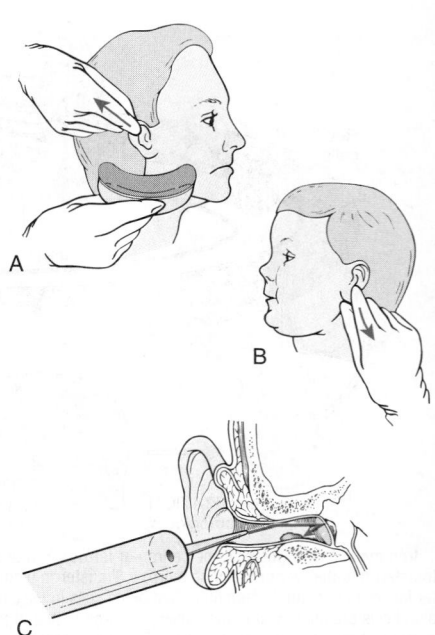

Irrigation of the ears. From Lammon et al., 1996.

irritable (ir'ĭ-tah-b'l) 1. capable of reacting to a stimulus. 2. abnormally sensitive to stimuli.

i. bowel syndrome the most common disorder presented by patients with gastrointestinal complaints, consisting of (1) altered bowel habits with diarrhea, constipation, or alternating diarrhea and constipation; (2) abdominal pain and intolerance to flatus; and (3) absence of detectable organic disease. Many inappropriate terms have been used to describe this disorder, including mucous colitis, nervous colon, spastic colon, and irritable colon. This syndrome should not be confused with COLITIS or other inflammatory diseases of the intestinal tract; in irritable bowel syndrome there is no inflammation, and it is not necessarily limited to the colon.

PATIENT CARE. Because of psychological factors that usually contribute to the disorder and its tendency to be chronic in nature, treatment should be holistic and individualized to meet the needs of each patient. In most cases, treatment is needed for an extended period of time. Patients should be assured that there is no relationship between their disorder and malignancy of the bowel. Modes of therapy include psychotherapy, biofeedback training, medications such as antidepressants, antispasmodics, and analgesics, and a diet that is high in bran and fiber.

Nursing care for the patient with irritable bowel syndrome is essentially the same as that for someone with DIARRHEA or CONSTIPATION. Patient teaching should include information about gas-forming foods such as legumes and those in the cabbage family. Milk and milk products are restricted in those patients who have shown an intolerance to milk.

Anxiety can often be mitigated by teaching the patient about the nature of the illness and reassurance that it is not related to malignancy of the bowel and can be managed by relatively simple, noninvasive measures. Ineffective coping patterns are not uncommon in these patients. When there is evidence that the patient is either unable to cope or is using harmful coping mechanisms such as smoking, drinking, or drug abuse, health teaching concerning relaxation techniques, wholesome diet, exercise, and recreation is appropriate.

irritant (ir'ĭ-tant) 1. causing irritation. 2. an agent that causes irritation.

irritation (ir''ĭ-ta'shun) 1. the act of stimulating. 2. a state of overexcitation and undue sensitivity. adj., **ir'ritative.**

IRV inspiratory reserve volume.

is(o)- word element [Gr.], *equal; alike; same.*

ischemia (is-ke'me-ah) deficiency of blood in a part, due to functional constriction or actual obstruction of a blood vessel. adj., **ische'mic.**

myocardial i. deficiency of blood supply to the heart muscle.

ischemic heart disease 1. heart disease that causes narrowing of coronary arteries, leading to inadequate blood supply to the myocardium. 2. heart disease that occurs as a result of inadequate blood supply to the myocardium, as in MYOCARDIAL INFARCTION and ANGINA PECTORIS.

ischesis (is-ke'sis) suppression of a discharge.

ischi(o)- word element [Gr.], *ischium.*

ischiadic (is''ke-ad'ik) 1. ischial. 2. sciatic (def. 2).

ischial (is'ke-al) pertaining to the ISCHIUM; called also ischiadic, ischiatic, and sciatic

ischialgia (is''ke-al'jah) pain in the ischium.

ischiatic (is''ke-at'ik) 1. ischial. 2. sciatic (def. 2).

ischiobulbar (is''ke-o-bul'bar) pertaining to the ischium and the bulb of the urethra.

ischiocapsular (is''ke-o-kap'su-lar) pertaining to the ischium and the capsular ligament of the hip joint.

ischiocele (is'ke-o-sēl'') hernia through the sacrosciatic notch.

ischiococcygeal (is''ke-o-kok-sij'e-al) pertaining to the ischium and coccyx.

ischiodidymus (is''ke-o-did'ĭ-mus) conjoined twins united at the pelvis.

ischiodynia (is''ke-o-din'e-ah) pain in the ischium.

ischiofemoral (is''ke-o-fem'o-ral) pertaining to the ischium and femur.

ischiopagus (is''ke-op'ah-gus) conjoined twins fused at the ischial region.

ischiopubic (is''ke-o-pu'bik) pertaining to the ischium and pubes.

ischiorectal (is''ke-o-rek'tal) pertaining to the ischium and rectum.

ischium (is'ke-um) the inferior, dorsal portion of the hip bone. See anatomic Table of Bones in the Appendices.

ischuria (is-ku're-ah) urinary RETENTION. adj., **ischuret'ic.**

iseikonia (i''si-ko'ne-ah) iso-iconia. adj., **iseikon'ic.**

isethionate (is''ĕ-thi'o-nāt) USAN contraction for 2-hydroxyethanesulfonate.

Ishihara test (ish''e-hah'rah) a test for color vision made by the use of a series of PSEUDOISOCHROMATIC plates or charts.

ISID International Society of Infectious Diseases.

island (i'land) a cluster of cells or an isolated piece of tissue.

blood i's aggregations of mesenchymal cells in the angioblast of the embryo, developing into vascular endothelium and blood cells.

i's of Langerhans islets of Langerhans.

i. of Reil insula.

islet (i'let) an island.

i's of Langerhans, pancreatic i's irregular microscopic structures scattered throughout the pancreas and comprising its endocrine portion. They contain the *alpha cells,* which secrete the hyperglycemic factor glucagon; the *beta cells,* which secrete insulin, and whose degeneration is one of the causes of DIABETES MELLITUS; and the *delta cells,* which secrete somatostatin.

Walthard's i's microscopic inclusions of the ovarian germinal epithelium, which have been implicated in the development of Brenner tumors.

Ismelin (is'mĕ-lin) trademark for a preparation of GUANETHIDINE monosulfate, an ANTIHYPERTENSIVE AGENT.

isoagglutinin (i″so-ah-gloo'tĭ-nin) an ISOANTIBODY capable of agglutinating cells of other individuals of the same species.

isoallele (i″so-ah-lēl') an allelic gene that is considered as being normal but can be distinguished from another allele by its differing phenotypic expression when in combination with a dominant mutant allele.

isoamylase (i″so-am'ĭ-lās) 1. any of the several isoenzymes of α-amylase. 2. a hydrolase that catalyzes the hydrolysis of 1,6-α-glycosidic branch linkages in glycogen and amylopectin.

isoantibody (i″so-an'tĭ-bod″e) an antibody produced by one individual that reacts with isoantigens of another individual of the same species; called also alloantibody.

isoantigen (i″so-an'tĭ-jen) an antigen existing in alternative (allelic) forms in a species, thus inducing an IMMUNE RESPONSE when one form is transferred to members of the species who lack it; typical isoantigens are the blood group antigens.

isobar (i'so-bahr) 1. one of two or more chemical species with the same atomic weight but different atomic numbers. 2. a line on a map or chart depicting the boundaries of an area of constant atmospheric pressure.

isobaric (i″so-bar'ik) having equal or constant pressure or weight across space or time.

isocarboxazid (i″so-kahr-bok'sah-zid) a monoamine oxidase INHIBITOR administered orally as an ANTIDEPRESSANT and in the prevention of MIGRAINE.

isocellular (i″so-sel'u-lar) made up of identical cells.

isochromatic (i″so-kro-mat'ik) of the same color throughout.

isochromatophil (i″so-kro-mat'o-fil) staining equally with the same stain.

isochromosome (i″so-kro'mo-sōm) an abnormal chromosome having a median centromere and two identical arms, formed by transverse, rather than normal longitudinal, splitting of a replicating chromosome.

isochronic (i″so-kron'ik) isochronous.

isochronous (i-sok'rŏ-nus) performed in equal times; said of motions and vibrations occurring at the same time and being equal in duration.

isocitric acid (i″so-sit'rik) an intermediate in the tricarboxylic acid CYCLE, formed from oxaloacetic acid and itself converted to ketoglutaric acid.

isocoria (i″so-ko're-ah) equality of size of the pupils of the two eyes.

isocortex (i″so-kor'teks) neocortex.

isocytolysin (i″so-si-tol'ĭ-sin) an ISOANTIBODY that causes destruction of the cells of animals of the same species.

isocytosis (i″so-si-to'sis) equality in size of cells, especially of erythrocytes.

isodactylism (i″so-dak'tĭ-lizm) relatively even length of the fingers.

isodiametric (i″so-di″ah-met'rik) measuring the same in all diameters.

isodontic (i″so-don'tik) having all the teeth of the same size and shape.

isodose (i'so-dōs) a radiation dose of equal intensity to more than one body area.

isoelectric (i″so-e-lek'trik) showing no variation in electric POTENTIAL.

isoenzyme (i″so-en'zīm) any of several forms of an ENZYME that all catalyze the same reaction but may differ in reaction rate, inhibition by various substances, electrophoretic mobility, or immunologic properties. Several enzymes, particularly alkaline phosphatase, lactate dehydrogenase, and creatine kinase, have clinically important isoenzymes. Isoenzymes are separated by electrophoresis, and the pattern indicates which damaged organ has released the enzymes.

isoetharine (i″so-eth'ah-rēn) a SYMPATHOMIMETIC amine having more effect on the β_2-adrenergic receptors of the bronchi and vascular smooth muscle than on the β_1-adrenergic receptors of the heart; used as a bronchodilator in bronchial asthma and for relief of BRONCHOSPASM in CHRONIC OBSTRUCTIVE PULMONARY DISEASE.

isoflurane (i″so-floo-rān) a potent inhalational ANESTHETIC similar to ENFLURANE, used

isogamety (i″so-gam′ĕ-te) production by an individual of one sex of gametes identical with respect to the sex chromosome. adj., **isogamet′ic.**

isogamy (i-sog′ah-me) reproduction resulting from union of two gametes identical in size and structure, as in protozoa. adj., **isog′amous.**

isogeneic (i″so-jĕ-ne′ik) syngeneic.

isogeneric (i″so-jĕ-ner′ik) of the same kind; belonging to the same species.

isogenesis (i″so-jen′ĕ-sis) similarity in the processes of development.

isograft (i′so-graft″) syngraft.

isohemagglutination (i″so-he″mah-gloo″tĭ-na′shun) agglutination of erythrocytes caused by an ISOHEMAGGLUTININ.

isohemagglutinin (i″so-he″mah-gloo′tĭ-nin) an ISOAGGLUTININ directed against antigenic determinants on the erythrocytes of an individual of the same species.

isohemolysin (i″so-he-mol′ĭ-sin) an ISOAN-TIBODY that causes hemolysis of erythrocytes of animals of the same species.

isohemolysis (i″so-he-mol′ĭ-sis) hemolysis produced by isohemolysin. adj., **isohemo-lyt′ic.**

isoiconia (i″so-i-ko′ne-ah) a condition in which the image of an object is the same in both eyes. adj., **iso-icon′ic.**

isoimmunization (i″so-im″u-nĭ-za′shun) development of antibodies in response to isoantigens.

isokinetic (i″so-kĭ-net′ik) pertaining to a concentric or eccentric CONTRACTION of a muscle in which the speed and tension are constant throughout the range of lengthening or contracting.

isolate (i′so-lāt) 1. to separate from others, or set apart. 2. a group of individuals prevented by geographic, genetic, ecologic, or social barriers from interbreeding with others of their kind. 3. a pure microbial strain that has been separated from a mixed laboratory culture.

isolation (i″so-la′shun) 1. the process of separating, or the state of being alone. 2. the physiologic separation of a part, as by tissue culture or by interposition of inert material. 3. the extraction and purification of a chemical substance of unknown structure from a natural source. 4. the separation of infected individuals from those uninfected for the period of communicability of a particular disease; see also QUARANTINE. 5. the separation of an individual with a radioactive implant from others to prevent unnecessary exposure to radioactivity. 6. the successive propagation of a growth of microorganisms until a pure culture is obtained. 7. in psychiatry, a DEFENSE MECHANISM in which emotions are separated from the ideas, impulses, or memories to which they usually connect, so that the idea or impulse enters consciousness detached from its unacceptable feeling.

i. precautions special precautionary measures, practices, and procedures used in the care of patients with contagious or communicable diseases. The CENTERS FOR DIS-EASE CONTROL AND PREVENTION (CDC) provides explicit and comprehensive guidelines for control of the spread of infectious disease in care of hospitalized patients. The type of infectious disease a patient has dictates the kind of isolation precautions necessary to prevent spread of the disease to others.

Isolation practices have evolved over the years. Changes have been based on new epidemiological data, emergence of new or drug-resistant organisms, and the need to protect patients and hospital personnel. The HOSPITAL INFECTION CONTROL PRACTICES ADVI-SORY COMMITTEE (HICPAC) advises the CDC on the need to update and revise guidelines and policies related to prevention of hospital acquired infections. Present guidelines distinguish two types of isolation precautions: (1) standard PRECAUTIONS, which synthesize major features of earlier practices of universal PRECAUTIONS and isolation of moist body substances; and (2) transmission-based PRECAUTIONS, based on routes of transmission, designed to be used together with the standard precautions, divided into the three subgroups of airborne, droplet, and contact PRECAUTIONS. These are identified for disorders associated with a high index of suspicion for infection.

The recommendations of the CDC for isolation practices are categorized as follows:

Category 1A: Strongly recommended for all hospitals and strongly supported by well designed experimental or epidemiological studies.

Category 1B: Strongly recommended for all hospitals and reviewed as effective by experts in the field and a consensus of HICPAC based on strong rationale and suggestive evidence, even though definitive scientific studies have not been done.

Category 2: Suggested for implementation in many hospitals; recommendations may be supported by suggestive clinical or epidemiological studies; a strong theoretical rationale or definitive studies may be applicable to some, but not all, hospitals.

General Principles of Patient Care. In addition to the specific measures taken to prevent the spread of certain types of infectious diseases, there are general principles that are basic to the care of any patient who is a source of infection to others or likely to become infected by coming in contact with others. Factors most important in preventing spread of infection are proper disinfection techniques and conscientious hand washing. The hands are used for many tasks in patient care and are therefore likely to be an excellent source of infection if they are not washed properly before and after each contact with the patient or with contaminated articles.

protective i., reverse i. a formerly common type of isolation designed to prevent contact between potentially pathogenic microorganisms and persons with seriously impaired resistance. The Centers for Disease Control and Prevention deleted this category in 1983, but a few institutions continue to use it. Several studies have demonstrated no significant reduction in infection rates when it was being used.

social i. a NURSING DIAGNOSIS approved by the North American Nursing Diagnosis Association, defined as aloneness experienced by an individual as a negative or threatening state. Contributing factors are many and varied and include delay in accomplishing developmental tasks, alterations in physical appearance or mental status, social behavior or social values that are not accepted, inadequate personal resources, and inability to engage in satisfying personal relationships. Negative feelings of aloneness are subjective, existing when the patient/client says they do. When one suspects that a patient/client is experiencing social isolation, the diagnosis must be validated by a thorough assessment. The individual may express feelings of abandonment, rejection, or dread, demonstrate or verbalize a desire for more contact with the nurse or with family members, become more irritable or restless or less physically active, or develop a sleep or eating disorder. See also impaired social INTERACTION.

isoleucine (i″so-lu′sēn) a naturally occurring AMINO ACID produced by hydrolysis of fibrin and other proteins, one of the essential amino acids, necessary for optimal infant growth and for nitrogen equilibrium in adults.

isologous (i-sol′o-gus) syngeneic.

isolysin (i-sol′ĭ-sin) a lysin acting on cells of animals of the same species as that from which it is derived.

isolysis (i-sol′ĭ-sis) lysis of cells by isolysins. adj., **isolyt′ic.**

isomer (i′so-mer) any compound exhibiting, or capable of exhibiting, ISOMERISM. adj., **isomer′ic.**

isomerase (i-som′er-ās) a major class of enzymes comprising those that catalyze the process of isomerization, such as the interconversion of aldoses and ketoses.

isomerism (i-som′ĕ-rizm) the possession by two or more distinct compounds of the same molecular formula, each molecule having the same number of atoms of each element, but in different arrangement.

isomerization (i-som″ĕ-rī-za′shun) the process whereby any isomer is converted into another isomer, usually requiring special conditions of temperature, pressure, or catalysts.

isometheptene mucate (i″so-mĕ-thep′tēn mu′kāt) a VASOCONSTRICTOR that acts on dilated carotid and cerebral vessels, used in combination with DICHLORALPHENAZONE and ACETAMINOPHEN in treatment of migraine and tension headache.

isometric (i″so-met′rik) maintaining, or pertaining to, the same length; of equal dimensions.

isometropia (i″so-mĕ-tro′pe-ah) equality in refraction of the two eyes.

isomorphism (i″so-mor′fizm) identity in form; in genetics, referring to genotypes of polyploid organisms that produce similar gametes even though containing genes in different combinations on homologous chromosomes. adj., **isomor′phic.**

isoniazid (i″so-ni′ah-zid) an antibacterial compound used in treatment of tuberculosis.

isophoria (i″so-fo′re-ah) correspondence of the visual axes of the two eyes; equality

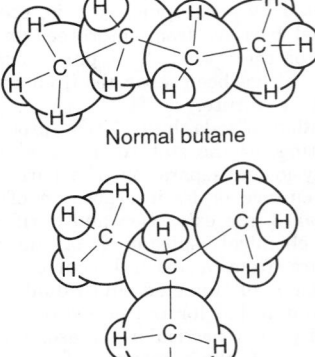

Normal butane

Isobutane

Chain isomerism. From Dorland's, 2000.

in the tension of the vertical muscles of the two eyes.

969 isoprecipitin – isozyme 969

isoprecipitin (i″so-pre-sip′ĭ-tin) an ISOANTIBODY that forms a precipitate when in the presence of antigens of animals of the same species.

isoprene (i′so-prēn) an unsaturated, branched-chain, five-carbon hydrocarbon that is the molecular unit of isoprenoid compounds.

isoprenoid (i″so-pre′noid) any compound biosynthesized from or containing isoprene units, including terpenes, carotenoids, fat-soluble vitamins, ubiquinone, rubber, and some steroids.

isopropamide (i″so-pro′pah-mīd) an ANTICHOLINERGIC and ANTIMUSCARINIC used in the form of the iodide to suppress gastric secretion and motility in the management of peptic ulcer and other intestinal ailments.

isopropanol (i″so-pro′pah-nol) isopropyl alcohol.

isoproterenol (i″so-pro-ter′ĕ-nol) a synthetic ADRENERGIC, used in the form of the hydrochloride and sulfate salts as a BRONCHODILATOR, and in the form of the hydrochloride salt as a cardiac stimulant.

isopter (i-sop′ter) a curve representing areas of equal visual acuity in the field of vision.

Isoptin (i-sop′tin) trademark for a preparation of VERAPAMIL, a coronary vasodilator.

Isopto-Carpine (i-sop′to-kahr″pēn) trademark for a preparation of PILOCARPINE hydrochloride, a MIOTIC agent.

isopyknosis (i″so-pik-no′sis) the quality of showing uniform density throughout, especially the uniformity of condensation observed in comparison of different chromosomes or in different areas of the same chromosome. adj., **isopyknot′ic.**

Isordil (i′sor-dil) trademark for preparations of ISOSORBIDE dinitrate, a coronary VASODILATOR.

isosensitization (i″so-sen″sĭ-tĭ-za′shun) allosensitization.

isosexual (i″so-sek′shoo-al) pertaining to the same sex; having secondary sex characters appropriate to one's sex.

isosmotic (i″soz-mot′ik) having the same osmotic pressure.

isosorbide (i″so-sor′bīd) an osmotic DIURETIC used to reduce intraocular pressure; its dinitrate and mononitrate esters are as coronary VASODILATORS in treatment of coronary INSUFFICIENCY and ANGINA PECTORIS.

Isospora (i-sos′po-rah) a genus of sporozoan parasites (order Coccidia), found in birds, amphibians, reptiles, and various mammals, including humans; *I. bel′li* is the etiologic agent of COCCIDIOSIS in humans. The former species *I. ho′minis* has been reclassified as two species, *Sarcocystis bovihominis* and *S. suihominis*.

isospore (i′so-spor) 1. a group of cells that conjugate or fuse with similar cells to reproduce a spore. 2. an asexual spore produced by spores that reproduce asexually.

isosthenuria (i″sos-thĕ-nu′re-ah) excretion of urine that has not been concentrated by the kidneys and has the same osmolality as that of plasma.

isotherm (i′so-therm) a line on a map or chart depicting the boundaries of an area in which the temperature is the same.

isotone (i′so-tōn) one of several nuclides having the same number of neutrons, but differing in number of protons in their nuclei.

isotonia (i″so-to′ne-ah) 1. a condition of equal tone, tension, or activity. 2. equality of osmotic pressure between two elements of a solution or between two different solutions.

isotonic (i″so-ton′ik) 1. of equal tension. 2. denoting a solution in which body cells can be bathed without net flow of water across the semipermeable cell membrane; also, denoting a solution having the same tonicity as another solution with which it is compared.

isotope (i′so-tōp) a chemical element having the same atomic number as another (i.e., the same number of nuclear protons), but having a different atomic mass (i.e., a different number of nuclear neutrons).

radioactive i. radioisotope.

stable i. one that does not transmute into another element with emission of corpuscular or electromagnetic radiations.

isotransplantation (i″so-trans-plan-ta′shun) syngeneic transplantation.

isotretinoin (i″so-tret′ĭ-no-in) a synthetic form of RETINOIC ACID (13-*cis*-retinoic acid), used orally to clear cystic and conglobate ACNE.

isotropic (i″so-trop′ik) 1. having the same value of a property, such as refractive index, in all directions, as in a cubic crystal or a piece of glass. 2. being singly refractive.

isotropy (i-sot′ro-pe) the quality or condition of being isotropic.

isotypical (i″so-tip′ĭ-kal) of the same kind.

isoxsuprine (i-sok′su-prēn) a beta-ADRENERGIC used as a VASODILATOR in peripheral vascular disease and cerebrovascular insufficiency.

isozyme (i′so-zīm) isoenzyme.

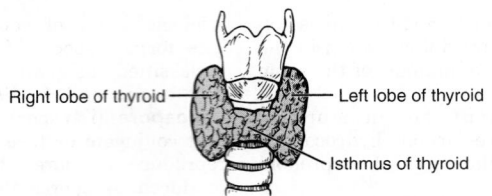

Isthmus of thyroid gland, connecting the two lobes. From Dorland's, 2000.

isradipine (is-rad′ĭ-pēn) a CALCIUM CHAN-NEL BLOCKING AGENT used alone or with a thiazide diuretic for the treatment of HYPERTENSION.

issue (ish′oo) a discharge of pus, blood, or other matter; a suppurating lesion emitting such a discharge.

isthmectomy (is-mek′to-me) surgical excision of an isthmus, especially of the isthmus of the thyroid.

isthmoparalysis (is″mo-pah-ral′ĭ-sis) **isthmoplegia** (is″mo-ple′jah) paralysis of the ISTHMUS OF THE FAUCES.

isthmus (is′mus) a narrow connection between two larger bodies or parts. adj., **isth′mian.**

i. of auditory tube, i. of eustachian tube the narrowest part of the eustachian tube at the junction of its bony and cartilaginous parts.

i. of fauces, i. fau′cium the constricted aperture between the cavity of the mouth and the pharynx.

i. of rhombencephalon the narrow segment of the fetal brain, forming the plane of separation between the rhombencephalon and cerebrum.

i. of thyroid the band of tissue joining the lobes of the thyroid.

i. of uterine tube the narrower, thicker-walled portion of the fallopian (uterine) tube closest to the uterus.

i. of uterus the constricted part of the uterus between the cervix and the body of the uterus.

Isuprel (i′su-prel) trademark for preparations of ISOPROTERENOL, a sympathomimetic BRONCHODILATOR and cardiac stimulant.

itch (ich) a skin condition accompanied by the desire to scratch an area of skin to relieve discomfort; see also PRURITUS.

bakers′ i. any of several inflammatory dermatoses of the hands and forearms, especially chronic candidal PARONYCHIA, seen with special frequency in bakers.

barbers′ i. 1. sycosis barbae. 2. tinea barbae. 3. pseudofolliculitis.

grain i. itching dermatitis due to a mite, *Pyemotes ventricosus,* which preys on certain insect larvae that live on straw, grain, and other plants.

grocers′ i. a vesicular dermatitis caused by certain mites found in stored hides, dried fruits, grain, copra, and cheese.

ground i. the itching eruption caused by entrance into the skin of the larvae of the hookworm *Ancylostoma duodenale* or *Necator americanus;* see also HOOKWORM DISEASE.

jock i. popular name for TINEA CRURIS.

seven-year i. popular name for SCABIES.

swimmers′ i. an itching dermatitis due to penetration into the skin of larval forms (cercaria) of SCHISTOSOMES, found in those who bathe in infested waters.

winter i. itching of the skin in cold weather, unassociated with structural lesions.

itching (ich′ing) pruritus.

-itis word element [Gr.], *inflammation.*

ITP idiopathic thrombocytopenic purpura.

itraconazole (it″rah-kon′ah-zōl) a triazole antifungal AGENT, used in a variety of infections; administered orally.

IU immunizing unit; International unit.

IUD intrauterine device.

IV intravenous; see also under INJECTION.

Ixodes (ik-so′dēz) a genus of arthropods, the hard TICKS (family Ixodidae); some species are vectors of disease.

ixodiasis (ik″so-di′ah-sis) any disease or lesion due to TICK bites; infestation with ticks.

ixodic (ik-sod′ik) pertaining to or caused by TICKS.

Ixodidae (iks-od′ĭ-de) a family of ticks (superfamily Ixodoidea); the hard TICKS.

Ixodides (iks-od′ĭ-dēz) the TICKS, a suborder of Acarina, including the superfamily Ixodoidea.

Ixodoidea (iks″o-doi′de-ah) a superfamily of arthropods (suborder Ixodides), comprising both the hard and soft TICKS.

J

J joule.

jacket (jak'et) an encasement or covering for the trunk, especially the thorax.

   plaster-of-Paris j. a casing of PLASTER OF PARIS enveloping the body, for the purpose of giving support or correcting deformities; see also CAST.

   Sayre's j. a plaster of Paris jacket used as a support for the vertebral column.

   strait j. popular name for CAMISOLE.

Jackson's syndrome (jak'sunz) paralysis of structures innervated by the tenth, eleventh, and twelfth cranial nerves, including the soft palate, larynx, half of the tongue, and the sternomastoid and trapezius muscles.

jactitation (jak″tĭ-ta'shun) restless tossing to and fro in acute illness.

jamais vu (zhah'ma voo) the sensation that familiar surroundings are strangely unfamiliar; the illusion that one has never seen anything like that before.

janiceps (jan'ĭ-seps) conjoined twins with a single head and faces on the anterior and posterior aspects.

Janský-Bielschowsky disease (yahn'ske byels-chov'ske) the late infantile form of neuronal ceroid lipofuscinosis, occurring between two to four years of age and characterized by abnormal accumulation of lipofuscin; it begins as myoclonic seizures and progresses to neurologic and retinal degeneration and death, usually by the age of 8 to 12 years.

Jarisch-Herxheimer reaction (yah'rish herks'hi-mer) a transient, short-term immunologic reaction commonly seen following antibiotic treatment of early and later stages of SYPHILIS and less often in other diseases, such as BORRELIOSIS, BRUCELLOSIS, TYPHOID FEVER, and TRICHINOSIS. Manifestations include fever, chills, headache, myalgias, and exacerbation of cutaneous lesions. The reaction has been attributed to liberation of ENDOTOXIN-like substances or ANTIGENS from the killed or dying microorganisms, but its exact pathogenesis is unclear.

jaundice (jawn'dis) yellowness of skin, sclerae, mucous membranes, and excretions due to hyperbilirubinemia and deposition of bile PIGMENTS. It is usually first noticeable in the eyes, although it may come on so gradually that it is not immediately noticed by those in daily contact with the jaundiced person. Called also icterus.

Jaundice is not a disease; it is a symptom of a number of different diseases and disorders of the LIVER and GALLBLADDER and of hemolytic blood disorders. One such disorder is the presence of a gallstone in the common bile duct, which carries bile from the liver to the intestine. This may obstruct the flow of bile, causing it to accumulate and enter the bloodstream. The obstruction of bile flow may cause bile to enter the urine, making it dark in color, and also decrease the bile in the stool, making it light and clay-colored. This condition requires surgery to remove the gallstone before it causes serious liver injury.

The pigment causing jaundice is called BILIRUBIN. It is derived from hemoglobin that

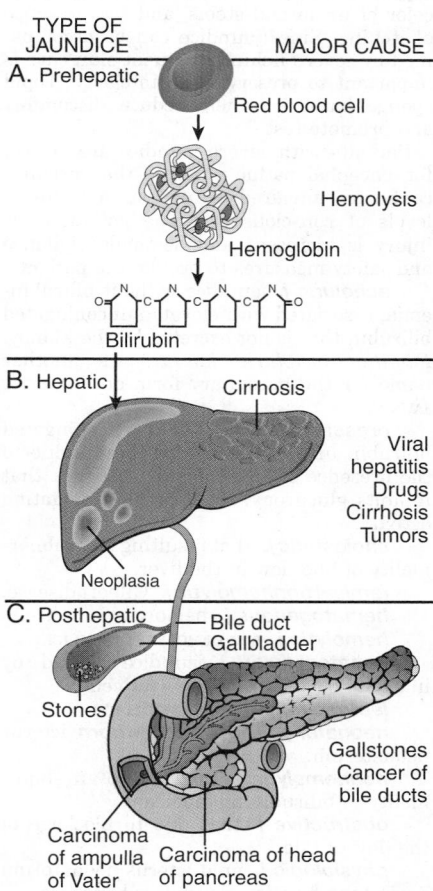

Jaundice may be attributable to prehepatic *(A)*, hepatic *(B)*, or posthepatic *(C)* causes. From Damjanov, 2000.

is released when erythrocytes are hemolyzed and therefore is constantly being formed and introduced into the blood as worn-out or defective erythrocytes are destroyed by the body. Normally the liver cells absorb the bilirubin and secrete it along with other bile constituents. If the liver is diseased, or if the flow of bile is obstructed, or if destruction of erythrocytes is excessive, the bilirubin accumulates in the blood and eventually will produce jaundice. Determination of the level of bilirubin in the blood is of value in detecting elevated bilirubin levels at the earliest stages before jaundice appears, when liver disease or hemolytic anemia is suspected.

Patient Care. Assessment of the patient with jaundice includes observations of the degree and location of yellowing, noting the color of urine and stools, and the presence of itching. Since jaundice can be accompanied by severe itching, frequent skin care is important to preserve skin integrity. Tepid sponge baths can help reduce discomfort and promote rest.

Patients with severe jaundice are at risk for encephalopathic changes that produce confusion, impaired mentation, and altered levels of consciousness. The potential for injury is increased and demands vigilance and safety measures to protect the patient.

acholuric j. jaundice without bilirubinemia, associated with elevated unconjugated bilirubin that is not excreted by the kidney. *Familial acholuric jaundice* is another name for the hereditary form of HEMOLYTIC JAUNDICE.

breast milk j. elevated unconjugated bilirubin in some breast-fed infants due to the presence of an abnormal PREGNANE that inhibits glucuronyl transferase conjugating activity.

cholestatic j. that resulting from abnormality of bile flow in the liver.

familial nonhemolytic j. Gilbert disease.

hematogenous j. hemolytic jaundice.

hemolytic j. see HEMOLYTIC JAUNDICE.

hepatocellular j. jaundice caused by injury to or disease of the liver cells.

leptospiral j. Weil's syndrome.

neonatal j., j. of the newborn icterus neonatorum.

nonhemolytic j. that due to an abnormality in bilirubin metabolism.

obstructive j. that due to blockage of the flow of bile.

physiologic j. mild icterus neonatorum during the first few days after birth.

jaw (jaw) either the MANDIBLE (lower jaw) or the MAXILLA (upper jaw), two opposing

CLASSIFICATION OF JAUNDICE

Category of Jaundice	Origin of the Problem	Type of Bilirubin Elevation
PREHEPATIC	Excessive hemolysis of erythrocytes Hemolytic jaundice	Indirect (unconjugated)
HEPATIC	Defect in transport or conjugation in hepatocytes Physiologic or neonatal jaundice	Indirect (unconjugated)
HEPATIC	Injury to or disease of hepatocytes Blockage of intrahepatic bile canaliculi Intrahepatic cholestasis	Direct (conjugated)
POSTHEPATIC	Blockage in the biliary ductal system Extrahepatic cholestasis	Direct (conjugated)

From Malarkey and McMorrow, 2000.

bony structures of the mouth of a vertebrate; they bear the teeth and are used for seizing prey, for biting, or for masticating food. See anatomic Table of Bones in the Appendices.

cleft j. a cleft between the median nasal and maxillary processes through the alveolus; see also CLEFT PALATE. Called also GNATHOSCHISIS.

Hapsburg j. a mandible that is PROGNATHOUS, often accompanied by Hapsburg LIP. See illustration.

phossy j. phosphonecrosis.

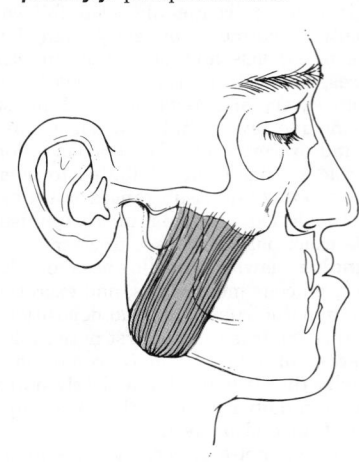

Hapsburg jaw with Hapsburg lip.

jaw-winking (jaw-wingk′ing) elevation of a congenitally ptotic eyelid when the mouth is opened, giving the appearance of constant winking.

JCAHO Joint Commission on the Accreditation of Healthcare Organizations.

jejunectomy (jĕ″joo-nek′to-me) excision of the jejunum.

jejunitis (jĕ″joo-ni′tis) inflammation of the jejunum.

jejunocecostomy (jĕ-joo″no-se-kos′tah-me) anastomosis of the jejunum to the cecum.

jejunocolostomy (jĕ-joo″no-kah-los′tah-me) anastomosis of the jejunum to the colon.

jejunoileal (je-joo″no-il′e-al) pertaining to the jejunum and ileum; connecting the proximal jejunum with the distal ileum.

jejunoileitis (jĕ-joo″no-il′e-i′tis) inflammation of the jejunum and ileum.

jejunoileostomy (jĕ-joo″no-il″e-os′tah-me) surgical creation of an anastomosis between the proximal jejunum and the terminal ileum; anastomosis of the jejunum to the ileum.

jejunojejunostomy (jĕ-joo″no-je″joo-nos′-tah-me) surgical anastomosis between two portions of the jejunum.

jejunorrhaphy (jĕ-joo-nor′ah-fe) operative repair of the jejunum.

jejunostomy (jĕ″joo-nos′tah-me) surgical creation of a permanent opening between the jejunum and the surface of the abdominal wall.

   needle-catheter j. insertion of a needle-catheter device to provide nutrition to patients undergoing major surgery of the esophagus, stomach, duodenum, pancreas, or hepatobiliary system. Since the small bowel regains normal motility and absorption capacity 8 to 12 hours postoperatively, this alternative method of feeding is an effective way to meet nutritional needs.

jejunotomy (jĕ″joo-not′ah-me) incision of the jejunum.

jejunum (jĕ-joo′num) that part of the small intestine extending from the duodenum to the ileum. adj., **jeju′nal.**

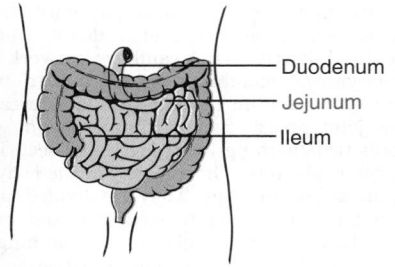

Jejunum. From Applegate, 2000.

jelly (jel′e) a soft, coherent, resilient substance; generally, a colloidal semisolid mass.

   cardiac j. a gelatinous substance present between the endothelium and myocardium of the embryonic heart that transforms into the connective tissue of the endocardium.

   contraceptive j. a nongreasy jelly containing a spermicide, used in the vagina for prevention of conception.

   petroleum j. petrolatum.

   Wharton's j. the soft, jelly-like intracellular substance of the umbilical cord.

Jenner (jen′er) Edward (1749–1823). English physician who discovered the principle of VACCINATION for SMALLPOX in 1796. By experimental demonstration, Jenner turned a local country tradition that dairymaids who had contracted cowpox did not acquire smallpox into a permanent working principle in science.

jennerian (jĕ-ne′re-an) relating to Edward Jenner, who developed smallpox vaccination.

jerk (jerk) a sudden reflex or involuntary movement.

   Achilles j., ankle j. plantar extension of the foot elicited by a tap on the ACHILLES TENDON, while the patient is seated on a bed or chair, with feet hanging freely; called also Achilles reflex and triceps surae jerk or reflex.

   biceps j. biceps reflex.

   elbow j. involuntary flexion of the elbow on striking the tendon of the biceps or triceps muscle.

   jaw j. jaw-jerk reflex.

   knee j. see KNEE JERK.

   tendon j. tendon reflex.

   triceps surae j. ankle jerk.

jet lag a condition of DESYNCHRONY with disruption of the normal circadian RHYTHM, caused by rapid travel across several time zones; it is characterized by fatigue, insomnia, and disturbances in body function, and lasts for several days.

Johnson (jon′son) Dorothy E. Nursing educator and developer of the BEHAVIORAL SYSTEM MODEL for nursing. Her chief interest has been in identifying the nature of service provided by nursing and in delineating the knowledge needed to provide that service.

joint (joint) the site of the junction or union of two or more bones of the body; its primary function is to provide motion and flexibility to the frame of the body. Some are immovable, such as the SUTURES where segments of bone are fused together in the skull. Others, such as those between the vertebrae, are *gliding joints* and have

J

limited motion. However, most joints allow considerable motion. The most common type are the *synovial joints*, which have a complex internal structure, composed not only of ends of bones but also of LIGAMENTS, CARTILAGE, the articular CAPSULE, the synovial MEMBRANE, and sometimes BURSAE.

acromioclavicular j. the point at which the clavicle joins with the acromion.

ankle j. the joint between the foot and the leg; see ANKLE.

arthrodial j. gliding joint.

ball-and-socket j. a synovial joint in which the rounded or spheroidal surface of one bone (the "ball") moves within a cup-shaped depression (the "socket") on another bone, allowing greater freedom of movement than any other type of joint. See illustration. Called also polyaxial or spheroidal joint.

bicondylar j. a condylar joint with a meniscus between the articular surfaces, as in the temporomandibular joint.

cartilaginous j. a type of SYNARTHROSIS in which the bones are united by cartilage, providing slight flexible movement; the two types are SYNCHONDROSIS and SYMPHYSIS.

composite j., compound j. a type of synovial joint in which more than two bones are involved.

condylar j., condyloid j. one in which an ovoid head of one bone moves in an elliptical cavity of another, permitting all movements except axial rotation; this type is found at the wrist, connecting the radius and carpal bones, and at the base of the index finger. See illustration.

diarthrodial j. synovial joint.

elbow j. the synovial joint between the HUMERUS, ULNA, and RADIUS. See also ELBOW.

ellipsoidal j. condylar joint.

facet j's the articulations of the vertebral column.

fibrous j. a joint in which the union of bony elements is by continuous intervening fibrous tissue, which makes little motion possible; the three types are SUTURE, SYNDESMOSIS, and GOMPHOSIS. Called also immovable or synarthrodial joint and synarthrosis.

flail j. an unusually mobile joint, such as results when joint resection is done to relieve pain.

glenohumeral j. the synovial joint formed by the head of the HUMERUS and the glenoid CAVITY of the SCAPULA. Called also humeral joint and shoulder joint.

gliding j. a synovial joint in which the opposed surfaces are flat or only slightly curved, so that the bones slide against each other in a simple and limited way. The intervertebral joints are this type, and many of the small bones of the wrist and ankle also meet in gliding joints. (See illustration.) Called also arthrodial joint and plane joint.

hinge j. a synovial joint that allows movement in only one plane, forward and backward. Examples are the elbow and the interphalangeal joints of the fingers. The jaw is primarily a hinge joint but it can also move somewhat from side to side. The knee and ankle joints are hinge joints that also allow some rotary movement. See illustration. Called also ginglymus.

hip j. the synovial joint formed at the head of the FEMUR and the ACETABULUM of the hip. See illustration at HIP.

humeral j. glenohumeral JOINT.

immovable j. fibrous j.

knee j. the compound joint between the FEMUR, PATELLA, and TIBIA.

pivot j. a synovial joint in which one bone pivots within a bony or an osseoligamentous ring, allowing only rotary movement; an example is the joint between the first and second cervical vertebrae (the atlas and axis). See illustration. Called also rotary or trochoid joint.

plane j. gliding joint.

polyaxial j. ball-and-socket joint.

rotary j. pivot joint.

sacroiliac j. the joint between the sacrum and ilium in the lower back; see also SACROILIAC JOINT.

saddle j. a synovial joint whose movement resembles that of a rider on horseback, who can shift in several directions at will; there is a saddle joint at the base of the thumb, so that the thumb is more flexible and complex than the other fingers but is also more difficult to treat if injured. (See illustration.)

shoulder j. humeral joint.

simple j. a type of synovial joint in which only two bones are involved.

spheroidal j. ball-and-socket joint.

synarthrodial j. fibrous j.

synovial j. a specialized joint that permits more or less free movement, the union of the bony elements being surrounded by an articular CAPSULE enclosing a cavity lined by synovial MEMBRANE. Called also articulation and diarthrosis. A capillary network in the synovial membrane provides nutrients and synovial fluid to nourish and lubricate the joint space. Strong fibrous bands or cords (LIGAMENTS) give strength and security to synovial joints. The majority of the body's joints are of this type. They are divided into five types according to structure and motion: ball and socket, gliding, saddle, hinge, and pivot. (See accompanying illustration.)

trochoid j. pivot joint.

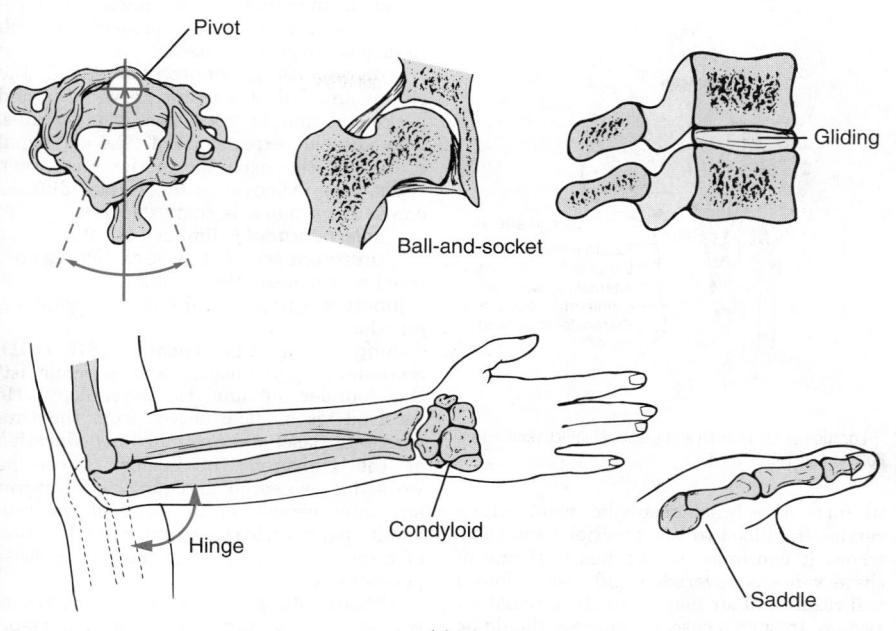

Pivot

Gliding

Ball-and-socket

Hinge

Condyloid

Saddle

Joints.

temporomandibular j. (TMJ) a bicondylar joint formed by the head of the MANDIBLE and the mandibular fossa, and the articular tubercle of the temporal BONE. See also TEMPOROMANDIBULAR JOINT DISORDER.

Joint Commission on the Accreditation of Healthcare Organizations (JCAHO) a private, nonprofit organization whose mission is to continuously improve the safety and quality of care provided to the public; it does this through the provision of health accreditation and related services that support performance improvement in health care organizations. JCAHO is governed by a 28-member Board of Commissioners that includes nurses, physicians, consumers, medical directors, administrators, providers, employers, labor representatives, health plan leaders, quality experts, ethicists, health insurance administrators, and educators. The corporate members of JCAHO are the American College of Physicians-American Society of Internal Medicine, the American College of Surgeons, the American Dental Association, the American Hospital Association, and the American Medical Association.

Jones-Mote reaction (jōnz mōt) a mild skin reaction of type IV delayed HYPERSENSITIVITY seen after challenge with a protein antigen in aqueous solution.

joule (J) (jōōl) the SI unit of energy, being the work done by a force of 1 newton acting over a distance of 1 meter.

judgment (juj'ment) the ability to make logical, rational decisions and decide whether a given action is right or wrong.

clinical j. the process by which the nurse decides on data to be collected about a client, makes an interpretation of the data, arrives at a NURSING DIAGNOSIS, and identifies appropriate nursing actions; this involves problem solving, decision making, and critical thinking.

jugal (joo'gal) 1. pertaining to the cheek. 2. zygomatic.

jugale (joo-ga'le) jugal point.

jugular (jug'u-lar) 1. cervical (def. 1). 2. pertaining to a JUGULAR VEIN. 3. a jugular vein.

j. veins large veins that return blood to the heart from the head and neck; each side of the neck has two jugular veins, external and internal. The external jugular carries blood from the face, neck, and scalp and has two branches, posterior and anterior. The internal jugular vein receives blood from the brain, the deeper tissues of the neck and the interior of the skull. The external jugular vein empties into the subclavian vein, and the internal jugular vein joins it

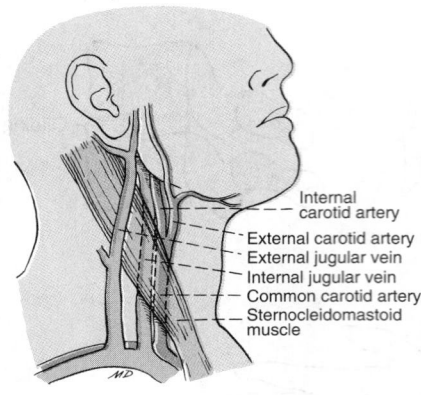

Location of the internal and external jugular veins. From Polaski and Tatro, 1996.

to form the brachiocephalic vein, which carries the blood to the superior vena cava, where it continues to the heart. If one of these veins is severed, rapid loss of blood will result and air may enter the circulatory system. In such a case, a compress should be applied to the wound with pressure. See anatomic Table of Veins in the Appendices and see color plates.

jugum (joo′gum) [L.] a depression or ridge connecting two structures; called also yoke.

j. pe′nis a forceps for compressing the penis.

juice (jōōs) any fluid from animal or plant tissue.

gastric j. see GASTRIC JUICE.

intestinal j. the liquid secretion of glands in the intestinal lining.

pancreatic j. the enzyme-containing secretion of the pancreas, conducted through its ducts to the duodenum.

prostatic j. the liquid secretion of the prostate, which contributes to semen formation.

junction (jungk′shun) a place of meeting or coming together. adj., **junc′tional.**

atrioventricular j. in the conduction system of the heart, the junction between the atrioventricular node and the non-branching portion of the bundle of His.

cementoenamel j. the line at which the cementum covering the root of a tooth meets the enamel covering the crown.

gap j. a narrowed portion of the intercellular space, containing channels linking adjacent cells and through which can pass ions, most sugars, amino acids, nucleotides, vitamins, hormones, and cyclic AMP. In electrically excitable tissues the gap junctions serve to transmit electrical impulses via ionic currents and are known as electrotonic SYNAPSES; they are present in such tissues as myocardial tissue.

myoneural j., neuromuscular j. the site of junction of a motor nerve FIBER and a skeletal muscle FIBER that it innervates. The discoid expansion of the terminal branch of the axon forms the motor END PLATE, the NEUROTRANSMITTER that diffuses across the synapse is ACETYLCHOLINE.

sclerocorneal j. limbus (def. 2).

ureteropelvic j. the area where the renal PELVIS meets the URETER.

junctura (jungk-tu′rah) [L.] 1. joint. 2. junction.

Jung (yoong) Carl Gustav (1875–1961). Swiss-born psychologist and psychiatrist; the founder of analytic psychology. He received his medical degree from the University of Basel and continued his education at the University of Zurich, where he worked as research assistant and lecturer and later served on the staff of the university psychiatric clinic under the direction of Eugen Bleuler, another important Swiss psychologist.

Although Jung corresponded with FREUD, who at first saw him as a possible successor, their relationship was short-lived, primarily because of Jung's rejection of Freud's concept of the LIBIDO. It is perhaps their differing concepts of the unconscious mental life that distinguishes freudian and jungian psychology the most. In regard to technique, analytical psychotherapy as formulated by Jung attaches more importance to an analysis and interpretation of certain aspects of the subject's dreams and fantasies and far less emphasis on free association than does freudian psychoanalysis.

Jung's view of the dynamics of personality represents an attempt to interpret human behavior from a philosophic, religious, and mystical, as well as scientific, viewpoint. Many of his concepts deal with disciplines and phenomena outside the field of psychology. Among these is the notion of a "collective unconscious," which is said to permeate each "personal unconscious" psyche and which enters consciousness only in symbolic form to indirectly influence thought and behavior. The whole personality (psyche) consists of these three interacting systems: the collective unconscious, the personal unconscious, and the conscious mind (ego).

The *ego* is the center of the conscious; it comprises the conscious perceptions, thoughts, and feelings, and is the focal point for individual identity. It stands between the inner and outer world and permits the individual to adapt to the environment. Much of the psychic activity within an individual involves the ego's interaction with internal and external reality.

The *personal unconscious* consists of the individual's experiences, wishes, and impulses, which were once conscious but have been repressed or forgotten, but can be brought to consciousness once again.

The *collective unconscious* is the most influential of the psychic systems. It is distinguished from the personal unconscious by images and symbols that do not originate in the personal acquisitions of an individual's life. The collective unconscious operates wholly without the conscious awareness of the individual. Whereas the personal unconscious has to do with an individual's personal history and experiences, the collective unconscious is that part of the psyche which retains and transmits the cumulative experience of all previous generations. The structural components of the collective unconscious are the ARCHETYPES, the universal patterns of behavior, inherited dispositions that dispose an individual to experience and behave in eternally recurrent situations (birth, death, marriage, war, religious customs, initiations, and so on) similarly to how the ancestors in that culture experienced and behaved in them. Archetypes are displayed in patterns and images that are the subject matter of dreams and visions and in mythology, legends, religion, fairy tales, and art.

The primary archetype from which all others come is the *self,* the organizing center from which all the regulatory forces of the psyche emanate. It is responsible for the integration and stability of personality, the hidden tendency directing the process of psychic growth. The self is central to jungian personality theory and is expressed in the innate striving of each person toward psychic wholeness, a process Jung calls INDIVIDUATION, or the striving for self-realization. Jung viewed neurosis as a disturbance of the process of individuation; hence, his analytical therapy aims at a restoration of the process of self-realization.

In Jung's 1921 work *Psychological Types,* he proposed personality *types* (INTROVERSION and EXTRAVERSION) and the four mental processes or *functions* of thinking, feeling, sensation, and intuition. The extraverted personality type is described by Jung as one whose philosophy of life is markedly collective and based only on what others say and do. Psychic energy (LIBIDO) is directed

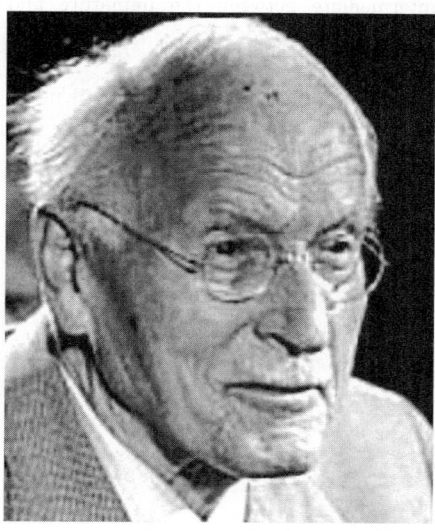
Carl G. Jung.

toward external happenings. The introverted personality type is characterized by an inward turning of libido, a focusing of interest on the subjective, inner aspects of life. There are many degrees of extraversion and introversion and pure types are rare. The four functions are seen as the natural aspects of conscious orientation: the means by which one gets one's bearings in the midst of an abundance of impressions from the environment.

jurisprudence (jōōr″is-proo′dens) the science of the law.

  medical j. the science of the law as applied to the practice of medicine; see also forensic MEDICINE.

justice (jus′tis) a principle of BIOETHICS that means giving others what is due to them; it is comprised of a group of norms for the fair distribution of benefits, risks, and costs. The terms *fairness, desert,* and *entitlement* have been used by philosophers to explicate the idea of justice, while *equitability* and *appropriateness of treatment* are used in interpretations. A situation involving justice is present whenever persons are due to receive benefits or burdens because of their particular circumstances. Justice may be *distributive, criminal* or *punitive,* or *rectificatory.*

juvenile (ju′vĕ-nīl) 1. pertaining to youth or childhood; young or immature. 2. a youth or child; a young animal; a cell or organism intermediate between the immature and mature forms.

juxta- word element [L.], *situated near; adjoining.*

juxta-articular (juks″tah-ahr-tik′u-lar) periarticular.

juxtaglomerular (juks″tah-glo-mer′u-lar) near to or adjoining a glomerulus of the kidney.

juxtaposition (juks″tah-po-zish′un) apposition; a placing side by side or close together; the condition of being side by side or close together.

juxtapyloric (juks″tah-pi-lor′ik) peripyloric.

juxtaspinal (juks″tah-spi′nal) paravertebral.

juxtavesical (juks″tah-ves′ĭ-kal) perivesical.

K

K kelvin; potassium (L. *ka'lium*).

k kilo-.

kak(o)- for words beginning thus, see those beginning CAC(O)-.

kakosmia (kak-oz'me-ah) cacosmia.

kala-azar (kah″lah-ah-zahr′) visceral leishmaniasis.

kalemia (kah-le'me-ah) the presence of potassium in the blood; see also HYPERKALEMIA.

kaliemia (ka″le-e'me-ah) kalemia.

kaliuresis (ka″le-u-re'sis) excretion of POTASSIUM in the urine.

kaliuretic (ka″le-u-ret'ik) 1. promoting KALIURESIS. 2. an agent that so acts.

kallidin (kal'ĭ-din) lysyl-bradykinin, a kinin produced by the action of tissue and glandular kallikreins on low-molecular-weight kininogen and having physiologic effects similar to those of bradykinin. Formerly, the term was applied to several different peptides: BRADYKININ was called kallidin I or 9 and lysyl-bradykinin was called kallidin II or 10.

kallikrein (kal″ĭ-kre'in) any of several serine ENDOPEPTIDASES that cleave kininogens to form kinins.

plasma k. a hydrolytic enzyme of the plasma that cleaves HMW (high-molecular-weight) KININOGEN to produce BRADYKININ. It also activates several blood coagulation factors and PLASMINOGEN. It is formed from PREKALLIKREIN by activated coagulation factor XII.

tissue k. a hydrolytic enzyme that cleaves LMW kininogen to produce kallidin. It and closely related forms are found in tissues and various glandular secretions such as lymph, pancreatic juice, urine, and saliva.

kallikreinogen (kal″ĭ-kre-in'ah-jen) prekallikrein.

Kallmann syndrome (kahl'mahn) a type of hypogonadotropic HYPOGONADISM caused by failure of fetal gonadotropin-releasing hormone neurons to migrate to the thalamus, usually associated with ANOSMIA or HYPOSMIA. It is usually passed by autosomal recessive inheritance, and some cases are x-linked.

kanamycin (kan″ah-mi'sin) a broad-spectrum aminoglycoside ANTIBIOTIC derived from *Streptomyces kanamyceticus;* effective against many gram-negative bacteria, and some gram-positive bacteria, including mycobacteria; used as the sulfate salt, administered orally, parenterally, or by inhalation.

Kantrex (kan'treks) trademark for preparations of KANAMYCIN, an ANTIBIOTIC.

kaolin (ka'o-lin) native hydrated ALUMINUM SILICATE, powdered and freed from gritty particles by elutriation; used as an adsorbent and, often with pectin, an antidiarrheal.

kaolinosis (ka″o-lin-o'sis) a type of SILICATOSIS due to inhaling particles of kaolin.

karaya gum (kar'a-ah) the dried gummy exudation from *Sterculia urens* or other species of *Sterculia,* which becomes gelatinous when moisture is added; used as a bulk CATHARTIC and dental adhesive. It is available in rings that can be molded into any desired shape. Products containing karaya gum are often used as protective skin barriers in the care of COLOSTOMY and other conditions in which there is a STOMA. Called also sterculia gum.

Kartagener's syndrome (kahr-tag′ĕ-nerz) a hereditary syndrome consisting of dextrocardia, bronchiectasis, and sinusitis.

kary(o)- word element [Gr.], *nucleus.*

karyocyte (kar'e-o-sīt″) a nucleated cell.

karyogenesis (kar″e-o-jen'ĕ-sis) the formation of a cell nucleus. adj., **karyogen'ic.**

karyokinesis (kar″e-o-ki-ne'sis) division of the nucleus, usually an early stage in the process of cell division, or mitosis. adj., **karyokinet'ic.**

karyolymph (kar'e-o-limf″) the fluid portion of the nucleus of a cell, in which the other elements are dispersed.

karyolysis (kar″e-ol'ĭ-sis) the dissolution of the nucleus of a cell. adj., **karyolyt'ic.**

karyomegaly (kar″e-o-meg'ah-le) abnormal enlargement of the nucleus of a cell.

karyomorphism (kar″e-o-mor'fizm) the shape of a cell nucleus.

karyophage (kar'e-o-fāj″) a protozoon that phagocytizes the nucleus of the cell it infects.

karyopyknosis (kar″e-o-pik-no'sis) shrinkage of a cell nucleus, with condensation of the chromatin. adj., **karyopyknot'ic.**

karyorrhexis (kar″e-o-rek'sis) rupture of the cell nucleus in which the chromatin disintegrates into formless granules that are extruded from the cell. adj., **karyorrhec'tic.**

karyotheca (kar″e-o-the'kah) the nuclear membrane.

karyotype (kar'e-o-tīp) the chromosomal constitution of the cell nucleus; by extension, the photomicrograph of chromosomes arranged. See also illustration at CHROMOSOME.

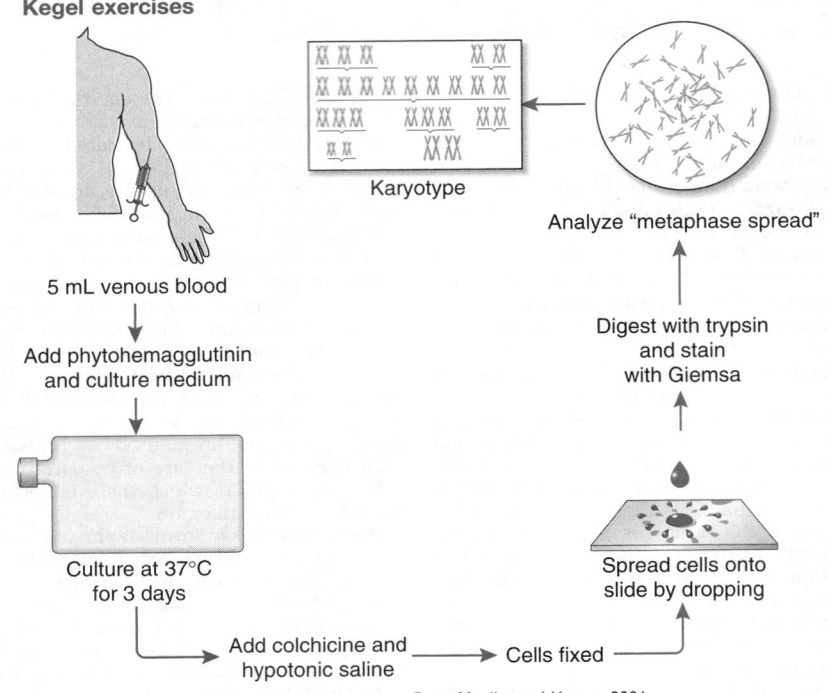

Karyotype

Analyze "metaphase spread"

5 mL venous blood

Add phytohemagglutinin
and culture medium

Digest with trypsin
and stain
with Giemsa

Culture at 37°C
for 3 days

Spread cells onto
slide by dropping

Add colchicine and ——→ Cells fixed ——
hypotonic saline

Preparation of a karyotype. From Mueller and Young, 2001.

Kashin-Beck disease (kah′shĕn bek) a disabling degenerative disease of the peripheral joints and spine, endemic in eastern Siberia, northern China, and Korea; believed to be caused by ingestion of cereal grains infected with the fungus *Fusarium sporotrichiella.*

kat katal.

kat(a)- word element [Gr.], *down; against.* See also words beginning CAT(A)-.

katal (kat′al) a unit of measurement proposed to express activities of all catalysts, including enzymes, being that amount of a catalyst that catalyzes a reaction rate of 1 mole of substrate per second. Symbol kat.

katathermometer (kat″ah-ther-mom′ĕ-ter) a thermometer with a wet bulb and a dry bulb, for detecting cooling rates.

Katayama fever acute systemic SCHISTOSOMIASIS causing a distinct serum sickness–like syndrome, usually associated with heavy infection by *Schistosoma japonicum,* characterized by fever, chills, nausea and vomiting, cough, headache, urticaria, hepatosplenomegaly, lymphadenopathy, marked eosinophilia, and usually increased levels of IgE and IgG. It was first reported from the Katayama River Valley in Japan.

Kawasaki disease (kah″wah-sah′ke) an illness of unknown etiology affecting primarily children, and characterized by high fever, polymorphous rash, cervical lymph node swelling, and pain. Treatment is largely supportive; corticosteroids are contraindicated. Death may occur as a result of cardiomyopathy and vasculitis. Called also mucocutaneous lymph node syndrome.

kcal kilocalorie.

Keflex (kef′lex) trademark for preparations of CEPHALEXIN, an oral CEPHALOSPORIN ANTIBIOTIC.

Kegel exercises (ka′gul) specific exercises named after Dr. Arnold H. Kegel, a gynecologist who first developed the exercises to strengthen the pelvic-vaginal muscles as a means of controlling stress INCONTINENCE in women. He later learned from patients who had been performing the exercises that strengthening of the pubococcygeus muscle, a sphincteric muscle that surrounds the vagina, also improved feminine sexual response and contributed to the attainment of orgasm. Research has since demonstrated that this muscle contains specialized nerve endings which contribute to a satisfactory sexual experience.

A third area in which the Kegel exercises are important is in pregnancy and childbirth. The exercises strengthen the pelvic floor and therefore are helpful in reducing discomfort and congestion during pregnancy and in providing support for the pelvic organs before and after birth. During delivery the mother who has developed good tone and conscious control over the pubococcygeus muscle is able to release the muscle and thereby facilitate the passage of the infant through the birth canal. After delivery the exercises maintain the strength of the muscle and greatly diminish the possibility of RECTOCELE and CYSTOCELE, DYSPAREUNIA, and other aftereffects of delivery.

Most patients must be taught an awareness of the muscle and how to control it. This usually can be done by having the woman shut off urine flow while sitting on the commode. After a few trials the sensation of control is recognized and the patient is able to perform the exercise on her own. Usually the exercises are begun with five or ten contractions before arising in the morning and also during each voiding of urine. Gradually the number of sessions and the number of contractions are increased until ultimately a pattern of three hundred daily contractions is reached. The exercises require concentration but a small expenditure of energy. Once the muscle has been strengthened it tends to maintain its strength and state of partial contraction at all times. Sexual activity helps preserve the muscle tone.

Keith-Wagener-Barker classification (kēth wag'ĕ-ner bahr'ker) a classification of hypertension and arteriolosclerosis based on retinal changes.

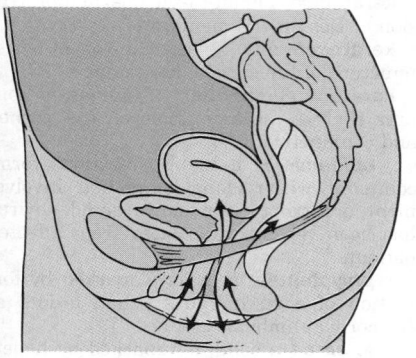

Contraction and release of the pubococcygeus muscle (Kegel exercises) can improve muscle tone, thereby providing better support to the pelvic organs. From Nichols and Zwelling, 1997.

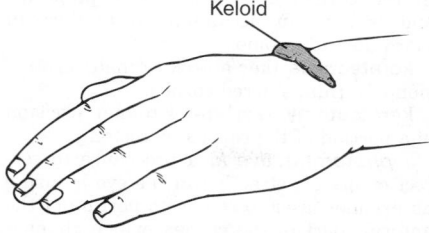

Keloid. From Dorland's, 2000.

keloid (ke'loid) a sharply elevated, irregularly shaped, progressively enlarging scar, due to excessive collagen formation in the corium during connective tissue repair. It is a benign tumor that usually has its origin in a scar from surgery or a burn or other injury; keloids are generally considered harmless and noncancerous, although they may produce contractures or cosmetic alterations that affect body image. Ordinarily they cause no trouble beyond an occasional itching sensation. Surgical removal is not usually effective because it results in a high rate of recurrence. However, intralesional injection of steroids, cryotherapy, and x-ray therapy often are of substantial help. When x-ray therapy is employed, care must be taken not to destroy the surrounding healthy tissue. adj., **keloid'al.**

kelvin (K) (kel'vin) the base SI unit of temperature, equal to 1/273.16 of the absolute temperature of the triple point of water.

Kemadrin (kem'ah-drin) trademark for a preparation of PROCYCLIDINE hydrochloride, used as an ANTIDYSKINETIC.

Kenalog (ken'ah-log) trademark for preparations of TRIAMCINOLONE acetonide, an ANTIINFLAMMATORY glucocorticoid.

Kepone (ke'pōn) trademark for a polychlorinated ketone used as an insecticide; workers exposed to this nonbiodegradable compound have suffered neurologic symptoms, such as tremors and slurred speech.

kerasin (ker'ah-sin) a cerebroside from brain tissue, yielding galactose, sphingosine, and lignoceric acid on hydrolysis.

kerat(o)- word element [Gr.], *horny tissue; cornea.*

keratalgia (ker″ah-tal'jah) pain in the cornea.

keratan sulfate (ker'ah-tan) either of two sulfated mucopolysaccharides (I and II). Keratan sulfate is an important component of the proteoglycan of cartilage, and occurs

K

in the cornea and the nucleus pulposus, and is also an accumulation product in Morquio's syndrome.

keratectasia (ker″ah-tek-ta′zhah) protrusion of a thin, scarred cornea.

keratectomy (ker″ah-tek′to-me) excision of a portion of the cornea; kerectomy.

　photorefractive k. a procedure to correct errors of refraction in the eye by using an excimer laser to remove a portion of the anterior part of the cornea, which changes the refraction by creating a new radius of curvature.

keratic (kĕ-rat′ik) 1. keratinous. 2. corneal.

keratin (ker′ah-tin) a scleroprotein that is the principal constituent of epidermis, hair, nails, horny tissues, and the organic matrix of the enamel of the teeth. Its solution is sometimes used in coating pills when the latter are desired to pass through the stomach unchanged.

keratinase (ker′ah-tin-ās″) a proteolytic enzyme that hydrolyzes keratin.

keratinization (ker″ah-tin″ĭ-za′shun) the development of or conversion into keratin.

keratinocyte (kĕ-rat′ĭ-no-sīt″) the cell of the epidermis that synthesizes keratin, known in its successive stages in the various layers of the skin as basal cell, prickle cell, and granular cell.

keratinosome one of the spherical granules formed near the Golgi apparatus in the skin, migrating to the cytoplasm and discharging its contents into the intercellular space, where the granules are believed to function as a barrier to penetration by foreign substances. Called also lamellar body or granule.

keratinous (kĕ-rat′ĭ-nus) containing KERATIN or of the nature of keratin; called also keratic.

keratitis (ker″ah-ti′tis) inflammation of the CORNEA. It may be deep, when the infection causing it is carried in the blood or spreads to the cornea from other parts of the eye, or superficial, caused by bacterial or viral infection or by allergic reaction. Agents causing the inflammation can be introduced into the cornea during the removal of foreign bodies from the eye. All infections of the eye are potentially serious because opaque fibrous tissue or scar tissue may form on the cornea during the healing process and cause partial or total loss of vision. See also KERATOCONJUNCTIVITIS.

　Causes. There are several kinds of keratitis. *Dendritic keratitis* is a viral form caused by the herpes simplex virus; it usually affects only one eye. *Acute serpiginous keratitis* is a bacterial form that may result from infection by pneumococci, streptococci, or staphylococci. *Dendritic keratitis* and certain other kinds may follow symptoms of upper respiratory tract infection, such as fever. Burns of the cornea, such as those produced by chemicals or ULTRAVIOLET RAYS, can also cause keratitis. In TRACHOMA, a contagious disease of the conjunctiva, the eyes become inflamed, and small, gritty particles develop on the cornea. *Herpetic keratitis* may accompany HERPES ZOSTER. *Interstitial keratitis* is a type usually caused by congenital SYPHILIS, appearing in children between ages 5 and 15; occasionally it may result from acquired syphilis. In rare cases it may result from tuberculosis or rheumatic infection in other parts of the body.

　Symptoms. Symptoms vary somewhat among the different forms of keratitis, but pain, which may be severe, and PHOTOPHOBIA (inability to tolerate light) are usual. There may also be considerable effusion of tears and a conjunctival discharge.

　Treatment. Antibiotics are the usual treatment for keratitis caused by an infectious organism. CORTISONE is used for other forms, but may be dangerous in some patients. Antiviral agents such as IDOXURIDINE have been used to treat herpes simplex (dendritic) keratitis. In cases of syphilitic interstitial keratitis, the syphilis is treated. Congenital interstitial keratitis can be prevented if syphilis is detected early in pregnancy by means of blood tests and the mother is treated.

keratoacanthoma (ker″ah-to-ak″an-tho′mah) a rapidly growing, benign papular lesion, with a superficial crater filled with a keratin plug, usually on the face; it resolves spontaneously.

keratocele (ker′ah-to-sēl″) hernial protrusion of Descemet's membrane.

keratocentesis (ker′ah-to-sen-te′sis) puncture of the cornea, keratonyxis.

keratoconjunctivitis (ker″ah-to-konjunk″tĭ-vi′tis) inflammation of the cornea and conjunctiva.

　epidemic k. a highly infectious form, commonly with regional lymph node involvement, occurring in epidemics; an adenovirus has been repeatedly isolated from affected patients.

　phlyctenular k. a form marked by formation of a PHLYCTENULE (small lesion) at the corneal limbus.

　k. sic′ca a condition marked by hyperemia of the conjunctiva, thickening and drying of the corneal epithelium, and itching and burning of the eye. Called also dry eye.

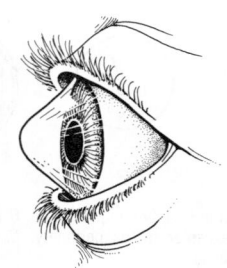

Keratoconus. From Dorland's, 2000.

keratoconus (ker″ah-to-ko′nus) conical protrusion of the central part of the cornea, resulting in an irregular astigmatism.

keratoderma (ker″ah-to-der′mah) hypertrophy of the horny layer of the skin.

    k. blennorrha′gicum a cutaneous manifestation of REITER'S DISEASE, most often involving the palms, soles, toes, and glans penis, and characterized by development of thick keratotic coverings; the lesions resemble those of pustular psoriasis. The disorder was formerly thought to be associated with gonorrhea.

    k. climacte′ricum an acquired form of keratoderma that affects the palms of the hands and soles of the feet; it occurs in women about the time of menopause and may be associated with fissuring of the thickened patches.

    palmoplantar k. a group of mostly inherited disorders characterized by the excessive formation of keratin, localized or diffuse, on the palms and soles, sometimes with painful lesions resulting from fissuring of the skin; it may occur alone or may accompany or be part of another disease.

keratodermia (ker″ah-to-der′me-ah) keratoderma.

keratogenous (ker″ah-toj′ĕ-nus) giving rise to a growth of horny material.

keratoglobus (ker″ah-to-glo′bus) megalocornea.

keratohelcosis (ker″ah-to-hel-ko′sis) ulceration of the cornea.

keratohemia (ker″ah-to-he′me-ah) deposition of blood in the cornea.

keratohyalin (ker″ah-to-hi′ah-lin) the substance in the granules in the stratum granulosum of the epidermis. adj., **keratohy′aline.**

keratoid (ker′ah-toid) resembling horn or corneal tissue.

keratoiridoscope (ker″ah-to-ĭ-rid′o-skōp) a compound microscope for examining the cornea and iris.

keratoiritis (ker″ah-to-i-ri′tis) inflammation of the cornea and iris; corneoiritis.

keratoleptynsis (ker″ah-to-lep-tin′sis) removal of the anterior portion of the cornea and replacement with bulbar conjunctiva.

keratoleukoma (ker″ah-to-loo-ko′mah) a white opacity of the cornea.

keratolysis (ker″ah-tol′ĭ-sis) loosening or separation of the horny layer of the epidermis.

    pitted k., k. planta′re sulca′tum a tropical disease marked by thickening and deep fissuring of the skin of the soles, occurring during the rainy season.

keratolytic (ker″ah-to-lit′ik) 1. pertaining to or promoting KERATOLYSIS. 2. an agent that so acts.

keratoma (ker″ah-to′mah), pl. *keratomas, keratoma′ta* [Gr.] a callus or callosity.

    k. heredita′rium mu′tilans an autosomal dominant, progressive, dystrophic form of palmoplantar KERATODERMA beginning in childhood, sometimes associated with scarring alopecia and deafness.

keratomalacia (ker″ah-to-mah-la′she-ah) softening and necrosis of the cornea associated with vitamin A deficiency.

keratome (ker′ah-tōm) a knife for incising the cornea.

keratometer (ker″ah-tom′ĕ-ter) an instrument for measuring the curves of the cornea.

keratometry (ker″ah-tom′ĕ-tre) measurement of the anterior curvature of the cornea with a keratometer.

keratomileusis (ker″ah-to-mĭ-loo′sis) keratoplasty in which a slice of the patient's cornea is removed, shaped to the desired curvature, and then sutured back on the remaining cornea to correct optical error.

    ***laser-assisted in-situ k.* (LASIK)** keratoplasty in which the excimer laser and microkeratome are combined for vision correction; the microkeratome is used to shave a thin slice and create a hinged flap in the cornea, the flap is reflected back, the exposed cornea is reshaped by the laser, and the flap is replaced, without sutures, to heal back into position.

keratomycosis (ker″ah-to-mi-ko′sis) fungal disease of the cornea.

keratonyxis (ker″ah-to-nik′sis) puncture of the cornea; keratocentesis.

keratopathy (ker″ah-top′ah-the) noninflammatory disease of the cornea.

    band k. a condition characterized by an abnormal gray circumcorneal band.

keratophakia (ker″ah-to-fa′ke-ah) keratoplasty in which a slice of donor's cornea is shaped to a desired curvature and inserted between layers of the recipient's cornea to change its curvature.

keratoplasty (ker'ah-to-plas"te) CORNEAL TRANSPLANTATION.

optic k. transplantation of corneal material to replace scar tissue that interferes with vision.

refractive k. removal of a section of cornea from a patient or donor, which is shaped to the desired curvature and inserted either between layers of the recipient's cornea (KERATOPHAKIA) or over the cornea (KERATOMILEUSIS) in order to change the corneal curvature and correct optical errors.

tectonic k. transplantation of corneal material to replace tissue that has been lost.

keratorhexis (ker"ah-to-rek'sis) rupture of the cornea.

keratorrhexis (ker"ah-to-rek'sis) keratorhexis.

keratoscleritis (ker"ah-to-sklĕ-ri'tis) inflammation of cornea and sclera.

keratoscope (ker'ah-to-skōp") a device consisting of alternate black and white concentric circles and used for examining corneal curvature.

keratoscopy (ker"ah-tos'kah-pe) inspection of the cornea.

keratosis (ker"ah-to'sis) any horny growth, such as a wart or callosity.

actinic k. a sharply outlined wartlike or keratotic growth, which may develop into a cutaneous horn, and may become malignant; it usually occurs in the middle aged or elderly and is due to excessive exposure to the sun. Called also senile or solar keratosis. (See Atlas 3, Part F).

k. follicula'ris a slowly progressive autosomal dominant disorder of KERATINIZATION characterized by pinkish to tan or skin-colored papules on the seborrheic areas of the body that coalesce to form plaques, which may become crusted and secondarily infected; over time, the lesions may become darker and may fuse to form papillomatous and warty malodorous growths. Called also Darier's disease and Darier-White disease.

k. palma'ris et planta'ris palmoplantar keratoderma.

k. pharyn'gea horny projections from the tonsils and pharyngeal walls. Called also pharyngokeratosis.

k. pila'ris HYPERKERATOSIS limited to the hair follicles.

k. puncta'ta a hereditary HYPERKERATOSIS in which the lesions are localized in multiple points on the palms and soles.

seborrheic k., k. seborrhe'ica a benign, noninvasive tumor of epidermal origin, marked by numerous yellow or brown, sharply marginated, oval, raised lesions.

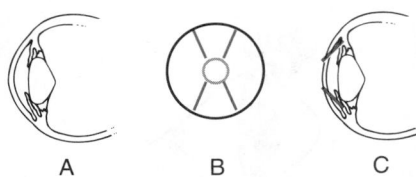

Radial keratotomy. *A*, Before procedure. *B*, Incisions are made from the center to the periphery. *C*, The corneal contour is flattened.

senile k., solar k. actinic keratosis.

keratotomy (ker"ah-tot'ah-me) incision of the cornea.

radial k. an operation in which a series of incisions is made in the cornea from its outer edge toward its center in a spokelike fashion; done to flatten the cornea and thus to correct myopia.

kerectomy (kĕ-rek'to-me) keratectomy.

kerion (ke're-on) a boggy, exudative swelling or mass covered with pustules, as may occasionally occur in TINEA infections.

kernicterus (ker-nik'ter-us) a condition in the newborn marked by severe neural symptoms, associated with high levels of bilirubin in the blood; it is commonly a sequela of icterus gravis neonatorum.

Kernig's sign (ker'nigz) in the supine position the patient can easily and completely extend the leg; in the sitting posture or when lying with the thigh flexed upon the abdomen the leg cannot be completely extended; it is a sign of meningitis.

ket(o)- word element, *ketone group.*

ketamine (ke'tah-mēn) a nonbarbiturate anesthetic related to PHENCYCLIDINE, administered intravenously or intramuscularly to produce dissociative anesthesia. Approximately 12 per cent of patients experience emergence reactions, which can include frightening hallucinations and dreams.

keto acid (ke'to) a carboxylic acid that also contains a carbonyl (CO) group.

ketoacidosis (ke"to-as"ĭ-do'sis) the accumulation of ketone bodies in the blood, which results in metabolic ACIDOSIS; it is

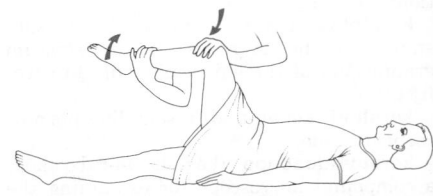

Kernig's sign, which indicates meningitis. Flexion of the hip and knee causes pain. From Ignatavicius and Workman, 2002.

ketoaciduria (ke″to-as″ĭ-du′re-ah) the presence of ketone bodies in the urine; this condition is common in uncontrolled DIABETES MELLITUS but can also occur anytime the body begins to break down fatty tissue to provide energy, as in starvation. Called also ketonuria.

branched-chain k. maple syrup urine disease.

ketoconazole (ke″to-kon′ah-zōl) a synthetic IMIDAZOLE that is a broad-spectrum antifungal AGENT used for treatment of chronic mucocutaneous candidiasis and systemic fungal infections due to species of *Candida, Epidermophyton, Microsporum, Trichophyton,* and others.

Keto-Diastix trademark for a reagent strip for detection of KETONES and GLUCOSE in the urine.

ketogenesis (ke″to-jen′ĕ-sis) the production of ketone bodies. adj., **ketogen′ic, ketogenet′ic.**

ketogenic (ke″to-jen′ik) forming or capable of being converted into ketone bodies.

α-ketoglutarate (ke″to-gloo′tah-rāt) a salt or anion or α-ketoglutaric acid.

α-ketoglutaric acid (ke″to-gloo′tar-ik) a metabolic intermediate involved in the tricarboxylic acid CYCLE, in amino acid metabolism, and as an amino group acceptor in TRANSAMINATION reactions.

ketolysis (ke-tol′ĭ-sis) the splitting up of ketone bodies. adj., **ketolyt′ic.**

ketone (ke′tōn) any compound containing the carbonyl group, $C=O$, and having hydrocarbon groups attached to the carbonyl carbon, i.e., the carbonyl group is within a chain of carbon atoms.

k. bodies the substances ACETONE, ACETOACETIC ACID, and β-HYDROXYBUTYRIC ACID; except for acetone (which may arise spontaneously from acetoacetic acid), they are normal metabolic products of lipid and pyruvate within the liver, and are oxidized by muscles. Excessive production leads to urinary excretion of these bodies, as in diabetes mellitus; see also KETOSIS. Called also acetone bodies.

ketonemia (ke″to-ne′me-ah) an excess of ketone bodies in the blood.

ketonuria (ke″to-nu′re-ah) ketoaciduria.

ketoprofen (ke″to-pro′fen) a NONSTEROIDAL ANTIINFLAMMATORY DRUG used in the treatment of various rheumatic and nonrheumatic inflammatory disorders, pain, dysmenorrhea, and vascular headaches; administered orally or rectally.

ketorolac (ke″to-ro′lak) a NONSTEROIDAL ANTIINFLAMMATORY DRUG available as the tromethamine salt; used systemically for short-term management of pain; also applied topically to the conjunctiva in the treatment of allergic conjunctivitis and of ocular inflammation following cataract surgery.

ketose (ke′tōs) one of the two main types of MONOSACCHARIDE sugars; those that contain a ketone group, such as FRUCTOSE.

ketosis (ke-to′sis) accumulation in the blood and tissues of large quantities of the KETONE BODIES: beta-hydroxybutyric acid, acetoacetic acid, and acetone. Because the first two are acids, this results in metabolic ACIDOSIS. Thus, the condition is often referred to as KETOACIDOSIS. adj., **ketot′ic.** When fatty acids are metabolized in the liver, an intermediate, acetylcoenzyme A (acetyl CoA), is produced. Normally, acetyl CoA is condensed with oxaloacetic acid, a product of carbohydrate metabolism, to form citric acid. This then enters the tricarboxylic acid CYCLE, the final common pathway of cellular energy metabolism.

When oxaloacetate is not present, acetyl CoA is converted by another pathway to ketone bodies. These compounds cannot be metabolized by the liver and are released into the blood stream. Other tissues, including muscle, brain, heart, and kidneys, can convert ketone bodies back to acetyl CoA and metabolize them as an energy source.

In acute starvation or in uncontrolled DIABETES MELLITUS, there is a great increase in fatty acid metabolism and impaired or absent carbohydrate metabolism, which results in a greatly increased production of ketone bodies. This can also occur when the diet is composed almost entirely of fat. The production of ketone bodies is reduced to the normal low level and the ketoacidosis is reversed when adequate carbohydrate metabolism is restored.

The patient with ketosis often has a sweet or "fruity" odor to his breath. This is produced by acetone, a ketone body that is highly volatile and is blown off in small amounts with air exhaled from the lungs.

K

CLINICAL SYMPTOMS ASSOCIATED WITH KETOSIS
Polyuria
Thirst
Depressed eyeballs
Fruity or acetone odor of breath
Kussmaul's respirations
Complaints of nausea
Vomiting
Stupor or coma (late sign)

ketosteroid (ke″to-ste′roid) a steroid having ketone groups on functional carbon atoms.

17-k's steroids found in normal urine and in excess in certain tumors, which have a ketone group on the 17th carbon atom, and include certain androgenic and adrenocortical hormones.

Ketostix (ke′to-stiks) trademark for a reagent strip for detection of KETONE BODIES in the urine.

ketotifen (ke″to-ti′fen) a noncompetitive H_1-receptor ANTAGONIST and mast cell stabilizer; used as the fumarate salt, administered orally in the chronic treatment of children with mild atopic ASTHMA and topically to the conjunctiva as an antipruritic in the treatment of allergic CONJUNCTIVITIS.

keV kiloelectron volt.

Kew Gardens spotted fever rickettsialpox.

kg kilogram.

kHz kilohertz.

kidney (kid′ne) either of the two bean-shaped organs in the lumbar region that filter the blood, excreting the end-products of body metabolism in the form of urine, and regulating the concentrations of hydrogen, sodium, potassium, phosphate, and other ions in the extracellular fluid.

Physiology. In an average adult each kidney is about 10 cm long, 5 cm wide, and 2.5 cm thick, and weighs 120 to 175 g. In this small area the kidney contains over a million microscopic filtering units, the NEPHRONS. Blood arrives at the kidney by way of the renal artery, and is distributed through arterioles into many millions of capillaries which lead into the nephrons. Fluids and dissolved salts in the blood pass through the walls of the capillaries and are collected within the malpighian CAPSULE, the central capsule of each nephron. Within the capsule is a tuft of capillaries called the GLOMERULUS that acts as a semipermeable membrane permitting a protein-free ultra-filtrate of plasma to pass through. This filtrate is forced into the renal TUBULES, hairpin-shaped collecting channels in the nephrons. Capillaries in the walls of the tubules reabsorb the water and the salts required by the body and deliver them to a system of small kidney veins which, in turn, carry them into the renal vein and return them to the general circulation. Excess water and other waste materials remain in the tubules as URINE. The urine contains, besides water, a quantity of UREA, URIC ACID, yellow pigments, amino acids, and trace metals. The urine moves through a system of ducts into the funnel-shaped renal PELVIS in each kidney, through which it is led into the two URETERS.

Filtering Capacity. About 1500 ml of urine are excreted daily by the average adult. The efficiency of the normal kidney is one of the most remarkable aspects of the body. Ordinarily it draws off from the blood about 164 liters of fluid daily, and usually returns 98 to 99 per cent of the water plus the useful dissolved salts, according to the body's changing needs.

Maintaining Acid-Base Balance. The kidneys help control the body's acidity by re-absorbing filtered bicarbonate ions in exchange for chloride and by secreting hydrogen ions. When there is ALKALOSIS, the kidney compensates by reabsorbing less bicarbonate ions and more hydrogen ions.

Regulation of Sodium-Water Balance. Normal OSMOLALITY and volume of body fluids are preserved by the normally functioning kidney. It does this by actively reabsorbing sodium and, by OSMOSIS, reabsorbing more water, thus varying the urine concentration. The regulation of the sodium level in the blood is influenced by ALDOSTERONE, which increases sodium reabsorption; it is secreted by the ADRENAL GLAND in response to low serum sodium levels and the presence of angiotensin II. The reabsorption of water is affected not only by the reabsorption of sodium but also by antidiuretic hormone, which is secreted by the pituitary gland in response to high serum osmolality.

Endocrine Functions. In response to renal ischemia the kidneys regulate blood pressure by the RENIN-ANGIOTENSIN-ALDOSTERONE SYSTEM. Also, when kidney cells become hypoxic they release a hormone called ERYTHROPOIETIN, which stimulates the maturation of oxygen-bearing red blood cells in the bone marrow. The kidneys also are involved in the conversion of inactive vitamin D to the active form, which increases calcium absorption in the intestine and calcium uptake by the bones.

Disorders of the Kidneys. Disorders of the kidney include inflammation, infection, obstruction, structural defects, injuries, calculus formation, and tumors. Specific disorders include types of GLOMERULONEPHRITIS, NEPHRITIS, NEPHROPATHY, and PYELITIS; KIDNEY STONES; POLYCYSTIC KIDNEY DISEASE; and NEPHROPTOSIS. See also RENAL FAILURE.

amyloid k. one with AMYLOIDOSIS; called also waxy kidney.

artificial k. popular name for an extra-corporeal HEMODIALYZER, a device used as a substitute for nonfunctioning kidneys.

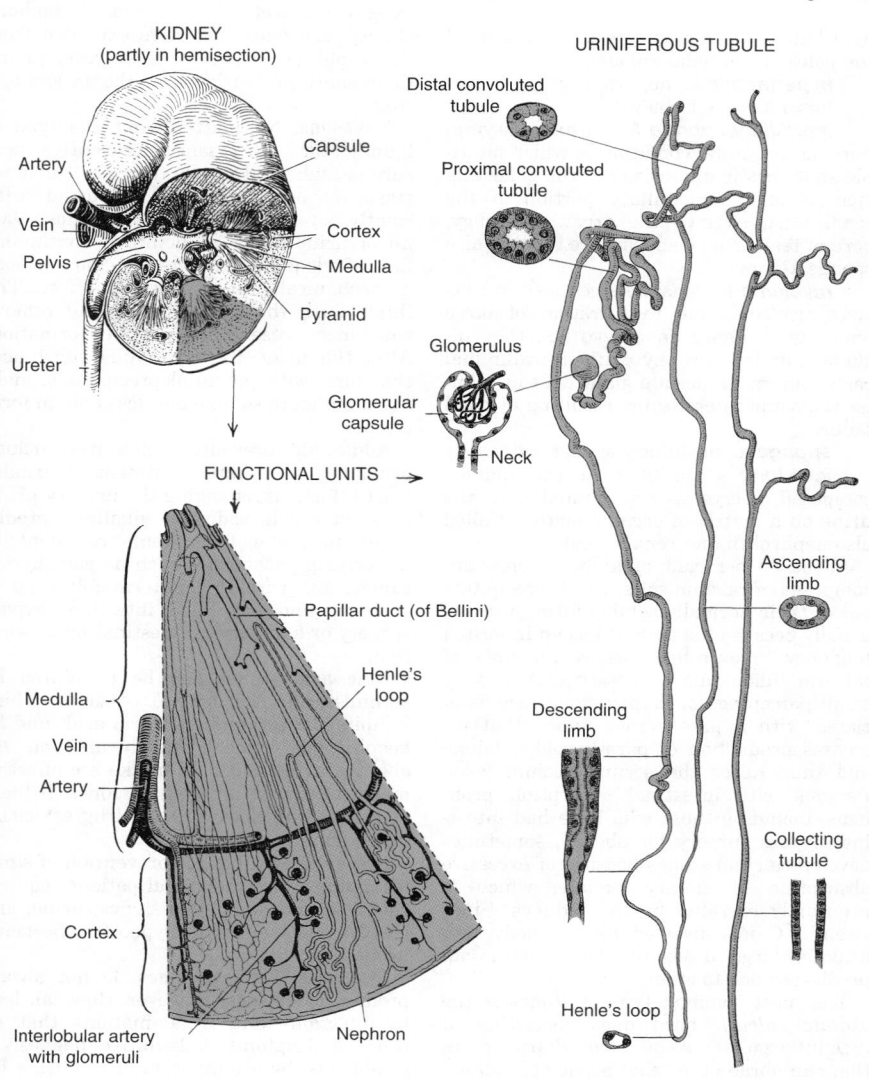

KIDNEY
(partly in hemisection)

Artery
Vein
Pelvis
Ureter

Capsule
Cortex
Medulla
Pyramid

FUNCTIONAL UNITS →

Medulla
Vein
Artery
Cortex
Interlobular artery
with glomeruli

Papillar duct (of Bellini)
Henle's loop
Nephron

URINIFEROUS TUBULE

Distal convoluted tubule
Proximal convoluted tubule
Glomerulus
Glomerular capsule
Neck
Ascending limb
Descending limb
Collecting tubule
Henle's loop

Details of structure of the kidney.

Ask-Upmark k. a hypoplastic kidney with fewer lobules than usual and fissures on its surface; most affected persons have severe HYPERTENSION, sometimes with hypertensive ENCEPHALOPATHY and RETINOPATHY. The condition may be either congenital or secondary to vesicoureteral REFLUX with PYELONEPHRITIS.

cake k. a solid, irregularly lobed organ of bizarre shape, formed by fusion of the two renal anlagen; called also lump kidney.

cicatricial k. a shriveled, irregular, and scarred kidney due to suppurative pyelonephritis.

fatty k. one with fatty DEGENERATION.

flea-bitten k. one with small, randomly scattered petechiae on its surface.

floating k. nephroptosis.

fused k. a single anomalous organ developed as a result of fusion of the renal anlagen.

horseshoe k. an anomaly in which the right and left kidneys are linked at one end by a band of tissue as a result of fusion of the poles of the renal anlagen.

hypermobile k. nephroptosis.

lump k. cake kidney.

medullary sponge k. a usually asymptomatic congenital condition in which multiple small cystic dilatations of the collecting TUBULES of the medullary portion of the renal PYRAMIDS give the organ a spongy, porous feeling and appearance. Called also sponge kidney.

myeloma k. renal changes seen in MULTIPLE MYELOMA, due to filtration of large amounts of Bence Jones PROTEIN; they include tubular atrophy with intraluminal casts and multinucleate giant cells in tubular walls and interstitium, resulting in renal failure.

sponge k. medullary sponge kidney.

k. stone a CALCULUS in the kidney, composed of crystals precipitated from the urine on a matrix of organic matter. Called also nephrolith and renal calculus.

About 80 per cent of kidney stones are composed of calcium salts, which precipitate out of their normally soluble form in urine, usually because the patient has an inherited tendency to excrete excessive amounts of calcium (idiopathic HYPERCALCEMIA). A very small percentage of kidney stones are associated with a parathyroid tumor that increases production of parathyroid HORMONE and thus raises the serum calcium level. Persons with intestinal absorption problems, including those who have had intestinal bypass surgery for obesity, sometimes develop calcium stones because of excessive absorption of dietary oxalate, which is eventually excreted by the kidneys. Since vitamin C is converted by the body into oxalate, large doses of the vitamin can predispose one to stone formation.

The most common type of stones is the *oxalate calculi,* hard ones consisting of CALCIUM OXALATE; some have sharp spines that can abrade the renal pelvic epithelium, and others are smooth. Another common type is the *phosphate calculi,* which contain CALCIUM PHOSPHATE in a mineral form such as brushite or whitlockite; they may be hard, soft, or friable and range from small to so large that they fill the renal pelvis. *Struvite stones* are composed of the salt magnesium ammonium phosphate and form in alkaline urine such as that produced in URINARY TRACT INFECTIONS. *Uric acid stones* form when there is an increased excretion of URIC ACID, as in GOUT or certain malignancies. An acid urine favors their formation. *Cystine stones* are associated with CYSTINURIA, a

hereditary kidney disorder in which there is excessive excretion of CYSTINE. "Staghorn stones" are ones that have extended from the renal pelvis into the calyces, giving them sharp protrusions like the antlers of a stag.

Prevention. No matter what the type of kidney stone, an essential preventive measure is high fluid intake to prevent urinary stasis. In order to dilute the urine sufficiently, an adult must put out almost 4000 ml of urine every 24 hours. A continuous flow of adequate amounts of urine has both a mechanical and a chemical effect. The fluids flush the urinary tract and remove substances essential to stone formation. Also, the urine itself contains substances that bind with potential precipitates, making them more soluble and less able to form a mass.

Additional preventive measures include avoidance or prompt treatment of urinary tract infections, changing the urinary pH in cases in which acidity or alkalinity predisposes to stone formation, treatment of underlying pathologies such as parathyroid tumor, and careful long-term follow-up of patients who have had intestinal bypass surgery or a history of intestinal malabsorption.

Uric acid stones can be prevented by administering the drug ALLOPURINOL, which inhibits the formation of uric acid, and by keeping the urine relatively alkaline. An alkaline urine and high intake are effective means of preventing cystine stones. If these measures fail, however, the drug PENICILLAMINE may be prescribed.

A specific strategy for prevention of stone formation in an individual patient requires chemical analysis of the stones, urine, and blood to determine the type of stone being formed.

Symptoms. Kidney stones do not always produce symptoms. However, they can lead to infections and inflammations that do produce symptoms. A definitive diagnosis is established by examination of the urine for HEMATURIA, an abdominal x-ray (which can detect stones of calcium salts), or an intravenous or retrograde PYELOGRAM using a radiopaque dye. The pyelogram will not show the stone itself but there will be a gap in the stream of dye as it courses down the ureter.

The classic symptoms of renal COLIC occur when a small calculus is dislodged from the renal pelvis and begins to travel down the ureter. Many stones have sharp spicules or spikes on their surfaces; as they roll along the ureter they can scrape the lining, causing excruciating pain and bleeding.

The pain is typically felt in the flank over the affected kidney and ureter and radiates downward toward the genitalia and inner thigh. Nausea and vomiting can occur as a result of the severe pain. If an infection is present the patient experiences fever and chills.

Treatment. Stones that are less than 5 mm can usually be eliminated with the normal passage of urine; this is the most desirable method of treatment. Adequate medication is given to relieve pain and relax the muscular walls of the ureter, thus easing passage of the stone. Fluids are given orally or intravenously to aid mechanical flushing. During this period the urine is strained in order to determine whether the stone is passed and, if it is, to collect it for laboratory analysis.

If the stone is not passed, the traditional treatment has been surgical intervention to remove it via URETEROSCOPY. A newer non-invasive technique is LITHOTRIPSY, which involves crushing the stone into fragments small enough to be passed in the urine; this is done using any of a variety of techniques, the most common being ULTRASOUND.

Patient Care. Prevention of kidney stones requires a knowledge of patients most at risk. Males are much more at risk than females for development of calcium stones; also at high risk are those of either sex who have a family history of stone formation. Other persons at risk are those who are immobilized for any reason, have a urinary tract infection, or have a history of intestinal bypass or malabsorption.

Analgesics should be administered promptly to provide relief of pain and facilitate passage of the stone. Fluid intake and output are measured; the intake is encouraged to be 4000 ml every 24 hours. Characteristics of the urine are noted, and all urine is strained until the stone is either passed or removed surgically. Dietary restrictions and recommendations to alter urinary pH and the reason for increased fluid intake are explained to the patient and family members as appropriate. The patient also is taught to take prescribed medications faithfully and to report symptoms of urinary tract infection promptly.

 wandering k. nephroptosis.

 waxy k. amyloid kidney.

Kienböck's disease (kēn'berks) 1. slowly progressive osteochondrosis of the lunate bone; it may affect other wrist bones. 2. traumatic cavitation of the spinal cord.

kilo- word element [Gr.], *one thousand;* used in naming units of measurement to designate an amount 10^3 times the size of the unit to which it is joined. Symbol k.

kilocalorie (kil'o-kal"o-re) a unit of heat equal to 1000 calories; symbol kcal.

kilogram (kg) (kil'o-gram) the basic SI UNIT of mass, being 1000 grams, or one cubic decimeter of water; equivalent to 2.205 pounds avoirdupois.

kilohertz (kHz) (kil'o-hertz) one thousand (10^3) HERTZ.

kilometer (km) (kĭ-lom'ĕ-ter, kil'o-me"ter) a unit of linear measurement of the metric system, being 1000 (10^3) meters, or the equivalent of 3280.83 feet, or about five-eighths of a mile.

kilovolt (kV) (kil'o-volt) one thousand (10^3) VOLTS.

 k's peak **(kVp)** the highest kilovoltage used in producing a radiograph.

kilovoltage (kil"o-vol'tij) in radiography, the x-ray tube peak voltage during an exposure, measured in kilovolts.

Kimmelstiel-Wilson syndrome (kim'el-stēl wil'sun) intercapillary GLOMERULOSCLEROSIS with nodular lesions.

kinanesthesia (kin"an-es-the'zhah) loss of the power of perceiving sensations of movement.

kinase (ki'nās) 1. a subclass of the transferases, comprising the enzymes that catalyze the transfer of a high-energy group from a donor (usually ATP) to an acceptor, and named, according to the acceptor, as creatine kinase, fructokinase, etc. 2. an enzyme that activates a zymogen, named, according to its source, such as enterokinase, streptokinase, etc.

kine- word element [Gr.], *movement.* See also words beginning CINE-.

kinematics (kin"ĕ-mat'iks) that phase of mechanics which deals with the possible motions of a material body.

kineplasty (kin'ĕ-plas"te) amputation in which the stump is so formed as to be usable for producing motion of a prosthesis; see discussion at PROSTHESIS. Called also cineplastic or kineplastic amputation.

kinesalgia (kin"ĕ-sal'jhah) pain on muscular exertion.

kinescope (kin'ĕ-skōp) an instrument for ascertaining ocular refraction.

kinesi(o)- word element [Gr.], *movement.*

kinesia (kĭ-ne'zhah) motion sickness.

kinesialgia (kĭ-ne"se-al'jhah) kinesalgia.

kinesiatrics (kĭ-ne"se-at'riks) kinesitherapy.

kinesics (kĭ-ne'siks) the scientific study of the role of body movements, such as facial expressions, gestures, and eye movements, in interpersonal communication.

kinesimeter (kin"ĕ-sim'ĕ-ter) 1. an instrument for quantitative measurement of

K

motions. 2. an instrument for exploring the body surface to test cutaneous sensibility.

kinesiology (kĭ-ne″se-ol′o-je) the scientific study of movement of the human body or its parts. See also BIOMECHANICS.

kinesis (ki-ne′sis) [Gr.] movement, such as the activity of an organism in response to a STIMULUS; the direction of the response is not controlled by the direction of the stimulus (in contrast to a TAXIS).

-kinesis word element [Gr.], *movement, activation.*

kinesitherapy (kĭ-ne″sĭ-ther′ah-pe) treatment of disease by movements or exercise.

kinesthesia (kin″es-the′zhah) the sense by which position, weight, and movement are perceived. adj., **kinesthet′ic.**

kinesthesiometer (kin″es-the″ze-om′ē-ter) an apparatus for testing kinesthesia.

kinesthesis (kin″es-the′sis) kinesthesia.

kinet(o)- word element [Gr.], *motion.*

kinetic (kĭ-net′ik) pertaining to or producing motion.

kinetics (kĭ-net′iks; ki-net′iks) the scientific study of the turnover, or rate of change, of a specific factor in the body, commonly expressed as units of amount per unit time.

 chemical k. the scientific study of the rates and mechanisms of chemical reactions.

 urea k. the movement of UREA in the body and its excretion through the KIDNEYS or DIALYSIS apparatus; see also urea CLEARANCE.

kinetocardiogram (kĭ-ne″to-kahr′de-o-gram″) the record produced by kinetocardiography.

kinetocardiography (kĭ-ne″to-kahr″de-og′rah-fe) the graphic recording of the slow vibrations of the anterior chest wall in the region of the heart, representing the absolute motion at a given point on the chest.

kinetochore (kĭ-ne′to-kōr) a centromere.

kinetogenic (kĭ-ne″to-jen′ik) causing or producing movement.

kinetoplast (kĭ-ne′to-plast) an accessory body found in many protozoa, primarily the Mastigophora; it contains DNA and replicates independently.

kinetosis (kĭ″nĕ-to′sis) any disorder due to unaccustomed motion; see also MOTION SICKNESS.

kinetotherapy (kĭ-ne″to-ther′ah-pe) kinesitherapy.

King (king) Imogene M. Nursing educator, administrator, researcher, and practitioner. She developed a conceptual framework for nursing at a time when nursing was striving for status as a science and for recognition as a legitimate profession. From her conceptual system, a theory of GOAL ATTAINMENT was derived, within which she developed a transaction process model that makes her theory a middle range THEORY. Her ideas have been tested in research and used by practitioners and educators. Several other theories have been derived from her conceptual system.

King-Devick test (king dev′ik) a tool for evaluation of SACCADE, consisting of a series of charts of numbers; the charts become progressively more difficult to read in a flowing manner because of increasing space between the numbers. Both errors in reading and speed of reading are included in deriving a score.

kingdom (king′dum) 1. in the classification of living organisms, the highest of the categories; the most widely used classification system lists five kingdoms: MONERA, PROTISTA, FUNGI, Planta (the PLANTS), and Animalia (the ANIMALS). 2. traditionally, one of three major categories into which natural objects may be classified, consisting of the animal, plant, and mineral kingdoms.

kinin (ki′nin) the generic term for any of the polypeptides related in amino acid sequence and physiological activity to BRADYKININ and KALLIDIN, formed by kallikrein-mediated cleavage of kininogens. Kinins are plasma proteins that increase vascular permeability, interact with prostaglandins to cause pain and smooth muscle contraction and to increase the migration of white blood cells during the inflammatory process, and act as potent renal vasodilators to increase the renal excretion of sodium.

kininogen (ki-nin′o-jen″) either of two plasma α_2-globulins that are KININ precursors. High-molecular-weight (HMW) kininogen (also called *Fitzgerald factor*) is split by plasma KALLIKREIN to produce BRADYKININ; low-molecular-weight (LMW) kininogen is split by tissue KALLIKREIN to produce KALLIDIN. Deficiency of HMW kallikrein is a rare condition but may be considered when prolonged activated partial thromboplastin TIME cannot be explained by deficiencies of other more common factors.

kinlein (kin′lin) a system of professional health care developed by M. Lucille Kinlein; it was formerly considered part of nursing but separated from nursing in 1979. The governing philosophy is called ESCA (exercise of self care agency). The residential care centers are called detente CENTERS. Called also kinlein care.

kinleiner (kin′lin-er) a practitioner of KINLEIN.

kinocilium (ki″no-sil′e-um), pl. *kinocil′ia* a motile, protoplasmic filament on the free surface of a cell.

WINDOW ON A CONCEPTUAL SYSTEM AND THEORY OF GOAL ATTAINMENT

In the formulation of my conceptual system, from which a theory of goal attainment was developed within which a transaction process model was derived, my concept of human beings, of health, of environment, and of nursing have been defined and discussed for the last thirty years of the twentieth century and into the present one. In the last few years of the twentieth century, these four abstract concepts were identified in the nursing literature as the metaparadigm of nursing.

My conceptual system is comprised of three dynamic interacting systems, personal systems (individuals), interpersonal systems (dyads, triads, small groups, such as nurses, physicians, pharmacists) and social systems (large groups, such as the educational system, the government system, health care systems, with specific concepts related to each system). These three interacting systems define the physical and social environments within which all individual human beings function.

Human beings are the primary focus of nursing. My personal philosophy about human beings influenced the development of my ideas, since we are all human beings who function in a variety of roles within the three interacting systems. Philosophical assumptions about human beings are that individuals are sentient, rational, social, perceiving, purposeful, action-oriented, time-oriented, and spiritual. When human beings function in role of nurse and role of patient, the primary goal is health.

My concept of health has been defined as dynamic life experiences of a human being, which implies continuous adjustment to stressors in the internal and external environment through optimum use of one's resources to achieve maximum potential for daily living. Illness has been defined as an interference, that is, an imbalance, in a person's biological structure or in psychological makeup, or a conflict in a person's social relationships. Because human beings are the primary focus of nursing, and health is the primary goal within the three interacting systems, my definition of nursing is that it is a process of action, reaction, interaction, and transaction whereby nurses assist individuals of any age and socioeconomic group to meet their basic needs in performing activities of daily living and to cope with health and illness at some particular point in the life cycle.

A study has been conducted to classify the elements in the nurse-patient interactions that lead to transaction. A critical variable in this process is mutual goal setting. My goal-oriented nursing record system begins with an assessment to gather a database about the patient from which nursing diagnoses are identified and patient goals are stated, resulting in a plan of care. Progress notes are recorded that relate to patient goals. Flow sheets provide a record of data essential for monitoring patient progress. The discharge summary shows patient attainment of goals, and if they have not been attained, why not, and reassessment takes place. This type of documentation system records data that are patient centered, goal directed, and written in terms that represent patient outcomes, which is evidence-based practice.

Some nurses who function within a health team in several hospitals have explained to me that they have introduced the health team members to my transaction process and that this has helped the team in identifying goals to be achieved by patients but has also clarified overall goals mutually agreed upon with patients. Theoretical knowledge of the concepts in the theory of goal attainment has been used by professionals in concrete situations in health care systems.

Use of my conceptual system and middle range theory of goal attainment in nursing practice has shown health care outcomes as evidence-based practice, cost containment, and a health team approach in using basic theoretical knowledge in health care.

IMOGENE M. KING, RN, EDD, FAAN

K

kinship (kin′ship) a group of individuals of varying degrees of descent from a common ancestor.

Klebsiella (kleb″se-al′ah) a genus of gram-negative, facultatively anaerobic rod-shaped bacteria that are widely distributed in nature and commonly found in the intestinal tract. They are a frequent cause of nosocomial urinary and pulmonary infections and wound infections. Species include *K. pneumo′niae* (also called *K. friedlän′deri*), the etiologic agent of Friedländer's PNEUMONIA; *K. pneumo′niae ozae′nae*, which occurs in OZENA and other respiratory diseases; and *K. rhinosclero′matis*, a species isolated from patients with RHINOSCLEROMA.

kleeblattschädel (kla″blaht-sha′del) [Ger.] cloverleaf skull; a congenital anomaly in which there is intrauterine SYNOSTOSIS of multiple or all cranial sutures.

Kleine-Levin syndrome (klīn′ĕ lev′in) episodic periods of excessive sleep and overeating lasting for several weeks, usually in adolescent boys.

kleptomania (klep″to-ma′ne-ah) an IMPULSE CONTROL DISORDER consisting of an abnormal, uncontrollable desire to steal.

kleptomaniac (klep″to-ma′ne-ak) a person exhibiting kleptomania.

Klinefelter's syndrome (klīn′fel-terz) a condition in males characterized by small testes, with fibrosis and hyalinization of seminiferous tubules, impairment of function and clumping of Leydig cells, and an increase in urinary gonadotropins, associated with an abnormality of the sex chromosomes. It is associated typically with an XXY chromosome complement.

Klippel-Feil syndrome (klī-pel′ fīl) shortness of the neck due to reduction in the number of cervical vertebrae or the fusion of multiple hemivertebrae into one osseous mass, with limitation of neck motion and low hairline.

Klonopin (klon′o-pin) trademark for a preparation of CLONAZEPAM, an ANTICONVULSANT and antipanic agent.

Kluyvera (kli′ver-ah) a genus of gram-negative, facultatively anaerobic, rod-shaped bacteria that are occasional opportunistic pathogens and cause respiratory and urinary infections.

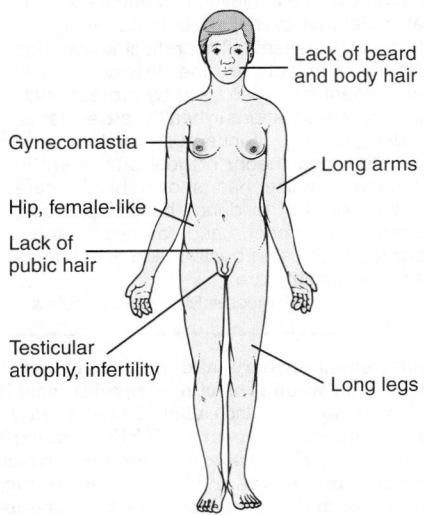

Klinefelter's syndrome. Redrawn from Damjanov, 2000.

Lack of beard and body hair
Gynecomastia
Long arms
Hip, female-like
Lack of pubic hair
Testicular atrophy, infertility
Long legs

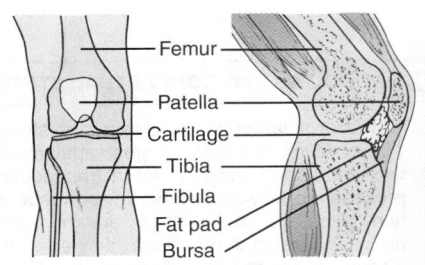

Left: Knee joint, front view. *Right:* Knee joint, flexed in profile.

Femur — Patella — Cartilage — Tibia — Fibula — Fat pad — Bursa

km kilometer.

knee (ne) the area around the knee JOINT, a hinge joint that is one of the largest joints of the body, sustaining great pressure. The knee is formed by the proximal portion of the TIBIA, the distal end of the FEMUR, and the PATELLA, or kneecap. The bones are joined by ligaments, and the patella is secured to the adjacent bones by powerful tendons. The FIBULA is attached at the side of the knee to the tibia. Two crescent-shaped pads of cartilage, one medial and one lateral, called MENISCI, lying on top of the tibia cushion it from the femur and form the gliding surfaces of the joint in motion. Further cushioning is supplied by bursae, which are located around the main joint, between it and the patella and on the outside of the patella. A capsule of ligaments binds the whole assembly together. The capsule is lined with synovial membrane, which secretes a lubricating synovial FLUID that makes possible a smooth, gliding motion. Traumatic disorders of the knee are common and include DISLOCATION, SPRAIN, and FRACTURE.

k. jerk, k. reflex a kick reflex produced by sharply tapping the patellar ligament. To test this reflex, the lower part of the leg is allowed to hang relaxed (such as by crossing the legs at the knees) and the examiner taps the ligament below the patella with a small rubber hammer. The normal reaction is contraction of the quadriceps muscle, causing involuntary extension of the lower leg. This is a stretch reflex; striking the patellar ligament stretches the quadriceps muscle at the front of the thigh and causes it to contract. Two nerves are involved; one receives the stimulus and transmits the impulse to the spinal cord, and the other, a motor nerve, receives the impulse and relays it to the quadriceps muscle. Inadequate response to the knee jerk test may mean that the reflex mechanism involved is in some way impaired. In some people with normal reflexes the jerk of the knee is so light as to be nearly imperceptible, and the examiner must make other tests to check the reflex mechanism. Called also patellar or quadriceps reflex.

kneecap (ne′kap) patella.

knock-knee (nok′ne) a childhood deformity, developing gradually, in which the knees rub together or "knock" in walking and the ankles are far apart; the most common causes are irregularity in growth of the long bones of the lower limb (sometimes from injury to the bone ends at the knee) and weak ligaments. The weight of the body, which is not supported properly, turns the knees in and the weak lower legs buckle until the ankles are spread far apart. Called also genu valgum.

Knock-knee in young children varies in seriousness. Milder cases may disappear after early childhood as bones, ligaments, and muscles strengthen and coordination improves. More serious cases can often be corrected by strengthening exercises and by proper manipulation of the joints. Sometimes braces are used to ensure the proper alignment of growing legs.

In a very young child, knock-knee involves only the soft bone ends where the bone grows. If allowed to continue for a number of years, the condition can lead to abnormal developments in body structure. The sooner corrective measures are taken, the more effective the treatment is likely to be.

knot (not) 1. an intertwining of the ends or parts of one or more threads, sutures, or strips of cloth. 2. in anatomy, a knoblike swelling or protuberance.

    surgeon's k., surgical k. a knot in which the thread is passed twice through the first loop and once through the second loop in square knot fashion.

knowledge (nŏ′lej) the ability of a client to remember and interpret information.

    k. deficit (specify) a NURSING DIAGNOSIS approved by the North American Nursing Diagnosis Association, defined as the absence or deficiency of cognitive information related to a specific topic. For purposes of assessing knowledge deficit, setting objectives, and planning and implementing patient teaching, three broad areas or domains are recognized: the *cognitive,* the *affective,*

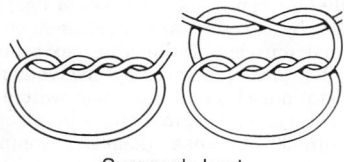

Surgeon's knot

From Dorland's, 2000.

and the *psychomotor* domains. These were devised by Benjamin S. Bloom and colleagues as a part of a taxonomy of educational objectives, whose purpose is to classify and better identify specific goals for teaching, learning, and evaluation of outcomes of the process.

The *cognitive domain* deals with the recall or recognition of knowledge and the development of intellectual abilities and skills. The *affective domain* encompasses interest, attitudes, and values. The *psychomotor domain* is the manipulative or motor-skill area of learning.

Learning objectives in each of these domains should be stated in behavioral terms. Educators contend that a change in behavior is evidence that learning has taken place. Hence, criteria by which one judges whether learning has occurred are written in terms of what the learner is able to do as a result of instruction. In the cognitive domain a goal of learning might be that the patient verbalizes dosage of prescribed medication, its expected actions, and any untoward reactions to be reported. In the affective domain, a change in attitude or value is observed as a change in behavior. Thus the fact that a patient loses the desired amount of weight in a specific period of time while following a special diet is evidence that the diet is valued and therefore has been followed. In the psychomotor domain a goal could be that the patient is able to take and record his or her own blood pressure accurately each day.

The overall purposes of assessing and implementing plans for correction of a knowledge deficit are to assist the patient and family members (1) to promote their own health and that of family members, (2) to maintain current health status and improve it as much as possible according to each person's capabilities, and (3) to improve to the fullest one's self-care abilities.

knuckle (nuk″l) the dorsal aspect of any interphalangeal joint, or any similarly bent structure.

Koch's law (kawks) see Koch's POSTULATES.

Kock pouch (kok) 1. the most common kind of continent ileal RESERVOIR; see also ILEOSTOMY. 2. a surgically created urinary bladder made from a segment of isolated ileum. It consists of an afferent nipple, into which the ureters are implanted in a manner that prevents reflux of urine, and a continent efferent nipple. It is drained by catheterization.

Köhler's bone disease (ker′lerz) 1. osteochondrosis of the tarsal navicular bone in

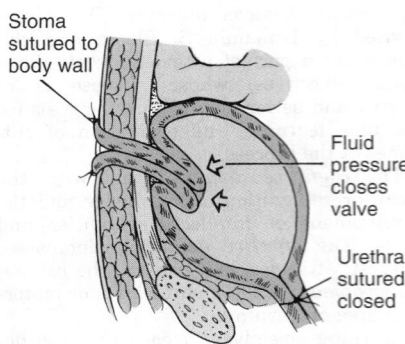

Kock pouch. From Polaski and Tatro, 1996.

children. 2. thickening of the shaft of the second metatarsal bone and changes about its articular head, with pain in the second metatarsophalangeal joint on walking or standing.

koil(o)- word element [Gr.], *hollowed; concave.*

koilonychia (koi″lo-nik′e-ah) dystrophy of the nails in which they are abnormally thin and concave from side to side, with the edges turned up.

koilorrhachic (koi″lo-rak′ik) having a vertebral column in which the lumbar curvature is anteriorly concave.

koilosternia (koi″lo-ster′ne-ah) pectus excavatum.

kolp- for words beginning thus, see those beginning *colp-.*

kolypeptic (ko″lĕ-pep′tik) hindering or checking digestion.

Korsakoff's syndrome (kor′sah-kofs) a mental disorder associated with chronic ALCOHOLISM and caused by vitamin B_1 (thiamine) deficiency; it is the amnestic component of the WERNICKE-KORSAKOFF SYNDROME. Characteristics include retrograde and anterograde amnesia, sometimes with disorientation, confabulation, and lack of insight into the memory deficit; there may also be signs of polyneuritis. Only about 20 percent of those affected recover completely or almost completely; confinement to an

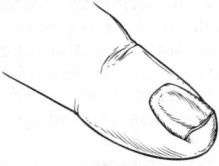

Koilonychia. From Dorland's, 2000.

institution is a frequent outcome of this condition. See also AMNESTIC SYNDROME. Called also Korsakoff's psychosis.

Kostmann's syndrome (kost′mahnz) infantile genetic AGRANULOCYTOSIS.

Kr krypton.

Krabbe's disease (krah′bez) a familial form of leukoencephalopathy beginning in infancy, in which the sphingolipid ceramide galactoside accumulates in the tissues due to a deficiency of β-galactosidase, marked pathologically by cerebral demyelination and by the presence of large globoid bodies in the white substance.

kraurosis (kraw-ro′sis) a dried, shriveled condition.

k. vul′vae atrophy of the female external genitalia, resulting in drying and shriveling, with leukoplakic patches on the mucosa and intense itching.

Krukenberg's tumor (kroo′ken-bergz) a type of carcinoma of the ovary, usually metastatic from cancer of the gastrointestinal tract, especially of the stomach. It is characterized by areas of mucoid degeneration and the presence of signet-ring–like cells.

krypton (Kr) (krip′ton) a chemical element, atomic number 36, atomic weight 83.80. (See Appendix 6.)

k. 81m an unstable radioactive isotope of krypton having a half-life of 13 seconds and emitting gamma rays. It is used in pulmonary ventilation studies to evaluate regional function.

KUB [*k*idneys, *u*reters, and *b*ladder] a plain film of the abdomen, providing information about abdominal organs including the kidneys, ureters, and bladder.

Kufs' disease (koofs) the rare adult form of NEURONAL CEROID-LIPOFUSCINOSIS, usually seen before age 40. Clinical findings include progressive neurologic degeneration, excessive storage of LIPOFUSCIN in the central nervous system, and shortened life expectancy. Unlike the late infantile (JANSKÝ-BIELSCHOWSKY DISEASE), and juvenile forms (VOGT-SPIELMEYER DISEASE), it is not associated with ocular lesions.

Kugelberg-Welander syndrome (koo′gelberg vel′an-der) a hereditary form of muscular atrophy due to lesions of the anterior horns of the spinal cord, with onset usually between 2 and 17 years of age; it is marked by atrophy and weakness of the proximal muscles of the lower extremities and pelvic girdle, followed by involvement of the distal muscles and muscular twitchings. Called also juvenile spinal muscular atrophy.

Kümmell's disease (kĕm′elz) compression fracture of a vertebra, with symptoms occurring a few weeks after injury, including spinal pain, intercostal neuralgia, motor disturbances of the lower limbs, and kyphosis that is painful on pressure and easily reduced by extension. Called also Kümmell's or post-traumatic spondylitis.

kurtosis (ker-to'sis) the degree of peakedness or flatness of a probability distribution, relative to the normal distribution with the same variance. See illustration.

kuru (koo'roo) an infectious form of prion disease with a long incubation period found only among the Fore and neighboring peoples of New Guinea and thought to be associated with ritual cannibalism. It is always fatal and is manifested by truncal and limb ataxia, a shivering-like tremor ("kuru" is the Fore word for "shivering"), and dysarthria. Amyloid plaques are present in about two thirds of affected individuals.

Kussmaul's disease (koos'moulz) polyarteritis nodosa.

kV kilovolt.

KVO keep vein open.

kVp kilovolts peak.

kwashiorkor (kwahsh"e-or'kor) a syndrome occurring in infants and young children soon after weaning. It is due to severe protein deficiency, and the symptoms include edema, pigmentation changes of skin and hair, impaired growth and development, distention of the abdomen, and pathologic liver changes.

Kyasanur Forest disease (ki-ah'sah-noor for'est) a highly fatal viral disease of monkeys in the Kyasanur Forest of India, communicable to humans, in whom it produces a type of HEMORRHAGIC FEVER.

kymatism (ki'mah-tizm) myokymia; quivering of muscles.

kynocephalus (ki"no-sef'ah-lus) a malformed fetus with a head like that of a dog.

kynurenine (kin"u-re'nin) a metabolite of tryptophan found in microorganisms and in the urine of normal animals; it is a precursor of kynurenic acid and an intermediate in the conversion of tryptophan to niacin.

kyphos (ki'fos) the hump in the spine in kyphosis.

kyphoscoliosis (ki"fo-sko"le-o'sis) backward (kyphosis) and lateral (scoliosis) curvature of the spine, in vertebral osteochondrosis (Scheuermann's disease).

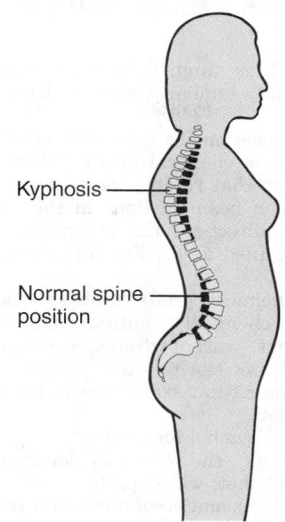

Kyphosis. From Frazier et al., 1996.

kyphosis (ki-fo'sis) abnormally increased convex curvature of the thoracic spine as seen from the side; it may be the result of an acquired disease, an injury, or a congenital disorder or disease. It never develops from poor posture. One of the most common causes is postmenopausal OSTEO-POROSIS accompanied by anterior vertebral body wedge-compression fractures. adj., **kyphot'ic.** Kyphosis sometimes occurs with certain forms of poliomyelitis and with diseases that cause bone destruction, as happens in osteitis deformans (PAGET'S DISEASE). An injury, such as a fracture of the spine, treated improperly or not at all, may also result in hunchback. Some rare cases are caused by congenital deformities and diseases. One example, ACHONDROPLASIA, or fetal rickets, is a congenital bone disorder that affects growth and bone formation. There are no specific symptoms besides back pain and increasing immobility of the spine. Symptoms vary with the cause, and any back pain or injury should be investigated.

kyrtorrhachic (kir"to-rak'ik) having a vertebral column in which the lumbar curvature is anteriorly convex.

kyt(o)- for words beginning thus, see those beginning *cyt(o)-*.

Kytril (ki'tril) trademark for preparations of GRANISETRON, an ANTIEMETIC used with antineoplastic AGENTS. or cancer RADIOTHERAPY.

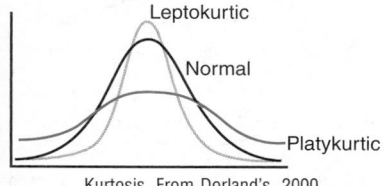

Kurtosis. From Dorland's, 2000.

L

L left; liter; lung; light chain (see IMMU-NOGLOBULIN); lumbar vertebra, L1–L5 (see vertebra).

l- abbreviation for *levo*- (left or counter-clockwise); a chemical prefix indicating an ENANTIOMER that rotates the plane of polar-ization of a beam of light in the counter-clockwise direction, the other enantiomer being specified as *d*-. For further explana-tion, see *d*-.

L- a chemical prefix that specifies the relative chemical configuration of an enantiomer, carbohydrates corresponding to L-GLYCERALDEHYDE and amino acids corresponding to L-SERINE; see D- for further explanation.

l former symbol for LITER.

λ (lambda, the eleventh letter of the Greek alphabet) wavelength.

L & A light and accommodation (reaction of the pupils).

La lanthanum.

label (la′b′l) something that identifies; an identifying mark or tag.

radioactive *l*. a radioisotope that is incorporated into a compound to mark it.

labetalol (la-bet′ah-lol) a BETA-ADRENERGIC BLOCKING AGENT with some ALPHA-ADRENERGIC BLOCKING AGENT activity, administered orally or intravenously as the hydrochloride salt as an ANTIHYPERTENSIVE AGENT.

labia (la′be-ah) [L.] plural of LABIUM.

labial (la′be-al) 1. pertaining to or directed toward a lip. 2. pertaining to a labium.

labialism (la′be-ah-lizm) defective speech with use of labial sounds.

labile (la′bīl) 1. gliding; moving from point to point over the surface. 2. unstable; fluctuating. 3. chemically unstable.

lability (lah-bil′ĭ-te) 1. the quality of being labile. 2. in psychiatry, emotional instabil-ity; rapidly changing emotions.

labio- word element [L.], *lip*.

labioglossolaryngeal (la′be-o-glos″o-lah-rin′je-al) pertaining to the lips, tongue, and larynx.

labioglossopharyngeal (la″be-o-glos″o-fah-rin′je-al) pertaining to the lips, tongue, and pharynx.

labiograph (la′be-o-graf″) an instrument for recording movements of the lips in speaking.

labioincisal (la″be-o-in-si′zal) pertaining to or formed by the labial and incisal surfaces of a tooth.

labiomental (la″be-o-men′t′l) pertaining to the lips and chin.

labionasal (la″be-o-na′zal) pertaining to the lips and nose.

labiopalatine (la″be-o-pal′ah-tīn) pertain-ing to the lips and palate.

labioplasty (la′be-o-plas″te) plastic repair of a lip; cheiloplasty.

labium (la′be-um), pl. *la′bia* [L.] lip. adj. **la′bial.**

 l. ma′jus (pl. *la′bia majo′ra*), an elon-gated fold in the female, one on either side of the rima pudendi.

 l. mi′nus (pl. *la′bia mino′ra*), the small fold of skin on either side, between the labia majora and the opening of the vagina.

 la′bia o′ris the lips of the mouth.

labor (la′ber) the physiologic process by which the uterus expels the products of CONCEPTION (FETUS or NEWBORN and PLA-CENTA), after 20 or more weeks of GESTATION. It may be divided into three stages: The *first stage (dilatation)* begins with the onset of regular uterine contractions and ends when the cervical os is completely dilated and flush with the vagina, thus completing the birth canal. The *second stage (expul-sion)* extends from the end of the first stage until the expulsion of the infant is completed. The *third stage (placental stage)* extends from the expulsion of the child until the placenta and membrane are expelled and contraction of the uterus is completed. Called also accouchement and parturition.

Labor is believed to be triggered by the release of oxytocin and prostaglandins, after

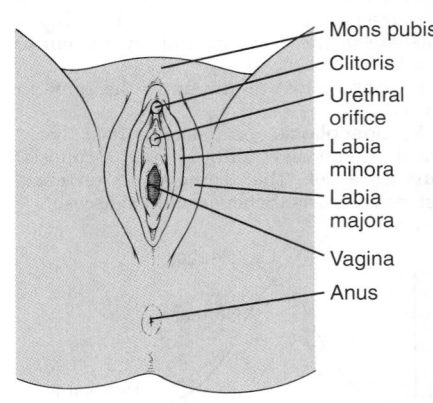

Female external genitalia. From Applegate, 2000.

a fall in the levels of other hormones. Normally at the end of pregnancy oxytocin, which is stored in the posterior lobe of the pituitary gland, is released and stimulates contraction of the uterine muscles.

The progress and final outcome of labor are influenced by four factors: (1) the "passage" (the soft and bony tissues of the maternal pelvis); (2) the "powers" (the contractions or forces of the uterus); (3) the "passenger" (the fetus); and (4) the "psyche" (mother's emotional state, e.g., anxiety).

The mechanisms of labor (for a vertex presentation) consist of the following sequence of events: ENGAGEMENT (posterior occiput of fetus enters the pelvic outlet); FLEXION (of fetal head); DESCENT (fetal head descends lower into the midpelvis); internal ROTATION (fetal head and body rotate so that the occiput is more anterior); EXTENSION (fetal head extends once the occiput is beneath the symphysis pubis); and *external rotation* (fetal head rotates back to position it had at engagement).

First Stage of Labor. The beginning of labor is usually indicated by one or more of the following signs: (1) *show* (passage from the vagina of small quantities of blood-tinged mucus); (2) *breaking the "bag of waters"* (normal rupture of membranes, indicated by a gush or slow leakage of amniotic fluid from the vagina); and (3) true labor *contractions*. The first two of these signs are almost always unmistakable. The contractions, however, can be confusing. BRAXTON-HICKS CONTRACTIONS, or "false labor pains," can be distinguished from true labor contractions by the irregular time intervals between them and by their tendency to disappear when the patient changes position or gets up and walks about. True labor contractions are regularly spaced and usually start in the small of the back, or as a feeling of tightness in the abdomen, or of pressure in the pelvis. The contractions recur at shorter and shorter intervals, every three to five minutes, and become progressively stronger and longer lasting. The increase in the strength of contractions usually is accompanied by an increase in the amount of show because of rupture of capillaries in the dilating cervix.

This first stage of childbirth is known as the dilatation period. The uterus is like a large rubber bottle with a half-inch long neck that is almost closed. As the uterine muscles contract, the cervix becomes thinner (effacement) and more open (dilated) so that the neck of the uterus eventually resembles that of a jar more than that of a bottle.

The length of the first stage of labor varies with each individual patient, with an average of 8 to 12 hours in primiparous and 6 to 8 hours in multiparous women. It is related to the strength and effectiveness of the contractions and is a period when the mother is instructed to relax as much as possible and let the uterus do the work. Pushing or bearing down is not effective during this stage and is harmful in that it may cause a tearing of the cervix and will only serve to exhaust the woman. She is encouraged to rest and possibly to nap between contractions.

The second stage of labor may be heralded by symptoms of nausea, vomiting, irritability, the urge to bear down, or periods of feeling hot and then cold, signs of the period of transition from the first to the second stage.

Second Stage of Labor. This period, called the expulsion stage, usually is characterized by intense contractions that last for about one full minute and occur at 2 to 3 minute intervals. The cervix is fully dilated and the woman is able to help with this process by bearing down with each uterine contraction, using her abdominal muscles to help expel the infant. This stage varies from a few minutes to one to two hours.

Third Stage of Labor. In this stage the placenta detaches itself from the uterine wall and is expelled. The process takes about 15 minutes, and is painless.

Fourth Stage of Labor. This final stage is the stage of recovery and lasts 2 to 4 hours.

Patient Care. Once labor has begun the patient should have someone in constant attendance. She will derive much emotional support from one who is warm, kind, and understanding, and displays a genuine interest in her welfare and that of her infant. It is best to have the same person care for her through the entire labor and birth process.

During labor the strength, frequency, and duration of contractions are noted and recorded. It is expected that the contractions will increase in all three characteristics, but a sudden change in any one should be reported to the health care provider immediately. The rate, regularity, and volume of the fetal heart tones are checked and recorded periodically. Some apprehensive patients may be helped by allowing them to listen to the infant's heartbeat.

Food and fluids are withheld during active labor, but thirst may cause some discomfort and may be lessened by allowing the patient to moisten her lips with a gauze

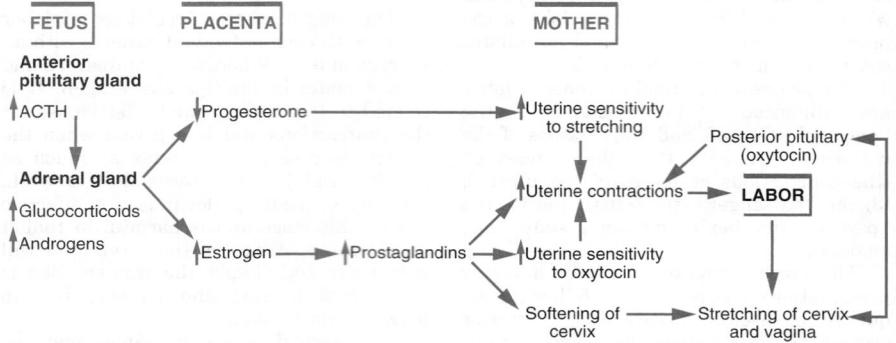

Schematic representation of factors believed to have a role in starting labor. From Gorrie et al., 1994.

sponge or to suck on ice chips. Intravenous fluids are usually given. Frequent bathing of the face with a cool washcloth often helps relieve the flushed feeling brought about by the actual hard work being done by the mother. Frequent changing of her gown and of the pad protecting the bed linens may be necessary to keep her clean, dry, and comfortable.

If there is a support person with the woman during labor, that person should be instructed in ways he or she can help the patient and at the same time feel that he or she is making some contribution in this very important event. The support person may wish to participate in keeping a record of the contractions, or might appreciate the opportunity to listen to the fetal heart tones occasionally. If the patient feels that sacral support during each contraction helps mitigate the pain, the support person can be shown how to do this. Some supporters have attended classes for expectant parents and are prepared for their role during labor and delivery. Both the patient and the support person should be informed of the progress during labor so they can feel that something is being accomplished by their efforts.

The patient is encouraged to rest and relax between contractions so as to conserve her strength. She should not bear down until the cervix is fully dilated, since this effort will only serve to exhaust her and may cause lacerations of the cervix. After the cervix is fully dilated she can speed the birth process by holding her breath and contracting her abdominal muscles. Controlled breathing exercises learned in classes for expectant parents promote relaxation and aid labor.

Although serious complications rarely develop during labor, they can occur and must be watched for. Observations to report immediately include hyperactivity of the fetus; vaginal bleeding in excess of a heavy show; a rapid and irregular pulse and drop in blood pressure; sudden rise in blood pressure; and headache, visual disturbances, extreme restlessness, or rapidly developing edema. A sudden cessation of contractions or a contraction that does not relax may indicate a serious disturbance in the labor process. The appearance of meconium in the vaginal discharge may indicate fetal distress unless the infant is in a breech position. (See also FETAL MONITORING.)

artificial l. induced labor.

dry l. a lay term indicating that in which the amniotic fluid escapes before contraction of the uterus begins.

false l. false pains.

induced l. that which is brought on by extraneous means, e.g., by the use of drugs that cause uterine contractions; called also artificial labor.

instrumental l. delivery facilitated by the use of instruments, particularly forceps.

missed l. that in which contractions begin and then cease, the fetus being retained for weeks or months.

precipitate l. delivery accomplished with undue speed.

premature l. expulsion of a viable infant before the normal end of gestation; usually applied to interruption of pregnancy between the twenty-eighth and thirty-seventh weeks.

preterm l. labor commencing before the end of 37 completed weeks of gestation; it can be arrested (see TOCOLYSIS) and does not necessarily lead to preterm delivery. Preterm labor can be treated by bed rest at home and use of a tokodynamometer with a recording unit that transmits data about uterine activity over the telephone to a monitoring station. Tocolytic drugs, including ritodrine hydrochloride and terbutaline, may be used to relax the uterine muscles.

spontaneous *l.* delivery occurring without artificial aid.

laboratory (lab′rah-tor″e) a place equipped for making tests or doing experimental work.

clinical *l.* 1. one for examination of materials derived from the human body (such as fluids, tissues, or cells) for the purpose of providing information on diagnosis, prognosis, prevention, or treatment of disease. 2. a setting in which learners can apply to clients skills learned in a clinical laboratory.

college *l.* a comprehensive college learning environment to acquire necessary skills; a well-equipped college laboratory for students of health care professions will include audiovisual learning modules and computer-aided instruction and will provide the opportunity to practice skills on simulated clients.

labrum (la′brum) [L.] a rim or LIP.

labyrinth (lab′ĭ-rinth) the inner EAR, consisting of the VESTIBULE, COCHLEA, and SEMICIRCULAR CANALS. The cochlea is concerned with HEARING and the vestibule and semicircular canals with the sense of EQUILIBRIUM. (See also color plates.) adj., **labyrin′thine.**

The bony portion of the labyrinth (*osseous labyrinth*) is composed of a series of canals tunneled out of the temporal bone. Inside the osseous labyrinth is the *membranous labyrinth,* which conforms to the general shape of the osseous labyrinth but is much smaller. A fluid called PERILYMPH fills the space (perilymphatic space) between the osseous and membranous labyrinths. Fluid inside the membranous labyrinth is called ENDOLYMPH. These fluids play an important role in the transmission of sound waves and the maintenance of body balance. The membranous labyrinth is divided into two parts: the *cochlear labyrinth,* which includes the perilymphatic space and the cochlear duct, and the *vestibular labyrinth,* which includes the UTRICLE, SACCULE, and semicircular CANALS.

Disorders of the inner ear, such as LABYRINTHITIS and MENIERE'S DISEASE, are characterized by episodes of dizziness, TINNITUS, and HEARING LOSS.

ethmoid *l.,* **ethmoidal** *l.* either of the paired lateral masses of the ethmoid BONE, consisting of numerous thin-walled cellular cavities, the ethmoidal CELLS.

labyrinthectomy (lab′ĭ-rin-thek′to-me) excision of the labyrinth.

labyrinthitis (lab″ĭ-rin-thi′tis) inflammation of the labyrinth; called also otitis interna.

acute serous *l.* a type caused by chemical or toxic irritants that invade the labyrinth, usually from the middle ear. Called also sterile or toxic labyrinthitis.

acute suppurative *l.* a type in which pus enters the labyrinth, usually through a fistula after middle ear infection or through temporal bone erosion from meningitis; it results in severe and often permanent vertigo and hearing loss. Called also bacterial or purulent labyrinthitis.

bacterial *l.* acute suppurative labyrinthitis.

circumscribed *l.* acute serous labyrinthitis in a discrete area, due to erosion of the bony wall of a semicircular canal with exposure of the membranous labyrinth; called also perilabyrinthitis.

meningogenic *l.* acute suppurative labyrinthitis that results from invasion of meningitis through an erosion of the temporal bone.

l. **ossi′ficans** abnormal ossification in the labyrinth after a trauma or an infection with inflammation.

purulent *l.* acute suppurative labyrinthitis.

sterile *l.,* **toxic** *l.* acute serous labyrinthitis.

labyrinthotomy (lab″ĭ-rin-thot′ah-me) incision of the labyrinth.

laceration (las″ĕ-ra′shun) 1. the act of tearing. 2. a wound produced by the tearing of body tissue, as distinguished from a cut or incision. External lacerations may be small or large and may be caused in many ways, such as a blow from a blunt instrument, a fall against a rough surface, or an accident with machinery. Lacerations within the body occur when an organ is compressed or moved out of place by an external or internal force. This may result from a blow that does not penetrate the skin, and surgical repair is usually necessary.

lacertus (lah-ser′tus) [L.] a name given certain fibrous attachments of muscles.

lacrimal (lak′rĭ-mal) pertaining to tears.

l. **apparatus** a group of organs concerned with the production and drainage of tears; it is a protective device that helps keep the eye moist and free of dust and other irritating particles. The lacrimal gland, which secretes tears, lies over the upper, outer corner of the eye; its excretory ducts branch downward toward the eyeball. A constant stream of tears washes down

L

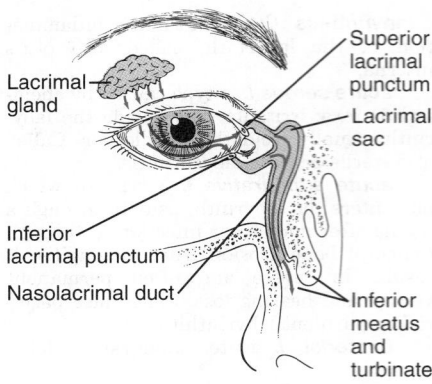

Lacrimal gland

Superior lacrimal punctum

Lacrimal sac

Inferior lacrimal punctum

Nasolacrimal duct

Inferior meatus and turbinate

The lacrimal apparatus. From Jarvis, 1996.

over the front of the eye and is drained off through two small openings located in the inner corner of the eye. Through these openings the tears pass into the lacrimal canaliculus, then through the lacrimal sac into the nasolacrimal duct and finally into the nasal cavity.

lacrimation (lak″rĭ-ma′shun) secretion and discharge of tears.

lacrimator (lak′rĭ-ma″ter) an agent, as a gas, that induces the flow of tears, usually due to local irritation of the conjunctivae.

lacrimatory (lak′rĭ-mah-tor″e) causing a flow of tears.

lacrimonasal (lak″rĭ-mo-na′zal) pertaining to the lacrimal sac and nose.

lacrimotomy (lak″rĭ-mot′ah-me) incision of the lacrimal gland, duct, or sac.

lact(o)- word element [L.], *milk.*

lactaciduria (lak-tas″ĭ-du′re-ah) lactic acid in the urine.

lactagogue (lak′tah-gog) galactagogue.

lactam (lak′tam) a cyclic amide formed from aminocarboxylic acids by elimination of water; lactams are isomeric with LACTIMS, which are their enol forms.

β-*l.* see under *antibiotic.*

β-lactamase (lak′tah-mās) either of two enzymes: β-lactamase I is penicillinase; β-lactamase II is cephalosporinase.

lactase (lak′tās) β-D-galactosidase; an enzyme in the intestinal mucosa that hydrolyzes lactose, producing glucose and galactose.

l. **deficiency** a deficiency of intestinal lactase, which causes abdominal distention and cramping and often diarrhea when milk is drunk. The condition is usually hereditary with an onset between infancy and early adulthood, and is more common in Blacks, American Indians, and East Asians (70 to 90 per cent) than in Whites (10 to 15 per cent). It may also occur secondary to massive small bowel resection or to diseases involving the mucosa, such as celiac disease, Crohn's disease, tropical sprue, and ulcerative colitis.

lactate (lak′tāt) 1. any salt of lactic acid or the anion of lactic acid. 2. to secrete milk.

lactate dehydrogenase (LD, LDH) (lak′-tāt de-hi′dro-jĕ-nās) an enzyme that catalyzes the interconversion of lactate and pyruvate. It is widespread in tissues and is particularly abundant in kidney, skeletal muscle, liver, and myocardium. It has five isoenzymes denoted LD_1 to LD_5. The "flipped" pattern in which the serum LD_1 level is greater than the LD_2 level is indicative of an acute myocardial infarction. This pattern occurs within 12 to 24 hours after the attack.

lactation (lak-ta′shun) 1. the secretion of milk by the breasts; it is thought to be brought about by action of progesterone and estrogen and specific pituitary hormones, such as lactogenic hormone (prolactin). It does not begin until at least 3 days after the birth of the baby; before that, and immediately after birth, the breast secretes COLOSTRUM. 2. the period of weeks or months during which a woman is lactating and a baby can be breast-fed; see BREASTFEEDING.

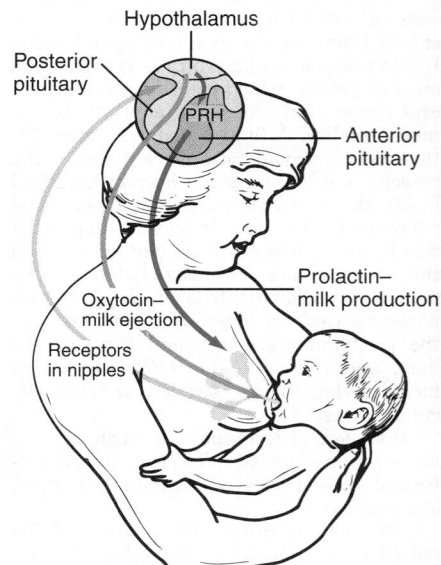

Hypothalamus

Posterior pituitary

PRH

Anterior pituitary

Oxytocin– milk ejection

Prolactin– milk production

Receptors in nipples

PRH = Prolactin-releasing hormone

Stimuli for lactation. From Applegate, 2000.

lacteal (lak'tēl) 1. pertaining to milk. 2. any of the intestinal lymphatics that transport chyle.

lactescence (lak-tes'ens) resemblance to milk.

lactic (lak'tik) pertaining to milk.

l. acid a metabolic intermediate involved in many biochemical processes; it is the end product of glycolysis, which provides energy anaerobically in skeletal muscle during heavy exercise, and it can be oxidized aerobically in the heart for energy production or can be converted back to glucose (gluconeogenesis) in the liver. Moderate elevations of blood lactate occur during heavy exercise; severe elevations (lactic acidosis) can occur in diabetes mellitus and in genetic deficiencies of enzymes involved in gluconeogenesis. Lactate is also the end product of fermentation in several bacterial species. The sodium salt of racemic or inactive lactic acid (sodium lactate) is used as an electrolyte and fluid replenisher.

lacticemia (lak"tĭ-se'me-ah) an excess of lactic acid in the blood; muscular damage is a common cause.

lactiferous (lak-tif'er-us) conveying milk.

lactifuge (lak'tĭ-fūj) antigalactic.

lactigenous (lak-tij'ĕ-nus) producing milk.

lactigerous (lak-tij'er-us) lactiferous.

lactim (lak'tim) see LACTAM.

lactitol (lak'-tĭ-tol) a disaccharide analogue of LACTULOSE, used as a sweetener; it is also laxative and is used to treat constipation.

lactivorous (lak-tiv'o-rus) feeding or subsisting upon milk.

Lactobacillus (lak"to-bah-sil'us) a genus of bacteria, some of which are considered to be etiologically related to dental caries, but are otherwise nonpathogenic. They produce lactic acid by fermentation.

lactobacillus (lak"to-bah-sil'us) any individual organism of the genus *Lactobacillus*.

lactocele (lak'to-sēl) galactocele.

lactoferrin (lak'to-fer"in) an iron-binding protein found in the granules of neutrophils where it apparently exerts an antimicrobial activity by withholding iron from ingested bacteria and fungi; it also occurs in many secretions and exudates, such as milk, tears, mucus, saliva, and bile.

lactogen (lak'to-jen) any substance that enhances lactation.

human placental l. (HPL) (hPL) a hormone secreted by the placenta, which disappears from the blood immediately after delivery. It has lactogenic, luteotropic, and growth-promoting activity, and inhibits maternal insulin activity during pregnancy.

lactogenesis (lak"to-jen'ĕ-sis) galactopoiesis.

lactogenic (lak"to-jen'ik) galactopoietic.

lactoglobulin (lak"to-glob'u-lin) a globulin occurring in milk.

immune l's antibodies (immunoglobulins) occurring in the colostrum of mammals.

lactone (lak'tōn) a cyclic organic compound in which the chain is closed by ester formation between a carboxyl and a hydroxyl group in the same molecule.

lactorrhea (lak"to-re'ah) excessive or spontaneous milk flow; persistent secretion of milk irrespective of nursing; galactorrhea.

lactose (lak'tōs) a sugar derived from the milk of mammals, which on hydrolysis yields GLUCOSE and GALACTOSE; used as a tablet and capsule diluent, a powder bulking agent, and as a component of infant feeding formulas. Many persons are intolerant to lactose as a result of hereditary deficiency of LACTASE.

lactoside (lak'to-sīd) glycoside in which the sugar constituent is lactose.

lactosuria (lak"to-su're-ah) elevated levels of lactose, as seen in lactose intolerance or during lactation.

lactotrope (lak'to-trōp") lactotroph.

lactotroph (lak'to-trōf") a type of ACIDOPHIL in the adenohypophysis that secretes PROLACTIN. Called also lactotrope, luteotroph, and mammotroph.

lactovegetarian (lak"to-vej"ĕ-tar'e-an) 1. a person who excludes from the diet all animal flesh (meats and fish), but will eat foods of vegetable origin as well as milk and milk products. 2. pertaining to such a diet.

lactulose (lak'tu-lōs) a synthetic disaccharide used as a CATHARTIC and to enhance the excretion of ammonia in treatment of hepatic ENCEPHALOPATHY.

lacuna (lah-ku'nah) [L.] 1. a small pit or hollow cavity. 2. a defect or gap, as in the field of vision (scotoma). adj., **lacu'nar.**

absorption l. resorption lacuna.

bone l. a small cavity within the bone matrix, containing an osteocyte, and from which slender canaliculi radiate and penetrate the adjacent lamellae to anastomose with the canaliculi of neighboring lacunae, thus forming a system of cavities interconnected by minute canals.

cartilage l. any of the small cavities within the cartilage matrix, containing a chondrocyte.

Howship's l. resorption lacuna.

intervillous l. one of the spaces of the placenta occupied by maternal blood, into which the fetal villi project.

L

osseous l. bone lacuna.

l. pharyn′gis a depression of the pharyngeal end of the eustachian tube.

resorption l. a pit or concavity found in bones undergoing resorption, frequently containing osteoclasts. Similar lacunae also may be found in eroding surfaces of cementum.

lacunule (lah-ku′nūl) a minute lacuna.

lacus (la′kus) [L.] lake.

l. lacrima′lis lacrimal lake.

lae- for words beginning thus, see those beginning *le-*.

Laënnec (la-nek′) René Théophile Hyacinthe (1781–1826). French physician. He is known for the invention of the stethoscope in 1819 and his *De l'auscultation médiate,* from which much of our knowledge of chest diseases is derived.

Laetrile (la′ĕ-tril) trademark for a semisynthetic derivative of amygdalin, alleged to have antineoplastic properties.

laetrile (la′ĕ-tril) AMYGDALIN derived from crushed pits of certain fruits.

Lafora's disease (lah-fo′rahz) a slowly progressive autosomal recessive form of myoclonus EPILEPSY beginning in childhood and characterized by attacks of intermittent or continuous clonus of muscle groups, resulting in difficulties in voluntary movement; there is mental deterioration, sometimes progressing to complete dementia, and the presence of Lafora's BODIES in various cells, including those of the nervous system, retina, heart, muscle, and liver.

lag (lag) 1. the time elapsing between application of a stimulus and the resulting reaction. 2. the early period after inoculation of bacteria into a culture medium, in which the growth or cell division is slow.

l. of accommodation the extent to which the eyes fail to focus accurately.

anaphase l. delayed movement during anaphase of one homologous chromosome in mitosis or of one chromatid in meiosis, so that the chromosome is not incorporated into the nucleus of one of the daughter cells; the result is one normal cell and one cell with MONOSOMY.

jet l. see JET LAG.

lageniform (lah-jen′ĭ-form) flask-shaped.

lagophthalmos (lag″of-thal′mos) inability to shut the eyes completely.

lake (lāk) 1. to undergo separation of hemoglobin from erythrocytes. 2. a circumscribed collection of fluid in a hollow or depressed cavity; see also lacuna.

lacrimal l. the triangular space at the medial angle of the eye, where the tears collect. See also LACRIMAL APPARATUS.

lal(o)- word element [Gr.], *speech; babbling.*

La Leche League (lah la′cha) a voluntary organization formed in 1957 that encourages BREASTFEEDING and offers support and guidance to nursing mothers. Local chapters may be listed in the telephone book, or their national office can be contacted by calling 1-800-LALECHE in the USA or 1-800-665-4324 in Canada. The web site for La Leche League International is http://www.lalecheleague.org.

lallation (lah-la′shun) a babbling, infantile form of speech.

lalognosis (lal″og-no′sis) the understanding of speech.

lalopathy (lah-lop′ah-the) speech disorder.

lalophobia (lal″o-fo′be-ah) irrational fear of speaking.

laloplegia (lal″o-ple′jah) logoplegia.

lalorrhea (lal″o-re′ah) logorrhea.

Lamaze method (lah-mahz′) a method of preparation for childbirth developed by the French obstetrician Fernand Lamaze, and based on the Russian psychoprophylactic technique of training the mind and body for the purpose of modifying the perception of pain during labor and delivery. The Lamaze method of prepared childbirth involves class sessions for the mother and her partner in which they learn about the birth process and the mechanisms of labor, are taught what to expect and what is expected of them during the birth of their child, and are trained in special exercises that develop neuromuscular control, promote physical conditioning, and eliminate or reduce the need for drugs and instruments during delivery. Advocates of the Lamaze method do not claim complete absence of pain during labor and delivery in every case, but they do feel that the method enriches the lives of the parents in many ways and provides for them a means of sharing the birth experience that is denied to them in the other methods of hospital deliveries.

lambda (lam′dah) 1. the eleventh letter of the Greek alphabet, or λ. 2. the point of union of the lambdoid and sagittal sutures.

lambdacism (lam′dah-sizm) inability to utter the *l* sound.

lambdoid (lam′doid) shaped like the Greek letter LAMBDA.

lame (lām) incapable of normal locomotion; deviation from the normal GAIT. See also CLAUDICATION.

lamella (lah-mel′ah) [L.] 1. a thin scale or plate, as of bone. 2. a medicated disk or wafer to be inserted under the eyelid. adj., **lamel′lar.**

circumferential l. one of the bony plates that underlie the periosteum and endosteum.

concentric l. haversian lamella.

endosteal l. one of the bony plates lying beneath the endosteum.

ground l. interstitial lamella.

haversian l. one of the concentric bony plates surrounding a haversian canal.

intermediate l., interstitial l. one of the bony plates that fill in between the haversian systems.

lamellipodia (lah-mel″ĭ-po′de-ah), sing. *lamellipo′dium.* Delicate sheetlike extensions of cytoplasm that form transient adhesions with the cell substrate and wave gently, enabling the cell to move along the substrate.

lamina (lam′ĭ-nah) [L.] 1. a thin, flat PLATE or STRATUM of a composite structure; called also layer. 2. vertebral lamina.

basal l., l. basa′lis the layer of the basement MEMBRANE lying next to the basal surface of the adjoining cell layer composed of an electron-dense LAMINA DENSA and an electron-lucent LAMINA LUCIDA.

l. basila′ris the posterior wall of the cochlear DUCT, separating it from the scala tympani.

l. choroidocapilla′ris the inner layer of the choroid, composed of a single-layered network of small capillaries.

l. cribro′sa 1. fascia cribrosa. 2. (of ethmoid bone) the horizontal plate of ethmoid bone forming the roof of the nasal cavity, and perforated by many foramina for passage of olfactory nerves. 3. (of sclera) the perforated part of the sclera through which pass the axons of the retinal ganglion cells.

l. den′sa an electron-dense layer of the basal lamina, consisting mainly of collagen fibrils and proteoglycans; it closely follows the plasma membrane of the basal aspect of the adjacent cell layer, from which it is separated by the LAMINA LUCIDA (or the LAMINA RARA in the renal glomerulus and pulmonary alveolus).

l. du′ra a layer of the alveolar bone that is thin and particularly compact and appears as a line on dental x-rays. Called also bundle bone.

epithelial l. the layer of ependymal cells covering the choroid plexus.

l. fus′ca the pigmentary layer of the sclera.

l. lu′cida an electron-dense layer of the basal LAMINA lying between the LAMINA DENSA and the adjoining cell layer; in the pulmonary alveolus and renal glomerulus it is divided into the internal and external LAMINAE RARAE.

l. pro′pria 1. the connective tissue layer of mucous membrane. 2. the middle fibrous layer of the tympanic membrane.

l. ra′ra 1. in the renal glomerulus and pulmonary alveolus, one of the layers of LAMINA LUCIDA surrounding the LAMINA DENSA; the *lamina rara externa* is on the epithelial side and the *lamina rara interna* is on the endothelial side. 2. a term sometimes used as a synonym for LAMINA LUCIDA.

reticular l. a layer of the basement MEMBRANE, adjacent to the connective tissue, seen in some epithelia; it is of variable thickness and is composed of condensed connective tissue with a reticulum of collagen fibers.

Rexed's laminae an architectural scheme used to classify the structure of the spinal cord, based on the cytological features of the neurons in different regions of the gray substance. It consists of nine laminae (I–IX) that extend throughout the cord, roughly paralleling the dorsal and ventral columns of the gray substance, and a tenth region (lamina X) that surrounds the central canal and consists of the dorsal and ventral commissures and the central gelatinous substance.

spiral l., l. spira′lis 1. a double plate of bone winding spirally around the modiolus, dividing the spiral canal of the cochlea into the scala tympani and scala vestibuli. 2. a bony projection on the outer wall of the cochlea in the lower part of the first turn.

terminal l. of hypothalamus the thin plate derived from the telencephalon, forming the anterior wall of the third ventricle of the cerebrum.

vertebral l., l. of vertebral arch either of the pair of broad plates of bone flaring out from the PEDICLES OF THE VERTEBRAL ARCHES and fusing together at the midline to complete the dorsal part of the arch and provide a base for the spinous PROCESS of the vertebra.

laminagraphy (lam″ĭ-nag′rah-fe) a special technique of body-section ROENTGENOGRAPHY.

laminaplasty (lam′in-ah-plas″te) incision completely through one lamina of a vertebral arch with creation of a trough in the contralateral lamina; the vertebral arch is then opened like a door, with the trough acting as a hinge; performed to relieve compression of the spinal cord or nerve roots.

laminar (lam′ĭ-nar) made up of laminae or layers; pertaining to a lamina.

l. flow hood a device that separates the air flowing through it into layers, cleansing the air of microorganisms. It is used to protect patients with compromised immune systems and is also used in operating rooms and pharmacies to provide a clean environment.

laminated (lam′ĭ-nāt″ed) made up of laminae or thin layers.

lamination (lam″ĭ-na′shun) a laminar structure or arrangement.

laminectomy (lam″ĭ-nek′to-me) surgical excision of the LAMINA OF A VERTEBRAL ARCH, usually done to relieve the symptoms of a HERNIATED DISK by disk excision. The spinal canal is exposed and the portion of the nucleus pulposus that has herniated through the ruptured disk is removed. This is indicated when conservative treatment is not effective and nerve damage is becoming progressively worse or when the patient is suffering from repeated attacks of leg pain. Laminectomy is sometimes followed by spinal FUSION in the area to stabilize that part of the spinal column. Bone grafts, usually taken from the iliac crest, are applied to fuse the affected vertebrae permanently, resulting in limitation of movement of this portion of the spine. Laminectomy is also performed for adequate visualization for the removal of an intervertebral or spinal cord tumor.

Patient Care. Prior to surgery the procedure and its expected outcome are explained to the patient and family. Patients will also need to know about intravenous fluids, a urinary catheter, and any other devices that may be used postoperatively. In most cases postlaminectomy patients are allowed out of bed one to three days after surgery. A back brace may be prescribed for spinal fusion patients when they are standing and walking. Fluids by mouth are usually allowed after bowel sounds reappear, which should be one to three days postoperatively.

Patients with this type of surgery have experienced significant long-term pain before surgery and may be apprehensive about perioperative pain, or they may expect to be completely free of discomfort after surgery. They should know that there probably will be some discomfort and that analgesic medications will be given promptly when requested.

Immediately after surgery the vital signs are noted and recorded and level of consciousness assessed. Peripheral pulses are palpated, and color, range of motion, temperature, and sensation in the feet and toes are checked. Dressings are checked for unusual drainage. Evidence of spinal fluid leakage on the dressing is immediately reported. Patients who have had a spinal fusion will have two dressings, one at the spinal column where the affected disk is located and one at the iliac crest where bone was removed for the graft.

The patient is assessed frequently and regularly for pain. In general, patients with laminectomies have less pain after than before surgery because pressure on the nerve root has been relieved. In contrast, those who have had spinal fusion often experience more postoperative pain at both operative sites. In keeping with the preoperative promise of prompt response to a request for relief, analgesics are given as needed. Transcutaneous electrical nerve stimulation (TENS) may be prescribed to provide relief and facilitate ambulation and recovery.

Positioning after surgery will depend on the preference of the surgeon. In general, the patient's head is not raised beyond a 45-degree angle. This avoids placing a strain on the lumbar region. Log-rolling spinal fusion patients while they are in bed prevents twisting of the spine and nonsetting or failure of the fusion. When these patients are allowed up they are instructed to avoid sudden movements and twisting of the spine. They also must wear lumbar orthoses to stabilize the spine when walking. They should be watched for orthostatic hypotension, which can occur if sympathetic nerves were traumatized during surgery.

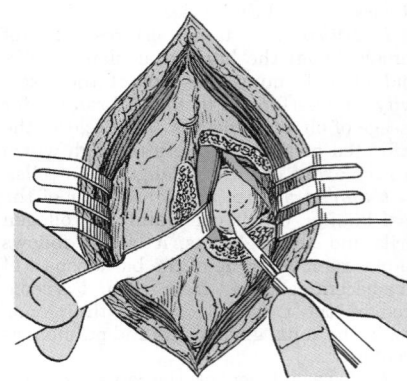

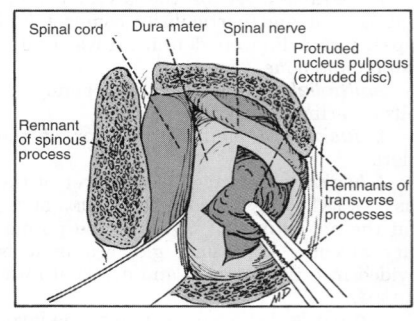

Laminectomy for the interlaminal removal of a herniated disk. From Polaski and Tatro, 1996.

Physical therapy and exercises to strengthen abdominal, back, and leg muscles are begun as soon as permitted by the surgeon. These usually are carried out under the direction of a physical therapist. Several months of rehabilitation and recuperation are usually needed to completely rehabilitate the spinal fusion patient. Patients who have had a diskectomy or laminectomy typically return to sedentary work in one month. If lifting or manual labor are necessary on the job, the patient should be able to resume work in three to six months.

laminotomy (lam″ĭ-not′ah-me) transection of a vertebral lamina.

lamivudine (lah-miv′u-dēn) a nucleoside ANALOGUE that inhibits reverse TRANSCRIPTASE and is used as an ANTIVIRAL agent in treatment of HEPATITIS B infection and, in combination with ZIDOVUDINE, in treatment of HIV infection and AIDS. Administered orally

lamotrigine (lah-mo′trĭ-jēn) an ANTICONVULSIVE used in treatment of certain forms of EPILEPSY.

lamp (lamp) an apparatus for furnishing heat or light.

    Gullstrand's slit l. an apparatus for projecting a narrow flat beam of intense light into the eye. See also slit lamp.

    slit l. one embodying a diaphragm containing a slitlike opening, by means of which a narrow, flat beam of intense light may be projected into the eye. It gives intense illumination so that microscopic study may be made of the conjunctiva, cornea, iris, lens, and vitreous, the special feature being that it illuminates a section through the substance of these structures.

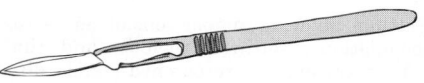

Lancet. From Dorland's, 2000.

    sun l., ultraviolet l. an electric light that transmits ULTRAVIOLET RAYS; used as a therapeutic device and as a means of obtaining an artificial suntan. See also ULTRAVIOLET THERAPY.

lamprophonia (lam″pro-fo′ne-ah) clearness of voice.

lanatoside C (lah-nat′o-sīd) a glycoside obtained from *Digitalis lanata,* with CARDIOTONIC uses similar to those of DIGITALIS.

lance (lans) 1. lancet. 2. to cut or incise with a lancet or similar instrument.

Lancefield classification (lans′fēld) the classification of hemolytic streptococci into groups on the basis of serologic action; there are currently 18 groups. Most of the infection-causing streptococci are in Group A.

lanceolate (lan′se-o-lát) shaped like a small blade or lance.

lancet (lan′set) a small, pointed, two-edged surgical knife.

lancinating (lan″sĭ-nāt″ing) tearing, darting, or sharply cutting; used to describe pain.

language (lang′gwij) 1. the use of a meaningful pattern of vocal sounds (or corresponding written symbols) to convey thoughts and feelings, or a system of such patterns that is understood by a group of people. 2. by extension, any of various other systems of communication that use sets of discrete symbols. 3. any of numerous sets of standardized vocabulary terms for use among health care providers in a variety of

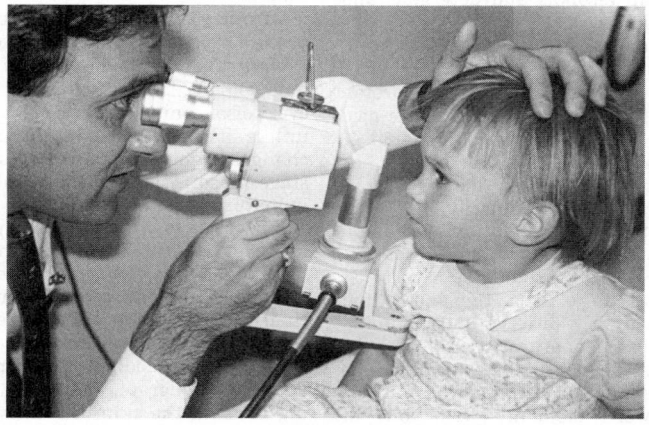

Examiner using hand-held slit lamp. (Photography by Leslie MacKeen.) From Stein et al., 2000.

settings allowing comparisons of care across populations, settings, regions, and time. There are over 30 researched standardized health care languages. Called also standardized vocabulary.

body l. the expression of thoughts or emotions by means of posture or gesture.

International Sign L. a sign language composed of a blending of vocabulary signs from numerous different countries, sometimes used at international meetings and events of DEAF persons; formerly called Gestuno.

natural l. ordinary language as used by the speakers of that language, as opposed to a language made up for a special purpose (as for use by a computer system).

nursing l. any of various sets of standardized terms and definitions for use in nursing to provide standardized descriptions, labels, and definitions for expressing the phenomena of nursing; some include category groupings of terms. The American Nurses Association has recognized twelve official languages.

lanolin (lan′o-lin) wool fat or wool grease that is refined and incorporated into many commercial preparations. Lanolin is a by-product of the process that accompanies the removal of sheep's wool from the pelt. In its crude form it is a greasy yellow wax of unpleasant odor. This odor disappears when the lanolin is emulsified and made into salves, creams, ointments, and cosmetics. Although lanolin is slightly antiseptic, it has no other medicinal benefits and is valuable principally because of the ease with which it penetrates the skin, and because it does not turn rancid. Modified lanolin has been additionally processed to reduce the amount of free lanolin alcohols and detergent and pesticide residues.

Lanoxin (lah-nok′sin) trademark for preparations of DIGOXIN, a CARDIOTONIC.

lansoprazole (lan-so′prah-zōl) a proton pump INHIBITOR used to inhibit gastric acid secretion for the treatment of duodenal or gastric ULCER, GASTROESOPHAGEAL REFLUX DISEASE, or other conditions due to gastric hyperacidity; administered orally.

lanthanum (La) (lan′thah-num) a chemical element, atomic number 57, atomic weight 138.91. (See Appendix 6.)

lanugo (lah-nu′go) the fine hair that covers the body of the fetus and begins to disappear during maturation so that by nine months' gestation it is usually seen only on the shoulders of the newborn.

lapar(o)- word element [Gr.], *loin* or *flank; abdomen.*

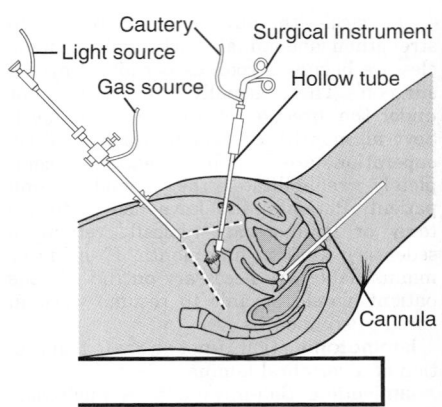

Laparoscopy. From Frazier et al., 2000.

laparohysterectomy (lap″ah-ro-his″ter-ek′tah-me) abdominal hysterectomy.

laparohysterotomy (lap″ah-ro-his″ter-ot′ah-me) abdominal hysterotomy.

laparorrhaphy (lap″ah-ror′ah-fe) suture or repair of the abdominal wall.

laparoscope (lap′ah-ro-skōp″) an endoscope for examining the peritoneal cavity; called also celioscope.

laparoscopy (lap″ah-ros′kah-pe) examination by means of the laparoscope; called also celioscopy. adj., **laparoscop′ic.**

laparotomy (lap″ah-rot′ah-me) incision through the abdominal wall.

laparotrachelotomy (lap″ah-ro-tra″kĕ-lot′ah-me) low cervical cesarean section, in which the lower uterine segment is incised.

lapinization (lap″in-ī-za′shun) serial passage of a virus or vaccine through rabbits to modify its characteristics.

lapinize (lap″in-īz) to attenuate (as a virus or vaccine) by serial passage through rabbits.

Larotid (lar′o-tid) trademark for a preparation of AMOXICILLIN, an ANTIBIOTIC.

larva (lahr′vah), pl. *lar′vae* [L.] 1. an independent, immature stage in the life cycle of an animal, in which it is markedly unlike the parent and must undergo changes in form and size to reach the adult stage. 2. something that resembles such an immature animal.

l. cur′rens a rapidly progressive creeping ERUPTION caused by autoinoculation of larvae of *Strongyloides stercoralis* that migrate to and mature at the anus in intestinal infections with the parasite.

cutaneous l. mi′grans, l. mi′grans a convoluted threadlike skin eruption that appears to migrate, caused by the burrowing beneath the skin of roundworm larvae, particularly of the species *Ancylostoma*;

similar lesions are caused by the larvae of BOTFLIES. Called also creeping eruption.

ocular l. migrans infection of the eye with larvae of the roundworm *Toxocara canis* or *T. cati,* which may lodge in the choroid or retina or migrate to the vitreous; on the death of the larvae, a granulomatous inflammation occurs, the lesion varying from a translucent elevation of the retina to massive retinal detachment and pseudoglioma.

visceral l. migrans a condition due to prolonged migration by the skin larvae of animal nematodes in human tissue other than skin; commonly caused by larvae of the roundworms *Toxocara canis* and *T. cati.*

larval (lahr′val) 1. pertaining to larvae. 2. larvate.

larvate (lahr′vāt) masked; concealed: said of a disease or of a symptom of a disease.

larvicide (lahr′vĭ-sīd) an agent that kills insect larvae.

laryng(o)- word element [Gr.], *larynx.*

laryngalgia (lar″in-gal′jah) pain in the larynx.

laryngeal (lah-rin′je-al) pertaining to the larynx.

laryngectomee (lar″in-jek′to-me) a person whose larynx has been removed.

laryngectomy (lar″in-jek′to-me) partial or total removal of the LARYNX by surgery. It is usually performed as treatment for cancer of the larynx. Depending on the type of surgical procedure, the patient's speech may change in quality or be lost entirely. Speech THERAPY is thus an important component of the treatment plan. There are three methods of speaking without use of the larynx. Esophageal speech is one method the patient may learn. The patient is taught to trap air in the esophagus. As an alternative to laryngeal voice, air vibrates the upper esophagus, providing a usable sound for speech. The patient modifies this sound into words by moving lips, tongue, and jaw.

An artificial LARYNX is a battery-operated device that projects sound into the oral cavity when words are formed. The tracheoesophageal PUNCTURE is a newer technique that is now widely used. It consists of a valve being placed in the tracheal stoma to permit air to be diverted into the esophagus and out through the mouth, with placement of a voice prosthesis to allow speech.

Patient Care. Because of the physical and emotional adjustments that patients and their families must make to the surgical procedure and its aftermath, it is especially important that they receive instruction and counseling prior to surgery. They will need help in coping with their fears and anxieties

about the patient's ability to communicate after surgery, and they must know that the members of the health care team are available to listen to them uncritically and answer their questions honestly. Patients should be given an explanation about the type of equipment to be used in the immediate postoperative period and the purpose of each procedure. They are assured that a pencil and paper or other means of communicating by writing will be at the bedside at all times after surgery and that they will not be left without some means of summoning help. It is understandable that one of the greatest fears of these patients is that, since they will be unable to cry out or speak, they will be left alone and might suffocate.

There is some justification for a patient's fear of suffocation; this is the major hazard during the immediate postoperative period. Turning, coughing, and deep breathing are important in maintaining a patent airway. Suctioning may be required, and humidification is also important. An extra tracheostomy tube is kept at the bedside in case an emergency arises and for daily changing of the outer tube if the surgeon so chooses. After a variable period of time, the tracheostomy tube may be removed permanently. Feedings usually begin at 1 to 2 weeks.

In preparation for discharge, patients are taught self-care of their laryngectomy. They are warned against aspirating water into the lungs during bathing or showering. Although a dressing is not necessary for covering the tracheal opening in the neck, the patient may wish to conceal it with a small square of cotton material or wear a collar or scarf of porous material to hide the wound. These types of covering are useful in that they act as filters and remove dust and other irritants from the air being inhaled through the stoma.

Printed material about self-care is available from the local Cancer Society. Many communities have a laryngectomee club, which offers much moral support and information that are valuable to patients and families during the period of adjustment. Information regarding these laryngectomee clubs and other aspects of postlaryngectomy rehabilitation can be obtained by writing to the American Speech Language Hearing Association, 10801 Rockville Pike, Department AP, Rockville, MD 20852; telephone (301) 897–5700.

laryngemphraxis (lar″in-jem-frak′sis) obstruction or closure of the larynx.

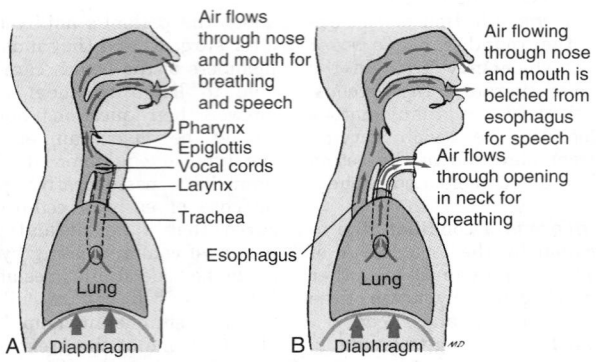

A, Prior to laryngectomy, air flow is through the nose and mouth. B, Surgical removal of the larynx requires that a new opening be made for air passage. The trachea and esophagus are separated. From Polaski and Tatro, 1996.

laryngismus (lar″in-jiz′mus) spasm of the larynx. adj., **laryngis′mal.**

l. stri′dulus sudden laryngeal spasm with crowing inhalations, usually seen in children at night; called also pseudocroup.

laryngitis (lar″in-ji′tis) inflammation of the mucous membrane of the larynx, characterized by dryness and soreness of the throat, hoarseness, cough, and dysphagia.

Acute Laryngitis. Acute laryngitis may be caused by overuse of the voice, allergies, irritating dust or smoke, hot or corrosive liquids, or even violent weeping. It also occurs in viral or bacterial infections, and is frequently associated with other diseases of the respiratory tract. In adults, a mild case begins with a dry, tickling sensation in the larynx, followed quickly by partial or complete loss of the voice. There may be a slight fever, minor discomfort, and poor appetite, with recovery after a few days. Other more uncomfortable symptoms can include a feeling of heat and pain in the throat, difficulty in swallowing, and dry cough followed by expectoration; the voice may be either painful to use or absent. Swelling of the larynx and epiglottis may impair breathing. Increasing difficulty in breathing may be a sign of edematous laryngitis, or CROUP.

Treatment requires that the patient refrain from talking. The room temperature should be steady and warm. The air is kept moist with a humidifier or vaporizer. An ice bag on the throat often is soothing. In some cases, antibiotics may be necessary.

Children are especially vulnerable to laryngitis because of the smallness of their air passages. Most cases in children subside within a few days, but if inflammation and swelling continue to increase, severe dyspnea occurs.

Chronic Laryngitis. After repeated attacks of the acute type, chronic laryngitis may develop. This is caused mostly by continual irritation from overuse of the voice, tobacco smoke, dust, or chemical vapors, or by a chronic nasal or sinus disorder. Often the moist mucous membrane lining the larynx becomes granulated. The granulation can proceed to thickening and hardening of the mucous membrane, which changes the voice or makes it hoarse. There is little or no pain, though there may be tickling in the throat and a slight cough. Chronic laryngitis that has persisted for a number of years may result in chronic hypertrophic laryngitis, a condition in which there is a permanent change in the voice because of hypertrophy of the membrane lining the larynx.

Treatment for chronic laryngitis is the same as for the acute form, with elimination of all sources of irritation and reinfection. Hoarseness that lasts longer than 2 weeks may be a warning of tumor or cancer of the larynx, or of a tumor in the thorax that presses on the recurrent laryngeal nerve, which controls the larynx.

Other Forms of Laryngitis. Paroxysmal laryngitis is a nervous disorder affecting infants that seems to be associated with enlarged adenoids and rickets. It consists of unexplained spasms in which the larynx closes, cutting off the air passage, and then suddenly opens. Sometimes the condition may be fatal. Treatment of this form of laryngitis calls for removal of adenoids.

Other types include diphtheritic laryngitis, tuberculous laryngitis, traumatic laryngitis, and allergic laryngitis. Treatment of diphtheritic and traumatic laryngitis often involves intubation or tracheostomy in order to admit air. Allergic laryngitis, often caused by smoking or other irritants, is treated in the same way as other allergies.

laryngocele (lah-ring′go-sēl) a congenital anomalous air sac communicating with a cavity of the larynx; it may produce a tumorlike lesion visible on the outside of the neck.

laryngocentesis (lah-ring″go-sen-te′sis) surgical puncture of the larynx, with aspiration.

laryngofissure (lah-ring″go-fish′er) median laryngotomy.

laryngogram (lah-ring′go-gram) a radiograph of the larynx.

laryngography (lar″ing-gog′rah-fe) radiography of the larynx.

laryngology (lar″ing-gol′o-je) the branch of medicine that deals with the throat, pharynx, larynx, nasopharynx, and tracheobronchial tree.

laryngopathy (lar″ing-gop′ah-the) any disorder of the larynx.

laryngophantom (lah-ring″go-fan′tom) an artificial model of the larynx.

laryngopharyngeal (lah-ring″go-fah-rin′je-al) pertaining to the larynx and pharynx.

laryngopharyngectomy (lah-ring″go-far″in-jek′to-me) excision of the larynx and pharynx.

laryngopharyngitis (lah-ring″go-far″in-ji′tis) inflammation of the larynx and pharynx.

laryngopharynx (lah-ring″go-far′ingks) the portion of the pharynx below the upper edge of the epiglottis, opening into the larynx and esophagus.

laryngophony (lar″ing-gof′o-ne) a voice SOUND heard over the larynx.

laryngoplasty (lah-ring′go-plas″te) plastic repair of the larynx.

laryngoplegia (lah-ring″go-ple′jah) paralysis of the larynx.

laryngoptosis (lah-ring″go-to′sis) a lowering and mobilization of the larynx, as sometimes seen in the aged.

laryngoscleroma (lah-ring″go-skle-ro′mah) scleroma of the larynx.

laryngoscope (lah-ring′go-skōp) an endoscope equipped with a light and mirrors for illumination and examination of the larynx.

laryngoscopy (lar″ing-gos′kah-pe) visual examination of the LARYNX with a LARYNGOSCOPE. With *direct* visualization, the patient is given a mild sedative to promote relaxation, because the procedure, though not uncomfortable, may be frightening and exhausting. Immediately before insertion of the laryngoscope, the throat is anesthetized

locally with cocaine spray. Following the procedure, fluids and foods are withheld until the effects of the anesthetic have worn off and the gag REFLEX has returned. Visualization may also be *indirect,* which means examination is done by observation of the reflection of the larynx in a laryngeal mirror. adj., **laryngoscop′ic.**

laryngospasm (lah-ring′go-spazm) spasmodic closure of the larynx.

laryngostenosis (lah-ring″go-stĕ-no′sis) narrowing or stricture of the larynx.

laryngostomy (lar″ing-gos′tah-me) surgical creation of an artificial opening into the larynx.

laryngotomy (lar″ing-got′ah-me) incision of the larynx.

inferior l. incision of the larynx through the lower part of the fibroelastic membrane of the larynx (cricothyroid membrane).

median l. incision of the larynx through the thyroid cartilage; called also thyrotomy and thyroidotomy.

subhyoid l., superior l. incision of the larynx through the fibroelastic membrane attached to the hyoid bone and the thyroid cartilage (thyrohyoid membrane).

laryngotracheal (lah-ring″go-tra′ke-al) pertaining to the larynx and trachea; called also tracheolaryngeal.

laryngotracheitis (lah-ring″go-tra″ke-i′tis) inflammation of the larynx and trachea.

laryngotracheobronchitis (lah-ring″go-tra″ke-o-brong-ki′tis) inflammation of the larynx, trachea, and bronchi; an acute form is the most common cause of CROUP.

laryngotracheotomy (lah-ring″go-tra″ke-ot′ah-me) incision of the larynx and trachea.

larynx (lar′ingks) [Gr.] the muscular and cartilaginous structure, lined with mucous membrane, situated at the top of the trachea and below the root of the tongue and the hyoid bone; it contains the VOCAL CORDS and is the source of the sound heard in speech. The larynx is part of the respiratory SYSTEM; air passes through it traveling from the pharynx to the trachea on its way to the lungs and again returning to the exterior.

The larynx is composed of nine cartilages that are held together by muscles and ligament: the single thyroid, cricoid, and epiglottic cartilages and the paired arytenoid, corniculate, and cuneiform cartilages. (See also color plates.) The largest of these, the thyroid cartilage, forms the Adam's apple, which protrudes in the front of the neck. Two flexible vocal cords reach from

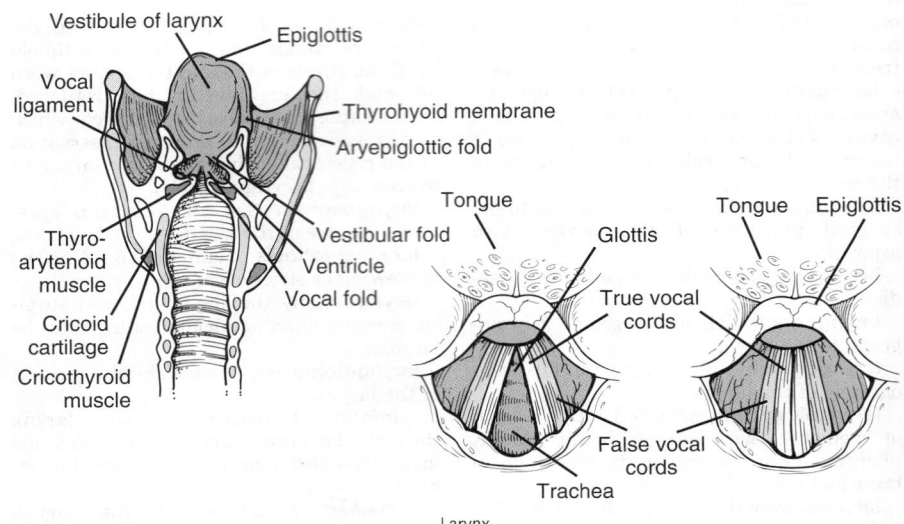

Larynx.

the back to the front wall of the larynx and are manipulated by small muscles to produce sound. The epiglottis, a flap or lid at the base of the tongue, closes the larynx as it is lifted up during swallowing and so prevents passage of food or drink into the larynx and trachea.

artificial l. an electromechanical device that enables a person after LARYNGECTOMY to produce speech. When the device is placed against the region of the laryngectomy a buzzing sound is made that can be converted into simulated speech by movements of the lips, tongue, and glottis. Called also electrolarynx.

LAS lymphangioscintigraphy.

Lasègue's sign (lah-segz′) in SCIATICA, aggravation of pain in the lower limb and back elicited by passive raising of the heel from the bed with the knee straight; no pain is produced when the knee is flexed.

laser (la′zer) a device that transfers light of various frequencies into an extremely intense, small, and nearly nondivergent beam of monochromatic radiation in the visible or invisible spectrum, with all the waves in phase; capable of mobilizing immense heat and power when focused at close range, lasers act on tissues by PHOTOCOAGULATION and PHOTODISRUPTION and are used in surgery, in diagnosis, and in physiological studies.

argon l. a laser with ionized argon as the active medium and with a beam in the blue and green visible light spectrum; used for PHOTOCOAGULATION.

carbon-dioxide l. a laser with carbon dioxide gas as the active medium and that produces infrared radiation at 10,600 nm; used to excise and incise tissue and to vaporize.

excimer l. [*exci*ted di*mer*] a laser with rare gas halides as the active medium, used in ophthalmological procedures and ANGIOPLASTY. The beam is in the ultraviolet spectrum and penetrates tissues only a small distance; it breaks chemical bonds instead of generating heat to destroy tissue.

holmium:YAG l. a laser whose active medium is a crystal of yttrium, aluminum, and garnet DOPED with holmium ions, and whose beam is in the near infrared spectrum at 2100 nm; used for PHOTOCOAGULATION and PHOTOABLATION.

neodymium:yttrium-aluminum-garnet (Nd:YAG) l. a laser whose active medium is a crystal of yttrium, aluminum, and garnet DOPED with neodymium ions, and whose beam is in the near infrared spectrum at approximately 1060 nm; used for PHOTOCOAGULATION and PHOTOABLATION.

LASIK laser-assisted in-situ keratomileusis.

Lasix (la′ziks) trademark for preparations of FUROSEMIDE, a diuretic.

Lassa fever (las′ah) a highly fatal acute type of HEMORRHAGIC FEVER caused by a virulent ARENAVIRUS, occurring in West Africa, and characterized by progressive prostration, sore throat, ulcerations of the mouth or throat, rash, and general aches and pains, which may be followed by serous effusions, generalized hemorrhages, and fatal shock.

lassitude (las′ĭ-tood) weakness; exhaustion.

latanoprost (lah-tan′o-prost″) an agent applied topically to the conjunctiva in treatment of open-angle GLAUCOMA and ocular hypertension.

latency (la′ten-se) 1. a state of seeming inactivity or being LATENT. 2. the time between the instant of stimulation and the beginning of a response. 3. latency STAGE.

latent (la′tent) dormant or concealed; not manifest; potential.

laterad (lat′er-ad) toward the lateral aspect.

lateral (lat′er-al) 1. denoting a position farther from the median plane or midline of the body or a structure. 2. pertaining to a side.

lateralis (lat″er-a′lis) [L.] lateral.

laterality (lat″er-al′ĭ-te) a tendency to use preferentially in voluntary motor acts the parts along one side of the body, such as the ear, eye, hand, or leg; see also DEXTRALITY, SINISTRALITY, and HANDEDNESS.

crossed l. the preferential use of contralateral members of the different pairs of organs in voluntary motor acts, e.g., right eye and left hand.

dominant l. the preferential use of ipsilateral members of the different pairs of organs in voluntary motor acts, e.g., right (dextrality) or left (sinistrality) ear, eye, hand, and leg.

lateroduction (lat″er-o-duk′shun) movement of an eye or limb to one side.

lateroflexion (lat″er-o-flek′shun) flexion to one side.

laterotorsion (lat″er-o-tor′shun) turning of the eyeball to the left or right on its anteroposterior axis.

lateroversion (lat″er-o-ver′zhun) abnormal turning to one side.

latex (la′teks) [L. "fluid"] 1. any of various white viscid fluids secreted by certain plants; the variety from *Hevea brasiliensis,* the rubber tree, was formerly

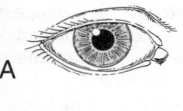
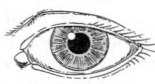

A

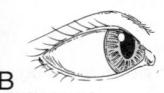
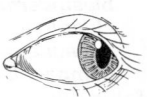

B

Forward gaze *A* contrasted with laterotorsion *B*. From Dorland's, 2000.

the main source of commercial rubber. Allergic reactions to natural latex are an important cause of type IV HYPERSENSITIVITY REACTIONS. See also latex ALLERGY. 2. any of several synthetic fluids resembling natural latex, including POLYSTYRENE and POLYVINYL CHLORIDE; these are not causes of latex ALLERGY.

l. agglutination test, l. fixation test a diagnostic study used to detect certain antibodies in body fluids; latex particles are used as passive carriers, and particles clump together following the addition of the antibody. One use is as a serologic test for rheumatoid FACTOR in diagnosis of rheumatoid ARTHRITIS.

lathyrism (lath′ĭ-rizm) a morbid condition caused by ingestion of the seeds of leguminous plants of the genus *Lathyrus,* which includes many kinds of peas; characteristics include spastic paraplegia, pain, hyperesthesia, and paresthesias. Chronic exposure is associated with dissecting ANEURYSMS due to the adverse effect on COLLAGEN formation. Fatal lathyrism has been seen in rats and nonhuman primates. adj., **lathyrit′ic.**

latissimus (lah-tis′ĭ-mus) [L.] widest; in anatomy, denoting a broad structure.

latitude (lat′ĭ-tood) the recording capability of x-ray film.

contrast l. the ability of a film to record differences in density.

film l. the ability of an emulsion to record a wide range of densities.

latrodectism (lat″ro-dek′tizm) the morbid condition caused by the venomous bite of spiders of the genus *Latrodectus;* see SPIDER BITE.

Latrodectus (lat″ro-dek′tus) a genus of poisonous spiders. *L. mac′tans* is the black widow spider. See also SPIDER BITE.

L. mac′tans a species found in the United States; commonly known as the black widow. Its bite may cause severe symptoms or even death. (For first aid, see SPIDER BITE.)

LATS (lats) long-acting thyroid stimulator.

LATS protector an antibody found in HYPERTHYROID patients with the capacity to block the LONG-ACTING THYROID STIMULATOR (LATS) from combining with thyroid MICROSOMES.

latus[1] (la′tus) [L.] broad, wide.

latus[2] (la′tus) [L.] the side or flank.

Launois' syndrome (lo-nwah′) pituitary GIGANTISM.

Laurence-Moon-Biedl syndrome (law′-rens moon′ be′d′l) a hereditary autosomal recessive syndrome characterized by obesity, HYPOGENITALISM, RETINITIS PIGMENTOSA, mental retardation, skull defects, and sometimes webbed FINGERS or TOES.

laureth-9 (law′reth) a compound used as a SPERMICIDE, SURFACTANT, and sclerosing AGENT.

lavage (lah-vahzh′) 1. irrigation or washing out of an organ or cavity, as of the stomach or intestine. 2. to wash out, or irrigate.

bronchoalveolar l. a technique by which cells and fluid from bronchioles and lung alveoli are removed for diagnosis of disease or evaluation of treatment; a bronchoscope is wedged into a bronchus and sterile saline is pumped in and then removed along with the fluid and cells to be analyzed.

Lavoisier (lah-vwah-zya′) Antoine Laurent (1743–1794). French chemist, born in Paris and later guillotined by the French Revolutionists. Lavoisier demolished the phlogiston theory (a theory of combustion) and explained the true nature of respiration by his introduction of quantitative relations in chemistry. He was secretary and treasurer of a committee seeking the uniformity of weights and measures in France, which led to the establishment of the metric system.

law (law) a uniform or constant fact or principle. For specific named laws, see under the name.

l. of independent assortment the members of gene pairs segregate independently during meiosis; see also MENDEL'S LAWS.

inverse square l. the intensity of radiation is inversely proportional to the square of the distance from the source of radiation.

l. of segregation in each generation the ratio of (a) pure dominants, (b) dominants giving descendants in the proportion of three dominants to one recessive, and (c) pure recessives is 1:2:1. This ratio follows from the fact that the two alleles of a gene cannot be a part of a single gamete, but must segregate to different gametes. See also MENDEL'S LAWS.

lawrencium (Lw) (law-ren′se-um) a chemical element, atomic number 103, atomic weight 257. (See Appendix 6.)

laxative (lak′sah-tiv) a medicine that loosens the bowel contents and encourages evacuation. One with a mild or gentle effect is also known as an APERIENT; one with a strong effect is referred to as a CATHARTIC or PURGATIVE. Bland laxatives may be used temporarily in treatment of CONSTIPATION along with other measures. MINERAL OIL and olive oil act as lubricants; sometimes mineral oil is used in combination with AGAR, which is bulk-producing. CASCARA SAGRADA aromatic fluid extract and MILK OF MAGNESIA are two other mild laxatives. Psyllium hydrophilic MUCILLOID, a preparation from a plant seed, helps elimination by encouraging peristaltic movements. Saline purges, such as SODIUM PHOSPHATE and MAGNESIUM SULFATE (Epsom salt), flush the intestinal tract by preventing the intestines from absorbing water; evacuation takes place as soon as water accumulates. CASTOR OIL is a strong cathartic that causes complete evacuation of the bowels. Its administration is followed by temporary constipation.

Dangers of Laxatives. Laxatives should be used only with the advice of a health care provider. Constipation may be a symptom of serious organic illness as well as the result of improper diet and habits. Also, laxatives taken regularly tend to deprive the colon of its natural muscle tone and thus can be the cause of chronic constipation rather than its cure. Mineral oil taken regularly interferes with the absorption of certain vitamins, especially those that are fat soluble. It can also seep into the lungs, causing a reaction resembling PNEUMONIA, especially in older people. Purgative salts can produce DEHYDRATION. Laxatives that produce bulk may cause stonelike balls (BEZOARS) to develop. A strong cathartic such as castor oil can have fatal results if used when there is nausea, vomiting, abdominal pain, or other symptoms of APPENDICITIS. It is also dangerous to use during pregnancy. Children cannot use as large dosages or as strong laxatives as adults.

laxator (lak-sa′ter) that which slackens or relaxes.

layer (la′er) a thin, flat PLATE or STRATUM of a composite structure; called also lamina.

ameloblastic l. the inner layer of cells of the enamel organ, which forms the enamel prisms of the teeth.

abrasion l. a protective covering of gelatin enclosing an emulsion on x-ray film; called also overcoat.

bacillary l. layer of rods and cones.

basal l. of endometrium the deepest layer of the uterine ENDOMETRIUM; it provides the regenerative endometrium after menstrual loss of the functional LAYER.

basal l. of epidermis stratum basale.

blastodermic l. germ layer.

clear l. stratum lucidum.

columnar l. mantle layer.

compact l. of endometrium a sublayer of the functional LAYER of endometrium, which faces the lumen of the uterus and contains the necks of the uterine GLANDS.

enamel l. the outermost layer of cells of the enamel organ.

functional l. of endometrium the layer of ENDOMETRIUM facing the lumen of the uterus; its cells are cast off at menstruation and childbirth. Sublayers are the compact LAYER and the spongy LAYER. It is known as the DECIDUA during pregnancy.

ganglionic l. of cerebellum the thin middle gray layer of the cortex of the cerebellum, consisting of a single layer of Purkinje cells.

germ l., germ cell l. any of the three primary layers of cells formed in the early development of the embryo (ECTODERM, ENTODERM, and MESODERM), from which the organs and tissues develop.

germinative l. stratum germinativum.

granular l. 1. stratum granulosum. 2. the deep layer of the cortex of the cerebellum. 3. the layer of follicle cells lining the theca of the vesicular ovarian follicle.

half-value l. the thickness of a given substance which, when introduced in the path of a given beam of rays, will reduce its intensity by one half.

Henle's l. the outermost layer of the inner root sheath of the hair follicle.

horny l. 1. stratum corneum. 2. the outer, compact layer of the nail.

malpighian l. stratum germinativum.

mantle l. the middle layer of the wall of the primordial neural tube, containing primordial nerve cells and later forming the gray matter of the central nervous system.

nervous l. all of the retina except the pigment layer; the inner layer of the optic cup.

odontoblastic l. the epithelioid layer of odontoblasts in contact with the dentin of teeth.

Ollier's l. the innermost layer of the periosteum.

prickle-cell l. stratum spinosum.

l. of rods and cones the layer of the nervous part of the RETINA, located between the pigmented part and the external limiting membrane, containing the sensory elements, the RODS and CONES.

spinous l. stratum spinosum.

spongy l. of endometrium a sublayer of the functional LAYER of endometrium, underlying the compact layer and containing the tortuous portions of the uterine GLANDS.

subendocardial l. the layer of loose fibrous tissue uniting the endocardium and myocardium.

subepicardial l. the layer of loose connective tissue uniting the epicardium and myocardium.

zonal l. of thalamus a layer of myelinated fibers covering the dorsal surface of the thalamus.

lazeroids (la′zer-oidz) drugs that are classified as oxygen-free-radical scavengers that work at the cellular level. They have been under investigation for preventing secondary injury after brain trauma.

lazy leukocyte syndrome a syndrome occurring in children, marked by recurrent low-grade infections, associated with a defect in neutrophil chemotaxis and deficient random mobility of neutrophils.

lb pound (L. *libra*).

LBW low birth weight; see under INFANT.

LD lethal DOSE.

LD$_{50}$ median lethal DOSE.

LDH lactate dehydrogenase.

LDL low-density LIPOPROTEIN.

LDL-C low-density-lipoprotein cholesterol; see CHOLESTEROL.

L-dopa levodopa.

LDR labor, delivery, recovery; see under ROOM.

LDRP labor, delivery, recovery, postpartum; see under ROOM..

LE lupus erythematosus.

lead[1] (Pb) (led) a chemical element, atomic number 82, atomic weight 207.19. Excessive ingestion or absorption causes LEAD POISONING. (See also Appendix 6.)

l. poisoning poisoning caused by the presence of lead or lead salts in the body; it affects the brain, nervous system, blood, and digestive system and can be either chronic or acute. Called also plumbism and saturnism.

Chronic Lead Poisoning. This was once fairly common among painters, and was called "painter's colic." It became less frequent as lead-free paints were substituted for lead-based ones and as plastic toys replaced lead ones. The disease is still seen among children with PICA (a craving for unnatural articles of food) who may eat lead paint chips or coatings. The Centers for Disease Control and Prevention defines an elevated blood lead level as >10 μg/dL for children younger than six years of age. However, there is evidence that there are subtle effects even at lower levels

Symptoms include weight loss, anemia, stomach cramps (lead colic), a bluish black line at the edge of the gums, and constipation. Other symptoms may be mental depression and, in children, irritability and convulsions. In addition to the poisoning, the anemia and weight loss must also be treated, usually by providing an adequate diet. In serious cases, EDTA (calcium disodium edetate) may be prescribed.

L

Acute Lead Poisoning. This rare condition can be caused in two ways: lead may accumulate in the bones, liver, kidneys, brain, and muscles and then be released suddenly to produce an acute condition; or large amounts of lead may be inhaled or ingested at one time. Symptoms are a metallic taste in the mouth, vomiting, bloody or black diarrhea, and muscle cramps. Diagnosis is made by examination of the blood and urine.

Treatment. Immediate removal of unabsorbed lead in the intestinal tract through the administration of mild saline cathartics and enemas. EDTA is given and in most cases measures must be taken to reduce the increased intracranial pressure that accompanies acute lead poisoning.

Prevention. An awareness of the prevalence of lead poisoning among children of preschool age who live in poorly maintained housing has led to neighborhood screening surveys in high-risk areas.

An important aspect of prevention of lead poisoning is determination of sources of lead in the environment and efforts to remove them. Sources include peeling paint from window sills, walls, floors, and bannisters, and from soil around old houses that have shed exterior paint through the years. An often unsuspected source is the glaze of certain pottery and "leaded glass;" lead can leach out into food and beverages from such vessels. A vital factor in coping with the problem of lead contamination is public education and development of a community awareness of possible sources and of the need for elimination of these hazards from the environment.

lead² (lēd) a pair of electrodes attached to a wire, used in recording changes in electric POTENTIAL, created by activity of an organ, such as the heart (ELECTROCARDIOGRAPHY) or brain (ELECTROENCEPHALOGRAPHY). Also, the particular segment of the TRACING produced by the potential registered through the specific electrodes; in electrocardiography, lead I records the potential differences between the two arms, lead II between the right arm and left leg, lead III between the left arm and left leg, and V leads from various sites over the heart and a composite reference point.

bipolar l. a configuration in which two electrodes are in contact with the organ being stimulated; this type is less susceptible to external electromagnetic interference than a unipolar LEAD is.

esophageal l. an electrode attached to a wire and inserted in the esophagus.

horizontal plane l. a unipolar precordial lead; it includes six of the 12 ECG leads whose positive electrodes are on the precordium and give information about right, left, anterior, or posterior current flow in the heart.

limb l's electrodes placed on the arms and left leg.

precordial l's leads recording electric POTENTIAL from various sites over the heart, designated V with a subscript numeral indicating the exact site: V_1, fourth intercostal space immediately to the right of the sternum; V_2, fourth intercostal space immediately to the left of the sternum; V_3, midway between V_2 and V_4; V_4, fifth intercostal space in the midclavicular line (the imaginary vertical line on the anterior surface of the body), passing through the center of the nipple; V_5, at the same horizontal level as V_4, in the left anterior axillary line (the imaginary vertical line passing through the middle of the axilla); V_6, left midaxillary line at the same horizontal level as V_4 and V_5.

unipolar l. a configuration of two electrodes, an active or therapeutic electrode in contact with the organ being stimulated and the other (the reference or indifferent electrode) at a distant site, usually the surface of the pulse GENERATOR.

leakage (le′kaj) the escape of something through a break in a barrier or wall.

radiation l. RADIATION going out through the x-ray TUBE housing in all directions other than that of the useful BEAM.

learning (lern′ing) the acquisition of knowledge.

l. disorders a group of disorders characterized by academic functioning that is substantially below the level expected on the basis of the patient's chronological age, measured intelligence, and age-appropriate education.

lifelong l. the continuation of the process of education throughout life.

Leber's disease (la-berz′) Leber's optic NEUROPATHY.

LE cell a neutrophil or macrophage that has ingested the nuclear material of an injured cell, converted to a dense, homogeneous mass by reaction with ANTINUCLEAR ANTIBODIES; this mass of nuclear material is called a hematoxylin body. This is a characteristic of SYSTEMIC LUPUS ERYTHEMATOSUS, but also found in analogous connective tissue disorders.

lecithin (les′ĭ-thin) phosphatidylcholine.

lecithinase (les′ĭ-thin-ās″) an enzyme that splits up LECITHIN; called also phospholipase.

lecithin/sphingomyelin ratio (L-S ratio) the ratio of lecithin to sphingomyelin in amniotic fluid, the determination of which is helpful in establishing the maturity of the fetus and its susceptibility to *hyaline membrane disease* after birth.

lecithoblast (les'ĭ-tho-blast") the primordial ENDODERM of a two-layered BLASTODISC.

lectin (lek'tin) a term applied to hemagglutinating substances present in saline extracts of certain plant seeds, which specifically agglutinate erythrocytes of certain blood groups or stimulate lymphocyte proliferation.

leech (lēch) any of the annelids of the class Hirudinea, especially *Hirudo medicinalis;* some species are bloodsuckers. Leeches were used extensively to treat various disorders and are still used occasionally to reduce postsurgical venous congestion, as in tissue flaps, grafts, or transplants.

Leeuwenhoek (la'ven-hōōk) Anton (or Anthony) van (1632–1723). Dutch microscopist. Born in Delft, Holland, he made many interesting discoveries through his careful observations even though his work was not conducted on a definite scientific plan. He gave the first accurate description of the red blood cells in 1674, and in 1677 he described and illustrated the spermatozoa in animals. He investigated the structure of muscle, the crystalline lens, and teeth, and was the first to see protozoa and bacteria under the microscope.

leflunomide (lĕ-floo'no-mīd) an IMMUNOMODULATOR used as a disease-modifying antirheumatic DRUG in treatment of rheumatoid ARTHRITIS, administered orally.

leg (leg) 1. that section of the lower LIMB between the knee and ankle; called also crus. 2. in common usage, the entire lower LIMB (in which case, the part below the knee is called the *lower leg*). 3. any of the four limbs of a quadruped.

> **bayonet l.** ankylosis of the knee after backward displacement of the tibia and fibula.

> **bow l.** see BOWLEG.

> **milk l.** phlegmasia alba dolens.

> **restless l's** restless legs syndrome.

Legg's disease (legz) Legg-Calvé-Perthes disease.

Legg-Calvé-Perthes disease (leg-kal-va'-per'tez) OSTEOCHONDROSIS of the epiphysis of the head of the femur.

Legg-Calvé-Waldenström disease (leg-kal-va'-vahl'den-strerm) Legg-Calvé-Perthes disease.

Legionella (le"jun-el'ah) a genus of gram-negative, aerobic rod-shaped bacteria, the cause of LEGIONELLOSIS. Species include *L. micda'dei,* the etiologic agent of Pittsburgh PNEUMONIA, and *L. pneumo'phila,* the

etiologic agent of LEGIONNAIRES' DISEASE and PONTIAC FEVER.

legionellosis (le"jun-el-o'sis) disease caused by infection with *Legionella* species, such as *L. pneumophila.*

legionnaires' disease (le-jun-ārz') a pulmonary form of LEGIONELLOSIS, resulting from infection with *Legionella pneumophila.* The disease acquired its name from an outbreak that occurred during the 1976 convention of the American Legion in Philadelphia. The gram-negative bacillus causing the disease was isolated from the lungs of four persons who attended the convention, contracted the disease, and died from it. The prevalence of legionnaires' disease is not certain but it is estimated that about 7 per cent of the annual cases of pneumonia in the United States are caused by *L. pneumophila.* Approximately 70 per cent of those cases occur in epidemic form, while the remainder are sporadic infections. The disease is seen most often in middle-aged to elderly men who are cigarette smokers or are IMMUNOCOMPROMISED. OSHA has published guidelines to protect workers at risk of being exposed in the workplace.

Specific diagnostic tests include both direct and indirect fluorescent testing for antibodies against *L. pneumophila.* Other laboratory tests reveal mild leukocytosis; elevated erythrocyte sedimentation rate; increased liver enzymes, especially lactate dehydrogenase; elevated blood urea nitrogen; and abnormal blood gases showing hypoxemia and hypocarbia.

The pulmonary symptoms are typical of pneumonia, but patients do not respond to the usual therapy for pneumonia and there can be permanent lung damage. Possible nonpulmonary complications include liver damage, altered levels of consciousness owing to neuronal involvement, and renal abnormalities that can require renal dialysis.

Treatment consists of antibiotic therapy with MACROLIDES and QUINOLONES. Other antibiotics may also be effective. ERYTHROMYCIN was formerly often used but is no longer the drug of choice. Severe hypoxia requires mechanical ventilation and oxygen therapy. Isolation of the patient is not considered to be necessary; however, respiratory precautions are indicated. Supportive measures to help the patient cope with high fever, nausea and vomiting, and RENAL FAILURE are essential components of patient care. See also PNEUMONIA.

legume (leg'ūm) 1. any plant of the large family Leguminosae. 2. the pod or fruit of one of these plants, such as a pea or bean;

this is an important source of PROTEIN in a VEGETARIAN DIET.

Leiner's disease (li′nerz) a condition resembling and probably identical with severe SEBORRHEIC DERMATITIS, affecting newborn breast-fed infants, characterized by generalized exfoliative dermatitis and marked erythroderma.

Leininger (li′nin-jer) Madeleine M. Nursing theorist, author, educator, researcher, and consultant. She formulated the field of TRANSCULTURAL NURSING in the mid 1950s and broadened the theoretical frameworks nurses use to care for individuals of diverse cultural backgrounds by developing the CULTURAL CARE DIVERSITY AND UNIVERSALITY theory of nursing. She discovered that cultural aspects were the critical missing link in nursing knowledge and practice and has advanced the goal "that the cultural needs of people in the world will be met by nurses prepared in transcultural nursing" by numerous scholarly presentations, books, book chapters, and articles pertaining to transcultural nursing theory, practice, and research.

leiodermia (li″o-der′me-ah) abnormal smoothness and glossiness of the skin.

leiomyofibroma (li″o-mi-o-fi-bro′mah) epithelioid leiomyoma.

leiomyoma (li″o-mi-o′mah) a benign tumor derived from smooth muscle, most often of the uterus (leiomyoma uteri).

bizarre l. epithelioid leiomyoma.

l. cu′tis one arising from cutaneous or subcutaneous smooth muscle fibers, found singly or multiply, usually as lesions arising from arrectores pilorum muscles; it may also occur as a solitary genital lesion or a solitary ANGIOLEIOMYOMA arising from the muscle of veins.

epithelioid l. one in which the cells are polygonal rather than spindle shaped, usually found in the stomach. Called also bizarre leiomyoma and leiomyofibroma.

l. u′teri, uterine l. leiomyoma of the UTERUS; called also uterine myoma and, colloquially, fibroids. It is the most common of all tumors found in women. It may occur in any part of the uterus, although it is most frequently in the body of the organ.

Leiomyomas usually occur during the third and fourth decades, and are often multiple, although a single tumor may occur. They are usually small but may grow quite large and occupy most of the uterine wall; after menopause, growth usually ceases. Symptoms vary according to the location and size of the tumors. As they grow they may cause pressure on neighboring organs, painful menstruation, profuse

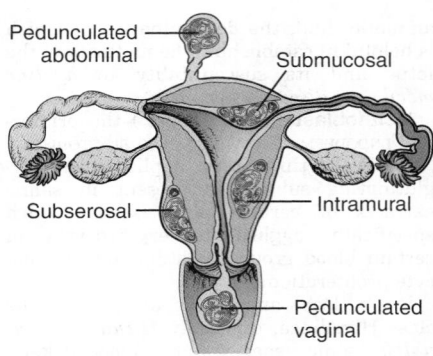

Leiomyoma of the uterus. The tumors may be subserosal, intramural, or submucosal. Subserosal and submucosal tumors may be pedunculated and may protrude from the uterine surface or into the uterine cavity, respectively. The stalk of pedunculated tumors may also become twisted. From Damjanov, 2000.

and irregular menstrual bleeding, vaginal discharge, or frequent urination, as well as enlargement of the uterus.

In pregnancy, the tumors may interfere with natural enlargement of the uterus with the growing fetus. They may also cause spontaneous abortion and death of the fetus.

Small leiomyomas are usually left undisturbed and are checked at frequent intervals. Larger tumors may be removed surgically, sometimes accompanied by a hysterectomy, or medication may be prescribed to induce a temporary menopause.

leiomyosarcoma (li″o-mi″o-sahr-ko′mah) a SARCOMA containing cells of smooth muscle.

Leishmania (lēsh-ma′ne-ah) a genus of protozoa comprising parasites of worldwide distribution, several species of which are pathogenic for humans. All species are morphologically indistinguishable, and therefore the organisms have usually been assigned to species and subspecies according to their geographic origin, the clinical syndrome they produce, and their ecologic characteristics. They have also been separated based on their tendency to cause visceral, cutaneous, or mucocutaneous leishmaniasis. In some classifications, *Leishmania* is grouped in four complexes comprising species and subspecies: *L. donovani, L. tropica, L. mexicana,* and *L. viannia.*

L. brazilien′sis Leishmania viannia.

L. donova′ni donova′ni a subspecies of the *L. donovani* complex causing the classic form of visceral leishmaniasis in India. It is transmitted by the sandfly *Phlebotomus argentipes,* with humans being the only major reservoir hosts. Called also *L. donovani.*

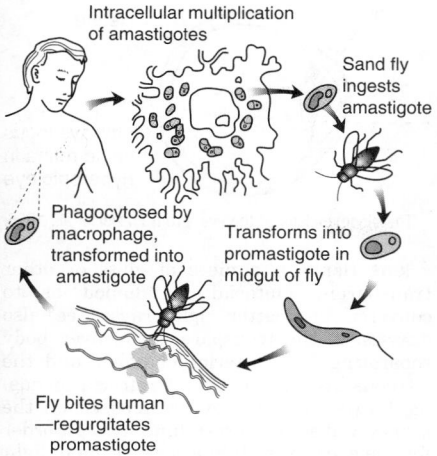

Intracellular multiplication of amastigotes

Sand fly ingests amastigote

Phagocytosed by macrophage, transformed into amastigote

Transforms into promastigote in midgut of fly

Fly bites human —regurgitates promastigote

Life cycle of *Leishmania*. From Mahon and Manuselis, 2000.

L. ma′jor a species of the *L. tropica* complex, transmitted by *Phlebotomus papatasi,* causing the rural form of Old World cutaneous leishmaniasis. Called also *L. tropica major.*

L. mexica′na a complex comprising the species and subspecies causing the New World form of cutaneous leishmaniasis in humans: *L. m. mexicana, L. m. amazonensis,* and *L. pifanoi.*

L. tro′pica 1. a complex comprising the species causing the Old World form of cutaneous leishmaniasis: *L. tropica, L. major,* and *L. aethiopica.* 2. a species of the *L. tropica* complex causing the urban form of Old World cutaneous leishmaniasis. It is found in Iran, Iraq, and India, transmitted by *Phlebotomus sergenti;* and in southern France, Italy and certain Mediterranean islands, transmitted by *P. papatasi.* Human to human transmission may also occur.

L. vian′nia a taxonomic complex comprising the subspecies that cause mucocutaneous leishmaniasis in its various forms; all of the subspecies develop in the midgut, foregut, and hindgut of their sandfly vectors. Formerly called *L. braziliensis.*

leishmaniasis (lēsh″mah-ni′ah-sis) any disease due to infection with *Leishmania.*

American l. forms of cutaneous leishmaniasis and visceral leishmaniasis found in the Americas.

cutaneous l. an endemic disease transmitted by the sandfly and characterized by the development of cutaneous papules that evolve into nodules, break down to form ulcers, and heal with scarring. It has been divided into Old World and New World forms, and the Old World form is subdivided into urban and rural types. The Old World form is caused by organisms of the *Leishmania tropica* complex; the New World form is caused by organisms of the *L. mexicana* and *L. viannia* complexes. It is endemic in the tropics and subtropics, and has been called by various names such as Aleppo boil, Delhi sore, Baghdad sore, and Oriental sore. Treatment consists of injections of pentavalent antimonial compounds. Antibiotics are used to combat secondary infection. Simple lesions may be cleaned, curetted, and left to heal.

cutaneous l., diffuse a rare chronic form of cutaneous leishmaniasis caused by *Leishmania aethiopica* in Ethiopia and Kenya, *L. pifanoi* in Venezuela, and species of the *L. viannia* and *L. mexicana* subclass in South and Central America, respectively, in which the lesions resemble those of nodular leprosy or of keloid. Pentavalent antimonial compounds are useful in some forms, while others are antimony-resistant. The prognosis for a complete cure is not good; relapses are common.

mucocutaneous l. a disease endemic in South and Central America caused by *Leishmania viannia,* marked by ulceration of the mucous membranes of the nose, mouth, and pharynx; widespread destruction of soft tissues in nasal and oral regions may occur. Called also espundia. Treatment consists of injections of pentavalent antimonial compounds.

l. reci′divans a prolonged, relapsing form of cutaneous leishmaniasis resembling tuberculosis of the skin; it may last for many years.

visceral l. a chronic, highly fatal if untreated, infectious disease endemic in the tropics and subtropics, caused by the protozoon *Leishmania donovani.* Sandflies of the genus *Phlebotomus* are the vectors. Called also kala-azar.

Symptoms. Symptoms are usually vague, resembling those of incipient pulmonary tuberculosis; the disease is often confused with malaria. There may be fever, chills, malaise, cough, anorexia, anemia, and wasting. The *Leishmania* organisms multiply in the cells of the reticuloendothelial system, eventually causing hyperplasia of the cells, especially those of the liver and spleen. Diagnosis is confirmed by demonstration of the parasite.

Treatment. Two groups of compounds are recommended: pentavalent organic antimonials, such as sodium antimony gluconate, and aromatic diamidines, such as pentamidine, if the antimonials are ineffective. Rest is prescribed for patients debilitated by anemia. A decrease in white cell count (leukopenia) often accompanies the disease, and therefore the patient's resistance to secondary infections is lowered. In some cases transfusion may be necessary to bring blood values back to normal. The patient is given a well balanced diet and liberal amounts of fluids. Special mouth care and attention to the skin are necessary to avoid complications.

leishmanin (lēsh′mah-nin) a suspension of killed leishmania promastigotes; used in a skin test for cutaneous leishmaniasis.

Lemierre syndrome (lĕ-myer′) thrombophlebitis of the internal jugular vein with secondary spread of infection, resulting from an acute oropharyngeal infection.

lemmoblastic (lem″o-blas′tik) forming or developing into a neurolemma cell.

lemmocyte (lem′o-sīt) a cell that develops into a neurolemma cell.

lemniscus (lem-nis′kus), pl. *lemnis′ci* [L.] a ribbon or band; in anatomy, a band of sensory nerve fibers in the central nervous system. Called also fillet.

length (length) an expression of the longest dimension of an object, or of the measurement between its two ends.

crown-heel l. **(CHL)** the distance from the crown of the head to the heel in embryos, fetuses, and infants; the equivalent of standing height in older persons.

crown-rump l. **(CRL)** the distance from the crown of the head to the breech in embryos, fetuses, and infants; the equivalent of sitting height in older subjects.

cycle l. in cardiac PACING terminology, the time interval in milliseconds from one event to the next; it is the inverse of the intrinsic RATE (beats per minute) or the paced RATE (pulses per minute).

focal l. the distance between a lens and an object from which all rays of light are brought to a focus.

lengthening reaction (leng′then-ing) reflex elongation of extensor muscles that permits flexion of a limb.

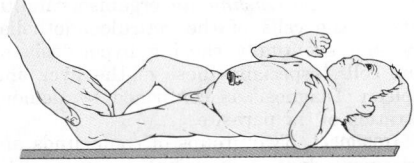

Measuring an infant's crown-heel length. From Lammon et al., 1996.

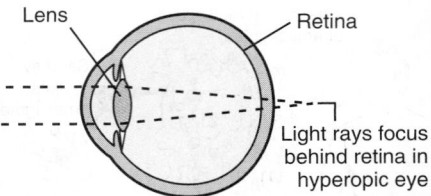

Light rays focus behind retina in hyperopic eye

The biconvex lens of the eye. From Frazier et al., 1996.

lens (lenz) 1. a piece of glass or other transparent material so shaped as to converge or scatter light rays. See also GLASSES. 2. the transparent, biconvex body separating the posterior chamber and the vitreous body of the eye; it refracts (bends) light rays so that they are focused on the RETINA. Called also crystalline lens. In order for the eye to see objects close at hand, light rays from the objects must be bent more sharply to bring them to focus on the retina; light rays from distant objects require much less REFRACTION. It is the function of the lens to do ACCOMMODATION, making of adjustments for viewing both near objects and more distant ones. To accomplish this it must be highly elastic so that its shape can be changed and made more or less CONVEX. The more convex the lens, the greater the refraction. Small ciliary muscles create tension on the lens, making it less convex; as the tension is relaxed the lens becomes more spherical in shape and hence more convex.

With increasing age the lenses lose their elasticity; thus their ability to focus light rays in the retina becomes impaired. This condition is called PRESBYOPIA. In farsightedness (HYPEROPIA) the image is focused behind the retina because the refractive power of the lens is too weak or the eyeball axis is too short. Nearsightedness (MYOPIA) occurs when the refractive power of the lens is too strong or the eyeball is too long, so that the image is focused in front of the retina.

achromatic l. one corrected for chromatic (color) aberration.

apochromatic l. one corrected for chromatic (color) and spheric aberration.

biconcave l. one concave on both faces.

biconvex l. one convex on both faces.

bifocal l. one having two segments with different refracting power, the upper for far vision and the lower for near vision. See also BIFOCAL GLASSES.

concave l. one curved like a section of the interior of a hollow sphere; it disperses light rays. Called also diverging lens.

contact l's corrective lenses that fit directly over the cornea of the eye; see also CONTACT LENSES.

converging l., convex l. one curved like the exterior of a hollow sphere; it brings light to a focus.

convexoconcave l. one that has one convex and one concave face.

crystalline l. lens (def. 2).

cylindrical l. one with at least one non-spherical surface, used to correct ASTIGMATISM.

diverging l. concave lens.

honeybee l. a magnifying eyeglass lens designed to resemble the multifaceted eye of the honeybee. It consists of three or six small telescopes mounted in the upper portion, directed toward the center and right and left visual fields. Prisms are included to provide a continuous, unbroken magnified field of view.

omnifocal l. one whose power increases continuously and regularly in a downward direction, avoiding the discontinuity in field and power inherent in bifocal and trifocal lenses.

orthoscopic l. one that gives a flat and undistorted field of vision, especially at the periphery.

planoconcave l. a lens with one plane and one concave side.

planoconvex l. a lens with one plane and one convex side.

Stokes's l's an apparatus used in the diagnosis of ASTIGMATISM.

trial l's ones used in testing the vision.

trifocal l. one having three segments of different refracting powers, the upper for distant, the middle for intermediate, and the lower for near vision.

lenticonus (len″tĭ-ko′nus) a congenital conical bulging, anteriorly or posteriorly, of the lens of the eye.

lenticular (len-tik′u-ler) 1. pertaining to or shaped like a lens. 2. pertaining to the lens of the eye. 3. pertaining to the lenticular nucleus.

lenticulostriate (len-tik″u-lo-stri′āt) pertaining to the lenticular nucleus and corpus striatum.

lenticulothalamic (len-tik″u-lo-thah-lam′-ik) relating to the lenticular nucleus and the thalamus.

lentiform (len′tĭ-form) lens-shaped.

lentiglobus (len″tĭ-glo′bus) exaggerated curvature of the lens of the eye, producing an anterior spherical bulging.

lentigo (len-ti′go) [L.] a flat, brownish pigmented spot on the skin due to increased deposition of melanin and an increased number of melanocytes; a freckle. (See Atlas 2, Part O.)

l. malig′na, malignant l. see lentigo maligna MELANOMA.

senile l., l. seni′lis, solar l. a small smooth round brownish patch appearing on the face, neck, or back of the hands of many older people, caused by an increase in pigment; these are entirely harmless. Although these spots are associated with aging, it is not age that is the principal cause but many years of exposure to sun and wind. Called also liver spot.

lentivirus (len′tĭ-vi″rus) any member of a genus of RETROVIRUSES that have long incubation periods and cause chronic, progressive, usually fatal diseases in humans and other animals. Species include the types of human immunodeficiency VIRUS.

leontiasis (le″on-ti′ah-sis) the leonine FACIES (lionlike face) of a person with lepromatous LEPROSY, due to nodular invasion of the subcutaneous tissue.

Leopold's maneuvers (le′ŏ-pōldz) gentle palpation of the lateral, upper, and lower borders of the uterus to determine the position of the fetus.

leper (lep′er) a person with leprosy; a term now in disfavor.

LE phenomenon the formation of LE CELLS on incubation of normal neutrophils with the serum of patients with systemic LUPUS ERYTHEMATOSUS; see also LE TEST.

lepidic (lĕ-pid′ik) pertaining to scales.

lepirudin (lep″ĭ-roo′din) a recombinant form of HIRUDIN used as an ANTICOAGULANT in

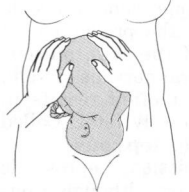 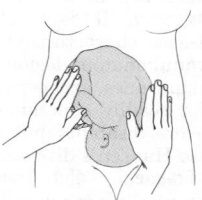

A First maneuver   B Second maneuver

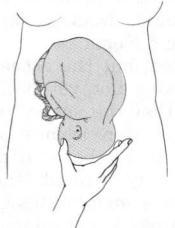 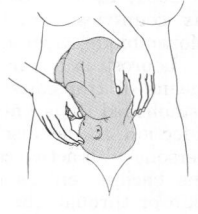

C Third maneuver   D Fourth maneuver

Leopold's maneuvers. From Lammon et al., 1996.

patients with HEPARIN-induced thrombocytopenia and associated thromboembolic disease; administered intravenously.

lepra (lep'rah) leprosy.

leprechaunism (lep're-kon"izm) a lethal familial congenital condition in which the infant is small and has an elfin face and severe endocrine disorders, such as enlargement of the clitoris in a female or of the penis in a male.

leprid (lep'rid) the cutaneous lesion or lesions of tuberculoid leprosy: hypopigmented or erythematous maculae or plaques, lacking bacilli.

leproma (lep-ro'mah) a superficial granulomatous nodule, rich in bacilli, the characteristic lesion of lepromatous leprosy. adj., **lepro'matous.**

lepromin (lep'ro-min) a repeatedly boiled, autoclaved, gauze-filtered suspension of finely ground lepromatous tissue and leprosy bacilli, used in the skin test for tissue resistance to leprosy.

leprosarium (lep"ro-sar'e-um) a hospital or colony for treatment and isolation of patients with leprosy.

leprostatic (lep"ro-stat'ik) 1. inhibiting the growth of the bacillus that causes LEPROSY. 2. an agent that has this effect.

leprosy (lep'ro-se) an inflammatory disease caused by *Mycobacterium leprae*, manifested in various ways, depending on the host's ability to develop cell-mediated IMMUNITY. It is a chronic communicable disease characterized by the production of granulomatous lesions of the skin, mucous membranes, and peripheral nervous system. Not readily contagious, it often results in severe disability but is rarely fatal. Called also Hansen's disease. adj., **lep'rous.**

Frequency and Transmission. Leprosy is essentially a tropical disease, although it has occurred in every country in the world. According to the World Health Organization, the number of leprosy patients in the world was less than 600,000 at the beginning of 2001. Its control remains a problem in six countries: Brazil, India, Madagascar, Mozambique, Myanmar, and Nepal.

Leprosy is not inherited, but the actual means of transmission have not yet been established. It is known that the source of infection is the discharge from lesions of persons with active cases. It is believed that the bacillus enters the body through the skin or through the mucous membranes of the nose and throat. Leprosy is considered one of the least contagious of infectious diseases; only 3 to 5 per cent of those exposed to it ever contract it.

Symptoms. The average incubation period of leprosy is 3 years. Initially, the infection is confined to the sheaths of nerves in the dermis. The disease progresses by spreading up the nerve sheath, resulting in loss of sensation, or by forming subcutaneous nodules and skin lesions.

In the *lepromatous type*, open sores later appear on the face, earlobes, and forehead, with tests showing large numbers of bacilli in the discharge from these lesions. If progress of the disease is not checked by treatment, the fingers and toes disintegrate and there may be other disfiguring due to trauma to the insensitive extremities. Death may occur in extreme cases of this type, but more often it is due to a secondary infection, such as tuberculosis or pneumonia.

In the *tuberculoid type*, there is loss of sensation on sections of the skin and atrophy of muscles. This often results in contraction of the hand into a claw.

Leprosy is further classified as either *paucibacillary* or *multibacillary* according to whether there are fewer or more than five lesions or patches present.

Treatment. Leprosy is most effectively and inexpensively treated with sulfone medications, such as dapsone, developed around 1950. In cases of sulfone resistance, the drug clofazimine (Lamprone) may be prescribed. A semisynthetic antibacterial, rifampin, is very effective in killing leprosy bacilli rapidly, so that patients receiving it may be considered minimal public health risks within a few days after treatment is begun. However, these drugs are expensive, have serious side effects, and are not readily available in many countries.

Treatment continues for several years at least, and sometimes indefinitely. In addition to specific medical therapy, adequate rest, diet, and exercise are provided. Physical therapy is employed to retrain affected muscles. Psychiatric help, not only for leprosy patients but for their close contacts and those who only imagine they have been exposed, is invaluable in relieving the anxieties arising from the age-old misconceptions about the disease.

Prevention. Preventive measures include establishment of clinics and hospitals for diagnosis and treatment. Early diagnosis and prompt treatment with multidrug therapy are key to prevention. Many patients return to their homes completely free of symptoms and are able to resume normal lives. Cure has been most successful in cases that were diagnosed and treated at an early stage, especially among the young.

Among the public health measures used to prevent leprosy are the laws in most countries requiring that all cases be reported to the local authorities and that all discharged leprous patients be examined at six-month intervals. Most countries also refuse entry to immigrants known to be infected. In the United States, information about leprosy, as well as treatment, can be obtained from the Gillis Long Hansen's Disease Center, Carville, LA 70721, telephone 800-642-2477.

lept(o)- word element [Gr.], *slender; delicate.*

leptocephalus (lep″to-sef′ah-lus) a person with an abnormally tall, narrow skull.

leptocyte (lep′to-sīt) target cell.

leptocytosis (lep″to-si-to′sis) the presence of target CELLS in the blood.

leptodactyly (lep″to-dak′tĭ-le) abnormal slenderness of fingers or toes. adj., **leptodac′tylous.**

leptomeninges (lep″to-mĕ-nin′jēz) (plural of leptomeninx) the two more delicate components of the meninges: the pia mater and arachnoid considered together; the piaarachnoid. adj., **leptomenin′geal.**

leptomeningitis (lep″to-men″in-ji′tis) inflammation of the leptomeninges.

leptomeningopathy (lep″to-men″ing-gop′-ah-the) any disease of the leptomeninges.

leptomonad (lep″to-mo′nad) 1. of or pertaining to *Leptomonas,* a genus of protozoa parasitic in the digestive tract of insects. 2. denoting the leptomonad form (see PROMASTIGOTE). 3. a protozoon exhibiting the leptomonad (promastigote) form.

leptopellic (lep″to-pel′ik) having a narrow pelvis.

leptophonia (lep″to-fo′ne-ah) weakness or feebleness of the voice. adj., **leptophon′ic.**

Leptospira (lep″to-spi′rah) a genus of aerobic, finely coiled spirochete bacteria with hooked ends. *L. inter′rogans* is the causative agent of LEPTOSPIROSIS.

leptospirosis (lep″to-spi-ro′sis) any of a group of infectious diseases due to certain serotypes of *Leptospira.* The best known is WEIL'S DISEASE (called also *leptospiral jaundice*); others are MUD FEVER (called also *autumn fever*) and SWINEHERD'S DISEASE. The etiologic agent is a spiral organism that infects the kidneys of cattle, swine, dogs, cats, rats, and other animals. The organisms are spread through the animals' urine. The portal of entry is usually through abrasions. The disease is most common among people who handle infected animals or the kidneys and other infected tissues of such animals.

Symptoms. Leptospirosis is usually a short illness that produces a variety of symptoms. It begins with fever, acute headache, chills, and sometimes nausea and vomiting. Later, other symptoms may be caused by the effects of the disease upon the kidneys, liver, skin, blood, and other organs. These symptoms can include jaundice, skin rashes, hemorrhages of the skin and mucous membranes, inflammation of the eye, hematuria, and oliguria.

Diagnosis is often difficult because the symptoms resemble those of several other diseases. Jaundice is a key symptom that, when present, aids in diagnosis.

Most cases are mild, consisting only of the early symptoms and having a duration of 1 to 2 weeks. In a few cases, a severe infection may cause damage to the kidneys, liver, or heart. Only rarely is the disease fatal.

Treatment and Prevention. The treatment of choice is doxycycline. Sanitation measures can reduce the spread of the disease in humans and other animals. Vaccines for animals are available, but provide only partial immunity to the disease. At the present time there are no vaccines of established value for human beings.

leptotene (lep′to-tēn) the stage of meiosis in which the chromosomes are threadlike in shape.

Leptotrichia (lep″to-trik′e-ah) a genus of gram-negative, anaerobic, straight or slightly curved, rod-shaped bacteria; *L. bucca′lis* is sometimes associated with oral or urogenital infections.

leptotrichosis (lep″to-trī-ko′sis) infection with a species of *Leptotrichia.*

l. **conjuncti′vae** name given to PARINAUD'S OCULOGLANDULAR SYNDROME when caused by infection with *Leptotrichia.*

Leriche syndrome (lĕ-rēsh′) fatigue in the hips, thighs, or calves on exercising, absence of femoral pulsations, impotence, and often pallor and coldness of the lower limbs, usually affecting males and due to chronic obstruction of the aortic bifurcation.

lesbian (lez′be-an) 1. pertaining to lesbianism. 2. a female homosexual.

lesbianism (lez′be-ah-nizm) homosexuality between women.

Lesch-Nyhan syndrome a hereditary disorder of purine metabolism transmitted as an X-linked recessive trait with physical and mental retardation, compulsive self-mutilation of fingers and lips by biting, choreoathetosis, spastic cerebral palsy, and impaired renal function.

lesion (le′zhun) any pathological or traumatic discontinuity of tissue or loss of function of a part. Lesion is a broad term, including wounds, sores, ulcers, tumors, cataracts, and any other tissue damage.

They range from the skin sores associated with eczema to the changes in lung tissue that occur in tuberculosis.

Kimmelstiel-Wilson l. a microscopic spherical hyaline mass surrounded by capillaries, found in the kidney glomerulus in the nodular form of intercapillary GLOMERULOSCLEROSIS.

let-down (let′down) the transport of milk from the alveoli of the breast to the ducts; called also milk let-down.

LE test a formerly common test for systemic LUPUS ERYTHEMATOSUS: serum from patients with lupus is combined with normal leukocytes; following incubation at 37° C., polymorphonuclear leukocytes engulf nuclei or nuclear fragments of cells to form LE CELLS.

lethal (le′thal) fatal.

lethargy (leth′er-je) 1. a lowered level of CONSCIOUSNESS marked by listlessness, drowsiness, and apathy. 2. a condition of indifference. adj., **lethar′gic.**

letrozole (let′rah-zōl) a nonsteroidal aromatase INHIBITOR used in treatment of advanced breast cancer in postmenopausal women; administered orally.

Letterer-Siwe disease (let′er-er si′we) a hereditary LANGERHANS CELL HISTIOCYTOSIS of early childhood, characterized by cutaneous lesions resembling seborrheic dermatitis, hemorrhagic tendency, hepatosplenomegaly with lymph node enlargement, and progressive anemia. If untreated it is rapidly fatal. Called also acute disseminated Langerhans cell histiocytosis.

letter of medical need a document required by insurance companies prior to the approval of HOME HEALTH CARE; it must be written by the physician and must include information about the patient's prognosis, diagnosis, current hospitalization status, equipment needs, and estimated hours of nursing care needed.

leuc(o)- for words beginning thus, see also those beginning LEUK(O)-.

leucine (loo′sēn) a naturally occurring AMINO ACID, one of the essential amino acids, necessary for growth in infants and for nitrogen equilibrium in adults.

leucovorin (loo″ko-vor′in) folinic acid.

l. calcium the calcium salt of FOLINIC ACID, used as an antidote for folic acid antagonists, e.g., methotrexate, when there is need to reverse the toxic effects of the latter, in the treatment of megaloblastic ANEMIAS due to folic acid deficiency, and as an adjunct in the palliative treatment of colorectal carcinoma; administered orally, intramuscularly, or intravenously.

leuk(o)- word element [Gr.], *white; leukocyte.*

leukapheresis (loo″kah-fĕ-re′sis) the selective removal of leukocytes from withdrawn blood, which is then retransfused into the donor.

leukemia (loo-ke′me-ah) a progressive, malignant neoplasm of the blood-forming organs, marked by diffuse replacement of the bone marrow development of leukocytes and their precursors in the blood and bone marrow. It is accompanied by a reduced number of erythrocytes and blood platelets, resulting in anemia and increased susceptibility to infection and hemorrhage. Other typical symptoms include fever, pain in the joints and bones, and swelling of the lymph nodes, spleen, and liver. adj., **leuke′mic.**

Types of Leukemia. Leukemia is classified clinically in several ways: (1) *acute* versus *chronic,* terms that have become altered from their usual meanings and refer to the degree of cell differentiation; (2) the predominant proliferating cells: myelocytic, granulocytic, or lymphocytic; and (3) increase in or maintenance of the number of abnormal cells in the blood—preleukemic.

Acute leukemia is characterized by fatigue, headache, sore throat, and dyspnea, followed by symptoms of acute tonsillitis, stomatitis, bleeding from the mucous membranes of the mouth, alimentary canal, and rectum, and pain in the bones and joints. There eventually is enlargement of the lymph nodes, liver, and spleen. Common to all leukemias are the tendency to bleed and the resultant anemia and increased susceptibility to infection. The diagnosis of leukemia requires confirmation of leukemic cells in the bone marrow by bone marrow biopsy and aspiration. Abnormalities may also be seen in peripheral blood smears.

Treatment. The treatment of choice is systemic combination chemotherapy with a variety of antineoplastic drug regimens. The disease can also be treated by a bone marrow transplant after a remission is achieved with chemotherapy.

Patient Care. Leukemia affects almost every system within the body and can present a variety of patient care problems. Of primary concern are those symptoms attendant to suppression of normal bone marrow function, particularly susceptibility to infection due to the predominance of immature and abnormally functioning white blood cells, bleeding tendency owing to decreased platelet count, and anemia due to decreased erythrocyte count. Chronic abnormal tissue perfusion, increased need for rest, and decreased sensitivity to heat and cold require careful planning and intervention.

TREATMENT PROTOCOL FOR ACUTE LEUKEMIA

The three phases in the treatment protocol for acute leukemia are:

Induction:	Intensive chemotherapy designed to achieve a complete remission.
Consol- idation:	Modified courses of chemotherapy to eradicate remaining disease.
Maintenance:	Small doses of chemotherapy administered every three to four weeks, may last up to a year.

Additionally, the patient will need relief from pain and discomfort arising from enlargement of the lymph nodes and distention of the liver and spleen.

Because of the malignant nature of leukemia and the fear and anxiety created by the knowledge that one has a form of cancer, patients and their families and significant others will need help in coping with anxiety, mental depression, and realistic fears about dying and death. The financial burden of the illness and disruption of the life of the individual and the family also impose a special burden on them. Referral to appropriate persons and agencies that can help meet their needs is an essential part of the holistic care of the patient with leukemia.

acute l. leukemia in which the involved cell line shows little or no differentiation, usually consisting of blast cells; two types are distinguished, acute lymphoblastic leukemia and acute myelogenous leukemia.

acute granulocytic l. acute myelogenous leukemia.

acute lymphoblastic l. (ALL), acute lymphocytic l. acute leukemia of the lymphoblastic type, one of the two major categories of acute leukemia, primarily affecting young children. Symptoms include anemia, fatigue, weight loss, easy bruising, thrombocytopenia, granulocytopenia with bacterial infections, bone pain, lymphadenopathy, hepatosplenomegaly, and sometimes spread to the central nervous system (MENINGISM) or to other organs. There are three major subtypes: The *pre–B-cell* is the most common, consisting of small uniform lymphoblasts that do not synthesize complete functional IMMUNOGLOBULINS or synthesize heavy chains only. The *B-cell type* is rare and consists of lymphoblasts that express surface immunoglobulins and have a surface translocation similar to that of Burkitt's LYMPHOMA. The *T-cell type* has cells that express surface antigens characteristic of T cells.

acute megakaryoblastic l., acute megakaryocytic l. a form of acute myelogenous leukemia in which MEGAKARYOCYTES are predominant and platelets are increased in the blood, often with fibrosis; it can occur at any age. Called also megakaryoblastic or megakaryocytic leukemia.

acute monocytic l. an uncommon form of acute myelogenous leukemia in which the predominating cells are identified as MONOCYTES; a few MYELOCYTES may also be present. It can affect any age group. Called also monocytic leukemia.

acute myeloblastic l. 1. a common kind of acute myelogenous leukemia, in which MYELOBLASTS predominate; it usually occurs in infants and middle-aged to older adults. Two types are distinguished; those that have minimal cell differentiation or maturation and those that have more advanced differentiation. Called also myeloblastic leukemia and acute myeloid leukemia. 2. acute myelogenous leukemia.

acute myelocytic l. acute myelogenous leukemia.

acute myelogenous l. (AML) acute leukemia of the myelogenous type, one of the two major categories of acute leukemia; most types affect primarily middle-aged to elderly people. Symptoms include anemia, fatigue, weight loss, easy bruising, thrombocytopenia, and granulocytopenia that leads to persistent bacterial infections. Several types are distinguished, named according to the stage in which abnormal proliferation begins: *acute undifferentiated l., acute myeloblastic l., acute promyelocytic l., acute myelomonocytic l., acute monocytic l., acute erythroleukemia,* and *acute megakaryocytic l.* Called also *acute myelocytic l.* and *acute nonlymphocytic l.*

acute myeloid l. 1. acute myeloblastic leukemia (def. 1). 2. acute myelogenous leukemia.

acute myelomonocytic l. one of the more common types of acute myelogenous leukemia, characterized by both malignant monocytes and myeloblasts; it usually affects middle aged to older adults. See also *chronic myelomonocytic leukemia.* Called also myelomonocytic or Naegeli's leukemia.

acute nonlymphocytic l. acute myelogenous leukemia.

acute promyelocytic l. acute myelogenous leukemia in which more than half the cells are malignant PROMYELOCYTES, often associated with abnormal bleeding secondary to thrombocytopenia, hypofibrinogenemia, and decreased levels of coagulation factor V; it usually occurs in young adults. Called also promyelocytic leukemia.

acute undifferentiated l. acute myelogenous leukemia in which the predominating cell is so immature and primitive that it cannot be classified. Called also stem cell leukemia and undifferentiated cell leukemia.

adult T-cell l., adult T-cell l./lymphoma a form of leukemia with onset in adulthood, leukemic cells with T-cell properties, frequent dermal involvement, lymphadenopathy and hepatosplenomegaly, and a subacute or chronic course; it is associated with human T-cell leukemia-lymphoma virus.

aleukemic l. leukemia in which the leukocyte count is normal or below normal; it may be lymphocytic, monocytic, or myelocytic.

basophilic l. a rare type of leukemia in which BASOPHILS predominate; both acute and chronic varieties have been observed.

blast cell l. acute undifferentiated leukemia.

chronic l. leukemia in which the involved cell line is well-differentiated, usually B-LYMPHOCYTES, but immunologically incompetent; types distinguished include *chronic granulocytic, chronic lymphocytic, chronic myelomonocytic, eosinophilic,* and *hairy cell leukemia.*

chronic granulocytic l. chronic leukemia of the myelogenous type, occurring mainly between the age of 25 and 60, usually associated with a unique chromosomal abnormality. The major clinical manifestations of malaise, hepatosplenomegaly, anemia, and leukocytosis are related to abnormal, excessive, unrestrained overgrowth of GRANULOCYTES in the bone marrow. Called also chronic myelocytic or chronic myeloid leukemia.

chronic lymphocytic l. chronic leukemia of the lymphoblastic type, a common form mainly seen in the elderly; symptoms include lymphadenopathy, fatigue, renal involvement, and pulmonary leukemic infiltrates. Circulating malignant cells are usually differentiated B-LYMPHOCYTES; a minority of cases have mixed T and B lymphocytes or entirely T-LYMPHOCYTES.

chronic myelocytic l., chronic myelogenous l., chronic myeloid l. chronic granulocytic leukemia.

chronic myelomonocytic l. a slowly progressing form of chronic leukemia that usually affects the elderly and sometimes progresses to acute myelomonocytic leukemia. Symptoms include splenomegaly, monocytosis with granulocytosis, and thrombocytopenia.

l. cu′tis leukemia with leukocytic invasion of the skin marked by pink, reddish brown, or purple macules, papules, and tumors.

eosinophilic l. a form of leukemia in which the EOSINOPHIL is the predominating cell. Although resembling chronic granulocytic leukemia in many ways, this form may follow an acute course despite the absence of predominantly blast forms in the peripheral blood.

granulocytic l. myelogenous leukemia.

hairy cell l. a form of chronic leukemia marked by splenomegaly and by an abundance of abnormal large mononuclear cells covered with hairlike villi (hairy CELLS) in the bone marrow, spleen, liver, and peripheral blood. Called also leukemic reticuloendotheliosis.

leukopenic l. aleukemic leukemia.

lymphatic l., lymphoblastic l. leukemia associated with hyperplasia and overactivity of the lymphoid tissue; there are increased numbers of circulating malignant lymphocytes and lymphoblasts. See also acute lymphoblastic leukemia and chronic lymphocytic leukemia.

lymphocytic l., lymphogenous l. lymphoid l. lymphoblastic leukemia.

lymphosarcoma cell l. the B-cell type of acute lymphoblastic leukemia.

mast cell l. a rare type marked by overwhelming numbers of tissue mast cells in the peripheral blood.

megakaryoblastic l. acute megakaryocytic leukemia.

megakaryocytic l. 1. hemorrhagic thrombocythemia. 2. acute megakaryocytic leukemia.

micromyeloblastic l. a form of myelogenous leukemia in which the immature, nucleoli-containing cells are small and are distinguishable from lymphocytes only by special staining.

monocytic l. acute monocytic leukemia.

myeloblastic l. 1. myelogenous leukemia. 2. acute myeloblastic leukemia.

myelocytic l., myelogenous l. myeloid granulocytic l. a form arising from myeloid tissue in which polymorphonuclear LEUKOCYTES and their precursors predominate.

myelomonocytic l., Naegeli's l. acute myelomonocytic leukemia.

plasma cell l., plasmacytic l. a rare type in which the predominating cell in the peripheral blood is the plasma cell; it is often seen in asociation with MULTIPLE MYELOMA.

prolymphocytic l. a type of chronic leukemia marked by large numbers of circulating lymphocytes, predominantly prolymphocytes, with massive splenomegaly and occasionally lymphadenopathy; prognosis is often poor.

promyelocytic l. acute promyelocytic leukemia.

Rieder cell l. a form of acute myelogenous leukemia in which the blood contains the abnormal cells called Rieder's LYMPHO-CYTES, asynchronously developed lymphocytes that have immature cytoplasm and a lobulated, indented, comparatively more mature nucleus.

stem cell l. acute undifferentiated leukemia.

subleukemic l. aleukemic leukemia.

undifferentiated l. acute undifferentiated leukemia.

leukemid (loo-ke'mid) any of the polymorphic skin eruptions associated with leukemia; clinically, they may be nonspecific (papular, macular, purpuric, etc.), but histopathologically they may represent true leukemic infiltrations.

leukemogen (loo-ke'mo-jen) any substance that produces leukemia. adj., **leukemogen'ic.**

leukemogenesis (loo-ke"mo-jen'ĕ-sis) the induction or development of leukemia.

leukemoid (loo-ke'moid) having blood counts and sometimes other clinical findings resembling those of leukemia but not due to uncontrolled proliferation of leukocytes.

l. reaction a peripheral blood picture resembling that of LEUKEMIA or indistinguishable from it on the basis of morphologic appearance alone, with leukocytosis of varying degrees and increased numbers of immature cells in circulation. It may be seen with infections such as TUBERCULOSIS,

BRUCELLOSIS, TOXOPLASMOSIS, staphylococcal infections, and streptococcal infections; with inflammatory disorders such as glomerulonephritis, rheumatoid arthritis, liver failure, and diabetic acidosis; with tumors and granulomatous infiltration of bone marrow; and with intoxications such as eclampsia, severe burns, and mercury poisoning.

Leukeran (loo'ker-an) trademark for a preparation of CHLORAMBUCIL, an antineoplastic AGENT.

leukoagglutinin (loo"ko-ah-gloo'tĭ-nin) an AGGLUTININ that acts upon leukocytes.

leukoblastosis (loo"ko-blas-to'sis) abnormal proliferation of LEUKOCYTES, as seen in LEUKEMIA.

leukocidin (loo"ko-si'din) 1. a substance toxic to leukocytes, killing the cells with or without lysis. 2. a type of EXOTOXIN produced by pathogenic bacteria such as STAPHYLO-COCCI or STREPTOCOCCI; it destroys LEUKOCYTES and may also damage MONOCYTES and MACROPHAGES.

leukocyte (loo'ko-sīt) a type of blood cell that lacks hemoglobin and is therefore colorless. Leukocytes are larger in size and fewer in number than ERYTHROCYTES; normally the blood has about 8000 of them per mm³. In contrast to erythrocytes, leukocytes can move about under their own power with ameboid MOVEMENT. Their chief functions are to act as scavengers and to help fight infections. Called also white cell or corpuscle and white blood cell or corpuscle. adj.,

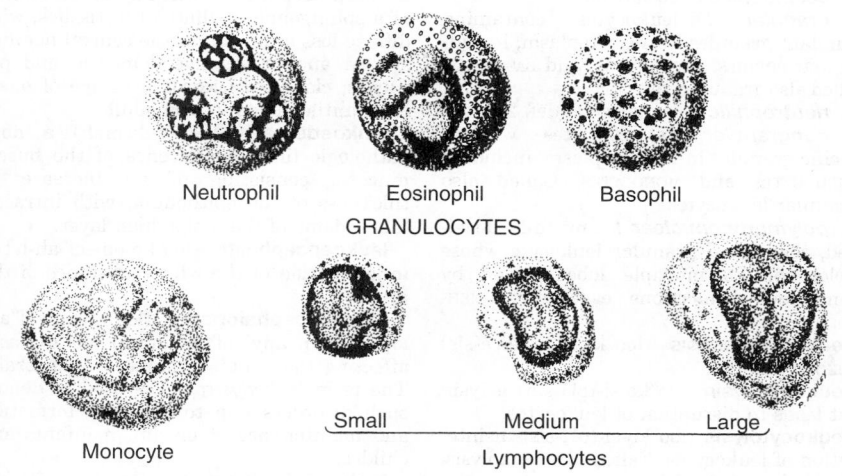

Neutrophil   Eosinophil   Basophil
GRANULOCYTES

Monocyte   Small   Medium   Large
                    Lymphocytes
AGRANULOCYTES

Types of leukocytes.

leukocyt′ic. Leukocytes may be classified in two main groups: the *granular leukocytes* are the BASOPHILS, EOSINOPHILS, and NEUTROPHILS, and the *nongranular leukocytes* are the LYMPHOCYTES and MONOCYTES. About 63 per cent of all leukocytes are neutrophils; 2.5 per cent are eosinophils; and the remaining types constitute less than 1 per cent each.

Leukocytes are actively engaged in the destruction or neutralization of invading microorganisms and are quickly transported to the vicinity of infection or inflammation, so that they can move through the blood vessel wall to reach the site of injury. For this reason, their life span in the blood is usually very short. When infection is present their numbers are greatly increased and they also become more mobile and move back and forth between the blood, lymph, and tissues. The granulocytes and monocytes are phagocytic, swallowing or ingesting the foreign particles with which they come in contact. During the process of phagocytosis the phagocytes themselves are destroyed. The two types of lymphocytes involved in immunity are B LYMPHOCYTES (B cells), which play a role in humoral immunity, and T LYMPHOCYTES (T cells), which are important in cell-mediated immunity. Plasma cells are activated B cells that secrete antibodies. Monocytes are also involved in some immune processes.

agranular *l′s* nongranular leukocyte.

basophilic *l.* BASOPHIL (def. 2).

eosinophilic *l.* EOSINOPHIL.

granular *l′s* leukocytes containing abundant granules in the cytoplasm, including NEUTROPHILS, EOSINOPHILS, and BASOPHILS. Called also granulocyte.

neutrophilic *l.* NEUTROPHIL (def. 2).

nongranular *l′s* leukocytes without specific granules in the cytoplasm, including LYMPHOCYTES and MONOCYTES. Called also agranular leukocytes.

polymorphonuclear *l.* any fully developed, segmented granular leukocyte whose nuclei contain multiple lobes joined by filamentous connections, especially a NEUTROPHIL.

leukocytogenesis (loo″ko-si″to-jen′ĕ-sis) LEUKOPOIESIS.

leukocytolysin (loo″ko-si-tol′ĭ-sin) a lysin that leads to disruption of leukocytes.

leukocytolysis (loo″ko-si-tol′ĭ-sis) disintegration of leukocytes. Called also leukolysis. adj., **leukocytolyt′ic.**

leukocytoma (loo″ko-si-to′mah) a tumor-like mass of LEUKOCYTES.

leukocytopenia (loo″ko-si″to-pe′ne-ah) leukopenia.

leukocytoplania (loo″ko-si″to-pla′ne-ah) wandering of leukocytes; passage of leukocytes through a membrane.

leukocytopoiesis (loo″ko-si″to-poi-e′sis) LEUKOPOIESIS.

leukocytosis (loo″ko-si-to′sis) a transient increase in the number of LEUKOCYTES in the blood, due to various causes.

basophilic *l.* basophilia (def. 1).

eosinophilic *l.* eosinophilia (def. 1).

mononuclear *l.* mononucleosis.

neutrophilic *l.* neutrophilia.

pathologic *l.* that due to some morbid condition, such as infection or trauma.

physiologic *l.* that caused by nonpathologic factors such as strenuous exercise.

leukocytotaxis (loo″ko-si″to-tak′sis) leukotaxis.

leukocyturia (loo″ko-si-tu′re-ah) the discharge of leukocytes in the urine, such as in kidney disease or urinary tract infections.

leukoderma (loo″ko-der′mah) an acquired condition with localized loss of pigmentation of the skin.

l. **acquisi′tum** **centri′fugum** a pigmented nevus surrounded by a ring of depigmentation; see also halo NEVUS.

syphilitic *l.* indistinct, coarsely mottled hypopigmentation, usually on the sides of the neck, in late secondary syphilis.

leukodystrophy (loo″ko-dis′tro-fe) disturbance of the white substance of the brain. See also ADRENOLEUKODYSTROPHY and LEUKOENCEPHALOPATHY.

metachromatic *l.* a hereditary leukoencephalopathy, marked by accumulation of a sphingolipid (sulfatide) in tissues, with diffuse loss of myelin in the central nervous system and progressive dementia and paralysis; classified according to age of onset as infantile, juvenile, and adult.

leukoedema (loo″ko-ĕ-de′mah) a nonpathologic filmy opalescence of the buccal mucosa, consisting of an increase in thickness of the epithelium, with intracellular edema of the malpighian layer.

leukoencephalitis (loo″ko-en-sef″ah-li′tis) inflammation of the white substance of the brain.

leukoencephalopathy (loo″ko-en-sef″ah-lop′ah-the) any of a group of diseases affecting the white substance of the brain. The term *leukodystrophy* is used to denote such disorders due to defective formation and maintenance of myelin in infants and children.

leukoerythroblastosis (loo″ko-ĕ-rith″ro-blas-to′sis) anemia due to destruction or crowding out of hematopoietic tissues in the bone marrow by a space-occupying lesion; reduction in normal marrow cells induces release of immature hematopoietic cells, especially nucleated erythrocytes, into the bloodstream. Called also myelopathic or myelophthisic anemia.

leukokeratosis (loo″ko-ker″ah-to′sis) leukoplakia.

leukokoria (loo″ko-kor′e-ah) any condition marked by the appearance of a whitish reflex or mass in the pupillary area behind the lens.

leukolymphosarcoma (loo″ko-lim″fo-sahr-ko′mah) lymphosarcoma cell leukemia.

leukolysin (loo-kol′ĭ-sin) leukocytolysin.

leukolysis (loo-kol′ĭ-sis) leukocytolysis.

leukoma (loo-ko′mah), pl. *leuko′mata* A dense, white corneal opacity. Causes include untreated syphilis, corneal inflammation or ulceration, and trachoma. Called also walleye.

l. adhae′rens a white tumor of the cornea enclosing a prolapsed adherent iris.

leukomyelitis (loo″ko-mi″ĕ-li′tis) inflammation of white matter of the spinal cord.

leukomyelopathy (loo″ko-mi″ĕ-lop′ah-the) disease of the white matter of the spinal cord.

leukonecrosis (loo″ko-nĕ-kro′sis) gangrene with formation of a white slough.

leukonychia (loo″ko-nik′e-ah) abnormal whiteness of the nails, either total or in spots or streaks.

leukopathia (loo″ko-path′e-ah) 1. leukoderma. 2. any disease of the leukocytes.

l. un′guium leukonychia.

leukopedesis (loo″ko-pĕ-de′sis) diapedesis of leukocytes through blood vessel walls.

leukopenia (loo″ko-pe′ne-ah) reduction of the number of leukocytes in the blood below about 5000 per mm³. Called also aleukemia, aleukocytosis, and leukocytopenia. adj., **leukope′nic.**

malignant l., pernicious l. agranulocytosis.

leukoplakia (loo″ko-pla′ke-ah) a disease marked by the development of white thickened patches on the mucous membranes of the cheeks (leukoplakia buccalis), gums, or tongue (leukoplakia lingualis); the patches sometimes form fissures and often become malignant. They may grow into larger patches or form ulcers. Those in the mouth may in time cause pain during swallowing of food or speaking. Leukoplakia affects mostly middle-aged to elderly men, often after prolonged irritation of the mouth from such varying factors as badly fitting dentures or immoderate use of tobacco. Treatment is aimed at removing any possible cause of physical or chemical irritation; the patient should give up tobacco and possibly also alcohol and extremely hot food. Dental attention may be necessary if teeth are uneven or dentures do not fit properly. Surgical removal of the affected area is relatively simple and may be the best means of preventing further development of the condition.

oral hairy l. a white filiform to flat patch occurring on the tongue or, rarely, on the buccal mucosa, caused by infection with Epstein-Barr virus and associated with human immunodeficiency virus infection.

l. vul′vae the presence of hypertrophic grayish-white infiltrated patches on the vulvar mucosa; specific diagnosis is determined by biopsy.

leukopoiesis (loo″ko-poi-e′sis) the production of leukocytes; called also leukocytogenesis and leukocytopoiesis.

leukorrhagia (loo″ko-ra′je-ah) profuse leukorrhea.

leukorrhea (loo″ko-re′ah) a white to yellow viscid discharge from the vagina or uterine cavity, which may be a symptom of a disorder either in the reproductive organs or elsewhere in the body. The glands of the vagina normally secrete a certain amount of mucuslike fluid that moistens the vaginal membranes. This is often increased at the time of ovulation and before a menstrual period, and it is also stimulated by sexual excitement, whether or not coitus takes place. Excessive discharge, however, may indicate an abnormal condition. A yellow or creamy white discharge, especially if it is thick, often contains pus and provides evidence of an infection. A thinner discharge, such as one that seems to be clear mucus, usually indicates that the disorder is chronic, but of less significance.

Causes. Frequent causes are TRICHOMONIASIS, CANDIDIASIS, and bacterial VAGINOSIS. The discharge of trichomoniasis is usually yellowish, odorous, and pruritic. Candidiasis is distinguished by a thin to thick white discharge with irritation and itching. Women with bacterial vaginosis often complain of a gray to yellow discharge with an offensive, fishy odor.

Another cause of leukorrhea is infection of the cervix during childbirth. The infection irritates the mucous glands of the cervix, causing them to secrete excessive mucus. SEXUALLY TRANSMITTED DISEASES, especially GONORRHEA and CHLAMYDIOSIS, are also common causes of leukorrhea. When the discharge is profuse, thick, and yellowish and there is a burning sensation during urination, gonorrhea or chlamydiosis should be suspected. Other bacteria and fungi may also be causes of leukorrhea, such as infections of the genital tract originating from foreign bodies like tampons, diaphragms, and pessaries that are left in the vagina too long.

Leukorrhea sometimes is an early indication of CERVICAL CANCER, or of benign conditions, such as POLYPS or LEIOMYOMA UTERI. It may also be caused by pelvic congestion associated with heart disease, by malnutrition, or by inflammation of the fallopian tubes as a result of tuberculosis. In later years, the disorder may be caused by simple debility; see also atrophic VAGINITIS.

leukosarcoma (loo″ko-sahr-ko′mah) the development of leukemia in patients originally having a well-differentiated, lymphocytic type of malignant lymphoma.

leukosis (loo-ko′sis) proliferation of leukocyte-forming tissue.

leukostasis increased blood viscosity and tendency to clotting, seen in leukemia that is accompanied by HYPERLEUKOCYTOSIS.

leukotaxis (loo″ko-tak′sis) cytotaxis of leukocytes; the tendency of leukocytes to collect in regions of injury and inflammation. adj., **leukotac′tic.**

leukotomy (loo-kot′ah-me) prefrontal lobotomy; see LOBOTOMY.

leukotoxic (loo′ko-tok″sik) destructive to leukocytes.

leukotoxin (loo′ko-tok″sin) a toxin that destroys leukocytes.

leukotrichia (loo″ko-trik′e-ah) whiteness of the hair in a circumscribed area. See also CANITIES and POLIOSIS.

leukotriene (loo″ko-tri′ēn) any of a group of compounds derived from unsaturated fatty acids, primarily arachidonic acid, that are extremely potent mediators of immediate hypersensitivity reactions and inflammation, producing smooth muscle contraction, especially bronchoconstriction, increased vascular permeability, and migration of leukocytes to areas of inflammation. Certain leukotrienes are collectively known as SRS-A (slow reacting substance of anaphylaxis), the name given to their potent bronchoconstrictor activity 30 years before their structure was elucidated; they also cause leakage of fluid and proteins from the microvasculature.

leuprolide (loo-pro′līd) a synthetic analogue of gonadotropin-releasing HORMONE, used in the form of the acetate ester as an antineoplastic AGENT, treatment for ENDOMETRIOSIS, and GONADOTROPIN inhibitor. Administered subcutaneously or intramuscularly.

Leustatin (loo-sta′tin) trademark for a preparation of CLADRIBINE, an antineoplastic AGENT.

lev(o)- word element [L.], *left.*

levalbuterol (lev″al-bu′ter-ol) *R*-albuterol; a β-adrenergic agent used as the hydrochloride salt as a BRONCHODILATOR for treatment and prophylaxis of bronchospasm in REVERSIBLE OBSTRUCTIVE AIRWAY DISEASE.

levallorphan (lev″ah-lor′fan) an analogue of LEVORPHANOL, which acts as an antagonist to opioid ANALGESICS; used in the treatment of respiratory depression produced by opioid analgesics.

levamisole (le-vam′ĭ-sōl) an oral IMIDAZOLE that enhances the immune response and is used as the hydrochloride salt as an adjuvant to FLUOROURACIL in ANTINEOPLASTIC THERAPY after surgery in patients with Dukes' stage C colon cancer.

levarterenol (lev″ahr-tĕ-re′nol) the levorotatory form of NOREPINEPHRINE, a much more potent PRESSOR agent than the natural dextrorotatory isomer.

levator (lĕ-va′ter) [L.] 1. a muscle that elevates an organ or structure. 2. an instrument for raising depressed osseous fragments in fractures.

level (lev′el) relative position, rank, or concentration.

l's of care the six divisions of the HEALTH CARE SYSTEM: preventive care, primary care, secondary or acute care, tertiary care, restorative care, and continuing care.

background l. the usual intensity of a chemical or other stimulus in the environment.

confidence l. the probability that a confidence interval does not contain the population parameter.

l's of consciousness see levels of CONSCIOUSNESS.

lowest observed adverse effect l. (LOAEL), lowest observed effect l. (LOEL) in studies of the toxicity of chemicals, the lowest dosage level at which chronic exposure to the substance shows adverse effects; usually calculated for laboratory animals.

no observed adverse effect l. (NOAEL), no observed effect l. (NOEL) in studies of the toxicity of chemicals, the highest dosage level at which chronic exposure to the substance shows no adverse effects; usually calculated for laboratory animals.

l. of significance a statistical measure that serves as the cutoff point used to determine whether a null HYPOTHESIS is retained or rejected; the probability of incorrectly rejecting the null hypothesis (see Type I ERROR).

sterility assurance l. (SAL) the probability that a process makes something

STERILE (see STERILIZATION). An SAL of 10^{-6} is the recommended probability of survival for organisms on a sterilized device. This level means that there is less than or equal to one chance in a million that an item remains contaminated or nonsterile.

levetiracetam (le″vĕ-ti-ras′ē-tam) an ANTICONVULSANT administered orally as an adjunct in the treatment of partial seizures in adults with EPILEPSY.

levigation (lev′ĭ-ga′shun) the grinding to a powder of a moist or hard substance.

Levine (lĕ-vēn′) Myra Estrin. Nursing educator, administrator, and practitioner (died 1996). In 1964 Levine presented the foundations of her conceptual model for nursing, the CONSERVATION MODEL. She published over 50 articles and was the recipient of numerous awards for her accomplishments.

levobetaxolol (le″vo-ba-tak′sah-lol) a cardioselective BETA-ADRENERGIC BLOCKING AGENT, used in the form of the hydrochloride salt; administered topically to the conjunctiva in treatment of GLAUCOMA and ocular hypertension.

levobunolol (le″vo-bu′no-lol) a BETA-ADRENERGIC BLOCKING AGENT used in treatment of GLAUCOMA and ocular HYPERTENSION; applied topically to the conjunctiva as the hydrochloride salt.

levobupivacaine (le″vo-bu-piv′ah-kān) a local ANESTHETIC used as the hydrochloride salt for local infiltration ANESTHESIA, peripheral nerve block, and epidural ANESTHESIA during surgical procedures and for postoperative pain management.

levocabastine (le″vo-kab′ah-stēn) an ANTIHISTAMINE applied topically to the conjunctiva as the hydrochloride salt to treat seasonal allergic conjunctivitis.

levocardia (le″vo-kahr′de-ah) a term denoting normal position of the heart associated with transposition of other viscera (situs inversus).

levocarnitine (le″vo-kahr′nĭ-tēn) a preparation of the biologically active L-isomer of CARNITINE, used to treat carnitine deficiency, either primary or secondary to an inborn error of metabolism, and to prevent and treat carnitine deficiency associated with HEMODIALYSIS in END-STAGE RENAL DISEASE; administered orally.

levoclination (le″vo-klĭ-na′shun) rotation of the upper poles of the vertical meridians of the two eyes to the left.

levodopa (le″vo-do′pah) L-dopa, the levorotatory isomer of dopa; used in treatment of PARKINSON'S DISEASE and other forms of parkinsonism, administered orally.

levoduction (le″vo-duk′shun) movement of an eye to the left.

levofloxacin (le″vo-flok′sah-sin) a broad-spectrum antibacterial agent, administered orally, intravenously, or topically to the conjunctiva.

levogyration (le″vo-ji-ra′shun) levorotation.

levomethadyl (le″vo-meth′ah-dil) an opioid ANALGESIC used as an adjunct in the treatment of OPIOID addiction; administered orally as the acetate hydrochloride salt.

levonorgestrel (le″vo-nor-jes′trel) the levorotatory form of NORGESTREL; used in CONTRACEPTION, either in combination with an estrogen component as an oral contraceptive or alone as a subdermal implant (see NORPLANT). It is also used alone as an oral emergency postcoital contraceptive, popularly called a "morning-after pill."

levorotary (le″vo-ro′tah-re) levorotatory.

levorotation (le″vo-ro-ta′shun) a turning to the left; levogyration.

levorotatory (le″vo-ro′tah-tor″e) turning the plane of polarized light to the left (counterclockwise).

levorphanol (lēv-or′fah-nol) a potent synthetic opioid ANALGESIC with properties and actions similar to those of morphine; used as the bitartrate salt as an analgesic and an anesthesia adjunct, administered orally, subcutaneously, intramuscularly, or intravenously.

levothyroxine (le″vo-thi-rok′sin) L-THYROXINE, obtained from the thyroid gland of domesticated food animals or prepared synthetically; used for replacement THERAPY in HYPOTHYROIDISM and for the prophylaxis and treatment of GOITER and of thyroid cancer; administered orally, intravenously, or intramuscularly as the sodium salt.

levoversion (le″vo-ver′zhun) a turning toward the left.

levulose (lev′u-lōs) fructose.

LFA left frontoanterior (position of the fetus).

LFP left frontoposterior (position of the fetus).

LFT left frontotransverse (position of the fetus).

LH luteinizing hormone.

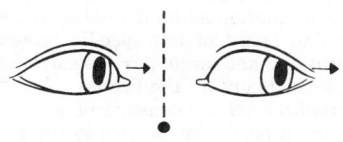

Levoversion of the eyes. From Stein et al., 2000.

Lhermitte's sign (lār′-mĕts′) a sensation like an electric shock coursing down the spine when the neck is flexed; a fairly common sign in MULTIPLE SCLEROSIS.

LH-RH (gonadotropin releasing hormone) luteinizing hormone releasing hormone.

Li lithium.

liberal individualism (lib′er-al in-dǐ-vid′u-al-izm) rights-based theory.

libido (lǐ-be′do, lǐ-bi′do) [L.] 1. sexual desire. 2. the psychic energy derived from instinctive biological drives; in early freudian theory it was restricted to the sexual drive, then expanded to include all expressions of love and pleasure, but the concept has evolved to include also the death instinct. FREUD postulated that libido development occurs in distinct stages: the oral STAGE, anal STAGE, and genital STAGE. Mental illnesses are therefore considered disturbances of libido development, such as regression to an earlier phase. JUNG proposed that although libido can be viewed according to the freudian pattern, it can also be desexualized and viewed as an undifferentiated energy that is at the basis of such mental processes as thinking, feeling, sensation, and intuition. adj., **libid′inal.**

Libman-Sacks disease (lib′man saks′) atypical verrucous ENDOCARDITIS.

Librax (lib′raks) trademark for a combination preparation of CHLORDIAZEPOXIDE hydrochloride and CLIDINIUM bromide, used as an ANTISPASMODIC in treatment of gastrointestinal disorders.

Librium (lib′re-um) trademark for preparations of CHLORDIAZEPOXIDE hydrochloride, an ANTIANXIETY AGENT.

lice (līs) plural of LOUSE.

licensure (li′sen-shur) the granting of a permit to perform acts which, without it, would be illegal. The licensure of health care personnel traditionally has been the responsibility of the state licensing boards, governed by licensing statutes enacted by the state.

individual l. the granting of a legal permit that is personal and cannot be transferred to another. The individual seeking the licensure must meet standards for practice as established by the state licensing statutes. In most instances the initial license is granted upon successful completion of an examination administered by the state examining board of the specific profession or vocation, and annual re-registration is required to maintain the license.

institutional l. licensure of an agency providing a particular service to the public. In the health field the licensure of health care agencies, such as hospitals and clinics has been common practice for many years.

licentiate (li-sen′she-āt) one holding a license from an authorized agency giving the right to practice a particular profession

lichen (li′ken) 1. any of certain plant formed by the mutualistic combination o an alga and a fungus. 2. any of various papular skin diseases in which the lesion are typically small, firm papules set ver close together.

l. amyloido′sus a condition character ized by localized cutaneous AMYLOIDOSIS.

l. fibromucinoido′sus, l. myxedemato′sus a condition resembling myxedema bu unassociated with hypothyroidism, marke by MUCINOSIS and a widespread eruption o asymptomatic, soft, pale red or yellowish discrete papules.

l. ni′tidus a usually asymptomati chronic inflammatory eruption consisting o numerous glistening, flat-topped, discrete smooth, commonly skin-colored micropap ules, located most often on the penis, lowe abdomen, inner thighs, flexor aspects of th wrists and forearms, breasts, and buttocks Widespread involvement may produce con fluence of the lesions, with formation o scaly plaques.

l. pila′ris lichen spinulosus.

l. planopila′ris a variant of lichen pla nus characterized by formation of cone shaped horny papules around the hai follicles, in addition to the typical lesions o ordinary lichen planus.

l. pla′nus an inflammatory skin diseas with wide, flat, purplish, shiny papules i circumscribed patches; it may involve th hair follicles, nails, and buccal mucosa called also lichen ruber planus.

l. ru′ber monilifor′mis a generalized o localized eruption with either round, dome shaped, waxy, dark or bright red papules, o waxy, yellow, milia-like papules, often form ing a moniliform (string-of-beads) pattern sometimes arranged in keloidal bands Some authorities consider the condition t be a variant of lichen simplex chronicus.

l. ru′ber pla′nus lichen planus.

l. sclero′sus, l. sclero′sus et atro′phi cus a chronic atrophic skin disease marke by white papules with an erythematous hal and keratotic plugging. It sometimes affect the vulva (kraurosis vulvae) or penis (bala nitis xerotica obliterans).

l. scrofuloso′rum, l. scrofulo′sus form of tuberculid manifested as an erup tion of clusters of lichenoid papules on th trunk of children with tuberculous disease.

l. sim′plex chro′nicus DERMATOSIS o psychogenic origin, marked by a pruriti discrete, or more often, confluent lichenoid papular eruption, usually confined to a localized area. Mechanical trauma, such as scratching or rubbing the area, is a factor in its development. The lesions may arise from normal skin or they may occur as a complication of other forms of DERMATITIS. Called also circumscribed or localized neurodermatitis and lichen chronicum simplex.

Treatment consists of administration of corticosteroids applied locally as a cream or given by intralesional injection to relieve the pruritus. The area should be protected by light dressings and the patient encouraged to avoid mental stress, emotional upsets, and irritation of the affected area. The application of very hot or very cold compresses may afford temporary relief of the itching. The condition tends to become chronic with unexplained remissions and reappearance of lesions in a different part of the body.

l. spinulo′sus a condition in which there is a horn or spine in the center of each hair follicle; called also lichen pilaris.

l. stria′tus a self-limited condition characterized by a linear lichenoid eruption, usually in children.

l. urtica′tus papular urticaria.

lichenification (li-ken″ĭ-fĭ-ka′shun) thickening and hardening of the skin, with exaggeration of its normal markings.

lichenoid (li′kĕ-noid) resembling lichen.

Lichtheim's syndrome (likt′hīmz) subacute combined degeneration of spinal cord.

licorice (lik′ah-ris) glycyrrhiza; the dried rhizome, roots, and stolons of various species of the perennial herb *Glycyrrhiza glabra,* used as a flavoring agent for various substances including drugs, tobacco, and candy. It has mineralocorticoid effects and can cause sodium and water retention and hypokalemia.

Lidex (li′deks) trademark for preparations of FLUOCINONIDE, a synthetic GLUCOCORTICOID used to treat dermatoses.

lidocaine (li′do-kān) an anesthetic with sedative, analgesic, and cardiac depressant properties, applied topically in the form of the base or hydrochloride salt as a local anesthetic; also used in the latter form to treat cardiac ARRHYTHMIAS and to produce infiltration anesthesia and various nerve blocks.

lie (li) the relationship of the long axis of the fetus to that of the mother; see also PRESENTATION.

longitudinal l. a situation in which the long axis of the fetus is parallel to that of the mother; in PRESENTATION, either the head or breech presents first. See accompanying illustration.

oblique l. a situation in which the long axis of the fetal body crosses that of the maternal body at an angle close to 45 degrees; in PRESENTATION, the shoulder usually presents first, but the arm or part of the trunk may also come first.

transverse l. a situation in which the long axis of the fetus is transverse to that of the mother; see illustration.

lien (li′en) [L.] spleen. adj., **lie′nal.**

l. accesso′rius an accessory spleen.

l. mo′bilis floating spleen.

lien(o)- word element [L.], *spleen;* see also words beginning SPLEN(O)-.

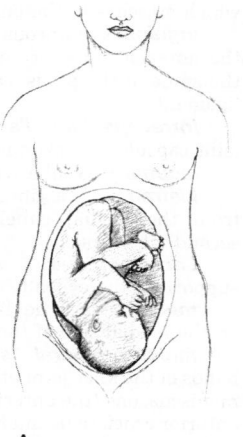
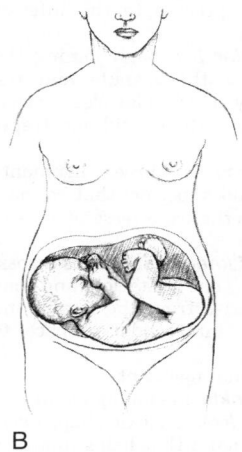

A   B
Longitudinal lie   Transverse lie

A, Longitudinal lie. *B,* Transverse lie.

lienocele (li-e′no-sēl) splenocele.

lienography (li″ĕ-nog′rah-fe) radiography of the spleen; splenography.

lienomalacia (li-e″no-mah-la′she-ah) splenomalacia.

lienomedullary (li-e″no-med′u-lar″e) splenomedullary.

lienomyelogenous (li-e″no-mi″ĕ-loj′ĕ-nus) splenomyelogenous.

lienomyelomalacia (li-e″no-mi″ĕ-lo-mah-la′she-ah) splenomyelomalacia.

lientery (li′en-ter″e) diarrhea with passage of undigested food. adj., **lienter′ic.**

lifeway (līf′wa) a manner of living, particularly one associated with a specific time, location, or group.

ligament (lig′ah-ment) 1. a band of fibrous tissue connecting bones or cartilages, serving to support and strengthen joints. See also SPRAIN. 2. a double layer of peritoneum extending from one visceral organ to another. 3. cordlike remnants of fetal tubular structures that are nonfunctional after birth. adj., **ligament′ous.**

> **accessory l.** one that strengthens or supports another.

> **arcuate l′s** the arched ligaments that connect the diaphragm with the lowest ribs and the first lumbar vertebra.

> **broad l. of uterus** a broad fold of peritoneum supporting the uterus, extending from the side of the uterus to the wall of the pelvis.

> **capsular l.** the fibrous layer of a joint capsule.

> **conoid l.** the posteromedial portion of the coracoclavicular ligament, extending from the coracoid process to the inferior surface of the clavicle.

> **coracoclavicular l.** a band joining the coracoid process of the scapula and the acromial extremity of the clavicle, consisting of two ligaments, the conoid and trapezoid.

> **costotransverse l.** three ligaments (lateral, middle, and superior) that connect the neck of a rib to the transverse process of a vertebra.

> **cruciate l′s of knee** more or less cross-shaped ligaments, one anterior and one posterior, which arise from the femur and pass through the intercondylar space to attach to the tibia.

> **crural l.** inguinal ligament.

> **deltoid l. of ankle** medial ligament.

> **falciform l. of liver** a sickle-shaped sagittal fold of peritoneum that helps to attach the liver to the diaphragm and separates the right and left lobes of the liver. Called also broad ligament of liver.

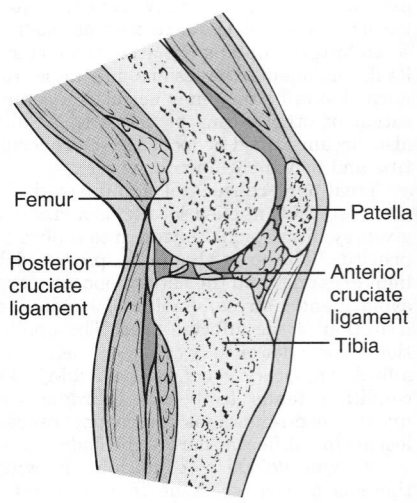

Cruciate ligaments of the knee. From Jarvis, 2000.

> **gastrosplenic l.** a peritoneal fold extending from the greater curvature of the stomach to the hilum of the spleen.

> **Gimbernat's l.** a membrane with its base just lateral to the femoral ring, one side attached to the inguinal ligament and the other to the pectineal line of the pubis. Called also lacunar ligament.

> **glenohumeral l′s** bands, usually three, on the inner surface of the articular capsule of the humerus, extending from the glenoid lip to the anatomical neck of the humerus.

> **Henle's l.** a lateral expansion of the lateral edge of the rectus abdominis muscle which attaches to the pubic bone.

> **inguinal l.** a fibrous band running from the anterior superior spine of the ilium to the spine of the pubis; called also Poupart's ligament.

> **intracapsulary l′s** ligaments of the joint capsule that are inside the capsule.

> **lacunar l.** Gimbernat's ligament.

> **Lisfranc's l.** a fibrous band extending from the medial cuneiform bone to the second metatarsal.

> **Lockwood's l.** a suspensory sheath supporting the eyeball.

> **medial l.** a large fan-shaped ligament on the medial side of the ankle.

> **meniscofemoral l′s** two small fibrous bands of the knee joint attached to the lateral meniscus, one (the anterior) extending to the anterior cruciate ligament and the other (the posterior) to the medial femoral condyle.

> **nephrocolic l.** fasciculi from the fatty capsule of the kidney passing down on the right side to the posterior wall of the

ascending colon and on the left side to the posterior wall of the descending colon.

nuchal l. a broad, fibrous, roughly triangular sagittal septum in the back of the neck, separating the right and left sides.

patellar l. the continuation of the central portion of the tendon of the quadriceps femoris muscle distal to the patella, extending from the patella to the tuberosity of the tibia; called also patellar tendon.

pectineal l. a strong aponeurotic lateral continuation of the lacunar ligament along the pectineal line of the pubis.

periodontal l. the connective tissue structure that surrounds the roots of the teeth and holds them in place in the dental alveoli.

Petit's l. uterosacral ligament.

phrenicocolic l. costocolic fold.

Poupart's l. inguinal ligament.

pulmonary l. a vertical fold extending from the hilus to the base of the lung.

rhomboid l. the ligament connecting the cartilage of the first rib to the undersurface of the clavicle.

round l. of femur a broad ligament arising from the fatty cushion of the acetabulum and inserted on the head of the femur.

round l. of liver a fibrous cord from the navel to the anterior border of the liver.

round l. of uterus a fibromuscular band attached to the uterus near the fallopian tube, passing through the abdominal ring, and into the labium majus.

splenorenal l. a peritoneal fold that passes from the diaphragm to the concave surface of the spleen.

suspensory l. of axilla a layer ascending from the axillary fascia and ensheathing the smaller pectoral muscle.

suspensory l. of lens ciliary zonule.

sutural l. a band of fibrous tissue between the opposed bones of a suture or immovable joint.

tendinotrochanteric l. a portion of the capsule of the hip joint.

transverse humeral l. a band of fibers bridging the intertubercular groove of the humerus and holding the tendon in the groove.

trapezoid l. the anterolateral portion of the coracoclavicular ligament, extending from the upper surface of the coracoid process to the trapezoid line of the clavicle.

umbilical l., medial a fibrous cord, the remains of the obliterated umbilical artery, running cranialward beside the bladder to the umbilicus.

uteropelvic l's expansions of muscular tissue in the broad ligament of the uterus, radiating from the fascia over the internal

obturator muscle to the side of the uterus and the vagina.

uterosacral l. a part of the thickening of the visceral pelvic fascia beside the cervix and vagina; called also Petit's ligament.

ventricular l. vestibular ligament.

vesicouterine l. a ligament that extends from the anterior aspect of the uterus to the bladder.

vestibular l. the membrane extending from the thyroid cartilage in front to the anterolateral surface of the arytenoid cartilage behind; called also ventricular ligament.

vocal l. the elastic tissue membrane extending from the thyroid cartilage in front to the vocal process of the arytenoid cartilage behind.

Weitbrecht's l. a small ligamentous band extending from the ulnar tuberosity to the radius.

ligamentopexy (lig″ah-men′to-pek″se) fixation of the uterus by shortening the round ligament.

ligamentum (lig″ah-men′tum) [L.] ligament.

ligand (li′gand, lig′and) an organic molecule that donates the necessary electrons to form coordinate covalent bonds with metallic ions. Also, an ion or molecule that reacts to form a complex with another molecule.

ligase (li′gās, lig′ās) any of a class of enzymes that catalyze the joining together of two molecules coupled with the breakdown of a pyrophosphate bond in ATP or a similar triphosphate.

DNA l. either of two enzymes that join two double-helical molecules of DNA together to make a longer DNA molecule.

l. chain reaction a type of DNA AMPLIFICATION that uses DNA LIGASE to link chains and amplify the template containing the sequence in question.

ligate (li′gāt) to apply a ligature.

ligation (li-ga′shun) application of a ligature.

Barron l., rubber band l. surgical treatment of HEMORRHOIDS by binding them with rubber bands so that the ligated portion sloughs away after several days.

tubal l. sterilization of the female by constricting, severing, or crushing the FALLOPIAN TUBES; constriction may be with an encircling ring or other ligature.

ligature (lig′ah-chur) any material, such as a thread or wire, used in surgery to tie off blood vessels to prevent bleeding, or to treat abnormalities in other parts of the body by constricting the tissues; see also STRANGULATION. Ligatures are used both inside and outside the body. If one must be left within the body after an operation, the type used will usually be of animal tissue or synthetic material that will dissolve or become incorporated in the patient's own body tissue. Those used on the outside of the body for stitches of cuts or incisions can be of any durable material and are removed after they have served their purpose. Special instruments have been developed for the application of ligatures to parts of the body that are difficult for the surgeon's hands to reach or to work in.

light (līt) electromagnetic radiation with a range of wavelength between 390 (violet) and 770 (red) nanometers, capable of stimulating the subjective sensation of sight; sometimes considered to include ultraviolet and infrared RADIATION as well.

idioretinal l., intrinsic l. the sensation of light in the complete absence of external stimuli.

polarized l. light of which the vibrations are made over one plane or in circles or ellipses.

Wood's l. ultraviolet RADIATION from a mercury vapor source, transmitted through a nickel-oxide filter (Wood's filter or glass), which holds back all but a few violet rays and passes ULTRAVIOLET RAYS of wavelength around 365 nm; used in diagnosis of fungal infections of the scalp and ERYTHRASMA, and to reveal the presence of PORPHYRINS and fluorescent minerals.

Lightcast (līt′kast) trademark for a fiberglass bandage that is used instead of a plaster cast. Lightcasts harden very quickly, weigh significantly less than plaster casts, and are water resistant.

lightening (līt′en-ing) the sensation of decreased abdominal distention caused by descent of the uterus into the pelvic cavity, 2 or 3 weeks before labor begins.

Lignac-Fanconi disease (lēn-yak′ fan-ko′ne) Fanconi syndrome.

lignin (lig′nin) a woody substance closely associated with cellulose in plants and grouped with the polysaccharides, although it is not actually a carbohydrate; it combines with bile acids to prevent their absorption. Lignin fibers are less digestible by gut bacteria than other polysaccharides.

lignoceric acid (lig″no-ser′ik) a saturated fatty acid found in wood tar, various cerebrosides, and in small amounts in most natural fats.

limb (lim) 1. one of the paired appendages of the body used in locomotion and grasping; see ARM and LEG. Called also member, membrum, and extremity. 2. a structure or part resembling an arm or leg.

anacrotic l. ascending limb (def. 2).

artificial l. a replacement for a missing limb; see also PROSTHESIS.

ascending l. 1. the distal part of Henle's LOOP. 2. the ascending portion of an arterial pulse tracing; called also anacrotic limb.

catacrotic l. descending limb (def. 2).

descending l. 1. the proximal part of Henle's LOOP. 2. the descending portion of an arterial pulse tracing; called also catacrotic limb.

lower l. the limb of the body extending from the gluteal region to the foot; it is specialized for weight-bearing and locomotion. See also LEG.

pectoral l. the arm (upper LIMB), or a homologous part.

pelvic l. the leg (lower LIMB), or a homologous part.

phantom l. the sensation, after amputation of a limb, that the absent part is still present; there may also be paresthesias, transient aches, and intermittent or continuous pain perceived as originating in the absent limb.

residual l. stump.

thoracic l. pectoral limb.

upper l. the limb of the body extending from the deltoid region to the hand; it is specialized for functions requiring great mobility, such as grasping and manipulating. See also ARM.

limbic (lim′bik) pertaining to a limbus, or margin.

Limbitrol (lim′bĭ-trol) trademark for a combination preparation of CHLORDIAZEPOXIDE and AMITRIPTYLINE hydrochloride, an ANTIDEPRESSANT and ANTIANXIETY AGENT.

limbus (lim′bus) [L.] 1. a BORDER or MARGIN. 2. the edge of the cornea, where it joins the sclera. Called also limbus corneae.

lime (līm) 1. calcium oxide, a corrosively alkaline and caustic earth, CaO; having various industrial uses and also a pharmaceutic NECESSITY. 2. the acid fruit of *Citrus aurantifolia,* which contains ASCORBIC ACID.

limen (li′men) [L.] a threshold or boundary.

l. of insula, l. in′sulae the point at which the cortex of the insula is continuous with the cortex of the frontal lobe.

l. na′si the ridge marking the boundary between the vestibule of the nose and the nasal cavity proper.

liminal (lim′ĭ-nal) barely perceptible; pertaining to a threshold.

liminometer (lim″ĭ-nom′ĕ-ter) an instrument for measuring the strength of a stimulus that just induces a tendon reflex.

limitans (lim′ĭ-tanz) [L.] limiting.

limitation (lim″ĭ-ta′shun) 1. a restriction on an individual's activities. 2. (in plural) factors in a research study that may decrease the generalizability of the findings; they may be of either a *conceptual* or a *methodological* type.

chronic airflow *l.* see CHRONIC AIRFLOW LIMITATION.

limp (limp) an abnormal gait pattern in which one side of the body dips or moves slightly downward with ambulation.

lincomycin (lin′ko-mi″sin) an ANTIBIOTIC produced by *Streptomyces lincolnensis;* used as the hydrochloride salt in infections with gram-positive cocci and gram-negative bacilli.

lindane (lin′dān) the gamma isomer of BENZENE HEXACHLORIDE, used as a topical treatment for lice and SCABIES.

Lindau's disease (lin′dowz), **Lindau-von Hippel disease** (lin′dow von hip′el) von Hippel-Lindau disease.

line (līn) 1. a STRIPE, STREAK, or narrow RIDGE; sometimes only an imaginary connector between two anatomic landmarks. Called also linea. adj., **lin′ear.** 2. tubing on a catheter.

absorption *l's* dark lines in the spectrum due to absorption of light by the substance through which the light has passed.

arterial *l.* a monitoring system that uses an artery for access and consists of a catheter in the artery, pressure tubing, a transducer, and an electronic monitoring device. The most common uses of arterial lines are for monitoring of systemic blood pressure and obtaining arterial blood for analysis.

Beau's *l's* transverse lines or grooves in the nail plate caused by various systemic and local traumatic factors.

bismuth *l.* a thin blue-black line along the gingival margin in BISMUTH poisoning.

blue *l.* lead line.

cement *l.* a line visible in microscopic examination of bone in cross section, marking the boundary of an osteon (haversian system).

cervical *l.* anatomical designation for the cementoenamel JUNCTION.

cleavage *l's* Langer's lines.

***l.* of Douglas** a crescentic line marking the termination of the posterior layer of the sheath of the rectus abdominis muscle.

***l's* of election** lines of expression.

Beau's line

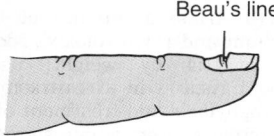

Beau's line. From Polaski and Tatro, 1996.

epiphyseal *l.* one on the surface of an adult long bone, marking the junction of the epiphysis and diaphysis.

***l's* of expression** the natural skin lines and creases of the face and neck; the preferred lines of incision in facial and cervical surgery.

gingival *l.* 1. a line determined by the level to which the gingiva extends on a tooth; called also gum line. 2. any linear mark visible on the surface of the gingiva.

gluteal *l.* any of the three rough curved lines (anterior, inferior, and posterior) on the gluteal surface of the ala of the ilium.

gum *l.* gingival line (def. 1).

hot *l.* see HOT LINE.

iliopectineal *l.* the ridge on the ilium and pubes showing the brim of the true pelvis.

incremental *l's* lines supposedly showing the successive layers deposited in a tissue, as in the tooth enamel.

intertrochanteric *l.* one running obliquely from the greater to the lesser trochanter on the anterior surface of the femur.

Langer's *l's* linear clefts in the skin indicative of the direction of the fibers; they correspond closely to the creases of the body but vary with body configuration. Lines of incision made parallel to them are thought to heal more efficiently. Called also cleavage lines.

lead *l.* a purple-blue line at the edge of the gums in chronic LEAD POISONING; called also blue line.

lip *l.* a line on the teeth at the level to which the margin of either lip extends.

median *l.* an imaginary vertical line dividing the body equally into right and left parts.

milk *l.* the line of thickened epithelium in the embryo along which the mammary glands are developed.

mylohyoid *l.* a ridge on the inner surface of the lower jaw from the base of the symphysis to the ascending rami behind the last molar tooth.

nuchal *l's* three lines (inferior, superior, and highest) on the outer surface of the occipital bone.

pectinate *l.* one marking the junction of the zone of the anal canal lined with stratified squamous epithelium and the zone lined with columnar epithelium.

semilunar *l.* a curved line along the lateral border of each rectus abdominis muscle, marking the meeting of the aponeuroses of the internal oblique and transverse abdominal muscles.

Shenton's l. a curved line seen in radiographs of the normal hip, formed by the top of the obturator foramen; it is used to determine the relationship between the head of the femur and the acetabulum.

temporal l's curved ridges, inferior and superior, on the external surface of the parietal bone, continuous with the temporal line of the frontal bone, a ridge that extends upward and backward from the zygomatic process of the frontal bone.

terminal l. one on the inner surface of each pelvic bone, from the sacroiliac joint to the iliopubic eminence anteriorly, separating the false from the true pelvis.

visual l. a line from the point of vision of the retina to the object of vision; called also visual axis.

linea (lin′e-ah) [L.] line.

l. al′ba white line; the tendinous median line on the anterior abdominal wall between the two rectus muscles.

li′neae albican′tes white or colorless lines on the abdomen, breasts, or thighs caused by mechanical stretching of the skin, with weakening of the elastic tissue; see also atrophic STRIAE.

l. as′pera a rough longitudinal line on the back of the femur for muscle attachments.

l. ni′gra the linea alba when it has become pigmented in pregnancy.

liner (lin′er) material applied to the inside of the walls of a cavity or container for protection or insulation.

cavity l. an agent used to line a tooth cavity for protection of the pulp from irritation and for neutralization of the free acids of zinc phosphate cements.

linezolid (li-nez′o-lid) a synthetic ANTIBACTERIAL of the OXAZOLIDINONE class, effective against gram-positive organisms; used for the treatment of community-acquired and nosocomial PNEUMONIA, skin and soft tissue infections, and BACTEREMIA, administered orally or intravenously.

lingu(o)- word element [L.], *tongue.*

lingua (ling′gwah) [L.] tongue.

l. geogra′phica geographic tongue.

l. ni′gra black tongue.

lingual (ling′gwal) 1. pertaining to or near the tongue; called also glossal. 2. in dental anatomy, facing the tongue or oral cavity; called also oral.

lingula (ling′gu-lah) [L.] a small, tongue-like anatomical structure. adj., **ling′ular.**

l. of cerebellum the most ventral part of the anterior lobe of the CEREBELLUM.

l. of left lung a small projection from the lower portion of the upper lobe of the left lung.

l. of sphenoid the bony ridge between the body and the great wing of the sphenoid bone.

lingulectomy (ling″gu-lek′to-me) excision of the lingula of the left lung.

linguoincisal (ling″gwo-in-si′zal) pertaining to or formed by the lingual and incisal surfaces of a tooth.

linguo-occlusal (ling″gwo-ŏ-kloo′zal) pertaining to or formed by the lingual and occlusal surfaces of a tooth.

linguopapillitis (ling″gwo-pap″ĭ-li′tis) inflammation or ulceration of the papillae of the edges of the tongue.

linguoversion (ling″gwo-ver′zhun) displacement of a tooth lingually from the line of occlusion.

liniment (lin′ĭ-ment) a medicinal preparation in an oily, soapy, or alcoholic vehicle, intended to be rubbed on the skin as a COUNTERIRRITANT or ANODYNE.

linitis (li-ni′tis) inflammation of gastric cellular tissue.

l. plas′tica diffuse fibrous proliferation of the submucous connective tissue of the stomach, resulting in thickening and fibrosis so that the organ is constricted, inelastic, and rigid (like a leather bottle). Called also leather bottle stomach.

linkage (lingk′ij) 1. the connection between different atoms in a chemical compound, or the symbol representing it in structural formulas; see also BOND. 2. in genetics, the association of genes having loci on the same chromosome, which results in the tendency of a group of such nonallelic genes to be associated in inheritance.

linoleic acid (lin″o-le′ik) an essential FATTY ACID that cannot be synthesized by animal tissues and must be obtained in the diet.

linolenic acid (lin″o-len′ik) an essential FATTY ACID that cannot be synthesized by animal tissues and must be obtained in the diet.

lint (lint) an absorbent surgical dressing material.

liothyronine (li″o-thi′ro-nēn) a synthetic pharmaceutical preparation of the levo-rotatory isomer of TRIIODOTHYRONINE; used for replacement THERAPY in HYPOTHYROIDISM and for the prophylaxis and treatment of GOITER and of thyroid cancer; administered orally or intravenously as the sodium salt.

liotrix (li′o-triks) a mixture of LIOTHYRONINE sodium and LEVOTHYROXINE sodium in a ratio of 1:4 by weight; used for replacement THERAPY in HYPOTHYROIDISM and for the prophylaxis and treatment of GOITER and of thyroid cancer; administered orally as the sodium salt.

lip (lip) 1. the upper or lower fleshy margin of the mouth. 2. any liplike part; called also labium.

cleft l. see CLEFT LIP AND CLEFT PALATE.

double l. redundancy of the submucous tissue and mucous membrane of the lip on either side of the median line.

glenoid l. a ring of fibrocartilage joined to the rim of the glenoid cavity.

Hapsburg l. a thick, overdeveloped lower lip that often accompanies Hapsburg JAW.

lip(o)- word element [Gr.], *fat; lipid.*

lipacidemia (lip″as-ĭ-de′me-ah) an excess of fatty acids in the blood.

lipaciduria (lip″as-ĭ-du′re-ah) FATTY ACIDS in the urine.

lipase (li′pās, lip′ās) fat-splitting enzyme; any enzyme that catalyzes the splitting of fats into GLYCEROL and FATTY ACIDS. Measurement of the serum lipase level is an important diagnostic test for acute and chronic PANCREATITIS.

lipectomy (lĭ-pek′to-me) excision of a mass of subcutaneous adipose tissue.

lipedema (lip″ĕ-de′mah) an accumulation of excess fat and fluid in subcutaneous tissues.

lipemia (lĭ-pe′me-ah) hyperlipidemia.

alimentary l. that occurring after eating.

l. retina′lis a milky appearance of the veins and arteries of the retina, occurring when the lipids of the blood exceed 5 per cent and in diabetes mellitus and leukemia.

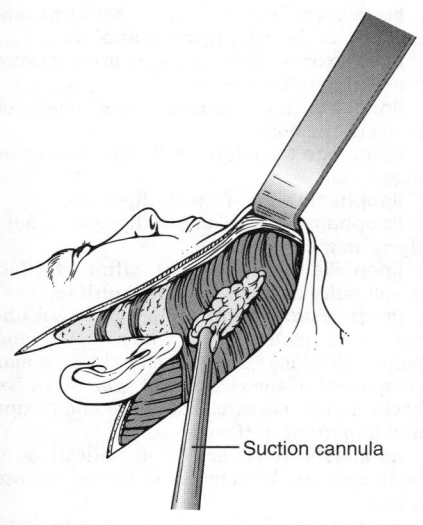

— Suction cannula

Suction assisted lipectomy.

lipid (lip′id) a group of substances comprising fatty, greasy, oily, and waxy compounds that are insoluble in water and soluble in nonpolar solvents, such as hexane, ether, and chloroform.

Simple lipids are the triglycerides or neutral fats. Each triglyceride molecule is composed of one molecule of glycerol joined by ester linkages to three fatty acid molecules. They are an important source of fuel to the body and a much lighter form of energy storage than carbohydrate.

Compound lipids are important structural components of cell membranes. Phospholipids include lecithin and the cephalins, which are composed of fatty acids linked to phosphatidic acid, and the sphingomyelins, which are composed of fatty acids linked to sphingosine. Glycolipids are composed of a carbohydrate chain and fatty acids linked to sphingosine or ceramide. Cholesterol is a steroid alcohol. Another important function of the phospholipids is as lung surfactants.

Intravenous lipid emulsions can be administered to patients with a deficiency of essential fatty acids.

lipidosis (lip″ĭ-do′sis), pl. *lipido′ses* any disorder of lipid metabolism involving abnormal accumulation of lipids, including HAND-SCHÜLLER-CHRISTIAN DISEASE, NIEMANN-PICK DISEASE, TAY-SACHS DISEASE, GAUCHER'S DISEASE, and other conditions.

lipiduria (lip″ĭ-du′re-ah) the presence of oil or fat in the urine, such as in the NEPHROTIC SYNDROME or after skeletal trauma; called also lipuria.

lipoarthritis (lip″o-ahr-thri′tis) inflammation of the fatty tissue of a joint.

lipoatrophy (lip″o-at′ro-fe) 1. atrophy of subcutaneous fat. 2. lipodystrophy.

insulin l. lipoatrophy in the subcutaneous tissues because of repeated injection of insulin at the same site.

lipoblast (lip′o-blast) a connective tissue cell that develops into a fat cell.

lipocardiac (lip″o-kahr′de-ak) pertaining to fatty degeneration of the heart.

lipochondroma (lip″o-kon-dro′mah) a tumor composed of mature lipomatous and cartilaginous elements.

lipochrome (lip″o-krōm) any of a group of fat-soluble hydrocarbon pigments, such as CAROTENE, LUTEIN, and the natural yellow coloring material of butter, egg yolk, and yellow corn. Called also carotenoid.

lipocyte (lip′o-sīt) 1. a fat cell. 2. a fat-storing cell of the liver.

lipodystrophy (lip″o-dis′tro-fe) 1. any disturbance of fat metabolism. 2. a group of conditions due to defective metabolism of fat, resulting in absence of subcutaneous fat; they may be congenital or acquired and partial or total. (See Atlas 2, Part F.)

congenital generalized l. an autosomal recessive condition marked by the virtual absence of subcutaneous adipose tissue, large body size, splenomegaly, hirsutism, acanthosis nigricans, and reduced glucose tolerance in the presence of high insulin levels.

intestinal l. former name for Whipple's disease.

partial l. a condition seen mainly in females in the first decade of life, characterized by symmetrical loss of subcutaneous fat, usually beginning on the face and gradually extending to the chest, neck, back, and upper limbs; this gives the lower part of the body an apparent, and possibly real, adiposity of the buttocks and lower limbs. Some affected patients develop insulin-resistant diabetes mellitus, triglyceridemia, and renal disease.

progressive l. progressive and symmetrical loss of subcutaneous fat from the parts above the pelvis, facial emaciation, and abnormal accumulation of fat about the thighs and buttocks.

total l. an autosomal recessive disorder occurring mainly in females, characterized by a generalized loss of subcutaneous fat and extracutaneous adipose tissue, present at birth or appearing later in life, and associated with hepatomegaly with abdominal protuberance, hypoglycemia and insulin-resistant nonketotic diabetes, hyperlipemia, marked elevation of the basal metabolic rate, accelerated somatic growth, advanced bone age, acanthosis nigricans and hirsutism.

lipofibroma (lip″o-fi-bro′mah) a LIPOMA containing fibrous elements.

lipofuscin (lip″o-fu′sin) 1. a yellow to brown, granular, iron-negative lipid pigment found particularly in muscle, heart, liver, and nerve cells; it is the product of cellular wear and tear, accumulating in lysosomes with age. 2. lipochrome.

lipofuscinosis (lip″o-fu″sin-o′sis) any disorder due to abnormal storage of LIPO-FUSCINS.

neuronal ceroid-l. any of several genetic lipidoses characterized by progressive neurodegeneration, loss of vision, and a fatal course; included are JANSKÝ-BIELSCHOWSKY DISEASE, VOGT-SPIELMEYER DISEASE, and KUFS' DISEASE. Formerly known as amaurotic familial idiocy.

lipogenesis (lip″o-jen′ĕ-sis) the formation of fat; the transformation of nonfat food materials into body fat. adj., **lipogenet′ic.**

lipogenic (lip″o-jen′ik) producing, forming, or caused by fat.

lipogenous (lĭ-poj′ĕ-nus) producing fatness.

lipogranuloma (lip″o-gran″u-lo′mah) a nodule of lipoid material associated with granulomatous inflammation.

lipogranulomatosis (lip″o-gran″u-lo″-mah-to′sis) a condition of faulty lipid metabolism in which yellow nodules of lipoid material are deposited in the skin and mucosae, giving rise to granulomatous reactions.

lipohypertrophy (lip″o-hi-per′tro-fe) hypertrophy of subcutaneous fat.

insulin l. localized hypertrophy of subcutaneous fat at insulin injection sites, caused by the lipogenic effect of insulin.

lipoid (lip′oid) 1. fatlike. 2. lipid.

lipoidosis (lip″oi-do′sis) a disturbance of lipid metabolism with abnormal deposit of lipids in the cells.

lipolysis (lĭ-pol′ĭ-sis) 1. the splitting up or decomposition of fat. 2. suction lipoplasty; lipoplasty by means of suction. adj., **lipolyt′ic.**

lipoma (lĭ-po′mah) a benign fatty tumor usually composed of mature fat cells.

lipomatosis (lip″o-mah-to′sis) abnormal localized or tumorlike accumulations of fat in the tissues. Called also liposis.

lipomatous (lĭ-po′mah-tus) affected with or of the nature of LIPOMA.

lipomeningocele (lip″o-mĕ-ning′go-sēl) meningocele associated with an overlying lipoma, as in spina bifida.

lipomeria (li″po-me′re-ah) congenital absence of a limb.

lipometabolism (lip″o-mĕ-tab′o-lizm) metabolism of fat. adj., **lipometabol′ic.**

lipomyxoma (lip″o-mik-so′mah) a MYXOMA containing fatty elements.

lipopenia (lip″o-pe′ne-ah) deficiency of lipids in the body.

lipophage (lip′o-fāj) a cell that absorbs or ingests fat.

lipophagia (lip″o-fa′je-ah) lipolysis.

lipophagy (lĭ-pof′ah-je) lipolysis. adj., **lipopha′gic.**

lipophilia (lip″o-fil′e-ah) 1. affinity for fat. 2. solubility in lipids. adj., **lipophil′ic.**

lipopolysaccharide (lip″o-pol″e-sak′ah-rīd) 1. a molecule in which lipids and polysaccharides are linked. 2. a major component of the cell wall of gram-negative bacteria; lipopolysaccharides are endotoxins and important antigens.

lipoplasty (lip′o-plas″te) modification of body contours by removal of excess adipose tissue.

lipoprotein (lip″o-pro′tēn, li″po-pro′tēn) any of the macromolecular complexes that are the form in which LIPIDS are transported in the blood. They consist of a core of hydrophobic lipids covered by a layer of PHOSPHOLIPIDS and APOPROTEINS, which make the complex water soluble. There are four main classes of lipoproteins: CHYLOMICRONS in which lipids are transported after a meal from the intestine to tissues where they are stored or used; *very-low-density lipoproteins* (VLDL); *low-density lipoproteins* (LDL); and *high-density lipoproteins* (HDL). VLDL and HDL are produced by both the liver and intestine; LDL is produced by the metabolism of VLDL (and perhaps that of HDL also).

LDL transports 60 to 75 per cent of the serum cholesterol, and is believed to carry cholesterol from the liver to body cells, including those of the blood vessels. HDL transports 20 to 25 per cent of the plasma cholesterol, and is believed to collect excess cholesterol from the body cells and carry it to the liver to be excreted.

It has long been known that high levels of serum cholesterol are associated with an increased risk of coronary heart disease. Because LDL carries most of the cholesterol, the serum LDL level is directly associated with heart disease risk. The higher the LDL level, the greater the incidence of heart attacks or angina pectoris.

Clinical findings indicate that the HDL level is inversely related to risk of heart disease. This suggests that HDL may in some way protect against the development of atherosclerosis and heart disease. It is also possible that there is no cause-and-effect relationship between risk of heart disease and HDL, because other factors that increase the risk of heart disease, including lack of exercise, obesity, smoking, poor control of diabetes, and use of oral contraceptives, are also correlated with HDL levels. LDL levels are directly related to the ingestion of saturated fats and cholesterol and inversely related to ingestion of polyunsaturated fats. Therefore, stopping smoking, taking regular exercise, losing weight, and reducing the consumption of animal fat and cholesterol can reduce the risk of developing heart disease.

lipoproteinemia (lip″o-pro″tēn-e′me-ah) hyperlipoproteinemia.

liposarcoma (lip″o-sahr-ko′mah) a malignant tumor characterized by large anaplastic LIPOBLASTS, sometimes with foci of normal fat cells.

liposis (lǐ-po′sis) lipomatosis.

liposoluble (lip″o-sol′u-b'l) soluble in fats.

liposome (lip′o-sōm) a microscopic spherical particle formed by a lipid bilayer enclosing an aqueous compartment.

LIPOPROTEINS: NORMAL VALUES	
LIPIDS, TOTAL	400–800 mg/dl *or* SI 4.0–8.0 g/L
CHOLESTEROL, TOTAL	120–200 mg/dl *or* SI 3.11–5.18 mmol/L
LOW-DENSITY LIPOPROTEIN (LDL)	< 130 mg/dl *or* SI < 3.37 mmol/L
HIGH-DENSITY LIPOPROTEIN (HDL)	**Male:** 44–45 mg/dl *or* SI 1.24–1.27 mmol/L **Female:** 55 mg/dl *or* SI 1.425 mmol/L
LDL:HDL RATIO	< 3
TRIGLYCERIDES	**Male:** < 40 years 46–316 mg/dl *or* SI 0.52–3.57 mmol/L > 50 years 75–313 mg/dl *or* SI 0.85–3.5 mmol/L **Female:** < 40 years 37–174 mg/dl *or* SI 0.42–1.97 mmol/L > 50 years 52–200 mg/dl *or* SI 0.59–2.26 mmol/L

lipotroph (lip′o-trōf) any of the acidophils of the anterior lobe of the pituitary gland that contain β-lipotropin; see also CORTICOTROPH.

lipotrophy (lǐ-pot′ro-fe) increase of bodily fat. adj., **lipotroph′ic.**

lipotropic (lip″o-trop′ik) 1. acting on fat metabolism by hastening removal, or decreasing the deposit, of fat in the liver. 2. an agent that so acts.

β-lipotropin (lip″o-tro′pin) a polypeptide synthesized by cells of the adenohypophysis which promotes fat mobilization and skin darkening by stimulation of melanocytes. It is the precursor molecule of β-endorphin and a melanocyte-stimulating hormone (β-MSH).

lipotropism (lǐ-pot′ro-pizm), **lipotropy** (lǐ-pot′rah-pe), the condition of being lipotropic.

lipovaccine (lip″o-vak′sēn) a vaccine in a vegetable oil vehicle.

lipoxidase (lǐ-pok′sǐ-dās) lipoxygenase.

lipoxygenase (lǐ-poks′ĭ-jĕ-nās) an enzyme that catalyzes the oxidation of polyunsaturated fatty acids to form a peroxide of the acid.

lipping (lip′ing) 1. a wedge-shaped shadow in the radiograph of chondrosarcoma between the cortex and the elevated periosteum. 2. the development of a bony overgrowth in osteoarthritis; see illustration.

lipuria (lǐ-pu′re-ah) lipiduria.

liquefacient (lik″wĕ-fa′shent) 1. producing or pertaining to liquefaction. 2. an agent that so acts.

liquefaction (lik″wĕ-fak′shun) conversion into a liquid form. adj., **liquefac′tive.**

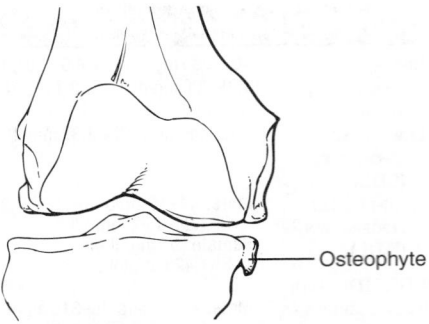

— Osteophyte

Lipping manifest as an osteophyte on the medial condyle of the right tibia. From Dorland's, 2000.

liquescent (lĭ-kwes′ent) tending to become liquid or fluid.

liquid (lik′wid) 1. a substance that flows readily in its natural state. 2. flowing readily; neither solid nor gaseous.

l. diet a diet limited to the intake of liquids or foods that can be changed to a liquid state; it may be restricted to clear liquids or it may be a full liquid diet.

Clear Liquid Diet. This is a temporary diet of clear liquids without residue. It is not nutritionally adequate, and is used in some acute illnesses and infections, postoperatively (especially after gastrointestinal surgery), and to reduce fecal matter in the colon. Foods allowed include water, tea, coffee, fat-free broth, carbonated beverages, synthetic fruit juices, plain gelatin, and sugar.

Full Liquid Diet. This diet can be nutritionally adequate with careful planning. It is used for acute GASTRITIS, as a transition between clear liquid and soft diet, and in conditions in which there is intolerance to solid food. Milk, strained soups, and fruit juices are allowed. Foods that liquefy at body temperature, such as ice cream, flavored gelatin, and soft custards, can be included. Cereal gruels and eggnogs are allowed. When a full liquid diet is used as a TUBE FEEDING it must be of a consistency that will allow easy passage through the tube. Most full liquid diets are given in feedings every 2 to 4 hours.

liquor (lik′er, li′kwor) 1. a liquid, especially an aqueous solution, containing medicinal substances. 2. a term applied to certain body fluids.

l. am′nii amniotic fluid.

l. cerebrospina′lis cerebrospinal fluid.

l. folli′culi the fluid in the cavity of a developing graafian follicle.

l. pu′ris the fluid portion of PUS.

lisinopril (li-sin′o-pril) a derivative of the active form of enalapril; an ANGIOTENSIN-CONVERTING ENZYME INHIBITOR used in the treatment of HYPERTENSION, congestive HEART FAILURE, and acute MYOCARDIAL INFARCTION, administered orally.

lisping (lisp′ing) faulty enunciation of *s* and *z* sounds; called also parasigmatism.

lissencephaly (lis″en-sef′ah-le) agyria. adj., **lissencephal′ic.**

listening (lis′en-ing) paying attention through hearing.

active l. in the NURSING INTERVENTIONS CLASSIFICATION, a nursing INTERVENTION defined as attending closely to and attaching significance to a patient's verbal and nonverbal messages.

Lister (lis′ter) Baron Joseph (1827–1912). Founder of modern antiseptic surgery. Born at Upton, Essex, England, Lister set out in a scientific manner to apply Pasteur's discoveries to the prevention of the development of microorganisms in wounds. His research was on the early stages of inflammation and blood coagulation, and in 1865 he successfully used carbolic acid in the treatment of an open fracture. Next he turned his attention to the arrest of hemorrhage in aseptic wounds, which led him to adopt a sulfochromic catgut for tying arteries, a material capable of more speedy absorption than silk or flax, which had long been employed. He wrote articles on amputation and anesthetics. Lister was created a baronet in 1883 and raised to the peerage in 1893, but perhaps the greatest memorial to him is the Lister Institute of Preventive Medicine in London.

Listeria (lis-tēr′e-ah) a genus of gram-positive bacteria (family Corynebacterium). *L. monocyto′genes* causes LISTERIOSIS.

listeriosis (lis-tēr″e-o′sis) infection caused by *Listeria monocytogenes.* In humans, in utero infections occur transplacentally and result in abortion, stillbirth, and premature birth; infections acquired during birth cause cardiorespiratory distress, diarrhea, vomiting, and meningitis. Infection in adults produces meningitis, endocarditis, and disseminated granulomatous lesions. Infection in cattle and sheep causes encephalitis and abortion. Nervous signs are common in ruminants, and necrosis of the liver in monogastric animals. Because affected animals tend to move in circles, it is also known as *circling disease.*

listerism (lis′ter-izm) the principles and practice of antiseptic and aseptic surgery.

liter (L) (le′ter) a basic unit of volume used for liquids with the SI system, equal to 1000 cubic centimeters, or 1 cubic decimeter, or to 1.0567 quarts liquid measure.

lith(o)- word element [Gr.], *stone; calculus.*

lithiasis (lǐ-thi'ah-sis) 1. a condition marked by formation of CALCULI and concretions. 2. sometimes used as a synonym for one of the specific types of lithiasis, such as UROLITHIASIS, NEPHROLITHIASIS, or CHOLELITHIASIS.

gallbladder l. cholecystolithiasis.

pancreatic l. pancreatolithiasis.

renal l. nephrolithiasis.

urinary l. urolithiasis.

lithium (Li) (lith'e-um) a chemical element, atomic number 3, atomic weight 6.939. (See Appendix 6.)

l. carbonate a psychotropic drug used to treat acute manic attacks in bipolar disorder and, when given on a maintenance basis, to prevent the recurrence of manic-depressive episodes. The desired serum levels are in the range 0.5–1.5 mEq/L. Life-threatening central nervous system effects and kidney damage occur at levels above 3.0 mEq/L. It is very important that the levels be carefully controlled. Lithium should not be given to patients with severe renal or cardiovascular disease or taken with diuretics because the potential for toxicity is very high. It is suspected of causing birth defects and should not be used during pregnancy.

l. citrate the citrate salt of lithium, having the same actions and uses as the carbonate salt.

lithocholic acid a secondary BILE ACID formed by dehydroxylation of CHENODEOXYCHOLIC ACID in the intestine; some is reabsorbed and forms conjugates with GLYCINE and TAURINE.

lithoclast (lith'o-klast) lithotrite.

lithogenesis (lith″o-jen'ĕ-sis) formation of calculi, or stones. adj., **lithog'enous.**

litholapaxy (lǐ-thol'ah-pak″se) the crushing of a stone in the bladder and washing out of the fragments.

litholysis (lǐ-thol'ǐ-sis) dissolution of calculi.

lithonephritis (lith″o-nĕ-fri'tis) inflammation of the kidney due to irritation by calculi.

lithopedion (lith″o-pe'de-on) calcified FETUS.

Lithostat (lith'o-stat) trademark for a preparation of ACETOHYDROXAMIC ACID, a UREASE inhibitor used in treatment of kidney stones and urinary tract infections.

lithotomy (lǐ-thot'ah-me) 1. incision of a duct or organ for removal of calculi. 2. cystolithotomy.

lithotripsy (lith'o-trip″se) the crushing of CALCULI in the bladder, urethra, kidney, or gallbladder.

electrohydraulic l. a method used for large upper urinary tract calculi: a high-capacity condenser creates a high-voltage spark between two electrodes at the tip of a probe; in a fluid-filled organ this creates a hydraulic shock wave that can be directed toward a calculus, causing it to cavitate and fragment.

extracorporeal shock-wave l. (ESWL) a noninvasive fragmentation of KIDNEY STONES or GALLSTONES with shock waves generated outside the body. It requires no incisions, catheters, or nephroscopes. The technique is based on the principle that shock waves are not destructive until they reach a surface in which there is a change in *acoustical impedance,* which is a form of resistance to the passage of sound waves. The impedance of calculi is different from that of water, bone, and soft tissue; therefore, tissue through which the wave travels as well as tissues surrounding the stone are not harmed.

For kidney stones, ESWL shatters the calculi into particles small enough to be passed in the urine. The procedure takes no longer than one to two hours, permits a shorter hospital stay, and allows the patient to return to normal life without delay.

ESWL is not appropriate for every patient with kidney stones. Body structure may prohibit proper positioning in the tank of water in which the patient must be submerged. Other contraindications include calcium deposits in the arteries, obstruction to urine flow, which is depended upon to flush out the fragments, and exaggerated spinal curvature, which interferes with visualization on x-ray. Stones that are not radiopaque cannot be treated by ESWL unless a radiopaque contrast medium is used because otherwise they cannot be seen and the shock waves cannot be properly focused on them. Very large stones (over one and a quarter inches in diameter) are not amenable to ESWL because they require more energy than the equipment can generate to break them into pieces small enough to travel through the urinary tract.

Complications such as obstruction to urine flow, bleeding, infection, and pain are less for ESWL than for other modes of therapy. The most formidable obstacle to widespread use of ESWL is the cost of the equipment.

For treatment of gallstones, the lithotriptor is used in combination with an ultrasound probe. The probe locates the calculi and the lithotriptor is fired. The fragments of gallstone traverse the biliary tract and are excreted via the intestines.

percutaneous ultrasonic l. (PUL) surgical removal of KIDNEY STONES via an

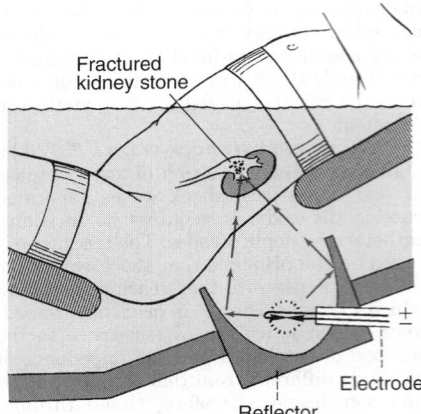

Fractured
kidney stone

Electrode

Reflector

Extracorporeal shock-wave lithotripsy. Electrically generated shock waves can fracture renal calculi. From Polaski and Tatro, 1996.

incision and insertion of a nephroscope into the portion of the kidney where the stone is lodged. An attempt is first made to remove the calculus through the endoscope by basket or forceps. If this is not successful, an ultrasonic lithotrite that sends out high-frequency sound waves is used to break up the stone. A continuous saline irrigation flushes out the particles, which are removed by suction. The drainage is filtered to trap the particles so that they can be sent to the laboratory for analysis.

Advantages of PUL over conventional surgical procedures for removal of kidney stones are fewer complications, a surgical incision less than 1 to 2 cm long as compared to one 20 cm long, shorter hospital stay, and more rapid recovery.

Patient Care. Preoperative care is fairly routine. The procedure usually is done in the radiology department and may be done in one or two stages. In the first stage the incision is made under local anesthesia and the nephrostomy catheter is inserted. In the second stage a general or epidural anesthetic is used and the ultrasonic lithotrite or "wand" is passed through the nephroscope. Ultrasonic waves of approximately 25,000 hertz are thus focused on the stone, breaking up its crystalline structure.

After surgery the vital signs are monitored to detect evidence of bleeding or infection. Some bright red blood in the urine passing through the nephrostomy can be expected for one to three days, but the amount of blood should gradually diminish.

As bleeding subsides the urine becomes smoky and tinged with old blood. The kidney is a highly vascular organ and postoperative hemorrhage is always a threat.

If the patient has either a Foley catheter or a ureteral catheter or both remaining in place after surgery, they must be kept open and draining. Irrigations, if ordered, are done gently to avoid excessive bleeding. A decrease in drainage and flank pain may indicate obstruction in the urinary tract. Other complications to be watched for include retroperitoneal bleeding, infection, delayed allergic reaction, and pneumothorax or hemothorax.

If the patient goes home with the catheter in place, instruction in self-care is necessary. The patient and family will need to know how to care for the incision site and the urine collection device. They should be taught how to note and record urine volume and evaluate its color and to report to the physician any leakage of urine from the incision site that persists after four days. They also will need to report any symptoms of infection, development of pain, or bright red hematuria. The importance of taking antibiotics precisely as prescribed is stressed. Antibiotic therapy is usually continued for two weeks after surgery. If no complications develop, the patient is able to return to normal daily activities within a week after drainage stops.

lithotrite (lith′o-trīt) an instrument for crushing calculi; called also lithoclast.

lithotrity (lĭ-thot′rĭ-te) lithotripsy.

lithuresis (lith″u-re′sis) passage of gravel in the urine.

litmus (lit′mus) a blue pigment prepared from *Rocella tinctoria* and other lichens.

l. paper absorbent paper impregnated with a solution of litmus, dried and cut into strips. It is used to indicate the acidity or alkalinity of solutions. If dipped into alkaline solution it remains blue; acid solution turns it red. It is used to test urine and other body fluids; it has a pH range of 4.5 to 8.3.

litter (lit′er) stretcher.

Little's disease (lit″lz) congenital spastic stiffness of the limbs, a form of cerebral spastic paralysis due to lack of development of the pyramidal tracts.

livedo (lĭ-ve′do) a discolored patch on the skin, usually associated with cold weather. adj., **liv′edoid.**

l. racemo′sa, l. reticula′ris reddish blue, netlike mottling of the skin; it is exacerbated by exposure to cold.

liver (liv′er) the large, dark-red gland located in the upper right portion of the abdomen, just beneath the diaphragm (see also color plates). Its manifold functions nclude storage and filtration of blood; secretion of BILE; conversion of sugars into GLYCOGEN; the synthesis and breakdown of fats and the temporary storage of fatty acids; and the synthesis of serum PROTEINS such as certain of the alpha and beta globulins, albumin (which helps regulate blood volume), and fibrinogen and prothrombin (which are essential COAGULATION FACTORS).

Storage Functions. The liver can store up to 20 per cent of its weight in glycogen and up to 40 per cent of its weight in fats. The basic fuel of the body is a simple form of sugar called glucose. This comes to the liver as one of the products of digestion, and is converted into glycogen for storage. It is reconverted to glucose, when necessary, to keep up a steady level of sugar in the blood. This is normally a slow, continuous process, but in emergencies the liver, responding to epinephrine in the blood, releases large quantities of this fuel into the blood for use by the muscles.

As the chief supplier of glucose in the body, the liver is sometimes called on to convert other substances into sugar. The liver cells can make glucose out of protein and fat. This may also work in reverse: the liver cells can convert excess sugar into fat and send it for storage to other parts of the body.

In addition to these functions, the liver builds many essential proteins and stores up certain necessary vitamins until they are needed by other organs in the body.

Protective Functions. The liver disposes of worn-out blood cells by breaking them down into their different elements, storing some and sending others to the kidneys for disposal in the urine. It also filters and destroys bacteria. One of the most important functions of the liver is the detoxification of drugs, alcohol, and environmental poisons.

The liver also helps to maintain the balance of sex hormones in the body. A certain amount of female hormone is normally produced in males, and male hormone in females. When the level of this opposite sex hormone rises above a certain point, the liver takes up the excess and disposes of it.

Finally, the liver polices the proteins that have passed through the digestive system. Some of the amino acids derived from protein metabolism cannot be used by the body; the liver rejects and neutralizes these acids and sends them to the kidneys for disposal.

Liver Function Tests. There are many laboratory procedures that measure some aspect of liver functions. Serum BILIRUBIN and urine bilirubin and urobilinogen levels provide information about the metabolism and excretion of bile pigments. Albumin and many of the alpha and beta globulins are synthesized by the liver. Disease that impairs their synthesis is shown by serum protein electrophoresis. Blood-clotting tests, such as one-stage prothrombin time, demonstrate a reduced synthesis of vitamin K–dependent COAGULATION FACTORS by the liver.

There are many enzymes that occur in the liver and are released into the blood when there is liver damage or biliary obstruction. The ones most commonly determined in the laboratory are alkaline phosphatase, aspartate transaminase (AST), and alanine transaminase (ALT). AST and ALT are also commonly called (serum) glutamic-oxaloacetic transaminase (GOT or SGOT) and (serum) glutamic-pyruvic transaminase (GPT or SGPT). Alkaline phosphatase is elevated in patients with intrahepatic or extrahepatic obstruction of bile flow, as in cholestatic jaundice or in primary or

L

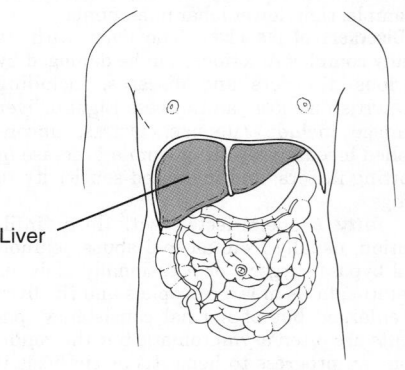

Liver

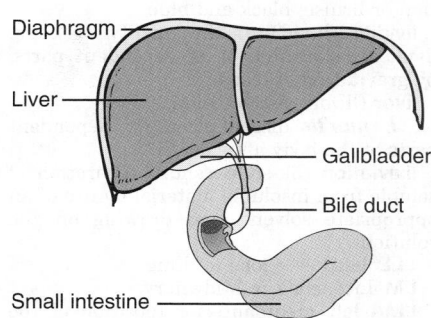

Diaphragm

Liver

Gallbladder

Bile duct

Small intestine

Liver. Bile, manufactured in the liver, is stored in the gallbladder; it passes through the bile duct into the duodenum, the upper end of the small intestine, where it aids in digestion.

metastatic carcinoma. AST and ALT are elevated in patients with hepatocellular injury as in acute viral or toxic hepatitis.

Both ULTRASONOGRAPHY and radioisotope scans (scintiscans) are useful in demonstrating space-occupying lesions of the liver, such as cysts, abscesses, and tumors. Ultrasonography is an excellent tool for evaluating ascites or preparing for a liver biopsy. The scintiscans use technetium-99m sulfur colloid, which is taken up by the reticuloendothelial cells of the liver and spleen, or gallium-67, which has an affinity for abscesses and certain tumors. On a colloid scan, abscesses and tumors appear as filling defects or "cold spots"; on the gallium scan, they appear as "hot spots."

A needle biopsy of the liver is useful in demonstrating the presence of cirrhosis, steatosis, alcoholic hepatitis, chronic hepatitis, and carcinoma. Liver biopsy is contraindicated in patients who have clotting defects, severe anemia, or a bacterial infection in an area to be traversed by the biopsy needle, for example, right lower lobar pneumonia.

Disorders of the Liver. The liver, with its many complex functions, can be damaged by various disorders and diseases, including HEPATITIS, CIRRHOSIS, and abscess. Signs of liver damage include JAUNDICE, ASCITES, uncontrolled bleeding resulting from a decrease in clotting factors, and increased sensitivity to drugs.

fatty l. one affected with fatty infiltration, usually from alcohol abuse, jejunoileal bypass surgery, or occasionally diabetes mellitus; fat is in large droplets and the liver is enlarged but of normal consistency; patients are often asymptomatic but the condition can progress to hepatitis or cirrhosis if the underlying cause is not removed.

livid (liv'id) discolored, as from a contusion or bruise; black and blue.

lividity (lĭ-vid'ĭ-te) the quality of being livid; discoloration, as of dependent parts, by gravitation of blood.

livor (li'vor) discoloration.

l. mor'tis discoloration on dependent parts of the body after death.

lixiviation (lik-siv″e-a'shun) separation of soluble from insoluble material by use of an appropriate solvent, and drawing off the solution.

LLL left lower lobe (of lung).

LM Licenciate in Midwifery.

LMA left mentoanterior (position of the fetus).

LMF lymphocyte mitogenic factor.

LMP left mentoposterior (position of the fetus).

LMT left mentotransverse (position of the fetus).

LNPF lymph node permeability factor.

LOA left occipitoanterior (position of the fetus).

Loa (lo'ah) a genus of filarial nematodes.

L. lo'a a threadlike species found in West Africa, 2–5 cm (1–2 in) long, that inhabits the subcutaneous connective tissue of the body, which it traverses freely (see LOIASIS). It is seen especially about the orbit including under the conjunctiva, causing itching and occasionally edematous swellings. The immature forms, or microfilariae are diurnal, being found in the peripheral circulation in greatest concentrations during the day. Flies of the genus *Chrysops* are the intermediate hosts and vectors.

load (lōd) the quantity of something that is carried or borne.

case l. the number of patients under the care of an individual health care worker.

viral l. the number of copies of RNA of a given virus per milliliter of blood.

loading (lōd'ing) 1. administering sufficient quantities of a substance to test a subject's ability to metabolize or absorb it. 2. the exertion of lengthening force on a body part such as a muscle or ligament.

LOAEL lowest observed adverse effect level.

loaiasis (lo″ah-i'ah-sis) loiasis.

lobar (lo'ber) pertaining to a lobe.

lobate (lo'bāt) divided into lobes.

lobe (lōb) 1. a more or less well defined portion of an organ or gland. 2. one of the main divisions of a tooth crown.

azygos l., l. of azygos vein a small anomalous lobe situated at the apex of the right lung, produced when the azygos vein arches over the upper part of the lung instead of at the hilus and presses deeply into the lung tissue to form a fissure that isolates a medial part of the lung.

caudate l. a small lobe of the liver between the inferior vena cava on the right and the left lobe.

ear l. the lower fleshy, noncartilaginous portion of the external ear.

flocculonodular l. one of the main subdivisions of the CEREBELLUM, located inferiorly, consisting of the paired FLOCCULI, their PEDUNCLES, and the NODULE OF THE VERMIS.

frontal l. the anterior portion of the gray MATTER of each cerebral HEMISPHERE.

hepatic l. one of the lobes of the liver, designated the right and left and the caudate and quadrate.

l's of lung the five major subdivisions of the lungs. see accompanying illustration and see LUNG.

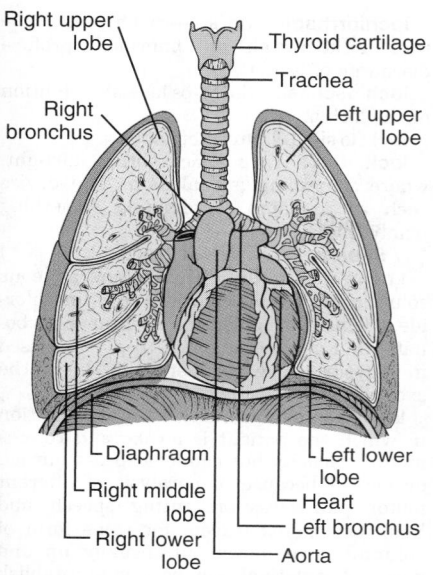

The lobes of the lungs. From Frazier et al., 2000.

Right upper lobe — **Thyroid cartilage** — **Trachea** — **Right bronchus** — **Left upper lobe** — **Aorta** — **Diaphragm** — **Left lower lobe** — **Right middle lobe** — **Heart** — **Right lower lobe** — **Left bronchus** — **Aorta**

occipital l. the most posterior portion of each cerebral HEMISPHERE, forming a small part of its posterolateral surface. See illustration.

parietal l. the upper central portion of the gray MATTER of each cerebral HEMISPHERE, between the frontal lobe and the occipital lobe and above the temporal lobe. It is the receptive area for fine sensory stimuli, and the highest integration and coordination of sensory information is carried on here. Damage to it can produce defects in vision or APHASIA.

polyalveolar l. a congenital disorder characterized in early infancy by the presence of far more than the normal number of alveoli in a lobe of the lungs; thereafter, normal multiplication of alveoli does not take place and they become enlarged, i.e., emphysematous.

quadrate l. 1. precuneus. 2. a small lobe of the liver, between the gallbladder on the right, and the left lobe.

Riedel's l. an anomalous tongue-shaped mass of tissue projecting from the right lobe of the liver in some individuals.

spigelian l. caudate lobe.

temporal l. a long tongue-shaped process that is the lower lateral portion of each cerebral HEMISPHERE.

lobectomy (lo-bek′to-me) surgical excision of a lobe, as of the lung, brain, liver, or thyroid. See also LOBOTOMY.

lobitis (lo-bi′tis) inflammation of a lobe, as of the lung.

lobotomy (lo-bot′ah-me) a form of PSYCHOSURGERY consisting of cutting of nerve fibers connecting a lobe of the brain with the thalamus. In most cases the affected parts are the prefrontal or frontal lobes, the areas of the brain involved with emotion; thus the operation is referred to as *prefrontal* or *frontal lobotomy*. Once fairly common as a method of controlling violent behavior, in recent decades its use has become rare because of the development of medications for treatment of severe mental illness, such as the ANTIPSYCHOTICS that suppress violent symptoms of psychosis.

Lobstein's disease (lōb′stīnz) see OSTEOGENESIS IMPERFECTA.

lobulated (lob′u-lāt″ed) made up of lobules.

lobule (lob′ūl) a small segment or lobe, especially one of the smaller divisions making up a lobe. adj., **lob′ular.**

l's of epididymis the wedge-shaped parts of the head of the epididymis, each comprising an efferent ductule of the testis.

hepatic l. one of the small vascular units composing the substance of the liver.

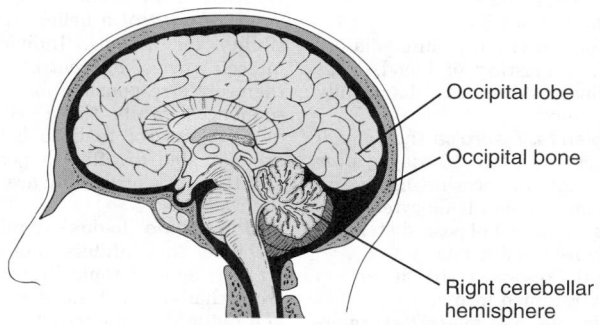

The occipital lobe of the brain. From Applegate, 2000.

Occipital lobe — Occipital bone — Right cerebellar hemisphere

l. of pancreas any of the distinct lobules into which the pancreas is divided by extension of septa of the capsule into the gland.

paracentral l. a lobule on the medial surface of the cerebral HEMISPHERE, continuous with the precentral GYRUS and the postcentral GYRUS.

parietal l. one of two divisions, inferior and superior, of the parietal lobe of the brain.

portal l. a polygonal mass of liver tissue containing portions of three adjacent hepatic lobules, and having a portal vein at its center and a central vein peripherally at each corner.

primary l. of lung, primary respiratory l. the functional unit of the lung; terminal respiratory unit.

lobulus (lob'u-lus) [L.] lobule.

lobus (lo'bus) [L.] lobe.

local (lo'k'l) restricted to or pertaining to one spot or part; not general.

localization (lo″kah-lĭ-za'shun) 1. restriction to a circumscribed or limited area. 2. the determination of a site or place of any process or lesion.

cerebral l. determination of areas of the cortex involved in performance of certain functions.

germinal l. the location on a blastoderm of prospective organs.

lochia (lo'ke-ah) a vaginal discharge occurring after childbirth. Lochia discharge should be checked every 15 minutes for the first hour after delivery, once every hour for the first 8 hours, and then every 8 hours. adj., **lo'chial.**

l. al'ba the final vaginal discharge after childbirth, largely mucus, when the amount of blood is decreased and the leukocytes are increased; it is usually of 10 to 14 days' duration but may last for 6 weeks.

l. cruen'ta lochia rubra.

l. purulen'ta lochia alba.

l. ru'bra that occurring immediately after childbirth, consisting of blood, fragments of decidua, and mucus. It usually lasts from 1 to 3 days.

l. sanguinolen'ta, l. sero'sa the vaginal discharge occurring 3 to 10 days after delivery. It is pink or brown-tinged and contains blood, mucus, and leukocytes.

lochiocolpos (lo″ke-o-kol'pos) distention of the vagina by retained lochia.

lochiometra (lo″ke-o-me'trah) distention of the uterus by retained lochia.

lochiometritis (lo″ke-o-me-tri'tis) puerperal metritis.

lochiorrhagia (lo″ke-o-ra'jah), **lochiorrhea** (lo″ke-o-re'ah) an abnormally profuse discharge of lochia.

lochioschesis (lo″ke-os'kĕ-sis) retention of the lochia.

loci (lo'si) [L.] plural of LOCUS.

lock (lok) 1. a place, often airtight, where something is sealed in. 2. a device such as a clamp for holding something firmly in place.

heparin l. see HEPARIN LOCK.

Locke's solution (loks) an aqueous solution of sodium chloride, calcium chloride, potassium chloride, sodium bicarbonate, and glucose adjusted to pH 7.4; used in physiologic experiments to keep the excised heart beating.

locked-in syndrome (lok't in) a condition in which the patient is awake and retains mental capacity but cannot express himself or herself because of paralysis of afferent motor pathways, preventing speech and limb movements (except for some form of voluntary eye movement, usually up and down). The patient may be able to establish effective communication through eye movements and specially adapted computers or letter boards.

lockjaw (lok'jaw) 1. tetanus. 2. trismus.

locomotion (lo″ko-mo'shun) movement, or the ability to move, from one place to another. adj., **locomo'tive.**

locomotor (lo″ko-mo'tor) of or pertaining to locomotion.

loculus (lok'u-lus) [L.] 1. a small space or cavity. 2. a local enlargement of the uterus in some mammals, containing an embryo. adj., **loc'ular.**

locum tenens (lo'kum ten'ens) a physician who temporarily takes the place of another.

locus (lo'kus) [L.] 1. a place or site. 2. in genetics, the specific site of a gene on a chromosome.

l. ceru'leus a pigmented eminence in the superior angle of the floor of the fourth ventricle of the brain.

l. of control a belief regarding responsibility for actions. Individuals with an *internal locus of control* generally hold themselves responsible for actions and consequences, while those with an *external locus of control* tend to believe that they are not able to affect a personal outcome and that luck or destiny are responsible for their actions.

Iodoxamide (lo-dok'sah-mīd) a mast CELL stabilizer that inhibits immediate HYPERSENSITIVITY, applied topically to the eye as the tromethamine salt for treatment of allergen-induced conjunctivitis, keratitis, and keratoconjunctivitis.

Löffler's disease (lef'lerz) Löffler's EN-DOCARDITIS.

löffleria (lef-le′re-ah) the presence of *Corynebacterium diphtheriae* (diphtheria bacillus) without the ordinary symptoms of diphtheria.

LOEL lowest observed effect level.

log(o)- word element [Gr.], *words; speech.*

logadectomy (log″ah-dek′to-me) excision of a portion of the conjunctiva.

logagraphia (log″ah-graf′e-ah) agraphia.

logamnesia (log″am-ne′zhah) receptive aphasia.

logaphasia (log″ah-fa′zhah) motor apha-sia.

logasthenia (log″as-the′ne-ah) easy fatig-ability of speaking.

logoclonia (log″o-klo′ne-ah) spasmodic repetition of words or parts of words, particularly the end syllables, as may occur in Alzheimer's disease.

logopathy (log-op′ah-the) speech disorder.

logopedia (log″o-pe′de-ah) logopedics.

logopedics (log″o-pe′diks) the study and treatment of speech defects. See also speech PATHOLOGY.

logoplegia (log″o-ple′jah) paralysis of the speech organs.

logorrhea (log″o-re′ah) excessive volubil-ty, with rapid, pressured speech, as in manic episodes of bipolar disorder and some cases of schizophrenia. Called also lalorrhea, pres-sured speech, tachylalia, and tachyphasia.

logospasm (log′o-spazm) 1. logoclonia. 2. stuttering.

log rolling a method of turning patients following neurosurgical procedures when the spine must be maintained in alignment. Two persons use a sheet to turn the patient as a unit; if the patient is unable to support the head, a third person is necessary.

-logy word element [Gr.], *science; treat-se; sum of knowledge in a particular subject.*

loiasis (lo-i′ah-sis) infection with nema-odes of the genus *Loa;* called also loaiasis.

loin (loin) the part of the back between the thorax and pelvis; called also lumbus.

lomefloxacin (lo″mĕ-flok′sah-sin) a broad-spectrum ANTIBIOTIC effective against a wide range of aerobic gram-negative and gram-positive organisms; used as the hydro-chloride salt.

Lomotil (lo′mo-til) trademark for combi-nation preparations of DIPHENOXYLATE hydro-chloride and ATROPINE sulfate, used in treatment of diarrhea.

lomustine (lo-mus′tēn) a nitrosourea ALKYLATING AGENT used as an antineoplastic AGENT in treatment of Hodgkin's disease and

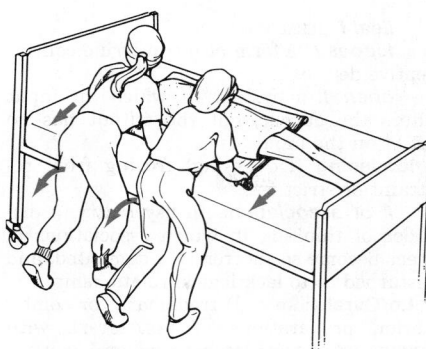

Log rolling a patient as a unit. Redrawn from Bolander, 1994.

brain tumors, administered orally. Called also CCNU.

loneliness (lōn′le-nes) a sense of dejection because of being alone.

  risk for l. a NURSING DIAGNOSIS accepted by the North American Nursing Diagnosis Association, defined as being at risk for experiencing vague DYSPHORIA.

Long (long) Crawford Williamson (1815–1878). American physician, born at Daniels-ville, Georgia, who in 1842 administered ether to a patient before removing a neck tumor, the first recorded use of an anesthetic in surgery.

long-acting thyroid stimulator (LATS) a substance occurring in the blood in HYPERTHYROIDISM, having a stimulating effect on the THYROID of longer duration than that of THYROTROPIN. It is associated with IMMUNOGLOBULIN IgG and may function as an AUTOANTIBODY.

longissimus (lon-jis′ĭ-mus) [L.] longest.

longitudinalis (lon″jĭ-tu″dĭ-na′lis) length-wise; in official anatomic nomenclature it designates a structure that is parallel to the long axis of the body or an organ.

long QT syndrome a combination of prolonged Q–T INTERVAL and TORSADES DE POINTES; it may be congenital or acquired, the latter usually being the result of drug administration.

longus (long′gus) [L.] long.

loop (lo͞op) a turn or sharp curve in a cordlike structure.

  capillary l's minute endothelial tubes that carry blood in the papillae of the skin.

  closed l. a system in which the input to one or more of the subsystems is affected by its own output.

  Henle's l. the U-shaped part of the NEPH-RON extending from the proximal to the distal convoluted tubule.

ileal l. ILEAL CONDUIT.

Lippes l. a form of intrauterine contraceptive device.

open l. a system in which an input alters the output, but the output has no effect on the input.

loosening (loo′sen-ing) freeing from restraint or strictness.

l. of associations in psychiatry, a disorder of thinking in which associations of ideas become so shortened, fragmented, and disturbed as to lack logical relationship.

Lo/Ovral (lo-o′vral) trademark for combination preparations of NORGESTREL with ETHINYL ESTRADIOL; used as an oral CONTRACEPTIVE.

LOP left occipitoposterior (position of the fetus).

loperamide (lo-per′ah-mīd) an agent used for its ANTIPERISTALTIC action for treatment of DIARRHEA and reduction of the volume of discharge from ILEOSTOMIES, administered orally.

lophotrichous (lo-fot′rĭ-kus) having two or more flagella at one end; said of bacterial cells.

Lopid (lo′pid) trademark for a preparation of GEMFIBROZIL, an ANTILIPIDEMIC agent.

lopinavir (lo-pin′ah-vir) an HIV protease inhibitor, an antiviral agent used in combination with ritonavir in the treatment of human immunodeficiency virus infection; administered orally.

Lopressor (lo-pres′er) trademark for preparations of METOPROLOL tartrate, used to treat HYPERTENSION, ANGINA PECTORIS, and MYOCARDIAL INFARCTION.

loracarbef (lor″ah-kahr′bef) a CARBACEPHEM ANTIBIOTIC closely related to CEFACLOR and with similar antimicrobial activity and uses.

loratadine (lah-rat′ah-dēn) a nonsedating antihistamine (H₁ receptor ANTAGONIST) used for treatment of allergic RHINITIS and chronic idiopathic urticaria and as a treatment adjunct in ASTHMA; administered orally.

lorazepam (lor-az′ĕ-pam) a BENZODIAZEPINE derivative used as an ANTIANXIETY AGENT, sedative-hypnotic, preanesthetic medication, and anticonvulsant, and as an antiemetic in cancer chemotherapy; administered orally, intravenously, or intramuscularly.

lordoscoliosis (lor″do-sko″le-o′sis) lordosis complicated with scoliosis.

lordosis (lor-do′sis) 1. the anterior concavity in the curvature of the lumbar and cervical spine as viewed from the side. 2. abnormal increase in this curvature. See also KYPHOSIS and SCOLIOSIS. adj., **lordot′ic.**

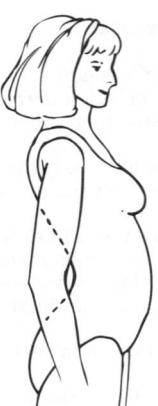

Abnormally increased curvature of the lower spine characteristic of lordosis. From Dorland's, 2000.

Lorelco (lo-rel′ko) trademark for a preparation of PROBUCOL, an ANTICHOLESTEREMIC.

losartan (lo-sahr′tan) an ANGIOTENSIN II receptor antagonist used as an ANTIHYPERTENSIVE; used as the potassium salt.

loss (laws) the amount by which a quantity or group is diminished; something that escapes from its owner's possession.

hearing l. see HEARING LOSS.

insensible l., insensible water l. the amount of fluid lost on a daily basis from the lungs, skin, and respiratory tract, as well as water excreted in the feces; the exact amount cannot be measured, but it is estimated to be between 40 cc and 600 cc in an adult under normal circumstances. See also SWEATING.

LOT left occipitotransverse (position of the fetus).

loteprednol (lo″tĕ-pred′nol) a CORTICOSTEROID applied topically to the conjunctiva in the treatment of seasonal allergic CONJUNCTIVITIS, postoperative inflammation, and ocular inflammatory disorders.

lotion (lo′shun) a liquid suspension, solution, or emulsion for external application to the body.

calamine l. a mixture of CALAMINE, ZINC OXIDE, GLYCERIN, bentonite magma (a suspending agent), and CALCIUM HYDROXIDE solution; used as a skin protectant.

Lotrimin (lo′trĭ-min) trademark for preparations of CLOTRIMAZOLE, an antifungal AGENT.

Lou Gehrig's disease (loo gar′igz) amyotrophic lateral sclerosis.

Louis-Bar's syndrome (loo-e-bahrz′) ataxia-telangiectasia.

loupe (loop) a magnifying lens.

louse (lows), pl. *lice* any of various grayish, wingless insects parasitic on birds and mammals, including humans; they are usually one sixteenth to one sixth of an inch (0.15 to 0.4 cm) long. Lice are classified into two orders, Anoplura (the sucking lice) and Mallophaga (the bird lice or biting lice). The causal organisms of TYPHUS, RELAPSING FEVER, TRENCH FEVER, and other diseases are transmitted by the bites of lice. The most important species parasitic on humans are *Pediculus humanus capitis,* the head louse, which attaches itself to the hairs of the head; *P. humanus corporis,* the body or clothes louse; and *Phthirus pubis,* the crab louse, which lives in the pubic hair, eyelashes, and eyebrows. Endemics of head lice infestations occur most frequently in school children. Pubic lice are often sexually transmitted. Louse infestation is called PEDICULOSIS.

lovastatin (lo'vah-stat″in) an ANTIHYPER-LIPIDEMIC agent that acts by inhibiting cholesterol synthesis, used in the treatment of HYPERCHOLESTEROLEMIA and other forms of DYSLIPIDEMIA and to lower the risks associated with ATHEROSCLEROSIS and CORONARY HEART DISEASE; administered orally.

Lowe disease (lō) oculocerebrorenal syndrome.

low-grade (lo'grād') occurring near the low end of a range, as of a fever or malignancy.

Lown-Ganong-Levine syndrome (lown'-gah-nong' lĕ-vēn') an electrocardiographic abnormality consisting of a short PR interval and normal QRS complex associated with paroxysmal supraventricular TACHYCARDIA. Called also short PR syndrome.

loxapine (loks'ah-pēn) a tricyclic ANTIPSY-CHOTIC AGENT, used as the hydrochloride and succinate salts; administered orally or intramuscularly.

loxoscelism (lok-sos'sĕ-lizm) a morbid condition resulting from the bite of the spiders *Loxosceles reclusa* and *L. laeta,* beginning with a painful inflamed vesicle and progressing to a gangrenous slough of skin that can be fatal. It is more common with the South American spider than with the North American one. See also SPIDER BITE.

Loxosceles (lok-sos'ĕ-lēz) a genus of six-eyed spiders, some of which have poisonous bites (see SPIDER BITE). *L. lae′ta* is a brown spider of South America and *L. reclu′sa* is the brown recluse spider of North America.

lozenge (loz'enj) a medicinal preparation for solution in the mouth, consisting of an active ingredient incorporated in a mass made of sugar and mucilage or fruit base. Called also troche.

LPN licensed practical nurse.

LSA left sacroanterior (position of the fetus).

LScA left scapuloanterior (position of the fetus).

LScP left scapuloposterior (position of the fetus).

LSD lysergic acid diethylamide, a HALLUCI-NOGEN derived from lysergic acid, a constituent of ERGOT alkaloids. It has consciousness-expanding effects and is capable of producing a state of mind in which there are HALLUCINATIONS (false sense perceptions). Called also lysergide. The perceptual changes brought about by LSD in normal persons are extremely variable and depend on factors such as age, personality, education, physical make-up, and state of health. The danger of the drug lies in the fact that it loosens control over impulsive behavior and may lead to a full-blown psychosis or less serious mental disorder in persons with latent mental illness. See also DRUG ABUSE.

LSP left sacroposterior (position of fetus).

L-spine lumbar spine.

LST left sacrotransverse (position of the fetus).

LT lymphotoxin.

LTF lymphocyte-transforming factor.

Lu lutetium.

lubb (lub) a syllable used to represent, or mimic, the first HEART SOUND.

lubb-dupp (lub'dup) syllables used to represent, or mimic, the combination of the first (lubb) and second (dupp) HEART SOUNDS.

lucidity (loo-sid'ĭ-te) clearness of mind. adj., **lu'cid.**

lucifugal (loo-sif'u-gal) avoiding, or repelled by, bright light.

lucipetal (loo-sip'ĕ-tal) seeking, or attracted to, bright light.

Ludiomil (loo'de-o-mil″) trademark for a preparation of MAPROTILINE hydrochloride, a tetracyclic ANTIDEPRESSANT.

Ludwig's angina (lōōd'vigz) a severe form of cellulitis of the submaxillary space and secondary involvement of the sublingual and submental spaces, usually resulting from an infection in the mandibular molar area or a penetrating injury of the floor of the mouth. Elevation of the tongue, difficulty in eating and swallowing, edema of the glottis, fever, rapid breathing, and moderate leukocytosis are the most common symptoms.

Luer-Lok (lōōr'lok) a syringe tip that contains grooves so that a needle can be securely screwed to it.

Lugol's solution (loo-golz') a solution of IODINE with POTASSIUM IODIDE, used as a source of iodine in preparation for THYROID surgery and in various staining methods.

lumb(o)- word element [L.], *loin.*

lumbago (lum-ba′go) pain in the lumbar region of the back, an old popular term for lower back pain. It includes various different conditions caused by factors such as injury, back strain, arthritis, abuse of the back muscles (such as from poor posture, a sagging mattress, or ill-fitting shoes), or any of a number of other disorders.

lumbar (lum′bahr) pertaining to the LOINS.

  l. puncture introduction of a hollow needle into the subarachnoid space of the spinal canal, usually between the fourth and fifth lumbar vertebrae; see also CISTERNAL PUNCTURE. Called also spinal puncture.

  It may be done for diagnostic purposes to determine the pressure within the cerebrospinal cavities, to determine presence of an obstruction to flow of CEREBROSPINAL FLUID, to remove a specimen of cerebrospinal fluid for laboratory examination, or to inject air or other contrast medium into the spinal canal to take an x-ray of the cerebrospinal system.

  Patient Care. Before the procedure is begun the patient is given a simple explanation of the nature and purpose of the test and is told that there is no danger of damage to the spinal cord during a lumbar puncture because the spinal cord does not extend below the second lumbar vertebra. For a cisternal puncture, the back of the neck may be shaved.

  The patient is positioned so that the knees and head are flexed as much as possible and is assisted in maintaining this position during the entire procedure. A local anesthetic is injected subcutaneously to anesthetize the skin and underlying tissues. The patient should be warned not to move suddenly and told there may be a slight feeling of pressure when the puncture needle is inserted.

  Strict adherence to the rules of aseptic technique is necessary to avoid the possibility of introducing microorganisms into the spinal canal. The attendant may be asked to assist in the Queckenstedt test during the lumbar puncture. This test involves compression of the veins of the neck, first on one side, then on the other and finally on both sides at once. The cerebrospinal fluid pressure is measured each time the veins are compressed. This test determines whether there is an obstruction in the spinal canal. Care must be taken that the trachea is not constricted while the neck veins are being compressed.

  After the procedure the patient is observed for signs of pulse changes, respiratory difficulty, or cyanosis. These rarely

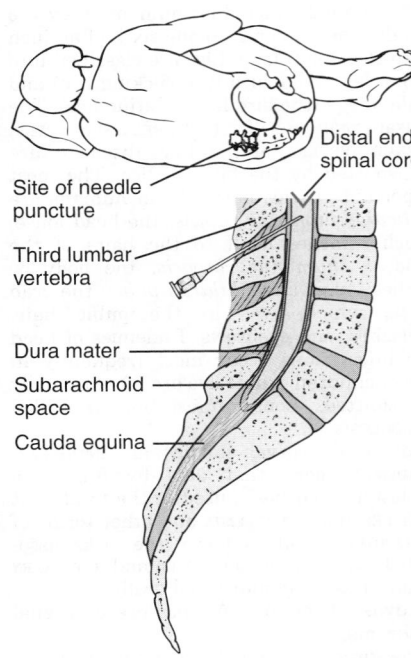

Technique of lumbar puncture. Needle is inserted between vertebrae and advanced through dura mater to the subarachnoid space. Cerebrospinal fluid is thus withdrawn from the spinal cavity.

occur, but headache is common and may be partially relieved by keeping the patient flat in bed for 8 hours after the procedure. An ice cap and aspirin may help alleviate the discomfort.

lumbarization (lum″bahr-ĭ-za′shun) nonfusion of the first and second segments of the sacrum so that there is one additional articulated vertebra, the sacrum consisting of only four segments.

lumbocostal (lum″bo-kos′t'l) pertaining to the loin and ribs.

lumbodynia (lum″bo-din′e-ah) lumbago.

lumbosacral (lum″bo-sa′kr'l) pertaining to the lumbar and sacral region, or to the lumbar vertebrae and sacrum.

lumbricoid (lum′brĭ-koid) resembling an earthworm; said of ASCARIDS, or intestinal roundworms.

lumbricosis (lum″brĭ-ko′sis) ascariasis.

lumbricus (lum′brĭ-kus), pl. *lum′brici* [L.] 1. the earthworm. 2. old term for ASCARIS.

lumbus (lum′bus) [L.] loin.

lumen (lu′men) [L.] 1. the cavity or channel within a tube or tubular organ, as a blood vessel or the intestine. 2. the SI unit of rate of flow of radiant energy, specifically that of the visible spectrum. adj., **lu′minal.**

luminescence (lu″mĭ-nes′ens) the property of giving off light without a corresponding degree of heat.

luminophor (lu′mĭ-no-for) a chemical group that gives the property of luminescence to organic compounds.

lumirhodopsin (loo″mĭ-ro-dop′sin) an intermediate product of exposure of rhodopsin to light.

lumpectomy (lump-ek′to-me) 1. surgical excision of only the palpable lesion in carcinoma of the breast; called also tylectomy. 2. surgical removal of a mass; see also excisional BIOPSY.

lunate (loo′nāt) 1. moon-shaped or crescentic. 2. the lunate bone; see anatomic Table of Bones in the Appendices.

Lund-Browder classification (lund brow′-der) a method for estimating the extent of burns that allows for the varying proportion of body surface in persons of different ages. It is used instead of the RULE OF NINES for children, in whom the head occupies a larger area and the lower limbs a smaller area than in adults. See illustration.

lung (lung) either of two large organs lying within the chest cavity on either side of the heart; they supply the blood with oxygen inhaled from the outside air and dispose of waste carbon dioxide in the exhaled air, as a part of the process known as RESPIRATION. Other functions include filtration of blood, serving as reservoirs to store blood, and playing a role in metabolic activities. See also color plates.

The lungs are made of elastic tissue filled with interlacing networks of tubes and sacs carrying air, and with blood vessels carrying blood. The BRONCHI, which bring air to the lungs, branch out within the lungs into many smaller tubes, the BRONCHIOLES, which culminate in clusters of tiny air sacs called ALVEOLI, whose total runs into millions. The alveoli are surrounded by a network of capillaries. Through the thin membranes of the capillaries, the air and blood make their exchange of oxygen and carbon dioxide.

The lungs are divided into lobes, the left lung having two (the *left upper lobe* and the *left lower lobe*) and the right having three (the *right upper lobe,* the *right middle lobe,* and the *right lower lobe);* these are further subdivided into bronchopulmonary segments, of which there are about 20. Protecting each lung is the pleura, a two-layered membrane that envelops the lung and contains lubricating fluid between its inner and outer layers.

Mechanics of Inflation and Deflation. The lungs are inflated by action of the diaphragm and the intercostal muscles. The diaphragm, a large dome-shaped muscle, forms the bottom of the thoracic cage. As it contracts it flattens, increasing the diameter of the thorax and elevating the lower ribs. Both of these actions increase the space for expansion of the lungs. The external intercostal muscles provide flexibility to the thoracic cage and allow more room for lung expansion by elevating the anterior end of each rib, thereby increasing the anterior-posterior diameter of the chest wall.

Deflation of the lungs is chiefly a passive maneuver. The major muscles involved in exhalation are the abdominal muscle group. As these muscles contract, they depress the lower ribs, and, through an increase in abdominal pressure, move the diaphragm upward.

As the lungs are compressed and distended by the respiratory muscles, the pressure within the alveoli (intra-alveolar pressure) rises and falls. During inhalation the pressure becomes slightly negative (-3 mm Hg) in relation to atmospheric pressure. During exhalation the intra-alveolar pressure rises to approximately $+3$ mm Hg. The effect of negative pressure within the alveoli is to cause air under atmospheric pressure to flow into the lungs (inhalation). The condition of positive pressure creates the opposite effect, causing air to flow outward (exhalation).

The lungs are surrounded by an airtight compartment, the pleural space within the pleural membrane. The intrapleural pressure is less than atmospheric pressure and is expressed as negative pressure. Normally the intrapleural pressure is about -4 mm Hg. When the lungs are fully expanded this pressure may be as great as -9 mm Hg. Under normal conditions, however, the intrapleural pressure fluctuates between -4 and -6 mm Hg.

If anything should penetrate the walls of the pleura, the negative pressure is lost as air rushes into the pleural cavity in response to atmospheric pressure. This condition is called PNEUMOTHORAX. The walls of the alveoli also must remain intact in order to maintain normal intrapleural pressure. If a lesion causes a break in the alveolar membranes, air enters the pleural cavity through the break and produces pneumothorax. Relief of pneumothorax and collapse of the lung from accumulations of either air or fluids within the pleural space may be provided by aspiration of the air or fluid from the thoracic cavity (THORACENTESIS) or by insertion of CHEST TUBES to provide for a gradual reexpansion of the lung. (Specific tests to determine

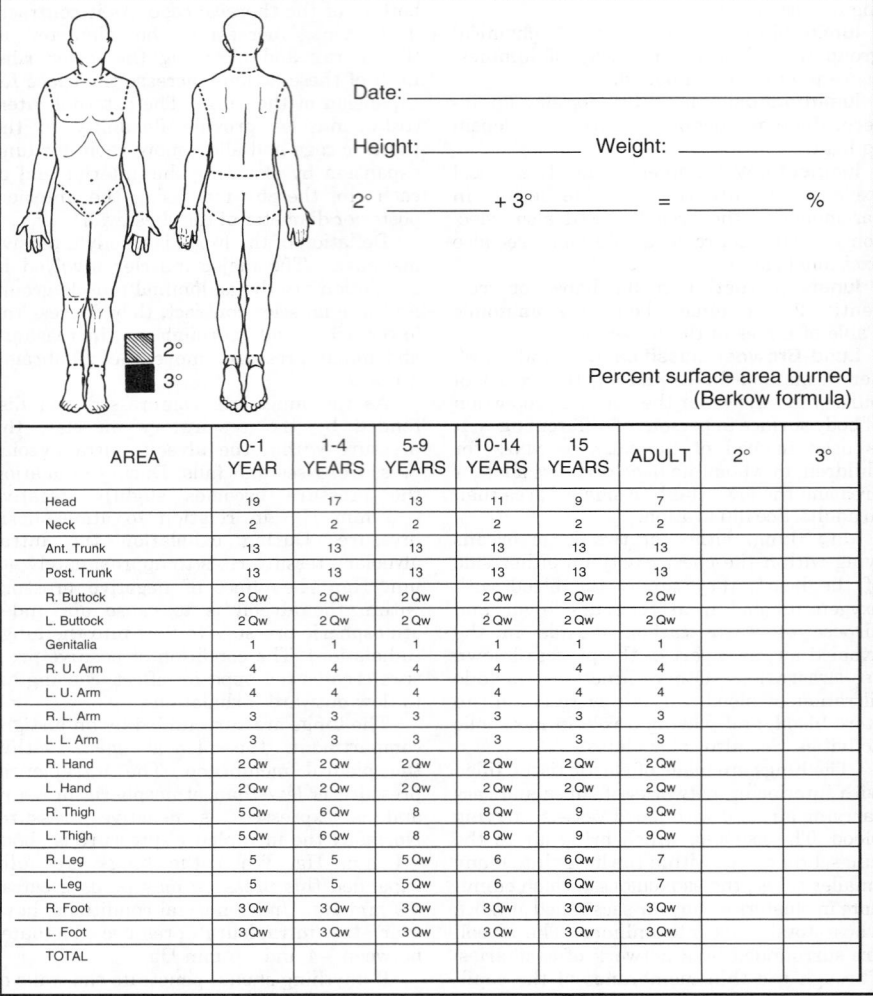

AREA	0-1 YEAR	1-4 YEARS	5-9 YEARS	10-14 YEARS	15 YEARS	ADULT	2°	3°
Head	19	17	13	11	9	7		
Neck	2	2	2	2	2	2		
Ant. Trunk	13	13	13	13	13	13		
Post. Trunk	13	13	13	13	13	13		
R. Buttock	2 Qw	2 Qw	2 Qw	2 Qw	2 Qw	2 Qw		
L. Buttock	2 Qw	2 Qw	2 Qw	2 Qw	2 Qw	2 Qw		
Genitalia	1	1	1	1	1	1		
R. U. Arm	4	4	4	4	4	4		
L. U. Arm	4	4	4	4	4	4		
R. L. Arm	3	3	3	3	3	3		
L. L. Arm	3	3	3	3	3	3		
R. Hand	2 Qw	2 Qw	2 Qw	2 Qw	2 Qw	2 Qw		
L. Hand	2 Qw	2 Qw	2 Qw	2 Qw	2 Qw	2 Qw		
R. Thigh	5 Qw	6 Qw	8	8 Qw	9	9 Qw		
L. Thigh	5 Qw	6 Qw	8	8 Qw	9	9 Qw		
R. Leg	5	5	5 Qw	6	6 Qw	7		
L. Leg	5	5	5 Qw	6	6 Qw	7		
R. Foot	3 Qw	3 Qw	3 Qw	3 Qw	3 Qw	3 Qw		
L. Foot	3 Qw	3 Qw	3 Qw	3 Qw	3 Qw	3 Qw		
TOTAL								

A sample chart for recording the extent and depth of a burn injury using the Lund-Browder formula. From Polaski and Tatro, 1996.

Disorders of the Lungs. The air brought to the lungs is filtered, moistened, and warmed on its way along the respiratory tract but it can nevertheless bring irritants and infectious organisms, and when the body resistance is low for any reason the lungs may suffer diseases of some seriousness. Such diseases include TUBERCULOSIS and PNEUMONIA. Other disorders of the lungs include pulmonary EDEMA, PLEURISY, ASTHMA, BRONCHIECTASIS, ATELECTASIS, EMPHYSEMA, and PNEUMOCONIOSIS. Still other diseases enter the lungs via pathogens in the circulation and the lungs may also be affected by pulmonary EMBOLISM and CHRONIC OBSTRUCTIVE PULMONARY DISEASE.

l. abscess an infection of the lung characterized by a localized accumulation of pus and destruction of tissue. It may be a complication of pneumonia or tuberculosis. A lung abscess may also follow a period of excessive drinking by an alcoholic. Infected

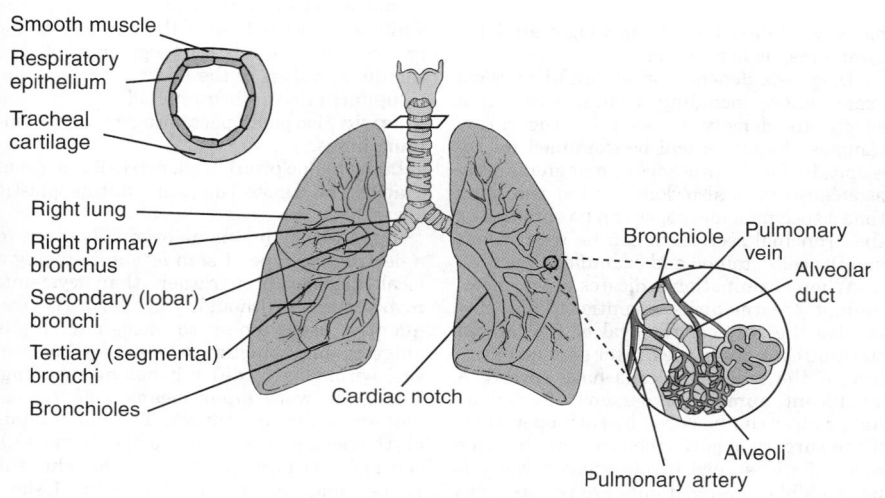

Structure of the lung. From Applegate, 2000.

matter that has been aspirated (usually in a drunken stupor) may lodge in a bronchiole and produce inflammation. Lung cancer may also be responsible for formation of an abscess.

The first symptoms include a dry cough and chest pain. Later these may be followed by fever, chills, productive cough, headache, perspiration, foul-smelling sputum, and sometimes dyspnea. If the abscess is a complication of pneumonia, the symptoms tend to be moderated to an exaggeration of the pneumonia symptoms.

When a lung abscess forms, it is in the acute stage and treatment with antibiotics usually is effective. POSTURAL DRAINAGE may be prescribed to assist in drainage of exudate from lungs and bronchioles. In most cases, this treatment produces a cure. If the abscess becomes chronic, surgery may be necessary and usually involves removal of the portion of the lung containing the abscess.

accessory l. pulmonary SEQUESTRATION.

bird breeder's l. pigeon breeder's lung.

black l. coal workers' PNEUMOCONIOSIS.

brown l. byssinosis.

l. cancer malignant growths of the lung. Although the exact cause of lung cancer is not known, inhaled carcinogens are known to be important predisposing causes. Cancer in the lungs may also be a metastasis of malignancy elsewhere in the body. Many years ago it was realized that miners of certain ores who inhaled the mine dust developed lung cancer much more often than workers in other occupations. Later, other carcinogens of lung tissue, such as air polluted by fumes from burning fuels or motor exhausts, were singled out as probable causes of the increasing number of cases of the disease in urban and industrial areas. The most obvious carcinogen, however, and the one most widely encountered, is tobacco smoke, especially cigarette smoke, which is much more frequently and deeply inhaled than the smoke of pipes or cigars.

A study based on autopsies of the lungs of individuals who had died from many varied causes, but whose SMOKING history was known, showed that unrecognized cancer and precancerous changes in tissue were numerous among smokers and rare among nonsmokers. These findings led the Surgeon General of the United States to appoint an investigative committee, which ultimately issued a report stating that "cigarette smoking is a health hazard of sufficient importance in the United States to warrant appropriate action."

Since the factors causing lung cancer act slowly and may produce a tumor near the periphery of the lung, early symptoms are vague or may not appear at all, and nearly a third of the cases are in an advanced stage when they are discovered. The earliest and most common symptom is a cough. Dry at first, this cough later produces sputum, which eventually becomes blood-streaked. An isolated persistent wheeze in the chest is frequently a symptom and indicates a partial obstruction in a bronchus. Chest pains, weakness, and loss of weight are later symptoms, as is dyspnea.

Diagnosis depends on a careful physical examination, including a chest x-ray. If a suspicious density is seen on the x-ray, samples of sputum will be examined microscopically for the presence of malignant cells. BRONCHOSCOPY is also done, and at the same time a specimen for biopsy can be obtained or the bronchial secretions can be washed out and the cells stained and examined.

When examination indicates lung cancer, prompt treatment is essential. This may involve the surgical removal of the lobe of the lung containing the cancer or of an entire lung if the malignant cells have spread. A significant number of persons affected by lung cancer can be cured by such operations if the surgery is performed in time. In some cases of widespread involvement surgery is not possible; these patients are treated with radiation therapy and ANTINEOPLASTIC drugs.

Carcinogens that can trigger lung cancer must be avoided and, when possible, eliminated. Mine workers should take adequate precautions to avoid inhaling harmful dusts. Public health authorities and industry must act more effectively to control air pollution. The most important step toward protection against lung cancer is elimination of cigarette smoking. State and local units of the American Lung Association are excellent sources of information about lung disease and its prevention.

Lung cancer clinical guidelines have been published in both the United States and Canada. In Canada they are available at the web site of Cancer Care Ontario, http://www.cancercare.on.ca. and in the United States they are available at the web site of the National Guideline Clearinghouse, http://www.guideline.gov.

coal miner's l. coal workers' PNEUMO-CONIOSIS.

farmer's l. hypersensitivity PNEUMONITIS caused by inhalation of moldy hay dust.

iron l. popular name for Drinker RESPIRATOR.

pigeon breeder's l. hypersensitivity PNEUMONITIS caused by inhalation of particles of bird feces, seen in those who work closely with pigeons or other birds; it may eventually result in pulmonary fibrosis.

shock l. acute respiratory distress syndrome.

wet l. 1. pulmonary edema. 2. acute respiratory distress syndrome.

lungworm (lung′werm) any parasitic worm that invades the lungs, such as *Paragonimus westermani* in humans.

lunula (loo′nu-lah) [L.] a small, crescentic or moon-shaped area or structure, e.g., the white area at the base of the nail of a finger or toe, or one of the segments of the semilunar valves of the heart.

lupiform (loo′pĭ-form) lupoid.

lupoid (loo′poid) pertaining to or resembling lupus.

Lupron (loo′pron) trademark for a preparation of LEUPROLIDE, an antineoplastic AGENT.

lupus (loo′pus) a name originally given to a destructive type of skin lesion, implying a local degeneration rather than systemic involvement. Although the term is frequently used alone to designate lupus vulgaris and sometimes lupus erythematosus, without a modifier it has no meaning. The Latin word *lupus* means wolf; *erythematosus* refers to redness. The name lupus erythematosus has been used since the 13th century because physicians thought the shape and color of the skin lesions resembled the bite of a wolf. Currently, there are at least two recognized manifestations of the disease: discoid lupus erythematosus and systemic lupus erythematosus.

chilblain l. erythematosus a form of discoid lupus erythematosus aggravated by cold, initially resembling CHILBLAINS, in which the lesions consist of reddened infiltrated patches on the exposed areas of the body, especially the finger knuckles.

cutaneous l. erythematosus one of the two main types of lupus erythematosus; it may involve only the skin or may precede involvement of other body systems. It may be chronic (discoid lupus erythematosus); subacute (systemic lupus erythematosus); or acute (characterized by an acute edematous, erythematous eruption, often with systemic exacerbations). The acute form may be the presenting symptom of systemic lupus erythematosus, such as after sun exposure.

discoid l. erythematosus (DLE) a superficial inflammation of the skin, marked by red macules up to 3 to 4 cm in width, and covered with scanty adherent scales, which extend into spreading follicles that fall off and leave scars. The lesions typically form a butterfly pattern over the bridge of the nose and cheeks, but other areas may be involved, notably the scalp and other areas that are exposed to light.

drug-induced l. a syndrome closely resembling systemic lupus erythematosus, precipitated by prolonged use of certain drugs, most commonly HYDRALAZINE, ISONIAZID, various ANTICONVULSANTS, and PROCAINAMIDE.

l. erythemato′sus (LE) a group of connective tissue disorders primarily affecting women aged 20 to 40, comprising a spectrum of clinical forms in which cutaneous disease may occur with or without systemic involvement.

l. per′nio 1. soft, purplish skin lesions on the cheeks, forehead, nose, ears, and digits, frequently associated with bone cysts, which may be the first manifestation of sarcoidosis or occur in the chronic stage of the disease. 2. chilblain lupus erythematosus.

systemic l. erythematosus (SLE) a chronic inflammatory disease, usually febrile and characterized by injury to the skin, joints, kidneys, nervous system, and mucous membranes. It can, however, affect any organ of the body and usually has periods of remissions and exacerbations. (See plate in Dermatology Atlas.)

It was once thought that this was a fairly rare disease, but improved immunologic testing procedures have shown that it is not. It is primarily a disease of women, occurring five to ten times more often in females than in males. Although the peak incidence is between 30 and 40 years of age, the condition has also been diagnosed in the very young and the very old.

SLE is the classic prototype of AUTOIMMUNE DISEASE of connective tissue. Its etiology is unknown, but the high level of AUTOANTIBODIES in persons with the condition indicates a defect in the regulatory mechanisms that sustain self-tolerance and prevent the body from attacking its own cells, cell constituents, and proteins. Patients with SLE can have a wide variety of autoantibodies against nuclear and cytoplasmic cellular components. The presence of high levels of antinuclear ANTIBODY (ANA) in SLE patients with glomerulonephritis indicates a *pathogenic* role for that antibody. The antibodies are directed against deoxyribonucleoprotein, DNA, histone, and a soluble non–nucleic acid molecule called Sm antigen.

Factors that appear to contribute to the development of SLE include exposure to sunlight or ultraviolet radiation from sunlamps, a genetic predisposition to the disease, certain drugs, viral infections, and hormonal influences.

Clinical manifestations of SLE are confusingly diverse owing to the involvement of connective tissue throughout the body. Typically, the patient seeks medical help for relief of fever, weight loss, joint pain, the characteristic butterfly rash, pleural effusion and pleuritic pain, and nephritis. The detection of ANA by microscopic immunofluorescence is supportive evidence for the presence of SLE.

Either glomerulonephritis, which is usually mild, or cardiovascular manifestations

such as MYOCARDITIS, ENDOCARDITIS, or PERICARDITIS, are found in about half the patients with SLE. Pulmonary disease, especially PLEURISY, is also relatively common, as are gastrointestinal disturbances and lymph node involvement. Organic neurologic disturbances produce behavioral aberrations and frank PSYCHOSIS in some patients; in a few others, there are peripheral NEUROPATHIES, motor weakness, and DIPLOPIA.

Supportive measures are used to prevent or minimize acute relapses and exacerbations of symptoms. The patient is instructed to avoid exposure to sunlight and ultraviolet radiation from other sources, blood transfusions, penicillin, and the sulfonamides. Active disease is treated with topical STEROIDS, NONSTEROIDAL ANTI-INFLAMMATORY DRUGS for fever and joint pain, CORTICOSTEROIDS, and IMMUNOSUPPRESSANTS. The goal of drug therapy is suppression of the immune system. Treatment of specific manifestations of SLE is aimed at prevention of complications. Physical therapy may be required to alleviate muscle weakness and prevent orthopedic deformities.

l. vulga′ris the most common and severe form of TUBERCULOSIS of the skin, most often affecting the face, with formation of reddish brown patches of nodules in the CORIUM, which progressively spread peripherally with central atrophy, causing ulceration and scarring and destruction of cartilage in involved sites.

lute (loot) 1. a substance such as cement, wax, or clay that coats a joint area to make a tight seal; called also luting agent. 2. to coat with such a substance.

luteal (loo′te-al) pertaining to or having the properties of the corpus luteum or its active principle.

lutein (loo′te-in) 1. a LIPOCHROME from the CORPUS LUTEUM, fat cells, and egg yolk. 2. any lipochrome.

luteinic (loo″te-in′ik) 1. pertaining to LUTEIN or to LUTEINIZATION. 2. luteal.

luteinization (loo″te-in″ĭ-za′shun) the process taking place in the luteal CELLS of GRAAFIAN FOLLICLES that have matured and discharged their eggs: the cells become hypertrophied and there is vascularization and lipid accumulation (the latter in some species giving a yellow color), the follicles then become corpora lutea.

Lutembacher's syndrome (loo′tem-bak″erz) mitral stenosis associated with atrial septal defect.

luteolysin (loo″te-ol′ĭ-sin) a substance that causes degeneration of corpus luteum.

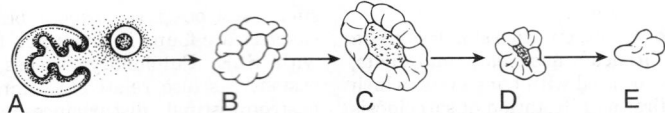

A   B   C   D   E

Luteinization, beginning after rupture of the ovarian follicle in ovulation *(A)* and progressing through vascularization and hypertrophy of the maturing corpus *(B, C);* it is followed by regression *(D)* to the corpus albicans *(E).* From Dorland's, 2000.

luteolysis (loo″te-ol′ĭ-sis) degeneration of corpus luteum.

luteoma (loo″te-o′mah) 1. a luteinized GRANULOSA-THECA CELL TUMOR. 2. nodular hyperplasia of ovarian lutein cells sometimes occurring in the last trimester of pregnancy.

luteotrope (loo′te-o-trōp″) lactotroph.

luteotroph (loo′te-o-trōf″) lactotroph.

luteotropic (loo″te-o-trop′ik) stimulating formation of the corpus luteum.

lutetium (Lu) (loo-te′she-um) a chemical element, atomic number 71, atomic weight 174.97. (See Appendix 6.)

Lutz-Splendore-Almeida disease paracoccidioidomycosis.

Luvox (loo′voks) trademark for a preparation of FLUVOXAMINE maleate, an ANTIDEPRESSANT.

lux (lx) (luks) the SI UNIT of illumination, being 1 lumen per square meter.

luxation (luk-sa′shun) dislocation.

luxus (luk′sus) [L.] excess.

LVN Licensed Vocational Nurse.

Lw lawrencium.

lyase (li′ās) any of a class of enzymes that remove groups from their substrates (other than by hydrolysis), leaving double bonds, or that conversely add groups to double bonds.

lycanthropy (li-kan′thro-pe) a delusion in which the patient believes that he is a wolf or other animal or that he can change into one.

lycoperdonosis (li″ko-per″do-no′sis) hypersensitivity PNEUMONITIS due to inhalation of spores of the puffball fungus, *Lycoperdon.*

lye (li) an alkaline percolate from wood ashes; household lye is a crude mixture of sodium hydroxide with some sodium carbonate.

lying-in (li′ing-in) 1. puerperal. 2. puerperium.

Lyme disease (līm) a recurrent multisystemic disease named for Old Lyme, Connecticut where a well-publicized outbreak occurred in 1975; the first report of the disease was actually from Europe in 1883. Its symptoms closely resemble those of many other disorders, making diagnosis difficult. There is now a direct detection test to confirm the presence of active disease.

Lyme disease is present worldwide, having been reported in 47 states in the United States, several provinces in Canada, and 20 countries on six continents. Called also Lyme arthritis.

Lyme disease is caused by *Borrelia burgdorferi,* with the vector being the ticks *Ixodes scapularis* and *I. pacificus;* tick control is one of the most important aspects of control of the disease. Tick bites can be avoided by wearing light colored long-sleeved shirts and long pants tucked into the socks and by using a tick repellent. After being in an area where ticks may be present, such as a grassy or woodland area, the body should be checked carefully for ticks and any that are attached should be removed immediately.

The person infected with Lyme disease will often initially experience flulike symptoms. Sixty per cent will experience a rash that is usually circular, but may be oblong and may be hot to the touch; it appears red on light skin and may look like a bruise on dark skin. Early symptoms disappear and are followed by a variety of multisystem complications that may include arthritis of the large joints, myalgia, malaise, and neurologic and cardiac manifestations. Early treatment with antibiotics will help to prevent long term complications.

Information and support for health care professionals and for patients with Lyme disease can be obtained from The Lyme Disease Foundation, Inc., One Financial Plaza, Hartford, CT 06103.

lymph (limf) a transparent, usually slightly yellow, often opalescent liquid found

LABORATORY TESTS TO SUPPORT THE DIAGNOSIS OF LYME DISEASE

Antibody Tests
  Titer tests (ELISA or IFA)
  Western blots

Direct Detection Tests
  Urine antigen detection
  Polymerase chain reaction (PCR)
  Antigen capture and detection (Gold stain)

within the lymphatic vessels, and collected from tissues in all parts of the body and returned to the blood via the lymphatic system. It is about 95 per cent water; the remainder consists of plasma proteins and other chemical substances contained in the blood plasma, but in slightly smaller percentage than in plasma. Its cellular component consists chiefly of lymphocytes.

The body contains three main kinds of fluid: blood, tissue fluid, and lymph. The blood consists of the blood cells and platelets, the plasma, or fluid portion, and a variety of chemical substances dissolved in the plasma. When the plasma, without its solid particles and some of its dissolved substances, seeps through the capillary walls and circulates among the body tissues, it is known as tissue fluid. When this fluid is drained from the tissues and collected by the lymphatic system, it is called lymph. The LYMPHATIC SYSTEM eventually returns the lymph to the blood, where it again becomes plasma. This movement of fluid through the body is described under CIRCULATORY SYSTEM.

l. node any of the accumulations of lymphoid tissue organized as definite lymphoid organs along the course of lymphatic vessels (see accompanying illustration); they consist of an outer cortical and an inner medullary part. Lymph nodes are the main source of lymphocytes of the peripheral blood and, as part of the reticuloendothelial system, serve as a defense mechanism by removing noxious agents such as bacteria and toxins, and probably play a role in antibody formation. Sometimes called, incorrectly, lymph gland. Called also lymph or lymphatic follicle and lymphatic nodule.

lymph(o)- word element [L.], *lymph; lymphoid tissue; lymphatics; lymphocytes.*

lympha (lim'fah) [L.] lymph.

lymphadenectomy (lim-fad″ĕ-nek'to-me) excision of one or more LYMPH NODES, usually for the purpose of examination. Called also lymph node dissection.

retroperitoneal l. surgical removal of lymph nodes in the retroperitoneal space, usually because of cancer metastasis, such as from carcinomas of the genital organs in men. Called also retroperitoneal lymph node dissection.

lymphadenitis (lim″fad-ĕ-ni'tis) inflammation of one or more LYMPH NODES, usually caused by a primary focus of infection elsewhere in the body.

cervical l. cervical adenitis.

cervical l., tuberculous tuberculosis of the cervical lymph nodes, formerly called scrofula. Called also tuberculous cervical adenitis.

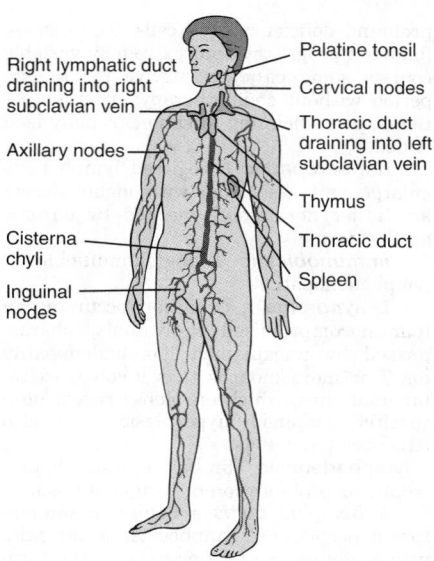

Right lymphatic duct draining into right subclavian vein
Axillary nodes
Cisterna chyli
Inguinal nodes
Palatine tonsil
Cervical nodes
Thoracic duct draining into left subclavian vein
Thymus
Thoracic duct
Spleen

Location of clusters of superficial lymph nodes. From Applegate, 2000.

tuberculous l. tuberculosis of lymph nodes, usually either cervical (*tuberculous cervical lymphadenitis*) or mediastinal. See also SCROFULODERMA.

lymphadenocele (lim-fad'ĕ-no-sēl) a cyst of a lymph node.

lymphadenogram (lim-fad'ĕ-no-gram″) the film produced by lymphadenography.

lymphadenography (lim″fad-ĕ-nog'rah-fe) radiography of lymph nodes after injection of a contrast medium in a lymphatic vessel.

lymphadenoid (lim-fad'ĕ-noid) resembling the tissues of the lymph nodes. Lymphadenoid tissue includes the spleen, bone marrow, tonsils, and the lymphoid tissues of the organs and mucous membranes.

lymphadenoma (lim-fad″ĕ-no'mah) lymphoma.

lymphadenopathy (lim-fad″ĕ-nop'ah-the) disease of the LYMPH NODES; called also adenopathy.

angioimmunoblastic l., angioimmunoblastic l. with dysproteinemia (AILD) a systemic disorder resembling lymphoma characterized by fever, night sweats, weight loss, generalized lymphadenopathy, hepatosplenomegaly, macropapular rash, polyclonal hypergammaglobulinemia, and Coombs'-positive hemolytic anemia. It is considered to be a nonmalignant hyperimmune reaction to chronic antigenic stimulation; there is proliferation of B cells accompanied by profound deficiency of T cells. The disease follows a progressive but extremely variable course: some patients survive for a long period without chemotherapy; in other patients, overwhelming infections rapidly lead to death

dermatopathic *l.* regional lymph node enlargement associated with melanoderma and other dermatoses marked by chronic erythroderma.

immunoblastic *l.* angioimmunoblastic lymphadenopathy.

l. **syndrome** a condition occurring in immunocompromised individuals, characterized by unexplained lymphadenopathy for 3 or more months that involves extrainguinal sites, which on biopsy reveal nonspecific lymphoid hyperplasia. See also AIDS-related COMPLEX.

lymphadenosis (lim-fad″ĕ-no′sis) hypertrophy or proliferation of lymphoid tissue.

l. **benig′na cu′tis** a benign inflammatory hyperplasia of lymphocytes in the skin, principally on the face or ears, in the form of solitary or disseminated yellowish brown to bluish red nodules that usually disappear spontaneously.

lymphadenotomy (lim-fad″ĕ-not′ah-me) incision of a lymph node.

lymphagogue (lim′fah-gog) something that promotes production of lymph.

lymphangial (lim-fan′je-al) pertaining to a lymphatic vessel.

lymphangiectasia (lim″fan-je-ek-ta′zhah) lymphangiectasis.

lymphangiectasis (lim-fan″je-ek′tah-sis) dilatation of the lymphatic vessels. adj., **lymphangiectat′ic.**

lymphangiectomy (lim-fan″je-ek′to-me) excision of one or more lymphatic vessels.

lymphangiitis (lim-fan″je-i′tis) lymphangitis.

lymphangioendothelioma (lim-fan″je-en″do-the′le-o′mah) LYMPHANGIOMA in which endothelial cells are the main component.

lymphangiofibroma (lim-fan″je-o-fi-bro′-mah) a fibrosing LYMPHANGIOMA.

lymphangiogram (lim-fan′je-o-gram″) the film produced by lymphangiography.

lymphangiography (lim-fan″je-og′rah-fe) ANGIOGRAPHY of lymphatic channels.

lymphangioleiomyomatosis (lim-fan″je-o-li″o-mi″o-mah-to′sis) lymphangiomyomatosis.

lymphangiology (lim-fan″je-ol′o-je) the scientific study of the lymphatic system.

lymphangioma (lim-fan″je-o′mah) a benign tumor composed of newly formed lymph spaces and channels. adj., **lymphangio′matous.**

l. **caverno′sum, cavernous** *l.* 1. a deeply situated lymphangioma, composed of cavernous lymphatic spaces, and always occurring in the neck or axilla. 2. cystic hygroma.

l. **circumscrip′tum** a cutaneous lymphangioma more superficial than the cavernous type, usually localized upper portion of the limbs, the axillary or inguinal folds, or the oral mucosa, especially the tongue; it consists of a grapelike group of thin-walled translucent lymph-filled vesicles that sometimes have a wartlike surface.

cystic *l.,* *l.* **cys′ticum** cystic HYGROMA.

simple *l.,* *l.* **sim′plex** one composed of small lymphatic channels that occurs subcutaneously in the head and neck region, in the axilla, and sometimes in internal organs. Superficial lesions are slightly raised or sometimes nodular; deeper lesions are sharply circumscribed, compressible, and gray to pink in color.

lymphangiomyomatosis (lim-fan″je-o-mi″o-mah-to′sis) a progressive disorder of women of child-bearing age, marked by nodular and diffuse interstitial proliferation of smooth muscle in the lungs, lymph nodes, and thoracic duct. Called also lymphangioleiomyomatosis.

lymphangiophlebitis (lim-fan″je-o-flĕ-bi′tis) inflammation of lymphatic vessels and veins.

lymphangiosarcoma (lim-fan″je-o-sahr-ko′mah) a malignant tumor of lymphatic vessels, usually arising in a limb that is the site of chronic lymphedema.

lymphangioscintigraphy (LAS) (lim-fan″je-o-sin-tig′rah-fe) SCINTIGRAPHIC evaluation of primary and secondary LYMPHEDEMA using radioactive tracers.

lymphangiotomy (lim-fan″je-ot′ah-me) incision of a lymphatic vessel.

lymphangitis (lim″fan-ji′tis) inflammation of a lymphatic vessel.

lymphapheresis (lim″fah-fĕ-re′sis) lymphocytapheresis.

lymphatic (lim-fat′ik) 1. pertaining to lymph or to a lymphatic vessel. 2. a lymphatic vessel.

l. **ducts** the two large vessels into which all lymphatic vessels converge. The right lymphatic duct joins the venous system at the junction of the right internal jugular and subclavian veins and carries lymph from the upper right side of the body. The left lymphatic duct, or thoracic duct, enters the circulatory system at the junction of the left internal jugular and subclavian veins; it returns lymph from the upper left side of the body and from below the diaphragm.

l. **system** the lymphatic VESSELS and lymphoid TISSUES considered collectively.

(See also CIRCULATORY SYSTEM.) Several diseases affect the lymphatic system. LYMPHOGRANULOMA VENEREUM is a viral disease that attacks lymph nodes in the groin and usually is transmitted by sexual contact. LYMPHADENITIS is an inflammation of the lymph nodes, particularly in the neck; swollen tonsils is an example. Generalized lymphadenitis can be a symptom of the secondary stage of SYPHILIS. Cancer attacks the lymphatic system, as it does other systems of the body; a tumor of the lymphoid tissue is known as a LYMPHOMA. The general term LYMPHOSARCOMA refers to malignant neoplastic disorders of lymphoid tissue.

lymphaticostomy (lim-fat″ĭ-kos′tah-me) surgical creation of a permanent opening into a lymphatic duct, usually the thoracic duct.

lymphatism (lim′fah-tizm) a morbid state due to excessive production or growth of lymphoid tissues, resulting in impaired development and lowered vitality. Called also status lymphaticus.

lymphatolysis (lim″fah-tol′ĭ-sis) destruction of lymphoid tissue. adj., **lymphatolyt′ic.**

lymphectasia (lim′fek-ta′zhah) distention with lymph.

lymphedema (lim″fĕ-de′mah) chronic swelling of a part due to accumulation of interstitial fluid (edema) secondary to obstruction of lymphatic vessels or lymph nodes.

congenital l. Milroy disease.

primary l. lymphedema that appears spontaneously without known cause. See table.

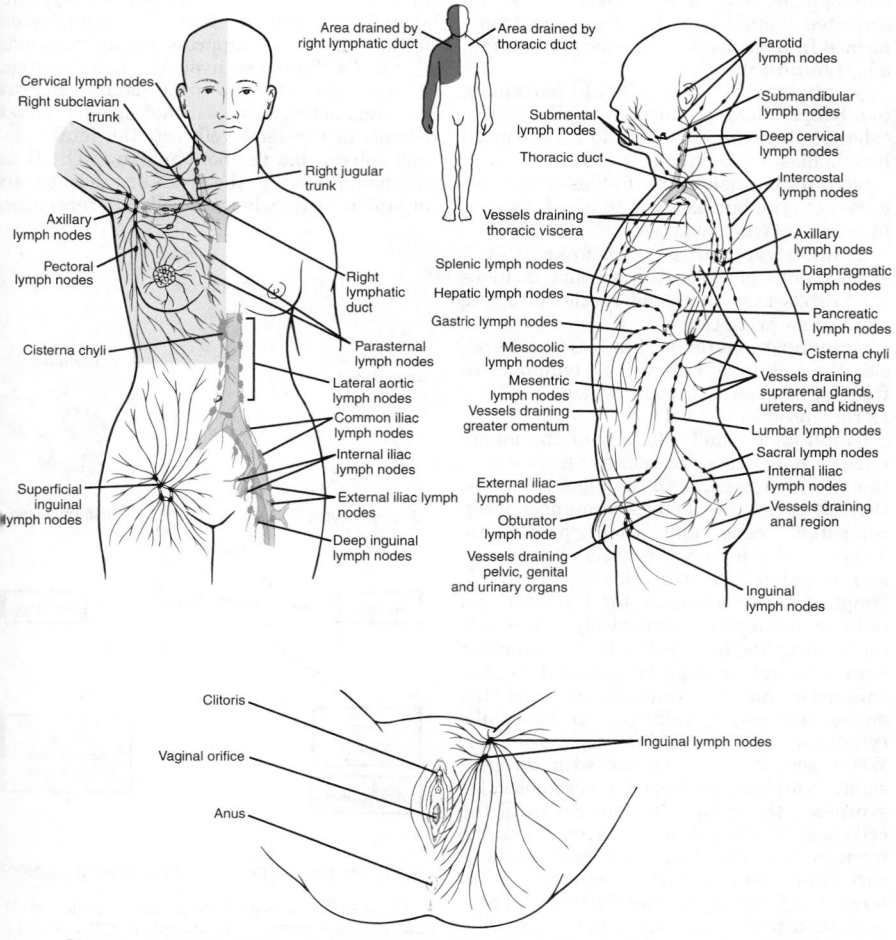

Diagrammatic representation of lymphatic drainage of various parts of the body. From Dorland's, 2000.

lymphenteritis (lim″fen-ter-i′tis) enteritis with serous infiltration.

lymphnoditis (limf″no-di′tis) inflammation of a lymph node.

lymphoblast (lim′fo-blast) a morphologically immature lymphocyte, once thought to represent an early stage in lymphocyte development but now known to be an activated lymphocyte that has been transformed in response to antigenic stimulation. adj., **lymphoblas′tic.**

lymphoblastic (lim″fo-blas′tik) pertaining to a lymphoblast; producing lymphocytes.

lymphoblastoma (lim″fo-blas-to′mah) lymphoblastic lymphoma.

lymphoblastosis (lim″fo-blas-to′sis) an excess of lymphoblasts in the blood, as seen in lymphoblastic LEUKEMIA.

Lymphocryptovirus (lim″fo-krip′to-vi″rus) a genus of HERPESVIRUSES that includes the EPSTEIN-BARR VIRUS and species affecting nonhuman primates.

lymphocytapheresis (lim″fo-si″tah-fē-re′sis) the selective removal of lymphocytes from withdrawn blood, which is then retransfused into the donor.

lymphocyte (lim′fo-sīt) any of the mononuclear nonphagocytic LEUKOCYTES found in the blood, lymph, and lymphoid tissues; they comprise the body's immunologically competent cells and their precursors. They are divided on the basis of ontogeny and function into two classes, B and T lymphocytes, responsible for humoral and cellular immunity, respectively. Most are *small lymphocytes* 7–10 μm in diameter with a round or slightly indented heterochromatic nucleus that almost fills the entire cell and a thin rim of basophilic cytoplasm that contains few granules. When activated by contact with antigen, small lymphocytes begin macromolecular synthesis, the cytoplasm enlarges until the cells are 10–30 μm in diameter, and the nucleus becomes less completely heterochromatic; they are then referred to as *large lymphocytes* or *lymphoblasts.* These cells then proliferate and differentiate into B and T memory cells and into the various effector cell types, B cells into plasma cells and T cells into helper, cytotoxic, and suppressor cells. See subentries here and under *cell.* adj., **lymphocyt′ic.**

l. activation stimulation of lymphocytes by specific antigen or nonspecific mitogens resulting in synthesis of RNA, protein, and DNA and production of lymphokines; it is followed by proliferation and differentiation of various effector and memory cells. Activation is accompanied by morphologic changes known as lymphocyte transformation, in which small, resting lymphocytes are transformed into large, active lymphocytes (LYMPHOBLASTS); the formation of lymphoblasts is referred to as BLASTOGENESIS.

amplifier T l's a T lymphocyte of the CD8 CELL type that modifies a developing IMMUNE RESPONSE by releasing nonspecific signals to which other T lymphocytes (either effector or suppressor cells) respond.

B l's "bursa-equivalent" lymphocytes; a type that develop from stem cells in hematopoietic tissue, including the blood islands of the fetal yolk sac, the fetal liver and spleen, and the bone marrow. The *B* in the name refers to the BURSA OF FABRICIUS, an organ in birds where B cell differentiation

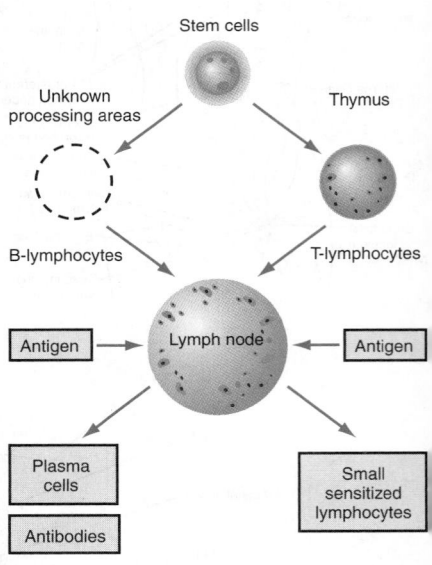

HUMORAL IMMUNITY   CELLULAR IMMUNITY

Origin of B- and T-lymphocytes responsible for cellular and humoral immunity. In response to antigens, B- and T-lymphocytes are sensitized by lymphoid tissue.

occurs; however, no analogous organ has been found in mammals. Called also B cells.

B lymphocytes are involved in humoral IMMUNITY, the secretion of ANTIBODIES. A mature B lymphocyte can be activated by the binding of an antigen to cell surface receptors. This induces proliferation of the cell, resulting in a clone of cells specific for that antigen. These cells can then differentiate and begin to secrete IMMUNOGLOBULIN (Ig) molecules; this step involves interaction with helper T lymphocytes. All the cells of a clone secrete Ig with identical antigen binding sites. Antibody-secreting cells can have the morphology of plasma CELLS, large lymphocytes, or LYMPHOBLASTS.

CD4 T l's, CD4⁺ T l's CD4 cells.

CD8 T l's, CD8⁺ T l's CD8 cells.

cytotoxic T l's differentiated T lymphocytes, marked by CD4 and CD8 ANTIGENS, able to recognize and lyse target cells bearing specific antigens recognized by their antigen receptors. The cytotoxic activity requires firm binding of the lymphocyte to the target cell to produce holes in its plasma membrane with loss of its cellular contents and osmotic lysis. These lymphocytes are important in graft rejection and killing of tumor cells and virus-infected host cells. Called also killer or killer T cells.

l. proliferation test a functional test of the ability of lymphocytes to respond to mitogens, specific antigens, or allogenic cells. The test with allogenic cells, called a mixed lymphocyte culture (MLC), is commonly performed for transplantation tissue typing; all three types of stimulants are used in investigation of immunodeficiency. Commonly used mitogens are phytohemagglutinin (PHA), concanavalin A (ConA), and pokeweed mitogen (PWM); commonly used antigens are PPD (tuberculin), *Candida* antigen, and streptokinase-streptodornase.

Rieder's l. a MYELOBLAST with a nucleus and several wide, deep indentations suggesting lobulation, seen in Rieder's cell LEUKEMIA and sometimes chronic lymphocytic LEUKEMIA. Called also Rieder's cell.

T l's "thymus-dependent" lymphocytes; a type that originates from a stem cell in hematopoietic tissue and undergoes differentiation in the THYMUS when triggered by THYMOPOIETIN. Called also T cells.

When activated by antigens such as the CD4 antigen or the CD8 antigen, T lymphocytes differentiate into the various types of regulatory and effector T cells (see CD4 CELLS and CD8 CELLS).

The CD8 cells called cytotoxic T CELLS or killer T CELLS are responsible for cell-mediated CYTOTOXICITY, which is the killing of cells bearing specific antigens, the

mechanism involved in cell-mediated IMMUNITY, delayed hypersensitivity, and killing of tumor cells and transplant tissue cells. A subpopulation, the LAK CELLS, is involved in the production of LYMPHOKINES, substances released into the blood that cause activation or inhibition of MACROPHAGES, destroy target cells, or are CHEMOTACTIC for the various types of leukocytes. The CD4 cells called helper T cells help B LYMPHOCYTES recognize certain antigens. Amplifier T LYMPHOCYTES are CD8 cells that enhance the activity of cytotoxic T cells. Suppressor T CELLS are CD8 cells that suppress antibody synthesis by their action on helper cells and B lymphocytes.

lymphocytoblast (lim″fo-si′to-blast) lymphoblast.

lymphocytoma (lim″fo-si-to′mah) pseudolymphoma.

lymphocytopenia (lim″fo-si″to-pe′ne-ah) reduction of the number of lymphocytes in the blood; called also lymphopenia.

lymphocytopheresis (lim″fo-si″to-fĕ-re′-sis) lymphocytapheresis.

lymphocytopoiesis (lim″fo-si″to-poi-e′sis) the formation of lymphocytes. adj., **lymphocytopoiet′ic.**

lymphocytosis (lim″fo-si-to′sis) increase in the number of normal lymphocytes in the blood or in an effusion.

lymphocytotoxicity (lim″fo-si″to-tok-sis′ĭ-te) the quality or capability of lysing lymphocytes, as in procedures in which lymphocytes having a specific cell surface antigen are lysed when incubated with antiserums and complement.

lymphoduct (lim′fo-dukt) lymphatic vessel.

lymphogenous (lim-foj′ĕ-nus) 1. producing lymph. 2. produced from lymph or in the lymph vessels.

lymphoglandula (lim″fo-glan′du-lah) [L.] lymph node.

lymphogram (lim′fo-gram) a radiograph of the lymphatic channels and lymph nodes.

lymphogranuloma (lim″fo-gran″u-lo′mah) Hodgkin's disease.

l. ingu ina′le, venereal l. l. vene′reum a SEXUALLY TRANSMITTED DISEASE caused by a strain of *Chlamydia trachomatis,* which affects the lymph organs in the genital area. It occurs most frequently in tropical and semitropical regions. Three to 21 days after the body is infected, a small, hard sore appears in the genital area. The disease soon spreads from the local sore to the LYMPH NODES, particularly those in the groin; nodes may swell to the size of a walnut. Since they seldom break open and drain

pus, the swellings may remain for months
unless aspirated. In women with the disease, the vulva may become greatly enlarged. The rectum may become narrowed,
so that surgery is necessary for relief. In the
early stages of the disease, there may also
be inflammation of the joints, skin rashes,
and fever. Sometimes the brain and meninges are affected. It is thought that after
the initial sore heals, men may no longer
transmit the disease. Women, however, may
infect sexual partners for years. The condition may be successfully treated with
DOXYCYCLINE or ERYTHROMYCIN.

lymphogranulomatosis (lim″fo-gran″u-
lo″mah-to′sis) 1. infectious granuloma of
the lymphatic system. 2. Hodgkin's disease.

lymphography (lim-fog′rah-fe) radiography of the lymphatic channels and lymph
nodes after injection of radiopaque material
in a lymphatic vessel.

lymphoid (lim′foid) resembling or pertaining to lymph or to tissue of the
lymphatic system.

lymphoidectomy (lim″foi-dek′to-me) excision of lymphoid tissue, such as tonsils and
adenoids.

lymphokine (lim′fo-kīn) any of various
soluble protein mediators released by sensitized lymphocytes on contact with antigen,
and believed to play a role in macrophage
activation, lymphocyte transformation, and
cell-mediated IMMUNITY. It regulates IMMUNE
RESPONSES through differentiation, amplification, and inhibition of cell functions.
Lymphokines may also have a cytotoxic
effector function. Used as biologic response
modifiers in the treatment of cancer.

lymphokinesis (lim″fo-ki-ne′sis) 1. movement of endolymph in the semicircular
canals. 2. the circulation of lymph in the body.

lymphology (lim-fol′o-je) the study of the
lymphatic system.

lympholytic (lim″fo-lit′ik) causing destruction of lymphocytes.

lymphoma (lim-fo′mah) any neoplastic
disorder of lymphoid tissue, including
HODGKIN'S DISEASE. Often used to denote
malignant LYMPHOMA, classifications of
which are based on predominant cell type
and degree of differentiation; various
categories may be subdivided into nodular
and diffuse types depending on the predominant pattern of cell arrangement.

    adult T-cell l., adult T-cell leukemia/l.
adult T-cell LEUKEMIA/lymphoma.

    African l. Burkitt's lymphoma.

    B-cell l's a heterogeneous group of
lymphoid malignancies including most non-
Hodgkin's LYMPHOMAS, representing clonal

expansions of malignant B LYMPHOCYTES
that have been arrested at a particular stage
in their differentiation from primitive stem
cells. B-cell lymphoma usually appears as a
painless lymph node enlargement, although
extranodal sites of origin are not uncommon. These lymphomas have been classified
on the basis of morphologic features characteristic of the different stages of normal B
lymphocyte differentiation.

    Burkitt's l. see BURKITT'S LYMPHOMA.

    l. cu′tis primary skin involvement by a
B-cell LYMPHOMA without demonstrable systemic disease.

    diffuse l. malignant LYMPHOMA in which
the neoplastic cells infiltrate the entire
lymph node without any organized pattern.

    follicular l. malignant LYMPHOMA in
which the lymphomatous cells are clustered
into identifiable nodules within the lymph
nodes that somewhat resemble the germinal
centers of lymphatic NODULES. Follicular
lymphomas usually occur in older persons
and commonly involve many or all nodes as
well as extranodal sites. Called also nodular
lymphoma.

    follicular center cell l. any of a large
group of B-cell LYMPHOMAS, comprising four
subtypes classified on the basis of the
predominant cell type (resembling small
cleaved, large cleaved, small noncleaved,
and large noncleaved follicular center
CELLS). Because of the wide variety of
prognostic levels and the existence of
tumors with several types of cells, the
original four categories have now been
divided up and scattered among several
new categories of follicular and diffuse
LYMPHOMAS.

    giant follicular l. follicular lymphoma.

    granulomatous l. Hodgkin's disease.

    histiocytic l. a rare type of non-Hodg-
kin's lymphoma of intermediate to high
malignancy, characterized by large tumor
cells that resemble histiocytes morphologically but are considered to be of lymphoid
origin. Many tumors formerly placed in this
category are now considered to belong in
one of the large cell lymphoma groups.

    Hodgkin's l. Hodgkin's disease.

    large cell l. any of several types of
lymphoma characterized by formation of
malignant large lymphocytes in a diffuse
pattern; some varieties contain exclusively
one type of cell, such as lymphoblasts or
cleaved or uncleaved follicular center cells,
and others have a mixture of cells, sometimes including ones that cannot be characterized as to lineage.

    Lennert's l. a type of non-Hodgkin's
LYMPHOMA with a high content of epithelioid
HISTIOCYTES; bone marrow involvement is

common and response to CHEMOTHERAPY is often poor.

lymphoblastic *l.* a highly malignant type of non-Hodgkin's LYMPHOMA composed of a diffuse, relatively uniform proliferation of cells with round or convoluted nuclei and scanty cytoplasm, which are cytologically similar to the lymphoblasts seen in acute lymphoblastic LEUKEMIA.

malignant *l.* a group of malignant neoplasms characterized by the proliferation of cells native to the lymphoid TISSUES, i.e., LYMPHOCYTES, HISTIOCYTES, and their precursors and derivatives. The group is divided into two major categories: HODGKIN'S DISEASE and non-Hodgkin's LYMPHOMA.

mixed lymphocytic-histiocytic *l.* non-Hodgkin's LYMPHOMA characterized by a mixed population of cells, with the smaller cells resembling LYMPHOCYTES and the larger ones HISTIOCYTES, usually occurring in a nodular histologic pattern but sometimes evolving into a diffuse pattern.

nodular *l.* follicular lymphoma.

non-Hodgkin's *l.'s* a heterogeneous group of malignant LYMPHOMAS whose common feature is absence of the giant Reed-Sternberg CELLS characteristic of HODGKIN'S DISEASE. They arise from the lymphoid components of the immune system, and present a clinical picture broadly similar to that of Hodgkin's disease except that these diseases are initially more widespread, with the most common manifestation being painless enlargement of one or more peripheral lymph nodes. The nomenclature and classification of these lymphomas has been a subject of controversy. One widely accepted classification is based on two criteria: cytologic characteristics of the constituent cells and type of cell growth pattern (defined as either nodular [follicular] or diffuse). Another system of classification is based on the cell type of origin: T- or B-LYMPHOCYTES or HISTIOCYTES. Still another formulation has been proposed, separating non-Hodgkin's lymphomas into major histopathologic subtypes using only morphologic criteria.

Diagnostic procedures used to confirm suspected non-Hodgkin's lymphoma include PET scans, gallium scans, and occasionally LYMPHANGIOGRAMS. If lymphoma is diagnosed, it will be staged using the same system as for Hodgkin's disease.

Treatment will depend on the type and stage. It may be single agent or multiagent CHEMOTHERAPY, radiation THERAPY, BIOTHERAPY, or a combination. Blood transfusions and bone marrow TRANSPLANTATION have shown efficacy for some types of lymphoma.

Patient care: major problems presented by the patient with non-Hodgkin's lym-

phoma include the management of side effects associated with treatment and the prevention of infection.

small lymphocytic *l.* a diffuse form of non-Hodgkin's lymphoma with a low grade of malignancy; it represents the neoplastic proliferation of well-differentiated B lymphocytes and may present with either focal lymph node enlargement or generalized lymphadenopathy and splenomegaly. The predominant cell type is a compact, small, normal-appearing lymphocyte with a dark-staining round nucleus, scanty cytoplasm, and little size variation. It nearly always involves the bone marrow, and often malignant cells are found in the blood, so that its clinical picture is similar to that of chronic lymphocytic leukemia. Called also well-differentiated lymphocytic lymphoma.

T-cell *l's* a heterogeneous group of lymphoid tumors representing malignant transformation of the T LYMPHOCYTES. Types include convoluted T-cell lymphomas, cutaneous T-cell lymphomas, adult T-cell LEUKEMIA, and certain other conditions.

undifferentiated *l.* malignant lymphoma composed of undifferentiated cells, i.e., cells that do not show morphologic evidence of maturation toward lymphocytes or histiocytes, which vary in size and may include bizarre giant forms.

well-differentiated lymphocytic *l.* small lymphocytic lymphoma.

lymphomatosis (lim″fo-mah-to′sis) the formation of multiple malignant cell infiltrations of the LYMPHATIC SYSTEM.

lymphomatous (lim-fo′mah-tus) pertaining to, or of the nature of, lymphoma.

lymphopathia (lim″fo-path′e-ah) lymphopathy.

***l.* vene′reum** lymphogranuloma venereum.

lymphopathy (lim-fop′ah-the) any disease of the lymphatic system.

lymphopenia (lim″fo-pe′ne-ah) lymphocytopenia.

lymphoplasia (lim″fo-pla′zhah) accumulation of lymphoreticular cells in the tissues.

lymphopoiesis (lim″fo-poi-e′sis) the development of lymphocytes or of lymphoid tissue. adj., **lymphopoiet′ic.**

lymphoproliferative (lim″fo-pro-lif′er-ah″-tiv) pertaining to or characterized by proliferation of lymphoid tissue.

***l.* disorders** a group of malignant neoplasms arising from cells related to the common multipotential, primordial lymphoreticular cell that includes among others the lymphocytic, histiocytic, and monocytic leukemias, multiple myeloma,

L

plasmacytoma, Hodgkin's disease, all lymphocytic lymphomas, and immunosecretory disorders associated with monoclonal gammopathy. An interrelationship with the MYELOPROLIFERATIVE DISORDERS is thought to exist.

lymphoreticular (lim″fo-rĕ-tik′u-ler) pertaining to the reticuloendothelial cells of lymph nodes.

l. disorders a group of disorders of the lymphoreticular SYSTEM, characterized by the proliferation of LYMPHOCYTES or lymphoid tissues; they may be either benign (such as LYMPHOCYTOSIS) or malignant (such as lymphoblastic LEUKEMIAS, MULTIPLE MYELOMA, or non-Hodgkin's LYMPHOMAS). See also LYMPHOPROLIFERATIVE DISORDERS.

lymphoreticulosis (lim″fo-rĕ-tik″u-lo′sis) proliferation of the reticuloendothelial cells of the lymph nodes.

benign l. cat-scratch disease.

lymphorrhagia (lim″fo-ra′jah) lymphorrhea.

lymphorrhea (lim″fo-re′ah) flow of lymph from cut or ruptured lymphatic vessels.

lymphorrhoid (lim′fo-roid) a localized dilatation of a perianal lymph channel, resembling a hemorrhoid.

lymphosarcoma (lim″fo-sahr-ko′mah) a diffuse lymphoma.

lymphosarcomatosis (lim″fo-sahr-ko″-mah-to′sis) a condition characterized by the presence of multiple lesions of lymphosarcoma.

lymphoscintigraphy (lim″fo-sin-tig′rah-fe) SCINTIGRAPHIC detection of metastatic tumors in radiolabeled LYMPH NODES, particularly that using radiolabeled COLLOID (radiocolloid lymphoscintigraphy). The colloid is taken up by MACROPHAGES in the lymph nodes, with depressed uptake in tumor-containing nodes.

lymphostasis (lim-fos′tah-sis) stoppage of lymph flow.

lymphotaxis (lim″fo-tak′sis) the property of attracting or repulsing lymphocytes.

lymphotoxin (lim′fo-tok″sin) a LYMPHOKINE containing 171 amino acids, one of the tumor necrosis FACTORS, produced by activated T lymphocytes. It inhibits the growth of tumors by causing lysis or stasis of sensitive cells, and also blocks transformation of cells. Called also tumor necrosis factor β.

lymphotropic (lim″fo-trop′ik) having an affinity for lymphatic tissue.

Lyon hypothesis (li′on) the random and fixed inactivation (in the form of sex chromatin) of all X chromosomes in excess of one in mammalian cells at an early stage of embryogenesis, leading to mosaicism for X-linked genes in the female, since the paternal X chromosome is inactivated in some cells and the maternal one in the remainder.

lyonization (li″on-ĭ-za′shun) the process by which or the condition in which all X chromosomes of the cells in excess of one are inactivated on a random basis.

lyophil (li′o-fil) a lyophilic substance.

lyophile (li′o-fil) lyophil.

lyophilic (li″o-fil′ik) having an affinity for or stable in, solution.

lyophilization (li-of″ĭ-lĭ-za′shun) the creation of a stable preparation of a biologic substance by rapid freezing and dehydration of the frozen product under high vacuum. See also FREEZE-DRYING.

lyophobe (li′o-fōb) a lyophobic substance.

lyophobic (li″o-fo′bik) not having an affinity for, or unstable in, solution.

lyotropic (li″o-trop′ik) lyophilic.

lypressin (li-pres′in) a synthetic preparation of lysine vasopressin, used as an antidiuretic and vasoconstrictor to treat central DIABETES INSIPIDUS when desmopressin is too potent; administered by intranasal spray.

lyse (līz) 1. to cause or produce disintegration of a compound, substance, or cell. 2. to undergo lysis.

lysergic acid diethylamide LSD.

lysergide (li′ser-jīd) LSD.

lysin (li′sin) 1. an ANTIBODY that causes complement-dependent lysis of cells; often used with a prefix indicating the target cells, as hemolysin or bacteriolysin. 2. any substance that causes cell lysis.

lysine (li′sēn) a naturally occurring AMINO ACID, one of those essential for human metabolism, necessary for optimal growth in human infants and for maintenance of nitrogen equilibrium in adults. The acetate and hydrochloride salts are used for dietary supplementation and the hydrochloride salt is used for the treatment of severe metabolic acidosis refractory to other treatment.

lysinogen (li-sin′o-jen) lysogen.

lysinuria (li″sĭ-nu′re-ah) an AMINOACIDURIA consisting of excessive LYSINE in the urine such as in HYPERLYSINEMIA.

lysis (li′sis) 1. destruction, as of cells by a specific LYSIN. 2. decomposition, as of a chemical compound by a specific agent. See also DEGRADATION. 3. mobilization of an organ by division of restraining adhesions. 4. the gradual abatement of the symptoms of a disease.

-lysis word element [Gr.], *dissolution.* adj., **-lyt′ic.**

lysogen (li′so-jen) 1. an antigen causing the formation of LYSIN; called also lysinogen 2. an agent that causes LYSIS.

lysogenicity (li″so-jĕ-nis′ĭ-te) 1. the ability to produce lysins or cause lysis. 2. the potentiality of a bacterium to produce BACTERIOPHAGE. 3. the specific association of the phage GENOME (PROPHAGE) with the bacterial GENOME in such a way that only a few, if any, phage genes are transcribed.

lysogeny (li-soj′e-ne) the phenomenon in which a bacterium is infected by a temperature bacteriophage, the viral DNA is integrated in the chromosome of the host cell and replicated along with the host chromosome for many generations (the lysogenic cycle), and then production of virions and lysis of host cells (the lytic cycle) begins again. The lytic cycle is initiated spontaneously about once in 10,000 cell divisions or may be induced by ultraviolet light or chemical agents.

lysosomal storage disease any inborn ERROR of metabolism in which the deficiency of a lysosomal enzyme results in accumulation of the substance normally degraded by that enzyme in the lysosomes of certain cells. These diseases are further classified, depending on the nature of the stored substance, as GLYCOGEN STORAGE DISEASES (GLYCOGENOSES), SPHINGOLIPIDOSES, MUCOPOLY-SACCHARIDOSES, and MUCOLIPIDOSES.

Lysol (li′sol) trademark for a solution containing PHENOL derivatives, used as a disinfectant and antiseptic.

lysosome (li′so-sōm) one of the minute bodies occurring in many types of cells, containing various hydrolytic enzymes and normally involved in the process of localized intracellular digestion. adj., **lyso-so′mal.**

lysotype (li′so-tīp) phage type.

lysozyme (li′so-zim) a crystalline, basic protein present in saliva, tears, egg white, and many animal fluids, which functions as an antibacterial enzyme.

lysozymuria (li″so-zi-mu′re-ah) urinary excretion of elevated levels of lysozyme.

lyssa (lis′ah) former term for rabies. adj., **lys′sic.**

Lyssavirus (lis′ah-vi′rus) a genus of RHABDOVIRUSES that includes the rabies VIRUS and other related viruses.

lyssoid (lis′oid) resembling rabies.

lyssophobia (lis″o-fo′be-ah) irrational fear of rabies.

lytic (lit′ik) pertaining to lysis or a lysin.

lyze (līz) lyse.

L

M

M mega-; molar[1](used with a number designating the strength of the solution relative to one molar, e.g., M/2 or 0.5M for half-molar); molar[2]; myopia.

M. [L.] mis'ce (mix); mistu'ra (a mixture).

M molar[1].

m median; meter; milli-.

m. [L.] mus'culus (muscle); minim.

m mass; molal.

m- met(a)- (def. 2).

μ (mu, the twelfth letter of the Greek alphabet) micro-; the heavy chain of IgM (see *immunoglobulin*).

MA Master of Arts; mental age; meter angle.

mA milliampere.

Maalox (ma'loks) any of various trademark preparations of magnesium and aluminum salts (usually MAGNESIUM HYDROXIDE and ALUMINUM HYDROXIDE) used as ANTACIDS.

Maass (mahs) Clara Louise (1876–1901). A graduate of the Christina Trefz Training School for Nurses in Newark who worked as a U.S. Army nurse during the Spanish-American War in Florida, Cuba, and the Philippines. In 1900 she returned to Cuba, where she was one of seven volunteers who were bitten by mosquitoes to test the theory that yellow fever is carried by mosquitoes. She survived an attack of yellow fever and volunteered to be bitten again; the second attack of fever proved fatal and she died at the age of 25 in Havana.

MAC membrane attack complex; minimal alveolar concentration; *Mycobacterium avium* complex (disease).

McArdle disease (mik-ar'd'l) GLYCOGEN STORAGE DISEASE (type V), a condition in which deficiency of muscle phosphorylase results in accumulation of glycogen in skeletal muscles, with muscle cramps and a depressed blood lactate level during exercise. Called also myophosphorylase deficiency glycogenosis.

McBurney sign (mik-ber'nēz) special tenderness at the McBurney point, indicating appendicitis.

MAC disease *Mycobacterium avium* complex disease.

McDonald's rule (mik-don'aldz) the length in centimeters of the abdominal contour from the upper margin of the pubic symphysis to the fundus of the uterus, divided by 3.5, gives the duration of pregnancy in lunar months; applicable only after the sixth month of pregnancy.

Mace (mās) trademark for an aerosol mixture of CS, a common tear GAS.

macerate (mas'er-āt) to soften by wetting or soaking.

maceration (mas"ĕ-ra'shun) the softening of a solid by soaking. In histology, the softening of a tissue by soaking, especially in acids, until the connective tissue fibers are dissolved so that the tissue components can be teased apart. In obstetrics, the degenerative changes with discoloration and softening of tissues, and eventual disintegration, of a fetus retained in the uterus after its death.

McMillan (mik-mil'in) Mary (1880–1959) early American PHYSICAL THERAPIST and a founder of the American Physical Therapy Association. She was educated in England and was employed in the Children's Hospital in Liverpool treating patients with poliomyelitis and spastic paralysis. She returned to America in 1915 and became an influential force in the development of the profession of physical therapy.

McMurray's sign (mik-mur'ēz) occurrence of a cartilage click during manipulation of the knee; indicative of meniscal injury.

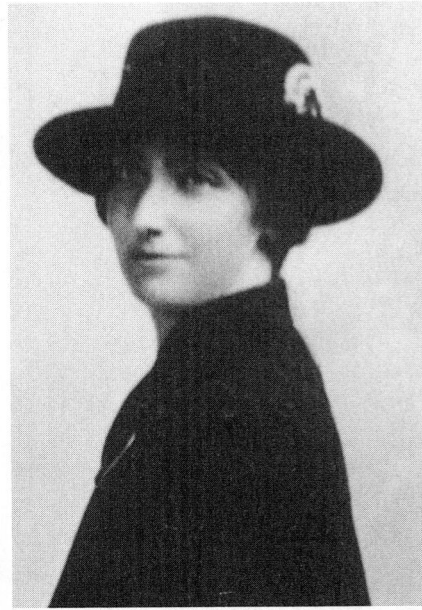

Mary McMillan. Courtesy of the American Physical Therapy Association.

McMurray's test (mik-mur'ēz) as the patient lies supine with one knee fully flexed, the examiner rotates the patient's foot fully outward and the knee is slowly extended; a painful "click" indicates a tear of the medial meniscus of the knee joint; if the click occurs when the foot is rotated inward, the tear is in the lateral meniscus.

macr(o)- word element [Gr.], *large; long.*

macrencephalia (mak″ren-sě-fa′le-ah) hypertrophy of the brain.

macroamylase (mak″ro-am′ĭ-lās) a complex in which normal serum amylase is bound to a variety of specific binding proteins, forming a complex too large for renal excretion. It is not correlated with any specific disease state; however, in hyperamylasemia or pancreatitis, it can result in urinary amylase levels not rising concomitantly with serum levels.

macroamylasemia (mak″ro-am″ĭ-lase′me-ah) the presence of macroamylase in the blood. adj., **macroamylase′mic.**

macroblast (mak′ro-blast) an abnormally large, nucleated erythrocyte; a large young erythroblast with megaloblastic features. Called also macronormoblast.

macroblepharia (mak″ro-blě-far′e-ah) abnormal largeness of the eyelid.

macrocardius (mak″ro-kahr′de-us) a fetus with an extremely large heart.

macrocephaly (mak″ro-sef′ah-le) megalocephaly. adj., **macroceph′ous.**

macrocheilia (mak″ro-ki′le-ah) excessive size of the lip.

macrocheiria (mak″ro-ki′re-ah) megalocheiria.

macrocolon (mak″ro-ko′lon) megacolon.

macrocrania (mak″ro-kra′ne-ah) abnormal increase in size of the skull in relation to the face.

macrocyte (mak′ro-sīt) an abnormally large erythrocyte. adj., **macrocyt′ic.**

macrocythemia (mak″ro-si-the′me-ah) the presence of macrocytes in the blood, as in macrocytic ANEMIA and some types of liver disease. Called also macrocytosis.

macrocytosis (mak″ro-si-to′sis) macrocythemia.

macrodactyly (mak″ro-dak′tĭ-le) megalodactyly.

Macrodantin (mak″ro-dan′tin) trademark for a preparation of NITROFURANTOIN, an ANTIBACTERIAL agent.

macrodontia (mak″ro-don′she-ah) abnormal increase in size of one or more teeth. adj., **mac′rodont, macrodon′tic.**

macroelement (mak″ro-el′ě-ment) a chemical element that has a minimal daily requirement greater than 100 mg; calcium, phosphorus, magnesium, potassium, sodium, and chloride are macroelements.

macrogamete (mak″ro-gam′ēt) 1. the larger, less active female gamete in sexual REPRODUCTION, which is fertilized by the smaller male gamete (MICROGAMETE). 2. the larger of two types of malarial parasites; see GAMETE (def. 2).

macrogametocyte (mak″ro-gah-me′to-sīt) a cell that produces macrogametes. 1. the female gametocyte of certain Sporozoa, such as malarial plasmodia, which matures into a macrogamete.

macrogenitosomia (mak″ro-jen″ĭ-to-so′me-ah) excessive bodily development, with unusual enlargement of the genital organs.

m. prae′cox macrogenitosomia occurring at an early age due to excessive ANDROGENS. In the female, PSEUDOHERMAPHRODITISM is apparent and in the male the external genitalia are enlarged.

macroglia (mah-krog′le-ah) neuroglia cells of ectodermal origin, i.e., the ASTROCYTES and OLIGODENDROCYTES considered together.

macroglobulin (mak″ro-glob′u-lin) a protein (globulin) of high molecular weight, in the range of 1,000,000; observed in the blood in a number of diseases.

α_2-*m.* a plasma protein that inhibits a wide variety of proteolytic enzymes, including trypsin, plasmin, thrombin, kallikrein, and chymotrypsin, by entrapping and reducing the accessibility of their functional sites to large molecules. Written also alpha$_2$-macroglobulin.

macroglobulinemia (mak″ro-glob″u-lin-e′me-ah) increased levels of macroglobulins in the blood.

Waldenström's m. a type of plasma cell DYSCRASIA with cells having lymphocytic, plasmacytic, or intermediate morphology and secreting IgM M-component. There is diffuse infiltration of bone marrow and in many cases also of the spleen, liver, or lymph nodes. The circulating macroglobulin produces symptoms of HYPERVISCOSITY SYNDROME: weakness, fatigue, bleeding disorders, and visual disturbances. Peak incidence is in the sixth and seventh decades.

macroglossia (mak″ro-glos′e-ah) excessive size of the tongue; called also megaloglossia.

macrognathia (mak″ro-nath′e-ah) abnormal overgrowth of the jaw. adj., **macrognath′ic.**

macrogyria (mak″ro-ji′re-ah) moderate reduction in the number of sulci of the

M

cerebrum, sometimes with increase in the brain substance, resulting in excessive size of the gyri.

macrolide (mak′ro-līd) 1. a chemical compound characterized by a large lactone ring containing multiple keto and hydroxyl groups. 2. any of a group of antibacterial ANTIBIOTICS containing such a ring linked to one or more sugars.

macromastia (mak″ro-mas′te-ah) excessive size of the breasts.

macromelia (mak″ro-me′le-ah) megalomelia.

macromelus (mah-krom′ĕ-lus) a fetus with abnormally large or long limbs.

macromere (mak′ro-mēr) one of the large BLASTOMERES formed at the vegetal pole in unequal cleavage of the fertilized ovum; see also MICROMERE.

macromineral (mak″ro-min′er-al) macroelement.

macromolecule (mak″ro-mol′ĕ-kūl) a very large molecule having a polymeric chain structure, as in proteins, polysaccharides, and certain other substances. adj., **macromolec′ular.**

macromonocyte (mak″ro-mon′o-sīt) an abnormally large monocyte.

macromyeloblast (mak″ro-mi′ĕ-lo-blast″) an abnormally large myeloblast.

macronormoblast (mak″ro-nor′mo-blast) macroblast.

macronutrient (mak″ro-noo′tre-ent) an essential nutrient that has a large minimal daily requirement, including proteins, fats, carbohydrates, and water. The term sometimes specifically includes, and sometimes specifically excludes, minerals required in amounts greater than 100 mg daily: calcium, chloride, magnesium, potassium, phosphorus, sodium, and sulfur.

macronychia (mak″ro-nik′e-ah) megalonychia.

macro-orchidism (mak-ro-or′kĭ-dizm) abnormal enlargement of the testis.

macro-ovalocyte (mak″ro-o′vah-lo-sīt) an enlarged, oval erythrocyte seen in MEGALOBLASTIC ANEMIA.

macropenis abnormal largeness of the penis; called also macrophallus and megalopenis.

macrophage (mak′ro-fāj) any of the large, mononuclear, highly phagocytic cells derived from MONOCYTES, occurring in the walls of blood vessels (adventitial cells) and in loose connective tissue (histiocytes, phagocytic reticular cells). They are components of the RETICULOENDOTHELIAL SYSTEM. Macrophages have their origin in the bone marrow, where they pass through the monoblast and promonocyte stages to the monocyte stage; the monocytes enter the blood and then the tissues, where they become macrophages. Macrophages are usually immobile but become actively mobile when stimulated by INFLAMMATION. Their functions include PHAGOCYTOSIS and PINOCYTOSIS, presentation of antigens to T and B lymphocytes, and secretion of a variety of products, including enzymes several complement components and coagulation factors, some prostaglandins and leukotrienes, and several regulatory molecules. See also IMMUNITY.

alveolar m′s rounded, granular, mononuclear phagocytes within the alveoli of the lungs that ingest inhaled particulate matter.

armed m′s those capable of inducing cytotoxicity as a consequence of antigen binding by cytophilic antibodies on their surfaces or by factors derived from T LYMPHOCYTES.

macrophallus macropenis.

macrophthalmia (mak″rof-thal′me-ah) megalophthalmos.

macropodia (mak″ro-po′de-ah) megalopodia.

macropolycyte (mak″ro-pol′e-sīt) a hypersegmented polymorphonuclear leukocyte of greater than normal size.

macroprosopia (mak″ro-pro-so′pe-ah) excessive size of the face.

macropsia (mah-krop′se-ah) an illusion in which objects appear larger than their actual size.

macroreentry (mak″ro-re-en′tre) REENTRY involving a circuit of electrical current that uses the bundle branches to rapidly activate

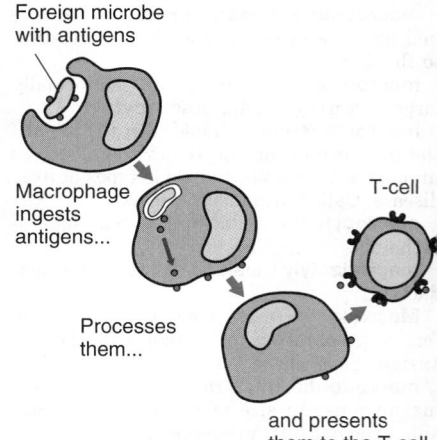

Foreign microbe with antigens

Macrophage ingests antigens...

Processes them...

T-cell

and presents them to the T-cell

A macrophage ingests an antigen. From Polaski and Tatro, 1996.

the heart, causing ventricular TACHYCARDIA
with a pattern like bundle branch block and
a relatively narrow QRS component.

macrorrhinia (mak″ro-rin′e-ah) excessive
size of the nose.

macroscopic (mak″ro-skop′ik) of large
size; visible to the unaided eye.

macroscopy (mah-kros′kah-pe) examination with the unaided eye.

macroshock (mak′ro-shok″) a strong
electric shock resulting from current that
has passed through the trunk, with contact
to the source through intact skin.

macrosigmoid (mak″ro-sig′moid) excessive size of the sigmoid colon.

macrosomatia (mak″ro-so-ma′shah)
macrosomia.

macrosomia (mak″ro-so′me-ah) great
bodily size; see also GIGANTISM. Called also
macrosomatia.

    neonatal m. excessive birth weight in
a neonate, seen most often in children
of diabetic mothers or those with cerebral
GIGANTISM.

macrostomia (mak″ro-sto′me-ah) excessive width of the mouth.

macrotia (mah-kro′she-ah) abnormal enlargement of the pinna of the ear.

macula (mak′u-lah) [L.] 1. a stain, spot,
or thickening; in anatomy, an area distinguishable by color or otherwise from its
surroundings. Often used alone to refer to
the macula retinae. 2. a discolored spot on
the skin that is not raised above the surface;
called also macule. 3. a corneal scar that can
be seen without special optical aids; it
presents as a gray spot intermediate
between a NEBULA and a LEUKOMA. 4. macula
lutea. adj., **mac′ular, mac′ulate.**

    acoustic maculae, ma′culae acus′ticae
the MACULA SACCULI and MACULA UTRICULI
considered together.

    m. atro′phica a white atrophic patch
on the skin.

    m. ceru′lea a blue patch on the skin
seen in pediculosis.

    m. cribro′sa a perforated spot or area;
one of three perforated areas (inferior,
medial, and superior) in the wall of the
vestibule of the ear through which branches
of the vestibulocochlear nerve pass to the
saccule, utricle, and semicircular canals.

    m. den′sa a zone of heavily nucleated
cells in the distal renal tubule that feed
information to the juxtaglomerular CELLS.

    m. fla′va a yellow nodule at one end of
a vocal cord.

    m. folli′culi follicular stigma.

    m. germinati′va germinal area; the part
of the ovum where the embryo is formed.

    m. lu′tea, m. lu′tea re′tinae m. re′tinae
an irregular yellowish depression on the

retina, lateral to and slightly below the optic
disk; receives and analyzes light only from
the center of the visual field.

    m. sac′culi a thickening on the wall of
the SACCULE where the epithelium contains
hair CELLS that receive and transmit vestibular impulses.

    m. utri′culi a thickening in the wall of
the UTRICLE where the epithelium contains
hair CELLS that are stimulated by linear
acceleration and deceleration and by gravity.

macular degeneration breakdown of
cells in the MACULA LUTEA, resulting in a loss
of central vision in the affected eye;
peripheral vision is not affected. There are
several varieties; most appear in persons 50
to 60 years of age (*age-related macular
degeneration*), but one variety is congenital
and is seen in younger people (STARGARDT'S
DISEASE or *Stargardt's macular degeneration*). In about 75 per cent of cases the cause
is not known, and nothing can be done to
prevent, arrest, or reverse the process.

Patient Care. Since a large majority of
cases of macular degeneration cannot be
arrested or treated, care is aimed at making
the most of the vision that the patient has.
The condition does not progress to total
blindness and usually is self-limiting. The
inability to perceive detail can be compensated for in part by using large-type books
and magazines and a magnifying lens for
reading, and having adequate lighting
whenever detail work is necessary.

    Patients with macular degeneration are
given a sheet of paper on which is printed a
grid of horizontal and vertical lines. They
are instructed to look at this grid daily and
note whether there is any change in distortion of lines in the center of vision. This
same technique can be used as a screening
test to evaluate central vision. However,
seeing distorted lines in the grid is not
necessarily symptomatic of macular degeneration. Further examination by an ophthalmologist is necessary for a definitive
diagnosis.

    age-related m. d. (ARMD) a type hav-
ing its onset between the ages of 50 and 60,
the leading cause of blindness in persons
over the age of 65. There are two main
types, *involutional* and *exudative age-
related macular degeneration.*

    The *involutional (dry* or *non-exudative)*
type accounts for 90 per cent of cases and is
characterized by the gradual wearing out of
the cells in the retinal pigment epithelium,
resulting in a slow, progressive loss of
central vision. Although visual acuity loss

M

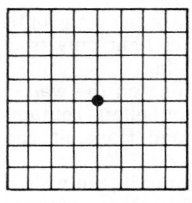 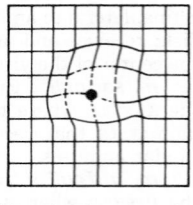

Normal   Macular degeneration

Grid for evaluating macular degeneration.

usually does not progress beyond the 20/200 level, this is a significant disability. Treatment is not generally available.

The *exudative (neovascular* or *wet) type* is characterized by the growth of a neovascular membrane within or very close to the macula, resulting in distorted and blurred vision. The vision loss from this type of macular degeneration may be only of hand movements. Laser photocoagulation of this form of macular degeneration is aimed at destroying the neovascular membrane; if diagnosed and treated very early when the membrane is small, significant loss of central vision may be avoided.

Patient Care. Health care providers can be of great help for early diagnosis of this devastating disease through ongoing patient education programs. After laser treatment, which is performed under a retrobulbar anesthetic, the patient should be instructed to leave the patch in place for at least six hours. Any increase in distortion or blurred vision should be immediately reported and followed up by an urgent outpatient exam. Low vision aids and services can improve quality of life for persons with this disorder.

Stargardt's m. d. Stargardt's disease.

maculate (mak'u-lāt) spotted or blotched.

macule (mak'ūl) a macula.

maculocerebral (mak″u-lo-ser'ĕ-bral) cerebromacular.

maculopapular (mak″u-lo-pap'u-ler) both macular and papular.

madarosis (mad″ah-ro'sis) loss of eyelashes or eyebrows.

mad cow disease bovine spongiform encephalopathy.

Madelung's disease (mah'dĕ-lo͞ongz) 1. Madelung's deformity. 2. Madelung's neck.

maduromycosis (mah-du″ro-mi-ko'sis) mycetoma.

mafenide (maf'en-īd) a compound used in the form of the acetate and hydrochloride salts for topical treatment of infections.

magaldrate (mag'al-drāt) a chemical combination of aluminum and magnesium hydroxides and sulfate; used as an oral ANTACID.

magenta (mah-jen'tah) fuchsin or other salt of rosaniline.

maggot (mag'ot) the soft-bodied larva of an insect, especially one living in decaying flesh.

magma (mag'mah) 1. a thick, viscous, aqueous suspension of finely divided, insoluble, inorganic material. 2. a thin, pastelike substance composed of organic material.

magnesia (mag-ne'zhah) magnesium oxide. See also MILK OF MAGNESIA.

magnesium (Mg) (mag-ne'ze-um) a chemical element, atomic number 12, atomic weight 24.312. (See Appendix 6.) Its salts are essential in nutrition, being required for the activity of many enzymes, especially those concerned with oxidative PHOSPHORYLATION. It is found in the intra- and extracellular fluids and is excreted in urine and feces. The normal serum level is approximately 2 mEq/L. Magnesium deficiency causes irritability of the nervous system with tetany, vasodilation, convulsions, tremors, depression, and psychotic behavior.

m. carbonate an ANTACID.

m. chloride an electrolyte replenisher and a pharmaceutic NECESSITY for HEMODIALYSIS and PERITONEAL DIALYSIS fluids.

m. citrate a saline laxative used for bowel evacuation before diagnostic procedures or surgery of the colon; administered orally.

m. hydroxide an ANTACID and CATHARTIC.

m. oxide an ANTACID and a sorbent in pharmaceutical preparations; called also magnesia.

m. salicylate see SALICYLATE.

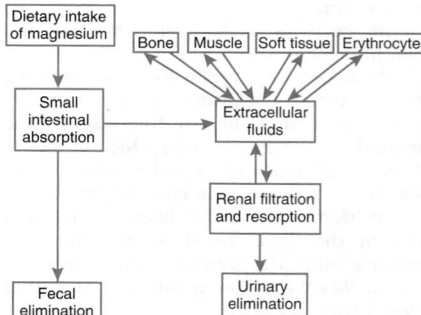

Homeostasis of magnesium in extracellular fluids. The normal serum magnesium level is regulated by intestinal and renal function. Most of the body's magnesium is stored in bones, muscle, and soft tissue. From Malarkey and McMorrow, 2000.

m. silicate MgSiO₃, a silicate salt of magnesium; the most common hydrated forms found in nature are ASBESTOS and TALC.

m. sulfate Epsom salt; an anticonvulsant and electrolyte replenisher, also used as a laxative and local antiinflammatory.

m. trisilicate a combination of magnesium oxide and silicon dioxide with varying proportions of water; used as a gastric ANTACID.

magnet (mag′net) an object having POLARITY (oppositely charged ends) and capable of attracting iron.

magnetic resonance imaging (MRI) a noninvasive nuclear procedure for imaging tissues of high fat and water content that cannot be seen with other radiologic techniques. The MRI image gives information about the chemical makeup of tissues, thus making it possible to distinguish normal, cancerous, atherosclerotic, and traumatized tissue masses in the image.

The patient having an MRI procedure lies in the bore of the cylindrical magnetic resonance machine; therefore, the test can induce claustrophobia. Furthermore, the person must lie motionless during the test, which can last from 15 to 90 minutes. If patients are susceptible to claustrophobia or cannot tolerate the tedium of lying still in a confined space, a sedative can be given without compromising test results.

magnetism (mag′nĕ-tizm) the attraction or repulsion characteristic of a MAGNET.

magnetoencephalography (MEG) (mag-ne″to-en-sef″ah-log′ra-fe) a noninvasive diagnostic technique that directly measures

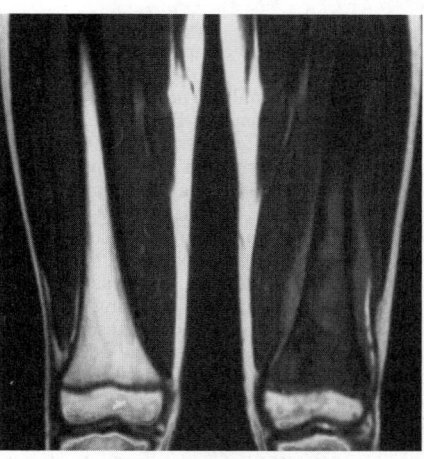

Coronal view from magnetic resonance imaging (MRI). The MRI study provides anatomical information about the osseous and soft tissue extent of a tumor. From Thrall and Ziessman, 2001.

the magnetic fields produced by electrical currents in the brain. A vaultlike device is necessary to ensure that the accuracy of the test is not affected by interference from magnetic fields produced by electrical wires and radio and television transmissions.

magnetropism (mag-net′ro-pizm) TROPISM in response to a magnetic field.

magnification (mag″nĭ-fĭ-ka′shun) 1. apparent increase in size, as under the microscope. 2. the process of making

M

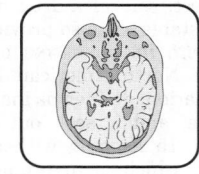

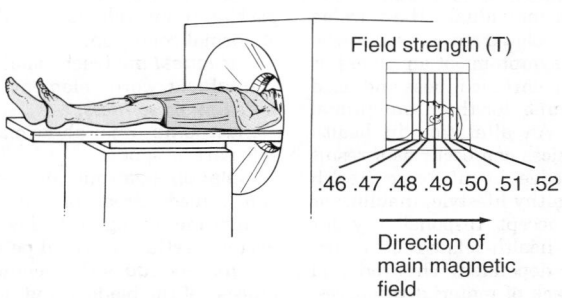

Field strength (T)

.46 .47 .48 .49 .50 .51 .52

Direction of main magnetic field

Magnetic resonance imaging. The patient enters a cylinder, which serves as a magnet. Radiofrequency coils within the cylinder emit signals that are transformed into an image of a display unit.

something appear larger, as by use of lenses. 3. the ratio of apparent (image) size to real size.

Mahoney (mah-ho′ne) Mary Eliza (1845–1926). America's first African American professional nurse. One of only four members of her class to complete the rigorous program at the training school of the New England Hospital for Women and Children, she was highly praised for the expert care she gave patients throughout her career. In addition, she was active in many local and national nursing organizations. In 1936, the National Association of Colored Graduate Nurses initiated the Mary Mahoney Medal, which is now awarded by the American Nurses' Association for contributions in intergroup relations.

main (măn) [Fr.] hand.

m. en griffe (man-ong-grēf′) clawhand.

mainstreaming (mān′strēm-ing) the placement of children with disabilities in classes with the general population of school children; special services tailored to the student's educational needs may still be provided.

maintainer (mān-tān′er) something that keeps or maintains existence or continuity in another thing.

space m. an orthodontic appliance, fixed or removable, that maintains the space left by a prematurely lost tooth or space that will be filled by a tooth not yet erupted.

maintenance (mā′ten-ans) providing a stable state over a long period as distinguished from a short-term remedial or prophylactic effect; said of a drug or treatment. Also, the stable state so provided.

altered health m. a NURSING DIAGNOSIS accepted by the North American Nursing Diagnosis Association, defined as inability to identify, manage, and/or seek out help to maintain health. In keeping with a major goal of nursing, which is to promote and maintain health in individuals, the nursing diagnosis can be related to persons who currently have no symptoms of an illness or to those who have a chronic illness and need assistance in attaining, for them, an optimal level of wellness. An alteration in health maintenance practices can occur as a result of lack of knowledge about basic health practices and a healthy lifestyle, inability or unwillingness to accept responsibility for one's health and health-related behaviors or those of one's dependent children and elderly relatives, lack of material resources, or unavailability of adequate health care services.

family process m. in the NURSING INTERVENTIONS CLASSIFICATION, a nursing INTERVENTION defined as minimization of family process disruption effects. See also interrupted family PROCESSES.

impaired home m. see HOME MAINTENANCE, IMPAIRED.

oral health m. in the NURSING INTERVENTIONS CLASSIFICATION, a nursing INTERVENTION defined as maintenance and promotion of oral HYGIENE and dental health for the patient at risk for developing oral or dental lesions.

venous access device m. in the NURSING INTERVENTIONS CLASSIFICATION, a nursing INTERVENTION defined as the management of the patient with prolonged vascular ACCESS via a catheter, shunt, or implanted port.

Majocchi's disease (mah-yok′ēz) annular telangiectatic PURPURA.

major depressive disorder a MOOD DISORDER characterized by the occurrence of one or more major depressive EPSIODES and the absence of any history of manic, mixed, or hypomanic EPISODES.

major mood disorders severe, full-blown MOOD DISORDERS, namely MAJOR DEPRESSIVE DISORDER and BIPOLAR DISORDERS.

mal (mal) [Fr. and Sp.] disease.

grand m. grand mal EPILEPSY.

m. de Meleda symmetrical keratosis of the palms and soles associated with a dry scaly thickening of the wrists and ankles.

m. de mer seasickness.

petit m. petit mal EPILEPSY.

mala (ma′lah) 1. cheek (def. 1). 2. zygomatic BONE; see anatomic Table of Bones in the Appendices. adj., **ma′lar.**

malabsorption (mal″ab-sorp′shun) impaired intestinal absorption of nutrients.

m. syndrome a group of disorders marked by subnormal intestinal absorption of dietary constituents, and thus excessive loss of nutrients in the stool; it may be due to a digestive defect, a mucosal abnormality, or lymphatic obstruction.

malacia (mal-la′she-ah) softening of a part or tissue related to a disease or other abnormal condition.

tracheal m. tracheomalacia.

-malacia word element [Gr.], *morbid softening or softness.*

malacoma (mal″ah-ko′mah) a morbidly soft spot or spot.

malacoplakia (mal″ah-ko-pla′ke-ah) a circumscribed area of softening on the membrane lining a hollow organ, as the ureter, urethra, or renal pelvis.

m. vesi′cae a flat yellow growth on the mucosa of the bladder and ureters, resulting from infection.

malacosis (mal″ah-ko′sis) malacia.

malacosteon (mal″ah-kos′te-on) soften-ing of the bones; osteomalacia.

malacotic (mal″ah-kot′ik) soft.

maladjustment (mal″ad-just′ment) in psy-chiatry, failure to fit one's inner needs to the environment; inability to meet the challenges of daily life.

malady (mal′ah-de) disease.

malaise (mal-āz′) [Fr.] a feeling of uneasiness or indisposition.

malalignment (mal″ah-līn′ment) displace-ment, especially of the teeth from their normal relation to the line of the dental arch.

malaria (mah-lar′e-ah) a serious infec-tious, sometimes fatal disease caused by a protozoal infection, characterized by peri-odic chills and high fever. It is endemic in many warm regions of the world and is estimated to occur at the rate of 500 million cases each year worldwide. It is one of the world's major causes of death, causing about a million deaths a year, and the number is increasing. Drug resistance is a growing problem. Epidemics of malaria usually occur in areas where mosquitoes infected with the protozoal parasite are found in large numbers and there are persons not immune to malaria. Acute cases occur when nonimmune persons travel to regions where the disease is

endemic. Called also paludism. adj., **malar′-ial.** A joint African-American-European project called the Multilateral Initiative on Malaria is attempting to increase coordi-nation of research efforts. Some difficulties encountered in malaria control have been resistance of mosquitoes to insecticides, insufficient funding in some developing countries, development of strains of proto-zoa that are resistant to antimalarial drugs, and the fact that malaria in monkeys can be transmitted to humans. As a result, recent efforts have been toward malaria control rather than eradication.

Cause. Malaria is caused by the protozoan parasite *Plasmodium,* which is carried by mosquitoes of the genus *Anopheles*. When the mosquito bites an infected person, it sucks in the parasites residing in the person's blood. In the mosquito the plasmo-dia multiply and travel to the salivary glands, from which they are transmitted to the bloodstream of the next person the mosquito bites. Inside the human host they first enter hepatic parenchymal cells and later are released to enter the bloodstream, where they penetrate the ERYTHROCYTES. There they mature, reproduce, and at com-plete maturity burst out of the blood cell. The life cycle varies according to the species of *Plasmodium*. For *P. vivax* it is 48 hours, for *P. malariae* 72 hours, and for *P. falciparum* 36 to 48 hours.

Symptoms. There are usually no symptoms until several cycles have been completed. Then there is a simultaneous rupturing of erythrocytes by the entire brood, causing the characteristic chills followed in a few hours by fever. The temperature may rise to 40° to 40.5°C (104° to 105°F). As it subsides, there is profuse perspiring. Other symptoms are headache, nausea, body pains and, after the attack, exhaustion. The symp-toms last from 4 to 6 hours and recur at regular intervals, depending upon the para-sitic species and its cycle. If the attack occurs every other day, the disease is called *tertian malaria,* and if it occurs at 3-day intervals it is called *quartan malaria.*

As the disease progresses, the attacks occur less frequently. Bouts of malaria may last from 1 to 4 weeks but usually about 2 weeks. Relapses are common, with attacks ceasing and recurring at irregular intervals for several years, especially if untreated. Malaria is not usually fatal; when it is, it is almost always caused by the falciparum species.

Treatment. For many years, QUININE was the standard treatment for malaria, and it

M

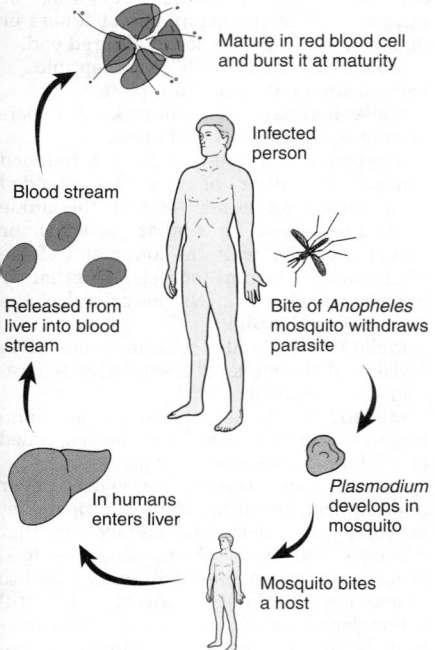

Mature in red blood cell and burst it at maturity

Blood stream

Infected person

Released from liver into blood stream

Bite of *Anopheles* mosquito withdraws parasite

In humans enters liver

Plasmodium develops in mosquito

Mosquito bites a host

Life cycle of malarial parasite.

is still important in treatment of infection with drug-resistant strains of the protozoa. Other medications include MAL-ARONE and MEFLOQUINE. Drug therapy will depend on a variety of factors including (but not limited to) availability of the medication.

Prevention. There is no effective inoculation against malaria, but antimalarial drugs may be given prophylactically to persons traveling to areas where the disease is widespread, or to pregnant women in areas in which the disease is endemic. Preventive measures are concentrated on destroying the mosquito by filling in swamps and other places containing stagnant water where mosquitoes breed, and by use of insecticides and natural biologic predators of mosquitoes.

Malaria information is available from the Fax Information Service of the Centers for Disease Control and Prevention (1-888-232-3299) or on the web site of the CDC at http://www.cdc.gov.

malariacidal (mah-lar″e-ah-si′d′l) plasmodicidal.

Malarone (mal′ah-rōn) trademark for a combination preparation of PROGUANIL and ATOVAQUONE, an antimalarial AGENT.

Malassezia (mal″ah-se′ze-ah) a genus of yeastlike fungi. *M. fur′fur* is a species normally found on normal skin but capable of causing TINEA VERSICOLOR in susceptible hosts. Called also Pityrosporon.

malassimilation (mal″ah-sim″ĭ-la′shun) 1. imperfect, faulty, or disordered assimilation. 2. the inability of the gastrointestinal tract to take up one or more ingested nutrients, whether due to faulty digestion (maldigestion) or to impaired intestinal mucosal transport (malabsorption).

malate (ma′lāt) a salt of malic acid.

malathion (mal-ah-thi′on) an ORGANOPHOS-PHORUS INSECTICIDE used in topical applications for lice.

malaxate (mal′ak-sāt) to knead, as in making pills.

malaxation (mal″ak-sa′shun) an act of kneading.

maldevelopment (mal″de-vel′op-ment) abnormal growth or development.

male (māl) an individual of the sex that produces spermatozoa.

m. **erectile disorder** the psychiatric term for PSYCHOGENIC IMPOTENCE; a SEXUAL DYSFUNCTION involving failure by a male to attain or maintain erection until completion of sexual relations causing significant distress or interpersonal difficulty. See also FEMALE SEXUAL AROUSAL DISORDER.

m. **orgasmic disorder** persistently delayed or absent orgasm in a man after a normal sexual excitement phase that is adequate in focus, intensity, and duration. The most common form involves inability to achieve orgasm during intercourse although it can be achieved by manual or oral stimulation. See also FEMALE ORGASMIC DISORDER.

maleruption (mal′e-rup′shun) eruption of a tooth out of its normal position.

malformation (mal″for-ma′shun) deformity.

malic acid (ma′lik) a compound that is found in the juices of many fruits and plants, and is an intermediate in the tricarboxylic ACID.

malignancy (mah-lig′nan-se) a tendency to progress in virulence. In popular usage any condition that, if uncorrected, tends to worsen so as to cause serious illness or death. Cancer is the best known example.

malignant (mah-lig′nant) tending to become progressively worse and to result in death; having the properties of anaplasia, invasiveness, and metastasis; said of tumors.

malignin (mah-lig′nin) a protein fragment present in the serum of patients with malignant glial tumors.

malingerer (mah-ling′ger-er) one who is guilty of malingering.

malingering (mah-ling′ger-ing) willful, deliberate, and fraudulent feigning or exaggeration of the symptoms of illness or injury to attain a consciously desired end.

malleable (mal′e-ah-b′l) susceptible of being beaten out into a thin plate.

malleoincudal (mal″e-o-ing′ku-d′l) pertaining to the malleus and incus.

malleolus (mah-le′o-lus) [L.] 1. a rounded process. 2. either of the two rounded prominences on either side of the ankle joint; the *lateral* (or fibular, external, or outer) malleolus is at the lower end of the fibula and the *medial* (or tibial, internal, or inner) malleolus is at the lower end of the tibia. adj. **malle′olar.**

malleotomy (mal″e-ot′ah-me) operative division of the malleus. 1. operative separation of the malleoli.

malleus (mal′e-us) the outermost and largest of the three ossicles of the EAR; called also hammer. See also color plates.

malnutrition (mal″noo-trish′un) poor nourishment resulting from improper diet or from some defect in metabolism that prevents the body from using its food properly. Extreme malnutrition may lead to STARVATION. Although poverty is still the major cause of malnutrition, the condition is by no means confined to the underdeveloped parts of the world. Anyone can become undernourished by seriously neglecting the diet. A well balanced diet, which varies slightly with a person's age, should include adequate amounts of protein, vitamins, minerals, and carbohydrates. For an explanation of the value of properly balanced diets and guidelines for a healthy diet, see NUTRITION.

Ignorance of the basic principles of nutrition is probably almost as great a cause of undernourishment as poverty. Misplaced faith in vitamin pills as a substitute for food, for example, can cause undernourishment if carried to extremes. So can overreliance on excessively processed foods. Modern methods of processing and refining foods can sometimes cause a loss of valuable nutrients, as happens in the refining of certain grains, such as rice. However, this danger is recognized by both the government and the manufacturers who try to retain or restore the nutritional value of many foods. ALCOHOLISM, which frequently leads a person to rely on alcohol at the expense of food, is another cause of malnutrition.

People who want to gain or lose weight, or who avoid certain foods, may endanger their health by following an unbalanced diet that lacks essential nutrients. Anyone who plans to follow a special diet should consult with a Registered Dietitian. Malnutrition can also stem from disease. If the organs of the digestive system that transform food into bone, tissue, blood, and energy fail to function properly, the body will not receive adequate nourishment. Such deficiencies can cause certain liver diseases, and some anemias. The ENDOCRINE GLANDS and enzymes are also vital to the proper use of food by the body, and defects in their functioning may cause forms of malnutrition.

Symptoms. In general, the symptoms of malnutrition are physical weakness, lassitude, and an increasing sense of detachment from the world. There are also specific symptoms that vary according to the essential substance lacking in the diet. For example, lack of vitamin A can result in NIGHT BLINDNESS, or poor vision in dim light. In the absence of adequate exposure to sunlight, a lack of vitamin D can cause RICKETS, which results in malformed limbs in infants and children because the bones fail to harden properly. A lack of vitamin C causes SCURVY, with symptoms of bleeding gums and easily bruised skin. Other vitamin deficiency diseases are BERIBERI and PELLAGRA. If there is not enough iron in the diet, iron deficiency ANEMIA develops. Malnutrition can also result from allergic reactions to foods, as in CELIAC DISEASE.

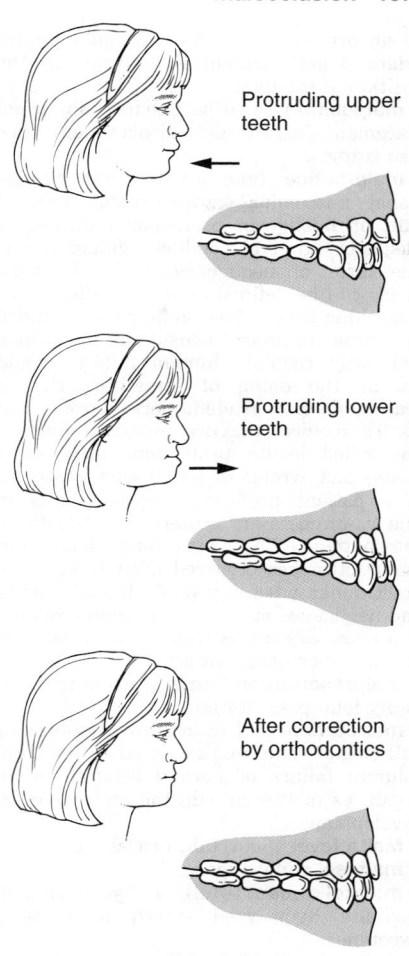

Protruding upper teeth

Protruding lower teeth

After correction by orthodontics

Malocclusion.

In starvation there are signs of multiple vitamin deficiency. There may be edema, abdominal distention, and excessive loss of weight. As starvation progresses, fat cells become small and accumulations of fat are depleted. The liver is reduced in size, the muscles shrivel, and the lymphoid tissue, gonads, and blood deteriorate.

malocclusion (mal″ŏ-kloo′zhun) malposition of the teeth resulting in the faulty meeting of the teeth or jaws. The condition should be corrected because it predisposes to dental caries, may lead to digestive disorders and inadequate nutrition because of difficulty in chewing, and can cause serious psychologic effects if there is facial distortion. Corrective treatment is provided by an orthodontist, who may apply appropriate dental appliances to improve the position of the teeth.

malposition (mal″po-zish′un) abnormal placement; called also displacement. See also ECTOPIA.

malpractice (mal″prak′tis) any professional misconduct, unreasonable lack of skill or fidelity in professional duties, or illegal or immoral conduct. Malpractice is one form of negligence, which in legal terms can be defined as the omission to do something that a reasonable person, guided by those ordinary considerations which ordinarily regulate human affairs, would do, or the doing of something that a reasonable and prudent person would not do. In medical practice, nursing practice, and allied health professions malpractice means bad, wrong, or injudicious treatment of a patient professionally; it results in injury, unnecessary suffering, or death to the patient. The court may hold that malpractice has occurred even though the practitioner acted in good faith. Malpractice and negligence may occur through omission of a necessary act as well as commission of an unwise or negligent act.

malpresentation (mal″prez-en-ta′shun) faulty fetal presentation.

malrotation (mal″ro-ta′shun) abnormal or pathologic rotation, as of the vertebral column; failure of normal rotation of an organ, as of the gut, during embryological development.

Malta fever (mawl′tah) brucellosis.

maltase α-glucosidase.

maltitol (mawl′tĭ-tol) a hydrogenated, partially hydrolyzed starch used as a sweetener.

maltose (mawl′tōs) a DISACCHARIDE formed when starch is hydrolyzed by amylase.

malum (ma′lum) [L.] disease.

  m. per′forans pe′dis perforating ulcer of the foot.

malunion (mal-ūn′yun) faulty union of the fragments of a fractured bone.

mamelon (mam′ĕ-lon) 1. one of three tubercles on the cutting edge of a newly erupted incisor tooth. 2. the nipple-like elevation in the umbilicus.

mamilla (mah-mil′ah) mammilla.

mamillitis (mam′ĭ-li′tis) mammillitis.

mamm(o)- word element [L.], *breast; mammary gland.*

mamma (mam′ah) [L.] breast.

mammal (mam′al) an individual of the Mammalia, a division of vertebrates, including all that possess hair and suckle their young. adj., **mammal′ian.**

mammalgia (mah-mal′jah) mastalgia.

mammaplasty (mam′ah-plas″te) plastic surgery of the breast; called also mammoplasty.

  augmentation m. plastic surgery to increase the size of the female breast, or sometimes to uplift pendulous breasts. It can be done for purely cosmetic purposes, as when a woman wants larger breasts, or following MASTECTOMY to replace surgically removed tissue (see *reconstructive mammaplasty*).

  reconstructive m. breast reconstruction after MASTECTOMY, done as an alternative to breast forms and specially designed brassieres to achieve a more normal appearance of the breast. If this procedure is chosen, it is usually considered to be just one stage in the total plan of treatment for breast cancer. It has both a psychologic and physiologic impact on the patient. Criteria used to determine whether reconstructive surgery is appropriate postmastectomy include the amount of tissue remaining after mastectomy, e.g., pectoral muscles, skin, and nipple; the probability of recurrent metastatic disease; appearance and size of the unoperated breast; and size and angle of the mastectomy scar. Adjuvant cancer therapy with radiation does not necessarily preclude additional plastic breast surgery.

  reduction m. plastic surgery to reduce the size of the female breast. Physical and psychological problems that may be amenable to this include fatigue or a dragging sensation caused by the weight of the breasts, breast tenderness and discomfort, and difficulty obtaining adequate support even with a sturdy brassiere. Psychological stress can result from embarrassment over deep grooves created by the shoulder straps of brassieres, fear of ridicule, and difficulty in finding suitable clothing. Reduction mammaplasty usually involves removal of excess breast tissue by way of a curved incision under the breast. The skin is pulled taut and the nipple transplanted to its normal position in the center of the newly formed breast. After surgery the patient may need help in adjusting to a new body image. If she is of childbearing age she should be informed that normal lactation is no longer possible after this procedure.

mammary (mam′ah-re) pertaining to the mammary gland or breast.

mammatroph (mam′ah-trōf) lactotroph.

mammectomy (mah-mek′to-me) mastectomy.

mammilla (mah-mil′ah), pl. *mamil′lae* 1. nipple (def. 1). 2. papilla. adj., **mam′millary.**

mammillated (mam′ĭ-lāt″ed) having nipple-like projections or prominences.

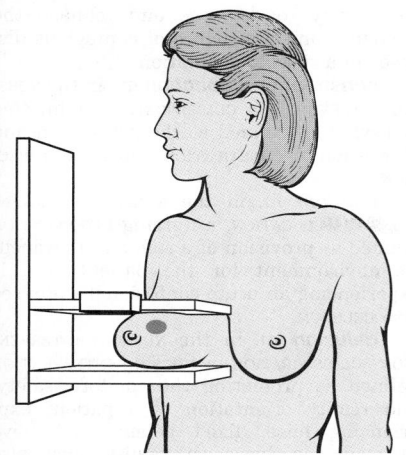

Mammograhy. From Damjanov, 2000.

mammillation (mam″ĭ-la′shun) 1. the condition of being mammillated. 2. a nipple-like elevation or projection.

mammilliform (mah-mil′i-form) shaped like a nipple.

mammillitis (mam″ĭli′tis) thelitis; inflammation of the nipple. Also spelled mamillitis.

mammiplasia (mam″ĭ-pla′zhah) mammoplasia.

mammitis (mah-mi′tis) mastitis.

mammogram (mam′o-gram) a radiograph of the breast.

mammography (mah-mog′rah-fe) radiography of the breast. The procedure involves exposure to less than one rad of radiation and is considered to have benefits that outweigh the relatively small risk to the patient. During mammography the patient's breasts are placed alternately on a metal plate and radiographs are taken from the side and above.

The American Cancer Society recommends that a baseline mammogram be done between the ages of 35 and 40 for later comparisons if needed. A yearly mammogram is recommended for women over the age of 50 to screen for breast cancer that may not be discovered during other types of breast examination.

mammoplasia (mam″o-pla′zhah) development of breast tissue.

mammoplasty (mam′o-plas″te) mammaplasty.

mammose (mam′ōs) 1. having unusually large breasts. 2. mammillated.

mammotomy (mah-mot′ah-me) mastotomy.

mammotrope (mam′o-trōp″) lactotroph.

mammotroph (mam′o trōf″) lactotroph.

mammotrophic (mam″o-trof′ik) mammotropic.

mammotropic (mam″o-trop′ik) having a stimulating effect on the mammary gland.

mammotropin (mam′o-tro″pin) prolactin.

management (man′ij-ment) the process of controlling how something is done or used.

acid-base m. in the NURSING INTERVENTIONS CLASSIFICATION, a nursing INTERVENTION defined as the promotion of ACID-BASE BALANCE and prevention of complications resulting from acid-base imbalance.

acid-base m.: metabolic acidosis in the NURSING INTERVENTIONS CLASSIFICATION, a nursing INTERVENTION defined as the promotion of acid-base balance and prevention of complications resulting from serum bicarbonate levels lower than desired. See also metabolic ACIDOSIS.

acid-base m.: metabolic alkalosis in the NURSING INTERVENTIONS CLASSIFICATION, a nursing INTERVENTION defined as the promotion of acid-base balance and prevention of complications resulting from serum bicarbonate levels higher than desired. See also metabolic ALKALOSIS.

acid-base m.: respiratory acidosis in the NURSING INTERVENTIONS CLASSIFICATION, a nursing INTERVENTION defined as the promotion of acid-base balance and prevention of complications resulting from serum pCO_2 levels higher than desired. See also respiratory ACIDOSIS.

acid-base m.: respiratory alkalosis in the NURSING INTERVENTIONS CLASSIFICATION, a nursing INTERVENTION defined as the promotion of acid-base balance and prevention of complications resulting from serum pCO_2 levels lower than desired. See also respiratory ALKALOSIS.

airway m. in the NURSING INTERVENTIONS CLASSIFICATION, a nursing INTERVENTION defined as insertion or assisting with insertion and stabilization of an artificial AIRWAY. See also artificial airway MANAGEMENT.

allergy m. in the NURSING INTERVENTIONS CLASSIFICATION, a nursing INTERVENTION defined as the identification, treatment, and prevention of allergic responses to food, medications, insect bites, contrast material, blood or other substances.

anaphylaxis m. in the NURSING INTERVENTIONS CLASSIFICATION, a nursing INTERVENTION defined as the promotion of adequate ventilation and tissue perfusion for a patient with severe allergic (antigen-antibody) reaction.

artificial airway m. in the NURSING INTERVENTIONS CLASSIFICATION, a nursing

M

INTERVENTION defined as the maintenance of endotracheal and tracheostomy tubes and preventing complications associated with their use. See also airway MANAGEMENT.

behavior m. in the NURSING INTERVENTIONS CLASSIFICATION, a nursing INTERVENTION defined as helping a patient to manage negative BEHAVIOR.

behavior m.: overactivity/inattention in the NURSING INTERVENTIONS CLASSIFICATION, a nursing INTERVENTION defined as the provision of a therapeutic milieu which safely accommodates the patient's attention deficit and/or overactivity while promoting optimal function.

behavior m.: self-harm in the NURSING INTERVENTIONS CLASSIFICATION, a nursing INTERVENTION defined as assisting the patient to decrease or eliminate self-mutilating or self-abusive behavior.

behavior m.: sexual in the NURSING INTERVENTIONS CLASSIFICATION, a nursing INTERVENTION defined as delineation and prevention of socially unacceptable sexual behaviors.

bowel m. in the NURSING INTERVENTIONS CLASSIFICATION, a nursing INTERVENTION defined as establishment and maintenance of a regular pattern of bowel elimination.

case m. 1. an approach to health care delivery that focuses on the complex needs of the patient and emphasizes the coordination and prioritization of all needed services. See also case MANAGER. 2. in the NURSING INTERVENTIONS CLASSIFICATION, a nursing INTERVENTION defined as coordinating care and advocating for specified individuals and patient populations across settings to reduce cost, reduce resource use, improve quality of health care, and achieve desired outcomes.

cerebral edema m. in the NURSING INTERVENTIONS CLASSIFICATION, a nursing INTERVENTION defined as limitation of secondary cerebral injury resulting from swelling of brain tissue. See also cerebral EDEMA.

chemotherapy m. in the NURSING INTERVENTIONS CLASSIFICATION, a nursing INTERVENTION defined as assisting the patient and family to understand the action and minimize side effects of CHEMOTHERAPY with antineoplastic AGENTS.

code m. in the NURSING INTERVENTIONS CLASSIFICATION, a nursing INTERVENTION defined as coordination of emergency measures to sustain life.

communicable disease m. in the NURSING INTERVENTIONS CLASSIFICATION, a nursing INTERVENTION defined as working with a community to decrease and manage the incidence and prevalence of contagious diseases in a specific population.

constipation/impaction m. in the NURSING INTERVENTIONS CLASSIFICATION, a nursing INTERVENTION defined as the prevention and alleviation of CONSTIPATION and FECAL IMPACTION.

delirium m. in the NURSING INTERVENTIONS CLASSIFICATION, a nursing INTERVENTION defined as provision of a safe and therapeutic environment for the patient who is experiencing an acute confusional state; see also DELIRIUM.

delusion m. in the NURSING INTERVENTIONS CLASSIFICATION, a nursing INTERVENTION defined as promoting the comfort, safety and reality orientation of a patient experiencing false, fixed beliefs that have little or no basis in reality. See also DELUSION.

dementia m. in the NURSING INTERVENTIONS CLASSIFICATION, a nursing INTERVENTION defined as provision of a modified environment for the patient who is experiencing a chronic confusional state; see also DEMENTIA.

diarrhea m. in the NURSING INTERVENTIONS CLASSIFICATION, a nursing INTERVENTION defined as the prevention and alleviation of DIARRHEA.

dysreflexia m. in the NURSING INTERVENTIONS CLASSIFICATION, a nursing INTERVENTION defined as prevention and elimination of stimuli that cause hyperactive reflexes and inappropriate autonomic responses in a patient with a cervial or high thoracic cord lesion. See also DYSREFLEXIA.

dysrhythmia m. in the NURSING INTERVENTIONS CLASSIFICATION, a nursing INTERVENTION defined as preventing, recognizing, and facilitating treatment of abnormal cardiac rhythms. See also DYSRHYTHMIA.

eating disorders m. in the NURSING INTERVENTIONS CLASSIFICATION, a nursing INTERVENTION defined as prevention and treatment of severe diet restriction and over-exercising or bingeing and purging of food and fluids. See also EATING DISORDER.

electrolyte m. in the NURSING INTERVENTIONS CLASSIFICATION, a nursing INTERVENTION defined as promotion of ELECTROLYTE balance and prevention of complications resulting from abnormal or undesired serum electrolyte levels.

electrolyte m.: hypercalcemia in the NURSING INTERVENTIONS CLASSIFICATION, a nursing INTERVENTION defined as promotion of calcium balance and prevention of complications resulting from serum calcium levels higher than desirable. See also HYPERCALCEMIA.

electrolyte m.: hyperkalemia in the NURSING INTERVENTIONS CLASSIFICATION, a nursing INTERVENTION defined as promotion of potassium balance and prevention of complications resulting from serum potassium levels higher than desirable. See also HYPERKALEMIA.

electrolyte m.: hypermagnesemia in the NURSING INTERVENTIONS CLASSIFICATION, a nursing INTERVENTION defined as promotion of magnesium balance and prevention of complications resulting from serum magnesium levels higher than desirable. See also HYPERMAGNESEMIA.

electrolyte m.: hypernatremia in the NURSING INTERVENTIONS CLASSIFICATION, a nursing INTERVENTION defined as promotion of sodium balance and prevention of complications resulting from serum sodium levels higher than desirable. See also HYPERNATREMIA.

electrolyte m.: hyperphosphatemia in the NURSING INTERVENTIONS CLASSIFICATION, a nursing INTERVENTION defined as promotion of phosphate balance and prevention of complications resulting from serum phosphate levels higher than desirable. See also HYPERPHOSPHATEMIA.

electrolyte m.: hypocalcemia in the NURSING INTERVENTIONS CLASSIFICATION, a nursing INTERVENTION defined as promotion of calcium balance and prevention of complications resulting from serum calcium levels lower than desirable. See also HYPOCALCEMIA.

electrolyte m.: hypokalemia in the NURSING INTERVENTIONS CLASSIFICATION, a nursing INTERVENTION defined as promotion of potassium balance and prevention of complications resulting from serum potassium levels lower than desirable. See also HYPOKALEMIA.

electrolyte m.: hypomagnesemia in the NURSING INTERVENTIONS CLASSIFICATION, a nursing INTERVENTION defined as promotion of magnesium balance and prevention of complications resulting from serum magnesium levels lower than desirable. See also HYPOMAGNESEMIA.

electrolyte m.: hyponatremia in the NURSING INTERVENTIONS CLASSIFICATION, a nursing INTERVENTION defined as promotion of sodium balance and prevention of complications resulting from serum sodium levels lower than desirable. See also HYPONATREMIA.

electrolyte m.: hypophosphatemia in the NURSING INTERVENTIONS CLASSIFICATION, a nursing INTERVENTION defined as promotion of phosphate balance and prevention of complications resulting from serum phosphate levels lower than desirable. See also HYPOPHOSPHATEMIA.

energy m. in the NURSING INTERVENTIONS CLASSIFICATION, a nursing INTERVENTION defined as regulating energy use to treat or prevent fatigue and optimize function.

environmental m. in the NURSING INTERVENTIONS CLASSIFICATION, a nursing INTERVENTION defined as manipulation of the patient's surroundings for therapeutic benefit.

environmental m.: attachment process in the NURSING INTERVENTIONS CLASSIFICATION, a nursing INTERVENTION defined as manipulation of the patient's surroundings to facilitate the development of the parent-infant relationship.

environmental m.: comfort in the NURSING INTERVENTIONS CLASSIFICATION, a nursing INTERVENTION defined as manipulation of the patient's surroundings for promotion of optimal comfort.

environmental m.: community in the NURSING INTERVENTIONS CLASSIFICATION, a nursing INTERVENTION defined as monitoring and influencing of the physical, social, cultural, economic, and political conditions that affect the health of groups and communities.

environmental m.: home preparation in the NURSING INTERVENTIONS CLASSIFICATION, a nursing INTERVENTION defined as preparing the home for safe and effective delivery of care.

environmental m.: safety in the NURSING INTERVENTIONS CLASSIFICATION, a nursing INTERVENTION defined as monitoring and manipulation of the physical environment to promote safety.

environmental m.: violence prevention in the NURSING INTERVENTIONS CLASSIFICATION, a nursing INTERVENTION defined as monitoring and manipulation of the physical environment to decrease the potential for violent behavior directed toward self, others, or environment.

environmental m.: worker safety in the NURSING INTERVENTIONS CLASSIFICATION, a nursing INTERVENTION defined as monitoring and manipulation of the worksite environment to promote safety and health of workers.

fiscal resource m. in the NURSING INTERVENTIONS CLASSIFICATION, a nursing INTERVENTION defined as procuring and directing the use of financial resources to assure the development and continuation of programs and services.

fluid m. in the NURSING INTERVENTIONS CLASSIFICATION, a nursing INTERVENTION defined as the promotion of FLUID BALANCE and prevention of complications resulting from abnormal or undesired fluid levels.

M

fluid/electrolyte m. in the NURSING INTERVENTIONS CLASSIFICATION, a nursing INTERVENTION defined as the regulation and prevention of complications from altered fluid and/or electrolyte levels.

hallucination m. in the NURSING INTERVENTIONS CLASSIFICATION, a nursing INTERVENTION defined as promoting the safety, comfort, and reality orientation of a patient experiencing HALLUCINATIONS.

hyperglycemia m. in the NURSING INTERVENTIONS CLASSIFICATION, a nursing INTERVENTION defined as preventing and treating above-normal glucose levels. See also HYPERGLYCEMIA.

hypervolemia m. in the NURSING INTERVENTIONS CLASSIFICATION, a nursing intervention defined as the reduction in extracellular and/or intracellular fluid volume and prevention of complications in a patient who is fluid overloaded. See also HYPERVOLEMIA.

hypoglycemia m. in the NURSING INTERVENTIONS CLASSIFICATION, a nursing INTERVENTION defined as preventing and treating low blood glucose levels. See also HYPOGLYCEMIA.

hypovolemia m. in the NURSING INTERVENTIONS CLASSIFICATION, a nursing INTERVENTION defined as the expansion of intravascular fluid volume in a patient whose volume is depleted. See also HYPOVOLEMIA.

immunization/vaccination m. in the NURSING INTERVENTIONS CLASSIFICATION, a nursing INTERVENTION defined as monitoring immunization status, facilitating access to immunizations, and provision of immunizations to prevent communicable disease.

ineffective community therapeutic regimen m. a NURSING DIAGNOSIS accepted by the North American Nursing Diagnosis Association, defined as a pattern of regulating and integrating into community processes of programs for treatment of illness and the sequelae of illness that are unsatisfactory for meeting health-related goals.

ineffective family therapeutic regimen m. a NURSING DIAGNOSIS accepted by the North American Nursing Diagnosis Association, defined as a pattern of regulating and integrating into family processes of a program for treatment of illness and its sequelae that is unsatisfactory for meeting specific health goals for a family member.

ineffective therapeutic regimen m. a NURSING DIAGNOSIS accepted by the North American Nursing Diagnosis Association, defined as a pattern of regulation and integration into daily living of a treatment program for illness and its sequelae that is unsatisfactory for meeting specific health goals.

medication m. in the NURSING INTERVENTIONS CLASSIFICATION, a nursing INTERVENTION defined as facilitation of safe and effective use of prescription and over-the-counter drugs.

mood m. in the NURSING INTERVENTIONS CLASSIFICATION, a nursing INTERVENTION defined as providing for safety and stabilization of a patient who is experiencing a dysfunctionally depressed MOOD or elevated mood.

nausea m. in the NURSING INTERVENTIONS CLASSIFICATION, a nursing INTERVENTION defined as prevention and alleviation of NAUSEA.

nutrition m. in the NURSING INTERVENTIONS CLASSIFICATION, a nursing INTERVENTION defined as assisting with or providing a balanced dietary intake of foods and fluids.

pain m. in the NURSING INTERVENTIONS CLASSIFICATION, a nursing INTERVENTION defined as alleviation of PAIN or a reduction in pain to a level of comfort that is acceptable to the patient.

peripheral sensation m. in the NURSING INTERVENTIONS CLASSIFICATION, a nursing INTERVENTION defined as prevention or minimization of injury or discomfort in the patient with altered sensation.

pessary m. in the NURSING INTERVENTIONS CLASSIFICATION, a nursing INTERVENTION defined as placement and monitoring of a vaginal device for treating stress urinary incontinence, uterine retroversion, genital prolapse, or incompetent cervix. See also PESSARY.

pressure m. in the NURSING INTERVENTIONS CLASSIFICATION, a nursing INTERVENTION defined as minimizing pressure to body parts.

program m. a system of health CARE delivery in an institution or agency whereby staff are divided by broad patient categories rather than by professional groups.

pruritus m. in the NURSING INTERVENTIONS CLASSIFICATION, a nursing INTERVENTION defined as preventing and treating itching.

radiation therapy m. in the NURSING INTERVENTIONS CLASSIFICATION, a nursing INTERVENTION defined as assisting the patient to understand and minimize the side effects of radiation treatments. See also RADIATION THERAPY.

rectal prolapse m. in the NURSING INTERVENTIONS CLASSIFICATION, a nursing INTERVENTION defined as the prevention and/or manual reduction of rectal PROLAPSE.

reproductive technology m. in the NURSING INTERVENTIONS CLASSIFICATION, a nursing INTERVENTION defined as assisting a

patient through the steps of complex INFER-
TILITY treatment.

risk m. the assessment and removal or
control of hazard to patients, employees, or
institutions.

seizure m. in the NURSING INTERVEN-
TIONS CLASSIFICATION, a nursing INTERVENTION
defined as care of a patient during a SEIZURE
and the POSTICTAL state.

shock m. in the NURSING INTERVENTIONS
CLASSIFICATION, a nursing INTERVENTION defined as facilitation of the delivery of oxygen
and nutrients to systemic tissue with removal of cellular waste products in a patient
with severely altered tissue perfusion. See
also SHOCK.

shock m.: cardiac in the NURSING INTER-
VENTIONS CLASSIFICATION, a nursing INTERVEN-
TION defined as the promotion of adequate
tissue perfusion for a patient with severely
compromised pumping function of the
heart.

shock m.: vasogenic in the NURSING
INTERVENTIONS CLASSIFICATION, a nursing IN-
TERVENTION defined as the promotion of
adequate tissue perfusion for a patient with
severe loss of vascular tone.

shock m.: volume in the NURSING INTER-
VENTIONS CLASSIFICATION, a nursing INTERVEN-
TION defined as the promotion of adequate
tissue perfusion for a patient with severely
compromised intravascular volume. See also
hypovolemic SHOCK.

specimen m. in the NURSING INTER-
VENTIONS CLASSIFICATION, a nursing INTERVEN-
TION defined as obtaining, preparing,
and preserving a SPECIMEN for a laboratory
test.

supply m. in the NURSING INTERVENTIONS
CLASSIFICATION, a nursing INTERVENTION defined as ensuring acquisition and maintenance of appropriate items for providing
care.

technology m. in the NURSING INTERVEN-
TIONS CLASSIFICATION, a nursing INTERVENTION
defined as the use of technical equipment
and devices to monitor patient condition or
sustain life.

time m. the effective planning and
balancing of activities such as self-care,
work, leisure, and rest in order to promote
satisfaction and health.

unilateral neglect m. in the NURSING
INTERVENTION CLASSIFICATION, a nursing IN-
TERVENTION defined as protecting and safely
reintegrating the affected part of the body
while helping the patient adapt to disturbed
perceptual abilities. See also unilateral
NEGLECT.

urinary elimination m. in the NURSING
INTERVENTIONS CLASSIFICATION, a nursing IN-
TERVENTION defined as the maintenance of

an optimum urinary elimination pattern.
See also URINATION.

vomiting m. in the NURSING INTERVEN-
TIONS CLASSIFICATION, a nursing INTERVENTION
defined as prevention and alleviation of
VOMITING.

weight m. in the NURSING INTERVENTIONS
CLASSIFICATION, a nursing INTERVENTION defined as facilitating maintenance of optimal
weight and percent body fat.

manager (man'ah-jer) one who controls
how something is done or used.

case m. the health care professional
responsible for formulating a coordinated,
comprehensive plan for individuals who
need long-term health care supervision. It is
the responsibility of the case manager to
work with all health care providers, the
patient, the patient's significant others, third
party payers, and health care facilities in
order to identify and meet the patient's
needs.

mandible (man'dĭ-b'l) the horseshoe-
shaped bone forming the lower jaw. adj.,
mandib'ular. It consists of a central
portion, which forms the chin and supports
the lower teeth, and two perpendicular
portions, or rami, which point upward from
the back of the chin on either side and
articulate with the temporal bones.

Mandol (man'dol) trademark for a preparation of CEFAMANDOLE, a broad-spectrum
CEPHALOSPORIN ANTIBIOTIC.

mandrin (man'drin) a firm stylet or guide
for a flexible catheter.

maneuver (mah-noo'ver) any dexterous
procedure; see also METHOD, OPERATION, PROCE-
DURE, SURGERY, and TECHNIQUE. For names of
specific maneuvers, see under the name.

mangafodipir (mang″gah-fo'dĭ-pir) a con-
trast-enhancing agent used to improve the
images obtained in MAGNETIC RESONANCE
IMAGING (MRI) of hepatic lesions; administered intravenously as the trisodium salt.

manganese (Mn) (mang'gah-nēs) a chemical element, atomic number 25, atomic
weight 54.938. (See Appendix 6.) Its salts
occur in the body tissue in very small
amounts and serve as activators of liver
arginase and other enzymes.

m. poisoning a condition usually
caused by inhalation of manganese dust;
symptoms of chronic exposure include mental disorders accompanying a syndrome
resembling Parkinson's disease, and inflammation throughout the respiratory system.

mange (mānj) a skin disease of domestic
animals, due to mites.

mania (ma'ne-ah) [Gr.] a phase of BIPOLAR
DISORDERS characterized by expansiveness,

elation, agitation, hyperexcitability, hyperactivity, and increased speed of thought or speech (FLIGHT OF IDEAS). adj., **man′ic.**

-mania word element [Gr.], *obsessive preoccupation with something.*

manic-depressive marked by alternating periods of mania and depression.

   m.-d. disorders former name for the BIPOLAR DISORDERS.

manipulation (mah-nip″u-la′shun) skillful or dexterous treatment by the hands. In PHYSICAL THERAPY, the forceful passive movement of a joint beyond its active limit of motion.

   joint m. the attempt to restore the full joint mobility by a single forceful movement. It may be performed with the patient under anesthesia, as when restoring knee or shoulder motion after prolonged loss of motion with formation of adhesions that limit joint PLAY. Joint manipulation applied to a spinal joint (usually referred to as high-velocity) is a short-amplitude thrust that is beyond the patient's voluntary control; it is always performed with the patient conscious.

man-living-health: a theory of nursing former name for the nursing theory now called THEORY OF HUMAN BECOMING.

mannitol (man′ĭ-tol) a sugar alcohol widely distributed in plants and fungi; it is an osmotic DIURETIC administered to prevent and treat acute RENAL FAILURE, to reduce cerebral edema or elevated intraocular or cerebrospinal fluid pressure, and to reduce renal damage due to toxic substances; also used as an irrigating solution to prevent hemolysis during transurethral resection of the prostate and similar transurethral procedures.

mannose (man′ōs) a monosaccharide sugar of the ALDOSE group, found as part of many GLYCOLIPIDS and GLYCOPROTEINS.

mannosidosis (man″o-sī-do′sis) an inborn ERROR of metabolism, thought to be an autosomal recessive trait, marked by a defect in alpha-mannosidase activity, resulting in lysosomal accumulation of MANNOSE-rich substrates. Clinically, there are coarse features, upper respiratory congestion and infections, profound mental retardation, hepatosplenomegaly, cataracts, radiographic signs of defective ossification, and a gibbus deformity (hump). A much milder form also occurs.

manometer (mah-nom′ĕ-ter) an instrument for ascertaining the pressure of liquids or gases.

manometry (mah-nom′ĕ-trē) the measurement of pressure by means of a manometer.

   esophageal m. a diagnostic study to assess the competence of the lower esophageal sphincter. A catheter sheathed with a water-filled balloon is inserted nasally and advanced into the esophagus; a series of measurements reflecting esophageal resting pressures are taken as the catheters are moved.

Mansonella (man″so-nel′ah) a genus of nematode parasites of the superfamily Filarioidea. *M. ozzar′di* is found in the mesentery and visceral fat of humans in Central and South America.

Mansonia (man-so′ne-ah) a genus of mosquitoes comprising some 55 species, distributed primarily in tropical regions, important as vectors of microfilariae and viruses.

mantle (man′t'l) an enveloping structure or layer, especially the brain mantle, or pallium.

Mantoux test (man-too′) a tuberculin skin test in which a solution of 0.1 mL of PPD-tuberculin containing 5 tuberculin units is injected intradermally into either the anterior or posterior surface of the forearm. The test is read 48 to 72 hours after injection. The size of the area of any induration at the site of injection, in combination with patient risk factors, is used to determine whether the test is positive, that is, whether exposure to or infection with MYCOBACTERIUM tuberculosis (the agent causing tuberculosis) or a related organism has occurred.

manubrium (mah-noo′bre-um) [L.] 1. the uppermost portion of the STERNUM; called also manubrium sterni. 2. the largest process of the MALLEUS, giving attachment to the tendon of the tensor muscle of the tympanum; called also manubrium mallei.

manus (ma′nus) [L.] hand.

MAO monoamine oxidase.

MAOI monoamine oxidase inhibitor.

MAP mean arterial pressure.

maple bark disease a granulomatous interstitial pneumonitis due to inhalation of the spores from *Cryptostroma corticale*, a mold found beneath the bark of maple logs.

maple syrup urine disease a genetic disorder involving deficiency of an enzyme necessary in the metabolism of branched-chain amino acids, marked clinically by mental and physical retardation, feeding difficulties, and a characteristic odor of the urine.

mapping (map′ing) the creation on a flat surface of a representation of an area, showing the relative position of various features.

   cardiac m. an electrophysiological procedure in which electric POTENTIALS recorded by electrodes placed directly on the heart are processed to give a two-dimensional display of the origin and path of an electrical impulse as it depolarizes the heart.

genetic m. determination of the location of genes on chromosomes.

intraoperative lymphatic m. sentinel node biopsy.

maprotiline (mah-pro′tĭ-lēn) a tetracyclic ANTIDEPRESSANT administered orally as the hydrochloride salt for relief of symptoms of depression. It acts by blocking the reuptake of NOREPINEPHRINE at nerve terminals; unlike tricyclic ANTIDEPRESSANTS, it has no effect on serotoninergic transmission.

marasmus (mah-raz′mus) a form of protein-calorie malnutrition occurring chiefly in the first year of life, with growth retardation and wasting of subcutaneous fat and muscle, but usually with retention of appetite and mental alertness. It is considered to be related to KWASHIORKOR. Infectious disease may be a precipitating factor. adj., **maran′tic, maras′mic.**

Marax (mar′aks) trademark for a preparation of EPHEDRINE sulfate, THEOPHYLLINE, and HYDROXYZINE hydrochloride; used for control of bronchospasm.

Marburg virus disease (mahr′boork) a severe, often fatal, type of HEMORRHAGIC FEVER first reported in Marburg, Germany, among laboratory workers exposed to African green monkeys.

march (mahrch) the progression of electrical activity through the motor cortex.

cortical m., epileptic m. jacksonian m. the spread of abnormal electrical activity from one area of the cerebral cortex to adjacent areas, characteristic of jacksonian EPILEPSY.

Marchiafava-Micheli syndrome (mar″ke-ah-fah′vah me-ka′le) paroxysmal nocturnal hemoglobinuria.

Marfan syndrome (mar-fahn′) a hereditary disorder of connective tissue characterized by abnormal length of the extremities, especially of the fingers and toes, subluxation of the lens, congenital anomalies of the heart, and other deformities.

margin (mahr′jin) an edge or BORDER.

gingival m. gum margin.

gum m. the border of the gingiva surrounding, but unattached to, the substance of the teeth.

m. of safety a calculation that takes the highest animal no observed adverse effect LEVEL and estimates a maximum safe level of exposure for humans. It is now generally superseded by the reference DOSE.

margination (mar″jĭ-na′shun) accumulation and adhesion of leukocytes to the epithelial cells of blood vessel walls at the

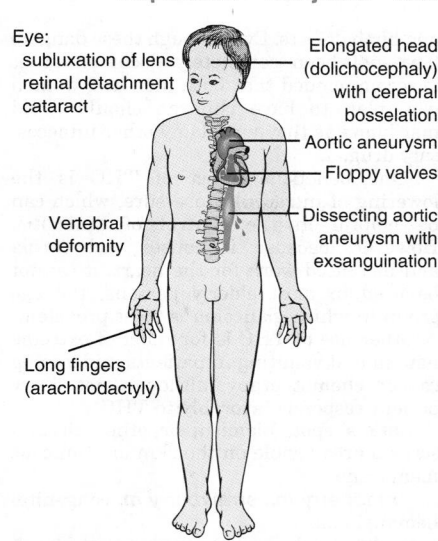

Eye:
subluxation of lens
retinal detachment
cataract

Elongated head (dolichocephaly) with cerebral bosselation

Aortic aneurysm

Floppy valves

Vertebral deformity

Dissecting aortic aneurysm with exsanguination

Long fingers (arachnodactyly)

Typical features of Marfan syndrome. From Damjanov, 2000.

site of injury in the early stages of inflammation.

margo (mar′go) [L.] margin.

Marie's disease (mah-rēz′) acromegaly.

Marie-Bamberger disease (mah-re′bahm′ber-ger) hypertrophic pulmonary osteoarthropathy.

Marie-Strümpell disease (mah-re′strim′pel) ankylosing spondylitis.

Marie-Tooth disease (mah-re′tooth′) progressive neuromuscular atrophy.

marihuana (mar″ĭ-wahn′ah) marijuana.

marijuana (mar″ĭ-wahn′ah) a preparation of the leaves and flowering tops of *Cannabis sativa,* the hemp plant, which contains a number of pharmacologically active principles (CANNABINOIDS). HASHISH, also derived from the hemp plant, is obtained from the clear resin secreted by the flowering tops of the plant and is four to eight times as potent as marijuana. Both drugs are used for their euphoric properties and are considerably more potent when smoked and inhaled than when simply eaten.

TETRAHYDROCANNABINOL (THC), the most active ingredient of marijuana, can, with heavy smoking, narrow the bronchi and bronchioles and produce inflammation of the mucous membranes. In addition, marijuana smoke contains many of the same chemicals and "tars" as tobacco smoke and, therefore, increases the risk of lung cancer. There is some evidence that marijuana increases the risk for miscarriage and birth defects. Even though these dangers have not been completely documented, it is recommended that both men and women who plan to have children should avoid marijuana as they would any other unnecessary drug.

One beneficial effect of THC is the lowering of intraocular pressure, which can be helpful in the control of GLAUCOMA. However, because it causes tachycardia and increased work for the heart, it cannot be used in most elderly persons, the age group in which glaucoma is most prevalent. Another use of THC is for relief of extreme nausea and vomiting in patients undergoing cancer chemotherapy, although not every patient responds favorably to THC.

mark a spot, blemish, or other circumscribed area visible on the skin or a mucous membrane.

raspberry m., strawberry m. congenital hemangioma.

marker (mahr′ker) something that identifies or that is used to identify; see also DETERMINANT.

cell-surface m. an antigenic DETERMINANT found on the surface of a specific type of cell.

tumor m. a biochemical substance indicative of presence of a TUMOR; ideally, it should be specific, sensitive, and proportional to tumor load. Called also biomarker.

Marplan (mahr′plan) trademark for a preparation of ISOCARBOXAZID, an ANTIDEPRESSANT.

marrow (mar′o) soft spongy material; called also medulla. The term is often restricted to mean bone MARROW.

bone m. the soft, organic, spongelike material in the cavities of bones; called also medulla ossium. It is a network of blood vessels and special connective tissue fibers that hold together a composite of fat and blood-producing cells. Its chief function is to manufacture ERYTHROCYTES, LEUKOCYTES, and PLATELETS. These blood cells normally do not enter the bloodstream until they are fully developed, so that the marrow contains cells in all stages of growth. If the body's demand for leukocytes is increased because of infection, the marrow responds immediately by stepping up production. The same is true if more erythrocytes are needed, as in hemorrhage or anemia.

There are two types of marrow, red and yellow. The former produces the blood cells; the latter, which is mainly formed of fatty tissue, normally has no blood-producing function. During infancy and early childhood all bone marrow is red. But gradually, as one gets older and less blood cell production is needed, the fat content of the marrow increases as some of it turns from red to yellow. Red marrow is present in adulthood only in the flat bones of the skull, the sternum, ribs, vertebral column, clavicle, humerus, and part of the femur. However, under certain conditions, as after hemorrhage, yellow marrow in other bones may again be converted to red and resume its cell-producing functions.

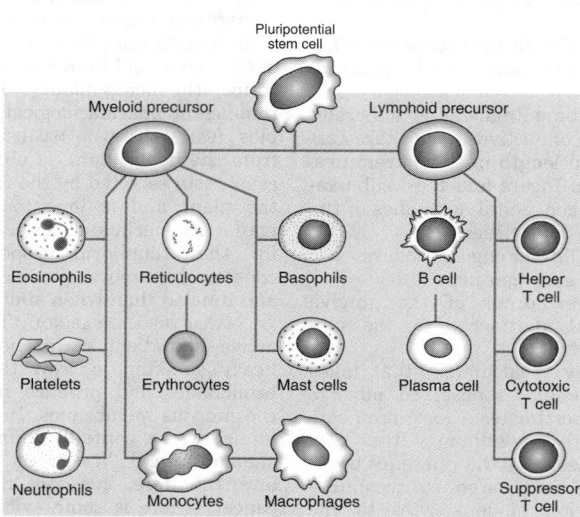

Cells of the bone marrow and the blood. From Malarkey and McMorrow, 2000.

The marrow is occasionally subject to disease, as in APLASTIC ANEMIA, which may be caused by destruction of the marrow by chemical agents or excessive x-ray exposure. Other diseases that affect the bone marrow are leukemia, pernicious anemia, myeloma, and metastatic tumors.

marsupialization (mar-soo″pe-ah-lĭ-za′-shun) conversion of a closed cavity, such as an abscess or cyst, into an open pouch, by incising it and suturing the edges of its wall to the edges of the wound.

mAs milliampere-second.

masculine (mas′ku-lin) having qualities usually associated with the male sex.

masculinity (mas″ku-lin′ĭ-te) the possession of masculine qualities.

masculinization (mas″ku-lin-ĭ-za′shun) 1. the normal induction or development of male secondary sex CHARACTERS in the male. 2. the induction or development of male secondary sex CHARACTERS in the female or prepubertal male. 3. the condition of having such sex characters. Called also virilization.

masculinize (mas′ku-lĭ-nīz) to produce normal secondary sex CHARACTERS in a male. 1. to produce male secondary sex CHARACTERS in a female.

maser (ma′zer) a device that produces an extremely intense, small and nearly nondivergent beam of monochromatic radiation in the microwave region, with all the waves in phase.

mask (mask) 1. a covering for the face, as a bandage, an apparatus for administering anesthesia or oxygen, or a cloth that prevents droplets from the mouth and nose from spreading in the air. 2. to cover or conceal, as the masking of the nature of a disorder by unassociated signs or organisms. 3. in audiometry, to obscure or diminish a sound by the presence of another sound of different frequency.

   m. of pregnancy popular term for MELASMA GRAVIDARUM.

Venturi m. see VENTURI MASK.

Maslow's hierarchy of needs see NEED.

masochism (mas′o-kizm) the act or instance of gaining pleasure experiencing physical or psychological pain. The term is usually used to denote sexual m. adj., **masochis′tic.**

   sexual m. a PARAPHILIA in which sexual gratification is derived from being hurt, humiliated, or otherwise made to suffer physically or psychologically.

masochist (mas′o-kist) a person exhibiting or characterized by masochism.

mass (mas) 1. a lump or collection of cohering particles. 2. that characteristic of matter that gives it inertia. Symbol *m*.

   atomic m. atomic WEIGHT; see also atomic mass UNIT.

   inner cell m. an internal cluster of cells at the embryonic pole of the blastocyst which develops into the body of the embryo.

   lean body m. that part of the body including all its components except neutral storage lipid; in essence, the fat-free mass of the body.

   relative molecular m. technically preferable term for molecular WEIGHT.

massa (mas′ah) [L.] mass (def. 1).

massage (mah-sahzh′) systematic therapeutic stroking or kneading of the body.

   cardiac m. intermittent compression of the heart by pressure applied either over the sternum (closed cardiac massage) or directly to the heart through an opening in the chest wall (open cardiac massage).

   simple m. in the NURSING INTERVENTIONS CLASSIFICATION, a nursing INTERVENTION defined as stimulation of the skin and underlying tissues with varying degrees of hand pressure to decrease pain, produce relaxation, and/or improve circulation.

   vibratory m. massage by rapidly repeated light percussion with a vibrating hammer or sound.

masseur (mah-ser′) [Fr.] a man who performs massage.

masseuse (mah″sōōs′) [Fr.] a woman who performs massage.

massotherapy (mas″o-ther′ah-pe) treatment of disease by massage.

MAST military anti-shock trousers; see under SUIT.

mast(o)- word element [Gr.], *mammary gland; breast.*

mastadenitis (mas″tad-ĕ-ni′tis) mastitis.

mastalgia (mas-tal′jah) pain in the breast; called also mammalgia and mastodynia.

mastatrophy (mas-tat′ro-fe) atrophy of the breast.

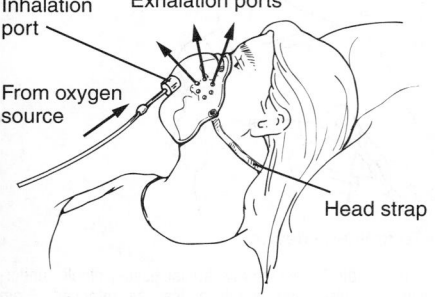

Inhalation port

Exhalation ports

From oxygen source

Head strap

A standard face mask. From Lammon et al., 1996.

mastectomy (mas-tek´to-me) surgical removal of breast tissue, usually for treatment of malignant breast tumors, although occasionally this may be advisable for benign tumors, other diseases of the breast such as FIBROCYSTIC DISEASE OF THE BREAST, or prophylaxis. Patients with breast disorders should be informed about all the options for treatment including alternatives to mastectomy. Types of mastectomy include the *simple* or *total mastectomy* and *radical, modified radical,* and *extended radical mastectomies.*

Patient Care. The psychological aspects of the breast must always be considered in the care of women who face the prospect of loss of breast tissue through surgery. The breast is symbolic of femininity, motherhood, and sexual attractiveness for some individuals. Psychological problems likely to be associated with mastectomy include disturbance in self-concept related to changes in body image, self-esteem, role performance, and personal identity. Newer, less mutilating surgical procedures and cosmetically successful reconstructive plastic surgery (MAMMAPLASTY) to replace surgically removed breast tissue have diminished some of the emotional trauma formerly associated with mastectomy.

Following mastectomy the patient is likely to experience such physical problems as pain, numbness, tingling, and weakness related to nerve damage and muscle atrophy. Additionally, the patient is subject to lymphedema and collections of serous fluid (seroma) associated with interruption of the flow of lymph.

In addition to routine postoperative care to prevent pulmonary and circulatory complications, the patient must be watched for the development of localized edema, especially if lymph nodes have been removed. In order to provide adequate drainage of serosanguineous fluid that could delay healing of the operative site, the surgeon may insert a flat, narrow drain with multiple openings. The device is part of a portable self-contained closed-suction system that exerts negative pressure. Systems of this kind include Hemovac and Reliavac.

The patient receives routine postoperative care, including coughing and deep-breathing exercises, to prevent respiratory complications and early ambulation to avoid circulatory stasis. When helping the patient from bed it is important to realize that her sense of balance may be impaired because of changes in upper body structures and some hesitancy to use the arm on the operative side to support herself and maintain balance.

Postoperative care should include periodic assessment of sensations (e.g. "phantom breast" sensations) and of functional limitations in the chest wall and affected arm. Additionally numbness, patterns of weakness, and paresthesias are evaluated. The patient should be taught how to recognize and report these symptoms and any changes noted, as they could indicate progressive nerve damage.

Impairment of lymph flow increases the risk of infection. Loss of sensation could predispose the patient to injury from burns, cuts, and other accidental trauma. Venipunctures are not done and blood pressure cuffs are not applied on the arm on the affected side. Prior to discharge the patient is given instruction in ways to avoid trauma: for example, do not carry a heavy handbag or other heavy articles with the affected arm, avoid excessive exposure to sun, do not pick or cut cuticles, and consult the physician or nurse before having vaccinations or injections in the affected arm. Exercises to improve mobility and lymphatic drainage are begun while the patient is in the hospital and continued by her after discharge. These exercises are described and illustrated in the booklet "Help Yourself to Recovery," which is available from local offices of the American Cancer Society. The Cancer Society also has self-help support groups, called Reach for Recovery, for women following mastectomy.

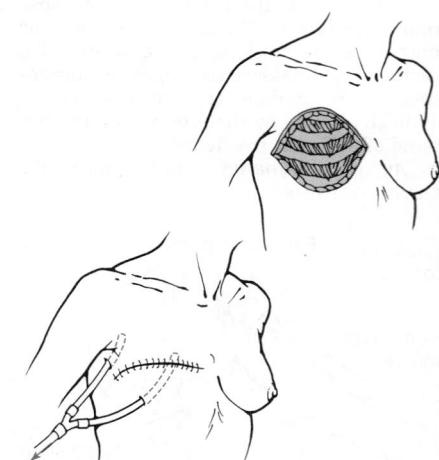

To drainage device

In a radical mastectomy, breast tissue, nipple, underlying muscles, and lymph nodes are removed. From Ignatavicius and Workman, 2001.

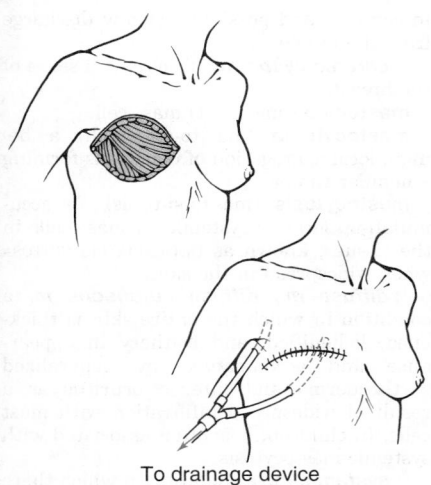

To drainage device

In a modified radical mastectomy, breast tissue, nipple, and lymph nodes are removed, but muscles are left intact. From Ignatavicius and Workman, 2001.

The woman is encouraged to continue follow-up care, including a clinical breast exam every 3 to 4 months for the first 3 years, then every 6 months for 2 years, and thereafter every 6 to 12 months. Annual mammograms should be obtained and the woman should perform breast self-exams monthly.

Halsted m. radical mastectomy.

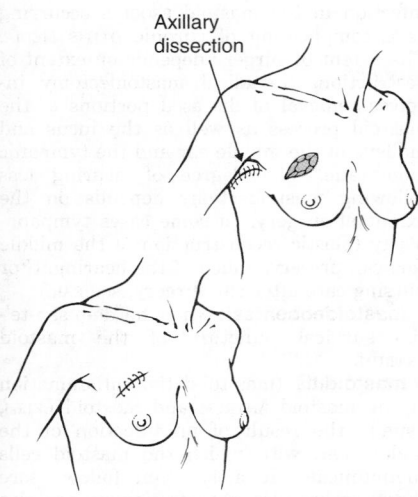

Axillary dissection

In a simple mastectomy, breast tissue and (usually) nipple are removed, but lymph nodes are left intact. From Ignatavicius and Workman, 2001.

partial m. removal of the tumor, along with varying amounts of surrounding normal tissue. See also LUMPECTOMY and QUADRANTECTOMY. Called also segmental mastectomy.

radical m. removal of the breast, pectoral muscles, axillary lymph nodes, and associated skin and subcutaneous tissue in treatment of breast cancer.

radical m., extended supraradical mastectomy; surgical removal of the internal mammary chain of lymph nodes, the entire involved breast, the underlying chest muscles, and the lymph nodes in the axilla.

radical m., modified surgical removal of the entire involved breast, and many lymph nodes in the axilla. The underlying chest muscles are removed in part or are left in place after removal of axillary lymph nodes.

segmental m. partial mastectomy.

simple m. surgical removal of the entire involved breast; the underlying chest muscles and axillary lymph nodes are not removed. More recently called total mastectomy.

subcutaneous m. excision of breast tissue with preservation of overlying skin, nipple, and areola so that the breast form may be reconstructed.

supraradical m. extended radical mastectomy.

total m. simple mastectomy.

Master "2-step" exercise test (mas′ter) a type of EXERCISE TESTING; electrocardiographic tracings are recorded first while the subject repeatedly ascends and descends two steps, then immediately after exercise cessation, and then 2 and 6 minutes after cessation. The amount of work (number of trips) is standardized for age, weight, and sex. TREADMILL EXERCISE TESTS are now more commonly used.

mastication (mas″tĭ-ka′shun) the act of chewing.

masticatory (mas′tĭ-kah-tor″e) 1. pertaining to mastication. 2. a substance to be chewed, but not swallowed.

Mastigophora (mas″tĭ-gof′o-rah) a subphylum of PROTOZOA, including all those that have one or more FLAGELLA throughout most of their life cycle, and a simple, centrally located nucleus; many are parasitic in both invertebrates and vertebrates, including humans.

mastigote (mas′tĭ-gōt) mastigophoran.

mastigophoran (mas″tĭ-gof′ah-rahn) any member of the subphylum MASTIGOPHORA; called also mastigote.

M

mastitis (mas″ti′tis) inflammation of the BREAST, occurring in a variety of forms and degrees of severity. FIBROCYSTIC DISEASE OF THE BREAST (called also *chronic cystic mastitis*) is the most common disorder of the breast resulting from hormonal imbalance. It generally occurs in women between the ages of 35 and 50, is probably related to the activity of the ovaries, and is rare after menopause. Occasionally mastitis becomes so severe as to require a MASTECTOMY.

Young girls whose breasts are maturing sometimes experience a painful swelling and hardness of the breast, known as *puberty mastitis;* this is rarely serious and usually resolves within a few weeks. Occasionally a cloudy liquid may be squeezed from the nipples. It is best to wear a brassiere that gives mild support but does not irritate.

A mild inflammation known as *stagnation mastitis*, or caked breast, may occur during the early lactation period. Glands of the breast can become congested with milk, with formation of painful lumps.

Acute mastitis may occur after childbirth, when it is known as *puerperal mastitis*. This is an infection that usually results from the presence of staphylococci, or occasionally streptococci, which enter through cracks in the skin of the breast, particularly of the nipples. The breasts are tender, red, and warm and become swollen and painful. The inflammation responds quickly to sulfonamide medicines or other antibiotics, but in some cases an abscess may develop which must be incised and drained.

A GALACTOCELE, or milk cyst, sometimes develops during lactation. It is probably caused by obstruction of a duct and can be removed after the baby has been weaned.

There are other types of infectious mastitis not related to lactation. Inflammation of the breast sometimes accompanies mumps, particularly in adults. *Tuberculous mastitis* usually occurs in young women and accompanies tuberculosis of the lungs or of the cervical lymph nodes. Treatment is with antibiotics, although surgery is sometimes necessary.

A condition that may occur at the time of menopause or later in women who have had children is mammary duct ECTASIA, or COMEDOMASTITIS, which is distention of the milk-producing ducts caused by the caking of secretions; some of the material may be discharged from the nipple. Eventually this may develop into *plasma cell mastitis*. The breast may be tender and painful, with lump formation, nipple retraction, change in contour, and possibly a cloudy discharge from the nipple.

chronic cystic m. fibrocystic disease of the breast.

mastocyte (mas′to-sīt) mast cell.

mastocytoma (mas″to-si-to′mah) a benign, local aggregation of mast cells forming a nodular tumor.

mastocytosis (mas′to-si-to′sis) an accumulation, local or systemic, of mast cells in the tissues; known as URTICARIA PIGMENTOSA when widespread in the skin.

diffuse m., diffuse cutaneous m. a condition in which the entire skin is thickened, lichenified, and leathery in appearance and accompanied by generalized erythroderma and intense pruritus as a result of widespread infiltration with mast cells. In children, it is often associated with systemic mastocytosis.

systemic m. a condition in which there are mast cell infiltrates in noncutaneous tissues, occurring with or without cutaneous lesions, and usually involving the liver, spleen, bone, lymph nodes, and gastrointestinal tract.

mastodynia (mas″to-din′e-ah) mastalgia.

mastography (mas-tog′rah-fe) mammography.

mastoid (mas′toid) 1. breast shaped. 2. mastoid PROCESS. 3. pertaining to the mastoid process.

mastoidalgia (mas″toi-dal′jah) pain in the mastoid region.

mastoidectomy (mas″toi-dek′to-me) surgical removal of mastoid CELLS; the most frequent indication for this is chronic infection in the mastoid PROCESS occurring as a complication of chronic OTITIS MEDIA. The extent of surgery depends on extent of destruction. A radical mastoidectomy involves removal of diseased portions of the mastoid process as well as the incus and malleus of the middle ear and the tympanic membrane. The degree of hearing loss following mastoidectomy depends on the extent of surgery. In some cases tympanoplasty (plastic reconstruction of the middle ear) can preserve much of the hearing. (For nursing care after ear surgery, see EAR.)

mastoideocentesis (mas-toi″de-o-sen-te′sis) surgical puncture of the mastoid ANTRUM.

mastoiditis (mas″toi-di′tis) inflammation of the mastoid ANTRUM and mastoid CELLS, usually the result of an infection of the middle ear, with which the mastoid cells communicate. It most often follows sore throat and respiratory infection but can also be caused by diseases such as diphtheria, measles, and scarlet fever. Symptoms include earache and a ringing in the ears.

WINDOW ON MATERNAL PKU SYNDROME

The maternal PKU syndrome is an adverse fetal outcome associated with mental retardation, microcephaly, cardiac defects, and other abnormalities, found in the offspring of women who have elevated levels of phenylalanine during pregnancy. Excessive phenylalanine in utero exerts a teratogenic effect on the developing fetus. As the levels of phenylalanine increase in the mother, the likelihood of severe fetal defects increases. Because the genetic defect of PKU is autosomal recessive, the mother with PKU can give birth to a child who does not have the metabolic defect if her mate does not have PKU or a carrier state of PKU.

The genetic defect of PKU can be treated with dietary restrictions, thus avoiding adverse effects, but the effects of the untreated maternal PKU syndrome are irreversible. Even moderately elevated levels of phenylalanine, as are found in variant PKUs, have been linked with some birth defects. It is still important for a woman with non-PKU hyperphenylalaninemia to contact a specialty clinic to evaluate her personal need for dietary treatment, even if she was never on a diet.

Management of the maternal PKU syndrome consists of identification of at-risk women and early initiation of dietary interventions to promote optimal fetal outcome.

It is very important that the woman with PKU or hyperphenylalaninemia plan all pregnancies and maintain near to normal levels of phenylalanine (2–6 mg/dL) prior to conception. As this management is complex, the assistance of a specialized clinic is required. A PKU Clinic or Inherited Metabolic Disease Clinic usually consists of a team of professionals such as a nutritionist, nurse, and physician. A reliable laboratory is necessary to frequently evaluate the mother's blood levels of phenylalanine. An individualized plan is needed for every woman according to her phenylalanine levels and response to treatment.

Despite the obvious advantage to the fetus of maternal dietary adherence, many women with PKU have not followed the recommended guidelines. Barriers such as lack of understanding, unpalatability of diet, expense of diet, and poor access to tertiary care centers may contribute to the problem of untreated maternal PKU. Thus, it remains a goal of health care professionals to locate, screen, and educate, and to provide access to specialty care for women with PKU or variant PKU in an effort to promote healthy babies. Assistance in locating PKU clinics can be found at the website, http://www.unco.edu/HHS/son/sonpku.htm.

TERESA HERGERT, MS, RN, FNP-C

The mastoid process may become painful and swollen. Treatment formerly was limited to MASTOIDECTOMY, in which infected cells were removed surgically. Today, however, use of antibiotics has made it possible to check most cases at an early stage, so that surgery can be avoided.

mastoidotomy (mas″toi-dot′ah-me) incision of the mastoid PROCESS.

masto-occipital (mas″to-ok-sip′ĭ-t'l) pertaining to the mastoid PROCESS and occipital BONE.

mastoparietal (mas″to-pah-ri′ĕ-t'l) pertaining to the mastoid PROCESS and parietal BONE.

mastopathy (mas-top′ah-the) any disease of the mammary gland.

mastopexy (mas′to-pek″se) surgical fixation of a pendulous breast.

mastoplasia (mas″to-pla′zhah) mammoplasia.

mastoplasty (mas′to-plas″te) mammaplasty.

mastoptosis (mas″to-to′sis, mas″top-to′sis) a pendulous condition of the breast.

mastorrhagia (mas″to-ra′jah) hemorrhage from the mammary gland.

mastoscirrhus (mas″to-skir′us) hardening of the mammary gland.

mastosquamous (mas″to-skwa′mus) pertaining to the mastoid and squama of the temporal bone.

mastotomy (mas-tot′ah-me) incision of a mammary gland.

masturbation (mas″tur-ba′shun) self-stimulation of the genitals for sexual pleasure.

matching (mach′ing) 1. comparison and selection of objects having similar or identical characteristics. 2. the selection of compatible donors and recipients for transfusion or transplantation. See also TYPING. 3. the selection of subjects for clinical trials or other studies so that the different groups being compared are similar in specified characteristics, e.g., age, sex, or race, in order to reduce bias caused by comparison of dissimilar

M

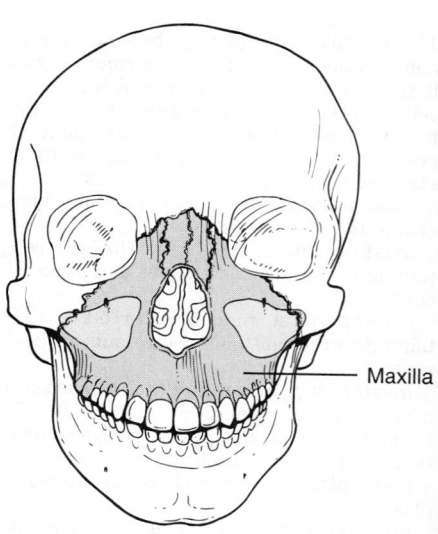

A   **B**

Matrices: *A*, Simple metal strip with a wooden wedge. *B*, Circumferential band of copper to encase the entire crown. From Baum et al., 1995.

groups. Matching may be on an individual (matched pairs) or a group-wide basis.

 cross m. crossmatching.

 materia medica (mah-tēr′e-ah med′ĭ-kah) pharmacology.

 maternal (mah-ter′nal) pertaining to the female parent.

 m. deprivation syndrome FAILURE TO THRIVE with severe growth retardation, unresponsiveness to the environment, depression, retarded mental and emotional development, and behavioral problems as a result of loss, absence, or neglect of the mother or other primary caregiver.

 maternity (mah-ter′nĭ-te) motherhood.

 matrix (ma′triks), pl. *ma′trices* [L.] 1. the intercellular substance of a tissue, as bone matrix, or the tissue from which a structure develops, as hair or nail matrix. 2. a metal or plastic band used to provide proper form to a dental restoration, such as amalgam in a prepared cavity.

 bone m. the intercellular substance of bone, consisting of collagenous fibers, ground substance, and inorganic salts.

 cartilage m. the intercellular substance of cartilage consisting of cells and extracellular fibers embedded in an amorphous ground substance.

 nail m., m. un′guis the nail bed.

 matter (mat′er) 1. physical material having form and weight under ordinary conditions; called also substance. 2. pus.

 gray m. areas of the nervous system where the nerve fibers are unmyelinated (not enveloped by a MYELIN SHEATH); it contains the bodies of the nerve cells. Tissue composed of myelinated fibers is called white matter. The cerebral cortex is entirely composed of gray matter and the cerebellum also contains some deep-seated masses of it. The spinal cord has a central core of gray matter surrounded by white matter; in cross section, its gray matter is shaped approximately like the letter H. Called also substantia grisea and gray substance.

 white m. areas of the nervous system composed mostly of myelinated nerve fibers (those having MYELIN SHEATHS) constituting the conducting portion of the brain and spinal cord. Tissue composed of unmyelinated fibers is called gray matter. Called also substantia alba and white substance.

 Matulane (mat′u-lān) trademark for a preparation of PROCARBAZINE, an antineoplastic AGENT.

 maturation (mach″u-ra′shun) 1. the stage or process of attaining maximal development; attainment of maximal intellectual and emotional development. 2. in biology, a process of cell division during which the number of chromosomes in the germ cell is reduced to half the number characteristic of the species.

 maxilla (mak-sil′ah) [L.] one of two identical bones that form the upper jaw. The maxillae meet in the midline of the face and often are considered as one bone. They have been described as the architectural key of the face because all bones of the face except the mandible touch them. Together the maxillae form the floor of the orbit for each eye, the sides and lower walls of the nasal cavities, and the hard palate. The lower border of the maxilla supports the upper teeth. Each maxilla contains an air space called the maxillary sinus.

 maxilloethmoidectomy (mak″sil-o-eth″-moi-dek′to-me) excision of the portion of the maxilla surrounding the maxillary sinus and of the cribriform plate and anterior ethmoid cells.

 maxillofacial (mak-sil″o-fa′shal) pertaining to the maxilla and the face.

 maxillomandibular (mak-sil″o-man-dib′u-ler) pertaining to the upper and lower jaws.

—— Maxilla

Maxilla.

maxillotomy (mak″sĭ-lot′ah-me) surgical sectioning of the maxilla, which allows movement of all or part of the maxilla into the desired position.

maximum (mak′sĭ-mum) the greatest quantity, effect, or value possible or achieved under given circumstances. adj., **max′imal.**

transport m., tubular m. T_m, the highest rate in milligrams per minute at which the renal tubules can transfer a substance either from the tubular luminal fluid to the interstitial fluid or from the interstitial fluid to the tubular luminal fluid, beyond which it may be excreted in the urine. In kidney function tests, it is expressed as T_m with inferior letters representing the substance used in the test, such as $T_{m_{PAH}}$ (transport maximum for *p*-aminohippuric acid).

maze (māz) a complicated system of intersecting paths used in intelligence tests and in demonstrating learning in experimental animals.

mazindol (ma′zin-dol) a SYMPATHOMIMETIC AMINE having amphetamine-like actions; used as an oral appetite suppressant.

MC[1] [L.] Ma′gister Chirur′giae (Master of Surgery).

MC[2] Medical Corps.

mcg microgram.

MCH mean corpuscular HEMOGLOBIN.

MCHB Maternal and Child Health Bureau, an agency of the Health Resources and Services Administration.

MCHC mean corpuscular hemoglobin CONCENTRATION.

mCi millicurie.

μCi microcurie.

MCT mean circulation time.

MCV mean corpuscular VOLUME.

MD [L.] Medici′nae Doc′tor (Doctor of Medicine).

Md mendelevium.

MDA methylenedioxyamphetamine.

MDMA 3,4-methylenedioxymethamphetamine.

meal (mēl) a portion of food or foods taken at some particular and usually stated or fixed time.

barium m. gastrointestinal series.

congregate m's a group nutritional program for socially isolated individuals whose nutritional problems are related more to access and to lack of social stimulation than to mechanical eating difficulties.

test m. see TEST MEAL.

mean (mēn) an average; a number that in some sense represents the central value of a set of numbers.

measles (me′z′lz) a highly contagious illness caused by a virus; it is usually a childhood disease but can be contracted at any age. Epidemics usually recur every 2 or 3 years and are most common in the winter and spring. In spite of the availability of a vaccine and intensive effort on the part of public health personnel to eradicate the disease, measles continues to occur in the United States. Called also rubeola.

Cause. The virus that causes measles is spread by droplet infection and can also be picked up by touching an article, such as a handkerchief, that an infected person has recently used. The incubation period is usually 11 days, although it may be as few as 9 or as many as 14. The patient can transmit the disease from 3 or 4 days before the rash appears until the rash begins to fade, a total of about 7 or 8 days. One attack of measles usually gives lifetime immunity to rubeola, although not to German measles (RUBELLA), a somewhat similar disease.

Symptoms. Measles symptoms generally appear in two stages. In the first stage the patient feels tired and uncomfortable, and may have a running nose, a cough, a slight fever, and pains in the head and back. The eyes may become reddened and sensitive to light. The fever rises a little each day.

The second stage begins at the end of the third or beginning of the fourth day. The patient's temperature is generally between 38° and 40°C (103° and 104°F). Koplik's spots, small white dots like grains of salt surrounded by inflamed areas, can often be seen on the gums and the inside of the cheeks. A rash appears, starting at the hairline and behind the ears and spreading downward, covering the body in about 36 hours. At first the rash consists of separate pink spots, about a quarter of an inch in diameter, but later some of the spots may run together, giving the patient a blotchy look. The fever usually subsides after the rash has spread. The rash turns brownish and fades after 3 or 4 days.

The most serious complication of rubeola is encephalitis, which occurs in about 0.1 per cent of all cases and is responsible for an estimated 600 cases of mental retardation each year. Other complications include pneumonia, otitis media, and mastoiditis.

Patient Care. The patient should be kept in bed as long as the rash and fever continue, and should get as much rest as possible. Aspirin, nose drops, and cough medicine may be prescribed during this stage. Water and fluids can be given for fever. The sickroom should be well ventilated and fairly warm. If the patient's eyes are sensitive to light, strong sunlight should be kept

M

out of the room. The rash may itch a great deal and prevent the patient from resting. If so, calamine lotion, cornstarch solution, or plain cool water will afford some relief. If the itching continues, antihistamine drugs may be necessary.

Measles can greatly lower resistance to other infections such as bronchitis, pneumonia, and ear infection. If the patient's temperature remains high for more than 2 days after the rash fades, or if he complains of pain in the ear, throat, chest, or abdomen, medical attention should be obtained without delay.

The person with measles should be placed under respiratory precautions until the fifth day of the rash. Anyone with a cold or cough should be kept away from the patient because another infection can cause serious complications. The Centers for Disease Control and Prevention recommend continuing respiratory isolation precautions for 4 days after start of the rash, except in immunocompromised patients, with whom precautions should be maintained for the duration of the illness.

Prevention. The first measles vaccine was developed and made available in the early 1960s. It consisted of killed virus and is now known to have conferred little or no immunity and, in addition, made the person susceptible to the development of atypical measles when exposed to the disease. Children who received this type of vaccine should be given the newer live vaccine in order to be protected against the disease. The live measles virus vaccine confers lifelong immunity in 95 per cent of those who receive potent vaccine. A 12 to 20 per cent potency failure can occur when the vaccine is not stored and refrigerated properly.

The live vaccine usually is given when the child is 15 months of age. Until then the child is protected by the temporary immunity acquired from its mother. If the vaccine is given before 15 months, the temporary immunity of the mother may prevent active immunity from taking place in the child. Children must be given the vaccine before exposure to measles, or within 48 hours after exposure; otherwise the vaccine is ineffective. If the vaccine cannot be given to a child exposed to measles, measles immune globulin (MIG) or the standard immune serum globulin is given; a waiting period of 3 months is then necessary before the measles vaccine is given. The vaccine is contraindicated during pregnancy.

German m., three-day m. rubella.

measure (mezh′er) 1. to determine the extent or quantity of a substance. 2. a specific extent or quantity of a substance. 3. a graduated scale by which the dimensions or mass of an object or substance may be determined. See Tables of Weights and Measures in Appendix. 4. a PROCEDURE or INTERVENTION.

assistive m. a nursing INTERVENTION in the NURSING MINIMUM DATA SET, in which the nurse facilitates ACTIVITIES OF DAILY LIVING (such as hygiene, exercise, rest, or grooming), provides physical comfort, and maintains a therapeutic environment.

m's of central tendency statistical procedures for determining the center of a distribution of scores; they include the MODE, the MEAN, and the MEDIAN.

m's of dispersion statistical procedures for examining how scores vary or are dispersed around the mean. These include the RANGE, the difference scores, the sum of squares, the VARIANCE, and the standard DEVIATION.

Functional Independence M. FIM; a standardized assessment instrument of functional status that is part of the Uniform Data Set for Medical Rehabilitation; it tests 23 items in seven areas of function and uses a seven-point scale for each item. It can be used clinically as an outcome measure, and a data pool is being established that will be large enough for prediction and comparison of functional outcomes. A pediatric version called the Wee-FIM is also available.

supportive m. a nursing INTERVENTION in the NURSING MINIMUM DATA SET, defined as action through which the nurse provides support of life functions and needed sustenance such as oxygen, nutrition, or fluids.

measurement (mĕzh′er-ment) 1. determination of the extent or quantity of something. 2. the assigning of numbers to objects, events, or situations in accord with some rule.

interval level m. measurement of data on an interval SCALE.

nominal level m. the lowest level of measurement, used when data can be organized into categories that are exclusive and exhaustive but the categories cannot be compared. Examples are gender, race, and marital status.

ordinal level m. measurement of data that can be assigned to categories of numerical rank; it must be kept in mind that the intervals between the ranked categories may not be equal, for example, levels of education, degrees of coping, and levels of mobility.

physiologic m. techniques used to measure bodily variations either directly or indirectly; examples are measurements of heart rate, mean arterial pressure, and total lung capacity.

ratio level m. the highest form of measurement that meets all the rules of other forms of measure; it includes mutually exclusive categories, exhaustive categories, rank ordering, equal spacing between intervals, and a continuum of values. Ratio level measurement also includes a value of zero. An example is weight.

meatoscopy (me″ah-tos′kah-pe) visual examination of a meatus, especially the urinary meatus or a ureteral orifice.

meatotomy (me″ah-tot′ah-me) incision of an acoustic or urinary meatus in order to enlarge it.

meatus (me-a′tus), pl. *mea′tus* [L.] an OPENING or passage, especially one leading to the body surface. adj., **mea′tal.**

acoustic m., m. acus′ticus either of two passages in the ear; the *external acoustic meatus* leads from the AURICLE to the TYMPANIC MEMBRANE (eardrum) and the *internal acoustic meatus* is for passage of nerves and blood vessels.

auditory m. acoustic meatus.

m. na′si, m. of nose one of the three portions of the nasal cavity on either side of the septum: inferior (*meatus nasi inferior*), middle (*meatus nasi medius*), and superior (*meatus nasi superior*).

ureteral m. ureteral orifice.

m. urina′rius, urinary m. the opening of the URETHRA on the body surface, through which urine is discharged.

mebendazole (mě-ben′dah-zōl) an ANTHELMINTIC used in the treatment of TRICHURIASIS, ENTEROBIASIS, ASCARIASIS, and HOOKWORM DISEASE.

mecamylamine (mek″ah-mil′ah-min) a ganglionic blocking AGENT administered orally as the hydrochloride salt as an ANTIHYPERTENSIVE AGENT.

mechanics (mě-kan′iks) the science dealing with the motions of material bodies.

body m. the application of kinesiology to use of the body in daily life activities and to the prevention and correction of problems related to posture.

mechanism (mek′ah-nizm) 1. a machine or machinelike structure. 2. the manner of combination of parts, processes, or other aspects that carry out a common function. 3. the theory that the phenomena of life are based on the same physical and chemical laws that govern inorganic matter, as opposed to *vitalism.*

coping m's conscious or unconscious strategies or mechanisms that a person uses to cope with stress or anxiety including turning to a comforting person for love and support, self-discipline, acting out or working off tension, talking and expressing feelings by crying or laughing, and also unconscious DEFENSE MECHANISMS, such as avoidance and rationalization.

defense m. see DEFENSE MECHANISM.

mechanoreceptor (mek″ah-no-re-sep′ter) a nerve ending sensitive to mechanical pressures or distortions, as those responding to touch and muscle contractions.

mechanotherapy (mek″ah-no-ther′ah-pe) use of mechanical apparatus in treatment of disease or its results, especially in therapeutic exercises.

mechlorethamine (mek″lor-eth′ah-mēn) an ALKYLATING AGENT that produces interstrand and intrastrand cross-linkages in DNA with resultant miscoding, breakage, and failure of replication. Used primarily for the treatment of disseminated HODGKIN'S DISEASE, especially in the MOPP treatment regimen, and for other lymphomas, including mycosis fungoides; administered intravenously as the hydrochloride salt. Called also nitrogen mustard.

Meckel's syndrome (mek′elz) Meckel-Gruber syndrome.

Meckel-Gruber syndrome (mek′el groo′-ber) a hereditary autosomal recessive syndrome in which infants are usually born with a sloping forehead, posterior MENINGOENCEPHALOCELE, POLYDACTYLY (extra fingers or toes), and polycystic kidneys; most die soon after birth. Called also Gruber's syndrome.

Meclan (mek′lan) trademark for a preparation of MECLOCYCLINE sulfosalicylate, a topical ANTIBACTERIAL.

meclizine (mek′lĭ-zēn) an ANTIHISTAMINE used orally as the hydrochloride salt to counteract the nausea of MOTION SICKNESS and to treat and prevent vertigo associated with diseases affecting the vestibular system.

meclocycline (mě″klo-si′klēn) a TETRACYCLINE ANTIBIOTIC used topically as *meclocycline sulfosalicylate* for treatment of ACNE VULGARIS.

meclofenamate (mek″lo-fen′ah-māt) a NONSTEROIDAL ANTIINFLAMMATORY DRUG used as the sodium salt in the treatment of rheumatic and nonrheumatic inflammatory disorders, pain, dysmenorrhea, hypermenorrhea, and vascular headaches; administered orally or rectally.

meconium (mě-ko′ne-um) dark green mucilaginous material in the intestine of the full-term fetus; this is the first type of feces passed by the newborn infant.

MED minimal effective dose; minimal erythema dose.

M

Medex (med′eks) a physician assistant program for former military medical corpsmen; also, a graduate of such a program.

media (me′de-ah) [L.] 1. plural of MEDIUM. 2. middle. 3. tunica media.

medial (me′de-al) pertaining to or situated toward the midline.

medialis (me″de-a′lis) [L.] medial.

median (me′de-an) 1. situated in the median plane or in the midline of a body or structure. 2. any value that divides the probability DISTRIBUTION of a random VARIABLE in half; that is, the probability of observing a value above the median and the probability of observing a value below the median are both less than or equal to one-half. For a finite population or sample, the median is the middle value of an odd number of values (arranged in ascending value) or any value between the two middle values of an even number of values; in the latter case it is conventional to use the average of the two middle values.

mediastinal (me″de-as-ti′n'l) of or pertaining to the mediastinum.

m. flutter movement of the tissues and organs of the mediastinum back and forth with each movement of air into and out of an open sucking wound in the thoracic cavity. The condition can produce serious impairment of cardiopulmonary function and is fatal if not treated promptly. Symptoms are similar to those of mediastinal shift.

m. shift a shifting or moving of the tissues and organs that comprise the mediastinum (heart, great vessels, trachea, and esophagus) to one side of the chest cavity. The condition occurs when a severe injury to the chest causes the entrapment of air in the pleural space (tension PNEUMOTHORAX). As the volume of air increases on the affected side, the lung collapses and the organs and tissues of the mediastinum are crowded to the opposite side of the chest. This can produce compression of the other lung and kinking or twisting of one or more of the great blood vessels, which in turn seriously impairs blood flow to and from the heart.

Symptoms of mediastinal shift include severe dyspnea, cyanosis, displacement of the trachea to one side, and distended neck veins. The immediate treatment is insertion of a hollow needle or trochar into the pleural space (THORACENTESIS) to provide an outlet for the escape of air and fluid. After the trapped air is released, closed chest drainage is initiated to allow for reexpansion of the lung.

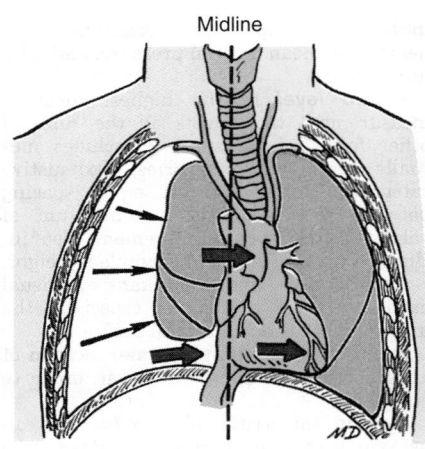

Midline

Mediastinal shift. As air from a pneumothorax is drawn into the chest cavity, it places pressure on the trachea, heart, and great vessels, causing them to shift from their normal anatomic positions. From Polaski and Tatro, 1996.

mediastinitis (me″de-as″ti-ni′tis) inflammation of the mediastinum.

fibrosing m., fibrous m. mediastinal fibrosis.

mediastinography (me″de-as″ti-nog′rah-fe) radiography of the structures of the mediastinum.

mediastinopericarditis (me″de-as″ti-no-per″i-kar-di′tis) inflammation of the mediastinum and pericardium.

mediastinoscope (me″de-ah-sti′no-skōp) a specially designed endoscope used in mediastinoscopy.

mediastinoscopy (me″de-as″ti-nos′kah-pe) examination of the mediastinum by means of an endoscope inserted through an anterior midline incision just above the thoracic inlet.

mediastinotomy (me″de-as″ti-not′ah-me) incision of the mediastinum.

mediastinum (me″de-ah-sti′num) [L.] 1. a median septum or partition. 2. the mass of tissues and organs separating the sternum in front and the vertebral column behind, containing the heart and its large vessels, trachea, esophagus, thymus, lymph nodes, and other structures and tissues. It is divided into anterior, middle, posterior, and superior regions.

m. tes′tis a partial septum of the testis formed near its posterior border by a continuation of the TUNICA ALBUGINEA.

mediation (me″de-a′shun) the act of intervening or serving as an intermediary.

conflict m. in the NURSING INTERVENTIONS CLASSIFICATION, a nursing INTERVENTION defined as facilitation of constructive dialogue between opposing parties with a goal of resolving disputes in a mutually acceptable manner.

medicable (med′ĭ-kah-b'l) subject to treatment with medicine with reasonable expectation of cure.

Medicaid (med′ĭ-kād) a state-operated program providing medical care to certain low-income persons; the state programs receive federal aid and are subject to federal guidelines.

medical (med′ĭ-kal) pertaining to medicine or to the treatment of diseases; pertaining to medicine as opposed to surgery.

m. assistant a person who, under the direction of a qualified physician, performs a variety of routine administrative and clinical tasks in a physician's office, a hospital, or some other clinical facility.

m. laboratory technician (MLT) see CLINICAL LABORATORY TECHNICIAN/MEDICAL LABORATORY TECHNICIAN.

m. record administrator one responsible for the indexing, recording, and storage of medical records and reports of patients admitted to hospitals and other health care agencies, and who also prepares reports of births, deaths, transfers, and discharges of patients, and of treatments received.

There are two levels of qualification for the medical record practitioner: Registered Record Administrator (RRA) and Accredited Record Technician (ART). Only those persons who have passed the registration examination of the AMERICAN HEALTH INFORMATION MANAGEMENT ASSOCIATION are entitled to use the professional designation of Registered Record Administrator or the job titles of medical record administrator and health record administrator. Only individuals who have passed the accreditation examination of the Association are entitled to use the designation of Accredited Record Technician. Suitable job titles for the RRA might include: Medical Record Administrator; Director, Medical Record Administration Program; Director, Medical Record Services; Instructor; Coordinator; and Research Associate. Suitable job titles for the ART might include: Medical Record Technician; Director; Assistant Director; Supervisor; and Instructor.

m. technologist (MT) CLINICAL LABORATORY SCIENTIST/MEDICAL TECHNOLOGIST.

MedicAlert (med″ik-ah-lert′) a necklace or bracelet identifying a medical problem of the wearer and a phone number to call in an emergency. It can be obtained for a small fee from the nonprofit MedicAlert

---

WINDOW ON MEDICAL TECHNOLOGIST

The need for laboratory professionals is acute and job openings abound, not only in hospital laboratories, but also in industry, research, public health, the military, and other settings. The generalist background that laboratory science (medical technology) provides is ideal for those who wish to work in traditional clinical laboratories, and also for those who want to move into other arenas. In a recent survey of over 2000 of our graduates, we found that they had assumed over 130 different positions—from forensic testing to infection control, to managing a clinic, to developing new laboratory products. One of five of our graduates has earned an advanced degree, the most common being the MD degree. The medical technologist, then, has excellent career possibilities, and opportunity and versatility mark the outlook for the laboratory professional—the medical technologist.

KAREN R. KARNI, PhD

M

Foundation International, P.O. Box 1009, Turlock, CA 95380.

Medicare (med′ĭ-kar) a program of the Social Security Administration which provides funding for medical care to the aged and to certain others.

medicated (med′ĭ-kāt″ed) imbued with a medicinal substance.

medication (med″ĭ-ka′shun) 1. administration of remedies. 2. medicine (def. 1). 3. impregnation with a medicine.

nonprescription m's NONPRESCRIPTION DRUGS.

over the counter m's see OVER THE COUNTER MEDICATIONS.

transdermal m. medication administered using a self-adhesive, premedicated patch applied to the skin. One side of the patch has an impermeable backing and the other side, which rests against the skin, has a membrane that is permeable to the drug.

medicinal (mě-dis′ĭ-nal) having healing qualities; pertaining to a medicine.

medicine (med′ĭ-sin) 1. any drug or remedy. 2. the art and science of the diagnosis and treatment of disease and the maintenance of health. 3. the nonsurgical treatment of disease.

alternative m. see complementary and alternative MEDICINE.

aviation m. the branch of medicine that deals with the physiologic, medical, psychologic, and epidemiologic problems involved in flying.

ayurvedic m. the traditional medicine of India, done according to Hindu scriptures and making use of plants and other healing materials native to India.

behavioral m. a type of psychosomatic medicine focused on psychological means of influencing physical symptoms, such as BIOFEEDBACK or relaxation.

clinical m. 1. the study of disease by direct examination of the living patient. 2. the last two years of the usual curriculum in a medical college.

complementary m., complementary and alternative m. (CAM) a large and diverse set of systems of diagnosis, treatment, and prevention based on philosophies and techniques other than those used in conventional Western medicine, often derived from traditions of medical practice used in other, non-Western cultures. Such practices may be described as *alternative,* that is, existing as a body separate from and as a replacement for conventional Western medicine, or *complementary,* that is, used in addition to conventional Western practice. CAM is characterized by its focus on the whole person as a unique individual, on the energy of the body and its influence on health and disease, on the healing power of nature and the mobilization of the body's own resources to heal itself, and on the treatment of the underlying causes, rather than symptoms, of disease. Many of the techniques used are the subject of controversy and have not been validated by controlled studies.

emergency m. the medical specialty that deals with the acutely ill or injured who require immediate medical treatment. See also EMERGENCY and emergency CARE.

experimental m. study of the science of healing diseases based on experimentation in animals.

family m. family practice.

forensic m. the application of medical knowledge to questions of law; see also medical JURISPRUDENCE. Called also legal medicine.

group m. the practice of medicine by a group of physicians, usually representing various specialties, who are associated together for the cooperative diagnosis, treatment, and prevention of disease.

internal m. the medical specialty that deals with diagnosis and medical treatment of diseases and disorders of internal structures of the body.

legal m. forensic medicine.

nuclear m. the branch of medicine concerned with the use of radionuclides in diagnosis and treatment of disease.

patent m. a drug or remedy protected by a trademark, available without a prescription.

physical m. physiatry.

preclinical m. the subjects studied in medicine before the student observes actual diseases in patients.

preventive m. the branch of medical study and practice aimed at preventing disease and promoting health.

proprietary m. any chemical, drug, or similar preparation used in the treatment of diseases, if such article is protected against free competition as to name, product, composition, or process of manufacture by secrecy, patent, trademark, or copyright, or by other means.

psychosomatic m. the study of the interrelations between bodily processes and emotional life.

socialized m. a system of medical care regulated and controlled by the government; called also state medicine.

space m. the branch of aviation MEDICINE concerned with conditions encountered by human beings in space.

sports m. the field of medicine concerned with injuries sustained in athletic endeavors, including their prevention, diagnosis, and treatment.

state m. socialized medicine.

travel m., travelers' m. the subspecialty of tropical MEDICINE consisting of the diagnosis and treatment or prevention of diseases of travelers.

tropical m. medical science as applied to diseases occurring primarily in the tropics and subtropics.

veterinary m. the diagnosis and treatment of diseases of animals other than humans.

medicolegal (med″ĭ-ko-le′g'l) pertaining to medicine and law, or to forensic medicine.

medicosocial (med″ĭ-ko-so′shal) having both medical and social aspects.

MEDICUS a patient classification system.

medionecrosis (me″de-o-nĕ-kro′sis) focal areas of destruction of the elastic tissue and smooth muscle of the TUNICA MEDIA of a blood vessel, especially of the aorta or its major branches.

mediotarsal (me″de-o-tahr′sal) pertaining to the center of the tarsus.

MedisGroups (med′is-grōōps″) [*Med*ical *I*llness *S*everity *Group*ing *S*ystem] a patient classification system based on key clinical findings from evidence in the patient record; it can be used as a tool for quality assurance.

Mediterranean disease (med″ĭ-tĕ-ra′ne-an) thalassemia major.

medium (me′de-um), pl. *mediums, me′dia* [L.] 1. an agent by which something is accomplished or an impulse is transmitted. 2. culture medium. 3. a preparation used in treating histologic specimens.

    contrast m. a radiopaque substance used in radiography to permit visualization of body structures. Called also contrast agent.

    culture m. a substance or preparation used to support the growth of microorganisms or other cells; called also medium.

    dioptric media refracting media.

    disperse m. dispersive m.

    dispersion m. dispersive m.

    dispersive m. the continuous phase of a colloid system; the medium in which the particles of the disperse phase are distributed, corresponding to the solvent in a true solution.

    refracting media the transparent tissues and fluid in the eye through which light rays pass and by which they are refracted and brought to a focus on the retina.

medius (me′de-us) [L.] middle.

MEDLARS (med′larz) acronym for *Medical Literature Analysis and Retrieval System*, a computerized bibliographic system of the NATIONAL LIBRARY OF MEDICINE, from which the INDEX MEDICUS is produced.

MEDLINE (med′līn) acronym for *MEDLARS on-line,* a computerized bibliographical retrieval system, an on-line segment of MEDLARS.

Medrol (med′rol) trademark for preparations of METHYLPREDNISOLONE, a steroid ANTIINFLAMMATORY agent.

medroxyprogesterone (med-rok″sĭ-pro-jes′tĕ-rōn) a progestational AGENT administered orally as the acetate ester for treatment of secondary amenorrhea and dysfunctional uterine bleeding, in the induction of menses, in the prevention and treatment of endometrial hyperplasia, in postmenopause hormone replacement THERAPY, and as a test for endogenous estrogen production; orally or intramuscularly as an antineoplastic in the treatment of metastatic endometrial, breast, and renal carcinoma, and intramuscularly as a long-acting contraceptive.

medrysone (med′rĭ-sōn″) a synthetic GLUCOCORTICOID used topically in treatment of allergic and inflammatory conditions of the eye.

medulla (mĕ-dul′ah) [L.] 1. the inmost part of a structure or organ. 2. medulla oblongata. 3. marrow. adj., **med′ullary.**

    adrenal m. the inner portion of the ADRENAL GLAND, where EPINEPHRINE and NOREPINEPHRINE are produced.

    m. of bone bone MARROW.

    m. oblonga′ta that part of the hindbrain continuous with the pons above and the spinal cord below; it houses nerve centers for both motor and sensory nerves, where such functions as breathing and the beating of the heart are controlled. See also BRAIN.

    m. os′sium bone MARROW.

    renal m. the inner part of the substance of the kidney, composed chiefly of collecting TUBULES, and organized into a group of structures called the renal PYRAMIDS.

    m. spina′lis, m. spina′lis SPINAL CORD.

    m. of thymus the central portion of each lobule of the thymus; it contains many more reticular cells and far fewer lymphocytes than does the surrounding cortex.

medullary (med′u-ler″e) 1. pertaining to a medulla. 2. myeloid (def. 1). 3. myeloid (def. 2).

medullated (med′u-lāt″ed) myelinated.

medullization (med″u-lĭ-za′shun) the enlargement of the haversian canals in rarefying osteitis followed by their conversion into marrow channels; also, the replacement of bone by marrow cells.

medulloadrenal (mĕ-dul″o-ah-dre′nal) adrenomedullary.

medulloblast (mĕ-dul′o-blast) an undifferentiated cell of the neural tube that may develop into either a neuroblast or a spongioblast.

medulloblastoma (mĕ-dul″o-blas-to′mah) a brain tumor composed of medulloblasts.

medulloepithelioma (mĕ-dul″o-ep″ĭ-the″le-o′mah) a brain tumor composed of primitive neuroepithelial cells lining the tubular spaces.

mefenamic acid (mĕ″fĕ-nam′ic) a NONSTEROIDAL ANTIINFLAMMATORY DRUG used to treat and prevent mild to moderate pain, inflammation, dysmenorrhea, and vascular headache.

mefloquine (mef′lo-kwin) an antimalarial AGENT effective against CHLOROQUINE-resistant strains of *Plasmodium falciparum* and *P. vivax;* used as the hydrochloride salt.

MEFR maximal expiratory flow rate.

MEG magnetoencephalography.

mega- (M) word element [Gr.], *large;* meaning large, enlarged, or of abnormally large size; also used in naming units of measurement (symbol M) to designate an amount one million (10^6) times the size of the unit to which it is joined.

M

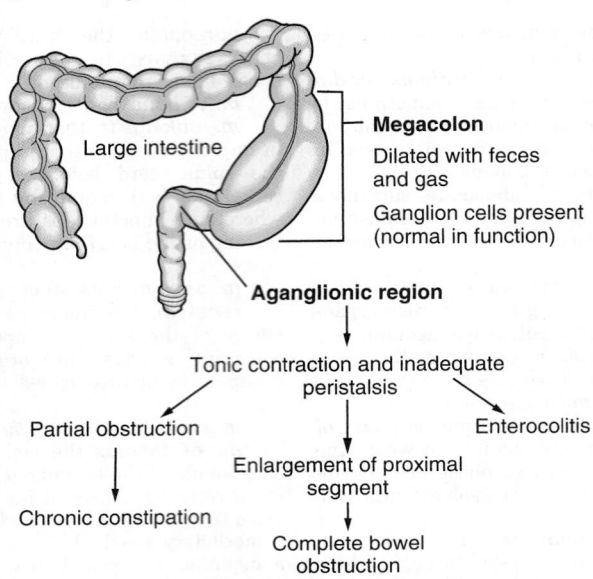

Megacolon. From McKinney et al., 2000

megabladder (meg″ah-blad′er) mega-cystis.

megacalicosis (meg″ah-kal″ĭ-ko′sis) nonobstructive dilatation of the renal calices due to malformation of the renal papillae. Spelled also *megacalycosis*.

megacaryocyte (meg″ah-kar′e-o-sīt″) megakaryocyte.

Megace (mĕ-gās′) trademark for a preparation of MEGESTROL acetate, a steroid used as a palliative antineoplastic AGENT and in treatment of anorexia and cachexia.

megacolon (meg″ah-ko′lon) dilatation and hypertrophy of the colon.

  acquired m. colonic enlargement associated with chronic constipation, but with normal ganglion cell innervation.

  acute m. toxic megacolon.

  aganglionic m., congenital m. Hirschsprung's disease.

  toxic m. acute dilatation of the colon associated with AMEBIC DYSENTERY or ULCERATIVE COLITIS; called also acute megacolon.

megacystis an abnormally enlarged urinary BLADDER; called also megabladder and megalocystis.

megacystis-megaureter   syndrome (meg″ah-sis′tis meg″ah-u-re′ter) chronic ureteral dilatation associated with hypotonia and dilatation of the bladder *(megacystis)* and gaping of the ureteral orifices *(megaureter),* permitting vesicoureteric REFLUX of urine, and resulting in chronic PYELONEPHRITIS.

megaesophagus (meg″ah-e-sof′ah-gus) dilatation and muscular hypertrophy of most of the ESOPHAGUS, above a constricted, often atrophied, distal segment. See also ACHALASIA.

megahertz (MHz) (meg′ah-hertz) one million (10^6) HERTZ.

megakaryoblast (meg″ah-kar′e-o-blast″) the earliest cytologically identifiable precursor in the thrombocytic series, which matures to form the promegakaryocyte.

megakaryocyte (meg″ah-kar′e-o-sīt″) the giant cell of bone marrow; it is a large cell with a greatly lobulated nucleus, and is generally supposed to give rise to blood platelets.

megakaryocytopoiesis (meg″ah-kar″e-o-si″to-poi-e′sis) the production of megakaryocytes.

megakaryocytosis (meg″ah-kar″e-o-si-to′-sis) the presence of megakaryocytes in the blood or of excessive numbers in the bone marrow, as in POLYCYTHEMIA vera.

megal(o)- word element [Gr.], *large; abnormal enlargement.*

megalencephaly (meg″ah-len-sef′ah-le) macrencephalia; hypertrophy of the brain.

megalgia (meg-al′jah) a severe pain.

megaloblast (meg′ah-lo-blast″) a large, nucleated immature progenitor of an abnormal erythrocytic SERIES, an abnormal counterpart to the NORMOBLAST; megaloblasts are present in the blood in certain ANEMIAS. adj., **megaloblas′tic.**

megalocardia (meg″ah-lo-kahr′de-ah) cardiomegaly.

megalocephaly (meg″ah-lo-sef′ah-le) abnormally increased size of the head; called also macrocephaly. adj., **megalocephal′ic.**

megalocheiria (meg″ah-lo-ki′re-ah) abnormal largeness of the hands.

megalocornea (meg″ah-lo-kor′ne-ah) a developmental anomaly of the cornea, which is of abnormal size at birth and continues to grow, sometimes reaching a diameter of 14 or 15 mm in the adult.

megalocystis (meg″ah-lo-sis′tis) megacystis.

megalocyte (meg′ah-lo-sīt″) macrocyte.

megalodactyly (meg″ah-lo-dak′tĭ-le) excessive size of the fingers or toes; called also macrodactyly.

megaloesophagus (meg″ah-lo-e-sof′ah-gus) megaesophagus.

megalogastria (meg″ah-lo-gas′tre-ah) gastromegaly.

megaloglossia (meg″ah-lo-glos′e-ah) macroglossia.

megalohepatia (meg″ah-lo-hĕ-pat′e-ah) hepatomegaly.

megalomania (meg″ah-lo-ma′ne-ah) a mental state characterized by delusions of exaggerated personal importance, wealth, power, or goodness. adj., **megaloma′niac.**

megalomelia (meg″ah-lo-me′le-ah) abnormal largeness of the limbs; called also macromelia.

megalonychia (meg″ah-lo-ni′-ke-ah) hypertrophy of the nails and their matrices; called also macronychia.

megalopenis (meg″ah-lo-pe′nis) macropenis.

megalophthalmos (meg″ah-lof-thal′mos) macrophthalmia.

megalopodia (meg″ah-lo-po′de-ah) abnormal largeness of the feet; called also macropodia.

megalopsia (meg″ah-lop′se-ah) macropsia.

megalosplenia (meg″ah-lo-sple′ne-ah) splenomegaly.

megalosyndactyly (meg″ah-lo-sin-dak′tĭ-le) a condition in which the digits are large and more or less webbed or fused together; see also SYNDACTYLY.

megaloureter (meg″ah-lo-u-re′ter) megaureter.

-megaly word element [Gr.], *enlargement.*

megarectum (meg″ah-rek′tum) a greatly dilated rectum.

megaureter congenital dilatation of the URETER; it may be either a primary condition or secondary to something else. Called also megaloureter.

megavitamin (meg″ah-vi′tah-min) a term denoting massive doses of vitamins far exceeding the recommended daily allowances.

megavolt (MV) (meg′ah-volt) one million (10^6) VOLTS.

megavoltage (meg′ah-vōl″taj) in RADIATION THERAPY, voltage greater than 1 megavolt, as contrasted to ORTHOVOLTAGE and SUPERVOLTAGE.

megestrol (mě-jes′trōl) a synthetic progestational AGENT administered orally as an antineoplastic AGENT for palliative treatment of recurrent, inoperable, or metastatic carcinoma of the breast or endometrium and for the treatment of anorexia, cachexia, and weight loss in patients with cancer or ACQUIRED IMMUNODEFICIENCY SYNDROME.

meglumine (meg′loo-mēn) a crystalline base used in preparing salts of certain acids for use as diagnostic radiopaque media. Meglumine diatrizoate is used in angiocardiography and excretory urography; meglumine iodipamide is used in cholecystography; and meglumine iothalamate is used in cerebral angiography, excretory urography, and peripheral arteriography. Called also methylglucamine.

megohm (megōm) one million (10^6) OHMS.

megophthalmos (meg″of-thal′mos) hydrophthalmos.

meiogenic (mi″o-jen′ik) promoting meiosis.

meiosis (mi-o′sis) the process of cell division by which reproductive cells (gametes) are formed. There are two successive divisions, meiosis I and meiosis II, in which four daughter cells that have the haploid chromosome number (23 in humans) are formed. As in MITOSIS (somatic cell division), meiosis I and II are each divided into four phases: *prophase, metaphase, anaphase,* and *telophase.* adj., **meiot′ic.** The first meiotic prophase is a complex process separated into five stages. During *leptotene* the chromosomes coil and contract; each consists of two chromatids joined along their length. During *zygotene* pairs of homologous chromosomes come into point-to-point contact along their length. This process is called *synapsis* and the structure formed is called a *bivalent.* The X and Y chromosomes synapse only at the ends of the short arms. During *pachytene* the chromosomes thicken, and the chromatids of each chromosome separate except at the centromeres. The bivalent is now a tetrad of four chromatids. During this stage crossing over occurs, in which the chromatids of homologous chromosomes break and rejoin, resulting in chromatids that contain sections derived

M

from both the mother and the father. During *diplotene* the two chromosomes of each bivalent separate except for X-shaped chiasmata where crossover has occurred. In the female, this stage (called *dictyotene*) is prolonged; the oocyte remains in this stage from late fetal life until the time of ovulation. In the last stage, *diakinesis,* the chiasmata move to the ends of the chromosomes.

The other phases of meiosis I and II resemble those of mitosis, except that in meiosis I the two chromosomes of each bivalent separate and move to opposite poles. Thus, each daughter cell receives the haploid number of chromosomes, each with two chromatids. The assortment is random; either the maternal or the paternal chromosome can go to a daughter cell. Meiosis II then follows immediately without DNA replication. Both daughter cells formed by meiosis I divide again and the two chromatids of each chromosome separate and go to separate daughter cells. This produces four haploid daughter cells with chromosomes composed of single chromatids.

melalgia (mel-al′jah) pain in the limbs.

melan(o)- word element [Gr.], *black; melanin.*

melancholia (mel″an-ko′le-ah) DEPRESSION; currently used particularly to describe severe cases of MAJOR DEPRESSIVE DISORDER. adj., **melanchol′ic.**

melaniferous (mel″ah-nif′er-us) containing melanin or other black pigment.

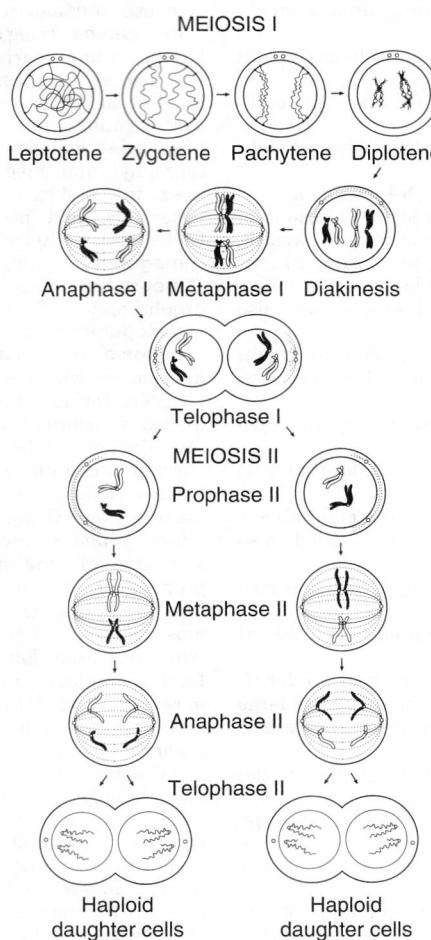

Meiosis (only two of the 23 human chromosome pairs are shown, the chromosomes from one parent in black, those from the other parent in outline). From Dorland's, 2000.

melanin (mel′ah-nin) any of several closely related dark, sulfur-containing pigments normally found in the hair, skin, ciliary body, choroid of the eye, pigment layer of the retina, and certain nerve cells. They occur abnormally in the tumors known as MELANOMAS and may be excreted in the urine when such tumors are present (MELANURIA).

melanism (mel′ah-nizm) melanosis.

melanoameloblastoma (mel″ah-no-ah-mel″o-blas-to′mah) melanotic neuroectodermal tumor.

melanoblast (mel′ah-no-blast″) a cell that develops into a melanocyte.

melanoblastoma mel″ah-no-blas-to′mah) malignant melanoma.

melanocarcinoma (mel″ah-no-kahr″sī-no′mah) malignant melanoma.

melanocyte (mel′ah-no-sīt″, mĕ-lan′o-sīt) any of the dendritic clear cells of the epidermis that synthesize tyrosinase and, within their melanosomes, the pigment melanin; the melanosomes are then transferred from melanocytes to keratinocytes. adj., **melanocyt′ic.**

melanoderma (mel″ah-no-der′mah) an abnormally increased amount of melanin in the skin due either to an increase in production of melanin by the melanocytes normally present or to an increase in the number of melanocytes, with production of hyperpigmented patches.

melanodermatitis (mel″ah-no-der″mah-ti′tis) dermatitis with a deposit of melanin in the skin.

melanogen (mĕ-lan′o-jen) a colorless chromogen, convertible into melanin, which may occur in the urine in certain diseases.

melanogenesis (mel″ah-no-jen′ĕ-sis) the production of melanin.

melanoglossia (mel″ah-no-glos′e-ah) black tongue.

melanoid (mel′ah-noid) 1. resembling MELANIN. 2. a substance resembling melanin.

melanoleukoderma (mel″ah-no-loo″ko-der′mah) a mottled appearance of the skin.

m. col′li a mottled appearance of the skin of the neck and adjacent regions, a rare manifestation of syphilis.

melanoma (mel″ah-no′mah) a tumor arising from the melanocytic system of the skin and other organs. When used alone, the term refers to malignant melanoma.

acral-lentiginous m. an uncommon type of melanoma, although it is the most common type seen in nonwhite individuals, occurring chiefly on the palms and soles, and sometimes involving mucosal surfaces, such as the vulva or vagina. The characteristic lesion is an irregular, enlarging black macule, which has a prolonged noninvasive stage.

juvenile m. spindle and epithelioid cell nevus.

lenti′go malig′na m. a cutaneous malignant melanoma found most often on the sun-exposed areas of the skin, especially the face. It begins as a circumscribed macular patch of mottled pigmentation, showing shades of dark brown, tan, or black (*lentigo maligna* or *melanotic freckle of Hutchinson*), and enlarges by lateral growth before dermal invasion occurs. This type seems to be the least aggressive form of malignant melanoma.

malignant m. a malignant skin tumor, usually developing from a NEVUS and consisting of dark masses of cells with a marked tendency to metastasis. It is not common, but its incidence is increasing and it is the most aggressive type of skin cancer. It arises from pigment- (MELANIN-) producing cells and varies in course and prognosis according to type; types include superficial spreading melanoma, nodular malignant melanoma, and lentigo maligna melanoma. In general, the superficial lesions can be cured by surgical excision of the mole and adjacent tissues. Deeper lesions tend to metastasize rapidly through the lymphatic and circulatory systems. In some cases the condition has a genetic component. Early detection and skin protection are key in its control.

melanomatosis (mel″ah-no″mah-to′sis) the formation of MELANOMAS throughout the body.

melanonychia (mel″ah-no-nik′e-ah) blackening of the nails by melanin pigmentation.

melanophage (mel′ah-no-fāj″) a histiocyte laden with phagocytosed melanin.

melanoplakia (mel″ah-no-pla′ke-ah) pigmented patches on the mucous membrane of the mouth.

melanosis (mel″ah-no′sis) 1. disordered MELANIN production, with darkening of the skin; called also melanism. 2. a disorder of pigment metabolism.

m. co′li brown-black discoloration of the mucosa of the colon.

m. i′ridis, m. of the iris abnormal pigmentation of the iris by infiltration of melanoblasts.

melanosome (mel′ah-no-sōm″) any of the granules that contain melanin. The melanin is synthesized within melanocytes; then the melanosomes are transferred to keratinocytes.

melanotic (mel″ah-not′ik) characterized by the presence of melanin; pertaining to melanosis.

M

melanotrichia (mel″ah-no-trik′e-ah) abnormally increased pigmentation of the hair.

melanuria (mel″ah-nu′re-ah) the discharge of darkly stained urine.

melarsoprol (mel-ahr′so-prol) an antiprotozoal AGENT effective against TRYPANOSOMES.

melasma (mĕ-laz′mah) MELANOSIS with sharply demarcated blotchy, brown macules usually in a symmetric distribution over the cheeks and forehead and sometimes on the upper lip and neck. It is most often seen in women during pregnancy (*melasma gravidarum* or "mask of pregnancy"), at menopause, and while taking oral contraceptives; it occasionally occurs in women who are not pregnant or taking oral contraceptives, as well as in men. A similar pattern of facial hyperpigmentation may be associated with chronic liver disease. Called also chloasma.

  m. **addiso′nii** Addison's disease.

  m. **gravida′rum** melasma occurring during pregnancy.

MELAS syndrome *m*itochondrial *e*ncephalopathy, *l*actic *a*cidosis, and *s*troke-like episodes; a familial type of mitochondrial encephalopathy, of maternal (mitochondrial) inheritance.

melatonin (mel″ah-to′nin) an indoleamine hormone synthesized and released by the pineal body during the hours of darkness; it may have a role in the control of the regulation of gonadotropin release.

melena (mĕ-le′nah) darkening of the feces by blood pigments.

melioidosis (mel″e-oi-do′sis) a glanders-like disease of rodents, caused by *Pseudomonas pseudomallei* and occasionally transmitted to humans; it is most commonly seen in China and Southeast Asia. Two forms are noted in humans: the *acute form* is characterized by pulmonary, liver, and spleen involvement with septicemia; and the *chronic form* leads to osteomyelitis and formation of abscesses and fistulas.

melituria (mel″ĭ-tu′re-ah) sugar in the urine; specific types are named for the sugar in question, such as FRUCTOSURIA, GALACTOSURIA, GLYCOSURIA, and LACTOSURIA.

Mellaril (mel′ah-ril) trademark for preparations of THIORIDAZINE, an ANTIPSYCHOTIC AGENT and sedative.

melomelus (mĕ-lom′ĕ-lus) a fetus with supernumerary limbs.

meloplasty (mel′o-plas″te) plastic surgery of the cheek.

melorheostosis (mel″o-re″os-to′sis) a form of osteosclerosis, with linear tracks extending through the long bones.

melotia (mĕ-lo′she-ah) congenital displacement of the auricle of the ear onto the cheek.

meloxicam (mĕ-lok′sĭ-kam) a NONSTEROIDAL ANTIINFLAMMATORY DRUG used in the treatment of OSTEOARTHRITIS; administered orally.

melphalan (mel′fah-lan) a cytotoxic ALKYLATING AGENT derived from NITROGEN MUSTARD, used as an antineoplastic AGENT, primarily for treatment of MULTIPLE MYELOMA; administered orally or intravenously.

member (mem′ber) 1. a distinct part of the body. 2. limb.

membra (mem′bra) [L.] plural of MEMBRUM.

membrana (mem-bra′nah) [L.] membrane.

membrane (mem′brān) a thin layer of tissue that covers a surface, lines a cavity, or divides a space or organ. adj., **membranous.**

  alveolar-capillary m., alveolocapillary m. a thin tissue barrier through which gases are exchanged between the alveolar air and the blood in the pulmonary capillaries. Called also blood-air barrier and blood-gas barrier.

  alveolodental m. periodontium.

  arachnoid m. arachnoid.

  basement m. a sheet of amorphous extracellular material upon which the basal surfaces of epithelial cells rest; it is also associated with muscle cells, Schwann cells, fat cells, and capillaries, interposed between the cellular elements and the underlying connective tissue. It comprises two layers, the basal LAMINA and the reticular LAMINA and is composed of Type IV collagen (which is unique to basement membranes), laminin, fibronectin, and heparan sulfate proteoglycans.

  basilar m. the lower boundary of the scala media of the ear.

  Bowman's m. a thin layer of basement membrane between the outer layer of stratified epithelium and the substantia propria of the cornea.

  Bruch's m. the inner layer of the choroid, separating it from the pigmented layer of the retina.

  cell m. plasma membrane.

  decidual m's, deciduous m's decidua.

  Descemet's m. the posterior lining membrane of the cornea; it is a thin hyaline membrane between the substantia propria and the endothelial layer of the cornea.

  diphtheritic m. the peculiar false membrane characteristic of diphtheria, formed by coagulation necrosis.

  drum m. TYMPANIC MEMBRANE.

  epiretinal m. a pathologic membrane partially covering the surface of the retina probably originating chiefly from the retinal pigment epithelial and glial cells; membranes peripheral to the macula are generally asymptomatic, while those involving the macula or adjacent to it may cause reduction in vision, visual distortion, and diplopia.

extraembryonic m's those that protect the embryo or fetus and provide for its nutrition, respiration, and excretion; the yolk sac (umbilical vesicle), allantois, amnion, chorion, decidua, and placenta. Called also fetal membranes.

false m. a membranous exudate, such as the diphtheritic membrane; called also neomembrane.

fenestrated m. one of the perforated elastic sheets of the tunica intima and tunica media of arteries.

fetal m's extraembryonic membranes.

hemodialyzer m. the semipermeable membrane that filters the blood in a HEMODIALYZER, commonly made of cuprophane, cellulose acetate, polyacrylonitrile, polymethyl methacrylate, or polysulfone.

Henle's m. fenestrated membrane.

high efficiency m. a hemodialyzer membrane that has clearance characteristics that increase progressively with increases in dialysis blood flow rates; this usually implies that the membrane is not a high flux membrane.

high flux m. a hemodialyzer membrane that has a high permeability to fluids and solutes and thus a high rate of clearance of fluids and solutes composed of large molecules.

hyaline m. 1. a membrane between the outer root sheath and inner fibrous layer of a hair follicle. 2. basement membrane. 3. a homogeneous eosinophilic membrane lining alveolar ducts and alveoli, frequently found at autopsy of infants that were preterm. See also HYALINE MEMBRANE DISEASE.

hyoglossal m. a fibrous lamina connecting the undersurface of the tongue with the hyoid bone.

impaired oral mucous m. a NURSING DIAGNOSIS approved by the North American Nursing Diagnosis Association, defined as disruptions of the lips and soft tissue of the oral cavity. Changes in the integrity and health of the oral mucous MEMBRANE can occur as a characteristic of such medical disorders as periodontal disease, uncontrolled diabetes mellitus, oral cancer, and infection with herpes. Chemical irritants such as alcohol and tobacco can also adversely affect the oral mucous membrane, as can mechanical trauma due to broken teeth, poorly fitting dentures, and endotracheal intubation. Other etiologic factors include dehydration, mouth breathing, poor

oral hygiene, radiation to the head or neck, and antineoplastic AGENTS.

Preventive measures that can help maintain the health and integrity of the oral mucosa will depend on the cause. Routinely brushing and flossing the teeth during the day and at bedtime can help avoid dental caries and periodontal disease. Some patients may need instruction in the proper procedure for cleaning the teeth and removing debris and plaque, or they may need assistance in devising ways to cope with physical disabilities that make good oral hygiene difficult for them. Patients who are unconscious or unable to perform self-care activities should have MOUTH CARE as often as needed to keep the mouth clean and moist and avoid aspiration of debris and infectious microorganisms. Adequate hydration and a lip lubricant can help avoid alterations in the oral mucosa and promote comfort.

limiting m. one that constitutes the border of some tissue or structure.

mucous m. the membrane covered with epithelium that lines the tubular organs of the body.

Nasmyth's m. primary cuticle.

nuclear m. 1. either of the membranes, inner and outer, comprising the nuclear envelope. 2. nuclear envelope.

olfactory m. the olfactory portion of the mucous membrane lining the nasal fossa.

placental m. the membrane that separates the fetal from the maternal blood in the placenta.

plasma m. the membrane that encloses a cell; it is composed of phospholipids, glycolipids, cholesterol, and proteins. The primary structure is a lipid bilayer. Phospholipid molecules have an electrically charged "head" that attracts water and a hydrocarbon "tail" that repels water; they line up side by side in two opposing layers with their heads on the inner or outer surface of the membrane and their tails in the core, from which water is excluded. The other lipids affect the structural properties of the membrane. Proteins embedded in the membrane transport specific molecules across the membrane, act as hormone receptors, or perform other functions.

Reissner's m. the thin anterior wall of the cochlear duct, separating it from the scala vestibuli.

m. of round window secondary tympanic membrane.

Scarpa's m. tympanic membrane, secondary.

M

semipermeable m. one permitting passage through it of some but not all substances.

serous m. the membrane lining the walls of the body cavities and enclosing the contained organs; it consists of mesothelium lying upon a connective tissue layer and it secretes a watery fluid.

synovial m. the inner of the two layers of the articular capsule of a synovial joint; composed of loose connective tissue and having a free smooth surface that lines the joint cavity.

tympanic m. see TYMPANIC MEMBRANE.

tympanic m., secondary the membrane enclosing the round WINDOW; called also Scarpa's membrane.

unit m. the trilaminar structure of all cellular membranes (such as the plasma membrane, nuclear membranes, mitochondrial membranes, endoplasmic reticulum, lysosomes) as they appear in electron micrographs. The biochemical structure is a lipid bilayer.

virginal m. hymen.

vitelline m. the external envelope of an OVUM.

vitreous m. 1. Descemet's membrane. 2. hyaline membrane (def. 1). 3. Bruch's membrane. 4. a delicate boundary layer investing the vitreous body.

membraniform (mem-bran′ĭ-form) resembling a membrane.

membranocartilaginous (mem″brah-no-kahr″tĭ-laj′ĭ-nus) 1. developed in both membrane and cartilage. 2. partly cartilaginous and partly membranous.

membranoid (mem′brah-noid) resembling a membrane.

membrum (mem′brum) [L.] 1. member. 2. limb.

memory (mem′o-re) the mental faculty that enables one to retain and recall previously experienced sensations, impressions, information, and ideas. The ability of the BRAIN to retain and to use knowledge gained from past experience is essential to the process of learning. Although the exact way in which the brain remembers is not completely understood, it is believed that a portion of the temporal lobe of the brain, lying in part under the temples, acts as a kind of memory center, drawing on memories stored in other parts of the brain.

impaired m. a NURSING DIAGNOSIS accepted by the North American Nursing Diagnosis Association, defined as inability to remember bits of information or behavioral skills.

immunologic m. the capacity of the IMMUNE SYSTEM to respond more rapidly and strongly to a subsequent antigenic CHALLENGE than to the first exposure. See also memory CELLS and IMMUNE RESPONSE.

long-term m. the aspect of memory in which knowledge is stored permanently, to be activated when cued; it is theoretically unlimited in capacity.

recent m. the ability to recall events from the immediate past.

remote m. the ability to recall events from the distant past.

screen m. a consciously tolerable memory serving to conceal or "screen" another memory that might be disturbing or emotionally painful if recalled.

short-term m. what one is conscious of at a given moment; in contrast to long-term memory it is of limited capacity (about seven items) and will be lost unless rehearsed and related to information in long-term memory.

menacme (mĕ-nak′me) the period of a woman's life during which there is MENSTRUATION.

menadiol (men″ah-di′ol) a VITAMIN K analogue; its sodium diphosphate salt is used as a prothrombinogenic vitamin, administered orally, intramuscularly, or subcutaneously.

menadione (men″ah-di′ōn) vitamin K_3. 1. a synthetic fat-soluble vitamin that can be converted in the body to active vitamin K; administered orally or intramuscularly. See VITAMIN. 2. the basic double ring quinone structure that is the parent structure of the related compounds with vitamin K activity, which can be formed by addition of long side chain substituents.

menaquinone (men″ah-kwin′ōn) any of a series of compounds having vitamin K activity, in which the phytyl side chain of phytonadione (vitamin K_1) is replaced by a side chain of prenyl units.

menarche (mĕ-nahr′ke) establishment or beginning of the menstrual function. adj., **menar′cheal.**

Mendel's laws (men′delz) in the inheritance of certain traits or characters, offspring are not intermediate in type between the parents, but inherit from one or the other parent in this respect. Thus, if a plant with the factor tallness (TT) is mated with one with the factor shortness (SS), then the offspring will inherit these factors in the ratio TT, 2Ts, SS. This law is usually expressed as the law of independent assortment and the law of segregation.

mendelevium (Md) (men″dĕ-le′ve-um) a chemical element, atomic number 101, atomic weight 256. (See Appendix 6.)

Ménétrier's disease (men″ĕ-tre-ārz′) excessive proliferation of the gastric mucosa, producing diffuse thickening of the wall; inflammatory changes may be associated. Called also giant hypertrophic gastritis.

Meniere's disease (mĕ-nyārz′) a disorder of the LABYRINTH of the inner ear, believed to result from dilation of the lymphatic channels in the cochlea. Called also labyrinthine vertigo; sometimes spelled Menière's or Ménière's. In about 90 per cent of cases only one ear is affected. The usual symptoms are TINNITUS, heightened sensitivity to loud sounds, progressive HEARING LOSS, HEADACHE, and VERTIGO. In the acute stage there may be severe nausea with vomiting, profuse sweating, disabling dizziness, and nystagmus. Some attacks last only minutes, and others continue for hours; they may occur frequently or only several weeks apart.

The disease usually lasts a few years, with progressive loss of hearing in the affected ear; sometimes the symptoms stop before all hearing is lost. If loss of hearing in the affected ear does become complete, nausea symptoms are likely to disappear. Ménière's disease sometimes develops after an injury to the head or infection of the middle ear, but most cases have no apparent cause. It is most common among men between the ages of 40 and 60.

A low salt diet, elimination or restriction of fluids, and vasodilating drugs are used to treat it. Sedatives are usually ordered to promote sleep and rest. If the ringing sensation becomes too disturbing to the patient, it may be masked (for example, by music piped in through earphones) to make sleeping easier. Surgical treatment involves relief from accumulation of inner ear fluid in the endolymphatic sac. Procedures may be directed toward relief of pressure by the bony structures surrounding the sac, or toward opening the sac and diverting the flow of endolymph by means of a shunt to the mastoid bone or to the subarachnoid space.

mening(o)- word element [Gr.], *meninges; membrane.*

meningeal (mĕ-nin′je-al) pertaining to the meninges.

meningeorrhaphy (mĕ-nin″je-or′ah-fe) suture of membranes, especially the meninges.

meninges (mĕ-nin′jēz) [Gr.] plural of MENINX; the three membranes covering the brain and spinal cord: the DURA MATER, ARACHNOID, and PIA MATER. adj., **menin′geal.**

meningioma (mĕ-nin″je-o′mah) a hard, usually vascular tumor occurring mainly along the meningeal vessels and superior

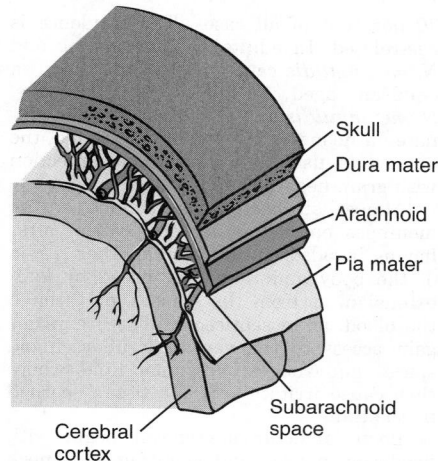

Skull
Dura mater
Arachnoid
Pia mater
Subarachnoid space
Cerebral cortex

Meninges of the central nervous system. From Applegate, 2000.

longitudinal sinus, invading the dura and skull and leading to erosion and thinning of the skull.

angioblastic m. angioblastoma (def. 2).

meningism (men′in-jizm) the symptoms and signs of meningitis associated with acute febrile illness or dehydration but without actual inflammation of the meninges.

meningitis (men″in-ji′tis), pl. *meningi′-tides* inflammation of the MENINGES, usually by either a bacterium *(bacterial m.)* or a virus *(viral m.).* When it affects the dura mater it is termed PACHYMENINGITIS; when the arachnoid and pia mater are involved, it is called LEPTOMENINGITIS. The term *meningitis* does not refer to a specific disease entity but rather to the pathologic condition of inflammation of the tissues of the meninges. The etiologic agent can be anything that activates an inflammatory RESPONSE, including both pathogenic and nonpathogenic organisms, such as bacteria, viruses, and fungi; chemical toxins such as lead and arsenic; contrast media used in myelography; and metastatic malignant cells. Enteroviruses are the most common causes of aseptic meningitis.

Bacterial Meningitis. This form occurs when pathogenic bacteria enter the subarachnoid space and cause a pyogenic inflammatory response. The most common causes are *Streptococcus pneumoniae* (pneumococcus), *Neisseria meningitidis* (meningococcus), and *Haemophilus influenzae,* which are responsible for approximately

70 per cent of all cases. The incidence is age-related. In adults, *S. pneumoniae* and *N. meningitidis* cause most of the cases; in children aged 1 month to 15 years, *N. meningitidis* and *H. influenzae* predominate; in neonates less than 1 month old, the disease is usually a nosocomial infection with gram-negative enteric bacilli.

Almost all bacterial infections of the meninges enter the nervous system after having invaded and infected another region of the body and then are spread by local extension, as from the sinuses, or through the blood, as in septicemia. The organisms gain access to the ventriculosubarachnoid spaces and the cerebrospinal fluid where they cause irritation of the tissues bathed by the fluid.

Bacterial meningitis typically begins with headache, nausea and vomiting, stiff neck (nuchal rigidity), and chills and fever. Irritability and confusion occur early in the course of the disease, and convulsive seizures occur in about 25 per cent of patients. As the disease progresses the patient becomes less rational, has decreasing levels of consciousness, and lapses into coma. Inability to straighten the knee when the hip is flexed (a positive KERNIG'S SIGN) and involuntary flexing of the hip and knee when the neck is flexed forward (a positive BRUDZINSKI'S SIGN) are indicative of meningeal irritation.

A diagnosis of bacterial meningitis is verified by isolation of the organism from a specimen of cerebrospinal fluid obtained by lumbar puncture. Treatment with the appropriate antibacterial agent is begun at once to reduce the numbers of proliferating bacteria attacking the central nervous system. Supportive measures include rest, maintenance of fluid and electrolyte balance, and prevention or control of convulsions with anticonvulsant drugs.

The prognosis is generally good, especially for meningococcal meningitis in which residual neurologic deficits and persistent convulsive seizures are rare. Pneumococcal meningitis and meningitis due to *Haemophilus influenzae* are more likely to be complicated by these sequelae as well as by septic shock and hydrocephalus.

Benign Viral Meningitis. This term encompasses a group of disorders in which there is some meningeal irritation but no pyogenic organism can be found in the cerebrospinal fluid. It is, therefore, called also *aseptic meningitis complex,* which is somewhat misleading because the meningeal irritation often follows infection with the mumps virus or with one of the picornaviruses.

The patient with this disorder typically complains of headache and signs characteristic of meningeal irritation, intolerance to light, and pain when the eyes are moved from side to side. Most of the symptoms are mild, and treatment is largely supportive and symptomatic; the disease is self-limiting.

Patient Care. Assessment of the patient with meningitis includes monitoring vital signs, neurologic status, and fluid and electrolyte status. The plan of care should include provisions for rest and relief from discomfort, a quiet and nonstimulating environment, protection from injury during convulsions, control of elevated body temperature, and isolation precautions as indicated by the specific causative organism. In general, enteric precautions are indicated for patients with aseptic meningitis caused by an enterovirus. Fungal and meningococcal meningitis require respiratory precautions. Antibiotics must be given precisely as ordered so as to avoid further damage to the central nervous system. Early signs of increased INTRACRANIAL PRESSURE from brain edema are reported promptly so that measures to reduce pressure can be taken as soon as possible. During the acute phase and convalescence the patient is watched for signs of complications such as septic shock, vascular collapse, and hydrocephalus. Nutritional status must be maintained throughout the course of illness to reinforce the patient's natural resources for combating infection and recovering from its deleterious effects.

aseptic m. any of several mild types of meningitis, most of which are caused by viruses; see viral MENINGITIS.

bacterial m. meningitis caused by bacteria; common pathogens are *Haemophilus influenzae, Neisseria meningitidis, Streptococcus pneumoniae,* and *Mycobacterium tuberculosis.* Some types may be serious, acute, or even fulminating. See also viral MENINGITIS.

cerebrospinal m. an inflammation of the brain and spinal cord; it may be caused by any of numerous different organisms.

epidemic cerebrospinal m. an acute infectious disease with seropurulent inflammation of the membranes of the brain and spinal cord, due to infection by *Neisseria meningitidis* (meningococcus). It usually occurs in epidemics, and symptoms are those of acute cerebral and spinal meningitis. There is also usually an eruption of erythematous, herpetic, or hemorrhagic spots on the skin. The fulminating or malignant form is known as Waterhouse-Friderichsen syndrome.

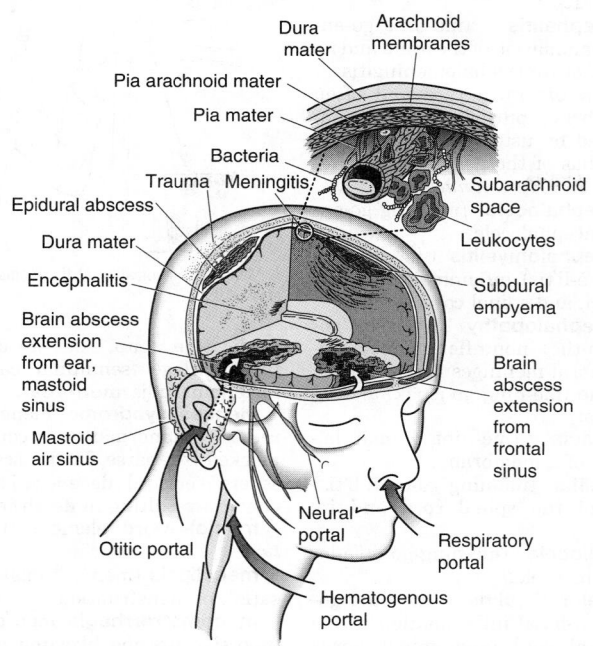

Dura mater
Arachnoid membranes
Pia arachnoid mater
Pia mater
Bacteria
Trauma Meningitis
Epidural abscess
Dura mater
Encephalitis
Brain abscess extension from ear, mastoid sinus
Mastoid air sinus
Otitic portal
Neural portal
Hematogenous portal
Subarachnoid space
Leukocytes
Subdural empyema
Brain abscess extension from frontal sinus
Respiratory portal

Portals of entry resulting in meningitis, meningoencephalitis, and intracranial mass lesions. From Mahon and Manuselis, 2000.

spinal m. inflammation of the meninges of the spinal cord.

viral m. meningitis due to any of various viruses, such as a COXSACKIEVIRUS or the mumps VIRUS, with lymphocytes in the cerebrospinal fluid. It usually has a short uncomplicated course characterized by malaise, fever, headache, stiffness of neck and back, and nausea. See also aseptic MENINGITIS.

meningocele (mĕ-ning′go-sēl) hernial protrusion of meninges through a defect in the bony spine. See also NEURAL TUBE DEFECT.

meningocerebritis (mĕ-ning″go-ser″ĕ-bri′tis) inflammation of the brain and meninges.

meningococcemia (mĕ-ning″go-kok-se′me-ah) the presence of meningococci in the blood, producing an acute fulminating disease or an insidious disorder persisting for months or years.

acute fulminating m. Waterhouse-Friderichsen syndrome.

meningococcus (mĕ-ning″go-kok′us) a microorganism of the species *Neisseria meningitidis,* the cause of some types of meningitis. adj., **meningococ′cal.**

meningocortical (mĕ-ning″go-kor′tĭ-k′l) pertaining to the meninges and cortex of the brain.

meningocyte (mĕ-ning′go-sīt) a histiocyte of the meninges.

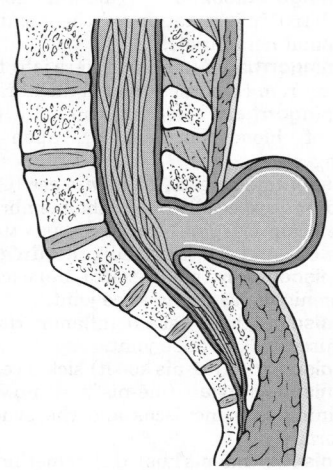

Meningocele: External protruding sac contains meninges and cerebrospinal fluid. From Frazier et al., 2000.

meningoencephalitis (mĕ-ning″go-en-sef″ah-li′tis) inflammation of the brain and its meninges; called also encephalomeningitis.

primary amebic m. a rare and often fatal acute, febrile, purulent meningoencephalitis caused by usually free-living soil and water amebas of the genera *Naegleria, Acanthamoeba,* and *Hartmannella.*

meningoencephalocele (mĕ-ning″go-en-sef′ah-lo-sēl″) encephalocele.

meningoencephalomyelitis (mĕ-ning″go-en-sef″ah-lo-mi″ĕ-li′tis) inflammation of the meninges, brain, and spinal cord.

meningoencephalopathy (mĕ-ning″go-en-sef″ah-lop′ah-the) noninflammatory disease of the cerebral meninges and brain.

meningogenic (mĕ-ning″go-jen′ik) arising in the meninges.

meningomalacia (mĕ-ning″go-mah-la′-shah) softening of a membrane.

meningomyelitis (mĕ-ning″go-mi″ĕ-li′tis) inflammation of the spinal cord and its meninges.

meningomyelocele (mĕ-ning-go-mi′e-lo-sēl″) myelomeningocele.

meningomyeloradiculitis (mĕ-ning″go-mi″ĕ-lo-rah-dik″u-li′tis) inflammation of the meninges, spinal cord, and spinal nerve roots.

meningopathy (men″in-gop′ah-the) any disease of the meninges.

meningorachidian (mĕ-ning″go-rah-kid′e-an) pertaining to the spinal cord and meninges.

meningoradicular (mĕ-ning″go-rah-dik′u-ler) pertaining to the meninges and the cranial or spinal nerve roots.

meningoradiculitis (mĕ-ning″go-rah-dik″u-li′tis) inflammation of the meninges and spinal nerve roots.

meningorrhagia (mĕ-ning″go-ra′jah) hemorrhage from cerebral or spinal membranes.

meningorrhea (mĕ-ning″go-re′ah) effusion of blood between or upon the meninges.

meninx (me′ningks), pl. *menin′ges* [Gr.] a membrane, especially one of the membranes of the brain or spinal cord; see DURA MATER, ARACHNOID, and PIA MATER. adj., **menin′geal.**

meniscectomy (men″ĭ-sek′to-me) excision of a meniscus, as of the knee joint.

meniscitis (men″ĭ-si′tis) inflammation of a meniscus of the knee joint.

meniscocyte (mĕ-nis′ko-sīt) sickle cell.

meniscosynovial (mĕ-nis″ko-sin-o′ve-al) pertaining to a meniscus and the synovial membrane.

meniscus (mĕ-nis′kus) [L.] something of crescent shape, as the concave or convex surface of a column of liquid in a pipet or

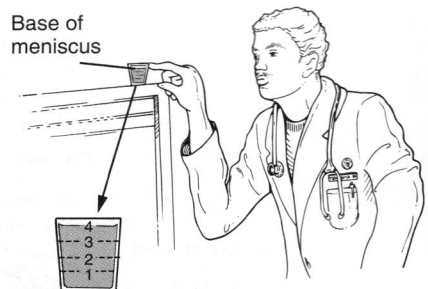

Base of
meniscus

Measuring medication at the meniscus. From Lammon et al., 1996.

medication cup, or a crescent-shaped fibrocartilage (semilunar cartilage) in the knee joint. adj., **menis′cal.**

Menkes' syndrome (mengks) an X-linked recessive abnormality in copper absorption marked by sparse, brittle scalp hair and by severe cerebral degeneration and arterial changes resulting in death in infancy.

men(o)- word element [Gr.], *menstruation.*

menolipsis (men″o-lip′sis) temporary cessation of menstruation.

menometrorrhagia men″o-met″ro-ra′jah excessive uterine bleeding at and between menstrual periods.

menopause (men′o-pawz) cessation of menstruation, defined as being when menstruation has not occurred for 6 to 12 months. The *climacteric* is that phase of life during which a woman passes from the reproductive to the non-reproductive stage. adj., **menopau′sal.** Menopause is a natural physiologic process that results from the normal aging of the ovaries. It occurs when the ovaries can no longer perform the function of ovulation and estrogen production. Because estrogen secretion stops, physiologic changes occur in the woman's body. The uterine tubes shrink in size and become less capable of movement. The uterus, the cavity of the uterus, and the cervix also decrease in size. The vagina contracts and its folds become shallower. The clitoris and external sexual organs become smaller. There may be some thinning of the pubic and axillary hair. The breasts usually become less full and firm.

OSTEOPOROSIS is one of the important health hazards associated with the climacteric. After cessation of ovarian function, bone loss (reduction in bone quantity without chemical change) is accelerated and fractures can more easily occur. In addition, after menopause women's risk of heart attack increases progressively until age 70, when it becomes equal to the risk for men.

Recent research questions the use of hormone replacement THERAPY for healthy postmenopausal women.

Menopause normally takes place between the ages of 40 and 58. If it occurs before age 40 it is *premature menopause;* after 58 it is called *delayed menopause.* Both premature and delayed menopause should be evaluated by a health care provider, because they can be inherited or be indicative of a primary endocrine disorder or gynecologic dysfunction.

About 25 per cent of American women reach menopause by the age of 47, half by the age of 50, 75 per cent by age 52, and 95 per cent by age 55. The climacteric period can last from 6 months to 3 years or more. There does not seem to be a relationship between age at menarche and age at menopause. Marriage, childbearing, height, weight, and prolonged use of oral contraceptives also do not seem to influence age at menopause. Smoking, however, is associated with earlier menopause. If for medical reasons surgery or radiation of the reproductive organs becomes necessary, *artificial* or *surgical menopause* can occur if both ovaries are removed or rendered dysfunctional. The symptoms usually are more severe than in natural menopause because of the sudden rather than gradual diminution of hormonal secretion.

Symptoms. The most readily recognized sign that a woman has entered the perimenopausal period is menstrual irregularity. The most common pattern is a gradual decrease in both amount and duration of flow during menses, tapering gradually to spotting and then cessation. In some cases there may be more frequent and heavier bleeding or bleeding between periods.

Menopause has taken place when periods have ceased for 6 to 12 months. Hormonal changes in menopause, which are responsible for many of its physical and psychological symptoms, include overproduction of both follicle-stimulating hormone (FSH) and luteinizing hormone (LH), and increased testosterone production by the ovaries.

The symptoms most commonly reported by menopausal women are hot flushes (flashes) of the face, neck, and upper body, excessive perspiration, especially at night, vaginal dryness, stress incontinence or urinary frequency, joint pain and backache, and insomnia, which is usually due to hot flashes. From 40 to 70 per cent of women experience hot flashes and 25 to 49 per cent have episodes of sweating during menopause.

There is variability in women's responses to menopause. Individual characteristics and self-perceptions, as well as sociopolitical factors, are important determinants of each woman's experience of the climacteric. Sexual function is affected by three components: motivation (desire and libido), endocrine function, and sociocultural beliefs. The decreased estrogen after menopause leads to atrophy of the internal genitalia, diminished genital secretion, less vasocongestion, and decreased vaginal expansion. These may not be experienced as discrete symptoms, but may influence a woman's perception that she is less responsive. Genital atrophy, however, does respond to estrogen therapy.

Treatment. Hormonal replacement therapy with estrogen is prescribed with caution because of contraindications and the possibility of complications. The health care provider prescribing estrogen replacement therapy takes into account such risk factors as potential for malignancy, thrombophlebitis or thromboembolism, or liver disease; obesity; varicosities; hypertension; and heavy smoking. Malignancy is a primary concern. The overall risk of breast cancer with estrogen use has not been shown to be increased, although long-term use has been associated with a mildly increased risk (1.2 to 1.5) in some meta-analyses. The greatest risk for malignancy is the link noted between endometrial cancer and unopposed estrogen therapy. The addition of at least 10 days of progestin therapy along with estrogen therapy eliminates the increased risk of endometrial cancer but may cause withdrawal bleeding. Less bleeding usually occurs with combined, continuous administration of both.

Alternatives to hormonal replacement include limitation of foods high in saturated fat and nitrites and avoiding red meat, coffee, tea, chocolate, colas, and alcohol. Vitamins E and D, vitamins of the B complex, calcium gluconate or carbonate, and magnesium may be prescribed by some health care providers. Regular exercise is especially important during and after the climacteric years. Exercise stimulates the production of endorphins, which increase one's sense of well-being, improve circulation, and help prevent osteoporosis.

Patient Care. Patient education is extremely important in the management of perimenopausal symptoms. Many times the patient suffers because of misinformation and lack of understanding that menopause is a natural process in the life of every woman. The manner in which she reacts to the changes taking place at this period of

M

her life depends to a great extent on her feelings of self-esteem. Knowing what to expect, having a knowledgeable and empathetic person who takes her symptoms seriously and offers support and guidance, and being able to get some control over what is happening to herself can significantly improve the menopausal woman's physical and mental health.

menorrhagia (men″o-ra′je-ah) hypermenorrhea.

menorrhalgia (men″o-ral′jah) dysmenorrhea.

menoschesis (mĕ-nos′kĕ-sis, men″o-ske′sis) suppression of menstruation.

menostaxis (men″o-stak′sis) a prolonged menstrual period; see also HYPERMENORRHEA.

menotropins (men″o-tro′pinz) a purified preparation of GONADOTROPINS extracted from the urine of postmenopausal women, containing follicle-stimulating HORMONE and luteinizing HORMONE; used to treat male hypogonadism, to induce ovulation and pregnancy in certain infertile, anovulatory women, and to increase the numbers of oocytes for patients attempting conception using assisted reproductive TECHNOLOGIES such as gamete intrafallopian TRANSFER (GIFT) or in vitro FERTILIZATION; administered intramuscularly.

menouria (men″o-u′re-ah) the flowing of menstrual blood through a fistula into the bladder.

menses (men′sēz) menstruation.

menstrual (men′stroo-al) pertaining to MENSTRUATION.

m. cycle the regularly recurring physiologic changes in the ENDOMETRIUM that culminate in its shedding (MENSTRUATION). Menstrual cycles vary in length, with the average being about 28 days. The length of time of menstrual flow is also variable, with an average of about 5 days. Women menstruate from PUBERTY to MENOPAUSE, except during pregnancy. The first 14 days of the cycle are called the *follicular phase;* a FOLLICLE containing an OVUM is developing in one of the OVARIES. It begins as the menstrual flow ceases; the lining of the uterus is stimulated by ESTROGEN and begins to increase in thickness to prepare for the possibility of REPRODUCTION. On the twelfth or thirteenth day of the cycle, the *ovulatory phase* begins with a surge in levels of luteinizing HORMONE and follicle-stimulating HORMONE; OVULATION then takes place and the ovary discharges the ovum. The ruptured follicle is transformed into a yellowish material called the CORPUS LUTEUM; the *luteal phase* begins as the corpus luteum secretes

PROGESTERONE. Progesterone acts on the endometrium, building up tissues with an enriched supply of blood to nourish the future embryo. If FERTILIZATION and CONCEPTION do not take place, the estrogen level in the blood falls, the endometrium is no longer stimulated, and the uterus again becomes thinner. Blood circulation slows, blood vessels contract, and the *menstrual phase* begins; unused tissue breaks down into the bloody discharge known as MENSTRUATION. The cycle then starts again.

menstruation (men″stroo-a′shun) the periodic discharge from the vagina of blood and tissues from a nonpregnant uterus; the culmination of the MENSTRUAL CYCLE. Menstruation occurs every 28 days or so between puberty and menopause, except during pregnancy, and the flow lasts about 5 days, the times varying from woman to woman.

Menstrual Difficulties. Some menstrual discomfort is common, but acute discomfort is usually indicative of some disorder. Among the disorders sometimes causing DYSMENORRHEA are leiomyoma uteri, endometrial cysts, and displacement of the uterus. Menstrual pain may in some cases be related to tension or anxiety. Excessive bleeding or prolonged periods (HYPERMENORRHEA) are sometimes an indication of tumors, polyps, cancer, or inflammation.

Menstruation usually starts between the ages of 11 and 14 and continues into the forties or fifties. At first the periods may be irregular, but once they are established they usually occur in a fairly definite rhythm, at intervals of 21 to 35 days. In these regular cycles, there may be monthly variations of a few days, which are considered normal. Cycle length may be influenced by changes in climate or living conditions, or by emotional factors. Slight irregularities, especially if they occur over a period of time, may be warnings of disturbance of either the thyroid or pituitary glands, or of tumors of the uterus or ovaries.

Occasionally menstruation does not occur at puberty; this is known as *primary amenorrhea.* It may be caused by underdevelopment or malformation of the reproductive organs, or by glandular disturbances, which generally can be corrected by the administration of hormones.

General ill health, a change in climate or living conditions, emotional shock, or, frequently, either the hope or fear of becoming pregnant can sometimes stop menstruation after it has begun (*secondary amenorrhea*). If this cessation is of short duration, it is not a cause for alarm. If it continues over a long

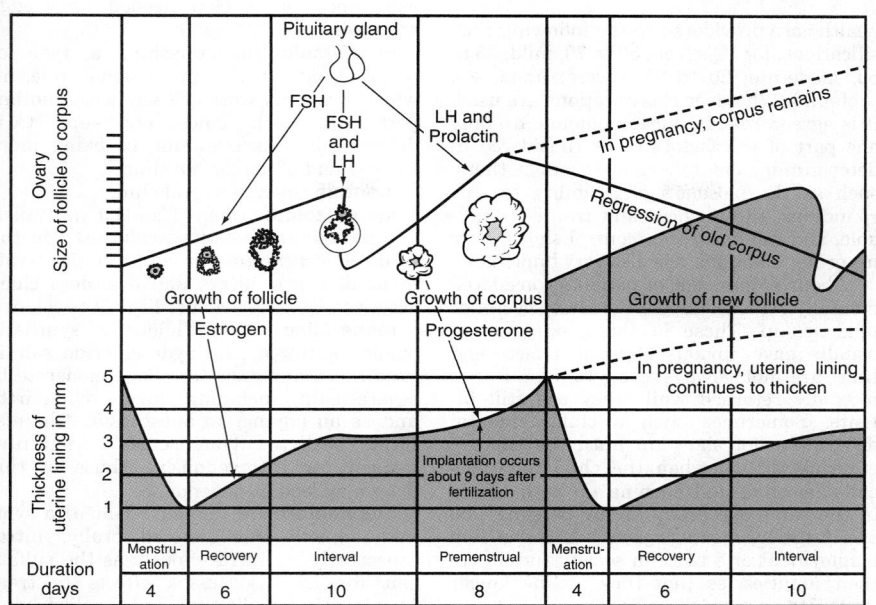

Average 28-day menstrual cycle. The cycle begins when hormones from the pituitary gland stimulate the development of an egg in a follicle inside one of the ovaries. About the fourteenth day, ovulation occurs: The follicle bursts, and the egg is discharged from the ovary. If the egg is not fertilized, the cycle ends in menstruation on the twenty-eighth day. If the egg is fertilized, pregnancy begins.

period of time, and there is also the problem of infertility, hormone treatments may be necessary.

anovular m., anovulatory m. periodic uterine bleeding without preceding ovulation.

vicarious m. bleeding from extragenital mucous membrane at the time one would normally expect the menstrual period.

menstruum (men′stroo-um) a solvent medium.

mensuration (men″su-ra′shun) the process of measuring.

mental (men′tal) 1. pertaining to the mind. 2. pertaining to the chin.

m. disorder any clinically significant behavioral or psychological syndrome characterized by distressing symptoms, significant impairment of functioning, or significantly increased risk of death, pain, or other disability. Mental disorders are assumed to result from some behavioral, psychological, or biological dysfunction in the individual. The concept does not include deviant behavior, disturbances that are essentially conflicts between the individual and society, or expected and culturally sanctioned responses to particular events.

m. retardation less than average general intellectual functioning that brings with it some degree of impaired adaptation in learning, social adjustment, or maturation, or in all three areas; it is now classified as a DEVELOPMENTAL DISABILITY.

Mental retardation is a relative term. Its meaning depends on what society demands of the individual in learning, skills, and social responsibility. Many people who are considered developmentally challenged in the complex modern world would get along normally in a simpler society.

Diagnosis: There is no absolute measurement for retardation. At one time the different types were classified only according to the apparent severity of the retardation. Since the most practical standard was intelligence, the degree of retardation was based on the score of the patient on INTELLIGENCE TESTS such as the INTELLIGENCE QUOTIENT (IQ). The average person is considered to have an IQ of between 90 and 110, and those who score below 70 are considered mentally retarded.

In the past, the different groupings were classified in terms such as feebleminded, idiot, imbecile, and moron. Today, most health care providers use the following classifications: for IQ's from 50 to 70, mild; 35 to 50, moderate; 20 to 35, severe; under 20, profound. Whatever classifications are used, it is agreed that IQ measurements are only one part of the factors to be considered in determining mental retardation. Others, such as the patient's adaptability to surroundings, the services and training available, and the amount of control shown over his or her emotions, are also very important.

About 85 per cent of patients considered mentally retarded are in the least severe, or mild, group. Those in this group do not usually have obvious physical defects and thus are not always easy to identify as mentally retarded while they are still infants. Sometimes such a child's mental defects do not show up until the time of entering school, when the child has difficulty learning and keeping up with others in the same age group. Many persons who are in the mild category, as adults can find employment or a place in society suitable to their abilities, so that they are no longer identified as mentally retarded.

Cause: The cause of mental retardation is often unidentifiable; known ones are classified as either *genetic* or *acquired.* Genetic conditions include chromosomal abnormalities such as DOWN SYNDROME and KLINEFELTER'S SYNDROME and errors of metabolism such as PHENYLKETONURIA, HYPOTHYROIDISM, and TAY-SACHS DISEASE. *Acquired conditions* may be prenatal, perinatal, or postnatal. Prenatal conditions include RUBELLA and other viral infections, toxins, placental insufficiency, and blood type incompatibility. Perinatal causes are anoxia, birth injury, and prematurity. Postnatal causes may include infections, poisons, poor nutrition, trauma, and sociocultural factors such as deprivation.

Many conditions that can cause severe retardation can be diagnosed during pregnancy, and in some cases proper treatment can lessen or even prevent retardation. Proper care for the mother during pregnancy and for the baby in the first months of life is also important.

menthol (men′thol) an alcohol from various mint oils or produced synthetically, used locally to relieve itching and by inhalation for treatment of upper respiratory tract disorders.

mentoplasty (men′to-plas″te) plastic surgery of the chin; surgical correction of deformities and defects of the chin.

mentor (men′tor) a person with more experience in a given area who takes responsibility for helping someone with less experience to develop needed knowledge and skills.

mentorship (men′tor-ship) a type of preparation for the professional role, in which a MENTOR works closely with another person to teach, guide, and support; it differs from PRECEPTORSHIP in being more intense and of longer duration.

mentum (men′tum) [L.] chin.

mepenzolate (me-pen′zo-lāt) an ANTICHOLINERGIC and ANTIMUSCARINIC used in the form of *mepenzolate bromide* in the treatment of peptic ulcers and disorders characterized by excessive motility of the colon.

meperidine (mĕ-per′ĭ-dēn) a synthetic opioid ANALGESIC; the hydrochloride salt is used as an analgesic to relieve moderate to severe pain, including during childbirth and as an adjunct to anesthesia. Administered orally, intramuscularly, subcutaneously, or intravenously. Abuse of this drug may lead to dependence.

mephentermine (mĕ-fen′ter-mēn) a sympathomimetic administered orally, intramuscularly, or intravenously as the sulfate salt for its VASOPRESSOR effects to treat hypotensive conditions, and applied topically to the nasal mucosa as a decongestant.

mephenytoin (mef″en-ĭ′to-in) an ANTICONVULSANT administered orally in treatment of several types of EPILEPSY when the seizures are refractory to other drugs.

mephitic (mĕ-fit′ik) noxious; foul smelling.

mephobarbital (mef″o-bar′bĭ-tal) a long acting BARBITURATE used as an ANTICONVULSANT in epilepsy.

mepivacaine (mĕ-piv′ah-kān) a LIDOCAINE analogue used in the form of the hydrochloride salt as a local ANESTHETIC.

meprednisone (mĕ-pred′nĭ-sōn) a GLUCOCORTICOID used as an antiinflammatory, antiallergic, and antineoplastic AGENT; administered orally.

meprobamate (mĕ-pro′bah-māt, mep″ro-bam′āt) an ANTIANXIETY AGENT and skeletal muscle RELAXANT; administered orally.

mEq milliequivalent.

mer(o)- word element [Gr.], 1. *part.* 2. *thigh.*

meradimate (mer-ad′ĭ-māt) an absorber of ultraviolet A radiation, used topically as a SUNSCREEN.

meralgia (mĕ-ral′jah) pain in the thigh.

m. paresthe′tica a condition of numbness and tingling on the anterolateral aspect of the thigh, rarely accompanied by pain; it is due to entrapment of the lateral femoral cutaneous nerve at the inguinal ligaments.

merbromin (mer-bro′min) a mercurial antiseptic that has been used topically for the disinfection of skin and wounds.

mercaptan (mer-kap′tan) thiol.

mercaptopurine (mer-kap″to-pu′rēn) a PURINE analogue in which sulfur replaces the oxygen atom of purine; it is used as an antineoplastic AGENT primarily for treatment of acute lymphoblastic leukemia. It is also used an IMMUNOSUPPRESSANT in the treatment of Crohn's disease and ulcerative colitis. Called also 6-mercaptopurine and 6-MP.

mercurial (mer-ku′re-al) 1. pertaining to mercury. 2. a preparation containing mercury. 3. pertaining to behavior patterns that change rapidly.

mercurialism (mer-ku′re-al-izm) MERCURY POISONING.

mercuric (mer-ku′rik) pertaining to mercury as a bivalent element; containing bivalent mercury.

Mercurochrome (mer-ku′ro-krōm) trademark for preparations of MERBROMIN, a topical antibacterial.

mercurous (mer′ku-rus) pertaining to mercury as a monovalent element; containing monovalent mercury.

mercury (Hg) (mer′ku-re) a chemical element, atomic number 80, atomic weight 200.59. (See Appendix 6.) Mercury forms two sets or classes of compounds: MERCUROUS, in which a single atom of mercury combines with a monovalent radical, and MERCURIC, in which a single atom of mercury combines with a bivalent radical. Mercury and its salts can be absorbed by the skin and mucous membranes, causing chronic poisoning (see MERCURY POISONING). The mercuric salts are more soluble and irritant than the mercurous.

ammoniated m. a compound used as an antiseptic skin and ophthalmic ointment. It should be applied with caution, as excessive use may irritate the skin and cause dermatitis.

m. bichloride an extremely poisonous compound formerly used in treatment of syphilis but now used only as a disinfectant.

m. poisoning acute or chronic disease caused by exposure to mercury or its salts; an important aspect is its toxic effect on the brain, causing impaired judgment, memory loss, sleeplessness, and nervousness. The *acute* form, due to ingestion, is marked by severe abdominal pain, metallic taste in the mouth, vomiting, oliguria or anuria at onset, followed by bloody diarrhea, and corrosion and ulceration of the entire digestive tract. The *chronic*, due to absorption by the skin and mucous membranes, inhalation of vapors, or ingestion of mercury salts, is marked by stomatitis, metallic taste in the mouth, a blue line along the border of the gum, sore hypertrophied gums that bleed easily, loosening of the teeth, excessive salivation, tremors and incoordination, and psychiatric symptoms including abnormal excitability, anxiety, and social withdrawal. A common cause of chronic mercury poisoning is the ingestion of contaminated fish. Because of this, some fishing areas are posted with signs recommending limiting consumption of fish caught there. See also MINAMATA DISEASE.

Treatment. Treatment consists of removal of the source of exposure and administration of a chelating AGENT. Exchange transfusions and removal of mercury by surgery are options in selected patients. Consultation with a toxicologist is warranted.

meridian (mĕ-rid′e-an) an imaginary line on the surface of a globe or sphere, connecting the opposite ends of its axis. adj., **merid′ional.**

meroblastic (mer″o-blas′tik) partially dividing; undergoing cleavage in which only part of the egg participates.

merocrine (mer′o-krin) partly secreting: denoting that type of glandular secretion in which the secreting cell remains intact throughout the process of formation and discharge of the secretory products, as in the salivary and pancreatic glands. See also APOCRINE and HOLOCRINE.

merogenesis (mer″o-jen′ĕ-sis) cleavage of a zygote.

merogony (mĕ-rog′o-ne) the development of only a portion of an ovum. adj., **merogon′ic.**

meromelia (mer″o-me′le-ah) congenital absence of a part, but not all, of a limb.

meromicrosomia (mer″o-mi″kro-so′me-ah) unusual smallness of some part of the body.

meromyosin (mer″o-mi′o-sin) a fragment of the myosin molecule isolated by treatment with proteolytic enzyme; there are two types, heavy (H-meromyosin) and light (L-meromyosin).

meropenem (mer″o-pen′em) a broad-spectrum β-lactam antibiotic effective against a wide variety of gram-positive and gram-negative organisms; used in treatment of intra-abdominal infections and bacterial meningitis.

meropia (mĕ-ro′pe-ah) partial blindness.

merorachischisis (me″ro-rah-kis′kĭ-sis) fissure of part of the spinal cord.

merosmia (mĕ-roz′me-ah) inability to perceive certain odors.

M

merotomy (mĕ-rot'ah-me) a cutting into segments.

merozoite (mer"o-zo'ĭt) one of the organisms formed by multiple fission (schizogony) of a sporozoite within the body of the host.

MERRF syndrome *m*yoclonus with *e*pilepsy and *r*agged *r*ed *f*ibers; a familial type of mitochondrial ENCEPHALOPATHY, of maternal (mitochondrial) inheritance.

Merthiolate (mer-thi'o-lāt) trademark for preparations of THIMEROSAL, a topical antibacterial.

mes(o)- word element [Gr.], *middle*.

mesalamine (mĕ-sal'ah-mēn) an active metabolite of SULFASALAZINE, used in prophylaxis and treatment of INFLAMMATORY BOWEL DISEASE; administered orally or rectally. Called also 5-aminosalicylic acid.

mesalazine (mĕ-sal'ah-zēn) mesalamine.

mesangiocapillary (mes-an"je-o-kap'ĭ-lar"e) pertaining to or affecting the mesangium and the associated capillaries.

mesangium (mes-an'je-um) the thin membrane supporting the capillary loops in renal glomeruli. adj., **mesan'gial.**

Mesantoin (mĕ-san'toin) trademark for a preparation of MEPHENYTOIN, an ANTICONVULSANT.

mesarteritis (mes"ahr-ter-i'tis) inflammation of the TUNICA MEDIA of an artery.

mesatipellic (mes-at"ĭ-pel'ik) having a round pelvis.

mescaline (mes'kah-lēn) a poisonous alkaloid derived from the flowering heads (mescal buttons) of a Mexican cactus; it is a HALLUCINOGEN, producing hallucinations of sound and color.

mescalism (mes'kah-lizm) intoxication due to mescal buttons or mescaline.

mesencephalitis (mes"en-sef"ah-li'tis) inflammation of the mesencephalon, or midbrain.

mesencephalon (mes"en-sef'ah-lon) 1. the short part of the BRAINSTEM just above the PONS; it contains the nerve pathways between the cerebral hemispheres and the medulla oblongata, as well as nuclei (relay stations or centers) of the third and fourth cranial nerves. The center for visual reflexes, such as moving the head and eyes, is located here. 2. the middle of the three primary brain vesicles of the embryo; called also midbrain. adj., **mesencephal'ic.**

mesencephalotomy (mez"en-sef'ah-lot'-ah-me) surgical production of lesions in the midbrain for the relief of intractable pain.

mesenchyma (mĕ-seng'kĭ-mah) the meshwork of embryonic connective tissue in the MESODERM; from it are formed the connective tissues of the body as well as blood vessels and lymph vessels. adj., **mesen'chymal.**

mesenchyme (mes'eng-kīm) mesenchyma.

mesenchymoma (mes"eng-ki-mo'mah) a mixed mesenchymal tumor composed of two or more cellular elements that are not commonly associated, exclusive of fibrous tissue.

mesenterectomy (mes"en-tĕ-rek'to-me) resection of the mesentery.

mesenteriopexy (mes"en-ter'e-o-pek"se) fixation or suspension of a torn mesentery.

mesenteriorrhaphy (mes"en-ter"e-or'ah-fe) suture of the mesentery.

mesenteriplication (mes"en-ter"ĭ-plĭ-ka'-shun) the operation of taking a tuck in the mesentery to shorten it.

mesenteritis (mes"en-tĕ-ri'tis) inflammation of the mesentery.

mesenterium (mes"en-te're-um) mesentery (def. 2).

mesenteron (mes-en'ter-on) the midgut.

mesentery (mes'en-ter"e) 1. a membranous fold attaching an organ to the body wall. 2. the peritoneal fold attaching the

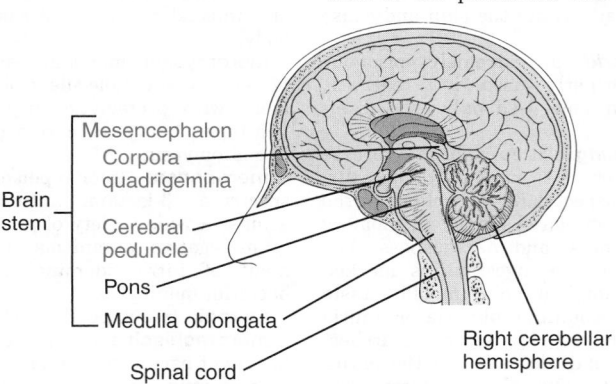

Brain stem
Mesencephalon
Corpora quadrigemina
Cerebral peduncle
Pons
Medulla oblongata
Spinal cord
Right cerebellar hemisphere

The mesencephalon (midbrain). From Applegate, 2000.

small intestine to the dorsal body wall; called also mesenterium. adj., **mesenter′ic.**

MeSH (mesh) [*M*edical *S*ubject *H*eadings] a THESAURUS published by the NATIONAL LIBRARY OF MEDICINE for use in MEDLARS.

mesiad (me′ze-ad) toward the middle or center.

mesial (me′ze-al) situated in the middle; median; nearer the middle line of the body or nearer the center of the dental arch.

mesially (me′ze-al″e) toward the median line.

mesiobuccal (me″ze-o-buk″l) pertaining to or formed by the mesial and buccal surfaces of a tooth, or the mesial and buccal walls of a tooth cavity.

mesiobucco-occlusal (me″ze-o-buk″o-ŏ-kloo′zal) pertaining to or formed by the mesial, buccal, and occlusal surfaces of a tooth.

mesiocervical (me″ze-o-ser′vĭ-kal) pertaining to the mesial surface of the neck of a tooth.

mesioclusion (me″ze-o-kloo′zhun) anteroclusion; malrelation of the dental arches with the mandibular arch anterior to the maxillary arch (prognathism).

mesiodistal (me″ze-o-dis′tal) pertaining to the mesial and distal surfaces of a tooth.

mesiolabial (me″ze-o-la′be-al) pertaining to the mesial and labial surfaces of a tooth or a tooth cavity.

mesiolabioincisal (me″ze-o-la″be-o-in-si′zal) pertaining to or formed by the mesial, labial, and incisal surfaces of a tooth.

mesiolingual (me″ze-o-ling′gwal) pertaining to or formed by the mesial and lingual surfaces of a tooth, or the mesial and lingual walls of a tooth cavity preparation.

mesiolinguoincisal (me″ze-o-ling′gwo-in-si′zal) pertaining to or formed by the mesial, lingual, and incisal surfaces of a tooth.

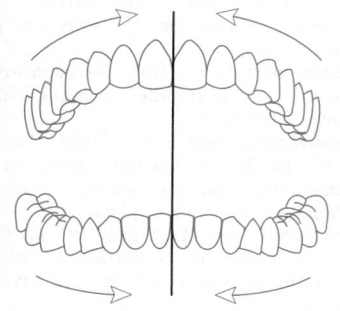

The mesial surfaces are those closest to the midline of the dental arch. From Darby and Walsh, 1994.

mesiolinguo-occlusal (me″ze-o-ling″gwo-ŏ-kloo′zal) pertaining to or formed by the mesial, lingual, and occlusal surfaces of a tooth.

mesion (me′ze-on) the plane dividing the body into right and left symmetrical halves.

mesio-occlusal (me″ze-o-o-ŏ-kloo′zal) pertaining to or formed by the mesial and occlusal surfaces of a tooth, or the mesial and occlusal walls of a tooth cavity.

mesmerism (mez′mer-izm) hypnotism.

mesna (mes′nah) a sulfhydryl compound given orally or intravenously together with a urotoxic antineoplastic AGENT such as IFOSFAMIDE or CYCLOPHOSPHAMIDE because it inactivates some of their metabolites and thus lessens damage to the bladder.

mesoappendix (mez′o-ah-pen′diks) the peritoneal fold connecting the appendix to the ileum.

mesoblast (mez′o-blast) the mesoderm, especially in the early stages.

mesocardia (mez″o-kahr′de-ah) location of the apex of the heart in the midline of the thorax.

mesocardium (mez″o-kahr′de-um) the part of the embryonic mesentery that connects the embryonic heart with the body wall in front and the foregut behind.

mesocecum (mez″o-se′kum) the occasionally occurring mesentery of the cecum.

mesocephalon (mez″o-sef′ah-lon) mesencephalon, or midbrain.

mesocolon (mez″o-ko′lon) the peritoneal process attaching the colon to the posterior abdominal wall, and called ascending, descending, or transverse, according to the portion of the colon to which it attaches.

   pelvic m., sigmoid m. the peritoneum attaching the sigmoid colon to the posterior abdominal wall.

mesocolopexy (mez″o-ko′lo-pek″se) suspension or fixation of the colon.

mesocoloplication (mes″o-ko″lo-pli-ka′shun) plication of the mesocolon to limit its mobility.

mesocord (mez′o-kord) an umbilical cord adherent to the placenta.

mesoderm (mez′o-derm) the middle of the three primary germ layers of the embryo, lying between the ectoderm and entoderm; from it are derived the connective tissue, bone, cartilage, muscle, blood and blood vessels, lymphatics, lymphoid organs, notochord, pleura, pericardium, peritoneum, kidneys, and gonads. adj., **mesoder′mal, mesoder′mic.**

   somatic m. the outer layer of the developing mesoderm.

M

splanchnic m. the inner layer of the developing mesoderm.

mesoduodenum (mez″o-doo′o-de′num) the mesenteric fold that in early fetal life encloses the duodenum.

mesoepididymis (mez″o-ep′ĭ-did′ĭ-mis) a fold of the TUNICA VAGINALIS TESTIS that connects the epididymis and testis.

mesogastrium (mez″o-gas′tre-um) the portion of the primordial mesentery that encloses the stomach and from which the greater omentum develops. adj., **mesogas′-tric.**

mesoileum (mez″o-il′e-um) the mesentery of the ileum.

mesojejunum (mez″o-jĕ-joo′num) the mesentery of the jejunum.

mesomere (mez′o-mēr) 1. a blastomere of size intermediate between a macromere and a micromere. 2. a midzone of the mesoderm between the epimere and hypomere.

mesomerism (mĕ-som′er-iz′m) the existence of organic chemical structures that cannot be accurately represented by a single structural formula, the actual formula lying intermediate between several possible representations that differ only in the position of electrons.

mesometrium (mez″o-me′tre-um) the portion of the broad ligament below the mesovarium.

mesomorph (mez′o-morf, mes′o-morf) an individual having a type of body build in which mesodermal tissues predominate: there is relative preponderance of muscle, bone, and connective tissue, usually with heavy, hard physique of rectangular outline; a somatotype classified between ECTOMORPH and ENDOMORPH.

mesomorphy (mez″o-mor′fe) the condition of being a mesomorph. adj., **mesomor′phic.**

meson (me′zon, mes′on) 1. mesion. 2. any elementary particle having a mass intermediate between the mass of the electron and that of the proton.

mesonephroma (mez″o-nĕ-fro′mah) clear cell ADENOCARCINOMA.

mesonephron (mez″o-nef′ron) mesonephros.

mesonephros (mez″o-nef′ros), pl. *mesoneph′roi* [Gr.] the excretory organ of the embryo, arising caudad to the pronephros and using its duct. adj., **mesoneph′ric.**

mesopexy (mez′o-pek″se) repair of the mesentery; mesenteriopexy.

mesophile (mez′o-fīl) a microorganism that grows best at 20° to 55°C.

mesophlebitis (mez″o-flĕ-bi′tis) inflammation of the TUNICA MEDIA of a vein.

mesorchium (mes-or′ke-um) the portion of the primordial mesentery enclosing the fetal testis, represented in the adult by a fold between the testis and epididymis. adj. **mesor′chial.**

mesorectum (mez″o-rek′tum) the fold of peritoneum connecting the upper portion of the rectum with the sacrum.

mesoridazine (mes″o-rid′ah-zēn) a PHENOTHIAZINE used in the form of the besylate salt as an ANTIPSYCHOTIC AGENT.

mesoropter (mez″o-rop′ter) the normal position of the eyes with their muscles at rest.

mesorrhaphy (mez-or′ah-fe) suture of the mesentery.

mesosalpinx (mez″o-sal′pinks) the part of the broad ligament above the mesovarium investing the fallopian tube.

mesosigmoid (mez″o-sig′moid) the peritoneal fold by which the sigmoid flexure is attached to the abdominal wall.

mesosigmoidopexy (mez″o-sig-moi′do-pek″se) fixation of the mesosigmoid in prolapse of the rectum.

mesosome (mes′o-sōm) an invagination of the bacterial cell membrane. Various mesosomes are associated with DNA replication, cell secretion, and electron transport.

mesosternum (mez″o-ster′num) the middle piece or body of the sternum.

mesotendineum (mez″o-ten-din′e-um) mesotendon.

mesotendon (mez″o-ten′don) the connective tissue sheath attaching a tendon to its fibrous sheath.

mesothelial (mez″o-the′le-al) pertaining to the mesothelium.

mesothelioma (mez″o-the″le-o′mah) a malignant tumor made up of cells derived from the mesothelium.

mesothelium (mez″o-the′le-um) the layer of flat cells, derived from the mesoderm, that lines the body cavity of the embryo. In the adult it forms the simple squamous epithelium that covers the surface of all true serous membranes (peritoneum, pericardium, pleura).

mesotympanum (mes″o-tim′pah-num) the portion of the middle ear medial to the tympanic membrane.

mesovarium (mez″o-var′e-um) the portion of the broad ligament between the mesometrium and mesosalpinx, enclosing and holding the ovary in place.

mestranol (mes′trah-nol) a synthetic ESTROGEN used in combination with a progestational AGENT as an oral CONTRACEPTIVE.

mesylate (mes′ĭ-lāt) USAN contraction for methanesulfonate.

met (met) a unit of measurement of heat production by the body, being the metabolic heat produced by a resting-sitting subject; it is equal to 50 kilogram calories per square meter of body surface per hour.

met(a)- word element [Gr.] (1) a prefix indicating *(a)* change; transformation; exchange; *(b)* after; next; (2) symbol *m*-, a prefix indicating a 1,3-substituted position in derivatives of benzene. (3) a prefix indicating a polymeric acid anhydride.

meta-analysis (met″ah-ah-nal′ĭ-sis) any systematic method that uses statistical analysis to integrate the data from a number of independent studies.

metabasis (mĕ-tab′ah-sis) change in the manifestations or course of a disease.

metabiosis (met″ah-bi-o′sis) the dependence of one organism upon another for its existence; commensalism.

metabolic (met″ah-bol′ik) pertaining to or of the nature of metabolism.

m. disease a disease caused by some defect in the chemical reactions of the cells of the body.

m. syndrome a combination including at least three of the following: abdominal obesity, HYPERTRIGLYCERIDEMIA, low level of high-density LIPOPROTEINS, HYPERTENSION, and high fasting plasma GLUCOSE level. It is associated with an increased risk for development of DIABETES mellitus and cardiovascular disease.

metabolism (mĕ-tab′o-lizm) 1. biotransformation. 2. the sum of the physical and chemical processes by which living organized substance is built up and maintained (ANABOLISM), and by which large molecules are broken down into smaller molecules to make energy available to the organism (CATABOLISM). Essentially these processes are concerned with the disposition of the nutrients absorbed into the blood following digestion.

There are two phases of metabolism: the anabolic and the catabolic phases. The anabolic, or constructive, phase is concerned with the conversion of simpler compounds derived from the nutrients into living, organized substances that the body cells can use. In the catabolic, or destructive, phase these organized substances are reconverted into simpler compounds, with the release of energy necessary for the proper functioning of the body cells.

The rate of metabolism can be increased by exercise; by elevated body temperature, as in a high fever, which can more than double the metabolic rate; by hormonal activity, such as that of thyroxine, insulin, and epinephrine; and by specific dynamic action that occurs following the ingestion of a meal.

The basal metabolic rate refers to the lowest rate obtained while an individual is at complete physical and mental rest. Metabolic rate usually is expressed in terms of the amount of heat liberated during the chemical reactions of metabolism. About 25 per cent of all energy from nutrients is utilized by the body to carry on its normal function; the remainder becomes heat.

basal m. the minimal energy expended for the maintenance of respiration, circulation, peristalsis, muscle tonus, body temperature, glandular activity, and the other vegetative functions of the body.

metabolite (mĕ-tab′o-līt) any substance produced during metabolism.

metabolize (mĕ-tab′o-līz) to subject to or be transformed by metabolism.

metacarpal (met″ah-kahr′p'l) 1. pertaining to the metacarpus. 2. a bone of the metacarpus.

metacarpectomy (met″ah-kahr-pek′to-me) excision or resection of a metacarpal bone.

metacarpophalangeal (met″ah-kahr″po-fah-lan′je-al) pertaining to the metacarpus and phalanges of the fingers.

metacarpus (met″ah-kahr′pus) the part of the hand between the wrist and fingers, its skeleton being five bones (metacarpals) extending from the carpus to the phalanges. See appendix 3-3.

metacentric (met″ah-sen′trik) having the centromere almost at the middle of the replicating chromosome.

metacercaria (met″ah-ser-kar′e-ah), pl. *metacerca′riae* The encysted resting or maturing stage of a trematode parasite in the tissues of an intermediate host.

metachromasia (met″ah-kro-ma′zhah) 1. failure to stain true with a given stain. 2. the different coloration of different tissues produced by the same stain. 3. change of color produced by staining. adj., **metachromat′ic.**

metachromatism (met″ah-kro′mah-tizm) metachromasia.

metachromophil (met″ah-kro′mo-fil) not staining normally.

metacognition (met″ah-kog-nish′un) an educational process that incorporates knowledge about one's abilities, the demands of given tasks, and potentially effective learning strategies; it involves self-regulation via planning, predicting, monitoring, regulating, evaluating, and revising strategies.

M

metaethics (met″ah-eth′iks) analysis of the language, concepts, and methods of reasoning in ethics. It studies the meanings of such ethical terms as right, obligation, virtue, principle, justification, sympathy, morality, and responsibility. It also includes study of *moral epistemology* (the theory of moral knowledge) and the logic and patterns of moral reasoning and justification. Questions for analysis include whether social morality is objective or subjective, relative or nonrelative, and rational or emotive. adj., **metaeth′ical.**

metagenesis (met″ah-jen′ĕ-sis) alternation in regular sequence of asexual and sexual methods of reproduction in the same species, as in certain FUNGI. Called also alternation of generations and heterogenesis.

Metagonimus (met″ah-gon′ĭ-mus) a genus of trematodes, including *M. yokoga′-wai,* which is parasitic in the small intestine of humans and other mammals in Japan, China, Indonesia, the Balkans, and Israel.

metal (met″l) any chemical element marked by luster, malleability, ductility, and conductivity of electricity and heat, and which will ionize positively in solution. adj., **metal′lic.**

alkali m. one of a group of monovalent elements including lithium, sodium, potassium, rubidium, and cesium.

m. fume fever an occupational disorder with malaria-like symptoms occurring in those engaged in welding and other metallic operations and due to the volatilized metals. It includes brassfounder's fever (brass chill, brazier's chill) and spelter's fever (zinc chill, zinc fume fever).

heavy m. one with a high specific gravity, usually defined to be above 5.0.

heavy m. poisoning poisoning with any of the heavy metals, particularly antimony, arsenic, cadmium, lead, mercury, thallium, or zinc.

noble m. a metal that is highly resistant to oxidation and corrosion.

metalloenzyme (mĕ-tal″o-en′zīm) any enzyme containing tightly bound metal atoms, e.g., the cytochromes.

metalloid (met″ah-loid) 1. any element with both metallic and nonmetallic properties. 2. any metallic element that does not have all the characters of a typical metal.

metalloporphyrin (mĕ-tal″o-por′fĭ-rin) a combination of a metal with porphyrin, e.g., heme.

metalloprotein (mĕ-tal″o-pro′tēn) a protein molecule bound to a metal ion, e.g., hemoglobin.

metallurgy (met′ah-lur″je) the science and art of using metals.

metamere (met′ah-mēr) one of a series of homologous segments of the body of an animal.

metamorphopsia (met″ah-mor-fop′se-ah) defective vision, with distortion of the shape of objects seen.

metamorphosis (met″ah-mor′fo-sis) change of structure or shape; particularly, transition from one developmental stage to another, as from larva to adult form. adj., **metamor′phic.**

fatty m. any normal or pathologic transformation of fat, including fatty infiltration and fatty degeneration.

Metamucil (met″ah-mu′sil) trademark for preparations of psyllium hydrophilic MUCILLOID, a bulk LAXATIVE.

metamyelocyte (met″ah-mi′ĕ-lo-sīt″) a precursor in the granulocytic series, being a cell intermediate in development between a promyelocyte and the mature, segmented (polymorphonuclear) granular leukocyte, and having a U-shaped nucleus.

metanephrine (met″ah-nef′rin) a urinary metabolite of epinephrine.

metanephros (met″ah-nef′ros), pl. *metaneph′roi* [Gr.] the permanent embryonic kidney, developing later than and caudad to the mesonephros. adj., **metaneph′ric.**

metaparadigm (met″ah-par′ah-dīm) a set of concepts and propositions that sets forth the phenomena with which a discipline is concerned. A metaparadigm is the most general statement of a discipline and functions as a framework in which the more restricted structures of conceptual models develop.

metaphase (met′ah-fāz) the second stage of cell division (mitosis or meiosis), in which the chromosomes, each consisting of two chromatids, are arranged in the equatorial plane of the spindle prior to separation.

Metaphen (met′ah-fen) trademark for preparations of NITROMERSOL, a disinfectant used as a topical antiinfective agent and for sterilizing instruments and other equipment.

metaphysis (mĕ-taf′ĭ-sis) [Gr.] the wider part at the end of the shaft of a long bone, adjacent to the epiphyseal disk. adj., **metaphys′eal.**

metaplasia (met″ah-pla′zhah) the change in the type of adult cells in a tissue to a form abnormal for that tissue. adj., **metaplas′tic.**

agnogenic myeloid m. the primary or idiopathic form of myeloid metaplasia, which is often accompanied by MYELOFIBROSIS; it is considered one of the MYELOPROLIFERATIVE DISORDERS. Called also aleukemic or nonleukemic myelosis.

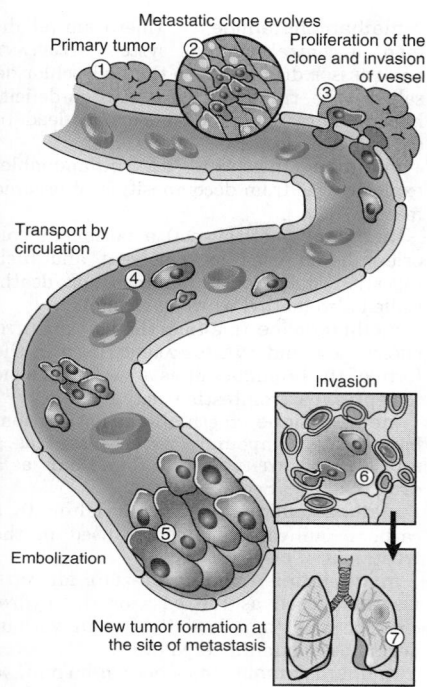

Metastasis: A metastatic cascade occurs in several steps, marked 1 through 7. From Damjanov, 2000.

myeloid m. the occurrence of myeloid tissue in extramedullary sites; specifically, a syndrome characterized by splenomegaly, anemia, nucleated erythrocytes and immature granulocytes in the circulating blood, and extramedullary hematopoiesis in the liver and spleen. The primary form is called *agnogenic myeloid metaplasia*. The secondary or symptomatic form may be associated with various diseases, including carcinomatosis, tuberculosis, leukemia, and polycythemia vera.

metapneumonic   (met″ah-noo-mon′ik) succeeding or following pneumonia.

metaproterenol (met″ah-pro-ter′ĕ-nol) a beta₂-adrenergic receptor agonist which also has significant beta₁-adrenergic activity; used in the form of the sulfate salt as a BRONCHODILATOR.

metapsychology (met′ah-si-kol′o-je) the branch of psychology that deals with the theoretical or speculative aspects of a particular subject of psychology, and the significance of mental processes that are beyond empirical verification.

metaraminol (met″ah-ram′ĭ-nol) a sympathomimetic agent acting mainly as an α-adrenergic agonist but also stimulating the β₁-adrenergic receptors of the heart and having potent VASOPRESSOR activity; administered intravenously, intramuscularly, or subcutaneously as the bitartrate salt for prevention and treatment of acute hypotensive states.

metarubricyte (met″ah-roo′brĭ-sīt) orthochromatic erythroblast.

metastasis (mĕ-tas′tah-sis) 1. the transfer of disease from one organ or part to another not directly connected with it. It may be due either to the transfer of pathogenic microorganisms (e.g., tubercle bacilli) or to the transfer of cells, as in malignant tumors. See also CANCER. 2. a growth of pathogenic microorganisms or of abnormal cells distant from the site primarily involved by the morbid process. adj., **metastat′ic.**

metastasize (mĕ-tas′tah-sīz) to form new foci of disease in a distant part by metastasis.

metasternum (met″ah-ster′num) the xiphoid process.

metatarsal (met″ah-tahr′sal) 1. pertaining to the metatarsus. 2. a bone of the metatarsus.

metatarsalgia (met″ah-tahr-sal′jah) pain and tenderness in the metatarsal region.

metatarsectomy (met″ah-tahr-sek′to-me) excision or resection of a metatarsal bone.

metatarsophalangeal (met″ah-tahr″so-fah-lan′je-al) pertaining to the metatarsus and the phalanges of the toes.

metatarsus (met″ah-tahr′sus) the part of the foot between the ankle and the toes, its skeleton being the five bones (metatarsals) extending from the tarsus to the phalanges. See appendix 3-3.

m. pri′mus va′rus angulation of the first metatarsal bone toward the midline of the body, producing an angle sometimes of 20 degrees or more between its base and that of the second metatarsal bone.

metathalamus (met″ah-thal′ah-mus) the part of the diencephalon inferior to the caudal end of the dorsal thalamus, comprising the lateral and medial geniculate bodies.

metathesis (mĕ-tath′ĕ-sis) 1. artificial transfer of a morbid process. 2. a chemical reaction in which an element or radical in one compound exchanges places with another element or radical in another compound.

metatrophic (met″ah-trof′ik) utilizing organic matter for food.

metaxalone (mĕ-taks′ah-lōn) a centrally acting skeletal muscle RELAXANT used for

M

relief of painful musculoskeletal conditions; administered orally.

Metazoa (met″ah-zo′ah) the division of the animal kingdom that includes the multicellular animals, i.e., all animals except the Protozoa. adj., **metazo′al, meta-zo′an.**

metazoon (met″ah-zo′on), pl. *metazo′a* [Gr.] an individual organism of the Metazoa.

Metchnikoff theory (mech′nĭ-kof) the theory that bacteria and other harmful elements in the body are attacked and destroyed by cells called phagocytes, and that the contest between such harmful elements and the phagocytes produces inflammation. Named for Elie Metchnikoff (1845–1916), Russian zoologist in Paris and winner, with Ehrlich, of the Nobel prize for medicine and physiology in 1908.

metencephalon (met″en-sef′ah-lon) [Gr.] 1. the anterior part of the RHOMBENCEPHALON, comprising the pons and cerebellum. 2. the anterior of two brain vesicles formed by specialization of the rhombencephalon in the developing embryo.

met-enkephalin (met″en-kef′ah-lin) see *enkephalin.*

meteorism (me′te-o-rizm) tympanites.

meteorotropism (me″te-o-rot′ro-pizm) the response to influence by meteorologic factors noted in certain biologic events, such as sudden death, attacks of angina, joint pain, insomnia, and traffic accidents. adj., **meteorotrop′ic.**

meter (me′ter) 1. the base SI UNIT of linear measure, approximately equivalent to 39.37 inches. Symbol m. 2. an apparatus for measuring the quantity of something passing through it, such as a gas or an electric current.

metformin (met-for′min) a hypoglycemic AGENT that potentiates the action of INSULIN; used in treatment of type 2 DIABETES MELLITUS.

-meter word element [Gr.], *instrument for measuring.*

methacholine (meth″ah-ko′lēn) a cholinergic agonist, having a longer duration of action than ACETYLCHOLINE and predominantly MUSCARINIC effects; it has VASODILATOR and cardiac VAGOMIMETIC effects but has largely been replaced by other drugs. It is also used in BRONCHIAL CHALLENGE TESTS.

methadone (meth′ah-dōn) a synthetic opioid ANALGESIC with pharmacologic properties similar to those of MORPHINE and HEROIN and equal potential for addiction; used as an analgesic and as a substitute opiate in the treatment of heroin addiction.

methamphetamine (meth″am-fet′ah-mēn) a central nervous system STIMULANT and PRESSOR drug, used as the hydrochloride salt in the treatment of attention-deficit/hyperactivity disorder. Abuse may lead to dependence. See also AMPHETAMINE.

methane (meth′ān) an inflammable, explosive gas from decomposition of organic matter.

methanol (meth′ah-nol) a poisonous colorless liquid used as a solvent and fuel; ingestion may cause blindness or death. Called also methyl or wood alcohol.

methantheline (mě-than′thě-lēn) an ANTICHOLINERGIC and ANTIMUSCARINIC, used in the form of the bromide salt as an ANTISPASMODIC to depress gastrointestinal activity.

methaqualone (meth″ah-qua′lōn) a nonbarbiturate compound formerly used as a SEDATIVE and HYPNOTIC; now found only as a drug of abuse. See DRUG ABUSE.

methazolamide (meth″ah-zo′lah-mīd) a carbonic anhydrase INHIBITOR used in the treatment of GLAUCOMA.

methdilazine (meth-di′lah-zēn) an ANTIHISTAMINE used as the base or the hydrochloride salt to relieve itching in various dermatoses; administered orally.

methemalbumin (met″he-mal-bu′min) a brownish pigment formed in the blood by the binding of albumin with heme; indicative of intravascular hemolysis.

methemalbuminemia (met″he-mal-bu″min-e′me-ah) the presence of methemalbumin in the blood.

methemoglobin (met-he′mo-glo′bin) a hematogenous pigment formed from hemoglobin by oxidation of the iron atom from the ferrous to the ferric state. A small amount is found in the blood normally, but injury or toxic agents convert a larger proportion of hemoglobin into methemoglobin, which does not function as an oxygen carrier.

methemoglobinemia (met-he″mo-glo″bĭ-ne′me-ah) the presence of excessive METHEMOGLOBIN in the blood, resulting in cyanosis and headache, dizziness, fatigue, ataxia, dyspnea, tachycardia, nausea, vomiting, and drowsiness, which can progress to stupor, coma, and occasionally death. It may be either chemical- or drug-induced *(acquired* or *toxic methemoglobinemia)* or hereditary *(congenital* or *hereditary methemoglobinemia).*

methemoglobinuria (met-he″mo-glo″bĭ-nu′re-ah) METHEMOGLOBIN in the urine, as in METHEMOGLOBINEMIA.

methenamine (mě-the′nah-mēn) a urinary antiseptic, administered orally as the hippurate and mandelate salts.

methicillin (meth″ĭ-sil′in) a semisynthetic PENICILLIN that is highly resistant to inactivation by penicillinase; its sodium salt is used parenterally as an antibacterial.

methimazole (meth-im'ah-zōl) a thyroid inhibitor used in treatment of HYPERTHYROID-ISM.

methionine (mĕ-thi'o-nēn) a sulfur-containing AMINO ACID, one of the essential amino acids, furnishing both methyl groups and sulfur necessary for metabolism.

methocarbamol (meth"o-kahr'bah-mol) a compound used as a skeletal muscle RELAXANT administered orally, intramuscularly, or intravenously in the treatment of painful musculoskeletal conditions.

method (meth'od) a manner of performing something; see also MANEUVER, OPERATION, PROCEDURE, SURGERY, and TECHNIQUE. For names of specific methods, see under the name.

methodology (meth"o-dol'o-je) the science dealing with principles of procedure in research and study.

methohexital (meth"o-hek'sĭ-tal) an ultra-short-acting BARBITURATE; its sodium salt is used as a general anesthetic, a general and local anesthesia adjunct, and a sedative for certain diagnostic procedures in children.

methotrexate (meth"o-trek'sāt) an ANTI-METABOLITE antineoplastic AGENT that inhibits the conversion of FOLIC ACID to tetrahydrofolic acid by binding the enzyme dihydrofolate reductase, thus inhibiting DNA synthesis; it is specific for the S phase of the cell cycle. Used as the base and the sodium salt in the treatment of leukemias, lymphomas, sarcomas, and cancer of the head and neck, breast, colon, lung, testes, and other organs. Called also MTX. It is also used in the treatment of psoriasis and rheumatoid arthritis. Administered orally, intravenously, intramuscularly, intrathecally, or intra-arterially.

methoxamine (mĕ-thok'sah-mēn) a sympathomimetic amine used as a VASOPRESSOR in the treatment of acute hypotensive states, particularly to maintain blood pressure during anesthesia, and also to treat paroxysmal supraventricular TACHY-CARDIA; administered intramuscularly or intravenously.

methoxsalen (mĕ-thok'sah-len) an acrylic acid compound that induces MELANIN production on exposure of the skin to ultraviolet RADIATION; used orally and topically in the treatment of idiopathic VITILIGO, MYCOSIS FUNGOIDES, and PSORIASIS.

methoxyflurane (mĕ-thok"se-floo'rān) a highly potent inhalational anesthetic agent, used primarily to produce analgesia during the first stage of labor; its use in surgery is limited by a dose-related nephrotoxicity to procedures of short duration.

methoxyphenamine (mĕ-thok"se-fen'ah-mēn) a sympathomimetic drug used as a BRONCHODILATOR.

methsuximide (meth-suk'sĭ-mīd) an ANTI-CONVULSANT used in the treatment of petit mal EPILEPSY; administered orally.

methyclothiazide (meth"ĭ-klo-thi'ah-zīd) a thiazide DIURETIC used for the treatment of hypertension and edema.

methyl (meth'il) the chemical group or radical —CH$_3$.

m. salicylate a natural or synthetic oil with a characteristic wintergreen odor and taste; used as a COUNTERIRRITANT in ointments or liniments for muscle pain and also as a flavoring agent. Called also wintergreen oil.

methylate (meth'ĭ-lāt) 1. a compound of methyl alcohol and a base. 2. to add a methyl group to a substance.

methylation (meth"ĭ-la'shun) the addition of methyl groups.

methylbenzethonium (meth"il-ben"zĕ-tho'ne-um) an ammonium compound used in the form of the chloride salt as a disinfectant and local antiinfective agent; it is applied topically to skin coming in contact with urine, feces, or perspiration, and used in a rinse for diapers and linens of babies and incontinent patients. Soap inhibits its action.

methylcellulose (meth"il-sel'u-lōs) a methyl ester of cellulose, used as a bulk LAXATIVE, as a suspending agent for drugs, and applied topically to the cornea during certain ophthalmic procedures to protect and lubricate the cornea.

methylcytosine (meth"il-si'to-sin) a pyrimidine occurring in deoxyribonucleic acid.

methyldopa (meth"il-do'pah) a phenyl-alanine derivative administered orally or intravenously as an ANTIHYPERTENSIVE AGENT.

methyldopate (meth"il-do'pāt) an ethyl ester of METHYLDOPA; its hydrochloride salt is given by intravenous infusion for acute hypertensive CRISIS.

methylene blue (meth'ĭ-lēn) a synthetic organic compound, in dark green crystals or lustrous crystalline powder, used in treatment of methemoglobinemia, as a stain in pathology and bacteriology, and as a diagnostic aid in the detection of the premature rupture of fetal membranes.

methylenedioxyamphetamine **(MDA)** (meth"il-di-ok"se-am-fet'ah-mēn) a hallucinogenic compound chemically related to AMPHETAMINE and MESCALINE; it is widely abused and causes dependence.

3,4-methylenedioxymethamphetamine (meth"ĭ-lēn"di-ok"se-meth"am-fet'ah-mēn) a compound chemically related to AMPHET-AMINE and having HALLUCINOGENIC proper-ties; it is widely abused. Popularly called Ecstasy.

methylergonovine (meth″il-er″go-no′vin) an OXYTOCIC used as the maleate salt especially to prevent or combat postpartum hemorrhage or atony.

methylglucamine (meth″il-gloo′kah-mēn) meglumine.

methylmalonic acid (meth″il-mah-lon′ik) a carboxylic acid that is a structural isomer of succinic acid; occurring in excess in the blood and other body fluids in methylmalon-icacidemia.

methylmalonicacidemia (meth″il-mah-lon″ik-as″ĭ-de′me-ah) 1. an inborn ERROR of metabolism characterized by excessive amounts of METHYLMALONIC ACID in the blood and urine, with developmental retardation, hepatomegaly, intermittent neutropenia, thrombocytopenia, and severe metabolic ACIDOSIS. It is due to any of various defects causing deficiency of activity of an enzyme necessary for using as fuel ISOLEUCINE, THREONINE, VALINE, PROPIONIC ACID, and other fatty acids with odd number chain lengths. 2. excess of methylmalonic acid in the blood.

methylmalonicaciduria (meth″il-mah-lon″ik-as″ĭ-du′re-ah) excess of methylmalo-nic acid in the urine. 1. methylmalonic-acidemia (def. 1).

methylphenidate (meth″il-fenĭ-dāt) a mild central nervous system STIMULANT; the hydrochloride salt is administered orally in the treatment of ATTENTION-DEFICIT/HYPER-ACTIVITY DISORDER and NARCOLEPSY.

methylprednisolone (meth″il-pred-nis′o-lōn) a synthetic GLUCOCORTICOID derived from progesterone, used in replacement therapy for adrenocortical insufficiency and as an antiinflammatory and immunosup-pressant; also used as *m. acetate* and *m. sodium succinate*.

methyltestosterone (meth″il-tes-tos′tĕ-rōn) a synthetic ANDROGEN having actions similar to those of TESTOSTERONE; used in males in the treatment of hypogonad-ism and delayed puberty, and in post-menopausal females in the palliation of metastatic breast carcinoma; administered orally.

methyltransferase (meth″il-trans′fer-ās) any enzyme that catalyzes transmethyla-tion.

methysergide (meth″ĭ-ser′jīd) a potent serotonin antagonist and VASOCONSTRICTOR, used in the prophylaxis of MIGRAINE; also available as the maleate salt.

Meticorten (met″ĭ-kor′ten) trademark fo. a preparation of PREDNISONE, an ANTIINFLAM[MATORY agent.

metipranolol (met″ĭ-pran′ah-lol) a BETA-ADRENERGIC BLOCKING AGENT, applied topically to the conjunctiva as the hydrochloride sal in the treatment of GLAUCOMA and ocula: HYPERTENSION.

metmyoglobin (met-mi″o-glo′bin) a com pound formed from myoglobin by oxidatioɪ of the ferrous to the ferric state witl essentially ionic bonds.

metoclopramide (met″o-klo-prah′mīd a DOPAMINE receptor antagonist and PRO KINETIC agent that stimulates gastriᴄ motility, used as the hydrochloride sal as an ANTIEMETIC, an aid in gastrointes tinal radiology and intestinal intuba ion, and in treatment of GASTROPARESI and gastroesophageal REFLUX; adminis tered orally, intravenously, or intramuscu larly.

metocurine (met″o-ku′rēn) a neuromus cular blocking AGENT used as *metocurinᴇ iodide* to induce skeletal muscle relaxatioɪ during surgery and in convulsive therapy administered intravenously.

metolazone (mĕ-tol′ah-zōn) a diureti(ᴄ with pharmacologic actions similar to thᴇ thiazide DIURETICS; used for treatment o hypertension and edema.

metonymy (mĕ-ton′ĭ-me) a disturbance o language seen in schizophrenia in which aɪ inappropriate but related term is usec instead of the correct one.

metopic (mĕ-top′ik) frontal (def. 1).

metoprolol (mĕ-to′pro-lol) a cardioselec tive BETA-ADRENERGIC BLOCKING AGENT havinɡ a greater effect on β_1-adrenergic receptor of the heart than on the β_2-adrenergiᴄ receptors of the bronchi and blood vessels the tartrate and succinate salts are used iɪ the treatment of HYPERTENSION, ANGIN/ PECTORIS, and MYOCARDIAL INFARCTION; admin istered orally or intravenously.

metoxenous (mĕ-tok′sĕ-nus) requirinɡ two hosts for the entire life cycle; said o parasites.

metr(o)- word element [Gr.], *uterus*.

metra (me′trah) uterus.

metratrophia (me″trah-tro′fe-ah) atrophy of the uterus.

metreurynter (me″troo-rin′ter) an inflat able bag for dilating the cervical canal of thᴇ uterus.

metric (met′rik) 1. pertaining to measures or measurement. 2. having the METER as ε basis.

m. system the system of units of measurement that is based on the METER GRAM, and LITER and in which new units are formed from the basic terms by prefixes denoting multiplication by a power of ten. See also SI UNITS.

metrifonate (met″rĭ-fo′nāt) an organophosphorous compound having potent ANTICHOLINESTERASE activity; used topically against ECTOPARASITES and internally as an ANTHELMINTIC, especially effective against *Schistosoma haematobium*.

metritis (me-tri′tis) inflammation of the uterus.

   m. dis′secans metritis with necrosis of portions of the uterine wall.

   puerperal m. infection of the uterus of the puerperal woman.

metrizamide (mĕ-triz′ah-mīd) a nonionic, water-soluble, iodinated radiographic contrast medium used in myelography and cisternography.

metrocele (me′tro-sēl) hysterocele.

metrocolpocele (me″tro-kol′po-sēl) hernia of the uterus with vaginal prolapse.

metrocystosis (me″tro-sis-to′sis) formation of cysts in the uterus.

metroleukorrhea (me″tro-lu″ko-re′ah) leukorrhea of uterine origin.

metrolymphangitis (me″tro-limf″an-ji′tis) inflammation of the uterine lymphatic vessels.

metromalacia abnormal softening of the uterus.

metronidazole (mĕ″tro-nid′ah-zōl) an ANTIBACTERIAL and antiprotozoal AGENT effective against obligate anaerobes; used as the base, administered orally and intravaginally in *Trichomonas vaginalis* infection in females and orally in *T. vaginalis* infection in males and in intestinal AMEBIASIS. It is used orally or intravenously in extraintestinal amebiasis and infection by obligate anaerobic bacteria and intravenously for the prophylaxis of colonic perioperative infection. It is also used topically in the treatment of ROSACEA. The hydrochloride salt is administered intravenously for the same indications for which the base is used intravenously.

metropathy (me-trop′ah-the) hysteropathy. adj., **metropath′ic.**

metroperitoneal (me″tro-per″ĭ-to-ne′al) pertaining to the uterus and peritoneum.

metroperitonitis (me″tro-per″ĭ-to-ni′tis) inflammation of the peritoneum about the uterus.

metrophlebitis (me″tro-flĕ-bi′tis) inflammation of the uterine veins.

metroplasty (me′tro-plas″te) plastic surgery on the uterus; called also *uteroplasty*.

metroptosis (me″tro-to′sis) prolapse of uterus.

metrorrhagia (me″tro-ra′je-ah) uterine bleeding, usually of normal amount, occurring at completely irregular intervals, the period of flow sometimes being prolonged.

metrorrhea (me″tro-re′ah) abnormal uterine discharge.

metrorrhexis (me″tro-rek′sis) rupture of the uterus.

metrosalpingitis (me″tro-sal″pin-ji′tis) inflammation of the uterus and fallopian tubes.

metroscope (me′tro-skōp) hysteroscope.

metrostaxis (me″tro-stak′sis) slight but persistent uterine bleeding.

metrostenosis (me″tro-stĕ-no′sis) stenosis of the uterus.

-metry word element [Gr.], *measurement.*

metyrapone (mĕ-tēr′ah-pōn) a synthetic compound that selectively inhibits an enzyme responsible for the biosynthesis of CORTICOSTEROIDS; it is used as a diagnostic aid in a test of pituitary reserve.

metyrosine (mĕ-ti′ro-sēn) α-methyl-L-tyrosine, an inhibitor of CATECHOLAMINE synthesis used to control hypertensive attacks in PHEOCHROMOCYTOMA.

MeV megaelectron volt.

mexiletine (mek′sĭ-lĕ-tēn) an agent used as the hydrochloride salt in treatment of ventricular ARRHYTHMIAS.

Meyer (mi′er) Adolf (1866–1950). Swiss-born psychiatrist in the United States who directed the development of the Henry Phipps Psychiatric Clinic at Johns Hopkins University. His major contributions include propounding the theory of PSYCHOBIOLOGY, standardizing case histories, and reforming mental health institutions (which were called "insane asylums" at that time).

mezlocillin (mez″lo-sil′in) a broad-spectrum PENICILLIN antibiotic used parenterally for treatment of serious infections due to susceptible organisms.

μF microfarad.

MFD minimum fatal dose.

Mg magnesium.

mg milligram.

μg microgram.

MHA-TP microhemagglutination assay–*Treponema pallidum.*

MHC major histocompatibility complex.

MHz megahertz.

mication (mi-ka′shun) a quick motion, such as winking.

micelle (mi-sel′) a supermolecular colloid particle, most often a packet of chain molecules in parallel arrangement.

miconazole (mi-kon′ah-zōl) an imidazole antifungal AGENT used as the nitrate salt, topically to treat cutaneous dermatophytic infections such as ATHLETE'S FOOT and intravaginally to treat vulvovaginal CANDIDIASIS.

micr(o)- word element [Gr.], *small;* also used in naming units of measurement (symbol μ) to designate an amount one millionth (10^{-6}) the size of the unit to which it is joined, e.g., microgram.

micrencephaly (mi″kren-sef′ah-le) abnormal smallness and underdevelopment of the brain.

microabrasion (mi′kro-ə-bra″zhun) removal of minute amounts of dental enamel using an ABRASIVE compound in order to correct enamel defects.

microabscess (mi″kro-ab′ses) an abscess visible only under a microscope.

Pautrier's m. one of the well-defined collections of mycosis cells located within the epidermis in T-cell lymphoma and mycosis fungoides.

microaerophilic (mi″kro-ar″o-fil′ik) requiring oxygen for growth but at lower concentration than is present in the atmosphere; said of bacteria.

microaggregate (mi″kro-ag′rĕ-gat) a microscopic collection of particles, as of platelets, leukocytes, and fibrin, that occurs in stored blood.

microalbuminuria (mi″kro-al-bu″min-u′re-ah) an increase in urinary ALBUMIN excretion too subtle to be measured by conventional means, often seen with the HYPERFILTRATION of DIABETES MELLITUS.

microanalysis (mi″kro-ah-nal′ĭ-sis) the chemical analysis of minute quantities of material.

microanatomy (mi″kro-ah-nat′o-me) histology.

microaneurysm (mi″kro-an′u-rizm) a minute aneurysm occurring on a vessel of small size, or such as occurs in thrombotic purpura.

microangiopathy (mi″kro-an″je-op′ah-the) a disorder involving the small blood vessels. adj., **microangiopath′ic.**

thrombotic m. formation of thrombi in the arterioles and capillaries; proposed name for a syndrome that would include both thrombotic thrombocytopenic PURPURA and HEMOLYTIC UREMIC SYNDROME.

microbe (mi′krōb) a MICROORGANISM, especially a pathogenic one such as a BACTERIUM, PROTOZOAN, or FUNGUS. adj., **micro′bial, micro′bic.**

microbicide (mi-kro′bĭ-sīd) an agent that destroys microbes; see also ANTIMICROBIAL AGENT. adj., **microbici′dal.**

microbiologist (mi″kro-bi-ol′o-jist) a specialist in microbiology.

microbiology (mi″kro-bi-ol′o-je) the study of microorganisms, including algae, bacteria, fungi, viruses, and protozoa. adj., **microbiolog′ical.**

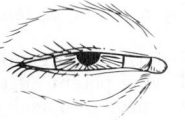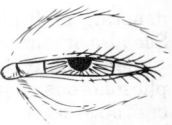

Microblepharia. From Dorland's, 2000.

microbiota (mi″kro-bi-o′tah) the microscopic living organisms of a region. adj., **microbiot′ic.**

microblast (mi′kro-blast) an erythroblast of 5 μm or less in diameter.

microblepharia (mi″kro-blĕ-far′e-ah) abnormal shortness of the vertical dimensions of the eyelids.

microbody (mi′kro-bod″e) any of the cytoplasmic particles found in kidney and liver cells and in certain other cells, surrounded by a limiting membrane, and containing dense crystalline-like inclusions and oxidases.

microbrachius (mi″kro-bra′ke-us) a fetus with abnormally small or rudimentary upper limbs.

microcardia (mi″kro-kahr′de-ah) abnormal smallness of the heart.

microcephalus (mi″kro-sef′ah-lus) an individual with a very small head.

microcephaly (mi″kro-sef′ah-le) small size of the head in relation to the rest of the body. adj., **microcephal′ic.**

microcheilia (mi″kro-ki′le-ah) abnormal smallness of the lip.

microcheiria (mi″kro-ki′re-ah) abnormal smallness of the hands.

microcirculation (mi″kro-ser″ku-la′shun) the flow of blood through the MICROVASCULATURE. adj., **microcir′culatory.**

Micrococcaceae (mi″kro-kok-a′se-e) a family of gram-positive, aerobic or facultatively anaerobic bacteria containing the genera *Staphylococcus* and *Micrococcus.*

Micrococcus (mi″kro-kok′us) a genus of gram-positive bacteria of the family Micrococcaceae, usually found in soil, water, dust, or dairy products.

micrococcus (mi″kro-kok′us) [Gr.] 1. any organism of the genus *Micrococcus.* 2. a very small, spherical microorganism.

microcolon (mi″kro-ko′lon) abnormal smallness of the colon.

microcoria (mi″kro-ko′re-ah) smallness of the pupil.

microcornea (mi″kro-kor′ne-ah) unusual smallness of the cornea, usually bilateral.

microcrystalline (mi″kro-kris′tah-lin) made up of minute crystals.

microcurie (μCi) (mi″kro-ku′re) one millionth (10^{-6}) of a CURIE.

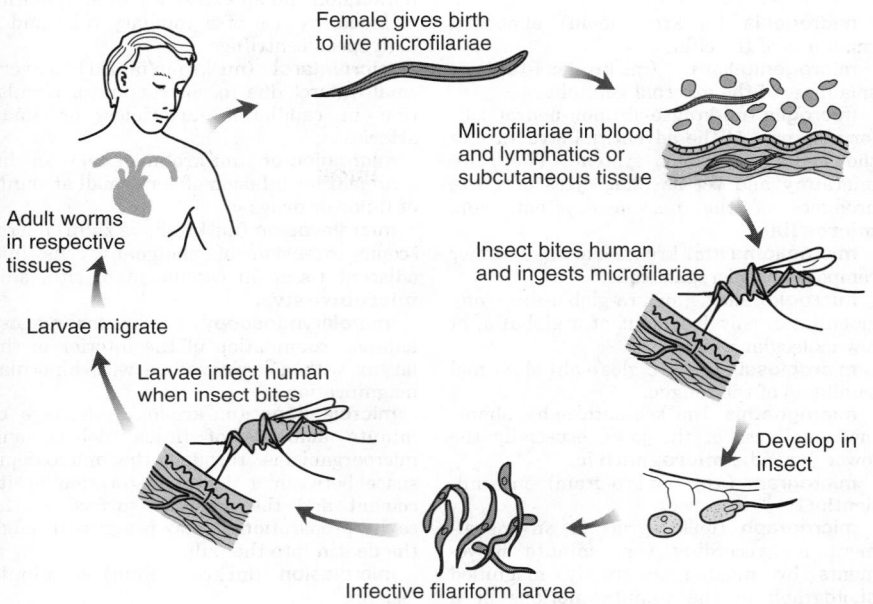

Female gives birth
to live microfilariae

Microfilariae in blood
and lymphatics or
subcutaneous tissue

Adult worms
in respective
tissues

Insect bites human
and ingests microfilariae

Larvae migrate

Larvae infect human
when insect bites

Develop in
insect

Infective filariform larvae
migrate to insect salivary gland

Generalized life cycle of microfilariae. From Mahon and Manuselis, 2000.

M

microcyst (mi′kro-sist) a cyst visible only under a microscope.

microcyte (mi′kro-sīt) an erythrocyte 5 μm or less in diameter. adj., **microcyt′ic.**

microcythemia (mi″kro-si-the′me-ah) a condition in which the erythrocytes are smaller than normal; see also microcytic ANEMIA. Called also microcytosis.

microcytosis microcythemia.

microdactyly (mi″kro-dak′tĭ-le) abnormal smallness of the fingers or toes.

microdissection (mi″kro-dĭ-sek′shun) dissection of tissue or cells under the microscope.

microdiskectomy (mi″kro-dis-kek′tah-me) debulking of a HERNIATED DISK using an operating microscope or loupe for magnification.

microdontia (mi″kro-don′she-ah) abnormal smallness of the teeth.

microdrepanocytic (mi″kro-drep″ah-no-sit′ik) containing microcytic and drepanocytic elements, as in sickle cell–thalassemia disease.

microembolus (mi″kro-em′bo-lus) [L.] an embolus of microscopic size.

microerythrocyte (mi″kro-ĕ-rith′ro-sīt) microcyte.

microfarad (μF) (mi″kro-far′ad) one millionth (10^{-6}) of a FARAD.

microfibril (mi″kro-fi′bril) an extremely small fibril.

microfilament (mi″kro-fil′ah-ment) any of the submicroscopic filaments, composed chiefly of actin, found in the cytoplasmic matrix of almost all cells, often in close association with the microtubules.

microfilaremia (mi″kro-fil′ah-re′me-ah) the presence of microfilariae in the circulating blood.

microfilaria (mi″kro-fi-lar″e-ah) the pre-larval stage of Filarioidea in the blood of humans and in the tissues of the vector. This term is sometimes incorrectly used as a genus name, and is then spelled with a capital M.

microflora (mi′kro-flor″ah) bacteria present in the large intestine.

microgamete (mi″kro-gam′ēt) 1. the smaller, actively motile male gamete that fertilizes the female gamete (MACROGAMETE) in sexual REPRODUCTION. 2. the smaller of two types of malarial parasites; see GAMETE (def. 2).

microgametocyte (mi″kro-gah-me′to-sīt) a cell that produces microgametes. 1. the male gametocyte of certain Sporozoa, such as malarial plasmodia.

microgastria (mi″kro-gas′tre-ah) congenital smallness of the stomach.

microgenia (mi″kro-je′ne-ah) abnormal smallness of the chin.

microgenitalism (mi″kro-jen′ĭ-tal-izm) smallness of the external genitalia.

microglia (mi-krog′le-ah) non-neural cells forming part of the adventitial structure of the central nervous system. They are migratory and act as phagocytes of waste products of the nervous system. adj., **microg′lial.**

microglioma (mi″kro-gli-o′mah) a tumor composed of microglial cells.

microglobulin (mi″kro-glob′u-lin) any globulin, or any fragment of a globulin, of low molecular weight.

microglossia (mi″kro-glos′e-ah) abnormal smallness of the tongue.

micrognathia (mi″kro-nath′e-ah) abnormal smallness of the jaws, especially the lower jaw. adj., **micrognath′ic.**

microgram (μg) (mi′kro-gram) one millionth (10^{-6}) of a GRAM.

micrograph (mi′kro-graf) 1. an instrument for recording very minute movements by making a greatly magnified photograph of the minute motions of a diaphragm. 2. a photograph of a minute object or specimen as seen through a microscope.

 electron m. a graphic reproduction of an object as viewed with an electron microscope.

microgyria (mi″kro-ji′re-ah) abnormal smallness of convolutions of the brain.

microgyrus (mi″kro-ji′rus) an abnormally small, malformed convolution of the brain.

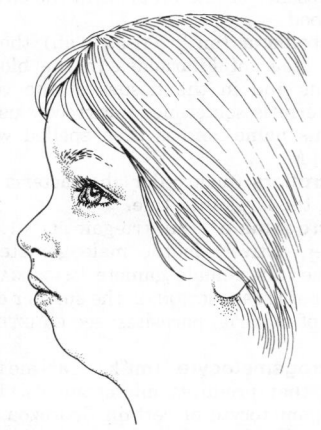

Micrognathia. This characteristic is the hallmark of the child with arthritis of the neck or joints of the jaw. From Betz et al., 1994.

microhematocrit a hematocrit determination done on an extremely small quantity of blood, by use of a capillary tube and a high speed centrifuge.

microinfarct (mi″kro-in′fahrkt) a very small infarct due to obstruction of circulation in capillaries, arterioles, or small arteries.

microinjector (mi″kro-in-jek′ter) an instrument for infusion of very small amounts of fluids or drugs.

microinvasion (mi″kro-in-va′zhun) microscopic extension of malignant cells into adjacent tissue in carcinoma in situ. adj., **microinva′sive.**

microlaryngoscopy (mi″kro-lar″ing-gos′-kah-pe) examination of the interior of the larynx with a laryngoscope with binocular magnification.

microleakage (mi″kro-lēk′aj) leakage of minute amounts of fluids, debris, and microorganisms through the microscopic space between a dental restoration or its cement and the adjacent surface of the cavity preparation; it may progress through the dentin into the pulp.

microlesion (mi′kro-le″zhun) a minute lesion.

microliter (μL) (mi′kro-le″ter) one millionth (10^{-6}) of a LITER.

microlith (mi′kro-lith″) a minute concretion or calculus.

microlithiasis (mi″kro-lĭ-thi′ah-sis) the formation of minute concretions in an organ.

 m. alveola′ris pulmo′num, pulmonary alveolar m. a condition simulating pulmonary tuberculosis, with deposition of minute calculi in the alveoli of the lungs.

micrology (mi-krol′o-je) the science dealing with the handling and preparation of materials for microscopic study.

micromanipulation (mi″kro-mah-nip″u-la′shun) 1. surgery, injection, dissection, or other techniques done with MICROMANIPULATORS. 2. in male factor INFERTILITY, the processing of GAMETES, as by partial removal of the ZONA PELLUCIDA or direct injection of sperm into the egg, in order to increase the possibility of FERTILIZATION.

micromanipulator (mi″kro-mah-nip′u-la″-ter) an instrument for moving, dissecting, or otherwise manipulating minute specimens under the microscope.

micromastia (mi″kro-mas′te-ah) abnormal smallness of the breast.

micromelia (mi″kro-me′le-ah) abnormal smallness of one or more limbs.

micromelus (mi-krom′ĕ-lus) an individual with abnormally small limbs.

micromere (mi′kro-mēr) one of the small BLASTOMERES formed at the animal pole by unequal cleavage of a fertilized ovum; see also MACROMERE.

micrometer[1] (mi-krom′ĕ-ter) an instrument for making minute measurements.

micrometer[2] **(μm)** (mi′kro-me″ter) one millionth (10^{-6}) of a METER.

micromethod (mi″kro-meth″od) a technique dealing with exceedingly small quantities of material.

micrometry (mi-krom′ĕ-tre) measurement of microscopic objects.

micromolar (mi″kro-mo′ler) denoting a concentration of one millionth (10^{-6}) of a mole per liter.

micromyelia (mi″kro-mi-e′le-ah) abnormal smallness or shortness of the spinal cord.

micromyeloblast (mi″kro-mi′ĕ-lo-blast″) a small, immature myelocyte. adj., **micro-myeloblas′tic.**

Micronase (mi′kro-nās) trademark for a preparation of GLYBURIDE, an oral HYPOGLY-CEMIC used for type 2 DIABETES MELLITUS.

microneedle (mi″kro-ne′d′l) a fine glass needle used in micromanipulation.

microneurosurgery (mi″kro-nŏŏ″ro-ser′-jer-e) surgery conducted under high magnification with miniaturized instruments on microscopic vessels and structures of the nervous system.

micronodular (mi″kro-nod′u-ler) marked by the presence of small nodules.

micronucleus (mi″kro-noo′kle-us) 1. in ciliate protozoa, the kinetoplast, the smaller of two types of nucleus in each cell, which functions in sexual reproduction. 2. a small nucleus. 3. nucleolus.

micronutrient (mi″kro-noo′tre-ent) a dietary element essential only in small quantities, such as SELENIUM, COPPER, or MANGANESE.

micronychia (mi″kro-nik′e-ah) abnormal smallness of the nails of the fingers or toes.

micro-orchidism (mi″kro-or′kĭ-dizm) abnormal smallness of the testis.

microorganism (mi″kro-or′gah-nizm) a microscopic organism; those of medical interest include bacteria, fungi, and protozoa. Viruses are often classified as microorganisms, although they are sometimes excluded because they are not cellular and they are unable to replicate without a host cell.

micropathology (mi″kro-pah-thol′o-je) 1. the sum of what is known about minute pathologic change. 2. pathology of diseases caused by microorganisms.

micropenis (mi″kro-pe′nis) abnormal smallness of the penis; called also microphallus.

microphage (mi′kro-fāj) a small PHAGO-CYTE; an actively motile NEUTROPHIL capable of phagocytosis.

microphakia (mi″kro-fa′ke-ah) abnormal smallness of the crystalline lens.

microphallus (mi″kro-fal′us) micropenis.

microphone (mi′kro-fōn) a device to pick up sound for purposes of amplification or transmission.

microphonic (mi″kro-fon′ik) 1. serving to amplify sound. 2. cochlear microphonic.

  cochlear m. any of the electrical PO-TENTIALS generated in the hair CELLS of the organ of Corti in response to acoustic stimulation.

microphotograph (mi″kro-fo′to-graf) a photograph of small size.

microphthalmia (mi″krof-thal′me-ah) microphthalmos.

microphthalmos (mi″krof-thal′mus) a developmental defect causing moderate or severe reduction in size of the eye.

micropinocytosis (mi″kro-pi″no-si-to′sis) the taking up into a cell of specific macromolecules by invagination of the plasma membrane, which is then pinched off, resulting in small vesicles in the cytoplasm.

micropipet (mi″kro-pi-pet′) a pipet for handling small quantities of liquids (up to 1 mL).

microplethysmography (mi″kro-pleth″iz-mog′rah-fe) the recording of minute changes in the size of a part as produced by circulation of blood.

micropodia (mi″kro-po′de-ah) abnormal smallness of the feet.

microprobe (mi′kro-prōb″) a minute probe, as one used in microsurgery.

micropsia (mi-krop′se-ah) a disorder of visual perception in which objects appear smaller than their actual size.

micropuncture (mi′kro-punk″cher) 1. the creation of minute openings by piercing. 2. in renal physiology, the process by which nephron segments are pierced.

microradiography (mi″kro-ra″de-og′rah-fe) radiography under conditions that permit subsequent microscopic examination or enlargement of the radiograph up to several hundred linear magnifications.

microreentry (mi″kro-re-en′tre) REENTRY involving a small circuit, such as one within the atrioventricular node or Purkinje fibers.

microrespirometer (mi″kro-res″pĭ-rom′ĕ-ter) an apparatus for investigating oxygen utilization in isolated tissues.

microscope (mi′kro-skōp) an instrument used to obtain an enlarged image of small objects and reveal details of structure not otherwise distinguishable.

  acoustic m. one using very high frequency ultrasound waves, which are

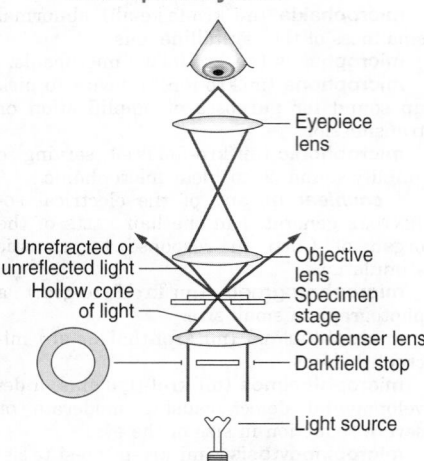

Eyepiece
lens

Unrefracted or
unreflected light
Hollow cone
of light

Objective
lens
Specimen
stage
Condenser lens
Darkfield stop

Light source

The light path of a darkfield microscope. From Hart and
Shears, 1997.

focused on the object; the reflected beam is
converted to an image by electronic processing.

binocular m. one with two eyepieces,
permitting use of both eyes simultaneously.

compound m. one consisting of two
lens systems whereby the image formed by
the system near the object is magnified by
the one nearer the eye.

darkfield m. one so constructed that
illumination is from the side of the field so
that details appear light against a dark
background.

electron m. one in which an electron
beam, instead of light, forms an image for
viewing, allowing much greater magnification and resolution. The image may be
viewed on a fluorescent screen or may be
photographed. Types include *scanning* and
transmission electron microscopes.

fluorescence m. one used for the examination of specimens stained with fluor-
ochromes or fluorochrome complexes, e.g., a
fluorescein-labeled antibody, which fluo-
resces in ultraviolet light.

light m. one in which the specimen is
viewed under ordinary illumination.

operating m. one designed for use in
performance of delicate surgical procedures,
e.g., on the middle ear or small vessels of
the heart.

phase m., phase-contrast m. a microscope that alters the phase relationships
of the light passing through and that passing around the object, the contrast permitting visualization of the object without the

necessity for staining or other special
preparation.

scanning electron m. (SEM) an electron microscope that produces a high magnification image of the surface of a metal-
coated specimen by scanning an electron
beam and building an image from the
electrons reflected at each point.

simple m. one that consists of a single
lens.

slit lamp m. a corneal microscope with
a special attachment that permits examination of the endothelium on the posterior
surface of the cornea.

stereoscopic m. a binocular microscope modified to give a three-dimensional
view of the specimen.

transmission electron m. (TEM) an electron microscope that produces highly magnified images of ultrathin tissue sections or
other specimens. An electron beam passes
through the metal-impregnated specimen
and is focused by magnetic lenses into an
image.

x-ray m. one in which x-rays are used
instead of light, the image usually being
reproduced on film.

microscopic (mi″kro-skop′ik) 1. of extremely small size; visible only by the aid of
a microscope. 2. pertaining or relating to a
microscope or to microscopy.

microscopist (mi-kros′ko-pist) a person
skilled in using the microscope.

microscopy (mi-kros′kah-pe) examination with a microscope.

fluorescence m. conjugation of antibodies with fluorescent dyes in order to identify specific microorganisms or tissue constituents; see also FLUORESCENCE MICROSCOPY.

microsecond (μs) (mi′kro-sek″ond) one
millionth (10^{-6}) of a second.

microshock (mi′kro-shok″) a small electric shock resulting from current that has
passed directly into the cardiac tissue from
an electrode in contact with it; in this
situation extremely small amounts of
current may produce FIBRILLATION.

microsome (mi′kro-sōm) any of the
vesicular fragments of endoplasmic reticulum produced during disruption and centrifugation of cells. adj., **microso′mal.**

microsomia (mi″kro-so′me-ah) abnormally small size of the body.

microspectroscope (mi″kro-spek′tro-
skōp) a spectroscope and microscope combined.

microspherocyte (mi″kro-sfēr′o-sīt) an
erythrocyte whose diameter is less than
normal, but whose thickness is increased.

microspherocytosis (mi″kro-sfēr′ro-si-
to′sis) the presence in the blood of an
excessive number of microspherocytes.

microsphygmia (mi″kro-sfig′me-ah) that condition of the pulse in which it is perceived with difficulty by the finger.

microsplenia (mi″kro-sple′ne-ah) smallness of the spleen.

microsporid (mi-kros′po-rid) a secondary skin eruption that is an expression of hypersensitivity to *Microsporum* infection.

Microsporum (mi″kro-spor′um) a genus of fungi that cause diseases of the skin and hair such as TINEA CAPITIS and TINEA CORPORIS. Species include *M. audoui′nii, M. ca′nis (M. lano′sum)*, and *M. ful′vum (M. gyp′seum)*.

Microstix-3 (mi′kro-stiks) trademark for a reagent strip with a chemical test area for recognition of nitrite in urine that turns pink on contact with nitrate, and two culture areas for semiquantification of bacterial growth after 18 to 24 hours of incubation; one culture area supports both gram-negative and gram-positive organisms; the other, only gram-negative organisms.

microstomia (mi″kro-sto′me-ah) abnormally decreased size of the mouth.

microsurgery (mi″kro-ser′jer-e) dissection of minute structures under the microscope with the use of extremely small instruments. With increasingly sophisticated operating microscopes surgeons are able to perform tissue transfers without the cumbersome standard transfer procedures, such as the tubed pedicle graft and cross-leg flap, that were once necessary to ensure adequate blood supply to the grafted part. Microvascular surgery permits anastomosis of peripheral blood vessels less than 2 mm in diameter. Similarly, microneural techniques allow the surgeon to reestablish sensation by repairing or replacing severed and damaged peripheral nerves. Because of the advances in microsurgery, it is possible to reattach amputated parts, provided the health status of the patient and the condition of the amputated part are favorable.

microsyringe (mi″kro-sĭ-rinj′) a syringe fitted with a screw-threaded micrometer for accurate measurement of minute quantities.

microtia (mi-kro′she-ah) abnormal smallness of the pinna of the ear.

microtiter (mi″kro-ti′ter) a titer of minute quantity.

microtome (mi′kro-tōm) an instrument for making thin sections for microscopic study.

   freezing m. one for cutting frozen tissues.

   rotary m. one in which wheel action is translated into a back-and-forth movement of the specimen being sectioned.

   sliding m. one in which the specimen being sectioned is made to slide on a track.

microtomy (mi-krot′ah-me) the cutting of thin sections.

microtrauma (mi″kro-traw′mah) a microscopic lesion or injury.

microtubule (mi″kro-tu′būl) any of the slender, tubular structures, composed chiefly of tubulin, found in the cytoplasmic ground substance of nearly all cells; they are involved in maintenance of cell shape and in the movements of organelles and inclusions, and form the spindle fibers of mitosis.

microvasculature (mi″kro-vas′ku-lah-chur″) the finer vessels of the body, such as the arterioles, capillaries, and venules. adj., **microvas′cular.**

microvillus (mi″kro-vil′us) a minute process or protrusion from the free surface of a cell, found especially in the proximal convolution of renal tubules and the intestinal epithelium. See illustration.

microvolt (μV) (mi′kro-vōlt) one millionth (10^{-6}) of a VOLT.

microwave (mi′kro-wāv) a wave typical of electromagnetic radiation between far infrared and radiowaves.

micrurgy (mi′krur-je) manipulative technique in the field of a microscope. adj., **micrur′gic.**

Micruroides (mi″kroo-roi′dēz) a genus of venomous coral SNAKES found in Mexico and the southwestern United States. See also SNAKEBITE.

Micrurus (mi-kroo′rus) a genus of venomous coral SNAKES, including a species found in the southeastern United States and south into Central America. See also SNAKEBITE.

micturate (mik′tu-rāt) urinate.

M

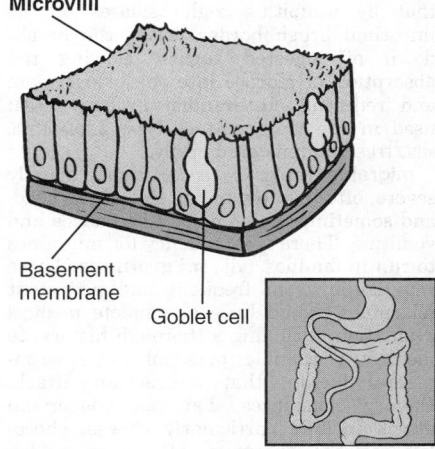

Microvilli

Basement membrane

Goblet cell

Microvilli in the intestinal tract. From Applegate, 1992.

micturition (mik″tu-rish′un) urination.

Midamor (mi′dah-mor) trademark for a preparation of AMILORIDE hydrochloride; a potassium sparing DIURETIC.

midazolam (mid-az′o-lam) a sedative of the BENZODIAZEPINE class used in the induction of anesthesia.

midbrain (mid′brān) mesencephalon.

middle lobe syndrome lobar ATELECTASIS in the right middle lobe of the lung, with chronic pneumonitis; called also Brock syndrome.

midget (mij′et) old term for a normal DWARF.

midgut (mid′gut) the region of the embryonic digestive tube into which the yolk sac opens; ahead of it is the foregut and caudal to it is the hindgut.

midline (mid′līn) the imaginary line that divides the body into right and left halves.

midodrine (mi′do-drēn″) a VASOPRESSOR used as the hydrochloride salt in treatment of orthostatic HYPOTENSION; administered orally.

midwife (mid′wīf) a person who assists at childbirth but who is not a physician.

    nurse-m. see NURSE-MIDWIFE.

midwifery (mid′wif-re, mid′wi-fer-e) the practice of assisting at childbirth.

MIF (mif) migration inhibition factor; migration inhibitory factor.

    MIF test migration inhibitory factor test.

mifepristone (mif″ĕ-pris′tōn) an ANTIPROGESTIN used with MISOPROSTOL or other prostaglandin to terminate pregnancy in the first trimester; administered orally. Called also RU-486.

miglitol (mig′lĭ-tol) an ANTIDIABETIC agent that by inhibiting α-glucosidases of the intestinal brush border delays the breakdown of ingested sugars, slowing the absorption of glucose into the bloodstream and reducing postprandial HYPERGLYCEMIA; used in the treatment of type 2 DIABETES MELLITUS, administered orally.

migraine (mi′grān) a HEADACHE, usually severe, often limited to one side of the head, and sometimes accompanied by nausea and vomiting. There is a tendency for migraines to run in families. adj., **mi′grainous.** Those who suffer from frequent and persistent migraines should have a complete medical evaluation, including a thorough history, to identify, if possible, personal and environmental factors that trigger an attack. Dietary substances that can trigger an attack include particularly cheese, chocolate, alcohol, excessive caffeine or sudden withdrawal from caffeine-rich foods, and some food preservatives, such as monosodium glutamate, and artificial flavorings. Skipping meals and fasting can also trigger a headache in certain people. Drugs that are known to precipitate migraines include hormonal CONTRACEPTIVES and the ANTIHYPERTENSIVE AGENT RESERPINE.

The selection of medications for relief of migraines should be based on the individual patient's history, symptoms, and needs. There are a wide variety of medications available; analgesics may or may not be effective. Nonpharmaceutical methods are preferred by some patients. The patient should be involved in the choice of treatment.

A consortium of experts has developed evidence-based guidelines for the diagnosis, treatment, and prevention of migraine. Those are available by writing the American Academy of Neurology, 1080 Montreal Ave., St. Paul MN 55116 or referring to their web site at http://www.aan.org. Additional information about migraines can be obtained by writing to The National Headache Foundation, 428 W. James Place, Chicago, IL 60614, or referring to their web site at http://www.headaches.org.

    abdominal m. migraine in which abdominal symptoms are prominent.

migration inhibitory factor test an *in vitro* test for the production of migration inhibitory FACTOR (MIF) by LYMPHOCYTES in response to specific antigens; used for evaluation of cell-mediated IMMUNITY. MIF production is absent in certain IMMUNODEFICIENCY disorders, such as WISKOTT-ALDRICH SYNDROME and HODGKIN'S DISEASE. Called also MIF test.

Mikulicz's disease (mik′u-lich″ez) originally, a chronic, benign, and usually painless inflammatory swelling of the lacrimal and salivary glands; some authorities have broadened the entity to include lacrimal and salivary gland enlargement associated with other diseases, such as SJÖGREN'S SYNDROME, SARCOIDOSIS, LUPUS ERYTHEMATOSUS, LEUKEMIA, LYMPHOMA, and TUBERCULOSIS, which they designate *Mikulicz's syndrome.*

miliaria (mil″e-ar′e-ah) a cutaneous condition with retention of sweat, which is extravasated at different levels in the skin. Treatment is directed at reducing sweating by reducing the external heat load and avoiding irritating agents and tight clothing. Bland powders may be helpful. Called also prickly heat and heat rash.

miliary (mil′e-ar″e) 1. like millet seeds. 2. characterized by the formation of lesions resembling millet seeds.

milieu (me-lyuh′) [Fr.] surroundings; environment.

m. extérieur (me-lyuh′ ek-sta″re-ur′) external environment.

m. intérieur (me-lyuh′ an-ta″re-ur′) internal environment; the blood and lymph in which the cells are bathed.

milium (mil′e-um) [L.] a white nodule in the skin, especially of the face, usually 1 to 4 mm in diameter, a spheroidal epithelial cyst of lamellated keratin lying just under the epidermis, often associated with vellus hair follicles. Those in the newborn usually appear on the nose and sometimes the cheeks for several weeks after birth. Popularly called whitehead.

milk (milk) 1. a nutrient fluid produced by the mammary gland of many animals for nourishment of young mammals. 2. a liquid (emulsion or suspension) resembling the secretion of the mammary gland.

acidophilus m. milk fermented with cultures of *Lactobacillus acidophilus;* used in gastrointestinal disorders to modify the bacterial flora of the intestinal tract.

m.-alkali syndrome ingestion of milk and absorbable alkali in excess amounts, resulting in kidney damage and elevated blood calcium levels.

casein m. a prepared milk containing very little salt or sugar and a large amount of fat and casein.

condensed m. milk that has been partly evaporated and sweetened with sugar.

dialyzed m. milk from which the sugar has been removed by dialysis through a parchment membrane.

evaporated m. milk prepared by evaporation of half of its water content.

m. fever an endemic fever said to be due to the use of unwholesome cow's milk.

fortified m. milk made more nutritious by addition of milk protein, vitamin A, or vitamin D.

homogenized m. milk treated so the fats form a permanent emulsion and the cream does not separate.

m. of magnesia a suspension of magnesium hydroxide, used as an ANTACID and LAXATIVE.

modified m. cow's milk made to correspond to the composition of human milk.

protein m. milk modified to have a relatively low content of carbohydrate and fat and a relatively high protein content.

witch's m. milk secreted in the breast of a newborn infant.

Milkman syndrome (milk′man) a generalized bone disease marked by multiple transparent stripes of absorption in the long and flat bones.

Miller-Abbott tube (mil′er-ab′ot) a double-channel intestinal tube with an inflatable balloon at its distal end, used for diagnosing and treating obstructive lesions of the small intestine. The tube is inserted via a nostril and gently passed through the stomach and into the small intestine.

The Miller-Abbott tube is often used in the treatment of INTESTINAL OBSTRUCTION. Care must be used in irrigating the tube and in attaching it to a suction apparatus because of the possibility of confusing the two lumina. The lumen marked "suction" is used for irrigations and suction; the other lumen leads to the small rubber bag intended to hold the tube in place. The introduction of too large an amount of fluid into the bag could lead to rupture of the intestine.

milli- word element [L.], *one thousand;* also used in naming units of measurement (symbol m) to designate an amount 10^{-3} the size of the unit to which it is joined, e.g., milligram.

milliamperage (mil″e-am′per-ij) in radiography, the x-ray tube current during an exposure, measured in milliamperes.

milliampere (mA) (mil″e-am′pēr) one thousandth (10^{-3}) of an AMPERE.

milliampere-second a unit of radiographic exposure equal to the product of the milliamperage and the exposure time in seconds. Abbreviated mAs.

milliequivalent (mEq) (mil″e-e-kwiv′ah-lent) one thousandth (10^{-3}) of a chemical equivalent (see equivalent WEIGHT). Concentrations of electrolytes are often expressed as milliequivalents per liter, which is an expression of the chemical combining power of the electrolyte in a fluid.

milligram (mg) (mil′ĭ-gram) one thousandth (10^{-3}) of a GRAM.

milliliter (mL) (mil′ĭ-le″ter) one thousandth (10^{-3}) of a liter.

millimeter (mm) (mil′ĭ-me″ter) one thousandth (10^{-3}) of a METER; equivalent to 0.039 inch.

millimolar (mM) (mil′ĭ-mo″ler) denoting a concentration of 1 millimole per liter.

millimole (mmol) (mil′ĭ-mōl) one thousandth (10^{-3}) of a mole (see MOLE[1]).

milliosmole (mOsm) (mil″e-oz′mōl) one thousandth (10^{-3}) of an OSMOLE.

Millipore filter (mil′ĭ-por) trademark for a device used to filter nutrient solutions as they are administered intravenously.

millirad (mrad) (mil′ĭ-rad) one thousandth (10^{-3}) of a RAD.

millirem (mrem) (mil′ĭ-rem) one thousandth (10^{-3}) of a REM.

M

milliroentgen (mR) (mil'ĭ-rent″gen) one thousandth (10^{-3}) of a ROENTGEN.

millisecond (ms) (mil' ĭ -sek″ und) one thousandth (10^{-3}) of a second.

millivolt (mV) (mil'ĭ-vōlt) one thousandth (10^{-3}) of a VOLT.

milphosis (mil-fo'sis) the falling out of the eyelashes.

milrinone (mil'rĭ-nōn) a CARDIOTONIC used in treatment of congestive HEART FAILURE.

Milroy disease (mil'roi) hereditary permanent LYMPHEDEMA of the lower limbs due to lymphatic obstruction; called also congenital lymphedema.

Miltown (mil'town) trademark for a preparation of MEPROBAMATE, an ANTIANXIETY AGENT.

min. minim; minimum; minute.

Minamata disease (min″ah-mah'tah) a severe neurologic disorder due to alkyl MERCURY POISONING, leading to severe permanent neurologic and mental disabilities or death; once common among those who ate contaminated seafood from Minamata Bay, Japan.

mind (mīnd) 1. the organ or seat of CONSCIOUSNESS; the faculty by which one is aware of surroundings and by which one is able to experience emotions, remember, reason, and make decisions. 2. the organized totality of an organism's mental and psychological processes, conscious and unconscious. 3. the characteristic thought process of a person or group.

mineral (min'er-al) any naturally occurring nonorganic homogeneous solid substance. There are 19 or more that form the mineral composition of the body; at least 13 are essential to health. These must be supplied in the diet and generally can be supplied by a varied or mixed diet of animal and vegetable products that meet energy and protein needs. For the recommended dietary ALLOWANCES of common minerals in the United States and Canada, see Appendices 4 and 5. Calcium, iron, and iodine are the ones most frequently missing in the diet. Zinc, copper, magnesium, and potassium are minerals that are frequently involved in disturbances of metabolism. Other essential minerals include selenium, phosphorus, manganese, fluoride, chromium, and molybdenum. Minerals are either electropositive or electronegative; combinations of electropositive and electronegative elements lead to the formation of salts such as sodium chloride and calcium phosphate.

m. oil a mixture of liquid hydrocarbons from petroleum, available in both light grade (light liquid petrolatum) and heavier grades (liquid or heavy liquid petrolatum). Light mineral oil is used chiefly as a vehicle for drugs, but it may also be used as a CATHARTIC and skin emollient and cleansing agent. Heavy mineral oil is used as a cathartic, solvent, and oleaginous vehicle. Prolonged use of mineral oil as a cathartic should be avoided because it prevents absorption of the fat-soluble vitamins. Lipid PNEUMONIA caused by aspiration of the oil has been shown to occur in those who habitually take it, especially the elderly.

mineralization (min″er-al-ĭ-za'shun) the addition of mineral matter to the body.

mineralocorticoid (min″er-al-o-kor'tĭ-koid) any of a group of hormones elaborated by the cortex of the ADRENAL GLAND, so called because of their effects on sodium, chloride, and potassium concentrations in the extracellular fluid. They are the adrenocortical hormones that are essential to the maintenance of adequate fluid volume in the extracellular and intravascular fluid compartments, normal cardiac output, and adequate levels of blood pressure. Without sufficient supply of the mineralocorticoids, fatal shock from diminished cardiac output can occur very quickly.

The principal mineralocorticoid is *aldosterone,* which accounts for most of the activities of this group of hormones. The primary effects of the mineralocorticoids are increasing the reabsorption of sodium and the secretion of potassium in the renal tubules. Secondary effects are related to the reabsorption of water, serum levels of sodium and potassium, anion reabsorption, and secretion of hydrogen ions. The net result of these activities is maintenance of fluid and electrolyte balance and, therefore, adequate cardiac output.

minim (m.) (min'im) in the apothecaries' system, the smallest unit of volume (liquid measure), equivalent to 0.0616 mL.

minimal change disease subtle alterations in kidney function demonstrable by clinical albuminuria and the presence of lipid droplets in cells of the proximal tubules; abnormalities of foot processes of the glomerular epithelial cells are present but too subtle to be seen with light microscopy. It is seen primarily in children under 6 but sometimes in adults with the NEPHROTIC SYNDROME and may or may not progress to glomerulosclerosis or glomerulonephritis.

Minipress (min'ĭ-pres) trademark for a preparation of PRAZOSIN hydrochloride, an ANTIHYPERTENSIVE AGENT.

Minocin (mĭ-no'sĭn) trademark for preparations of MINOCYCLINE hydrochloride, a TETRACYCLINE ANTIBIOTIC.

minocycline (mĭ-no-si'klēn) a semisynthetic broad-spectrum ANTIBIOTIC of the TETRACYCLINE group; administered orally or intravenously as the hydrochloride salt

minoxidil (mi-noks'ĭ-dil) a potent, long-acting VASODILATOR, acting primarily on arterioles; administered orally as an ANTI-HYPERTENSIVE AGENT and topically in treatment of androgenetic alopecia.

miocardia (mi"o-kahr'de-ah) systole.

miopus (mi'o-pus) deformed conjoined twins with two fused heads, one face being rudimentary.

miosis (mi-o'sis) excessive contraction of the pupil.

miotic (mi-ot'ik) 1. pertaining to, characterized by, or causing MIOSIS (contraction of the pupil). 2. an agent that so acts.

miracidium (mi"rah-sid'e-um) [Gr.] the free-swimming larva of a trematode parasite which emerges from an egg and penetrates the body of a snail host.

mire (mēr) [Fr.] a figure on the arm of an ophthalmometer, the image of which is reflected on the cornea; used to measure corneal astigmatism.

MIRL membrane inhibitor of reactive lysis; see PROTECTIN.

mirtazapine (mir"taz-ah-pēn) an ANTIDE-PRESSANT that is not structurally related to any of the classes of antidepressants.

miscarriage (mis-kar'ij) the lay term for spontaneous ABORTION.

miscible (mis'ĭ-b'l) susceptible of being mixed.

misogamy (mĭ-sog'ah-me) aversion to marriage.

misogyny (mĭ-soj'ĭ-ne) aversion to women.

misoprostol (mi"so-pros'tol) a synthetic PROSTAGLANDIN E₁ analogue used to treat gastric irritation resulting from long-term therapy with NONSTEROIDAL ANTIINFLAMMA-TORY DRUGS. It is also used in conjunction with MIFEPRISTONE for termination of pregnancy in the first trimester. Administered orally.

Mitchell's disease (mich'elz) erythromelalgia.

mite (mīt) any arthropod of the order Acarina except the ticks; they are characterized by minute size, usually transparent or semitransparent body, and other features distinguishing them from the ticks. They may be free living or parasitic on animals or plants, and may produce various irritations of the skin.

chigger m., harvest m. chigger.

itch m., mange m. Sarcoptes scabiei.

mithramycin (mith"rah-mi'sin) plica-mycin.

miticide (mi'tĭ-sīd) an agent destructive to mites.

mitochondrion (mi"to-kon'dre-ah), pl. *mitochon'dria* [Gr.] a small, spherical to rod-shaped, membrane-bounded cytoplasmic organelle, the principal sites of ATP synthesis; mitochondria also contain enzymes of the citric acid CYCLE and ones for FATTY ACID oxidation, oxidative PHOSPHORYLATION, and other biochemical pathways. They also contain DNA, RNA, and ribosomes; they replicate independently and synthesize some of their own proteins. adj., **mitochon'drial.**

mitogen (mi'to-jen) a substance that induces blast transformation; DNA, RNA, and protein synthesis; and proliferation of lymphocytes; e.g., concanavalin A, phytohe-magglutinin, or lipopolysaccharide.

mitogenesis (mi"to-jen'ĕ-sis) the induction of mitosis in a cell.

mitomycin (mi"to-mi'sin) 1. any of a group of antitumor antibiotics (e.g., mito-mycin A, B, C) produced by *Streptomyces caespitosus.* 2. mitomycin C, which inhibits DNA and RNA synthesis by causing cross-linking of DNA. It is effective against cancers of the breast, lung, cervix, bladder, and gastrointestinal tract but because of its toxicity is mainly used for palliative treatment of patients who have not responded to other treatment. Administered intravenously.

mitosis (mi-to'sis) the ordinary process of cell division resulting in the formation of two daughter cells, by which the body

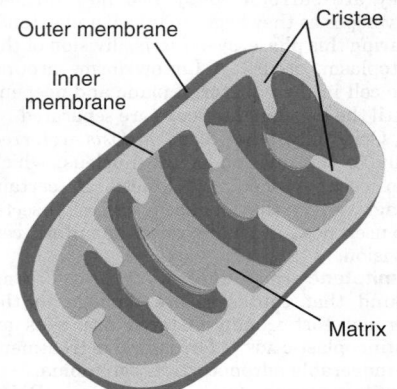

Mitochondrion. This organelle has a double membrane that unfolds and forms cristae. The membrane and cristae serve as attachment sites for oxidative enzymes. From Damjanov, 2000.

replaces dead cells. The daughter cells have identical diploid complements of chromosomes (46 in human somatic CELLS). Cell division that results in haploid reproductive cells is known as MEIOSIS. The period between mitotic divisions is called *interphase,* and mitosis itself occurs in four phases: *prophase, metaphase, anaphase,* and *telophase.* adj., **mitot'ic.** During *interphase* the chromosomes are extended long threads that cannot be visibly identified. The DNA of the chromosomes is replicated during this phase, resulting in duplication of the genetic material.

During *prophase* the chromosomes coil up and contract, becoming short rods. Each chromosome consists of a pair of strands, called *chromatids,* held together at the centromere. At the same time the nuclear envelope disappears, and the centriole divides and the two daughter centrioles move toward opposite poles of the cell.

During *metaphase* the chromosomes move so that their centromeres are aligned in the equatorial plane of the cell (the metaphase plate), and the mitotic spindle forms. The mitotic spindle is formed of fibers composed of microtubules, which extend from the centrioles to the metaphase plate and to the centromeres of the chromosomes.

During *anaphase* the chromatids of each chromosome separate, becoming new daughter chromosomes, which are drawn to opposite poles of the cell by the spindle fibers.

During *telophase* the daughter chromosomes arrive at the poles of the cell, where they are surrounded by two new nuclear envelopes as they begin to uncoil and extend. During this phase, *cytokinesis,* division of the cytoplasm, occurs. A furrow forms around the cell in the equatorial plane and deepens until the two daughter cells are separated.

Originally, the term *mitosis* referred only to the division of the nucleus, which can occur without cytokinesis in certain fungi and in the fertilized eggs of insects. As used now, it usually refers to mitotic cell division.

mitotane (mi'to-tān) a CYTOTOXIC compound that causes severe damage to the adrenal cortex; administered orally as an antineoplastic AGENT for palliative treatment of inoperable adrenocortical carcinoma.

mitoxantrone (mi″to-zan'trōn) a DNA-reactive agent of the ANTHRACENEDIONE group that inserts into DNA, causing crosslinks and strand breaks; administered intravenously as the hydrochloride salt as an

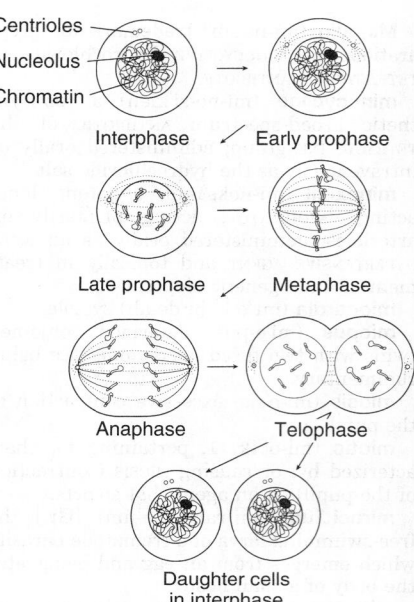

Centrioles
Nucleolus
Chromatin

Interphase   Early prophase

Late prophase   Metaphase

Anaphase   Telophase

Daughter cells
in interphase

Mitosis shown as occurring in a cell of a hypothetical animal with a diploid chromosome number of six (haploid number three); one pair of chromosomes is short, one pair is long and hooked, and one pair is long and knobbed. From Dorland's, 2000.

antitumor ANTIBIOTIC for the treatment of acute myelogenous LEUKEMIA and advanced, hormone-refractory prostate cancer. It is also used to reduce the frequency and severity of relapses in patients with secondary MULTIPLE SCLEROSIS.

mitral (mi'tral) 1. shaped like a miter (tall pointed hat worn by Roman Catholic bishops). 2. pertaining to the left atrioventricular VALVE.

m. valve prolapse (MVP) a condition in which some portion of the mitral VALVE is pushed back into the left atrium during ventricular contraction. For reasons not fully understood (there is no evident disease process) there is redundant tissue on one or both leaflets of the valve. The prolapsed portion of the valve causes a clicking sound halfway through the ventricular contraction, which is followed by a systolic murmur as blood is regurgitated back through the mitral valve into the left atrium. Echocardiography can demonstrate the mitral valve as it prolapses into the left atrium. Called also click-murmur syndrome and Barlow's syndrome.

The condition was first noted in association with potentially serious complications such as infective endocarditis, transient ischemic attack, and arrhythmias. However, in the vast majority of persons in whom mitral valve prolapse is detected by auscultation, the condition is benign and there are no other symptoms.

Mitral valve prolapse is found in persons of all ages and is fairly common, particularly in women. The few who have problems usually experience chest pain, dyspnea, palpitations, fatigue, and sometimes syncope. Electrocardiographic studies may show some premature ventricular contractions, but unlike those in coronary heart disease, these do not indicate injury to the heart muscle.

Persons who suffer from the above symptoms may require administration of a BETA-ADRENERGIC BLOCKING AGENT such as PROPRANOLOL, restriction of CAFFEINE intake, and avoidance of heavy meals. Those with severe symptoms may require repair or replacement of the mitral valve. It is recommended that patients with mitral valve prolapse take antibiotics prior to dental procedures.

mitralization (mi″tral-ĭ-za′shun) a straightening of the left border of the cardiac shadow, commonly seen radiographically in mitral stenosis.

Mitrolan (mi-trol′an) trademark for a preparation of CALCIUM POLYCARBOPHIL, a bulk LAXATIVE.

mittelschmerz (mit′el-shmerts) [Ger.] pain at the time of ovulation, midway between the menstrual periods.

mivacurium (mi″vah-ku′re-um) a nondepolarizing neuromuscular blocking AGENT of short duration, administered intravenously as the chloride salt as an adjunct to anesthesia.

mixed connective tissue disease a combination of scleroderma, myositis, systemic lupus erythematosus, and rheumatoid arthritis, and marked serologically by the presence of antibody against extractable nuclear antigen.

mixture (miks′chur) a combination of different drugs or ingredients, as a fluid with other fluids or solids, or of a solid with a liquid.

Miyagawanella (mi″yah-gah″wah-nel′ah) Chlamydia.

mL, ml milliliter.

μL microliter.

MLA Medical Library Association.

MLD minimum lethal dose.

MLT medical laboratory technician; see CLINICAL LABORATORY TECHNICIAN/MEDICAL LABORATORY TECHNICIAN.

MLVA multiple-locus variable number of tandem repeat analysis.

mM millimolar.

mm millimeter.

μM micromolar.

μm micrometer^2.

MMF maximal midexpiratory flow.

MMFR maximal midexpiratory flow rate.

mm Hg millimeters of mercury; a unit of pressure equal to 1 torr, or 133.3 pascals.

mmol millimole.

MMR measles-mumps-rubella (vaccine); see measles, mumps, and rubella VACCINE.

Mn manganese.

M'Naghten rule (mik-naw′ton) a definition of criminal responsibility formulated in 1843 by English judges questioned by the House of Lords as a result of the acquittal of Daniel M' Naghten on grounds of insanity. It holds that "to establish a defense on the ground of insanity, it must be clearly proved that, at the time of committing the act, the party accused was laboring under such a defect of reason, from disease of the mind, as not to know the nature and quality of the act he was doing, or, if he did know it, he did not know he was doing what was wrong" and further that a defendant who "labors under partial delusions only and is not in other respects insane must be considered in the same situation as to responsibility as if the facts with respect to which the delusion exists were real." These rules are still used in many American jurisdictions.

mnemonics (ne-mon′iks) improvement of memory by special methods or techniques. adj., **mnemon′ic.**

MO Medical Officer.

Mo molybdenum.

MOAB monoclonal antibody.

mobility (mo-bil′i-te) the ability to move in one's environment with ease and without restriction.

impaired bed m. a NURSING DIAGNOSIS approved by the North American Nursing Diagnosis Association, defined as the limitation of independent movement from one bed position to another.

impaired physical m. a NURSING DIAGNOSIS approved by the North American Nursing Diagnosis Association, defined as the state in which an individual has a limitation in independent, purposeful physical movement of the body or of one or more extremities. Related factors arising from within the person include pain or fear of discomfort, anxiety or depression, and physical limitations due to neuromuscular or musculoskeletal impairment. External factors include enforced rest for therapeutic purposes, as in the case of immobilization of a fractured limb. The human body is designed for motion; hence, any restriction of movement will take its toll on every major anatomic system.

The goals of interventions are to avoid the hazards of immobility, prevent dependent disabilities, and assist the patient in restoring, preserving, or maintaining as much mobility and functional independence as possible. Activities to accomplish these goals include proper positioning and repositioning of the patient, special skin care, coughing and deep breathing, active and passive exercises including range of motion exercises, and maintenance of adequate nutrition and bowel and urine elimination. Impaired physical mobility represents a complex health care problem that involves many different members of the health care team.

   impaired wheelchair m. a NURSING DIAGNOSIS approved by the North American Nursing Diagnosis Association, defined as limitation of independent operation of a wheelchair within the environment.

   tooth m. physiologic movement of a tooth, varying in degree for different teeth and different times of day; that exceeding a normal range is pathological.

   mobilization (mo″bĭ-lĭ-za′shun) 1. the process of making a fixed part movable by separating it from surrounding structures so that it is accessible for an operative procedure. 2. the release of a substance stored in the body into the circulation for bodily use. 3. the assembling or preparation of something in response to a need.

   family m. in the NURSING INTERVENTIONS CLASSIFICATION, a nursing INTERVENTION defined as making use of family strengths to influence patient's health in a positive direction.

   joint m. passive movement of a joint to restore motion or relieve pain. Small oscillatory motions that do not stretch the capsular or other soft tissue structures are often used for reducing pain, while larger (grade III or IV) oscillatory or sustained motions are used to stretch structures and restore accessory or joint PLAY motions. Movements are slow enough that the patient can voluntarily stop them. See also joint MANIPULATION.

   stapes m. surgical correction of immobility of the stapes in treatment of deafness.

   moccasin (mok′ah-sin) any of several species of snakes of the genus *Agkistrodon*.

   highland m. copperhead.

   water m. *Agkistrodon piscivorus,* a venomous semiaquatic pit VIPER with an olive or brown back, found in the southern United States. Called also cottonmouth.

   modafinil (mo-daf′ĭ-nil″) a central nervous system STIMULANT used in the treatment of NARCOLEPSY.

   Möbius disease (mer′be-oos) periodic migraine with paralysis of the oculomotor muscles.

   Möbius syndrome (mer′be-oos) a hereditary defect of the motor nuclei of cranial nerves, which causes bilateral facial paralysis in various combinations, such as paralysis of the abductors of the eye; persons with this syndrome cannot smile. Anomalies of the limbs are often present, such as missing or webbed fingers. There may or may not be mental retardation. Current treatment is supportive rather than curative. (See Atlas 1, Part C.)

   modality (mo-dal′ĭ-te) 1. in homeopathy, a condition that modifies drug action; a condition under which symptoms develop, becoming better or worse. 2. a method of application of, or the employment of, any therapeutic agent; limited usually to physical agents. 3. a specific sensory entity, such as taste.

   mode (mōd) in statistics, the most frequently occurring value or item in a distribution. 1. pacing mode. 2. the manner of interaction between a VENTILATOR and the person being ventilated, usually defined in terms of what the stimulus is that starts the ventilation.

   assist m. a mode of positive pressure VENTILATION in which the patient initiates and terminates all or most breaths and the ventilator gives some amount of support. See also control mode and assist-control mode.

   assist-control m. a mode of positive pressure VENTILATION in which the ventilator is in assist mode unless the patient's respiration rate falls below a certain amount, in which case the ventilator switches to a control mode. When the strength or rate of respiration increases again, the ventilator goes back into assist mode.

   assisted m. assist mode.

   asynchronous m. a pacing mode in which there is regular stimulation without regard to sensed cardiac signals.

   control m., controlled m. a mode of positive pressure VENTILATION in which the ventilator controls the initiation and volume of breaths. See also assist mode and assist-control mode.

   inhibited m. a pacing mode in which a sensed event prevents or stops a pacing stimulus and starts a timing cycle.

pacing m. in cardiac PACING terminology, the manner of stimulation of a cardiac chamber by an artificial PACEMAKER, referring to whether or not sensed cardiac signals (events) are used to inhibit or trigger stimulation. Types include asynchronous, inhibited, and triggered MODES.

pressure control m. a mode of positive pressure VENTILATION in which each breath is augmented by air at a fixed rate and amount of pressure, with tidal volume not being fixed. See also under VENTILATION.

pressure support m. a mode of positive pressure VENTILATION similar to the assist mode; the patient breathes spontaneously and breathing is augmented by air at a preset amount of pressure. See also under VENTILATION.

triggered m. a pacing mode in which the stimulus is emitted in response to a sensed event.

model (mod″l) 1. something that represents or simulates something else; a replica. 2. a reasonable facsimile of the body or any of its parts; used for demonstration and teaching purposes. 3. to initiate another's behavior; see MODELING. 4. a hypothesis or theory. 5. in nursing theory, an abstract conceptual framework used to organize knowledge and serve as a guide for observation and interpretation; see also CONCEPTUAL MODEL.

articulation m's a process of educational mobility in which programs work together to enable students to progress between levels of nursing education programs with the fewest possible barriers and repetitions of content.

conceptual m. see CONCEPTUAL MODEL.

PLISSIT m. a progressive design of sexual counseling that contains the four steps of permission, limited information, specific suggestions, and intensive therapy.

modeling (mod″ling) learning vicariously by observation and imitation, which can be used as a form of behavior therapy.

modem (mo′dem) a hardware device that converts digital signals from a computer or computer terminal to and from analog signals for transmission along communication lines.

modifier (mod′ĭ-fi-er) 1. an agent or method that causes something else to change. 2. problem modifier.

biologic response m. (BRM), biological response m. a method or agent, such as a cytokine, monoclonal antibody, or vaccine, that alters host-tumor interaction. This is usually accomplished by amplifying the antitumor mechanisms of the immune system, but it also may be effected by mechanisms that affect host or tumor cell characteristics, either directly or indirectly. Called also biomodulator.

modiolus (mo-di′o-lus) the central pillar or columella of the cochlea.

MODS multiple organ dysfunction syndrome.

modulation (mod″u-la′shun) the normal capacity of cell adaptability to its environment.

antigenic m. the alteration of antigenic determinants in a living cell surface membrane following interaction with antibody.

modulator (mod′u-la″ter) a specific inductor or agent that brings out characteristics peculiar to a definite region.

selective estrogen receptor m. (SERM) an agent that activates some estrogen RECEPTORS but not others, thereby having estrogenlike effects on target tissues (such as bone) without affecting other tissues that have estrogen receptors.

MODY maturity-onset diabetes of youth.

moexipril (mo-ek′sĭ-pril″) an ANGIOTENSIN-CONVERTING ENZYME INHIBITOR used as the hydrochloride salt as an ANTIHYPERTENSIVE.

Mohs' technique (mōz) a technique of microscopically controlled serial excision of skin cancers; the tissue to be removed is first fixed in situ with zinc chloride paste (*Mohs' chemosurgery*), or only serial excisions of fresh tissue are used for microscopic analysis (*Mohs' surgery*).

moiety (moi′ĕ-te) any equal part; a half; also any part or portion, as a portion of a molecule.

mol (mol) mole[1].

molal (*m*) (mo′lal) containing one mole of solute per kilogram of solvent. (See also MOLAR[1].)

molality (mo-lal′ĭ-te) the number of MOLES of a solute per kilogram of solvent. See also MOLARITY.

molar[1] (mo′lar) 1. pertaining to a mole of a substance. 2. containing one mole of solute per liter of solution. Symbol M, *M,* or mol/L. NOTE: *molal* refers to the mass of the *solvent, molar* to the volume of the *solution.*

molar[2] (M) (mo′lar) a molar tooth; see TOOTH. 1. pertaining to a molar tooth.

molarity (mo-lar′ĭ-te) the number of MOLES of a solute per liter of solution; see also MOLALITY.

mold (mōld) any of a group of parasitic and saprobic fungi causing a cottony growth on organic substances; also, the deposit of growth produced by such fungi.

M

molding (mōld′ing) the shaping of the fetal head to the size and shape of the birth canal.

mole[1] (mōl) the base SI UNIT of amount of matter. It is the amount of a substance that contains as many elementary entities (atoms, ions, molecules, or free radicals) as there are atoms in 0.012 kg of carbon 12 (^{12}C), i.e., AVOGADRO'S NUMBER, 6.023×10^{23}, of elementary entities.

mole[2] (mōl) 1. nevocytic NEVUS. 2. any of various other pigmented skin lesions.

 pigmented m. nevus pigmentosus.

mole[3] (mōl) a fleshy mass formed in the uterus by degeneration or abnormal development of a fertilized ovum.

 hydatid m., hydatidiform m. an abnormal pregnancy resulting from a pathologic ovum, with proliferation of the epithelial covering of the chorionic villi and dissolution and cystic cavitation of the avascular stroma of the villi. It results in a mass of cysts resembling a bunch of grapes.

molecular (mo-lek′u-ler) of, pertaining to, or composed of molecules.

 m. disease any disease in which the pathogenesis can be traced to a single chemical substance, usually a protein, which is either abnormal in structure or present in reduced amounts.

molecule (mol′ĕ-kūl) a group of atoms joined by chemical bonds; the smallest amount of a substance that possesses its characteristic properties.

 adhesion m's, cell adhesion m's **(CAM)** cell surface GLYCOPROTEINS that mediate intercell adhesion in vertebrates.

 middle m. any molecule that has an atomic mass between 350 and 2000 daltons; these accumulate in the body fluids of patients with uremia.

molimen (mo-li′men) [L.] a laborious effort made for the performance of any normal body function, especially that manifested by a variety of unpleasant symptoms preceding or accompanying menstruation.

molindone (mo-lin′dōn) a SEDATIVE used as an ANTIPSYCHOTIC AGENT in management of schizophrenia.

mollities (mo-lish′e-ēz) [L.] abnormal softening.

 m. os′sium osteomalacia.

molluscum (mŏ-lus′kum) 1. any of various skin diseases marked by the formation of soft rounded cutaneous tumors. 2. molluscum contagiosum. adj., **mollus′cous.**

 m. contagio′sum a common, benign, usually self-limited viral disease of the skin marked by the formation of firm, rounded, translucent, crateriform papules containing caseous matter and intracytoplasmic inclusions (molluscum bodies), which contain replicating virions. The disease is spread by contact and is common in young children. In adults, lesions in the pubic area indicate sexual transmission.

 Treatment consists of curettage or light cauterization with an electric cautery.

Mol wt, mol wt molecular weight.

molybdenum (Mo) (mah-lib′dĕ-num) a hard, silvery-white, metallic element, atomic number 42, atomic weight 95.94. (See Appendix 6.) It is an essential trace element, being a component of the enzymes xanthine oxidase, aldehyde oxidase, and nitrate reductase.

momentum (mo-men′tum) the quantity of motion; the product of mass by velocity.

mometasone (mo-met′ah-sōn) a synthetic CORTICOSTEROID; as *m. furoate* it is used topically for the relief of inflammation and pruritus in dermatoses and intranasally in the treatment of allergic rhinitis and other inflammatory nasal conditions.

mon(o)- word element [Gr.], *one; single; limited to one part; combined with one atom.*

monad (mo′nad) 1. a single-celled PROTOZOON or COCCUS. 2. a univalent radical or element. 3. in meiosis, one member of a TETRAD.

monarthric (mon-ahr′thrik) pertaining to a single joint.

monarthritis (mon″ahr-thri′tis) inflammation of a single joint.

monarticular (mon″ahr-tik′u-ler) pertaining to a single joint.

monathetosis (mon-ath″ĕ-to′sis) athetosis of one limb.

monatomic (mon″ah-tom′ik) 1. containing one atom. 2. univalent.

Mondor's disease (mon′dorz) phlebitis affecting the large subcutaneous veins normally crossing the lateral chest wall and breast from the epigastric or hypochondriac region to the axilla.

Monera (mo-ne′rah) in the classification of living organisms, a KINGDOM comprising all unicellular organisms that lack true nuclei (the PROKARYOTE), including principally the BACTERIA. Formerly called Procaryotae.

monesthetic (mon″es-thet′ik) affecting a single sense or sensation.

Monge's disease (mōn′hāz) the chronic form of ALTITUDE SICKNESS.

mongolian spot (mon-gōl′e-an) a smooth brown to grayish blue nevus consisting of an excess of melanocytes, typically found at birth in the sacral region in East Asians Blacks, American Indians, and many southern Europeans; it usually disappears during childhood.

mongolism (mon′go-lizm) old term for DOWN SYNDROME; now considered offensive.

mongoloid (mon′go-loid) 1. pertaining to or resembling the Mongols, a group in Central Asia. 2. old term for certain features characteristic of an individual with DOWN SYNDROME.

monilethrix (mo-nil′ĕ-thriks) a hereditary condition in which the hair is brittle and beaded.

Monilia (mo-nil′e-ah) 1. former name for *Candida*. 2. a genus of imperfect fungi of the family Moniliaceae.

monilial (mo-nil′e-al) pertaining to or caused by *Monilia* (*Candida*).

moniliasis (mo″nĭ-li′ah-sis) candidiasis.

moniliform (mo-nil′ĭ-form) beaded; having the appearance of a string of beads.

Monistat (mo′nĭ-stat) trademark for preparations of MICONAZOLE, an antifungal AGENT.

monitor (mon′ĭ-ter) 1. to check constantly on a given condition or phenomenon, e.g., blood pressure or heart or respiration rate. 2. an apparatus by which such conditions or phenomena can be constantly observed and recorded.

ambulatory ECG m. a portable continuous ELECTROCARDIOGRAPH recorder, typically monitoring two channels for 24 hours; it is used to detect the frequency and duration of cardiac rhythm disturbances and to assess PACEMAKER programming. The term is sometimes used synonymously with Holter MONITOR.

apnea m. a device with alarms, used to detect cessation of breathing, most commonly used in neonates and infants who have demonstrated apnea or who may be at risk for developing apnea. These monitors can be used in the hospital or in the patient's home.

Holter m. a type of ambulatory ECG monitor.

monitoring (mon′ĭ-ter-ing) constant checking on a patient's condition, either personally or by means of a mechanical MONITOR.

acid-base m. in the NURSING INTERVENTIONS CLASSIFICATION, a nursing INTERVENTION defined as the collection and analysis of patient data to regulate ACID-BASE BALANCE.

biological m. examination of materials such as blood or urine that come from living organisms, to determine if there has been exposure to given chemical substances.

electrolyte m. in the NURSING INTERVENTIONS CLASSIFICATION, a nursing INTERVENTION defined as collection and analysis of patient data to regulate electrolyte balance.

electronic fetal m.: antepartum in the NURSING INTERVENTIONS CLASSIFICATION, a nursing INTERVENTION defined as electronic evaluation of fetal heart rate response to movement, external stimuli, or uterine contractions during antepartal testing.

electronic fetal m.: intrapartum in the NURSING INTERVENTIONS CLASSIFICATION, a nursing INTERVENTION defined as electronic evaluation of heart rate response to uterine contractions during INTRAPARTAL care.

fetal m. see FETAL MONITORING.

fluid m. in the NURSING INTERVENTIONS CLASSIFICATION, a nursing INTERVENTION defined as the collection and analysis of patient data to regulate FLUID BALANCE.

health policy m. in the NURSING INTERVENTIONS CLASSIFICATION, a nursing INTERVENTION defined as surveillance and influence of government and organization regulations, rules, and standards that affect nursing systems and practices to ensure quality care of patients.

hemodynamic m. see HEMODYNAMIC MONITORING.

intracranial pressure m. see INTRACRANIAL PRESSURE MONITORING.

invasive hemodynamic m. in the NURSING INTERVENTIONS CLASSIFICATION, a nursing INTERVENTION defined as the measurement and interpretation of invasive hemodynamic parameters to determine cardiovascular function and regulate therapy as appropriate.

neurologic m. in the NURSING INTERVENTIONS CLASSIFICATION, a nursing INTERVENTION defined as the collection and analysis of patient data to prevent or minimize neurologic complications.

newborn m. in the NURSING INTERVENTIONS CLASSIFICATION, a nursing INTERVENTION defined as the measurement and interpretation of the physiologic status of the NEONATE in the first 24 hours after delivery.

nutritional m. in the NURSING INTERVENTIONS CLASSIFICATION, a nursing INTERVENTION defined as the collection and analysis of patient data to prevent or minimize malnourishment.

quality m. in the NURSING INTERVENTIONS CLASSIFICATION, a nursing INTERVENTION defined as the systematic collection and analysis of an organization's quality indicators for the purpose of improving patient care.

respiratory m. in the NURSING INTERVENTIONS CLASSIFICATION, a nursing INTERVENTION defined as the collection and analysis of patient data to ensure airway patency and adequate gas EXCHANGE.

transcutaneous oxygen m. see transcutaneous OXYGEN MONITORING.

vital signs m. in the NURSING INTERVENTIONS CLASSIFICATION, a nursing INTERVENTION defined as the collection and analysis of cardiovascular, respiratory, and body temperature data to determine and prevent complications. See also vital SIGNS.

monitrice (mon′ĭ-trēs) a trained individual who supports women in labor using the PSYCHOPROPHYLAXIS method of PREPARED CHILDBIRTH.

monoamine (mon″o-am′ēn) an amine containing only one amino group.

m. oxidase (MAO) a copper-containing enzyme that deaminates monoamines such as DOPAMINE, EPINEPHRINE, NOREPINEPHRINE, and SEROTONIN. See also monoamine oxidase INHIBITOR.

monoaminergic (mon″o-am″in-er′jik) of or pertaining to neurons that secrete the monoamine neurotransmitters dopamine, norepinephrine, and serotonin.

monoamniotic (mon″o-am″ne-ot′ik) having or developing within a single amniotic cavity; said of monozygotic TWINS.

monobasic (mon″o-ba′sik) having but one atom of replaceable hydrogen.

monobenzone (mon″o-ben′zōn) a MELANIN-inhibiting agent used for skin depigmentation in VITILIGO.

monoblast (mon′o-blast) the earliest precursor in the monocytic series, which develops into the promonocyte.

monoblastoma (mon″o-blas-to′mah) a tumor containing monoblasts and monocytes.

monoblepsia (mon″o-blep′se-ah) 1. a condition in which vision is better when only one eye is used. 2. blindness to all colors but one.

monobrachius (mon″o-bra′ke-us) a fetus with only one upper limb.

monocephalus (mon″o-sef′ah-lus) a malformed fetus with two bodies and one head.

monochorea (mon″o-ko-re′ah) chorea affecting but one part.

monochorionic (mon″o-kor″e-on′ik) having or developing in a common chorionic sac; said of monozygotic TWINS.

monochromat (mon″o-kro′mat) a person with monochromatic VISION.

monochromatic (mon″o-kro-mat′ik) 1. existing in or having only one color. 2. able to see only one color; see monochromatic VISION. 3. staining with only one dye at a time.

monochromatism (mon″o-kro′mah-tizm), (mon″o-kro″mah-top′se-ah) **monochromatopsia** monochromatic VISION.

cone m. that in which there is some cone function.

rod m. that in which there is complete absence of cone function.

monoclonal (mon″o-klo′nal) derived from a single cell; pertaining to a single clone.

monococcus (mon″o-kok′us) a form of COCCUS consisting of single cells.

monocontaminated (mon″o-kon-tam′ĭ-nāt″ed) infected by only one species of microorganisms or a single contaminating agent.

monocular (mon-ok′u-ler) 1. pertaining to one eye. 2. having but one eyepiece, as in a microscope.

monoculus (mon-ok′u-lus) a bandage for one eye. 1. cyclops.

monocyte (mon′o-sīt) a mononuclear, phagocytic leukocyte, 13 μm to 25 μm in diameter, having an ovoid or kidney-shaped nucleus and azurophilic cytoplasmic granules. Monocytes are derived from PROMONOCYTES in the bone marrow and circulate in the blood for about 24 hours before migrating to the tissues, such as the lung and liver, where they develop into MACROPHAGES. adj., **monocyt′ic.**

monocytopenia (mon″o-si-to-pe′ne-ah) deficiency of monocytes in the blood.

monocytosis (mon″o-si-to′sis) excess of monocytes in the blood.

monodactyly (mon″o-dak′tĭ-le) the presence of only one finger or toe on a hand or foot.

monodermoma (mon″o-der-mo′mah) a tumor developed from one germinal layer.

monodiplopia (mon″o-dĭ-plo′pe-ah) double vision in one eye.

monoecious (mon-e′shus) having reproductive organs typical of both sexes in a single individual.

monoethanolamine (mon″o-eth″ah-nōl′ah-mēn) an amino alcohol occurring in PHOSPHATIDYLETHANOLAMINES; used as a pharmaceutical SURFACTANT. The oleate salt, a sclerosing AGENT, is called ETHANOLAMINE OLEATE. Called also ethanolamine.

monogerminal (mon″o-jer′mĭ-nal) monozygotic.

monokine (mon′o-kīn) any of various soluble mediators of IMMUNE RESPONSES that are not antibodies or complement components and that are produced by mononuclear phagocytes (monocytes or macrophages).

monolayer (mon″o-la′er) pertaining to or consisting of a single layer of molecules.

monolocular (mon″o-lok′u-ler) having but one cavity, as a cyst.

monomania (mon″o-ma′ne-ah) a form of mental disorder characterized by preoccupation with one subject or idea.

monomelic (mon″o-mel′ik) affecting one limb.

monomer (mon′o-mer) 1. a simple molecule of relatively low molecular weight, which is capable of reacting chemically with other molecules to form a dimer, trimer, or polymer. 2. some basic unit of a molecule, either the molecule itself or some structural or functional subunit of it, e.g., an individual polypeptide in a multi-subunit protein.

fibrin m. the material resulting from the action of thrombin on fibrinogen, which then polymerizes to form the fibrin clot.

monomeric (mon″o-mer′ik) 1. pertaining to, comprising, or affecting a single segment. 2. in genetics, determined by a gene or genes at a single locus.

monomolecular (mon″o-mo-lek′u-ler) pertaining to a single molecule or to a layer one molecule thick.

monomorphic (mon″o-mor′fik) existing in only one form.

monomphalus (mon-om′fah-lus) conjoined twins attached in the umbilical region.

monomyoplegia (mon″o-mi″o-ple′jah) paralysis of a single muscle.

monomyositis (mon″o-mi″o-si′tis) inflammation of a single muscle.

mononeural (mon″o-noor′al) supplied by a single nerve.

mononeuritis (mon″o-nōō-ri′tis) inflammation of a single nerve.

m. mul′tiplex simultaneous inflammation of several nerves remote from one another.

mononuclear (mon″o-noo′kle-ar) having only one nucleus.

mononucleosis (mon″o-noo″kle-o′sis) excess of MONOCYTES in the blood; frequently used alone to refer to infectious mononucleosis.

cytomegalovirus m. a syndrome similar to infectious mononucleosis but caused by infection with CYTOMEGALOVIRUS.

infectious m. an acute infectious disease that causes changes in the leukocytes; it is caused by the Epstein-Barr virus and is usually transmitted by direct oral contact (which is why it is sometimes called the "kissing disease"). It occurs more frequently in the spring and affects primarily children and young adults. Although epidemics have been reported, some authorities doubt that the disorder has been the same in all instances. Called also glandular fever.

Symptoms. Generally, after an incubation period of one week to several weeks, headache, sore throat, fatigue, severe weakness, and influenzalike symptoms occur. Skin

rashes may also occur. Diagnosis can be confirmed by the finding of a marked increase in the number of monocytes in the patient's blood. Besides these normal cells of the lymphocyte class, there is often an increase in atypical lymphocytes. Another diagnostic test that indicates mononucleosis is the PAUL-BUNNELL TEST, which demonstrates the presence of certain antibodies capable of causing clumping of cells in a sample of sheep's blood.

In about 8 to 10 per cent of all cases, the liver is involved and jaundice occurs, resulting in a condition that resembles infectious hepatitis. In rare cases, the heart, lungs, and central nervous system may also be affected. The spleen may become enlarged; one of the complications, serious but rare, is rupture of the spleen. The lymph nodes and spleen may both remain enlarged for sometime after other symptoms have disappeared.

Treatment. Treatment is chiefly symptomatic. Rest is especially important in the early stages of the disease, or later if the liver is involved. There is as yet no specific treatment for mononucleosis, and no immunization is available. Headache and sore throat may be relieved by aspirin and gargles. Although the more obvious symptoms may disappear after a period of rest, sufficient rest and curtailed activities must be maintained in order to improve the patient's severely weakened condition and prevent recurrence. There is often mental as well as physical fatigue, especially among students, and in these cases some mental depression may accompany convalescence.

Chronic, lingering infectious mononucleosis occurs in some patients. They experience profound fatigue, low-grade fever, swollen lymph glands, a sore throat, and aching muscles and joints. These symptoms can persist for months or years, and often cause the patient to be labeled neurotic because of a lack of objective evidence of disease. The condition can be definitively diagnosed by blood testing for antibodies to the Epstein-Barr virus. Unfortunately, diagnosis can provide psychological relief only, as there is no effective treatment or cure for the disorder.

monooctanoin (-ok″tah-no′in) a semisynthetic glycerol derivative used to dissolve cholesterol GALLSTONES in the common and intrahepatic bile ducts.

monoparesis (mon″o-pah-re′sis) paresis of a single part.

monoparesthesia (mon″o-par″es-the′-zhah) paresthesia of a single part.

monopathy (mo-nop'ah-the) a disease affecting a single part.

monophthalmus (mon''of-thal'mus) cyclops.

monophyletic (mon''o-fi-let'ik) descended from a common ancestor or stem cell.

monoplegia (mon''o-ple'je-ah) paralysis of a single part. adj., **monople'gic**.

monopoiesis (mon''o-poi-e'sis) the development of monocytes.

monopolar (mon''o-po'ler) having a single pole.

monops (mon'ops) cyclops.

monopus (mon'o-pus) a malformed fetus with only one foot; see also SYMMELIA.

monorchid (mon-or'kid) 1. having only one testis in the scrotum. 2. a male having only one testis in the scrotum.

monorchidism (mon-or'kid-izm) monorchism.

monorchism (mon'or-kizm) the condition of having only one testis or one descended testis.

monosaccharide (mon''o-sak'ah-rīd) a simple sugar; a carbohydrate that cannot be broken down to simpler substances by hydrolysis. Subgroups include the ALDOSES and the KETOSES.

monosodium glutamate (mon''o-so'de-um) a salt of GLUTAMIC ACID, used as a pharmaceutic NECESSITY, and also used to enhance the flavor of foods. See also Chinese restaurant syndrome.

monosomy (mon''o-so'me) existence in a cell of only one instead of the normal diploid pair of a particular chromosome, seen in TURNER'S SYNDROME, MONOSOMY 9P⁻ DISEASE, and various other conditions. adj., **monoso'mic**.

m. 9p⁻ syndrome a rare chromosomal disorder in which a piece of the short arm of the ninth chromosome is broken and often lost. Symptoms include mental retardation, a triangular head with forward angulation of the frontal bone, and various other physical deformities. A support group for more information on this syndrome can be reached at 43304 Kipton Nickel Plate Road, La Grange, OH 44050.

monospecific (mon''o-spĕ-sif'ik) having an effect only on a particular kind of cell or tissue, or reacting with a single antigen, as a monospecific antiserum.

Monosporium (mon''o-spor'e-um) a genus of fungi. *M. apiosper'mum* is one of the causative organisms of MADUROMYCOSIS.

Monospot (mon'o-spot'') trademark for a test kit used to determine the presence or absence of HETEROPHIL ANTIBODIES.

monostotic (mon''os-tot'ik) affecting a single bone.

monosymptomatic (mon''o-simp''to-mat'ik) manifested by only one symptom.

monosynaptic (mon''o-sī-nap'tik) pertaining to or passing through a single synapse.

monothermia (mon''o-ther'me-ah) a condition in which the body temperature remains the same throughout the day.

monotrichous (mon-ot'rī-kus) having a single FLAGELLUM; said of bacterial cells.

monovalent (mon''o-va'lent) 1. having a valence of one; called also univalent. 2. denoting an antiserum, vaccine, or antitoxin specific for a single antigen or organism.

monoxenous (mo-nok'sĕ-nus) requiring only one host to complete the life cycle.

monozygotic (mon''o-zi-got'ik; mon''o-zi'gus) **monozygous** pertaining to or derived from a single ZYGOTE (fertilized ovum); said of TWINS. See also DIZYGOTIC. (See accompanying illustration.)

mons (mons) [L.] an elevation or eminence.

m. pu'bis the rounded fleshy prominence over the symphysis pubis in the female.

m. ve'neris mons pubis.

Monsel's solution (mon-selz') a reddish brown aqueous solution of basic ferric sulfate, prepared from ferrous sulfate and nitric acid; used as an astringent and hemostatic.

monster (mon'ster) a term formerly used to denote a fetus or infant with such pronounced developmental ANOMALIES as to be grotesque and usually nonviable. More appropriate terms are *congenitally deformed, malformed,* or *abnormal fetus* especially when discussing these individuals with loved ones.

monstrosity (mon-stros'ĭ-te) 1. great congenital deformity; see MONSTER. 2. teratism.

montelukast (mon''tĕ-loo'kast) a LEUKOTRIENE antagonist used as the sodium salt in prophylaxis and chronic treatment of ASTHMA.

monticulus (mon-tik'u-lus) [L.] a small eminence.

m. cerebel'li the projecting part of the superior vermis cerebelli.

mood (mood) a pervasive and sustained emotion that, when extreme, can color one's whole view of life; in psychiatry and psychology the term is generally used to refer to either ELATION or DEPRESSION. See also MOOD DISORDERS.

m.-congruent consistent with one's mood, a term used particularly in the classification of MOOD DISORDERS. In disorders with psychotic features, *mood-congruent*

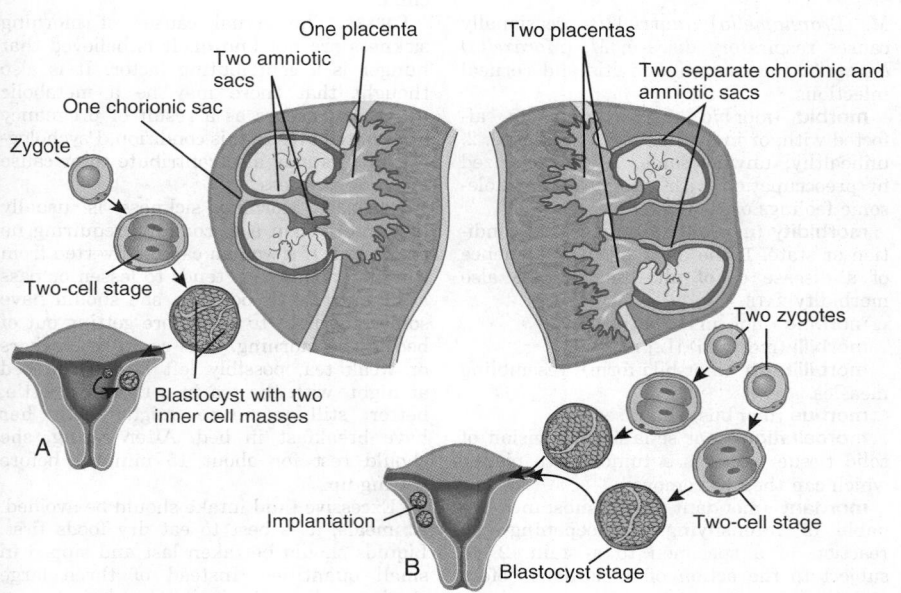

A, Monozygotic twinning. The single inner cell mass divides into two inner cell masses during the blastocyst stage. These twins have a single placenta and chorion, but each twin develops in its own amnion. B, Dizygotic twinning. Two ova are released during ovulation, and each is fertilized by a separate spermatozoon. The ova may implant near each other in the uterus, or they may be far apart. From McKinney et al., 2000.

psychotic features are grandiose delusions or related hallucinations occurring in a manic episode or depressive delusions or related hallucinations in a major depressive episode, while *mood-incongruent psychotic features* are delusions or hallucinations that either contradict or are inconsistent with the prevailing emotions, such as delusions of persecution or of thought insertion in either a manic or a depressive episode.

m. disorders MENTAL DISORDERS whose essential feature is a disturbance of MOOD manifested by episodes of manic, hypomanic, or depressive symptoms, or some combination of these. The two major categories are BIPOLAR DISORDERS and DEPRESSIVE DISORDERS.

m.-incongruent not MOOD-CONGRUENT.

Moore (mor) Ruth Ella (1903–1994). The first African American woman to earn a Ph.D. in bacteriology. Her areas of research were BLOOD GROUPS and the family ENTEROBACTERIACEAE.

MOPP a regimen of MECHLORETHAMINE, ONCOVIN (VINCRISTINE), PROCARBAZINE, and PREDNISONE, used in ANTINEOPLASTIC THERAPY.

morality (mo-ral′ĭ-te) accordance with widely shared conventions of right or good conduct that form a stable, but usually incomplete, social consensus; it includes the concept of moral ideals. See also VIRTUE.

principle-based common m. a type of ethical thinking based on premises that are unphilosophical common sense and tradition and come from the morality shared by members of a society. Principle-based theories have an emphasis on obligation and are *pluralistic* (in contrast to teleological and deontological theories, which are *monistic,* i.e., have one supreme, absolute principle supporting all other guides in the system). The principles are generally accepted in most types of ethical theory and are what are called "middle level" principles in that they are not the most general principles but are those likely to be acceptable to proponents of different normative theories. This type of thinking has been most influential in bioethics and in nursing.

Moraxella (mo″-rak-sel′ah) a genus of gram-negative, aerobic bacteria found as parasites on the mucous membranes of mammals. There are two subgenera: M. (Moraxella), occurring as rods, and M. (Branhamella), occurring as cocci.

M. (Branhamella) catarrha'lis occasionally causes respiratory disease; *M. (Moraxella) lacuna'ta* causes conjunctivitis and corneal infections.

morbid (mor'bid) 1. pertaining to, affected with, or inducing disease; diseased. 2. unhealthy; unwholesome. 3. characterized by preoccupation with gloomy or unwholesome feelings or thoughts.

morbidity (mor-bid'i-te) a diseased condition or state. 1. the incidence or prevalence of a disease or of all diseases. See also morbidity RATE.

morbific (mor-bif'ik) pathogenic.

morbilli (mor-bil'i) [L.] measles.

morbilliform (mor-bil'i-form) resembling measles.

morbus (mor'bus) [L.] disease.

morcellation (mor″sĕ-la'shun) division of solid tissue (such as a tumor) into pieces, which can then be removed.

mordant (mor'dant) 1. a substance capable of intensifying or deepening the reaction of a specimen to a stain. 2. to subject to the action of a mordant before staining.

Morganella (mor-gah-nel'ah) a genus of gram-negative, facultatively anaerobic, rod-shaped bacteria. The single species is *M. morga'nii,* which is a primary cause of urinary tract infections and is an opportunistic pathogen, causing secondary infections of the respiratory tract, blood, and wounds.

morgue (morg) a place where dead bodies may be temporarily kept, for identification or until claimed for burial.

moribund (mor'i-bund) in a dying state.

moricizine (mor-ĭ'sĭ-zēn) a PHENOTHIAZINE derivative used as the hydrochloride salt in treatment of ventricular ARRHYTHMIAS.

morning sickness nausea and vomiting occurring during pregnancy, usually during the early months. Between 50 and 65 per cent of all women experience some degree of this during pregnancy, and about one third are affected to the point of vomiting. Morning sickness usually begins during the fifth or sixth week of pregnancy. Some cases may clear up in 1 to 3 weeks; others may persist until the fourteenth or sixteenth week. In most cases, morning sickness begins with a feeling of nausea on arising. Despite its name, morning sickness is not always limited to the morning. In rare cases, about one woman in 200, HYPEREMESIS GRAVIDARUM, or pernicious vomiting of pregnancy, may develop. If unchecked, it may result in such symptoms as dehydration and weight loss, and may threaten the life of both the mother and the unborn child.

Causes. The actual causes of morning sickness are not known. It is believed that hunger is a contributing factor. It is also thought that there may be a metabolic upset that occurs as a result of pregnancy and contributes to this condition. Psychological factors may also contribute to or cause morning sickness.

Treatment. Morning sickness is usually little more than a discomfort, requiring no treatment. If a woman can be diverted from thinking about it, it tends to lessen or pass away entirely. If possible, she should have something light to eat before getting out of bed in the morning. This could be crackers or weak tea, possibly left beside the bed at night, with the tea in a thermos bottle; better still, someone might help her have breakfast in bed. After eating, she should rest for about 15 minutes before getting up.

Excessive fluid intake should be avoided. At meals, it is best to eat dry foods first. Liquids should be taken last and sipped in small quantities. Instead of three large meals, small meals should be eaten at more frequent intervals. It is also advisable to rest after each meal. Dry foods, such as crackers, or soft foods eaten every 2 hours until the nausea is over can also be helpful.

Sights, smells, and foods that may be disturbing should be avoided, as should greasy foods, fats, and butter. Also to be avoided are those vegetables which are hard to digest, such as cabbage, cauliflower, cucumbers, and onions. Antiemetics should be avoided during the first trimester because of the possible risks of teratogenesis.

Moro reflex (mo'ro) flexion of an infant's thighs and knees, fanning and then clenching of fingers, with arms first thrown outward and then brought together as though embracing something; produced by a sudden stimulus, such as striking the table on either side of the child, and seen normally in the newborn. Called also embrace reflex.

moron (mo'ron) obsolete term for a person with the highest grade of MENTAL RETARDATION, equivalent to the modern classification "mild mental retardation."

morphea (mor-fe'ah) [Gr.] a type of localized SCLERODERMA in which connective tissue replaces the skin and sometimes subcutaneous tissues, with formation of ivory white or pink patches, bands, or lines that are sometimes bordered by a purple areola. The lesions are firm but not hard and are usually depressed; they may remain localized or may involute, leaving atrophy

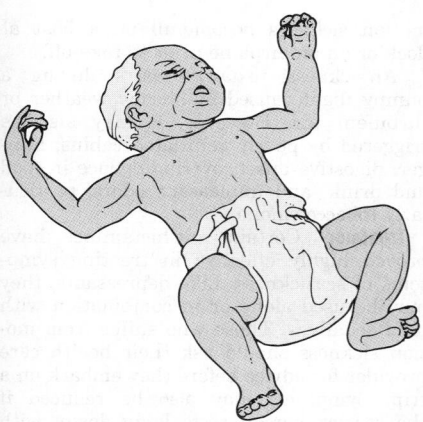

The Moro reflex occurs when the infant is startled.

and scarring. Called also circumscribed or localized scleroderma.

linear m. linear scleroderma.

morphine (mor'fēn) the principal and most active OPIUM alkaloid, an opioid ANALGESIC and respiratory depressant, usually used as the sulfate salt and administered orally, parenterally, or rectally. It is used as an analgesic for relief of severe pain, antitussive, adjunct to anesthesia, and adjunct to treatment of pulmonary edema caused by left ventricular failure. Its use carries with it the dangers of addiction (see DRUG DEPENDENCE), as well as drug TOLERANCE (the need for increasingly larger doses over time to achieve the desired effect). Since morphine is a powerful respiratory depressant, it should be withheld and the patient carefully assessed if the patient's respirations are less than 12 per minute.

morphinism (mor'fin-izm) 1. a pathological state due to habitual misuse of morphine. 2. morphine addiction.

morphogenesis (mor″fo-jen'ĕ-sis) the developmental changes of growth and differentiation occurring in the organization of the body and its parts. adj., **morphogenet'ic.**

morphology (mor″fol'o-je) 1. the science of the form and structure of organisms. 2. the form and structure of a particular organism, organ, tissue, or cell. adj., **morpholog'ic.**

morphometry (mor-fom'ĕ-tre) the measurement of forms.

morphotype (mor'fo-tīp) a group of bacterial strains within a single species that are distinguishable from other such strains because of morphological characteristics that may or may not indicate differing serological states.

-morphous word element [Gr.], *shape; form.*

Morquio's disease (syndrome) (mor-ke'ōz) a form of MUCOPOLYSACCHARIDOSIS becoming evident when the affected infant starts to walk, marked by severe dwarfism, prominent sternum, short neck, kyphosis, genu valgum, and waddling gait; mental retardation is absent or slight. Called also osteochondrodystrophy and familial osteochondrodystrophy.

Morquio-Ullrich disease (mor-ke'o ool'-rik) Morquio's disease.

morrhuate (mor'u-āt) the fatty acids of cod liver oil; the sodium salt is used as a sclerosing AGENT.

mors (mors) [L.] death.

morsus (mor'sus) [L.] bite.

m. dia'boli the fimbriated end of a fallopian tube.

mortal (mor't'l) 1. destined to die. 2. fatal.

mortality (mor-tal'ĭ-te) the quality of being mortal. 1. death rate. 2. the ratio of actual deaths to expected deaths.

mortar (mor'ter) a vessel with a rounded internal surface, used with a PESTLE, for reducing a solid to a powder or producing a homogeneous mixture of solids.

mortification (mor″tĭ-fĭ-ka'shun) gangrene.

morula (mor'u-lah) a solid mass of cells (BLASTOMERES) resembling a mulberry, formed by cleavage of a ZYGOTE (fertilized ovum).

Morvan's syndrome (mor-vahz') 1. syringomyelia. 2. a form of syringomyelia with painless ulceration of the fingertips and analgesic paralysis and atrophy of the forearms and hands.

mosaic (mo-za'ik) a pattern made of numerous small pieces fitted together; in genetics, occurrence in an individual of two or more cell populations each having a different chromosome complement.

mosaicism (mo-za'ĭ-sizm) the presence in an individual of cells derived from the same zygote, but differing in chromosomal constitution.

Moschcowitz's disease (mosh'ko-wit″-zez) thrombotic thrombocytopenic purpura.

mOsm milliosmole.

mosquito (mos-ke'to) any of various small winged insects, many of which are bloodsucking and important vectors of disease. The most important genera are AEDES, ANOPHELES, and CULEX, which are responsible for the transmission of YELLOW FEVER, MALARIA, DENGUE, and other diseases.

mother (moth'er) a female parent. With techniques of ASSISTED FERTILITY, three types of mother can be defined: (1) genetic, (2) gestational, and (3) social. A woman may be one, two, or all three types of mother to a child.

genetic m. a woman whose contribution to the child was the ovum, and hence genes.

gestational m. a woman whose uterus was used for the nurturing and development of an embryo into a baby.

social m. a woman who rears the baby after birth.

motile (mo′til) having spontaneous but not conscious or volitional movement.

motilin (mo-til′in) a polypeptide hormone secreted by enterochromaffin cells of the gut; it causes increased motility of several portions of the gut and stimulates pepsin secretion. Its release is stimulated by the presence of acid and fat in the duodenum.

motility (mo-til′ĭ-te) the ability or power to move spontaneously.

motion (mo′shun) movement.

m. sickness discomfort felt by some people on a moving boat, train, airplane, or automobile, or even on an elevator or a swing. The discomfort is caused by irregular and abnormal motion that disturbs the organs of balance located in the inner ear. There may be mild symptoms of nausea, dizziness, or headache, as well as pallor and cold perspiration. In more acute cases, there may be vomiting and sometimes prostration. Though most people quickly adapt to travel by airplane, ship, and automobile, few are wholly immune to motion sickness. Even astronauts become ill if the inner ear organs of balance are continuously stimulated by unusual motion. Fortunately, most cases of motion sickness vanish quickly once the journey is over, leaving no ill effects.

Causes. The inner ear possesses three semicircular canals, located at right angles in three different planes. People are accustomed to movement in the horizontal plane, which stimulates certain semicircular canals, but not to vertical movements such as the motion of an elevator or a ship pitching at sea. These vertical movements stimulate the semicircular canals in an unusual way, producing the sensation of nausea, or motion sickness.

Anxiety, grief, or other emotions can also cause motion sickness. A person unaccustomed to traveling by boat or airplane may be apprehensive or nervous and therefore may develop symptoms of nausea. Some individuals with previous experience of motion sickness become ill on a boat at dock or on an airplane prior to take-off.

Airsickness usually occurs during a bumpy flight caused by stormy weather or turbulent air. However, it may also be triggered by poorly ventilated cabins, hunger, digestive upset, overindulgence in food and drink, and unpleasant odors, particularly tobacco smoke.

Treatment. Certain antihistamines have proved highly effective in treating symptoms of seasickness. Like depressants, they may be used alone or in combination with mild sedatives. Those who suffer from motion sickness should ask their health care provider for advice before they embark on a trip. Symptoms may also be reduced if the seasick person rests lying down, with the head low, in a comfortable, well aired place.

Prevention. Being rested and in good health prior to a journey helps to prevent motion sickness. During a voyage by boat, it is advisable for the passenger to remain near the center of the ship, where there will be the least motion. Ample fresh air and exercise and avoidance of stuffy rooms and disagreeable smells are also good precautions. The traveler should keep comfortably warm and avoid overeating and eating rich foods.

For those traveling by air, adequate hydration and small, easily digested meals taken during the flight help to prevent airsickness. The passenger who experiences motion sickness may benefit from reclining in the seat as far as possible and closing the eyes.

Carsickness is often relieved if the journey is interrupted for short walks in the fresh air and by keeping a window open Children will frequently find it helpful to glance down, and to refrain from reading Tobacco smoke can also be an aggravating factor.

motoceptor (mo′to-sep″ter) any muscle sense receptor.

motoneuron (mo″to-noor′on) a neuron having a motor function; an efferent neuron conveying motor impulses. Called also motor neuron.

lower m. a peripheral neuron whose cell body lies in the ventral gray columns of the spinal cord and whose termination is in a skeletal muscle.

peripheral m's neurons in a peripheral reflex arc that receive impulses from interneurons and transmit them to voluntary muscles.

upper m. a neuron in the cerebral cortex that conducts impulses from the motor cortex to a motor nucleus of one of

motor (mo′ter) 1. pertaining to motion. 2. a muscle, nerve, or center that effects movements.

m. neuron disease any disease of the motor NEURONS, including spinal muscular ATROPHY, progressive bulbar PARALYSIS, AMYOTROPHIC LATERAL SCLEROSIS, and lateral SCLEROSIS.

Motrin (mo′trin) trademark for preparations of IBUPROFEN, a NONSTEROIDAL ANTIINFLAMMATORY DRUG.

mottle (mot″l) a disturbance in a recorded radiographic image.

grid m. in radiology, a widening of grid lines when the grid is in motion.

quantum m. variations in optical density on a radiograph.

mottling (mot′ling) discoloration in irregular areas.

moulage (moo-lahzh′) [Fr.] a wax model of a structure or lesion.

mould (mōld) mold.

mounding (mownd′ing) the rising in a lump of a wasting muscle when struck.

mount (mownt) to prepare specimens and slides for study.

mountain sickness altitude sickness.

mourning (mor′ning) 1. the normal psychological processes that follow the loss of a loved one; grief is the accompanying emotional state (see GRIEVING). Four phases have been described: a short phase of numbness and denial, followed by a phase of yearning and protest marked by intense pining for the dead, followed by a phase of disorganization marked by pain and despair, ending in a phase of detachment and reorganization of love relationships that completes the work of mourning. 2. social expressions of grief, such as funeral and burial services, prayers, the wearing of black or other specific garments, or other rituals.

mouse (mows) a small rodent, various species of which are used in laboratory experiments. 1. a small loose body. 2. a computer pointing device.

joint m. a movable fragment of synovial membrane, cartilage, or other body within a joint; usually associated with degenerative osteoarthritis and osteochondritis dissecans.

knockout m. a mouse that has had a specific gene artificially deleted from its genome.

nude m. a mouse homozygous for the *nu* gene; these mice are hairless, lack a THYMUS, and thus lack T LYMPHOCYTES.

peritoneal m. a free body in the peritoneal cavity, probably a small detached mass

or omentum, sometimes visible radiographically.

SCID m. (severe combined *i*mmuno*d*eficiency) a strain of mice lacking in T and B LYMPHOCYTES and IMMUNOGLOBULINS, either from inbreeding with an autosomal recessive trait or from genetic engineering, used as a model for studies of the IMMUNE SYSTEM.

mouth (mowth) 1. an opening or aperture. 2. the oral cavity, which forms the beginning of the DIGESTIVE SYSTEM and in which the chewing of food takes place. The mouth is also the site of the organs of TASTE and of the TEETH, TONGUE, and LIPS. It is not only the entrance to the body for food and sometimes air, but also a major organ of SPEECH and emotional expression.

Structure. Except for the teeth, the interior of the mouth is covered with mucous membrane. This thin lining extends out from the front of the mouth to form the lips. Salivary glands lie above and below the mouth and produce saliva, a liquid that protects the delicate membranes and mixes with food in the first step of digestion of food.

The PALATE forms the roof of the mouth. The front two thirds of the palate comprises the hard palate, and the back third, the soft palate. The soft palate is hinged to the hard palate and is flanked on both sides by the TONSILS. In the middle of the soft palate is the UVULA, a projection pointing down to the tongue. At the root of the tongue, below the uvula, lies the EPIGLOTTIS.

Disorders. Because of its special functions the mouth is constantly exposed to infection and irritation. These can affect the whole mouth generally or only certain parts, such as the tongue. Inflammation of the mouth, or STOMATITIS, can indicate the presence of either a mild or severe disease. Local conditions include THRUSH, GINGIVITIS, and HERPES SIMPLEX. Generalized diseases can also give rise to inflammation of the mouth; these include diphtheria, tuberculosis, blood dyscrasias, vitamin deficiencies, and syphilis.

Cancer can afflict the sides of the mouth, the lips, the tongue, and occasionally the salivary glands. Continued irritation, such as pipe smoking, is thought to be a cause of many mouth cancers. Any persistent sore or swelling should be promptly examined by a health care worker.

Birth defects affecting the mouth include CLEFT LIP and CLEFT PALATE. Both have the same cause: failure of adjacent parts of the body to unite properly in fetal life. A cleft lip (popularly called "harelip") involves a split in the upper lip. Sometimes the cleft extends into the upper jaw, the floor of the nose, and the palate. The resulting deformity of nose and mouth interferes with sucking and speech unless corrected by surgery. A cleft palate, which may cause difficulties in speaking and eating, signifies a cleavage in the uvula and the soft palate. Both conditions can be successfully corrected by surgery.

m. care techniques of oral HYGIENE whose purpose is to preserve or restore and maintain normal physiology and function of the oral cavity. These include assessment of the mouth, cleaning, and removal of debris from the teeth, palate, tongue, and sides of the mouth. Periodically and systematically cleaning the mouth, brushing the teeth, and flossing help prevent DENTAL CARIES, inflammatory PERIODONTAL DISEASE, and HALITOSIS. Mouth care also promotes a sense of cleanliness and well-being, facilitates speech, and helps overcome loss of appetite. Additionally, a healthy oral mucosa is the first line of defense against infection in the oral cavity.

In the normal mouth a healthy oral mucosa is maintained in part by movements of the tongue, lips, and cheeks during speech, chewing, and swallowing. Salivation and the mechanical action of chewing foods also help keep the mucosa soft and moist. Brushing and flossing or other less forceful measures facilitate removal of debris, bacteria, and plaque and preserve the integrity of the teeth and gums.

Patients most in need of special mouth care include those who (1) breathe through their mouths because of nasal obstruction or other conditions, (2) are receiving nasal oxygen, (3) have a restricted oral intake or are being fed by tube, (4) are comatose or otherwise unable to care for their teeth and mouth, (5) are receiving radiation therapy to the head and neck, or (6) are receiving chemotherapy for a malignancy. Both radiation and chemotherapy can cause severe STOMATITIS and XEROSTOMIA.

Initial and ongoing assessment of the oral cavity can establish the type and frequency of mouth care needed. In general, the more easily damaged the integrity of the oral mucosa, the more gentle the chemical and mechanical cleansing. If brushing with a soft nylon toothbrush and nonabrasive toothpaste and flossing cannot be tolerated, the teeth can be cleaned with unflavored oral care sponges dipped into plain water or a physiologic saline solution. Flossing is contraindicated if the patient has a low platelet count or low white cell count. Mouthwashes are not a substitute for toothbrushing.

XEROSTOMIA (excessive dryness of the mouth) can be relieved by artificial SALIVA or by application of a water soluble lubricant such as KY jelly. If the patient is able to eat and drink, fluids and moist foods are encouraged. Dry, cracked lips respond best to petroleum JELLY or a camphor-based lip balm. Lemon juice and GLYCERIN are not recommended in patients with MUCOSITIS because when used over a period of time glycerin tends to dry oral tissues.

Thick and tenacious mucus in the oral cavity can be removed by diluted HYDROGEN PEROXIDE or SOCIUM BICARBONATE solution. The hydrogen peroxide solution is prepared by mixing equal parts hydrogen peroxide (USP 3 per cent) and water just before application. A peroxide solution is contraindicated if the patient has LEUKEMIA or there are freshly granulating surfaces or exposed bone in the oral cavity. Sodium bicarbonate solution is made by adding one teaspoon of sodium bicarbonate to one pint (half a liter) of water. The same proportions of salt and water are used to prepare a 0.9 per cent solution of normal SALINE.

If pain in the mouth prevents a patient from eating comfortably, it may be possible to provide temporary relief by rinsing the mouth with a solution of one part LIDOCAINE viscous 2 per cent added to two parts water. However, since this solution diminishes sensitivity to heat, the patient must not be fed hot food or drinks that could cause burns.

Diligent, systematic mouth care is an integral part of hospital care. Research has shown that such care prevents many problems of nutrition, infection, and pain associated with stomatitis, especially those occurring as a complication of chemotherapy and radiation therapy. Moreover, routine care of the mouth, teeth, and gums, no matter what the health status of the patient, can prevent many problems, maintain a healthy oral cavity, and do much to make the patient more comfortable.

denture sore m. denture stomatitis.

trench m. name given to necrotizing ulcerative GINGIVITIS during World War I, when it was common among soldiers in the trenches.

mouthwash a solution for rinsing the mouth.

movement (mo͞ov′ment) 1. an act of moving; called also motion. 2. an act of DEFECATION.

active m. movement produced by the person's own muscles.

ameboid m. movement like that of an ameba, accomplished by protrusion of cytoplasm of the cell.

associated m. movement of parts that act together, as the eyes.

brownian m. the peculiar, rapid, oscillatory movement of fine particles suspended in a fluid medium; called also molecular movement.

circus m. the propagation of an impulse again and again through tissue already previously activated by it; the term is usually reserved for the REENTRY involving an accessory PATHWAY.

molecular m. brownian movement.

passive m. a movement of the body or of the extremities of a patient performed by another person without voluntary motion on the part of the patient.

vermicular m's the wormlike movements of the intestines in peristalsis.

moxa (mok′sah) a tuft of soft, combustible material to be burned upon the skin as a CAUTERY and COUNTERIRRITANT.

moxalactam (mok′sah-lak″tam) a third generation CEPHALOSPORIN ANTIBIOTIC having a broad spectrum of activity, effective against β-lactamase–producing strains of *Haemophilus influenzae* and gram-negative enteric bacilli, including multiple drug-resistant strains.

Moxam (mok′sam) trademark for a preparation of MOXALACTAM disodium, a broad-spectrum antibiotic.

moxibustion (mok″sĭ-bus′chun) COUNTER-IRRITATION produced by igniting a cone or cylinder of MOXA placed on the skin.

moxifloxacin (mok″sĭ-flok′sah-sin) a broad-spectrum ANTIBIOTIC effective against many gram-positive and gram-negative bacteria; administered orally as the hydrochloride salt in the treatment of bacterial complication of chronic BRONCHITIS, acute SINUSITIS, community-acquired PNEUMONIA, and skin and skin structure infections due to susceptible organisms.

6-MP mercaptopurine.

MPD maximum permissible dose.

MPH Master of Public Health.

mR milliroentgen.

MRA Medical Record Administrator.

mrad millirad.

MRCP Member of the Royal College of Physicians.

MRCS Member of the Royal College of Surgeons.

mrem millirem.

MRI magnetic resonance imaging.

MRL Medical Record Librarian, former name for MEDICAL RECORD ADMINISTRATOR.

mRNA messenger RNA; see RIBONUCLEIC ACID.

MS Master of Science; Master of Surgery; mitral stenosis; multiple sclerosis.

ms millisecond.

μs microsecond.

MSH melanocyte-stimulating hormone.

MSN Master of Science in Nursing.

MT medical technologist; see CLINICAL LABORATORY SCIENTIST/MEDICAL TECHNOLOGIST.

MTX methotrexate.

mu chain disease (mu chān) the rarest form of HEAVY CHAIN DISEASE, found in patients with chronic lymphocytic leukemia; symptoms include hepatomegaly and splenomegaly.

muciferous (mu-sif′er-us) muciparous.

muciform (mu′sĭ-form) mucoid (def. 1).

mucigen (mu′sĭ-jen) a substance present in mucous cells, convertible into mucin and mucus.

mucilage (mu′sĭ-lij) an aqueous solution of a gummy substance, used as a vehicle or soothing agent. adj., **mucilag′inous.**

mucilloid (mu′sil-oid) a preparation of a mucilaginous substance.

psyllium hydrophilic m. a powdered preparation of the mucilaginous portion of blond PSYLLIUM seeds, used in treatment of constipation.

mucin (mu′sin) a mucopolysaccharide or glycoprotein that is the chief constituent of mucus.

mucinase (mu′sĭ-nās) an enzyme that acts upon mucin.

mucinogen (mu-sin′o-jen) a precursor of mucin.

mucinoid (mu′sĭ-noid) 1. resembling mucin. 2. mucoid (def. 2).

mucinosis (mu″si-no′sis) a state with abnormal deposits of mucin in the skin, often associated with hypothyroidism (myxedema).

follicular m. a disease of the pilosebaceous unit, presenting clinically as grouped follicular papules or plaques with associated hair loss, caused by mucinous infiltration of tissues, and usually involving the scalp, face, and neck. It may be primary (idiopathic), occurring most often in children, or it may be secondary to mycosis fungoides or reticulosis.

muciparous (mu-sip′ah-rus) secreting MUCUS.

mucocele (mu′ko-sēl) 1. dilation of a cavity with accumulated mucous secretion. 2. a mucous polyp.

mucocutaneous (mu″ko-ku-ta′ne-us) pertaining to mucous membrane and skin.

m. lymph node syndrome Kawasaki's disease.

mucoepidermoid (mu″ko-ep″ĭ-der′moid) composed of mucus-producing epithelial cells.

mucoid (mu′koid) 1. resembling mucus. 2. resembling mucus; called also myxoid.

M

3. a mucus-like conjugated protein of animal origin, differing from mucin in solubility.

mucokinetic (mu″ko-kĭ-net′ik) a drug that facilitates removal of mucus from the respiratory tract.

mucolipidosis (mu″ko-lip″ĭ-do′sis), pl. *mucolipido′ses* any of a group of genetic disorders in which both GLYCOSAMINOGLYCANS (GAGs) and LIPIDS accumulate in tissues, but without excess of GAG in the urine.

m. I sialidosis (type I).

m. II a rapidly progressing disease of young children, histologically characterized by abnormal fibroblasts containing a large number of dark inclusions which fill the central part of the cytoplasm except for the juxtanuclear zone (I-cells), and clinically by severe growth impairment, minimal hepatic enlargement, extreme mental and motor retardation, and clear corneas; inherited as an autosomal recessive trait, it is due to deficiency of multiple lysosomal hydrolases. Called also I-cell disease.

m. III a disorder similar to but milder than mucolipidosis II, and thought to be due to the same enzyme deficiency but to a lesser extent. Called also pseudo-Hurler polydystrophy.

m. IV a form marked by early corneal clouding, psychomotor retardation, and the presence of lysosomal storage bodies; thought to be transmitted as an autosomal recessive trait.

mucolytic (mu″ko-lit′ik) 1. capable of reducing the viscosity of mucus. 2. an agent that so acts.

mucomembranous (mu″ko-mem′brah-nus) pertaining to or composed of mucous membrane.

mucoperiosteum (mu″ko-per″e-os′te-um) periosteum having a mucous surface, as in parts of the auditory apparatus. adj., **mucoperios′teal.**

mucopolysaccharide (mu″ko-pol″ĭ-sak′-ah-rīd) a group of polysaccharides that contain hexosamine, that may or may not be combined with protein and that, dispersed in water, form many of the mucins.

mucopolysaccharidosis (mu″ko-pol″ĭ-sak″ah-rĭ-do′sis), pl. *mucopolysaccharido′ses* any of a group of genetically determined disorders due to a defect in mucopolysaccharide metabolism, marked by skeletal changes, mental retardation, visceral involvement, and corneal clouding, with widespread tissue deposits and mucopolysacchariduria. HURLER'S SYNDROME is the prototype of this disorder.

mucoprotein (mu″ko-pro′tēn) a compound present in all connective and supporting tissues, containing, as prosthetic groups (non–amino acid components), mucopolysaccharides; soluble in water and relatively resistant to denaturation.

Tamm-Horsfall m. a substance produced by cells of the ascending limb of the loop of Henle; it is a normal constituent of urine and is the major protein constituent of urinary casts.

mucopurulent (mu″ko-pu′roo-lent) marked by an exudate containing both mucus and pus.

mucopus (mu′ko-pus) mucus blended with pus.

Mucor (mu′kor) a genus of perfect fungi; several species are molds and saprobes on fruits, vegetables, or baked goods and can cause MUCORMYCOSIS.

Mucorales an order of perfect fungi of the class Zygomycetes, made up of bread molds and related fungi; genera *Absidia, Mucor,* and *Rhizopus* can cause opportunistic MUCORMYCOSIS in humans.

mucormycosis (mu″kor-mi-ko′sis) a MYCOSIS due to fungi of the order Mucorales, such as species of *Rhizopus* and less often *Mucor* or *Absidia.* In humans it is usually an OPPORTUNISTIC INFECTION in IMMUNOCOMPROMISED patients or those with a chronic debilitating disease such as uncontrolled diabetes mellitus. Organisms enter through the respiratory tract, digestive tract, or a skin lesion, and then invade blood vessel walls and are disseminated in the blood; spread along nerve trunks also occurs. The disease may affect the head and neck, the respiratory tract, the digestive tract, or more rarely the skin. Clinical manifestations range from chronic to fulminant. Related fungi in the class Entomophthorales cause a similar condition called ENTOMOPHTHOROMYCOSIS. Called also phycomycosis and zygomycosis.

cerebral m. fulminant, usually fatal mucormycotic infection of the brain, usually seen in IMMUNOCOMPROMISED patients or those with acidotic diabetes or leukemia; it may be caused by dissemination of fungi from a distant site or by direct extension of rhinocerebral mucormycosis.

cutaneous m. mucormycosis of the skin, usually seen in weak, diabetic, or IMMUNOCOMPROMISED patients.

pulmonary m. mucormycosis of the lung, usually seen in weak or IMMUNOCOMPROMISED patients; symptoms include bronchitis, cavitation, hemoptysis, and often death within a month.

rhinocerebral m. cerebral mucormycosis in which the original site of infection is in the ethmoid, sphenoid, or maxillary sinuses, or, in some cases, the palate or pharynx.

mucosa (mu-ko′sah) [L.] mucous membrane. adj., **muco′sal.**

alveolar m. the mucosal lining of the dental alveoli; a thin, soft, fragile continuation of the mucous membrane of the cheek, lips, and floor of the mouth.

mucosal neuroma syndrome (mu-ko′sahl nōō-ro′mah) multiple endocrine NEOPLASIA, type III.

mucosanguineous (mu″ko-sang-gwin′e-us) composed of mucus and blood.

mucosectomy (mu-ko-sek′tah-me) excision of mucosa, such as in the colon in treatment of INFLAMMATORY BOWEL DISEASE.

mucoserous (mu″ko-sēr′us) composed of mucus and serum.

mucositis (mu″ko-si′tis) inflammation of a mucous membrane.

mucosocutaneous (mu-ko″so-ku-ta′ne-us) pertaining to a mucous membrane and the skin.

mucous (mu′kus) pertaining to or secreting MUCUS.

mucoviscidosis (mu″ko-vis″ĭ-do′sis) cystic fibrosis.

mucus (mu′kus) the free slime of the mucous membrane, composed of the secretion of its glands, various salts, desquamated cells, and leukocytes.

cervical m. that constituting the mucous membrane of the uterine CERVIX; it undergoes chemical and physical changes owing to hormone stimulation during the MENSTRUAL CYCLE and plays an important role in helping SPERMATOZOA travel inwards after COITUS. See also discussion of the *cervical mucus method* of contraception, under CONTRACEPTION.

fertile m. see ovulation method of CONTRACEPTION.

mud fever a type of LEPTOSPIROSIS occurring in the summer and autumn in Germany and Russia, caused by *Leptospira interrogans*; it is transmitted to humans by the field mouse *Microtus arvalis* and affects mainly workers in swamps or flooded fields. Called also autumn fever.

Müller's maneuver (mil′erz) an effort at inhalation with a closed glottis after exhalation, used during fluoroscopic examination to cause a negative intrathoracic pressure with engorgement of intrathoracic vascular structures, which is helpful in recognizing esophageal varices, and in distinguishing vascular from nonvascular structures.

multi- word element [L.], *many.*

multiallelic (mul″te-ah-lel′ik) pertaining to or occupied by many different genes

affecting the same or different hereditary characters.

multiarticular (mul″te-ahr-tik′u-ler) pertaining to or affecting many joints.

multibacillary (mul″tĭ-bas′ĭla-re) having numerous BACILLI; see LEPROSY.

multicapsular (mul″tĭ-kap′su-ler) having many capsules.

multicellular (mul″tĭ-sel′u-ler) composed of many cells.

multicuspidate (mul″tĭ-kus′pĭ-dāt) having numerous cusps.

multicystic (mul″ti-sis′tik) polycystic.

multifactorial (mul″tĭ-fak-to′re-al) 1. of or pertaining to, or arising through the action of, many factors. 2. in genetics, arising as the result of the interaction of several genes.

multifocal (mul″tĭ-fo′k′l) arising from or pertaining to many sites or locations.

multiform (mul′tĭ-form) occurring in many forms; polymorphic.

multiglandular (mul″tĭ-glan′du-ler) pluriglandular.

multigravida (mul″tĭ-grav′ĭ-dah) a woman pregnant for at least the third time; called also plurigravida.

grand m. a woman who has had six or more previous pregnancies.

multilobar (mul″tĭ-lo′ber) having numerous lobes.

multilobular (mul″tĭ-lob′u-ler) having many lobules.

multilocular (mul″tĭ-lok′u-ler) having many compartments.

multinodular (mul″tĭ-nod′u-ler) having many nodules.

multinucleate (mul″tĭ-noo′kle-āt) polynuclear.

multipara (mul-tip′ah-rah) a woman who has had two or more pregnancies resulting in viable offspring; called also pluripara. adj., **multip′arous.**

grand m. a woman who has had six or more pregnancies that resulted in viable offspring.

multiparity (mul″tĭ-par′ĭ-te) the condition of being a MULTIPARA; called also PLURIPARITY.

multiple (mul′tĭ-p′l) manifold; occurring in various parts of the body at once.

m. myeloma a malignant neoplasm of plasma CELLS in which the plasma cells proliferate and invade the bone marrow, causing destruction of the bone and resulting in pathologic fracture and bone pain. It is the most common type of monoclonal GAMMOPATHY, characterized by presence of a monoclonal IMMUNOGLOBULIN (immunoglobulin recognized as a single protein), Bence Jones PROTEINS in the urine, anemia, and

M

lowered resistance to infection. Called also plasma cell myeloma.

Diagnostic procedures to confirm suspected multiple myeloma include blood analyses, quantitative immunologic assays of serum and urine, urinalysis, bone marrow aspiration and biopsy, and skeletal x-rays. Findings indicative of the disease are an increased number of plasma cells in the bone marrow (usually over 10 per cent of the total), ANEMIA, HYPERCALCEMIA due to release of calcium from deteriorating bone tissue, and elevated BLOOD UREA NITROGEN, Bence Jones protein in the urine, and osteolytic lesions that give the bone a honeycomb appearance on x-ray and lead to vertebral collapse.

Treatment. Treatment of multiple myeloma involves chemotherapy and radiation to relieve pain and manage the acute lesions of the spinal column. High-dose chemotherapy followed by blood cell rescue has shown some efficacy in certain situations. Individuals diagnosed with multiple myeloma who show no symptoms do not usually receive treatment.

Patient Care. Major problems presented by the patient with multiple myeloma are related to anemia, hypercalcemia, bone pain and pathologic fractures, and emotional distress created by trying to cope with the day-to-day physiologic and emotional aspects associated with the diagnosis of a malignant disease. The more common complications to be avoided are infection, RENAL FAILURE, and the sequelae of spinal cord compression.

Transfusions with packed red blood CELLS can help alleviate and minimize some of the more severe symptoms of anemia. It is important that the patient be adequately hydrated to improve viscosity of the blood and circulation, to help avoid hypercalcemia, and to maintain kidney function for excretion of the products of protein metabolism. Continued ambulation and moderate exercise help slow down the loss of minerals, especially calcium, from the bones. Other problems are related to the administration of highly toxic antineoplastic drugs.

m. organ dysfunction syndrome, m. organ failure failure of two or more organ systems in a critically ill patient because of a complex and interrelated series of events. See accompanying illustration.

m. personality disorder dissociative identity disorder.

m.-puncture test an intracutaneous test in which the material used (such as

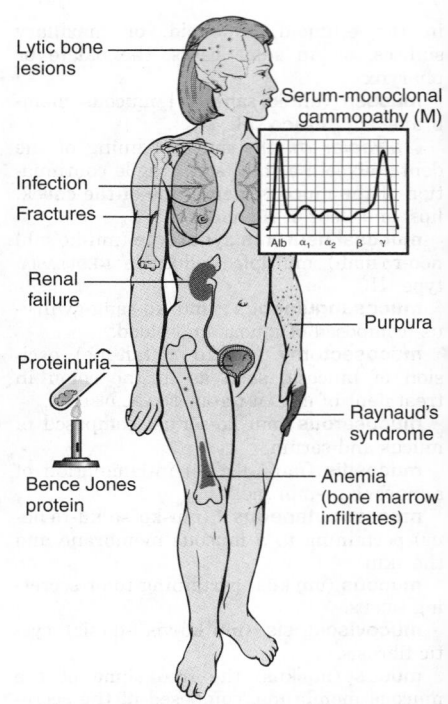

Multiple myeloma. Radiographs of the skull, ribs, and vertebrae show multiple punched out lesions. There is anemia secondary to bone marrow lesions that replace red blood cell precursors. Kidney failure is the most common cause of death. The urine contains Bence Jones protein. From Damjanov, 2000.

TUBERCULIN) is introduced into the skin by pressure of several needles or pointed tines or prongs. This procedure is used in mass screenings, but it is not as accurate as other tests because of lack of precise measurement of the amount of medication actually entering the skin.

m. sclerosis (MS) a chronic neurologic disease in which there are patches of DEMYELINATION scattered throughout the WHITE MATTER of the central nervous system, sometimes extending into the GRAY MATTER. The disease primarily affects the MYELIN and not the nerve cells themselves; any damage to the neurons is secondary to destruction of the myelin covering the axon. The symptoms caused by these lesions are typically weakness, incoordination, paresthesias, speech disturbances, and visual disturbances, particularly diplopia. More specific signs and symptoms depend on the location of the lesions and the severity and destructiveness of the inflammatory and sclerotic processes.

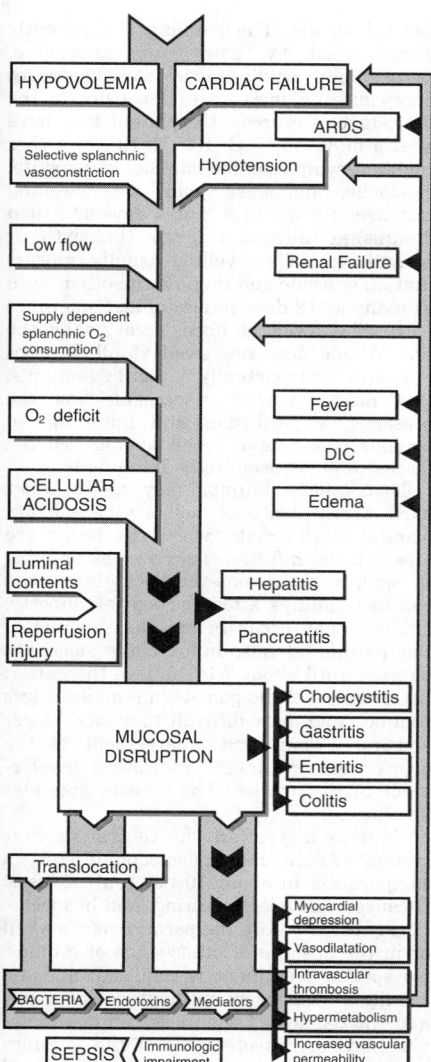

The pathogenesis of multiple organ failure. From Datex Medical Instrumentation, Inc., Tewksbury, MA.

The course of the disease is usually prolonged, with remissions and relapses over many years. Brief exacerbations, even with acute and severe symptoms, are thought to be the result of a transient inflammatory depression of neural transmission. Recovery occurs when there has been no permanent damage to the myelin sheath during the attack. Repeated attacks can, however, eventually permanently denude the axons and leave the yellow sclerotic plaques that are characteristic of the disease. Once the disease process reaches the stage of sclerosis the affected axons cannot recover and there is permanent damage.

The prevalence of MS is not certain because the disease is not one that is reported, and mild cases can be either misdiagnosed or never brought to the attention of a health care provider. It is far more common in the temperate zones of the world than in tropical and subtropical climates. The onset of symptoms most often occurs between the ages of 20 and 40 years, and the disease affects both sexes about equally.

The cause of multiple sclerosis is unknown. It is likely that an inherited IMMUNE RESPONSE is somehow responsible for the production of AUTOANTIBODIES that attack the myelin sheath. Some authorities believe that infection by one of the slow viruses occurs during childhood and after some years of latency the virus triggers an autoimmune response. Others believe there is an antigen or environmental trigger for the disease.

The diagnosis of multiple sclerosis is difficult because of the wide variety of possible clinical manifestations and the resemblance they bear to other neurological disorders. There is no definitive diagnostic test for the condition, but persons with objectively measured abnormalities of the central nervous system, a history of exacerbation and remission of symptoms, and demonstrable delayed blink reflex and evoked visual response are diagnosed as having either possible or probable multiple sclerosis. With time and progressive worsening of symptoms the diagnosis can become definite.

Treatment. A multidisciplinary approach is required to diagnose the condition and help patients and their families cope with the attendant problems. Multiple sclerosis has an impact on physical activity and life style, role, and interpersonal relationships; therefore, vocational guidance, counseling, and group therapy are helpful. It is important that the patient with severe disability maintain a positive attitude, focusing on functional abilities rather than disabilities. Regeneration of the damaged neural tissue is not possible but retraining and adaptation are. Stress due to trauma, infection, overexertion, surgery, or emotional upset can aggravate the condition and precipitate a flare-up of symptoms.

Supportive measures include a regimen of rest and exercise, a well-balanced diet, avoidance of extremes of heat and cold, avoidance of known sources of infection, and adaptation of a life style that is relatively unstressful while still being as productive as possible.

Therapeutic measures include medications to diminish muscle spasticity; measures to overcome urinary retention (such as CREDÉ'S METHOD or intermittent CATHETERIZATION); speech therapy; and physical therapy to maintain muscle tone and avoid orthopedic deformities. Management of MS has been greatly enhanced by the availability of INTERFERONS BETA-1A and BETA-1B. Research support is strong that these medications reduce the frequency and severity of relapses.

Many multiple sclerosis patients and their families receive valuable support and encouragement from communication with others coping with the condition. A local chapter of the National Multiple Sclerosis Society is within reach of most persons in the United States. Information and assistance in all phases of the disease are available by writing to The National Multiple Sclerosis Society, 733 Third Ave., 6th floor, New York, NY 10017, or consulting their web site at http://www.nmss.org.

multipolar (mul″tĭ-po′ler) having more than two poles or processes.

multisynaptic (mul″tĭ-sĭ-nap′tik) pertaining to or relayed through two or more synapses.

multivalent (mul″ti-va′lent) 1. having a valence of two or more. 2. denoting an antiserum, vaccine, or antitoxin specific for more than one antigen or organism; called also polyvalent.

multivariate (mul″tĭ-var′e-āt) involving more than one variable (usually taken to mean three or more variables).

mumps (mumps) a communicable PARA-MYXOVIRUS disease that attacks one or both of the parotid glands, the largest of the salivary glands. Occasionally the submandibular glands are also affected. Although older people may contract the disease, mumps usually strikes children between the ages of 5 and 15. It is spread by droplet infection and is contagious in the infected person from 1 to 2 days before symptoms appear until 1 or 2 days after they disappear. The incubation period is usually 18 days, although it may vary from 12 to 26 days. One attack usually gives immunity. Called also contagious or epidemic parotitis.

Symptoms. Often the first noticeable symptom of mumps is a swelling of one of the parotid glands. The swelling is frequently accompanied by pain and tenderness. Occasionally acidic foods and beverages may cause an increase in the pain. In the first stage of mumps, the patient may have a fever of 38° to 40°C (100° to 104°F). Other common symptoms include loss of appetite, headache, and back pain. The swelling increases for the first 2 or 3 days and then diminishes, disappearing by the sixth or seventh day. The swelling usually appears first on one side and then on the other, with as many as 12 days intervening. Sometimes both sides swell at once; occasionally the second side does not swell at all. Mumps may also occur virtually without symptoms; this mild form is responsible for the presence of antibodies and immunity in persons who cannot recall having had the disease and yet seem to be immune to it.

Complications. Mumps may affect other parts of the body as well as the salivary glands. In the male, when the testes are affected, the infection is known as orchitis. It strikes about one-third of those who contract mumps after the age of puberty. Orchitis may occur before the swelling of the parotid glands, but usually does not develop until about 7 to 10 days thereafter. Involvement of the gonads in females is less common and more difficult to detect. Lower abdominal pain and enlargement of the ovaries are symptoms indicating involvement of the ovaries. The breasts may also be affected.

Mumps may affect the central nervous system. Acute meningoencephalitis is a complication in about 10 per cent of cases. It causes dizziness, vomiting, and headache. It may occur before the parotid glands swell or in the absence of other signs of mumps. No specific treatment is required, and the condition disappears without causing permanent damage. Other less common complications are involvement of the auditory nerve (resulting in deafness), myelitis, and facial neuritis.

Treatment. Most children with mumps do not feel ill enough to be confined to bed, and it is sufficient if they remain quietly at home, unless there is a rise in temperature or a complication develops. The Centers for Disease Control and Prevention recommend droplet PRECAUTIONS for 9 days after the onset of swelling. Persons who are not susceptible need not wear masks while in contact with the person who has mumps.

Prevention. Men over the age of puberty who are still susceptible to mumps should avoid contact with the patient. The mumps virus cannot survive for any length of time in open air, so it is unnecessary to take special precautions with the patient's clothing, bedding, dishes, or utensils. The mumps vaccine induces antibodies in 95 per cent of those inoculated, but it does not afford protection if given during the incubation period following exposure, and it is contraindicated if another infection is present. Children should receive the mumps vaccine with measles and rubella vaccination at 12 to 15 months of age, with a second immunization when they are 4 to 6 years old. It is not given to infants under one year of age and is not recommended for persons allergic to eggs or NEOMYCIN. Mumps immune globulin may afford short-term immunity when there is an extraordinary need for protection, but the extent of its effectiveness is not known.

Munchausen syndrome (mun′chow-zen) habitual seeking of hospital treatment for apparent acute illness, the patient giving a plausible and dramatic history, all of which is false. It is a subtype of FACTITIOUS DISORDER.

Munchausen syndrome by proxy (mun′chow-zen) see FACTITIOUS DISORDER BY PROXY.

mupirocin (mu-pir′o-sin) an antibacterial derived from *Pseudomonas fluorescens,* effective against staphylococci and non-enteric streptococci; used in the treatment of impetigo and, as the calcium salt, in the treatment of nasal colonization by *Staphylococcus aureus.*

mural (mu′ral) pertaining to or occurring in a wall of an organ or cavity.

muramidase (mu-ram′ĭ-dās) lysozyme.

Murchison-Pel-Ebstein fever (mur′chĭ-son-pel-eb′stīn) a type of fever typical of Hodgkin's disease, marked by irregular episodes of pyrexia of several days' duration, with intervening periods in which the temperature is normal.

murine (mu′rēn) pertaining to or affecting mice or rats.

murmur (mer′mer) an auscultatory sound, benign or pathologic, loud or soft, particularly a periodic sound of short duration of cardiac or vascular origin.

    aortic m. a sound indicative of disease of the aortic valve.

    apex m., apical m. a HEART MURMUR heard over the apex of the heart.

    arterial m. one in an artery, sometimes aneurysmal and sometimes constricted.

    Austin Flint m. a loud presystolic MURMUR at the apex heard when aortic REGURGITATION is preventing the mitral valve from closing; called also Flint's murmur.

    blood m. one due to an abnormal, commonly anemic, condition of the blood. Called also hemic murmur.

    cardiac m. HEART MURMUR.

    cardiopulmonary m. one produced by the impact of the heart against the lung.

    continuous m. a humming HEART MURMUR heard throughout systole and diastole.

    crescendo m. one marked by progressively increasing loudness that suddenly ceases.

    Cruveilhier-Baumgarten m. one heard at the abdominal wall over veins connecting the portal and caval systems.

    diastolic m. a HEART MURMUR heard at DIASTOLE, due to mitral obstruction or to aortic or pulmonic REGURGITATION with forward flow across the atrioventricular valve; it has a rumbling quality.

    Duroziez's m. a double murmur during systole and diastole, palpated over the femoral or another large peripheral artery; due to aortic INSUFFICIENCY.

    ejection m. a systolic MURMUR heard predominantly in midsystole, when ejection volume and velocity of blood flow are at their maximum; it is produced by ejection of blood into the pulmonary artery and aorta.

    Flint's m. Austin Flint murmur.

    friction m. friction rub.

    functional m. a HEART MURMUR occurring in the absence of structural changes in the heart, usually due to high cardiac output states. Called also innocent murmur and physiologic murmur.

    Gibson m. a long rumbling sound occupying most of systole and diastole, usually localized in the second left interspace near the sternum, and usually indicative of PATENT DUCTUS ARTERIOSUS. Called also machinery murmur.

    Graham Steell m. a high-pitched diastolic MURMUR due to pulmonic REGURGITATION in patients with pulmonary hypertension and mitral stenosis.

    heart m. see HEART MURMUR.

    hemic m. blood murmur.

    innocent m. functional murmur.

    machinery m. Gibson murmur.

    mitral m. a HEART MURMUR due to disease of the mitral valve; it can be either obstructive or regurgitant.

    musical m. one that has a periodic harmonic pattern; it may be either a HEART MURMUR or a vascular MURMUR.

    organic m. one due to a lesion in the organ or organ system being examined, e.g., in the heart, in a blood vessel, or in lung tissue.

    pansystolic m. a regurgitant MURMUR heard throughout systole, due to blood flow between two chambers normally of very

M

different pressures in systole; the most common causes are mitral REGURGITATION, tricuspid REGURGITATION, and VENTRICULAR SEPTAL DEFECTS.

physiologic m. functional murmur.

prediastolic m. one occurring just before and with DIASTOLE, due to aortic REGURGITATION or pulmonic REGURGITATION.

presystolic m. one shortly before the onset of ventricular ejection, usually associated with a narrowed atrioventricular valve.

pulmonic m. one due to disease of the pulmonary valve or artery.

regurgitant m. a HEART MURMUR due to a dilated valvular orifice with consequent valvular REGURGITATION.

seagull m. a raucous murmur resembling the call of a seagull, frequently heard in aortic STENOSIS or mitral REGURGITATION.

Still's m. a functional HEART MURMUR of childhood, with a buzzing or vibratory tone heard in midsystole; it usually disappears by puberty.

systolic m. a HEART MURMUR heard at SYSTOLE, usually due to mitral or tricuspid REGURGITATION or to aortic or pulmonary obstruction.

to-and-fro m. a friction sound or murmur heard with both SYSTOLE and DIASTOLE.

tricuspid m. a HEART MURMUR caused by disease of the tricuspid valve; it may be either obstructive or regurgitant.

vascular m. one heard over a blood vessel.

vesicular m. vesicular breath SOUNDS.

muromonab-CD3 (mu″ro-mo′nab) a murine monoclonal ANTIBODY to the CD3 antigen of human T cells, functioning as an IMMUNOSUPPRESSANT in treatment of acute rejection of renal, hepatic, and cardiac transplants.

Murphy's sign (mur′fēz) a sign of gallbladder disease consisting of pain on taking a deep breath when the examiner's fingers are on the approximate location of the gallbladder.

Musca (mus′kah) a genus of flies, including the common housefly, *M. domes′-tica.*

musca (mus′kah) [L.] fly.

mus′cae volitan′tes specks seen as floating before the eyes.

muscarine (mus′kah-rin) a deadly alkaloid from various mushrooms, e.g., *Amanita muscaria* (the fly agaric), and also from rotten fish. See also muscarinic RECEPTORS.

muscarinic (mus″kah-rin′ik) pertaining to the transmission of nerve impulses mediated by muscarinic RECEPTORS.

muscle (mus″l) a bundle of long slender cells (muscle FIBERS) that have the power to contract and hence to produce movement. Muscles are responsible for locomotion and play an important part in performing vital body functions. They also protect the contents of the abdomen against injury and help support the body. See appendix 3-4 and see color plates.

Muscle fibers range in length from a few hundred thousandths of a centimeter to several centimeters. They also vary in shape, and in color from white to deep red. Each fiber receives its own nerve impulses, so that fine and varied motions are possible. Each has its small stored supply of GLYCOGEN, which it uses as fuel for energy. Muscles, especially the heart, also use free fatty acids as fuel. At the signal of an impulse traveling down the nerve, the muscle fiber changes chemical energy into mechanical energy, and the result is muscle contraction.

Some muscles are attached to bones by TENDONS. Others are attached to other muscles, or to skin (producing the smile, the wink, and other facial expressions, for example). All or part of the walls of hollow internal organs, such as the heart, stomach, intestines, and blood vessels, are composed of muscles. The last stages of swallowing and of peristalsis are actually series of contractions by the muscles in the walls of the organs involved.

Types of Muscle. There are three types of muscle: *involuntary, voluntary,* and *cardiac,* composed respectively of *smooth, striated,* and *mixed* smooth and striated tissue. (See illustration.)

Involuntary muscles are those not under the control of the conscious part of the brain; they respond to the nerve impulses of the autonomic nervous system. They include the countless short-fibered, or smooth, muscles of the internal organs and power the digestive tract, the pupils of the eyes, and all other involuntary mechanisms.

Voluntary muscles are those controlled by the conscious part of the brain, and are striated. These are the skeletal muscles that enable the body to move, and there are more than 600 of them in the human body. Their fibers are grouped together in sheaths of muscle cells. Groups of fibers are bundled together into FASCICLES, surrounded by a tough sheet of connective tissue to form a muscle group such as the biceps. Unlike the involuntary muscles, which can remain in a state of contraction for long periods without tiring and are capable of sustained rhythmic contractions,

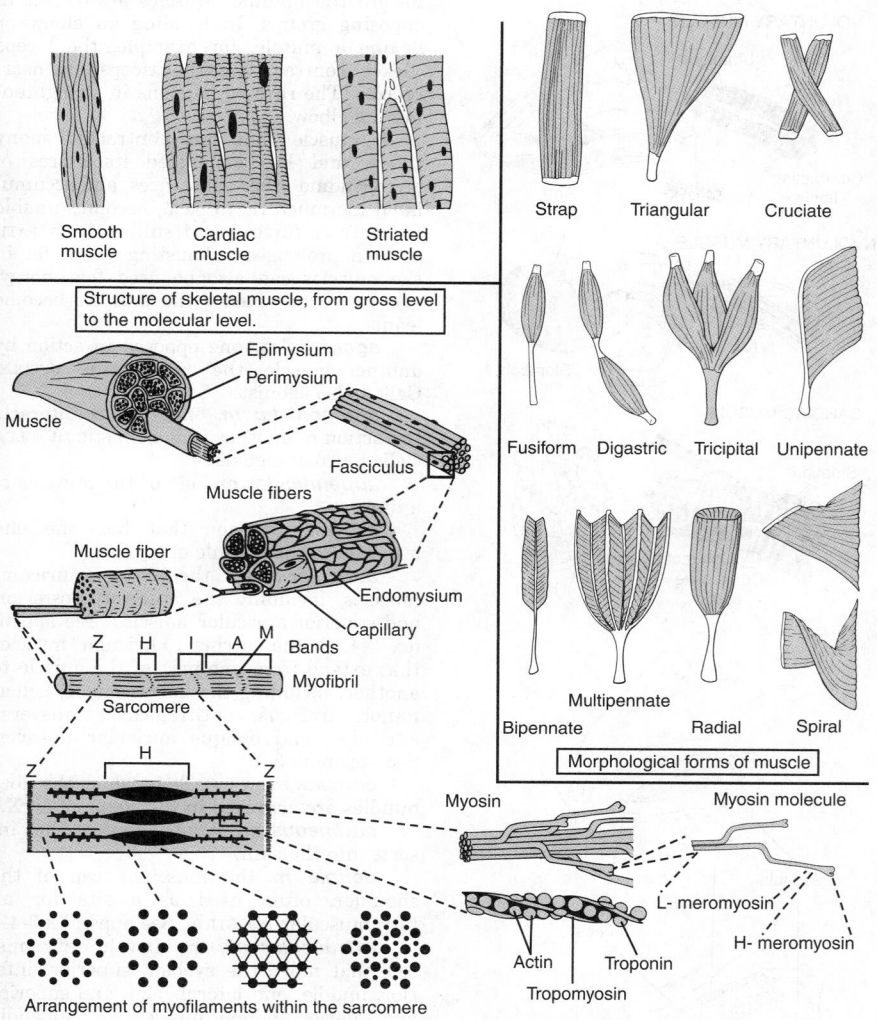

Smooth muscle

Cardiac muscle

Striated muscle

Strap Triangular Cruciate

Structure of skeletal muscle, from gross level to the molecular level.

Epimysium

Perimysium

Muscle

Fasciculus

Muscle fibers

Muscle fiber

Endomysium

Capillary

Z H I A M Bands

Myofibril

Sarcomere

Fusiform Digastric Tricipital Unipennate

Multipennate

Bipennate Radial Spiral

Morphological forms of muscle

H

Z Z

Myosin

Myosin molecule

L- meromyosin

H- meromyosin

Actin Troponin

Tropomyosin

Arrangement of myofilaments within the sarcomere

Types and structure of muscle. From Dorland's, 2000.

M

the voluntary muscles are readily subject to fatigue.

Cardiac muscles (the muscles of the heart) are the third kind; they are involuntary and consist of striated fibers different from those of voluntary muscle. The contraction and relaxation of cardiac muscle continues at a rhythmic pace until death unless the muscle is injured in some way. (See also HEART.)

Physiology of Muscles. No muscle stays completely relaxed, and as long as a person is conscious, it remains slightly contracted.

This condition is called TONUS, or TONE. It keeps the bones in place and enables a posture to be maintained. It allows a person to remain standing, sitting up straight, kneeling, or in any other natural position. Muscles also have elasticity. They are capable of being stretched and of performing reflex actions. This is made possible by the motor and sensory nerves which serve the muscles.

Muscles enable the body to perform different types of movement. Those that bend a limb at a joint, raising a thigh or

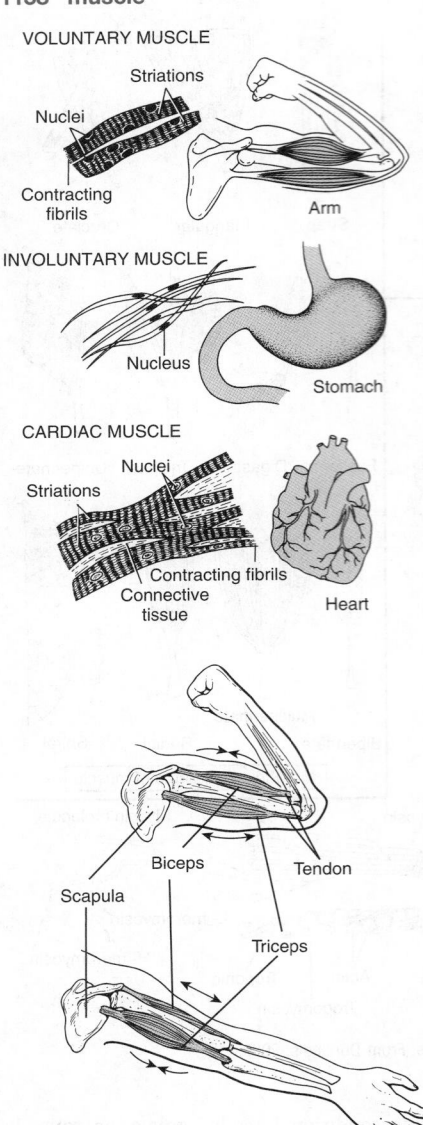

VOLUNTARY MUSCLE

Striations

Nuclei

Contracting fibrils

Arm

INVOLUNTARY MUSCLE

Nucleus

Stomach

CARDIAC MUSCLE

Nuclei

Striations

Contracting fibrils

Connective tissue

Heart

Biceps

Tendon

Scapula

Triceps

Voluntary muscles extend from one bone to another, cause movements by contraction, and work on the principle of leverage. For every direct action made by a muscle, an antagonistic muscle can cause an opposite movement. To flex the arm, the biceps contracts and the triceps relaxes; to extend the arm, the triceps contracts and the biceps relaxes.

bending an elbow, are called FLEXORS. Those that straighten a limb are called EXTENSORS. Others, the ABDUCTORS, make possible movement away from the midline of the body,

whereas the ADDUCTORS permit movement toward the midline. Muscles always act in opposing groups. In bending an elbow or flexing a muscle, for example, the biceps (flexor) contracts and the triceps (extensor) relaxes. The reverse happens in straightening the elbow.

A muscle that has contracted many times, and has exhausted its stores of glycogen and other substances, and accumulated too much LACTIC ACID, becomes unable to contract further and suffers from FATIGUE. In prolonged exhausting work, fat in the muscles can also be used for energy, and as a consequence the muscles become leaner.

agonistic m. one opposed in action by another muscle, the antagonistic MUSCLE. Called also agonist.

antagonistic m. one that counteracts the action of another (the agonistic MUSCLE). Called also antagonist.

appendicular m. one of the muscles of a limb.

articular m. one that has one end attached to the capsule of a joint.

auricular m's 1. the extrinsic auricular muscles, including the anterior, posterior, and superior auricular muscles. See appendix 3-4. 2. the intrinsic auricular muscles that extend from one part of the auricle to another, including the helicis major, helicis minor, tragicus, antitragicus, transverse auricular, and oblique auricular muscles. See appendix 3-4.

cruciate m. a muscle in which the fiber bundles are arranged in the shape of an X.

cutaneous m. striated muscle that inserts into the skin.

deltoid m. the muscular cap of the shoulder, often used as a site for an intramuscular INJECTION. See appendix 3-4.

extraocular m's the six voluntary muscles that move the eyeball: superior, inferior, middle, and lateral recti, and superior and inferior oblique muscles. See appendix 3-4.

extrinsic m. one that originates in another part than that of its insertion, as those originating outside the eye, which move the eyeball.

fixation m's, fixator m's accessory muscles that serve to steady a part.

gluteal m's three muscles, the greatest, middle, and least, that extend, abduct, and rotate the thigh. See appendix 3-4.

hamstring m's the muscles of the back of the thigh, including the biceps femoris, semitendinosus, and semimembranosus. See appendix 3-4.

intraocular m's the intrinsic muscles of the eyeball. See appendix 3-4.

intrinsic m. one whose origin and insertion are both in the same part or organ, as those entirely within the eye.

multipennate m. a muscle in which the fiber bundles converge to several tendons.

palatine m's the intrinsic and extrinsic muscles that act upon the soft palate.

pectoral m's four muscles of the chest; See appendix 3-4.

quadrate m. a square-shaped muscle; see appendix 3-4.

quadriceps m. a name applied collectively to four muscles of the thigh; see anatomic Table of Muscles in the Appendices.

scalene m's four muscles of the upper thorax that raise the first two ribs, aiding in respiration. See appendix 3-4.

skeletal m's striated muscles that are attached to bones and typically cross at least one joint.

sphincter m. a ringlike muscle that closes a natural orifice; called also sphincter.

synergic m's, synergistic m's those that assist one another in action.

thenar m's the abductor and flexor muscles of the thumb. See appendix 3-4.

triangular m. a muscle that is triangular in shape.

yoked m's those that normally act simultaneously and equally, as in moving the eyes.

muscular (mus′ku-lar) 1. pertaining to a muscle. 2. having well-developed muscles.

m. dystrophy a group of genetically determined, painless, degenerative MYOPATHIES that are progressively crippling because muscles are gradually weakened and eventually atrophy. At present there is no specific cure. Not all forms are totally disabling, and it can sometimes be arrested temporarily.

The word DYSTROPHY means faulty or imperfect nutrition. In muscular dystrophy the muscles suffer a vital loss of protein, and muscle fibers are replaced gradually by fat and connective tissue until, in the late stages of the disease, the voluntary muscle system becomes virtually useless. In muscular dystrophy all visible damage occurs in the muscles themselves, and thus the disease is markedly different from MULTIPLE SCLEROSIS, in which the muscles are rendered impotent by damage to the nerves that control them.

Muscular dystrophy is believed to be hereditary, although the way it is inherited is not the same for all types of the disease. The disease (or a propensity for it) seems to be carried mainly by women who, while not suffering from it themselves, may pass it on to their offspring, usually their sons. A woman who has conceived a child with muscular dystrophy is probably a carrier, as is a woman who has a relative with the condition.

Childhood Muscular Dystrophy. Muscular dystrophy cannot be detected at birth; in most cases symptoms begin to be noticeable about the second or third year. The child gradually finds it more difficult to play and walk, and as the weakening process continues, a wheelchair becomes necessary. In many cases death comes before the age of 20 from respiratory ailments or heart failure. This childhood type of disease (unfortunately the most common type) is known as the *Duchenne type* or *progressive muscular dystrophy*. It is also called *pseudohypertrophic muscular dystrophy* because at the beginning the muscles, especially those in the calves, appear healthy and bulging when actually they are already weakened and their size is due to an excess of fat.

Other Types. Another type sometimes begins in childhood but is much more likely to appear during the teens or twenties. When the first symptom is a failure of the musculature of the pelvic girdle, this type is referred to as *limb-girdle muscular dystrophy*. It usually proceeds more slowly than the childhood form. This same type may take the form of *facioscapulohumeral muscular dystrophy* (referring to the face, shoulder, and upper arm muscles), which is likely to manifest itself first in an almost imperceptible weakening of the facial muscles. It is also known as *Landouzy-Dejerine muscular dystrophy*. Muscle deterioration starts in childhood or early adulthood but it may proceed very gradually over a number of years, sometimes until late in life. Some patients may be only slightly disabled. Other, rarer types of muscular dystrophy have been identified, including a distal type that begins in the peripheral muscles of the extremities and one that affects only muscles of the eye. Sometimes two or more forms are present in the same patient.

Management. There is almost never any pain in muscular dystrophy. The mind is not affected; patients have normal intelligence. As the small muscles often are the last to be damaged, patients may continue to use their fingers. Children with muscular dystrophy are able to enjoy many recreations, even when they must rely on crutches or wheelchairs. Physical therapy, including exercise of the lungs by deep breathing, is important. The aim of such exercise is not to restore muscle power (which cannot be

M

done) but to ensure that the patient makes the best use of the good muscle tissue remaining and does not develop CONTRACTURES. The more active patients are, the better they will be physically and mentally. Obesity should be avoided. Splints, braces, and, occasionally, corrective orthopedic surgery are sometimes helpful.

The Muscular Dystrophy Association of America has many local chapters and is concerned both with research and with every aspect of the care and comfort of patients with the disease. They can be contacted at Muscular Dystrophy Association of America, 3300 East Sunrise Drive, Tucson, AZ 85718, or through their web site at http://www.mdausa.org. The Muscular Dystrophy Association of Canada also has information available and has many local chapters. Their national office can be contacted by writing to Muscular Dystrophy Association of Canada, 2345 Yonge Street, Suite 900, Toronto ON M4P 2E5 or consulting their web site at http://www.mdac.ca.

muscularis (mus″ku-lar′ris) [L.] 1. muscular. 2. pertaining to a muscular layer or coat; see TUNICA MUSCULARIS.

musculature (mus′ku-lah-chur) the muscular system of the body, or the muscles of a particular region.

musculocutaneous (mus″ku-lo-ku-ta′ne-us) pertaining to muscle and skin.

musculomembranous (mus″ku-lo-mem′-brah-nus) pertaining to muscle and membrane.

musculophrenic (mus″ku-lo-fren′ik) pertaining to (chest) muscles and the diaphragm.

musculoskeletal (mus″ku-lo-skel′ĕ-t'l) pertaining to muscle and skeleton.

musculotendinous (mus″ku-lo-ten′dĭ-nus) pertaining to muscle and tendon.

musculotropic (mus″ku-lo-trop′ik) exerting its principal effect upon muscle.

musculus (mus′ku-lus) [L.] muscle.

mushroom (mush′rōōm) the fruiting body of any of a variety of fleshy fungi of the order Agaricales, especially one that is edible. Poisonous species are popularly called TOADSTOOLS.

m. poisoning poisoning resulting from ingestion of mushrooms; potentially deadly mushrooms include _Amanita phalloides, A. verna, A. virosa,_ and certain other species that contain neurotoxins. Rapid identification of mushroom poisoning and treatment is critical. According to the Center for Food Safety and Applied Nutrition of the Food and Drug Administration, persons who have ingested poisonous mushrooms and are treated immediately have a mortality rate of 10 per cent, whereas those who are treated 60 or more hours later have a 60 to 90 per cent mortality rate.

Musset's sign (mu-sāz′) de Musset's sign.

mustard (mus′terd) 1. a plant of the genus _Brassica._ 2. the ripe seeds of _Brassica alba_ (white mustard) and _B. nigra_ (black mustard), whose oils have irritant, stimulant, and emetic properties. 3. resembling, or something resembling, mustard in one or more of its properties.

nitrogen m. 1. mechlorethamine. 2. see NITROGEN MUSTARDS.

Mustargen (mus′ter-jen) trademark for a preparation of MECHLORETHAMINE hydrochloride, an antineoplastic AGENT.

mutagen (mu′tah-jen) an agent that induces genetic mutation.

mutagenesis (mu″tah-jen′ĕ-sis) the induction of genetic mutation.

mutagenic (mu″tah-jen′ik) inducing genetic MUTATION.

mutagenicity (mu″tah-jĕ-nis′ĭ-te) the property of being able to induce genetic MUTATION.

mutant (mu′tant) 1. in genetics, a variation that breeds true, owing to genetic changes. 2. produced by mutation.

mutase (mu′tās) any of a group of enzymes (transferases) that catalyze the intramolecular shifting of a chemical group from one position to another.

mutation (mu-ta′shun) 1. a permanent transmissible change in the genetic material. 2. an individual exhibiting such a change.

point m. a mutation resulting from a change in a single base pair in the DNA molecule.

somatic m. a genetic mutation occurring in a somatic cell, providing the basis for mosaicism.

suppressor m. the correction of the effect of a mutation at one locus by a mutation at another locus.

mute (mūt) 1. unable or unwilling to speak, such as because of DEAFNESS. 2. to muffle or soften a sound.

mutism (mu′tizm) inability or refusal to speak, most often because DEAFNESS has prevented the person from hearing the spoken word. SPEECH is learned by imitating the speech of others. The child who is born with normal hearing and then loses it may lose part or all of the power of speech through loss of contact with the speech of others. Mutism may also occur because the voice organs themselves have been damaged or removed, such as when a LARYNGECTOMY is performed for throat cancer. In other cases loss of speech may be psychogenic in nature. Called also aphonia.

akinetic m. a state in which the person makes no spontaneous movement or vocal sound, because of either neurologic or psychologic reasons. Called also abulia.

selective m. a mental disorder of childhood characterized by continuous refusal to speak in social situations when the child is able and willing to speak to selected persons.

mutualism (mu′choo-al-izm) the biologic association of two individuals or populations of different species, both of which are benefited by the relationship and sometimes unable to exist without it. adj., **mutualis′- tic.**

mutualist (mu′choo-al-ist) one of the organisms or species living in a state of mutualism.

MV¹ [L.] *Medicus Veterinarius* (veterinary physician).

MV² megavolt; minute volume.

mV millivolt.

μV microvolt.

MVV maximal voluntary ventilation.

MWIA Medical Women's International Association.

Mx Medex.

my(o)- word element [Gr.], *muscle.*

myalgia (mi-al′jah) muscular pain.

epidemic m. epidemic pleurodynia.

myasthenia (mi″as-the′ne-ah) muscular debility or weakness. adj., **myasthen′ic.**

m. gas′trica weakness and loss of tone in the muscular coats of the stomach; atony of the stomach.

m. gra′vis an AUTOIMMUNE DISEASE manifested as fatigue and exhaustion of the muscles, aggravated by activity and relieved by rest; the weakness ranges from mild to life-threatening. There is no muscular atrophy or loss of sensation. It characteristically affects the ocular and other cranial muscles and tends to fluctuate in severity. The muscular weakness is believed to be caused by the presence of circulating antibodies directed against the postsynaptic ACETYLCHOLINE receptors at the neuromuscular JUNCTION; it is not clear what initiates formation of the antibodies. There also is evidence of altered cellular IMMUNITY.

Symptoms of myasthenia gravis include PTOSIS, DIPLOPIA, and difficulty in chewing and swallowing. Weakness of the upper and lower limbs usually is first noted when the patient tries to walk upstairs, gets up from a sitting position, raises arms over the head, or lifts a heavy object. Ventilatory deficiency due to weakness of the respiratory muscles occurs in those with a severe form of the

disease. About 20 per cent of all affected patients have only ocular myasthenia; the others have some form of generalized weakness. The presence of ACETYLCHOLINE receptor antibodies is elevated in patients with myasthenia gravis. Diagnosis is established when there is a favorable response to cholinergic drugs, which are inhibitors of ACETYLCHOLINESTERASE (an enzyme that breaks down acetylcholine); their action permits acetylcholine levels to become high enough to stimulate the postsynaptic receptors.

Children born of mothers with the disease exhibit a transient weakness that is evident at birth or may appear in the first day or so, with feeding difficulties manifested by poor sucking and swallowing abilities. They rarely have bulbar involvement, and usually recover in a week or so after birth. This condition is called *neonatal myasthenia,* and is related to circulating antibodies acquired from the mother while the fetus was *in utero. Congenital myasthenia* is also present at birth, but it may not be evident until after the first year of life. The child produces antibodies against acetylcholine receptor sites and experiences symptoms similar to those presented by myasthenia gravis patients of all ages.

The patient is started on ANTICHOLINESTERASE drugs, such as NEOSTIGMINE or PYRIDOSTIGMINE, as soon as the diagnosis is confirmed. The steroid PREDNISONE and other IMMUNOSUPPRESSIVE drugs provide some relief of symptoms and longer periods of remission. THYMECTOMY is an alternative treatment for those patients whose weakness and debility do not respond adequately to cholinergic drug therapy. PLASMA EXCHANGE to remove the circulating autoantibodies provides some clinical improvement. High-dose intravenous immune GLOBULIN may also be used to temporarily improve immune function.

Myasthenic CRISIS can develop suddenly after a systemic infection, surgery, or some other stressful event. The crisis usually is transient, but during the critical phase assisted ventilation and intensive care are needed to assure survival of the patient with respiratory failure.

neonatal m. transient MYASTHENIA GRAVIS (lasting a week to a month) in infants born to myasthenic women.

myatonia (mi″ah-to′ne-ah) defective muscular tone.

myatrophy (mi-at′ro-fe) atrophy of a muscle.

myc(o)- word element [Gr.], *fungus.*

M

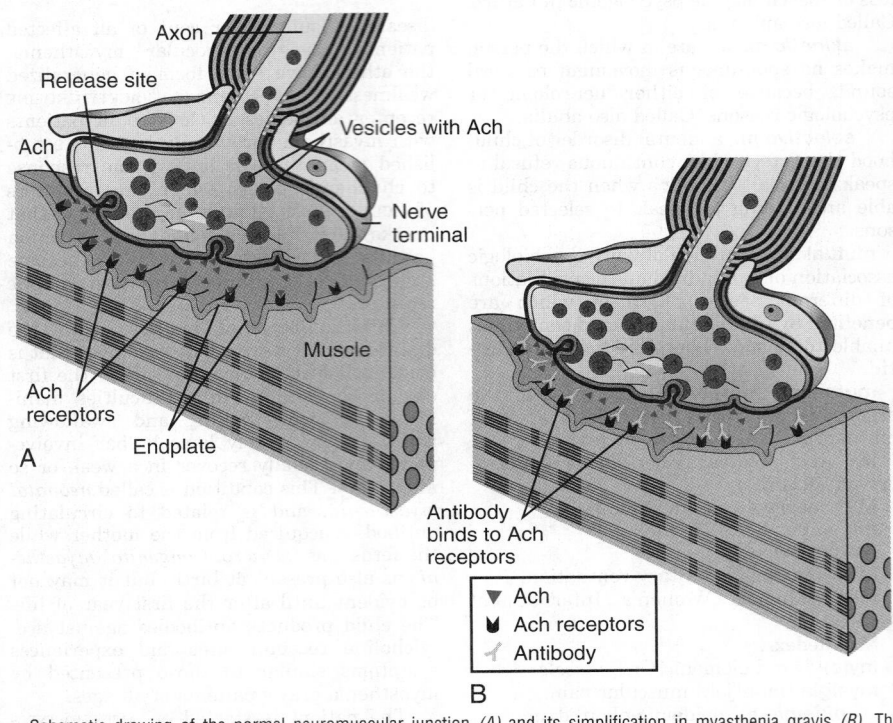

Schematic drawing of the normal neuromuscular junction *(A)* and its simplification in myasthenia gravis *(B)*. The antibodies bind to the acetylcholine (Ach) receptor preventing binding of the neurotransmitter (Ach). From Damjanov, 2000.

mycelium (mi-se′le-um) the mass of threadlike processes (hyphae) constituting the THALLUS of a fungus. adj., **myce′lial.**

mycetismus (mi″sĕ-tiz′mus) mushroom poisoning.

mycetogenic (mi-se″to-jen′ik) caused by fungi.

mycetoma (mi″sĕ-to′mah) an initially localized, slowly progressive, destructive infection of the cutaneous and subcutaneous tissues, fascia, and bone, caused by certain ACTINOMYCETES (*actinomycotic mycetoma*) or true FUNGI (*eumycotic mycetoma*). It usually involves the leg or foot (Madura FOOT), but the hand or any other site may be affected. There is swelling accompanied by formation of granulomas, suppurating abscesses, and multiple sinuses. Called also maduromycosis.

Mycobacterium (mi″ko-bak-tēr′e-um) a genus of gram-positive, aerobic, acid-fast bacteria, occurring as slightly curved or straight rods. It contains many species, including the highly pathogenic organisms that cause TUBERCULOSIS (*M. tuberculo′sis*) and LEPROSY (*M. lep′rae*). *M. a′vium* causes tuberculosis in birds and pigs and pulmonary disease in humans. *M. bo′vis* is the bovine tubercle bacillus and can cause tuberculosis in humans who drink infected milk (strict testing of cattle makes this uncommon in developed countries); an attenuated strain is used to prepare BCG VACCINE. *M. chelo′nae* is an opportunistic pathogen that causes synovial lesions, gluteal abscesses, and gross lesions in various organs. *M. fortu′itum* causes lesions of the lung, bone, or soft tissue following trauma. *M. haemo′philum* causes skin lesions. *M. ho′minis* is a common inhabitant of the vagina and cervix and causes infections of the male and female reproductive tracts, as well as respiratory disease and pharyngitis. *M. intracellula′re* occasionally causes chronic pulmonary disease in adults and lymph node infection in children. *M. kansa′sii* causes a tuberculosis-like disease. *M. mari′num* (also known as *M. bal′nei*) is the agent of swimming pool GRANULOMA.

mycobacterium (mi″ko-bak-tē″re-um) [L.] 1. an individual organism of the genus *Mycobacterium.* 2. a slender, acid-fast microorganism resembling the bacillus that causes tuberculosis.

nontuberculous mycobacteria mycobacteria other than *M. tuberculosis* or *M. bovis,* consisting of nonpathogens and pathogens causing opportunistic infections in immunocompromised patients and infections in otherwise normal individuals.

Mycobacterium avium **complex disease** a systemic disease caused by infection with organisms of the *Mycobacterium avium-intracellulare* complex in patients with human immunodeficiency VIRUS (HIV) infection. Signs and symptoms include bacteremia, fever, chills, fatigue, night sweats, weight loss, abdominal pain, anemia, and elevated alkaline phosphatase. Called also MAC disease

mycodermatitis (mi″ko-der″mah-ti′tis) fungal infection of the skin.

mycologist (mi-kol′o-jist) a specialist in mycology.

mycology (mi-kol′o-je) the study of fungi and fungus diseases.

mycomyringitis (mi″ko-mir″in-ji′tis) fungus inflammation of the eardrum.

mycophenolate (mi″ko-fen′o-lāt) an IMMUNOSUPPRESSANT used as *mycophenolate mofetil* to prevent rejection of allogeneic cardiac, hepatic, and renal transplants; administered orally or intravenously.

Mycoplasma (mi′ko-plaz″mah) a genus of highly pleomorphic, gram-negative, aerobic or facultatively anaerobic bacteria that lack cell walls, including the PLEUROPNEUMONIA-LIKE ORGANISMS and other species.

M. ho′minis a species found associated with nongonococcal URETHRITIS and mild pharyngitis.

M. pneumo′niae a cause of primary atypical PNEUMONIA; called also Eaton agent.

mycosis (mi-ko′sis) any disease caused by fungi.

m. fungoi′des a chronic or rapidly progressive form of cutaneous T-cell lymphoma (formerly thought to be of fungal origin), which in some cases evolves into generalized lymphoma. It may be divided generally into three successive stages: *premycotic,* associated with intensely pruritic eruptions; *infiltrated plaques,* or *mycotic,* characterized by the presence of abnormal mononuclear cells (*Sézary cells*); and mushroom-like *tumors* that often ulcerate. The tumor stage (*d'emblée type*) may develop without preceding lesions or prodromal symptoms.

opportunistic m. a fungal or fungus-like disease occurring as an opportunistic INFECTION. Fungi that may become opportunistic pathogens include species of *Aspergillus, Candida, Mucor,* and *Cryptococcus.* Successful treatment of opportunistic mycoses depends on identification of the specific organism causing the infection. Without effective therapy a systemic infection of this type can be fatal.

mycostasis (mi-kos′tah-sis) prevention of growth and multiplication of fungi.

mycostat (mi′ko-stat) an agent that inhibits the growth of fungi.

Mycostatin (mi′ko-stat″in) trademark for preparations of NYSTATIN, an antifungal AGENT.

mycotic (mi-kot′ik) pertaining to a mycosis; caused by fungi.

mycotoxicosis (mi″ko-tok-sĭ-ko′sis) 1. poisoning due to a fungal or bacterial toxin. 2. poisoning due to ingestion of toxic fungi such as mushrooms; see MUSHROOM POISONING.

mydriasis (mĭ-dri′ah-sis) great dilatation of the pupil.

mydriatic (mid″re-at′ik) 1. dilating the pupil. 2. a drug that dilates the pupil.

myectomy (mi-ek′to-me) surgical excision of a muscle.

myectopia (mi″ek-to′pe-ah) displacement of a muscle or a portion of a muscle.

myel(o)- word element [Gr.], *marrow; spinal cord.*

myelalgia (mi″ĕ-lal′jah) pain in the spinal cord.

myelapoplexy (mi″el-ap′o-plek″se) hematomyelia; hemorrhage in the spinal cord.

myelatelia (mi″el-ah-te′le-ah) atelomyelia.

myelatrophy (mi″el-at′ro-fe) atrophy of the spinal cord.

myelemia (mi″el-e′me-ah) myelocytosis.

myelencephalon (mi″el-en-sef′ah-lon) 1. the posterior part of the RHOMBENCEPHALON, comprising the medulla oblongata and lower part of the fourth ventricle. 2. the posterior of the two brain vesicles formed by specialization of the rhombencephalon in the developing embryo.

myelin (mi′ĕ-lin) the lipid substance forming a sheath (the myelin SHEATH) around the axons of certain nerve fibers; it is an electrical insulator that serves to speed the conduction of nerve impulses in these nerve fibers, which are called myelinated or medullated FIBERS. adj., **myelin′ic.**

Myelinated nerve fibers occur predominantly in the cranial and spinal nerves and compose the WHITE MATTER of the brain and spinal cord. Unmyelinated fibers are abundant in the autonomic

M

NERVOUS SYSTEM. The term GRAY MATTER refers to areas in the nervous system in which the nerve fibers are unmyelinated. In unmyelinated nerves impulses are conducted by the propagation of the ACTION POTENTIAL along the membrane of the axon. In myelinated nerves impulses are transmitted by an entirely different process, called *saltatory conduction,* in which the impulse jumps from one NODE OF RANVIER to the next. Impulses in myelinated nerves are transmitted hundreds of times faster and require much less energy than in unmyelinated nerves.

myelinated (mi′ĕ-lĭ-nāt′ed) having a myelin SHEATH.

myelination (mi-ĕ-lin-a′shun) myelinization.

myelinization (mi″ĕ-lin″ĭ-za′shun) production of MYELIN around an axon. Called also myelination.

myelinolysis (mi″ĕ-lin-ol′ĭ-sis) demyelination.

myelinosis (mi″ĕ-lĭ-no′sis) fatty degeneration, with formation of myelin.

myelinotoxic (mi″ĕ-lin′o-tok″sik) having a deleterious effect on MYELIN; causing DEMYELINATION.

myelitis (mi″ĕ-li′tis) 1. inflammation of the spinal cord; see also POLIOMYELITIS. 2. inflammation of the bone marrow; see also OSTEOMYELITIS. adj., **myelit′ic.**

   bulbar m. that involving the medulla oblongata.

myeloablation (mi″ĕ-lo-ab-la′shun) severe MYELOSUPPRESSION. adj., **myeloab′lative.**

myeloblast (mi′ĕ-lo-blast″) an immature cell of bone marrow, not normally found in peripheral blood; it is the most primitive precursor in the granulocytic series, which develops into the promyelocyte and eventually into a granulocyte.

myeloblastemia (mi″ĕ-lo-blas-te′me-ah) myeloblasts in the peripheral blood, as seen in MYELOBLASTIC LEUKEMIA.

myeloblastoma (mi″ĕ-lo-blas-to′mah) a focal malignant tumor composed of MYELOBLASTS or early myeloid precursors occurring outside of the bone marrow; observed in acute myelogenous LEUKEMIA.

myeloblastosis (mi″ĕ-lo-blas-to′sis) excess of myeloblasts in the blood, as seen in MYELOBLASTIC LEUKEMIA.

myelocele (mi′ĕ-lo-sēl″) protrusion of the spinal cord through a defect in the vertebral column.

myelocyst (mi′ĕ-lo-sist) a cyst developed from rudimentary medullary canals.

myelocystocele (mi″ĕ-lo-sis′to-sēl) myelomeningocele.

myelocystomeningocele (mi″ĕ-lo-sis″to-mĕ-ning′go-sēl) myelomeningocele.

myelocyte (mi′ĕ-lo-sīt″) 1. a precursor in the granulocytic series intermediate between a PROMYELOCYTE and a METAMYELOCYTE, normally occurring only in the bone marrow. In this stage, differentiation into specific cytoplasmic granules has begun. 2. any cell of the gray matter of the nervous system. adj., **myelocyt′ic.**

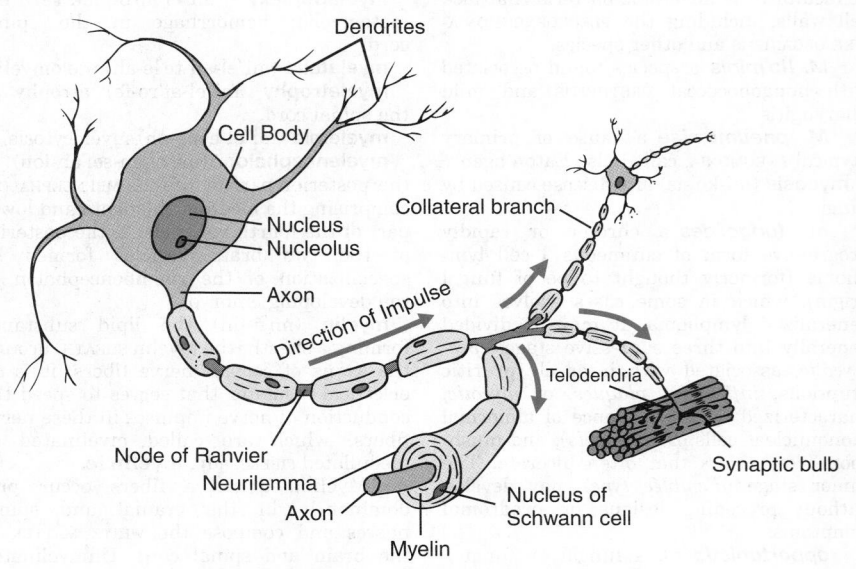

Structure of a typical myelin sheath. From Applegate, 2000.

myelocythemia (mi″ĕ-lo-si-the′me-ah) an excess of myelocytes in the circulating blood.

myelocytoma (mi″ĕ-lo-si-to′mah) myeloma.

myelocytosis (mi″ĕ-lo-si-to′sis) increase of myelocytes in the blood.

myelodysplasia (mi″ĕ-lo-dis-pla′zhah) 1. a NEURAL TUBE DEFECT consisting of defective development of part of the spinal cord. See also SPINA BIFIDA. 2. dysplasia of MYELOCYTES and other elements of the bone marrow, a chronic disease that in time may evolve into acute myelogenous LEUKEMIA. adj., **myelodysplas′tic.**

myeloencephalic (mi″ĕ-lo-en″sĕ-fal′ik) cerebrospinal.

myeloencephalitis (mi″ĕ-lo-en-sef″ah-li′-tis) inflammation of the spinal cord and brain.

myelofibrosis (mi″ĕ-lo-fi-bro′sis) replacement of bone marrow by fibrous tissue.

myelogenesis (mi″ĕ-lo-jen′ĕ-sis) 1. development of the central nervous system. 2. the deposition of myelin around the axon.

myelogenic (mi″ĕ-lo-jen′ik) produced in the bone marrow.

myelogenous (mi-ĕ-loj′ĕ-nus) myelogenic.

myelogeny (mi″ĕ-loj′ĕ-ne) development of the myelin sheaths of nerve fibers.

myelogram (mi′ĕ-lo-gram) 1. the film produced by myelography. 2. a graphic representation of the differential count of cells found in a stained representation of bone marrow.

myelography (mi″ĕ-log′rah-fe) radiography of the spinal cord after injection of a contrast medium into the subarachnoid space.

myeloid (mi′ĕ-loid) 1. pertaining to, derived from, or resembling bone marrow. 2. pertaining to the spinal cord. defs. 1 and 2 called also medullary. 3. having the appearance of myelocytes, but not derived from bone marrow.

myeloidosis (mi″ĕ-loi-do′sis) formation of myeloid tissue, especially hyperplastic development of such tissue.

myelolipoma (mi″ĕ-lo-lip′o-mah) a rare benign tumor of the adrenal gland composed of adipose tissue, lymphocytes, and primitive myeloid cells.

myeloma (mi″ĕ-lo′mah) 1. a tumor composed of plasma cells of the type normally found in the bone marrow. 2. multiple myeloma.

　　giant cell m. giant cell tumor (def. 1).

　　multiple m. see MULTIPLE MYELOMA.

　　plasma cell m. multiple myeloma.

　　solitary m. a variant of MULTIPLE MYELOMA in which there is a single localized tumor focus. Called also plasma cell tumor.

myelomalacia (mi″ĕ-lo-mah-la′she-ah) morbid softening of the spinal cord.

myelomatosis (mi″ĕ-lo-mah-to′sis) multiple myeloma.

myelomeningitis (mi″ĕ-lo-men″in-ji′tis) meningomyelitis.

myelomeningocele (mi″ĕ-lo-mĕ-ning′go-sēl) hernial protrusion of the spinal cord and its meninges through a defect in the vertebral arch (SPINA BIFIDA); see also NEURAL TUBE DEFECT. Called also meningomyelocele.

M

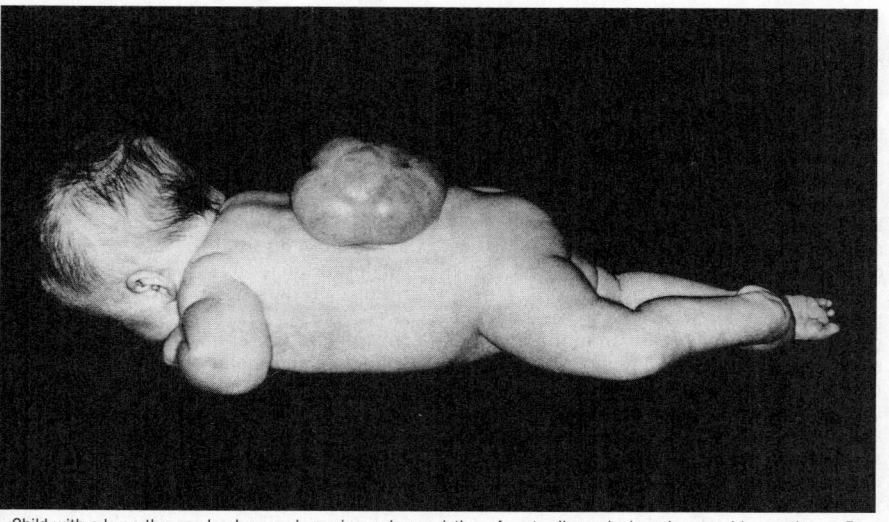

Child with a large thoraco-lumbar myelomeningocele consisting of protruding spinal cord covered by meninges. From Mueller and Young, 2001.

myeloneuritis (mi″ĕ-lo-noo-ri′tis) inflammation of the spinal cord and peripheral nerves.

myelopathy (mi″ĕ-lop′ah-the) 1. any functional disturbance or pathological change in the spinal cord; often used to denote nonspecific lesions, as opposed to myelitis. 2. pathological bone marrow changes. adj., **myelopath′ic.**

ascending m. myelopathy that progresses along the spinal cord towards the head.

cervical m. compression MYELOPATHY of the cervical spinal cord, a common complication of rheumatoid ARTHRITIS and OSTEOARTHRITIS.

compression m. myelopathy due to pressure on the spinal cord, as from a tumor.

cystic m. syringomyelia.

descending m. myelopathy that progresses along the spinal cord towards the hips.

spondylotic cervical m. myelopathy secondary to encroachment of cervical spondylosis upon a congenitally small cervical spinal canal.

myeloperoxidase (mi″ĕ-lo-per-ok′sĭ-dās) a hemoprotein having peroxidase activity, occurring in the primary granules of promyelocytes, myelocytes, and neutrophils, and that exhibits bactericidal, fungicidal, and viricidal properties.

myelopetal (mi″ĕ-lop′ĕ-t'l) moving toward the spinal cord.

myelophthisis (mi″ĕ-lo-thi′sis) 1. wasting of the spinal cord. 2. bone marrow SUPPRESSION.

myeloplast (mi′ĕ-lo-plast″) any leukocyte of the bone marrow.

myelopoiesis (mi″ĕ-lo-poi-e′sis) the formation of marrow or the cells arising from it.

ectopic m., extramedullary m. formation of myeloid tissue outside bone marrow.

myeloproliferative (mi″ĕ-lo-pro-lif′er-ah″-tiv) pertaining to or characterized by abnormal proliferation of bone marrow constituents.

m. disorders a group of usually neoplastic diseases, which may be related histogenetically by a common multipotential stem cell; it includes among others acute myelogenous LEUKEMIA, chronic granulocytic LEUKEMIA, acute and chronic myelomonocytic LEUKEMIAS, and POLYCYTHEMIA vera. An interrelationship with the LYMPHOPROLIFERATIVE DISORDERS is thought to exist.

myeloradiculitis (mi″ĕ-lo-rah-dik″u-li′tis) inflammation of the spinal cord and posterior nerve roots.

myeloradiculodysplasia (mi″ĕ-lo-rah-dik″u-lo-dis-pla′zhah) abnormal development of the spinal cord and spinal nerve roots.

myeloradiculopathy (mi″ĕ-lo-rah-dik″u-lop′ah-the) disease of the spinal cord and spinal nerve roots.

myelorrhagia (mi″ĕ-lo-ra′jah) hematomyelia; spinal hemorrhage.

myelosarcoma (mi″ĕ-lo-sahr-ko′mah) a sarcomatous growth made up of myeloid tissue or bone marrow cells.

myelosclerosis (mi″ĕ-lo-sklĕ-ro′sis) 1. sclerosis of the spinal cord. 2. obliteration of the marrow cavity by small spicules of bone. 3. myelofibrosis.

myelosis (mi″ĕ-lo′sis) myelocytosis. 1. formation of a tumor of the spinal cord.

aleukemic m. agnogenic myeloid metaplasia.

erythremic m. erythroleukemia.

nonleukemic m. agnogenic myeloid metaplasia.

myelospongium (mi″ĕ-lo-spun′je-um) a network developing into the neuroglia.

myelosuppression (mi″ĕ-lo-soo-presh′un) bone marrow suppression.

myelosuppressive (mi″ĕ-lo-soo-pres′iv) 1. causing bone marrow SUPPRESSION. 2. an agent that so acts.

myelotomy (mi″ĕ-lot′ah-me) severance of nerve fibers in the spinal cord.

myelotoxic (mi″ĕ-lo-tok″sik) 1. destructive to bone marrow. 2. myelosuppressive. 3. arising from diseased bone marrow.

myenteron (mi-en′ter-on) the muscular coat of the intestine. adj., **myenter′ic.**

Myerson's sign (mi′er-sunz) in Parkinson's disease, repeated blinking of the eyes on tapping the forehead.

myesthesia (mi″es-the′zhah) muscle sensibility.

myiasis (mi-i′ah-sis) invasion of the body by the larvae of flies, characterized as cutaneous (subdermal tissue), gastrointestinal, nasopharyngeal, ocular, or urinary, depending on the region invaded.

myk(o)- for words beginning thus, see those beginning MYC(O)-.

Myleran (mi′ler-an) trademark for a preparation of BUSULFAN, an antineoplastic AGENT.

mylohyoid (mi″lo-hi′oid) pertaining to the hyoid bone and molar teeth.

myoatrophy (mi″o-at′ro-fe) muscular atrophy.

myoblast (mi′o-blast) an embryonic cell that becomes a cell of muscle fiber. adj., **myoblas′tic.**

myoblastoma (mi″o-blas-to′mah) a benign circumscribed tumorlike lesion of soft tissue.

myobradia (mi″o-bra′de-ah) slow reaction of muscle to stimulation.

myocardial (mi″o-kahr′de-al) pertaining to the muscular tissue of the heart (the myocardium).

m. infarction (MI) death of the cells of an area of the heart muscle (MYOCARDIUM) as a result of oxygen deprivation, which in turn is caused by obstruction of the blood supply; commonly referred to as a "heart attack."

The myocardium receives its blood supply from the two large coronary arteries and their branches. Occlusion of one or more of these blood vessels (CORONARY OCCLUSION) is one of the major causes of myocardial infarction. The occlusion may result from the formation of a clot that develops suddenly when an atheromatous plaque ruptures through the sublayers of a blood vessel, or when the narrow, roughened inner lining of a sclerosed artery leads to complete thrombosis. Coronary artery disease is the most common type of heart disease in the United States and many other countries. The risk rises rapidly with age, women tending to develop the disease 15 to 20 years later than men.

Other causes of MI may be attributed to a sudden increased unmet need for blood supply to the heart, as in shock, hemorrhage, and severe physical exertion, and to restriction of blood flow through the aorta, as in aortic stenosis.

Pathology. The most common sites of myocardial infarction are in the left ventricle, that chamber of the heart which has the greatest workload. Tissue changes that occur in the myocardium are related to the extent to which the cells have been deprived of oxygen. Total deprivation results in an *area of infarction,* in which the cells die and the tissue becomes necrotic. Necrosis in this area is evident within 5 to 6 hours after the occlusion. In response to this necrosis the body increases its production of leukocytes,

ELECTROCARDIOGRAPHIC CHANGES WITH ACUTE MYOCARDIAL INFARCTION

	Lead Changes	Reciprocal Changes
ANTERIOR WALL	V2, V3, V4	II, III, aVF
ANTEROSEPTAL	V1, V2, V3, V4	II, III, aVF
INFERIOR WALL	II, III, aVF	I, aVL
LATERAL WALL	I, aVL, V5, V6	V1, V2, V3
POSTERIOR WALL		V1, V2, V3, V4

which aid in removal of the dead cells. As collateral circulation enlarges, it brings fibroblasts, which form a connective tissue scar within the area of infarction. Usually, the formation of fibrous scar tissue is complete within 2 to 3 months.

Immediately surrounding the area of infarction is a less seriously damaged *area of injury.* It may deteriorate and thus extend the area of infarction or, with adequate collateral circulation, it may regain its function within 2 to 3 weeks.

The outermost area of damage is the *zone of ischemia,* which borders the area of injury. The cells in this area are weakened by decreased oxygen supply, but function can return usually within two to three weeks after the onset of occlusion.

All of the pathological changes described above can be identified by electrocardiography. The information thus obtained is used to prescribe the varying degrees of physical activity allowed the patient during convalescence.

Risk Factors. Unavoidable traits that increase a person's chances for coronary artery disease include genetic susceptibility, sex, increasing age, and diabetes mellitus. Factors that can be controlled to some extent in order to ameliorate the risk include hypertension, cigarette smoking, and elevated serum lipids. Almost half of the persons who have suffered heart attacks have a history of one or more of these latter three risk factors. Minimizing or eliminating these avoidable factors can reduce the incidence and severity of ischemic heart disease. Preventive measures are discussed more fully under HEART.

Symptoms. The most outstanding symptom of acute myocardial infarction is a sudden painful sensation of pressure, often described as a "crushing pain" in the chest, occasionally radiating to the arms, throat, and back, and persisting for hours. Pallor, profuse perspiration, and other signs of shock are present. There may be nausea

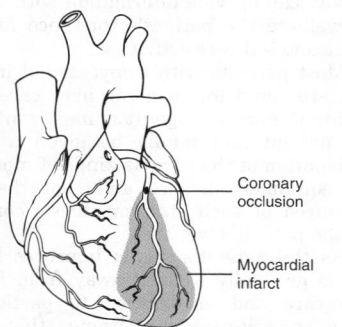

Myocardial infarction. From Frazier et al., 2000.

Coronary occlusion

Myocardial infarct

and vomiting, leading to the mistaken impression that the victim is suffering from acute indigestion. In almost all cases of severe MI the patient is extremely apprehensive and has a sense of impending death.

Severity of symptoms may depend on the size of the artery at the point of occlusion and the amount of myocardial tissue served by the artery. In some instances the artery may be small and the symptoms mild. In other cases the extent of damage is quite large and the attack is fatal.

Within 24 hours of the initial attack there is an elevated temperature and increased white cell count in response to the inflammatory process arising from necrosis of myocardial tissue. Death of the cells also brings about the release of certain enzymes that enter the general circulation. The levels of these enzymes in the blood can be determined by clinical laboratory tests. Within 2 to 4 hours after infarction the level of CREATINE KINASE (CK) is increased; it reaches its peak within 24 hours and subsides to normal level within 48 hours. The level of serum ASPARTATE TRANSAMINASE (AST) increases rapidly in 4 to 6 hours, reaches its peak in 24 to 48 hours, and returns to normal in five days. In contrast to the rapid rise and decline of these two enzyme levels, LACTATE DEHYDROGENASE (LD) levels begin to increase the first day after attack and persist at high levels for 10 to 20 days. TROPONIN is another enzyme that is a sensitive marker of myocardial infarction. Tests can be made more specific by measuring the LD_1 and CK_2 isoenzymes, which are found in the heart. Diagnosis of MI is based on the presenting symptoms and evidence of impaired heart function found by physical examination and electrocardiography and on abnormal serum enzyme levels.

Treatment and Patient Care. Immediate care of acute myocardial infarction is concerned with combatting SHOCK, relieving respiratory difficulty, and preventing further circulatory collapse. The victim should be kept lying down, and all tight clothing should be loosened to relieve dyspnea and promote comfort. Supplemental oxygen should be supplied, and oxygen consumption should be reduced by relieving anxiety and pain and supporting respiration. Without delay, but in a calm manner, the patient is transported to a medical care facility. If the victim shows signs of CARDIAC ARREST, efforts at CARDIOPULMONARY RESUSCITATION are begun immediately.

Medical treatment includes administration of thrombolytic therapy and an analgesic such as MORPHINE sulfate or MEPERIDINE (Demerol). On occasion the physician may order ATROPINE sulfate with morphine to counteract serious bradycardia. In almost all cases oxygen is administered for at least the first 24 hours.

Intravenous thrombolytic therapy using tissue plasminogen ACTIVATOR or STREPTOKINASE should be considered for all patients presenting within 12 hours of onset of pain. Maximum potential benefit occurs when these drugs are administered within 4 to 6 hours. Nursing considerations include the early accurate assessment of potential candidates for thrombolytic therapy, prompt administration of medication, and careful monitoring of complications such as arrhythmias, hypotension, allergic reactions, reocclusion, and hemorrhage. Early catheterization and angioplasty with a stent may also be done and may be superior to intravenous thrombolytic therapy.

Rest is essential for repair of damaged myocardial cells, but that does not necessarily mean absolute bed rest. Whether the patient is placed on bed rest or allowed up in a chair depends on symptoms and nursing judgments. During the acute stage some physicians may prefer that the patient rest in a chair at the bedside. The patient is permitted to get out of bed with assistance and sit in the chair until he begins to feel fatigued. The amount of time the patient is allowed to sit up and become more physically active is gradually increased.

Adequate rest can be achieved more easily if mental anxiety is reduced; a restful environment is thought to enhance the ability to rest. The amount of rest needed and the degree of physical activity allowed depends on how extensive the area of infarction is thought to be, whether cardiac arrhythmias and other complications develop, and the response of the patient to increased physical activity. Careful monitoring of the pulse rate and blood pressure before and after each activity can provide information with which to evaluate the patient's tolerance for exercise and self-care activities.

Most patients with a myocardial infarction are cared for in a coronary care unit during the acute stage. It is important that the patient and family be given a brief explanation of the various kinds of monitoring equipment in use and that they be reassured of each staff member's concern for the patient's welfare.

As the patient's status improves he or she is gradually weaned away from intensive care and encouraged to participate more in self-care. For some, this is a traumatic experience and they become very apprehensive about leaving the security of the monitors and the attention of the staff. Cardiac rehabilitation is also an important aspect of care. In some hospitals the transition from coronary care unit to home is made easier by transfer to a "step-down" or intermediate care unit where the patient's response to activities is monitored and instructions are given regarding care for himself or herself after discharge. Information about local coronary clubs, assistance in patient education, and availability of a Cardiac Work Evaluation Unit to determine the patient's readiness to return to work can be obtained by contacting the local unit of the American Heart Association.

myocardiograph (mi″o-kahr′de-o-graf′) an instrument for making tracings of movements of heart muscles.

myocardiopathy (mi″o-kar″de-op′ah-the) any noninflammatory disease of the myocardium.

myocarditis (mi″o-kahr-di′tis) inflammation of the muscular walls of the heart (the MYOCARDIUM); it may result from bacterial or viral infections or it may be a toxic inflammation caused by drugs or toxins from infectious agents. Other systemic diseases that may be accompanied by myocarditis are TRICHINOSIS, SERUM SICKNESS, RHEUMATIC FEVER, and COLLAGEN DISEASES. In many cases the etiology is unknown.

Symptoms. Symptoms are flulike; in acute myocarditis there is usually pain in the epigastric region or under the sternum (either ischemic, atypical, or pericardial), as well as dyspnea and cardiac arrhythmias. If the condition persists and becomes chronic, there is pain in the right upper quadrant of the abdomen, owing to hepatic congestion. The latter symptom is a sign of left biventricular failure and often is accompanied by edema and other signs of congestive heart failure.

Treatment (for both symptoms and underlying cause). Acute myocarditis usually subsides when the primary illness improves. It is considered incidental to the systemic disease and, though it may be a serious manifestation of a systemic illness, acute myocarditis often does not require specific treatment. Steroids may be used to reduce the inflammatory process. Antiarrhythmic drugs may be required, as well as therapy to combat congestive heart failure.

If the heart involvement becomes chronic, treatment then must be aimed at management of the chronic heart failure. See also congestive HEART FAILURE.

myocardium (mi″o-kar′de-um) the middle and thickest layer of the heart wall,

composed of cardiac muscle. adj., **myocar′-dial.**

myocele (mi′o-sēl) hernia of muscle through its sheath.

myocellulitis (mi″o-sel″u-li′tis) myositis with cellulitis.

myoceptor (mi′o-sep″ter) the end-plate.

myoclonus (mi″o-klo′nus) shocklike contractions of part of a muscle, an entire muscle, or a group of muscles; usually a manifestation of a convulsive disorder. adj., **myoclon′ic.**

> *palatal m.* a condition characterized by a rapid rhythmic movement of one or both sides of the palate.

myocyte (mi′o-sīt) muscle cell.

myocytoma (mi″o-si-to′mah) a tumor composed of myocytes.

myodystonia (mi″o-dis-to′ne-ah) disorder of muscular tone.

myoedema (mi″o-ĕ-de′mah) 1. mounding. 2. edema of a muscle.

myoelectric (mi″o-e-lek′trik) pertaining to the electric properties of muscle.

myoendocarditis (mi″o-en″do-kahr-di′tis) inflammation of the muscular wall and membrane lining the heart; combined myocarditis and endocarditis.

myoepithelioma (mi″o-ep″ĭ-the″le-o′mah) a benign tumor predominantly composed of myoepithelial cells; a pure myoepithelial neoplasm is rare.

myoepithelium (mi″o-ep″ĭ-the′le-um) tissue made up of contractile epithelial cells. adj., **myoepithe′lial.**

myofascitis (mi″o-fah-si′tis) inflammation of a muscle and its fascia.

myofibril (mi″o-fi′bril) one of the slender threads of a muscle FIBER, composed of numerous MYOFILAMENTS; called also muscle fibril. adj., **myofi′brillar.**

myofibroblast (mi″o-fi′bro-blast) an atypical fibroblast combining the ultrastructural features of a fibroblast and a smooth muscle cell.

myofibroma (mi″o-fi-bro′mah) myoma combined with fibroma.

myofibrosis (mi″o-fi-bro′sis) replacement of muscle tissue by fibrous tissue.

myofibrositis (mi″o-fi″bro-si′tis) inflammation of the sheath of a muscle FIBER.

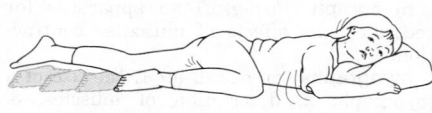

A single myoclonic arm or leg jerk is normal when the person is falling asleep. Myoclonic jerks are severe with grand mal seizures. From Jarvis, 1996.

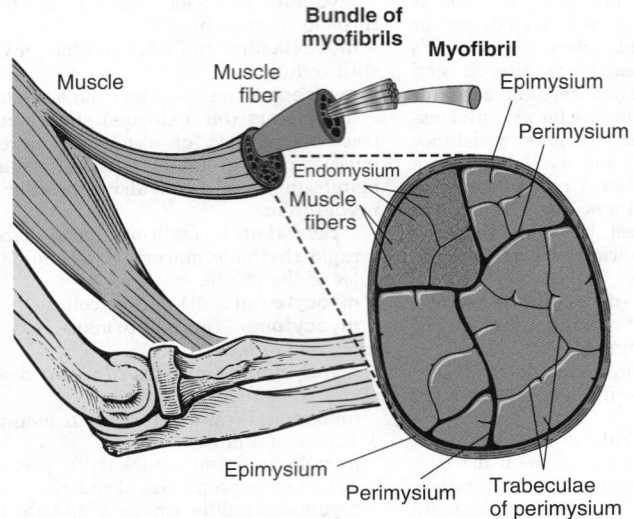

Bundles of myofibrils in a muscle. From Damjanov, 2000.

myofilament (mi″o-fil′ah-ment) any of the ultramicroscopic threadlike structures composing the MYOFIBRILS of striated muscle FIBERS.

myogenesis (mi″o-jen′ĕ-sis) the formation of muscle fibers and muscles in embryonic development. adj., **myogenet′ic.**

myogenic (mi″o-jen′ik) giving rise to or forming muscle tissue.

myogenous (mi-oj′ĕ-nus) originating in muscular tissue.

myoglobin (mi′o-glo″bin) the oxygen-transporting pigment of muscle, a type of HEMOPROTEIN resembling a single subunit of HEMOGLOBIN, being composed of one globin polypeptide chain and one heme group.

myoglobinuria (mi″o-glo″bin-u′re-ah) the presence of myoglobin in the urine.

myoglobulin (mi″o-glob′u-lin) a globulin from muscle serum.

myogram (mi′o-gram) a record produced by myography.

myograph (mi′o-graf) an apparatus for recording the effects of muscular contraction.

myography (mi-og′rah-fe) 1. the use of a myograph. 2. description of muscles. 3. radiography of muscle tissue after injection of a radiopaque medium. adj., **myograph′ic.**

myoid (mi′oid) resembling muscle.

myoischemia (mi″o-is-ke′me-ah) local deficiency of blood supply in muscle.

myokinesimeter (mi″o-kin″ĕ-sim′ĕ-ter) an apparatus for measuring muscular contraction induced by electrical stimulation.

myokinetic (mi″o-kĭ-net′ik) pertaining to the motion or kinetic function of muscle, as contrasted with the myotonic or tonic function.

myokymia (mi″o-ki′me-ah) a benign condition in which there is persistent quivering of the muscles.

myolipoma (mi″o-lĭ-po′mah) myoma with fatty elements.

myology (mi-ol′o-je) scientific study or description of the muscles and accessory structures (bursae and synovial sheath).

myolysis (mi-ol′ĭ-sis) degeneration of muscle tissue.

myoma (mi-o′mah) a tumor formed of muscle tissue. adj., **myo′matous.**

   uterine m., m. of uterus leiomyoma uteri.

myomalacia (mi″o-mah-la′she-ah) morbid softening of a muscle.

myomatosis (mi″o-mah-to′sis) the formation of multiple MYOMAS.

myomectomy (mi″o-mek′to-me) 1. surgical excision of a myoma. 2. myectomy.

uterine m. surgical removal of a uterine MYOMA (leiomyoma); called also fibroidectomy and fibromyomectomy.

myomelanosis (mi″o-mel″ah-no′sis) MELANOSIS of muscle.

myomere (mi′o-mēr) myotome; the muscle plate or portion of a somite that develops into voluntary muscle.

myometer (mi-om′ĕ-ter) an apparatus for measuring muscle contraction.

myometritis (mi″o-me-tri′tis) inflammation of the myometrium.

myometrium (mi″o-me′tre-um) the smooth muscle coat of the uterus. adj., **myome′trial.**

myonecrosis (mi″o-nĕ-kro′sis) necrosis or death of individual muscle fibers.

myoneural (mi″o-noor′al) pertaining to nerve terminations in muscles.

myoneuralgia (mi″o-nŏo-ral′jah) neuralgic pain in a muscle.

myopalmus (mi″o-pal′mus) muscle twitching.

myoparalysis (mi″o-pah-ral′ĭ-sis) paralysis of a muscle.

myoparesis (mi″o-pah-re′sis) slight muscle paralysis.

myopathy (mi-op′ah-the) any disease of a muscle. adj., **myopath′ic.**

    centronuclear m. myotubular myopathy.

    distal m. an autosomal dominant form of MUSCULAR DYSTROPHY, appearing in two types. The first has onset in infancy, does not progress past adolescence, and is not incapacitating. The second has onset in adulthood and is called late distal hereditary MYOPATHY. Called also distal muscular dystrophy.

    glycolytic m. any metabolic MYOPATHY resulting from a defect of glycolytic enzyme activity, marked by exercise intolerance and cramping, the accumulation of GLYCOGEN in muscle, and recurrent MYOGLOBINURIA.

    late distal hereditary m. distal MYOPATHY that sets in usually after age 40, does not affect life span and first affects the

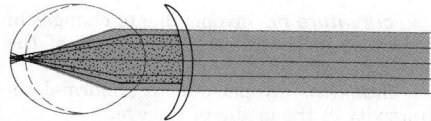

Refraction and correction in myopia. From Ignatavicius and Workman, 2000.

small muscles of the hands and feet and then spreads proximally.

    metabolic m. myopathy due to disordered metabolism, usually caused by genetic defects or hormonal dysfunction.

    mitochondrial m. any of a group of myopathies associated with an increased number of enlarged, often abnormal, MITOCHONDRIA in muscle fibers, manifested by exercise intolerance, generalized weakness, lactic ACIDOSIS, infantile TETRAPARESIS, OPHTHALMOPLEGIA, and cardiac abnormalities.

    myotubular m. a form marked by myofibers resembling the MYOTUBULES of early fetal muscle.

    nemaline m. a congenital abnormality of myofibrils in which small threadlike fibers are scattered through the muscle fibers; marked by hypotonia and proximal muscle weakness.

    ocular m. a slowly progressive form affecting the extraocular muscles, with ptosis and progressive immobility of the eyes.

myope (mi′ōp) a person affected with myopia.

myopericarditis (mi″o-per″ĭ-kahr-di′tis) inflammation of both the myocardium and pericardium.

myopia (M) (mi-o′pe-ah) a defect of VISION consisting of an error of refraction in which rays of light entering the eye parallel to the optic axis are brought to a focus in front of the retina, so that vision for near objects is better than for far. This results from the eyeball being too long from front to back. Called also nearsightedness. adj., **myop′ic.**

Myopia generally appears before the age of 8, often becoming gradually worse until about the age of 20, when it ceases to change much. In later years the nearsighted person may find he or she can read comfortably without glasses. In children the most frequent symptoms of myopia are attempts to brush away blurriness, frequent rubbing of the eyes, and squinting at distant objects. Myopia can almost always be corrected with eyeglasses or contact lenses. Surgical procedures to correct it include radial KERATOTOMY, photorefractive KERATECTOMY, and LASIK.

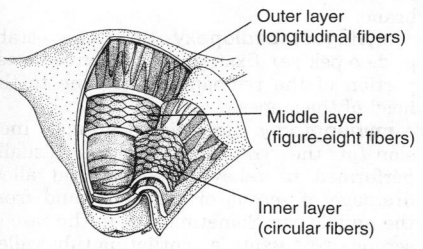

Layers of myometrium showing the three layers of smooth muscle fiber. From Gorrie et al., 1994.

Outer layer (longitudinal fibers)

Middle layer (figure-eight fibers)

Inner layer (circular fibers)

M

curvature m. myopia due to changes in curvature of the refracting surfaces of the eye, especially of the cornea.

index m. myopia due to abnormal refractivity of the media of the eye.

malignant m., pernicious m. progressive myopia with disease of the choroid, leading to retinal detachment and blindness.

progressive m. myopia that continues to increase in adult life.

myoplasm (mi′o-plazm) the contractile part of the muscle cell.

myoplasty (mi′o-plas″te) plastic surgery on muscle whereby portions of detached muscles are used, especially in the field of defects or deformities. adj., **myoplas′-tic.**

myoreceptor (mi″o-re-sep′ter) a receptor situated in skeletal muscle that is stimulated by muscular contraction, providing information to higher centers regarding muscle position.

myorrhaphy (mi-or′ah-fe) suture of a muscle.

myorrhexis (mi″o-rek′sis) rupture of a muscle.

myosarcoma (mi″o-sahr-ko′mah) a malignant tumor derived from myogenic cells.

myosclerosis (mi″o-skle-ro′sis) hardening of muscle tissue.

myosin (mi′o-sin) one of the two main proteins of muscle. Myosin and ACTIN are the proteins involved in contraction of muscle FIBERS.

myositis (mi″o-si′tis) inflammation of a voluntary muscle; called also initis.

m. fibro′sa a type in which there is a formation of connective tissue in the muscle.

multiple m. polymyositis.

m. ossi′ficans myositis marked by bony deposits in muscle.

trichinous m. that which is caused by the presence of *Trichinella spiralis.*

myospasm (mi′o-spazm) spasm (def. 1).

myotactic (mi″o-tak′tik) pertaining to the proprioceptive sense of muscles.

myotasis (mi-ot′ah-sis) stretching of muscle. adj., **myotat′ic.**

myotenositis (mi″o-te″no-si′tis) inflammation of a muscle and tendon.

myotenotomy (mi″o-te-not′ah-me) surgical division of the tendon of a muscle.

myotome (mi′o-tōm) 1. an instrument for dividing muscles. 2. the muscle plate or portion of a somite that develops into voluntary muscle. 3. a group of muscles innervated from a single spinal nerve. adj., **myotom′ic.**

myotomy (mi-ot′ah-me) cutting or dissection of muscular tissue or of a muscle.

Myotonachol (mi″o-tōn-ah-kol) trademark for preparations of BETHANECHOL chloride, a smooth muscle RELAXANT used to treat urinary retention.

myotonia (mi″o-to′ne-ah) any disorder involving tonic spasm of muscle. adj., **myoton′ic.**

m. atro′phica myotonic DYSTROPHY.

m. conge′nita a hereditary disease marked by tonic spasm and rigidity of certain muscles when attempts are made to move them. The stiffness tends to disappear as the muscles are used.

m. dystro′phica myotonic DYSTROPHY.

myotonus (mi-ot′o-nus) tonic spasm of a muscle or a group of muscles.

myotrophic (mi′o-tro″fik) 1. increasing the weight of muscle. 2. pertaining to myotrophy.

myotrophy (mi-ot′ro-fe) nutrition of muscle.

myotropic (mi″o-trop′ik) having a special affinity for muscle.

myotube (mi′o-tōōb) myotubule.

myotubule (mi″o-too′būl) a developing skeletal muscle fiber with a centrally located nucleus. adj., **myotu′bular.**

myovascular (mi″o-vas′ku-ler) pertaining to muscle and blood vessels.

Myriapoda (mir″e-ap′o-dah) a class of arthropods, including the millipedes and centipedes.

myring(o)- word element [L.], *tympanic membrane.*

myringa (mi-ring′gah) TYMPANIC MEMBRANE.

myringectomy (mir″in-jek′to-me) tympanectomy.

myringitis (mi-rin-ji′tis) inflammation of the tympanic membrane.

m. bullo′sa, bullous m. a form of viral otitis media in which serous or hemorrhagic blebs appear on the tympanic membrane and adjacent wall of the acoustic meatus.

myringomycosis (mi-ring″go-mi-ko′sis) OTOMYCOSIS of the tympanic membrane.

myringoplasty (mi-ring′go-plas″te) surgical reconstruction of the tympanic membrane.

myringostapediopexy (mi-ring″go-stah″pe′de-o-pek″se) fixation of the large lower portion of the tympanic membrane to the head of the stapes.

myringotomy (mir″ing-got′ah-me) incision of the TYMPANIC MEMBRANE, usually performed to relieve pressure and allow drainage of serous or purulent fluid from the middle ear. Sometimes, as in the case of serous OTITIS MEDIA, a ventilating tube called a GROMMET is inserted to permit continuous ventilation and avoid a chronic middle ear problem with fluid accumulation, pain, and loss of hearing. When a simple myringotomy is done for purposes of draining purulent material resulting from recurrent suppurative otitis media, care should be taken to avoid contamination by the fluid. Eardrops may be prescribed if there is fluid in the ear. The ear should be kept dry for two weeks after the procedure, with no fluid entering the ear until the myringotomy site in the eardrum is healed.

Mysoline (mi′so-lēn) trademark for preparations of PRIMIDONE, an ANTICONVULSANT.

mysophilia (mi″so-fil′e-ah) abnormal interest in dirt or filth, with a desire for contact with it that may encompass a paraphilia.

mysophobia (mi″so-fo′be-ah) irrational fear of dirt and contamination.

myx(o)- word element [Gr.], *mucus; slime.*

myxadenitis (mik″sad-ĕ-ni′tis) inflammation of a mucus-secreting gland.

myxadenoma (mik″sad-ĕ-no′mah) an epithelial tumor with the structure of a mucous gland.

myxasthenia (mik″sas-the′ne-ah) deficient secretion of mucus.

myxedema (mik″sĕ-de′mah) a condition resulting from advanced HYPOTHYROIDISM, or deficiency of THYROXINE; it is the adult form of the disease whose congenital form is known as CRETINISM. adj., **myxedem′atous.**

Myxedema may be caused by lack of iodine in the diet; by atrophy, surgical removal, or a disorder of the thyroid gland; by destruction of the gland by radioactive iodine; or by deficient excretion of thyrotropin by the pituitary gland. It is marked primarily by a growing puffiness or "sogginess" of the skin, nonpitting EDEMA, abnormal deposits of mucin in the skin, and distinctive facial changes such as swollen lips and a thickened nose.

Because thyroxine plays such an important role in the body's metabolism, lack of this hormone seriously upsets the balance of body processes. Among the symptoms associated with myxedema are excessive fatigue and drowsiness, headaches, weight gain, dryness of the skin, sensitivity to cold, and increasing thinness and brittleness of the nails. In women, menstrual bleeding may become irregular. Medical tests reveal slow tendon reflexes, low blood iodine, below-normal metabolism, and abnormal uptake of radioactive iodine by the thyroid.

The body's defenses against infection also are weakened. If the patient has heart disease, it may worsen. Upset of the functions of the adrenal glands may become critical. In time, if myxedema is not brought under control, progressive mental deterioration may result in a psychosis marked by paranoid delusions.

Myxedema is treated by administration of thyroid extract or similar synthetic preparations. If treatment is begun soon after the symptoms appear, recovery may be complete. Delayed or interrupted treatment may mean permanent deterioration. In most instances, treatment with thyroid hormones or synthetics must be continued throughout the patient's lifetime.

pretibial m. localized skin lesions associated with preceding HYPERTHYROIDISM, found most often on the front of the legs. It is almost always associated with GRAVES′ DISEASE, occurring in 0.5 to 5 per cent of patients. Called also thyroid dermopathy.

myxedematoid (mik″sĕ-dem′ah-toid) resembling myxedema.

myxochondroma (mik″so-kon-dro′mah) CHONDROMA with stroma resembling primitive MESENCHYMAL tissue.

myxocyte (mik″so-sīt) one of the cells of mucous tissue.

myxofibroma (mik″so-fi-bro′mah) a FIBROMA containing myxomatous tissue; called also fibroma myxomatodes and fibromyxoma.

myxofibrosarcoma (mik″so-fi″bro-sahr-ko′mah) fibrosarcoma with myxomatous areas.

myxoid (mik′soid) mucoid (def. 1).

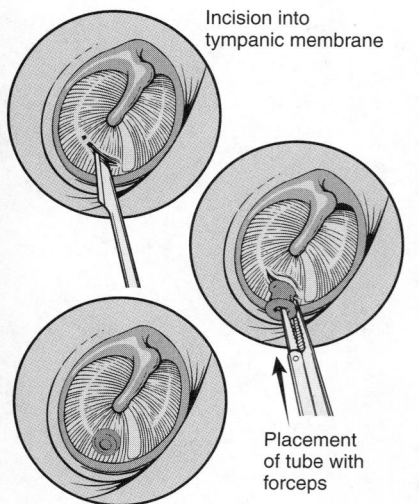

Incision into tympanic membrane

Placement of tube with forceps

Tube in place

Myringotomy and insertion of a tympanoplasty tube as treatment for otitis media. From Frazier et al., 2000.

M

myxolipoma (mik″so-lĭ-po′mah) lipoma with foci of myxomatous degeneration.

myxoma (mik-so′mah) a tumor composed of primitive connective tissue cells and stroma resembling MESENCHYMA. adj., **myxo′matous.**

myxomatosis (mik″so-mah-to′sis) 1. the development of multiple myxomas. 2. myxomatous degeneration.

myxomyoma (mik″so-mi-o′mah) a myoma with myxomatous degeneration.

myxopoiesis (mik″so-poi-e′sis) the formation of mucus.

myxosarcoma (mik″so-sahr-ko′mah) a sarcoma containing myxomatous tissue.

myxovirus (mik′so-vi″rus) any of numerous RNA viruses, some of which cause disease, now distinguished as either ORTHOMYXOVIRUSES or PARAMYXOVIRUSES.

N

N newton; nitrogen; normal (solution), used with a number designating the strength of the solution relative to the normal, e.g., N/2 or 0.5 N for half-normal.

N normal (see N); number; Avogadro's number.

N_A Avogadro's number.

n nano-; refractive index.

NA Nomina Anatomica.

Na sodium (L. *na'trium*).

nabumetone (nah-bu'mĕ-tōn) a NONSTEROIDAL ANTIINFLAMMATORY DRUG used in treatment of rheumatoid ARTHRITIS and OSTEOARTHRITIS.

NACA National Advisory Council on Aging, an organization of the Canadian federal government.

nacreous (na'kre-us) having a pearl-like luster.

NAD nicotinamide-adenine dinucleotide.

nadolol (na-do'lol) a BETA-ADRENERGIC BLOCKING AGENT that affects both β_1- and β_2-receptors; administered orally as an ANTIHYPERTENSIVE AGENT and for treatment of ANGINA PECTORIS.

nafarelin (naf'ah-rel''in) a synthetic preparation of gonadotropin-releasing HORMONE, used as the acetate ester in treatment of central precocious PUBERTY and ENDOMETRIOSIS; administered by nasal spray.

NADONA/LTC National Association of Directors of Nursing Administration Long Term Care.

NADP nicotinamide adenine dinucleotide phosphate.

nafcillin (naf-sil'in) a semisynthetic, acid- and penicillinase-resistant PENICILLIN antibiotic effective against staphylococcal infections; administered orally or parenterally as the sodium salt.

naftifine (naf'tĭ-fēn) a broad-spectrum antifungal AGENT, applied topically as the hydrochloride salt.

Nägele's rule (na'gĕ-lēz) a method for calculating the estimated (or expected) date of confinement (EDC) or of delivery (EDD): count back three months from the first day of the last menstrual period, and then add one year and seven days. An unavoidable error of plus or minus two weeks may occur.

NAHC National Association for Home Care.

nail (nāl) 1. a rod of metal, bone, or other material used for fixation of the ends of fractured bones. 2. a hardened or horny cutaneous plate overlying the dorsal surface

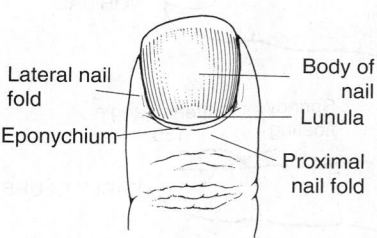

Parts of the nail. From Dorland's, 2000.

of the distal end of a finger or toe. The nails are part of the outer layer of the skin and are composed of hard tissue formed of KERATIN. Called also unguis.

ingrown n. see INGROWN NAIL.

spoon n. a nail with a concave surface.

naïve (nah-ēv') not previously exposed to therapy or treatment.

nalbuphine (nal-bu'fēn) a potent opioid ANALGESIC used as the hydrochloride salt for relief of moderate to severe pain and as an adjunct to anesthesia; administered intravenously, intramuscularly, and subcutaneously.

Nalfon (nal'fon) trademark for a preparation of FENOPROFEN calcium, a NONSTEROIDAL ANTIINFLAMMATORY DRUG.

nalidixic acid (nal''ĭ-dik'sik) a QUINOLONE antibacterial agent, active against most gram-negative bacteria causing urinary tract infection including *Escherichia coli*, *Klebsiella* and *Enterobacter* species, and some *Proteus* species. *Pseudomonas* species are generally resistant.

nalmefene (nal'mĕ-fēn'') an OPIOID antagonist, used as the hydrochloride salt in the treatment of opioid overdose and postoperative opioid depression.

nalorphine (nal'or-fēn) a semisynthetic congener of MORPHINE, used as an antagonist to morphine and related narcotics and in the diagnosis of narcotic addiction.

naloxone (nal-oks'ōn) an opioid antagonist structurally related to OXYMORPHONE, used in the diagnosis and treatment of opioid toxicity, to reverse opioid-induced respiratory depression, and as an adjunct in the treatment of hypotension associated with septic SHOCK; administered parenterally.

naltrexone (nal-trek'sōn) an OPIOID antagonist used as the hydrochloride salt in treatment of opioid or alcohol abuse.

NAMI National Alliance for the Mentally Ill.

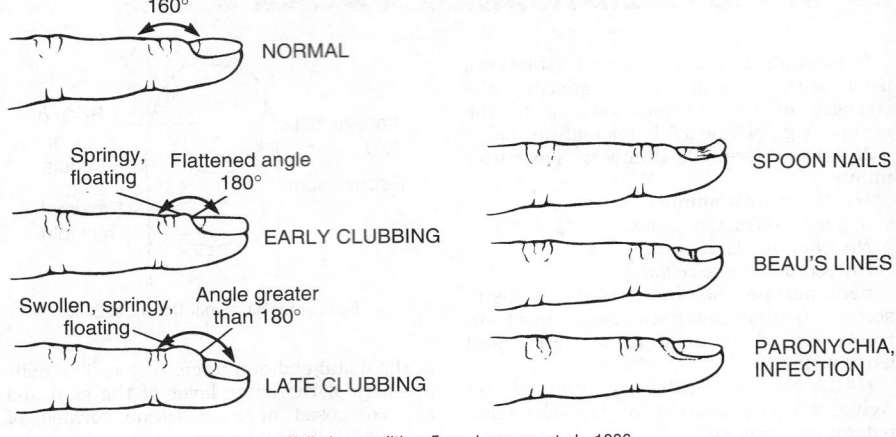

Nail abnormalities. From Lammon et al., 1996.

nan(o)- word element [Gr.], *dwarf; small size;* also used in naming units of measurement (symbol n) to designate an amount one billionth (10^{-9}) the size of the unit to which it is joined, e.g., nanocurie.

NANDA North American Nursing Diagnosis Association.

nandrolone (nan'dro-lōn) an anabolic STEROID with lesser androgenic effects; used as *n. decanoate* and *n. phenpropionate* in the treatment of severe growth retardation in children and of metastatic breast cancer and as an aid in the treatment of chronic wasting diseases and anemia associated with renal insufficiency.

nanism (na'nizm) dwarfism.

nanocephaly (nan″o-sef'ah-le) microcephaly.

nanocormia (nan″o-kor'me-ah) abnormal smallness of the body or trunk.

nanocurie (nCi) (nan'o-ku″re) a unit of radioactivity, being one billionth (10^{-9}) of a CURIE.

nanogram (nan'o-gram) one billionth (10^{-9}) of a GRAM.

nanoid (nan'oid) dwarfish.

nanomelus (nan-om'ĕ-lus) micromelus.

nanometer (nm) (nan'o-me″ter) one billionth (10^{-9}) of a METER.

nanophthalmia (nan″of-thal'me-ah) nanophthalmos.

nanophthalmos (nan″of-thal'mus) abnormal smallness in all dimensions of one or both eyes in the absence of other ocular defects; see MICROPHTHALMOS.

nanophthalmus (nan″of-thal'mus) 1. nanophthalmos. 2. a person affected with nanophthalmos.

nanosecond (ns) (nan'o-sek″ond) one billionth (10^{-9}) of a second.

nanosomia (nan″o-so'me-ah) dwarfism.

nanous (nan'us) dwarfish.

NANT National Association of Nephrology Technologists.

nanus (nan'us) dwarf.

nape (nāp) the back of the neck; called also NUCHA.

naphazoline (naf-az'o-lēn) a sympathomimetic used in the form of the hydrochloride salt as a VASOCONSTRICTOR to decongest nasal and ocular mucosae.

naphthalene (naf'thah-lēn) a hydrocarbon from coal tar oil, used as a moth repellent, fungicide, and preservative; it is toxic by ingestion, inhalation, and ingestion.

naphthol (naf'thol) a phenol occurring in coal tar in two forms: α- or 1-naphthol and β- or 2-naphthol. It is used in dyes, insecticides, and pharmaceutical compounds. If excessive amounts are ingested poisoning may result, characterized by anemia, jaundice, convulsions, and coma.

NAPNES National Association for Practical Nurse Education and Services.

Naprosyn (nah-pro'sin) trademark for preparations of NAPROXEN, a NONSTEROIDAL ANTIINFLAMMATORY DRUG.

naproxen (nah-prok'sen) a NONSTEROIDAL ANTIINFLAMMATORY DRUG that is a PROPIONIC ACID derivative with analgesic, antipyretic and antiinflammatory activity; used for treatment of rheumatoid ARTHRITIS, OSTEO ARTHRITIS, GOUT, CALCIUM PYROPHOSPHATE DEPOSITION DISEASE, fever, and dysmenorrhea, and in the prophylaxis and suppression of vascular HEADACHE; administered orally or rectally, as the base or the sodium salt.

napsylate (nap′sĭ-lāt) USAN contraction for 2-naphthalenesulfonate.

naratriptan (nar″ah-trip′tan) a selective SEROTONIN receptor agonist used as the hydrochloride salt in the acute treatment of MIGRAINE; administered orally.

narcissism (nahr′sĭ-sizm) dominant interest in oneself; self-love. adj., **narcis′sis′tic.**

  primary n. that occurring in the early infantile phase of object relationship development, when the child has not differentiated himself from the outside world and regards all sources of pleasure as originating within himself.

  secondary n. that in which the libido, once attached to external love objects, is redirected back to the self.

  narc(o)- word element [Gr.], *stupor; stuporous state.*

narcissistic personality disorder a PERSONALITY DISORDER marked by a grandiose sense of self-importance. Patients are preoccupied with fantasies of unlimited success, power, brilliance, beauty, or ideal love. In spite of these fantasies, they are troubled by a sense of inadequacy and respond to criticism, defeat, or rejection either by indifference or by feelings of rage, shame, humiliation, or emptiness. Their relationships with others are disturbed by expectations of special favors, exploitativeness, overidealization and devaluation of others, and a lack of empathy.

narcoanalysis (nahr″ko-ah-nal′ĭ-sis) a controversial method of psychotherapy that uses administration of medications to release suppressed or repressed thoughts or affect-laden and unacceptable ideas.

narcohypnosis (nahr″ko-hip-no′sis) hypnotic suggestions made while the patient is narcotized.

narcolepsy (nahr′ko-lep″se) recurrent, uncontrollable, brief episodes of sleep, often associated with HALLUCINATIONS just beforehand or just afterward, or CATAPLEXY or sleep PARALYSIS. adj., **narcolep′tic.**

narcosis (nahr-ko′sis) a reversible state of central nervous system depression induced by a drug.

  basal n. narcosis with complete unconsciousness, amnesia, and analgesia.

  carbon dioxide n. respiratory acidosis.

  nitrogen n. a state resembling drunkenness, with euphoria and disorientation, seen in divers below about 30 meters (100 feet) who are breathing compressed air, because of the high nitrogen content of air; some of the nitrogen enters the bloodstream and acts as a narcotic.

narcotic (nahr-kot′ic) 1. pertaining to or producing NARCOSIS. 2. an agent that produces insensibility or stupor, applied especially to the OPIOIDS, i.e., to any natural or synthetic drug that has actions like those of MORPHINE. See also DRUG ABUSE.

narcotize (nahr′ko-tīz) to put under the influence of a narcotic.

Nardil (nahr′dil) trademark for a preparation of PHENELZINE sulfate, an ANTIDEPRESSANT.

nares (na′rēz) [L.] plural of *na′ris*, the external openings of the nasal cavity; called also nostrils.

nas(o)- word element [L.], *nose.*

nasal (na′zal) pertaining to the nose.

Nasalide (na′zal-īd) trademark for a preparation of FLUNISOLIDE, an ANTIINFLAMMATORY agent used for allergic RHINITIS and other inflammatory nasal conditions.

nascent (nas′ent, na′sent) 1. being born; just coming into existence. 2. just liberated from a chemical combination, and hence more reactive because uncombined.

nasion (na′ze-on) the middle point of the junction of the frontal and the two nasal bones (frontonasal suture).

nasoantral (na″zo-an′tral) pertaining to the nose and maxillary antrum.

nasoantrostomy (na″so-an-tros′tah-me) surgical formation of a nasoantral window for drainage of an obstructed maxillary sinus.

nasociliary (na″zo-sil′e-er″e) pertaining to the eyes, brow, and root of the nose.

nasofrontal (na″zo-frun′tal) pertaining to the nose and forehead or to the nasal and frontal bones.

nasogastric tube (na″zo-gas′trik) NG tube; a tube of soft rubber or plastic that is inserted through a nostril and into the stomach for instilling liquid foods or other substances or for gastric decompression. Both medications and nutritive feedings can be given through the tube; see also TUBE FEEDING. Prior to insertion of the tube a measurement is made to assure that the distal end of the tube will be positioned in the stomach. This is done by placing the tip of the tube on the bridge of the patient's nose and then marking on the tube the point at which it touches the tip of the xiphoid process. Once the tube is inserted its position should be checked to be sure it is in the stomach and not the trachea or bronchi. This is done by aspirating for stomach contents, using a bulb syringe or 50-ml aspirating syringe. Alternatively, the syringe can be used to inject air into the tube while at the same time listening through a stethoscope for a "whooshing"

N

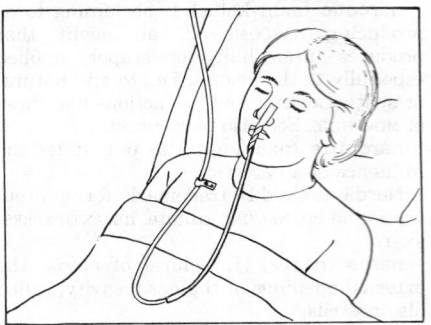

Nasogastric tube. From Lammon et al., 1996.

sound made by the air being injected. The tube should be anchored so that it points downward away from the nares. It is *not* brought up over the nose and anchored by tape over the bridge of the nose. This increases irritation of the nasal mucosa, impedes circulation, and causes unnecessary discomfort. To avoid tension and drag on the tube a pin and rubber band can be used to secure the tube to the shoulder of the patient's gown or pajama top. MOUTH CARE is of particular importance while a nasogastric tube is in place.

nasolabial (na″zo-la′be-al) pertaining to, or extending between, the nose and lip.

nasolacrimal (na″zo-lak′rĭ-mal) pertaining to the nose and lacrimal apparatus.

naso-oral (na″zo-or′al) pertaining to the nose and mouth.

nasopalatine (na″zo-pal′ah-tīn) pertaining to the nose and palate.

nasopharyngitis (na″zo-far″in-ji′tis) inflammation of the nasopharynx.

nasopharyngolaryngoscope (na″zo-fah-ring″go-lah-ring′go-skōp) a flexible fiber-

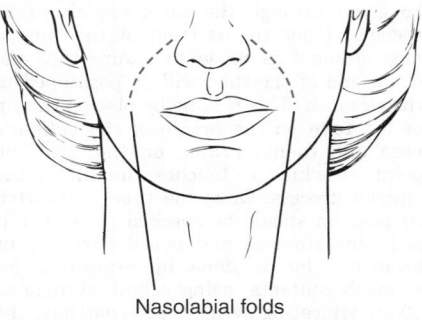

Nasolabial folds

In the nasolabial region are lines or creases that run between the nose and mouth and should be assessed for symmetry. From Lammon et al., 1996.

optic endoscope for examining the nasopharynx and larynx.

nasopharynx (na″zo-far′ingks) the part of the pharynx above the soft palate. adj., **nasopharyn′geal.**

nasosinusitis (na″zo-si″nŭ-si′tis) rhinosinusitis.

nasus (na′sus) [L.] nose.

natal (na′tal) 1. pertaining to birth. 2. gluteal.

natality (na-tal′ĭ-te) the birth rate.

natamycin (nat″ah-mi′sin) a POLYENE antibiotic used in topical treatment of fungal keratitis, blepharitis, and conjunctivitis.

nateglinide (nah-teg′lĭ-nīd) an antidiabetic AGENT that lowers blood glucose concentrations by stimulating the release of INSULIN from pancreatic islet beta cells; administered orally in the treatment of type 2 DIABETES MELLITUS, either alone or in combination with METFORMIN.

nates (na′tēz) [L., pl.] buttocks.

natimortality (na″tĭ-mor-tal′ĭ-te) fetal death rate.

National Academies of Practice (NAP) ten organizations, the first of which were founded in 1981, limited to 100 Distinguished Practitioners in each of the ten major health professions as recognized by the Congress of the United States: Dentistry, Medicine, Nursing, Optometry, Osteopathic Medicine, Pharmacy, Podiatric Medicine, Psychology, Social Work, and Veterinary Medicine. The purpose of the Academies is to advise Congress in matters of health care practice and delivery.

Patterned after the National Academy of Sciences, which advises Congress on matters of science, membership in the National Academies of Practice is contingent upon election as a Distinguished Practitioner in one of the Academies. Chosen by their peers as persons who have made a significant and enduring contribution to practice, these Distinguished Practitioners have spent an important part of their lives in the practice of their profession. By their very stature, they have transcended the turf interests of their respective professions and are prepared to address the issue of national health. The National Academies of Practice differ from the National Academy of Sciences in that their members are practitioners who have been nationally recognized primarily for their contributions to professional practice rather than achievements in science, although many are renowned scientists as well. It is the only interdisciplinary group of practitioners dedicated to addressing the problems of practice in the interests of the citizens of the United States. It is the goal and the objective of this self-supported organization to constitute itself as the nation's interdisciplinary health policy forum.

National Alliance for the Mentally Ill (NAMI) a national self-help and advocacy group composed of persons with mental illness and their family members. Its work includes developing new treatment approaches and advocating problems to legislators and the public.

National Association for Practical Nurse Education and Service (NAPNES) the first national organization concerned solely with practical nurse education and the services rendered by the practical nurse, organized in 1941. Members include professional and practical nurses, physicians, hospital administrators, other health and welfare workers, and interested lay citizens.

The organization maintains an accrediting program for state-approved schools of practical nursing, provides a consulting service for groups interested in starting a practical nurse program, prepares and publishes leaflets, booklets, and other educational materials for practical nurses, and sponsors regional workshops and summer school courses on practical nurse education and services.

National Cancer Institute (NCI) an institute of the NATIONAL INSTITUTES OF HEALTH that leads a national effort to reduce the burden of cancer morbidity and mortality by stimulating and supporting scientific discoveries through basic and clinical biomedical research and training. It conducts and supports programs to understand the causes of cancer; prevent, detect, diagnose, treat, and control cancer; and disseminate information to the practitioner, patient, and public in general.

National Center for Chronic Disease Prevention and Health Promotion (NCCDPHP) an organizational component of the CENTERS FOR DISEASE CONTROL AND PREVENTION, charged with preventing premature death and DISABILITY from chronic diseases and promoting healthy personal behaviors.

National Center for Complementary and Alternative Medicine (NCCAM) an institute of the NATIONAL INSTITUTES OF HEALTH, dedicated to exploring complementary and alternative MEDICINE practices in the context of rigorous science, training researchers in the field, and disseminating authoritative information.

National Center for Environmental Health (NCEH) an organizational component of the CENTERS FOR DISEASE CONTROL AND PREVENTION, charged with providing national leadership in prevention and control of disease and death resulting from the interaction between people and their environment.

National Center for Health Statistics (NCHS) an organizational component of the CENTERS FOR DISEASE CONTROL AND PREVENTION, charged with providing statistical information that will guide actions and policies to improve the health of the American people.

National Center for HIV, STD, and TB Prevention (NCHSTP) an organizational component of the CENTERS FOR DISEASE CONTROL AND PREVENTION, charged with providing national leadership in preventing and controlling human immunodeficiency VIRUS infection, SEXUALLY TRANSMITTED DISEASES, and TUBERCULOSIS.

National Center for Infectious Diseases (NCID) an organizational component of the CENTERS FOR DISEASE CONTROL AND PREVENTION, charged with preventing illness, DISABILITY, and death caused by INFECTIOUS DISEASES in the United States and around the world.

National Center for Injury Prevention and Control (NCIPC) an organizational component of the CENTERS FOR DISEASE CONTROL AND PREVENTION, charged with preventing death and DISABILITY from nonoccupational injuries, including those that are unintentional and those that result from violence.

National Center for Research Resources an institute of the NATIONAL INSTITUTES OF HEALTH that advances biomedical research and improves human health through research projects and shared resources that create, develop, and provide a comprehensive range of human, animal, technological, and other resources.

National Center on Birth Defects and Developmental Disabilities (NCBDDD) an organizational component of the CENTERS FOR DISEASE CONTROL AND PREVENTION, charged with providing national leadership for preventing birth defects and developmental DISABILITIES and for improving the health and wellness of people with DISABILITIES.

National Center on Minority Health and Health Disparities an institute of the NATIONAL INSTITUTES OF HEALTH whose mission is to reduce and ultimately eliminate health disparities between racial and ethnic minorities (and other groups such as the urban and rural poor) and society as a whole. It does this by conducting and supporting basic, clinical, and behavioral research, emerging programs, training, and information dissemination in this area.

National Council of State Boards of Nursing, Inc. an organization through which boards of nursing from all 50 states, the District of Columbia, Guam, American Samoa, the Commonwealth of the Northern Mariana Islands, Puerto Rico, and the Virgin Islands act and counsel together on matters of common interest and concern related to the safe and effective practice of nursing in the interest of public health, safety, and welfare, including the development of nurse licensure examinations (NCLEX-RN and NCLEX-PN).

National Eye Institute (NEI) an institute of the NATIONAL INSTITUTES OF HEALTH whose mission is to conduct and support research that helps prevent and treat eye diseases and other disorders of vision.

National Federation of Licensed Practical Nurses (NFLPN) the only national organization with a membership consisting solely of licensed practical-vocational nurses.

National Formulary (NF) a book of standards for certain pharmaceuticals and preparations not included in the USP; revised every 5 years, and recognized as a book of official standards by the Pure Food and Drug Act of 1906.

National Heart, Lung, and Blood Institute (NHLBI) an institute of the NATIONAL INSTITUTES OF HEALTH whose mission is to provide leadership for a national program in diseases of the heart, blood vessels, lungs, and blood, as well as of blood resources and sleep disorders. It also has administrative responsibility for the NIH Women's Health Initiative.

National Human Genome Research Institute an institute of the NATIONAL INSTITUTES OF HEALTH that supports the NIH component of the HUMAN GENOME PROJECT.

National Immunization Program (NIP) an organizational component of the CENTERS FOR DISEASE CONTROL AND PREVENTION, charged with preventing disease, DISABILITY, and death from VACCINE-preventable diseases in children and adults.

National Institute for Occupational Safety and Health (NIOSH) an organizational component of the CENTERS FOR DISEASE CONTROL AND PREVENTION, charged with ensuring safety and health for all people in the workplace through research and prevention.

National Institute of Allergy and Infectious Diseases (NIAID) an institute of the NATIONAL INSTITUTES OF HEALTH; its research strives to understand, treat, and ultimately prevent infectious, immunologic, and allergic disorders affecting human beings.

National Institute of Arthritis and Musculoskeletal and Skin Diseases (NIAMS) an institute of the NATIONAL INSTITUTES OF HEALTH that supports research into the causes, treatment, and prevention of ARTHRITIS, musculoskeletal diseases, and skin diseases.

National Institute of Biomedical Imaging and Bioengineering an institute of the NATIONAL INSTITUTES OF HEALTH whose mission is to improve health by promoting fundamental discoveries, design and development, translation, and assessment of technological capabilities in biomedical imaging and BIOENGINEERING.

National Institute of Child Health and Human Development (NICHD) an institute of the NATIONAL INSTITUTES OF HEALTH; it conducts research on FERTILITY, PREGNANCY, growth, development, and medical rehabilitation, striving to ensure that every child is born healthy and wanted and grows up free from disease and DISABILITY.

National Institute of Dental and Craniofacial Research (NIDCR) an institute of the NATIONAL INSTITUTES OF HEALTH; it provides leadership for a national research program designed to understand, treat, and ultimately prevent infectious and inherited craniofacial, oral, and dental diseases and disorders.

National Institute of Diabetes and Digestive and Kidney Diseases (NIDDK) an institute of the NATIONAL INSTITUTES OF HEALTH; it conducts and supports basic and applied research and provides leadership for a national program in diabetes, endocrinology, and metabolic diseases; digestive diseases and nutrition; and kidney, urologic, and hematologic diseases.

National Institute of Environmental Health Sciences (NIEHS) an institute of the NATIONAL INSTITUTES OF HEALTH whose mission is to reduce the burden of human illness and dysfunction from environmental causes by defining how environmental exposures, genetic susceptibility, and age interact to affect the individual's health.

National Institute of General Medical Sciences (NIGMS) an institute of the NATIONAL INSTITUTES OF HEALTH whose mission is to support biomedical research that is not targeted at specific diseases, resulting in increased understanding of life and laying the foundation for advances in disease diagnosis, treatment, and prevention.

National Institute of Mental Health (NIMH) an institute of the NATIONAL INSTITUTES OF HEALTH whose mission is to provide national leadership in the understanding, treatment, and prevention of mental illnesses through basic research on the brain and behavior, as well as through clinical, epidemiological, and services research.

National Institute of Neurological Disorders and Stroke an institute of the NATIONAL INSTITUTES OF HEALTH whose mission is to reduce the burden of neurological diseases by supporting and conducting research (both basic and clinical) on the normal and diseased nervous system, fostering the training of investigators in the neurosciences, and seeking better understanding, diagnosis, treatment, and prevention of neurological disorders.

National Institute of Nursing Research an institute of the NATIONAL INSTITUTES OF HEALTH that supports clinical and basic research to establish a scientific basis for the care of individuals across the life span in a variety of ways.

National Institute on Aging (NIA) an institute of the NATIONAL INSTITUTES OF HEALTH that leads a national program of research on the biomedical, social, and behavioral aspects of the AGING process; the prevention of age-related diseases and disabilities; and the promotion of a better quality of life for older Americans.

National Institute on Alcohol Abuse and Alcoholism an institute of the NATIONAL INSTITUTES OF HEALTH that conducts research focused on improving the treatment and prevention of ALCOHOLISM and alcohol-related problems.

National Institute on Deafness and Other Communication Disorders an institute of the NATIONAL INSTITUTES OF HEALTH that conducts and supports biomedical research and research training on normal mechanisms as well as diseases and disorders of HEARING, BALANCE, SMELL, TASTE, VOICE, SPEECH, and LANGUAGE.

National Institute on Drug Abuse (NIDA) an institute of the NATIONAL INSTITUTES OF HEALTH that seeks to bring the power of science to bear on DRUG ABUSE and addiction through support and conduct of research across a broad range of disciplines, with rapid and effective dissemination of results of the research.

National Institutes of Health (NIH) a health agency of the United States Public Health Service, composed of numerous different component institutes and centers, many of which are dedicated to medical research.

National League for Nursing (NLN) a national organization concerned with improving nursing education and nursing service at all levels. In 1952 three existing national organizations and four committees agreed to combine and form the NLN: the National League of Nursing Education (founded in 1893), National Organization

for Public Health Nursing (founded in 1912), Association of Collegiate Schools of Nursing (founded in 1933), Joint Committee on Practical Nurses and Auxiliary Workers in Nursing (founded in 1945), Joint Committee on Careers in Nursing (founded in 1948), National Committee for the Improvement of Nursing Services (founded in 1949), and the National Accrediting Service (founded in 1949). The focus of the League is to "foster the development of hospital, industrial, public health, and other organized nursing service and of nursing education through the coordinated action of nurses, allied professional groups, citizens, agencies, and schools to the end that the nursing needs of the people will be met."

The official publication of the National League for Nursing is *Nursing Perspectives on Community Health Care.* The national office is located at 350 Hudson St., New York, NY 10014, and its telephone number is 212-989-9393.

National League for Nursing Accrediting Commission (NLNAC) a corporation established in 2001 that is a wholly-owned subsidiary of the NATIONAL LEAGUE FOR NURSING and is responsible for accreditation of nursing education schools and programs in the United States.

National Library of Medicine (NLM) a library and information resource center that is part of the NATIONAL INSTITUTES OF HEALTH; it collects, organizes, and makes available biomedical science information to investigators, educators, and practitioners and carries out programs designed to strengthen medical library services in the United States. It publishes the INDEX MEDICUS, and its electronic databases include MEDLINE and MEDLINEplus.

National Practitioner Data Bank (NPDB) a computerized information system that contains a record of malpractice claims, privileges actions, and other disciplinary actions. It was created to ensure that incompetent health care professionals do not move from one state to another.

natremia (na-tre′me-ah) hypernatremia.

natriuresis (na″tre-u-re′sis) the excretion of SODIUM in the urine; see also salt WASTING and SALT-LOSING CRISIS (SYNDROME).

natriuretic (na″tre-u-ret′ik) 1. pertaining to natriuresis. 2. promoting NATRIURESIS. 3. an agent that so acts.

naturopath (na′chur-o-path″) a practitioner of naturopathy.

naturopathy (na″chur-op′ah-the) a drugless system of healing by the use of physical methods, such as light, air, or water.

N

nausea (naw′ze-ah) 1. an unpleasant sensation vaguely referred to the epigastrium and abdomen, with a tendency to vomit. Nausea may be a symptom of a variety of disorders, some minor and some more serious.

Nausea is usually felt when nerve endings in the stomach and other parts of the body are irritated. The irritated nerves send messages to the center in the brain that controls the vomiting reflex. When the nerve irritation becomes intense, vomiting results.

Nausea and vomiting may be set off by nerve signals from many other parts of the body besides the stomach. For example, intense pain in almost any part of the body can produce nausea. The reason is that the nausea-vomiting mechanism is part of the involuntary autonomic nervous system. Nausea can also be precipitated by strong emotions. 2. a NURSING DIAGNOSIS accepted by the North American Nursing Diagnosis Association, defined as an unpleasant, wavelike sensation in the back of the throat or epigastrium, or throughout the abdomen, that may or may not lead to VOMITING.

nauseant (naw′ze-ant) 1. inducing nausea. 2. an agent causing nausea.

nauseate (naw′ze-āt) to affect with nausea.

nauseous (naw′shus) pertaining to or producing nausea or disgust.

navel (na′vel) umbilicus.

navicular (nah-vik′u-lar) scaphoid.

Nb niobium.

NCBDDD National Center on Birth Defects and Developmental Disabilities.

NCCAM National Center for Complementary and Alternative Medicine, part of the NATIONAL INSTITUTES OF HEALTH.

NCCDPHP National Center for Chronic Disease Prevention and Health Promotion.

NCEH National Center for Environmental Health.

NCHS National Center for Health Statistics.

NCHSTP National Center for HIV, STD, and TB Prevention.

NCI National Cancer Institute.

nCi nanocurie.

NCID National Center for Infectious Diseases.

NCIPC National Center for Injury Prevention and Control.

NCLEX (en′kleks) [National Council Licensure Examination for Nurses] a standardized national examination designed to test the entry-level nursing competence of candidates for licensure as registered nurses and as practical/vocational nurses. The NCLEX is administered by the individual boards of nursing that are members of the NATIONAL COUNCIL OF STATE BOARDS OF NURSING, INC.

NCLEX CAT administration of NCLEX through computerized adaptive testing.

NCMHD National Center on Minority Health and Health Disparities.

NCRR National Center for Research Resources, part of the NATIONAL INSTITUTES OF HEALTH.

ND Doctor of Nursing; a doctoral level program that leads to an entry-level nursing degree. Individuals with an academic baccalaureate degree complete three years or so of professional education leading to a Doctor of Nursing degree as the first professional degree. Students may then choose to continue their graduate education by pursuing either the degree of Doctor of Nursing Science (D.N.Sc.), a Ph.D. in nursing, or a Doctor of Education (Ed.D.) in nursing.

Nd neodymium.

NDA National Dental Association.

NDHA National Dental Hygienists Association.

Nd:YAG neodymium:yttrium-aluminum-garnet; see under LASER.

Ne neon.

ne(o)- word element [Gr.], *new; recent.*

nearsightedness (nēr′sīt′ed-nes) myopia.

nearthrosis (ne″ahr-thro′sis) 1. pseudarthrosis. 2. an artificial joint used in total joint ARTHROPLASTY.

Nebcin (neb′sin) trademark for preparations of TOBRAMYCIN sulfate, an AMINOGLYCOSIDE ANTIBIOTIC.

nebula (neb′u-lah) 1. slight corneal opacity. 2. an oily preparation for use in a NEBULIZER.

nebulization (neb″u-lĭ-za′shun) 1. conversion into a spray; called also atomization. 2. treatment by a spray.

nebulizer (neb′u-līz″er) a device for dispensing liquid in a fine spray; types used include *jet* and *ultrasonic* nebulizers. Called also atomizer.

  small volume n. a pneumatically powered device used to aerosolize medications for delivery to patients.

  ultrasonic n. an electronic device that generates ultrasound waves that break up water into an aerosol mist.

  Venturi n. a type of nebulizer used in AEROSOL THERAPY. The pressure drop of gas flowing through the VENTURI MASK draws liquid from a capillary tube; as the liquid enters the gas stream it breaks up into a spray of small droplets.

Necator (ne-ka′tor) a genus of HOOKWORMS. *N. america′nus* is the New World or

American hookworm, a species widely distributed in the southern United States, the Caribbean, and Central and South America.

necatoriasis (ne-ka″to-ri′ah-sis) HOOKWORM DISEASE caused by species of *Necator*.

necessity (nĕ-ses′ĭ-te) something necessary or indispensable.

pharmaceutic n., pharmaceutical n. a substance having slight or no value therapeutically, but used in the preparation of various pharmaceuticals, including preservatives, solvents, ointment bases, and flavoring, coloring, diluting, emulsifying, and suspending agents.

neck (nek) 1. the constricted part connecting the head with the trunk of the body. 2. the constricted part of an organ or other structure; called also cervix and collum.

anatomic n. of humerus the constriction of the HUMERUS just below its proximal articular surface.

bladder n. a constricted portion of the urinary BLADDER where its inferolateral surfaces meet at the opening of the URETHRA.

n. of femur the heavy column of bone connecting the head of the FEMUR and the shaft.

Madelung's n. diffuse symmetrical lipomas of the neck.

n. of spermatozoon a short portion of the TAIL OF A SPERMATOZOON immediately posterior to the HEAD, aterior to the middle PIECE. See illustration at SPERMATOZOON.

surgical n. of humerus the constricted part of the HUMERUS just below the tuberosities.

n. of tooth the narrowed part of a tooth between the crown and the root; called also cervix dentis and collum dentis.

uterine n., n. of uterus cervix uteri.

webbed n. a thick skin fold on the side of the neck, from the mastoid region to the acromion. Called also pterygium colli.

wry n. torticollis.

necr(o)- word element [Gr.], *death.*

necrobiosis (nek″ro-bi-o′sis) the physiologic death of cells; a normal mechanism in the constant turnover of many cell populations. Called also bionecrosis. adj., **necrobiot′ic.**

n. lipoi′dica a dermatosis characterized by patchy degeneration of the elastic and connective tissue of the skin with degenerated collagen occurring in irregular patches, especially in the dermis, most often on the mid or lower shins; usually associated with diabetes.

necrocytosis (nek″ro-si-to′sis) death and decay of cells.

necrogenic (nek″ro-jen′ik) productive of necrosis or death.

necrogenous (nĕ-kroj′ĕ-nus) originating or arising from dead matter.

necrology (nĕ-krol′o-je, ne-krol′o-je) statistics or records of death. adj., **necrolog′ic.**

necrolysis (nĕ-krol′ĭ-sis) separation or exfoliation of necrotic tissue.

toxic epidermal n. an exfoliative skin disease in which erythema spreads rapidly over the body, followed by blisters much like those seen in a second degree burn. It may be caused by drug reactions, infections (viral, bacterial, or fungal), neoplastic disease, graft-versus-host reaction, and chemical exposure.

necrophagous (nĕ-krof′ah-gus) feeding upon dead flesh.

necrophilia (nek″ro-fil′e-ah) sexual attraction to or sexual contact with dead bodies.

necrophilic (nek″ro-fil′ik) 1. pertaining to necrophilia. 2. showing a preference for dead tissue; said of certain microorganisms.

necrophilous (nĕ-krof′ĭ-lus) necrophilic.

necrophobia (nek″ro-fo′be-ah) irrational fear of death or of dead bodies.

necropsy (nek′rop-se) autopsy.

necrose (nek′rōs) to become necrotic or to undergo necrosis.

necrosis (nĕ-kro′sis, ne-kro′sis) [Gr.] the morphological changes indicative of cell death caused by enzymatic degradation.

aseptic n. necrosis without infection or inflammation.

acute tubular n. acute RENAL FAILURE with mild to severe damage or necrosis of tubule cells, usually secondary to either NEPHROTOXICITY, ischemia after major surgery, trauma (see CRUSH SYNDROME), severe HYPOVOLEMIA, sepsis, or burns. See also *lower nephron nephrosis.*

Balser's fatty n. gangrenous pancreatitis with omental bursitis and disseminated patches of necrosis of fatty tissues.

bridging n. septa of confluent necrosis bridging adjacent central veins of hepatic lobules and portal triads characteristic of subacute hepatic necrosis.

caseous n. caseation (def. 2).

central n. necrosis affecting the central portion of an affected bone, cell, or lobule of the liver.

cheesy n. caseation (def. 2).

coagulation n. death of cells, the protoplasm of the cells becoming fixed and opaque by coagulation of the protein elements, the cellular outline persisting for a long time.

colliquative n. liquefactive necrosis.

fat n. necrosis in which fat is broken down into fatty acids and glycerol, usually occurring in subcutaneous tissue as a result of trauma.

liquefactive n. necrosis in which the necrotic material becomes softened and liquefied.

massive hepatic n. massive, usually fatal, necrosis of the liver, a rare complication of viral HEPATITIS (fulminant HEPATITIS) that may also result from exposure to HEPATOTOXINS or from drug hypersensitivity.

moist n. necrosis in which the dead tissue is wet and soft.

postpartum pituitary n. see POSTPARTUM PITUITARY NECROSIS.

selective myocardial cell n. myofibrillar degeneration.

subcutaneous fat n. of newborn a benign, self-limited disease affecting term newborns and young infants, characterized by circumscribed, indurated, nodular areas of fat necrosis. It is thought to be related to trauma on bony prominences during delivery, hypothermia, asphyxia, or maternal diabetes; it usually resolves spontaneously by 2 to 4 weeks with no scarring. Called also adiponecrosis neonatorum or subcutanea.

Zenker's n. hyaline DEGENERATION and necrosis of striated muscle; called also Zenker's degeneration.

necrospermia (nek″ro-sper′me-ah) a condition in which the spermatozoa of the semen are dead or motionless.

necrotizing (nek′ro-tīz″ing) causing necrosis.

n. enterocolitis (NEC) the development of necrotic patches in the intestine that interfere with digestion and absorption and can lead to a paralytic ileus, perforation, and peritonitis. The entire bowel may be affected, or the ischemic necrosis may be localized.

NEC is a serious condition that occurs most often in preterm and very immature neonates; it develops in about 5 per cent of all neonates in neonatal intensive care units. The exact cause of the condition is not known, but it is related to ischemia or poor perfusion of blood vessels in sections of the bowel. The ischemia is thought to occur when an earlier oxygen depletion in the heart and brain, as in anoxia or shock, causes blood to be shunted away from less vital organs such as the intestine.

Since the incidence of NEC is low in neonates who are breast-fed, it is likely that the necrotizing process is initiated by a response to the protein in cow's milk and the profuse multiplication of bacteria that thrive more readily in cow's milk than in breast milk. The gas-forming bacteria invade the damaged intestinal cells, causing them to rupture and producing *pneumatosis intestinalis,* that is, the presence of air in the submucosal or subserosal surfaces of the colon.

Abdominal x-rays will show a characteristic invasion of air in the intestinal wall. If perforation has occurred, the x-ray will reveal free air in the abdominal cavity. Nonspecific symptoms of NEC usually appear in the first week of life and may be overlooked when caregivers are preoccupied with more obvious life-threatening problems. Typically, the neonate exhibits lethargy, vomiting, distended abdomen, signs of intestinal bleeding, and absence of bowel sounds.

Once the condition is diagnosed, all oral feedings are stopped to rest the intestinal tract. Feeding must then be accomplished intravenously. Gastrointestinal decompression via nasogastric suction may be instituted to relieve distention, and antibiotics administered to limit secondary bacterial infection. Progressive deterioration or evidence of perforation are indications for surgery to remove the diseased portion of the bowel. If damage is extensive an ileostomy or colostomy may be necessary.

necrotomy (ně-krot′ah-me) 1. dissection of a dead body. 2. excision of a sequestrum.

necrotoxin (nek′ro-tok″sin) a toxin that kills tissue cells, such as one of the EXOTOXINS secreted by species of *Clostridium* or by *Staphylococcus aureus*

nedocromil (ned″o-kro′mil) a NONSTEROIDAL ANTIINFLAMMATORY DRUG administered by inhalation in the treatment of bronchial ASTHMA. It is also administered topically to the conjunctiva as the sodium salt in the treatment of allergic CONJUNCTIVITIS.

need (nēd) something that is required or necessary. Basic human needs are those things that are required for complete physical and mental well-being. Needs vary greatly in the degree to which they are necessary for survival. For this reason, they are often classified into a hierarchy according to their relative urgency. Those on lower levels must be met before attention can be paid to needs on higher levels. The most widely used classification is called *Maslow's hierarchy of needs,* devised by Abraham H. Maslow, shown in the accompanying figure.

Physiologic Needs. These are the needs that are essential for the maintenance of biological homeostasis and the survival of the individual and the species. They include needs for oxygen, water, food, elimination of

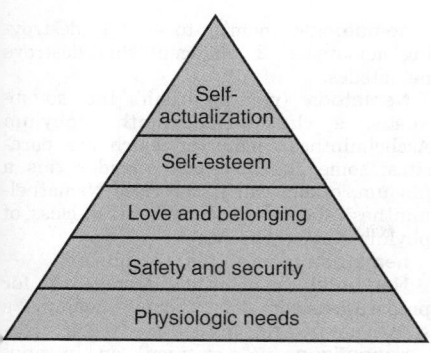

Maslow's hierarchy of needs.

wastes, temperature regulation, avoidance of pain, rest and sleep, exercise and sex.

Needs for Safety and Security. These include needs for protection from physical harm, for order, consistency, and familiarity in one's surroundings, and for some degree of control over matters concerning oneself.

Needs for Love and Belonging. These include needs for giving and receiving love and affection and for sexual intimacy, for friendship and companionship, and to identify with a group.

Needs for Esteem and Self-Esteem. These are the needs that are necessary for a person to have a basic sense of self-respect and self-acceptance and to be self-sufficient. Self-esteem requires an understanding of oneself and one's limitations and the ability to face and cope with stress and painful realities. Persons in whom these needs have been met are relatively free of feelings of inferiority or inadequacy. This level also includes needs for approval and recognition from others.

Need for Self-Actualization. This is the need to make full use of one's talents, capabilities, and potential. Self-actualizing persons tend to be dedicated, realistic, autonomous, creative, and open. They are not in conflict with themselves and are motivated by their own values and goals.

needle (ne′d′l) a sharp instrument used for suturing, for puncturing, or for the guiding of ligatures.

aneurysm n. a blunt-pointed, curved needle with the eye at the point; used for passing ligatures around aneurysms or vessels.

aspirating n. a long, hollow needle for removing fluid from a cavity.

atraumatic n. an eyeless surgical needle with the suture attached to a hollow end.

biopsy n. a hollow needle with an inner needle that detaches tissue for biopsy and brings it to the surface of its lumen;

types include the Menghini and Silverman needles. See also needle BIOPSY.

cataract n. one used in removing a cataract.

discission n. a special form of cataract needle.

fine n. a very thin, highly flexible steel needle with a narrow inner core used to cannulate very small bile ducts to perform transhepatic cholangiography (fine needle transhepatic cholangiography).

Hagedorn's n. a form of flat suture needle.

hypodermic n. a hollow, sharp-pointed needle to be attached to a hypodermic syringe for injection of solutions.

knife n. a slender knife with a needle-like point, used in ophthalmic operations.

ligature n. a long-handled, slender steel needle having an eye in its curved end, used for passing a ligature underneath an artery.

Menghini n. a needle for liver biopsy, not requiring rotation to cut loose the tissue specimen.

Reverdin's n. a surgical needle with an eye that can be opened and closed by means of a slide.

scalp vein n. a short rigid needle with flexible wings on each side; used to infuse IV fluids for short periods of time, in patients with small veins or in children.

Silverman n. a biopsy needle for taking tissue specimens, consisting of an outer cannula and an inner split needle with a longitudinal groove in which tissue is retained when the needle is withdrawn.

skinny n. fine needle.

spatula n. a minute needle with a flat or slightly curved concave surface that does not cut or pierce.

stop n. one with a shoulder that prevents too deep penetration.

swaged n. a needle with no eye, having suture attached to a hollow end.

nefazodone (nĕ-fa′zo-dōn) an ANTIDEPRESSANT, used as the hydrochloride salt.

negativism (neg′ah-tĭ-vizm″) opposition to suggestion or advice; an attitude or behavior opposite to that appropriate to a specific situation. A tendency to do the opposite of what most people would do under similar circumstances, of what one is told to do, or of what physiologic needs would suggest; e.g., it is not uncommon in catatonic schizophrenia for the patient to feel compelled to lower his arms if asked to raise them or to clench his fists if asked to open his hands.

N

negativistic personality disorder passive-aggressive personality disorder.

negatron (neg'ah-tron) a negatively charged electron.

NegGram (neg'gram) trademark for preparations of NALIDIXIC ACID, a urinary tract antiseptic.

neglect (ně-glekt') disregard of or failure to perform some task or function.

unilateral n. 1. HEMIAPRAXIA with failure to pay attention to bodily grooming and stimuli on one side but not on the other, usually due to a lesion in the central nervous system, as after a STROKE. Called also selective inattention. 2. a NURSING DIAGNOSIS accepted by the North American Nursing Diagnosis Association, defined as a state in which there is a lack of awareness and attention to one side of the body.

negligence (neg'lĭ-jens) in law, the failure to do something that a reasonable person of ordinary prudence would do in a certain situation or the doing of something that such a person would not do. Negligence may provide the basis for a lawsuit when there is a legal duty, as the duty of a physician or nurse to provide reasonable care to patients and when the negligence results in damage to the patient.

NEI National Eye Institute.

Neisseria (ni-se're-ah) a genus of gram-negative, aerobic or facultatively anaerobic cocci, which are a part of the normal flora of the oropharynx, nasopharynx, and genitourinary tract. Pathogenic species include *N. gonorrhoe'ae,* the etiologic agent of GONORRHEA; *N. meningi'tidis,* a prominent cause of meningitis and the specific agent of meningococcal MENINGITIS; and *N. muco'sa,* which is found in the nasopharynx and occasionally causes PNEUMONIA.

Neisseriaceae (ni-se″re-a'se-e) a family of parasitic bacteria (order Eubacteriales).

neisserial (nīs-se're-al) of, relating to, or caused by *Neisseria.*

nelfinavir (nel-fin'ah-vir) an HIV protease INHIBITOR used as the mesylate salt in treatment of human immuno deficiency virus infection and ACQUIRED IMMUNODEFICIENCY SYNDROME; administered orally.

Nelson's syndrome (nel'sunz) the development of an ACTH-producing pituitary tumor after bilateral adrenalectomy in Cushing's syndrome; it is characterized by aggressive growth of the tumor and hyperpigmentation of the skin.

Nemathelminthes (nem″ah-thel-min'thēz) in some classifications, a phylum including the Acanthocephala and Nematoda.

nematocide (nem'ah-to-sīd″) 1. destroying nematodes. 2. an agent that destroys nematodes.

Nematoda (nem″ah-to'dah) the ROUNDWORMS, a class of helminths (phylum Aschelminthes), many of which are parasites; some classifications consider this a phylum, others call it the class Nemathelminthes, and others consider it a class of phylum Nemathelminthes.

nematode (nem'ah-tōd) roundworm.

Nembutal (nem'bu-tal) trademark for preparations of PENTOBARBITAL sodium, a SEDATIVE, HYPNOTIC, and ANTICONVULSANT.

neoantigen (ne″o-an'tĭ-jen) an intranuclear antigen, e.g., a T antigen, present in cells infected by oncogenic viruses.

neoarthrosis (ne″o-ahr-thro'sis) nearthrosis.

neobladder (ne″o-blad'er) a continent urinary RESERVOIR made from a detubularized segment of bowel or stomach, with implantation of ureters and urethra; used to replace the bladder after cystectomy.

neoblastic (ne″o-blas'tik) originating in or of the nature of new tissue.

neocerebellum (ne″o-ser″ĕ-bel'um) phylogenetically, the newer parts of the cerebellum, consisting of those parts predominately supplied by corticopontocerebellar fibers.

neocortex (ne″o-kor'teks) the newer, six layered portion of the cerebral CORTEX showing stratification and organization characteristic of the most highly evolved type of cerebral tissue.

neodymium (Nd) (ne″o-dim'e-um) a chemical element, atomic number 60, atomic weight 144.24. (See Appendix 6.)

neogenesis (ne″o-jen'ĕ-sis) tissue regeneration. adj., **neogenet'ic.**

neoglottis (ne″o-glot'is) a glottis created by suturing the pharyngeal mucosa over the superior end of the transected trachea above the primary tracheostoma and making a permanent stoma in the mucosa; done to permit phonation after laryngectomy. adj., **neoglot'tic.**

neokinetic (ne″o-kĭ-net'ik) pertaining to the nervous motor mechanism regulating voluntary muscular control.

neologism (ne-ol'o-jizm) a newly coined word; in psychiatry, a word whose meaning may be known only to the patient using it; see also WORD SALAD.

neomembrane (ne″o-mem'brān) false membrane.

neomycin (ne″o-mi'sin) a broad-spectrum AMINOGLYCOSIDE antibiotic produced by *Streptomyces fradiae,* effective against a wide range of gram-negative bacilli and some gram-positive bacteria. It is used, as the sulfate salt, for urinary tract irrigation, administered orally to prepare the bowel for surgery, and applied to the skin, eyes, and ears to treat infections due to susceptible organisms. In topical preparations it is often combined with other antibiotics or anti-inflammatory steroids.

neon (Ne) (ne′on) a chemical element, atomic number 10, atomic weight 20.183. (See Appendix 6.)

neonatal (ne″o-na′tal) newborn (def. 1).

neonate (ne′o-nāt) newborn INFANT.

neonatologist (ne″o-na-tol′o-jist) a physi-cian who specializes in neonatology. Before becoming a board-certified neonatologist, one must be a pediatrician.

neonatology (ne″o-na-tol′o-je) the branch of health science dealing with disorders of the neonate; a subspecialty of pediatrics.

neopallium (ne″o-pal′le-um) neocortex.

neoplasia (ne″o-pla′zhah) the formation of a neoplasm.

> ***cervical intraepithelial n.* (CIN)** dyspla-sia of the cervical epithelium, often prema-lignant, characterized by various degrees of hyperplasia, abnormal keratinization, and the presence of condylomata.

> ***multiple endocrine n.* (MEN)** a group of rare hereditary disorders of autonomous hyperfunction of more than one endocrine gland. In *Type I* (MEN I), called also Wermer's syndrome, there are tumors of the pituitary, parathyroid gland, and pan-creatic islet cells in association with a high incidence of peptic ulcer. *Type II* (MEN II), called also Sipple's syndrome, is character-ized by medullary carcinoma of the thyroid, pheochromocytoma, often bilateral and mul-tiple, and parathyroid hyperplasia. *Type III* (MEN III), called also mucosal neuroma syndrome, resembles Type II except that parathyroid hyperplasia is rare, the mean survival time is shorter, and there may be neuromas and neurofibromas. All forms are transmitted as autosomal dominant traits.

neoplasm (ne′o-plazm) TUMOR; any new and abnormal growth, specifically one in which cell multiplication is uncontrolled and progressive. Neoplasms may be benign or malignant.

neoplastic (ne″o-plas′tik) pertaining to neoplasia or neoplasm.

Neosporin (ne″o-spor′in) trademark for combination preparations of NEOMYCIN sul-fate, POLYMYXIN B sulfate, and (in some preparations) either BACITRACIN zinc or GRAMICIDIN; an antibiotic.

neostigmine (ne″o-stig′mēn) an ANTI-CHOLINESTERASE and PROKINETIC agent used for the symptomatic treatment of MYASTHENIA GRAVIS, for prevention and treatment of postoperative stasis and atony of the

gastrointestinal tract or urinary bladder, and for reversal of the effects of certain neuromuscular blocking AGENTS, such as TUBOCURARINE, after surgery. Available as *neostigmine bromide* and *neostigmine methylsulfate.*

neostriatum (ne″o-stri-a′tum) the more recently developed part of the corpus striatum, comprising the caudate nucleus and the putamen.

neoteny (ne-ot′ĕ-ne) prolongation of the larval form in a sexually mature organism. adj., **neoten′ic.**

neothalamus (ne″o-thal′ah-mus) the part of the thalamus connected to the neopal-lium.

neovascularization (ne″o-vas″ku-lar-ĭ-za′-shun) 1. new blood vessel formation in abnormal tissue or in abnormal positions; see also ANGIOGENESIS. 2. revascularization.

nephelometer (nef′ĕ-lom′ĕ-ter) an instru-ment for measuring the concentration of substances in suspension by the amount of light that is scattered by the suspended particles.

nephelometry (nef″ĕ-lom′ĕ-tre) measure-ment of the concentration of a suspension by means of a nephelometer. adj., **nephelo-met′ric.**

nephr(o)- word element [Gr.], *kidney.*

nephralgia (nĕ-fral′jah) pain in a kidney.

nephrectasia (nef″rek-ta′zhah) distention of the kidney.

nephrectomy (nĕ-frek′to-me) surgical re-moval of a KIDNEY, a procedure indicated when chronic disease or severe injury produces irreparable damage to the renal cells. Tumors, multiple cysts, and congeni-tal anomalies may also necessitate removal of a kidney.

Patient Care. The surgical incision for nephrectomy can be lumbar, retroperito-neal, transabdominal, thoracic, or thoracic abdominal. Upon the patient's return from the operating room the location of the surgical wound is immediately noted, as well as whether there are any tubes or drains exiting the wound. If the thoracic cavity has been entered, the patient will have one or more chest tubes. There may also be surgical drains for removal of sero-sanguineous fluid from the operative site.

Dressings over the wound are checked frequently and may be reinforced to keep the patient dry, but they are not changed without a written prescription to do so. The drainage on the dressings will be blood-tinged at first but should gradually become clearer. Hemorrhage is a major complica-tion; hence, any appearance of bright red blood or a change in the amount of drainage is reported immediately. The kidney has a very rich supply of blood directly from the vena cava and aorta, so that if a ligature should slip, there could be substantial blood loss. The vital signs are therefore monitored closely and any signs of shock reported promptly. An intravenous line · should be kept open in the event a transfusion is needed.

Sometimes the drain will have a safety pin attached to its end. The pin is kept closed at all times and is never attached to the dressings, the patient's gown, or the bedclothes. When dressings are reinforced or changed, care must be taken that drains and tubes are not dislodged or pulled from the surgical incision. All tubes and drains are checked frequently to assure that they are patent and draining freely. The exception, of course, is a chest tube attached to a closed system.

Positioning of the patient will depend on the site of the incision and the preference of the physician. Some may prefer that the patient lie only on the affected side to facilitate drainage and protect the remaining kidney. Turning, coughing, and deep breathing will produce some discomfort because of the location of the incision. However, adequate aeration of the lungs is essential. One also should watch for spontaneous pneumothorax, which can occur if the thoracic cavity has been entered accidentally during surgery.

Adequate drainage from the unaffected kidney is of extreme importance. Urinary output is monitored hourly at first and then at longer intervals to be sure there is normal renal function. Fluids may be restricted immediately after surgery and gradually increased as the remaining kidney compensates for the loss of its partner. A single kidney can carry out the work of two kidneys; thus a patient can survive a nephrectomy in good health.

    radical n. removal of a kidney with its fascia, the adjacent adrenal gland, and all lymph nodes in the region; done for renal cell CARCINOMA.

  nephric (nef′rik) renal.

  nephritic (nĕ-frit′ik) pertaining to or affected with NEPHRITIS.

  nephritis (nĕ-fri′tis), pl. *nephri′tides* inflammation of the KIDNEY; a focal or diffuse proliferative or destructive disease that may involve the glomerulus, tubule, or interstitial renal tissue. Called also Bright's disease. The most usual form is GLOMERULO-NEPHRITIS, that is, inflammation of the glomeruli, which are clusters of renal capillaries. Damage to the membranes of the glomeruli results in impairment of the filtering process, so that blood and proteins such as albumin pass out into the urine. Depending on the symptoms it produces, nephritis is classified as acute nephritis, chronic nephritis, or NEPHROSIS (called also the nephrotic syndrome).

  Acute Nephritis. This occurs most frequently in children and young people and seems to strike those who have recently suffered from sore throat, scarlet fever, and other infections caused by streptococci; it is believed to originate as an IMMUNE RESPONSE on the part of the kidney. An attack may produce no symptoms, but more often there are headaches, a rundown feeling, back pain, and perhaps slight fever. The urine may look smoky, bloody, or wine-colored. Analysis of the urine shows the presence of erythrocytes, albumin, and casts. Another symptom is edema of the face or ankles, more common in the morning than in the evening. The blood pressure usually rises during acute nephritis, and in severe cases hypertension may be accompanied by convulsions.

Treatment consists chiefly of bed rest and a carefully controlled diet. Penicillin is often used if an earlier streptococcal infection is still lingering. Recovery is usually complete. In a small percentage of cases, however, acute nephritis resists complete cure. It may subside for a time and then become active again, or it may develop into chronic nephritis. Dialysis may be indicated in patients with fluid overload that is refractory to diuretics, or who become clinically uremic.

  Chronic Nephritis. Chronic nephritis may follow a case of acute nephritis immediately or it may develop after a long interval during which no symptoms have been present. Many cases of chronic nephritis occur in people who have never had the acute form of the disease. Symptoms are often unpredictable and variable from case to case, but there is almost always steady, progressive, permanent damage to the kidneys.

Chronic nephritis generally moves through three stages. In the first stage, the latent stage, there are few outward symptoms. There may be slight malaise, but often the only indication of the disease is the presence of albumin and other abnormal substances in the urine. If a blood count is made during this stage, anemia may be found. There is no special treatment during the latent stage of chronic nephritis. The patient can live a normal life but should avoid extremes of fatigue and exposure and should eat a well balanced diet.

The first stage may be followed by a second stage, in which edema occurs in the face, legs, or arms. The main treatment in this stage consists of a low-protein, low-sodium diet and diuretics. Steroid hormones may be helpful.

At the final stage of chronic nephritis is END-STAGE RENAL DISEASE. Treatments are kidney transplant and DIALYSIS. At any stage of chronic nephritis it is particularly important to avoid other infections, which will aggravate the condition.

There is no known cure for chronic nephritis, although the progress of the disease can be delayed, so that the patient can live an almost normal life for years. Many patients are being helped by repeated purification of their uremic blood by HEMODIALYSIS or PERITONEAL DIALYSIS, or by TRANSPLANTATION.

glomerular n. glomerulonephritis.

interstitial n. nephritis with increase of interstitial tissue and thickening of vessel walls and malpighian corpuscles; it may be due to overuse of analgesics, mercury poisoning, gout, or any of various other conditions.

lupus n. GLOMERULONEPHRITIS associated with systemic LUPUS ERYTHEMATOSUS.

potassium-losing n. see under *nephropathy*.

radiation n. kidney damage caused by ionizing radiation; symptoms include glomerular and tubular damage, hypertension, and proteinuria, sometimes leading to RENAL FAILURE. It may be acute or chronic, and some varieties do not manifest until years after the radiation exposure.

salt-losing n. salt-losing nephropathy.

transfusion n. nephropathy following transfusion from an incompatible donor as a result of the hemoglobin of the hemolyzed red blood cells being deposited in the renal tubules.

tubulointerstitial n. nephritis of the renal TUBULES and interstitial tissues, usually seen secondary to a drug sensitization, systemic infection, graft rejection, or AUTOIMMUNE DISEASE. Characteristics include lymphocytes in interstitial infiltrate and within tubules, mild hematuria, and pyuria. *Acute tubulointerstitial nephritis* is usually seen as a complication of infection or allergy. *Chronic tubulointerstitial nephritis* is when the condition has progressed to interstitial fibrosis with shrunken kidneys, a lowered glomerular filtration RATE, and danger of RENAL FAILURE.

nephritogenic (nĕ-frit″o-jen′ik) causing nephritis.

nephroblastoma (nef″ro-blas-to′mah) Wilms' tumor.

nephrocalcinosis (nef″ro-kal″sĭ-no′sis) deposition of calcium phosphate in the renal tubules, resulting in renal insufficiency.

nephrocardiac (nef″ro-kahr′de-ak) cardiorenal.

nephrocele (nef′ro-sēl) hernia of a kidney.

nephrocolic (nef″ro-kol′ik) pertaining to or connecting the kidney and colon, such as a FISTULA.

nephrocoloptosis (nef″ro-ko″lop-to′sis) downward displacement of the kidney and colon.

nephrocystitis (nef″ro-sis-ti′tis) inflammation of the kidney and bladder.

nephrogenic (nef″ro-jen′ik) producing kidney tissue.

nephrogenous (nĕ-froj′ĕ-nus) arising in a kidney.

nephrogram (nef′ro-gram) a radiograph of the kidney.

nephrography (nĕ-frog′rah-fe) radiography of the kidney; see also PYELOGRAPHY.

nephroid (nef′roid) resembling a kidney.

nephrolith (nef′ro-lith) kidney stone.

nephrolithiasis (nef″ro-lĭ-thi′ah-sis) 1. the formation of KIDNEY STONES. 2. a condition marked by the presence of KIDNEY STONES.

nephrolithotomy (nef″ro-lĭ-thot′ah-me) incision of kidney for removal of KIDNEY STONES.

nephrology (nĕ-frol′o-je) the branch of medicine dealing with the kidneys.

nephrolysin (nĕ-frol′ĭ-sin) 1. nephrotoxin. 2. an antibody that causes destruction of kidney cells.

nephrolysis (nĕ-frol′ĭ-sis) 1. freeing of a kidney from adhesions. 2. destruction of kidney substance. adj., **nephrolyt′ic.**

nephroma (nĕ-fro′mah) a tumor of kidney tissue.

nephromegaly (nef″ro-meg′ah-le) enlargement of the kidney.

nephron (nef′ron) the structural and functional unit of the KIDNEY, each nephron being capable of forming urine by itself. The nephron consists of the renal corpuscle, the proximal convoluted tubule, the descending and ascending limbs of the loop of Henle, the distal convoluted tubule, and the collecting tubule. Each kidney is an aggregation of about a million nephrons. The specific function of the nephron is to remove from the blood plasma certain end products of metabolism, such as urea, uric acid, and creatinine, and also any excess sodium, chloride, and potassium ions. By allowing for reabsorption of water and some electrolytes back into the blood, the nephron also plays a vital role in the

N

maintenance of normal fluid balance in the body.

The nephron is a complex system of arterioles, capillaries, and tubules. Blood is brought to the nephron via the afferent arteriole. As the blood flows through the glomerulus (a network of capillaries), about one-fifth of the plasma is filtered through the glomerular membrane and collects in the malpighian (Bowman's) capsule, which encases the glomerulus. The fluid then passes through the proximal tubule, from there into the loop of Henle, then into the distal tubule, and finally into the collecting tubule. As the fluid is making its tortuous journey through these various tubules, most of its water and some of the solutes are reabsorbed into the blood via the peritubular capillaries. The water and solutes remaining in the tubules become urine.

nephronophthisis   (nef″ron-of-thĭ-sis) wasting disease of the kidney substance.

familial juvenile n. a progressive hereditary kidney disease marked by anemia, polyuria, renal loss of sodium, progressing to chronic renal failure, tubular atrophy, interstitial fibrosis, glomerular sclerosis, and medullary cysts.

nephropathy (nĕ-frop'ah-the) 1. any disease of the kidneys. adj., **nephropath'ic.** 2. any disease of the kidneys; see also NEPHRITIS. Called also nephrosis. adj., **nephropath'ic.**

AIDS n. former name for HIV-associated NEPHROPATHY.

analgesic n. interstitial nephritis with renal papillary necrosis, seen in patients with a history of abuse of analgesics such as aspirin or acetaminophen alone or in combination.

diabetic n. the nephropathy that commonly accompanies later stages of DIABETES MELLITUS; it begins with hyperfiltration, renal hypertrophy, microalbuminuria, and hypertension; in time proteinuria develops, with other signs of decreasing function leading to END-STAGE RENAL DISEASE.

gouty n. any of a group of chronic kidney diseases associated with the abnormal production and excretion of URIC ACID.

heavy metal n. the kidney damage resulting from any of various forms of heavy metal poisoning, usually in the form of tubulointerstitial nephritis. The most common metals involved are CADMIUM, LEAD, and MERCURY.

HIV-associated n. renal pathology in patients infected with the human immunodeficiency VIRUS, similar to focal segmental GLOMERULOSCLEROSIS, with proteinuria, enlarged kidneys, and dilated tubules

containing proteinaceous casts; it may progress to END-STAGE RENAL DISEASE within weeks.

hypokalemic n. nephropathy with HYPOKALEMIA, interstitial NEPHRITIS, swelling and vacuolization of proximal renal TUBULES, and progressive RENAL FAILURE, resulting from conditions such as oncotic overloading of the kidney filtration mechanisms by sugars. See also potassium-losing nephropathy.

IgA n. a chronic form marked by hematuria and proteinuria and by deposits of IgA immunoglobulin in the mesangial areas of the renal glomeruli, with subsequent reactive hyperplasia of mesangial cells. Called also Berger's disease and IgA glomerulonephritis.

ischemic n. nephropathy resulting from partial or complete obstruction of a renal artery with ISCHEMIA, accompanied by a significant reduction in the glomerular filtration RATE.

lead n. the kidney damage that accompanies LEAD POISONING; lead deposits appear in the epithelium of the proximal tubules and as nuclear inclusions in cells. In time this leads to tubulointerstitial nephritis with chronic renal failure and other symptoms.

membranous n. membranous glomerulonephritis.

minimal change n. minimal change disease.

obstructive n. nephropathy caused by obstruction of the urinary tract (usually the ureter), with HYDRONEPHROSIS, slowing of the glomerular filtration RATE, and tubular abnormalities.

potassium-losing n. hypokalemic nephropathy after persistent potassium loss; it may be seen in metabolic alkalosis, adrenocortical hormone excess, or in intrinsic renal disease such as renal tubular acidosis or hyperplasia of juxtaglomerular cells. Called also potassium-losing nephritis.

reflux n. childhood PYELONEPHRITIS in which the renal scarring results from vesicoureteric REFLUX, with radiological appearance of intrarenal REFLUX.

salt-losing n. intrinsic renal disease causing abnormal urinary sodium loss in persons ingesting normal amounts of sodium chloride, with vomiting, dehydration, and vascular collapse. Called also salt-losing nephritis.

urate n., uric acid n. any of a group of kidney diseases occurring in patients with HYPERURICEMIA, including an acute form, a chronic form (gouty NEPHROPATHY), and NEPHROLITHIASIS with formation of uric acid CALCULI.

nephropexy (nef'ro-pek"se) surgical fixation of a floating or hypermobile kidney NEPHROPTOSIS). The care of a patient having his type of surgery is generally the same as that for any type of surgery of the kidney. One important point is that after nephropexy the patient is positioned so that the chest is lower than the hips; this position relieves strain on the sutures and helps to maintain the kidney in a normal position.

nephroptosis (nef'rop-to'sis) downward displacement of a kidney, usually found in young adult women, especially those who are thin and long-waisted; it can occur when kidney supports are weakened by a sudden strain or blow, or are congenitally defective. Although it may not produce serious symptoms, if there is kinking of the ureters, this could cause an obstruction to their urinary flow, and some patients also have increased susceptibility to infection. Treatment is usually by NEPHROPEXY (surgical fixation). Called also floating, hypermobile, or wandering kidney.

nephropyelitis (nef"ro-pi"ĕ-li'tis) pyelonephritis.

nephropyelography (nef"ro-pi"ĕ-log'rah-e) radiography of the kidney and renal pelvis; see also PYELOGRAPHY.

nephropyosis (nef"ro-pi-o'sis) pyonephrosis.

nephrorrhagia (nef"ro-ra'jah) hemorrhage from the kidney.

nephrorrhaphy (nef-ror'ah-fe) suture of the kidney.

nephrosclerosis (nef"ro-sklĕ-ro'sis) hardening of the kidney, usually associated with hypertension and disease of the renal arterioles. It is characterized as benign or malignant depending on the severity and rapidity of the hypertension and arteriolar changes.

 arteriolar n. that involving chiefly the arterioles, with degeneration of the renal tubules and fibrotic thickening of the glomeruli; it has an insidious onset and is characterized by cylindruria, edema, hypertrophy of the heart, degeneration of the renal tubules, and GLOMERULONEPHRITIS. Types include benign and malignant arteriolar nephrosclerosis.

 benign n., benign arteriolar n. arteriolar nephrosclerosis usually seen in patients over 60 years old and associated with benign HYPERTENSION and hyaline ARTERIOLOSCLEROSIS. In younger persons, it may occur in diabetics with a predisposition to arteriolosclerosis and in those who have hypertension resulting from an apparent underlying disease, such as pheochromocytoma.

 hypertensive n. the most common kind of arteriolar nephrosclerosis, due to hypertension of the renal arterioles.

 malignant n., malignant arteriolar n. an uncommon form of arteriolar nephrosclerosis affecting all the vessels of the body, especially the small arteries and arterioles of the kidneys, and frequently associated with malignant HYPERTENSION and hyperplastic ARTERIOLOSCLEROSIS. Renal changes include arteriolar necrosis with red blood cells and casts in the urine. It may occur in the absence of previous history of hypertension, or may be superimposed on benign hypertension or primary renal disease, especially glomerulonephritis, benign nephrosclerosis, and pyelonephritis.

nephroscope (nef'ro-skōp) an instrument inserted into an incision in the renal pelvis for viewing the inside of the kidney, equipped with three channels for telescope, fiberoptic light input, and irrigation.

nephroscopy (nĕ-fros'kah-pe) visualization of the kidney by means of the nephroscope.

nephrosis (nĕ-fro'sis) 1. nephropathy. 2. any kidney disease, especially one marked by purely degenerative lesions of the renal TUBULES. adj., **nephrot'ic.** Often the cause is not known. When a viral infection precedes the symptoms, it is probably a precipitating rather than a causative factor. There may be not one but several pathologic processes involved, all of which affect the glomerular membranes, increasing their permeability to protein.

The loss of proteins, especially ALBUMIN, by leakage from the capillaries into the urine, produces a shift of fluids from the intravascular fluid compartment into the interstitial spaces. The result is EDEMA and HYPOVOLEMIA, which stimulates tubular reabsorption of SODIUM and water to increase intravascular volume. These pathologic processes and others that are less well understood bring about the group of symptoms known as the NEPHROTIC SYNDROME.

The first sign noted is usually swelling about the eyes on rising in the morning that subsides during the day. As edema worsens there is a gradual weight gain, which parents may mistake for healthy growth. The fluid shift progresses and eventually causes abdominal swelling from ascites, respiratory difficulty from pleural effusion, and generalized edema. ANASARCA (severe generalized swelling) sometimes occurs in association with an acute infection. Intestinal edema can cause diarrhea and anorexia.

N

There is also a diminished output of urine, which is dark and frothy.

Diagnosis and Treatment. Laboratory analyses of urine and blood reveal proteinuria, elevated specific gravity of the urine, decreased serum proteins, and elevated serum cholesterol levels. Renal biopsy and the appearance of renal tissue under microscopic examination can establish the diagnosis and identify the type of nephrotic syndrome present.

Treatment includes rest during the edema phase, management of fluid balance, and administration of CORTICOSTEROIDS such as PREDNISONE. Corticosteroid therapy is gradually decreased until the urine is free of proteins and edema subsides. About 80 per cent of children with nephrosis have a favorable prognosis. Cases resistant to this therapy may be given an IMMUNOSUPPRESSANT such as CYTOXAN, which is alternated with prednisone every other day.

Patient Care. The acutely ill child is hospitalized for diagnostic testing and placed on bed rest until there is remission of symptoms. In the presence of massive edema, sodium is restricted but water usually is not. While on bed rest the child will need diligent skin care to prevent breakdown of the skin over edematous tissues. Measures are taken to avoid respiratory infections to which these children are especially susceptible.

Monitoring includes measurement of vital signs, daily weight, fluid intake and output, and abdominal girth. The progress of edema is assessed daily or more often as indicated. Once the swelling subsides the child usually is less lethargic and should be ready and eager to resume usual activities.

In preparation for discharge the parents are taught how to test urine for albumin, the purpose and untoward side effects of prescribed medications, signs of relapse, and the techniques and importance of avoiding infection. Referral to a home health care nurse or visiting nurse may be appropriate if the parents have a need for continued support and guidance.

amyloid n. chronic nephrosis with amyloid degeneration of the median coat of the arteries and glomerular capillaries.

lipid n., lipoid n. minimal change disease.

lower nephron n. renal insufficiency leading to uremia, due to necrosis of the lower nephron cells that blocks the tubular lumens of this region; seen after severe injuries, especially crushing injury to muscles. See also CRUSH SYNDROME.

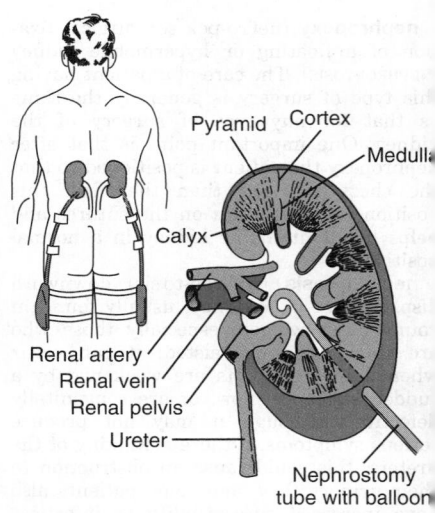

Positioning of a percutaneous nephrostomy tube. From Bolander, 1994.

nephrosonephritis (nĕ-fro″so-nĕ-fri′tis) renal disease with nephrotic and nephritic components.

nephrostolithotomy (nĕfros″to-lĭ-thot′ah me) removal of KIDNEY STONES through a NEPHROSTOMY tube inserted through th abdominal wall into the renal pelvis.

nephrostoma (nĕ-fros′to-mah) one o the ciliated funnel-shaped orifices of th excretory tubules that open into the coelon in the embryo; best seen in lower verte brates.

nephrostomy (nĕ-fros′tah-me) creatio of a permanent opening into the rena PELVIS.

percutaneous n. insertion of a cathe ter through the skin and into the rena pelvis under the guidance of fluorography o ultrasonography; performed for relief o obstruction and to gain access to the uppe urinary tract for a variety of procedures such as dilation of strictures or removal o calculi.

nephrotic syndrome (nĕ-frot′ik) any o several conditions marked by massive edema, heavy proteinuria, hypoalbumin emia, and unusual susceptibility to inter current infections. See also NEPHROSIS.

nephrotome (nef′ro-tōm) one of th segmented divisions of the embryoni mesoderm connecting the somite with th lateral plates of unsegmented mesoderm the source of much of the urogenital system

nephrotomogram (nef′ro-to′mo-gram) tomogram of the kidney obtained b nephrotomography.

nephrotomography (nef″ro-to-mog′rah-fe) radiologic visualization of the kidney by TOMOGRAPHY after introduction of a contrast medium. adj., **nephrotomograph′ic.**

nephrotomy (ně-frot′ah-me) incision of a kidney.

nephrotoxic (nef′ro-tok″sik) pertaining to or characterized by NEPHROTOXICITY.

nephrotoxicity the quality of being destructive to KIDNEY cells.

nephrotoxin (nef′ro-tok″sin) a toxin having a specific destructive effect on kidney tissue.

nephrotropic (nef′ro-trop′ik) having a special affinity for kidney tissue.

nephrotuberculosis (nef″ro-too-ber″ku-lo′sis) renal tuberculosis.

neptunium (Np) (nep-too′ne-um) a chemical element, atomic number 93, atomic weight 237. (See Appendix 3.)

nerve (nerv) a macroscopic cordlike structure of the body, comprising a collection of nerve FIBERS that convey impulses between a part of the central NERVOUS SYSTEM and some other body region. See Appendix 2-6 and see color plates.

Depending on their function, nerves are known as *sensory, motor,* or *mixed.* Sensory nerves, sometimes called *afferent nerves,* carry information from the outside world, such as sensations of heat, cold, and pain, to the brain and spinal cord. Motor nerves, or *efferent nerves,* transmit impulses from the brain and spinal cord to the muscles. Mixed nerves are composed of both motor and sensory fibers, and transmit messages in both directions at once.

Together, the nerves make up the peripheral nervous system, as distinguished from the central nervous system (brain and spinal cord). There are 12 pairs of CRANIAL NERVES, which carry messages to and from the brain. *Spinal nerves* arise from the spinal cord and pass out between the vertebrae; there are 31 pairs, 8 cervical, 12 thoracic, 5 lumbar, 5 sacral, and 1 coccygeal. The various nerve fibers and cells that make up the autonomic nervous system innervate the glands, heart, blood vessels, and involuntary muscles of the internal organs.

accelerator *n's* the cardiac sympathetic nerves, which, when stimulated, accelerate the action of the heart.

acoustic *n.* VESTIBULOCOCHLEAR NERVE; see anatomic Table of Nerves in the Appendices.

afferent *n.* any nerve that transmits impulses from the periphery toward the central nervous system, such as a sensory nerve. See also NEURON.

articular *n.* any mixed peripheral nerve that supplies a joint and its associated structures.

auditory *n.* VESTIBULOCOCHLEAR NERVE; see anatomic Table of Nerves in the Appendices.

autonomic *n.* any nerve of the AUTONOMIC NERVOUS SYSTEM; called also visceral nerve.

cranial *n's* see CRANIAL NERVES.

cutaneous *n.* any mixed peripheral nerve that supplies a region of the skin. See anatomic Table of Nerves in the Appendices.

depressor *n.* 1. a nerve that lessens the activity of an organ. 2. an afferent nerve whose stimulation causes a fall in blood pressure.

efferent *n.* any nerve that carries impulses from the central nervous system toward the periphery, such as a motor nerve. See also NEURON.

excitor *n.* one that transmits impulses resulting in an increase in functional activity.

excitoreflex *n.* a visceral nerve that produces reflex action.

fusimotor *n's* those that innervate the intrafusal fibers of the muscle spindle.

gangliated *n.* any nerve of the sympathetic nervous system.

inhibitory *n.* one that transmits impulses resulting in a decrease in functional activity.

medullated *n.* myelinated nerve.

mixed *n., n.* of mixed fibers a nerve composed of both sensory (afferent) and motor (efferent) fibers.

motor *n.* a peripheral efferent nerve that stimulates muscle contraction.

myelinated *n.* one whose axons are encased in a myelin sheath; called also medullated nerve.

peripheral *n.* any nerve outside the central nervous system.

pilomotor *n's* those that supply the arrector muscles of hair.

pressor *n.* an afferent nerve whose irritation stimulates a vasomotor center and increases intravascular tension.

sciatic *n.* see SCIATIC NERVE.

secretory *n.* an efferent nerve whose stimulation increases vascular activity.

sensory *n.* a peripheral nerve that conducts impulses from a sense organ to the spinal cord or brain. See also NEURON.

somatic *n's* the sensory and motor nerves supplying skeletal muscle and somatic tissues.

spinal *n's* the 31 pairs of nerves arising from the spinal cord and passing out

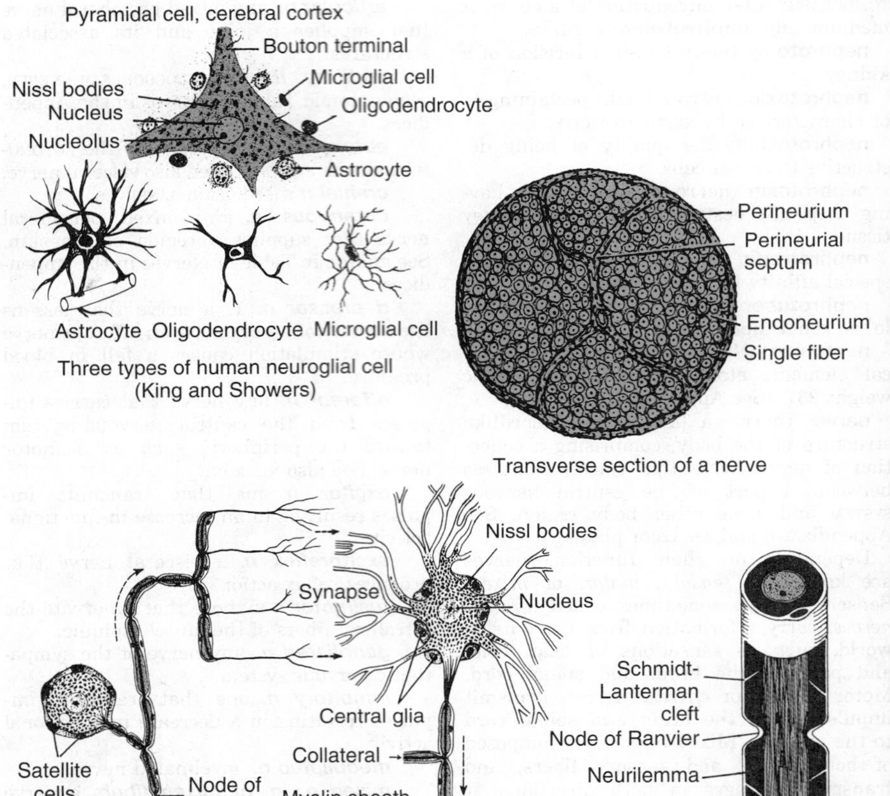

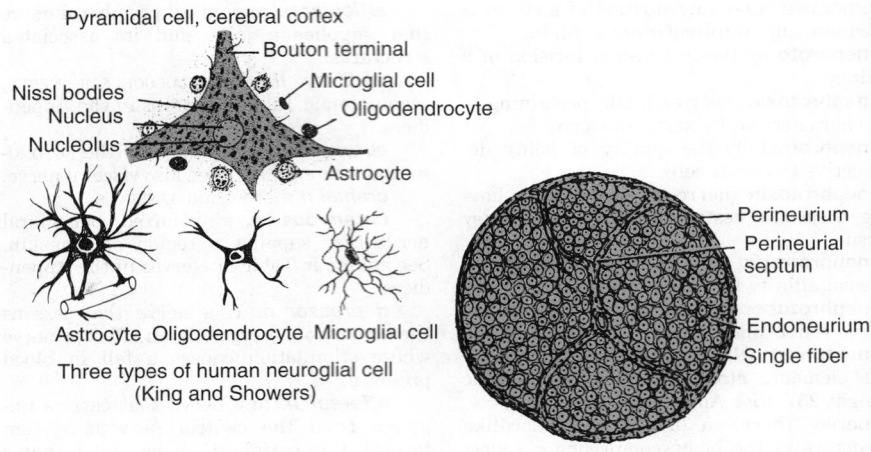

Pyramidal cell, cerebral cortex
Bouton terminal
Nissl bodies
Microglial cell
Nucleus
Oligodendrocyte
Nucleolus
Astrocyte

Astrocyte Oligodendrocyte Microglial cell

Three types of human neuroglial cell
(King and Showers)

Perineurium
Perineurial septum
Endoneurium
Single fiber

Transverse section of a nerve

Nissl bodies
Synapse
Nucleus

Central glia
Collateral →
Satellite cells
Node of Ranvier
Myelin sheath
Axon
Neurolemma
Free nerve ending
Skin
Motor end plate
Muscle

Schmidt-Lanterman cleft
Node of Ranvier
Neurilemma
Nucleus of neurilemmal cell
Mitochondria
Axon (composed of fibrils)
Myelin (here dissolved, above blackened by fixation)

Longitudinal section of a nerve fiber
(Leeson and Leeson)

SENSORY NEURON   MOTOR NEURON

Diagrammatic representation of two types of neurons
(King and Showers)

Details of structure of components of nerve tissue.

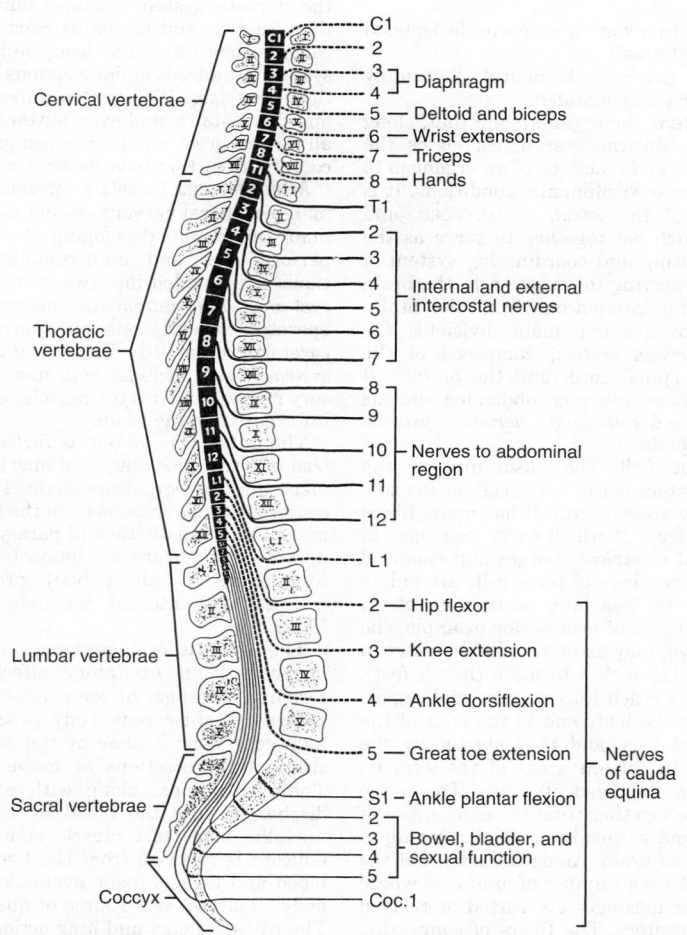

C1
2
3 ⎱ Diaphragm
4 ⎰
5 — Deltoid and biceps
6 — Wrist extensors
7 — Triceps
8 — Hands
T1
2
3
4
5 Internal and external
6 intercostal nerves
7
8
9
10 ⎱ Nerves to abdominal
11 ⎰ region
12
L1
2 — Hip flexor
3 — Knee extension
4 — Ankle dorsiflexion
5 — Great toe extension
S1 — Ankle plantar flexion
2
3 ⎱ Bowel, bladder, and
4 ⎰ sexual function
5
Coc.1

Cervical vertebrae

Thoracic vertebrae

Lumbar vertebrae

Sacral vertebrae

Coccyx

Nerves of cauda equina

Spinal nerves emerging from the spinal cord through the intervertebral foramina with muscles or muscle movements listed for specific levels. From McQuillan et al., 2002.

through the vertebrae; there are eight cervical, twelve thoracic, five lumbar, five sacral, and one coccygeal. See accompanying illustration, and see anatomic Table of Nerves in the Appendices.

splanchnic n's those of the blood vessels and viscera, especially the visceral branches of the thoracic, abdominal (lumbar), and pelvic parts of the sympathetic trunks. See Appendix 3-5.

sudomotor n's those that innervate the sweat glands.

sympathetic n's 1. see sympathetic TRUNK. 2. any nerve of the sympathetic nervous system.

trophic n. one concerned with regulation of nutrition.

unmyelinated n. one whose axons are not encased in a myelin sheath.

vasoconstrictor n. one whose stimulation causes contraction of blood vessels.

vasodilator n. one whose stimulation causes dilation of blood vessels.

vasomotor n. one concerned in controlling the caliber of vessels, whether as a vasoconstrictor or vasodilator.

vasosensory n. any nerve supplying sensory fibers to the vessels.

visceral n. autonomic nerve.

nervimotor (ner″vĭ-mo′tor) pertaining to a motor nerve.

nervone (ner′vōn) a cerebroside isolated from nerve tissue.

nervous (ner′vus) 1. neural. 2. unduly excitable or easily agitated.

n. system the organ system that, along with the endocrine SYSTEM, correlates the adjustments and reactions of an organism to internal and environmental conditions. It is composed of the BRAIN, SPINAL CORD, and NERVES, which act together to serve as the communicating and coordinating system of the body, carrying information to the brain and relaying instructions from the brain. The system has two main divisions: the *central nervous system,* composed of the brain and spinal cord; and the *peripheral nervous system,* which is subdivided into the *voluntary* and *autonomic nervous systems.* (See color plates.)

The Nerve Cell. The basic unit of the nervous system is the nerve cell, or NEURON. This highly specialized cell has many fibers extending from it which carry messages in the form of electrical charges and chemical changes. The fibers of some cells are only a centimeter or less long (a fraction of an inch), but those of others (for example, the sciatic nerve) may extend for half a meter to one meter (18 inches to more than 3 feet). These fibers reach into muscles and organs throughout the body and to the ends of the fingers and toes, and they cluster by the thousands in certain areas of the skin no larger than the head of a pin. The nerve fibers come together from the extremities of the body and gather into cables running to and from the brain. Along the length of the spinal cord are a number of junctions where impulses or messages are sorted or relayed to higher centers. The fibers of connecting nerve cells do not touch each other. Impulses are relayed from one to another by chemical means across the gap or synapse between them. In most cases an impulse must cross more than one synapse to cause the desired action.

In a REFLEX, the impulse is relayed from one nerve to another by a shortcut that produces a reaction without involving the brain. The KNEE JERK is an example of the simplest sort of reflex reaction. When the knee is tapped, the impulse travels through the sensory nerve that receives the tap, crosses a single synapse, and activates the motor nerve that controls the quadriceps muscle in the thigh, causing the leg to jerk up automatically.

A very different sort of reflex is the *conditioned reflex.* CONDITIONING is the process of building links or paths in the nervous system. When an action is done repeatedly the nervous system becomes familiar with the situation and learns to react automatically. A new reflex has been built into the system. Hundreds of daily actions are conditioned reflexes. Walking, running, going up and down stairs, and even buttoning a shirt all involve great numbers of complex muscle coordinations that have become automatic.

Autonomic and Voluntary Systems. The human peripheral nervous system evolved over many millennia, developing the ability to perform more and more complicated functions. It is divided into two specialized subsystems. The *autonomic nervous system* operates without conscious control as the caretaker of the body. The *voluntary nervous system,* which includes both motor and sensory nerves, controls the muscles and carries information to the brain.

The autonomic system is further specialized into two subsidiary systems: the *sympathetic* and the *parasympathetic.* The control centers of these systems lie in the hypothalamus. The sympathetic and parasympathetic nervous systems are continuously operative, functioning to adjust body processes to external and internal demands. (See also Plates.)

The sympathetic nervous system has in general an excitatory effect, and in response to danger or some other challenge, almost instantly puts body processes into high gear. This is done by the discharge of stimulating secretions at nerve junctions. These secretions, along with epinephrine discharged into the blood by the adrenal medulla, help start muscle action quickly. Glucose is released from the liver into the blood and thus is made available to all the body's muscles as a source of quick energy. The rates of heart and lung action increase, digestive activity slows down, blood vessels constrict, and sweating begins so that the body will be kept cool while under stress. Thus the body is prepared for an extraordinary effort.

The parasympathetic nervous system prevents body processes from accelerating to extremes. Acting more slowly than the sympathetic system, it causes the discharge of secretions that slow the heartbeat and lung action, restore digestive functioning, and limit the constriction of the blood vessels. Generally it acts as a damper, so that unless the challenge demands a prolonged effort, body processes will begin returning to normal.

The *voluntary nervous system* has nerves of two kinds, sensory and motor. The sensory nerves bring messages to the brain from all parts of the body. They are sorted in the spinal cord and sent on to the brain to be analyzed, acted upon, associated with other information and stored as MEMORY. Messages from the brain, often in response to information received by way of the sensory nerves, are delivered to the muscles by the motor nerves. One motor nerve with its branching fibers may control thousands of muscle fibers.

The different parts of the nervous system are constantly interacting, and are so well coordinated that humans can think, feel, and act on many different levels and without serious confusion, all at the same time. (See also NEUROLOGIC ASSESSMENT.)

nervousness (ner'vus-nes) a state of excitability, with great mental and physical unrest.

nervus (ner'vus) [L.] nerve (see also anatomic Table of Nerves in the Appendices).

nesidiectomy (ně-sid″e-ek'to-me) excision of the pancreatic islets.

nesidioblast (ně-sid'e-o-blast″) any of the cells giving rise to islet cells of the pancreas.

netilmicin (net″il-mi'sin) a semisynthetic aminoglycoside antibiotic having a wide range of activity; used as the sulfate salt in the treatment of infection caused by susceptible gram-negative organisms.

network (net'werk) 1. a meshlike structure of interlocking fibers, strands, or tubules. See also PLEXUS and RETE. 2. a group of people who have a connectedness; connectedness may be close-knit, with many relationships between the individuals, or loose-knit, with few relationships between individuals. Networks are classified as strong (marked by interdependence on a relatively small number of people) or as weak (marked by little interdependence and a wide range of diverse and superficial contacts).

venous n. rete venosum.

Neuman (noo'man) Betty. Nursing educator and developer of NEUMAN'S SYSTEMS MODEL for nursing. Her conceptual model was first presented in a 1972 article entitled *A Model for Teaching Total Person Approach to Patient Problems* and has since been further refined.

Neuman's systems model a CONCEPTUAL MODEL of nursing, formulated by Betty NEUMAN, concerned with variances from wellness, the presence of stressors, and the need of the client system to attain and maintain stability.

Neupogen (noo'po-jen) trademark for a preparation of filgrastim, a granulocyte colony-stimulating FACTOR that stimulates HEMATOPOIESIS and decreases NEUTROPENIA.

neur(o)- word element [Gr.], *nerve.*

neurad (noor'ad) toward the neural axis or aspect.

neural (noor'al) pertaining to a NERVE or to the nerves; called also nervous.

n. tube defect a congenital defect in closure of the bony encasement of the spinal cord or of the skull. The most severe defects are a fissure along the entire length of the spinal column that leaves the meninges and spinal cord exposed (RACHISCHISIS), or herniation through the skull of a saclike structure containing brain tissue and meninges (ENCEPHALOCELE). ANENCEPHALY is a major defect in which the brain is absent and there is only an exposed vascular mass with no bony covering.

Classification and nomenclature of spinal column defects are based on the extent to which the meninges and spinal cord are involved. SPINA BIFIDA refers to abnormal closure with or without visible protrusion of the meninges and spinal cord through the cleft in the spinal column. If there is no visible protrusion, the condition is called *spina bifida occulta*. An external protrusion consisting of a saclike structure is called *spina bifida cystica*. Two subtypes of spina bifida cystica are MENINGOCELE, which involves the meninges surrounded by spinal fluid, and MYELOMENINGOCELE (or *meningomyelocele*), in which the sac contains meninges, spinal fluid, and a portion of the spinal cord with its nerves.

Developmental defects of the neural tube tend to run in families and are believed by most authorities to occur during early development of the embryo. Prenatal detection of some major open neural tube defects is possible through ultrasonic scanning of the uterus and laboratory evaluation of the amniotic fluid. In the presence of anencephaly and meningomyelocele there are elevated concentrations of alpha-fetoprotein in the amniotic fluid.

Genetic predisposition to neural tube defects is inheritable; thus family history is significant in predicting the risk of recurrence. For example, a couple who has had one child with such a defect has a one in twenty (5 per cent) probability of having a second child with the disorder. The risk is doubled to one in ten (10 per cent) if two of their children are so affected. Siblings of an affected child who are themselves normal are at greater than average risk of producing a child with a similar problem.

Treatment. Immediate care of the neonate with a neural tube defect includes prevention of infection and assessment of neurological involvement. Later, an orthopedic assessment is done to identify problems related to locomotion. Corrective procedures such as casting, bracing, and traction are indicated if there is hope for some functioning of the lower extremities. Associated anomalies of the hip, knee, and foot may require correction by orthopedic surgery.

Meningoceles usually are repaired to prevent infection, especially if there is danger of rupture of the sac. Most authorities recommend closure within the first 24 to 48 hours after birth. However, authorities do not agree on whether an attempt should be made to perform skin closure over a myelomeningocele. If HYDROCEPHALUS develops, the treatment of choice is a ventriculoperitoneal shunt or some other procedure to drain spinal fluid and decompress the fluid-filled ventricles.

Bowel and bladder dysfunction usually occur as a result of myelomeningocele. Management of neurogenic bladder and incontinence includes preventing urinary stasis and infection and providing some means for collecting urine. Fecal incontinence may be amenable to bowel training and modification of the diet. In some children a colostomy is the most desirable way to handle the problem.

Patient Care. Immediate concerns in the care of the newborn with a neural tube defect center on protection of the fragile sac from trauma and infection, observation for complications, and support and guidance for parents and family members. Positioning before and after surgery is critical. Preoperatively, the goal is to minimize tension on and trauma to the sac. The baby may be placed in a prone position with head slightly lower than body to reduce spinal fluid pressure in the sac. The hips are slightly flexed to relieve tension on the spine. After surgery, it may be desirable to elevate the head because of increased intracranial pressure and impending hydrocephalus. Many surgeons allow a side-lying position postoperatively because of diapering and feeding problems associated with the prone position. The variety of allowable positions permits frequent position changes to avoid pressure sores. As soon as the operative site is sufficiently healed, the baby can be held for feeding and receiving the body contact every neonate needs. If a baby with inoperable myelomeningocele cannot be held and cuddled, stroking, fondling, and other comfort measures can be used to meet the need for tactile stimulation.

Long-term care will depend on the specific orthopedic, urologic, and neurologic problems each child has. Patients will require continued guidance and support. Comprehensive care for the patient and family can only be provided by a coordinated team of health care providers, including physicians, nurses, physical therapists, rehabilitation specialists, and social workers. The familial tendency toward neural tube defects demands that genetic counseling be available to the family.

neuralgia (noo-ral′jah) pain in a nerve or along the course of one or more nerves, usually consisting of a sharp, spasmlike pain that may recur at intervals. It is caused by inflammation of or injury to a nerve or group of nerves. Inflammation of a nerve, or NEURITIS, may affect different parts of the body, depending upon the location of the nerve. Two common types of neuralgia are that of the trigeminal nerve (see TIC DOULOUREUX) and that of the sciatic nerve (see SCIATICA). adj., **neural′gic.**

n. facia′lis ve′ra Ramsay Hunt syndrome.

Fothergill's n. tic douloureux (trigeminal neuralgia).

geniculate n. Ramsay Hunt syndrome.

glossopharyngeal n. that affecting the petrosal and jugular ganglion of the glossopharyngeal nerve, marked by severe paroxysmal pain originating on the side of the throat and extending to the ear.

Hunt's n. Ramsay Hunt syndrome.

idiopathic n. neuralgia of unknown etiology, not accompanied by any structural change.

intercostal n. neuralgia of the intercostal nerves, causing pain in the side.

mammary n. neuralgic pain in the breast.

Morton's n. tenderness or pain in the metatarsal area of the foot and in the third and fourth toes caused by pressure on a neuroma of the branch of the medial plantar nerve supplying these toes. The neuroma is produced by chronic compression of the nerve between the metatarsal heads. Called also Morton's foot or toe.

nasociliary n. pain in the eyes, brow, and root of the nose.

postherpetic n. persistent burning pain and tingling along the distribution of a cutaneous nerve following an attack of HERPES ZOSTER.

trifacial n., trigeminal n. tic douloureux.

neuraminic acid (noor″ah-min′ik) a nine-carbon amino acid formed from mannosamine and pyruvate; see also SIALIDASE.

neuraminidase (noor″ah-min′ĭ-dās) sialidase.

neuranagenesis (noor″an-ah-jen′ĕ-sis) regeneration of nerve tissue.

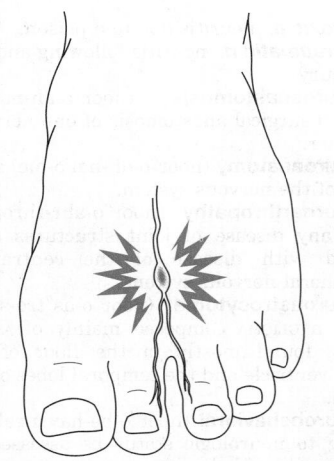

The pain of Morton's neuroma is frequently made worse with prolonged standing or walking. From Waldman, 2002.

neurapophysis (noor″ah-pof′ĭ-sis) a structure forming either side of the neural arch; also, the part supposedly homologous with this structure in a so-called cranial vertebra.

neurapraxia (noor″ah-prak′se-ah) failure of nerve conduction in the absence of structural changes, due to blunt injury, compression, or ischemia.

neurarthropathy (noor″ahr-throp′ah-the) neuroarthropathy.

neurasthenia (noor″as-the′ne-ah) a virtually obsolete term formerly used to describe a vague disorder marked by chronic abnormal fatigability, moderate depression, inability to concentrate, loss of appetite, insomnia, and other symptoms. Popularly called nervous prostration. adj., **neurasthen′ic.**

neuraxis (noo-rak′sis) 1. axon. 2. central nervous system. adj., **neurax′ial.**

neurectasia (noor″ek-ta′zhah) neurotony.

neurectomy (noo-rek′to-me) excision of a part of a nerve.

neurectopia (noor″ek-to′pe-ah) displacement or abnormal situation of a nerve.

neurenteric (noor″en-ter′ik) pertaining to the neural tube and archenteron of the embryo.

neurergic (noo-rer′jik) pertaining to or dependent on nerve action.

neurexeresis (noor″ek-ser′ĕ-sis) the operation of tearing out (avulsion) of a nerve.

neurilemma (noor″ĭ-lem′ah) the plasma membrane of a Schwann cell, forming the sheath of Schwann of a myelinated or unmyelinated peripheral nerve. adj., **neurilem′mal.**

neurilemmitis (noor″ĭ-lĕ-mi′tis) inflammation of the neurilemma.

neurilemoma (noor″ĭ-lĕ-mo′mah) a tumor of a NEURILEMMA (peripheral nerve sheath); called also schwannoma and neurinoma.

neurinoma (noor″ĭ-no′mah) neurilemoma.

neuritis (noo-ri′tis) inflammation of a nerve; also used to denote certain noninflammatory lesions of the peripheral nervous system. There are many forms with different effects; some increase or decrease sensitivity of the body part served by the nerve, others produce paralysis, and some cause pain and inflammation. The cases in which pain is the chief symptom are generally called NEURALGIA. See also NEUROPATHY. adj., **neurit′ic.** Neuritis and neuralgia attack the peripheral nerves, the nerves that link the brain and spinal cord with the muscles, skin, organs, and all other parts of the body. These nerves usually carry both sensory and motor fibers; hence both pain and some paralysis may result. Treatment varies with the specific form of neuritis involved.

Generalized Neuritis. Certain toxic substances such as lead, arsenic, and mercury may produce a generalized poisoning of the peripheral nerves, with tenderness, pain, and paralysis of the limbs. Other causes of generalized neuritis include alcoholism, vitamin-deficiency diseases such as beriberi, and diabetes mellitus, thallium poisoning, some types of allergy, and some viral and bacterial infections, such as diphtheria, syphilis, and mumps. Some attacks begin with fever and other symptoms of an acute illness. However, neuritis caused by lead or alcohol poisoning comes on very slowly over the course of weeks or months. Usually an attack of generalized neuritis will subside by itself when the toxic substance is eliminated. Rest and a nutritious diet containing extra vitamins, especially of the B group, are helpful. Physical therapy may relieve the pain and paralysis. Generalized neuritis may be prevented through knowledge of the dangers of poor nutrition, industrial hazards, chronic alcoholism, and infections.

Special Types of Neuritis. Frequently, instead of a generalized irritation of the nerves, only one nerve is affected. BELL'S PALSY, or facial paralysis, results when the facial nerve is affected. It usually lasts only a few days or weeks. Sometimes, however, the cause is a tumor pressing on the nerve, or injury to the nerve by a blow, cut, or bullet. In that event, recovery depends on the success in treating the tumor or injury.

Sciatica is inflammation of or injury to the sciatic nerve, a large nerve running downward from the spinal cord into the lower limb. The most common cause is probably a

HERNIATED DISK. Back injury, irritation from arthritis of the spine, or pressure on the nerve from certain types of work are other causes. Certain diseases such as diabetes mellitus or gout may also be inciting factors. (See also SCIATICA.)

Neuritis of the Spinal Nerves. Injury or disease may affect any of the many nerves traveling out from the spine. For example, inflammation of the nerves between the ribs causes pain in the chest that may resemble pleurisy or even coronary occlusion (heart attack). This is called intercostal neuritis or intercostal neuralgia. Similarly, the nerves traveling down the neck to the arm may be subject to various injuries or diseases. For example, too vigorous pulling on the nerves in the neck of a fetus, as in difficult obstetrical deliveries, causes the condition known as brachial paralysis.

Neuritis of the Cranial Nerves. Bell's palsy results from inflammation of the seventh cranial, or facial, nerve. The fifth cranial, or trigeminal, nerve, also ends in the face and jaws, and may be the source of a neuralgia that causes spasms of pain on one side of the face, called TIC DOULOUREUX or trigeminal neuralgia. It may be set off by a draft of cold air, by chewing, or by other factors. Medicines and, if necessary, surgery can relieve this painful malady.

Optic neuritis refers to any of various conditions in the nerves leading to the retina of the eye; this is potentially dangerous to vision and requires immediate treatment. Any of the other cranial nerves may be affected by infections, tumors, and toxins. The antibiotic streptomycin occasionally causes damage to the eighth cranial nerve, which helps control the sense of balance in the inner ear. Any disturbance of vision, hearing, balance, swallowing, taste, or speech may be a sign of trouble in the cranial nerves, and should be immediately brought to the attention of a health care provider.

   endemic n. beriberi.

   interstitial n. inflammation of the connective tissue of a nerve trunk.

   multiple n. polyneuritis.

   optic n. inflammation of the optic nerve; it may affect the part of the nerve within the eyeball (NEUROPAPILLITIS) or behind the eyeball (retrobulbar NEURITIS).

   parenchymatous n. neuritis affecting primarily the axons and the myelin of the peripheral nerves.

   retrobulbar n. OPTIC NEURITIS affecting the part of the optic nerve behind the eyeball.

   serum n. serum neuropathy.

   toxic n. neuritis due to a poison.

   traumatic n. neuritis following and due to injury.

neuroanastomosis (noor″o-ah-nas″to-mo′sis) surgical anastomosis of one nerve to another.

neuroanatomy (noor″o-ah-nat′o-me) anatomy of the nervous system.

neuroarthropathy (noor″o-ahr-throp′ah-the) any disease of joint structures associated with disease of the central or peripheral nervous system.

neuroastrocytoma (noor″o-as″tro-si-to′mah) a GLIOMA composed mainly of ASTROCYTES, found mostly in the floor of the third ventricle and the temporal lobes of the brain.

neurobehavioral (noor″o-be-hāv′u-ral) relating to neurologic status as assessed by observation of behavior.

neurobiologist (noor″o-bi-ol′o-jist) a specialist in neurobiology.

neurobiology (noor″o-bi-ol′o-je) biology of the nervous system.

neuroblast (noor′o-blast) an embryonic cell from which nervous tissue is formed.

neuroblastoma (noor″o-blas-to′mah) SARCOMA of nervous system origin, composed chiefly of NEUROBLASTS, affecting mostly infants and children up to 10 years of age, usually arising in the autonomic nervous system (SYMPATHICOBLASTOMA) or in the adrenal medulla.

neurocanal (noor″o-kah-nal′) vertebral canal.

neurocardiac (noor″o-kahr′de-ak) pertaining to the nervous system and the heart.

neurocentrum (noor″o-sen′trum) one of the embryonic vertebral elements from which the spinous PROCESSES of the vertebrae develop. adj., **neurocen′tral.**

neurochemistry (noor″o-kem′is-tre) the branch of NEUROLOGY dealing with the chemistry of the nervous system.

neurochorioretinitis (noor″o-kor″e-o-ret′ĭ-ni′tis) inflammation of the optic nerve, choroid, and retina.

neurochoroiditis (noor″o-kor″oi-di′tis) inflammation of the optic nerve and choroid.

neurocirculatory (noor″o-ser″ku-lah-tor″e) pertaining to the nervous and circulatory systems.

neurocladism (noo-rok′lah-dizm) the formation of new branches by the process of a neuron; especially the force by which, in regeneration of divided nerves, the newly formed axons become attracted by the peripheral stump, so as to form a bridge between the two ends.

neuroclonic (noor″o-klon′ik) marked by nervous spasm.

neurocommunications (noor″o-kŏ-mu″nĭ-ka′shunz) the branch of neurology dealing with the transfer and integration of information within the nervous system.

neurocranium (noor″o-kra′ne-um) the part of the cranium enclosing the brain. adj., **neurocra′nial.**

neurocrine (noor′o-krīn) 1. denoting an endocrine influence on or by the nerves. 2. pertaining to neurosecretion.

neurocristopathy (noor″o-kris-top′ah-the) any disease arising from maldevelopment of the neural crest.

neurocutaneous (noor″o-ku-ta′ne-us) pertaining to nerves and skin, or the cutaneous nerves.

neurocyte (noor′o-sīt) a nerve cell of any kind.

neurocytoma (noor″o-si-to′mah) a brain tumor consisting of undifferentiated cells of nervous origin, i.e., cells resembling medullary neural epithelium. Called also neuro-epithelioma.

neurodendrite (noor″o-den′drīt) dendrite.

neurodendron (noor″o-den′dron) dendrite.

neurodermatitis (noor″o-der″mah-ti′tis) an extremely variable eczematous dermatosis presumed to be a cutaneous response to prolonged vigorous scratching, rubbing, or pinching to relieve intense pruritus. It is believed by some authorities to be a psychogenic disorder. The term is also used to refer to LICHEN SIMPLEX CHRONICUS *(circumscribed neurodermatitis)* and sometimes to atopic DERMATITIS *(disseminated neurodermatitis).*

neurodynamic (noor″o-di-nam′ik) pertaining to nervous energy.

neurodynia (noor″o-din′e-ah) pain in a nerve.

neuroectoderm (noor″o-ek′to-derm) the portion of the ectoderm of the early embryo which gives rise to the central and peripheral nervous systems, including some glial cells. adj., **neuroectoder′mal.**

neuroeffector (noor″o-ĕ-fek′tor) of or relating to the junction between a neuron and the effector organ it innervates.

neuroencephalomyelopathy (noor″o-en-sef″ah-lo-mi″ĕ-lop′ah-the) disease involving the nerves, brain, and spinal cord.

neuroendocrine (noor″o-en′do-krin) pertaining to neural and endocrine influence, and particularly to the interaction between the nervous and endocrine systems.

neuroendocrinology (noor″o-en″do-krĭ-nol′o-je) the study of the interactions of the nervous and endocrine systems.

neuroendoscope (noor″o-en′do-skōp″) an endoscope for examining and performing various interventions in the central nervous system.

neuroepithelioma (noor″o-ep″ĭ-the″le-o′mah) neurocytoma.

neuroepithelium (noor″o-ep″ĭ-the′le-um) 1. epithelium made up of cells specialized to serve as sensory cells for reception of external stimuli. Called also sense or sensory epithelium. 2. the ectodermal epithelium, from which the central nervous system develops.

neurofiber (noor″o-fi′ber) nerve fiber.

neurofibril (noor″o-fi′bril) one of the delicate threads running in every direction through the cytoplasm of a nerve cell, extending into the axon and dendrites.

neurofibroma (noor″o-fi-bro″mah) a tumor of peripheral nerves due to abnormal proliferation of Schwann CELLS; called also fibroneuroma.

neurofibromatosis (noor″o-fi″bro-mah-to′sis) a genetic disorder characterized by tumor growth along various types of nerves; bone, muscle, and skin may also be affected. There are two types: *Type I* (called also Recklinghausen's or von Recklinghausen's disease) is characterized by developmental changes in the nervous system, muscles, bones, and skin with formation of neurofibromas over the entire body and patches of pigmentation; scoliosis may also be associated. Half of those with the disorder have some form of learning disability. (See accompanying illustration.) *Type II* (called also bilateral acoustic neurofibromatosis) is a benign tumor that forms intracranially or intraspinally, usually associated with the eighth cranial nerve (see also acoustic NEUROMA). Information and support for individuals with neurofibromatosis and those caring for them can be obtained by writing to the National Neurofibromatosis Foundation, 95 Pine St., 16th Floor, New York, NY 10005 or consulting their web site at http://www.nf.org.

neurofilament (noor″o-fil′ah-ment) any of the slender, fibrillar elements which, along with the neurotubules, forms a neurofibril.

neurogenesis (noor″o-jen′ĕ-sis) the development of nervous tissue.

neurogenic (noor″o-jen′ik) 1. forming nervous tissue, or stimulating nervous energy. 2. originating in the nervous system.

neurogenous (noo-roj′ĕ-nus) arising from the nervous system, or from some lesion of the nervous system.

neuroglia (noo-rog′le-ah) the supporting structure of nervous tissue, consisting, in the central nervous system, of ASTROCYTES, OLIGODENDROCYTES, and MICROGLIA; called also glia. adj., **neurog′lial.**

N

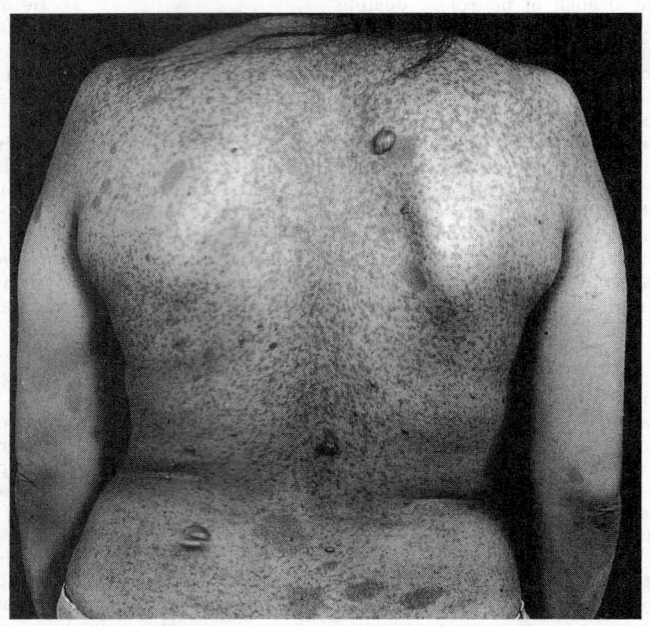

A patient with neurofibromatosis type I showing truncal freckling, café au lait spots, and multiple neurofibromas. From Mueller and Young, 2001.

neurogliocyte (noo-rog'le-o-sīt) one of the cells composing the neuroglia.

neuroglioma (noor″o-gli-o'mah) glioma.

n. gangliona're ganglioneuroma.

neurogliosis (noo-rog″le-o'sis) a condition marked by numerous NEUROGLIOMAS.

neurohistology (noor″o-his-tol'o-je) histology of the nervous system.

neurohormone (noor'o-hor″mōn) a hormone that stimulates neural mechanisms or is released when activated by neural stimuli.

neurohumor (noor″o-hu'mor) a chemical substance formed in a neuron and able to activate or modify the function of a neighboring neuron, muscle, or gland. adj., **neurohu'moral.**

neurohypophysis (noor″o-hi-pof'ĭ-sis) the posterior lobe of the PITUITARY GLAND. adj., **neurohypophys'eal.**

neuroid (noor'oid) resembling a nerve.

neuroimmunology (noor″o-im″u-nol'o-je) the branch of biomedical science that deals with the interaction of the nervous and immune systems in health and disease, such as the effect of autonomic nervous activity on the IMMUNE RESPONSE and the role of antibodies in myasthenia gravis. adj., **neuroimmunolog'ic.**

neurolemma (noor″o-lem'ah) neurilemma.

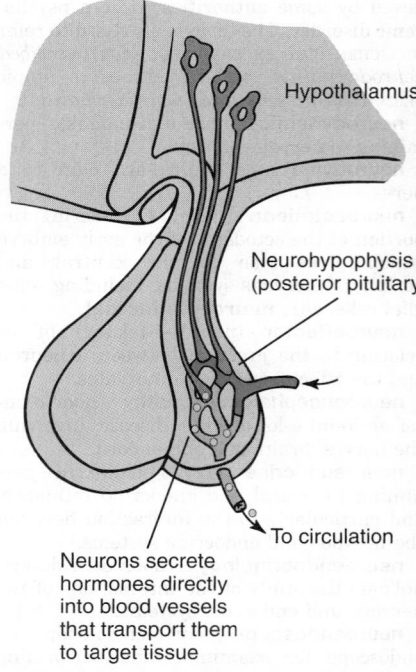

The neurohypophysis (posterior pituitary gland). From Applegate, 2000.

Hypothalamus

Neurohypophysis (posterior pituitary)

To circulation

Neurons secrete hormones directly into blood vessels that transport them to target tissue

neurolemmitis (noor″o-lĕ-mi′tis) neurilemmitis.

neurolemmoma (noor″o-lĕ-mo′mah) neurilemoma.

neuroleptic (noor″o-lep′tik) a term coined to refer to the effects on cognition and behavior of the original ANTIPSYCHOTIC AGENTS, which produced a state of apathy, lack of initiative, and limited range of emotion and in psychotic patients caused a reduction in confusion and agitation and normalization of psychomotor activity. The term is still used to refer to agents, such as droperidol, used to produce such effects as part of anesthesia or analgesia; however, it is outdated as a synonym for antipsychotic agents because newer agents do not necessarily have such effects.

n. malignant syndrome a rare but dramatic condition that occurs in severely ill patients being treated with high-potency antipsychotics (neuroleptics); symptoms include diaphoresis, muscle rigidity, and hyperpyrexia. It is believed to be caused by dopamine blockade in the hypothalamus.

neuroleptanalgesia (noor″o-lep″tan-al-je′zhah) a state of quiescence, altered awareness, and analgesia produced by the administration of a combination of an opioid ANALGESIC and a neuroleptic (ANTIPSYCHOTIC AGENT).

neuroleptanesthesia (noor″o-lep″tan-es-the′zhah) a state of NEUROLEPTANALGESIA and unconsciousness, produced by the combined administration of an opioid ANALGESIC and a neuroleptic (ANTIPSYCHOTIC AGENT), together with the inhalation of nitrous oxide and oxygen.

neurologic assessment evaluation of the health status of a patient with a nervous system disorder or dysfunction. Purposes of the assessment include establishing a medical DIAGNOSIS to guide the physician in prescribing medical and surgical treatments, and a NURSING DIAGNOSIS to guide the nurse in planning and implementing nursing measures to help the patient cope effectively with daily living activities. Important parts of the neurologic assessment include a general physical examination and a detailed neurologic examination; these may be conducted by either a physician or a nurse practitioner. A neurologic history must also be obtained, as well as any necessary special neurologic diagnostic studies. The neurologic physical examination involves evaluation of the patient's level of consciousness, mood, orientation, speech, content of thought, and memory; gait while walking and ability to stand quietly with feet together; physical status of the head, neck, and spine as determined by palpation, inspection, and auscultation; function of the cranial nerves; sensory and motor function; and reflex activity.

Nursing assessment of a patient's neurologic status is concerned with identifying functional disabilities that interfere with the person's self-care ability and ability to lead an active life. A functionally oriented nursing assessment includes: (1) consciousness, (2) mentation, (3) motor function, and (4) sensory function. Evaluation of these functions gives the nurse information about the patient's ability to perform everyday activities such as thinking, remembering, seeing, eating, speaking, moving, smelling, feeling, and hearing. Some patients should also be assessed for signs of hallucinations, delusions, delirium, and convulsive seizures.

A patient with an acute and life-threatening alteration in neurologic function is evaluated and monitored in four general areas: (1) level of consciousness, (2) sensory and motor function, (3) pupillary changes and extraocular movements, and (4) vital signs and pattern of respiration. (See also INTRACRANIAL PRESSURE.) In many institutions a checklist for "neuro checks" is available to the nursing staff to be used as a guide for objective assessment of a patient with an altered level of CONSCIOUSNESS such as COMA.

neurologist (noo-rol′o-jist) a specialist in NEUROLOGY.

neurology (noo-rol′o-je) the branch of health science that deals with the NERVOUS SYSTEM, both normal and in disease. adj., **neurolog′ic.**

clinical n. that especially concerned with the diagnosis and treatment of disorders of the nervous system.

neurolysin (noo-rol′ĭ-sin) a cytolysin with a specific destructive action on neurons.

neurolysis (noo-rol′ĭ-sis) 1. release of a nerve sheath by cutting it longitudinally. 2. operative breaking up of perineural adhesions. 3. relief of tension upon a nerve obtained by stretching. 4. exhaustion of nervous energy. 5. destruction or dissolution of nerve tissue. adj., **neurolyt′ic.**

neuroma (noo-ro′mah) a tumor or new growth largely made up of nerve cells and nerve fibers. adj., **neurom′atous.**

acoustic n. a benign tumor within the auditory canal arising from the eighth cranial (acoustic) nerve. HEARING LOSS begins in the teens or early 20's and may be surgically managed. Acoustic neuroma is a manifestation of Type II NEUROFIBROMATOSIS.

amputation n. traumatic neuroma occurring after amputation of a limb or other part.

n. cu′tis neuroma in the skin.

false n. one that does not contain nerve elements.

plexiform n. one made up of contorted nerve trunks.

n. telangiecto′des one containing an excess of blood vessels.

traumatic n. an unorganized bulbous or nodular mass of nerve fibers and Schwann cells produced by hyperplasia of nerve fibers and their supporting tissues after accidental or purposeful sectioning of the nerve.

neuromalacia (noor″o-mah-la′shah) morbid softening of the nerves.

neuromatosis (noor″o-mah-to′sis) a condition characterized by the presence of many neuromas.

neuromere (noor′o-mēr) 1. any of a series of transitory segmental elevations in the wall of the neural tube in the developing embryo; also, such elevations in the wall of the mature rhombencephalon. 2. a part of the spinal cord to which a pair of dorsal roots and a pair of ventral roots are attached.

neuromodulation (noor″o-mod″u-la′shun) electrical stimulation of a peripheral nerve, the spinal cord, or the brain for relief of pain; it may be done transcutaneously or with an implanted stimulator.

neuromuscular (noor″o-mus′ku-ler) pertaining to the nerves and muscles.

neuromyelitis (noor″o-mi″ĕ-li′tis) inflammation of nervous and medullary substance; myelitis attended with neuritis.

n. op′tica combined demyelination of the optic nerve and spinal cord, with diminution of vision and possible blindness, flaccid paralysis of extremities, and sensory and genitourinary disturbances.

neuromyopathy (noor″o-mi-op′ah-the) any disease of both muscles and nerves,

especially a muscular disease of nervous origin.

carcinomatous n. a paraneoplastic syndrome of neuromyopathy in patients with carcinoma, usually of the lung.

neuromyositis (noor″o-mi″o-si′tis) neuritis blended with myositis.

neuron (noor′on) a highly specialized cell of the NERVOUS SYSTEM, having two characteristic properties: IRRITABILITY (ability to be stimulated) and CONDUCTIVITY (ability to conduct impulses). They are composed of a cell body (called also neurosome or perikaryon), containing the nucleus and its surrounding cytoplasm, and one or more processes (nerve FIBERS) extending from the body. Called also nerve cell. adj., **neuro′nal.**

The nerve fibers are actually extensions of the cytoplasm surrounding the nucleus of the neuron. A nerve cell may have only one such slender fiber extending from its body, in which case it is classified as *unipolar.* A neuron having two processes is *bipolar,* and one with three or more processes is *multipolar.* Most neurons are multipolar; this type is widely distributed throughout the central nervous system and autonomic ganglia. The multipolar neurons have a single process called an AXON and several branched extensions called DENDRITES. The dendrites receive stimuli from other nerves or from a receptor organ, such as the skin or ear, and transmit them through the neuron to the axon. The axon conducts the impulses to the dendrite of another neuron or to an effector organ that is thereby stimulated to action. Many processes are covered with a layer of lipid material called the myelin SHEATH. Peripheral nerve fibers have a thin outer covering called NEURILEMMA.

Types of Neurons. Neurons that receive stimuli from the outside environment and transmit them toward the brain are called *afferent* or *sensory neurons.* Those that carry impulses in the opposite direction, away from the brain and other nerve centers to muscles, are called *efferent neurons, motor neurons,* or *motoneurons.* Another type, the *interneuron,* found in the brain and spinal cord, conducts impulses from afferent to efferent neurons.

Synapses. The point at which an impulse is transmitted from one neuron to another is called a synapse. The transmission is chemical in nature; that is, there is no direct contact between the axon of one neuron and the dendrites of another. The *cholinergic nerves* (PARASYMPATHETIC NERVOUS SYSTEM) liberate at their axon endings a substance called ACETYLCHOLINE, which acts as a stimulant to the dendrites of adjacent

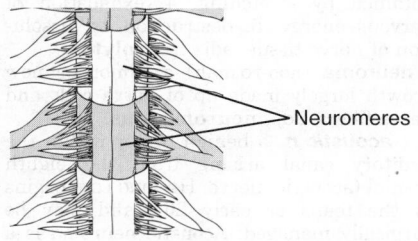

Neuromere. From Dorland's, 2000.

Neuromeres

neurons. In a similar manner, the *adrenergic nerves* (SYMPATHETIC NERVOUS SYSTEM) liberate EPINEPHRINE or related substances. The synapse may involve one neuron in chemical contact with many adjacent neurons, or it may involve the axon terminals of one neuron and the dendrites of a succeeding neuron in a nerve pathway. There are many different patterns of synapses.

Receptor End-Organs. The dendrites of the sensory neurons are designed to receive stimuli from various parts of the body. These dendrites are called receptor endorgans and are of three general types: *exteroceptors, interoceptors,* and *proprioceptors.* The exteroceptors are located near the external surface of the body, receive impulses from the skin, and transmit information about the senses of touch, heat, cold, and other factors in the external environment. The interoceptors are located in the internal organs and receive information from the viscera, e.g., pressure, tension, and pain. The proprioceptors are found in muscles, tendons, and joints and transmit "muscle sense," by which one is aware of the position of one's body in space.

Neurons and Effectors. The axons of motor neurons form synapses with skeletal fibers to produce motion. These junctions are called *motor end-plates* or *myoneural junctions.* The axon of a motor neuron divides just before it enters the muscle fibers and forms synapses near the nuclei of muscle fibers. These motor neurons are called somatic efferent neurons. Visceral efferent neurons form synapses with smooth muscle, cardiac muscle, and glands.

   Golgi n's 1. (type I): pyramidal cells with long axons, which leave the gray matter of the central nervous system, traverse the white matter, and terminate in the periphery. 2. (type II): stellate neurons with short axons in the cerebral and cerebellar cortices and in the retina.

   motor n. motoneuron.

   postganglionic n's neurons whose cell bodies lie in the autonomic ganglia and whose purpose is to relay impulses beyond the ganglia.

   preganglionic n's neurons whose cell bodies lie in the central nervous system and whose efferent fibers terminate in the autonomic ganglia.

   neuronevus (noor″o-ne′vus) a cellular or nevocytic nevus, especially a mature one with differentiation toward neural skin structures.

   neuronophage (noŏ-ron′o-fāj) a phagocyte that destroys nerve cells.

   neuronophagia (noor″on-o-fa′jah) phagocytic destruction of nerve cells.

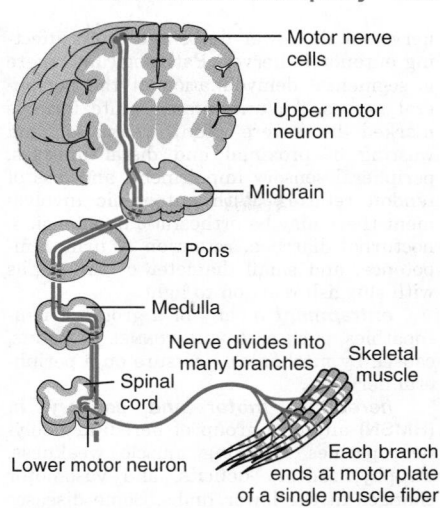

Upper and lower motor neurons. From Damjanov, 2000.

   neuro-oncology (noor″o-on-kol′ah-je) the field of specialization dealing with tumors of the nervous system.

   neuro-ophthalmology (noor″o-of″thal-mol′o-je) the branch of OPHTHALMOLOGY dealing with portions of the nervous system related to the eye.

   neuropapillitis (noor″o-pap″ĭ-li′tis) optic NEURITIS affecting the part of the optic nerve within the eyeball.

   neuropathogenicity (noor″o-path″o-jĕ-nis′ĭ-te) the quality of producing or the ability to produce pathologic changes in nerve tissue.

   neuropathology (noor″o-pah-thol′o-je) pathology of the nervous system.

   neuropathy (noŏ-rop′ah-the) any of numerous functional disturbances and pathologic changes in the peripheral nervous system. The etiology may be known (e.g., arsenical, diabetic, ischemic, or traumatic neuropathy) or unknown. ENCEPHALOPATHY and MYELOPATHY are corresponding terms relating to involvement of the brain and spinal cord. The term is also used to designate noninflammatory lesions in the peripheral nervous system, in contrast to inflammatory lesions (NEURITIS). adj., **neuropath′ic.**

   alcoholic n. neuropathy due to thiamine deficiency in chronic ALCOHOLISM.

   Denny-Brown's sensory n. hereditary sensory radicular neuropathy.

   diabetic n. a complication of DIABETES MELLITUS consisting of chronic symmetrical sensory polyneuropathy affecting first the

N

nerves of the lower limbs and often affecting autonomic nerves. Pathologically, there is segmental demyelination of the peripheral nerves. An uncommon, acute form is marked by severe pain, weakness, and wasting of proximal and distal muscles, peripheral sensory impairment, and loss of tendon reflexes. With autonomic involvement there may be orthostatic hypotension, nocturnal diarrhea, retention of urine, impotence, and small diameter of the pupils with sluggish reaction to light.

entrapment n. any of a group of neuropathies, such as CARPAL TUNNEL SYNDROME, caused by mechanical pressure on a peripheral nerve.

hereditary motor and sensory n. (HMSN) any of a group of hereditary polyneuropathies involving muscle weakness, atrophy, sensory deficits, and vasomotor changes in the lower limbs. Some diseases in this group have been numbered: types I and II are varieties of CHARCOT-MARIE-TOOTH DISEASE and type III is progressive hypertrophic NEUROPATHY.

hereditary sensory n. hereditary sensory radicular neuropathy.

hereditary sensory and autonomic n. (HSAN) any of several inherited neuropathies that involve slow ascendance of lesions of the sensory nerves, resulting in pain, distal trophic ulcers, and a variety of autonomic disturbances. Types include hereditary sensory radicular NEUROPATHY and familial DYSAUTONOMIA.

hereditary sensory radicular n. a dominantly inherited polyneuropathy characterized by signs of radicular sensory loss in both the upper and lower limbs; shooting pains; chronic, indolent, trophic ulceration of the feet; and sometimes deafness. Called also hereditary sensory neuropathy and Denny-Brown's sensory neuropathy or SYNDROME.

Leber's optic n. a maternally transmitted disorder characterized by bilateral progressive optic atrophy, with onset usually at about the age of twenty. Degeneration of the optic nerve and papillomacular bundle results in progressive loss of central vision that may remit spontaneously. It is much more common in males. Called also Leber's disease and Leber's optic atrophy.

progressive hypertrophic n. a slowly progressive familial disease beginning in early life, marked by hyperplasia of interstitial connective tissue, causing thickening of peripheral nerve trunks and posterior roots, and by sclerosis of the posterior columns of the spinal cord, with atrophy of distal parts of the legs and diminution of tendon reflexes and sensation. Called also Dejerine's disease and Dejerine-Sottas disease.

serum n. a neurologic disorder, usually involving the cervical nerves or brachial plexus, occurring two to eight days after the injection of foreign protein, as in immunization or serotherapy for tetanus, diphtheria, or scarlet fever, and characterized by local pain followed by sensory disturbances and paralysis. Called also serum neuritis.

neuropeptide (noor″o-pep′tīd) any of several types of molecules found in brain tissue, composed of short chains of amino acids; they include endorphins, enkephalins, vasopressin, and others.

neuropharmacology (noor″o-fahr″mah-kol′o-je) scientific study of the effects of drugs on the nervous system.

neurophthisis (noo-rof′thĭ-sis) wasting of nerve tissue.

neurophysin (noor″o-fi′sin) any of a group of soluble proteins secreted in the hypothalamus that serve as binding proteins for vasopressin and oxytocin, playing a role in their transport in the neurohypophyseal tract and their storage in the posterior pituitary.

neurophysiology (noor″o-fiz″e-ol′o-je) physiology of the nervous system.

neuropil (noor′ro-pil) a dense feltwork of interwoven cytoplasmic processes of nerve cells (dendrites and axons) and of neuroglial cells in the central nervous system and some parts of the peripheral nervous system.

neuroplasm (noor′o-plazm) the protoplasm of a nerve cell. adj., **neuroplas′mic.**

neuroplasty (noor′o-plas″te) plastic repair of a nerve.

neuropodium (noor″o-po′de-um) a bulbous termination of an axon in one type of synapse.

neuropore (noor′o-pōr) an opening in the anterior (rostral) or posterior (caudal) end of the neural tube of the developing embryo; the rostral neuropore is normally closed by 25 to 26 days and the caudal neuropore is usually closed by the end of the fourth week.

neuroprotective (noor″o-pro-tek′tiv) guarding or protecting against neurotoxicity.

neuropsychiatrist (noor″o-si-ki′ah-trist) a physician specializing in neuropsychiatry.

neuropsychiatry (noor″o-si-ki′ah-tre) a branch of health science combining neurology and psychiatry.

neuroradiology (noor″o-ra″de-ol′o-je) radiology of the nervous system

neuroretinitis (noor″o-ret″ĭ-ni′tis) inflammation of the optic nerve and retina.

neuroretinopathy (noor″o-ret″ĭ-nop′ah-the) pathologic involvement of the optic disk and retina.

neurorrhaphy (noo-ror′ah-fe) suture of a divided nerve.

neurosarcocleisis (noor″o-sahr″ko-kli′sis) an operation for neuralgia, done by relieving pressure on the affected nerve by partial resection of the bony canal through which it passes and transplanting the nerve among soft tissues.

neurosarcoma (noor″o-sahr-ko′mah) a SARCOMA with neuromatous elements.

neuroscience (noor″o-si′ens) the embryology, anatomy, physiology, biochemistry, and pharmacology of the nervous system.

neurosclerosis (noor″o-sklĕ-ro′sis) hardening of nerve tissue.

neurosecretion (noor″ro-sĕ-kre′shun) 1. secretory activities of nerve cells. 2. a substance secreted by nerve cells. adj., **neurosecre′tory.**

neurosis (noo-ro′sis), pl. *neuro′ses* former name for a category of MENTAL DISORDERS characterized by ANXIETY and avoidance behavior. In general, the term has been used to refer to disorders in which the symptoms are distressing to the person, reality TESTING does not yield unusual results, behavior does not violate gross social norms, and there is no apparent organic etiology. Such disorders are currently classified as ANXIETY DISORDERS, DISSOCIATIVE DISORDERS, MOOD DISORDERS, SEXUAL DISORDERS, and SOMATOFORM DISORDERS.

anxiety n. an obsolete term (Freud) for conditions now reclassified as PANIC DISORDER and GENERALIZED ANXIETY DISORDER.

hysterical n. a former classification of mental disorders, now divided into CONVERSION DISORDER and DISSOCIATIVE DISORDERS.

obsessive-compulsive n. former name for OBSESSIVE-COMPULSIVE DISORDER.

prison n. CHRONOPHOBIA occurring in prisoners having trouble adjusting to a long prison sentence, characterized by feelings of restlessness, panic, anxiety, and CLAUSTROPHOBIA.

transference n. a phenomenon occurring in most PSYCHOANALYSES, in which the patient undergoes, with the analyst as the object, an intense repetition of childhood conflicts, reexperiencing impulses, feelings, and fantasies that originally developed in relation to the parent.

neurosome (noor′o-sōm) perikaryon.

neurospasm (noor′o-spazm) nervous twitching of a muscle.

neurosplanchnic (noor″o-splangk′nik) pertaining to the cerebrospinal and sympathetic nervous systems.

neurospongioma (noor″o-spun″je-o′mah) glioma.

neurospongium (noor″o-spun′je-um) 1. the fibrillar component of neurons. 2. a meshwork of nerve fibrils, especially the inner reticular layer of the retina.

Neurospora (noo-ros′po-rah) a genus of fungi, comprising the bread molds, capable of converting tryptophan to niacin; used in genetic and enzyme research.

neurosurgeon (noor″o-ser′jun) a physician who specializes in neurosurgery.

neurosurgery (noor″o-ser′jer-e) surgery of the nervous system.

neurosuture (noor″o-soo″chur) neurorrhaphy.

neurosyphilis (noor″o-sif′ĭ-lis) the central nervous system manifestations of tertiary syphilis, which may be divided into two groups, asymptomatic and symptomatic; see also general PARESIS and TABES DORSALIS.

neurotendinous (noor″o-ten′dĭ-nus) pertaining to both nerve and tendon.

neurotensin (noor″o-ten′sin) a tridecapeptide that induces vasodilation and hypotension; present in the brain and intestine and postulated to be a neurotransmitter.

neurotic (noo-rot′ik) 1. pertaining to or characterized by neurosis. 2. a person affected with a neurosis.

n. disorder neurosis.

neurotization (noo-rot″ĭ-za′shun) 1. regeneration of a nerve after its division. 2. the implantation of a nerve into a paralyzed muscle.

neurotmesis (noor″rot-me′sis) partial or complete severance of a nerve, with disruption of the axon and its myelin sheath and the connective tissue elements.

neurotome (noor′o-tōm) 1. a needle-like knife for dissecting nerves. 2. neuromere (def. 1).

neurotomy (noo-rot′ah-me) dissection or cutting of nerves.

radiofrequency n. interruption of spinal nerve roots by coagulation with RADIOFREQUENCY waves.

neurotony (noo-rot′o-ne) the surgical stretching of a nerve; called also neurectasia.

neurotoxicity (noor″o-tok-sis′ĭ-te) the ability to exert a destructive or poisonous effect upon nerve tissue. adj., **neurotox′ic.**

neurotoxin (noor′o-tok″sin) a substance that is poisonous or destructive to nerve tissue.

neurotransmitter (noor″o-trans′mit-er) a substance (e.g., norepinephrine, acetylcholine, dopamine) that is released from the axon terminal of a presynaptic neuron on

---

WINDOW ON NEUROTRAUMA

Over one half of all neurotrauma occurs in or by motor vehicles. The other causes of neurotrauma are falls, violent assaults, sports and recreation, and firearms. The victims who survive are left with paralysis, disfigurement, loss of sight and hearing, seizures, epilepsy, psychiatric disorders, amnesia—in short, significant and often permanent impairment. To permanently prevent this human destruction, health care providers should have a prevention agenda that includes advocating for air bags in all cars, helmet use for all motorcyclists, the elimination of handguns, and the regionalization of all trauma care. After this is accomplished, we can continue working on preventing other neurotrauma problems.

ANDREW McGUIRE, BA

---

excitation, and that travels across the synaptic cleft to either excite or inhibit the target cell.

neurotrauma (noor″o-traw′mah) mechanical injury to nerve.

neurotrophy (noo-rot′ro-fe) nutrition and maintenance of tissues as regulated by nervous influence. adj., **neurotroph′ic.**

neurotropism (noo-rot′ro-pizm) 1. the quality of having a special affinity for nervous tissue. 2. the alleged tendency of regenerating nerve fibers to grow toward specific portions of the periphery. adj., **neurotrop′ic.**

neurotubule (noor″o-too′būl) any of the long, straight, parallel tubules within neurons, which along with neurofilaments form neurofibrils.

neurovaccine (noor″o-vak′sēn) vaccine virus prepared by growing the virus in the brain of a rabbit.

neurovascular (noor″o-vas′ku-ler) pertaining to both nervous and vascular elements, or to nerves controlling the caliber of blood vessels.

neurovisceral (noor″o-vis′er-al) neurosplanchnic.

neurula (noor′oo-lah) the early embryonic stage following the gastrula, marked by the first appearance of the nervous system.

neurulation (noor″oo-la′shun) formation in the early embryo of the neural plate and neural folds, followed by its closure with development of the neural tube.

neutral (noo′tral) neither basic nor acid.

neutralization test one for the bacterial neutralization power of a substance by testing its action on the pathogenic properties of the organism concerned.

neutralize (noo′tral-īz) to render neutral.

neutrino (noo-tre′no) a subatomic particle with an extremely small mass and no electric charge.

neutrocyte (noo′tro-sīt) neutrophil (def. 2).

neutron (noo′tron) an electrically neutral or uncharged particle of matter existing along with protons in the atoms of all elements except the mass 1 isotope of hydrogen.

neutropenia (noo″tro-pe′ne-ah) diminished numbers of NEUTROPHILS in the blood.

   congenital n. infantile genetic AGRANU-LOCYTOSIS.

   cyclic n. a chronic form marked by regular, periodic episodic recurrences, associated with malaise, fever, stomatitis, and various infections. Called also periodic neutropenia.

   drug-induced n. that caused by medications; the most common mechanisms are immunological (formation of antibodies destructive to neutrophils or of immune complexes that bind to neutrophils), followed by inhibition of granulopoiesis and direct damage to bone marrow or precursor cells of the granulocytic series.

   idiopathic n. agranulocytosis.

   Kostmann's n. infantile genetic AGRAN-ULOCYTOSIS.

   malignant n. agranulocytosis.

   neonatal n., alloimmune neutropenia in the newborn due to in utero incompatibility between its immunoglobulin G antigens and those of the mother's blood; the mother's blood produces antibodies that cross the placenta and sensitize fetal neutrophils. Affected infants may have fever, pneumonia, septicemia, and other infections that can be fatal. The condition eventually resolves as the infant's immunoglobulin replaces that from the mother.

   periodic n. cyclic neutropenia.

neutrophil (noo′tro-fil) 1. any cell, structure, or histologic element readily stainable with neutral dyes. 2. a granular LEUKOCYTE having a nucleus with three to five lobes connected by threads of chromatin, and cytoplasm containing very fine granules; called also polymorphonuclear LEUKOCYTE and neutrophilic leukocyte. See also HETERO-PHIL.

   band n. band cell.

   stab n. band cell.

neutrophilia (noo″tro-fil′e-ah) increase in the number of neutrophils in the blood; called also neutrophilic leukocytosis.

Neutrophil maturation. From Ignatavicius and Workman, 2002.

neutrophilic (noo″tro-fil′ik) 1. pertaining to neutrophils. 2. stainable by neutral dyes.

nevirapine (ně-vir′ah-pēn) a nonnu-cleoside human immunodeficiency VIRUS-1 (HIV-1) reverse transcriptase INHIBITOR that acts by interfering with the ability of the virus to replicate; used in combination with other ANTIRETROVIRAL agents in treatment of HIV-1 infection, administered orally.

nevocyte (ne″vo-sīt) nevus cell.

nevoid (ne′void) resembling a nevus.

nevoxanthoendothelioma (ne″vo-zan″-tho-en″do-the″le-o′mah) a condition in which groups of yellow-brown papules or nodules occur on the extensor surfaces of the extremities of infants.

nevus (ne′vus), pl. *ne′vi* [L.] a circumscribed stable malformation of the skin or sometimes the oral mucosa, which is not due to external causes; the excess (or deficiency) of tissue may involve epidermal, connective tissue, adnexal, nervous, or vascular elements. Most are either brown, black, or pink; they may appear on any part of the skin, vary in size and thickness, and occur either in groups or alone. See also mole.

A nevus is usually not troublesome unless it is unsightly or disfiguring or becomes inflamed. If it changes noticeably, malignancy may be suspected, especially if any of the following are present: a highly irregular border, an uneven (pebbly) surface, or a mixture of colors (especially black, gray, or blue). Any change in size, color, or texture, or any bleeding or excessive itching, should be reported to a health care provider. Nevi can be removed by surgery or by other methods such as the application of solid carbon dioxide, injections, or radiotherapy.

n. ara′neus vascular SPIDER.

blue n. a dark blue nodular lesion composed of closely grouped MELANOCYTES and MELANOPHAGES in the mid-dermis.

blue rubber bleb n. a hereditary condition marked by multiple bluish cutaneous HEMANGIOMAS with soft raised centers, frequently associated with hemangiomas of the gastrointestinal tract.

n. comedo′nicus a rare epidermal nevus marked by one or more patches 2 to 5 cm or more in diameter, in which there are collections of large comedones or comedolike lesions. This condition is occasionally associated with other lesions such as ICHTHYOSIS, vascular NEVI, and CATARACTS.

compound n. a nevocytic nevus composed of fully formed nests of nevus cells in the epidermis and newly forming ones in the dermis.

connective tissue n. any nevus found in the dermal connective tissue with nodules, papules, plaques, or combinations of such lesions. Histologically, there is inconstant focal or diffuse thickening and abnormal staining of collagen.

epidermal n., epithelial n. a circumscribed congenital developmental anomaly resulting in faulty production of mature or nearly mature cutaneous structures; such nevi vary widely in appearance, size, and distribution and are commonly hyperkeratotic.

n. flam′meus a congenital vascular malformation involving mature capillaries, present at birth. It consists of a reddish purple lesion that is flat or barely elevated and does not fade with age. It is a benign condition but may be associated with other syndromes such as STURGE-WEBER SYNDROME. The dark variety is called a port-wine STAIN and a light variety is called a salmon PATCH. (See Atlas 1, Part E).

giant congenital pigmented n., giant hairy n. giant pigmented n. any of a group of large, darkly pigmented hairy nevi, usually bilaterally symmetrical and present at birth; the most common locations are the chest, upper back, shoulders, arms, legs, and or hip and groin area. These nevi are associated with other cutaneous and subcutaneous lesions, as well as neurofibromatosis and other developmental anomalies, and they exhibit a predisposition to development of malignant melanoma.

halo n. a pigmented nevus surrounded by a ring of depigmentation; called also leukoderma acquisitum centrifugum, Sutton's disease, and Sutton's nevus.

intradermal n. a type of nevocytic nevus clinically indistinguishable from compound nevus, in which the nests of nevus cells lie exclusively within the dermis.

n. of Ito a mongolian spot–like lesion having the same features as nevus of Ota except for localization to the areas of distribution of the posterior supraclavicular and lateral cutaneous brachial nerves, involving the shoulder, side of the neck, supraclavicular areas, and upper arm.

junction n., junctional n. a brownish, smooth, flat or slightly raised nevocytic nevus; histologically, there are nests of melanin-containing nevus cells at the dermo-epidermal junction. (See Atlas 2, Part N.)

n. lipomato′sus one that contains much fibrofatty tissue.

melanocytic n. any nevus, usually pigmented, composed of MELANOCYTES.

nevocytic n., n. cell n. the most common type of nevus, usually more or less hyperpigmented, initially flat but soon becoming elevated, composed of nests of nevus cells. These nevi are classified as compound, intradermal, or junction according to the histologic pattern and location of nevus cells. Called also mole.

n. of Ota, Ota's n. a persistent mongolian spot–like lesion, usually present at birth and unilateral, involving the conjunctiva and skin about the eye, as well as the sclera, ocular muscles, retrobulbar fat, periosteum, and buccal mucosa. It is a blue or gray-brown patchy area of pigmentation that grows slowly and becomes deeper in color. Although the lesion is benign, malignant MELANOMA occasionally develops, usually in the iris.

pigmented n., n. pigmento′sus one containing MELANIN; the term is usually restricted to nevocytic nevi (moles), but may be applied to other nevi that have pigmentation.

sebaceous n., n. sebaceus of Jadassohn an epidermal nevus of the scalp or less often the face, frequently growing larger during puberty or early adult life. In later life, some lesions may give rise to a variety of new growths, including basal cell CARCINOMA.

n. sim′plex salmon patch.

spider n. vascular SPIDER.

n. spi′lus a smooth, tan to brown macular nevus composed of MELANOCYTE and speckled with smaller, darker macules.

spindle and epithelioid cell n. a benign compound nevus occurring most often in children before puberty, composed of spindle and epithelioid cells located mainly in the dermis, sometimes in association with large atypical cells and multinucleate cells and having a close histopathological resemblance to malignant melanoma.

n. spongio′sus al′bus muco′sae white sponge nevus.

Sutton's n. halo nevus.

n. uni′us la′teris a wartlike epidermal nevus, ranging from flesh colored to brown, found in a linear, unilaterally distributed pattern; on the extremities, the lesion usually follow the long axis, and on the trunk, they usually have a transverse orientation.

vascular n., n. vascula′ris n. vasculo′sus any of various reddish swellings or patches on the skin due to hypertrophy of capillaries; the term includes NEVUS FLAMMEUS, strawberry HEMANGIOMA, blue rubber bleb NEVUS, vascular SPIDER, and cavernous HEMANGIOMA.

white sponge n. a spongy white nevus of a mucous membrane, occurring as a hereditary condition.

newborn (noo′born) 1. recently born; called also neonatal. 2. newborn INFANT.

postmature n., post-term n. post-term INFANT.

premature n., preterm n. preterm INFANT.

Newcastle disease (noo′kas-el) a viral disease of birds, including domestic fowl, characterized by respiratory and gastrointestinal or pneumonic and encephalitic symptoms; it is also transmissible to humans.

Newman (noo′man) Margaret. Nursing educator, theorist, and researcher. Her interest in time, movement, and health began in rehabilitation nursing and is based on Martha ROGERS' conceptual system of nursing. This laid the groundwork for the development of her theory, HEALTH AS EXPANDING CONSCIOUSNESS, proposed as a paradigm of health for nursing practice.

newton (N) (noo′ton) the SI UNIT of force, being that when applied in a vacuum to a body having a mass of 1 kilogram accelerates it at the rate of 1 meter per second squared.

nexus (nek′sus) 1. a bond, as between members of a series or group. 2. gap junction.

NF National Formulary.

NFLPN National Federation of Licensed Practical Nurses.

ng nanogram.

NHGRI National Human Genome Research Institute.

NHLBI National Heart, Lung, and Blood Institute.

Ni nickel.

NIA National Institute on Aging.

NIAAA National Institute on Alcohol Abuse and Alcoholism.

niacin (ni′ah-sin) a water-soluble vitamin of the B complex (see VITAMIN), found in various animal and plant tissues, especially liver, yeast, bran, peanuts, lean meats, fish, and poultry. A well balanced diet usually supplies more than the daily requirement. It is required by the body for the synthesis of the coenzymes NAD and NADP, which are required for many oxidation-reduction reactions. Deficiency of niacin produces PELLAGRA, and administration of niacin is used to prevent and treat that condition. It is also used to treat HYPERLIPIDEMIA. Called also NICOTINIC ACID.

niacinamide (ni″ah-sin-am′ĭd) the amide of NIACIN, occurring naturally in the body and interconvertible with niacin; used in prophylaxis and treatment of PELLAGRA, administered orally, intravenously, or intramuscularly. Called also nicotinamide.

NIAID National Institute of Allergy and Infectious Diseases.

NIAMSD National Institute of Arthritis and Musculoskeletal and Skin Diseases.

NIBIB National Institute of Biomedical Imaging and Bioengineering.

NIC Nursing Interventions Classification.

nicardipine (ni-kahr′dĭ-pēn) a CALCIUM CHANNEL BLOCKING AGENT that acts as a vasodilator; administered orally as the hydrochloride salt in the treatment of angina pectoris and hypertension.

niche (nich) a small recess, depression or indentation, especially a recess in the wall of a hollow organ that tends to retain contrast media, as revealed by radiographs.

NICHHD National Institute of Child Health and Human Development.

nickel (Ni) (nik′el) a chemical element, atomic number 28, atomic weight 58.71. (See Appendix 6.) It is a major component of some alloys used in dentistry and is also found in stainless steel. Prolonged exposure to nickel, such as in jewelry, can cause nickel DERMATITIS.

nicking (nik′ing) localized constriction of the retinal blood vessels.

niclosamide (ni-klo′sah-mīd) one of the most effective ANTHELMINTIC agents for use against TAPEWORM infections, including most

species that infect humans; it acts by inhibiting anaerobic metabolism.

Nicolas-Favre disease (ne-ko-lah′ fahv′) lymphogranuloma venereum.

nicotinamide (nik″o-tin′ah-mīd) niacinamide.

   ***n.-adenine dinucleotide* (NAD)** a coenzyme that is involved in many biochemical oxidation-reduction reactions. The symbols for the oxidized and reduced forms are NAD and NADH.

   ***n.-adenine dinucleotide phosphate* (NADP)** a coenzyme similar to nicotinamide-adenine dinucleotide but involved in fewer reactions. The symbols for the oxidized and reduced forms are NADP and NADPH.

nicotine (nik′o-tēn, nik′o-tin) a very poisonous alkaloid that in its pure state is a colorless, pungent, oily liquid, having an acrid burning taste. It is a constituent of TOBACCO, and is also produced synthetically. It is administered orally, intranasally, or by inhalation as an aid to smoking cessation. In water solution, it is sometimes used as an insecticide and plant spray.

Although nicotine is highly toxic, the amount inhaled while smoking tobacco is too small to cause death. The nicotine in tobacco can, however, cause indigestion and increase in blood pressure, and dull the appetite. It also acts as a vasoconstrictor. Researchers link SMOKING with heart disease, lung cancer, and other diseases.

   n. poisoning poisoning by NICOTINE, such as in children who eat cigarettes, workers who handle wet TOBACCO leaves, or persons who overuse nicotine gums or patches. Symptoms include stimulation followed by depression of the central and autonomic nervous systems and occasionally death due to respiratory paralysis. Called also nicotinism.

   n. polacrilex nicotine bound to a cation exchange RESIN; used in nicotine chewing gum as an aid to smoking cessation.

nicotinic (nik″o-tin′ik) pertaining to the transmission of nerve impulses mediated by NICOTINIC RECEPTORS.

nicotinic acid (nik″o-tin′ik) niacin.

nicotinism (nik′o-tin-izm″) nicotine poisoning.

nictitation (nik″tĭ-ta′shun) winking.

NICU neonatal INTENSIVE CARE UNIT.

NIDA National Institute on Drug Abuse.

NIDCD National Institute on Deafness and Other Communication Disorders.

nidation (ni-da′shun) implantation (def. 1).

Nidation, occurring over the period between 7 to 10 days after fertilization. From Dorland's, 2000.

NIDCR National Institute of Dental and Craniofacial Research.

NIDDKD National Institute of Diabetes and Digestive and Kidney Diseases.

NIDDM non–insulin-dependent diabetes mellitus, former name for type 2 DIABETES MELLITUS.

nidus (ni′dus) [L.] 1. a nest or cluster. 2. the point of origin or focus of a disease process. 3. nucleus (def. 2). adj., **ni′dal.**

NIEHS National Institute of Environmental Health Sciences.

Niemann-Pick disease (ne′mahn pik′) a lysosomal storage disease due to sphingomyelin accumulation in the reticuloendothelial system; there are five types distinguished by age of onset, amount of central nervous system involvement, and degree of enzyme deficiency. At least some types are characterized by foamy reticular cells containing phospholipids which infiltrate the liver, spleen, lungs, lymph nodes, and bone marrow.

nifedipine (ni-fed′ĭ-pēn) a CALCIUM CHANNEL BLOCKING AGENT administered orally as a coronary VASODILATOR in the treatment of ANGINA PECTORIS; also used in the treatment of HYPERTENSION.

night blindness inability or a reduced ability to see in dim light; the eyes not only see more poorly in dim light, but are slower to adjust from brightness to dimness. Called also nyctalopia.

Depending on its brightness, light is perceived by either of two sets of visual cells located in the retina of the eye. One set, the cones, perceive bright light primarily; the other set, the rods, perceive dim light primarily. Dim light produces a change in a pigment called rhodopsin in the rods. This change causes nerve impulses to travel to the brain, where they register as visual impressions. Night blindness occurs when the rods lack rhodopsin.

One cause of night blindness is a deficiency of vitamin A—the primary source of rhodopsin. The defect in vision usually can be cured by proper diet plus therapeutic doses of the deficient vitamin.

In the elderly, there is sometimes a diminution of rhodopsin, with resulting night blindness. Other losses in vision may follow. Diminished blood supply to the eyes is thought to be a cause of this form of the condition. Treatment generally is only of limited effectiveness.

Night blindness sometimes accompanies glaucoma.

Nightingale (nīt′in-gāl″) Florence (1820–1910). Founder of modern nursing. She was born in Florence, Italy, of English parents. In 1854 she led a group of nurses to the Crimea to care for English troops, and later she reorganized military nursing and sanitation in England and then India. She also contributed to the field of dietetics, and her skill as a statistician in gathering data won her election to the Royal Statistical Society and honorary membership in the American Statistical Association.

Nightingale Pledge an oath written in 1893 by a committee of which Mrs. Lystra E. Gretter was chairman. It was first administered to the 1893 graduating class of the Farrand Training School, Harper Hospital, Detroit, Michigan. It is as follows:

I solemnly pledge myself before God and in the presence of this assembly:

To pass my life in purity and to practice my profession faithfully.

I will abstain from whatever is deleterious and mischievous, and will not take or knowingly administer any harmful drug.

I will do all in my power to elevate the standard of my profession, and will hold in confidence all personal matters committed to my keeping and all family affairs coming to my knowledge in the practice of my profession.

With loyalty will I endeavor to aid the physician in his work, and devote myself to the welfare of those committed to my care.

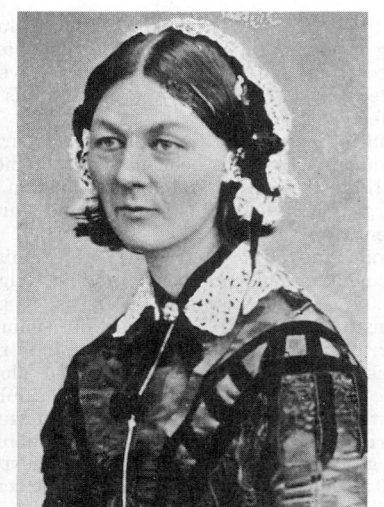

Florence Nightingale. Courtesy of Florence Nightingale Museum, London, U.K.

nightmare (nīt′mār) a terrifying dream; an anxiety attack during dreaming, accompanied by mild autonomic reactions and usually awakening the dreamer, who recalls the dream but is oriented.

    n. disorder a sleep disorder of the parasomnia group, consisting of repeated episodes of nightmares.

NIGMS National Institute of General Medical Sciences.

nigra (ni′grah) substantia nigra. adj., **ni′gral.**

nigrities (ni-grish′e-ēz) blackness.

    n. lin′guae black tongue.

nigrostriatal (ni″gro-stri-a′tal) projecting from the substantia nigra to the corpus striatum; said of a bundle of nerve fibers.

NIH National Institutes of Health.

nihilism (ni′ĭ-lizm) 1. an attitude of skepticism regarding traditional values and beliefs or their frank rejection. 2. a delusion of nonexistence of part or all of the self or the world. adj., **nihilis′tic.**

Nikolsky's sign (nĭ-kol′skēz) in pemphigus vulgaris and some other bullous diseases, the outer epidermis separates easily from the basal layer on exertion of firm sliding manual pressure.

nilutamide (ni-loo′tah-mīd) a nonsteroidal antiandrogen used as an antineoplastic, in combination with measures to lower testosterone levels such as bilateral orchiectomy, in treatment of prostatic carcinoma; administered orally.

NIMH National Institute of Mental Health.

nimodipine (ni-mo′dĭ-pēn) a CALCIUM CHANNEL BLOCKING AGENT used as a vasodilator in the treatment of neurologic deficits associated with subarachnoid hemorrhage from a ruptured intracranial aneurysm; administered orally.

NINDS National Institute of Neurological Disorders and Stroke.

NINR National Institute of Nursing Research.

niobium (Nb) (ni-o′be-um) a chemical element, atomic number 1, atomic weight 92.906. (See Appendix 6.)

NIOSH National Institute for Occupational Safety and Health.

NIP National Immunization Program.

nipple (nip′l) 1. the pigmented projection at the tip of each BREAST; it is smaller in men than women. In women it gives outlet to the lactiferous DUCTS. Called also mammary papilla, mammilla, and teat. 2. any structure shaped like the nipple of the breast; see PAPILLA.

The nipples are located slightly to the side rather than in the middle of the breasts. Usually, the size of the nipple is in proportion to the size of the breast, but large nipples may be found on small breasts and vice versa.

Surrounding the nipple is a pigmented area called the areola. The color of the areola varies with the complexion. In childless women, it is usually reddish. During pregnancy it increases in size and darkens in color, becoming almost black in brunettes. The color fades after the milk-producing period ends. The tip of the female nipple contains tiny depressions that are openings of the lactiferous ducts. During pregnancy special care should be given the nipples. Any secretion that accumulates should be gently washed off. If the nipples are tender, the physician will advise the use of cold cream, cocoa butter, lanolin, or another emollient to increase their pliability.

nisoldipine (ni-sol′dĭ-pēn) a CALCIUM CHANNEL BLOCKING AGENT used in the treatment of hypertension; administered orally.

NISS New Injury Severity Score, a patient classification system.

Nissen procedure (nis′en) fundoplication.

nisus (ni′sus) [L.] an effort, strong tendency, or endeavor to achieve an outcome or aim.

nit (nit) the egg of a LOUSE.

nitrate (ni′trāt) any salt or ester of nitric acid; organic nitrates are used in the treatment of angina pectoris and as preservatives in meat products. Some individuals have sensitivity to nitrates and may suffer from headache, diarrhea, or urticaria after ingesting them.

nitric (ni′trik) pertaining to or containing nitrogen in one of its higher valences.

n. acid a highly caustic, fuming acid that has a characteristic choking odor and can be fatal if swallowed. It is sometimes used as a cauterizing agent in the eradication of warts; large amounts of it on the skin can cause necrosis. It is also used in the form of its potassium and sodium salts. The antidote for nitric acid poisoning is liberal application of an alkali or sodium bicarbonate.

n. oxide 1. NO, a naturally occurring gas that in the body is a short-lived dilator released from vascular epithelial cells in response to the binding of vasodilators to endothelial cell receptors; it causes inhibition of muscular contraction, and thus relaxation. Excesses of nitric oxide are toxic to cells of the central nervous system and also cause the drop in blood pressure seen in septic shock. Called also endothelial- or endothelium-derived relaxing factor. 2. a preparation of nitric oxide used together with ventilatory support or other agents in the treatment of respiratory failure due to persistent fetal circulation in term and near-term neonates; administered by inhalation.

nitride (ni′trīd) a binary compound of nitrogen with a metal.

nitrification (ni″trĭ-fĭ-ka′shun) the bacterial oxidation of ammonia and organic nitrogen to nitrites and nitrates in the soil.

nitrifying (ni′trĭ-fi″ing) oxidizing ammonia into nitrites and then into nitrates; said of certain bacteria.

nitrile (ni′tril) an organic compound containing trivalent nitrogen attached to one carbon atom, —C≡N.

nitrocellulose (ni″tro-sel′u-lōs) pyroxylin.

Nitrodisc (ni′tro-disk) trademark for a preparation of NITROGLYCERIN, a VASODILATOR used in treatment of ANGINA PECTORIS.

Nitro-Dur (ni′tro-dur) trademark for a preparation of NITROGLYCERIN, a VASODILATOR used in treatment of ANGINA PECTORIS.

nitrofuran (ni″tro-fu′ran) any of a group of antibacterials, including NITROFURANTOIN, NITROFURAZONE, and others, that are effective against a wide range of bacteria.

nitrofurantoin (ni″tro-fu-ran′to-in) a broad-spectrum ANTIBACTERIAL agent used in treatment of urinary tract infections.

nitrofurazone (ni″tro-fu′rah-zōn) an ANTIBACTERIAL agent effective against a wide variety of organisms, used as a topical antiinfective agent for skin lesions including wounds, burns, skin infections, and ulcers and to aid healing and prevent infection of skin grafts and other kinds of infections.

nitromersol (ni″tro-mer′sol) a mercurial compound that has been used as a topical antiinfective agent and for disinfection of surgical and dental instruments and equipment.

nitrogen (N) (ni′tro-jen) a chemical element, atomic number 7, atomic weight 14.007. (See Appendix 6.) It is a gas constituting about four-fifths of common air; chemically it is almost inert. It is not poisonous but is fatal if breathed alone because of oxygen deprivation. It is soluble in the blood and body fluids, and can cause serious symptoms when released as bubbles of gas by rapid decompression (see BENDS). Nitrogen occurs in proteins and amino acids and is thus present in all living cells.

n. 13 a radioactive isotope of nitrogen having a half-life of 9.97 minutes and decaying by positron emission; it is used as a TRACER in positron emission TOMOGRAPHY.

n. balance the state of the body in regard to the rate of PROTEIN intake and protein utilization. When protein is metabolized, about 90 per cent of its nitrogen is excreted in the urine in the form of UREA, URIC ACID, CREATININE, and other nitrogen end-products. The remaining 10 per cent of the nitrogen is eliminated in the feces. A *negative nitrogen balance* occurs when more protein is used by the body than is taken in. A *positive nitrogen balance* implies a net gain of protein in the body. Negative nitrogen balance can be caused by such factors as MALNUTRITION, debilitating diseases, blood loss, and GLUCOCORTICOIDS. A positive balance can be caused by exercise, growth HORMONE, and TESTOSTERONE.

liquid n. nitrogen in liquid form, i.e., below −195.79°C; used as a coolant, such as in thermographic equipment.

n. mustards a group of toxic, blistering ALKYLATING AGENTS that are cell cycle phase nonspecific; it includes nitrogen mustard itself (MECHLORETHAMINE hydrochloride), CHLORAMBUCIL, CYCLOPHOSPHAMIDE, IFOSFAMIDE, and MELPHALAN. Some have been used as antineoplastic AGENTS in certain forms of cancer; they do not cure these conditions, but ease their effects by destroying mitotic cells (those newly formed by division), thereby affecting malignant tissue in its early stage of development, and leaving normal tissue unaffected. They are especially useful in treatment of leukemia, in which they reduce the leukocyte count, and in cases in which the malignant disease is widespread throughout the body and therefore cannot be effectively treated locally by surgery or radiotherapy. In cases of lung cancer, mechlorethamine hydrochloride is usually injected directly into the lungs via the pulmonary circulation. Side effects, which tend to limit the usefulness of these drugs, include nausea, vomiting, and a decrease in bone marrow production.

nonprotein n. (NPN) the nitrogenous constituents of the blood exclusive of the protein bodies, consisting of the nitrogen of urea, uric acid, creatine, creatinine, amino acids, polypeptides, and an undetermined part known as rest nitrogen. Measurement of this is used as a test of renal function, but has been largely replaced by measurement of specific substances, such as UREA and CREATININE.

n. washout test a test for VITAL CAPACITY of lungs; with the patient inhaling pure oxygen, the volume of exhaled nitrogen is obtained for each breath until it falls below 1 per cent of the gas being exhaled (usually about seven minutes' time); the total volume of nitrogen that has been exhaled at this point is assumed to be 0.8 of the vital capacity.

n. washout test, single breath the patient inhales a vital capacity's volume of pure oxygen and then slowly exhales. The nitrogen content of the exhalation is measured over the entire breath and a curve is generated; different parts of the curve represent nitrogen concentrations of gas in different components of the total lung capacity, and can be analyzed for irregularities. Called also single breath test.

nitrogenous (ni-troj′ĕ-nus) containing nitrogen.

nitroglycerin (ni″tro-glis′er-in) a chemical well known as an explosive but also having medical uses; it is a vasodilator and is used medically especially in the prophylaxis and treatment of ANGINA PECTORIS. Called also glyceryl trinitrate.

The most common means of administration has been the sublingual tablet, which is placed under the tongue when the attack occurs; it is not effective if swallowed. Under the tongue, it quickly dissolves and should give relief within 1 or 2 minutes. It may cause transient palpitation, flushing, faintness, and perhaps headache. The patient who is taking nitroglycerin should keep it nearby at all times, stored in a tightly closed dark glass container free from heat and moisture. It is not addicting and there is no limit to the number that may be taken in a 24-hour period; however, no more than three tablets should be taken at 5 minute intervals during an attack. If no relief is obtained 15 minutes after the third tablet is taken, the physician should be notified immediately.

Several alternatives to sublingual tablets have been developed that also are absorbed through the oral mucosa, including extended release buccal tablets, which are held between the lip or cheek and upper gum, and a lingual aerosol, which is sprayed on or under the tongue.

Oral administration is now also possible, by means of extended-release tablets or capsules.

Nitroglycerin is injected intravenously for prophylaxis and long-term treatment of angina pectoris, control of blood pressure during surgery or creation of controlled hypotension during surgery, and as an adjunct in the treatment of congestive HEART FAILURE.

An alternative to sublingual administration of nitroglycerin is application in an ointment to a hairless site on the body surface. Rotation of sites helps eliminate minor skin irritation which is a common problem. The drug is applied by using a manufacturer-supplied measuring applicator paper. A measured amount of ointment is squeezed onto the paper (never directly on the skin) in a thin uniform layer and the paper is placed on the site. The paper is then covered with plastic wrap and held in place with tape or an elastic bandage.

The usual dosage is a 1- to 2-inch strip, but 5-inch strips are also available. Most patients need several applications per day. The area is cleansed of any remaining ointment and a new site chosen when the next dose is due. Patients who are to use the nitroglycerin ointment at home must be given detailed instructions in its use and should be aware of its expected results and local and systemic side effects.

Nitroglycerin is also available as a transdermal patch.

nitrosourea (ni-tro″so-u-re′ah) any of a group of cell cycle phase nonspecific, lipid soluble biological ALKYLATING AGENTS, including CARMUSTINE, LOMUSTINE, SEMUSTINE, and STREPTOZOCIN; they cross the blood-brain barrier and are used as antineoplastic AGENTS. Streptozocin is an antibiotic that contains a nitrosourea group and differs somewhat in action from the other three.

Nitrostat (ni′tro-stat) trademark for a preparation of NITROGLYCERIN, a VASODILATOR used in treatment of ANGINA PECTORIS.

nitrous (ni′trus) pertaining to or containing nitrogen in its lowest valence.

N

n. oxide a colorless, odorless gas that is a weak inhalational anesthetic, usually used in combination with a potent halogenated inhalational anesthetic to produce general ANESTHESIA or briefly for dental surgery. Its use as a sole agent requires high concentrations that may cause HYPOXIA. ABUSE poses the risk of anoxic death from ASPHYXIA. Popularly known as laughing gas.

nizatidine (nĭ-za'tĭ-dēn) a histamine H_2 receptor antagonist, used to inhibit gastric acid secretion in the treatment of gastric and duodenal ulcer, gastroesophageal reflux disease, and conditions that cause gastric hypersecretion; administered orally.

Nizoral (niz-or'al) trademark for preparations of KETOCONAZOLE, an antifungal AGENT.

NKF National Kidney Foundation.

NLM NATIONAL LIBRARY OF MEDICINE, part of the NATIONAL INSTITUTES OF HEALTH.

NLN National League for Nursing.

NLNAC National League for Nursing Accrediting Commission.

nm nanometer.

NMDS Nursing Minimum Data Set.

NMR nuclear magnetic resonance.

No nobelium.

Noack syndrome (no'ak) Pfeiffer's syndrome.

NOAEL no observed adverse effect level.

nobelium (No) (no-be'le-um) a chemical element, atomic number 102, atomic weight 253. (See Appendix 6.)

NOC Nursing Outcomes Classification.

Nocardia (no-kahr'de-ah) a genus of gram-negative, aerobic, spore-forming bacteria, including *N. asteroi'des,* a species of opportunistic pathogens that cause NOCARDIOSIS and actinomycotic MYCETOMA.

nocardial (no-kahr'de-al) pertaining to or caused by *Nocardia*.

Nocardiopsis (no-kahr″de-op'sis) a genus of gram-positive, aerobic soil bacteria; they resemble *Nocardia* but differ in cell wall type and are not resistant to lysozymes. They are potential pathogens, causing abscesses and pulmonary lesions.

nocardiosis (no-kahr″de-o'sis) infection with *Nocardia*.

nocebo (no-se'bo) [L.] an adverse, nonspecific side effect occurring in conjunction with a medication but not directly resulting from the pharmacologic action of the medication.

noci- word element [L.], *harm; injury.*

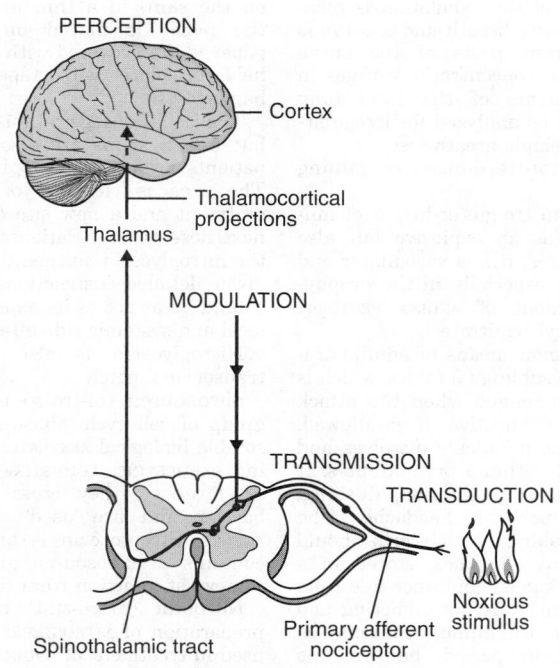

The four processes that make up nociception: transduction, transmission, modulation, and perception. From Ferrante and VadeBoncouer, 1993.

nociassociation (no″se-ah-so″se-a′shun) unconscious discharge of nervous energy under the stimulus of trauma.

nociception (no″se-sep′shun) the ability to feel PAIN, caused by stimulation of a NOCICEPTOR. Physiologically, it is composed of four processes: TRANSDUCTION, TRANSMISSION, MODULATION, and PERCEPTION. (See illustration.) Called also pain sense, algesia, and algesthesia.

nociceptor (no″se-sep′tor) a receptor for PAIN, stimulated by various kinds of tissue injury. adj., **nocicep′tive.**

noci-influence (no″se-in′floo-ens) injurious or traumatic influence.

nociperception (no″se-per-sep′shun) nociception.

noctalbuminuria (nok″tal-bu″mĭ-nu′re-ah) ALBUMINURIA in urine secreted at night.

noctiphobia (nok″tĭ-fo′be-ah) irrational fear of night and darkness.

nocturia (nok-tu′re-ah) urinary FREQUENCY at night; called also nycturia.

node (nōd) a small mass of tissue in the form of a swelling, knot, or protuberance, either normal or pathological. adj., **no′dal.**

n. of Aschoff and Tawara atrioventricular node.

atrioventricular n., AV n. a collection of cardiac fibers at the base of the interatrial septum that transmits the cardiac impulse initiated by the SINOATRIAL NODE.

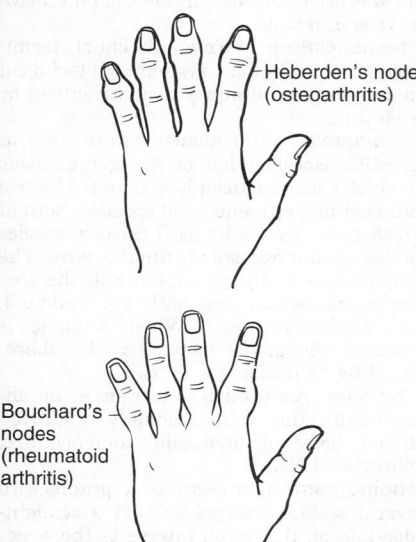

Heberden's nodes (osteoarthritis)

Bouchard's nodes (rheumatoid arthritis)

Comparison of Heberden's nodes (seen in patients with osteoarthritis) with Bouchard's nodes (seen in patients with rheumatoid arthritis). From Copstead and Banasik, 2000.

Bouchard's n's cartilaginous and bony enlargements of the proximal interphalangeal joints of the fingers in degenerative joint disease; such nodes on the distal joints are called Heberden's nodes. See accompanying illustration.

Delphian n. a lymph node encased in the fascia in the midline just above the thyroid isthmus, so called because it is exposed first at operation and, if diseased, is indicative of disease of the thyroid gland.

Flack's n. sinoatrial node.

Heberden's n's nodular protrusions on the phalanges at the distal interphalangeal joints of the fingers in osteoarthritis. Similar nodes on the proximal joints are called BOUCHARD'S NODES.

hemal n's nodes with a rich content of erythrocytes within sinuses, found near large blood vessels along the ventral side of the vertebrae and near the spleen and kidneys in various mammals, especially ruminants, having functions probably like those of the spleen; their presence in humans is doubtful.

Keith's n., Keith-Flack n. sinoatrial node.

Legendre's n's Bouchard's nodes.

lymph n. see LYMPH NODE.

Osler's n's small, raised, swollen, tender areas, bluish or sometimes pink or red, due to inflammation around the site of lodgement of small infected emboli in distal arterioles; they occur commonly in the pads of the fingers or toes, in the palms, or in the soles and are practically pathognomonic for subacute bacterial ENDOCARDITIS.

Parrot's n's bony nodes on the outer table of the skull of infants with congenital syphilis.

n's of Ranvier constrictions of myelinated nerve fibers at regular intervals at which the myelin SHEATH is absent and the axon is enclosed only by Schwann CELL processes.

SA n. sinoatrial node.

Schmorl's n. an irregular or hemispherical bone defect in the upper or lower margin of the body of a vertebra into which the nucleus pulposus of the intervertebral disk herniates.

sentinel n. 1. the first LYMPH NODE to receive drainage from a tumor; used to determine whether there is lymphatic metastasis in certain types of cancer. If this node is negative for malignancy, others "upstream" from it are usually also negative. 2. signal n.

signal n. an enlarged supraclavicular lymph node; often the first sign of a malignant abdominal tumor.

N

singer's n's vocal cord nodules.

sinoatrial n. a collection of atypical muscle fibers in the wall of the right atrium where the rhythm of cardiac contraction is usually established; therefore also referred to as the pacemaker of the heart. Called also SA node.

syphilitic n. a swelling on a bone due to syphilitic periostitis.

n. of Tawara atrioventricular node.

teacher's n's vocal cord nodules.

Troisier's n., Virchow's n. sentinel node.

nodi (no'di) [L.] plural of NODUS.

nodose (no'dōs) having nodes or projections.

nodosity (no-dos'ĭ-te) 1. a node. 2. the quality of being nodose.

nodular (nod'u-lar) marked with, or resembling, nodules.

nodulation (nod″u-la'shun) the formation of or presence of nodules.

nodule (nod'ūl) a small node that is solid and can be detected by touch.

Albini's n's gray nodules of the size of small grains, sometimes seen on the free edges of the atrioventricular valves of infants; they are remains of fetal structures.

apple jelly n's minute, yellowish or reddish brown, translucent nodules, seen on diascopic examination of the lesions of LUPUS VULGARIS.

Aschoff's n's Aschoff's bodies.

Gamna n's brown or yellow pigmented nodules seen in the spleen in certain cases of enlargement, such as Gamna's disease and siderotic splenomegaly.

Jeanselme's n's, juxta-articular n's gummata of tertiary syphilis and of nonvenereal treponematoses, located on joint capsules, bursae, or tendon sheaths.

lymphatic n. 1. lymph node. 2. a small dense accumulation of LYMPHOCYTES found within the cortex of a LYMPH NODE, expressing the cytogenic and defense functions of the tissue. Called also lymph or lymphatic follicle.

milker's n's hard circumscribed nodules on the hands of those who milk cows affected with cowpox.

rheumatic n's small, round or oval, mostly subcutaneous nodules made up chiefly of a mass of Aschoff's bodies and seen in rheumatic fever.

Schmorl's n. Schmorl's node.

singer's n's vocal cord nodules.

surfer's n's hyperplastic, fibrosing granulomas occurring over bony prominences of the lower limbs and feet as a result of repeated trauma from kneeling on surfboards.

teacher's n's vocal cord nodules.

typhus n's minute nodules produced by perivascular infiltration of polymorphonuclear leukocytes and mononuclear cells in rickettsial disease; they were originally described in typhus.

n. of vermis the part of the VERMIS OF THE CEREBELLUM, on the ventral surface, where the inferior medullary velum attaches.

vocal n's, vocal cord n's small white nodules appearing on the vocal cords in chorditis tuberosa with excessive use of the voice; called also singer's nodes or nodules and teacher's nodes or nodules.

nodulus (nod'u-lus) [L.] nodule.

nodus (no'dus) [L.] node.

NOEL no observed effect level.

noise (noiz) 1. unwanted variations in a signal that result from imperfections in transmission; see also signal-to-noise RATIO. 2. any disturbance in a visual signal being recorded in radiography; see also MOTTLE.

Nolvadex (nol'vah-deks) trademark for a preparation of TAMOXIFEN, an ANTIESTROGEN used for breast cancer.

noma (no'mah) gangrenous processes of the mouth or genitalia. In the mouth (*cancrum oris, gangrenous stomatitis*), it begins as a small gingival ulcer and results in gangrenous necrosis of surrounding facial tissues. The condition on the genitalia is called erosive BALANITIS in males and erosive VULVITIS in females.

nomenclature (no'men-kla″chur) terminology; a classified system of technical names, such as of anatomical structures or organisms.

binomial n. the nomenclature used in scientific classification of living organisms in which each organism is designated by two latinized names (genus and species), both of which must always be used because species names are not necessarily unique. NOTE: The genus name is always capitalized, the species name is not, and both are italicized, e.g., *Escherichia coli*. When a name is repeated the genus name may be abbreviated by its initial, e.g., *E. coli*.

Nomina Anatomica (no'mi-nah an″ah-tom'ĭ-kah) the internationally approved official body of anatomic nomenclature; abbreviated NA.

nomogram (nom'o-gram) a graph with several scales arranged so that a straight-edge laid on the graph intersects the scales at related values of the variables; the values of any two variables can be used to find the values of the others.

nomotopic (no″mo-top'ik) occurring at a normal place.

non- word element [L.] *not*.

nonan (no'nan) recurring on the ninth day (every eight days).

noncompliance (non″kom-pli'ans) 1. failure or refusal to conform to or follow rules, regulations, or the advice or wishes of another. 2. a NURSING DIAGNOSIS approved by the North American Nursing Diagnosis Association, defined as a behavior of person and/or caregiver that fails to coincide with a health-promoting or therapeutic plan agreed on by the person (and/or family or community) and the health care professional. In the presence of an agreed-on, health-promoting or therapeutic plan, the person's or caregiver's behavior is fully or partially nonadherent and may lead to clinically ineffective or only partially effective outcomes.

The cause or causes may be difficult to ascertain. The patient/client may have values and beliefs about health that are different from those of the health care provider, or there may be other conflicts in their relationship that work against following the advice offered. In some cases the patient/client may not have the financial resources, family support, physical ability, or emotional stability to perform the prescribed tasks. Poor self-esteem, negative side effects of drugs and other forms of treatment, and lack of progress after adhering to the prescribed regimen can also lead to noncompliance. Since it is assumed that the individual has sufficient knowledge to make an informed decision, lack of knowledge is not considered a likely cause of failure to comply. The nurse also should be aware that the patient/client may have the necessary knowledge and resources but have made an autonomous decision not to comply.

Statements by the patient/client or family member, direct observation of patient/client behaviors, objective measurement of physiologic signs, failure to record self-care activities or to keep appointments, and development of preventable complications are all characteristics indicative of noncompliance. Nursing interventions to improve compliance might include more extensive assessment activities to determine the reason for noncompliance, involving the patient/client in goal-setting, improving the nurse-patient relationship and interaction, and identifying alternative therapies that are more acceptable to the patient/client.

non compos mentis (non kom'pos men'tis) [L.] not of sound mind, and so not legally responsible.

nonconductor (non″kon-duk'tor) a substance that does not readily transmit electricity, light, or heat.

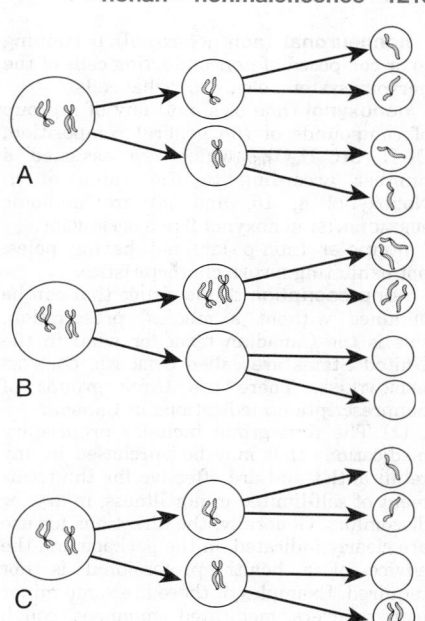

Nondisjunction. Normal meiosis *(A)* is contrasted with failure of homologous chromosomes to separate in meiosis I *(B)* or of sister chromatids to separate in meiosis II *(C)*. From Dorland's, 2000.

nondisjunction (non″dis-jungk'shun) failure either of two homologous chromosomes to pass to separate cells during the first meiotic division, or of the two chromatids of a chromosome to pass to separate cells during mitosis or during the second meiotic division. As a result, one daughter cell has two chromosomes or two chromatids, and the other has none. If this happens during meiosis, an aneuploid individual (for example, a child with Down syndrome) may develop following fertilization.

nonelectrolyte (non″e-lek'tro-līt) a compound which, dissolved in water, does not separate into charged particles and is incapable of conducting an electric current.

noninvasive (non″in-va'siv) not involving puncture of the skin or other entry into the body; said of diagnostic studies and procedures.

nonmaleficence (non-mah-lef'ĭ-sens) a principle of bioethics that asserts an obligation not to inflict harm intentionally. It is useful in dealing with difficult issues surrounding the terminally or seriously ill and injured. Some philosophers combine nonmaleficence and BENEFICENCE, considering them a single principle.

nonneuronal (non″noo-ro′nal) pertaining to or composed of nonconducting cells of the nervous system, e.g., neuroglial cells.

nonoxynol (non-ok′sĭ-nol) any of a group of compounds of the general composition, $C_{15}H_{24}O(C_2H_4O)_n$, which are assigned a number according to the value of n. Nonoxynol 4, 15, and 30 are nonionic SURFACTANTS; nonoxynol 9 is a SPERMICIDE.

nonpolar (non-po′lar) not having poles; not exhibiting DIPOLE characteristics.

nonprescription drugs drugs that can be obtained without a medical prescription; this is the Canadian term for what in the United States are called OVER THE COUNTER MEDICATIONS. There are three groups of nonprescription medications in Canada:

(1) The first group includes proprietary medications that may be purchased in any retail outlet and are effective for the treatment of self-limited minor illness, injury, or discomfort. Generally, the directions for use are clearly indicated on the package and the advice of a health professional is not required. Examples of these are some minor pain relievers, medicated shampoos, cough drops.

(2) The second group of drugs is generally available only in pharmacies and is commonly referred to as over the counter (OTC) medications. These are also intended for the treatment of self-limiting problems but may require the advice of a health professional for proper use. Examples include laxatives, cough and cold medicines, and vitamins.

(3) The third group is the smallest; it consists of medications available only in the pharmacy and used only upon the recommendation of a physician. Insulin, nitroglycerin, and muscle relaxants are common examples. This category also includes certain drugs that are kept in a place of limited public access and can be purchased only if the pharmacist personally dispenses them after a consultation with the patient. They include analgesic compounds that contain low doses of codeine.

nonresponder (non-re-spon′der) an individual who after vaccination against a given virus does not show any IMMUNE RESPONSE when challenged with the virus.

nonsecretor (non″se-kre′tor) a person with A or B type blood whose body secretions do not contain the particular (A or B) substance.

nonself (non′self) in immunology, pertaining to foreign antigens; see also SELF.

nonspecific (non-spĕ-sif′ik) 1. not due to any single known cause. 2. not directed against a particular agent, but rather having a general effect.

nonsteroidal antiinflammatory drug (NSAID) any in a large group of drugs having ANALGESIC, ANTIPYRETIC, and ANTIINFLAMMATORY activity due to their ability to inhibit the synthesis of PROSTAGLANDINS. Examples are ASPIRIN, IBUPROFEN, INDOMETHACIN, NAPROXEN, PHENYLBUTAZONE, SULINDAC, and TOLMETIN. Called also nonsteroidal antiinflammatory agent.

nonstress test (NST) (non-stres′) evaluation of fetal well being during the intrauterine period. Observations of fetal heart rate response to fetal movements are made: a reactive pattern of more than 15 beats per minute above the baseline heart rate twice in 10 minutes is indicative of well being; a nonreactive pattern may indicate asphyxia, maternal medication, fetal anomalies, or a prolonged rest state. See also FETAL MONITORING.

nontreponemal antigen test any of various tests detecting serum antibodies to REAGIN (cardiolipin and lecithin) derived from host tissues in the diagnosis of the *Treponema pallidum* infection of SYPHILIS.

nonunion (non-ūn′yun) failure of the ends of a fractured bone to unite.

nonviable (non-vi′ah-b′l) not capable of living.

Noonan's syndrome (noo′nanz) the male phenotype of TURNER'S SYNDROME, with short stature, webbed NECK, low nuchal hairline, low-set ears, and the elbow deformity CUBITUS VALGUS; valvular pulmonary STENOSIS, rather than COARCTATION OF THE AORTA, is often present.

nor- a chemical prefix denoting either (a) a compound of normal structure (having an unbranched chain of carbon atoms) that is isomeric with one having a branched chain, or (b) a compound whose chain or ring contains one less methylene (CH_2) group than that of its homologue.

noradrenaline (nor″ah-dren′ah-lin) norepinephrine.

noradrenergic (nor″ah-dren-er′jik) activated by or secreting norepinephrine.

no-reflow phenomenon (no re′flo) when cerebral blood flow is restored following prolonged global cerebral ischemia, there is initial hyperemia followed by a gradual decline in perfusion until there is almost no blood flow.

norepinephrine (nor″ep-ĭ-nef′rin) a CATECHOLAMINE that is the NEUROTRANSMITTER of most sympathetic postganglionic neurons and also of certain tracts in the central nervous system. It is also a NEUROHORMONE stored in the chromaffin granules of the adrenal medulla and released in response to sympathetic stimulation, primarily in response to HYPOTENSION. It produces vaso-constriction, an increase in heart rate, and elevation of blood pressure. It is administered intravenously in the form of the bitartrate salt as a VASOPRESSOR to restore blood pressure in certain cases of acute hypotension and to improve cardiac function during decompensation associated with congestive heart failure or cardiovascular surgery. Called also nor-adrenaline.

norethindrone (nor-eth'in-drōn) a proges-tational agent having some anabolic, estro-genic, and androgenic properties; used as the base or the acetate ester in the treatment of amenorrhea, dysfunctional uterine bleeding, and endometriosis, and as an oral contraceptive.

norethynodrel (nor″ĕ-thi'no-drel) a PRO-GESTIN used in treatment of abnormal uterine bleeding, amenorrhea, and endome-triosis and, in combination with an ESTRO-GEN, as an oral CONTRACEPTIVE.

norfloxacin (nor-flok'sah-sin) a broad-spectrum QUINOLONE antibacterial agent effective against penicillin-resistant gram-negative and gram-positive bacteria.

norgestimate (nor-jes'tĭ-māt) a synthetic progestational AGENT used in combination with an estrogen component as an oral CONTRACEPTIVE.

norgestrel (nor-jes'trel) a potent syn-thetic progestational agent used, alone or in combination with an estrogen compo-nent, as an oral contraceptive.

Norinyl (nor'ĭ-nil) trademark for oral CONTRACEPTIVE preparations containing NOR-ETHINDRONE as the progestational agent and either ETHINYL ESTRADIOL or MESTRANOL as the estrogenic agent.

norm (norm) 1. a fixed ideal or standard. 2. in particular, any of the rules by which human behavior is evaluated and which provide direction for achieving the values of a culture; the norms for a culture are usually learned in childhood.

n. referenced test a standardized test that has been carefully developed and has extensive reliability and validity data avail-able.

norm(o)- word element [L.], *normal; usual; conforming to the rule.*

normal (nor'mal) agreeing with the regular and established type. When said of a solution, it denotes one containing one chemical equivalent of solute per liter of solution; e.g., a 0.5 normal (0.5 N) solution has a concentration of 0.5 Eq/l. The use of standard units (Eq/l) is now preferred.

n. saline solution, n. salt solution physiologic salt solution.

normetanephrine (nor-met″ah-nef'rin) metabolite of norepinephrine excreted in the urine and found in certain tissues.

normoblast (nor'mo-blast) a nucleated precursor cell in the erythrocytic SERIES, specifically one in a normal course of erythrocyte maturation, as opposed to a MEGALOBLAST. The four developmental stages of the series are called *pronormoblasts* or *proerythroblasts, basophilic normoblasts* or *erythroblasts, polychromatophilic* (or *poly-chromatic*) *normoblasts* or *erythroblasts,* and *orthochromatic normoblasts* or *erythro-blasts.* adj., **normoblas'tic.**

normoblastosis (nor″mo-blas-to'sis) ex-cessive production of normoblasts by the bone marrow.

normocalcemia (nor″mo-kal-se'me-ah) a normal level of calcium in the blood. adj., **normocalce'mic.**

normochromia (nor″mo-kro'me-ah) nor-mal color of erythrocytes.

normocyte (nor'mo-sīt) an erythrocyte that is normal in size, shape, and color.

normocytosis (nor″mo-si-to'sis) a nor-mal state of the blood in respect to erythrocytes.

normoglycemia (nor″mo-gli-se'me-ah) normal glucose content of the blood. adj., **normoglyce'mic.**

normokalemia (nor″mo-kah-le'me-ah) a normal level of potassium in the blood. adj., **normokale'mic.**

normospermic (nor″mo-sper'mik) pro-ducing spermatozoa normal in number, morphology, and motility.

normotensive (nor″mo-ten'siv) 1. charac-terized by normal tension, tone, or pres-sure, as by normal blood pressure. 2. a person with normal blood pressure.

normothermia (nor″mo-ther'me-ah) a normal state of temperature. adj., **nor-mother'mic.**

normotonia (nor″mo-to'ne-ah) normal tone or tension. adj., **normoton'ic.**

normovolemia (nor″mo-vo-le'me-ah) nor-mal blood volume.

Norpace (nor'pās) trademark for a prep-aration of DISOPYRAMIDE, an ANTIARRHYTHMIC agent.

Norplant (nor'plant) trademark for a preparation of the CONTRACEPTIVE LEVONOR-GESTREL in the form of an implant that can be inserted beneath a woman's skin.

Norpramin (nor'prah-min) trademark for a preparation of DESIPRAMINE, a tricyclic ANTIDEPRESSANT.

Norrie's disease (nor'rēz) an X-linked disorder, present from birth, con-sisting of bilateral blindness from retinal

N

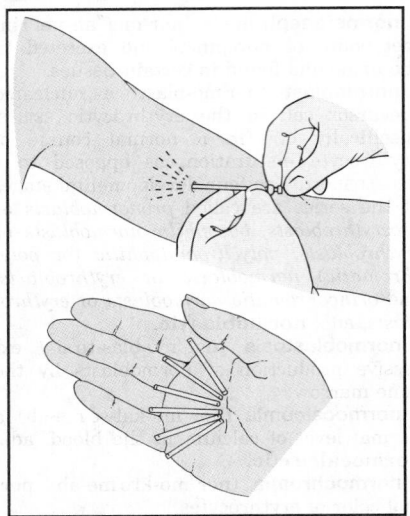

Insertion of Norplant capsules beneath the skin. From Nichols and Zwelling, 1997.

malformation with possible mental retardation and deafness developing later.

nortriptyline (nor-trip′tĭ-lēn) a tricyclic ANTIDEPRESSANT, administered orally as the hydrochloride salt; it is also used to treat panic disorder and chronic severe pain.

nos(o)- word element [Gr.], *disease.*

noscapine (nos′kah-pēn) an alkaloid present in OPIUM; used as a nonaddictive antitussive.

nose (nōz) the specialized structure of the face that serves both as the organ of smell and as a means of bringing air into the lungs. (See also Plates.) Air breathed in through the nose is warmed, filtered, and humidified; that breathed through the mouth is not.

The NOSTRILS, which form the external entrance of the nose, lead into the two nasal CAVITIES, which are separated from each other by the nasal SEPTUM, a partition formed of cartilage and bone. Three bony ridges project from the outer wall of each nasal cavity and partially divide the cavity into three air passages. At the back of the nose these passages lead into the PHARYNX. The passages also are connected by openings with the paranasal SINUSES. One of the functions of the nose is to drain fluids discharged from the sinuses. The nasal cavities also have a connection with the ears by the EUSTACHIAN TUBES, and with the region of the eyes by the nasolacrimal DUCTS.

The interior of the nose is lined with mucous membrane, and most of the membrane is covered with minute hairlike projections called CILIA. Moving in waves these cilia sweep out from the nasal passages the nasal mucus, which may contain pollen, dust, and bacteria from the air. The mucous membrane also acts to warm and moisten the inhaled air.

High in the interior of each nasal cavity is a small area of mucous membrane that is not covered with cilia. In this pea-sized area are located the endings of the nerves of smell, the olfactory RECEPTORS. These receptors sort out odors. Unlike the taste BUDS of the tongue, which distinguish between only four different tastes (salt, sweet, sour, and bitter), the olfactory receptors can detect innumerable different odors. This ability to smell contributes greatly to what we usually think of as taste, because much of what we consider flavor is really odor. (See also SMELL.)

Disorders of the Nose. The mucous membrane of the nose is subject to inflammation; any such inflammation is called RHINITIS, which may be caused by the COMMON COLD, or by an allergy, particularly HAY FEVER. Nasal POLYPS may obstruct the nasal passages. EPISTAXIS, or nosebleed, may be caused by an injury to the nose or may be a symptom of other diseases. The nasal septum may grow irregularly or be deflected to one side by injury; this condition is called deviated SEPTUM.

Surgery of the Nose. Nasal surgery is indicated in disorders of the nasal septum, polyps and other growths, and traumatic injury to the structures that interfere with normal nasal breathing. Cosmetic plastic surgery is also done to correct disfigurement that is disturbing to the patient.

Patient Care. Prior to surgery the patient is instructed in the kind of surgery anticipated and is informed of the immediate aftereffects of swelling and discoloration. He is told that the residual swelling may last for several weeks and success of the operation cannot be assessed until after that time.

Immediately after surgery the greatest danger is hemorrhage. If the patient swallows repeatedly or spits up blood, excessive bleeding should be suspected. A Teflon splint or intranasal packing often is used to support the nasal structures and prevent the formation of hematoma, another complication that may develop.

Ice compresses are applied for 24 hours after surgery to reduce swelling and minimize bleeding. The patient is placed in semi-Fowler position during this time.

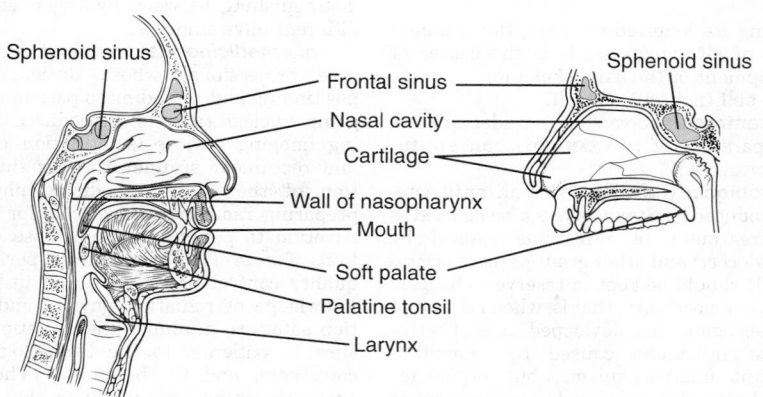

Nose and related structures.

During convalescence the patient should avoid blowing his nose and picking at crusts. A lubricant may be used to soften the crusts, but no swabs or other objects should be used to clean the nose. A humidifier in the room may help reduce drying and irritation of the mucous membranes during healing.

artificial n. 1. a device placed between the endotracheal tube and the breathing apparatus to trap the heat and humidity in the exhaled gas and use it to warm and humidify subsequently inhaled gas. 2. an electronic system used to monitor and classify odors and gases, consisting of a sensor and a pattern recognition system; called also electric nose.

nosebleed (nōz′blēd) epistaxis.

nosocomial (nos″o-ko′me-al) pertaining to or originating in a hospital.

n. infection an infection acquired during hospitalization. More than one third of all such infections are easily preventable without sophisticated and expensive equipment or procedures. In most cases washing the hands after each patient contact is the most effective way to prevent the spread of infections. Other measures include basic cleanliness and sanitation in handling and storing of equipment, and particularly careful handling of urinary catheters and drainage bags. In addition to the urinary tract, other common sites of infection are the respiratory tract and surgical wounds. The Joint Commission on the Accreditation of Health Care Organizations sets specific standards for in-house control of infection. See also INFECTION CONTROL.

nosogeny (no-soj′ĕ-ne) pathogenesis.

nosoparasite (nos″o-par′ah-sīt) an organism found in a disease that it is able to modify, but not to produce.

nosophobia (nos″o-fo′be-ah) irrational fear of sickness or of a specific disease.

nostril (nos′tril) either aperture of the nose; see NARES.

nostrum (nos′trum) a quack, patent, or secret remedy.

not(o)- word element [Gr.], *the back.*

notalgia (no-tal′jah) pain in the back.

notch (noch) an indentation, especially one on the edge of a bone or other organ; called also incisure.

aortic n., dicrotic n. a small downward deflection in the arterial pulse or pressure contour immediately following the closure of the semilunar valves, sometimes used as a marker for the end of systole or the ejection period.

parotid n. the notch between the RAMUS OF THE MANDIBLE and the mastoid PROCESS of the temporal bones.

Rivinus' n., tympanic n. a defect in the upper tympanic part of the temporal bone, filled by the upper portion of the tympanic membrane. Called also Rivinus' or tympanic incisure.

notencephalocele (no″ten-sef′ah-lo-sēl″) occipital encephalocele.

notencephalus (no″ten-sef′ah-lus) a fetus with an occipital ENCEPHALOCELE.

notifiable (no″tĭ-fi′ah-b'l) necessary to be reported to the board of health.

n. disease one required to be reported to federal, state, or local health officials when diagnosed, because of infectiousness, severity, or frequency of occurrence.

notochord (no′to-kord) a cylindrical cord of cells on the dorsal aspect of an embryo, marking its longitudinal axis; the common factor of all CHORDATES. It is the center of development of the axial skeleton.

not-self (not'self) nonself.

Novantrone (no-van'trōn) trademark for a preparation of MITOXANTRONE, an antitumor ANTIBIOTIC.

novobiocin (no″vo-bi'o-sin) an antibacterial produced by *Streptomyces niveus,* used in the treatment of infections caused by staphylococci and other gram-positive organisms. It should be kept in reserve to be used only when necessary, that is, when resistance to other agents has developed. It is effective against infections caused by penicillin-resistant microorganisms, but organisms have been able to develop resistance to novobiocin rapidly. Leukopenia in some patients and jaundice in infants have been observed after novobiocin administration.

Novocain (no'vo-kān) trademark for preparations of procaine, a local anesthetic.

noxious (nok'shus) hurtful; injurious; pernicious.

Np neptunium.

NPA National Perinatal Association.

NPDB National Practitioner Data Bank.

NPN nonprotein nitrogen.

NPO [L.] nil per os (nothing by mouth).

NREM non–rapid eye movement; see SLEEP.

ns nanosecond.

NSAIA nonsteroidal antiinflammatory analgesic (or agent); see NONSTEROIDAL ANTIINFLAMMATORY DRUG.

NSAID nonsteroidal antiinflammatory drug.

NSNA National Student Nurses' Association.

NSPB National Society for the Prevention of Blindness.

N-terminal (ter'min-al) the amino (NH_2) end of a polypeptide chain, conventionally written to the left.

Nubain (nu'bān) trademark for a preparation of NALBUPHINE hydrochloride, an opioid ANALGESIC.

nucha (noo'kah) nape. adj., **nu'chal.**

nuclear (noo'kle-ar) pertaining to a nucleus.

   n. magnetic resonance a phenomenon exhibited by many atomic nuclei: when placed in a constant magnetic field, the nuclei absorb electromagnetic radiation at a few characteristic frequencies. By applying an external magnetic field to a solution in a constant radio frequency field, it is possible to determine the structure of an unknown compound. An application of this technique, called MAGNETIC RESONANCE IMAGING, permits imaging of soft tissues of the body by distinguishing between hydrogen atoms in different environments.

   n. medicine technologist a health care professional whose duties include positioning and attending to patients undergoing nuclear MEDICINE procedures, operating imaging devices (scintillation cameras and rectilinear scanners) under the direction of the nuclear medicine physician, preparing radiopharmaceuticals for administration to patients, making dose calculations for *in vivo* procedures, performing quality control procedures, and utilizing a knowledge of radiation physics and radiation safety to minimize the radiation exposure to patients, to the technologist and coworkers, and to the public. There are currently three organizations that certify nuclear medicine technologists: the American Registry of Radiologic Technologists (ARRT), the American Society of Clinical Pathologists (ASCP), and the Nuclear Medicine Technology Certification Board (NMTCB). Individuals certified by the ARRT are designated RT(N)(ARRT); those certified by the ASCP are designated NM(ASCP); and those certified by the NMTCB are designated CNMT.

nuclease (noo'kle-ās) any of a group of enzymes that split nucleic acids into nucleotides and other products.

nucleated (noo'kle-āt″ed) having a nucleus or nuclei.

nuclei (noo'kle-i) [L.] plural of NUCLEUS.

nucleic acids (noo-kle'ik) extremely complex, long-chain compounds of high molecular weight that occur naturally in the cells of all living organisms and constitute the non–amino acid components of NUCLEOPROTEINS. They form the genetic material of the cell and direct the synthesis of protein within the cell.

Nucleic acids are composed of repeating smaller units, called NUCLEOTIDES, which are made up of a pentose sugar, a nitrogenous base, and a phosphate group. There are two major classes of nucleic acids: DEOXYRIBONUCLEIC ACID (DNA) whose pentose sugar is deoxyribose, and RIBONUCLEIC ACID (RNA) whose pentose sugar is ribose. The major purine and pyrimidine bases in the nucleic acids are adenine (A), guanine (G), and cytosine (C), which occur in both, and thymine (T) in DNA and uracil (U) in RNA.

RNA is present in both the nucleus and the cytoplasm of many cells. Most of the cytoplasmic RNA is associated with ribosomes, which are the site of protein synthesis. RNA molecules perform several functions in the cell, depending on the type of RNA molecule and its specific properties. DNA is a major constituent of chromosomes in the nuclei of all cells. Its chief function is to provide a genetic message that is encoded in the sequence of bases.

nucleocapsid (noo″kle-o-kap′sid) a unit of viral structure, consisting of a CAPSID with the enclosed NUCLEIC ACID; it is generally inside the CYTOPLASM.

nucleofugal (noo″kle-of′u-gal) moving away from a nucleus.

nucleohistone (noo″kle-o-his′tōn) the nucleoprotein complex made up of deoxyribonucleic acid (DNA) and histones. It is the principal constituent of chromatin.

nucleoid (noo′kle-oid) 1. resembling a NUCLEUS. 2. a nucleus-like body sometimes seen in the center of an ERYTHROCYTE. 3. the central region of a bacterium, consisting of a dense irregularly shaped region containing DNA material without a surrounding nuclear MEMBRANE. 4. the genetic material (NUCLEIC ACID) of a virus, situated in the center of the VIRION.

nucleolonema (noo″kle-o″lo-ne′mah) a network of strands formed by organization of a finely granular substance, perhaps containing RNA, in the nucleolus of a cell.

nucleolus (noo-kle′o-lus) [L.] a rounded refractile body in the nucleus of most cells, which is the site of synthesis of ribosomal RNA, becoming enlarged during periods of synthesis and smaller during quiescent periods; multiple nucleoli occur in some cells.

nucleon (noo′kle-on) a PROTON or NEUTRON; one of the particles of an atomic nucleus.

nucleonics (noo″kle-on′iks) nuclear physics.

nucleopetal (noo″kle-op′ĕ-tal) moving toward a nucleus.

nucleophile (noo′kle-o-fīl″) an electron donor in chemical reactions involving covalent catalysis in which the donated electrons bond other chemical groups (electrophiles). adj., **nucleophil′ic.**

nucleoplasm (noo′kle-o-plazm″) the protoplasm of the nucleus of a cell.

nucleoprotein (noo″kle-o-pro′tēn) any of a class of conjugated proteins, consisting of nucleic acids and simple proteins (e.g., a histone).

nucleosidase (noo″kle-o-si′dās) an intracellular enzyme that is capable of causing the decomposition of nucleosides.

nucleoside (noo′kle-o-sīd) any of a class of compounds produced by hydrolysis of NUCLEOTIDES, consisting of a sugar (a pentose or a hexose) and a purine or pyrimidine BASE.

nucleosome (noo′kle-o-sōm″) any of the complexes of histone and DNA in eukaryotic cells, seen under the electron microscope as beadlike bodies on a string of DNA.

nucleotidase (noo″kle-o-ti′dās) an enzyme that splits nucleotides into nucleosides and phosphoric acid.

nucleotide (noo′kle-o-tīd) any of a group of compounds obtained by hydrolysis of NUCLEIC ACIDS, consisting of a purine or pyrimidine BASE linked to a sugar (RIBOSE or DEOXYRIBOSE), which in turn is esterified with PHOSPHORIC ACID.

cyclic n's those in which the phosphate group bonds to two atoms of the sugar forming a ring, as in cyclic AMP and cyclic GMP, which act as intracellular second messengers.

nucleotidyl (nu″kle-o-tīd′il) a nucleotide residue.

nucleotoxin (noo′kle-o-tok″sin) a toxin from cell nuclei, or one that affects cell nuclei.

nucleus (noo′kle-us), pl. *nu′clei* [L.] 1. cell nucleus; a spheroid body within a cell, contained in a double membrane, the nuclear envelope, and containing the CHROMOSOMES and one or more nucleoli. The contents are collectively referred to as *nucleoplasm.* The chromosomes contain DEOXYRIBONUCLEIC ACID (DNA), which is the genetic material that codes for the structure of all the proteins of the cell. 2. a mass of gray MATTER in the central nervous system, especially such a mass marking the central termination of a CRANIAL NERVE. 3. in organic chemistry, the combination of atoms forming the central element or basic framework of the molecule of a specific compound or class of compounds. 4. the dense core of an atom, made of protons and neutrons held together by the strong nuclear force. Traveling in orbit around it is a cloud of negatively charged particles called ELECTRONS. The number of protons in the atomic nucleus gives a substance its identity as a particular ELEMENT. Called also atomic nucleus. adj., **nu′clear.**

n. ambi′guus the nucleus of origin of motor fibers of the glossopharyngeal, vagus, and accessory nerves in the medulla oblongata.

n. an′sae lenticula′ris, n. of ansa lenticularis a collection of neurons in the ansa lenticularis as it curves around the medial edge of the globus pallidus.

arcuate nuclei of medulla oblongata, nu′clei arcua′ti medul′lae oblonga′tae small irregular areas of gray substance on the ventromedial aspect of the pyramid of the medulla oblongata.

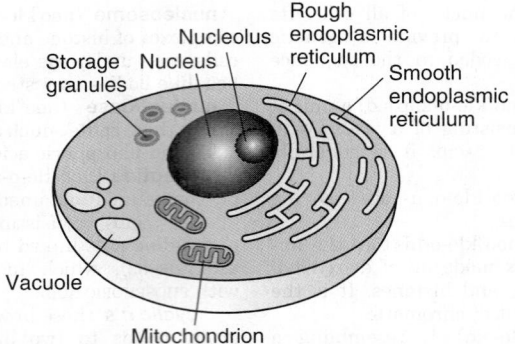

The nucleus and nucleolus of a cell. From Mahon and Manuselis, 2000.

atomic n. nucleus (def. 3).

basal nuclei, nu'clei basa'les specific interconnected subcortical masses of gray MATTER embedded in each cerebral HEMISPHERE and in the upper BRAINSTEM, comprising the CORPUS STRIATUM (caudate and lentiform nuclei), amygdaloid BODY, CLAUSTRUM, and external, extreme, and internal CAPSULES. Called also basal ganglia.

caudal olivary n. a folded band of gray substance enclosing a white core, which produces the elevation on the medulla oblongata known as the olive.

caudate n., n. cauda'tus an elongated, arched gray mass closely related to the lateral ventricle throughout its entire extent, which, together with the putamen, forms the neostriatum.

n. ceru'leus a compact aggregation of pigmented neurons lying below the locus ceruleus.

cochlear nuclei, anterior and posterior the nuclei of termination of sensory fibers of the cochlear nerve (see anatomic Table of Nerves in the Appendices); they partly encircle the inferior cerebellar peduncle at the junction of the medulla oblongata and pons.

dentate n., n. denta'tus the largest of the deep cerebellar nuclei, lying in the white MATTER of the cerebellum just lateral to the emboliform NUCLEUS.

droplet nuclei small particles of pathogen-containing respiratory secretions expelled into the air by coughing, which are reduced by evaporation to small, dry particles that can remain airborne for long periods; one possible mechanism for transmission of infection from one individual to another.

emboliform n., n. embolifor'mis a small cerebellar nucleus lying between the dentate NUCLEUS and the globose NUCLEUS and contributing to the superior cerebellar PEDUNCLES.

fastigial n., n. fasti'gii the most medial of the deep cerebellar nuclei, near the midline in the roof of the fourth ventricle.

globose n., n. globo'sus a cerebellar nucleus lying between the emboliform NUCLEUS and the NUCLEUS FASTIGII and projecting its fibers via the superior cerebellar PEDUNCLE.

intracerebellar nuclei four accumulations of gray MATTER embedded in the white MATTER of the cerebellum, comprising the dentate NUCLEUS, emboliform NUCLEUS, NUCLEUS FASTIGII, and globose NUCLEUS.

lenticular n., lentiform n. the part of the corpus striatum somewhat resembling a biconvex lens, divided into a larger external or lateral part called the putamen and a smaller light colored internal or medial part called the globus pallidus.

motor n. any collection of cells in the central nervous system giving origin to a motor nerve.

olivary n. a folded band of gray matter that encloses a white core and produces the elevation called the OLIVE on the medulla oblongata; it receives heavy projections from the spinal cord, mesencephalon, and cerebral cortex and projects fibers via the contralateral inferior cerebellar peduncle.

nuclei of origin, nu'clei ori'ginis groups of nerve cells in the central nervous system from which arise the motor, or efferent, fibers of the cranial nerves.

paraventricular n., n. paraventricula'ris a band of cells in the wall of the third ventricle in the supraoptic part of the hypothalamus; many of its cells are neurosecretory in function and project to the

cin (and, to a lesser extent, antidiuretic
hormone).

pontine nuclei, nu'clei pon'tis masses
of nerve cells scattered throughout the ventral part of the pons, in which the longitudinal fibers of the pons terminate,
and whose axons in turn cross to the opposite side and form the middle cerebellar
peduncle, which projects fibers to the neocerebellum.

n. pro'prius a column of large neurons
that extends throughout the posterior horn
of the spinal cord.

n. pulpo'sus, pulpy n. a semifluid mass
of fine white elastic fibers forming the
center of an intervertebral disk.

red n., n. ru'ber an oval mass of gray
matter (pink in fresh specimens) in the
anterior part of the tegmentum and
extending into the posterior part of the
hypothalamus; it receives fibers from the
cerebellum.

sensory n. the nucleus of termination
of the afferent (sensory) fibers of a peripheral nerve.

supraoptic n., n. supraop'ticus one
just above the lateral part of the optic
chiasm; many of its cells are neurosecretory
in function and project to the neurohypophysis, where they secrete antidiuretic
hormone (ADH) and, to a lesser extent,
oxytocin; other cells are osmoreceptors that
stimulate ADH release in response to increased osmotic pressure.

tegmental n., laterodorsal several nuclear masses of the reticular formations of
the pons and midbrain, especially of the
latter, where they are in close approximation to the superior cerebellar peduncles.

**vestibular nuclei, nu'clei vestibula'-
res** the four cellular masses in the floor of
the fourth ventricle: *superior* (rostral or
cranial), *lateral, medial,* and *inferior* (caudal)
vestibular nuclei; in them are the terminations of the branches of the vestibular nerve
(see anatomic Table of Nerves in the Appendices). The nuclei give rise to a widely
dispersed special sensory system through
projections to motor nuclei in the brain
stem and cervical cord, to the cerebellum,
and to motor cells throughout the spinal
cord; they also have connections that
provide for conscious perception of, and
autonomic reactions to, labyrinthine stimulation.

nuclide (noo'klīd) a species of atom
characterized by the charge, mass, number,
and quantum state of its nucleus, and
capable of existing for a measurable lifetime
(usually more than 10^{-10} sec).

nullipara (nŭ-lip'ah-rah) a woman who
has not produced a viable offspring; PARA 0.
adj., **nullip'arous.**

nulliparity (nul"ĭ-par'ĭ-te) the state of
being a nullipara.

number (num'ber) a symbol, as a figure
or word, expressive of a certain value or a
specified quantity determined by count.

atomic n. (Z) a number expressive of
the number of protons in an atomic nucleus,
or the positive charge of the nucleus expressed in terms of the electronic charge.

Avogadro's n. (N) (N_A) the number
of molecules in one mole of a substance:
6.023×10^{23}. Called also Avogadro's constant.

CT n. the density assigned to a VOXEL in
a CAT SCAN on an arbitrary scale on which air
has a density -1000; water, 0; and compact
bone $+1000$. See also HOUNSFIELD UNIT.

mass n. (A) the number of nucleons
(protons plus neutrons) in the atom of a
nuclide; generally indicated by a super-
script preceding the symbol of a chemical
element (e.g., ^{131}I), denoting a specific isotope.

oxidation n. a number assigned to each
atom in a molecule or ion that represents
the number of electrons theoretically gained
(positive oxidation numbers) or lost (negative numbers) in converting the atom to the
elemental form.

numbness (num'nes) a lack or diminution of sensation in a part.

nummular (num'u-lar) 1. coin-sized and
coin-shaped. 2. made up of round, flat disks.
3. arranged like a stack of coins.

nunnation (nun-a'shun) the too frequent
use of *n* sounds.

nurse (ners) 1. a person trained in the
scientific basis of NURSING, meeting certain
prescribed standards of education and
clinical competence; see also NURSING PRAC-
TICE. 2. to provide services that are essential
to or helpful in the promotion, maintenance, and restoration of health and well-
being. 3. to breast-feed an infant; see
BREASTFEEDING.

advanced practice n. a registered
NURSE having education beyond the basic
nursing education and certified by a nationally recognized professional organization in
a nursing specialty, or meeting other criteria
established by a Board of Nursing. The Board
of Nursing establishes rules specifying which
professional nursing organization certifications can be recognized for advanced practice
nurses and sets requirements of education,
training, and experience. Designations
recognized as advanced practical nursing

N

include clinical NURSE SPECIALIST, NURSE PRAC-
TITIONER, certified registered NURSE ANESTHE-
TIST, and certified NURSE-MIDWIFE.

n. anesthetist an advanced practice
NURSE who administers intravenous, spinal,
and other ANESTHETICS during surgical operations, deliveries, and other medical and
dental procedures. The certified registered
nurse anesthetist (CRNA) has completed
postgraduate training and been certified in
the administration of anesthetics. The address of the American Association of Nurse
Anesthetists is 222 S. Prospect Ave., Park
Ridge, IL 60068.

certified n. (CN) a registered nurse who
has met the criteria established by the
American Nurses' Association for certification in one or more specialized areas of
nursing practice.

Certified Postanesthesia N. (CPAN) a
postanesthesia nurse who has been certified
by the American Board of Postanesthesia
Nursing Certification.

charge n. a registered nurse responsible for the management of a patient care
unit.

circulating n. a nurse member of the
surgical team, responsible for activities of
the operating room outside the sterile field
and for managing nursing care of the
surgical patient in the room. Responsibilities include application of the nursing
process in coordinating care and support of
the patient; maintenance of a safe, comfortable environment; assistance to members of
the surgical team; identification of potential
environmental hazards; maintenance of
communication between the surgical team,
the surgical staff, and the patient's family
or significant other; and representation of
the patient by acting as advocate during the
period of patient dependence.

clinical n. specialist an advanced practice NURSE with a graduate-level degree in
nursing and competence in a specialized
area of nursing, such as gerontology, pediatrics, or psychiatric nursing. Functions of
the clinical nurse specialist include providing direct patient care, teaching patients
and their families, guiding and planning
care with other personnel, and conducting
research. These skills are made directly
available through the provision of nursing
care to clients and indirectly available
through guidance and planning of care with
other nursing personnel. Clinical nurse
specialists hold a master's degree in nursing, preferably with an emphasis in a
specific clinical area of nursing. Called also
nurse specialist.

n. clinician a registered nurse who
has well-developed competencies such as
for prescribing and implementing direct
and indirect nursing care and articulating nursing therapies with other planned therapies. Nurse clinicians have
expertise in nursing practice and ensure
continuing expertise through clinical
experience and continuing education. Generally, minimal preparation is the baccalaureate degree.

community n. in Great Britain, a public health nurse.

community health n. an especially prepared registered nurse whose work combines elements of both PRIMARY CARE nursing
and PUBLIC HEALTH practice and takes place
primarily outside the therapeutic institution. Emphasis is on disease prevention and
health promotion by measures such as early
detection of disease and prompt intervention in cases of disease or high-risk behavior. See also PUBLIC HEALTH NURSING and
community health NURSING.

consultation-liaison n. liaison nurse.

flight n. a registered nurse who accompanies seriously ill patients during air
transport.

general duty n. a registered nurse,
usually one who has not had formal education beyond the basic nursing program,
who sees to the general nursing care of
patients in a hospital or other health
agency.

graduate n. a graduate of a school of
nursing; often used to designate one who
has not been registered or licensed.

liaison n. 1. a nurse specialist with
a master's degree who provides psychiatric nursing services in nonpsychiatric
settings. 2. in Europe, a nurse who provides information and reassurance to
patients in any of various different settings.

**licensed practical n., licensed voca-
tional n.** a graduate of a school of practical
nursing whose qualifications have been
examined by a state board of nursing and
who has been legally authorized to practice
as a licensed practical or vocational nurse
(L.P.N. or L.V.N.). According to the role
definition proposed as a model by the
American Nurses' Association, the definition of L.P.N. practice has been updated to
include "the performance under the supervision of a registered nurse of those
services required in observing and caring
for the ill, injured, or infirm, in promoting
preventive measures in community health,
in acting to safeguard life and health, in
administering treatment and medication
prescribed by a physician or dentist or in

performing other acts not requiring the skill, judgment, and knowledge of a registered nurse."

n.-midwife a professional nurse who specializes in the care of women throughout pregnancy, delivery, and the postpartum period. The official organization, established in 1955, is the American College of Nurse-Midwives.

n.-midwife, certified (CNM) an advanced practice NURSE who has completed a nurse-midwifery program approved by the American College of Nurse-Midwives (ACNM) and passed the ACNM National Certification Examination.

operating room n. perioperative nurse.

perioperative n. a registered nurse specializing in perioperative nursing practice; the professional organization AORN defines perioperative nurses as "those who provide, manage, teach, and study the care of patients undergoing operative or other invasive procedures." This includes a variety of nursing roles that incorporate both behavioral and technical components; they may include, but are not limited to, roles such as scrub nurse, circulating nurse, and educator. Formerly called operating room nurse.

In the preoperative period, nursing activities can range from a beginning assessment of the patient in the clinic or home, through the preoperative interview, to preoperative assessment and care planning in the holding area or surgical suite. In the intraoperative period, beginning when the patient is transferred to the operating room bed and ending when he or she is admitted to the postanesthesia care unit, the nurse's activities include implementation of planned nursing care and evaluation of appropriateness and effectiveness of care. In the postoperative phase, which begins with admission to the postanesthesia care unit and ends with resolution of the surgical sequelae, nursing activities can range from communicating information to personnel in the postanesthesia care unit to a postoperative evaluation in the clinic or the patient's home.

The perioperative nurse delivers care using the nursing process as described in *Standards of Perioperative Nursing Practice,* published in the United States by the professional organization, the Association of Perioperative Registered Nurses (AORN); in Canada, standards are published by the Operating Room Nurses' Association of Canada.

pool n. an employee of the hospital who is not assigned to a specific patient care unit and is available to work in (float to) units with the greatest need.

n. practice acts laws regulating the practice of nursing. They are included in the codes of all 50 states, the District of Columbia, Puerto Rico, Guam, and the Virgin Islands. Each state and territory has its own statute, yet most have many features in common. The similarities among the various nurse practice acts and the National Council Licensure Examination permits Registered Nurses to move relatively easily from one state to another and continue practicing.

Recently, revisions and amendments to nurse practice acts have facilitated expansion of the role of the Registered Nurse. The revisions and amendments interpret nursing in a broader context than older practice acts that were based on physician delegatory statutes in which the role of the professional nurse was as assistant to the physician rather than as colleague. Newer definitions of nursing view the practice of nursing as including both independent nursing functions and delegated medical functions that may be performed autonomously or in collaboration with other members of the health care team.

n. practitioner an advanced practice NURSE trained in assessment of the physical and psychosocial health-illness status of individuals, families, or groups in a variety of settings through health and development history taking and physical examination. Specialties include family NURSE PRACTITIONER and pediatric NURSE PRACTITIONER.

n. practitioner, family (FNP) a nurse practitioner specializing in the provision of primary care to families.

n. practitioner, pediatric (PNP) a nurse practitioner who specializes in pediatric care.

private n., private duty n. one who attends an individual patient, usually on a fee-for-service basis, and who may specialize in a specific class of diseases.

public health n. community health nurse.

Queen's N. in Great Britain, a district nurse who has been trained at or in accordance with the regulations of the Queen Victoria Jubilee Institute for Nurses.

registered n. a graduate NURSE registered and licensed to practice by a State Board of Nurse Examiners or other state authority.

scrub n. one who directly assists the surgeon in the operating room, being responsible for setting up sterile instruments and supplies and handing them to the surgeon or surgical assistant during the operative procedure. This role may be filled by a registered nurse, a licensed practical or vocational nurse, or a surgical technologist.

n. specialist clinical nurse specialist.

transcultural n. a nurse who is certified by the Transcultural Nursing Society; see also TRANSCULTURAL NURSING.

transcultural n. specialist a nurse prepared in TRANSCULTURAL NURSING through post-baccalaureate education, having studied selected cultures and become knowledgeable about care, health, and environmental factors related to transcultural nursing perspectives. The specialist serves as an expert in selected cultures as a NURSE PRACTITIONER, teacher, researcher, and consultant.

visiting n. community health nurse.

wet n. a woman who breast-feeds the infant of another.

nurse-midwifery (ners-mid'wi-fer-e) the independent management of care of essentially normal newborns and women, antepartally, intrapartally, postpartally, and/or gynecologically, occurring within a health care system which provides for medical consultation, collaborative management, or referral.

nursery (ner'sĕ-re) the department in a hospital where newborn infants are cared for.

nursing (ners'ing) 1. the profession of performing the functions of a NURSE. Nursing is defined by the American Nurses' Association as "the diagnosis and treatment of human responses to actual or potential health problems." See also NURSING PRACTICE. 2. breastfeeding.

n. assessment in the NURSING PROCESS, gathering of information about the health status of the patient/client, analysis and synthesis of these data, and the making of a clinical judgment. The outcome of this assessment is the establishment of a NURSING

WINDOW ON NURSING

Nursing has always been fluid and evolutionary. However, in the past two decades, while the "nature" of nursing has not changed, the practice of nursing has been revolutionized. As long as the nature of nursing has been defined it has included the care of people with actual or potential health problems and the manipulation of the environment to contribute to optimal health. Nursing is defined as including the promotion and maintenance of health, prevention of illness, care of persons during acute phases of illness, rehabilitation or restoration of health, and where all of these are not possible helping to sustain the individual through a dignified death.

More recently nursing has been seen as a vital part of the solution to the almost insurmountable problems our society faces in caring for the elderly, for the chronically ill of all ages, for victims of AIDS, and for those who have little access to health care. New research tells us that nurses can provide excellent and affordable care to many segments of the population—young mothers and children, adults with common health problems, people with chronic illnesses who are trying to get along as best they can with the strengths they have, and the elderly and their families. Nursing's dominant focus is the caring process. Whether involved in high technological interventions in hospital or home, or in lower technological, high interpersonal interventions in hospital, nursing home, and community, nurses have a common definition for success. They define success by the extent to which they can help others. The patients they serve are energizing, particularly when they can serve them well.

Nurses are in practice in the widest variety of health care and health care–related positions imaginable: in hospitals, in community health settings, in entrepreneurial firms of their own and others, in the military, and in governmental positions reviewing and monitoring care. Nurses are educators working with students at all levels. Nurses are researchers studying the human phenomena central to the nursing role. Nurses are in policy positions, helping to influence solutions to America's health problems. Nurses are committed to improving access for all to health care, and they play an important role in health policy in order to effect the changes necessary to move toward this goal. As the 21st century begins, nursing is poised to bring to the public wider recognition and understanding of the benefits of its knowledge. Nursing is a national resource and when properly used can help solve the problems we are facing today and anticipating tomorrow.

CLAIRE FAGIN, PhD, RN

DIAGNOSIS. Data-gathering techniques and sources of objective and subjective data for nursing assessment are both formal and informal. The means by which data can be collected include interview, observation, physical examination, review of laboratory data, review of nursing history and medical history of previous admissions or visits to the clinic, current physician's orders, and consultation with other health care providers.

Objective data are bits of information obtained through the senses (such as a rash) or measurable by instrumentation (such as arterial blood gases). *Subjective data* include information that the subject or patient provides, for example, itching, pain, or depression. The patient or client is the primary source of data, giving firsthand information that has not been filtered through someone or something else.

Assessment and reassessment are ongoing activities. An *initial assessment* is made during the nurse's first contact with the patient. Information gathered at this time establishes a data base, which can be used later to determine whether the patient is progressing toward achievement of specified goals.

In addition to data collection, the assessment phase of the nursing process includes processing or interpreting the data. This too is an ongoing activity as more data are collected. The nurse utilizes herself, her knowledge, and nursing responsibilities to translate the data and make decisions about the areas of care in which the patient can benefit from assistance from the nurse. Once nursing diagnoses are made, a plan of care is developed to set goals or objectives and nursing orders.

n. audit a systematic procedure for assessing the quality of nursing care rendered to a specific patient population. The nursing audit developed partly in response to public demand for accountability for the kind of health care being provided, and partly as the result of a growing recognition among nurses of the need for professional self-regulation.

Concurrent audits are conducted at the time the care is being provided to clients/patients. They may be conducted by means of observation and interview of clients/patients, review of open charts, or conferences with groups of consumers and providers of nursing care.

Retrospective audits are conducted after the patient's discharge. Methods include the study of closed patients' charts and nursing care plans, questionnaires, interviews, and surveys of patients and families.

In any type of audit, the nursing audit involves a thorough and systematic examination of patient records and other sources of information for the purpose of acquiring specific and relevant data. The observable data related to nursing activities are then applied to previously established criteria stated in terms of patient-centered outcomes. Deficiencies in patient care can thus be identified by comparing the actual nursing practice and the effects of the NURSING PROCESS to the established criteria. If deficiencies are identified, appropriate correction can then be taken. This may involve a change in staffing patterns, inservice education programs for members of the nursing staff, patient education programs, a change in available resources (both human and material), and a host of other actions designed to cope with the specific problems identified through the nursing audit.

The nursing audit provides a means of evaluating both the nursing process and the changes in the patient's health status that are a result of nursing interventions. Because the implementation of an audit is greatly facilitated by the development of a data base, the identification of major problems the patient is experiencing, the recording of a plan of action, and the maintenance of progress notes to determine whether the plan of action is effectively achieving desired outcomes, it is clear that a PROBLEM-ORIENTED RECORD is essential to the assessment and improvement of patient care through nursing audits. (See also AUDIT and EVALUATION.)

community health n. a branch of nursing that combines primary CARE and NURSING PRACTICE with PUBLIC HEALTH NURSING done outside of the tertiary care institution; it may involve either individual or aggregate services. See also community health NURSE.

n. diagnosis a concise problem-centered description of actual or potential health problems that alter a person's life processes (physiological, psychological, sociocultural, developmental, or spiritual), and that the nurse is legally allowed and professionally prepared to treat. It is one of the Uniform Nursing Languages.

Diagnosis as PROCESS involves collecting, analyzing, clustering (recognizing a pattern in), and validating clinical data. After the first conference on nursing diagnosis in 1973, the term nursing diagnosis was used to denote an OUTCOME of the problem-solving process rather than the process itself. Hence, a nursing diagnosis identifies specific kinds of health-related problems that are within the domain of nursing. It excludes medical problems that require surgery, prescription drugs, and other modes of therapy that are the prerogative of and legally defined as medical practice. The concept of nursing diagnosis was introduced by V.S. Fry in 1953. Since then it has undergone evolutionary changes in definition and implementation. The First National Conference on Classification of Nursing Diagnoses was held in St. Louis in 1973. In later years there have been additional conferences to revise and define diagnostic terminology. The group is representative of nurses from many different countries and actively solicits input from professional nurses interested in developing and implementing nursing diagnoses.

The three major components of each nursing *diagnostic category* approved by the North American Nursing Diagnosis Association (NANDA) are the title or label, related factors, and defining characteristics. The *title* gives a concise description of the individual's actual or potential health problem.

Related factors help explain physiological, situational, and other factors that can cause the problem or influence its development. *Defining characteristics* are signs and symptoms noted in the individual with the problem. The diagnostic statement itself has two parts, the title or label and the related factors, which are linked to each other by the words "related to." An exception to the use of the words "related to" occurs when using them would describe a clinical situation that a nurse cannot legally diagnose and treat, such as *decreased cardiac output, related to congestive heart failure.* In such cases, a colon replaces the phrase "related to" and is followed by a description of the patient's response. Thus the nursing diagnosis might be *decreased cardiac output: pain secondary to myocardial ischemia.*

Nursing diagnoses are limited to problems amenable to NURSING INTERVENTION and are an integral part of the NURSING PROCESS. They can greatly facilitate written and verbal communication, give direction to NURSING ASSESSMENT activities, and provide a basis for effective nursing care. Nursing diagnosis reflects changes in nursing practice and research and therefore is updated often. Current information on nursing diagnosis definitions, related factors, and defining characteristics can be obtained for a small fee from the North American Nursing Diagnosis Association, 1211 Locust Street, Philadelphia, PA 19107; telephone (800) 647-9002.

n. home an institution that cares for individuals with chronic illnesses and physical impairments. The focus of care is on those not requiring hospitalization but unable to care for themselves. There are officially two types of nursing homes, the *skilled nursing* FACILITY and the *intermediate care* FACILITY. The term *nursing home* is often loosely applied to any residential care home that delivers personal care and other non-health care services.

A *teaching nursing home* is one affiliated with a school of nursing; faculty serve as educators, consultants, and clinical experts in gerontology. The nursing home staff serve as role models and expand the educational opportunities for students in gerontological nursing. Linkages between schools of nursing and nursing facilities also provide the opportunity for nursing research and improvement of patient care.

N. Interventions Classification (NIC) 1. any of a specific group of nursing INTERVENTIONS, defined as "any treatment, based upon clinical judgment and knowledge, that a NURSE performs to enhance patient/client OUTCOMES." 2. a standardized nursing LANGUAGE describing treatments that NURSES perform in all settings and specialties. (See Appendix on Nursing Languages.) This is a research-based language developed as a component of an active and ongoing research program at The Center for Nursing Classification at the University of Iowa College of Nursing. Additional information may be obtained from The Center for Nursing Classification, College of Nursing, University of Iowa, 407 Nursing Building, Iowa City IA 52242-1121. Phone: 319-335-7051; fax: 319-335-6820 or 319-335-9990; e-mail: classification-center@iowa.edu; web site: http://www.nursing.uiowa.edu/nic.

N. Minimum Data Set (NMDS) a nursing LANGUAGE consisting of a minimum set of items of information with uniform definitions and categories concerning the specific dimensions of NURSING, meeting the information needs of multiple data users in the health care system. It includes those specific items of information that are used on a regular basis by the majority of nurses across all types of settings in the delivery of care. It has three categories of elements: (1) nursing care; (2) patient or client demographics; and (3) service elements. (See Appendix on Nursing Languages.)

modular n. a method of care delivery by which a group of nursing staff has 24-hour responsibility for a caseload of patients.

N. Outcomes Classification (NOC) a standardized nursing LANGUAGE of patient/client OUTCOMES developed to evaluate the effects of nursing INTERVENTIONS. (See Appendix on Nursing Languages.)

n. practice the definition of professional nursing practice suggested by the American Nurses' Association is as follows: "The practice of nursing means the performance for compensation of professional services requiring substantial specialized knowledge of the biological, physical, behavioral, psychological, and sociological sciences and of nursing theory as a basis for assessment, diagnosis, planning, intervention, and evaluation in the promotion and maintenance of health; the casefinding and management of illness, injury, or infirmity; the restoration of optimum function; or the achievement of a dignified death. Nursing practice includes but is not limited to administration, teaching, counseling, supervision, delegation, and evaluation of practice and the execution of the medical regimen, including the administration of medications and treatments prescribed by any person authorized by state law to prescribe. Each registered nurse is directly accountable and responsible to the consumer for the quality of nursing care rendered."

Professional nurses are prepared for these special skills by formal continuing education that adheres to the guidelines approved by the American Nurses' Association or in a baccalaureate nursing program.

Nursing Care Delivery Systems. In response to social, political, technological, and professional forces of change and the demands of clients and patients, professional nursing offers a variety of modalities for the delivery of nursing care. Some of the more commonly used models are *case method, functional method, team nursing,* and *primary nursing.* Each of these models is currently employed in a variety of settings.

The *case method* is one of the oldest modalities; a nurse is assigned to one patient or to a caseload of patients for comprehensive care. The assigned nurse is responsible for total care of the patient while on duty. The case method is currently used in private duty nursing and in settings of intensive care. It is the precursor of primary nursing. Prior to World War II, when the supply of professional nurses was diverted from civilian to military hospitals, the case method was the most commonly used way in which nursing services were organized. During and after the war, increasing numbers of nonprofessional ancillary nursing personnel were utilized to provide nursing care, thus forcing nursing administrators to consider alternative modalities.

The *functional method* focuses on the tasks to be completed. It fragments nursing care by dividing total care of the patient into specific procedures and jobs and assigning the less complicated of these to people with less educational preparation. Advantages of the functional method are that it is economical and efficient and that it may permit centralized direction and control of patient care. It requires clearly defined protocols and job descriptions and demands a high level of communication among the various caregivers. Disadvantages of this task-oriented system are that it cannot accommodate the holistic approach to nursing and, further, that it damages continuity of care by putting patients and clients in the position of being served by a number of people with confusing titles and responsibilities and a sense that there is no one person to whom they can relate with consistency. While a functional modality may serve a product-oriented agency or corporation very well, it is not appropriate for a service-oriented profession that purports to meet the needs of people.

Team nursing developed as a means of bringing together a diversified work force and overcoming the fragmentation associated with a task-oriented system. It is an attempt to meet the needs of employees who work best in whole-task jobs, as well as the needs of patients who need continuity and consistency. A major disadvantage is that this modality places the professional nurse in the position of team leader, a task for which the nurse may not be prepared by education or by experience. It is part of the responsibilities of the professional nurse to be able to make assignments of available personnel and match each person's skills with patient needs, hold conferences for discussion of patient care, individualize patient care and prepare nursing care plans, instruct personnel, and perform follow-up evaluations of the care delivered. Additionally, the nurse invariably must deal with the more complex aspects of patient care while less educationally prepared personnel attend to routine tasks.

Primary nursing is similar to the case method modality. The nurse assigned to a patient has full responsibility and accountability for the quality of nursing care provided. Associates may share in the planning and implementation phases of the nursing process, but it is the primary nurse

---

WINDOW ON PRIMARY NURSING

When I launched this form of care in 1953 in a psychiatric hospital I called it nurse-physician team management of patients. It was an indication that the same nurse and same physician were to manage the patient from the time that each patient entered the hospital until discharge. The concept was based on the usual pattern of care of all other major clinical professions. Nurses were to have much more visibility, especially to patients and their families, and interdisciplinary care was to be facilitated. The structure of care is a crucial variable in how care will be delivered. Thus nurses were made as accountable as physicians, dentists, clinical psychologists, and others for the planning and outcomes of care for specific patients.

In this posture of perfect accountability every error of omission or commission could be traced unerringly to each primary nurse. The other side of the coin is more interesting. Every act of clinical competence and excellence in care could be identified with the same accuracy. Thus professional pride and the incentive toward competency could be nourished in a way that was very different from functional, team nursing or any other global concept no matter how it was labeled. The clinical competence of each nurse was now much more visible and could be rewarded. The economic incentive helped feed the growth of clinical abilities by allocating salaries according to professional growth rather than by blunting the desire to grow when every category of nurse receives the same salary. Theoretically, every nurse on the staff should receive a different salary.

This approach also had the seeds for acquiring more education. In an experiment conducted many years later we found that the errors of omission in nursing care were one to one with the level of preparation. Nurses with graduate education made the fewest errors of omission while those with less than baccalaureate preparation made the most. Costs of care followed the same pattern. The more the education the less the cost to the organization because of efficiency and effectiveness. In addition, this form of care reduces the tendency of nurses to gravitate to nonclinical tasks. Thus nursing time is conserved and shortages reduced as well as economic costs contained. This is a major means of building a constituency with patients because of the time- and space-binding relationships.

LUTHER CHRISTMAN, PhD, RN

---

who is responsible for coordinating and evaluating all aspects of care. (See also PRIMARY NURSING.)

primary n. a form of nursing service organization in which the nursing care of a specific patient is under the continuous guidance of one nurse from admission through discharge. The primary nurse is accountable for every phase of the nursing process from assessment through evaluation of the effectiveness of care. Since the primary nurse cannot give direct patient care 24 hours a day, seven days a week, other nurses function as associates, contributing to and implementing the primary nurse's plan of care by accepting responsibility for delegated nursing tasks and evaluating and reporting to the primary nurse the patient's status and response to nursing interventions and medical treatment.

n. process a goal-directed series of activities whereby the practice of nursing is approached in a systematic and orderly way. The goal of the nursing process is to alleviate, minimize, or prevent actual or potential health problems. The problems identified and dealt with in the nursing process are those which the nurse is qualified to diagnose and treat by virtue of education, experience, and commitment to the goals of nursing.

The nursing process is based on some fundamental beliefs about the nature of humans, the role of nursing, and the delivery of health care. It is assumed that nurses believe that every person is endowed with personal worth and dignity and has a right to service of a high quality regardless of socioeconomic status, cultural background, or religious beliefs.

Further, it is assumed every person has basic needs common to all humans and that these needs must be satisfied to some degree if a person is to survive and enjoy an acceptable level of wellness. Meeting one's needs may require assistance from someone else until one is able to resume or begin to accept responsibility for oneself.

Another assumption is that a patient or client and family prefer a patient-centered approach that actively seeks their input and respects their thoughts, feelings, and needs. Such an approach encourages them to enter into a fruitful and mutually beneficial relationship with health care providers.

Components. The components of a system are its structural parts or elements. The components of the nursing process are phases or stages through which one moves toward achievement of goals. Although there is a beginning and an end to each phase, none stands alone. Each phase is dependent on the others and there is continuous interaction among them as energy and information flow through them. Because the nursing process is dynamic, its components represent points at which action can take place in response to feedback.

The five major components of the nursing process are NURSING ASSESSMENT, NURSING DIAGNOSIS, PLANNING, IMPLEMENTATION (or nursing INTERVENTION), and EVALUATION.

Criteria by which the nursing process can be measured have been formulated by the American Nurses' Association. They include the following Standards of Nursing Practice:

I. The collection of data about the health status of the client/patient is systematic and continuous. The data are accessible, communicated, and recorded.

II. Nursing diagnoses are derived from health status data.

III. The plan of nursing care includes goals derived from the nursing diagnoses.

IV. The plan of nursing care includes priorities and the prescribed nursing approaches or measures to achieve the goals derived from the nursing diagnoses.

V. Nursing actions provide for client/patient participation in health promotion, maintenance, and restoration.

VI. Nursing actions assist the client/patient to maximize health capabilities.

VII. The client's/patient's progress or lack of progress toward goal achievement is determined by the client/patient and the nurse.

VIII. The client's/patient's progress or lack of progress toward goal achievement directs reassessment, reordering of priorities, new goal setting, and revision of the plan of nursing care.

public health *n.* see PUBLIC HEALTH NURSING.

team *n.* a method of organizing the care of a group of patients such that each staff member is responsible for certain tasks for all the patients.

transcultural *n.* see TRANSCULTURAL NURSING.

nurturance (nur'chur-ans) a fostering of learning, growing, and healing.

nutation (noo-ta'shun) the act of nodding, especially involuntary nodding.

nutraceuticals (noo″trah-soo'tĭ-kalz) functional foods.

nutrient (noo'tre-ent) 1. nourishing; aiding NUTRITION. 2. a FOOD or biochemical substance used by the body that must be supplied in adequate amounts from foods consumed. There are six classes of nutrients: WATER, PROTEINS, CARBOHYDRATES, FATS, MINERALS, and VITAMINS.

nutriment (noo'trĭ-ment) NUTRIENT (def. 2). 1. nourishment; food and other nourishing materials.

nutrition (nu-trĭ'shun) the sum of the processes involved in taking in nutrients, assimilating them, and using them. adj., **nutri'tional.** It is particularly concerned with those properties of food that build sound bodies and promote health. Good nutrition means a balanced diet containing adequate amounts of the essential nutritional elements that the body must have to function normally.

To form the foundation for a balanced diet, the Institute of Home Economics, United States Department of Agriculture, recommends selection of foods from the Food Pyramid (see illustration). The essential ingredients of a balanced diet are PROTEINS, VITAMINS, MINERALS, FATS, and CARBOHYDRATES. The body can manufacture sugars from fats, and fats from sugars and proteins, depending on the need, but it cannot manufacture proteins from sugars and fats.

Because the body's needs change as it grows and develops, good nutrition for a child or teenager is not the same as good nutrition for a mature or older person. Growing bodies need plentiful supplies of calcium, phosphorus, and other minerals to build strong bones and teeth, and abundant protein for firm muscles, energy, and stamina. For children especially, breakfast is the key meal of the day. Expending as much energy as they do, children need a hearty morning meal, rich in vitamin C, calcium, iron, and thiamine, in order to offset the physical and mental fatigue that they usually feel before lunch time.

Dietitians generally consider breakfast the most important meal of the day because it ends the body's overnight fast and supplies the "fuel" for a person to get under way at top efficiency. If possible, meals should be spaced at regular intervals. They should never be rushed; this is especially true of the main daily meal.

Dietary Guidelines. Typical North American diets have been implicated in the development of many so-called "killer diseases." Therefore, in consultation with nutrition scientists, the Department of Agriculture and the Department of Health and Human Services in the USA, and Health Canada in Canada, have periodically issued dietary guidelines for people in those countries. The guidelines are developed and recommended for the purpose of reducing the mortality and morbidity rates for conditions such as coronary artery disease, hypertension, cancer, and diabetes mellitus. Another target disease, dental caries, is not a potentially fatal disease, but it is costly in terms of general health and expenditure of money for health care.

In spite of controversy over whether there is sufficient validated evidence for a cause and effect relationship between diet and specific diseases, the general public seems to have become more aware of the benefits of eating sensibly and exercising regularly, and many are changing their eating habits and lifestyles. Current dietary guidelines for the United States and Canada are shown in the Appendices. They are similar to recommendations made by the American Heart Association and the American Cancer Society.

enteral n. foods and liquids provided via TUBE FEEDING. See illustration.

imbalanced n.: less than body requirements a NURSING DIAGNOSIS approved by the North American Nursing Diagnosis Association, defined as a state in which an individual has an intake of nutrients insufficient to meet metabolic needs. Etiologic factors include DYSPHAGIA, ANOREXIA, ALLERGY, NAUSEA, fad diets, depression, and social isolation. Patients with CANCER are at risk for nutritional deficits because of the catabolic nature of the illness as well as side effects of radiation therapy or chemotherapy. See also MALNUTRITION.

imbalanced n.: more than body requirements a NURSING DIAGNOSIS approved by the North American Nursing Diagnosis Association, defined as a state in which an individual has an intake of nutrients in excess of metabolic needs. Related factors include cultural values that encourage eating and large body size; emotional factors such as depression, boredom, or guilt; lack of exercise appropriate for caloric intake; aging and decreased physical activity; and reported deleterious eating patterns. Defining characteristics include a body weight of

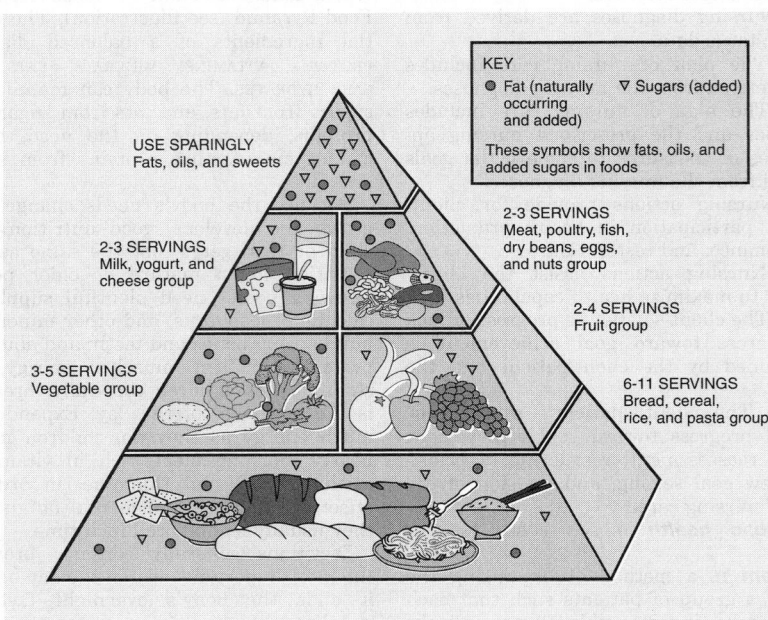

The food pyramid. From USDA's Food Guide Pyramid Booklet, 1996.

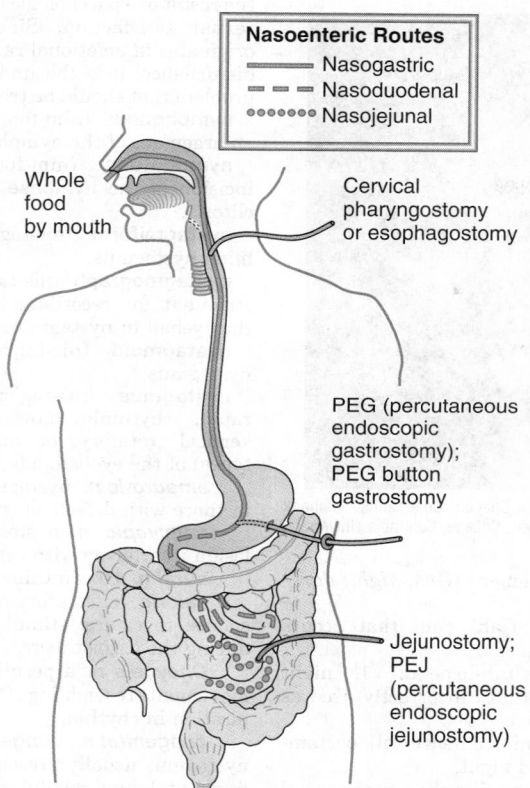

Nasoenteric Routes
——— Nasogastric
— — — Nasoduodenal
•••••• Nasojejunal

Whole food by mouth

Cervical pharyngostomy or esophagostomy

PEG (percutaneous endoscopic gastrostomy); PEG button gastrostomy

Jejunostomy; PEJ (percutaneous endoscopic jejunostomy)

Diagram of enteral tube placement. From Mahan and Escott-Stump, 2000.

more than 20 per cent above ideal weight for height and frame and triceps skin fold greater than 15 mm in men and 25 mm in women. See also OBESITY.

parenteral n. see PARENTERAL NUTRITION.

risk for imbalanced n.: more than body requirements a NURSING DIAGNOSIS approved by the North American Nursing Diagnosis Association, defined as a state in which an individual is at risk of having an intake of nutrients that exceeds metabolic needs. See also OBESITY.

nutritionist (noo-trī'shun-ist) a person who uses the science of NUTRITION to help individuals improve their health. There is often no accreditation process for nutritionists, and those using the services of one should examine his or her qualifications carefully. In contrast, a Registered DIETITIAN (RD) has been certified as qualified by the American Dietetic Association.

nutritious (noo-trish'us) affording nourishment.

nutritive (noo'trĭ-tiv) nutritional.

nutriture (noo'trĭ-chur) the status of the body in relation to nutrition.

Nutting (nut'ing) M. Adelaide (1858–1948). A pioneer in establishing the foundations on which nursing as a modern profession rests. She was in the first graduating class at Johns Hopkins Hospital School of Nursing and eventually became Superintendent of Nurses and Principal of the School of Nursing. At Johns Hopkins, Miss Nutting instituted many reforms and advances in nursing education. She eliminated the 12-hour-duty day, abolished the monthly stipend for students, and instituted a 3-year course. Her purposes in instigating these changes were to release the student from financial obligation to the hospital so that exploitation of the student as a source of cheap labor could be abolished, and to provide the student with more time for study and learning.

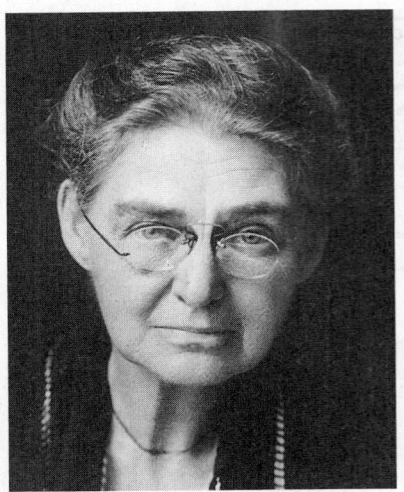

M. Adelaide Nutting. Special Collections, Milbank Memorial Library, Teachers College, Columbia University.

nyct(o)- word element [Gr.], *night; darkness.*

nyctalgia (nik-tal′jah) pain that occurs only in sleep.

nyctalopia (nik″tah-lo′pe-ah) 1. night blindness. 2. sometimes incorrectly used as a synonym for HEMERALOPIA.

nyctohemeral (nik″to-hem′er-al) pertaining to both day and night.

nyctophilia (nik″to-fil′e-ah) an abnormal preference for darkness or for night; called also scotophilia.

nyctophobia (nik″to-fo′be-ah) irrational fear of darkness.

nyctophonia (nik″to-fo′ne-ah) loss of voice during the day but not at night.

nycturia (nik-tu′re-ah) nocturia.

nylidrin (nil′ĭ-drin) a β-adrenergic receptor stimulant used as a peripheral VASODILATOR.

nymph (nimf) a developmental stage in certain arthropods (e.g., ticks) between the larval form and the adult; it resembles an adult but does not have fully developed wings or genitalia.

nymph(o)- word element [Gr.], *nymphae* (labia minora).

nympha (nim′fah), pl. *nym′phae* [Gr.] labium minus.

nymphectomy (nim-fek′to-me) excision of the nymphae (labia minora).

nymphitis (nim-fi′tis) inflammation of the nymphae (labia minora).

nymphomania (nim″fo-ma′ne-ah) a former term for excessive sexual desire in a woman, which may lead to promiscuous sexual behavior; a form of paraphilia that is usually the result of a psychologic inability to achieve sexual satisfaction. Since the condition originates in emotional rather than physical disturbance, it is the underlying emotional problem that should be treated.

nymphoncus (nim-fong′kus) swelling or enlargement of the nymphae (labia minora).

nymphotomy (nim-fot′ah-me) surgical incision of the nymphae (labia minora) or clitoris.

nystagmiform (nis-tag′mĭ-form) resembling nystagmus.

nystagmograph (nis-tag′mo-graf) an instrument for recording the movements of the eyeball in nystagmus.

nystagmoid (nis-tag′moid) resembling nystagmus.

nystagmus (nis-tag′mus) involuntary, rapid, rhythmic movement (horizontal, vertical, rotatory, or mixed, i.e., of two types) of the eyeball. adj., **nystag′mic.**

amaurotic n. nystagmus in the blind or in those with defects of central vision.

amblyopic n. nystagmus due to any lesion interfering with central vision.

aural n. labyrinthine nystagmus.

caloric n. rotatory nystagmus in response to caloric stimuli in the ear, seen during the CALORIC TEST.

Cheyne's n. a peculiar rhythmical eye movement resembling Cheyne-Stokes respiration in rhythm.

congenital n., congenital hereditary n. nystagmus usually present at birth, usually horizontal and pendular, but occasionally jerky and pendular; the nystagmus may be caused by or associated with optic atrophy, coloboma, albinism, bilateral macular lesions, congenital cataract, severe astigmatism, and glaucoma.

dissociated n. that in which the movements in the two eyes are dissimilar.

end-position n. that occurring only at extremes of gaze.

fixation n. that occurring only on gazing fixedly at an object.

gaze n. nystagmus made apparent by looking to the right or to the left.

labyrinthine n. vestibular nystagmus due to labyrinthine disturbance.

latent n. that occurring only when one eye is covered.

lateral n. involuntary horizontal movement of the eyes.

optokinetic n. nystagmus induced by looking at objects moving across the visual field.

pendular n. nystagmus in which the oscillations of the eyes have an equal rate, amplitude, direction, and type of movement.

positional n. that which occurs, or is altered in form or intensity, on assumption of certain positions of the head.

retraction n., n. retracto′rius a spasmodic backward movement of the eyeball occurring on attempts to move the eye; a sign of midbrain disease.

rotatory n. involuntary rotation of the eyes about the visual axis.

secondary n. nystagmus occurring after the abrupt cessation of rotation of the head, caused by the labyrinthine fluid continuing to move.

spontaneous n. that occurring without specific stimulation of the vestibular system.

vertical n. involuntary up-and-down movement of the eyes.

vestibular n. nystagmus due to disturbance of the labyrinth or of the vestibular nuclei; the movements are usually jerky.

nystatin (ni-stat′in) an antibiotic produced by *Streptomyces noursei;* used as an antifungal AGENT in treatment of infections due to *Candida albicans* and other *Candida* species; administered orally or topically.

nystaxis (nis-tak′sis) nystagmus.

nyxis (nik′sis) paracentesis.

O

O oxygen.

O. [L.] o'culus (eye).

o- symbol used in chemistry for *ortho-*.

Ω ohm.

oasthouse urine disease (ōst'hows) methionine malabsorption syndrome.

OB obstetrics.

ob- word element [L.], *against; in front of; toward.*

obcecation (ob"sĕ-ka'shun) incomplete blindness.

obesity (o-be'sĭ-te) excessive accumulation of fat in the body; increase in weight beyond that considered desirable with regard to age, height, and bone structure. Called also adiposity, adiposis, and corpulency. adj., **obese'.** The NATIONAL INSTITUTES OF HEALTH considers obesity as existing when the body mass INDEX is 30 kg/m² or more. The NATIONAL HEART, LUNG, AND BLOOD INSTITUTE has published *The Practical Guide: Identification, Evaluation, and Treatment of Overweight and Obesity in Adults.* This is available either online at http://www.nhlbi.nih.gov/guidelines or by calling the NHLBI Health Information Center at 1-301-592-8573.

adult-onset o. that beginning in adulthood and characterized by increase in size (hypertrophy) of adipose cells with no increase in number.

o.-hypoventilation syndrome the specific association of extreme obesity, excessive sleepiness, polycythemia, chronic alveolar hypoventilation, and excessive appetite; sometimes called *pickwickian syndrome* because it affected the character Fat Joe in Dickens' *Pickwick Papers.* Respiratory problems are caused by the increased work of ventilation in moving the ponderous thorax and abdomen.

lifelong o. that beginning in childhood and characterized by an increase both in number (hyperplasia) and in size (hypertrophy) of adipose cells.

obex (o'beks) the ependyma-lined junction of the teniae of the fourth ventricle of the brain at the inferior angle.

objection (ob-jek'shun) opposition, or a reason for opposition.

objective (ob-jek'tiv) 1. perceptible by the external senses. 2. a clear, concise declarative statement that directs action toward a specific goal. 3. the lens or system of lenses of a microscope nearest the object that is being examined.

achromatic o. one in which the chromatic aberration is corrected for two colors and the spherical aberration for one color.

affective o. a statement of expectations regarding changes in attitude or feelings.

apochromatic o. one in which chromatic aberration is corrected for three colors and the spherical aberration for two colors.

behavioral o. a written statement identifying an action or pattern of actions to be expected after an intervention.

cognitive o. a statement of expectations regarding knowledge.

flat field o. a microscopic objective that provides an image in which all parts of the field are simultaneously in focus.

immersion o. one designed to have its tip and the coverglass over the specimen connected by a liquid instead of air.

psychomotor o. a statement of expectations regarding the acquisition of skills.

obligate (ob'lĭ-gāt) not facultative; necessary; compulsory; pertaining to or characterized by the ability to survive only in a particular environment or to assume only a particular role, as an obligate anaerobe.

oblique (o-blēk') slanting; inclined.

obliquity (o-blik'wĭ-te) the state of being oblique or slanting.

obliteration (ob-lit"er-a'shun) complete removal, as by disease, degeneration, surgical procedure, or irradiation, or by the filling up of a space with fibrous tissue or inflammation.

oblongata (ob"long-gah'tah) oblong; see MEDULLA OBLONGATA.

obsession (ob-sesh'un) a recurrent, persistent thought, image, or impulse that is unwanted and distressing (ego-dystonic) and comes involuntarily to mind despite attempts to ignore or suppress it. Common obsessions involve violence, contamination, and doubts. See also OBSESSIVE-COMPULSIVE DISORDER and OBSESSIVE-COMPULSIVE PERSONALITY DISORDER. adj., **obses'sive.**

obsessive-compulsive (ob-ses'iv-kom-pul'siv) pertaining to obsessions and compulsions, to obsessive-compulsive disorder, or to obsessive-compulsive personality disorder.

o.-c. disorder OCD; an ANXIETY DISORDER consisting of two symptoms, obsession and compulsion; although they are different, they are closely related and often occur in the same person. An obsession is a recurrent and persistent thought or desire. It is not voluntary and is distressing to the patient, but although the patient tries to suppress or ignore it, it is very difficult to eliminate from

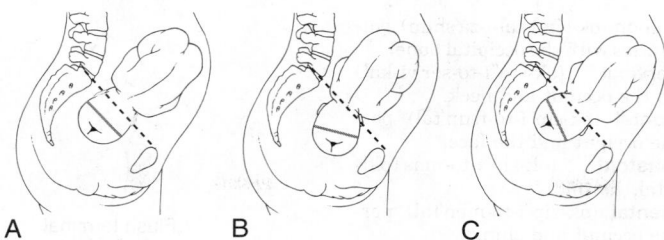

Obliquity *A*, Concordance of the fetal and pelvic planes (synclitism); *B*, Litzmann's obliquity (posterior asynclitism); *C*, Nägele's obliquity (anterior asynclitism), From Dorland's, 2000.

the mind. A compulsion is an uncontrollable urge to perform some repetitive and stereotyped action. This action is not an end in itself but serves as a substitute for unacceptable unconscious ideas and impulses. Although the patient does not know the reason for this action, failure to perform it leads to increasing anxiety, which can be relieved by giving in to the compulsion. Eventually, after repeatedly failing to resist the compulsion, the patient may lose the desire to resist it.

The mild forms of these three symptoms are familiar to most people. For example, most children play the game of avoiding the cracks in the sidewalk. As adults, they find themselves doing this occasionally, perhaps when thinking over a problem. Individuals with obsessive-compulsive disorder, however, might feel real anxiety if they step on a crack in the sidewalk.

In obsessive-compulsive disorder, the patient deflects, or displaces the unresolved conflict onto an external object or action as a substitute. By doing this, the person tries to control the conflict magically and eliminate anxiety. The obsession or ritual represents a smokescreen which the mind throws up to keep the inner conflict from becoming conscious. This is not the same as OBSESSIVE-COMPULSIVE PERSONALITY DISORDER, which is a PERSONALITY DISORDER.

o.-c. personality disorder a PERSONALITY DISORDER characterized by an emotionally constricted manner that is unduly conventional, serious, rigid, stubborn, and stingy, by preoccupation with trivial details, rules, order, organization, schedules, and lists to the point that the major point of an activity is lost or task completion is delayed, by reluctance to delegate tasks or work cooperatively unless everything is done one's own way, and by excessive devotion to work and productivity to the detriment of interpersonal relationships. This is not the same as OBSESSIVE-COMPULSIVE DISORDER, which is an ANXIETY DISORDER.

obstetrician (ob″stĕ-trǐ′shun) a physician who specializes in obstetrics.

obstetrics (ob-stet′riks) the branch of health science dealing with pregnancy, labor, and the puerperium. adj., **obstet′ric, obstet′rical.**

obstipation (ob″stǐ-pa′shun) intractable constipation.

obstruction (ob-struk′shun) 1. the act of blocking or clogging. 2. the state or condition of being clogged; see also ATRESIA. Called also blockade, closure, and occlusion.

chronic airflow o., chronic airway o. name given to a group of disorders in which the upper or lower airways are chronically obstructed; it includes chronic BRONCHITIS, ASTHMA, EMPHYSEMA, PNEUMOCONIOSIS, and any other type of CHRONIC OBSTRUCTIVE PULMONARY DISEASE.

intestinal o. see INTESTINAL OBSTRUCTION.

obstructive small airways disease chronic bronchitis with irreversible narrowing of the bronchioles and small bronchi with hypoxia and often hypercapnia.

obstruent (ob′stroo-ent) 1. causing obstruction or blocking. 2. an agent that so acts.

obtund (ob-tund′) to render dull or blunt.

obtundation (ob-tun-da′shun) CLOUDING OF CONSCIOUSNESS. adj., **obtun′dent.**

obturation (ob′too-ra′shun) obstruction.

canal o. filling of a root canal completely and densely with a nonirritating hermetic sealing agent.

obturator (ob′too-ra″tor) 1. a disk or plate that closes an opening. 2. a prosthesis for closing an acquired or congenital opening of the palate (CLEFT PALATE).

o. sign pain on outward pressure on the obturator foramen as a sign of inflammation in the sheath of the obturator nerve, probably caused by appendicitis.

obtusion (ob-too′zhun) blunting of sensation and perception.

occipital (ok-sip′ĭ-tal) pertaining to the occiput; see occipital BONE and occipital LOBE.

occipitalization (ok-sip″ĭ-tal-ĭ-za′shun) synostosis of the atlas with the occipital bone.

occipitocervical (ok-sip″ĭ-to-ser′vĭ-kal) pertaining to the occiput and neck.

occipitofrontal (ok-sip″ĭ-to-frun′tal) pertaining to the occiput and the face.

occipitomastoid (ok-sip″ĭ-to-mas′toid) masto-occipital.

occipitomental (ok-sip″ĭ-to-men′tal) pertaining to the occiput and chin.

occipitoparietal (ok-sip″ĭ-to-pah-ri′ĕ-tal) pertaining to the occipital and parietal bones or lobes of the brain.

occipitotemporal (ok-sip″ĭ-to-tem′po-ral) pertaining to the occipital and temporal bones.

occipitothalamic (ok-sip″ĭ-to-thah-lam′ik) pertaining to the occipital lobe and thalamus.

occiput (ok′sĭ-put) the back part of the head.

occlude (ŏ-klood′) 1. to fit close together. 2. to close tight. 3. to obstruct.

occlusal (ŏ-kloo′zal) pertaining to closure. 1. pertaining to the masticating surfaces of the premolar and molar teeth, or to the contacting surfaces of opposing occlusion rims. 2. designating a position toward the hypothetical plane passing between the mandibular and maxillary teeth when the jaws are brought into approximation.

occlusion (ŏ-kloo′zhun) 1. obstruction. 2. the trapping of a liquid or gas within cavities in a solid or on its surface. 3. the relation of the teeth of both jaws when in functional contact during activity of the mandible. 4. momentary complete closure of some area in the vocal tract, causing breathing to stop and pressure to accumulate.

   abnormal o. malocclusion.

   central o., centric o. occlusion of the teeth when the mandible is in centric relation to the maxilla, with full occlusal surface contact of the upper and lower teeth in habitual occlusion.

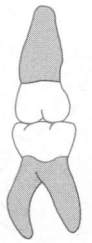

Flush terminal
plane

Normal occlusion of the primary molars. From Darby and Walsh, 1994.

   coronary o. see CORONARY OCCLUSION.

   eccentric o. occlusion of the teeth when the lower jaw has moved from the centric position.

   functional o. contact of the maxillary and mandibular teeth that provides the highest efficiency in the centric position and during all exclusive movements of the jaw that are essential to mastication without producing trauma.

occlusive (ŏ-kloo′siv) pertaining to or effecting occlusion.

occult (ŏ-kult′) obscure or hidden from view.

   o. blood test examination by microscope or chemical test of a specimen (such as feces, urine, or gastric juice) for presence of blood that is not otherwise detectable. Feces are tested when intestinal bleeding is suspected but there is no visible evidence of blood.

occupational (ok″u-pa′shun-al) 1. pertaining to a vocation or source of livelihood. 2. pertaining to the skills a person needs to live independently and carry on a desired lifestyle; see also occupational performance AREAS.

   o. diseases diseases caused by any of various factors involved in a person's occupation; there are many types. Dusts are a common cause; fine particles of silica can lead to SILICOSIS among miners, glassworkers, and persons involved in the manufacture of cement and similar materials. Another cause is toxic gases and vapors, which can result in respiratory disorders and may also involve the blood and other body systems. Many different substances are toxic, including some usually considered therapeutic when in sufficient doses. Certain kinds of chemicals can affect the skin, causing some forms of DERMATITIS. Working conditions, such as high temperatures or humidity, excessive noise, changes in air pressure, or continuous exposure to sun and

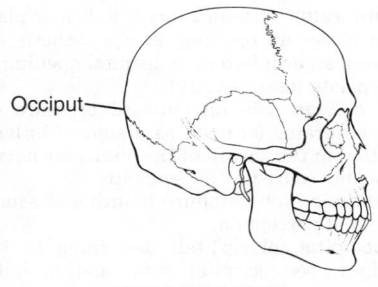

Occiput

From Dorland's, 2000.

wind, can cause varied disorders such as HEAT EXHAUSTION, impaired hearing or vision, DECOMPRESSION SICKNESS, or skin conditions.

Control and prevention of occupational diseases is very much a major concern of the individual worker, management, the community health service, and the state and federal governments. It involves education on how to protect oneself against occupational hazards; management's cooperation in supplying proper equipment and conditions; inspection and testing services performed by the government; the existence of adequate medical and first-aid services at the location of the work; adequate hospitalization facilities, insurance and compensation; and research into methods to provide safety and good health.

o. therapist a health care professional who provides services designed to restore self-care, work, and leisure skills to patients/clients who have specific performance incapacities or deficits that reduce their abilities to cope with the tasks of everyday living. The occupational therapist evaluates and treats problems arising from developmental deficits, physical illness or injury, emotional disorders, the aging process, and psychological or social disability. Graduates of an accredited degree program who have completed field work requirements and are eligible for the certification examination given by the National Board for Certification in Occupational Therapy (NBCOT).

o. therapy the use of purposeful ACTIVITY to help individuals acquire the knowledge, skills, and attitudes necessary for the performance of life tasks. It is defined by the American Occupational Therapy Association as "the art and science of directing man's participation in selected tasks to restore, reinforce, and enhance performance, facilitate learning of those skills and functions essential for adaptation and productivity, diminish or correct pathology, and promote and maintain health. Its fundamental concern is the development and maintenance of the capacity, throughout the life span, to perform with satisfaction to self and others those tasks and roles essential to productive living and to the mastery of self and environment."

The broad concerns of occupational therapy include all factors that facilitate the development of adaptive skills and increase performance capacity, and also those factors that may impede or restrict an individual's ability to function. In addition to those persons recovering from physical injury or

illness, occupational therapy serves others who because of age, poverty, cultural differences, or psychologic and social disability, have difficulty coping with the tasks of living. The reference to occupation in the title is to be understood in the context of goal-directed use of time, energy, interest, and attention.

As is true of all types of therapeutic measures, the skills that are taught and the tasks prescribed for the client take into account his individual needs, abilities, and interests. This implies a thorough evaluation of his physical, mental, and emotional status and an acceptance of him as a person. In consultation with other members of the health care team, the occupational therapist designs a program of therapy that will lead to the goal of a productive life and satisfactory adjustment on the part of the patient. The address of the American Occupational Therapy Association is 4720 Montgomery Lane, P.O. Box 31220, Bethesda, MD 20824-1220.

o. therapy assistant a health care professional who works under the supervision of an occupational therapist in planning and implementing programs to restore the self-care, work, and leisure skills of clients/patients. Those certified by the American Occupational Therapy Association are designated Certified Occupational Therapy Assistant (COTA).

Occupational Safety and Health Administration (OSHA) the United States government agency that administers the Occupational Safety and Health Act of 1970. This act of the United States Congress established minimum health and safety standards for workers and provides for the inspection of places of employment and the penalizing of employers who do not provide conditions that meet the established standards. Further information on OSHA can be obtained by writing to Office of Information Services, OSHA, U.S. Department of Labor, 200 Constitution Ave. NW, Washington, DC 20210.

OCD obsessive-compulsive disorder.

ochrometer (ŏ-krom′ĕ-ter) an instrument for measuring capillary blood pressure.

ochronosis (ok″ro-no′sis) a peculiar discoloration of body tissues caused by deposit of alkapton bodies as the result of a metabolic disorder.

ocular o. brown or gray discoloration of the sclera, sometimes involving also the conjunctivae and eyelids.

oct(a)- word element [Gr., L.], *eight*.

WINDOW ON OCCUPATIONAL THERAPY

Occupational therapy is an invisible profession. It is not easily recognized because its science and practice are ordinary activities of daily living—eating, working, playing, and caring for oneself, others, and the environment. Because of and in spite of its very nature, occupational therapy has since the early part of the last century become one of the fastest growing health care fields in America.

Individuals who presently survive catastrophic physical injury (such as head injury) because of advanced medical technology, are seeking ways to lead meaningful lives with considerable limitations in abilities to process information, make choices, and act upon personal wishes. Infants with developmental and social disadvantages stemming from birth trauma, parental substance abuse, and diseases such as AIDS require occupational therapy. Elderly individuals are now living longer, often with less social support from family, and require modifications to living spaces to remain independent and social in the community. Americans have now won the right to fair and reasonable accommodation in the workplace, school, and community regardless of differences due to physical limitation or disability. We are now also in a better position to understand prevention and adaptation to disability through social and technological interventions.

The range of settings and work of an occupational therapist is varied and flexible. Thanks to public legislation, many therapists now work in early intervention programs and schools. Private practice in areas such as wellness programs and home care for the elderly has seen tremendous growth in the past few years. Challenging opportunities now exist in industry, for example in injury prevention, work hardening programs to prepare injured workers for entry or reentry into the job market, and in modifying work as well as home and school environments for individuals requiring assistive devices such as grab bars.

Occupational therapists can do this work because they begin their education in the liberal arts and health sciences. With this foundation they are prepared to study human occupation and the impact of disease, injury, and social deprivation. They learn to investigate, reason, and intervene through therapeutic relationships and by adapting basic activities that enable patients to perform selective risks such as driving, dressing and grooming, eating, socializing, and communicating with others. Finally, to be consultants they develop skills to assist families, schools, industry, and other caregivers to enable individuals to function with meaning and dignity through purposeful action.

SHARAN L. SCHWARTZBERG, EdD, OTR, FAOTA

octan (ok′tan) occurring on the eighth day (every seven days).

octavalent (ok″tah-va′lent) having a valency of eight.

octinoxate (ok-tin′ok-sāt) an absorber of ultraviolet B radiation, used topically as a SUNSCREEN.

octisalate (ok″tĭ-sal′āt) a substituted salicylate that absorbs ultraviolet light in the UVB range, used as a SUNSCREEN.

octocrylene (ok′to-kril″ēn) a SUNSCREEN that absorbs ULTRAVIOLET RAYS in the UVB range.

octreotide (ok-tre′o-tīd) a synthetic analogue of SOMATOSTATIN, used as the acetate ester in palliative treatment of symptoms of gastrointestinal endocrine tumors and in treatment of ACROMEGALY; administered subcutaneously, intragluteally, or intravenously.

octyl methoxycinnamate (ok′til mĕ-thok″se-sin′ah-māt) octinoxate.

ocul(o)- word element [L.], *eye.* See also words beginning OPHTHALM(O)-.

ocular (ok′u-lar) 1. pertaining to the eye; called also ophthalmic and optic. 2. eyepiece.

oculist (ok′u-list) ophthalmologist.

oculocerebrorenal syndrome (ok″u-lo-sĕ-re″bro-re′nal) a rare X-linked genetic syndrome of males, characterized by vitamin D–refractory rickets, distention of the eyeball, congenital glaucoma and cataracts, mental retardation, and renal tubule dysfunction as evidenced by hypophosphatemia, acidosis, and aminoaciduria. Called also Lowe disease.

oculocutaneous (ok″u-lo-ku-ta′ne-us) pertaining to or affecting both the eyes and the skin.

oculofacial (ok″u-lo-fa′shal) pertaining to the eyes and face.

oculogyration (ok″u-lo-ji-ra′shun) the movement of the eyeball about the anteroposterior axis. adj., **oculogy′ric.**

oculomotor (ok″u-lo-mo′tor) pertaining to or affecting eye movements.

o. nerve the third CRANIAL NERVE; it is mixed, that is, it contains both sensory and motor fibers. Various branches of the oculomotor nerve provide for muscle sense and movement in most of the muscles of the eye, for constriction of the pupil, and for accommodation of the eye. See anatomic Table of Nerves in the Appendices.

oculomotorius (ok″u-lo-mo-to′re-us) the oculomotor nerve.

oculomycosis (ok″u-lo-mi-ko′sis) any fungal disease of the eye.

oculonasal (ok″u-lo-na′zal) pertaining to the eye and the nose.

oculopupillary (ok″u-lo-pu′pĭ-ler″e) pertaining to the pupil of the eye.

oculovestibular test (ok″u-lo-ves-tib′u-ler) caloric test.

oculozygomatic (ok″u-lo-zi″go-mat′ik) pertaining to the eye and the zygomatic ARCH or BONE.

oculus (ok′u-lus) [L.] eye.

OD¹ [L.] o′culus dex′ter (right eye).

OD² optical density; Doctor of Optometry; outside diameter; popular term for *overdose*.

odont(o)- word element [Gr.], *tooth.*

odontalgia (o″don-tal′jah) toothache.

odontectomy (o″don-tek′to-me) tooth extraction.

odontic (o-don′tik) pertaining to the teeth.

odontoblast (o-don′to-blast) one of the connective tissue cells that deposit dentin and form the outer surface of the dental pulp adjacent to the dentin.

odontoblastoma (o-don″to-blas-to′mah) a tumor made up of odontoblasts.

odontoclast (o-don′to-klast) cementoclast.

odontogenesis (o-don″to-jen′ĕ-sis) the origin and development of the teeth. adj., **odontogenet′ic.**

o. imperfec′ta dentinogenesis imperfecta.

odontogenic (o-don″to-jen′ik) 1. forming teeth. 2. arising in tissues that give origin to the teeth.

odontogeny (o″don-toj′ĕ-ne) odontogenesis.

odontoid (o-don′toid) like a tooth.

odontology (o″don-tol′o-je) 1. scientific study of the teeth. 2. dentistry.

odontolysis (o″don-tol′ĭ-sis) tooth resorption.

odontoma (o″don-to′mah) any odontogenic tumor, especially a composite odontoma.

ameloblastic o. a rare, slow-growing, mixed tumor of odontogenic origin that combines the characteristics of composite odontoma and ameloblastoma.

composite o. one consisting of both enamel and dentin in an abnormal pattern.

radicular o. one associated with a tooth root, or formed when the root was developing.

odontopathy (o″don-top′ah-the) any disease of the teeth.

odontosis (o″don-to′sis) formation or eruption of the teeth.

odontotomy (o″don-tot′ah-me) incision of a tooth.

odorant (o′dor-ant) any substance capable of stimulating the sense of smell.

odynacusis (o-din″ah-ku′sis) painful hearing.

-odynia word element [Gr.], *pain.*

odynometer (o″din-om′ĕ-ter) an instrument for measuring pain.

odynophagia (o-din″o-fa′jah) a DYSPHAGIA in which swallowing causes pain.

oe- for most words beginning thus, see those beginning *e-.*

oedipal (ed′ĭ-pal) pertaining to the Oedipus complex.

Oedipus complex (ed′ĭ-pus) a term used originally in PSYCHOANALYSIS to signify the complicated conflicts and emotions felt by a child when, during a stage of his normal development as a member of the family circle, he becomes aware of a particularly strong, sexually tinged attachment to his mother; the term also applies to a similar attachment felt by a girl to her father (called also Electra complex). At the same time, the child tends to view the other parent as a rival and yearns to take that parent's place. This pattern, which was described by Sigmund Freud, is named from the legend of the mythical Greek hero, King Oedipus of Thebes, who was raised by foster parents, unknowingly killed his real father in a quarrel, and later married his mother. When he learned of his unwitting incestuous relationship with his wife he blinded himself.

According to psychoanalysts, a child enters the oedipal phase at about the third year and usually has solved his largely unconscious conflicts in a satisfactory way by the age of 5 or 6. He does this by turning his feelings of possessiveness toward one parent and competitiveness toward the other into a wish to be liked by both of them. Eventually, a child who has worked out his conflicts well can focus his affection on members of the opposite sex outside the family circle and can establish satisfactory marital relationships as an adult.

Freud's theory is generally accepted by psychiatrists, although many have developed supplementary theories for the behavior pattern he described.

Oestrus (es′trus) a genus of botflies. *O. o′vis* deposits its larvae in the nostrils of sheep and goats and can cause ocular MYIASIS in humans.

official (ŏ-fī′shal) authorized by pharmacopeias and recognized formularies.

ofloxacin (o-flok′sah-sin) a broad-spectrum QUINOLONE ANTIBACTERIAL agent with actions similar to those of norfloxacin, effective against a wide variety of aerobic gram-negative and gram-positive organisms; administered orally in the treatment of prostatitis, sexually transmitted diseases, and infections of the lower respiratory tract, urinary tract, and skin and soft tissues, and applied topically in the treatment of bacterial corneal ulcers and ear infections.

Ogen (o′jen) trademark for preparations of ESTROPIPATE, an estrone used in the treatment of ESTROGEN deficiency.

Oguchi's disease (o-goo′chēz) a form of hereditary night blindness occurring in Japan.

ohm (Ω) (ōm) the SI UNIT of electrical RESISTANCE, named for Georg Simon Ohm; one ohm is produced when a current of 1 AMPERE flowing through a conductor produces a potential difference of 1 VOLT. IMPEDANCE is also measured in ohms.

Ohm's law (ōmz) a mathematical relationship formulated by the German physicist Georg Simon Ohm in 1826, comparing VOLTAGE (V), CURRENT (I), and RESISTANCE (R), usable for either alternating CURRENT or direct CURRENT. It originally applied only to situations of steady direct current, with the formula V = IR; with alternating current, the electrical circuit contains resistors, inductors, and capacitors and the formula becomes V = IZ, where Z is a complex number representing the IMPEDANCE.

ohmmeter (ōm′me-ter) an instrument that measures electrical resistance in ohms.

OHNAC Occupational Health Nurses in Agricultural Communities, a program of the National Institute for Occupational Safety and Health (NIOSH) that places public health nurses in rural communities and hospitals in ten states to conduct surveillance of agriculture-related illnesses and injuries among farmers and their families in order to reduce the risk of occupational disease and injury in agricultural populations.

oil (oil) 1. an unctuous, combustible substance that is liquid, or easily liquefiable, on warming, and is not miscible with water, but is soluble in ether. Such substances, depending on their origin, are classified as animal, mineral, or vegetable oils. Depending on their behavior on heating, they are classified as volatile or fixed. For specific oils, see under the name, as CASTOR OIL. 2. a fat that is liquid at room temperature.

essential o. volatile o.

expressed o., fatty o. fixed o. one that is not volatile, i.e., does not evaporate on warming; such oils consist of a mixture of FATTY ACIDS and their esters, and are classified as solid, semisolid, and liquid, or as drying, semidrying, and nondrying as a function of their tendency to solidify on exposure to air.

volatile o. an oil that evaporates readily; such oils occur in aromatic plants, to which they give odor and other characteristics.

ointment (oint′ment) a semisolid preparation for external application to the skin or mucous membranes. Official ointments consist of medicinal substances incorporated in suitable vehicles (bases). Called also salve and unguent.

OL [L.] o′culus lae′vus (left eye).

-ol word termination indicating that the substance is a hydroxyl derivative of a hydrocarbon, e.g., an alcohol or a phenol.

olanzapine (o-lan′zah-pēn) a monoaminergic antagonist used as an ANTIPSYCHOTIC AGENT; administered orally.

ole(o)- word element [L.], *oil.*

oleaginous (o′le-aj′ĭ-nus) oily; greasy.

oleate (o′le-āt) 1. a salt or ester of oleic acid. 2. a solution of an alkaloid or other basic drug in oleic acid.

olecranarthritis   (o-lek″ran-ahr-thri′tis) anconitis.

olecranoid (o-lek′rah-noid) resembling the olecranon.

olecranon (o-lek′rah-non) the bony projection of the ULNA at the elbow. adj., **olec′ranal.**

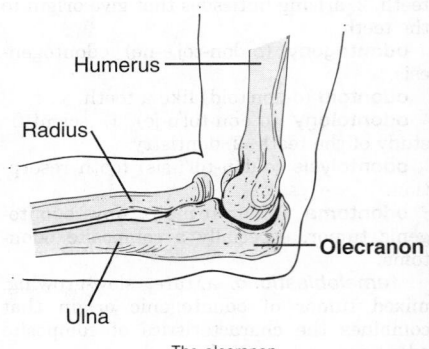

The olecranon.

oleic acid (o-le′ik) a long-chain unsaturated fatty acid found in most animal fats and vegetable oils; used in pharmacy as an emulsifier and to assist absorption of some drugs by the skin.

oleoresin (o″le-o-rez′in) 1. a natural combination of a resin and a volatile oil, such as exudes from pines, etc. 2. a compound extracted from a drug, containing both volatile oil and resin, by percolation with a volatile solvent, such as acetone, alcohol, or ether, and removal of the solvent.

oleotherapy (o″le-o-ther′ah-pe) treatment by injections of oil.

oleovitamin (o″le-o-vi′tah-min) a preparation of fat-soluble vitamins in fish liver or edible vegetable oil.

olfact (ol′fakt) a unit of odor, the minimal perceptible odor, being the minimal concentration of a substance in solution that can be perceived by a large number of normal individuals, expressed in terms of grams per liter.

olfaction (ol-fak′shun) smell.

olfactology (ol″fak-tol′o-je) the science of the sense of SMELL.

olfactometer (ol″fak-tom′ĕ-ter) an instrument for testing the sense of smell.

olfactory (ol-fak′tŏ-re) pertaining to SMELL.

 o. nerve the first CRANIAL NERVE; it is purely sensory and is concerned with the sense of SMELL. The nerve cell bodies are situated in the olfactory area of the mucous membrane of the nose. The nerve fibers lead upward through openings in the ethmoid bone, connect with the cells of the olfactory bulb, and then pass inward to the cerebrum. See Appendix 2-5.

olig(o)- word element [Gr.], *few; little; scanty.*

oligocythemia (ol″ĭ-go-si-the′me-ah) deficiency of the cellular elements of the blood. adj., **oligocythe′mic.**

oligodactyly (ol″ĭ-go-dak′ĭ-le) congenital absence of one or more fingers or toes.

oligodendrocyte (ol″ĭ-go-den′dro-sīt) a cell of OLIGODENDROGLIA.

oligodendroglia (ol″ĭ-go-den-drog′le-ah) 1. the non-neural cells of ectodermal origin forming part of the adventitial structure of the central nervous system. 2. the tissue composed of such cells.

oligodendroglioma (ol″ĭ-go-den″dro-gli-o′mah) a neoplasm derived from and composed of oligodendroglia.

oligodipsia (ol″ĭ-go-dip′se-ah) hypodipsia.

oligodontia (ol″ĭ-go-don′shah) congenital absence of some of the teeth.

oligodynamic (ol″ĭ-go-di-nam′ik) active in small quantities or at low concentrations.

oligogalactia (ol″ĭ-go-gah-lak′shah) deficient secretion of milk.

oligohydramnios (ol″ĭ-go-hi-dram′ne-os) deficiency in the amount of AMNIOTIC FLUID, defined as 500 mL or less at term and smaller amounts at earlier gestational ages.

oligomeganephronia (ol″ĭ-go-meg″ah-nĕ-fro′ne-ah) congenital renal hypoplasia in which there is a reduced number of lobes and NEPHRONS, with hypertrophy of the nephrons. adj., **oligomeganephron′ic.**

oligomenorrhea (ol″ĭ-go-men″o-re′ah) scanty or infrequent menstruation.

oligonucleotide (ol″ĭ-go-noo′kle-o-tīd) a polymer made up of a few (2 to 10) nucleotides.

oligospermia (ol″ĭ-go-sper′me-ah) deficiency of spermatozoa in the semen.

oligotrophia (ol″ĭ-go-tro′fe-ah) malnutrition.

oliguria (ol″ĭ-gu′re-ah) diminished urine secretion in relation to fluid intake. adj., **oligu′ric.**

olivary (ol′ĭ-ver″e) 1. shaped like an olive. 2. pertaining to the OLIVE.

olive (ol′iv) the tree *Olea europaea* or its fruit. A rounded elevation lateral to the upper part of each pyramid of the medulla oblongata; it is formed by the olivary nucleus just beneath its surface and is linked by fiber systems to the pons and cerebellum. Called also olivary body.

 o. oil a fixed oil obtained from ripe fruit of *Olea europaea;* used as a setting retardant for dental cements, topical EMOLLIENT, pharmaceutic NECESSITY, and sometimes as a LAXATIVE.

olivifugal (ol″ĭ-vif′u-gal) moving or conducting away from the olive.

olivipetal (ol″ĭ-vip′e-tal) moving or conducting toward the olive.

olivopontocerebellar (ol″ĭ-vo-pon″to-ser″ĕ-bel′ar) pertaining to the olive, the middle peduncles, and the cerebellar cortex.

Ollier's disease (o-le-āz′) enchondromatosis.

olopatadine (o″-lo-pat′ah-dēn) a histamine H_1 RECEPTOR antagonist used as the hydrochloride salt in the topical treatment of allergic CONJUNCTIVITIS.

olsalazine (ol-sal′ah-zēn) a derivative of mesalamine used as the sodium salt as an antiinflammatory in ulcerative colitis.

-oma word element [Gr.], *tumor; neoplasm.*

omagra (o-mag′rah) gout in the shoulder.

Omaha System (o'ma-hah) a research-based and comprehensive practice, documentation, and information management framework based on the nursing or problem-solving process, the clinician-client relationship, and concepts of diagnostic reasoning, clinical judgment, and quality improvement. It was designed for members of various disciplines, including nurses, other health care professionals, and students. It consists of three relational, reliable, and valid clinical components useful from the time of client admission until discharge from service. The components are designed for classifying assessment (PROBLEM CLASSIFICATION SCHEME), interventions (INTERVENTION SCHEME), and outcomes measurement (PROBLEM RATING SCALE FOR OUTCOMES). See Appendix on the Omaha System.

omalgia (o-mal'jah) pain in the shoulder; called also omodynia.

omarthritis (o″mahr-thri'tis) inflammation of the shoulder joint.

omentectomy (o″men-tek'to-me) excision of all or part of the omentum.

omentitis (o″men-ti'tis) inflammation of the omentum.

omentofixation (o-men″to-fik-sa'shun) omentopexy.

omentopexy (o-men'to-pek″se) an operation in which omentum is fastened to some other tissue, especially one in which the omentum is being used as a circulatory bridge to reduce congestion or provide vascular nutrition. Called also omentofixation.

omentorrhaphy (o″men-tor'ah-fe) suture or repair of the omentum.

omentum (o-men'tum) [L.] a fold of peritoneum extending from the stomach to adjacent abdominal organs. adj., **omen'tal.**

   gastrocolic o. greater omentum.

   gastrohepatic o. lesser omentum.

   greater o. a peritoneal fold attached to the anterior surface of the transverse colon.

   lesser o. a peritoneal fold joining the lesser curvature of the stomach and the first part of the duodenum to the porta hepatis.

   o. ma'jus greater omentum.

   o. mi'nus lesser omentum.

omeprazole (o-mep'ra-zōl) a proton pump INHIBITOR, used in treatment of DYSPEPSIA, GASTROESOPHAGEAL REFLUX DISEASE, disorders of gastric hypersecretion, and peptic ULCER, including that associated with *Helicobacter pylori* infection; administered orally.

omitis (o-mi'tis) inflammation of the shoulder.

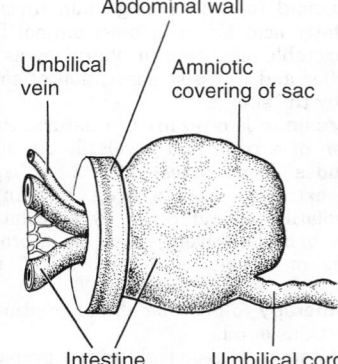

A large omphalocele with structure and contents of the hernial sac. From Betz et al., 1994.

Omnipen (om'nĭ-pen) trademark for preparations of AMPICILLIN, a broad-spectrum ANTIBIOTIC.

omnivorous (om-niv'ŏ-rus) eating both plant and animal foods.

omoclavicular (o″mo-klah-vik'u-lar) pertaining to the shoulder and clavicle.

omodynia (o″mo-din'e-ah) omalgia.

omohyoid (o″mo-hi'oid) pertaining to the shoulder and the hyoid bone.

omphal(o)- word element [Gr.], *umbilicus.*

omphalectomy (om″fah-lek'to-me) excision of the umbilicus.

omphalic (om-fal'ik) umbilical.

omphalitis (om″fah-li'tis) inflammation of the umbilicus.

omphaloangiopagus (om″fah-lo-an″je-op'ah-gus) conjoined twin fetuses, one of which derives its blood supply from the umbilicus or placenta of the other.

omphalocele (om'fah-lo-sēl″) protrusion, at birth, of part of the intestine through a defect in the abdominal wall at the UMBILICUS; see also UMBILICAL HERNIA.

omphalomesenteric (om″fah-lo-mes″enter'ik) pertaining to the umbilicus and mesentery.

omphalophlebitis (om″fah-lo-flĕ-bi'tis) inflammation of the umbilical veins.

omphalorrhagia (om″fah-lo-ra'jah) hemorrhage from the umbilicus.

omphalorrhea (om″fah-lo-re'ah) effusion of lymph at the umbilicus.

omphalorrhexis (om″fah-lo-rek'sis) rupture of the umbilicus.

omphalosite (om'fah-lo-sīt″) the underdeveloped parasitic member of pair of monochorionic twins, joined to the more developed member (autosite) by the vessels of the umbilical cord and not capable of sustaining life after separation from the placenta.

omphalotomy (om″fah-lot′ah-me) the cutting of the umbilical cord.

onanism (o′nah-nizm) 1. coitus interruptus. 2. masturbation.

onc(o)- word element [Gr.], *tumor; swelling; mass.*

Onchocerca (ong″ko-ser′kah) a genus of parasitic FILARIA. *O. vol′vulus* is a common parasite of humans, breeding in fast-flowing rivers and streams in tropical parts of the Americas and equatorial Africa, particularly West Africa. It is the etiologic agent of human ONCHOCERCIASIS and is transmitted by the bites of blackflies (buffalo gnats) of the genus *Simulium,* in which the parasite passes part of its life cycle.

onchocerciasis (ong″ko-ser-ki′ah-sis) infection with worms of the genus *Onchocerca.* Human infection is caused by *O. volvulus,* with heavy infestations usually being characterized by subcutaneous nodules (onchocercomas) containing tangled masses of adult worms, a persistent dermatitis, lymphadenitis, and ocular lesions related to the invasion and death of microfilariae, which may progress to optic neuritis, optic atrophy, and blindness. The condition is also known by many local and regional names (craw-craw, Robles' disease) and by various names descriptive of the manifestations of the disease (coast erysipelas, river blindness, blinding filarial disease).

onchocercoma (ong″ko-ser-ko′mah) one of the dermal or subcutaneous nodules containing *Onchocerca volvulus* in human onchocerciasis.

oncogene (ong′ko-jēn) a gene found in the chromosomes of tumor cells whose activation is associated with the initial and continuing conversion of normal cells into cancer cells.

oncogenesis (ong″ko-jen′ĕ-sis) the production or causation of tumors; called also tumorigenesis. adj., **oncogenet′ic.**

oncogenic (ong″ko-jen′ik) giving rise to tumors or causing tumor formation; said especially of tumor-inducing viruses.

oncogenous (ong-koj′ĕ-nus) arising in or originating from a tumor.

oncology (ong-kol′ŏ-je) 1. the sum of knowledge regarding TUMORS and CANCER, or the study of these conditions. 2. the care and treatment of patients with TUMORS or CANCER.

oncolysate (ong-kol′ĭ-sāt) any agent that lyses or destroys tumor cells. See also CYTOTOXICITY.

oncolysis (ong-kol′ĭ-sis) destruction or dissolution of tumor cells. adj., **oncolyt′ic.**

oncoma (ong-ko′mah) a tumor.

oncosis (ong-ko′sis) a morbid condition marked by the development of tumors.

oncosphere (ong′ko-sfēr) the larva of the tapeworm contained within the external embryonic envelope and armed with six hooks.

oncotherapy (ong″ko-ther′ah-pe) the treatment of tumors.

oncotic (ong-kot′ik) pertaining to swelling.

oncotropic (ong″ko-trop′ik) having special affinity for tumor cells.

Oncovin (ong′ko-vin) trademark for a preparation of VINCRISTINE sulfate, an antineoplastic AGENT.

oncovirus (ong′ko-vi″rus) any virus that promotes cancer.

ondansetron (on-dan′sĕ-tron) an antiemetic used as the hydrochloride salt, in conjunction with cancer chemotherapy, radiotherapy, or after surgery; administered orally or intravenously.

Ondine's curse (on′dēnz) a condition in which patients have lost autonomic control of respiration and become apneic upon falling asleep; it is due to lesions or surgery of the high spinal cord or brainstem; named after Ondine, a water nymph in Greek mythology who caused a mortal who loved her to sleep forever.

oneir(o)- word element [Gr.], *dream.*

oneiric (o-ni′rik) pertaining to or characterized by dreaming or oneirism.

oneirism (o-ni′rizm) an abnormal dreamlike state of CONSCIOUSNESS.

oneirology (o″ni-rol′ŏ-je) the science of dreams and their interpretation.

onlay (on′la) 1. a graft applied or laid on the surface of an organ or structure. 2. a cast metal restoration that overlays cusps, thus restoring the occlusal and proximal surfaces and lending strength to the tooth.

onomatology (on″o-mah-tol′ŏ-je) the science of names and nomenclature.

onomatomania (on″ah-mat″ah-ma′ne-ah) irresistible preoccupation with specific names or words.

onomatophobia (on″o-mat″o-fo′be-ah) irrational fear of hearing a particular word or name.

ontogeny (on″toj′ĕ-ne) the complete developmental history of an individual organism. adj., **ontogenet′ic, ontogen′ic.**

onyalai (o″ne-al′a-e) a form of thrombopenic purpura occurring in Central Africa, due to a nutritional disorder; characteristics include blebs on the buccal and palatal mucosa, containing semicoagulated blood.

onych(o)- word element [Gr.], *the nails*.

onychatrophia (on″ik-ah-tro′fe-ah) atrophy of a nail or the nails.

onychauxis (on″ĭ-kawk′sis) hypertrophy of the nail(s) without deformity.

onychectomy (on″ĭ-kek′to-me) excision of a nail or nail bed.

onychia (o-nik′e-ah) inflammation of the nail bed, resulting in loss of the nail.

onychitis (on″ĭ-ki′tis) onychia.

onychocryptosis (on″ĭ-ko-krip-to′sis) ingrown nail.

onychodystrophy (on″ĭ-ko-dis′trŏ-fe) malformation of a nail.

onychogenic (on″ĭ-ko-jen′ik) producing nail substance.

onychograph (o-nik′o-graf) an instrument for observing and recording the nail pulse and capillary circulation.

onychogryphosis (on″ĭ-ko-grĭ-fo′sis) abnormal hypertrophy and curving of the nails, giving them a clawlike appearance.

onychogryposis (on″ĭ-ko-grĭ-po′sis) onychogryphosis.

onychoheterotopia (on″ĭ-ko-het″er-o-to′pe-ah) abnormal location of the nails.

onycholysis (on″ĭ-kol′ĭ-sis) loosening or separation of a nail from its bed.

onychomadesis (on″ĭ-ko-mah-de′sis) periodic separation of the proximal portions of the nail plate from the matrix and bed with subsequent shedding of the nails.

onychomalacia (on″ĭ-ko-mah-la′shah) softening of the nail(s).

onychomycosis (on″ĭ-ko-mi-ko′sis) fungal disease of the nails; the nails become opaque, white, thickened, and friable.

onychopathy (on″ĭ-kop′ah-the) any disease or deformity of the nails.

onychophagia (on″ĭ-ko-fa′jah) biting of the nails.

onychorrhexis (on″ĭ-ko-rek′sis) spontaneous splitting or breaking of the nails.

onychoschizia (on″ĭ-ko-skiz′e-ah) splitting or lamination of the nail plate, usually in the horizontal plane at the free edge.

onychosis (on″ĭ-ko′sis) onychopathy.

onychotillomania (on″ĭ-ko-til″o-ma′ne-ah) compulsive picking or tearing at the nails.

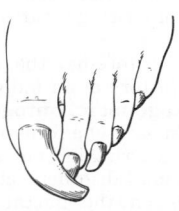

Onychogryphosis. From Dorland's, 2000.

onychotomy (on″ĭ-kot′ah-me) incision into a fingernail or toenail.

onyx (on′iks) 1. nail (def. 2). 2. a variety o HYPOPYON.

oo- word element [Gr.], *egg; ovum*. See also words beginning OV(O)-.

ooblast (o′o-blast) a primordial cell from which an OOCYTE (OVUM) ultimately develops.

oocyst (o′o-sist) the encysted or encapsulated ookinete in the wall of a mosquito's stomach; also, the analogous stage in the development of any sporozoon.

oocyte (o′o-sīt) an immature ovum; it is derived from an OOGONIUM, and is called a *primary oocyte* prior to completion of the first maturation division, and a *secondary oocyte* between the first and second maturation division.

oogamous (o-og′ah-mus) 1. pertaining to or produced by OOGAMY. 2. heterogamous.

oogamy (o-og′ah-me) 1. fertilization of a large nonmotile egg by a small, motile male gamete or sperm, as seen in certain algae. 2. heterogamy.

oogenesis (o″o-jen′ĕ-sis) the development of mature ova from oogonia. adj. **oogenet′ic.**

oogonium (o″o-go′ne-um) [Gr.], a primordial OOCYTE during fetal development; near the time of birth it becomes a primary OOCYTE.

ookinesis (o″o-kĭ-ne′sis) the mitotic movements of an OOCYTE during maturation and fertilization.

ookinete (o″o-kĭ-nēt′) the fertilized form of the malarial parasite in a mosquito's body, formed by fertilization of a macrogamete by a microgamete and developing into an oocyst.

oolemma (o″o-lem′ah) zona pellucida (def 1).

oophor(o)- word element [Gr.], *ovary*. See also words beginning OVARI(O)-.

oophorectomy (o″of-o-rek′to-me) removal of one or both OVARIES; done for tumors severe infection, or certain other ovarian disorders. If this is done to a girl who has not yet reached puberty, it prevents the development of secondary sex CHARACTERS. If both ovaries are removed from an adult woman, reproduction is not possible and the female sex hormones ESTROGEN and PROGESTERONE are no longer produced. Called also ovariectomy.

oophoritis (o″of-o-ri′tis) inflammation of an OVARY; called also ovaritis.

oophorocystectomy (o-of″o-ro-sis-tek′to-me) excision of an ovarian cyst.

oophorocystosis (o-of″o-ro-sis-to′sis) the formation of an ovarian cyst.

oophorohysterectomy (o-of″o-ro-his″ter-ek′to-me) excision of the ovaries and uterus.

oophoron (o-of′o-ron) an ovary.

oophoropexy (o-of′o-ro-pek″se) ovariopexy.

oophoroplasty (o-of′o-ro-plas″te) plastic repair of an ovary.

oophorostomy (o-of″o-ros′tah-me) incision of an ovarian cyst for drainage purposes; called also ovariostomy.

oophorotomy (o-of″ah-rot′ah-me) incision of an ovary.

ooplasm (o′o-plazm) cytoplasm of an OOCYTE.

oosperm (o′o-sperm) a recently fertilized OOCYTE.

ootid (o′o-tid) a mature OOCYTE (OVUM); the cell produced by meiotic division of a secondary oocyte. In mammals, this second maturation division is not completed unless FERTILIZATION occurs.

opacification (o-pas″ĭ-fĭ-ka′shun) the development of an opacity.

opacity (o-pas′ĭ-te) 1. the condition of being opaque. 2. an opaque area.

opalescent (o″pal-es′ent) showing a milky iridescence, like an opal.

opaque (o-pāk) impervious to light rays or, by extension, to x-rays or other electromagnetic radiation; neither translucent nor transparent.

open (o′pen) 1. not obstructed or closed. 2. exposed to the air; not covered by unbroken skin. 3. pertaining to a clinical trial or other experiment in which both subjects and observers know which treatment is administered to each subject, as opposed to a SINGLE BLIND, DOUBLE BLIND, or TRIPLE BLIND study.

opening (o′pen-ing) a gap or open space; anatomic nomenclature for various types of openings includes ADITUS, APERTURE, FORAMEN, FOSSA, HIATUS, INLET, MEATUS, ORIFICE, OSTIUM, and OUTLET.

    aortic o. 1. the aperture in the diaphragm for passage of the descending aorta. 2. aortic orifice.

    cardiac o. the opening from the esophagus into the stomach.

    pulmonary o., o. of pulmonary trunk pulmonary orifice.

    pyloric o. the opening between the stomach and duodenum.

open systems model former name for the GENERAL SYSTEMS FRAMEWORK AND THEORY OF GOAL ATTAINMENT.

operable (op′er-ah-b'l) subject to being operated upon with a reasonable degree of safety; appropriate for surgical intervention with a reasonable expectation of cure or relief.

operant (op′er-ant) in psychology, said of a response not elicited by specific external

stimuli but that recurs at a given rate under particular circumstances. See operant CONDITIONING.

operate (op′er-āt) 1. to perform an operation. 2. the subject of an experiment who has undergone a specific surgical procedure.

operation (op″er-a′shun) 1. any action performed with instruments or by the hands of a surgeon; see also METHOD, PROCEDURE, SURGERY, and TECHNIQUE. For specific operations, see the specific name, such as BLALOCK-TAUSSIG OPERATION. 2. the performance of a mental or physical task in an orderly manner.

    cosmetic o. one intended to remove or correct a deformity in an esthetically acceptable manner.

    exploratory o. incision into the body for determination of the cause of otherwise unexplainable symptoms.

    flap o. any operation involving the raising of a flap of tissue.

    intellectual o's in space the mental manipulation of spatial relationships, a cognitive PERFORMANCE COMPONENT of occupational therapy.

    radical o. one involving extensive resection of tissues for the complete extirpation of disease.

operative (op′er-ah-tiv) 1. pertaining to an operation. 2. effective; not inert.

operculum (o-per′ku-lum) [L.] 1. a lid or covering. 2. the folds of pallium from the frontal, parietal, and temporal lobes of the cerebrum overlying the insula. adj., **oper′-cular.**

    dental o. the hood of gingival tissue overlying the crown of an erupting tooth.

    trophoblastic o. the plug of trophoblast that helps close the gap in the endometrium made by the implanting blastocyst.

operon (op′er-on) a segment of a chromosome comprising an operator gene and closely linked structural genes having related functions, the activity of the latter being controlled by the operator gene through its interaction with a regulator gene.

ophiasis (o-fi′ah-sis) a form of alopecia areata involving the temporal and occipital margins of the scalp in a continuous band.

ophidism (o′fi-dizm) poisoning by snake venom.

ophryosis (of″re-o′sis) spasm of the eyebrow.

ophthalm(o)- word element [Gr.] *eye.* See also words beginning OCUL(O)-.

ophthalmagra (of″thal-mag′rah) sudden pain in the eye.

ophthalmalgia (of″thal-mal′jah) pain in the eye; called also ophthalmodynia.

ophthalmectomy (of″thal-mek′to-me) excision of an eye; ENUCLEATION of the eyeball.

ophthalmencephalon (of″thal-men-se-f′ah-lon) the retina, optic nerve, and visual apparatus of the brain.

ophthalmia (of-thal′me-ah) severe inflammation of the eye or of the conjunctiva or deeper structures of the eye.

   Egyptian o. trachoma.

   gonorrheal o. gonorrheal conjunctivitis.

   o. neonato′rum any hyperacute purulent conjunctivitis, such as gonorrheal CONJUNCTIVITIS, occurring during the first 10 days of life, usually contracted during birth from infected vaginal discharge of the mother. The term formerly referred only to gonorrheal conjunctivitis, but now other types are recognized. It is prevented by instilling silver nitrate or other medication in the eyes of the newborn, although in an occasional infant silver nitrate may cause iatrogenic ophthalmia. Called also neonatal conjunctivitis.

   phlyctenular o. phlyctenular keratoconjunctivitis.

   sympathetic o. granulomatous inflammation of the uveal tract of the uninjured eye following a wound involving the uveal tract of the other eye, resulting in bilateral granulomatous inflammation of the entire uveal tract. Called also sympathetic uveitis.

ophthalmic (of-thal′mik) ocular (def. 1).

ophthalmitis (of″thal-mi′tis) inflammation of the eyeball. adj., **ophthalmit′ic.**

ophthalmoblennorrhea (of-thal″mo-blen″o-re′ah) gonorrheal conjunctivitis.

ophthalmocele (of-thal′mo-sēl) exophthalmos.

ophthalmodonesis (of-thal″mo-do-ne′sis) trembling motion of the eyes.

ophthalmodynamometry (of-thal″mo-di″-nah-mom′ē-tre) determination of the blood pressure in the retinal artery.

ophthalmodynia (of-thal″mo-din′e-ah) ophthalmalgia.

ophthalmoeikonometer (of-thal″mo-i″ko-nom′-ē-ter) an instrument used to determine both the refraction of the eye and the relative size and shape of the ocular images.

ophthalmography (of″thal-mog′rah-fe) description of the eye and its diseases.

ophthalmogyric (of-thal″mo-ji′rik) oculogyric.

ophthalmolith (of-thal′mo-lith) dacryolith.

ophthalmologist (of″thal-mol′ŏ-jist) a physician who specializes in diagnosing and prescribing treatment for defects, injuries, and diseases of the EYE, and is skilled at delicate eye surgery, such as that required to remove cataracts; called also oculist.

ophthalmology (of″thal-mol′ŏ-je) the branch of health science dealing with the eye, including its anatomy, physiology, pathology, and other aspects. adj., **ophthalmolog′ic.**

ophthalmomalacia (of-thal″mo-mah-la′-shah) abnormal softness of the eyeball.

ophthalmometer (of″thal-mom′ē-ter) an instrument used in ophthalmometry.

ophthalmometry (of″thal-mom′ē-tre) determination of the refractive powers and defects of the eye.

ophthalmomycosis (of-thal″mo-mi-ko′sis) any disease of the eye caused by a fungus.

ophthalmomyotomy (of-thal″mo-mi-ot′-ah-me) surgical division of the muscles of the eyes.

ophthalmoneuritis (of-thal″mo-nōō-ri′tis) inflammation of the optic nerve.

ophthalmopathy (of″thal-mop′ah-the) any disease of the eye.

   infiltrative o. ocular changes, most often seen in thyroid disorders, caused by increased water content of the orbital contents, including discomfort, lacrimation, edema, chemosis, and conjunctival infection; if the changes are severe, exophthalmos results.

ophthalmoplasty (of-thal″mo-plas″te) plastic surgery of the eye or its appendages.

ophthalmoplegia (of-thal″mo-ple′jah) paralysis of the eye muscles. adj., **ophthalmople′gic.**

   o. exter′na paralysis of the extraocular muscles.

   o. inter′na paralysis of the iris and ciliary apparatus.

   nuclear o. that due to a lesion of nuclei of motor nerves of eye.

   Parinaud's o. Parinaud syndrome.

   partial o. that affecting some of the eye muscles.

   progressive o. gradual paralysis of all the eye muscles.

   total o. paralysis of all the eye muscles, both intraocular and extraocular.

ophthalmoptosis (of-thal″mop-to′sis) exophthalmos.

ophthalmorrhagia (of-thal″mo-ra′jah) hemorrhage from the eye.

ophthalmorrhea (of-thal″mo-re′ah) oozing of blood from the eye.

ophthalmorrhexis (of-thal″mo-rek′sis) rupture of an eyeball.

ophthalmoscope (of-thal″mo-skōp) an instrument for examining the interior of the eye.

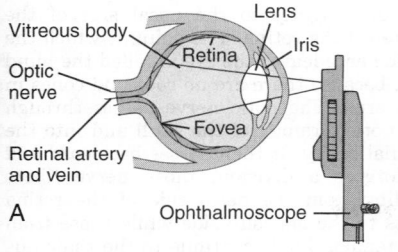

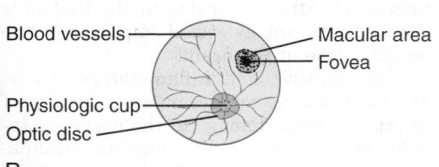

A, Inspection of the eye with a direct ophthalmoscope.
B, Structures that are visualized. From Polaski and Tatro, 1996.

direct o. one that produces an upright, or unreversed, image of approximately 15 times magnification. The direct ophthalmoscope is used to inspect the fundus of the eye, which is the back portion of the interior eyeball. Examination is best carried out in a darkened room. The examiner looks for changes in the color or pigment of the fundus, changes in the caliber and shape of retinal blood vessels, and any abnormalities in the macula lutea, the portion of the retina that receives and analyzes light only from the very center of the visual field. Macular degeneration and opacities of the lens can be seen through direct ophthalmoscopy.

indirect o. one that produces an inverted, or reversed, direct image of two to five times magnification. An indirect ophthalmoscope provides a stronger light source, a specially designed objective lens, and opportunity for stereoscopic inspection of the interior of the eyeball. It is invaluable for diagnosis and treatment of retinal tears, holes, and detachments. The pupils must be fully dilated for satisfactory indirect ophthalmoscopy.

scanning laser o. (SLO) an instrument for retinal imaging in which light from a low-power laser beam that scans the retina is reflected back to a sensor; the light detected by the sensor is used to create a full-color composite digital image.

ophthalmoscopy (of″thal-mos′kah-pe) examination of the eye by means of the ophthalmoscope.

medical o. that performed for diagnostic purposes.

metric o. that performed for measurement of refraction.

ophthalmostasis (of″thal-mos′tah-sis) fixation of the eye with the ophthalmostat.

ophthalmostat (of-thal′mo-stat) an instrument for holding the eye steady during operation.

ophthalmosteresis (of-thal″mo-stĕ-re′sis) loss of an eye.

ophthalmosynchysis (of-thal″mo-sin′kĭ-sis) effusion into the eye.

ophthalmotomy (of″thal-mot′ah-me) incision of the eye.

ophthalmotrope (of-thal′mo-trōp) a mechanical eye that moves like a real eye.

ophthalmoxerosis (of-thal″mo-ze-ro′sis) xerophthalmia.

opiate (o′pe-at) 1. any sedative narcotic containing OPIUM or any of its derivatives; the most common ones are CODEINE, HEROIN, METHADONE, and MORPHINE. 2. hypnotic (def. 2).

endogenous o's ENDORPHINS and EN-KEPHALINS that are released by the body as a defense against pain or during physical exercise, deep relaxation, sexual activity, crying, and laughing.

opioid (o′pe-oid) 1. any synthetic narcotic that has opiate-like activities but is not derived from opium. 2. denoting naturally occurring peptides, such as ENKEPHALINS, that exert OPIATE-like effects by interacting with opiate RECEPTORS of cell membranes. See also opioid ANALGESIC.

opisthorchiasis (o″pis-thor-ki′ah-sis) infection of the biliary tract by the liver flukes *Opisthorchis felineus* or *O. viverrini.*

Opisthorchis (o″pis-thor′kis) a genus of flukes parasitic in the liver and biliary tract of various birds and mammals, including humans; see OPISTHORCHIASIS. *O. feli′neus* is found from the Philippines, Japan, and Vietnam across Asia to Eastern Europe. *O. viverri′ni* is found in Southeast Asia.

opisthotonos (o″pis-thot′o-nos) a form of spasm in which the head and heels are bent backward and the body bowed forward. adj., **opisthoton′ic.**

opium (o′pe-um) the air-dried milky exudation from unripe capsules of *Papaver somniferum* and *P.album* (the opium poppies). It contains some 25 alkaloids, the most important being CODEINE, MORPHINE (from which HEROIN is derived), NOSCAPINE, PAPAVERINE, and THEBAINE, all of which can be used for their narcotic and analgesic effects. Opium is poisonous in large doses; because it is highly addictive, production and cultivation of the poppies is prohibited by most nations by international agreement, and its

O

sale or possession for other than medical uses is strictly prohibited by federal, state, and local laws. See also DRUG ABUSE.

opocephalus (o″po-sef′ah-lus) a malformed fetus with ears fused to the head, one orbit, no mouth, and no nose.

opodidymus (o″po-did′ĭ-mus) conjoined twins with one body, two fused heads, and sense organs partly fused.

Oppenheim sign (op′en-hīm) dorsiflexion of the big toe on stroking the medial aspect of the tibia in a downward motion; seen in pyramidal tract disease.

opportunistic (op″or-too-nis′tik) 1. denoting a microorganism that does not ordinarily cause disease but becomes pathogenic under certain circumstances. 2. denoting a disease or infection caused by such an organism.

oppositional defiant disorder a type of DISRUPTIVE BEHAVIOR DISORDER characterized by a recurrent pattern of defiant, hostile, disobedient, and negativistic behavior directed toward those in authority.

oprelvekin (o-prel′vĕ-kin″) recombinant INTERLEUKIN-11, used as a stimulator of HEMATOPOIESIS to prevent THROMBOCYTOPENIA following MYELOSUPPRESSIVE chemotherapy.

opsiuria (op″se-u′re-ah) excretion of urine more rapidly during fasting than after a meal.

opsoclonia (op″so-klo′ne-ah) opsoclonus.

opsoclonus (op″so-klo′nus) involuntary, nonrhythmic horizontal and vertical oscillations of the eyes, seen in certain disorders of the brainstem or cerebellum.

opsonin (op′so-nin) an antibody that renders bacteria and other cells susceptible to phagocytosis. adj., **opson′ic.**

 immune o. an antibody that sensitizes a particulate antigen to phagocytosis.

opsonization (op″so-nĭ-za′shun) the rendering of bacteria and other cells subject to phagocytosis.

opsonize (op′so-nīz) to subject to opsonization.

opsonocytophagic (op″so-no-si″to-faj′ik) denoting the phagocytic activity of blood in the presence of serum opsonins and homologous leukocytes.

opt(o)- word element [Gr.], *visible; vision; sight.*

optic (op′tik) ocular (def. 1).

 o. nerve the second CRANIAL NERVE; it is purely sensory and is concerned with carrying impulses for the sense of sight (see VISION). See anatomic Table of Nerves in the Appendices.

 The rods and cones of the RETINA are connected with the optic nerve which leaves

the eye slightly to the nasal side of the center of the retina. The point at which the optic nerve leaves the eye is called the blind spot because there are no rods and cones in this area. The optic nerve passes through the optic foramen of the skull and into the cranial cavity. It then passes backward and undergoes a division; those nerve fibers leading from the nasal side of the retina cross to the opposite side while those from the temporal side continue to the thalamus uncrossed. After synapsing in the thalamus the neurons convey visual impulses to the occipital lobe of the brain.

 Degenerative and inflammatory lesions of the optic nerve occur as a result of infections, toxic damage to the nerve, metabolic or nutritional disorders, or trauma. Syphilis is the most frequent cause of infectious disorders of the optic nerve. Methanol (methyl alcohol) is highly toxic to the optic nerve and can cause total blindness. Diabetes mellitus and anemia are examples of metabolic and nutritional disorders that can lead to damage to the optic nerve and produce serious loss of vision.

 Treatment of optic neuritis is aimed at control of the primary cause of the disorder. Cortisone and similar steroids are often used to relieve symptoms; however, nothing can be done to regain sight lost through damage to the nerve.

optical (op′tĭ-kal) visual; see VISION.

optician (op-tish′an) a specialist in OPTICIANRY. Although this is an exact and intricate science, the optician does not need a state license to practice and is not qualified to examine eyes or prescribe eyeglasses.

opticianry (op-tish′an-re) the translation, filling, and adapting of ophthalmic prescriptions, products, and accessories.

opticociliary (op″tĭ-ko-sil′e-er″e) pertaining to the optic and ciliary nerves. See anatomic Table of Nerves in the Appendices.

opticopupillary (op″tĭ-ko-pu′pĭ-ler″e) pertaining to the optic nerve and pupil.

optics (op′tiks) the science of light and vision.

optogram (op′to-gram) the visual image formed on the retina by bleaching of visual purple under the influence of light.

optokinetic (op″to-kĭ-net′ik) pertaining to movement of the eyes in response to the movement of objects across the visual field, as in optokinetic NYSTAGMUS.

optometer (op-tom′ĕ-ter) a device for measuring ocular refraction.

optometric vision therapy technician (OVTT) an allied health professional, supervised by an OPTOMETRIST, who participates in evaluating clients and in planning and implementing optometric vision THERAPY programs.

optometrist (op-tom′ĕ-trist) a specialist in OPTOMETRY; an independent primary health care provider who examines the eyes to evaluate health and visual abilities, diagnoses eye diseases and conditions of the eye and visual system, and provides necessary treatment such as eyeglasses, contact lenses, vision therapy, and low vision aids; optometrists may also perform certain surgical procedures. In most states, they may use drugs to treat eye disease. Optometrists are not medical doctors and are educated and licensed in accordance with state laws. Preparation includes a preprofessional undergraduate degree and four years of professional education at a college of optometry, leading to a degree of Doctor of Optometry (OD); some optometrists also complete a residency.

optometry (op-tom′ĕ-tre) the professional practice of eye and vision care for the diagnosis, treatment, and prevention of diseases and conditions of the eye and visual system. See OPTOMETRIST.

optomyometer (op″to-mi-om′ĕ-ter) a device for measuring the power of ocular muscles.

OPV poliovirus vaccine live oral.

OR operating room.

ora¹ (o′rah), pl. *o′rae* [L.] an edge or margin.

o. serra′ta re′tinae the zigzag margin of the RETINA.

ora² (o′rah) [L.] plural of OS, mouth.

orad (o′rad) toward the mouth.

oral (o′ral) 1. pertaining to the mouth; taken through or applied in the mouth. 2. denoting that aspect of the teeth that faces inward towards the oral cavity or tongue.

orality (o-ral′ĭ-te) the psychic organization of all the sensations, impulses, and personality traits derived from the oral stage of psychosexual development.

orange (or′anj) 1. the trees *Citrus aurantium* and *Citrus sinensis* or their fruits; the flowers and peels are used in pharmaceutical preparations. 2. a color between red and yellow, produced by energy of wavelengths between 590 and 630 nm.. 3. a dye or stain with this color.

methyl o. an orange-yellow aniline dye, used as an indicator with a pH range of 3.2–4.4 and a color change from pink to yellow.

orbicular (or-bik′u-lar) circular; rounded.

orbit (or′bit) 1. the bony cavity containing the eyeball and its associated muscles, vessels, and nerves; the ethmoid, frontal, lacrimal, nasal, palatine, sphenoid, and zygomatic

bones and the maxilla contribute to its formation. 2. the path of an electron around the nucleus of an atom. adj., **or′bital.**

orbitonasal (or″bĭ-to-na′zal) pertaining to the orbit and nose.

orbitonometer (or″bĭ-to-nom′ĕ-ter) an instrument for measuring backward displacement of the eyeball produced by a given pressure on its anterior aspect.

orbitopathy (or″bĭ-top′ah-the) disease affecting the orbit and its contents.

orbitotomy (or″bĭ-tot′ah-me) incision into the orbit.

orbivirus (or′bĭ-vi″rus) any member of a genus of RNA viruses, some of which have been found to cause disease in areas of the world such as Central Africa and Siberia. Mosquitoes, ticks, and sandflies are vectors.

orcein (or-se′in) a brownish-red coloring substance obtained from orcinol; used as a stain for elastic tissue.

orchi(o)- word element [Gr.], *testis*.

orchialgia (or″ke-al′jah) pain in a testis; called also testalgia.

orchidectomy (or″kĭ-dek′to-me) orchiectomy.

orchiectomy (or″ke-ek′to-me) excision of one or both TESTES, done when a testis is seriously injured or diseased (as in testicular cancer).

If both testes are removed (*bilateral orchiectomy* or CASTRATION), the ability to reproduce is ended. There is also a decrease in production of TESTOSTERONE, and although bilateral orchiectomy does not interfere with the ability to have sexual intercourse, the loss of both testes can reduce sexual desire. When this occurs before puberty, it prevents the development of secondary sex CHARACTERS because of testosterone deficit. Replacement therapy may be necessary to maintain a desirable level of the hormone. If the procedure is done after puberty, when the masculine characters have already developed, the effects are much less extreme.

Patient Care. The patient having orchiectomy for treatment of testicular cancer will have special needs in addition to those expected in a cancer patient. He will need help in dealing with problems related to his masculinity, self-concept, and sexual activity. He should be given time to think about and discuss the effects of his surgery. The surgeon is responsible for informing the patient about the procedure and its anticipated long-term effects. The nurse and other health care personnel can clarify any information the patient and his family may have been unable to assimilate during their

O

conference with the surgeon. All members of the health care team should know the expected prognosis and be prepared to answer the patient's questions truthfully and matter-of-factly. He will need an optimistic outlook and encouragement to deal with the future without being given false hope and unreasonable expectations for recovery from the effects of his therapy.

orchiepididymitis (or″ke-ep′ĭ-did″ĭ-mi′tis) epididymo-orchitis.

orchiocele (or′ke-o-sēl″) 1. hernial protrusion of a testis. 2. scrotal hernia. 3. tumor of a testis.

orchiopathy (or″ke-op′ah-the) any disease of the testes.

orchiopexy (or′ke-o-pek″se) surgical fixation of an undescended TESTIS in the scrotum. An incision is made over the inguinal canal and the testis is brought down. In most cases the surgeon applies traction by placing a suture in the lower scrotum and attaching the suture to the inner thigh with adhesive tape. This traction is continued for about a week. Alternatively, a surgeon may prefer to suture the undescended testis to surrounding tissue in the scrotum. **Patient Care.** Preoperative care of the child is routine. During the postoperative period care must be taken to avoid disturbing the tension mechanism. Contamination of the suture line should be avoided, and if the boy is not toilet trained, he usually must have an indwelling catheter in place until his incision has healed.

orchioplasty (or′ke-o-plas″te) plastic surgery of a testis.

orchiotomy (or″ke-ot′ah-me) incision and drainage of a testis.

orchitis (or-ki′tis) inflammation of a testis. Orchitis is not a common disorder, but it can occur in a variety of infectious diseases, including syphilis, tuberculosis, glanders, leprosy, and certain of the parasitic diseases. It usually accompanies EPIDIDYMITIS. Acute orchitis may also occur in such diseases as typhoid fever, pneumonia, or mumps in adult males. The symptoms of acute orchitis are swelling of one or both testes with pain and sensitivity to touch. In chronic orchitis there is no pain but the testes swell slowly and become hard. adj., **orchit′ic.**

order (or′der) 1. a taxonomic category subordinate to a class and superior to a family (or suborder). 2. the prescription of a physician regarding treatment of a patient.

  standing o. a physician's order that can be exercised by other health care workers when predetermined conditions have been met.

orderly (or′der-le) an attendant in a hospital who works under the direction of a nurse.

ordinate (or′dĭ-nat) the vertical line in a graph along which is plotted one of the variables considered in the study, as temperature in a time-temperature study. The other line is called the ABSCISSA.

Orem (or′em) Dorothea E. A leader in nursing service and nursing education, whose concept of nursing was first published in 1959 in a government publication entitled *Guides for Developing Curricula for the Education of Practical Nurses.* Development of a SELF-CARE MODEL for nursing was continued by Orem and other members of the Nursing Model Committee of the Catholic University Faculty.

orexigenic (o-rek″sĭ-jen′ik) increasing or stimulating the appetite.

orf (orf) a contagious pustular viral dermatitis of sheep, sometimes communicable to humans.

organ (or′gan) organum.

  accessory digestive o's, accessory o's of digestive system organs and structures not part of the alimentary canal that aid in digestion; they include the teeth, salivary glands, liver, gallbladder, and pancreas.

  o. of Corti the organ lying against the basilar membrane in the cochlear DUCT, containing special sensory receptors for HEARING, and consisting of neuroepithelial hair CELLS and several types of supporting cells.

  effector o. a muscle or gland that contracts or secretes, respectively, in direct response to nerve impulses.

  enamel o. a process of epithelium forming a cap over a dental papilla and developing into the enamel.

  end o. end-organ.

  Golgi tendon o. any of the mechanoreceptors arranged in series with muscle in the tendons of mammalian muscles, being the receptor for stimuli responsible for the lengthening reaction.

  reproductive o's see REPRODUCTIVE ORGANS, FEMALE and REPRODUCTIVE ORGANS, MALE.

  sense o's, sensory o's organs that receive stimuli that give rise to sensations, i.e., organs that translate certain forms of energy into nerve impulses that are perceived as special sensations.

  spiral o. organ of Corti.

  target o. the organ affected by a particular hormone.

  vestigial o. an undeveloped organ that, in the embryo or in some remote ancestor, was well developed and functional.

o's of Zuckerkandl para-aortic bodies.

organ(o)- word element [Gr.], *organ.*

organelle (or"gah-nel') any of the organized cytoplasmic structures of distinctive morphology and function present in all eukaryotic cells, including such structures as the NUCLEUS, MITOCHONDRIA, LYSOSOMES, PEROXISOMES, Golgi APPARATUS, and endoplasmic RETICULUM, as well as CHLOROPLASTS in plants and CILIA and FLAGELLA in protozoa.

organic (or-gan'ik) 1. pertaining to an organ or organs. 2. having an organized structure. 3. arising from an organism. 4. pertaining to substances derived from living organisms. 5. denoting chemical substances containing covalently bonded carbon atoms. 6. pertaining to or cultivated by use of animal or vegetable fertilizers, rather than synthetic chemicals.

o. anxiety syndrome a term used in a former system of classification for an OR-GANIC MENTAL SYNDROME characterized by prominent, recurrent panic attacks or generalized anxiety caused by a specific organic factor and not associated with DELIRIUM. Such disorders are now mainly classified as substance-induced anxiety disorders and anxiety disorders due to a general medical condition. See also SUBSTANCE-INDUCED DISORDERS.

o. brain syndrome organic mental syndrome.

o. delusional syndrome a term used in a former system of classification, denoting an ORGANIC MENTAL SYNDROME characterized by DELUSIONS caused by a specific organic factor and not associated with CLOUDING OF CONSCIOUSNESS (DELIRIUM), intellectual impairment (DEMENTIA), or prominent hallucinations (organic HALLUCINOSIS). The disorders are now mainly classified as substance-induced psychotic disorders and psychotic disorders due to a general medical condition. See also SUBSTANCE-INDUCED DISORDERS.

o. disease a disease due to or accompanied by structural changes in organs or tissues.

o. mental disorder a term formerly used to denote any mental disorder with a specifically known or presumed organic etiology; now discouraged because of the implication that other disorders do not have an organic basis. The term was sometimes used as a synonym of ORGANIC MENTAL SYNDROME.

o. mental syndrome former term for a constellation of psychological or behavioral signs and symptoms associated with brain dysfunction of unknown or unspecified etiology, grouped according to symptoms (see also ORGANIC MENTAL DISORDER). The

designating of certain conditions as having an organic basis, possibly implying that other conditions do not, is currently discouraged.

o. mood syndrome a term used in a former system of classification, denoting an ORGANIC MENTAL SYNDROME characterized by manic or depressive mood disturbance caused by a specific organic factor and not associated with CLOUDING OF CONSCIOUSNESS (DELIRIUM), intellectual impairment (DEMENTIA), or prominent delusions or hallucinations (ORGANIC DELUSIONAL SYNDROME or organic HALLUCINOSIS). Such disorders are now mainly classified as substance-induced MOOD DISORDERS and mood disorders due to a general medical condition. See also SUBSTANCE-INDUCED DISORDERS.

o. personality syndrome former term for an ORGANIC MENTAL SYNDROME characterized by a marked change in behavior or personality, e.g., emotional instability, marked apathy, or impaired impulse control, caused by a specific organic factor and not associated with DELIRIUM, prominent mood disturbance, DELUSIONS, or HALLUCINATIONS. Such disorders are now mainly classified on the basis of etiology, such as those that are substance-induced or are due to a general medical condition.

organism (or'gah-nizm) an individual animal or plant.

pleuropneumonia-like o's PPLO; originally, a group of filtrable microorganisms similar to *Mycoplasma mycoides*, the causative agent of PLEUROPNEUMONIA in cattle, which have been isolated from humans and other animals such as sheep, goats, dogs, rats, mice. They are now classified as bacteria and have been assigned to various species of the genus *Mycoplasma.*

organization (or"gah-nĭ-za'shun) 1. the process of organizing or being organized. 2. an organized body, group, or structure. 3. the replacement of blood clots by fibrous tissue.

comprehensive health o. (CHO) a non-profit health care agency in Canada, formed jointly by representatives of the community and of health care providers. The aim is to provide a variety of health promotion and treatment services and to unify different elements of health care for a defined member population.

health maintenance o. see HEALTH MAINTENANCE ORGANIZATION.

professional review o. (PRO) a program on multiple governmental levels (local, state, and federal) that regulates the quality and cost of federally funded medical care.

See also PROFESSIONAL STANDARDS REVIEW ORGANIZATION.

Professional Standards Review O. (PSRO) see PROFESSIONAL STANDARDS REVIEW ORGANIZATION.

organizer (or'gah-nīz"er) a special region of the embryo that is capable of determining the differentiation of other regions.

  primary o. the dorsal lip region of the blastopore.

organogenesis (or"gah-no-jen'ē-sis) the origin or development of organs.

organogeny (or"gah-noj'ē-ne) organogenesis.

organoid (or'gah-noid) 1. resembling an organ. 2. a structure that resembles an organ.

organology (or"gah-nol'ŏ-je) the sum of what is known regarding the body organs.

organomegaly (or"gah-no-meg'ah-le) visceromegaly.

organomercurial (or"gah-no-mer-ku're-al) any mercury-containing organic compound.

organometallic (or"gah-no-mē-tal'ik) consisting of a metal combined with an organic radical, particularly when the metal is linked directly to a carbon atom.

organon (or'gah-non) [Gr.] organ.

organophosphate (or"gah-no-fos'fāt) an organic ester of a PHOSPHATE such as PHOSPHORIC ACID with an organic compound such as GLUCOSE or SORBITOL; see also ORGANOPHOSPHORUS. adj., **organophos'phorous.**

organophosphorus (or"gah-no-fos'fah-rus) a compound containing phosphorus bound to an organic molecule. Some are used as insecticides and others are nerve gases; they are highly toxic acetylcholinesterase inhibitors.

  o. compound poisoning poisoning by excessive exposure to an organophosphorus compound; there are usually neurologic symptoms such as axonopathy and paralysis, and it often ends fatally.

organotherapy (or"gah-no-ther'ah-pe) therapeutic administration of animal endocrine organs or their extracts.

organotrophic (or"gah-no-trof'ik) heterotrophic.

organotropism (or-gah-not'rŏ-pizm) the special affinity of chemical compounds or pathogenic agents for particular tissues or organs of the body. adj., **organotrop'ic.**

organ-specific (or'gan-spē-sif'ik) restricted to, or having an effect only on, a particular organ, as an organ-specific antigen.

organum (or'gah-num) [L.] organ.

orgasm (or'gazm) the apex and culmination of sexual excitement.

orgasmic disorders SEXUAL DYSFUNCTION characterized by inhibited or premature orgasm; see FEMALE ORGASMIC DISORDER, MALE ORGASMIC DISORDER, and PREMATURE EJACULATION.

orientation (o"re-en-ta'shun) 1. awareness of one's environment, with reference to place, time, and people. 2. attraction or tendency. 3. the relative positions of atoms or groups in chemical compounds. 4. a planned series of classes and educational experiences on patient care units to acquaint a newly employed health care provider with routines, protocols, and expectations.

  reality o. see REALITY ORIENTATION.

  topographical o. determination of the location of objects and settings and the route to the location.

orifice (or'ĭ-fis) 1. the entrance or outlet of any body cavity. 2. any OPENING or MEATUS. adj., **orific'ial.**

  aortic o. the opening of the left ventricle into the aorta; called also aortic opening.

  external urethral o. urinary meatus.

  internal urethral o. the opening from the urinary BLADDER into the urethra at one corner of the TRIGONE OF THE BLADDER.

  left atrioventricular o., mitral o. the opening between the left atrium and ventricle of the heart.

  pulmonary o., o. of pulmonary trunk the opening between the pulmonary TRUNK and the right ventricle of the heart; called also opening of pulmonary trunk.

  right atrioventricular o., tricuspid o. the opening between the right atrium and ventricle of the heart.

  ureteral o. the opening of a URETER into the urinary BLADDER at one corner of the TRIGONE OF THE BLADDER. Called also ureteral meatus.

origin (or'ĭ-jin) the source or beginning of anything, especially the more fixed end or attachment of a muscle (as distinguished from its insertion), or the site of emergence of a peripheral nerve from the central nervous system.

Orinase (or'ĭ-nās) trademark for a preparation of TOLBUTAMIDE, an oral hypoglycemic AGENT.

orlistat (or'lĭ-stat) an inhibitor of gastrointestinal lipases that prevents the digestion, and therefore absorption, of dietary fat, used in the treatment of obesity administered orally. Because it interferes with the absorption of some fat-soluble vitamins and beta carotene, persons taking orlistat should also take a dietary supplement containing fat-soluble vitamins and beta carotene.

Ormond disease (or'mond) retroperitoneal fibrosis.

ORNAC Operating Room Nurses' Association of Canada.

Ornade (or'nād) trademark for combination preparations of CHLORPHENIRAMINE maleate and PHENYLPROPANOLAMINE hydrochloride; a cold and allergy preparation.

ornithine (or'nĭ-thēn) an amino acid obtained from arginine by splitting of urea; it is an intermediate in urea biosynthesis.

   o. carbamoyltransferase, o. transcarbamylase an enzyme that catalyzes a reaction occurring in the liver mitochondria as part of the urea CYCLE.

Ornithodoros (or″nĭ-thod'o-ros) a genus of soft-bodied ticks, many species of which are reservoirs and vectors of the spirochetes (*Borrelia*) of relapsing fevers.

ornithosis (or″nĭ-tho'sis) a term that has been used in various ways, including: (1) to replace the term psittacosis (originally thought to affect only parrots); (2) to refer to *Chlamydia psittaci* infection in other birds, with the term psittacosis being reserved for infection in parrots and humans; and (3) to refer to *Chlamydia psittaci* infection in all birds, with the term psittacosis being reserved for human infection.

orofaciodigital syndrome (or″o-fa'sho-dij'ĭ-tal) a syndrome seen only in females, with mental retardation and anomalies of the mouth, tongue, fingers, and frequently the face.

orolingual (or″o-ling'gwal) pertaining to the mouth and tongue.

oronasal (or″o-na'zal) pertaining to the mouth and nose.

oropharyngeal (o″ro-fah-rin'je-al) 1. pertaining to the mouth and the pharynx. 2. pertaining to the OROPHARYNX.

oropharynx (or″o-far'ingks) the part of the pharynx between the soft palate and the upper edge of the epiglottis.

orosomucoid (or″ŏ-so-mu'koid) α₁-acid GLYCOPROTEIN.

orotic acid (o-rot'ik) an intermediate in the biosynthesis of pyrimidine nucleotides.

oroticaciduria (o-rot″ik-as'ĭ-du're-ah) a hereditary defect of PYRIMIDINE metabolism associated with excessive urinary excretion of OROTIC ACID, and characterized by megaloblastic ANEMIA, CRYSTALLURIA, and frequently physical and mental retardation.

Oroya fever (o-ro'yah) the acute febrile anemic stage of BARTONELLOSIS.

orphenadrine (or-fen'ah-drēn) an anticholinergic AGENT used as the citrate salt as a skeletal muscle RELAXANT for relief of muscle spasms; administered orally, intramuscularly, or intravenously.

ORS oral rehydration salts.

ORT oral rehydration therapy.

orth(o)- word element [Gr.], *straight; normal; correct.* In chemistry, *ortho-* indicates an isomer; also, a cyclic derivative having two substitutes in adjacent positions.

orthesis (or-the'sis) [Gr.] orthosis.

orthetics (or-thet'iks) orthotics.

orthetist (or'thĕ-tist) orthotist.

orthocephalic (or″tho-sĕ-fal'ik) having a head with a vertical index of 70.1 to 75.

orthochorea (or″tho-ko-re'ah) choreic movements in the erect posture.

orthochromatic (or″tho-kro-mat'ik) staining normally.

orthodeoxia (or″tho-de-ok'se-ah) accentuation of arterial hypoxemia in the erect position.

orthodontia (or″tho-don'shah) orthodontics.

orthodontics (or″tho-don'tiks) the branch of DENTISTRY concerned with growth and development of orofacial structures, including irregularities of teeth, malocclusion, and associated facial problems.

orthodontist (or″tho-don'tist) a dentist who specializes in orthodontics.

orthodromic (or″tho-drom'ik) conducting impulses in the normal direction; said of nerve fibers.

orthognathia (or″thog-nath'e-ah) the science dealing with the cause and treatment of malposition of the bones of the jaw. adj., **orthogna'thic.**

orthograde (or'tho-grād) carrying the body upright in walking.

Orthohepadnavirus (or″tho-hep-ad'nah-vi″rus) a genus of HEPADNAVIRUSES that includes the hepatitis B VIRUS infecting humans.

orthometer (or-thom'ĕ-ter) an instrument for determining the relative protrusion of the eyeballs.

orthomyxovirus (or″tho-mik″so-vi'rus) any of a family of RNA VIRUSES that cause INFLUENZA. Replication occurs in the nucleus and cytoplasm, and assembly is by budding on the plasma membrane. Genera include *Influenzavirus A, Influenzavirus B,* and *Influenzavirus C.*

Ortho-Novum (or″tho-no'vum) trademark for preparations of NORETHINDRONE with MESTRANOL or with ETHINYL ESTRADIOL, used as an oral CONTRACEPTIVE.

orthopedic (or″tho-pe'dik) 1. pertaining to the correction of deformities of the musculoskeletal system. 2. pertaining to orthopedics.

orthopedics (or″tho-pe'diks) the branch of SURGERY dealing with the preservation and restoration of the function of the

O

skeletal system, its articulations, and associated structures.

orthopedist (or″tho-pe′dist) an orthopedic surgeon.

orthopercussion (or″tho-per-kush′un) percussion with the distal phalanx of the finger held perpendicularly to the body wall.

orthophoria (or″tho-fo′re-ah) normal equilibrium of the eye muscles, or muscular balance. adj., **orthophor′ic.**

orthopnea (or″thop-ne′ah) DYSPNEA that is relieved in the upright position; see also PLATYPNEA.

orthopoxvirus (or′tho-poks-vi″rus) any member of a genus of POXVIRUSES, including the viruses that cause human SMALLPOX and VACCINIA.

orthopraxis (or″tho-prak′sis) orthopraxy.

orthopraxy (or″tho-prak″se) mechanical correction of deformities.

orthopsychiatry (or″tho-si-ki′ah-tre) an interdisciplinary field that combines psychiatry with principles of psychology, sociology, social work, and other fields in the study and practice of maintaining or restoring mental health, emphasizing a prophylactic approach to mental disease.

orthoptic (or-thop′tik) correcting obliquity of one or both visual axes.

orthoptics (or-thop′tiks) treatment of STRABISMUS by exercise of the ocular muscles.

orthoscope (or′tho-skōp) an apparatus that neutralizes corneal refraction by means of a layer of water; used in ocular examinations.

orthoscopic (or″tho-skop′ik) 1. pertaining to orthoscopy or an orthoscope. 2. having normal, undistorted vision. 3. pertaining to an optical system that produces undistorted images.

orthoscopy (or-thos′kah-pe) examination by means of an orthoscope.

orthosis (or-tho′sis) [Gr.] an orthopedic appliance or apparatus used to support, align, prevent, or correct deformities or to improve function of movable parts of the body. See also BRACE and SPLINT.

   cervical o. a rigid plastic orthosis that encircles the neck and supports the chin and the back of the head; used in the treatment of injuries to the cervical spine.

   dynamic o. an orthosis that both gives support and aids in the initiation and performance of movement by a body part.

   flexion o., flexor o. tenodesis splint.

orthostatic (or″tho-stat′ik) pertaining to or caused by standing erect; see also orthostatic HYPOTENSION.

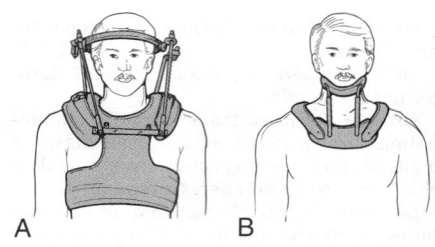

Cervical orthoses offering rigid support to the cervical spine: *A,* Halo-type cervical orthosis attached to a polyethylene jacket. *B,* Four poster orthosis.

orthostatism (or′tho-stat″izm) an erect standing position of the body.

orthotic (or-thot′ik) serving to protect or to restore or improve function; pertaining to the use or application of an orthosis.

orthotics (or-thot′iks) the field of knowledge relating to orthoses and their use.

orthotist (or′tho-tist) a person skilled in orthotics and practicing its application in individual cases.

orthotonos (or-thot′ŏ-nus) tetanic spasm that fixes the head, body, and limbs in a rigid straight line.

orthotonus (or-thot′ŏ-nus) orthotonos.

orthotopic (or″tho-top′ik) 1. occurring at the normal place in the body. 2. pertaining to a tissue transplant grafted into its normal place in the body.

orthovoltage (or′tho-vōl″taj) in RADIATION THERAPY, voltage in the range of 140 to 400 kilovolts, as contrasted to SUPERVOLTAGE and MEGAVOLTAGE.

OS [L.] o′culus sinis′ter (left eye).

Os osmium.

os[1] (os) [L.] 1. any body orifice. 2. the mouth.

os[2] (os) [L.] bone (see anatomic Table of Bones in the Appendices).

Osborne (oz′born) Estelle M. (1901–1981). American nursing educator, administrator, and consultant, and the first black nurse in the United States to earn a master's degree. She was also the first black instructor at New

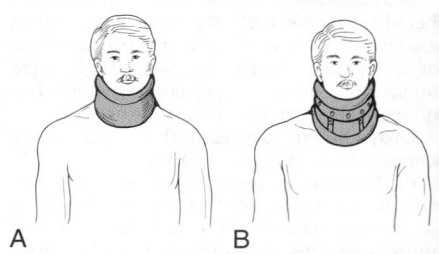

Cervical orthoses. *A,* Soft foam collar. *B,* Firm plastic collar.

WINDOW ON ORTHOTICS

An orthotist is dedicated to the mobility of people. Practitioners and technical staff maintain high standards of knowledge with continuing education programs, insuring that the patient receives the latest technology available. Practitioners can achieve the designation of ABC, which indicates American Board Certification.

The orthotist utilizes a team approach, applying knowledge, biomechanical principles, and compassion to aid patients in achieving a successful outcome. Experience and advanced technology help to provide the best clinical care possible.

Orthotic care can range from custom arch and knee supports to acute care fracture bracing and postsurgical supports. Practitioners have established relationships with the rehabilitation community as part of the team approach. Orthotics and prosthetics are designed with one purpose in mind: to allow people to reach their potential.

DAVID OSBORNE, CPO
KATE ALLYN, CPEDCO

York University. Ms. Osborne was concerned with increasing opportunities for black nurses in professional nursing and was active in a number of professional and civil rights groups; she served as president of the National Association of Colored Graduate Nurses from 1934 to 1939.

osche(o)- for terms beginning thus, see those beginning *scrot(o)-*.

oscill(o)- word element [L.], *oscillation.*

oscillation (os″ĭ-la′shun) a backward and forward motion, like that of a pendulum; also vibration, fluctuation, or variation.

   high frequency o. a type of high frequency VENTILATION characterized by the use of active EXPIRATION.

oscillometer (os″ĭ-lom′ĕ-ter) an instrument for measuring oscillations.

oscillopsia (os″ĭ-lop′se-ah) a visual sensation that stationary objects are swaying back and forth.

oscilloscope (ŏ-sil′o-skōp) an instrument that displays a visual representation of electrical variations on the fluorescent screen of a cathode-ray tube.

oscitation (os″ĭ-ta′shun) yawning.

osculum (os′ku-lum) a minute opening.

oseltamivir (o″sel-tam′ĭ-vir) an inhibitor of viral neuraminidase, used as the phosphate salt in the treatment of influenza.

Osgood-Schlatter disease (oz′good shlaht′er) OSTEOCHONDROSIS of the tuberosity of the tibia; called also Schlatter-Osgood disease.

OSHA Occupational Safety and Health Administration.

-osis word element [Gr.], *disease, morbid state; abnormal increase.*

Osler's disease (ōs′lerz) 1. polycythemia vera. 2. hereditary hemorrhagic telangiectasia.

Osler-Vaquez disease (ōs′ler vah-kāz′) polycythemia vera.

osmatic (oz-mat′ik) olfactory.

osmidrosis (oz″mĭ-dro′sis) bromhidrosis.

osmium (Os) (oz′me-um) a chemical element, atomic number 76, atomic weight 190.2. (See Appendix 6.)

osmolality (oz″mo-lal′ĭ-te) the concentration of a solution in terms of osmoles of solutes per kilogram of solvent.

   serum o. a measure of the number of dissolved particles per unit of water in serum. In a solution, the fewer the particles of solute in proportion to the number of units of water (solvent), the less concentrated the solution. A low serum osmolality means a higher than usual amount of water in relation to the amount of particles dissolved in it, and accompanies overhydration, or EDEMA. An increased serum osmolality indicates deficient fluid VOLUME. Measurement of the serum osmolality gives information about the hydration status within the cells because of the osmotic equilibrium that is constantly being maintained on either side of the cell membrane (HOMEOSTASIS). Water moves freely back and forth across the membrane in response to the osmolar pressure being exerted by the molecules of solute in the intracellular and extracellular fluids. Serum osmolality reflects the status of hydration of the intracellular as well as the extracellular compartments and thus describes total body hydration. The normal value for serum osmolality is 270–300 mOsm/kg water.

   urine o. a measure of the number of dissolved particles per unit of water in the urine. A more accurate measure of urine concentration than specific gravity, urine osmolality is useful in diagnosing renal disorders of urinary concentration and dilution and in assessing status of hydration. The normal value is 500 to 800 mOsm/L.

osmolar (oz-mo′lar) pertaining to the concentration of osmotically active particles in solution.

osmolarity (oz″mo-lar′ĭ-te) the concentration of a solution in terms of osmoles of solutes per liter of solution.

osmole (oz′mōl) a unit of osmotic pressure equivalent to the amount of solute that

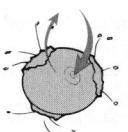
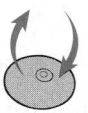
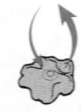

| Hypotonic (Swollen cell) | Isotonic (Normal looking cell) | Hypertonic (Shrivelled cell) |

If the solution surrounding a cell has the same solute concentration as the internal environment of the cell (isotonic), the flow rates in and out of the cell are the same, and the cell remains the same size. If the solute concentration outside the cell is lower (hypotonic), more water will flow into the cell than out, and the cell will swell and perhaps burst. If the solute concentration outside the cell is greater (hypertonic), more water will flow out of the cell than into it, and the cell will shrivel.

dissociates in solution to form one mole (Avogadro's number) of particles (molecules and ions). Symbol Osm.

osmometer (oz-mom′ĕ-ter) an instrument for measuring osmotic concentration or pressure.

osmophilic (oz″mo-fil′ik) having an affinity for solutions of high osmotic pressure.

osmophobia (oz″mo-fo′be-ah) irrational fear of odors.

osmophore (oz′mo-fōr) the group of atoms in a molecule of a compound that is responsible for its odor.

osmoreceptor (oz″mo-re-sep′tor) 1. any of a group of specialized neurons of the supraoptic nuclei of the thalamus that are stimulated by increased extracellular fluid osmolality to cause the release of antidiuretic hormone (ADH) from the posterior pituitary. 2. olfactory receptor.

osmoregulation (oz″mo-reg″u-la′shun) adjustment of internal osmotic pressure of a simple organism or body cell in relation to that of the surrounding medium. adj., **osmoreg′ulatory.**

osmose (oz′mōs) to diffuse by osmosis.

osmosis (oz-mo′sis, os-mo′sis) the diffusion of pure solvent across a membrane in response to a concentration gradient, usually from a solution of lesser to one of greater solute concentration. adj., **osmot′ic.**

The process of osmosis and the factors that influence it are important clinically in the maintenance of adequate body fluids and in the proper balance between volumes of extracellular and intracellular fluids.

The term osmotic pressure refers to the amount of pressure necessary to stop the flow of water across the membrane. The hydrostatic pressure of the water exerts an opposite effect; that is, it exerts pressure in favor of the flow of water across the membrane. The osmotic pressure of the particles in a solute depends on the relative concentrations of the solutions on either side of the membrane, and on the area of the membrane. The osmotic pressure exerted by the nondiffusible particles in a solution is determined by the numbers of particles in a unit of fluid and not by the mass of the particles.

osmostat (oz′mo-stat″) the regulatory centers that control the osmolality of the extracellular fluid.

ossein (os′e-in) the collagen of bone.

osseocartilaginous (os″e-o-kahr″tĭ-laj′ĭnus) osteochondral.

osseofibrous (os″e-o-fi′brus) made up of fibrous tissue and bone.

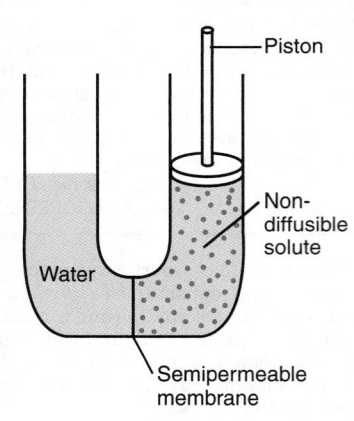

Piston

Non-diffusible solute

Water

Semipermeable membrane

Time

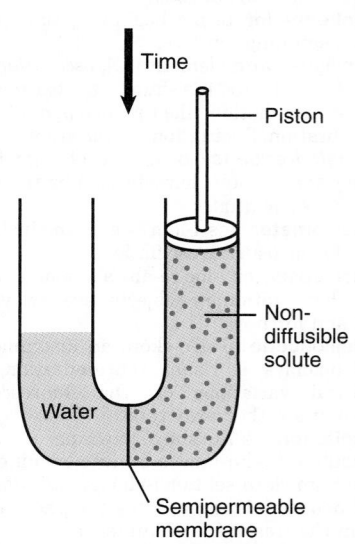

Piston

Non-diffusible solute

Water

Semipermeable membrane

Demonstration of osmotic pressure on the two sides of a semipermeable membrane.

osseointegration (os″e-o-in″tĕ-gra′shun) the formation of a direct interface between an orthopedic or dental implant and bone, without intervening soft tissue.

osseomucin (os″e-o-mu′sin) the ground substance that binds together the collagen and elastin fibrils of bone.

osseous (os′e-us) of the nature or quality of bone; bony.

ossicle (os′ĭ-k'l) a small bone, especially one of those in the middle ear. adj., **ossic′ular.**

   auditory o′s the small bones of the middle ear, the INCUS, MALLEUS, and STAPES. (See Plates.)

ossicular (ŏ-sik′u-ler) pertaining to an ossicle.

ossiculectomy (os″ĭ-ku-lek′to-me) surgical excision of one or more of the ossicles of the middle ear.

ossiculotomy (os″ĭ-ku-lot′ah-me) incision of the auditory ossicles.

ossiculum (ŏ-sik′u-lum) ossicle.

ossiferous (ŏ-sif′er-us) producing bone.

ossific (ŏ-sif′ik) forming or becoming bone.

ossification (os″ĭ-fĭ-ka′shun) formation of or conversion into BONE or a bony substance.

   ectopic o. a pathological condition in which bone arises in tissues not in the osseous system and in connective tissues usually not manifesting osteogenic properties.

   endochondral o. ossification that occurs in and replaces cartilage.

   heterotrophic o. metaplastic ossification.

   intramembranous o. ossification of bone that occurs in and replaces connective tissue.

   metaplastic o. the development of bony substance in normally soft body structures; called also heterotrophic ossification.

ossify (os′ĭ-fi) to change or develop into bone.

oste(o)- word element [Gr.], *bone.*

ostealgia (os″te-al′jah) pain in the bones; called also osteodynia.

ostearthritis (os″te-ahr-thri′tis) osteoarthritis.

ostearthrotomy (os″te-ahr-throt′ah-me) excision of an articular end of a bone.

ostectomy (os-tek′to-me) excision of a bone or part of a bone.

osteectopia (os″te-ek-to′pe-ah) displacement of a bone.

ostein (os′te-in) ossein.

osteitis (os″te-i′tis) inflammation of bone, often with enlargement, tenderness, and a dull, aching pain.

   alveolar o. dry socket.

   condensing o. osteitis with hard deposits of earthy salts in affected bone.

   o. defor′mans rarefying osteitis of unknown cause resulting in deformed bones of increased mass leading to bowing of the long bones and deformation of the flat bones. See also PAGET'S DISEASE.

   o. fibro′sa cys′tica rarefying osteitis with fibrous degeneration and the formation of cysts and the presence of fibrous nodules on the affected bones, due to osteoclastic activity secondary to HYPERPARATHYROIDISM. If a tumor of the parathyroid gland is the cause of the hyperparathyroidism, treatment includes removal of the tumor. When the disease is generalized, all the bones are affected (VON RECKLINGHAUSEN'S DISEASE). Orthopedic surgery may be necessary to correct severe bone deformities.

   o. fragi′litans osteogenesis imperfecta.

   o. fungo′sa chronic osteitis in which the haversian canals are dilated and filled with granulation tissue.

   rarefying o. a bone disease in which the inorganic matter is diminished and the hard bone becomes cancellced.

   sclerosing o. 1. sclerosing nonsuppurative osteomyelitis. 2. condensing osteitis.

ostempyesis (ost″em-pi-e′sis) suppuration within a bone.

osteoarthritis (os″te-o-ahr-thri′tis) a noninflammatory degenerative joint disease marked by degeneration of the articular cartilage, hypertrophy of bone at the margins, and changes in the synovial membrane. Primary osteoarthritis, as part of the normal aging process, is most likely to strike the joints that receive the most use or stress over the years. These include the knees, the joints of the big toes, and those of the lower part of the spine. Another common form of osteoarthritis affects the distal joints of the fingers; this form usually occurs in women. Called also degenerative joint disease.

   Symptoms vary from mild to severe, depending on the amount of degeneration that has taken place. Osteoarthritis is caused by disintegration of the cartilage that covers the ends of the bones. As the cartilage wears away, the roughened surface of the bone is exposed, and pain and stiffness result. In severe cases the center of the bone wears away and a bony ridge is left around the edges. This ridge may restrict movement of the joint. Osteoarthritis is less crippling than rheumatoid ARTHRITIS, in which two bone surfaces may fuse, completely immobilizing the joint.

   Treatment is aimed at preventing crippling deformities, relieving pain, and

O

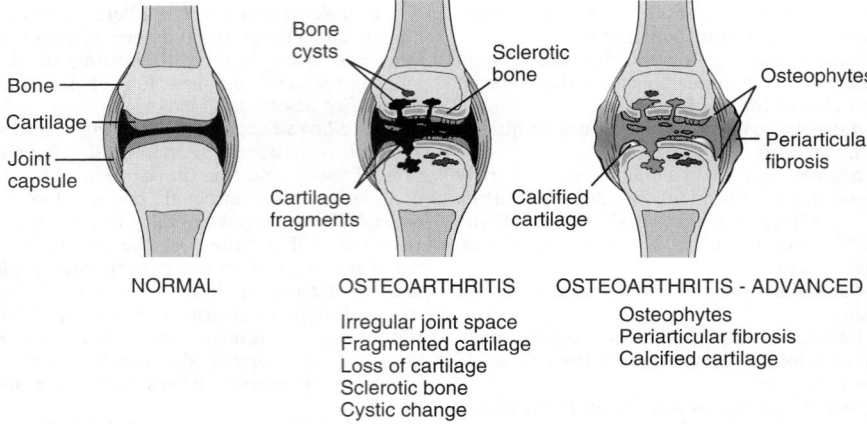

NORMAL

OSTEOARTHRITIS

OSTEOARTHRITIS - ADVANCED

Irregular joint space
Fragmented cartilage
Loss of cartilage
Sclerotic bone
Cystic change

Osteophytes
Periarticular fibrosis
Calcified cartilage

Osteoarthritis. Schematic presentation of the pathologic changes in osteoarthritis. Fragmentation and loss of cartilage denude the subchondral bone, which undergoes sclerosis and cystic change. Osteophytes form on the lateral sides and protrude into the adjacent soft tissues, causing irritation, inflammation, and fibrosis. From Damjanov, 2000.

maintaining motion of the joint; see also treatment of ARTHRITIS.

osteoarthropathy (os″te-o-ahr-throp′ah-the) any disease of the joints and bones.

hypertrophic pulmonary o., secondary hypertrophic o. symmetrical osteitis of the four limbs, chiefly localized to the phalanges and terminal epiphyses of the long bones of the forearm and lower leg; it is often secondary to chronic lung and heart conditions.

osteoarthrosis (os″te-o-ahr-thro′sis) chronic noninflammatory bone disease.

osteoarthrotomy (os″te-o-ahr-throt′ah-me) osteoarthrotomy.

osteoblast (os′te-o-blast″) a cell arising from a fibroblast, which, as it matures, is associated with bone production.

osteoblastoma (os″te-o-blas-to′mah) a benign, painful, rather vascular tumor of bone marked by formation of osteoid tissue and primitive bone.

osteocampsia (os″te-o-kamp′se-ah) curvature of a bone.

osteochondral (os″te-o-kon′dral) pertaining to or composed of bone and cartilage; called also osseocartilaginous.

osteochondritis (os″te-o-kon-dri′tis) inflammation of bone and cartilage.

o. defor′mans juveni′lis osteochondritis of the capitular head of the epiphysis of the femur.

o. defor′mans juveni′lis dor′si osteochondrosis of vertebrae.

o. dis′secans osteochondritis resulting in the splitting of pieces of cartilage into the joint, particularly the knee joint or shoulder joint. The fragment of cartilage is called a joint mouse.

osteochondrodysplasia (os″te-o-kon″dro-dis-pla′zhah) any disorder of cartilage and bone growth.

osteochondrodystrophy (os″te-o-kon″dro-dis′trö-fe) Morquio's disease.

familial o. Morquio's disease.

osteochondrolysis (os″te-o-kon-drol′ĭ-sis) osteochondritis dissecans.

osteochondroma (os″te-o-kon-dro′mah) a benign bone tumor consisting of projecting adult bone capped by cartilage.

osteochondromatosis (os″te-o-kon-dro″mah-to′-sis) the occurrence of multiple OSTEOCHONDROMAS.

osteochondromyxoma (os″te-o-kon″dro-mik-so′-mah) OSTEOCHONDROMA blended with MYXOMA.

osteochondrosarcoma (os″te-o-kon″dro-sahr-ko′-mah) SARCOMA blended with OSTEOMA and CHONDROMA.

osteochondrosis (os″te-o-kon-dro′sis) a disease of the growth ossification centers in children, beginning as a degeneration or necrosis followed by regeneration or recalcification; known by various names, depending on the bone involved.

o. defor′mans ti′biae tibia vara.

osteoclasis (os″te-ok′lah-sis) surgical fracture or refracture of a bone.

osteoclast (os′te-o-klast″) 1. a large multinuclear cell frequently associated with resorption of bone. 2. a surgical instrument used for osteoclasis. adj., **osteoclas′tic.**

osteoclastoma (os″te-o-klas-to′mah) a giant cell TUMOR of bone.

osteocope (os′te-o-kōp″) severe ostealgia.

osteocranium (os″te-o-kra′ne-um) the fetal skull during the period of ossification, from early in the third month of gestation.

osteocystoma (os″te-o-sis-to′mah) a bone cyst.

osteocyte (os′te-o-sīt″) an osteoblast that has become embedded within the bone matrix, occupying a bone lacuna, and sending, through the canaliculi, cytoplasmic processes that connect with other osteocytes in developing bone.

osteodentin (os″te-o-den′tin) dentin that resembles bone.

osteodermia (os″te-o-der′me-ah) osteoma cutis.

osteodiastasis (os″te-o-di-as′tah-sis) the separation of two adjacent bones.

osteodynia (os″te-o-din′e-ah) ostealgia.

osteodystrophy (os″te-o-dis′trŏ-fe) abnormal development of bone.

    renal o. a condition due to chronic kidney disease and RENAL FAILURE, marked by impaired vitamin D metabolism, elevated serum phosphorus levels, low or normal serum calcium levels, and stimulation of PARATHYROID function. There may be any of various bone diseases, including OSTEITIS FIBROSA CYSTICA, OSTEOMALACIA, OSTEOPOROSIS, and sometimes OSTEOSCLEROSIS. If onset is in childhood, renal DWARFISM may result.

osteoepiphysis (os″te-o-ĕ-pif′ĭ-sis) any bony epiphysis.

osteofibroma (os″te-o-fi-bro′mah) OSTEOMA blended with FIBROMA.

osteogen (os′te-o-jen″) the substance composing the inner layer of the periosteum, from which bone is formed.

osteogenesis (os″te-o-jen′ĕ-sis) the formation of bone; the development of bones.

    o. imperfec′ta an inherited condition marked by abnormally brittle bones that are subject to fracture. The most common kind is *osteogenesis imperfecta tarda,* in which the fractures occur when the child begins to walk; it is usually attended by blue coloration of the sclera (Lobstein's disease) and sometimes by otosclerotic deafness (van der Hoeve's syndrome). A less common, usually lethal type is *osteogenesis imperfecta congenita,* in which deformities occur in utero and the child is born with them. (See Atlas 1, Part B).

osteogenic (os″te-o-jen′ik) derived from or composed of any tissue concerned in bone growth or repair.

osteogeny (os″te-oj′ĕ-ne) osteogenesis.

osteography (os″te-og′rah-fe) description of the bones.

osteohalisteresis (os″te-o-hah-lis″ter-e′sis) deficiency in mineral elements of bone.

osteoid (os′te-oid) 1. resembling bone. 2. the organic matrix of bone; young bone that has not undergone calcification.

    o. osteoma a benign HAMARTOMATOUS lesion of cortical bone in young persons. There are small sclerotic bone-forming areas visible on technetium diphosphate bone scan. The small central nidus produces large amounts of PROSTAGLANDIN. There is often night pain, which may be responsive to NONSTEROIDAL ANTIINFLAMMATORY DRUGS. Lesions may be excised in toto or may be treated with nonsteroidal antiinflammatory drugs, and often undergo involution in 5 to 7 years.

osteoinduction (os″te-o-in-duk′shun) the act or process of stimulating osteogenesis.

osteolipochondroma (os″te-o-lip″o-kon-dro′mah) OSTEOCHONDROMA with fatty elements.

osteologist (os″te-ol′ŏ-jist) a specialist in osteology.

osteology (os″te-ol′ŏ-je) scientific study of the bones.

osteolysis (os″te-ol′ĭ-sis) dissoluton of bone; applied especially to the removal or loss of calcium from the bone. adj., **osteolyt′ic.**

osteoma (os″te-o′mah) a tumor, benign or malignant, composed of bony tissue; a hard tumor of bonelike structure developing on a bone (homoplastic osteoma) or other structures (heteroplastic osteoma).

Symptoms. Symptoms of bone cancer are pain, swelling, and disability in the area of the diseased bone. The pain at first is mild, stops and starts again, and then becomes increasingly severe. Swelling may appear soon after the first signs of pain, but often it cannot be seen until later. The disability may affect a nearby joint, such as the knee, shoulder, or hip. There may also be a hard, painful lump over which the skin moves freely. The skin temperature in the area may be slightly elevated.

Diagnosis and Treatment. Diagnosis of bone tumor is made after examination of x-ray film and a microscopic study of the suspected tissue. Malignant tumors can be treated by radiotherapy and surgery during the early stage of development. The prognosis for these tumors is grave, however. Hormone therapy and medication can also be helpful in certain types of the disease.

    o. cu′tis progressive dermal ossification during childhood, with development of hard,

O

round to irregular nodules representing islands of heterotopic bone within the dermis or subcutis, followed by coalescence of the lesions into plaques, and later by invasion of ossification into deep connective tissues. It may be sporadic or inherited as an autosomal dominant trait. Called also progressive osseous heteroplasia.

o. du'rum, o. ebur'neum one containing hard bony tissue.

o. medulla're one containing marrow spaces.

osteoid o. see OSTEOID OSTEOMA.

o. spongio'sum, spongy o. one containing cancellated bone.

osteomalacia (os″te-o-mah-la′shah) softening of the bones, resulting from impaired mineralization, with excess accumulation of OSTEOID, caused by a VITAMIN D deficiency in adults. A similar condition in children is called RICKETS. The deficiency may be due to lack of exposure to ultraviolet rays, inadequate intake of vitamin D in the diet, or failure to absorb or utilize vitamin D. There is decalcification of the bones, particularly those of the spine, pelvis, and lower extremities. X-ray examination reveals transverse, fracture-like lines in the affected bones and areas of demineralization in the matrix of the bone. As the bones soften they become bent, flattened, or otherwise deformed. Treatment consists of administration of large daily doses of vitamin D and dietary measures to insure adequate calcium and phosphorus intake. adj., **osteomala′cic.**

antacid-induced o. osteomalacia in which the combination of low dietary phosphorus intake and chronic excessive consumption of aluminum hydroxide–containing antacids has led to phosphate depletion; characteristics include hypophosphatemia, nephrolithiasis, anorexia, muscle weakness, and bone loss.

anticonvulsant o. 1. osteomalacia occurring in anticonvulsant RICKETS of children. 2. anticonvulsant RICKETS in adults.

hepatic o. osteomalacia as a complication of cholestatic liver disease, which may lead to severe bone pain and multiple fractures.

oncogenic o. a type seen in association with usually benign mesenchymal neoplasms. The tumors appear to produce a substance that impairs renal tubular functions and leads to HYPOPHOSPHATEMIA. Called also tumor-induced osteomalacia.

puerperal o. a type resulting from exhaustion of skeletal stores of calcium and phosphorus by repeated pregnancies and lactation.

renal tubular o. a type resulting from acidosis and hypercalciuria when deficient renal tubular activity has caused inability to produce acid urine or ammonia.

senile o. softening of bones in old age due to VITAMIN D deficiency.

tumor-induced o. oncogenic osteomalacia.

osteomatoid (os″te-o′mah-toid) resembling an osteoma.

osteomere (os′te-o-mēr″) one of a series of similar bony structures, such as the vertebrae.

osteometry (os″te-om′ĕ-tre) measurement of the bones.

osteomyelitis (os″te-o-mi′ĕ-li′tis) inflammation of bone, localized or generalized, due to an infection, usually by a pyogenic organism. It may result in bone destruction in stiffening of joints if the infection spreads to the joints, and, in extreme cases occurring before the end of the growth period, in the shortening of a limb if the growth center is destroyed.

Acute osteomyelitis is caused by bacteria that enter the body through a wound, spread from an infection near the bone (*exogenous osteomyelitis*), or come from a skin or throat infection (*endogenous osteomyelitis*). The infection usually affects the long bones of the upper and lower limbs and causes acute pain and fever. It most often occurs in children and adolescents. Onset may be sudden, with chills, high fever, and severe pain. Signs and symptoms include a marked increase in leukocytes; tenderness swelling, and redness of the skin over the bone involved; and bacteremia. About 10 to 14 days after the onset of symptoms, x-rays show signs of the bone infection.

Intravenous antibiotic treatment is usually effective. If not, the infection destroys areas of the bone and an abscess forms. Acute osteomyelitis may become chronic, especially if the patient has a low resistance to infection. Bone metabolizes more slowly than other organs and its blood supply is less generous than that to other organs. Aggressive intravenous antibiotic therapy is essential.

Treatment. Treatment of acute osteomyelitis consists of administration of antibiotics and sometimes surgical drainage of the abscess. Fragments of dead bone (sequestra) that remain and prevent healing must be removed surgically. If the blood supply to the bone is not obstructed, the bone can grow back. Treatment of chronic osteomyelitis is similar to that for the acute type.

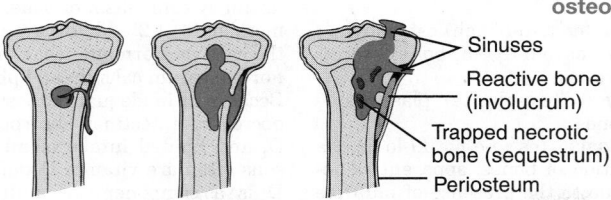

Sinuses
Reactive bone
(involucrum)
Trapped necrotic
bone (sequestrum)
Periosteum

Osteomyelitis. The bacteria reach the metaphysis through the nutrient artery. Bacterial growth results in bone destruction and formation of an abscess. From the abscess cavity, the pus spreads between the trabeculae into the medulla, through the cartilage into the joints, or through the haversian canals of the compact bones to the outside. These sinuses traversing the bone persist for a long time and heal slowly. The pus destroys the bone and sequesters parts of it in the abscess cavity. Reactive new bone is formed around the focus of inflammation. From Damjanov, 2000.

Garré's o. sclerosing nonsuppurative osteomyelitis.

salmonella o. osteomyelitis due to salmonella organisms; it occurs more frequently than normal in SICKLE CELL DIS-EASE.

sclerosing nonsuppurative o. a chronic form involving the long bones, especially the tibia and femur, marked by a diffuse inflammatory reaction, increased density and spindle-shaped sclerotic thickening of the cortex, and an absence of suppuration.

osteomyelodysplasia (os″te-o-mi″ĕ-lo-dis-pla′zhah) a condition characterized by thinning of the osseous tissue of bones, increase in size of the marrow cavities, and associated leukopenia and fever.

osteomyxochondroma (os″te-o-mik″so-kon-dro′-mah) osteochondromyxoma.

osteon (os′te-on) [Gr.] the basic unit of structure of compact bone, comprising a haversian canal and its concentrically arranged lamellae.

osteonecrosis (os″te-o-nĕ-kro′sis) necrosis of bone due to obstruction of its blood supply.

osteoneuralgia (os″te-o-noor-al′jah) neuralgia of a bone.

osteopath (os′te-o-path″) a practitioner of OSTEOPATHY.

osteopathia (os″te-o-path′e-ah) osteopathy (def. 1).

o. conden′sans dissemina′ta osteopoikilosis.

o. stria′ta an asymptomatic condition characterized radiographically by multiple condensations of cancellous bone tissue, giving a striated appearance.

osteopathology (os″te-o-pah-thol′ŏ-je) any disease of bone.

osteopathy (os″te-op′ah-the) 1. any disease of a bone. 2. a system of therapy that uses generally accepted physical, medicinal, and surgical methods of diagnosis and therapy, and emphasizes the importance of normal body mechanics and manipulative methods of detecting and correcting faulty structure. adj., **osteopath′ic.**

Osteopathy is founded on the theory that the body is capable of producing the remedies necessary to protect itself against disease and other toxic conditions when it is in normal structural relationship and has favorable environmental conditions and adequate nutrition.

Osteopaths hold to the tenet that the body is a unit that has the inherent ability to overcome most curable diseases. They recognize that physical, chemical, and nutritional factors influence the state of health and that medicines and surgery are necessary in treatment of disease. Disorders that can be recognized are treated as distinct diseases, and manipulation may or may not be used as an adjunct to other treatment.

osteopenia (os″te-o-pe′ne-ah) reduced bone mass due to a decrease in the rate of osteoid synthesis to a level insufficient to compensate normal bone lysis. The term is also used to refer to any decrease in bone mass below the normal. adj., **osteopen′ic.**

osteoperiosteal (os″te-o-per″e-os′te-al) pertaining to bone and its periosteum.

osteoperiostitis (os″te-o-per″e-os-ti′tis) inflammation of a bone and its periosteum.

osteopetrosis (os″te-o-pĕ-tro′sis) a rare hereditary, congenital condition in which there are bandlike areas of condensed bone at the epiphyseal lines of long bones and condensation of the edges of smaller bones. Fractures occur frequently and deformities of the head, chest, or spine develop. There is no treatment and the prognosis is unfavorable. There may be obliteration of the marrow spaces, causing anemia. Called also Albers-Schönberg disease and marble bones.

osteophage (os′te-o-fāj) osteoclast.

osteophlebitis (os″te-o-flĕ-bi′tis) inflammation of the veins of a bone.

osteophony (os″te-of′ŏ-ne) bone conduction.

osteophyma (os″te-o-fi′mah) osteophyte.

osteophyte (os′te-o-fīt) a bony excrescence or outgrowth.

osteoplasty (os′te-o-plas″te) plastic surgery of the bones.

osteopoikilosis (os″te-o-poi″kĭ-lo′sis) a mottled condition of bones, apparent radiographically, due to the presence of multiple sclerotic foci and scattered stippling. adj., **osteopoikilot′ic.**

osteoporosis (os″te-o-po-ro′sis) a decreased mass per unit volume of normally mineralized bone, calculated in comparison to age- and sex-matched controls; it is the most prevalent bone disease worldwide. There are many etiologic factors of osteoporosis, which give the various types their names.

Postmenopausal, estrogen-deficient osteoporosis is the most common type; more than half the women in the United States 50 years of age or older are likely to have radiologically detectable evidence of abnormally decreased bone mass (OSTEOPENIA) in the spine, and in more than a third, major orthopedic problems related to osteoporosis will eventually occur. Most fractures sustained by women over the age of 50 are secondary to osteoporosis. Women at risk for this disorder can reduce that risk by maintaining adequate calcium levels with dietary calcium or calcium supplements (see diet-related bone loss below), and taking estrogen in the perimenopausal period when indicated. Estrogen replacement therapy is especially recommended for women whose ovaries were removed before age 50.

Age-related osteoporosis is a type that occurs in both men and women and is caused by bone loss that normally accompanies aging.

Diet-related bone loss is caused by chronic dietary deficiencies in calcium and protein, as well as deficiency in vitamin C, which is an essential cofactor in collagen metabolism. Intestinal absorption of calcium becomes less efficient with age; hence older persons need more rather than less dietary calcium to maintain a positive calcium balance. Although dairy products are the primary source of dietary calcium, supplementary calcium is needed by some women. Healthy premenopausal women over the age of 30 may need as much as 1000 mg of calcium a day, which is the amount supplied by a quart of milk. However, for pregnant women and those over the age of 50, the recommended daily intake increases to more than 1500 mg. Lactating women need 2000 mg of calcium daily to prevent untimely catabolism of bone. The vitamin D metabolite 1,25-dihydroxycholecalciferol is the active hormone that helps maintain normal serum calcium and phosphate levels. Because of inadequate exposure to sunlight, decreased intestinal absorption of vitamin D, and limited intake of milk, elderly persons often are vitamin D–deficient. Vitamin D is a component of multivitamins, and health care providers often recommend supplemental multivitamins for the elderly.

Disuse osteoporosis is related to the response of bone mass change to mechanical stress. Net bone mass does not change throughout much of adult life; however, living bone is never metabolically at rest and constantly remodels and reappropriates its mineral stores along lines of mechanical stress. Without weight-bearing stress, bone mass diminishes. As much as 30 to 40 per cent of initial bone mass may be lost after six months of total immobilization, as in PARAPLEGIA and QUADRIPLEGIA due to spinal cord injury. Movement alone is not sufficient to prevent osteoporosis. There must be weight-bearing activity and the use of antigravity muscles to maintain healthy bones.

Heritable osteoporosis includes at least four types of congenital diseases grouped under the term OSTEOGENESIS IMPERFECTA. Symptoms of varying severity that are characteristic of these disorders include skeletal fragility, multiple pathologic fractures, generalized osteoporosis, and scoliosis. All of the diseases included under osteogenesis imperfecta are thought to be associated with defective bone matrix formation.

Endocrine-mediated bone loss can produce osteoporosis because numerous endocrine hormones affect skeletal remodeling and hence skeletal mass. Examples of endocrine disorders that can produce associated osteopenia include HYPOGONADISM, HYPERTHYROIDISM, HYPERPARATHYROIDISM, and HYPERADRENALISM or chronic GLUCOCORTICOID hormone excess.

Disease-related bone loss can occur with almost any kind of chronic disease that is associated with malnutrition and disuse. Osteopenia is also a common complication of most tumors of the bone marrow. Leukemia, lymphoma, and the extremely rare mast cell tumor also may be associated with osteoporosis.

Idiopathic osteoporosis, in both the adult and juvenile form, is extremely uncommon. *Drug-induced bone loss* may be associated with long-term use of heparin for anticoagulation therapy or with the administration of methotrexate, which has both cytotoxic and calciuric effects.

Diagnosis. Osteoporosis is an insidious disease that silently robs the skeleton of its banked resources. Sometimes it is decades before the bone is weak enough to sustain a spontaneous fracture. The most common sites for such bone loss and consequent fractures are the thoracic and lumbar vertebral bodies, ribs, proximal femur, and distal radius. The earliest signs of osteoporosis are often associated with compression fracture of the spine characterized by an episode of acute pain in the middle to low thoracic or high lumbar region. Prevention of osteoporosis through diet, exercise, and the reduction of risk factors should be a priority. The critical years for building bone mass are before the age of 30. Maintenance of skeletal mass is accomplished by oral calcium supplementation, vitamin D therapy, weight-bearing activity through a daily exercise program, and sodium fluoride therapy.

During the intervals between compression fractures, the patient may be symptom-free, but kyphosis, decrease in height, and appearance of a "dowager's hump" are reliable indicators of the early progress of the disease. Two other associated effects of vertebral compression are the result of a decrease in the size of the thoracic and abdominal cavities. The patient experiences diminished activity tolerance as a result of disease-related postural changes and often reports early satiety and a bloated feeling after eating only a small amount of food.

Radiographs of the thoracic and lumbar spine show a visible loss of bone density. In general, as much as 30 to 50 per cent of the bone mass must be lost before the decrease can be seen on x-ray. Bone density measurement can help in evaluation of this disease and prediction of the likelihood of fracture.

Treatment and Patient Care. The management of osteoporosis is concerned with treatment of symptomatic disease and its sequelae and with maintenance of skeletal mass and integrity. Treatment of acute symptoms is aimed at relieving pain, providing comfortable mechanical support for the spine, arranging assistance in activities of daily living, coordinating a rehabilitation program, and providing encouragement and

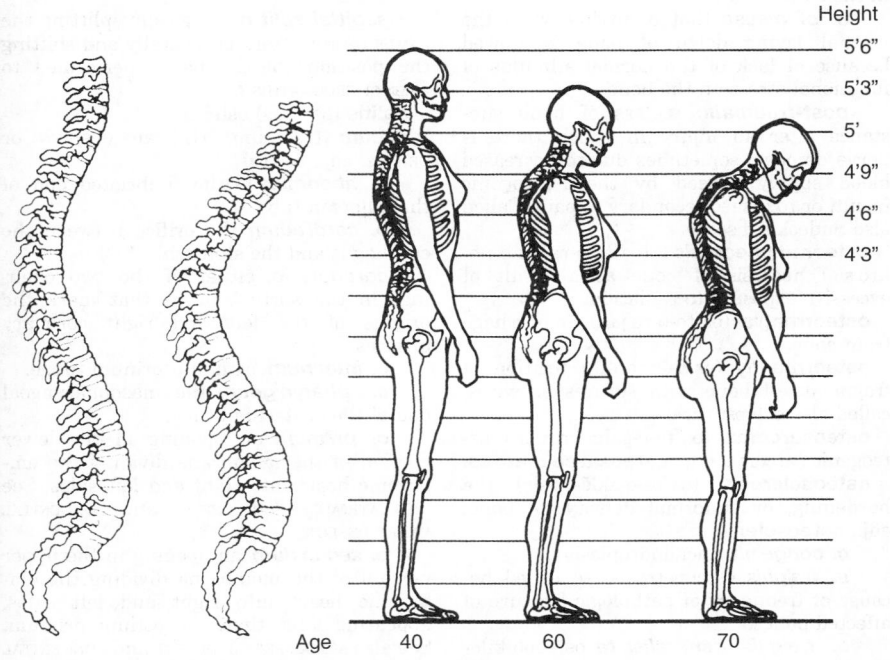

Loss of bone mass due to osteoporosis produces characteristic changes in the curvature of the spine. At far left are normal curvatures compared with those typical of osteoporosis. Figures to the right show the normal spine at age 40 and osteoporotic changes at 60 and 70 years of age. As shown, these changes bring about a loss of as much as 6 to 9 inches in height, and the so-called dowager's hump in the upper thoracic vertebrae.

reassurance to the patient and family. The rehabilitation process must include instruction in proper back care, and especially in how to avoid unnecessary spinal compression forces while lifting or bending.

Estrogen replacement therapy is often prescribed for women at menopause. Because it increases the risk for breast and gynecologic malignancies, careful assessment of these patients is necessary. Pharmacologic agents approved by the Food and Drug Association for osteoporosis treatment or treatment include the BISPHOSPHONATES ALENDRONATE and RISEDRONATE; CALCITONIN, estrogen replacement THERAPY, and selective estrogen receptor MODULATORS such as RALOXIFENE.

Information on osteoporosis can be obtained by writing the National Osteoporosis Foundation, 1232 22nd St. NW, Washington, DC 20037-1292 or consulting their web site at http://www.nof.org. They have also published clinical guidelines for the prevention and treatment of osteoporosis on their web site.

o. circumscrip′ta demineralization occurring in localized areas of bone, especially in the skull.

o. of disuse that occurring when the normal laying down of bone is slowed because of lack of the normal stimulus of functional stress on the bone.

post-traumatic o. loss of bone substance after an injury in which there is nerve damage, sometimes due to decreased blood supply caused by the neurogenic insult, or to disuse secondary to pain. Called also Sudeck's disease.

osteoradionecrosis (os″te-o-ra″de-o-nĕ-kro′sis) necrosis of bone as a result of excessive exposure to radiation.

osteorrhagia (os″te-o-ra′jah) hemorrhage from bone.

osteorrhaphy (os″te-or′ah-fe) fixation of fragments of bone with sutures or wires; called also osteosuture.

osteosarcoma (os″te-o-sahr-ko′mah) osteogenic sarcoma. adj., **osteosarco′matous.**

osteosclerosis (os″te-o-sklĕ-ro′sis) the hardening, or abnormal density, of bone. adj., **osteosclerot′ic.**

o. conge′nita achondroplasia.

o. fra′gilis osteopetrosis; so called because of frequency of pathologic fracture of affected bones.

o. fra′gilis generalisa′ta osteopoikolosis.

osteosis (os″te-o′sis) the formation of bony tissue.

o. cu′tis osteoma cutis.

osteosuture (os″te-o-soo′chur) osteorrhaphy.

osteosynovitis (os″te-o-sin″o-vi′tis) synovitis with osteitis of neighboring bones.

osteosynthesis (os″te-o-sin′thĕ-sis) surgical fastening of the ends of a fractured bone.

osteotabes (os″te-o-ta′bēz) a disease chiefly of infants, in which bone marrow cells are destroyed and the marrow disappears.

osteothrombosis (os″te-o-throm-bo′sis) thrombosis of the veins of a bone.

osteotome (os′te-o-tōm″) a chisel-like knife for cutting bone.

osteotomy (os″te-ot′ah-me) incision or transection of a bone.

cuneiform o. removal of a wedge of bone.

displacement o. surgical division of a bone and shifting of the divided ends to change the alignment of the bone or to alter weight-bearing stresses.

Le Fort o. transverse sectioning and repositioning of the MAXILLA; the incision for each of the three types (Le Fort I, II, and III o's) is placed along the line defined by the corresponding Le Fort's FRACTURE.

linear o. the sawing or simple cutting of a bone.

sagittal split o. surgically splitting the RAMUS OF THE MANDIBLE sagitally and shifting the positions of the parts, performed to correct PROGNATHISM.

ostitis (os-ti′tis) osteitis.

ostium (os′te-um) [L.] an OPENING or ORIFICE. adj., **os′tial.**

o. abdomina′le the fimbriated end of the fallopian tube.

o. cardi′acum the orifice between the esophagus and the stomach.

coronary o. either of the two openings in the aortic sinuses that mark the origins of the left and right coronary arteries.

o. inter′num ostium uterinum tubae.

o. pharyn′geum the nasopharyngeal end of the eustachian tube.

o. pri′mum an opening in the lower portion of the membrane dividing the embryonic heart into right and left sides. See also ATRIAL SEPTAL DEFECT and CONGENITAL HEART DEFECT.

o. secun′dum an opening in the upper portion of the membrane dividing the embryonic heart into right and left sides, appearing later than the ostium primum. See also ATRIAL SEPTAL DEFECT and CONGENITAL HEART DEFECT.)

tympanic o., o. tympa′nicum the opening of the eustachian tube on the carotid wall of the tympanic cavity.

o. u'teri the external opening of the cervix of the uterus into the vagina.

o. uteri'num tu'bae the uterine end of the fallopian tube; the point where the cavity of the tube becomes continuous with that of the uterus.

o. vagi'nae the external orifice of the vagina.

ostomate (os'to-māt) one who has undergone enterostomy or ureterostomy.

ostomy (os'tah-me) an operation in which an artificial opening is formed, such as a COLOSTOMY or URETEROSTOMY; see also STOMA.

-ostomy word element [Gr.], *surgical creation of an artificial opening.*

OT occupational therapy; Old tuberculin.

ot(o)- word element [Gr.], *ear.*

otalgia (o-tal'jah) earache.

OTC over the counter; see OVER THE COUNTER MEDICATIONS.

otic (o'tik) auditory (def. 1).

otitis (o-ti'tis) inflammation of the ear. adj., **otit'ic.**

aviation o. a symptom complex due to difference between atmospheric pressure of the environment and air pressure in the middle ear; called also barotitis media.

o. exter'na inflammation of the external ear, usually caused by a bacteria or fungus. See also OTOMYCOSIS.

o. externa, circumscribed acute bacterial otitis externa in a limited area, with formation of a furuncle that may obstruct the canal; usually due to a staphylococcal infection. Called also furuncular otitis externa.

o. externa, diffuse otitis externa involving a relatively wide area, without formation of a furuncle.

o. externa, furuncular circumscribed otitis externa.

o. externa, malignant a progressive, necrotizing infection of the external auditory canal caused by *Pseudomonas aeruginosa* and affecting chiefly elderly diabetic and immunocompromised patients. It begins with the formation of granulation tissue in the external auditory canal, followed by localized chondritis and osteomyelitis, extension to the tissues surrounding the ear with destruction of involved bone, and involvement of the cranial nerves at the base of the skull; mortality in patients with nerve involvement is high.

furuncular o. circumscribed otitis externa.

o. inter'na labyrinthitis.

o. me'dia inflammation of the middle ear, usually seen in infants and young children, and classified as either *serous* (or *secretory*) or *suppurative* (or *purulent*). Both types characteristically result in

accumulations of fluid behind the tympanic membrane with some degree of HEARING LOSS.

Serous Otitis Media. In this condition the eustachian tube fails to maintain equality of the barometric pressure within and outside the middle ear. When the tube fails to open and close as it should, air within the middle ear is under negative pressure. This causes inward retraction of the eardrum and movement of serous fluid from the mucosal capillaries into the middle ear space. The serous fluid can fill up the space and cause conductive hearing loss.

Acute serous otitis media usually follows an upper respiratory infection or trauma to the ear or may be associated with an allergy or enlarged adenoids. Symptoms are mild and may consist only of a feeling of fullness in the ear and some evidence of hearing loss. *Otitis media with effusion* is fluid in the middle ear with no signs or symptoms of infection.

Suppurative Otitis Media. The introduction of pus-producing bacteria into the middle ear causes this condition. It usually is associated with an upper respiratory infection, particularly when organisms from the nasopharynx find their way into the middle ear via the eustachian tube.

Symptoms include irritability, difficulty in sleeping, some pain, and loss of hearing. If sufficient pressure builds up behind the tympanic membrane it may rupture spontaneously and exude a purulent discharge. If the pus-laden fluid breaks through internally it can result in intracranial abscess, meningitis, and mastoiditis. Acute suppurative otitis media is treated aggressively with antibacterials and tympanocentesis to relieve pressure and obtain fluid for culturing. If the condition becomes chronic there is continuous otorrhea and hearing loss. Treatment includes systemic antibacterials, topical therapy with ear drops, tympanoplasty to repair a ruptured ear drum and damaged ossicles, and, sometimes, mastoidectomy to eliminate all sources of infection.

Otitis Media with Effusion. is fluid in the middle ear with no signs or symptoms of infection. MANAGEMENT. The American Academy of Pediatrics MANAGEMENT has developed clinical guidelines called *Managing Otitis Media With Effusion in Young Children.* They recommend the use of pneumatic otoscopy to assess middle ear status and tympanometry. Children who have had fluid in both middle ears for a total of three months should undergo hearing evaluation. Observation or antibiotic therapy are treatment options if the effusion has been present for less than four to six

O

months. Most cases of otitis media with effusion resolve spontaneously.

Three sets of guidelines are available: the aforementioned (AHCPR Publication 94-0623); *Otitis Media with Effusion in Young Children* (AHCPR Publication 94-0622); and *Middle Ear Fluid in Children: Parent Guide* (AHCPR Publication 94-0624). Copies can be obtained by writing the AHCPR Publications Clearinghouse, P.O. Box 8547, Silver Spring, MD 20907, calling 1-800-358-9295, or consulting their web site at http://www.ahcpr.gov.

Otobius (o-to′be-us) a genus of soft-bodied ticks parasitic in the ears of various animals, sometimes including humans.

otocephalus (o″to-sef′ah-lus) an individual exhibiting otocephaly.

otocephaly (o″to-sef′ah-le) a developmental ANOMALY consisting of absence of the lower jaw with the ears united below the face.

otoconia (o″to-ko′ne-ah) statoconia.

otocranium (o″to-kra′ne-um) the area of the petrous part of the temporal bone surrounding the osseous labyrinth. adj., **otocra′nial.**

otocyst (o′to-sist) 1. the auditory vesicle of the embryo. 2. the organ of hearing in certain animals.

otodynia (o″to-din′e-ah) earache.

otoencephalitis (o″to-en-sef″ah-li′tis) inflammation of brain extending from an inflamed middle ear.

otogenic (o″to-jen′ik) otogenous.

otogenous (o-toj′ĕ-nus) originating within the ear.

otography (o-tog′rah-fe) description of the ear.

otolaryngology (o″to-lar″ing-gol′ŏ-je) the branch of medicine dealing with disease of the ear, nose, and throat; called also otorhinolaryngology.

otolith (o′to-lith) statolith.

otologist (o-tol′ŏ-jist) a specialist in otology.

otology (o-tol′ŏ-je) the branch of medicine dealing with the ear and its anatomy, physiology, and pathology. adj., **otolog′ic.**

otomucormycosis (o″to-mu″kor-mi-ko′-sis) a fungal disease (MUCORMYCOSIS) of the ear.

otomycosis (o″to-mi-ko′sis) OTITIS EXTERNA caused by a fungal infection; it thrives in warm, moist climates and is encouraged by poor local hygiene and swimming. Symptoms include itching, which may be intense, pain, and a stinging sensation in the external acoustic meatus. It is treated with antibiotics to prevent

secondary infection and the administration of ear drops containing neomycin or poly myxin B sulfate. The area should be cleaned locally with dilute aluminum ace tate solution combined with acetic acid before ear drops are applied.

otoneurology (o″to-noo-rol′ŏ-je) the branch of OTOLOGY dealing especially with those portions of the nervous system related to the ear. adj., **otoneurolog′ic.**

otopharyngeal (o″to-fah-rin′je-al) pertaining to the ear and pharynx.

otoplasty (o′to-plas″te) plastic surgery of the external ear.

otopyorrhea (o″to-pi″o-re′ah) otorrhea that is purulent.

otorhinolaryngology (o″to-ri″no-lar″ing-gol′ŏ-je) otolaryngology.

otorhinology (o″to-ri-nol′ŏ-je) the branch of medicine dealing with ear and nose.

otorrhea (o″to-re′ah) a discharge from the ear.

otosclerosis (o″to-sklĕ-ro′sis) the formation of spongy bone in the capsule of the labyrinth of the ear, often causing the auditory ossicles to become fixed and less able to pass on vibrations when sound enters the ear. Approximately 10 per cent of adults have otosclerosis, but in only 1 per cent does it affect the STAPES, which becomes fixed to the oval window and causes symptoms. adj., **otosclerot′ic.**

The cause is still unknown; it may be hereditary or related to vitamin deficiency or OTITIS MEDIA. An early symptom is ringing in the ears, but the most noticeable symptom is progressive loss of hearing. It usually begins in the teens or early twenties, strikes women about twice as often as men, and may be worsened by pregnancy. Although no cure is known, surgical techniques can often restore hearing by freeing the stapes or replacing it with other tissue. In this operation (STAPEDECTOMY), the stapes is removed and replaced with grafted tissue attached to a stainless steel wire or plastic tube. Patients who do not desire surgery may have their hearing loss relieved by the use of a hearing aid. Large but uncontrolled research studies have suggested that SODIUM FLUORIDE may decrease the rate of hearing loss; this dietary supplement along with VITAMIN D is used to slow the disease in selected patients.

otoscope (o′to-skōp) an instrument for inspecting the ear.

otoscopy (o-tos′kah-pe) examination of the external acoustic meatus with an otoscope.

otospongiosis (o″to-spon″je-o′sis) the formation of spongy bone in the bony labyrinth of the ear.

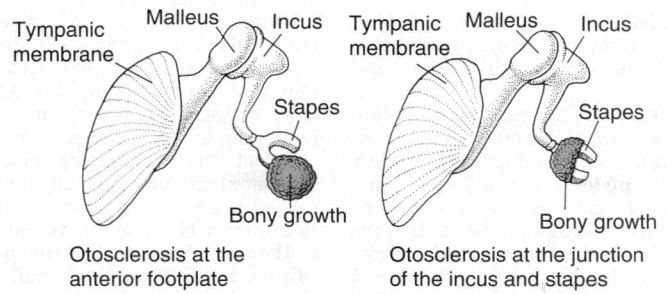

Common sites of otosclerosis. Otosclerosis can cause fixation of the stapes by spongy growth of bone around the anterior footplate or at the junction of the incus and stapes. From Ignatavicius et al., 1995.

otosteal (o-tos′te-al) pertaining to the ossicles of the ear.

ototoxic (o′to-tok″sik) having a damaging effect upon the eighth cranial (vestibulocochlear) nerve or on the organs of hearing and balance.

ototoxicity (o″to-tok-sis′ĭ-te) the property of being ototoxic.

OTR Registered Occupational Therapist.

OU [L.] o′culus uter′que (each eye).

ounce (oz) (owns) 1. in the APOTHECARIES′ SYSTEM, a unit of weight equal to $\frac{1}{12}$ of a POUND or 480 GRAINS (31.103 GRAMS); symbol ℥. See also Table of Weights and Measures in the Appendix. 2. in the AVOIRDUPOIS SYSTEM, a unit of weight equal to $\frac{1}{16}$ POUND (28.3495 GRAMS).

  fluid o. a unit of capacity (liquid measure) of the apothecaries′ system. In the United States, it is 8 fluid drams, one sixteenth of a pint, or the equivalent of 29.57 mL. In Great Britain, it is an *imperial ounce* and is 8 (imperial) fluid drams but is one twentieth of an (imperial) pint, or 28.41 mL. See also Table of Weights and Measures in the Appendix.

outcome criteria (owt′kum kri-te′re-ah) measurable changes in the conditions or behavior of an individual as a result of a specific intervention or action.

outcome (owt′kum) a patient behavior or attitude that results from the interventions of the health care team.

  nursing o. an aspect of patient or client health status that is influenced by nursing INTERVENTION and recorded at specific times for an episode of care; it is measured by the resolution status of each NURSING DIAGNOSIS as being either resolved or not resolved. The term is used in both the NURSING MINIMUM DATA SET and the NURSING OUTCOMES CLASSIFICATION (see Appendices).

outlet (owt′let) a means or route of exit or egress.

  pelvic o. the inferior opening of the pelvis minor.

outlier (out′li-er) an observation so distant from the central mass of the data that it noticeably influences results and must be carefully checked to ensure it is not an error.

outpatient (owt′pa-shent) a patient who comes to the hospital, clinic, or dispensary for diagnosis or treatment but is not admitted for an overnight stay.

outpocketing (owt-pok′et-ing) evagination.

output (owt′poot) the yield or total of anything produced by any functional system of the body. When measuring output for a patient record, the volume of urine, drainage from tubes, vomitus, and any other measurable liquid should be recorded.

  cardiac o. the effective volume of blood expelled by either ventricle of the heart per unit of time (generally per minute); it usually refers to left ventricle output. It is equal to the stroke VOLUME multiplied by the heart RATE. Normal values are 4 to 8 liters per minute.

  decreased cardiac o. a NURSING DIAGNOSIS accepted by the North American Nursing Diagnosis Association, defined as a state in which inadequate blood is pumped by the heart to meet the metabolic demands of the body. The most obvious causative factors are pathologic changes in the heart′s muscle or electrical conduction system, congenital heart defects, electrolyte imbalances (as of calcium or potassium), blood dyscrasias, and chronic pulmonary disease. Factors that could lead to changes in a patient′s functional capacities because of decreased cardiac output might include physical exercise of a type or intensity that the patient cannot tolerate because of diminished oxygen supply, ingestion of large meals that place an

O

added workload on the heart, obesity, retention of fluid (edema), hypovolemia or hypervolemia, emotional stress, and smoking.

Patient Care. Nursing interventions are planned only after a thorough nursing assessment has been conducted to collect the relevant subjective and objective data. For example, it may be that the patient will need instruction and guidance in limiting sodium intake, reducing caloric intake to lose excess fat and maintain normal body weight, decreasing fat consumption to reduce blood lipid levels, or otherwise striving for dietary management of the problem.

energy o. the energy a body is able to manifest in work or activity.

stroke o. stroke volume.

urinary o. the amount of urine secreted by the kidneys. See also FLUID BALANCE.

ov(o)- word element [L.], *egg; ovum.* See also words beginning OO-.

ova (o'vah) [L.] plural of OVUM.

ovalocyte (o'vah-lo-sīt") elliptocyte.

ovalocytosis (o-val"o-si-to'sis) elliptocytosis.

ovari(o)- word element [L.], *ovary.* See also words beginning OOPHOR(O)-.

ovarialgia (o-var"e-al'jah) pain in an ovary.

ovarian (o-var'e-an) pertaining to an ovary.

o. cancer cancer of the ovary, one of the leading causes of cancer-related death in women in the United States. Despite advances in treatment, the survival rate has risen only slightly since 1950. Although aggressive treatment in the early stages offers the best prognosis, detection before the malignancy reaches an advanced stage is difficult.

Signs and symptoms become more apparent as the tumor grows. The first finding is usually a pelvic mass noted on pelvic examination. However, if the patient is obese or has difficulty relaxing and cooperating with the examiner, the mass may not be felt. With increased size, the tumor compresses the surrounding pelvic structures, which may cause a feeling of fullness and pain in the pelvis or abdomen, abnormal uterine bleeding, urinary complaints, dyspareunia, and later ascites. Gastrointestinal symptoms such as heartburn, nausea, and anorexia may also be associated. Diagnosis is established when the mass is found during exploratory surgery and peritoneal cytology.

A plan of treatment is developed according to the stage of the disease. The modes of therapy include total abdominal hysterectomy, bilateral salpingo-oophorectomy, and a partial or complete omentectomy. Radiation and chemotherapy are administered after surgery to destroy malignant cells remaining in the abdominal cavity.

Patient Care. Among the major problems associated with ovarian malignancy are those related to abdominopelvic surgery, and the side effects of radiation therapy and chemotherapy. Additionally, the patient with advanced malignancy may suffer from the effects of ASCITES, which can cause discomfort and shortness of breath, and PLEURAL EFFUSION, which can produce cough, dyspnea, and chest pain. Nutritional problems and emaciation can occur because of a host of factors such as nausea and anorexia, fullness and discomfort of ascites, and tumor involvement of the intestines. Moreover, cancer itself interferes with normal metabolism of nutrients. Intestinal obstruction or other complications related to digestion, absorption, and excretion are the major causes of death in the patient with ovarian cancer.

While specific measures to prevent ovarian cancer are not known, health care providers can encourage early detection by stressing the importance of regular gynecologic examinations and teaching women to recognize the signs and symptoms of ovarian tumors.

o. vein syndrome obstruction of the ureter, usually on the right side, due to compression by an enlarged or varicose ovarian vein; typically the vein becomes enlarged during pregnancy, the symptoms being those of obstruction or infection of the upper urinary tract.

ovariectomy (o-var"e-ek'to-me) oophorectomy.

ovariocele (o-var'e-o-sēl") hernia of an ovary.

ovariocentesis (o-var"e-o-sen-te'sis) surgical puncture of an ovary or an ovarian cyst.

ovariocyesis (o-var"e-o-si-e'sis) ovarian pregnancy.

ovariopexy (o-var"e-o-pek'se) the operation of elevating and fixing an ovary to the abdominal wall.

ovariorrhexis (o-var"e-o-rek'sis) rupture of an ovary.

ovariosalpingectomy (o-var"e-o-sal"pin-jek'to-me) salpingo-oophorectomy.

ovariostomy (o-var"e-os'tah-me) incision of an ovary, with drainage; oophorostomy.

ovariotomy (o-var"e-ot'ah-me) surgical removal of an ovary, or removal of an ovarian tumor.

ovariotubal (o-var″e-o-too′bal) tubo-ovarian.

ovaritis (o″vah-ri′tis) oophoritis.

ovarium (o-var′e-um) [L.] ovary.

ovary (o′vah-re) the female gonad; either of the sex glands in the female in which the ova are formed. Ovaries are paired oval organs approximately 3 cm long, 2 cm wide, and 1 cm thick, one on either side of the uterus, usually near the lateral pelvic wall adjacent to the anterior superior iliac spine. They have two basic functions: OVULATION and the production of hormones, chiefly ESTROGEN and PROGESTERONE, which influence a woman's feminine physical characteristics and affect the process of REPRODUCTION. OVARIAN CANCER is the fifth leading cause of death among women in the United States. adj., ovar′ian.

overanxious disorder former name for an anxiety disorder of childhood or adolescence, now subsumed by GENERALIZED ANXIETY DISORDER.

overbite (o′ver-bīt) extension of incisal RIDGES of the upper anterior teeth below the incisal ridges of the corresponding lower teeth when the jaws are closed normally.

overcoat (o′ver-kōt) abrasion layer.

overcompensation (o″ver-kom″pen-sa′-shun) conscious or unconscious exaggerated correction for a real or imagined physical or psychological deficiency.

overdenture (o″ver-den′chur) a complete denture supported both by mucosa and by a few remaining natural teeth that have been altered, as by insertion of a long or short coping, to permit the denture to fit over them.

overdosage (o″ver-do′saj) 1. the administration of an excessive dose. 2. the condition resulting from an excessive dose.

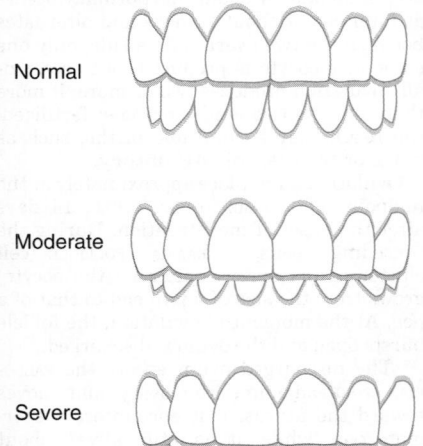

Normal

Moderate

Severe

Classification of overbite. From Darby and Walsh, 1994.

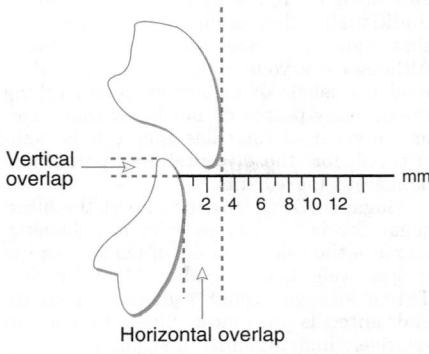

Vertical overlap

Horizontal overlap

mm

2 4 6 8 10 12

Vertical overlap (overbite) and horizontal overlap (overjet).

overdose (o′ver-dōs″) 1. to administer an excessive dose. 2. an excessive dose.

overhydration (o″ver-hi-dra′shun) hyperhydration.

overjet (o′ver-jet) extension of the incisal or buccal cusp ridges of the upper teeth horizontally (labially or buccally) beyond the ridges of the teeth in the lower jaw when the jaws are closed normally.

overload (o′ver-lōd) an excess over what is normal or needed.

iron o. an excess of IRON in the body; see HEMOCHROMATOSIS, HEMOSIDEROSIS, and SIDEROSIS.

sensory o. a condition in which an individual receives an excessive or intolerable amount of sensory stimuli, as in a busy hospital or clinic or an INTENSIVE CARE UNIT; the effects of sensory overload are similar to those of sensory DEPRIVATION, including confusion and hallucination.

overriding (o″ver-rīd′ing) 1. the slipping of either part of a fractured bone past the other. 2. extending beyond the usual position.

over the counter medications (OTCs) 1. drugs that can be purchased by a lay person without a prescription. When obtaining the drug history, it is important to ascertain if a patient is taking such medications. Some patients do not consider them significant and do not report them because they do not require a prescription. Over the counter medications are chemically active agents that may interact with prescribed drugs. 2. in Canada, a subgroup of NONPRESCRIPTION DRUGS available only in pharmacies.

Over the counter drugs have the potential for initiating drug-drug interactions with prescription drugs and thereby

O

enhancing or inhibiting their desired effect. Additionally, they often contain substances that can aggravate an existing illness. Although everyone should be cautioned to read the labels of medicines before taking them, many people do not know that there are alternative remedies that can be substituted for those containing potentially dangerous ingredients.

Sugar in OTC drugs can upset the blood sugar levels of persons who are diabetic, increase the caloric intake of persons trying to lose weight, and promote dental caries. Throat lozenges, cough remedies, laxatives, and antacids are most likely to contain relatively high amounts of sugar.

Sodium intake is especially important for patients who have hypertension, heart disease, premenstrual syndrome, or other disorders associated with fluid retention. Cold products, analgesic powders, antacids, and laxatives frequently contain amounts of sodium that are prohibitive for the person who is trying to avoid this substance.

Potassium is another electrolyte that can cause problems if taken in excessive amounts. For patients taking a potassium-sparing diuretic, or those with renal disease in which potassium is not excreted in normal amounts by the kidney, an extra amount of potassium taken in non-prescription drugs can produce hyperkalemia. Sources of potassium include salt substitutes, which are often almost pure potassium chloride, laxatives, and sleep aids containing potassium bromide and potassium salicylate.

Caffeine is often a major ingredient in analgesics, products that are taken to manage menstrual pain, in cold remedies, and in products to induce wakefulness. Increased amounts of caffeine can be harmful to persons with peptic ulcer or cardiac disease, those who are under a great deal of stress, and persons who are especially sensitive to caffeine. These persons, as well as patients on long-term theophylline or aminophylline therapy, can experience elevated blood pressure, tachycardia, and other symptoms associated with caffeine overdose.

overventilation (o″ver-ven″tĭ-la′shun) hyperventilation.

overwear syndrome (o′ver-wār) extreme photophobia, pain, and lacrimation associated with contact lenses, particularly non–gas permeable hard lenses, usually caused by wearing them excessively. Prolonged lens-induced corneal hypoxia results in corneal epithelial edema and eventually erosion; it can be a chronic condition or an acute episode that usually occurs several hours after lenses are removed.

ovi- word element [L.], *egg; ovum.* See also words beginning oo- and ov(o)-.

ovicide (o′vī-sīd) an agent destructive to ova, such as of parasites.

oviduct (o′vī-dukt) 1. FALLOPIAN TUBE. 2. in nonmammals, a passage through which ova leave the maternal body or pass to an organ communicating with the exterior of the body. adj., **ovidu′cal, oviduc′tal.**

oviferous (o-vif′er-us) producing ova.

ovigenesis (o″vĭ-jen′ĕ-sis) oogenesis.

ovine (o′vīn) pertaining to, characteristic of, or derived from sheep.

oviparous (o-vip′ah-rus) capable of producing eggs in which the embryo develops outside of the maternal body, as in birds.

oviposition (o″vĭ-pŏ-zish′un) the act of laying or depositing eggs.

ovipositor (o″vĭ-pos′ĭ-tor) a specialized organ by which many female insects deposit their eggs.

ovoplasm (o′vo-plazm) ooplasm.

ovotestis (o″vo-tes′tis) a gonad containing both testicular and ovarian tissue.

ovoviviparous (o″vo-vi-vip′ah-rus) bearing living young that hatch from eggs inside the maternal body, the embryo being nourished by food stored in the egg; lizards are one example.

Ovral (ōv′ral) trademark for a combination preparation of NORGESTREL and ETHINYL ESTRADIOL, used as an oral CONTRACEPTIVE.

OVTT optometric vision therapy technician.

ovular (ov′u-lar) 1. pertaining to an OVULE. 2. pertaining to an OOCYTE (OVUM).

ovulation (ov″u-la′shun) the discharge of a secondary OOCYTE from the GRAAFIAN FOLLICLE; in an adult woman this normally occurs at intervals of about 28 days and alternates between the two ovaries. As a rule, only one secondary oocyte is produced, but occasionally ovulation produces two or more; if more than one subsequently become fertilized, the result may be multiple births, such as twins or triplets. adj., **ov′ulatory.**

Ovulation takes place approximately at the midpoint of the MENSTRUAL CYCLE, 14 days after the onset of menstruation. During the preceding weeks, a GRAAFIAN FOLLICLE (cell cluster in the ovary containing the oocyte) grows from the size of a pinhead to that of a pea. At the moment of ovulation, the follicle bursts open and the ovum is discharged.

The discharged ovum enters the FALLO-PIAN TUBE adjoining the ovary and moves toward the uterus; if it encounters a spermatozoon while it is still alive (about 48 hours), the two merge and FERTILIZATION takes place, usually in the fallopian tube.

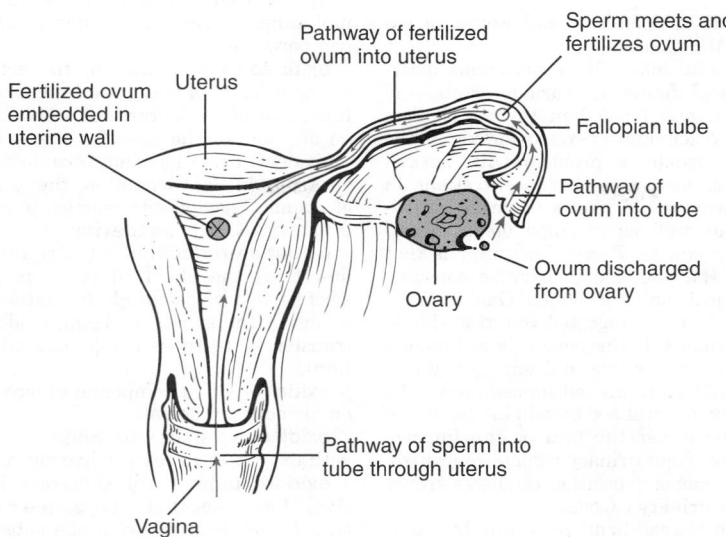

Ovulation.

The fertilized ovum then makes its way to the uterus, where it becomes embedded in the prepared wall as the first stage of growth of the fetus (see illustration, and see also REPRODUCTION). If fertilization does not take place the ovum loses its vitality and the blood and tissue lining the uterus are shed in the menstrual flow.

o. method CERVICAL MUCUS METHOD; see discussion under CONTRACEPTION.

ovule (ov′ūl) 1. the ovum within the graafian follicle. 2. any small, egglike structure.

ovum (o′vum), pl. *o′va* [L.] the female reproductive or germ CELL which after fertilization is capable of developing into a new member of the same species; called also egg. The term is sometimes applied to any stage of the fertilized germ cell during cleavage and even until hatching or birth of the new individual. The human ovum consists of protoplasm that contains some yolk, enclosed by a cell wall consisting of two layers, an outer one (ZONA PELLUCIDA) and an inner, thin one (vitelline MEMBRANE). There is a large nucleus (germinal vesicle) within which is a nucleolus (germinal spot). adj., **o′vular.**

centrolecithal o. one with the yolk concentrated at the center of the egg, surrounded by a peripheral shell of cytoplasm, and with an island of cytoplasm surrounding the nucleus, such as that of an arthropod.

holoblastic o. one that undergoes total cleavage.

isolecithal o. one with a small amount of yolk evenly distributed throughout the cytoplasm.

meroblastic o. one that undergoes partial cleavage.

primitive o., primordial o. any OOCYTE very early in its development.

telolecithal o. one with a comparatively large amount of yolk massed at one pole, such as that of a reptile or bird.

Owren's disease (ow′renz) parahemophilia.

ox- see OXY-.

oxacillin (ok″sah-sil′in) a semisynthetic penicillinase-resistant PENICILLIN used orally or parenterally as the sodium salt in infections due to penicillin-resistant, gram-positive organisms.

oxalate (ok′sah-lāt) any salt of oxalic acid.

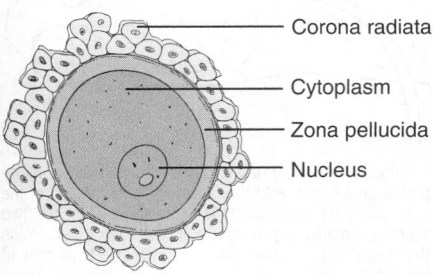

Corona radiata

Cytoplasm

Zona pellucida

Nucleus

Ovum.

oxalemia (ok″sah-le′me-ah) excess of oxalates in the blood.

oxalic acid (ok-sal′ik) a poisonous dicarboxylic acid found in various fruits and vegetables, and formed in the metabolism of ASCORBIC ACID and ETHYLENE GLYCOL. While it is not usually a problem with normal diets, it is seen in high concentrations in certain ornamental plants (such as *Diffenbachia*), as well as in some bleaches and antirust products. Persons or animals that chew on the plants or otherwise consume the chemical can be poisoned. Oxalic acid is highly toxic and if ingested vomiting should not be induced. If the person is at home, a POISON CONTROL CENTER and emergency services should be contacted immediately. The acid can be neutralized by administration of CALCIUM by either the oral or the intravenous route. High urinary oxalate concentrations may cause deposition of KIDNEY STONES and other urinary CALCULI.

oxalism (ok′sah-lizm) poisoning by oxalic acid or by an oxalate.

oxaloacetate (ok″sah-lo-as′ĕ-tāt) a salt or ester of oxaloacetic acid.

oxaloacetic acid (ok″sah-lo-ah-se′tik) a metabolic intermediate in the tricarboxylic acid CYCLE, which is also a substrate of aspartate transaminase.

oxalosis (ok″sah-lo′sis) generalized deposition of calcium oxalate, in renal and extrarenal tissues, as may occur in primary hyperoxaluria.

oxaluria (ok″sah-lu′re-ah) hyperoxaluria.

oxamniquine (ok-sam′nĭ-kwin) an ANTHELMINTIC agent effective against all stages of infection with *Schistosoma mansoni.*

oxandrolone (ok-san′dro-lōn) an androgenic and anabolic STEROID that is administered orally in the treatment of catabolic or tissue-wasting diseases or states.

oxaprozin (ok″sah-pro′zin) a NONSTEROIDAL ANTIINFLAMMATORY DRUG, used in treatment of ARTHRITIS.

oxazepam (ok-saz′ĕ-pam) a benzodiazepine used as an ANTIANXIETY AGENT and sometimes used for relief of symptoms of acute alcohol WITHDRAWAL.

oxazolidinone (ok″sah-zo-lid′ĭ-nōn) any of a class of synthetic antibacterial agents effective against gram-positive organisms.

oxcarbazepine (oks″kahr-baz′ĕ-pēn) an ANTICONVULSANT used in the treatment of partial SEIZURES, administered orally.

oxiconazole (ok″sĭ-kon′ah-zōl) a topical antifungal AGENT used as the nitrate salt in treatment of ATHLETE'S FOOT and RINGWORM.

oxidant (ok′sĭ-dant) the electron acceptor in an oxidation-reduction (redox) reaction.

oxidase (ok″sĭ-dās) any of a class of enzymes that catalyze the reduction of molecular oxygen independently of hydrogen peroxide.

oxidation (ok″sĭ-da′shun) the act of oxidizing or state of being oxidized. Chemically it consists of the increase of positive charges on an atom or the loss of negative charges. Univalent oxidation indicates loss of one electron; divalent oxidation, the loss of two electrons. The opposite reaction to oxidation is REDUCTION. adj., **ox′idative.**

oxidation-reduction (ok″sĭ-da′shun-re-duk′shun) the chemical reaction whereby electrons are removed (oxidation) from atoms of the substance being oxidized and transferred to those being reduced (reduction).

oxide (ok′sīd) a compound of oxygen with an element or radical.

oxidize (ok′sĭ-dīz) to cause to combine with oxygen or to remove hydrogen.

oxidoreductase (ok″sĭ-do-re-duk′tās) a class of enzymes that catalyze the reversible transfer of electrons from one substance to another (oxidation-reduction, or redox reaction).

oxime (ok′sēm) any of a series of compounds containing the CH(=NOH) group, formed by action of hydroxylamine on an aldehyde or ketone.

oximeter (ok-sim′ĕ-ter) a photoelectric device that measures oxygen saturation of the blood by recording the amount of light transmitted or reflected by deoxygenated versus oxygenated hemoglobin.

finger o. a pulse OXIMETER whose sensor is attached to a finger, so that the oxygenation of blood flowing through the finger can be determined. See illustration.

pulse o. an oximeter that permits measurement of oxygen saturation in an artery by recording the different modulations of a transmitted beam of light by reduced hemoglobin and oxyhemoglobin as seen during

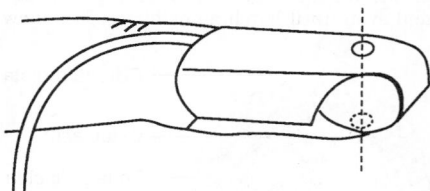

Finger oximeter. Pulse oximetry transducer properly placed on a finger. Fold the Oxisensor over the end of the digit. Align the other end of the sensor so that the two alignment marks are directly opposite each other. Press the sensor into the skin. Wrap the adhesive flaps around the digit. Courtesy of Nellcor Puritan Bennett Corp., Pleasanton, CA.

the pulse. A component of the oximeter analyzes the variations in light absorption and provides a readout of the per cent of saturation of the hemoglobin. A saturation above 90 per cent corresponds to a Pa_{O_2} of 60 torr or higher. The presence of fetal hemoglobin, carboxyhemoglobin, or intravascular dyes may alter the accuracy of a pulse oximeter. In these instances a Sa_{O_2} of 90 per cent may not be associated with a Pa_{O_2} of greater than 60 torr.

oximetry (ok-sim′ĕ-tre) measurement of oxygen saturation of the blood using an OXIMETER.

   pulse o. a noninvasive method of indicating the arterial oxygen saturation of functional HEMOGLOBIN, using a pulse OXIMETER.

oxolinic acid (ok″so-lin′ik) a long-acting antibacterial agent, used orally in the treatment of urinary tract infections caused by susceptible gram-negative organisms.

oxprenolol (oks-pren′ah-lol) a nonselective BETA-ADRENERGIC BLOCKING AGENT, administered orally as the hydrochloride salt in the treatment of HYPERTENSION, hypertrophic CARDIOMYOPATHY, cardiac ARRHYTHMIAS, and MYOCARDIAL INFARCTION.

5-oxoproline (ok″so-pro′lēn) a modified amino acid occurring in several proteins; called also pyroglutamic acid.

5-oxoprolinuria (ok″so-pro″lin-u′re-ah) an inborn ERROR of metabolism marked by abnormally increased levels of 5-OXOPROLINE in the urine, metabolic acidosis, and an increase in the rate of hemolysis. Called also pyroglutamicaciduria.

oxtriphylline (oks-trif′ĭ-lēn) the choline salt of THEOPHYLLINE, used as a BRONCHODILATOR.

oxy- word element [Gr.], *sharp; quick; sour; presence of oxygen in a compound.* Also OX-.

oxybenzone (ok″se-ben′zōn) a topical SUNSCREEN that absorbs ultraviolet B and some ultraviolet A rays.

oxyblepsia (ok″se-blep′se-ah) oxyopia.

oxybutynin (ok″se-bu′tĭ-nin) an ANTICHOLINERGIC and ANTIMUSCARINIC having direct ANTISPASMODIC effects on smooth muscle; used orally as the chloride salt in treatment of uninhibited neurogenic bladder and reflex neurogenic bladder.

oxycephaly (ok-se-sef′ah-le) a condition in which the top of the skull is pointed or conical owing to premature closure of the coronal and lambdoid sutures. adj., **oxycephal′ic.**

oxychlorosene (ok″se-klor′o-sēn) a stabilized organic complex of hypochlorous acid used as a topical antiseptic in the treatment of localized infections.

oxycinesia (ok″se-si-ne′zhah) kinesalgia.

oxycodone (ok″se-ko′dōn) an opioid ANALGESIC derived from MORPHINE; used in the form of the hydrochloride and terephthalate salts, administered orally or rectally.

oxygen (O) (ok′sĭ-jen) a chemical element, atomic number 8, atomic weight 15.999. (See Appendix 6.) It is a colorless and odorless gas that makes up about 20 per cent of the atmosphere. In combination with hydrogen, it forms water; by weight, 90 per cent of water is oxygen. It is the third most abundant of all the elements of nature. Large quantities of it are distributed throughout the solid matter of the earth because it combines readily with many other elements. With carbon and hydrogen, oxygen forms the chemical basis of much organic material. Oxygen is essential in sustaining all kinds of life. Among the land animals, it is obtained from the air and drawn into the lungs by the process of RESPIRATION. See also BLOOD GAS ANALYSIS.

Oxygen Balance and "Oxygen Debt." The need of every cell for oxygen requires a balance in supply and demand. But this balance need not be exact at all times. In fact, in strenuous exercise the oxygen needs of muscle cells are greater than the amount the body can absorb even by the most intense breathing. Thus, during athletic competition, the participants make use of the capacity of muscles to function even though their needs for oxygen are not fully met. When the competition is over, however, the athletes will continue to breathe heavily until the muscles have been supplied with sufficient oxygen. This temporary deficiency is called oxygen debt.

Severe curtailment of oxygen, as during ascent to high altitudes or in certain illnesses, may bring on a variety of symptoms of HYPOXIA, or oxygen lack. A number of poisons, such as CYANIDE and CARBON MONOXIDE,, as well as large overdoses of SEDATIVES, disrupt the oxygen distribution system of the body. Such disruption occurs also in various illnesses, such as ANEMIA and diseases of lungs, heart, kidneys, and liver.

   o. 15 an artificial radioactive isotope of oxygen having a half-life of 2.04 minutes and decaying by positron emission. It is used as a TRACER in the measurement of regional blood volume and flow and oxygen metabolism by positron emission TOMOGRAPHY.

   o. analyzer an instrument that measures the concentration of oxygen in a gas mixture. There are three types of handheld analyzers: *physical/paramagnetic, electric,* and *electrochemical* analyzers.

o. blender a device used to mix oxygen with other gases to any concentration between 21 per cent and 100 per cent.

o. concentrator an electronic device that removes nitrogen from room air, thus increasing the oxygen concentration; commonly used by patients who require long-term oxygen administration at home.

o. consumption the amount of oxygen consumed by the tissues of the body, usually measured as the oxygen uptake in the lung. The normal value is 250 ml/min (or 3.5 to 4.0 ml/kg/min), and it increases with increased metabolic rate.

o. hood a device that fits over the head of an infant or small child for administration of oxygen or aerosolized medications.

hyperbaric o. oxygen under greater than atmospheric pressure.

liquid o. oxygen in liquid form, a common storage form of oxygen; one liter of liquid oxygen will produce 860 liters of gas.

o. tent a large plastic canopy that encloses the patient in a controlled environment, formerly much used for OXYGEN THERAPY, HUMIDITY THERAPY, or AEROSOL THERAPY.

o. therapy 1. in the NURSING INTERVENTIONS CLASSIFICATION, a nursing INTERVENTION defined as administration of oxygen and monitoring of its effectiveness. 2. a form of RESPIRATORY CARE involving administration of supplemental oxygen for relief of hypoxemia and prevention of damage to the tissue cells as a result of oxygen lack (HYPOXIA). Oxygen can be toxic and therefore, as with a drug, its dosage and mode of administration are based on an assessment of the needs of the individual patient. Although many types of hypoxia can be treated successfully by the administration of oxygen, not all cases respond to this therapy. There also is the possibility that the injudicious use of oxygen can produce serious and permanent damage to the body tissues. The administration of oxygen should never be considered a "routine" or harmless procedure.

Adverse Effects of Oxygen. Although it is true that all living organisms require oxygen to maintain life, an environment of 100 per cent oxygen inhibits growth of living tissue cultures, and laboratory experiments have shown that hyperoxygenation of body tissues can cause irreversible damage. It is known that high concentrations of inhaled oxygen can result in collapse of alveoli because of displacement of nitrogen by oxygen. RETINOPATHY OF PREMATURITY in premature infants was found to be caused in part by excessively high levels of oxygen in the blood.

Another serious complication of high-oxygen concentration therapy is the development of a hyaline MEMBRANE because of a deficiency of pulmonary SURFACTANT; surfactant is vitally important to normal expansion and deflation of the alveoli. Prolonged exposure to inspired oxygen concentrations in excess of 50 per cent can impair the production of this surfactant in a patient of any age. The result is a loss of lung compliance and reduction of the transport of oxygen across the alveolar membrane.

The danger of oxygen toxicity can be minimized by careful assessment of each patient's need for oxygen therapy and systematic BLOOD GAS ANALYSIS to determine patient response and effectiveness of treatment. Symptoms of oxygen toxicity are substernal distress, nausea and vomiting, malaise, fatigue, and numbness and tingling of the extremities.

Indications for Oxygen Therapy. In general, the clinical situations in which the administration of supplemental oxygen is indicated are: (1) Profound but potentially reversible hypoxia that appears amenable to the short-term administration of high concentrations of oxygen. Examples would include the patient who is apneic, is suffering from cardiovascular collapse, or is a victim of carbon monoxide poisoning. (2) Conditions in which there is a need to reduce the work load of the cardiovascular and pulmonary systems and at the same time assure an adequate supply of oxygen to the tissues. Congestive heart failure, myocardial infarction, and such acute pulmonary diseases as pulmonary embolism and pneumonia are examples of the types of clinical situations that are best treated by the administration of moderate levels of oxygen concentration. (3) Evidence of hypoventilation, whether from anesthesia and sedation, CHRONIC OBSTRUCTIVE PULMONARY DISEASE, or other conditions. The patient who is hypoventilating is in danger of suffering from an adverse effect of oxygen therapy because increased oxygenation can lead to decreased respiratory effort. In other words, the oxygen acts as a respiratory depressant and may produce an increase in partial pressure of carbon dioxide in the arterial blood, thus contributing to rather than overcoming the problem of hypoxia. If there is evidence that the patient is hypoventilating, it may be necessary to administer the oxygen by assisted or controlled ventilation.

The delivery of appropriate and effective oxygen therapy requires frequent monitoring of arterial blood gases. An initial blood gas analysis at the time the therapy is started provides baseline data with which to evaluate changes in the patient's status.

In addition to monitoring blood gases to assess the patient's need for and response to supplemental oxygen, it is helpful to observe the patient closely for signs of hypoxemia. However, these signs are not as reliable as blood gas analysis because the clinical manifestations of hypoxemia vary widely in individual patients. The typical clinical manifestations of hypoxemia are confusion, impaired judgment, restlessness, tachycardia, central cyanosis, and loss of consciousness.

Dosage and Method of Administration. It must be kept in mind that oxygen is considered a drug and should be prescribed and administered as such; thus it is apparent that vague orders about its administration are never acceptable. There must be specific written orders for flow rate and mode of administration. Decisions about the initial dosage, as well as any changes in mode of administration and dosage, including the discontinuance of oxygen therapy, should be based on evaluation of the P_{O_2}, the P_{CO_2}, and the blood pH. (See also TRANSCUTANEOUS OXYGEN MONITORING and pulse OXIMETER.)

The clinical signs and symptoms of hypoxemia may vary from patient to patient, and they should not be depended upon as valid indications of oxygen insufficiency. This is especially true of cyanosis, a symptom that depends on local circulation to the area, the red cell count, and hemoglobin level. In addition to the data obtained from blood gas analyses, an oxygen analyzer should be used occasionally to check inspired oxygen concentration.

In general, the dosage and mode of administration fall into the following categories. *High concentrations* above 50 per cent usually are prescribed when there is a need for the delivery of high levels of oxygen for a short period of time to overcome acute hypoxemia, as in cardiovascular failure and pulmonary edema. The flow rate may be as high as 12 liters per minute, administered through a close-fitting face mask with or without a rebreathing bag, or via an endotracheal tube.

Moderate concentrations of oxygen are indicated when the patient is suffering from impaired circulation of oxygen, as in congestive heart failure and pulmonary embolism, or from increased need for oxygen, as in thyrotoxicosis, in which the increased metabolic rate creates a need for more oxygen. The rate of flow should be 4 to 8 liters per minute, administered through an air entrainment mask that delivers concentrations above 23 per cent, or in a dosage of 3 to 5 liters per minute through a nasal cannula.

Low concentrations of oxygen are indicated when the patient is receiving oxygen therapy over an extended period of time, as in chronic obstructive pulmonary disease, and there is the possibility of hypoventilation and the danger of increased CO_2 retention. The rate of flow should be 1 to 2 liters per minute, administered through a nasal cannula, or via an air entrainment mask that delivers 24 to 35 per cent oxygen.

Other methods of oxygen administration include the nasal catheter and the oxygen tent. The nasal catheter can cause some discomfort to the patient, and since it is no more and no less effective than the cannula, most therapists and patients prefer not to use it. The oxygen tent is considered by many to be obsolete, its use being limited to the administration of oxygen to children who cannot or will not tolerate other modes of delivery, and to children in whom the objective is to provide oxygen and humidity or humidity alone.

Patient Care. No matter what mode of administration is used, it is essential that the inspired air be moisturized. This is necessary to prevent drying of the respiratory mucosa and thickening of secretions that can further inhibit the flow of air through the air passages. Humidity may be provided by humidifying the oxygen with water, or by aerosoling the water into fine particles and adding it to the oxygen. Most patients need 60 to 65 per cent relative humidity at room temperature. Patients with endotracheal tubes require as close to 100 per cent humidity as possible.

Oxygen is not an explosive gas, but it does support combustion and presents a serious fire hazard. All electrical equipment should be checked for defects that could produce sparks. All appliances that transmit house current must be kept outside an oxygen tent, and all equipment with exposed switches and meters must be considered potential sources of fire. Static electricity is a minimal risk which can be further reduced by maintaining a relatively high humidity in the oxygen tent. Smoking in the immediate area of oxygen administration is prohibited and there should be signs informing visitors and others of this restriction.

When the patient is wearing a mask for an extended period of time, discomfort can be minimized by removing the mask and washing and drying the face at least every eight hours. To be effective the mask must fit snugly and follow the contour of the face. This means that reddened areas will appear where the mask has pressed against the skin. These areas should be gently massaged and the skin lightly powdered to reduce friction.

A program of infection control is especially important in the prevention of cross-infection from the equipment that is used to administer oxygen. Humidifiers and nebulizers may serve as sources of infection because they provide a medium for the growth of bacteria and molds. There is less danger of this happening when disposable equipment is used, but this does not preclude the need for a systematic development of policies and procedures to prevent and control the spread of infection. Every person involved in the care of the patient must be aware of this program and cooperate in its implementation.

transcutaneous o. monitoring a method for obtaining data about oxygen levels through electrodes attached to the skin. This method is preferred for ill neonates who cannot tolerate frequent drawing of blood samples for blood gas analysis. The P_{O_2} levels obtained by cutaneous monitoring correlate with those obtained from samples of arterial blood and spare the neonate blood loss and interruption of rest.

The transcutaneous electrodes are heated to encourage an adequate supply of blood to the area of skin to which they are attached and remain in place to permit continuous monitoring of arterial oxygen levels. To avoid burns, the electrode site can be changed every two hours. An ongoing record provides information about the neonate's oxygen level at any given moment. It allows caregivers to observe the neonate's response to handling and other procedures that may require modification to avoid severe anoxia. Placing the electrodes at specific sites can also aid the diagnosis of patent ductus arteriosus.

oxygenase (ok′sĭ-jen-ās″) any enzyme of the oxidoreductase class that catalyzes the incorporation of both atoms of molecular oxygen into the substrate.

oxygenation (ok″sĭ-jĕ-na′shun) saturation with oxygen.

extracorporeal membrane o. (ECMO) a technique of providing respiratory support; the blood is circulated through an artificial lung consisting of two compartments separated by a gas-permeable membrane, with the blood on one side and the ventilating gas on the other. It was originally used exclusively in newborns but is now being used more and more in adults.

high pressure o., hyperbaric o. (HBO) see HYPERBARIC OXYGENATION.

pulsed o. a technique by which oxygen is delivered to the patient only during inhalation rather than continuously during the respiratory cycle; used to conserve oxygen in patients using chronic low-flow oxygen therapy at home.

transtracheal o. a technique of oxygen administration for patients requiring chronic oxygen therapy, in which oxygen is administered at low flow through a catheter passing directly into the trachea. This may be more cosmetic for patients and may require a lower flow of oxygen than other methods such as the use of a nasal cannula.

oxygenator (ok′sĭ-jĕ-na″tor) an apparatus by which oxygen is introduced into the blood during circulation outside the body, as during open-heart surgery. See also HEART-LUNG MACHINE.

bubble o. a device in which pure oxygen is bubbled through an extracorporeal reservoir of blood, either directly or through a filter.

film o. a device, encased in a container of oxygen, that makes possible reduction of a thin film of blood to facilitate the exchange of gases.

pump o. heart-lung machine.

rotating disk o. a type of film oxygenator in which a series of parallel disks rotate through an extracorporeal pool of venous blood in a container of oxygen; gaseous exchange occurs between the thin film of blood on the exposed surface of the disks and the oxygen in the container.

screen o. a type of film oxygenator in which the venous blood is passed over a series of screens in a container of oxygen, gaseous exchange taking place in the thin film of blood produced on the screens.

oxyhemoglobin (ok″se-he′mo-glo″bin) hemoglobin combined with molecular oxygen, the form in which oxygen is transported in the blood.

oxymetazoline (ok″se-mĕ-taz′o-lēn) a VASOCONSTRICTOR used topically as the hydrochloride salt in nasal congestion and conjunctival congestion.

oxymetholone (ok″se-meth′o-lōn) an anabolic STEROID used to treat patients with ANEMIA due to bone marrow failure or deficient red blood cell production and for prophylaxis and treatment of hereditary ANGIOEDEMA; administered orally.

oxymorphone (ok″se-mor′fōn) an opioid ANALGESIC, used as the hydrochloride salt as an analgesic and adjunct to anesthesia; administered parenterally or rectally.

oxymyoglobin (ok″se-mi′o-glo′bin) myoglobin charged with oxygen.

oxyntic (ok-sin′tik) secreting acid, as the parietal (oxyntic) cells.

oxyopia (ok″se-o′pe-ah) abnormal acuteness of sight; called also oxyblepsia.

oxyphencyclimine (ok″se-fen-si′klĭ-mēn) an ANTICHOLINERGIC and ANTIMUSCARINIC with antisecretory, antimotility, and antispasmodic actions; the hydrochloride salt is used in treatment of peptic ulcer and other gastrointestinal disorders.

oxyphil (ok′se-fil) an Askanazy cell.

oxyphonia (ok″se-fo′ne-ah) an abnormally sharp quality or pitch of the voice.

oxyquinoline (ok″sĭ-kwin′o-lēn) a dicyclic aromatic compound used as a chelating agent; also used in the form of the base or the sulfate salt as a bacteriostatic, fungistatic, antiseptic, and disinfectant.

oxytalan (ok-sit′ah-lan) a connective tissue fiber found in the periodontal membrane.

oxytetracycline (ok″se-tet-rah-si′klēn) a broad-spectrum ANTIBIOTIC of the TETRACYCLINE group produced by *Streptomyces rimosus;* used as the base or the hydrochloride salt, administered orally or intramuscularly.

oxytocia (ok″se-to′se-ah) rapid labor.

oxytocic (ok″se-to′sik) 1. pertaining to, marked by, or promoting OXYTOCIA. 2. an agent that promotes rapid LABOR by stimulating contractions of the myometrium.

oxytocin (ok″se-to′sin) a hypothalamic hormone stored in and released from the posterior pituitary; it may also be prepared synthetically or obtained from the posterior pituitary of domestic animals. It acts as a powerful stimulant to the pregnant uterus, especially toward the end of gestation, and also causes milk to be expressed from the alveoli into the lactiferous ducts during breastfeeding. Injection of oxytocin may be used to induce labor or strengthen uterine contractions during labor, to contract uterine muscle after delivery of the placenta, and to control postpartum hemorrhage. It must be administered with care to avoid trauma to the mother or infant by hyperactivity of uterine muscles during labor. Oxytocin also may be administered intravenously by slow drip or applied to the mucous membranes of the nasal cavity to be absorbed into the bloodstream.

o. challenge test (OCT) a type of CONTRACTION STRESS TEST to assess placental reserve for transmitting oxygen to the fetus and detecting insufficiency by observing the fetal heart rate response to oxytocin-induced contraction. See also FETAL MONITORING.

oxyuriasis (ok″se-u-ri′ah-sis) 1. infection with oxyurids such as *Enterobius vermicularis.* 2. enterobiasis.

oxyuricide (ok″se-u′rĭ-sīd) an ANTHELMINTIC agent that kills OXYURIDS.

oxyurid (ok″se-u′rid) an individual organism of the superfamily OXYUROIDEA; called also pinworm.

Oxyuroidea (ok″se-u″roi-de′ah) the OXYURIDS or PINWORMS, a superfamily of small NEMATODES; they are usually parasitic in the cecum and colon of vertebrates, but may infect invertebrates.

oz ounce.

ozena (o-ze′nah) an atrophic rhinitis marked by a thick mucopurulent discharge, mucosal crusting, and a strong odor.

ozone (o′zōn) a bluish explosive gas or blue liquid, being an allotropic form of oxygen, O_3; it is antiseptic and disinfectant, and irritating and toxic to the pulmonary system. Ozone that is carried in the air is odorless and colorless.

Ozone is artificially produced when automobile exhaust fumes combine with nitrogen oxide in the presence of sunlight and high temperatures. This leads to ozone pollution. Federal standards have been established to determine when the level of ozone in atmospheric air is unhealthful.

o. alert a warning issued by health and environmental officials during periods of excessive ozone pollution for those individuals most sensitive to ozone, such as the very young, the elderly, and ill individuals, especially those with respiratory conditions. Advice is to remain indoors and limit physical activity. Healthy individuals are also advised to limit outdoor activity.

ozostomia (o″zo-sto′me-ah) halitosis.

P

P para; peta-; phosphate (group); phosphorus; posterior; premolar; proline; pupil.

P power; pressure.

P₁ parental generation.

P₂ pulmonic second sound; the pulmonic component of the second HEART SOUND.

p pico-; proton; the short arm of a chromosome.

p- para- (def. 2).

PA physician assistant.

Pa protactinium; pascal.

Pa$_{CO_2}$ symbol for partial pressure of carbon dioxide in the arterial blood; see also BLOOD GAS ANALYSIS.

Pa$_{O_2}$ symbol for partial pressure of oxygen in arterial blood; see also BLOOD GAS ANALYSIS.

PAB, PABA *p*-aminobenzoic acid.

pacemaker (pās′māk-er) 1. an object or substance that controls the rate at which a certain phenomenon occurs. 2. cardiac pacemaker. 3. in biochemistry, a substance whose rate of reaction sets the pace for a series of interrelated reactions.

artificial p. an electronic cardiac pacemaker that has a pulse GENERATOR to generate an extrinsic electrical impulse, causing the heart muscle to depolarize and then contract; its rate is preset regardless of the heart's intrinsic activity. It can be either temporary (transcutaneous, transvenous, or epicardial) or implanted.

asynchronous p. an implanted pacemaker that delivers stimuli at a fixed rate, independent of any atrial or ventricular activity; this type is now rarely used except to initiate or terminate some TACHYCARDIAS.

AV sequential p. an implanted pacemaker with dual chamber pacing that maintains the atrial part of ventricular filling by stimulating the atrium if it does not respond at the proper interval after ventricular activity; used for patients with abnormal sinus node function or decreased atrioventricular conduction.

cardiac p. a small mass of specialized muscle tissue in the heart that sets a rhythm of contraction and relaxation for the other parts of the heart, resulting in the HEARTBEAT. Usually the pacemaker site is the sinoatrial NODE, near the junction with the superior vena cava. The normal rhythm, 60 to 100 contractions per minute, increases during physical or emotional stress and decreases during rest. The pace varies from person to person and is affected by abnormal conditions such as heart injuries and generalized infections. If the normal pacemaker fails to function, its regulating task may be taken over by another small mass of special muscular tissue, the ATRIOVENTRICULAR NODE.

DDD p. dual chamber pacemaker.

demand p. an artificial pacemaker that activates only when it receives sensations indicating a lack of adequate spontaneous rhythm by the heart. It thus avoids competition with the patient's own natural pacemaker.

diaphragmatic p. phrenic pacemaker.

dual chamber p. an implanted pacemaker having two leads, one in the atrium and one in the ventricle, so that electromechanical synchrony between the chambers can be approximated. Called also DDD pacemaker.

ectopic p. any biological cardiac PACEMAKER other than the sinoatrial NODE; under normal conditions it is not active.

electronic p. artificial pacemaker.

epicardial p. a temporary pacemaker whose leads are attached to the epicardial surface; usually used in the diagnosis and treatment of postoperative DYSRHYTHMIAS.

escape p. an ectopic PACEMAKER that assumes control of cardiac impulse propagation because of failure of the sinoatrial node to generate one or more normal impulses.

Pacemaker lead enters external jugular vein

Pacemaker placed beneath skin in pectoral region

Tip of lead lodged in apex of right ventricle

A dual chamber pacemaker senses and paces in both the atrium and the ventricle.

external p. an artificial pacemaker located outside the body; the primary types are transcutaneous and transvenous. See also temporary pacemaker.

gastric p. a saddle-shaped area of the greater curvature of the stomach at the junction of its proximal and middle thirds, which regulates the frequency of gastric contractions.

implantable p., implanted p. an artificial pacemaker implanted within the body.

phrenic p. the device used in electrophrenic RESPIRATION; it converts radiofrequency signals into electrical impulses that stimulate the phrenic nerve, resulting in descent and flattening of the diaphragm and improved inhalation of air. Called also diaphragmatic pacemaker.

synchronous p. an implanted pacemaker that synchronizes the physiological events in the atrium with those of the ventricle; it stimulates the ventricle when triggered by the P wave from the atrium.

temporary p. an artificial pacemaker in which the pulse GENERATOR is not implanted, usually either a transcutaneous or transvenous PACEMAKER. See also external pacemaker.

transcutaneous p. a temporary pacemaker in which large surface, high impedance electrodes are applied to the anterior and posterior chest walls to deliver high current stimuli of long duration for pacing of the ventricles.

transvenous p. an artificial pacemaker, either external or implanted, that is connected to the heart by pacing leads passed through the venous circulation to make contact with the endocardium of the right atrium or right ventricle.

uterine p. either of the two regulating centers that control uterine contractions, located near the openings of the fallopian tubes. When the fetus is ready to be born the pacemakers set off a series of rhythmic contractions in the uterine muscle that gradually force the infant out into the birth canal.

wandering p. a condition in which the site of origin of the impulses controlling the heart rate shifts from the head of the sinoatrial node to a lower part of the node or to another part of the atrium.

pachy- word element [Gr.], *thick.*

pachyblepharon (pak″e-blef′ah-ron) thickening of the eyelids.

pachycephaly (pak″e-sef′ah-le) abnormal thickness of the bones of the skull. adj., **pachycephal′ic.**

pachycheilia (pak″e-ki′le-ah) thickening of the lips.

pachychromatic (pak″e-kro-mat′ik) having the chromatin in thick strands.

pachydactyly (pak″e-dak′tĭ-le) megalodactyly.

pachyderma (pak″e-der′mah) abnormal thickening of the skin. adj., **pachyder′matous.**

p. circumscrip′tum, p. laryn′gis localized warty epithelial thickenings on the vocal cords.

pachydermatocele (pak″e-der-mat′o-sēl) plexiform neuroma attaining a large size, producing an elephantiasis-like condition.

pachydermoperiostosis (pak″e-der″mo-per″e-os-to′sis) a condition believed to be inherited as an autosomal dominant trait, chiefly characterized by thickening of the skin of the head and distal extremities, deep folds and furrows of the skin of the forehead, cheeks, and scalp, seborrhea, hyperhidrosis, periostosis of the long bones, digital clubbing, and spadelike enlargement of the hands and feet.

pachyglossia (pak″e-glos′e-ah) abnormal thickness of the tongue.

pachygyria (pak″e-ji′re-ah) macrogyria.

pachyleptomeningitis (pak″e-lep″to-men″in-ji′tis) inflammation of the dura mater and pia mater.

pachymeningitis (pak″e-men″in-ji′tis) inflammation of the dura mater; called also perimeningitis.

pachymeningopathy (pak″e-men″in-gop′-ah-the) noninflammatory disease of the dura mater.

pachymeninx (pak″e-men′ingks), pl. *pachymenin′ges.* The dura mater.

pachynsis (pah-kin′sis) an abnormal thickening. adj., **pachyn′tic.**

pachyonychia (pak″e-o-nik′e-ah) abnormal thickening of the nails.

p. conge′nita a congenital autosomal dominant syndrome primarily affecting males, characterized by increased thickness of the nails, hyperkeratosis involving the palms, soles, knees, and elbows, widespread tiny cutaneous horns, leukoplakia of the mucous membranes, and usually excessive sweating of the hands and feet; sometimes associated with development of bullae on palms and soles after trauma.

pachyperiostitis (pak″e-per″e-os-ti′tis) periostitis of long bones resulting in abnormal thickness of affected bones.

pachyperitonitis (pak″e-per″ĭ-to-ni′tis) inflammation and thickening of the peritoneum.

pachypleuritis (pak″e-plŏŏ-ri′tis) 1. fibrothorax. 2. pleural fibrosis.

pachysalpingitis (pak″e-sal″pin-ji′tis) chronic interstitial inflammation of the

P

muscular coat of the FALLOPIAN TUBE, producing thickening; called also mural salpingitis and parenchymatous salpingitis.

pachysalpingo-ovaritis (pak″e-sal-ping″-go-o″vah-ri′tis) chronic inflammation of the ovary and fallopian tube, with thickening.

pachytene (pak′e-tēn) in prophase of meiosis, the stage following zygotene, during which the chromosomes shorten, thicken, and separate into two sister chromatids joined at their centromeres. Paired homologous chromosomes, which were joined by synapsis, now form a tetrad of four chromatids. Where crossing over has occurred between nonsister chromatids, they are joined by X-shaped chiasmata.

pachyvaginalitis (pak″e-vaj″ĭ-nal-i′tis) inflammation and thickening of the TUNICA VAGINALIS TESTIS.

pachyvaginitis (pak″e-vaj″ĭ-ni′tis) chronic VAGINITIS with thickening of the vaginal walls.

pacing (pās′ing) 1. regulation of the rate of a physiologic process, such as by providing timed stimuli. 2. cardiac pacing.

  biventricular p. that in which a lead is used to deliver current directly to the left ventricle, in addition to those used to deliver current to the right atrium and ventricle, so that the ventricles can be induced to pump in synchrony.

  cardiac p. regulation of cardiac rhythm (or the rate of contraction of the heart muscle) with electrical stimuli from a pulse GENERATOR or an artificial PACEMAKER.

  diaphragm p., diaphragmatic p. electrophrenic respiration.

  dual chamber p. control of the heart rate by means of an artificial PACEMAKER that paces, senses, or does both in the atria and in the ventricles.

  phrenic p. electrophrenic respiration.

  single chamber p. control of the heart rate by an artificial PACEMAKER that paces and senses in either atria or ventricles, usually in the latter.

  transthoracic p. a system of single or dual chamber epicardial pacing in which the electrode wires are sewn directly onto the epicardium and brought out through an incision in the chest wall. See also epicardial PACEMAKER.

  transvenous p. a system of single or dual chamber endocardial pacing in which the electrode wires are passed through veins into the right atrium or ventricle. See also transvenous PACEMAKER.

pack (pak) 1. treatment by wrapping a patient in blankets or sheets, or a limb in towels, wet or dry and either hot or cold; referred to as wet, dry, hot, or cold pack respectively. 2. the blankets, sheets, or towels used for this treatment. 3. TAMPON. 4. a type of dressing used for hemostasis, such as in the nose (*nasal pack*) or vagina (*vaginal pack*). See also PACKING.

packing (pak′ing) 1. the filling of a wound or cavity with gauze, sponge, or other material. 2. the material used for this purpose.

paclitaxel (pak″lĭ-tak′sel) an antineoplastic AGENT that acts by promoting and stabilizing the polymerization of microtubules, isolated from the Pacific yew tree (*Taxus brevifolia*); used in the treatment of advanced ovarian or breast carcinoma, non-small cell lung carcinoma, and AIDS-related Kaposi's sarcoma. Administered intravenously.

PACU postanesthesia care UNIT.

pad (pad) a cushion-like mass of soft material.

  abdominal p. a pad for the absorption of discharges from abdominal wounds, or for packing off abdominal viscera to improve exposure during surgery. Called also laparotomy pad.

  dinner p. a pad placed over the stomach before a plaster jacket is applied; the pad is then removed to leave space under the jacket to take care of expansion of the stomach after eating.

  infrapatellar fat p. a large pad of fat lying behind and below the patella.

  knuckle p's nodular thickenings of the skin on the dorsal surface of the interphalangeal joints.

  laparotomy p. abdominal p.

  sucking p., suctorial p. a lobulated mass of fat that occupies the space between the masseter muscle and the external surface of the buccinator muscle. It is well developed in infants.

padimate O (pad′ĭ-māt) a substituted AMINOBENZOATE used as a SUNSCREEN, absorbing ULTRAVIOLET RAYS of the UVB type.

pae- for words beginning thus, see those beginning *pe-*.

PAF platelet-activating factor.

Paget's disease (paj′ets) any of three diseases named after Sir James Paget (1814–1889): Paget's disease of bone, Paget's disease of the breast, and extramammary Paget's disease.

  Paget's disease of bone is a localized bone disorder that is also called osteitis deformans. It is relatively common, particularly in the United States, United Kingdom, Australia, France, and Germany, occurring in 3 per cent of the population over the age of 40 and 10 per cent of those over the age of 70. It occurs more often in males than in females. Once thought to be a rare form of localized bone disease, the disorder is now diagnosed more frequently because of newer diagnostic techniques, such as bone scanning, and routine testing of plasma alkaline phosphatase.

Symptoms of Paget's disease of bone depend on the site of the bone lesions and their severity. In 20 per cent of diagnosed cases there are no symptoms at all, and in others the symptoms are very mild. Lesions in the long bones seem to cause the most difficulty. The disease disturbs the growth of new bone tissue with the result that the bones often thicken, become soft, and coarsen in texture. In an advanced case, the weakened bone may be fractured by even a light blow, or, as in the case of the vertebrae, may collapse.

Lesions in the long bones can cause pain, deformity from bowing, and disability due to the arthritic changes that are a complication of the disease. When the disease process affects the skull the patient may complain of headaches, intermittent ringing in the ears and dizziness, and hearing loss. Severe involvement of the occipital region can cause pressure on the pons and cerebellum and compression of the spinal cord. These pathologic changes produce loss of coordination, muscle weakness, diplopia, ataxia, and other signs of neurologic dysfunction.

Diagnosis of this disease is verified by radiologic studies of the affected bones and by laboratory tests. The serum alkaline phosphatase and urinary hydroxyproline levels are elevated. Drugs of choice for its treatment are calcitonin, mithramycin, and etidronate disodium.

Paget's disease of the breast is an erythematous scaling lesion of the breast, involving the nipple and areola unilaterally, and associated with an underlying malignancy. It usually appears around the age of 55 in women, but can also affect males. (See Atlas 2, Part I.)

Extramammary Paget's disease is characterized by similar lesions occurring in middle-aged women and men, but the lesions are located in the anogenital area. The skin disorder is not always associated with malignancy, as it is when affecting the breast, but in almost half the cases there is an underlying carcinoma.

pagetoid (paj′ĕ-toid) resembling or characteristic of PAGET'S DISEASE.

pagophagia (pag″o-fa′jah) the habit of eating large amounts of ice, a form of PICA sometimes linked to iron deficiency.

-pagus word element [Gr.], *conjoined twins*.

PAH, PAHA *p*-aminohippuric acid.

PAI plasminogen activator inhibitor.

pain (pān) a feeling of distress, suffering, or agony, caused by stimulation of specialized nerve endings. Its purpose is chiefly protective; it acts as a warning that tissues are being damaged and induces the sufferer to remove or withdraw from the source. The North American Nursing Diagnosis Association has accepted pain as a NURSING DIAGNOSIS, defining it as a state in which an individual experiences and reports severe discomfort or an uncomfortable sensation; the reporting of pain may be either by direct verbal communication or by encoded descriptors.

Pain Receptors and Stimuli. All receptors for pain stimuli are free nerve ENDINGS of groups of myelinated or unmyelinated neural fibers abundantly distributed in the superficial layers of the skin and in certain deeper tissues such as the periosteum, surfaces of the joints, arterial walls, and the falx and tentorium of the cranial cavity. The distribution of pain receptors in the gastrointestinal mucosa apparently is similar to that in the skin; thus, the mucosa is quite sensitive to irritation and other painful stimuli. Although the parenchyma of the liver and the alveoli of the lungs are almost entirely insensitive to pain, the liver and bile ducts are extremely sensitive, as are the bronchi and parietal pleura.

Some pain receptors are selective in their response to stimuli, but most are sensitive to more than one of the following types of excitation: (1) mechanical stress of trauma; (2) extremes of heat and cold; and (3) chemical substances, such as histamine, potassium ions, acids, prostaglandins, bradykinin, and acetylcholine. Pain receptors, unlike other sensory receptors in the body, do not adapt or become less sensitive to repeated stimulation. Under certain conditions the receptors become more sensitive over a period of time. This accounts for the fact that as long as a traumatic stimulus persists the person will continue to be aware that damage to the tissues is occurring.

The body is able to recognize tissue damage because when cells are destroyed they release the chemical substances previously mentioned. These substances can stimulate pain receptors or cause direct damage to the nerve endings themselves. A lack of oxygen supply to the tissues can also produce pain by causing the release of chemicals from ischemic tissue. Muscle spasm is another cause of pain, probably because it has the indirect effect of causing ischemia and stimulation of chemosensitive pain receptors.

Transmission and Recognition of Pain. When superficial pain receptors are excited the impulses are transmitted from these surface receptors to synapses in the gray matter (*substantia gelatinosa*) of the dorsal horns of the spinal cord. They then travel upward along the sensory pathways to the thalamus, which is the main sensory relay station of the brain. The dorsomedial nucleus of the thalamus projects to the prefrontal cortex of the brain. The conscious perception of pain probably takes place in the thalamus and lower centers; interpretation of the quality of pain is probably the role of the cerebral cortex.

The perception of pain by an individual is highly complex and individualized, and is subject to a variety of external and internal influences. The cerebral cortex is concerned with the appreciation of pain and its quality, location, type, and intensity; thus, an intact sensory cortex is essential to the perception of pain. In addition to neural influences that transmit and modulate sensory input, the perception of pain is affected by psychological and cultural responses to pain-related stimuli. A person can be unaware of pain at the time of an acute injury or other very stressful situation, when in a state of depression, or when experiencing an emotional crisis. Cultural influences also precondition the perception of and response to painful stimuli. The reaction to similar circumstances can range from complete stoicism to histrionic behavior.

Pain Control. There are several theories related to the physiologic control of pain but none has been completely verified. One of the best known is that of Mellzak and Wall, the *gate control theory,* which proposed that pain impulses were mediated in the substantia gelatinosa of the spinal cord with the dorsal horns acting as "gates" that controlled entry of pain signals into the central pain pathways. Also, pain signals would compete with tactile signals with the two constantly balanced against each other.

Since this theory was first proposed, researchers have shown that the neuronal circuitry it hypothesizes is not precisely correct. Nevertheless, there are internal systems that are now known to occur naturally in the body for controlling and mediating pain. One such system, the opioid system, involves the production of morphinelike substances called ENKEPHALINS and ENDORPHINS. Both are naturally occurring analgesics found in various parts of the brain and spinal cord that are concerned with pain perception and the transmission of pain signals. Signals arising from stimulation of neurons in the gray matter of the brain stem travel downward to the dorsal horns of the spinal cord where incoming pain impulses from the periphery terminate. The descending signals block or significantly reduce the transmission of pain signals upward along the spinal cord to the brain where pain is perceived by releasing these substances.

In addition to the brain's opioid system for controlling the transmission of pain impulses along the spinal cord, there is another mechanism for the control of pain. The stimulation of large sensory fibers extending from the tactile receptors in the skin can suppress the transmission of pain signals from thinner nerve fibers. It is as if the nerve pathways to the brain can accommodate only one type of signal at a time, and when two kinds of impulses simultaneously arrive at the dorsal horns, the tactile sensation takes precedence over the sensation of pain.

The discovery of endorphins and the inhibition of pain transmission by tactile signals has provided a scientific explanation for the effectiveness of such techniques as relaxation, massage, application of liniments, and acupuncture in the control of pain and discomfort.

Assessment of Pain. Pain is a subjective phenomenon that is present when the person who is experiencing it says it is. The person reporting personal discomfort or pain is the most reliable source of information about its location, quality, intensity, onset, precipitating or aggravating factors, and measures that bring relief.

Objective signs of pain can help verify what a patient says about pain, but such data are not used to prove or disprove whether it is present. Physiologic signs of moderate and superficial pain are responses of the sympathetic nervous system. They include rapid, shallow, or guarded respiratory movements, pallor, diaphoresis, increased pulse rate, elevated blood pressure, dilated pupils, and tenseness of the skeletal muscles. Pain that is severe or located deep in body cavities acts as a stimulant to parasympathetic neurons and is evidenced by a drop in blood pressure, slowing of pulse, pallor, nausea and vomiting, weakness, and sometimes a loss of consciousness.

Behavioral signs of pain include crying, moaning, tossing about in bed, pacing the floor, lying quietly but tensely in one position, drawing the knees upward toward the abdomen, rubbing the painful part, and a pinched facial expression or grimacing. The person in pain also may have difficulty concentrating and remembering and may be totally self-centered and preoccupied with the pain.

Psychosocial aspects of tolerance for pain and reactions to it are less easily identifiable and more complex than physiologic responses. An individual's reaction to pain is subject to a variety of psychologic and cultural influences. These include previous experience with pain, training in regard to how one should respond to pain and discomfort, state of health, and the presence of fatigue or physical weakness. One's degree of attention to and distraction from painful stimuli can also affect one's perception of the intensity of pain. A thorough assessment of pain takes into consideration all of these psychosocial factors.

Management of Pain. Among the measures employed to provide relief from pain, administration of analgesic drugs is probably the one that is most often misunderstood and abused. When an analgesic drug has been ordered "as needed," the patient should know that the drug is truly available when needed and that it will be given promptly when asked for. If the patient is forced to wait until someone else decides when an analgesic is needed, the patient

COMMON MISCONCEPTIONS ABOUT PAIN

Myth	Fact
There must be a demonstrable cause for pain to occur.	Pain can be very real even if no cause can be found. Cellular damage need not be present for pain to occur. Although damage to cells does lead to the release of chemicals that stimulate pain receptors, in many cases no cellular pathology can be demonstrated; nevertheless, the pain exists.
Persons who have a low tolerance for pain have poor self-control and probably are emotionally insecure. It may also be said that such a person has "dependent" personality.	Tolerance is defined as that duration or intensity of pain that a person is willing to endure without seeking relief. It is a physiologic response to pain that is made more complex by psychosocial factors, many of which can be beyond the control of the person who is in pain.
Causes of and reactions to acute and chronic pain are essentially the same. Treatment of one type will be effective for the other.	Physiologic and emotional responses to acute pain and chronic pain differ; therefore management and measures for relief differ. In general, acute pain is more often associated with anxiety, and chronic pain with reactive depression.
Addiction to pain-relieving drugs is always a hazard. For the sake of the patient it is often necessary to withhold an analgesic.	Studies have repeatedly shown that only a small percentage of patients become addicted to drugs administered for the relief of pain. Patients should be assured that pain can and will be relieved.
Health care providers are experts in patient pain.	Pain is experienced in many different ways. The patient should be considered the expert in defining the pain.
Pain perception decreases with aging.	In the older adult with an intact central nervous system there is no alteration in pain perception. The response to pain may be affected by a variety of factors; for example, in an individual with aphasia the ability to communicate discomfort verbally is impaired.
Placebos are useful in assessing pain.	There is no basis for believing that a patient who experiences pain relief from a placebo is not experiencing real pain. Additionally, the administration of a placebo is an ethically questionable practice for the nurse.
Narcotics should never be given to older patients.	The appropriate drug to treat severe pain should always be administered. The older person may have more difficulty with biotransforming and excreting narcotics and the dosage should be adjusted based on the patient's level of pain and metabolism of the medication.
Pain medication should not be administered to confused patients.	Pain can cause confusion, especially in the older person. Pain often interferes with sleep and rest, leading to confusion. Following assessment, if it is determined that the patient is in pain and there is no other cause for the confusion, pain medication should be administered. This will often cause the confusion to clear.

P

may become angry, resentful, and tense, thus diminishing or completely negating the desired effect of the drug. Studies have shown that when analgesics are left at the bedside of terminally ill cancer patients to be taken at their discretion, fewer doses are taken than when they must rely on someone else to make the drug available. Habituation and addiction to analgesics probably result as much from not using other measures along with analgesics for pain control as from giving prescribed analgesics when they are ordered. Patient-controlled ANAL-GESIA has been used safely and effectively.

When analgesics are not appropriate or sufficient or when there is a real danger of addiction, there are noninvasive techniques that can be used as alternatives or adjuncts to analgesic therapy. The selection of a particular technique for the management of pain depends on the cause of the pain, its intensity and duration, whether it is acute or chronic, and whether the patient perceives the technique as effective.

Distraction techniques provide a kind of sensory shielding to make the person less aware of discomfort. Distraction can be effective in the relief of brief periods of acute pain, such as that associated with minor surgical procedures under local anesthesia, wound débridement, and venipuncture.

Massage and gentle pressure activate the thick-fiber impulses and produce a preponderance of tactile signals to compete with pain signals. It is interesting that stimulation of the large sensory fibers leading from superficial sensory receptors in the skin can relieve pain at a site distant from the area being rubbed or otherwise stimulated. Since ischemia and muscle spasm can both produce discomfort, massage to improve circulation and frequent repositioning of the body and limbs to avoid circulatory stasis and promote muscle relaxation can be effective in the prevention and management of pain. Transcutaneous electrical nerve stimulation (TENS) units enhance the production of endorphins and enkephalins and can also relieve pain.

Specific relaxation techniques can help relieve physical and mental tension and stress and reduce pain. They have been especially effective in mitigating discomfort during labor and delivery but can be used in a variety of situations. Learning proper relaxation techniques is not easy for some people, but once these techniques have been mastered they can be of great benefit in the management of chronic ongoing pain. The intensity of pain also can be reduced by stimulating the skin through applications of either heat or cold, menthol ointments, and liniments. Contralateral stimulation involves stimulating the skin in an area on the side opposite a painful region. Stimulation can be done by rubbing, massaging, or applying heat or cold.

Since pain is a symptom and therefore of value in diagnosis, it is important to keep accurate records of the observations of the patient having pain. These observations should include the following: the nature of the pain, that is, whether it is described by the patient as being sharp, dull, burning, aching, etc.; the location of the pain, if the patient is able to determine this; the time of onset and the duration, and whether or not certain nursing measures and drugs are successful in obtaining relief; and the relation to other circumstances, such as the position of the patient, occurrence before or after eating, and stimuli in the environment such as heat or cold that may trigger the onset of pain.

acute p. 1. one of the three categories of pain established by the International Association for the Study of Pain, denoting pain that is caused by occurrences such as traumatic injury, surgical procedures, or medical disorders; clinical symptoms often include increased heart rate, blood pressure, and respiratory rate, shallow respiration, agitation or restlessness, facial grimaces, or splinting. 2. a NURSING DIAGNOSIS accepted by the North American Nursing Diagnosis Association, defined as an unpleasant sensory and emotional experience arising from actual or potential tissue damage or described in terms of such damage, with sudden or slow onset of any intensity from mild to severe with an anticipated or predictable end and a duration of less than 6 months.

bearing-down p. pain accompanying uterine contractions during the second stage of LABOR.

cancer p. one of the three categories of pain established by the International Association for the Study of Pain, denoting pain associated with malignancies and perceived by the individual patient; there are various scales ranking it from 0 to 10 according to level of severity.

chronic p. 1. one of the three categories of pain established by the International Association for the Study of Pain, denoting pain that is persistent, often lasting more than six months; clinical symptoms may be the same as for acute pain, or there may be no symptoms evident. The North American Nursing Diagnosis Association has accepted chronic pain as a NURSING DIAGNOSIS. 2. a

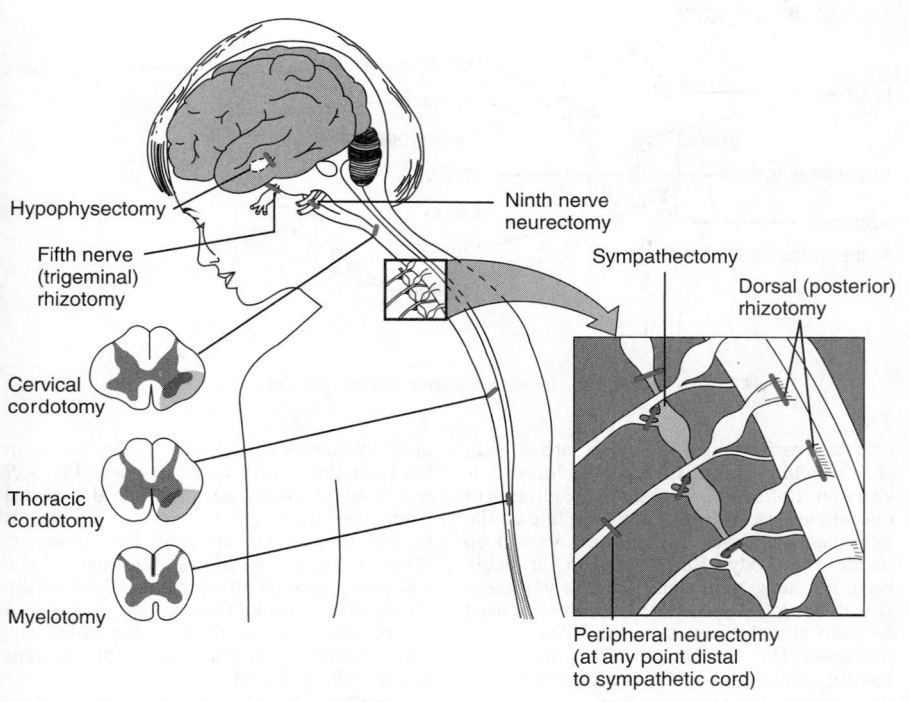

Surgical procedures designed to alleviate pain. From Ignatavicius et al., 1999.

NURSING DIAGNOSIS accepted by the North American Nursing Diagnosis Association, defined as an unpleasant sensory and emotional experience arising from actual or potential tissue damage or described in terms of such damage, with sudden or slow onset of any intensity from mild to severe, without an anticipated or predictable end, and with a duration of greater than 6 months.

p. disorder a SOMATOFORM DISORDER characterized by a chief complaint of severe chronic pain that causes substantial distress or impairment in functioning; the pain is neither feigned nor intentionally produced, and psychological factors appear to play a major role in its onset, severity, exacerbation, or maintenance. The pain is related to psychological conflicts and is made worse by environmental stress; it enables the patient to avoid an unpleasant activity or to obtain support and sympathy. Patients may visit many health care providers searching for relief and may consume excessive amounts of analgesics without any effect. They are difficult to treat because they strongly resist the idea that their symptoms have a psychological origin.

false p's ineffective pains during pregnancy that resemble labor pains, not accompanied by cervical dilatation; see also BRAXTON-HICKS CONTRACTIONS. Called also false labor.

gas p's see GAS PAINS.

growing p's any of various types of recurrent limb pains resembling those of rheumatoid conditions, seen in early youth and formerly thought to be caused by the growing process.

hunger p. pain coming on at the time for feeling hunger for a meal; a symptom of gastric disorder.

intermenstrual p. pain accompanying ovulation, occurring during the period between the menses, usually about midway.

labor p's the rhythmic pains of increasing severity and frequency due to contraction of the uterus at childbirth; see also LABOR.

lancinating p. sharp darting pain.

phantom p. pain felt as if it were arising in an absent or amputated limb or organ; see also AMPUTATION.

psychogenic p. symptoms of physical pain having psychological origin; see PAIN DISORDER.

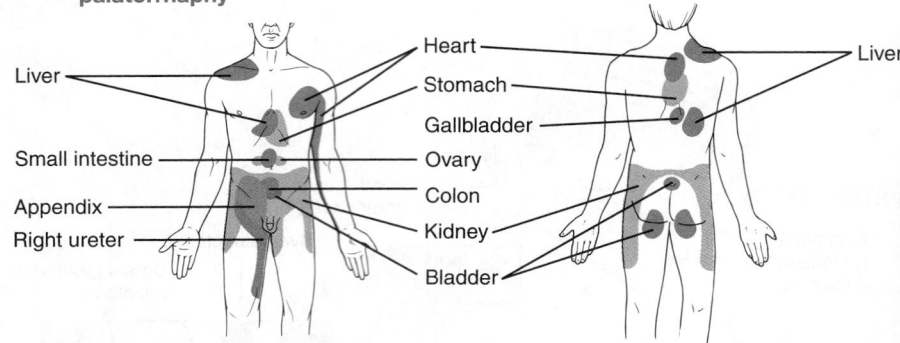

Area of referred pain, anterior and posterior views.

referred p. pain in a part other than that in which the cause that produced it is situated. Referred pain usually originates in one of the visceral organs but is felt in the skin or sometimes in another area deep inside the body. Referred pain probably occurs because pain signals from the viscera travel along the same neural pathways used by pain signals from the skin. The person perceives the pain but interprets it as having originated in the skin rather than in a deep-seated visceral organ.

rest p. a continuous unrelenting pain due to ischemia of the lower leg, beginning with or being aggravated by elevation and being relieved by sitting with legs in a dependent position or by standing.

root p. pain caused by disease of the sensory nerve roots and occurring in the cutaneous areas supplied by the affected roots.

painful bruising syndrome a purpuric reaction seen chiefly in young to middle-aged women in which spontaneous, chronic recurring painful ecchymoses occur on the body without antecedent trauma or after insufficient trauma; these may be precipitated by emotional stress. Based on studies that show that certain patients exhibit autoerythrocyte sensitization in which intradermal injection of their own erythrocytes produces a painful ecchymosis, the etiology of the condition has been ascribed by some to an autosensitivity to a component of the erythrocyte membrane; others consider it to be of psychosomatic or factitious origin. Called also autoerythrocyte sensitization syndrome.

palat(o)- word element [L.], *palate.*

palate (pal′at) the roof of the mouth. The *hard palate* is the front portion braced by the upper jaw bones (maxillae); it has a bony framework and forms the partition between the mouth and the nose. The *soft palate* is the fleshy part arching downward from the hard palate to the throat; it separates the mouth and the pharynx. When a person swallows, the rear of the soft palate swings up against the back of the pharynx and blocks the passage of food and air to the nose. A fleshy lobe called the UVULA hangs from the middle of the soft palate. adj., **pal′atal.**

cleft p. see CLEFT LIP AND CLEFT PALATE.

premaxillary p., primary p. that portion of the palate that was the median nasal process during early development.

secondary p. that portion of the palate that was the lateral nasal processes during early development.

palatitis (pal″ah-ti′tis) inflammation of the palate.

palatoglossal (pal″ah-to-glos′al) pertaining to the palate and tongue.

palatognathous (pal″ah-tog′nah-thus) having a congenitally cleft palate.

palatomaxillary (pal″ah-to-mak′sĭ-ler-e) pertaining to the palate and maxilla.

palatopharyngeal (pal″ah-to-fah-rin′je-al) pertaining to the palate and pharynx.

palatopharyngoplasty (pal″ah-to-fah-ring′go-plas″te) a trimming back of excess palatal and pharyngeal tissue, done in order to widen the airway and relieve obstructive sleep apnea or severe snoring.

palatoplasty (pal′ah-to-plas″te) plastic reconstruction of the palate, such as to repair a CLEFT PALATE. See also STAPHYLOPLASTY and PALATORRHAPHY.

palatoplegia (pal″ah-to-ple′jah) paralysis of the palate.

palatorrhaphy (pal″ah-tor′ah-fe) surgical correction of a CLEFT PALATE; see also PALATOPLASTY.

palatoschisis (pal″ah-tos′kĭ-sis) cleft palate.

palatum (pal-ah′tum) [L.] palate.

pale(o)- word element [Gr.], *old.*

paleencephalon (pa″le-en-sef′ah-lon) the (phylogenetically) old brain; all of the brain except the cerebral cortex and its dependences.

paleocerebellum (pa″le-o-ser″ĕ-bel′um) originally, the phylogenetically older parts of the cerebellum; the term is now applied specifically to those parts whose afferent inflow is predominantly supplied by spinocerebellar fibers. adj., **paleocerebel′lar.**

paleocortex (pa″le-o-kor′teks) that portion of the cerebral CORTEX that, with the ARCHEOCORTEX, develops in association with the olfactory system, and which is phylogenetically older and less stratified than the neocortex. It is composed chiefly of the piriform cortex and the parahippocampal gyrus.

paleogenetic (pa″le-o-jĕ-net′ik) originated in the past; said of traits, structures, and other aspects of species that are not newly acquired.

paleopathology (pa″le-o-pah-thol′ŏ-je) study of disease in bodies that have been preserved from ancient times.

paleostriatum (pa″le-o-stri-a′tum) the phylogenetically older portion of the corpus striatum, represented by the globus pallidus. adj., **paleostria′tal.**

paleothalamus (pa″le-o-thal′ah-mus) the phylogenetically older part of the thalamus, i.e., the medial portion which lacks reciprocal connections with the neopallium.

pali(n)- word element [Gr.], *again; pathologic repetition.*

palikinesia (pal″ĭ-kĭ-ne′zhah) pathologic repetition of movements.

palilalia (pal″ĭ-la′le-ah) a condition in which a phrase or word is repeated with increasing rapidity.

palindromia (pal″in-dro′me-ah) a recurrence or relapse. adj., **palindrom′ic.**

palingraphia (pal″in-graf′e-ah) pathologic repetition of words or phrases in writing.

palinopsia (pal″in-op′se-ah) visual perseveration; the pathologic continuance or recurrence of a visual sensation after the stimulus is gone.

palinphrasia (pal″in-fra′zhah) pathologic repetition of words or phrases in speaking.

palivizumab (pal″ĭ-viz′u-mab) a monoclonal ANTIBODY against respiratory syncytial VIRUS, used as a passive immunizing agent against infection with the virus in susceptible infants and children; administered intramuscularly.

palladium (Pd) (pah-la′de-um) a chemical element, atomic number 46, atomic weight

106.4. (See Appendix 6.) It is used in alloys for dental and orthodontic appliances.

pallanesthesia (pal″an-es-the′zhah) loss or absence of PALLESTHESIA.

pallesthesia (pal″es-the′zhah) sensibility to vibrations; the peculiar vibrating sensation felt when a vibrating tuning-fork is placed against a subcutaneous bony prominence of the body. adj., **pallesthet′ic.**

palliate (pal′e-āt) to relieve symptoms.

palliative (pal′e-ah-tiv) 1. giving relief but not curing. 2. a drug with this effect.

pallidectomy (pal″ĭ-dek′to-me) complete removal of the globus pallidus.

pallidotomy (pal″ĭ-dot′ah-me) creation of lesions by stereotaxic surgery in the globus pallidus for treatment of extrapyramidal disorders.

pallidum (pal′ĭ-dum) the globus pallidus of the brain. adj., **pal′lidal.**

pallium (pal′e-um) 1. cerebral cortex. 2. the cerebral cortex during its development.

pallor (pal′or) paleness, as of the skin.

palm (pahm) the hollow or flexor surface of the hand. adj., **pal′mar.**

palma (pahl′mah) [L.] palm.

palmaris (pahl-mar′is) palmar.

Palmer (pahl′mer) Sophia E. (1853–1920). American nursing writer and organizer; first editor of the *American Journal of Nursing.* She campaigned for state registration of nursing and assisted in drafting much of the legislation. She served as first president of the New York State Board of Examiners and helped to organize the American Nurses' Association and the American Society of Superintendents of Training Schools for Nurses.

palmitic acid (pal-mit′ik) a saturated fatty acid from animal and vegetable fats.

palpable (pal′pah-b'l) perceptible by touch.

palpate (pal′pāt) to perform palpation.

palpation (pal-pa′shun) the act of feeling with the hand; the application of the fingers with light pressure to the surface of the body for the purpose of determining the condition of the parts beneath in physical diagnosis.

  bimanual p. palpation with both hands in the physical examination of a patient.

palpebra (pal′pĕ-brah) [L.] eyelid. adj., **pal′pebral.**

palpebritis (pal″pĕ-bri′tis) blepharitis.

palpitation (pal″pĭ-ta′shun) a heartbeat that is unusually rapid, strong, or irregular enough to make a person aware of it, usually over 120 beats per minute, as opposed to the normal 60 to 100 per minute. In most cases, it is the result of excitement,

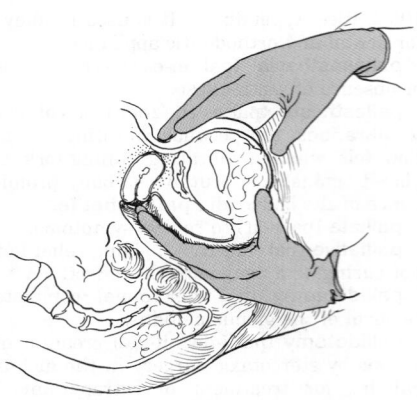

Bimanual palpation. From Gorrie et al., 1994.

nervousness, strong exertion, or taking of certain medications (including CAFFEINE and NICOTINE). There are also palpitations that result from heart disorders such as paroxysmal TACHYCARDIA, FLUTTER, abnormal rhythms in which the heart has runs of rapid beats, and atrial FIBRILLATION (in which the beats are rapid but irregular or seemingly random).

Palpitations may be caused by organic heart disease, but they also can result from other factors. Similarly, emotional pressures rather than organic changes may cause the so-called "nervous heart," or functional heart disease.

PALS pediatric advanced life support.

palsy (pawl′ze) paralysis.

    Bell's p. see BELL'S PALSY.

    birth p. birth paralysis.

    cerebral p. see CEREBRAL PALSY.

    crossed leg p. palsy of the fibular nerve, caused by sitting with one leg crossed over the other.

    Erb's p., Erb-Duchenne p. Erb-Duchenne paralysis.

    facial p. Bell's palsy.

    shaking p. Parkinson's disease.

paludism (pal′u-dizm) old name for malaria.

pamabrom (pam′ah-brom) a mild diuretic used in preparations for the relief of premenstrual symptoms.

Pamelor 1. pam′ĕ-lor 2. trademark for a preparation of NORTRIPTYLINE hydrochloride, a tricyclic ANTIDEPRESSANT.

pamidronate (pam″ĭdro′nāt) an inhibitor of bone resorption, used to treat malignancy-associated hypercalcemia, Paget's disease of bone, and osteolytic metastasis secondary to breast cancer or myeloma;

used as the disodium salt. Complexed with TECHNETIUM 99m it is used in bone imaging.

pamoate (pam′o-āt) USAN contraction for 4,4′-methylenebis[3-hydroxy-2-naphtho-ate].

pampiniform (pam-pin′ĭ-form) shaped like a tendril.

pan- word element [Gr.], *all.*

panacea (pan″ah-se′ah) a remedy for all diseases.

panacinar (pan-as′ĭ-ner) affecting many acini or alveoli.

panagglutinin (pan″ah-gloo′tĭ-nin) an agglutinin that agglutinates the erythrocytes of all human blood groups.

panangiitis (pan″an-je-i′tis) diffuse necrotizing inflammation involving all the coats of a vessel.

panarthritis (pan″ahr-thri′tis) inflammation of all the joints.

panatrophy (pan-at′rŏ-fe) atrophy of several parts; diffuse atrophy.

panautonomic (pan-aw″to-nom′ik) pertaining to or affecting the entire autonomic (sympathetic and parasympathetic) nervous system.

pancarditis (pan″kahr-di′tis) diffuse inflammation of the heart.

Pancoast's syndrome (pan′kōsts) 1 radiographic shadow at the apex of the lung, neuritic pain in the upper limb, atrophy of the muscles of the arm and hand, and HORNER'S SYNDROME, observed with a tumor near the apex of the lung, due to involvement of the brachial plexus. 2 osteolysis in the posterior part of one or more ribs and sometimes involving also the corresponding vertebra.

pancolectomy (pan″ko-lek′to-me) excision of the entire colon, with creation of an outlet from the ileum on the body surface.

pancreas (pan′kre-as), pl. *pancre′ata* [Gr.] a large, elongated, racemose gland located transversely behind the stomach, between the spleen and duodenum. (See also Plate 11.) It is composed of both exocrine and endocrine tissue. The ACINI secrete digestive enzymes, and small ductules leading from the acini secrete sodium bicarbonate solution. The combined product, *pancreatic juice,* enters a long pancreatic duct and from there is transported through the hepatic duct to the duodenum. The pancreatic juice contains enzymes for the breakdown of proteins, carbohydrates, and fats. The bicarbonate ions in the pancreatic secretion help neutralize the acidic chyme that is passed along from the stomach to the duodenum.

Regulation of pancreatic secretion of enzymes and bicarbonate ions is both neural and hormonal; however, the influences of the hormones SECRETIN and

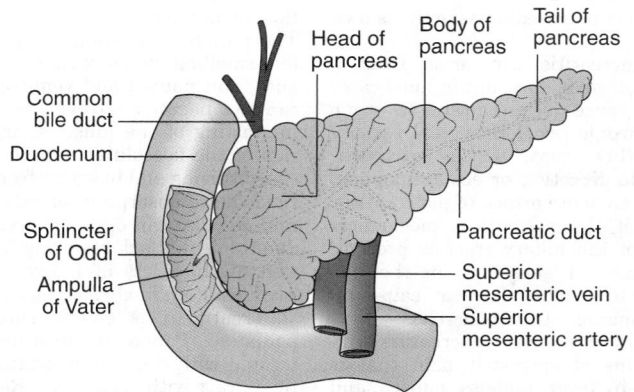

The anatomical relations of the pancreas. From Aspinal and Taylor-Robinson, 2001.

CHOLECYSTOKININ are more important than vagal stimulation. The entry of chyme into the small intestine causes the transformation of an inactive proenzyme, PROSECRETIN, into active secretin that is released from the mucosa of the upper portion of the duodenum. The composition of the partially digested food entering the duodenum influences the amount of each hormone that is released and, therefore, the characteristics of the pancreatic juice.

The endocrine functions of the pancreas are related to the islets of Langerhans located on the surface of the pancreas. These small islands contain three major types of cells: the *alpha, beta,* and *delta* cells. The alpha cells secrete the hormone GLUCAGON, which elevates blood sugar. The beta cells secrete INSULIN, which affects the metabolism of carbohydrates, proteins, and fats. The delta cells secrete SOMATOSTATIN, the functions of which are not fully understood, but it is known that it can inhibit the secretion of both glucagon and insulin and may act as a controller of metabolic processes. The somatostatin produced by the delta cells of the pancreas is the same as that produced by the hypothalamus as an inhibitor of the release of growth hormone from the pituitary gland.

Disorders of the Pancreas. Failure of the islets of Langerhans to produce sufficient amounts of insulin results in DIABETES MELLITUS. Disturbances in the exocrine functions of the pancreas produce serious digestive disorders. The pancreas can also be the seat of cancerous growth, and occasionally the pancreatic ducts are blocked by stones. Various factors, not yet fully understood, may result in acute PANCREATITIS, a condition

in which the fluids digest the tissue of the organ itself. CYSTIC FIBROSIS, a serious congenital disease, is characterized by a deficiency in the secretion of pancreatic juice, and an increase in its viscosity.

  annular p. a developmental anomaly in which the pancreas forms a ring entirely surrounding the duodenum.

  pancreat(o)- word element [Gr.], *pancreas.*

  pancreatalgia (pan″kre-ah-tal′jah) pain in the pancreas.

  pancreatectomy (pan″kre-ah-tek′to-me) excision of the pancreas.

  pancreatic (pan″kre-at′ik) pertaining to the pancreas.

  pancreatic(o)- word element [Gr.], *pancreatic duct.*

  pancreaticoduodenal (pan″kre-at″ĭ-ko-doo″o-de′nal) pertaining to the pancreas and duodenum.

  pancreaticoduodenostomy (pan″kre-at″ĭ-ko-doo″o-dĕ-nos′tah-me) anastomosis of the pancreatic duct to a different site on the duodenum.

  pancreaticoenterostomy (pan″kre-at″ĭ-ko-en″ter-os′tah-me) anastomosis of the pancreatic duct to the intestine.

  pancreaticogastrostomy (pan″kre-at″ĭ-ko-gas-tros′tah-me) anastomosis of the pancreatic duct to the stomach.

  pancreaticojejunostomy (pan″kre-at″ĭ-ko-jĕ-joo-nos′tah-me) anastomosis of the pancreatic duct to the jejunum.

  pancreatin (pan′kre-ah-tin) a substance from the pancreas of the hog or ox containing enzymes, principally AMYLASE, PROTEASE, and LIPASE; used as a digestive aid.

  pancreatitis (pan″kre-ah-ti′tis) inflammation of the PANCREAS, which is due to

P

autodigestion of pancreatic tissue by its own enzymes.

Acute pancreatitis can arise from a variety of etiologic factors, but in most cases the specific cause is unknown. In some instances chronic alcoholism or toxicity from some other agent, such as glucocorticoids, thiazide diuretics, or acetaminophen, can bring on an acute attack of pancreatitis. In about half the patients a mechanical obstruction of the biliary tract is present, usually because of gallstones in the bile ducts. Viral infections also can cause an acute inflammation of the pancreas.

The patient with acute pancreatitis typically complains of epigastric pain that is accompanied by fever, malaise, nausea, and vomiting. Very mild cases can be overlooked or misdiagnosed quite easily. There is no specific laboratory diagnostic test for acute pancreatitis.

Treatment is largely symptomatic and designed to provide rest for the organ. Oral intake may be restricted and intravenous fluids given to maintain an adequate blood volume. Analgesic administration and other noninvasive techniques are necessary for the management of pain, which can be quite severe in some patients. Surgical removal of gallstones often has an excellent prognosis in acute pancreatitis related to obstruction of the biliary system by the stones. Alcoholic pancreatitis responds relatively well to conservative treatment if the patient stops drinking; however, there is a tendency toward recurrent attacks. Surgical removal of the pancreas is a drastic measure usually reserved for the severe form of the disease with life-threatening complications.

Chronic pancreatitis is characterized by progressive loss of the exocrine functions of the pancreas, that is, the production of pancreatic enzymes essential for normal digestion. There is relative preservation of the organ's endocrine functions until late in the disease. The specific cause of chronic pancreatitis can rarely be identified, but most of the factors that produce the acute form of the disease can also cause the chronic form. Alcoholism is considered by many to be one of the primary causes now that prompt diagnosis and treatment of biliary obstruction have reduced the incidence of pancreatitis secondary to obstruction.

Chronic pancreatitis can lead to pancreatic insufficiency as a result of the replacement of acinar tissue with fibrous tissue. Because the acini secrete pancreatic enzymes necessary for the digestion of proteins, carbohydrates, and fats, dysfunction of acinar tissue results in malabsorption of nutrients from the small intestine. The patient may complain of bulky, fatty, foul-smelling stools, weight loss, fever, malaise, and nausea and vomiting. There also can be a negative nitrogen balance resulting in wasting of the muscles, and malabsorption of the fat-soluble vitamins resulting in easy bruising and bleeding from mild injury. Inadequate absorption of calcium and vitamin B_{12} also can occur. Glucose intolerance due to insulin lack resulting from degeneration of the islets of Langerhans is a late manifestation of chronic pancreatitis.

Treatment is chiefly substitutive and palliative. Pancreatic insufficiency can be treated with the administration of pancreatic extract with each meal. Relief of pain is not so easily accomplished and often necessitates the use of addictive narcotic analgesics such as codeine, morphine, and meperidine. Symptomatic relief can make the patient more comfortable and substitutive therapy can help maintain adequate nutrition and strengthen the patient's resources so that he can continue most everyday activities of living, but there is no cure for chronic pancreatitis and the long-term prognosis is not good.

Pancreatectomy and islet cell autotransplantation are being done experimentally as an alternative mode of therapy for patients who continue to have chronic pancreatitis. Oral replacement of digestive enzymes and management of diabetes mellitus are necessary after the pancreas is removed. Transplantation of pancreatic islet cells is an attempt to overcome the problem of insulin deficit and diabetes.

acute hemorrhagic p. a condition due to autolysis of pancreatic tissue caused by escape of enzymes into the substance, resulting in hemorrhage into the parenchyma and surrounding tissues.

chronic calcifying p. a form accompanying chronic hepatitis and precipitated by chronic alcohol abuse.

pancreatoduodenectomy (pan″kre-ah-to-doo″o-dĕ-nek′to-me) excision of the head of the pancreas along with the encircling loop of the duodenum.

pancreatogenous (pan″kre-ah-toj′ĕ-nus) arising in the pancreas.

pancreatogram (pan″kre-at′o-gram) the x-ray film produced by pancreatography.

pancreatography (pan″kre-ah-tog′rah-fe) radiography of the pancreas, performed during surgery by injecting contrast medium into the pancreatic duct.

endoscopic retrograde p. that in which the radiopaque medium is injected into the pancreatic duct at the ampulla of Vater via a cannula introduced through a fiberoptic endoscope; see also GALLBLADDER and endoscopic retrograde CHOLANGIOPAN-CREATOGRAPHY.

pancreatolithectomy (pan″kre-ah-to-lĭ-thek′to-me) excision of a calculus from the pancreas.

pancreatolithiasis (pan″kre-ah-to-lĭ-thi′ah-sis) the presence of calculi in the ductal system or parenchyma of the pancreas.

pancreatolithotomy (pan″kre-ah-to-lĭ-thot′ah-me) incision of the pancreas for the removal of calculi.

pancreatolysis (pan″kre-ah-tol′ĭ-sis) destruction of pancreatic tissue. adj., **pancreatolyt′ic.**

pancreatotomy (pan″kre-ah-tot′ah-me) incision of the pancreas.

pancreatotropic (pan″kre-ah-to-trop′ik) having a special affinity for the pancreas.

pancrelipase (pan″kre-li′pās) a preparation of hog pancreas containing enzymes, principally AMYLASE, PROTEASE, and LIPASE; used as a digestive aid in treatment of pancreatic insufficiency.

pancreolithotomy (pan″kre-o-lĭ-thot′ah-me) pancreatolithotomy.

pancreolysis (pan″kre-ol′ĭ-sis) pancreatolysis.

pancreozymin (pan′kre-o-zi″min) cholecystokinin.

pancuronium (pan″ku-ro′ne-um) a neuromuscular blocking AGENT used as an anesthesia adjunct in the form of the bromide salt.

pancystitis (pan″sis-ti′tis) cystitis involving the entire thickness of the wall of the urinary bladder, as occurs in interstitial cystitis.

pancytopenia (pan″si-to-pe′ne-ah) abnormal depression of all the cellular elements of the blood.

pandemic (pan-dem′ik) 1. a widespread epidemic of a disease. 2. widely epidemic.

panencephalitis (pan″en-sef″ah-li′tis) encephalitis, probably of viral origin, that produces intranuclear or intracytoplasmic inclusion bodies that result in parenchymatous lesions of both the gray and white matter of the brain.

panendoscope (pan-en′do-skōp) 1. an endoscope for wide-angle viewing. 2. a cystoscope that gives a wide-angle view of the bladder.

panesthesia (pan″es-the′zhah) the sum of the sensations experienced. adj., **panesthet′ic.**

panhypopituitarism (pan-hi″po-pĭ-too′ĭ-tar-izm″) generalized HYPOPITUITARISM due to absence of or damage to the pituitary gland; in its complete form it leads to

absence of gonadal function, loss of secondary sex CHARACTERS, and insufficiency of thyroid and adrenal function. When cachexia is a prominent feature, it is called SIMMONDS' DISEASE.

panhysterectomy (pan″his-ter-ek′to-me) total hysterectomy.

panhysterosalpingectomy (pan-his″ter-o-sal″pin-jek′to-me) excision of the uterus, cervix, and fallopian tubes.

panhysterosalpingo-oophorectomy (pan-his″ter-o-sal-ping″go-o″of-o-rek′to-me) excision of the uterus, cervix, fallopian tubes, and ovaries.

panic (pan′ik) acute, extreme anxiety with disorganization of personality and function; panic attacks are characteristic of panic disorder (see ANXIETY DISORDERS) and may also occur in other mental disorders.

p. disorder an ANXIETY DISORDER characterized by recurrent attacks of panic, episodes of intense apprehension, fear, or terror associated with somatic symptoms such as dyspnea, palpitations, dizziness, vertigo, faintness, or shakiness and with psychological symptoms such as feelings of unreality, fear of dying, going crazy, or losing control; there is usually chronic nervousness between attacks. It is almost always associated with AGORAPHOBIA and is officially classified as either *panic disorder with agoraphobia* or *panic disorder without agoraphobia.* This disorder does not include panic attacks that may occur in PHOBIAS when the patient is exposed to the phobic stimulus.

homosexual p. a severe episode of anxiety due to unconscious conflicts involving sexual identity; see also HOMOSEXUAL PANIC.

panimmunity (pan″ĭ-mu′nĭ-te) immunity to several bacterial and viral infections.

panmyeloid (pan-mi′ĕ-loid) pertaining to all elements of the bone marrow.

panmyelophthisis (pan-mi″ĕ-lof′thĭ-sis) APLASTIC ANEMIA.

panniculectomy (pah-nik″u-lek′to-me) surgical excision of the abdominal apron of superficial fat in the obese.

panniculitis (pah-nik″u-li′tis) inflammation of the subcutaneous fat, characterized by development of single or multiple cutaneous nodules. See also STEATITIS.

nodular nonsuppurative p., relapsing febrile nonsuppurative p. Weber-Christian disease.

panniculus (pah-nik′u-lus) [L.] a layer of membrane.

p. adipo′sus the subcutaneous fat; a layer of fat underlying the corium.

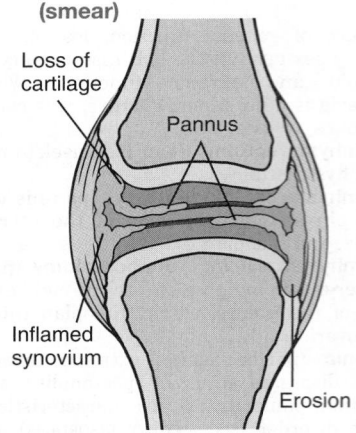

Loss of cartilage

Pannus

Inflamed synovium

Erosion

Schematic presentation of the pathologic changes in rheumatoid arthritis. The inflammation (synovitis) leads to pannus formation, obliteration of the articular space. From Damjanov, 2000.

p. carno′sus a muscular layer in the superficial fascia, well developed in certain animals; represented in humans mainly by the PLATYSMA.

pannus (pan′us) 1. superficial vascularization of the cornea with infiltration of granulation tissue. 2. an inflammatory exudate overlying synovial cells on the inside of a joint capsule, usually occurring in rheumatoid arthritis or related articular rheumatism. 3. panniculus adiposus.

panophthalmitis (pan″of-thal-mi′tis) inflammation of all the eye structures or tissues.

panosteitis (pan″os-te-i′tis) inflammation of every part of a bone.

panotitis (pan″o-ti′tis) inflammation of all the parts or structures of the ear.

panphobia (pan-fo′be-ah) fear of everything; a vague and persistent dread of some unknown evil.

pansinusitis (pan″si-nŭ-si′tis) inflammation involving all the paranasal sinuses.

pant(o)- word element [Gr.], *all; the whole.*

pantalgia (pan-tal′jah) pain over the whole body.

panthenol (pan′thĕ-nol) an alcohol oxidized in the body to pantothenic acid; administered as a source of this vitamin. The term is sometimes used specifically for the isomer called DEXPANTHENOL.

pantomography (pan″to-mog′rah-fe) a method of tomography for visualization of body curved surfaces at any depth. In dentistry, it may be used for radiography of the maxillary and mandibular dental arches

and their associated structures. Called also *panoramic radiography.*

pantoprazole (pan-to′prah-zōl) a gastric acid pump inhibitor with properties similar to those of omeprazole, administered orally and intravenously as the sodium salt in the treatment of erosive esophagitis associated with GASTROESOPHAGEAL REFLUX DISEASE and intravenously as the sodium salt in the treatment of hypersecretion associated with ZOLLINGER-ELLISON SYNDROME or other neoplastic condition.

pantothenate (pan-to′then-āt) any salt of pantothenic acid.

pantothenic acid (pan″to-then′ik) a vitamin of the B complex present in all living tissues, almost entirely in the form of a coenzyme A (CoA). (See also VITAMIN.) This coenzyme has many metabolic roles in the cell, and a lack of pantothenic acid can lead to depressed metabolism of both carbohydrates and fats. The daily requirement for this vitamin has not been established, and no definite deficiency syndrome has been recognized in humans, perhaps because of its wide occurrence in almost all foods. Intakes of 4 to 7 mg/day are safe and adequate for adults. Some symptoms attributed to deficiency of other B complex vitamins may be due to a lack of pantothenic acid.

pantotropic (pan″to-trop′ik) pantropic.

pantropic (pan-trop′ik) having affinity for tissues derived from all three of the germ layers (ectoderm, entoderm, and mesoderm); called also pantotropic.

panzootic (pan″zo-ot′ik) occurring among animals over a wide geographical area.

Pap test (smear) (pap) Papanicolaou test.

papain (pah-pa′in, pah-pi′in) a proteolytic enzyme from the latex of papaw, *Carica papaya,* the active ingredient of meat tenderizers. In medicine, it is used as a protein digestant and for enzymatic débridement and promotion of normal healing of surface lesions.

Papanicolaou test (smear) (pap″ah-nik″o-la′oo) a simple, painless test used most commonly to detect cancer of the uterus and cervix; it is based on the discovery by Dr. George N. Papanicolaou (1883–1962) that malignant uterine tumors slough off cancerous cells into surrounding vaginal fluid. Called also Pap test and Pap smear.

The Papanicolaou technique, an exfoliative cytological staining procedure, is used also in diagnosis of lung, stomach, and bladder cancers. It can be performed on any body excretion (urine, feces), secretion (sputum, prostatic fluid, vaginal fluid), or tissue scraping (as from the uterus, cervix,

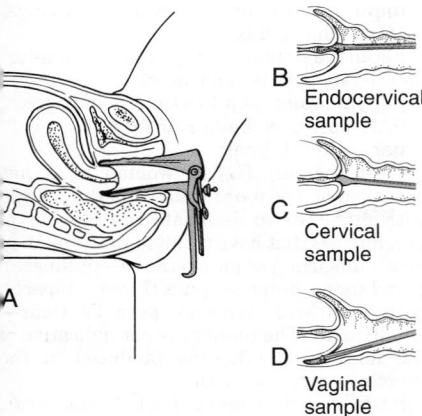

B Endocervical sample

C Cervical sample

D Vaginal sample

Pap smear. From Lammon et al., 1995.

r stomach). The sample is removed from he area being examined, placed on a glass slide, stained, and then studied under a microscope for evidence of abnormal or cancerous cells.

In five minutes the Pap test can reveal uterine or cervical cancer at a stage in which it produces no visible symptoms, has done no damage, and usually can be completely cured. It is recommended that all women over age 18, and younger women who have been sexually active, should have an annual Pap test and pelvic examination.

papaverine (pah-pav′er-in) an alkaloid obtained from OPIUM or prepared synthetically; the hydrochloride salt has been used as a smooth muscle RELAXANT and VASODILATOR to relieve arterial spasms causing cerebral, peripheral, or myocardial ischemia and is also injected into the penis in the diagnosis and treatment of erectile DYSFUNCTION.

papilla (pah-pil′ah) [L.] a small, nipple-shaped projection or elevation. adj., **pap′-llary.**

circumvallate p. 1. vallate papilla. 2. one of the papillae in the area next to a vallate papilla.

THE PAPANICOLAOU SMEAR	
Class I	Normal
Class II	Atypical
Class III	Suggestive for cancer
Class IV	Strongly suggestive for cancer
Class V	Conclusive for cancer

conical p. one of the sparsely scattered elevations on the tongue, often considered to be modified filiform papillae.

papillae of corium conical extensions of the fibers, capillary blood vessels, and sometimes nerves of the corium into corresponding spaces among downward- or inward-projecting rete ridges on the undersurface of the epidermis.

dental p., dentinal p. the small mass of condensed mesenchyme capped by each of the enamel organs.

duodenal p. either of the small elevations (major and minor) on the mucosa of the duodenum, the major at the entrance of the conjoined pancreatic and common bile ducts, the minor at the entrance of the accessory pancreatic duct.

filiform p. one of the threadlike elevations covering most of the tongue surface.

foliate p. one of the parallel mucosal folds on the tongue margin at the junction of its body and root.

fungiform p. one of the knoblike projections of the tongue scattered among the filiform papillae.

gingival p. the triangular pad of the gingiva filling the space between the proximal surfaces of two adjacent teeth.

hair p. the fibrovascular mesodermal papilla enclosed within the hair bulb.

incisive p. an elevation at the anterior end of the raphe of the palate.

lacrimal p. an elevation on the margin of either eyelid, near the medial angle of the eye.

lingual papillae elevations on the surface of the tongue, containing the taste buds; the conical, filiform, foliate, fungiform, and vallate papillae.

mammary p. nipple (def. 1).

optic p. optic disk.

palatine p. incisive papilla.

p. pi′li hair papilla.

renal p. the blunted apex of a renal PYRAMID.

tactile p. tactile CORPUSCLE.

urethral p. a slight elevation in the vestibule of the vagina at the external orifice of the urethra.

vallate p. one of the 8 to 12 large papillae arranged in a V near the base of the tongue.

p. of Vater, Vater's p. major duodenal papilla.

papillectomy (pap″ĭ-lek′to-me) excision of a papilla.

papilledema (pap″il-ĕ-de′mah) edema and hyperemia of the optic disk, usually associated with increased intracranial pressure; called also choked disk.

P

papillitis (pap″ĭ-li′tis) inflammation of a papilla, especially of the optic disk.

papilloadenocystoma (pap″ĭ-lo-ad″ĕ-no-sis-to′mah) papillary cystadenoma.

papillocarcinoma (pap″ĭ-lo-kahr″sĭ-no′-mah) papillary carcinoma.

papilloma (pap″ĭ-lo′mah) a benign tumor derived from epithelium. Papillomas may arise from skin, mucous membranes, or glandular ducts. adj., **papillo′matous.**

papillomatosis (pap″ĭ-lo″mah-to′sis) development of multiple papillomas.

papillomavirus (pap″ĭ-lo′mah-vi″rus) any member of a genus of viruses that cause PAPILLOMAS in humans and various other animals.

   human p. any of numerous species that cause warts, particularly plantar and venereal WARTS, on the skin and mucous membranes in humans, transmitted by either direct or indirect contact. They have also been associated with cervical cancer.

papilloretinitis (pap″ĭ-lo-ret″ĭ-ni′tis) inflammation of the optic nerve and disk.

papillotomy (pap″ĭ-lot′ah-me) incision of a papilla, as of a duodenal papilla.

papovavirus (pah-po′vah-vi″rus) any member of a group of small ether-resistant DNA viruses; this term is no longer used in official viral nomenclature. The species that infect humans are all PAPILLOMAVIRUSES.

Papovaviridae (pah-po′vah-vir″ĭ-de) the PAPOVAVIRUSES, a family of DNA viruses having a VIRION 40 to 55 nm in diameter with 72 CAPSOMERS in skew arrangement. Replication and assembly occur in the nucleus; virions are released by cell destruction. Host range is generally narrow; transmission is by contact or by airborne particles, and many species are ONCOGENIC. There are two genera, *Papovavirus* and *Polyomavirus.*

papulation (pap″u-la′shun) the formation of papules.

papule (pap′ūl) a small circumscribed, superficial, solid elevation of the skin with a diameter less than 1 cm (0.5 cm according to some authorities). (See plate in Dermatology Atlas.) See also PLAQUE.

   piezogenic p's transitory, noninflammatory, soft, sometimes painful, large papules appearing above the heel on the side of one or both feet, elicited by weight bearing associated with prolonged standing or running. They disappear when the pressure is removed.

papulopustular (pap″u-lo-pus′tu-lar) marked by papules and pustules.

papulosis (pap″u-lo′sis) the presence of multiple papules.

papulosquamous (pap″u-lo-skwa′mus) both papular and scaly.

papulovesicular (pap″u-lo-vĕ-sik′u-lar) marked by papules and vesicles.

papyraceous (pap″ĭ-ra′shus) like paper.

PAR post-anesthesia recovery.

par (pahr) [L.] pair.

para (par′ah) [L.] a woman who has produced one or more viable offspring. Used with numerals to designate the number of pregnancies that have resulted in the birth of viable offspring, as para 0 (none—nullipara), para I (one—unipara), para II (two—bipara), para III (three—tripara), para IV (four—quadripara). The number is not indicative of the number of offspring produced in the event of a multiple birth.

para-¹ word element [Gr.], *beside, near; resembling; accessory to; beyond; apart from; abnormal.*

para-² symbol *p-*. In organic chemistry, indicating a substituted benzene ring whose substituents are on opposite carbon atoms in the ring.

para-aminobenzoic acid (par″ah-ah-me″no-ben-zo′ik) *p*-aminobenzoic acid.

para-aminohippuric acid (par″ah-ah-me″-no-hĭ-pūr′ik) *p*-aminohippuric acid.

para-aminosalicylic acid (par″ah-ah-me″no-sal″ĭ-sil′ik) *p*-aminosalicylic acid.

para-anesthesia (par″ah-an″es-the′zhah) anesthesia of the lower part of the body.

para-aortic bodies (par″ah-a-or′tik) small masses of chromaffin CELLS near the sympathetic ganglia along the abdominal aorta that secrete norepinephrine. They reach their maximum size during fetal life and then degenerate during childhood as the adrenal medulla matures. Tumors of these structures produce symptoms similar to those of PHEOCHROMOCYTOMA. Called also organs of Zuckerkandl.

parabiosis (par″ah-bi-o′sis) 1. the union of two individuals, as conjoined twins, or of experimental animals by surgical operation. 2. temporary suppression of conductivity and excitability. adj., **parabiot′ic.**

parabulia (par″ah-bu′le-ah) perversion of the will, as when an individual intends to perform a particular action but halts and substitutes either an opposite action or an unrelated alternative. It is often seen in schizophrenics.

paracasein (par″ah-ka′se-in) the chemical product of the action of rennin on casein.

paracenesthesia (par″ah-sen″es-the′-zhah) any disturbance of the general sense of well-being.

paracentesis (par″ah-sen-te′sis) surgical PUNCTURE of a cavity for the aspiration of fluid. adj., **paracentet′ic.**

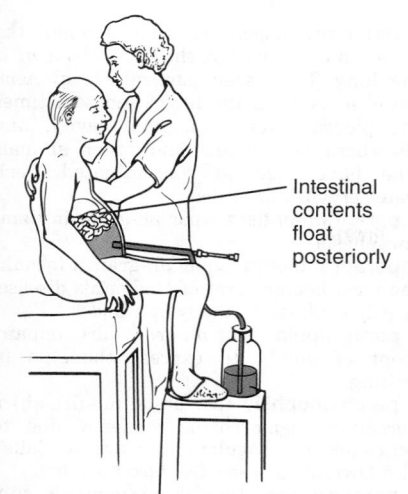

Intestinal
contents
float
posteriorly

Client position for paracentesis. From Lammon et al., 1995.

abdominal p. insertion of a TROCAR through a small incision and into the peritoneal CAVITY to remove ascitic fluids or inject a therapeutic agent. This is most often done to remove excess fluid in a patient with CIRRHOSIS of the liver. Called also abdominocentesis and peritoneocentesis.

Before the procedure the patient is instructed to empty the bladder to reduce the danger of accidental puncture of the bladder. The skin below the umbilicus and overlying the rectus muscle is cleansed with an antiseptic. A local anesthetic is used to anesthetize the skin and underlying tissues at the site of insertion of the trocar. During the procedure the patient may be placed in a sitting position with the feet resting on a foot stool or on the floor. The back and arms should be well supported. The container for collecting the drainage is placed at the patient's feet. As the fluid is being withdrawn the patient is observed for symptoms of fainting or shock.

The amount and character of the fluid obtained are recorded and a specimen is saved if the physician requests laboratory examination of the fluid. After the trocar is removed a sterile dressing is applied to the site. A more permanent procedure for relief of accumulations of excess fluid in the peritoneal cavity is insertion of a peritoneovenous SHUNT.

thoracic p. thoracentesis.

paracephalus (par″ah-sef′ah-lus) a malformed fetus with a rudimentary head and imperfect sense organs.

parachlorophenol (par″ah-klo″ro-fe′nol) a local antiinfective agent used in dentistry.

paracholera (par″ah-kol′er-ah) a disease resembling Asiatic cholera but not caused by *Vibrio cholerae.*

parachordal (par″ah-kor′dal) beside the notochord.

parachromatopsia (par″ah-kro″mah-top′-se-ah) dichromatic VISION.

paraclinical (par″ah-klin′ĭ-kal) pertaining to abnormalities (e.g., morphological or biochemical) underlying clinical manifestations (e.g., chest pain or fever).

Paracoccidioides (par″ah-kok-sid″e-oi′-dēz) a genus of imperfect fungi that proliferate by multiple budding yeast cells in the tissues. *P. brasilien′sis* causes PARACOCCIDIOIDOMYCOSIS.

P. brasilien′sis the etiologic agent of PARACOCCIDIOIDOMYCOSIS. Called also *Blastomyces brasiliensis.*

paracoccidioidomycosis (par″ah-kok-sid″e-oi″do-mi-ko′sis) an often fatal, chronic granulomatous disease caused by *Paracoccidioides brasiliensis;* it is endemic in Brazil and also occurs elsewhere in South and Central America and in arid regions of the southwestern United States. Infection primarily involves the lungs, but spreads to the skin, mucous membranes, lymph nodes, and internal organs. Amphotericin B is the specific drug used for treatment. Called also South American blastomycosis.

paracolitis (par″ah-ko-li′tis) inflammation of the outer coat of the colon.

paracrine (par′ah-krin) denoting a type of hormone function in which hormone synthesized in and released from endocrine cells binds to its receptor in nearby cells and affects their function.

paracusia 1. any deficiency in the sense of hearing; see also DEAFNESS. Called also paracusis. 2. auditory hallucination.

paracusis (par″ah-ku′sis) paracusia.

paracystic (par″ah-sis′tik) situated near the bladder.

paracystitis (par″ah-sis-ti′tis) inflammation of tissues around the bladder.

paradental (par″ah-den′tal) 1. having some association with dentistry. 2. periodontal.

paradidymis (par″ah-did′ĭ-mis) a small, vestigial structure found occasionally in the adult in the anterior part of the spermatic cord.

paradigm (par′ah-dīm) a shared understanding among scientists or scholars working in a discipline regarding the important problems, structures, values, and assumptions determining that discipline.

paradipsia (par″ah-dip′se-ah) an abnormally increased appetite for fluids, which are ingested without relation to bodily need.

paradoxical respiration (par″ah-dok′sĭ-kal) breathing in which all or part of the chest wall moves in during inhalation and out during exhalation; there is also dyssynchrony between rib cage and abdomen, causing a "seesaw" type motion. The condition seriously inhibits the movement of gases during respiration and can produce severe and even fatal cardiovascular disturbances and respiratory insufficiency if not quickly relieved by emergency treatment. It usually results from traumatic injury to the thorax (FLAIL CHEST), in which several ribs are fractured in two or more places and are no longer attached by bony cartilage to the rest of the rib cage. It can also be seen following surgical removal of several ribs, in paralysis of the diaphragm, and secondary to respiratory muscle fatigue in patients with acute ventilatory failure.

paraffin (par′ah-fin) 1. a purified mixture of solid hydrocarbons from petroleum, used for embedding histological specimens and as a stiffening agent in pharmaceutical preparations. 2. alkane.

  liquid p. see MINERAL OIL.

paraffinoma (par″ah-fĭ-no′mah) a chronic granuloma produced by prolonged exposure to paraffin.

Paraflex (par′ah-fleks) trademark for preparations containing CHLORZOXAZONE, a skeletal muscle RELAXANT.

Parafon (par′ah-fon) trademark for preparations containing CHLORZOXAZONE, a skeletal muscle RELAXANT.

paragammacism (par″ah-gam′ah-sizm) faulty enunciation of *g, k,* and *ch* sounds.

paraganglioma (par″ah-gang″gle-o′mah) a tumor of the tissue composing the paraganglia.

paraganglion (par″ah-gang′gle-on), pl. *paragan′glia* a collection of chromaffin cells, derived from neural ectoderm, occurring outside of the adrenal medulla, most commonly near the sympathetic ganglia and in relation to the aorta and its branches. Most, if not all, of the paraganglia secrete EPINEPHRINE or NOREPINEPHRINE.

parageusia (par″ah-goo′zhah) perversion of the sense of taste. adj., **parageu′sic.**

paragonimiasis (par″ah-gon″ĭ-mi′ah-sis) infection with flukes of the genus *Paragonimus.*

Paragonimus (par″ah-gon′ĭ-mus) a genus of trematode parasites, having two invertebrate hosts, the first a snail, the second a crab or crayfish. *P. westerma′ni* is the lung fluke, seen particularly in Asia, found in cysts in the lungs and sometimes the pleura, liver, abdominal cavity, and elsewhere in humans and other animals who have ingested contaminated fresh water crayfish or crabs.

paragrammatism (par″ah-gram′ah-tizm) paraphasia.

paragranuloma (par″ah-gran″u-lo′mah) the most benign form of Hodgkin's disease, largely confined to the lymph nodes.

paragraphia (par″ah-graf′e-ah) impairment of ability to express thoughts in writing.

parahemophilia (par″ah-he″mo-fil′e-ah) a hereditary hemorrhagic tendency due to deficiency of coagulation factor V. Called also Owren's disease. See also CLOTTING.

parahormone (par″ah-hōr′mon) a substance, not a true hormone, that has a hormone-like action in controlling the functioning of some distant organ.

parainfectious (par″ah-in-fek′shus) pertaining to manifestations of infectious disease that are caused by the IMMUNE RESPONSE to the infectious agent.

parainfluenza virus (par″ah-in″floo-en′zah) one of a group of viruses isolated from patients with upper respiratory tract disease of varying severity.

parakeratosis (par″ah-ker″ah-to′sis) persistence of the nuclei of keratinocytes as they rise into the horny layer of the skin; it occurs normally in the epithelium of the true mucous membrane of the mouth and vagina.

parakinesia (par″ah-kĭ-ne′zhah) perversion of motor powers; in ophthalmology, irregular action of an individual ocular muscle.

paralalia (par″ah-la′le-ah) a disorder of speech, especially the production of a vocal sound different from the one desired, or the substitution in speech of one letter for another.

paralambdacism (par″ah-lam′dah-sizm) faulty enunciation of the *l* sound.

paraldehyde (pah-ral′dĕ-hīd) a SEDATIVE and HYPNOTIC; because of its low therapeutic index and certain unpleasant side effects, its use has declined in recent years.

paralexia (par″ah-lek′se-ah) dyslexia.

paralgesia (par″al-je′zhah) an abnormal and painful sensation.

parallagma (par″ah-lag′mah) displacement of a bone or of the fragments of broken bone.

parallax (par′ah-laks) an apparent displacement of an object due to change in the observer's position.

parallergy (par-al'er-je) a condition in which an allergic state, produced by specific sensitization, predisposes the body to react to other allergens with clinical manifestations that differ from the original reaction. adj., **paraller'gic.**

paralogia (par"ah-lo'jah) disturbance of the reasoning faculty, marked by illogical or delusional speech.

paralysis (pah-ral'ĭ-sis), pl. *paral'yses.* Loss or impairment of motor function in a part due to a lesion of the neural or muscular mechanism; also, by analogy, impairment of sensory function (sensory paralysis). Paralysis is a symptom of a wide variety of physical and emotional disorders rather than a disease in itself. Called also palsy.

Types of Paralysis. Paralysis results from damage to parts of the nervous system. The kind of paralysis resulting, and the degree, depend on whether the damage is to the central nervous system or the peripheral nervous system.

If the central nervous system is damaged, paralysis frequently affects the movement of a limb as a whole, not the individual muscles. The more common forms of central paralysis are HEMIPLEGIA (in which one entire side of the body is affected, including the face, arm, and leg) and PARAPLEGIA (in which both legs and sometimes the trunk are affected). In *central paralysis* the tone of the muscles is increased, causing SPASTICITY.

If the peripheral nervous system is damaged, individual muscles or groups of muscles in a particular part of the body, rather than a whole limb, are more likely to be affected. The muscles are flaccid, and there is often impairment of sensation.

Causes of Central Paralysis. STROKE SYNDROME is one of the most common causes of central paralysis. Although there is usually some permanent disability, much can be done to rehabilitate the patient. Paralysis produced by damage to the spinal cord can be the result of direct injuries, tumors, and infectious diseases. Paralysis in children may be a result of failure of the brain to develop properly in intrauterine life or of injuries to the brain, as in the case of CEREBRAL PALSY. Congenital SYPHILIS may also leave a child partially paralyzed. Paralysis resulting from HYSTERIA has no organic basis and is a result of emotional disturbance or mental illness.

Causes of Peripheral Paralysis. Until the recent development of immunizing vaccines, the most frequent cause of peripheral paralysis in children was POLIOMYELITIS. NEURITIS, inflammation of a nerve, can also produce paralysis. Causes can be physical, as with cold or injury; chemical, as in lead

poisoning; or disease states, such as diabetes mellitus or infection. Paralysis caused by neuritis frequently disappears when the disorder causing it is corrected.

p. of accommodation paralysis of the ciliary muscles of the eye so as to prevent accommodation.

p. a'gitans Parkinson's disease.

ascending p. spinal paralysis that progresses upward.

birth p. that due to injury received at birth.

brachial p. paralysis of an upper limb from damage to the BRACHIAL PLEXUS.

bulbar p. that due to changes in motor centers of the medulla oblongata; the chronic form is marked by progressive paralysis and atrophy of the lips, tongue, pharynx, and larynx, and is due to degeneration of the nerve nuclei of the floor of the fourth ventricle.

central p. any paralysis due to a lesion of the brain or spinal cord.

cerebral p. paralysis caused by an intracranial lesion; see also CEREBRAL PALSY.

compression p. that caused by pressure on a nerve.

conjugate p. loss of ability to perform some parallel ocular movements.

crossed p. paralysis affecting one side of the face and the other side of the body.

crutch p. brachial paralysis caused by pressure from a crutch.

decubitus p. paralysis due to pressure on a nerve from lying for a long time in one position.

divers' p. decompression sickness.

Duchenne's p. 1. Erb-Duchenne paralysis. 2. progressive bulbar paralysis.

Erb-Duchenne p. paralysis of the upper roots of the BRACHIAL PLEXUS due to destruction of the fifth and sixth cervical roots, without involvement of the small muscles of the hand. Called also Erb's palsy.

facial p. weakening or paralysis of the facial nerve, as in BELL'S PALSY.

familial periodic p. a hereditary disease with recurring attacks of rapidly progressive flaccid paralysis, associated with a fall in (hypokalemic type), a rise in (hyperkalemic type), or normal (normokalemic type) serum potassium levels; all three types are inherited as autosomal dominant traits.

flaccid p. paralysis with loss of muscle tone of the paralyzed part and absence of tendon REFLEXES.

immunologic p. former name for immunologic TOLERANCE.

infantile p. the major form of POLIOMYELITIS.

infantile cerebral ataxic p. a congenital condition due to defective development of the frontal regions of the brain, affecting all extremities.

ischemic p. local paralysis due to stoppage of circulation.

Klumpke's p., Klumpke-Dejerine p. atrophic paralysis of the lower arm and hand, due to lesion of the eighth cervical and first dorsal thoracic nerves.

Landry's p. Guillain-Barré syndrome.

lead p. severe peripheral NEURITIS with WRISTDROP, due to LEAD POISONING.

mixed p. combined motor and sensory paralysis.

motor p. paralysis of the voluntary muscles.

musculospiral p. Saturday night paralysis.

obstetric p. birth paralysis.

periodic p. 1. any of various diseases characterized by episodic flaccid paralysis or muscular weakness. 2. familial periodic paralysis.

progressive bulbar p. the chronic form of bulbar paralysis; called also Duchenne's disease or paralysis.

pseudobulbar muscular p. pseudohypertrophic muscular dystrophy.

pseudohypertrophic muscular p. pseudohypertrophic muscular dystrophy.

radial p. Saturday night paralysis.

Saturday night p. paralysis of the extensor muscles of the wrist and fingers, so called because of its frequent occurrence in alcoholics. It is most often due to prolonged compression of the radial (musculospiral) nerve, and, depending upon the site of nerve injury, is sometimes accompanied by weakness and extension of the elbow. Called also musculospiral or radial paralysis.

sensory p. loss of sensation resulting from a morbid process.

sleep p. paralysis occurring at awakening or sleep onset; it represents extension of the atonia of REM SLEEP into the waking state and is often seen in those suffering from NARCOLEPSY or sleep APNEA. Called also waking paralysis.

spastic p. paralysis with rigidity of the muscles and heightened deep muscle reflexes and tendon REFLEXES.

spastic spinal p. lateral sclerosis.

tick p. progressive ascending flaccid motor paralysis following the bite of certain ticks, usually *Dermacentor andersoni;* first seen in children and domestic animals in the northern Pacific region of North America, and now seen in other parts of the world.

Volkmann's p. ischemic paralysis.

waking p. sleep paralysis.

paralytic (par″ah-lit′ik) 1. pertaining to paralysis. 2. a person affected with paralysis.

paralyzant (par′ah-līz″ant) causing paralysis. 1. a drug that causes paralysis.

paramagnetic (par″ah-mag-net′ik) being attracted by a magnet and assuming a position parallel to that of a magnetic force, but not becoming permanently magnetized.

paramastigote (par′ah-mas′tĭ-gōt) having an accessory flagellum by the side of a larger one.

paramastitis (par″ah-mas-ti′tis) inflammation of tissues around the mammary gland.

parameatal (par″ah-me-a′tal) situated near or around a meatus.

Paramecium (par″ah-me′she-um) a genus of ciliate protozoa.

paramecium (par″ah-me′she-um) any organism of the genus *Paramecium.*

paramedic (par″ah-med′ik) a person trained to manage the emergency CARE of sick or injured persons during transport to a hospital, including administration of injections and intravenous fluids, reading of electrocardiograms, and performance of DEFIBRILLATION and other advanced life-support measures if ordered by a physician. See also EMERGENCY MEDICAL TECHNICIAN.

paramedical (par″ah-med′ĭ-kal) connected with the science or practice of medicine; adjunctive to the practice of medicine in maintenance or restoration of health and normal functioning. See ALLIED HEALTH.

parameter (pah-ram′ĕ-ter) 1. in a mathematical expression, a constant that distinguishes specific cases, having a definite fixed value in one case but different values in other cases. 2. in statistics, a value that specifies one of the members of a family of probability DISTRIBUTIONS, such as the MEAN or the standard DEVIATION. 3. a variable whose measure is indicative of a quantity or function that cannot itself be directly determined precisely.

paramethasone (par″ah-meth′ah-sōn) a glucocorticoid used as the 21-acetate ester for its ANTIINFLAMMATORY effects.

parametrial (par″ah-me′tre-al) 1. parametric. 2. pertaining to the parametrium.

parametric[1] (par″ah-met′rik) situated near the uterus; parametrial.

parametric[2] (par″ah-met′rik) pertaining to or defined in terms of a parameter.

parametritis (par″ah-mĕ-tri′tis) inflammation of the parametrium.

parametrium (par″ah-me′tre-um) the extension of the subserous coat of the supracervical portion of the uterus laterally between the layers of the broad ligament.

paramnesia (par″am-ne′zhah) a disturbance of memory in which reality and fantasy are confused.

paramyloidosis (par-am″ĭ-loi-do′sis) accumulation of an atypical form of amyloid in tissues.

paramyoclonus (par″ah-mi-ok′lŏ-nus) a condition characterized by myoclonic contractions of various muscles.

p. mul′tiplex a condition characterized by sudden shocklike contractions.

paramyotonia (par″ah-mi″o-to′ne-ah) a disease marked by tonic spasms due to disorder of muscular tonicity, especially a hereditary and congenital affectation.

p. conge′nita a condition similar to MYOTONIA CONGENITA, except that the precipitating factor is exposure to cold, the myotonia is aggravated by activity, and only the proximal muscles of the limbs, eyelids, and tongue are affected.

paramyxovirus (par″ah-mik′so-vi″rus) any of a family of viruses, including those that cause MUMPS, MEASLES, and NEWCASTLE DISEASE, and the parainfluenza VIRUSES.

paraneoplastic syndrome (par″ah-ne″o-plas′tik) a collective term for disorders arising from metabolic effects of cancer on tissues remote from the tumor; such disorders may, for example, appear as primary endocrine, hematologic, or neuromuscular disorders.

paranephric (par″ah-nef′rik) near the kidney.

paranephritis (par″ah-ně-fri′tis) 1. inflammation of the adrenal gland. 2. inflammation of the connective tissue around the kidney.

paranesthesia (par″an-es-the′zhah) paraanesthesia.

paraneural (par″ah-noo′ral) alongside a nerve.

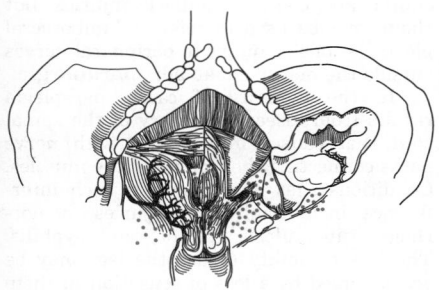

Parametritis. Infection spreads via lymphatics through uterine wall to connective tissue of broad ligament or entire pelvis. From Gorrie et al., 1994.

paranoia (par″ah-noi′ah) 1. in current usage, a descriptive term limited to the characterization of behavior that is marked by well-systematized delusions of persecution, delusions of grandeur, or a combination of the two. adj., **paranoi′ac** or **par′anoid.** There are several disorders in which paranoia may occur; see DELUSIONAL DISORDER, SHARED PSYCHOTIC DISORDER, PARANOID PERSONALITY DISORDER, and SCHIZOPHRENIA (paranoid type). 2. former name for what is now called DELUSIONAL DISORDER.

paranoid (par′ah-noid) resembling paranoia. 1. a person suffering from PARANOIA; called also paranoiac.

p. disorder older term for DELUSIONAL DISORDER.

p. personality disorder a PERSONALITY DISORDER in which the patient views other people as hostile, devious, and untrustworthy and reacts in a combative manner to disappointments or to events that he or she considers rebuffs or humiliations. Notable are a questioning of the loyalty of friends, the bearing of grudges, a tendency to read threatening meanings into benign remarks, and unfounded suspicions about the fidelity of a partner. Unlike DELUSIONAL DISORDERS or paranoid SCHIZOPHRENIA, in which delusional or hallucinatory persecution occurs, it is not characterized by psychosis.

paranomia (par″ah-no′me-ah) amnestic aphasia.

paranucleus (par″ah-noo′kle-us) a body sometimes seen in cell protoplasm near the nucleus. adj., **paranu′clear.**

paraparesis (par″ah-pah-re′sis) a partial paralysis of the lower extremities.

parapertussis (par″ah-per-tus′is) an acute respiratory disease clinically indistinguishable from mild or moderate pertussis, caused by *Bordetella parapertussis.*

parapharyngeal (par″ah-fah-rin′je-al) situated beside the pharynx.

paraphasia (par″ah-fa′zhah) partial APHASIA in which the patient uses wrong words, or uses words in wrong and senseless combinations. Called also paragrammatism, paraphemia, and paraphrasia.

paraphemia (par″ah-fe′me-ah) paraphasia.

paraphia (pah-ra′fe-ah) perversion of the sense of touch; called also parapsis.

paraphilia (par″ah-fil′e-ah) a SEXUAL DISORDER characterized by recurrent intense sexual urges, sexually arousing fantasies, or behavior involving use of a nonhuman object, the suffering or humiliation of oneself or one's partner, or children or

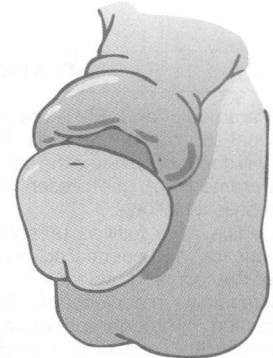

Paraphimosis. From Copstead and Banasik, 2000.

other nonconsenting partners. Paraphilias include TRANSVESTIC FETISHISM, other types of FETISHISM, FROTTEURISM, PEDOPHILIA, EXHIBITIONISM, VOYEURISM, sexual MASOCHISM, and sexual SADISM.

paraphimosis (par″ah-fi-mo′sis) retraction of a phimotic foreskin, causing swelling of the glans.

paraphrasia (par″ah-fra′zhah) paraphasia.

paraplasm (par′ah-plazm) any abnormal growth.

paraplastic (par″ah-plas′tik) exhibiting an abnormal formative power; of the nature of a PARAPLASM.

Paraplatin (par″ah-pla′tin) trademark for a preparation of CARBOPLATIN, an antineoplastic AGENT.

paraplectic (par″ah-plek′tik) paraplegic.

paraplegia (par″ah-ple′jah) impairment or loss of motor or sensory function in areas of the body served by the thoracic, lumbar, or sacral neurological segments owing to damage of neural elements in those parts of the spinal column. It spares the upper limbs but, depending on the level, may involve the trunk, pelvic organs, or lower limbs. This term is correctly used for describing cauda equina and conus medullaris injuries, but should not be used to refer to lumbosacral plexus lesions or injury to peripheral nerves outside the neural canal. adj., **paraple′gic.**

In the majority of cases, paraplegia results from disease or injury of the spinal cord that causes interference with nerve paths connecting the brain and the muscles. Conditions that may result in such interference include physical injuries, hemorrhage, tuberculosis, tumor, and syphilis. The loss of ability to use the legs may be accompanied by a loss of sensation in them and, in some cases, by loss of control over the bowel and bladder. Fortunately, much has been learned about the techniques of restoring paraplegics to normal activity, and today many are able to resume useful and productive lives.

Patient Care. Because rehabilitation is the ultimate goal for a paraplegic patient, the patient care during the early stages of the disorder must be particularly concerned with preventing complications that may stand in the way of successful rehabilitation. These complications include pressure ulcers, respiratory disorders, orthopedic deformities, urinary tract infections or calculi, and gastrointestinal disorders. The psychological and emotional aspects of paraplegia also must be considered. Many times the paraplegic patient is suddenly thrust into the role of dependence because of accidental injury to the spinal cord. This means that a tremendous adjustment to the condition must be made in a short time. Mental attitude and emotional response to paralysis will greatly affect the success of attempts at rehabilitation.

During the early stages of their illness patients may not be able to assist in their daily personal care, but as their condition improves and they are able to have more physical activity, they are encouraged to do as much as possible for themselves. As they learn to become less dependent on others, their attitude toward the future will improve. If it is anticipated that the patient will be confined to a wheelchair or will use crutches, transfer techniques for moving from bed to chair and from chair to other surfaces are taught. Wheelchairs and crutches are prescribed according to the individual patient's body build and weight, and the purpose for which they are to be used. The patient is instructed in correct CRUTCH walking if crutches are to be used; if using a wheelchair, the patient is taught how to operate the chair to receive maximum benefit from it. Mastering these techniques can enhance mobility, increase independence, and give a degree of confidence that can greatly improve one's outlook.

Care of the Skin. The type of bed used and the positioning of the patient with paraplegia will depend on the cause and extent of the paralysis and the preference of the health care provider. Patients with spinal cord injuries may be placed in traction or the spinal cord may be hyperextended by placing the patient's head at the foot of the bed and adjusting the bed. In some cases the health care provider may request a special orthopedic frame or specialized bed. These devices facilitate daily care but the patient still must be turned frequently (as allowed by the physician) and receive special skin care to avoid the development of pressure ulcers. Since these patients have no feeling below the point of damage to the spinal cord, they will not be aware of discomfort or other signs of pressure.

Respiratory Disorders. Hypostatic pneumonia and other respiratory problems are guarded against by deep breathing exercises. The patient should be protected from respiratory infections, such as the COMMON COLD, which can have serious complications in a paraplegic who is confined to bed.

Orthopedic Deformities. Until the patient is allowed out of bed and can engage in some form of physical activity, range of motion EXERCISES for all joints should be performed frequently. Proper positioning of the feet and legs will help prevent contractures, footdrop, and ankylosis. A program of therapeutic EXERCISE, including passive and active exercises, is initiated to maintain any remaining muscle function and to restore as much muscle activity in the affected parts as possible. If the patient is to use crutches or wheelchair he must strengthen his arm and shoulder muscles in preparation for transfer techniques. HYDROTHERAPY and DIATHERMY may be used to promote relaxation of muscle spasms and tension and to facilitate implementation of the exercise program.

Urinary Problems. URINARY TRACT INFECTIONS and the formation of CALCULI, particularly in the bladder, present real problems for the patient with paralysis. If there is no control over urination, an indwelling CATHETER may be the technique of choice for keeping the patient dry, but it also predisposes to infection. A thorough assessment of the patient's status and potential for achieving bladder control should be made before a final choice is made.

Ideally, the patient learns to achieve bladder control through an intensive bladder TRAINING program designed to fit individual needs. Whether this can be accomplished depends on the extent of nerve damage and the degree of success in avoiding such complications as infection and calculi. The achievement of bladder control is more difficult than bowel control. Patients with neurogenic BLADDER are unaware of the need to urinate and therefore require training to initiate urination. In some patients the bladder empties by reflex, and training involves techniques to make reflex emptying more effective. Intermittent catheterization may also be used. If the lesion causing paralysis is at the second, third, or fourth sacral segment, the bladder is flaccid and training must be aimed at avoiding overdistention and dribbling. Some may never be able to achieve bladder control to any appreciable degree, requiring the use of catheters, penile clamps, or other collecting devices. URETEROSTOMY or URETEROILEOSTOMY may be required in some cases.

The formation of bladder stones results from incomplete emptying of the bladder, with pooling of urine and inadequate elimination of wastes. To minimize the formation of stones it is recommended that the patient receive between 2500 and 3000 ml of fluid every 24 hours. Medications are often needed to change the urinary pH. The high calcium content of milk also may foster stone formation, and carbonated drinks irritate the bladder. A wide variety of liquids can be most effective in avoiding the formation of stones.

Gastrointestinal Complications. A flaccid bowel produces abdominal distention and predisposes the patient to fecal impaction. The patient may have fecal INCONTINENCE as well as frequent accumulations of flatus and fecal material in the lower intestine. Rehabilitation of the patient then requires working out some method of bowel control so that regularity of defecation can be accomplished.

As in bladder training, the program for BOWEL TRAINING is designed according to the individual needs of the patient and ability to work with those who are developing the program. It is essential that an assessment be made of the patient's status in regard to nerve damage and potential for rehabilitation. In addition, it is important to know about the patient's previous bowel habits in regard to frequency and time of day for a movement.

The training program also should include attention to fluid and food intake. The patient learns to avoid foods that produce diarrhea and flatus, and to rely upon a daily intake of fluids sufficient to insure soft, formed stools. Adequate physical exercise also is helpful in establishing regularity of defecation. Rectal suppositories and digital stimulation at regular intervals may be necessary to stimulate evacuation at a time convenient for the patient.

paraplegiform (par″ah-ple′jĭ-form) resembling paraplegia.

parapoplexy (par-ap′o-plek″se) a condition resembling apoplexy.

parapraxia (par″ah-prak′se-ah) parapraxis.

parapraxis (par″ah-prak′sis), pl. *paraprax′es.* a lapse of memory or mental error, such as a slip of the tongue or misplacement of an object, which, in psychoanalytic theory, is due to unconscious associations and motives; commonly called a "freudian slip."

paraprofessional (par″ah-pro-fesh′un-al) 1. a person specially trained in a particular field or occupation to assist a professional such as a physician. 2. pertaining to such a person or occupation.

paraprotein (par″ah-pro′tēn) a normal or abnormal plasma protein appearing in large quantities as a result of some pathologic condition, now replaced in most contexts by the term M COMPONENT.

paraproteinemia (par″ah-pro″te-ne′me-ah) a plasma cell DYSCRASIA.

parapsis (par-ap′sis) paraphia.

parapsoriasis (par″ah-so-ri′ah-sis) any of a group of slowly developing, persistent, maculopapular scaly erythrodermas, devoid of subjective symptoms and resistant to treatment.

parapsychology (par″ah-si-kol′ŏ-je) the branch of psychology dealing with psychic effects and experiences that appear to fall outside the scope of physical law, e.g., telepathy and clairvoyance.

paraquat (par′ah-kwat) a poisonous compound some of whose salts are used as contact HERBICIDES. Concentrated solutions cause skin irritation, cracking and shedding of nails, and delayed healing of cuts and wounds. After ingestion of large doses, renal and hepatic failure may develop, followed by pulmonary insufficiency, sometimes ending

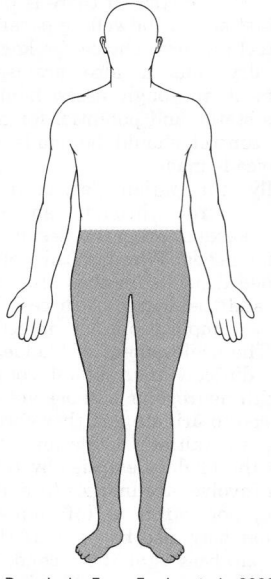

Paraplegia. From Frazier et al., 2000.

fatally; it may also be accidentally inhaled. Since it is absorbed slowly from the gastrointestinal tract, the best treatment for poisoning is administration of a large amount of an absorbent such as activated CHARCOAL to bind with the paraquat, followed by a CATHARTIC to shorten transit time.

parareflexia (par″ah-re-flek′se-ah) any disorder of the reflexes.

pararhotacism (par″ah-ro′tah-sizm) faulty enunciation of the *r* sound.

pararosaniline (par″ah-ro-zan′ĭ-lin) a basic dye; a triphenylmethane derivative, one of the components of basic fuchsin.

pararrhythmia (par″ah-rith′me-ah) parasystole.

parasacral (par″ah-sa′kral) situated near the sacrum.

parasigmatism (par″ah-sig′mah-tizm) lisping.

parasinoidal (par″ah-si-noi′d'l) situated along the course of a sinus.

parasite (par′ah-sīt) 1. a plant or animal that lives upon or within another living organism at whose expense it obtains some advantage; see also SYMBIOSIS. Parasites include multicelled and single-celled animals, fungi, and bacteria, and some authorities also include viruses. Those that feed upon human hosts can cause diseases ranging from the mildly annoying to the severe or even fatal. (See accompanying table.) 2. parasitic FETUS. adj., **parasit′ic.**

accidental p. one that parasitizes an organism other than the usual host.

facultative p. one that may be parasitic upon another organism but can exist independently.

incidental p. accidental parasite.

malarial p. Plasmodium.

obligate p., obligatory p. one that is entirely dependent upon a host for its survival.

periodic p. one that parasitizes a host for short periods.

temporary p. one that lives free of its host during part of its life cycle.

parasitemia (par″ah-si-te′me-ah) the presence of parasites, especially malarial forms, in the blood.

parasiticide (par″ah-sit′ĭ-sīd) antiparasitic (def. 2).

parasitism (par′ah-si″tizm) 1. symbiosis in which one population (or individual) adversely affects another, but cannot live without it. 2. infection or infestation with parasites.

parasitize (par′ah-sĭ-tīz″) to live on or within a host as a parasite.

parasitogenic (par″ah-si″to-jen′ik) due to parasites.

parasitologist (par″ah-si-tol′o-jist) a person skilled in parasitology.

parasitology (par″ah-si-tol′o-je) the scientific study of parasites and parasitism.

parasitotropic (par″ah-si″to-trop′ik) having affinity for parasites.

parasomnia (par″ah-som′ne-ah) a category of primary SLEEP DISORDERS in which abnormal events occur during sleep, due to inappropriately timed activation of physiological systems. Included are NIGHTMARE DISORDER, SLEEP TERROR DISORDER, and SLEEP-WALKING DISORDER. See also DYSSOMNIA.

paraspadias (par″ah-spa′de-as) a congenital condition in which the urethra opens on one side of the penis.

parasternal (par″ah-ster′nal) beside the sternum.

parasuicide (par″ah-soo′ĭ-sīd) attempted suicide, emphasizing that in most such attempts death is not the desired outcome.

parasympathetic nervous system part of the AUTONOMIC NERVOUS SYSTEM, the preganglionic fibers of which leave the central nervous system with cranial nerves III, VII, IX, and X and the first three sacral nerves; postganglionic fibers are distributed to the heart, smooth muscles, and glands of the head and neck, and thoracic, abdominal, and pelvic viscera. (See also Color Plates.) Almost three-fourths of all parasympathetic

P

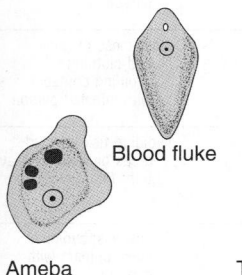
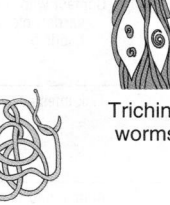
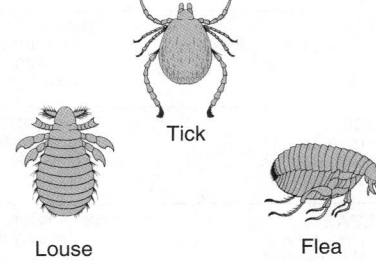

Blood fluke

Trichina worms

Tick

Ameba

Tapeworm

Louse

Flea

Types of parasites.

Parasite (Approximate Length) Areas of Occurrence	Conditions Caused	Usual Source of Infection	Prevention
Internal Parasites			
AMEBA (1/25,000 in.—microscopic) Tropics: occasionally U.S.	Amebic dysentery	Contaminated food and drink	Avoiding unsanitary food and drink
MALARIA PARASITE (1/3,000 in.—microscopic) Tropics; southern U.S.	Malaria	Mosquito bites	Mosquito control; protection against bites
BLOOD FLUKE (1/4–1/2 in.) Tropics; rare in U.S.	Schistosomiasis (disease of liver, intestine, bladder)	Water (organism can penetrate skin)	Avoiding contaminated water
TAPEWORM (6–60 ft.) Most contries; beef tapeworm common in U.S.	Tapeworm (in intestine)	Raw or poorly cooked beef, pork, or fish	Cooking meat and fish
HOOKWORM (1/4–1/2 in.) Warm regions; common in southern U.S.	Hookworm disease (ancylostomiasis)	Contaminated soil	Wearing shoes; avoiding direct contact with infected soil
ASCARIS ROUNDWORM (6–12 in.) Parts of southern U.S.; wherever sanitation is poor	Intestinal disorders (ascariasis)	Raw vegetables and fruits	Cooking fruits and vegetables
PINWORM (1/12–1/2 in.) Throughout world	Pinworm infection (enterobiasis)	Contaminated food; contact with infected person	Personal cleanliness
TRICHINA WORM (1/16–1/6 in.) Throughout world; common in U.S.	Trichinosis	Poorly cooked pork	Thorough cooking of pork products
FILARIA WORM (1-1/2–4 in.) Tropics	Filariasis	Mosquito bites	Avoiding mosquito bites
Skin Parasites			
ITCH MITE (1/100 in.) Most countries, including U.S.	Scabies	Contact with infected person	Cleanliness of body and clothing; avoiding contact with infected person
LICE (1/25–1/8 in.) Most countries, including U.S.	Itching of skin (pediculosis); also may carry disease germ	Contact with human carrier, clothing, bedding	Cleanliness of body and clothing; avoiding contact with infected person
TICKS (1/10–1/2 in.) Most countires, including U.S.	Skin infestation; also may carry rabbit fever, Lyme disease, other diseases	Tick-infested areas	Avoiding tick-infested areas or wearing heavy tight-fitting clothing
FLEAS (1/12–1/8 in.) Most countries, including U.S.	Skin irritation; also may carry disease germs	Animal and human carriers	Cleanliness; avoiding close contact with carriers

nerve fibers are in the VAGUS NERVES, which serve the entire thoracic and abdominal regions of the body.

The predominant secretion of the nerve endings of the parasympathetic nervous system is ACETYLCHOLINE, which acts on organs of the body to either excite or inhibit certain activities. For example, stimulation of the parasympathetic system causes constriction of the pupil of the eye and contraction of the ciliary muscle; increase of the glandular secretion of enzymes, as in the case of the pancreas; increased peristalsis; and a slowed heart rate. It often happens that excitation of the sympathetic nervous system results in an effect opposite that of the parasympathetic system; however, most organs are under the almost exclusive control of either one or the other of the two nervous systems that compose the autonomic nervous system.

parasympatholytic (par″ah-sim″pah-tho-lit′ik) 1. producing effects resembling those of interruption of the parasympathetic nerve supply of a part; having a destructive effect on the parasympathetic nerve fibers or blocking the transmission of impulses by them. 2. anticholinergic (def. 2).

parasympathomimetic (par″ah-sim″pah-tho-mi-met′ik) producing effects resembling those of stimulation of the parasympathetic nerve supply of a part. 1. cholinergic (def. 2).

parasynapsis (par″ah-sĭ-nap′sis) the union of chromosomes side by side during meiosis.

parasynovitis (par″ah-sin″o-vi′tis) inflammation of the tissues about a synovial sac.

parasystole (par″ah-sis′to-le) a cardiac arrhythmia attributed to the interaction of two foci independently initiating cardiac impulses at different rates; it cannot be discharged by impulses of the dominant rhythm but it may be modulated by electrotonic influences. The two independent rhythms coexist but not as a result of atrioventricular block. It is an abnormality of both AUTOMATICITY and impulse conduction. See also entrance BLOCK.

paratenon (par″ah-ten′on) the fatty areolar tissue filling the interstices of the fascial compartment in which a tendon is situated.

parathion (par″ah-thi′on) an ORGANO-PHOSPHATE agricultural insecticide, highly toxic to humans and other animals and the cause of many accidental poisonings.

parathormone (par″ah-thor′mōn) parathyroid hormone.

parathymia (par″ah-thi′me-ah) an abnormal, contrary, or inappropriate mood, as seen in SCHIZOPHRENIA.

parathyroid (par″ah-thi′roid) 1. near the THYROID GLAND. 2. a parathyroid gland. 3. a preparation containing parathyroid hormone from animal parathyroid glands; used for diagnosis and treatment of HYPOPARA-THYROIDISM.

p. glands four small endocrine bodies in the region of the thyroid gland; they contain two types of cells: *chief cells* and *oxyphils*. Chief cells are the major source of parathyroid hormone (PTH), the secretion of which is dependent on the serum calcium level. Through a closed-loop feedback mechanism a low serum calcium level stimulates secretion of PTH; conversely, a high serum calcium level inhibits its secretion. The essential role of PTH is maintenance of a normal serum calcium level in association with vitamin D and calcitonin. It does this by exerting its effects on bone, kidney, and gastrointestinal tract. In bone, it enhances bone resorption by increasing digestion of the bone matrix by osteoclasts, which produces calcium that gets released into the bloodstream. In the kidney, PTH increases the excretion of phosphate and the reabsorption of filtered calcium. In the intestine, it increases intestinal absorption of calcium. The parathyroid glands may be subject to either HYPERPARATHYROIDISM or HYPOPARATHY-ROIDISM.

parathyroidectomy (par″ah-thi″roi-dek′-to-me) excision of one or more of the parathyroid glands.

parathyrotropic (par″ah-thi″ro-trop′ik) having an affinity for the parathyroid glands.

paratope (par′ah-tōp) an antigen-binding site of an antibody molecule; see also antigenic DETERMINANT.

paratrophy (par-at′ro-fe) dystrophy.

paratuberculosis (par″ah-too-ber″ku-lo′-sis) a tuberculosis-like disease not due to *Mycobacterium tuberculosis*.

paratyphoid (par″ah-ti′foid) 1. resembling TYPHOID FEVER. 2. paratyphoid fever.

p. fever infection caused by *Salmonella* of all groups except *S. typhosa*. The disease is usually milder than TYPHOID FEVER and has a shorter incubation period, more abrupt onset, and a lower mortality rate. Clinically and pathologically, however, the two diseases cannot be distinguished.

paraurethral (par″ah-u-re′thral) near the urethra.

paravaccinia (par″ah-vak-sin′e-ah) an infection due to the paravaccinia virus, a species of the genus *Parapoxvirus* that produces lesions similar to those of cowpox and orf on the udders and teats of milk cows. Paravaccinia may be transmitted to humans during milking, producing purple nodules on the fingers or adjacent areas; the lesions break down and crust and heal without scarring.

paravaginitis (par″ah-vaj″ĭ-ni′tis) perivaginitis.

paravertebral (par″ah-ver′tĕ-bral) near the vertebral column; called also juxtaspinal.

Paré (pah-ra′) Ambroise (1510–1590). French surgeon. As an army surgeon treating gunshot wounds, Paré discontinued the application of boiling oils as was customary at that time. He invented many new surgical instruments and reintroduced the use of ligatures to tie off the blood vessels for amputation. He described carbon monoxide poisoning and has been cited as probably the first to think of flies as transmitters of infectious disease. In obstetrics he did podalic versions and induced labor for uterine hemorrhage. He introduced reimplantation of the teeth in dentistry, and wrote a book on medical jurisprudence.

paregoric (par″ĕ-gor′ik) a mixture of powdered OPIUM, anise oil, BENZOIC ACID, CAMPHOR, and GLYCERIN in alcohol, used as an ANTIPERISTALTIC agent for treatment of DIARRHEA and as a mild pain reliever.

parenchyma (pah-reng′kĭ-mah) the essential or functional elements of an organ, as distinguished from its framework, which is called the STROMA. adj., **paren′chymal, parenchym′atous.**

p. of prostate glandular substance consisting of small compound tubulosaccular or tubuloalveolar glands, making up the bulk of the PROSTATE; it is surrounded by muscular substance and permeated by muscular strands.

renal p. the functional tissue of the KIDNEY, consisting of the NEPHRONS.

parenchymatitis (par″eng-kim″ah-ti′tis) inflammation of a parenchyma.

parenteral (pah-ren′ter-al) by some route other than through the alimentary canal, such as by subcutaneous, intramuscular, intrasternal, or intravenous injection.

p. nutrition a technique for meeting a patient's nutritional needs by means of intravenous feedings; sometimes called *hyperalimentation,* even though it does not provide excessive amounts of nutrients. Nutrition by intravenous feeding may be either *total parenteral nutrition* or only supplemental.

Total parenteral nutrition provides all of the carbohydrates, proteins, fats, water, electrolytes, vitamins, and minerals needed for the building of tissue, expenditure of energy, and other physiologic activities. The procedure originated as an emergency life-saving technique following surgery for severe and massive trauma of the gastrointestinal tract but has now become a relatively common means of providing bowel rest and nutrition in a variety of conditions in spite of inherent risks. Although primarily used as a short-term temporary measure until either surgical or medical treatment corrects the gastrointestinal dysfunction, it has also been used with some success as a long-term therapy for selected patients on an outpatient basis.

Parenteral nutrition may be used in the following conditions: malnutrition from such acute and chronic inflammatory bowel diseases as regional ileitis (CROHN'S DISEASE) and ULCERATIVE COLITIS, partial or total obstruction of the gastrointestinal tract that cannot be relieved immediately by surgery, congenital anomalies in the newborn prior to surgery, massive burns that produce critical protein loss, and other disorders in which malnutrition is a threat to the life of the patient who cannot receive nutrients via the digestive tract.

The nutrient mix is tailored to the individual needs and tolerance of the patient. There is not complete agreement among the experts as to the ideal mix, especially of amino acids. The nutrient solutions usually are prepared in clean-air rooms in the pharmacy of a hospital under aseptic conditions to avoid contamination.

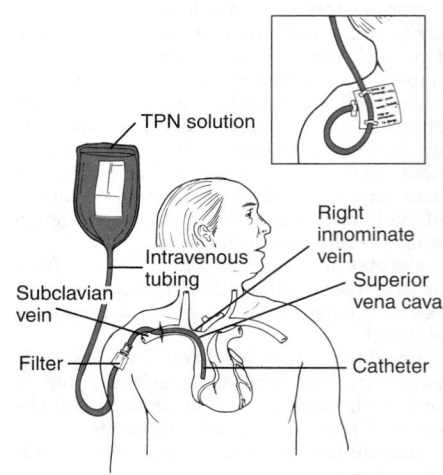

Superior vena cava administration of parenteral nutrition through a subclavian venous line. From Lammon et al., 1996.

Administration of the nutrients is accomplished via a CENTRAL VENOUS CATHETER, usually inserted in the superior vena cava. The route of administration, constant rate of flow required, and potential patient sensitivity to the elements administered, all contribute to the potential complications of parenteral nutrition.

Of the many complications that may develop, the most common are febrile reactions arising from patient intolerance to the required rate of flow, reactions due to individual sensitivity to some of the elements in the nutrient mix, and infection from contamination of either the site of insertion of the catheter or the apparatus used to administer the nutrients. Other complications that may develop include phlebitis and thrombosis of the vena cava, electrolyte imbalance, hyperglycemia, cardiac overload, dehydration, metabolic acidosis, and mechanical trauma to the heart.

Patient Care. Principles of strict aseptic technique must be followed in the daily changing of dressings and in handling the nutrient solution and the administration equipment. The catheter through which the nutrients are administered should not be used for administration of medication, blood, or any other substance that may induce clotting in the vein.

parentification (pah-ren″tĭ-fĭ-ka′shun) the assumption of a parentlike (or adult) role by a child.

parenting (par′ent-ing) providing a nurturing and constructive environment that promotes growth and development in a child or children; see also ATTACHMENT.

impaired p. a NURSING DIAGNOSIS accepted by the North American Nursing Diagnosis Association, defined as inability of the primary caregiver to create, maintain, or regain an environment that promotes the optimum growth and development of the child.

risk for impaired p. a NURSING DIAGNOSIS accepted by the North American Nursing Diagnosis Association, defined as risk for inability of the primary caretaker to create, maintain, or regain an environment that promotes the optimum growth and development of the child.

parepididymis (par″ep-ĭ-did′ĭ-mis) paradidymis.

paresis (pah-re′sis, par′ĕ-sis) slight or incomplete paralysis. adj., **paret′ic.**

general p. chronic MENINGOENCEPHALITIS from a syphilitic infection that is causing gradual loss of cortical function, resulting in progressive dementia and generalized paralysis; this may occur 10 to 20 years after an initial infection of SYPHILIS in untreated

individuals. Called also Bayle's disease and dementia paralytica.

paresthesia (par″es-the′zhah) a morbid or abnormal sensation, such as burning, prickling, or formication.

postoperative p. prolonged paresthesia after surgery done with a local anesthetic, especially around the mouth due to injury of the mental nerve or mandibular nerve.

paricalcitol (par″ĭ-kal′sĭ-tol) a synthetic analogue of VITAMIN D, used for prevention and treatment of HYPERPARATHYROIDISM secondary to chronic RENAL FAILURE; administered intravenously.

paries (pa′re-ez) [L.] wall.

parietal (pah-ri′ĕ-t'l) 1. of or pertaining to the walls of an organ or cavity. 2. pertaining to or located near the parietal bone. See anatomic Table of Bones in the Appendices.

parietofrontal (pah-ri″ĕ-to-frun′t'l) pertaining to the parietal and frontal bones, gyri, or fissures.

parietography (pah-ri″ĕ-tog′rah-fe) radiographic visualization of the walls of an organ.

Parinaud oculoglandular syndrome (pah-rĭ-no′) a general term applied to conjunctivitis, usually unilateral and of the follicular type, followed by tenderness and enlargement of the preauricular lymph nodes; often due to LEPTOTRICHOSIS but sometimes associated with other infections.

Parinaud syndrome (pah-rĭ-no′) paralysis of conjugate upward movement of the eyes without paralysis of convergence, associated with midbrain lesions. Called also Parinaud's ophthalmoplegia.

parity (par′ĭ-te) 1. para; the condition of a woman with respect to her having borne viable offspring. 2. equality; close correspondence or similarity.

Parkinson's disease (pahr′kin-sunz) a slowly progressive disease usually occurring in later life, characterized pathologically by degeneration within the nuclear masses of the extrapyramidal system, and clinically by a masklike face (parkinson's FACIES), a characteristic tremor of resting muscles, a slowing of voluntary movements, a festinating GAIT, peculiar posture, and muscular weakness. Called also paralysis agitans and shaking palsy. When the symptom complex occurs secondarily to another disorder, the condition is called PARKINSONISM.

Symptoms. Parkinson's disease usually appears gradually and progresses slowly. At first the victim may be troubled by "resting tremors" of the hands and feet that diminish or disappear when the patient begins to move. Hypokinesia (reduced

P

movement) is the most disabling feature of Parkinson's disease. A minor feeling of sluggishness may progress to inability to get up from a chair or even change position in bed. However, once the patient gets into motion, prolonged walking is possible. The gait is shuffling and festinating as the person attempts to regain his center of gravity. Rigidity of muscles in the arms, legs, and face is due to an increase in the tone of skeletal muscles. Loss of mobility in the face produces the characteristic mask-like expression. Parkinson's disease does not adversely affect mental capacity.

Treatment. In general, treatment is symptomatic, supportive, and palliative. Most patients require lifelong management consisting of drug therapy, supportive psychotherapy, physical therapy, and rarely, surgical intervention. Newer forms of treatment now give hope for freedom from the progressive disability that once was almost inevitable. The biochemical basis of parkinsonism is a loss or inhibition of DOPAMINE activity in the corpus striatum, resulting from degeneration of the dopaminergic nigrostriatal pathway. Normally, the two opposing neurotransmitters in this structure, DOPAMINE and ACETYLCHOLINE, are in balance. When dopamine is depleted, the functional overactivity of acetylcholine produces the symptoms of parkinsonism.

In patients with mild symptoms and little functional impairment, some relief from symptoms can be obtained with anticholinergic AGENTS, such as TRIHEXYPHENIDYL (ARTANE), or with ANTIHISTAMINES with anticholinergic properties, such as DIPHENHYDRAMINE (BENADRYL). These drugs block the muscarinic effects of ACETYLCHOLINE in the central nervous system. Tricyclic ANTIDEPRESSANTS, such as IMIPRAMINE or AMITRIPTYLINE, are also effective; they block the reuptake of dopamine from nerve synapses and also have anticholinergic effects.

In patients with more severe symptoms and difficulty with routine daily activities, it is necessary to augment the dopamine level in the brain. This is done by administering LEVODOPA, which crosses the blood-brain barrier and is converted to dopamine by decarboxylation. This reaction also occurs in the peripheral tissues, and the dopamine produced may cause side effects such as cardiac stimulation (tachycardia and arrhythmias) and also nausea and vomiting. A newer drug called SINEMET, which combines CARBIDOPA with levodopa, is now being used to counteract the undesirable effects that may occur when levodopa

is used alone. Carbidopa inhibits production of dopamine outside the brain, thus allowing more effective relief of symptoms. A disadvantage to the combination drug is that in some patients it may have only a limited span of effectiveness; therefore, it is usually reserved for more severe cases.

Patients receiving levodopa alone or in combination with carbidopa require nutritional counseling because dietary habits can greatly affect the action of the drug. Protein intake requires special attention because levodopa, an amino acid, must compete with the dietary amino acids for transport through the intestinal epithelium and across the blood-brain barrier. Alcohol intake also must be limited because in large amounts it can antagonize the effects of dopamine. Although the newer combined form of medication offers relief to many persons with Parkinson's disease, it must be given with caution and under continued supervision. Fewer than 10 per cent of patients with Parkinson's fail to respond to some combination of individual drugs.

Patient Care. Since these patients' mental outlook and motivation can affect the extent to which they can successfully cope with their disability, it is important that they receive psychological support. They should know the nature of the disease affecting them and be given realistic hopes for forestalling or preventing its more serious effects.

Some benefits can be derived from physical therapy in the form of applications of heat and massage to alleviate muscle cramps and relieve the tension headaches that often accompany rigidity of the cervical muscles. The patient also is instructed in simple EXERCISES to perform at home. Although depression often accompanies the physical limitations of Parkinson's disease, much psychological benefit can be derived from maintaining mobility and observing social and emotional ties. Patients can be taught to initiate walking by leaning forward to stimulate intact walking reflexes. Family members will need help in dealing with the patient's slowness of speech and communication difficulties. Some minor changes in the home, such as railings and support bars, can encourage independent movement.

parkinsonian (pahr″kin-so′ne-an) pertaining to parkinsonism.

p. syndrome any disorder manifesting the symptoms of PARKINSON'S DISEASE.

parkinsonism (pahr′kin-sun-izm) any disorder manifesting the symptoms of PARKINSON'S DISEASE or any such symptom complex occurring secondarily to another disorder, such as encephalitis, cerebral arteriosclerosis, poisoning with certain toxins, and neurosyphilis.

Parlodel (pahr'lo-del) trademark for a preparation of BROMOCRIPTINE mesylate, a DOPAMINE agonist used to suppress PROLACTIN secretion and to treat PARKINSONISM and ACROMEGALY.

Parnate (pahr'nāt) trademark for a preparation of TRANYLCYPROMINE, an ANTIDE-PRESSANT.

paroccipital (par″ok-sip'ĭ-t'l) beside the occipital bone.

paromomycin (par′ah-mo-mi″sin) a broad-spectrum ANTIBIOTIC derived from *Streptomyces rimosus* var. *paromomycinus;* the sulfate salt is used as an ANTIAMEBIC.

paronychia (par″o-nik′e-ah) inflammation involving folds of tissue surrounding a NAIL or nails. The causative organisms may be bacteria or fungi, which usually gain entrance through a hangnail or break in the skin due to improper manicuring. Acute infections are treated with hot compresses and the application of an antibiotic or fungicidal ointment. A pocket of purulent material may require incision with a scalpel to promote drainage and healing. Chronic infections are more difficult to cure and may require the application of a corticosteroid ointment. If the infection is widespread and difficult to treat topically, removal of the nail may be necessary.

paroöphoron (par″o-of′o-ron) an inconstantly present, small group of coiled tubules between the layers of the mesosalpinx, being a remnant of the excretory part of the mesonephros.

parophthalmia (par″of-thal′me-ah) inflammation of the connective tissue around the eye.

paropsis (par-op′sis) a disorder of vision.

parorexia (par″o-rek′se-ah) disordered appetite, with craving for unusual foods. The term is sometimes used synonymously with pica.

parosmia (par-oz′me-ah) perversion of the sense of smell.

parostosis (par″os-to′sis) ossification of tissues outside of the periosteum.

parotid (pah-rot′id) near the ear.

p. glands the largest of the three main pairs of salivary glands, located on either side of the face, just below and in front of the ears. From each gland a duct, the parotid duct (sometimes called Stensen's duct), runs forward across the cheek and opens on the inside surface of the cheek opposite the second molar of the upper jaw.

The parotid glands are made up of groups of cells clustered around a globular cavity, resembling a bunch of grapes. Small ducts draining each cavity join the ducts of neighboring cavities to form large ducts, which in turn join the parotid duct.

From the system of ducts flows the thin, watery secretion of the parotid glands called saliva, which plays an important role in the process of digestion. As food is chewed the saliva with which it is mixed and moistened makes it possible for the food to be reduced to a substance that can be swallowed.

Controlled by the autonomic nervous system, the secretion of the salivary glands begins whenever the sensory nerves of the mouth, or in some cases nerves located elsewhere in the body, are stimulated.

Salivation may be an involuntary reflex, as when food or even inedible material placed in the mouth starts the flow of the secretion from the glands, or it may be a conditioned reflex, as when the flow is started by the sight, smell, or thought of food.

Disorders of the Parotid Glands. The most common disease affecting the parotid glands is MUMPS, or epidemic parotitis.

Swelling and tenderness may also result from infections caused by other viruses or bacteria in the glands. Less often, these symptoms indicate a blockage of a duct by either infection or a calculus, in which case the swelling is likely to fluctuate, especially at mealtimes. Though stubborn or recurring cases sometimes require surgery, stones often can be removed by massage. For infections, antibiotics and warm compresses are the usual treatment.

Occasionally additional glandular masses grow in or near a parotid gland. The majority of such growths are mixed tumors, so called because they contain cartilage or other material as well as the usual glandular material. Usually they are benign; occasionally they may be malignant and require surgery.

parotidectomy (pah-rot″ĭ-dek′to-me) excision of a parotid gland.

parotiditis (pah-rot″ĭdi′tis) parotitis.

parotitis (par″o-ti′tis) inflammation of the parotid gland.

  contagious p., epidemic p. mumps.

parovarian (par″o-va′re-an) 1. beside the ovary. 2. pertaining to the epoöphoron.

parovarium (par″o-var′e-um) epoöphoron.

paroxetine (pah-rok′sĕ-tēn) a selective serotonin reuptake INHIBITOR administered orally as the hydrochloride salt as an ANTIDEPRESSANT and to treat obsessive-compulsive, panic, and social anxiety disorders.

paroxysm (par'ok-sizm) 1. a sudden recurrence or intensification of symptoms. 2. a spasm or seizure. adj., **paroxys'mal.**

parrot fever psittacosis.

Parry's disease (par'ēz) Graves' disease.

pars (pahrs), pl. *par'tes* [L.] part.

p. mastoi'dea os'sis tempora'lis mastoid part of temporal bone; see under PART.

p. petro'sa os'sis tempora'lis petrous part of temporal bone; see under PART.

p. pla'na the thin part of the ciliary body; the ciliary disk.

p. squamo'sa os'sis tempora'lis squamous part of temporal bone; see under PART.

p. tympa'nica os'sis tempora'lis tympanic part of temporal bone.

Parse (pahr'se) Rosemarie Rizzo. Nursing educator, researcher, theorist, and consultant. She drew on the work of Martha ROGERS and on existential phenomenology to develop the conceptual model THEORY OF HUMAN BECOMING. She posits a conception of nursing grounded in the human sciences rather than the natural sciences, focusing on man's total experience with health.

part a division of a larger structure.

mastoid p. of temporal bone the posterior portion of the petrous (or petromastoid) part. Called also mastoid bone.

petromastoid p. of temporal bone see *petrous part of temporal bone.*

petrous p. of temporal bone the part of the temporal bone located at the base of the cranium, containing the inner ear. Some anatomists divide it into two separate subparts, calling the posterior section the *mastoid part,* reserving the term *petrous part* for the anterior section only, and calling the entire area the *petromastoid part.* Called also petrous bone.

squamous p. of temporal bone the flat, scalelike, anterior superior portion of the temporal bone. Called also squamous bone.

tympanic p. of temporal bone the part of the temporal bone forming the anterior and inferior walls and part of the posterior wall of the external acoustic meatus. Called also tympanic bone.

parthenogenesis (pahr''thĕ-no-jen'ĕ-sis) a modified form of sexual reproduction in which a gamete develops into a new individual without the fertilization of an oocyte by a spermatozoon, as in certain arthropods and other animals; it may occur as a natural phenomenon or be induced by chemical or mechanical stimulation (artificial parthenogenesis). adj., **parthenogenet'ic.**

particle (pahr'tĭ-k'l) an extremely small mass of material.

alpha p's see ALPHA PARTICLES.

beta p's see BETA PARTICLES.

Dane p. an intact hepatitis B virion.

elementary p. any of the subatomic particles, including electrons, protons, neutrons, positrons, neutrinos, and muons.

particulate (pahr-tik'u-lāt) composed of separate particles.

parturient (pahr-tu're-ent) giving birth or pertaining to birth; by extension, a woman in LABOR.

parturiometer (pahr-tu''rĭ-om'ĕ-ter) a device used in measuring the expulsive power of the uterus.

parturition (pahr''tu-rish'un) childbirth.

parulis (pah-roo'lis) an elevated nodule at the site of a fistula draining a chronic periapical ABSCESS; called also gum boil or gumboil.

parumbilical (par''um-bil'ĭ-k'l) periumbilical.

parvicellular (par''vĭ-sel'u-ler) composed of small cells.

parvovirus (pahr'vo-vi''rus) a group of extremely small, morphologically similar, ether-resistant DNA viruses, including the adeno-associated viruses.

human p. B19 B19 virus.

PAS, PASA *p*-aminosalicylic acid.

pascal (Pa) (pas-kal', pas'kal) the SI UNIT of pressure, which corresponds to a force of one newton per square meter.

PASG pneumatic antishock garment.

passive-aggressive personality disorder a PERSONALITY DISORDER whose essential features are resistance to the demands of others that is expressed indirectly under the cover of obstructionism, procrastination, stubbornness, dawdling, forgetfulness, and intentional inefficiency combined with negative, defeatist attitudes. The behavior pattern persists even when more effective behavior is possible. Such people are manipulative and attempt to make themselves dependent on others; they are often pessimistic and resentful but do not realize that their ineffective behavior is the source of their problems. Called also negativistic personality disorder.

paste (pāst) a semisolid preparation containing one or more drug substances, for topical application.

Pasteur (pas-ter') Louis (1822–1895). French chemist and bacteriologist, founder of microbiology and developer of the method of vaccination by attenuated virus. By optical investigation of racemic acid, he discovered a new class of isomeric substances which led to work by others on stereochemistry and for which he received the ribbon of the Legion of Honor. Pasteur came to the rescue of the wine industry by his interest in fermentation, and showed that spoiling of wine caused by microorganisms could be prevented by partial heat sterilization (pasteurization), a process now applied to many perishable foods. Experimental foundation was given to his ideas of fermentation and the long-accepted theory of spontaneous generation was disposed of once and for all. Later he came to the rescue of the silkworm industry and found methods for detecting and preventing pébrine and flâcherie, the two diseases that were destroying it. He turned his attention then to anthrax, chicken cholera, and hydrophobia (rabies), and developed preventive inoculations against them. The Pasteur Institute was opened shortly thereafter and institutions were founded all over the world for inoculation against rabies.

Pasteurella (pas″tĕ-rel′ah) a genus of gram-negative, nonmotile, facultatively anaerobic, ovoid to rod-shaped bacteria. *P. multoci′da* is the etiologic agent of hemorrhagic septicemia. *P. haemoly′tica* and *P. pneumotro′pica* are animal pathogens that sometimes cause infection in humans.

pasteurellosis (pas″ter-ĕ-lo′sis) infection with organisms of the genus *Pasteurella*.

pasteurization (pas″ter-i-za′shun) the process of heating milk or other liquids, e.g., wine or beer, to destroy microorganisms that would cause spoilage. The milk is held at 62°C for 30 minutes (LTHM, low temperature holding method, holding method), or heated rapidly to 80°C and held for 15–30 seconds (HTST, high temperature short time, flash method), and then chilled. The procedure kills most pathogenic bacteria while retaining the flavor of the liquid.

Patau's syndrome (pah-tōz′) trisomy 13 syndrome.

patch (pach) a small area differing from the rest of a surface.

Peyer's p's whitish, oval, elevated patches of closely packed lymph follicles in mucous and submucous layers of the small intestine.

salmon p. a salmon-colored NEVUS FLAMMEUS usually found over the eyelids, between the eyes, or on the forehead. It is the most common vascular lesion of infancy, found in 40 per cent of newborns, and usually fades in the first year of life. Called also nevus simplex.

p. test a type of SKIN TEST for hypersensitivity in which filter paper or gauze saturated with the substance in question is applied to the skin, usually on the forearm; a positive reaction is reddening or swelling at the site.

patella (pah-tel′ah) [L.] a triangular bone at the knee; see anatomic Table of Bones in the Appendices. Called also kneecap.

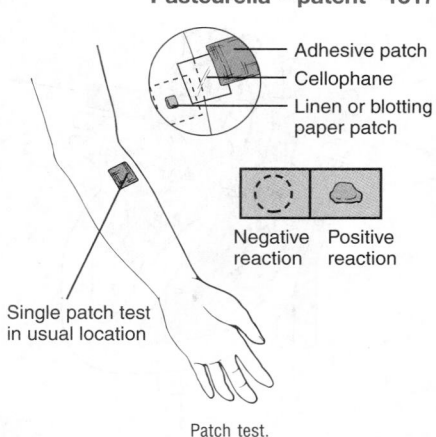

Patch test.

patellar (pah-tel′er) of or pertaining to the patella.

patellectomy (pat″ĕ-lek′to-me) excision of the patella.

patelliform (pah-tel′ĭ-form) shaped like the patella.

patellofemoral (pah-tel″o-fem′o-ral) pertaining to the patella and femur.

patency (pa′ten-se) the condition of being wide open.

patent (pa′tent) 1. open, unobstructed, or not closed. 2. apparent, evident.

p. ductus arteriosus abnormal persistence of an open lumen in the ductus arteriosus, between the aorta and the pulmonary artery, after birth. The ductus arteriosus is open during prenatal life, allowing most of the blood of the fetus to bypass the lungs, but normally this channel closes shortly after birth and changes into a fibrous cord called the ligamentum arteriosum. When it remains open, it places special burdens on the left ventricle, since much of the ventricular output is being shunted from the aorta into the pulmonary artery. The condition may coexist with other congenital malformations.

The symptoms of patent ductus arteriosus are usually so slight that they are not noticed until the child is older and more active. He then begins to experience dyspnea on exertion. If the ductus is large there may be retardation of growth. Pulmonary congestion may result from poor left ventricular function. The heart compensates through hypertrophy and dilation.

Treatment is surgical ligation of the open ductus, preferably when the child is from 4 to 10 years of age. Prognosis, when

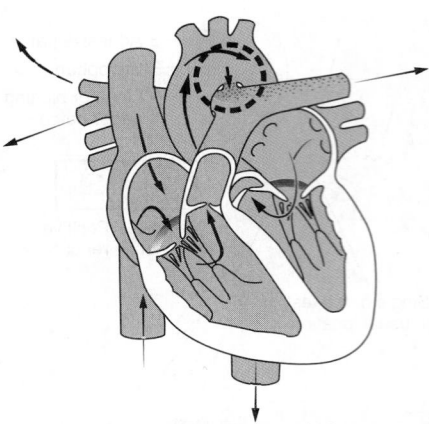

Patent ductus arteriosus. The shunt is from aorta to pulmonary artery. From Betz et al., 1994.

the condition is not accompanied by other congenital heart defects, is excellent.

The ductus may remain open in as many as 10 per cent of preterm infants, especially those under 1500 grams. If the shunt across the ductus is large, heart failure can occur and surgical repair may be necessary. Investigators into the effects of the PROSTA-GLANDINS have reported that closure of a patent ductus arteriosus can be produced in preterm infants by administration of an inhibitor of prostaglandin formation. Conversely, in neonates suffering from severe complex congenital heart defects in which an open ductus arteriosus could be beneficial, injections of prostaglandins have been used to keep the channel open.

path(o)- word element [Gr.], *disease.*

pathergy (path'er-je) 1. an abnormal reaction to an allergen, either a subnormal reaction or an excessive reaction. 2. a condition of being allergic to several antigens. adj., **pather'gic.**

pathfinder (path'fīnd-er) an instrument for locating urethral strictures. 1. root canal probe.

pathobiology (path″o-bi-ol'o-je) pathology.

pathoclisis (path″o-klis'is) a specific sensitivity to specific toxins, or a specific affinity of certain toxins for certain systems or organs.

pathogen (path'o-jen) any disease-producing agent or microorganism. adj., **pathogen'ic.**

pathogenesis (path″o-jen'ĕ-sis) the development of morbid conditions or of disease; more specifically the cellular events and reactions and other pathologic mechanisms

occurring in the development of disease. adj., **pathogenet'ic.**

pathogenic disease causing.

pathogenicity (path″o-jĕ-nis'ĭ-te) the quality of producing or the ability to produce pathologic changes or disease.

pathogeny (pah-thoj'ĕ-ne) pathogenesis.

pathognomonic (path″og-no-mon'ik) specifically distinctive or characteristic of a disease or pathologic condition; denoting a sign or symptom on which a diagnosis can be made.

pathologist (pah-thol'o-jist) a specialist in some kind of PATHOLOGY; for specific types, see under the name.

pathology (pah-thol'o-je) 1. the branch of medicine treating of the essential nature of disease, especially of the changes in body tissues and organs that cause or are caused by disease. 2. the structural and functional manifestations of a disease. adj., **patholog'ic, patholog'ical.**

clinical p. pathology applied to the solution of clinical problems, especially the use of laboratory methods in clinical diagnosis.

comparative p. that which considers human disease processes in comparison with those of other animals.

experimental p. the study of artificially induced pathologic processes.

oral p. that which treats of conditions causing or resulting from morbid anatomic or functional changes in the structures of the mouth.

speech p., speech-language p. a field of the health sciences dealing with the evaluation of speech, language, and voice disorders and the rehabilitation of patients with such disorders not amenable to medical or surgical treatment. See also SPEECH-LANGUAGE PATHOLOGIST.

surgical p. the pathology of disease processes that are surgically accessible for diagnosis or treatment.

pathomimesis (path″o-mi-me'sis) mimicry of a disease or disorder, particularly malingering.

pathomorphism (path″o-mor'fizm) abnormal morphology.

pathonomia (path″o-no'me-ah) the science of the laws of disease.

pathophysiology (path″o-fiz″e-ol'o-je) the physiology of disordered function.

pathopsychology (path″o-si-kol'o-je) the psychology of mental disease.

pathway (path'wa) a course usually followed. In neurology, the nerve structures through which a sensory impression is conducted to the cerebral cortex (afferent pathway), or through which an impulse passes from the brain to the skeletal musculature (efferent pathway). Also used alone to indicate a sequence of reactions that convert one biological material to another (metabolic pathway).

accessory p., accessory conduction p. extra muscle tissue between the atrium and ventricle that bypasses all or part of the normal conduction SYSTEM. When the ventricles are activated prematurely via this pathway, initial forces are slow, producing the delta wave of WOLFF-PARKINSON-WHITE SYNDROME, and PREEXCITATION is said to exist; the delta wave causes the PR interval to shorten and the QRS interval to broaden.

alternative complement p. see COMPLEMENT.

amphibolic p. a group of metabolic reactions with a dual function, providing small metabolites for further catabolism to end products or for use as precursors in synthetic, anabolic reactions. The tricarboxylic acid CYCLE is an example. See also ANABOLISM and CATABOLISM.

biosynthetic p. the sequence of enzymatic steps in the synthesis of a specific end-product in a living organism.

classical complement p. see COMPLEMENT.

coagulation p's see common p. of coagulation, extrinsic p. of coagulation, and intrinsic p. of coagulation.

common p. of coagulation the steps in the mechanism of coagulation (see CLOTTING) from the activation of FACTOR X through the conversion of FIBRINOGEN to FIBRIN. See also intrinsic PATHWAY of coagulation and extrinsic PATHWAY of coagulation.

concealed accessory p. an accessory PATHWAY that has only retrograde conduction; thus its PR and QRS complexes are normal on the electrocardiogram, but there is a tendency to develop premature supraventricular TACHYCARDIA. If atrial FIBRILLATION develops, conduction will proceed across the atrioventricular node.

Embden-Meyerhof p. the series of enzymatic reactions in the anaerobic conversion of glucose to lactic acid, resulting in energy in the form of adenosine triphosphate (ATP).

extrinsic p. of coagulation the mechanism that produces FIBRIN following tissue injury, beginning with formation of an activated complex between tissue FACTOR and FACTOR VII and leading to activation of FACTOR X, which induces the reactions of the common PATHWAY of coagulation. See also intrinsic PATHWAY of coagulation.

final common p. 1. the motor neurons by which nerve impulses from many central sources pass to a muscle or gland in the periphery. 2. any mechanism by which several independent effects exert a common influence.

intrinsic p. of coagulation a sequence of reactions leading to FIBRIN formation, beginning with the contact activation of FACTOR XII. This is followed by the sequential activation of FACTORS XI and IX, which results in the activation of FACTOR X. Activated factor X (factor Xa) initiates the common PATHWAY of coagulation. See also extrinsic PATHWAY of coagulation.

pentose phosphate p. a pathway of hexose oxidation in which glucose-6-phosphate undergoes two successive oxidations by NADP, the final forming a pentose phosphate.

-pathy word element [Gr.], morbid condition or disease; generally used to designate a noninflammatory condition.

patient (pa'shent) a person who is ill or is undergoing treatment for disease. There is considerable debate regarding the appropriate use of this term. In some institutional settings it is not used because it is thought to denote a dependent relationship on the part of the person undergoing treatment. The words client, resident, and at times guest can also be used to refer to a person receiving treatment.

p's rights those rights attributed to a person seeking health care. In 1973 the American Hospital Association approved a statement called the "Patient's Bill of Rights," regarding a patient's rights during hospitalization. (A revised document was subsequently approved in 1992.) This was published with the expectation that observance of patient's rights would contribute to more effective care and greater satisfaction for the patient, health care providers, and the hospital organization in general. Although it is recognized that a personal relationship between the health care provider and the patient is essential for provision of care, legal precedent has established that the hospital itself also has a responsibility to the patient.

In general, the rights of a patient are concerned with the patient being fully informed about his or her illness, the diagnostic and therapeutic measures anticipated, and the written records of the care received. The patient has the right to considerate and respectful care, delivered in response to a request for services and in a manner that provides continuity of care. In regard to payment for services, the patient has the right to examine and receive an explanation of the bill regardless of source of payment.

P

Patrick's test (pat′riks) the thigh and knee of the supine patient are flexed, the external malleolus rests on the patella on the opposite leg, and the knee is depressed; production of pain indicates arthritis of the hip. Called also fabere sign.

patrilineal (pah-trĭ-lin′e-al) descended through the male line.

pattern (pat′ern) 1. a design to be followed or a device to be used in the construction or fabrication of something. 2. a characteristic set of traits or actions. 3. In the conceptual model HEALTH AS EXPANDING CONSCIOUSNESS, information that depicts the whole rather than its separated parts and that gives an understanding of the meaning of relationships.

capsular p. the predictable loss of RANGE OF MOTION in a joint following injury or a degenerative process such as ARTHRITIS; this often occurs in a limb when it is continually held in a position of comfort. When the limb is held against the body and internally rotated, the greatest loss of motion will be external rotation, followed by abduction, then flexion, then internal rotation.

disturbed sleep p. a NURSING DIAGNOSIS approved by the North American Nursing Diagnosis Association, defined as a time-limited disruption of sleep (the natural, periodic suspension of consciousness) amount and quality. Many factors in an individual's life can disrupt the usual sleep pattern; some common factors include physical illness, discomfort, psychological stress, anxiety, change in accustomed place for sleep, and the side effects of medications. Defining characteristics include reported difficulty falling asleep, awakening earlier or later than desired, interrupted sleep, and not feeling rested after sleeping. Changes in a person's sleep pattern can also lead to behavioral changes, as well as such physical signs as slight hand tremor, drooping eyelids, yawning, dozing during the day, and decreased attention span. Formerly called sleep pattern disturbance.

ineffective breathing p. see BREATHING PATTERN, INEFFECTIVE.

ineffective infant feeding p. a NURSING DIAGNOSIS accepted by the North American Nursing Diagnosis Association, defined as a state in which an infant demonstrates impaired ability to suck or to coordinate the suck-swallow REFLEX.

ineffective sexuality p's a NURSING DIAGNOSIS accepted by the North American Nursing Diagnosis Association, defined as a state in which an individual expresses concern regarding his or her sexuality. See also SEXUAL DYSFUNCTION.

patulous (pat′u-lus) spread widely apart; open; distended.

paucibacillary (paw″sĭ-bas′ĭ-la-re) containing just a few BACILLI; see LEPROSY.

Paul-Bunnell test (pawl bun-el′) a method of testing for the presence of heterophil antibodies in the blood for the diagnosis of infectious mononucleosis, based on the agglutination of sheep erythrocytes by the inactivated serum of patients with the disease.

pause (pawz) an interruption or rest.

compensatory p. the period following a premature ventricular contracture, which causes the R-R cycles of the premature and normal beats to equal the length of two normal beats when added together.

pavor (pa′vor) [L.] terror.

p. diur′nus attacks of anxiety in children during a daytime nap.

p. noctur′nus a sleep disturbance usually occurring in children and characterized by extreme anxiety occurring shortly after sleep onset, with panicky awakening, fear and signs of autonomic arousal, inability to be comforted, poor recall of any dream, and later amnesia for the event. Repeated occurrences are called SLEEP TERROR DISORDER.

Paxil (pak′sil) trademark for preparations of PAROXETINE hydrochloride, an ANTIDEPRESSANT and ANTIANXIETY agent.

payment (pa′ment) remuneration in exchange for goods or services.

prospective p. payment to a health care facility at a predetermined rate for treatment regardless of the cost of care for a specific individual patient.

third party p. payment of hospital or other health care bills by a source other than the patient; the most common sources are private or governmental insurance. Called also third party reimbursement.

PB *Pharmacopoeia Britannica* (British Pharmacopoeia).

Pb lead[1] (L. *plum′bum*).

PBB polybrominated biphenyl.

PBI protein-bound iodine.

p.c. [L.] *post ci′bum (after meals).*

PCA patient-controlled analgesia.

PCB polychlorinated biphenyl.

PCC prothrombin complex concentrate.

PCG phonocardiogram.

PCI percutaneous coronary intervention.

PCO_2 carbon dioxide partial pressure or tension; also written P_{CO_2}, pCO_2, or pCO_2 (see RESPIRATION and BLOOD GAS ANALYSIS).

PCOS polycystic ovary syndrome.

PCP phencyclidine.

PCR polymerase chain reaction.

PCV packed-cell volume.

PD PERITONEAL DIALYSIS.

Pd palladium.

PDA personal digital assistant.

pd potential difference; prism diopter.

PDR *Physicians' Desk Reference.*

PEA pulseless electrical activity.

peanut oil (pe′nut) a refined fixed oil from seed kernels of cultivated varieties of *Arachis hypogaea;* used as a solvent for drugs.

pearl (perl) 1. a smooth lustrous deposit found in certain mollusks, valued as a gem. 2. something resembling this structure, either because of being round and hard or because of being considered valuable. 3. a small medicated granule, or a glass globule with a single dose of volatile medicine, as amyl nitrite. 4. a rounded mass of tough sputum, as seen in the early stages of an attack of ASTHMA.

   clinical **p.** a short, straightforward piece of clinical advice.

   epidermic p's, epithelial p's rounded concentric masses of epithelial cells found in certain papillomas and epitheliomas.

   Laënnec's p's soft casts of the smaller bronchial tubes expectorated in bronchial asthma; see also Curschmann's SPIRALS.

pecten (pek′ten) [L.] 1. a comb; in anatomy, applied to certain comblike structures. 2. a narrow zone in the anal canal, bounded above by the pectinate line. adj., **pectin′eal.**

   p. os′sis pu′bis pectineal line.

pectenitis (pek″tĕ-ni′tis) inflammation of the pecten of the anus.

pectenosis (pek″tĕ-no′sis) stenosis of the anal canal due to an inelastic ring of tissue between the anal groove and anal crypts.

pectin (pek′tin) a one-sugar polymer of sugar acids of fruit that forms gels with sugar at the proper pH. A purified form from the rind of citrus fruits or from apple pomace is used as the protective component of formulations used in treatment of diarrhea and as a suspending agent in pharmaceutical preparations. It is also used in preparation of foods such as jams and jellies.

pectinate (pek′tĭ-nāt) comb-shaped.

pectineal (pek-tin′e-al) pertaining to the os pubis.

pectiniform (pek-tin′ĭ-form) comb-shaped.

pectoral (pek′tor-al) thoracic.

pectoralis (pek″to-ra′lis) [L.] thoracic.

pectoriloquy (pek″to-ril′o-kwe) voice sounds of increased resonance heard through the chest wall, such as EGOPHONY and BRONCHOPHONY.

pectus (pek′tus) thorax.

   p. carina′tum a malformation of the chest wall in which the sternum is abnormally prominent. Moderate cases cause no difficulties and require no treatment; in severe cases the deformity may interfere with lung and heart action, causing dyspnea on exercise and increased susceptibility to respiratory infections. Serious malformations can usually be corrected by surgery. Called also pigeon breast or chest and chicken breast.

   p. excava′tum a congenital malformation of the chest wall characterized by a funnel-shaped depression with its apex over the lower end of the sternum; it is caused by shortening of the central portion of the diaphragm, which pulls the sternum backward during inhalation, and by the growth of ribs. Except in mild cases, it decreases the ability of the child to engage in sustained exercise. It also delays recovery from coughs and colds, reduces the ability to eat a full meal (so that most patients are underweight), and often produces a functional heart murmur. Noisy breathing may occur during sleep. A child may develop an emotional problem because of embarrassment over the deformity. It can be satisfactorily corrected by surgery. Called also funnel breast or chest and koilosternia.

ped(o)- 1. [Gr.] *child.* 2. [L.] *foot.*

pedagogy (ped′ah-go″je) the teaching of children; the teacher often has full responsibility for making decisions about what will be learned, how it will be learned, when it will be learned, and determining if it has been learned. See also ANDRAGOGY.

pedal (ped″l) pertaining to the foot or feet.

pederast (ped′er-ast) one who practices pederasty.

pederasty (ped″er-as′te) anal intercourse between a man and a boy.

pedi- word element [Gr.], *child.* See also PED(O)- (def. 1).

pediatrician (pe″de-ah-trish′un) a physician specializing in PEDIATRICS.

pediatrics (pe″de-at′riks) the branch of medicine dealing with the child, development and care of children, and the nature and treatment of diseases of children. adj., **pediat′ric.**

pedicellation (ped″ĭ-sĕ-la′shun) pediculation (def. 1).

pedicle (ped′ĭ-k′l) a footlike, stemlike, or narrow basal part or structure, such as a narrow strip by which a graft of tissue remains attached to the donor site.

p. of vertebral arch one of the paired parts of the vertebral arch that connect a lamina to the vertebral body.

pediculation (pĕ-dik″u-la′shun) 1. the process of forming a pedicle. 2. pediculosis.

pediculicide (pĕ-dik′u-lĭ-sīd) destroying lice. 1. an agent that destroys lice.

pediculosis (pĕ-dik″u-lo′sis) infestation with lice (see LOUSE). Lice live on the host's blood, obtained by piercing the skin and sucking the blood through the mouth part. The area bitten itches and may become sore and infected from scratching. Not only are lice an annoyance, but they also transmit some diseases, such as typhus.

Treatment. Head lice hatch eggs in silvery oval-shaped envelopes that attach to the shafts of the hairs. The eggs, called nits, can be removed with some difficulty by combing with a very fine-toothed comb. The lice and nits are effectively killed by applications of 1 per cent gamma benzene hexachloride (Kwell) in a cream or shampoo, lindane, permethrin cream or rinse, or pyrethrins and piperonyl butoxide liquid, gel, or shampoo.

p. pu′bis infestation with lice of the species *Phthirus pubis*, the crab louse, usually limited to the pubic hairs but sometimes involving other hairy areas such as the eyelashes, eyebrows, or axillae. It is usually transmitted sexually but may be contracted from bedding and clothing. On the body, it can be treated with a special cream, lotion, or shampoo, such as Kwell, twice daily for two weeks. If the eyelashes are involved, a thick layer of petrolatum should be applied. Called also crabs and phthiriasis.

pediculous (pĕ-dik′u-lus) infested with lice.

Pediculus (pĕ-dik′u-lus) a genus of lice.

P. huma′nus a species that feeds on human blood and is an important vector of relapsing fever, typhus, and trench fever; two subspecies are recognized: *P. humanus* var. *capitis* (head louse) found on the scalp hair, and *P. humanus* var. *corporis* (body, or clothes, louse) found elsewhere on the body.

pedigree (ped′ĭ-gre″) a table, chart, diagram, or list of an individual's ancestors, used in genetics in the analysis of mendelian inheritance.

pedodynamometer (pe″do-di″nah-mom′ĕ-ter) an instrument for measuring leg strength.

pedograph (ped′o-graf) 1. the analysis of a footprint. 2. a device used to obtain footprints for analysis.

pedophilia (pe″do-fil′e-ah) a PARAPHILIA in which an adult desires or engages in sexual relations with a child; it may be either homosexual or heterosexual in nature. adj., **pedophil′ic.**

pedorthics (pĕ-dor′thiks) the design, manufacture, fitting, and modification of shoes and related foot appliances as prescribed for the amelioration of painful or disabling conditions of the lower limb and foot. adj., **pedor′thic.**

pedorthist (pe-dor′thist) a person skilled in pedorthics and practicing its application.

peduncle (pe-dung′k'l) 1. a stemlike connecting part. 2. a collection of nerve fibers connecting between different regions in the central nervous system. 3. the stalk by which a nonsessile tumor is attached to normal tissue. adj., **pedun′cular.**

cerebellar p's three sets of paired bundles (superior, middle, and inferior) connecting the cerebellum to the midbrain, pons, and medulla oblongata, respectively.

cerebral p. the anterior half of the MIDBRAIN, divisible into a posterior part (TEGMENTUM) and an anterior part (CRUS CEREBRI), which are separated by the SUBSTANTIA NIGRA.

inferior cerebellar p. a large bundle of nerve fibers serving to connect the medulla oblongata and spinal cord with the cerebellum (especially the archicerebellum and paleocerebellum); it courses along the lateral border of the fourth ventricle and turns dorsally into the cerebellum. Formerly called caudal cerebellar peduncle.

middle cerebellar p. a large bundle of projection fibers originating in the contralateral pontine nuclei and entering the cerebellum, conveying impulses from the cerebral cortex to the neocerebellum.

pineal p. habenula (def. 2).

superior cerebellar p. a large bundle of projection fibers arising chiefly in the dentate nucleus of each cerebellar hemisphere (neocerebellum) and ascending to decussate in the mesencephalon; its fibers end mostly in the red nucleus and thalamus. Spinocerebellar fibers to the paleocerebellum lie adjacent to each peduncle. Formerly called rostral cerebellar peduncle.

p's of thalamus the four two-way radiations of thalamocortical fibers that connect the dorsal thalamus with many parts of the cerebral cortex, which together form a major portion of the internal capsule and the corona radiata.

pedunculated (pe-dung′ku-lāt″ed) having a peduncle.

pedunculus (pe-dung′ku-lus) peduncle.

peel (pēl) 1. the outer covering of something. 2. to remove such an outer covering.
   chemical p. chemabrasion.
PEEP positive end-expiratory pressure.
peer review 1. a basic component of a QUALITY ASSURANCE program in which the results of health care given to a specific patient population are evaluated according to health-wellness outcome criteria established by peers of the professionals delivering the care. Peer review is focused on the patient and on the results of care given by a group of professionals rather than on individual professional practitioners. Review by peer groups is promoted by professional organizations as a means of maintaining standards of care. *Retrospective review* critically evaluates the results of work that has been completed; it is done for purposes of improving future practice. The source of data is medical records which document the full continuum of care provided and each patient's response to that care. *Concurrent review* takes place at the time the care is being given. It critically examines each patient's progress toward desired health-wellness outcomes. Sources of data for concurrent review are the patient's record and interview, observation, and inspection of the patient. A major advantage of concurrent review is that it provides the opportunity to improve care so that patients benefit from the review and recommended changes in ongoing care. 2. in the NURSING INTERVENTIONS CLASSIFICATION, a nursing INTERVENTION defined as the systematic evaluation of a peer's performance compared with professional standards of practice. 3. Evaluation of a manuscript or research proposal by professional colleagues.
peg (peg) a projecting structure.
   rete p's inward projections of the epidermis into the dermis, as seen histologically in vertical sections.
pegademase (peg-ad′ĕ-mās) adenosine DEAMINASE derived from bovine intestine and attached covalently to POLYETHYLENE GLYCOL, used in replacement therapy for adenosine deaminase deficiency in immuno-compromised patients.
Peganone (peg′ah-nōn) trademark for a preparation of ETHOTOIN, an ANTICONVULSANT.
pegaspargase (peg-as′pahr-jās) L-ASPARA-GINASE derived from *Escherichia coli* and covalently linked to POLYETHYLENE GLYCOL; used as an antineoplastic in the treatment of acute lymphoblastic LEUKEMIA, administered intramuscularly or intravenously.
pegfilgrastim (peg″-fil-gras′tim) a long-acting colony-stimulating FACTOR produced by recombinant technology and used as an adjunct in patients with bone marrow SUPPRESSION caused by ANTINEOPLASTIC therapy.

peginterferon alfa-2b (peg″in″ter-fēr′on) a covalent conjugate of recombinant interferon alfa-2b and polyethylene glycol; a biologic response modifier administered subcutaneously in the treatment of chronic hepatitis C virus infection.
Pel-Ebstein fever (pel′ eb′stīn) a cyclic fever occasionally seen in HODGKIN'S DISEASE and other diseases, characterized by irregular episodes of fever of several days' duration.
pelage (pel′ij, pĕ-lahzh′) [Fr.] the hairy coat of mammals; the hairs of the body, limbs, and head, collectively.
peliosis (pe″le-o′sis) purpura.
pellagra (pĕ-la′grah, pĕ-lag′rah) a syndrome caused by a diet seriously deficient in NIACIN (or by failure to convert TRYPTOPHAN to niacin). Most persons with pellagra also suffer from deficiencies of RIBOFLAVIN (vitamin B_2) and other essential vitamins and minerals. adj., **pellag′rous.**
Pellagra occurs in many areas of the world. In the early 1900s it was the major form of acute vitamin deficiency in the southeastern United States. It is now no longer a problem because of enrichment of cereal, grain, and bread products. Pellagra also occurs in persons suffering from alcoholism and drug addiction.
Symptoms. Chief symptoms of pellagra are various skin, digestive, and mental disturbances. The mouth becomes inflamed and the tongue red and sore; cracks and sores appear in the skin around the mouth. The skin on the back of the hands may become red, thick, and scaly, as may that of the neck and chest, areas exposed to sunlight and the chafing of clothes. Vomiting and loss of appetite occur. Diarrhea often appears early and becomes worse as the disease progresses, thus hampering treatment by preventing effective absorption of essential vitamins. Mental symptoms are variable. In some cases, there may be only insomnia and minor depression. In other cases, the sufferer may become stuporous, or on the contrary become violent and irrational. Headache, irritability, and general anxiety may also be present.
Treatment. Treatment of pellagra consists of an improved diet, often combined with large doses of niacinamide. In acute cases, niacinamide must be administered by injection and must be accompanied by large doses of other vitamins. The diet should include meat (particularly liver), whole grain cereals, and peanuts, all of which are especially good sources of niacin. In severe

cases of pellagra, bed rest is required. Skin lesions are treated with antibiotics.

pellagroid (pĕ-lag′roid) resembling pellagra.

Pellegrini's disease (pel″ĕ-gre′nēz), **Pellegrini-Stieda disease** (pel″ĕ-gre′ne shte′-dah) calcification of the medial collateral ligament of the knee due to trauma.

pellet (pel′et) a small pill or granule.

pellicle (pel′ĭ-k'l) a thin scum forming on the surface of liquids.

   acquired p. a colorless acellular bacteria-free film composed of salivary glycoproteins, deposited on the teeth within minutes after eruption or cleaning.

pellucid (pĕ-lu′sid) translucent.

pelvic (pel′vik) pertaining to the pelvis.

   p. diameter any diameter of the pelvis. The *diagonal conjugate* joins the posterior surface of the pubis to the tip of the sacral promontory; the *external conjugate* joins the depression under the last lumbar spine to the upper margin of the pubis; the *true* or *internal conjugate* is the anteroposterior diameter of the pelvic inlet, measured from the upper margin of the pubic symphysis to the sacrovertebral angle; the *oblique* joins one sacroiliac articulation to the iliopubic eminence of the other side; the *transverse diameter of the inlet* joins the two most widely separated points of the pelvic inlet; and the *transverse diameter of the outlet* joins the medial surfaces of the ischial tuberosities.

   p. inflammatory disease any pelvic infection involving the upper female genital tract beyond the cervix; such diseases are a major cause of female INFERTILITY.

pelvicaliceal (pel″ve-kal″ĭ-se′al) pertaining to the renal PELVIS and CALICES.

pelvicephalometry (pel″vĭ-sef″ah-lom′ĕ-tre) measurement of the fetal head in relation to the maternal pelvis.

pelvifixation (pel″vĭ-fik-sa′shun) surgical fixation of a displaced pelvic organ.

pelvimeter (pel-vim′ĕ-ter) an instrument for measuring the pelvis.

pelvimetry (pel-vim′ĕ-tre) measurement of the capacity and diameter of the pelvis, either internally or externally or both, with the hands or with a pelvimeter.

pelviotomy (pel″ve-ot′ah-me) incision or transection of a pelvic (hip) bone.

pelviperitonitis (pel″vĭ-per″ĭ-to-ni′tis) inflammation of the pelvic peritoneum.

pelvirectal (pel″vĭ-rek′t'l) pertaining to the pelvis and rectum.

pelvis (pel′vis) [L.] 1. any basinlike structure in the body. 2. the bony pelvis, the lower (caudal) portion of the trunk of the body, forming a basin bounded anteriorly and laterally by the hip bones and posteriorly by the SACRUM and COCCYX; it is formed by the sacrum, the coccyx, and the ILIUM, PUBIS, and ISCHIUM, bones that also form the HIP and the pubic ARCH. These bones are separate in the child, but become fused by adulthood. The pelvis is subjected to more stress than any other body structure. Its upper part, which is somewhat flared, supports the weight of internal organs in the upper part of the body. The *floor of the pelvis* or *pelvic floor* is the layer of tissue just below the outlet, formed by the coccygeal and levator ani muscles and the perineal fascia.

   Pelvic structures in men and women differ both in shape and in relative size. The male pelvis is heart-shaped and narrow and proportionately heavier and stronger than that of the female, so that it is better suited for lifting and running. The female pelvis is constructed to accommodate the fetus during pregnancy and to facilitate its downward passage through the pelvic cavity in childbirth. The most obvious difference between the male and female pelvis is in the shape. A woman's hips are wider and her pelvic cavity is round and relatively large. There are differences in the shape of the female pelvis, which must be taken into account in childbirth. During PREGNANCY the capacity of the pelvis and the PELVIC DIAMETERS are measured, so that possible complications during labor can be anticipated.

   android p. one with a wedge-shaped inlet and narrow anterior segment typically found in the male.

   anthropoid p. one whose anteroposterior diameter equals or exceeds the transverse diameter.

   assimilation p. one in which the ilia articulate with the vertebral column higher (*high assimilation pelvis*) or lower (*low assimilation pelvis*) than normal, the number of lumbar vertebrae being correspondingly decreased or increased.

   beaked p. one with the pelvic bones laterally compressed and their anterior junction pushed forward.

   brachypellic p. a short oval type of pelvis, in which the transverse diameter exceeds the anteroposterior diameter by 1 to 3 cm.

   contracted p. one showing a decrease of 1.5 to 2 cm in an important diameter; when all dimensions are proportionately diminished, it is a generally contracted pelvis.

   cordate p. a heart-shaped pelvis.

   dolichopellic p. a long, oval pelvis with the anteroposterior diameter greater than the transverse diameter.

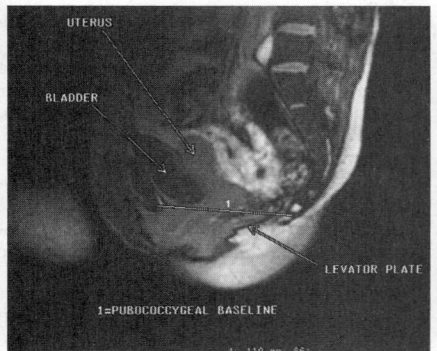

A

1=PUBOCOCCYGEAL BASELINE

UTERUS

BLADDER

LEVATOR PLATE

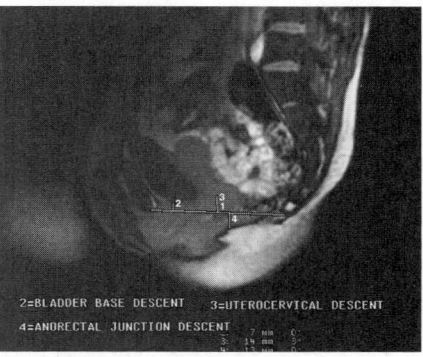

B

2=BLADDER BASE DESCENT   3=UTEROCERVICAL DESCENT
4=ANORECTAL JUNCTION DESCENT

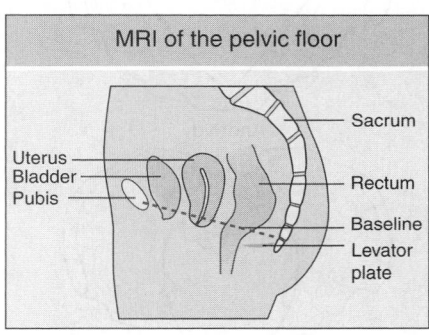

C

MRI of the pelvic floor

Sacrum

Uterus
Bladder
Pubis

Rectum

Baseline

Levator
plate

Dynamic pelvic floor imaging using MRI. MR sequences can now be acquired every half-second or so and this rapidity allows functional studies of the gastrointestinal tract to be undertaken. *A* and *B*, These sagittal views can be used to measure pelvic floor descent as well as to give valuable information on the local anatomy. *C*, Diagrammatic baseline sagittal view. (1 = pubococcygeal baseline; 2 = bladder base descent; 3 = uterocervical descent; 4 = anorectal junction descent.) From Aspinal and Taylor-Robinson, 2001.

extrarenal p. see renal PELVIS.

false p. pelvis major.

flat p. one in which the anteroposterior dimension is abnormally reduced.

frozen p. a condition, due to infection or carcinoma, in which the adnexa and uterus are fixed in the pelvis.

funnel p. one with a normal inlet but a greatly narrowed outlet.

greater p. pelvis major.

gynecoid p. the normal female pelvis: a rounded oval pelvis with well rounded anterior and posterior segments.

infantile p. a generally contracted pelvis with an oval shape, a high sacrum, and inclination of the walls; called also juvenile pelvis.

p. jus'to ma'jor an unusually large gynecoid pelvis, with all dimensions increased.

p. jus'to mi'nor a small gynecoid pelvis, with all dimensions symmetrically reduced.

juvenile p. infantile pelvis.

kyphotic p. a deformed pelvis marked by increase of the conjugate diameter at the brim with decrease of the transverse diameter at the outlet.

lesser p. pelvis minor.

p. ma'jor the part of the pelvis superior to a plane passing through the ileopectineal lines. Called also false pelvis and greater pelvis.

p. mi'nor the part of the pelvis inferior to a plane passing through the ileopectineal lines. Called also lesser pelvis and true pelvis.

Nägele's p. one contracted in an oblique diameter, with complete ankylosis of the sacroiliac synchondrosis on one side and imperfect development of the sacrum and coxa on the same side.

Otto p. one in which the acetabulum is depressed, accompanied by protrusion of the femoral head into the pelvis.

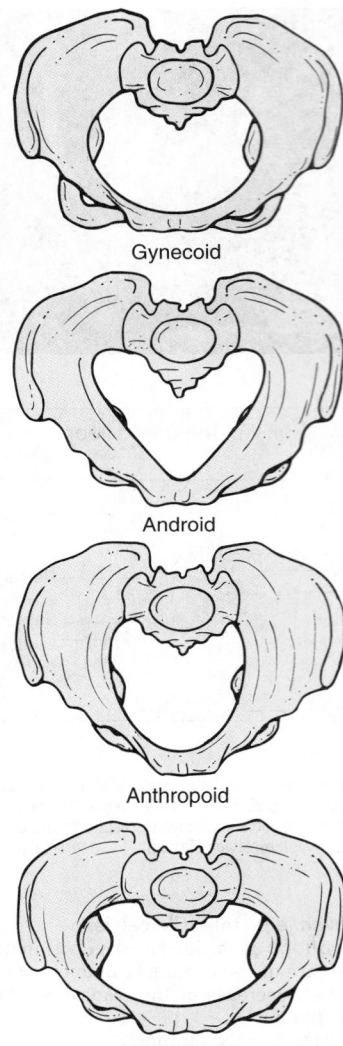

Gynecoid

Android

Anthropoid

Platypelloid

Various types of pelvic inlets.

platypellic p., platypelloid p. one shortened in the anteroposterior aspect, with a flattened transverse, oval shape.

rachitic p. one distorted as a result of rickets.

renal p. the funnel-shaped expansion of the upper end of the URETER into which the renal CALICES open; it is usually within the renal SINUS, but under certain conditions a large part of it may be outside the kidney (*extrarenal pelvis*).

scoliotic p. one deformed as a result of scoliosis.

split p. one with a congenital separation at the symphysis pubis.

spondylolisthetic p. one in which the last, or rarely the fourth or third, lumbar vertebra is dislocated in front of the sacrum, more or less occluding the pelvic brim.

true p. pelvis minor.

pelviureteral (pel″ve-u-re′ter-al) ureteropelvic.

pelvospondylitis (pel″vo-spon″dī-li′tis) inflammation of the pelvic portion of the spine.

p. ossi′ficans ankylosing spondylitis.

pemirolast (pĕ-mir′o-last″) a mast cell stabilizer that inhibits type I hypersensitivity REACTIONS; administered topically to the conjunctiva as the potassium salt to prevent pruritus associated with allergic CONJUNCTIVITIS.

pemoline (pem′o-lēn) a central nervous system STIMULANT used in treatment of ATTENTION-DEFICIT/HYPERACTIVITY DISORDER.

pemphigoid (pem′fĭ-goid) 1. resembling PEMPHIGUS. 2. any of a group of skin disorders similar to but clearly distinguishable from pemphigus.

benign mucosal p. a chronic bullous disease of elderly persons, involving primarily the mucous membranes, particularly the conjunctiva and oral mucosa, with scarring.

bullous p. a usually mild, relatively benign, self-limited blistering skin disease, predominantly affecting elderly persons. IgE antibodies are found at the basement membrane.

localized chronic p. a form in which bulla formation is confined for many years to a circumscribed region, with scarring but without affecting the mucous membranes.

pemphigus (pem′fĭ-gus) any of a group of diseases characterized by successive crops of large bullae ("water blisters"). Although rare, they are serious and require prompt treatment. The cause is unknown; they seem to occur only in adults and can occur in acute or chronic form. The term is often used alone to refer to PEMPHIGUS VULGARIS.

Clusters of blisters usually appear first near or inside the nose and mouth and then gradually spread over the skin of the rest of the body. When the blisters burst, they leave round patches of raw and tender skin. The skin itches, burns and gives off an offensive odor. The patient loses appetite and weight. If the disease is allowed to progress, it may cause extreme weakness, prostration and shock, accompanied by chills, sweating, fever, and often pneumonia.

The patient must be hospitalized from the beginning and given antibiotics and sometimes blood transfusions. Intense discomfort is present and the patient may need to suck anesthetic tablets to allay pain around the mouth while eating. Progress has been made in the treatment of this disease through the persistent use of cortisone, administered orally, and of the pituitary extract ACTH, administered intramuscularly. Fatalities, once fairly common, now can usually be averted. The disease is difficult to control, however, and therapy sometimes must be maintained for years to prevent continuing attacks.

benign familial p. a hereditary, recurrent vesiculobullous dermatitis, usually involving the axillae, groin, and neck, with crops of lesions that regress over several weeks or months. Called also Hailey-Hailey disease.

p. erythemato'sus a variant of pemphigus foliaceus in which the lesions, limited to the face and chest, resemble those of disseminated lupus erythematosus.

p. folia'ceus a superficial, relatively mild and chronic form of pemphigus, usually occurring in the fourth and fifth decades of life, and characterized by the development of small flaccid bullae that rupture and crust and localized or generalized exfoliation. The lesions may be found on the scalp, face, and trunk, or they may spread to become generalized.

p. ve'getans a variant of pemphigus vulgaris in which the bullae are replaced by large wartlike vegetative masses.

p. vulga'ris the most common and severe form of pemphigus, usually occurring between the ages of 40 and 60, characterized by the chronic development of flaccid, easily ruptured bullae upon apparently normal skin and mucous membranes, beginning focally but progressing to become generalized, leaving large, weeping, denuded surfaces that become partially crusted over with little or no tendency to heal and that enlarge by confluence. In untreated cases, sepsis, cachexia, and electrolyte imbalance may occur and lead to death.

penbutolol (pen-bu'tah-lol) a BETA-ADRENERGIC BLOCKING AGENT with intrinsic sympathomimetic activity; used as an ANTIHYPERTENSIVE in the form of the sulfate salt.

penciclovir (pen-si'klo-vir) a compound that inhibits viral DNA synthesis in HERPESVIRUSES 1 and 2, used in the treatment of recurrent herpes labialis; applied topically.

pendelluft (pen'del-looft'') the movement of air back and forth between the lungs, resulting in increased dead space ventilation.

pendulous (pen'du-lus) hanging loosely; dependent.

penectomy (pe-nek'to-me) surgical removal of the penis.

penetrability (pen''ĕ-trah-bil'ĭ-te) the ability of x-rays to penetrate matter.

penetrance (pen'ĕ-trans) the frequency with which a heritable trait is manifested by individuals carrying the principal gene or genes conditioning it.

penetrometer (pen''ĕ-trom'ĕ-ter) an instrument for measuring the penetrating power of x-rays; qualimeter.

-penia word element [Gr.], *deficiency.*

penicillamine (pen''ĭ-sil'ah-mēn) a degradation product of PENICILLIN that chelates certain heavy metals; used orally to reduce the blood COPPER level in WILSON'S DISEASE and to promote excretion of CYSTINE in patients with CYSTINURIA or recurrent cystine renal calculus formation, by helping to solubilize cystine. It is also used as a disease-modifying antirheumatic DRUG in treatment of refractory rheumatoid ARTHRITIS.

penicillin (pen''ĭ-sil'in) any of a large group of natural or semisynthetic antibacterial ANTIBIOTICS derived directly or indirectly from strains of fungi of the genus *Penicillium* and other soil-inhabiting fungi grown on special culture media. Penicillins exert a bacteriocidal as well as a bacteriostatic effect on susceptible bacteria by interfering with the final stages of the synthesis of peptidoglycan, a substance in the bacterial cell wall. Despite their relatively low toxicity for the host, they are active against many bacteria, especially gram-positive pathogens (streptococci, staphylococci, pneumococci); clostridia; certain gram-negative forms (gonococci and meningococci); certain spirochetes (*Treponema pallidum* and *T. pertenue*); and certain fungi. Certain strains of some target species, for example staphylococci, secrete the enzyme PENICILLINASE, which inactivates penicillin and confers resistance to the antibiotic. Some of the newer penicillins, such as METHICILLIN, are more effective against penicillinase-producing organisms. A class of extended-spectrum penicillins includes PIPERACILLIN and MEZLOCILLIN. Penicillin is administered intramuscularly, orally, in liquid or tablet form, and topically in ointments. Oral administration requires larger doses of the drug because absorption is incomplete. Allergic reactions occur in some persons. The reaction may be slight—a stinging or burning sensation at the site of injection—or it can be more serious—severe dermatitis or even anaphylactic shock, which may be fatal.

p. G the most widely used penicillin, used principally in the treatment of infections due to gram-positive organisms, gram-negative cocci, *Treponema pallidum* and *Actinomyces israelii.* The usual forms are salts such as *penicillin benzathine, potassium, procaine,* or *sodium.* Called also benzylpenicillin.

p. V a biosynthetically or semisynthetically produced ANTIBIOTIC similar to PENICILLIN G, used orally in the form of the benzathine or potassium salt for mild to moderately severe infections due to susceptible gram-positive bacteria.

penicillinase (pen″ĭ-sil′ĭ-nās) an enzyme produced by certain bacteria that inactivates PENICILLIN, so that such bacteria have increased resistance to the antibiotic; a purified form from *Bacillus cereus* is used in treatment of reactions to penicillin.

Penicillium a genus of imperfect fungi of the form-class Hyphomycetes; many species are commonly found in the human environment. Some are toxic, and others are sources of PENICILLINS.

penicilliosis (pen″ĭ-sil″e-o′sis) infection by species of *Penicillium,* usually consisting of a pulmonary infection with fever, coughing, and leukocytosis.

penicilloyl polylysine (pen″ĭ-sil′oil pol″ĕ-li′sēn) benzylpenicilloyl polylysine.

penicillus (pen″ĭ-sil′us) [L.] any of the brushlike groups of arterial branches in the lobules of the spleen.

penile (pe′nīl) of or pertaining to the penis.

p. prosthesis a device that is surgically implanted to overcome the problem of IMPOTENCE. Several different designs are currently available; some are semirigid, others can be inflated when an erection is desired and deflated after intercourse. A penile prosthesis does not interfere with the physiologic mechanisms of sexual intercourse, orgasm, or ejaculation.

penis (pe′nis) the external male organ of urination and copulation.

The body of the penis consists of three cylindrical-shaped masses of erectile tissue which run the length of the penis. Two of the masses lie alongside each other and end behind the head of the penis. The third mass lies underneath them. This latter mass contains the urethra. The penis terminates in an oval or cone-shaped body, the glans penis, which contains the exterior opening of the urethra.

The glans penis is covered by a loose skin, the foreskin or prepuce, which enables it to expand freely during erection. The skin ends just behind the glans penis and folds forward to cover it. The inner surface of the foreskin contains glands that secrete a lubricating fluid called smegma which makes it easy for the penis to expand and retract past the foreskin.

buried p. concealed penis.

clubbed p. penile curvature.

concealed p. a small penis concealed beneath a fat pad or the skin of the scrotum, abdomen, or thigh; called also buried penis.

double p. diphallus.

webbed p. a penis enclosed by the skin of the scrotum.

penitis (pe-ni′tis) inflammation of the penis.

penniform (pen′ĭ-form) shaped like a feather.

pent(a)- word element [Gr.], *five.*

pentaerythritol (pen″tah-e-rith′rĭ-tol) a coronary VASODILATOR used in treatment of ANGINA PECTORIS, used as the tetranitrate ester.

pentagastrin (pen″tah-gas′trin) a synthetic pentapeptide consisting of β-alanine and C-terminal tetrapeptide of gastrin; used as a test of gastric secretory function.

pentamidine (pen-tam′ĭ-dēn) an anti-infective used as the isethionate salt, administered intravenously or intramuscularly in treatment of early African TRYPANOSOMIASIS and LEISHMANIASIS, and intravenously, intramuscularly, or by oral inhalation in treatment and prophylaxis of *Pneumocystis carinii* PNEUMONIA.

pentasomy (pen″tah-so′me) the presence of three additional chromosomes of one type (e.g., 5 X chromosomes) in an otherwise diploid cell (2n + 3).

pentavalent (pen″tah-va′lent) having a valence of five.

pentazocine (pen-taz′o-sēn) a synthetic opioid ANALGESIC, used in the form of the hydrochloride and lactate salts as an analgesic and anesthesia adjunct; administered orally or parenterally.

pentetate (pen′tĕ-tāt) a salt, anion, ester, or complex of pentetic acid.

pentetic acid (pen-te′tik) diethylenetriamine pentaacetic acid, DTPA; a chelating agent (iron) with the general properties of the edetates; used in preparing RADIOPHARMACEUTICALS.

Penthrane (pen′thrān) trademark for a preparation of methoxyflurane, an inhalation anesthetic.

pentobarbital (pen″to-bahr′bĭ-tal) a short- to intermediate-acting BARBITURATE used in the form of the sodium salt as a SEDATIVE AND HYPNOTIC, usually presurgery, and as an ANTICONVULSANT.

pentosan (pen′to-san″) a carbohydrate derivative used as an ANTIINFLAMMATORY, in the form of *pentosan polysulfate sodium*, in the treatment of interstitial cystitis; administered orally.

pentose (pen′tōs) a monosaccharide containing five carbon atoms in a molecule.

pentoside (pen′to-sīd) a compound (glycoside) of pentose with another substance.

pentostatin (pen″to-stat′in) a highly toxic antitumor ANTIBIOTIC administered intravenously in the treatment of refractory hairy cell LEUKEMIA.

pentosuria (pen″to-su′re-ah) excretion of PENTOSES in the urine; *benign pentosuria* is an inborn ERROR of metabolism due to a defect in the activity of the enzyme L-xylulose dehydrogenase, resulting in high levels of L-xylulose in the urine.

Pentothal (pen′to-thal) trademark for a preparation of thiopental sodium, used as an anesthetic.

pentoxifylline (pen″tok-sif′ah-lin) a XANTHINE derivative that reduces blood viscosity; used for the symptomatic relief of INTERMITTENT CLAUDICATION in peripheral vascular disease.

penumbra (pě-num′brah) 1. the part of a shadow in which there is a small amount of illumination from a light source. 2. blurring at the edges of a structure on a radiograph.

Pen Vee K (pen′ve) trademark for preparations of PENICILLIN V potassium, an ANTIBIOTIC.

peplomer (pep′lo-mer) a subunit of a peplos.

peplos (pep′los) envelope (def. 2).

peppermint oil a volatile oil from fresh overground parts of the flowering plant of peppermint *(Mentha piperita);* used as a flavoring agent for drugs, and as a gastric stimulant and carminative.

pepsin (pep′sin) a proteolytic enzyme that is the principal digestive component of gastric juice. It acts as a catalyst in the chemical breakdown of protein to form a mixture of polypeptides; it is formed from pepsinogen in the presence of acid or, autocatalytically, in the presence of pepsin itself. Pepsin also has milk-clotting action similar to that of rennin and thereby facilitates the digestion of milk protein.

pepsinogen (pep-sin′o-jen) a zymogen secreted by the chief cells of the gastric glands and converted into pepsin in the presence of gastric acid or of pepsin itself.

peptic (pep′tik) 1. pertaining to PEPSIN. 2. pertaining to digestion by or other action of GASTRIC JUICES.

   p. ulcer a loss of tissues lining the lower esophagus, stomach, or duodenum; an acute lesion that does not extend through the muscularis mucosae is simply called an EROSION. Chronic ulcers involve the muscular coat, destroying the musculature and replacing it with permanent scar tissue at the site of healing.

   Cause. While it is known that gastric HYDROCHLORIC ACID and PEPSIN are responsible for ulcer formation, it is not known why mucosal resistance to them should become impaired. Duodenal ulcers and some prepyloric gastric ulcers are associated with an increased amount or hyperacidity of the gastric juice. Gastric ulcers, on the other hand, are not associated with excessive acid levels. Theories about genetic and environmental causes of peptic ulcer abound. Both gastric and duodenal ulcers tend to occur in families. Relatives of persons with gastric ulcers have three times the expected number of gastric ulcers. The same is true of duodenal ulcers. There is evidence that the increased familial incidence of both gastric and duodenal ulcers is not just due to a shared environment. An infection with *Helicobacter pylori* may contribute to ulceration, particularly in persons with a history of chronic GASTRITIS.

   Psychosomatic factors are known to play some role in the development of peptic ulcers. Psychologic stress can and does alter gastric function. Prolonged psychologic or physiologic stress produces what is known as a *stress ulcer,* which differs pathologically and clinically from a chronic peptic ulcer in being more acute and more likely to produce hemorrhage; perforation occurs occasionally and pain is rare. Conditions often associated with stress ulcers include severe trauma, surgery, advanced malignancy, extensive burns (Curling's ulcer), and brain injury.

   Drug-induced ulcers are most commonly caused by the ingestion of ASPIRIN, with ALCOHOL running a close second. Other drugs that are strongly suspected of being ulcerogenic include the GLUCOCORTICOIDS, INDOMETHACIN, and PHENYLBUTAZONE.

   Symptoms. The cardinal symptom of peptic ulcer is epigastric pain that may be described as burning, gnawing, cramping, or aching, and usually comes in waves that last several minutes. The daily pattern of pain is related to the secretion of acid and the presence of food in the stomach to act as a buffer. This pain is diminished in the morning when secretion is low and after meals when food is present. The pain is most severe before meals and at bedtime. It often appears for three or four days or

P

weeks and then subsides only to reappear weeks or months later. Other symptoms of uncomplicated peptic ulcer include nausea, loss of appetite, and sometimes weight loss.

Complications. The three major complications of ulcer are hemorrhage, perforation, and obstruction. Bleeding may be manifested by emesis of bright red blood or of coffee-ground vomitus, and by tarry feces. The bleeding may vary from massive hemorrhage to occult (hidden) bleeding that occurs over a period of time. Perforation frequently is a surgical emergency because of the possibility of a chemical peritonitis caused by spilling of the gastric and intestinal contents into the peritoneal cavity. Obstruction of the upper intestinal tract occurs as a result of scarring and loss of musculature at the pylorus. It is manifested by persistent vomiting that can quickly bring on ALKALOSIS because of the loss of gastric acid in the vomitus. The obstruction is treated by surgical removal of the scar tissue.

Diagnosis. The most commonly used technique in the diagnosis of peptic ulcers is an upper gastrointestinal series with a BARIUM TEST (barium swallow). Double contrast films are sometimes done to clearly define the mucosal pattern in the upper gastrointestinal tract. GASTROSCOPY may be helpful in establishing the site of bleeding in a gastric ulcer, in differentiating between benign and malignant ulcerations based on biopsies, and between esophageal ulcer and diverticulum. Gastric analysis to determine level of acidity may be helpful in some cases but there is much individual variation in gastric acid secretions among patients with ulcer.

Treatment. The primary goals of medical treatment of peptic ulcers are: (1) relief of symptoms, (2) promotion of healing, (3) prevention of complications, and (4) prevention of recurrences. Because each patient responds differently to various modes of treatment, the medical regimen is planned according to individual needs and responses.

In general the medical management of ulcers hinges on ANTACIDS, drugs such as CIMETIDINE that are antagonistic to histamine H_2 RECEPTORS, anticholinergic drugs, and sedatives; this is also accompanied by dietary modification and identifying and relieving sources of psychologic stress. Antacids such as MAGNESIUM HYDROXIDE and ALUMINUM HYDROXIDE relieve the pain of ulcer by decreasing the levels of gastric hydrochloric acid and pepsin.

CIMETIDINE is an antagonist of histamine H_2 RECEPTORS and inhibits gastric acid secretion; it is easier to take than liquid antacids. It is an effective treatment for peptic ulcers but produces side effects in some patients, e.g., breast enlargement in men, mental confusion in elderly patients, and delayed hepatic metabolism of other drugs. SUCRALFATE, which is not absorbed into the body, is an alternative drug that has fewer side effects and is also effective. Another drug, RANITIDINE, has action similar to that of cimetidine, but has greater potency, can be taken less frequently, and has fewer side effects.

If *Helicobacter pylori* is found in the ulcer, the patient is treated with antibiotics.

Most ulcers can be treated without surgery when patients cooperate fully; however, surgery may be necessary in certain cases, such as when there is scarring of the ulcer (producing obstruction), recurrent bleeding, extreme pain, and perforation. Gastric ulcers

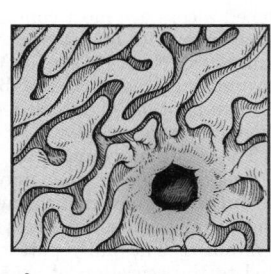

A ENDOSCOPIC VIEW

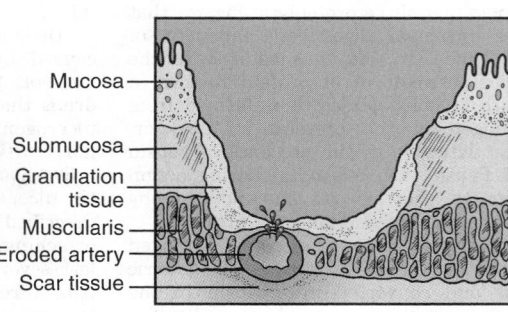

B HISTOLOGIC CROSS SECTION

Mucosa
Submucosa
Granulation tissue
Muscularis
Eroded artery
Scar tissue

Peptic ulcer. *A,* Gross appearance of the ulcer as seen by endoscopy. *B,* Histologically, the bottom of the ulcer replacing the mucosa consists mostly of granulation tissue and admixed necrotic cell debris and inflammatory cells. Peptic ulcer may bleed from eroded mucosa blood vessels. The tissue underlying the ulcer shows fibrosis and scarring. From Damjanov, 2000.

are more likely to require surgery than are duodenal ulcers. The operative procedure most frequently done for a gastric ulcer is subtotal GASTRECTOMY, in which the ulcerous portion of the stomach is removed (see also surgery of the STOMACH). This procedure is often done in conjunction with VAGOTOMY, division of the vagus nerve, which eliminates cerebral stimuli of the stomach muscle and glands, thereby reducing gastric motility and secretion.

Patient Care. Assessment data pertinent to peptic ulcer patients include information about (1) family history of peptic ulcer, (2) the patient's eating habits and how eating affects symptoms, (3) whether the patient drinks or smokes and to what extent, (4) any history of psychological or physical stress such as severe trauma, burns, or other conditions that might produce a stress ulcer, and (5) any drugs the patient might be taking that are irritants to the gastrointestinal tract.

Dietary restrictions are usually limited to those foods, if any, that an individual identifies with the onset or worsening of symptoms. Exceptions are alcohol and caffeine, both of which are capable of inducing gastritis and promoting erosion of the gastric mucosa. It is generally agreed that what the patient with an ulcer eats is not as important as when it is eaten. Frequent and regular feedings throughout the day, rather than two or three large meals, are encouraged. Patients should not skip meals and should try to have some nonirritating food in the stomach at all times.

Patient education includes the following: (1) Regulate the types of foods eaten and the manner in which they are eaten. Meals should be unhurried, relaxed, and spaced at regular intervals. (2) Try to avoid situations of stress and anxiety and develop some effective skills for coping with stress. (3) Drink water at least once every hour when awake. This acts to dilute gastric juices, making them less corrosive. (4) Stop or at least cut down on smoking. (5) Keep alcohol intake to a minimum. (6) Report any side effects of antacids or other drugs to the health care provider. There are alternative drugs if the side effects of one are worrisome. (7) Take prescribed medications exactly as ordered and do not discontinue them without consulting the health care provider. (8) Avoid taking aspirin; develop the habit of reading labels of nonprescription drugs to ascertain whether they contain acetylsalicylic acid. Since some prescription drugs also contain aspirin, inform any health care provider treating a coexisting condition that aspirin cannot be tolerated.

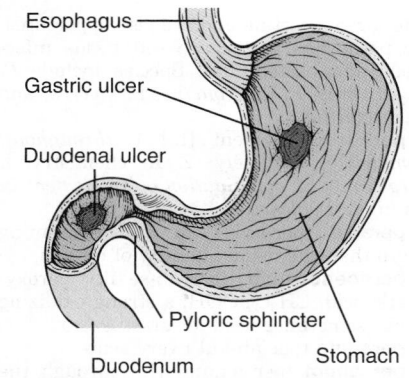

Most common sites for peptic ulcer disease. From Frazier et al., 2000.

peptidase (pep'tĭ-dās) any of a subclass of proteolytic enzymes that catalyze the hydrolysis of peptide linkages.

peptide (pep'tīd) any member of a class of compounds of low molecular weight that yield two or more AMINO ACIDS on hydrolysis. They are the constituent parts of PROTEINS and are formed by loss of water from the NH_2 and COOH groups of adjacent amino acids. Peptides are known as dipeptides, tripeptides, tetrapeptides, and so on depending on the number of amino acids in the molecule. See also POLYPEPTIDE.

vasoactive intestinal p. vasoactive intestinal polypeptide.

peptidergic (pep″tĭ-der'jik) of or pertaining to neurons that secrete peptide hormones.

peptidoglycan (pep″tĭ-do-gli'kan) a glycan (polysaccharide) attached to short crosslinked peptides; found in bacterial cell walls.

peptidyl-dipeptidase A (pep'tĭdil di-pep'tĭ-dās) angiotensin-converting enzyme.

Peptococcus (pep″to-kok'us) a genus of gram-positive, anaerobic, coccoid bacteria; they are part of the flora of the mouth, upper respiratory tract, and large intestine, and also cause soft tissue infection and bacteremias. *P. mag'nus* is the species most often recovered from clinical specimens.

peptogenic (pep″to-jen'ik) 1. producing pepsin or peptones. 2. promoting digestion.

peptolysis (pep-tol'ĭ-sis) the splitting up of peptone. adj., **peptolyt'ic.**

Peptostreptococcus (pep″to-strep″to-kok'us) a genus of gram-positive, aerobic, coccoid bacteria; they are part of the normal flora of the mouth, upper respiratory tract,

P

and large intestine and are also opportunistic pathogens that cause soft tissue infections and bacteremias. Species include *P. anaero'bius, P. lanceola'tus, P. mi'cros,* and *P. produc'tus.*

per- word element [L.] 1. *throughout; completely; extremely.* 2. in chemistry, *a large amount; combination of an element in its highest valence.*

peracid (per-as'id) an acid containing more than the usual quantity of oxygen.

peracetic acid (per″ah-se'tik) peroxyacetic acid, CH₃COOOH, a strong oxidizing agent sometimes used for STERILIZATION.

peracute (per″ah-kūt′) very acute.

per anum (per a'num) [L.] through the anus.

percentile (per-sen'tīl) any one of the 99 values that divide the RANGE of a probability DISTRIBUTION or sample into 100 intervals of equal probability or frequency; for example, 45 per cent of a population scores below the 45th percentile.

percept (per'sept) the object perceived; the mental image of an object in space perceived by the senses.

perception (per-sep'shun) the conscious mental registration of a sensory stimulus. adj., **percep'tive.**

depth p. the ability to recognize depth or the relative distances to different objects in space.

disturbed sensory p. a NURSING DIAGNOSIS accepted by the North American Nursing Diagnosis Association, defined as a change in the amount of patterning of incoming stimuli, accompanied by a diminished, exaggerated, distorted, or impaired response to such stimuli.

extrasensory p. **(ESP)** knowledge of, or response to, an external thought or objective event not achieved as the result of stimulation of the sense organs.

perceptivity (per″sep-tiv′ĭ-te) ability to receive sense impressions.

Percocet (per'ko-set) trademark for a combination preparation of OXYCODONE hydrochloride WITH ACETAMINOPHEN, an opioid ANALGESIC

Percodan (per-ko'dan) trademark for a combination preparation of OXYCODONE hydrochloride, OXYCODONE terephthalate, and ASPIRIN, used as an opioid analgesic.

percolate (per'ko-lāt) 1. to strain; to submit to percolation. 2. a liquid that has been submitted to percolation. 3. to trickle slowly through a substance.

percolation (per″ko-la'shun) the extraction of soluble parts of a drug by passing a solvent liquid through it.

percolator (per″ko-la'ter) a vessel used in percolation.

percuss (per-kus′) to perform percussion.

percussible (per-kus'ĭ-b'l) detectable on percussion.

percussion (per-kush'un) 1. in physical examination, striking a part of the body with short, sharp blows of the fingers in order to determine the size, position, and density of the underlying parts by the sound obtained. Percussion is most commonly used on the chest and back for examination of the heart and lungs. For example, since the heart is not resonant and the adjacent lungs are, when the examiner's fingers strike the chest over the heart the sound waves will change in pitch. This serves as a guide to the precise location and size of the heart. 2. the rhythmic clapping of cupped hands over various segments of the lungs to mobilize secretions; called also cupping.

auscultatory p. auscultation of the sound produced by percussion.

immediate p. that in which the blow is struck directly against the body surface.

mediate p. that in which a pleximeter is used.

palpatory p. a combination of palpation and percussion, affording tactile rather than auditory impressions.

percussor (per-kus'er) an instrument for performing percussion.

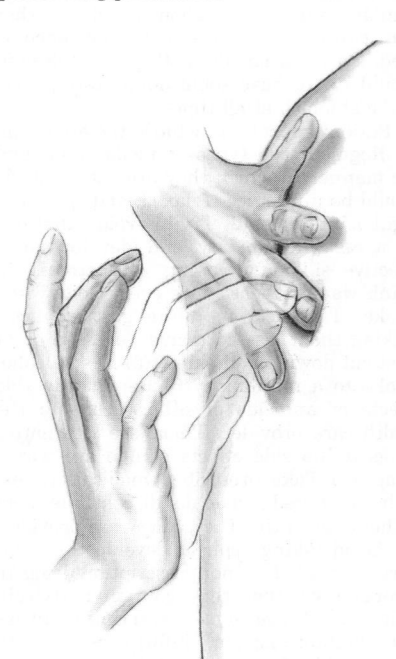

Percussion. (def. 1) From Jarvis, 1996.

percutaneous (per″ku-ta′ne-us) performed through the skin; see also TRANSDERMAL.

perencephaly (per″en-sef′ah-le) porencephaly.

Pereyra procedure (colposuspension) (pĕ-ra′rah) 1. a surgical technique for the correction of stress incontinence: a loop of suture or other material is inserted through the paraurethral tissue near the bladder neck and attached to the abdominal fascia in order to elevate the bladder. 2. a type of bladder neck suspension similar to the Burch procedure; a loop of suture or other material is inserted through the paraurethral tissue near the bladder neck and attached to the abdominal fascia.

perfectionism (per-fek′shun-izm) the setting for oneself or others of a standard of flawless work or performance, or at least of one that is higher than the situation requires.

perfluorocarbon (per-floor′o-kahr″bon) any of various substances chemically related to a HYDROCARBONS but with the hydrogen atoms replaced by fluorine atoms. In gaseous form they cause environmental damage by collecting in the upper atmosphere; in liquid form, some are used in partial liquid VENTILATION.

perforans (per′fo-rans) [L.] penetrating or perforating; a term applied to various muscles and nerves.

perforation (per″fo-ra′shun) a hole or break in the containing walls or membranes of an organ or structure of the body. Perforation occurs when erosion, infection, or other factors create a weak spot in the organ and internal pressure causes a rupture. It also may result from a deep penetrating wound caused by trauma.

performance (per-form′ans) action taken to fulfill a task.

p. **components** formerly, in OCCUPATIONAL THERAPY, aspects of functional ability required for occupational PERFORMANCE; they were grouped into sensorimotor, cognitive, and psychological subcategories.

ineffective role p. a NURSING DIAGNOSIS accepted by the North American Nursing Diagnosis Association, defined as patterns of behavior and self-expression that do not match the environmental context, norms, and expectations; this may be a change in self-perception or perception by someone else, a denial of role, a conflict between roles, a change in capacity to perform a role, or some other change.

occupational p. in OCCUPATIONAL THERAPY, performance of all the activities that make up the individual's lifestyle; see also PERFORMANCE COMPONENTS.

role p. the fulfilling of an expected pattern of behavior.

perfusate (per-fu′zāt) a liquid that has been subjected to perfusion.

perfusion (per-fu′zhun) 1. the act of pouring through or over; especially the passage of a fluid through the vessels of a specific organ. 2. a liquid poured through or over an organ or tissue.

tissue p. the circulation of blood through the vascular bed of tissue.

ineffective tissue p. (specify type) (renal, cerebral, cardiopulmonary, gastrointestinal, peripheral) a NURSING DIAGNOSIS accepted by the North American Nursing Diagnosis Association, defined as a state in which an individual has a decrease in oxygen resulting in failure to nourish the tissues at the capillary level.

perfusionist (per-fu′zhun-ist) a technologist who operates the heart-lung machine during cardiopulmonary bypass.

pergolide (per′go-līd) a long-acting ERGOT derivative with DOPAMINERGIC properties; used as the mesylate salt in treatment of PARKINSONISM, administered orally.

peri- word element [Gr.], *around; near.* See also PARA-[1].

periacinal (per″e-as′ĭ-nal) around an ACINUS; called also periacinous.

periacinous (per″e-as′ĭ-nus) periacinal.

Periactin (per″e-ak′tin) trademark for preparations of CYPROHEPTADINE hydrochloride, an ANTIHISTAMINE used for relief of allergy and itching.

periadenitis (per″e-ad″ĕ-ni′tis) inflammation of tissues around a gland.

p. muco′sa necro′tica recur′rens the more severe form of aphthous STOMATITIS, marked by recurrent attacks of aphthalike lesions that begin as small, firm nodules that later enlarge, ulcerate, and heal by scar formation, leaving atrophied scars on the oral mucosa. Called also Sutton's disease.

periampullary (per″e-am′pu-lar″e) around an AMPULLA.

perianal (per″e-a′nal) around the anus.

periangiitis (per″e-an″je-i′tis) inflammation of the tissue around a blood or lymph vessel.

periangiocholitis (per″e-an″je-o-ko-li′tis) inflammation of tissues around the bile ducts; pericholangitis.

periaortitis (per″e-a″or-ti′tis) inflammation of tissues around the aorta.

periapical (per″e-a′pĭ-k'l) surrounding the apex of the root of a tooth.

periappendicitis (per″e-ah-pen″dĭ-si′tis) inflammation of the vermiform appendix and surrounding tissues.

periarterial (per″e-ahr-tēr′e-al) around an artery.

periarteritis (per″e-ahr″ter-i′tis) inflammation of the outer coat of an artery and of the tissues surrounding it.

p. gummo′sa accumulation of gummas on the blood vessels in syphilis.

p. nodo′sa polyarteritis nodosa.

periarthritis (per″e-ahr-thri′tis) inflammation of the tissues around a joint.

periarticular (per″e-ahr-tik′u-ler) around a joint; called also juxta-articular.

periaxial (per″e-ak′se-al) around an axis.

periaxillary (per″e-ak′sĭ-lar″e) around the axilla.

periblast (per′ĭ-blast) the portion of the BLASTODERM of a telolecithal OVUM, in which cells lack complete cell membranes.

peribronchial (per″ĭ-brong′ke-al) around a bronchus or bronchi.

peribronchiolar (per″ĭ-brong″ke-o′ler) around the bronchioles.

peribronchiolitis (per″ĭ-brong″ke-o-li′tis) inflammation of the tissues around the bronchioles.

peribronchitis (per″ĭ-brong-ki′tis) a form of bronchitis consisting of inflammation and thickening of the tissues around the bronchi.

pericaliceal (per″ĭ-kal″ĭ-se′al) near or around a renal CALIX; also spelled pericalyceal.

pericallosal (per″ĭ-kah-lo′sal) situated around the corpus callosum.

pericalyceal (per″ĭ-kal″ĭ-se′al) pericaliceal.

pericardiac (per″ĭ-kahr′de-ak) 1. pericardial. 2. pertaining to the PERICARDIUM.

pericardial (per″ĭ-kahr′de-al) pertaining to the area around the heart.

pericardicentesis (per″ĭ-kahr″dĭ-sen-te′-sis) pericardiocentesis.

pericardiectomy (per″ĭ-kahr″de-ek′to-me) excision of a portion of the pericardium.

pericardiocentesis (per″ĭ-kahr″de-o-sen-te′sis) surgical puncture into the pericardial space and aspiration of fluid for therapeutic or diagnostic purposes. Therapeutically, the procedure is used as an emergency measure to relieve life-threatening cardiac tamponade. Other clinical situations in which it may be done include pericardial effusion, traumatic perforation or rupture of the myocardium, and effusion secondary to a tumor or chest injury. Since serious dysrhythmias can develop, cardiac monitoring is necessary throughout the procedure. Blood pressure, pulse, and heart rhythm also are monitored during it and for 24 hours afterwards. Serious and life-threatening immediate complications are possible, such as perforation of a ventricle, laceration

of a coronary artery, aspiration of blood from a heart chamber, or air embolism. Infection and hydropneumothorax can develop later.

pericardiolysis (per″ĭ-kahr″de-ol′ĭ-sis) the operative freeing of adhesions between the visceral and parietal pericardium.

pericardiophrenic (per″ĭ-kahr″de-o-fren′-ik) pertaining to the pericardium and diaphragm.

pericardiopleural (per″ĭ-kahr″de-o-ploo′ral) pertaining to the pericardium and pleura.

pericardiorrhaphy (per″ĭ-kahr″de-or′ah-fe) suture of the pericardium.

pericardiostomy (per″ĭ-kahr″de-os′tah-me) creation of an opening into the pericardium, usually for drainage of effusions.

pericardiotomy (per″ĭ-kahr″de-ot′ah-me) incision of pericardium.

pericarditis (per″ĭ-kahr-di′tis) inflammation of the pericardium. adj., **pericardit′ic.**

Types of Pericarditis. There are many forms of pericarditis. *Acute pericarditis* is usually secondary to some other bacterial infection, such as osteomyelitis, lung abscess, or pneumonia. It may also occur without bacterial infection, resulting from a tumor, rheumatic heart disease, uremia, coronary thrombosis, myocardial infarction, chest wound, or surgery in which the pericardium is pierced. It may be dry, or fibrinous, with a fibrinous exudate on the serous membrane, or accompanied by effusion, accumulation of fluid in the pericardial cavity.

Occasionally the pericardium is affected directly by what appears to be a virus; this condition is called *acute nonspecific pericarditis.*

Another form, *chronic pericarditis,* is usually adhesive; that is, the heart is anchored to surrounding tissues by adhesions. It sometimes follows acute pericarditis, but often the cause is unknown. In its constrictive form (*chronic constrictive pericarditis*), which may be tuberculous in origin, calcium and fibrous deposits may form around the heart and interfere with its movements. This form may be extremely serious and difficult to cure.

Symptoms and Treatment. The symptoms of acute pericarditis vary with the cause but usually include chest pain and dyspnea, an increase in the pulse rate, and a rise in temperature. There is often a pericardial friction rub with serial changes on the electrocardiogram. In dry pericarditis the friction rub is distinct, caused by deposits of fibrin, and may be heard through a stethoscope. In the effusive form, the excess accumulation of pericardial fluid can be detected by x-rays or electrocardiography. The excess fluid is sometimes drained by PERICARDIOCENTESIS.

Treatment of acute pericarditis is directed mainly at curing its original cause. Antibiotics have proved successful in treating bacterial pericarditis. Many patients with nonspecific pericarditis with effusion are helped dramatically by cortisone medications.

In the constrictive form of chronic pericarditis there may be dyspnea and pain in the heart region, plus symptoms elsewhere in the body, such as edema, enlargement of the liver, or distention of the neck veins. The best means of treatment is surgery to remove the constrictions and permit free heart action.

pericardium (per″ĭ-kahr′de-um) the fibroserous sac enclosing the heart and the roots of the great vessels, composed of external (fibrous) and internal (serous) layers.

   adherent p. one abnormally connected with the heart by dense fibrous tissue.

   fibrous p. the external layer of the pericardium, consisting of dense fibrous tissue.

   parietal p. the parietal layer of the serous pericardium, which is in contact with the fibrous pericardium.

   serous p. the inner, serous portion of pericardium, consisting of two layers, visceral and parietal; the space between the layers is the pericardial CAVITY.

   visceral p. the inner layer of the serous pericardium, which is in contact with the heart and roots of the great vessels. Called also epicardium.

pericecal (per″ĭ-se′kal) around the CECUM.

pericecitis (per″ĭ-se-si′tis) inflammation of the tissues around the cecum.

pericellular (per″ĭ-sel′u-lar) surrounding a cell.

pericholangitis (per″ĭ-ko″lan-ji′tis) inflammation of tissues surrounding the bile ducts; periangiocholitis.

pericholecystitis (per″ĭ-ko″le-sis-ti′tis) inflammation of tissues around the gallbladder.

perichondritis (per″ĭ-kon-dri′tis) inflammation of the perichondrium.

perichondrium (per″ĭ-kon′dre-um) the layer of fibrous connective tissue investing all cartilage except the articular cartilage of synovial joints. adj., **perichon′dral.**

perichordal (per″ĭ-kor′dal) surrounding the NOTOCHORD.

perichoroidal (per″ĭ-kor-oi′dal) surrounding the choroid coat of the eye.

pericolic (per″ĭ-kol′ik) around the colon.

pericolitis (per″ĭ-ko-li′tis) inflammation around the colon, especially of its peritoneal coat.

pericolonitis (per″ĭ-ko″lon-i′tis) pericolitis.

pericolpitis (per″ĭ-kol-pi′tis) perivaginitis.

periconchal (per″ĭ-kong′kal) around a CONCHA.

pericorneal (per″ĭ-kor′ne-al) around the cornea.

pericoronal (per″ĭ-kor′o-nal) around the crown of a tooth.

pericranitis (per″ĭ-kra-ni′tis) inflammation of the pericranium.

pericranium (per″ĭ-kra′ne-um) the periosteum of the skull. adj., **pericra′nial.**

pericystitis (per″ĭ-sis-ti′tis) inflammation of tissues about the bladder.

pericyte (per′ĭ-sīt) one of the peculiar elongated, contractile cells found wrapped about precapillary arterioles outside the basement membrane.

pericytial (per″ĭ-si′te-al) around a cell.

periderm (per′ĭ-derm) the outer layer of the bilaminar fetal epidermis; it generally disappears before birth. Called also epitrichium.

peridesmitis (per″ĭ-dez-mi′tis) inflammation of the peridesmium.

peridesmium (per″ĭ-dez′me-um) the areolar membrane that covers the ligaments.

perididymis (per″ĭ-did′ĭ-mis) tunica vaginalis testis.

perididymitis (per″ĭ-did′ĭ-mi′tis) periorchitis.

peridiverticulitis (per″ĭ-di″ver-tik″u-li′tis) inflammation around an intestinal diverticulum.

periductal (per″ĭ-duk′tal) around a duct.

periduodenitis (per″ĭ-doo″o-dĕ-ni′tis) inflammation around the duodenum.

periencephalitis (per″e-en-sef″ah-li′tis) inflammation of the surface of the brain.

perienteritis (per″e-en″ter-i′tis) inflammation of the peritoneal coat of the intestines.

periesophagitis (per″e-e-sof″ah-ji′tis) inflammation of the tissues around the esophagus.

perifistular (per″ĭ-fis′tu-lar) around a fistula.

perifollicular (per″ĭ-fŏ-lik′u-lar) surrounding a follicle.

perifolliculitis (per″ĭ-fŏ-lik″u-li′tis) inflammation around the hair follicles.

perigangliitis (per″ĭ-gang″gle-i′tis) inflammation around a ganglion.

perigastric (per″ĭ-gas′trik) around the stomach; pertaining to the peritoneal coat of the stomach.

perigastritis (per″ĭ-gas-tri′tis) inflammation of the peritoneal coat of the stomach.

P

perigraft (per′ĭ-graft) situated or occurring around a graft.

perihepatic (per″ĭ-hĕ-pat′ik) around the liver.

perihepatitis (per″ĭ-hep″ah-ti′tis) inflammation of the peritoneal coat of the liver and the surrounding tissue.

peri-islet (per″e-i′let) situated around the islets of Langerhans.

perijejunitis (per″ĭ-je″joo-ni′tis) inflammation around the jejunum.

perikaryon (per″ĭ-kar′e-on) the cell body of a NEURON; called also neurosome.

perikymata (per″ĭ-ki′mah-tah) the numerous small transverse ridges on the surface of the enamel of permanent teeth, representing overlapping prism groups; continued abrasion erodes the enamel surface and obliterates them.

perilabyrinthitis (per″ĭ-lab″ĭ-rin-thi′tis) circumscribed labyrinthitis.

perilesional (per″ĭ-le′zhun-al) located or occurring around a lesion.

perilymph (per′e-limf) the fluid contained within the space separating the membranous labyrinth from the osseous labyrinth; it is entirely separate from the ENDOLYMPH.

perilympha (per″e-lim′fah) perilymph.

perilymphangitis (per″ĭ-lim″fan-ji′tis) inflammation around a lymphatic vessel.

perimeningitis (per″ĭ-men″in-ji′tis) pachymeningitis.

perimenopause (per″e-men′o-pawz) the time just before and just after MENOPAUSE. adj., **perimenopau′sal.**

perimeter (pĕ-rim′ĕ-ter) 1. the boundary of a two-dimensional figure. 2. an apparatus for determining the extent of the peripheral visual field.

perimetrium (per″ĭ-me′tre-um) the TUNICA SEROSA surrounding the UTERUS.

perimetry (pĕ-rim′ĕ-tre) determination of the extent of the peripheral visual field. adj., **perimet′ric.**

perimyelitis (per″ĭ-mi″ĕ-li′tis) 1. inflammation of the pia mater of the spinal cord. 2. inflammation of the endosteum.

perimyositis (per″ĭ-mi″o-si′tis) inflammation of connective tissue around a muscle.

perimysiitis (per″ĭ-mis″e-i′tis) inflammation of the perimysium; myofibrositis.

perimysium (per″ĭ-mis′e-um) connective tissue demarcating a fascicle of skeletal muscle FIBERS. adj., **perimys′ial.**

perinatal (per″ĭ-na′t′l) relating to the period shortly before and after birth; from the twentieth to twenty-ninth week of gestation to 1 to 4 weeks after birth.

perinatologist (per″ĭ-na-tol′o-jist) a specialist in perinatology.

perinatology (per″ĭ-na-tol′o-je) the branch of medicine (obstetrics and pediatrics) dealing with the fetus and infant during the perinatal period.

perineal (per″ĭ-ne′al) pertaining to the perineum.

perineocele (per″ĭ-ne′o-sēl) a hernia between the rectum and the prostate or between the rectum and the vagina.

perineometer (per″in-e-om′ĕ-ter) a device inserted into the vagina to measure the strength of muscular contractions when KEGEL EXERCISES are performed. It is also frequently used to monitor the patient's progress in bladder reeducation programs.

perineoplasty (per″ĭ-ne′o-plas″te) plastic repair of the perineum.

perineorrhaphy (per″ĭ-ne-or′ah-fe) suture of the PERINEUM. The term is most often used to denote repair of an EPISIOTOMY done during childbirth, but it also can mean repair of any tear or laceration of the perineum.

Patient Care. Care of the wound and suture line is done as a clean rather than a sterile procedure. The wound should be kept clean and dry to avoid infection and promote healing. Most obstetrical patients prefer to do this for themselves if they are able; they must be taught how to do it correctly in order to avoid infection and trauma. They are told to work from front to back when removing soiled perineal pads and washing the site. The hands are washed before and after each cleansing as well as after urination, defecation, and replacement of a pad. Constipation and resultant straining at stool should be avoided as it can cause pain and injury to the suture line.

The suture line should be inspected periodically by the caregiver to be sure there is adequate healing of the suture line as well as a normal flow of lochia. Discomfort can be relieved by a cream or suture line spray and application of intermittent cold packs or ice for the first 24 hours, then applications of heat in the form of sitz baths, a heat lamp, or a rubber K-pad through which warm water circulates. Kegel's exercises also help relieve discomfort and promote healing by increasing circulation to and relieving edema of the operative site. If an analgesic cream or spray is prescribed the patient is taught how to apply it correctly.

To avoid discomfort while sitting, patients can be taught to squeeze the buttocks before being seated and to sit with them in that position. Perineorrhaphy sutures do not have to be removed because they are made of a material that is completely absorbed in about ten days. The discomfort associated with perineorrhaphy should subside in four or five days.

perineotomy (per″ĭ-ne-ot′ah-me) incision of the perineum.

perineovaginal (per″ĭ-ne″o-vaj′ĭ-nal) pertaining to or communicating with the perineum and vagina.

perinephric (per″ĭ-nef′rik) around the kidney; called also perirenal.

perinephritis (per″ĭ-nĕ-fri′tis) inflammation of the perinephrium.

perinephrium (per″ĭ-nef′re-um) the peritoneal envelope and other tissues around the kidney. adj., **perineph′rial.**

perineum (per″ĭ-ne′um) the pelvic floor and associated structures occupying the pelvic outlet, bounded anteriorly by the pubic symphysis, laterally by the ischial tuberosities, and posteriorly by the coccyx. During childbirth the perineum may be torn, resulting in possible damage to the urinary meatus and anal sphincter. To avoid a perineal tear, the obstetrician often cuts the perineum just before delivery and sutures the incision after delivery of the infant and the placenta. This procedure is called an episiotomy. Surgical repair of an episiotomy or of a torn or lacerated perineum is called perineorrhaphy.

perineuritis (per″ĭ-noo-ri′tis) inflammation of the perineurium.

perineurium (per″ĭ-noor′e-um) the connective tissue sheath surrounding each bundle of nerve fibers (fascicle) in a peripheral nerve. adj., **perineu′rial.**

periocular (per″e-ok′u-ler) around the eye.

period (pēr′e-od) an interval or division of time; the time for the regular recurrence of a phenomenon.

absolute refractory p. the part of the refractory PERIOD from phase 0 to approximately −60 mV during phase 3; during this time it is impossible for the MYOCARDIUM to respond with a propagated ACTION POTENTIAL, even with a strong stimulus. Called also effective refractory period.

blanking p. a period of time during and after a pacemaker stimulus when the unstimulated chamber is insensitive to avoid sensing the electronic event in the stimulated chamber.

effective refractory p. absolute refractory period.

ejection p. the second phase of ventricular SYSTOLE (0.21 to 0.30 sec), between the opening and closing of the semilunar valves, while the blood is discharged into the aorta and pulmonary artery. Called also sphygmic period.

gestation p. see GESTATION PERIOD.

incubation p. see INCUBATION PERIOD.

isoelectric p. the moment in muscular contraction when no deflection of the GALVANOMETER is produced.

latency p. 1. latent period. 2. latency STAGE.

latent p. a seemingly inactive period, as that between exposure to an infection and the onset of illness (INCUBATION PERIOD) or that between the instant of stimulation and the beginning of response (LATENCY, def. 2).

refractory p. the period of DEPOLARIZATION and REPOLARIZATION of the cell membrane after excitation; during the first portion (absolute refractory PERIOD), the nerve or muscle fiber cannot respond to a second stimulus, whereas during the relative refractory PERIOD it can respond only to a strong stimulus.

relative refractory p. the part of the refractory PERIOD from approximately −60 mV during phase 3 to the end of phase 3; during this time a depressed response to a strong stimulus is possible.

safe p. the period during the MENSTRUAL CYCLE when CONCEPTION is considered least likely to occur; it comprises approximately the ten days after MENSTRUATION begins and the ten days preceding menstruation. See the section on *fertility awareness methods,* under CONTRACEPTION.

sphygmic p. ejection period.

supernormal p. in electrocardiography, a period at the end of phase 3 of the ACTION POTENTIAL during which activation can be initiated with a milder stimulus than is required at maximal REPOLARIZATION, because at this time the cell is excitable and closer to threshold than at maximal diastolic POTENTIAL.

vulnerable p. that time at the peak of the T wave during which serious arrhythmias are likely to result if a stimulus occurs.

Wenckebach's p. a usually repetitive sequence seen in partial HEART BLOCK, marked by progressive lengthening of the P–R INTERVAL; see also dropped BEAT.

periodic (pe″re-od′ik) repeated or recurring at intervals.

p. fever a hereditary condition characterized by repetitive febrile episodes and systemic symptoms, occurring in precise or irregular cycles of days, weeks, or months. See also FAMILIAL PERIODIC FEVER.

periodicity (pēr″e-o-dis′ĭ-te) recurrence at regular intervals of time.

periodontal (per″e-o-don′t′l) around a tooth; pertaining to the periodontium.

p. disease any disease of the PERIODONTIUM, such as PERIODONTITIS or GINGIVITIS.

CLASSIFICATION OF PERIODONTAL DISEASES*

I. Gingival Diseases
  A. **Dental plaque-induced gingival diseases**†
    1. Gingivitis associated with dental plaque only
      a. without other local contributing factors
      b. with local contributing factors (see VIII A)
    2. Gingival diseases modified by systemic factors
      a. associated with the endocrine system
        1) puberty-associated gingivitis
        2) menstrual cycle–associated gingivitis
        3) pregnancy-associated
          a) gingivitis
          b)pyogenic granuloma
        4) diabetes mellitus–associated gingivitis
      b. associated with blood dyscrasias
        1) leukemia-associated gingivitis
        2) other
    3. Gingival diseases modified by medications
      a. drug-influenced gingival diseases
        1) drug-influenced gingival enlargements
        2) drug-influenced gingivitis
          a) oral contraceptive–associated gingivitis
          b) other
    4. Gingival diseases modified by malnutrition
      a. ascorbic acid deficiency gingivitis
      b. other
  B. **Non—plaque-induced gingival lesions**
    1. Gingival diseases of specific bacterial origin
      a. *Neisseria gonorrhea*–associated lesions
      b. *Treponema pallidum*–associated lesions
      c. streptococcal species–associated lesions
      d. other
    2. Gingival diseases of viral origin
      a. herpesvirus infections
        1) primary herpetic gingivostomatitis
        2) recurrent oral herpes
        3) varicella-zoster infections
      b. other

  3. Gingival diseases of fungal origin
    a. *Candida*-species infections
      1) generalized gingival candidosis
    b. linear gingival erythema
    c. histoplasmosis
    d. other
  4. Gingival lesions of genetic origin
    a. hereditary gingival fibromatosis
    b. other
  5. Gingival manifestations of systemic conditions
    a. mucocutaneous disorders
      1) lichen planus
      2) pemphigoid
      3) pemphigus vulgaris
      4) erythema multiforme
      5) lupus erythematosus
      6) drug-induced
      7) other
    b. allergic reactions
      1) dental restorative materials
        a) mercury
        b) nickel
        c) acrylic
        d) other
      2) reactions attributable to
        a) toothpastes/dentifrices
        b) mouthrinses/mouthwashes
        c) chewing gum additives
        d) foods and additives
      3) other
  6. Traumatic lesions (factitious, iatrogenic, accidental)
    a. chemical injury
    b. physical injury
    c. thermal injury
  7. Foreign body reactions
  8. Not otherwise specified (NOS)

*Official classification of the American Academy of Periodontology (1999).
†Can occur on a periodontium with no attachment loss or on a periodontium with attachment loss that is not progressing.

Sometimes it is a manifestation of a systemic disease.

periodontics (per″e-o-don′tiks) the branch of dentistry dealing with the study and treatment of diseases of the periodontium.

periodontist (per″e-o-don′tist) a dentist who specializes in periodontics.

periodontitis (per″e-o-don-ti′tis) inflammation of the PERIODONTIUM, usually caused by specific pathologic bacteria that grow in the spaces between the gum and lower part of the tooth crown, and the host response to inflammation. If it continues unchecked the infection will spread to the bone in which the teeth are rooted. The bone then resorbs and the teeth slowly become detached from their supporting tissues. Periodontitis is the major cause of tooth loss after the age of 35. It can be prevented or controlled by good dental hygiene such as proper brushing and interdental cleaning, or by nonsurgical or surgical periodontal therapy. It is treated with local cleansing and DÉBRIDEMENT of the area, establishment of drainage for exudate, and use of antimicrobial agents. Antibiotic drugs and host modulating THERAPY are indicated if the symptoms are severe and unresponsive to other treatments. Extraction of the affected teeth may be necessary if the lesion is advanced.

periodontium (per″ĭ-o-don′she-um), pl. *periodon′tia* [L.] the tissues investing and supporting the teeth, including the cementum, periodontal ligament, alveolar bone, and gingiva. In official nomenclature, restricted to the periodontal LIGAMENT.

periomphalic (per″e-om-fal′ik) periumbilical.

perionychium (per″e-o-nik′e-um) cuticle.

perioophoritis (per″e-o″of-o-ri′tis) inflammation of the tissues around the ovary.

CLASSIFICATION OF PERIODONTAL DISEASES*—cont'd

II. Chronic Periodontitis†
   A. Localized
   B. Generalized
III. Aggressive Periodontitis†
   A. Localized
   B. Generalized
IV. Periodontitis as a Manifestation of
   Systemic Diseases
   A. Associated with hematological disorders
      1. Acquired neutropenia
      2. Leukemias
      3. Other
   B. Associated with genetic disorders
      1. Familial and cyclic neutropenia
      2. Down syndrome
      3. Leukocyte adhesion deficiency syndromes
      4. Papillon-Lefèvre syndrome
      5. Chediak-Higashi syndrome
      6. Histiocytosis syndromes
      7. Glycogen storage disease
      8. Infantile genetic agranulocytosis
      9. Cohen syndrome
      10. Ehlers-Danlos syndrome (Types IV and VIII)
      11. Hypophosphatasia
      12. Other
   C. Not otherwise specified (NOS)
V. Necrotizing Periodontal Diseases
   A. Necrotizing ulcerative gingivitis (NUG)
   B. Necrotizing ulcerative periodontitis (NUP)
VI. Abscesses of the Periodontium
   A. Gingival abscess
   B. Periodontal abscess
   C. Pericoronal abscess
VII. Periodontitis Associated with Endodontic
   Lesions
   A. Combined periodontic-endodontic lesions

VIII. Developmental or Acquired Deformities
   and Conditions
   A. Localized tooth-related factors
      that modify or predispose to
      plaque-induced gingival
      diseases/periodontitis
      1. Tooth anatomic factors
      2. Dental restorations/appliances
      3. Root fractures
      4. Cervical root resorption and
         cemental tears
   B. Mucogingival deformities and conditions
      around teeth
      1. Gingival/soft tissue recession
         a. facial or lingual surfaces
         b. interproximal (papillary)
      2. Lack of keratinized gingiva
      3. Decreased vestibular depth
      4. Aberrant frenum/muscle position
      5. Gingival excess
         a. pseudopocket
         b. inconsistent gingival margin
         c. excessive gingival display
         d. gingival enlargement
         (See I.A.3. and I.B.4)
      6. Abnormal color
   C. Mucogingival deformities and conditions
      on edentulous ridges
      1. Vertical and/or horizontal
         ridge deficiency
      2. Lack of gingiva/keratinized tissue
      3. Gingival/soft tissue enlargement
      4. Aberrant frenum/muscle position
      5. Decreased vestibular depth
      6. Abnormal color
   D. Occlusal trauma
      1. Primary occlusal trauma
      2. Secondary occlusal trauma

†Can be further classified on the basis of extent and severity. As a general guide, extend can be characterized as Localized ≤ 30% of sites involved and Generalized ≥ 30% of sites involved. Severity can be characterized on the basis of the amount of clinical attachment loss (CAL) as follows: Slight = 1 or 2 mm CAL, Moderate = 3 or 4 mm CAL, and Severe ≥ 5 mm CAL.

---

perioophorosalpingitis (per″e-o-of″o-ro-sal″pin-ji′tis) inflammation of the tissues around the ovary and fallopian tube.

perioperative (per″ĕ-op′er-ah-tiv″) pertaining or relating to the period of time surrounding a surgical procedure, including the preoperative, intraoperative, and postoperative periods.

p. nursing data set a nursing LANGUAGE specialized for vocabulary that addresses the perioperative patient experience from preadmission until discharge. See also perioperative NURSE.

periophthalmic (per″e-of-thal′mik) around the eye.

perioptometry (per″e-op-tom′ĕ-tre) measurement of acuity of peripheral vision or of the limits of the visual field.

perioral (per″e-o′ral) around the mouth.

periorbita (per″e-or′bĭ-tah) the periosteum of the bones forming the orbit, or eye socket. adj., **perior′bital.**

periorbititis (per″e-or-bĭ-ti′tis) inflammation of the periorbita.

periorchitis (per″e-or-ki′tis) inflammation of the TUNICA VAGINALIS TESTIS; called also perididymitis and vaginalitis.

periosteitis (per″e-os′te-i′tis) periostitis.

periosteoma (per″e-os-te-o′mah) a morbid bony growth surrounding a bone.

periosteomyelitis (per″e-os″te-o-mi″ĕ-li′-tis) inflammation of the entire bone, including periosteum and marrow.

periosteophyte (per″e-os′te-o-fīt″) a bony growth on the periosteum.

periosteotomy (per″e-os″te-ot′ah-me) incision of the periosteum.

periosteum (per″e-os′te-um) a specialized connective tissue covering all bones of the body, and possessing bone-forming potentialities. Periosteum also serves as a point of attachment for certain muscles. The connective tissues of the muscle fuse with the fibrous layers of periosteum. adj., **perios′-teal.**

periostitis (per″e-os-ti′tis) inflammation of the periosteum.

diffuse p. widespread periostitis of the long bones.

periostosis (per″e-os-to′sis) abnormal deposition of periosteal bone, manifested by the growth of PERIOSTEOMAS.

periotic (per″e-o′tik) 1. situated about the ear, especially the internal ear. 2. the petrous and mastoid portions of the temporal bone, at one stage a distinct bone.

peripachymeningitis (per″ĭ-pak″ĭ-men″in-ji′tis) inflammation of the substance between the dura mater and the bony covering of the central nervous system.

peripancreatitis (per″ĭ-pan″kre-ah-ti′tis) inflammation of tissues around the pancreas.

peripapillary (per″ĭ-pap′ĭ-ler″e) around the optic papilla.

peripartum (per″ĭ-pahr′tum) occurring during the last month of gestation or the first few months after delivery, with reference to the mother.

periphacitis (per″ĭ-fah-si′tis) inflammation of the capsule of the eye lens.

peripherad (pĕ-rif′er-ad) toward the periphery.

peripheral (pĕ-rif′er-al) pertaining to or situated at or near the periphery.

p. vascular disease (PVD) any disorder affecting blood flow through the veins and arteries distal to the heart. Disruption of circulation in the peripheral veins can be caused by venous stasis, hypercoagulability, or injury to the vein wall secondary to immobility, orthopedic surgery, aging, and dehydration. Arterial insufficiency in the peripheral vessels is most often due to atherosclerosis, blood clots, trauma, spasms of smooth muscles in the arterial walls, and congenital structural defects in the arteries.

Diminished or interrupted flow of blood through peripheral arteries can eventually lead to ischemic necrosis and gangrene. Sluggish venous flow leads to increased pressure within the vessels, causing varicose veins and sometimes thrombophlebitis. When blood is not moved out of the veins of the lower limbs, it accumulates there and serves as an excellent medium for bacterial growth and contributes to the formation of leg ulcers. Treatment is aimed at improving blood flow by removing or mitigating the cause of impaired circulation.

Assessment of Arterial Circulation. Arterial insufficiency is characterized by two types of pain. The first is a cramping pain in the muscles brought on by exercise and relieved by rest (INTERMITTENT CLAUDICATION). The pain is most often felt in the calves of the legs, but it may also affect the thighs and buttocks. A second type of pain is characteristic of advanced chronic occlusive arterial disease. It occurs when the patient is at rest, usually at night while lying down. The sensation is described as burning and tingling, with numbness of the toes.

Assessment includes noting the color and temperature of the skin in the affected areas and any signs of trophic changes. Epidermoid tissues that are chronically malnourished because of poor blood supply appear shiny, smooth, and thin, with little or no hair on the surface. The nails are thick, with deposits of cornlike material under them. With time, a decreased blood supply produces ischemic changes that cause the skin to assume a purple-black color that is characteristic of cyanosis and gangrene. Additional assessment data include the rate, rhythm, and force of the peripheral pulses.

Assessment of Venous Circulation. Assessment of venous circulation focuses on changes in the hydration status (edema) and pigmentation of the skin. Chronic edema can lead to ulceration. Venous insufficiency also produces a darkened color, dryness, and scaling of the skin in the affected areas. Venography, a radiologic test in which the vein is injected with a radiopaque dye prior to filming, can also demonstrate engorged and tortuous veins.

Patient Teaching. In order to prevent or mitigate the effects of arterial insufficiency or venous stasis, patients must be taught techniques of self-care. Exercises such as the BUERGER-ALLEN EXERCISES are often prescribed. Additionally, patients need to know how to take care of their feet and legs (see FOOT CARE), the reasons for avoiding smoking and keeping warm, and the importance of taking prescribed medications.

periphery (pĕ-rif′er-e) an outward structure or surface; the portion of a system outside the central region.

periphlebitis (per″ĭ-flĕ-bi′tis) inflammation of the tissues around a vein, or the external coat of a vein.

periplasmic (per″ĭ-plas′mik) around the plasma membrane; between the plasma membrane and the cell wall of a bacterium.

periportal (per″ĭ-por′t'l) situated around the portal vein.

periproctitis (per″ĭ-prok-ti′tis) inflammation of tissues around the rectum and anus.

periprostatic (per″ĭ-pros-tat′ik) around the prostate.

periprostatitis (per″ĭ-pros″tah-ti′tis) inflammation of the tissues around the prostate.

peripylephlebitis (per″ĭ-pi″le-flĕ-bi′tis) inflammation of tissues around the portal vein.

peripyloric (per″ĭ-pi-lor′ik) around the PYLORUS; called also juxtapyloric.

periradicular (per″ĭ-rah-dik′u-lar) around a root, such as the root of a tooth.

perirectal (per″ĭ-rek′t'l) around the rectum.

perirectitis (per″ĭ-rek-ti′tis) periproctitis.

perirenal (per″ĭ-re′nal) perinephric.

perirhinal (per″ĭ-ri′nal) around the nose.

perisalpingitis (per″ĭ-sal″pin-ji′tis) inflammation of tissues around the fallopian tube.

periscopic (per″ĭ-skop′ik) affording a wide range of vision.

perisigmoiditis (per″ĭ-sig″moi-di′tis) inflammation of the peritoneum of the sigmoid flexure.

perisinusitis (per″ĭ-si″nŭ-si′tis) inflammation of the tissues around a sinus.

perisplanchnic (per″ĭ-splangk′nik) around a viscus or the viscera.

perisplanchnitis (per″ĭ-splangk-ni′tis) inflammation of tissues around the viscera.

perisplenic (per″ĭ-splen′ik) around the spleen.

perisplenitis (per″ĭ-sple-ni′tis) inflammation of the peritoneal surface of the spleen.

perispondylitis (per″ĭ-spon″dĭ-li′tis) inflammation of tissues around a vertebra.

peristalsis (per″ĭ-stal′sis) the wormlike movement by which the alimentary canal or other tubular organs with both longitudinal and circular muscle fibers propel their contents, consisting of a wave of contraction passing along the tube. adj., **peristal′tic.**

When food is swallowed, it passes into the esophagus. Muscular contractions in the wall of the esophagus work the food downward, pushing it into the stomach. Here peristaltic contractions not only move the food in small amounts into the intestine but also aid in the disintegration of the food and help mix it with gastric juice. Peristalsis forces the food into and through the intestine for further digestion until the food waste finally reaches the rectum, from which it is periodically discharged from the body. The waves of peristalsis are irregular; they are stronger at some times than at others. They are also weaker in some people, notably the elderly.

Although the normal peristaltic wave is downward, it is sometimes reversed. Reverse peristaltic action may be triggered by mild digestive upsets or more serious disorders, such as an obstruction in the stomach or intestines.

peristaphyline (per″ĭ-staf′ĭ-līn) around the uvula.

perisynovial (per″ĭ-sĭ-no′ve-al) around a synovial structure.

peritectomy (per″ĭ-tek′to-me) excision of a ring of conjunctiva around the cornea in treatment of pannus.

peritendineum (per″ĭ-ten-din′e-um) connective tissue investing larger tendons and extending between the fibers composing them.

peritendinitis (pĕr″e-ten-dĭ-ni′tis) tenosynovitis.

peritenonitis (pĕr″e-ten-o-ni′tis) tenosynovitis.

perithelioma (per″ĭ-the″le-o′mah) hemangiopericytoma.

perithelium (per″ĭ-the′le-um) the connective tissue layer surrounding the capillaries and smaller vessels.

perithyroiditis (per″ĭ-thi″roi-di′tis) inflammation of the capsule of the thyroid.

peritomy (pĕ-rit′ŏ-me) 1. surgical incision of the conjunctiva and subconjunctival tissue about the whole circumference of the cornea. 2. circumcision.

peritoneal (per″ĭ-to-ne′al) pertaining to the peritoneum.

P

p. dialysis a type of HEMODIALYSIS in which the PERITONEUM surrounding the abdominal cavity is used as a dialyzing membrane for removal of waste products or toxins accumulated as a result of RENAL FAILURE. Substances that can be removed in this way include crystalloids such as UREA, CREATININE, ELECTROLYTES, and drugs such as the SALICYLATES, BROMIDES, and BARBITURATES.

The exchange of substances across this type of semipermeable membrane involves three physical processes: diffusion, osmosis, and solvent drag. In *diffusion* the random motion of the molecules of solids, liquids, or gases in solution causes a flow of each solute from regions of high concentration to regions of low concentration. Diffusible solutes, those with molecules small enough to pass through the pores of the membrane, flow from the side on which the concentration is high to the side on which it is low. *Osmosis* is a flow of water molecules (or some other solvent) through the membrane. The flow moves from the side on which the concentration of nondiffusible solutes, those with molecules too large to pass through the membrane pores, is low (and thus there is more water) to the side on which the concentration is high (and there is less water). Solutes with molecules of intermediate size are not retarded in their flow through the membrane, but their flow is subject to *solvent drag,* that is, the rate at which a solute flows through the membrane is increased by a solvent flow in the same direction and decreased by a solvent flow in the opposite direction.

Indications and Contraindications. Peritoneal dialysis has the advantage of being more quickly initiated than hemodialysis because a dialyzing machine is not needed, anticoagulants are not necessary, and there is no need for vascular cannulization. Also, since chemical and fluid exchanges occur more slowly, there is less stress on internal organs.

Acute and chronic renal failure are among the most common indications for peritoneal dialysis. Other indications are congestive HEART FAILURE and difficult or absent vascular ACCESS. Since certain drugs can be removed by this method of dialysis, some types of drug poisoning can be treated in this way. Peritoneal dialysis cannot be used when there is severe abdominal trauma, multiple abdominal surgical procedures, adhesions, severe coagulation defects, paralytic ileus, or previous diffuse peritonitis.

The Procedure. Fluid equal in osmolarity and similar in chemical composition to normal body fluid is introduced into the peritoneal cavity via a catheter. The fluid infuses by gravity; its rate of flow can be controlled by lowering or raising the container of dialysate or by manipulating the occlusive clamp on the tubing.

The length of time the dialyzing solution is left in the peritoneal cavity depends on the molecular weight of the substance to be removed and the amount of dialyzing solution used. Substances with low molecular weights equilibrate in two to three hours, while those with high molecular weights can take more than 12 hours to move across the membrane and equalize the concentrations of the two solutions. This period of equalization is sometimes called the "dwell time." It is followed by a period of drainage to complete the dialysis or to prepare for instillation of fresh dialysate.

Peritoneal dialysis is done in one of three ways: *Intermittent peritoneal dialysis* (IPD) can be done manually or with an automated cycling machine. The dialysate is introduced, allowed to dwell for a specified number of minutes, and then drained. Automated IPD is usually done while the patient sleeps. *Continuous ambulatory peritoneal dialysis* (CAPD) is performed continuously by the patient on an outpatient basis. The dialysate fluid dwells for four to eight hours: the drainage bag is clamped, folded and held in the person's clothing during this time. When the dwell period is over, the catheter to the drainage bag is unclamped and the dialysate fluid is drained by gravity. A new bag of dialysate is then started and the process goes on over a 24-hour period. *Continuous cycling peritoneal*

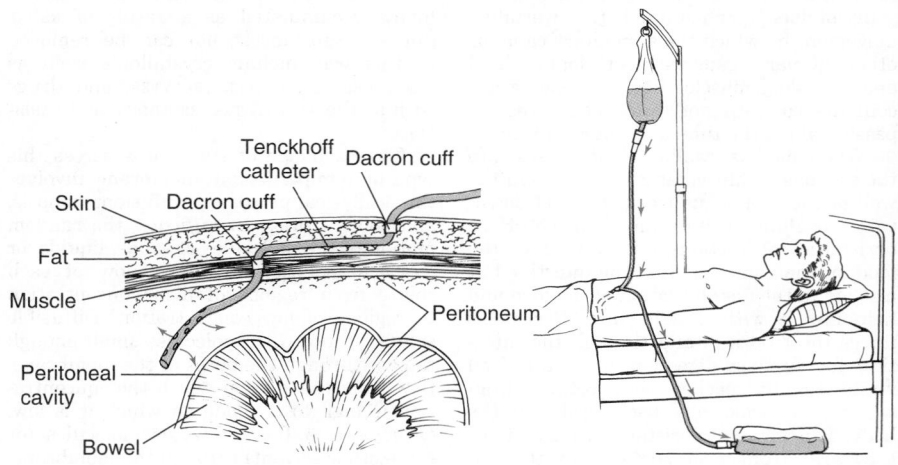

Manual peritoneal dialysis via an implanted abdominal catheter (Tenckhoff's catheter). From Ignatavicius and Workman, 2002.

dialysis (CCPD) involves the use of a cycler
for exchanges while the client sleeps. The

peritonealgia – peritonitis   1343

last exchange before the patient arises for
the day is allowed to dwell for the day,
avoiding the interruption of daily activities
for maintenance of the system.

Because HEMODIALYSIS is more efficient in
removing toxins from the blood and body
fluids, it has always been the treatment of
choice for END-STAGE RENAL DISEASE. There are
certain patients, however, who fare better on
less drastic and gentler dialytic therapy and
who can benefit from continuous ambulatory
peritoneal dialysis. The procedure is becoming an accepted alternative for persons with
either chronic or acute renal failure.

Complications. The most obvious complication of peritoneal dialysis is PERITONITIS,
which is a real danger to any patient
receiving this treatment. Contamination of
some part of the system, a malfunctioning
piece of equipment, contamination of the
fluid, and infection of the catheter site are
all possible sources of peritonitis. The
catheter itself can cause complications
through leakage at the site of insertion,
infection, and occlusion of the perforations
on the catheter. Respiratory difficulty can
occur as a result of fluid retention that
increases pressure against the diaphragm,
and fluid overload that requires the more
frequent use of hypertonic solutions. Fluid
depletion and hypotension are also possible
complications.

Patient Care. To avoid complications strict
adherence to aseptic technique is essential.
If there is any break in the tubing connections during the procedure the peritoneal
cavity must be considered contaminated. If
the tubing becomes blocked the physician
should be notified immediately.

An *exchange record* is kept of the fluid
that is introduced into and withdrawn from
the peritoneal cavity. The amount withdrawn is expected to closely approximate or
be slightly more than the amount introduced. The exchange record contains information about the starting time of infusion,
amount infused, concentration of fluid and
drugs added, finishing time of infusion,
starting time of drainage, volume of drainage, and total patient fluid loss (−) or
retention (+) up to the time of recording.
Since this last item is frequently a source of
error, it is essential that all personnel
involved in the dialysis procedure know
how the recording is done. Daily weight on
a stretcher scale facilitates calculation of
fluid loss or gain.

The peritoneal drainage fluid is observed
for cloudiness and the presence of blood or
other abnormal constituents. The vital signs

are recorded at frequent intervals so that
early signs of shock or the development of
an infection can be discovered. Respiratory
difficulty may develop as a result of pressure of the fluid against the diaphragm.
Mild dyspnea may be relieved by elevating
the head of the bed. Severe dyspnea may
necessitate immediate drainage of the fluid
from the peritoneal cavity and collaboration
among health care professionals to ensure
the patient's safety.

peritonealgia (per″ĭ-to″ne-al′jah) pain in
the peritoneum.

peritoneocentesis (per″ĭ-to″ne-o-sen-te′-
sis) abdominal PARACENTESIS.

peritoneoclysis (per″ĭ-to″ne-ok′ĭ-sis) injection of fluid into the peritoneal cavity.

peritoneopathy (per″ĭ-to″ne-op′ah-the)
any disease of the peritoneum.

peritoneopericardial (per″ĭ-to-ne″o-per″ĭ-
kahr′de-al) pertaining to the peritoneum
and pericardium.

peritoneovenous (per″ĭ-to-ne″o-ve′nus)
communicating with the peritoneal cavity
and the venous system, such as a peritoneovenous SHUNT.

peritoneum (per″ĭ-to-ne′um) the serous
membrane lining the walls of the abdominal
and pelvic cavities (parietal peritoneum)
and investing contained viscera (visceral
peritoneum), the two layers enclosing a
potential space, the peritoneal cavity.

peritonitis (per″ĭ-to-ni′tis) inflammation
of the peritoneum. (See accompanying
illustration.)

Acute Peritonitis. Acute peritonitis may be
produced by inflammation of abdominal
organs, by irritating substances from a
perforated gallbladder or gastric ulcer, by
rupture of a cyst, or by irritation from
blood, as in cases of internal bleeding.

Symptoms and Diagnosis. Immediate and
intense pain is felt at the site of infection,
followed usually by fever, vomiting, and
extreme weakness. The abdomen becomes
rigid and sensitive to the touch. The patient
may suffer mental confusion, fever, prostration, or shock. Although antibiotics have
greatly reduced the mortality rate of acute
peritonitis, the infection should be treated
and controlled immediately; it can be fatal if
neglected.

Diagnosis is based on manual examination, x-ray films, and blood tests.

Treatment. The basic treatment for acute
peritonitis is a combination of surgery,
antibiotics, and other measures. The peritoneal cavity often must be opened and the
toxic material removed. The original source
of infection, such as an inflamed appendix,

P

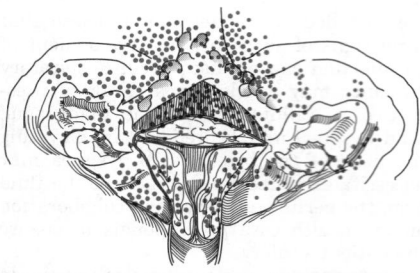

Peritonitis. Infection spreads via lymphatics to peritoneum; formation of a pelvic abscess may occur. From McKinney et al., 2000.

may have to be removed, or an abscess caused by the peritonitis may have to be drained. Antibiotics are used to fight the infection itself.

The patient usually takes nothing by mouth. Fluids are given intravenously. Narcotics and sedatives are often used to relieve pain and ensure rest. Treatment may also include blood transfusions and suction through a nasogastric tube to relieve abdominal pressure and to prevent accumulation of gas in the intestines.

Chronic Peritonitis. The chronic form of this disease is comparatively rare, and is often associated with tuberculosis. Less frequently it may result from longstanding irritation caused by the presence in the abdomen of a foreign body such as gunshot.

In general, symptoms of chronic peritonitis are milder than those of acute peritonitis. Symptoms of tuberculous peritonitis are abdominal pain, low-grade fever, constipation, and general ill health, including loss of weight and appetite. Treatment depends on the underlying cause and the severity of the condition.

   adhesive p. peritonitis characterized by adhesions between adjacent serous structures.

   bile p., biliary p. that due to the presence of bile in the peritoneum; choleperitoneum.

   gas p. peritonitis with the accumulation of gas in the peritoneum.

   septic p. peritonitis caused by a pyogenic microorganism.

   silent p. asymptomatic peritonitis.

peritonsillar (per″ĭ-ton′sĭ-ler) around a tonsil.

peritonsillitis (per″ĭ-ton″sĭ-li′tis) inflammation of peritonsillar tissues.

peritracheal (per″ĭ-tra′ke-al) around the trachea.

Peritrate (per′ĭ-trāt) trademark for a preparation of PENTAERYTHRITOL, a VASODILATOR used in treatment of ANGINA PECTORIS.

peritrichous (pĕ-rit′rĭ-kus) 1. having FLAGELLA around the entire surface; said of bacteria. 2. of flagella, occurring around the entire surface of a bacterial cell. 3. having flagella around the CYTOSTOME only; said of CILIOPHORA.

periumbilical (per″e-um-bil′ĭ-k'l) near or around the UMBILICUS.

periureteral (per″ĭ-u-re′ter-al) around the ureter.

periureteritis (per″ĭ-u-re″ter-i′tis) inflammation of tissues around the ureter.

periurethral (per″ĭ-u-re′thral) around the urethra.

periurethritis (per″ĭ-u″rĕ-thri′tis) inflammation of the tissues around the urethra; spongiositis.

periuterine (per″ĭ-u′ter-in) around the uterus.

perivaginal (per″ĭ-vaj′ĭ-nal) around the vagina.

perivaginitis (per″ĭ-vaj″ĭ-ni′tis) inflammation of tissues around the vagina; called also pericolpitis.

perivascular (per″ĭ-vas′ku-ler) around a vessel.

perivasculitis (per″ĭ-vas″ku-li′tis) inflammation of a perivascular sheath and surrounding tissue.

perivesical (per″ĭ-ves′ĭ-k'l) next to the urinary BLADDER; called also juxtavesical.

perivesiculitis (per″ĭ-vĕ-sik″u-li′tis) inflammation of tissues around the seminal vesicles.

perlèche (per-lesh′) angular cheilitis.

PermCath (perm′kath) trademark for a type of cuffed hemodialysis CATHETER that may remain in place for several months.

permeability (per″me-ah-bil′ĭ-te) the property or state of being permeable.

permeable (per′me-ah-b'l) not impassable; pervious; permitting passage of a substance.

permeate (per′me-āt″) 1. to penetrate or pass through, as through a filter. 2. the constituents of a solution or suspension that pass through a filter.

permethrin (per-meth′rin) a topical insecticide used in the treatment of SCABIES and head LOUSE or TICK infestation. It is also applied to objects such as furniture and bedding.

pernicious (per-nish′us) tending to a fatal outcome.

   p. anemia a type of megaloblastic ANEMIA seen most often in older adults, caused by lack of intrinsic FACTOR, which normally is produced by the stomach mucosa. The deficiency results in inadequate and abnormal formation of erythrocytes, leukocytes, and platelets, with failure to absorb vitamin B$_{12}$. Some patients show only mild symptoms and are not particularly aware of the illness; in others it becomes very serious and if untreated can lead to permanent neurologic impairment and even death. It may be caused by deficient vitamin B$_{12}$ intake, impaired absorption due to intrinsic factor deficiency or intrinsic intestinal disease or increased requirements and impaired utilization.

Symptoms. A pale, colorless, or lemon-yellow complexion is typical. JAUNDICE also occurs, with soreness and reddening of the tongue, difficulty in swallowing, and digestive disturbances such as diarrhea. Other symptoms may include fatigability, heart palpitation, and dyspnea. Changes in the nerves and spinal cord may produce numbness and tingling in the fingers and toes, and the gait may become unsteady; involvement of the nerves can be avoided if the condition is detected and treated in the early stages. Laboratory tests reveal abnormalities in the erythrocytes in the blood and in the bone marrow. Gastric analysis shows an absence of hydrochloric acid and perhaps even an absence of gastric juice.

Treatment. Pernicious anemia is successfully treated by regular injections of vitamin B$_{12}$, given several times a week at first and monthly after the condition has been brought under control. This treatment must be lifelong to prevent relapse. The injections do not cure the disease but arrest it by providing the body directly with the necessary vitamin that it fails to absorb from the digestive tract. Special diets, liver extract, and other medications taken by mouth usually are not required since the basic defect is not dietary deficiency but improper use of food ingested. The etiology of pernicious anemia is unknown although there appears to be an autoimmune component, as anti–intrinsic factor antibodies are often found. For patient care, see also ANEMIA.

pernio (per'ne-o) chilblain.

pero- word element [Gr.], *deformity; maimed.*

perobrachius (pe″ro-bra'ke-us) an individual with deformed upper limbs; see also DYSMELIA.

perocephalus (pe″ro-sef'ah-lus) an individual with a congenitally deformed head and face.

perochirus (pe″ro-ki'rus) an individual with congenitally deformed hands.

peromelia (pe″ro-me'le-ah) severe DYSMELIA.

peromelus (pe″rom'ĕ-lus) an individual with severe DYSMELIA (congenitally deformed limbs).

peroneal (per″o-ne'al) 1. fibular. 2. pertaining to the outer aspect of the leg.

peropus (pe'ro-pus) an individual with congenitally malformed lower limbs and feet.

peroral (per-or'al) performed or administered through the mouth.

per os (per os) [L.] by mouth.

peroxidase (pĕ-rok'sĭ-dās) any of a group of iron-porphyrin enzymes that catalyze the oxidation of some organic substrates in the presence of hydrogen peroxide.

peroxide (pĕ-rok'sīd) that oxide of any element containing more oxygen than any other; more correctly applied to compounds having such linkage as —O—O—.

peroxisome (pĕ-roks'ĭ-sōm) a microbody found in vertebrate animal cells, especially kidney and liver cells, that contains urate oxidase, amino acid oxidase, catalase, and other enzymes.

perphenazine (per-fen'ah-zēn) a PHENOTHIAZINE compound used orally and intramuscularly as an ANTIPSYCHOTIC AGENT and ANTIEMETIC.

per primam (intentionem) (per pri'mam in-ten″she-o'nem) [L.] by first intention (see HEALING).

per rectum (per rek'tum) by way of the rectum.

Persantine (per-san'tēn) trademark for preparations of DIPYRIDAMOLE, a coronary VASODILATOR used to prevent clotting associated with mechanical heart valves and as an adjunct in radionuclide myocardial perfusion imaging.

per secundam (intentionem) (per se-kun'dam in-ten″she-o'nem) [L.] by second intention (see HEALING).

perseveration (per-sev″er-a'shun) the inappropriate persistence or repetition of a thought or action after the causative stimulus has ceased or in response to different stimuli; for example, a patient answers a question correctly but incorrectly gives the same answer to succeeding questions. Perseveration is most often associated with brain lesions but is also seen in schizophrenia.

persona (per-so'nah) Jung's term for the personality mask or facade presented by a person to the outside world, as opposed to the ANIMA, the inner being.

personality (per″sŭ-nal'ĭ-te) the characteristic way that a person thinks, feels, and behaves; the relatively stable and predictable part of a person's thought and behavior; it includes conscious attitudes, values, and styles as well as unconscious conflicts and defense mechanisms. *Personality traits* are simple features of normal and abnormal personalities. *Personality types* are categories applicable to both normal and abnormal personalities; usually they belong to a coherent typology, such as introvert/extrovert or oral/anal/phallic.

Early Life and Personality. The newborn comes into the world completely dependent on others for satisfying individual basic human needs. Feelings of security in a relationship with the mother, or an adequate substitute, is the cornerstone of mental health in later years.

As children develop, they need to learn and to meet the day-to-day problems of life, and to master them. In resolving these challenges, one chooses solutions from many possibilities. Psychologists have studied how these choices are made and use technical terms to describe them, such as repression and sublimation. The behavior patterns chosen result in certain character traits which will influence a child's way of meeting the world—whether the child will lead or follow, be conscientious or reckless, imitate his or her parents or prefer to be as different from them as possible, or take a realistic, flexible path between these extremes. The sum total of these traits represents the personality.

The Well-Adjusted Personality. A well-adjusted individual is one who adapts to surroundings. If adaptation is not possible, the individual makes realistic efforts to change the situation, using personal talents and abilities constructively and successfully. The well-adjusted person is realistic and able to face facts whether they are pleasant or unpleasant, and deals with them instead of merely worrying about them or denying them. Well-adjusted mature persons are independent. They form reasoned opinions and then act on them. They seek a reasonable amount of information and advice before making a decision, and once the decision is made, they are willing to face the consequences of it. They do not try to force others to make decisions for them. An ability to love others is typical of the well-adjusted individual. In addition, the mature well adjusted person is also able to enjoy receiving love and affection and can accept a reasonable dependence on others.

alternating p. multiple personality disorder.

compulsive p. obsessive-compulsive personality disorder.

cyclothymic p. a temperament characterized by rapid, frequent swings between sad and cheerful moods; see also CYCLOTHYMIC DISORDER.

p. disorders a group of MENTAL DISORDERS characterized by enduring, inflexible, and maladaptive personality traits that deviate markedly from cultural expectations, pervade a broad range of situations, and are either a source of subjective distress or a cause of significant impairment in social, occupational, or other functioning. In general, they are difficult both to diagnose and to treat.

Although individuals with a personality disorder can function in day-to-day life, they are hampered both emotionally and psychologically by the maladaptive nature of their disorder, and their chances of forming good relationships and fulfilling their potentialities are poor. In spite of their problems, these patients refuse to acknowledge that anything is wrong and insist that it is the rest of the world that is out of step. Very often their behavior is extremely annoying to those around them.

Personality disorders result from unresolved conflicts, often dating back to childhood. To alleviate the anxiety and depression that accompany these conflicts, the ego uses DEFENSE MECHANISMS. Although defense mechanisms are not pathological in themselves, they become maladaptive in individuals with personality disorders.

The category includes: ANTISOCIAL PERSONALITY DISORDER, AVOIDANT PERSONALITY DISORDER, BORDERLINE PERSONALITY DISORDER, DEPENDENT PERSONALITY DISORDER, HISTRIONIC PERSONALITY DISORDER, NARCISSISTIC PERSONALITY DISORDER, OBSESSIVE-COMPULSIVE PERSONALITY DISORDER, PARANOID PERSONALITY DISORDER, SCHIZOID PERSONALITY DISORDER, and SCHIZOTYPAL PERSONALITY DISORDER. Distinguishing one disorder from another can be difficult because the various traits can occur in more than one disorder. For example, patients with borderline personality disorder and those with narcissistic personality disorder both may have a tendency to angry outbursts and may be hindered in forming interpersonal relationships because they often exploit, idealize, or devalue others. The symptoms of a personality disorder may also occur as features of another mental disorder. More than one personality disorder can exist in the same person.

Because patients refuse to admit that there is anything wrong, personality disorders are more difficult to treat than other mental disorders. However, a great deal can be done in many cases, if the therapist can break through a patient's defense mechanisms and help the patient resolve the underlying conflict.

double p., dual p. dissociative identity disorder.

hysterical p. former name for HISTRIONIC PERSONALITY DISORDER.

multiple p. a DISSOCIATIVE DISORDER in which an individual adopts two or more personalities alternately. See MULTIPLE PERSONALITY DISORDER.

split p. an obsolete term formerly used colloquially to refer to either SCHIZOPHRENIA or DISSOCIATIVE IDENTITY DISORDER.

perspiration (per″spĭ-ra′shun) 1. sweating. 2. sweat.

per tertiam (intentionem) (per ter′she-am in-ten″she-o′nem) [L.] by third intention (see HEALING).

Perthes' disease (per′tēz) LEGG-CALVÉ-PERTHES DISEASE.

per tubam (per tu′bam) [L.] through a tube.

pertussis (per-tus′is) WHOOPING COUGH.

pertussoid (per-tus′oid) resembling whooping cough.

per vaginam (per vah-ji′nam) [L.] through the vagina.

pervasive developmental disorders a group of disorders characterized by impairment of development in multiple areas, including the acquisition of reciprocal social interaction, verbal and nonverbal communication skills, and imaginative activity, and by stereotyped interests and behaviors; included are AUTISTIC DISORDER and various less common conditions.

perversion (per-ver′zhun) 1. deviation from the normal course; a morbid alteration of function which may occur in emotional, intellectual, or volitional fields. 2. sexual DEVIATION.

sexual p. sexual deviation.

pes (pes), pl. *pe′des* [L.] 1. foot. 2. any footlike part.

p. abduc′tus talipes valgus.

p. adduc′tus talipes varus.

p. ca′vus TALIPES cavus.

p. hippocam′pi a formation of two or three elevations on the ventricular surface of the HIPPOCAMPUS.

p. pla′nus, p. val′gus flatfoot.

p. va′rus TALIPES varus.

pessary (pes′ah-re) 1. an instrument placed in the vagina to support the uterus or rectum or as a CONTRACEPTIVE device. 2. a medicated vaginal suppository.

pesticide (pes′tĭ-sīd) a poison used to destroy pests of any sort.

pestilence (pes′tĭ-lens) a virulent contagious epidemic or infectious epidemic disease. adj., **pestilen′tial.**

pestle (pes″l) an instrument with a rounded end, used in a mortar to reduce a solid to a powder or produce a homogeneous mixture of solids.

PET positron emission tomography.

peta- (P) a word element used in naming units of measurement to designate a quantity 10^{15} (a quadrillion) times the unit to which it is joined.

-petal word element [L.], *directed* or *moving toward.*

petaling (pet′al-ing) applying small curved pieces of moleskin to a dry plaster of Paris cast to create a smooth edge that is less likely to crumble and injure the skin.

petechia (pe-te′ke-ah) [L.] a minute, pinpoint, nonraised, perfectly round, purplish red spot caused by intradermal or submucous hemorrhage, which later turns blue or yellow. adj., **pete′chial.**

petiole (pet′e-ōl) a stem, stalk, or pedicle.

epiglottic p. the pointed lower end of the epiglottic cartilage, attached to the thyroid cartilage.

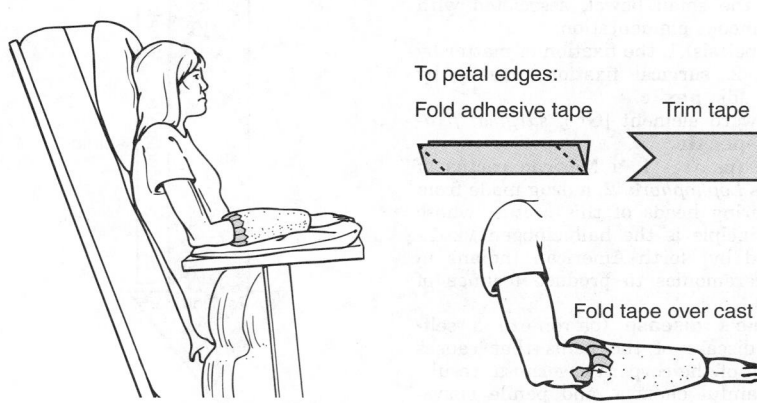

To petal edges:

Fold adhesive tape   Trim tape

Fold tape over cast

Petaling of the edges of a cast. From Lammon et al., 1995.

petiolus (pĕ-ti′ŏ-lus) petiole.

Petri dish (pe′tre) a round, shallow, flat-bottomed transparent glass or plastic dish with vertical sides and a similar but slightly larger dish that forms a cover; used for the culture of microorganisms on solid media and for tissue cell cultures.

petrichloral (pet″rĭ-klor′al) a nonbarbiturate SEDATIVE and HYPNOTIC.

pétrissage (pa-tre-sahzh′) [Fr.] foulage.

petrolatum (pet″ro-la′tum) a purified mixture of semisolid hydrocarbons obtained from petroleum, used as a base for ointments, protective dressings, and soothing applications to the skin. Called also petroleum jelly.

liquid p. see MINERAL OIL.

petroleum (pĕ-tro′le-um) a thick natural oil obtained from beneath the earth. It consists of a mixture of various hydrocarbons of the paraffin and olefin series.

petromastoid (pet″ro-mas′toid) 1. pertaining to the petrous PART of the temporal bone and its mastoid PROCESS. 2. otocranium (def. 2).

petrosal (pĕ-tro′sal) pertaining to the pars petrosa, or petrous portion of the temporal bone.

petrositis (pet″ro-si′tis) inflammation of the pars petrosa or petrous portion of the temporal bone.

petrosphenoid (pet″ro-sfe′noid) pertaining to the petrous portion of the temporal bone and to the sphenoid bone.

petrosquamous (pet″ro-skwa′mus) pertaining to the petrous and squamous portions of the temporal bone.

petrous (pet′rus) resembling rock or stone; stony.

Peutz-Jeghers syndrome (pertz ya′gerz) familial gastrointestinal polyposis, especially in the small bowel, associated with mucocutaneous pigmentation.

pexis (pek′sis) 1. the fixation of matter by a tissue. 2. surgical fixation, usually by suturing. adj., **pex′ic.**

-pexy word element [Gr.], *surgical fixation.* adj. **-pec′tic.**

peyote (pa-o′te) 1. a Mexican cactus of the genus *Lophophora.* 2. a drug made from the flowering heads of this cactus, whose active principle is the hallucinogen MESCALINE; used by North American Indians in certain ceremonies to produce feelings of ecstasy.

Peyronie's disease (pa-ron-ēz′) a self-limiting disease of the penis that causes hardening of the corpora cavernosa, resulting in painful CHORDEE and penile CURVATURE.

Pfeiffer's disease (glandular fever) (fī′ferz) infectious mononucleosis.

Pfeiffer syndrome (fī′fer) a hereditary autosomal dominant disorder characterized by conical deformity of the head, extra fingers and toes, webbed fingers and TOES, and broad short thumbs and big toes. Called also acrocephalosyndactyly type V and acrocephalopolysyndactyly type I.

PG prostaglandin.

pg picogram.

pH the negative logarithm of the hydrogen ion concentration, [H^+], a measure of the degree to which a solution is acidic or alkaline. An ACID is a substance that can give up a hydrogen ion (H^+); a BASE is a substance that can accept H^+. The more acidic a solution the greater the hydrogen ion concentration and the lower the pH; a pH of 7.0 indicates neutrality, a pH of less than 7 indicates acidity, and a pH of more than 7 indicates alkalinity. The pH is used as a measure of whether the body is maintaining a normal ACID-BASE BALANCE. A favorable

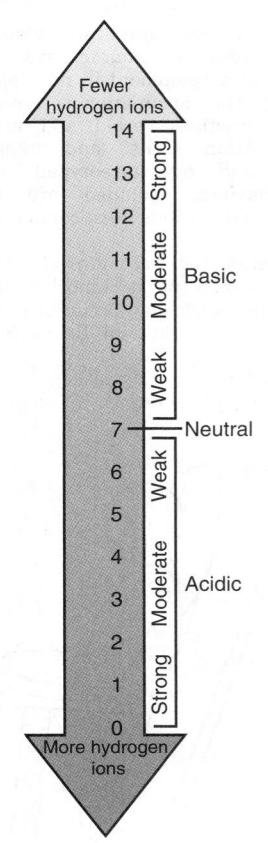

pH scale. From Applegate, 2000.

pH is essential to the functioning of enzymes and other biochemical systems. The body's fluids are normally somewhat alkaline, the pH being between 7.35 and 7.45. A pH above 7.8 or below 6.8 is generally fatal. See also ACIDOSIS and ALKALOSIS.

phac(o)- word element [Gr.], *lens.* See also words beginning PHAK(O)-.

phacitis (fah-si′tis) phakitis.

phacoanaphylaxis (fak″o-an″ah-fĭ-lak′sis) hypersensitivity to the protein of the crystalline lens of the eye, induced by escape of material from the lens capsule.

phacocele (fak′o-sēl) hernia of the eye lens.

phacocystectomy (fak″o-sis-tek′to-me) excision of part of the lens capsule for cataract.

phacocystitis (fak″o-sis-ti′tis) inflammation of the capsule of the eye lens.

phacoemulsification (fak″o-e-mul″sĭ-fĭ-ka′shun) a technique of CATARACT extraction, utilizing high-frequency ultrasonic vibrations to fragment the lens combined with controlled irrigation to maintain normal pressure in the anterior chamber, and suction to remove lens fragments and irrigating fluid.

phacoerysis (fak″o-er′ĭ-sis) removal of the eye lens in cataract by suction.

phacoid (fak′oid) shaped like a lens.

phacoiditis (fak″oi-di′tis) phakitis.

phacolysis (fah-kol′ĭ-sis) dissolution or discission of the crystalline lens. adj., **phacolyt′ic.**

phacomalacia (fak″o-mah-la′she-ah) softening of the eye lens; a soft cataract, that is, one without a hard nucleus.

phacometachoresis (fak″o-met″ah-ko-re′-sis) displacement of the eye lens.

phacosclerosis (fak″o-sklĕ-ro′sis) hardening of the eye lens; a hard cataract, that is, one with a hard nucleus.

phacoscope (fak′o-skōp) an instrument for viewing accommodative changes of the eye lens.

phacotoxic (fak′o-tok″sik) exerting a deleterious effect upon the crystalline lens.

phaeohyphomycosis (fe″o-hi″fo-mi-ko′-sis) a HYPHOMYCOSIS in which the infecting fungus is dark in color; most are opportunistic infections.

phag(o)- word element [Gr.], *eating; ingestion.*

phage (fāj) bacteriophage.

-phage word element [Gr.] *one that eats or destroys.*

phagedena (faj″ē-de′nah) rapidly spreading and sloughing ulceration. adj., **phage-de′nic.**

-phagia word element [Gr.], *eating; swallowing.*

phagocyte (fag′o-sīt) any cell capable of ingesting particulate matter, usually referring to a MICROPHAGE, MACROPHAGE, or MONOCYTE. They ingest microorganisms and other particulate antigens that are coated with antibody or complement (OPSONIZED), a process mediated by specific cell-surface receptors. Other cell types exhibit phagocytosis, but not specific phagocytosis of opsonized particles.

phagocytic dysfunction disorders a group of IMMUNODEFICIENCY conditions characterized by disordered phagocytic activity; they may be *extrinsic* (e.g. suppression of the number of phagocytes by immunosuppressive agents, or dysfunction caused by corticosteroids) or *intrinsic* (related to enzyme deficiencies); they are marked by bacterial or fungal infections that range from mild recurrent skin infection to fatal systemic infection.

phagocytin (fag″o-si′tin) a bactericidal substance from neutrophilic leukocytes.

phagocytize (fag′o-sī-tīz) phagocytose.

phagocytolysis (fag″o-si-tol′ĭ-sis) destruction of phagocytes. adj., **phagocytolyt′ic.**

phagocytose (fag″o-si′tōs) to envelop and destroy bacteria and other foreign material; phagocytize.

phagocytosis (fag″o-si-to′sis) the engulfing of microorganisms or other cells and foreign particles by phagocytes. adj., **phagocytot′ic.**

phagosome (fag′o-sōm) a membrane-bound vesicle in a phagocyte containing the phagocytized material.

phagotype (fag′o-tīp) phage type.

-phagy see *-phagia.*

phak(o)- see *phac(o)-.*

phakitis (fa-ki′tis) inflammation of the crystalline lens of the eye.

phakoma (fah-ko′mah) 1. an occasional small, grayish white tumor seen

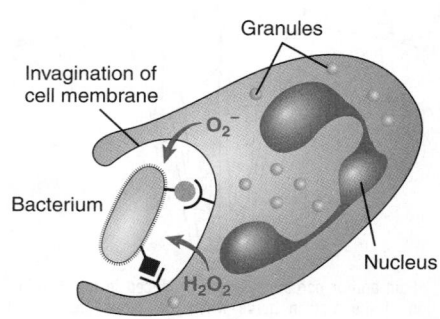

Phagocytosis. From Damjanov, 2000.

P

microscopically in the retina in tuberous sclerosis. 2. a patch of myelinated nerve fibers seen very infrequently in the retina in neurofibromatosis.

phakomatosis (fak″o-mah-to′sis) any of five hereditary syndromes (neurofibromatosis, tuberous sclerosis, Sturge-Weber syndrome, and von Hippel-Lindau disease, and ataxia-telangiectasia) marked by disseminated hamartomas of the eye, skin, and brain.

phalangeal (fah-lan′je-al) pertaining to a phalanx.

phalangectomy (fal″an-jek′to-me) excision of a phalanx.

phalanges (fah-lan′jēz) sing., *pha′lanx* [Gr.] the bones of the fingers and toes; see anatomic Table of Bones in the Appendices. adj., **phalan′geal.**

phalangitis (fal″an-ji′tis) inflammation of one or more phalanges.

Phalen's maneuver (fa′lenz) to detect CARPAL TUNNEL SYNDROME, the size of the carpal tunnel is reduced by flexion (or extension) of the affected wrist for 30 to 60 seconds, or by inflating a SPHYGMOMANOMETER cuff around the involved hand to a point between diastolic and systolic pressure for 30 to 60 seconds. Pain or paresthesias occur along the distribution of the median nerve when the patient has carpal tunnel syndrome.

phallectomy (fal-ek′to-me) penectomy.

phallic (fal′ik) penile.

phallitis (fal-i′tis) penitis.

phallocampsis (fal″o-kamp′sis) penile curvature.

phalloidin (fah-loid′in) a hexapeptide poison from the mushroom *Amanita*

Phalen's Maneuver

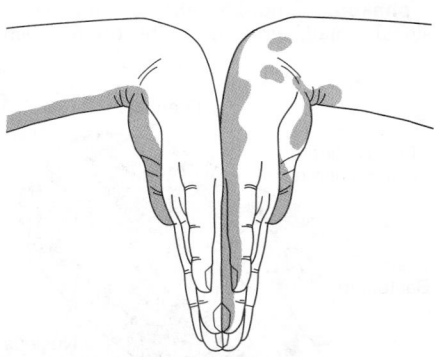

Pain and/or paresthesias are produced in the distribution of the median nerve when the hands are held in flexion for 30 to 60 seconds. From Goldman and Bennett, 2000.

phalloides, which causes asthenia, vomiting, diarrhea, convulsions, and death.

phallus (fal′us) the penis. adj., **phal′lic.**

phanerosis (fan″er-o′sis) the process of becoming visible.

phantasm (fan′tazm) phantom (def. 1).

phantogeusia (fan″to-gu′ze-ah) continuous abnormal taste in the mouth, usually metallic or salty.

phantom (fan′tom) 1. an image or impression not evoked by actual stimuli. 2. a model of the body or of a specific part thereof. 3. a device for simulating the in vivo effect of radiation on tissues.

phar pharmacy; pharmaceutical; pharmacopeia.

pharm pharmacy; pharmaceutical; pharmacopeia.

pharmac(o)- word element [Gr.], *drug; medicine.*

pharmaceutical (fahr″mah-soo′tĭ-k′l) 1. pertaining to pharmacy or drugs. 2. a medicinal drug.

pharmaceutics (fahr″mah-soo′tiks) 1. pharmacy (def. 1). 2. pharmaceutical preparations.

pharmacist (fahr′mah-sist) a person licensed to prepare, compound, and dispense drugs upon written order (PRESCRIPTION) from a licensed practitioner such as a physician, dentist, or advanced practice nurse. A pharmacist is a health care professional who cooperates with, consults with, and sometimes advises the licensed practitioner concerning drugs.

For a licensed pharmacist, five years of education is a minimum, and some curricula require six years. This gives the pharmacist advanced knowledge of the chemical and physical properties of drugs and their available dosage forms, and he or she is thus qualified to play a key role in supplying information about drugs (both prescription and over-the-counter) to patients—those to whom such information is most important. Since the pharmacist may be the last health care professional to communicate with the patient or a significant other before the medication is taken, he or she is therefore in an ideal position to discuss the drug with those concerned. The discussion may include any side effects associated with the drug, its stability under various conditions, its toxicity, its dosage, and its route of administration, all of which may be reassuring to the patient and be of benefit in helping insure patient compliance with the drug regimen.

pharmacoangiography (fahr″mah-ko-an-je-og′rah-fe) ANGIOGRAPHY in which visualization is enhanced by manipulating the

WINDOW ON PHARMACIST

The pharmacist is a licensed health care professional who assumes responsibility for the monitoring and appropriate use of patients' medications through the practice of pharmacy. Pharmacy is a science that involves the preparation, compounding, and dispensing of drugs for use in patients, the monitoring of patients' drug therapy for both efficacy and adverse effects, and the provision of recommendations to ensure proper therapeutic outcomes. In addition, the profession of pharmacy includes the provision of drug and therapeutic information to other members of the health care team and the public.

There are two professional degrees in pharmacy that allow an individual to complete the licensure requirements and practice as a pharmacists, the baccalaureate degree (BS) in pharmacy and the Doctor of Pharmacy degree (PharmD). The BS degree is generally awarded after five years of study in a school or college of pharmacy. The PharmD degree is generally awarded after six or seven years of study in a school or college of pharmacy. Currently, most schools/colleges of pharmacy either offer or are planning to offer the PharmD degree as the first (entry-level) professional degree, with the elimination of the BS degree in pharmacy program.

Contemporary pharmacists have a wide variety of career opportunities available to them. These include: community pharmacy, e.g., practice in retail or home health care pharmacies or as consultants to extended care facilities; institutional pharmacy, e.g., practice in hospitals, health maintenance organizations (HMOs), or clinics; industrial practice, e.g., practice in the pharmaceutical industry; government service, e.g., practice in governmental agencies such as the Food and Drug Administration, the Indian Health Service, the Public Health Service, or the Armed Forces; pharmacy education, e.g., full-time, part-time, or adjunct faculty members in schools/colleges of pharmacy; and organization service, e.g., practice in various local, state, or national professional pharmacy organizations.

Individuals with either a BS or a PharmD degree can also further their education and pursue a master of science (MS) degree or a doctor of philosophy (PhD) degree in the pharmaceutical sciences, which include the disciplines of pharmacology, pharmaceutics, medicinal chemistry, natural products, biopharmaceutics and pharmacokinetics, and behavioral and administrative pharmacy.

The profession of pharmacy has undergone considerable change since the days of the old "corner drug store" in which pharmacists primarily compounded and dispensed drug products. Pharmacists today currently embrace and practice the concept of "pharmaceutical care," and take responsibility for all aspects of a patient's medication therapy. They are members of the most respected profession, according to recent Gallup polls, and continue to be highly utilized members of the health care team.

MARIE A. ABATE, PHARMD

---

flow of blood by administration of vasodilating and vasoconstricting agents.

pharmacodiagnosis (fahr″mah-ko-di″ag-no′sis) use of drugs in diagnosis.

pharmacodynamics (fahr″mah-ko-di-nam′iks) the study of the biochemical and physiological effects of drugs and the mechanisms of their actions, including the correlation of their actions and effects with their chemical structure. adj., **pharmacodynam′ic.**

pharmacogenetics (fahr″mah-ko-jĕ-net′-iks) the study of the relationship between genetic factors and the nature of responses to drugs.

pharmacognosy (fahr″mah-kog′no-se) the branch of pharmacology dealing with natural drugs and their constituents.

pharmacokinetics (fahr″mah-ko-kĭ-ne-t′iks) the study of the movement of drugs in the body, including the processes of absorption, distribution, localization in tissues, biotransformation, and excretion. adj., **pharmacokinet′ic.**

pharmacologist (fahr″mah-kol′o-jist) a specialist in pharmacology.

pharmacology (fahr″mah-kol′o-je) the science that deals with the origin, nature, chemistry, effects, and uses of drugs; it includes pharmacognosy, pharmacokinetics, pharmacodynamics, pharmacotherapeutics, and toxicology. adj., **pharmacolog′ic.**

pharmacomania (fahr″mah-ko-ma′ne-ah) uncontrollable desire to take or to administer drugs.

pharmacopeia (fahr″mah-ko-pe′ah) an authoritative treatise on drugs and their preparations; see also USP. adj., **pharmacopei′al.**

pharmacophobia (fahr″mah-ko-fo′be-ah) irrational fear of medicines or drugs.

pharmacophore (fahr′mah-ko-for″) the group of atoms in the molecule of a drug responsible for the drug's action.

pharmacopoeia (fahr″mah-ko-pe′ah) pharmacopeia.

pharmacotherapy (fahr″mah-ko-ther′ah-pe) treatment of disease with medicines.

pharmacy (fahr′mah-se) 1. the branch of the health sciences dealing with the preparation, dispensing, and proper utilization of drugs. 2. a place where drugs are compounded or dispensed.

Pharm D [L.] Pharma′ciae Doc′tor (Doctor of Pharmacy).

pharyng(o)- word element [Gr.], *pharynx.*

pharyngalgia (far″ing-gal′jah) pharyngodynia.

pharyngeal (fah-rin′je-al) pertaining to the pharynx.

pharyngectomy (far″in-jek′to-me) excision of part of the pharynx.

pharyngismus (far″in-jiz′mus) pharyngospasm.

pharyngitis (far″in-ji′tis) inflammation of the PHARYNX; called also sore throat. adj., **pharyngit′ic.** *Acute pharyngitis* usually appears suddenly and runs its course in a few days or a week. Symptoms, more severe in children, are dry, sore throat, fatigue, and mild fever. Often, swallowing is painful, the head aches, and there is a harsh cough and a persistent desire to clear the throat. The throat frequently becomes swollen and covered with a thick mucous material. Sometimes there is pain in the ears, or hoarseness.

The American College of Physicians and American Society of Internal Medicine have published *Clinical Practice Guidelines on Principles of Appropriate Antibiotic Use for Acute Pharyngitis in Adults.* They recommend that any adult with pharyngitis should be offered ANALGESICS, ANTIPYRETICS, and other supportive care. Prescriptions of ANTIMICROBIALS should be limited to those patients most likely to have group A beta-hemolytic *Streptococcus.*

Chronic pharyngitis is the result of continuous reinfection or chronic irritation of exposed parts of the throat. It is similar to acute pharyngitis, but less severe. The simple catarrhal form can be caused by smoking, dust, smog, or constant breathing through the mouth.

Pharyngitis may also occur as part of an early stage of a disease such as SCARLET FEVER, MEASLES, or WHOOPING COUGH. Symptomatic treatment includes hot saline gargles, liquid diet, and an increase in fluid intake. Antibiotics may be prescribed when a bacterial infection is present.

pharyngocele (fah-ring′go-sēl) a herniation or cystic deformity of the pharynx.

pharyngoconjunctival fever (fah-ring″go-kon″jung-ti′val) an epidemic disease due to an adenovirus, occurring chiefly in school children, with fever, pharyngitis, conjunctivitis, rhinitis, and enlarged cervical lymph nodes.

pharyngodynia (fah-ring″go-din′e-ah) pain in the pharynx.

pharyngoesophageal (fah-ring″go-e-sof″-ah-je′al) pertaining to the pharynx and esophagus.

pharyngoglossal (fah-ring″go-glos′al) glossopharyngeal.

pharyngokeratosis (fah-ring″go-ker″ah-to′sis) keratosis pharyngea.

pharyngolaryngitis (fah-ring″go-lar″in-ji′-tis) laryngopharyngitis.

pharyngomycosis (fah-ring″go-mi-ko′sis) any fungal infection of the pharynx.

pharyngonasal (fah-ring″go-na′zal) nasopharyngeal.

pharyngoparalysis (fah-ring″go-pah-ral′ĭ-sis) paralysis of the pharyngeal muscles; pharyngoplegia.

pharyngoplasty (fah-ring′go-plas″te) plastic repair of the pharynx.

pharyngoplegia (fah-ring″go-ple′jah) pharyngoparalysis.

pharyngoscleroma (fah-ring″go-sklĕ-ro′-mah) scleroma of the pharynx.

pharyngoscope (fah-ring′go-skōp) an instrument for inspecting the pharynx.

pharyngoscopy (far″ing-gos′kah-pe) direct visual examination of the pharynx.

pharyngospasm (fah-ring′go-spazm) spasm of the pharyngeal muscles; called also PHARYNGISMUS.

pharyngostenosis (fah-ring″go-stĕ-no′sis) narrowing of the pharynx.

pharyngotomy (far″ing-got′ah-me) incision of the pharynx.

pharynx (far′ingks) the throat; the musculomembranous cavity, about 5 inches (12.5 cm) long, behind the nasal cavities, mouth, and larynx, communicating with them and with the esophagus. It includes many individual structures and may be divided into three areas: the NASOPHARYNX (top), OROPHARYNX (center, behind the mouth), and LARYNGOPHARYNX (bottom). The nasopharynx, connected with the nasal cavities, provides a passage for air during breathing and contains the openings of the eustachian tubes through which air enters the middle ear. The oropharynx and laryngopharynx provide passageways for both air and food. The pharynx also functions as a resonating organ in speech.

The pharynx is separated from the mouth by the soft palate and its fleshy V-shaped extension or flap, the UVULA, which hangs from the top of the back of the mouth, above the root of the tongue. In swallowing, the uvula lifts up, closing off the nasopharynx as food passes from the mouth through the lower parts of the pharynx to the esophagus. On each side of the entrance to the pharynx from the mouth, and behind the nasal passage, are the TONSILS and ADENOIDS, masses of lymphoid tissue.

phase (fāz) 1. one of the aspects or stages through which a varying entity may pass. 2. In physical chemistry, any physically or chemically distinct, homogeneous, and mechanically separable part of a system.

p. 0 in cardiac physiology, the phase representing the upstroke of the ACTION POTENTIAL, in which rapid DEPOLARIZATION occurs after the cell reaches or is driven to threshold POTENTIAL. It is the result of the opening of fast sodium CHANNELS and calcium CHANNELS.

p. 1 in cardiac physiology, the initial rapid REPOLARIZATION phase of the ACTION POTENTIAL, caused by the closure of the fast sodium CHANNELS and an exodus of potassium from the cell.

p. 2 in cardiac physiology, the phase representing the plateau of the ACTION POTENTIAL, which contributes to the refractory PERIOD of the heart; there is a slow entry of calcium into the cell. It is the result of a balance between inward and outward currents and is particularly long in Purkinje and ventricular cells.

p. 3 in cardiac physiology, the terminal rapid REPOLARIZATION phase of the ACTION POTENTIAL; it begins with the closing of the slow channels, resulting in an exodus of potassium from the cell and the activation of the sodium-potassium PUMP. The result is reestablishment of the normal resting POTENTIAL.

p. 4 in cardiac physiology, the phase representing electrical DIASTOLE, i.e. the time between ACTION POTENTIALS. It is the resting phase of the electrical cardiac cycle and is steadily maintained in nonpacemaker cells. In pacemaker CELLS, the membrane POTENTIAL is normally reduced slowly until threshold POTENTIAL is reached; if there is an outside stimulus, it may be driven down more rapidly.

continuous p. in a heterogeneous system, the component in which the disperse phase is distributed, corresponding to the solvent in a true solution. See also COLLOID.

disperse p. the discontinuous portion of a heterogeneous system, corresponding to the solute in a true solution.

G₁ p. a part of the cell CYCLE during INTERPHASE, lasting from the end of cell division (the M phase) until the start of DNA synthesis (the S phase).

G₂ p. a relatively quiescent part of the cell CYCLE during INTERPHASE, lasting from the end of DNA synthesis (the S phase) until the start of cell division (the M phase).

M p. the part of the cell CYCLE during which MITOSIS occurs; subdivided into PROPHASE, METAPHASE, ANAPHASE, and TELOPHASE.

S p. a part of the cell CYCLE near the end of INTERPHASE, during which DNA is synthesized; it comes between the G₁ and G₂ phases.

phaseolamin (fah-se″o-lam′in) 1. an alpha-amylase inhibitor purified from the kidney bean (*Phaseolus vulgaris*); it is the basis of starch-blocker tablets. 2. an α-AMYLASE inhibitor purified from the kidney bean (*Phaseolus vulgaris*); it has been used in preparations alleged to enhance weight control by preventing absorption of ingested carbohydrate.

phasmid (faz′mid) either of the two caudal chemoreceptors occurring in certain nematodes (Phasmidia). 1. any nematode containing phasmids.

Phe phenylalanine.

phen(o)- word element [Gr.], 1. *showing; displaying.* 2. *a compound derived from benzene.*

phenacemide (fĕ-nas′ĕ-mīd) an ANTICONVULSANT used in psychomotor and grand mal EPILEPSY.

phenanthrene (fĕ-nan′thrĕn) a tricyclic aromatic hydrocarbon occurring in coal tar and isomeric with anthracene; it is toxic and CARCINOGENIC.

phenazone antipyrine.

phenazopyridine (fen″ah-zo-pēr′ĭ-dēn) a urinary tract ANALGESIC, used as the hydrochloride salt; administered orally.

phencyclidine (fen-si′klĭ-dēn) a central nervous system DEPRESSANT, introduced as an anesthetic in the early 1950s but later abandoned because of unpredictable side effects such as agitation, disorientation, and hallucination. The drug is easily synthesized by anyone with a basic knowledge of chemistry and has become one of the drugs most frequently used by drug abusers. (See DRUG ABUSE.) It has a variety of street names, including "angel dust," "animal tranquilizer," "PCP," "peace pill," "crystal joints," and "peace weed," with the name often reflecting the form in which it is taken. It can be smoked, "snorted" through the nose, ingested, or taken intravenously. There is always danger from the poor and erratic quality of the product illegally sold on the streets. It can produce a schizophrenia-like syndrome, neurologic and cognitive dysfunction, coma, convulsions, and respiratory arrest.

phendimetrazine (fen″di-met′rah-zēn) a sympathomimetic amine with pharmacologic actions similar to those of the AMPHET-AMINES, used as the tartrate salt as an appetite suppressant.

phenelzine (fen′el-zēn) a monoamine oxidase INHIBITOR, administered orally as the sulfate salt as an ANTIDEPRESSANT and in the prevention of MIGRAINE.

Phenergan (fen′er-gan) trademark for preparations of PROMETHAZINE, an ANTIHISTAMINE, ANTIEMETIC, and SEDATIVE.

phenindamine (fĕ-nin′dah-min) an ANTIHISTAMINE with sedative and anticholinergic effects; used as the tartrate salt in the treatment of nasal, eye, and skin manifestations of allergic reactions, including allergic rhinitis, conjunctivitis, and itching, and also as an ingredient in some cough and cold preparations, administered orally.

pheniramine (fĕ-nir′ah-min) an ANTIHISTAMINE with sedative properties, used as the maleate salt in the treatment of allergic disorders, including rhinitis, conjunctivitis, and pruritic skin disorders; administered orally, intranasally, or topically to the conjunctiva. It is also used as an ingredient in cough and cold preparations, administered orally.

Phenistix (fen′ĭ-stiks) trademark for a reagent strip impregnated with ferric chloride and glacial acetic acid; used in screening tests for phenylketonuria and in detection of salicylates and chlorpromazine in the urine.

phenmetrazine (fen-met′rah-zēn) a central nervous system STIMULANT, used as an appetite suppressant in the form of the hydrochloride salt; abuse may lead to habituation.

phenobarbital (fe″no-bahr′bĭ-tal) a long-acting BARBITURATE used as the base or the sodium salt as an ANTICONVULSANT, SEDATIVE, and HYPNOTIC.

phenocopy (fe′no-kop″e) 1. an environmentally induced phenotype mimicking one usually produced by a specific genotype. 2.

an individual exhibiting such a phenotype; the simulated trait in a phenocopy.

phenodeviant (fe″no-de′ve-ant) an individual whose phenotype differs significantly from that of the typical phenotype in the population.

phenol (fe′nol) 1. an extremely poisonous compound, used in dilute solution as an antimicrobial, anesthetic, and antipruritic. Ingestion or absorption through the skin causes symptoms including colic, local irritation, corrosion, seizures, cardiac arrhythmias, shock, and respiratory arrest. Phenol should be properly labeled and stored to avoid accidental poisoning. Called also carbolic acid. 2. any of various related organic compounds containing one or more hydroxyl groups attached to an aromatic carbon ring.

p. coefficient a measure of the bactericidal activity of a chemical compound in relation to phenol. The activity of the compound is expressed as the ratio of dilution in which it kills in 10 minutes but not in 5 minutes under the specified conditions. It can be determined in the absence of organic matter, or in the presence of a standard amount of added organic matter.

phenolphthalein (fe″nol-thal′ēn) a CATHARTIC and pH indicator.

phenomenology (fĕ-nom″ĕ-nol′o-je) the study of phenomena in their own right rather than inferring causes; in psychiatry, the theory that behavior is determined by the way the person perceives reality rather than by objective external reality.

phenomenon (fĕ-nom′ĕ-non), pl. *phenom′-ena* any sign or objective symptom; any observable occurrence or fact. For names of specific phenomena, see under the name.

phenothiazine (fe″no-thi′ah-zēn) any of a group of having a similar tricyclic structure and acting as potent dopaminergic and alpha-ADRENERGIC BLOCKING AGENTS, as well as having hypotensive, antispasmodic, antihistaminic, analgesic, sedative, and antiemetic activity.

phenotype (fe′no-tīp) 1. the outward, visible expression of the hereditary constitution of an organism. 2. an individual exhibiting a certain phenotype; a trait expressed in a phenotype. adj., **phenotyp′ic.**

phenoxybenzamine (fĕ-nok″se-ben′zah-mēn) an ADRENERGIC BLOCKING AGENT; the hydrochloride salt is used to control HYPERTENSION in PHEOCHROMOCYTOMA and to treat urinary symptoms in benign prostatic HYPERPLASIA.

phenozygous (fe″no-zi′gus) having the calvaria narrower than the face, so that the zygomatic ARCHES are visible when the head is viewed from above.

phensuximide (fen-suk′sĭ-mīd) an ANTI-
CONVULSANT used in the treatment of petit
mal EPILEPSY; administered orally.

phentermine (fen′ter-mēn) a SYMPATHOMI-
METIC AMINE related to AMPHETAMINE, used as
an appetite suppressant either as the hydrochloride salt or as the base in a complex
with a resin, which has a sustained action.

phentolamine (fen-tol′ah-mēn) a potent
ALPHA-ADRENERGIC BLOCKING AGENT that blocks
the hypertensive action of epinephrine and
norepinephrine and most responses of
smooth muscles that involve alpha-adrenergic RECEPTORS. Its mesylate salt is used
intravenously or intramuscularly to prevent
and treat HYPERTENSION occurring before and
during surgery for PHEOCHROMOCYTOMA and is
also used intravenously to prevent and treat
cutaneous necrosis and sloughing when
extravasation of NOREPINEPHRINE occurs after
intravenous administration.

Phenurone (fen′u-rōn) trademark for a
preparation of PHENACEMIDE, an ANTICONVUL-
SANT.

phenyl (fen′il, fe′nil) the monovalent
radical, C_6H_5— derived from benzene by
removal of hydrogen. adj., **phenyl′ic.**

phenylacetic acid (fen″il-ah-se′tik) a
CATABOLITE of PHENYLALANINE; it is excessively
formed and excreted, sometimes conjugated
with GLUTAMINE, in PHENYLKETONURIA.

phenylalanine (fen″il-al′ah-nīn) a naturally occurring AMINO ACID, one of the
essential amino acids, necessary for optimal
growth in infants and for nitrogen equilibrium in adults.

phenylalaninemia (fen″il-al″ah-nĭ-ne′me-
ah) hyperphenylalaninemia.

phenylbutazone (fen″il-bu′tah-zōn) a
NONSTEROIDAL ANTIINFLAMMATORY DRUG administered orally in the short-term treatment of
severe rheumatoid disorders unresponsive
to less toxic agents. It is given for periods of
less than one week because it can cause
aplastic anemia and agranulocytosis.

phenylephrine (fen″il-ef′rin) an adrenergic with potent VASOCONSTRICTOR properties;
used as the hydrochloride salt for various
purposes: topically to decongest nasal and
laryngeal mucous membranes or to produce
mydriasis without cycloplegia; intravenously to maintain blood pressure during
spinal and inhalation anesthesia, to treat
vascular failure in drug-induced shock,
shocklike states, and hypotension, to prolong spinal anesthesia, and to treat
paroxysmal supraventricular tachycardia;
and orally as a component of combination
antihistaminic-decongestant preparations.

phenylketonuria (PKU or PKU1) (fen″il-
ke″to-nu′re-ah) a congenital disease due to a
defect in metabolism of the amino acid

PHENYLALANINE. The condition is hereditary
and transmitted as a recessive trait.
Symptoms result from lack of an enzyme,
phenylalanine hydroxylase, necessary for
the conversion of phenylalanine to TYROSINE.
Phenylalanine collects in the blood and
there is eventual excretion of PHENYLPYRUVIC
ACID in the urine (See accompanying
illustration.) If untreated, the condition
results in mental retardation and other
abnormalities. adj., **phenylketonu′ric.**

The carrier state for PKU can be detected
by enzyme assay. The widespread success of
screening programs introduced in the 1960s
has led to parents who are carriers to be
successfully treated and go through childbearing years avoiding either transmitting
the disease or affecting the unborn fetus.
(See Window on Maternal PKU Syndrome.)

Persons with phenylketonuria are
usually blue-eyed and blond with defective
pigmentation; the skin is excessively sensitive to light and susceptible to eczema.
Other manifestations include tremors,
poor muscular coordination, and excessive
perspiration. A characteristic "mousy odor"
may be present due to PHENYLACETIC
ACID in the breath, skin, and urine. Convulsions may also be associated with the
disease.

Diagnosis. Screening of newborns for
PKU entails a simple heel-stick blood sampling test called the GUTHRIE TEST, which is
routinely performed in the United States,
Canada, and many other countries. The test
should be done within two weeks of birth,
preferably soon after the infant has been
fed. Variants of PKU have been named
*hyperphenylalaninemia without phenylketo-
nuria* and *atypical phenylketonuria.* Criteria for establishment of a diagnosis of
classic PKU vary from state to state and
country to country. The most common blood
phenylalanine recommendations in U.S.
laboratories are 2 to 6 mg/dL for individuals
under age 12 and 2 to 10 mg/dL for those
aged 12 and up. Diagnosis of variants of
the disease depends in part on values of
plasma phenylalanine, family history, clinical course, and the infant's response to
ingestion of natural protein.

Treatment. Restriction of the infant's diet
to control the effects of PKU is prescribed
on the basis of his or her requirements
for phenylalanine, protein, and calories.
Effectiveness of the special diet must be
evaluated by frequent determinations of
phenylalanine blood levels; otherwise the
child may suffer from serious dietary deficiencies. The development of palatable

P

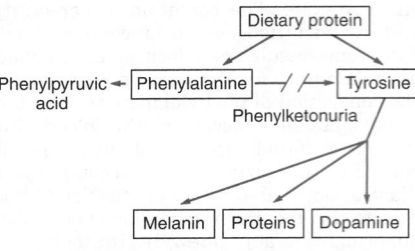

Phenylketonuria. Lack of phenylalanine hydroxylase blocks the transformation of phenylalanine into tyrosine. Unmetabolized phenylalanine is shunted into the pathway that leads to the formation of phenylketones. Excess phenylalanine also inhibits formation of melanin from tyrosine. From Damjanov, 2000.

HYDROLYSATE preparations such as Lofenalac has made treatment easier. About 90 per cent of the protein requirement is derived from this dietary protein substitute.

The National Institutes of Health Consensus Development Conference in October, 2000 identified the need for more research on PKU to develop better treatments than the dietary restrictions that are now the mainstay of therapy. Among other recommendations were the development of standard screening procedures, equal access to culturally sensitive, age-appropriate treatment programs, and appropriate family education. Infants with blood phenylalanine levels greater than 10 mg/dL should be started on treatment as soon as possible, no later than 7 to 10 days after birth. Frequent monitoring of blood levels is required. It was also recommended that those affected stay on the restricted diet for life. Treatment should be multidisciplinary and lifelong. The full NIH Consensus Statement on Phenylketonuria (PKU): Screening and Management is available by calling 1-888-NIH-CONSENSUS (1-888-644-2667) or accessing the NIH Consensus Development Program web site at http://consensus.nih.gov.

phenylmercuric (fen″il-mer-ku′rik) denoting a compound containing the radical C_6H_5Hg—, forming various antiseptic, antibacterial, and fungicidal salts; compounds of the acetate and nitrate salts are used as bacteriostatics, and the former is also used as an herbicide.

phenylpropanolamine (fen″il-pro″pah-nol′ah-min) an adrenergic used in the form of the hydrochloride salt as a nasal and sinus DECONGESTANT, as an appetite suppressant, and in the treatment of mild to moderate stress incontinence.

phenylpyruvic acid (fen″il-pi-roo′vik) an intermediate product of the metabolism of phenylalanine in the body.

phenyltoloxamine (fen″il-to-lok′sah-mēn) a sedating ANTIHISTAMINE, used as the citrate salt in cough and cold preparations.

phenytoin (fen′ĭ-toin″) an ANTICONVULSANT used in the treatment of EPILEPSY other than the petit mal type, the treatment of STATUS EPILEPTICUS, and the prevention and treatment of seizures associated with neurosurgery; administered orally. Called also diphenylhydantoin.

pheochrome (fe′o-krōm) chromaffin.

pheochromoblast (fe″o-kro′mo-blast) any of the embryonic structures that develop into chromaffin (pheochrome) cells.

pheochromocyte (fe″o-kro′mo-sīt) a chromaffin CELL.

pheochromocytoma (fe″o-kro″mo-si″to′-mah) a small chromaffin CELL tumor, usually in the adrenal medulla but occasionally in chromaffin tissue of the sympathetic paraganglia. It is relatively rare and tends to occur in families. It can be cured if diagnosed early, but can be fatal once it causes irreparable damage to the cardiovascular system.

Symptoms. Because it is composed of cells similar to the secreting cells of the adrenal medulla, it often secretes EPINEPHRINE and NOREPINEPHRINE, so that the cardinal symptom is HYPERTENSION. In some cases the blood pressure is consistently high with slight fluctuations, and in others it is intermittently high with normal periods. Other symptoms include severe headache, sweating, visual blurring, apprehension, tachycardia, and postural hypotension.

Diagnosis. Pheochromocytoma must be differentiated from several other disorders that it closely resembles, such as essential HYPERTENSION and THYROTOXICOSIS. Studies have shown that over 20 per cent of patients with this condition are carriers of associated familial disorders, such as cerebellar HEMANGIOBLASTOMA, STURGE-WEBER SYNDROME, tuberous SCLEROSIS, or VON HIPPEL-LINDAU DISEASE. Diagnosis is based on the patient's symptoms and the findings of specific chemical and pharmacologic tests. A test involving measurement of VANILLYLMANDELIC ACID, METANEPHRINE, and NORMETANEPHRINE in urine is most commonly used. The level of these substances in the urine of patients with pheochromocytoma is almost twice the upper limits of normal.

Treatment. Surgical removal of the tumor or tumors is necessary for complete remission of symptoms. There are two possible sets of complications of surgery: (1) a sudden rise in BLOOD PRESSURE with development of TACHYCARDIA due to discharge of pressor

SUBSTANCES as the tumor is being manipulated; and (2) severe HYPOTENSION and SHOCK following removal of the tumor. These hazards can be substantially reduced by the preoperative administration of SEDATIVES and ANTIHYPERTENSIVE AGENTS, and the use of blood or plasma to maintain adequate blood volume. If surgery has involved resection of a portion of the adrenal CORTEX, it may be necessary for the patient to receive adrenocortical HORMONES by injection. With proper treatment, up to 90 per cent of patients are curable.

Patient Care. Once the diagnosis of pheochromocytoma has been established, the patient is prepared for surgery. The preoperative period may extend for several weeks while attempts are made to stabilize the blood pressure and hormonal imbalances. The patient should be kept in a quiet atmosphere and usually is given sedatives, such as phenobarbital, to promote rest. Blood pressure is taken at frequent intervals and recorded. These readings are used later as a basis for comparison during the postoperative period. They also alert the physician to extremes in blood pressure that are characteristic in this disorder.

A day or two before surgery the patient may be given repeated doses of PHENTOLAMINE to block the vasoconstricting effects of epinephrine and norepinephrine. The blood pressure may be drastically affected and therefore must be monitored frequently for signs of instability and dangerous extremes.

Postoperatively the patient must again be watched for development of severe hypertension, which can lead to STROKE SYNDROME, and for extreme hypotension with circulatory collapse and profound shock.

If the adrenal cortex has been resected during surgery, hormonal imbalances are likely to occur. These include HYPOGLYCEMIA, addisonian crisis and extreme DIURESIS, and electrolyte and fluid imbalance. The hypoglycemia is most likely to occur in patients who have had symptoms of diabetes mellitus prior to surgery and is treated with infusions of glucose solution. Adrenocortical hormones may be administered intravenously. The patient's status is closely monitored so that disturbances in electrolyte and FLUID BALANCE, extremes in blood pressure, and disorders of metabolism can be recognized early and treated promptly.

pheresis (fĕ-re′sis) apheresis.

pheromone (fer′o-mōn) a substance secreted to the outside of the body and perceived (as by smell) by other individuals of the same species, releasing specific behavior in the percipient.

PhG Graduate in Pharmacy.

Phialophora (fi″ah-lof′o-rah) a genus of imperfect fungi. *P. verruco′si* is a cause of CHROMOBLASTOMYCOSIS and *P. jeansel′mi* is a cause of MADUROMYCOSIS.

-phil word element [Gr.], *one having an affinity for something.* Also, *-phile.* adj., **-phil′ic.**

-phile see *-phil.*

-philia word element [Gr.], *affinity for; morbid fondness of.* adj., **-phil′ic.**

philosophy (fĭ-los′ŏ-fe) a system of beliefs and principles.

   concordant p. a philosophical system used in KINLEIN, concerned with the practical aspects of a person on a day to day basis; a central principle is that of CORDISING. See also ESCA.

philtrum (fil′trum) the vertical groove in the median portion of the upper lip.

phimosis (fi-mo′sis) constriction of the orifice of the prepuce so that it cannot be drawn back over the glans. adj., **phimot′ic.**

pHisoHex (fi′so-heks) trademark for an emulsion containing HEXACHLOROPHENE; used as a skin cleanser.

phleb(o)- word element [Gr.], *vein.* See also words beginning VEN(O)-.

phlebangioma (fleb″an-je-o′mah) a venous aneurysm.

phlebarteriectasia (fleb″ahr-tēr″e-ek-ta′-zhah) general dilatation of veins and arteries.

phlebectasia (fleb″ek-ta′zhah) varicosity (def. 1).

phlebectomy (flĕ-bek′to-me) excision of a vein, or a segment of a vein.

phlebemphraxis (fleb″em-frak′sis) stoppage of a vein by a plug or clot.

phlebismus (flĕ-biz′mus) obstruction and consequent dilation of veins.

phlebitis (flĕ-bi′tis) inflammation of a VEIN, especially one in a lower limb. It is usually not serious in a superficial vein, since these veins are numerous enough to permit blood flow to be rechanneled so that it bypasses the inflamed vein. When a deep vein is involved, however, it may be more dangerous. It can also have serious consequences in certain areas such as the veins of the cranium, where it may lead to cerebral abscess. adj., **phlebit′ic.**

The causes of phlebitis are uncertain; it often occurs for no apparent reason. At other times, it seems to follow some other disorder, such as a circulatory difficulties like venous STASIS, a blood disorder such as a MYELOPROLIFERATIVE DISORDER, or OBESITY with concomitant lack of activity and venous stasis. It may also be a result of injury to a vein, either after an accident or occasionally as an aftermath of surgery.

Once in about a hundred births phlebitis develops in a newly delivered mother; in such cases it usually appears about 10 days after delivery. This form of phlebitis is commonly called "milk leg," because it is associated with the onset of milk production by the mother. It may also develop when circulation is sluggish after long periods of staying in bed without proper exercising of the limbs and frequent changing of position.

Symptoms and Treatment. When phlebitis occurs in a superficial vein, there is usually pain and tenderness. This may be so slight at first that it is felt only when pressure is applied. As the inflammation increases, the pain becomes more acute, especially during walking or other exercise. The inflamed area swells and becomes red and warm. A tender cordlike mass may form under the skin; it may grow smaller as the condition subsides, but occasionally lasts for some time. When the inflammation occurs in a deep vein and affects the tunica intima, there may be formation of a thrombus on the vein wall, a condition known as THROMBOPHLEBITIS. When clots in the veins interfere with the normal flow of blood, fluid accumulates and causes edema.

If phlebitis is superficial, the patient usually does not have to be confined to bed. When deeper veins are affected, however, or if the inflammation is severe, bed rest may be required. Antibiotics are sometimes prescribed to combat infection. In some extreme cases, or when an EMBOLISM is likely to occur, surgery with removal of the clot may be necessary as a preventive measure. In persons prone to thrombophlebitis, ANTICOAGULANTS are used as a preventive measure along with graduated elastic stockings, particularly when long periods of bed rest are required.

phleboclysis (flĕ-bok′lĭ-sis) injection of fluid into a vein; see also INTRAVENOUS INFUSION. Called also venoclysis.

phlebogram (fleb′o-gram) 1. a radiograph of a vein filled with contrast medium. 2. a phlebographic or sphygmographic tracing of the venous pulse.

phlebograph (fleb′o-graf) an instrument for recording the venous pulse.

phlebography (flĕ-bog′rah-fe) 1. ANGIOGRAPHY of a vein or veins. 2. the graphic recording of the venous pulse; called also venography.

phlebolith (fleb′o-lith) a calculus in a vein.

phlebolithiasis (fleb″o-lĭ-thi′ah-sis) the development of phleboliths.

phlebomanometer (fleb″o-mah-nom′ĕ-ter) an instrument for the direct measurement of venous blood pressure.

phlebophlebostomy (fleb″o-flĕ-bos′tah-me) operative anastomosis of one vein to another, as of the portal vein and inferior vena cava.

phleboplasty (fleb′o-plas″te) plastic repair of a vein.

phleborrhaphy (flĕ-bor′ah-fe) suturing of a vein.

phleborrhexis (fleb″o-rek′sis) rupture of a vein.

phlebosclerosis (fleb″o-sklĕ-ro′sis) fibrous thickening of the walls of veins; called also venosclerosis.

phlebostasis (flĕ-bos′tah-sis) 1. venous stasis. 2. temporary sequestration of a portion of blood from the general circulation by compressing the veins of a limb.

phlebothrombosis (fleb″o-throm-bo′sis) the development of venous thrombi in the absence of associated inflammation of the vessel wall; it is to be distinguished from THROMBOPHLEBITIS, in which there are inflammatory changes in the vessel wall. Called also venous thrombosis.

phlebotomist a health professional trained in the opening of veins for the withdrawal of blood.

Phlebotomus (flĕ-bot′o-mus) a genus of biting flies, called sandflies, the females of which are blood sucking. They are vectors of various diseases, including visceral leishmaniasis (*P. argen′tipes, P. chinen′sis, P. marti′ni, P. pernicio′sus*), Carrión's disease (*P. nogu′chi, P. verruca′rum*), cutaneous leishmaniasis (*P. lon′gipes, P. pe′difer, P. sergen′ti*), and phlebotomus fever (*P. papata′sii*).

phlebotomus fever (flĕ-bot′o-mus) a febrile viral disease of short duration, transmitted by the sandfly *Phlebotomus papatasii,* with symptoms like those of DENGUE, occurring in Mediterranean and Middle East countries. Called also sandfly fever.

phlebotomy (flĕ-bot′ah-me) incision of a vein for the removal or withdrawal of blood; called also venesection and venotomy.

arterial blood sample p. in the NURSING INTERVENTIONS CLASSIFICATION, a nursing INTERVENTION defined as obtaining a blood sample from an uncannulated artery to assess oxygen and carbon dioxide levels and ACID-BASE BALANCE.

p.: blood unit acquisition in the NURSING INTERVENTIONS CLASSIFICATION, a nursing INTERVENTION defined as procuring blood and blood products from donors.

p.: venous blood sample in the NURS-ING INTERVENTIONS CLASSIFICATION, a nursing INTERVENTION defined as removal of a sample of venous blood from an uncannulated vein.

phlegm (flem) viscid mucus excreted in abnormally large quantities from the respiratory tract.

phlegmasia (fleg-ma′zhah) old term for INFLAMMATION.

p. al′ba do′lens phlebitis of the femoral vein, with swelling of the lower limb, usually without redness, a condition that sometimes follows childbirth or an acute febrile illness. Called also milk leg.

p. ceru′lea do′lens an acute fulminating form of deep venous THROMBOSIS, with pronounced edema and severe cyanosis of the limb.

phlegmatic (fleg-mat′ik) of dull and sluggish temperament.

phlegmon (fleg′mon) diffuse inflammation of the soft or connective tissue due to infection with microaerophilic streptococci. adj., **phleg′monous.**

pancreatic p. a solid, swollen, inflamed mass of pancreatic tissue occurring as a complication of acute pancreatitis.

phlogogenic (flo″go-jen′ik) producing inflammation.

phlyctena (flik-te′nah) 1. a small blister made by a burn. 2. a small vesicle containing lymph seen on the conjunctiva in certain conditions. adj., **phlyc′tenar.**

phlyctenoid (flik′tĕ-noid) resembling a phlyctena.

phlyctenular (flik-ten′u-lar) associated with formation of PHLYCTENULES.

phlyctenule (flik′ten-ūl) a minute vesicle; an ulcerated nodule of the cornea or conjunctiva.

phlyctenulosis (flik-ten″u-lo′sis) a condition marked by formation of PHLYCTENULES.

phobia (fo′be-ah) a persistent, irrational, intense fear of a specific object, activity, or situation (the phobic stimulus), fear that is recognized as being excessive or unreasonable by the individual himself. When a phobia is a significant source of distress or interferes with social functioning, it is considered a mental disorder (sometimes called a PHOBIC DISORDER). Some typical phobias are: acrophobia (fear of heights), astraphobia (fear of lightning), cenotophobia (fear of new things or new ideas), claustrophobia (fear of closed places), hemophobia (fear of blood), and xenophobia (dread of strangers). Phobias are subclassified as AGORAPHOBIA, social PHOBIAS, and specific PHOBIAS. See also ANXIETY DISORDERS. adj., **pho′bic.**

simple p. specific phobia.

social p. an ANXIETY DISORDER characterized by fear and avoidance of social or

performance situations in which the individual fears possible embarrassment and humiliation, for example, fear of speaking, performing, or eating in public.

specific p. an ANXIETY DISORDER characterized by persistent and excessive or unreasonable fear of a circumscribed, well-defined object or situation, in contrast to fear of being alone or of public places (AGORAPHOBIA) or of embarrassment in social situations (SOCIAL PHOBIA). Common specific phobias involve fear of animals, particularly dogs, snakes, insects, and mice; fear of closed spaces (claustrophobia); and fear of heights (acrophobia).

-phobia word element [Gr.], *fear of; aversion to.*

phobic disorder see PHOBIA.

phobophobia (fo″bo-fo′be-ah) irrational fear of one's own fears or of acquiring a phobia.

phocomelia (fo″ko-me′le-ah) congenital absence of the proximal portion of a limb or limbs, the hands or feet being attached to the trunk by a small, irregularly shaped bone. adj., **phocome′lic.**

phocomelus (fo-kom′ĕ-lus) an individual exhibiting phocomelia.

phon(o)- word element [Gr.], *sound; voice; speech.*

phonal (fo′nal) 1. pertaining to sound. 2. vocal.

phonasthenia (fo″nas-the′ne-ah) weakness of the voice or difficulty speaking owing to fatigue; called also vocal fatigue.

phonation (fo-na′shun) the utterance of vocal sounds.

phonatory (fo′nah-tor″e) subserving or pertaining to phonation.

phoneme (fo′nēm) the smallest distinct unit of sound in speech; the basic unit of spoken language.

phonendoscope (fo-nen′do-skōp) a stethoscopic device that intensifies auscultatory sounds.

phonetic (fo-net′ik) pertaining to the voice or to articulate sounds.

phonetics (fo-net′iks) the science of vocal sounds.

phoniatrics (fo″ne-at′riks) the treatment of speech defects.

phonic (fon′ik, fo′nik) 1. vocal. 2. phonetic.

phonism (fo′nizm) a sensation of hearing produced by the effect of something seen, felt, tasted, smelled, or thought of.

phonoangiography (fo″no-an″je-og′rah-fe) the recording and analysis of arterial bruits to estimate the extent of arterial stenosis.

phonocardiogram (fo″no-kahr′de-o-gram″) the record produced by phonocardiography.

phonocardiograph (fo″no-kahr′de-o-graf″) the instrument used in phonocardiography to record heart sounds.

phonocardiography (fo″no-kahr″de-og′rah-fe) the graphic recording of heart sounds and murmurs; by extension, the term includes pulse tracings (carotid, apex, and venous pulse). adj., **phonocardiograph′ic.**
Phonocardiography involves picking up, through a highly sensitive microphone, sonic vibrations from the heart which are then converted into electrical energy and fed into a galvanometer, where they are recorded on paper. The procedure is most useful when there is evidence of heart murmurs or unusual heart sounds, such as gallops, that are difficult to discern by the human ear.

phonocatheter (fo″no-kath′ĕ-ter) a catheter with a device in its tip for picking up and transmitting sounds from within the heart and great vessels.

phonogram (fo′no-gram) a graphic record of a sound.

phonomyoclonus (fo″no-mi-ok′lŏ-nus) myoclonus in which a sound is heard on auscultation of an affected muscle, indicating fibrillar contractions.

phonomyogram (fo″no-mi′o-gram) a record produced by phonomyography.

phonomyography (fo″no-mi-og′rah-fe) the recording of sounds produced by muscle contraction.

phonophoresis (fo″no-fo-re′sis) the transdermal introduction of a topical agent into the body using mechanical energy supplied by ULTRASOUND.

phonophotography (fo″no-fo-tog′rah-fe) photographic recording of the movements of a diaphragm set up by sound waves.

phonopsia (fo-nop′se-ah) a visual sensation caused by the hearing of sounds.

phonostethograph (fo″no-steth′o-graf) an instrument by which chest sounds are amplified, filtered, and recorded.

-phore word element [Gr.], *a carrier.*

-phoresis word element [Gr.], *transmission.*

phoria (for′e-ah) any tendency to deviation of the eyes from the normal when fusional stimuli are absent or fusion is otherwise prevented; a latent or usually unmanifested TROPIA; see also HETEROPHORIA.

phorometer (fo-rom′ĕ-ter) 1. an instrument to test oculomotor balance. 2. phoro-optometer.

phoro-optometer (for″o-op-tom′ĕ-ter) an instrument to test ocular ductions, phorias, refractions, and vergences.

phoropter (for-op′ter) an instrument for evaluation of vision, with lenses placed on dials in a unit that is positioned in front of the patient. See illustration.

phoroscope (for′o-skōp) a fixed trial frame for eye testing, with a head rest that may be fastened to the table or the wall.

phose (fōz) a subjective visual sensation, as of light or color.

phosgene (fos′jēn) a suffocating and highly poisonous war gas, carbonyl chloride, $COCl_2$.

phosphatase (fos′fah-tās) any of a group of enzymes capable of catalyzing the hydrolysis of esterified phosphoric acid, with liberation of inorganic phosphate, found in practically all tissues, body fluids, and cells, including erythrocytes and leukocytes.
acid p. see ACID PHOSPHATASE.
alkaline p. see ALKALINE PHOSPHATASE.

phosphate (fos′fāt) any salt or ester of phosphoric acid. adj., **phosphat′ic.** Phosphates are widely distributed in the body, the largest amounts being in the bones and teeth. They are continually excreted in the urine and feces and must be replaced in the diet. Inorganic phosphates function as buffer salts to maintain the ACID-BASE BALANCE in blood, saliva, urine, and other body fluids. The principal phosphates in this buffer system are monosodium and disodium phosphate. Organic phosphates, in particular adenosine triphosphate (ATP), take part in a series of reversible reactions involving phosphoric acid, lactic acid, glycogen, and other substances, which furnish the energy expended in muscle contraction. This is thought to occur through the hydrolysis of the so-called high-energy phosphate bond present in ATP, phosphocreatine, and certain other body compounds.

phosphatemia (fos″fah-te′me-ah) an excess of phosphates in the blood.

phosphatidylcholine (PC) (fos″fah-ti″dil-ko′lēn) a phospholipid containing choline that is a major component of cell membranes and is localized preferentially in the outer surface of the plasma membrane; it is found in animal tissues, especially nerve tissue, the liver, semen, and egg yolk. Called also lecithin.

phosphatidylethanolamine (fos″fah-ti″-dil-eth″ah-nol′ah-mēn) a phospholipid containing ethanolamine that is a major constituent of cell membranes and is localized preferentially in the inner surface of the plasma membrane. Abbreviated PE.

phosphatidylserine (fos″fah-ti″dil-ser′ēn) a phospholipid containing serine that is an important constituent of cell membranes and is localized preferentially in the inner surface of the plasma membrane. Abbreviated PS.

phosphaturia (fos″fah-tu′re-ah) 1. excretion of PHOSPHATES in the urine. 2. hyperphosphaturia.

phosphene (fos′fēn) an objective visual sensation that occurs with the eyes closed, and in the absence of retinal stimulation by visible light.

phosphoamidase (fos″fo-am′ĭ-dās) an enzyme that catalyzes the conversion of phosphocreatine to creatine and orthophosphate.

phosphocreatine (PC) (fos″fo-kre′ah-tin) a compound of creatine and phosphoric acid occurring in muscle, being the most important storage form of high-energy phosphate, the energy source in muscle contraction.

phosphofructokinase (fos″fo-fruk″to-ki′nās) an enzyme of the glycolytic (Embden-Meyerhof) pathway that catalyzes the conversion of fructose-6-phosphate to fructose-1,6-bisphosphate.

phosphoglyceride (fos″fo-glis′er-īd) a class of phospholipids, including lecithin and cephalin, consisting of a glycerol backbone, two fatty acids, and a phosphorylated alcohol, e.g., choline, ethanolamine, serine, or inositol. They are a major component of cell membranes.

phosphokinase (fos″fo-ki′nās) kinase.

phospholipase (fos″fo-lip′ās) any of four enzymes (phospholipase A to D) that catalyze the hydrolysis of a phospholipid.

phospholipid (fos″fo-lip′id) any lipid that contains phosphorus, including those with a glycerol backbone (phosphoglycerides and plasmalogens) or a backbone of sphingosine or a related substance (sphingomyelins). They are the major lipids in cell membranes.

phosphonecrosis (fos″fo-nĕ-kro′sis) necrosis of the mandible due to excessive exposure to PHOSPHORUS; this was a common occupational illness in the 1800s among workers in the match industry and was an early example of the demonstrated need to protect workers from detrimental conditions by applying simple safety measures. Called also phossy jaw.

phosphoprotein (fos″fo-pro′tēn) a protein to which one or more phosphate groups are attached at serine or threonine (rarely tyrosine) residues.

phosphorated (fos′fo-rāt″ed) charged or combined with phosphorus.

phosphorescence (fos″fo-res′ens) the emission of light without appreciable heat; it is characterized by the emission of absorbed light after a delay and at a considerably longer wavelength than that of the absorbed light. adj., **phosphores′cent.**

phosphoribulokinase (fos″fo-ri″bu-lo-ki′-nās) an enzyme that catalyzes the conversion of ATP and D-ribulose 5-phosphate to ADP and D-ribulose 1,5-diphosphate.

phosphoric acid (fos-for′ik) a crystalline acid formed by oxidation of phosphorus; its salts are called phosphates.

phosphorism (fos′fo-rizm) chronic phosphorus poisoning; see also PHOSPHORUS.

phosphorolysis (fos″fo-rol′ĭ-sis) cleavage of a chemical bond with simultaneous addition of the elements of phosphoric acid to the residues.

phosphorus (P) (fos′for-us) a chemical element, atomic number 15, atomic weight 30.974. (See Appendix 6.) Phosphorus is an essential element in the diet; in the form of phosphates it is a major component of the mineral phase of bone and is involved in almost all metabolic processes. It also plays an important role in cell metabolism. It is obtained by the body from milk products, cereals, meat, and fish, and its use by the body is controlled by vitamin D and calcium.

Free phosphorus is very inflammable and exceedingly poisonous; ingestion causes fatty degeneration of the liver and other viscera. Inhalation of its vapor by workers in chemical industries may cause necrosis of the mandible (PHOSPHONECROSIS). adj., **phosphor′ous.**

p. 32 a radioisotope of phosphorus having a half-life of 14.28 days and emitting only beta particles, used as a RADIOPHARMACEUTICAL. As the sodium salt its therapeutic uses include treatment of POLYCYTHEMIA vera, chronic granulocytic LEUKEMIA, chronic lymphocytic LEUKEMIA, and palliation of metastatic skeletal disease. As a colloid with chromium its uses include treatment of certain ovarian and prostate carcinomas and of intraperitoneal and intrapleural malignant effusions resulting from metastatic disease. Symbol ^{32}P.

phosphorylase (fos-for′ĭ-lās) an enzyme that, in the presence of inorganic phosphate, catalyzes the conversion of glycogen into glucose-1-phosphate.

phosphorylation (fos″for-ĭ-la′shun) the process of introducing a phosphate group into an organic molecule.

oxidative p. the final common pathway of aerobic energy metabolism in which high-energy phosphate bonds are formed by

P

phosphorylation of ADP to ATP coupled with the transfer of electrons along a chain of carrier proteins with molecular oxygen as the final acceptor. It occurs in mitochondria.

phosphotransacetylase (fos″fo-trans″ah-set′ĭ-lās) an enzyme that catalyzes the transfer of an acetyl group between acetylphosphate and acetylcoenzyme A.

phosphotransferase (fos″fo-trans′fer-ās) any of a class of enzymes that catalyze the transfer of a phosphate group.

phot(o)- word element [Gr.], *light.*

photalgia (fo-tal′jah) ocular pain caused by light.

photic (fo′tik) pertaining to light.

photism (fo′tizm) a visual sensation produced by the effect of something heard, felt, tasted, smelled, or thought of.

photoablation (fo″to-ab-la′shun) volatilization of tissue by ultraviolet rays emitted by a laser.

photoactive (fo″to-ak′tiv) reacting chemically to sunlight or ultraviolet RADIATION.

photoaging (fo″to-āj′ing) premature aging of the skin due to long-term exposure to sunlight or other ultraviolet RADIATION. See also *actinic elastosis.*

photoallergen (fo″to-al′er-jen) an agent that elicits an allergic response to light.

photoallergic (fo″to-ah-ler′jik) pertaining to, characterized by, or producing PHOTO-ALLERGY.

photoallergy (fo″to-al′er-je) a delayed immunologic type of photosensitivity involving both a chemical substance to which the individual has become previously sensitized and radiant energy.

photobiology (fo″to-bi-ol′o-je) the branch of biology dealing with the effect of light on organisms. adj., **photobiolog′ic, photobiolog′ical.**

photobiotic (fo″to-bi-ot′ik) living only in the light.

photocatalysis (fo″to-kah-tal′ĭ-sis) promotion or stimulation of a chemical reaction by light. adj., **photocatalyt′ic.**

photocatalyst (fo″to-kat′ah-list) a substance, e.g., chlorophyll, that brings about a chemical reaction on exposure to light.

photochemistry (fo″to-kem′is-tre) the branch of chemistry that deals with the chemical properties or effects of light rays or other radiation. adj., **photochem′ical.**

photochemotherapy (fo″to-ke″mo-ther′-ah-pe) treatment by means of drugs (such as METHOXSALEN) that react to ultraviolet RADIATION or sunlight.

photochromogen (fo″to-kro′mo-jen) a microorganism whose pigmentation develops

as a result of exposure to light. adj., **photochromogen′ic.**

photocoagulation (fo″to-ko-ag″u-la′shun) condensation of protein material by the controlled use of an intense beam of light (e.g., argon laser); used especially in the treatment of retinal detachment and destruction of abnormal retinal vessels or intraocular tumor masses.

photoconvulsive (fo″to-kon-vul′siv) photoparoxysmal.

photodermatitis (fo″to-der″mah-ti′tis) an abnormal state of the skin in which light is an important causative factor.

photodermatosis (fo″to-der-mah-to′sis) photodermatitis.

photodisruption (fo″to-dis-rup′shun) disruption of tissues by laser-produced rapid ionization of molecules.

photodynia (fo″to-din′e-ah) photalgia.

photofluorography (fo″to-floor-og′rah-fe) the photographic recording of fluoroscopic images on small films, using a fast lens; used in mass radiography of the chest. Called also fluorography and fluororadiography.

photogenic (fo″to-jen′ik) 1. produced by light. 2. emitting or producing light.

photokinetic (fo″to-kĭ-net′ik) moving in response to the stimulus of light.

photolysis (fo-tol′ĭ-sis) chemical decomposition or change by the action of light or other radiant energy. adj., **photolyt′ic.**

photolyte (fo′to-līt) a substance decomposed by light.

photometer (fo-tom′ĕ-ter) 1. a device for measuring the intensity of infrared, ultraviolet, or visible light. 2. a device for testing the sensitivity of the eye to light by determining the light minimum.

photometry (fo-tom′ĕ-tre) measurement of the intensity of light.

photomicrograph (fo″to-mi′kro-graf) a photograph of an object as seen through an ordinary light microscope.

photomyoclonic (fo″to-mi″o-klon′ik) photomyogenic.

photomyogenic (fo″to-mi″o-jen′ik) photomyoclonic; denoting an electroencephalographic response to photic stimulation (brief flashes of light) marked by myoclonus of the facial muscles.

photon (fo′ton) a discrete particle (QUANTUM) of radiant energy.

photo-onycholysis (fo″to-o″nĭ-kol′ĭ-sis) ONYCHOLYSIS resulting from exposure to sunlight or ULTRAVIOLET RAYS, such as after treatment with TETRACYCLINES or METHOXSALEN.

photoparoxysmal (fo″to-par″ok-siz′mal) photoconvulsive; denoting an abnormal electroencephalographic response to photic stimulation (brief flashes of light), marked by diffuse paroxysmal discharge recorded as spike-wave complexes; the response may be accompanied by minor seizures.

photoperceptive (fo″to-per-sep′tiv) able to perceive light.

photoperiod (fo′to-pēr″e-od) the period of time per day that an organism is exposed to daylight (or to artificial light). adj., **photoperiod′ic.**

photoperiodism (fo″to-pēr′e-o-dizm) the physiologic and behavioral reactions brought about in organisms by changes in the duration of daylight and darkness.

photopheresis (fo″to-fĕ-re′sis) a technique for treating cutaneous T-cell LYMPHOMA, in which a PHOTOACTIVE chemical is administered, and the blood is removed and circulated through a source of ultraviolet RADIATION, then returned to the patient; it is believed to stimulate the IMMUNE SYSTEM.

photophilic (fo″to-fil′ik) thriving in light.

photophobia (fo″to-fo′be-ah) abnormal visual intolerance to light. adj., **photopho′-bic.**

photophthalmia (fo″tof-thal′me-ah) ophthalmia caused by intense light or glare.

photopia (fo-to′pe-ah) day vision. adj., **photop′ic.**

photopsia (fo-top′se-ah) an appearance as of sparks or flashes, in retinal irritation.

photoptarmosis (fo″to-tahr-mo′sis) sneezing caused by the influence of light.

photoptometer (fo″top-tom′ĕ-ter) an instrument for measuring visual acuity by determining the smallest amount of light that will render an object just visible.

photoreactivation (fo″to-re-ak″tī-va′shun) reversal of the biological effects of ultraviolet RADIATION on cells by subsequent exposure to visible light.

photoreceptive (fo″to-re-sep′tiv) sensitive to stimulation by light.

photoreceptor (fo″to-re-sep′tor) a nerve end-organ or receptor sensitive to light.

photorefractive (fo″to-re-frak′tiv) pertaining to the refraction of light; see photorefractive KERATECTOMY.

photoretinitis (fo″to-ret″ĭ-ni′tis) retinitis due to exposure to intense light.

photosensitive (fo″to-sen′sĭ-tiv) exhibiting PHOTOSENSITIVITY.

photosensitivity (fo″to-sen″sĭ-tiv′ĭ-te) 1. sensitivity of a cell to light. 2. abnormally heightened sensitivity to sunlight, such as of the eyes or skin. See also PHOTOSENSITIZATION.

photosensitization (fo″to-sen″sĭ-tī-za′-shun) the development of abnormally heightened reactivity of the skin or eyes to sunlight; it can be caused by a wide variety of drugs and chemicals. PHOTOTOXIC

reactions occur when a given drug absorbs ultraviolet RADIATION from the sun and a sunburnlike response occurs in a short period of time. Within hours there is a burning sensation of the exposed skin, followed by redness and swelling. Within a day or two the skin becomes heavily pigmented and begins to peel; a severe reaction can cause scarring. Phototoxic reactions are more likely to occur in light-skinned persons than in those with darkly pigmented skin that can block harmful radiation.

PHOTOALLERGIC reactions occur after an initial exposure to the drug or chemical which triggers the production of antibodies. On second exposure a skin eruption appears and there may be intense itching. It is possible for the eruption to appear on unexposed areas of skin as well as exposed areas. There is a long list of drugs that can cause this type of reaction; antineoplastics, antimicrobials, diuretics, hypoglycemic agents, and even antihistamines may trigger it in certain individuals.

photostable (fo′to-sta″b′l) unchanged by the influence of light.

photosynthesis (fo″to-sin′thĕ-sis) a chemical combination caused by the action of light; specifically the formation of carbohydrates from carbon dioxide and water in the chlorophyll tissue of plants under the influence of light. adj., **photosynthet′ic.**

phototaxis (fo″to-tak′sis) TAXIS of cells and microorganisms under the influence of light. adj., **phototac′tic.**

phototherapy (fo″to-ther′ah-pe) treatment of disease by exposure to light; one example is the treatment of nonhemolytic HYPERBILIRUBINEMIA IN THE NEWBORN. Phototherapy reduces bilirubin levels in the blood by decomposing unconjugated bilirubin into colorless compounds excreted in the bile. Photodecomposition is a normal alternative route for the excretion of bilirubin; the use of artificial light hastens this process. Either sunlight or an ultraviolet LAMP is effective; the distance of the ultraviolet lamp from the subject is important.

Patient Care. Although phototherapy is inexpensive and relatively easy to use, it is not without danger to the newborn. Damage to the retina by prolonged exposure to the bright light, as well as drying of the cornea, can lead to permanent impairment of vision. To protect the newborn the eyes must be covered for the entire time the child is under the light. The use of eyedrops every two hours can help prevent excessive drying. Insensible water loss due to rapid

P

evaporation of water from the skin can cause a fluid volume deficit. Hence the newborn must be assessed periodically for signs of fluid volume deficit; the monitoring of fluid intake and output and the status of skin turgor are especially important. Because increased body heat is also possible, careful attention must be paid to thermoregulation in order to avoid hyperthermia.

neonate p. in the NURSING INTERVENTIONS CLASSIFICATION, a nursing INTERVENTION defined as the use of light therapy to reduce bilirubin levels in newborn infants; see PHOTOTHERAPY.

ultraviolet p. the use of ultraviolet RADIATION (which may be type A, B, or C, or a combination of types) in the treatment of skin diseases. The radiation is generated by an artificial source such as an arc lamp and may be used in combination with photosensitizing drugs; see also PHOTOCHEMOTHERAPY.

phototoxic (fo'to-tok"sik) having a toxic effect triggered by exposure to light.

phototrophic (fo"to-trof'ik) capable of deriving energy from light.

phototropism (fo-tot'ro-pizm) 1. TROPISM of an organism in response to light; it may be either *positive* (toward the light) or *negative* (away from the light). 2. change of color produced in a substance by the action of light. adj., **phototrop'ic.**

photuria (fo-tu're-ah) excretion of urine having a luminous appearance.

phren(o)- word element [Gr.] 1. *diaphragm.* 2. *mind.*

phrenalgia (frĕ-nal'jah) pain in the diaphragm.

phrenic (fren'ik) 1. pertaining to the diaphragm or to the mind. 2. diaphragmatic. 3. mental (def. 1).

p. nerve a major branch of the cervical plexus, extending through the thorax to provide innervation of the diaphragm. Nerve impulses from the inspiratory center in the brain travel down it, causing contraction of the diaphragm, so that inhalation can occur.

phrenitis (frĕ-ni'tis) inflammation of the diaphragm; called also diaphragmitis.

phrenocolic (fren"o-kol'ik) pertaining to the diaphragm and colon.

phrenogastric (fren"o-gas'trik) pertaining to the diaphragm and stomach.

phrenohepatic (fren"o-hĕ-pat'ik) pertaining to the diaphragm and liver.

phrenoplegia (fren"o-ple'jah) paralysis of the diaphragm.

phrenotropic (fren"o-trop'ik) exerting its principal effect upon the mind.

phronesis (fro-ne'sis) in bioethics, the virtue of practical wisdom, the capacity for moral insight to discern what moral choice or course of action is most conducive to the good of the agent or the activity in which the agent is engaged.

phrynoderma (frin"o-der'mah) follicular hyperkeratosis.

phthiriasis (thĭ-ri'ah-sis) pediculosis pubis.

Phthirus (thir'us) a genus of lice. *P. pu'bis* is the pubic or crab louse, a species that infests human pubic hair and sometimes other hairy areas; see also PEDICULOSIS PUBIS.

P. pu'bis the pubic LOUSE or crab louse, a species that infests the pubic hair and sometimes other hairy areas of the body of humans. See also PEDICULOSIS PUBIS.

phthisis (thi'sis; ti'sis) WASTING of the body.

p. bul'bi shrinkage of the eyeball.

grinder's p. a combination of tuberculosis and pneumoconiosis occurring in grinders in the cutlery trade.

miner's p. pneumoconiosis of coal workers.

Phycomycetes (fi"ko-mi-se'tēz) in some systems of classification, a class of fungi comprising the common water, leaf, and bread molds and including the medically important Zygomycetes as a subclass.

phycomycosis (fi"ko-mi-ko'sis) 1. any of a group of acute fungal diseases caused by members of the class Phycomycetes. 2. mucormycosis.

phylogeny (fi-loj'ĕ-ne) the complete developmental history of a group of organisms. adj., **phylogenet'ic, phylogen'ic.**

phylum (fi'lum), pl. *phy'la* [L., Gr.] a primary division of the plant or animal kingdom, including organisms that are assumed to have a common ancestry.

phyma (fi'mah) [Gr.] a skin swelling or tumor larger than a tubercle.

phys(o)- word element [Gr.], *air; gas.*

physi(o)- word element [Gr.], *nature; physiology; physical.*

physiatrics (fiz"e-at'riks) physiatry.

physiatrist (fiz"e-at'rist) a physician who specializes in PHYSIATRY.

physiatry (fiz"e-at're) the branch of medicine that uses PHYSICAL THERAPY, physical agents, such as light, heat, water, and electricity, and mechanical apparatus, in the diagnosis, prevention, and treatment of bodily disorders. Called also physiatrics and physical medicine.

physical (fiz'ĭ-kal) pertaining to the body, to material things, or to physics.

p. fitness a state of physiologic well being that is achieved through a combination of good diet, regular physical exercise, and other practices that promote good health.

p. therapist a rehabilitation professional who promotes optimal health and functional independence through the application of scientific principles to prevent, identify, assess, correct, or alleviate acute or chronic movement dysfunction, physical disability, or pain. A physical therapist is a graduate of a PHYSICAL THERAPY program approved by a nationally recognized accrediting body or has achieved the documented equivalent in education, training, or experience; in addition, the therapist must meet any current legal requirements of licensure or registration and be currently competent in the field.

Persons wishing to practice as qualified physical therapists must be licensed. All 50 states of the United States, the District of Columbia, and the Commonwealth of Puerto Rico require such licensure. All applicants for licensure must have a degree or certificate from an accredited physical therapy educational program. To qualify for licensure they must pass a state licensure examination.

Physical therapy assistants and aides work under the supervision of professional physical therapists. Training requirements for physical therapy assistants are not uniform throughout the United States. In 39 of the states licensure is available to graduates of an accredited two-year associate degree program; some require the passing of a written examination. Physical therapy aides can qualify for that position by training on the job in hospitals and other health care facilities.

Further information about the curriculum for physical therapists and physical therapist assistants, available programs of study, requirements for practice, and other relevant information can be obtained by contacting the American Physical Therapy Association, 1111 N. Fairfax St., Alexandria, VA 22314, telephone (703) 684-2782.

p. therapy the profession practiced by licensed PHYSICAL THERAPISTS. According to guidelines published by the American Physical Therapy Association, physical therapy should be defined as the examination, treatment, and instruction of persons in order to detect, assess, prevent, correct, alleviate, and limit physical disability and bodily malfunction. The practice of physical therapy includes the administration, interpretation, and evaluation of tests and measurements of bodily functions and structures and the planning, administration, evaluation, and modification of treatment and instruction, including the use of physical measures,

WINDOW ON PHYSICAL THERAPIST

Physical therapists (PTs) are health care professionals who manage the care of individuals with problems that may result from diseases, disorders, conditions, or injuries. PTs diagnose and manage movement dysfunction and enhance physical and functional abilities; restore, maintain, and promote not only optimal physical function but also optimal wellness and fitness and optimal quality of life as it relates to movement and health; and prevent the onset, symptoms, and progression of impairments, functional limitations, and disabilities. Interventions used by PTs might include therapeutic exercise to address goals such as aerobic conditioning, balance, flexibility, or strength; manual therapy techniques; and functional training including reintegration into home, work, and leisure settings.

The majority of PTs practice in traditional settings such as private outpatient offices or group practices (32%), hospital/health system–based outpatient clinics (17%), and acute care hospitals (16%). But PTs can also be found in a variety of other settings such as community health and wellness centers, industrial settings, nursing homes, home care, and school systems, in addition to research institutions and academic settings.

The "Scope of Physical Therapist Practice," adopted by the American Physical Therapy Association, states that physical therapist practice includes:

- Examining individuals with impairment, functional limitation, and disability or other health-related conditions in order to determine a diagnosis, prognosis, and intervention.
- Alleviating impairment and functional limitation by designing, implementing, and modifying therapeutic interventions.
- Preventing injury, impairment, functional limitation, and disability, including the promotion and maintenance of health, wellness, fitness, and quality of life in all age populations.
- Engaging in consultation, education, and research.

AMERICAN PHYSICAL THERAPY ASSOCIATION

activities, and devices, for preventive and therapeutic purposes. Additionally, it provides consultative, educational, and other advisory services for the purpose of reducing the incidence and severity of physical disability, bodily malfunction, movement dysfunction, and pain.

chest p. therapy a form of RESPIRATORY THERAPY in which the patient is positioned to facilitate removal of secretions (POSTURAL DRAINAGE) and the chest wall is clapped to help loosen the secretions (PERCUSSION).

physician (fĭ-zish′un) an authorized practitioner of medicine, as one graduated from a college of medicine or osteopathy and licensed by the appropriate board; see also DOCTOR.

attending p. one who attends a hospital at stated times to visit the patients and give directions as to their treatment.

emergency p. a specialist in emergency MEDICINE.

family p. a medical specialist who plans and provides the comprehensive primary health care of all members of a family, regardless of age or sex, on a continuous basis. See also family PRACTICE.

resident p. a graduate and licensed physician learning a specialty through in-hospital training.

physician assistant a health care professional who is able to perform certain of a physician's duties, serving in either of two roles: assistant to the primary care physician (PA) or SURGEON ASSISTANT (SA). The PA possesses the knowledge and skill to perform history taking, physical examination, drawing of blood samples, urinalysis, electrocardiographic examination, and routine therapeutic procedures, such as injections, immunizations, and suturing of wounds, all under the supervision of a physician. Graduates of accredited physician assistant programs who successfully complete the National Certifying Examination for Primary Care Physician Assistants are designated PA-C, Physician Assistant–Certified. The address of the American Academy of Physician Assistants is 950 N. Washington Ave., Alexandria, VA 22314.

Physicians' Desk Reference (PDR) a reference book published yearly that contains drug monographs and an illustrated section for drug identification; it is also available on CD-ROM.

physicochemical (fiz″ĭ-ko-kem′ĭ-kal) pertaining to both physics and chemistry.

WINDOW ON PHYSICIAN

Physicians are responsible for preventing disease, and maintaining or restoring the health of the patients they treat. There are 119 different specialties or subspecialties that physicians can be trained in (36 primary specialties and 83 subspecialties), including such narrow disciplines as undersea medicine and cardiac electrophysiology. Although most physicians specialize in one of these 119 areas, a good health care system depends on a large number of personal or primary care physicians to manage the majority of health care problems. Primary care physicians are family physicians, general internists, and pediatricians.

Personalized, accessible, cost-effective, quality health care is the aim of every physician. Although the goal is to prevent disease entirely due to good hygiene and effective public health measures, we must also focus on the early detection of disease, called secondary prevention. This is much more cost-effective than treating advanced disease. Detecting potentially serious disease at its early stage when the symptoms are undifferentiated and could be due to a variety of less serious problems is one of the most difficult challenges in medicine.

A physician is best able to assess these problems when there has been a long-standing relationship with the patient. Care is also more effective when a patient has the confidence and trust that comes from a continuing relationship with a personal physician. Unfortunately, in today's health care system, employers often shift health plans in attempts to lower costs, forcing the patient to change physicians due to requirements of the plan. This often leads to more expensive health care as the unfamiliar physician, in order to rule out disease, performs more tests than may be necessary.

The physician's greatest ally in combating disease is a knowledgeable, informed patient. Increased emphasis is being placed on educating the public to stop harmful practices such as smoking, to prevent disease through immunization, to recognize that depression and the toll that stress takes in our lives is treatable, and to modify sexual patterns to combat AIDS.

ROBERT E. RAKEL, MD

WINDOW ON PHYSICIAN ASSISTANT

Physician Assistants (PAs) traditionally have served in areas of need, providing care to those who might otherwise have little or no access to quality medical care. However, PAs work in many settings, from remote rural areas to major urban medical centers, private physicians' offices, hospitals, public health clinics, Health Maintenance Organizations, the Armed Forces, and other federal agencies.

The majority of PAs work in family medicine and other primary care areas. Utilization of PAs is increasing to include every field and subspeciality found in medicine because PAs have proven their effectiveness and ability to provide quality care. Other nonclinical fields such as research and administration are also open to physician assistants. National employment trends indicate there are 7.5 positions available for every new graduate. The PA profession is one of the top 15 career choices. Graduates can expect a very satisfying career for many years, helping meet the nation's health needs.

The maldistribution and shortage of health manpower in the 1960s gave rise to the concept of the physician assistant. The concept was addressed in 1961 by Charles L. Hudson, past president of the American Medical Association, when he called for the establishment of an advanced medical assistant, an intermediate between the technician and the physician. This assistant would be able to handle technical procedures and exercise some degree of medical responsibility. In 1965, Dr. Eugene Stead, Jr. launched the first PA program at Duke University with the admission of four ex-military corpsmen to be educated as assistants to the primary care physician. Since then, under the impetus of the Comprehensive Health Manpower Training Act of 1971, the number of programs has increased to 81 with approximately 2500 PAs graduating annually.

A commitment to quality patient care is the foundation of the physician assistant profession. Whether working in a satellite rural health clinic in the mountains of North Carolina or assisting in cardiothoracic surgery in a major medical center, PAs are making a difference. By assuming some of the duties traditionally performed by a physician, the PA enables the supervising physician to spend time with patients with serious or complicated medical problems.

GLEN COMBS

---

physics (fiz'iks) the study of the laws and phenomena of nature, especially of forces and general properties of matter and energy.

   nuclear p. the study of atomic nuclei and their reactions.

physiochemical (fiz″e-o-kem'ĭ-kal) pertaining to both physiology and chemistry.

physiognomy (fiz″e-og'no-me) 1. facial expression and appearance as a means of diagnosis. 2. the attempt to determine temperament and character on the basis of facial features.

physiologic (fiz″e-o-loj'ik) pertaining to physiology; normal; not pathologic.

   p. saline solution, p. salt solution p. sodium chloride solution a 0.9 per cent solution of sodium chloride and water; it is isotonic, i.e., of the same osmotic pressure as blood serum. It is sometimes given intravenously to replace lost sodium and chloride. Excessive quantities may cause edema, elevated blood sodium levels, and loss of potassium from the tissue fluid. Called also normal saline or normal salt solution.

physiological (fiz″e-o-loj'ĭ-kal) physiologic.

physiologist (fiz″e-ol'o-jist) a specialist in physiology.

physiology (fiz″e-ol'o-je) 1. the science that treats of the functions of the living organism and its parts, and of the physical and chemical factors and processes involved. 2. the basic processes underlying the functioning of a species or class of organism, or any of its parts or processes.

   cell p. the scientific study of phenomena involved in cell growth and maintenance, self-regulation and division of cells, interactions between nucleus and cytoplasm, and general behavior of protoplasm.

   morbid p., pathologic p. the study of disordered functions or of function in diseased tissues.

physiopathologic (fiz″e-o-path″o-loj'ik) pertaining to pathologic physiology.

physiotherapist (fiz″e-o-ther'ah-pist) physical therapist.

physiotherapy (fiz″e-o-ther'ah-pe) physical therapy.

   chest p. 1. chest PHYSICAL THERAPY. 2. in the NURSING INTERVENTIONS CLASSIFICATION, a

P

nursing INTERVENTION defined as assisting the patient to move airway secretions from peripheral airways to more central airways for expectorating and/or suctioning.

physique (fĭ-zēk′) the body organization, development, and structure.

physohematometra (fi″so-hem″ah-to-me′-trah) gas and blood in the uterine cavity.

physohydrometra (fi″so-hi″dro-me′trah) gas and serum in the uterine cavity.

physometra (fi″so-me′trah) gas in the uterine cavity.

physopyosalpinx (fi″so-pi″o-sal′pinks) gas and pus in a FALLOPIAN TUBE.

physostigmine (fi″zo-stig′mēn) a cholinergic alkaloid having anticholinesterase activity, obtained from the dried ripe seed (Calabar bean) of *Physostigma venenosum*; used topically to produce miosis and to decrease intraocular pressure in glaucoma. It may also be applied parenterally to reverse the central nervous system effects produced by overdosage of anticholinergic drugs.

phyt(o)- word element [Gr.], *plant; an organism of the vegetable kingdom.*

phytoagglutinin (fi″to-ah-gloo′tĭ-nin) an agglutinin of plant origin.

phytobezoar (fi″to-be′zor) a bezoar composed of vegetable fibers.

phytogenous (fi-toj′ĕ-nus) derived from plants, or caused by a vegetable growth.

phytohemagglutinin (fi″to-he″mah-gloo′tĭ-nin) a lectin isolated from the red kidney bean (*Phaseolus vulgaris*); it is a hemagglutinin that agglutinates mammalian erythrocytes and a mitogen that stimulates predominantly T lymphocytes. Abbreviated PHA.

phytoid (fi′toid) resembling a plant.

phytonadione (fi″to-nah-di′ōn) a fat-soluble vitamin of the VITAMIN K group; used to promote PROTHROMBIN formation in HYPOPROTHROMBINEMIA of various causes, administered orally or parenterally.

phytoparasite (fi″to-par′ah-sīt) any parasitic vegetable organism.

phytophotodermatitis (fi″to-fo″to-der″-mah-ti′tis) phototoxic dermatitis due to contact with certain plants and subsequent exposure to sunlight.

phytoprecipitin (fi″to-pre-sip′ĭ-tin) a precipitin formed in response to vegetable antigen.

phytosis (fi-to′sis) any disease caused by a phytoparasite.

phytosterol (fi″to-ste′rol) a sterol of vegetable origin.

phytotoxic (fi′to-tok″sik) 1. pertaining to phytotoxin. 2. poisonous to plants.

phytotoxin (fi′to-tok″sin) an EXOTOXIN produced by certain species of higher plants; any toxin of plant origin.

pia-arachnitis (pi″ah-ar″ak-ni′tis) leptomeningitis.

pia-arachnoid (pi″ah-ah-rak′noid) the pia mater and arachnoid considered together as one functional unit; the leptomeninges.

pial (pi′al) pertaining to the pia mater.

pia mater (pi′ah ma′ter) [L.] the innermost of the three meninges covering the brain and spinal cord.

piarachnitis (pi″ar-ak-ni′tis) leptomeningitis.

piarachnoid (pi″ah-rak′noid) pia-arachnoid.

pica (pi′kah) [L.] compulsive eating of nonnutritive substances, such as ice (PAGOPHAGIA), dirt (GEOPHAGIA), gravel, flaking paint or plaster, clay, hair (TRICHOPHAGIA), or laundry starch (AMYLOPHAGIA). It is often seen during pregnancy and also occurs in some patients with iron or zinc deficiencies. In children this syndrome, classified with the EATING DISORDERS in DSM-IV, is a rare mental disorder with onset typically in the second year of life; it usually remits in childhood but may persist into adolescence.

Pick's disease (piks) a rare progressive degenerative disease of the brain very similar in clinical manifestations and course to ALZHEIMER'S DISEASE but differing in histopathology; cortical atrophy is confined to the frontal and temporal lobes and degenerating neurons contain globular filamentous inclusions (Pick bodies) in their cytoplasm.

pickwickian syndrome (pik-wik′e-an) obesity-hypoventilation syndrome.

pico- word element [It.] designating one trillionth (10^{-12}) part of the unit to which it is joined. Symbol p.

picogram (pg) (pi′ko-gram) one trillionth (10^{-12}) of a GRAM.

picornavirus (pi-kor′nah-vi″rus) any member of a family of extremely small, ether-resistant RNA viruses, including the ENTEROVIRUSES and RHINOVIRUSES.

picric acid (pik′rik) trinitrophenol.

picrocarmine (pik″ro-kahr′min) a histological stain consisting of a mixture of carmine, ammonia, distilled water, and aqueous solution of picric acid.

PID pelvic inflammatory disease.

PIE pulmonary interstitial emphysema.

piebaldism (pi′bawld-izm) a congenital autosomal dominant pigmentary disorder of the skin due to absence of functioning melanocytes and melanin, resulting in patchy areas of depigmentation or hypopigmentation, often occurring in association with white forelock.

piece (pēs) a part or portion.

end p. the terminal portion of the TAIL OF THE SPERMATOZOON. See illustration at SPERMATOZOON.

middle p. an anterior portion of the TAIL OF THE SPERMATOZOON, between the NECK and the ANULUS. See illustration at SPERMATOZOON.

principal p. the main portion of the TAIL OF A SPERMATOZOON, beginning at the ANULUS and gradually tapering toward the end PIECE. See illustration at SPERMATOZOON.

piedra (pe-a'drah) a fungal disease of the hair in which white or black nodules of fungi form on the shafts.

Pierre Robin syndrome (pyār ro-ban') an autosomal recessive disorder characterized by smallness of the mandible, CLEFT PALATE, and often drooping of the tongue, backward and upward displacement of the larynx, and angulation of the MANUBRIUM sterni. Cleft palate makes sucking and swallowing difficult, permitting easy access of fluids into the larynx.

piesesthesia (pi-e"zes-the'zhah) the sense by which pressure stimuli are felt.

piesimeter (pi"e-sim'ĕ-ter) an instrument for testing the sensitiveness of the skin to pressure.

-piesis word element [Gr.], *pressure.*

piggyback (pig'e-bak") supplementary or added on; used to refer to an INTRAVENOUS INFUSION.

pigment (pig'ment) 1. any coloring matter of the body. 2. a stain or dyestuff. 3. a paintlike medicinal preparation applied to the skin. adj., **pig'mentary.**

bile p. any of the coloring matters of the BILE, derived from HEME, including BILIRUBIN, BILIVERDIN, and several others.

blood p., hematogenous p. any of the pigments derived from HEMOGLOBIN, such as HEMATOIDIN, HEMATOPORPHYRIN, HEMOFUSCIN, and METHEMOGLOBIN.

lipid p. any of various pigments having lipid characteristics, some of which also contain protein or iron, the most important one being LIPOFUSCIN.

respiratory p's substances, e.g., hemoglobin, myoglobin, or cytochromes, which take part in the oxidative processes of the animal body.

retinal p's the photopigments in retinal RODS and CONES that respond to certain colors of light and initiate the process of vision.

pigmentation (pig"men-ta'shun) the deposition of coloring matter; the coloration or discoloration of a part by a pigment.

pigmented (pig'ment-ed) colored by deposit of pigment.

pigmentophage (pig-men'to-fāj) any pigment-destroying cell, especially such a cell of the hair.

piitis (pi-i'tis) inflammation of the pia mater.

pil(o)- word element [L.], *hair; composed of hair.*

pilar (pi'ler) pertaining to the hair.

pile (pīl) 1. hemorrhoid. 2. in nucleonics, a chain-reacting fission device for producing slow neutrons and radioisotopes.

sentinel p. a hemorrhoid-like thickening of the mucous membrane at the lower end of an anal fissure.

pileus (pil'e-us) caul.

pili (pi'li) [L.] plural of PILUS.

pill (pil) tablet.

morning-after p. popular name for an emergency postcoital contraceptive containing a high dose of the hormones usually found in an oral CONTRACEPTIVE, either an estrogen plus a progestational agent, or the latter alone; used to prevent pregnancy after unprotected intercourse occurs, or after a contraceptive method fails during intercourse, administered orally.

pillar (pil'er) a supporting column, usually occurring in pairs.

p's of fauces folds of mucous membrane at the sides of the fauces.

pillion (pil'yon) a temporary artificial lower limb.

pilocarpine (pi"lo-kahr'pin) a cholinergic alkaloid from leaves of *Pilocarpus jaborandi* and *P. microphyllus;* used topically in the eye as the base or the hydrochloride or nitrate salt as an ANTIGLAUCOMA agent and MIOTIC; the hydrochloride salt is also used orally to treat mouth dryness resulting from radiotherapy or associated with SJÖGREN'S SYNDROME. The nitrate salt has also been administered by iontophoresis to produce sweating in a test for CYSTIC FIBROSIS.

pilocystic (pi"lo-sis'tik) hollow or cystlike, and containing hair; said of dermoid tumors.

piloerection (pi"lo-e-rek'shun) erection of the hair.

piloleiomyoma (pi"lo-li"o-mi-o'mah) leiomyoma cutis, single or multiple, arising from the arrectores pilorum muscles.

pilomatricoma (pi"lo-ma-trĭ-ko'mah) a solitary benign calcifying tumor of hair follicle origin manifested as a sharply circumscribed, firm, intracutaneous nodule, usually on the face, neck, or upper limb and presenting before age 20. Histological features include a fibrous stroma surrounding nests of basophilic cells and ghost, or shadow, cells.

pilomotor (pi"lo-mo'ter) causing movement of the HAIRS; pertaining to the arrector muscles, the contraction of which produces goose FLESH (cutis anserina) and PILOERECTION.

pilonidal (pi″lo-ni′d'l) having a nidus of hairs.

p. cyst, p. sinus a hair-containing sacrococcygeal dermoid cyst or sinus, often opening at a postanal dimple, believed to result from an infolding of skin in which hair continues to grow. These cysts cause no symptoms unless they become infected, which is likely because of their location. Pain and swelling, with the formation of an abscess, are the symptoms of infection. Treatment consists of surgical removal.

Patient Care. Postoperative care includes dressing changes and wound care to avoid contamination and promote healing. A lubricating laxative and an oil enema are usually given before the first bowel movement to avoid strain on the suture line. Patients are taught handwashing and toileting to prevent infection until the wound is completely healed.

pilose (pi′lōs) hairy; covered with hair.

pilosebaceous (pi″lo-sĕ-ba′shus) pertaining to the hair follicles and sebaceous glands.

pilus (pi′lus) [L.] 1. hair. adj., **pi′lial.** 2. one of the minute filamentous appendages of certain bacteria associated with antigenic properties and sex functions of the cell. Called also fimbria. adj., **pi′liate.**

pi′li cunicula′ti a condition characterized by burrowing HAIRS.

F p. in bacterial genetics, a hollow tubular pilus possessed by (male) F⁺ cells, the carrier of the F PLASMID (fertility plasmid). It forms a connection with a (female) F⁻ cell in bacterial CONJUGATION to allow the transfer of genetic material.

pi′li incarna′ti a condition characterized by ingrown HAIRS.

pi′li tor′ti a condition characterized by twisted HAIRS.

pimelitis (pim″ĕ-li′tis) inflammation of the adipose tissue.

pimelopterygium (pim″ĕ-lo-ter-ij′e-um) a fatty outgrowth on the conjunctiva.

pimozide (pi′mah-zīd) an ANTIPSYCHOTIC AGENT and ANTIDYSKINETIC agent used in the treatment of GILLES DE LA TOURETTE'S SYNDROME; administered orally.

pimple (pim′p'l) a papule or pustule.

pin (pin) a slender, elongated piece of metal used for securing fixation of parts.

Steinmann p. a metal rod for the internal fixation of fractures; see also nail EXTENSION.

pincement (pans-maw′) [Fr.] pinching of the flesh in massage.

pindolol (pin′dah-lol) a nonselective BETA-ADRENERGIC BLOCKING AGENT with intrinsic sympathomimetic activity; administered orally as an ANTIHYPERTENSIVE AGENT.

pineal (pin′e-al) 1. shaped like a pine cone. 2. pertaining to the pineal body.

p. body a small, conical structure attached by a stalk to the posterior wall of the third ventricle of the cerebrum, believed by many to be an endocrine gland. In certain amphibians and reptiles the gland is thought to function as a light receptor. In most mammals, including humans, it appears to be the major or unique site of melatonin biosynthesis; the effect of melatonin on the body and the exact function of the pineal body remain obscure. Called also epiphysis cerebri and pineal gland.

pinealectomy (pin″e-ah-lek′to-me) excision of the pineal body.

pinealism (pin′e-al-izm) the condition due to deranged secretion of the pineal body.

pinealoblastoma (pin″e-ah-lo-blas-to′-mah) pinealoma in which the pineal cells are not well differentiated.

pinealocyte (pin′e-ah-lo-sīt) an epithelioid cell of the pineal body.

pinealoma (pin″e-ah-lo′mah) a tumor of the pineal body composed of neoplastic nests of large epithelial cells; it may cause hydrocephalus, precocious puberty, and gait disturbances.

Pinel (pe-nel′) Philippe (1745–1826). French physician and philosopher who worked with the mentally ill; he is credited with the development of the foundations of occupational therapy.

pinguecula (ping-gwek′u-lah), pl. *pingue′-culae* [L.] a small, benign, yellowish spot on the bulbar conjunctiva, seen usually in the elderly.

piniform (pin′ĭ-form) conical or cone-shaped.

pink disease acrodynia.

pinkeye (pink′i) popular term for acute contagious conjunctivitis.

pinna (pin′ah) auricle (def. 1).

pinocyte (pin′o-sīt) a cell that exhibits pinocytosis.

pinocytosis (pin″o-si-to′sis) a mechanism by which cells ingest extracellular fluid and its contents; it involves the formation of invaginations by the cell membrane, which close and break off to form fluid-filled vacuoles in the cytoplasm (see accompanying illustration). adj., **pinocytot′ic.**

pinosome (pin′o-sōm) the intracellular vacuole formed by pinocytosis.

pint (pīnt) a unit of liquid measure; in the United States it is 16 fluid ounces, or the equivalent of 0.473 liter. In Great Britain, it

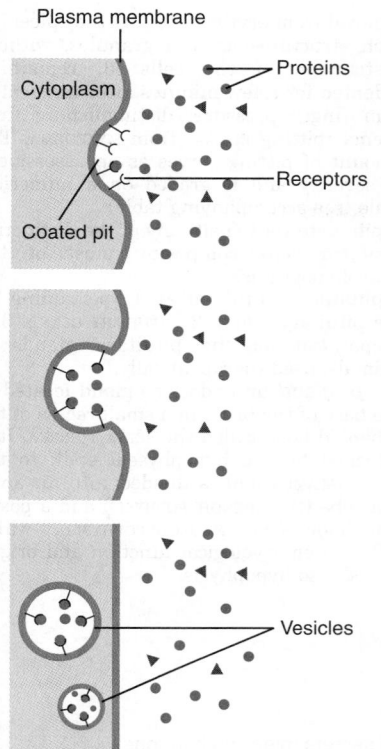

Mechanism of pinocytosis. Tiny droplets of fluid are trapped by the folds of the plasma membrane and engulfed as fluid-filled vesicles into the cytoplasm.

is the *imperial pint* and is 20 fluid ounces, or the equivalent of 0.568 liter.

pinta (pin'tah) a treponemal infection characterized by bizarre pigmentary changes in the skin occurring in tropical America; it is effectively treated by penicillin.

p. fever a disease observed in northern Mexico, identical with Rocky Mountain spotted fever.

pinworm (pin'werm) oxyurid.

pioglitazone (pi"o-glit'ah-zōn) an agent used in treatment of type 2 DIABETES MELLITIS, decreasing insulin resistance in the peripheral tissues and liver, used orally as the hydrochloride salt.

pipecuronium (pip"ě-ku-ro'ne-um) a non-depolarizing neuromuscular blocking AGENT used in the bromide salt as an adjunct to anesthesia, inducing skeletal muscle relaxation and facilitating management of patients on mechanical ventilation; administered intravenously.

piperacillin (pi-per'ah-sil"in) a broad-spectrum semisynthetic PENICILLIN active against a wide variety of gram-positive and gram-negative bacteria; administered intramuscularly or intravenously as the sodium salt.

piperazine (pi-per'ah-zēn) an ANTHELMINTIC used in various salts against *Ascaris lumbricoides* and *Enterobius vermicularis*.

piperocaine (pi'per-o-kān) a local anesthetic, used as the hydrochloride salt.

pipet (pi-pet') pipette.

pipette (pi-pet') [Fr.] 1. a glass or transparent plastic tube used in measuring or transferring small quantities of liquid or gas. 2. to dispense by means of such a tube.

Pipracil (pi'prah-sil) trademark for a preparation of PIPERACILLIN sodium, an antibacterial.

pirbuterol (pir-bu'ter-ol) a beta₂-adrenergic RECEPTOR agonist, administered by oral inhalation in the form of the acetate ester as a BRONCHODILATOR.

piriform (pir'ĭ-form) pear-shaped.

piroxicam (pēr-ok'sī-kam) a NONSTEROIDAL ANTIINFLAMMATORY DRUG with a long plasma half-life; used in treatment of ARTHRITIS and related conditions, GOUT, CALCIUM PYROPHOSPHATE DEPOSITION DISEASE, and DYSMENORRHEA.

Pirquet's reaction (per-kāz') appearance of a papule with a red areola 24–48 hours after introduction of two small drops of Old tuberculin by slight scarification of the skin; a positive test indicates previous infection with tubercle bacilli.

pisiform (pi'sī-form) resembling a pea in size and shape.

pit (pit) 1. a hollow fovea or indentation. 2. a pockmark. 3. to indent, or to become and remain for a few minutes indented, by pressure.

anal p. proctodeum.

auditory p. a distinct depression in each auditory placode, marking the beginning of the embryonic development of the internal ear.

lens p. a pitlike depression in the fetal head where the lens develops.

nasal p., olfactory p. a depression appearing in the olfactory placodes in the early stages of development of the nose.

p. of stomach the epigastric fossa or epigastric region.

pitch (pich) 1. a dark, more or less viscous residue from distillation of tar and other substances. 2. any of various bituminous substances such as natural asphalt. 3. a resin from the sap of some coniferous trees. 4. the quality of sound dependent on the frequency of vibration of the waves producing it.

pithecoid (pith'ě-koid) apelike.

Although many practitioners discourage the use of a scale to grade the degree of pitting because of a lack of standardization, in clinical practice it is common to assign a positive number for the severity of pitting edema in the lower extremities, as follows:

+ 1—a normal foot and leg contour with a barely perceptible pit
+ 2—fairly normal lower extremity contours with a moderately deep pit
+ 3—obvious foot and leg swelling with a deep pit
+ 4—severe foot and leg swelling distorting normal contours with a deep pit

pithing (pith′ing) destruction of the brain and spinal cord by thrusting a blunt needle into the vertebral canal and cranium, done on animals to destroy sensibility preparatory to experimenting on their living tissue.

pitting (pit′ing) 1. the formation, usually by scarring, of a small depression. 2. the removal from erythrocytes, by the spleen, of such structures as iron granules, without destruction of the cells. 3. remaining indented for a few minutes after removal of firm finger pressure, distinguishing fluid edema (pitting EDEMA) from MYXEDEMA. The amount of pitting serves as an assessment of severity and is graded on a numerical scale (see accompanying table).

pituicyte (pĭ-tu′ĭ-sīt) any of the distinctive fusiform cells composing most of the neurohypophysis.

pituitary (pĭ-tu′ĭ-tar″e) 1. pertaining to the pituitary gland. 2. PITUITARY GLAND. 3. a preparation of the pituitary glands of animals, used therapeutically.

   p. gland an endocrine gland located at the base of the brain in a small recess of the sphenoid bone called the SELLA TURCICA. It is attached by the hypophyseal stalk to the HYPOTHALAMUS and is divided into an anterior lobe (the ADENOHYPOPHYSIS) and a posterior lobe (the NEUROHYPOPHYSIS), which differ in embryological function and origin. Called also hypophysis.

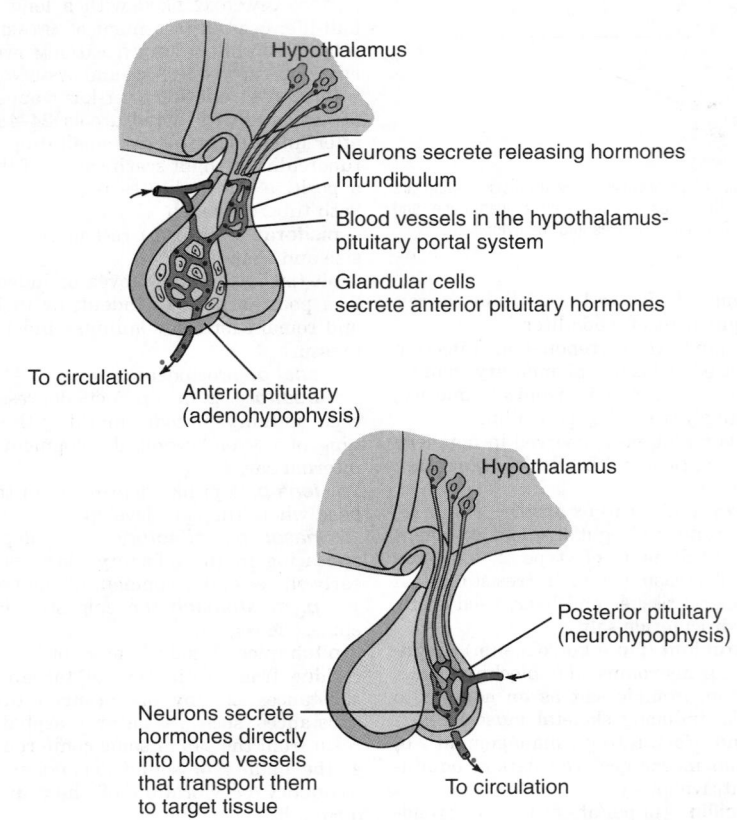

The pituitary gland and its relationship to the hypothalamus.

The *adenohypophysis* originates from epithelial tissue. The adenohypophysis secretes six important hormones: growth HORMONE, thyroid-stimulating HORMONE or THYROTROPIN, adrenocorticotropic HORMONE or CORTICOTROPIN, PROLACTIN, follicle-stimulating HORMONE, and luteinizing HORMONE. Most of these hormones are *tropic hormones,* which regulate the growth, development, and proper functioning of other endocrine glands and are of vital importance to the growth, maturation, and reproduction of the individual. Secretion of the anterior pituitary hormones is controlled by *releasing* and *inhibiting hormones* produced by the hypothalamus. Information gathered by the nervous system about the well-being of an individual is collected in the hypothalamus and used to control the secretion of hormones by the pituitary gland. The hypothalamic releasing and inhibiting hormones are transported to the pituitary gland by way of the hypothalamic-hypophyseal portal system in which the hypothalamic venules connect with the capillaries of the anterior pituitary.

The *neurohypophysis* originates from neural tissue; it stores and secretes two hormones, OXYTOCIN and VASOPRESSIN (antidiuretic HORMONE). These hormones are synthesized in the cell bodies of neurons located in the hypothalamus and transported along the axons to the terminals located in the neurohypophysis and are released in response to neural stimulation.

Surgical removal of part or all of the pituitary gland is called *hypophysectomy* and is usually done for treatment of a pituitary tumor. Because of its influence on the adrenal cortex and other endocrine glands, removal of the pituitary gland has widespread effects on the body. See HYPOPHYSECTOMY.

posterior p. neurohypophysis.

pityriasis (pit″ĭ-ri′ah-sis) any of various skin diseases characterized by the formation of fine, branny scales.

acute lichenoid p. an acute or subacute, sometimes relapsing, widespread macular, papular, or vesicular eruption that tends to crusting, necrosis, and hemorrhage; when it heals it leaves pigmented depressed scars, followed by a new crop of lesions. Progression to the chronic lichenoid form occasionally occurs.

p. al′ba a chronic condition with patchy scaling and hypopigmentation of the skin of the face.

chronic lichenoid p. a chronic brown to red-brown scaly macular eruption, seen mainly on the trunk, with epidermal changes and a perivascular lymphocytic infiltrate.

It may arise independently or happen as a progression of the acute lichenoid form.

p. ro′sea a common acute or subacute, self-limited exanthematous disease of unknown etiology. It begins with a solitary red to tan plaque (herald plaque), usually on the trunk, arms, or thighs, which is followed by similar but smaller papular or macular lesions; these later may peel and leave a scaly collarette.

p. ru′bra pila′ris a chronic inflammatory skin disease marked by pink scaling macules and cone-shaped horny follicular papules; it usually begins with severe seborrhea of the scalp and face, associated with keratoderma of palms and soles.

p. versi′color tinea versicolor.

pityroid (pit′ĭ-roid) scaly or branny; called also furfuraceous.

Pityrosporon (pit″ĭ-ros′po-ron) *Malassezia.*

pivalate (piv′ah-lāt) USAN contraction for trimethylacetate.

pixel (pik′sel) a picture element; a CT SCAN or PET scan is composed of an array of squares (pixels), each of which is colored a uniform shade of gray or another color. The corresponding region in the tissue slice that is imaged is called a VOXEL (volume element).

pK_a the negative logarithm of the ionization constant (K) of an acid, the pH of a solution in which half of the acid molecules are ionized.

PKU phenylketonuria.

PKU1 phenylketonuria.

placebo (plah-se′bo) [L.] 1. a supposedly inert substance such as a sugar pill or injection of sterile water, given under the guise of effective treatment. Paradoxically, it may exert either a positive or a negative effect on the recipient (see placebo EFFECT). A positive placebo effect can occur when caregiver and patient believe and expect a medication or procedure will relieve symptoms. Placebos are sometimes used in controlled clinical trials of new drugs; while some patients selected at random are given the new drug, others are given a placebo. It may be an active placebo that mimics the new drug's side effects. The patients taking the new drug must have significantly more relief of symptoms than the control group taking the placebo for the new drug to be considered to be effective. See also SINGLE BLIND, DOUBLE BLIND, and TRIPLE BLIND. 2. the term has been extended to mean virtually any type of ineffective treatment, including surgery and psychotherapy. Use of placebos is ethically problematic because it deceives

P

the patient. Ethical questions regarding the use of placebos include: (1) Is deception necessary to produce benefit? and (2) Do placebos have a nondeceptive use?

placenta (plah-sen′tah), pl. *placentas, placen′tae* [L.] an organ characteristic of true mammals during pregnancy, joining mother and offspring, providing endocrine secretion and selective exchange of soluble bloodborne substances through apposition of uterine and trophoblastic vascularized parts. See also afterbirth. adj., **placen′tal.**

In anatomic nomenclature the placenta consists of a uterine and a fetal portion. The chorion, the superficial or fetal portion, is surfaced by a smooth, shining membrane continuous with the sheath of the umbilical cord (amnion). The deep, or uterine, portion is divided by deep sulci into lobes of irregular outline and extent (the cotyledons). Over the maternal surface of the placenta is stretched a delicate, transparent membrane of fetal origin. Around the periphery of the placenta is a large vein (the marginal sinus), which returns a part of the maternal blood from the organ.

The major function of the placenta is to allow diffusion of nutrients from the mother's blood into the fetus's blood and diffusion of waste products from the fetus back to the mother. This two-way exchange takes place across the placental membrane, which is semipermeable; that is, it acts as a selective filter, allowing some materials to pass through and holding back others.

In the early months of pregnancy the placenta acts as a nutrient storehouse and helps to process some of the food substances that nourish the fetus. Later, as the fetus grows and develops, these metabolic functions of the placenta are gradually taken on by the fetal liver.

The placenta secretes both estrogens and progesterone. After birth of the infant the placenta is cast off from the uterus and expelled via the birth canal.

p. accre′ta one abnormally adherent to the myometrium, with partial or complete absence of the decidua basalis.

battledore p. one with the umbilical cord inserted at the edge.

p. circumvalla′ta one encircled with a dense, raised, white nodular ring, the attached membranes being doubled back over the edge of the placenta.

p. fenestra′ta one that has spots where placental tissue is lacking.

p. incre′ta placenta accreta with penetration of the myometrium.

p. membrana′cea one that is abnormally thin and spread over an unusually large area of the myometrium.

p. percre′ta placenta accreta with invasion of the myometrium to the peritoneal covering, sometimes causing rupture of the uterus.

p. pre′via low implantation of the placenta so that it partially or completely covers the cervical os. Percentages are used to designate the amount of obstruction; e.g., 100 per cent is total placenta previa, and 50 per cent indicates that about half the opening is obstructed. The condition occurs with greater frequency in women who have had multiple pregnancies or are over 35. The exact cause is not known.

With the onset of any contractions and cervical dilation, or when the cervix begins to dilate at the onset of labor and the upper and lower uterine segments differentiate, the placenta is stretched and pulled from the uterine wall, producing bleeding. The bleeding usually is abrupt and painless and may stop on its own. However, if it continues it can be life-threatening for the mother since it is maternal blood that is being lost. The life of the fetus is in jeopardy because of anoxia resulting from separation of the placenta from its blood supply.

Diagnosis can be established by ultrasonography or radiologic placentography. Once diagnosis is made, treatment will depend on the gestational age of the fetus and the percentage of placenta covering the cervical os. Cesarean delivery is recommended if 30 per cent or more of the opening is obstructed by the placenta. If there is minimal bleeding that stops on its own, the fetus is not in distress, and if the gestational age is such that continuing the pregnancy is necessary for delivery of a viable fetus, the pregnancy may be continued under careful monitoring in the hospital, or at home if the mother is able to stay in bed. However, if the life of the mother or fetus is threatened by continued and excessive bleeding, delivery is indicated.

Vaginal examinations are carried out in an operating room so that if hemorrhage does occur as a result of manipulation of the uterus, a cesarean section can be done immediately to remove the placenta, stop the bleeding, and deliver the child safely.

Patient Care. Premature separation of the placenta is an emergency. The maternal signs are monitored every 15 minutes and blood loss is evaluated. Fetal heart tones also are monitored to detect fetal distress. The amount of bleeding is estimated and documented. Oxygen equipment should be at hand in the event signs of fetal distress indicate anoxia.

Postpartal hemorrhage and infection are more likely in women who have had placenta previa. Placement of the placenta in the lower segment predisposes to more bleeding because that portion of the uterus does not contract as forcefully as the upper segment. Additionally, the misplaced placenta has enlarged its bed to compensate for its poor location, so that there is a larger denuded area after delivery of the placenta. The same denuded area is also more susceptible to infection because it is located near the cervical opening where infectious organisms may enter.

Vaginal bleeding during pregnancy or labor is frightening for the mother. She will need reassurance and frequent explanations of what is happening to her throughout the period of monitoring and delivery. Some emotional stress can be alleviated by encouraging the mother to be aware of fetal movements and allowing her to listen to normal fetal heart sounds.

p. reflex′a one in which the margin is thickened, appearing to turn back on itself.

p. spu′ria an accessory portion without blood vessels connecting it with the main placenta.

p. succenturia′ta an accessory portion with an artery and a vein connecting it with the main placenta.

placentation (plas″en-ta′shun) the series of events following implantation of the embryo and leading to development of the placenta.

placentitis (plas″en-ti′tis) inflammation of the placenta.

placentography (plas″en-tog′rah-fe) radiological visualization of the placenta after injection of a contrast medium.

placentoid (plah-sen′toid) resembling the placenta.

Placidyl (plas′ĭ-dil) trademark for a preparation of ETHCHLORVYNOL, a SEDATIVE and HYPNOTIC.

placode (plak′ōd) a platelike structure, especially a thickening of the ectoderm marking the site of future development in the early embryo of an organ of special sense, e.g., the *auditory placode* (ear), *lens placode* (eye), and *olfactory placode* (nose).

placoid (plak′oid) platelike or plaquelike.

plagiocephaly (pla″je-o-sef′ah-le) distortion of the shape of the skull resulting from premature closure of the cranial sutures. adj., **plagiocephal′ic.**

plague (plāg) an acute febrile, infectious, highly fatal disease caused by the bacillus *Yersinia pestis.* It is primarily a disease of rats and other rodents and is usually spread to human beings by fleas. The most common form is *bubonic plague. Pneumonic plague* is a second type, which can be spread directly between humans by droplet infection.

Plague is a devastating disease; three outbreaks in history wiped out whole populations. The first of these spread over Europe in the sixth century A.D. in a tremendous cycle of pestilence that lasted for more than 50 years. The second, called the "Black Death," was perhaps the most deadly outbreak the world has ever known. It swept over Europe in the 14th century, and in many areas up to three quarters of the population perished; perhaps 25 million Europeans died. The "Great Plague of London" in 1665 was actually a relatively minor outbreak. A third great epidemic raged in Asia at the turn of the 20th century. The greatest toll was in India, where there were more than 12 million deaths from 1896 to 1933.

Some cases have occurred in the United States. Extensive epidemics have been prevented in this country by strict quarantines and by sanitation measures that have been enforced since the disease was traced to rat and wild rodent fleas.

Bubonic Plague. Bubonic plague is characterized by acutely inflamed and painful swellings of the lymph nodes, or buboes, usually in the groin. The disease strikes suddenly with chills and fever. Children may have convulsions. There is vomiting and thirst, generalized pain, headache, and mental dullness. Delirium may also be present. After the third day, black spots, which give the disease the name "black death," may appear on the skin. Tender, enlarged lymph nodes are usually seen between the second and fifth days. Some cases of bubonic plague are mild. The more virulent cases last 5 or 6 days and are usually fatal. If the patient survives past the tenth or twelfth day, there is a good chance of recovery. The mortality rate for untreated cases is usually between 25 and 50 per cent, but has reached as high as 90 per cent. When antibiotic therapy is administered promptly (see *Treatment*), the mortality rate can be as low as 5 per cent.

Pneumonic Plague. Pneumonic plague usually occurs during outbreaks of bubonic plague and may be a direct complication of it. There is extensive involvement of the lungs, and the sputum contains many organisms. At one time, pneumonic plague was always fatal. Now, when antibiotic therapy is administered promptly (see *Treatment*), the mortality rate is much lower.

Prevention. The most important measure in controlling plague is the extermination of rats. This is especially necessary around shipping areas, in warehouses, and on docks. Rat control for ships arriving from plague areas is vital. Where there is an outbreak of plague, strict quarantine measures are called for, as well as the use of insecticides to protect inhabitants of the stricken area against fleas. Immunization with plague vaccine is recommended only for persons whose occupation requires contact with possibly infected rodents.

A consensus statement called "Plague as a Biological Weapon" has been issued by the Working Group on Civilian Biodefense. It notes the danger that would be associated with an aerosol plague weapon.

Treatment. Prompt treatment is essential with antibiotics, which can also be used for prophylaxis. Antibiotics of choice are STREPTOMYCIN, GENTAMICIN, TETRACYCLINE, and FLUOROQUINOLONES.

plan (plan) a detailed method worked out in advance for the attainment of a goal; see also PLANNING.

Baylor p. a method of staffing nursing units developed at Baylor University Medical Center; nurses work only 12-hour shifts on the weekend and are paid for a standard work week.

care p. a document that identifies nursing orders for a patient and serves as a guide to nursing care. It can either be written for an individual patient, be retrieved from a computer and individualized, or be preprinted for a specific disease, condition, or nursing diagnosis and individualized to the specific patient. Standardized care plans are available for a number of patient conditions.

plane (plān) 1. a flat surface determined by the position of three points in space. 2. an imaginary flat surface that divides the body into sections (see accompanying figure). adj., **pla′nar.** 3. a specified level, as the plane of anesthesia. 4. to rub away or abrade; see also PLANING and PLASTIC SURGERY. 5. a superficial incision in the wall of a cavity or between tissue layers, especially in plastic surgery, made so that the precise point of entry into the cavity or between the layers can be determined.

coronal p's frontal p's.

datum p. a given horizontal plane from which craniometric measurements are made.

frontal p's those planes passing longitudinally through the body, an organ, or a

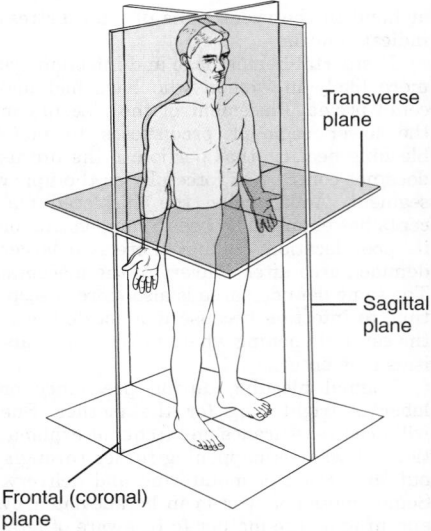

Frontal (coronal) plane

Planes of section. Transverse, sagittal, and frontal planes of the body. From Applegate, 2000.

part, at right angles to the median plane and dividing into front and back portions. Called also coronal planes.

horizontal p. transverse plane.

median p. one passing longitudinally through the body, an organ, or a part from front to back, dividing it into right and left halves.

sagittal p's vertical planes through the body parallel to the median plane or the sagittal suture, dividing the body into unequal left and right portions.

transverse p. one passing horizontally through the body, an organ, or a part at right angles to the median and frontal planes, dividing it into upper and lower portions. Called also horizontal plane.

vertical p. one perpendicular to a horizontal plane, such as a sagittal plane, median plane, or frontal plane.

planigraphy (plah-nig′rah-fe) a method of body section radiography that shows in detail structures lying in a predetermined plane of the body while blurring structures in other planes, produced by movement of the film and x-ray tube in certain specified directions. adj., **planigraph′ic.**

planing (pla′ning) 1. abrasion of disfigured skin to promote reepithelization with minimal scarring; done by mechanical means (DERMABRASION) or by application of a caustic (CHEMABRASION). See also PLASTIC SURGERY. 2. root planing.

root p. smoothing of the root surface of a tooth after subgingival scaling or DÉBRIDEMENT.

Planned Parenthood an organization that provides reproductive health care services, including the promotion of accessible means of voluntary fertility control, operation of clinics, conduction of educational programs, conduction of research, and dissemination of information.

planner (plan′er) one who does or that which assists PLANNING.

discharge p. the worker who coordinates discharge PLANNING; in a hospital this person may also be in a position to evaluate which patients exceed length of stay requirements and to provide data for re-evaluation according to DIAGNOSIS-RELATED GROUP.

planning (plan′ing) consciously setting forth a scheme to achieve a desired end or goal. The planning phase of the NURSING PROCESS provides a blueprint for nursing INTERVENTIONS to achieve specified goals. A plan of nursing care includes NURSING DIAGNOSES arranged in order of priority, goals or objectives that give direction and purpose to nursing intervention, nursing orders that encompass nursing activities necessary to achieve specified goals, and criteria by which it is possible to evaluate the effectiveness of nursing intervention and the plan of care. In most instances the goals or objectives can be used as outcome criteria for the evaluation phase of the process.

Goals or objectives in the care PLAN should be stated in behavioral terms, that is, they should describe what the patient will be able to do as a result of nursing interventions. If they are to be useful as criteria for evaluation, they should be measurable and realistic. *Nursing orders* are the nursing actions and patient activities prescribed by the nurse to achieve the stated goals and objectives.

discharge p. in the NURSING INTERVENTIONS CLASSIFICATION, a nursing INTERVENTION defined as preparation for moving a patient from one level of care to another within or outside the current health care agency. See also discharge PLANNER.

family p. the practice of BIRTH CONTROL measures within the context of family values, attitudes, and beliefs; including oral contraceptives, diaphragm, condom, and natural family PLANNING; see also CONTRACEPTION.

family p., natural methods of avoiding CONCEPTION without the use of artificial contraceptive means; see discussion under CONTRACEPTION. Called also fertility awareness methods.

family p.: contraception in the NURSING INTERVENTIONS CLASSIFICATION, a nursing

INTERVENTION defined as facilitation of pregnancy prevention by providing information about the physiology of reproduction and methods to control conception. See also CONTRACEPTION.

family p.: infertility in the NURSING INTERVENTIONS CLASSIFICATION, a nursing INTERVENTION defined as management, education, and support of the patient and significant other undergoing evaluation and treatment for INFERTILITY.

family p.: unplanned pregnancy in the NURSING INTERVENTIONS CLASSIFICATION, a nursing INTERVENTION defined as facilitation of decision making regarding pregnancy outcome.

planoconcave (pla″no-kon′kāv) flat on one side and concave on the other.

planoconvex (pla″no-kon′veks) flat on one side and convex on the other.

planography (plah-nog′rah-fe) planigraphy.

plant (plant) any multicellular EUKARYOTIC organism that performs PHOTOSYNTHESIS to obtain its nutrition; plants comprise one of the five KINGDOMS in the most widely used classification of living organisms.

planta (plan′tah) the bottom of the foot; called also sole. adj., **plan′tar.**

Plantago (plan-ta′go) a genus of herbs, including *P. in′dica, P. psyl′lium* (Spanish psyllium), and *P. ova′ta* (blond psyllium); see also psyllium hydrophilic MUCILLOID, plantago SEED, and psyllium HUSK.

plantalgia (plan-tal′jah) pain in the sole of the foot.

plantar (plan′ter) pertaining to the sole of the foot.

plantaris (plan-tar′is) [L.] plantar.

plantigrade (plan′tĭ-grād) walking or running flat on the full sole of the foot; characteristic of humans and of such quadrupeds as the bear.

planula (plan′u-lah) a larval coelenterate.

planum (pla′num) [L.] plane.

plaque (plak) 1. any patch or flat area. 2. a superficial, solid, elevated skin lesion with a diameter equal to or greater than 1.0 cm (0.5 cm according to some authorities); see also PAPULE. 3. dental plaque.

atheromatous p. fibrous plaque.

dental p. a dense, nonmineralized, highly organized BIOFILM of microbes, organic and inorganic material derived from the saliva, gingival crevicular fluid, and bacterial byproducts. It plays an important etiologic role in the development of dental caries and periodontal and gingival diseases; calcified plaque forms dental CALCULUS.

P

fibrous p. the lesion of atherosclerosis, a white to yellow area within the wall of an artery that causes the intimal surface to bulge into the lumen; it is composed of lipid, cell debris, smooth muscle cells, collagen, and, in older persons, calcium. Called also atheromatous plaque.

Hollenhorst p's atheromatous emboli containing cholesterol crystals in the retinal arterioles.

pleural p's opaque white plaques on the parietal pleura, visible radiographically in cases of ASBESTOSIS.

senile p's microscopic lesions composed of fragmented axon terminals and dendrites surrounding a core of amyloid seen in the cerebral cortex in Alzheimer's disease.

Plaquenil (pla′kwĕ-nil) trademark for a preparation of HYDROXYCHLOROQUINE, an ANTI-INFLAMMATORY and antiprotozoal AGENT used for treatment of malaria, lupus erythematosus, rheumatoid arthritis, and giardiasis.

plasm (plazm) 1. plasma. 2. a formative substance; used as a word element in terms such as CYTOPLASM and HYALOPLASM.

plasma (plaz′mah) 1. the fluid portion of the lymph. 2. the fluid portion of the BLOOD, in which the formed elements (blood CELLS) are suspended. Plasma is to be distinguished from SERUM, which is plasma from which the FIBRINOGEN has been separated in the process of clotting. Called also blood plasma. adj., **plasmat′ic, plas′mic.** Of the total volume of blood, 55 per cent is made up of plasma. It is a clear, straw-colored liquid, 92 per cent water, in which are contained plasma PROTEINS, inorganic salts, nutrients, gases, waste materials from the cells, and various hormones, secretions, and enzymes. These substances are transported to or from the tissues of the body by the plasma.

Plasma obtained from blood donors is given to persons suffering from loss of blood or from shock to help maintain adequate blood pressure. Since plasma can be dried and stored in bottles, it can be transported almost anywhere, ready for immediate use after addition of the appropriate fluid. Plasma can be given to anyone, regardless of blood type. (See also TRANSFUSION.)

Plasma volume is sometimes measured in order to calculate the total BLOOD VOLUME. The most common method for determining plasma volume is by injection of a dye (T-1824, called Evans blue) into the circulating blood and, after the dye has been dispersed throughout the body, using the dilution of the dye to calculate the total blood volume.

antihemophilic human p. normal human plasma that has been processed promptly to preserve the ANTIHEMOPHILIC properties of the original blood; used for temporary correction of bleeding tendency in HEMOPHILIA.

blood p. plasma (def. 2).

citrated p. blood plasma treated with SODIUM CITRATE, which prevents clotting.

p. exchange the removal of plasma from withdrawn blood (PLASMAPHERESIS) and retransfusion of the formed elements and type-specific fresh frozen PLASMA into the donor; done for removal of circulating antibodies or abnormal plasma components.

fresh frozen p. plasma separated from whole blood and frozen within 8 hours; it contains all the COAGULATION FACTORS.

p. thromboplastin antecedent deficiency hemophilia C.

plasmablast (plaz′mah-blast) the immature precursor of a plasmacyte, or plasma cell.

plasmacyte (plaz′mah-sīt) plasma cell. adj., **plasmacyt′ic.**

plasmacytoma (plaz″mah-si-to′mah) 1. a plasma cell DYSCRASIA. 2. a discrete, presumably solitary, plasma cell tumor mass.

plasmacytosis (plaz″mah-si-to′sis) an excess of plasmacytes in the blood.

plasmalemma (plaz″mah-lem′ah) plasma membrane.

plasmapheresis (plaz″mah-fĕ-re′sis) the removal of PLASMA from withdrawn blood, with retransfusion of the formed elements into the donor; generally, type-specific fresh frozen PLASMA or ALBUMIN is used to replace the withdrawn plasma. The procedure may be done for purposes of collecting plasma components or for therapeutic purposes.

plasmatorrhexis (plaz″mah-to-rek′sis) bursting of a cell from internal pressure.

plasmid (plaz′mid) an extrachromosomal self-replicating structure found in bacterial cells that carries genes for a variety of functions not essential for cell growth. Plasmids consist of cyclic double-stranded DNA molecules, replicating independently of the chromosomes and transmitting through successive cell divisions genes specifying such functions as antibiotic resistance (R plasmid); conjugation (F plasmid); the production of enzymes, toxins and antigens; and the metabolism of sugars and other organic compounds. Plasmids can be transferred from one cell to another by conjugation and by transduction. Some plasmids may also become integrated into the bacterial chromosome; these are known as EPISOMES.

conjugative p. a plasmid that is transferred from one bacterial cell to another during conjugation.

F p. a conjugative plasmid found in F^+ (male) bacterial cells that leads with high frequency to its transfer and much less often to transfer of the bacterial chromosome. A cell possessing the F plasmid (F^+, male) can form a conjugation bridge (F pilus) to a cell lacking the F plasmid (F^-, female), through which genetic material may pass from one cell to another.

F' p. a hybrid F plasmid that contains also a segment of the host chromosome.

R p. a conjugative factor in bacterial cells that promotes resistance to agents such as antibiotics, metal ions, ultraviolet radiation, and bacteriophage.

plasmin (plaz′min) the active principle of the fibrinolytic or clot-lysing system, a proteolytic enzyme with a high specificity for fibrin and the particular ability to dissolve formed fibrin clots.

plasminogen (plaz-min′o-jen) the inactive precursor of PLASMIN, occurring in plasma and converted to plasmin by the action of UROKINASE; called also profibrinolysin.

plasminogen activator (plaz-min′o-jen ak′tĭ-va″tor) any of a group of substances that cleave plasminogen and convert it to plasmin, its active form, e.g., tissue plasminogen activator.

plasmocyte (plaz′mo-sīt) plasma cell.

plasmocytoma (plaz″mo-sī-to′mah) 1. a plasma cell DYSCRASIA. 2. plasmacytoma (def. 2).

plasmodicidal (plaz-mo″dĭ-si′d′l) destructive to PLASMODIA; see also antimalarial. Called also malariacidal.

Plasmodium (plaz-mo′de-um) a genus of sporozoa (family Plasmodiidae) parasitic in the red blood cells of humans and other animals; the malarial parasite. The organism is transmitted to the bloodstream of man by the bite of anopheline mosquitoes. The sporozoites migrate directly to the liver, where they develop and multiply within the parenchymal cells as MEROZOITES, which then burst the liver cells and invade erythrocytes. Some of the merozoites develop into GAMETOCYTES, which are ingested by mosquitoes, beginning the sexual stage, which ends with the development of sporozoites. Four species, *P. falci′parum, P. mala′riae, P. ova′le,* and *P. vi′vax,* cause the four specific types of human MALARIA. (See accompanying illustration.)

plasmodium (plaz-mo′de-um) 1. a parasite of the genus *Plasmodium.* 2. a multinucleate continuous mass of protoplasm. adj., **plasmo′dial.**

plasmogen (plaz′mo-jen) the more vital or essential part of the cytoplasm.

plasmolysis (plaz-mol′ĭ-sis) contraction of cell protoplasm due to loss of water by osmosis. adj., **plasmolyt′ic.**

plasmoma (plaz-mo′mah) 1. a plasma cell DYSCRASIA. 2. plasmacytoma (def. 2).

plasmon (plaz′mon) the hereditary factors of the cytoplasm of an oocyte.

plasmorrhexis (plaz″mo-rek′sis) a morphologic change in ERYTHROCYTES, consisting in the escape from the cells of round, shiny granules and splitting off of particles; called also erythrocytorrhexis.

plasmoschisis (plaz-mos′kĭ-sis) the splitting up of cell protoplasm.

plaster (plas′ter) 1. a mixture of materials that hardens; used for immobilizing or making impressions of body parts. 2. an adhesive substance spread on fabric or other suitable backing material, for application to the skin, often containing some medication, such as an analgesic or local vasodilator.

p. of Paris calcium sulfate dihydrate, reduced to a fine powder; the addition of water produces a porous mass used in making casts and bandages to support or immobilize body parts, and in dentistry for making study models.

Plastibell (plas′tĭ-bel) trademark for a bell-shaped device used as a guide in the removal of the foreskin in CIRCUMCISION. The Plastibell is slipped over the glans, and the foreskin is then pulled over and secured tightly around the bell. After the tissue is trimmed from the glans, the handle of the Plastibell is snapped off, leaving the bell in place; within 5 to 10 days the bell and the remnant of the foreskin become detached, leaving a healed edge.

plastic (plas′tik) 1. tending to build up tissues or to restore a lost part. 2. capable of being molded. 3. a high-molecular-weight polymeric material, usually organic, capable of being molded, extruded, drawn, or otherwise shaped and then hardened into a form. 4. material that can be molded.

p. surgery surgery concerned with the restoration, reconstruction, correction, or improvement in the shape and appearance of body structures that are defective, damaged, or misshapen by injury, disease, or anomalous growth and development. This kind of surgery has been practiced for thousands of years. Artificial noses and ears have been found on Egyptian mummies. Medical records show that the ancient Hindus reconstructed noses by using skin flaps lifted from the cheek or forehead—a technique that was often practiced, since it was a custom to mutilate the noses of persons who broke the laws.

Skin Grafting. This is the most common procedure of plastic surgery, consisting of

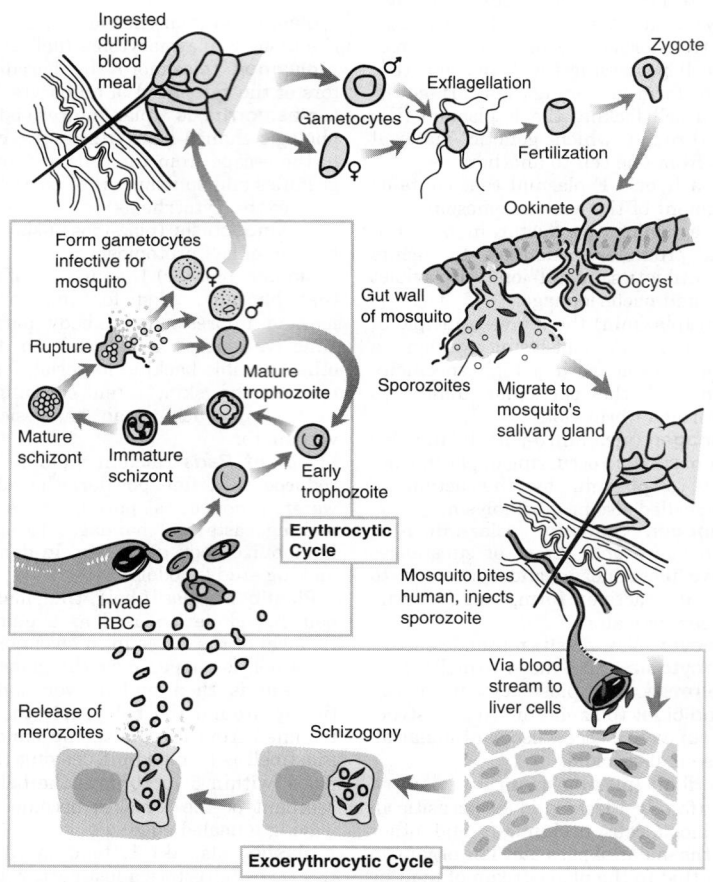

Life cycle of *Plasmodium* spp. From Mahon and Manuselis, 2000.

the replacement of severely damaged skin in one area with healthy skin from another area of the patient's body or from the body of a skin donor. (See further discussion at GRAFTING.) With the advent of MICROSURGERY, much of the inconvenience and lengthy waiting necessary for successful grafting of skin flaps has been eliminated.

The transplanting of tissues other than skin also is possible through microsurgery. Free-bone grafts can be used to provide rapid replacement of long bone defects, and free muscle transfers permit restoration of muscle function.

Repairing Mouth and Other Defects. Among common defects that can be corrected by plastic surgery are CLEFT LIP and CLEFT PALATE. Others are webbed FINGERS and TOES, protruding or missing ears, receding chins, and injured noses. In addition, the shape of various types of noses can be altered for the sake of appearance. RHYTI-DECTOMY is another common type of plastic surgery, done on the face to improve the aging patient's appearance. It is popularly known as a face lift.

Facial Reconstruction. In facial reconstruction, missing bone and muscle, and sometimes skin, are replaced by substitutes. Sometimes the reconstruction is made with bone or cartilage taken from another part of the body, or sometimes it is made by artificial means.

Use of Prostheses. Often the substitute for missing tissue is a PROSTHESIS, a replacement not made from living tissue. It may be inserted beneath the skin (such as to build out a receding chin) or attached to the skin surface (for example, to replace an ear). Prostheses attached to, not inserted beneath, the skin frequently are employed to fill out depressed or missing facial areas, the aftereffects of accidents, cancer, or war injuries. In building such a replacement, the surgeon first makes an impression of the face and a plaster cast of the impression. The substitute part is molded in wax or clay in the plaster cast, and from this model the actual replacement part is made. Such parts, molded and painted to match the texture and color of the skin, have been used to replace many structures, including missing ears and noses.

Use of Cartilage, Skin, and Bone. Noses and ears also have been reconstructed with rib cartilage and skin grafts. Eyebrows have been made by the use of skin grafts from the scalp, and chest deformities repaired by the use of bone chips from other parts of the body.

Sometimes a nose is remodeled to correct a hump or hook, or a saddle nose (a depression on the ridge), or a twisted nose. Incisions are made inside to avoid causing outside scars, and the surgeon either removes excess cartilage or bone, or inserts it, according to the improvement wanted. Cartilage and bone may be obtained from other parts of the body, usually the ribs or hip. After the operation, the skin over the nose adapts to the new structure.

Dermabrasion. Skin blemishes such as acne scars and pits can be "sandpapered" or planed. This technique, called dermabrasion, seeks to correct superficial blemishes and to remove superficial accumulations of pigment. However, as dermabrasion can occasionally cause increased scarring or introduce variation in skin color and texture, such treatment is infrequently performed today.

plasticity (plas-tis′ĭ-te) the quality of being plastic, or capable of being molded.

plastid (plas′tid) 1. any elementary constructive unit, as a cell. 2. any specialized organ of the cell other than the nucleus and centrosome, such as chloroplast or amyloplast.

-plasty word element [Gr.], *formation* or *plastic repair of.*

plate (plāt) 1. a flat STRATUM or LAYER. 2. dental plate; sometimes, by extension, incorrectly used to designate a complete denture. 3. a flat vessel, usually a PETRI DISH, containing sterile solid medium for the culture of microorganisms. 4. to prepare a culture medium in a PETRI DISH, or to inoculate such a medium with a bacterial culture.

axial p. primitive streak.

bite p. biteplate.

cortical p. a layer of compact bone overlying the spongiosa of the alveolar process on the vestibular and oral aspects of the mandible and maxilla.

deck p. roof plate.

dental p. a plate of acrylic resin, metal, or other material that is fitted to the shape of the mouth, and serves for the support of artificial teeth.

dorsal p. roof plate.

end p. see END PLATE.

epiphyseal p. the thin plate of cartilage between the epiphysis and the shaft of a long bone; it is the site of growth in length and is obliterated by epiphyseal closure.

equatorial p. the collection of chromosomes at the equator of the spindle in mitosis.

floor p. the unpaired ventral longitudinal zone of the neural TUBE; called also ventral plate.

foot p. footplate.

force p. force platform.

medullary p. neural plate.

muscle p. myotome (def. 2).

neural p. a thickened band of ectoderm in the midbody region of the developing embryo, which develops into the neural TUBE; called also medullary plate.

roof p. the unpaired dorsal longitudinal zone of the neural TUBE; called also dorsal plate and deck plate.

tarsal p. tarsus (def. 2).

ventral p. floor plate.

platelet (plāt′let) the smallest of the formed elements in blood, a disk-shaped, non-nucleated blood element with a fragile membrane, formed in the red bone marrow by fragmentation of MEGAKARYOCYTES. Platelets tend to adhere to uneven or damaged surfaces, and there are an average of about 250,000 per mm^3 of blood. The bone marrow produces from 30,000 to 50,000 platelets per mm^3 of blood daily, which means that in any ten-day period all the platelets in the body are completely replaced. Called also thrombocyte.

The rate of platelet formation seems to be governed by the amount of oxygen in the blood and the presence of nucleic acid derivatives from injured tissue. At any given time about one-third of the total blood platelets can be found in the spleen; the remaining two-thirds are in the circulating blood. Their primary functions are related to COAGULATION of blood. Because of their adhesion and aggregation capabilities they can occlude small breaks in blood vessels and prevent escape of blood (See accompanying illustration). They also are able to take up, store, transport, and release SEROTONIN and PLATELET FACTOR 3. Abnormally high numbers

P

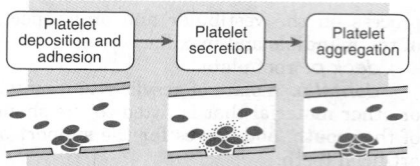

Platelet response to vascular injury. From Malarkey and McMorrow, 2000.

of platelets occur in the presence of malignancy, splenectomy, asphyxiation, polycythemia vera, and acute infections. A very low count can occur as a result of idiopathic thrombocytopenic purpura, pernicious anemia, and allergic conditions, and during cancer chemotherapy. Many drugs can cause a toxic decrease in the number of platelets.

p. factors factors important in hemostasis which are contained in or attached to the platelets: platelet factor 1 is adsorbed COAGULATION FACTOR V from the plasma; platelet factor 2 is an accelerator of the thrombin-fibrinogen reaction; platelet factor 3 is a lipoprotein with roles in the activation of both coagulation factor X and prothrombin; platelet factor 4 is capable of inhibiting the activity of heparin.

plateletpheresis (plāt″let-fĕ-re′sis) thrombocytapheresis.

platform (plat′form) a flat horizontal surface higher than the level of the areas around it.

force p. a small platform that measures variations in downward force between different points on its surface, for assessing stability of stance and posture as a person stands on it. Called also force plate.

Platinol (plat′ĭ-nol) trademark for a preparation of CISPLATIN, an antineoplastic AGENT.

platinum (Pt) (plat′ĭ-num) a chemical element, atomic number 78, atomic weight 195.09. (See Appendix 6.)

platy- word element [Gr.], *broad; flat.*

platybasia (plat″ĭ-ba′zhah) malformation of the base of the skull due to softening of skull bones or a developmental anomaly, with bulging upwards of the floor of the posterior cranial fossa adjacent to the foramen magnum, upward displacement of the upper cervical vertebrae, and bony impingement on the brainstem, accompanied by neurologic signs referable to the medulla oblongata. See also basilar INVAGINATION. Called also basilar impression.

platycelous (plat″ĭ-se′lus) having one surface flat and the other concave, referring to vertebrae.

platycephalic (plat″ĭ-sĕ-fal′ik) having wide, flat head.

platycoria (plat″ĭ-kor′e-ah) a dilated condition of the pupil of the eye.

platyhelminth (plat″ĭ-hel′minth) flatworm.

Platyhelminthes (plat″ĭ-hel-min′thēz) the FLATWORMS, a phylum of acoelomate, dorsoventrally flattened, bilaterally symmetrical animals; it includes the classes CESTOIDEA (TAPEWORMS) and TREMATODA (FLUKES).

platyhieric (plat″ĭ-hi-er′ik) having a wide sacrum, with a sacral index above 100.

platypellic (plat″ĭ-pel′ik) having a broad PELVIS.

platypelloid (plat″ĭ-pel′oid) platypellic.

platypnea (plat″e-ne′ah) DYSPNEA that is relieved when the patient is lying flat; see also ORTHOPNEA.

platypodia (plat″ĭ-po′de-ah) flatfoot.

platyrrhine (plat′ĭ-rīn) having a broad nose, with a nasal index above 53.

platysma (plah-tiz′mah) a subcutaneous neck muscle extending from the neck to the clavicle, acting to wrinkle the skin of the neck and to depress the jaw. See Appendix 3-4.

play (pla) 1. involvement in enjoyable recreational activities; see also PLAY THERAPY. 2. the extent to which mechanical movement is available.

joint p. the accessory movement available within a JOINT, which is not under voluntary control but is needed for proper functioning of the joint.

p. therapy 1. a technique used in child psychotherapy in which play is used to reveal unconscious material. Play is the natural way in which children express and work through unconscious conflicts; thus play therapy is analogous to the technique of free association used in PSYCHOANALYSIS of adults. The therapy is done in a playroom containing toys such as dolls, a doll house, and furniture; blocks; art materials; toy animals, cars, trucks, guns, soldiers, and telephone; and games. As the child plays he expresses his fantasies and gives the therapist clues about his family relationships and unconscious conflicts. For example, the child may be unable to verbally express hostile feelings about a parent or sibling but be able to act out these feelings playing with a doll. The role of the therapist is nondirective. The therapist provides an accepting, understanding adult relationship that allows the child to work through his conflicts and to experiment with new ways of relating to himself and other people. 2. in the NURSING INTERVENTIONS CLASSIFICATION, a nursing INTERVENTION defined as the purposeful and directive use of toys and other materials to assist children in communicating their perception and knowledge of their world and to help in gaining mastery of their environment.

playing (pla′ing) engaging in enjoyable, recreational activity. 1. acting or behaving in a specified way.

   role p. a technique used in family therapy and group therapy, particularly PSYCHODRAMA, in which members of the group act out the behavior of others in specific roles in order to recognize the roles and to clarify role responses and choices.

pledget (plej′et) a small compress or tuft.

-plegia word element [Gr.], *paralysis; a stroke.*

pleiotropism (pli-ot′rŏ-pizm) pleiotropy.

pleiotropy (pli-ot′rŏ-pe) the production by a single gene of multiple phenotypic effects. The term is often used to refer to a single gene defect that is expressed as problems in multiple systems of the body, such as in OSTEOGENESIS IMPERFECTA, where the gene causes defects in several different systems that contain COLLAGEN.

plenary session the portion of a professional meeting or convention that all members attend.

pleocytosis (ple″o-si-to′sis) more than the normal number of lymphocytes in cerebrospinal fluid.

pleomastia (ple″o-mas′te-ah) polymastia.

pleomorphism (ple″o-mor′fizm) the assumption of various distinct forms by a single organism or within a species. adj., **pleomor′phic, pleomor′phous.**

pleonasm (ple′o-nazm) an excess of parts.

pleonectic (ple″o-nek′tik) characterized by having a higher than normal O_2 content at a given Po_2; said of blood.

pleonexia (ple″o-nek′se-ah) 1. a psychiatric disorder characterized by greediness; excessive desire for acquisition of wealth or objects. 2. the condition of being pleonectic.

pleonosteosis (ple″on-os″te-o′sis) abnormally increased ossification.

   Léri's p. a hereditary syndrome of premature and excessive ossification, with short stature, limitation of movement, broadening and deformity of digits, and a face similar to that seen with DOWN SYNDROME.

plessesthesia (ples″es-the′zhah) palpatory percussion.

plessimeter (plĕ-sim′ĕ-ter) pleximeter.

plessor (ples′er) plexor.

plethora (pleth′o-rah) 1. an excess of blood in a part. 2. by extension, a red florid complexion. adj., **pletho′ric.**

plethysmograph (plĕ-thiz′mo-graf) any device for measuring and recording

variations in the volume of an organ, part, or limb.

   body p. a device used in PULMONARY FUNCTION TESTS to measure parameters such as functional residual capacity (FRC) and lung-thorax compliance (C_{LT}). It consists of a large box in which the subject can be sealed so that volume of the thorax can be determined from pressure changes in the box.

plethysmography (plĕth″iz-mog′rah-fe) the determination of changes in volume by means of a plethysmograph.

   air-cuff p. a technique for measuring changes in the circumference of a limb by recording the changes in pressure in an air-filled cuff surrounding the limb.

   respiratory inductive p. a technique that uses elastic bands around the chest and abdomen of the patient to calculate chest and abdominal expansion, respiratory rate, respiratory pattern, and tidal volume.

pleur(o)- word element [Gr.], *pleura; rib; side.*

pleura (ploor′ah) [Gr.] the serous membrane investing the lungs (*visceral* or *pulmonary pleura*) and lining the walls of the thoracic cavity (*parietal pleura*); the two layers enclose a potential space, the pleural CAVITY. adj., **pleu′ral.**

pleuracotomy (ploor″ah-kot′ah-me) thoracotomy.

pleural effusion the presence of fluid in the pleural space, between the membrane encasing the lung and that lining the thoracic cavity; types include CHYLOTHORAX, HEMOTHORAX, HYDROTHORAX, and PYOTHORAX (EMPYEMA). Conditions that may lead to it include trauma, infections, inflammatory processes, malignancies affecting the pulmonary structures, kidney disease, and cardiac disease. The normal pleural space contains only a small amount of fluid to prevent friction as the lung expands and deflates. If, however, there is a disturbance in either the production of this fluid or its removal, the fluid accumulates and threatens collapse of the lung. In extreme cases there is total collapse of the lung and MEDIASTINAL SHIFT. Excess fluid in the pleural space may be removed by THORACENTESIS or by insertion of CHEST TUBES to allow for drainage of the fluid and, through a closed-drainage system, gradual reexpansion of the lung. See also PLEURISY.

pleuralgia (ploor-al′jah) pleurodynia. adj., **pleural′gic.**

pleurapophysis (ploor″ah-pof′ĭ-sis) a rib, or a vertebral process corresponding to a rib.

pleurectomy (plōo-rek′to-me) excision of a portion of the pleura.

Pleur-Evac trademark for a disposable underwater-seal unit designed for drainage of the pleural cavity; it has a graduated collection chamber, permitting immediate and accurate measurement of the amount of drainage from the pleural cavity via the CHEST TUBE.

pleurisy (ploor′ĭ-se) inflammation of the PLEURA; it may be caused by infection, injury, or tumor. It may be a complication of lung diseases, particularly of pneumonia, or sometimes of tuberculosis, lung abscess, or influenza. The symptoms are cough, fever, chills, sharp, sticking pain that is worse on inhalation, and rapid shallow breathing. Called also pleuritis. adj., **pleurit′ic.**

Types of Pleurisy. The membranous pleura that encases each lung is composed of two close-fitting layers; between them is a lubricating fluid. If the fluid content remains unchanged by the disease, it is called *dry, adhesive,* or *fibrinous pleurisy.* If the fluid increases abnormally, it is called *pleurisy with effusion* or *wet pleurisy.* (See also PLEURAL EFFUSION.) In *dry* or *fibrinous pleurisy* the two layers of membrane may become congested and swollen and rub against each other, which can be painful. Although only the outer layer causes pain (the inner layer has no pain nerves), the pain may be severe enough to necessitate the use of a strong analgesic.

Pleurisy with effusion is less likely to cause pain, because there usually is no chafing, but the fluid may interfere with breathing by compressing the lung. In some cases the lung is permanently displaced, failing to return to full capacity because of thickening of the pleura. If the excess fluid of wet pleurisy becomes infected, with formation of pus, the condition is known as *purulent* or *suppurative pleurisy* or EMPYEMA. Inflammation of the part of the pleura that covers the diaphragm is called *diaphragmatic pleurisy.*

Treatment. The most effective measures against pleurisy are those directed at the cause of the inflammation, such as administration of antibiotics and antiinflammatory medications.

blocked p., circumscribed p. encysted pleurisy.

encysted p. a form with adhesions that surround the effused material; called also blocked or circumscribed pleurisy.

interlobular p. encysted pleurisy between the lobes of the lung; called also interlobitis.

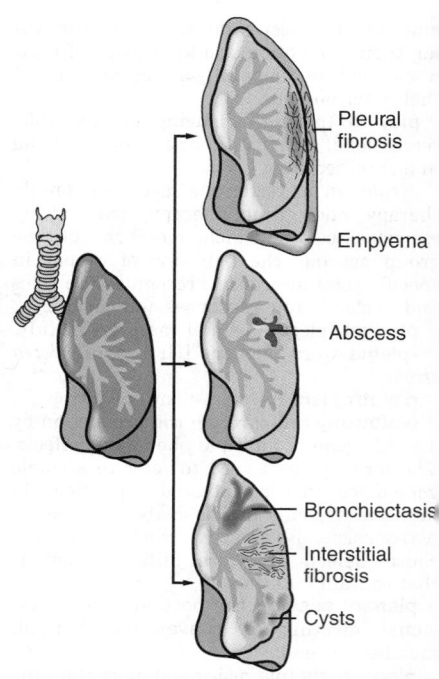

Pleurisy. Pneumonia may extend to the pleura and cause pleurisy, which may heal in the form of pleura fibrosis. Persistence of pus in the pleural cavity is called empyema. Suppurative pneumonia results in abscess formation. Bronchiectasis is a consequence of chronic lung infection. Interstitial fibrosis with cysts accounts for the honeycomb appearance of lungs in chronic lung disease. From Damjanov, 2000.

pleuritis (plōo-ri′tis) pleurisy.

lupus p. pleurisy, pleural effusion, and fever in patients with systemic lupus erythematosus.

rheumatoid p. pleurisy, pleural effusion, and often empyema in patients with rheumatoid arthritis.

tuberculous p. pleurisy with pleural effusion and tubercles on the pleura in patients with primary tuberculosis.

uremic p. pleurisy, usually of the fibrinous type, with pleural effusion in patients with uremia, often accompanying uremic PERICARDITIS.

pleurocele (ploor′o-sēl) pneumonocele (def. 1).

pleurocentesis (ploor″o-sen-te′sis) thoracentesis.

pleurocentrum (ploor″o-sen′trum) the lateral element of the vertebral column.

pleurodesis (plōo-rod′ĕ-sis) the artificial production of adhesions between the parietal and the visceral pleura for treatment of persistent PNEUMOTHORAX or severe PLEURAL

EFFUSION; formerly done by physically irritating the pleural surface, it is now usually done with a chemical sclerosing AGENT.

pleurodynia (ploor″o-din′e-ah) 1. pain in the pleural cavity; called also pleuralgia. 2. costalgia (def. 2).

epidemic p. an epidemic disease usually caused by group B coxsackieviruses and sometimes by group A coxsackieviruses, echoviruses, and other enteroviruses, marked by a sudden attack of violent pain in the chest, fever, and a tendency to recurrence on the third day. Called also devil's grip and Bornholm disease.

pleurogenic (ploor″o-jen′ik), **pleurogenous** (ploo-roj′ĕ-nus) originating in the pleura.

pleurography (ploor-og′rah-fe) radiography of the pleural cavity.

pleurohepatitis (ploor″o-hep″ah-ti′tis) hepatitis with inflammation of a portion of the pleura near the liver.

pleurolith (ploor′o-lith) a hard mass or CONCRETION in the pleura.

pleurolysis (ploor-ol′ĭ-sis) surgical separation of pleural adhesions.

pleuroparietopexy (ploor″o-pah-ri′ĕ-to-pek″se) the operation of fixing the visceral pleura to the parietal pleura, thus binding the lung to the chest wall.

pleuropericardial (ploor″o-per″ĭ-kahr′de-al) pertaining to the pleura and pericardium.

pleuropericarditis (ploor″o-per″ĭ-kahr-di′-tis) inflammation involving the pleura and the pericardium.

pleuroperitoneal (ploor″o-per″ĭ-to-ne′al) pertaining to the pleura and peritoneum.

pleuropneumonia (ploor″o-noo-mo′nyah) 1. pneumonia accompanied by pleurisy; called also pneumopleuritis. 2. an infectious disease of cattle, combining pneumonia and pleurisy, due to *Mycoplasma mycoides;* see also pleuropneumonia-like ORGANISMS.

pleurothotonos (ploor″o-thot′o-nos) tetanic bending of the body to one side.

pleurotomy (ploor-ot′ah-me) thoracotomy.

pleurovisceral (ploor″o-vis′er-al) pertaining to the pleura and viscera.

plexiform (plek′sĭ-form) resembling a plexus or network.

pleximeter (plek-sim′ĕ-ter) 1. a plate to be struck in mediate percussion. 2. diascope.

plexitis (plek-si′tis) inflammation of a nerve plexus.

plexopathy (pleks-op′ah-the) any disorder of a plexus, especially of nerves.

lumbar p. neuropathy of the lumbar plexus.

plexor (plek′ser) a hammer used in diagnostic percussion; plessor.

plexus (plek′sus), pl. *plex′us, plexuses* [L.] a network or tangle, chiefly of veins or nerves; see also RETE. adj., **plex′al.**

p. basila′ris a venous plexus of the dura mater located over the basilar part of the occipital bone and the posterior part of the body of the sphenoid bone, extending from the cavernous sinus to the foramen magnum.

brachial p. see BRACHIAL PLEXUS.

cardiac p. the plexus around the base of the heart, chiefly in the epicardium, formed by cardiac branches from the vagus nerves and the sympathetic trunks and ganglia, and made up of sympathetic, parasympathetic, and visceral afferent fibers that innervate the heart.

carotid p's nerve plexuses surrounding the common, external, and internal carotid arteries.

celiac p. SOLAR PLEXUS.

cervical p. a nerve plexus formed by the ventral branches of the first four cervical spinal nerves and supplying the structures in the region of the neck. One important branch is the phrenic nerve, which supplies the diaphragm.

choroid p. infoldings of blood vessels of the pia mater covered by a thin coat of ependymal cells that form tufted projections into the third, fourth, and lateral ventricles of the brain; they secrete the cerebrospinal fluid.

coccygeal p. a nerve plexus formed by the ventral branches of the coccygeal and fifth sacral nerve and by a communication from the fourth sacral nerve, giving off the anococcygeal nerves.

cystic p. a nerve plexus near the gallbladder.

dental p. either of two plexuses (inferior and superior) of nerve fibers, one from the inferior alveolar nerve, situated around the roots of the lower teeth, and the other from the superior alveolar nerve, situated around the roots of the upper teeth.

lumbar p. one formed by the ventral branches of the second to fifth lumbar nerves in the psoas major muscle (the branches of the first lumbar nerve often are included).

lumbosacral p. the lumbar and sacral plexuses considered together, because of their continuous nature.

lymphatic p. an interconnecting network of lymph vessels that provides drainage of lymph in a one-way flow. An example is the lymphocapillary vessels, collecting vessels, and trunks.

P

myenteric p. a nerve plexus situated in the muscular layers of the intestines.

nerve p. a plexus composed of intermingled nerve fibers.

pampiniform p. 1. in the male, a plexus of veins from the testis and the epididymis, constituting part of the spermatic cord. 2. in the female, a plexus of ovarian veins draining the ovary.

sacral p. a plexus arising from the ventral branches of the last two lumbar and first four sacral spinal nerves.

solar p. see SOLAR PLEXUS.

tympanic p. a network of nerve fibers supplying the mucous lining of the tympanum, mastoid air cells, and pharyngotympanic tube.

plica (pli′kah) [L.] a ridge or FOLD on some body structure.

plicamycin (pli″kah-mi′sin) an antineoplastic ANTIBIOTIC produced by *Streptomyces plicatus* that binds to DNA and inhibits RNA synthesis; it is used for treatment of advanced testicular carcinoma; major side effects are thrombocytopenia and hemorrhagic diathesis that can be life-threatening. It also has an inhibiting effect on osteoclasts and is used to treat hypercalcemia and hypercalciuria caused by metastatic malignancy. Administered intravenously. Formerly called mithramycin.

plicate (pli′kāt) plaited or folded.

plication (pli-ka′shun) the operation of taking tucks in a structure to shorten it.

plicotomy (pli-kot′ah-me) surgical division of the posterior fold of the tympanic membrane.

plinth (plinth) 1. a padded table for a patient to sit on or lie on while performing exercises, receiving a massage, or undergoing other PHYSICAL THERAPY treatments. 2. a waterproof table used in a HYDROTHERAPY tub to facilitate exercise and movement in the water.

PLT *p*sittacosis–*l*ymphogranuloma venereum–*t*rachoma; see under *group*.

plug (plug) an obstructing mass.

epithelial p. mass of ectodermal cells that temporarily closes the external naris of the fetus.

mucous p. 1. a plug formed by secretions of mucous glands of the cervix uteri and closing the cervical canal during pregnancy. 2. abnormally thick mucus occluding the bronchi and bronchioles, as in ASTHMA or bronchopulmonary ASPERGILLOSIS.

plugger (plug′er) a dental instrument for packing, condensing, and compacting filling material into a tooth cavity.

plumbic (plum′bik) pertaining to lead.

plumbism (plum′bizm) lead poisoning.

Plummer-Vinson syndrome (plum′er vin′sun) a syndrome usually seen in middle-aged women with hypochromic anemia, chiefly characterized by cracks or fissures at the corners of the mouth, painful tongue with atrophy of filiform and later fungiform papillae, and dysphagia due to esophageal stenosis or webs.

pluri- word element [L.], *many*.

pluriglandular (ploor″ĭ-glan′du-ler) pertaining to several glands or their secretions.

plurigravida (ploor″ĭ-grav′ĭ-dah) multigravida.

plurilocular (ploor″ĭ-lok′u-ler) multilocular; having many cells or compartments.

pluripara (ploo-rip′ah-rah) multipara.

pluriparity (ploor″ĭ-par′ĭ-te) multiparity.

pluripotentiality (ploor″ĭ-po-ten″she-al′ĭ-te) ability to develop in any one of several different ways, or to affect more than one organ or tissue. adj., **pluripo′tent, pluripoten′tial.**

plutonium (Pu) (ploo-to′ne-um) a chemical element, atomic number 94, atomic weight 242. (See Appendix 6.)

Pm promethium.

PMD personal medical doctor.

P-mitrale (pe-mi-tra′le) a left atrial ABNORMALITY evident on the electrocardiograph as broad notched P waves in v_1 and v_2.

PMN polymorphonuclear.

-pnea word element [Gr.], *respiration, breathing.* adj., **-pne′ic.**

pneum(o)- word element [Gr.], *air or gas; lung.*

pneumarthrogram (noo-mahr′thro-gram) a film obtained by pneumarthrography.

pneumarthrography (noo″mahr-throg′rah-fe) radiography of a joint after it has been injected with air or gas as a contrast medium; pneumoarthrography.

pneumarthrosis (noo″mahr-thro′sis) gas or air in a joint.

pneumat(o)- word element [Gr.], *air or gas; lung.*

pneumatic (noo-mat′ik) 1. pertaining to air. 2. respiratory.

pneumatization (nu″mah-tĭ-za′shun) the formation of air cavities in tissue, especially such formation in the temporal bone.

pneumatocele (noo-mat′o-sēl) 1. a tumor or cyst formed by air or other gas filling an adventitious pouch, such as a LARYNGOCELE, TRACHEOCELE, or gaseous swelling of the scrotum. Called also aerocele and pneumocele. 2. a usually benign, thin-walled, air-containing cyst of the lung, as in staphylococcal pneumonia. Called also pneumatocele and pneumonocele.

pneumatosis (noo″mah-to′sis) air or gas in an abnormal location in the body.

p. cystoi′des intestina′lis a condition characterized by the presence of thin-walled, gas-containing cysts in the wall of the intestines. Called also intestinal emphysema.

pneumaturia (noo″mah-tu′re-ah) passage of gas in the urine, usually as a result of a fistula between the bladder and intestine.

pneumectomy (noo-mek′to-me) pneumonectomy.

pneumoangiogram (noo″mo-an′je-o-gram″) a composite of radiographs obtained by pneumoencephalography and cerebral angiography.

pneumoangiography (noo″mo-an″je-og′rah-fe) radiography of the blood vessels of the lungs.

pneumoarthrography (noo″mo-ahr-throg′rah-fe) pneumarthrography.

pneumobilia (noo″mo-bil′e-ah) the presence of gas in the biliary system.

pneumocele (noo′mo-sēl) 1. pneumonocele (def. 1). 2. pneumatocele (def. 1). 3. pneumatocele (def. 2).

pneumocephalus (noo″mo-sef′ah-lus) air in the intracranial cavity.

pneumococcemia (noo″mo-kok-se′me-ah) pneumococci in the blood.

pneumococcidal (noo″mo-kok-si′d′l) destroying pneumococci.

pneumococcosis (noo″mo-kok-o′sis) infection with pneumococci.

pneumococcosuria (noo″mo-kok″o-su′re-ah) BACTERIURIA with PNEUMOCOCCI in the urine.

pneumococcus (noo″mo-kok′us) *Streptococcus pneumoniae.* adj., **pneumococ′cal.**

pneumoconiosis (noo″mo-ko″ne-o′sis) any of a group of lung diseases resulting from inhalation of particles of industrial substances, particularly inorganic dusts such as the dust of iron ore or coal, and permanent deposition of substantial amounts of such particles in the lungs. The diseases vary in severity but all are occupational diseases, acquired by workers in the course of their jobs. Symptoms include shortness of breath, chronic cough, and expectoration of mucus containing the offending particles.

SILICOSIS is probably the best known and most severe of these diseases. ASBESTOSIS, caused by inhalation of asbestos fibers, is probably second only to silicosis in severity. Prevention and early diagnosis are important, for no effective treatment is available. *Coal workers' pneumoconiosis,* or *black lung,* usually in the form of BITUMINOSIS or ANTHRACOSILICOSIS, is caused by the inhalation of coal dust, often with silica, and is

similar in its development and its effects to silicosis. BERYLLIOSIS is a variety found in workers exposed to beryllium in the manufacture of fluorescent lamps, and in members of their families who are contaminated by the chemicals in the worker's clothing. Other types of pneumoconiosis include ALUMINOSIS, CADMIOSIS, and SIDEROSIS.

talc p. a type of SILICATOSIS caused by the inhalation of TALC; symptoms include shortness of breath, cough, fatigue, weakness, and weight loss. Prolonged exposure may result in pulmonary FIBROSIS. Called also talcosis.

Pneumocystis (noo″mo-sis′tis) a genus of yeastlike fungi. *P. cari′nii* is the causative agent of interstitial plasma cell PNEUMONIA.

pneumocystography (noo″mo-sis-tog′rah-fe) radiography of the urinary bladder after injection of air or gas.

pneumocystosis (noo″mo-sis-to′sis) interstitial plasma cell pneumonia.

pneumocyte (noo′mo-sīt) alveolar cell.

pneumoderma (noo″mo-der′mah) subcutaneous emphysema; air or gas in subcutaneous tissues.

pneumodynamics (noo″mo-di-nam′iks) 1. the dynamics of the respiratory process. 2. the study of the forces exerted in the process of breathing.

pneumoencephalogram (noo″mo-en-sef′-ah-lo-gram″) the film produced by pneumoencephalography.

pneumoencephalography (PEG) (noo″-mo-en-sef″ah-log′rah-fe) radiographic visualization of the fluid-containing structures of the brain after cerebrospinal fluid is intermittently withdrawn by lumbar puncture and replaced by air, oxygen, or helium.

pneumoenteritis (noo″mo-en″ter-i′tis) inflammation of the lungs and intestine.

pneumogram (noo′mo-gram″) 1. a radiogram made after the injection of air into the part. 2. spirogram.

pneumography (noo-mog′rah-fe) 1. radiography of a part after injection of a gas. 2. spirography.

pneumohemopericardium (noo″mo-he″mo-per″ĭ-kahr′de-um) hemopneumopericardium.

pneumohemothorax (noo″mo-he″mo-thor′aks) hemopneumothorax.

pneumohydrometra (noo″mo-hi″dro-me′-trah) gas and fluid in the uterus.

pneumohydropericardium (noo″mo-hi″-dro-per″ĭ-kahr′de-um) hydropneumopericardium.

pneumohydrothorax (noo″mo-hi″dro-thor′aks) hydropneumothorax.

P

pneumolith (noo'mo-lith) LUNG CALCULUS.

pneumolithiasis (noo"mo-lĭ-thi'ah-sis) the presence of concretions in the lungs.

pneumomediastinum (noo"mo-me"de-as-ti'num) the presence of air or gas in the mediastinum, which may interfere with respiration and circulation, and may lead to such conditions as pneumothorax or pneumopericardium. It may occur spontaneously or as a result of trauma or a pathologic process, or it may be induced deliberately as a diagnostic procedure.

pneumomycosis (noo"mo-mi-ko'sis) any fungal disease of the lungs.

pneumomyelography (noo"mo-mi"ĕ-log'-rah-fe) radiography of the spinal canal after withdrawal of cerebrospinal fluid and injection of air or gas.

pneumon(o)- word element [Gr.], *lung*.

pneumonectomy (noo"mo-nek'to-me) excision of lung tissue, of an entire lung (total pneumonectomy) or less (partial pneumonectomy), or of a single lobe (LOBECTOMY).

Patient Care. Pneumonectomy is most often done as a treatment for lung cancer; it is also done with less common diseases such as extensive unilateral tuberculosis, bronchiectasis, and multiple abscesses of the lung. Thus patients who have a pneumonectomy are likely to have suffered some chronic and debilitating illness prior to surgery and will have special needs to avoid complications and promote healing and recovery.

After surgical removal of a lung, the chest is closed and there is no closed drainage of the thoracic cavity. Instead, pressure within the pleural space is adjusted by using a simple thoracentesis and manometer, which help maintain the mediastinum midline. Fluid and air are allowed to accumulate in the space left by the excised lung to prevent shift of the mediastinum to the operative side. A second reason for not inserting a chest tube and drainage is the danger of contamination and possible empyema.

The patient is not allowed to lie on the operative side. If the operative lung is permitted to be dependent, fluid can enter the space, causing tension pneumothorax secondary to mediastinal shift; should the bronchial stump rupture, drowning in the accumulated fluid could occur.

Fluid balance is watched closely by pressure monitoring to avoid overhydrating the patient. A central venous line or Swan-Ganz catheter may be used to guide fluid replacement. Serial blood gases and chest x-rays are done to detect early signs of respiratory complications. Additionally, blood tests are done and electrolyte levels are evaluated to detect problems of infection and imbalance.

The most common postoperative complication is respiratory insufficiency, especially in patients who have had poor pulmonary function before surgery. Signs of respiratory problems include a change in mental status related to hypoxia, fever, tachycardia, and tachypnea. Pain is managed with analgesics on a routine basis. In addition to providing comfort and rest for the patient, analgesics allow the patient to move more freely and cough up accumulated secretions more effectively. Pulmonary hygiene is a vital component of postoperative care as it helps the remaining lung increase its vital capacity and total lung capacity and avoid atelectasis.

In patients who are over 60 years of age or have a preexisting cardiac disease, there is the possibility that cardiac arrhythmias can develop. Pain, hypoxemia, hypovolemia, and acid-base imbalance can contribute to this complication. A fistula between the bronchus and pleura sometimes occurs, leading to subcutaneous emphysema and mediastinal shift caused by a massive air leak. If the fistula is evident on the first or second postoperative day, it is probably due to a slipped ligature on the bronchial stump. An air leak that occurs later, on the fifth to tenth postoperative day, is probably due to an infection and poor wound healing. A ruptured bronchial stump must be repaired surgically as soon as possible. Signs that a stump has ruptured include dyspnea, change in mental status, and expectoration of serosanguineous fluid.

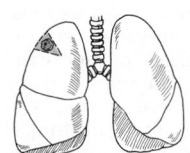

WEDGE RESECTION

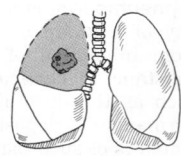

LOBECTOMY

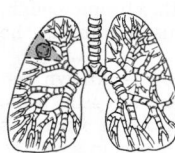

SEGMENTAL RESECTION

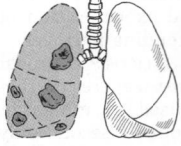

PNEUMONECTOMY

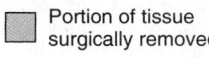

Portion of tissue surgically removed

Pneumonectomy. From Polaski and Tatro, 1996.

Hemorrhage, usually due to a slipped ligature on a major artery, is a relatively rare complication, but when it occurs it can be fatal. The patient rapidly goes into profound shock from circulatory collapse. This complication must be detected early and corrected promptly.

Patients recovering from pneumonectomy require intensive care to avoid the life-threatening complications listed above. Central pressure monitoring, continuous cardiac monitoring, serial laboratory testing of arterial blood gases and electrolyte levels, and frequent periodic checking of vital signs are all necessary either to avoid or to detect and manage these complications in their earliest stages. Additionally, expert care by each member of an interdisciplinary team is necessary to assure an uneventful recovery and restoration of patients to their former daily activities.

pneumonia (noo-mo′nyah) inflammation of the lung with consolidation and exudation, formerly a common cause of death that killed one out of four victims. It is still a serious disease, especially in infants and the elderly. In spite of the advent of antibiotic therapy in the 1940s and a reduction in the mortality rate for all infectious diseases, pneumonia and influenza still account for over 67,000 deaths per year in the United States and consistently rank among the ten leading causes of death.

Types and Symptoms. Infectious pneumonia may be caused by bacteria, viruses, fungi, or protozoa. It may be primary or secondary (a complication of another disease) and may involve one or both lungs. It is most frequently in the form of *lobar pneumonia* caused by the pneumococcus, *Streptococcus pneumoniae (pneumococcal pneumonia);* this one type represents 90 per cent of all bacterial pneumonias. *Pneumocystis carinii* causes a condition called *interstitial plasma cell pneumonia* in debilitated or immunocompromised persons, such as those with ACQUIRED IMMUNODEFICIENCY SYNDROME (AIDS). Other causative agents are *Mycoplasma* spp., *Legionella pneumophila,* influenza A virus, gramnegative bacteria, and *Staphylococcus aureus.* The microorganisms that give rise to pneumonia are often normal flora in the upper respiratory tract. They cause no harm unless resistance is severely lowered by some other factor, such as a severe cold, disease, alcoholism, or general poor health. Age is also a factor. Nosocomial pneumonia is common in hospitalized patients. When resistance is lowered or the conditions are favorable, the infectious agents invade the lungs.

Lobar pneumonia is a common type that affects a segment or an entire lobe of the lung and is usually caused by pneumococci (pneumococcal pneumonia). Whole sections of the lung tissue become solidified by inflammatory material, so that air cannot enter the alveoli. A chest x-ray is usually made to confirm the diagnosis and determine the extent of the disease. Sputum cultures may be done to identify the causative organism. Lobar pneumonia strikes suddenly. The symptoms are a cough, sharp chest pains (due to accompanying PLEURISY), blood-streaked or brownish sputum, and a high fever that generally starts with a chill. Pulse and respiration increase to almost twice their normal rates.

Bronchial pneumonia (or bronchopneumonia) is a less dramatic form that is even more prevalent than lobar pneumonia. The area affected is usually smaller than in the lobar type. The inflammation is localized in or around the bronchi, and causes the lung to be spotted with clusters of infected tissue. The symptoms appear gradually and are usually milder than in lobar pneumonia. The temperature rises more slowly and does not go as high, and there is no crisis as in lobar pneumonia. Bronchopneumonia is rarely fatal except in patients with heart disease or other underlying disorders. It is often more difficult to treat, however; relapses are common and can be serious. Diagnosis is also more difficult because the causes are varied.

Staphylococcal pneumonia refers to any type caused by a species of *Staphylococcus,* some of which are antibiotic resistant. It may be very serious and occasionally even fatal.

Primary atypical pneumonia (called also *atypical* or *atypical bronchial pneumonia*) is a type that occurs chiefly in young adults who are otherwise healthy. It is often found in military camps and is due to various viruses or to *Mycoplasma pneumoniae.* In the past it often went undetected. The symptoms are similar to those of a cold; there may be headache, fever, a dry cough, myringitis, generalized aches, and a feeling of extreme fatigue. X-ray examination of the lungs will reveal evidence of infection.

Other Types. Other kinds of pneumonia (see separate entries) include aspiration pneumonia, lipid pneumonia, traumatic pneumonia, and hypostatic pneumonia.

Prevention. Many debilitated and elderly patients are prime candidates for the development of pneumonia, as are those who are physically inactive and immobile and those who suffer from acute and chronic

P

pulmonary disease. It is possible to prevent pneumonia in many susceptible persons by being aware of factors that predispose one to the disease and by taking precautionary measures.

In the postoperative period it is important to position patients properly and watch them closely while they are recovering from anesthesia so that they do not aspirate vomitus or other material into the lungs. The same precautions are essential for all patients in varying stages of unconsciousness and coma and in those who have a poorly functioning gag reflex. Early ambulation is another preventive measure to be used in postoperative and postpartum patients unless contraindicated. All patients who are immobilized for any reason should be turned regularly to avoid atelectasis. Oversedation and overenthusiastic use of cough depressants can make a person more susceptible to pneumonia. The infectious agents that can cause pneumonia must be considered a constant hazard; vigorous adherence to the principles of cleanliness and personal hygiene are necessary to avoid the introduction of these agents into the respiratory tract of the susceptible person.

A vaccine can provide protection from pneumococcal disease for a period of 3 to 5 years in 80 per cent of vaccinated persons. Those who can benefit most from a pneumonia vaccine are the elderly; persons suffering from chronic disorders of the lungs, heart, liver, or kidneys; patients with poorly controlled diabetes mellitus; and those whose immune system has been impaired by disease or the loss of the spleen.

Patient Care. Rest is of primary importance in assisting the body to combat the infection and in preventing unnecessary strain on the lungs and respiratory system. The fever presents problems of dehydration as does diaphoresis. Fluids are given frequently by mouth, or intravenously if necessary. An accurate record must be kept of the patient's intake and output (although it should be kept in mind that most of the fluid loss in patients with pneumonia may be due to insensible water loss). Bowel elimination must be checked regularly since the peristaltic action of the intestines may be affected in severe pneumonia. Delirium frequently occurs because of the high fever; thus, careful observation of the patient is necessary, with measures to prevent self-injury. A liquid diet may be best if the patient is experiencing dyspnea. MOUTH CARE is given regularly to combat dryness and cracking of the lips, which occur as a result of fever and dehydration.

To relieve the chest pain caused by pleurisy, it may help to have the patient lie on the affected side so that the side is splinted during coughing episodes. Coughing and deep breathing exercises are helpful in removing mucus from the respiratory tract. Temperature, pulse, and respiration are checked and recorded at least every 4 hours. When the temperature falls the patient usually perspires profusely, requiring frequent changing of gown and bed linens. The patient must be protected from drafts and kept warm during this time.

A research study supported by the Agency for Health Care Policy and Research was conducted and developed a clinical prediction model to determine the most appropriate care for community-acquired pneumonia. The results and recommendations can be found online at web site http://www.ahcpr.gov.

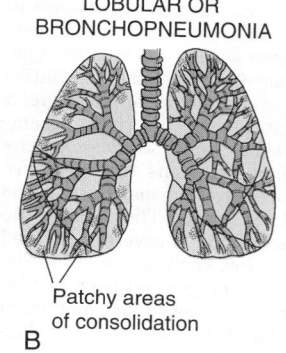

LOBAR PNEUMONIA

Consolidation of one lobe

A

LOBULAR OR BRONCHOPNEUMONIA

Patchy areas of consolidation

B

Two types of pneumonia. *A*, Lobar pneumonia with consolidation in one lobe of one lung. *B*, Lobular, or bronchopneumonia, with patchy consolidation throughout both lungs. From Polaski and Tatro, 1996.

p. al'ba a fatal desquamative pneumonia of the newborn due to congenital syphilis, with fatty degeneration of the lungs, which appear pale and virtually airless.

anaerobic p. any pneumonia caused by anaerobic bacteria, usually due to aspiration of contaminated secretions from the mouth, pharynx, or paranasal sinuses, such as with the increased bacterial load of periodontal disease or some other infection. It usually runs a protracted course, progressing to lung cavitation with abscesses and putrid or bloody expectorations.

aspiration p. pneumonia due to the entrance of foreign matter, such as food particles, into the respiratory passages or lungs.

atypical p., atypical bronchial p. primary atypical pneumonia.

bacterial p. pneumonia caused by bacteria, such as *Streptococcus pneumoniae, S. hemolytica, Staphylococcus aureus, Klebsiella pneumoniae, Mycoplasma pneumoniae,* and others.

bronchial p. bronchopneumonia; see PNEUMONIA.

Candida p. pulmonary candidiasis.

cytomegalovirus p. viral pneumonia caused by infection with a CYTOMEGALOVIRUS, an often fatal disease seen in IMMUNOCOMPROMISED patients; symptoms include fever, a nonproductive cough, and dyspnea.

desquamative p. chronic pneumonia with hardening of the fibrous exudate and proliferation of the interstitial tissue and epithelium.

desquamative interstitial p. chronic pneumonia with desquamation of large alveolar cells and thickening of the walls of distal air passages; marked by dyspnea and nonproductive cough.

eosinophilic p., chronic a chronic interstitial lung disease characterized by cough, dyspnea, malaise, fever, night sweats, weight loss, eosinophilia, and a chest film revealing nonsegmental, nonmigratory infiltrates in the lung periphery.

Friedländer's p., Friedländer's bacillus p. Klebsiella pneumonia.

fungal p. pneumonia caused by inhaled fungi, usually *Histoplasma capsulatum, Blastomyces dermatitidis,* or *Coccidioides immitis;* in Central and South America it may be caused by *Paracoccidioides brasiliense.* See also HISTOPLASMOSIS, North American BLASTOMYCOSIS, COCCIDIOIDOMYCOSIS, and PARACOCCIDIOIDOMYCOSIS. Numerous other fungi, such as *Aspergillus* and *Candida,* infect immunocompromised patients.

hypostatic p. pneumonia due to dorsal DECUBITUS in weak or aged persons.

influenzal p., influenza virus p. viral pneumonia caused by an influenza virus, usually the type A virus; some cases are mild, but it can develop into a fulminant condition characterized by high fever, prostration, severe dyspnea, and massive (sometimes rapidly fatal) pulmonary hemorrhagic edema with consolidation. It may be accompanied by a superinfection with bacterial pneumonia.

interstitial p. 1. any of various types of pneumonia characterized by thickening of the interstitial tissue. 2. idiopathic pulmonary fibrosis.

interstitial plasma cell p. a pulmonary disease caused by *Pneumocystis carinii,* occurring in premature infants and immunocompromised persons, including those who are receiving cytotoxic or immunosuppressive drugs or who are affected by immunodeficiency disorders including the acquired immunodeficiency syndrome. It is characterized by dyspnea, tachypnea, fever, cough, and cyanosis, with cellular detritus containing plasma cells appearing in the lungs; if untreated it leads to pulmonary consolidation, hypoxemia, and death. Called also pneumocystosis and *Pneumocystis carinii* pneumonia.

Klebsiella p. an acute type of bacterial pneumonia characterized by massive mucoid inflammatory exudates in a lobe of the lung, due to *Klebsiella pneumoniae.* Called also Friedländer's or Friedländer's bacillus pneumonia.

Legionella p. pneumonia caused by a species of *Legionella;* see LEGIONNAIRES' DISEASE.

lipid p., lipoid p. a rare type of aspiration pneumonia caused by aspiration of oil; mineral oils and vegetable oils usually cause lower grade, chronic inflammation while animal fats tend to cause more acute inflammation and sometimes pulmonary hemorrhage. Called also oil-aspiration pneumonia.

lobar p. see PNEUMONIA.

Mycoplasma p., mycoplasmal p. the most common form of primary atypical pneumonia, caused by *Mycoplasma pneumoniae* and occurring most frequently in young adults.

nosocomial p. pneumonia acquired by the patient in the hospital, which the patient did not have at the time of admission.

oil-aspiration p. lipid pneumonia.

Pittsburgh p. a type of pneumonia resembling LEGIONNAIRES' DISEASE, caused by *Legionella micdadei,* and occurring as a nosocomial infection especially in immuno-compromised patients.

pneumococcal p. the most common type of lobar pneumonia; see PNEUMONIA.

pneumocystis p., Pneumocystis carinii p. interstitial plasma cell pneumonia.

primary atypical p. see PNEUMONIA.

rheumatic p. a rare, usually fatal complication of acute rheumatic fever, characterized by extensive pulmonary consolidation and rapidly progressive functional deterioration and by alveolar exudate, interstitial infiltrates, and necrotizing arteritis.

staphylococcal p. see PNEUMONIA.

traumatic p. pneumonia following injury to the thorax.

varicella p. a type of viral pneumonia developing after the skin eruption in varicella (chickenpox) and apparently due to the same virus; symptoms may be severe, with violent cough, hemoptysis, and severe chest pain.

ventilator-associated p. a frequently fatal type of pneumonia seen in patients breathing with a ventilator; it is the most common type of nosocomial pneumonia and may be bacterial, viral, or fungal.

viral p. any of numerous pneumonias caused by a virus, such as an adenovirus, influenza virus, parainfluenza virus, respiratory syncytial virus, or varicella virus.

pneumonic (noo-mon′ik) 1. pertaining to pneumonia. 2. pulmonary.

pneumonitis (noo″mo-ni′tis) inflammation of the lung; see also PNEUMONIA.

hypersensitivity p. a respiratory HYPERSENSITIVITY REACTION to repeated inhalation of organic particles, usually in an occupational setting, with onset a few hours after exposure to the allergen. Many different substances are potential causes of the condition; see BAGASSOSIS, farmer's LUNG, and pigeon breeder's LUNG. Characteristics include fever, fatigue, chills, unproductive cough, tachycardia, and tachypnea; in the chronic form there is interstitial fibrosis with collagenous thickening of the alveolar septa. Called also extrinsic allergic alveolitis.

radiation p. lung inflammation resulting from radiation exposure, usually RADIATION THERAPY, with coughing, dyspnea, and alveolar infiltration of secretions, leading to mild to severe or even fatal fibrosis 6 to 9 months after the exposure.

pneumonocele (noo-mon′o-sēl) 1. hernial protrusion of lung tissue, as through a fissure in the chest wall. Called also pleurocele, pneumatocele, and pneumocele. 2. pneumatocele (def. 2).

pneumonocentesis (noo-mo″no-sen-te′sis) PARACENTESIS of a lung.

pneumonocyte (noo-mon′o-sīt) alveolar cell.

pneumonolysis (noo″mo-nol′ĭ-sis) a form of collapse THERAPY involving surgical separation of tissues attaching the lung to the wall of the chest cavity.

pneumonopathy (noo″mo-nop′ah-the) any lung disease; called also pneumonosis.

pneumonopexy (noo-mo′no-pek″se) fixation of the lung to the thoracic wall.

pneumonorrhaphy (noo″mo-nor′ah-fe) suture of the lung.

pneumonosis (noo″mo-no′sis) pneumonopathy.

pneumonotomy (noo″mo-not′ah-me) incision of the lung; called also pneumotomy.

pneumopericardium (noo″mo-per″ĭ-kahr′de-um) the presence of air or gas in the pericardial cavity.

pneumoperitoneum (noo″mo-per″ĭ-to-ne′um) the presence of air or gas in the peritoneal cavity, occurring pathologically or introduced intentionally.

pneumoperitonitis (noo″mo-per″ĭ-to-ni′-tis) peritonitis with accumulation of air or gas in the peritoneal cavity.

pneumopleuritis (noo″mo-ploo-ri′tis) pleuropneumonia (def. 1).

pneumopyelography (noo″mo-pi″ĕ-log′rah-fe) radiography after injection of oxygen or air into the renal pelvis.

pneumopyopericardium (noo″mo-pi″o-per″ĭ-kar′de-um) air or gas and pus in the pericardium.

pneumopyothorax (noo″mo-pi″o-thor′aks) pyopneumothorax.

pneumoradiography (noo″mo-ra″de-og′rah-fe) radiography of a part after injection of oxygen or other gas as contrast material.

pneumoretroperitoneum (noo″mo-ret″ro-per″ĭ-to-ne′um) the presence of air or gas in the retroperitoneal space.

pneumorrhagia (noo″mo-ra′jah) hemorrhage from the lungs; severe hemoptysis.

pneumotachograph (noo″mo-tak′o-graf) an instrument for recording the velocity of respired air.

pneumotachometer (noo″mo-tah-kom′e-ter) a transducer for measuring exhaled air flow.

pneumotaxic (noo″mo-tak′sik) regulating the respiratory rate.

pneumotherapy (noo″mo-ther′ah-pe) treatment of disease of the lungs.

pneumothorax (noo″mo-thor′aks) accumulation of air or gas in the pleural cavity, resulting in collapse of the lung on the affected side. The condition may occur spontaneously (*spontaneous pneumothorax*), as in the course of a pulmonary disease, or it may follow perforating trauma to the chest wall or lung parenchyma (*traumatic* or *open pneumothorax*).

Spontaneous Pneumothorax. This condition occurs when there is an opening on the surface of the lung allowing leakage of air from the airways or lung parenchyma into the pleural cavity. Most often it occurs when an emphysematous bulla or other weakened area on the lung ruptures. Normally the pleural cavity is an airtight compartment with a negative pressure. When air enters the pleural cavity the lung collapses, producing shortness of breath and mediastinal shift toward the unaffected side (see also MEDIASTINAL SHIFT). Other signs and symptoms are a sudden sharp chest pain, fall in blood pressure, weak and rapid pulse, and cessation of normal respiratory movements on the affected side of the chest.

A small spontaneous pneumothorax may require no specific treatment beyond rest and administration of oxygen for relief of DYSPNEA. Chest x-rays should be obtained. The patient usually is more comfortable if allowed to sit up. A larger spontaneous pneumothorax may require a more aggressive approach such as ASPIRATION to allow for reexpansion of the lung. If air continues to leak from the defect in the lung surface a continuous closed-drainage apparatus is set up (see CHEST TUBE). As soon as the lung lesion heals and the lung is reexpanded, the patient is allowed to resume usual daily activities. Guidelines for the treatment of spontaneous pneumothorax have been published by the American College of Chest Physicians and are available on their web site at http://www.chestnet.org.

Tension pneumothorax. This is a particularly dangerous form that occurs when air escapes into the pleural cavity from a bronchus but cannot regain entry into the bronchus. As a result, continuously increasing air pressure in the pleural cavity causes progressive collapse of the lung tissue. Emergency ASPIRATION of air from the pleural cavity is necessary in this disorder. If untreated, increased pressure within the pleural cavity will cause lung collapse and MEDIASTINAL SHIFT.

pneumotomy (noo-mot'ah-me) pneumonotomy.

pneumoventriculography (noo″mo-ven-trik″u-log′rah-fe) pneumoencephalography.

PO [L.] per os (by mouth, orally).

Po polonium.

Po₂ oxygen partial pressure (tension); also written P_{O_2}, pO_2, and pO_2. See also BLOOD GAS ANALYSIS.

pock (pok) a pustule, especially of smallpox.

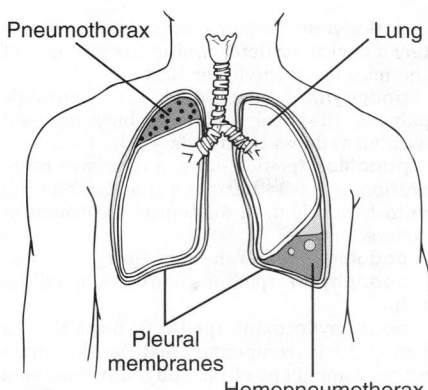

Pneumothorax. Air within the pleural cavity has entered some of the space normally occupied by the lung, thus preventing its expansion and causing partial collapse.

pocket (pok'et) a bag or pouch; see also CAVITY, RECESS, and SAC.

 infrabony p., intra-alveolar p. intrabony p. a periodontal pocket in which the bottom is apical to the level of the adjacent alveolar bone.

 periodontal p. a gingival sulcus that extends abnormally deep into the periodontal ligament apically to the original level of the resorbed alveolar crest.

 suprabony p., supracrestal p. a periodontal pocket in which the bottom is coronal to the underlying bone.

pockmark (pok'mahrk) a depressed scar left by a pustule.

pod(o)- word element [Gr.], *foot.*

podagra (po-dag'rah) gouty pain in the great toe.

podalgia (po-dal'jah) pain in the feet.

podalic (po-dal'ik) pertaining to or by means of the feet, as podalic version.

podarthritis (pod″ahr-thri'tis) inflammation of the joints of the feet.

podencephalus (pod″en-sef'ah-lus) a deformed fetus without a cranium, the brain hanging by a pedicle.

podiatrist (po-di'ah-trist) chiropodist; a specialist in podiatry.

podiatry (po-di'ah-tre) the specialized field dealing with the study and care of the foot, including its anatomy, pathology, medical and surgical treatment, and other aspects. adj., **podiat'ric.**

podocyte (pod'o-sīt) an epithelial cell of the visceral layer of a renal glomerulus, having a number of footlike radiating processes (pedicles).

pododynamometer (pod″o-di″nah-mom′ĕ-ter) a device for determining the strength of the muscles of the lower limb.

pododynia (pod″o-din′e-ah) neuralgic pain of the heel and sole; burning pain without redness in the sole of the foot.

podofilox (po-dof′ĭ-loks) a corrosive preparation of PODOPHYLLOTOXIN that inhibits cell mitosis and is used for topical treatment of venereal WARTS.

podology (po-dol′ah-je) podiatry.

podophyllin (pod″ah-fil′in) podophyllum resin.

podophyllotoxin (pod″o-fil″o-tok′sin) a highly toxic compound that is the main active component of podophyllum RESIN and has CATHARTIC and CAUSTIC properties. Some of its less toxic derivatives, such as ETOPOSIDE and TENIPOSIDE, are used as antineoplastic AGENTS.

podophyllum (pod″o-fil′um) the dried rhizome and roots of *Podophyllum peltatum.* See also PODOPHYLLOTOXIN and podophyllum RESIN.

pogoniasis (po″go-ni′ah-sis) excessive growth of the beard, or growth of a beard on a woman.

pogonion (po-go′ne-on) the anterior midpoint of the chin.

-poiesis word element [Gr.], *formation.*

poikil(o)- word element [Gr.], *varied; irregular.*

poikiloblast (poi′kĭ-lo-blast″) an abnormally shaped erythroblast.

poikilocyte (poi′kĭ-lo-sīt″) an abnormally shaped erythrocyte, such as a burr cell, sickle cell, target cell, acanthocyte, elliptocyte, schistocyte, spherocyte, or stomatocyte.

poikilocytosis (poi″kĭ-lo-si-to′sis) the presence of poikilocytes in the blood.

poikiloderma (poi″kĭ-lo-der′mah) a condition characterized by pigmentary and atrophic changes in the skin, giving it a mottled appearance.

poikilotherm (poi′kĭ-lo-therm″) 1. an animal that exhibits poikilothermy; a cold-blooded animal. 2. ectotherm.

poikilothermal (poi″kĭ-lo-ther′m'l) poikilothermic.

poikilothermic (poi″kĭ-lo-ther′mik) 1. pertaining to or characterized by poikilothermy. 2. ectothermic.

poikilothermy (poi″kĭ-lo-ther′me) the state of having a body temperature that varies with that of the environment. 1. the ability of organisms to adapt themselves to variations in the temperature of the environment. 2. ectothermy.

point (point) 1. a small area or spot; the sharp end of an object. 2. to approach the surface, like the pus of an abscess, at definite spot or place. 3. a tapered, pointe endodontic instrument used for explorin the depth of the root canal in root cana THERAPY; called also root canal point.

p. A a radiographic, cephalometri landmark, determined on the lateral hea film; it is the most retruded part of th curved bony outline from the anterior nasa spine to the crest of the maxillary alveola process.

absorbent p. in root canal therapy, cone of variable width and taper, usuall made of paper or a paper product, used t dry or maintain a liquid disinfectant in th canal. Called also paper point.

p. B a radiographic, cephalometri landmark, determined on the lateral hea film; it is the most posterior midline poin in the concavity between the infradental and pogonion.

boiling p. the temperature at which liquid will boil; at sea level the boiling poin of water is 100°C (212°F).

cardinal p's 1. the points on the differ ent refracting media of the eye that deter mine the direction of the entering o emerging light rays. 2. four points withi the pelvic inlet— the two sacroiliac articula tions and the two iliopectineal eminences.

craniometric p's the established point of reference for measurement of the skull.

dew p. the temperature at whic moisture in the atmosphere is deposited a dew.

far p. the most remote point at whic an object is clearly seen when the eye is a rest.

p. of fixation 1. the point or object o which one's sight is fixed and throug which the axis opticus passes. 2. the poin on the retina, usually the fovea, on whic are focused the rays coming from an objec directly regarded.

freezing p. the temperature at which liquid begins to freeze, for water, 0°C (32°F); it is often used interchangeabl with melting POINT, but should be use for substances being cooled while meltin point is reserved for substances bein heated.

gutta-percha p. gutta-percha cone.

ice p. the true melting point of ice being the temperature of equilibrium be tween ice and air-saturated water under on atmosphere pressure.

isoelectric p. (pI) the pH of a solutio in which molecules of a specific substance such as a protein, have equal numbers o positively and negatively charged group and therefore do not migrate in an electri field.

J p. on an electrocardiogram, the junction between the end of the QRS segment and the beginning of the ST segment.

jugal p. the point at the angle formed by the masseteric and maxillary edges of the zygomatic bone; called also jugale.

lacrimal p. a small aperture on a slight elevation at the medial end of the eyelid margin, through which tears from the lacrimal lake enter the lacrimal canaliculi. See also LACRIMAL APPARATUS.

p. of maximal impulse the point on the chest where the impulse of the left ventricle is sometimes felt or seen most strongly, normally in the fifth costal interspace inside the mammillary line.

McBurney p. a point of special tenderness in APPENDICITIS, about 4 to 5 cm from the right anterior iliac spine on a line between the spine and the navel; it corresponds to the normal position of the appendix. (See accompanying illustration.)

melting p. (mp) the minimum temperature at which a solid begins to liquefy; see also freezing POINT.

near p. the nearest point of clear vision, the absolute near point being that for either eye alone with accommodation relaxed, and the relative near point being that for the two eyes together with employment of accommodation.

nodal p's two points on the axis of an optical system situated so that a ray falling on one will produce a parallel ray emerging through the other.

paper p. absorbent point.

pressure p. 1. a point of extreme sensitivity to pressure. 2. one of various locations on the body at which digital pressure may be applied for the control of hemorrhage. (See accompanying illustration.)

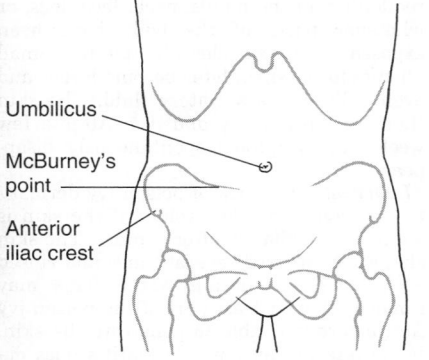

Umbilicus
McBurney's point
Anterior iliac crest

McBurney's point is located midway between the anterior iliac crest and the umbilicus in the right lower quadrant. From Ignatavicius and Workman, 2002.

root canal p. point (def. 3).

silver p. in root canal THERAPY, a tapered and elongated silver plug that is cemented into the canal as a filling. Called also silver cone.

trigger p. a spot on the body at which pressure or other stimulus gives rise to specific sensations or symptoms.

triple p. the temperature and pressure at which the solid, liquid, and gas phases of a substance are in equilibrium.

pointillage (pwahn-te-yahzh′) [Fr.] massage with the points of the fingers.

Poiseuille's law (pwah-zwēz′) at a constant driving pressure the flow rate of liquid through a capillary tube is directly proportional to the fourth power of the radius of the tube and inversely proportional to the length and viscosity of the tube.

poison (poi′zun) a substance that, on ingestion, inhalation, absorption, application, injection, or development within the body, in relatively small amounts, may cause structural or functional disturbance. Called also toxin and venom. adj., **poisonous.**

Corrosives are poisons that destroy tissues directly. They include the mineral acids, such as nitric acid, sulfuric acid, and hydrochloric acid; the caustic alkalis, such as ammonia, sodium hydroxide (lye), sodium carbonate, and sodium hypochlorite; and carbolic acid (phenol). *Irritants* are poisons that inflame the mucous membranes by direct action. These include arsenic, copper sulfate, salts of lead, zinc, and phosphorus, and many others. NEUROTOXINS or nerve toxins act on the nerves or affect some of the basic cell processes. This large group includes the narcotics, such as opium, heroin, and cocaine, and the barbiturates, anesthetics, and alcohols. HEMOTOXINS or blood toxins act on the blood and deprive it of oxygen. They include carbon monoxide, carbon dioxide, hydrocyanic acid, and the gases used in chemical warfare. Some blood toxins destroy the blood cells or the platelets. See also POISONING and names of individual poisons.

p. ivy, oak, and sumac common plants of the genus *Rhus* that cause allergic skin reactions. The poison contained in their leaves, roots, and berries is an oily substance called urushiol. It has no effect on some people; in others, momentary or even indirect contact may cause itching and even painful rashes, blisters, and swelling; see *Rhus* DERMATITIS.

Poison Ivy. Poison ivy (*Rhus radicans*) grows in the form of climbing vines, shrubs

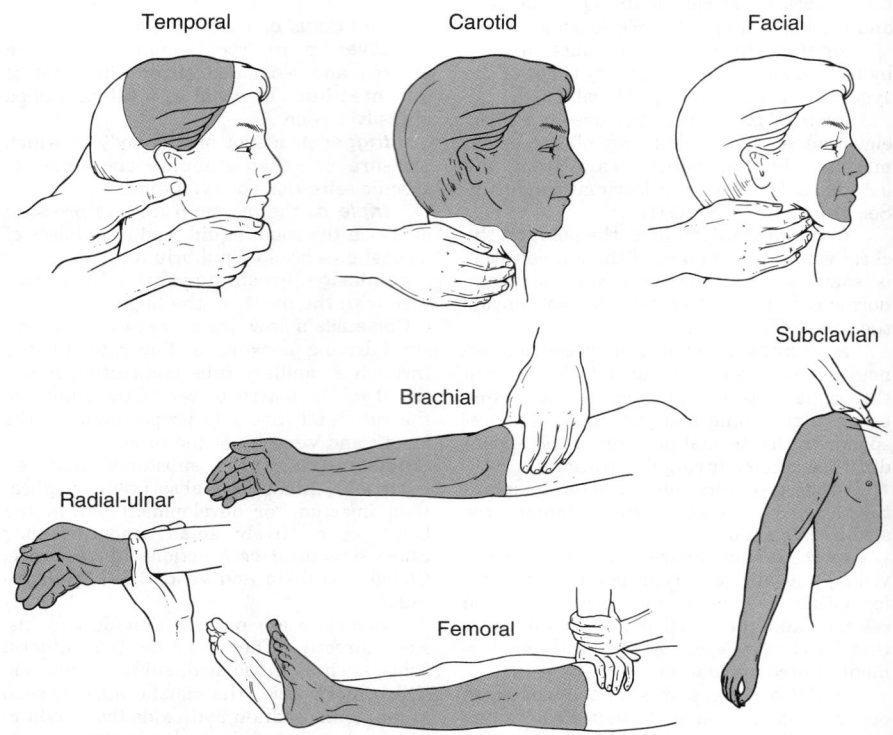

Locations of pressure points. Shaded areas show the regions in which hemorrhage may be controlled by pressure at the points indicated.

that trail on the ground, and shrubbery that grows upright without any support. The vine clings to stone and brick houses and climbs trees and poles. It flourishes abundantly along fences, paths, and roadways, and is often partly hidden by other foliage.

Recognition. The poison ivy plant is attractive and is often picked as a decoration by unsuspecting flower gatherers. Although poison ivy comes in many forms and displays seasonal changes, it has one constant characteristic: The leaves always grow in clusters of three, one at the end of the stalk, the other two opposite one another.

Transmission. The plant is particularly potent in the spring and early summer when it is full of oily resinous sap. This forms an invisible film upon the human skin on contact. Direct contact is not always necessary. Some cases of poison ivy dermatitis are caused by the handling of clothing or garden implements that have been contaminated by the sap, sometimes months earlier; dogs and cats may carry it on their fur. Many people are so sensitive that

smoke from a brush fire containing poison ivy brings on a rash.

Symptoms. After exposure, the symptoms of poison ivy dermatitis may develop in a matter of hours, though sometimes they do not appear for several days. There is reddening on the hands, neck, face, legs, or whatever parts of the body have been exposed, with considerable itching. Small blisters form which later become larger and eventually exude a watery fluid. The skin then becomes crusty and dry. After a few weeks all symptoms spontaneously disappear.

Treatment. An attack of poison ivy dermatitis can sometimes be avoided if the skin is washed immediately after contact. The skin should be lathered several times and rinsed each time in running water. This may remove all or at least part of the poison ivy film before it is able to penetrate the skin. If, despite precautions, dermatitis does develop, various treatments may relieve the itching. An old standard remedy is calamine lotion. If the inflammation becomes unusually severe or is accompanied by fever, a health care provider should be consulted. A cortisone preparation may be prescribed, which can be taken orally, injected, or applied locally as a cream.

Poison Oak. Poison oak (*Rhus diversiloba* or *R. toxicodendron*), sometimes known as oakleaf ivy, is related to poison ivy and not to the oak tree; its eastern and western varieties resemble each other closely. It is usually a low-growing shrub and seldom a climbing vine. It has three leaves, like poison ivy, but they are lobed and bear a slight resemblance to small oak leaves. Its berries are white and small, like those of poison ivy. Poison oak causes the same symptoms as poison ivy. Prevention and treatment are the same as for poison ivy.

Poison Sumac. Although poison sumac (*Rhus vernix*) goes by other names, such as swamp sumac, poison elder, poison ash, poison dogwood, and thunderwood, there is only one variety of it. Sometimes, however, poison sumac is confused with the several harmless kinds of sumac. Poison sumac is a coarse woody shrub or small tree, and it has white berries, distinguishing it from the harmless varieties of sumac, which have red berries. Symptoms and treatment are the same as for poison ivy.

p. center, p. control center a telephone service with toxicology experts providing emergency treatment advice for all kinds of POISONINGS, 24 hours a day. Poison control centers also provide poison prevention information to the community and education about recognition and treatment of poison exposures for health care providers. By gathering data about the outcomes of poison exposures, they also identify new or unexpected toxic hazards, allowing for product recalls, reformulations, or repackaging. Their staffs include physicians, nurses, and pharmacists with training in toxicology. There are more than 500 poison control centers in the United States; 65 of them are officially certified and are members of the American Association of Poison Control Centers. All of these provide 24-hour service and can be reached by calling 1-800-222-1222. See the Appendix of Poison Control Centers, which lists the certified ones.

poisoning (poi′zun-ing) development of symptoms after contact with a potentially toxic substance (see also POISON). Such substances can enter the body by several routes: oral (medicines, household products, etc.); nasal (carbon monoxide, pesticides, etc.); through the eyes (household products and industrial chemicals, etc.); through the skin (caustics, pesticides, etc.); and

parenteral (bites, stings, injected drugs, etc.). Children account for about half of all exposures to poisons, but most fatalities are in teenagers and adults who abuse drugs or commit suicide with drugs, chemicals, or gases.

Symptoms. Symptoms vary widely depending on the type and amount of substance involved, the route of exposure, and the age, weight, and medical condition of the victim. Some poisons are associated with characteristic clusters of symptoms called TOXIDROMES. For example, OPIOID poisoning causes constricted pupils, depressed respirations, and coma. Poisoning by organophosphate INSECTICIDES causes tearing, salivation, loss of bowel and bladder control, and copious bronchial secretions. (See ORGANOPHOSPHORUS COMPOUND POISONING). However, many poisonings result in very general symptoms; for example, the headache, nausea, and lethargy of CARBON MONOXIDE poisoning often are misdiagnosed as a viral illness. For some poisonings, such as METHANOL and ETHYLENE GLYCOL, symptoms are delayed for many hours after exposure. Suspect a possible poisoning when someone has unexplained illness, seizures, cardiac arrhythmias, change in mental status, or loss of consciousness. Of course, also consider poison exposure in the face of obvious burns to the skin, evidence of medicine or foreign substance around the mouth or on the skin, or unexpectedly empty bottles or containers.

First Aid. If the victim is unconscious, having seizures, or not breathing, call 911 or the local emergency ambulance number immediately. Otherwise, the immediate goal is to prevent or decrease further contact with the poison. After immediate measures are taken, always call the POISON CENTER at 1-800-222-1222. The poison center staff of physicians, nurses, and pharmacists, all with special training in toxicology, will provide both immediate and ongoing treatment advice.

Swallowed poison: dilute by having the victim drink a small amount of milk or water.

Inhaled poison: remove victim to fresh air if it is safe for the rescuer to enter.

Poison on the skin: rinse with running water for a minimum of 15–20 minutes.

Poison in the eyes: rinse with running water for a minimum of 15–20 minutes.

Treatment for poisoning. A careful history plus consultation with the poison center will allow a determination of how dangerous the situation may be. Next steps may

Millions of poisoning exposures occur each year in the United States, resulting in nearly 900,000 visits to emergency departments. About 90% of poisonings happen in the home, and more than half of them involve children under age 6. Many poisonings can be prevented if safety precautions are taken around the home. If a poisoning occurs, calling a poison control center can help ensure rapid, appropriate treatment.

Safety Tips

Preventing Poisonings in the Home

The simple steps that follow, provided by the American Association of Poison Control Centers, can help you protect children from poisons:

- Post the telephone number for your poison control center near your phone, in a place where all family members would be able to find it quickly in an emergency.
- Remove all nonessential drugs and household products from your home. Discard them according to the manufacturer's instructions.
- If you have small children, avoid keeping highly toxic products, such as drain cleaners, in the home, garage, shed or other place children can access.
- Buy medicines and household products in child-resistant packaging and be sure that caps are always on tight. Do not remove child-safety caps. Avoid keeping medicines, vitamins, or household products in anything but their original packaging.
- Store all of your medicines and household products in a locked closet or cabinet—including products and medicines with child-resistant containers.
- Crawl around your house, including inside your closets, to inspect it from a child's point of view. You'll likely find a poisoning hazard you hadn't noticed before.
- Never refer to medicine or vitamins as "candy."
- Make sure visiting grandparents, family friends, or other care givers keep their medications away from children. For example, if Grandma keeps pills in her purse, make sure the purse is out of children's reach.
- Keep a bottle of syrup of ipecac in your home—this can be used to induce vomiting. Use it only when the poison control center tells you to.
- Avoid products such as cough syrup or mouth wash that contain alcohol—these are hazardous for young children. Look for alcohol-free alternatives.
- Keep cosmetics and beauty products out of children's reach. Remember that hair permanents and relaxers are toxins as well.

Carbon Monoxide Poisoning

Carbon monoxide (CO) is an invisible, odorless, poisonous gas that can cause sickness and death. The gas is produced by the incomplete burning of fuels such as natural gas, oil, kerosene, coal, and wood. Fuel-burning appliances that are not working properly or are installed incorrectly can produce fatal concentrations of carbon monoxide in your home. Other hazards include burning charcoal indoors and running a car in the garage, both of which can lead to dangerous levels of CO in your home.

Every year, more than 200 Americans die from CO produced by fuel-burning appliances, and several thousand go to emergency departments for treatment for CO poisoning. You can prevent carbon monoxide poisonings in your home by following a few simple tips.

- Install carbon monoxide alarms near bedrooms and on each floor of your home. If your alarm sounds, the U.S. Consumer Product Safety Commission suggests that you press the reset button, call emergency services (911 or your local fire department), and immediately move to fresh air (either outdoors or near an open door or window). If you learn that fuel-burning appliances were the most likely cause of the poisoning, have a serviceperson check them for malfunction before turning them back on. Refer to the instructions on your CO alarm for more specific information about what to do if your alarm goes off.
- Symptoms of CO poisoning are similar to the flu, only without a fever (headache, fatigue, nausea, dizziness, shortness of breath). If you experience any of these symptoms, get fresh air immediately and contact a physician for proper diagnosis. Also, open windows and doors, turn off combustion appliances, contact emergency services, and take the steps listed above to ensure your home's safety.
- To keep carbon monoxide from collecting in your home, make sure that any fuel-burning equipment, such as a furnace, stove, or heater, works properly, and never use charcoal or other grills indoors or in the garage. Do not leave your car's engine running while it's in the garage, and consider putting weather stripping around the door between the garage and the house.

The Problem

Who Is Affected?

Millions of poisoning exposures occur each year in the United States, resulting in nearly 900,000 visits to the emergency department. About 90 percent of poisonings happen in the home, and common household items are often the cause. The poisons involved most often are cleaning products, pain relievers, cosmetics, personal care products, plants, and cough and cold medicines.

(continued)

POISONING PREVENTION—cont'd

Children—especially those under age six—are at highest risk for unintentional poisoning. Adolescents are also at risk for poisonings, both intentional and unintentional. About half of all poisonings among teens are classified as suicide attempts.

Poison control centers help millions of people each year, ensuring that poisonings are treated rapidly and correctly. Poison control centers managed more than 2 million cases of poison exposure in 1996. About three-quarters of these cases were managed at home over the telephone with the help of specialists trained in poison information. Poison control centers are extremely cost effective. For every $1 spent on poison control centers, an estimated $7 is saved in medical care costs. By helping people manage emergencies at home, these centers prevent about 50,000 hospitalizations and 400,000 trips to doctors' offices each year.

Safety Resources

American Academy of Pediatrics

AAP's National Poison Prevention Week site, www.aap.org/family/poisonwk.htm
includes links to poisoning prevention tips.
You can call AAP at 847-228-5097.

American Association of Poison Control Centers

Find your local poison control center and poison prevention tips through this web site, www.aapcc.org, or call the SafeUSA hotline at 1-888-252-7751.

Centers for Disease Control and Prevention

CDC's spotlight on National Poison Prevention Week, www.cdc.gov/ncipc/dacrrdp/spotlite/poi2.htm,
offers safety tips and data about poisonings. CDC also offers information for parents about lead poisoning.
www.cdc.gov/nceh/programs/lead/faq/cdc97a.htm.
For more information, call the SafeUSA hotline at 1-888-252-7751.

U.S. Consumer Product Safety Commission

CPSC offers extensive information on carbon monoxide poisoning—what causes it and how to prevent it—at www.cpsc.gov/cpscpub/pubs/466.html. CPSC's phone number is 1-800-638-2772.

National SAFE KIDS Campaign

On the SAFE KIDS web site, http://www.safekids.org/tier3_cd.cfm?folder id=540&content_item_id=1152, you'll find poisoning data and prevention tips. You can call SAFE KIDS at 202-662-0600.

References

The data and safety tips in this fact sheet were obtained from the following sources:

Poisoning Prevention: Know the Facts.

American Association of Poison Control Centers. Prevention Tips. Available at www.aapcc.org/preventi.htm. Accessed September 10, 1999.

Burt CW, Fingerhut LA. Injury visits to hospital emergency departments: United States, 1992–95. Vital and Health Statistics 13(131). DHHS publication no. 98–1792. Hyattsville, MD: National Center for Health Statistics, 1998.

Committee on Injury and Poison Control Prevention, American Academy of Pediatrics. Injury Prevention and Control for Children and Youth. Elk Grove Village, IL: The Academy, 1997.

Litovitz TL, Smilkstein M, Felberg L, Klein-Schwartz W, Berlin R, Morgan JL. 1996 annual report of the American Association of Poison Control Centers Toxic Exposure Surveillance System. American Journal of Emergency Medicine 1997;15(5):447–500.

Miller TR, Lestina DC. Costs of poisoning in the United States and savings from poison control centers: A benefit-cost analysis. Annals of Emergency Medicine 1997;29(2):239–245.

U.S. Consumer Product Safety Commission. Carbon Monoxide Factsheet. Available at www.cpsc.gov/cpscpub/pubs/466.html. Accessed September 23, 1999.

From http://www.cdc.gov/safeusa/poison/htm.
SafeUSA is a trademark name and subject to protection under trademark law.

P

include: decontamination of the gastrointestinal tract or further irrigation of eyes or skin; stabilization of the airway, breathing, and circulation; and treatment of seizures, if present. Supportive care, which may be as simple as observation or may be extremely complex, is sufficient for most poisonings. Few substances have specific antidotes, but the poison center will recommend when one is indicated and can help locate unusual antidotes.

Poison Prevention.

1. Use child-resistant packaging for medicines and household products.

2. Keep potential poisons locked out of sight and reach of children.

3. Store medicines and household products in their original, labeled containers.

4. Call medicines by their proper names.

5. Take medicines where children cannot watch, as children learn by imitation.

6. Read the label before giving or taking any medicine.

7. Read the label and follow precautions when using any household products.

8. Wear personal protective equipment as indicated when working with industrial and household chemicals.

9. Put the poison center number on the phone: 1-800-222-1222.

10. Call the poison center immediately for any possible poison exposure.

risk for p. a NURSING DIAGNOSIS accepted by the North American Nursing Diagnosis Association, defined as an accentuated risk of accidental exposure to or ingestion of drugs or dangerous products in doses sufficient to cause poisoning.

Polaramine (po-lar′ah-mēn) trademark for preparations of DEXCHLORPHENIRAMINE maleate, an ANTIHISTAMINE.

polarimeter (po″lah-rim′ĕ-ter) a device for measuring the rotation of plane polarized light.

polarimetry (po″lah-rim′ĕ-tre) measurement of the rotation of plane polarized light.

polarity (po-lar′ĭ-te) the condition of having poles or of exhibiting opposite effects at the two extremities.

polarization (po″lar-ĭ-za′shun) 1. the presence or absence of polarity. 2. the production of that condition in light in which its vibrations are parallel to each other in one plane or in circles and ellipses. 3. the separation of electric charge so that there is directionality of flow, as in a body, cell, atom, or molecule.

polarizer (po′lah-rīz″er) an appliance for polarizing light.

polarography (po″lar-og′rah-fe) an electrochemical technique for identifying and estimating the concentration of reducible elements in an electrochemical cell by means of the dual measurement of the CURRENT flowing through the cell and the electrical POTENTIAL at which each element is reduced. adj., **polarograph′ic.**

pole (pōl) 1. either extremity of any axis, as of the fetal ellipse or a body organ. 2. either one of two points that have opposite physical qualities (electric or other). adj., **po′lar.**

cephalic p. the end of the fetal ellipse at which the head of the fetus is situated.

frontal p. the most prominent part of the anterior end of each cerebral HEMI-SPHERE.

occipital p. the posterior end of the occipital lobe of the brain.

pelvic p. the end of the fetal ellipse at which the breech of the fetus is situated.

temporal p. the prominent anterior end of the temporal lobe of the brain.

poli(o)- word element [Gr.], *gray matter.*

policy (pol′ĭ-se) a plan of activity or behavior that serves some end such as being expedient or beneficial.

health care p. subfield of political science covering the making and implementing of decisions by public administrators and elected legislators to improve the health and well-being of the public.

polio (po′le-o) poliomyelitis.

polioclastic (po″le-o-klas′tik) destroying the gray matter of the nervous system.

poliodystrophia (po″le-o-dis-tro′fe-ah) poliodystrophy.

p. ce′rebri a rare disease of young children, marked by neuron degeneration of the cerebral cortex and elsewhere, with progressive mental deterioration, motor disturbances, sometimes cortical deafness and blindness, and early death. Called also Alpers' disease.

poliodystrophy (po″le-o-dis′trah-fe) atrophy of the cerebral gray matter.

polioencephalitis (po″le-o-en-sef″ah-li′tis) inflammatory disease of the gray matter of the brain.

inferior p. bulbar paralysis.

polioencephalomeningomyelitis (po″le-o-en-sef″ah-lo-mĕ-ning″go-mi″ĕ-li′tis) inflammation of the gray matter of the brain and spinal cord and of the meninges.

polioencephalomyelitis (po″le-o-en-sef″-ah-lo-mi″ĕ-li′tis) inflammation of the gray matter of the brain and spinal cord.

polioencephalopathy (po″le-o-en-sef″ah-lop′ah-the) any disease of the gray matter of the brain.

poliomyelitis (po″le-o-mi″ĕ-li′tis) an acute infectious disease occurring sporadically or in epidemics and caused by a virus, usually a POLIOVIRUS but occasionally a COXSACKIEVIRUS or ECHOVIRUS. Called also polio.

Initial clinical characteristics include fever, sore throat, headache, and vomiting, often with stiffness of the neck and back. In the *minor illness* these may be the only symptoms. The *major illness* (called also infantile paralysis), which may or may not be preceded by the minor illness, is characterized by involvement of the central nervous system, stiff neck, PLEOCYTOSIS in the spinal fluid, and perhaps paralysis within a week. *Bulbar poliomyelitis* is a serious form involving the medulla oblongata and usually becomes evident within three days. The muscles of swallowing and breathing are affected, so that the patient has difficulty swallowing, speaking, and breathing. In all forms, there may be subsequent atrophy of groups of muscles, ending in contraction and permanent deformity.

There are three known types of poliovirus, each causing a different type of the disease. Most paralytic cases are caused by type 1. Poliovirus is found in the throat of a patient for the first few days of the disease, and in the intestines for a longer period, sometimes as long as 17 weeks. The disease spreads by means of droplets of moisture from an infected person's throat or by waste products from the intestines. The contagious period is 7 or more days from the time of onset of the disease. The poliovirus is short-lived, and cannot survive long in the air. The incubation period of polio is from 1 to 2 weeks, and occasionally as long as 3 weeks. Members of the family or other contacts may be carriers, but only for a short period of time.

Treatment. There is at present no cure for polio; once the disease begins it must be allowed to run its course. Supportive care is important, however, and proper symptomatic treatment can reduce discomfort and prevent some crippling aftereffects. Applications of heat in the form of hot wet packs, DIATHERMY, warm baths in the form of HYDROTHERAPY, and gentle exercising can reduce pain caused by muscle spasms and prevent deformities. During the acute stage of the disease bed rest is essential and the patient is kept warm and quiet.

Postpolio Weakness. Although immunization efforts to eradicate polio have reduced its current incidence in the United States to fewer than 10 cases each year, survivors of previous epidemics are experiencing a second encounter with the illness. Weakness in one or more muscles appears to be a late complication of the infection. The weakness can affect muscles that were first involved in the disease or it can affect those that were not formerly weakened. The cause of this phenomenon is not yet known and there is no treatment available, other than medications known to be effective in combating AUTOIMMUNE DISEASES. It is hoped that this form of therapy will

retard or arrest the process causing the weakness.

Prevention. The first safe, effective vaccine against polio used killed polioviruses to stimulate production and release of antibodies. It was developed under the direction of Dr. Jonas E. Salk, and was nicknamed the Salk VACCINE; its proper name is poliovirus VACCINE inactivated (IPV). It was later replaced by an oral preparation of attenuated viruses called poliovirus VACCINE live oral, nicknamed the Sabin VACCINE after its discoverer, Dr. Albert Sabin. In recent years in the United States, the Salk vaccine has come back into use. It does not induce intestinal immunity and so is not effective for poliovirus eradication in areas where wild-type polioviruses still exist in large numbers. However, it does not cause vaccine-associated paralytic poliomyelitis and so is preferred for routine immunization in areas where the risk of infection by a wild-type polivirus is very low.

poliomyelopathy (po″le-o-mi″ĕ-lop′ah-the) any disease of the gray matter of the spinal cord.

poliosis (po″le-o′sis) circumscribed depigmentation of the hair, particularly of the scalp, occurring in association with or following various pathologic conditions. See also LEUKOTRICHIA and CANITIES.

poliovirus (po′le-o-vi″rus) a species of ENTEROVIRUS that is the etiologic agent of POLIOMYELITIS. It is separable into three serotypes, designated types 1, 2, and 3, with type 1 being responsible for about 85 per cent of all cases of paralytic poliomyelitis and for most epidemics.

polishing (pol′ish-ing) creation of a smooth and glossy finish on a surface, as of a tooth or denture.

pollen (pol′en) the male fertilizing element of flowering plants.

pollenosis (pol″ĕ-no′sis) pollinosis.

pollex (pol′eks) [L.] thumb.

pollinosis (pol″ĭ-no′sis) an allergic reaction to pollen; hay fever.

pollution (pah-loo′shun) defiling or making impure, especially contamination by noxious substances.

polonium (Po) (pah-lo′ne-um) a chemical element, atomic number 84, atomic weight 210. (See Appendix 6.)

poloxamer (pol-ok′sah-mer) any of a series of nonionic SURFACTANTS, also used as emulsifiers, stabilizers, and food additives.

polus (po′lus) [L.] pole.

poly- word element [Gr.], *many; much.*

polyadenitis (pol″e-ad″ĕ-ni′tis) inflammation (ADENITIS) of several glands.

polyadenosis (pol″e-ad″ĕ-no′sis) disorder of several glands, particularly endocrine glands.

polyalveolar (pol″e-al-ve′o-ler) having more than the usual number of alveoli, such as a polyalveolar lobe of a lung.

polyandry (pol′e-an″dre) a form of marriage in which one woman has two or more husbands at the same time.

polyangiitis (pol″e-an″je-i′tis) inflammation involving multiple blood or lymph vessels.

polyarteritis (pol″e-ahr″tĕ-ri′tis) multiple sites of inflammatory and destructive lesions in the arterial system.

p. nodo′sa a form of systemic necrotizing vasculitis involving the small and medium-sized arteries with signs and symptoms resulting from infarction and scarring of the affected organ system. Called also Kussmaul's disease and periarteritis nodosa.

polyarthric (pol″e-ahr′thrik) polyarticular.

polyarthritis (pol″e-ahr-thri′tis) inflammation of several joints.

chronic villous p. chronic inflammation of the synovial membrane of several joints.

polyarticular (pol″e-ahr-tik′u-lar) affecting many joints; polyarthric.

polyatomic (pol″e-ah-tom′ik) made up of several atoms.

polybasic (pol″e-ba′sik) having several replaceable hydrogen atoms.

polycarbophil (pol″e-kahr′bo-fil) a bulk-forming LAXATIVE that also acts as a gastrointestinal absorbent in the treatment of DIARRHEA; often used as the calcium salt (calcium polycarbophil).

polychemotherapy (pol″e-ke″mo-ther′ah-pe) CHEMOTHERAPY involving simultaneous administration of several agents.

polycholia (pol″e-ko′le-ah) excessive flow or secretion of bile.

polychondritis (pol″e-kon-dri′tis) inflammation of many cartilages of the body.

chronic atrophic p., p. chro′nica atro′-phicans relapsing p. an acquired disease of unknown origin, chiefly involving various cartilages and showing both chronicity and a tendency to recurrence; it is marked by inflammatory and degenerative lesions of various cartilaginous structures.

polychromasia (pol″e-kro-ma′ze-ah) 1. variation in the hemoglobin content of erythrocytes. 2. polychromatophilia.

polychromatic (pol″e-kro-mat′ik) many-colored.

polychromatocyte (pol″e-kro-mat′o-sīt) a cell stainable with various kinds of stains.

polychromatophil (pol″e-kro-mat′o-fil) a structure stainable with many kinds of stains.

polychromatophilia (pol″e-kro″mah-to-fil′e-ah) 1. the property of being stainable with various stains; affinity for all sorts of stains. 2. a condition in which the erythrocytes, on staining, show various shades of blue combined with tinges of pink. adj., **polychromatophil′ic.**

polychromemia (pol″e-kro-me′me-ah) HYPERHEMOGLOBINEMIA.

polyclinic (pol″e-klin′ik) a hospital and school where diseases and injuries of all kinds are studied and treated.

polyclonal (pol″e-klōn′al) derived from different cells; pertaining to several clones.

polyclonia (pol″e-klo′ne-ah) a disease marked by many clonic spasms; called also polymyoclonus.

polycoria (pol″e-kor′e-ah) more than one pupil in an eye.

polycrotism (pol-ik′rah-tizm) the quality of having several waves to each beat of the pulse. adj., **polycrot′ic.**

polycyesis (pol″e-si-e′sis) multiple pregnancy.

polycystic (pol″e-sis′tik) containing many cysts.

p. kidney disease either of two unrelated hereditary diseases in which there is massive enlargement of the kidney with cyst formation. It occurs in two forms, distinguished by age of onset and other characteristics.

Autosomal dominant polycystic kidney disease (ADPKD, formerly called *adult polycystic kidney disease*) is the most common type of cystic disease of the kidneys. It is usually manifested during the third decade of life. Renal failure may appear by the fifth decade, with terminal failure occurring in the next ten years, although in some cases it never appears. Although there is rarely any liver dysfunction accompanying this disorder, cyst formation in the liver does occur.

Autosomal recessive polycystic kidney disease (ARPKD), formerly called *childhood polycystic kidney disease*, is diagnosed at birth or in the first ten years of life and is much less common than the autosomal dominant form. Both the kidney and the liver are involved, causing RENAL FAILURE and liver failure with portal hypertension. Characteristic symptoms early in the process include pain, hematuria, urinary tract infection, KIDNEY STONES, and obstructive uropathy with anuria.

Treatment of both types of polycystic kidney disease is largely symptomatic. Renal DIALYSIS and kidney transplantation during END-STAGE RENAL DISEASE can prolong life but offer no cure. Families with histories of polycystic kidney disease require genetic counseling and may need help in coping with the prospect of future offspring afflicted with the disease.

p. ovary syndrome (PCOS) a clinical symptom complex associated with polycystic ovaries and characterized by oligomenorrhea or amenorrhea, anovulation (hence infertility), and hirsutism. Both hyperestrogenism (from peripheral conversion of androgen) and hyperandrogenism are present. Excretion of follicle-stimulating hormone and 17-ketosteroids is normal, but infertility is usually persistent, requiring treatment with wedge resection, clomiphene, or gonadotropins. Called also Stein-Leventhal syndrome.

p. renal disease polycystic kidney disease.

polycythemia (pol″e-si-the′me-ah) an increase in the total red blood cell mass of the blood; called also erythrocythemia, hypercythemia, and hypererythrocythemia.

There are two distinct forms of the disease: *Primary polycythemia (polycythemia vera)* is a MYELOPROLIFERATIVE DISORDER of unknown etiology. It is characterized by hyperplasia of the cell-forming tissues of the bone marrow, with resultant elevation of the erythrocyte count and hemoglobin level, and an increase in the number of leukocytes and platelets.

Secondary polycythemia is a physiologic condition resulting from a deficient oxygen supply to the tissues. The body attempts to compensate for the deficiency by manufacturing more hemoglobin and erythrocytes. Living at high altitudes can produce polycythemia, as can severe chronic lung and heart disorders, especially congenital heart defects.

Absolute polycythemia refers to an increase in red cell mass from any cause. *Relative polycythemia* refers to a loss of PLASMA volume causing an elevated HEMATOCRIT.

Symptoms. The symptoms of primary and secondary polycythemia are much the same. The increased erythrocyte production results in thickening of the blood and an increased tendency toward clotting. The viscosity of the blood limits its ability to flow properly, so that the supply to the brain and other vital tissues is diminished. This may cause sluggishness, irritability, headache, dizziness, fainting, disturbances of sensation in the hands and feet, and a feeling of fullness in the head. There may be episodes of acute pain as spontaneous clots occur in the blood vessels. The spleen becomes enlarged and the smaller veins become more prominent, so that the skin has a bluish hue.

The secondary form is often accompanied by enlargement of the tips of the fingers (CLUBBING).

Treatment. Treatment of polycythemia vera is aimed at reducing the red cell count and decreasing the blood volume. Mild cases can be managed by periodic PHLEBOTOMY. More serious cases may require MYELOSUPPRESSIVE therapy; INTERFERON and large-dose ASPIRIN therapy may also be used. Research on treatment modalities is ongoing. In secondary polycythemia, successful treatment of the causative illness will relieve the polycythemia.

polydactylism (pol″e-dak′til-iz′m) polydactyly.

polydactyly (pol″e-dak′tĭ-le) the presence of more than the usual number of fingers or toes; called also hyperdactyly and polydactylism.

polydipsia (pol″e-dip′se-ah) excessive thirst and fluid intake. It may be due to an organic lesion or have a psychological cause.

polydysplasia (pol″e-dis-pla′zhah) faulty development of several tissues, organs, or systems.

polydystrophy (pol″e-dis′trah-fe) degeneration, dysfunction, or atrophy of several tissues or organs, as in some congenital syndromes.

pseudo-Hurler p. mucolipidosis III.

polyendocrine (pol″e-en′do-krin) pertaining to several endocrine glands.

p. autoimmune disease the combination of endocrine and nonendocrine AUTOIMMUNE DISEASES. In type I, which usually begins at age 10 to 12 years, symptoms include candidiasis, hypoparathyroidism, and primary adrenal insufficiency. Pernicious anemia, vitiligo, gonadal failure, alopecia, and chronic hepatitis may also occur. Type II is better known as SCHMIDT'S SYNDROME.

polyene (pol′e-ēn) 1. a chemical compound with a carbon chain of four or more atoms and several conjugated double bonds. 2. any of a group of antibiotic antifungal AGENTS with similar structure, such as AMPHOTERICIN B, CANDICIDIN, or NYSTATIN; they are produced by species of *Streptomyces* that damage cell membranes by forming complexes with sterols.

polyesthesia (pol″e-es-the′zhah) a sensation as if several points were touched on application of a stimulus to a single point.

polyestradiol phosphate (pol″e-es″trah-di′ol) a polymer of ESTRADIOL phosphate having estrogenic activity similar to that of estradiol; used in the palliative therapy of prostatic carcinoma.

polyethylene (pol″e-eth′ĭ-lēn) polymerized ethylene, $(—CH_2—CH_2—)_n$, a synthetic

P

plastic material, forms of which have been used in reparative surgery.

p. glycol a polymer of ETHYLENE OXIDE and water, available in liquid form (polyethylene glycol 300 or 400) or as waxy solids (polyethylene glycol 1540 or 4000), used in various pharmaceutical preparations as a water-soluble ointment base. Polyethylene glycol is also used as a laxative.

polygalactia (pol″e-gah-lak′she-ah) excessive secretion of milk.

polygamy (pah-lig′ah-me) the practice of having two or more spouses at one time.

polygene (pol′e-jēn) a group of nonallelic genes that interact to influence the same character with additive effect.

polygenic (pol″e-jēn′ik) pertaining to or determined by several different genes.

polyglactin (pol″e-glak′tin) a filamentous material that is braided and used for absorbable SUTURES.

polyglandular (pol″e-glan′du-lar) pluriglandular.

polyglycolic acid (pol″e-gli-kol′ik) a polymer of glycolic acid used for absorbable SUTURES.

polygnathus (po-lig′nah-thus, pol″e-nath′us) a fetal malformation in which a parasitic twin is attached to the autosite's jaw.

polygram (pol′e-gram) a tracing made by a polygraph.

polygraph (pol′e-graf) an apparatus for simultaneously recording several mechanical or electrical impulses, such as blood pressure, pulse, and respiration, and variations in electrical resistance of the skin; popularly known as a lie detector.

polygyny (pah-lij′ĭ-ne) a form of marriage in which a man has two or more wives at the same time.

polygyria (pol″e-ji′re-ah) polymicrogyria.

polyhedral (pol″e-he′dral) having many sides or surfaces.

polyhidrosis (pol″e-hi-dro′sis) hyperhidrosis.

polyhydramnios (pol″e-hi-dram′ne-os) hydramnios; an excessive amount (more than 2000 ml) of amniotic fluid.

polyhydric (pol″e-hi′drik) containing more than two hydroxyl groups.

polyinfection (pol″e-in-fek′shun) infection with more than one organism.

polyisoprenoid (pol″e-i′so-pre-noid″) any isoprenoid that contains multiple isoprene units, such as rubber.

polyleptic (pol″e-lep′tik) having many remissions and exacerbations.

polymastia (pol″e-mas′te-ah) the presence of supernumerary mammary glands or nipples; called also pleomastia.

polymelus (pah-lim′ĕ-lus) an individual with supernumerary limbs.

polymenorrhea (pol″e-men″o-re′ah) abnormally frequent menstruation.

polymer (pol′ĭ-mer) a compound, usually of high molecular weight, formed by combination of simpler molecules (monomers).

polymerase (pah-lim′er-ās) an enzyme that catalyzes POLYMERIZATION.

p. chain reaction a rapid technique for in vitro amplification of specific DNA or RNA sequences, allowing small quantities of short sequences to be analyzed without cloning.

polymer fume fever an occupational disorder due to exposure to the products of combustion of polymers such as Teflon; the manifestations are quite similar to those of metal fume fever.

polymeric (pol″ĭ-mer′ik) exhibiting the character of a polymer.

polymerization (pah-lim″er-ĭ-za′shun) the combining of several simpler molecules (monomers) to form a polymer.

polymerize (pah-lim′er-īz) to subject to or to undergo polymerization.

polymicrobial (pol″e-mi-kro′be-al), **polymicrobic** (pol″e-mi-kro′bik) marked by the presence of several species of microorganisms.

polymicrogyria (pol″e-mi″kro-ji′re-ah) a brain malformation marked by development of numerous microgyri.

polymorph (pol′e-morf) a colloquial term for a polymorphonuclear leukocyte.

polymorphic (pol″e-mor′fik) occurring in several or many forms; appearing in different forms in different developmental stages.

polymorphism (pol″e-mor′fizm) the ability to exist in several different forms.

balanced p. an equilibrium mixture of homozygotes and heterozygotes maintained by natural selection against both homozygotes.

genetic p. the occurrence together in the same population of two or more genetically determined phenotypes in such proportions that the rarest of them cannot be maintained merely by recurrent mutation.

single nucleotide p. (SNP) a genetic polymorphism between two genomes that is based on deletion, insertion, or exchange of a single nucleotide.

polymorphocellular (pol″e-mor″fo-sel′u-lar) having cells of many forms.

polymorphonuclear (pol″e-mor″fo-noo′kle-ar) having a nucleus so deeply lobed or so divided as to appear to be multiple; see under LEUKOCYTE.

polymorphous (pol″e-mor′fus) polymorphic.

polymyalgia (pol″e-mi-al′jah) pain involving many muscles.

polymyoclonus (pol″e-mi-ok′lo-nus) 1. a fine or minute muscular tremor. 2. polyclonia.

polymyopathy (pol″e-mi-op′ah-the) any disease affecting several muscles simultaneously.

polymyositis (pol″e-mi″o-si′tis) a chronic, progressive inflammatory disease of skeletal muscle, occurring in both children and adults, and characterized by symmetrical weakness of the limb girdles, necks, and pharynx, usually associated with pain and tenderness, and sometimes preceded or followed by manifestations typical of scleroderma, arthritis, systemic lupus erythematosus, or Sjögren's syndrome. It is also sometimes associated with malignancy, and may be accompanied by characteristic skin lesions.

polymyxin (pol″e-mik′sin) a generic term for ANTIBIOTICS derived from various strains of *Bacillus polymyxa,* several closely related compounds being designated by letters.

p. B a bacteriostatic and bactericidal ANTIBIOTIC, effective mainly against gramnegative organisms. It is used as the sulfate salt, and is especially effective against *Pseudomonas aeruginosa,* which may cause septicemia, meningitis, urinary tract infections, and middle ear infections. Toxicity is low but there is sometimes damage to kidney and nerve cells. The route of administration is parenteral, oral, or topical to the ear or eye. Oral preparations are not used for systemic infections because the drug is poorly absorbed from the intestinal tract.

polynesic (pol″ĭ-ne′sik) occurring in many foci.

polyneural (pol″e-noor′al) pertaining to or supplied by many nerves.

polyneuralgia (pol″e-noo-ral′jah) neuralgia of several nerves.

polyneuritis (pol″e-noo-ri′tis) inflammation of many nerves simultaneously.

acute febrile p., acute idiopathic p., acute infectious p., acute postinfectious p. Guillain-Barré syndrome.

polyneuromyositis (pol″e-noor″o-mi″o-si′tis) inflammation involving the muscles and peripheral nerves, with loss of reflexes, sensory loss, and paresthesias.

polyneuropathy (pol″e-noo-rop′ah-the) a disease involving several nerves.

amyloid p. polyneuropathy caused by AMYLOIDOSIS; symptoms may include dysfunction of the autonomic nervous system, CARPAL TUNNEL SYNDROME, and sensory disturbances in the extremities.

familial amyloid p. autosomal dominant amyloid polyneuropathy occurring in

hereditary amyloidosis; subtypes include *Finnish type, Indiana type, Iowa type,* and *Portuguese type.* The Finnish and Indiana types are slowly progressive, whereas in the Portuguese and Iowa types death may occur within 7 to 10 years.

erythredema p. acrodynia.

polyneuroradiculitis (pol″e-noor″o-rah-dik″u-li′tis) inflammation of spinal ganglia, nerve roots, and peripheral nerves.

polynuclear (pol″e-noo′kle-ar) having several nuclei; called also polynucleate.

polynucleate (pol″e-noo′kle-āt) polynuclear.

polynucleotide (pol″e-noo′kle-o-tīd) a compound formed by the joining of more than one NUCLEOTIDE.

polyodontia (pol″e-o-don′shah) the presence of supernumerary teeth.

polyonychia (pol″e-o-nik′e-ah) the presence of supernumerary nails.

polyopia (pol″e-o′pe-ah) visual perception of several images of a single object.

polyorchidism (pol″e-or′kĭ-dizm) the presence of more than two testes.

polyorchism (pol″e-or′kizm) polyorchidism.

polyostotic (pol″e-os-tot′ik) affecting several bones.

polyotia (pol″e-o′shah) the presence of more than two ears.

polyovular (pol″e-ov′u-lar) pertaining to or produced from more than one ovum, as in dizygotic TWINS.

polyovulatory (pol″e-ov′u-lah-tor″e) discharging several ova in one ovarian cycle.

polyoxyl (pol″e-ok′sil) a group of SURFACTANTS numbered according to the average polymer length of oxyethylene units; polyoxyl 40 stearate and many others are used in pharmaceutical preparations.

polyp (pol′ip) any growth or mass protruding from a mucous membrane. Polyps may be attached to a membrane by a thin stalk (*pedunculated polyps*), or they may have a broad base (*sessile polyps*). They are usually an overgrowth of normal tissue, but sometimes they are true tumors (masses of new tissue separate from the supporting membrane). Usually benign, they may lead to complications or eventually become malignant. They can occur wherever there is mucous membrane: in the nose, ears, mouth, lungs, heart, stomach, intestines, urinary bladder, uterus, and cervix.

intestinal p's polyps in the intestines, usually found in middle age although some infants are born with them in the large intestine. Multiple intestinal polyps may be a hereditary disorder. In most cases they

P

cause no symptoms unless they become large enough to obstruct the intestine or become ulcerated so that they bleed. When they do, symptoms may include cramping pains in the lower abdomen, diarrhea, and the passage of blood and mucus. Whether or not they cause symptoms, intestinal polyps should be removed, since any one of them may become malignant. Although all causes of intestinal cancer have not yet been discovered, it is believed that polyps are often a contributing factor.

nasal p's polyps in the nasal cavity or sinuses, usually produced by local irritation, sometimes as a result of an allergy. They are not dangerous, but if they grow large enough to extend into the nose, they may cause stuffiness and headaches. The allergy or other source of irritation responsible for the polyps should be treated; if the polyps continue to be troublesome, surgery may be necessary.

polypathia (pol″e-path′e-ah) the presence of several diseases at one time.

polypectomy (pol″ĭ-pek′tah-me) excision of a polyp.

polypeptide (pol″e-pep′tīd) a PEPTIDE containing two or more amino acids linked by a peptide bond; called dipeptide, tripeptide, etc., depending on the number of amino acids present.

vasoactive intestinal p. see VASOACTIVE INTESTINAL POLYPEPTIDE.

polypeptidemia (pol″e-pep″tĭ-de′me-ah) the presence of polypeptides in the blood.

polyphagia (pol″e-fa′jah) excessive eating; see also BULIMIA.

polyphalangia (pol″e-fah-lan′je-ah), **polyphalangism** (pol″e-fah-lan′jizm) excess of phalanges in a finger or toe.

polypharmacy (pol″e-fahr′mah-se) 1. the administration of many drugs together. 2. administration of excessive medication.

polyphobia (pol″e-fo′be-ah) irrational fear of many things.

polyplastic (pol″e-plas′tik) 1. containing many structural or constituent elements. 2. undergoing many changes of form.

polyplegia (pol″e-ple′jah) paralysis of several muscles.

polyploid (pol′e-ploid) 1. characterized by POLYPLOIDY. 2. an individual or cell characterized by polyploidy.

polyploidy (pol′e-ploi″de) the state of having more than two sets of homologous chromosomes.

polypnea (pol″ip-ne′ah) hyperpnea.

polypodia (pol″e-po′de-ah) the presence of supernumerary feet.

polypoid (pol′ĭ-poid) resembling a polyp.

polyporous (pol-ip′ah-rus) having many pores.

polyposia (pol″ĭ-po′ze-ah) ingestion of abnormally increased amounts of fluids for long periods of time.

polyposis (pol″ĭ-po′sis) the formation of numerous polyps.

familial p., familial adenomatous p. (FAP) a hereditary condition marked by multiple adenomatous polyps with high malignant potential, lining the intestinal mucosa, especially that of the colon. Polyps are first seen around puberty, and by age 35 years 95 per cent of patients have polyps. Without colectomy, colon cancer is inevitable. Extracolonic manifestations may also be present. It occurs as part of several different conditions, including GARDNER'S, PEUTZ-JEGHERS, CANADA-CRONKHITE, and TURCOT'S SYNDROMES.

polypous (pol′ĭ-pus) pertaining to or like a POLYP.

polyptychial (pol″e-ti′ke-al) arranged in several layers.

polyradiculitis (pol″e-rah-dik″u-li′tis) inflammation of the nerve roots.

polyradiculoneuritis (pol″e-rah-dik″u-lo-noo̅-ri′tis) acute infectious polyneuritis that involves the peripheral nerves, the spinal nerve roots, and the spinal cord.

polyribosome (pol″e-ri′bo-sōm) a cluster of ribosomes connected with messenger RNA; they play a role in peptide synthesis.

polysaccharide (pol″e-sak′ah-rīd) a carbohydrate which, on acid hydrolysis, yields many monosaccharides.

polyscelia (pol″e-se′le-ah) the presence of more than two lower limbs.

polyserositis (pol″e-se″ro-si′tis) general inflammation of serous membranes, with effusion.

polysinusitis (pol″e-si″nŭ-si′tis) inflammation of several sinuses.

polysome (pol′e-sōm) polyribosome.

polysomia (pol″e-so′me-ah) doubling or tripling of the fetal body.

polysomnography (pol″e-som-nog′rah-fe) the polygraphic recording during sleep of multiple physiological variables that are directly or indirectly related to the state and stages of sleep; done to assess possible biological causes of sleep disorders.

polysomus (pol″e-so′mus) a fetus exhibiting polysomia. adj., **polyso′mic.**

polysomy (pol″e-so′me) an excess of a particular chromosome.

polysorbate (pol″e-sor′bāt) a generic name for esters of SORBITOL and its anhydrides condensed with polymers of ETHYLENE OXIDE, used as SURFACTANTS; polysorbates 20, 40, 60, and 80 are official in NF.

polyspermia (pol″e-sper′me-ah) 1. excessive secretion of semen. 2. polyspermy.

polyspermy (pol″e-sper′me) FERTILIZATION of an OVUM by more than one SPERMATOZOON; occurring normally in certain species *(physiologic polyspermy)* but only abnormally in species such as humans *(pathologic polyspermy)*.

polysplenia (pol″e-sple′ne-ah) the presence of multiple spleens or accessory spleens.

polystichia (pol″e-stik′e-ah) two or more rows of eyelashes on an eyelid.

polystyrene (pol″e-sti′rēn) the resin produced by polymerization of styrol, a clear resin of the thermoplastic type, used in the construction of denture bases.

polysynaptic (pol″e-sĭ-nap′tik) pertaining to or relayed through two or more synapses.

polysyndactyly (pol″e-sin-dak′tĭ-le) hereditary association of POLYDACTYLY (extra fingers or toes) and SYNDACTYLY (webbed FINGERS or TOES).

polytef (pol′ĕ-tef) the pharmaceutical name for Teflon, a polymer of tetrafluoroethylene, used as a surgical implant material for many prostheses, such as artificial vessels and orbital floor implants, and for many applications in skeletal augmentation and skeletal fixation.

polytenosynovitis (pol″e-ten″o-sin″o-vi′-tis) inflammation of several or many tendon sheaths at the same time.

polythelia (pol″e-the′le-ah) the presence of supernumerary nipples.

polythiazide (pol″e-thi′ah-zīd) a thiazide DIURETIC used as an ANTIHYPERTENSIVE AGENT and for treatment of EDEMA.

polytocous (po-lit′ŏ-kus) giving birth to several offspring at one time.

Polytome (pol′e-tōm) trademark name for a tomographic machine that can achieve a multidimensional motion.

polytomogram (pol″e-to′mo-gram) the record produced by polytomography.

polytomography (pol″e-to-mog′rah-fe) tomography of tissue at several predetermined planes.

polytrichia (pol″e-trik′e-ah) hypertrichosis; excessive hairiness.

polyunsaturated (pol″e-un-sach′er-a-ted) denoting a fatty acid, e.g., linoleic acid, having more than one double bond in its hydrocarbon chain.

polyuria (pol″e-u′re-ah) excessive excretion of urine, such as with DIABETES MELLITUS.

polyvalent (pol″e-va′lent) multivalent; having more than one valence.

polyvinyl chloride a tasteless, odorless, clear hard resin with many industrial uses, including as packaging, clothing, and insulation of pipes and wires. Workers in

its manufacture are at risk primarily because of the toxicity of its parent compound, vinyl chloride. Excessive inhalation of its dust can cause PNEUMOCONIOSIS.

polyvinylpyrrolidone (pol″e-vi″nil-pi-rol′ĭ-dōn) povidone.

Pompe's disease (pom′pez) GLYCOGEN STORAGE DISEASE (type II), a condition in which deficiency of the enzyme α-1,4-glucosidase results in generalized glycogen accumulation, with cardiomegaly and usually fatal cardiorespiratory failure; children affected with this disease are mentally retarded and hypotonic. Called also generalized glycogenosis.

pompholyx (pom′fo-liks) an intensely pruritic skin eruption on the sides of the digits or on the palms and soles, consisting of small, discrete, round vesicles, accompanied by pruritus, a burning sensation, and excessive sweating. It is a self-limited condition usually lasting a few weeks.

POMR Problem-Oriented Medical Record (see PROBLEM-ORIENTED RECORD).

pons (ponz), pl. *pon′tes* [L.] 1. that part of the metencephalon lying between the medulla oblongata and the midbrain, ventral to the cerebellum; see also BRAINSTEM. 2. any slip of tissue connecting two parts of an organ.

Ponstel (pon′stel) trademark for a preparation of MEFENAMIC ACID, an ANALGESIC and ANTIINFLAMMATORY.

Pontiac fever (pon′te-ak) an influenzalike illness with little or no pulmonary involvement, caused by *Legionella pneumophila* and first observed in Pontiac, Michigan. It is not life-threatening as is the pulmonary form known as LEGIONNAIRES' DISEASE. The syndrome appears within 2 to 3 hours of contact with an infected person and lasts 2 to 5 days. There is complete recovery without residual effects, with or without antimicrobial therapy.

pontic (pon′tik) an artificial tooth on a fixed partial DENTURE, usually occupying the space previously occupied by the crown of a natural tooth.

ponticulus (pon-tik′u-lus), pl. *ponti′culi* [L.] a small ridge or bridgelike structure. adj., **pontic′ular.**

pontine (pon′tīn) pertaining to the pons.

pontobulbar (pon″to-bul′bar) pertaining to the pons and the region of the medulla oblongata dorsal to it.

pontocerebellar (pon″to-ser″ĕ-bel′ar) pertaining to the pons and cerebellum.

pontomesencephalic (pon″to-mes″en-sĕ-fal′ik) pertaining to or involving the pons and the mesencephalon.

P

popliteal (pop″lĭ-te′al) pertaining to the area behind the knee.

population (pop″u-la′shun) 1. the individuals collectively constituting a certain category or inhabiting a specified geographic area. 2. in genetics, a stable group of randomly interbreeding individuals. 3. in statistics, a theoretical concept used to describe an entire group or collection of units, finite or infinite; from it a sample can be drawn.

POR Problem-Oriented Record.

poractant alfa (por-ak′tant al′fah) an extract of porcine lung SURFACTANT administered by instillation via the endotracheal tube in treatment of RESPIRATORY DISTRESS SYNDROME OF THE NEWBORN.

poradenitis (por″ad-ĕ-ni′tis) inflammation of lymph nodes with formation of small abscesses.

porcine (por′sīn) pertaining to swine.

pore (por) a small opening or empty space.

porencephalia (por″en-sĕ-fal′e-ah) porencephaly.

porencephalitis (por″en-sef″ah-li′tis) porencephaly with inflammation of the brain.

porencephalous (por″en-sef′ah-lus) characterized by porencephaly.

porencephaly (por″en-sef′ah-le) development or presence of abnormal cysts or cavities in the brain tissue, usually communicating with a lateral ventricle; they may or may not cause symptoms. adj., **porencephal′ic, porenceph′alous.**

porfimer (por′fĭ-mer″) a light-activated antineoplastic AGENT related to PORPHYRIN, used as the sodium salt in the treatment of esophageal carcinoma and non–small cell lung carcinoma; administered intravenously.

porokeratosis (por″o-ker″ah-to′sis) a rare, chronic, progressive autosomal dominant skin disorder, seen most often in males, usually first appearing in early childhood, and characterized clinically by the presence of craterlike patches that have central atrophy with an elevated thick keratotic border and enlarge to form lesions. adj., **porokeratot′ic.**

poroma (pō-ro′mah) a tumor arising in a pore.

eccrine p. a benign tumor arising from the intradermal portion of an eccrine sweat duct, usually on the sole.

porosis (pŏ-ro′sis) 1. formation of the callus in repair of a fractured bone. 2. cavity formation.

porosity (pŏ-ros′ĭ-te) the condition of being porous; a pore.

porous (por′us) penetrated by pores and open spaces.

porphin (por′fin) the fundamental ring structure of four linked pyrrole nuclei around which porphyrins, hemin, cytochromes, and chlorophyll are built.

porphobilinogen (por″fo-bĭ-lin′o-jen) an intermediary product in the biosynthesis of heme.

porphyria (por-fēr′e-ah) a genetic disorder characterized by a disturbance in PORPHYRIN metabolism with resultant increase in the formation and excretion of porphyrins (UROPORPHYRIN and COPROPORPHYRIN) or their precursors; called also hematoporphyria. Porphyrins, in combination with iron, form HEMES, which in turn combine with specific proteins to form HEMOPROTEINS. HEMOGLOBIN is a hemoprotein, as are many other substances essential to normal functioning of the cells and tissues of the body.

Two general types are known: the *erythropoietic porphyrias,* which are concerned with the formation of erythrocytes in the bone marrow; and the *hepatic porphyrias,* which are responsible for liver dysfunction. Manifestations of porphyria include gastrointestinal, neurologic, and psychologic symptoms, cutaneous photosensitivity, pigmentation of the face (and later of the bones), and anemia with enlargement of the spleen. Large amounts of porphyrins are excreted in the urine and feces.

Treatment of this condition has been primarily symptomatic and varies in its effectiveness. Emphasis is on prevention of attacks by avoiding fasting and drugs that precipitate the symptoms. Photosensitivity may be controlled by avoiding exposure to light. Removal of the spleen is useful in some cases of the erythropoietic type of porphyria. Drug therapy includes the use of phenothiazines, chlorpromazine and promazine in particular. These drugs allay pain and nervousness and apparently allow a period of remission from symptoms. Meperidine hydrochloride (Demerol) may be given for pain and hydroxypheme (Hemetin) is given intravenously to compensate for genetic impairment of heme synthesis.

Patients with porphyria must not be given barbiturates, sulfonamides, alcohol, or chloroquine as these chemicals may precipitate or intensify attacks. It is recommended that persons with this disease carry with them at all times identification saying that they have porphyria so that in an emergency they will not be given medication that could precipitate an attack or even death.

acute intermittent p. **(AIP)** a hereditary, autosomal dominant, form of hepatic porphyria manifested by recurrent attacks of abdominal pain, gastrointestinal dysfunction, and neurologic disturbances, and by excessive amounts of δ-aminolevulinic acid and porphobilinogen in the urine; it is due to an abnormality of pyrrole metabolism. Called also intermittent acute porphyria.

congenital erythropoietic p. (CEP) a form of erythropoietic porphyria, with cutaneous photosensitivity leading to mutilating lesions, hemolytic anemia, splenomegaly, excessive urinary excretion of uroporphyrin and coproporphyrin, and invariably erythrodontia and hypertrichosis. Called also Günther disease.

p. cuta′nea tar′da (PCT) the most common form of porphyria, characterized by cutaneous photosensitivity that causes scarring bullae, discoloration, growth of facial hair, and sometimes sclerodermatous thickenings and alopecia; it is frequently associated with alcohol abuse, liver disease, or hepatic siderosis. Urinary levels of uroporphyrin and coproporphyrin are increased. There are two main types: an autosomal dominant (or *familial*) form in which activity of the affected enzyme is reduced to half normal in liver, erythrocytes, and fibroblasts; and a *sporadic* (but probably also familial) form in which the reduction is confined to the liver. Both types are believed to be heterozygous and clinical expression occurs in adulthood, precipitated by disease or environmental factors. A more severe homozygous form begins in childhood and is called hepatoerythropoietic porphyria.

erythropoietic p. porphyria in which excessive formation of porphyrin or its precursors occurs in bone marrow erythroblasts; the group includes congenital erythropoietic porphyria and erythropoietic protoporphyria.

hepatic p. porphyria in which the excess formation of porphyrin or its precursors is found in the liver; it includes acute intermittent porphyria, variegate porphyria, and hereditary coproporphyria.

hepatoerythropoietic p. (HEP) a severe homozygous form of porphyria cutanea tarda believed to result from an autosomal dominant defect in the same enzyme as is affected in porphyria cutanea tarda; it is clinically identical to that disease but onset is in early childhood and enzyme activity in liver, erythrocytes, and fibroblasts is virtually absent.

intermittent acute p. acute intermittent porphyria.

p. variega′ta, variegate p. (VP) a hereditary, autosomal dominant, type of hepatic porphyria characterized by chronic cutaneous manifestations, notably extreme

mechanical fragility of the skin, particularly areas exposed to the sunlight, and by episodes of abdominal pain and neuropathy. There is typically an excess of coproporphyrin and protoporphyrin in the bile and feces.

porphyrin (por′fĭ-rin) any of a group of iron- or magnesium-free cyclic tetrapyrrole derivatives, occurring universally in protoplasm, and forming the basis of the respiratory pigments of animals and plants; in combination with iron they form HEMES. Examples include COPROPORPHYRIN, HEMATOPORPHYRIN, PROTOPORPHYRIN, and UROPORPHYRIN. See also PORPHYRIA.

porphyrinogen (por″fĭ-rin′o-jen) the reduced form of a PORPHYRIN. The porphyrinogens are the functional intermediates in the biosynthesis of heme and if oxidized to their corresponding porphyrins, such as occurs in PORPHYRIAS, are irreversibly removed from the biosynthetic pathway and accumulate in tissues. Their nomenclature corresponds to that of the porphyrins.

porphyrinuria (por″fĭ-rĭ-nu′re-ah) excessive excretion of one or more PORPHYRINS in the urine; see PORPHYRIA.

porta (por′tah) [L.] an entrance or gateway, especially the site where blood vessels and other supplying or draining structures enter an organ; called also portal.

p. he′patis the transverse fissure on the visceral surface of the LIVER, where the portal vein and hepatic artery enter and the hepatic ducts leave. Called also portal fissure and transverse fissure.

portacaval (por″tah-ka′val) pertaining to or connecting the portal vein and inferior vena cava.

portal (por′tal) 1. porta. 2. pertaining to an entrance, especially the porta hepatis.

p. vein a short, thick trunk formed by the union of the superior mesenteric, inferior mesenteric, and splenic veins behind the neck of the pancreas; it ascends to the right end of the porta hepatis, where it divides into successively smaller branches, following branches of the hepatic artery, until it forms a capillary system of sinusoids that permeates the entire substance of the liver.

portio (por′she-o) [L.] a part or division.

p. vagina′lis cer′vicis ectocervix.

portoenterostomy (por″to-en″ter-os′tah-me) surgical anastomosis of the jejunum to a decapsulated area of liver in the porta hepatis region, and to the duodenum; done to establish a conduit from the intrahepatic bile ducts to the intestine in biliary atresia.

portogram (por′to-gram) the film obtained by portography.

POSITIONS OF THE FETUS IN VARIOUS PRESENTATIONS

Cephalic Presentation

Vertex—occiput the point of direction
Left occipitoanterior (LOA)
Left occipitotransverse (LOT)
Right occipitoposterior (ROP)
Right occipitotransverse (ROT)
Right occipitoanterior (ROA)
Left occipitoposterior (LOP)

Face—chin the point of direction
Right mentoposterior (RMP)
Left mentoanterior (LMA)
Right mentotransverse (RMT)
Right mentoanterior (RMA)
Left mentotransverse (LMT)
Left mentoposterior (LMP)

Brow—the point of direction
Right frontoposterior (RFP)
Left frontoanterior (LFA)
Right frontotransverse (RFT)
Right frontoanterior (RFA)
Left frontotransverse (LFT)
Left frontoposterior (LFP)

Breech or Pelvic Presentation

Complete breech—sacrum the point of direction (feet crossed and thighs flexed on abdomen)
Left sacroanterior (LSA)
Left sacrotransverse (LST)
Right sacroposterior (RSP)
Right sacroanterior (RSA)
Left sacroposterior (LSP)

Incomplete breech—sacrum the point of direction
Some designations as above, adding the qualifications footling, knee, etc.

Transverse Lie or Shoulder Presentation

Shoulder—scapula the point of direction
Left scapuloanterior (LScA)   Back
Right scapuloanterior (RScA)   anterior
                                 positions

Right scapuloposterior (RScA)   Back
Left scapuloposterior (LScA)   posterior
                                 positions

portography (por-tog′rah-fe) radiography of the portal vein after injection of opaque material.

portal p. portography after injection of opaque material into the superior mesenteric vein or one of its branches, the abdomen being opened.

splenic p. portography after percutaneous injection of opaque material into the substance of the spleen.

portosystemic (por″to-sis-tem′ik) connecting the portal and systemic venous circulation.

Porto-Vac (por′to-vak) trademark for a portable wound suction device that is compressed to create a gentle suction; as the unit expands a negative pressure is created, allowing fluids and debris to be evacuated.

porus (por′us) [L.] pore.

p. acus′ticus exter′nus the outer end of the external acoustic meatus.

p. acus′ticus inter′nus the opening of the internal acoustic meatus in the cranial cavity.

p. op′ticus the opening in the sclera for passage of the optic nerve.

-posia word element [Gr.], *intake of fluids.*

position (pŏ-zish′un) 1. a bodily posture or attitude. 2. the relationship of a given point on the presenting part of the fetus to a designated point of the maternal pelvis; see accompanying table. See also PRESENTATION.

anatomical p. that of the human body standing erect, palms facing forward; it is the position of reference in designating site or direction of structures of the body. The anatomical position for quadrupeds is standing with all four feet on the ground; the difference between animal and human anatomical position leads to confusion among terms indicating position and direction. (See accompanying illustration.)

batrachian p. a lying position of infants in which the lower limbs are flexed, abducted, and resting on the bed on their outer aspects, resembling the legs of a frog.

Bozeman's p. the knee-elbow position with straps used for support.

decubitus p. that of the body lying on a horizontal surface, designated according to the aspect of the body touching the surface as *dorsal decubitus* (on the back), *left* or *right lateral decubitus* (on the left or right side), and *ventral decubitus* (on the anterior surface). In radiology, the patient is placed in either the right or left lateral decubitus position with the beam perpendicular to the long axis of the body.

dorsal recumbent p. position of patient on the back, with lower limbs flexed and rotated outward; used in vaginal examination, application of obstetrical forceps, and other procedures. See illustration.

Fowler's p. a position in which the head of the patient's bed is raised 30 to 90

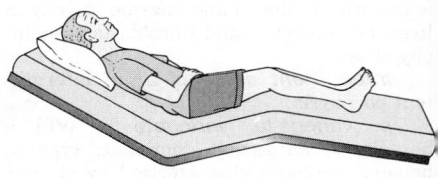

Low Fowler's.

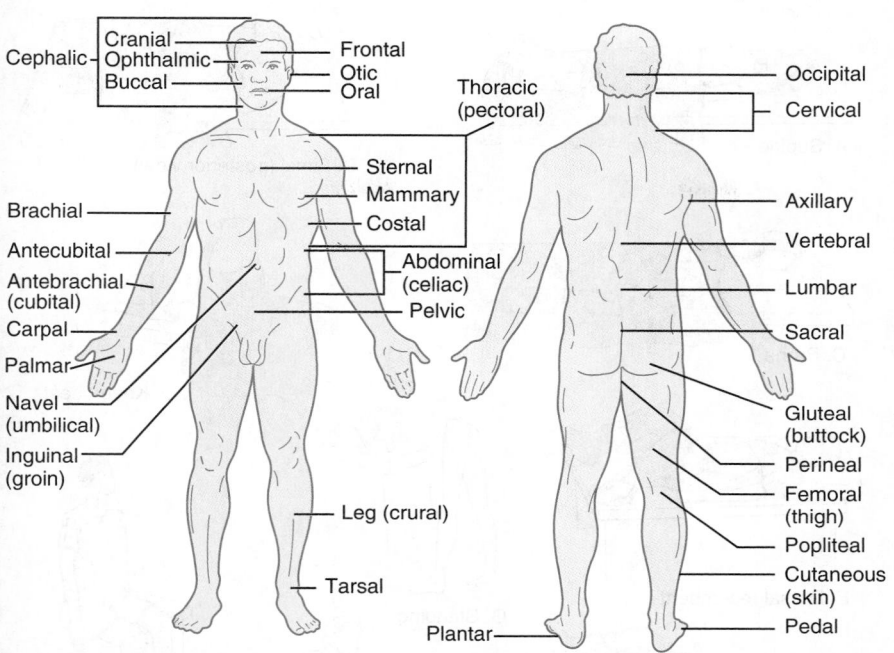

Cephalic { Cranial · Ophthalmic · Buccal
Frontal
Otic
Oral
Thoracic (pectoral)
Occipital
Cervical
Sternal
Mammary
Costal
Brachial
Antecubital
Antebrachial (cubital)
Carpal
Palmar
Abdominal (celiac)
Pelvic
Axillary
Vertebral
Lumbar
Sacral
Navel (umbilical)
Inguinal (groin)
Gluteal (buttock)
Perineal
Femoral (thigh)
Leg (crural)
Popliteal
Cutaneous (skin)
Tarsal
Pedal
Plantar

The body in the anatomical poisition, showing regions of the body. From Applegate, 2000.

degrees above the level, with the knees sometimes also elevated. See illustration.

froglike p. batrachian position.

knee-chest p. the patient rests on the knees and chest with head is turned to one side, arms extended on the bed, and elbows flexed and resting so that they partially bear the patient's weight; the abdomen remains unsupported, though a small pillow may be placed under the chest. See illustration.

knee-elbow p. the patient resting on the knees and elbows with the chest elevated.

lateral p. Sims' position.

lithotomy p. the patient lies on the back with the legs well separated, thighs acutely flexed on the abdomen, and legs on thighs; stirrups may be used to support the feet and legs. See illustration.

orthopneic p. a position assumed to relieve ORTHOPNEA (difficulty breathing except when in an upright position); the patient assumes an upright or semivertical position by using pillows to support the head and chest, or sits upright in a chair.

prone p. a position with the patient lying face down with arms bent comfortably at the elbow and padded with the arm-boards positioned forward. See accompanying illustration.

reverse Trendelenburg p. a supine position with the patient on a plane inclined with the head higher than the rest of the body and appropriate safety devices such as a footboard.

Rose's p. one intended to prevent aspiration or swallowing of blood, as from an injured lip: the patient is supine with head hanging over the end of the table in full extension so as to enable bleeding to be over the margins of the inverted upper incisors.

semi-Fowler p. a position similar to Fowler's POSITION but with the head less elevated.

Sims p. the patient lies on the left side with the left thigh slightly flexed and the right thigh acutely flexed on the abdomen; the left arm is behind the body with the body inclined forward, and the right arm is positioned according to the patient's comfort. See illustration. Called also lateral position.

Sims recumbent p. a variant of the Sims POSITION in which the patient lies on the left side in a modified left lateral position; the upper leg is flexed at hip and knees, the lower leg is straight, and the upper arm rests in a flexed position on the bed.

P

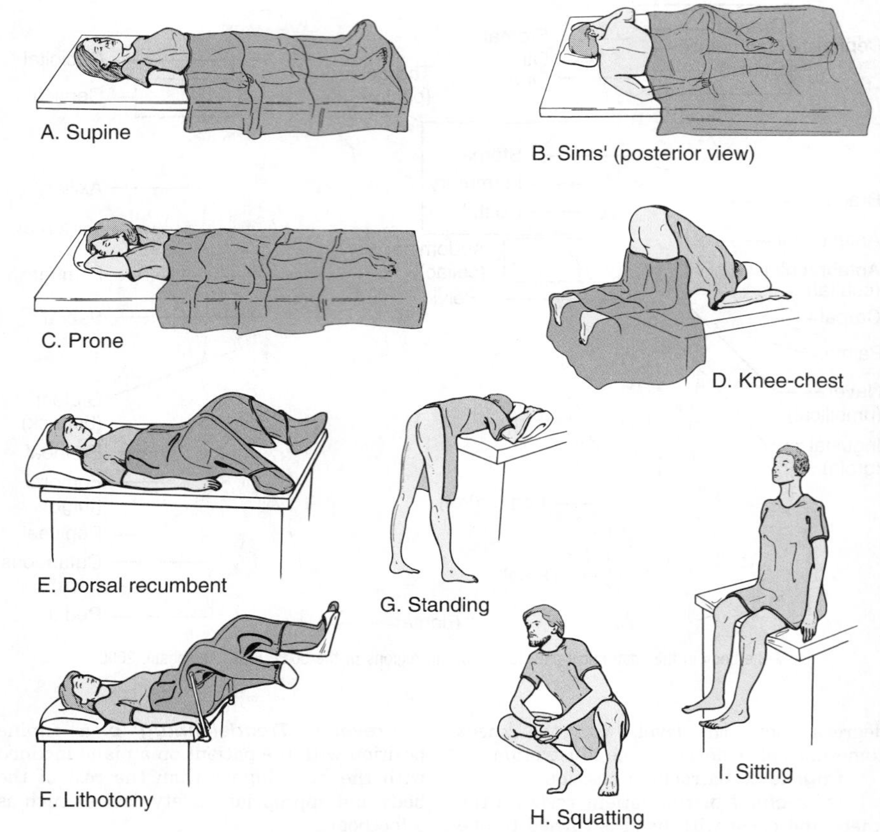

A. Supine

B. Sims' (posterior view)

C. Prone

D. Knee-chest

E. Dorsal recumbent

G. Standing

F. Lithotomy

H. Squatting

I. Sitting

Common examination positions. From Lammon et al., 1995.

Trendelenburg's p. the patient is on the back on a table or bed whose upper section is inclined 45 degrees so that the head is lower than the rest of the body; the adjustable lower section of the table or bed is bent so that the patient's legs and knees are flexed. There is support to keep the patient from slipping. See illustration.

positioning (pŏ-zĭ′shun-ing) in the NURSING INTERVENTIONS CLASSIFICATION, a nursing INTERVENTION defined as deliberate placement of the patient or a body part to promote physiological and/or psychological well-being.

intraoperative p. in the NURSING INTERVENTIONS CLASSIFICATION, a nursing INTERVENTION defined as moving the patient or body part to promote surgical exposure while reducing the risk of discomfort and complication.

neurologic p. in the NURSING INTERVENTIONS CLASSIFICATION, a nursing INTERVENTION defined as the achievement of optimal, appropriate body alignment for the patient experiencing or at risk for spinal cord injury or vertebral irritability.

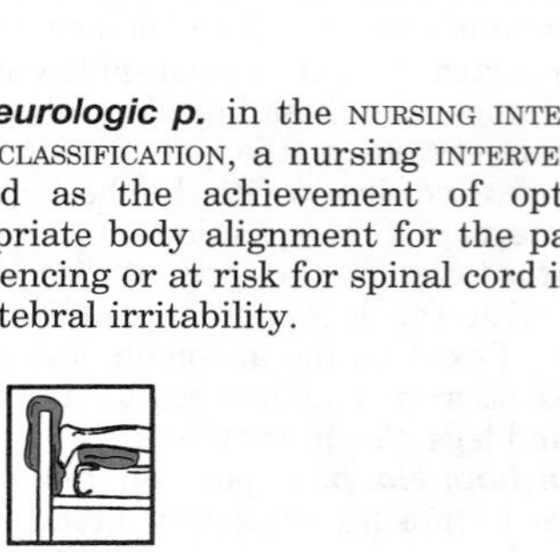

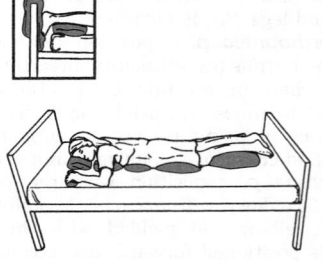

Prone position. From Lammon et al., 1995.

wheelchair p. in the NURSING INTERVENTIONS CLASSIFICATION, a nursing INTERVENTION defined as the placement of a patient in a properly selected wheelchair to enhance comfort, promote skin integrity, and foster independence.

positive (poz'ĭ-tiv) 1. having a value greater than zero. 2. indicating existence or presence, as chromatin-positive or Wassermann-positive. 3. characterized by affirmation or cooperation.

positron (poz'ĭ-tron) the antiparticle of the ELECTRON. When a positron is emitted by a radionuclide it combines with an electron and both undergo annihilation, producing two 511-keV gamma RAYS traveling in opposite directions. This effect is used in positron emission TOMOGRAPHY.

posology (po-sol'ah-je) the science of dosage or a system of dosage. adj., **posolog'ic.**

post- word element [L.], *after; behind.*

postauricular (pōst″aw-rik'u-lar) located or performed behind the auricle of the ear.

postaxial (pōst-ak'se-al) behind an axis; in anatomy, referring to the medial (ulnar) aspect of the upper limb, and the lateral (fibular) aspect of the lower limb.

postbrachial (pōst-bra'ke-al) on the posterior part of the upper limb.

postcapillary (pōst-kap'ĭ-lar″e) 1. located just to the venous side of a capillary. 2. venous capillary.

postcardiotomy (pōst-kahr″de-ot'ah-me) occurring after open-heart surgery.

postcava (pōst-ka'vah) inferior VENA CAVA. adj., **postca'val.**

postcibal (pōst-si'bal) postprandial.

postcoital (pōst-koi'tahl) after COITUS.

postcommissurotomy syndrome (pōst-kom″ĭ-sher-ot'ah-me) fever, chest pain, pleuritis, pericarditis, and pneumonia, occurring frequently in patients who have undergone mitral commissurotomy, and sometimes related to cytomegalic inclusion disease.

postconcussional syndrome physical and personality changes that may occur following a head injury. They may include amnesia, headache, dizziness, difficulty concentrating, restlessness, depression, irritability, sweating, heart palpitations, and insomnia.

postcordial (pōst-kor'de-al) behind the heart.

postcornu (pōst-kor'nu) the posterior horn of the lateral ventricle.

postdiastolic (pōst-di″as-tol'ik) after diastole.

postdicrotic (pōst″di-krot'ic) after the dicrotic wave of the sphygmogram.

poster(o)- word element [L.], *the back; posterior to.*

posterior (pos-tēr'e-or) directed toward or situated at the back; opposite of ANTERIOR. Called also dorsal.

posteroanterior (pos″ter-o-an-tēr'e-or) directed from the back toward the front; called also dorsoventral.

posteroexternal (pos″ter-o-ek-ster'nal) situated on the outside of a posterior aspect.

posteroinferior (pos″ter-o-in-fe're-or) behind and below.

posterolateral (pos″ter-o-lat'er-al) situated on the side and toward the posterior aspect.

posteromedian (pos″ter-o-me'de-an) situated on the middle of a posterior aspect.

posterosuperior (pos″ter-o-soo-pe're-or) situated behind and above.

postganglionic (pōst″gang-gle-on'ik) distal to a ganglion.

posthioplasty (pos'the-o-plas″te) plastic repair of the prepuce.

posthitis (pos-thi'tis) inflammation of the prepuce.

posthypnotic (pōst″hip-not'ik) following the hypnotic state.

postictal (pōst-ik'tal) following a seizure.

postmaturity (pōst″mah-chu'rĭ-te) the condition of an infant after a prolonged gestation period. adj., **postmature'.**

postmenopausal (pōst″men-o-paw'zal) after the menopause.

postmitotic (pōst″mi-tot'ik) occurring after or pertaining to the time following mitosis.

post mortem (pōst mor'tem) [L.] after death.

postmortem (pōst-mor'tem) performed or occurring after death.

Care of the body after death (postmortem care) is an essential component of the total care of the patient and surviving family members and friends. Specific policies and procedures for postmortem care are a matter of agency policy, local customs, and cultural and religious ritual.

Physical care of the body is based on certain changes that take place at a fairly predictable rate, depending on body temperature at the time of death, and environmental temperature once death has taken place. The size of the body and the presence or absence of bacterial infection also influence these changes.

Rigor mortis is the first of these changes after cessation of circulation and respiration. Within two to four hours after death depletion of glycogen stores prevents synthesis of adenosine triphosphate (ATP). Without ATP the muscle fibers do not relax, resulting in rigid contraction of the fibers and immobilization of the joints. The rigor first occurs in the involuntary muscles and then involves the voluntary musculature, starting with the head and neck and descending gradually to the trunk and lower extremities. The process usually takes about 45 hours and continues for about 96 hours.

Another noticeable change is cooling of the body, which occurs rather rapidly once circulation stops and the heat-regulating center in the brain no longer is functioning. This postmortem loss of body heat is called *algor mortis.*

Decomposition of the tissues begins almost as soon as blood supply stops. With the breakdown of hemoglobin, discoloration, or *livor mortis,* appears as mottled, reddened areas that can be mistaken for bruises, particularly in the extremities or other parts of the body where there is pooling of blood. As deterioration of tissues continues and bacterial fermentation occurs, the tissues soften and then liquefy. Refrigeration or some other method of cooling the body inhibits this process.

postnatal (pōst-na′tal) occurring after birth, with reference to the newborn.

postoperative (pōst-op′er-ah-tiv) after a surgical operation.

p. care care of the patient following a surgical procedure. Immediately after surgery the patient usually is transferred to a postanesthesia care UNIT (PACU), a special unit designed to facilitate management of the patient recovering from anesthesia and staffed with personnel experienced in this.

Immediately after surgery, the patient requires constant attendance. A patent AIRWAY must be maintained so that respiration is adequate. An ENDOTRACHEAL TUBE and VENTILATOR may be used to assist the patient with respiratory difficulties. The skin is observed for color, turgor, and dryness. A flaccid, parchmentlike skin indicates dehydration, cold clammy skin may be symptomatic of shock, and cyanosis and local discoloration are indicative of oxygen deficiency occurring as a result of an obstructed airway or impaired circulation. The pulse, respirations, and blood pressure are checked every 15 minutes or more often; notes are made as to their quality, rate, and rhythm. (See accompanying table.)

The position of the patient is governed by the type of surgery done, but ideally the patient should be placed in a lateral or side-lying position with a pillow to the back for support. The uppermost leg is slightly flexed to relieve tension on the abdominal muscles and may be supported with a small pillow. The side-lying position allows for drainage of mucus or other material in the mouth and lessens the danger of aspiration of vomitus. During vomiting the head is kept turned to the side and suctioning is used as necessary to clear the air passages. The patient's position should be changed at least every 2 hours unless there is a contra-indication, and pressure areas are gently massaged. In repositioning the patient, all movements should be gentle and slow, as sudden overstimulation can cause a drop in blood pressure.

While the patient is awakening from anesthesia the hospital personnel must use caution in their conversations and statements made about the patients in the unit. With the senses dulled and reasoning hampered by drugs and anesthesia, the patient may misinterpret the sounds and statements that are overheard. Noise must be kept at a minimum and voices should be kept low. Whispering (which is rude at any time) is especially disturbing to the patient recovering from anesthesia.

In many cases a catheter, nasogastric tube, or surgical drain is inserted during surgery. The purposes of these should be understood by the nurse and it is usually the nurse's responsibility to connect them to the proper drainage and suction apparatus. Dressings around drainage tubes should be observed for excess drainage or bleeding and reinforced as necessary.

Common problems, goals, and interventions are shown in the accompanying table. For complications that may arise during the postoperative period, see also SHOCK, HEMORRHAGE, THROMBOSIS, EMBOLISM, and CARDIAC ARREST.

postparalytic (pōst″par-ah-lit′ik) following an attack of paralysis.

post partum (pōst″ pahr′tum) [L.] after childbirth.

postpartum (pōst-pahr′tum) occurring after childbirth, with reference to the mother.

p. pituitary necrosis necrosis of the pituitary during the postpartum period, resulting from an infarct; it is often associated with shock and excessive uterine bleeding during delivery, and leads to variable patterns of hypopituitarism. Called also Sheehan's syndrome.

postpericardiectomy syndrome (pōst-per″e-kahr″de-ek′tah-me) delayed pericardial or pleural reaction, with fever, chest pains, and signs of pleural and/or pericardial inflammation, following opening of the pericardium.

postphlebitic syndrome (pōst-flĕ-bit′ik) a form of chronic venous stasis that follows an episode of PHLEBITIS, owing to

POSTOPERATIVE CARE: COMMON PROBLEMS AND INTERVENTIONS

Problem	Goal	Intervention
Potential for injury related to infection of surgical wound	Infection will be avoided	Dressings changed under sterile technique; reinforced using clean technique; soiled dressings promptly removed from room; hands washed before and after each contact with patient; drainage maintained via surgical drain, tubes; wound cleansed as indicated; patient and wound assessed regularly for symptoms and signs of infection
Potential for delay in healing related to circulatory and respiratory stasis; nutrients deficient	Healing will occur as expected	Reinforce preoperative teaching: encourage deep breathing, coughing, leg exercises, ambulation; monitor vital signs q4h; encourage patient to eat nutritious foods and supplements that are served
Potential for fluid and electrolyte imbalance	Fluid and electrolyte balance restored and maintained as evidenced by clinical signs and symptoms, measured fluid intake and output, and laboratory test data	Monitor incisional drainage; evaluate amount, color of drainage in suction apparatus and on dressing; measure fluid intake and output; monitor IVs; monitor laboratory data; encourage oral intake of fluids when allowed
Alteration in comfort related to surgical trauma	Comfort expressed verbally and nonverbally	Assess pain location, type, intensity; administer analgesics as prescribed and promptly when requested or need is apparent
Potential for grieving over loss of body part Potential for alteration in self-concept, self-esteem, personal identity	Verbalization by patient of feelings of self-worth and confidence; ability to use effective coping mechanisms to deal with loss of body part	Have patient list strengths and positive aspects of life situation; have patient make list of positive self-statements; e.g., "I am the same person I was before surgery"; "My family and significant others love me and can show that love to me"; encourage assertive behavior in patient; involve family members in care

incompetent valves or occlusion in the veins. The patient usually experiences edema, lower limb discoloration, and pain. The most serious sequela of this condition is a stasis ULCER; poor circulation to the area makes such a lesion difficult to heal.

postpolio syndrome postpoliomyelitis syndrome.

postpoliomyelitis syndrome (pōst-po″le-o-mi-ĕ-li′tis) a group of symptoms of unknown etiology seen in patients several years to many years after they have recovered from the major illness of POLIOMYELITIS; it includes new weakness, fatigue, and pain, either generalized or limited to the parts that were affected by the poliomyelitis. Called also postpoliomyelitis sequela.

postprandial (pōst-pran′de-al) after a meal; called also postcibal.

postpuberal (pōst-pu′ber-al), **postpubertal** (pōst-pu′ber-t'l) occurring in or pertaining to the period following puberty.

postpubescent (pōst″pu-bes′ent) after puberty.

postrenal (pōst-re′nal) 1. located behind a kidney. 2. occurring after leaving a kidney, such as renal failure that results from processes impairing normal excretion of urine after it has been formed. See also PRERENAL.

postsinusoidal (pōst″si-nŭ-soi′d'l) located beyond a sinusoid or affecting the circulation beyond a sinusoid; used especially to denote the location of vascular resistance in portal hypertension.

poststenotic (pōst″stĕ-not′ik) located or occurring distal to or beyond a stenosed segment.

postsynaptic (pōst″sĭ-nap′tik) distal to or occurring beyond a synapse.

post-trauma syndrome a NURSING DIAGNOSIS accepted by the North American Nursing Diagnosis Association, defined as the experiencing by an individual of a sustained maladaptive response to an overwhelming traumatic event or events such as a natural disaster, war, epidemic, rape, assault, or catastrophic illness or accident. See also POSTTRAUMATIC STRESS DISORDER.

risk for p.-t. s. a NURSING DIAGNOSIS accepted by the North American Nursing Diagnosis Association, defined as being at risk for sustained maladaptive response to a traumatic, overwhelming event.

posttraumatic (pōst″traw-mat′ik) following injury.

p. stress disorder PTSD; an ANXIETY DISORDER caused by exposure to an intensely traumatic event, such as rape or assault, military combat or bombing of civilians, torture, death camps, natural disasters, terrible accidents, developmentally inappropriate sexual experiences, or life-threatening illness. Characteristics include reexperiencing the traumatic event in recurrent intrusive recollections, nightmares, or flashbacks; avoidance of trauma-associated stimuli and a generalized numbing of emotional responsiveness; and hyperalertness with difficulty in sleeping, remembering, or concentrating. The onset of symptoms may be delayed for months to years after the event.

postulate (pos′tu-lat) anything assumed or taken for granted.

p. of causality the postulate that every phenomenon has a cause or causes; i.e., that events do not occur at random but in accordance with physical laws so that in principle causes can be found for each effect.

Koch's p's a statement of the kind of experimental evidence required to establish the causative relation of a given microorganism to a given disease. The conditions are: 1, the microorganism is present in every case of the disease; 2, it is to be cultivated in pure culture; 3, inoculation of such culture must produce the disease in susceptible animals; 4, it must be obtained from such animals, and again grown in a pure culture.

postural (pos′chur-al) pertaining to posture or position.

p. drainage a technique in which the patient assumes one or more positions that will facilitate the drainage of secretions from the bronchial airways. The procedure uses gravity to move secretions toward the trachea, where they can be coughed up more easily. Choice of position is based on radiologic studies and auscultatory evidence of pooled secretions. Variations of the most effective position are adapted to the patient's general physical condition, tolerance, and pulmonary status.

External manipulation of the thorax includes PERCUSSION (or "clapping,") and VIBRATION, often done in conjunction with postural drainage; they may be done either manually or with mechanical devices. Percussion involves rhythmic striking of the chest wall over the area being drained. The manual method is done with hands cupped, fingers flexed, and thumbs held tightly against index fingers. If done properly, a hollow sound is heard and there is no discomfort to the patient.

Vibration is done immediately after percussion and is directed to the same area. While the patient performs a prolonged exhalation through pursed lips, the therapist presses the flat of the hands or the mechanical device against the thorax in a downward movement toward the midline of the body. This is repeated four or five times. While neither percussion nor vibration is a difficult technique to master, anyone attempting to assist the patient in this manner should have instruction and practice beforehand. The purpose of both activities is to dislodge plugs of mucus, allowing air to penetrate behind them and thus aid in their removal.

The American Association for Respiratory Care has published clinical guidelines, which are available on their web site at http://www.aarc.org. These indicate that BRONCHOSPASM is sometimes a complication of external manipulation of the thorax.

posture (pos′chur) an attitude of the body. Good posture cannot be defined by a rigid formula; it is usually considered to be the natural and comfortable bearing of the body in normal, healthy persons. This means that in a standing position the body is naturally, but not rigidly, straight, and that in a sitting position the back is comfortably straight. Good standing and sitting posture helps promote normal functioning of the body's organs and increases the efficiency of the muscles, thereby minimizing fatigue. (See illustration.) Maintenance of good posture for a patient confined to bed or wheelchair is essential to the patient's general wellbeing and also is important in the prevention of deformities of the muscles and bones. The patient should be observed for evidence of "slumping," in which the normal curves of the spine are exaggerated. The rib cage should be supported so that the ribs are elevated and there is no constriction of the chest wall. Pillows are arranged under the shoulders and head so that the chin is not forced downward on the chest. Excessive extension of the ankles

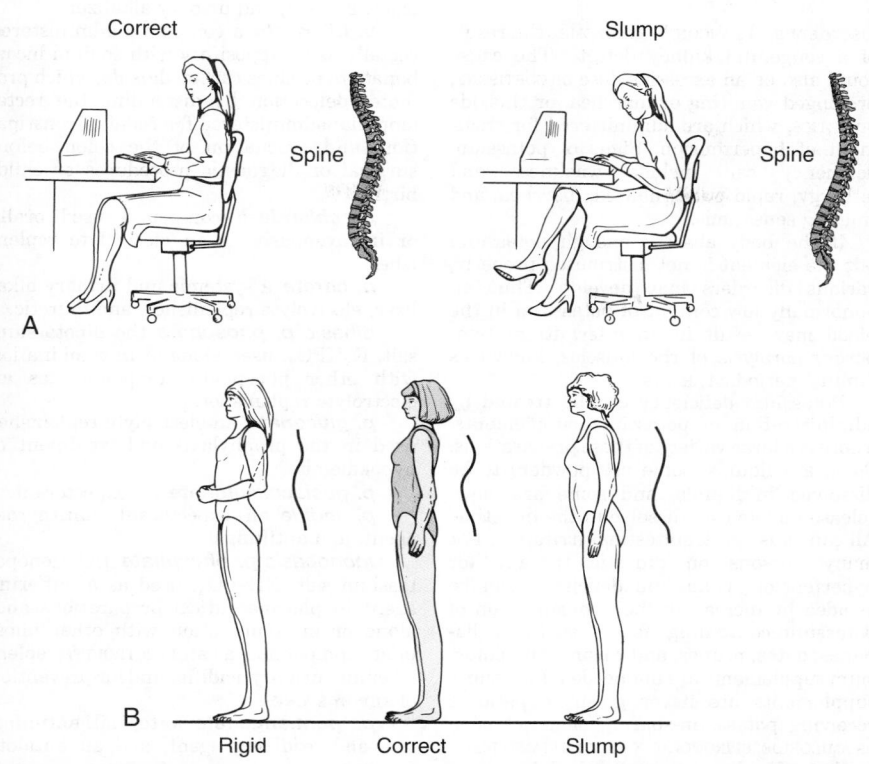

Correct   Slump

Spine   Spine

A

Rigid   Correct   Slump

A, Left, Good sitting posture: the spine and feet are in normal positions and the weight of the body is equally distributed. *Right,* Slouching puts too much weight on the end of the spine, compresses internal organs, strains muscles, and interferes with the circulation in the legs. *B,* Correct standing posture, *center,* is easy and natural. The chest is slightly raised and the buttocks are tucked in. *Left,* Too rigid posture. Keeping the spine unnaturally straight can cause strain on the knees and back muscles. *Right,* Slumping can lead to backache and round shoulders.

should be avoided by adequate support against the soles of the feet. The legs should be supported so that the weight of one does not fall on the other. The arms are supported so that they do not lie across the chest or pull the shoulders into a rounded position. Frequent changing of position and adequate exercise of the limbs are also essential to the maintenance of good posture and the prevention of deformities.

posturing (pos'chur-ing) the assumption of abnormal patterns of flexion and extension in a patient with severe brain injury. See also DECEREBRATE RIGIDITY and DECORTI-CATE RIGIDITY.

    decerebrate p. see DECEREBRATE RIGID-ITY.

posturography (pos″cher-og′rah-fe) testing procedures for upright posture, balance, and sense of equilibrium, done with the patient standing on a force PLATFORM.

potable (po′tah-b'l) fit to drink.

potassemia (pot″ah-se′me-ah) hyperkalemia.

potassium (K) (po-tas′e-um) a chemical element, atomic number 19, atomic weight 39.102. (See Appendix 6.) In combination with other minerals in the body, potassium forms alkaline salts that are important in body processes and play an essential role in maintenance of the acid-base and water balance in the body. All body cells, especially muscle tissue, require a high content of potassium. A proper balance between SODIUM, CALCIUM, and potassium in the blood plasma is necessary for proper cardiac function.

    Since most foods contain a good supply of potassium, potassium deficiency (HYPOKA-LEMIA) is unlikely to be caused by an unbalanced diet. Possible causes include CUSHING'S SYNDROME (due to an adrenal gland disorder) and FANCONI'S SYNDROME (the result of a congenital kidney defect). The cause could also be an excessive dose of CORTISONE, prolonged vomiting or diarrhea, or thiazide DIURETICS, which are administered for treatment of hypertension. Signs of potassium deficiency can include weakness and lethargy, rapid pulse, nausea, diarrhea, and tingling sensations.

If the body absorbs enough potassium but the element is not distributed properly, various disorders may develop. Thus an abnormally low content of potassium in the blood may result in an intermittent temporary paralysis of the muscles, known as familial periodic PARALYSIS.

Potassium deficiency can be treated by administration of potassium supplements. There is a large variety of these preparations. Some are liquids, some are powders to be dissolved in liquids, and some are slow-release tablets that dissolve in the intestine. All can cause gastrointestinal irritation. For many persons on diuretic therapy for hypertension, potassium deficiency can be avoided by increasing their consumption of potassium-containing foods, such as bananas, dates, prunes, and raisins, and potassium supplements are not needed. Potassium supplements are never given to patients receiving potassium-sparing DIURETICS such as AMILORIDE, SPIRONOLACTONE, or TRIAMTERENE. If the difficulty lies in the body's use of potassium, treatment is concerned with the primary cause of the deficiency.

p. acetate an electrolyte replenisher and systemic and urinary alkalizer.

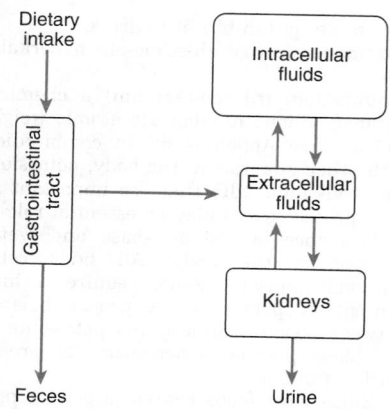

Dietary intake

Intracellular fluids

Gastrointestinal tract

Extracellular fluids

Kidneys

Feces

Urine

Homeostatic balance of potassium. Through the functions of resorption and excretion, the kidneys are the best regulator of potassium balance in the extracellular fluids. From Malarkey and McMorrow, 2000.

p. bicarbonate an electrolyte replenisher, antacid, and urinary alkalizer.

p. bitartrate a compound administered rectally as a suppository with sodium bicarbonate to produce carbon dioxide, which promotes defecation by distending the rectal ampulla; administered for relief of constipation, and evacuation of the colon before surgical or diagnostic procedures or childbirth.

p. chloride a compound used orally or intravenously as an electrolyte replenisher.

p. citrate a systemic and urinary alkalizer, electrolyte replenisher, and diuretic.

dibasic p. phosphate the dipotassium salt, K_2HPO_4; used alone or in combination with other phosphate compounds as an electrolyte replenisher.

p. gluconate an electrolyte replenisher used in the prophylaxis and treatment of hypokalemia.

p. guaiacolsulfonate an expectorant.

p. iodide an expectorant, antithyroid agent, and antifungal.

monobasic p. phosphate the monopotassium salt, KH_2PO_4; used as a buffering agent in pharmaceutical preparations and, alone or in combination with other phosphate compounds, as an ELECTROLYTE replenisher and urinary acidifier and for prevention of KIDNEY STONES.

p. permanganate a topical antiinfective and oxidizing agent, and an antidote for many poisons.

p. phosphate a compound combining potassium and phosphoric acid, usually dibasic potassium phosphate.

p. sodium tartrate a compound used as a saline cathartic.

potency (po'ten-se) 1. power. 2. the ability of the male to perform coitus; see also IMPOTENCE. 3. the power of a medicinal agent to produce the desired effects. 4. the ability of an embryonic part to develop and complete its destiny. adj., **po'tent.**

potential (po-ten'shal) existing and ready for action, but not active. 1. electric tension or pressure.

action p. see ACTION POTENTIAL.

after-p. the period following termination of the spike POTENTIAL.

auditory evoked p. in electroencephalography, changes in waves in response to sound; see also brainstem auditory evoked POTENTIAL.

brainstem auditory evoked p. that portion of the auditory evoked POTENTIAL that comes from the BRAINSTEM; abnormalities can be analyzed to evaluate comas, to support diagnosis of multiple sclerosis, and to detect early posterior fossa tumors.

cognitive event–related p's a diagnostic study that uses electroencephalographic equipment and a computer dedicated to analyze brain wave P300; this wave is a measure of the brain's active cognitive processing of information. The patient is instructed to complete a task that requires attention and information processing. A recording of brain wave activity as well as information related to cognitive function is produced.

diastolic p. the transmembrane potential of the cell during electrical DIASTOLE.

maximal diastolic p. the most negative level attained during the cardiac CYCLE by the cell membrane of a fiber that does not have a constant resting potential, occurring at the end of phase 3 of the action potential. In pacemaker cells this is a point of hyperpolarization.

membrane p. the electric potential that exists on the two sides of a membrane or across the wall of a cell.

resting p., resting membrane p. the difference in potential across the membrane of a cell when it is at rest, i.e., fully repolarized. In cardiac physiology this occurs during electrical DIASTOLE in pacemaker cells and continuously in nonpacemaker cells.

spike p. the initial, very large change in potential of the membrane of an excitable CELL during excitation.

threshold p. the transmembrane potential that must be achieved before a membrane channel can open; it differs among the various cardiac membrane channels.

potentialization (po-ten″shal-ĭ-za′shun) potentiation (def. 1).

potentiation (po-ten″she-a′shun) enhancement of one agent by another so that the combined effect is greater than the sum of the effects of each one alone.

Pott's curvature (pots) abnormal posterior curvature of the spine occurring as a result of Pott's disease.

Pott's disease (pots) tuberculosis of the spine, usually beginning as a tuberculous OSTEOMYELITIS of the vertebrae and progressing to damage of the intervertebral disks. If erosion continues unchecked, there is complete destruction of the affected vertebrae. Symptoms include stiffness of the back, pain on motion, prominence of the spinous PROCESS of certain vertebrae, and occasionally abscess formation, paralysis, and abdominal pain. Diagnosis is confirmed by demonstration of *Mycobacterium tuberculosis* in the affected bone. Treatment includes administration of antibacterial

drugs such as isoniazid and streptomycin. Para-aminosalicylic acid (PAS) may be used instead of streptomycin if streptomycin is contraindicated. Surgical fixation of the affected vertebrae (spinal FUSION) may be required for correction of orthopedic deformities such as KYPHOSIS that may occur as a result of Pott's disease.

pouch (powch) a BAG or POCKET; see also CAVITY, RECESS, and SAC.

abdominovesical p. the pouchlike reflection of the peritoneum from the abdominal wall to the anterior surface of the bladder.

craniobuccal p., craniopharyngeal p. Rathke's pouch.

Douglas' p. Douglas' cul-de-sac.

Indiana p. a bladder surgically created using a segment of isolated, detubularized colon that may or may not be patched with small bowel. The ureters are implanted into the pouch in a non-refluxing manner. A continence stoma to the abdomen is created by intussusception of a small segment of bowel.

Kock p. see KOCK POUCH.

Prussak's p. a recess in the tympanic membrane between the flaccid part of the membrane and the neck of the malleus.

Rathke's p. a diverticulum from the embryonic buccal cavity from which the anterior lobe of the PITUITARY GLAND is developed. Called also craniobuccal or craniopharyngeal pouch.

rectouterine p. Douglas' cul-de-sac.

Seessel's p. an outpouching of the embryonic pharynx rostrad to the pharyngeal membrane and caudal to Rathke's pouch.

poudrage (poo-drahzh′) [Fr.] the application of powder to a surface, as between the visceral and parietal layers of the pericardium or pleura to promote their fusion in PLEURODESIS.

poultice (pōl′tis) a soft, moist mass about the consistency of cooked cereal, spread between layers of muslin, linen, gauze, or towels and applied hot to a given area in order to create moist local heat or COUNTERIRRITATION.

pound (lb) (pownd) 1. in the AVOIRDUPOIS SYSTEM, a unit of weight equal to 16 OUNCES (453.6 GRAMS). 2. in the APOTHECARIES' SYSTEM, a unit of weight equal to 12 OUNCES (373.2 GRAMS).

povidone (po′vĭ-dōn) a synthetic polymer used as a dispersing and suspending agent. Called also polyvinylpyrrolidone.

p.-iodine (PVP-I) a complex produced by reacting IODINE with the polymer

P

povidone; it slowly releases iodine and is used as a topical ANTIINFECTIVE agent.

powder (pow'der) an aggregation of particles, as that obtained by grinding or rubbing a solid.

power 1. capability; the ability to act. 2. the ability of a statistical test to detect statistically significant differences when they exist.

   durable p. of attorney for health care advance directives.

powerlessness (pow'er-les-nes'') a NURSING DIAGNOSIS accepted by the North American Nursing Diagnosis Association, defined as the perception that one's own action will not dignificantly affect an outcome; a perceived lack of control over a current situation or immediate happening. Factors leading to this feeling may include the patient's usual pattern of dealing with stress and conflict (such as dependence on others for decision-making), a lifelong sense of helplessness, an inability to use resources, and a lack of personal resources. The environment in which health care is provided can influence the recipient's perception of personal control. Institutional rules and regulations, autocratic caregivers, and social isolation can increase one's sense of powerlessness. Finally, inability to communicate because of a neurologic disorder, inability to care for oneself, and progressive debilitating disease in spite of compliance with prescribed regimen can contribute to a feeling that one has no control over what is happening.

   risk for p. a NURSING DIAGNOSIS accepted by the North American Nursing Diagnosis Association, defined as being at risk for perceived lack of control over a situation and/or one's ability to significantly affect an outcome.

pox (poks) any eruptive or pustular disease, especially one caused by a virus, such as CHICKENPOX, COWPOX, or SMALLPOX.

poxvirus (poks'vi''rus) any member of a family of morphologically similar and immunologically related DNA viruses, including the disease-causing ORTHOPOXVIRUSES.

PPD purified protein derivative (tuberculin).

PPLO pleuropneumonia-like organisms.

ppm 1. parts per million. 2. pulses per minute.

P-pulmonale (pul-mŏ-nă'le) an abnormal pattern seen on an electrocardiogram, associated with diffuse lung disease and acute pulmonary embolism; it consists of tall peaked P waves in the inferior leads and P axis to the right of + 70°.

Pr praseodymium.

practice (prak'tis) the exercise of a profession.

   collaborative p. communication, sharing, and problem solving between the physician and nurse as peers; this pattern of practice also implies a shared responsibility and accountability for patient care.

   differentiated p. the use of nursing staff in an acute care setting according to their expertise and qualifications.

   evidence-based p. provision of health care that incorporates the most current and valid research results.

   family p. the medical specialty of a family PHYSICIAN, concerned with the planning and provision of comprehensive primary health care, regardless of age or sex, on a continuing basis. Called also family medicine.

   general p. old term for comprehensive medical care regardless of age of the patient or presence of a condition that may require the services of a specialist; this term has now largely been replaced by the term *family practice.*

   nursing p. see NURSING PRACTICE.

practitioner (prak-tish'un-er) a person who practices a profession.

   multiskilled health p. a person who is cross-trained to provide more than one function, often in more than one discipline. These combined functions can be found in a broad spectrum of health-related jobs, ranging in complexity from the nonprofessional to the professional level and including both clinical and management functions. The additional functions added to the original health care worker's job may be of a higher, lower, or parallel level.

   nurse p. see NURSE PRACTITIONER.

Prader-Willi syndrome (prah'der vil'e) a congenital syndrome consisting of obesity, short stature, lack of muscle tone, hypogonadism, and central nervous system dysfunction. Information and support for families and individuals affected by this syndrome can be obtained from the Prader-Willi Syndrome Association U.S.A., 5700 Midnight Pass Road, Sarasota, FL 34242, telephone (800) 926–4797.

prae- for words beginning thus, see those beginning *pre-*.

pralidoxime (pral''ĭ-doks'ēm) a cholinesterase reactivator whose salts are used in treatment of ORGANOPHOSPHORUS COMPOUND POISONING; it also has limited value in counteracting overdosage of carbamate-type cholinesterase INHIBITORS in persons being treated for MYASTHENIA GRAVIS.

pramipexole (pram″ĭ-pek′sōl) a DOPAMINE agonist used in the form of the dihydrochloride salt in treatment of PARKINSON'S DISEASE, administered orally.

pramoxine (pră-mok′sēn) a local ANESTHETIC applied topically as the hydrochloride salt for temporary relief of pain and pruritus associated with skin and anorectal disorders.

prandial (pran′de-al) pertaining to a meal.

praseodymium (Pr) (pra″ze-o-dim′e-um) a chemical element, atomic number 59, atomic weight 140.907. (See Appendix 6.)

Prausnitz-Küstner reaction (prowz′nits kĕst′ner) an immediate HYPERSENSITIVITY reaction produced in a nonatopic subject by intradermal injection of serum from an atopic subject followed 12 or more hours later by an injection of antigen. Formerly the standard method of demonstrating reaginic antibody, this test is no longer used because of the risk of transmitting serum HEPATITIS and because serum IMMUNOGLOBULIN E can now be measured by in vitro assays.

pravastatin (prav′ah-stat″in) an ANTIHYPERLIPIDEMIC agent that acts by inhibiting cholesterol synthesis, used as the sodium salt in the treatment of HYPERCHOLESTEROLEMIA and other forms of DYSLIPIDEMIA and to lower the risks associated with ATHEROSCLEROSIS and CORONARY HEART DISEASE; administered orally.

praxiology (prak″se-ol′o-je) the science or study of conduct.

praxis (prak′sis) the conception and planning of a new action in response to an environmental demand.

feminist p. praxis done from a belief system involving ideas of mutual nurturance, nonviolence, and small groups working for change, with attention to emotions, communal life, reciprocity, and the development of persons over time. See also feminist THEORY.

praziquantel (pra″zĭ-kwon′tel) a broad-spectrum ANTHELMINTIC used for treatment of a wide variety of parasitic FLUKE and TAPEWORM infections; administered orally.

prazosin (prah′zo-sin) a postsynaptic ALPHA-ADRENERGIC BLOCKING AGENT that acts as a peripheral VASODILATOR; administered orally as the hydrochloride salt as an oral ANTIHYPERTENSIVE AGENT.

pre- word element [L.], *before* (in time or space).

preanesthetic (pre″an-es-thet′ik) 1. pertaining to preanesthesia. 2. an agent that produces preanesthesia. 3. occurring before the administration of an anesthetic.

preauricular (pre″aw-rik′u-ler) in front of the auricle of the ear.

preaxial (pre-ak′se-al) situated before an axis; in anatomy, referring to the lateral (radial) aspect of the upper limb, and the medial (tibial) aspect of the lower limb.

prebetalipoproteinemia (pre″ba″tah-lip″o-pro″tēn-e′me-ah) hyperprebetalipoproteinemia.

precancer (pre′kan-ser) a condition that tends to become malignant (see CANCER). adj., **precan′cerous.**

precapillary (pre-kap′ĭ-lar″e) 1. located just to the arterial side of a capillary. 2. arterial capillary.

precaution (pre-kaw′shun) a protective measure taken in advance.

airborne p's a group of transmission-based PRECAUTIONS used when caring for patients who have diseases that spread through the air, such as TUBERCULOSIS, CHICKENPOX, and MEASLES. The patient should be in a private room.

aspiration p's in the NURSING INTERVENTIONS CLASSIFICATION, a nursing INTERVENTION defined as the prevention or minimization of risk factors in the patient at risk for ASPIRATION.

bleeding p's in the NURSING INTERVENTIONS CLASSIFICATION, a nursing INTERVENTION defined as reduction of stimuli that may induce bleeding or HEMORRHAGE in at-risk patients.

cardiac p's in the NURSING INTERVENTIONS CLASSIFICATION, a nursing INTERVENTION defined as the prevention of an acute episode of impaired cardiac function by minimizing myocardial oxygen consumption or increasing myocardial oxygen supply. See also MYOCARDIAL INFARCTION.

circulatory p's in the NURSING INTERVENTIONS CLASSIFICATION, a nursing INTERVENTION defined as the protection of a localized area with limited PERFUSION.

contact p's a group of transmission-based PRECAUTIONS used when caring for patients who have diseases that spread through direct skin to skin contact or through indirect contact with contaminated equipment.

droplet p's a group of transmission-based PRECAUTIONS used when caring for patients who have diseases that spread by droplets or dust particles, such as by coughing, sneezing, or talking or during procedures such as suctioning and bronchoscopy. The diseases include RUBELLA, MUMPS, DIPHTHERIA, and INFLUENZA.

elopement p's in the NURSING INTERVENTIONS CLASSIFICATION, a nursing INTERVENTION defined as minimizing the risk of a patient leaving a treatment setting without

P

authorization when departure presents a threat to the safety of the patient or others.

embolus p's in the NURSING INTERVENTIONS CLASSIFICATION, a nursing INTERVENTION defined as the reduction of the risk of an EMBOLUS in a patient with thrombi or at risk for developing THROMBUS formation.

fire-setting p's in the NURSING INTERVENTIONS CLASSIFICATION, a nursing INTERVENTION defined as the prevention of fire-setting behaviors.

isolation p's see ISOLATION PRECAUTIONS.

laser p's in the NURSING INTERVENTIONS CLASSIFICATION, a nursing INTERVENTION defined as limiting the risk of injury to the patient related to use of a LASER.

latex p's in the NURSING INTERVENTIONS CLASSIFICATION, a nursing INTERVENTION defined as reducing the risk of systemic reaction to LATEX. See also latex ALLERGY.

malignant hyperthermia p's in the NURSING INTERVENTIONS CLASSIFICATION, a nursing INTERVENTION defined as prevention or reduction of malignant HYPERTHERMIA (hypermetabolic response to pharmacologic agents used during surgery).

pneumatic tourniquet p's in the NURSING INTERVENTIONS CLASSIFICATION, a nursing INTERVENTION defined as applying a pneumatic TOURNIQUET while minimizing the potential for patient injury from use of the device.

seizure p's in the NURSING INTERVENTIONS CLASSIFICATION, a nursing INTERVENTION defined as prevention or minimization of potential injuries sustained by a patient with a known SEIZURE disorder.

standard p's a classification of ISOLATION PRECAUTIONS that replaces the former classifications of universal PRECAUTIONS and measures used for isolation of moist body products.

subarachnoid hemorrhage p's in the NURSING INTERVENTIONS CLASSIFICATION, a nursing intervention defined as the reduction of internal and external stimuli or stressors to minimize the risk of rebleeding prior to ANEURYSM surgery.

surgical p's in the NURSING INTERVENTIONS CLASSIFICATION, a nursing INTERVENTION defined as minimizing the potential for iatrogenic injury to the patient related to a surgical procedure.

transmission-based p's ISOLATION PRECAUTIONS used when caring for patients with highly transmissible or epidemiologically important pathogens; these constitute additional measures beyond standard PRECAUTIONS. There are three types, depending on the type of disease the patient has: airborne PRECAUTIONS, droplet PRECAUTIONS, and contact PRECAUTIONS.

universal p's a group of measures formerly recommended for protection of noninfected individuals against bloodborne infections such as hepatitis B VIRUS and human immunodeficiency VIRUS, now replaced by the measures called standard PRECAUTIONS.

precava (pre-ka′vah) superior VENA CAVA. adj., **preca′val.**

preceptor (pre-sep′ter) a person who guides, tutors, and provides direction aimed at a specific performance.

employee p. in the NURSING INTERVENTIONS CLASSIFICATION, a nursing INTERVENTION defined as assisting and supporting a new or transferred employee through a planned orientation to a specific clinical area.

student p. in the NURSING INTERVENTIONS CLASSIFICATION, a nursing INTERVENTION defined as assisting and supporting learning experiences for a student.

preceptorship (pre-sep′ter-ship) a shorter-term relationship between a student as novice and an experienced staff person (such as a professional nurse) as the PRECEPTOR who provides individual attention to the student's learning needs and feedback regarding performance; students experience relative independence in making decisions, setting priorities, management of time, and patient care activities.

prechordal (pre-kor′d'l) in front of the notochord.

precipitant (pre-sip′ĭ-tant) a substance that causes precipitation.

precipitate (pre-sip′ĭ-tāt) 1. to cause settling in solid particles of a substance in solution. 2. a deposit of solid particles settled out of a solution. 3. to cause an event or occurrence. 4. (pre-sip′i-tat) occurring with undue rapidity, as precipitate labor.

precipitation (pre-sip″ĭ-ta′shun) the act or process of precipitating.

p. test precipitin test.

precipitin (pre-sip′ĭ-tin) an antibody to antigen that specifically aggregates the antigen in vivo or in vitro to give a visible precipitate.

p. reaction a reaction involving the specific serologic precipitation of an antigen in solution with its specific antiserum in the presence of electrolytes. The reaction is used in the typing of PNEUMOCOCCUS strains, in testing whether blood is human or animal, and for diagnostic purposes.

p. test any test in which the positive reaction consists of the formation and deposit of a precipitate in the fluid being tested. See also precipitin REACTION.

precipitinogen (pre-sip″ĭ-tin′o-jen) an antigen that stimulates the formation of and reacts with a precipitin.

precision (pre-sizh′un) 1. the quality of being sharply or exactly defined. 2. in statistics, the extent to which a measurement procedure gives the same results each time it is repeated under identical conditions.

preclinical (pre-klin′ĭ-k′l) before a disease becomes clinically recognizable.

preclotting (pre-klot′ing) the forcing of a patient's blood through the interstices of a knitted vascular prosthesis prior to implantation to render the graft temporarily impervious to blood by disposition of fibrin and platelets in the interstices; after implantation, fibrous ingrowth from the recipient replaces the fibrin-platelet network.

precocity (pre-kos′ĭ-te) unusually early development of mental or physical traits. adj., **preco′cious.**

precognition (pre″kog-nish′un) the extrasensory perception of a future event.

precoma (pre-ko′mah) the neuropsychiatric state preceding coma, as in hepatic encephalopathy. adj., **precom′atose.**

preconscious (pre-kon′shus) the part of the mind that is not in immediate awareness but can be consciously recalled with effort, one of the systems of Freud's topographic model of the mind.

precordium (pre-kor′de-um), pl. *precor′-dia* [L.] the region over the heart and lower thorax; adj., **precor′dial.**

precostal (pre-kos′t′l) in front of the ribs.

precuneus (pre-ku′ne-us) [L.] a small convolution on the medial surface of the parietal lobe of the cerebrum.

precursor (pre-ker′ser) something that precedes. In biological processes, a substance from which another, usually more active or mature substance, is formed. In clinical medicine, a sign or symptom that heralds another.

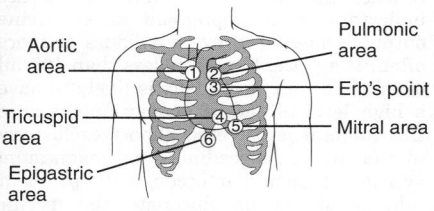

Precordial points of the heart. From Lammon et al., 1995.

prediabetes (pre-di″ah-be′tēz) a state of latent impairment of carbohydrate metabolism in which the criteria for diabetes mellitus are not all satisfied.

prediastole (pre″di-as′to-le) the interval immediately preceding diastole. adj., **prediastol′ic.**

predicrotic (pre″di-krot′ik) occurring before the dicrotic wave of the sphygmogram.

predigestion (pre″di-jes′chun) partial artificial digestion of food before its ingestion into the body.

predisposition (pre-dis″po-zish′un) a latent susceptibility to disease which may be activated under certain conditions.

prediverticular (pre-di″ver-tik′u-ler) denoting a condition of thickening of the muscular wall of the colon and increased intraluminal pressure without evidence of diverticulosis.

prednicarbate (pred″nĭ-kahr′bāt) a synthetic corticosteroid used topically for the relief of inflammation and pruritus in certain dermatoses.

prednisolone (pred-nis′o-lōn) a synthetic GLUCOCORTICOID used in the form of the base or the acetate, sodium phosphate, or tebutate ester in replacement therapy for adrenocortical INSUFFICIENCY, as an ANTIINFLAMMATORY agent, and as an IMMUNOSUPPRESSANT.

prednisone (pred′nĭ-sōn) a synthetic GLUCOCORTICOID used as an ANTIINFLAMMATORY and IMMUNOSUPPRESSANT.

preeclampsia (pre″ĕ-klamp′se-ah) a pathologic condition of late pregnancy characterized by edema, proteinuria, and hypertension; it is a precursor to eclampsia if not successfully treated. Called also toxemia of pregnancy and gestosis.

p.-eclampsia syndrome a group of symptoms associated with late pregnancy and encompassing both nonconvulsive and convulsive stages. Although the condition occurs in only 5 to 7 per cent of all pregnancies in the United States, it is the third most common cause of maternal mortality. Fetal mortality is also high because of the high incidence of premature delivery in these cases.

Etiologic Factors. This condition has sometimes been called TOXEMIA OF PREGNANCY because it was once believed that a toxin produced by the mother in response to a foreign protein from the fetus was responsible for the symptoms. This is not the case, although the cause of the syndrome is not known. Inadequate prenatal care and poor nutrition are suspected as contributing factors because the condition is more common in women who have a history of inadequate dietary intake, especially protein. It is also seen more often in primigravidas under the age of 20 or over 30, and in those who have had 5 or more pregnancies. Women who have a preexisting heart disease, diabetes mellitus with renal or vessel involvements, or essential hypertension are also at high risk for developing symptoms of hypertension, edema, and proteinuria.

Essentially, the pathology responsible for the elevation of blood pressure is spasm of the blood vessels. Normally, the blood vessels of a pregnant woman have a diminished response to the effects of such pressor substances as angiotensin and norepinephrine. In pregnancy-induced hypertension, resistance to vasospasm is somehow comprised and so blood pressure increases. It is not known whether the change in responsiveness to pressors is a cause or a result of vasospasm and elevated blood pressure.

Stages. For purposes of assessment and management, preeclampsia-eclampsia syndrome can be classified according to three stages: mild preeclampsia, severe preeclampsia, and eclampsia.

Mild Preeclampsia. This condition is characterized by a blood pressure reading of 140 mm Hg systolic, or an elevation of 30 mm Hg or more systolic or 15 mm Hg diastolic above the patient's prepregnancy level. The blood pressure readings are taken on two occasions 6 hours apart, with special attention to the diastolic pressure, which reflects peripheral vascular spasm.

Blood pressure can also be evaluated by determining the mean arterial pressure on two occasions at least 6 hours apart. A pregnant patient is considered hypertensive when her mean arterial pressure rises 15 mm Hg from her baseline or is over 100 mm Hg.

Pathologic changes in the glomeruli of the kidney produce proteinuria, oliguria, and edema. Increased permeability of the glomerular membrane allows passage of serum proteins into the urine (PROTEINURIA), diminished glomerular filtration lowers urine output, and increased reabsorption of sodium causes fluid retention and edema and weight gain.

Mild preeclampsia is said to be present when the patient has elevated blood pressure, proteinuria of 1+ or 2+ on a reagent test strip or 500 mg/24 hours or more, swelling in the upper part of her body rather than the usual ankle edema associated with pregnancy, and a weight gain of more than 1 kg (2 pounds) a week in the second trimester and 0.5 kg (1 pound) a week in the third trimester.

Mild preeclampsia is managed by bed rest to facilitate sodium excretion, which takes place more rapidly when the body is at rest. While resting in bed the patient is positioned on her left side to avoid pressure of the uterus against the vena cava and supine hypotension syndrome. Rest is often all that is needed to relieve the symptoms of mild preeclampsia. Some physicians also prescribe a high-protein diet to compensate for the protein lost in the urine and, perhaps, mild restriction of sodium intake. However, restriction of sodium can activate the angiotensin system and cause an undesirable elevation in blood pressure.

Diuretics are not used for control of edema because they can only aggravate the condition by increasing glomerular vessel permeability and stimulating angiotension activity.

Severe Preeclampsia. Preeclampsia becomes severe when systolic blood pressure is over 160 mm Hg or the diastolic pressure is over 110 mm Hg. To help establish the diagnosis two blood pressure readings are taken 6 hours apart after the woman has been on bed rest. Other symptoms are a marked increase in proteinuria, a 24-hour urinary output of 400 ml or less, visual disturbances, and marked hyperreflexia. Hospitalization is recommended to assure adequate rest, provide a quiet, nonstimulating environment, and monitor the progress of the mother and fetus. If more conservative measures fail, MAGNESIUM SULFATE is given to promote excretion of fluid, reduce blood pressure, and forestall convulsive seizures. In addition to its cathartic properties, magnesium sulfate acts as a central nervous system depressant and therefore reduces the possibility of convulsions. The serum level of magnesium must be kept fairly constant between 4.0 and 7.5 mEq/L to achieve the desired anticonvulsant effect.

While magnesium sulfate is being administered, whether intravenously or intramuscularly, the patient must be monitored at frequent intervals to assess deep tendon reflexes and respiratory rate, which are indicators of its depressant effect. Urine output is measured every 4 hours or more often. If a patient excretes less than 100 ml of urine in four hours, she is likely to have a high level of serum magnesium because this mineral is excreted almost exclusively in the urine. In readiness for magnesium overdosage should it occur, a 10 per cent solution of calcium gluconate, the specific antidote for magnesium toxicity, should be on hand.

Other drugs that may be prescribed include hypotensive drugs to reduce blood pressure and sedatives such as PHENOBARBITAL to manage central nervous system irritability. Because of the high fetal and maternal morbidity and mortality associated with preeclampsia and eclampsia, the pregnancy is terminated as soon as feasible.

Eclampsia. If the patient's condition continues to deteriorate and edema worsens, she becomes eclamptic. Cerebral edema predisposes her to CONVULSIONS and COMA. Signs and symptoms that may signal progression to eclampsia include elevated body temperature, sudden rise in blood pressure, gastrointestinal symptoms produced by congestion of portal circulation, and severe headache, blurred vision, and other signs of increased central nervous system irritability. The patient with eclampsia is critically ill. She is kept under constant surveillance, with her vital signs recorded at least every hour. All of the measures presented above for severe preeclampsia are instituted for management of eclampsia. Because of the potential for injury during convulsions, safety measures must be taken and preparations made for the possibility of a seizure. The comatose patient must be given the special care needed by anyone in a coma.

Maternal mortality from eclampsia is distressingly high. The cause of death can be cerebral HEMORRHAGE, circulatory COLLAPSE, or RENAL FAILURE. Mothers who survive eclampsia and the birth of their babies can continue to have hypertension for 10 to 14 days after delivery. Follow-up care is needed to evaluate residual or preexisting hypertension and renal disease and to initiate long-term management as indicated.

Infant mortality also is high when the mother is eclamptic. The status of the fetus is closely monitored before delivery to assure that HYPOXIA and life-threatening ACIDOSIS do not develop. When it is necessary to deliver the infant before term, problems of low birth weight and prematurity must be managed.

preexcitation (pre-ek″si-ta′shun) abnormal premature activation of part of the ventricular myocardium, signifying conduction of some of the activating impulses by routes outside the normal ones.

prefrontal (pre-frun′t′l) 1. situated in the anterior part of the frontal region or lobe. 2. the central part of the ethmoid bone.

preganglionic (pre″gang-gle-on′ik) proximal to a ganglion.

pregenital (pre-jen′ĭ-t′l) pertaining to the early stages of psychosexual development (oral and anal), before the genitals have become the dominant influence on sexual behavior.

pregnancy (preg′nan-se) the condition of having a developing EMBRYO or FETUS in the body, after union of an OOCYTE (OVUM) and SPERMATOZOON. The average GESTATION PERIOD for a human pregnancy is 10 lunar months (280 days) from the first day of the last menstrual period.

Conception. Once a month an ovum (secondary oocyte) matures in one of the OVARIES and travels down the nearby FALLOPIAN TUBE to the UTERUS; this process is called OVULATION. At FERTILIZATION, which must take place within a day or two of ovulation, one of the spermatozoa unites with the ovum to form a ZYGOTE. The zygote then implants itself in the wall of the uterus, which is richly supplied with blood, and begins to grow. (See also REPRODUCTION.)

Signs of Pregnancy. Usually the first indication of pregnancy is a missed menstrual period. Unless the period is more than 10 days late, however, this is not a definite indication, since many factors, including a strong fear of pregnancy, can delay menstruation. Nausea, or MORNING SICKNESS, usually begins in the fifth or sixth week of pregnancy. About 4 weeks after conception, changes in the breasts become noticeable: there may be a tingling sensation in the breasts, the nipples enlarge, and the areolae (dark areas around nipples) may become darker. Frequent urination, another early sign, is the result of expansion of the uterus, which presses on the bladder.

Other signs of pregnancy include softening of the cervix and filling of the cervical canal with a plug of mucus. Early in labor this plug is expelled and there is slight bleeding; expulsion of the mucous plug is known as SHOW and indicates the beginning of cervical dilatation. CHADWICK'S SIGN of pregnancy refers to a bluish color of the vagina which is a result of increased blood supply to the area.

When the abdominal wall becomes stretched there may be a breaking down of elastic tissues, resulting in depressed areas in the skin which are smooth and reddened. These markings are called STRIAE GRAVIDARUM. In subsequent pregnancies the old striae appear as whitish streaks and frequently do not disappear completely.

There are several fairly accurate laboratory tests for pregnancy; all are designed to detect human chorionic GONADOTROPIN (hCG), a hormone produced by living chorionic placental tissue and evident in the blood and urine of pregnant women. See also PREGNANCY TESTS.

P

Growth of the Fetus. The average pregnancy lasts about 280 days, or 40 weeks, from the date of conception to childbirth. Since the exact date of conception usually is not known, the *estimated date of delivery* can be calculated using NÄGELE'S RULE. This is approximate, since pregnancy may be shorter than the average or can last as long as 300 days. (For stages of growth of the fetus, see FETUS.)

Care of the Fetus. A host of influences can adversely affect the growth and development of the fetus and his or her chances for survival and good health after birth. The diet of the mother should be nutritious and well-balanced so that the fetus receives the necessary food elements for development and maturity of body structures. It is especially important that the mother receive adequate protein in her diet, because a protein deficiency can hamper fetal intellectual development. Supplemental iron and vitamins usually are recommended during pregnancy.

There is now less emphasis on severe restriction of the mother's dietary intake to maintain a limited weight gain. The average gain is about 28 lb during pregnancy, and either starvation diets or forced feedings can be unhealthy for the mother and hazardous for the fetus. Ideally, the mother should achieve normal weight before she becomes pregnant because obesity increases the possibility of ECLAMPSIA and other serious complications of pregnancy. Mothers who are underweight are more likely to deliver immature babies who, by virtue of their physiologic immaturity, are more likely to suffer from birth defects, HYALINE MEMBRANE DISEASE, and other developmental disorders of the newborn.

Other factors affecting the fetus include certain drugs taken by the mother during pregnancy. A well-known example is thalidomide, which inhibits the growth of the extremities of the fetus, resulting in gross deformities. Many drugs, including prescription as well as nonprescription medications, are now believed to be capable of causing fetal abnormalities. In addition, consumption of alcohol during pregnancy may result in FETAL ALCOHOL SYNDROME. Most health care providers recommend that all drugs be avoided during pregnancy except those essential to the control of disease in the mother.

Diseases that increase the risk of obstetrical complications include diabetes, heart disease, hypertension, kidney disease, and anemia. RUBELLA (German measles) can be responsible for many types of birth defects, particularly if the mother contracts it in the first 3 months of pregnancy. Sexually transmitted diseases can have tragic effects on the baby, even though the symptoms in the mother are minor at the time of pregnancy. SYPHILIS is particularly dangerous because it is one of the few diseases that can be transmitted to the fetus in utero. The baby is either stillborn or born infected, and rarely escapes physical or mental defects or both. Successful treatment of the mother before the fifth month of pregnancy will prevent infection in the infant.

During the birth process the infant may be infected with GONORRHEA as it passes through the birth canal. Gonorrheal infection of the eyes can cause blindness. HERPES SIMPLEX Type II involving the genitals of the mother can also be transmitted to the infant at birth. The mortality and morbidity rates for such infected infants are high.

The age of the mother is also an important factor in the well-being of the fetus. The mortality and morbidity rate for infants born of mothers below age 15 and above 40 are higher than for those of mothers between these ages.

Recently developed tests to monitor fetal health have taken much of the guesswork out of predicting the chances of survival and health status of the fetus after birth. Such tests and evaluation techniques include AMNIOCENTESIS, chemical and hormonal assays, biophysical profiles, testing for alpha-fetoprotein, ultrasound examinations, electronic surveillance of fetal vital signs and reaction to uterine contractions, and analyses of the infant's blood during labor.

Prenatal Care. The care of the mother during her entire pregnancy is important to her well-being and that of the fetus she is carrying. It will help provide ease and safety during pregnancy and childbirth. The health care provider learns about the patient's physical condition and medical history, and can detect possible complications before they become serious.

On the first prenatal visit the patient's medical history is taken in considerable detail, including any diseases or operations she has had, the course of previous pregnancies, if any, and whether there is a family history of multiple births or of diabetes mellitus or other chronic diseases. The first visit also includes a thorough physical examination and measurement of the pelvis. Blood samples are taken for screening for rubella and sexually transmitted diseases such as syphilis, hepatitis B, chlamydiosis, infection by the human immunodeficiency virus, and other conditions.

A complete blood count is also needed. Urine is tested for albumin and sugar and examined microscopically. On subsequent visits the patient brings a urine specimen, collected upon arising that morning, to be tested for albumin and glucose. At each prenatal visit her blood pressure is taken and recorded and she is weighed. In the second trimester, when the uterus becomes an abdominal organ, the height of the fundus is measured at each visit. After the sixth month a rule such as MCDONALD'S RULE can be applied to assess fetal growth.

Patients who are considered high-risk mothers usually are sent to a specialist and the infant is delivered at a regional hospital where sophisticated monitoring equipment and laboratory tests are available, and specially trained personnel can attend to the needs of the mother and her infant.

Discomforts and Complications. MORNING SICKNESS usually appears in the early months of pregnancy and rarely lasts beyond the third month. Often it requires no treatment or can be relieved by such simple measures as eating dry crackers and tea before rising. Indigestion and heartburn are best prevented by avoiding foods that are difficult to digest, such as cucumbers, cabbage, cauliflower, spinach, onions, and rich foods. Constipation usually can be corrected by diet or a mild laxative; strong laxatives should not be used unless prescribed by the health care provider.

A visit to a dentist early in pregnancy is a good idea to forestall any possibility of infection arising from tooth decay. Pregnancy does not encourage tooth decay. Hemorrhoids sometimes occur in pregnancy because of pressure from the enlarged uterus on the veins in the rectum. The health care provider should be consulted for treatment. VARICOSE VEINS also result from pressure of the uterus, which restricts the flow of blood from the legs and feet. Lying flat with the feet raised on a pillow several times a day will help relieve swelling and pain in the legs. In more difficult cases the health care provider may prescribe an elastic bandage or support stockings.

Backache during pregnancy is caused by the heavy abdomen pulling on muscles that are not normally used, and can be relieved by rest, sensible shoes, and good posture. Swelling of the feet and ankles usually is relieved by rest and by remaining off the feet for a day or two. If the swelling does not disappear, the health care provider should be informed since it may be an indication of a more serious complication.

Shortness of breath is common in the later stages of pregnancy. If at any time it

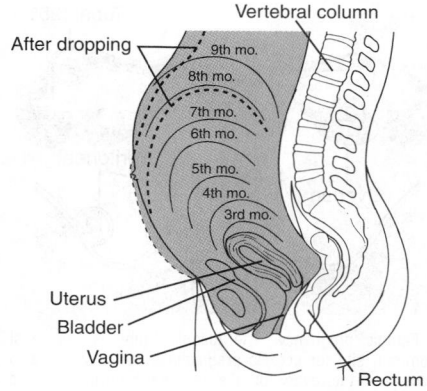

Uterine levels in pregnancy.

becomes so extreme that the woman cannot climb a short flight of stairs without discomfort, the health care provider should be consulted. If a mild shortness of breath interferes with sleep, lying in a half-sitting position, supported by several pillows, may help.

The more serious complications of pregnancy include PYELITIS, HYPEREMESIS GRAVIDARUM, ECLAMPSIA, and PLACENTA PREVIA and ABRUPTIO PLACENTAE.

abdominal p. ectopic pregnancy within the peritoneal cavity.

ampullar p. ectopic pregnancy in the ampulla of the fallopian tube.

cervical p. ectopic pregnancy within the cervical canal.

combined p. simultaneous intrauterine and extrauterine pregnancies.

cornual p. pregnancy in a horn of the uterus.

ectopic p. pregnancy in which the fertilized ovum becomes implanted outside the uterus instead of in the wall of the uterus; this is almost always in a fallopian tube *(tubal pregnancy)*, although occasionally the ovum develops in the abdominal cavity, ovary, or cervix uteri. Called also extrauterine pregnancy.

In a tubal pregnancy a spontaneous abortion may occur, but more often the fetus will grow to a size large enough to rupture the tube. This is an emergency situation requiring immediate treatment. The symptoms of such a tubal rupture are vaginal bleeding and severe pain in one side of the abdomen. Prompt surgery is necessary to remove the damaged tube and the fetus, and to stop the bleeding. Fortunately, the removal of one tube usually leaves the

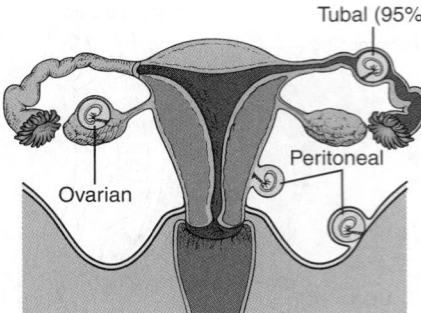

Ectopic pregnancy. The fallopian tube is the most common site for ectopic pregnancies but they can also occur on the ovary or the peritoneal surface of the abdominal cavity. From Damjanov, 2000.

other one intact, so that future pregnancy is possible. Patients who are Rh-negative should be given Rh₀ (D) immune globulin (RhoGAM) after ectopic pregnancy for iso-immunization protection in future pregnancies.

extrauterine p. ectopic pregnancy.

false p. development of all the signs of pregnancy without the presence of an embryo; called also pseudocyesis and pseudopregnancy.

interstitial p. pregnancy in that part of the fallopian tube within the wall of the uterus.

intraligamentary p., intraligamentous p. ectopic pregnancy within the broad ligament.

molar p. conversion of the fertilized ovum into a mole.

multiple p. the presence of more than one fetus in the uterus at the same time.

mural p. interstitial pregnancy.

ovarian p. pregnancy occurring in an ovary.

phantom p. false pregnancy due to psychogenic factors.

surrogate p. one in which a woman other than the female partner is artificially impregnated with the male partner's sperm. The resultant child represents only the male of the marital unit, and may be adopted by the female.

p. tests procedures for early determination of pregnancy. By the first missed menstrual period or shortly thereafter, human CHORIONIC GONADOTROPIN (hCG), a hormone secreted by the placenta, is present in the blood and urine of a pregnant woman. It was formerly determined by bioassay in which a urine or serum specimen was injected into a laboratory animal and the response of ovarian tissue was noted. All testing now uses immunologic techniques based on antigen-antibody binding between hCG and anti-hCG antibody. There are several commercial kits available (see EARLY PREGNANCY TESTS), based on the agglutination of hCG-coated latex particles by anti-hCG serum, which is inhibited if the urine specimen added to the serum contains hCG. Clinical laboratories generally use RADIO-IMMUNOASSAY or radioreceptor ASSAY to determine serum hCG levels. These methods are more accurate and less likely to produce false-positive results.

tubal p. the most common type of ectopic PREGNANCY, occurring within a FALLOPIAN TUBE.

tuboabdominal p. ectopic pregnancy occurring partly in the fimbriated end of the fallopian tube and partly in the abdominal cavity.

tubo-ovarian p. pregnancy at the fimbriae of the fallopian tube.

pregnane (preg′nān) a crystalline saturated steroid hydrocarbon; β-*pregnane* is the form from which several hormones, including progesterone, are derived; α-*pregnane* is the form excreted in the urine.

pregnanediol (preg″nān-di′ol) a crystalline, biologically inactive end product of PROGESTERONE metabolism, found especially in the urine of pregnant women and during the premenstrual and luteal phases of the menstrual cycle.

pregnanetriol (preg″nān-tri′ol) a metabolite of 17-hydroxyprogesterone; its excretion in the urine is greatly increased in disorders of the adrenal cortex such as adrenal hyperplasia.

pregnant (preg′nant) with child; having a developing embryo or fetus within the uterus; called also gravid.

prehallux (pre-hal′uks) a supernumerary bone of the foot growing from the medial border of the scaphoid.

prehensile (pre-hen′sil) adapted for grasping or seizing.

prehension (pre-hen′shun) the act of grasping.

prehormone (pre-hor′mōn) prohormone.

prehypophysis (pre″hi-pof′ĭ-sis) the anterior lobe of the PITUITARY GLAND.

preictal (pre-ik′t'l) occurring before a stroke, seizure, or attack.

preicteric (pre″ik-ter′ik) preceding the appearance of jaundice (icterus).

preinvasive (pre″in-va′siv) not yet invading tissues outside the site of origin.

prekallikrein (pre-kal″ĭ-kre′in) a plasma protein that is the proenzyme of plasma KALLIKREIN; it is cleaved to its active enzyme form by activated COAGULATION FACTOR XII.

preleukemia (pre″loo-ke′me-ah) a stage of bone marrow dysfunction preceding the development of acute myelogenous leukemia. adj., **preleuke′mic.**

prelimbic (pre-lim′bik) in front of a limbus.

preload (pre′lōd) the volume of blood in the ventricle at the end of diastole.

premalignant (pre″mah-lig′nant) precancerous.

Premarin (prem′ah-rin) trademark for preparations of conjugated ESTROGENS.

premature (pre″mah-chur′) born or interrupted before the state of maturity; occurring before the proper time.

prematurity (pre″mah-chur′ĭ-te) underdevelopment; the condition of a premature infant.

premaxilla (pre-mak′sĭ-lah) a separate element derived from the median nasal processes in the embryo, which later fuses with the maxilla.

premaxillary (pre-mak′sĭ-lar″e) 1. situated in front of the maxilla proper. 2. incisive bone.

premedication (pre″med-ĭ-ka′shun) preliminary medication, particularly that administered to produce reversible central nervous system depression prior to general ANESTHESIA.

premenarchal (pre″mĕ-nar′k′l) occurring before establishment of menstruation.

premenstrual (pre-men′stroo-al) preceding MENSTRUATION.

    p. dysphoric disorder PREMENSTRUAL SYNDROME viewed as a psychiatric disorder.

    p. syndrome **(PMS)** the presence of symptoms in the period before menstruation or in the early days of the menstrual period; also called premenstrual tension. Definition and diagnosis depend on the timing and the cyclic nature of symptoms rather than on specific clinical manifestations, which can vary greatly from one patient to another but follow a consistent pattern in the individual from cycle to cycle.

    Various psychological and emotional causes of this syndrome have been proposed; only recently has serious attention been paid to it as a physical as well as a psychological phenomenon. Research has shown that onset and increased severity of symptoms often occur when rapid hormonal changes are taking place, e.g., at puberty, after a pregnancy, or when oral contraceptives are discontinued. A transient increase in water retention seems to account for edema, weight gain, bloating, and breast changes. Other etiologic factors may be an estrogen-progesterone imbalance, hypoglycemia, vitamin deficiencies, prostaglandins, and psychogenic disturbances.

Symptoms. Symptoms may begin at the time of ovulation and increase until the menses, or they may appear at ovulation, abate, and then reappear and increase until menses. In some cases they arise only a few days before the onset of menstruation. In true PMS the symptoms cease with the onset of menses or last no more than a few days into the cycle.

    Premenstrual syndrome can affect virtually every system of the body and produce behavioral changes that have significant psychosocial impact. Physical symptoms may include headache, vertigo, or paresthesias; common colds, rhinitis, asthma, sinusitis, or sore throat; abdominal bloating, nausea, or food cravings; breast tenderness and engorgement; backache, joint pain, and edema; and others. Psychological or emotional symptoms may include irritability, tiredness with sleep disturbance, mood swings, depression, and altered libido.

Treatment. Successful management of the syndrome is difficult and protocols vary greatly, probably because there is no clear understanding of the causes. Therapies include progesterone therapy, administration of vitamin B_6 daily, and curtailment of intake of sodium, methylxanthines (coffee, tea, and chocolate), and nicotine. Additionally, the patient may be advised to restrict the intake of refined sugar, alcohol, and animal fats. Increasing the intake of vegetable oils may be recommended in order to enhance prostaglandin formation.

Patient Care. A major goal of intervention is the promotion of self-care strategies. For example, the patient is encouraged to keep a menstrual calendar to validate cyclic changes and to give her a sense of purposeful management of her life. She may then plan to avoid stressful events during the time symptoms are present. Counseling can help identify sources of stress and effective mechanisms to deal with stressful situations. Sufficient sleep and rest are needed because fatigue tends to exaggerate the symptoms. Moderate exercise can increase the patient's sense of well-being. A nutritious diet is also helpful, especially the inclusion of foods that are natural sources of the B vitamins and magnesium. The intake of sodium, caffeine, and refined sugar should be limited and alcohol and tobacco avoided.

    Severe premenstrual symptoms can seriously disrupt vital human relationships, leading to domestic problems including child abuse and other acts of violence. Health care providers will need to be aware

P

of the psychosocial ramifications of premenstrual syndrome and to facilitate positive coping behaviors, make referrals to agencies prepared to deal with these kinds of problems, and provide support and counseling when indicated.

premenstruum (pre-men'stroo-um) the period immediately before menstruation.

premolar (pre-mo'ler) 1. in front of the molar teeth. 2. premolar tooth; see TOOTH. Called also bicuspid.

premorbid (pre-mor'bid) occurring before the development of disease.

premunition (pre″mu-nish'un) resistance to infection by the same or closely related pathogen established after an acute infection has become chronic, and lasting as long as the infecting organisms are in the body. adj., **premu'nitive.**

premyeloblast (pre-mi'ĕ-lo-blast″) a precursor of a myeloblast.

prenatal (pre-na't'l) preceding birth.

preoperative (pre-op'er-ah-tiv) preceding an operation.

p. care the psychologic and physiologic preparation of a patient before an operation. The preoperative period may be extremely short, as with an emergency operation, or it may encompass several weeks during which diagnostic tests, specific medications and treatments, and measures to improve the patient's general well-being are employed in preparation for surgery. (See accompanying tables.)

Psychologic Aspects. Although patients react in their own unique ways to the news that they are going to have surgery, all patients experience some degree of anxiety and fear—fear of the unknown, worry over disability or death, and apprehension about the insecurity of their own and their family's future.

Much of this anxiety can be relieved if the various aspects of preoperative and postoperative care and the type of surgery planned are explained to the patient. The

PREOPERATIVE CARE: COMMON PROBLEMS AND INTERVENTIONS

Problem	Goal	Intervention
Anxiety, fear of disfigurement, diagnosis and prognosis, death	Patient and family can openly discuss fears and anxieties; patient will verbalize feeling less afraid of diagnosis and surgical procedure; preoperative and postoperative diagnosis will be accepted and dealt with by positive coping mechanisms	Encourage patient and family members to discuss fears and anxieties about surgery, diagnosis, and death; establish rapport with patient and family; answer questions honestly; help patient identify specific fears and deal with each one separately; assist with identification of irrational thoughts; encourage patient to stop irrational and anxiety-producing thoughts; teach patient relaxation and deep-breathing techniques to reduce anxiety
Spiritual distress	Patient and family able to identify and utilize resources for spiritual support and consolation	Notify pastoral counselor of patient's desire to see him or her; provide time and privacy for family prayer; join them when invited; encourage patient to talk about and use sources of spiritual strength and consolation
Lack of knowledge about surgical routines and what is expected of patient and family	Patient and family can verbalize anticipated routines and expectations for their participation in postoperative care	Provide information to patient about: Routine preoperative procedures for physical preparation; technical information about surgical procedure, location of incision, dressings, drains, wound suction; Expected time of surgery, probable length of procedure, where family will wait, and other concerns of family; Information about recovery room; postoperative pain and availability of relief; daily care routines; coughing, deep breathing, exercises, ambulation; participation of family in postoperative care

surgeon usually explains the surgical procedure and assists the patient in planning rehabilitation. The anesthesiologist usually reviews the type of anesthesia to be used and the general effects it will have on the patient. The nursing staff explains the hospital routine, specific nursing procedures necessary, the purpose of diagnostic tests required, and the types of equipment that will be used during the preoperative and postoperative periods. The nurse can demonstrate interest in the patient and family by answering questions (or referring them to the surgeon), and giving them a general idea of how long the patient will be away from his or her room during surgery and recovery from anesthesia. It is reassuring for patients to know, for example, that oxygen administration, blood transfusions, and the use of a nasogastric tube or catheter do not necessarily indicate a critical situation. The use of various pieces of equipment that seem "routine" to the hospital staff may be extremely upsetting to patients and their families if they do not understand why the equipment is necessary.

Spiritual reinforcement during this period may be very important to some patients, and without giving the impression of prying into the patient's private affairs, the nurse must also show a willingness to assist patient and family in obtaining a spiritual advisor if they indicate such a desire. The nurse must always respect the individual patient's beliefs and convictions whether sharing them or not, and must support patients in their search for spiritual reassurance and guidance.

Legal Aspects. Any patient undergoing surgery, whether it is expected to be major or minor surgery, must sign an operative permit. Patients have the right to know the type of surgery intended and its expected outcome, aftereffects, and possible complications. If an individual is underage, mentally incompetent, or unconscious, the permit is signed by a relative or guardian. The permit protects the patient against unwanted surgery and operative procedures the patient does not understand. It protects the hospital staff and surgeon from legal claims that the surgery was done without the patient's permission or knowledge of what was to be done. The signed operative permit is placed in the patient's chart and is sent to the operating room with the patient.

Preventive Aspects. During the preoperative period the patient is instructed in coughing, turning, deep breathing, and exercises of the extremities. These techniques can be most effective in preventing many of the complications of surgery. Exercises to strengthen specific muscles in preparation for rehabilitation, as following AMPUTATION, for example, are begun well in advance so that the patient is in optimal condition to begin a program of rehabilitation as soon after surgery as possible. Other topics of instruction will depend on the anticipated needs of the patient during recovery from surgery.

PREOPERATIVE DIAGNOSTIC TESTS		
Test	Normal Ranges*	Purpose
Blood urea nitrogen	10 to 20 mg/dL	To identify impaired liver or kidney function or excessive protein or tissue catabolism
Chest x-ray study	No abnormal heart or lung lesions	To determine size and contour of heart, lungs, and major vessels
Creatinine	0.7 to 1.4 mg/dL	To identify acute or chronic renal disease
Electrocardiogram	Baseline rate and rhythm	To determine the electrical activity of the heart
Glucose	60 to 100 mg/dL	To identify hypoglycemia or hyperglycemia
Hematocrit	Female: 36 to 45 per cent Male: 39 to 51 per cent	To identity the presence and extent of anemia
Hemoglobin	Female: 12.0 to 15.0 g/dL Male: 13.0 to 17.0 g/dL	To identify the presence and extent of anemia
Partial thromboplastin time	35 to 45 seconds	To identify deficiencies of coagulation factors
Prothrombin time	11 to 18 seconds	To identify dysfunction of blood clotting (prothrombin level)
Serum chloride	96 to 106 mEq/L	To identify hyperchloremia, hypochloremia, or metabolic alkalosis
Serum potassium	3.5 to 5.0 mEq/L	To identify hyperkalemia or hypokalemia
Serum sodium	136 to 145 mEq/L	To identify hypernatremia, hyponatremia, dehydration, or overhydration

*May vary with different laboratories.

Physiologic Aspects. Except in emergency situations every effort is made to have the patient in a state of optimal health before surgery is performed. Specific diets, protein and vitamin supplements, and other measures to improve the nutritional status may be employed. Intravenous infusions and transfusions of whole blood or plasma may be necessary to improve the fluid and electrolyte status and blood volume. Infections should be brought under control before surgery if they cannot be eliminated completely. Accurate records of the patient's vital signs, blood pressure, and urinary output will assist the surgeon in diagnosing and correcting conditions that may adversely affect the patient's physiologic response to an operative procedure.

Physical Preparation. Hospital protocol and the preference of the surgeon dictate the procedures for physical preparation prior to surgery. Although studies have repeatedly shown that the removal of hair is not effective in preventing infection and actually may contribute to it by damaging the skin, some surgeons still order removal of hair from the operative site.

Restriction of food and fluids varies. Usually the patient is allowed a light evening meal and then given nothing by mouth after midnight the night before surgery. Other procedures for preparation of the gastrointestinal tract may include enemas and insertion of a nasogastric tube.

Preoperative Medications. Generally there are three types of drugs used prior to surgery: sedatives, such as one of the barbiturates, to promote relaxation and rest and to stabilize the blood pressure and pulse; drying agents, such as atropine and scopolamine, which decrease secretion of mucus in the mouth and throat; and narcotics, such as morphine and meperidine hydrochloride (Demerol), which promote relaxation and enhance the effects of the anesthetic.

Preoperative medications must be given at the exact time ordered because their strength, action, and duration are planned according to the type of anesthesia used.

Immediate Preoperative Care. Most institutions use a check list or clearance record for surgical procedures. This eliminates the danger of overlooking some aspect of the immediate preoperative preparation. Such an omission might delay surgery or result in legal problems. The operative permit must be signed by the patient or guardian or legal representative. This permit is necessary to protect the surgeon against claims of unauthorized surgery, and to protect the patient against surgery he would not willingly endorse.

The preoperative check list includes such items as laboratory tests and their findings, history and physical examination records, disposal of valuables, removal of dentures and their disposition, vital signs and blood pressure of the patient immediately before going to the operating room, and other specific information such as consultation for sterilization.

Unless a urinary catheter has been inserted, the patient is offered the bedpan just before being taken to the operating room. Hairpins, bobby pins, and combs are removed from the hair and the head is covered with a cap or scarf.

preparation (prep″ah-ra′shun) the act or process of making ready.

 childbirth p. in the NURSING INTERVENTIONS CLASSIFICATION, a nursing INTERVENTION defined as providing information and support to facilitate CHILDBIRTH and to enhance the ability of an individual to develop and perform the role of parent.

 surgical p. in the NURSING INTERVENTIONS CLASSIFICATION, a nursing INTERVENTION defined as providing care to a patient immediately prior to surgery and verification of required procedures or tests and documentation in the clinical record.

prepared childbirth an educational approach to LABOR and DELIVERY in which the parents are specially prepared for the event. The aim is for the mother to be awake and cooperative and for the father to assume an active and supportive role during the birth of their child. Called also natural, educated, or cooperative childbirth.

The underlying concept for all methods of prepared childbirth is education of the parents so that they can actively participate in and share the experience of childbirth. The methods of instruction may vary, but all proponents advocate a family-centered maternity care program. The benefits of this approach are believed to be a more comfortable pregnancy, a shorter period of labor, less trauma during birth, and a decrease in the morbidity and mortality rates among newborn infants.

Methods. One of the most widely used methods of prepared childbirth is the LAMAZE METHOD, named after the French obstetrician Fernand Lamaze, who adapted the Russian method of PSYCHOPROPHYLAXIS to his practice. The overall goal of psychoprophylaxis is use of the mind in prevention of pain and, more specifically, the modification of the perception of pain. The Read method of preparation, based on the teaching of Dr. Grantly Dick-Read, had its beginning earlier than the Lamaze method; its emphasis is on passivity of the mother and an interruption of the fear-tension-pain cycle. Another method is the psychosexual method of Sheila Kitzinger, which includes marriage counseling and encompasses all family interrelationships and their effect on childbirth and feminine sexual response.

Although there are variations in the underlying philosophies and the specific techniques that are characteristic of each method, all are concerned with helping both parents understand the birth process and their expected role during labor and delivery, with giving instruction in exercises to develop neuromuscular control and physical conditioning, and with teaching specific breathing patterns to be employed during the three stages of labor. The father is given instruction in the ways he can support his partner and promote her comfort during labor. Many of the techniques learned in childbirth classes can be used to reduce the effects of stress and to relieve the discomfort associated with tension in situations not related to childbirth. Most parents who have chosen prepared childbirth describe it as an exhilarating and emotionally satisfying experience.

preparedness (pre-păr′ed-nes) the state of being ready beforehand for a given event.

community disaster p. in the NURSING INTERVENTIONS CLASSIFICATION, a nursing INTERVENTION defined as preparing for an effective response to a large-scale DISASTER.

prepartal (pre-pahr′tal) antepartal.

prepatellar (pre″pah-tel′er) in front of the patella.

preprandial (pre-pran′de-al) before meals.

preproinsulin (pre″pro-in′soo-lin) the precursor of proinsulin, containing an additional polypeptide sequence at the N-terminal.

preproprotein (pre″-pro-pro′tēn) any precursor of a proprotein.

preprotein (pre-pro′tēn) a protein precursor that contains a signal peptide sequence; it is a nonpolar sequence at the head of the growing polypeptide chain and is required for its transfer into the cistern of the endoplasmic reticulum; the signal sequence is then cleaved to form the protein or proprotein.

prepuberal (pre-pu′ber-al), **prepubertal** (pre-pu′ber-t'l) before puberty; pertaining to the period of accelerated growth preceding gonadal maturity.

prepubescent (pre″pu-bes′ent) prepubertal.

prepuce (pre′pūs) foreskin. adj., **prepu′tial.**

p. of clitoris a fold capping the clitoris formed by union of the LABIA MINORA and the CLITORIS.

preputiotomy (pre-pu″she-ot′ah-me) incision of the prepuce of the penis to relieve PHIMOSIS.

preputium (pre-pu′she-um) foreskin.

prepyloric (pre″pi-lor′ik) just proximal to the pylorus.

prerenal (pre-re′nal) 1. located in front of a kidney. 2. pertaining to a process that occurs before the kidney is reached, such as acute renal failure in which the kidney does not receive adequate blood flow. See also *postrenal.*

presacral (pre′sa-kral) anterior to the sacrum.

presby- word element [Gr.], *old age.*

presbyatrics (pres″be-at′riks) geriatrics.

presbycardia (pres″be-kahr′de-ah) impairment of cardiac function attributed to aging, with senescent changes in the body and no evidence of other cause of heart disease.

presbycusis (pres″be-ku′sis) progressive, bilaterally symmetrical perceptive HEARING LOSS occurring with age; it usually occurs after age 50 and is caused by structural changes in the organs of hearing. Initially, changes in the inner ear, such as degeneration of hair cells and changes in the basilar membrane, lead to decreased hearing at higher tones and a decline in pitch discrimination. As hearing continues to be lost, even lower pitch tones become harder to hear.

presbyope (pres′be-ōp) one who is affected with presbyopia.

presbyopia (pres″be-o′pe-ah) diminution of accommodation of the lens of the eye occurring normally with aging, and usually resulting in hyperopia, or farsightedness. adj., **presbyop′ic.** Presbyopia is caused by a loss of elasticity in the crystalline lens of the eye. The lens focuses images on the retina with the aid of muscles that stretch it to make it less convex or relax it to make it more spherical and thus more convex. As it ages, the lens may lose its ability to become convex enough to accommodate to nearby objects. This condition usually begins around the age of 40. Presbyopia can most often be comfortably corrected through the use of eyeglasses.

prescribing (pre-skrīb′ing) making a PRESCRIPTION.

medication p. in the NURSING INTERVENTIONS CLASSIFICATION, a nursing INTERVENTION defined as prescribing medication for a health problem.

prescription (pre-skrip′shun) a written directive, as for the compounding or dispensing and administration of drugs, or for other service to a particular patient.

Federal law divides medicines into two main classes: prescription medicines and over-the-counter medicines. Dangerous, powerful, or habit-forming medicines to be used under a health care provider's supervision can be sold only by prescription. The prescription must be written by a physician, dentist, or advanced practice nurse; otherwise the pharmacist is forbidden to prepare and fill it.

There are four parts to a drug prescription. The first is the SUPERSCRIPTION, the symbol ℞ from the Latin *recipe,* meaning "take." The second part is the INSCRIPTION, specifying the ingredients and their quantities. The third part is the SUBSCRIPTION, which tells the pharmacist how to compound the medicine. The fourth and last part is the SIGNATURE; it is usually preceded by an S to represent the Latin *signa,* meaning "mark." The signature is where the health care provider indicates what instructions are to be put on the outside of the package to tell the patient when and how to take the medicine and in what quantities. The pharmacist keeps a file of all the prescriptions filled.

presence (prez′ens) in the NURSING INTERVENTIONS CLASIFICATION, a nursing INTERVENTION defined as being with another, both physically and psychologically, during times of need.

presenile (pre-se′nīl) pertaining to a condition resembling senility, but occurring in early or middle life.

presentation (prez″en-ta′shun) that part of the fetus lying over the pelvic inlet; the presenting body part of the fetus. See also POSITION and LIE.

breech p. presentation of the fetal buttocks, knees, or feet in labor; the feet may be alongside the buttocks (complete breech presentation); the legs may be extended against the trunk and the feet lying against the face (frank breech presentation); or one or both feet or knees may be prolapsed into the maternal vagina (incomplete breech presentation).

antigen p. presentation of ingested antigens on the surface of macrophages near histocompatibility antigens; see also ANTIGEN PRESENTATION.

cephalic p. presentation of any part of the fetal head in labor, whether the vertex, face, or brow.

compound p. prolapse of one of the limbs of the fetus alongside the head in cephalic PRESENTATION or of one or both arms

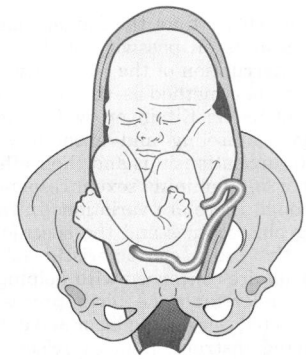

Breech presentation. From McKinney et al., 2000.

alongside a presenting breech at the beginning of labor.

footling p. presentation of the fetus with one foot (single footling) or two feet (double footling) prolapsed into the maternal vagina.

funic p. presentation of the umbilical cord in labor.

placental p. placenta praevia.

shoulder p. presentation with the fetal shoulder as the presenting part; see oblique LIE and transverse LIE.

transverse p. transverse lie.

preservation (prĕ-zer-va′shun) maintenance.

fertility p. in the NURSING INTERVENTIONS CLASSIFICATION, a nursing INTERVENTION defined as providing information, counseling, and treatment that facilitates reproductive

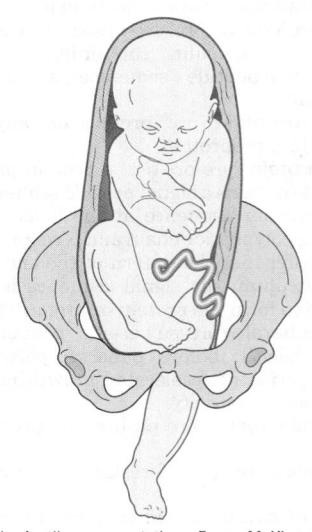

Single footling presentation. From McKinney et al., 2000.

preservative (pre-zer′vah-tiv) a substance added to a product to destroy or inhibit multiplication of microorganisms.

presinusoidal (pre″si-nŭ-soi′d′l) located in front of a sinusoid or affecting the circulation before the sinusoids are reached; used especially to denote the location of vascular resistance in portal hypertension.

presomite (pre-so′mīt) referring to embryos before the appearance of somites.

presphenoid (pre-sfe′noid) the anterior portion of the body of the sphenoid bone.

prespinal (pre-spi′nal) in front of the spine.

pressor (pres′er) tending to increase blood pressure.

pressoreceptive (pres″o-re-sep′tiv) sensitive to stimuli due to vasomotor activity; called also pressosensitive.

pressoreceptor (pres″o-re-sep′ter) baroreceptor.

pressosensitive (pres″o-sen′sĭ-tiv) pressoreceptive.

pressure (P) (presh′ur) force per unit area.

   arterial p., arterial blood p. BLOOD PRESSURE (def. 2).

   atmospheric p. the pressure exerted by the atmosphere, usually considered as the downward pressure of air onto a unit of area of the earth's surface; the unit of pressure at sea level is one ATMOSPHERE. Pressure decreases with increasing altitude.

   barometric p. atmospheric p.

   blood p. 1. see BLOOD PRESSURE. 2. pressure of blood on walls of any blood vessel.

   capillary p. the blood pressure in the capillaries.

   central venous p. see CENTRAL VENOUS PRESSURE.

   cerebral perfusion p. the mean arterial pressure minus the intracranial pressure; a measure of the adequacy of cerebral blood flow.

   cerebrospinal p. the pressure of the cerebrospinal fluid, normally 100 to 150 mm Hg.

   continuous positive airway p. see CONTINUOUS POSITIVE AIRWAY PRESSURE.

   filling p. see mean circulatory filling PRESSURE.

   high blood p. hypertension.

   intracranial p. see INTRACRANIAL PRESSURE.

   intraocular p. the pressure exerted against the outer coats by the contents of the eyeball.

   intrapleural p., intrathoracic p. pleural pressure.

   intrinsic positive end-expiratory p. elevated positive end-expiratory PRESSURE and dynamic pulmonary HYPERINFLATION caused by insufficient expiratory time or a limitation on expiratory flow. It cannot be routinely measured by a ventilator's pressure monitoring system but is measurable only using an expiratory hold maneuver done by the clinician. Its presence increases the work needed to trigger the ventilator, causes errors in the calculation of pulmonary compliance, may cause hemodynamic compromise, and complicates interpretation of hemodynamic measurements. Called also auto-PEEP and intrinsic PEEP.

   maximal expiratory p. maximum expiratory pressure.

   maximal inspiratory p. the pressure during inhalation against a completely occluded airway; used to evaluate inspiratory respiratory muscle strength and readiness for WEANING from mechanical ventilation. A maximum inspiratory pressure above -25 cm H_2O is associated with successful weaning.

   maximum expiratory p. (MEP) a measure of the strength of respiratory muscles, obtained by having the patient exhale as strongly as possible against a mouthpiece; the maximum value is near total lung CAPACITY.

   maximum inspiratory p. (MIP) the inspiratory pressure generated against a completely occluded airway; used to evaluate inspiratory respiratory muscle strength and readiness for weaning from mechanical ventilation. A maximum inspiratory pressure above -25 cm H_2O is associated with successful WEANING.

   mean airway p. the average pressure generated during the respiratory cycle.

   mean circulatory filling p. a measure of the average (arterial and venous) pressure necessary to cause filling of the circulation with blood; it varies with blood volume and is directly proportional to the rate of venous return and thus to cardiac output.

   negative p. pressure less than that of the atmosphere.

   oncotic p. the osmotic pressure of a colloid in solution.

   osmotic p. the pressure required to stop osmosis through a semipermeable membrane between a solution and pure solvent; it is proportional to the osmolality of the solution. Symbol π.

   partial p. the pressure exerted by each of the constituents of a mixture of gases.

   peak p. in mechanical ventilation, the highest pressure that occurs during inhalation.

P

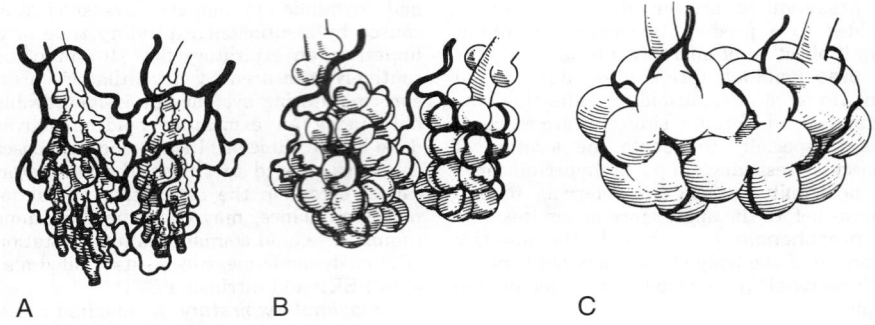

Effects of the application of positive end-expiratory pressure (PEEP) on the alveoli. *A,* Atelectatic alveoli before PEEP application. *B,* Optimal PEEP application has reinflated alveoli to normal volume. *C,* Excessive PEEP application overdistends the alveoli and compresses adjacent pulmonary capillaries, creating dead space with its attendant hypercapnia. From Pierce, 1995.

plateau p. in mechanical ventilation, the pressure measured at the proximal airway during an end-inspiratory pause; a reflection of alveolar pressure.

pleural p. the pressure between the visceral pleura and the thoracic pleura in the pleural cavity. Called also intrapleural or intrathoracic pressure.

positive p. pressure greater than that of the atmosphere.

positive end-expiratory p. (PEEP) a method of control mode ventilation in which positive pressure is maintained during expiration to increase the volume of gas remaining in the lungs at the end of expiration, thus reducing the shunting of blood through the lungs and improving gas exchange. A PEEP higher than the critical closing pressure prevents alveolar collapse and can markedly improve the arterial Po_2 in patients with a lowered functional residual capacity, as in acute respiratory failure.

pulmonary artery wedge p. (PAWP), pulmonary capillary wedge p. (PCWP) intravascular pressure, reflecting the left ventricular end diastolic pressure, measured by a SWAN-GANZ CATHETER wedged into a small pulmonary artery to block the flow from behind.

pulse p. the difference between the systolic and diastolic pressures. If the systolic pressure is 120 mm Hg and the diastolic pressure is 80 mm Hg, the pulse pressure is 40 mm Hg; the normal pulse pressure is between 30 and 40 mm Hg.

urethral p. the pressure inwards exerted by the walls of the urethra, which must be counteracted in order for urine to flow through; see also urethral pressure PROFILE.

venous p. the blood pressure in the veins; see also CENTRAL VENOUS PRESSURE.

water vapor p. the tension exerted by water vapor molecules, 47 mm Hg at normal body temperature.

wedge p. BLOOD PRESSURE measured by a small catheter wedged into a vessel, occluding it; see also pulmonary capillary wedge pressure and wedged hepatic vein pressure.

wedged hepatic vein p. the venous pressure measured with a catheter wedged into the hepatic vein. The difference between wedged and free hepatic vein pressures is used to locate the site of obstruction in portal hypertension; it is elevated in that due to cirrhosis, but low in cardiac ascites or portal vein thrombosis.

pressure ulcer an ulcer due to local interference with circulation; persons most at risk are those who are emaciated (nutritionally deficient in protein), obese, immobilized by traction or anything else, diabetic, or suffering from a circulatory disorder. Because urine and feces contribute to skin breakdown, incontinent patients are at high risk. Absence of sensation, advanced age, and immunodeficiency are also risk factors. Called also decubitus ulcer and, popularly, bedsore or pressure sore.

Three major factors in the development of pressure ulcers are (1) prolonged pressure on a part due to the weight of the body or a limb; (2) a SHEARING force that exerts downward and forward pressure on tissues beneath the skin (this can occur when the patient slides downward while sitting in a bed or chair, or when bedclothes are forcibly pulled from under the patient); and (3) nutritional status: good nutrition is essential for preventing pressure ulcers and healing already existing ones; a dietary deficiency should be suspected with a loss of 5 per cent or more of body weight or a serum albumin level below 3.5 mg/dl.

A pressure ulcer usually occurs over a bony prominence at the sacrum, hip (trochanter), heel, shoulder, or elbow. The lesion begins as a reddened area, which can quickly involve deeper structures and become an ulcer. (See accompanying illustration.)

Prevention. Repositioning the patient must be done as often as necessary to prevent impairment of circulation to any one part. For some patients this may mean turning and repositioning every hour. Gentle massage of the area stimulates circulation to the areas most likely to be affected, but reddened areas should never be massaged, because massage encourages tissue breakdown. Thorough cleansing, especially to remove perspiration, urine, and feces, helps prevent chemical breakdown of the skin and aids in the removal of bacteria. Numerous different pressure-relieving devices are available.

Stages. For purposes of assessment, treatment, and evaluation of effectiveness of nursing and medical intervention, the pathologic changes occurring in the development of a pressure ulcer are divided into four stages.

In *Stage 1* the area of skin is deep pink, red, or mottled. Digital pressure on the area will cause temporary blanching for up to 15 minutes after pressure is released. The skin will feel very warm and firm or tightly stretched across the area. At this stage no destruction of tissue has occurred and the condition is reversible. It is essential that the area be relieved of prolonged pressure, and that shearing forces be avoided. The reddened area may need protection by covering it with either a transparent film or a skin barrier.

Stage 2 is characterized by blistering, cracking, or abrasion of the skin. The surrounding skin is reddened and probably will feel hot or warmer than normal. Since there is now an opening in the skin for the entrance of bacteria, treatment must include cleaning the wound and providing some type of dressing or cover in addition to relieving pressure on the area.

Stage 3 is characterized by a craterlike sore with involvement of the underlying structures. Bacterial infection is almost always present at this stage and accounts for continued erosion of the ulcer and the production of drainage. Irrigation of the wound usually is done each time the dressing is changed. Wound débridement may be necessary to promote healing.

At *Stage 4* there is deep ulceration and necrosis involving underlying muscle and possibly bone tissue. At this point the ulcer usually is extensively infected. It can be dry, black in color, and covered with a tough accumulation of necrotic tissue, or it can be wet and oozing dead cells and purulent exudate. Deep and extensive ulceration and tissue loss may require surgical repair with myocutaneous flaps to close the defect.

Topical applications vary widely. The diligence with which the prescribed regimen is carried out greatly influences its effectiveness. Guidelines summarizing current recommended practice for the treatment of pressure ulcers (publication number 95-0653) are available from the Agency for Health Care Policy and Research, P.O. Box 8547, Silver Spring, MD 20907-8547 (telephone 800-358-9295).

presymptomatic (pre″simp-to-mat′ik) existing before the appearance of symptoms.

presynaptic (pre″sī-nap′tik) situated or occurring proximal to a synapse.

presystole (pre-sis′to-le) the interval just before systole.

presystolic (pre″sis-tol′ik) preceding systole.

preterm (pre-term) before completion of the full term of pregnancy.

WINDOW ON PRESSURE ULCERS

Pressure sore prevention is the desired goal to maintain skin integrity. It is a challenging nursing responsibility. The process of pressure sore prevention requires skilled nursing assessment of the integumentary system and knowledge of risk factors, as well as an ongoing evaluation plan to monitor incidence and efficacy of nursing care.

Pressure sore assessment is greatly aided by the availability of several research-based instruments, such as the Norton Scale, the Gosnell Instrument, and the Braden Scale. Assessment instruments grounded in research are rather unique because few nursing problems, other than pressure sores, have such instruments available. Further testing of predictive validity of risk factors is needed even though instruments have already proved valuable in delineating high risk patients. Well-designed programs of process and outcome evaluation can result in lower incidence rates and reduced severity of pressure sores. Assessment and evaluation are essential to quality nursing care.

DAVINA J. GOSNELL, PhD, RN, FAAN

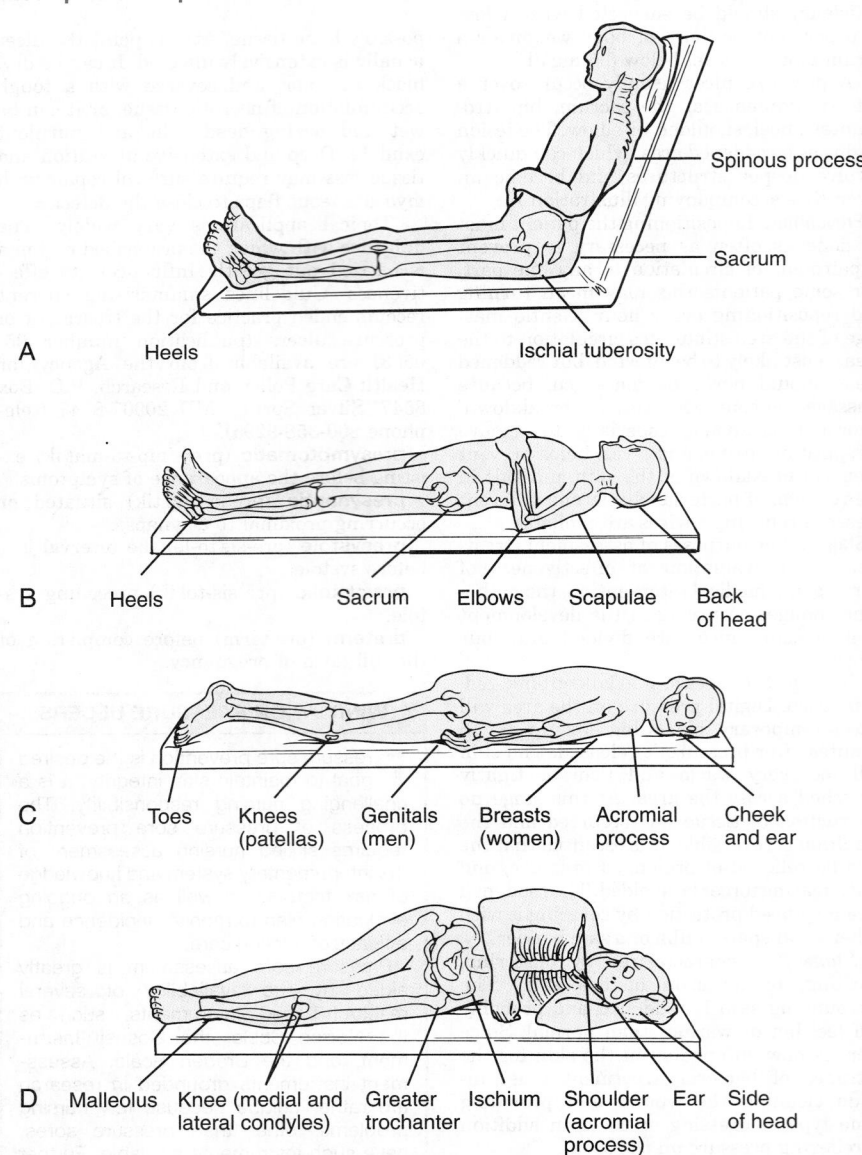

A   Heels   Spinous process   Sacrum   Ischial tuberosity

B   Heels   Sacrum   Elbows   Scapulae   Back of head

C   Toes   Knees (patellas)   Genitals (men)   Breasts (women)   Acromial process   Cheek and ear

D   Malleolus   Knee (medial and lateral condyles)   Greater trochanter   Ischium   Shoulder (acromial process)   Ear   Side of head

Pressure areas in common resting positions: *A,* Fowler's; *B,* supine; *C,* prone; and *D,* side-lying.

pretibial (pre-tib′e-al) in front of the TIBIA.

p. fever LEPTOSPIROSIS due to *Leptospira interrogans* serogroup *autumnalis,* marked by a rash on the pretibial region, with lumbar and postorbital pain, malaise, nasal inflammation, and fever. Also known as Fort Bragg fever because it was observed at Fort Bragg, North Carolina.

prevalence (prev′ah-lens) the number of cases of a specific disease present in a given population at a certain time; see also prevalence RATE.

prevention (pre-ven′shun) the keeping of something (such as an illness or injury) from happening.

fall p. in the NURSING INTERVEN-TIONS CLASSIFICATION, a nursing INTERVENTION defined as instituting special precautions with the patient at risk for injury from falling.

pressure ulcer p. in the NURSING INTERVENTIONS CLASSIFICATION, a nursing INTERVENTION defined as the prevention of PRESSURE ULCERS for a patient at high risk for developing them.

primary p. the first level of health care, designed to prevent the occurrence of disease and promote health.

religious addiction p. in the NURSING INTERVENTIONS CLASSIFICATION, a nursing INTERVENTION defined as prevention of a self-imposed controlling religious lifestyle. See also ADDICTION.

secondary p. the second level of health care, based on the earliest possible identification of disease so that it can be more readily treated or managed and adverse sequelae can be prevented.

shock p. in the NURSING INTERVENTIONS CLASSIFICATION, a nursing INTERVENTION defined as detecting and treating a patient at risk for impending SHOCK.

sports-injury p.: youth in the NURSING INTERVENTIONS CLASSIFICATION, a nursing INTERVENTION defined as reducing the risk of sport-related injury in young athletes.

substance use p. in the NURSING INTERVENTIONS CLASSIFICATION, a nursing INTERVENTION defined as the prevention of an ALCOHOLIC or drug use lifestyle. See also substance ABUSE.

suicide p. in the NURSING INTERVENTIONS CLASSIFICATION, a nursing INTERVENTION defined as reducing risk of self-inflicted harm with intent to end life. See also SUICIDE.

tertiary p. the third phase or level of health care, concerned with promotion of independent function and prevention of further disease-related deterioration.

preventive (pre-ven′tiv) serving to avert the occurrence of; prophylactic.

prevesical (pre-ves′ĭ-k'l) anterior to the urinary BLADDER.

prezygotic (pre″zi-got′ik) occurring before completion of FERTILIZATION.

priapism (pri′ah-pizm) persistent abnormal erection of the penis, accompanied by pain and tenderness. It is seen in diseases and injuries of the spinal cord, and may be caused by vesical calculus and certain injuries to the penis.

prilocaine (pril′o-kān) a local anesthetic, used parenterally as the hydrochloride salt or topically, together with lidocaine, as the base.

primaquine (pri′mah-kwin) an antimalarial AGENT effective against the extraerythrocytic forms of *Plasmodium vivax* and *P. ovale* and the gametocytes of

P. falciparum, used especially in the treatment of relapsing vivax MALARIA; used orally as the phosphate salt.

primate (pri′māt) an individual belonging to the highest order of mammals, Primates, which includes human beings, apes, monkeys, and lemurs.

prime mover a muscle that acts directly to bring about a desired movement.

primidone (pri′mĭ-dōn) an ANTICONVULSANT used in the treatment of EPILEPSY; administered orally.

primigravida (pri″mĭ-grav′ĭ-dah) a woman pregnant for the first time; gravida I.

priming (prīm′ing) the preparation of tubing that will transport fluids.

primipara (pri-mip′ah-rah) a woman who has had one pregnancy that resulted in a fetus that attained a weight of 500 g or a gestational age of 20 weeks, regardless of whether the infant was living at birth or whether it was a single or multiple birth. Also written para I or I-para. adj., **primip′arous.**

primiparity (pri″mĭ-par′ĭ-te) the state of being a primipara.

primitive (prim′ĭ-tiv) first in point of time; existing in a simple or early form that shows little complexity.

primordial (pri-mor′de-al) original or primitive; of the simplest and most undeveloped character.

primordium (pri-mor′de-um) the first beginnings of an organ or part in the developing embryo.

principle (prin′sĭ-p'l) 1. a chemical component. 2. a substance on which certain of the properties of a drug depend. 3. an accepted or professed rule of action or conduct; in a given philosophical system it is a fundamental or general law or truth from which others are derived. In bioethics some important principles are BENEFICENCE, JUSTICE, NONMALEFICENCE, and respect for AUTONOMY; these are derived in part from professional roles and traditions.

active p. any constituent of a drug that helps to confer upon it a medicinal property.

Bobath p's a type of neurophysiological rehabilitation; see BOBATH METHOD.

Bohr's p. of complementarity reflexes do not independently account for the complex nature of infant behavior.

negentropic p. a principle of GENERAL SYSTEMS THEORY stating that open systems have mechanisms that slow down or arrest the process of movement toward less efficiency and growth. Negentropy (negative entropy) is the tendency toward order and organization.

P

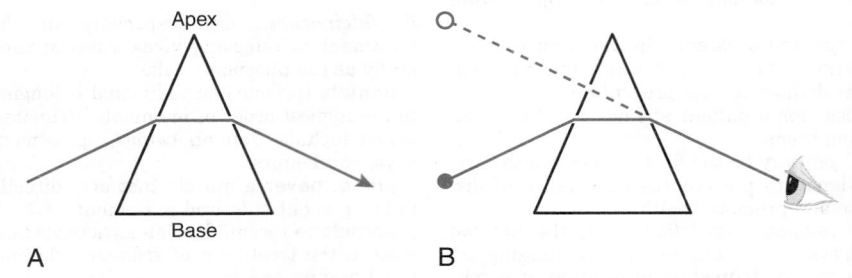

A, Light is deviated by the prism toward its base. B, The observer views an object through the prism and the object appears displaced toward its apex. From Stein et al., 2000.

pleasure p., pleasure-pain p. in psychoanalytic theory, an inborn tendency to avoid pain and seek pleasure through the immediate reduction of tension by either direct or fantasied gratification.

reality p. in psychoanalytic theory, the ego functions that modify the demands of the pleasure principle to meet the demands and requirements of the external world.

prion (pri′on) any of several pathogenic, transmissible forms of the core of PRION PROTEIN that cause a group of degenerative diseases of the nervous system known as PRION DISEASES. Prions have a structure different from that of normal prion protein, lack detectable nucleic acid, and do not elicit an IMMUNE RESPONSE.

p. disease any of a group of fatal degenerative diseases of the nervous system caused by abnormalities in the metabolism of prion PROTEIN. These diseases are unique in that they may be transmitted genetically as an autosomal dominant trait, or by infection with abnormal forms of the protein (PRIONS). Inherited forms result from mutations in the gene that codes for prion protein; such mutations may also occur sporadically. Hereditary forms include some forms of CREUTZFELDT-JAKOB DISEASE, GERSTMANN-STRÄUSSLER SYNDROME, and FATAL FAMILIAL INSOMNIA. Infectious forms of the disease result from ingestion of infected tissue or the introduction of infected tissue into the body (KURU and some forms of Creutzfeldt-Jakob disease). The latter has occasionally occurred during surgical procedures; it has also occurred as the result of injection of human growth hormone prepared from infected pituitary glands. Prion diseases also occur in animals. Called also transmissible neurodegenerative disease and subacute spongiform or transmissible spongiform encephalopathy.

prism (priz″əm) a solid of glass, plastic, or a similar substance with a triangular or polygonal cross section, which splits up a ray of light into its constituent colors and turns or deflects light rays toward its base. Prisms are used to correct deviations of the eyes, since they alter the apparent situation of objects.

PRK photorefractive keratectomy.

PRL, Prl prolactin.

p.r.n. [L.] *pro re na′ta* (according to circumstances).

PRO professional review organization.

pro- word element [L., Gr.], *before; in front of; favoring.*

proaccelerin (pro″ak-sel′er-in) factor V, one of the COAGULATION FACTORS.

proactivator (pro-ak′tĭ-va″ter) a precursor of an activator; a factor that reacts with an enzyme to form an activator.

proatlas (pro-at′las) a rudimentary vertebra that lies in front of the atlas in some animals; sometimes seen in humans as an anomaly in the lower posterior part of the skull.

probability (prob″ah-bil′ĭ-te) the likelihood of occurrence of a specified event, which is often represented as a number between 0 (never) and 1 (always) that corresponds to the long-run frequency at which the event occurs in a sequence of random independent trials under identical conditions, as the number of trials approaches infinity.

proband (pro′band) propositus.

probang (pro′bang) a flexible rod with a ball, tuft, or sponge at the end; used to apply medications to or remove matter from the esophagus or larynx.

Pro-Banthine (pro-ban-thīn′) trademark for preparations of PROPANTHELINE bromide, an ANTICHOLINERGIC used to treat peptic ulcers.

probe (prōb) 1. a long, slender instrument for exploring wounds, body cavities, passages, or periodontal pockets. 2. a radioactive or chemiluminescent DNA or

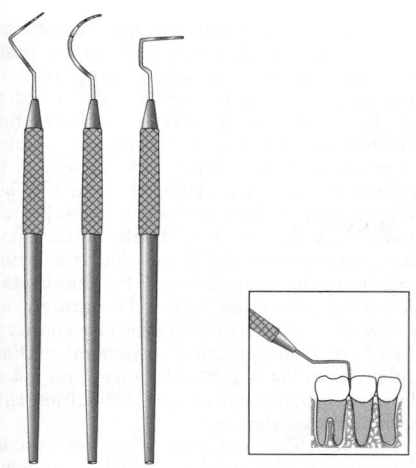
Dental probes are marked in millimeters to measure the depth of periodontal pockets. From Novak, 2001.

RNA fragment used to detect the presence of a complementary fragment. The labeled sequence is added to a specimen, where it forms a complex with the DNA in the sample, which has previously been treated to separate the DNA into single strands. DNA probes are used clinically to detect and identify infectious disease agents.

root canal p. in root canal THERAPY, an instrument for tracing the course of the root canal. Called also pathfinder, pathfinder broach, and smooth broach.

probenecid (pro-ben′ĕ-sid) a compound used in treatment of GOUT to promote excretion of uric acid; also used to increase serum concentration of certain antibiotics and other drugs.

problem (prob′lem) something of difficulty or concern.

Problem Classification Scheme one of the three clinical components of the OMAHA SYSTEM; it is a client-focused taxonomy used by nurses and other health care professionals to standardize the assessment process. It consists of four domains (the *environmental, psychosocial, physiological,* and *health-related behaviors* domains), 40 problems or NURSING DIAGNOSES, two sets of modifiers, and signs and symptoms. See Appendix on the Omaha System.

Problem-Oriented Record (POR) an approach to patient care record keeping that focuses on the patient's specific health problems requiring immediate attention, and the structuring of a cooperative health care plan designed to cope with the identified problems. In contrast to the

traditional "diary" method of record keeping organized according to the source of information (such as a physician or nurse), the POR uses progress sheets that integrate all written notes under labeled problems. Called also Problem-Oriented Medical Record (POMR).

This system of record keeping was first introduced in the late 1960's by Dr. Lawrence L. Weed for the purpose of improving patient care through systematic analysis and logical documentation of the care rendered by various members of the health care team. When properly implemented, the approach should provide a more effective means of communication among the members of the health care team (including the patient), and facilitate coordination of preventive care, health maintenance, and continuity of care. Other areas affected by the POR include cost of health care delivery, evaluation and control of quality of care rendered, and medical-legal aspects related to informed consent by the patient.

By eliminating much of the duplication of time and effort spent by health care professionals in acquiring and recording patient care data, this system can reduce significantly the overall cost of health care. Other costs related to the preparation of insurance forms, record reviews for quality control, and duplication of patient records can be reduced substantially by the more efficient and less cumbersome problem-oriented system. The accumulation of specific and objective data relative to patient care is a major step toward the establishment of explicit criteria against which the performance of health care providers can be measured. The objective evaluation of performance is especially important in the certification and recertification of health care personnel.

Although the details of implementing a POR system may vary according to the setting in which it is to be used and the type of clientele being served, there are four components that are basic to the problem-oriented record. These are the *database, problem list, plan,* and *notes.*

The Database. In the traditional system of recording, pertinent information about the patient's history and present status is scattered throughout the patient's chart. The POR system contains only one database section in which input from a variety of sources is recorded. The information recorded in the database section pertains to the particular patient in the particular setting, that is, hospital, outpatient clinic, or other health care setting, and includes his general history, physical examination findings, physiologic and laboratory data, nursing history, and observations about lifestyle and current status. Data are acquired for the purpose of identifying current (active) major problems, which are *flagged* in the database and then described under a titled *Notes* section. Minor and inactive problems are described within the database.

As time goes on, the acquisition of new information about the patient requires additional notes on the database forms. In the event such additions become extensive, the original database form may be "retired" to an inactive record and a new database generated for the active record. The active database serves as a concise and relevant record of the patient's current status, and thus facilitates continuity of care and coordination of plans for his care as he moves through various inpatient and outpatient agencies and institutions.

The patient's contribution to the database usually involves the completion of any of a number of forms designed to elicit information about his personal and family medical history. The patient accepts responsibility for answering the questions presented as accurately as possible; however, he may need assistance in completing the forms so as to avoid trivial and "false-positive" clues to the exact nature of his problems.

The database and the more extensive data about his major problems constitute the "complete data set," that is, a complete work-up.

The Problem List. The active problem list contains those major problems currently needing attention for further observation, diagnosis, management, or patient education. It serves as the basis for a plan of care. The problems may fall into the area of psychologic, social, and economic factors, as well as the more familiar physical diagnosis. For example, the problem identified could be congestive heart failure, if this has been established previously as a documented diagnosis, or it may be only a symptom, an abnormal laboratory finding, a risk factor, or some other problem that must be dealt with. As problems are resolved or new problems added, the problem list may be retired to an inactive record and a new list prepared.

The problem list is the first document encountered in the patient's chart. It serves as a guide to the current and important health problems of the patient. Its purpose is to draw attention to the problem areas so that they will not be overlooked. In order for the problem list to serve the purpose for which it is intended, it is necessary to use language that is concise and explicit. If a diagnosis has been made, that should be written, but if there are several manifestations of an illness, they should be incorporated into a single definition that is as brief and accurate as possible. The manifestations themselves may be listed separately on a flow sheet or narrative notes elsewhere in the chart. It is important to remember that the problem list is just that, a list, and not a detailed explanation of the difficulties the patient is experiencing.

The Plan. This is a plan of action that is derived from the problems which have been identified and that serves as a focus for patient care. The written plan is entered on the progress notes under each labeled problem. Specific physicians' plans and nursing plans should be integrated to avoid duplication and to provide a means of coordinating and communicating the care plan. The physician-generated plans are those related to diagnostic studies and therapy, the traditional physician's "orders." The nurse-generated plans are concerned with observations, interventions, diet, and patient education.

The plan as recorded in the problem-oriented record is intended to eliminate the unnecessary writing of trivia and is focused on the reporting of exceptional and relevant information only. Routine procedures and data such as the daily bath, respiratory rate, and bowel movements can be deleted from the permanent record if they are not related to the patient's problems. They may be entered on work sheets that are discarded at the time of discharge. Should an abnormality or difficulty in carrying out routine care be detected, it is entered as a problem on the problem list.

Notes. In the problem-oriented approach there is only one section for progress notes. Physicians, nurses, and all other health care personnel directly participating in the care of the patient use the progress notes to document their observations, assessments, nursing care plans, physician's orders, and so on. As a device for conceptualizing the process of recording progress notes, Weed and others suggest the SOAP structuring of notes: *S* stands for *subjective data* obtained from the patient and his significant others; *O* stands for *objective data* obtained by observation, physical examination, diagnostic studies, and so on; A stands for *assessment of the patient's status* through analysis of the problem, possible interaction of problems, and changes in status of problems; and P stands for *plan.* Progress notes need not be daily records of each problem. It usually is not necessary to record every problem every day, and all four components of SOAP need not be written daily. The goal of problem-oriented recording is to keep writing at a minimum and record only what is relevant to the patient's problems and important to communication and continuity of care.

Problem Rating Scale for Outcomes one of the three clinical components of the OMAHA SYSTEM; it is an organized framework used by nurses and other health care professionals to standardize outcomes measurement. It consists of three five-point Likert-type scales of knowledge, behavior, and status. See Appendix on the Omaha System.

problem solving the process of recognizing a problem, defining it, identifying alternative plans to resolve the problem, selecting a plan, organizing steps of the plan, implementing the plan, and evaluating the outcome; a PERFORMANCE COMPONENT of occupational therapy.

probucol (pro′bu-kol) a bis-phenol compound used as an ANTICHOLESTEREMIC; taken orally.

procainamide (pro-kān′ah-mīd) a cardiac DEPRESSANT used as the hydrochloride salt in the treatment of cardiac ARRHYTHMIAS, administered orally, intramuscularly, or intravenously.

procaine (pro′kān) a local anesthetic; the hydrochloride salt is used for infiltration and spinal anesthesia and peripheral nerve block.

Procanbid (pro′kan-bid″) trademark for a preparation of PROCAINAMIDE hydrochloride, a cardiac DEPRESSANT.

procarbazine (pro-kahr′bah-zēn) an antineoplastic AGENT used primarily in combination with MECHLORETHAMINE, VINCRISTINE, and PREDNISONE in the regimen called MOPP for treatment of advanced HODGKIN'S DISEASE; it also has activity against non-Hodgkin's lymphomas and brain tumors.

procarboxypeptidase (pro″kahr-bok″se-pep′tĭ-dās) the inactive precursor of carboxypeptidase, which is converted to the active enzyme by the action of trypsin.

procarcinogen (pro″kahr-sin′o-jen) a chemical substance that becomes a CARCINOGEN only after it is altered by metabolic processes.

Procardia (pro-kahr′de-ah) trademark for preparations of NIFEDIPINE, a coronary VASODILATOR used in treatment of ANGINA PECTORIS and HYPERTENSION.

Procaryotae (pro-kar″e-o′te) former name for MONERA.

procedure (pro-se′jer) a series of steps for doing something; see also MANEUVER, METHOD, OPERATION, SURGERY, and TECHNIQUE. For specific types of procedures, see under the name.

procelous (pro-se′lus) having the anterior surface concave; said of vertebrae.

procentriole (pro-sen′tre-ōl) the immediate precursor of centrioles and ciliary basal bodies.

procephalic (pro″sĕ-fal′ik) pertaining to the anterior part of the head.

procercoid (pro-ser′koid) a larval stage of fish tapeworms.

process (pros′es) 1. a prominence or projection, as from a bone. 2. a series of operations or events leading to achievement of a specific result. 3. to subject to such a series to produce desired changes.

acromial p. acromion.

altered family p's former name for the nursing diagnosis interrupted family PROCESSES.

alveolar p. the part of the bone in either the maxilla or mandible that surrounds and supports the teeth.

basilar p. a quadrilateral plate of the occipital bone projecting superiorly and anteriorly from the foramen magnum.

calcaneal p. of cuboid bones a process projecting posteriorly from the inferomedial angle of the cuboid bone that supports the anterior calcaneus.

caudate p. the right of the two processes on the caudate lobe of the liver.

ciliary p's meridionally arranged ridges or folds projecting from the crown of the ciliary body.

clinoid p. any of three processes of the sphenoid bone (anterior, medial, and posterior).

coracoid p. a curved process arising from the upper neck of the scapula and overhanging the shoulder joint; called also coracoid.

coronoid p. 1. the anterior part of the upper end of the RAMUS OF THE MANDIBLE. 2. a projection at the proximal end of the ULNA.

disturbed thought p's a NURSING DIAGNOSIS approved by the North American Nursing Diagnosis Association, defined as the experiencing by an individual of disruption in cognitive operations and activities; it is related to various mental and

P

personality disorders. Contributing factors include physiologic changes, psychologic conflicts, memory loss, impaired judgment, and sleep deprivation. Defining characteristics include inaccurate interpretation of the environment; cognitive dissonance; distractibility; decreased ability to grasp ideas; impaired ability to make decisions, solve problems, or reason; disorientation to time, place, person, circumstances, or events; and inappropriate or nonreality-based thinking.

dysfunctional family p's: alcoholism a NURSING DIAGNOSIS approved by the North American Nursing Diagnosis Association, defined as psychosocial, spiritual, and physiological functions of the family unit that are chronically disorganized, leading to conflict, denial of problems, resistance to change, ineffective problem solving, and a series of self-perpetuating crises. See also ALCOHOLISM.

ensiform p. xiphoid process.

ethmoid p. a bony projection above and behind the maxillary process of the inferior nasal CONCHA.

family p's the psychosocial, physiological, and spiritual functions and relationships within the family unit; nursing diagnoses include dysfunctional family PROCESSES: alcoholism and interrupted family PROCESSES.

frontonasal p. frontonasal prominence.

interrupted family p's a NURSING DIAGNOSIS accepted by the North American Nursing Diagnosis Association, defined as a change in family relationships and/or functioning.

malar p. zygomatic process of the maxilla.

mammillary p. a tubercle on each superior articular process of a lumbar vertebra.

mandibular p. mandibular prominence.

mastoid p. a conical projection at the base of the mastoid portion of the temporal bone.

maxillary p. 1. maxillary prominence. 2. a bony process descending from the ethmoid process of the inferior nasal concha.

nursing p. see NURSING PROCESS.

odontoid p. a toothlike projection of the axis that articulates with the atlas.

pterygoid p. either of the two processes of the sphenoid bone, descending from the points of junction of the great wings and the body of the bone, and each consisting of a lateral and a medial plate.

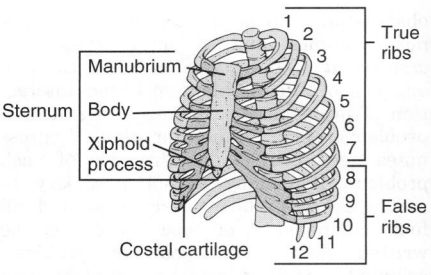

The xiphoid process. Redrawn from Applegate, 1995.

spinous p. of vertebra a part of a vertebra projecting backward from the arch, giving attachment to muscles of the back.

styloid p. a long, pointed projection, particularly a long spine projecting downward from the inferior surface of the temporal bone.

temporal p. the posterior blunt process of the zygomatic BONE that articulates with the zygomatic PROCESS of the temporal bone to form the zygomatic ARCH.

uncinate p. any hooklike process, as of vertebrae, the lacrimal bone, or the pancreas.

xiphoid p. the pointed process of cartilage, supported by a core of bone, connected with the lower end of the sternum; called also xiphoid.

zygomatic p. a projection in three parts, from the frontal bone, temporal bone, and maxilla, by which they articulate with the zygomatic bone (see Appendix 3-3).

processing (pros'es-ing) the subjecting of something to a series of operations or events to produce desired changes.

sensory p. the ability to interpret sensory stimuli, a PERFORMANCE COMPONENT of occupational therapy.

processus (pro-ses'us) [L.] process.

prochlorperazine (pro″klor-per'ah-zēn) a PHENOTHIAZINE derivative used as an ANTIEMETIC and sometimes as an ANTIPSYCHOTIC AGENT; used as the base or as the edisylate or mesylate salts, administered orally, intravenously, intramuscularly, or rectally.

prochondral (pro-kon'dral) occurring before the formation of cartilage.

procidentia (pro″sĭ-den'she-ah) prolapse (def. 1).

procoagulant (pro″co-ag'u-lant) 1. tending to promote coagulation. 2. a precursor of a natural substance necessary to coagulation of the blood.

proconvertin (pro″kon-ver'tin) factor VII, one of the COAGULATION FACTORS.

procreation (pro″kre-a'shun) the act of begetting or generating.

Procrit (pro'krit) trademark for a preparation of EPOETIN alfa, used to treat ANEMIA from various causes.

proct(o)- word element [Gr.], *rectum;* see also words beginning RECT(O)-.

proctalgia (prok-tal'jah) pain in the rectum; proctodynia.

proctatresia (prok"tah-tre'zhah) imperforate anus.

proctectasia (prok"tek-ta'zhah) dilatation of the rectum or anus.

proctectomy (prok-tek'to-me) excision of the rectum.

procteurynter (prok"tu-rin'ter) a baglike device used to dilate the rectum.

proctitis (prok-ti'tis) inflammation of the rectum.

ulcerative p. recurrent ulceration of the mucosa of the rectum, probably a variant of ULCERATIVE COLITIS.

proctocele (prok'to-sēl) hernial protrusion of part of the rectum into the vagina; rectocele.

proctocolonoscopy (prok"to-ko"lon-os'-kah-pe) inspection of the interior of the rectum and lower colon.

proctocolpoplasty (prok"to-kol'po-plas"te) repair of a rectovaginal fistula.

proctocystotomy (prok"to-sis-tot'ah-me) incision into the bladder from the rectum.

proctodeum (prok"to-de'um) the ectodermal depression of the caudal end of the embryo, which becomes the anal CANAL; called also anal pit.

proctodynia (prok"to-din'e-ah) pain in the rectum; proctalgia.

proctology (prok-tol'o-je) the branch of medicine concerned with disorders of the rectum and anus. adj., **proctolog'ic.**

proctoparalysis (prok"to-pah-ral'ĭ-sis) paralysis of the anal and rectal muscles; called also proctoplegia.

proctoplasty (prok'to-plas"te) plastic repair of the rectum and anus.

proctoplegia (prok"to-ple'jah) proctoparalysis.

proctoptosis (prok"top-to'sis) prolapse of the rectum.

proctorrhaphy (prok-tor'ah-fe) suture of the rectum.

proctorrhea (prok"to-re'ah) a mucous discharge from the anus.

proctoscope (prok'to-skōp) a speculum or tubular instrument with illumination for inspecting the rectum.

proctoscopy (prok-tos'kah-pe) inspection of the rectum with a proctoscope. The examination is usually done prior to rectal surgery, and it may be a part of the physical examination of a patient with hemorrhoids, rectal bleeding, or other symptoms of a rectal disorder.

proctosigmoidectomy (prok"to-sig"moi-dek'to-me) excision of the rectum and sigmoid colon; rectosigmoidectomy.

proctosigmoiditis (prok"to-sig"moi-di'tis) inflammation of the rectum and sigmoid colon.

proctosigmoidoscopy (prok"to-sig"moi-dos'kah-pe) examination of the rectum and sigmoid colon with the sigmoidoscope.

proctospasm (prok'to-spazm) spasm of the rectum.

proctostenosis (prok"to-stĕ-no'sis) stricture of the rectum.

proctostomy (prok-tos'tah-me) surgical creation of a permanent artificial opening from the body surface into the rectum.

proctotomy (prok-tot'ah-me) incision of the rectum, usually for anal or rectal stricture.

procumbent (pro-kum'bent) prone.

procurement (pro-kūr'ment) the obtaining of something.

organ p. in the NURSING INTERVENTIONS CLASSIFICATION, a nursing INTERVENTION defined as guiding families through the donation process to ensure timely retrieval of vital organs and tissue for TRANSPLANTATION.

procursive (pro-ker'siv) tending to run forward.

procyclidine (pro-si'klĭ-dēn) an ANTIDYSKINETIC used as the hydrochloride salt in the treatment of PARKINSONISM and for the control of drug-induced extrapyramidal reactions (except tardive dyskinesia); administered orally.

prodrome (pro'drōm) a premonitory symptom; a symptom indicating the onset of a disease. adj., **prodro'mal, prodro'mic.**

prodrug (pro'drug) a compound that, on administration, must undergo chemical conversion by metabolic processes before becoming an active pharmacological agent; a precursor of a drug.

product (prod'ukt) 1. something created or yielded. 2. the mathematical result of multiplying two or more quantities together.

fibrinogen degradation p's see FIBRINOGEN DEGRADATION PRODUCTS.

pressure rate p. the heart rate multiplied by the systolic blood pressure and divided by 100; this value correlates well with myocardial oxygen consumption.

production (pro-duk'shun) the creation or bringing forth of something.

carbon dioxide p. the amount of carbon dioxide produced by the tissues, measured as the amount of carbon dioxide given off by the lungs; normally 200 ml/min (or 3.0 ml/kg/min), but increased with increased metabolic rate.

P

productive (pro-duk′tiv) producing or forming; said especially of an inflammation that produces new tissue or of a cough that brings forth sputum or mucus.

proencephalus (pro″en-sef′ah-lus) a malformed fetus with a protrusion of the brain through a frontal fissure.

proenzyme (pro-en′zīm) zymogen; an inactive precursor of an enzyme.

proerythroblast (pro″ĕ-rith′ro-blast) the earliest erythrocyte precursor in the erythrocytic SERIES, preceding the basophilic erythroblast and having a large nucleus containing several nucleoli, surrounded by a small amount of cytoplasm. The term may encompass both normal and abnormal red cell precursors, in which case the two types may be called PRONORMOBLAST and PROMEGALOBLAST, or it may be used to mean a normal precursor only, as synonymous with pronormblast. Called also rubriblast.

proestrogen (pro-es′tro-jen) a substance without estrogenic activity but which is metabolized in the body to active estrogen.

proestrus (pro-es′trus) the period of heightened follicular activity preceding estrus.

profession (pro-fesh′un) 1. an avowed, public declaration or statement of intention or purpose. 2. a calling or vocation requiring specialized knowledge, methods, and skills, as well as preparation, in an institution of higher learning, in the scholarly, scientific, and historical principles underlying such methods and skills. A profession continously enlarges its body of knowledge, functions autonomously in formulation of policy, and maintains by force of organization or concerted opinion high standards of achievement and conduct. Members of a profession are committed to continuing study, place service above personal gain, and are committed to providing practical services vital to human and social welfare.

professional (pro-fesh′un-al) pertaining to one's profession or occupation. 1. one who is a specialist in a particular field or occupation.

allied health p. a person with special training, certification, and licensing with responsibilities bearing on patient care. See also ALLIED HEALTH.

impaired p. a professional who has gotten involved in substance ABUSE.

Professional Standards Review Organization (PSRO) an organization established to monitor health care services paid for through Medicare, Medicaid, and Maternal and Child Health programs to assure that services provided are medically necessary, meet professional standards, and are provided in the most economic medically appropriate health care agency or institution.

The PSROs are an outcome of the Social Security Amendment of 1972 (Public Law 92-603), which requires the setting up of PSROs to monitor health care services paid for, wholly or in part, under provisions of the Social Security Act. Each PSRO serves a specific geographic area and develops or selects its own norms of care, diagnosis, and treatment. The norms are based on typical patterns of practice in the area being served, including typical lengths of stay for institutional care by age and diagnosis.

profibrinolysin (pro-fi″brĭ-nol′ĭ-sin) plasminogen, the precursor of fibrinolysin.

profile (pro′fīl) 1. a simple outline, as of the side view of the head or face. 2. a graph representing quantitatively a set of characteristics determined by tests.

biophysical p. a numeric scoring system used to assess the well-being of the fetus in high-risk pregnancies, based on the nonstress test combined with sonographic evaluation of fetal breathing, fetal movements, fetal tone, amniotic fluid volume, and, sometimes, the echogenicity of the placenta.

PULSES p. a tool for early functional ASSESSMENT, comprising assessment of *p*hysical condition, *u*pper limb function, *l*ower limb function, *s*ensory components, *e*xcretory function, and *e*motional or mental *s*tatus.

urethral pressure p. **(UPP)** a record of the resistance of the urethra to fluid flow, measured as variations in urethral PRESSURE. A liquid or gas is pumped into the bladder with a catheter in place and the catheter is slowly withdrawn while measurements are taken of the pressure at various points in the urethra. It is usually done from the internal orifice to the external orifice in females and from the internal orifice to the sphincter urethrae muscle in males.

profundaplasty (pro-fun′dah-plas″te) reconstruction of the occluded or stenosed deep femoral artery (arteria profunda femoris).

profundus (pro-fun′dus) [L.] deep.

progastrin (pro-gas′trin) an inactive precursor of gastrin.

progeria (pro-jēr′e-ah) premature old age, a condition occurring in childhood marked by small stature, absence of facial and pubic hair, wrinkled skin, gray hair, and eventual development of atherosclerosis. Called also Hutchinson-Gilford syndrome.

progestagen (pro-jes′tah-jen) progestational AGENT.

progestational (pro″jes-ta′shun-al) 1. favoring GESTATION; referring to the phase of the MENSTRUAL CYCLE just before MENSTRUATION, when there are changes in the ENDOMETRIUM preparatory to implantation of the zygote should fertilization occur. 2. having effects similar to those of PROGESTERONE; see under AGENT.

progesterone (pro-jes′tĕ-rōn) a steroid sex hormone that is the principal progestational agent; it plays a major part in the MENSTRUAL CYCLE. During the maturation of the secondary OOCYTE (OVUM), ESTROGEN, the principal female sex hormone, is produced at a high rate. At ovulation estrogen production is sharply reduced, and the ovary then creates within itself a special endocrine structure called the CORPUS LUTEUM whose sole function is to produce progesterone. Unless fertilization takes place, the corpus luteum disappears when it has performed its function. The progesterone it has produced is promptly carried by the blood to the uterus, as was the estrogen previously. Both hormones now work to prepare the uterus for possible conception.

In pregnancy progesterone acts in a way that protects the embryo and fosters growth of the placenta. By decreasing the frequency of uterine contractions it helps to prevent expulsion of the implanted ZYGOTE. It also promotes secretory changes in the mucosa of the fallopian tubes, thereby helping to provide nutrition for the fertilized ovum as it travels through the tube on its way to the uterus.

Another function of progesterone is promotion of the development of the mammary glands in preparation for lactation. PROLACTIN, from the anterior lobe of the PITUITARY GLAND, stimulates production of milk, and progesterone prepares the glands for milk secretion. Progesterone also has an indirect effect on the fluid and electrolyte balance of the body by blocking the effect of ALDOSTERONE. Diminished secretion of progesterone can lead to menstrual difficulties in nonpregnant women and spontaneous abortion in pregnant women.

Progesterone is used medically in the treatment of dysfunctional uterine bleeding and abnormalities of the menstrual cycle, as part of postmenopausal hormone replacement therapy, as a test for endogenous estrogen production, and as an adjunct in the treatment of infertility associated with partial or complete ovarian failure; administered orally, intramuscularly, or intravaginally.

progestin (pro-jes′tin) 1. progestational agent. 2. a progestational AGENT secreted by the CORPUS LUTEUM and stimulating release of proteolytic enzymes in preparation for OVULATION and maturation of the ENDOMETRIUM.

progestogen (pro-jes′to-jen) progestational agent.

proglossis (pro-glos′is) the tip of the tongue.

proglottid (pro-glot′id) one of the segments making up the body of a TAPEWORM.

proglottis (pro-glot′is), pl. *proglot′tides* proglottid.

Proglycem (pro-gli′sem) trademark for a preparation of oral DIAZOXIDE, used in treatment of HYPOGLYCEMIA.

prognathism (prog′nah-thizm) abnormal protrusion of one or both jaws, especially the lower jaw, the gnathic index being above 103. adj., **prognath′ic, prog′nathous.**

prognose (prog-nōs′) prognosticate.

prognosis (prog-no′sis) a forecast of the probable course and outcome of an attack of disease and the prospects of recovery as indicated by the nature of the disease and the symptoms of the case. adj., **prognos′tic.**

dental p. forecast of the results to be achieved from any oral treatment.

medical p. an evaluation of the results to be achieved from any medical treatment.

nursing p. the application of information obtained during a NURSING ASSESSMENT in order to determine the prospect for altering, through nursing intervention, a client's/patient's response to illness or injury. The prognosis provides a rationale for setting priorities for meeting a particular client's/patient's nursing care needs and enhances continuity of nursing care by clearly indicating the agreed upon priorities.

prognosticate (prog-nos′tĭ-kāt) to give a PROGNOSIS; called also prognose.

program (pro′gram) 1. a set of organized procedures. 2. a list describing such procedures.

early intervention p. a multidisciplinary approach to assess and treat the problems of children who are at developmental risk or who have handicaps. The setting of the program will vary and is often dependent on the age of the child.

independent living p. a residential facility providing rehabilitative services for the individual with a disability.

twelve step p's self-help groups for people dealing with addictions, based on the twelve steps of ALCOHOLICS ANONYMOUS.

programmability (pro-gram″ah-bil′ĭ-te) in cardiac PACING terminology, the quality in an implanted PACEMAKER by which it can be changed in MODE (such as rate, impulse, or amplitude) by noninvasive means.

progranulocyte (pro-gran′u-lo-sīt″) promyelocyte.

progravid (pro-grav′id) denoting the phase of the endometrium in which it is prepared for pregnancy.

progressive (pro-gres′iv) 1. advancing. 2. increasing in scope or severity.

proguanil (pro-gwahn′il) an antimalarial AGENT, administered orally as the hydrochloride salt; its use in the United States is limited because of the development of drug-resistant malarial parasites.

prohormone (pro-hor′mōn) a precursor of a HORMONE, such as a polypeptide that is cleaved to form a shorter polypeptide hormone or a steroid that is converted to an active hormone by peripheral metabolism. Called also prehormone.

proinsulin (pro-in′soo-lin) a precursor of insulin, having low biologic activity.

projection (pro-jek′shun) 1. a throwing forward, especially the reference of impressions made on the sense organs to their proper source, so as to locate correctly the objects producing them. 2. a connection between the cerebral cortex and other parts of the nervous system or organs of special sense. 3. the condition of extending or jutting out, or a part that juts out. 4. in psychiatry, an unconscious DEFENSE MECHANISM whereby emotionally unacceptable traits are denied in oneself and are regarded (projected) as belonging to the external world or to someone else. It is often called the "blaming" mechanism because in using it the person seeks to place the blame for personal inadequacies upon someone else. In its extreme form projection can lead to hostility and physical attack upon others when one mistakenly perceives other persons as responsible for one's own mental anguish. 5. the orientation of a radiographic machine in relation to the body or a body part; called also view.

projective test any of various tests in which an individual interprets ambiguous stimulus situations, e.g., a series of inkblots (Rorschach t.), according to his own unconscious dispositions, thus yielding information about his personality structure, its underlying dynamics, and possible psychopathology.

prokaryon (pro-kar′e-on) 1. nuclear material scattered in the cytoplasm of the cell, rather than bounded by a nuclear membrane; found in some unicellular organisms, such as bacteria. 2. prokaryote.

Prokaryotae (pro-kar″e-o′te) Monera.

prokaryote (pro-kar′e-ōt) any member of the kingdom MONERA; a unicellular organism lacking a true nucleus and nuclear membrane, having genetic material composed of a single loop of naked double-stranded DNA. The microorganisms, comprising the bacteria and blue-green bacteria (formerly blue-green algae), are predominantly unicellular but may have filamentous, mycelial, or colonial forms. Prokaryotes, with the exception of genus *Mycoplasma,* have a rigid cell wall. adj., **prokaryot′ic.**

prokinetic (pro″kĭ-net′ik) stimulating movement or MOTILITY, such as a drug that promotes gastrointestinal motility.

prolabium (pro-la′be-um) the prominent central part of the upper lip.

prolactin (pro-lak′tin) a hormone secreted by the anterior PITUITARY GLAND that promotes the growth of breast tissue and stimulates and sustains milk production in postpartum mammals, and shows luteotropic activity in certain mammals. Called also lactogenic hormone and mammotropin.

prolactinoma (pro-lak″tĭ-no′mah) a pituitary adenoma made up of LACTOTROPHS that secretes excessive amounts of PROLACTIN; this may delay puberty in either sex, cause galactorrhea-amenorrhea syndrome in women, or decrease libido and fertility in men. Called also prolactin cell or prolactin-secreting adenoma and lactotrope or lactotroph adenoma.

prolapse (pro′laps) 1. the falling down or downward displacement of a part or viscus; called also procidentia and ptosis. 2. to undergo such displacement.

p. of cord protrusion of the umbilical cord ahead of the presenting part of the fetus in labor. (See accompanying illustration.)

p. of the iris protrusion of the iris through a wound in the cornea.

mitral valve p. see MITRAL VALVE PROLAPSE.

rectal p., p. of rectum protrusion of the rectal mucous membrane through the anus.

p. of uterus downward displacement of the uterus so that the cervix is within the vaginal orifice (first-degree prolapse), the cervix is outside the orifice (second-degree prolapse), or the entire uterus is outside the orifice (third-degree prolapse).

prolepsis (pro-lep′sis) recurrence of a paroxysm before the expected time. adj., **prolep′tic.**

prolidase (pro′lĭ-dās) an enzyme that catalyzes the hydrolysis of the imide bond between an α-carboxyl group and proline or hydroxyproline.

Occult (hidden) prolapse

Cord prolapsed in front of the fetal head

Complete cord prolapse

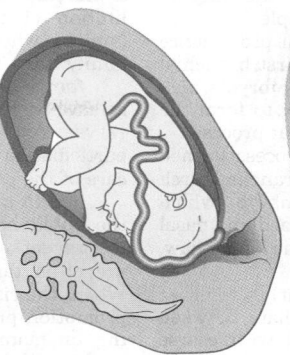
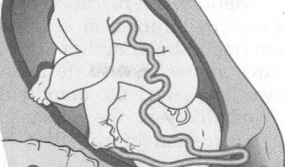

The cord can be seen protruding from the vagina.

The cord cannot be seen but can probably be felt as a pulsating mass during vaginal examination.

The cord is compressed between the fetal presenting part and pelvis but cannot be seen or felt during vaginal examination.

Variations of prolapsed umbilical cord. From McKinney et al., 2000.

proliferation (pro-lif″ĕ-ra′shun) the reproduction or multiplication of similar forms, especially of cells. See also *hyperplasia* and *hypertrophy.* adj., **prolif′erative, prolif′- erous.**

proligerous (pro-lij′er-us) producing offspring.

prolinase (pro′lĭ-nās) an enzyme that catalyzes the hydrolysis of dipeptides containing proline or hydroxyproline as N-terminal groups.

proline (pro′lēn) a cyclic, nonessential AMINO ACID; it is a major constituent of collagen.

Prolixin (pro-lik′sin) trademark for preparations of FLUPHENAZINE, an ANTIPSYCHOTIC AGENT.

prolymphocyte (pro-lim′fo-sīt) a cell of the lymphocytic series intermediate between the lymphoblast and the lymphocyte.

promastigote (pro-mas′tĭ-gōt) the morphologic stage in the development of certain protozoa, characterized by a free anterior flagellum and resembling the typical adult form of *Leptomonas.*

promazine (pro′mah-zēn) a phenothiazine derivative used as an ANTIPSYCHOTIC AGENT in the form of the hydrochloride salt; administered orally, intramuscularly, and intravenously.

promegakaryocyte (pro″meg-ah-kar′e-o-sīt″) a precursor in the thrombocytic series that is a developmental form intermediate between the megakaryoblast and the megakaryocyte.

promegaloblast (pro-meg′ah-lo-blast″) the earliest form in the abnormal erythrocyte maturation sequence occurring in vitamin B$_{12}$ and folic acid deficiencies; it corresponds to the pronormoblast, and develops into a megaloblast.

promethazine (pro-meth′ah-zēn) a PHENO-THIAZINE derivative having marked antihistaminic activity as well as sedative and antiemetic actions; used to provide bedtime, surgical, and obstetrical sedation, to treat allergic conditions including rhinitis, conjunctivitis, and itching, to manage nausea, vomiting, and vertigo associated with surgery, pregnancy, or motion sickness, and as an ingredient in cough and cold preparations; administered orally, rectally, intramuscularly, and intravenously as the hydrochloride salt.

promethium (Pm) (pro-me′the-um) a chemical element, atomic number 61, atomic weight 147. (See Appendix 6.)

prominence (prom′ĭ-nens) a protrusion or projection.

frontonasal p. an expansive facial process in the embryo that develops into the forehead and bridge of the nose; called also frontonasal process.

P

laryngeal p. a subcutaneous prominence at the front of the throat produced by the thyroid cartilage of the larynx; popularly known as Adam's apple.

mandibular p. the ventral prominence formed by bifurcation of the first branchial arch (mandibular arch) in the embryo, which unites ventrally with its fellow to form the lower jaw; called also mandibular process.

maxillary p. the dorsal process formed by bifurcation of the first branchial arch (mandibular arch) in the embryo, which joins with the ipsilateral median nasal process in the formation of the upper jaw. Called also maxillary process.

promonocyte (pro-mon′o-sīt) a cell of the monocytic series intermediate between the monoblast and monocyte, with coarse chromatin structure and one or two nucleoli.

promontory (prom′on-tor″e) a projecting process or eminence.

promotion (pro-mo′shun) encouragement or ENHANCEMENT.

attachment p. in the NURSING INTERVENTIONS CLASSIFICATION, a nursing INTERVENTION defined as facilitation of the development of the parent-infant relationship.

body mechanics p. in the NURSING INTERVENTIONS CLASSIFICATION, a nursing INTERVENTION defined as facilitating the use of posture and movement in daily activities to prevent fatigue and musculoskeletal strain or injury.

cerebral perfusion p. in the NURSING INTERVENTIONS CLASSIFICATION, a nursing INTERVENTION defined as the promotion of adequate perfusion and limitation of complications for a patient experiencing or at risk for inadequate cerebral perfusion. See also cerebral INFARCTION.

exercise p. in the NURSING INTERVENTIONS CLASSIFICATION, a nursing INTERVENTION defined as facilitation of regular physical EXERCISE to maintain or advance to a higher level of fitness and health.

exercise p.: strength training in the NURSING INTERVENTIONS CLASSIFICATION, a nursing INTERVENTION defined as facilitating regular resistive muscle training to maintain or increase muscle strength.

exercise p.: stretching in the NURSING INTERVENTIONS CLASSIFICATION, a nursing INTERVENTION defined as facilitation of systematic slow-stretch-hold muscle exercises to induce relaxation, to prepare muscles/joints for more vigorous exercise, or to increase or maintain body flexibility.

family integrity p. in the NURSING INTERVENTIONS CLASSIFICATION, a nursing INTERVENTION defined as the promotion of FAMILY cohesion and unity.

family integrity p.: childbearing family in the NURSING INTERVENTIONS CLASSIFICATION, a nursing INTERVENTION defined as facilitation of the growth of individuals or families who are adding an infant to the family unit.

family involvement p. in the NURSING INTERVENTIONS CLASSIFICATION, a nursing INTERVENTION defined as facilitating family participation in the emotional and physical care of the patient.

health p. programs designed to inform the public about health risks and methods to prevent or reduce them; the programs are often targeted at specific populations. Where the risk cannot be eliminated, health promotion programs may focus on improving or maintaining the affected person's quality of life.

normalization p. in the NURSING INTERVENTIONS CLASSIFICATION, a nursing INTERVENTION defined as assisting parents and other family members of children with chronic illnesses or disabilities in providing normal life experiences for their children and families.

oral health p. in the NURSING INTERVENTIONS CLASSIFICATION, a nursing INTERVENTION defined as promotion of oral HYGIENE and dental care for a patient with normal oral and dental health.

parenting p. in the NURSING INTERVENTIONS CLASSIFICATION, a nursing INTERVENTION defined as providing parenting information, support and coordination of comprehensive services to high-risk families.

resiliency p. in the NURSING INTERVENTIONS CLASSIFICATION, a nursing INTERVENTION defined as assisting individuals, families, and communities in development, use, and strengthening of protective factors to be used in coping with environmental and societal stressors.

vehicle safety p. in the NURSING INTERVENTIONS CLASSIFICATION, a nursing INTERVENTION defined as assisting individuals, families, and communities to increase awareness of measures to reduce unintentional injuries in motorized and non-motorized vehicles.

promyelocyte (pro-mi′ĕ-lo-sīt″) a precursor in the granulocytic series, intermediate between myeloblast and myelocyte, containing a few undifferentiated cytoplasmic granules.

pronate (pro′nāt) to subject to pronation.

pronation (pro-na′shun) the act of assuming the prone position, or the state of being prone. Applied to the hand, turning the palm backward (posteriorly) or downward.

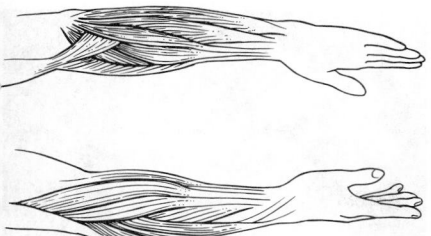

Pronation (top) versus supination (bottom).

performed by medial rotation of the forearm. Applied to the foot, a combination of eversion and abduction movements taking place in the tarsal and metatarsal joints and resulting in lowering of the medial margin of the foot, hence of the longitudinal arch.

pronator (pro-na′tor) a muscle that pronates.

prone (prōn) lying face downward, or on the ventral surface; see also prone POSITION. Called also procumbent.

pronephros (pro-nef′ros) [Gr.] the primordial KIDNEY; an excretory structure or its rudiments developing in the embryo before the mesonephros; its duct is later used by the mesonephros, which arises caudal to it.

Pronestyl (pro-nes′til) trademark for preparations of PROCAINAMIDE, a cardiac DEPRESSANT.

prong (prong) a conical projection.

nasal p's nasal cannula.

pronormoblast (pro-nor′mo-blast) a term often considered a synonym of PROERYTHRO-BLAST; sometimes limited to one in the course of normal erythrocyte maturation, as opposed to a PROMEGALOBLAST.

pronucleus (pro-noo′kle-us) the haploid nucleus of a germ CELL.

female p. the haploid nucleus of the fully mature OOCYTE, which loses its nuclear envelope and liberates its chromosomes to meet the synapsis with those from the male pronucleus.

male p. the nuclear material of the HEAD OF A SPERMATOZOON, after it has penetrated the oocyte and acquired a pronuclear membrane.

pro-otic (pro-ot′ik) preauricular.

propafenone (pro″pah-fe′nōn) a sodium channel blocking AGENT that acts on the Purkinje fibers and the myocardium; used as the hydrochloride salt in treatment of life-threatening ARRHYTHMIAS, administered orally.

propagation (prop″ah-ga′shun) reproduction. adj., **prop′agative.**

propantheline (pro-pan′thĕ-lēn) an ANTICHOLINERGIC and ANTIMUSCARINIC used as

the bromide salt for its ANTISPASMODIC effects, especially in the treatment of peptic ulcer.

proparacaine (pro-par′ah-kān) a topical ophthalmic anesthetic; used as the hydrochloride salt.

propepsin (pro-pep′sin) pepsinogen; the inactive precursor of pepsin.

properdin (pro′per-din) a protein of the alternative COMPLEMENT pathway, augmenting complement activation. Called also factor P.

prophage (pro′fāj) the latent stage of a BACTERIOPHAGE in a lysogenic BACTERIUM, in which the viral GENOME becomes inserted into a specific portion of the host CHROMOSOME and is duplicated into each cell generation.

prophase (pro′fāz) the first stage of cell replication in either meiosis or mitosis.

prophylactic (pro″fĭ-lak′tik) 1. pertaining to PROPHYLAXIS. 2. tending to ward off disease. 3. an agent that so acts. 4. condom.

prophylaxis (pro″fĭ-lak′sis) disease PREVENTION; called also preventive treatment.

dental p. oral prophylaxis.

oral p. cleaning of the teeth by a dentist or dental hygienist, including removal of plaque, materia alba, calculus, and extrinsic stains; done as a preventive measure for control of GINGIVITIS. Called also dental prophylaxis.

propiolactone (pro″pe-o-lak′tōn) a disinfectant effective against bacteria, fungi, and viruses.

Propionibacterium (pro″pe-on″ĭ-bak-te′-re-um) a genus of gram-positive, anaerobic, rod-shaped bacteria, found as saprophytes in humans, animals, and dairy products. *P. ac′nes* (also known as *Corynebacterium acnes*) is a normal skin inhabitant and can cause chronic infections of the blood and bone marrow. *P. granulo′sum* (also known as *Corynebacterium granulosum*) causes abscesses.

propionic acid (pro″pe-on′ik) a FATTY ACID found in chyme and sweat, and one of the products of bacterial fermentation of wood pulp waste; its salts (CALCIUM PROPIONATE and SODIUM PROPIONATE) are antifungal AGENTS and inhibitors of mold on foods.

propofol (pro′pah-fol) a short-acting SEDATIVE and HYPNOTIC used as a general anesthetic and adjunct to anesthesia; administered intravenously.

propositus (pro-poz′ĭ-tus) [L.] the original person presenting a mental or physical disorder who serves as the basis for a hereditary or genetic study; called also proband.

propoxyphene (pro-pok′sĭ-fēn) an OPIOID ANALGESIC administered orally as the hydrochloride and napsylate salts; called also dextropropoxyphene.

propranolol (pro-pran′o-lol) a BETA-ADRENERGIC BLOCKING AGENT used as the hydrochloride salt in treatment of hypertension, cardiac arrhythmias, and hypertrophic subaortic stenosis, tremors, and inoperable pheochromocytoma, in prophylaxis of migraine, and for reducing the long-term risk of mortality and reinfarction after the acute phase of a myocardial infarction. Administered orally or intravenously.

proprietary (pro-pri′ĕ-tar-e) protected against free competition as to name, product, composition, or process of manufacture by secrecy, patent, trademark, copyright, or other means; see also proprietary MEDICINE.

proprioception (pro″pre-o-sep′shun) perception mediated by proprioceptors or proprioceptive tissues.

proprioceptor (pro″pre-o-sep′tor) any of the sensory nerve endings that give information concerning movements and position of the body; they occur chiefly in muscles, tendons, and the labyrinth. adj., **propriocep′tive.**

proprotein (pro-pro′tēn) a protein precursor that is cleaved to form an active protein, e.g., proinsulin, the precursor of insulin.

proptometer (pro-tom′ĕ-ter) an instrument for measuring the degree of exophthalmos.

proptosis (prop-to′sis) forward displacement or bulging, especially of the eye.

propulsion (pro-pul′shun) 1. a tendency to fall forward in walking. 2. festination.

propyl (pro′pil) the univalent radical $CH_3CH_2CH_2$—, from propane.

propylene glycol (pro′pĭ-lēn gli′kol) a clear viscous liquid used as a moistening agent and solvent in pharmaceutical preparations.

propylhexedrine (pro″pil-hek′sĕ-drēn) an adrenergic given by inhalation to decongest nasal mucosa.

propyliodone (pro″pil-i′o-dōn) a radiopaque medium used in bronchography.

propylthiouracil (pro″pil-thi″o-u′rah-sil) a THYROID inhibitor used to treat HYPERTHYROIDISM; administered orally.

pro re nata (p.r.n.) (pro re na′tah) [L.] according to circumstances.

prorenin (pro-ren′in) the inactive precursor of RENIN, stored in the juxtaglomerular CELLS of the kidney and activated by cleavage to renin. Called also big renin.

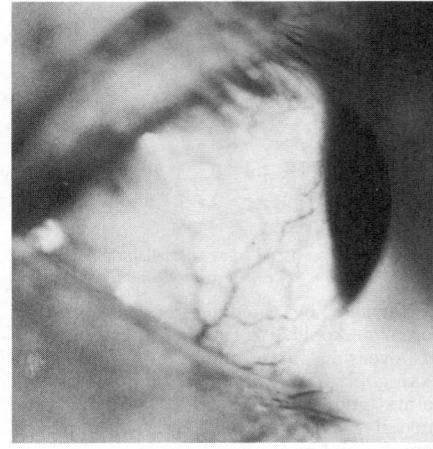

Proptosis of eye. Note lid retraction and exposed sclera above and below cornea. From Stein et al., 2000.

prorubricyte (pro-roo′brĭ-sīt) basophilic erythroblast.

pros(o)- word element [Gr.], *forward; anterior.*

prosecretin (pro″se-kre′tin) the precursor of secretin.

prosection (pro-sek′shun) carefully programmed dissection for demonstration of anatomic structure.

prosector (pro-sek′tor) one who performs prosection.

prosencephalon (pros″en-sef′ah-lon) 1. the portion of the brain developed from the anterior of the three primary brain vesicles in the early embryo, comprising the DIENCEPHALON and TELENCEPHALON. 2. the most anterior of the primary brain vesicles; called also forebrain.

prosodemic (pros″o-dem′ik) pertaining to or denoting a disease transmitted directly from person to person rather than spread generally (as by a contaminated water supply).

prosop(o)- word element [Gr.], *face.*

prosopagnosia (pros″o-pag-no′se-ah) inability to recognize the faces of other people or one's own features in a mirror, due to damage to the underside of both occipital lobes.

prosopectasia (pros″o-pek-ta′zhah) oversize of the face.

prosoplasia (pros″o-pla′zhah) 1. abnormal differentiation of tissue. 2. development into a higher state of organization or function.

prosopoplegia (pros″o-po-ple′jah) facial paralysis.

prosoposchisis (pros″o-pos′kĭ-sis) facial cleft (def. 2).

prosoposternodymus (pros″o-po-ster″no-dim′us) conjoined twins joined face to face and sternum to sternum.

prosopothoracopagus (pros″o-po-thor″-ah-kop′ah-gus) conjoined twins fused from the face to the thorax.

prostacyclin (pros″tah-si′klin) a PROSTA-GLANDIN, PGI$_2$, synthesized by endothelial cells lining the walls of arteries and veins; it is a potent vasodilator and a potent inhibitor of platelet aggregation. When used pharmaceutically it is called EPOPROSTENOL.

prostaglandin (pros″tah-glan′din) any of a group of naturally occurring, chemically related, long-chain hydroxy fatty acids that stimulate contractility of the uterine and other smooth muscle and have the ability to lower blood pressure, regulate acid secretion of the stomach, regulate body temperature and platelet aggregation, and control inflammation and vascular permeability. They also affect the action of certain hormones. First found in semen, they have since been found in cells throughout the body and in menstrual fluid. There are nine types, designated by the letters A to I, the degree of saturation of the side chain of each being designated by subscripts 1, 2, and 3.

Prostaglandins are used clinically to control postpartum hemorrhage, to temporarily manage patent ductus arteriosus, and to treat impotence in men; prostaglandin injections into the amniotic sac, an in-hospital procedure, have been used as an ABORTION technique in pregnancies after the 16th week. About 30 minutes after an injection of prostaglandin F$_{2\alpha}$, contractions begin, and abortion takes place within 19 to 20 hours.

prostaglandin endoperoxide synthase (pros″tah-glan′din en″do-per-ok′sīd sin′thās) an enzyme of the OXIDOREDUCTASE class that has both CYCLOOXYGENASE and PEROXIDASE activities, which together catalyze part of the synthesis of PROSTAGLANDINS and THROMBOX-ANES from ARACHIDONIC ACID.

prostatalgia (pros″tah-tal′jah) pain in the prostate.

prostate (pros′tāt) a gland in the male that surrounds the bladder NECK and URETHRA; it consists of a median lobe and two lateral lobes and is made up partly of glandular matter (whose ducts empty into the prostatic portion of the urethra) and partly of muscular fibers that encircle the urethra. It contributes to the seminal fluid a secretion containing acid phosphatase, citric acid, and proteolytic enzymes, which account for the liquefaction of the coagulated semen. The rate of secretion increases greatly during sexual stimulation. Called

also prostate gland. adj., **prostat′ic.** (See accompanying illustration.)

Disorders of the Prostate. Enlargement of the prostate (benign prostatic HYPERTROPHY) is a common complaint in men over 50 years of age. Because of its position around the urethra, enlargement of the prostate quickly interferes with the normal passage of urine from the bladder. Urination becomes increasingly difficult, and the bladder never feels completely emptied. If the condition is left untreated, continued enlargement of the prostate eventually obstructs the urethra completely, and emergency measures become necessary to empty the bladder. If the prostate is markedly enlarged, chronic constipation may result. The usual remedy is prostatectomy. In men over 60 years of age, cancer of the prostate may occur. PROSTATITIS is a relatively common inflammation of the prostate and may be acute or chronic.

Surgery of the Prostate. Malignancy of the prostate and intractable prostatic infection are treated by PROSTATECTOMY, which is removal of the entire gland and its capsule. Benign prostatic hypertrophy can be treated by either a closed or open approach to the gland and removal of only the hyperplastic tissue (ENUCLEATION).

The closed method of treatment is TRANSURETHRAL RESECTION OF THE PROSTATE (TURP); it is preferred when there is relatively minor enlargement of the gland, and the patient is elderly and a poor surgical risk. A resectoscope is inserted through the penis and along the urethra in a manner similar to that for cystoscopy. When the site of the hyperplasia is reached an electrical cutting loop is inserted, excess tissue is resected, and bleeders are cauterized. Other techniques that can be used with the transurethral approach are the cold punch technique, using a hollow sliding knife to scoop out tissue, and cryosurgery, in which the tissue is frozen and thereby destroyed. A TURP removes only the enlarged tissue; normal prostatic tissue and its outer capsule are left intact. The procedure is less traumatic, requires less time, and requires a shorter postoperative recovery period than any of the open methods of surgery.

There are essentially three approaches to prostatic tissue that involve a surgical incision. In the *suprapubic* approach, an incision is made through the abdominal walls and the bladder, and the prostatic tissue is enucleated. In the *retropubic* approach, a low abdominal incision is made between the pubic arch and the bladder. The bladder is left intact but the prostatic

P

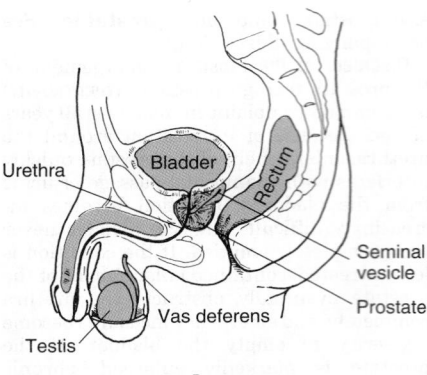

Urethra

Bladder

Rectum

Seminal vesicle

Prostate

Vas deferens

Testis

Prostate.

capsule is incised and the glandular tissue removed. The *perineal* approach requires an incision between the anus and scrotum. The prostatic capsule is opened and the prostatic tissue removed.

The aftereffects of surgery of the prostate vary according to the surgical procedure, the age of the patient, and other factors related to his general state of health. Almost all postprostatectomy patients experience a backflow of semen into the bladder (retrograde EJACULATION) during sexual intercourse. The semen is thus eliminated in the urine rather than being expelled during ejaculation. Studies show that about 6 per cent of men who have had a transurethal resection experience impotence, though there is no known physiologic cause for failure to have an erection postoperatively. The incidence of impotence is slightly higher in men who have had suprapubic and retropubic surgical approaches to the prostate.

Other consequences of prostatic surgery include urinary incontinence, which affects fewer than 1 per cent, urethral scarring and strictures, which affect from 3 to 15 per cent, and regrowth of prostatic tissue, which occurs in about 3 per cent of prostatectomy patients. The urethral strictures can usually be relieved by periodic enlargement of the urethral passage. In general, more than 90 per cent of postprostatectomy patients whose condition is not malignant have successful and uncomplicated surgery.

prostatectomy (pros″tah-tek′to-me) surgical removal of the PROSTATE.

radical p. removal of the prostate with its capsule, seminal vesicles, ductus deferens, some pelvic fasciae, and sometimes pelvic lymph nodes; performed via either the retropubic or the perineal route.

prostatism (pros′tah-tizm) a symptom complex resulting from compression or obstruction of the urethra, due most commonly to hyperplasia of the PROSTATE; symptoms include diminution in the caliber and force of the urinary stream, hesitancy in initiating URINATION, inability to terminate urination abruptly (with resultant dribbling), a sensation of incomplete bladder emptying, and occasionally, urinary retention.

prostatitis (pros″tah-ti′tis) inflammation of the PROSTATE. adj., **prostatit′ic.**

allergic p., eosinophilic p. a condition seen in certain allergies, characterized by diffuse infiltration of the prostate by eosinophils, with small foci of fibrinoid necrosis.

nonspecific granulomatous p. prostatitis characterized by focal or diffuse tissue infiltration by peculiar, large, pale macrophages.

prostatocystitis (pros″tah-to-sis-ti′tis) inflammation of the urinary BLADDER, the bladder NECK and the prostatic part of the URETHRA.

prostatocystotomy (pros″tah-to-sis-tot′-ah-me) incision of the bladder and prostate.

prostatodynia (pros″tah-to-din′e-ah) pain in the prostate.

prostatolith (pros-tat′o-lith) a calculus in the prostate.

prostatolithotomy (pros″tah-to-lĭ-thot′ah-me) incision of the prostate for removal of a calculus.

prostatomegaly (pros″tah-to-meg′ah-le) hypertrophy of the prostate.

prostatorrhea (pros″tah-to-re′ah) a discharge from the prostate.

prostatotomy (pros″tah-tot′ah-me) surgical incision of the prostate.

prostatovesiculectomy (pros″tah-to-vĕ-sik″u-lek′to-me) excision of the prostate and seminal vesicles.

prostatovesiculitis (pros″tah-to-vĕ-sik″u-li′tis) inflammation of the prostate and seminal vesicles.

prosthesis (pros-the′sis), pl. *prosthe′ses* [Gr.] an artificial substitute for a missing part, such as an eye, limb, or tooth, used for functional or cosmetic reasons, or both.

Artificial Limb. Advances in the field of surgical AMPUTATION and the art of designing artificial limbs have made it possible for persons who have lost a limb to be equipped with a prosthesis that functions so efficiently, and so closely resembles the original in appearance, that they can resume normal activities with the disability passing almost unnoticed.

Materials Used in the Prosthesis. A variety of materials can be used for the manufacture of artificial limbs. Wood, especially willow, is the most popular because it is comparatively light and resilient, and is easily shaped. Aluminum or an aluminum alloy is used when lightness is particularly desirable, such as in a limb for an aged person. Plastic limbs are also available. Leather and various metals are used for reinforcement and control.

Powering the Limb. Most artificial limbs are powered by the muscles, either those remaining in the residual limb or other available muscles. The muscles of the residual limb often can be considerably strengthened by physical therapy. Muscle power can be reinforced by means of springs, straps, gears, locks, levers, or, in some cases, hydraulic mechanisms.

The Artificial Lower Limb. The most commonly fitted artificial limb is the knee-jointed leg, used by persons whose lower limbs have been amputated above the knee. This prosthesis is powered by the hip and remaining thigh muscles, which kick the leg forward. The key points in such a limb are the socket, where it fits onto the residual limb, the knee, and the ankle. The possibility of walking with a normal gait depends primarily on the successful alignment of the socket joint; the knee usually consists of a joint centered slightly behind that of the natural leg, as this has been found to afford greater stability; sometimes the ankle joint is omitted and flexibility of the ankle achieved by the use of a rubber foot.

The Artificial Upper Limb. The choice of a particular artificial upper limb depends largely on the person's occupation. There are many different types, ranging from the purely functional, which will enable a person to perform heavy work, to the purely cosmetic, which aims only at looking as natural as possible. Those persons whose work requires them to do heavy lifting are often fitted with a "pegarm," a short limb without an elbow joint, which is easily controlled and has great leverage.

The Artificial Hand. There are many different types of artificial hands. Many artificial upper limbs are so constructed that they can be fitted with a selection of different hands, depending on the type of work to be done. Researchers generally agree that the various types of hooks offer the greatest functional efficiency. These reproduce the most powerful function of natural hands—the pressure between thumb and forefinger. There are also artificial hands that combine a certain amount of utility with cosmetic value, often by means of a cosmetic glove covering a mechanical hand; others are designed simply for appearance, though they may offer some support as well.

Most hooks and hands are mechanically connected to the opposite shoulder and operated by a shrugging motion. However, a procedure known as KINEPLASTY uses the person's own arm and chest muscles to work the device. In this method, selected muscles are tunneled under by surgery and lined by skin. Pegs adapted to the tunnels can then be made to move an artificial hand mechanism. Kineplasty is used when skill rather than strength is desired.

Protecting the Residual Limb (Stump). In a person with an artificial limb, there is always a danger of irritation or infection. A sock is worn to cover the residual limb, and

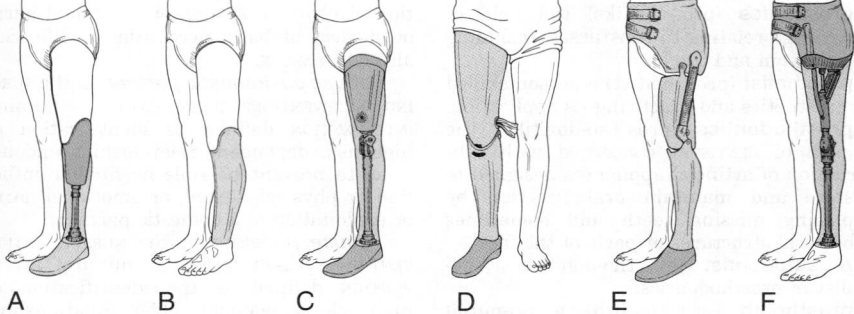

Types of lower limb prostheses. *A,* Below-knee endoskeletal prosthesis. The strength is derived from the inner endoskeleton. *B,* Below-knee exoskeletal prosthesis. The strength is derived from the outer exoskeleton. *C,* Above-knee endoskeletal prosthesis. *D,* Above-knee exoskeletal prosthesis. Exoskeletal (*E*) and endoskeletal (*F*) hip disarticulation prostheses. From Myers, 1995.

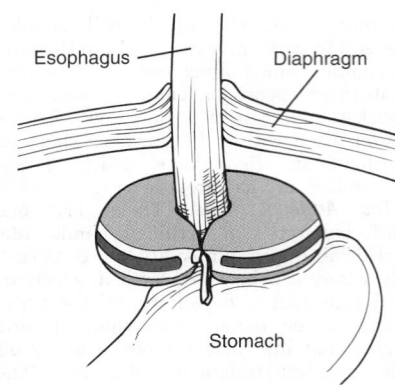

Esophagus — Diaphragm

Stomach

Placement of the Angelchik antireflux prosthesis. From Ignatavicius and Workman, 2002.

this should be washed daily; the residual limb itself should also be washed regularly and carefully, particularly between skin folds. When the artificial limb is not being used, the residual limb should be exposed to the air if possible.

Angelchik p. a -shaped silicone device used in the management of reflux ESOPHAGITIS; it can also be placed around the distal esophagus during a LAPAROTOMY. (See accompanying illustration.)

Austin Moore p. a metallic implant used in hip ARTHROPLASTY.

Charnley p. an implant for hip ARTHROPLASTY consisting of an acetabular cup and a relatively small femoral head component that form a low-friction joint.

penile p. see PENILE PROSTHESIS.

prosthetic (pros-thet′ik) 1. serving as a substitute. 2. pertaining to a PROSTHESIS or to PROSTHETICS. 3. see prosthetic GROUP.

prosthetics (pros-thet′iks) the field of knowledge relating to PROSTHESES, including their design and use.

prosthetist (pros′thĕ-tist) a person skilled in prosthetics and practicing its application.

prosthodontics (pros″tho-don′tiks) the branch of DENTISTRY concerned with construction of artificial appliances designed to restore and maintain oral function by replacing missing teeth and sometimes other oral structures or parts of the face.

prosthodontist (pros″tho-don′tist) a specialist in prosthodontics.

prostholith (pros′tho-lith) a preputial concretion or calculus.

prostration (pros-tra′shun) extreme exhaustion or lack of energy or power.

heat p. HEAT EXHAUSTION.

prot(o)- word element [Gr.], *first.*

protactinium (Pa) (pro″tak-tin′e-um) a chemical element, atomic number 91, atomic weight 231. (See Appendix 6.)

protamine (pro′tah-min) any of a class of simple proteins, soluble in water, not coagulated by heat, and precipitated from aqueous solution by addition of alcohol. Protamines neutralize HEPARIN, and protamine sulfate is used as an antidote in heparin overdosage, administered intravenously.

protanomaly (pro″tah-nom′ah-le) a type of anomalous trichromatic VISION in which the first, red-sensitive, cones have decreased sensitivity.

protanopia (pro″tah-no′pe-ah) imperfect perception of red, with confusion of reds and greens; called also red blindness. adj., **protanop′ic.**

protean (pro′te-an) changing form or assuming different shapes.

protease (pro′te-ās) endopeptidase.

protectant (pro-tek′tant) protective.

protectin (pro-tek′tin) a membrane-bound protein, CD59 (see CD ANTIGEN), which protects normal bystander cells from lysis after COMPLEMENT activation in nearby bacteria or immune complexes. Called also membrane inhibitor of reactive lysis.

protection (pro-tek′shun) defense or immunity against harmful influences.

abuse p. in the NURSING INTERVENTIONS CLASSIFICATION, a nursing INTERVENTION defined as the identification of high-risk, dependent relationships and actions to prevent further infliction of physical or emotional harm. See also physical ABUSE and sexual ABUSE.

abuse p.: child in the NURSING INTERVENTIONS CLASSIFICATION, a nursing INTERVENTION defined as the identification of high-risk, dependent child relationships and actions to prevent possible or further infliction of physical, sexual, or emotional harm or neglect of basic necessities of life. See also CHILD ABUSE.

abuse p.: domestic partner in the NURSING INTERVENTIONS CLASSIFICATION, a nursing INTERVENTION defined as identification of high-risk, dependent relationships and actions to prevent possible or further infliction or physical, sexual, or emotional harm or exploitation of a domestic partner.

abuse p.: elder in the NURSING INTERVENTIONS CLASSIFICATION, a nursing INTERVENTION defined as the identification of high-risk, dependent elder relationships and actions to prevent possible or further infliction of physical, sexual, or emotional harm; neglect of basic necessities; or exploitation. See also elder ABUSE.

abuse p.: religious in the NURSING INTERVENTIONS CLASSIFICATION, a nursing INTERVENTION defined as identification of high-risk, controlling religious relationships and actions to prevent infliction of physical, sexual, or emotional harm and/or exploitation.

environmental risk p. in the NURSING INTERVENTIONS CLASSIFICATION, a nursing INTERVENTION defined as preventing and detecting disease and injury in populations at risk from environmental hazards.

ineffective p. a NURSING DIAGNOSIS accepted by the North American Nursing Diagnosis Association, defined as a decrease in the ability of an individual to guard the self from internal or external threats such as illness or injury.

infection p. in the NURSING INTERVENTIONS CLASSIFICATION, a nursing INTERVENTION defined as prevention and early detection of infection in a patient at risk. See also ISOLATION PRECAUTIONS.

patient rights p. in the NURSING INTERVENTIONS CLASSIFICATION, a nursing INTERVENTION defined as protection of PATIENT'S RIGHTS, the health care rights of the patient, especially one who is a minor, incapacitated, or incompetent and unable to make decisions.

protective (pro-tek′tiv) 1. affording PROTECTION. 2. an agent that provides defense against harmful influences; called also screen.

protein (pro′tēn) any large organic compound made from one or more polypeptides, which are chains of AMINO ACIDS joined by peptide linkages between the amino group of one amino acid and the carboxylic acid group of the next. The primary structure of a polypeptide chain (the sequence of amino acids) is determined by the sequence of bases in the DNA of the gene for that polypeptide (see DEOXYRIBONUCLEIC ACID).

The genetic code of the gene is first transcribed into messenger RNA (mRNA). Then the mRNA is "read" (translated) by a ribosome to produce the polypeptide. The genetic code contains 20 different α-amino acids that can be incorporated into polypeptides by ribosomes. In some proteins other amino acids are produced by post-translational enzymatic modification. As the protein is synthesized it folds up into a unique three-dimensional structure with polar (hydrophilic) side chains of amino acids on the surface and nonpolar (hydrophobic) side chains in the interior. In this way the structure and function of a protein are entirely determined by the genes.

Protein substances in the body are essential to its structure and function. For example, such structures as cell walls, various membranes, connective tissue, and muscles are mainly protein. None of the cells of the body can survive without an adequate supply of protein; in fact, proteins constitute about 20 per cent of the cell mass. Some hormones, which are important in the regulation of metabolism, are proteins, as are the ENZYMES that act as catalysts in the chemical reactions of metabolism.

The proteins in blood plasma are divided into four major classes: transport PROTEINS, such as ALBUMIN, which are involved in the transport of hormones and other substances; *acute phase reactants,* such as ALPHA₁-ANTITRYPSIN or FIBRINOGEN, which are involved in INFLAMMATION or in CLOTTING; COMPLEMENT components; and IMMUNOGLOBULINS. Albumin plays an important role in the maintenance of normal distribution of water in the various compartments of the body by exerting osmotic pressure at the capillary membrane. This pressure prevents fluid of the plasma from leaking out of the capillaries and into the space between the tissue cells. (See also body FLUIDS.)

Food proteins are of great nutritional importance since they are necessary for the building and repair of all kinds of body tissues, especially of muscles and organs such as the heart, liver, and kidneys. Major sources of protein are animal products such as meat, eggs, fish, and milk.

The digestion of protein foods begins in the stomach, is continued in the duodenum, and is completed in the small intestine. The end products of protein digestion, amino acids, pass into the blood, some to be used as structural proteins for the building of body tissues, others to be used as enzymes, and the rest to be carried to various parts of the body as a reserve. If a ready supply of carbohydrates is not available, some proteins may be converted into needed energy.

Symptoms of Protein Deficiency. Severe protein deficiency undermines general health, and is usually manifest in weakness, poor resistance, and swelling of body tissues (nutritional edema) due to accumulation of fluid in the tissue spaces. Protein starvation can result from lack of protein in the diet, such as in persons who, from lack of available supplies of protein foods or through ignorance, satisfy their hunger with large amounts of carbohydrates and little else.

KWASHIORKOR is a disorder of infants and young children whose diet is deficient in protein. The illness develops soon after weaning when the child no longer receives a protein supply from the mother's milk. Sometimes deficiency develops when digestive disorders or infections interfere with proper digestion. A congenital defect in metabolism such as PHENYLKETONURIA may lead to inability to make proper use of the protein that is available in the diet. The first step in treatment of protein deficiency is correction of the deficiency in the diet. If the protein deficiency is secondary to another disorder, treatment is aimed at relief of the primary cause of the deficiency.

AA p. amyloid A protein.

acute phase p. any of the non-antibody proteins found in increased amounts in serum during the acute phase RESPONSE; they include C-reactive PROTEIN, serum amyloid A PROTEIN, FIBRINOGEN, and α1-acid GLYCOPROTEIN.

amyloid A p. a pathological fibrillar low-molecular-weight protein occurring in reactive systemic AMYLOIDOSIS and FAMILIAL MEDITERRANEAN FEVER; it is antigenically related to the high-molecular-weight serum amyloid A PROTEIN. Called also AA protein. See also AMYLOID (def. 2).

Bence Jones p. an abnormal low-molecular weight, heat-sensitive plasma and urinary protein found in multiple myeloma; it coagulates when heated to 45°C–55°C and redissolves partially or wholly on boiling.

binding p. 1. transport protein. 2. any protein able to specifically and reversibly bind other substances, such as ions, sugars, nucleic acids, or amino acids; they are believed to function in transport.

p. C a vitamin K–dependent plasma protein that, when activated by thrombin, inhibits the clotting cascade at the levels of factor V and factor VIII by enzymatic cleavage of the activated forms of these clotting factors; it also enhances fibrinolysis. Deficiency of protein C results in recurrent venous thrombosis. The activated form is abbreviated APC.

carrier p. 1. one which, when coupled to a hapten, renders it capable of eliciting an IMMUNE RESPONSE. 2. transport protein.

C4 binding p. a COMPLEMENT system regulatory protein that inhibits activation of the classical pathway.

complete p. one containing the essential AMINO ACIDS in the proportion required in the human diet.

conjugated p's those in which the protein molecule is united with nonprotein molecules or prosthetic groups, such as GLYCOPROTEINS, LIPOPROTEINS, and METALLOPROTEINS.

C-reactive p. a globulin that forms a precipitate with the somatic C-polysaccharide of the pneumococcus in vitro; the most predominant of the acute phase PROTEINS.

G p. any of a family of similar proteins of the intracellular portion of the plasma membrane that bind activated receptor complexes and cause alterations in the movement of ions across plasma membrane CHANNELS, thus coupling cell surface receptors to intracellular responses. Some G proteins are named for their activities; for example, G_s stimulates and G_i inhibits enzyme activity.

incomplete p. one having a ratio of essential AMINO ACIDS different from that of the average body protein. Called also partial protein.

membrane cofactor p. (MCP) an inhibitor of COMPLEMENT activation found in most blood cells, endothelial and epithelial cells, and fibroblasts.o

myeloma p. a monoclonal immunoglobulin or immunoglobulin fragment produced in multiple myeloma or other plasma cell dyscrasias.

partial p. incomplete protein.

plasma p's the hundreds of different proteins present in blood PLASMA, including transport proteins such as ALBUMIN, TRANSFERRIN, and HAPTOGLOBIN; FIBRINOGEN and other COAGULATION FACTORS; COMPLEMENT components; IMMUNOGLOBULINS; enzyme inhibitors; precursors of substances such as ANGIOTENSIN and BRADYKININ; and many others. See table.

prion p. a protein of uncertain function, in humans coded for by a gene on

SOME PLASMA PROTEINS AND THEIR FUNCTIONS		
Protein	Total Plasma Protein, %	Function
Albumin	60	Maintains blood osmotic pressure
Globulin	36	
α		Transport of lipids and fat-soluble vitamins
β		Transport of lipids and fat-soluble vitamins
γ		Immunity; these are the antibodies
Fibrinogen	4	Blood clotting

From Polaski and Tatro, 1996.

the short arm of chromosome 20. The protease-resistant core is the functional, and perhaps only, component of prions; several abnormal forms have been identified and are responsible for prion DISEASE.

p. S a vitamin K–dependent plasma protein that inhibits blood clotting by serving as a cofactor for activated PROTEIN C. Not to be confused with S p.

S p. see VITRONECTIN.

SAA p. serum amyloid A protein.

serum p's proteins of the blood serum, which include all the plasma proteins except fibrinogen, factor V, and factor VIII.

serum amyloid A p. a high-molecular-weight protein antigenically related to amyloid A PROTEIN; it is an acute phase PROTEIN and apparently suppresses antibody formation. Called also SAA protein.

Tamm-Horsfall p. Tamm-Horsfall MU-COPROTEIN.

transport p. a protein that binds to another protein and provides a transport system for it, either in the plasma or across a plasma membrane. Called also carrier and carrier protein.

proteinaceous (pro″tēn-a′shus) pertaining to or of the nature of protein.

proteinase (pro′tēn-ās) endopeptidase.

protein-bound iodine test a laboratory test done to determine thyroid function by measuring the amount of iodine contained in compounds bound to plasma proteins. It has been largely replaced by radioimmunoassay for the thyroid hormones thyroxine (T_4) and triiodothyronine (T_3).

proteinemia (pro″tēn-e′me-ah) excess of protein in the blood.

Bence Jones p. the presence of monoclonal IMMUNOGLOBULIN light chains in serum.

proteinosis (pro″tēn-o′sis) the accumulation of excess protein in the tissues.

alveolar p. pulmonary alveolar proteinosis.

lipid p. a hereditary defect of lipid metabolism marked by yellowish deposits of hyaline lipid carbohydrate mixture on the inner surface of the lips, under the tongue, and on the oropharynx and larynx, and in skin lesions.

pulmonary alveolar p. see PULMONARY ALVEOLAR PROTEINOSIS.

proteinuria (pro″te-nu′re-ah) an excess of serum proteins in the urine, such as in renal disease, after strenuous exercise, or in dehydration.

accidental p., adventitious p. proteinuria due not to a kidney disease but to some other condition such as hemorrhage in the urinary tract; called also false proteinuria.

athletic p. effort proteinuria.

dietetic p., digestive p. functional proteinuria produced by the eating of certain foods.

effort p. functional PROTEINURIA occurring as a result of vigorous and prolonged exercise of the lower limbs; called also athletic proteinuria.

false p. adventitious proteinuria.

functional p. any proteinuria that is not due to renal disease, such as the transient proteinuria of pregnancy, effort proteinuria, and orthostatic proteinuria.

glomerular p. the most common kind of proteinuria, being due to glomerular disease and abnormal permeability of the glomerular capillaries to protein.

orthostatic p. a form of functional PROTEINURIA, usually seen between the ages of ten and twenty, that occurs on standing erect and disappears on lying down.

overflow p. that due to hemoglobin, myoglobin, or immunoglobulin loss into the urine due to excessive amounts in the bloodstream, such as in multiple myeloma; it is not usually associated with glomerular or tubular disease.

tubular p. proteinuria due to excretion of proteins of low molecular weight such as immunoglobulins, which normally should be reabsorbed.

proteoglycan (pro″te-o-gli′kan) any of a group of GLYCOPROTEINS found primarily in connective tissue and formed of subunits of glycosaminoglycans (long polysaccharide chains containing amino sugars) linked to a protein core like bristles on a bottle brush. Hydrated proteoglycans form the highly viscous fluid of mucus and the matrix of the intercellular ground substance of connective tissue. Called also MUCOPOLYSACCHARIDE.

proteolipid (pro″te-o-lip′id) a combination of a peptide or protein with a lipid, having the solubility characteristics of lipids.

proteolysis (pro″te-ol′ĭ-sis) the splitting of proteins by hydrolysis of the peptide bonds, with formation of smaller polypeptides.

proteolytic (pro″te-o-lit′ik) 1. pertaining to, characterized by, or promoting proteolysis. 2. a proteolytic enzyme.

proteometabolism (pro″te-o-mĕ-tab′o-lizm) the metabolism of protein.

proteopeptic (pro″te-o-pep′tik) digesting protein.

Proteus (pro′te-us) a genus of gram-negative, facultatively anaerobic, motile, rod-shaped bacteria. Organisms are found in fecal material, especially in patients treated with oral antibiotics. P. mira′bilis is a leading cause of urinary tract infections. P. morga′nii is found in the intestines and is associated with summer DIARRHEA of infants. *P. vulga'ris* is a common cause of CYSTITIS and PYELONEPHRITIS and is associated with eye and ear infections, PLEURITIS, PERITONITIS, and suppurative abscesses.

prothrombin (pro-throm'bin) a glycoprotein present in the plasma that is converted into THROMBIN by extrinsic THROMBOPLASTIN during the second stage of blood CLOTTING; called also factor II.

    p. consumption a clinical laboratory test done to determine THROMBOPLASTIN generating capacity, which provides information about the first stage of blood CLOTTING. When clotting of a normal blood sample occurs, prothrombin is converted to THROMBIN; thus there should be little or no prothrombin in the serum after the clot is formed. If, however, there is deficiency of blood clotting (coagulation), some of the prothrombin will not be utilized (consumed). Abnormal results of the test are found in deficiencies of the first-stage COAGULATION FACTORS (factors VIII and IX), and in the presence of circulating ANTICOAGULANTS, THROMBOCYTOPENIA, and any other condition leading to inadequate generation of THROMBOPLASTIN.

    p. consumption test a test to measure the formation of intrinsic THROMBOPLASTIN by determining the residual serum prothrombin after blood CLOTTING is complete.

    p. time a test to measure the activity of COAGULATION FACTORS I, II, V, VII, and X, which participate in the extrinsic pathway of coagulation; abbreviated Pro time or PT. Called also one-stage prothrombin time and Quick's test. Deficiency of any of these factors leads to a prolongation of the one-stage prothrombin times, as will circulating anticoagulants that are active against factors V and VII or against thromboplastin.

    The test is considered basic to any study of the CLOTTING process and is also widely used for guidance in establishing and maintaining anticoagulant therapy. Test results are best understood when both the patient's and the control times are reported. The therapeutic range for coagulation therapy is usually 2 to 3 times that of the normal (12 to 15 sec.) control.

prothrombinase (pro-throm'bin-ās) 1. thromboplastin. 2. the complex formed between activated FACTOR X and calcium, phospholipid, and modified FACTOR V; it can cleave and activate PROTHROMBIN to THROMBIN in the common PATHWAY of coagulation. The term is sometimes used to refer specifically to the active enzyme center of the complex, which is activated FACTOR X.

prothrombinogenic (pro-throm''bī-no-je-n'ik) promoting the production of prothrombin.

protirelin (pro-ti'rĕ-lin) a synthetic tripeptide used pharmaceutically and believed to be structurally identical to thyrotropin-releasing HORMONE.

protist (pro'tist) any member of the Protista.

    eukaryotic p. the higher protists, comprising those organisms having a true nucleus.

    prokaryotic p. the lower protists, comprising those organisms lacking a true nucleus.

Protista (pro-tis'tah) in the classification of living organisms, a KINGDOM comprising unicellular organisms with distinct nuclei (the EUKARYOTES), including PROTOZOA, ALGAE (except blue-green "algae," which are now classified as bacteria), and certain intermediate forms.

protium (pro'te-um) the mass 1 isotope of hydrogen, symbol ^{1}H; ordinary, or light, hydrogen.

protoblast (pro'to-blast) a blastomere from which a particular organ or part develops. adj., **protoblas'tic.**

protocol (pro'to-kol) 1. an explicit, detailed plan of an experiment. 2. the original notes made on an autopsy, an experiment, or a case of disease. 3. a detailed written set of instructions to guide the care of a patient or to assist the practitioner in the performance of a procedure.

protodiastolic (pro''to-di''ah-stol'ik) pertaining to early diastole, i.e., immediately following the second heart sound.

protoduodenum (pro''to-doo''o-de'num) the first or proximal portion of the duodenum, extending from the pylorus to the duodenal papilla.

protofibril (pro''to-fi'bril) the first elongated unit appearing in formation of any type of fiber.

protogaster (pro''to-gas'ter) archenteron.

proton (pro'ton) an elementary particle of mass number 1, with a positive charge equal to the negative charge of the electron; a constituent particle of every nucleus, the number of protons in the nucleus of each ATOM of a chemical element being indicated by its atomic number.

protoneuron (pro''to-noo'ron) the first neuron in a peripheral reflex arc.

proto-oncogene (pro''to-ong'ko-jēn) a normal gene that with slight alteration by mutation or other mechanism becomes an ONCOGENE.

protoplasm (pro'to-plazm) the viscid, translucent colloid material, the essential constituent of the living cell, including cytoplasm and nucleoplasm. adj., **protoplas'-mic.**

protoplast (pro'to-plast) a bacterial, yeast, or fungal cell deprived of its rigid wall but with its plasma membrane intact; the cell is dependent for its integrity on an isotonic or hypertonic medium.

protoporphyria (pro"to-por-fir'e-ah) erythropoietic p.

   erythropoietic p. **(EPP)** an autosomal dominant disorder, a form of erythropoietic PORPHYRIA, characterized by increased levels of protoporphyrin in the erythrocytes, plasma, liver, and feces and a wide variety of photosensitive skin changes, ranging from a burning or pruritic sensation to erythema, plaquelike edema, and wheals.

protoporphyrin (pro'to-por'fĭ-rin) a porphyrin whose iron complex united with protein occurs in hemoglobin, myoglobin, and certain respiratory pigments. It is accumulated and excreted excessively in the feces in erythropoietic protoporphyria and variegate porphyria.

protoporphyrinemia (pro"to-por"fĭ-rĭ-ne'me-ah) PROTOPORPHYRIN in the urine; see PROTOPORPHYRIA.

Prototheca (pro"to-the'kah) a genus of ubiquitous yeastlike organisms generally considered as being achloric algae, occurring as spherical to elliptical cells containing thick-walled autospores. *P. wickerha'mii* and *P. zop'fii* are the species involved in human and animal infection. See also PROTOTHECOSIS.

protothecosis (pro"to-the-ko'sis) an infection caused by organisms of the genus *Prototheca*, especially *P. wickerhamii* or *P. zopfii,* varying from cutaneous and subcutaneous lesions to systemic invasion involving several internal organs, which may occur as an opportunistic infection or as a result of traumatic implantation of the pathogen into the tissues.

prototroph (pro'to-trōf) an organism with the same growth factor requirements as the ancestral strain; said of microbial mutants. adj., **prototroph'ic.**

prototype (pro'to-tīp) the original type or form that is typical of later individuals or species.

protovertebra (pro"to-ver'tĕ-brah) 1. somite. 2. the caudal half of a somite forming most of the vertebra.

Protozoa (pro"to-zo'ah) a subkingdom (formerly a phylum) comprising the unicellular eukaryotic organisms; most are free-living, but some lead commensalistic, mutualistic, or parasitic existences. According to newer classifications, the Protozoa

are divided into seven phyla: Sarcomastigophora, Labyrinthomorpha, Apicoplexa, Microspora, Acetospora, Myxozoa, and Aliophora. Pathogenic protozoa include *Plasmodium* species, the cause of human MALARIA; *Trypanosoma gambiense,* the cause of African TRYPANOSOMIASIS; *Toxoplasma gondii,* of which house cats are the reservoir and humans the intermediate host; *Entamoeba histolytica,* the cause of amebic DYSENTERY; and *Balantidium coli* and *Isospora belli,* both of which cause diarrhea in humans.

Protozoa can be ingested and transmitted through contaminated feces. Prevention of transmission is extremely important; handwashing and stool precautions are recommended. Other necessary precautions (see INFECTION CONTROL) should be carried out according to directions from the Centers for Disease Control and Prevention. Protozoal infections are occurring more frequently in North America and other industrialized countries because of increased world travel.

protozoa (pro"to-zo'ah) plural of PROTOZOON.

protozoacide (pro"to-zo'ah-sīd) antiprotozoal AGENT.

protozoal (pro"to-zo'al) pertaining to or caused by protozoa.

protozoan (pro"to-zo'an) 1. of or pertaining to protozoa. 2. an organism belonging to the Protozoa.

protozoiasis (pro"to-zo-i'ah-sis) any disease caused by protozoa.

protozoology (pro"to-zo-ol'o-je) the scientific study of protozoa.

protozoon (pro"to-zo'on) [Gr.] any member of the PROTOZOA.

protozoophage (pro"to-zo'o-fāj) a cell having phagocytic action on protozoa.

protraction (pro-trak'shun) a forward projection of a facial structure; in mandibular protraction the gnathion is anterior to the orbital plane; in maxillary protraction the subnasion is anterior to the orbital plane.

protractor (pro-trak'ter) 1. a muscle that pulls a part forward; see also RETRACTOR. 2. a semicircular device for measuring and constructing angles.

protransglutaminase (pro-tranz"glootam'in-ās) the inactive precursor of transglutaminase; called also coagulation factor XIII.

protriptyline (pro-trip'tĭ-lēn) a tricyclic ANTIDEPRESSANT, also used in the treatment of attention-deficit/hyperactivity disorder, and narcolepsy; administered orally as the hydrochloride salt.

protrusion (pro-troo′zhun) extension beyond the usual limits, or above a plane surface.

protuberance (pro-too′ber-ans) a projecting part, or prominence.

Proventil (pro-ven′til) trademark for preparations of ALBUTEROL, a BRONCHODILATOR.

Provera (pro-ver′ah) trademark for preparations of MEDROXYPROGESTERONE acetate, a progestational AGENT.

provertebra (pro-ver′tĕ-brah) protovertebra.

Providencia (prov″ĭ-den′shah) a genus of gram-negative, facultatively anaerobic, motile, rod-shaped bacteria, occurring in normal urine and feces. Organisms are potential pathogens associated with urinary tract and secondary tissue infections. *P. stuar′tii* causes nosocomial infections and is a major agent in burn infections.

provirus (pro-vi′rus) a DNA transcript of an RNA VIRUS that migrates from the cytoplasm into the nucleus and integrates into the host GENOME by CROSSING OVER so that it will be thus replicated in the daughter cells.

provitamin (pro-vi′tah-min) a substance, e.g., ergosterol, from which the animal organism can form a vitamin.

provocation (prov″ah-ka′shun) challenge (def. 3).

proximad (prok′sĭ-mad) in a proximal direction.

proximal (prok′sĭ-mal) nearest to a point of reference, as to a center or median line or to the point of attachment or origin.

proximalis (prok″sĭ-ma′lis) [L.] proximal.

proximate (prok′sĭ-māt) immediate; nearest.

proximoataxia (prok″sĭ-mo-ah-tak′se-ah) ataxia of the proximal part of a limb.

proximobuccal (prok″sĭ-mo-buk′al) pertaining to the proximal and buccal surfaces of a posterior tooth.

Prozac (pro′zak) trademark for preparations of FLUOXETINE hydrochloride, an ANTIDEPRESSANT.

prozone (pro′zōn) in an agglutination or precipitation reaction, the zone of relatively high antibody concentrations within which no reaction occurs. As the antibody concentration is lowered below the prozone, the reaction occurs. This phenomenon may be due simply to antibody excess or it may be due to blocking antibody or to nonspecific inhibitors in serum.

prurigo (proo-ri′go) any of several itchy skin eruptions in which the characteristic lesion is dome-shaped with a small transient vesicle on top, followed by crusting or lichenification. adj., **prurig′inous.**

p. gestatio′nis, p. gestationis of Besnier an extremely pruritic condition of unknown etiology occurring in the third trimester of pregnancy, characterized by the development of tiny crust-covered excoriated papules mainly on the extensor surfaces of the limbs but also found on the upper trunk and other areas of the body, and leaving a postinflammatory residue on resolution of the lesions. It tends to clear after delivery and to recur with subsequent pregnancies.

p. mi′tis prurigo of a mild type.

p. nodula′ris a form of neurodermatitis, usually occurring on the extremities in middle-aged women, marked by discrete, firm, rough-surfaced, dark brownish-gray, intensely itchy nodules.

p. sim′plex papular urticaria.

pruritogenic (proo″rit-o-jen′ik) causing pruritus, or itching.

pruritus (proo-ri′tus) an unpleasant sensation of the skin, provoking the desire to scratch or rub it; called also itching. adj., **prurit′ic.** It is common in many types of skin disorders, especially allergic inflammation and parasitic infestations. Systemic diseases that may cause pruritus include DIABETES MELLITUS (pruritus vulvae) and liver disorders with jaundice. Hemorrhoids are often accompanied by rectal pruritus. Emotional distress plays an important role in the development and control of this disturbing symptom. Unless pruritus is relieved the patient may become exhausted from lack of sleep. Cleanliness, soothing ointments or lotions, sodium bicarbonate baths, and sometimes tranquilizing drugs are used in the relief of pruritus. Since it is a symptom of some other disorder, complete cure of pruritus depends on control of the primary illness.

p. a′ni intense chronic itching in the anal region.

p. seni′lis itching in the aged, due to degeneration of the skin.

uremic p. generalized itching associated with chronic renal failure and not attributable to other internal or skin disease.

p. vul′vae intense itching of the external genitalia in the female.

psammoma (sah-mo′mah) a tumor, especially a MENINGIOMA, that contains psammoma BODIES.

psammosarcoma (sam″o-sahr-ko′mah) a SARCOMA containing granular material.

PSE portal-systemic encephalopathy.

pseud(o)- word element [Gr.], *false.*

pseudoainhum (soo″do-īn′yoom) ringlike constrictions around the digits, limbs, or trunk; it occurs both congenitally and in in association with a wide variety of hereditary and nonhereditary disorders. The most severe cases of congenital pseudoainhum result in AUTOAMPUTATION in utero.

pseudarthrosis (soo″ahr-thro′sis) a pathologic entity characterized by deossification of a weight-bearing long bone, followed by bending and pathologic fracture, with inability to form normal callus; this leads to existence of the "false joint" that gives the condition its name.

pseudencephalus (soo″den-sef′ah-lus) a malformed fetus with a tumor in place of the brain.

pseudesthesia (soo″des-the′zhah) a subjective sensation occurring in the absence of the appropriate stimuli; an imaginary sensation.

pseudoacanthosis nigricans (soo″do-ak″an-tho′sis ni′grĭ-kans) a benign form of ACANTHOSIS NIGRICANS associated with obesity; the obesity is sometimes due to endocrine disturbance.

pseudoagraphia (soo″do-ah-graf′e-ah) a condition in which the patient can copy writing, but cannot write except in a meaningless and illegible manner.

pseudoallele (soo″do-ah-lēl′) one of two or more genes that are seemingly allelic, but which can be shown to have distinctive but closely linked loci. adj., **pseudoallel′ic.**

pseudoanemia (soo″do-ah-ne′me-ah) marked pallor with no evidence of anemia.

pseudoaneurysm (soo″do-an′u-rizm) a condition resembling an ANEURYSM, but due to dilation or tortuosity of a vessel. Called also false or spurious aneurysm.

pseudoangina (soo″do-an-ji′-nah) a nervous disorder resembling angina, consisting of slight chest or breast pain, usually with pallor followed by cyanosis and coldness or numbness of the extremities.

pseudoankylosis (soo″do-ang″kĭ-lo′sis) a false ankylosis.

pseudoapoplexy (soo″do-ap′o-plek″se) a condition resembling apoplexy, but without cerebral hemorrhage.

pseudobulbar (soo″do-bul′bar) apparently, but not really, due to a bulbar lesion.

pseudocartilaginous (soo″do-kahr″tĭ-laj′ĭ-nus) chondral.

pseudocast (soo′do-kast) an accidental formation of urinary sediment resembling a true cast.

pseudocele (soo′do-sēl) cavity of septum pellucidum.

pseudochancre (soo″do-shang′ker) an indurated lesion resembling a chancre.

pseudochromesthesia (soo″do-krōm″es-the′zhah) a synesthesia in which certain sounds induce sensations of color.

pseudochromhidrosis (soo″do-krōm″hĭ-dro′sis) discoloration of sweat caused by the action of pigment-producing bacteria.

pseudocoarctation (soo″do-ko″ahrk-ta′-shun) a condition radiographically resembling coarctation but without compromise of the lumen, as occurs in a congenital anomaly of the aortic arch.

pseudocoele (soo″do-sēl) cavity of septum pellucidum.

pseudocolloid (soo″do-kol′oid) a mucoid substance sometimes found in ovarian cysts.

pseudocoloboma (soo″do-kol″o-bo′mah) a line or scar on the iris resembling a coloboma.

pseudocoma (soo″do-ko′mah) locked-in syndrome.

pseudocoxalgia (soo″do-kok-sal′jah) osteochondrosis of the capitular epiphysis of the femur.

pseudocrisis (soo″do-kri′sis) sudden but temporary abatement of febrile symptoms.

pseudocroup (soo″do-krōōp) laryngismus stridulus.

pseudocyesis (soo″do-si-e′sis) false pregnancy.

pseudocylindroid (soo″do-sĭ-lin′droid) a shred of mucin in the urine resembling a cylindroid.

pseudocyst (soo′do-sist) 1. an abnormal or dilated cavity resembling a true cyst but not lined with epithelium; called also adventitious or false cyst. 2. a cystic collection of fluid and necrotic debris whose walls are formed by the pancreas and other surrounding organs. It occurs as a complication of acute PANCREATITIS and may subside spontaneously or become secondarily infected and develop into an abscess. 3. a cluster of small comma-shaped forms of *Toxoplasma gondii,* sometimes containing thousands of organisms within an irregular wall; it represents a resting stage, as opposed to the active, motile stage. Pseudocysts are found in the tissues, especially muscles and the brain, in chronic (latent) TOXOPLASMOSIS.

pseudodementia (soo″do-dĕ-men′shah) a disorder resembling dementia but not due to organic brain disease and is potentially reversible by treatment; one form is the depressive symptoms seen in some older adults.

pseudodiphtheria (soo″do-dif-the′re-ah) any of a group of infections resembling diphtheria but not caused by *Corynbacterium diphtheriae;* called also diphtheroid.

P

pseudodominant (soo″do-dom′ĭ-nant) the rarely observed pattern of inheritance of a recessive genetic trait in the offspring of parents one of whom is homozygous and the other heterozygous for the gene. Half the offspring are affected as in the common pattern of dominant inheritance seen when only one parent, who is heterozygous, carries the gene.

pseudoedema (soo″do-ĕ-de′mah) a puffy state resembling edema

pseudoemphysema (soo″do-em″fĭ-ze′-mah) a condition resembling emphysema, but due to temporary obstruction of the bronchi.

pseudoephedrine (soo″do-ĕ-fed′rin) one of the optical isomers of EPHEDRINE, used in the form of the hydrochloride and sulfate salts as a nasal DECONGESTANT; administered orally.

pseudoexstrophy (soo″do-ek′stro-fe) a developmental anomaly marked by the characteristic musculoskeletal defects of exstrophy of the bladder, but with no major defect of the urinary tract.

pseudofolliculitis (soo″do-fŏ-lik″u-li′tis) a chronic disorder, usually caused by *Staphylococcus aureus,* occurring chiefly in the beards of men of African descent, most often in the submandibular region of the neck; the characteristic lesions are erythematous papules, less commonly pustules, containing buried hairs whose tips can easily be freed up; in contrast to SYCOSIS BARBAE, it affects exclusively those who shave.

pseudofracture (soo″do-frak′chur) radiographic appearance of a thickened periosteum and new bone formation over what looks like an incomplete fracture.

pseudoganglion (soo″do-gang′gle-on) an enlargement on a nerve resembling a ganglion.

pseudogeusesthesia (soo″do-goos″es-the′zhah) a false sensation of taste associated with a sensation of another modality.

pseudogeusia (soo″do-goo′zhah) a sensation of taste occurring in the absence of a stimulus or inappropriate to the exciting stimulus.

pseudoglioma (soo″do-gli-o′mah) any condition mimicking retinoblastoma, e.g., retrolental fibroplasia or exudative retinopathy.

pseudoglottis (soo″do-glot′is) 1. the aperture between the false vocal cords. 2. neoglottis. adj., **pseudoglot′tic.**

pseudogout (soo′do-gout) CALCIUM PYROPHOSPHATE DEPOSITION DISEASE, especially the acute and subacute forms.

pseudohematuria (soo″do-he″mah-tu′re-ah) the presence in the urine of pigments that give it a pink or red color in absence of detectable hemoglobin or blood cells.

pseudohemophilia (soo″do-he″mo-fil′e-ah) von Willebrand's disease.

pseudohermaphrodite (soo″do-her-maf′ro-dīt) an individual exhibiting pseudohermaphroditism.

pseudohermaphroditism (soo″do-her-maf′ro-dit-izm″) a congenital abnormality in which an individually is genetically and gonadally of one sex but has significant contradictions in the morphologic criteria of sex, often including ambiguous external genitalia. In *female pseudohermaphroditism,* the individual is a genetic and gonadal female with partial MASCULINIZATION such as an enlarged clitoris resembling a penis and labia majora resembling a scrotum. In *male pseudohermaphroditism,* the individual is a genetic and gonadal male with FEMINIZATION or incomplete masculinization, including a small penis, perineal hypospadias, and a scrotum that lacks testes. Pseudohermaphroditism is not to be confused with HERMAPHRODITISM, in which the individual has both ovarian and testicular tissue.

pseudohernia (soo″do-her′ne-ah) an inflamed sac or gland simulating strangulated hernia.

pseudohypertrophy (soo″do-hi-per′tro-fe) increase in size without true hypertrophy. adj., **pseudohypertroph′ic.**

pseudohypoaldosteronism (soo″do-hi″po-al-dos′ter-ōn-izm) a hereditary disorder of infancy, characterized by severe salt loss by the kidneys despite elevated secretion and urinary excretion of aldosterone; it is thought to be due to unresponsiveness of the distal renal tubule to aldosterone.

pseudohyponatremia (soo″do-hi″po-nah-tre′me-ah) a decreased serum sodium concentration that does not correspond to a real hypotonic disorder, i.e., the serum osmolality is normal. It occurs when hyperlipemia increases the serum non-water volume or hyperproteinemia increases the serum non-sodium solute.

pseudohypoparathyroidism (soo″do-hi″po-par″ah-thi′roi-dizm) a hereditary condition clinically resembling HYPOPARATHYROIDISM, but caused by failure of response to, rather than deficiency of, parathyroid hormone; it is marked by hypocalcemia and hyperphosphatemia and often by short stature, obesity, short metacarpals, and ectopic calcification. Mental retardation, cataracts, tetany, and convulsions may also occur.

pseudoisochromatic (soo″do-i″so-kro-mat′ik) seemingly of the same color throughout, referring to a solution or chart for testing color BLINDNESS, having two pigments or colors that are distinguished by the normal eye but not by the color blind eye.

pseudojaundice (soo″do-jawn′dis) yellowness of the skin due to blood changes and not to liver disease.

pseudologia (soo″do-lo′je-ah) lying; falsehood.

p. fantas′tica a tendency to tell extravagant and fantastic falsehoods centered about the storyteller, who often comes to believe in and may act on them.

pseudolymphoma (soo″do-lim-fo′mah) any of a group of disorders having a benign course but exhibiting clinical and histologic features suggestive of malignant lymphoma. Called also lymphocytoma.

pseudomelanoma (soo″do-mel″ah-no′-mah) a benign melanotic lesion resembling a superficial spreading melanoma occurring at the site of an incompletely removed melanocytic nevus.

pseudomelanosis (soo″do-mel″ah-no′sis) pigmentation of tissues after death by blood pigments.

pseudomembrane (soo″do-mem′brān) false membrane.

Pseudomonas (soo″do-mo′nas) a genus of gram-negative, strictly aerobic, motile, straight or curved rod-shaped bacteria. Most species are saprophytic, but some are pathogenic for plants and animals. *P. aerugino′sa* (which produces the pigments pyocyanin and fluorescein that give a characteristic blue color to the pustular discharge of some suppurative infections) is a major agent of severe or fatal nosocomial infections in debilitated patients. Some species are opportunistic pathogens in humans; these include *P. alcali′genes, P. cepa′cia, P. fluores′cens, P. mal′lei* (which also causes glanders in horses), *P. maltophi′lia, P. pseudomal′lei,* and *P. stut′zeri.*

pseudomucin (soo″do-mu′sin) a mucinlike substance found in ovarian cysts. adj., **pseudomu′cinous.**

pseudomyxoma (soo″do-mik-so′mah) 1. a mass of epithelial mucus resembling a MYXOMA. 2. pseudomyxoma peritonei.

p. peritone′i the presence in the peritoneal cavity of mucoid material from a ruptured ovarian cyst or a ruptured mucocele of the appendix.

pseudoneuritis (soo″do-noŏ-ri′tis) a congenital hyperemic condition of the optic papilla.

pseudopapilledema (soo″do-pap″il-ĕ-de′-mah) anomalous elevation of the optic disk.

MEMBERS OF *PSEUDOMONAS* GENUS	
P. acidovorans	Occasionally opportunistic
P. aeruginosa	Most common isolate; blue-green pigment; grapelike odor; causes pneumonia, blue plus, urinary tract infection
P. alcaligenes	Occasionally opportunistic
P. diminuta	In clinical specimens; nonpathogenic
P. fluorescens	Fluorescent pigments; occasionally opportunistic
P. mendocina	In urine; nonpathogenic
P. paucimohilis	Sometimes opportunistic
P. pseudo-alcaligenes	Sometimes pathogenic
P. putida	Fluorescent; occasionally opportunistic
P. putrefaciens	Food spoilage; occasionally pathogenic
P. stutzeri	Occasionally opportunistic
P. vesicularis	Genitourinary tract infections

pseudoparalysis (soo″do-pah-ral′ĭ-sis) apparent loss of muscular power without real paralysis.

Parrot's p., syphilitic p. pseudoparalysis of one or more extremities in infants, due to syphilitic osteochondritis of an epiphysis.

pseudoparaplegia (soo″do-par″ah-ple′jah) spurious paralysis of the lower limbs, as in CONVERSION DISORDER or MALINGERING.

pseudoparesis (soo″do-pah-re′sis) a conversion or nonorganic condition simulating paresis.

pseudopelade (soo″do-pe′lād) an uncommon type of alopecia characterized by the asymptomatic development of a distinctive scarlike patchy alopecia in adults.

pseudoplegia (soo″do-ple′jah) paralysis due to a CONVERSION DISORDER.

pseudopodium (soo″do-po′de-um) a temporary protrusion of the cytoplasm of an ameba, serving for purposes of locomotion or to engulf food.

pseudopolyp (soo″do-pol′ip) a hypertrophied tab of mucous membrane resembling a polyp, but caused by ulceration surrounding intact mucosa.

pseudopolyposis (soo″do-pol″ĭ-po′sis) numerous pseudopolyps in the colon and rectum, due to longstanding inflammation.

pseudopregnancy (soo″do-preg′nan-se) false pregnancy.

pseudoprognathism (soo″do-prog′nah-thizm) protruding mandible resembling prognathism but due to altered tooth alignment, resulting from malocclusion.

P

pseudopseudohypoparathyroidism (soo″do-soo″do-hi″po-par″ah-thi′roi-dizm) an incomplete form of pseudohypoparathyroidism, marked by the same constitutional features but by normal levels of calcium and phosphorus in the blood serum.

pseudopterygium (soo″do-tĕ-rij′e-um) an adhesion of the conjunctiva to the cornea following a burn or other injury.

pseudoptosis (soo″do-to′sis) decrease in the size of the palpebral aperture.

pseudoreaction (soo″do-re-ak′shun) a false or deceptive reaction; in intradermal skin tests, a reaction not due to the specific test substance but to protein in the medium employed in producing the toxin.

pseudorickets (soo″do-rik′ets) renal osteodystrophy.

pseudosarcoma (soo″do-sahr-ko′mah) sarcomatoid transformation of a carcinoma histologically resembling a sarcoma.

pseudoscarlatina (soo″do-skahr″lah-te′-nah) a septic condition with fever and eruption resembling scarlet fever.

pseudosclerosis (soo″do-sklĕ-ro′sis) a condition with the symptoms but without the lesions of multiple sclerosis.

Westphal-Strümpell p. hepatolenticular degeneration.

pseudosmia (soo″doz′me-ah) a sensation of odor without the appropriate stimulus.

pseudotetanus (soo″do-tet′ah-nus) persistent muscular contractions resembling tetanus but not associated with *Clostridium tetani.*

pseudotruncus arteriosus (soo″do-trunk′us ahr-te″re-o′sus) the most severe form of TETRALOGY OF FALLOT, consisting of atresia of the pulmonic valve and absence of the main pulmonic artery; the lungs are supplied through a patent ductus arteriosus or from bronchial arteries arising from the aorta.

pseudotumor (soo″do-too′mer) an enlargement that resembles a tumor; it may result from inflammation, accumulation of fluid, or other causes, and may or may not regress spontaneously.

p. ce′rebri cerebral edema and raised intracranial pressure without neurological signs except occasional sixth-nerve palsy.

inflammatory p. a tumorlike mass resulting from an inflammatory reaction; it may occur in a variety of organs and is composed of granulation tissue with leukocyte infiltration.

pseudovertigo (soo″do-ver′tĭ-go) any dizziness or other form of lightheadedness that resembles vertigo but does not involve a sense of rotation. Among many possible causes are hyperventilation, orthostatic hypotension, and panic disorder.

pseudoxanthoma elasticum (soo″do-zan-tho′mah e-las′tĭ-kum) a dermatosis marked clinically by small yellowish macules and papules, individual or confluent, or massed into plaques, and histologically by masses of swollen, calcified elastic fibers with degeneration of the collagen fibers in the lower and middle dermis and in the gastrointestinal tract and heart.

psi pounds per square inch.

psicofuranine (si-ko-fūr′ah-nēn) a nucleoside ANTIBIOTIC produced by *Streptomyces hygroscopicus,* having antibacterial and antitumor activity.

psilocin (si′lo-sin) a HALLUCINOGENIC substance closely related to PSILOCYBIN.

psilocybin (si′lo-si′bin) a HALLUCINOGEN having indole characteristics, isolated from the mushroom *Psilocybe mexicana.*

psittacosis (sit″ah-ko′sis) a disease due to a strain of *Chlamydia psittaci;* it was first seen in parrots and later was found in other birds and domestic fowl (in which it is called *ornithosis*). It is transmissible to humans. The etiologic organism is inhaled into the body and attacks the respiratory tract. The first symptoms appear after an incubation period of 6 to 15 days and include fever, sore throat, headache, loss of appetite, chills, and profuse sweating. Later there may be coughing, difficulty in breathing, abdominal distress, and often splenomegaly. Prostration may occur. Infiltrates may appear in the chest x-ray. Special laboratory tests are necessary for accurate diagnosis. Psittacosis usually runs its course in 2 or 3 weeks. Complications may be avoided by the administration of such antibiotics as tetracycline and penicillin. Fatalities are uncommon.

psoitis (so-i′tis) inflammation of a psoas muscle or its sheath.

psoralen (sor′ah-len) any of the constituents of certain plants, such as *Psoralea corylifolia,* that have the ability to produce phototoxic DERMATITIS when an individual is first exposed to it and then to sunlight; certain perfumes and drugs, such as METHOXSALEN, contain psoralens.

psoriasis (so-ri′ah-sis) a chronic, recurrent skin disease marked by discrete bright red macules, papules, or patches covered with lamellated silvery scales. There are also guttate, erythrodermic (exfoliative), and pustular forms. adj., **psoriat′ic.**

Any body surface can be affected, but lesions appear most often on the scalp, knees, and elbows. Sometimes the nails are affected, causing pitting and scaling of the base, or ridging and furrowing with an alteration in transparency. Emotional response to the persistence and cosmetically disfiguring effects can be severe. Psoriasis can occur in either sex at any age, but is most often seen in persons 15 to 35 years of age. It affects about 2 per cent of white adults and is less common in blacks and Asians. About 10 per cent of patients have arthritis associated with their psoriasis (psoriatic ARTHRITIS). The cause is not known; psoriasis is not an infectious disease and cannot be transmitted from one person to another. Recent research has established that it is an immune-mediated disorder. It tends to occur in families; about one third of the cases are believed to be related to a hereditary factor. Skin injury (such as from scratching or surgery) or inflammation (as from over-exposure to ultraviolet light) can lead to the development of more lesions. Certain drugs are known to exacerbate psoriasis. Early attacks respond well to treatment, only to reappear within weeks or months. Complete and permanent remission is rare.

Treatment. There is at present no curative agent available; some topical treatments currently in use must be prescribed with caution to avoid permanent damage to the skin. Recommended topical agents include moisturizers, keratolytics, coal tar, anthralin, steroids, and vitamin D derivatives. Exposure to the sun or artificial ultraviolet light can be helpful. The oldest form of therapy is the Goeckerman routine, which combines crude coal tar with increasing exposure to ultraviolet B. PHOTOCHEMOTHER-APY (PSORALEN and ultraviolet light [PUVA]) is a newer form of treatment. With this therapy the combination of a photosensitizing agent (psoralen) with long-wave ultraviolet light (UVA) reduces cellular proliferation by inhibiting DNA synthesis. The folic acid antagonist METHOTREXATE controls psoriasis by inhibiting cell reproduction. Retinoids (acitretin, etretinate, isotretinoin) are used alone or in combination with PUVA and are often effective against pustular forms of the disease. Methotrexate, retinoids, and PUVA have potentially serious side effects and are therefore usually given only to those patients with severe psoriasis that is not controlled by other forms of treatment. Cyclosporine is used in severe cases. Topical, systemic, and ultraviolet therapies are sometimes combined; the patient may be rotated from one therapy to another in succession to reduce cumulative side effects and forestall resistance to therapy.

Extensive information about psoriasis can be obtained from the National Psoriasis Foundation, 6600 S.W. 92nd Ave., Suite 300, Portland, OR 97223 (telephone 800-723-9166). (See Atlas 2, Part J.)

PSRO Professional Standards Review Organization.

PSVT paroxysmal supraventricular tachycardia.

psych(o)- word element [Gr.], *mind.*

psychalgia (si-kal′jah) 1. pain, usually in the head and perceived as being of emotional origin, that may accompany intolerable ideas, obsessions, or hallucinations. 2. psychogenic pain. adj., **psychal′-gic.**

psychataxia (si″kah-tak′se-ah) a disordered mental state with confusion and inability to concentrate.

psyche (si′ke) 1. the human faculty for thought, judgment, and emotion; the

---

OVERVIEW OF PSORIASIS AND PSORIASIS THERAPIES

Affects
 Skin, joints, nails, mucous membranes
 All age groups

Severity and Location
 Scattered lesions to full body involvement
 Lesions may itch, burn, and bleed
 Erythrodermic and pustular forms may be life threatening
 Location of lesions is a better predictor of disability than extent

Impairment
 Decreased skin function and flexibility
 Difficulty in walking, climbing, grasping
 Restricted bending or crouching
 Limited stretching because of splitting and bleeding of skin
 Types of clothing that can be worn limited because of lesions on the trunk
 Inability to sit because of lesions on the buttocks
 Chills and fever resulting from poor control of body temperature in erythrodermic psoriasis
 Joint disability resulting from psoriatic arthritis
 Life-threatening systemic infections and cardiac and pulmonary complications in erythrodermic and generalized pustular psoriasis
 Sleep deprivation caused by itching
 Depression resulting from disfigurement and social rejection

Therapy
 No cure
 Therapy aims to restore function and maintain health during periods of clearance
 No universally effective therapy
 Response varies from one person to another
 Psoriasis may return after treatment is discontinued, possibly more severely than before treatment
 The most potent treatments have the most dangerous side effects
 Most patients receive most therapies during their lives

mental life, including both conscious and unconscious processes; the mind in its totality, as distinguished from the body. 2. the soul or self. adj., **psy′chic.**

psychedelic (si″kĕ-del′ik) pertaining to or characterized by hallucinations, distortions of perception and awareness, and sometimes psychotic-like behavior; also, a drug producing such effects (see also HALLUCINOGEN). Psychedelic drugs include LSD and MESCALINE.

psychiatrist (si-ki′ah-trist) a physician who specializes in psychiatry.

psychiatry (si-ki′ah-tre) the branch of health science that deals with the study, treatment, and prevention of mental disorders. adj., **psychiat′ric.**

> **biological p.** that which emphasizes biochemical, pharmacological, and neurological causes and treatment approaches.

> **community p.** the branch of psychiatry concerned with the detection, prevention, and treatment of mental disorders in a designated geographical area, with emphasis on environmental factors.

> **descriptive p.** psychiatry based on the study of observable symptoms and behavioral phenomena, rather than underlying psychodynamic processes.

> **dynamic p.** psychiatry based on the study of the mental mechanisms and emotional processes that govern and motivate human behavior, rather than observable behavioral phenomena.

> **forensic p.** that dealing with the legal aspects of mental disorders.

> **geriatric p.** geropsychiatry.

> **preventive p.** a broad term referring to the amelioration, control, and limitation of psychiatric disability.

> **social p.** that concerned with the cultural and social factors that engender, precipitate, intensify, or prolong maladaptive patterns of behavior and complicate treatment.

psychic (si′kik) 1. pertaining to the PSYCHE. 2. mental (def. 1).

psychoactive (si″ko-ak′tiv) affecting the mind or behavior; see psychoactive SUBSTANCE. Called also psychotropic.

> **p. substance–induced organic mental disorders** former name for substance-induced disorders.

> **p. substance use disorders** substance use disorders.

psychoanaleptic (si″ko-an″ah-lep′tik) exerting a stimulating effect on the mind.

psychoanalysis (si″ko-ah-nal′ĭ-sis) a system of theoretical psychology and psychotherapy formulated by Sigmund FREUD

to analyze mental processes and mental disorders, based on recognition of unconscious mental processes such as resistance repression, and transference, and of the importance of infantile experience as a determinant of adult behavior; techniques used include free association, interpretation, and dream analysis. This theory has increased our understanding of the causes of many different mental phenomena, such as NEUROSES and PERSONALITY DISORDERS. Called also psychoanalytic psychotherapy adj., **psychoanalyt′ic.**

Neurotic patterns of behavior have their origin in conflicts, feelings, and attitudes that arise in childhood. Children have many desires, impulses, and thoughts that are in conflict with the expectations of their parents. In order to avoid the unbearable anxiety of direct conflict with their parents, which they fear would result in loss of affection or other forms of punishment, these conflicts are *repressed;* the anxiety-producing thoughts or feelings are excluded from conscious awareness. Normally, the conflict is resolved unconsciously by acting out the repressed wish in a disguised form in play, fantasy, or dreams in order to come to terms with it.

When unconscious conflicts are not resolved, the repressed wishes and fantasies may continue to be acted out in daily life, producing neurotic symptoms. A neurotic adult will tend to respond to people in terms of childhood feelings toward members of the family, even though these responses are not appropriate to the situation. Without realizing it, the person is going through adult life still acting out fantasies of childhood. The unresolved conflicts prevent the person from seeing others as they are and reacting to them in an appropriate way.

Psychoanalytic PSYCHOTHERAPY. Psychoanalysis is an insight-oriented type of PSYCHOTHERAPY. Its goal is to uncover unconscious psychologic patterns and enable the patient to discover the influence of these patterns in daily life. As the patient acquires self-knowledge, the unconscious patterns are undone and areas of behavior come under conscious control. For a person who has the required maturity and intelligence and who is motivated to accomplish a thorough reconstruction of the personality, psychoanalysis is the psychotherapy of choice. The treatment is usually prolonged, such as with four or five analytic sessions a week, lasting 45 minutes to an hour, for two to five years. Many analysts also conduct less intensive treatment with two or three sessions a week with patients who might not be suitable for the more intensive treatment, such as those with severe personality disorders, or those unable to afford the time or expense for the more extensive treatment.

Key techniques include free ASSOCIATION and description of DREAMS by the patient and periodic INTERPRETATION by the psychoanalyst. Other concepts in psychoanalytic theory include RESISTANCE and TRANSFERENCE on the part of the patient.

psychoanalyst (si″ko-an′ah-list) a practitioner of psychoanalysis.

psychobiology (si″ko-bi-ol′o-je) 1. biopsychology; a field of study examining the relationship between brain and mind, studying the effect of biological influences on psychological functioning or mental processes. 2. a psychiatric theory in which the human being is viewed as an integrated unit, incorporating psychological, social, and biological functions, with behavior a function of the total organism. adj., **psychobiolog′ical.**

psychocortical (si″ko-kor′tĭ-kal) pertaining to the mind and to the cortex of the brain as the site of mental functions.

psychodiagnosis (si″ko-di″ag-no′sis) the diagnostic use of psychologic testing.

Psychodopygus (si″ko-do-pi′gus) a genus of sandflies of the family Psychodidae. *P. wellco′mei* is a vector of *Leishmania donovani,* the etiologic agent of visceral leishmaniasis.

psychodrama (si″ko-drah′mah) a form of group psychotherapy in which patients dramatize their own or assigned life situations in order to achieve insight into personalities, relationships, conflicts, and emotional problems, and to alter faulty behavior patterns.

psychodynamics (si″ko-di-nam′iks) the science of mental forces and motivations that influence human behavior and mental activity, including recognition of the role of unconscious motivation in human behavior.

psychogenesis (si″ko-jen′ĕ-sis) 1. mental development. 2. the production of a symptom or illness by psychic factors.

psychogenic (si″ko-jen′ik) having an emotional or psychologic origin. See also *psychosomatic.*

psychogram (si′ko-gram) 1. psychograph. 2. a visual sensation associated with a mental idea, such as a certain number which appears visualized when it is thought of.

psychograph (si′ko-graf) 1. a chart for recording graphically the personality traits of an individual. 2. a written description of the mental functioning of an individual.

psychokinesis (si″ko-kĭ-ne′sis) the postulated production or alteration of motion by directed thought processes.

P

PSYCHODRAMA TECHNIQUES

Task	Procedure
Setting the scene	The protagonist chooses and sets the scene by describing what is happening. Strategic questions include "Where did this situation occur?" Who was with you at the time?" "What did they say to you?" "Where were the other people who were with you?"
Role reversals	Role reversals are conducted by the director. Moreno(1964) believed that the protagonist should take the role of all significant persons so that distortions may be explored and reintegrated.
Soliloquy and aside	The actor or actress speaks aloud the thoughts and feelings that go unspoken.
Doubling	The double becomes an auxiliary ego that represents a part or parts of the protagonist.
Concretization	Concretization makes visible through deliberate action and visual stimuli what otherwise exists only as symbol or feeling. For example, an authority figure might be placed on a higher level than the protagonist, or physically hanging onto someone can represent clinging behaviors.
Mirroring	Mirroring is similar to the role of double, except that the auxiliary ego actually replaces the protagonist in the scene and mirrors observed behavior. By observing an auxiliary ego acting out his or her own situation, the protagonist frequently is able to develop alternative solutions that were unavailable when he or she was enmeshed in his or her own situation.
Self-counseling	Self-counseling requires the protagonist to take the role of counselor to the individual playing his or her auxiliary ego. The protagonist gains enough distance to reality-test resistances, and offers practical solutions to his or her auxiliary ego. The result is greater insight about what might work in his or her own situation.

From Carson and Arnold, 1996.

psycholinguistics (si″ko-ling-gwis′tiks) the study of psychological factors involved in the development and use of language.

psychological tests (si″ko-loj′ĭ-kal) any test to measure such factors as one's development, achievement, personality, intelligence, and thought processes.

psychologist (si-kol′ŏ-jist) a qualified specialist in PSYCHOLOGY.

psychology (si-kol′o-je) the science dealing with the mind and mental processes, especially in relation to human and animal behavior. adj., **psycholog′ic, psycholog′ical.**

analytic p., analytical p. the system of psychology founded by Carl Gustav Jung, based on the concepts of the collective unconscious and the complex.

clinical p. the use of psychologic knowledge and techniques in the treatment of persons with emotional difficulties.

WINDOW ON PSYCHOLOGIST

Psychology is a science that seeks to understand the relationships among the causes and dynamics of behavior patterns, and it is a profession that applies knowledge, skills, and specialized techniques to the solutions of individual and social problems. Individuals may work in the mental health field with a bachelor's, master's, or doctoral degree.

There are many categories of study in psychology, the most common ones being biopsychology and experimental, developmental, social, cognitive, clinical, counseling, school, and organizational psychology (also known as industrial-organizational psychology, or simply "I.O."). These last four (clinical, counseling, school, and organizational) are considered by the American Psychological Association (APA) to be the four distinct areas of applied psychology. Other more specialized graduate programs might be devoted to such areas as sports psychology, psychology and law, or behavioral medicine.

A few people may find employment with a BA. These are usually specialized programs—e.g., programs for chronic psychiatric patients, prison settings, drug addictions, etc. There are a variety of master's level programs in fields related to clinical and counseling psychology. Usually these programs train people in basic counseling skills. Some programs may have specialized areas of training such as marriage and family counseling, drug addiction counseling, group counseling, vocational counseling, family therapy, child therapy, divorce mediation, prison counseling, etc. Professionals with master's degrees usually work in group counseling practices, clinics, programs for specific populations (drug abusers, battered wives, chronic psychiatric patients, etc.), and employee assistance programs.

At the doctoral level, counseling psychology programs usually emphasize training in counseling/psychotherapy methods. Counseling psychologists tend to work in group counseling practices, private practice, and programs for special populations. The PhD in clinical psychology is educated about issues related to mental health and mental health treatment. Many programs emphasize research, and all clinical programs require an internship. Clinical psychologists often teach at universities, work in hospitals and clinics, or are in private practice. The PsyD in clinical psychology is designed for people who specifically want to practice psychology and are not as interested in quantitative research. The school psychologist is trained to do counseling and psychological testing in the school setting. Their strength, therefore, is their understanding of school systems and education. They may work with the children in the school or the staff. Some school psychology programs offer the EdD. Other psychologists work in the business world doing psychological assessments, testing, interpersonal mediation, group dynamic assessments, and workshops (on stress, depression, communication skills, etc.)

In order to practice psychology you must be licensed by the state. Most states require approximately two years of supervised experience after earning the doctoral degree. You must also pass a national multiple choice examination and, in many states, present a case study to a board of psychologists. You cannot advertise yourself as a "psychologist" or say that psychological services are offered unless you are licensed.

A psychologist works with people from all walks of life. A good psychotherapist is someone who is well rounded in his or her knowledge.

JOHN SULER, PhD

community p. the application of psychological principles to the study and support of the mental health of individuals in their social sphere.

criminal p. the study of the mentality, the motivation, and the social behavior of criminals.

depth p. the study of unconscious mental processes.

developmental p. the study of changes in behavior that occur with age.

dynamic p. psychology stressing the causes and motivations for behavior.

environmental p. study of the effects of the physical and social environment on behavior.

experimental p. the study of the mind and mental operations by the use of experimental methods.

forensic p. psychology dealing with the legal aspects of behavior and mental disorders.

gestalt p. gestaltism; the theory that the objects of mind, as immediately presented to direct experience, come as complete unanalyzable wholes or forms that cannot be split into parts.

individual p. the psychiatric theory of Alfred ADLER, stressing compensation and overcompensation for feelings of inferiority and the interpersonal nature of a person's problems.

physiologic p., physiological p. the branch of psychology that studies the relationship between physiologic and psychologic processes.

social p. psychology that focuses on social interaction, on the ways in which actions of others influence the behavior of an individual.

psychometrician (si″ko-mĕ-trish′an) a person skilled in psychometry.

psychometrics (si″ko-met′riks) psychometry.

psychometry (si-kom′et-re) the testing and measuring of mental and psychological ability, efficiency, potentials, and functioning. adj., **psychomet′ric.**

psychomotor (si″ko-mo′tor) pertaining to motor effects of cerebral or psychic activity.

p. test a test that assesses the subject's ability to perceive instructions and perform motor responses often including measurement of the speed of the reaction.

psychoneural (si″ko-noor′al) relating to the totality of neural events initiated by a sensory input and leading to storage, to discrimination, or an output of any kind.

psychoneurosis (si″ko-noo-ro′sis) neurosis. adj., **psychoneurot′ic.**

psychonomy (si-kon′o-me) the science of the laws of mental activity.

psychopath (si′ko-path) old term for a person with an ANTISOCIAL PERSONALITY DISORDER.

psychopathology (si″ko-pah-thol′o-je) 1. the branch of medicine dealing with the causes and processes of mental disorders. 2. abnormal, maladaptive behavior or mental activity.

psychopathy (si-kop′ah-the) older term for a mental disorder, sometimes specifically ANTISOCIAL PERSONALITY DISORDER. adj., psychopath′ic.

psychopharmacology (si″ko-fahr″mah-kol′o-je) 1. the study of the action of drugs on psychological functions and mental states. 2. the use of drugs to modify psychological functions and mental states. adj., **psychopharmacolog′ic.**

psychophysical (si″ko-fiz′ĭ-kal) pertaining to the mind and its relation to physical manifestations.

psychophysics (si″ko-fiz′iks) scientific study of the quantitative relations between characteristics or patterns of physical stimuli and the sensations induced by them.

psychophysiology (si″ko-fiz″e-ol′o-je) physiologic psychology. adj., **psychophysiolog′ic.**

psychoplegic (si″ko-ple′jik) an agent lessening cerebral activity or excitability.

psychoprophylaxis (si″ko-pro″fĭ-lak′sis) a method of PREPARED CHILDBIRTH using mental and physical training aimed at preventing pain and modifying the perception of painful sensations associated with normal uncomplicated childbirth; see also LAMAZE METHOD. adj., **psychoprophylac′tic.**

psychosensory (si″ko-sen′so-re) perceiving and interpreting sensory stimuli.

psychosexual (si″ko-sek′shoo-al) pertaining to the mental or emotional aspects of sex.

p. disorders sexual disorders (def. 2).

psychosis (si-ko′sis), pl. *psycho′ses* a state in which a person's mental capacity to recognize reality, communicate, and relate to others is impaired, thus interfering with the capacity to deal with life demands. adj. **psychot′ic.** Mental disorders in which psychotic symptoms may be present include MOOD DISORDERS, SCHIZOPHRENIA, BRIEF PSYCHOTIC DISORDER, DELUSIONAL DISORDERS, SCHIZOPHRENIFORM DISORDER, SCHIZOAFFECTIVE DISORDER, SHARED PSYCHOTIC DISORDER, and PERVASIVE DEVELOPMENTAL DISORDERS.

alcoholic p's psychoses associated with alcohol use and involving organic brain damage, a category that includes alcohol withdrawal delirium, Korsakoff's syndrome, alcoholic hallucinosis, and alcoholic paranoia (concurrent paranoia and alcoholism).

brief reactive p. an episode of BRIEF PSYCHOTIC DISORDER that is a reaction to a recognizable and distressing life event.

depressive p. older term for a psychosis characterized by severe depression, which is now more commonly described as a form of major depressive disorder.

Korsakoff's p. Korsakoff's syndrome.

postpartum p. a psychotic episode occurring during the postpartum period.

senile p. depressive or paranoid delusions or hallucinations or similar mental disorders due to degeneration of the brain in old age, as in senile dementia.

toxic p. that due to ingestion of toxic agents or to the presence of toxins within the body.

psychosocial (si″ko-so′shal) pertaining to or involving both psychic and social aspects.

psychosomatic (si″ko-so-mat′ik) pertaining to the interrelations of mind and body; having bodily symptoms of psychic, emotional, or mental origin.

p. disorder, p. illness a disorder in which the physical symptoms are caused or exacerbated by psychological factors, such as migraine headache, lower back pain, or irritable bowel syndrome; see also SOMATOFORM DISORDERS. It is now recognized that emotional factors play a role in the development of nearly all organic illnesses and that the physical symptoms experienced by the patient are related to many interdependent factors, including psychological and cultural. The physical manifestations of an illness, unless caused by mechanical trauma, cannot be divorced from a person's emotional life. Each person responds in a unique way to stress; emotions affect one's sensitivity to trauma and to irritating elements in the environment, susceptibility to infection, and ability to recover from the effects of illness. Physical conditions to which psychological factors are shown to be contributory are currently classified as *psychological factors affecting medical condition.* Any physical condition can be so classified, but the most frequently included are ASTHMA, PEPTIC ULCER, bowel disorders, cardiovascular disorders, ARTHRITIS, ALLERGY, HEADACHE, and certain endocrine disorders. In recent years there has been some success in using behavior therapy to treat these and other illnesses whose symptoms are related to the autonomic nervous system. Clients are taught new ways of coping with stress and new patterns of behavior. Among the techniques used are BIOFEEDBACK, relaxation training, classical CONDITIONING, and operant CONDITIONING using social and material reinforcement.

psychostimulant (si″ko-stim′u-lant) 1 producing a transient increase in psychomotor activity. 2. a drug that produces such effects, such as AMPHETAMINE, METHYLPHENIDATE, or CAFFEINE.

psychosurgery (si″ko-ser′jer-e) brain surgery done to treat psychiatric disorders. adj., **psychosur′gical.**

psychotherapy (si″ko-ther′ah-pe) any of a number of related techniques for treating mental illness by psychologic methods. These techniques are similar in that they all rely mainly on establishing a relationship between the therapist and the patient as a means of developing the patient's insight into the motivation behind his or her behavior. On occasion, drugs may be used, but only in order to make this communication easier.

Forms of PSYCHOTHERAPY. Perhaps the best known form of psychotherapy is PSYCHOANALYSIS, the technique developed by Dr. Sigmund Freud. Psychoanalysis attempts, through free association and dream interpretation, to reveal and resolve the unconscious conflicts that are at the root of mental illness.

Closely related to psychoanalysis is analytically oriented therapy, or "brief therapy." This uses some of the techniques of psychoanalysis, but tends to concentrate on the patient's present-life difficulties rather than on the unconscious roots of these difficulties.

One widely used technique is group therapy. Six to ten patients meet regularly to discuss their problems under the guidance of a group therapist. Group therapy is based on the principle of transference— that is, a patient tends to react to others in terms of his childhood attitudes toward family members. During group therapy, he may react to one member of the group as a hated rival brother, and to another as a dominating mother. In the give-and-take of discussion, he will begin to recognize the distortions in these reactions, and to see similar distortions in his day-to-day relationships with other people. Group therapy may be combined with individual therapy. Group therapy can help reduce the cost to each patient. It is also widely used in mental health centers, where it has helped relieve the great shortage of trained therapists.

Adjunctive therapy, such as occupational therapy and music therapy, is helpful in relieving tensions and emotional problems that are associated with a feeling of uselessness. Psychodrama, in which patients act out fantasies or real-life situations, may provide a means of communication for patients who are not capable of expressing their problem by speech.

Play therapy is a form of psychotherapy adapted to children. It is very difficult to induce an emotionally disturbed or even a normal child to talk about his problems. Play therapy provides an alternative. Children reveal themselves when they play with toys provided by the therapist and act out their fantasies. The therapist helps them "get things out of their system," accepting them warmly as they are, and guiding them toward a solution to their problems. Since these are closely related to the way children are treated at home, play therapy is usually combined with some form of therapy for the parents. Family group therapy, in which the entire family meets regularly with the therapist, can be particularly effective.

Cognitive therapy is based on the idea that a person's feelings and behavior result from that person's perceptions of the world and that psychological disturbances result from faulty ways of thinking. The therapist is active in helping the patient to restructure his or her distorted perceptions, using a combination of verbal and behavior modification techniques.

brief p. psychotherapy limited to a pre-agreed number of sessions, generally 10 to 20, or termination date. It is usually active and directive, and often oriented toward a specific problem or symptom.

psychoanalytic p. psychoanalysis (def. 3).

psychotic (si-kot′ik) 1. pertaining to, characterized by, or caused by psychosis. 2. a person exhibiting psychosis.

p. disorder psychosis.

psychotogenic (si-kot″o-jen′ik) psychotomimetic.

psychotomimetic (si-kot″o-mi-met′ik) 1. characterized by or producing symptoms similar to those of a psychosis. 2. a drug or other agent that has such effects; called also psychotogenic.

psychotropic (si″ko-trop′ik) psychoactive. 1. psychoactive SUBSTANCE.

psychr(o)- word element [Gr.], *cold.* See also words beginning CRY(O)-.

psychroalgia (si″kro-al′jah) a painful sensation of cold.

psychrometer (si-krom′ĕ-ter) an instrument for measuring the moisture of the atmosphere.

psychrophile (si′kro-fīl) a psychrophilic organism.

psychrophilic (si″kro-fil′ik) fond of cold; said of bacteria that grow best in the cold (15° – 20°C).

psychrotherapy (si″kro-ther′ah-pe) treatment of disease by applying cold.

psyllium (sil′e-um) 1. a plant of the genus *Plantago.* 2. the husk (*psyllium husk*) or seed (*plantago*) or (*psyllium* SEED) of various species of *Plantago*; used as a bulk-forming LAXATIVE. See also psyllium hydrophilic MUCILLOID.

Pt platinum.

pt pint.

PTA plasma thromboplastin antecedent (factor XI, one of the COAGULATION FACTORS).

PTA deficiency hemophilia C.

ptarmic (tahr′mic) causing sneezing.

ptarmus (tahr′mus) spasmodic sneezing.

PTC plasma thromboplastin component (factor IX, one of the COAGULATION FACTORS.

PTCA percutaneous transluminal coronary angioplasty.

pteroylglutamic acid (ter″o-il-gloo-tam′-ik) folic acid.

pterygium (tĕ-rij′e-um) a winglike structure, especially an abnormal triangular fold of membrane in the interpalpebral fissure, extending from the conjunctiva to the cornea.

p. col′li webbed neck.

pterygoid (ter′ĭ-goid) shaped like a wing.

pterygomandibular (ter″ĭ-go-man-dib′u-lar) pertaining to the pterygoid process and the mandible.

pterygomaxillary (ter″ĭ-go-mak′sĭ-ler″e) pertaining to a pterygoid process and the maxilla.

pterygopalatine (ter″ĭ-go-pal′ah-tīn) pertaining to a pterygoid process and the palatine bone.

ptomaine (to′mān, to-mān′) any of several toxic bases formed by decarboxylation of an

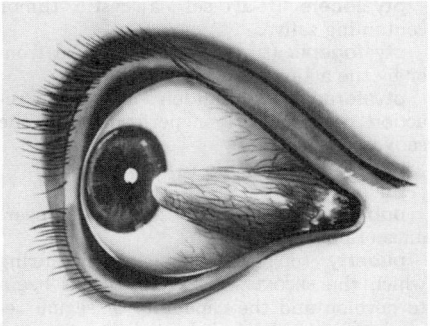

Pterygium. From Stein et al., 2000.

P

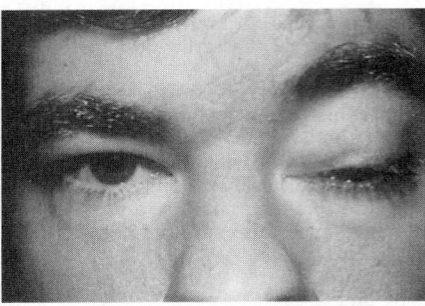

Primary ptosis associated with left third nerve paralysis.
From McQuillan et al., 2002.

amino acid, often by bacterial action, such as CADAVERINE, MUSCARINE, and PUTRESCINE.

p. poisoning a term commonly misapplied to FOOD POISONING. Contrary to popular belief, ptomaines are not injurious to the human digestive system, which is quite capable of reducing them to harmless substances.

ptosed (tōst) affected with ptosis.

ptosis (to'sis) 1. prolapse (def. 1). 2. paralytic drooping of the upper eyelid; called also blepharoptosis. adj., **ptot'ic.** (See Atlas 3, Part D).

-ptosis word element [Gr.], *downward displacement.* adj., **-ptot'ic.**

PTSD posttraumatic stress disorder.

PTT partial thromboplastin time; see activated partial thromboplastin TIME.

ptyal(o)- word element [Gr.], *saliva.*

ptyalagogue (ti-al'ah-gog) sialagogue.

ptyalectasis (ti″ah-lek'tah-sis) 1. a state of dilatation of a salivary duct. 2. surgical dilation of a salivary duct.

ptyalin (ti'ah-lin) α-amylase occurring in saliva.

ptyalism (ti'ah-lizm) excessive SALIVATION; called also hypersalivation and sialorrhea.

ptyalocele (ti-al'o-sēl) a cystic tumor containing saliva.

ptyalogenic (ti″ah-lo-jen'ik) formed from or by the action of saliva.

ptyaloreaction (ti″ah-lo-re-ak'shun) a reaction occurring in or performed on the saliva.

ptyalorrhea (ti″ah-lo-re'ah) ptyalism.

Pu plutonium.

pubarche (pu-bahr'ke) the first appearance of pubic hair.

puberty (pu'ber-te) the period during which the SECONDARY SEX CHARACTERS begin to develop and the capability of sexual reproduction is attained. In girls it is marked by broadening of the hips, development of the breasts, appearance of pubic hair, and onset of MENSTRUATION. In boys it is marked by broadening of the shoulders, deepening of the voice, and appearance of pubic and facial hair. Girls usually reach puberty between age 11 and 13, and boys between 13 and 15, although the timing varies widely.

precocious p. unusually early sexual maturation, defined as before age 8 in girls and 9 in boys; both ISOSEXUAL and CONTRASEXUAL types occur. It is usually hormonal (*central* or *true precocious p.,*) although occasionally it occurs in otherwise normal children, such as those with a family history of it *(constitutional precocious p.).*

pubes (pu'bēz) [L.] 1. the hairs growing over the pubic region. 2. the pubic region.

pubescence (pu-bes'ens) the state of approaching PUBERTY.

pubescent (pu-bes'ent) 1. arriving at the age of PUBERTY. 2. covered with down or LANUGO.

pubic (pu'bik) pertaining to or lying near the pubes.

pubiotomy (pu″be-ot'ah-me) surgical separation of the pubis (pubic bone) lateral to the symphysis.

pubis (pu'bis) [L.] pubic bone; see Appendix 3-3.

public health the field of health science that is concerned with safeguarding and improving the physical, mental, and social well-being of the community as a whole. The UNITED STATES PUBLIC HEALTH SERVICE (USPHS) is a federal health agency that is part of the United States Department of Health and Human Services. State and county public health agencies function under the supervision of and with financial support from the Department of Health and Human Services.

p. h. nursing the branch of nursing concerned with providing nursing care and health guidance to individuals, families, and other population groups in settings such as the home, school, workplace, and other community settings such as medical and health centers. The nurse in this field, a COMMUNITY HEALTH NURSE, must have a baccalaureate degree and training in public health nursing theory and practice; employment is typically with a local agency such as a nonprofit proprietary organization or with an agency under the United States Department of Health and Human Services. The work involves implementing such programs as school and preschool health programs, immunization and treatment of communicable diseases, maternal and child health clinics, and home visits for the purpose of providing health education and nursing care. There is also frequent participation in educational programs for nurses, allied professional workers, and civic organizations, and involvement in studying, planning, formulating public policy, and putting into action local and national health programs.

pubofemoral (pu″bo-fem′o-ral) pertaining to the pubis and femur.

puboprostatic (pu″bo-pros-tat′ik) pertaining to the pubis and prostate.

pubovesical (pu″bo-ves′ĭ-kal) vesicopubic.

pudendal (pu-den′dal) pertaining to or supplying the PUDENDUM, such as pudendal nerves (see Appendix 3-5) or a pudendal BLOCK.

pudendum (pu-den′dum) [L.] 1. the external genitalia of humans. 2. the pudendum femininum or external genitalia of the female, including the mons pubis, labia majora and minora, vestibule, and clitoris; see also VULVA.

puerile (pu′er-il) pertaining to a child or to childhood; childish.

puerpera (pu-er′per-ah) a woman who has just given birth to a child.

puerperal (pu-er′per-al) pertaining to a puerpera or to the puerperium.

p. fever an infectious, sometimes fatal, disease of childbirth; until the mid-19th century, this dreaded, then-mysterious illness could sweep through a hospital maternity ward and kill most of the new mothers. Today strict aseptic hospital techniques have made the condition uncommon in most parts of the world, except in unusual circumstances such as illegally induced abortion. Called also puerperal sepsis and childbed fever.

Puerperal fever results from an infection, usually streptococcal, originating in the birth canal and affecting the endometrium. This infection can spread throughout the body, causing septicemia. The preliminary symptoms are fever, chills, excessive bleeding, foul lochia, and abdominal and pelvic pain. In acute stages, the pain spreads to the legs and chest; complications may be serious or even fatal. Treatment consists mainly of administration of antibiotics, which in most instances promptly clear up the infection. If the disease has progressed to an acute stage before treatment begins, blood transfusions may be necessary.

puerperalism (pu-er′per-al-izm″) a morbid condition incident to childbirth.

puerperium (pu″er-pēr′e-um) the period from the end of the third stage of LABOR until involution of the uterus is complete, usually lasting between 3 and 6 weeks.

puffer fish (puf′er fish) any of several species of marine fish of genera *Fugu,*

Sphaeroides, Tetraodon, and others, which when disturbed can inflate themselves to a spherical shape. Their flesh contains TETRODOTOXIN and can cause fatal TETRODOTOXISM.

Pulex (pu′leks) a genus of fleas, several species of which transmit the microorganism causing plague.

P. ir′ritans a widely distributed species, known as the human flea, which infests domestic animals as well as humans, and may act as an intermediate host of certain helminths.

pulicicide (pu-lis′ĭ-sīd) an agent destructive to fleas.

pullulation (pul″u-la′shun) development by sprouting, or budding.

pulm(o)- word element [L.], *lung.*

pulmo (pul′mo) [L.] lung.

pulmoaortic (pul″mo-a-or′tik) aorticopulmonary.

pulmonary (pul′mo-ner″e) 1. pertaining to the LUNGS; called also pulmonic and pneumonic. 2. pertaining to the pulmonary artery.

p. acid aspiration syndrome a disorder produced as a complication of inhalation of gastric contents; it may progress to a syndrome resembling ACUTE RESPIRATORY DISTRESS SYNDROME.

p. alveolar proteinosis a disease of unknown etiology marked by chronic filling of the alveoli with a proteinaceous, lipid-rich, granular material consisting of surfactant and the debris of necrotic cells. Some patients have a history of exposure to irritating dusts or fumes. The condition is treated by whole lung lavage with balanced salt solution; most patients need repeated lavage.

p. artery the large artery originating from the superior surface of the right ventricle of the heart and carrying deoxygenated blood to the lungs for oxygenation; it starts as the pulmonary trunk, which divides between the fifth and sixth thoracic vertebrae to form the right pulmonary artery that enters the right lung and the left pulmonary artery that enters the left lung. See Appendix 3-1.

p. circulation the circulation of blood to and from the lungs. Unoxygenated blood from the right ventricle flows through the right and left pulmonary arteries to the right and left lungs. After entering the lungs, the branches subdivide, finally emerging as capillaries which surround the alveoli and release the carbon dioxide in exchange for a fresh supply of oxygen. The capillaries unite gradually and assume the characteristics of veins. These veins join to form the pulmonary veins, which return the oxygenated blood to the left atrium. See also CIRCULATORY SYSTEM.

p. function tests tests used to evaluate lung mechanics, gas exchange, pulmonary blood flow, and blood gases and pH. They are used to evaluate patients in the diagnosis of pulmonary disease, assessment of disease development, or evaluation of the risk of pulmonary complications from surgery.

Lung VOLUMES AND CAPACITIES. The total lung capacity (TLC) is divided into four volumes. The tidal volume (V_T) is the volume inhaled or exhaled in normal quiet breathing. The inspiratory reserve volume (IRV) is the maximum volume that can be inhaled following a normal quiet inhalation. The expiratory reserve volume (ERV) is the maximum volume that can be exhaled following a normal quiet exhalation. The residual volume (RV) is the volume remaining in the lungs following a maximal exhalation. The vital capacity (VC) is the maximum volume that can be exhaled following a maximal inhalation; VC = IRV $+ V_T +$ ERV. The inspiratory capacity (IC) is the maximum volume that can be inhaled following a normal quiet exhalation; IC = IRV $+ V_T$. The functional residual capacity (FRC) is the volume remaining in the lungs following a normal quiet exhalation; FRC = ERV + RV.

The vital capacity and its components are measured using a SPIROMETER, which measures the volumes of air inhaled and exhaled. The functional residual capacity is usually measured by the helium dilution method using a closed spirometry system. A known amount of helium is introduced into the system at the end of a normal quiet exhalation. When the helium equilibrates throughout the volume of the system, which is equal to the FRC plus the volume of the spirometer and tubing, the FRC is determined from the helium concentration. This test may underestimate the FRC of patients with emphysema. The FRC can be determined quickly and more accurately by body PLETHYSMOGRAPHY. The residual volume and total lung capacity are determined from the functional reserve capacity.

Forced VITAL CAPACITY **(FVC).** In the forced vital capacity maneuver, the patient exhales as forcefully and rapidly as possible, beginning at maximal exhalation. Several parameters are determined from the spirogram. The forced vital capacity is the total volume of air exhaled during the maneuver; it is

normally equal to the vital capacity. The forced expiratory volume (FEV) is the volume expired during a specified time period from the beginning of the test. The times used are 0.5, 1, 2, and 3 seconds; corresponding parameters are $FEV_{0.5}$, $FEV_{1.0}$, $FEV_{2.0}$, and $FEV_{3.0}$. The maximal expiratory flow is the slope of the line connecting the points where 200 ml and 1200 ml have been exhaled; it is also called $FEF_{200-1200}$ (forced expiratory flow). The maximal midexpiratory flow is the slope of the line connecting the points where 25 per cent and 75 per cent of the forced vital capacity have been exhaled; it is also called $FEF_{25-75\%}$.

Maximal Voluntary Ventilation (MVV). This is the maximal volume of air that can be breathed by the patient, expressed in liters per minute; it was formerly called maximal breathing capacity. The patient breathes as rapidly and deeply as possible for 12 to 15 seconds and the volume exhaled is determined by spirometry.

Predicted VALUES. Because the results of pulmonary function tests vary with size and age, the normal values are calculated using prediction equations or nomograms, which give the normal value for a specific age, height, and sex. The prediction equations are derived using linear regression on the data from a population of normal subjects. The observed values are usually reported as a percentage of the predicted value.

Interpretation. These tests provide evidence of impairment of ventilatory function; they do not point to specific disease processes. Abnormal test results may show either an obstructive or a restrictive pattern; sometimes both are present.

The Obstructive Pattern. This pattern occurs when there is airway obstruction from any cause, as in asthma, bronchitis, emphysema, or advanced bronchiectasis; these conditions are grouped together in the nonspecific term CHRONIC OBSTRUCTIVE PULMONARY DISEASE. In this pattern, the residual volume is increased and the PV/TLC ratio is markedly increased. Owing to increased airway resistance, the flow rates are decreased. The FEV/FVC ratios, maximal midexpiratory flow, and maximal expiratory flow are all decreased; $FEV_{1.0}$/FVC is less than 75 per cent.

The Restrictive Pattern. This pattern occurs when there is a loss of lung tissue or when lung expansion is limited as a result of decreased compliance of the lung or thorax or of muscular weakness. This pattern occurs in conditions such as pectus excavatum, myasthenia gravis, diffuse idiopathic interstitial fibrosis, and space-occupying lesions (tumors, effusions). The vital capacity and forced vital capacity are less than 80 per cent of the predicted value, but the FEV/FVC ratios are normal. The total lung capacity is decreased and the RV/TLC ratio is normal.

p. vein any of the four large veins (two right and two left branches) that carry oxygenated blood from the lungs to the left atrium of the heart. See anatomic Table of Veins in the Appendices.

pulmonic (pul-mon′ik) pulmonary.

pulmonitis (pul″mo-ni′tis) pneumonitis.

pulp (pulp) any soft, juicy animal or vegetable tissue. adj., **pul′pal.**

dental p. the richly vascularized and innervated connective tissue inside the pulp cavity of a tooth.

digital p. a cushion of soft tissue on the palmar or plantar surface of the distal phalanx of a finger or toe.

p. test a diagnostic test to determine whether the pulp of a tooth is vital (alive) or nonvital (dead); called also pulp vitality test.

red p., splenic p. the dark reddish brown substance filling the interspaces of the splenic sinuses.

tooth p. dental pulp.

p. vitality test pulp test.

white p. sheaths of lymphatic tissue surrounding the arteries of the spleen.

pulpectomy (pul-pek′to-me) root canal THERAPY involving complete removal of dental PULP from a tooth.

pulpitis (pul-pi′tis) inflammation of dental PULP.

irreversible p. severe pulpitis with minimal chance of spontaneous recovery, accompanied by an exudate and often pain.

reversible p. pulpitis in which the pulp may recover spontaneously; it is usually asymptomatic until pain is caused by some external stimulus.

pulpotomy (pul-pot′ah-me) root canal THERAPY involving partial removal of dental PULP from a tooth.

pulpy (pul′pe) soft; of the consistency of pulp.

pulsatile (pul′sah-tīl) characterized by a rhythmic pulsation.

pulsation (pul-sa′shun) a rhythmic beat, as of the heart.

pulse (puls) 1. pulsation. 2. the beat of the heart as felt through the walls of a peripheral artery, such as that felt in the radial artery at the wrist. Other sites for pulse measurement include the side of the neck (carotid artery), the antecubital fossa (brachial artery), the temple (temporal artery), the anterior side of the hip bone (femoral artery), the back of the knee (popliteal artery), and the instep (dorsalis pedis artery). (See accompanying illustration.)

What is felt is not the blood pulsing through the arteries (as is commonly supposed) but a shock wave that travels along the walls of the arteries as the heart contracts. This shock wave is generated by the pounding of the blood as it is ejected from the heart under pressure. It is analogous to the hammering sound heard in steam pipes as the steam is forced into the pipes under pressure. A pulse in the veins is too weak to be felt, although sometimes it is measured by SPHYGMOGRAPH (see below); the tracing obtained is called a PHLEBOGRAM.

The pulse is usually felt just inside the wrist below the thumb by placing two or three fingers lightly upon the radial artery. The examiner's thumb is never used to take a pulse because its own pulse is likely to be confused with that of the patient. Pressure should be light; if the artery is pressed too hard, the pulse will disappear entirely. The number of beats felt in exactly 1 minute is the pulse rate.

In taking a pulse, the rate, rhythm, and strength or amplitude of the pulse are noted. The average rate in an adult is between 60 and 100 beats per minute. The rhythm is checked for possible irregularities, which may be an indication of the general condition of the heart and the circulatory system.

The amplitude of a pulse can range from totally impalpable to bounding and full; however, such terms are vague and subject to misinterpretation. To provide a more standardized description of pulse amplitude some agencies and hospitals use a scale that provides a more objective evaluation and reporting of the force of a pulse. On such a scale zero would mean that the pulse cannot be felt; +1 would indicate a thready, weak pulse that is difficult to palpate, fades in and out, and is easily obliterated with slight pressure; +2 would be a pulse that requires light palpation but once located would be stronger than a +1; +3 would be considered normal; and a +4 pulse would be one that is strong, bounding, easily palpated, and perhaps hyperactive, and could indicate a pathological condition such as aortic regurgitation.

If a pulse is noted to be weaker during inhalation and stronger during exhalation (*pulsus paradoxus*), this could indicate either greater reduction in the flow of blood to the left ventricle than is normal, as in constrictive PERICARDITIS or pericardial EFFUSION, or a grossly exaggerated inspiratory

P

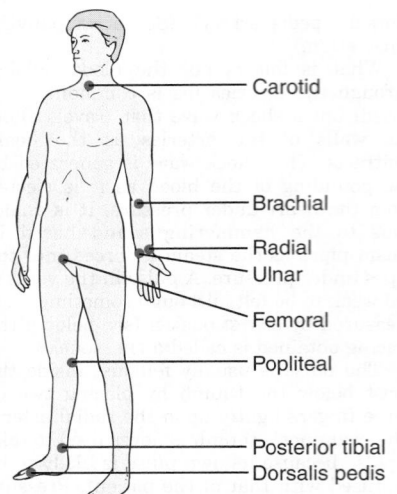

Carotid

Brachial

Radial
Ulnar

Femoral

Popliteal

Posterior tibial
Dorsalis pedis

Pulses palpated during assessment of the arterial system.

maneuver, as in tracheal obstruction, ASTHMA, or EMPHYSEMA.

An instrument for registering the movements, form, and force of the arterial pulse is called a SPHYGMOGRAPH. The sphygmographic tracing (or pulse tracing) consists of a curve having a sudden rise (primary elevation) followed by a sudden fall, after which there is a gradual descent marked by a number of secondary elevations.

abdominal p. that over the abdominal aorta.

alternating p. one with regular alteration of weak and strong beats without changes in cycle length. Called also pulsus alternans.

anacrotic p. one in which the ascending limb of the tracing shows a transient drop in amplitude, or a notch.

anadicrotic p. one in which the ascending limb of the tracing shows two extra small waves or notches.

anatricrotic p. one in which the ascending limb of the tracing shows three extra small waves or notches.

apical p. the pulse over the apex of the heart, as heard through a stethoscope or palpated.

atrial venous p., atriovenous p. a venous pulse in the neck that has an accentuated a wave during atrial systole, owing to increased force of contraction of the right atrium; a characteristic of tricuspid stenosis.

bigeminal p. one in which two beats occur in rapid succession, the groups of two

being separated by a longer interval, usually related to regularly occurring ventricular premature beats. Called also pulsus bigeminus.

bisferious p. pulsus bisferiens.

brachial p. that which is felt over the brachial artery at the inner aspect of the elbow; palpated before taking BLOOD PRESSURE to determine location for the stethoscope.

capillary p. Quincke's pulse.

carotid p. the pulse felt over the carotid artery, which lies between the larynx and the sternocleidomastoid muscle in the neck; frequently used to assess effectiveness of cardiac massage during CARDIOPULMONARY RESUSCITATION. It can be felt by pushing the muscle to the side and pressing against the larynx, or, if the patient is dyspneic, by palpating the pulse at the groove in the muscle.

catadicrotic p. one in which the descending limb of the tracing shows two small notches.

catatricrotic p. one in which the descending limb of the tracing shows three small additional waves or notches.

Corrigan's p. a jerky pulse with full expansion and sudden collapse occurring in aortic REGURGITATION; called also waterhammer pulse.

dicrotic p. a pulse characterized by two peaks, the second peak occurring in DIASTOLE and being an exaggeration of the dicrotic WAVE; called also pulsus bisferiens.

dorsalis pedis p. the pulse felt on the top of the foot, between the first and second metatarsal bones. In 8 to 10 per cent of the population this pulse cannot be detected.

entoptic p. a subjective sensation of seeing a flash of light in the dark with each heart beat.

femoral p. one located where the femoral artery passes through the groin in the femoral triangle.

funic p. the arterial tide in the umbilical cord.

hard p., high-tension p. one with a gradual impulse, long duration, slow subsidence, and a firm state of the artery between beats.

jerky p. one in which the artery is suddenly and markedly distended.

paradoxical p. one that markedly decreases in amplitude during inhalation, as often occurs in constrictive PERICARDITIS.

pistol-shot p. Corrigan's pulse.

plateau p. one that is slowly rising and sustained.

popliteal p. one palpated in the popliteal fossa, most easily detected when the

posterior tibial p. a pulse felt over the posterior tibial artery just posterior to the ankle bone on the inner aspect of the ankle.

quick p. one that strikes the finger smartly and leaves it quickly; called also pulsus celer.

Quincke's p. alternate blanching and flushing of the skin that may be elicited in several ways, such as by pressing on the end of the nail and observing the nail bed or skin at the root of the nail. It is caused by pulsation of subpapillary arteriolar and venous plexuses and is sometimes seen in aortic insufficiency, although it may occur in normal persons under certain conditions. Called also capillary pulse (because it was formerly thought to be due to pulsations in the capillaries) and Quincke's sign.

radial p. that felt over the radial artery at the wrist.

Riegel's p. one that is diminished during respiration.

slow p. one with less than the usual number of pulsations per minute; called also vagus pulse and pulsus tardus.

thready p. one that is very fine and scarcely perceptible.

tricrotic p. one in which the tracing shows three marked expansions in one beat of the artery.

trigeminal p. one with a pause after every third beat.

vagus p. slow pulse.

venous p. the pulsation over a vein, especially over the right jugular vein.

water-hammer p. Corrigan's pulse.

wiry p. a small, tense pulse.

pulseless disease an inflammatory and stenotic disease of medium and large arteries, with a strong predilection for the aortic arch and its branches (brachiocephalic trunk, left subclavian artery, and left common carotid artery). Pulses are commonly absent in involved vessels, leading to symptoms associated with ischemia of the brain, eyes, face, and upper limbs. Called also Takayasu's arteritis or disease, aortic arch arteritis, and brachiocephalic arteritis.

pulsion (pul′shun) a pushing outward.

pulsus (pul′sus) [L.] pulse.

p. alter′nans alternating pulse.

p. bige′minus bigeminal pulse.

p. bisfe′riens a pulse characterized by two strong systolic peaks separated by a midsystolic dip, most commonly occurring in pure aortic REGURGITATION with stenosis.

p. ce′ler quick pulse.

p. dif′ferens inequality of the pulse observable at corresponding sites on either side of the body.

p. paradox′us paradoxical pulse.

p. par′vus et tar′dus a small hard pulse that rises and falls slowly.

p. tar′dus slow pulse.

pultaceous (pul-ta′shus) like a poultice; pulpy.

pulverulent (pul-ver′u-lent) powdery; dusty.

pulvinar (pul-vi′nar) the prominent, cushionlike mass of nuclei that forms the medial portion of the posterior extremity of the thalamus, which partly overhangs the rostral colliculus and its brachium and is separated inferiorly from the geniculate body by the brachium of the rostral colliculus; it receives fibers from other thalamic nuclei and gives off widespread cortical projections.

pumice (pum′is) a substance consisting of silicates of aluminum, potassium, and sodium; used in dentistry as an abrasive.

pump (pump) 1. an apparatus for drawing or forcing liquid or gas. 2. to draw or force liquids or gases.

blood p. a machine used to propel blood through the tubing of extracorporeal circulation devices.

breast p. a pump for taking milk from the breast.

calcium p. the mechanism of active transport of calcium (Ca^{2+}) across a membrane, as of the sarcoplasmic reticulum of muscle cells, against a concentration gradient; the mechanism is driven by hydrolysis of ATP.

enteral feeding p. an infusion pump specifically designed for administration of a solution through a feeding TUBE.

insulin p. see INSULIN PUMP.

intra-aortic balloon p. see INTRA-AORTIC BALLOON PUMP.

muscle p. compression of veins by the contraction of skeletal muscles, forcing blood towards the heart against the flow of gravity; seen particularly in the deep veins of the lower limbs. Called also venous pump.

Na^+-K^+ p. sodium-potassium pump.

proton p. a system for transporting protons across cell membranes, often exchanging them for other positively charged ions.

sodium p., sodium-potassium p. the mechanism of active transport driven by the energy generated by Na^+,K^+-ATPASE, by which sodium (Na^+) is extruded from a cell and potassium (K^+) is brought in, so as to maintain the low concentration of sodium and the high concentration of potassium within the cell with respect to the

P

surrounding medium. A high concentration of intracellular potassium is necessary for vital processes such as protein biosynthesis, certain enzyme activities, and maintenance of the membrane potential of excitable CELLS. Called also Na^+-K^+ pump.

   stomach p. see STOMACH PUMP.

   venous p. muscle pump.

punchdrunk (punch´drunk) a traumatic encephalopathy of prizefighters resulting from cumulative cerebral concussions, with general slowing of mental functions, bouts of confusion, and scattered memory loss.

punctate (pungk´tāt) spotted; marked with points or punctures.

punctiform (pungk´tĭ-form) like a point.

punctograph (pungk´to-graf) an instrument for radiographic localization of foreign bodies.

punctum (pungk´tum) [L.] a point or small spot.

   p. cae´cum blind spot.

   p. lacrima´le (pl. *punc´ta lacrima´lia*), an opening of a lacrimal duct on the edge of the eyelid.

   p. prox´imum near point.

   p. remo´tum far point.

   punc´ta vasculo´sa minute red spots that mark the cut surface of white matter of the brain.

puncture (pungk´chur) 1. the act of piercing or penetrating with a pointed object. 2. a wound so made.

   cisternal p. see CISTERNAL PUNCTURE.

   lumbar p., spinal p. see LUMBAR PUNCTURE.

   sternal p. see STERNAL PUNCTURE.

   tracheoesophageal p. surgical creation of a tracheoesophageal fistula to hold a one-way plastic valve to restore speech after LARYNGECTOMY.

Punnett square (pun´et) a graphic depiction in grid form of how genes from each parent might combine in an offspring.

PUO pyrexia of unknown origin.

pupa (pu´pah) [L.] the second stage in the development of an insect, between the larva and the imago. adj., **pu´pal.**

pupil (P) (pu´pil) the opening in the center of the iris through which light enters the eye; see also Plate 17.

   Adie's p. tonic pupil.

   Argyll Robertson p. one that is miotic and responds to accommodation effort, but not to light.

   fixed p. a pupil that does not react either to light or on convergence, or in accommodation.

   Hutchinson's p. one that is dilated while the other is not.

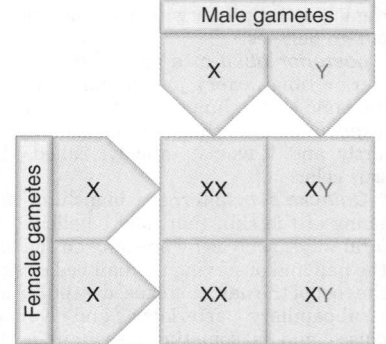

Punnett square showing sex chromosome combinations for male and female gametes. From Mueller and Young, 2001.

   tonic p. a usually unilateral condition of the eye in which the affected pupil is larger than the other, responds to accommodation and convergence in a slow, delayed fashion, and reacts to light only after prolonged exposure to dark or light; see also ADIE'S SYNDROME. Called also Adie's pupil.

pupilla (pu-pil´ah) [L.] pupil.

pupillometer (pu˝pĭ-lom´ĕ-ter) an instrument for measuring the width or diameter of the pupil.

pupillometry (pu˝pĭ-lom´ĕ-tre) measurement of the diameter or width of the pupil of the eye.

pupilloplegia (pu˝pĭ-lo-ple´jah) Adie's pupil.

pupilloscopy (pu˝pĭ-los´kah-pe) skiametry; retinoscopy.

pupillostatometer (pu˝pĭ-lo-stah-tom´ĕ-ter) an instrument for measuring the distance between the pupils.

purgation (per-ga´shun) catharsis (def. 1).

purgative (per´gah-tiv) cathartic.

purge (perj) 1. to cleanse or purify; to remove undesirable substances from something. 2. to cause free evacuation of feces. 3. a cathartic.

purine (pu´rēn) a heterocyclic compound that is the nucleus of the purine bases such as ADENINE and GUANINE (which occur in DNA and RNA), and XANTHINE and HYPOXANTHINE.

Purinethol (pu´rēn-thol) trademark for a preparation of MERCAPTOPURINE, an antineoplastic AGENT and IMMUNOSUPPRESSANT.

purple (pur´p'l) 1. a color between blue and red. 2. a substance of this color used as a dye or indicator.

   visual p. rhodopsin.

purpura (per´pu-rah) a hemorrhagic disease characterized by extravasation of blood into the tissues, under the skin, and through the mucous membranes, and producing spontaneous bruises, ecchymoses, and petechiae (small hemorrhagic spots) on the skin. (See plate in Dermatology Atlas.) When accompanied by a decrease in the circulating platelets, it is called *thrombocytopenic purpura*; when there is no decrease in the platelet count, it is called *nonthrombocytopenic purpura*. adj., **purpu'ric.** There are two general types of thrombocytopenic purpura: *primary* or *idiopathic,* in which the cause is unknown, and *secondary* or *symptomatic,* which may be associated with exposure to drugs or other chemical agents, systemic diseases such as multiple myeloma and leukemia, diseases affecting the bone marrow or spleen, and infectious diseases such as rubella (German measles).

Symptoms. The outward manifestations and laboratory findings of primary and secondary thrombocytopenic purpura are similar. There is evidence of bleeding under the skin, with easy bruising and the development of petechiae. In the acute form there may be bleeding from any of the body orifices, such as hematuria, nosebleed, vaginal bleeding, and bleeding gums. The platelet COUNT is below 100,000 per cubic millimeter of blood and may go as low as 10,000 per cubic millimeter (normal count is about 250,000 per cubic millimeter). The bleeding time is prolonged and clot retraction is poor. Coagulation time is normal.

Treatment. Differential diagnosis is necessary to determine the type of purpura present and to eliminate the cause if it can be determined. General measures include protection of the patient from trauma, elective surgery, and tooth extractions, any one of which may lead to severe or even fatal hemorrhage. In the thrombocytopenic form, corticosteroids may be administered when the purpura is moderately severe and of short duration. Splenectomy is indicated when other, more conservative measures fail and is successful in a majority of cases. In some instances, especially in children, there may be spontaneous and permanent recovery from idiopathic purpura. (See Atlas 2, Part Q.)

allergic p., anaphylactoid p. Henoch-Schönlein purpura.

annular telangiectatic p. a rare form in which pinpoint reddened lesions coalesce to form a ring-shaped or continuously linked pattern, commonly beginning in the lower extremities and becoming generalized. Called also Majocchi's disease.

fibrinolytic p. purpura associated with increased fibrinolytic activity of the blood.

p. ful'minans a form of nonthrombocytopenic purpura seen mainly in children, usually after an infectious disease, marked by fever, shock, anemia, and sudden, rapidly spreading symmetrical skin hemorrhages of the lower limbs, often associated with extensive intravascular thromboses and gangrene.

p. hemorrha'gica primary thrombocytopenic purpura.

Henoch's p. a type of Henoch-Schönlein purpura in which abdominal symptoms predominate.

Henoch-Schönlein p. a type of nonthrombocytopenic purpura, of unknown cause but thought to be due to a vasculitis; it is most often seen in children and is associated with clinical symptoms such as urticaria and erythema, arthritis and other joint diseases, gastrointestinal symptoms, and renal involvement. Called also Schönlein-Henoch purpura or syndrome and allergic or anaphylactoid purpura.

idiopathic thrombocytopenic p. thrombocytopenic purpura not directly associated with any definable systemic disease, although it often follows a systemic infection; the cause is thought to be an IgG immunoglobulin that acts as an antibody against platelets, causing ecchymoses, petechiae, and other bleeding. There are both acute and chronic forms: the *acute form* has a sudden onset, is more common in children, and usually resolves spontaneously within a few months; the *chronic form* has a slower onset, is more common in adults, and may be recurrent.

nonthrombocytopenic p. purpura without any decrease in the platelet count of the blood. In such cases the cause is either abnormal capillary fragility or a clotting factor deficiency.

Schönlein p. a type of Henoch-Schönlein purpura in which articular systems predominate; called also Schönlein's disease.

Schönlein-Henoch p. Henoch-Schönlein purpura.

p. seni'lis dark purplish red ecchymoses occurring on the forearms and backs of the hands in the elderly.

thrombocytopenic p. purpura associated with a decrease in the number of platelets in the blood; see PURPURA.

thrombotic thrombocytopenic p. a form of thrombotic MICROANGIOPATHY characterized by THROMBOCYTOPENIA, HEMOLYTIC ANEMIA, bizarre neurological manifestations, UREMIA (AZOTEMIA), fever, and thromboses in terminal arterioles and capillaries; some

P

authorities consider it identical to the HEMOLYTIC UREMIC SYNDROME. Called also microangiopathic hemolytic anemia and Moschcowitz's disease.

purulence (pu′roo-lens) suppuration.

purulent (pu′roo-lent) 1. pertaining to or consisting of pus. 2. containing pus. 3. suppurative. 4. caused by pus.

puruloid (pu′roo-loid) pyoid.

pus (pus) a protein-rich liquid INFLAMMATION product made up of LEUKOCYTES, cellular debris, and a thin fluid called LIQUOR PURIS.

blue p. pus with a bluish tint, seen in certain suppurative infections, the color occurring as a result of the presence of an antibiotic pigment (pyocyanin) produced by *Pseudomonas aeruginosa.*

pustula (pus′tu-lah) [L.] pustule.

pustular (pus′tu-lar) 1. pertaining to or of the nature of a PUSTULE. 2. consisting of pustules.

pustulation (pus″tu-la′shun) the formation of pustules.

pustule (pus′tūl) a small, elevated, circumscribed, pus-containing lesion of the skin.

pustulosis (pus″tu-lo′sis) a condition marked by an eruption of pustules.

putamen (pu-ta′men) the larger, darker, and more lateral part of the lentiform nucleus, separated from the lateral globus pallidus by the lateral medullary lamina.

Putnam-Dana syndrome (put′nam da′-nah) subacute combined degeneration of spinal cord.

putrefaction (pu″trĕ-fak′shun) enzymatic decomposition, especially of proteins, with the production of foul-smelling compounds, such as hydrogen sulfide, ammonia, and mercaptans. adj., **putrefac′tive.**

putrefy (pu′trĕ-fi) to undergo putrefaction.

putrescence (pu-tres′ens) the condition of undergoing putrefaction. adj., **putres′-cent.**

putrescine (pu-tres′in) a polyamine first found in decaying meat; small quantities occur in most cells.

putrid (pu′trid) rotten; putrified.

PVP polyvinylpyrrolidone (see POVIDONE).

PVP-I povidone-iodine.

PWA person with AIDS.

py(o)- word element [Gr.], *pus.*

pyarthrosis (pi″ahr-thro′sis) acute suppurative arthritis.

pyel(o)- word element [Gr.], *renal pelvis.*

pyelectasis (pi″ĕ-lek′tah-sis) dilatation of the renal PELVIS.

pyelitis (pi″ĕ-li′tis) inflammation of the renal PELVIS, a fairly common disease that usually can be diagnosed and cured without great difficulty. Prompt and effective treatment is necessary to prevent the spread of infection and the development of PYELONEPHRITIS, which in its chronic form is a severely disabling disease in which damage to the kidney cells may lead to high blood pressure and UREMIA. adj., **pyelit′ic.**

Cause. Pyelitis is usually caused by a microorganism such as *Escherichia coli* or (less often) streptococci or staphylococci, which may invade the kidneys by way of the blood. It may also arise from an infection of the bladder (CYSTITIS). It is most common among young children, affecting females far more often than males because the urethra is shorter in the female than in the male. This favors the entrance of ascending infections from the outside into the bladder. Female children not properly trained in their toilet habits will, after bowel movements, rub the toilet tissue from the anus forward toward the urethra rather than vice versa. In this way the bacteria commonly found in fecal matter can find their way into the urinary bladder and from there to the renal pelvis.

Any urinary obstruction can sharply increase the chances of the development of pyelitis, since obstruction interferes with the normal ability of the kidney to rid the body of harmful bacteria.

Symptoms. Probably the most common symptoms of pyelitis are frequency and urgency of urination and dysuria. Other possible symptoms include fever, chills, headache, and pain in one or both sides of the lower back. Pyelitis may also be present without any outward symptoms, but urinalysis will reveal many pus cells and occasionally erythrocytes.

Treatment. Pyelitis and pyelonephritis can usually be treated successfully with sulfonamides. Certain antibiotics and the urinary antiseptics are also helpful. If the disease is treated promptly, the patient can look forward to early and complete recovery.

cystic p. pyelitis with formation of multiple submucosal cysts.

pyelocaliectasis (pi″ĕ-lo-kal″e-ek′tah-sis) dilation of the renal PELVIS and CALICES.

pyelocystitis (pi″ĕ-lo-sis-ti′tis) inflammation of the renal PELVIS and BLADDER; called also cystopyelitis.

pyelogram (pi′ĕ-lo-gram″) the film produced by pyelography.

pyelography (pi″ĕ-log′rah-fe) radiography of the renal PELVIS and URETER after injection of a contrast medium; there are two methods: the *intravenous method* and the *retrograde method*. Preparation of the patient for pyelography includes clearing the intestinal tract of as much fecal material and gas as possible so that there can be adequate visualization of the urinary tract structures. Usually this is accomplished by administration of a laxative. The evening before the examination the patient is given a light meal and then all foods and fluids are restricted after 9:00 PM. In the intravenous method the contrast medium is injected intravenously at designated intervals and x-ray films are taken to observe the rate of excretion, the concentration of the contrast medium in the pelvis and calices of the kidney, and the outline of the ureters and urinary bladder. The possibility of an allergic reaction to the contrast medium must always be considered. Drugs such as epinephrine and hydrocortisone should be on hand for use in the event of a serious allergic reaction. The patient may experience a mild transitory sensation of warmth, flushing of the face, or a salty taste in the mouth, but these should last only a few moments. Symptoms of ANAPHYLAXIS demand immediate treatment.

The retrograde method involves introduction of the contrast medium by way of ureteral catheters. This procedure may be done when special studies of certain parts of the urinary tract are indicated, when adequate concentration of the contrast medium cannot be achieved by the intravenous method, or when a chronic illness, such as diabetes mellitus, affects renal arterioles and prevents intravenous injection of contrast medium.

pyelointerstitial (pi″ē-lo-in″ter-stish′al) pertaining to the interstitial tissue of the renal pelvis.

pyelolithotomy (pi″ē-lo-lĭ-thot′ah-me) incision of the renal PELVIS for removal of a CALCULUS.

pyelonephritis (pi″ē-lo-nĕ-fri′tis) inflammation of the kidney and renal pelvis; see also PYELITIS and NEPHRITIS. Called also nephropyelitis.

pyelonephrosis (pi″ē-lo-nĕ-fro′sis) any disease of the kidney and renal pelvis.

pyeloplasty (pi′ē-lo-plas″te) plastic repair of the renal pelvis.

pyelostomy (pi″ē-los′tah-me) the operation of forming an opening in the renal PELVIS in order to temporarily divert the urine from the URETER.

pyelotomy (pi″ē-lot′ah-me) incision of the renal pelvis.

pyelovenous (pi″ē-lo-ve′nus) pertaining to the renal pelvis and renal veins.

pyemesis (pi-em′ĕ-sis) the vomiting of pus.

pyemia (pi-e′me-ah) septicemia in which secondary foci of pus formation occur and multiple abscesses are formed. adj., **pye′mic.**

  arterial p. a form due to the dissemination of septic emboli from the heart.

  cryptogenic p. that in which the source of infection is in an unidentified tissue.

pyencephalus (pi″en-sef′ah-lus) abscess of the brain.

pygal (pi′gal) gluteal.

pygalgia (pi-gal′jah) pain in the buttocks.

pygoamorphus (pi″go-ah-mor′fus) asymmetrical conjoined twins, in which the parasite is an amorphous mass attached to the sacral region of the autosite.

pygodidymus (pi″go-did′ĭ-mus) conjoined twins fused in the cephalothoracic region, with double hips and pelvis.

pygomelus (pi-gom′ĕ-lus) a fetus with a supernumerary limb or limbs attached to or near the buttocks.

pygopagus (pi-gop′ah-gus) conjoined twins fused in the sacral region.

pykn(o)- word element [Gr.], *thick; compact; frequent.*

pyknic (pik′nik) having a short, thick, stocky build.

pyknocyte (pik′no-sīt) a distorted and contracted, occasionally spiculed erythrocyte.

pyknocytosis (pik″no-si-to′sis) conspicuous increase in the number of pyknocytes.

pyknodysostosis (pik″no-dis″os-to′sis) a hereditary syndrome of dwarfism, osteopetrosis, and skeletal anomalies of the cranium, digits, and mandible.

pyknometer (pik-nom′ĕ-ter) an instrument for determining the specific gravity of fluids.

pyknomorphous (pik″no-mor′fus) having the stained portions of the cell body compactly arranged.

pyknophrasia (pik″no-fra′zhah) thickness of speech.

pyknosis (pik-no′sis) a thickening, especially the degeneration of a cell in which the nucleus shrinks in size and the chromatin condenses to a solid, structureless mass or masses. adj., **pyknot′ic.**

pyle- word element [Gr.], *portal vein.*

pylephlebectasis (pi″le-flĕ-bek′tah-sis) dilatation of the portal vein.

pylephlebitis (pi″le-flĕ-bi′tis) inflammation of the portal vein.

pylethrombophlebitis (pi″le-throm″bo-flĕ-bi′tis) thrombosis and inflammation of the portal vein.

pylethrombosis (pi″le-throm-bo′sis) thrombosis of the portal vein.

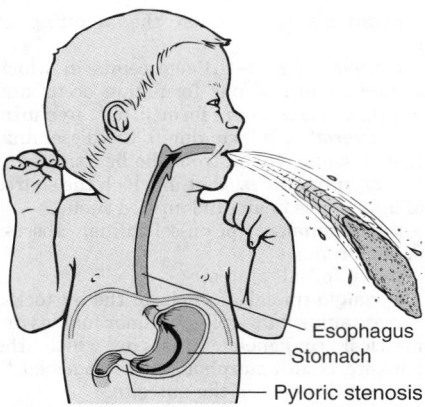

Congenital pyloric stenosis. The abnormal narrowing of the opening of the pylorus causes episodes of projectile vomiting. From Frazier et al., 2000.

pylor(o)- word element [Gr.], *pylorus.*

pyloralgia (pi″lo-ral′jah) pain in the region of the pylorus.

pylorectomy (pi″lo-rek′to-me) excision of the pylorus.

pyloric (pi-lor′ik) pertaining to the pylorus or to the pyloric part of the stomach.

   p. stenosis obstruction of the pyloric orifice of the stomach; it may be congenital, as in hypertrophic pyloric stenosis, or acquired, due to peptic ulceration or prepyloric carcinoma.

   The initial symptom is vomiting, mild at first but becoming increasingly more forceful. It can occur both during and after feedings. Diagnosis may be confirmed by x-ray examination using a barium meal.

   Treatment is usually surgical, involving longitudinal splitting of the muscle (pyloromyotomy).

pylorodiosis (pi-lor″o-di-o′sis) dilatation of a pyloric stricture with the fingers during a surgical operation.

pyloroduodenitis (pi-lor″o-doo″o-dĕ-ni′tis) inflammation of the pyloric and duodenal mucosa.

pylorogastrectomy (pi-lor″o-gas-trek′to-me) excision of the pylorus.

pyloromyotomy (pi-lor″o-mi-ot′ah-me) incision of the longitudinal and circular muscles of the pylorus.

pyloroplasty (pi-lor′o-plas″te) plastic surgery of the pylorus, especially for pyloric stricture, to provide a larger communication between the stomach and duodenum.

Finney p. enlargement of the pyloric canal by establishment of an inverted U-shaped anastomosis between the stomach and duodenum after longitudinal incision.

   Heineke-Mikulicz p. enlargement of a pyloric stricture by incising the pylorus longitudinally and suturing the incision transversely.

pyloroscopy (pi-lor-os′kah-pe) endoscopic inspection of the pylorus.

pylorospasm (pi-lor′o-spazm) spasm of the pylorus or of the pyloric portion of the stomach.

pylorostenosis (pi-lor″o-stĕ-no-sis) pyloric stenosis.

pylorostomy (pi″lor-os′tah-me) surgical formation of an opening through the abdominal wall into the stomach near the pylorus.

pylorotomy (pi″lor-ot′ah-me) incision of the pylorus.

pylorus (pi-lor′us) the distal aperture of the stomach, opening into the duodenum. The term has also been used to mean the pyloric part of the stomach, and the pyloric antrum, canal, opening, or sphincter. A ring of muscles, the pyloric SPHINCTER, serves as a "gate," closing the opening from the stomach to the intestine. It opens periodically, allowing the contents of the stomach to move into the duodenum. The pylorus contains many glands that help produce HYDROCHLORIC ACID. Occasionally, in infants, the pyloric muscle is greatly enlarged and thickened, so that emptying of the stomach is prevented. This condition, hypertrophic pyloric obstruction or pyloric STENOSIS, can be corrected by surgery.

pyocele (pi′o-sēl) a collection of pus, as in the scrotum.

pyocephalus (pi″o-sef′ah-lus) BRAIN ABSCESS.

pyochezia (pi″o-ke′ze-ah) the presence of pus in the feces.

pyococcus (pi″o-kok′us) a pus-forming COCCUS.

pyocolpocele (pi″o-kol′po-sēl) a vaginal tumor or cyst containing pus.

pyocolpos (pi″o-kol′pos) pus in the vagina.

pyocyanic (pi″o-si-an′ik) pertaining to blue pus, or to *Pseudomonas aeruginosa.*

pyocyanin (pi″o-si′ah-nin) a blue-green pigment produced by *Pseudomonas aeruginosa;* it gives the color to blue PUS.

pyocyst (pi′o-sist) a cyst containing pus.

pyoderma (pi″o-der′mah) any purulent skin disease.

   p. gangreno′sum a rapidly evolving cutaneous ulcer or ulcers, with undermining of the border. Once regarded as a complication peculiar to ulcerative colitis, it is

pyodermia (pi″o-der′me-ah) pyoderma.

pyogenesis (pi″o-jen′ĕ-sis) suppuration (def. 1).

pyogenic (pi″o-jen′ik) producing pus.

pyohemia (pi″o-he′me-ah) pyemia.

pyohemothorax (pi″o-he″mo-tho′raks) a PLEURAL EFFUSION containing pus and blood.

pyohydronephrosis (pi″o-hi″dro-nĕ-fro′-sis) the accumulation of pus and urine in the kidney.

pyoid (pi′oid) resembling or like pus; called also puruloid.

pyometra (pi″o-me′trah) an accumulation of pus within the uterus.

pyometritis (pi″o-me-tri′tis) purulent inflammation of the uterus.

pyomyoma (pi″o-mi-o′mah) a LEIOMYOMA that has undergone suppuration.

pyonephritis (pi″o-nĕ-fri′tis) purulent inflammation of the kidney.

pyonephrolithiasis (pi″o-nef″ro-lĭ-thi′ah-sis) calculous pyonephrosis.

pyonephrosis (pi″o-nĕ-fro′sis) suppurative destruction of the renal PARENCHYMA, often with kidney FAILURE; called also nephropyosis.

   calculous p. pus and calculi in the kidney.

pyo-ovarium (pi″o-o-va′re-um) an abscess of the ovary.

pyopericarditis (pi″o-per″ĭ-kahr-di′tis) purulent pericarditis.

pyopericardium (pi″o-per″ĭ-kahr′de-um) pus in the pericardium.

pyoperitoneum (pi″o-per″ĭ-to-ne′um) pus in the peritoneal cavity.

pyoperitonitis (pi″o-per″ĭ-to-ni′tis) purulent inflammation of the peritoneum.

pyophthalmitis (pi″of-thal-mi′tis) purulent inflammation of the eye.

pyophysometra (pi″o-fi″so-me′trah) pus and gas in the uterus.

pyopneumocholecystitis (pi″o-noo″mo-ko″le-sis-ti′-tis) distention of the gallbladder, with the presence of pus and gas.

pyopneumohepatitis (pi″o-noo″mo-hep″-ah-ti′tis) abscess of the liver with pus and gas in the abscess cavity.

pyopneumopericardium (pi″o-noo″mo-per″ĭ-kahr′de-um) pus and gas in the pericardium.

pyopneumoperitonitis (pi″o-noo″mo-per″ĭ-to-ni′tis) peritonitis with the presence of pus and gas.

pyopneumothorax (pi″o-noo″mo-tho′raks) pus and air or gas within the pleural cavity; called also pneumopyothorax.

pyoptysis (pi-op′tĭ-sis) expectoration of purulent matter.

pyopyelectasis (pi″o-pi″ĕ-lek′tah-sis) dilatation of the renal PELVIS with pus.

pyorrhea (pi″o-re′ah) periodontitis.

pyosalpingitis (pi″o-sal″pin-ji′tis) purulent salpingitis.

pyosalpingo-oophoritis (pi″o-sal-ping″go-o″of-o-ri′-tis) purulent inflammation of the fallopian tube and ovary.

pyosalpinx (pi″o-sal′pinks) an accumulation of pus in a fallopian tube.

pyostatic (pi″o-stat′ik) 1. stopping or hindering pus formation. 2. an agent that has this effect.

pyostomatitis (pi″o-sto″mah-ti′tis) a suppurative inflammation of the mouth.

pyothorax (pi″o-thor′aks) empyema (def. 2).

pyoureter (pi″o-u-re′ter) pus in the ureter.

pyr(o)- word element [Gr.], *fire; heat;* (in chemistry) *produced by heating.*

pyramid (pir′ah-mid) a pointed or cone-shaped structure or part.

   p. of cerebellum pyramid of vermis.

   p. of light a triangular reflection seen upon the tympanic membrane.

   malpighian p's renal pyramids.

   p's of the medulla oblongata either of two rounded masses, one on either side of the median fissure of the medulla oblongata.

   renal p's the conical masses constituting the medulla of the kidney, the base toward the cortex and culminating at the summit in the renal papilla.

   p. of thyroid an occasional third lobe of the thyroid gland, extending upward from the isthmus.

   p. of tympanum the hollow elevation in the inner wall of the middle ear that contains the stapedius muscle.

   p. of vermis the part of the vermis cerebelli between the tuber vermis and the uvula.

pyramidal (pĭ-ram′ĭ-dal) shaped like a pyramid.

pyramis (pir′ah-mis) [Gr.] pyramid.

pyran (pi′ran) a cyclic compound in which the ring consists of 5 carbon atoms and 1 oxygen atom.

pyranose (pir′ah-nōs) a six-membered ring structure formed by the reaction of the carbonyl group and a hydroxy group of a sugar to form a hemiacetal.

pyrantel (pĭ-ran′tel) a broad-spectrum ANTHELMINTIC agent with activity against HOOKWORMS, PINWORMS, and ROUNDWORMS; used as the pamoate or tartrate salt for infections due to *Ascaris lumbricoides* or *Enterobius vermicularis.*

P

pyrazinamide (pir″ah-zin′ah-mīd) an antibacterial derived from nicotinic acid, used in treatment of TUBERCULOSIS.

pyrectic (pi-rek′tik) 1. febrile. 2. pyrogen.

pyretic (pi-ret′ik) febrile. 1. pyrogen.

pyretogenesis (pi-re″to-jen′ĕ-sis) the origin and causation of fever.

pyretogenous (pi″rĕ-toj′ĕ-nus) 1. caused by high fever. 2. pyrogenic.

pyretotherapy (pi-re″to-ther′ah-pe) treatment by artificially increasing the patient's body temperature. 1. the treatment of FEVER.

pyrexia (pi-rek′se-ah) fever. adj., **pyrex′-ial.**

Pyribenzamine (pir″ĭ-ben′zah-mēn) trademark for preparations of TRIPELENNAMINE, an ANTIHISTAMINE.

pyridine (pir′ĭ-dēn) 1. a toxic, colorless, liquid hydrocarbon usually derived from coal tar and used as a laboratory and industrial intermediate.

Pyridium (pĭ-rid′e-um) trademark for preparations of PHENAZOPYRIDINE hydrochloride; a urinary tract ANALGESIC.

pyridostigmine (pir″ĭ-do-stig′mēn) an anticholinesterase; used as the bromide salt in the treatment of MYASTHENIA GRAVIS and as an antidote to nondepolarizing neuromuscular blocking AGENTS such as TUBOCURARINE.

pyridoxal (pir″ĭ-dok′sal) a form of vitamin B₆.

p. phosphate a major coenzyme involved in amino acid metabolism.

pyridoxamine (pir″ĭ-doks′ah-mēn) one of the three active forms of vitamin B₆.

p. phosphate a coenzyme involved in amino acid metabolism.

pyridoxine (pir″ĭ-dok′sēn) one of the forms of vitamin B₆, used as the hydrochloride salt in the prophylaxis and treatment of vitamin B₆ deficiency. It is also used in counteracting the neurotoxic effects of ISONIAZID and as an antidote to CYCLOSERINE.

pyrilamine (pĭ-ril′ah-mēn) an ANTIHISTAMINE, administered orally as the maleate and tannate salts, usually in a combination cold or cough product together with a DECONGESTANT.

pyrimethamine (pir″ĭ-meth′ah-mēn) a FOLIC ACID ANTAGONIST used as an antimalarial AGENT, especially for suppressive prophylaxis, and also used concomitantly with a SULFONAMIDE in treatment of TOXOPLASMOSIS.

pyrimidine (pĭ-rim′ĭ-dēn) an organic compound that is the fundamental form of the pyrimidine bases, which include CYTOSINE, THYMINE, and URACIL.

pyrogen (pi′ro-jen) an agent that causes fever; called also pyretic and pyrectic. adj., **pyrogen′ic.**

endogenous p. a low-molecular-weight protein that is produced by phagocytic leukocytes in response to stimulation by exogenous pyrogens and released into the circulation; it induces fever by acting on the preoptic area of the hypothalamus to raise the set-point of the hypothalamic thermostat. The pyrogen produced by monocytes and macrophages is not identical to that produced by neutrophils and eosinophils; the mononuclear phagocytes also produce a greater amount of pyrogen for a longer period of time than do the polymorphonuclear cells.

exogenous p's fever-producing agents of external origin, e.g., bacterial endotoxins and other microbial products, antigen-antibody complexes, viruses and synthetic polynucleotides, incompatible blood and blood products, and androgen breakdown products such as etiocholanolone; the action is mediated by endogenous pyrogen.

pyroglobulin (pi″ro-glob′u-lin) a monoclonal immunoglobulin that precipitates irreversibly upon heating to 56°C (as opposed to Bence Jones proteins, which precipitate but redissolve on cooling).

pyroglobulinemia (pi″ro-glob″u-lĭ-ne′me-ah) the presence of pyroglobulin in the blood, occurring most frequently in multiple myeloma, Waldenström's macroglobulinemia, and other lymphoproliferative disorders, but also occasionally without known associated disease.

pyroglutamic acid (pi″ro-gloo-tam′ik) 5-oxoproline.

pyroglutamicaciduria 5-oxoprolinuria.

pyromania (pi″ro-ma′ne-ah) an IMPULSE CONTROL DISORDER consisting of a compulsion to set fires or watch fires, in the absence of monetary or other material gain to the person. The pyromaniac gets intense pleasure and emotional relief from these activities.

pyronin (pi′ro-nin) a red aniline histologic stain.

pyrophobia (pi″ro-fo′be-ah) irrational fear of fire.

pyrophosphatase (pi″ro-fos′fah-tās) any enzyme that catalyzes the hydrolysis of central pyrophosphate linkages.

pyrophosphate (pi″ro-fos′fāt) any salt of pyrophosphoric acid.

pyrophosphoric acid (pi″ro-fos-for′ik) a dimer of phosphoric acid, $H_4P_2O_7$.

pyrosis (pi-ro′sis) heartburn.

pyrotic (pi-rot′ik) 1. caustic. 2. pertaining to HEARTBURN (pyrosis).

pyroxylin (pi-rok′sĭ-lin) a product of the action of a mixture of nitric and sulfuric acids on cotton; used to make collodion.

pyrrobutamine (pir″o-bu′tah-min) an ANTIHISTAMINE.

pyrrole (pir′ōl) a basic, cyclic substance, obtained by destructive distillation of various animal substances.

pyrrolidine (pĭ-rol′ĭ-din) a simple base obtained from tobacco or prepared from pyrrole.

pyruvate (pi′roo-vāt) a salt, ester, or anion of pyruvic acid. Pyruvate is the end

product of glycolysis and may be metabolized to lactate or to acetyl CoA.

pyruvic acid (pi-roo′vik) a compound formed in the body in aerobic metabolism of carbohydrate; also formed by dry distillation of tartaric acid.

pyrvinium (pir-vin′e-um) an ANTHELMINTIC used for intestinal PINWORMS in the form of the pamoate salt.

pyuria (pi-u′re-ah) pus in the urine.

PZI protamine zinc insulin.

Q quadrant

q 1. symbol for (1) the long arm of a chromosome or (2) the frequency of the rarer allele of a pair. 2. the long arm of a chromosome.

q.d. [L.] qua′que di′e (every day).

Q fever a febrile rickettsial infection caused by *Coxiella burnetii.* The causative microorganisms are found on the hides of sheep and cattle, and human beings contract the disease by breathing in the dried microorganisms carried in dust particles in the air. Symptoms include sudden high fever, chills, headache, muscle pains, and coughing; pneumonitis, hepatitis, and endocarditis are occasional complications. The disease usually is quickly brought under control by antibiotics. The "Q" stands for *query.*

q.h. [L.] qua′que ho′ra (every hour).

q.i.d. [L.] qua′ter in di′e (four times a day).

q.q.h. [L.] qua′que quar′ta ho′ra (every four hours).

q.s. [L.] quan′tum sa′tis (sufficient quantity).

q-sort (ku′sort) a technique of personality assessment in which the subject (or an observer) indicates the degree to which a standardized set of descriptive statements applies to the subject.

qt quart.

quack (kwak) one who misrepresents ability and experience in diagnosis and treatment of disease or the effects to be achieved by treatment.

quackery (kwak′er-e) the practice or methods of a quack.

quadr(i)- word element [L.], *four.* See also words beginning TETRA-.

quadrangular (kwod-rang′gu-lar) having four angles; see QUADRILATERAL (def. 1).

quadrant (kwod′rant) 1. one fourth of the circumference of a circle. 2. one of four corresponding parts, as of the abdominal surface, the dentition, the field of vision, or the tympanic membrane.

quadrantanopia (kwod″ran-tah-no′pe-ah) defective vision or blindness in one fourth of the visual field.

quadrantanopsia (kwod″ran-tah-nop′se-ah) quadrantanopia.

quadrantectomy (kwod″ran-tek′tah-me) a form of partial MASTECTOMY involving en bloc excision of tumor in one quadrant of breast tissue, as well as the pectoralis major muscle fascia and overlying skin.

quadrate (kwod′rāt) square or squared.

quadriceps (kwod′rĭ-seps) having four heads; see table at MUSCLE.

quadrigeminal (kwod″rĭ-jem′ĭ-nal) fourfold; in four parts; forming a group of four.

quadrilateral (kwod″rĭ-lat′er-al) 1. having four sides. 2. a four-sided figure.

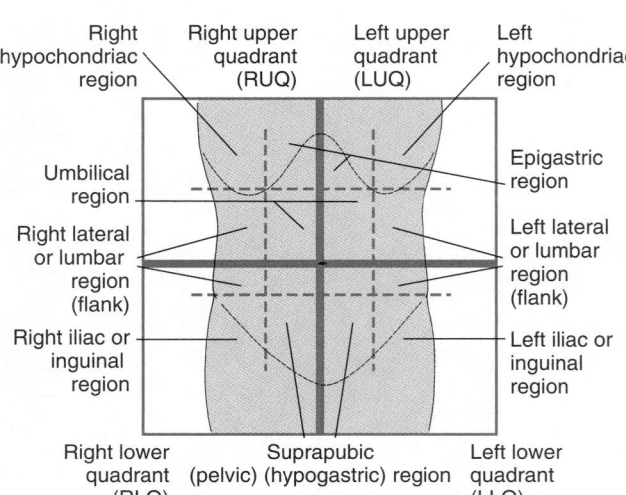

Quadrants of the abdomen. From Polaski and Tatro, 1996.

quadrilocular (kwod″rĭ-lok′u-lar) having four cavities.

quadripara (kwod-rip′ah-rah) a woman who has had four pregnancies that resulted in viable offspring; para IV.

quadripartite (kwod″rĭ-pahr′tīt) divided into four.

quadriplegia (kwod″rĭ-ple′jah) paralysis of all four limbs; motor and/or sensory function in the cervical spinal segments is impaired or lost due to damage to that part of the spinal cord, resulting in impaired function in the upper limbs, lower limbs, trunk, and pelvic organs. This term does not include conditions due to brachial plexus lesions or to injuries of peripheral nerves outside the spinal canal. Called also tetraplegia. adj., **quadriple′gic.**

Patient Care. The quadriplegic patient has major sensory and motor deficits and is therefore subject to the many problems associated with immobility and loss of sensation. (See HAZARDS OF IMMOBILITY.) The immediate goal of care is the prevention of complications that can affect all body systems, and maintenance of the integrity of the body systems so that optimum rehabilitation can be achieved. The extent to which the patient may eventually achieve mobility in a wheelchair and some degree of independence is greatly affected by the caliber of care received and the motivation and drive of the individual patient.

Mechanical devices such as braces are helpful in compensating for the loss of muscular function. PHYSICAL THERAPY procedures and techniques and OCCUPATIONAL THERAPY are essential aspects of patient care and are vital to the attainment of the goals of rehabilitation. (See also PARAPLEGIA.)

Patient education is especially important to the long-range goal of prevention of serious complications. Patients and their families should be aware of the early signs and symptoms of breakdown of the skin (PRESSURE ULCER), FECAL IMPACTION, a developing infection, and urinary difficulties. As with any type of long-term care, these patients should be medically evaluated periodically and their care should be under the supervision of a visiting nurse. In spite of the many difficulties that may be encountered by paralyzed patients, it is possible for them to lead useful and personally rewarding lives.

quadrisect (kwod′rĭ-sekt) to cut into four parts.

quadritubercular (kwod″rĭ-too-ber′ku-lar) having four tubercles or cusps.

quadrivalent (kwod″rĭ-va′lent) having a valence of four.

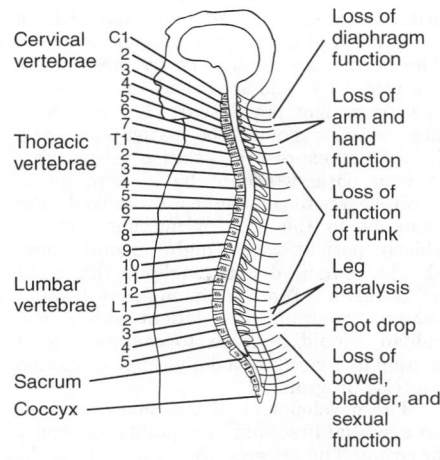

Quadriplegia.

quadruped (kwod′roo-ped) 1. four-footed. 2. an animal having four feet.

quadruplet (kwah-droop′let) one of four offspring produced at one birth.

quality assurance in the health care field, a pledge to the public by those within the various health disciplines that they will work toward the goal of an optimal achievable degree of excellence in the services rendered to every patient. Since the 1960s there has been an increasing emphasis on the individual citizen's right to health and the obligation of individual members of the health care team to hold themselves accountable to the public for the caliber of care they provide.

A quality assurance program takes into account the need to define that which is to be measured. Quality assurance implies a clear understanding of what is meant by "quality" and a valid and reliable method for evaluating the care that is provided. (See also EVALUATION.) In the health care field, evaluation of practice operates within the parameters of *outcome, cost-benefit,* and *access* to the health care delivery system. Outcome represents a measurable change in the health/illness status of the patient that is the end result of the care the patient received. Cost-benefit refers to the expenditure of money, time, and effort in providing health care and the relationship this cost bears to the actual benefits to the recipient. Access to health care refers to its availability or the ease with which one can obtain the kind of health care one needs.

Implementation of a quality assurance program involves the development of

Q

criteria based on acceptable standards of care and norms of professional behavior. The norms are established by members of the profession who are expert in the care of specific patient populations. The health/illness criteria should be patient-centered: they must express in positive terms what it is a patient should be able to do as a direct result of the care received. For example, in the area of nursing care, an elderly patient with "night incontinence" should remain dry throughout the night as a result of an individualized bladder TRAINING program, or a patient who is bedridden should be able to maintain joint motion as a result of a daily range-of-motion exercise program.

The development of outcome criteria is an essential first step in a quality assurance program. The criteria are then used as the "yardstick" against which actual practice and its results can be evaluated. Evaluation is conducted by a review committee, preferably one composed of practitioners in the area of health care being evaluated. A *retrospective review* measures actual documented outcomes against desirable and valued outcomes. Data for documentation of actual outcomes are obtained from the medical records of a specific patient population after the patients have been discharged. A *concurrent review* evaluates patient care while it is in progress. Documentation of the caliber of care being delivered is obtained through review of the patient's chart, interview, observation, and examination of the patient. The advantage of concurrent review is that it can provide opportunities for improvement of patient care while it is in progress.

The ultimate goal of both retrospective and concurrent review is improvement of patient care. If, at the time of review, a deficiency is detected in either the health care process or the health/illness status of the patient, an effort is made to correct the difference between "what should be" and "what actually is." It is this promise to evaluate thoroughly and to employ the results of the evaluation for continuous improvement of patient care that is the essence of quality assurance.

quality of life the degree of satisfaction an individual has regarding a particular style of life. Although assessment tools are available to evaluate physical and social dimensions, an individual's general sense of well being or satisfaction with the attributes of life is more difficult to evaluate.

quantimeter (kwon-tim′ĕ-ter) an instrument for measuring the quantity of x-ray generated by a Coolidge tube.

quantity (kwon′tĭ-te) 1. a characteristic, a of energy or mass, susceptible of precis physical measurement. 2. a measurabl amount. adj., **quan′titative.**

quantum (kwon′tum) [L.] an elementa unit of energy; the amount emitted o absorbed at each step when energy i emitted or absorbed by atoms or molecules.

quarantine (kwor′an-tēn) 1. restrictio of freedom of movement of apparentl well individuals who have been expose to infectious disease, which is impose for the usual maximal incubation perio of the disease (*quarantine period*). 2. a period of detention of vessels, vehicles or travelers coming from infected or sus pected ports or places. 3. the place wher persons are detained for inspection. 4. t detain or isolate on account of suspecte contagion.

quart (kwort) one fourth of a gallon; i the United States it is equal to 0.946 lite and in Great Britain it is an *imperial quar* and is equal to 1.14 liters.

quartan (kwor′tan) 1. recurring in four day cycles (i.e. on the third day after th previous episode). 2. a variety of intermit tent fever in which the paroxysms recur o every third day; see MALARIA.

quartile (kwor′tĭl) any of the three value that divide the RANGE of a probabilit DISTRIBUTION into four parts of equal prob ability; the first, second, and third quartile are the 25th, 50th, and 75th PERCENTILES.

quartipara (kwor-tip′ah-rah) quadripara a woman who has had four pregnancies tha resulted in viable offspring; para IV.

quasispecies (quah″zĭ-spe′sēz) a swarm of virus with similar genetic structure shar ing a host with other quasispecies of differ ent genetic makeup; usually all quasispecie in one host are descended from a singl ancestor strain.

quater in die (kwah′ter in de′a) [L.] fou times a day.

quaternary (kwah′ter-nar″e, kwah-ter′ nar-e) 1. fourth in a series. 2. made up o four elements or groups.

quazepam (kwah′zĕ-pam) a BENZODIAZE PINE used as a SEDATIVE and HYPNOTIC in th treatment of insomnia; administered orally

Queckenstedt's test (kwek′en-stets″ when the veins in the neck are compresse on one or both sides there is a rapid rise i the pressure of the cerebrospinal fluid o healthy persons, and this rise quickly dis appears when pressure is taken off the neck But when there is a block in the spina canal the pressure of the cerebrospinal flui

quenching (kwench'ing) extinguishing, suppressing, or diminishing a physical property, as the rapid chilling of a hot metal by plunging it into cold liquid. The term is frequently used to describe decrease of fluorescence from an excited molecule by other molecules that absorb some of the energy, which would otherwise be emitted as light. In several specific applications, it is used in liquid scintillation counting to denote any process that results in a decrease in number or intensity of the light flashes produced, thus lowering the amount of energy recorded, and it is also used to describe the termination of secondary and subsequent ionizations in a detector to give the detector time to become sensitive again.

Quervain's disease (kăr-vaz') inflammation of the long abductor and short extensor tendons of the thumb, with swelling and tenderness. Called also de Quervain's disease.

question (kwes'chun) an utterance about something unknown, seeking knowledge or other response.

research q. an interrogative phrase focused on what is to be described by a given research project and what relationships may be established.

quetiapine (kwĕ-ti'ah-pēn) a serotonin and dopamine antagonist used as the fumarate salt as an ANTIPSYCHOTIC AGENT; administered orally.

Quick's test (one-stage prothrombin time test) (kwik) PROTHROMBIN TIME.

Quick tourniquet test (kwik) estimation of capillary fragility by counting the number of petechiae appearing in a limited area on the flexor surface of the forearm after obstruction to the circulation for five minutes by a blood pressure cuff applied to the upper arm.

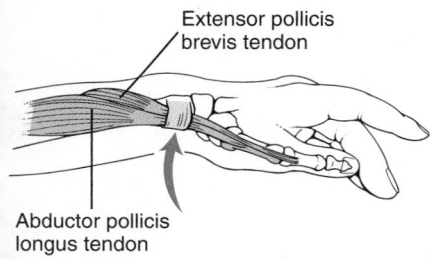

Extensor pollicis brevis tendon

Abductor pollicis longus tendon

Quervain's (or de Quervain's) disease, which involves tendons in the first dorsal compartment, the extensor pollicis brevis and abductor pollicis longus. From Myers, 1995.

quickening (kwik'en-ing) the first perceptible movement of the fetus in the uterus, appearing usually in the sixteenth to eighteenth week of pregnancy.

quinacrine (kwin'ah-krin) an ANTHELMINTIC and antiprotozoal AGENT used especially for treatment of MALARIA, GIARDIASIS, and TAPEWORM infestations. It is a yellow fluorescent dye also used in chromosome banding.

Quinaglute (kwin'ah-glo͞ot) trademark for a preparation of QUINIDINE gluconate, a cardiac ANTIARRHYTHMIC agent.

quinapril (kwin'ah-pril') an angiotensin-converting enzyme INHIBITOR used in the form of the hydrochloride salt in treatment of HYPERTENSION and congestive HEART FAILURE.

Quincke's disease (kwing'kez) angioedema.

Quincke's sign (kwin'kez) Quincke's pulse.

quinethazone (kwin-eth'ah-zōn) a diuretic with the same pharmacologic action as thiazide DIURETICS; used for treatment of hypertension and edema.

quinidine (kwin'ĭ-dēn) the dextrorotatory isomer of QUININE, administered orally as the gluconate, polygalacturonate, or sulfate salts, or intravenously as the gluconate salt in treatment of cardiac ARRHYTHMIAS. It is also administered intravenously as the gluconate salt in the treatment of life-threatening MALARIA caused by PLASMODIUM FALCIPARUM.

quinine (kwi'nīn) an alkaloid of CINCHONA that is an antimalarial AGENT; it suppresses the asexual erythrocytic forms of malarial parasites and has a slight effect on the gametocytes. It also has analgesic, antipyretic, mild oxytocic, cardiac depressant, and sclerosing properties, and it decreases the excitability of the motor endplate. It is administered orally as the dihydrochloride, hydrochloride or sulfate salt or parenterally as the dihydrochloride salt in the treatment of MALARIA caused by PLASMODIUM FALCIPARUM. It is also used orally as the sulfate salt in the treatment of leg and foot cramps.

quininism (kwin'ĭ-nizm) cinchonism.

quinoline (kwin'o-lēn) an amine or alkaloid derivable from QUININE, coal tar, and various other sources, which has antiseptic, antipyretic, and antimalarial properties.

quinolone (kwin'o-lōn) any of a group of synthetic ANTIBACTERIAL agents that includes CINOXACIN, CIPROFLOXACIN, NALIDIXIC ACID, NORFLOXACIN, and OFLOXACIN.

quinquevalent (kwing'kwĕ-va'lent) pentavalent; having a valence of five.

quinsy (kwin'ze) peritonsillar abscess.

Q

quint- word element [L.], *five*. See also words beginning PENT(A)-.

quintan (kwin'tan) recurring every five days (i.e., on the fourth day after the previous episode).

  q. fever trench fever.

quintile (kwin'tīl) any of the four values that divide the RANGE of a probability DISTRIBUTION distribution into five parts of equal probability; the first, second, third, and fourth quintiles are the 20th, 40th, 60th, and 80th PERCENTILES.

quintipara (kwin-tip'ah-rah) a woman who has had five pregnancies that resulted in viable offspring; para V.

quintuplet (kwin-tup'let) one of five offspring produced at one birth.

quinupristin (kwin-u'pris-tin) a semisynthetic ANTIBACTERIAL effective against a variety of gram-positive organisms. It is used in conjunction with DALFOPRISTIN in the treatment of serious BACTEREMIA caused by VANCOMYCIN-resistant ENTEROCOCCUS FAECIUM and complicated skin and skin structure infections caused by STREPTOCOCCUS PYOGENES or METHICILLIN-sensitive STAPHYLOCOCCUS AUREUS; administered intravenously.

quotid. *quotid'ie* (every day).

quotidian (kwo-tid'e-an) 1. recurring every day. 2. a form of intermittent malarial fever with daily recurrent paroxysms.

  q. fever a fever that recurs every day, such as with a type of MALARIA.

quotient (kwo'shent) a number obtained by division.

  achievement q. the achievement age divided by the mental age, indicating progress in learning.

  caloric q. the heat evolved (in calories) divided by the oxygen consumed (in milligrams) in a metabolic process.

  intelligence q. IQ; a numerical expression of intellectual capacity obtained by multiplying the mental age of the subject, ascertained by testing, by 100 and dividing by the chronological age.

  respiratory q. RQ; the ratio of the volume of carbon dioxide given off by the body tissues to the volume of oxygen absorbed by them; usually equal to the corresponding volumes given off and taken up by the lungs. It varies with the fuel source used: for carbohydrates it is 1.0; for lipids 0.7; for proteins 0.8; and with overfeeding (lipogenesis) 1.0–1.3.

R

R arginine; organic radical (in chemical formulas); respiration; rhythm; right; roentgen.

℞ [L.] re′cipe (take); prescription; treatment.

r ring chromosome.

Ra radium.

rabbit fever tularemia.

rabeprazole (rah-bep′rah-zōl) an inhibitor of stomach HYDROCHLORIC ACID secretion administered orally as the sodium salt in treatment of gastroesophageal reflux disease and similar conditions marked by excessive acid.

rabid (rab′id) affected with rabies; pertaining to rabies.

rabies (ra′bēz, ra′be-ēz) an acute infectious disease of the central nervous system, which affects all warm-blooded animals, including humans. It is caused by an RNA virus of the genus *Lyssavirus*. The virus is often present in the host's saliva, and human infection is usually transmitted by the bite or lick of a rabid animal, such as a bat, wolf, dog, cat, or other mammal; it is sometimes transmitted by the respiratory route. The incubation period in humans is from one to three months, being shorter following bites near the brain.

The earliest symptoms are intermittent pain, numbness, tingling, or burning around the site of infection; soon afterward, generalized hyperexcitability occurs, followed by fever, paralysis of the muscles of swallowing, and glottal spasm brought on by the sight of fluids or the drinking of fluids, and by maniacal behavior. Convulsions, tetany, and respiratory paralysis are the inevitable terminal events in untreated cases. The diagnosis can be determined by viral isolation (from saliva, cerebrospinal fluid, urine) or by demonstration of neutralizing antibody, and after death by the appearance of cytoplasmic inclusion bodies (Negri bodies) in degenerated neurons.

Without adequate immunization and treatment a person who has been infected with rabies is not likely to survive.

Prevention. All warm-blooded family pets (such as dogs, cats, and monkeys) should be vaccinated against rabies periodically.

It is also essential to learn to recognize a rabid animal. In the early "anxiety" stages, a rabid animal may have a change of temperament. Many, including wild animals, may become unusually friendly. The rabid animal may next enter a "furious" stage, in which it wanders about biting everything that moves, and even some things that do not move, such as sticks and stones. It then develops paralysis of the throat, which makes swallowing difficult. The name hydrophobia, "fear of water," was given to the disease because it was observed that stricken animals avoided water. Actually, this is not because of fear of water, but because they cannot swallow. Saliva often drips from the animal's mouth and may be whipped into a foam.

Some animals pass directly from the anxiety stage to paralysis without becoming violent. This is called the "dumb" form of rabies. The animal may appear to have something caught in its throat. A dog with something in its throat usually tries to remove it, but a rabid dog will not do this. Eventually all of the rabid animal's muscles become paralyzed and it dies.

Treatment. When a person is bitten by an animal, the wound should be washed thoroughly with soap and water, and then treated like any other wound. It is extremely important to seek emergency health care immediately. If possible, steps should be taken to find out if the biting animal has rabies, preferably by finding the animal and confining it for observation. When the biting animal must be killed in order to capture it, care must be taken to see that the head is not damaged, so that the brain can be examined to establish a diagnosis. If the biting animal cannot be caught for observation, the bitten person must be given antirabies treatment immediately.

Preventive treatment of suspected rabies is based on immunization by a series of vaccine and immune serum injections. When bites are in areas close to the head or in areas with many nerve endings, such as the hands, the virus may reach the brain quickly. In such cases treatment should start immediately, even though the suspected animal is still being observed.

Agents used to confer passive immunity are human rabies immune GLOBULIN and anitrabies SERUM. Allergic reactions to the immune globulin are rare, making it the preferred agent. In response to administration of antirabies serum, an occasional patient may experience severe anaphylaxis, while others develop serum sickness; hence, this agent is given only when human rabies immune globulin is not available. In many patients, the serum antibodies produce permanent immunity only after the last booster. If active immunity has been established, however, it lasts a lifetime. If a patient does not have permanent immunity established by the vaccine, the Centers for Disease Control and Prevention should be contacted.

A more effective and less troublesome immunizing agent is the newer human diploid cell VACCINE. It requires only five injections over 28 days.

There is no cure for rabies and once symptoms appear treatment can only be palliative. This includes sedation of the patient and provision of a quiet environment to reduce anxiety and relieve pain, administration of a powerful muscle relaxant (curare-like drugs) to reduce muscular contractions, and supportive measures to maintain urinary and respiratory function. Death occurs in 2 to 5 days.

race (rās) a class or breed of animals; a group of individuals having certain characteristics in common, owing to a common inheritance.

racemase (ra′sĕ-mās) an enzyme that catalyzes the RACEMIZATION of an optically active substance, such as L-lactic acid.

racemate (ra′sĕ-māt) a racemic mixture or compound.

racemethionine (rās″ĕ-mĕ-thi′o-nēn) a racemic mixture of D- and L-METHIONINE, used as a dietary supplement with lipotropic action.

racemic (ra-se′mik) optically inactive, being composed of equal amounts of DEXTRO-ROTATORY and LEVOROTATORY isomers.

racemization (ra″sĕ-mī-za′shun) the transformation of one-half of the molecules of an optically active compound into molecules that possess exactly the opposite (mirror-image) configuration, with complete loss of rotatory power because of the statistical balance between equal numbers of DEXTRO-ROTATORY and LEVOROTATORY molecules.

racemose (ra′sĕ-mōs) shaped like a bunch of grapes on its stalk.

rachi(o)- word element [Gr.], *spine.*

rachialgia (ra″ke-al′jah) rachiodynia.

rachicentesis (ra″ke-sen-te′sis) lumbar puncture.

rachidial (rah-kid′e-al) spinal (def. 2).

rachidian (rah-kid′e-an) spinal (def. 2).

rachigraph (ra′ke-graf) an instrument for recording the outlines of the spine and back.

rachilysis (rah-kil′ĭ-sis) correction of lateral curvature of the spine by combined traction and pressure.

rachiocampsis (ra″ke-o-kamp′sis) spinal curvature.

rachiodynia (ra″ke-o-din′e-ah) pain in the spine; called also rachialgia.

rachiometer (ra″ke-om′ĕ-ter) an apparatus for measuring spinal curvature.

rachiomyelitis (ra″ke-o-mi″ĕ-li′tis) myelitis (def. 1).

rachiotomy (ra″ke-ot′ah-me) incision of a vertebra or the vertebral column.

rachipagus (ra-kip′ah-gus) twin fetuses joined at the vertebral column.

rachis (ra′kis) SPINE (def. 2).

rachischisis (rah-kis′kĭ-sis) congenital fissure of the spinal COLUMN; see also SPINA BIFIDA.

   r. poste′rior spina bifida.

rachitic (rah-kit′ik) pertaining to RICKETS.

rachitis (rah-ki′tis) 1. rickets. 2. spondylitis.

rachitogenic (rah-kit″o-jen′ik) causing RICKETS.

rachitomy (rah-kit′ah-me) rachiotomy.

rad (rad) acronym for *r*adiation *a*bsorbed *d*ose; a unit of measurement of the absorbed dose of ionizing radiation. It corresponds to an energy transfer of 100 ergs per gram of any absorbing material (including tissue). The biological effect of 1 rad of radiation varies with the type of radiation. When the dose is in REMS, all types have the same biological effect.

rad. [L.] ra′dix (root).

radectomy (rah-dek′tah-me) root amputation.

radi(o)- word element [L.], *ray; radiation; emission of radiant energy; radium; radius* (bone of the forearm); affixed to the name of a chemical element to designate a radioactive isotope of that element.

radiability (ra″de-ah-bil′ĭ-te) the property of being readily penetrated by x-rays or other rays.

radiad (ra′de-ad) toward the radius or radial side.

radial (ra′de-al) 1. radiating; spreading outward from a common center. 2. pertaining to a RADIUS. 3. pertaining to the radial (lateral) aspect of the arm as opposed to the ulnar (medial) aspect.

   r. artery an artery in the forearm, wrist, and hand; the one usually used for taking the PULSE.

radialis (ra″de-a′lis) [L.] radial.

radiant (ra′de-ant) 1. diverging from a center. 2. emitting rays, as of light or heat.

radiate (ra′de-āt) 1. to diverge or spread from a common point. 2. arranged in a radiating manner.

radiathermy (ra-de″ah-ther′me) short wave diathermy.

radiatio (ra″de-a′she-o) [L.] RADIATION (def. 2).

radiation (ra″de-a′shun) 1. a proceeding outward from a common center. 2. a structure made up of parts that go outward from a center, especially a tract of the central

RADIATION SIDE EFFECTS, HEALING TIME, AND INTERVENTIONS

Effect	Healing Time	Interventions
Skin 1st to 4th degree inflammatory response	1st degree: within 7–10 days 2nd degree: within 1–2 weeks; hair may not grow back 3rd degree: 2–3 weeks; destruction of hair follicles and sweat glands can be permanent 4th degree: weeks to months: cancer can be long-term sequela	Assess skin daily; do not use alcohol or other drying agents, lotions, or salves; use only prescribed softening agent; wash gently with mild soap and tepid water and only as necessary; do not wash away markings for target area; avoid lying on area; wear loose-fitting clothing; do not expose area to direct sunlight, heat lamp, or other source of heat
Alopecia	Hair may grow back in several months	Shampoo with mild soap; brush and comb gently, hair pieces, wigs, and scarves can be worn if hair loss is extensive
Oral Mucosa	Within weeks if irritation not severe	Increase fluid intake to 2 liters daily; avoid hot and spicy foods and liquids; restrict smoking; frequent MOUTH CARE; apply lip balm; suck ice chips or hard candy to encourage salivation; use artificial saliva if mouth very dry; assess for oral candidiasis
Intestinal Mucosa	Several weeks or months, depending on degree of irritation	Check intake and output; assess for diarrhea, vomiting, anorexia; administer antidiarrheic agents; analgesic suppository for local irritation; encourage intake of foods rich in potassium to replace that lost in stools; small, frequent feedings; avoid milk and milk products if they worsen diarrhea; weigh daily; assess for nausea; advise patient not to eat for several hours prior to treatment; administer antiemetics before meals as needed
Urinary Mucosa	As above	Increase fluid intake to 2 liters daily orally or IV; measure urinary output, observe urine for blood, collect samples for urinalysis; ensure that clot formation has not obstructed bladder outlet; administer antibiotics for urinary tract infection
Bone Marrow and Lymphoid Tissue	Depends on dosage and degree of damage	Protect from infection, assess for early signs of infection; assess for anemia; watch for bleeding and other signs of thrombocytopenia; avoid trauma from injections and invasive procedures
Eyes	As above	Assess for drying, excessive tearing, conjunctivitis, damage to the lens and cataract formation; artificial tears if conjunctiva too dry; antibiotic eyedrops for infection
Ears	As above	Assess for blockage of eustachian tube and bulging of eardrum; protect from falls related to dizziness; assess for HEARING LOSS and implement appropriate care; administer antibiotics for ear infection
Nervous System	Necrosis of brain can develop as late as a year after treatment	Assess for level of mentation, dizziness, slurred speech, weakness and numbness of extremities; assess for spinal cord damage, e.g., changes in gait, pain, numbness, or tingling of extremities, incontinence; assess for Lhermitte's sign, which may occur months after treatments

nervous system made up of fibers that go out in different dfirections. 3. energy carried by waves or a stream of particles. One type is electromagnetic RADIATION, which consists of wave motion of electric and magnetic fields. The quantum THEORY is based on the fact that electromagnetic waves consist of discrete "packets" of electromagnetic radiation, called PHOTONS, which have neither mass nor charge and have an energy inversely proportional to the wavelength of the wave. In order of increasing photon energy and decreasing wavelength, the electromagnetic spectrum is divided into radio waves, infrared light, visible light, ultraviolet light, and x-rays.

Another type is the radiation emitted by radioactive materials. ALPHA PARTICLES are

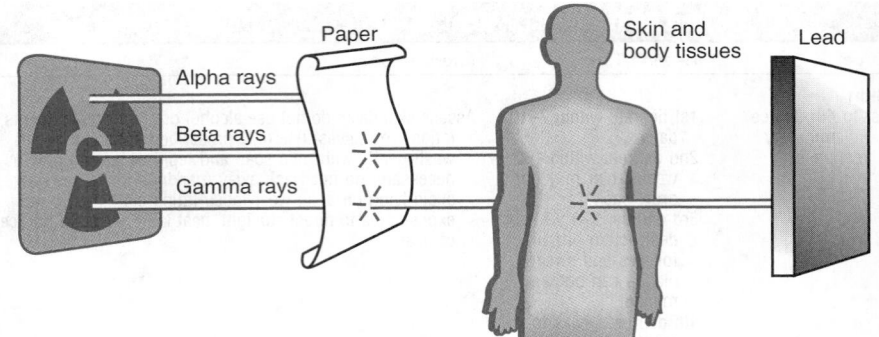

Penetrating capacity of different types of radiation. From Ignatavicius and Workman, 2002.

high-energy helium-4 nuclei consisting of two protons and two neutrons, emitted by radioisotopes of heavy elements such as uranium. BETA PARTICLES are high-energy electrons emitted by radioisotopes of lighter elements. GAMMA RAYS are high-energy photons emitted along with alpha and beta particles and also emitted alone by metastable radionuclides, such as technetium-99m. Gamma rays have energies in the x-ray region of the spectrum and differ from x-rays only in that they are produced by radioactive decay rather than by x-ray machines.

Radiation with enough energy to knock electrons out of atoms and produce ions is called ionizing RADIATION and includes alpha particles, beta particles, x-rays, and gamma rays. This kind of radiation can produce tissue damage directly by striking a vital molecule, such as DNA, or indirectly by striking a water molecule and producing highly reactive free radicals that chemically attack vital molecules. The effects of radiation can kill cells, make them unable to reproduce, or cause nonlethal mutations,

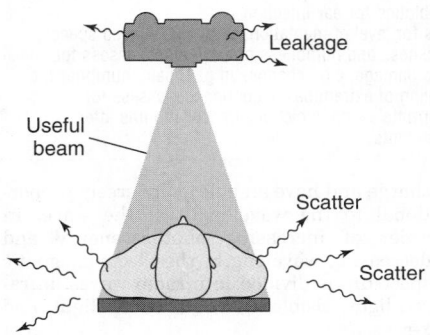

Three types of radiation—the useful beam, leakage radiation, and scatter radiation. From Bushong, 2001.

producing cancer cells or birth defects in offspring. The radiosensitivity of normal tissues or cancer cells increases with their rate of cell division and decreases with their rate of cell specialization. Highly radiosensitive cells include lymphocytes, bone marrow hematopoietic cells, germ cells, and intestinal epithelial cells. Radiosensitive cancers include leukemias and lymphomas, seminoma, dysgerminoma, granulosa cell carcinoma, adenocarcinoma of the gastric epithelium, and squamous cell carcinoma of skin, mouth, nose and throat, cervix, and bladder.

The application of radiation, whether by x-ray or radioactive substances, for treatment of various illnesses is called RADIATION THERAPY or RADIOTHERAPY.

Three types of units are used to measure ionizing radiation. The ROENTGEN (R) is a unit of exposure dose applicable only to x-rays and gamma rays. It is the amount of radiation that produces 2.58×10^{-4} coulomb of positive and negative ions passing through 1 kilogram of dry air. The RAD is a unit of absorbed dose equal to 100 ergs of energy absorbed per 1 g of absorbing material; the absorbed dose depends both on the type of radiation and on the material in which it is absorbed. The REM is a unit of absorbed dose equivalent that produces the same biologic effect as 1 rad of high-energy x-rays. For beta and gamma radiation, 1 rem is approximately equal to 1 rad; for alpha radiation, 1 rad is approximately 20 rem.

Previously, doses administered in radiation therapy were commonly specified as measured exposure doses in roentgens. The current practice is to specify the absorbed dose in the tissue or organ of interest in rads. Many personnel monitoring devices read out in rems. Eventually, the rad and rem may be replaced by the new SI units,

Radiation is emitted by radioactive material. Radiation quantity is measured in roentgens, rads, or rems, depending on precise use. From Bushong, 2001.

the gray and sievert; 1 gray equals 100 rad, and 1 sievert equals 100 rem.

Radiation Hazards. Harmful effects of radiation include serious disturbances of bone marrow and other blood-forming organs, burns, and sterility. There may be permanent damage to GENES, which results in genetic mutations. The mutations can be transmitted to future generations. Radiation also may produce harmful effects on the embryo or fetus, bringing about fetal death or malformations. Long-term studies of groups of persons exposed to radiation have shown that radiation acts as a carcinogen; that is, it can produce cancer, especially leukemia. It also may predispose persons to the development of cataracts.

Exposure to large doses of radiation over a short period of time produces a group of symptoms known as the acute radiation syndrome. These symptoms include general malaise, nausea, and vomiting, followed by a period of remission of symptoms. Later, the patient develops more severe symptoms such as fever, hemorrhage, fluid loss, anemia, and central nervous system involvement. The symptoms then gradually subside or become more severe, and may lead to death.

Radiation Protection. In order to avoid the radiation hazards mentioned above, one must be aware of the three basic principles of time, distance, and shielding involved in protection from radiation. Obviously, the longer one stays near a source of radiation the greater will be the exposure. The same is true of proximity to the source; the closer one gets to a source of radiation the greater the exposure.

Shielding is of special importance when time and distance cannot be completely utilized as safety factors. In such instances lead, which is an extremely dense material, is used as a protective device. The walls of diagnostic x-ray rooms are lined with lead, and lead containers are used for radium, cobalt-60, and other radioactive materials used in radiotherapy.

Monitoring devices such as the film badge, thermoluminescent dosimeter, or pocket monitor are worn by persons working near sources of radiation. These devices contain special detectors that are sensitive to radiation and thus serve as guides to the amount of radiation to which a person has been exposed. For monitoring large areas in which radiation hazards may pose a problem, survey meters such as the Geiger counter may be used. The survey meter also is useful in finding sources of radiation such as a radium implant, which might be lost.

Sensible use of these protective and monitoring devices can greatly reduce unnecessary exposure to radiation and allow for full realization of the many benefits of radiation.

corpuscular r. particles emitted in nuclear disintegration, including alpha and beta particles, protons, neutrons, positrons, and deuterons.

electromagnetic r. energy, unassociated with matter, that is transmitted through space by means of waves (electromagnetic waves) traveling in all instances at 3×10^{10} cm or 186,284 miles per second, but ranging in length from 10^{11} cm (electrical waves) to 10^{-12} cm (cosmic rays) and including radio waves, infrared, visible light and ultraviolet, x-rays, and gamma rays.

extrafocal r. radiation that arises from a source other than the focal spot of the x-ray tube.

infrared r. the portion of the spectrum of electromagnetic radiation of wavelengths between 0.75 and 1000 μm; see also INFRARED.

interstitial r. energy emitted by radium, radon, or some other RADIOPHARMACEUTICAL inserted directly into the tissue; see also RADIATION THERAPY.

ionizing r. corpuscular or electromagnetic radiation that is capable of producing ions, directly or indirectly, in its passage through matter. See also RADIATION.

optic r. either of two large fan-shaped fiber tracts in the brain extending from the lateral geniculate body on either side to the striate cortex

primary r. that coming directly from a source, such as a radioactive substance or an x-ray tube, without interactions with matter.

pyramidal r. fibers extending from the pyramidal tract to the cortex.

scatter r., secondary r. that generated by the interaction of primary RADIATION with matter. See illustration.

striothalamic r. a fiber system joining the thalamus and the hypothalamic region.

tegmental r. fibers radiating laterally from the nucleus ruber.

thalamic r's fibers streaming out through the lateral surface of the thalamus, through the internal capsule to the cerebral cortex.

ultraviolet r. the portion of the spectrum of electromagnetic radiation of wavelengths between 0.39 and 0.18 μm; see also ULTRAVIOLET RAYS.

radiation physicist a physicist who is responsible for certain technical aspects of RADIOLOGY and RADIATION THERAPY, such as computer estimations, preparation of isodose curves, preparation of wedge and compensating filters, and calibration of teletherapy equipment, and who supervises quality assurance and control and radiation safety procedures.

radiation sickness a condition sometimes seen in patients who have received therapeutic doses of radiation. Its severity varies according to factors such as the individual's physical condition, the body areas exposed, and the amount, kind, and intensity of the exposure. The disease may be so slight that it is scarcely noticeable, or it may cause severe symptoms. Modern techniques and increased knowledge about radiation have lowered the incidence of severe radiation sickness. Systemic reactions to radiation include a general feeling of malaise, loss of appetite or nausea and vomiting, and headache. The symptoms tend to subside when the therapy is discontinued, leaving no permanent effect on the patient.

radiation therapist a specialist in the treatment of disease by means of ionizing radiation; see RADIATION THERAPY.

radiation therapy the treatment of disease, usually cancer, by ionizing RADIATION in order to deliver an optimal dose of either particulate or electromagnetic radiation to a particular area of the body with minimal damage to normal tissues. The source of radiation may be outside the body of the patient (external beam IRRADIATION) or it may be an isotope that has been implanted or instilled into abnormal tissue or a body cavity. Called also radiotherapy and irradiation.

Because of improvements in tumor localization, beam direction, planning and prescribing the FIELD to be irradiated, and determining the precise dosage needed radiation therapy is far more effective and less harmful now than when it was first introduced.

External Beam Irradiation. Modern radiation therapy primarily uses high-energy x-rays or gamma rays with peak photon energies above 1 megavolt; this is called *megavoltage therapy*. These high voltages are produced by linear accelerators or by cobalt-60 teletherapy units. Megavoltage radiation is more penetrating than lower energy radiation. It produces less damage to the skin at the entry port, is absorbed less in bone, and is scattered less, thus reducing the exposure to tissues outside the x-ray beam Low-energy x-rays that do not penetrate are used for treatment of superficial skin lesions

Internal Radiation Therapy (brachytherapy). This can involve the implantation of sealed radiation sources in or near cancerous tissue. Isotopes, such as radium-226 cesium-137, iridium-192, and iodine-125, are introduced either temporarily or permanently into body tissues *(interstitial radiation therapy)* or body cavities *(intracavitary radiation therapy).* Permanent sources have a short half-life so that the dose received by the patient is limited.

Another form of internal radiation therapy is the administration of radioactive materials into the bloodstream or a body cavity. Iodine-131 is given orally in certain cases of hyperthyroidism and cancer of the thyroid; it is absorbed by the digestive system and concentrated in the thyroid Phosphorus-32, a pure beta emitter, is injected intravenously for the treatment of various myeloproliferative diseases, leukemias, and lymphomas.

Protection from Radiation. Hospital personnel concerned with the care of patients receiving radiation therapy must be aware of the hazards of radiation and the protective policies and procedures established to reduce these hazards. Most institutions and clinics provide a safety program under the leadership of a radiation physicist or radiation safety officer. Since radiation cannot be seen or felt, it is extremely important to observe all rules outlined in the program.

Sources of radiation that may be of particular concern to health care personnel include: radioactive substances such as radium and cobalt-60 that are used as implants and serve as internal sources of radiation; external sources of radiation such as x-ray machines and cobalt-60 therapy units; and liquid radioisotopes such as iodine-131 and suspensions of radioactive gold or phosphorus.

Generally speaking, the degree of exposure to radiation depends on three factors: (1) the distance between the source of radiation and the individual, (2) the amount of time an individual is exposed to radiation, and (3) the type of shielding provided. (See discussion at RADIATION.)

When a patient receives radiation therapy from an external source, therapists must be aware of, and observe carefully, the policies and procedures established for personnel in and around x-ray rooms and the rooms that house teletherapy units. After the treatment is finished, the patient will not serve as a hazard of radiation. This type of radiation therapy is often done on an outpatient basis.

Internal implants can present certain hazards for persons in contact with the patient for as long as the implant is in place. Visitors should sit at least six feet away from the patient and stay no longer than a total of one hour each day. Pregnant staff members and visitors should avoid all contact with the patient.

When administering direct patient care, staff members should plan interventions so that each task can be accomplished as quickly as possible. Since distance is a factor in protection, it is advisable to position oneself as far as is feasible from the source of radiation. For example, if the radioactive implant is in the pelvis, the caregiver might stand at the head or foot, rather than the side, of the bed. Protective lead aprons or portable shields may or may not be recommended by hospital protocol. Whatever the policies, every person caring for the patient should know and follow the recommended policies and procedures.

A film badge is worn on the outside of any protective devices worn by caregivers. The badge records the cumulative dose of radiation received by each person, and is used to monitor exposure over a period of time. It should be sent for monthly testing to be sure that no one is receiving more than the maximum allowable exposure. This amount should not exceed five rem per year. One should never lend one's badge to another staff member or borrow another staff member's badge.

Another factor to be considered is accidental removal or dislodgment of a radioactive implant. Most patients are confined to bed and refused bathroom privileges, but it is still possible for a radium needle or radon seeds, for example, to be accidentally removed from the body. Should an implant become dislodged the physician or radiation safety officer must be notified immediately. Under no circumstances should a radioactive substance be handled with the bare hands. A lead container and long-handled forceps should be kept at the patient's bedside in the event an implant should become dislodged. It can then be picked up immediately and placed in the container. Dressings, bed linen, bedpans, and emesis basins should be checked with a radiation detection instrument after each use or before disposal.

Liquid radioactive substances require additional precautions since these substances can enter the body of a worker through the skin, or by ingestion or inhalation. Not all types of radioactive materials require the same precautions. For example, iodine-131 is excreted in the urine for several days after it has been administered to the patient. In addition it appears in the patient's sweat, tears and saliva; thus all articles such as bed linens and toothbrush used by the patient must be considered a possible radiation hazard. Phosphorus-32 acts in the same way. Colloidal gold-98 usually is instilled into a body cavity and is not absorbed as are iodine and phosphorus. However, the radioactive gold emits gamma rays that penetrate beyond the patient's body and present a radiation hazard.

Patient Care. Specific goals for the care of a patient receiving radiation thearapy will depend on the location of the irradiated site, the patient's medical diagnosis, and the source of radiation, i.e., whether it is internal or external. Special precautions in regard to handling radioactive material have been presented above. In addition to the goal of protecting patients and caregivers from unnecessary exposure, goals of patient care include familiarizing patients and significant others with the purpose and therapeutic effects of radiation therapy and helping them recognize and deal with its expected side effects.

Most people have a limited knowledge of radiation and how it affects cells, both normal and malignant. This lack of knowledge can add to the anxiety and stress already being felt by patients and significant others. The kinds of information they will need include how radiation works, whether or not patients present a hazard to others while undergoing treatment, when they will begin to experience its effects, and how long it will be before they begin to recover from the effects.

Before treatment is initiated, the patient is told the expected therapeutic effects, what it is like to have a treatment, and what might be expected of the patient during the course of therapy. Most patients will receive external radiation therapy on an outpatient basis; hence, they will need to keep scheduled appointments or notify the clinic if they are unable to come when expected. They should be assured that the source of radiation is outside their bodies (if it is) and that they cannot serve as a source of radiation.

Teaching patients and significant others how to recognize expected side effects and participate in their management is especially important when patients are not hospitalized. Written information that is easily comprehended should be available to them, as well as sufficient time and personnel to answer any questions they may have after reading the instructions and attempting to follow them at home. They should be encouraged to write down questions that have arisen between visits and to bring these questions with them on their next visit.

In general, most side effects will not begin before a week to ten days after the first treatment. This allows time for patients to assimilate information given to them and to adjust to whatever changes they might experience. They can be told that side effects typically continue throughout the course of treatment and for several weeks after the last treatment. However, individual reactions can and do vary.

Although all body systems can be affected by radiation, the skin is the system most at risk for injury. The reaction results from an inflammatory process caused by breakdown of cells in the epidermis and is similar to a sunburn. In preparation for radiation therapy the physician will mark the target area with indelible ink.

Daily assessment of the skin for degree of reaction can be done by the patient or some other knowledgeable person.

First-degree reactions resemble a sunburn and can destroy hair roots, causing the hair to fall out. *Second-degree* reactions, also called dry desquamation, produce bright red erythema. Sweat glands and hair follicles are damaged and the hair falls out. This change can be irreversible. *Third-degree* reactions, also called moist desquamation, are characterized by a dark purple color and possibly formation of blisters and ulcers. If the area is exposed to air, scabbing over the exposed area can occur. *Fourth-degree* reactions are very rare and are the result of radiation overdose. They are characterized by tissue necrosis.

Effects of radiation on major systems of the body, healing time, and appropriate nursing interventions are summarized in the table at RADIATION.

radiation therapy technologist a health care professional who delivers courses of radiation therapy prescribed by a radiation therapist. Duties include positioning and caring for patients; calibration of teletherapy equipment; preparation of brachytherapy equipment and handling of radioactive materials; assisting the radiation physicist in preparation of isodose curves, performance of computer estimations, and preparation of wedge and compensating filters; observing the patient for signs of clinical progress or complications that require consultation with the physician; and observing radiation safety measures. Individuals completing an accredited program and passing the certification examination of the American Registry of Radiologic Technologists are designated RT(T)(ARRT), Registered Technologist. See also RADIOLOGIC TECHNOLOGIST.

radical (rad′ĭ-kal) 1. thorough or sweeping; directed to the cause or root of a morbid process. 2. a group of atoms that enters into and goes out of chemical combination without change and that forms one of the fundamental constituents of a molecule.

    color r. chromophore.

    free r. a radical that carries an unpaired electron; such radicals are extremely reactive, with a very short HALF-LIFE.

    oxygen r. a toxic metabolite of oxygen, such as superoxide or singlet oxygen, capable of damaging microorganisms and normal tissues.

radicle (rad′ĭ-k'l) one of the smallest branches of a vessel or nerve; called also ramulus.

radicotomy (rad″ĭ-kot′ah-me) rhizotomy; division or transection of a nerve root.

radiculalgia (rah-dik″u-lal′jah) pain due to disorder of the spinal nerve roots.

radicular (rah-dik′u-lar) pertaining to a root or radicle.

radiculitis (rah-dik″u-li′tis) inflammation of a spinal nerve root, especially of the portion of the root that lies between the spinal cord and the spinal canal.

radiculoganglionitis (rah-dik″u-lo-gang″-gle-o-ni′tis) inflammation of the posterior spinal nerve roots and their ganglia.

radiculomedullary (rah-dik″u-lo-med′u-lar″e) affecting the nerve roots and spinal cord.

radiculomeningomyelitis (rah-dik″u-lo-mĕ-ning″-go-mi″ĕ-li′tis) meningomyeloradiculitis.

radiculomyelopathy (rah-dik″u-lo-mi″ĕ-lop′ah-the) myeloradiculopathy.

radiculoneuritis (rah-dik″u-lo-noo-ri′tis) acute febrile polyneuritis.

radiculoneuropathy (rah-dik″u-lo-noo-rop′ah-the) disease of the nerve roots and spinal nerves.

radiculopathy (rah-dik″u-lop′ah-the) disease of the nerve roots.

spondylotic caudal r. compression of the cauda equina due to encroachment upon a congenitally small spinal canal by spondylosis, resulting in neural disorders of the lower limbs.

radiectomy (ra″de-ek′tah-me) root amputation.

radioactive (ra″de-o-ak′tiv) characterized by radioactivity.

r. iodine uptake test radioiodine uptake test.

radioactivity (ra″de-o-ak-tiv′ĭ-te) the emission of particulate or electromagnetic RADIATION as a result of decay of the nuclei of unstable elements, a property of all chemical elements of atomic number above 83, and possibly inducible in all other known elements. The chemical elements are made up of ATOMS, each consisting of a NUCLEUS around which orbits a cloud of negatively charged ELECTRONS. The nucleus itself is made up of two kinds of particles: NEUTRONS (which have no electrical charge) and PROTONS (each of which has a single positive charge). A neutral atom has an equal number of protons and electrons and no electric charge. The atomic NUMBER of an element is the number of protons in the nucleus of each of its atoms. The mass NUMBER of an element is the sum of the number of protons and neutrons in the nucleus.

All of the atoms of a particular element have the same atomic number, but they can have different numbers of neutrons (i.e., different mass numbers). ISOTOPES of a chemical element consist of atoms having different numbers of neutrons. When an atomic nucleus is unstable it decomposes or decays spontaneously, emitting high-energy particles. The emissions from radioactive decay,

called RADIATION, can consist of electrons (BETA PARTICLES), or electromagnetic energy in the form of PHOTONS, or helium ions (ALPHA PARTICLES). The process of decay can produce a product that is itself unstable, in which case it too will decay. The process continues until a stable nuclide is finally formed.

The radioactivity of a substance can be measured by finding the rate at which atoms decay in a given period of time. The basic unit of measurement of radioactivity is the CURIE (Ci), which equals 37 billion disintegrations per second. One thousandth of a curie is a *millicurie* and one millionth is a *microcurie;* these units are used to calculate the dosage of radioactivity administered for therapeutic procedures in much the same way that units such as the gram and milligram are used to measure dosages of medications. The curie may eventually be replaced by a new SI unit of radioactivity, the BECQUEREL (Bq), which is equal to 1 disintegration per second. One microcurie equals 37 kilobecquerels.

The HALF-LIFE of an element is the time necessary for one half of a given amount of the isotope to decay. Half-lives can range from billions of years to fractions of a second. The rate at which atomic decay occurs in a particular isotope cannot be altered by any outside force such as temperature, pressure, or chemical reaction. The knowledge of the half-life of a particular isotope is essential to the proper handling of the substance for the protection of the medical staff and the patient who is receiving some form of radiation therapy.

Both particulate and electromagnetic radiations are capable of penetrating matter and interacting with it by indiscriminately knocking out the electrons from atoms and molecules. The process of ionizing radiation produces ions (charged particles) and complex radicals (a group of charged atoms), which may combine to form different molecules. Radiation damage to the nuclei of cells interferes with their reproduction by changing their genetic structure. This ability to penetrate matter and change the basic structure and function of cells is used beneficially in the treatment of malignant tumors. (See also RADIATION THERAPY.)

Rendering an element radioactive by artificial means does not alter its chemical behavior within the body; therefore, the body's systems respond to a radioactive element as if it were stable. This phenomenon makes it possible to use radioactive elements for diagnostic as well as

R

therapeutic purposes. For example, the iodine isotope ^{131}I is readily taken up by the thyroid gland, permitting evaluation of iodine uptake of the gland by measuring the amount of radiation emitting from it. An isotope of technetium, ^{99m}Tc, is attached to many different compounds that localize in various organs. The organ or structure can then be imaged with a scintillation camera.

radioallergosorbent test (RAST) (ra″de-o-al″er-go-sor′bent) a radioimmunoassay for the measurement of extremely small amounts of specific IgE antibody to a variety of allergens in the serum of a patient, using an allergen complex fixed in a solid-phase matrix, passing the serum over the matrix so the allergen can catch and bind specific IgE antibodies, and detecting the antibody using radiolabeled anti–human IgE antibody. Uptake of the labeled antibody is proportional to the level of specific serum IgE antibodies to the allergen. RAST is used as an alternative to skin tests to determine sensitivity to suspected allergens.

radioautogram (ra″de-o-aw′to-gram) autoradiogram.

radioautography (ra″de-o-aw-tog′rah-fe) autoradiography.

radiobicipital (ra″de-o-bi-sip′ĭ-tal) pertaining to the radius and biceps muscle of the upper limb.

radiobiologist (ra″de-o-bi-ol′ah-jist) an expert in radiobiology.

radiobiology (ra″de-o-bi-ol′ah-je) the branch of science concerned with effects of light and of ultraviolet and ionizing radiations on living tissue or organisms. adj., **radiobiolog′ical.**

radiocardiogram (ra″de-o-kahr′de-o-gram″) the graphic record produced by radiocardiography.

radiocardiography (ra″de-o-kahr″de-og′rah-fe) 1. graphic recording of variation with time of the concentration, in a selected chamber of the heart, of a radioactive isotope, usually injected intravenously. 2. radioelectrocardiography.

radiocarpal (ra″de-o-kahr′pal) pertaining to the radius and carpus.

radiochemistry (ra″de-o-kem′is-tre) the branch of chemistry dealing with radioactive materials.

radiochemotherapy (ra″de-o-ke″mo-ther′-ah-pe) chemoradiotherapy.

radiocolloids (ra″de-o-kol′oidz) RADIOISOTOPES in pure form in solution, which tend to act more like COLLOIDS than solutes.

radiocurable (ra″de-o-kūr′ah-b'l) curable by radiation therapy.

radiocystitis (ra″de-o-sis-ti′tis) radiation cystitis.

radiodense (ra′de-o-dens″) radiopaque.

radiodensity (ra″de-o-den′sĭ-te) radiopacity.

radiodermatitis (ra″de-o-der″mah-ti′tis) a cutaneous inflammatory reaction to exposure to biologically effective levels of ionizing radiation; x-ray dermatitis.

radiodiagnosis (ra″de-o-di″ag-no′sis) diagnosis by means of x-rays or gamma rays.

radioelectrocardiogram (ra″de-o-e-lek″-tro-kahr′de-o-gram″) the graphic recording obtained by radioelectrocardiography.

radioelectrocardiograph (ra″de-o-e-lek″tro-kahr′de-o-graf″) the apparatus used in radio electrocardiography.

radioelectrocardiography (ra″de-o-e-lek″tro-kahr″de-og′rah-fe) a TELEMETRY technique of recording of alterations in the electric POTENTIAL of the heart, with impulses beamed by radio waves from the subject to the recording device by means of a small transmitter attached to the patient.

radioencephalogram (ra″de-o-en-sef′ah-lo-gram″) the graphic record obtained by radioencephalography.

radioencephalography (ra″de-o-en-sef″ah-log′rah-fe) 1. REG; the study of the passage of an injected TRACER through the cerebral blood vessels as revealed by an external scintillation COUNTER. 2. the recording of changes in the electric POTENTIAL of the brain without direct attachment between the recording apparatus and the subject, the impulses being beamed by radio waves from the subject to the receiver.

radiofrequency (ra″de-o-fre′kwen-se) radio FREQUENCY.

radiogold (ra′de-o-gold″) any of the radioactive isotopes of GOLD, especially ^{198}Au; used as SCINTISCANNING agents and antineoplastic AGENTS. See also GOLD 198.

radiogram (ra′de-o-gram″) radiograph.

radiograph (ra′de-o-graf″) an image or record produced on exposed or processed film by radiography.

bite-wing r. a type of dental radiograph that reveals the crowns, necks, and coronal thirds of the roots of both the upper and lower posterior teeth, as well as the dental arches, produced using bite-wing FILM.

cephalometric r. a radiograph of the head, including the mandible, in full lateral view; used to make measurements; called also cephalogram.

flat plate r. a radiograph that visualizes abdominal organs and some abnormalities. It is usually one of the first diagnostic studies performed in assessing a patient for gastrointestinal disorders; no special physical preparation of the patient is necessary.

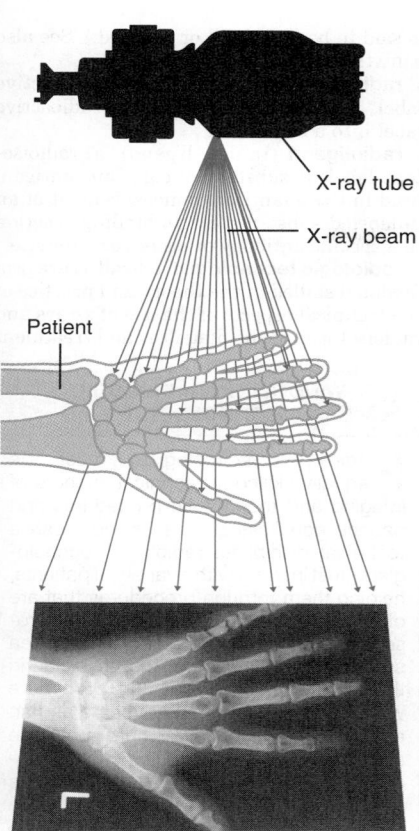

X-ray tube

X-ray beam

Patient

Image receptor (film)

Relative positions of x-ray tube, patient, and film necessary to make the radiograph shown. Bones tend to stop diagnostic x-rays, but soft tissue does not. This results in the light and dark regions that form the image. From Thompson et al., 1994.

panoramic r. a type of extraoral body-section radiograph on which the entire maxilla or mandible can be depicted on a single film.

radiographer (ra″de-og′rah-fer) a RADIOLO-GIC TECHNOLOGIST whose work is the making of diagnostic radiographs. Duties include positioning patients for radiologic examinations; determining the proper voltage, current, and exposure time for each radiograph and adjusting the x-ray equipment; the production of radiographs as requested; developing the x-ray film; and assisting the RADIOLOGIST in special procedures and in preparation of radiopaque contrast media. Graduates of approved programs who pass the certifying examination of the American Registry of Radiologic Technologists are designated (ARRT), Registered Technologist.

radiography (ra″de-og′rah-fe) the making of film records (radiographs) of internal structures of the body by exposure of film specially sensitized to x-rays or gamma rays. adj., **radiograph′ic.**

body section r. tomography.

double-contrast r. mucosal relief radiography.

electron r. radiography consisting of electronic images that can be computer enhanced, electronically reversed, stored, retrieved, transmitted, and/or printed on photographic film.

mass r. examination by x-rays of the general population or of large groups of the population.

mucosal relief r. a technique for revealing any abnormality of the intestinal mucosa, involving injection and evacuation of a barium enema, followed by inflation of the intestine with air under light pressure. The light coating of barium on the inflated intestine in the radiograph reveals clearly even small abnormalities; double-contrast r.

neutron r. that in which a narrow beam of neutrons from a nuclear reactor is passed through tissues; especially useful in visualizing bony tissue.

panoramic r. pantomography.

serial r. the making of several exposures of a particular area at arbitrary intervals.

spot-film r. the making of localized instantaneous radiographic exposures; see also spot FILM.

radiohumeral (ra″de-o-hu′mer-al) pertaining to the radius and humerus.

radioimmunity (ra″de-o-ĭ-mu′nĭ-te) diminished sensitivity to radiation.

radioimmunoassay (RIA) (ra″de-o-im″u-no-as′a) a sensitive assay method that can be used for the measurement of minute quantities of specific antibodies or any antigen, such as a hormone or drug, against which specific antibodies can be raised. An assay for a specific hormone uses antihormone antibody produced by injecting the human hormone into an animal, such as a rabbit, and hormone that has been labeled with a radioisotope. These are mixed with the assay specimen and the antigen (hormone) bound to antibody is separated from the unbound antigen by chromatography or other means. Because any hormone in the assay specimen competes with the radiolabeled hormone for antibody binding sites, the amount of hormone in the specimen is inversely proportional to the radioactivity of the bound fraction or directly proportional to the activity of the free fraction. This is the

R

standard method for clinical laboratory measurements of hormones and is also used for therapeutic drug monitoring, drug abuse screening, and other laboratory tests.

radioimmunodiffusion (ra″de-o-im″u-no-dĭ-fu′-zhun) immunodiffusion conducted with radioisotope-labeled antibodies or antigens.

radioimmunoelectrophoresis (ra″de-o-im″u-no-e-lek″tro-fah-re′sis) electrophoresis in which any layer of precipitate is identified by adding the corresponding radioactive-labeled antigen or antibody and subjecting it to autoradiography.

radioimmunotherapy (ra″de-o-im-mu″no-ther′ah-pe) use of RADIONUCLIDES to deliver monoclonal ANTIBODIES to targeted cancer cells.

radioimmunosorbent test (RIST) (ra″de-o-im″u-no-sor′bent) a radioimmunoassay technique for measuring serum IgE concentration, using radiolabeled IgE and anti–human IgE bound to an insoluble matrix. The patient's IgE competes with the radiolabeled IgE attached to the matrix, so that the decrease in radiolabel remaining attached to the matrix can be used to determine the total concentration of serum IgE in the patient.

radioiodine (ra″de-o-i′o-dīn) any radioactive isotope of iodine; of the nine isotopes, IODINE 123, IODINE 125, and IODINE 131 are the most commonly used in diagnosis and treatment of benign and malignant diseases of the THYROID GLAND and in SCINTISCANS of organs such as the lung, liver, and kidney. Called also radioactive iodine.

r. uptake test one of the most common THYROID FUNCTION TESTS; a known quantity of RADIOIODINE is administered and 24 hours later the per cent is calculated that has been absorbed by the THYROID GLAND. Patients who have recently been exposed to iodine compounds, such as in dietary supplements, contrast media, medications, or antiseptics may not be good candidates for this test.

radioisotope (ra″de-o-i′so-tōp) a radioactive form of an element, consisting of atoms with unstable nuclei, which undergo radioactive decay to stable forms, emitting characteristic alpha, beta, or gamma radiation. These may occur naturally, as in the cases of radium and uranium, or may be created artificially. Scientists create artificial radioisotopes by bombarding stable atoms of an element with subatomic particles in a nuclear reactor or in an atom smasher, or cyclotron. When the nucleus of a stable atom is charged by bombarding particles, the atom usually becomes unstable, or radioactive, and

is said to be "labeled" or "tagged." See also RADIATION THERAPY.

radiolabel (ra′de-o-la″b′l) 1. radioactive label. 2. to incorporate such a radioactive label into a compound.

radioligand (ra″de-o-li′gand) a radioisotope-labeled substance, e.g., an antigen, used in the quantitative measurement of an unlabeled substance by its binding reaction to a specific antibody or other receptor site.

radiologic technologist a health care professional skilled in the theory and practice of the technical aspects of the use of x-rays and radioisotopes in the diagnosis and treatment

---

WINDOW ON RADIOLOGIC TECHNOLOGIST

Radiologic technologists must be equally skilled in technical aspects of imaging and therapeutic procedures and patient care skills. This is not just a technical discipline; radiologic technologists must interact with a variety of patients, helping them through procedures that are often unpleasant. For example, in fluoroscopic procedures, a radiographer often serves as an assistant to the physician in the technical aspects of the procedure while serving as both an advocate and an educator to the patient. There are three accepted levels of radiologic technologists: (1) limited licensure—practitioners with approximately a year of education and training in radiology who are able to perform only certain procedures (e.g., chest or extremities), usually under the direct supervision of a physician; (2) entry-level—practitioners educated at the two-year (associate degree) level, able to perform a full range of radiologic procedures without supervision; and (3) professional—practitioners educated at the baccalaureate level, who typically assume a number of advanced roles, including CT, MRI, or cardiovascular-interventional (CVIT) technologist, quality assurance technologist, and so on. In addition to limited licensure and certification as a radiographer, radiation therapist, or nuclear medicine technologist by the American Registry of Radiologic Technologists (ARRT), there are a number of advanced examinations offered by the ARRT—CT, MRI, mammography, and CVIT. A test in quality assurance is under development. Given the multifaceted nature of their role and work settings, the occupational outlook for radiologic technologists, especially those with advanced education and training, is bright.

STEVEN B. DOWD, EDD, RT(R)

radiologic technologists can specialize in RADIOGRAPHY, RADIATION THERAPY, or NUCLEAR MEDICINE. (See also RADIOGRAPHER, RADIATION THERAPY TECHNOLOGIST, and NUCLEAR MEDICINE TECHNOLOGIST.) The address of the American Registry of Radiologic Technologists is 1255 Northland Drive, St. Paul, MN 55120. The address of the professional organization, the American Society of Radiologic Technologists, is 15000 Central Ave. SE, Albuquerque, NM 87123.

radiologist (ra″de-ol′ah-jist) a physician specializing in radiology.

radiology (ra″de-ol′ah-je) the branch of medical science dealing with use of x-rays, radioactive substances, and other forms of radiant energy in diagnosis and treatment of disease. adj., **radiolog′ic, radiolog′-ical.**

    interventional r. the branch of radiology concerned with providing diagnosis and treatment of disease by a variety of percutaneous procedures performed under the guidance of radiologic imaging.

radiolucency (ra″de-o-loo′sen-se) the quality of permitting the passage of radiant energy, such as X-RAYS, yet offering some resistance to it, the representative areas appearing dark on the exposed film. adj., **radiolu′cent.**

radiometer (ra″de-om′ĕ-ter) 1. an instrument for estimating x-ray quantity. 2. an instrument in which radiant heat and light may be directly converted into mechanical energy. 3. an instrument for measuring the penetrating power of radiant energy.

radiomimetic (ra″de-o-mi-met′ik) producing effects similar to those of ionizing radiations.

radionecrosis (ra″de-o-ně-kro′sis) tissue destruction due to radiant energy.

radioneuritis (ra″de-o-noo-ri′tis) neuritis from exposure to radiant energy.

radionuclide (ra″de-o-noo′klīd) a radioactive nuclide; one that disintegrates with the emission of corpuscular or electromagnetic radiations.

radiopacity (ra″de-o-pas′ĭ-te) the quality or property of being RADIOPAQUE.

radiopaque obstructing the passage of radiant energy, such as x-rays, the representative areas appearing light or white on the exposed film.

radiopathology (ra″de-o-pah-thol′ah-je) the pathology of radiation effects on tissues.

radiopharmaceutical (ra″de-o-fahr″mah-soo′tĭ-k'l) a radioactive pharmaceutical, nuclide, or other chemical used for diagnostic purposes or for RADIATION THERAPY.

radiophosphorus (ra″de-o-fos′fah-rus) either of two radioactive isotopes of PHOSPHORUS, ^{32}P and ^{33}P; see also PHOSPHORUS 32.

radiopotentiation (ra″de-o-po-ten″she-a′shun) the action of a drug in enhancing the effects of irradiation.

radioprotectant (ra″de-o-pro-tek′tant) 1. providing protection against the toxic effects of ionizing radiation. 2. radioprotector.

radioprotector (ra″de-o-pro-tek′ter) an agent that provides protection against the toxic effects of ionizing radiation.

radioreceptor (ra″de-o-re-sep′tor) 1. a receptor for the stimuli that are excited by radiant energy, such as light or heat. 2. a receptor that can bind to either a RADIOLIGAND or an unlabeled ligand; see also radioreceptor ASSAY.

radioresistance (ra″de-o-re″zis′tans) resisting the effects of radiation, especially in reference to the treatment of malignancy. adj., **radioresist′ant.**

radioresponsive (ra″de-o-re-spon′siv) reacting favorably to irradiation.

radioscopy (ra″de-os′kah-pe) fluoroscopy.

radiosensitivity (ra″de-o-sen″sĭ-tiv′ĭ-te) sensitivity of the skin, tumor tissue, or other tissue to radiant energy, such as x-ray or other radiations. adj., **radiosen′sitive.**

radiosensitizer (ra″de-o-sen′sĭ-ti″zer) a chemotherapeutic agent used to enhance the effect of radiation therapy.

radiosurgery (ra″de-o-ser′jer-e) surgery in which tissue destruction is performed by means of ionizing radiation rather than surgical incision; the radiation may originate from an implant of radioactive material or may be delivered from an external source.

    stereotaxic r. stereotaxic surgery in which lesions are produced by ionizing radiation.

radiotelemetry (ra″de-o-tě-lem′ĕ-tre) measurement based on data transmitted by radio waves from the subject to the recording apparatus.

radiotherapist (ra″de-o-ther′ah-pist) a specialist in radiotherapy.

radiotherapy (ra″de-o-ther′ah-pe) radiation therapy.

radiotoxemia (ra″de-o-tok-se′me-ah) TOXEMIA produced by a radioactive substance, or resulting from radiotherapy.

radiotracer (ra″de-o-tra′ser) radioactive tracer.

radiotransparent (ra″de-o-trans-par′ent) radiolucent.

radiotropic (ra″de-o-trop′ik) influenced by radiation.

radioulnar (ra″de-o-ul′nar) pertaining to the radius and ulna.

radium (ra′de-um) a chemical element, atomic number 88, atomic weight, 226, symbol Ra. (See Appendix 6.) Radium is highly

R

radioactive and is found in uranium minerals. Radium-226 has a half-life of 1622 years. It and its short-lived decay products emit alpha particles, beta particles, and gamma rays. One of the decay products, radon-222, is a radioactive gas. In clinical use, radium is contained in a metal container that stops alpha and beta particles and traps radon.

Radium is used in RADIATION THERAPY for malignant diseases, particularly those that are readily accessible, for example, tumors of the cervix uteri, mouth, or tongue. In the form of needles or pellets, it can be inserted in the tumorous tissue (interstitial implantation) and left in place until its rays penetrate and destroy malignant cells. It can also be used in the form of plaques applied to the diseased tissue. Large amounts of radium are used as a source of GAMMA RAYS, which are capable of deep penetration of matter. Radium rays have been used in the treatment of lupus erythematosus, eczema, psoriasis, xanthoma, mycosis fungoides, and other skin diseases; for the removal of papillomas, granulomas, and nevi; for palliative treatment in carcinoma and sarcoma; and in myelogenous and lymphatic leukemia.

radius (ra′de-us) [L.] 1. a line radiating from a center, or a circular limit defined by a fixed distance from an established point or center. 2. in anatomy, the bone on the outer or thumb side of the forearm.

   grid r. grid focus.

radix (ra′diks) [L.] root.

radon (ra′don) a chemical element, atomic number 86, atomic weight 222, symbol Rn. (See Appendix 6.) Radon is a colorless, gaseous, radioactive element produced by the disintegration of radium.

rage (rāj) a state of violent anger.

   sham r. an outburst of motor activity resembling the outward manifestations of fear and anger, occurring in decorticated animals and in certain pathologic conditions in humans.

ragocyte (rag′o-sīt) a cell found in the joints in rheumatoid arthritis. Such cells are produced when polymorphonuclear leukocytes ingest aggregated IgG immunoglobulin, rheumatoid factor, fibrin, and complement.

rale (rahl) a discontinuous SOUND heard on auscultation, primarily during inhalation; called also crackle.

   crackling r. subcrepitant rale.

   crepitant r. a fine sound like that of rubbing a hair between the fingers or by particles of salt thrown on fire; heard at the end of inhalation. Called also crepitus.

   dry r. a fine sound associated with any of various interstitial lung diseases, such as idiopathic pulmonary FIBROSIS.

   moist r. one heard over fluid in the bronchial tubes.

   subcrepitant r. a fine moist rale heard over liquid in the smaller tubes; called also crackling rale.

raloxifene (ral-ok′sī-fēn) a selective estrogen receptor MODULATOR that has estrogen-like effects on bone, increasing bone mineral density, and lipid metabolism, lowering total and LDL cholesterol; it has no effect on breast or uterine tissue. Administered orally as the hydrochloride salt for the prevention of postmenopausal OSTEOPOROSIS.

ramal (ra′mal) pertaining to a ramus.

rami (ra′mi) [L.] plural of RAMUS.

ramification (ram″ĭ-fĭ-ka′shun) 1. distribution in branches. 2. a branch or set of branches.

ramify (ram′ĭ-fi) 1. to branch; to diverge in different directions. 2. to traverse in branches.

ramipril (rah-mi′pril) an angiotensin converting enzyme INHIBITOR used in treatment of HYPERTENSION and congestive HEART FAILURE; administered orally.

ramisection (ram″ĭ-sek′shun) section of the appropriate rami communicantes of the sympathetic nervous system.

ramitis (ram-i′tis) inflammation of a ramus.

ramose (ra′mōs) branching; having many branches.

Ramsay Hunt syndrome (ram′ze-hunt) HERPES ZOSTER involving the facial and auditory nerves associated with ipsilateral facial paralysis, usually transitory, and herpetic vesicles of the external ear or tympanic membrane, which also may or may not be associated with tinnitus, vertigo, and hearing disorders. Called also herpes zoster auricularis or oticus, geniculate neuralgia, and Hunt's neuralgia.

ramulus (ram′u-lus) [L.] radicle.

ramus (ra′mus) [L.] branch.

   r. commu′nicans (pl. *ra′mi communican′tes*), a branch connecting two nerves or two arteries.

   r. of mandible a quadrilateral process projecting upwards from the posterior part of either side of the MANDIBLE.

rancid (ran′sid) having a musty, rank taste or smell; applied to fats that have undergone decomposition, with the liberation of fatty acids.

random (ran′dum) pertaining to a chance-dependent process.

randomization (ran″dom-ĭ-za′shun) random assignment.

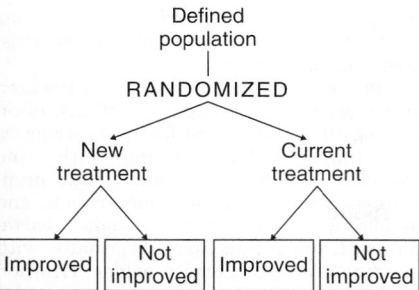

Defined
population
|
RANDOMIZED

New
treatment

Current
treatment

| Improved | Not improved | Improved | Not improved |

The use of randomization in the design of a clinical trial. From Gordis, 1996.

range (rānj) 1. the difference between the upper and lower limits of a variable or of a series of values. 2. an interval in which values sampled from a population, or the values in the population itself, are known to lie.

r. of accommodation the total amount of accommodative power of the eye; the difference in refractive power of the eye when adjusted for near and for far vision. The amplitude diminishes as age increases because elasticity of the lens is decreased.

r. of audibility the range between the extreme frequencies of sound waves beyond which the human ear perceives no sound: lower limit, 16 to 20 cycles per second; upper limit, 18,000 to 20,000 cycles per second.

r. of motion the range, measured in degrees of a circle, through which a joint can be extended and flexed; see also range of motion EXERCISES.

ranine (ra′nīn) 1. pertaining to a frog. 2. ranular. 3. sublingual.

ranitidine (rah-nit′ĭ-dēn) an antagonist of histamine H_2 RECEPTORS, used as the hydrochloride salt to inhibit stomach HYDROCHLORIC ACID secretion in treatment of PEPTIC ULCERS, gastroesophageal REFLUX, and conditions of gastric hypersecretion, administered orally, intramuscularly, or intravenously.

ranula (ran′u-lah) a cystic tumor beneath the tongue due to obstruction and dilatation of the sublingual or submaxillary gland or of a mucous gland. adj., **ran′ular.**

pancreatic r. a retention cyst of the pancreatic duct.

rape (rāp) sexual assault or abuse; sexual intercourse (vaginal or anal penetration) against the will and without the consent of the individual. The crime of rape continues to occur at an alarming rate. Many cases are not reported by victims because of feelings of shame, guilt, embarrassment, or fear. Most rape victims are girls or women, although rape or sexual assault can also occur between men (homosexual rape).

Immediately after the crime of rape has occurred, victims should be calmed as much as possible and assured that they are safe. Any bleeding wounds, fractures, or other existing injuries should be treated. They should be encouraged to obtain treatment as soon as possible and not to change clothes, bathe, douche, or urinate because that could destroy legal evidence needed to arrest and convict the attacker.

Rape is a physical and psychological emergency, and the victim must be treated with compassion as well as professional competence. The American College of Obstetricians and Gynecologists has provided guidelines for the physical care of a rape victim, identifying a twofold purpose for the physical examination: (1) to protect the victim against disease, pregnancy, and psychological trauma, and (2) to aid in the collection of legal evidence that could be used later in court.

Many hospitals have on call a rape counselor who can stay with the victim through emergency treatment and provide guidance and referral to a follow-up program of care. Recovery from rape is a difficult task. Some victims may appear to return to normal rather quickly, when in fact they are using temporary psychological mechanisms such as denial, suppression, and rationalization. Crisis intervention through all phases of the recovery period is a necessary component of the total care of a rape victim. The main purposes of follow-up are to keep channels of communication open to victims, assess their coping skills, to offer support and encouragement in efforts to resume life, and to provide assistance and referral if necessary. Rape is a crime of violence in which the sexual act is secondary to the brutality of the attack.

The American College of Emergency Physicians has published a consensus document called *Evaluation and Management of the Sexually Assaulted or Abused Patient.* It is available from ACEP Sales and Service, P.O. Box 619911, Dallas TX 75261-9911 or on their web site at http://www.acep.org. They can also be reached by telephone at 1-800-798-1822, ext. 6. A review of informative materials for women who have been raped or sexually assaulted, and practice guidelines for care, is available from the National Violence Against Women Prevention Research Center, whose web site is http://www.vawprevention.org.

acquaintance r., date r. rape by someone known to the victim.

r.-trauma syndrome 1. a group of symptoms caused by, or that are responses to,

R

RAPE. 2. a NURSING DIAGNOSIS approved by the North American Nursing Diagnosis Association, defined as a sustained maladaptive response to a forced, violent sexual penetration against the victim's will and consent. It includes an *acute phase* of disorganization of the victim's lifestyle, followed by a *long-term phase* of reorganization of lifestyle. Characteristics in the acute phase may include emotional reactions such as anger, humiliation, revenge, and self-blame, and multiple physical symptoms. In the long-term phase the victim must cope with changes in lifestyle that could include moving to another residence, changing telephone number, dealing with recurrent nightmares and phobias, and seeking support from individuals and groups.

There may also be either a *compound reaction* or a *silent reaction*. The nursing diagnosis *rape trauma syndrome: compound reaction* is identified as an acute stress reaction to a rape or attempted rape, experienced along with other major stressors that can include reactivation of symptoms of a previous condition. The victim suffers from the emotional and physiological manifestations listed above and may also resort to reliance on drugs or alcohol and experience reactivated symptoms of preexisting physical or psychiatric illnesses. The nursing diagnosis *rape trauma syndrome: silent reaction* is identified as a complex stress reaction to a rape in which an individual is unable to describe or discuss the rape. Characteristics can include sudden changes in relationships with men and in sexual behavior, increasing anxiety during interview, silence about the rape incident, and sudden onset of phobic reactions.

rapeseed oil (rāp′sēd) the oil expressed from the seeds of the rapeseed plant; used in the manufacture of soaps, margarines, and lubricants. See also *canola oil.*

raphe (ra′fe) a seam; anatomic nomenclature for the line of union of the halves of various symmetrical parts.

   abdominal r. linea alba.

rapid plasma reagin (RPR) test (rap′id plaz′mah re′ah-jin) any of a group of screening flocculation tests for syphilis, using a modified VDRL antigen.

rapport (rah-por′) a relation of harmony and accord, as between the patient and the health care provider.

rarefaction (rar″ĕ-fak′shun) the condition of being or becoming less dense.

rash (rash) a temporary eruption on the skin.

   butterfly r. a skin eruption across the nose and adjacent areas of the cheeks in the pattern of a butterfly, as in lupus erythematosus and seborrheic dermatitis. (See Atlas 2, Part B).

   diaper r. irritant DERMATITIS in the area in contact with the diaper in infants, often sparing the genitocrural folds, occurring as a reaction to prolonged contact with urine and feces, retained soaps and topical preparations, and friction and maceration, and commonly associated with secondary bacterial and yeast infections, especially with *Candida albicans.* Some consider irritation by the ammoniac decomposition products of urine to be a contributing factor. Called also diaper dermatitis.

   drug r. drug eruption.

   heat r. miliaria.

rasp (rasp) 1. a coarse file used in surgery; called also raspatory. 2. to file with such an instrument.

raspatory (ras′pah-to″re) rasp (def. 1).

RAST radioallergosorbent test.

rat-bite fever either of two distinct diseases transmitted to humans by the bite of an infected rat or less commonly of a squirrel, weasel, dog, cat, or pig. The more common of the two in the United States is HAVERHILL FEVER. The other form, SODOKU, rarely occurs in North America but is observed frequently in Japan and other countries around East Asia. Although when both diseases were originally identified they followed the bite of a rat or similar animal, there are also other modes of transmission.

Haverhill fever is caused by *Streptobacillus moniliformis.* If the disease follows a rat bite, a fluid-filled sore appears at the site of the bite within 10 days. High fever alternates with periods of normal temperature at intervals of 24 to 48 hours, and there is swelling of regional lymph nodes. The joints—usually the large joints—become reddened, swollen, and painful. There may be back pain, and a spotty, measles-like skin rash.

Sodoku, or spirillar rat-bite fever, is caused by *Spirillum minus.* The original bite heals promptly, but within 5 to 28 days the site becomes swollen and takes on a dusky, purplish hue. There is usually no joint inflammation and the rash is patchy rather than spotty. Otherwise the symptoms are similar to those characteristic of Haverhill fever.

Treatment for both forms of rat-bite fever is with PENICILLIN, TETRACYCLINE, or other antibiotics.

rate (rāt) the speed or frequency with which an event or circumstance occurs per unit of time, population, or other standard of comparison.

   adjusted r. a fictitious summary rate statistically adjusted to remove the effect of a variable, such as age or sex, to permit unbiased comparison between groups having different compositions with respect to these variables. See also crude RATE and specific RATE.

attack r. in the analysis of acute outbreaks of disease, the proportion of persons who are exposed to the disease during the outbreak who do become ill.

basal metabolic r. an expression of the rate at which oxygen is utilized in a fasting subject at complete rest as a percentage of a value established as normal for such a subject. Abbreviated BMR.

birth r. the number of live births in a geographic area in a defined period, usually one year, relative to some specified population. For the crude birth rate, it is the average total population or the midyear population in the area during the period. Specific birth rates for subsets of the population may also be calculated, for example, an age-specific birth rate is limited to the population of females of a defined age range.

case fatality r. the number of deaths due to a specific disease as compared to the total number of cases of the disease.

crude r. one giving the total number of events occurring in an entire population over a period of time, without reference to any of the individuals or subgroups within the population. See also adjusted RATE and specific RATE.

death r. the number of deaths in a certain period of time divided by the total of a given population. The *crude death rate* is the ratio of the number of deaths in a geographic area in one year divided by the average population in the area during the year. The *age-specific death rate* is the ratio

of the number of deaths occurring in a specified age group to the average population of that group. The *cause-specific death rate* is the ratio of the number of deaths due to a specified cause to the average total population. Called also mortality rate.

DEF r. an expression of dental caries experienced in primary teeth, calculated by adding number of those requiring filling (*D*), decayed teeth requiring extraction (*E*), and those that have already been successfully filled (*F*); missing primary teeth are not included in the calculation.

DMF r. an expression of the condition of the permanent teeth based on the number of teeth decayed, missing (or indicated for removal), and filled or bearing restorations. It is calculated by adding the number of carious permanent teeth requiring filling (*D*), carious ones requiring extraction (*Mr*), ones previously extracted because of caries (*Mp*), and permanent teeth (*F*).

dose r. the amount of any therapeutic agent administered per unit of time.

erythrocyte sedimentation r. (ESR) see ERYTHROCYTE SEDIMENTATION RATE.

fatality r. the death RATE in a specific group of persons simultaneously affected by some event or circumstances, such as a natural disaster.

fertility r. a measure of fertility in a defined population over a specified period of time, usually one year; particularly the general fertility RATE, but also including more specific rates such as those for females of a given parity or a particular age range or that describing the completed rate for females who have finished childbearing.

R

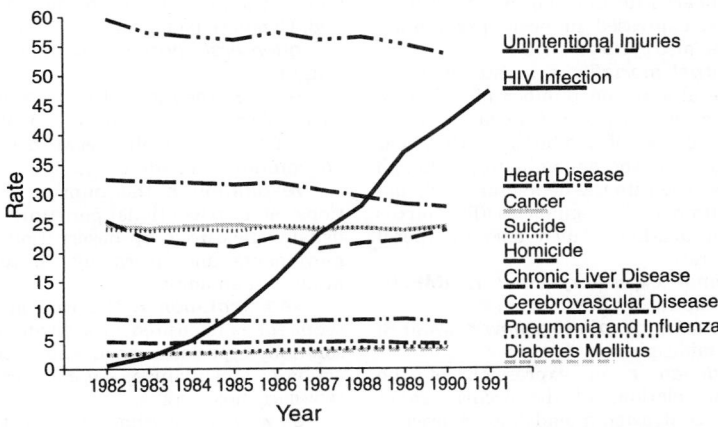

Death rates (per 100,000) for leading causes of death for men aged 25–44 years. From Centers for Disease Control and Prevention: *Morbidity and Mortality Weekly Report* 42:483, 1993.

fetal death r. the ratio of the number of fetal deaths in one year to the total number of both live births and fetal deaths in that year.

five-year survival r. an expression of the number of survivors with no trace of a given disease five years after each has been diagnosed or treated for the disease.

flow r. flow (def. 2).

forced expiratory flow r. forced expiratory flow.

general fertility r. the most widely used measure of fertility; the number of live births in a geographic area in a year per 1000 women of childbearing age, which is usually defined as age 15 to 44 years.

glomerular filtration r. an expression of the quantity of glomerular filtrate formed each minute in the nephrons of both kidneys, calculated by measuring the clearance of specific substances, e.g., inulin or creatinine.

growth r. an expression of the increase in size of an organic object per unit of time.

heart r. the number of contractions of the cardiac ventricles per unit of time (usually per minute).

incidence r. the risk of developing a particular disease during a given period of time; the numerator of the rate is the number of new cases during the specified time period and the denominator is the population at risk during the period. Compare PREVALENCE R.

infant mortality r. the ratio of the number of deaths in one year of children less than one year of age to the number of live births in that year.

intrinsic r. in cardiac PACING terminology, the heart rate unaided by an artificial PACEMAKER, expressed in beats per minute (bpm). See also cycle LENGTH.

maternal mortality r. a rate in which the numerator is the number of maternal deaths ascribed to puerperal causes in one year; the number of live births in that year is often used as the denominator, although to make a true rate the denominator should be the number of pregnancies (live births plus fetal deaths). Called also puerperal mortality rate.

maximal expiratory flow r. (MEFR) maximal expiratory flow.

maximal midexpiratory flow r. (MMFR) maximal midexpiratory flow.

mendelian r. an expression of the numerical relations of the occurrence of distinctly contrasted mendelian characteristics in succeeding generations of hybrid offspring.

metabolic r. an expression of the amount of oxygen consumed by the body cells.

morbidity r. an inexact term that can mean either the incidence RATE or the prevalence RATE.

mortality r. death rate.

neonatal mortality r. the ratio of the number of deaths in one year of children less than 28 days of age to the number of live births in that year.

paced r. in cardiac PACING terminology, the rate of PULSES of an artificial PACEMAKER, expressed as pulses per minute (ppm). See also cycle LENGTH.

perinatal mortality r. the ratio of the number of the sum of fetal deaths after 28 or more weeks of gestation (stillbirths) and deaths of infants less than 7 days of age in one time period and population to the sum of the number of live births and fetal deaths after 28 or more weeks of gestation (stillbirths) in that same time period and population.

postneonatal mortality r. the ratio of the number of deaths in a given year of children between the 28th day of life and the first birthday relative to the difference between the number of the live births and neonatal deaths in that year; the denominator is sometimes simplified, less correctly, to the number of live births. The ratio is sometimes approximated as the difference between the infant mortality rate and the neonatal mortality rate.

prevalence r. the number of people in a population who have a disease at a given time; the numerator is the number of existing cases of disease at a specified time and the denominator is the total population. Time may be a point or a defined interval and is traditionally the former if unspecified. Compare INCIDENCE R.

puerperal mortality r. maternal mortality r.

pulse r. the rate of the PULSE, measured as number of pulsations in an artery per unit of time; normally between 60 and 80 per minute in an adult.

respiration r. the number of inhalations and exhalations per unit of time, usually measured by observation of chest movements and averaging 16 to 20 per minute in an adult.

sedimentation r. the rate at which a sediment is deposited in a given volume of solution, especially when subjected to the action of a centrifuge; see also ERYTHROCYTE SEDIMENTATION RATE.

slew r. in cardiac PACING, the rate expressed in units of mV/msec, at which an R wave reaches peak amplitude; it represents the maximum rate of change of amplifier output voltage.

specific r. a rate that applies to a specific demographic subgroup, e.g., individuals of a specific age, sex, or race, giving the total number of events in relation only to that subgroup. See also adjusted RATE and crude RATE.

stillbirth r. fetal death rate.

ratio (ra'she-o) [L.] an expression of the quantity of one substance or entity in relation to that of another; the relationship between two quantities expressed as the quotient of one divided by the other.

A/D r. adult versus developmental toxicity ratio; the ratio between the toxic effects of a substance on adults (humans or animals, especially pregnant females) and such effects on developing embryos or fetuses.

A-G r., albumin-globulin r. the ratio of albumin to globulin in blood serum, plasma, cerebrospinal fluid, or urine.

arm r. a figure expressing the relation of the length of the longer arm of a mitotic chromosome to that of the shorter arm.

benefit-risk r. a determination of the potential of a research study for positive effects on patients compared to the risks of doing harm.

cardiothoracic r. on a chest radiograph, the ratio of the transverse diameter of the heart to the internal diameter of the chest at its widest point just above the dome of the diaphragm.

grid r. a ratio comparing the height of lead lines in an x-ray grid to the distance between the lead strips.

inspiratory-expiratory r. the ratio of the inspiratory time to the expiratory time during the breathing cycle. Normally, expiratory time will be longer than inspiratory time; if the inspiratory time is longer than the expiratory time, gas trapping may result.

lecithin/sphingomyelin r. see LECITHIN-SPHINGOMYELIN RATIO.

risk r. relative risk.

sex r. the proportion of one sex to the other; by tradition the number of males in a population to the number of females, usually stated as the number of males per 100 females.

signal-to-noise r. the ratio between the amplitude of a signal being measured and that of the NOISE.

urea excretion r. the ratio of the amount of urea in the urine excreted in one hour to the amount in 100 ml of blood. The normal ratio is 50.

zeta sedimentation r. (ZSR) a measurement comparable to the erythrocyte sedimentation rate, except that it is unaffected by anemia. The packed-cell volume (ZETACRIT) of a blood specimens is calculated by centrifuging the specimen in a ZETAFUGE, a specially designed instrument that produces controlled cycles of compaction and dispersion and allows rouleaux to form and sediment rapidly. The zetacrit divided into the true hematocrit gives the zeta sedimentation ratio.

rational (rash'un-al) based upon reason; characterized by possession of one's reason.

rationalization (rash"on-al-ĭ-za'shun) an unconscious DEFENSE MECHANISM in which a person finds logical reasons (justification) for his or her behavior while ignoring the real reasons. It is a form of self-deception unconsciously used to make tolerable certain feelings, behaviors, and motives that would otherwise be unacceptable. Everyone uses rationalization at some time or other and in most instances it is a relatively harmless behavior pattern; the danger lies in deceiving oneself habitually so that eventually harmful or destructive behavior comes to be justified in one's mind.

rattler (rat'ler) rattlesnake.

rattlesnake (rat't'l-snāk) any of numerous pit VIPERS, venomous snakes of North America of the genera *Crotalus* and *Sistrurus*. See also SNAKEBITE.

rauwolfia (raw-wol'fe-ah) 1. any member of the genus *Rauwolfia,* tropical trees and shrubs. 2. the dried root, or extract of the dried root, of one of these plants.

r. serpenti'na the dried root of *Rauwolfia serpentina,* sometimes with fragments of rhizome and other parts, used as an ANTIHYPERTENSIVE AGENT.

ray (ra) a line emanating from a center, as a more or less distinct portion of radiant energy (light or heat), proceeding in a specific direction.

α-r's high-speed helium nuclei ejected from radioactive substances; they have less penetrating power than beta rays. See also ALPHA PARTICLES.

actinic r's light rays that produce chemical action, especially those beyond the violet end of the spectrum.

alpha r's α-rays.

β-r's, beta r's electrons ejected from radioactive substances with velocities as high as 98 per cent of the velocity of light; they have more penetrating power than alpha rays but less than gamma rays. See also BETA PARTICLES.

cosmic r's very penetrating radiations that apparently move through interplanetary space in every direction.

digital r. a digit of the hand or foot and corresponding metacarpal or metatarsal bone, regarded as a continuous unit.

γ-r's, gamma r's a type of electromagnetic radiation emitted by an atomic nucleus during a nuclear reaction; see also GAMMA RAYS.

grenz r's very soft electromagnetic radiation of wavelengths of about 2 angstroms.

infrared r's radiations just beyond the red end of the visible spectrum, having wavelengths of 0.75–1000 μm; see also INFRARED.

medullary r. a cortical extension of a bundle of tubules from a renal PYRAMID.

roentgen r's x-rays.

ultraviolet r's radiant energy beyond the violet end of the visible spectrum, of wavelengths 0.39 to 0.18 μm; see also ULTRAVIOLET RAYS.

x-r's see X-RAYS.

Raynaud's disease (ra-nōz′) a primary or idiopathic VASOSPASTIC disorder characterized by bilateral and symmetrical pallor and cyanosis of the fingers, with or without local GANGRENE. In some cases both the hands and feet may be affected, and occasionally it may involve the nose, chin, or cheeks. The cause is unknown; attacks are precipitated by cold or emotional upset and relieved by warmth. It occurs almost exclusively in young women, especially those who are experiencing tension and emotional pressure.

Attacks often end spontaneously or upon application of warmth. As the disease progresses, however, small gangrenous ulcers may develop on the fingertips and, eventually, permanent disability of the hands can result from contractures, severe pain, and changes in the skin. The latter condition (SCLERODACTYLY) is characterized by tightening of the skin so that it appears stretched over the fingers, decreased mobility, and smooth, abnormally shiny skin.

Pharmacologic management of the symptoms of Raynaud's disease includes VASODILATORS such as RAUWOLFIA alkaloids (for example, RESERPINE) that decrease peripheral vasoconstriction. ALPHA-ADRENERGIC BLOCKING AGENTS may be prescribed to produce vasodilation and relax vasospasms. However, patients often discontinue taking these and other drugs because of unpleasant side effects, which may be as bothersome as the symptoms of the original disease.

Those who cannot find relief from persistent and severe symptoms may be candidates for surgical sympathectomy to prevent conduction of sympathetic nerve impulses that stimulate constriction of local peripheral vessels. Lumbar ganglion sympathectomy may be effective for cases that involve the feet, but success with surgical intervention for vasoconstriction of peripheral vessels of the hands is less predictable.

Patient Care. Those who choose to try managing their symptoms without medical or surgical treatment often can benefit from noninvasive interventions that minimize the incidence and severity of attacks. During initial assessment they are asked to identify specific factors and conditions that precipitate attacks or worsen symptoms. For most, exposure to cold is the major contributing factor. Although moving to a warm climate may be beneficial, this is not always feasible, and susceptible persons may continue to have attacks in any climate. All patients are advised to keep their entire bodies warm so as to prevent vasospasm of the digits. Layered clothing, mittens, and warm socks can greatly decrease heat loss. Fleece-lined footwear and innersoles made of reflective material can help retain heat normally lost while walking or standing on cold ground.

Drinking warm beverages helps some patients rewarm their bodies and extremities, thereby ending or avoiding an attack. Physical exercise does not generally seem to mitigate symptoms. Since nicotine is a vasoconstrictor, smoking is prohibited. There are no dietary restrictions, nor are there specific foods that are helpful in managing Raynaud's disease. Stress can trigger vasospasm; therefore patients may benefit from stress reduction strategies and relaxation techniques. Through biofeedback some patients can learn to raise the temperature of the hands consciously.

Arterial insufficiency predisposes these patients to ulceration and gangrene. Those who have severe disease in which sensation has been diminished must be careful to avoid trauma or excessive pressure. Activities that can precipitate an attack for them include typing, playing the piano or guitar, sewing, and chopping or dicing food. The use of vibratory tools such as a jackhammer, chainsaw, or drill can also precipitate an attack.

With effective interventions over a period of time, many patients can learn to avoid precipitating factors, relieve symptoms when an attack does occur, and gain some sense of control over their illness.

Raynaud's phenomenon (ra-nōz′) intermittent bilateral attacks of ischemia of the fingers or toes and sometimes the ears or nose, marked by severe pallor, and often accompanied by paresthesia and pain; it is brought on characteristically by cold or emotional stimuli and relieved by heat, and is due to an underlying disease or anatomical abnormality. When the condition is idiopathic or primary it is termed RAYNAUD'S DISEASE.

Rb rubidium.

RBC red blood CELL; red blood cell COUNT.

RBE relative biological effectiveness.

RD Registered Dietitian.

RDA recommended dietary allowance.

RDH Registered Dental Hygienist.

RDS respiratory distress syndrome.

Re rhenium.

reabsorb (re″ab-sorb′) to absorb again; to undergo or to subject to reabsorption; to resorb.

reabsorption (re″ab-sorp′shun) 1. the act or process of absorbing again, as the absorption by the kidneys of substances that were already secreted into the tubules, such as glucose, proteins, or sodium. 2. resorption.

react (re-akt′) 1. to respond to a stimulus. 2. to enter into chemical action.

reaction (re-ak′shun) 1. opposite action or counteraction; the response of a part to stimulation. 2. the phenomena caused by the action of chemical agents; a chemical process in which one substance is transformed into another substance or substances. 3. in psychology, the mental or emotional state that develops in any particular situation. 4. the specific cellular effect produced by foreign matter, as in testing for allergies. For specific reactions, see under the name, such as PIRQUET'S REACTION.

r. of degeneration the reaction to electrical stimulation of muscles whose nerves have degenerated, consisting of loss of response to a faradic stimulation in a muscle, and to galvanic and faradic stimulation in the nerve.

r. time the time elapsing between the application of a stimulus and the resulting reaction.

reaction-formation an unconscious DEFENSE MECHANISM in which a person assumes an attitude that is the reverse of some infantile wish or impulse the person harbors.

reactive attachment disorder a mental disorder of infancy or early childhood characterized by notably unusual and developmentally inappropriate social relatedness, usually associated with grossly pathological care. It may be the *inhibited type*, with failure to initiate or respond to social interactions, or the *disinhibited type*, with indiscriminate sociability or attachment.

reactivity (re″ak-tiv′ĭ-te) the process or property of reacting.

reading (rēd′ing) understanding of written or printed symbols representing words.

lip r., speech r. understanding of speech through observation of the speaker's lip movements.

reagent (re-a′jent) a substance used to produce a chemical reaction so as to detect, measure, or produce other substances.

reagin (re′ah-jin) antibody of a specialized immunoglobulin class (IgE) which attaches to tissue cells of the same species from which it is derived, and which interacts with its antigen to induce the release of histamine and other vasoactive amines. A form of cytotropic antibody, it is present in the serum of naturally hypersensitive individuals and can confer specific immediate (type I) hypersensitivity in nonreactive individuals. adj., **reagin′ic.**

reality orientation 1. a program designed to improve cognitive and psychomotor function in persons who are confused or disoriented. It is often employed in long-term facilities to create an environment in which perceptions of the environment in relation to the external world are directed toward the reality of that world. Aids such as calendars and clocks and sensory stimuli such as distinctive sights, sounds, and smells are used to improve sensory awareness. The expected outcome of such programs for severely impaired persons is improvement in intellect and language skills, and increased participation in ACTIVITIES OF DAILY LIVING. 2. in the NURSING INTERVENTIONS CLASSIFICATION, a nursing INTERVENTION defined as promotion of the patient's awareness of personal identity, time, and environment. See also reality TESTING.

reamer (rēm′er) in root canal THERAPY, an engine-driven or hand-operated instrument for canal enlargement, consisting of a serrated triangular shaft twisted in a loose spiral.

rebound (re′bound) a reversed response occurring upon withdrawal of a stimulus.

acid r. an increased rate of gastric acid secretion occurring 30 to 60 minutes after eating.

insulin r. see INSULIN REBOUND.

recall 1. (re-kawl′) to remember or recollect. 2. (re′kawl) the process of bringing information back into consciousness.

recanalization (re-kan″ə-lǐ-za′shun) formation of new CANALS or paths, especially blood vessels, through an obstruction such as a clot; called also canalization.

recapitulation theory ontogeny recapitulates phylogeny, i.e., an organism, in the course of its development, goes through the same successive stages (in abbreviated

R

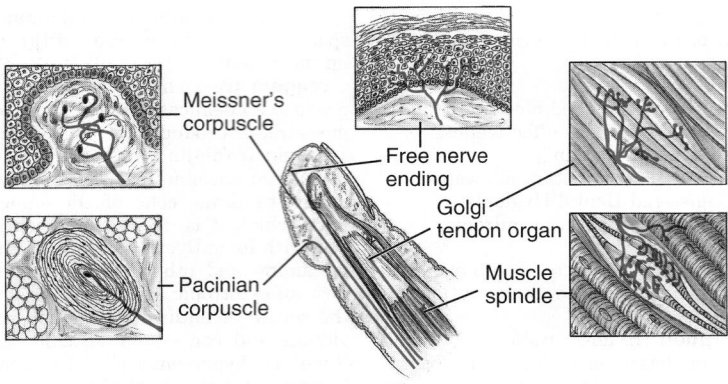

Meissner's corpuscle

Free nerve ending

Golgi tendon organ

Muscle spindle

Pacinian corpuscle

General sense receptors. (From Applegate, 2000.)

form) as did the species in its evolutionary development.

receptaculum (re″sep-tak′u-lum) [L.] a receptacle or container.

   r. chy′li cisterna chyli.

receptor (re-sep′tor) 1. a molecule on the cell surface *(cell-surface* or *membrane receptor)* or within a cell, usually in its nucleus *(nuclear receptor)* that recognizes and binds with specific molecules, producing some effect in the cell; e.g., the cell-surface receptors of immunocompetent cells that recognize antigens, complement components, or lymphokines; or those of neurons and target organs that recognize neurotransmitters or hormones. 2. a sensory nerve ending that responds to various stimuli.

   α-r′s, α-adrenergic r′s alpha-adrenergic receptors.

   adrenergic r′s receptors for EPINEPHRINE or NOREPINEPHRINE, such as those on effector organs innervated by postganglionic adrenergic fibers of the sympathetic nervous system. There are two types, alpha-adrenergic receptors and beta-adrenergic receptors.

   alpha r′s, alpha-adrenergic r′s adrenergic receptors found in cardiac muscle and vascular smooth muscle; they are stimulated by NOREPINEPHRINE and blocked by agents such as PHENOXYBENZAMINE. They are subdivided into two types: α_1, found in smooth muscle, heart, and liver, with effects including vasoconstriction, intestinal relaxation, uterine contraction and pupillary dilation, and α_2, found in platelets, vascular smooth muscle, nerve termini, and pancreatic islets, with effects including platelet aggregation, vasoconstriction, and inhibition of norepinephrine release and of insulin secretion. Called also α-receptors and α-adrenergic receptors.

   β-r′s, β-adrenergic r′s beta-adrenergic receptors.

   B cell antigen r′s monomeric IgM, IgD, and (on memory CELLS only) IgG that is attached to the cell membrane of B LYMPHOCYTES (B CELLS); in conjunction with helper T CELLS, it triggers B cell activation on contact with antigen.

   beta r′s, beta-adrenergic r′s adrenergic receptors that are stimulated by EPINEPHRINE and blocked by agents such as PROPRANOLOL. They are subdivided into two basic types: β_1-receptors are found in the myocardium and cause lipolysis and cardiac stimulation, and β_2-receptors are found in smooth and skeletal muscle and liver and cause bronchodilation and vasodilation. A third type, β_3, is atypical; it is more sensitive to norepinephrine than to epinephrine, relatively resistant to propranolol blockade, and may be involved in lipolysis regulation in adipose tissue. Called also β-receptors and β-adrenergic receptors.

   cell-surface r. membrane receptor.

   cholinergic r′s membrane receptors on cells of effector organs, innervated by cholinergic nerve fibers and responsive to the acetylcholine secreted by these fibers. There are two types, muscarinic receptors and nicotinic receptors.

   complement r. a membrane receptor that can bind activated COMPLEMENT components. For example, component C3b binds to complement receptors of NEUTROPHILS, B LYMPHOCYTES, and MACROPHAGES.

   estrogen r. a cellular regulatory protein that binds estrogenic hormones, found particularly in estrogen-sensitive tissues such as the uterus and breast. Cytoplasmic levels are measured in surgically removed breast carcinomas; high levels indicate that a positive response to endocrine therapy is likely.

Fc r's specific membrane receptors for antigen-antibody complexes or aggregated immunoglobulins that bind a site in the Fc portion of the immunoglobulin molecule and may exhibit specificity for particular immunoglobulin classes. Fc receptors are found on B cells, K cells, macrophages, neutrophils, and eosinophils, and, during some developmental stages, on T cells.

histamine r's receptors for HISTAMINE. *H₁-receptors* mediate contraction of smooth muscles and dilation of capillaries, causing effects such as BRONCHOCONSTRICTION and contraction of the intestine; they are blocked by ANTIHISTAMINES such as PYRILAMINE or CHLORPHENIRAMINE. *H₂-receptors* mediate acceleration of the heart rate and produce gastric acid secretion; they are blocked by agents such as CIMETIDINE.

IgE r's membrane receptors for IgE, found on mast cells and basophils.

insulin r's a type of membrane receptors specific for insulin, found on target cells.

LDL r's, low-density lipoprotein r's specific receptors for low-density lipoproteins found in coated pits on the surface of mammalian cells. The coated pits are internalized forming coated vesicles from which the receptors are recycled back to the plasma membrane while particles of low-density lipoprotein are transferred to lysosomes where they are degraded, releasing free cholesterol, phospholipids, and amino acids. Genetic defects in LDL receptors are responsible for familial HYPERCHOLESTEROLEMIA.

membrane r. a receptor located on or in the membrane of a cell. Called also cell-surface receptor.

muscarinic r's cholinergic receptors on autonomic effector cells (and also on some autonomic ganglion cells and in some central neurons) that are stimulated by MUSCARINE and parasympathomimetic drugs and blocked by ATROPINE.

nicotinic r's cholinergic receptors of autonomic ganglion cells and motor endplates of skeletal muscle that are stimulated by low doses of NICOTINE and blockaded by high doses of nicotine or by TUBOCURARINE.

olfactory r. a specialized sensory nerve-ending sensitive to stimulation giving rise to the sensation of odors; called also osmoreceptor.

opiate r's, opioid r's receptors that combine with particular opiates to create analgesia and certain other effects. Several different ones have been identified and assigned Greek letters; the μ receptor gives superior analgesia, and the κ receptor is

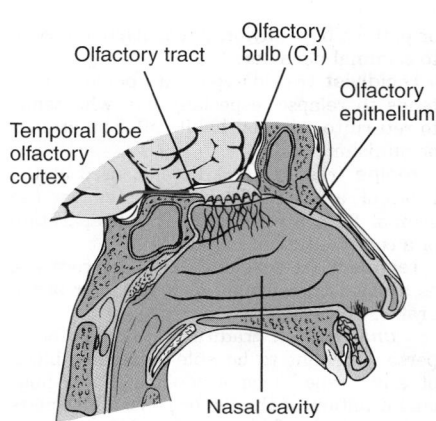

Structure of the olfactory receptors. (From Applegate, 2000.)

associated with a low degree of physical dependency.

pain r's free nerve endings that are receptors for PAIN.

stretch r. a sense organ in a muscle or tendon that responds to elongation.

T cell r's the characteristic marker of T LYMPHOCYTES (T cells) that recognize specific foreign antigens as well as self MHC antigens; both must be seen simultaneously to trigger T cell activation (see also LYMPHOCYTE ACTIVATION). The receptor is not a complete IMMUNOGLOBULIN molecule but may contain heavy and light chain variable regions.

recess (re′ses, re-ses′) a small, empty space or cavity.

epitympanic r. a small upper space of the middle ear, containing the head of the malleus and the body of the incus. Called also attic and epitympanum.

recession (re-sesh′un) the drawing away of a tissue or part from its normal position.

gingival r. the drawing back of the gingivae from the necks of the teeth, with exposure of root surfaces.

recessive (re-ses′iv) 1. tending to recede. 2. in genetics, incapable of expression unless the responsible allele is carried by both members of a set of homologous chromosomes. See also recessive GENE. 3. an allele or trait that has this characteristic.

recessus (re-ses′us) [L.] recess.

recidivation (re-sid″ĭ-va′shun) relapse, recurrence, or repetition, as of a disease or condition or of a pattern of behavior, particularly a criminal act.

recidivism (re-sid′ĭ-vizm) a tendency to relapse into a previous condition, disease, or pattern of behavior, particularly a return to criminal behavior.

recidivist (re-sid´ĭ-vist) a person who tends to relapse, especially one who tends to return to criminal habits after treatment or punishment.

recipe (res´ĭ-pe) [L.] 1. take: used at the head of a prescription, indicated by the symbol ℞. 2. a formula for the preparation of a combination of ingredients.

recipient (re-sip´e-ent) one who receives, as a blood transfusion, or a tissue or organ graft.

 universal r. traditional name for a person thought to be able to receive blood of any "type" (see BLOOD GROUP) without agglutination of the donor cells. This refers to individuals of blood group AB; however, research and clinical experience have now demonstrated that antibodies may be present to cause serious reactions. Therefore, prior to a blood TRANSFUSION, any recipient must be checked for COMPATIBILITY (see CROSSMATCHING).

recirculation (re-ser-ku-la´shun) in HEMO-DIALYSIS, circulation of part of the blood from the venous line to the arterial line and back into the patient's body without dialyzing it.

Recklinghausen's disease (rek´ling-how˝zenz) 1. type I NEUROFIBROMATOSIS. 2. see OSTEITIS FIBROSA CYSTICA.

recognin (re-kog´nin) any of a group of protein fragments produced from cancer cells that are capable of recognizing specific cells; they include astrocytin and malignin.

recognition (rek˝og-nish´un) 1. the act of recognizing (seeing something as familiar). 2. the state of being seen as familiar. 3. the interaction of immunologically competent cells with antigen that begins with the binding of the antigen to specific antigen receptors on B and T lymphocytes and results in an IMMUNE RESPONSE directed against the antigen. Called also antigen recognition.

recoil (re-koyl´) 1. to pull back quickly, such as towards a resting position upon removal of a strong opposing force. 2. (re´koil) a pulling back quickly.

 elastic r. the ability of a stretched elastic object or organ, such as the lung or bladder, to return to its resting position. See also ELASTANCE.

recombinant (re-kom´bĭ-nant) 1. the new entity (e.g., gene, protein, cell, individual) that results from genetic RECOMBINATION. 2. pertaining or relating to such an entity.

 r. DNA technology the process of taking a gene from one organism and inserting it into the DNA of another; called also gene splicing. One commonly used technique involves the insertion of a new fragment of DNA that codes for a specific protein such as human insulin into a bacterium such as *Escherichia coli*. The gene is first inserted into a PLASMID, a self-replicating ring of DNA involved in the transfer of genes between bacteria. The plasmid is cut at a specific site by using a special cutting enzyme called a *restriction endonuclease*. The same procedure is used to cut out a segment of DNA from another organism, for example, the gene for human INSULIN. This fragment of insulin DNA is inserted into the plasmid and then sealed into place by an annealing enzyme. The altered plasmid is then taken up by bacterium and incorporated into the GENOME. When the bacterial cells divide they pass on the new information to the next generation. This produces clones of bacteria that produce large quantities of the new protein, in this example, insulin.

This process has had great impact in the field of medicine. It has revolutionized the manufacture of pharmaceutical products, where it is used to manufacture a variety of proteins used in the treatment of disease, including hormones, vaccines, and interferons.

Recombinant DNA Advisory Committee (re-kom´bĭ-nant) RAC, a committee composed of scientists and ethicists, set up to review human gene therapy research in order to protect patients from unethical practices, procedures, and research. All research involving human gene therapy must comply with both the Common Federal Rule and the RAC.

recombination (re˝kom-bĭ-na´shun) 1. the reunion, in the same or different arrangement, of formerly united elements that have been separated. 2. in genetics, the process that creates new combinations of genes by shuffling the linear order of the DNA, such as occurs naturally by CROSSING OVER of homologous chromosomes during meiosis or of homologous DNA sequences in somatic cells during mitosis, or occurs in vitro when DNA or RNA is manipulated for genetic engineering.

 bacterial r. in bacterial genetics, the process of producing a new gene by any of several processes, e.g., the sexual union of two parents, molecular crossing over between two DNA chains, or transformation.

Recombivax HB (re-kom´bĭ-vaks˝) a trademark for a preparation of hepatitis B vaccine (recombinant).

recompression (re˝kom-presh´un) return to normal environmental pressure after exposure to greatly diminished pressure.

reconstruction (re″kon-struk′shun) 1. the reassembling or re-forming of something from constituent parts. 2. surgical restoration of function of a body part, such as with BYPASS or PLASTIC SURGERY.

   aortic r. restoration of function to a damaged aorta, as by BYPASS or AORTOPLASTY.

record (rek′ord) 1. a permanent or long-lasting account of something, such as in writing or on film. 2. in dentistry, a REGISTRATION.

   bibliographic r. an index record standing for or representing a journal article, book, or other document.

   Problem-Oriented R., Problem-Oriented Medical R. see PROBLEM-ORIENTED RECORD.

recrement (rek′rĕ-ment) saliva, or other secretion, that is reabsorbed into the blood. adj., **recrementi′tious.**

recrudescence (re″kroo-des′ens) recurrence of symptoms after temporary abatement; a recrudescence occurs after some days or weeks, a relapse after weeks or months. adj., **recrudes′cent.**

recruitment (re-kroot′ment) 1. the gradual increase to a maximum in a reflex when a stimulus of unaltered intensity is prolonged. 2. in AUDIOLOGY, an abnormal increase in loudness caused by a very slight increase in sound intensity, as in MENIERE'S DISEASE.

rect(o)- word element [L.], *rectum.* See also words beginning PROCT(O)-.

rectal (rek′tal) pertaining to the rectum.

rectalgia (rek-tal′jah) proctalgia; pain in the rectum.

rectectomy (rek-tek′tah-me) excision of the rectum.

rectification (rek″tĭ-fĭ-ka′shun) 1. the act of making straight, pure, or correct. 2. redistillation of a liquid to purify it. 3. the converting of alternating current to direct current.

rectified (rek′tĭ-fīd) refined; made straight.

rectify (rek′tĭ-fi) 1. to refine or make straight. 2. to convert alternating current to direct current.

rectitis (rek-ti′tis) proctitis; inflammation of the rectum.

rectoabdominal (rek″to-ab-dom′ĭ-nal) pertaining to the rectum and abdomen.

rectocele (rek′to-sēl) hernial protrusion of part of the rectum into the vagina.

rectocolitis (rek″to-co-li′tis) coloproctitis; inflammation of the rectum and colon.

rectocutaneous (rek″to-ku-ta′ne-us) pertaining to the rectum and the skin.

rectolabial (rek″to-la′be-al) relating to the rectum and a labium majus.

rectopexy (rek′to-pek″se) proctopexy.

rectoplasty (rek′to-plas″te) proctoplasty.

rectoscope (rek′to-skōp) proctoscope.

rectosigmoid (rek″to-sig′moid) the lower portion of the sigmoid colon and the upper portion of the rectum.

rectosigmoidectomy (rek″to-sig′moi-dek′tah-me) excision of the rectosigmoid colon; proctosigmoidectomy.

rectostomy (rek-tos′tah-me) the operation of forming a permanent opening into the rectum for the relief of stricture of the rectum.

rectourethral (rek″to-u-re′thral) pertaining to or communicating with the rectum and urethra.

rectouterine (rek″to-u′ter-in) pertaining to the rectum and uterus.

rectovaginal (rek″to-vaj′ĭ-nal) pertaining to the rectum and vagina.

rectovesical (rek″to-ves′ĭ-kal) pertaining to or communicating with the rectum and bladder.

rectovestibular (rek″to-ves-tib′u-lar) pertaining to or communicating with the rectum and the vestibule of the vagina.

rectovulvar (rek″to-vul′var) pertaining to or communicating with the rectum and vulva.

rectum (rek′tum) the distal portion of the large intestine, beginning anterior to the third sacral vertebra as a continuation of the sigmoid and ending at the anal canal. The feces, the solid waste products of digestion, are formed in the large intestine and are gradually pushed down into the rectum by the muscular action of the intestine. Distention of the rectum by the accumulating feces sets up nerve impulses that indicate to the brain the need to empty the bowels. The rectum is 15 to 20 cm (6 to 8 inches) long, with the anal canal making up the last segment. The anus is kept closed (except during the evacuation process) by muscular rings called the anal SPHINCTERS.

In a rectal examination, the examiner palpates the rectum by inserting a gloved and lubricated finger into the rectum. The examination helps in determining whether there are masses in the rectum or pelvic region, and in determining the size and texture of the prostate in men. More extensive examination of the interior surface of the rectum may be done by PROCTOSCOPY.

R

rectus (rek′tus) [L.] straight.

recumbent (re-kum′bent) lying down.

recuperation (re-koo″per-a′shun) recovery of health and strength.

recurrence (re-kur′ens) the return of symptoms after a remission.

recurrent (re-kur′ent) returning after a remission; reappearing.

   r. fever 1. relapsing fever. 2. recurrent paroxysmal fever occurring in various diseases, including tularemia, meningococcemia, malaria, and rat-bite fever.

recurvation (re″kur-va′shun) a backward bending or curvature.

red (red) 1. the color produced by the longest waves of the visible spectrum, approximately 630 to 750 nm. 2. a dye or stain with this color.

scarlet r. an azo dye used as a biological stain for fats.

redia (re′de-ah) [L.] a larval stage of certain TREMATODE parasites, which develops in the body of a snail host and gives rise to daughter rediae, or to the CERCARIAE.

redintegration (red″in-tĕ-gra′shun) 1. the restoration or repair of a lost or damaged part. 2. a psychic process in which part of a complex stimulus provokes the complete reaction that was previously made only to the complex stimulus as a whole. 3. reintegration (def. 2).

redox (re′doks) oxidation-reduction.

reduce (re-dōōs′) 1. to restore to the normal place or relation of parts, as to reduce a fracture. 2. to undergo reduction. 3. to decrease in weight or size.

reducible (re-doo′sĭ-b'l) permitting of reduction.

reductant (re-duk′tant) the electron donor in an oxidation-reduction (redox) reaction.

reductase (re-duk′tās) an enzyme that catalyzes a chemical reduction.

5α-r. an enzyme that catalyzes the irreversible reduction of testosterone to dihydrotestosterone.

reduction (re-duk′shun) 1. a lessening or diminishing. 2. the correction of a fracture,

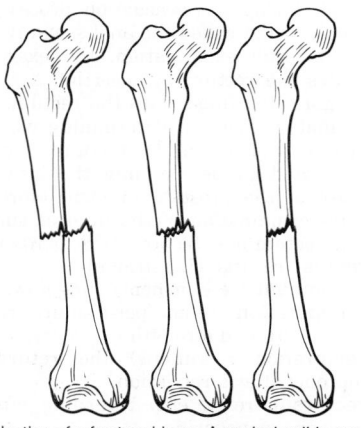

Reduction of a fractured bone. A gradual pull is exerted on the distal (lower) fragment of the bone until it is in alignment with the proximal fragment.

dislocation, or hernia. 3. the addition of hydrogen to a substance, or more generally, the gain of electrons; the opposite of OXIDATION.

anxiety r. in the NURSING INTERVENTIONS CLASSIFICATION, a nursing INTERVENTION defined as minimizing apprehension, dread, foreboding, or uneasiness related to an unidentified source of anticipated danger. See also ANXIETY.

bleeding r. in the NURSING INTERVENTIONS CLASSIFICATION, a nursing INTERVENTION defined as the limitation of loss of blood volume during an episode of BLEEDING.

bleeding r.: antepartum uterus in the NURSING INTERVENTIONS CLASSIFICATION, a nursing INTERVENTION defined as limitation of the amount of blood loss from the pregnant uterus during the third trimester of pregnancy.

bleeding r.: gastrointestinal in the NURSING INTERVENTIONS CLASSIFICATION, a nursing INTERVENTION defined as limitation of the amount of blood loss from the upper and lower gastrointestinal tract and related complications.

bleeding r.: nasal in the NURSING INTERVENTIONS CLASSIFICATION, a nursing INTERVENTION defined as the limitation of blood loss from the nasal cavity. See also EPISTAXIS.

bleeding r.: postpartum uterus in the NURSING INTERVENTIONS CLASSIFICATION, a nursing INTERVENTION defined as the limitation of blood loss from the postpartum uterus.

bleeding r.: wound in the NURSING INTERVENTIONS CLASSIFICATION, a nursing INTERVENTION defined as the limitation of the blood loss from a wound that may be a result of trauma, incisions, or placement of a tube or catheter.

closed r. the manipulative reduction of a fracture or dislocation without incision.

flatulence r. in the NURSING INTERVENTIONS CLASSIFICATION, a nursing INTERVENTION defined as the prevention of flatus formation and facilitation of the passage of excessive gas. See also FLATULENCE.

open r. reduction of a fracture or dislocation after incision into the fracture site.

reduplication (re-doo″plĭ-ka′shun) 1. a doubling back. 2. the recurrence of paroxysms of a double type. 3. a developmental ANOMALY resulting in doubling of an organ or part, with a connection between them at some point and the excess part usually a mirror image of the other.

Reed (rēd) Walter (1851–1902). American bacteriologist, born in Gloucester County, Virginia. As a military physician, Reed was appointed during the Spanish-American War chief of a committee to investigate typhoid fever epidemic in the army camps. In 1899, when yellow fever was particularly severe in Cuba, he again was appointed chairman of a committee to study its method of transmission, and he proved by thorough experimentation that yellow fever was carried only by a certain species of mosquito, *Aedes aegypti.*

reef (rēf) an infolding or tuck of tissue, as a tuck made in plication.

reentry (re-en′tre) in cardiology, reexcitation of a region of cardiac tissue by a single impulse, continuing for one or more cycles and sometimes resulting in ectopic BEATS or TACHYARRHYTHMIAS; see also circus MOVEMENT.

    atrioventricular (AV) nodal r. an arrhythmia-causing mechanism in which two opposing pathways are established within the atrioventricular node (longitudinal dissociation); the anterograde pathway, which is usually slower, activates the ventricles and the retrograde pathway, which is usually faster, activaties the atria. This mechanism is responsible for approximately half of symptomatic paroxysmal supraventricular TACHYCARDIAS.

refection (re-fek′shun) recovery; repair.

refeeding (re-fēd′ing) restoration of normal nutrition after a period of fasting or starvation.

    r. syndrome moderate to severe electrolyte and fluid shifts occurring during a period of REFEEDING; HYPOPHOSPHATEMIA is common, and HEART FAILURE sometimes occurs.

refereed (ref″er-ēd′) pertaining to a journal article or presentation that has been reviewed by the author's peers to determine its scientific merit and acceptability.

referral (re-fer′al) in the NURSING INTERVENTIONS CLASSIFICATION, a nursing INTERVENTION defined as arrangement for services by another care provider or agency.

refine (re-fīn′) to purify or free from foreign matter.

reflection (re-flek′shun) 1. a turning or bending back. 2. the folds produced when a membrane passes over the surface of an organ and then passes back to the body wall that it lines. 3. the turning back of a ray of light, sound, or heat when it strikes a surface it does not penetrate. 4. a communication skill in which a counselor or other professional reiterates either the content or the feeling message of the patient.

reflex (re′fleks) a reflected action or movement; the sum total of any particular automatic response mediated by the nervous system. A reflex is built into the nervous system and does not need the intervention of conscious thought to take effect.

The KNEE JERK is an example of the simplest type of reflex. When the knee is tapped, the nerve that receives this stimulus sends an impulse to the spinal cord, where it is relayed to a motor nerve. This causes the quadriceps muscle at the front of the thigh to contract and jerk the leg up. This reflex, or simple reflex ARC, involves only two nerves and one synapse. The leg begins to jerk up while the brain is just becoming aware of the tap.

Other simple reflexes, the *stretch reflexes*, help the body maintain its balance. Every time a muscle is stretched, it reacts with a reflex impulse to contract. As a person reaches or leans, the skeletal muscles tense and tighten, tending to hold him and keep him from falling. Even in standing still, the stretch reflexes in the skeletal muscles make many tiny adjustments to keep the body erect.

The "hot stove" reflex is more complex, calling into play many different muscles. Before the hand is pulled away, an impulse must go from the sensory nerve endings in the skin to a center in the spinal cord, from there to a motor center, and then out along the motor nerves to shoulder, arm, and hand muscles. Trunk and leg muscles respond to support the body in its sudden change of position, and the head and eyes turn to look at the cause of the injury. All this happens while the person is becoming aware of the burning sensation. A reflex that protects the body from injury, as this one does, is called a *nociceptive reflex.* Sneezing, coughing, and gagging are similar reflexes in response to foreign bodies in the nose and throat, and the wink reflex helps protect the eyes from injury.

A *conditioned reflex* is one acquired as the result of experience. When an action is done repeatedly the nervous system becomes familiar with the situation and learns to react automatically, and a new reflex is built into the system. Walking, running, and typewriting are examples of activities that require large numbers of complex muscle coordinations that have become automatic.

    abdominal r's contractions of the abdominal muscles about the navel on stimulating the abdominal skin. It indicates that the spinal cord from the eighth to the twelfth thoracic nerve is intact.

    accelerator r. an increase in heart rate in response to changes in intrathoracic pressure or respiratory rate; see also Bainbridge REFLEX and cardiac respiratory REFLEX.

    accommodation r. the coordinated changes that occur when the eye adapts

R

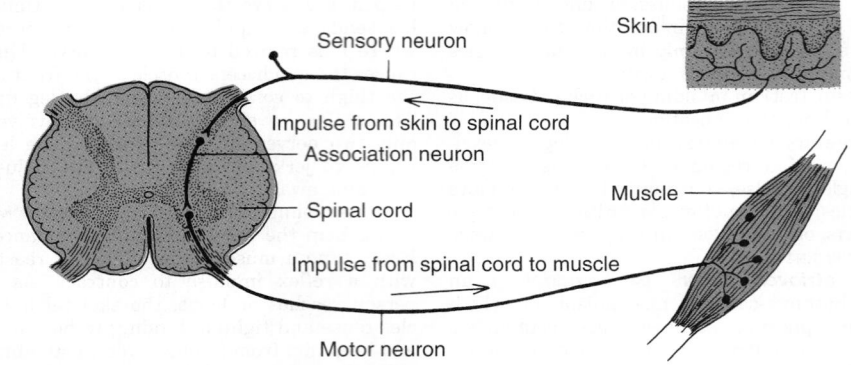

Nerve pathway of a simple reflex. When the sensory nerve ending is stimulated, a nerve impulse travels along a sensory (afferent) neuron to the spinal cord. Here an association neuron transfers the impulse to a motor (efferent) neuron. The motor neuron carries the impulse to a muscle, which contracts and moves a body part.

itself for near vision; they are constriction of the pupil, convergence of the eyes, and increased convexity of the lens.

Achilles r. ankle jerk.

acoustic r. contraction of the stapedius muscle in response to intense sound.

anal r. contraction of the anal sphincter on irritation of the anal skin.

ankle r. Achilles reflex.

auditory r. any reflex caused by stimulation of the vestibulocochlear nerve; especially momentary closure of both eyes produced by a sudden sound.

Babinski r. see BABINSKI REFLEX.

Babkin r. see BABKIN REFLEX.

Bainbridge r. a rise in pressure in, or increased distension of, the large somatic veins or the right atrium causes acceleration of the heart beat. Called also Bainbridge effect.

baroreceptor r. the reflex responses to stimulation of baroreceptors of the carotid sinus and aortic arch, regulating blood pressure by controlling heart rate, strength of heart contractions, and diameter of blood vessels.

biceps r. contraction of the biceps muscle when its tendon is tapped.

bite r. strong closure of the jaws when the teeth or gums are stimulated.

Brain's r. extension of a hemiplegic flexed upper limb when a person is in a quadrupedal posture; called also quadrupedal extensor reflex.

bulbocavernosus r., bulbospongiosus r. contraction of the bulbocavernous muscle in response to a tap on the dorsum of the penis; called also penile reflex.

cardiac respiratory r. an increase in heart rate caused by an increase in respiratory rate that reduces venous return.

carotid sinus r. slowing of the heartbeat when pressure is applied to the carotid artery at the level of the cricoid cartilage. See also CAROTID SINUS SYNDROME.

Chaddock's r. in lesions of the pyramidal tract, stimulation below the external malleolus causes extension of the great toe; called also Chaddock's sign.

chain r. a series of reflexes, each serving as a stimulus to the next, making a complete activity.

ciliary r. the movement of the pupil in accommodation.

ciliospinal r. dilation of the ipsilateral pupil on painful stimulation of the skin at the side of the neck.

clasp-knife r. clasp-knife rigidity.

conditioned r. CONDITIONED RESPONSE.

conjunctival r. closure of the eyelid when the conjunctiva is touched.

corneal r. see CORNEAL REFLEX.

cough r. the sequence of events initiated by the sensitivity of the lining of the airways and mediated by the medulla as a consequence of impulses transmitted by the vagus nerve, resulting in coughing, i.e., the clearing of the passageways of foreign matter.

cremasteric r. contraction of the ipsilateral cremaster muscle, drawing the testis upward, when the upper inner aspect of the thigh is stroked longitudinally.

deep r. one elicited by a sharp tap on the appropriate tendon or muscle to induce brief stretch of the muscle.

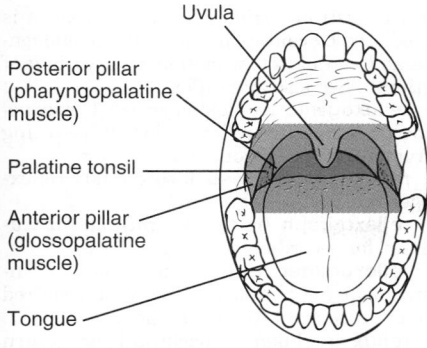

Uvula

Posterior pillar
(pharyngopalatine
muscle)

Palatine tonsil

Anterior pillar
(glossopalatine
muscle)

Tongue

Areas that react in a gag reflex when touched.

digital r. Hoffmann's sign (def. 2).

doll's eye r. doll's eye phenomenon.

embrace r. Moro reflex.

gag r. elevation of the soft palate and retching which is elicited by touching the back of the tongue or the wall of the pharynx; called also pharyngeal reflex.

gastrocolic r. increase in intestinal peristalsis after food enters the empty stomach.

gastroileal r. increase in ileal motility and opening of the ileocecal valve when food enters the empty stomach.

grasp r. flexion or clenching of the fingers or toes on stimulation of the palm of the hand or sole of the foot.

Hering-Breuer r's see HERING-BREUER REFLEXES.

Hoffmann's r. Hoffmann's sign (def. 2).

jaw r., jaw-jerk r. closure of the mouth caused by a downward blow on the passively hanging chin; rarely seen in health but very noticeable in corticospinal tract lesions.

knee r. KNEE JERK.

light r. 1. constriction of the pupil when a light is shone into the same (direct light reflex) or the opposite eye (indirect or consensual light reflex). 2. a luminous image reflected when light strikes the normal tympanic membrane.

lung r's Hering-Breuer reflexes.

Magnus and de Kleijn neck r's extension of both limbs on the same side, or one limb or part of a limb, with increase of tonus on the side to which the chin is turned when the head is rotated, and flexion with loss of tonus on the side to which the occiput points; it usually indicates DECEREBRATE RIGIDITY.

Mayer's r. opposition and adduction of the thumb combined with flexion at the metacarpophalangeal joint and extension at the interphalangeal joint, on downward pressure of the index finger.

Mendel-Bekhterev r. dorsal flexion of the second to fifth toes on percussion of the dorsum of the foot; in certain organic nervous disorders, plantar flexion occurs.

micturition r. any of the reflexes necessary for effortless urination and subconscious maintenance of continence.

Moro r. see MORO REFLEX.

myotatic r. stretch reflex.

neck righting r. rotation of the trunk in the direction in which the head of the supine infant is turned; this reflex is absent or decreased in infants with spasticity.

nociceptive r's reflexes initiated by painful stimuli; see also NOCICEPTOR and PAIN.

oculocephalic r. doll's eye phenomenon.

orbicularis pupillary r. unilateral contraction of the pupil, followed by dilatation after closure or attempted closure of eyelids that are forcibly held apart.

palatal r., palatine r. stimulation of the PALATE causes SWALLOWING. Called also swallowing reflex.

paradoxical pupillary r. reversed pupillary reflex.

patellar r. knee jerk.

penile r. bulbocavernosus reflex.

pharyngeal r. gag reflex.

pilomotor r. the production of goose FLESH on stroking of the skin.

placing r. flexion followed by extension of the leg when the infant is held erect and the dorsum of the foot is drawn along the under edge of a table top; it is obtainable in the normal infant up to the age of six weeks.

plantar r. plantar flexion of the foot when the ankle is grasped firmly and the lateral border of the sole is stroked or scratched from the heel toward the toes.

proprioceptive r. a reflex that is initiated by stimuli arising from some function of the reflex mechanism itself.

psychogalvanic r. decreased electrical resistance of the body due to emotional or mental agitation.

pupillary r. 1. contraction of the pupil on exposure of the retina to light. 2. any reflex involving the iris, resulting in change in the size of the pupil, occurring in response to various stimuli, e.g., change in illumination or point of fixation, sudden loud noise, or emotional stimulation.

quadriceps r. knee jerk.

quadrupedal extensor r. Brain's reflex.

red r. a luminous red appearance seen upon the retina in retinoscopy.

reversed pupillary r. any abnormal pupillary reflex opposite of that which occurs normally; e.g., stimulation of the retina by light dilates the pupil. Called also paradoxical pupillary reflex.

R

righting r. the ability to assume an optimal position when there has been a departure from it.

rooting r. a reflex in the newborn in which stimulation of the side of the cheek or upper or lower lip causes the infant to turn the mouth and face to the stimulus.

Rossolimo's r. in pyramidal tract lesions, plantar flexion of the toes on tapping their plantar surface.

spinal r. any reflex action mediated through a center of the spinal cord.

startle r. Moro reflex.

stepping r. movements of progression elicited when the infant is held upright and inclined forward with the soles of the feet touching a flat surface; it is obtainable in the normal infant up to the age of six weeks.

stretch r. reflex contraction of a muscle in response to passive longitudinal stretching.

sucking r. sucking movements of the lips of an infant elicited by touching the lips or the skin near the mouth.

suck-swallow r. rhythmical sucking and swallowing movements in an infant when a finger or nipple is placed in the mouth.

superficial r. any withdrawal reflex elicited by noxious or tactile stimulation of the skin, cornea, or mucous membrane, including the corneal, pharyngeal, and cremasteric reflexes.

swallowing r. palatal reflex.

tendon r. contraction of a muscle caused by percussion of its tendon.

tonic neck r. extension of the upper limb and sometimes the lower limb on the side to which the head is forcibly turned, with flexion of the contralateral limbs; seen normally in the newborn. If it persists into the second or third year of life, it indicates a neurologic disorder.

triceps r. contraction of the belly of the triceps muscle and slight extension of the upper limb when the tendon of the muscle is tapped directly, with the limb flexed and fully supported and relaxed.

triceps surae r. Achilles reflex.

vestibular r's the reflexes for maintaining the position of the eyes and body in relation to changes in orientation of the head.

vestibulo-ocular r. nystagmus or deviation of the eyes in response to stimulation of the vestibular system by angular acceleration or deceleration or when the CALORIC TEST is performed.

vomiting r. the reflex for VOMITING, caused by reflexive stimulation of muscles

of the gastrointestinal tract and throat; it is mediated by centers in the medulla oblongata and can be set in motion by a variety of stimuli. See also *gag reflex.*

reflexogenic (re-flek″so-jen′ik) 1. producing or increasing reflex action. 2. resulting from a reflex reaction.

reflexogenous (re-flek-soj′ĕ-nus) reflexogenic.

reflexograph (re-flek′so-graf) an instrument for recording a reflex.

reflexometer (re″flek-som′ĕ-ter) an instrument for measuring the force required to produce myotatic contraction.

reflux (re′fluks) a backward or return flow; see also BACKFLOW and REGURGITATION (def. 1).

esophageal r., gastroesophageal r. reflux of the stomach contents into the esophagus.

hepatojugular r. distention of the jugular vein induced by applying manual pressure over the liver; it suggests insufficiency of the right heart.

intrarenal r. reflux of urine into the renal PARENCHYMA.

vesicoureteral r., vesicoureteric r. backward flow of urine from the bladder into a ureter.

refract (re-frakt′) 1. to cause to deviate. 2. to ascertain errors of ocular refraction.

refraction (re-frak′shun) the act or process of refracting; specifically, the determination of the refractive errors of the eye and their correction with glasses. 1. the deviation of light in passing obliquely from one medium to another of different density.

cycloplegic r. a type of static REFRACTION, measured after lens ACCOMMODATION is paralyzed by administration of CYCLOPLEGIC eye drops.

double r. refraction in which incident rays are divided into two refracted rays.

dynamic r. refraction of the eye during accommodation.

ocular r. the refraction of light produced by the media of the normal eye and resulting in the focusing of images upon the retina.

static r. refraction of the eye when its accommodation is paralyzed.

refractionist (re-frak′shun-ist) one skilled in determining the refracting power of the eyes and correcting refracting defects.

refractive (re-frak′tiv) pertaining to or subserving a process of refraction; having the power to refract.

refractometer (re″frak-tom′ĕ-ter) 1. an instrument for measuring the refractive power of the eye. 2. an instrument for determining the indexes of refraction of various substances, particularly for determining the strength of lenses for spectacles.

refractoriness (re-frak′tah-re″nes) the state of being refractory.

    postrepolarization r. refractoriness to stimuli that exists even after a fiber has completely repolarized; see also absolute refractory PERIOD.

refractory (re-frak′tah-re) 1. not readily yielding to treatment. 2. not responding to a stimulus.

refrangible (re-fran′jĭ-b′l) susceptible of being refracted.

refresh (re-fresh′) 1. to freshen. 2. to make raw again; to denude a wound of epithelium to enhance tissue repair.

refrigeration (re-frij″er-a′shun) therapeutic application of low temperature; see also induced HYPOTHERMIA.

refusal (re-fu′zal) a declining to do something or to accept something.

    conscientious r. conscientious objection.

    informed r. refusal of treatment after one has been informed about it in an effort to gain informed CONSENT.

    r. of treatment a declining of treatment; it may be either informed REFUSAL or not fully informed.

refusion (re-fu′zhun) the return of blood to the circulation after its temporary removal or after stoppage of flow, as after LIGATURE of a part or passage through a HEART-LUNG MACHINE.

regeneration (re-jen″er-a′shun) the natural renewal of a structure, as of a lost tissue or part.

regio (re′je-o) [L.] region; anatomic nomenclature for any of various areas on the surface of the body.

region (re′jun) a plane with more or less definite boundaries; called also regio. adj., re′gional.

    abdominal r's the areas into which the anterior surface of the abdomen is divided, including the epigastric, hypochondriac (right and left), iliac (right and left), lumbar (right and left), hypogastric, and umbilical. See illustration.

    AN r. the area of the heart where the atrial fibers merge with the atrioventricular node.

    anal r. the part of the perineal REGION that surrounds the ANUS.

    axillary r. the area of the upper chest surrounding the AXILLA, lateral to the pectoral REGION.

    epigastric r. the abdominal region that is superior and central in location, above the umbilical region and between the two hypochondriac regions.

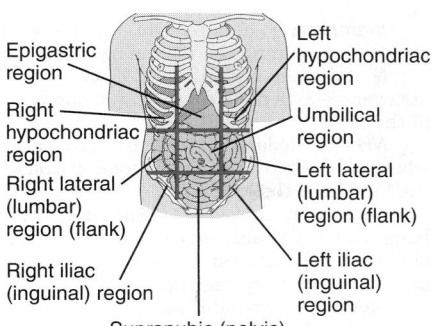

Epigastric region

Right hypochondriac region

Right lateral (lumbar) region (flank)

Right iliac (inguinal) region

Suprapubic (pelvic) (hypogastric) region

Left hypochondriac region

Umbilical region

Left lateral (lumbar) region (flank)

Left iliac (inguinal) region

Nine abdominopelvic regions. From Applegate, 2000.

    facial r. that comprising the various anatomical regions of the face, divided into *buccal* (side of oral cavity), *infraorbital* (below eye), *mental* (chin), *nasal* (nose), *oral* (lips), *orbital* (eye), *parotid* (angle of jaw), and *zygomatic* (cheek bone) regions.

    H r. the area of the bundle of His from its connection with the atrioventricular node to its branching portion.

    homology r's looped structures, comprising approximately 100 amino acid residues and fastened by disulfide bonds, that show similarities in primary structure from one region to another. They represent the building blocks or units of immunoglobulin molecules.

    hypochondriac r. either of the abdominal regions that are in superior lateral locations, one on the left (*left hypochondriac region*) and one on the right (*right hypochondriac region*) of the epigastric REGION; called also hypochondrium.

    hypogastric r. suprapubic region.

    I r. that part of the major histocompatibility complex where immune response genes are present.

    iliac r. inguen.

    inframammary r. the part of the pectoral REGION inferior to the breast, bordered inferiorly by the hypochondriac REGION of the abdomen.

    inguinal r. inguen.

    lateral r. either of the abdominal regions that are in central lateral locations, one to the left (*left lateral region*) and one to the right (*right lateral region*) of the umbilical REGION; called also flank and lumbar region.

    lateral pectoral r. the most lateral part of the pectoral REGION, bounded laterally by the axillary REGION.

    lumbar r. 1. the region of the back lying lateral to the lumbar vertebrae. See also LOIN. 2. lateral region.

R

mammary r. the part of the pectoral REGION surrounding the mammary GLAND.

N r. [*n*odal region] the region of the atrioventricular node consisting of the body of the node.

NH r. [*n*odal-*H*is region] the area where the atrioventricular node becomes the bundle of His.

pectoral r. the aspect of the chest overlying the pectoralis major muscle, subdivided into the lateral pectoral, mammary, and inframammary regions.

pelvic r. suprapubic region.

perineal r. the region underlying the pelvic outlet, subdivided into the anal and urogenital regions.

precordial r. the part of the anterior surface of the body covering the heart and the pit of the stomach.

presternal r. the region of the thorax overlying the STERNUM, bounded laterally by the pectoral REGIONS.

pubic r. suprapubic region.

suprapubic r. the abdominal region that is inferior and central in location, below the umbilical REGION and between the two iliac (inguinal) REGIONS; called also hypogastric or pelvic region.

umbilical r. the abdominal region that is most central in location, surrounding the UMBILICUS; it is bounded laterally by the two lateral or lumbar regions, superiorly by the epigastric region, and inferiorly by the suprapubic or hypogastric region.

urogenital r. the part of the perineal REGION that surrounds the external genital organs and the urethral orifice,

regionalization (re″jun-al-ĭ-za′shun) a HEALTH CARE SYSTEM under which all institutions and agencies in a given geographical area are organized under a single board and administration; it may involve the integration of some or all of the service providers in the region.

Registered Record Administrator (RRA) see MEDICAL RECORD ADMINISTRATOR.

Registered Respiratory Therapist (RRT) a RESPIRATORY THERAPIST who has passed the advanced level written and clinical simulation examinations of the National Board for Respiratory Care.

registrant (rej′is-trant) a nurse listed on the books of a registry as available for duty.

registrar (rej′is-trar) 1. an official keeper of records. 2. in British hospitals, a resident specialist who acts as assistant to the chief or attending specialist.

registration (rej″is-tra′shun) the act of recording; in dentistry, the making of a record of the jaw relations present or

desired, in order to transfer them to an articulator to facilitate proper construction of a dental prosthesis.

registry (rej′is-tre) 1. an office where a nurse's name may be listed as being available for duty. 2. a central agency for collection of pathologic material and related data in a specified field of pathology, so organized that the data can be properly processed and made available for study.

Reglan (reg′lan) trademark for preparations of METOCLOPRAMIDE hydrochloride, used to stimulate gastrointestinal motility.

Regonol (reg′o-nōl) trademark for preparations of PYRIDOSTIGMINE bromide, a cholinesterase inhibitor used in treatment of MYASTHENIA GRAVIS and as an antidote to nondepolarizing neuromuscular blocking AGENTS.

regression (re-gresh′un) 1. return to a former or earlier state. 2. subsidence of symptoms or of a disease process. 3. in biology, the tendency in successive generations toward the mean. 4. an unconscious DEFENSE MECHANISM used to resolve conflict or frustration by returning to a behavior that was effective in earlier years. Some degree of regression frequently accompanies physical illness. Patients who are mentally ill may exhibit regression to an extreme degree, reverting all the way back to infantile behavior; this is called *atavistic regression*. adj., **regres′sive.**

Regroton (reg′ro-ton) trademark for a preparation of CHLORTHALIDONE and RESERPINE, an ANTIHYPERTENSIVE AGENT.

regulation (reg″u-la′shun) 1. the act of adjusting or state of being adjusted to a certain standard. 2. in biology, the adaptation of form or behavior of an organism to changed conditions. 3. the power to form a whole embryo from stages before the gastrula. 4. the biochemical mechanisms that control the expression of genes.

hemodynamic r. in the NURSING INTERVENTIONS CLASSIFICATION, a nursing INTERVENTION defined as optimization of heart rate, preload, afterload and contractility. See also HEMODYNAMIC MONITORING.

temperature r. in the NURSING INTERVENTIONS CLASSIFICATION, a nursing INTERVENTION defined as attaining and/or maintaining body TEMPERATURE within a normal range.

temperature r.: intraoperative in the NURSING INTERVENTIONS CLASSIFICATION, a nursing INTERVENTION defined as attaining and/or maintaining desired intraoperative body TEMPERATURE.

regulator (reg′u-la″tor) in the ADAPTATION MODEL of nursing, one of two major internal processing subsystems by which an individual adapts to or copes with internal and external environmental stimuli. The regulator subsystem is related primarily to physiologic needs and includes neural, endocrine, and psychomotor inputs. These inputs are transformed into perception, thereby linking the regulator subsystem to the COGNATOR subsystem.

regurgitant (re-ger′jĭ-tant) flowing back.

regurgitation (re-ger″jĭ-ta′shun) 1. a backward flowing; see also BACKFLOW and REFLUX. 2. VOMITING.

  aortic r. backflow of blood from the aorta into the left ventricle, owing to insufficiency of the aortic VALVE; it may be chronic or acute.

  mitral r. backflow of blood from the left ventricle into the left atrium, owing to insufficiency of the mitral VALVE; it may be acute or chronic, and is usually due to mitral valve prolapse, rheumatic heart disease, or a complication of cardiac dilatation.

  pulmonic r. backflow of blood from the pulmonary artery into the right ventricle, owing to insufficiency of the pulmonic VALVE.

  tricuspid r. backflow of blood from the right ventricle into the right atrium, owing to imperfect functioning (INSUFFICIENCY) of the tricuspid VALVE.

  valvular r. backflow of blood through the orifice of one of the heart valves owing to imperfect closing of the valve (valvular INSUFFICIENCY); see aortic, mitral, pulmonic, and tricuspid regurgitation.

rehabilitation (re″hah-bil″ĭ-ta′shun) the process of restoring a person's ability to live and work as normally as possible after a disabling injury or illness. It aims to help the patient achieve maximum possible physical and psychologic fitness and regain the ability to be independent. It offers assistance with the learning or relearning of skills needed in everyday activities, with occupational training and guidance and with psychologic readjustment.

  Rehabilitation is an integral part of convalescence. Proper food, medication, and hygiene and suitable exercise provide the physical basis for recovery. The patient is encouraged to be active physically and mentally to the extent recommended by the health care team. Nursing care, PHYSICAL THERAPY, OCCUPATIONAL THERAPY, and vocational training are used extensively in the rehabilitation of the severely handicapped.

  cancer r. a process by which individuals in their own environments are assisted to achieve optimal functioning within the limits imposed by CANCER.

  rehabilitee (re″hah-bil′ĭ-te) the subject of rehabilitation.

  rehydration (re″hi-dra′shun) the restoration of water or fluid content to a body or to

---

WINDOW ON REHABILITATION

Rehabilitation is young compared with other specialties and has been influenced profoundly by the rapid changes impacting the general health care arena. Consequently, rehabilitationists are seeing greater complexity in patient care requirements, increased demand for rehabilitation services, and pressure for coordinated cost-effective programs.

  Perceptions that rehabilitation takes place only after discharge from the hospital, that it can be ensured by a simple referral, or that it occurs only in specialized facilities are inconsistent with the reality of today's rehabilitation arena. Currently, rehabilitationists participate in the acute care of patients with spinal cord injury (and others) and bring reality to the phrase "rehab begins at the time of admission." The rehabilitation team, consisting of specialists from a variety of professions, models an approach to comprehensive care that decreases fragmentation and discontinuity. The number of rehabilitation units in general hospitals has increased dramatically, and outpatient and home health services receive growing attention as treatment sites.

  Clearly, rehabilitation today begs acknowledgement as a process that occurs in a variety of settings and is directed by the belief that given the appropriate services and opportunities, the individual can achieve the maximum performance of which he/she is capable.

DOROTHY GORDON, DNSc, RN

---

a substance that has become dehydrated. See also oral rehydration THERAPY.

  reimbursement (re″im-bers′ment) a compensation or paying back; see also PAYMENT.

  third party r. third party payment.

  reimplantation (re″im-plan-ta′shun) replantation.

  reinfection (re″in-fek′shun) a second infection by the same agent.

  reinforcement (re″in-fors′ment) the increasing of force or strength. In the psychological theory of BEHAVIORISM, presentation of a stimulus following a response that increases the frequency of subsequent responses. This is central in operant CONDITIONING.

  Positive reinforcement consists of a stimulus that is added to the environment immediately after the desired response has been exhibited. It serves to strengthen the response, that is, to increase the likelihood of its occurring again. Examples of such reinforcement are food, money, a special privilege, or some other reward that is satisfying to the subject.

Negative reinforcement consists of a stimulus that is withdrawn (subtracted) from the environment immediately after the response, so that the withdrawal serves to strengthen the response.

r. of reflex strengthening of a reflex response by the patient's performance of some unrelated action during elicitation of the reflex.

reinforcer (re″in-for′ser) anything that produces reinforcement, whether POSITIVE to desirable events, or NEGATIVE to undesirable events which are reinforced in their removal.

reinfusate (re″in-fu′zāt) fluid for reinfusion into the body, usually after being subjected to a treatment process.

reinfusion (re″in-fu′zhun) infusion of body fluid that has previously been withdrawn from the same individual, e.g., reinfusion of ascitic fluid after ultrafiltration.

reinnervation (re″in-er-va′shun) restoration of nerve function to a part from which it was lost; it may occur spontaneously or be achieved by nerve grafting.

reintegration (re″in-tĕ-gra′shun) 1. biological integration. 2. the restoration of harmonious mental function after disintegration of the personality in mental illness.

Reiter (ri′ter) Frances (1904–1977). American nursing educator and researcher; first dean of the Graduate School of Nursing (later the Lienhard School of Nursing) at New York Medical College. She believed strongly in the supreme importance of practice in the nursing profession. She was an advocate of the education of nurse clinicians; the term NURSE CLINICIAN is her coinage.

Reiter's syndrome (ri′-terz) a triad of symptoms of unknown etiology comprising urethritis, conjunctivitis, and arthritis (the dominant feature), appearing concomitantly or sequentially associated with mucocutaneous manifestations of keratoderma blennorrhagicum, circinate balanitis, and stomatitis, chiefly affecting young men, and usually running a self-limited but relapsing course.

rejection (re-jek′shun) the IMMUNE RESPONSE of the recipient to foreign tissue cells (ANTIGENS) after homograft TRANSPLANTATION, with the production of antibodies and ultimate destruction of the transplanted organ. In *hyperacute rejection,* there is an immediate response against the graft because of the presence of preformed antibody, resulting in fibrin deposition, platelet aggregation, and neutrophilic infiltration. In *acute rejection,* the response occurs after the sixth day and then proceeds rapidly. It is characterized by loss of function of the transplanted organ and by pain and swelling, with leukocytosis and thrombocytopenia. In *chronic rejection,* there is gradual progressive loss of function of the transplanted organ with less severe symptoms than in the acute form.

relapse (re-laps′) the return of a disease weeks or months after its apparent cessation.

relapsing fever any of a group of similar infectious diseases transmitted to humans by the bites of lice and ticks, and marked by alternating periods of normal temperature and periods of fever relapse. The diseases in the group are caused by several different species of spirochetes belonging to the genus *Borrelia.* Called also recurrent fever.

Symptoms and Diagnosis. Generally, relapsing fever starts with a sudden high fever of 40° to 40.5°C (104° to 105°F), accompanied by chills, headache, muscle aches, nausea, and vomiting. There may also be jaundice and a rash. The attack lasts 2 or 3 days, after which the symptoms disappear by crisis, with profuse sweating accompanying the rapid drop in temperature. In elderly people this may be accompanied by collapse, in which the heart and respiratory system function poorly. After 3 or 4 days there is a relapse and the symptoms return in their former severity. The cycle continues through four or more attacks before the disease has run its course. Relapsing fevers are rarely fatal, but they can be serious.

Treatment and Prevention. Treatment is with antibiotics. Sponge baths and aspirin help to control the fever and comfort the patient. Although tickborne relapsing fever still occurs in the western United States as well as in other parts of the world, louseborne fever is now largely confined to underdeveloped parts of Asia, Africa, and Latin America. Improved public sanitation and louse and tick control account for the decline in the incidence of the disease.

relation (re-la′shun) the condition or state of one object or entity when considered in connection with another.

object r's the emotional bonds existing between an individual and another person, as contrasted with one's interest in, and love for, oneself; usually described in terms of one's capacity for loving and reacting appropriately to others.

relationship (re-la′shun-ship″) a state of being in relation with something.

causal r. an association between two variables in a research study such that the independent variable is shown to determine the value of the dependent variable.

relativism (rel′ah-tiv″izm) a philosophical system that considers truth to be dependent on individual persons, cultural contexts, times, or places.

cultural r. the understanding of distinct cultures and lifestyles within the context of each culture; the behaviors of a cultural group are evaluated in the context of that specific culture, from an impartial perspective, rather than according to the standards of some other culture.

relaxant (re-lak′sant) 1. causing relaxation. 2. an agent that causes relaxation.

muscle r. an agent that specifically aids in reducing muscle tension.

relaxation (re″lak-sa′shun) a lessening of tension.

force r. the decrease in the amount of force required to maintain a tissue at a set amount of displacement or deformation over time.

progressive r. a method of deep muscle relaxation based on the premise that muscle tension is the body's physiological response to anxiety-provoking thoughts and that muscle relaxation blocks anxiety.

progressive muscle r. 1. progressive relaxation. 2. in the NURSING INTERVENTIONS CLASSIFICATION, a nursing INTERVENTION defined as facilitating the tensing and releasing of successive muscle groups while attending to the resulting differences in sensation.

r. techniques methods used to promote lessening of tension, reduction of anxiety, and management of pain. Physiologic effects include a decrease in pulse rate, respiratory rate and oxygen consumption, carbon dioxide production and elimination, blood pressure, metabolic rate, and muscle tension. Additionally, relaxation can cause peripheral vasodilation and increased peripheral temperature.

Relaxation techniques include full-body relaxation, color exchange, in which a discomfort is given a color and eliminated, and listening to restful music or meditative sounds. Such techniques are helpful in many situations in which persons are tense, in pain, highly stressed, or anxious. They can be useful in the treatment of asthma, hyperventilation, high blood pressure, Raynaud's disease, headache, and peptic ulcers.

Though varied, techniques have several features in common: rhythmic breathing, reduced muscle tension, and an altered state of consciousness. In the latter, the relaxed person sinks into an alpha level of consciousness, which falls between full consciousness and unconsciousness. In this state thought processes become less logical and more associative and creative; hence, one is more receptive to positive suggestions, and better able to concentrate on a single mental image or idea. Upon returning from the alpha state of consciousness to full consciousness one feels rested and more alert.

release (re-lēs′) 1. a setting free. 2. surgical incision or cutting of soft tissue to bring about relaxation.

tendon r. tenotomy.

wheelchair pressure r. weight SHIFT of a person confined to a wheelchair.

reliability (re-li″ah-bil′ĭ-te) 1. in statistics, the tendency of a system to be resistant to failure. 2. precision (def. 2).

relocation stress syndrome a NURSING DIAGNOSIS accepted by the North American Nursing Diagnosis Association, defined as physiological or psychological disturbances following transfer from one environment to another.

REM *r*apid *e*ye *m*ovement; see SLEEP.

rem (rem) *r*oentgen *e*quivalent *m*an; the amount of any ionizing radiation which has the same biological effect as 1 rad of x-rays; 1 rem = 1 rad RBE (relative biological effectiveness).

remedy (rem′ĕ-de) anything that cures or palliates disease. adj., **reme′dial.**

remifentanil (rem″ĭ-fen′tah-nil) an opioid ANALGESIC used as the hydrochloride salt as an adjunct to anesthesia.

remineralization (re-min″er-al-ĭ-za′shun) restoration of mineral elements, as of calcium salts to bones or teeth.

remission (re-mish′un) diminution or abatement of the symptoms of a disease; the period during which such diminution occurs.

remittence (re-mit′ens) temporary abatement, without actual cessation, of symptoms.

remittent (re-mit′ent) having periods of abatement and of exacerbation.

r. fever elevated body temperature showing fluctuation each day, but never falling to normal.

remodeling (re-mod′el-ing) reorganization or renovation of an old structure.

bone r. absorption of bone tissue and simultaneous deposition of new bone; in normal bone the two processes are in dynamic equilibrium.

remotivation (re-mo″tĭ-va′shun) any of various group therapy techniques used with long-term, withdrawn patients in mental hospitals to stimulate their communication,

R

vocational, and social skills and interest in their environment.

ren (ren), pl. *re'nes* [L.] kidney.

renal (re'nal) pertaining to the KIDNEY; called also nephric.

   r. clearance tests laboratory tests that determine the ability of the kidney to remove certain substances from the blood. The most commonly used is the CREATININE CLEARANCE test, which is a measure of the glomerular filtration RATE.

   r. failure inability of the KIDNEY to maintain normal function, so that waste products and metabolites accumulate in the blood. This affects most of the body's systems because of its important role in maintaining fluid balance, regulating the electrochemical composition of body fluids, providing constant protection against acid-base imbalance, and controlling blood pressure. Called also kidney failure.

ACUTE RENAL FAILURE occurs suddenly and may be caused by physical trauma, infection, inflammation, or exposure to NEPHRO-TOXIC chemicals. Nephrotoxic agents include drugs such as PENICILLINS, SULFONAMIDES, AMINOGLYCOSIDES, and TETRACYCLINES; radiographic IODINE contrast materials; and heavy METALS. These agents inflict damage on the renal tubules, causing tubular necrosis, and may also indirectly harm the tubules by producing severe vasoconstriction of renal blood vessels with ischemia of kidney tissue. Other causes of tubular ischemia include circulatory collapse, severe dehydration, and hypotension in certain compromised surgical patients.

Acute renal failure may be classified as: *prerenal,* associated with poor systemic perfusion and decreased renal blood flow; *intrarenal,* associated with renal ischemia or toxins; or *postrenal,* resulting from the obstruction of urine flow out of the kidneys.

OLIGURIA is the hallmark of tubular necrosis, but it is not always present. Other symptoms besides a marked decrease in urinary output are related to fluid and electrolyte imbalances, anemia, hypertension, and UREMIA. In addition to supportive measures to restore and maintain a tolerable internal environment during acute renal failure, it may be necessary to remove toxic wastes by HEMODIALYSIS or PERITONEAL DIALYSIS.

CHRONIC RENAL FAILURE is a progressive loss of kidney function that may eventually progress to END-STAGE RENAL DISEASE. The clinical course is described in four stages. First there is *decreased renal reserve,* with diminishing renal function but without accumulation of the end products of protein metabolism; the patient has no symptoms. In the second stage, *renal insufficiency,* the glomerular filtration RATE (GFR) is depressed to about 30 ml per minute and plasma chemistry begins to show abnormalities as waste products accumulate. The third stage, *frank renal failure,* is characterized by steadily rising serum creatinine and blood urea nitrogen levels accompanying a drop in the GFR. The fourth and final stage is UREMIA; levels of protein end products continue to rise, residual urine function is less than 15 per cent, and all body systems are impaired.

Causes of renal failure are many and can be roughly divided into three groups: (1) those that directly affect the kidney by infection, inflammation, and upper urinary tract obstruction; (2) those in which there is an obstruction of the lower urinary tract; and (3) systemic diseases and toxicities, such as HYPERCALCEMIA, HYPERTENSION, disseminated LUPUS ERYTHEMATOSUS, ATHEROMA, and DIABETES MELLITUS.

Treatment. The treatment of chronic renal failure is highly complex owing to its impact on systems throughout the body. It involves prevention of imbalances in water and electrolytes whenever possible and correction of these imbalances when they do occur. Therapy may include phosphate BINDERS to prevent absorption of phosphorus from the intestinal tract, ANTIHYPERTENSIVE AGENTS to control high blood pressure, DIURETICS to manage hypervolemia, ERYTHROPOIETIN to manage anemia, and cardiac drugs to manage heart failure. Fluids often are restricted to a given amount during each 24-hour period. Dietary restrictions are aimed at minimizing urea toxicity, controlling various metabolic upheavals and providing optimal nutrition. Protein intake is an especially critical factor because the end products of the metabolism of protein and amino acids are excreted for the most part by the kidney.

Symptomatic relief of the many manifestations of end-stage renal disease is a challenge to every member of the health care team. Virtually every system within the body is adversely affected in some way. Pathophysiologic changes involve the gastrointestinal tract, the skin, the cardiovascular system, the lungs, bone, and blood, and the metabolism of glucose and protein.

HEMODIALYSIS or PERITONEAL DIALYSIS may be employed to rid the body of wastes that the kidney can no longer handle. For some patients TRANSPLANTATION of a human kidney is a viable alternative to continuous dialysis. Others who cannot withstand surgery and long-term immunosuppression are not good candidates for a kidney transplant.

Rendu-Osler-Weber   disease (ron-du′ oz′ler va′ber) hereditary hemorrhagic telangiectasia.

Renese (rĕ′nēs) trademark for preparations of POLYTHIAZIDE, a diuretic used for treatment of hypertension and edema. Renese-R also contains RESERPINE.

reniform (ren′ĭ-form) kidney-shaped.

renin (re′nin) a proteolytic enzyme synthesized, stored, and secreted by the juxtaglomerular CELLS of the kidney; it plays a role in regulation of blood pressure by catalyzing the conversion of the plasma glycoprotein ANGIOTENSINOGEN to ANGIOTENSIN I. This, in turn, is converted to ANGIOTENSIN II by an enzyme that is present in relatively high concentrations in the lung. Angiotensin II is one of the most potent VASOCONSTRICTORS known, and also is a powerful stimulus of ALDOSTERONE secretion. Stimuli to the secretion of renin include sodium depletion, dehydration, serum albumin depletion, cirrhosis of the liver, cardiac failure, renal artery stenosis, and renal nerve stimulation.

Whenever blood flow to the kidney diminishes, renin is secreted and angiotensin is formed. The angiotensin causes widespread VASOCONSTRICTION and elevation of blood pressure consequent to greatly increased total peripheral resistance. A second effect, the increased secretion of ALDOSTERONE, results in retention of salt and water by the kidneys and therefore increased extracellular fluid volume, cardiac output, and arterial pressure. Additionally, the angiotensin acts *directly* on the kidneys to cause salt and water retention, which causes a long-term increase in arterial blood pressure.

r.-angiotensin-aldosterone   system the regulation of sodium balance, fluid volume, and blood pressure by secretion of renin in response to reduced perfusion of the kidney. Renin hydrolyzes a plasma globulin to release ANGIOTENSIN I, which is rapidly hydrolyzed to angiotensin II, which in turn stimulates ALDOSTERONE secretion. Aldosterone brings about sodium retention, water retention, increase in blood pressure, and restoration of renal perfusion, which shuts off the signal for renin release. Angiotensin II is a potent VASOCONSTRICTOR, which also increases blood pressure.

big r. prorenin.

reninism (re′nin-izm) a condition marked by overproduction of renin.

primary r. a syndrome of hypertension, hypokalemia, hyperaldosteronism, and

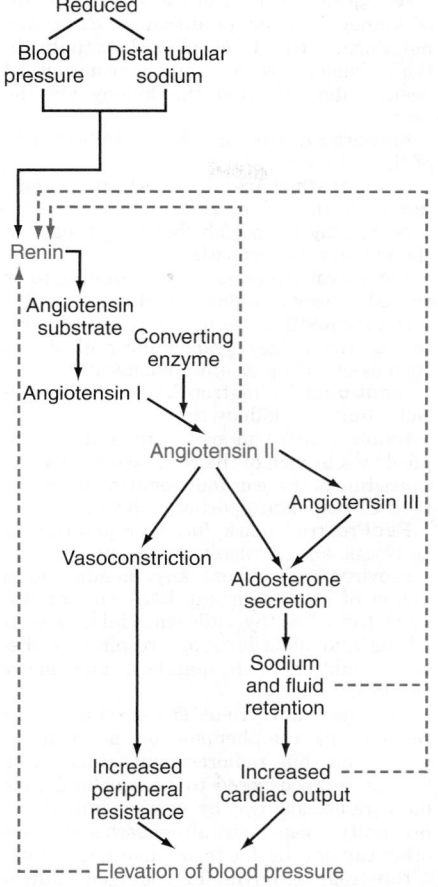

The role of the renin-angiotensin-aldosterone system in regulation of blood pressure. Solid lines represent positive interactions; broken lines show negative interactions or feedback inhibition. From Cotran et al., 1994.

elevated plasma renin activity, due to proliferation of juxtaglomerular CELLS.

renipelvic (ren″ĭ-pel′vik) pertaining to the renal PELVIS.

rennin (ren′in) the milk-curdling enzyme found in the gastric juice of human infants (before pepsin formation) and abundantly in that of the calf and other ruminants; a preparation from the stomach of the calf is used to coagulate milk protein to facilitate its digestion. Rennin catalyzes the conversion of casein from a soluble to an insoluble form (paracasein or curd).

renogastric (re″no-gas′trik) pertaining to the kidney and stomach.

renogram (re'no-gram) a graphic record of kidney function produced by externally monitoring the level of radioactivity in the bladder as a radiopharmaceutical agent enters it from the kidney via the ureters.

renography (re-nog'rah-fe) radiography of the kidney.

renointestinal (re"no-in-tes'tĭ-nal) pertaining to the kidney and intestine.

renopathy (re-nop'ah-the) any disease of the kidneys; nephropathy.

renoprival (re"no-pri'val) pertaining to or caused by lack of kidney function.

renoprotective (re"no-pro-tek'tiv) protecting the kidney against harmful effects such as of a drug or other chemical.

renotropic (re"no-trop'ik) having a special affinity for kidney tissue.

renule (ren'ūl) an area of the kidney supplied by a branch of the renal artery, usually consisting of three or four renal PYRAMIDS and their corresponding cortical substance.

ReoPro trademark for a preparation of ABCIXIMAB, an ANTITHROMBOTIC agent.

reovirus (re'o-vi"rus) any member of a family of ether-resistant RNA viruses isolated from healthy children, children with febrile and afebrile upper respiratory disease, children with diarrhea, and many animals.

reoxygenation (re-ok"sĭ-jĕ-na'shun) in radiobiology, the phenomenon in which hypoxic (and thus radioresistant) tumor cells become more exposed to oxygen (and thus more radiosensitive) by coming into closer proximity to capillaries after death and loss of other tumor cells due to previous irradiation.

rep (rep) acronym for *r*oentgen *e*quivalent *p*hysical, a unit of radiation equivalent to the absorption of 93 ergs per gram of water or soft tissue.

repaglinide (rĕ-pag'lĭ-nīd) an oral hypoglycemic AGENT used in treatment of type 2 DIABETES MELLITUS.

repair (re-pār') the physical or mechanical restoration of damaged tissues, especially the replacement of dead or damaged cells in a body tissue or organ by healthy new cells.

Hill's r. Hill posterior GASTROPEXY.

plastic r. restoration of anatomic structure by means of tissue transferred from other sites or derived from other individuals, or by other substance.

repeat (rĕ-pēt') something done or occurring more than once, particularly over and over.

long terminal r's identical NUCLEOTIDE sequences occurring at each end of a proviral GENOME or a TRANSPOSON and believed to be essential for integration of the molecule into host DNA.

tandem r. appearance of two or more identicle segments close to each other within a strand of DNA.

repellent (re-pel'ent) 1. able to repel or drive off. 2. an agent that so acts.

repercussion (re"per-kush'un) the driving in of an eruption or the scattering of a swelling.

reperfusion (re"per-fu'zhun) restoration of blood flow to an area or part that had had temporary ISCHEMIA.

replacement (re-plās'ment) 1. substitution; see also replacement THERAPY. 2. arthroplasty.

joint r. arthroplasty.

total hip r. total hip ARTHROPLASTY.

total joint r. total joint ARTHROPLASTY.

replantation (re"plan-ta'shun) the replacement of an organ or other structure, such as a digit, limb, or tooth, to the site from which it was previously lost or removed; called also reimplantation.

replication (rep'lĭ-ka'shun) 1. a turning back of a part so as to form a duplication. 2. repetition of an experiment to ensure accuracy. 3. the process of duplicating or reproducing, as replication of an exact copy of a polynucleotide strand of DNA or RNA.

repolarization (re"po-lah-rĭza'shun) 1. the reestablishment of POLARITY, especially the return of a cell's membrane POTENTIAL to resting POTENTIAL after DEPOLARIZATION. 2. in cardiac physiology, the restoration of the cell to its maximal diastolic POTENTIAL, represented by phase 0 to phase 3 of the ACTION POTENTIAL.

report (re-port') a prepared account of an event, investigation, or evaluation, usually for formal presentation to an authority or group.

accident r. incident report.

case r. a narrative in the professional literature that identifies a single incident and discusses pertinent factors related to the patient.

incident r. a written document describing inadvertent trauma to a patient, errors or omissions in care, or untoward events happening to staff or visitors. Such a report should be filed as soon after the event as possible. Called also accident report.

shift r. in the NURSING INTERVENTIONS CLASSIFICATION, a nursing INTERVENTION defined as exchanging essential patient care information with other nursing staff at change of shift.

reporting (re-port'ing) the making of a REPORT.

incident r. in the NURSING INTERVENTIONS CLASSIFICATION, a nursing INTERVENTION defined as written and verbal reporting of any vent in the process of patient care that is inconsistent with desired patient outcomes or routine operations of the health care facility. See also incident REPORT.

repositor (re-poz′ĭ-tor) an instrument used in returning a displaced organ, especially the uterus, to the normal position.

repression (re-presh′un) 1. the act of restraining, inhibiting, or suppressing. 2. in molecular genetics, inhibition of gene transcription by a repressor. 3. in psychiatry, a DEFENSE MECHANISM by which a person unconsciously banishes unacceptable ideas, feelings or impulses from consciousness. A person using repression to obtain relief from mental conflict is unaware of "forgetting" unpleasant situations as a way of avoiding them. If done to an extreme, repression may lead to increased tension and irresponsible behavior that the person himself cannot understand or explain.

enzyme r. interference, usually by the end product of a pathway, with synthesis of the enzymes of that pathway.

repressor (re-pres′or) that which restrains or inhibits; a specific protein molecule coded for by a regulatory gene, which acts through the cytoplasm to repress the synthesis of a specific protein.

reproduction (re″pro-duk′shun) 1. the creation of a similar object or situation; replication or duplication. 2. the process by which a living entity or organism produces a new individual of the same kind. The sex glands, or GONADS (the OVARIES in the female and the TESTES in the male) produce the germ cells (ova and sperm) that unite and grow into a new individual. Reproduction begins when the germ cells unite, a process called FERTILIZATION.

Production of Germ Cells. The germ cells are the male SPERMATOZOON and the female OVUM (secondary OOCYTE). The secondary oocyte (mature ovum) is a large round cell that is just visible to the naked eye. Spermatozoa, on the other hand, can be seen only under a microscope, where each appears as a small, flattened head with a long whiplike tail used for locomotion.

In the female, maturation of an ovum is a remarkable process controlled by hormones secreted by the endocrine glands. The MENSTRUAL CYCLE is ordinarily 28 days long, measured from the beginning of one menstrual period to the beginning of the next. During the first 2 weeks of the usual cycle, one of the ova becomes mature enough to be released from the ovary. At the time of OVULATION this mature ovum (secondary oocyte) is released and at this point can be fertilized. If FERTILIZATION occurs, the fertilized ovum (ZYGOTE) is then discharged into the abdominal cavity. Somehow, by mechanisms that are not clear, it moves into a FALLOPIAN TUBE and begins its descent toward the uterus. If the ovum remains unfertilized, menstrual bleeding occurs about 2 weeks later.

In the male there is no sexual cycle comparable to the cyclical activity of ovulation in the female. Mature sperm are constantly being made in the testes of the adult male and stored there in the duct system.

Fertilization, or Conception. During coitus, semen is ejaculated from the penis into the back of the vagina near the cervix uteri. About a teaspoonful of semen is discharged with each ejaculation, containing several hundred millions of spermatozoa. Of this enormous number of sperm, only one is needed to fertilize the ovum. Yet the obstacles to be overcome are considerable. Many of the sperm are deformed and cannot move. Others are killed by the acid secretions of the vagina (the semen itself is alkaline). The sperm must then swim against the current of secretions flowing out of the uterus.

The sperm swim an average of 0.4 to 2.5 cm (0.1 to 1.0 inch) per minute. When one or more vigorous sperm are able to reach the ovum, which is normally in the outer half of the fallopian tube, fertilization occurs. The head end of the sperm plunges through the thick wall of the ovum, leaving its tail outside. The genetic materials, the chromosomes, are injected into the ovum, where they unite with the chromosomes inherited from the mother (see HEREDITY). The sex of the child is determined at this instant; it depends on the sex chromosome carried by the sperm.

If by chance two ova have been released and are fertilized by two sperm, fraternal (dizygotic) TWINS are formed. Identical (monozygotic) TWINS are produced by a single fertilized ovum that divides into two early in its development.

Ovulation and Fertilization. Fertilization typically can occur only (on the average) on 4 days of every menstrual cycle. The mature ovum lives only 1 or 2 days after ovulation, and the sperm have only about the same amount of time before they perish in the female reproductive tract. To fertilize the ovum, coitus must take place within the time that begins 1 or 2 days before ovulation and lasts until 1 or 2 days after ovulation. There is much variation, however, in the time when ovulation occurs. Most women ovulate between 12 and 16 days after the beginning of the last period, but others ovulate as early as 8 or as late as 20 days after the last period began.

R

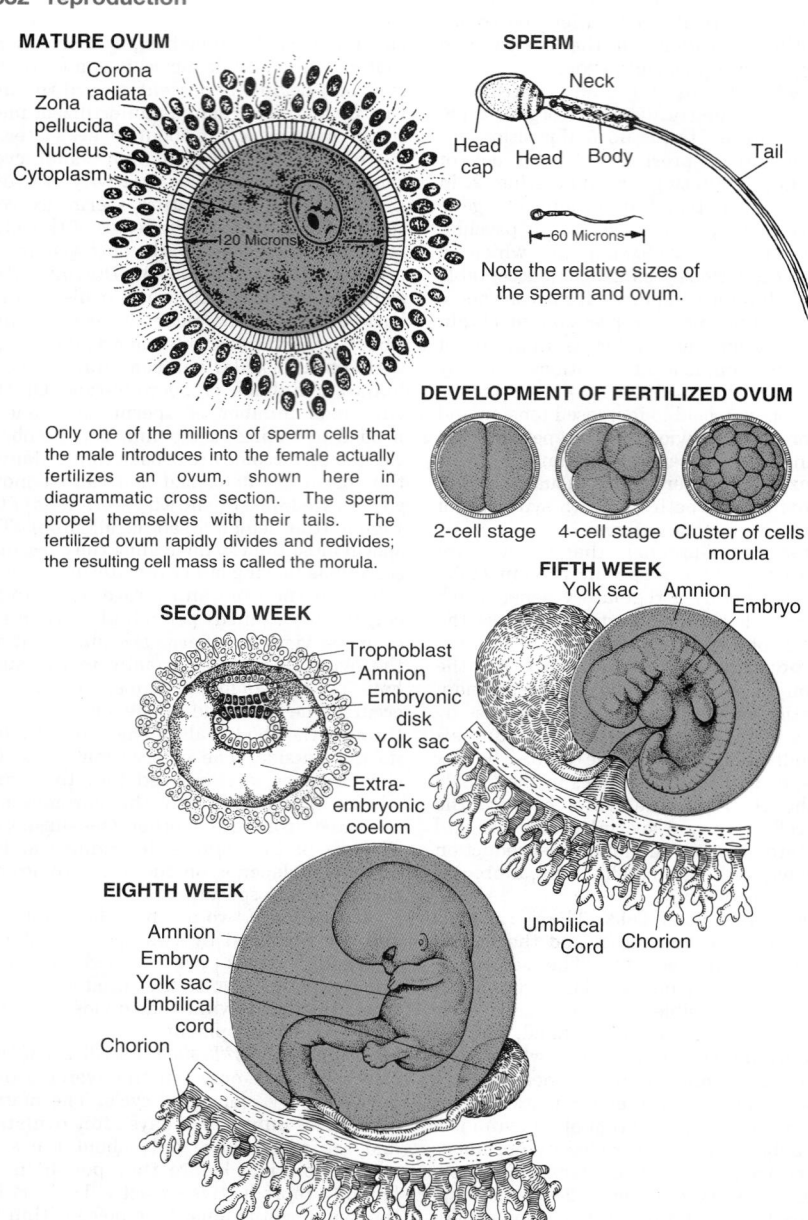

MATURE OVUM

Corona
radiata
Zona
pellucida
Nucleus
Cytoplasm

20 Microns

SPERM

Neck

Head
cap   Head   Body   Tail

60 Microns

Note the relative sizes of
the sperm and ovum.

Only one of the millions of sperm cells that
the male introduces into the female actually
fertilizes an ovum, shown here in
diagrammatic cross section. The sperm
propel themselves with their tails. The
fertilized ovum rapidly divides and redivides;
the resulting cell mass is called the morula.

DEVELOPMENT OF FERTILIZED OVUM

2-cell stage   4-cell stage   Cluster of cells
morula

FIFTH WEEK
Yolk sac   Amnion
Embryo

SECOND WEEK

Trophoblast
Amnion
Embryonic
disk
Yolk sac
Extra-
embryonic
coelom

EIGHTH WEEK

Amnion
Embryo
Yolk sac
Umbilical
cord
Chorion

Umbilical
Cord   Chorion

Reproduction.

Pregnancy. The ovum, now known as a ZYGOTE, begins to change immediately after fertilization. The membrane surrounding it becomes impenetrable to other sperm. Soon the zygote is dividing into a cluster of two, then four, then more cells, as it makes its way down the fallopian tube toward the uterus. At first it looks like a bunch of grapes. By the time it reaches the uterus, in 3 to 5 days, the cells are formed in the shape of a minute ball, the BLASTOCYST, which is hollow on the inside with an internal bump at one side where the embryo will form. The blastocyst quickly buries itself in the lining of the uterus (implantation). Occasionally implantation takes place not in the uterine lining, but elsewhere, producing an ECTOPIC PREGNANCY.

As soon as the blastocyst is implanted, its wall begins to change into a structure that eventually develops into the PLACENTA. Through the placenta the fetus secures nourishment from the mother and rids itself of waste products. Essentially the placenta is a filtering mechanism by which the mother's blood is brought close to the fetal blood without the actual mixing of blood cells.

During the early stages of pregnancy, the fetus grows at an extremely rapid rate. The mother's body must undergo profound changes to support this organism. The muscles of the uterus grow, vaginal secretions change, the blood volume expands, the work of the heart increases, the mother gains weight, the breasts prepare for nursing, and other adjustments are made throughout the mother's body.

   asexual r. reproduction without the fusion of germ CELLS.

   assisted r. assisted FERTILITY.

   cytogenic r. production of a new individual from a single germ cell or zygote.

   sexual r. reproduction by the fusion of female and male germ CELLS or by the development of an unfertilized ovum.

   somatic r. production of a new individual from a multicellular fragment by fission or budding.

   reproductive (re″pro-duk′tiv) subserving or pertaining to REPRODUCTION.

   r. organs, female the OVARIES, FALLOPIAN TUBES, UTERUS, VAGINA, and VULVA (external genitalia) of a female. The BREASTS are a secondary sex CHARACTER, enclosing the mammary glands (see also Plates).

The OVARIES link the reproductive system to the body's system of endocrine glands. Besides producing the ova, they secrete the female sex hormones ESTROGEN and PROGESTERONE, which influence the body's development and general functioning as well as the sexual function. The two ovaries, each about the size of a small plum, lie one on each side

of the pear-shaped uterus at its wide upper part. When a female is born, her undeveloped ovaries already contain the specialized cells that can eventually become ova. At puberty these ova begin to ripen, one a month; usually the ovaries alternate in producing them. As the undeveloped egg cell, called a follicle, begins to ripen, it makes its way to the ovary's surface, breaks through its own outer covering, and is released. Release of an egg cell, called OVULATION, occurs about once every 28 days.

After its separation from the ovary the ovum is drawn into the nearby FALLOPIAN TUBE through its fringed, flared opening, and is moved along by rhythmic contractions of the tube's walls and by the cilia of its mucous membrane lining. In the course of its passage the ovum ripens fully, and if fertilization occurs it usually takes place while the ovum is moving through the fallopian tube.

The other end of the tube opens directly into the UTERUS, a muscular organ capable of stretching to contain a fertilized ovum growing through the 9 months of pregnancy. The mucous membrane lining the uterus is also specially adapted to hold the fetus securely and nourish it. When the ovum arrives, the hormones estrogen and progesterone produced in the ovary have previously stimulated the uterus to prepare its lining with extra blood vessels. If the egg has not been fertilized, it loses its vitality, the hormone supply ceases, and the extra blood and tissues are discharged from the body through the vagina, in the menstrual flow. If FERTILIZATION has taken place, the growth of a new life has begun; menstruation does not occur, and in fact ceases entirely during the 9 months (approximately 280 days) of pregnancy.

The lower end of the uterus forms an opening called the CERVIX (neck), which protrudes into the VAGINA. Enclosed by muscles and lined with mucous membrane, the vagina measures on the average about 8 cm (3 in) in length. In coitus it receives the penis (male copulatory organ) and the discharge of sperm during ejaculation. Like the uterus, the vagina undergoes changes during pregnancy that enable it to stretch to many times its usual size, allowing the infant to pass through it in childbirth.

The exterior opening of the vagina and the surrounding organs make up the VULVA; this consists of the LABIA MAJORA, LABIA MINORA, VESTIBULE, and CLITORIS. Anterior to the vulva is a triangular fatty pad covered with pubic hair, the MONS PUBIS. Between the clitoris and the entry to the vagina is the opening of the urethra, from which urine is

R

excreted. The anus lies to the rear of the vaginal opening. In a virgin, a membrane called the HYMEN usually closes off a part of the opening to the vagina.

The labia majora envelop the labia minora, and these join together at the clitoris, a diminutive penislike organ that has a purely erotic function. Like the penis, the clitoris has a foreskin and many nerve endings. The vestibule is the area surrounding the entry to the vagina and within the labia minora; at each side of the vaginal opening and elsewhere in the vestibule, glands secrete lubricating fluids to facilitate coitus.

A woman's breasts serve to provide milk for the newborn infant. At puberty the breasts increase in size; during pregnancy they become much larger and start to secrete milk shortly after childbirth.

Disorders of the Female Reproductive Organs. Bacterial and other infections, tumors, and birth injuries can affect the female reproductive tract and organs. Growths or tumors can develop in any part of the tract; they are usually benign and may not require treatment but should be examined periodically in case they grow large and affect the organs, or become malignant. The most prevalent bacterial diseases of a woman's reproductive organs are the VENEREAL DISEASES (diseases usually contracted during coitus). The most serious of these are SYPHILIS and GONORRHEA.

r. organs, male that the external genitalia, accessory glands that secrete special fluids, and the accompanying ducts in the male (see also Plate 13).

External Genitalia. These include the PENIS, TESTES, and SCROTUM. The penis is the organ through which SEMEN is transferred into the female during coitus; semen is a carrier for the SPERMATOZOA produced in the testes. The testes also produce the male hormone TESTOSTERONE, which gives a sexually mature male his distinctively masculine characteristics and his sexual energy and drive. The testes are suspended from the spermatic cord, which also connects the testes with the other parts of the reproductive system. This cord consists of blood vessels, nerves and ducts, all enclosed in connective tissue.

ACCESSORY GLANDS. The accessory reproductive glands include the PROSTATE, two seminal VESICLES, and two bulbourethral GLANDS (also known as *Cowper's glands*). The prostate is located below and against the urinary bladder and completely surrounds the urethra. It produces a thin, clear, slightly alkaline fluid that neutralizes the normal acidity of the urethra caused by

the continual passage of urine and enables the spermatozoa to pass through the urethra unharmed. The seminal vesicles are two glands located just above and to the rear of the prostate; they consist of many small sacs, or pockets, in which is produced and stored the thick, milky fluid that is ejaculated during the male orgasm. The fluid serves as the carrier for the sperm and is the major constituent of the semen. The two bulbourethral glands, about the size of peas, secrete a clear, sticky fluid that lubricates the urethra and makes it easier for the semen to pass through it during the process of ejaculation.

DUCTS. The spermatozoa are led from the testes to the urethra through a system of ducts. First is a convoluted tube (one on top of each testis and connected directly to it), called an EPIDIDYMIS, where mature spermatozoa produced in the testes are stored. Each epididymis is connected to a DUCTUS DEFERENS (called also *vas deferens*), a part of the spermatic cord that conducts the spermatozoa to the duct lying close to the bladder. These ducts join with ducts leading from the seminal vesicles just before the urethra; the combined duct, called the ejaculatory DUCT, passes through the prostate and joins with the urethra. The urethra then conducts the semen through the penis.

Discharge of Semen. The tissues that form the mass of the penis are called erectile tissue. This tissue is spongy in nature and filled with innumerable hollow spaces. There is also a network of veins and arteries within the penis. Sexual excitement causes the muscles surrounding the veins to contract, thereby restricting the flow of blood from the penis. At the same time, the muscles surrounding the arteries relax, permitting the free flow of blood into the penis at the full pressure of the circulatory system. The result is that the spongy tissue fills with blood and the penis swells in size and becomes stiff and erect.

Sexual excitement also stimulates the accessory glands to secrete larger amounts of their fluids. When the sexual tension becomes acute enough, as a result of coitus, masturbation, or purely mental stimulation (as in nocturnal EMISSIONS or "wet dreams"), there is a series of reflex contractions of the reproductive organs. The muscles surrounding the seminal ducts, the prostate, and the seminal vesicles contract convulsively; this causes the semen to be ejaculated forcibly from the penis. There is first an ejaculation of the fluid from the prostate, followed immediately by the semen. About 2 or 3 ml of semen are ejaculated. This volume of semen is believed to contain between 200 and 500 million sperm, only one of which is necessary to fertilize the ovum.

Disorders of the Male Reproductive Organs. For disorders that affect particular organs, see PENIS, PROSTATE, and CRYPTORCHIDISM. Since the male reproductive organs are connected so closely with each other, an infection in one is likely to spread throughout the entire reproductive system. This is particularly true of VENEREAL DISEASES (those usually contracted through coitus), such as SYPHILIS and GONORRHEA.

reptilase (rep'til-ās) an enzyme from Russell's viper venom used in determining blood clotting time.

repulsion (re-pul'shun) 1. the act of driving apart or away; a force that tends to drive two bodies apart. 2. in genetics, the occurrence on opposite chromosomes in a double heterozygote of the two mutant alleles of interest.

RES reticuloendothelial system.

rescinnamine (re-sin'ah-min) a RAUWOLFIA alkaloid administered orally as an ANTIHYPERTENSIVE AGENT.

research the systematic, rigorous investigation of a situation or problem in order to generate new knowledge or validate existing knowledge. Research in health care takes place in a variety of areas and has many potential benefits; the areas include professional practice, environmental issues affecting health, vitality, treatments, theory development, health care economics, and many others. Health care research can be conducted by one group of professionals for generation of knowledge specific to that group, or by a diverse group of researchers collaborating on a given health care problem.

applied r. scientific investigations conducted to answer specific clinical questions or solve practice-related problems.

basic r. scientific investigation that involves the generation of new knowledge or development of new theories; its results often cannot be applied directly to specific clinical situations.

correlational r. the systematic investigation of relationships among two or more variables, without necessarily determining cause and effect.

descriptive r. research that provides an accurate portrayal of characteristics of a particular individual, situation, or group. These studies are a means of discovering new meaning, describing what exists, determining the frequency with which something occurs, and categorizing information.

ethnographic r. the investigation of a culture through an in-depth study of the members of the culture; it involves the systematic collection, description, and analysis of data for development of theories of cultural behavior.

experimental r. objective, systematic, controlled investigation for the purpose of predicting and controlling phenomena and examining probability and causality among selected variables.

exploratory r. studies that are merely formative, for the purpose of gaining new insights, discovering new ideas, and increasing knowledge of phenomena.

grounded theory r. a research approach designed to discover what problems exist in a given social environment and how the persons involved handle them; it involves formulation, testing, and reformulation of propositions until a theory is developed.

historical r. research involving analysis of events that occurred in the remote or recent past.

phenomenological r. an inductive, descriptive research approach developed from phenomenological philosophy; its aim is to describe an experience as it is actually lived by the person.

qualitative r. research dealing with phenomena that are difficult or impossible to quantify mathematically, such as beliefs, meanings, attributes, and symbols; it may involve content ANALYSIS.

quantitative r. research involving formal, objective information about the world, with mathematical quantification; it can be used to describe test relationships and to examine cause and effect relationships.

resect (re-sekt') to excise part of an organ or other structure.

resection (re-sek'shun) removal, as of an organ, by cutting; called also excision.

gastric r. gastrectomy.

root r., root-end r. apicoectomy.

transurethral r. of the prostate, transurethral prostatic r. see TRANSURETHRAL RESECTION OF THE PROSTATE.

wedge r. removal of a triangular mass of tissue.

resectoscope (re-sek'tah-skōp) an endoscope with a wide-angle telescope and an electrically activated wire loop for transurethral removal or biopsy of lesions of the bladder, prostate, or urethra.

resectoscopy (re″sek-tos'kah-pe) resection or biopsy of lesions by means of the resectoscope.

reserpine (res'er-pēn) a RAUWOLFIA alkaloid, administered orally and intramuscularly as an ANTIHYPERTENSIVE AGENT.

reserve (re-zerv') 1. to hold back for future use. 2. a supply beyond that ordinarily used, for use in an emergency.

alkali r., alkaline r. see ALKALI RESERVE.

R

cardiac r. an increase in cardiac output related to an increase in heart rate or stroke volume to meet body requirements.

reservoir (rez´er-vwahr) 1. a storage place or cavity. 2. an alternate or passive host or carrier that harbors pathogenic organisms without injury to itself and serves as a source from which other individuals can be infected.

cardiotomy r. in cardiopulmonary BY-PASS, a collection chamber for blood suctioned from the heart chambers and pericardium.

continent ileal r. an intra-abdominal pouch having a volume of at least 500 ml and a valve created from a portion of the ileum, pulled through the stoma, and lying flat against the abdominal wall; it maintains continence of feces and is emptied by a catheter when full. See also continent ILEOSTOMY and KOCK POUCH.

ileoanal r. see ILEOANAL RESERVOIR.

Ommaya r. a device implanted in the brain for instillation of medication or removal of fluid through a CATHETER in a lateral ventricle. When used for the direct administration of CHEMOTHERAPY, it enhances the concentration of medication in brain tissue.

residue (rez´ĭ-doo) a remainder; that which remains after the removal of other substances; in organic chemistry a portion of a molecule that is incorporated into another molecule, e.g., an amino acid residue of a polypeptide.

residuum (re-zid´u-um) [L.] residue.

resin (rez´in) 1. a solid or semisolid organic substance exuded by plants or by insects feeding on plants, or produced synthetically; they are insoluble in water but mostly soluble in alcohol or ether. adj., **res´inous.** 2. a compound made by condensation or polymerization of low-molecular-weight organic compounds.

acrylic r's products of the polymerization of acrylic or methacrylic acid or their derivatives, used in fabrication of medical prostheses and dental restorations and appliances.

anion exchange r. see ion-exchange resin.

cation exchange r. see ion-exchange resin.

cholestyramine r. a synthetic, strongly basic anion exchange resin in the chloride form which chelates bile salts in the intestine, thus preventing their reabsorption; used as an adjunctive therapy to diet in management of certain hypercholesterolemias and in the symptomatic relief of pruritus associated with bile stasis.

composite r. a synthetic resin, usually acrylic based, to which a high percentage of ceramic reinforcing filler has been added such as particles of glass or silica coated with a coupling agent to bind them to the matrix; used chiefly in dental restorations. Called also composite.

epoxy r. a tough, chemically resistant adhesive, flexible, dimensionally stable resin of EPOXY polymers; used as denture base material.

ion exchange r. a high-molecular-weight insoluble polymer of simple organic compounds capable of exchanging its attached ions for other ions in the surrounding medium; classified as *(a)* cation or anion exchange resins, depending on which ions the resin exchanges; and *(b)* carboxylic sulfonic, and so on depending on the nature of the active groups.

podophyllum r. a mixture of resins from PODOPHYLLUM, used as a topical caustic in treatment of laryngeal PAPILLOMAS, CONDYLOMATA ACUMINATA, and other EPITHELIOMAS.

resistance (re-zis´tans) 1. opposition, or counteracting force, as opposition of a conductor to passage of electricity or other energy or substance. 2. the natural ability of a normal organism to remain unaffected by noxious agents in its environment; see also IMMUNITY. 3. in psychology or psychiatry, conscious or unconscious defenses against change, preventing repressed material from coming into awareness; they can take such forms as forgetfulness, evasions, embarrassment, mental blocks, denial, anger, superficial talk, intellectualization, or intensification of symptoms. It occurs because the blocked association or understanding would be too threatening to face at this point in the therapy; identification of what point the resistance comes at can be an important indicator of the patient's unconscious patterns.

airway r. the opposition of the tissues of the air passages to air flow: the mouth-to-alveoli pressure difference divided by the rate of air flow. Symbol R_A or R_{AW}.

androgen r. resistance of target organs to the action of ANDROGENS, resulting in any of a spectrum of defects from a normal male phenotype in which men have normal genitalia but infertility to complete androgen resistance in which the individual has a female phenotype. *Complete androgen resistance* is an extreme form of male PSEUDO-HERMAPHRODITISM in which the individual is phenotypically female but is of XY chromosomal sex; there may be rudimentary uterus and tubes, but the gonads are typically testes, which may be abdominal or inguinal in position. Called also testicular feminization and testicular feminization syndrome. *Incomplete androgen resistance* is any of various forms less than the complete type, manifested by a male phenotype with various degrees of ambiguous genitalia such as hypospadias and a small vaginal pouch, a hooded phallus, or a bifid scrotum that may or may not contain gonads.

drug r. the ability of a microorganism to withstand the effects of a drug that are lethal to most members of its species.

insulin r. see INSULIN RESISTANCE.

multidrug r., multiple drug r. a phenomenon seen in some malignant cell lines: cells that have developed natural resistance to a single cytotoxic compound are also resistant to structurally unrelated CHEMOTHERAPY agents. Called also CROSS-RESISTANCE.

peripheral r. resistance to the passage of blood through the small blood vessels, especially the arterioles.

pulmonary vascular r. the vascular RESISTANCE of the pulmonary circulation; the difference between the mean pulmonary arterial pressure and the left atrial filling pressure divided by the cardiac output. Called also total pulmonary vascular resistance.

total peripheral r. the vascular RESISTANCE of the systemic circulation: the difference between the mean arterial PRESSURE and CENTRAL VENOUS PRESSURE divided by the cardiac OUTPUT.

total pulmonary r., total pulmonary vascular r. pulmonary vascular resistance.

vascular r. the opposition to blood flow in a vascular bed; the pressure drop across the bed divided by the blood flow, conventionally expressed in peripheral resistance units. Symbol R or *R*.

resolution (rez″o-loo′shun) 1. subsiding of a pathologic state, such as the reduction of inflammation or the softening and disappearance of swelling. 2. perception of two adjacent points as separate; in microscopy, the smallest distance at which two adjacent objects can be distinguished as separate. 3. in radiology, a measure of how much detail a device can print or display.

resolvent (re-zol′vent) 1. promoting resolution or the dissipation of a pathologic growth. 2. an agent that promotes resolution.

resolving power the ability of the eye or of a lens to make small objects that are close together separately visible, thus revealing the structure of an object.

resonance (rez′o-nans) 1. the prolongation and intensification of sound produced by transmission of its vibrations to a cavity, especially such a sound elicited by percussion. Decrease of resonance is called *dull-*

ness; its increase, *flatness.* 2. a vocal sound heard on auscultation. 3. mesomerism.

amphoric r. a sound resembling that produced by blowing over the mouth of an empty bottle.

nuclear magnetic r. see NUCLEAR MAGNETIC RESONANCE.

skodaic r. increased percussion resonance at the upper part of the chest, with flatness below it; heard over a large pleural effusion or area of consolidation.

tympanic r. tympanitic resonance (def. 2).

tympanitic r. 1. the peculiar sound elicited by percussing a tympanitic abdomen. 2. the drumlike reverberation of a cavity full of air; called also tympanic resonance.

vocal r. (**VR**) the sound of ordinary speech as heard through the chest wall.

resonancy (rez′o-nan-se) a principle of HOMEODYNAMICS in the SCIENCE OF UNITARY HUMAN BEINGS; the continuous change from lower to higher frequency wave patterns in human and environmental fields.

resonant (rez′o-nant) giving an intense, rich sound on percussion; exhibiting resonance.

resonator (rez′o-na″tor) 1. an instrument used to intensify sounds. 2. an electric circuit in which oscillations of a certain frequency are set up by oscillations of the same frequency in another circuit.

resorb (re-sorb′) to take up or absorb again; to undergo resorption.

resorcinism (rĕ-zor′sĭ-nizm) chronic poisoning by RESORCINOL, resulting in methemoglobinemia, paralysis, and damage to the capillaries, kidneys, heart, and nervous system.

resorcinol (rĕ-zor′sĭ-nol) a PHENOL with bactericidal, fungicidal, keratolytic, exfoliative, and antipruritic activity; used especially as a topical KERATOLYTIC in the treatment of acne and other dermatoses.

resorption (re-sorp′shun) 1. the lysis and assimilation of a substance, as of bone. 2. reabsorption.

resource (re′sors) a person or group of persons serving as an available support and source of aid because of intellectual or personal capabilities.

respirable (rĕ-spīr′ah-b'l) 1. suitable for respiration. 2. small enough to be inhaled, such as an irritating particle.

respiration (res″pĭ-ra′shun) 1. the exchange of OXYGEN and CARBON DIOXIDE between the atmosphere and the body cells, including INHALATION and EXHALATION, DIFFUSION of oxygen from the pulmonary alveoli to

R

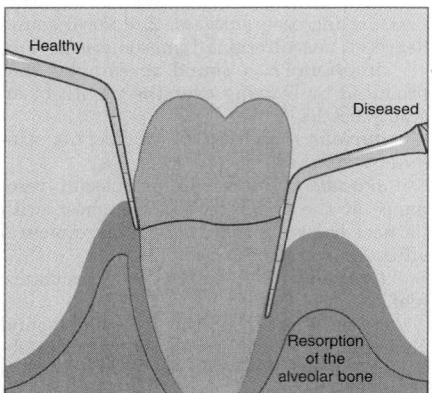

Alveolor Resorption of the alveolar bone in periodontitis. From Darby and Walsh, 1995.

the blood and of carbon dioxide from the blood to the alveoli, followed by the transport of oxygen to and carbon dioxide from the body cells. See also VENTILATION (def. 2) and see Plates. 2. the metabolic processes by which living cells break down carbohydrates, amino acids, and fats to produce energy in the form of ADENOSINE TRIPHOSPHATE (ATP); called also cell respiration.

The Respiratory Sequence. The sequence of the respiration process begins as air enters the corridors of the nose or mouth, where it is warmed and moistened. The air then passes through the pharynx, larynx, and trachea and into the bronchi.

The bronchi branch in the lungs into smaller and smaller bronchioles, ending in clusters of tiny air sacs called ALVEOLI; there are 750 million alveoli in the lungs. The blood flows through the lungs in the PULMONARY CIRCULATION. Through the thin membrane of the network of capillaries around the alveoli, the air and the blood exchange oxygen and carbon dioxide. The carbon dioxide molecules migrate from the erythrocytes in the capillaries through the porous membrane into the air in the alveoli, while the oxygen molecules cross from the air into the red blood cells.

The erythrocytes proceed through the circulatory system, carrying the oxygen in loose combination with HEMOGLOBIN and giving it up to the body cells that need it. In cellular respiration the blood cells release oxygen and pick up carbon dioxide. The lungs dispose of the carbon dioxide, left there by the red blood cells, in the process of breathing. With each breath, about one-sixth of the air in the lungs is exchanged for new air.

Breathing. The lungs inflate and deflate 16 to 20 times per minute in adults, 12 to 20 per minute in teenagers, 20 to 30 per minute in children 2 to 12 years old, and 30 to 50 per minute in newborns. Their elastic tissue allows them to expand and contract like a bellows worked by the diaphragm and the intercostal muscles. The diaphragm contracts, flattening itself downward, and thus enlarges the thoracic cavity. At the same time the ribs are pulled up and outward by the action of the narrow but powerful intercostal muscles that expand and contract the rib cage. As the chest expands, the air flows in. Exhalation occurs when the respiratory muscles relax and the chest returns automatically to its minimum size, expelling the air (see also LUNG).

Automatic Breathing Controls. The automatic control of breathing stems from poorly defined areas known as the respiratory CENTERS, located in the medulla oblongata and pons. From there, impulses are sent down the spinal cord to the nerves that control the diaphragm, and to the intercostal muscles. Chemical and reflex signals control these nerve centers. (See HERING-BREUER REFLEXES.) The chemical controls of breathing are mainly dependent on the level of CARBON DIOXIDE in the blood. The response is so sensitive that if the carbon dioxide level increases two-tenths of 1 per cent, the respiratory rate increases automatically to double the amount of air taken in, until the excess of carbon dioxide is eliminated. It is not lack of oxygen but excess of carbon dioxide that causes this instant and powerful reaction.

The carbon dioxide TENSION (P_{CO_2}), of arterial blood normally is 35 to 45 mm Hg. When the P_{CO_2} increases, the respiratory centers are stimulated and breathing becomes more rapid; conversely, decrease of the P_{CO_2} slows the rate of respiration. The P_{CO_2} acts both directly on the respiratory centers and on the carotid and aortic BODIES, chemoreceptors that are responsive to changes in blood P_{CO_2}, P_{O_2}, and pH (see also BLOOD GAS ANALYSIS).

Protective Respiratory Mechanisms. The lungs are constantly exposed to the surrounding atmosphere. Twenty times a minute, more or less, they take in a gaseous mixture, along with whatever foreign particles happen to be suspended in it and at whatever temperature it may be. To compensate, the lungs have some remarkable protective devices.

On its way through the nasal passage, the cold air from outside is preheated by a large supply of blood, which gives off warmth through the thin mucous membrane that lines the respiratory tract. This same mucous lining is always moist, and dry air picks up moisture as it passes.

Dust, soot, and bacteria are filtered out by a barrier of CILIA, tiny hairlike processes that line the passageways of the respiratory tract. The cilia trap not only foreign particles but also mucus produced by the respiratory passages themselves. Since the movement of the cilia is always toward the outside, they move the interfering matter upward, away from the delicate lung tissues, so that it can be expectorated or swallowed. Particles that are too large for the cilia to dispose of usually stimulate a sneeze or a cough, which forcibly expels them. Sneezing and coughing are reflex acts in response to stimulation of nerve endings in the respiratory passages. The stimulus for a cough comes from the air passages in the throat; for a sneeze, from those in the nose.

abdominal r. inspiration accomplished mainly by the diaphragm.

aerobic r. oxidative transformation of certain substrates into high-energy chemical compounds; see also ADENOSINE TRIPHOSPHATE.

artificial r. see ARTIFICIAL RESPIRATION.

Biot's r. breathing characterized by irregular periods of apnea alternating with periods in which four or five breaths of identical depth are taken; seen in patients with increased intracranial pressure associated with spinal meningitis and other central nervous system disorders.

cell r. respiration (def. 2).

Cheyne-Stokes r. see CHEYNE-STOKES RESPIRATION.

cogwheel r. breathing with jerky inhalation.

diaphragmatic r. that performed mainly by the diaphragm.

electrophrenic r. induction of respiration by electric stimulation of the phrenic nerve; see phrenic PACEMAKER. Called also diaphragmatic or phrenic pacing.

external r. the exchange of gases between the lungs and the blood.

internal r. the exchange of gases between the body cells and the blood.

Kussmaul's r. a distressing, paroxysmal dyspnea affecting both inspiration and expiration, characterized by increased respiratory rate (above 20 per minute), increased depth of respiration, panting, and labored respiration; seen in diabetic acidosis and coma and renal failure. Called also air hunger.

paradoxical r. see PARADOXICAL RESPIRATION.

tissue r. internal respiration.

respirator (res'pĭ-ra″tor) 1. an apparatus that qualifies air breathed through it, to be distinguished from a VENTILATOR. 2. frequently used misnomer for VENTILATOR (def. 2).

Drinker r. a formerly common but now rarely used type of VENTILATOR that provides controlled, automatic breathing for a patient whose respiratory muscles are paralyzed; it consists of a metal tank, enclosing the patient's body with the head outside, within which artificial respiration is maintained by alternating negative and positive pressure. It was instrumental in the treatment of the poliomyelitis epidemic of the early decades of the 20th century. Popularly known as iron lung.

respiratory (res'pir-ah-tor″e) pertaining to respiration.

acute r. distress syndrome, adult r. distress syndrome a group of symptoms accompanying fulminant pulmonary edema and resulting in acute respiratory failure; see also ACUTE RESPIRATORY DISTRESS SYNDROME.

r. care 1. the health care profession providing, under qualified supervision, diagnostic evaluation, therapy, monitoring, and rehabilitation of patients with cardiopulmonary disorders; it also employs educational activities to support patients and their families and to promote cardiovascular health among the general public. 2. the care provided by members of this profession. 3. the diagnostic and therapeutic use of medical gases and their administering apparatus, environmental control systems, humidification, aerosols, medications, ventilatory support, bronchopulmonary drainage, pulmonary rehabilitation, cardiopulmonary resuscitation, and airway management.

r. distress syndrome, neonatal, r. distress syndrome of the newborn (RDS) a condition of the newborn marked by dyspnea with cyanosis, heralded by such prodromal signs as dilatation of the nares, grunting on exhalation, and retraction of the suprasternal notch or costal margins. It usually occurs in newborns who are preterm, have diabetic mothers, or were delivered by cesarean section; sometimes there is no apparent predisposing cause.

This is the major cause of death in neonates and survivors have a high risk for chronic neurologic complications. No one factor is known to cause the condition; however, prematurity and interrupted development of the SURFACTANT system is thought to be the major causative factor. Surfactant is secreted by the epithelial cells of the alveoli. It acts as a detergent, decreasing the surface tension of fluids that line the alveoli and bronchioles and allowing for uniform expansion of the lung and maintenance of lung expansion. When there is an inadequate amount of surfactant, a

R

great deal of effort is required to re-expand the alveoli with air; thus the newborn must struggle for each breath. Insufficient expansion of the alveoli results in partial or complete collapse of the lung (ATELECTASIS). This in turn produces hypoxemia and elevated serum carbon dioxide levels.

The hypoxemia causes metabolic acidosis from increased production of lactic acid and respiratory acidosis due to the hypercapnia. The lowered pH constricts pulmonary blood vessels and inhibits intake of oxygen, thus producing more hypoxemia and interfering with the transport of substances necessary for the production of the sorely needed surfactant.

Patient Care. In order to minimize the hazards of oxygen toxicity and RETINOPATHY OF PREMATURITY, the blood gases of the newborn with respiratory distress syndrome must be carefully monitored to assess response to therapy. The goal is to administer only as much oxygen as is necessary to maintain an optimal level of oxygenation.

To improve respiratory function, intubation, suctioning of the air passages, and continuous positive airway PRESSURE via nasal prongs are commonly used, as well as instillation of artificial surfactant. Monitoring is conducted using transcutaneous oxygen MONITORING or a PULSE OXIMETER. To optimize breathing effort and facilitate air exchange, the newborn is positioned on the back with a shoulder support to keep the neck slightly extended, or on the side with the head supported. Because of the drying effect of oxygen therapy and the prohibition of oral fluids, mouth care must be given frequently to prevent drying and cracking of the lips and oral mucosa.

r. failure a life-threatening condition in which respiratory function is inadequate to maintain the body's need for oxygen supply and carbon dioxide removal while at rest; it usually occurs when a patient with CHRONIC AIRFLOW LIMITATION develops an infection or otherwise suffers an additional strain on already seriously impaired respiratory functions. Inadequate or unsuccessful treatment of RESPIRATORY INSUFFICIENCY from a variety of causes can lead to respiratory failure. Called also ventilatory failure.

Early symptoms include dyspnea, wheezing, and apprehension; cyanosis is rarely present. As the condition worsens the patient becomes drowsy and mentally confused and may slip into a coma. BLOOD GAS ANALYSIS is an important tool in diagnosing respiratory failure and assessing effectiveness of treatment. The condition is a medical emergency that can rapidly progress to irreversible cardiopulmonary failure and death. Treatment is concerned with improving ventilation and oxygenation of tissues, restoring and maintaining FLUID BALANCE and ACID-BASE BALANCE, and stabilizing cardiac function.

r. insufficiency a condition in which respiratory function is inadequate to meet the body's needs when increased physical activity places extra demands on it. Insufficiency occurs as a result of progressive degenerative changes in the alveolar structure and the capillary tissues in the pulmonary bed, as, for example, in CHRONIC AIRFLOW LIMITATION and pulmonary FIBROSIS. Treatment is essentially supportive and symptomatic. If the condition is not successfully managed it may progress to RESPIRATORY FAILURE.

r. therapist a health care professional skilled in the treatment and management of patients with respiratory problems, who administers RESPIRATORY CARE. The minimum educational requirement is an associate degree, providing knowledge of anatomy, physiology, pharmacology, and medicine sufficient to serve as a supervisor and consultant. Those registered by the National Board for Respiratory Therapy are designated Registered Respiratory Therapist (RRT).

r. therapy RESPIRATORY CARE.

r. therapy technician a health care professional who has completed a specialized one- or two-year educational program and who performs routine care, management, and treatment of patients with respiratory problems under the supervision of a RESPIRATORY THERAPIST. Such programs are usually found in community colleges and are accredited by the Joint Review Committee for Respiratory Therapy Education.

respirometer (res″pĭ-rom′ĕ-ter) an instrument for determining the nature of the respiration.

response (re-spons′) any action or change of condition evoked by a stimulus.

acute phase r. a group of physiologic processes occurring soon after the onset of infection, trauma, inflammatory processes and some malignant conditions. The most prominent change is a dramatic increase of acute phase PROTEINS in the serum, especially C-reactive PROTEIN. Also seen are fever, increased vascular permeability, and a variety of metabolic and pathologic changes.

anamnestic r. the rapid reappearance of antibody in the blood following introduction of an antigen to which the subject had previously developed a primary IMMUNE RESPONSE.

auditory brainstem r. ABR; a special hearing test that tracks the nerve signals

---

WINDOW ON RESPIRATORY THERAPIST

A decision to become a respiratory therapist should be made only after a very personal commitment is made to become a health care professional with direct patient contact. This decision should not be made lightly because it requires assuming the responsibility of caring for patients who are seriously ill. A career as a respiratory therapist provides exciting and intellectually challenging work with sophisticated life-support systems. Respiratory therapists are important members of the health care team, working with medical direction from pulmonologists and physicians specialized in trauma resuscitation, emergency and critical care, and pulmonary and cardiac rehabilitation. Respiratory care practitioners typically feel a strong sense of accomplishment and know that their work is important. Registered Respiratory Therapists (RRTs) have a well-defined scope of practice and have been identified by the Medical Board of the National Academy of Sciences as Type B Physician Assistants. Type B Physician Assistants are expected to have more knowledge about their medical specialty than the average physician who is not board certified in that area. Accordingly, RRTs are expected to make recommendations on the respiratory care of patients with pulmonary disorders. This level of interaction with physicians and other members of the health care team can be very rewarding. RRTs are considered to be authorities on the operation of life-support equipment used in critical care areas such as trauma centers and intensive care units. Interfacing mechanical ventilators to critically ill patients in respiratory failure, in order to provide life support, places great intellectual demands on the respiratory therapist. Accordingly, respiratory care professionals have high standards, with specialty board examinations provided by the National Board for Respiratory Care and licensure of respiratory care practitioners by 33 states in the USA. Career opportunities abound for both men and women as staff therapists or managers in critical care, rehabilitation, and education, or as technical specialists for high-tech equipment companies.

THOMAS A. BARNES, EdD, RRT

---

arising in the inner ear as they travel along the auditory nerve to the brain region responsible for hearing. A small speaker placed near the ear makes a clicking sound, and special electrodes record the nerve signal as it travels. The test can determine where along the nerve there is a lesion responsible for sensorineural HEARING LOSS. It is often used for individuals with such loss in just one ear; this is often caused by a benign tumor along the auditory nerve, but if the ABR reading is normal in a given region, the chances of there being a tumor there are small. This test can also be used on infants since it requires no conscious response from the person being tested.

autoimmune r. the IMMUNE RESPONSE in which antibodies or immune lymphoid cells are produced against the body's own tissues. See also AUTOIMMUNE DISEASE.

conditioned r. see CONDITIONED RESPONSE.

dysfunctional ventilatory weaning r. a NURSING DIAGNOSIS adopted by the North American Nursing Diagnosis Association, defined as inability of a patient to adjust to lowered levels of mechanical ventilator support, which interrupts and prolongs the process of weaning. See also mechanical ventilatory WEANING.

galvanic skin r. the alteration in the electrical resistance of the skin associated with sympathetic nerve discharge.

immune r. see IMMUNE RESPONSE.

inflammatory r. the various changes that tissue undergoes when it becomes inflamed; see INFLAMMATION.

post-trauma r. former name for the nursing diagnosis POST-TRAUMA SYNDROME.

reticulocyte r. increase in the formation of RETICULOCYTES in response to a bone marrow stimulus.

triple r. (of Lewis) a physiologic reaction of the skin to stroking with a blunt instrument: first a red line develops at the site of stroking, owing to the release of histamine or a histamine-like substance, then a flare develops around the red line, and lastly a wheal is formed as a result of local edema.

unconditioned r. an unlearned response, i.e., one that occurs naturally, in contrast to a CONDITIONED RESPONSE.

responsibility (re-spon″si-bil′-i-te)   accountability; the condition of being required to account for one's actions.

corporate social r. a set of generally accepted relationships, obligations, and duties that relate to an institution's impact on the welfare of society.

rest (rest) 1. repose after exertion. 2. a fragment of embryonic tissue retained within the adult organism.

restenosis (re″stĕ-no′sis) recurrent stenosis, especially of a cardiac valve or coronary artery after surgical correction of the primary condition.

false r. stenosis recurring after failure to divide either commissure of a cardiac valve beyond the area of incision of the papillary muscles.

restiform (res′tĭ-form) shaped like a rope.

restitution (res″tĭ-too′shun) the spontaneous realignment of the fetal head with the fetal body, after delivery of the head.

restless legs syndrome unpleasant deep discomfort inside the calves when sitting or lying down, especially just before sleep, producing an irresistible urge to move the legs.

restlessness (rest′les-nes) an inability to achieve relaxation; a feeling of mild mental discomfort. Restlessness is frequently an early, subtle sign of a patient's deterioration.

restoration (res″to-ra′shun) 1. induction of a return to a previous state, as a return to health or replacement of a part to normal position. 2. filling. 3. partial or complete reconstruction of a body part. 4. the device used for such a reconstruction.

oral health r. in the NURSING INTERVENTIONS CLASSIFICATION, a nursing INTERVENTION defined as promotion of healing for a patient who has an oral mucosa or dental lesion.

restorative (rĕ-stor′ah-tiv) 1. promoting a return to health or to consciousness. 2. a remedy that aids in restoring health, vigor, or consciousness.

restraint (re-strānt′) the forcible confinement or control of a subject, as of a confused, disoriented, psychotic, or irrational person; it may be either physical or chemical. Restraint of any kind is used only when the patient's behavior presents a danger to himself or herself or another person. It is never used for the convenience of staff or as a substitute for conscientious nursing care.

Chemical restraint refers to the quieting of a violently psychotic or irrational person by means of medication. *Physical restraints* include restraining mitts to prevent removal of drainage tubes, restraints of upper and lower limbs to limit mobility and prevent the patient from climbing out of bed or physically harming someone at the bedside, and waist and body restraints such as a CAMISOLE (STRAITJACKET). Even though the patient might not fully understand the

need for restraint, a brief explanation of why it is being done should be given.

Assessment of the need for physical restraint includes a systematic determination of the level of confusion or disorientation exhibited by the patient and objective observations of his behavior. If possible, the cause of the patient's behavior should be identified, e.g., trauma, drug or alcohol intoxication, electrolyte imbalance, elevated temperature, pain, fear, or mental exhaustion. Findings of the assessment should be well documented in specific terms for legal reasons as well as to inform other caretakers and provide continuity of care.

Alternatives to physical restraint include reality orientation for disoriented patients

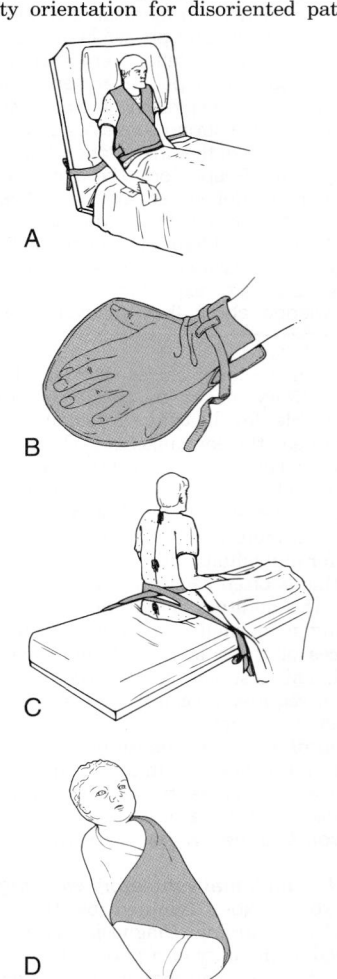

Types of restraints: *A,* Chest restraint; *B,* Hand mitt restraint; *C,* Belt restraint; *D,* Mummy restraint. From Lammon et al., 1996.

locks, radio, television, newspapers, and magazines will all aid patients to orient hemselves to reality); controlling the nvironment to minimize confusion and imulation (restraints can intensify anxiety nd confusion); and constant attendance at he bedside.

Since restraint of patients subjects them the HAZARDS OF IMMOBILITY, it is essential hat they be monitored closely, their vital gns checked regularly, and their position hanged at least every two hours. The use of estraints is an active area of nursing esearch. The most appropriate and least estrictive type of restraint should always e the one chosen.

jacket r. camisole.

physical r. 1. see RESTRAINT. 2. in the URSING INTERVENTIONS CLASSIFICATION, a ursing INTERVENTION defined as the applica- on, monitoring, and removal of mechanical estraining devices or manual restraints hich are used to limit the physical mobility f a patient.

restriction (re-strik′shun) 1. something hat limits; a limitation. 2. see restriction NDONUCLEASE.

area r. in the NURSING INTERVENTIONS LASSIFICATION, a nursing INTERVENTION de- ned as the limitation of patient mobility to specified area for purposes of safety or ehavior management.

fluid r. the limitation of oral fluid take to a prescribed amount for each 24- our period. This therapeutic measure is dicated in patients who have edema ssociated with kidney disease, such as ephrosis and glomerulonephritis, or Laën- ec's cirrhosis, and also in certain patients ith pulmonary edema.

PATIENT CARE. Approaches to the problem f discomfort from thirst and dryness of he mouth include careful distribution of the uid intake over the entire 24 hours in small, equent drinks; giving oral medications at ealtime, when not contraindicated, so as to low sips of liquid at other times; providing ld water for rinsing the mouth without wallowing between drinks; giving hard andy and chewing gum; and allowing atients to choose the fluids they prefer to rink. Frequent mouth care with a refresh- g mouthwash also is helpful.

restructuring (re-struk′choor-ing) alter- g the structure of something.

cognitive r. in the NURSING INTERVEN- IONS CLASSIFICATION, a nursing INTERVENTION efined as challenging a patient to alter istorted thought patterns and view self and he world more realistically.

resuscitation (re-sus″ĭ-ta′shun) 1. re- oration to life or CONSCIOUSNESS of one

apparently dead, or whose respirations had ceased; see also ARTIFICIAL RESPIRATION. 2. in the NURSING INTERVENTIONS CLASSIFICATION, a nursing INTERVENTION defined as administer- ing EMERGENCY measures to sustain life.

cardiopulmonary r. see CARDIOPULMO- NARY RESUSCITATION.

r.: fetus in the NURSING INTERVENTIONS CLASSIFICATION, a nursing INTERVENTION de- fined as administering emergency measures to improve placental perfusion or correct fetal acid-base status.

fluid r. 1. the correction of fluid volume imbalances, especially in patients with burn injuries. 2. in the NURSING INTERVENTIONS CLASSIFICATION, a nursing INTERVENTION de- fined as administering prescribed intrave- nous fluids rapidly.

mouth-to-mouth r. a method of ARTI- FICIAL RESPIRATION in which the rescuer covers the patient's mouth with his own and exhales vigorously, inflating the patient's lungs.

r.: neonate in the NURSING INTERVEN- TIONS CLASSIFICATION, a nursing INTERVENTION defined as administering EMERGENCY mea- sures to support adaptation of the NEONATE to extrauterine life.

resuscitator (rĕ-sus′ĭ-ta″tor) an appara- tus for initiating respiration in persons whose breathing has stopped.

retainer (re-tān′er) an appliance or device that keeps a tooth or partial denture in proper position.

matrix r. a mechanical device that clamps the ends of a matrix BAND and tightens it around a tooth.

Tofflemire r. a type of matrix retainer.

retardation (re″tahr-da′shun) delay; hin- drance; delayed development.

mental r. subnormal general intellec- tual development, associated with impair- ment of either learning and social adjustment, maturation, or both; see also MENTAL RETARDATION.

psychomotor r. a generalized slowing of physical and emotional reaction, such as that seen in major DEPRESSION and in cata- tonic SCHIZOPHRENIA.

retching (rech′ing) a strong involuntary effort to vomit.

rete (re′te) [L.] a NETWORK or PLEXUS.

arterial r., r. arterio′sum an anastomotic network of arterioles or minute arteries, just before they become capillaries.

articular r. a network of anastomosing blood vessels in or around a joint.

r. lymphocapilla′re any of the closed, freely communicating networks formed by the lymphocapillary vessels.

R

r. malpi'ghii the innermost stratum of epidermis.

r. mira'bile a vascular network formed by division of an artery or vein into many smaller vessels that reunite into a single vessel; in the human this occurs only in the arterioles that supply the glomeruli of the kidney.

r. tes'tis the network of channels formed in the mediastinum of the testis by the seminiferous tubules.

r. veno'sum an anastomotic network of small veins; called also venous network.

retention (re-ten'shun) 1. the process of holding back or keeping in a position. 2. persistence in the body of material normally excreted, such as from the bowel or bladder. 3. the number of staff members in a facility that remain in employment.

urinary r. a NURSING DIAGNOSIS accepted by the North American Nursing Diagnosis Association, defined as a state in which an individual has incomplete emptying of the bladder.

r. of urine accumulation of urine within the bladder because of inability to urinate.

reteplase (ret'ĕ-plās) a recombinant form of tissue plasminogen ACTIVATOR; used intravenously as a THROMBOLYTIC agent in treatment of myocardial infarction.

reticular (rĕ-tik'u-lar) resembling a net.

r. activating system the system of cells of the reticular formation of the medulla oblongata that receive collaterals from the ascending sensory pathways and project to higher centers; they control the overall degree of central nervous system activity, including wakefulness, attentiveness, and sleep; abbreviated RAS.

reticulated (rĕ-tik'u-lāt''ed) reticular.

reticulation (rĕ-tik''u-la'shun) the formation or presence of a network.

reticulin (rĕ-tik'u-lin) a scleroprotein present in the connective fibers of reticular tissue, closely related to collagen in composition.

reticulocyte (rĕ-tik'u-lo-sīt'') a young erythrocyte showing a basophilic reticulum under vital staining.

reticulocytopenia (rĕ-tik''u-lo-si''to-pe'ne-ah) a deficiency of reticulocytes in the peripheral blood.

reticulocytosis (rĕ-tik''u-lo-si-to'sis) an excess of reticulocytes in the peripheral blood.

reticuloendothelial (rĕ-tik''u-lo-en''do-the'le-al) pertaining to the reticuloendothelium or to the reticuloendothelial system.

r. system a network of cells and tissues found throughout the body, especially in the blood, general connective tissue, spleen, liver, lungs, bone marrow, and lymph node They have both endothelial and reticula attributes and the ability to take up colloid. dye particles. Some of the reticuloendothelia cells found in the blood and in the gener. connective tissue are unusually large in siz These cells are concerned with blood ce formation and destruction, storage of fatt materials, and metabolism of iron and pi; ment, and they play a role in inflammatio and immunity. Some of the cells are motile that is, capable of spontaneous motion—an phagocytic—they can ingest and destro unwanted foreign material.

The reticuloendothelial cells of the SPLEE possess the ability to dispose of disint grated erythrocytes. They do not, howeve destroy hemoglobin, which is liberated i the process.

The reticuloendothelial cells located i the blood cavities of the LIVER are calle Kupffer cells. These cells, together with th cells of the general connective tissue an bone marrow, are capable of transformir into bile pigment the hemoglobin release by disintegrated erythrocytes.

reticuloendothelioma (rĕ-tik''u-lo-en''de the''le-o'-mah) malignant lymphoma.

reticuloendotheliosis (rĕ-tik''u-lo-en''do the''le-o'sis) hyperplasia of reticuloendoth lial tissue.

leukemic r. hairy cell leukemia.

reticuloendothelium (rĕ-tik''u-lo-en''d the'le-um) the tissue of the RETICULOEI DOTHELIAL SYSTEM.

reticulohistiocytoma (rĕ-tik'u-lo-his''te-(si-to'-mah) a granulomatous aggregation (lipid-laden histiocytes and multinucleate giant cells.

reticuloma (rĕ-tik''u-lo'mah) histiocyt lymphoma.

reticulopenia (rĕ-tik''u-lo-pe'ne-ah) reti ulocytopenia.

reticulosis (rĕ-tik''u-lo'sis) an abnorm increase in cells derived from or related 1 the reticuloendothelial CELLS.

familial histiocytic r., histiocytic mec ullary r. a fatal hereditary disorder marke by anemia, granulocytopenia, thron bocytopenia, phagocytosis of blood cell diffuse proliferation of histiocytes, and e largement of the liver, spleen, and lymp nodes.

midline malignant r. lethal midlir granuloma thought to be due to lymphom

pagetoid r. a solitary skin lesion (long duration and slow growth characte ized histologically by large numbers (abnormal mononuclear cells infiltrating th epidermis with an underlying reactiv mixed dermal infiltrate.

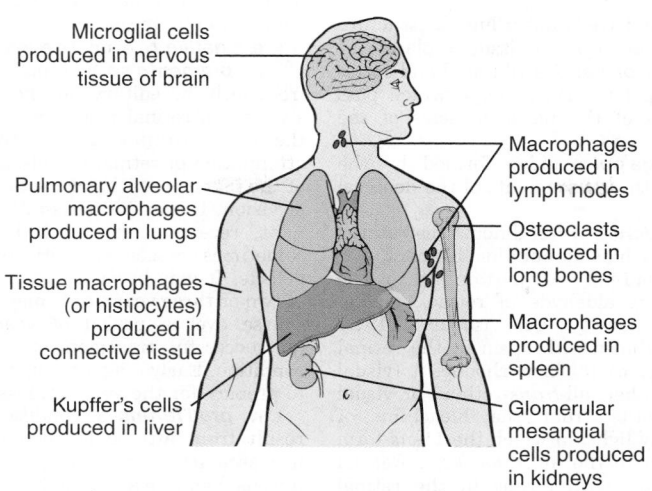

Microglial cells produced in nervous tissue of brain

Pulmonary alveolar macrophages produced in lungs

Tissue macrophages (or histiocytes) produced in connective tissue

Kupffer's cells produced in liver

Macrophages produced in lymph nodes

Osteoclasts produced in long bones

Macrophages produced in spleen

Glomerular mesangial cells produced in kidneys

Reticuloendothelial system. From Frazier et al., 1996.

reticulum (rĕ-tĭk′u-lum) [L.] 1. a small network, especially a protoplasmic network in cells. 2. reticular tissue.

agranular r. smooth-surfaced endoplasmic reticulum.

endoplasmic r. an ultramicroscopic organelle of nearly all higher plant and animal cells, consisting of a system of membrane-bound cavities in the cytoplasm, occurring in two types: granular or rough-surfaced, bearing large numbers of ribosomes on its outer surface, and agranular or smooth-surfaced.

granular r. rough-surfaced endoplasmic reticulum.

sarcoplasmic r. a form of agranular reticulum in the sarcoplasm of striated muscle, comprising a system of smooth-surfaced tubules surrounding each myofibril.

retiform (re′tĭ-form, ret′ĭ-form) reticular.

retina (ret′ĭ-nah) the innermost of the three tunics of the EYE, surrounding the vitreous body and continuous posteriorly with the optic nerve. The retina is composed of light-sensitive neurons arranged in three layers; the first layer is made up of rods and cones and the other two transmit impulses from the rods and cones to the OPTIC NERVE. The rods are sensitive in dim light, and the cones are sensitive in bright light and are responsible for color vision.

Disorders of the Retina. RETINOPATHIES are pathologic conditions of the retina; they occur in conjunction with certain systemic disorders, such as hypertension, nephritis, toxemia of pregnancy, and diabetes mellitus.

DETACHMENT OF THE RETINA is complete or partial separation of the retina from the choroid, the middle coat of the eyeball. It occurs most often in persons with MYOPIA (nearsightedness), but it also can result from trauma to the head.

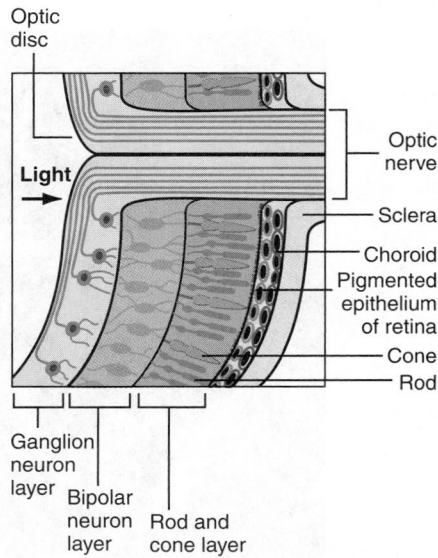

Optic disc

Light

Optic nerve

Sclera

Choroid

Pigmented epithelium of retina

Cone

Rod

Ganglion neuron layer

Bipolar neuron layer

Rod and cone layer

Structure of the retina showing the rods and cones. From Applegate, 2000.

R

retinaculum (ret″ĭ-nak′u-lum) a structure that retains an organ or tissue in place.

flexor r. of hand a fibrous band forming the carpal tunnel, through which pass the tendons of the flexor muscles of the hand and fingers.

r. morga′gni a ridge formed by the coming together of segments of the ileocecal valve.

r. ten′dinum a tendinous restraining structure, such as an annular ligament.

retinal (ret′ĭ-nal) 1. pertaining to the retina. 2. the aldehyde of retinol, having vitamin A activity. One isomer (11-*cis*-retinal) combines with opsin in the retinal rods (scotopsin) to form rhodopsin (visual purple); another, all-*trans*-retinal, or visual yellow, results from the bleaching of rhodopsin by light, in which the 11-*cis* form is converted to the all-*trans* form. Retinal also combines with opsins in the retinal cones to form the three pigments responsible for color vision.

retinene (ret′ĭ-nēn) an ocular pigment derived from vitamin A and formed by the bleaching action of light on rhodopsin. It occurs in two forms: retinene$_1$ is retinal (def. 2), and retinene$_2$ is dehydroretinal.

retinitis (ret″ĭ-ni′tis) inflammation of the retina.

r. circina′ta, circinate r. circinate retinopathy.

cytomegalovirus r. opportunistic infection of the retina by CYTOMEGALOVIRUS, seen in IMMUNOCOMPROMISED patients; symptoms include retinal necrosis and hemorrhage, leading to blindness.

exudative r. exudative RETINOPATHY.

r. pigmento′sa a group of diseases, frequently hereditary, marked by progressive loss of retinal response (as recorded by the ELECTRORETINOGRAPH), retinal atrophy, attenuation of retinal vessels, and clumping of the pigment, with contraction of the field of vision. It may be transmitted as a dominant, recessive, or X-linked trait and is sometimes associated with other genetic defects. It may become manifest at the age of two or three years, or it may follow a slow course over a period of years. There is no successful treatment or cure for the condition. Early diagnosis allows the patient to prepare for the eventual loss of vision.

r. proli′ferans a condition that may result from intraocular hemorrhage, with neovascularization and the formation of fibrous bands extending into the vitreous from the retina; retinal detachment may result.

suppurative r. retinitis due to pyemic infection.

retinoblastoma (ret″ĭ-no-blas-to′mah) a malignant congenital hereditary blastoma composed of retinal cells arising from the nuclear layers, appearing in one or both eyes in children under 5 years of age, and usually diagnosed initially by a bright white or yellow pupillary reflex (leukokoria).

retinochoroiditis (ret″ĭ-no-kor″oi-di′tis) inflammation of the retina and choroid.

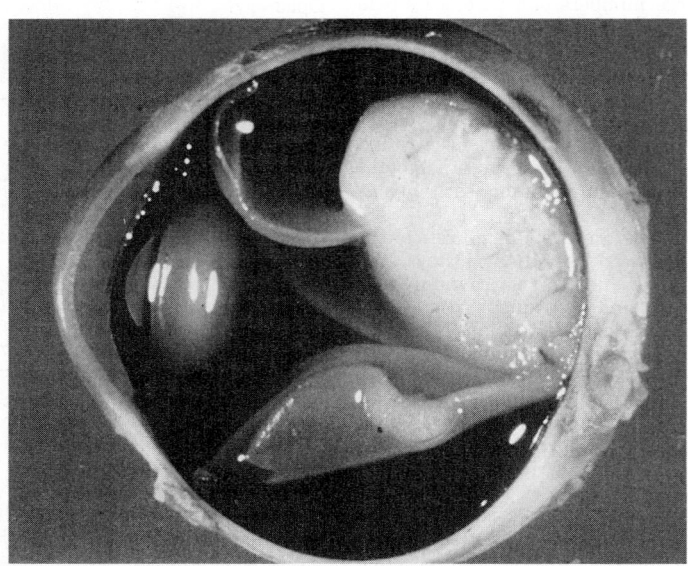

Section of an eye showing a retinoblastoma in situ. From Mueller and Young, 2001.

r. juxtapapilla′ris a small area of inflammation on the fundus of the eye near the papilla; seen in young healthy individuals.

retinoic acid (ret″ĭ-no′ik) an oxidized derivative of RETINOL, believed to be the form of vitamin A that plays a role in the development and growth of bone and in the maintenance of normal epithelial structures. The all-*trans* isomer is called TRETINOIN and used as a KERATOLYTIC and antineoplastic AGENT. The 13-*cis* isomer is called ISOTRETINOIN and used as a treatment for acne.

retinoid (ret′ĭ-noid) 1. resembling the retina. 2. RETINAL, RETINOL, or any structurally similar natural derivative or synthetic compound, with or without vitamin A activity.

retinol (ret′ĭ-nol) vitamin A_1; the form of vitamin A found in mammals, which is reversibly dehydrogenated by enzymatic action into its aldehyde, retinal. See VITAMIN.

retinomalacia (ret″ĭ-no-mah-la′shah) softening of the retina.

retinopapillitis(ret″ĭ-no-pap″ĭ-li′tis)inflammation of retina and optic disk (papilla).

retinopathy (ret″ĭ-nop′ah-the) any noninflammatory disease of the retina.

central serous r. a usually self-limiting condition marked by acute localized detachment of the neural retina or retinal pigment epithelium in the region of the macula, with hypermetropia.

circinate r. a condition marked by a circle of white spots enclosing the macular area, leading to complete foveal blindness.

diabetic r. retinal manifestations of DIABETES MELLITUS, including MICROANEURYSMS and punctate exudates. There are two major forms of diabetic retinopathy, *nonproliferative* and *proliferative*. The nonproliferative form is characterized by dilation of the retinal veins and microaneurysms which may leak blood cells and/or plasma, causing internal hemorrhaging or edema in the retina. Edema in peripheral areas of the retina goes unnoticed by the patient and may go untreated, whereas edema occurring in the central retina (macula) causes noticeably decreased vision and is the primary cause of vision loss in nonproliferative disease. (See Atlas 4, Part D.) Treatment by local laser PHOTOCOAGULATION is aimed at sealing shut the breaks in the blood vessels and preventing additional leakage of fluid into the area. Early diagnosis and treatment are essential in this disease to enhance a final visual outcome of stabilization and prevention of further loss of vision.

In proliferative diabetic retinopathy new blood vessels form near the optic disk, break through the inner membranous lining, and grow on the vitreous chamber and elsewhere in the retina and may rupture, causing gross vitreous hemorrhage. Additionally, fibrous tissue is generated secondary to the new blood vessel formation, and both the fibrous tissue and the new blood vessels become firmly attached to the posterior vitreous face. As the vitreous humor moves, the blood vessels and fibrous tissue cause tractional pulling on the retina and may result in separation or detachment of areas of retina. Panretinal laser photocoagulation is the definitive therapy. The study of early treatment for diabetic retinopathy proved the efficacy of this procedure in causing regression of the new blood vessels and prevention of vitreous hemorrhage and tractional retinal detachments, the two major causes of vision loss from this form of the disease.

exudative r. a condition marked by masses of white or yellowish exudate in the posterior part of the fundus oculi, with deposits of cholestrin and blood debris from retinal hemorrhage, and leading to destruction of the macula and blindness.

hemorrhagic r. retinopathy marked by profuse hemorrhaging in the retina, occurring in diabetes, occlusion of the central vein, and hypertension.

hypertensive r. that associated with essential HYPERTENSION; changes may include irregular narrowing of the retinal arterioles, hemorrhages in the nerve fiber layers and the outer plexiform layer, exudates and cotton-wool patches, arteriosclerotic changes, and, in malignant HYPERTENSION, PAPILLEDEMA. (See also Atlas 4, Part C.)

leukemic r. a condition occurring in leukemia, with paleness of the fundus resulting from infiltration of the retina and choroid with leukocytes, and swelling of the disk with blurring of its margin.

r. of prematurity a disease of the developing retinal vasculature of the premature newborn. The incidence correlates with degree of prematurity; that is, the more premature the infant is, the greater the possibility of this condition occurring. The cause is vasoconstriction of retinal capillaries due to the presence of very high concentrations of oxygen in these blood vessels, which produces an overgrowth of retinal blood vessels. The vascular proliferation and exudation of blood and serum detaches the retina and produces scarring and inevitable blindness. To prevent retinopathy of prematurity it is recommended that oxygen be administered to premature newborns in as low a concentration and for as short a time as feasible. Careful monitoring of the newborn and evaluation of oxygen tension level are essential because no totally safe dosage of oxygen that will prevent the retinal changes has been found. Called also retrolental fibroplasia.

proliferative r. the proliferative type of diabetic retinopathy.

retinopexy (ret′in-o-pek″se) restoring of the RETINA to its proper anatomical location.

pneumatic r. a treatment for retinal DETACHMENT involving injection of gas into the posterior vitreous cavity in such a way that the gas bubble presses against the area of torn retina, forcing it back into place.

retinoschisis (ret″ĭ-nos′kĭ-sis) splitting of the retina, occurring in the nerve fiber layer (in juvenile form), or in the external plexiform layer (in adult form).

retinoscope (ret′ĭ-no-skōp″) skiascope; an instrument used in retinoscopy.

retinoscopy (ret″ĭ-nos′kah-pe) an objective method of investigating, diagnosing, and evaluating refractive errors of the eye, by projection of a beam of light into the eye and observation of the movement of the illuminated area on the retinal surface and of the refraction by the eye of the emergent rays. Called also pupilloscopy and shadow test.

book r. a type in which the patient focuses on reading a book; commonly used with children.

dynamic r. a type in which the patient fixes the gaze on a target at a near distance; ACCOMMODATION is active.

mem r. a type of dynamic RETINOSCOPY in which the fixation target is a series of letters on the RETINOSCOPE, or a card with letters at a normal reading distance.

Nott r. a type of dynamic RETINOSCOPY in which the fixation target is 40 cm from the eye; the test is first done with the object farther away than the target distance, and then continued while moving it towards the patient until neutrality is observed.

static r. a type in which the patient fixes the gaze on a target at a long distance in order to relax ACCOMMODATION.

retinosis (ret″ĭ-no′sis) any degenerative, noninflammatory condition of the retina.

retinotopic (ret″ĭ-no-top′ik) relating to the organization of the visual pathways and visual area of the brain.

retothelium (re″to-the′le-um) reticuloendothelium.

retr(o)- word element [L.], *behind; backward.*

retractile (re-trak′til) susceptible of being drawn back.

retraction (re-trak′shun) the act of drawing back, or condition of being drawn back.

clot r. the drawing away of a blood clot from the wall of a vessel, a stage of wound healing caused by contraction of platelets; it is a function of blood platelets that can be tested to assess platelet viability.

retractor (re-trak′tor) 1. an instrument for holding open the edges of a wound or drawing back structures. 2. a muscle that draws a part back.

retrieval (re-tre′val) in psychology, the process of obtaining memory information from wherever it has been stored.

retroaction (ret″ro-ak′shun) action in a reversed direction; reaction.

retroauricular (ret″ro-aw-rik′u-lar) behind the auricle of the ear.

retrobulbar (ret″ro-bul′bar) 1. behind the pons. 2. behind the eyeball.

retrocervical (ret″ro-ser′vĭ-kal) behind the cervix uteri.

retrocession (ret″ro-sesh′un) a going backward; backward displacement.

retrocochlear (ret″ro-kok′le-ar) 1. behind the cochlea. 2. denoting the eighth cranial nerve and cerebellopontine angle as opposed to the cochlea.

retrocollic (ret″ro-kol′ik) 1. nuchal. 2. pertaining to torticollis.

retrocollis (ret″ro-kol′is) spasmodic torticollis in which the head is drawn back.

retrocursive (ret″ro-ker′siv) marked by stepping backward.

retrodeviation (ret″ro-de″ve-a′shun) any displacement backwards; the term includes RETROVERSION, RETROFLEXION, and other deviations. Called also retrodisplacement and retroposition.

retrodisplacement (ret″ro-dis-plās′ment) retrodeviation.

retrofilling (ret′ro-fil″ing) a method of root canal THERAPY in which the canal is filled from the apex, which has been surgically exposed.

retrofitting (ret′ro-fit″ing) the architectural modification of a building to meet current standards, particularly regarding access for the handicapped.

retroflexion (ret″ro-flek′shun) the bending of an organ or part so that its top is thrust backward, such as bending backward of the body of the uterus upon the cervix.

retrogasserian (ret″ro-gah-se′re-an) pertaining to the sensory (posterior) root of the trigeminal (gasserian) ganglion.

retrognathia (ret″ro-nath′e-ah) retrognathism.

retrognathism (ret″ro-nath′izm) retrusion of the mandible. Called also retrognathia. adj., **retrognath′ic.**

retrograde (ret′ro-grād) 1. moving backward or against the usual direction of flow 2. degenerating, deteriorating, or catabolic.

retrogression (ret″ro-gresh′un) degeneration; deterioration; regression; return to an earlier, less complex condition.

retrolental (ret″ro-len′tal) behind the lens of the eye.

retromorphosis (ret″ro-mor-fo′sis) retrograde metamorphosis.

retroparotid (ret″ro-pah-rot′id) behind the parotid gland.

retroperitoneal (ret″ro-per″ĭ-to-ne′al) behind the peritoneum.

retroperitoneum (ret″ro-per″ĭ-to-ne′um) the retroperitoneal space; the space between the peritoneum and the posterior abdominal wall.

retroperitonitis (ret″ro-per″ĭ-to-ni′tis) inflammation in the retroperitoneal space.

retropharyngitis (ret″ro-far″in-ji′tis) inflammation of posterior part of the pharynx.

retroplasia (ret″ro-pla′zhah) retrograde METAPLASIA; degeneration of a tissue or cell into a more primitive type.

retroposed (ret″ro-pōzd′) displaced backward.

retroposition (ret″ro-po-zish′un) retrodeviation.

retropulsion (ret″ro-pul′shun) 1. a driving back, as of the fetal head in labor. 2. tendency to walk backward, as in some cases of tabes dorsalis. 3. an abnormal gait in which the body is bent backward.

retroversion (ret″ro-ver′zhun) the tipping backward of an entire organ or part, as of the uterus.

retrovesical (ret″ro-ves′ĭ-kal) behind the urinary bladder.

Retrovir (ret′ro-vir) trademark for preparations of ZIDOVUDINE, an ANTIRETROVIRAL active against the human immunodeficiency VIRUS.

retrovirus (ret′ro-vi″rus) any member of a large family of RNA viruses that includes the LENTIVIRUSES and certain ONCOVIRUSES, given this name because they carry REVERSE TRANSCRIPTASE.

 human endogenous r's (HERV) retroviruslike sequences found in the human genome, thought to constitute the remains of true retroviruses that were absorbed through evolution; at least one is thought to be linked to expression of tumor cells.

retrusion (re-troo′zhun) the state of being located posterior to the normal position, such as the mandible or a tooth displaced in the line of occlusion.

Rett syndrome (ret) a PERVASIVE DEVELOPMENTAL DISORDER affecting the gray matter of the brain, occurring exclusively in females and present from birth; it is characterized by autistic behavior, ataxia, dementia, seizures, and loss of purposeful use of the hands, with cerebral atrophy, mild

hyperammonemia, and decreased levels of biogenic amines.

return (re-tern′) a coming back.

 venous r. the flow of blood into the heart from the peripheral vessels.

reuptake (re-up′tāk) reabsorption of a previously secreted substance.

revascularization (re-vas″ku-lah-rĭ-za′-shun) 1. the restoration of blood supply, as after a wound. 2. the restoration of an adequate blood supply to a part by means of a blood vessel graft, as in aortocoronary bypass.

reversal (re-ver′sal) a turning or change in the opposite direction.

 sex r. a change in characteristics from those typical of one sex to those typical of the other.

reverse transcriptase (re-vers′ tran-skrip′tās) an enzyme of RNA VIRUSES that catalyzes the transcription of RNA to DNA, which is then incorporated into the GENOME of the host cell. This is the reverse of the usual mechanism for replication of genetic information; in the presence of this enzyme it is the RNA that serves as the template for DNA copies. It is one mechanism by which reproduction of cancer cells is facilitated. Called also RNA-directed DNA polymerase.

reversible obstructive airway disease a condition characterized by bronchospasm reversible by intervention, as in ASTHMA.

reversion (re-ver′zhun) a returning to a previous condition; regression.

review (re-vu′) an assessment or appraisal.

 peer r. an evaluation by one's peers; see also PEER REVIEW.

 r. of symptoms a detailed assessment of each body system, performed to ascertain the presence of deviations from normal.

revulsion (re-vul′shun) the drawing of blood from one part to another, as occurs in COUNTERIRRITATION.

Reye's syndrome (rīz) an acute, potentially fatal disease of childhood, characterized by severe edema of the brain and increased intracranial pressure, hypoglycemia, and fatty infiltration and dysfunction of the liver. The cause is unknown, but it is almost always associated with a previous viral infection. In the United States, the most frequently reported viral diseases present prior to the development of Reye's syndrome are INFLUENZA type B and CHICKENPOX (varicella). At least 14 other viruses are known to have preceded Reye's syndrome. The relationship between these infections and the typical pathologic changes in the brain and liver is not yet clear. However,

R

there is an association between the administration of aspirin for acute febrile illnesses, particularly influenza and varicella, and the subsequent development of Reye's syndrome. Reye's syndrome was once among the ten major causes of death in children over one year of age. A massive public health campaign was undertaken to warn of the danger of giving aspirin to children with influenza or varicella, and Reye's syndrome now occurs only rarely. Some scientists believe that the disorder was misdiagnosed in the past and that it has always been a major viral disease of children. The prognosis for the disease has been greatly improved with better recognition in its earliest stages and improved modes of therapy.

SYMPTOMS. Within several hours to several days after a viral infection the child suddenly develops persistent vomiting, begins to show signs of encephalopathy, and becomes listless, lethargic, and unusually quiet. As intracranial pressure increases the child may become more agitated, irritable, and delirious. In its severest form the disorder causes convulsions and coma. There are no meningeal or focal neurologic signs present, and the cerebrospinal fluid is normal.

Treatment. Treatment is aimed at the correction of the hypoglycemia, acidosis, and electrolyte imbalance. Measures are employed to reduce intracranial pressure and to correct metabolic abnormalities. There is no specific medication or treatment that will cure the disease. The child must be monitored continuously, and the fluid imbalances and increased intracranial pressure must be corrected as soon as possible to avoid permanent brain damage. The sooner treatment is initiated the better the prognosis.

Reduction in the mortality rate, which has been reported as low as 25 per cent and as high as 80 per cent, is believed to be the result of increased awareness of the disease, earlier diagnosis, and improved modes of therapy.

Additional information about Reye's syndrome and medical facilities equipped to handle the disease can be obtained by calling or writing to the National Reye's Syndrome Foundation, P.O. Box 829, Bryan, OH 43805, (419) 636–2679.

RFA right frontoanterior (position of the fetus).

RfD reference dose.

RFP right frontoposterior (position of the fetus).

RFT right frontotransverse (position of the fetus).

Rh 1. rhodium. 2. symbol for Rhesus factor (see RH FACTOR).

Rh$_{null}$ symbol for a rare blood type in which all Rh factors are lacking.

rhabd(o)- word element [Gr.], *rod; rod-shaped.*

Rhabditis (rab-di'tis) a genus of minute nematodes found mostly in damp earth, and as an accidental PARASITE in humans.

rhabdoid (rab'doid) resembling a rod; rod-shaped.

rhabdomyoblastoma (rab″do-mi″o-blas-to'mah) rhabdomyosarcoma.

rhabdomyolysis (rab″do-mi-ol'ĭ-sis) disintegration of striated muscle FIBERS with excretion of MYOGLOBIN in the urine. See also CRUSH SYNDROME.

rhabdomyoma (rab″do-mi-o'mah) a tumor containing striated muscle fibers.

rhabdomyosarcoma (rab″do-mi″o-sahr-ko'mah) a highly malignant tumor arising in striated muscle or in embryonal mesenchymal cells that exhibit differentiation along rhabdomyoblastic lines, including but not limited to the presence of cells with recognizable cross striations. The pleomorphic form affects predominantly the skeletal muscles of adults; the embryonal-alveolar form occurs mainly in the skeletal muscles of children and young adults, and the embryonal-botryoid form occurs predominantly in tissues of the head, neck, orbit, and urogenital tract of children and young adults.

rhabdosarcoma (rab″do-sahr-ko'mah) rhabdomyosarcoma.

rhabdosphincter (rab'do-sfink″ter) a sphincter consisting of striated muscle fibers.

rhabdovirus (rab'do-vi″rus) any of a family of bullet-shaped or bacilliform RNA viruses;one genus, *Lyssavirus,* includes the rabies VIRUS.

rhachi- for words beginning thus, see those beginning *rachi-.*

rhagades (rag'ah-dēz) fissures, cracks, or fine scars in the skin, especially such lesions around the mouth or other regions subjected to frequent movement.

rhaphe (ra'fe) raphe.

rhe(o)- word element [Gr.], *electric current; flow* (as of fluids).

rhegma (reg'mah) a rupture, rent, or fracture.

rhegmatogenous (reg″mah-toj'ĕ-nus) arising from a rhegma, as rhegmatogenous detachment of the retina.

rhenium (re'ne-um) a chemical element, atomic number 75, atomic weight 186.2, symbol Re. (See Appendix 6.)

rheobase (re'o-bās) the minimal electric current of infinite duration necessary to produce a twitch in a muscle. In a

trength-duration CURVE for muscle stimula-
ion, it is the voltage at which there is no
urther decrease in threshold when the
ulse WIDTH or duration is increased.

rheology (re-ol′ah-je) the science of the
eformation and flow of matter, such as the
low of blood through the heart and blood
essels.

rheostat (re′o-stat) an apparatus for reg-
lating resistance in an electric circuit.

rheostosis (re″os-to′sis) a condition of
yperostosis marked by the presence of
treaks in the bones; melorheostosis.

rheotaxis (re″o-tak′sis) orientation of an
rganism in a stream of liquid, with its long
xis parallel with the direction of flow, desig-
ated negative (moving in the same direction)
r positive (moving in the opposite direction).

rheum (rōōm) any watery or catarrhal
ischarge.

rheumarthritis (roo″mahr-thri′tis) rheu-
natoid arthritis.

rheumatalgia (roo″mah-tal′jah) chronic
heumatic pain.

rheumatic (roo-mat′ik) pertaining to or
ffected with RHEUMATISM.

   r. fever a disease associated with the
resence of hemolytic STREPTOCOCCI in the
ody. It is called rheumatic fever because two
ommon symptoms are fever and pain in the
ints similar to that of RHEUMATISM. It is
elatively common, particularly in children
etween 5 and 15 years old; young adults in
he early twenties are also susceptible.

Causes. Rheumatic fever is a delayed se-
uela of an upper respiratory infection
aused by the Group A hemolytic streptococ-
us that causes such common childhood
lnesses as SCARLET FEVER, TONSILLITIS, STREP-
OCOCCAL SORE THROAT ("strep throat"), and
ar infections. It is only one of several com-
lications that can result from a strepto-
occal infection.

The connection between rheumatic fever
nd a previous streptococcal infection has
een proved only indirectly. In almost all
ases of rheumatic fever there is evidence of
revious streptococcal infection, and when
he infection is treated promptly, the like-
hood of rheumatic fever decreases sharply.
There is evidence that the symptoms of
heumatic fever may result from an
NTIGEN-ANTIBODY REACTION to one or more of
he products of the hemolytic streptococcus,
ut the exact way this happens is not
nown. Rheumatic fever has been classified
s an AUTOIMMUNE DISEASE. It tends to run in
amilies, indicating a possible hereditary
redisposition. Economic and environmen-
al conditions such as a damp, cold climate
nd poor health habits may also be con-
ributing factors.

Pathogenesis of rheumatic fever. Following infection
("strep throat"), an immune response elicited by the
streptococci acts on the heart and several other organs,
most notably the joints, skin, and central nervous system.
In the heart, it causes endocarditis, myocarditis, and
pericarditis. From Damjanov, 2000.

Symptoms. The initial symptoms usually
appear 1 to 4 weeks after the streptococcal
infection has occurred. The actual onset of
the disease may be either gradual or sudden.
The symptoms vary widely and may be of
any degree of severity. The most common
initial complaints are a slight fever, a
feeling of tiredness, a vague feeling of pain
in the limbs, and nosebleeds. If the disease
takes an acute form, the fever may reach
40°C (104°F) by the second day and continue for several weeks, although the usual
course of the fever is about 2 weeks. On the
other hand, the fever may be quite mild.

Joint pain develops at any stage of the
disease and lasts from a few hours to several
weeks. The joints swell and are tender to

the touch. The pain and swelling often subside in one group of joints and arise in another. As the pain subsides, the joints return to normal.

Other symptoms may include the spasmodic twitching movements known as SYDENHAM'S CHOREA, especially in girls between the ages of 6 and 11. A rash caused by the fever may appear upon the body. Nodules may be seen or felt under the skin at the elbow, knee, and wrist joints, and along the spine. Among the most serious signs is the development of a heart murmur and cardiac decompensation.

HEART DAMAGE. The seriousness of rheumatic fever lies primarily in the permanent damage it can do to the heart. The disease tends to recur, and the recurrent attacks may further weaken the heart. The usual cardiac complication is ENDOCARDITIS (inflammation of the inner lining of the heart, including the membrane over the valves). As a valve heals, its edges may become so scarred and stiff that they fail to close properly. As a result, blood leaks through the valve when it is closed, producing the sound characteristic of a heart murmur. The valves may become thickened with scar tissue, so that the amount of blood that can flow through the heart is restricted. If there is severe stenosis of the mitral valve and the patient develops symptoms of congestive HEART FAILURE, surgery to enlarge the valve (mitral COMMISSUROTOMY) may be indicated.

Treatment. The main purposes of treatment are reduction of fever and pain and promotion of the natural healing processes; no means have yet been discovered for fighting the disease directly. Until the introduction of antibiotics and steroids, the chief medications were aspirin and other salicylates. Penicillin is prescribed if there is evidence of an ongoing streptococcal infection or the chance of exposure to streptococcal infection. Prednisone may be prescribed to reduce the pain and swelling in the joints, but its effect on the ultimate course of the disease is controversial. If pain is severe, analgesic drugs may be given. Bed rest is an important part of the treatment, particularly if the disease has caused heart damage. Depending upon the severity of the disease, the patient may be kept in bed for months, and prolonged convalescence may be needed.

Patient Care. In the acute phase of rheumatic fever rest is most important to reduce the work load of the heart. The patient should be made as comfortable as possible and disturbed only when necessary. The care should be planned so that long periods of

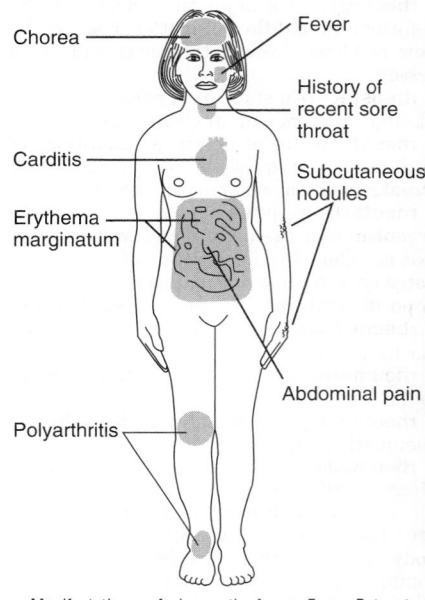

Manifestations of rheumatic fever. From Betz et al 1994.

complete rest are possible. Proper positioning with adequate support of the limbs and maintenance of good body alignment essential to rest and the prevention of complications.

The temperature, pulse, and respiration are checked and recorded at least every hours during the day. The volume and rhythm as well as the rate of the pulse should be noted. The blood pressure taken at least once a day. Fluid intake may be restricted if there is edema, and sodium intake may also be limited; in either case the reason for the restriction should be explained to the patient. A record is kept of the intake and output.

Frequent back care and good oral hygiene are needed to promote comfort and relaxation. When turning the patient, one should be gentle and slow, avoiding unnecessary handling of the joints, which may be tender and swollen.

During the convalescent period the patient is allowed a gradual return to physical activities. The amount of activity depends on the physician's orders and is based on the patient's pulse rate, erythrocyte sedimentation rate, and C-reaction protein test. Measures must be taken to avoid espiratory infections, which will retard the progress of the patient. Small, frequent feedings that provide a well-balanced diet re usually preferred to three meals a day, which may be only partially eaten by a patient who is not engaging in a normal mount of physical activity.

As the need for rest is decreased, some provision must be made for diversional activities that will help eliminate boredom and keep the child content. The psychologic effects of a prolonged period of enforced dependence on others must also be considered. The parents and the child will need encouragement and help in the transition from total dependence to relative independence. Parents and family members also will need support and guidance during adjustment to home care of the child. Referral to the public health nurse or home health care agency can help provide continuity of care and continued support.

Prevention. Preventive care is extremely important, especially when rheumatic fever has once occurred, since it tends to return unless precautionary steps are taken. The patient is given penicillin, orally every day or by intramuscular injection once a month, for many years in order to prevent streptococcal infection. A good nutritious diet and sufficient sleep are important. Administration of antibiotics to all patients with history of rheumatic fever undergoing even minor surgery, including tooth extraction, is important in preventing bacterial endocarditis. Prompt and effective treatment of "strep throat" among the general population has reduced the incidence of rheumatic fever.

    r. heart disease the most important and constant manifestation of RHEUMATIC FEVER, consisting of inflammatory changes with valvular deformities.

rheumatid (roo′mah-tid) any skin lesion biologically associated with rheumatism.

rheumatism (roo′mah-tizm) popular but indefinite term for any of a variety of disorders marked by inflammation, degeneration, or metabolic derangement of connective tissue structures (especially joints and related structures), with pain, stiffness, or limitation of motion; it includes such disorders as ARTHRITIS, OSTEOARTHRITIS, BURSITIS, and SCIATICA.

    desert r. the primary form of COCCIDIOIDOMYCOSIS.

    muscular r. fibrositis.

    palindromic r. repeated attacks of arthritis and periarthritis without fever and without causing irreversible joint changes.

rheumatoid (roo′mah-toid) resembling rheumatism.

    r. disease rheumatoid ARTHRITIS with emphasis on nonarticular changes, e.g., pulmonary interstitial fibrosis, pleural effusion, and lung nodules.

rheumatologist (roo″mah-tol′ah-jist) a specialist in rheumatology.

rheumatology (roo″mah-tol′ah-je) the branch of medicine dealing with rheumatic disorders, their causes, pathology, diagnosis, treatment, and other aspects.

rhexis (rek′sis) the rupture of a blood vessel or of an organ.

Rh factor genetically determined antigens (agglutinogens) present on the surface of ERYTHROCYTES. There are at least eight different variations, each being called an Rh factor (named for the rhesus monkey used in early experiments). If one of these factors is present in an individual's erythrocytes, the blood type is Rh positive (D positive, Rh_0); if the factor is absent the blood type is Rh negative (D negative, dd, or Hr_0). Approximately 85 per cent of all Caucasian people are Rh positive and 15 per cent are Rh negative; other races may have different percentages.

The presence or absence of an Rh factor is especially important in blood transfusions because mixing of two types of blood may result in the agglutination (clumping together) of red blood cells, with plugging of the capillaries and destruction of the red blood cells. This agglutination is an immune reaction and depends on the formation of antibodies against the specific agglutinogen (Rh factor) present on the erythrocytes and in transfused blood. It should be pointed out that this immune reaction does not occur immediately, but depends on the gradual formation of antibodies; the response also is more severe in some persons than in others. Thus there may be no difficulty in the first transfusion of Rh incompatible blood, but on repeated exposure to the Rh factor, the Rh-negative individual becomes "sensitized" to the agglutinogens in Rh positive blood and builds up a greater quantity of antibodies.

In pregnancy difficulty may arise when the mother is Rh negative and the fetus is Rh-positive. The Rh antigens (agglutinogens) in the fetal tissues diffuse through the placental membrane at birth and enter the mother's blood. Her body reacts by forming anti-Rh agglutinins; in future pregnancies these may diffuse back through the placental membrane into the fetal circulation and cause clumping of the fetal erythrocytes. This condition is called ERYTHROBLASTOSIS FETALIS, or hemolytic disease of the newborn. When the erythrocytes are

R

destroyed, hemoglobin leaks into the plasma, producing jaundice and anemia. *In utero,* the hemoglobin is metabolized by the mother mainly; however, post partum, the neonate cannot detoxify the excess hemoglobin pigments such as BILIRUBIN, and these may destroy nerve tissue and produce brain damage, a condition called KERNICTERUS. The antibodies also may damage many other cells of the body.

The fetal-maternal reaction is similar to an Rh-produced transfusion reaction in that the agglutination varies in severity and usually occurs gradually. An Rh-negative mother having her first Rh-positive child usually does not build up sufficient antibodies (agglutinins) to cause harm to the fetus, but in subsequent pregnancies with Rh-positive infants she may. The incidence of erythroblastosis fetalis in infants of Rh-negative mothers depends on the number of Rh-positive children she has. If the father of the children is Rh-positive and heterozygous (about 55 per cent are) about one fourth of the offspring will be Rh-negative and will not stimulate the production of antibodies in the mother.

Scientific advances have helped reduce the risk to the Rh-positive infants of Rh-negative mothers. (See also AMNIOCENTESIS, exchange TRANSFUSION, and intrauterine TRANSFUSION.) It is important to immunize Rh-negative mothers after their first pregnancy to guard against future Rh incompatibility reactions. Immediately after childbirth, anti-Rh antibody (RhoGAM) injected into the mother; it combines with Rh-positive erythrocytes or substances from the fetus that have entered the maternal circulation, and renders them inert (no longer capable of eliciting maternal antibody formation). Immunization must be repeated after each pregnancy, including ectopic pregnancies and miscarriages. The Institute for Clinical Systems Improvement has issued clinical practice guidelines for prenatal care that recommend RhoGAM immunization in the 28th week of the prenatal period.

rhigosis (rĭ-go'sis) the perception of cold.
rhin(o)- word element [Gr.], *nose; nose-like structure.*
rhinal (ri'nal) nasal.
rhinalgia (ri-nal'jah) pain in the nose; called also rhinodynia.
rhinencephalon (ri"nen-sef'ah-lon) 1. the part of the brain once thought to be concerned entirely with olfactory mechanisms, including olfactory nerves, bulbs, tracts, and subsequent connections (all olfactory in function) and the limbic system (not primarily olfactory in function); homologous with olfactory portions of the brain in certain other animals. 2. the area of the brain consisting of the substantia perforata rostralis, bandaletta diagonalis (Broca), area subcallosa, and gyrus paraterminalis. 3. one of the parts of the embryonic telencephalon.

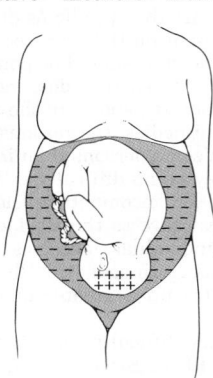 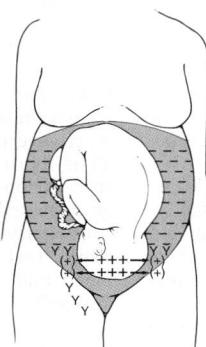 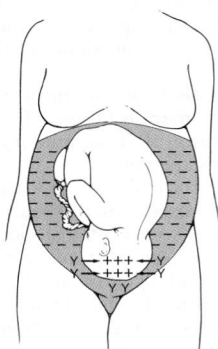

FIRST PREGNANCY

AT DELIVERY OF FIRST PREGNANCY

SECOND PREGNANCY

+ = Rh⁺ antigen baby's RBC's

− = Rh⁻ mother

(+) = Rh⁺ antigen passed from baby to mother

Y = Antibody made by mother in response to Rh⁺ antigen from baby

Y = Antibodies from mother pass to baby and destroy RBC's of baby

Maternal-fetal incompatibility. From Chabner, 1996.

rhinion (rin′e-on) a landmark in CEPHAL-OMETRY, the lower end of the suture between the nasal bones.

rhinitis (ri-ni′tis) inflammation of the mucous membrane of the nose; it may be either mild and chronic or acute. Viruses, bacteria, and allergens are responsible for its varied manifestations. Often a viral rhinitis is complicated by a bacterial infection caused by streptococci, staphylococci, and pneumococci or other bacteria. HAY FEVER, an acute type of allergic rhinitis, is also subject to bacterial complications. Many factors assist the invasion of the mucous membranes by bacteria, including allergens, excessive dryness, exposure to dampness and cold, excessive inhalation of dust, and injury to the nasal cilia due to viral infection.

It usually is not serious, but some forms may be contagious. The mucous membrane of the nose becomes swollen and there is a nasal discharge. Some types are accompanied by fever, muscle aches, and general discomfort with sneezing and running eyes. Breathing through the nose may become difficult or impossible. Often rhinitis is accompanied by inflammation of the throat and sinuses. If bacterial infection develops, the nasal discharge is thick and contains pus.

Acute rhinitis is the medical term for the COMMON COLD. *Chronic rhinitis* may result in permanent thickening of the nasal mucosa. Treatment of rhinitis is aimed at eliminating the primary cause and administration of decongestants to relieve nasal congestion.

    acute r. common cold.

    allergic r. any allergic reaction of the nasal mucosa, occurring perennially (nonseasonal allergic RHINITIS) or seasonally (HAY FEVER).

    atrophic r. a chronic form of nonallergic noninfectious rhinitis marked by wasting of the mucous membrane and the glands. It is sometimes the result of trauma, vascular damage by radiation therapy, and environmental irritants, and disease has also been implicated.

    r. caseo′sa that with a caseous, gelatinous, and fetid discharge.

    fibrinous r. membranous rhinitis.

    hypertrophic r. that with thickening and swelling of the mucous membrane.

    membranous r. chronic rhinitis with the formation of a false membrane, as in nasal DIPHTHERIA; called also fibrinous rhinitis.

    nonseasonal allergic r. allergic rhinitis occurring continuously or intermittently all year round, due to exposure to a more or less ever-present allergen, marked by sudden attacks of sneezing, swelling of the nasal mucosa with profuse watery discharge, itching of the eyes, and lacrimation. Called also nonseasonal or perennial hay fever.

    seasonal allergic r. hay fever.

    vasomotor r. 1. nonallergic rhinitis in which transient changes in vascular tone and permeability (with the same symptoms of allergic rhinitis) are brought on by such stimuli as mild chilling, fatigue, anger, and anxiety. 2. any condition of allergic or nonallergic rhinitis, as opposed to infectious rhinitis.

rhinoantritis (ri″no-an-tri′tis) inflammation of the nasal cavity and maxillary sinus.

rhinocanthectomy (ri″no-kan-thek′tah-me) rhinommectomy.

rhinocephalus (ri″no-sef′ah-lus) a fetus exhibiting rhinocephaly.

rhinocephaly (ri″no-sef′ah-le) a developmental ANOMALY characterized by the presence of a proboscis-like nose above eyes partially or completely fused into one.

rhinocheiloplasty (ri″no-ki′lo-plas″te) plastic surgery of the nose and lip.

rhinodynia (ri″no-din′e-ah) rhinalgia.

rhinoentomophthoromycosis (ri″no-en″to-mof″tho-ro-mi-ko′sis) the usual form of entomophthoromycosis conidiobolae, marked by development of large polyps in the subcutaneous tissues of the nose and paranasal sinuses; orbital involvement with unilateral blindness may follow. Sometimes, especially in weak or immunocompromised patients, it can spread to the central nervous system and cause fatal rhinocerebral zygomycosis. Called also rhinofacial zygomycosis.

rhinogenous (ri-noj′ĕ-nus) arising in the nose.

rhinokyphosis (ri″no-ki-fo′sis) an abnormal hump on the ridge of the nose.

rhinolalia (ri″no-la′le-ah) a nasal quality of speech from some disease or defect of the nasal passages; called also rhinophonia.

    r. aper′ta hypernasality.

    r. clau′sa hyponasality.

rhinolaryngitis (ri″no-lar″in-ji′tis) inflammation of the mucosa of the nose and larynx.

rhinolith (ri′no-lith) a calculus formed in the nose from mucous and nasal debris. Called also nasal calculus.

rhinolithiasis (ri″no-lĭ-thi′ah-sis) a condition associated with formation of rhinoliths.

rhinologist (ri-nol′ah-jist) a specialist in rhinology.

rhinology (ri-nol′ah-je) the medical specialty that deals with the nose and its diseases.

rhinomanometer (ri″no-mah-nom′ĕ-ter) a manometer used in rhinomanometry.

rhinomanometry (ri″no-mah-nom′ĕ-tre) measurement of the airflow and pressure

R

within the nose during respiration; nasal resistance or obstruction can be calculated from the figures obtained.

rhinometer (ri-nom′ĕ-ter) an instrument for measuring the nose or its cavities.

rhinommectomy (ri″nom-mek′tah-me) excision of the inner canthus of the eye.

rhinomycosis (ri″no-mi-ko′sis) fungal infection of the nasal mucosa.

rhinonecrosis (ri″no-nĕ-kro′sis) necrosis of the nasal bones.

rhinopathy (ri-nop′ah-the) any disease of the nose.

rhinopharyngitis (ri″no-far″in-ji′tis) nasopharyngitis.

rhinophonia (ri″no-fo′ne-ah) rhinolalia.

rhinophycomycosis (ri″no-fi″ko-mi-ko′-sis) a fungal disease caused by *Entomophthora coronata,* marked by formation of large polyps in the subcutaneous tissues of the nose and paranasal sinuses; orbital involvement and unilateral blindness may follow. Cerebral involvement is common.

rhinophyma (ri″no-fi′mah) a manifestation of severe rosacea involving the lower half of the nose and sometimes spreading to adjacent cheek areas, usually seen in adult males, and characterized by thickened, lobulated overgrowth of sebaceous glands and epithelial connective tissue.

rhinoplasty (ri′no-plas″te) plastic surgery of the nose.

rhinorrhagia (ri″no-ra′jah) epistaxis.

rhinorrhea (ri″no-re′ah) the free discharge of a thin nasal mucus.

cerebrospinal fluid r. discharge of cerebrospinal fluid through the nose, usually due to skull fracture.

rhinosalpingitis (ri″no-sal″pin-ji′tis) inflammation of the mucosa of the nose and eustachian tube.

rhinoscleroma (ri″no-sklĕ-ro′mah) a granulomatous disease involving the nose and nasopharynx, due to infection by *Klebsiella rhinoscleromatis,* seen mainly in Egypt, Eastern Europe, and Central and South America; the growth forms hard patches or nodules, which tend to enlarge and are painful to the touch.

rhinoscope (ri′no-skōp) a speculum for use in nasal examination.

rhinoscopy (ri-nos′kah-pe) examination of the nose with a speculum, through either the anterior nares or the nasopharynx.

rhinosinusitis (ri″no-si″nus-i′tis) inflammation of the paranasal sinuses; called also nasosinusitis.

rhinosporidiosis (ri″no-spor-id″e-o′sis) a chronic, localized granulomatous fungal infection of the mucocutaneous tissues, especially that of the nose, caused by *Rhinosporidium seeberi,* usually found in India and Sri Lanka but also seen in many temperate and tropical regions worldwide, characterized by the development of polyps, tumors, papillomas, or wartlike lesions.

rhinotomy (ri-not′ah-me) incision into the nose.

rhinovirus (ri′no-vi″rus) any member of a genus of PICORNAVIRUSES, considered to be etiologically associated with the COMMON COLD and certain other upper respiratory ailments. Over 90 antigenically different strains are known to cause the common cold. Called also coryza virus.

rhiz(o)- word element [Gr.], *root.*

rhizoid (ri′zoid) resembling a root.

rhizolysis (ri-zol′ĭ-sis) radiofrequency neurotomy; interruption of spinal nerve roots by coagulation with radiofrequency waves.

rhizomelic (ri″zo-mel′ik) pertaining to the hips and shoulders (the roots of the limbs).

rhizomeningomyelitis (ri″zo-mĕ-ning″go-mi″ĕ-li′-tis) meningomyeloradiculitis.

Rhizopoda (ri-zop′ah-dah) a superclass of protozoa comprising the amebae, which move about and acquire food by means of PSEUDOPODIA or by protoplasmic flow without production of discrete pseudopodia. The majority are free-living in soil or water, but some are parasitic and pathogenic in humans.

Rhizopus a genus of perfect fungi; several species are molds and saprobes on fruits, vegetables, or baked goods and can cause MUCORMYCOSIS.

rhizotomy (ri-zot′ah-me) division or transection of a nerve root, either within the spinal canal or outside it.

Rh-null syndrome chronic HEMOLYTIC ANEMIA affecting individuals who lack all RH FACTORS (Rh_{null}); it is marked by spherocytosis, stomatocytosis, and increased osmotic fragility.

rhodium (ro′de-um) a chemical element, atomic number 45, atomic weight 102.905, symbol Rh. (See Appendix 6.)

rhodogenesis (ro″do-jen′ĕ-sis) regeneration of rhodopsin after its bleaching by light.

rhodophylaxis (ro″do-fi-lak′sis) the property of the retinal epithelium of facilitating rhodogenesis. adj., **rhodophylac′tic.**

rhodopsin (ro-dop′sin) visual purple; a photosensitive purple-red chromoprotein in the retinal rods that is bleached to visual yellow (all-*trans*retinal) by light, thereby stimulating retinal sensory endings. Lack of rhodopsin results in NIGHT BLINDNESS. Vitamin A is the primary source of rhodopsin.

RhoGAM (ro′gam) trademark for a preparation of Rh_0 (D antigen) immune globulin. The gamma globulin is derived from the plasma of women previously immunized to the Rh_0 (D) antigen and is administered after each Rh-incompatible pregnancy. The gamma globulin prevents the formation of antibodies after delivery or abortion. See also RH FACTOR.

rhombencephalon (rom″ben-sef′ah-lon) 1. the portion of the brain developed from the most caudal of the three primary brain vesicles of the early embryo, comprising the METENCEPHALON and MYELENCEPHALON. 2. the most caudal of the three primary vesicles formed in embryonic development of the brain, which later divides into the metencephalon and the myelencephalon. Called also hindbrain.

rhombocoele (rom′bo-sēl) the terminal expansion of the canal of the spinal cord.

rhomboid (rom′boid) shaped like a rectangle that has been skewed to one side so that the angles are oblique.

rhonchus (rong′kus), pl. *rhon′chi* [L.] a continuous SOUND consisting of a dry whistlelike noise with a lower pitch than that of a WHEEZE, produced in the throat or bronchial tube due to a partial obstruction.

Rhus (rus) a genus of trees and shrubs, many of them poisonous. Contact with certain species produces a severe dermatitis in sensitive individuals. The most important poisonous species are *R. diversilo′ba* and *R. oxicoden′dron,* or poison oak, *R. ra′dicans,* or poison ivy, and *R. ver′nix,* or poison sumac. Most species of *Rhus* are sometimes classified in the genus *Toxicodendron.* See also *poison ivy, oak, and sumac.*

rhythm (rith′m) a measured movement; the recurrence of an action or function at regular intervals. adj., **rhyth′mic, rhyth′nical.**

   accelerated idiojunctional r. a junctional rhythm, without retrograde conduction to the atria, at a rate exceeding the normal firing rate of the junction; it is an ectopic rhythm located in the bundle of His and controlling ventricles at a rate of 60 to 100 beats per minute.

   accelerated idioventricular r. a rhythm of ectopic ventricular origin, faster than the normal rate of the His-Purkinje system but slower than 100 beats per minute, without retrograde conduction to the atria.

   accelerated junctional r. a rhythm emanating from a focus in the AV junction at a rate greater than its normal rate of 60 but less than 100 beats per minute; it may be due to altered automaticity secondary to disease or to triggered activity secondary to digitalis toxicity. There may or may not be retrograde conduction to the atria.

   alpha r. uniform rhythm of waves in the normal electroencephalogram, showing an average frequency of 10 per second, typical of a normal person awake in a quiet resting state. Called also Berger rhythm. See also ELECTROENCEPHALOGRAPHY.

   atrioventricular junctional r. a junctional rhythm originating in the bundle of His, with a heart rate of 40 to 60 beats per minute; called also nodal rhythm.

   automatic r. spontaneous rhythms initiated by the sinoatrial node, or by subsidiary atrial or ventricular pacemakers; in practice this refers to a normal sinus rhythm at a rate of 60 to 100 beats per minute.

   Berger r. alpha rhythm.

   beta r. a rhythm in the electroencephalogram consisting of waves smaller than those of the alpha rhythm, having an average frequency of 25 per second, typical during periods of intense activity of the nervous system. See also ELECTROENCEPHALOGRAPHY.

   biological r's the cyclic changes that occur in physiological processes of living organisms; these rhythms are so persistent in nature that they probably should be considered a fundamental characteristic of life, as are growth, reproduction, metabolism, and irritability. Many of the physiological processes that recur in humans about every 24 hours (with circadian RHYTHM) have been known for centuries. Examples include the peaks and troughs seen in body temperature, vital signs, brain function, and muscular activity. Biochemical analyses of urine, blood enzymes, and plasma serum also demonstrated circadian rhythms. Called also biorhythms.

   It has long been believed that the cyclic changes observed in plants and animals were totally in response to environmental changes and, as such, were exogenous or of external origin. This hypothesis has now been rejected by most CHRONOBIOLOGISTS, who hold that the biological rhythms are intrinsic to the organisms, and that the organisms possess their own physiological mechanism for keeping time. This mechanism has been called the "biological clock." An example of adjustment of the biological clock in humans is recovery from "jet lag." This phenomenon, also known as jet syndrome, occurs when humans are transported by jet plane across time zones. It is characterized by fatigue and lowered efficiency, which persist until the biological clock adjusts to the new environmental cycle.

R

Biological rhythms are responsive to, or synchronous with, environmental cycles, but it is generally agreed among chronobiologists that the rhythmic changes in environmental factors do not create biological rhythms, even though they are capable of influencing them. Even in the absence of such environmental stimuli as light, darkness, temperature, gravity, and electromagnetic field, biological rhythms continue to maintain their cyclic nature for a period of time.

circadian r. the regular recurrence in cycles of about 24 hours from one point to another, such as certain biological activities that do this regardless of long periods of darkness or other changes in environmental conditions.

circamensual r. recurrence in cycles of about one month (30 days).

circannual r. recurrence of a phenomenon in cycles of about one year.

circaseptan r. that which occurs in cycles of about seven days (one week).

coupled r. heart beats occurring in pairs, the second beat of the pair usually being a ventricular premature beat.

delta r. 1. electroencephalographic waves having a frequency below 312 per second, typical in deep sleep, in infancy, and in serious brain disorders. See also ELECTROENCEPHALOGRAPHY. 2. delta waves.

escape r. a heart rhythm initiated by lower centers when the sinoatrial node fails to initiate impulses, its rhythmicity is depressed, or its impulses are completely blocked.

gallop r. an auscultatory finding of three or four heart sounds, created by gushes of blood entering resistant or stiffened ventricles. This can happen at two different times during ventricular diastole: either at initial filling or at the time of ventricular contraction. Therefore, gallops occur during early and late ventricular diastole.

gamma r. a rhythm in the waves in the electroencephalogram having a frequency of 50 per second. See also ELECTROENCEPHALOGRAPHY.

idiojunctional r. a rhythm emanating from the atrioventricular junction but without retrograde conduction to the atria.

infradian r. the regular recurrence in cycles of more than 24 hours, as certain biological activities which occur at such intervals, regardless of conditions of illumination or other environmental conditions.

junctional r. an arrhythmia caused by an abnormality in the atrioventricular junction; see accelerated junctional rhythm and atrioventricular junctional rhythm.

r. method old popular name for natural family PLANNING.

nodal r. 1. atrioventricular junctional rhythm. 2. junctional rhythm.

nyctohemeral r. a day and night rhythm.

pendulum r. alternation in the rhythm of the heart sounds in which the diastolic sound is equal in time, character, and loudness to the systolic sound, the beat of the heart resembling the tick of a watch.

sinus r. normal heart rhythm originating in the sinoatrial node, with a normal rate of 60 to 100 beats per minute.

theta r. electroencephalographic waves having a frequency of 4 to 7 per second occurring mainly in children but also in adults under emotional stress. See also ELECTROENCEPHALOGRAPHY.

ultradian r. the regular recurrence in cycles of less than 24 hours, as certain biological activities which occur at such intervals, regardless of conditions of illumination or other environmental conditions.

ventricular r. the ventricular contractions which occur in cases of complete heart block.

rhythmicity (rith-mis′ĭ-te) in cardiology the ability to beat, or the state of beating rhythmically without external stimuli.

rhytid (ri′tid), pl. *rhy′tides* skin wrinkle.

rhytidectomy (rit″ĭ-dek′tah-me) PLASTIC SURGERY for the removal of wrinkles, done to make an aging face look younger. When done with skill, it can be moderately successful. However, the changes are not permanent and the patient may in time feel the need for another operation. The usual procedure is to open skin flaps in the region around the ears and to undermine the skin of the cheeks and jaws. Now this can be done with incisions adjacent to or within the hairline so that the scars are not noticeable. The area of the eyelids and eyebrows may also be operated on in association with the primary operation. Called also rhytidoplasty, and popularly known as a face-lift.

rhytidoplasty (rit″ĭ-do-plas″te) rhytidectomy.

rhytidosis (rit″ĭ-do′sis) a wrinkling, as of the cornea.

RIA radioimmunoassay.

rib (rib) any of the paired bones, 12 on either side, extending from the thoracic vertebrae toward the median line on the ventral aspect of the trunk, forming the major part of the thoracic skeleton. Called also costa. See anatomic Table of Bones in the Appendices.

abdominal r's, asternal r's false ribs.

cervical r. a supernumerary rib arising from a cervical vertebra.

false r's the five lower ribs on either side, not attached directly to the sternum.

floating r's the two lower false ribs on either side, usually without ventral attachment.

slipping r. one whose attaching cartilage is repeatedly dislocated.

true r's the seven upper ribs on either side, attached to both vertebrae and sternum.

vertebral r's floating ribs.

vertebrocostal r's the three upper false ribs on either side, attached to vertebrae and costal cartilages.

vertebrosternal r's true ribs.

ribavirin (ri″bah-vi′rin) a nucleoside ANALOGUE that acts as a broad-spectrum ANTIVIRAL; used in treatment of severe viral pneumonia caused by respiratory syncytial VIRUS, particularly in high-risk infants with underlying conditions such as cardiopulmonary disease; administered by oral inhalation. It is also used in conjunction with interferon alfa-2b in the treatment of chronic hepatitis C, administered orally.

riboflavin (ri′bo-fla″vin) vitamin B_2, a component of FLAVIN ADENINE DINUCLEOTIDE and FLAVIN MONONUCLEOTIDE, coenzymes that are prosthetic groups for FLAVOPROTEINS, enzymes that catalyze many oxidation-reduction reactions. Foods with the highest content of riboflavin are liver, kidney, heart, brewer's yeast, milk, eggs, greens, and enriched cereals, bread, and other grain products. Riboflavin deficiency (ARIBOFLAVINOSIS) is most common among people in regions such as Asia and the West Indies where the diet contains large quantities of corn, potatoes, or rice (white rice that is not enriched), which lack riboflavin. A well-balanced diet will prevent riboflavin deficiency; it will also correct the disorder, with the help of supplementary doses of riboflavin and other vitamins.

r. kinase a phosphotransferase enzyme that catalyzes the conversion of free riboflavin and ATP to FLAVIN MONONUCLEOTIDE and ADP.

ribonuclease (ri″bo-noo′kle-ās) an enzyme that catalyzes the depolymerization of ribonucleic acid.

ribonucleic acid (RNA) (ri″bo-noo-kle′ik) a NUCLEIC ACID that is present in all living cells and controls cellular protein synthesis; it replaces DEOXYRIBONUCLEIC ACID (DNA) as a carrier of genetic codes in some viruses. RNA is similar in composition to DNA with two exceptions: the sugar in RNA is RIBOSE, as opposed to the DEOXYRIBOSE of DNA, and in RNA the pyrimidine URACIL is found instead of the THYMINE of DNA. The structure of RNA varies from helical to uncoiled strands of varying lengths, depending on

the number of nucleotide units forming the strand. This variance in structure is evident in the different types of RNA. For example, transfer RNA (tRNA) contains only about 75 nucleotide units, while other types may contain thousands of units.

Messenger RNA (mRNA) receives its name from its function of carrying the genetic code from the nucleus of the cell to the cytoplasm, where most cellular functions take place. The transfer of the genetic code from DNA to mRNA is called transcription. Molecules of mRNA migrate to the ribosomes, where the manufacture of proteins occurs. The strands of RNA contain codons, some of which signal when formation of a particular protein should stop and the formation of another should start.

Transfer RNA (tRNA) brings about the transfer of specific amino acid molecules to protein molecules during the synthesis of proteins. Each of the 20 common amino acids found in protein molecules has a corresponding type of transfer RNA. Thus, a specific tRNA carries the appropriate amino acid to its appropriate place in the chain of the protein molecule being synthesized.

Ribosomal RNA (rRNA) is so called because it is found in the RIBOSOMES. It is the most abundant type of RNA and in some way affects the linking of amino acids into protein molecules.

ribonucleoprotein (ri″bo-noo″kle-o-pro′tēn) a substance composed of both protein and ribonucleic acid.

ribonucleoside (ri″bo-noo′kle-o-sīd) a nucleoside in which the purine or pyrimidine base is combined with ribose.

ribonucleotide (ri″bo-noo′kle-o-tīd) a nucleotide in which the purine or pyrimidine base is combined with ribose.

ribose (ri′bōs) 5-carbon sugar present in ribonucleic acid (RNA).

ribosome (ri′bo-sōm) any of the intracellular ribonucleoprotein ORGANELLES concerned with protein synthesis, found either bound to cell membranes or free in the cytoplasm. They may occur singly or in clusters (POLYRIBOSOMES). The GENETIC CODE is translated when ribosomes attach to messenger RNA.

ribosyl (ri′bo-sil) a glycosyl radical formed from ribose.

Richards (rich′ardz) Melinda Ann (1841–1930). "America's first trained nurse," the first graduate of the Training School of the New England Hospital in Boston, in 1873. She devoted her life to active nursing and to the training of other nurses.

R

ricin (ri′sin) a phytotoxin in the seeds of the castor oil plant *(Ricinus communis)*, inhalation or ingestion of which causes intoxication, producing superficial inflammation of the respiratory mucosa with hemorrhages into the lungs, or edema of the gastrointestinal tract with hemorrhages.

rickets (rik′ets) a condition of infancy and childhood caused by deficiency of vitamin D, which leads to altered calcium and phosphorus metabolism and consequent disturbance of ossification of bone. Because of the widespread use of vitamin D–fortified milk, and the giving of vitamin supplements to most infants, the disease is now uncommon in the United States. (A second disease, clinically indistinguishable from ordinary rickets but resistant to large doses of vitamin D, is called vitamin D–resistant rickets.) Since the action of sunlight on the skin produces vitamin D in the human body, rickets often occurs in parts of the world where the winter is especially long, or where smoke and fog constantly intercept the sun. Black and other dark-skinned people are somewhat more susceptible to the disease if they live in areas with little sunlight, since the pigment in the skin blocks absorption of the sun's rays. When a vitamin D deficiency occurs in adults, it produces OSTEOMALACIA.

Symptoms. A major symptom of rickets is softening (decalcification) of the bones. In children, this can produce various degrees of deformity, including nodules on the ribs and flexibility and bending of bones. Bowleg and knock-knee and an improperly developed or misshapen skull of a squared or boxed appearance are typical. The ability of the bones to support the body is seriously impaired.

Prevention. A proper diet that includes vitamin D–fortified milk is usually sufficient to prevent rickets. Ordinary milk contains adequate amounts of calcium but is a poor source of vitamin D. Small amounts of the vitamin are present in eggs, and in such fish as cod, herring, tuna, sardines, and salmon. Sunlight and other sources of ultraviolet light are beneficial.

Treatment. Treatment of an active case of rickets involves the administration of vitamin D concentrate. The response to treatment usually is rapid.

anticonvulsant r. rickets occurring in children receiving long-term anticonvulsant therapy; the drugs induce vitamin D deficiency (frequently compounded by dietary insufficiency of the vitamin) and hypocalcemia, hypophosphatemia, and secondary hyperparathyroidism by increasing the rate of conversion of the vitamin to inactive metabolites.

familial hypophosphatemic r. any of several inherited disorders of proximal renal tubular function causing phosphate loss, hypophosphatemia, and skeletal deformities, including rickets and OSTEOMALACIA.

hypophosphatemic r. any of a group of disorders characterized by rickets associated with hypophosphatemia, resulting from dietary phosphorus deficiency (antacid-induced osteomalacia) or due to defects in renal tubular function, either hereditary (familial hypophosphatemic rickets) or acquired. While skeletal deformities (e.g., bowleg, short stature) are present, neither hypocalcemia, myopathy, nor tetany occur, and serum parathyroid hormone is normal.

vitamin D–dependent r., type I an autosomal recessive disorder of rickets with myopathy, hypocalcemia, moderate hypophosphatemia, secondary hyperparathyroidism, and subnormal serum concentrations of 1,25-dihydroxyvitamin D. The disorder can be overcome by high doses of vitamin D or physiologic doses of calcitriol.

vitamin D–dependent r., type II an autosomal recessive disorder similar to type I but with elevated serum concentrations of 1,25-dihydroxyvitamin D. The disorder cannot be overcome by high levels of vitamin D or its metabolites and is believed to be due to defective receptor binding, absence of the receptors, or post-receptor defects. Multiple variants exist, subdivided as those with or without alopecia.

vitamin D–resistant r. a condition almost indistinguishable from ordinary rickets clinically but resistant to unusually large doses of vitamin D; it is often familial but may occur sporadically. In *hypophosphatemic vitamin D–resistant rickets*, hypophosphatemia is the main characteristic, while in *hypocalcemic vitamin D–resistant rickets*, the serum concentration of phosphate is within normal limits or nearly so, and the concentration of calcium is abnormally low.

Rickettsia (rĭ-ket′se-ah) a genus of bacteria of the tribe RICKETTSIAE, made up of small, gram-negative, rod-shaped to coccoid often pleomorphic microorganisms, which multiply only in host cells. Organisms occur in the cytoplasm of tissue cells or free in the gut lumen of lice, fleas, ticks, and mites and are transmitted by their bites. *R. cono′rii* is the etiologic agent of BOUTONNEUSE FEVER and is transmitted by the bite of ixodid ticks. *R prowaze′kii* is the agent of scrub TYPHUS and BRILL-ZINSSER DISEASE; it is transmitted between humans by the human body louse and from flying squirrels to humans by fleas and ce. *R. ty′phi* is the cause of murine TYPHUS, which is transmitted to humans chiefly by rat fleas. Rickettsial diseases are not common in communities with good sanitary standards, since prevention depends on controlling the rodent and insect populations. Major epidemics have occurred, especially in times of war when standards of sanitation drop.

rickettsia (rĭ-ket′se-ah), pl. *rickett′siae* An individual organism of the family Rickettsiaceae.

Rickettsiaceae (rĭ-ket″se-a′se-e) a family of the order Rickettsiales.

Rickettsiae (rĭ-ket′se-e) Rickettsieae.

rickettsial (rĭ-ket′se-al) pertaining to or caused by rickettsiae.

Rickettsiales (rĭ-ket″se-a′lez) an order of bacteria comprising small, gram-negative, rod-shaped or coccoid, often pleomorphic microorganisms occurring as elementary bodies that typically multiply only inside the cells of the host. Found as parasites in both vertebrates and invertebrates, which may serve as vectors, they may be pathogenic for both humans and other animals.

rickettsialpox (rĭ-ket′se-al-poks″) a febrile disease marked by a vesiculopapular eruption, resembling chickenpox clinically, caused by *Rickettsia akari* and transmitted by mites. Called also Kew Gardens spotted fever.

rickettsicidal (rĭ-ket″sĭ-si′dal) destructive to rickettsiae.

Rickettsieae (rik″et-si′e-e) a tribe of bacteria of the family Rickettsiaceae, order Rickettsiales, made up of small, pleomorphic, mostly intracellular organisms, which are classified in three genera, *Coxiella*, *Rickettsia*, and *Rochalimaea*. They occur as parasites in arthropods and cause disease in vertebrate hosts. Pathogenic species fall generally into four groups, based upon immunologic characterization: I, classic TYPHUS (also causing epidemic TYPHUS, BRILL-ZINSSER DISEASE, and murine TYPHUS); II, spotted fever causing ROCKY MOUNTAIN SPOTTED FEVER, BOUTONNEUSE FEVER, RICKETTSIALPOX, Siberian tick TYPHUS, and Queensland tick TYPHUS); III, scrub TYPHUS; and IV, miscellaneous organisms (including the causes of Q FEVER and TRENCH FEVER). Called also Rickettsiae.

ridge (rij) a linear projection or projecting structure; a crest.

alveolar r. a bony ridge of the maxilla or mandible, the part of the alveolar PROCESS that contains the alveoli; called also alveolar crest.

dental r. any linear elevation on the crown of a tooth.

dermal r's ridges of the skin produced by the projecting papillae of the corium on

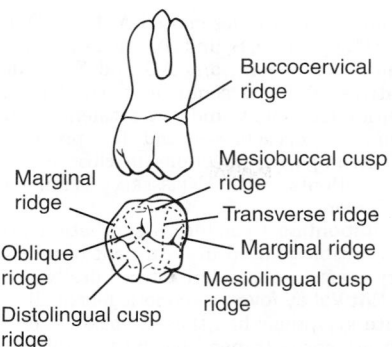

Dental ridges in a maxillary molar. From Dorland's, 2000.

the palm of the hand and sole of the foot, producing a fingerprint and footprint characteristic of the individual; called also cristae cutis.

genital r. the more medial part of the urogenital ridge, giving rise to the gonad.

healing r. an indurated ridge that normally forms deep to the skin along the length of a healing wound.

incisal r. the part of the crown of an anterior tooth that makes up the actual incisal portion; see *incisal surface,* under *surface.*

interureteric r. a fold on mucous membrane extending across the bladder between the ureteric orifices.

mammary r. an ectodermal thickening in early embryos, along which the mammary glands subsequently develop.

mesonephric r. the more lateral portion of the urogenital ridge, giving rise to the mesonephros.

oblique r. a variable linear elevation obliquely crossing the occlusive surface of a maxillary molar.

urogenital r. a longitudinal ridge in the embryo, lateral to the mesentery.

rifabutin (rif″ah-bu′tin) an antibacterial used for the prevention of disseminated *Mycobacterium avium* COMPLEX DISEASE in patients with advanced HIV infection; administered orally.

rifampicin (rif-am′pĭ-sin) rifampin.

rifampin (rif-am′pin) a semisynthetic derivative of RIFAMYCIN, with the antibacterial actions and uses of the rifamycin group; administered orally or intravenously.

rifamycin (rif″ah-mi′sin) any of a family of antibiotics biosynthesized by a strain of *Streptomyces mediterranei*, effective against a broad spectrum of bacteria. The five

R

components are designated A, B, C, D, and E; rifamycins O, S, and SV are derivatives of the B component, and AG and X are derivatives of the O component. Used for the initial treatment and retreatment of pulmonary TUBERCULOSIS and for prevention of meningoccal infections in close contacts of patients with NEISSERIA MENINGITIDIS infections.

rifapentine (-pen′tēn) a synthetic RIFAMYCIN antibiotic used in treatment of pulmonary TUBERCULOSIS, administered orally.

Rift Valley fever a zoonotic febrile disease with symptoms like those of DENGUE, due to an arbovirus transmitted by mosquitoes or by contact with diseased animals; first observed in the Rift Valley, Kenya.

right (rīt) something that is due to someone by law or by tradition.

    r. to fair treatment the fair selection and treatment of subjects during the course of a research study. Principles governing fairness include informed voluntary decision by the subjects to participate and selection according to criteria directly related to the study rather than according to artificial social or cultural biases.

    negative r. a right to refuse care or not to be interfered with; it obligates another to refrain from doing something. One example is the right to refuse treatment, which is grounded in the principle of respect for AUTONOMY. This is mentioned in the "Patient's Bill of Rights;" see PATIENT'S RIGHTS.

    patient's r's see PATIENT'S RIGHTS.

    positive r. a right to be provided with a good or service such as health care, usually grounded in the principle of JUSTICE. It is philosophically more difficult to justify than a negative right because it obligates another to do something.

righting reactions (rīt′ing) responses of the head and eyes that occur as the body processes sensory input from the visual and vestibular systems. Their purpose is to maintain the correct orientation of the head and body with respect to the vertical.

rigidity (rĭ-jid′ĭ-te) inflexibility or stiffness.

    clasp-knife r. increased tension in the extensor of a joint when it is passively flexed, giving way suddenly on exertion of further pressure; seen especially in upper motor neuron disease. Called also clasp-knife reflex.

    cogwheel r. tension in a muscle that gives way in little jerks when the muscle is passively stretched; seen in PARKINSON'S DISEASE.

    decerebrate r. see DECEREBRATE RIGIDITY.

    decorticate r. see DECORTICATE RIGIDITY.

    paratonic r. an intermittent abnormal increase in resistance to passive movement in a comatose patient.

rigor (rig′or, ri′gor) 1. a chill; rigidity. strict discipline or scrupulous adherence a given set of standards.

    r. mor′tis the stiffening of a dead body accompanying depletion of adenosine triphosphate in the muscle fibers.

Riley-Day syndrome (ri′le da′) 1. familial dysautonomia. 2. an autosomal recessive disease of childhood characterized by defective tear formation, skin blotching, emotional instability, motor incoordination total absence of pain sensation, and hyporeflexia; seen almost exclusively in Ashkenazi Jews. Called also familial dysautonomia

riluzole (ril′u-zōl) a compound used prolong survival time in the treatment amyotrophic lateral SCLEROSIS.

rima (ri′mah) [L.] a cleft or crack.

    r. glot′tidis the elongated opening between the true vocal cords and between the arytenoid cartilages; called also vocal area

    r. o′ris the opening of the mouth.

    r. palpebra′rum palpebral fissure.

    r. puden′di the space between the labia majora; called also pudendal fissure.

rimantadine (ri-man′tah-dēn) an ANTIVIRAL agent used in prophylaxis and treatment of INFLUENZA A.

rimexolone (rĭ-mek′sah-lōn″) a CORTICOSTEROID used in topical treatment of inflammation following eye surgery and of uveitis affecting the anterior structures of the eye

rimula (rim′u-lah) [L.] a minute fissure as of the spinal cord or brain.

ring (ring) 1. any annular or circular organ, structure, or area. 2. in chemistry, collection of atoms united in a continuous closed chain.

    abdominal r., external an opening the aponeurosis of the external oblique muscle for the spermatic cord or round ligament.

    abdominal r., internal an aperture the transverse fascia for the spermatic cord or round ligament.

    Albl's r. a ring-shaped shadow in radiographs of the skull, caused by aneurysm of cerebral artery.

    Bandl's r. see BANDL'S RING.

    benzene r. the hexagon representing the arrangement of carbon atoms in molecule of benzene, different compounds being derived by replacement of the hydrogen atoms by different elements compounds.

    Cannon's r. a focal contraction seen radiographically at the mid-third of the transverse colon, marking an area of overlap between the superior and inferior nerve plexuses.

conjunctival r. a ring at the junction of the conjunctiva and cornea.

constriction r. a contracted area of the uterus, where the resistance of the uterine contents is slight, as over a depression in the contour of the fetus, or below the presenting part.

fibrous r. of heart anulus fibrosus.

halo r. a metal ORTHOSIS used for traction in the treatment of spinal cord injuries. The halo apparatus can maintain stability and alignment of the cervical vertebrae while the patient is out of bed.

inguinal r., deep an aperture in the transverse fascia for the spermatic cord or the round ligament.

inguinal r., external superficial inguinal ring.

inguinal r., internal deep inguinal ring.

inguinal r., superficial an opening in the aponeurosis of the external oblique muscle for the spermatic cord or the round ligament.

Kayser-Fleischer r. a golden brown or green discoloration in the zone of Descemet's membrane in the limbic region of the cornea seen in WILSON'S DISEASE and other liver disorders.

pathologic retraction r. a complication of prolonged labor marked by failure of relaxation of the circular fibers at the internal opening of the cervix, obstructing delivery of the infant. See also BANDL'S RING.

physiologic retraction r. the demarcation between the upper, contracting portion of the uterus in labor and the lower, dilating part.

Schwalbe's r. a circular ridge composed of collagenous fibers surrounding the outer margin of Descemet's membrane.

tympanic r. the bony ring forming part of the temporal bone at birth and developing into the tympanic plate.

umbilical r. the orifice in the abdominal wall of the fetus for transmission of the umbilical vein and arteries.

vascular r. a congenital anomaly of the aortic arch and its tributaries, the vessels forming a ring about the trachea and esophagus and causing varying degrees of compression.

Ringer's solution (ring′erz) a sterile solution of SODIUM CHLORIDE, POTASSIUM CHLORIDE, and CALCIUM CHLORIDE in purified water, used as a fluid and electrolyte replenisher and an irrigating physiologic salt solution. A preparation for injection is known as *Ringer's injection,* and one for irrigation as *Ringer's irrigation. Lactated Ringer's solution* includes the above compounds plus sodium lactate.

ringworm (ring′werm) the popular name for TINEA, a fungal infection of the skin, even though it is not caused by a worm and is not always ring-shaped in appearance. (See types under TINEA.) It is caused by a group of related fungi that feed on the body's waste products of dead skin and perspiration; they attack the skin in various areas, especially body folds such as the armpit and crotch. One type found between the toes is tinea pedis or ATHLETE'S FOOT; another affects the soles and toenails. Some forms, usually found in children and traceable to exposure to infected pets, attack the scalp or exposed areas of the body such as the arms or legs. These infections appear as reddish patches, often scaly or blistered, with itching, soreness, and sometimes destruction of hair shafts. They may become ring-shaped as the infection spreads out while its center heals or seems to heal.

The fungi are highly contagious and are spread by humans, animals, and even objects, such as combs or towels handled by infected persons. Scratching is almost certain to pass the infection from one part of the body to another.

Ringworm is treated with antifungal drugs. Prevention is largely a matter of cleanliness. All parts of the body should be washed with soap and water, especially hairy areas and body folds where perspiration is likely to collect. Thorough drying is as important as bathing, for the fungi thrive in warm dampness.

Rinne test (rin′ĕ) a TUNING FORK TEST that compares the duration of perception by bone conduction and by air conduction. In the normal ear, the fork is heard twice as

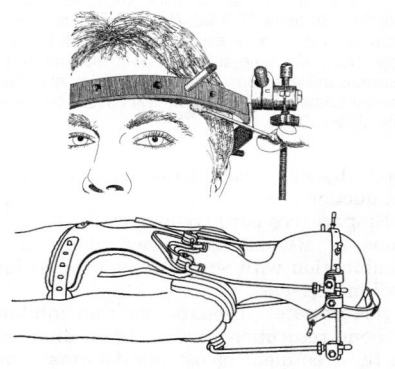

Halo ring. From Barker, 2002. Courtesy of Depuy Acromed, Rayham, MA.

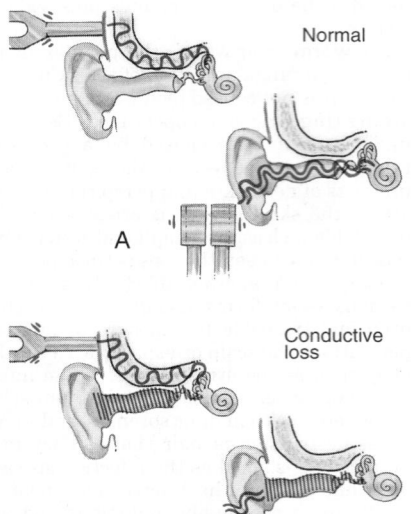

Normal

A

Conductive
loss

B

Sensorineural
loss

C

Rinne test: *A,* Normal: sound is heard twice as long by
air conduction (AC) as by bone conduction (BC); a
"positive" Rinne, or AC > BC. *B,* Conductive loss: person
hears as long by bone conduction (AC = BC) or even
longer (AC < BC), a "negative" finding on the Rinne test. *C,*
Sensorineural loss: normal ratio of AC > BC is intact but is
reduced overall . That is, person hears poorly both ways.
From Jarvis, 2000.

long by air conduction as by bone
conduction.

Riopan (ri′o-pan) trademark for preparations of MAGALDRATE, either alone or in
combination with SIMETHICONE, used as low-
sodium ANTACIDS.

risedronate (ris-ed′ro-naāt″) an inhibitor
of bone resorption used as the sodium salt
in the treatment of osteitis deformans and
for the prevention and treatment of osteoporosis, administered orally.

risk (risk) a danger or hazard; the probability of suffering harm.

  attributable r. the amount or proportion of incidence of disease or death (or risk
of disease or death) in individuals exposed
to a specific risk factor that can be attributed to exposure to that factor; the difference in the risk for unexposed versus
exposed individuals.

  empiric r. the probability that a trait
will occur or recur in a family based solely on
experience rather than on knowledge of the
causative mechanism. See also genetic RISK.

  genetic r. the probability that a trait
will occur or recur in a family, based on
knowledge of its genetic pattern of transmission. See also empiric RISK.

  relative r. for a disease, death, or other
outcome, the ratio of the incidence rate
among individuals with a given risk factor to
the incidence rate among those without it.

risperidone (ris-per′ĭ-dōn) an orally administered ANTIPSYCHOTIC AGENT; its mechanism of action is unknown, but it may
function as an antagonist to dopamine and
serotonin.

RIST radioimmunosorbent test.

risus (ri′sus) [L.] laughter.

  r. sardo′nicus a grinning expression
produced by spasm of the facial muscles; seen
in TETANUS and certain types of poisoning.

Ritalin (rit′ah-lin) trademark for preparations of METHYLPHENIDATE hydrochloride, a
mild central nervous system STIMULANT.

ritodrine (rit′oh-drēn) a β₂-adrenergic RE-
CEPTOR agonist used in the form of the
hydrochloride salt as a smooth muscle
(uterine muscle) relaxant to decrease uterine activity and delay uncomplicated premature labor.

ritonavir (rĭ-ton′ah-vir) an HIV protease
INHIBITOR that causes the human immunodeficiency VIRUS to form noninfectious particles; used to treat HIV infection and AIDS,
administered orally.

Ritter's disease (rit′erz) dermatitis exfo-
liativa neonatorum.

rituximab (rĭ-tuk′sĭ-mab) a monoclonal
ANTIBODY that binds CD20 antigen; used as
an antineoplastic AGENT in treatment of
B-cell non-Hodgkin's LYMPHOMA positive for
that antigen, administered intravenously.

rivalry (ri′val-re) a state of competition or
antagonism.

  sibling r. competition between siblings
for the love, affection, and attention of one
or both parents or for other recognition or
gain.

rivastigmine (riv″ah-stig′mēn) a reversible inhibitor of CHOLINESTERASE, believed to
increase the level of ACETYLCHOLINE available
in the central nervous system; administered

orally as the tartrate salt as an adjunct in the treatment of mild to moderate DEMENTIA OF THE ALZHEIMER TYPE.

rizatriptan (ri″zah-trip′tan) a selective SEROTONIN receptor agonist used as the benzoate salt in the acute treatment of MIGRAINE.

riziform (riz′ĭ-form) resembling grains of rice.

RLL right lower lobe (of lung).

RLQ right lower quadrant (of abdomen).

RMA right mentoanterior (position of the fetus).

RMP right mentoposterior (position of the fetus).

RMT right mentotransverse (position of the fetus).

RN Registered Nurse.

Rn radon.

RNA ribonucleic acid.

   messenger RNA (mRNA) see RIBONU-CLEIC ACID.

   ribosomal RNA (rRNA) see RIBONUCLEIC ACID.

   transfer RNA (tRNA) see RIBONUCLEIC ACID.

RNA-directed DNA polymerase reverse transcriptase.

RNase ribonuclease.

ROA right occipitoanterior (position of the fetus).

Robaxin (ro-bak′sin) trademark for preparations of METHOCARBAMOL, a skeletal muscle RELAXANT.

Robb (rob) Isabel Hampton (1860–1910). An early leader in nursing education, the first "principal" of Johns Hopkins School of Nursing in Baltimore and a founder of the forerunner of the American Nurses' Association.

Roberts (rob′erts) Mary M. (1877–1959). Nursing editor and writer, editor of the *American Journal of Nursing* and author of a number of books on the nursing profession. Concerned with the need for a public relations program for nursing, she founded the Nursing Information Bureau in 1934.

robotics (ro-bot′iks) the science of designing exact mechanical, computerized instruments for procedures.

Rocaltrol (ro-kal′trōl) trademark for preparations of CALCITRIOL, a form of VITAMIN D.

Rocephin (ro-sef′in) trademark for a preparation of CEFTRIAXONE sodium, a CEPHALOSPORIN antibiotic.

Rochalimaea (ro″kah-li-me′ah) a genus of bacteria of the family Rickettsiaceae resembling the genus *Rickettsia,* but usually found extracellularly in the arthropod host; *R. quinta′na* is the etiologic agent of TRENCH

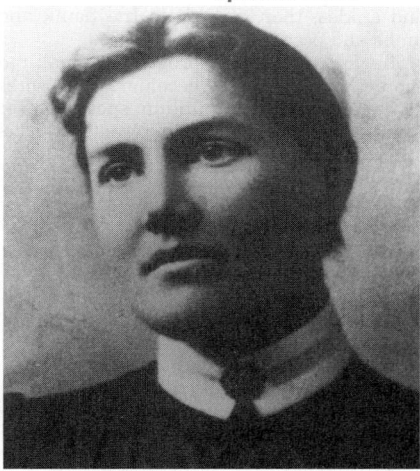

Isabel Hampton Robb. The Alan Mason Chesney Medical Archives of the Johns Hopkins Medical Institutions.

FEVER, transmitted by the body louse *Pediculus humanus.*

Rocky Mountain spotted fever an infectious TICK FEVER originally seen in the Rocky Mountains of North America but now recognized in various other parts of North and South America. Characteristics include fever, headache, muscle pain, and rash. It was originally called "black measles" because of the appearance of the rash, and it is known by various other names in specific geographic areas.

Rocky Mountain spotted fever belongs to a group of insect-borne fevers caused by microscopic parasites known as RICKETTSIAE, which attack the cells lining small blood vessels. The species *Rickettsia rickettsii,* responsible for Rocky Mountain spotted fever, is transmitted from rodent to humans by various ticks.

Symptoms. After the bite of the infected tick, there is an incubation period of 3 to 10 days before the major symptoms set in. Within a day or two after the bite, victims may feel somewhat ill and lose their appetite. The actual onset is marked by chills or chilly sensations, fever, headache, pain behind the eyes, joint and muscle pain, and photophobia. Other symptoms are nausea, vomiting, sore throat, and abdominal pain. Some patients become highly irritable and delirious, or so lethargic that they may lapse into a stupor or coma. Usually 3 to 5 days after the onset a rash appears on the wrists

R

and ankles, then spreads to the trunk and limbs and occasionally to the face.

The appearance and progress of small red spots that eventually become larger sores distinguish Rocky Mountain spotted fever from the several diseases it resembles in its other symptoms (measles, typhoid fever, typhus).

Treatment and Prevention. Like other rickettsial diseases, Rocky Mountain spotted fever responds readily to treatment with tetracyclines and chloramphenicol. If untreated, it can be serious and often fatal. Preventive measures are directed mainly against the disease-carrying ticks and rodents.

rocuronium (ro″ku-ro′ne-um) a neuromuscular blocking AGENT, used as the bromide salt as an adjunct in general ANESTHESIA to facilitate endotracheal intubation and as a skeletal muscle relaxant during surgery or mechanical ventilation; administered intravenously.

rod (rod) 1. a straight, slim mass of substance. 2. one of two types of visual cells, cylindrical segments that contain RHODOPSIN; together with the CONES they form the light-sensitive elements of the RETINA. See also EYE and VISION. Called also retinal rod.

Corti's r's pillar cells.

Harrington r. a rigid contoured metal rod used in Harrington INSTRUMENTATION.

olfactory r. the slender apical portion of an olfactory bipolar neuron, a modified dendrite extending to the surface of the epithelium.

retinal r. ROD (def. 2).

rodenticide (ro-den′tĭ-sīd) 1. destructive to rodents. 2. an agent with this effect.

r. poisoning poisoning by the effects of rodenticides; in humans it is rarely accidental but may occur in cases such as suicide attempts. Domestic animals may sicken and even die after either eating the poison directly or consuming rodents that have died from the poison. Poisoning by anticoagulant rodenticides such as INDANEDIONE and derivatives of WARFARIN occurs most often.

roentgen (rent′gen) the international unit of x- or γ-radiation; it is the quantity of x- or γ-radiation such that the associated corpuscular emission per 0.001293 g of air produces, in air, ions carrying 1 electrostatic unit of electrical charge of either sign. Abbreviated R.

roentgenograph (rent′gen-o-graf″) radiograph.

roentgenography (rent″gĕ-nog′rah-fe) radiography. adj., **roentgenograph′ic.**

roentgenologist (rent″gĕ-nol′ah-jist) radiologist.

roentgenology (rent″gĕ-nol′ah-je) radiology.

roentgenoscope (rent′gen-o-skōp″) fluoroscope.

roentgenoscopy (rent″gĕ-nos′kah-pe) fluoroscopy.

rofecoxib (ro″fĕ-cok′sib) a NONSTEROIDAL ANTIINFLAMMATORY DRUG of the COX-2 INHIBITORS group, used in treatment of OSTEOARTHRITIS, acute pain, and DYSMENORRHEA.

Roger's disease (ro-zhāz′) a ventricular septal defect; the term is usually restricted to small, asymptomatic defects.

Rogers (roj′erz) Martha E. (died 1994). A leader in community health nursing, visiting lecturer, research associate, nursing educator, author, and developer of the SCIENCE OF UNITARY HUMAN BEINGS, a conceptual model of nursing. She was a pioneer in the development of a body of knowledge that is specific and unique to nursing. This recognition of the need for an organized body of nursing knowledge was evident in her early writing on nursing education. Her goal was "to evolve a conceptual system that would give identity to nursing as a knowledgeable endeavor."

role (rōl) a pattern of behavior developed in response to the demands or expectations of others; the pattern of responses to the persons with whom an individual interacts in a particular situation.

caregiver r. the functions performed by a CAREGIVER; see also under FATIGUE and STRAIN.

gender r. the public expression of GENDER; the image projected by a person that identifies their maleness or femaleness, which need not correspond to their gender IDENTITY.

impaired r. the role played by a person who is disabled or chronically ill and who is experiencing a state of wellness and realization of potential commensurate with the condition. Unlike the sick person, the impaired person cannot be expected to "want to get well" but is expected to resume as much normal behavior as is possible.

sick r. the role played by a person who has defined himself or herself as ill, with or without validation of the role by health care providers or family members. Adoption of the sick role changes the behavioral expectations of others toward sick persons. They are exempted from normal social responsibilities and not held responsible for the condition; they are obliged to "want to get well" and to seek competent medical help. The sick role also involves behavioral changes, including increased attention to the body and bodily functions, regression (increase in dependen

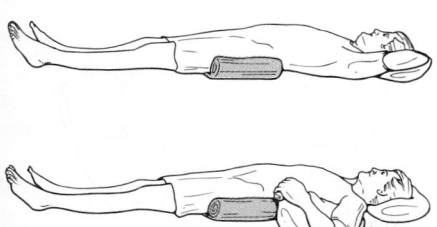

Use of trochanter roll to prevent external rotation of hip.

behavior), narrowing of interests, and emotional overreactions.

roll (rōl) 1. to turn along an axis while moving forward along a surface. 2. the act of rolling. 3. an object that has been rolled into a cylindrical shape.

pelvic r. pelvic rotation.

trochanter r. a wedge (usually a rolled towel) placed from the crest of the ilium to midthigh to prevent external rotation of the hip when the patient is in a recumbent position. See illustration.

rollover test (rōl′o-ver) a test to assess the risk of toxemia in pregnant women. A comparison of blood pressure is made with the woman lying on her left side and on her back; an excessive increase in blood pressure when she rolls to the supine position indicates increased risk of toxemia.

ROM range of motion.

Romano-Ward syndrome (ro-mah′no ward′) prolongation of the Q–T INTERVAL with SYNCOPE, sometimes with ventricular FIBRILLATION and sudden death; it is inherited as an autosomal dominant trait and can be triggered by stress or exercise. See also LONG QT SYNDROME.

rombergism (rom′berg-izm) the tendency of a patient to sway while standing still with feet close together and eyes closed; associated with loss of position sense.

rongeur (ron-zher′) [Fr.] a forcepslike instrument for cutting tough tissue, particularly bone.

Röntgen (rent′gen) Wilhelm Conrad (1845–1923). German physicist, born at

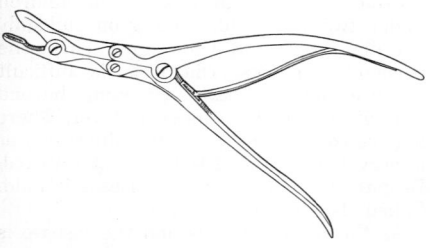

Rongeur. From Dorland's, 2000.

Lennep (Rheinland). For his discovery of x-rays while experimenting with a cathode-ray tube in 1895, he received the first Nobel prize for physics in 1901.

Rood method (rōōd) a method of neuromuscular treatment that views the nervous system as hierarchical and is used for individuals with mobility problems. It emphasizes the use of sensory inputs to produce and modify motor responses; the developmental stage and abilities of the patient are used in developing purposeful responses.

room (rōōm) a place in a building enclosed and set apart for occupancy or for the performance of certain procedures.

birthing r. a hospital room that is utilized for labor and delivery. It is decorated in a homelike, comfortable fashion and contains a specially equipped bed that can be adjusted for delivery. Specialized equipment is often concealed.

emergency r. popular term for EMERGENCY DEPARTMENT.

labor, delivery, recovery r. a birthing room or suite so equipped that a patient can remain in the same room throughout the birthing experience.

labor, delivery, recovery, postpartum r. a birthing room or suite so equipped that a patient can remain in the same room throughout the birthing experience and into the postpartum period.

LDR r. labor, delivery, recovery room.

LDRP r. labor, delivery, recovery, postpartum room.

operating r. one especially equipped for the performance of surgical operations.

recovery r. postanesthesia care UNIT.

rooming in the placement of a mother and newborn child in the same hospital room to facilitate attachment and the acquisition of skills of caring for the newborn.

root (rōōt) 1. the descending and subterranean part of a plant. 2. that portion of an organ, such as a tooth, hair, or nail, that is buried in the tissues, or by which it arises from another structure, or the part of a nerve that is adjacent to the center to which it is connected.

anterior r. the anterior, or motor, division of each spinal nerve, attached centrally to the spinal cord and joining peripherally with the posterior root to form the nerve before it emerges from the intervertebral foramen; it conveys motor fibers to skeletal muscle and contains preganglionic autonomic fibers at the thoracolumbar and sacral levels. Called also ventral root.

dorsal r. posterior root.

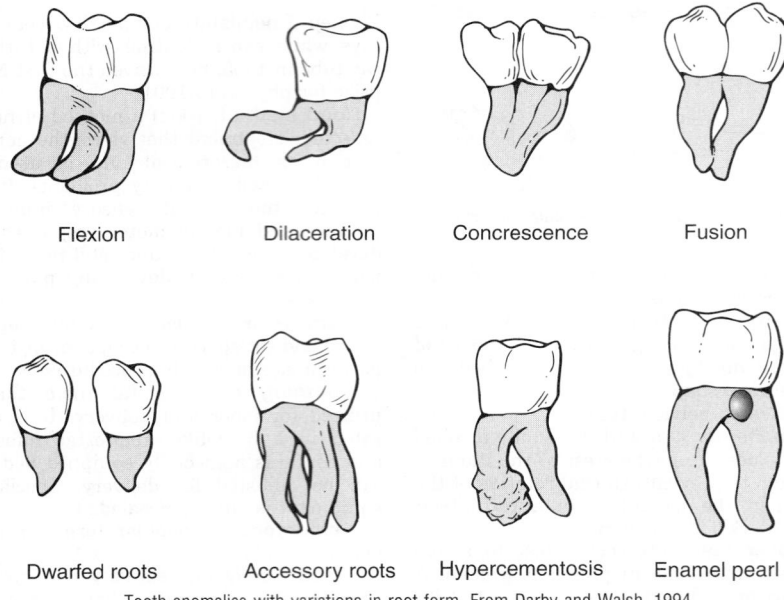

Flexion   Dilaceration   Concrescence   Fusion

Dwarfed roots   Accessory roots   Hypercementosis   Enamel pearl

Tooth anomalies with variations in root form. From Darby and Walsh, 1994.

motor r. anterior root.

nerve r's the series of paired bundles of nerve fibers which emerge at each side of the spinal cord, termed dorsal (or posterior) or ventral (or anterior) according to their position. There are 31 pairs (8 cervical, 12 thoracic, 5 lumbar, 5 sacral, and 1 coccygeal), each corresponding dorsal and ventral root joining to form a spinal nerve. Certain cranial nerves, e.g., the trigeminal, also have nerve roots.

posterior r. the posterior, or sensory, division of each spinal nerve, attached centrally to the spinal cord and joining peripherally with the anterior root to form the nerve before it emerges from the intervertebral foramen; each posterior root bears a spinal ganglion that conveys sensory fibers to the spinal cord. Called also dorsal root.

sensory r. posterior root.

ventral r. anterior root.

ropinirole (ro-pin'ĭ-rōl″)   a   DOPAMINE agonist used as the hydrochloride salt in treatment of PARKINSON'S DISEASE; administered orally.

ropivacaine (ro-piv'ah-kān) a local ANESTHETIC used as the hydrochloride salt for percutaneous infiltration anesthesia, peripheral nerve block, and epidural block.

ROP right occipitoposterior (position of the fetus).

Rorschach test (ror'shahk) one for disclosing personality traits and conflicts by the patient's interpretation of 10 cards bearing symmetrical ink blots in various colors and shadings.

rosacea (ro-za'she-ah) acne rosacea.

rosaniline (ro-zan'ĭ-lin) a triphenylmethane derivative, the basis of various dyes and a component of basic fuchsin.

rosary (ro'zah-re) a structure resembling a string of beads.

rachitic r. a succession of beadlike prominences along the costal cartilages, in rickets.

Rosenthal syndrome (ro″zen-thawl) hemophilia C.

roseola (ro-ze'o-lah, ro″ze-o'lah) [L.] 1. any rose-colored rash. 2. roseola infantum.

r. infan'tum a common acute disease caused by infection with the HERPESVIRUS *Roseolovirus.* It usually occurs in children under two years old, coming on suddenly and disappearing in 3 to 5 days, leaving no permanent marks. Diagnosis is difficult because the sole early symptom, beyond irritability and drowsiness, is fever. There may be convulsions, and generally the fever is very high; 40°C (104°F) is not unusual. Despite the high fever, the disease is mild. Called also exanthem subitum.

As the fever subsides and the disease is apparently at an end, a rash breaks out, usually on the body. This is unlike the course of other childhood diseases such as measles, scarlet fever, and chickenpox, in which the rash is present during the most intense phase; the rash of roseola infantum lasts only a few days and may disappear within hours (often it is so transitory that it is missed). Treatment consists only of such standard measures as antipyretics and tepid sponge baths to allay the fever. Rest and fluids are also recommended.

Once it is over, the child is believed to be permanently immune from further attacks. Roseola is sometimes confused with RUBELLA, but is distinguished by having no lymph node involvement. Blood antibody titers are sometimes used when symptoms appear, to determine which disease it is.

syphilitic r. an eruption of rose-colored spots in early secondary SYPHILIS.

Roseolovirus (ro″ze-o′lo-vi″rus) a genus of HERPESVIRUSES closely related to the genus *Cytomegalovirus*, containing the single species human HERPESVIRUS 6, which is the etiologic agent of ROSEOLA INFANTUM.

rosette (ro-zet′) 1. any structure or formation resembling a rose. 2. the clusters of polymorphonuclear leukocytes around a globule of lipid nuclear material, as observed in the test for disseminated lupus erythematosus. 3. a figure formed by the chromosomes in an early stage of mitosis.

rosiglitazone (ro-sig-lit′ah-zōn) an antidiabetic agent that increases insulin sensitivity, used orally as the maleate salt in the treatment of type 2 diabetes mellitus.

rosin (roz′in) the solid resin obtained from species of pines, used in preparation of ointments and plasters, but potentially a cause of contact allergy.

rostellum (ros-tel′um) a small protuberance or beak, especially the fleshy protuberance of the scolex (mouth) of a TAPEWORM, which may or may not bear hooks.

rostrad (ros′trad) 1. toward a rostrum; nearer the rostrum in relation to a specific point of reference. 2. cephalad.

rostral (ros′tral) 1. pertaining to, resembling, or having a rostrum or beak. 2. situated toward a rostrum (oral and nasal region). In humans this may mean superior (in relationships of areas of the spinal cord) or anterior (in relationships of brain areas).

r. spread the distribution of a NARCOTIC within the cerebrospinal fluid during epidural administration; it is determined by fat and water solubility properties of the narcotic.

rostrate (ros′trāt) beaked.

rostrum (ros′trum) [L.] 1. a beak-shaped process. 2. the oral and nasal region.

ROT right occipitotransverse (position of the fetus).

rotation (ro-ta′shun) 1. the process of turning around an axis. 2. in obstetrics, the turning of the fetal head (or presenting part) for proper orientation to the pelvic axis. It should occur naturally, but if it does not it must be accomplished manually or instrumentally by the OBSTETRICIAN or manually by the nurse-MIDWIFE. 3. a clinical assignment for students in a specific clinical area. 4. in dentistry, the turning of a malturned tooth into its proper position.

pelvic r. movement of the pelvis around an imaginary axis.

site r. the selection of sequential injection locations for a patient receiving multiple injections. A chart is frequently utilized to guide the nurse in rotating sites so that the same location is not used repeatedly, which would lead to tissue damage and irregular absorption of drugs.

rotavirus (ro′tah-vi″rus) any member of a genus of REOVIRUSES that have a wheellike appearance; they are transmitted by the fecal-oral route and cause acute gastroenteritis and diarrhea in infants and young children. There are 6 different antigenic groups.

rotenone (ro′tĕ-nōn) a poisonous compound from derris root and other roots; used as an INSECTICIDE.

roughage (ruf′ij) coarse, largely indigestible material, such as bran, cereals, fruit, and vegetable fibers, that acts as an irritant to stimulate intestinal evacuation.

rouleau (roo-lo′) [Fr.] an abnormal group of red blood cells adhering together like a pile of coins.

roundworm (round′werm) any member of the class NEMATODA, somewhat resembling common earthworms in appearance; many are found as parasites in humans or other animals. Those most frequently infecting humans include *Ascaris lumbricoides* (see ASCARIASIS); *Enterobius vermicularis*

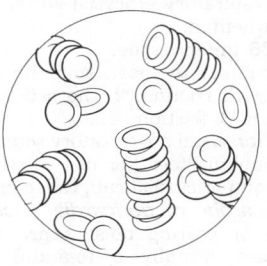

Human red blood cells arranged in rouleaux. From Dorland's, 2000.

(the PINWORM; see ENTEROBIASIS); the HOOK-WORM (see HOOKWORM DISEASE); the FILARIA (see FILARIASIS); and the TRICHINA (see TRICHI-NOSIS).

Roux-en-Y (roo-en-wi; Fr. roo-ahn-e-grek′) denoting any Y-shaped anastomosis in which the small intestine is included.

Rovsing sign (rov′sing) pressure on the left side over the point corresponding to the McBurney point will elicit pain at the McBurney point typical of appendicitis.

Roy (roy) Sister Callista. Nursing educator, lecturer, and developer of the ADAPTATION MODEL for nursing. In more recent years she has given attention to the development of a nursing taxonomy and nursing diagnoses, actively participating in regional conferences on the classification of nursing diagnoses. She continues research on the elements of her conceptual model, including clinical research on it.

RPF renal plasma FLOW.

R Ph Registered Pharmacist.

rpm revolutions per minute.

RPR test rapid plasma reagin test.

RQ respiratory quotient.

RRA Registered Record Administrator.

-rrhage, -rrhagia word element [Gr.], *excessive flow.* adj., **-rrha′gic.**

-rrhea word element [Gr.], *profuse flow;* adj., **-rrhe′ic.**

rRNA ribosomal RNA; see RIBONUCLEIC ACID.

RRT Registered Respiratory Therapist.

RSA right sacroanterior (position of the fetus).

RScA right scapuloanterior (position of the fetus).

RScP right scapuloposterior (position of the fetus).

RSNA Radiological Society of North America.

RSP right sacroposterior (position of the fetus).

RST right sacrotransverse (position of the fetus).

RSV respiratory syncytial virus.

Ru ruthenium.

RU-486 mifepristone.

rub (rub) 1. to move something over a surface with friction. 2. the action of such movement. 3. friction rub.

friction r. an auscultatory sound caused by the rubbing together of two serous surfaces, as in pericardial rub; called also rub.

pericardial r., pericardial friction r. a scraping or grating noise heard with the heart beat, usually a to-and-fro sound, associated with an inflamed pericardium. Patients often complain of pleuritic discomfort that radiates in the chest, especially during inhalation. This condition must be distinguished from ANGINA PECTORIS.

pleural r., pleuritic r. a friction rub caused by friction between the visceral and costal pleurae.

rubefacient (roo″bĕ-fa′shent) 1. reddening the skin by producing local VASODILATION with HYPEREMIA. 2. an agent that so acts.

rubella (roo-bel′ah) a mild systemic disease caused by a virus and characterized by a fever and a transient rash. It is not as contagious as CHICKENPOX or MEASLES, but there are frequent epidemics among schoolchildren, usually during the spring and early summer. The virus is spread by direct contact and by droplet infection. Rubella begins with a slight cold, fever, and sore throat. The lymph nodes behind the ears and at the back of the neck may swell, causing soreness or pain when the head is moved. The rash appears first on the face and scalp, and spreads to the body and arms the same day; it is similar to the rash of measles, although the spots usually do not run together. It fades after 2 or 3 days, although in a few cases the disease may last as long as a week. Called also German measles and three-day measles If a pregnant woman contracts rubella, especially during the first trimester, the virus can damage the developing offspring. The location and extent of the resulting congenital anomaly are determined in large part by the developmental stage of the embryo at the time of the attack. Congenital heart defects, cataracts, mental retardation, and deafness are some of the more common defects resulting from maternal rubella.

TREATMENT AND PREVENTION. Except for complications that may result if the disease is contracted during pregnancy, other complications are rare. No special treatment, medicine, or diet is necessary unless the patient has a high fever. One attack usually gives lifetime immunity to the disease, although a second attack does occasionally occur. The Centers for Disease Control and Prevention recommends two doses of rubella vaccine for all children, given as combination measles-mumps-rubella VACCINE, with doses at least four weeks apart. The first dose should be given when the child is 12 months old. Vaccine is also recommended for susceptible nonpregnant adolescents and adults who do not have rubella immunity.

congenital r. syndrome, r. syndrome transplacental infection of the fetus with rubella usually in the first trimester of pregnancy, as a consequence of maternal infection (which may or may not be

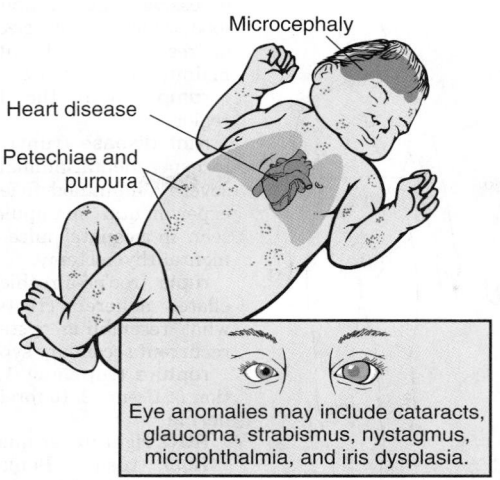

Microcephaly

Heart disease

Petechiae and
purpura

Eye anomalies may include cataracts,
glaucoma, strabismus, nystagmus,
microphthalmia, and iris dysplasia.

Congenital rubella syndrome is marked by a triad that includes microcephaly, microphthalmia, and congenital heart disease. From Damjanov, 2000.

clinically apparent), resulting in various developmental abnormalities in the newborn infant. They include cardiac and ocular lesions, deafness, microcephaly, mental retardation, and generalized growth retardation, which may be associated with acute self-limited conditions such as thrombocytopenic purpura, anemia, hepatitis, encephalitis, and radiolucencies of long bones. Infected infants may shed the virus to all contacts for extended periods of time.

rubeola (roo-be′o-lah, roo″be-o′lah) a synonym of measles in English and of German measles in French and Spanish.

rubeosis (roo″be-o′sis) redness.

r. i′ridis a condition characterized by a new formation of vessels and connective tissue on the surface of the iris, frequently seen in diabetics.

ruber (roo′ber) [L.] red.

rubescent (roo-bes′ent) growing red; reddish.

rubidium (roo-bid′e-um) a chemical element, atomic number 37, atomic weight 85.47, symbol Rb. (See Appendix 6.)

r. 82 a radioactive isotope of rubidium having a half-life of 1.273 minutes and decaying by positron emission. It is used as a TRACER in positron emission TOMOGRAPHY.

Rubin's test (roo′binz) a test for patency of the FALLOPIAN TUBES, made by transuterine inflation with carbon dioxide gas; called also tubal insufflation.

rubor (roo′bor) [L.] redness, one of the cardinal signs of INFLAMMATION.

rubriblast (roo′brĭ-blast) proerythroblast.

rubric (roo′brik) red; specifically, pertaining to the red nucleus.

rubricyte (roo′brĭ-sīt) polychromatophilic erythroblast.

rubrospinal (roo″bro-spi′nal) pertaining to the red nucleus and the spinal cord.

rubrothalamic (roo″bro-thah-lam′ik) pertaining to the red nucleus and the thalamus.

rubrum (roo′brum) [L.] red.

rudiment (roo′dĭ-ment) 1. an organ or part having little or no function but which has functioned at an earlier stage in the same individual or in his ancestors. 2. primordium.

rudimentary (roo″dĭ-men′tar-e) 1. imperfectly developed. 2. vestigial.

rudimentum (roo″dĭ-men′tum) rudiment; in NA, the first indication of a structure in the course of its embryonic development.

ruga (roo′gah) [L.] a ridge, wrinkle, or fold.

rugose (roo′gōs) marked by ridges; wrinkled.

rugosity (roo-gos′ĭ-te) 1. the condition of being rugose. 2. a fold, wrinkle, or ruga.

RUL right upper lobe (of lung).

rule (rool) a statement of conditions commonly observed in a given situation, or of a prescribed procedure to obtain a given result. For specific rules, see specific name, as M′NAGHTEN RULE.

r. of nines a method of estimating the extent of burns, expressed as a percentage of total body surface. In this method, the body is divided into sections of 9 per cent, or

R

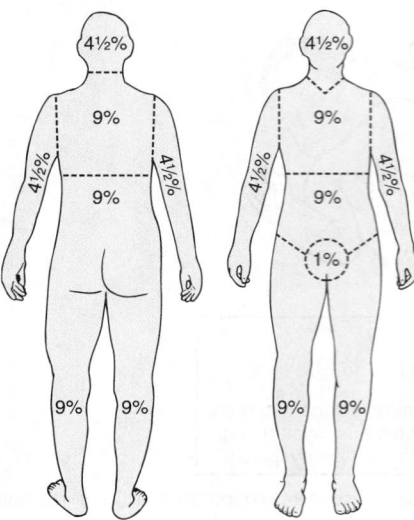

Rule of nines.

multiples of 9 per cent, each: head and neck, 9 per cent; anterior trunk, 18 per cent; posterior trunk, 18 per cent; upper limbs, 18 per cent; lower limbs, 36 per cent; genitalia and perineum, 1 per cent. (See accompanying illustration.) The rule of nines is fairly accurate for adults but does not allow for differences in proportion in children, for whom the LUND AND BROWDER CLASSIFICATION is generally used.

ruminant (roo′mĭ-nant) 1. chewing the cud. 2. an animal that has a stomach with four complete cavities, and that characteristically regurgitates undigested food from the rumen, the first stomach, and masticates it when at rest.

rumination (roo″mĭ-na′shun) 1. in ruminants, the casting up of food out of the rumen and chewing of it a second time. 2. in humans, the regurgitation of food after almost every meal, part of it being vomited and the rest swallowed; this is sometimes seen in infants (RUMINATION DISORDER OF INFANCY) and in individuals with MENTAL RETARDATION. 3. persistent meditation on a subject, particularly thinking about and reviewing one's past.

r. disorder an EATING DISORDER seen in infants under one year of age; after a period of normal eating habits, the child begins excessive regurgitation and rechewing of food, which is then ejected from the mouth or reswallowed; if untreated, death from malnutrition may occur.

rump (rump) the buttock or gluteal region.

runt disease (runt) a clinical syndrome in experimental animals that is a result of severe immunodeficiency produced by experimental manipulation; it was first seen in neonatal mice subjected to experimental thymectomy.

rupia (roo′pe-ah) thick, dark, raised, lamellated, adherent crusts on the skin, somewhat resembling oyster shells, as in late recurrent secondary syphilis. adj., **ru′pial.**

rupture (rup′chur) 1. tearing or disruption of tissue. 2. to forcibly disrupt tissue. 3. hernia.

RUQ right upper quadrant (of abdomen).

Rush (rush) Benjamin (1745–1813). American physician, born in Philadelphia, and educated at Princeton and the University of Edinburgh. He helped found the Philadelphia Dispensary in 1786, and was physician to Pennsylvania Hospital, where he introduced clinical instruction. Rush protested against improper treatment of the insane until the legislature made provision for construction of a ward for them at Pennsylvania Hospital. He served as a surgeon in the Continental Army, and with James Pemberton founded the first anti-slavery society in America. As a member of the Continental Congress, Rush was a signer of the Declaration of Independence, and in 1787 he was a member of the Pennsylvania convention that adopted the Federal Constitution.

rush (rush) peristaltic rush; a powerful wave of contractile activity that travels very long distances down the small intestine, caused by intense irritation or unusual distention.

ruthenium (roo-the′ne-um) a chemical element, atomic number 44, atomic weight 101.07, symbol Ru. (See Appendix 6.)

rutherford (ruth′er-ford) a unit of radioactive disintegration, representing one million disintegrations per second.

RV residual volume.

Rx re′cipe (take); prescription; treatment.

rye (ri) the cereal plant *Secale cereale,* and its nutritious seed.

S

S siemens; substrate; sulfur; Svedberg unit; sacral vertebrae (S1–S5).

S. [L.] sig′na (mark).

S₁ first heart sound; see HEART SOUNDS.

S₂ second heart sound; see HEART SOUNDS.

S₃ third heart sound; see HEART SOUNDS.

S₄ fourth heart sound; see HEART SOUNDS.

S_f Svedberg flotation unit.

s second.

s. [L.] sinis′ter (left); se′mis (half).

s̄ [L.] si′ne (without).

SA SURGEON ASSISTANT.

Sabin (sa′bin) Albert Bruce (1906–1993). American virologist, born in Bialystok, Poland; he developed an oral vaccine against poliomyelitis; see poliovirus VACCINE live oral.

sabulous (sab′u-lus) gritty or sandy.

saburra (sah-bur′ah) sordes; foulness of the mouth or stomach.

saburral (sah-bur′al) 1. pertaining to saburra. 2. gritty, gravelly.

sac (sak) a baglike organ or structure; see also BAG, POCKET, and POUCH.

   air s′s, alveolar s′s the spaces into which the alveolar ducts open distally, and with which the alveoli communicate; see also LUNG.

   amniotic s. the sac formed by the amnion, enclosing the fetus suspended in amniotic fluid; popularly known as the bag of waters.

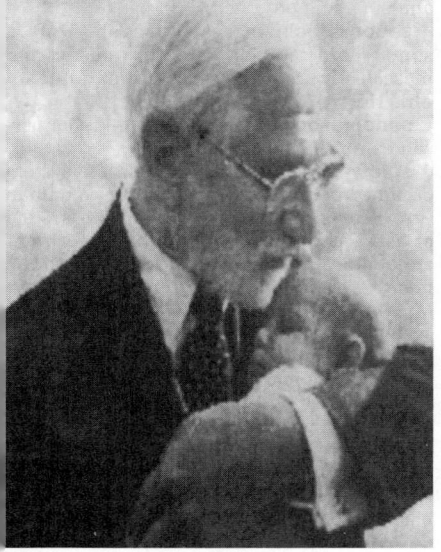

Albert Bruce Sabin. Courtesy Sabin Vaccine Institute.

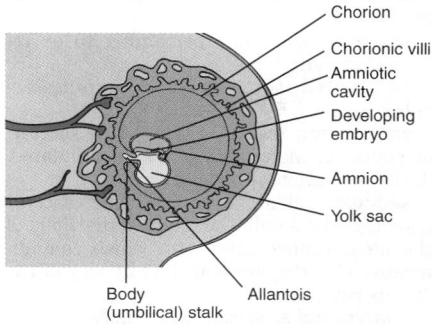

Yolk sac in a developing embryo. From Applegate, 2000.

   conjunctival s. the potential space, lined by conjunctiva, between the eyelids and the eyeball.

   endolymphatic s. the blind, flattened cerebral end of the endolymphatic duct.

   hernial s. the peritoneal pouch that encloses protruding intestine.

   lacrimal s. the dilated upper end of the nasolacrimal duct; see also LACRIMAL APPARATUS.

   yolk s. the extraembryonic membrane connected with the midgut; in vertebrates below true mammals, it contains a yolk mass.

saccade (sah-kād′) the series of involuntary, abrupt, rapid, small movements or jerks of both eyes simultaneously in changing the point of fixation. adj., **saccad′ic.**

saccate (sak′āt) 1. saccular. 2. contained in a bag or sac.

saccharide (sak′ah-rīd) one of a series of carbohydrates, including the sugars; they are divided into monosaccharides, disaccharides, trisaccharides, and polysaccharides according to the number of saccharide groups composing them.

sacchariferous (sak″ah-rif′er-us) containing sugar.

saccharin (sak′ah-rin) a white, crystalline compound several hundred times sweeter than SUCROSE; used as a noncaloric sweetening agent, but now proved to be CARCINOGENIC in test animals.

saccharogalactorrhea (sak″ah-ro-gah-lak″-to-re′ah) secretion of milk containing an excess of sugar.

saccharolytic (sak″ah-ro-lit′ik) capable of splitting up sugar.

saccharometabolic (sak″ah-ro-met″ah-bol′ik) pertaining to the metabolism of sugar.

saccharometabolism (sak″ah-ro-mĕ-tab′-o-lizm) the metabolism of sugar.

sacciform (sak′sĭ-form) shaped like a bag or sac.

saccular (sak′u-lar) pertaining to or resembling a sac.

sacculated (sak′u-lāt″ed) containing saccules.

sacculation (sak″u-la′shun) 1. a saccule, or pouch. 2. the quality of being sacculated. 3. the formation of pouches.

saccule (sak′ūl) 1. a little bag, sac, or pouch. 2. the smaller of the two divisions of the membranous LABYRINTH, which communicates with the cochlear duct by way of the ductus reuniens.

laryngeal s. sacculus laryngis.

sacculus (sak′u-lus), pl. *sac′culi* [L.] saccule.

s. laryn′gis a diverticulum extending upward from the front of the ventricle of the larynx.

saccus (sak′us) [L.] sac.

sacr(o)- word element [L.], *sacrum.*

sacrad (sa′krad) toward the sacrum.

sacral (sa′kral) pertaining to the sacrum.

sacralgia (sa-kral′jah) pain in the sacrum.

sacralization (sa″kral-ĭ-za′shun) anomalous fusion of the fifth lumbar vertebra with the first segment of the sacrum.

sacrectomy (sa-krek′tah-me) excision or resection of the sacrum.

sacrococcygeal (sa″kro-kok-sij′e-al) pertaining to the sacrum and coccyx.

sacrocoxalgia (sa″kro-kok-sal′jah) a painful condition of the sacrum and coccyx.

sacrocoxitis (sa″kro-kok-si′tis) sacroiliitis.

sacrodynia (sa″kro-din′e-ah) pain in the sacral region.

sacroiliac (sa″kro-il′e-ak) pertaining to the SACRUM and ILIUM, or the joint formed between them, or to the lower part of the back where they meet.

s. disease chronic tuberculous inflammation of the SACROILIAC JOINT.

s. joint the joint formed by the sacrum and ilium where they meet on either side of the lower back. The tight joint allows little motion and is subject to great stress, as the body's weight pushes downward and the legs and pelvis push upward against the joint. The sacroiliac joint must also bear the leverage demands made by the trunk of the body as it turns, twists, pulls, and pushes. When these motions place an excess of stress on the ligaments binding the joint and on the connecting muscles (such as during weight lifting), strain may result.

sacroiliitis (sa″kro-il″e-i′tis) inflammation (ARTHRITIS) of the sacroiliac joint.

sacrolumbar (sa″kro-lum′bar) pertaining to the sacrum and loins.

sacrosciatic (sa″kro-si-at′ik) pertaining to the sacrum and ischium.

sacrosidase (sak-ro′sĭ-dās) an enzyme used as a substitute to replace the sucrase activity lacking in sucrase-isomaltase deficiency, administered orally.

sacrospinal (sa″kro-spi′nal) pertaining to the sacrum and vertebral column.

sacrouterine (sa″kro-u′ter-in) pertaining to the sacrum and uterus.

sacrovertebral (sa″kro-ver′tĕ-bral) pertaining to the sacrum and vertebrae.

sacrum (sa′krum) the triangular bone at the base of the spine formed by usually five fused vertebrae wedged dorsally between the two hip bones. See Appendix 3-3.

SAD seasonal affective disorder.

sadism (sa′dizm) the act or instance of gaining pleasure from inflicting physical or psychological pain on another. The term is usually used to denote sexual s. adj., **sadis′-tic.**

sexual s. a PARAPHILIA in which sexual gratification is derived from hurting, humiliating, or otherwise inflicting physical or psychological suffering on another.

sadist (sa′dist) a person who practices sadism.

sadistic personality disorder a PERSONALITY DISORDER marked by a pervasive pattern of cruel, demeaning, and aggressive behavior. Satisfaction is gained in intimidating, coercing, humiliating, and inflicting pain and suffering on others.

sadomasochism (sa″do-mas′ah-kizm) a state characterized by both sadistic and masochistic tendencies. adj., **sadomaso-chis′tic.**

sadomasochist (sa″do-mas′ah-kist) a person exhibiting sadomasochism.

safety system (sāf′te sis′tem) a system designed to minimize hazards due to human error; in RESPIRATORY THERAPY it is a system of connections designed to help prevent accidental interchanging of incorrect equipment or gases.

American Standard Safety System a system of specifications for threaded high-pressure connections between compressed gas cylinders and their attachments.

Diameter-Indexed Safety System a system of specifications for threaded low-pressure connections between station outlets, flowmeters, and other devices such as nebulizers, ventilators, and anesthesia apparatus.

Pin-Indexed Safety System a subsection of the American Standard Safety

SYSTEM that applies only to valve outlets of small cylinders and employs a joke and pin connection.

sagittal (saj´ĭ-tal) 1. shaped like an arrow. 2. situated in the direction of the sagittal suture; said of an anteroposterior plane or section parallel to the median plane of the body.

sagittalis (saj˝ĭ-ta´lis) [L.] sagittal.

Saint Anthony's fire 1. ergotism. 2. erysipelas.

Saint John's wort (sānt jonz wort) any of various species of the genus *Hypericum; H. perforatum* is the medicinal herb, which is used as a mild antidepressant, sedative, and anxiolytic; it is also used topically for inflammation of the skin, contusions, myalgia, and first-degree burns.

Saint Vitus's dance Sydenham's chorea.

Sakati-Nyhan syndrome (sah-kah´te ni´-han) a hereditary autosomal dominant disorder characterized by conical deformity of the head, extra fingers or toes, webbed FINGERS and TOES, hypoplastic tibias, and deformed, displaced fibulas. Called also acrocephalopolysyndactyly, type III.

SAL sterility assurance level.

salicylamide (sal´˝ĭ-sil´ah-mīd) the amide of SALICYLIC ACID, a component of some over-the-counter ANALGESICS and ANTIPYRETICS.

salicylate (sah-lis´ĭ-lāt) any salt or ester of SALICYLIC ACID; those used as drugs for their ANALGESIC, ANTIPYRETIC, and ANTIINFLAMMATORY effects include ASPIRIN, choline salicylate, magnesium salicylate, and sodium salicylate. Low dosages of salicylates are used primarily for the relief of mild to moderate pain or fever; high dosages are particularly useful for treatment of rheumatoid arthritis and other rheumatoid disorders.

The mechanism of most of the effects of aspirin and other salicylates is inhibition of PROSTAGLANDIN synthesis, thus blocking pyretic and inflammatory processes that are mediated by prostaglandins. Aspirin also prolongs bleeding time through its effects on platelets owing to both inhibition of prostaglandin synthesis and acetylation of platelet structures. Salicylates also cause ulceration and hemorrhagic lesions of the gastric mucosa. They act by interfering with the stomach's mucosal barrier (either directly or possibly by an effect on prostaglandins when given parenterally) so that H$^+$ ions leak and there is subsequent damage. Aspirin should not be taken with alcohol, because this increases gastrointestinal damage. Aspirin should be avoided by persons with gastric ulcers, hemophilia, or hemorrhagic states, and by children with a viral illness.

Another problem associated with the use of salicylates is hypersensitivity. This most commonly occurs with aspirin and is less common with other salicylates. Aspirin-sensitive individuals often also react to other antiinflammatory agents, such as INDOMETHACIN, and to a yellow dye used to color foods and drugs called tartrazine or FD & C Yellow No. 5. The allergic reaction usually takes the form of edema of the face and intestinal tract and asthma. Aspirin sensitivity occurs in about 0.25–1.0 per cent of the population and is more common in persons with a history of asthma or other allergic disorders. There is a common association with nasal polyps.

Salicylate Poisoning. Mild salicylate toxicity, which can occur from high dosage therapy, has symptoms that include headache, dizziness, tinnitus, deafness, nausea, vomiting, and acid-base disturbances. If the poisoning occurs in the home, a POISON CONTROL CENTER should be contacted immediately. Large overdoses produce acute poisoning that is a medical emergency. Treatment consists of gastrointestinal decontamination, administration of intravenous fluids to correct dehydration and acid-base imbalance, and hemodialysis if serum salicylate levels are very high. Body sponging with cool water is done for HYPERPYREXIA. Blood salicylate levels and blood gases and electrolytes are periodically determined by laboratory tests. Life-threatening poisoning may require exchange transfusion or renal dialysis.

methyl s. see under METHYL.

salicylic acid (sal´˝ĭ-sil´ik) a KERATOLYTIC and caustic, used to treat a variety of skin conditions, such as dandruff, seborrheic dermatitis, acne, and psoriasis, and to remove calluses, corns, and warts. Its salts are the SALICYLATES.

salicylism (sal´ĭ-sil˝izm) toxic effects of overdosage with SALICYLIC ACID or SALICYLATES, usually marked by tinnitus, nausea, and vomiting.

saline (sa´lēn, sa´līn) salty; of the nature of a salt.

s. solution a solution of salt (sodium chloride) in purified water. See also PHYSIOLOGIC SALINE SOLUTION.

saliva (sah-li´vah) the enzyme-containing secretion of the salivary glands.

salivant (sal´ĭ-vant) causing flow of saliva.

salivary (sal´ĭ-ver-e) pertaining to the saliva.

s. glands the glands in the mouth that secrete SALIVA. The major ones are the three pairs known as the parotid, submaxillary, and sublingual GLANDS (see Plates); there are other smaller salivary glands within the cheeks and tongue. The largest are the

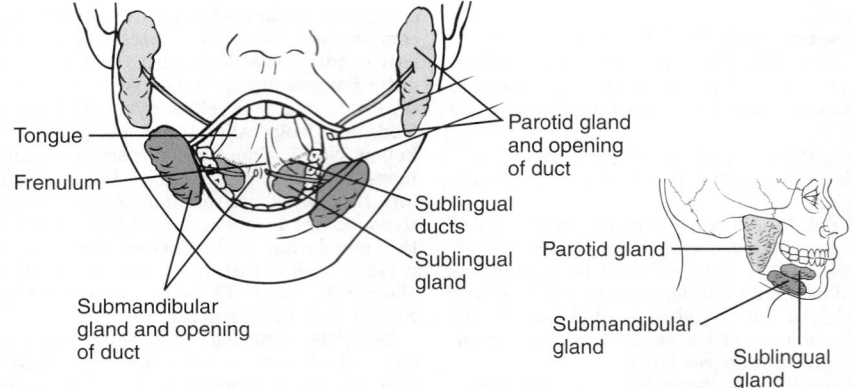

The salivary glands. From Jarvis, 2000.

parotids, located below and in front of each ear. Saliva secreted by these glands is discharged into the mouth through openings in the cheeks on each side opposite the upper teeth. The submaxillary glands, located inside the lower jaw, discharge saliva upward through openings into the floor of the mouth. The sublingual glands, beneath the tongue, also discharge saliva into the floor of the mouth.

The saliva is needed to moisten the mouth, lubricate food for easier swallowing, remineralize the tooth surface, and provide the enzyme (PTYALIN) necessary to begin food breakdown in the preliminary stage of digestion. The salivary glands produce about 1.5 liters of saliva daily.

The salivary glands are controlled by the nervous system. Normally they respond by producing saliva within 2 or 3 seconds after being stimulated by the sight, smell, or taste of food. This quick response is a reflex action.

In mumps (parotitis), the parotids become inflamed and swollen. Occasionally, salivary glands produce too much saliva; this condition is called ptyalism, and is the result of local irritation from dental appliances or of disturbances of digestion or of the nervous system or other causes. Certain diseases, drugs such as morphine or atropine, and nutritional deficiency of vitamin B can result in decreased secretion of saliva.

s. gland inclusion disease cytomegalic inclusion disease.

salivation (sal″ĭ-va′shun) 1. the secretion of saliva. 2. ptyalism.

Salk (sawlk) Jonas Edward (1914–1995). American physician, born in New York City. He developed a vaccine for the prevention of poliomyelitis; see poliovirus VACCINE inactivated.

salmeterol (sal-met′er-ol) a beta₂-adrenergic RECEPTOR agonist, used as s. xinafoate as an orally inhaled BRONCHODILATOR.

Salmonella (sal″mo-nel′ah) a genus of gram-negative, facultatively anaerobic, usually motile, rod-shaped bacteria; this genus is very complex and has been described by several different systems of nomenclature. Clinical laboratories frequently report salmonellae as one of three species, differentiated on the basis of serologic and biochemical reactions: S. ty′phi, S. cho′leraesu′is, and S. enteri′tidis; the last contains all serotypes except the first two. In this system (the Ewing scheme) many strains familiarly named as species are designated as serotypes of S. enteritidis (for example, S. paraty′phi becomes S. enteri′tidis serotype paraty′phi A).

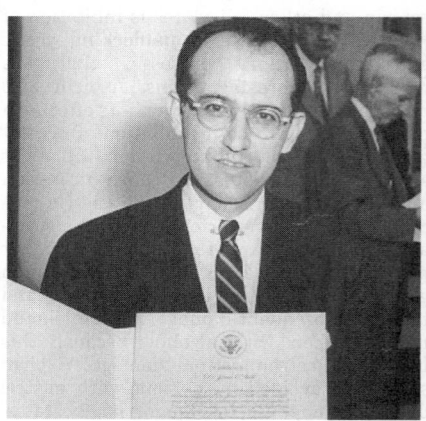

Dr. Jonas Salk with Presidential citation. Courtesy Dwight D. Eisenhower Library Abilene, Kansas. Original photo by National Park Service.

Salmonellae may also be grouped into five subgenera (I–V) on the basis of biochemical reactions and further into species on the basis of antigenic reactions: subgenus I contains most of the species.

Salmonella species are widely distributed in other animals, frequently producing disease that can be transmitted to humans. In humans pathogenic species cause enteric fevers (TYPHOID FEVER and PARATYPHOID FEVER), SEPTICEMIA, and GASTROENTERITIS. The most frequent manifestation is FOOD POISONING. Pathogenic species include *S. arizo'nae* (SALMONELLOSIS), *S. cho'lerae-su'is* (a strain pathogenic for pigs that may infect humans), *S. enteri'tidis* (gastroenteritis; also see discussion of Ewing scheme above), *S. paraty'phi* (or *S. enteri'tidis* serotype *para-y'phi* A) (paratyphoid fever), *S. ty'phi* (typhoid fever), and *S. typhimu'rium* (or *S. enteri'tidis* serotype *typhimu'rium* (food poisoning and paratyphoid fever).

salmonella (sal″mo-nel'ah) any organism of the genus *Salmonella*. adj., **salmonel'lal.**

salmonellosis (sal″mo-nel-o'sis) infection with certain species of the genus *Salmonella,* usually caused by the ingestion of food containing salmonellae or their products. The organisms can be found in raw meats, raw poultry, eggs, and dairy products; they multiply rapidly at temperatures between 7° and 46°C (45° and 115°F). Symptoms of salmonellosis include violent diarrhea attended by abdominal cramps, nausea and vomiting, and fever. It is rarely fatal and can be prevented by adequate cooking. Normal cooking temperatures destroy bacteria, even in rare roast beef. In order to avoid salmonellosis, frozen meat should be thawed in the refrigerator rather than at room temperature, leftovers should be refrigerated promptly, and raw eggs should be avoided. In the care of patients with *Salmonella* infections, enteric precautions are recommended for the duration of the illness.

salping(o)- word element [Gr.] *tube (eustachian tube* or *fallopian tube).*

salpingectomy (sal″pin-jek'tah-me) excision of a FALLOPIAN TUBE; called also tubectomy.

salpingemphraxis (sal″pin-jem-frak'sis) obstruction of a eustachian tube.

salpingian (sal-pin'je-an) tubal.

salpingion (sal-pin'je-on) a point at the apex of the petrous bone on the lower surface.

salpingitis (sal″pin-ji'tis) 1. inflammation of a FALLOPIAN TUBE. 2. inflammation of the EUSTACHIAN TUBE.

    mural s., parenchymatous s. pachysalpingitis.

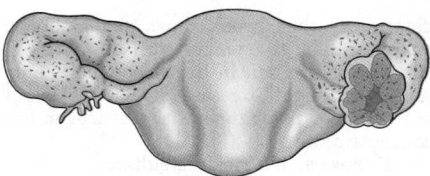

Salpingitis. Infection in fallopian tubes causes them to become enlarged, hyperemic, and tender. McKinney et al., 2000.

salpingocele (sal-ping'go-sēl) hernial protrusion of a fallopian tube.

salpingography (sal″ping-gog'rah-fe) radiography of the fallopian tubes after intrauterine injection of a radiopaque medium.

salpingolithiasis (sal-ping″go-lĭ-thi'ah-sis) the presence of calcareous deposits in the wall of the fallopian tubes.

salpingolysis (sal″ping-gol'ĭ-sis) surgical separation of adhesions involving the fallopian tubes.

salpingo-oophorectomy (sal-ping″go-o″-of-o-rek'tah-me) excision of a fallopian tube and ovary; called also ovariosalpingectomy.

salpingo-oophoritis (sal-ping″go-o″of-o-ri'tis) inflammation of a fallopian tube and ovary.

salpingo-oophorocele (sal-ping″go-o-of'-o-ro-sēl″) hernia of a fallopian tube and ovary.

salpingopexy (sal-ping′go-pek″se) fixation of a fallopian tube.

salpingopharyngeal (sal″ping-go-fah-rin'-je-al) pertaining to the auditory tube and the pharynx.

salpingoplasty (sal-ping′go-plas″te) plastic repair of a fallopian tube.

salpingostomy (sal″ping-gos'tah-me) 1. surgical creation of an opening or formation of a fistula into a fallopian tube for the purpose of drainage. 2. surgical restoration of the patency of a fallopian tube.

salpingotomy (sal″ping-got'ah-me) surgical incision of a fallopian tube.

salpinx (sal'pinks) 1. fallopian tube. 2. eustachian tube.

salsalate (sal'sah-lāt) an ester formed from two molecules of SALICYLIC ACID, used in treatment of rheumatoid ARTHRITIS and osteoarthritis.

salt (sawlt) 1. any compound of a base and an acid. 2. sodium chloride. 3. in the plural, a saline CATHARTIC.

    bile s's GLYCINE or TAURINE conjugates of BILE ACIDS, which are formed in the liver and secreted in the bile. They are powerful

S

detergents that break down fat globules, enabling them to be digested.

buffer s. a salt in the blood that is able to absorb slight excesses of acid or alkali with little or no change in the hydrogen ion concentration.

Epsom s. magnesium sulfate.

Glauber's s. sodium sulfate.

***oral rehydration s's* (ORS)** a dry mixture of sodium chloride, potassium chloride, dextrose, and either sodium citrate or sodium bicarbonate; dissolved in water for use in oral rehydration THERAPY.

smelling s's aromatic AMMONIUM CARBONATE, a stimulant and restorative.

saltation (sal-ta′shun) 1. the action of leaping. 2. the dancing that sometimes accompanies chorea. 3. conduction along myelinated nerves. 4. in genetics, an abrupt variation in species; a mutation. adj., **sal′tatory.**

salting out (sawl′ting out) the separation of protein fractions in the serum or plasma by precipitation in increasing concentrations of neutral salts.

salt-losing crisis (syndrome) vomiting, dehydration, hypotension, and sudden death due to very large sodium losses from the body (see salt WASTING). It may be seen in abnormal losses of SODIUM into the urine (as in congenital adrenal hyperplasia, adrenocortical insufficiency, or one of the forms of salt-losing NEPHRITIS) or in large extrarenal sodium losses, usually from the gastrointestinal tract.

salubrious (sah-loo′bre-us) conducive to health; wholesome.

saluresis (sal″u-re′sis) excretion of sodium and chloride in the urine.

A linear incision is made in the intact tube

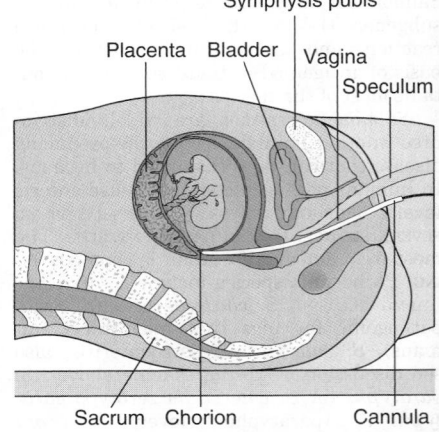

Forceps are used to remove products of conception

The incision is left to heal without being sutured

Linear salpingostomy. From Gorrie et al., 1994.

A diagram of the technique of transvaginal chorionic villus sampling. From Mueller and Young, 2001.

saluretic (sal″u-ret′ik) 1. pertaining to or promoting SALURESIS. 2. an agent that so acts.

salutary (sal′u-tar″e) healthful.

Salutensin (sal″u-ten′sin) trademark for a preparation of HYDROFLUMETHIAZIDE and RESERPINE; an ANTIHYPERTENSIVE AGENT.

salve (sav) ointment.

SAMA Student American Medical Association.

samarium (sah-ma′re-um) a chemical element, atomic number 62, atomic weight 150.35, symbol Sm. (See Appendix 6.) The complex *samarium Sm 153 lexidronam* is used in the palliative treatment of bone pain associated with osteoblastic metastatic bone lesions, administered intravenously.

SAMHSA Substance Abuse and Mental Health Services Administration.

sample 1. a representative part taken to typify the whole. 2. a subset of a population that is selected for inclusion in a research study.

sampling (sam′pling) the selection or making of a sample. 1. the selection of a group of people, events, behaviors, or other elements that are representative of the population being studied in order to derive conclusions about the entire population from a limited number of observations.

accidental s. a type of nonprobability SAMPLING in which the population selected is easily accessible to the researcher; available subjects are simply entered into the study without any attempt at randomization. Called also convenience sampling.

***chorionic villus s.* (CVS)** sampling of CHORIONIC VILLI from the villous area of the CHORION, a procedure used for prenatal diagnosis at nine to 12 weeks of gestation

A catheter is inserted either through the cervix or through the abdominal wall and fetal chorionic villus tissue for analysis is aspirated under ultrasonic guidance. This has been used for the prenatal diagnosis of fetal trisomies, hemoglobinopathies, and biochemical disorders. It allows first trimester diagnosis and direct chromosomal and biochemical analysis but does not screen for neural tube defects or certain other anomalies; some of those may be identified by maternal serum and amniotic fluid ALPHA-FETOPROTEIN measurements.

cluster s. a type of probability sampling in which the population is divided into groups on the basis of some shared characteristic (such as hospitals grouped by geographic region) and a random sample is drawn from each of these groups.

convenience s. accidental sampling.

nonprobability s. sampling in which not every element of the population has an opportunity of being selected for the sample; the sample is not representative of the population and generalizations cannot be made to the population.

percutaneous umbilical blood s. a procedure used to obtain fetal blood for examination; a sterile needle is inserted through the mother's abdomen and uterus, and guided to one of the umbilical veins via ultrasound. This procedure has begun to replace FETOSCOPY because it has a lower complication rate. Direct sampling of fetal blood provides more rapid test results than

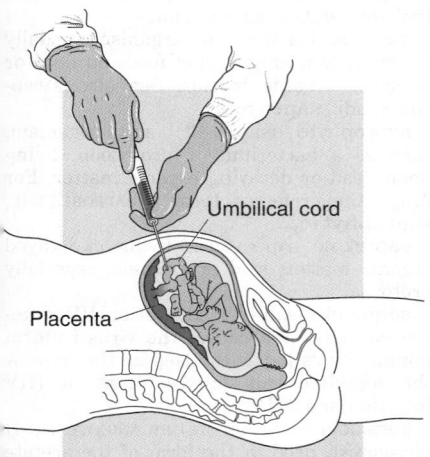

Percutaneous umbilical cord sampling, also known as cordocentesis. The needle is advanced through the skin and into the uterus. Once the needle punctures the umbilical cord and one of the uterine veins, cord blood is aspirated by the syringe. From Malarkey and McMorrow, 2000.

AMNIOCENTESIS, and a more definitive diagnosis. It can be used to identify chromosomal abnormalities, detect a fetal infection, and assess fetal growth and development. Called also cordocentesis.

probability s. sampling in which each element of a population has an opportunity of being selected for the sample; its purpose is to obtain a sample that is representative of the population and from which generalizations to the population can be made.

purposive s. a type of nonprobability sampling in which the researcher consciously selects specific elements or subjects for inclusion in a study in order to ensure that the elements will have certain characteristics relevant to the study.

quota s. a type of nonprobability sampling in which an accidental sample is adjusted to ensure that certain subgroups are not underrepresented; its purpose is to obtain a sample that is representative of the population to which the researcher wishes to make generalizations.

random s. probability sampling.

stratified random s. sampling in which the population is divided into several groups that are alike in certain ways and a random selection is made from each group.

systematic s. the selection of study objects conducted when an ordered list of all members of the population is available; subjects are chosen from the list at a given uniform interval from each other, using a starting point that is selected randomly.

sanative (san′ah-tiv) curative; healing.

sanatorium (san″ah-to′re-um) an institution for treatment of sick persons, especially a private hospital for convalescents or patients who are not extremely ill; often applied to an institution for the treatment of tuberculosis.

sanatory (san′ah-tor″e) conducive to health.

sanctuary (sangk′choo-ar″e) an area in the body where a drug tends to collect and to escape metabolic breakdown.

sand (sand) material occurring in fine gritty particles.

brain s. sandy matter about the pineal gland and other parts of the brain.

sandfly (sand′fli) any of various two-winged flies, especially those of the genus *Phlebotomus*, which are important vectors in the transmission of LEISHMANIASIS and PHLEBOTOMUS FEVER.

s. fever phlebotomus fever.

Sandhoff's disease (sand′hofz) a variant of TAY-SACHS DISEASE not restricted to particular ethnic groups and marked by a progressively more rapid course; it is due to a defect in the enzymes hexosaminidase A and B.

Sandifer's syndrome (san'diferz) intermittent TORTICOLLIS in children as a symptom of reflux ESOPHAGITIS or hiatal HERNIA.

sane (sān) sound in mind.

Sanfilippo's syndrome (san-fil'ĭ-pōz) a form of MUCOPOLYSACCHARIDOSIS, transmitted as an autosomal recessive trait, resembling HURLER'S SYNDROME, except that most of the somatic and skeletal changes are less severe. It occurs in two clinically indistinguishable types: type A, due to deficiency of heparan sulfate sulfamidase, and type B, due to deficiency of N-acetyl-α-D-glucosaminidase. (See Atlas 1, Part F).

Sanger (sang'er) Margaret H. (1883–1966). Founder of the American birth control movement. Her early practice among poor families in New York City led her to recognize the relationship between overpopulation, high infant and maternal mortality, and poverty. As a result she began publishing information on contraception and opened the nation's first birth control clinic.

sangui- word element [L.], *blood.*

sanguifacient (sang″gwĭ-fa'shent) HEMATOPOIETIC.

sanguine (sang'gwin) 1. plethoric. 2. ardent; hopeful.

sanguineous (sang-gwin'e-us) 1. bloody. 2. plethoric.

sanguinolent (sang-gwin'o-lent) of a bloody tinge.

sanguinopurulent (sang″gwĭ-no-pu'ru-lent) containing both blood and pus.

sanguis (sang'gwis) [L.] blood.

sanguivorous (sang-gwiv'ah-rus) bloodeating; said of female mosquitoes that prefer blood to other nutrients.

sanies (sa'ne-ēz) a foul-smelling watery discharge containing serum, pus, and blood. adj., **sa′nious.**

saniopurulent (sa″ne-o-pu'roo-lent) partly sanious and partly purulent.

sanioserous (sa″ne-o-se'rus) partly sanious and partly serous.

sanitarian (san″ĭ-tar'e-an) a PUBLIC HEALTH worker skilled in surveillance of food services, water and air pollution, and sewage planning and control.

sanitarium (san″ĭ-ta're-um) an institution for the promotion of health. The word was originally coined to designate the institution established by the Seventh Day Adventists at Battle Creek, Michigan, to distinguish it from institutions providing care for mental or tuberculous patients.

sanitary (san'ĭ-tar″e) promoting or pertaining to health.

sanitization (san″ĭ-tĭ-za'shun) the process of making or the quality of being made sanitary.

sanitize (san'ĭ-tīz) to clean and sterilize.

sanity (san″ĭ-te) soundness, especially soundness of mind.

San Joaquin Valley fever the primary form of COCCIDIOIDOMYCOSIS.

Sa$_{O_2}$ symbol for percentage of available hemoglobin that is saturated with oxygen; see also BLOOD GAS ANALYSIS.

saphena (sah-fe'nah) the small saphenous or the great saphenous vein.

saphenous (sah-fe'nus) pertaining to or associated with a SAPHENA, such as certain arteries, nerves, and veins.

sapo (sa'po) [L.] soap.

saponaceous (sa″po-na'shus) soapy; of soaplike feel or quality.

saponification (sah-pon″ĭ-fĭ-ka'shun) conversion of an oil or fat into a soap by combination with an alkali. In chemistry, the term now denotes the hydrolysis of an ester by an alkali, resulting in the production of a free alcohol and an alkali salt of the ester acid.

saponin (sap'o-nin) any of a group of glycosides widely distributed in the plant world; they are powerful SURFACTANTS, form durable foam when their watery solutions are shaken, and can dissolve erythrocytes even when highly diluted.

sapophore (sap'o-for) the group of atoms in the molecule of a compound that gives the substance its characteristic taste.

sapr(o)- word element [Gr.], *rotten; putrid; decay; decayed material.*

saprobe (sa'prōb) an organism, usually referring to a fungus, that feeds on dead or decaying organic matter. See also SAPROPHYTE. adj., **sapro′bic.**

saprophyte (sap'ro-fīt) any organism, such as a bacterium or protozoon, living upon dead or decaying organic matter. For fungi, the preferred term is SAPROBE. adj., **saprophyt′ic.**

saprozoic (sap″ro-zo'ik) living on decayed organic matter; said of animals, especially protozoa.

saquinavir (sah-kwin'ah-vir) an HIV protease INHIBITOR that causes the virus to form noninfectious particles; used as the base or the mesylate salt in treatment of HIV infection and AIDS.

saralasin (sar-al'ah-sin) an ANGIOTENSIN II antagonist, used in the form of the acetate ester as an ANTIHYPERTENSIVE in treatment of severe hypertension and in diagnosis of renin-dependent hypertension.

sarc(o)- word element [Gr.], *flesh.*

sarcoblast (sahr'ko-blast) a primordial cell that develops into a muscle cell.

sarcocele (sahr′ko-sēl) any fleshy swelling or tumor of the testis.

sarcocyst (sahr′ko-sist) 1. any member of the genus *Sarcocystis*. 2. a cylindrical cyst containing parasitic spores, found in the muscles of those infected with *Sarcocystis*.

Sarcocystis (sahr″ko-sis′tis) a genus of coccidian protozoa parasitic in birds, reptiles, and mammals, including humans, cattle, horses, sheep, swine, and rabbits and other rodents, occurring as elongated cylindrical bodies (sarcocysts) in the host's muscles. They have an obligatory two-host life cycle, involving sexual reproduction in the definitive host (a carnivore) and asexual reproduction, including schizogony and sarcocyst formation, which occurs in the intermediate host. Infection is transmitted by ingestion of the sporocysts in the feces passed by infected animals. See also SARCO-CYSTOSIS.

S. boviho′minis a species for which cattle are the specific intermediate hosts and humans the definitive hosts; it causes intestinal SARCOCYSTOSIS in humans. It was formerly considered to be combined with *S. suihominis* in a single species, *S. hominis* (*Isospora hominis*).

S. lindeman′ni a species causing human infection, most cases of which are asymptomatic, although it may cause polymyositis sometimes associated with eosinophilia.

S. suiho′minis a species for which swine are the specific intermediate hosts and humans the definitive hosts; it causes intestinal SARCOCYSTOSIS in humans. It was formerly considered to form a single species with *S. bovihominis,* called *S. hominis* (*Isospora hominis*).

sarcocystosis (sahr″ko-sis-to′sis) infection with protozoa of the genus *Sarcocystis;* in humans it is usually asymptomatic but may be manifested either by muscle cysts associated with myositis or myocarditis or by intestinal infection. It is usually transmitted by the eating of raw or undercooked beef or pork containing sporocysts of the parasites or by ingestion of sporocysts from the feces of an infected animal, usually in contaminated soil.

Sarcodina (sahr″ko-di′nah) a subphylum of Protozoa, including all the amebae, both free-living and parasitic, characterized by the ability to produce PSEUDOPODIA during most of the life cycle; flagella, when present, develop only during the early stages.

sarcoid (sahr′koid) 1. fleshlike. 2. sarcomalike. 3. a sarcomalike tumor. 4. sarcoidosis.

Boeck's s. sarcoidosis.

sarcoidosis (sahr″koi-do′sis) a chronic, progressive, generalized granulomatous

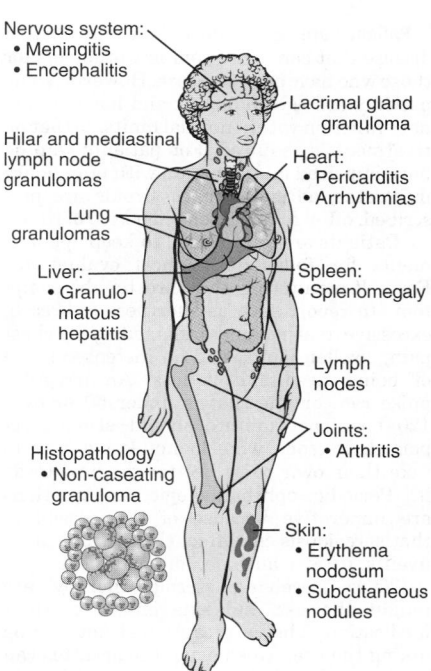

Sarcoidosis. The most common sites of granulomas are the lungs and thoracic lymph nodes. Other extrathoracic sites are less commonly involved. Also shown is a granuloma composed primarily of epithelioid cells, macrophages, and lymphocytes. From Damjanov, 2000.

RETICULOSIS that may affect any part of the body but most frequently involves the lymph nodes, liver, spleen, lungs, skin, eyes, and small bones of the hands and feet, characterized by the presence in all affected organs or tissues of epithelioid cell tubercles, which become converted, in the older lesions, into a rather hyaline featureless fibrous tissue.

As there is no specific test for sarcoidosis, diagnosis is based on clinical examination, x-rays, fiberoptic bronchoscopy, gallium-67 scan, serum ANGIOTENSIN-CONVERTING ENZYME, and a skin test called the Kveim test.

Blood studies may reveal blood dyscrasias such as anemia, leukopenia, eosinophilia, hypergammaglobulinemia, and a reduction in serum albumin. In a small percentage of patients there may be a transient hypercalcemia and hypercalciuria in the early stages of the disease. Patients have a delayed skin reactivity to tuberculin and other antigens such as candidiasis and mumps.

Patient Care. Sarcoidosis is a multisystem disease that can cause complex problems for those who have an active case. However, some patients are asymptomatic and have pulmonary function within normal limits, so that no treatment is required. For patients who do have impaired lung function with pulmonary infiltrates, adrenal corticosteroids are prescribed, often for an extended period of time.

Patients are encouraged to keep appointments for follow-up medical evaluations. For self-monitoring they are taught symptoms to report such as shortness of breath, excessive tearing and inflamed eyes, chest pain, swollen joints, and an increased sense of being tired and listless. An irregular pulse rate or one that is under 50 or over 120 beats per minute should also be reported. Persons who do not know how to take their own pulse are taught how to do it. Periodic ophthalmologic examinations are imperative because of the possibility that sarcoidosis can affect the eye and cause uveitis, iritis, glaucoma, and cataracts.

Those receiving steroid therapy are taught the use and side effects of their medication. They are cautioned not to stop taking the prescribed drug, because this can produce a drop in blood pressure with fever, nausea, vomiting, and diarrhea.

Smoking is harmful because it aggravates impaired lung function; hence patients are encouraged to seek help if they need to quit smoking. Prolonged exposure to direct sunlight should be avoided because vitamin D aids absorption of calcium, which can contribute to elevated serum and urinary calcium levels and the formation of kidney stones. Well-informed patients can contribute a great deal to the management of their disease and enhance their sense of self-esteem and control, as well as avoid serious complications.

cardiac s. involvement of the heart in sarcoidosis, with lesions ranging from a few asymptomatic granulomas to widespread infiltration of the myocardium by large masses of sarcoid tissue; it is characterized by a high incidence of atrioventricular BLOCK as well as right bundle branch BLOCK and ventricular ARRHYTHMIAS.

muscular s. sarcoidosis involving the skeletal muscles, with sarcoid tubercles, interstitial inflammation with fibrosis, and disruption and atrophy of the muscle fibers.

sarcolemma (sahr″ko-lem′ah) the delicate elastic sheath covering every striated muscle FIBER. adj., **sarcolem′mic, sarcolem′mous.**

sarcoma (sahr-ko′mah), pl. *sarcomas, sarco′mata.* A tumor, often highly malignant, composed of cells derived from connective tissue such as bone, cartilage, muscle, blood vessel, or lymphoid tissue; sarcomas usually develop rapidly and metastasize through the lymph channels. Different types are named for the specific tissue they affect: FIBROSARCOMA in fibrous connective tissue; LYMPHOSARCOMA in lymphoid tissues; OSTEOSARCOMA in bone; CHONDROSARCOMA in cartilage; RHABDOSARCOMA in muscle; and LIPOSARCOMA in fat cells. adj., **sarco′matous.**

Abernethy's s. a malignant fatty tumor occurring mainly on the trunk.

alveolar soft part s. one with a reticulated fibrous stroma enclosing groups of sarcoma cells enclosed in alveoli walled with connective tissue.

botryoid s., s. botryoi′des an embryonal RHABDOMYOSARCOMA arising in submucosal tissue, usually in the upper vagina, cervix uteri, or bladder neck in young children and infants, presenting grossly as a polypoid grapelike structure.

endometrial stromal s. a pale, polypoid, fleshy, malignant tumor of the endometrial stroma.

Ewing's s. a malignant tumor of the bone that arises in medullary tissue, usually found in cylindrical bones, with pain, fever, and leukocytosis as prominent symptoms; called also Ewing's tumor.

giant cell s. a malignant form of giant cell TUMOR of bone.

granulocytic s. chloroma.

immunoblastic s. of B cells an aggressive B-cell lymphoma believed to arise from transformed interfollicular B lymphocytes, which in many cases is associated with a preexisting immunologic disorder, e.g., Sjögren's syndrome, systemic lupus erythematosus, or Hashimoto's thyroiditis, or with an immunocompromised state.

immunoblastic s. of T cells a group of T-cell lymphomas comprising tumors derived from T lymphocytes in the paracortical area arising from a mixture of small lymphocytes and many large transformed cells; the latter are characterized by one or more small but distinctly eosinophilic nucleoli.

Kaposi s. a multicentric, malignant neoplastic vascular proliferation characterized by bluish red cutaneous nodules, usually on the lower extremities, most often on the toes or feet; the nodules slowly increase in size and number and spread to more proximal sites. Tumors often remain confined to skin and subcutaneous tissue, but widespread visceral involvement may occur. The condition occurs endemically in certain parts of Central Africa and Central and Eastern Europe, and a particularly virulent and disseminated form occurs in

MMUNOCOMPROMISED patients such as transplant recipients and those with ACQUIRED MMUNODEFICIENCY SYNDROME. Human HERPESVIRUS 8 has been implicated as a causative gent.

lymphatic s. diffuse lymphoma.

osteogenic s. a malignant primary umor of bone composed of a malignant connective tissue stroma with evidence of osteoid, one, and/or cartilage formation; depending upon the dominant component, classified as osteoblastic, fibroblastic, or chondroblastic.

pseudo–Kaposi s. unilateral subacute o chronic dermatitis, often with postinflammatory hyperpigmentation, occurring in association with underlying arteriovenous istula, which closely resembles Kaposi sarcoma both clinically and histologically.

reticulum cell s. histiocytic lymphoma.

sarcomatoid (sahr-ko″mah-toid) resembling a SARCOMA.

sarcomatosis (sahr-ko″mah-to′sis) a condition characterized by development of many SARCOMAS.

sarcomatous (sahr-ko′mah-tus) pertaining to or of the nature of a SARCOMA.

sarcomere (sahr′ko-mēr) the contractile unit of a myofibril; sarcomeres are repeating units, delimited by the Z bands along the length of the myofibril.

sarcoplasm (sahr′ko-plazm) the interfibrillary matter of striated muscle. adj., **sarcoplas′mic.**

sarcoplast (sahr′ko-plast) an interstitial cell of a muscle, itself capable of being transformed into a muscle.

sarcopoietic (sahr″ko-poi-et′ik) forming muscle.

sarcosine (sahr′ko-sēn) an amino acid occurring as an intermediate in the metabolism of CHOLINE in the kidney and liver;

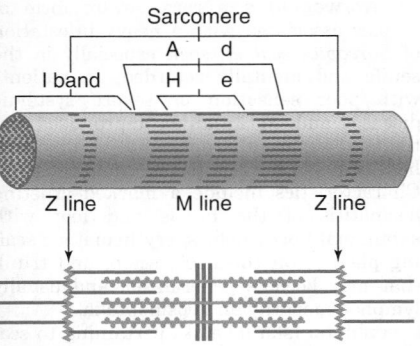

Thick and thin filaments are organized into contractile units called sarcomeres. A sarcomere extends from one Z line to the next and represents the fundamental unit of muscle contraction. From Copstead, 1995.

it is normally not detectable in human blood or urine.

sarcosinemia (sahr″ko-sī-ne′me-ah) an inborn ERROR of metabolism due to a defect of the enzyme that breaks down SARCOSINE, resulting in elevated levels of sarcosine in the blood. Clinical manifestations include poor feeding in an infant with FAILURE TO THRIVE and developmental delays; however, no consistent clinical syndrome has been reported. Called also hypersarcosinemia.

Sarcoptes (sahr-kop′tēz) a widely distributed genus of mites, including the species *S. scabie′i*, the itch mite, the cause of scabies in man; different varieties of the organism cause mange in different animals.

sarcosis (sahr-ko′sis) abnormal increase of flesh.

Sarcosporidia (sahr″ko-spō-rid′e-ah) in former systems of classification, an order of sporozoan protozoa that included the genus *Sarcocystis*.

sarcosporidiosis (sahr″ko-spor-id″e-o′sis) sarcocystosis.

sarcostosis (sahr″kos-to′sis) ossification of fleshy tissue.

sarcotubules (sahr″ko-too′būlz) the membrane-limited structures of the sarcoplasm, forming a canalicular network around each myofibril.

sarcous (sahr′kus) pertaining to flesh or muscle tissue.

sardonic (sahr-don′ik) denoting a kind of spasmodic or satanic grin or involuntary smile; see RISUS SARDONICUS.

Sargent (sahr′jent) Emilie G. (1894–1977). Public health nurse and director of the Detroit Visiting Nursing Association. Under her directorship, the Visiting Nursing Association greatly expanded both its range of services and the area it served. She was also a leader in many professional organizations at the state and national levels and made significant contributions to the improvement of health care for the elderly and the chronically ill.

sargramostim (sahr-gram′o-stim) granulocyte-macrophage colony-stimulating factor produced by recombinant technology; used to enhance neutrophil function, stimulating HEMATOPOIESIS and decreasing NEUTROPENIA; administered intravenously or subcutaneously.

sat. saturated.

satellite (sat′ĕ-līt) 1. in genetics, a knob of CHROMATIN connected by a stalk to the short arm of certain CHROMOSOMES. 2. a minor, or attendant, lesion situated near a large one. 3. a vein that closely accompanies an artery. 4. exhibiting SATELLITISM. 5. satellite CLINIC.

satellitism (sat′ĕ-li-tizm) the phenomenon in which certain bacterial species grow more vigorously in the immediate vicinity of colonies of other unrelated species, owing to the production of an essential metabolite by the latter species.

satellitosis (sat″ĕ-li-to′sis) accumulation of neuroglial cells about neurons; seen whenever neurons are damaged.

saturated (sach′er-āt-ed) 1. denoting an organic compound that has only single bonds between carbon atoms. 2. holding all of a solute that can be held in a solution by the solvent (saturated solution).

saturation (sach″er-a′shun) the state of being saturated, or the act of saturating.

   oxygen s. the amount of oxygen bound to hemoglobin in the blood, expressed as a percentage of the maximal binding capacity.

saturnine (sat′ur-nīn) pertaining to lead.

saturnism (sat′ur-nizm) lead poisoning.

satyriasis (sat″ĭ-ri′ah-sis) pathologic or exaggerated sexual desire in the male; the corresponding term in the female is NYMPHOMANIA.

saucerization (saw″ser-ĭ-za′shun) 1. the excavation of tissue to form a shallow shelving depression, usually performed to facilitate drainage from infected areas of bone. 2. the shallow saucer-like depression on the upper surface of a vertebra that has suffered a compression fracture.

saxitoxin (sak′sī-tok″sin) a powerful heat-stable low molecular weight neurotoxin synthesized and secreted by certain dinoflagellates, such as species of *Gonyaulax*, which accumulates in the tissue of bivalve mollusks feeding on the dinoflagellates; it may cause a severe toxic reaction called SHELLFISH POISONING in those who ingest contaminated mollusks.

Sb antimony (L. *sti′bium*).

SC secretory component; closure of semilunar valves; subcutaneous.

Sc scandium.

scab (skab) 1. the crust of a superficial sore. 2. to become covered with a crust or scab.

scabicide (ska′bĭ-sīd) 1. lethal to *Sarcoptes scabiei,* the cause of SCABIES. 2. an agent that has this quality.

scabies (ska′bēz, ska′be-ēz) a contagious skin disease caused by the itch mite, *Sarcoptes scabiei*. Scabies, sometimes popularly called "seven-year itch," is most likely to erupt in folds of the skin, such as in the groin, beneath the breasts, or between the toes or fingers. It is classified as a SEXUALLY TRANSMITTED DISEASE.

The adult itch mite has a rounded body about one-fiftieth of an inch long. The skin lesions are caused by the female, which burrows beneath the skin and digs a short tunnel parallel to the surface, in which it lays its eggs. The eggs hatch in a few days after which the baby mites find their way to the skin surface, where they mate and complete the life cycle.

Symptoms. During the initial tunnel digging and egg laying, the human host may be oblivious to what is happening. There is little itching and there are few lesions. In about a month, the itching becomes intense because of hypersensitivity to the mite. The itch is often worse at night. The tunnels in the skin can now be discerned as slightly elevated grayish white lines. The mite itself can often be seen—with the aid of a magnifying glass—as a tiny black speck at the end of the tunnel. Blisters and pustules also may develop in the skin near the tunnel.

Transmission. Scabies is usually transmitted from person to person by direct skin contact. Transmission via clothing and other inanimate objects is uncommon. Epidemics are fairly common in such places as camps, barracks, and institutions. It is unusual for one member of a family not to communicate it to the others. The Centers for Disease Control and Prevention recommend the wearing of gowns and gloves for close contact with an infested person. Masks are not necessary. All contacts that the patient has had should be treated at the same time.

Treatment and Prevention. Scabies treatment consists of topical permethrin cream (Elimite), lindane, or crotamiton (Eurax) applied from the neck down and then washed off. For infants, 5 to 6 per cent precipitated sulfur in petrolatum, applied twice daily for a week, is usually adequate.

   Norwegian s. a rare, severe form of scabies associated with a heavy infestation of *Sarcoptes scabiei*, seen especially in the senile and mentally retarded, in patients with poor sensation or severe systemic disease, and in immunocompromised patients; it apparently represents an abnormal host IMMUNE RESPONSE to the etiologic agent. Characteristics include a marked crusting dermatitis of the hands and feet with subungual horny debris, erythematous scaling plaques on the neck, scalp, and trunk that may become generalized, and usually lymphadenopathy and eosinophilia.

scabietic (ska″be-et′ik) pertaining to scabies.

scala (ska′lah) [L.] a ladderlike structure, especially any of various passages of the COCHLEA.

s. me'dia cochlear duct.

s. tym'pani the part of the cochlea below the spiral lamina.

s. vesti'buli the part of the cochlea above the spiral lamina.

scalar (ska'lar) 1. a physical quantity specified by a single number (a magnitude or point on a scale), such as mass or temperature. See also VECTOR. 2. pertaining to a scalar quantity.

scald (skawld) a burn caused by a hot liquid or a hot, moist vapor; to burn in such fashion.

scale (skāl) 1. a thin flake or compacted platelike body, as of cornified epithelial cells. See also SQUAMA. 2. a scheme or device by which some property may be measured (as hardness, weight, linear dimension). 3. to remove incrustations or other material from a surface, as from the enamel of teeth.

absolute s., absolute temperature s. 1. one with its zero at absolute zero (−273.15°C, −459.67°F). 2. Kelvin s.

ASIA s. a descriptive tool developed by the American Spinal Injury Association (ASIA) as a part of the complete classification of patients with spinal cord injuries. Called also Frankel Classification. See accompanying table.

Bayley S's of Infant Development a psychological test for assessing development of infants, using motor, mental, and behavioral developmental scales.

Borg s. a numerical scale for assessing DYSPNEA, from 0 representing no dyspnea to 10 as maximal dyspnea.

Brazelton Neonatal Behavioral Assessment S. a behavioral assessment scale used to evaluate the interactive behavior of a newborn by its responses to environmental stimuli.

Celsius s. (C) a temperature scale with zero at the freezing point of water and the normal boiling point of water at 100 degrees. The abbreviation 100°C should be read "one hundred degrees Celsius." (For equivalents of Celsius and Fahrenheit temperatures, see Appendix.)

centigrade s. one with 100 gradations or steps between two fixed points, as the Celsius scale.

Fahrenheit s. (F) a temperature scale with the freezing point of water at 32 degrees and the normal boiling point of water at 212 degrees. The abbreviation 100°F should be read "one hundred degrees Fahrenheit." (For equivalents of Fahrenheit and Celsius temperatures, see Appendix.)

ASIA SCALE OF SPINAL CORD INJURY

A. *Complete*: All motor and sensory function is absent below the zero of partial preservation.

B. *Incomplete, preserved sensation only*: Preservation of any demonstrable, reproducible sensation, excluding phantom sensations. Voluntary motor functions are absent.

C. *Incomplete, preserved motor (nonfunctional)*: Preservation of voluntary motor function which is minimal and performs no useful purpose. Minimal is defined as preserved voluntary motor ability below the level of injury where the majority of key muscles test less than a grade of 3.

D. *Incomplete, preserved motor (functional)*: Preservation of voluntary motor function which is useful functionally. This is defined as preserved voluntary motor ability below the level of injury, where the majority of the key muscles test at least a grade of 3.

E. *Normal*

WINDOW ON ASIA SCALE

Better. Worse. Improved. Unimproved. Same. These terms in this computerized age are still used to describe treatment results. It was early recognized by physicians managing spinal cord injury that these words were not accurate enough. With paralysis, especially if quadriplegia, a single muscle improving, and certainly regaining an additional nerve root, can cause significant functional improvement. In the 1970s, Dr. Hans Frankel introduced 5 grades: A—motor and sensory complete; B—motor complete, sensory incomplete; C—useless distal motor function, sensory incomplete; D—useful distal motor function, sensory incomplete; and E—normal. This system permitted a better but still gross ability to assess improvement. Subsequently, the American Spinal Injury Association (ASIA) developed a motor index score which has improved the accuracy for assessing neurological improvement. The score is obtained by grading, from 0 to 5, the major muscle of the corresponding nerve segment, with 100 being the score for normal function. Using this scoring, even a small change in muscle function can be documented. A patient with a 6th cervical spinal cord level injury will have a score of 20, and if one nerve root recovers the score would increase to 26 and possibly 30. Thus improvement has a numerical meaning and treatment effectiveness can be judged.

DAVID F. APPLE, JR., MD

GLASGOW COMA SCALE

Test	Response	Score
Eyes Open (E)	Spontaneous	4
	To voice	3
	To pain	2
	None	1
Best Verbal Response (V)	Oriented	5
	Confused	4
	Inappropriate words	3
	Incomprehensible sounds	2
	None	1
Best Motor Response (M)	Obeys commands	6
	Localizes pain	5
	Flexion withdrawal	4
	Abnormal flexion	3
	Abnormal extension (decerebrate posturing)	2
	None (flaccid)	1

French s. one used for denoting the size of catheters, sounds, and other tubular instruments, each French unit (symbol F) being approximately 0.33 mm in diameter.

Glasgow Coma S. a standardized system for assessing response to stimuli in a neurologically impaired patient, assessing eye opening, verbal response, and motor ability. Reaction scores are depicted in numerical values, thus minimizing the problem of ambiguous and vague terms to describe the patient's neurologic status. (See accompanying Table.) The total score is obtained by adding E, M, and V; a score of 7 or less indicates coma and a score of 9 or more rules out coma.

Global Assessment of Functioning (GAF) s. a hundred-point scale used as axis V of DSM-IV to assess a client's recent and current levels of social, psychological, and occupational functioning.

gray s. a representation of intensities in shades of gray, as in gray-scale ULTRA-SONOGRAPHY.

interval s. a scale having equal numerical distances between intervals in addition to mutually exclusive categories, exhaustive categories, and rank ordering but no zero point.

Karnofsky s., Karnofsky performance s. a widely used performance SCALE, assigning scores ranging from 0 for a nonfunctional or dead patient to 100 for one with completely normal functioning.

Kelvin s. an absolute scale in which the unit of measurement, the kelvin, corresponds to that of the Celsius scale; therefore the ice point is at 273.15 kelvins.

Likert s. a tool used to determine opinions or attitudes; it contains a list of declarative statements, each followed by a scale on which the subject is to indicate degrees of intensity of a given feeling.

Neonatal Behavior Assessment S Brazelton Neonatal Behavioral Assessment Scale.

performance s. a scale that measures a patient's performance STATUS, serving as a prognostic indicator of seriousness of disease or disability. The most widely used scale is the Karnofsky SCALE.

Problem Rating S. for Outcomes see PROBLEM RATING SCALE FOR OUTCOMES.

semantic differential s. a measurement device that consists of two opposite adjectives with a seven-point scale between them; each item under examination is assigned to a specific point on the scale.

temperature s. one for expressing degree of heat, based on absolute zero as a reference point, or with a certain value arbitrarily assigned to such temperatures as the ice point and boiling point of water.

scalenectomy (ska'le-nek'tah-me) resection of a scalene muscle.

scalenus syndrome, scalenus anterior syndrome, scalenus anticus syndrome THORACIC OUTLET SYNDROME caused by compression or friction on nerves and blood vessels due to abnormality of position or insertion of the anterior scalene muscle. The term may be used as a synonym of thoracic outlet syndrome.

scaler (ska'ler) a dental instrument for removal of PLAQUE, bacterial ENDOTOXINS, and CALCULUS from teeth.

ultrasonic s. an ultrasonic instrument with a tip for supplying high-frequency vibrations, used to remove plaque and

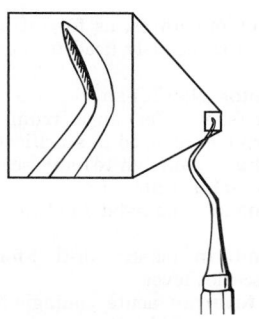

Scaler. From Dorland's, 2000.

calculus from teeth and bits of inflamed tissue from the walls of the gingival crevice.

scaling (skāl'ing) 1. the removal of PLAQUE, bacterial ENDOTOXINS, and CALCULUS from a tooth with a SCALER. 2. measurement of something using a SCALE.

hand s. scaling and oral DÉBRIDEMENT using a manual scaler.

ultrasonic s. scaling using an ultrasonic SCALER.

scalp (skalp) that part of the skin of the head (exclusive of the face) which is usually covered by a growth of hair.

scalpel (skal'p'l) a small surgical knife with a convex or concave sharp edge; there are now types consisting of a handle with a disposable blade.

scaly (ska'le) characterized by scales; scalelike.

scan (skan) 1. to examine or map the body, or one or more organs or regions of it, by gathering information with a sensing device, such as a moving detector or a sweeping beam of radiation. 2. the data or image so obtained, often designated according to the organ under examination, such as a *brain scan, kidney scan,* or *thyroid scan.* 3. shortened form of SCINTISCAN.

A-s. display on a cathode ray tube of ultrasonic echoes, in which one axis represents the time required for return of the echo and the other corresponds to the strength of the echo.

B-s. display on a cathode ray tube of ultrasonic echoes, in which the position of a bright dot on the tube corresponds to the

time elapsed and the brightness of the spot to the strength of the echo; movement of the transducer across the skin surface yields a two-dimensional cross-sectional display.

CAT s., CT s. the image generated by computerized axial TOMOGRAPHY.

HIDA s. a type of scan using a technetium 99m complex to assess hepatobiliary function.

thallium s. a SCINTISCAN involving use of thallium 201; see also THALLIUM SCAN.

ventilation-perfusion s., V/Q s. a scintigraphic technique for demonstrating perfusion defects in normally ventilated areas of the lung in the diagnosis of pulmonary embolism, consisting of the imaging of the distribution of an inhaled radionuclide followed by the imaging of the perfusion of the lungs by an injected radionuclide.

scandium (skan'de-um) a chemical element, atomic number 21, atomic weight 44.956, symbol Sc. (See Appendix 6.)

scanner (skan'er) 1. a device that converts an image, such as from a patient, to a format appropriate for viewing on a computer or being transmitted electronically. 2. equipment used for producing a SCAN or SCANNING.

scanning (skan'ing) 1. close visual examination of a small area or of different isolated areas. 2. any of several diagnostic radiologic techniques, including computed TOMOGRAPHY, MAGNETIC RESONANCE IMAGING, and positron emission TOMOGRAPHY. 3. a manner of utterance characterized by somewhat regularly recurring pauses.

brain s. see BRAIN SCANNING.

MUGA s., multiple gated acquisition s. equilibrium radionuclide angiocardiography.

radioisotope s. production of a two-dimensional record or image of the GAMMA RAYS emitted by a radioactive isotope concentrated in a specific organ or tissue of the body, as brain, kidney, or thyroid gland.

scintillation s. the process resulting in a SCINTISCAN.

thallium s. production of a scintillation scan involving the use of THALLIUM 201; see also THALLIUM SCAN.

total body s. use of computed TOMOGRAPHY to examine a cross section of the entire body. The scanner produces an image of tissue density in a complete cross section of the part of the body being scanned. Total body scanning does not require the injection of a radiopaque substance, nor is there a need for use of a radioactive material to produce a record of the findings. The total body scanner is particularly useful in visualizing organs in the retroperitoneal space, for example, the

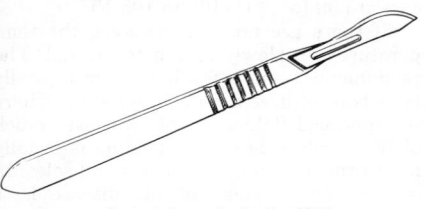

Scalpel. From Dorland's, 2000.

pancreas, liver, spleen, and ovaries, and the abdominal section of the aorta.

scanography (skan-og′rah-fe) a method of making radiographs by the use of a narrow slit beneath the tube, so that, as the x-ray tube moves over the target, all the rays of the central beam pass through the part being radiographed at the same angle.

scapegoating (skāp′gōt-ing) a process by which an individual or group is identified as being different from others and becomes the focus of the group's fears, anger, or aggression.

scapha (ska′fah) [L.] the curved depression separating the HELIX and ANTIHELIX of the ear.

scaphocephaly (skaf″o-sef′ah-le) abnormal length and narrowness of the skull as a result of premature closure of the sagittal suture. adj., **scaphocephal′ic, scaphoceph′alous.**

scaphoid (skaf′oid) boat-shaped; called also navicular. See anatomic Table of Bones in the Appendices.

scaphoiditis (skaf″oi-di′tis) inflammation of the scaphoid bone.

scapula (skap′u-lah) [L.] the flat triangular bone in the back of the shoulder. See anatomic Table of Bones in the Appendices.

  winged s. one having a prominent vertebral border usually owing to weakness of one of the muscles holding the scapula in place.

scapulalgia (skap″u-lal′jah) pain in the scapular region.

scapular (skap′u-lar) pertaining to the scapula.

scapulectomy (skap″u-lek′tah-me) excision or resection of the scapula.

scapuloclavicular (skap″u-lo-klah-vik′u-lar) pertaining to the scapula and clavicle.

scapulohumeral (skap″u-lo-hu′mer-al) pertaining to the scapula and humerus.

scapulopexy (skap′u-lo-pek″se) surgical fixation of the scapula.

scapulothoracic (skap″u-lo-thŏ-ras′ik) pertaining to the scapula and thorax.

scar (skar) a mark remaining after the healing of a wound, such as one caused by injury, illness, smallpox vaccination, or surgery. (See also HEALING and KELOID.) Beneath the skin is a fibrous connective tissue known as subcutaneous tissue, composed of cells called fibroblasts, which after injury are stimulated to grow into granulation tissue, knitting the wound together. Scar tissue is formed by dense masses of granulation tissue. Called also CICATRIX.

scarification (skar″ĭ-fĭ-ka′shun) production in the skin of many small superficial scratches or punctures, as for introduction of vaccine. Erroneously used to mean scarring.

scarificator (skar′ĭ-fĭ-ka″tor) scarifier.

scarifier (skar′ĭ-fĭ″er) an instrument with many sharp points, used in scarification.

scarlatina (skahr″lah-te′nah) scarlet fever. adj., **scarlat′inal.**

scarlatinella (skahr-lat″ĭ-nel′ah) Duke's disease.

scarlatiniform (skahr″lah-tin′ĭ-form) resembling scarlet fever.

scarlet fever an acute contagious childhood disease caused by Group A beta-hemolytic streptococci or occasionally other serotypes of beta-hemolytic streptococci. It usually affects the pharynx but may also affect the skin (wound and burn scarlet fever) or the birth canal (puerperal scarlet fever). The disease is most common in late winter and spring. Called also scarlatina.

Scarlet fever is usually spread by droplet infection. Objects the infected person has used, such as clothes, dishes, or toys, may carry the streptococcus, but this mode of transmission is rare. Occasionally a widespread outbreak may be caused by milk or food that has been infected by a person carrying the streptococcus. It was formerly a very common and serious disease, but in recent decades the number and severity of cases have greatly decreased. Complications are much less common, largely as a result of the development and use of antibiotics.

Symptoms. The incubation period is usually 2 to 5 days, although it may be as few as 1 or as many as 7 days. Symptoms vary a great deal. In some patients there is only sore throat and swelling of the lymph nodes of the neck. The tonsils may be covered by a patchy purulent discharge. The bright red rash from which the disease takes its name appears on the second day; it may be mild or widely spread, depending on the strain of the causative streptococcus. The rash is caused by a toxin produced by scarlatinal strains. There may be nausea and vomiting. The skin usually feels hot and dry, and there also may be headache and chills. In mild cases the temperature may rise to about 38°C (101°F) and in severe cases to 39 to 40°C (103 to 105°F).

If there are no complications, the temperature will slowly return to normal. The rash may last only a few hours, but typically lasts two to three days before fading. There is superficial flaking of the skin over much of the involved area; this peeling is usually most pronounced on the palms and soles. In all, the active stage of the disease lasts about 7 days.

Treatment. Antibiotics are administered, usually penicillin; this is continued for about 10 days to avoid relapse. Eating may be painful if the throat infection is severe, so that soft foods and a liquid diet may be necessary. Drinking of fluids should be encouraged.

Complications. Among the possible complications are swelling of the lymph nodes of the neck, infection of the ears and sinuses, kidney disease, pneumonia, and rheumatic fever. Any of these complications may be serious. However, they are now rare in developed countries such as the United States and Canada. Prompt and adequate treatment greatly reduces the danger of complications.

SCAT sheep cell agglutination test.

scatology (skah-tol'ah-je) 1. study and analysis of feces, as for diagnostic purposes. 2. a preoccupation with feces and filth. adj., **scatolog'ic.**

scatoscopy (skah-tos'kah-pe) examination of the feces.

scatter (skat'er) the diffusion or deviation of x-rays produced by a medium through which the rays pass.

   back s. backward diffusion of x-rays.

scattergram (skat'er-gram) scatterplot.

scattering (skat'er-ing) a change in the direction of motion of a photon or subatomic particle as the result of a collision or interaction.

scatterplot (skat'er-plot) a plot in rectangular coordinates of paired observations of two random variables, each observation plotted as one point on the graph; the scatter or clustering of points provides an indication of the strength of the relationship between the two variables.

ScD Scien'tiae Doc'tor (Doctor of Science).

Scheie's syndrome (shāz) a type of MUCOPOLYSACCHARIDOSIS considered to be an atypical form of HURLER'S SYNDROME. The principal sign is marked progressive corneal clouding; other signs are hirsutism, joint stiffness, mild bone deformities (often only in the hands), disease of the aorta, and a wide-mouthed face. There is no mental retardation.

schema (ske'mah) a plan, outline, or arrangement.

scheme (skēm) 1. a calculated plan of action. 2. schema.

   body s. the acquisition of an internal awareness of the body and the relationship of body parts to one another; a sensorimotor PERFORMANCE COMPONENT of occupational therapy.

   Intervention S. see INTERVENTION SCHEME.

Problem Classification S. see PROBLEM CLASSIFICATION SCHEME.

Scheuermann's disease (shoi'er-manz) osteochondrosis of the vertebral epiphyses in juveniles.

Schick test (shik) intracutaneous injection of diluted diphtheria TOXIN equal to one-fiftieth of the minimum lethal dose. Lack of immunity to DIPHTHERIA is indicated by redness and edema appearing at the injection site in 24 to 36 hours and lasting four to five days. This test has now largely been replaced by HEMAGGLUTINATION INHIBITION TESTS.

Schilder's disease (shil'derz) a subacute or chronic LEUKOENCEPHALOPATHY of children and adolescents, closely related to ADRENOLEUKODYSTROPHY, with massive destruction of the white MATTER of the cerebral HEMISPHERES; clinical symptoms include blindness, deafness, bilateral spasticity, and mental deterioration. Called also encephalitis periaxialis diffusa and progressive subcortical encephalopathy.

Schilling test (shil'ing) a test for gastrointestinal absorption of vitamin B$_{12}$; a measured amount of radioactive vitamin B$_{12}$ (cyanocobalamin Co 57) is given orally, followed by a parenteral flushing dose of the nonradioactive vitamin, and the percentage of radioactivity is determined in the urine excreted over a 24-hour period. A low urinary excretion that becomes normal after the test is repeated with intrinsic factor is diagnostic of primary pernicious anemia.

Schimmelbusch's disease (shim'el-boosh''ez) cystic disease of the breast.

schindylesis (shin''dĭ-le'sis) an articulation in which a thin plate of one bone is received into a cleft in another, as in the articulation of the perpendicular plate of the ethmoid bone with the vomer.

Schirmer's test (sher'merz) a test for keratoconjunctivitis sicca; a piece of filter paper is inserted into the conjunctival sac over the lower eyelid with the end of the paper hanging down on the outside. If the projecting paper remains dry after 15 minutes, deficient tear formation is indicated.

-schisis word ending denoting a cleft or cleavage.

schist(o)- word element [Gr.], *split, cleft, divided.*

schistocelia (shis''to-se'le-ah) gastroschisis.

schistocephalus (shis''-, skis''to-sef'ah-lus) a fetus with cranium bifidum.

schistocoelia (shis''to-se'le-ah) gastroschisis.

S

schistocormus (shis″-, skis′to-kor′mus) a malformed fetus with a cleft abdomen, often with rudimentary lower limbs. Called also schistosomus.

schistocyte (shis′-, skis′to-sīt) a fragment of an erythrocyte, commonly observed in the blood in HEMOLYTIC ANEMIA; called also helmet cell and schizocyte.

schistocytosis (shis″-, skis″to-si-to′sis) an accumulation of schistocytes in the blood.

schistomelus (shis-, skis-tom′ĕ-lus) a malformed fetus with a cleft limb.

schistoprosopus (shis″-, skis″to-pros′o-pus) a fetus with a facial CLEFT.

Schistosoma (shis″-, skis″to-so′mah) a genus of trematodes, including several species parasitic in the blood of humans and domestic animals. The organisms are called schistosomes or blood flukes. Larvae (cercariae) enter the body of the host by way of the digestive tract, or through the skin from contact with contaminated water, and migrate in the blood to small blood vessels of organs of the intestinal or urinary tract; they attach themselves to the blood vessel walls and mature and reproduce. The intermediate hosts are snails of various species.

S. haemato′bium a species endemic in North, Central, and West Africa and the Middle East; the organisms are found in the venules of the urinary bladder wall, and eggs may be isolated from the urine.

S. japo′nicum a species geographically confined to China, Japan, and nearby countries; found chiefly in the venules of the intestine.

S. manso′ni a species widely distributed in Africa and parts of South America; the organisms are found in the host's mesenteric veins, and eggs may be found in the feces.

schistosome (shis-, skis′to-sōm) an individual worm of the genus Schistosoma.

schistosomiasis (shis″-, skis″to-so-mi′-ahsis) infection with flukes of the genus Schistosoma; called also bilharziasis. The disease is rare in North America, but is a significant health problem in many parts of the world, including the Middle East, Africa, East Asia, South America, and the Caribbean. Different species cause different forms of the disease: S. mansoni and S. japonicum produce intestinal symptoms, while S. haematobium produces hematuria and other urinary symptoms. The early stages of acute infection with S. japonicum produce KATAYAMA FEVER, a serum sickness–like illness. Initial treatment includes correction of anemia and other nutritional disorders caused by the parasites; definitive treatment may be delayed until acute symptoms subside. ANTHELMINTIC medications are administered, such as OXAMNIQUINE or PRAZIQUANTEL. Improvement in sanitation and snail control are the chief preventive measures.

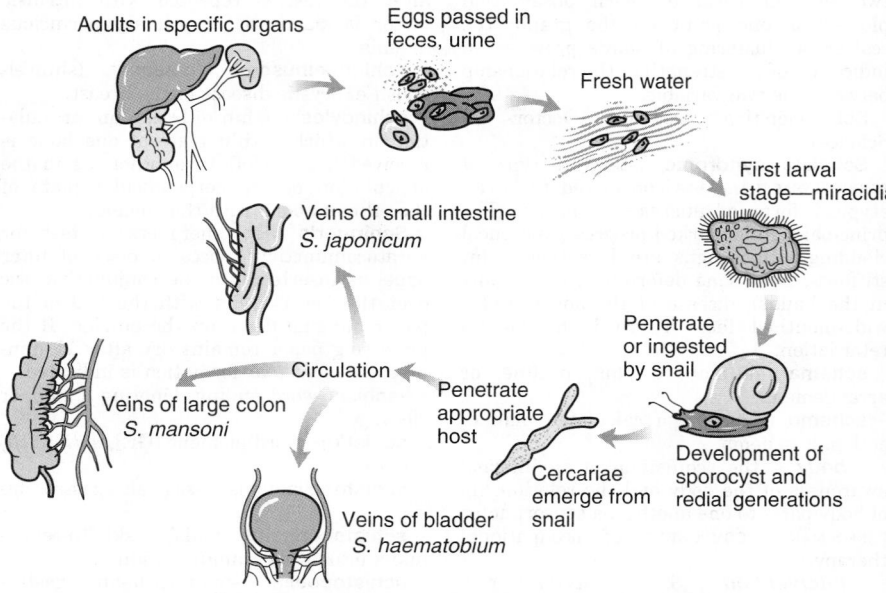

Adults in specific organs

Eggs passed in feces, urine

Fresh water

First larval stage—miracidia

Veins of small intestine
S. japonicum

Penetrate or ingested by snail

Veins of large colon
S. mansoni

Circulation

Penetrate appropriate host

Development of sporocyst and redial generations

Cercariae emerge from snail

Veins of bladder
S. haematobium

The life cycle of *Schistosoma*. From Mahon and Manuselis, 2000.

schistosomicide (shĭs″-, skĭs″to-so′mĭ-sīd) an ANTHELMINTIC agent that destroys species of *Schistosoma*.

schistosomus (shĭs″-, skĭs″to-so′mus) schistocormus.

schistothorax (shĭs″-, skĭs″to-thŏ′raks) thoracoschisis.

schiz(o)- word element [Gr.], *split, cleft, divided.*

schizaxon (skĭz-ak′son) an axon that divides into two nearly equal branches.

schizoaffective disorder (skĭz″o-ah-fek′-tiv) a mental disorder in which symptoms of a MOOD DISORDER occur along with prominent psychotic symptoms characteristic of SCHIZOPHRENIA, the symptoms of the mood disorder being present for a substantial portion of the illness, but not for its entirety.

schizocyte (skĭz′o-sīt) schistocyte.

schizogenesis (skĭz″o-jen′ĕ-sis) reproduction by fission.

schizogony (skĭ-zog′ah-ne) the asexual reproduction of a SPOROZOITE by multiple fission within the body of the host, giving rise to MEROZOITES, as in MALARIA. adj., **schizogon′ic.**

schizogyria (skĭz″o-ji′re-ah) a condition in which the cerebral convolutions have wedge-shaped cracks.

schizoid (skĭz′oid, skĭt′soid) 1. the traits of shyness, sensitivity, social withdrawal, and introversion that characterize a person with SCHIZOID PERSONALITY DISORDER. 2. a term used loosely to refer to any of a variety of characteristics related to SCHIZOPHRENIA, including schizophrenia-like traits said to indicate a predisposition to schizophrenia as well as any disorder other than schizophrenia either occurring in a relative of a schizophrenic or occurring more commonly than average in families of schizophrenics. 3. a person with SCHIZOID PERSONALITY DISORDER.

s. personality disorder a PERSONALITY DISORDER marked by withdrawal from social relationships and a restricted range of emotional experience and expression. An individual with a schizoid personality lacks the capacity for, or interest in, social relationships, is cold and aloof, consistently prefers solitary activities, appears to take pleasure in few activities, and is indifferent to praise, criticism, or the feelings of others. Such a person does not, however, show the eccentricities of speech or behavior found in the SCHIZOTYPAL PERSONALITY DISORDER.

schizomycete (skĭz″o-mi-sēt′) an organism of the class Schizomycetes.

Schizomycetes (skĭz″o-mi-se′tēz) a former taxonomic class comprising the bacteria, consisting of unicellular organisms that commonly multiply by cell division.

schizont (skĭz′ont) the stage in the development of the malarial parasite following the TROPHOZOITE whose nucleus divides into many smaller nuclei.

schizonychia (skĭz″o-nik′e-ah) splitting of the nails.

schizophasia (skĭz″o-fa′zhah) word salad.

schizophrenia (skĭt-so-, skĭz-o-fre′ne-ah) any of a large group of mental disorders (the schizophrenic disorders) characterized by mental deterioration from a previous level of functioning and characteristic disturbances of multiple psychological processes, including delusions, loosening of associations, poverty of the content of speech, auditory hallucinations, inappropriate affect, disturbed sense of self, and withdrawal from the external world. adj., **schizophren′ic.** Because the onset is usually in adolescence or early adulthood, schizophrenia was formerly called *dementia praecox,* a term still used by some European psychiatrists for process schizophrenia. The term *schizophrenia* literally means "split personality," referring to portions of the psyche that are contradictory; it does not mean MULTIPLE PERSONALITY DISORDER, which is the presence of distinct, autonomous alternate personalities.

There are various theories regarding causes of schizophrenia. Biologic theories include genetics, biochemicals, and structural alterations. It is generally accepted that schizophrenics inherit a genetic vulnerability for the disease, and this interacts with environmental factors in causation.

Classification. The current nomenclature classifies schizophrenia into five types. *Disorganized* (*hebephrenic*) schizophrenia is characterized by disorganized, incoherent thinking; shallow, inappropriate, and silly affect; and regressive behavior without systematized delusions. *Catatonic* schizophrenia is characterized by psychomotor disturbance which may involve stupor, rigidity, excitement, negativism, or posturing, or an alteration among these behaviors; associated features include mutism, stereotypy, and waxy flexibility. This type, once common, is now rare. *Paranoid* schizophrenia is characterized by persecutory or grandiose delusions, delusional jealousy, or hallucinations with persecutory or grandiose content. The *undifferentiated* type refers to cases in which there are prominent psychotic symptoms, such as delusions, hallucinations, incoherence, or grossly disorganized behavior, and which cannot be classified as one of the first three types. The *residual* type refers to cases in which the

S

prominent psychotic symptoms of a previous episode have disappeared but signs of the illness, such as inappropriate affect, social withdrawal, or loosening of associations, persist.

Treatment. A variety of therapeutic measures may be used to help the schizophrenic patient cope with reality and the demands of everyday living. The combination of therapies will depend on the needs of the individual patient, age and family background, and the environment in which the patient must live. Among the kinds of therapy are treatment with one of the ANTIPSYCHOTIC AGENTS (formerly called *neuroleptics*) and intensive psychotherapy for outpatients and various forms of group therapy and milieu therapy for hospitalized patients.

childhood s. see PERVASIVE DEVELOPMENTAL DISORDERS.

catatonic s. a type of schizophrenia characterized by marked psychomotor disturbance, which may include immobility (STUPOR or CATALEPSY), excessive motor activity, extreme negativism, MUTISM, ECHOLALIA, ECHOPRAXIA, and peculiar voluntary movements such as posturing, mannerisms, grimacing, or stereotyped behaviors.

latent s. older term for a type of schizophrenia characterized by clear symptoms of schizophrenia but no history of a psychotic schizophrenic episode; it includes conditions that have been called incipient, prepsychotic, prodromal, pseudoneurotic, and pseudopsychopathic schizophrenia. See SCHIZOID PERSONALITY DISORDER and SCHIZOTYPAL PERSONALITY DISORDER.

pseudoneurotic s. a form characterized by all-pervasive anxiety and a wide variety of neurotic symptoms that initially mask underlying psychotic tendencies, which may be manifest as occasional, brief psychotic episodes. It is usually considered to be more of a personality disorder; see also SCHIZOTYPAL PERSONALITY DISORDER.

pseudopsychopathic s. a term applied to patients in whom antisocial, impulsive, or sociopathic tendencies initially mask underlying psychotic tendencies typical of schizophrenia. It is often considered to be more of a personality disorder; see SCHIZOTYPAL PERSONALITY DISORDER.

schizoaffective s. schizoaffective disorder.

simple s. a form characterized by gradual loss of drive, social withdrawal, and emotional apathy, but without prominent psychotic features. It is often considered to be a form of personality disorder; see SCHIZOTYPAL PERSONALITY DISORDER.

schizophreniform disorder a mental disorder with the signs and symptoms of schizophrenia but duration of less than six months.

schizotrichia (skiz″o-trik′e-ah) splitting of the hairs at the ends.

schizotypal personality disorder a PERSONALITY DISORDER characterized by a pattern of social and interpersonal deficits with eccentricities of behavior, thought, and speech. People with schizotypal personalities may exhibit magical thinking, for example, claiming that they are clairvoyant or telepathic, may have recurrent illusions, or may exhibit derealization. Their speech is marked by vagueness, metaphors, odd usages of words, and other features that can make it difficult to understand. Persons with this disorder often are aloof and socially isolated with little capability or desire for close relationships, excessive social anxiety, suspiciousness, and disturbed affect. Although the disorder is related to SCHIZOPHRENIA, it differs in that any periods of psychosis are only transient.

Schlatter-Osgood disease (shlat′er oz′-good) OSTEOCHONDROSIS of the tuberosity of the tibia; called also Osgood-Schlatter disease.

Schmidt's syndrome (shmits) 1. paralysis on one side, affecting the vocal cord, soft palate, trapezius muscle, and sternocleidomastoid muscle, due to a lesion of the nucleus ambiguus and the nucleus accessorius. 2. hypofunction of more than one ENDOCRINE GLAND, which may include the THYROID, ADRENALS, GONADS, PARATHYROIDS, and endocrine PANCREAS, in any combination, along with nonendocrine abnormalities of presumed autoimmune origin, such as VITILIGO, ALOPECIA, and PERNICIOUS ANEMIA; it occurs primarily in adult females.

Schmorl's disease (shmorlz) herniation of the nucleus pulposus.

Schönlein's disease (shern′līnz) Schönlein purpura.

Schönlein-Henoch syndrome (shern′līn hen′ok) Henoch-Schönlein purpura.

Schüller's disease (shil′erz) Hand-Schüller-Christian disease.

Schüller-Christian disease (shil′er kris′chan) Hand-Schüller-Christian disease.

Schwabach test (shvah′bahk) a TUNING FORK TEST made, with the opposite ear masked, placing the stems of vibrating forks on the mastoid PROCESS first of the patient and then of the examiner. If heard longer by the patient it indicates that he or she has conductive HEARING LOSS and if heard longer by the examiner it indicates that the patient has sensorineural HEARING LOSS.

schwannoma (shwah-no′mah) 1. a neoplasm originating from Schwann cells of

MANIFESTATIONS OF FIELD PATTERNING IN UNITARY HUMAN BEINGS

The evolution of unitary human beings is a dynamic, irreducible, non-linear process characterized by increasing diversity of energy field patterning. Manifestations of patterning emerge out of human/environmental field mutual process and are continuously innovative. Pattern is an abstraction that reveals itself through its manifestations.

The nature of unitary field patterning is unpredictable and creative. Change is relative and increasingly diverse. Some manifestations of relative diversity in field patterning are noted below.

lesser diversity		greater diversity
longer rhythms	shorter rhythms	seem continuous
slower motion	faster motion	seems continuous
time experienced as slower	time experienced as faster	timelessness
pragmatic	imaginative	visionary
longer sleeping	longer waking	beyond waking

neurons; schwannomas include NEUROFIBROMAS and NEURILEMOMAS. 2. neurilemoma.

SCI spinal cord injury.

sciage (se-ahzh′) [Fr.] a sawing movement in massage.

sciatic (si-at′ik) 1. ischial. 2. pertaining to or located near the sciatic nerve or vein.

s. nerve a nerve extending from the base of the spine down the thigh, with branches throughout the lower leg and foot; it is the widest nerve of the body and one of the longest. SCIATICA is pain or inflammation along the course of this nerve. See anatomic Table of Nerves in the Appendices and see Plates.

sciatica (si-at′ĭ-kah) NEURALGIA along the course of the SCIATIC NERVE; the term is popularly used to describe a number of disorders directly or indirectly affecting the

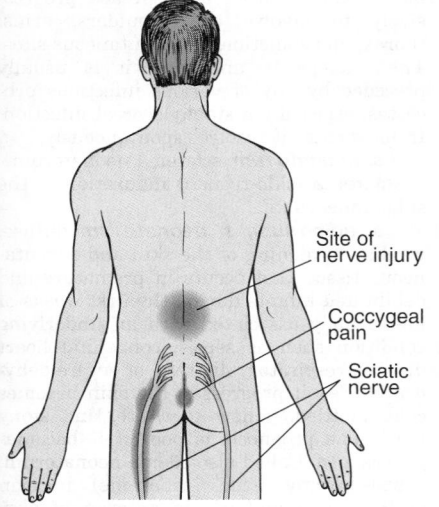

Site of nerve injury

Coccygeal pain

Sciatic nerve

Radiation of sciatic nerve pain. From Frazier et al., 2000.

nerve. Because of its length, the sciatic nerve is exposed to many different kinds of injury, and inflammation of the nerve or injury to it causes pain that travels down from the back or thigh along its course through the lower limb into the foot and toes. Certain leg muscles may be partly or completely paralyzed by such a disorder.

True sciatic neuritis is rare; it can be caused by a toxic substance such as lead or alcohol, and occasionally by other factors. Sciatic pain, however, can also be produced by conditions other than inflammation of the nerve. Probably the most common cause is a HERNIATED DISK. A back injury, irritation from arthritis of the spine, or pressure on the nerve from certain types of exertion may also be the cause. Occasionally diseases such as diabetes mellitus, gout, or vitamin deficiencies may be the inciting factor. In rare cases, pain may be referred over connected nerve pathways to the sciatic nerve from a disorder in another part of the body. Finally, some cases are idiopathic. Because of the long, painful, and disabling course of severe sciatica, the underlying cause should be investigated and corrected when possible.

SCID severe combined immunodeficiency disease.

science of unitary human beings a CONCEPTUAL MODEL of nursing, formulated by Martha E. ROGERS, concerned with nursing as the study of unitary, irreducible, indivisible human and environmental fields, people, and their world. See accompanying table.

scieropia (si″er-o′pe-ah) a defect of vision in which objects appear in a shadow.

scintigram (sin′tĭ-gram) the graphic record obtained by scintigraphy.

scintigraphy (sin-tig′rah-fe) production of two-dimensional images of the distribution of radioactivity in tissues after internal administration of a RADIOPHARMACEUTICAL

S

imaging agent, the images being obtained by a scintillation camera. adj., **scinti-graph′ic.**

exercise thallium s. myocardial perfusion using thallium 201 as a tracer and performed in conjunction with an exercise stress test.

gastroesophageal s. scintigraphy of the esophagus and stomach. A radioisotope is introduced into the stomach and scintillation measurements are taken over both the esophagus and the stomach; usually used to determine the degree of gastroesophageal REFLUX.

gated blood pool s. equilibrium radionuclide scintigraphy.

infarct avid s. that performed following myocardial infarction to confirm infarction as well as detect, localize, and quantify regions of myocardial necrosis. A radiotracer that concentrates in these regions, usually technetium ^{99m}Tc pyrophosphate, is administered intravenously and images are obtained with a gamma camera. For maximal sensitivity, the study is performed between 24 and 72 hours after infarction.

myocardial perfusion s. that performed using a radiotracer that traverses the myocardial capillary system and enters myocardial cells; after the radionuclide, usually thallium 201, is introduced into the bloodstream, regional myocardial blood flow and cell viability are assessed using immediate and delayed images. Scintigraphy is frequently combined with an exercise stress test (see EXERCISE TESTING) in the diagnosis of coronary artery disease.

scintillation (sin″tĭ-la′shun) 1. the emission of sparks. 2. the sensation of sparks before the eyes. 3. a particle emitted in disintegration of a radioactive element.

scintiscan (sin′tĭ-skan) a two-dimensional representation (map) of the radiation emitted by a radioisotope, revealing its concentration in specific organs or tissues.

scintiscanner (sin″tĭ-skan′er) the system of equipment used to make a scintiscan.

scirrhoid (skir′oid) resembling scirrhous CARCINOMA.

scirrhous (skir′us) hard or indurated.

scirrhus (skir′us) scirrhous carcinoma.

scler(o)- word element [Gr.], *hard; sclera.*

sclera (skle′rah) [L.] the tough, white outer coat of the eyeball, covering approximately the posterior five-sixths of its surface, continuous anteriorly with the cornea and posteriorly with the external sheath of the optic nerve. adj., **scle′ral.**

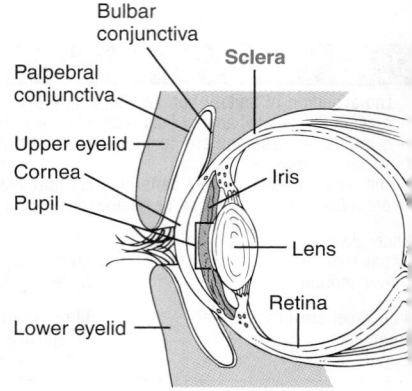

The sclera and other eye structures. From Lammon et al., 1995.

blue s. abnormal blueness of the sclera; it is a prominent feature of OSTEOGENESIS IMPERFECTA and is also seen in certain other conditions. (See Atlas 1, Part B.)

scleradenitis (sklēr″ad-ĕ-ni′tis) inflammation and hardening of a gland.

sclerectasia (sklēr″ek-ta′zhah) a bulging state of the sclera.

sclerectoiridectomy (skle-rek″to-ir″ĭ-dek′tah-me) excision of part of the sclera and of the iris.

sclerectoiridodialysis (skle-rek″to-ir″ĭ-do-di-al′ĭ-sis) sclerectomy and iridodialysis.

sclerectomy (sklĕ-rek′tah-me) excision of part of the sclera.

scleredema (sklē″rĕ-de′mah) diffuse symmetrical, woodlike, nonpitting induration of the skin; it typically begins on the face, head, or neck and spreads progressively to involve the shoulders, arms, thorax, and sometimes extracutaneous sites. The etiology is unknown; it is usually preceded by any of various infectious processes, especially a staphylococcal infection. In most cases it resolves spontaneously.

s. neonato′rum sclerema neonatorum.

sclerema (sklĕ-re′mah) induration of the subcutaneous fat.

s. adipo′sum, s. neonato′rum diffuse waxlike hardening of the skin and subcutaneous tissue that occurs in premature and debilitated infants during the first weeks of life, usually associated with an underlying condition such as sepsis, congenital heart disease, respiratory distress, or severe dehydration. As it progresses, the skin becomes cold, mottled, yellow to white, and stony hard. The prognosis is poor if it becomes generalized. Called also edema neonatorum.

scleriritomy (skle′rĭ-rit′ah-me) incision of the sclera and iris in anterior staphyloma.

scleritis (sklĕ-ri′tis) inflammation of the sclera. It may be superficial (episcleritis) or deep.

anterior s. inflammation of the sclera adjoining the limbus of the cornea.

posterior s. scleritis involving the retina and choroid.

scleroblastema (skle″ro-blas-te′mah) the embryonic tissue from which bone is formed.

sclerochoroiditis (skle″ro-ko″roi-di′tis) inflammation of the sclera and choroid.

sclerocornea (skle″ro-kor′ne-ah) the sclera and cornea regarded as one.

sclerodactyly (skle″ro-dak′tĭ-le) SCLERODERMA of the fingers and toes.

scleroderma (skle″ro-der′mah) chronic hardening and shrinking of the connective tissues of any organ of the body, including the skin, heart, esophagus, kidney, or lung. The skin may be thickened, hard, and rigid, and pigmented patches may occur. The two main types are systemic scleroderma and localized scleroderma. The milder forms are most often seen in women between the ages of 30 and 50; the more severe forms usually affect men, blacks, and older persons. The cause of scleroderma is not known. Current theories suggest three possibilities: an immunological reaction in which the skin attracts lymph cells which stimulate the production of collagen, hereditary factors related to abnormal serum proteins and antinuclear factors, and occupational exposure to silica dust.

Because the symptoms of scleroderma often mimic those of other diseases such as bursitis, osteoarthritis, rheumatoid arthritis, and other collagen disorders, it is difficult to diagnose. There is no test specific for confirmation of a diagnosis of scleroderma, but x-rays, skin biopsies, and tests for antinuclear antibodies, gamma globulin, sedimentation rate, and latex fixation can provide evidence that the disease is present.

Treatment. Treatment includes drugs such as penicillamine, immunosuppressives, and antiinflammatory agents. Ulcers that form on the knuckles, elbows, and other bony prominences as a result of calcium deposits are treated topically with ointments. Physiotherapy to restore and maintain musculoskeletal function as much as possible is indicated for certain patients. For others, diet therapy and small frequent feedings can help relieve the problems of malabsorption due to intestinal involvement.

Patient Care. Patients with scleroderma have especially thick skin that is hard to penetrate with a needle. Injections and venipunctures can be quite painful and should be done with as much care and

dispatch as possible. The site of venipuncture for intravenous therapy is monitored frequently, especially for infiltration, which can cause a painful swelling and pressure for weeks. The skin should be protected from irritation that could lead to breakdown and the introduction of infectious agents.

Calcium deposit sites are assessed regularly to note any signs of prolonged pressure, ulceration, or infection. Cool, moist compresses and a topical ointment can help relieve infections when they do develop at these sites. Protection of the respiratory tract includes stopping smoking, avoiding infectious agents, and getting adequate rest. Emotional stress can aggravate the condition; hence patients are taught effective coping strategies and relaxation techniques.

Mouth care and proper brushing and flossing, as well as periodic dental checks, are necessary to prevent cavities and periodontal disease. Patients with scleroderma have great difficulty opening their mouths wide enough to allow dental work to be done. Patients are encouraged to take prescribed medications exactly as ordered and are taught the names of their drugs, their expected action, and when and how to take them, that is, with meals and never with milk products.

Patients and their families can participate better in self-care and management of the illness if they are provided with continued support, either with a group or by a visiting nurse. Additional information about the disease can be obtained by contacting the United Scleroderma Foundation, P.O. Box 399, Watsonville, CA 95077-0399, telephone (800) 722-HOPE.

circumscribed s. 1. localized scleroderma. 2. morphea.

diffuse s., generalized s. systemic scleroderma.

linear s. localized scleroderma in a bandlike lesion with discoloration of the skin and atrophy of skin, subcutaneous tissue, muscle, and bone. See also COUP DE SABRE. Called also linear morphea.

localized s. 1. scleroderma confined to the skin and subcutaneous tissue or secondarily involving the musculoskeletal system. It occurs in three forms: MORPHEA, linear SCLERODERMA, and COUP DE SABRE. Called also circumscribed scleroderma. 2. morphea.

systemic s. a systemic disorder of the connective tissue characterized by hardening and thickening of the skin, with TELANGIECTASIAS, RAYNAUD'S PHENOMENON, and fibrotic degenerative changes in organs such as the heart, lungs, kidneys, and

S

gastrointestinal tract. It may remain confined to the face and hands for a long time or may spread diffusely to become generalized. Called also diffuse or generalized scleroderma and systemic sclerosis. See also CREST SYNDROME.

sclerogenous (skle̅-roj'e̅-nus) producing sclerosis or a hard tissue or material.

scleroiritis (skle″ro-i-ri'tis) inflammation of the sclera and iris.

sclerokeratitis (skle″ro-ker″ah-ti'tis) inflammation of the sclera and cornea.

scleroma (skle̅-ro'mah) a hardened patch or induration of skin or mucous membrane.

> **respiratory s.** rhinoscleroma.

scleromalacia (skle″ro-mah-la'shah) degeneration (softening) of the sclera, occurring in patients with rheumatoid arthritis.

scleromyxedema (skle″ro-mik″se̅-de'mah) a variant of LICHEN MYXEDEMATOSUS characterized by a generalized eruption of the nodules and diffuse thickening of the skin.

scleronyxis (skle″ro-nik'sis) surgical puncture of the sclera.

sclero-oophoritis (skle″ro-o″of-o-ri'tis) sclerosing inflammation of the ovary.

sclerophthalmia (skle″rof-thal'me-ah) encroachment of the sclera upon the cornea so that only a portion of the central part remains clear.

scleroprotein (skle″ro-pro'te̅n) a simple protein characterized by its insolubility and its fibrous structure; it usually serves a supportive or protective function in the body.

sclerosant (skle-ro'sant) sclerosing agent.

sclerose (skle-ro̅s) to become, or cause to become, hardened.

sclerosis (skle̅-ro'sis) an INDURATION or HARDENING, especially of a part from inflammation, or in disease of the interstitial substance. The term is used chiefly for such a hardening of the nervous system due to hyperplasia of the connective tissue or for hardening of the blood vessels. Called also induration. adj., **sclerot′ic.**

> **amyotrophic lateral s.** see AMYOTROPHIC LATERAL SCLEROSIS.

> **arteriolar s.** arteriolosclerosis.

> **disseminated s.** multiple sclerosis.

> **familial centrolobar s.** a progressive familial form of LEUKOENCEPHALOPATHY marked by nystagmus, ataxia, tremor, parkinsonian FACIES, dysarthria, and mental deterioration.

> **focal glomerular s.** focal segmental glomerulosclerosis.

> **glomerular s.** glomerulosclerosis.

> **hippocampal s.** loss of neurons in the region of the HIPPOCAMPUS, with GLIOSIS; sometimes seen in EPILEPSY.

> **lateral s.** a form seated in the lateral columns of the spinal cord. It may be primary, with spastic paraplegia, rigidity of the limbs, and increase of the tendon reflexes but no sensory disturbances, or secondary to myelitis, with paraplegia and sensory disturbance.

> **medial calcific s., Mönckeberg's s.** Mönckeberg's arteriosclerosis.

> **multiple s.** see MULTIPLE SCLEROSIS.

> **systemic s.** systemic scleroderma.

> **tuberous s.** a congenital heredofamilial disease, transmitted as an autosomal dominant trait, characterized principally by the presence of hamartomas of the brain (TUBERS), retina (PHAKOMAS), and viscera, mental retardation, seizures, and adenoma sebaceum, and often associated with other skin lesions.

scleroskeleton (skle″ro-skel'e̅-ton) the part of the bony skeleton formed by ossification in ligaments, fasciae, and tendons.

sclerostenosis (skle″ro-ste̅-no'sis) induration or hardening combined with contraction.

sclerostomy (skle̅-ros'tah-me) surgical creation of an opening through the sclera for the relief of glaucoma.

sclerotherapy (skle″ro-ther'ah-pe) injection of sclerosing AGENTS in the treatment of hemorrhoids, varicose veins, or esophageal varices.

sclerotitis (skle″ro-ti'tis) scleritis.

sclerotium (skle̅-ro'she-um) a hard blackish mass formed by certain fungi, as ergot.

sclerotome (skle'ro-to̅m) 1. an instrument used in incision of the sclera. 2. the area of a bone innervated from a single spinal segment. 3. one of the paired masses of mesenchymal tissue, separated from the ventromedial part of a somite, which develop into vertebrae and ribs.

sclerotomy (skle̅-rot'ah-me) incision of the sclera.

> **anterior s.** the opening of the anterior chamber of the eye, chiefly done for the relief of glaucoma.

> **posterior s.** an opening made into the vitreous through the sclera, as for correction of detachment of the retina or the removal of a foreign body.

sclerous (skle'rus) indurated.

scolex (sko'leks) [Gr.] the attachment organ (mouth) of a TAPEWORM, generally considered the anterior, or cephalic, end.

scoli(o)- word element [Gr.], *crooked; twisted.*

scoliokyphosis (sko″le-o-ki-fo'sis) combined lateral (scoliosis) and posterior (kyphosis) curvature of the spine.

scoliorachitic (sko″le-o-rah-kit'ik) affected with scoliosis and rickets.

measurement of spinal curvature.

scoliosis (sko″le-o′sis) lateral deviation in the normally straight vertical line of the spine; it may or may not include rotation or deformity of the vertebrae. Scoliosis occurs in both sexes, but girls are more likely to have more severe curvatures. It can occur at any age, and is most often noticed during adolescence when there is an accelerated growth rate and the deformity progresses to a severe curvature in a very short period of time. adj., **scoliot′ic.**

Classification. There are two major types of scoliosis: *postural* and *structural*. Postural scoliosis does not involve fixed rotation of the vertebrae, is not usually pronounced, and can be corrected by exercise. Structural scoliosis is the result of changes in the body structure with fixed rotation of the vertebrae in the direction of the convexity of the curve. This type is further divided into three categories based on the cause and kind of deformity presented: *congenital, neuromuscular,* and *idiopathic.*

Congenital scoliosis results from improper development of the spine during the third and fifth weeks of fetal life. Congenital abnormalities progress throughout early life and can interfere with normal growth of the trunk. Such defects rarely occur alone and are usually associated with other abnormalities in the newborn.

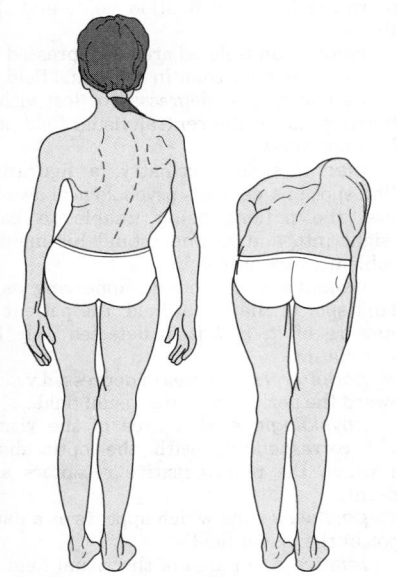

Structural scoliosis with vertebral rotation shown by rib rotation on bending forward. From Lissauer and Clayden, 2002.

Neuromuscular scoliosis results from muscular weakness, localized muscle imbalance, or neurologic dysfunction and paralysis. The curvature is flexible at first, with little rotation, but as the disease progresses, the curves become more pronounced and more rigid.

Idiopathic scoliosis has no known cause. The most severe cases usually appear before puberty, but it can appear at any time from infancy to adulthood. It tends to run in families; the mode of inheritance is thought to be multifactorial.

Detection. Most cases of scoliosis can be corrected if detected early and treated promptly before inflexible structural changes occur and cardiopulmonary complications develop. Since the early 1960's, screening programs for detection of scoliosis in school children have been initiated and several states now require periodic screening of all children in the public schools. Parents also are encouraged to look for early signs of the disorder in their children.

The signs of scoliosis include: (1) one shoulder higher than the other or one scapula more prominent, (2) abnormal waistline tilt with more indentation on one side, (3) a tilting of the hips with one hip more prominent, and (4) a prominence of the posterior chest or the shoulder when the child bends over. (See illustration.) Inspection of the adolescent child for these signs should be made every few months.

Treatment. There are several ways in which scoliosis can be treated and corrected. Milder forms respond well to active and passive exercise, but the more severe structural defects require either nonsurgical immobilization or surgical correction. Nonsurgical modes of therapy involve some form of bracing of the spine, using either a special brace that consists of a leather girdle and neck ring connected by metal struts (the Milwaukee brace); or a less cumbersome molded plastic jacket. Rigid casting is also used, but less frequently than other methods. Application of a localizer cast is another orthopedic procedure that is sometimes used preoperatively to stretch muscles, and also after surgery to maintain alignment until the bone graft is healed.

Various surgical techniques, determined by the type of structural defects present, are employed to realign the spine through the use of external or internal fixation and instrumentation in combination with spinal fusion to maintain normal curvature. Surgical intervention is indicated when the curve is more than 40 degrees or when a congenital curvature will inevitably progress if not treated by early stabilization.

scopolamine (sko-pol′ah-mēn) an ANTI-CHOLINERGIC and ANTIMUSCARINIC alkaloid derived from various plants, having a depressant effect on the central nervous system. Used as an antisialagogue preanesthetic medication and as an adjunct to general anesthesia, administered parenterally; as an antiemetic, administered orally or parenterally; and as a cycloplegic and mydriatic, applied topically to the conjunctiva. Called also hyoscine.

scopometer (sko-pom′ĕ-ter) an instrument for measuring the turbidity of a solution by comparing the contrast between an illuminated line viewed through the solution and an illuminated field of the same brightness.

scopometry (sko-pom′ĕ-tre) measurement of the turbidity of a solution using a scopometer.

scopophilia (sko″po-fil′e-ah) usually, voyeurism, but the disorder is sometimes divided into active and passive forms, *active scopophilia* being *voyeurism* and *passive scopophilia* being *exhibitionism.*

scopophobia (sko″po-fo′be-ah) irrational dread of being seen.

-scopy word element [Gr.], *examination of.*

scorbutic (skor-bu′tik) pertaining to scurvy.

scorbutigenic (skor-bu″tĭ-jen′ik) causing scurvy.

scordinema (skor″dĭ-ne′mah) yawning and stretching with a feeling of lassitude, a precursor of various diseases.

score (skor) a rating, usually expressed numerically, based on specific achievement or the degree to which certain qualities are manifest.

APACHE s. [*a*cute *p*hysiological *a*ssessment and *c*hronic *h*ealth *e*valuation] a widely used method for assessing severity of illness in acutely ill patients in INTENSIVE CARE UNITS, taking into account a variety of routine physiological parameters.

Apgar s. a numerical expression of an infant's condition at birth, based on heart rate, respiratory effort, muscle tone, reflex irritability, and color; see also APGAR SCORE.

Bishop s. a score for estimating the prospects of induction of labor, arrived at by evaluating the extent of cervical dilatation, effacement, the station of the fetal head, consistency of the cervix, and the cervical position in relation to the vaginal axis.

Silverman-Andersen s. a system for evaluating the breathing of premature infants; see also SILVERMAN-ANDERSEN SCORE.

stroke s. any of various scoring systems that seek to characterize a patient's clinical state following a STROKE.

trauma s. a rating system used in the evaluation of patients with traumatic injury. Scores range from 1 to 15, with lower scores being associated with higher mortality rates.

scot(o)- word element [Gr.], *darkness.*

scotochromogen (sko″to-kro′mah-jen) a microorganism whose pigmentation develops in the dark as well as in the light; specifically, a member of a group of the anonymous mycobacteria. adj., **scotochromogen′ic.**

scotodinia (sko″to-din′e-ah) dizziness with headache, dimness of vision, and sometimes black spots in the visual field.

scotoma (sko-to′mah) [Gr.] 1. an area of lost or depressed vision within the visual field, surrounded by an area of less depressed or of normal vision. 2. mental scotoma. adj., **scotom′atous.**

absolute s. an area within the visual field in which perception of light is entirely lost.

annular s. a circular area of depressed vision surrounding the point of fixation.

arcuate s. an arc-shaped defect of vision arising in an area near the blind spot and extending toward it.

central s. an area of depressed vision corresponding with the fixation point and interfering with or abolishing central vision.

centrocecal s. a horizontal oval defect in the visual field situated between and embracing both the fixation point and the blind spot.

color s. an isolated area of depressed or defective vision for color in the visual field.

hemianopic s. depressed or lost vision affecting half of the central visual field; see also HEMIANOPIA.

mental s. in psychiatry, a figurative blind spot in a person's psychological awareness, the patient being unable to gain insight into and to understand his mental problems; lack of insight.

negative s. a scotoma appearing as a blank spot in the visual field; the patient is unaware of it, and it is detected only by examination.

peripheral s. an area of depressed vision toward the periphery of the visual field.

physiologic s. that area of the visual field corresponding with the optic disk, in which the photosensitive receptors are absent.

positive s. one which appears as a dark spot in the visual field.

relative s. an area of the visual field in which perception of light is only diminished, or loss is restricted to light of certain wavelengths.

ring s. annular s.

scintillating s. blurring of vision with the sensation of a luminous appearance before the eyes, with a zigzag, wall-like outline; called also teichopsia.

scotomagraph (sko-to'mah-graf) an instrument for recording the size and shape of a scotoma.

scotometer (sko-tom'ĕ-ter) an instrument for diagnosing and measuring scotomas.

scotometry (sko-tom'ĕ-tre) the measurement of isolated areas of depressed vision (scotomas) within the visual field.

scotophilia (sko''to-fil'e-ah) nyctophilia.

scotophobia (sko''to-fo'be-ah) irrational fear of darkness.

scotopia (sko-to'pe-ah) 1. night vision. 2. the adjustment of the eye for darkness; dark adaptation. adj., **scotop'ic.**

scotopsin (sko-top'sin) the protein moiety in the retinal rods that combines with 11-*cis*-retinal to form rhodopsin.

scr scruple.

scratch test (skrach) a SKIN TEST for HYPERSENSITIVITY in which a minute amount of the substance in question is inserted in small scratches made in the skin. A positive reaction is swelling and reddening at the site within 30 minutes. It is used in allergy testing and in testing for tuberculosis (PIRQUET'S REACTION).

screen (skrēn) 1. a framework or agent used as a shield or protector; called also protectant and protective. 2. to separate well individuals in a population from those who have an undiagnosed disease, defect, or other pathologic condition or who are at high risk by means of tests, examinations, or other procedures. See also SCREENING.

Bjerrum s. tangent screen.

fluoroscopic s. a phosphorescent screen that shows the movement and relationship of organs and structures in fluoroscopy.

intensifying s. a fluorescent screen used in conjunction with x-ray film to enhance the effect of the radiation and reduce dosage to the patient. The screen must be matched to the emissivity range; the emissivity of phosphorus is similar to that of the human eye, so that phosphors absorb x-ray energy and convert it to visible light.

tangent s. a large square of black cloth with a central mark for fixation; used with a campimeter in mapping the field of vision.

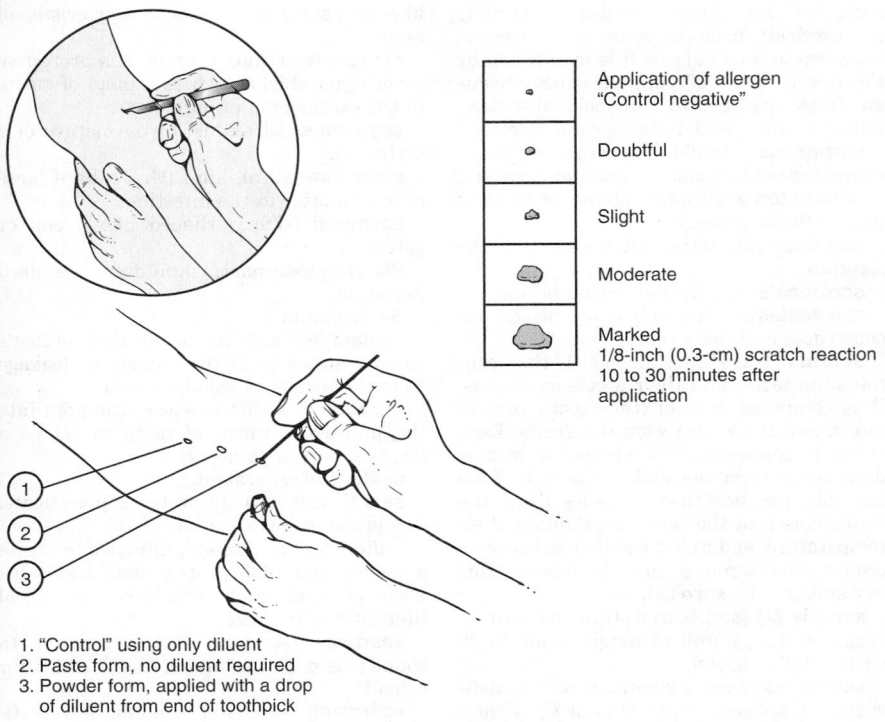

Application of allergen "Control negative"

Doubtful

Slight

Moderate

Marked
1/8-inch (0.3-cm) scratch reaction 10 to 30 minutes after application

1. "Control" using only diluent
2. Paste form, no diluent required
3. Powder form, applied with a drop of diluent from end of toothpick

Scratch test.

S

screening (skrēn'ing) examination or testing of a group of individuals to separate those who are well from those who have an undiagnosed disease or defect or who are at high risk.

health s. in the NURSING INTERVENTIONS CLASSIFICATION, a nursing INTERVENTION defined as detecting health risks or problems by means of history, examination, and other procedures.

multiphasic s., multiple s. that in which various diagnostic procedures are employed during the same screening program.

prescriptive s. that performed for the early detection of disease or disease precursors in apparently well individuals so that health care can be provided early in the course of the disease or before the disease becomes manifest.

scrobiculate (skro-bik'u-lāt) marked with pits.

scrofula (skrof'u-lah) former name for tuberculous cervical LYMPHADENITIS.

scrofuloderma (skrof''u-lo-der'mah) a tuberculous or nontuberculous mycobacterial infection affecting children and young adults, representing direct extension of tuberculosis into the skin from underlying structures such as the lymph nodes (especially the cervical), bone, or lung, or by contact exposure to tuberculosis. It is manifested by the development of painless subcutaneous swellings that evolve into cold abscesses, multiple ulcers, and draining sinus tracts.

scrofulous (skrof'u-lus) pertaining to or characterized by SCROFULODERMA or SCROFULA.

scrotectomy (skro-tek'tah-me) excision of part of the scrotum.

scrotitis (skro-ti'tis) inflammation of the scrotum.

scrotocele (skro'to-sēl) scrotal hernia.

scrotoplasty (skro'to-plas''te) plastic reconstruction of the scrotum.

scrotum (skro'tum) the pouch that contains the testes and their accessory organs. It is composed of skin, the TUNICA DARTOS, fascia, and the TUNICA VAGINALIS TESTIS. Each TESTIS is connected to a cremaster muscle descending from the abdominal wall. During cold weather these muscles draw the testes closer to the body to maintain their temperature, and in hot weather the reverse occurs; the scrotum usually follows this movement. adj., **scro'tal.**

scruple (℈) **(scr)** (skroo'pl) in the APOTHECARIES' SYSTEM, a unit of weight equal to 20 GRAINS (1.296 GRAMS).

scurvy (skur've) a condition due to deficiency of ASCORBIC ACID (vitamin C). Symptoms of infantile scurvy include poor appetite, digestive disturbances, failure to gain weight, increasing irritability, and bruises scattered over the skin. Severe deficiency may cause changes in bone structure. The only adults in the United States likely to develop scurvy are older people who live alone and neglect their diet. In adults, scurvy causes swollen and bleeding gums, looseness of the teeth, rupture of small blood vessels, and small bruises on the skin. Later symptoms may include anemia, extreme weakness, soreness of upper and lower limbs, tachycardia, and dyspnea.

Treatment of scurvy consists of supplying the missing vitamin in prescribed doses, and supplying the proper diet, including fresh fruits and vegetables. When this is done, the symptoms quickly disappear. Fruits and vegetables that are rich in vitamin C include grapefruit, oranges, lemons, limes, cantaloupes, strawberries, raspberries, turnips, raw cabbage, potatoes, and tomatoes.

scute (skūt) a squama or scalelike structure.

tympanic s. the bony plate which divides the upper part of the tympanic cavity from the mastoid cells.

scutiform (sku'tī-form) shaped like a shield.

scutulum (sku'tu-lum) one of the disklike or saucerlike crusts characteristic of FAVUS.

scutum (sku'tum) 1. scute. 2. a protective covering or shield, such as a plate of CHITIN in the exoskeleton of hard TICKS.

scybalous (sib'ah-lus) of the nature of a scybalum.

scybalum (sib'ah-lum) [Gr.] a hard mass of fecal matter in the intestine.

scyphoid (si'foid) shaped like a cup or goblet.

SD streptodornase; skin dose; standard deviation.

Se selenium.

sealant (sēl'ant) an agent that protects against access from the outside or leakage from the inside; called also sealer.

dental s. a thin plastic coating put into the pits and fissures of teeth to act as a physical barrier to decay.

sealer (sēl'er) sealant.

search (serch) 1. to probe or investigate. 2. a probe or investigation.

literature s. a search intended to create a customized bibliography that treats aspects of a research, scholarly, or topical literature of interest.

searcher (serch'er) an instrument (a sound) used in examining the bladder for calculi.

searching (serch'ing) probing or investigating.

titles, abstracts, full texts, or other natural language fields of bibliographic or source databases are searched for one or more words, whose proximity to each other may be specified in order to increase the specificity of the search.

seasickness (se'sik-nes) discomfort caused by the motion of a boat under way, a form of MOTION SICKNESS. The unusual motion disturbs the organs of balance located in the inner ear. Symptoms are nausea and vomiting, dizziness, headache, pallor, and cold perspiration. Ways to help ward off seasickness include staying in the fresh air instead of in a stuffy room, eating lightly, and avoiding fatty, fried, or spicy foods. Antinausea medicines may be effective. If seasickness occurs, the sufferer should rest lying down with the head low, in a comfortable well ventilated place. Also written *sea sickness*.

seasonal affective disorder (SAD) a MOOD DISORDER characterized by depression, extreme lethargy, increased need for sleep, overeating, and carbohydrate craving. It recurs each year in one or more specific seasons, most commonly the winter months, and is hypothesized to be related to MELATONIN levels.

seatworm (sēt'werm) pinworm.

sebaceous (sĕ-ba'-shus) pertaining to or secreting SEBUM.

s. cyst a benign retention cyst of a sebaceous gland containing the fatty secretion of the gland; this may occur anywhere on the body except the palms of the hands and soles of the feet, although such cysts are most common on the scalp, back, and scrotum. It may be a source of irritation or infection, and should be excised by a health care worker. Called also wen.

sebiferous (sĕ-bif'er-us) sebiparous.

sebiparous (sĕ-bip'ah-rus) secreting or producing a fatty substance.

sebolith (seb'o-lith) a calculus in a sebaceous gland.

seborrhea (seb"o-re'ah) excessive discharge from the sebaceous glands, forming greasy scales or cheesy plugs on the body; it is generally attended with itching or burning.

s. sic'ca dry, scaly, seborrheic dermatitis.

seborrheic (seb"o-re'ik) 1. affected with or of the nature of seborrhea. 2. pertaining to those areas of the body whose sebaceous glands are abundant, as the scalp, face, and axillae.

s. dermatitis an inflammatory condition, usually of the skin of the scalp, with yellowish greasy scaling of the skin and itching. A mild case in the scalp is called DANDRUFF. Seborrheic dermatitis can involve

other areas such as the face, neck, central part of the trunk, or axilla. The underlying cause is not known; the hair and scalp may be excessively oily, but the connection (if any) between this and the dermatitis is not known. Although there is no specific cure for dandruff, various measures are used to control and relieve it. Most patients can control scalp scaling by frequent use of a shampoo containing zinc pyrithione, selenium sulfide, or tar. The dermatitis responds well to hydrocortisone cream.

sebotropic (seb"o-trop'ik) having an affinity for or a stimulating effect on sebaceous glands; promoting the excretion of sebum.

sebum (se'bum) the oily secretion of the sebaceous glands, whose ducts open into the hair follicles. It is composed of fat and epithelial debris from the cells of the malpighian layer, and it lubricates the skin.

seclusion (sĕ-kloo'zhun) in the NURSING INTERVENTIONS CLASSIFICATION, a nursing INTERVENTION defined as solitary containment in a fully protective environment with close surveillance by nursing staff for purposes of safety or behavior management.

secobarbital (sek"o-bahr'bĭ-tal) a short-acting BARBITURATE used as the sodium salt as a SEDATIVE and HYPNOTIC, particularly as a presurgical aid to anesthesia, and as an ANTICONVULSANT in the treament of tetanus.

Seconal (sek'ŏ-nal) trademark for preparations of SECOBARBITAL sodium, a SEDATIVE and HYPNOTIC.

second (s) (sek'und) the base SI UNIT of time, equal to $\frac{1}{60}$ of a minute, and defined in terms of the periodicity of specific radiation of cesium 133.

secondary disease (sek'un-der"e) 1. a morbid condition subsequent to or a consequence of another disease. 2. a condition due to introduction of incompatible, immunologically competent cells into a host rendered incapable of accepting them by heavy exposure to ionizing radiation.

second-set phenomenon the accelerated and intensified rejection by the recipient of a second graft of tissue from the same donor as a consequence of the primary IMMUNE RESPONSE (i.e., antibody production and cell-mediated IMMUNITY) induced by the first graft.

secreta (se-kre'tah) [L., *pl.*] secretion (def. 2).

secretagogue (se-krēt'ah-gog) 1. causing a flow of secretion. 2. an agent that so acts.

secretary (sek'rĕ-tar"e) a person employed to do clerical work such as handling of correspondence, keeping of files, and similar duties.

S

unit s. ward clerk.

secrete (se-krēt′) to synthesize and release a substance.

secretin (se-kre′tin) a hormone secreted by the mucosa of the duodenum and jejunum when acid chyme enters the intestine; carried by the blood, it stimulates the secretion of pancreatic juice and, to a lesser extent, bile and intestinal secretion.

s. test an examination of the gastric and duodenal contents after intravenous administration of exogenous secretin; useful in the diagnosis of disorders affecting pancreatic exocrine function, for example, pancreatitis and neoplastic disease. Specimens are obtained via a Drieling TUBE, which is a double-lumen tube passed orally, and are analyzed for output (secretory rate), bicarbonate concentration, and amylase activity.

secretinase (se-kre′tin-ās) a substance in the serum that inactivates secretin.

secretion (se-kre′shun) 1. the cellular process of elaborating a specific product. This activity may range from separating a specific substance of the blood to the elaboration of a new chemical substance. 2. material that is secreted, such as SEBUM (the fatty substance produced by the sebaceous glands to lubricate the skin), SALIVA (produced by the salivary glands), and GASTRIC JUICE (secreted by specialized glands of the stomach). The secretions of the endocrine glands include various HORMONES and are important in the overall regulation of body processes.

secretoinhibitory (se-kre″to-in-hib′ĭ-tor″e) antisecretory.

secretomotor (se-kre″to-mo′tor) stimulating secretion; said of nerves.

secretor (se-kre′tor) in genetics, one who secretes the ABH antigens of the ABO blood group in the saliva and other body fluids; also, the gene determining this trait.

secretory (se-kre′tah-re) pertaining to secretion.

section (sek′shun) 1. an act of cutting. 2. a cut surface. 3. a segment or subdivision of an organ.

abdominal s. laparotomy; incision of the abdominal wall.

cesarean s. delivery of a fetus by incision through the abdominal wall and uterus; see also CESAREAN SECTION.

frontal s. a section through the body passing at right angles to the median plane, dividing the body into dorsal and ventral parts.

frozen s. a specimen cut by microtome from tissue that has been frozen; see also FROZEN SECTION.

perineal s. external urethrotomy.

sagittal s. a section through the body coinciding with the sagittal suture, thus dividing the body into right and left halves.

serial s's histologic sections of a specimen made in consecutive order and so arranged for the purpose of microscopic examination.

sectorial (sek-tor′e-al) cutting.

Sectral trademark for a preparation of ACEBUTOLOL hydrochloride, used in treatment of hypertension, arrhythmias, and angina pectoris.

secundigravida (sĕ-kun″dĭ-grav′ĭ-dah) a woman pregnant the second time; gravida II

secundines (se-kun′dīnz, dēnz) afterbirth.

secundipara (se″kun-dip′ah-rah) a woman who has had two pregnancies that resulted in viable offspring; para II.

sedation (sĕ-da′shun) 1. the allaying of irritability or excitement, especially by administration of a SEDATIVE. 2. the state so induced.

conscious s. in the NURSING INTERVENTIONS CLASSIFICATION, a nursing INTERVENTION defined as administration of SEDATIVES, monitoring of the patient's response, and provision of necessary physiological support during a diagnostic or therapeutic procedure

sedative (sed′ah-tiv) 1. allaying irritability, excitement, or nervousness. 2. an agent that does this. The usual mode of action is depression of the central nervous system, which tends to cause lassitude and reduced mental activity. Sedatives are distinct from TRANQUILIZERS, which also have a calming effect but unlike sedatives usually do not suppress bodily reactions. Sedatives may be classified according to the organ most affected, such as cardiac, gastric, and so on. Called also calmative.

The degree of relaxation produced varies with the kind of sedative, the dose, the means of administration, and the mental state of the patient. By causing relaxation, a sedative may help a patient go to sleep, but it does not put him to sleep. Medicines that induce sleep are known as HYPNOTICS (some drugs act as sedatives in small amounts and as hypnotics in large amounts). The BARBITURATES, such as PHENOBARBITAL, are the best known sedatives and are also widely used as hypnotics. Other effective sedatives include PARALDEHYDE and CHLORAL HYDRATE. Sedatives are useful in the treatment of any condition in which rest and relaxation are important to recovery. Some sedatives are also useful in treatment of convulsive disorders or epilepsy and in counteracting the effect of convulsion-producing drugs. They are used to calm patients before childbirth or surgery.

Restlessness in invalids, profound grief in adults, and overexcitement in children can be controlled by medically supervised sedation. Because many sedatives are habit-forming, they should be used with caution.

sedentary (sed′en-tar″e) of inactive habits; pertaining to a sitting posture.

sediment (sed′ĭ-ment) a precipitate, especially that formed spontaneously.

sedimentation (sed″ĭ-men-ta′shun) the settling out of sediment; see also sedimentation RATE.

seed (sēd) 1. the mature ovule of a flowering plant. 2. semen. 3. a small cylindrical shell of gold or other suitable material, used in application of radiation therapy. 4. to inoculate a culture medium with microorganisms.

plantago s., plantain s. , psyllium s. cleaned, dried ripe seed of species of *Plantago;* used as a bulk-forming LAXATIVE.

radon s. a small sealed container for radon, for insertion into the tissues of the body in radiotherapy.

segment (seg′ment) a demarcated portion of a whole. adj., **segmen′tal.**

behavior s. the smallest descriptive unit of a response to a stimulus.

bronchopulmonary s′s the smaller subdivisions of the lobe of a lung; each segment is separated from others by a connective tissue septum and supplied by its own branch of the bronchus leading to the particular lobe.

hepatic s′s subdivisions of the hepatic lobes based on arterial and biliary supply and venous drainage.

renal s′s subdivisions of the kidney that have independent blood supply from branches of the renal artery, including the *superior, anterior superior, inferior, anterior inferior,* and *posterior* segments.

uterine s. either of the two portions into which the uterus becomes differentiated early in labor; the upper contractile portion (corpus uteri) becomes thicker as labor approaches, and the lower noncontractile portion (the isthmus) is thin walled and passive in character.

segmentation (seg″men-ta′shun) 1. division into similar parts. 2. cleavage.

segregation (seg″rĕ-ga′shun) the separation of allelic genes during meiosis as homologous chromosomes begin to migrate toward opposite poles of the cell, so that eventually the members of each pair of allelic genes go to separate gametes.

segregator (seg′rĕ-ga′tor) an instrument for obtaining the urine from the ureter of each kidney separately.

seismotherapy (sīz″mo-ther′ah-pe) treatment of disease by mechanical vibration.

seizure (se′zhur) 1. the sudden attack or recurrence of a disease. 2. a CONVULSION or attack of EPILEPSY.

absence s. the seizure seen in petit mal EPILEPSY, marked by a momentary break in the stream of thought and activity, accompanied by a symmetrical spike and wave at 3 cycles per second on the electroencephalogram. Called also petit malseizure. See EPILEPSY.

atonic s. an absence seizure characterized by sudden loss of muscle tone.

complex partial s. see partial seizure.

febrile s. febrile CONVULSION.

focal s. partial seizure.

focal motor s. a simple partial seizure consisting of clonus or spasm of a muscle or muscle group, occurring either singly or in a continuous repetitive series.

generalized tonic-clonic s., grand mal s. the seizure seen in grand mal epilepsy, marked by loss of consciousness and generalized tonic convulsions followed by clonic convulsions. See EPILEPSY.

jackknife s′s infantile spasms.

myoclonic s. one characterized by a brief episode of MYOCLONUS.

partial s. any seizure due to a lesion in a specific, known area of the cerebral cortex; symptoms vary with different lesion locations. A *simple partial seizure* is the most localized type, with a discharge that is predominantly one-sided or presents localized features without loss of consciousness. A *complex partial seizure* is associated with disease of the temporal lobe and characterized by varying degrees of impairment of consciousness. See EPILEPSY.

petit mal s. absence seizure.

reflex s., sensory s. an epileptic seizure in response to a sensory stimulus, which may be tactile, visual, auditory, or musical.

simple partial s. see partial seizure.

tonic-clonic s. see generalized tonic-clonic SEIZURE.

selectivity (sĕ-lek-tiv′ĭ-te) in pharmacology, the degree to which a dose of a drug produces the desired effect in relation to adverse effects. adj., **selec′tive.**

grid s. a ratio comparing the transmitted primary radiation to the transmitted scatter radiation in an x-ray grid.

selegiline (sĕ-lej′ĭ-lēn) an agent used in treatment of PARKINSONISM; used as the hydrochloride salt in conjunction with LEVODOPA and CARBIDOPA.

selenious acid (sĕ-le′ne-us) monohydrated selenium dioxide, a source of elemental SELENIUM; administered intravenously.

S

selenium (sĕ-le′ne-um) a chemical element, atomic number 34, atomic weight 78.96, symbol Se. (See Appendix 6.) It is an essential mineral nutrient. Dietary sources of selenium include seafoods, kidney, and liver. Humans can adjust their homeostasis mechanism for selenium over a wide range of dietary intakes. Recommended intake levels are generally met from the diet, so that supplements are not necessary.

s. sulfide 1. the sulfide salt of selenium, a topical antiseborrheic and antifungal applied topically to the scalp to control seborrheic dermatitis and dandruff; also used topically in the treatment of tinea versicolor. 2. the sulfide salt of selenium, an antiseborrheic and antifungal; used topically in the treatment of seborrheic dermatitis and dandruff of the scalp and of tinea versicolor.

self (self) 1. a term used to denote an animal's own antigenic constituents, in contrast to "NONSELF" (which denotes foreign antigenic constituents). The self constituents are metabolized without antibody formation, whereas the antigens that are nonself are eliminated through the IMMUNE RESPONSE mechanism. It has been postulated that there is a mechanism of "self recognition" that enables the organism to distinguish between self and nonself. See also IMMUNITY. 2. the complete being of an individual, comprising both physical and psychological characteristics, and including both conscious and unconscious components. The concept of self is central to the jungian personality theory. See also JUNG.

therapeutic use of s. the ability to use theory, experiential knowledge, and self-awareness, and to explore one's impact on others.

self-antigen (self-an′ti-jen) any constituent of the body's own tissues capable of stimulating autoimmunity. See also IMMUNITY.

self-awareness (self″ah-wār′-nes) a sense of knowing and understanding what one is experiencing.

self-care model a CONCEPTUAL MODEL of nursing, formulated by Dorothea E. OREM, concerned with the individual's ability or inability to provide complete or effective self-care or care of dependent others.

self-defeating personality disorder a PERSONALITY DISORDER characterized by a persistent pattern of behavior detrimental to the self, including being drawn to problematic situations or relationships, failing to accomplish tasks crucial to life objectives, excessive self-sacrifice, inviting criticism and anger, undermining of pleasurable experiences, and inability to enjoy the reward of success.

self-disclosure (self″dis-klo′zhoor) sharing personal feelings and information with others.

self-effacement (self-ĕ-fās′ment) in bioethics, a virtue consisting of obligation of fidelity, or putting patients and their needs before the self-interest of the professional. Professionals give precedence or priority to the needs of patients rather than fulfilling their own needs; patients' interest take priority over the interests of others. Changes in the structure of health care have caused many stresses and divided loyalties for all health care professionals. Conflicts can be between the interests of patients and those of institutions, funding agencies, corporations, the state, and so forth.

self-esteem (self es-tēm′) respect for or pride about oneself; see also self-esteem ENHANCEMENT.

chronic low s.-e. a NURSING DIAGNOSIS accepted by the North American Nursing Diagnosis Association, defined as a longstanding negative self-evaluation or feeling about one's own self or self-capabilities.

risk for situational low s.-e. a NURSING DIAGNOSIS accepted by the North American Nursing Diagnosis Association, defined as being at risk for developing a negative perception of self-worth (situational low SELF-ESTEEM).

situational low s.-e. a NURSING DIAGNOSIS accepted by the North American Nursing Diagnosis Association, defined as a negative perception of self-worth in response to a current situation (specify).

self-limited (self-lim′ĭ-ted) limited by its own peculiarities, and not by outside influence.

s.-l. disease one that runs a definite limited course without treatment.

self-mutilation (self″mu′-tĭ-la′shun) 1. destructive, disfiguring actions toward one's own body. 2. a NURSING DIAGNOSIS accepted by the North American Nursing Diagnosis Association, defined as deliberate self-injurious behavior causing tissue damage with the intent of causing nonfatal injury to attain relief of tension.

risk for s.-m. a NURSING DIAGNOSIS accepted by the North American Nursing Diagnosis Association, defined as a state in which an individual is at high risk for deliberate self-injurious behavior (SELF-MUTILATION).

self-suspension (self″sus-pen′shun) suspension of the body by the head and axillae for the purpose of stretching the vertebral column.

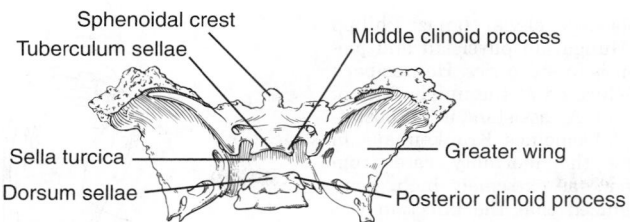

Sphenoidal crest
Tuberculum sellae
Middle clinoid process
Sella turcica
Dorsum sellae
Greater wing
Posterior clinoid process

Sella turcica in the superior aspect of the sphenoid bone. From Dorland's, 2000.

self-tolerance (self-tol′er-ans) immuno-logical tolerance to self-antigens.

sella (sel′ah) [L.] a saddle-shaped depres-sion. adj., **sel′lar.**

    empty s. see EMPTY-SELLA SYNDROME.

    s. tur′cica a depression on the upper surface of the sphenoid bone, lodging the pituitary gland.

semantics (sĕ-man′tiks) study of the meanings of words and the rules of their use; study of the relation between language and significance.

semelincident (sem″el-in′sĭ-dent) affect-ing a person only once.

semel in d. [L.] sem′el in di′e (once a day); written also *s.i.d.*

semen (se′men) fluid discharged at ejac-ulation in the male, consisting of spermato-zoa in their nutrient plasma, secretions from the prostate, seminal vesicles, and various other glands, epithelial cells, and minor constituents. adj., **sem′inal.**

semi- word element [L.], *half.*

semicanal (sem″e-kah-nal′) a trench or furrow open at one side.

semicircular (sem″e-ser′ku-lar) shaped like a half-circle.

    s. canals the passages in the bony LABYRINTH of the inner ear that control the SENSE OF EQUILIBRIUM. Each ear has three semicircular canals (anterior, lateral, and posterior), at approximately right angles to each other, which are filled with fluid and have AMPULLAE (enlarged portions) at one end that contain nerve endings. (See also Plates.) The semicircular canals respond to move-ment of the head. When the head changes position in any direction, the fluid in the canal that lies in the plane of movement also moves, but because of its inertia the fluid flow lags behind the head movement. Thus the fluid presses against the delicate hairs of the nerves in the ampulla, and the nerves then register the fact that the head is turning in a given direction so that the body can seek to maintain its equilibrium.

It is the fluid movement in the semi-circular canals that causes the feeling of dizziness or vertigo after spinning. When the spinning stops, the fluid in the horizon-tal canal continues to move for a moment in the direction of the spin, giving a temporary false reading that the head is turning in the other direction. MOTION SICKNESS is caused by the unusual and erratic motions of the head in an airplane, car, or ship, and the result-ing stimulation of the semicircular canals.

semicoma (sem″e-ko′mah) a stupor from which the patient may be aroused. adj., **semico′matose.**

semiflexion (sem″e-flek′shun) the position of a limb midway between flexion and exten-sion; the act of bringing to such a position.

semilunar (sem″e-loo′nar) shaped like a half-moon or crescent.

semination (sem″ĭ-na′shun) insemination.

seminiferous (sem″ĭ-nif′er-us) producing or carrying semen.

seminoma (sem″ĭ-no′mah) a malignant tumor of the testis thought to arise from primordial germ cells of the sexually un-differentiated embryonic gonad.

seminuria (se″mĭ-nu′re-ah) discharge of semen in the urine; called also spermaturia.

semiology (se″me-ol′ah-je) symptomatol-ogy.

semiotic (se″me-ot′ik) 1. pertaining to signs and symbols. 2. pertaining to the signs and symptoms of a disease. 3. pathogno-monic. Also spelled semeiotic.

semiotics (se″me-ot′iks) 1. the study of signs and symbols. 2. symptomatology.

semipermeable (sem″e-per′me-ah-bl) per-mitting passage only of certain molecules.

semiquantitative (sem″e-kwon′tĭ-ta′tiv) yielding an approximation of the quantity or amount of a substance; falling short of a quantitative result.

semis (ss.) (se′mis) [L.] half.

semisulcus (sem″e-sul′kus) a depression that, with an adjoining one, forms a sulcus.

semisupination (sem″e-soo″pĭ-na′shun) a position halfway toward supination.

semisynthetic (sem″e-sin-thet′ik) pro-duced by chemical manipulation of natu-rally occurring substances.

S

Semmelweis (sem′el-vīs) Ignaz Philipp (1818–1865). Hungarian physician and pioneer of antisepsis in obstetrics. He was born at Buda and educated at the universities of Pest and Vienna. As assistant in an obstetrics ward of Allgemeines Krankenhaus in Vienna, where the mortality rate from puerperal fever was extremely high, Semmelweis recognized that the infection was carried from patient to patient by the physicians, and he instituted preventive measures, such as cleansing of the physicians' hands with chlorinated lime. He met such fierce opposition from many of his colleagues that he left Vienna and returned to Pest to work as a physician in a maternity department.

semustine (sĕ-mus′tēn) the methyl analog of LOMUSTINE, a cytotoxic ALKYLATING AGENT used as an antineoplastic AGENT, primarily for treatment of brain tumors, colorectal carcinoma, gastric carcinoma, Hodgkin's disease, and malignant melanoma.

senescence (sĕ-nes′ens) the process of growing old; see also AGING. adj., **senes′-cent.**

Sengstaken-Blakemore tube (sengz′taken blāk′mōr) a device used for the TAMPONADE of bleeding esophageal VARICES, consisting of three tubes; one leading to a balloon that is inflated in the stomach, to retain the instrument in place and compress the vessels around the cardia; one leading to a long narrow balloon by which pressure is exerted against the wall of the esophagus; and the third attached to a suction apparatus for aspirating the contents of the stomach.

Patient Care. Prior to insertion the tube is held under water to check for leaks. It is then chilled to make it more firm, and lubricated to facilitate passage. After the tube is in place, ice water may be circulated through the stomach balloon to help control hemorrhage.

Mild traction is applied to the tubing at the point at which it enters the nose. Because of the danger of tissue erosion and necrosis of the gastric and esophageal mucosa, it is recommended that the tube be deflated for 5 minutes at 8 to 12 hour intervals. The tubing is removed in 24 hours if bleeding is controlled.

The patient must be watched continuously for signs of either injury to or rupture of the esophagus, respiratory distress, and shock. It is possible that the tube may be pulled upward into the oropharyngeal area, causing acute respiratory distress and asphyxiation. A pair of scissors are kept readily at hand so that the tube may be cut in the event this occurs.

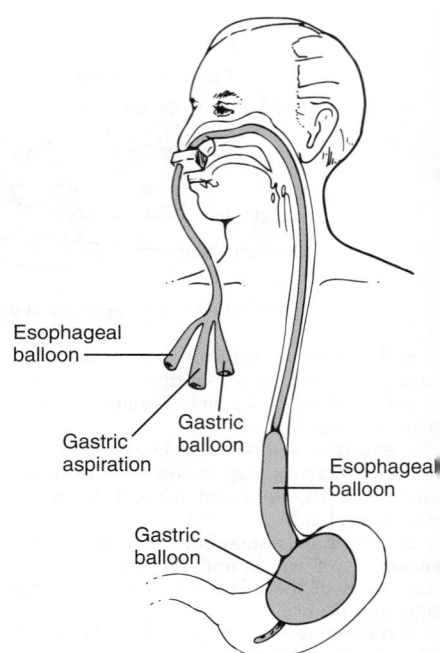

Esophageal balloon

Gastric aspiration

Gastric balloon

Esophageal balloon

Gastric balloon

Sengstaken-Blakemore tube. If bleeding site is in the esophagus, as from esophageal varices, the esophageal balloon is inflated. If bleeding site is in the stomach, the gastric balloon is inflated. Inflation creates pressure against bleeding vessels.

senile (se′nīl) pertaining to old age; see also AGED. Called also gerontic.

senilism (se′nil-izm) premature old age.

senility (sĕ-nil′ĭ-te) an obsolete and imprecise term used to denote a pronounced loss of mental or physical control in the AGED. Certain types of psychosis are associated with aging, such as senile DEMENTIA and DEMENTIA OF THE ALZHEIMER TYPE.

senna (sen′ah) the dried leaflets of *Cassia acutiflora;* used in a syrup, fluid extract, or compound powder as a CATHARTIC.

sennoside (sen′o-sīd) either of two anthraquinone glucosides, sennoside A and B, found in senna as the calcium salts; a mixture of the two is used as a cathartic.

senopia (se-no′pe-ah) improvement of vision, especially near vision, in the AGED, a sign of developing CATARACT; called also gerontopia.

sensation (sen-sa′shun) an impression produced by impulses conveyed by an afferent nerve to the sensorium.

girdle s. zonesthesia.

gnostic s's sensations perceived by the more recently developed senses, such as those of light touch and the epicritic sensibility to muscle, joint, and tendon vibrations.

primary s. that resulting immediately and directly from application of a stimulus.

referred s., reflex s. one felt elsewhere than at the site of application of a stimulus.

subjective s. one originating with the organism and not occurring in response to an external stimulus.

sense (sens) 1. a faculty by which the conditions or properties of things are perceived. Five major senses were traditionally considered: VISION, HEARING, SMELL, TASTE, and TOUCH. In addition, EQUILIBRIUM, HUNGER, THIRST, MALAISE, PAIN, and other types of senses have been distinguished. The operation of all senses involves the reception of stimuli by sense ORGANS, each of which is sensitive to a particular kind of stimulus. The eyes are sensitive to light; the ears, to sound; the olfactory organs, to odor; and the taste buds, to taste. Various sense organs of the skin and other tissues are sensitive to touch, pain, temperature, and other sensations. On receiving stimuli, the sense organ translates them into nerve impulses that are transmitted along the sensory nerves to the brain. In the cerebral cortex, the impulses are interpreted, or perceived, as sensations. The brain associates them with other information, acts upon them, and stores them as memory. See also NERVOUS SYSTEM and BRAIN. 2. pertaining to the sense STRAND of a nucleic acid.

s. of equilibrium the sense of maintenance of or divergence from an upright position, controlled by receptors in the vestibule of the ear.

kinesthetic s. muscle sense.

light s. the faculty by which degrees of brilliancy are distinguished.

muscle s., muscular s. the faculty by which muscular movements are perceived.

pain s. nociception.

position s., posture s. a variety of muscular sense by which the position or attitude of the body or its parts is perceived.

pressure s. the faculty by which pressure upon the surface of the body is perceived.

sixth s. the general feeling of consciousness of the entire body; cenesthesia.

somatic s's senses other than the special SENSES; these include TOUCH, KINESTHESIA, NOCICEPTION, pressure SENSE, temperature SENSE, and muscle SENSE, among others.

space s. the faculty by which relative positions and relations of objects in space are perceived.

special s's the senses of VISION, HEARING, TASTE, and SMELL; EQUILIBRIUM is sometimes considered a special sense, but TOUCH usually is not. See also somatic SENSES.

stereognostic s. the sense by which form and solidity are perceived.

temperature s. the ability to recognize differences in TEMPERATURE; called also thermesthesia.

sensibility (sen″sĭ-bil′ĭ-te) susceptibility of feeling; ability to feel or perceive.

deep s. the sensibility of deep tissue (such as muscles or tendons) to pressure, pain, and movement.

epicritic s. the sensibility to gentle stimulations permitting fine discriminations of touch and temperature, localized in the skin.

proprioceptive s. the sensibility afforded by receptors in muscles, joints, and other parts, by which one is made aware of their position and state.

protopathic s. the sensibility to strong stimulations of pain and temperature; it is low in degree and poorly localized, existing in the skin and in the viscera, and acting as a defensive agency against pathologic changes in the tissues.

somesthetic s. proprioceptive sensibility.

splanchnesthetic s. the sensibility to stimuli received by splanchnic receptors.

sensible (sen′sĭ-bl) perceptible to the senses; capable of sensation.

sensitive (sen′sĭ-tiv) 1. able to receive or respond to stimuli. 2. unusually responsive to stimulation, or responding quickly and acutely.

sensitivity (sen″sĭ-tiv′ĭ-te) 1. the state or quality of being sensitive; often used to denote a state of abnormal responsiveness to stimulation, or of responding quickly and acutely. 2. analytical sensitivity, the smallest concentration of a substance that can be reliably measured by a particular analytical method. 3. diagnostic sensitivity; the conditional probability that a person having a disease will be correctly identified by a clinical test, i.e., the number of true positive results divided by the total with the disease (which is the sum of the numbers of true positive plus false negative results). See also SPECIFICITY. 4. sensing threshold.

sensitization (sen″sĭ-tĭ-za′shun) 1. immunization. 2. exposure to allergen that results in the development of HYPERSENSITIVITY. 3. the coating of erythrocytes with antibody so that they are subject to lysis by complement in the presence of homologous antigen, the first stage of a complement fixation test.

autoerythrocyte s. see AUTOERYTHROCYTE SENSITIZATION SYNDROME.

sensitized (sen′sĭ-tīzd) rendered sensitive.

sensitometer (sen″sĭ-tom′ĕ-ter) a device used to produce a stepwedge of photographic density; used in quality assurance testing.

S

sensomobile (sen″so-mo′bĭl) moving in response to a stimulus.

sensomotor (sen″so-mo′tor) sensorimotor.

sensorial (sen-sor′e-al) pertaining to the sensorium.

sensorimotor (sen″sŏ-re-mo′tor) both sensory and motor.

sensorineural (sen″sŏ-re-noor′al) of or pertaining to a sensory nerve or sensory mechanism, as sensorineural deafness.

sensorium (sen-sor′e-um) 1. a primary receiving AREA. 2. the state of an individual as regards CONSCIOUSNESS or mental awareness.

sensory (sen′sŏ-re) pertaining to sensation or to the response of the senses (hearing, sight, touch, etc.) to incoming stimuli.

sentient (sen′she-ent) able to feel; sensitive.

separation anxiety disorder undue and prolonged distress and apprehension in a child concerning removal from parents, home, or familiar surroundings. Separation ANXIETY is common in children, especially infants, but in separation anxiety disorder the reaction is greater than what is expected for the child's developmental level.

separation-individuation the process usually seen in infants by which the child identifies itself as different from the primary caretaker while maintaining an emotional attachment.

sepsis (sep′sis) 1. the presence in the blood or other tissues of pathogenic microorganisms or their toxins. 2. septicemia.

puerperal s. sepsis after childbirth, due to putrefactive matter absorbed from the birth canal; see also PUERPERAL FEVER.

septa (sep′tah) [L.] plural of SEPTUM.

septal (sep′tal) pertaining to a septum.

septan (sep′tan) recurring on the seventh day (i.e., six days after the previous episode).

septate (sep′tāt) divided by a septum.

septectomy (sep-tek′tah-me) excision of part of the nasal septum.

septic (sep′tik) pertaining to sepsis.

septicemia (sep″tĭ-se′me-ah) the presence of infective agents or their toxins in the bloodstream, popularly known as blood poisoning. It is characterized by elevated body temperature, chills, and weakness. Small abscesses may form on the surface of the body and red and blue streaks become apparent along the pathway of surface blood vessels leading to and from the site of the primary infection. A blood culture confirms the diagnosis and helps identify the most effective antiinfective drug for therapy. This is a serious condition that must be treated promptly; otherwise the process of infection leads to circulatory collapse profound shock, and death. adj., **septice′mic.**

cryptogenic s. septicemia in which the focus of infection is not evident during life.

puerperal s. puerperal fever.

septicopyemia (sep″tĭ-ko-pi-e′me-ah) septicemia with pyemia.

septomarginal (sep″to-mar′jin-al) pertaining to the margin of a septum.

septonasal (sep″to-na′zal) pertaining to the nasal septum.

septoplasty (sep″to-plas′te) surgical reconstruction of the nasal septum.

septotomy (sep-tot′ah-me) incision of the nasal septum.

Septra (sep′trah) trademark for combination preparations of TRIMETHOPRIM and SULFAMETHOXAZOLE, an antimicrobial.

septulum (sep′tu-lum) [L.] a small separating wall or partition.

septum (sep′tum) [L.] 1. a wall or partition dividing a body space or cavity. Some are membranous, some are osseous, and some are cartilaginous; each is named according to its location. See also septal DEFECT. adj., **sep′tal.** 2. nasal septum.

alveolar s. interalveolar septum.

atrial s., s. atrio′rum cor′dis interatrial septum.

atrioventricular s. the part of the membranous portion of the interventricular septum between the left ventricle and the right atrium.

deviated s. an injury or malformation of the nasal SEPTUM so that one part of the nasal cavity is smaller than the other; this is fairly common and seldom causes complications. Occasionally the deviation may handicap breathing, block the normal flow of mucus from the sinuses during a cold, or prevent proper drainage of infected sinuses. In some cases surgery (called partial or complete submucous resection) may be necessary to relieve the obstruction and reduce irritation and infection in the nose and sinuses.

interalveolar s. 1. one of the thin plates of bone separating the ALVEOLI of the teeth in the mandible and maxilla. Called also interradicular septum. 2. one of the thin septa that separate adjacent pulmonary alveoli, containing connective tissue and the capillary network of the blood supply of the lung. Defs. 1 and 2 called also alveolar septum.

interatrial s., s. interatria′le cor′dis the partition separating the right and left atria of the heart; called also atrial septum.

interradicular s. interalveolar septum (def. 1).

interventricular s., s. interventricula're cor'dis the partition separating the right and left ventricles of the heart; called also ventricular septum.

nasal s. a plate of bone and cartilage covered with mucous membrane that divides the nasal cavity.

s. lu'cidum septum pellucidum.

pellucid s., s. pellu'cidum the triangular double membrane separating the anterior horns of the lateral ventricles of the brain; called also septum lucidum.

s. pri'mum a septum in the embryonic heart, dividing the primitive atrium into right and left chambers. See also CONGENITAL HEART DEFECT.

rectovaginal s. the membranous partition between the rectum and vagina.

rectovesical s. a membranous partition separating the rectum from the prostate and urinary bladder.

s. of ventricles of heart, ventricular s., s. ventriculo'rum cor'dis interventricular septum.

septuplet (sep-tup'let) one of seven offspring produced at one birth.

sequel (se'kwel) sequela.

sequela (sě-kwel'ah), pl. *seque'lae* [L.] a morbid condition following or occurring as a consequence of another condition or event.

postpolio s., postpoliomyelitis s. postpoliomyelitis syndrome.

sequencing (se'kwens-ing) the placement in order of information, concepts, or actions.

sequester (se-kwes'ter) 1. to detach or separate abnormally a small portion from the whole. 2. to isolate a portion of a chemical system by chelation or other means; see also SEQUESTRANT.

sequestrant (se-kwes'trant) a SEQUESTERING agent, such as cholestyramine RESIN (which binds bile acids in the intestine and prevents their absorption).

sequestration (se″kwes-tra'shun) 1. abnormal separation of a part from a whole, as a portion of a bone by a pathologic process, or a portion of the circulating blood in a specific part occurring naturally or produced by application of a tourniquet. 2. isolation of a patient.

pulmonary s. loss of connection of lung tissue, and sometimes bronchi, with the bronchial tree and pulmonary veins, the tissue receiving its arterial supply from the systemic circulation. It may be completely separated anatomically and physiologically from normally connected lung *(extralobar)* or contiguous to and partly surrounded by normal lung *(intralobar).* Called also accessory lung.

sequestrectomy (se″kwes-trek'tah-me) excision of a sequestrum.

sequestrum (se-kwes'trum) [L.] 1. a piece of dead bone that has become separated from sound bone during the process of necrosis. 2. any tissue that has become SEQUESTERED.

sequoiosis (se″kwoi-o'sis) a form of hypersensitivity PNEUMONITIS due to inhalation of and tissue reaction to dust from moldy redwood bark.

sera (se'rah) [L.] plural of SERUM.

Ser-Ap-Es (ser'ap-es) trademark for a preparation of HYDRALAZINE hydrochloride, RESERPINE, and HYDROCHLOROTHIAZIDE, an ANTIHYPERTENSIVE AGENT.

Serax (ser'aks) trademark for preparations of OXAZEPAM, an ANTIANXIETY AGENT.

SERM selective estrogen receptor modulator.

series (se'rēz) a group or succession of events, objects, or substances arranged in regular order or forming a kind of chain; in electricity, parts of a circuit connected successively to end to end to form a single path for the current. adj., **se'rial.**

erythrocyte s., erythrocytic s. the succession of morphologically distinguishable cells that that are stages in erythrocyte development: in order of maturity, the PROERYTHROBLAST, basophilic ERYTHROBLAST, polychromatophilic ERYTHROBLAST, orthochromatic ERYTHROBLAST, RETICULOCYTE, and ERYTHROCYTE.

gastrointestinal s., GI s. an examination of the upper gastrointestinal TRACT using BARIUM as the contrast medium for a series of x-ray films; see also BARIUM TEST. Called also barium meal.

granulocyte s., granulocytic s. the succession of morphologically distinguishable cells that are stages in granulocyte development: in order of maturity, the myeloblast, promyelocyte, myelocyte, metamyelocyte, the band or stab cell, which is the least mature form normally found in the peripheral blood, and the mature segmented (polymorphonuclear) granulocyte. Commitment to one of the granulocyte lines occurs in stem cells before the myeloblast stage is reached; thus there are distinct neutrophil, eosinophil, and basophil series; however, the morphologic stages are the same.

lymphocyte s., lymphocytic s. the succession of developing cells that ultimately culminates in mature lymphocytes. The morphologically distinguishable forms are lymphoblast, prolymphocyte, and lymphocyte.

monocyte s., monocytic s. the succession of developing cells that ultimately culminates in the monocyte.

The morphologically distinguishable forms are monoblast, promonoblast, and monocyte.

plasmacyte s., plasmacytic s. a series of morphologically distinguishable cells that are stages in plasma cell development: in order of maturity, the plasmablast (an activated B cell usually referred to as a large lymphocyte or lymphoblast), proplasmacyte, and plasmacyte.

thrombocyte s., thrombocytic s. the succession of developing cells that ultimately culminates in platelets (thrombocytes). The morphologically distinct cell types are megakaryoblast, promegakaryocyte, and megakaryocyte, which fragments to form platelets.

serine (sēr′ēn) a naturally occurring, nonessential AMINO ACID, used as a dietary supplement, in biological studies and tests, and in culture media.

sermorelin (ser″mo-rel′in) a synthetic peptide corresponding to a portion of growth hormone–releasing HORMONE; used as the acetate salt in treatment of growth HORMONE deficiency in prepubertal children, administered subcutaneously.

serocolitis (se″ro-ko-li′tis) inflammation of the serous coat of the colon.

seroconversion (se″ro-kon-ver′zhun) the change of a serologic test from negative to positive, indicating the development of antibodies in response to infection or immunization.

seroculture (se″ro-kul′chur) a bacterial culture on blood serum.

serodiagnosis (se″ro-di″ag-no′sis) diagnosis using serologic tests. adj., **serodiagnos′tic.**

seroenteritis (se″ro-en″tĕ-ri′tis) inflammation of the serous coat of the intestine.

serofibrinous (se″ro-fi′brĭ-nus) marked by both a serous exudate and precipitation of fibrin.

serogroup (sēr′o-grōōp) 1. a group of bacteria containing a common ANTIGEN, sometimes including more than one SEROTYPE, species, or genus. This is an unofficial designation, used in the classification of certain genera of bacteria, such as *Leptospira, Salmonella, Shigella,* and *Streptococcus.* 2. a group of viral species that are closely related antigenically.

serologic test (sēr″o-loj′ik) any laboratory test involving serologic reactions, such as PRECIPITIN REACTION, AGGLUTINATION, or complement FIXATION, especially any such test measuring serum antibody titer.

s. t. for syphilis (STS) any test for serum antibodies indicative of *Treponema pallidum* infection. There are two types,

NONTREPONEMAL ANTIGEN TESTS and TREPONEMAL ANTIGEN TESTS; the term is occasionally used with reference only to the former.

serologist (se-rol′ah-jist) a specialist in serology.

serology (se-rol′ah-je) originally, the study of the in vitro reactions of immune sera, e.g., precipitin, agglutination, and complement fixation reactions. Currently, the term is used to refer to the use of such reactions to measure serum antibody titers in infectious disease (SEROLOGIC TESTS), to the clinical correlations of the antibody titer (the serology of a disease), and to the use of serologic reactions to detect antigens (such as HLA ANTIGENS). adj., **serolog′ic.**

serolysin (se-rol′ĭ-sin) a lysin of the blood serum.

seroma (se-ro′mah) a collection of serum in the body, producing a tumorlike mass.

seromembranous (se″ro-mem′brah-nus) pertaining to or composed of serous membrane.

seromucous (se″ro-mu′kus) both serous and mucous.

seromuscular (se″ro-mus′ku-lar) pertaining to the serous and muscular coats of the intestine.

seronegative (se″ro-neg′ah-tiv) showing negative results on serologic examination; showing a low level of ANTIBODY.

seropositive (se″ro-poz′ĭ-tiv) showing positive results on serologic examination; showing a high level of ANTIBODY.

seroprognosis (se″ro-prog-no′sis) prognosis of disease based on serum reactions.

seropurulent (se″ro-pu′roo-lent) both serous and purulent.

seropus (se″ro-pus′) serum mingled with pus.

seroreaction (se″ro-re-ak′shun) a reaction demonstrating a specific antibody or antigen in serum.

seroresistant (se″ro-re-zis′tant) showing a seropositive reaction to a pathogen after treatment.

seroreversion (sēr″o-re-ver′zhun) spontaneous or induced conversion from a seropositive to a seronegative state.

serosa (se-ro′sah) any serous membrane. adj., **sero′sal.**

serosanguineous (se″ro-sang-gwin′e-us) composed of serum and blood.

seroserous (se″ro-se′rus) pertaining to two serous surfaces.

serositis (se″ro-si′tis) inflammation of a serous membrane.

serosity (se-ros′ĭ-te) the quality of serous fluids.

serosurvey (se″ro-sur′va) a screening test of the serum of persons at risk to determine susceptibility to a particular disease.

serosynovitis (se"ro-sin"o-vi'tis) synovitis with effusion of serum.

serotherapy (se"ro-ther'ah-pe) the treatment of infectious disease by the injection of immune serum or antitoxin.

serotonergic (ser"o-tōn-er'jik) containing or activated by serotonin.

serotonin (ser"o-to'nin) a hormone and neurotransmitter, 5-hydroxytryptamine (5-HT), found in many tissues, including blood platelets, intestinal mucosa, pineal body, and central nervous system; it has many physiologic properties, including inhibition of gastric secretion, stimulation of smooth muscles, and production of vasoconstriction.

serotoninergic (ser"o-to"nin-er'jik) pertaining to neurons that release SEROTONIN as a NEUROTRANSMITTER, such as those of the raphe nuclei of the brainstem, or neurons that secrete serotonin as a hormone.

serotype (se'ro-tīp) the type of a microorganism determined by its constituent antigens, or a taxonomic subdivision based thereon.

serous (se'rus) 1. pertaining to serum; thin and watery, like serum. 2. producing or containing serum.

serovaccination (se"ro-vak"sī-na'shun) injection of serum combined with bacterial vaccination to produce passive and active immunity.

serpiginous (ser-pij'ĭ-nus) creeping from part to part; having a wavy border.

serpin (ser'pin) any of a superfamily of inhibitors of serine endopeptidase (serine proteinase), found in plasma and tissues; all are similarly structured single-chain GLYCO-PROTEINS although each one acts specifically on particular endopeptidases. Among their targets are serine proteinases involved in coagulation, complement activation, fibrinolysis, inflammation, and tissue remodeling. The serpins include ALPHA₁-ANTITRYPSIN, ANTI-THROMBIN III, α₂-ANTIPLASMIN, C1 INHIBITOR, and plasminogen activator INHIBITOR 1 (PAI-1). Called also serine protease or proteinase inhibitor.

serrated (ser'āt-ed) having a sawlike edge or border.

Serratia (sĕ-ra'she-ah) a genus of gram-negative, facultatively anaerobic, motile bacteria, many species of which are opportunistic pathogens, causing infections of the endocardium, blood, wounds, and urinary and respiratory tracts. *S. marces'cens* is the most frequently isolated species.

serration (sĕ-ra'shun) 1. the state of being serrated. 2. a serrated structure or formation.

Sertoli-cell–only syndrome (ser-to'le) congenital absence of the germinal epithelium of the testes, the seminiferous tubules

containing only Sertoli cells, marked by testes slightly smaller than normal, azoospermia, and elevated titers of follicle-stimulating hormone or of general gonadotropins.

sertraline (ser'trah-lēn) a selective serotonin reuptake INHIBITOR administered orally as the hydrochloride salt as an ANTIDEPRESSANT and to treat obsessive-compulsive disorder and panic disorder.

serum (se'rum), pl. *serums, se'ra* [L.] the clear portion of any animal or plant fluid that remains after the solid elements have been separated out. The term usually refers to blood serum, the clear, straw-colored, liquid portion of the plasma that does not contain fibrinogen or blood cells, and remains fluid after clotting of blood. Blood serum from persons or animals whose bodies have built up antibodies is called *antiserum* or *immune serum*. Inoculation with such an antiserum provides temporary, or passive, immunity against the disease, and is used when a person has already been exposed to or has contracted the disease. Diseases in which passive immunization is sometimes used include diphtheria, tetanus, botulism, and gas gangrene.

***antilymphocyte s.* (ALS)** antiserum derived from animals that have been immunized against human lymphocytes, a powerful nonspecific immunosuppressive agent that causes destruction of circulating lymphocytes.

antirabies s. ANTISERUM obtained from the blood serum or plasma of animals immunized with rabies VACCINE; used for postexposure prophylaxis against RABIES if rabies immune GLOBULIN is unavailable.

blood grouping s's preparations containing particular antibodies against red cell antigens, used for blood typing. Those most commonly used are the anti-A and anti-B blood grouping serums used to determine ABO blood types and the anti-Rh blood grouping serums (anti-D, anti-C, anti-E, anti-c, and anti-e) used to determine Rh blood types.

***s. glutamic-oxaloacetic transaminase* (SGOT)** see ASPARTATE TRANSAMINASE.

***s. glutamic-pyruvic transaminase* (SGPT)** see ALANINE TRANSAMINASE.

immune s. antiserum.

pooled s. the mixed serum from a number of individuals.

s. sickness a HYPERSENSITIVITY REACTION following the administration of foreign serum or other antigens; it is marked by urticarial rashes, edema, adenitis, joint pains, high fever, and prostration. Reactions to tetanus ANTITOXIN derived from horse serum were

S

especially common but are now rare owing to refinement of the antigenic components.

s. sickness syndrome a serum sickness–like HYPERSENSITIVITY REACTION occurring after the administration of certain drugs. It is marked clinically by low-grade fever, urticaria, facial edema, pain and swelling of the joints, and lymphadenopathy, and occasionally may be associated with neuritis of the brachial plexus, GUILLAIN-BARRÉ SYNDROME, PERIARTERITIS NODOSA, and nephritis.

serumal (se-roo′mal) pertaining to or formed from serum.

serum-fast (se′rum-fast) resistant to the effects of serum.

service (ser′vis) the performance of work for others or the performance of an action for the benefit of others.

ancillary s′s tasks provided by hospital employees that are not directly related to health care, such as housekeeping and security.

sesamoid (ses′ah-moid) 1. denoting a small nodular bone embedded in a tendon or joint capsule. 2. a sesamoid bone; see anatomic Table of Bones in the Appendices.

sessile (ses′il) not pedunculated; attached by a broad base.

setaceous (se-ta′shus) bristle-like.

set-point (set′point) the target value of the controlled variable that is maintained by an automatic control system, e.g., the point at which body temperature is controlled by the hypothalamic thermostat. Written also set point.

setting (set′ing) establishment or creation of something.

limit s. in the NURSING INTERVENTIONS CLASSIFICATION, a nursing INTERVENTION defined as establishing the parameters of desirable and acceptable patient behavior.

mutual goal s. in the NURSING INTERVENTIONS CLASSIFICATION, a nursing INTERVENTION defined as collaborating with the patient to identify and prioritize care goals, then developing a plan for achieving those goals through the construction and use of goal attainment SCALING.

set test (set) a screening tool for the presence of dementia.

sevelamer (sĕ-vel′ah-mer) a phosphate BINDER used as the hydrochloride salt to reduce serum phosphorus concentrations in HYPERPHOSPHATEMIA associated with END-STAGE RENAL DISEASE; administered orally.

severe combined immunodeficiency disease (SCID) severe combined immunodeficiency.

sex (seks) 1. the fundamental distinction, found in most species of animals and plants,

based on the type of GAMETES produced by the individual; also the category to which the individual fits on the basis of that criterion. Called also gender. See also gender IDENTITY and gender ROLE. 2. to determine which of these categories an organism belongs in. 3. sexual INTERCOURSE.

chromosomal s. the sex as determined by the presence of the XX (female) or the XY (male) genotype in somatic cells, without regard to phenotypic manifestations. Called also genetic sex.

endocrinologic s. the phenotypic manifestations of sex determined by endocrine influences, such as development of breasts and genital organs.

genetic s. chromosomal sex.

gonadal s. the sex as determined on the basis of the gonadal tissue present (ovarian or testicular).

s. hormones glandular secretions involved in the regulation of sexual functions. The principal sex hormone in the male is TESTOSTERONE, produced by the testes. In the female the principal sex hormones are the ESTROGENS and PROGESTERONE, produced by the ovaries. These hormones influence the secondary sex characters, such as the shape and contour of the body, the distribution of body hair, and the pitch of the voice. The male hormones stimulate production of spermatozoa in men, and the female hormones control ovulation, pregnancy, and the menstrual cycle in women.

morphological s. sex determined on the basis of the morphology of the external genitals.

nuclear s. the sex as determined on the basis of the presence or absence of sex chromatin in somatic cells, its presence normally indicating the XX (female) genotype, and its absence the XY (male) genotype.

sex-conditioned (seks″kon-dish′und) sex-influenced.

sexduction (seks-duk′shun) F-duction.

sex-influenced (seks-in′floo-enst) denoting an autosomal trait that is expressed differently, either in frequency or degree, in males and females, as for example, male-pattern baldness.

sex-limited (seks-lim′ĭ-ted) affecting individuals of one sex only.

sex-linked (seks-linkt′) determined by a gene located on a sex chromosome; only X linkage has clinical significance.

sexology (sek-sol′ah-je) the scientific study of sex and sexual relations.

sextan (seks′tan) recurring on the sixth day (i.e., five days after the previous episode).

sextant (seks′tant) one of the six equal parts into which the dental arch may be divided: maxillary right, left, and anterior and mandibular right, left, and anterior.

sextipara (seks-tip′ah-rah) a woman who has had six pregnancies that resulted in viable offspring; para VI.

sextuplet (seks-tup′let) any one of six offspring produced at the same birth.

sexual (seks′shoo-al) 1. pertaining to, characterized by, involving, or endowed with sex, sexuality, the sexes, or the sex organs and their functions. 2. characterized by the property of maleness or femaleness. 3. pertaining to reproduction involving both male and female gametes. 4. implying or symbolizing erotic desires or activity.

   s. arousal disorders SEXUAL DYSFUNCTION characterized by alterations in sexual arousal; see FEMALE SEXUAL AROUSAL DISORDER and MALE ERECTILE DISORDER.

   s. aversion disorder feelings of repugnance for and active avoidance of genital contact with a partner, causing substantial distress or interpersonal difficulty.

   s. desire disorders SEXUAL DYSFUNCTIONS characterized by alteration in sexual desire; see HYPOACTIVE SEXUAL DESIRE DISORDER and SEXUAL AVERSION DISORDER.

   s. development the biologic and psychosocial changes that lead to sexual maturity. (Biologic changes in humans are discussed under REPRODUCTIVE ORGANS.) The basis for current study of the child's normal psychosexual development is a series of essays on sexuality published by Sigmund Freud in 1905. Although Freud failed to recognize differences in the sexual development of males and females and some parts of this theory have been questioned, his essays on sexuality, in which he describes three phases or stages of human sexual development (oral, anal, phallic), are considered classics in the fields of psychology and psychiatry.

   The *oral stage* of psychosexual development is the infantile period lasting from birth to 12 months, or even to 24 months of age, in which sensual pleasure is derived and sexual tensions are released through oral activities. It is followed by the *anal stage* at about the age of 18 months to 3 years, which is characterized by the libidinous experience of anal function. In this stage, the boy begins to identify with his father, brothers, and male peers and, after learning to stand and walk, can further fixate the image of his penis and control his urinary function; and the girl becomes aware of the differences between the sexes but is still unaware of her vagina. The female develops penis envy during the anal stage, which may be manifested through feelings of shame, inferiority, jealousy, and

perhaps rage. The anal stage is followed by the *phallic stage*, which usually is seen in boys between the ages of 3 and 4½ years and in girls a short time later. During this stage, sexual interest, curiosity, and pleasurable experiences center about the penis in boys, and in girls, to a lesser extent, the clitoris. Boys may develop castration anxiety during the phallic stage.

   The *latency period* in sexual development extends from about 6 years to 9 or 10 years of age. Children in this period form close relationships with those of the same sex. Masturbation is not uncommon, and is considered by some authorities to be useful in reinforcing the child's awareness of sexuality, to discharge sexual and aggressive impulses, and to contribute to continued sexual development.

   Adolescence is a time of rapid change in sexual development; puberty brings on the appearance of secondary sex characters. During puberty the *genital stage*, the final stage in psychosexual development, occurs, during which the person can achieve sexual gratification from genital-to-genital contact and is capable of a mature relationship with a person of the opposite sex. In midadolescence both sexes become more interested in members of the opposite sex and seek heterosexual experiences.

   s. disorders 1. any disorders involving sexual functioning, desire, or performance. 2. more specifically, any such disorders that are caused at least in part by psychological factors. Those characterized by decrease or other disturbance of sexual desire are called SEXUAL DYSFUNCTIONS, and those characterized by unusual or bizarre sexual fantasies or acts are called PARAPHILIAS. Called also psychosexual disorders.

   s. dysfunction 1. any of a group of SEXUAL DISORDERS characterized by disturbance of sexual desire or of psychophysiological changes that usually characterize sexual response. Included are SEXUAL DESIRE DISORDERS, SEXUAL AROUSAL DISORDERS, ORGASMIC DISORDERS, and SEXUAL PAIN DISORDERS. 2. a NURSING DIAGNOSIS accepted by the North American Nursing Diagnosis Association, defined as the experiencing by an individual of a change in sexual function that he or she feels is unsatisfying, unrewarding, or otherwise inadequate. The perception of the patient/client is a critical factor in determining whether the diagnosis is within the domain of nursing and amenable to nursing intervention in the form of teaching and counseling. Defining characteristics include verbalization of the problem, whether

S

actual or perceived, limitation imposed by disease or therapy, and reported inability to achieve desired satisfaction. See also ineffective sexuality PATTERNS.

The concept of human SEXUALITY is broad and complex. All persons are sexual beings from birth to death. Acute and chronic disorders, disabling neurologic injury and disease, and aging may necessitate adaptations in the ways in which sexuality is expressed, but the individual with a sexual dysfunction, no matter how severe, does not cease to be a sexual being.

Because of the complexity of human sexuality, specific etiologies of sexual dysfunction can be classified as pathophysiological, psychological, environmental, or maturational. Altered body function related to endocrine disease, surgery, trauma, radiation, or cancer can be a primary or secondary cause of dysfunction. Lack of information, misinformation, developmental disability, absence of an effective role model, and physical and sexual abuse can alter sexual function, as can lack of privacy, fear or guilt, an incompatible or abusive partner, and excessive stress.

s. health a concept defined in 1975 by the World Health Organization as "the integration of the somatic, emotional, intellectual, and social aspects of sexual being, in ways that are positively enriching and enhance personality, communication, and love."

s. pain disorders SEXUAL DYSFUNCTIONS characterized by pain associated with intercourse; it includes DYSPAREUNIA and VAGINISMUS not due to a general medical condition.

sexuality (sek″shoo-al′ĭ-te) 1. the characteristic quality of the male and female reproductive elements. 2. the constitution of an individual in relation to sexual attitudes or activity. This is a broad concept that includes aspects of the physical, psychological, social, emotional, and spiritual makeup of an individual. It is not limited to the physical or biological reproductive elements and behavior, but encompasses the manner in which individuals use their own roles, relationships, values, customs, and gender.

infantile s. in freudian theory, the erotic life of infants and children, encompassing the oral, anal, and phallic phases of psychosexual development.

sexually transmitted disease (STD) one that can be transmitted by means of sexual intercourse or by intimate contact with the genitals, mouth, or rectum. Called also venereal disease. Within this category are what are termed the five "classic venereal diseases" of GONORRHEA, SYPHILIS, CHANCROID,

EXAMPLES OF SEXUALLY TRANSMITTED DISEASES WITH CAUSATIVE ORGANISMS

Acquired immunodeficiency syndrome (AIDS)	HIV (virus)
Bacterial vaginosis	*Bacteroides* species, *Gardnerella vaginitis* *Mycoplasma homini.*
Chancroid	*Haemophilus ducreyi*
Gonorrhea	*Neisseria gonorrhoeae*
Syphilis	*Treponema pallidum*
Trichomoniasis	*Trichomonas vaginalis*

LYMPHOGRANULOMA VENEREUM, and GRANULOM; INGUINALE, as well as CHLAMYDIA infections genital HERPES, nonspecific URETHRITIS TRICHOMONIASIS, PEDICULOSIS PUBIS, SCABIES venereal WARTS, HEPATITIS B, MOLLUSCUM CONTAGIOSUM, and VAGINITIS caused by eithe *Corynebacterium vaginale* or *Haemophilu. vaginalis.* While sexual transmission is the only important means of spreading some o these diseases, others such as hepatitis car also be acquired by nonsexual means.

Sézary syndrome (sa′zah-re) a form o cutaneous T-cell lymphoma manifested by generalized exfoliative erythroderma, in tense pruritus, peripheral lymphadenopathy, and abnormal hyperchromatic mononuclear cells in the skin, lymph nodes, an peripheral blood (*Sézary cells*).

SGOT serum glutamic-oxaloacetic trans aminase; see ASPARTATE TRANSAMINASE.

SGPT serum glutamic-pyruvic transaminase; see ALANINE TRANSAMINASE.

shadow test (shad′o) retinoscopy.

shadow-casting (shad″o-kast′ing) application of a coating of gold, chromium, o other metal for the purpose of increasing the visibility of ultramicroscopic specimen: under the microscope.

shaft (shaft) a long slender part, such a: the DIAPHYSIS of a long bone.

shank (shangk) 1. leg (def. 1). 2. crus (def. 2).

shaping (shāp′ing) a technique in BEHAVIOR THERAPY in which new behavior i: produced by providing reinforcement for progressively closer approximations of the final desired behavior. Called also successive approximation.

shared governance an organizationa model used on nursing divisions, consisting of a decentralized system of management in which all of the nurses make decisions Managers advise, consult, coach, mentor and may or may not have veto power. This mandates collaboration among the nurse: on the unit and a high degree of autonomy.

shared psychotic disorder a delusiona system that develops in one or more persons as a result of a close relationship with someone who already has a psychotic disorder with prominent delusions. It most commonly involves only two people and then is usually called *folie à deux.*

shear (shēr) an applied force that tends to cause an opposite but parallel sliding motion of the planes of an object. Such motions cause tissues and blood vessels to move in such a way that blood flow may be interrupted, placing the patient at risk for pressure ulcers. An example of a shearing force is seen when a patient slumps in a chair; the skin around the buttocks is stretched by the movement and interferes with circulation.

sheath (shēth) a tubular case or envelope.

arachnoid s. the delicate membrane between the pial sheath and the dural sheath of the optic nerve.

carotid s. a portion of the cervical fascia enclosing the carotid artery, internal jugular vein, vagus nerve, and sympathetic nerves supplying the head.

WINDOW ON SHARED GOVERNANCE

As health care begins the 21st century, with newer models of work relationships, performance, and outcomes, innovative approaches to transforming the workplace must be designed and implemented. As with all major change, a vehicle for transformation must be constructed in order to give form and substance to the change process. Shared governance is such a vehicle. In health care, the concept was initiated in nursing services but has grown to influence the relationship between and among all the disciplines and roles in health care. It is a set of principles about collaboration, ownership, worker investment, and partnership between people necessary to achieve high quality patient care outcomes. Through redesigning the workplace structure, relationships, and processes, shared governance provides a vehicle for the transformation of health care in a way that is patient centered and service focused. Shared governance is the basis for emerging new models for health care for the 21st century. It provides a service based structure for organizing health professionals in a manner that promotes emphasis on team based relationships, quality outcomes, and patient participation. Shared governance creates a format for a collective service consciousness, resulting in improved health care services.

TIM PORTER-O'GRADY, EDD, PHD, FAAN

---

connective tissue s. of Key and Retzius endoneurium.

crural s. femoral sheath.

dural s. the external investment of the optic nerve.

femoral s. the fascial sheath of the femoral vessels.

Henle's s. endoneurium.

lamellar s. the perineurium.

medullary s. myelin sheath.

myelin s., nerve s. the sheath surrounding the axon of myelinated nerve cells, consisting of concentric layers of myelin formed in the peripheral nervous system by the plasma membrane of Schwann cells, and in the central nervous system by the plasma membrane of oligodendrocytes. It is interrupted at intervals along the length of the axon by gaps known as NODES OF RANVIER. Myelin is an electrical insulator that serves to speed the conduction of nerve impulses (see saltatory CONDUCTION).

pial s. the innermost of the three sheaths of the optic nerve.

root s. the epidermic layer of a hair follicle.

s. of Schwann neurilemma.

synovial s. synovial membrane lining the cavity of a bone through which a tendon moves.

tendon s. a lubricated fibrous or synovial layer of tissue in which the tendon is housed and through which it moves.

Sheehan's syndrome postpartum pituitary necrosis.

sheep cell agglutination test (SCAT) a laboratory test for infectious mononucleosis. When the antibody level of a person with this disease reaches a certain level, a sample of his blood will cause agglutination of sheep erythrocytes. If there is agglutination of these cells in concentrations up to 1:28, the findings are considered positive for infectious mononucleosis.

shellfish poisoning an acute intoxication caused by ingestion of bivalve mollusks contaminated with the neurotoxin (SAXITOXIN) secreted by certain dinoflagellates, protozoa that are an important component of marine plankton. One form, *paralytic shellfish poisoning,* is caused by species of *Gonyaulax,* and is characterized by paresthesias of the mouth, lips, face, and limbs, nausea, vomiting, and diarrhea; in rare severe cases muscle weakness or paralysis and respiratory embarrassment and death may occur. A self-limited milder form, *neurotoxic shellfish poisoning,* not associated with paralysis, is caused by species of *Gymnodinium.*

S

shield (shēld) 1. any protecting structure. 2. in radiology, a protective device, often made of lead, through which particualr types of rays cannot pass; used to avoid the effects of ionizing radiation.

shift (shift) a change or deviation.

antigenic s. a sudden, major change in the antigenicity of a virus, seen especially in influenza VIRUSES, resulting from the recombination of the GENOMES of two different strains; it is associated with pandemics because hosts do not have immunity to the new strain. See also antigenic DRIFT.

chloride s. the exchange of chloride and carbonate between the plasma and the erythrocytes that takes place when the blood gives up oxygen and receives carbon dioxide. It serves to maintain ionic equilibrium between the cell and surrounding fluid.

mediastinal s. a shifting to one side of the tissues and organs of the mediastinum; see also MEDIASTINAL SHIFT.

s. to the left 1. a change in the blood picture, with a preponderance of young neutrophils. 2. an increased oxygen affinity of hemoglobin.

s. to the right 1. a preponderance of older neutrophils in the blood picture. 2. a decreased oxygen affinity of hemoglobin.

weight s. 1. the frequent movement of a paralyzed or partially paralyzed patient to redistribute the patient's weight and prevent impairment of circulation, which leads to pressure sores. One variation is the wheelchair pressure RELEASE. 2. relocation of a patient's center of mass in order to allow movement; see also GAIT.

Shigella (shĭ-gel′ah) a genus of gram-negative, facultatively anaerobic, nonmotile, rod-shaped bacteria containing four species that are differentiated by biochemical reactions: *S. dysente′riae* (subgroup A), *S. flex′neri* (subgroup B), *S. boy′dii* (subgroup C), and *S. son′nei* (subgroup D). Their normal habitat is the intestinal tract of humans and higher monkeys; all species cause DYSENTERY.

shigella (shĭ-gel′ah) any individual organism of the genus *Shigella.*

shigellosis (shĭ-gel-o′sis) any infection with *Shigella,* such as BACILLARY DYSENTERY.

shin (shin) the prominent anterior edge of the TIBIA and lower leg.

saber s. marked anterior convexity of the TIBIA, seen in congenital SYPHILIS.

shingles (shing′gelz) herpes zoster.

shiver (shiv′er) 1. a slight tremor. 2. to tremble slightly, as from cold.

shivering (shiv′er-ing) involuntary shaking of the body, as with cold. It is caused by contraction or twitching of the muscles, and is a physiologic method of heat production in humans and other mammals. As a form of aerobic skeletal muscle activity, vigorous shivering uses about as much energy as riding a bicycle or shoveling snow. Weak or debilitated patients tolerate this activity poorly. Patients commonly feel helpless when experiencing contractions of muscles normally under voluntary control. Increased metabolic rate and oxygen demand caused by shivering are particularly stressful for patients with heart or lung disease. Cold-induced shivering is stimulated when body temperatures drop below the thermostatic range or "set point" governed by the HYPOTHALAMUS. Shivering in FEVER occurs not because body temperatures fall but because the set point range is driven by the PYROGEN. The more vigorous the shivering, the higher the fever is driven up. Heat loss from skin is a dominant stimulus.

shock (shok) 1. a sudden disturbance of mental equilibrium. 2. a condition of acute peripheral circulatory failure due to derangement of circulatory control or loss of circulating fluid. It is marked by hypotension and coldness of the skin, and often by tachycardia and anxiety. Untreated shock can be fatal. Called also circulatory collapse.

Mechanisms of Circulatory Shock. The essentials of shock are easier to understand if the circulatory system is thought of as a four-part mechanical device made up of a pump (the heart), a complex system of flexible tubes (the blood vessels), a circulating fluid (the blood), and a fine regulating system or "computer" (the nervous system) designed to control fluid flow and pressure. The diameter of the blood vessels is controlled by impulses from the nervous system which cause the muscular walls to contract. The nervous system also affects the rapidity and strength of the heartbeat, and thereby the blood pressure as well.

Shock, which is associated with a dangerously low blood pressure, can be produced by factors that attack the strength of the heart as a pump, decrease the volume of the blood in the system, or permit the blood vessels to increase in diameter.

Types of Circulatory Shock. There are five main types: *Hypovolemic (low-volume) shock* occurs whenever there is insufficient blood to fill the circulatory system. *Neurogenic shock* is due to disorders of the nervous system. *Anaphylactic (allergic) shock* and *septic shock* are both due to reactions that impair the muscular functioning of the blood vessels. And *cardiogenic shock* is caused by impaired function of the heart.

Hypovolemic (Low-Volume) Shock. This is a common type that happens when blood or

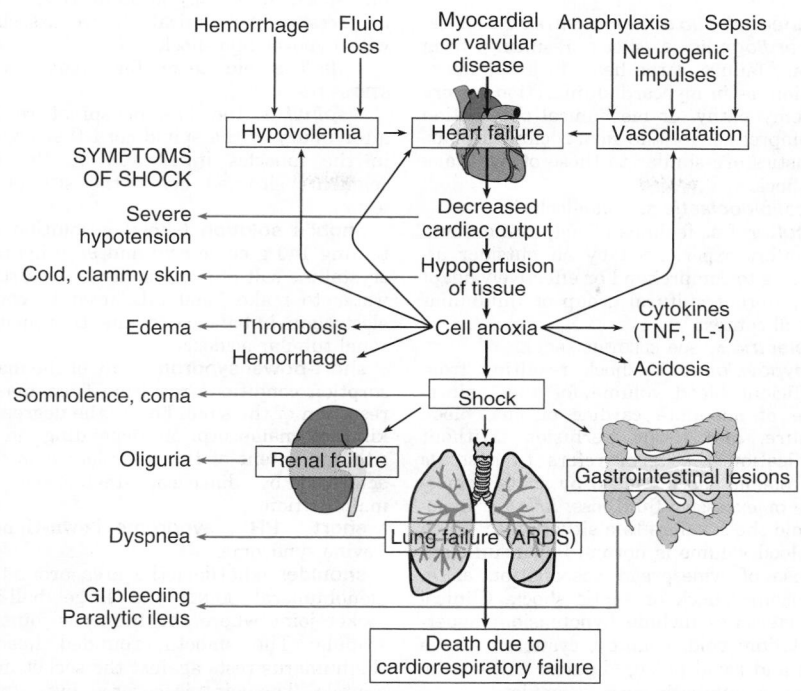

Pathogenesis of shock. (ARDS = adult respiratory distress syndrome, GI = gastrointestinal, IL = interleukin, TNF = tumor necrosis factor.) From Damjanov, 2000.

plasma is lost in such quantities that the remaining blood cannot fill the circulatory system despite constriction of the blood vessels. The blood loss may be external, as when a vessel is severed by an injury, or the blood may be "lost" into spaces inside the body where it is no longer accessible to the circulatory system, as in severe gastrointestinal bleeding from ulcers, fractures of large bones with hemorrhage into surrounding tissues, or major burns that attract large quantities of blood fluids to the burn site outside blood vessels and capillaries. The treatment of hypovolemic shock requires replacement of the lost volume.

Neurogenic Shock. This type, often accompanied by fainting, may be brought on by severe pain, fright, unpleasant sights, or other strong stimuli that overwhelm the usual regulatory capacity of the nervous system. The diameter of the blood vessels increases, the heart slows, and the blood pressure falls to the point where the supply of oxygen carried by the blood to the brain is insufficient, which can bring on fainting. Placing the head lower than the body is usually sufficient to relieve this form of shock.

Anaphylactic (Allergic) Shock. This type (see also ANAPHYLAXIS) is a rare phenomenon that occurs when a person receives an injection of a foreign protein but is highly sensitive to it. The blood vessels and other tissues are affected directly by the allergic reaction. Within a few minutes, the blood pressure falls and severe dyspnea develops. The sudden deaths that in rare cases follow bee stings or injection of certain medicines are due to anaphylactic reactions.

Septic Shock. This type, resulting from bacterial infection, is being recognized with increasing frequency. Certain organisms contain a toxin that seems to act on the blood vessels when it is released into the bloodstream. The blood eventually pools within parts of the circulatory system that expand easily, causing the blood pressure to drop sharply. Gram-negative shock is a form of septic shock due to infection with gram-negative bacteria.

Cardiogenic Shock. This type may be caused by conditions that interfere with the function of the heart as a pump, such as severe myocardial infarction, severe heart failure, and certain disorders of rate and rhythm.

anaphylactic s. see ANAPHYLACTIC SHOCK.

cardiogenic s. shock resulting from primary failure of the heart in its pumping function, as in myocardial infarction, severe cardiomyopathy, or mechanical obstruction or compression of the heart; clinical characteristics are similar to those of hypovolemic shock.

colloidoclastic s. colloidoclasia.

cultural s. feelings of helplessness and discomfort experienced by an outsider attempting to comprehend or effectively adapt to a different cultural group or unfamiliar cultural context.

electric s. see ELECTRIC SHOCK.

hypovolemic s. shock resulting from insufficient blood volume for the maintenance of adequate cardiac output, blood pressure, and tissue perfusion. Without modification the term refers to *absolute* hypovolemic shock caused by acute hemorrhage or excessive fluid loss. *Relative* hypovolemic shock refers to a situation in which the blood volume is normal but insufficient because of widespread vasodilation as in neurogenic shock or septic shock. Clinical characteristics include hypotension; hyperventilation; cold, clammy, cyanotic skin; a weak and rapid pulse; oliguria; and mental confusion, combativeness, or anxiety.

insulin s. a hypoglycemic reaction to overdosage of insulin, a skipped meal, or strenuous exercise in an insulin-dependent diabetic, with tremor, dizziness, cool moist skin, hunger, and tachycardia; if untreated it may progress to coma and convulsions.

respirator s. circulatory shock due to interference with the flow of blood through the great vessels and chambers of the heart, causing pooling of blood in the veins and the abdominal organs and a resultant vascular collapse. The condition sometimes occurs as a result of increased intrathoracic pressure in patients who are being maintained on a mechanical VENTILATOR.

septic s. shock associated with overwhelming infection, usually by gram-negative bacteria, although it may be produced by other bacteria, viruses, fungi, and protozoa. It is thought to result from the action of endotoxins or other products of the infectious agent on the vascular system causing large volumes of blood to be sequestered in the capillaries and veins; activation of the complement and kinin systems and the release of histamine, cytokines, prostaglandins, and other mediators may be involved. Clinical characteristics include initial chills and fever, warm flushed skin, increased cardiac output, and a lesser degree of hypotension than with hypovolemic shock; if therapy is ineffective, it may progress to the clinical picture associated with hypovolemic shock.

shell s. old term for POSTTRAUMATIC STRESS DISORDER.

spinal s. the loss of spinal reflexes after injury of the spinal cord that appears in the muscles innervated by the cord segments situated below the site of the lesion.

Shohl's solution (shōlz) a solution containing 140 g citric acid and 98 g hydrated crystalline salt of sodium citrate in distilled water to make 1000 mL; used to correct electrolyte imbalance in the treatment of renal tubular acidosis.

short-bowel syndrome any of the malabsorption conditions resulting from massive resection of the small bowel, the degree and kind of malabsorption depending on the site and extent of the resection; it is characterized by diarrhea, steatorrhea, and malnutrition.

short PR syndrome Lown-Ganong-Levine syndrome.

shoulder (shōl′der) the area around the glenohumeral JOINT, the large ball-and-socket joint where the humerus joins the scapula. The smooth, rounded head of the humerus rests against the socket in the scapula. The joint is covered by a tough, flexible protective capsule and is heavily reinforced by ligaments that stretch across the joint. The ends of the bones where they meet at the joint are covered with a layer of cartilage that reduces friction and absorbs shock. A thin membrane, the synovial membrane, lines the socket and lubricates the joint with synovia. Further cushioning and lubrication are provided by fluid-filled sacs called bursae. Disorders of the shoulder include BURSITIS and DISLOCATION.

frozen s. popular but misleading name for adhesive CAPSULITIS.

shoulder-hand syndrome a disorder of the upper limb characterized by pain and stiffness in the shoulder, with puffy swelling and pain in the ipsilateral hand; it sometimes occurs after myocardial infarction but can also be produced by other causes.

show (sho) appearance of blood forerunning labor or menstruation.

bloody s. vaginal discharge of blood-tinged mucus; it usually means that the cervix has dilated somewhat and the onset of labor is imminent.

shunt (shunt) 1. to turn to one side; to divert; to bypass. 2. a passage or anastomosis between two natural channels, especially between blood vessels. Such structures may be formed physiologically (e.g., to bypass a

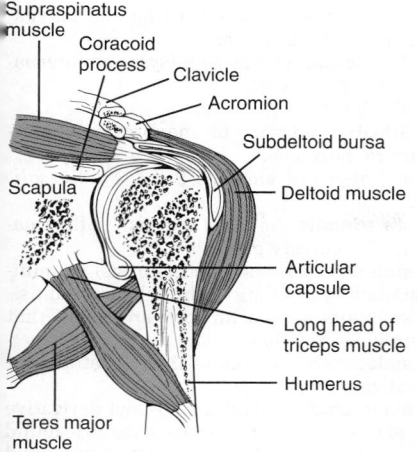

Supraspinatus muscle
Coracoid process
Clavicle
Acromion
Subdeltoid bursa
Scapula
Deltoid muscle
Articular capsule
Long head of triceps muscle
Humerus
Teres major muscle

Coronal section through the shoulder joint.

thrombosis), or they may be structural anomalies. 3. a surgical anastomosis.

arteriovenous s. a U-shaped plastic tube inserted between an artery and a vein (usually between the radial artery and cephalic vein), bypassing the capillary network, a formerly common means of arteriovenous ACCESS.

cardiovascular s. an abnormality of the blood flow between the sides of the heart or between the systemic and pulmonary circulation; see left-to-right SHUNT and right-to-left SHUNT.

jejunoileal s. an INTESTINAL BYPASS performed to control obesity.

left-to-right s. diversion of blood from the left side of the heart to the right side, or from the systemic to the pulmonary circulation through an anomalous opening such as a septal defect or patent ductus arteriosus.

LeVeen s. peritoneovenous shunt.

mesocaval s. a portosystemic shunt between the superior mesenteric vein and the inferior vena cava to reduce portal hypertension.

peritoneovenous s. a device whose purpose is to remove excess ascitic fluid from the peritoneal cavity and return it to the venous system; called also LeVeen shunt.

The shunt consists of a peritoneal tube, a one-way valve, and a tube leading to a large vein, usually the superior vena cava or the jugular vein. The perforated peritoneal tube is placed in the peritoneal cavity and attached to the one-way valve which opens at a pressure of 3 cm H_2O. The valve controls the direction of the flow of ascitic fluid and prevents a backflow of blood from the vein. A tube leading from the valve empties into the venous system.

The shunt is triggered into action by the patient's breathing. Upon inspiration, the diaphragm descends toward the abdominal cavity and causes a rise in fluid pressure in the thoracic superior vena cava. The difference in pressure, usually about 5 cm H_2O, opens the shunt valve, allowing the flow of ascitic fluid into the large vein. The action of the shunt can be enhanced by the

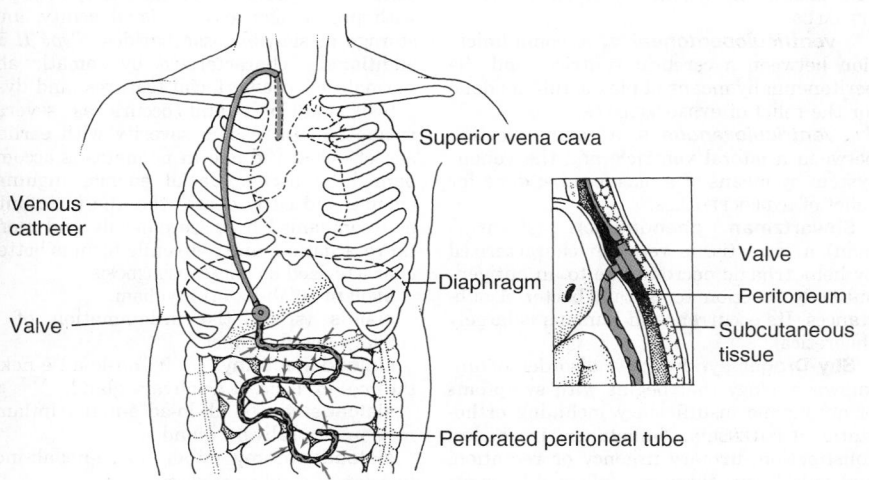

Superior vena cava
Venous catheter
Diaphragm
Valve
Valve
Peritoneum
Subcutaneous tissue
Perforated peritoneal tube

Peritoneovenous (LeVeen) shunt for chronic ascites moves fluid from the peritoneal (abdominal) cavity into the superior vena cava. From Ignatavicius and Workman, 2000.

patient's inspiring against pressure, as when using a blow bottle.

A disadvantage of the shunt is dilution of the blood and a resultant drop in hematocrit, which necessitates transfusion of packed cells and perhaps a slowing of the rate of flow of ascitic fluid into the venous system. Other inherent risks are infection, leakage of ascitic fluid from the operative site, elevated bilirubin, gastrointestinal bleeding, and disseminated intravascular coagulation.

portacaval s. a portosystemic shunt between the portal vein and the vena cava.

portosystemic s. a surgically created shunt that connects the portal and systemic circulations, such as a mesocaval, portacaval, or splenorenal shunt.

postcaval s. portacaval shunt.

pulmonary s. an anomaly in which blood moves from the venous circulation to the arterial circulation without participating in gas exchange, resulting in hypoxemia.

reversed s. right-to-left shunt.

right-to-left s. diversion of blood from the right side of the heart to the left side or from the pulmonary to the systemic circulation through an anomalous opening such as septal defect or patent ductus arteriosus.

splenorenal s. an anastomosis of the splenic vein and the left renal vein, created to lower portal hypertension following splenectomy.

ventriculoatrial s. the surgical creation of a communication between a cerebral ventricle and a cardiac atrium by means of a plastic tube; done for relief of HYDROCEPHALUS.

ventriculoperitoneal s. a communication between a cerebral ventricle and the peritoneum by means of plastic tubing; done for the relief of HYDROCEPHALUS.

ventriculovenous s. a communication between a lateral ventricle and the venous system by means of a plastic tube; done for relief of HYDROCEPHALUS.

Shwartzman phenomenon (shwarts'-man) a local tissue reaction characterized by hemorrhagic necrosis due to an antigen-antibody reaction to certain bacterial substances. Its occurrence in humans is largely theoretical.

Shy-Drager syndrome a disorder of unknown etiology that begins with symptoms of autonomic insufficiency including orthostatic HYPOTENSION, impotence in males, constipation, urinary urgency or retention, and anhidrosis; these are followed by signs of nervous system disturbance such as parkinsonian-like symptoms, cerebellar incoordination, muscle wasting and fasciculations, and leg tremors.

SI international system (système internationale); see SI UNITS.

Si silicon.

SIADH syndrome of inappropriate antidiuretic hormone.

sial(o)- word element [Gr.], *saliva; salivary glands.*

sialadenitis (si″al-ad″ĕ-ni′tis) inflammation of a salivary gland.

sialadenosis (si″al-ad″ĕ-no′sis) noninflammatory swelling of the salivary glands.

sialagogue (si-al′ah-gog) an agent that stimulates the flow of saliva.

sialectasia (si″al-ek-ta′zhah) dilatation of a salivary duct.

sialic acid (si-al′ik) any *N*-acyl derivative of NEURAMINIC ACID; various ones are found in polysaccharides, glycoproteins, and glycolipids.

sialidase (si-al′ĭ-dās) 1. an enzyme of the hydrolase class that catalyzes the cleavage of glucosidic linkages between a SIALIC ACID residue and a HEXOSE or HEXOSAMINE residue at the nonreducing terminal of oligosaccharides in glycoproteins, glycolipids, and proteoglycans. Deficiency of it is an autosomal recessive trait and is seen in SIALIDOSIS and GALACTOSIALIDOSIS. 2. the enzyme with this activity specifically cleaving sialic acid–containing gangliosides; it is deficient in MUCOLIPIDOSIS IV. Called also *neuraminidase.*

sialidosis (si-al″ĭ-do′sis) an autosomal recessive disorder due to a deficiency of SIALIDASE; there are two different types: *Type I* is of adolescent or adult onset and is characterized by myoclonus, ocular cherry red spot with progressive loss of visual acuity, and storage of sialyloligosaccharides. *Type II* is additionally characterized by somatic abnormalities, coarse facial features, and dysostosis multiplex and occurs as several variants of increasing severity with earlier age of onset; the one in neonates is accompanied by ascites, facial edema, inguinal edema, and early death; the one in infants is accompanied by visceromegaly and mental retardation; and a juvenile form is better characterized as GALACTOSIALIDOSIS.

sialism (si′ah-liz′m) ptyalism.

sialitis (si″ah-li′tis) inflammation of a salivary gland or duct.

sialoadenectomy (si″ah-lo-ad″ĕ-nek′tah-me) excision of a salivary gland.

sialoadenitis (si″ah-lo-ad″ĕ-ni′tis) inflammation of a salivary gland.

sialoadenotomy (si″ah-lo-ad′ĕ-not′ah-me) incision of a salivary gland.

sialoaerophagy (si″ah-lo-ār-of′ah-je) the swallowing of saliva and air.

sialoangiectasis (si″ah-lo-an″je-ek′tah-is) dilatation of a salivary duct.

sialoangiitis (si″ah-lo-an″je-i′tis) inflammation of a salivary DUCT; called also sialodochitis and sialoductitis.

sialoangiography (si″ah-lo-an″je-og′rah-e) radiography of the ducts of the salivary glands after injection of radiopaque material.

sialocele (si′ah-lo-sēl) a salivary cyst.

sialodochitis (si″ah-lo-do-ki′tis) sialoangiitis.

sialodochoplasty (si″ah-lo-do′ko-plas″te) plastic repair of a salivary duct.

sialoductitis (si″ah-lo-duk-ti′tis) sialoangiitis.

sialogenous (si″ah-loj′ĕ-nus) producing saliva.

sialogogue (si-al′o-gog) sialagogue.

sialogram (si-al′o-gram) a film obtained by sialography.

sialography (si″ah-log′rah-fe) radiographic demonstration of the salivary ducts by means of the injection of substances opaque to x-rays.

sialolith (si-al′o-lith) a calculus in a salivary gland or duct.

sialolithiasis (si″ah-lo-lĭ-thi′ah-sis) a condition characterized by the presence of SIALOLITHS.

sialolithotomy (si″ah-lo-lĭ-thot′ah-me) excision of a salivary calculus.

sialomucin (si″ah-lo-mu′sin) an acid mucopolysaccharide containing sialic acid, a component of airway secretions of the lungs.

sialorrhea (si″ah-lo-re′ah) ptyalism.

sialoschesis (si″ah-los′kĕ-sis) suppression of secretion of saliva.

sialostenosis (si″ah-lo-stĕ-no′sis) stenosis of a salivary duct.

sialosyrinx (si″ah-lo-sir′inks) 1. salivary fistula. 2. a syringe for washing out the salivary ducts, or a drainage tube for the salivary ducts.

Siamese twins (si″ah-mēz′) monozygotic TWINS whose bodies are joined. The connection may be slight or extensive; it may involve skin and muscles or cartilage of a limited region, such as the head, chest, hip, or buttock, or the twins may share an organ, such as an intestine or parts of the spine. If joined superficially, the twins may be easily separated by surgery soon after birth. If more deeply united, they may have to go through life with their handicap, if they survive. New techniques in surgery are making it possible to separate some Siamese twins whose physical links are highly complex. Called also conjoined twins.

sib (sib) 1. a blood relative; one of a group of persons all descended from a common ancestor. 2. sibling.

sibilant (sib′ĭ-lant) shrill, whistling, or hissing.

sibling (sib′ling) any of two or more offspring of the same parents; a brother or sister.

half s. an individual who shares just one parent with the person of reference.

sibship (sib′ship) a group of individuals born of the same parents.

sibutramine (si-bu′trah-mēn″) an appetite suppressant used as the hydrochloride salt in treatment of obesity; administered orally.

sicca syndrome (sik′ah) keratoconjunctivitis and xerostomia (dry mouth) without connective tissue disease.

siccative (sik′ah-tiv) 1. drying; removing moisture. 2. an agent that produces drying.

siccus (sik′us) [L.] dry.

sick (sik) not in good health; ill; afflicted with disease.

s. sinus syndrome a complex cardiac ARRHYTHMIA usually associated with SYNCOPE and manifested as severe sinus BRADYCARDIA alone, sinus bradycardia alternating with TACHYCARDIA (see BRADYCARDIA-TACHYCARDIA SYNDROME), or sinus bradycardia with atrioventricular BLOCK. It is a combination of sinoatrial NODE dysfunction and failure of an escape PACEMAKER.

sickle cell a crescentic or sickle-shaped ERYTHROCYTE, the abnormal shape caused by the presence of varying proportions of HEMOGLOBIN S. See illustration at CELL.

s. c. anemia an autosomal dominant, chronic form of HEMOLYTIC ANEMIA in which large numbers of sickle cells circulate in the blood; it is most common among persons of African and Mediterranean descent. Persons genetically homozygous have 85 to 95 per cent sickle cells and have the full-blown condition; see sickle cell disease. Those who are heterozygous are usually asymptomatic.

s. c. crisis a broad term describing several different acute conditions occurring as part of SICKLE CELL DISEASE, such as aplastic CRISIS, hemolytic CRISIS, and vaso-occlusive CRISIS.

s. c. disease any of the diseases associated with the presence of HEMOGLOBIN S, including SICKLE CELL ANEMIA, sickle cell–THALASSEMIA, and the conditions called sickle cell–hemoglobin C and D disease. They are found most often in those of black African descent, but they also occur in persons of Mediterranean (Southern European and North African), Middle Eastern, or Asian Indian ancestry. About 8 to 10 per cent of all African Americans carry the sickle cell gene. About 90 per cent of persons with the gene are HETEROZYGOUS for it, simply carriers

S

of the sickle cell trait and usually without symptoms. The remainder, or about 1 in 500 of an ethnic group where the gene occurs, are HOMOZYGOUS for hemoglobin S, actually having sickle cell disease and suffering from the effects of HEMOLYSIS. Sickle cell disease is a serious, hereditary, chronic disease in which the red blood cells have reduced life span and are rigid, with a crescent or sickle shape. The shape is the result of an abnormality in the hemoglobin, which alters the deformability of the cells under conditions of low oxygen tension. Because of their distorted shape the cells have difficulty passing through the small arterioles and capillaries and have a tendency to clump together and occlude the blood vessel. Some scientists believe that sickle cell disease developed as a defense against MALARIA. Malarial parasites do not grow in erythrocytes containing hemoglobin S. Therefore, carriers (heterozygotes) have an advantage in areas where malaria is prevalent (called the *heterozygote advantage*). (See accompanying figure.)

Symptoms. There are many symptoms of sickle cell disease, all of them related to the defective hemoglobin and its effect on red blood cells. Some persons with the condition suffer from only a few symptoms, while others are severely affected and have a short life span. Better understanding and management of the disease in recent decades has improved the prognoses for patients with it.

The major symptoms are anemia, periodic joint and limb pain and sometimes edema of the joints, chronic ulceration about the ankles, episodes of severe abdominal pain with vomiting, and abdominal distention. The spleen becomes infarcted so that it is essentially absent and predisposes the patient to infection with encapsulated organisms. Bone changes often can be seen on x-ray and are due to bone infarcts. Headache, paralysis, and convulsions may result from cerebral thrombosis, which can cause stroke, blindness, and other neurological disturbances. There is a tendency toward progressive renal disease and renal failure.

Sickle cell crisis is a broad term that describes several different conditions, particularly *aplastic crisis,* which is temporary bone marrow aplasia; *hemolytic crisis,* which is acute red cell destruction, leading to jaundice; and *vaso-occlusive crisis,* which is severe pain due to infarctions located in the bones, joints, lungs, liver, spleen, kidney, eye, or central nervous system. Factors that precipitate a crisis include infection, dehydration, trauma, strenuous physical

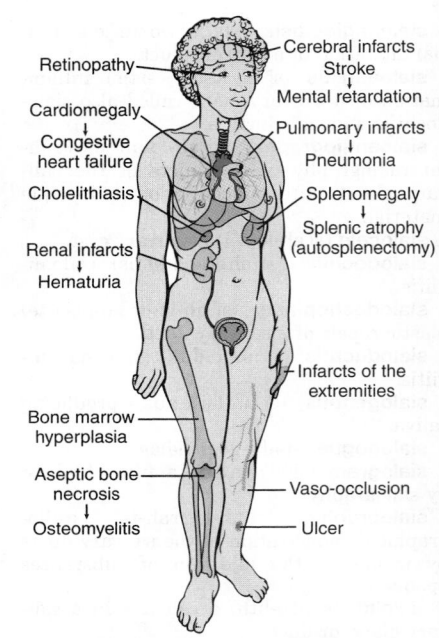

Clinicopathologic findings in sickle cell anemia. The findings are a consequence of infarctions, anemia hemolysis, and recurrent infection. From Damjanov, 2000

exertion, emotional stress, and extremes of heat and cold.

Treatment and Care. There is no cure for sickle cell disease. Treatment is symptomatic; preventive measures are employed to reduce the incidence of crises and to avoid infections. It is also important that the patient receive all available immunizing agents. Nutritional deficiencies should be corrected when present (FOLATE supplementation is especially important), and then a well-balanced dietary intake should be maintained. HYDROXYUREA and prophylactic PENICILLIN are administered according to therapeutic guidelines. Social service programs are required to facilitate adjustment to the disease and its sequelae. Control of pain associated with this condition should be a priority.

Patient Care. Sickle cell disease is a chronic condition with acute episodes related to vaso-occlusion. Virtually every system of the body can be affected by the ischemia resulting from obstruction of the blood vessels by clumps of deformed erythrocytes. Among the more common acute complications are inflammation of fingers and toes, aplastic anemia, splenic sequestration, and stroke. Chronic disorders include leg ulcers, renal complications, aseptic necrosis, and retinopathy. Bacterial infection is one of the major causes of morbidity and mortality in

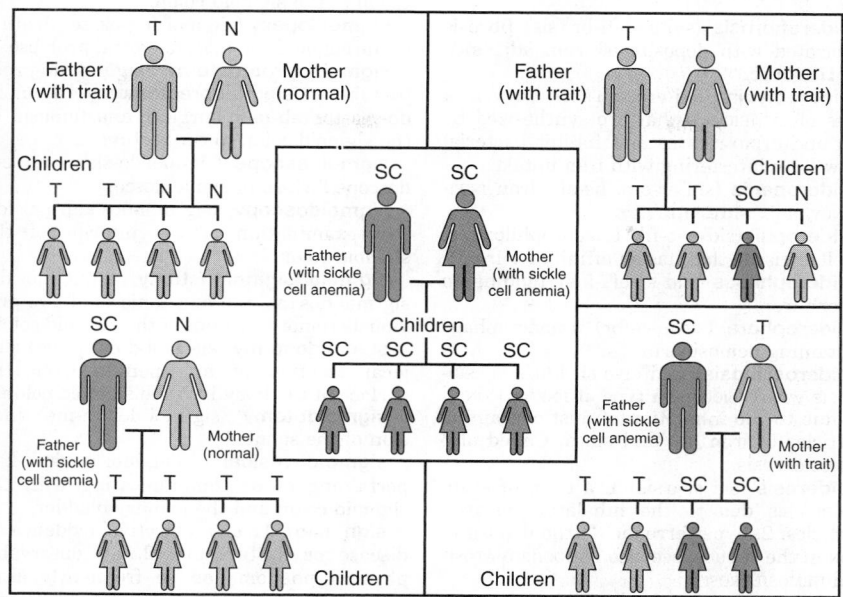

T- Trait
N- Normal
SC- Sickle cell

Statistical probabilities of inheriting sickle cell anemia.

patients with sickle cell disease.

Because of the potential for serious complications due to occlusion of blood vessels, patients with sickle cell disease should have regular physical examinations to detect early changes. Periodic eye examinations are necessary to monitor retinal changes due to vaso-occlusion of retinal vessels.

Measures to improve or maintain the general well-being of patients include preventing DEHYDRATION, maintaining adequate nutrition to optimize the patient's resistance to infection and resources for healing, and managing the anemia that is characteristic of sickle cell disease. Education of patients and their parents and family members is an essential component of care. Patient support groups can be an effective mechanism to diffuse fear. Guidelines for the management of acute and chronic PAIN are available from the American Pain Society. A comprehensive biopsychosocial clinical assessment should be performed at least yearly.

The National Heart, Lung, and Blood Institute of NIH has published a guide called *NIH Management and Therapy of Sickle Cell Disease.* A printed copy is available as NIH publication number 95-2117. The guidelines are available online at http://www.emory.edu/peds/sickle/nih1/htm.

s. c. disorders any blood disorders associated with the presence of hemoglobin S, including the SICKLE CELL DISEASES and SICKLE CELL TRAIT.

sicklemia (sik-le′me-ah) sickle cell anemia.

sickling (sik′ling) the development of sickle cells in the blood.

s. test a method of demonstrationg HEMOGLOBIN S and the sickling phenomenon in erythrocytes, performed by reducing the oxygen concentration to which the erythrocytes are exposed.

sickness (sik′nes) DISEASE. For specific conditions called sicknesses, see under the name of the condition.

s.i.d. [L.] sem′el in di′e (once a day); written also *semel in d.*

sider(o)- word element [Gr.], *iron.*

sideroblast (sid′er-o-blast″) an erythroblast containing ferritin granules in its cytoplasm. adj., **sideroblas′tic.**

siderocyte (sid′er-o-sīt″) a red blood cell containing nonhemoglobin iron.

sideroderma (sid″er-o-der′mah) bronzed coloration of the skin due to disordered iron metabolism.

S

siderofibrosis (sid″er-o-fi-bro′sis) fibrosis associated with deposits of iron. adj., **siderofibrot′ic.**

sideromycin (sid″er-o-mi′sin) any of a class of ANTIBIOTICS that are synthesized by certain ACTINOMYCETES and inhibit bacterial growth by interfering with iron uptake.

sideropenia (sid″er-o-pe′ne-ah) iron DEFICIENCY. adj., **siderope′nic.**

siderophil (sid′er-o-fil) 1. siderophilous. 2. a cell or tissue that has an affinity for iron.

siderophilous (sid″er-of′ĭ-lus) tending to absorb iron.

siderophore (sid′er-o-for) a macrophage containing hemosiderin.

siderosilicosis (sid″er-o-sil″ĭ-ko′sis) SIDEROSIS with SILICOSIS, a type of PNEUMOCONIOSIS due to the inhalation of dust containing particles of iron ore and silica. Called also silicosiderosis.

siderosis (sid″er-o′sis) 1. a form of PNEUMOCONIOSIS due to the inhalation of IRON particles. 2. hyperferremia. 3. the deposit of IRON in the tissues; see also HEMOCHROMATOSIS and HEMOSIDEROSIS.

   hepatic s. hepatic HEMOSIDEROSIS.

   urinary s. hemosiderinuria.

SIDS sudden infant death syndrome.

siemens (S) (se′menz) the SI unit of conductance; it is the conductance of one ampere per volt in a body with one ohm resistance.

sievert (se′vert) the SI unit of radiation absorbed dose equivalent, defined as that producing the same biologic effect in a specified tissue as 1 gray of high-energy x-rays; 1 sievert equals 100 rem.

sig. [L.] sig′na (mark).

sigh (si) 1. a long, audible exhalation. 2. an intermittent inflation of the lungs with a large volume from a mechanical VENTILATOR; this is essentially a deep breath that is incorporated into the ventilation cycle. The use of large tidal volumes has replaced the use of the sigh in many settings.

sight (sīt) vision. 1. a thing seen.

   far s. hyperopia.

   near s. myopia.

   night s. hemeralopia.

Sigma Theta Tau (sig′mah tha′tah taw′) the international honor society of nursing; its official magazine is called *The Journal of Nursing Scholarship.*

sigmatism (sig′mah-tizm) faulty enunciation or too frequent use of *s* sounds; see also LISPING.

sigmoid (sig′moid) 1. shaped like the letter C or S. 2. the sigmoid colon, the distal part of the colon from the level of the iliac crest to the rectum.

sigmoidectomy (sig″moi-dek′tah-me) excision of the sigmoid colon.

sigmoidopexy (sig-moi′do-pek″se) fixation of the sigmoid colon, as for rectal prolapse.

sigmoidoproctostomy (sig-moi″do-prok-tos′tah-me) **sigmoidorectostomy** (sig-moi″do-rek-tos′tah-me) surgical anastomosis of the sigmoid colon to the rectum.

sigmoidoscope (sig-moi′do-skōp) an endoscope for use in sigmoidoscopy.

sigmoidoscopy (sig″moi-dos′kah-pe) direct examination of the interior of the sigmoid colon.

sigmoidosigmoidostomy (sig-moi″do-sig″moi-dos′tah-me) anastomosis of two previously remote portions of the sigmoid colon.

sigmoidostomy (sig″moi-dos′tah-me) surgical creation of an opening from the surface of the body into the sigmoid colon.

sigmoidotomy (sig″moi-dot′ah-me) incision of the sigmoid.

sigmoidovesical (sig-moi″do-ves′ĭ-kal) pertaining to or communicating with the sigmoid colon and the urinary bladder.

sign (sīn) 1. any objective evidence of disease or dysfunction. 2. an observable physical phenomenon so frequently associated with a given condition as to be considered indicative of its presence. See also names of specific signs such as TINEL'S SIGN.

   vital s's the signs of life, namely pulse, respiration, and temperature.

signa (sig′nah) [L.] mark or write; abbreviated S. or sig. in prescriptions, followed by the signature.

signature (sig′nah-chur) the part of a drug prescription that gives directions to be followed by the patient in taking the medicine.

significant other a person who plays an important role in the life of an individual, such as a member of the immediate family, a lover, a close friend, or a role model.

signing (sīn′ing) communication between individuals, especially the DEAF, using a system of signs made with the hands and fingers. Called also dactylology.

Silastic (sĭ-las′tik) trademark for polymeric silicone substances that have the properties of rubber but are biologically inert; used in surgical prostheses.

sildenafil (sil-den′ah-fil″) an agent that relaxes the smooth muscle of the penis, facilitating blood flow to the corpus cavernosum; used as the citrate salt to treat erectile DYSFUNCTION.

silence absence of NOISE; a state of producing no detectable signs or symptoms.

   electrical s. in electroencephalography and electromyography, absence of measurable electrical activity in tissue.

silica (sil′ĭ-kah) silicon dioxide, which occurs in nature as agate, amethyst, and sand quartz, chalcedony, cristobalite, and flint; it is one of the major constituents of dental porcelain, and in granular form serves as a dental abrasive and polishing agent. See also SILICOSIS.

silicatosis (sil″ĭ-kah-to′sis) PNEUMOCONIOSIS caused by the inhalation of the dust of silicates, particularly aluminum silicate and magnesium silicate (e.g., ASBESTOS, KAOLIN, MICA, or TALC).

silicoanthracosis (sil″ĭ-ko-an″thrah-ko′-sis) anthracosilicosis.

silicon (sil′ĭ-kon) a chemical element, atomic number 14, atomic weight 28.086, symbol Si. (See Appendix 6.)

s. dioxide SILICA.

silicone (sil′ĭ-kōn) any of a large group of organic compounds comprising alternating silicon and oxygen atoms linked to organic radicals; uses have included wetting agents and surfactants, sealants, coolants, contact lenses, and surgical membranes and implants.

s. oil any of various fluid silicone polymers; some are injected into the vitreous of the eye to serve as a vitreous substitute during or after certain ophthalmologic surgical procedures, such as to prevent the reoccurrence of retinal detachment.

silicoproteinosis (sil″ĭ-ko-pro″tēn-o′sis) a rapidly fatal pneumoconiosis occurring several weeks to months after massive exposure to silica dust, characterized by the presence of proteinaceous fluid in the air spaces.

silicosiderosis (sil″ĭ-ko-sid″er-o′sis) siderosilicosis.

silicosis (sil″ĭ-ko′sis) a type of PNEUMOCO-NIOSIS caused by the prolonged inhalation of SILICA dust. adj., **silicot′ic**. In the past it was called such colorful names as potter's asthma, stonecutter's cough, miner's mold, and grinder's rot, according to the occupation in which it was acquired. Today silicosis is most likely to be contracted in such industrial jobs as sandblasting in tunnels and hardrock mining, but it can occur in anyone who is habitually exposed to the dust contained in silica, one of the most common minerals. All types of miners, for example, may be subject to it, from gold miners to coal miners.

Silicosis usually takes about 10 years of fairly constant exposure to develop. It may give few warning symptoms. As time goes on, an affected person experiences progressive shortness of breath, along with steady coughing which in the early stages is dry and unproductive of mucus. Later there may be mucus tinged with blood, loss of appetite, pain in the chest, and general weakness. The silica produces a nodular fibrotic reaction that scars the lungs and makes them receptive to the further complications of bronchitis and emphysema; persons with silicosis are also more susceptible to tuberculosis.

Since this is a serious disease, persons who must work near silica should take precautions to breathe as little of it as possible, such as by the use of face masks, proper ventilation, and other safety devices. The cooperation of industry, labor, and government in developing protective measures has made the condition much less common today than it used to be. The OCCUPATIONAL SAFETY AND HEALTH ADMINISTRATION (OSHA) notes that silicosis is 100 per cent preventable if employers, workers, and health care providers work together to reduce exposure to the dust. Regular chest x-rays are recommended for all workers at risk as the quickest and easiest way to detect silicosis. If discovered in its early stages, it can usually be arrested by a change of occupation or avoidance of dust inhalation. Once fully developed, however, it rarely yields to treatment.

Silicote (sil′ĭ-kōt) trademark for preparations of DIMETHICONE, a skin protective.

silicotuberculosis (sil″ĭ-ko-too-ber″ku-lo′-sis) SILICOSIS complicated by pulmonary TUBERCULOSIS; called also tuberculosilicosis.

silk the protein filament produced by the larvae of various insects; silk obtained from the cocoons of the silkworm *Bombyx mori* is washed to remove the gum and braided for use as a nonabsorbable suture material. Silk from which the gum has not been removed, known as virgin silk, is used for extremely fine sutures in ophthalmic surgery.

silo-filler's disease pulmonary inflammation, often with acute pulmonary edema, due to inhalation of the irritant gases (especially oxides of nitrogen) that collect in recently filled silos.

silver (sil′ver) a chemical element, atomic number 47, atomic weight 107.870, symbol Ag. (See Appendix 6.) It is used in medicine for its caustic, astringent, and antiseptic effects. It is also used in dentistry in alloys, in soldering, and as cones to obliterate the root canal.

s. nitrate colorless or white crystals, used as a caustic and local antiinfective; an important use is in prevention of OPHTHAL-MIA NEONATORUM.

s. protein silver made colloidal by the presence of, or combination with, protein; an active germicide with a local irritant and astringent effect.

s. sulfadiazine the silver derivative of sulfadiazine, having bactericidal activity

S

against many gram-positive and gram-negative organisms, as well as being effective against yeasts; used as a topical antiinfective for the prevention and treatment of wound sepsis in patients with second and third degree burns.

toughened s. nitrate a mixture of silver nitrate with hydrochloric acid, sodium chloride, or potassium nitrate, occurring as white crystalline masses molded into pencils or cones; a convenient means of applying silver nitrate locally.

Silverman-Andersen score (sil′ver-man an′der-sen) a system for evaluation of breathing performance of premature infants. It consists of five items: (1) chest retraction as compared with abdominal retraction during inhalation; (2) retraction of the lower intercostal muscles; (3) xiphoid retraction; (4) flaring of the nares with inhalation; and (5) grunting on exhalation. Each of the five factors is graded 0, 1, or 2. The sum of these factors yields the score. Adequate ventilation is indicated by a 0, severe respiratory distress is indicated by a score of 10.

simethicone (sĭ-meth′ĭ-kōn) an agent used as a remedy for FLATULENCE, and also used to prevent foaming in gastroscopy.

similitude (sĭ-mil′-ĭ-tōōd) a principle of motor development: it is necessary that change in form be in proportion to change in size.

Simmonds' disease (sim′ondz) panhypopituitarism in which cachexia is a prominent feature; it usually follows destruction of the pituitary gland by surgery, infection, injury, or tumor, but may also occur after difficult labor in childbirth. Symptoms, which vary in intensity, are extreme weight loss, debility, pallor, dry yellowish skin, a slow pulse, hypotension, and atrophy of the genitalia and breasts, progressing to premature senility. Treatment is by regular administration of the various hormones whose release is normally dependent on pituitary function. Called also pituitary CACHEXIA.

Simplexvirus (sim′pleks-vi″rus) the herpes simplex VIRUSES, a genus of HERPESVIRUSES that cause HERPES SIMPLEX; species pathogenic in humans include human HERPESVIRUS 1 and human HERPESVIRUS 2.

Sims (simz) James Marion (1813–1883). American surgeon and pioneer in gynecology. Born in South Carolina and graduated from Jefferson Medical College in Philadelphia, he is known chiefly for the semiprone position and the curved speculum that are named after him, and that contributed to his success in operating for vesicovaginal fistula. He established the State Hospital

for Women in New York, and was president of the American Medical Association and honorary president of the International Medical Congress.

simulation (sim″u-la′shun) 1. the act of counterfeiting a disease; malingering. 2. the imitation of one disease by another.

simulator (sim″u-la′tor) something that simulates, such as an apparatus that simulates conditions that will be encountered in real life.

simultanagnosia (si″mul-tān″ag-no′zhah) the inability to comprehend more than one element of a visual scene at the same time or to integrate the parts as a whole.

simvastatin (sim′vah-stat″in) an ANTIHYPERLIPIDEMIC agent that acts by inhibiting cholesterol synthesis, used in the treatment of HYPERCHOLESTEROLEMIA and other forms of DYSLIPIDEMIA and to lower the risks associated with ATHEROSCLEROSIS and CORONARY HEART DISEASE; administered orally.

SIMV synchronized intermittent mandatory ventilation.

sincalide (sin′kah-līd) the synthetic C-terminal octapeptide of CHOLECYSTOKININ, used to stimulate gallbladder contraction in order to be able to aspirate a bile specimen from the duodenum or to obtain postevacuation films in CHOLECYSTOGRAPHY.

sinciput (sin′sĭ-put) the upper and front part of the head. adj., **sincip′ital.**

Sinemet (sin′ĕ-met) trademark for a combination of CARBIDOPA and LEVODOPA used in treatment of PARKINSONISM.

Sinequan (sin′ĕ-kwan) trademark for a preparation of DOXEPIN hydrochloride, an ANTIDEPRESSANT.

sinew (sin′u) a tendon of a muscle.

weeping s. an encysted ganglion, chiefly on the back of the hand, containing synovial fluid.

single blind pertaining to a clinical TRIAL or other experiment in which no subject knows whether he or she is receiving particular treatments or even lack of treatment (see PLACEBO), but the administrator does have that information.

single breath test (sing′g'l breth) single breath NITROGEN WASHOUT TEST.

singultus (sing-gul′tus) hiccup.

sinister (sin′is-ter) [L.] left; on the left side.

sinistr(o)- word element [L.], *left; left side.*

sinistrad (sin′is-trad) to or toward the left.

sinistral (sin′is-tral) pertaining to the left side.

sinistrality (sin″is-tral′ĭ-te) the preferential use, in voluntary motor acts, of the left member of the major paired organs of the body, such as the ear, eye, hand, and leg. See also LATERALITY and HANDEDNESS

sinistraural (sin″is-traw′ral) hearing better with the left ear.

sinistrocardia (sin″is-tro-kahr′de-ah) levocardia.

sinistrocerebral (sin″is-tro-ser′ĕ-bral) located in the left cerebral HEMISPHERE.

sinistrocular (sin″is-trok′u-lar) having the left eye dominant.

sinistrocularity (sin″is-trok″u-lar′ĭ-te) dominance of the left eye.

sinistrogyration (sin″is-tro-ji-ra′shun) a turning to the left.

sinistromanual (sin″is-tro-man′u-al) left-handed.

sinistropedal (sin″is-trop′ĕ-dal) using the left foot in preference to the right.

sinistrotorsion (sin″is-tro-tor′shun) a twisting toward the left, as of the eye.

sinoatrial (si″no-a′tre-al) pertaining to the sinus venosus and the atrium of the heart.

sinobronchitis (si″no-brong-ki′tis) chronic paranasal sinusitis with recurrent bronchitis.

sinuous (sin′u-us) bending in and out; winding.

sinus (si′nus) 1. a recess, cavity, or channel, such as one in bone or a dilated channel for venous blood. 2. an abnormal channel or fistula, permitting escape of pus. 3. paranasal sinus.

anal s's furrows, with pouchlike recesses at the distal end, separating the rectal COLUMNS; called also anal crypts.

anterior s's, s. anterio′res the anterior air cells that together with the middle and posterior air cells form the ethmoidal sinus.

aortic s's pouchlike dilatations at the root of the aorta, one opposite each semilunar cusp of the aortic valve, from which the coronary arteries originate.

carotid s. a dilatation of the proximal portion of the internal carotid or distal portion of the common carotid artery, containing in its wall pressoreceptors that are stimulated by changes in blood pressure. See also CAROTID SINUS SYNDROME.

cavernous s. an irregularly shaped venous channel between the layers of dura mater of the brain, one on either side of the body of the sphenoid bone and communicating across the midline. Several cranial nerves course through this sinus.

cerebral s. one of the ventricles of the brain.

cervical s. a temporary depression in the neck of the embryo containing the branchial arches.

circular s. the venous channel encircling the pituitary gland, formed by the two cavernous sinuses and the anterior and posterior intercavernous sinuses.

coccygeal s. a sinus or fistula just over or close to the tip of the coccyx.

coronary s. the dilated terminal portion of the great cardiac vein, receiving blood from other veins draining the heart muscle and emptying into the right atrium.

dermal s. a congenital sinus tract extending from the surface of the body, between the bodies of two adjacent lumbar vertebrae, to the spinal canal.

ethmoid s's, ethmoidal s's ethmoid cells.

frontal s. one of the paired paranasal sinuses in the frontal bone, each communicating with the middle nasal meatus on the same side.

intercavernous s's channels connecting the two cavernous sinuses, one passing anterior and the other posterior to the stalk of the pituitary gland.

lymphatic s's irregular, tortuous spaces within lymphoid tissues through which lymph flows.

maxillary s. one of the paired paranasal sinuses in the body of the maxilla on either side, opening into the middle nasal meatus on the same side.

occipital s. a venous sinus between the layers of dura mater, passing upward along the midline of the cerebellum.

paranasal s's the eight cavities in the skull that are connected with the nasal cavity (see also Plates). They are arranged in four pairs, each of which has one member on the left and one on the right. The pairs are the maxillary SINUSES in the maxillae; the frontal SINUSES in the frontal bone; the sphenoid SINUSES in the sphenoid bone behind the nasal cavity; and the ethmoid CELLS (ethmoid SINUSES) in the ethmoid bone behind and below the frontal sinuses. The

S

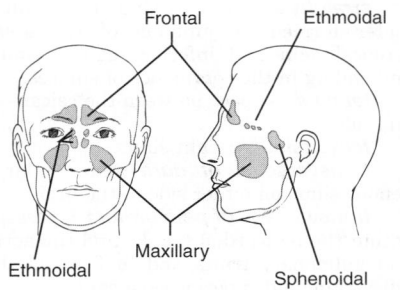

Sinus paranasal (Paranasal sinuses). From Dorland's, 2000.

functions of the sinuses are not certain. They are believed to help the nose in circulating, warming, and moistening the air as it is inhaled, thereby lessening the shock of cold, dry air to the lungs. They also are thought to have a minor role as resonating chambers for the voice.

petrosal s., inferior a venous channel arising from the cavernous sinus and draining into the internal jugular vein.

petrosal s., superior one arising from the cavernous sinus and draining into the transverse sinus of the dura mater.

pilonidal s. pilonidal cyst.

prostatic s. the posterolateral recess between the seminal colliculus and the wall of the urethra, where the prostatic ductules empty into the urethra.

s's of pulmonary trunk spaces between the wall of the pulmonary trunk and cusps of the pulmonary valve at its opening from the right ventricle.

renal s. a recess in the substance of the kidney, occupied by the renal pelvis, calices, vessels, nerves, and fat.

sagittal s., inferior a small venous sinus of the dura mater, opening into the straight sinus.

sagittal s., superior a venous sinus of the dura mater that ends in the confluence of sinuses.

sigmoid s. a venous sinus of the dura mater on either side, continuous with the straight sinus and draining into the internal jugular vein of the same side.

sphenoid s., sphenoidal s. one of the paired paranasal sinuses in the body of the sphenoid bone, opening into the superior nasal meatus on the same side.

sphenoparietal s. one of the venous sinuses of the dura mater, emptying into the cavernous sinus.

s's of spleen dilated venous sinuses found in the splenic pulp; they are not lined by ordinary endothelial cells.

straight s. a venous sinus of the dura mater formed by junction of the great cerebral vein and inferior sagittal sinus, and ending in the confluence of sinuses.

tarsal s. a space between the calcaneus and talus.

tentorial s. straight sinus.

transverse s. of dura mater a large venous sinus on either side of the brain.

transverse s. of pericardium a passage within the pericardial sac, behind the aorta and pulmonary trunk and in front of the left atrium and superior vena cava.

tympanic s. a deep recess on the medial wall of the middle ear.

urogenital s. an elongated sac that is formed by division of the cloaca in the early embryo, which ultimately forms most of the vestibule, urethra, and vagina in the female and some of the urethra in the male.

uterine s's venous channels in the wall of the uterus in pregnancy.

uteroplacental s's blood spaces between the placenta and uterine sinuses.

s. of venae cavae the posterior portion of the right atrium into which the inferior and the superior vena cava open; called also sinus venosus.

s. veno′sus, venous s. 1. see venous sinuses of dura mater and venous sinus of sclera. 2. the common venous receptacle in the early embryo attached to the posterior wall of the primitive atrium. 3. sinus of venae cavae.

venous s's of dura mater large channels for venous blood forming an anastomosing system between the layers of the dura mater of the brain, receiving blood from the brain and draining into the veins of the scalp or deep veins at the base of the skull.

venous s. of sclera a circular channel at the junction of the sclera and cornea, into which aqueous humor filters from the anterior chamber of the eye. Called also Schlemm's canal.

sinusitis (si″nŭ-si′tis) inflammation of one or more of the paranasal sinuses, often occurring during an upper respiratory tract infection when infection in the nose spreads to the sinuses (sometimes encouraged by excessively strong blowing of the nose). It also may be a complication of tooth infection, allergy, or certain infectious diseases such as pneumonia and measles. There are many other causes, including air pollution, diving and underwater swimming, sudden extremes of temperature, and structural defects of the nose that interfere with breathing, such as deviated septum.

As the mucous membranes of the sinus become inflamed and swollen, the openings that lead from each sinus into the nasal passages become partially or wholly blocked. The mucus that accumulates in the sealed-off sinus causes pressure on the sinus walls, resulting in discomfort, fever, pain, and difficult breathing.

Symptoms. The common symptoms of sinusitis are headache, usually located near the sinuses most involved, and nasal discharge. These may be accompanied by a slight rise in temperature, dizziness, and a general feeling of weakness and discomfort.

When sinusitis is suspected as the cause of such symptoms, the health care provider may use a light to evaluate the patency of the sinuses. A bright light is held against he forehead and cheeks to determine the mount of light transmitted through the inuses in these areas. If a sinus is filled vith fluid and inflamed it will transmit ittle or no light. Radiologic tests also are used to confirm a diagnosis of sinusitis and o locate the extent of involvement. Specialzed techniques such as multiple x-ray xposures (POLYTOMOGRAPHY) and computed OMOGRAPHY are sometimes used to pinpoint he nature and scope of a sinus disorder.

The American Academy of Pediatrics has leveloped clinical practice guidelines called *Management of Sinusitis*, applicable for any-ne up to age 21. They note that imaging tudies are not necessary to confirm a diagnosis of clinical sinusitis in children younger han age 6. They further recommend that CT cans be used only for those patients in whom urgery is a likely management strategy.

TREATMENT. Acute sinusitis usually reponds to antibiotic therapy and increased trainage from the sinuses through the use of lecongestants, which are applied locally in he form of nosedrops and also taken sysemically. Inhalation of steam or warm noisturized air and local applications of heat ncourage drainage and help relieve discomort. Because of the severe pain associated vith inflamed and swollen sinus membranes, otent analgesics may be needed for the first ew days to provide relief and permit rest.

Chronic sinusitis often develops follow-ng a particularly resistant case of acute inusitis. The mucous membranes in the inuses thicken and normal drainage is bstructed. If medical management such as hat described previously for acute sinusitis loes not relieve the condition, surgical ntervention may be necessary. In some ases, repair of a deviated nasal septum or emoval of nasal polyps may be all that is lecessary to eliminate the source of the roblem. Others may need to have a new utlet created in the sinus to allow for lrainage into the nose. More extensive urgery involves removal of the thickened nembranous lining of the sinus or oblitera-ion of the sinus itself in order to prevent efilling with purulent drainage.

Since sinusitis can lead to more serious nfections in nearby tissues, such as the ones of the ear and mastoid or the brain, t is important that it be treated aggres-ively to eliminate infection. Though a hange of climate can sometimes help in ases of chronic sinusitis, it rarely is a lecessity. Creating a better indoor climate vith such devices as air conditioners and umidifiers often is equally beneficial in educing the number and severity of sinus ttacks. Psychotherapy may be of help to

some patients with disabling, chronic sinusitis because continual emotional strain is one of the factors that can intensify the symptoms.

ethmoid s. inflammation of an ethmoid CELL (ethmoid SINUS); called also ethmoiditis.

maxillary s. inflammation of a maxillary SINUS; called also antritis.

sphenoid s. inflammation of a sphenoid SINUS; called also sphenoiditis.

sinusoid (si′nŭ-soid) 1. resembling a sinus. 2. a form of terminal blood channel consisting of a large, irregular, anastomosing vessel, having a lining of reticuloendothelium but little or no adventitia. Sinusoids are found in the liver, adrenal glands, heart, parathyroid glands, carotid bodies, spleen, hemolymph glands, and pancreas.

sinusotomy (si″nus-ot′ah-me) incision of a sinus.

siphon (si′fon) 1. a bent tube with arms of unequal length, for drawing liquid from a higher to a lower level by force of atmospheric pressure. 2. to draw liquid by means of a siphon.

siphonage (si′fon-ij) the use of the siphon, as in gastric lavage or in draining the bladder.

Sipple's syndrome (sip′l'z) multiple endocrine NEOPLASIA, Type II.

sirenomelus (si″ren-om′ĕ-lus) a fetus with SIRENOMELIA; see also SYMMELIA.

sirenomelia apodal SYMMELIA.

sirolimus (sī-ro′lĭ-məs) a macrolide antibiotic obtained from *Streptomyces hygroscopicus,* having immunosuppressant properties; used to prevent rejection of kidney transplants. Administered orally.

-sis word element [Gr.], *state; condition.* See also -ESIS, -IASIS, and -OSIS.

SISI short increment sensitivity index.

sister (sis′ter) the nurse in charge of a hospital ward (Great Britain).

Sistrurus (sis-troo′rus) a genus of small RATTLESNAKES widely distributed throughout the United States, having symmetrical plates covering their heads.

sitophobia (si″to-fo′be-ah) irrational fear of eating or of food.

sitosterol (si″tos′ter-ol) 1. any of a group of closely related plant sterols, designated by Greek letters according to distinguishing characteristics. 2. a preparation of β-sitosterol and certain saturated sterols, used to treat HYPERCHOLESTEROLEMIA.

sitosterolemia (si-tos″ter-ol-e′me-ah) the presence of excessive levels of sitosterols in the blood, especially β-sitosterol, absorbed from dietary vegetables due to an unknown intestinal defect. A rare form is associated

S

with xanthomatosis, with tuberous and tendon xanthomas appearing in childhood.

sitotropism (si-tot′ro-pizm) TROPISM in response to the presence or absence of food.

situs (si′tus) [L.] site or position.

s. inver′sus total or partial transposition of the body organs to the side opposite the normal.

SI units the units of measurement generally accepted for all scientific and technical uses; together they make up the International System of Units. (See also METRIC SYSTEM.) The abbreviation SI, from the French *Système International d'Unités,* is used in all languages. There are seven base SI units, defined by specified physical measurements, and two supplementary units. Units are derived for any other physical quantities by multiplication and division of the base and supplementary units. The derived units with special names are shown in the accompanying table.

SI is a *coherent* system. This means that units are always combined without conversion factors. The derived unit of velocity is the meter per second (m/s); the derived unit

of volume is the cubic meter (m^3). If you know that pressure is force per unit area then you know that the SI unit of pressure (the pascal) is the unit of force divided by the unit of area and is therefore equal to 1 newton per square meter.

The metric prefixes can be attached to any unit in order to make a unit of a more convenient size. The symbol for the prefix is attached to the symbol for the unit, e.g., nanometer (nm) = 10^{-9} m. The units of mass are specified in terms of the gram, e.g., microgram (µg) = 10^{-9} kg.

Only one prefix is used with a unit; the use of units such as the millimicrometer is no longer acceptable. When a unit is raised to a power, the power applies to the prefix as well, e.g., a cubic millimeter (mm^3) = 10^{-9} m^3. When a prefix is used with a ratio unit, it should be in the numerator rather than in the denominator, e.g., kilometers/second (km/s) rather than meters/millisecond (m/ms). Only prefixes denoting powers of 10^3 are normally used. Hecto-, deka-, deci-, and centi- are usually attached only to the metric system units gram, meter, and liter.

Owing to the force of tradition, one non coherent unit, the liter, equal to 10^{-3} m^3, or 1 dm^3, is generally accepted for use with SI

SI UNITS				
Quantity	Unit	Symbol	Pronunciation	Derivation
Base Units				
length	meter	m	me′ter	
mass	kilogram	kg	kil′o-gram	
time	second	s	sek′und	
electric current	ampere	A	am′pēr	
temperature	kelvin	K	kel′vin	
luminous intensity	candela	cd	kan-del′ah	
amount of substance	mole	mol	mōl	
Supplementary Units				
plane angle	radian	rad	ra′de-an	
solid angle	steradian	sr	stĕ-ra′de-an	
Derived Units				
force	newton	N	noo′ton	kg·m/s^2
pressure	pascal	Pa	pas′kal	N/m^2
energy, work	joule	J	jōōl	N·m
power	watt	W	waht	J/s
electric charge	coulomb	C	koo′lom	A·s
electric potential	volt	V	volt	J/C
electric capacitance	farad	F	far′ad	C/V
electric resistance	ohm	Ω	ōm	V/A
electric conductance	siemens	S	se′menz	Ω^{-1}
magnetic flux	weber	Wb	web′er	V·s
magnetic flux density	tesla	T	taes′lah	Wb/m^2
inductance	henry	H	hen′re	Wb/A
frequency	hertz	Hz	herts	s^{-1}
luminous flux	lumen	lm	loo′men	cd·sr
illumination	lux	lx	luks	lm/m^2
temperature	degree celsius	°C	sel′se-us	K−273.15
radioactivity	becquerel	Bq	bek-er-el′	s^{-1}
absorbed dose	gray	Gy	grā	J/kg
absorbed dose equivalent	sievert	Sv	se′vert	J/kg

PREFIXES FOR SI UNITS			
Multiplication	Prefix	Symbol	Pronunciation
$1\ 000\ 000\ 000\ 000\ 000\ 000 = 10^{18}$	exa	E	ek'sah
$1\ 000\ 000\ 000\ 000\ 000 = 10^{15}$	peta	P	pet'ah
$1\ 000\ 000\ 000\ 000 = 10^{12}$	tera	T	ter'ah
$p1\ 000\ 000\ 000 = 10^{9}$	giga	G	gig'ah
$1\ 000\ 000 = 10^{6}$	mega	M	meg'ah
$1\ 000 = 10^{3}$	kilo	k	kil'o
$100 = 10^{2}$	hecto	h	hek'to
$10 = 10$	deka	dk	dek'ah
$0.1 = 10^{-1}$	deci	d	des' ĭ
$0.01 = 10^{-2}$	centi	c	sen'tĭ
$0.001 = 10^{-3}$	milli	m	mil'ĭ
$0.000\ 001 = 10^{-6}$	micro	μ	mi'kro
$0.000\ 000\ 001 = 10^{-9}$	nano	n	nan'o
$0.000\ 000\ 000\ 001 = 10^{-12}$	pico	p	pi'ko
$0.000\ 000\ 000\ 000\ 001 = 10^{-15}$	femto	f	fem'to
$0.000\ 000\ 000\ 000\ 000\ 001 = 10^{-18}$	atto	a	at'o

The internationally accepted abbreviation for liter is the letter l; however, this can be confused with the numeral 1, especially in typescript. For this reason, the capital letter L is also used as a symbol for liter. The lower case letter is generally used with prefixes, e.g., dl, ml, fl. The symbols for all other SI units begin with a capital letter if the unit is named after a person and with a lower case letter otherwise. The name of a unit is never capitalized.

Sjögren's syndrome (sha'grenz) a symptom complex of unknown etiology, usually occurring in middle-aged or older women, marked by the triad of keratoconjunctivitis sicca with or without lacrimal gland enlargement, xerostomia with or without salivary gland enlargement, and the presence of a connective tissue disease, usually rheumatoid arthritis but sometimes systemic lupus erythematosus, scleroderma, or polymyositis. An abnormal IMMUNE RESPONSE has been implicated. The dryness and the discomfort related to the lack of secretions are treated symptomatically.

SK streptokinase.

skatole (skat'ōl) a compound formed in the putrefaction of proteins which contributes to the characteristic odor of the feces.

skatoxyl (skah-tok'sil) an oxidation product of skatole found in the urine in certain diseases of the large intestine.

skeletal (skel'ĕ-tal) pertaining to the skeleton.

s. system the body's framework of bones; there are 206 distinct bones in the body of an average adult human. (See anatomic Table of Bones in the Appendices and see Plates.) The bones give support and shape to the body, protect delicate internal organs, and provide sites of attachment for muscles to make motion possible. In addition, they store and help maintain the correct level of CALCIUM, and the bone MARROW manufactures blood cells. Called also skeleton.

Main Parts of the Skeleton. There are two main parts of the skeleton: the axial skeleton, including the bones of the head and trunk, and the appendicular skeleton, including the bones of the limbs. The axial skeleton has 80 bones and the appendicular skeleton has 126 bones.

Axial Skeleton. The axial skeleton includes the skull, the spine, and the ribs and sternum. The most important of these is the SPINE (called also the *spinal* or *vertebral column*), consisting of 26 separate bones. Twenty-four vertebrae have holes through them, which are lined up vertically to form a hollow tube called the spinal CANAL; the spinal cord runs through this canal and is protected by it.

The seven topmost vertebrae, in the neck, are the cervical vertebrae; they support the skull, which encloses and protects the brain and provides protection for the eyes, inner ears, and nasal passages. The skull includes the cranium, the facial bones, and the auditory ossicles. Of the 28 bones of the skull, only one, the mandible, is movable.

Below the cervical vertebrae are 12 thoracic vertebrae; attached to them are 12 pairs of RIBS, one pair to a vertebra. The ribs curve around to the front of the body, where most attach directly to the sternum or are indirectly attached to it by means of cartilage. The two bottom pairs of ribs are unattached in front and are called floating

S

ribs. Together, the thoracic vertebrae, the ribs, and the sternum form a bony basket called the thoracic (or rib) cage, which prevents the chest wall from collapsing and protects the heart and the lungs. The remaining bones of the spine include five lumbar vertebrae, which support the small of the back, and the sacrum and coccyx. The axial skeleton also includes a single bone in the neck, the hyoid bone, to which muscles of the mouth are attached. This is the only bone of the body that does not join with another bone.

Appendicular Skeleton. The appendicular skeleton includes the shoulder girdle, bones of the upper limb, pelvic girdle, and bones of the lower limb. The shoulder girdle, from which the arms hang, consists of two CLAVICLES and two SCAPULAE; the scapulae are joined to the sternum.

The upper LIMB has three long bones. The uppermost bone is the HUMERUS, whose upper (proximal) end fits into a socket in the shoulder girdle; its lower (distal) end is connected at the elbow to the ULNA and RADIUS, the two long bones of the forearm. Eight small bones, the carpals, compose the wrist. Five metacarpals form the palm of the hand, and the finger bones are made up of 14 phalanges in each hand.

At the lower end of the spine is the pelvic girdle; it, along with the last two bones of the spinal column (the SACRUM and COCCYX), forms the PELVIS. This part of the skeleton encircles and protects the internal organs of the genitourinary system. In each side of the pelvis is the ACETABULUM, a socket into which a femur fits.

The bones of the lower LIMB are similar in construction to those of the upper limb but are heavier and stronger. The FEMUR (thigh bone), which is the longest bone in the body, extends from the pelvis to the knee. The TIBIA and the FIBULA are long bones that extend from the knee to the ankle. On the knee is another single bone, the PATELLA or kneecap. In each leg there are seven ankle bones, or tarsals; five foot bones, or metatarsals; and 14 toe bones, or phalanges.

Joints and Movement. Anywhere in the skeleton that two or more bones come together is known as a JOINT. The way these bones are joined determines whether they can move and how they move. The elbow, for example, is a hinge joint, which allows bending in only one direction. In contrast, both bending and rotary movements are possible in the hip joint, a ball-and-socket joint. Many joints, such as most of those in the skull, are rigid and permit no movement whatsoever.

The force needed to move the bones is provided by MUSCLES, which are attached to the bones by tendons. A muscle typically spans a joint so that one end is attached by a tendon to one bone, and the other end to a second bone. Usually one bone serves as an anchor for the muscle, and the second bone is free to move. When the muscle contracts it pulls the second bone. Actually, two sets of muscles that pull in opposite directions take part in any movement. When one set contracts, the opposing set relaxes.

skeletization (skel″ĕ-tĭ-za′shun) 1. extreme emaciation. 2. removal of soft parts from the skeleton.

skeletogenous (skel″ĕ-toj′ĕ-nus) producing skeletal structures or tissues.

skeleton (skel′ĕ-ton) the hardened tissues forming the supporting framework of an animal body; see SKELETAL SYSTEM.

axial s., s. axia′le the bones of the cranium, vertebral column, ribs, and sternum.

skenitis (ske-ni′tis) inflammation of Skene's glands.

skill (skil) a talent or ability; dexterity or expertise.

coping s's the identification and management of stress and related reactors, a PERFORMANCE COMPONENT in occupational therapy.

functional s's tasks that are necessary to care for oneself; see also ACTIVITIES OF DAILY LIVING.

skin (skin) the outer covering of the body. The skin is the largest organ of the body and it performs a number of vital functions. It serves as a protective barrier against microorganisms. It helps shield the delicate sensitive tissues underneath from mechanical and other injuries. It acts as an insulator against heat and cold, and helps eliminate body wastes in the form of perspiration. It guards against excessive exposure to the ultraviolet rays of the sun by producing a protective pigmentation, and it helps produce the body's supply of vitamin D. Its sense receptors enable the body to feel pain, cold, heat, touch, and pressure. The skin consists of two main parts: an outer layer, the *epidermis*, and an inner layer, the *corium* (or *dermis*).

Epidermis. The epidermis is thinner than the corium, and is made up of several layers of different kinds of cells. The number of cells varies in different parts of the body; the greatest number is in the palms of the hands and soles of the feet, where the skin is thickest.

The cells in the outer or horny layer of the epidermis are constantly being shed and replaced by new cells from its bottom layers.

in the lower epidermis. The cells of the protective, horny layer are nonliving and require no supply of blood for nourishment. As long as the horny outer layer remains intact, microorganisms cannot enter.

Corium. Underneath the epidermis is the thicker part of the skin, the corium, or dermis, which is made up of connective tissue that contains blood vessels and nerves. It projects into the epidermis in ridges called *papillae of the corium.* The nerves that extend through the corium end in the papillae. The various skin sensations, such as touch, pain, pressure, heat, and cold, are felt through these nerves. The reaction to heat and cold causes the expansion and contraction of the blood capillaries of the corium. This in turn causes more or less blood to flow through the skin, resulting in greater or smaller loss of body heat (see TEMPERATURE).

The sweat glands are situated deep in the corium. They collect fluid containing water, salt, and waste products from the blood and carry it away in canals that end in pores on the skin surface, where it is deposited as sweat. Perspiration helps regulate body temperature as well, because cooling of the skin occurs when sweat evaporates. The sebaceous glands are also in the corium. They secrete the oil that keeps the skin surface lubricated.

Beneath the corium is a layer of subcutaneous tissue. This tissue helps insulate the body against heat and cold, and cushions it against shock.

The hair and nails are outgrowths of the skin. The roots of the hair lie in follicles, or pockets of epidermal cells situated in the corium. Hair grows from the roots, but the hair cells die while still in the follicles, and the closely packed remains that are pushed upward form the hair shaft that is seen on the surface of the skin.

The nails grow in much the same way as the hair. The nail bed, like the hair root, is situated in the corium. The pink color of the nails is due to their translucent quality which allows the blood capillaries of the corium to show through.

s. test application of a substance to the skin, or intradermal injection of a substance, to permit observation of the body's reaction to it. Such a test detects a person's sensitivity to such allergens as dust and pollen, or to preparations of microorganisms believed to be the cause of a disorder.

There are several types of skin tests, including the patch test, the scratch test, and the intradermal test.

Patch Test. This is the simplest type of skin test. A small piece of gauze or filter paper is impregnated with a minute quantity of the

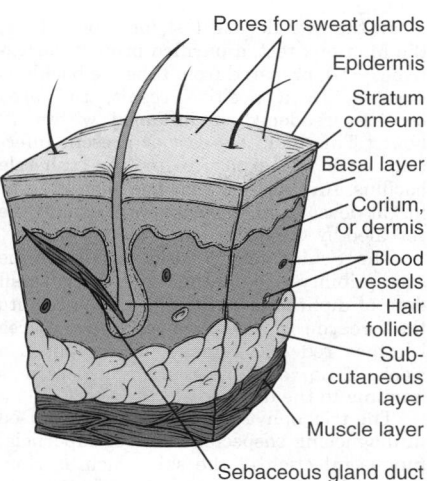

Pores for sweat glands
Epidermis
Stratum corneum
Basal layer
Corium, or dermis
Blood vessels
Hair follicle
Subcutaneous layer
Muscle layer
Sebaceous gland duct

Normal skin. From Frazier et al., 2000.

substance to be tested and is applied to the skin, usually on the forearm. After a certain length of time the patch is removed and the reaction observed. If there is no reaction, the test result is said to be negative; if the skin is reddened or swollen, the result is positive.

The patch test is used most often in testing for skin allergies, especially CONTACT DERMATITIS.

Scratch Test. In this test, one or more small scratches or superficial cuts are made in the skin, and a minute amount of the substance to be tested is inserted in the scratches and allowed to remain there for a short time. If no reaction has occurred after 30 minutes, the substance is removed and the test is considered negative. If there is redness or swelling at the scratch sites, the test is considered positive.

The scratch test is often used in testing for allergies. A complete screening for allergic sensitivity may require numerous skin tests. Only an extremely minute quantity of the substance can be used in each test since severe allergic reactions can occur.

The scratch test is also used in the diagnosis of tuberculosis. In Pirquet's reaction, for example, tuberculin is used, and the local inflammatory reaction that results is more marked in tuberculous persons than in normal ones.

Intradermal Tests. In these tests, the substance under study is injected between the layers of skin. Intradermal tests are used for diagnosis of infectious diseases and determination of susceptibility to a disease or sensitivity to an allergen.

S

In the intradermal test for tuberculosis, the Mantoux test, a purified protein derivative (PPD), prepared from tubercle bacilli, is injected. In a positive result, the area becomes reddened or inflamed within 72 hours. This indicates past or present infection with or exposure to the tubercle bacillus. An infection that has been present for at least 2 to 8 weeks will usually be revealed by the test.

The Schick test is used to determine susceptibility to diphtheria. A very small dose of diphtheria antitoxin is injected into the forearm. In a positive reaction the area becomes red and remains so for about a week. If no reaction occurs, the person is immune to the disease.

The trichophytin test is sometimes used in diagnosing suspected cases of superficial fungus infection of the skin, such as ringworm. In the presence of infection by the fungus *Trichophyton,* an injection of trichophytin, which is prepared from cultures of the fungus, will produce a reaction similar to the tuberculin reaction. Skin tests, of course, are always made in an area separate from the infected area.

In addition to their frequent use in testing for allergies, intradermal tests are employed in the diagnosis of parasitic infections, such as SCHISTOSOMIASIS, other fungus diseases besides trichophytosis, and mumps.

Skinner box (skin′er) an experimental enclosure for testing animal conditioning, in which the subject animal performs (such as by pressing a bar or lever) to obtain a reward; see also instrumental CONDITIONING.

skler(o)- for words beginning thus, see those beginning *scler(o)-*.

skot(o)- for words beginning thus, see those beginning *scot(o)-*.

skull (skul) the skeleton of the head, consisting of the CRANIUM and the MANDIBLE. The cranium forms the domed top, back, and sides of the skull; several of its bones are large, smooth, gently curved, and connected to each other by dovetailed joints called sutures, which permit no movement and make the mature skull rigid. They protect the brain, with their curved exterior serving to deflect blows; the eyes, ears, and nose are also protected by being recessed into the skull and surrounded by bone.

At birth the skull joints are flexible, so that the infant's head can be compressed as it emerges from the birth canal. The joints remain flexible to allow expansion until the cranial bones are fully formed, around the second year of life. An infant's skull contains soft areas, or FONTANELS, where the bones of the cranium do not meet.

The skull is supported by the highest vertebra, called the atlas. This joint permits a back-and-forth, nodding motion. The atlas turns on the vertebra below it, the axis, which allows the skull to turn from side to side.

Disorders of the Skull. The skull is rarely affected by disease. Uncommon ones like OSTEITIS DEFORMANS and ACROMEGALY cause the bones to increase in size. Like other

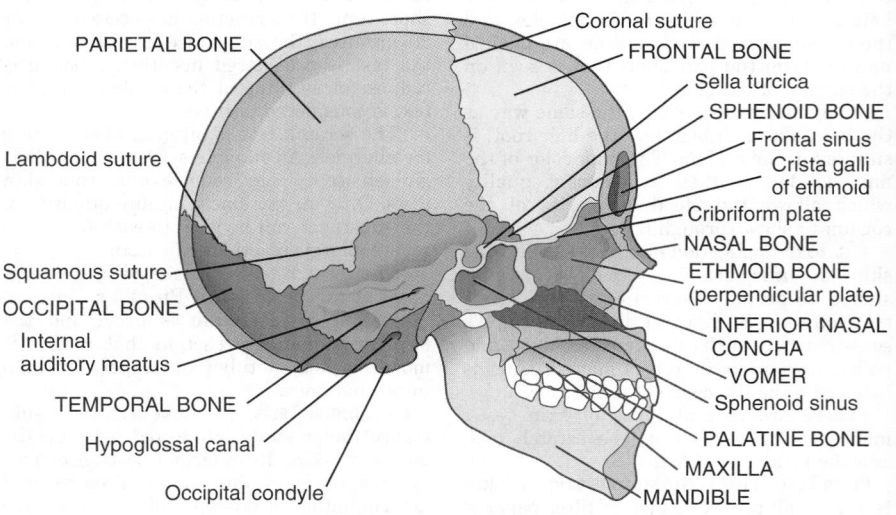

Skull, midsagittal section. From Applegate, 2000.

bones, the skull may be fractured by blows, falls, or other accidents, but skull fracture can be far more dangerous because of its proximity to the brain.

sleep (slēp) a period of rest for the body and mind, during which volition and CONSCIOUSNESS are in partial or complete abeyance and the bodily functions partially suspended. Sleep has also been described as a behavioral state marked by characteristic immobile posture and diminished but readily reversible sensitivity to external stimuli.

NREM and REM Sleep. Prior to the discovery and reporting of rapid eye movements during sleep, it was thought that sleep was a single state of passive recuperation in which the central nervous system was deactivated. Studies concerned with the measurement of central and autonomic activities during sleep have led to its division into two types: *non–rapid eye movement (NREM) sleep*, also called *orthodox* or *synchronized (S) sleep*; and *rapid eye movement (REM) sleep* (so called because of the rapid eye movements during this stage), also called *paradoxical* or *desynchronized (D) sleep.* On the basis of electroencephalographic (EEG) criteria, NREM sleep is subdivided into four stages. *Stage 1* is observed immediately after sleep begins or after momentary arousals and is characterized by low-voltage, mixed-frequency EEG tracing, with predominantly theta-wave activity (four to seven hertz, that is, cycles per second). *Stage 2* is characterized by intermittent waves of 12 to 16 hertz, known as *sleep spindles. Stages 3* and *4* consist of relatively high voltage EEG tracings with a predominance of delta wave activity (one to two hertz).

The EEG patterns of NREM sleep suggest that this is the kind of apparently restful state that supports the recuperative functions assigned to sleep. NREM sleep is increased after physical activity and has a relatively high priority among humans in the recovery sleep following extended periods of wakefulness.

Within 90 minutes after sleep begins, an adult progresses through all four stages of NREM sleep and then proceeds into the first of a series of REM periods of sleep. Brief cycles of about 10 to 30 minutes of REM sleep recur throughout the night, alternating with various stages of NREM sleep. With each cycle, NREM sleep decreases and REM sleep increases so that by the end of the night most of the sleep is REM sleep, which is when dreams occur. While everyone dreams every night, many do not remember dreaming; most people are aware, however, that they dream more just before rising.

In addition to the rapid eye movements that can be observed through closed eyelids, REM sleep can be recognized by complete relaxation of the lower jaw. Convulsions, myocardial infarction, and cardiac arrhythmias are more likely to occur during REM sleep. This is probably because of increased autonomic activity, irregular pulse, and fluctuations in blood pressure, which are all typical of REM sleep.

Patterns of Sleep. Although the average adult spends approximately 25 percent of total accumulated sleep in REM sleep and 75 percent in NREM sleep, the cyclic changes vary with individuals. The pattern of sleep, in addition to the REM and NREM states, also includes the periods of sleep and wakefulness within a 24-hour period.

Factors affecting the total sleep pattern include age, state of physical health, psychological state, and certain drugs. Newborns follow a pattern of several hours of sleep followed by a period of wakefulness. REM sleep occurs at the onset of sleep in infants; it rarely does in adults. As the child matures there is an increasing tendency toward longer periods of nocturnal sleep. Elderly persons sometimes return to the shorter periods of sleep that are typical of infants.

Benefits of Sleep. Sleep requirements vary greatly among individuals. Infants usually require 16 to 20 hours of total sleep during a 24-hour period, and the amount decreases as the child matures. An adult usually requires 6 to 9 hours of total sleep, and requirements continue to decrease with aging.

Most theorists agree that sleep has value as a recuperative and adaptive function in the lives of humans. The relatively high metabolic needs of mammals and birds to maintain a constant body temperature in a wide range of environmental temperatures suggests that the periodic decreases in metabolic rate and body temperature that occur in NREM sleep allow for recuperation and restitution of body tissues. For example, even though the function of stage 2 NREM sleep is not clear, approximately half of human sleep time is spent in this stage. It is also theorized that REM sleep provides a period of recuperation of mental activities and preparation for wakefulness. During REM sleep it is believed that there is increased metabolic activity in the brain so that during waking hours it is more receptive to new information and can assimilate it more easily.

s. apnea syndrome episodes of APNEA (cessation of breathing) occurring at the

transition from NREM to REM sleep, with
repeated wakening and excessive daytime
sleepiness; it occurs most often in middle-aged, obese males and is thought to
have several causes, one being collapse or
obstruction of the airway with the inhibition of muscle tone that characterizes REM
sleep. The condition is arbitrarily defined as
more than five cessations of airflow for at
least 10 seconds each per hour of sleep.

   s. disorders chronic disorders involving sleep; primary sleep disorders are classified as DYSSOMNIAS or PARASOMNIAS. Among
the minor disorders are SLEEPWALKING, SLEEP-
TALKING, ENURESIS, BRUXISM (tooth grinding),
and NIGHTMARES. Sleepwalking is not considered serious if it occasionally occurs in
childhood. It should be considered pathological, however, if it persists into adulthood. Sleeptalking is common to many
persons and, while it may annoy others
whose sleep it may disturb, it is not
considered pathological.

   A sleep disorder occurring in early childhood, and not to be confused with nightmares, is SLEEP TERROR DISORDER. The child
awakens with a scream, is in panic and
cannot be consoled, and often is incoherent;
the following morning, there is poor recall
of the event. Treatment usually involves
reassurance of the parents. Adults who
experience night terrors often have some
psychological problem requiring treatment.
More serious disorders of sleep include
persistent INSOMNIA, NARCOLEPSY, and chronic
HYPERSOMNIA. Hypersomnia can occur with
central nervous system damage or may be
secondary to some physical and mental
illnesses, particularly depression.

   s. terror disorder a sleep disorder of
the parasomnia group, consisting of repeated episodes of pavor nocturnus (sleep
terrors).

   sleeping sickness a disease characterized by increasing drowsiness and lethargy,
caused by a protozoal infection, such as
African trypanosomiasis, or by a viral infection, such as lethargic encephalitis, St.
Louis encephalitis, or eastern or western
encephalomyelitis.

   African s. s. African trypanosomiasis.

   sleeptalking (slēp′tok-ing) somniloquism.

   sleepwalking rising from bed and walking
or performing other complex motor behavior
during an apparent state of sleep; much
mystery has been attached to this, although
it is no more mysterious than dreaming. The
chief difference between the two is that the
sleepwalker, besides dreaming, is also using
the part of the brain that stimulates walking.

This usually occurs during the first third of
the night and lasts for a few minutes to a half
hour. The sleeper is relatively unresponsive,
not easily awakened, and usually amnesic for
the episode later. It is most likely to happen
during periods of emotional stress and
usually ceases when the source of anxiety is
removed. In many cases it occurs only once or
twice and does not happen again. If it recurs
frequently (called sleepwalking disorder) it
may stem from serious emotional distress
(see SLEEP DISORDERS). Called also somnambulism.

   s. disorder repeated episodes of sleepwalking.

   slide (slīd) a piece of glass or other
transparent substance on which material is
placed for examination under the microscope.

   sling (sling) a bandage or suspensory for
supporting a part.

   SLO scanning laser ophthalmoscope.

   slough (sluf) 1. a mass of dead tissue in,
or cast out from, living tissue; see also
GANGRENE. 2. to shed or cast off.

   sludge (sluj) a suspension of solid or
semisolid particles in a fluid.

   sludging (sluj′ing) settling out of solid
particles from solution.

   s. of blood intravascular agglutination
of erythrocytes into irregular masses, interfering with circulation of blood.

   slurry (sler′e) a mixture of a liquid,
usually water, and a fine insoluble particulate substance.

   slush (slush) an ice solution with a
consistency like that of snow, used for
preservation.

   Sm samarium.

   small airways disease chronic obstructive bronchitis with irreversible narrowing
of the bronchioles and small bronchi. See
also OBSTRUCTIVE SMALL AIRWAYS DISEASE.

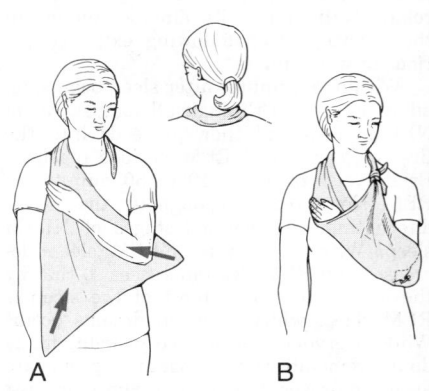

A   B

Applying an arm sling. From Lammon et al., 1995.

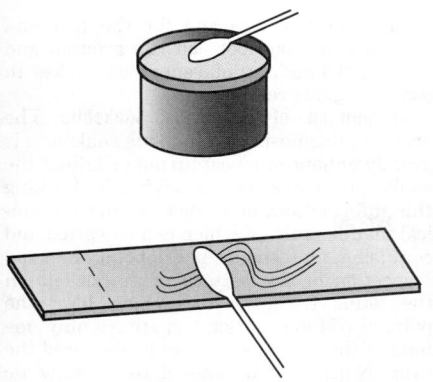

Smears from opaque thick liquids or semisolids, such as stool, can be made using a swab to sample and smear the material. From Mahon and Manuselis, 1995.

smallpox (smawl′poks) a highly contagious, often fatal disease caused by a poxvirus; its most noticeable symptom is the appearance of blisters and pustules on the skin. It formerly occurred in epidemics that killed millions but has now been eradicated throughout the world as a result of a global eradication program by the World Health Organization. Called also variola.

There are now concerns that the smallpox virus could be reintroduced for the purpose of bioterrorism. Because of this, the Centers for Disease Control and Prevention (CDC) has revised and updated its guidelines to help health care providers and public health officials respond to such an event. Information is available on the CDC website: http://www.cdc.gov.

smear (smēr) a specimen for microscopic study, the material being spread thinly and unevenly across the slide with a swab or loop, or with the edge of another slide.

Pap s., Papanicolaou s. see PAPANICOLAOU TEST.

smegma (smeg′mah) the secretion of sebaceous glands, especially the cheesy secretion, consisting principally of desquamated epithelial cells, found chiefly beneath the prepuce. adj., **smegmat′ic.**

smell (smel) the sense that enables one to perceive odors; it depends on the stimulation of sense organs in the nose by small particles carried in inhaled air. It is important not only for the detection of odors, but also for the enjoyment of food, since flavor is a blend of taste and smell. Taste registers only four qualities: salt, sour, bitter, and sweet; other qualities of flavor depend on smell. Called also olfaction.

The organs of smell are small patches of special cells (olfactory CELLS) in the nasal mucosa. One patch is located in each of the two main compartments of the back of the nose. The olfactory cells are connected to the brain by the first CRANIAL NERVE (olfactory nerve). Air currents do not flow directly over the patches in breathing; this is why one must sniff to detect a faint odor or to enjoy a fragrance to the fullest.

When one sniffs, air currents carrying molecules of odorous chemicals enter special compartments, called olfactory chambers, where the chemicals are dissolved in mucus. There they can act on the organs of smell in much the same way that solutions act on the taste buds of the tongue. The endings of the sensory nerves that detect odors, the olfactory receptors, can quickly adapt to an odor and cease to be stimulated by it after a few minutes of full exposure.

The sense of smell may be diminished or lost entirely, usually temporarily, as a result of an obstruction of the nose, nasal infection, injury or deterioration of the nasal tissue, brain tumor, or mental illness. In rare instances, injury or disease causes such damage to the olfactory nerve that loss of the sense of smell is permanent. Complete absence of the sense of smell is known as ANOSMIA.

Smith-Lemli-Opitz syndrome (smith′ lem′le o′pitz) a hereditary syndrome, transmitted as an autosomal recessive trait, characterized by microcephaly, mental retardation, hypotonia, incomplete development of male genitalia, short nose with anteverted nostrils, and syndactyly of the second and third toes.

Smith-Strang disease (smith′ străng) a methionine malabsorption syndrome that results in a characteristic smell of the urine; individuals with this condition have white hair and varying degrees of mental retardation.

smoking (smōk′ing) the act of drawing into the mouth and puffing out the smoke of TOBACCO contained in a cigarette, cigar, or pipe. For centuries, tobacco smoking was suspected of being a health hazard, and now a close relationship between smoking and LUNG CANCER and heart disease has definitely been established. While smoking is not the only cause of these diseases, its relationship to them and also to other diseases has been so strongly established that no smoker can afford to ignore the evidence. Parents especially owe it to their children to educate them in order that the cigarette habit will never begin.

General Effects on Health. Tobacco smoke contains a number of harmful substances, including poisons such as NICOTINE, various irritants, and carcinogenic compounds. Because cigarette smokers usually inhale this smoke, they are much more subject to its harmful effects than pipe and cigar smokers, who generally do not inhale. In pipe and cigar smoking, however, there is some danger to the heart because of the nicotine that is absorbed by the mouth. There is also the possibility of cancer of the lips, tongue, and mouth. Statistically, there is no question that nonsmokers are far less subject to the diseases that affect smokers. Passive smoke, that inhaled by individuals in close proximity to smokers, can also cause respiratory problems.

Among the respiratory diseases closely related to cigarette smoking are lung cancer, cancer of the larynx, chronic BRONCHITIS, and EMPHYSEMA. Coronary artery disease and hypertensive heart disease are also closely related to smoking, as are PEPTIC ULCERS, BUERGER'S DISEASE (THROMBOANGIITIS OBLITERANS), and BLADDER CANCER. Still other diseases are thought to be linked with smoking. The risk of incurring any of these diseases increases with the number of cigarettes smoked daily, the length of each cigarette consumed, and the length of time the smoking habit has persisted. In general, heavy smokers as a group die younger than do nonsmokers.

SMP Society of Medical Psychoanalysts.

Sn tin (L. *stan'num*).

SNA State Nurses Association.

snake (snāk) any of many limbless reptiles; numerous species have venomous bites. See also SNAKEBITE.

   coral s. any of various venomous pit VIPERS of the genera *Micrurus* and *Micruroides;* called also harlequin snake.

   harlequin s. coral snake.

snakebite (snāk'bīt) injury caused by the mouth parts of a snake, usually from VENOM. It is estimated that the worldwide number of deaths from venomous snakebites may be as high as 50,000 annually, with the greatest number being reported in the Indian subcontinent. In North America most poisonous snakes are pit VIPERS (RATTLESNAKES, COPPERHEADS, and water MOCCASINS). A few species of coral SNAKES are found from the southern and southwestern United States southward into Mexico and Central America. Major groups found in other parts of the world include the COBRAS and the ADDERS.

Not many snakebite deaths occur annually in North America; there are far more deaths from hypersensitivity to INSECT BITES AND STINGS. Practices that increase the incidence of snakebites include failure to wear protective covering for the feet and legs, sleeping outdoors on the ground, and the ritual handling of venomous snakes in some religious ceremonies.

Recognition of Venomous Snakebite. The accurate diagnosis of venomous snakebite is greatly enhanced by capturing or killing the snake and correctly identifying it. Lacking this information, one must depend on clinical manifestations, which can be varied and confusing. One should not depend on visual inspection of the pattern of marks left on the skin. Local swelling may blur the pattern of fang marks; sometimes only one fang of the venomous snake has entered the skin. Nonvenomous snakebites usually do not produce much local swelling or pain, and they bleed freely. These symptoms may, however, also occur in some types of venomous snakebites.

Symptoms. In general, venomous snakebites of the type found in the United States produce severe local pain, swelling that spreads from the site of puncture, and involvement of the lymph glands. The patient may experience nausea and vomiting, thirst, sweating, and a low grade fever. If no other symptoms develop, the prognosis is excellent. More serious symptoms indicating poisoning by a NEUROTOXIN include numbness and tingling of the face, hypotension, convulsions, and visual disturbances. If the snake is the type whose venom contains a HEMOTOXIN, the bite may produce hemorrhaging with hemoptysis, hematuria, and increased prothrombin time.

Treatment. There are conflicting opinions among experts as to the value of incisions over the fang marks and suctioning of venom from the wound if this is done outside a medical facility or by someone other than a specially trained health care provider. Some continue to recommend emergency treatment consisting of immediate application of a tourniquet, deep incisions over the fang marks, and suctioning. Others feel that the application of a tourniquet to reduce peripheral circulation and packing the affected part in ice to reduce absorption of the venom is the best first aid treatment. Some, however, do not recommend use of ice. In any case, the victim is kept calm and as physically inactive as possible and is quickly transported to a medical facility where adequate débridement of the wound and mechanical removal and neutralization of the venom can be done. This also minimizes the danger of introducing infectious agents into the wound.

In addition to local wound treatment, which may require skin grafting at a later date, treatment is concerned with administration of an immune serum (ANTI-SERUM or ANTIVENIN), counteraction of the specific pharmacologic effects of the venom, symptomatic relief, and prevention of complications.

Prevention of Snakebite. Most snakebites are inflicted on people who handle snakes or are foolishly careless in areas where there are known to be venomous snakes. Certain common-sense precautions should be taken when visiting such an area. Important facts to keep in mind are that most snakes are active in the early evening, that they often congregate on rocky slopes facing south or west in order to bask in the sunlight (especially in the spring and fall), and that they are not active at temperatures below 10°C (50°F).

snap (snap) a short, sharp sound.

opening s. a short, sharp, high-pitched click occurring in early diastole and caused by opening of the mitral cusps, a characteristic sound in mitral stenosis.

snapper (snap'er) any of various carnivorous marine fish of the family Lutjanidae found in tropical waters; they are often eaten by humans but sometimes contain CIGUATOXIN and can cause CIGUATERA.

snare (snār) a wire loop for removing polyps and other pedunculated growths by cutting them off at the base.

sneeze (snēz) 1. an involuntary, sudden, violent, and audible expulsion of air through the mouth and nose. 2. to expel air in such a manner. Sneezing is usually caused by the irritation of sensitive nerve endings in the mucous membrane that lines the nose. Allergies, drafts of cold air, and even bright light can produce sneezing. Sneezing and coughing are similar in that both are reflex actions and are preceded by quick inhalations, although a cough may also be deliberate, to clear the throat or bronchi. In a sneeze, the glottis is momentarily closed after air is inhaled and the tongue is pressed against the roof of the mouth. When the glottis is suddenly opened, part of the air goes through the nose and, when the tongue is released, part goes through the mouth; in this way mucus and other irritants are expelled from the nose.

SNF skilled nursing facility.

snoring (snor'ing) breathing during sleep accompanied by harsh sounds, occurring when inhaled air causes the soft palate to vibrate. This is common among persons who sleep with their mouths open. Called also stertor.

Although snoring is a sign of sound sleep, it is sometimes desirable to reduce or eliminate it. If the mouth breathing is stopped, the snoring will also stop. An obvious reason for mouth breathing is lying on the back, in which position the mouth tends to hang open. Further, when a person is in deep sleep and lying on the back, the tongue may rest back in the throat, partly blocking the air passage and helping to make the snoring sounds. Gently rolling the snorer onto the side can sometimes eliminate the snoring in these cases.

Snoring may be an indication of obstructive sleep APNEA. Other functional reasons for snoring include a common cold or allergy, causing mucus to stop up the nose. Growths, called polyps, may obstruct the nasal passages. A deformity of the nasal SEPTUM (the bony portion dividing the nasal cavity into two compartments) may make nose breathing difficult. Correction of sleeping habits and of nose or throat troubles may lessen snoring. However, there is little that can be done to change the sleeping habits of an elderly person who has been snoring regularly for many years.

snowblindness (sno'blīnd-nes) temporary loss of sight due to injury to superficial cells of the cornea caused by ULTRAVIOLET RAYS of the sun reinforced by those reflected by snow.

SNP single nucleotide polymorphism.

snuffles (snuf'l'z) catarrhal discharge from the nasal mucous membrane in congenital syphilis in infants.

S$_p$O$_2$ OXYGEN SATURATION measured by pulse oximetry.

SOAP acronym for *s*ubjective data, *o*bjective data, *a*ssessment, *p*lan, the way the progress notes are organized in PROBLEM-ORIENTED RECORD keeping.

soap (sōp) any compound of one or more fatty acids, or their equivalents, with an alkali. Soap is detergent and used as a cleanser.

green s., medicinal s., soft s. a soap made from vegetable oils other than coconut oil or palm kernel oil, potassium hydroxide as an alkali, and glycerin.

social (so'shal) pertaining to societies or other groups of people.

s. anxiety disorder social phobia.

s. breakdown syndrome deterioration of social and interpersonal skills, work habits, and behavior seen in chronically hospitalized psychiatric patients. Symptoms are due to the effects of long term hospitalization rather than the primary illness, and include excessive passivity, assumption of the chronic sick role, withdrawal, and apathy. Such effects are also seen in long term inmates of prisons or concentration camps. Called also institutionalism.

S

s. worker a professional trained in the treatment of psychosocial problems of patients and their families. *Family social workers* practice social case work. *Psychiatric social workers* practice various forms of counseling and group or individual psychotherapy. Most social workers have a master's degree in social work (M.S.W.). There are also bachelor's (B.S.W.) and doctoral (D.S.W.) degrees in social work.

socialization (so″shal-ĭ-za′shun) the process by which society integrates the individual, and the individual learns to behave in socially acceptable ways.

anticipatory s. the learning of expectations for a role prior to placement in a new situation where the role should be assumed.

sociobiology (so″se-o-bi-ol′ah-je) the branch of theoretical biology that proposes that animal (including human) behavior has a biological basis controlled by the genes. adj., **sociobiolog′ical.**

sociologist (so″se-ol′ah-jist) a specialist in sociology.

sociology (so″se-ol′ah-je) the scientific study of social relationships and phenomena.

sociometry (so″se-om′ĕ-tre) the branch of sociology concerned with the measurement of human behavior.

sociopath (so′se-o-path″) former term for a person with an ANTISOCIAL PERSONALITY DISORDER.

sociopathy (so″se-op′ah-the) former term for ANTISOCIAL PERSONALITY DISORDER. adj., **sociopath′ic.**

sociotherapy (so″se-o-ther′ah-pe) any treatment emphasizing socioenvironmental and interpersonal rather than intrapsychic factors.

socket (sok′et) a hollow into which a corresponding part fits.

dry s. a condition sometimes occurring after tooth extraction, particularly after traumatic extraction, resulting in a dry appearance of the exposed bone in the socket, due to disintegration or loss of the blood clot. It is basically a focal osteomyelitis without suppuration and is accompanied by severe pain (ALVEOLALGIA) and foul odor. Called also alveolar osteitis.

soda (so′dah) a term loosely applied to sodium bicarbonate, sodium hydroxide, or sodium carbonate.

baking s. sodium bicarbonate.

sodium (so′de-um) a chemical element, atomic number 11, atomic weight 22.990, symbol Na. (See Appendix 6.) Sodium is the major cation of the extracellular fluid, constituting 90 to 95 per cent of all cations in the blood plasma and interstitial fluid; it

---

WINDOW ON SOCIAL WORKER

Throughout the profession's history, social workers have tried creatively to help people shape and influence their environment, improve their lives, and fulfill their needs and aspirations. Although methods have varied and changed over the years, making change happen is the historical role of social workers. Social work's special contribution rests on a growing body of knowledge and skills pertinent to understanding human relationships and the interaction between people in families, groups, organizations, and communities and their social environments.

Since the social worker must be able to assess strengths and weaknesses in these relationships, the social worker learns and then teaches to others skills in problem-solving, resource identification and utilization, and planned change strategies.

In order to educate social workers who can help resolve problems and social inequities, the Bachelor's Degree in Social Work prepares students for entry-level professional social work practice. Programs leading to the Master of Science degree in Social Work provide the student with the knowledge and advanced skills necessary to assume leadership in the social work profession. The PhD in Social Welfare seeks to develop scholars and educators who will contribute to making social work a more effective profession.

WILLIAM A. HEISS, MSSW

---

thus determines the osmolality of the extracellular fluid. The serum sodium concentration is normally about 140 mEq/L. If the sodium level and osmolality fall, OSMORECEPTORS in the HYPOTHALAMUS are stimulated and cause the release of ANTIDIURETIC HORMONE from the posterior lobe of the PITUITARY GLAND. This hormone increases the absorption of water in the collecting ducts of the kidneys so that water is conserved while sodium and other electrolytes are excreted in the urine. If the sodium level and osmolality rise, neurons in the thirst center of the hypothalamus are stimulated. The thirsty person then drinks enough water to restore the osmolality of the extracellular fluid to the normal level.

A decrease in the serum sodium concentration (HYPONATREMIA) can occur in a variety of conditions. It is often associated with deficient fluid VOLUME due to diarrhea or vomiting when water is replaced faster than sodium. It can also occur in SYNDROME OF INAPPROPRIATE ANTIDIURETIC HORMONE, in the late stages of congestive HEART FAILURE or CIRRHOSIS of the liver, in acute or chronic RENAL FAILURE, and in DIURETIC therapy. An increase in the serum sodium concentration (HYPERNATREMIA) occurs when insensible water loss is not replaced by drinking, as in a comatose patient with diabetes insipidus.

s. acetate a source of sodium ions for HEMODIALYSIS and PERITONEAL DIALYSIS, as well as a systemic and urinary alkalizer.

s. ascorbate an ANTISCORBUTIC vitamin and nutritional supplement for parenteral administration. It is also used as an aid to DEFEROXAMINE therapy in the treatment of chronic iron toxicity.

s. benzoate an antifungal AGENT also used in a test of liver function.

s. bicarbonate $NaHCO_3$, a white powder commonly found in households. It has a wide variety of uses in chemistry, in pharmaceuticals, and in consumer products. It is sometimes taken in water as a remedy for acid indigestion but should not be used regularly since when taken in excess it tends to cause ALKALOSIS. It can be mixed with water and applied as a paste for relief of pain in treatment of minor BURNS and INSECT BITES AND STINGS. A cupful in the bath water may help relieve itching caused by an allergic reaction. Called also baking soda and bicarbonate of soda.

s. biphosphate monobasic sodium phosphate.

s. carbonate a compound now used primarily as an alkalizing agent in pharmaceuticals; it has been used as a lotion or bath in the treatment of scaly skin, and as a detergent.

s. chloride common table salt, a necessary constituent of the body and therefore of the diet, involved in maintaining osmotic tension of blood and tissues; uses include replenishment of electrolytes in the body, irrigation of wounds and body cavities, enema, inhaled mucolytic, topical osmotic ophthalmic agent, and preparation of pharmaceuticals. Called also salt.

s. citrate a sodium salt of citric acid, used as an ANTICOAGULANT for blood or plasma that is to be fractionated or for blood that is to be stored. It is also administered orally as a urinary alkalizer.

dibasic s. phosphate a salt of PHOSPHORIC ACID; used alone or in combination with other phosphate compounds, it is given intravenously as an electrolyte replenisher, orally or rectally as a LAXATIVE, and orally as a urinary acidifier and for prevention of KIDNEY STONES.

s. ferric gluconate a HEMATINIC used especially in treatment of HEMODIALYSIS patients with iron deficiency ANEMIA who are also receiving ERYTHROPOIETIN therapy. Administered by intravenous injection.

s. fluoride a DENTAL CARIES preventative used in FLUORIDATION of drinking water or applied topically to teeth. Topical preparations include gels (sodium fluoride and phosphoric acid gel, also called APF gel) and solutions (sodium fluoride and acidulated phosphate topical solution, also called APF solution).

s. glutamate monosodium glutamate.

s. hydroxide NaOH, a strongly alkaline and caustic compound; used as an alkalizing agent in pharmaceuticals.

s. hypochlorite a compound having germicidal, deodorizing, and bleaching properties; used in solution to disinfect utensils, and in diluted form (Dakin's solution) as a local antibacterial.

s. iodide a compound used as a source of IODINE.

s. lactate a compound used in solution to replenish body fluids and electrolytes.

monobasic s. phosphate 1. a monosodium salt of phosphoric acid; used in buffer solutions, as a urinary acidifier, as a LAXATIVE, and as a source of PHOSPHORUS in hypophosphatemia, often in combination with potassium phosphate. 2. a monosodium salt of phosphoric acid; used in buffer solutions. Used alone or in combination with other phosphate compounds, it is given intravenously as an electrolyte replenisher, orally or rectally as a laxative, and orally as a urinary acidifier and for prevention of KIDNEY STONES.

s. monofluorophosphate a DENTAL CARIES preventative applied topically to the teeth.

s. nitrite an antidote for CYANIDE POISONING; also used as a preservative in cured meats and other foods.

s. nitroprusside an ANTIHYPERTENSIVE AGENT used in the treatment of acute congestive heart failure and of hypertensive crisis and to produce controlled hypotension during surgery; also used as a reagent.

s. phenylbutyrate an agent used as adjunctive treatment to control the HYPERAMMONEMIA of pediatric urea cycle enzyme disorders.

s. phosphate any of various compounds of sodium and phosphoric acid; usually specifically dibasic sodium phosphate.

s. polystyrene sulfonate an ion-exchange RESIN used for removal of potassium ions in HYPERKALEMIA, administered orally or rectally.

s. propionate a salt used as an ANTI-FUNGAL preservative in foods and pharmaceuticals and as a topical antifungal AGENT.

s. salicylate see SALICYLATE.

s. sulfate a CATHARTIC and LAXATIVE.

s. thiosulfate a compound used intravenously as an antidote for CYANIDE POISONING, in foot baths for prophylaxis of RINGWORM, and as a topical antifungal AGENT for TINEA VERSICOLOR. Also used in measuring the volume of extracellular body fluid and the renal glomerular filtration RATE.

sodoku (so'do-koo) a relapsing type of infection due to *Spirillum minus*, an organism transmitted by the bite of an infected rat; a form of RAT-BITE FEVER.

sodomy (sod'ah-me) 1. anal intercourse. 2. old term for any form of HOMOSEXUALITY; sometimes extended to mean any of numerous PARAPHILIAS.

softening (sof'en-ing) a change of consistency, with loss of firmness or hardness; called also malacia.

software (soft'wār) a program written in a computer language telling a computer to perform a given task.

database access s. programs that make it easier to use regular online systems by providing an interface between the user and these systems. This interface can translate a search statement into the command language of the system, and sometimes provide automatic dialing, access, and so on. Called also front end or gateway software.

front end s., gateway s. database access software.

menu driven s. software aided by a menu of choices for commands and formats to be selected by the user.

sol (sol) a colloid system in which the dispersion is liquid or gas; the latter is usually called an AEROSOL.

sol. solution.

solar plexus a network of ganglia and nerves in the center of the abdomen, part of the AUTONOMIC NERVOUS SYSTEM and important in control of function of the liver, stomach, kidneys, and adrenal glands. A blow to it may cause great pain or render a person unconscious, because the organs are momentarily thrown out of gear. Although the plexus recovers quickly from this, its effects on the body as a whole last longer. Called also celiac plexus.

solation (so-la'shun) the conversion of a gel into a sol.

sole (sōl) planta pedis.

solid (sol'id) 1. not fluid or gaseous; not hollow. 2. a substance or tissue not fluid or gaseous.

solubility (sol″u-bil'ĭ-te) the quality of being soluble.

soluble (sol'u-b'l) susceptible of being dissolved.

solute (sol'ūt) the substance that is dissolved in a liquid (solvent) to form a solution.

solution (so-loo'shun) 1. a homogeneous mixture of one or more substances (solutes) dispersed molecularly in a sufficient quantity of dissolving medium (solvent). 2. in pharmacology, a liquid preparation of one or more soluble chemical substances, which are usually dissolved in water. For names of specific solutions, see under the name. 3. the process of dissolving or disrupting. 4. a loosening or separation.

Preparation of Solutions. Formula for preparing solutions from a pure drug:

pure drug : finished solution =
strength of solution
(expressed in percentage or ratio)

For example, to prepare 2000 mL of a 2 per cent solution from boric acid crystals, the proportion would be

$$x \text{ gram} : 2000 \text{ mL} = 2 \text{ g} : 100 \text{ mL}$$
$$x = 40 \text{ g pure drug}$$

Formula for preparing solutions from stock solutions:

lesser amount of stock solution : greater
× amount of stock solution = lesser
× strength : greater strength

For example, to prepare 1000 mL of a 2 per cent solution from a 4 per cent stock solution, the proportion would be

$$x \text{ mL} : 1000 \text{ mL} = 2 \text{ per cent} : 4 \text{ per cent}$$
$$x = 500 \text{ mL stock solution}$$

aqueous s. one in which water is used as the solvent.

BCG s. an aqueous suspension of BACILLE CALMETTE-GUÉRIN for instillation into the bladder to activate the IMMUNE SYSTEM in treatment of superficial bladder cancers. It reduces the risk of a subsequent bladder cancer developing, although the exact mechanism of action is unknown.

buffer s. one that resists appreciable change in its hydrogen ion concentration (pH) when acid or alkali is added to it.

colloid s., colloidal s. imprecise term for COLLOID (def. 3).

hyperbaric s. one having a greater specific gravity than a standard of reference.

hypertonic s. one having an osmotic pressure greater than that of a standard of reference.

hypobaric s. one having a specific gravity less than that of a standard of reference.

hypotonic s. one having an osmotic pressure less than that of a standard of reference.

isobaric s. a solution having the same specific gravity as a standard of reference.

isotonic s. one having an osmotic pressure the same as that of a standard of reference.

molar s. a solution in which each liter contains 1 mole of the dissolved substance; designated 1 M. The concentration of other solutions may be expressed in relation to that of molar solutions as tenth-molar (0.1 M), etc.

normal s. a solution in which each liter contains 1 equivalent weight of the dissolved substance; designated 1 N.

ophthalmic s. a sterile solution, free from foreign particles, for instillation into the eye.

saturated s. one in which the solvent has taken up all of the dissolved substance that it can hold in solution.

sclerosing s. one containing an irritant substance (sclerosing AGENT) that will cause obliteration of a space, as in SCLEROTHERAPY.

standard s. one that contains in each liter a definitely stated amount of reagent; usually expressed in terms of normality (equivalent weights of solute per liter of solution) or molarity (moles of solute per liter of solution).

supersaturated s. an unstable solution containing more of the solute than it can permanently hold.

volumetric s. one that contains a specific quantity of solvent per stated unit of volume.

solvent (sol'vent) 1. capable of dissolving other material. 2. the substance, usually a liquid, in which another substance (the solute) is dissolved to form a solution.

soma (so'mah) 1. the body as distinguished from the mind. 2. the body tissue as distinguished from the germ cells. 3. the cell body. adj., **so'mal, somat'ic.**

somasthenia (so″mas-the'ne-ah) bodily weakness with poor appetite and poor sleep.

somat(o)- word element [Gr.], *body*.

somatalgia (so″mah-tal'jah) bodily pain.

somatesthesia (so″mat-es-the'zhah) cenesthesia.

somatic (so-mat'ik) pertaining to or characteristic of the body (soma).

somatization (so″mah-tĭ-za'shun) in psychiatry, the conversion of mental experiences or states into bodily symptoms.

s. disorder a SOMATOFORM DISORDER characterized by multiple vague, recurring somatic complaints that cannot be fully explained by any known general medical condition or the direct effect of a chemical substance, but are not intentionally feigned

or produced; it usually begins before age 30 and persists for several years. The patient may simply complain of being ill or may have specific symptoms, but the complaints will include a combination of at least multiple pain symptoms, multiple gastrointestinal symptoms, a sexual symptom, and a neurological symptom. Typical complaints include double vision, fainting, abdominal pain, bowel problems, painful menstruation, and sexual indifference. The complaints are often presented in a dramatic and exaggerated manner, but the patient is vague about their exact nature. The patient may visit many health care providers, sometimes several simultaneously, and undergo numerous diagnostic procedures, unnecessary treatments, and even surgery. Most such patients are anxious and depressed and have difficulty in personal relationships; many have traits of HISTRIONIC PERSONALITY DISORDER. They are seldom free of symptoms in spite of frequent medical attention; in fact, the repeated, unnecessary diagnostic procedures or surgery may only add to their suffering. The outlook for these patients is poor. Called also Briquet's syndrome.

somatochrome (so-mat'o-krōm) any neuron which has a well marked cell body completely surrounding the nucleus, its colorable protoplasm having a distinct contour; used also adjectivally.

somatoform (so-mat'-o-form) denoting physical symptoms that can not be attributed to organic disease and appear to be of psychic origin.

s. disorders a group of mental disorders in which physical symptoms suggest the presence of a medical disorder but are not fully explained by a general medical condition, the direct effects of a psychoactive substance, or another mental disorder. Symptoms are not under voluntary control, unlike those occurring in FACTITIOUS DISORDERS. The category includes: BODY DYSMORPHIC DISORDER, CONVERSION DISORDER, HYPOCHONDRIASIS, PAIN DISORDER, SOMATIZATION DISORDER, and UNDIFFERENTIATED SOMATOFORM DISORDER.

s. pain disorder pain disorder.

undifferentiated s. disorder one or more persistent physical complaints, not intentionally produced or feigned, that can not be fully explained by a general medical condition or the direct effects of a substance; this category is the group of persisting disorders that do not completely satisfy the criteria for other somatoform disorders.

somatogenic (so″mah-to-jen'ik) originating in the cells of the body, as a disease process; the term contrasts with PSYCHOGENIC.

S

somatognosis (so″mah-tog-no′sis) cenesthesia.

somatology (so″mah-tol′ah-je) the sum of what is known about the body.

somatomedin (so″mah-to-me′din) any of a group of peptides found in the liver and in other tissues which mediate the effect of growth hormone (somatotropin) on cartilage; they are responsible for uptake of sulfate and increased synthesis of collagen and other proteins by cartilage. Somatomedins also have insulinlike biologic actions and increase RNA synthesis and promote DNA synthesis.

somatometry (so″mah-tom′ĕ-tre) measurement of the dimensions of the entire body.

somatopagus (so″mah-top′ah-gus) conjoined twins united at the trunks.

somatopathy (so″mah-top′ah-the) a bodily disorder rather than a mental one. adj., **somatopath′ic.**

somatoplasm (so-mat′o-plazm) the protoplasm of the body cells exclusive of the germ CELLS.

somatopsychic (so″mah-to-si′kik) pertaining to both mind and body; relating to the effects of the body on the mind.

somatoschisis (so″mah-tos′kĭ-sis) splitting of the bodies of the vertebrae.

somatoscopy (so″mah-tos′kah-pe) examination of the body.

somatosexual (so″mah-to-sek′shoo-al) pertaining to both physical and sex characteristics or to physical manifestations of sexual development.

somatostatin (SRIF, SS) (so″mah-to-stat′-in) a cyclic tetradecapeptide hormone and neurotransmitter that inhibits the release of peptide hormones in many tissues. It is released by the hypothalamus to inhibit the release of growth hormone (GH, somatotropin) and thyroid stimulating hormone (TSH) from the anterior pituitary; it is also released by the delta cells of the islets of Langerhans in the pancreas to inhibit the release of glucagon and insulin and by the similar D cells in the gastrointestinal tract.

somatostatinoma (so″mah-to-stat″ĭ-no′-mah) a rare SOMATOSTATIN-secreting tumor occurring primarily in the head of the pancreas and in the upper small intestine, associated with diabetes mellitus and gallbladder disease.

somatotherapy (so″mah-to-ther′ah-pe) biological treatment of mental disorders, such as by drug or electric shock therapy.

somatotonia (so″mah-to-to′ne-ah) a temperament type characterized by love of physical adventure, boundless energy, boldness, aggressiveness, and need for exercise

and activity; the behavior counterpart of MESOMORPHY.

somatotopic (so″mah-to-top′ik) related to particular areas of the body; describing the organization of the motor area of the brain, specific regions of the cortex being responsible for the motor control of different areas of the body.

somatotrope (so-mat′o-trōp) somatotroph.

somatotroph (so-mat′o-trof″) a type of ACIDOPHIL of the adenohypophysis that secretes growth HORMONE.

somatotrophin (so′mah-to-tro″fin) growth hormone. adj., **somatotroph′ic.**

somatotropin (so′mah-to-tro″pin) growth hormone. adj., **somatotro′pic.**

somatotype (so-mat′o-tīp) a particular type of body build.

somatotyping (so-mat″o-tīp′ing) objective classification of individuals according to type of body build.

somatrem (so′mah-trem) a biosynthetic pharmaceutical preparation of human growth hormone, prepared by recombinant technology and differing from the natural human hormone in containing an additional methionine residue at one end. It is used to treat growth failure and AIDS-associated cachexia or weight loss, administered intramuscularly or subcutaneously.

somatropin (so″mah-tro′pin) a pharmaceutical preparation of growth hormone, having the same amino acid sequence as the natural hormone. Originally derived from cadaver pituitary glands, the human form is now biosynthetic, prepared by recombinant means. It is used to treat growth failure and AIDS-associated cachexia or weight loss, administered intramuscularly or subcutaneously.

somesthesia (so″mes-the′zhah) cenesthesia.

SOMI sternal-occipital-mandibular immobilizer.

somite (so′mīt) one of the paired segments along the neural tube of a vertebrate embryo, formed by transverse subdivision of the thickened mesoderm next to the midplane, that develop into the vertebral column and muscles of the body.

somnambulism (som-nam′bu-lizm) sleepwalking.

somnifacient (som″nĭ-fa′shent) 1. hypnotic (def. 1). 2. hypnotic (def. 2).

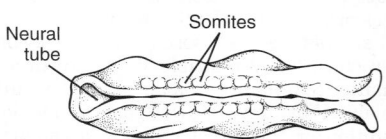

Somites in a 22-day embryo. From Dorland's, 2000.

somniferous (som-nif´er-us) hypnotic (def. 1).

somniloquism (som-nil´o-kwizm) talking in one's sleep.

somnolence (som´no-lens) drowsiness or sleepiness, particularly in excess.

somnolentia (som″no-len´shah) 1. incomplete sleep; drowsiness. 2. sleep drunkenness.

Somogyi effect (phenomenon) (so-mo´gee) a rebound phenomenon occurring in DIABETES MELLITUS; overtreatment with INSULIN induces HYPOGLYCEMIA, which initiates the release of epinephrine, ACTH, glucagon, and growth hormone, which stimulate lipolysis, gluconeogenesis, and glycogenolysis, which, in turn, result in rebound hyperglycemia and ketosis.

Indications that the Somogyi effect may be taking place include the following: (1) the appearance of strongly positive tests for sugar and acetone in the urine within a few hours after a period in which the urine had been negative for both tests, (2) a 2 per cent glycosuria all day preceded by nocturnal sweating, headaches, and other symptoms of hypoglycemia, (3) unresponsiveness of insulin during the period of rebound hyperglycosuria, (4) wide fluctuations in blood glucose levels, over several hours, and unrelated to meals, and (5) improved control of blood sugar levels and ketonuria with gradual reduction in the amount of insulin taken. Treatment consists of gradual reduction of the insulin dose until the optimum dose is reached.

sonicate (son´ĭ-kāt) 1. to expose to sound waves; to disrupt bacteria by exposure to high-frequency sound waves. 2. the products of such disruption.

sonication (son″ĭ-ka´shun) exposure to sound waves; disruption of bacteria by exposure to high-frequency sound waves.

sonogram (son´o-gram) a record or display obtained by ultrasonic scanning.

sonography (so-nog´rah-fe) ultrasonography. adj., **sonograph´ic.**

sonolucent (son″o-loo´sent) in ULTRASONOGRAPHY, permitting passage of ultrasound waves without reflecting them back to their source (without giving off echoes).

sonorous (sah-no´rus, son´ah-rus) resonant; sounding.

Sonata (so-nah´tah) trademark for a preparation of ZALEPLON, used to treat INSOMNIA.

sopor (so´por) [L.] unnaturally deep or profound sleep.

soporific (sop″o-rif´ik, so″po-rif´ik) 1. producing deep sleep. 2. hypnotic (def. 2).

soporous (so´por-us) associated with coma or deep sleep.

sorb (sorb) to attract and retain substances by absorption or adsorption.

sorbefacient (sor″bĕ-fa´shent) absorbefacient.

sorbic acid (sor´bik) an agent that inhibits growth of yeasts and molds and is used as an antimicrobial preservative.

sorbitol (sor´bĭ-tol) a six-carbon sugar alcohol from a variety of fruits, found in lens deposits in DIABETES MELLITUS. A pharmaceutical preparation is used as a sweetening agent and osmotic LAXATIVE, and in drugs as a tablet EXCIPIENT, moistening agent, and stabilizer.

Sorbitrate (sor´bĭ-trāt) trademark for preparations of ISOSORBIDE dinitrate, a coronary VASODILATOR.

sordes (sor´dēz) foul matter collected on the lips and teeth in low fevers, consisting of food, microorganisms, and epithelial elements.

s. gas´tricae undigested food, mucus, and other substances in the stomach.

sore (sor) a popular term for any lesion of the skin or mucous membrane.

bed s. popular term for PRESSURE ULCER.

canker s. recurrent aphthous stomatitis.

cold s's herpes febrilis.

desert s. a form of tropical phagedenic ULCER seen in desert areas of Africa, Australia, and the Middle East.

pressure s. pressure ulcer.

sore throat (sor thrōt) 1. inflammation of the THROAT; called also faucitis. 2. pharyngitis.

clergyman's s. t. loss of the voice from overuse, as by clergymen; called also dysphonia clericorum.

streptococcal s. t. a sore throat caused by a streptococcus; see also STREPTOCOCCAL SORE THROAT.

sorption (sorp´shun) the process or state of being sorbed; absorption or adsorption.

sorting test (sort´ing) a type of test for assessing abstract thinking; the patient must arrange objects or cards into groups based on some abstract relationship. Schizophrenics and patients with cortical lesions show impaired performance.

S.O.S. [L.] si o´pus sit (if necessary).

sotalol (so´tah-lol) a non-cardioselective BETA-ADRENERGIC BLOCKING AGENT, used as the hydrochloride salt in treatment of life-threatening ventricular ARRHYTHMIAS.

Sotos syndrome (so´tōs) cerebral GIGANTISM.

souffle (soo´f'l) a soft, blowing auscultatory sound.

cardiac s. any heart murmur of a blowing quality.

funic s., funicular s. a hissing souffle synchronous with fetal heart sounds, probably from the umbilical cord.

S

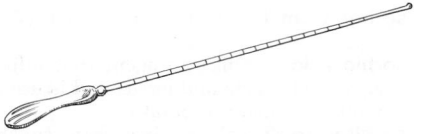

Sound. From Dorland's, 2000.

placental s. a souffle supposed to be produced by the blood current in the placenta; called also placental bruit.

uterine s. a sound made by the blood within the arteries of the gravid uterus.

sound (sownd) 1. a slender instrument to be introduced into body passages or cavities, especially for the dilatation of strictures or detection of foreign bodies. 2. the sensation resulting from stimulation of the ear by vibrations of air or some other elastic medium with a frequency between 20 and 20,000 Hz. 3. a noise, normal or abnormal, heard within the body; see also under BRUIT, FREMITUS, MURMUR, and RALE.

adventitious s's abnormal auscultatory sounds heard over the lungs, such as RALES, RHONCHI, or any of the abnormal types of RESONANCE; they are usually characterized as either *continuous* or *discontinuous sounds*. See also breath SOUNDS.

auscultatory s's sounds heard on AUSCULTATION, such as HEART SOUNDS, breath SOUNDS, adventitious SOUNDS, and Korotkoff SOUNDS.

bowel s's high-pitched abdominal sounds caused by propulsion of the contents of the intestines; see also BOWEL SOUNDS.

breath s's the sounds of air moving through the tracheobronchial tree, heard during auscultation of the chest. There are four main types: *bronchial breath sounds* are high-pitched ones heard normally over the manubrium sterni but indicative of consolidation or compression when heard elsewhere; *bronchovesicular breath sounds* are intermediate between bronchial and vesicular and are normal on certain peripheral parts of the thorax but indicative of partial consolidation if heard over a lung; *cavernous breath sounds* are abnormal ones with a hollow resonance heard over a cavity in a lung; and *vesicular breath sounds* are low-pitched ones heard over the normal lung during ventilation. Called also respiratory sounds.

continuous s's adventitious SOUNDS that last longer than 0.2 sec; they include WHEEZES and RHONCHI.

discontinuous s's adventitious SOUNDS that last less than 0.2 sec and come in a series; the most common kind are RALES (CRACKLES).

ejection s's high-pitched clicking sounds heard in septal defects just after the first HEART SOUND, attributed to sudden distention of a dilated pulmonary artery or aorta or to forceful opening of the pulmonic or aortic cusps.

friction s. friction rub.

heart s's see HEART SOUNDS.

Korotkoff s's sounds heard during auscultatory determination of BLOOD PRESSURE, thought to be produced by vibratory motion of the arterial wall as the artery suddenly distends when compressed by a pneumatic blood pressure cuff. Origin of the sound may be within the blood passing through the vessel or within the wall itself.

percussion s. any sound obtained by PERCUSSION.

physiological s's those heard when an external acoustic meatus is plugged, caused by the rush of blood through blood vessels in or near the inner ear and by adjacent muscles in continuous low-frequency vibration.

respiratory s's breath sounds.

succussion s's splashing sounds heard on SUCCUSSION over a distended stomach or in HYDROPNEUMOTHORAX.

to-and-fro s. to-and-fro MURMUR.

urethral s. a long, slender instrument for exploring and dilating the urethra.

voice s's auscultatory SOUNDS heard over the lungs or airways when the patient speaks; increased resonance indicates CONSOLIDATION or EFFUSION. Types include BRONCHOPHONY, EGOPHONY, LARYNGOPHONY, and TRACHEOPHONY.

white s. that produced by a mixture of all frequencies of mechanical vibration perceptible as sound.

space (spās) 1. a delimited area. 2. an actual or potential cavity of the body. 3. the areas of the universe beyond the earth and its atmosphere. adj., **spa′tial.**

danger s. a subdivision of the retropharyngeal space, extending from the base of the skull to the level of the diaphragm; so called because it provides a route by which infection of the pharynx can spread to the mediastinum.

dead s. see DEAD SPACE.

epidural s. the space between the dura mater and the lining of the spinal canal.

intercostal s. the space between two adjacent ribs.

interpleural s. mediastinum.

interproximal s., interproximate s. the space between the proximal SURFACES of adjoining teeth; called also proximal or proximate space.

intervillous s. the space of the placenta into which the chorionic villi project and through which the maternal blood circulates.

lymph s's open spaces filled with lymph in connective or other tissue, especially in the brain and meninges.

Meckel's s. a recess in the dura mater that lodges the trigeminal ganglion.

mediastinal s. mediastinum.

medullary s. the central cavity and the intervals between the trabeculae of bone that contain the marrow.

palmar s. a large fascial space in the hand, divided by a fibrous septum into a midpalmar and a thenar space.

parasinoidal s's spaces in the dura mater along the superior sagittal sinus which receive the venous blood.

perivascular s. a lymph space within the walls of an artery.

plantar s. a fascial space on the sole of the foot, divided by septa into the lateral, middle, and median plantar spaces.

pneumatic s. a portion of bone occupied by air-containing cells, especially the spaces constituting the paranasal sinuses.

proximal s., proximate s. interproximal space.

retroperitoneal s. the space between the peritoneum and the posterior abdominal wall.

retropharyngeal s. the space behind the pharynx, containing areolar tissue.

subarachnoid s. the space between the arachnoid and the pia mater, containing cerebrospinal fluid.

subdural s. a narrow fluid-containing space, often only a potential space, between the dura mater and the arachnoid.

subphrenic s. the space between the diaphragm and underlying organs.

subumbilical s. somewhat triangular space in the body cavity beneath the umbilicus.

Tenon's s. a lymph space between the sclera and Tenon's capsule.

sparfloxacin (spahr-flok'sah-sin) a synthetic, broad-spectrum antimicrobial agent.

spargana (spahr'gah-nah) plural of SPARGANUM.

sparganosis (spahr"gah-no'sis) infection with SPARGANA, which invade the subcutaneous tissues, causing inflammation and fibrosis. If the lymphatics are involved, ELEPHANTIASIS results.

sparganum (spahr'gah-num) [Gr.] a migrating larva of a TAPEWORM; see also SPARGANOSIS.

spasm (spazm) 1. a sudden involuntary contraction of a muscle or group of muscles. 2. a sudden, transitory constriction of a passage, canal, or orifice; spasms usually occur when the nerves supplying muscles are irritated, and are often accompanied by pain. A VASOSPASM is a rare type that occurs in

a blood vessel. Spasms vary from mild twitches to severe CONVULSIONS and may be the symptoms of any number of disorders. Usually, they will cease when the cause is corrected, but sometimes the only treatment is to suppress the symptoms, as in EPILEPSY.

Clonic Spasms. These are spasms in which contraction and relaxation of the muscle alternate; this is the most common type of spasm and usually is not severe. A typical clonic spasm is the HICCUP. Hiccups usually occur when the diaphragm is irritated, as by indigestion, although occasionally they may result from a serious condition such as a brain tumor; they generally disappear by themselves or after a drink of water.

Spasms may be repetitive twitching motions, some of which are called TICS. Tics often accompany other types of spasm, as in such diseases as CEREBRAL PALSY and SYDENHAM'S CHOREA, and may also be seen in neuralgia. In TIC DOULOUREUX the nerves of the face are involved.

Habit spasms are a type of repetitive twitching movements that seem purposeless or without a cause; they include twitching of the face, blinking of the eyes, and grimacing. The movements are rapid and always repeated in the same way, unlike the spasms associated with chorea. The motions are carried out automatically in response to a stimulus that once may have existed but no longer does.

In a *convulsive spasm* the entire body is jerked by sudden violent movements that may involve almost all the muscles. These spasms may last from a fraction of a second to several seconds, or even minutes. (See also CONVULSION.)

Tonic Spasms. If the contraction of a spasm is sustained or continuing, it is called a *tonic* or *tetanic spasm*. These are generally severe because they are caused by diseases that affect the central nervous system or brain, such as TETANUS, RABIES, and CEREBRAL PALSY. Severe tonic spasms can be fatal if not treated promptly; continued spasms can bring on exhaustion or asphyxiation. The treatment varies with the cause; if the disease is caused by a microorganism in the system, as in tetanus, antiserum must be administered immediately. Antibiotics are also used to help curb infection. In many cases tranquilizers, sedatives, and narcotics must be administered to help ease the spasms.

bronchial s. spasmodic contraction of the muscular coat of the smaller divisions of the bronchi, as occurs in ASTHMA; called also bronchospasm.

S

clonic s. a spasm consisting of clonic contractions; see also CLONUS.

infantile s's, infantile massive s's, jackknife s's a syndrome of severe MYOCLONUS appearing in the first 18 months of life, and associated with general cerebral deterioration; it is marked by severe flexion spasms of the head, neck, and trunk and extension of the arms and legs. Called also jackknife seizures.

nodding s. clonic spasm of the sternomastoid muscles, causing a nodding motion of the head.

saltatory s. clonic spasms of the muscles of the lower limbs, producing a peculiar jumping or springing action.

tetanic s., tonic s. physiological TETANUS.

spasmodic (spaz-mod′ik) of the nature of a spasm; occurring in spasms.

spasmolysis (spaz-mol′ĭ-sis) the arrest of spasm.

spasmolytic (spaz″mo-lit′ik) 1. arresting or checking spasms. 2. antispasmodic.

spasmophilia (spaz″mo-fil′e-ah) abnormal tendency to convulsions; abnormal sensitivity of motor nerves to stimulation with a resultant tendency to spasm.

spasmus (spaz′mus) [L.] spasm.

s. nu′tans nodding spasm.

spastic (spas′tik) characterized by SPASMS, or tightening of the muscles, causing stiff and awkward movements and in some cases a scissors-like gait. The term is sometimes used to describe a person suffering from CEREBRAL PALSY.

spasticity (spas-tis′ĭ-te) continuous resistance to stretching by a muscle due to abnormally increased tension, with heightened deep tendon reflexes.

clasp-knife s. clasp-knife rigidity.

spatial (spa′shal) pertaining to space.

spatium (spa′she-um) [L.] space.

spatula (spach′u-lah) a wide, flat, blunt, usually flexible instrument of little thickness, used for spreading material on a smooth surface or mixing.

spatulate (spach′ŭ-lāt) 1. having a flat blunt end. 2. to mix or manipulate with a spatula.

spatulation (spach″u-la′shun) the combining of materials into a homogeneous mixture by continuously heaping them together and smoothing the mass out on a smooth surface with a spatula.

spay (spa) to castrate a female animal, usually by OOPHOROHYSTERECTOMY.

SPCA serum prothrombin conversion accelerator (factor VII, one of the COAGULATION FACTORS).

specialist (spesh′ah-list) a health care professional whose practice is limited to a particular area, such as a branch of medicine, surgery, or nursing; especially, one who by virtue of advanced training is certified by a specialty board as being qualified to so limit his or her practice.

clinical nurse s. a clinician with a high degree of knowledge, skill, and competence in a specific area of nursing. See clinical NURSE SPECIALIST.

transcultural nurse s. transcultural NURSE SPECIALIST.

specialty (spesh′al-te) the field of practice of a specialist.

species (spe′shēz) a taxonomic category subordinate to a genus (or subgenus) and superior to a subspecies or variety; composed of individuals similar in certain morphologic and physiologic characteristics.

type s. the original species from which the description of the genus is formulated.

species-specific (spe′shēz-spē-sif′ik) characteristic of a particular species; having a characteristic effect on, or interaction with, cells or tissues of members of a particular species; said of an antigen, drug, or infective agent.

specific (spē-sif′ik) 1. pertaining to a species. 2. produced by a single kind of microorganism. 3. restricted to a particular structure or function, such as in application or effect. 4. a remedy specially indicated for a particular disease. 5. in immunology, pertaining to the special affinity of antigen for the corresponding antibody.

s. gravity the weight of a substance compared with the weight of an equal amount of some other substance taken as a standard. For liquids the usual standard is water. The specific gravity of water is 1; if a sample of urine shows a specific gravity of 1.025, this means that the urine is 1.025 times heavier than water. (The normal specific gravity of urine is 1.003–1.030.) Specific gravity is measured by means of a hydrometer.

specificity (spes″ĭ-fis′ĭ-te) 1. the quality of having a certain action, as of affecting only certain organisms or tissues, or reacting only with certain substances, as antibodies with certain antigens (antigen specificity). 2. diagnostic specificity; the probability that a person not having a disease will be correctly identified by a clinical test, i.e., the number of true negative results divided by the total number of all those without the disease (which is the sum of the number of true negative plus false positive results). See also SENSITIVITY.

host s. the natural adaptability of a particular parasite to a certain species or group of hosts.

specimen (spes'ĭ-men) a small sample or part taken to show the nature of the whole, such as a small quantity of urine for URINALYSIS or a small fragment of tissue for microscopic study.

clean-catch s., clean-voided s. a urine specimen obtained after the external urethral area is washed with a liquid soap and rinsed well; then the patient starts a urinary stream, stops it, and voids into a sterile specimen container. The purpose of obtaining such a specimen is to minimize contamination by external organisms. Called also midstream specimen.

midstream s. clean-catch specimen.

sputum s. a sample of mucous secretion from the bronchi and lungs; see also SPUTUM SPECIMEN.

spectacles (spek'tah-k'lz) glasses.

spectinomycin (spek″tĭ-no-mi'sin) an ANTIBIOTIC derived from *Streptomyces spectabilis,* used as the hydrochloride salt in treatment of GONORRHEA.

spectr(o)- word element [L.], *spectrum, image.*

spectra (spek'trah) [L.] plural of SPECTRUM.

spectrin (spek'trin) a contractile protein attached to glycophorin at the cytoplasmic surface of the cell membrane of erythrocytes, important in maintenance of cell shape.

Spectrobid (spek'tro-bid) trademark for a preparation of BACAMPICILLIN, an antibacterial.

spectrometry (spek-trom'ĕ-tre) determination of the place of lines in a spectrum.

spectrophotometer (spek″tro-fo-tom'ĕ-ter) 1. an apparatus for measuring light sense by means of a spectrum. 2. an apparatus for determining the quantity of coloring matter in a solution by measurement of transmitted light. See also *colorimeter.*

spectrophotometry (spek″tro-fo-tom'ĕ-tre) the use of the spectrophotometer.

spectroscope (spek'trah-skōp) an instrument for developing and analyzing the spectrum of a substance. adj., **spectroscop′ic.**

spectroscopy (spek-tros'kah-pe) examination by means of a spectroscope.

spectrum (spek'trum) [L.] 1. the series of images resulting from the refraction of electromagnetic radiation (e.g., light, x-rays) and their arrangement according to frequency or wavelength. 2. range of activity, as of an antibiotic, or of manifestations, as of a disease. adj., **spec′tral.**

absorption s. one obtained by passing radiation with a continuous spectrum through a selectively absorbing medium.

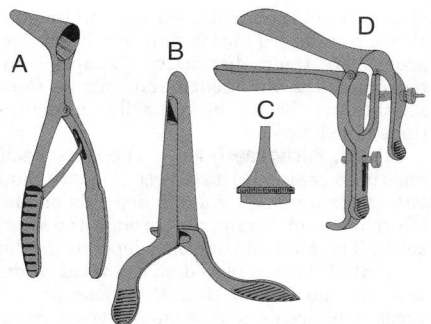

Speculums: *A,* nasal; *B,* rectal; *C,* ear (for otoscope); *D,* vaginal.

broad-s. effective against a wide range of microorganisms.

visible s. that portion of the range of wavelengths of electromagnetic vibrations (from 770 to 390 nanometers) which is capable of stimulating specialized sense organs and is perceptible as light.

speculum (spek'u-lum) an instrument for opening or distending a body orifice or cavity to permit visual inspection. See illustration.

speech (spēch) the utterance of vocal sounds conveying ideas; the faculty of conveying thoughts and ideas by vocal sounds. The process is controlled through motor speech AREAS located in the frontal lobe of the brain.

The Mechanics of Speech. The voice originates in the LARYNX, which is in the upper end of the air passage to the lungs and is behind the thyroid cartilage. The larynx, in cooperation with the mouth, throat, trachea, and lungs, works on the same principle as musical instruments such as organs and oboes, in which air is forced over a thin reed to produce sound. The VOCAL CORDS, two reedlike bands, are attached at one end to the wall of the larynx behind the laryngeal PROMINENCE or "Adam's apple"; the other ends are attached to movable cartilages. When the voice is not being used, muscles move these cartilages outward and hold the vocal cords against the sides of the larynx so that breathing is not obstructed. When a person starts to speak, sing, grunt, or shout, the ends of the vocal cords connected to the cartilages are brought across the larynx, so that they partly obstruct it. As air is forced through, the cords vibrate, producing sound waves, which are what is known as the VOICE. In speaking, the size and shape of the mouth and pharynx are varied as the sound goes through, by means

S

of muscles of the mouth, throat, and tongue. Vowel sounds are initiated in the throat and are given their distinctive "shapes" by movements of the mouth and tongue. Consonants are formed by controlled interruptions of exhaled air.

Volume, Pitch, and Timbre. The voice itself has three characteristics: VOLUME, PITCH, and TIMBRE (or quality). Volume depends on the effort made in forcing air through the vocal cords. The pitch of the voice depends on the amount of tension placed on the vocal cords, and on the length and thickness of the cords. Children's and women's vocal cords are short, giving them higher-pitched voices. A man's are longer and thicker and his voice is deeper. Timbre is affected by the size and shape of the individual's various resonating chambers (mouth, pharynx, chest, and others) and the way they are used. Bones in the head and chest also contribute to the quality of a voice. By long training in the use of the voice, singers are able to alter and control the mouth, throat, and chest cavities to produce a wide range of harmonics or overtones.

Speech Defects. Over 100 muscles are involved in the utterance of a simple word, and the construction of a simple sentence is a feat so complicated that it is beyond the capacity of any animal except the human being. The process of learning to talk is obviously a difficult task for children, and it is not surprising that 5 to 7 per cent of children reach adulthood with a serious speech disorder.

The baby learns to make specific sounds with the voice by babbling and cooing. Gradually he or she becomes able, more or less unconsciously, to put these sounds together to form intelligible speech in imitation of parents and other speakers in the environment. This complicated process is sometimes disturbed if the child has congenital physical defects, illness, or psychologic difficulties. As a result, speech disorders may occur.

Congenital Causes. Prominent among the congenital defects that may cause speech problems are CLEFT LIP and CLEFT PALATE. These abnormalities are evident at birth and should be corrected by surgery at an early age. Another congenital defect is ANKYLOGLOSSIA (TONGUE-TIE), abnormal shortness of the FRENULUM OF THE TONGUE. This condition, which if uncorrected may cause lisping and other awkwardness, is easily corrected by surgical cutting of the frenulum as soon as the difficulty becomes evident. Congenital DEAFNESS will prevent a child from learning to speak in the usual way and may result in MUTISM. However, if the speech mechanism are normal, the child can be taught to speak by a speech therapist. Malformations of th nasal passages, larynx, or other parts o the voice-producing tract may cause odditie in the sound of the voice. Such defects als can be corrected in many cases by mino surgery.

Other Causes. By the age of 5 or 6 years mos children have mastered the basic art o talking. Serious difficulties that persist o appear for the first time after this age, an that are not due to congenital defects, ar likely to arise from illness, injury, or psychologic disturbance. Damage to speec centers of the brain by MULTIPLE SCLEROSIS SYPHILIS, or PARKINSON'S DISEASE, for example may cause speech to be singsong, explosive mechanical, or slurred. In such instance improvement of speech follows treatment o the basic disorder. Poor alignment of th front teeth also may interfere with prope speech. Speech defects of psychologic rathe than physiologic origin include STAMMERIN and STUTTERING.

s. disorder defective ability to speak; i may be either psychogenic or neurogenic. Se also APHASIA, APHONIA, DYSPHASIA, an DYSPHONIA. Called also lalopathy and logopa thy.

esophageal s. speech produced by ex pelling swallowed air across one or mor constrictions in the pharyngoesophagea segment; used after LARYNGECTOMY.

explosive s. loud, sudden enunciation occurring in certain brain diseases.

mirror s. speech in which the order o syllables is reversed.

pressured s. logorrhea.

scanning s. speech in which syllable are separated by pauses.

telegraphic s. speech consisting of onl certain prominent words, without other such as modifiers; it is typical of childre around age two but in older persons it is form of AGRAMMATISM.

speech-language pathologist a profes sional trained to identify, assess, and reha bilitate persons with speech or languag disorders such as articulation problems language problems (e.g., aphasia, delaye language development), voice problems, o stuttering problems.

sperm (sperm) 1. the SEMEN or testicula secretion. 2. spermatozoon.

sperm(o)- word element [Gr.], *seed sperm.*

spermat(o)- word element [Gr.], *seed sperm.*

spermatic (sper-mat'ik) pertaining to the spermatozoa or to semen.

WINDOW ON SPEECH-LANGUAGE PATHOLOGY

It is commonly misassumed that good communication just happens. But there are many things that can interfere with naturally occurring, taken for granted, communication. As a result of these interferences, individuals can exhibit different types of speech, voice, language, or fluency problems that require diagnosis and remediation from a professional speech-language pathologist. For these individuals, good communication doesn't just happen, it needs special attention.

The professional discipline of speech-language pathology specializes in diagnosing and remediating communication difficulties. This professional field draws from a variety of conceptual frameworks. Speech-language pathologists may use biological frameworks when diagnosing and treating physical aspects of communication disabilities. They may use a linguistics framework when identifying and treating language-based disabilities and when differentiating normal language differences from those that require language therapy. They work within psychological frameworks when examining or treating memory, attention, or other psychological processes affecting communication. And they use social frameworks to analyze and facilitate individuals' integration into their social communities.

Speech-language pathologists collaborate with other professionals in a variety of employment settings. Some work in medical settings such as hospitals or medical clinics. Others work in agencies such as speech and hearing centers, day care centers, or nursing homes. Most work in public school settings where they provide services in separate facilities ("the speech room") or in the children's classroom. Speech-language pathologists are often on collaborative teams working to develop school inclusion programs for children with special communication needs.

In order to be a speech-language pathologist in America, professionals need to have a master's or doctoral degree from a university department specializing in communications disorders. They must also have a Certificate of Clinical Competence from the American Speech-Language-Hearing Association (www.asha.org). Many states in the US also require a state license to practice as a speech-language pathologist. Speech-language pathologists can now obtain specialty status from the American Speech-Language-Hearing Association in fields of neurogenic speech disorders (e.g., dysarthria, swallowing), fluency disorders (stuttering), and childhood language disorders (e.g., phonology, syntax, discourse).

JUDITH FELSON DUCHAN, CCC, PHD

spermatid (sper'mah-tid) a cell produced by meiotic division of a secondary spermatocyte; it develops into the spermatozoon.

spermatitis (sper″mah-ti'tis) inflammation of a vas deferens; deferentitis.

spermatoblast (sper-mat'o-blast) spermatid.

spermatocele (sper-mat'o-sēl) a cystic distention of the epididymis or rete testis, containing spermatozoa.

spermatocelectomy (sper″mah-to-se-lek'-tah-me) excision of a spermatocele.

spermatocyst (sper-mat'o-sist) spermatocele.

spermatocystectomy (sper″mah-to-sis-tek'tah-me) excision of a seminal vesicle.

spermatocystitis (sper″mah-to-sis-ti'tis) inflammation of a seminal vesicle.

spermatocystotomy (sper″mah-to-sis-tot'ah-me) incision of a seminal vesicle, for the purpose of drainage.

spermatocyte (sper-mat'o-sīt) the mother cell of a spermatid.

primary s. the original large diploid cell into which a SPERMATOGONIUM develops; it can later undergo the first meiotic division into the secondary spermatocyte.

secondary s. a haploid cell produced by meiotic division of the primary spermatocyte; it can then develop into the SPERMATID.

spermatocytogenesis (sper″mah-to-si″-to-jen'ĕ-sis) the first stage of formation of SPERMATOZOA, in which the SPERMATOGONIA develop into SPERMATOCYTES and then into SPERMATIDS.

spermatogenesis (sper″mah-to-jen'ĕ-sis) the development of mature spermatozoa from spermatogonia; it includes SPERMATOCYTOGENESIS and SPERMIOGENESIS.

spermatogenic (sper″mah-to-jen'ik) giving rise to sperm.

spermatogonium (sper″mah-to-go'ne-um) [Gr.] an undifferentiated male germ CELL, originating in a seminal tubule and dividing into two SPERMATOCYTES.

spermatoid (sper'mah-toid) resembling spermatozoa.

S

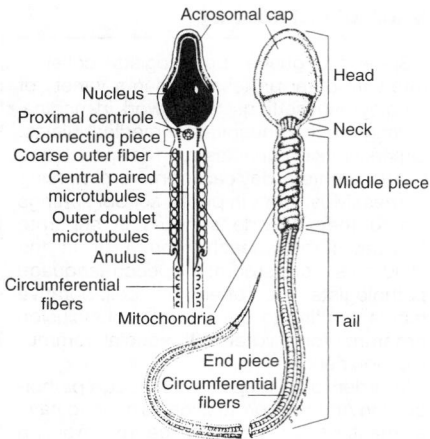

Human spermatozoon: side view (in cross-section) and flat view.

spermatolysis (sper″mah-tol′ĭ-sis) dissolution of spermatozoa. adj., **spermatolyt′ic.**

spermatopathia (sper″mah-to-path′e-ah) abnormality of the semen.

spermatorrhea (sper″mah-to-re′ah) old term for EMISSION (def. 2).

spermatozoon (sper″mah-to-zo′on), pl. *spermatozo′a* [Gr.] a mature male germ CELL, the specific output of the testes, which fertilizes the mature OVUM (secondary OOCYTE) in sexual REPRODUCTION. It is microscopic in size, looks like a translucent tadpole, and has a flat elliptical head containing a spherical center section, and a long tail by which it propels itself with a vigorous lashing movement. Spermatozoa are produced in the seminiferous tubules of the testes. The developmental stages of the germ cell are the SPERMATOGONIUM, SPERMATOCYTE, SPERMATID, and finally spermatozoon. When mature, the spermatozoa are carried in the SEMEN. At the climax of coitus, the semen is discharged into the vagina of the female. A single discharge (about a teaspoonful of semen on the average) may contain more than 250 million spermatozoa. Only a few of these will travel as far as the fallopian tubes; if an ovum is present there, and if the head of a single sperm penetrates the ovum, FERTILIZATION takes place. adj., **spermatozo′al.**

spermaturia (sper″mah-tu′re-ah) seminuria.

spermectomy (sper-mek′tah-me) excision of part of the spermatic cord.

spermicide (sper′mĭ-sīd) an agent destructive to spermatozoa. adj., **spermici′dal.**

spermidine (sper′mĭ-dēn) a polyamine first found in human semen but now known to occur in almost all tissues, in association with nucleic acids.

spermiduct (sper′mĭ-dukt) the ejaculatory duct and vas deferens together.

spermine (sper′mēn) a polyamine first found in human semen but now known to occur in almost all tissues, in association with nucleic acids.

spermiogenesis (sper″me-o-jen′ĕ-sis) the second stage in the formation of SPERMATOZOA, in which the SPERMATIDS transform into SPERMATOZOA.

spermotoxin (sper″mo-tok″sin) 1. a toxin destructive to spermatozoa; see also *spermicide.* 2. especially, a cytotoxic antibody produced by injecting an animal with spermatozoa.

SPF sun protection factor.

sp gr SPECIFIC GRAVITY.

sphaceloderma (sfas″ĕ-lo-der′mah) gangrene of the skin.

sphen(o)- word element [Gr.], *wedge-shaped; sphenoid bone.*

sphenion (sfe′ne-on) the point at the sphenoid angle of the parietal bone.

sphenoid (sfe′noid) 1. wedge-shaped. 2. pertaining to the sphenoid bone; see anatomic Table of Bones in the Appendices.

sphenoidal (sfe-noi′dal) sphenoid.

sphenoiditis (sfe″noi-di′tis) sphenoid sinusitis.

sphenoidotomy (sfe″noi-dot′ah-me) incision of a sphenoid sinus.

sphenomaxillary (sfe″no-mak′sĭ-lar″e) pertaining to the sphenoid bone and the maxilla.

sphenopalatine (sfe″no-pal′ah-tīn) pertaining to the sphenoid and palatine bones.

spher(o)- word element [Gr.], *round; a sphere.*

sphere (sfēr) a three dimensional round body; called also globus. adj., **spher′ical.**

   attraction s. centrosome.

   segmentation s. 1. morula. 2. blastomere.

spherocyte (sfēr′o-sīt) a small, globular, completely hemoglobinated erythrocyte without the usual central pallor, found in hereditary SPHEROCYTOSIS and acquired HEMOLYTIC ANEMIA. adj., **spherocyt′ic.**

spherocytosis (sfe″ro-si-to′sis) the presence of spherocytes in the blood.

   hereditary s. a congenital hereditary form of hemolytic anemia characterized by spherocytosis, abnormal fragility of erythrocytes, jaundice, and splenomegaly.

spheroid (sfēr′oid) a spherelike body.

spheroidal (sfe-roi′dal) resembling a sphere.

spherophakia (sfe″ro-fa′ke-ah) a developmental defect in which a smaller, more spherical optic lens than normal is formed, with partial or complete aplasia of the zonule.

spheroplast (sfēr′o-plast) a bacterial, yeast, or fungal cell that results after partial removal of the rigid cell wall, which forms a membrane-bound cell with a spherical shape that is dependent for its integrity on an isotonic or hypertonic medium.

sphincter (sfingk′ter) a circular muscle that constricts a passage or closes a natural orifice. When relaxed, a sphincter allows materials to pass through the opening. When contracted, it closes the opening. Four main sphincter muscles along the alimentary canal aid in digestion: the cardiac SPHINCTER, the pyloric SPHINCTER, and two anal SPHINCTERS. Other sphincters are found in the iris of the eye, the bile duct (SPHINCTER of Oddi), the urinary tract, and elsewhere.

    anal s., s. a′ni either of two sphincters (the *internal* and *external anal sphincters*) that open and close to control evacuation of feces from the ANUS.

    cardiac s. a sphincter between the esophagus and the stomach, opening at the approach of food that can then be swept into the stomach by rhythmic peristaltic waves.

    s. of Oddi a sheath of muscle fibers investing the associated bile and pancreatic passages as they traverse the wall of the duodenum.

    pyloric s. a sphincter at the opening from the stomach into the duodenum; it is usually closed, opening only for a moment when a peristaltic wave passes over it.

    urinary s., artificial a fluid-filled system that surrounds the urethra with a silicone cuff that functions as a sphincter; a pump is in the scrotum and a fluid reservoir is in the abdomen. For urination, the pump's release valve is squeezed to allow the fluid to leave the urethral cuff and return to the reservoir; after urination is complete, the pump is squeezed and the fluid returns to the cuff to occlude the urethra.

sphincteralgia (sfingk″ter-al′jah) pain in a sphincter muscle.

sphincterectomy (sfingk″ter-ek′tah-me) excision of a sphincter.

sphincterismus (sfingk″ter-iz′mus) spasm of a sphincter.

sphincteritis (sfingk″ter-i′tis) inflammation of a sphincter, particularly the sphincter of Oddi.

sphincterolysis (sfingk″ter-ol′ĭ-sis) surgical separation of the iris from the cornea in anterior synechia.

sphincteroplasty (sfingk′ter-o-plas″te) plastic reconstruction of a sphincter.

sphincterotomy (sfingk″ter-ot′ah-me) incision of a sphincter.

sphingolipid (sfing″go-lip′id) a phospholipid containing sphingosine (e.g., ceramides, sphingomyelins, gangliosides, and cerebrosides), occurring in high concentrations in the brain and other nerve tissue.

sphingolipidosis (sfing″go-lip″ĭ-do′sis) a general designation applied to diseases characterized by abnormal storage of SPHINGO-LIPIDS, such as GAUCHER'S DISEASE, NIEMANN-PICK DISEASE, HURLER'S SYNDROME, and TAY-SACHS DISEASE; all are associated with mental retardation and premature death.

sphingomyelin (sfing″go-mi′ĕ-lin) a group of phospholipids that on hydrolysis yield phosphoric acid, choline, sphingosine, and a fatty acid.

sphingosine (sfing′go-sēn) a basic amino alcohol present in sphingomyelin.

sphygm(o)- word element [Gr.], *the pulse.*

sphygmic (sfig′mik) pertaining to the PULSE.

sphygmobolometer (sfig″mo-bo-lom′-ĕ-ter) an instrument for recording the energy of the pulse wave, and so, indirectly, the strength of the systole.

sphygmochronograph (sfig″mo-kro′no-graf) a self-registering sphygmograph.

sphygmodynamometer (sfig″mo-di″nah-mom′ĕ-ter) an instrument for measuring the force of the pulse.

sphygmogram (sfig′mo-gram) the record or tracing made by a SPHYGMOGRAPH; called also pulse curve.

sphygmograph (sfig′mo-graf) an apparatus for registering the movements, form, and force of the arterial pulse. adj., **sphygmograph′ic.**

sphygmoid (sfig′moid) resembling the pulse.

sphygmomanometer (sfig″mo-mah-nom′-ĕ-ter) an instrument for measuring arterial blood pressure. (See accompanying illustration.)

sphygmometer (sfig-mom′ĕ-ter) an instrument for measuring the force and frequency of the pulse.

S

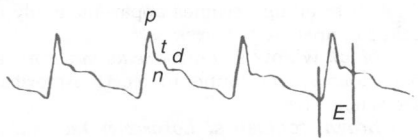

Radial sphygmogram from a healthy person. *p,* The percussion wave; *t,* tidal or predicrotic wave; *n,* dicrotic or aortic notch; *d,* dicrotic wave; *E,* the sphygmic period during which the semilunar valves are open.

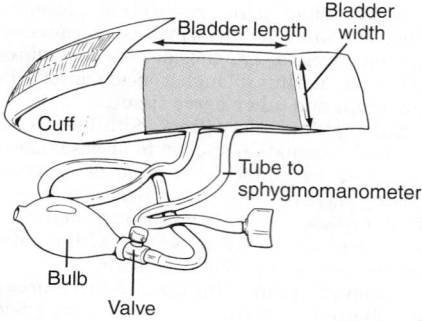

Sphygmomanometer. From Lammon et al., 1995.

sphygmoscope (sfig′mo-skōp) a device for rendering the pulse beat visible.

sphygmotonometer (sfig″mo-to-nom′-ĕ-ter) an instrument for measuring the elasticity of arterial walls.

spica (spi′kah) a figure-of-8 bandage, with turns crossing each other.

spiculated (spik′u-la″ted) having spicules.

spicule (spik′ūl) a sharp, needle-like body or spike.

spider (spi′der) 1. an arthropod of the class Arachnida. 2. vascular spider.

s. bite in the United States, the two spiders whose bites are most likely to cause a serious reaction are the black widow spider (*Latrodectus mactans*) and the brown recluse spider (*Loxosceles reclusa*). Signs and symptoms are associated with the effects of injection of the venom and include pain at the injection site, weakness, muscle pain and cramps, elevated blood pressure, and restlessness. Bites by these spiders must be treated promptly and effectively. First aid is the same as that for a SNAKEBITE and includes the following:

1. Wash the wound with soap and water and apply a clean dressing.

2. Apply a constricting band between the area of the bite and the heart.

3. Keep the person calm and transport him to the hospital or medical facility as soon as possible.

4. If swelling becomes apparent, apply a cold compress to the area.

black widow s. *Latrodectus mactans,* a poisonous spider found in North America; see SPIDER BITE.

brown recluse s. *Loxosceles reclusa,* a poisonous spider found in North America; see SPIDER BITE.

vascular s. a TELANGIECTASIS due to dilatation and branching of superficial cutaneous arteries, which presents as a bright red central portion with branching radiations, the whole somewhat resembling the configuration of a spider. The lesions may occur singly or in large numbers, and may be nevoid or acquired, being commonly associated with pregnancy and liver disease. Called also nevus araneus, spider nevus, and spider telangiectasia.

Spielmeyer-Vogt disease (spēl′mi-er fogt′) Vogt-Spielmeyer disease.

spike (spīk) 1. a sharp upward deflection in a curve or tracing, as on the encephalogram. 2. the attachment of an intravenous infusion set to the bag containing the solution.

spin(o)- word element [Gr.], *spine; spinal* or *vertebral column.* See also words beginning SPONDYL(O)- and VERTEBR(O)-.

spina (spi′nah) [L.] spine (def. 1).

s. bi′fida a developmental anomaly characterized by defective closure of the bony encasement of the spinal cord; the spinal cord and meninges may or may not protrude through the defect (see SPINA BIFIDA CYSTICA and SPINA BIFIDA OCCULTA). It is further classified according to the extent of neural involvement (see MENINGOCELE and MENINGOMYELOCELE). See also NEURAL TUBE DEFECT.

s. bi′fida ante′rior a defect of closure on the anterior surface of the bony spinal canal, often associated with defective development of the abdominal or thoracic viscera.

s. bi′fida cys′tica spina bifida in which there is protrusion through the defect of a cystic swelling that contains the meninges (MENINGOCELE) or the meninges and spinal cord (MENINGOMYELOCELE).

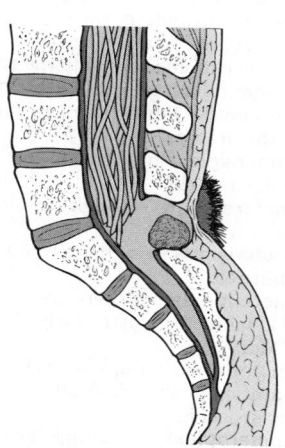

Spina bifida occulta. Posterior vertebral arches have not fused; there is no herniation of the spinal cord or meninges. From Frazier et al., 2000.

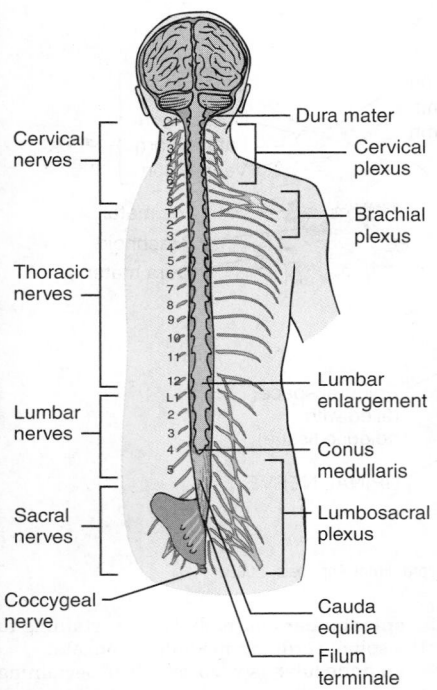

Cervical nerves

Thoracic nerves

Lumbar nerves

Sacral nerves

Coccygeal nerve

Dura mater

Cervical plexus

Brachial plexus

Lumbar enlargement

Conus medullaris

Lumbosacral plexus

Cauda equina

Filum terminale

Gross anatomy of the spinal cord. From Applegate, 2000.

s. bi′fida occul′ta spina bifida in which there is a defect in the bony spinal canal without protrusion of the cord or meninges.

s. vento′sa dactylitis of the bones of the hands or feet, occurring mostly in infants and children, with enlargement of digits, caseation, sequestration, and sinus formation.

spinal (spī′nal) 1. pertaining to a spine. 2. pertaining to the vertebral column.

s. cord that part of the central nervous system lodged in the spinal canal, extending from the foramen magnum to the upper part of the lumbar region. It is composed of an inner core of gray substance in which nerve cells predominate and an outer layer of white substance in which myelinated nerve fibers predominate. Called also medulla spinalis. (See Plates and see accompanying figures.)

spinate (spi′nāt) thorn-shaped; having thorns.

spindle (spin′d'l) 1. a pin tapered at one end or both ends, or something with this shape. 2. the thin, tapering figure occurring during metaphase of cell division, composed of microtubules radiating from the centrioles and connecting to the chromosomes at their centromeres. Called also mitotic spindle. 3. muscle spindle.

mitotic s. spindle (def. 2).

muscle s. a MECHANORECEPTOR found between the skeletal muscle FIBERS; the muscle spindles are arranged in parallel with muscle fibers, and respond to passive stretch of the muscle but cease to discharge if the muscle contracts isotonically, thus signaling muscle length. The muscle spindle is the receptor responsible for the stretch or myotatic REFLEX.

sleep s's bursts of activity of a particular waveform in the electroencephalogram in light or early SLEEP.

spine (spīn) 1. a thornlike process or projection; called also acantha and spina. 2. the rigid bony structure in the midline of the back, composed of the VERTEBRAE; called also backbone, spinal column, and vertebral column.

The spinal column is the axis of the skeleton; the skull and limbs are in a sense appendages. The vertebrae also provide the protective bony corridor (spinal CANAL) through which the SPINAL CORD passes; they can move to a certain extent and so give flexibility to the spine, allowing it to bend forward, sideways and, to a lesser extent, backward. In the areas of the neck and lower back, the spine also can pivot, which permits the turning of the head and torso.

There are usually 24 movable vertebrae and nine that are fused together. The topmost are the seven cervical vertebrae, which form the back of the neck, supporting the skull. The head turns from side to side by means of a pivotal motion between the two highest vertebrae. Below these are the 12 thoracic vertebrae, the supports on which the ribs are hinged, and then the five lumbar vertebrae, the largest movable vertebrae (the cervical are the smallest). Below the lumbar vertebrae, the spine terminates with two groups of vertebrae fused into single bones: the sacrum, composed of five vertebrae, and the coccyx, composed of four vertebrae. Viewed from the side of the body, the spine has the shape of a gentle double S curve.

Malformations of the Spine. Of the various types of spinal malformations, some are congenital and others the result of postural defects or injuries. SPINA BIFIDA is congenital. KYPHOSIS may occasionally be congenital but is more often caused by one of the diseases that attack the structure of the bones. The most common of these is POTT'S DISEASE, or tuberculosis affecting the vertebrae and soft tissues of the spine. Another is OSTEITIS DEFORMANS, a type of bone inflammation in which parts of the bone are replaced by

S

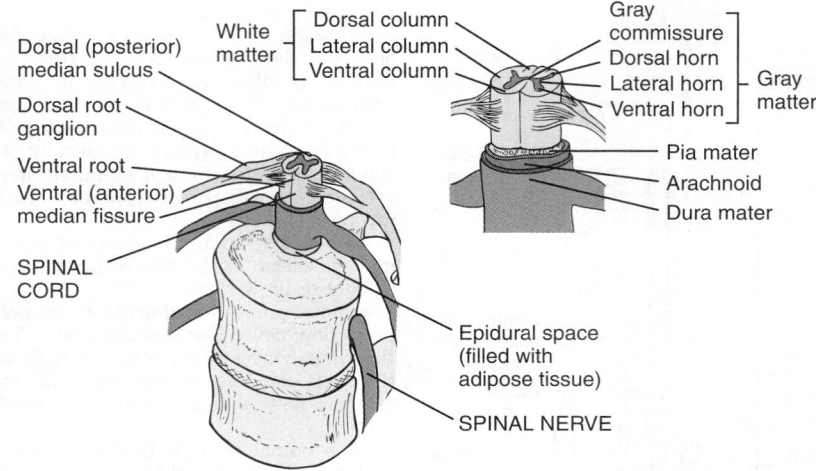

Cross section of the spinal cord. From Applegate, 2000.

softer tissue. SCOLIOSIS is a curvature of the spine toward one side.

cervical s. that portion of the spine comprising the cervical VERTEBRAE.

lumbar s. that portion of the spine comprising the lumbar VERTEBRAE.

thoracic s. that part of the spine comprising the thoracic VERTEBRAE.

spinifugal (spi-nif'u-gal) conducting or moving away from the spinal cord.

spinipetal (spi-nip'ĕ-tal) conducting or moving toward the spinal cord.

spinnbarkeit (spin'bahr-kīt) [Ger.] the formation of a thread by mucus from the cervix uteri when spread onto a glass slide and drawn out by a coverglass; the time at which it can be drawn to the maximum length usually precedes or coincides with the time of ovulation. (See accompanying illustration.)

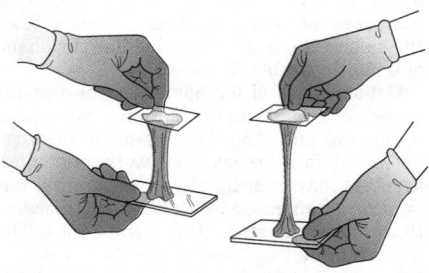

Cervical mucus changes throughout the menstrual cycle. Spinnbarkeit describes how much mucus can be stretched between two fingers or between a microscope slide and coverslip. From McKinney et al., 2000.

spinobulbar (spi″no-bul'bar) pertaining to the spinal cord and medulla oblongata.

spinocellular (spi″no-sel'u-lar) pertaining to prickle cells.

spinocerebellar (spi″no-ser″ĕ-bel'ar) pertaining to the spinal cord and cerebellum.

spinous (spi'nus) pertaining to or like a spine.

spir(o)- 1. [Gr.] a combining form denoting relationship to a coil or spiral. 2. [L.] a combining form denoting relation to the breath or to breathing.

spiradenoma (spi″rad-ĕ-no'mah) adenoma of the sweat glands.

spiral (spi'ral) 1. winding like the thread of a screw; called also helical. 2. a winding structure; see also COIL and HELIX.

Curschmann's s's coiled fibrils of mucin sometimes found in the sputum of patients with asthma. See also Laënnec's PEARLS.

spireme (spi'rēm) the threadlike continuous or segmented figure formed by the chromosome material during prophase.

spirilla (spi-ril'ah) [L.] plural of SPIRILLUM.

spirillicide (spi-ril'ĭ-sīd) an agent that destroys SPIRILLA. adj., **spirillici'dal..**

spirillosis (spi″rĭ-lo'sis) a disease caused by presence of spirilla, such as ratbite fever.

Spirillum (spi-ril'um) a genus of gram-negative, spiral, and curved bacteria, including one species, *S. mi'nus,* that is pathogenic for guinea pigs, rats, mice, and monkeys and is the cause of RAT-BITE FEVER in humans.

spirillum (spi-ril'um) [L.] 1. a spiral-shaped bacterium. 2. a member of the genus *Spirillum.*

spirit (spir'it) 1. a volatile or distilled liquid. 2. an alcoholic or hydroalcoholic solution of a volatile material.

aromatic ammonia s., aromatic s. of ammonia a mixture of ammonia, ammonium carbonate, and other agents for use as an inhalant to revive a person who has fainted.

spiritual care that aspect of health care that attends to spiritual and religious needs brought on by an illness or injury. Health care professionals profess a commitment to holistic care, in which the whole person is ministered to, yet they often leave spiritual problems to persons whom they consider better qualified than they to deal with problems of this kind. Thus patients often have deep concerns that are unspoken and suffering that is not shared.

Assessment of spiritual needs should go beyond a perfunctory question about religious affiliation at the time of admission. Questions about values and beliefs should be asked, preferably at the end of the assessment interview, when the patient shows trust and confidence in the nurse. It may be that patients will provide little information at first, but later on, when there is a more trusting relationship with the nurse, or when a frightening medical diagnosis has been made, assessment and interventions may be indicated. However, if patients remain reluctant to discuss personal beliefs and values, their right to privacy is respected.

Stoll has suggested that there are four general areas of concern to be addressed during spiritual assessment. These include (1) the person's concept of God or deity and how this concept is significant in his or her life; (2) sources of help and strength in times of spiritual crises; (3) religious practices; and (4) the relation between spiritual beliefs and health, sickness, and death.

Profound questions of the meaning of suffering and death may surface when a person is experiencing a serious illness or similar crisis of physical health. In the face of impending death or a radical change imposed by the loss of a body part or function, patients may experience panic, anxiety, depression, and feelings of guilt or abandonment. They need opportunities to express spiritual concerns to an attentive listener, to bring into focus and work through their questions and doubts, and to experience hope and support for the beliefs that give them strength and consolation.

While health care providers are not typically the primary source of spiritual counsel, they can contribute to the overall welfare of their patients by being alert for

expressions of spiritual distress, listening to the patients when they want to talk about spiritual concerns, and reading and praying with them when appropriate. Referral to the hospital chaplain or the patient's minister, priest, or other spiritual guide is an important part of meeting a patient's spiritual needs, but it does not relieve health care professionals of their responsibility for continued spiritual support.

Spirochaetales (spi″ro-ke-ta′lēz) the spirochetes, an order of bacteria in which some species are free-living and some parasitic; it includes the disease-causing genera *Borrelia, Leptospira,* and *Treponema.*

spirochete (spi′ro-kēt) a highly coiled bacterium; a general term applied to any organism of the order Spirochaetales, which includes the genera *Borrelia, Leptospira,* and *Treponema.* Spirochetes are the causative organisms of SYPHILIS, YAWS, LYME DISEASE, and various other diseases. adj., **spiroche′tal.**

spirocheticide (spi″ro-ke′tĭ-sīd) an agent that destroys SPIROCHETES.

spirochetolysis (spi″ro-ke-tol′ĭ-sis) the destruction of spirochetes by lysis.

spirochetosis (spi″ro-ke-to′sis) infection with spirochetes.

spirogram (spi′ro-gram) a graph of respiratory movements made by the SPIROMETER.

spirograph (spi′ro-graf) an apparatus for measuring and recording respiratory movements.

spirography (spi-rah′grah-fe) the graphic measurement of breathing, including breathing movements and breathing capacity; see also SPIROMETRY. Called also pneumography.

spiroid (spi′roid) resembling a spiral.

spirolactone (spi″ro-lak′tōn) any of a group of compounds capable of opposing the action of sodium-retaining steroids on renal transport of sodium and potassium.

spirometer (spi-rom′ĕ-ter) an instrument for measuring air inhaled into and exhaled out of the lungs; it provides a simple way of determining most of the lung volumes and capacities that are measured in PULMONARY FUNCTION TESTS. One type is the *water-seal spirometer,* which consists of a hollow drum floating over a chamber of water and counterbalanced by weights so that it can move freely up and down. Inside the drum is a mixture of gases, usually oxygen and air. Leading from the hollow space in the drum to the outside is a tube that has a mouthpiece through which the patient breathes. As one inhales and exhales

S

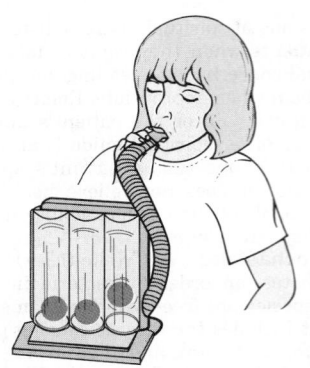

Using a flow spirometer. From Lammon et al., 1995.

through the tube the drum rises and falls, causing a needle to move on a nearby rotating chart. The tracing recorded on the chart is called a SPIROGRAM.

spirometry (spi-rom′ĕ-tre) measurement of the breathing capacity by means of a SPIROMETER; results can record total lung CAPACITY, VITAL CAPACITY, tidal VOLUME, functional residual CAPACITY, and residual VOLUME.

incentive s. a goal-oriented inhalation maneuver in which the patient is encouraged by visual feedback from a spirometer to execute sustained maximal inhalation. Patients usually perform 10 to 20 sustained deep breath exercises an hour until they can achieve their predicted inspiratory reserve volume. See illustration.

spironolactone (spi″rah-no-lak′tōn) one of the SPIROLACTONES, a competitive antagonist of ALDOSTERONE and a potassium-sparing DIURETIC; used in treatment of EDEMA, HYPOKALEMIA, primary ALDOSTERONISM,

and (usually in combination with other drugs) HYPERTENSION.

splanchn(o)- word element [Gr.], *viscus; splanchnic nerve.*

splanchnapophysis (splangk″nah-pof′ĭ-sis) a skeletal element, such as the lower jaw, connected with the alimentary canal.

splanchnectopia (splangk″nek-to′pe-ah) displacement of a viscus or of the viscera.

splanchnesthesia (splangk″nes-the′zhah) visceral sensation. adj., **splanchnesthet′ic.**

splanchnic (splangk′nik) pertaining to the viscera.

splanchnicectomy (splangk″nĭ-sek′tah-me) excision of part of the greater splanchnic nerve.

splanchnicotomy (splangk″nĭ-kot′ah-me) transection of a splanchnic nerve.

splanchnocele (splangk′no-sēl) hernial protrusion of a viscus.

splanchnocoele (splangk′no-sēl) the portion of the embryonic body cavity from which the abdominal, pericardial, and pleural cavities are formed.

splanchnodiastasis (splangk″no-di-as′-tah-sis) displacement of a viscus or viscera.

splanchnolith (splangk′no-lith) intestinal calculus.

splanchnology (splangk-nol′ah-je) scientific study or description of the organs of the body, as of the digestive, respiratory, and genitourinary systems.

splanchnomegaly (splangk″no-meg′ah-le) visceromegaly.

splanchnopathy (splangk-nop′ah-the) any disease of the viscera.

splanchnopleure (splangk′no-ploor) the embryonic layer formed by union of the splanchnic mesoderm with entoderm; from it are developed the muscles and the connective tissue of the digestive tube.

splanchnosclerosis (splangk″no-sklĕ-ro′-sis) hardening of the viscera.

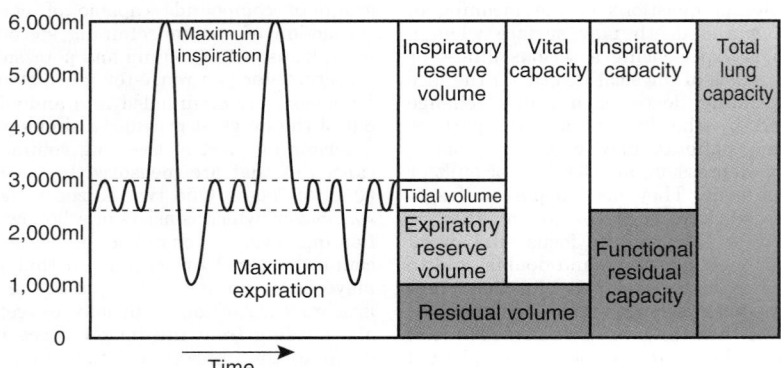

Spirometry, showing respiratory volumes and capacities as subdivisions of total lung capacity. From Applegate, 2000.

splanchnoskeleton (splangk″no-skel′ĕ-ton) skeletal structures connected with viscera.

splanchnotomy (splangk-not′ah-me) anatomy or dissection of the viscera.

splanchnotribe (splangk′no-trīb) an instrument for crushing the intestine to obliterate its lumen.

splayfoot (spla′foot) flatfoot.

spleen (splēn) a large glandlike but ductless organ in the upper part of the abdominal cavity on the left side, lateral to the cardiac end of the stomach. Called also lien. adj., **splen′ic**. It is the largest collection of reticuloendothelial CELLS in the body and is composed of spongelike tissue of two types: red PULP, which is the dark reddish brown substance filling the interspaces of the sinuses of the spleen, and white PULP, which consists of sheaths of lymphatic tissue surrounding the arteries of the spleen. It is enclosed in a dense capsule. In a normal adult the spleen is about 12.5 cm long and weighs about 140 to 210 g. After gastric digestion and in the presence of disease the spleen enlarges.

During fetal life the spleen and liver produce erythrocytes, but after birth that function is taken over by the bone marrow. However, if there is bone marrow failure, the spleen may again produce erythrocytes. In the normal adult the spleen is a reservoir for blood, and contains a high concentration of erythrocytes. In times of exertion, emotional stress, pregnancy, severe bleeding, carbon monoxide poisoning, or other occasions when the oxygen content of the blood must be increased, the spleen contracts rhythmically to release its store of erythrocytes into the bloodstream.

The spleen also acts to help keep the blood free of unwanted substances, including wastes and infecting organisms. The blood is delivered to it by the splenic artery, and passes through smaller branch arteries into a network of channels lined with leukocytes known as PHAGOCYTES (see RETICULOENDOTHELIAL SYSTEM). These clear the blood of old erythrocytes, damaged cells, parasites, and other toxic or foreign substances. Hemoglobin from the removed red cells is temporarily stored.

accessory s. a small mass of tissue elsewhere in the body, histologically and functionally identical with that composing the normal spleen.

splen(o)- word element [Gr.], *spleen*.

splenalgia (sple-nal′jah) pain in the SPLEEN; called also splenodynia.

splenectasis (sple-nek′tah-sis) splenomegaly.

splenectomy (sple-nek′tah-me) excision of the SPLEEN, done in cases of severe trauma to

or rupture of the spleen, enlargement (splenomegaly) when the destructive properties of the organ are greatly accelerated, and such blood disorders as idiopathic thrombocytopenic purpura and hereditary spherocytosis. The latter two conditions respond well to splenectomy. In blood dyscrasias in which parts of the reticuloendothelial system other than the spleen are involved, splenectomy may be of little value. Other indications include cancer of the lymph glands, transplant rejection, sickle cell disease, abscesses, a clot in a major blood vessel serving the spleen, and hepatic cirrhosis.

Although its known functions are important and many of its other functions are poorly understood, the spleen is not an indispensable organ. Normally, the other reticuloendothelial cells scattered throughout the body take over its chores once the spleen is removed. However, those persons who no longer have a functioning spleen, either as a result of splenectomy or because of a destructive disease process, are at very high risk for the development of life-threatening infections, especially those caused by pneumococci. With the recognition that the spleen has important immunologic functions, current therapy is often directed toward salvage of the injured spleen. Such efforts include longer observation of the injured patient, CAT scans, and radioisotope studies, and if surgery is needed, attempts are made to save the spleen with repair of the lacerations and control of bleeding with hemostatic agents.

splenectopia (splen″ek-to′pe-ah) displacement of the spleen.

splenectopy (splen-ek′tŏ-pe) splenectopia.

splenic (splen′ik) pertaining to the spleen.

splenitis (sple-ni′tis) inflammation of the spleen, a condition that is attended by enlargement of the organ and severe local pain.

splenium (sple′ne-um) 1. a compress or bandage. 2. a bandlike structure.

s. cor′poris callo′si the posterior, rounded end of the corpus callosum.

splenization (splen″ĭ-za′shun) the conversion of a tissue, as of the lung, into tissue resembling that of the spleen, due to engorgement and consolidation.

splenocele (sple′no-sēl) hernia of the spleen.

splenocolic (sple″no-kol′ik) pertaining to the spleen and colon.

splenocyte (sple′no-sīt) the monocyte characteristic of splenic tissue.

splenodynia (sple″no-din′e-ah) splenalgia.

S

splenography (sple-nog'rah-fe) 1. radiography of the spleen. 2. a description of the spleen.

splenohepatomegaly (sple″no-hep″ah-to-meg′ah-le) hepatosplenomegaly.

splenoid (sple′noid) resembling the spleen.

splenolysin (sple-nol′ĭ-sin) a lysin that destroys spleen tissue.

splenolysis (sple-nol′ĭ-sis) destruction of splenic tissue by a lysin.

splenoma (sple-no′mah) a splenic tumor.

splenomalacia (sple″no-mah-la′shah) abnormal softness of the SPLEEN; called also lienomalacia.

splenomedullary (sple″no-med′u-lar″e) of or pertaining to the spleen and bone marrow; called also lienomedullary.

splenomegaly (sple″no-meg′ah-le) enlargement of the spleen.

  congestive s. splenomegaly secondary to portal hypertension, with ascites, anemia, thrombocytopenia, leukopenia, and episodic hemorrhage from the intestinal tract. Called also Banti's disease.

  hemolytic s. enlargement of the spleen associated with hemolytic diseases of the blood.

  siderotic s. splenomegaly with deposit of iron and calcium.

splenometry (sple-nom′ĕ-tre) determination of the size of the spleen.

splenomyelogenous (sple″no-mi″ĕ-loj′ĕ-nus) formed in the spleen and bone marrow; called also lienomyelogenous.

splenomyelomalacia (sple″no-mi″ĕ-lo-mah-la′shah) softening of the spleen and bone marrow; called also lienomyelomalacia.

splenoncus (sple-nong′kus) splenoma.

splenopancreatic (sple″no-pan″kre-at′ik) pertaining to the spleen and pancreas.

splenopathy (sple-nop′ah-the) any disease of the spleen.

splenopexy (sple′no-pek″se) surgical fixation of the spleen.

splenoptosis (sple″nop-to′sis) downward displacement of the spleen.

splenorenal (sple″no-re′nal) pertaining to the spleen and kidney, or to splenic and renal veins.

splenorrhagia (sple″no-ra′jah) hemorrhage from the spleen.

splenorrhaphy (sple-nor′ah-fe) suture of the spleen.

splenotomy (sple-not′ah-me) incision of the spleen.

splenotoxin (sple′no-tok″sin) a toxin produced by or acting on the spleen.

splint (splint) 1. a rigid or flexible appliance for fixation of displaced or movable parts; see also ORTHOSIS. 2. to supply support for the purpose of immobilizing an injured or displaced body part.

Uses. Splints are most commonly used to immobilize broken bones or dislocated joints. When a broken bone has been properly set, a splint permits complete rest at the site of the fracture and thus allows natural healing to take place with the bone in the proper position. Splints are also necessary to immobilize unset fractures when a patient is moved after an accident; they prevent motion of the fractured bone, which might cause greater damage.

In a pelvic or spinal fracture, the effect of splinting is achieved by placing the patient on a stretcher or board. Breaks of the ribs and of face and skull bones usually do not require the use of splints, since these parts are naturally splinted by adjacent bone and tissue.

Making and Applying Splints. A splint can be improvised from a variety of materials, but should usually be light, straight, and rigid. It should be long enough to extend beyond the joint above the injury and below

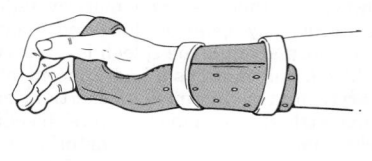
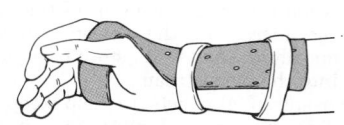

Wrist splint

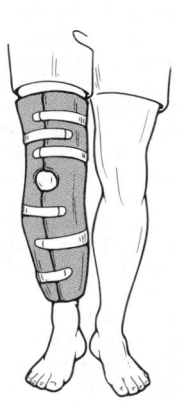

Knee splint

Types of splints. From Lammon et al., 1996.

the fracture site. A board used as a splint should be at least as wide as the injured part. Tightly rolled newspapers or magazines can be used to splint the arm or lower leg. Ice cream sticks have been used as splints for broken fingers.

Splints should be padded, at least on one side. Thick soft padding permits the injured part to swell and reduces interference with circulation. Bandages or strips of cloth or adhesive tape are used to hold splints in place. Pulses distal to the injury should be checked before and after splinting to determine whether the blood supply has been impaired. If the limb becomes cold, pale, or blue, or if the affected part becomes too painful, the splint should be loosened. Splints should never be tight.

Internal Splints. Internal splints, as well as pins, wires, and other devices for the fixation of fractures, are among the more spectacular advances in orthopedics. They have worked wonders in the setting of hip fractures, especially in older people. Internal splints are available for almost every type of fracture. Stainless steel, titanium, and Vitallium are the most commonly used materials. Splints and devices of this type require surgery for insertion, but are less cumbersome than external splints and permit earlier use of the fractured bone.

   airplane s. one that holds the splinted limb suspended in the air.

   anchor s. one for fracture of the jaw, with metal loops fitting over the teeth and held together by a rod.

   Balkan s. Balkan frame.

   coaptation s's small splints adjusted about a fractured limb to produce coaptation of fragments.

   Denis Browne s. a splint for the correction of CLUBFOOT, consisting of two metal footplates connected by a crossbar.

   dynamic s. a supportive or protective apparatus that aids in initiation and performance of motion by the supported or adjacent parts.

   flexion s. tenodesis splint.

   functional s. dynamic splint.

   shin s's strain of the long flexor muscle of the toes, occurring in athletes and marked by pain along the tibia.

   Taylor s. a horizontal pelvic band and long lateral posterior bars; used to apply traction to the lower limb.

   tenodesis s. an orthosis that allows pinch and grasp movements through the wrist extensors.

   Thomas s. two iron rods joined at the upper end by an oval iron ring or half-ring, and bent at the lower end to form a W shape; used to give support to the lower limb and

remove the weight of the body from the knee joint by transferring it to the pelvis.

splinting (splint'ing) 1. treatment by use of a SPLINT. 2. in dentistry, the application of a fixed restoration to join two or more teeth into a single rigid unit for stabilization. 3. in the NURSING INTERVENTIONS CLASSIFICATION, a nursing INTERVENTION defined as the stabilization, immobilization, and/or protection of an injured body part with a supportive appliance.

splitting (split'ing) in psychoanalytic theory, a primitive DEFENSE MECHANISM in which the self and internal and external objects are divided into parts that are either "all good" or "all bad." Characteristic of very young children, it is also seen in those with BORDERLINE PERSONALITY DISORDER and sometimes in those with other personality disorders or psychoses.

spodogenous (spo-doj'ĕ-nus) caused by accumulation of waste material in an organ.

spondyl(o)- word element [Gr.], *vertebra; vertebral column.* See also words beginning SPIN(O)- and VERTEBR(O)-.

spondylalgia (spon″dĭ-lal'jah) pain in the vertebrae.

spondylarthritis (spon″dil-ahr-thri'tis) arthritis of the spine.

spondylitic (spon″dĭ-lit'ik) pertaining to or marked by spondylitis.

spondylitis (spon″dĭ-li'tis) inflammation of the VERTEBRAE, usually a serious and chronic disorder. It may be associated with tuberculosis of the bones, in which case it is called POTT'S DISEASE. The vertebrae become eroded and collapse, causing KYPHOSIS. Spondylitis may also be associated with other infectious diseases, such as BRUCELLOSIS, in which the intervertebral disks and the vertebrae are affected and sometimes destroyed; this is one cause of ankylosing SPONDYLITIS, a particularly serious variety.

   ankylosing s., Bekhterev's s. a form of rheumatoid ARTHRITIS that affects the spine, characterized by inflammation of the facet joints and inflammatory changes of the stabilizing ligaments of the spine (ENTHESOPATHY). It affects males almost exclusively. There is stiffening of spinal joints and ligaments, so that movement becomes increasingly painful and difficult. When it runs its full course, it results in bony ankylosis of the vertebral joints, which may extend to the ribs and limit the flexibility of the rib cage, so that breathing is impaired. (See illustration.) Called also Marie-Strümpell disease or spondylitis and rheumatoid spondylitis.

S

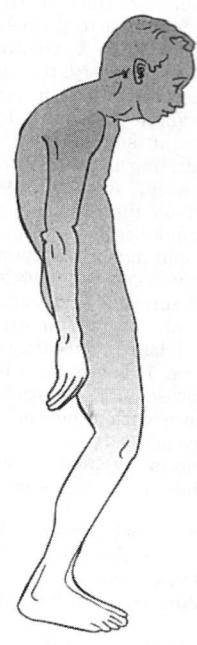

Typical posture of patient with ankylosing spondylitis. From Copstead and Banasik, 2000.

Kümmell's s. Kümmell's disease.

Marie-Strümpell s. ankylosing spondylitis.

post-traumatic s. Kümmell's disease.

rheumatoid s. ankylosing spondylitis.

spondylizema (spon″dĭ-li-ze′mah) downward displacement of a vertebra because of destruction or softening of the one below it.

spondyloarthropathy (spon″dĭ-lo-ahr-throp′ah-the) disease of the joints of the spine.

spondylocace (spon″dĭ-lok′ah-se) tuberculosis of the vertebrae.

spondylodymus (spon″dĭ-lod′ĭ-mus) conjoined twins united by the vertebrae.

spondylodynia (spon″dĭ-lo-din′e-ah) pain in a vertebra.

spondylolisthesis (spon″dĭ-lo-lis-the′sis) forward displacement of a vertebra over a lower segment due to a congenital defect or fracture in the pars interarticularis, usually of the fifth lumbar over the sacrum, or of the fourth lumbar over the fifth. adj., **spondylolisthet′ic.**

spondylolysis (spon″dĭ-lol′ĭ-sis) the breaking down of a vertebra. adj., **spondylolyt′ic.**

spondylopathy (spon″dĭ-lop′ah-the) any disease of the vertebrae.

spondylopyosis (spon″dĭ-lo-pi-o′sis) suppuration of a vertebra.

spondyloschisis (spon″dĭ-los′kĭ-sis) spina bifida.

spondylosis (spon″dĭ-lo′sis) 1. ankylosis of a vertebral joint. 2. degenerative spinal changes due to OSTEOARTHRITIS.

spondylosyndesis (spon″dĭ-lo-sin′dĕ-sis) spinal fusion.

sponge (spunj) a porous, absorbent mass, as a pad of gauze or cotton surrounded by gauze, or the elastic fibrous skeleton of certain species of marine animals.

absorbable gelatin s. a sterile, absorbable, water-insoluble, gelatin-base material used in the control of bleeding.

spongi(o)- word element [L., Gr.], *sponge; spongelike.*

spongiform (spun′jĭ-form) resembling a sponge.

spongioblast (spun′je-o-blast″) 1. any of the embryonic epithelial cells developed about the neural TUBE; they later become transformed, some into NEUROGLIAL and some into EPENDYMAL cells. 2. amacrine (def. 2).

spongioblastoma (spun″je-o-blas-to′mah) a tumor containing SPONGIOBLASTS; types include GLIOBLASTOMA and GLIOSARCOMA.

spongiocyte (spun′je-o-sīt″) 1. a NEUROGLIA cell. 2. one of the cells with spongy vacuolated protoplasm in the adrenal cortex.

spongioid (spun′je-oid) resembling a sponge.

spongioplasm (spun′je-o-plazm″) 1. a substance forming the network of fibrils pervading the cell substance and forming the reticulum of the fixed cell. 2. the granular material of an axon.

spongiosa (spun″je-o′sah) spongy; sometimes used alone to mean the spongy substance of bone (substantia spongiosa ossium).

spongiosaplasty (spun″je-o″sah-plas′te) autoplasty of the spongy substance of bone (substantia spongiosa ossium) to potentiate formation of new bone or to cover bone defects.

spongiosis (spun″je-o′sis) intercellular edema within the epidermis.

spongiositis (spun″je-o-si′tis) periurethritis.

spongy (spun′je) of spongelike appearance or texture.

sporadic (spŏ-rad′ik) occurring singly; widely scattered; not epidemic or endemic.

spore (spor) 1. a refractile, oval body formed within bacteria, especially *Bacillus* and *Clostridium*, which is regarded as a resting stage during the life history of the cell, and is characterized by its resistance to environmental changes. 2. the reproductive element, produced sexually or asexually, of one of the lower organisms, such as protozoa, fungi, or algae.

sporicide (spor'ĭ-sīd) an agent that kills spores. adj., **sporici'dal.**

sporocyst (spor'o-sist) 1. any cyst or sac containing spores or reproductive cells; the oocyst of certain protozoa in which sporozoites develop. 2. the larval stages of flukes in snails.

sporogenic (spor″o-jen'ik) producing spores.

sporogony (spŏ-rog'ah-ne) the sexual stage in the life cycle of a sporozoan parasite, with development of the zygote into one or several haploid spores, each containing a distinctive number of sporozoites. adj., **sporogon'ic.**

sporont (spor'ont) a mature protozoon in its sexual cycle.

sporoplasm (spor'o-plazm) the protoplasm of a spore.

Sporothrix (spor'o-thriks) a genus of fungi, including *S. schenck'ii,* which causes SPOROTRICHOSIS, and *S. car'nis,* which causes formation of white mold on meat in cold storage.

sporotrichosis (spor″o-trĭ-ko'sis) a chronic fungal infection caused by *Sporothrix schenckii,* occurring in three forms. The *cutaneous lymphatic form* is characterized by a single pustule, papule, or nodule at the site of invasion, followed by lymphatic spread and the development of multiple, painless, subcutaneous granulomas, which tend to break down and form often painless ulcers or cold abscesses. The *disseminated form* is marked by multiple, painless, cutaneous or subcutaneous nodules, which may form cold abscesses, ulcers, or fistulas; this form may involve the muscles, joints, bones, eyes, gastrointestinal system, mucous membranes, and nervous system. The *pulmonary form* results from the inhalation of spores and causes acute disease or chronic granulomas similar to those seen in other mycoses.

Sporozoa (spor″o-zo'ah) Sporozoea.

sporozoa (spor″o-zo'ah) [Gr.] plural of SPOROZOON.

sporozoan (spor″o-zo'an) 1. pertaining to the Sporozoa. 2. an individual of the Sporozoa.

Sporozoea (spor″o-zo'e-ah) a class of parasitic protozoa with both sexual and asexual phases; it contains the medically important subclass Coccidia. Called also Sporozoa.

sporozoite (spor″o-zo'īt) a spore formed after fertilization; any one of the sickle-shaped nucleated germs formed by division of the protoplasm of a spore of a sporozoan organism. In malaria, the sporozoites are

the forms of the plasmodium that are liberated from the oocysts in the mosquito, that accumulate in the salivary glands, and that are transferred to humans when the mosquito feeds.

sporozoon (spor″o-zo'on) [Gr.] an individual protozoon of the Sporozoea.

sporulation (spor″u-la'shun) formation of spores.

spot (spot) a circumscribed area or place, usually distinguished by its color; see also MACULA and TACHE.

actual focal s. the section of a focal spot on which there is intersection of an electron beam with an anode of an x-ray tube.

Bitot's s's foamy gray triangular spots of keratinized epithelium on the conjunctivae, a sign of vitamin A deficiency.

blind s. 1. optic disk. 2. mental scotoma.

café au lait s. a light brown pigmented macule seen in NEUROFIBROMATOSIS and ALBRIGHT'S SYNDROME.

cherry-red s. the choroid appearing as a red circular area surrounded by gray-white retina, as viewed throught the fovea centralis in TAY-SACHS DISEASE. Called also Tay's spot.

cotton-wool s. white or gray soft-edged opacities in the retina composed of cytoid bodies; seen in hypertensive retinopathy, lupus erythematosus, and numerous other conditions.

effective focal s. the size of a projected focal spot in a specified direction measured with a quality assurance test tool such as the slit camera.

focal s. 1. the object of a patient's gaze during distraction techniques. 2. a small area of an x-ray target that receives the main electron stream.

Forschheimer s's a fleeting skin eruption consisting of discrete rose spots on the soft palate sometimes seen in rubella just prior to the onset of the skin rash.

Koplik's s's small, irregular, bright red spots on the buccal and lingual mucosa, with a minute bluish white speck in the center of each; they are pathognomonic of beginning measles.

liver s. 1. a lay term for senile LENTIGO. 2. (in pl.) tinea versicolor.

mental blind s. mental scotoma.

mongolian s. a type of congenital brown to gray-blue nevus; see also MONGOLIAN SPOT.

Roth's s's round or oval white spots consisting of coagulated fibrin seen in the retina in a number of diseases in which a vascular insult resulting in hemorrhage is followed by healing.

S

Tay's s. cherry-red spot.

spotted fever a febrile disease characterized by a skin eruption, such as Rocky Mountain spotted fever, boutonneuse fever, and other infections due to tickborne rickettsiae.

sprain (sprān) wrenching or twisting of a joint, with partial rupture of its ligaments. There may also be damage to the associated blood vessels, muscles, tendons, and nerves. A sprain is more serious than a STRAIN, which is simply the overstretching of a muscle, without swelling. Severe sprains are so painful that the joint cannot be used. There is much swelling, with reddish to blue discoloration due to hemorrhage from ruptured blood vessels.

First aid for a sprain includes immediate rest with no weight bearing in order to prevent further damage. The injured part should be elevated to decrease swelling. Applications of ice or cold compresses (not heat) to the injured part during the first 24 hours also will relieve pain and help prevent swelling. If there is severe tearing or rupture of a ligament or tendon the condition will require immobilization in a cast or surgical repair or both.

spreader (spred'er) an instrument for distributing something over a broad area.

root canal filling s. in root canal THERAPY, a tapered metal instrument used to compress filling material against the sides of the canal to make room for additional CONES.

sprue (sproo) a chronic form of MALABSORPTION SYNDROME occurring in both tropical and nontropical forms.

celiac s., nontropical s. CELIAC DISEASE.

tropical s. a chronic disease affecting the digestive system, marked by imperfect absorption of food elements, especially fat, xylose, and vitamin B_{12}, from the small intestine. It is closely related to CELIAC DISEASE and may be identical to it.

The name sprue derives from a Dutch word describing inflammation of the mouth, which is a frequent symptom. The disease has been recognized for more than 2000 years. It occurs mostly, but not exclusively, in the tropics.

Symptoms and Treatment. Symptoms are loss of appetite, flatulence, anemia, diarrhea, stomach cramps, and extreme loss of weight. Stools are usually pale, greasy, unformed, and foul-smelling, but at times become watery. If a deficiency of vitamin B complex is also present, cracks develop at the corners of the mouth and the tongue becomes smooth, glossy, and bright red.

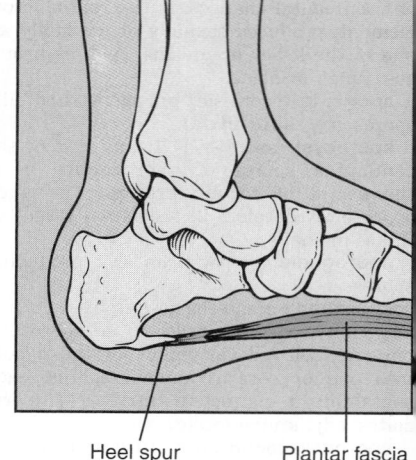

Heel spur   Plantar fascia

Calcaneal (heel) spur. From Frazier et al., 2000.

Treatment consists of a special diet of foods that are low in fat and high in protein. Diets free of gluten, a viscid grain protein, may be prescribed. Liver preparations, folic acid, calcium lactate tablets, vitamin B_{12}, and iron supplements to provide food elements that are not absorbed, as well as skim milk and ripe bananas, have produced favorable results. Antibiotics have proved temporarily successful, but their prolonged use is not recommended.

Cases of sprue that are recognized early respond better to treatment than do cases of long standing. Appetite and weight return rapidly. The time required for complete recovery is prolonged, however, especially in extreme cases.

spur (sper) 1. a spiked object or goad. 2. a projecting body, as from a bone; called also calcar.

spurious (spu're-us) simulated; not genuine; false.

sputum (spu'tum) mucous secretion from the lungs, bronchi, and trachea that is ejected through the mouth, in contrast to SALIVA, which is the secretion of the SALIVARY GLANDS. Called also expectoration.

induced s. a SPUTUM SPECIMEN produced for diagnostic tests by aerosol administration of a hypertonic saline solution.

s. specimen a sample of mucous secretion from the bronchi and lungs. The specimen may be examined microscopically for the presence of malignant cells (cytologic examination) or tested to identify pathogenic bacteria (bacteriologic examination). It is essential that the specimen obtained be mucus from the lungs and bronchi and not saliva. For those unable to produce sputum for examination, an AEROSOL may be used to increase the flow of secretions and stimulate coughing. The optimum time for collection of a sputum specimen is in the morning before eating or drinking anything. At this time secretions accumulated in the bronchi through the night are more readily available, and, should the coughing produce gagging, the patient is less likely to vomit if the stomach is empty. Specimens collected for bacteriologic culture must be placed in a sterile container and handled with care to avoid contamination from sources other than the sputum.

SQ subcutaneous.

squalene (skwaʹlēn) an unsaturated TERPENE that is an intermediate in cholesterol synthesis and occurs normally at low levels in blood plasma and at elevated levels in viral influenza; used as a vehicle for pharmaceuticals.

squama (skwaʹmah) [L.] a SCALE, or other thin, platelike structure.

squame (skwām) squama.

squamoparietal (skwaʺmo-pah-riʹĕ-tal) pertaining to the pars squamosa (squamous PART of the temporal bone) and the parietal bone.

squamosoparietal (skwa-moʺso-pah-riʹĕ-tal) squamoparietal.

squamous (skwaʹmus) scaly or platelike.

squatting (skwahtʹing) a position with the hips and knees flexed, the buttocks resting on the heels; sometimes adopted by a parturient woman at delivery or by a child with any of certain types of cardiac defects.

squeeze technique (skwēz) one used for the treatment of premature EJACULATION, in which a man is repeatedly aroused almost to the point of ejaculatory inevitability and then the thumb and first two fingers are used to forcibly squeeze the head of the penis, preventing ejaculation.

squill (skwil) 1. any of various plants of the genus *Urginea*, especially *U. maritima* or *U. indica*. 2. the fleshy inner scales of the bulb of *U. maritima* or *U. indica;* a distinction is made between those with white bulbs *(white squill)* and those with red bulbs *(red squill)*.

   red s. 1. a variety of *Urginea maritima* that has red bulbs. 2. the fleshy inner scales of the bulb of this plant, a source of the cardiac glycoside scilliroside; it can cause convulsions or cardiac arrest and is used as a RODENTICIDE.

   white s. 1. a variety of *Urginea maritima* that has white bulbs. 2. the fleshy inner scales of the bulb of this plant; it contains several cardioactive glycosides.

squint (skwint) strabismus.

SR sedimentation rate.

Sr strontium.

SRH somatotropin-releasing hormone (growth hormone–releasing hormone).

SRS-A slow-reacting substance of anaphylaxis.

ss. [L.] seʹmis (half).

SSRI selective serotonin reuptake inhibitor.

St stoke.

stability (stah-bilʹĭ-te) the quality of maintaining a constant character despite forces that threaten to disturb it.

stabilization (staʺbĭ-lĭ-zaʹshun) the process of making firm and steady.

stable (staʹb'l) not readily subject to change.

stactometer (stak-tomʹĕ-ter) a device for measuring drops.

staff (staf) 1. a wooden rod or rodlike structure. 2. a grooved director used as a guide for the knife in lithotomy. 3. the professional personnel of a health care facility or agency.

   s. of Aesculapius see AESCULAPIUS.

   attending s. the corps of attending physicians and surgeons of a hospital.

   consulting s. specialists associated with a hospital and acting in an advisory capacity to the attending staff.

   house s. the resident physicians and surgeons of a hospital.

   s. mix a term in the NURSING MINIMUM DATA SET, defined as the combination of all caregivers participating in nursing care for an individual patient or client.

stage (stāj) 1. a distinct period or phase, as of development of a disease or organism. For specific names of stages, see under the name. 2. the platform of a microscope on which the slide containing the object to be studied is placed.

   anal s. in psychoanalytic theory, the second stage of psychosexual DEVELOPMENT, occurring between the ages of 1 and 3 years, during which the infant's activities, interests, and concerns are on the anal zone. It is preceded by the oral stage and followed by the phallic stage. See also SEXUAL DEVELOPMENT.

   first s. of labor see LABOR.

   fourth s. of labor see LABOR.

   genital s. in psychoanalytic theory, the last stage in psychosexual development, occurring during puberty, during which the person can achieve sexual gratification from genital-to-genital contact and is capable of a mature relationship with a person of the opposite sex. It follows the latency stage. See also SEXUAL DEVELOPMENT.

S

latency s. 1. the INCUBATION PERIOD of any infectious disorder. 2. the quiescent period following an active period in certain infectious diseases, during which the pathogen remains dormant for a variable length of time before again initiating signs of active disease. 3. in psychoanalytic theory, the relatively quiescent period in psychosexual DEVELOPMENT following the phallic stage and lasting from age 5 or 6 years to adolescence. Energy is focused on learning and on more organized play. See also SEXUAL DEVELOPMENT.

oral s. in psychoanalytic theory, the earliest stage of psychosexual development, lasting from birth to about 18 months, during which the oral zone is the center of the infant's needs, expression, and pleasurable erotic experiences. It is followed by the anal stage. See also SEXUAL DEVELOPMENT.

phallic s. in psychoanalytic theory, the third stage in psychosexual DEVELOPMENT, lasting from age 2 or 3 years to 5 or 6 years, during which sexual interest, curiosity, and pleasurable experiences are centered on the penis in boys and the clitoris in girls. It is preceded by the anal stage and followed by the latency stage. See also SEXUAL DEVELOPMENT.

prodromal s. the period of early symptoms of a disease occurring after the incubation period and just before the appearance of the characteristic symptoms of the disease.

second s. of labor see LABOR.

third s. of labor see LABOR.

staging (stāj′ing) 1. the determination of distinct phases or periods in the course of a disease, the life history of an organism, or any biological process. 2. the classification of neoplasms according to the extent of the tumor. See also CANCER.

diet s. in the NURSING INTERVENTIONS CLASSIFICATION, a nursing INTERVENTION defined as instituting required DIET restrictions with subsequent progression of diet as tolerated.

TNM s. an international standard for the staging of tumors; the systems of the American Joint Committee on Cancer and the International Union Against Cancer are now identical. Staging is according to three basic components: primary tumor (T), regional nodes (N), and metastasis (M). Subscripts are used to denote size and degree of involvement; for example, 0 indicates undetectable, and 1, 2, 3, and 4 a progressive increase in size or involvement. Thus, a tumor might be described as $T_1N_2M_0$. See also CANCER.

stain (stān) 1. a substance used to impart color to tissues or cells, to facilitate microscopic study and identification. 2. an area of discoloration of the skin.

acid-fast s. a staining procedure for demonstrating acid-fast microorganisms.

differential s. one that facilitates differentiation of various elements in a specimen.

endogenous s. an intrinsic stain acquired during tooth development.

exogenous s. an intrinsic stain acquired after a tooth has erupted.

extrinsic s. a stain that can be removed from a tooth surface by polishing.

Giemsa s. a solution containing azure II-eosin, azure II-glycerin, and methanol; used for staining protozoan parasites such as *Plasmodium* and *Trypanosoma*, for *Chlamydia*, for differential staining of blood smears, and for viral inclusion bodies. Stained elements appear pink to purple to blue.

Gram s. a staining procedure in which bacteria are stained with crystal violet, treated with strong iodine solution, decolorized with ethanol or ethanol-acetone, and counterstained with a contrasting dye; those retaining the stain are called GRAM-POSITIVE, and those losing the stain but staining with the counterstain are called GRAM-NEGATIVE.

hematoxylin and eosin s. a mixture of hematoxylin in distilled water and aqueous eosin solution, employed universally for routine examination of tissues.

intrinsic s. a stain that is within the enamel of a tooth and cannot be removed by polishing.

metachromatic s. one that produces in certain elements a color different from that of the stain itself.

nuclear s. one that selectively stains cell nuclei, generally a basic stain.

port-wine s. a persistent dark red to purple NEVUS FLAMMEUS that grows proportionately with the affected child and is usually found on the face. Initially it is macular, but the surface may develop angiomatous overgrowths with time. Port-wine stains often occur in association with other congenital abnormalities.

supravital s. a stain introduced in living tissue or cells that have been removed from the body.

tumor s. an area of increased density in a radiograph, due to collection of contrast material in distorted and abnormal vessels, prominent in the capillary and venous phases of arteriography, and presumed to indicate neoplasm.

vital s. a stain introduced into the living organism, and taken up selectively by various tissue or cellular elements.

Wright's s. a mixture of eosin and methylene blue, used for demonstrating blood cells and malarial parasites.

staining (stān'ing) artificial coloration of a substance to facilitate examination of tissues, microorganisms, or other cells under the microscope. For various techniques, see under STAIN.

relief s. a method of staining that colors the background and leaves the cells uncolored.

stalagmometer (stal''ag-mom'ĕ-ter) an instrument for measuring surface tension by determining the exact number of drops in a given quantity of a liquid; the lower the surface tension, the smaller each drop will be, and the more drops will be in a given volume.

stammering (stam'er-ing) a SPEECH DISORDER characterized by involuntary pauses in speaking, often with repetition of sounds; see also STUTTERING.

standard (stan'dard) something established as a measure or model to which other similar things should conform. There are three types of standards in health care: structure, process, and outcome standards. *Structure* refers to evaluation of the setting in which care is rendered and the resources that are available. *Process* refers to evaluation of the actual activities carried out by the care giver. *Outcome* refers to evaluation of the results of activities in which the nurse has been involved (what the result is for the patient).

s's of practice a set of guidelines that identifies the content of practice and serves as a model to guide care towards excellence.

standardized test (stan'dard-īzd) a test that has already been used on a wide population of subjects; its results are not limited in application to a particular test group.

standstill (stand'stil) cessation of motion, as of the heart (cardiac standstill) or chest (respiratory standstill).

Stanford-Binet test a modification of BINET'S TEST, translated, adapted, and standardized on children in the United States; the information obtained estimates the mental AGE of the individual.

stannous (stan'us) containing tin as a bivalent element.

s. fluoride SnF_2, a substance used in prevention of DENTAL CARIES, applied topically to the teeth.

stanolone (stan'o-lōn) a semisynthetic form of dihydrotestosterone, which has been used as an androgenic and anabolic steroid.

stanozolol (stan'o-zo-lol'') an androgenic anabolic STEROID, used orally to prevent attacks of hereditary ANGIOEDEMA.

stapedectomy (sta''pe-dek'tah-me) surgical removal of the STAPES, which is then replaced with a prosthetic device composed of stainless steel, Teflon, or a similar substance. This is done for relief of deafness produced by OTOSCLEROSIS (fixation of the minute bones of the middle ear). Replacement of the fixed stapes with a device capable of vibrating permits transmission of sound waves from the outer ear to the inner ear so that hearing is restored.

Because the stapes is one of the smallest bones in the body, this procedure is delicate and must be performed under an operating microscope. Very fine instruments are used, designed specifically for this procedure.

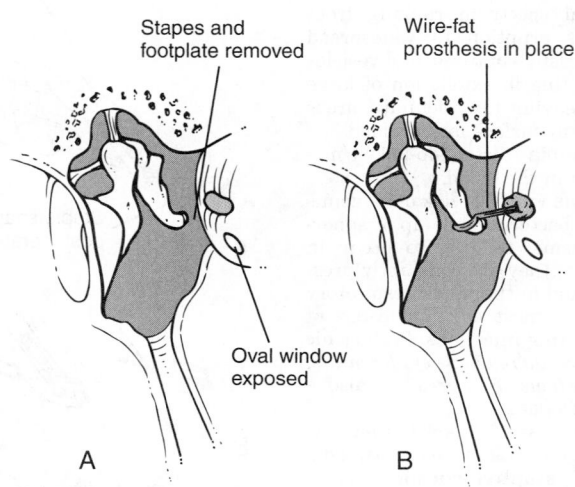

Stapedectomy to correct hearing loss caused by otosclerosis. *A*, Middle ear tissue has been removed. *B*, Prosthesis is in place.

Patient Care. The procedure is done under local anesthesia and the patient usually can go home on the first postoperative day. VERTIGO (dizziness) is common following stapedectomy but it is only temporary. The patient must be protected from falls and self-injury until the sense of balance is regained. Care must also be taken to prevent infection and the patient must be cautioned against blowing the nose and getting water in the ear while bathing until the operative site is completely healed.

stapedial (stah-pe′de-al) pertaining to the stapes.

stapediotenotomy (stah-pe″de-o-tĕ-not′-ah-me) cutting of the tendon of the stapedius muscle.

stapediovestibular (stah-pe″de-o-ves-tib′-u-lar) pertaining to the stapes and vestibule.

stapes (sta′pēz) the innermost of the three ossicles of the EAR; called also stirrup. See also Plates.

staphyl(o)- word element [Gr.], *uvula; resembling a bunch of grapes; staphylococci.*

staphyledema (staf″il-ĕ-de′mah) edema of the UVULA.

staphyline (staf′ĭ-līn) 1. uvular. 2. botryoid.

staphylitis (staf″ĭ-li′tis) uvulitis.

staphylococcal scalded skin syndrome an infectious disease of infants and young children and rarely of older children and adults occurring following infection with certain strains of *Staphylococcus aureus.* The organisms elaborate exfoliatin, an epidermolytic erythrogen endotoxin that causes a clinical spectrum ranging from localized bullous eruption to widespread development of easily ruptured fine vesicles and bullae, resulting in exfoliation of large sheets of skin, leaving raw, denuded areas that make the skin surface look scalded.

staphylococcemia (staf″ĭ-lo-kok-se′me-ah) staphylococci in the blood.

Staphylococcus (staf″ĭ-lo-kok′us) a genus of gram-positive bacteria made up of spherical microorganisms, tending to occur in grapelike clusters; they are constantly present on the skin and in the upper respiratory tract and are the most common cause of localized suppurating infections. Pathogenic species include *S. au′reus, S. epider′midis,* and *S. saprophy′ticus. S. aureus* is also a cause of FOOD POISONING.

staphylococcus (staf″ĭ-lo-kok′us) any organism of the genus *Staphylococcus.* adj., **staphylococ′cal, staphylococ′cic.**

staphyloderma (staf″ĭ-lo-der′mah) pyogenic skin infection by staphylococci.

staphylokinase (staf″ĭ-lo-ki′nās) a bacterial KINASE produced by certain strains of STAPHYLOCOCCUS; it induces fibrinolysis by converting plasminogen to plasmin.

staphylolysin (staf″ĭ-lol′ĭ-sin) a substance produced by staphylococci that causes hemolysis.

staphyloma (staf″ĭ-lo′mah) protrusion of the sclera or cornea, usually lined with uveal tissue, due to inflammation.

anterior s. staphyloma in the anterior part of the eye.

corneal s. 1. bulging of the cornea with adherent uveal tissue. 2. one formed by protrusion of the iris through a corneal wound.

posterior s., s. posti′cum backward bulging of sclera at the posterior pole of the eye.

scleral s. protrusion of the contents of the eyeball where the sclera has become thinned.

staphyloncus (staf″ĭ-long′kus) a tumor or swelling of the uvula.

staphyloplasty (staf′ĭ-lo-plas″te) plastic repair of the soft palate and uvula. See also PALATOPLASTY.

staphylorrhaphy (staf″ĭ-lor′ah-fe) palatorrhaphy.

staphyloschisis (staf″ĭ-los′kĭ-sis) bifid uvula.

staphylotomy (staf″ĭ-lot′ah-me) 1. uvulotomy. 2. excision of a STAPHYLOMA.

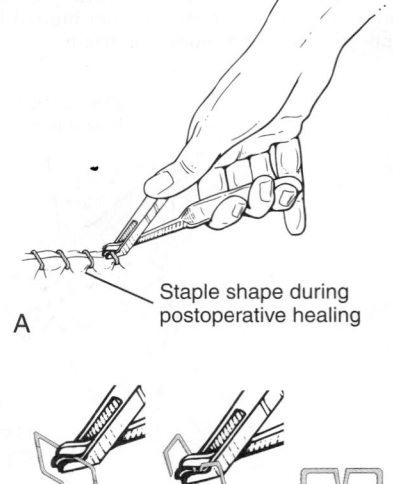

A   Staple shape during postoperative healing

B

Staple shape after extraction

Removing staples. From Lammon et al., 1995.

staple (sta′p'l) a stainless steel wound closure device, usually removed 7 to 10 days after the surgical procedure.

starch (starch) 1. any of a group of polysaccharides of the general formula, $(C_6H_{10}O_5)_n$; it is the chief storage form of CARBOHYDRATES in plants. 2. granular material separated from mature corn (*Zea mays*), wheat, or potatoes; used as a dusting powder and pharmaceutic aid.

Stargardt's disease (stahr′gahrts) a congenital form of MACULAR DEGENERATION that first appears between the ages of 6 and 20 and is marked by rapid loss of visual acuity with a cystlike macular lesion that in the early stages resembles egg yolk. Called also Stargardt's macular degeneration.

startle reaction (stahr′t'l) the various psychophysiological phenomena, including involuntary motor and autonomic reactions, evidenced by an individual in reaction to a sudden, unexpected stimulus, as a loud noise.

starvation (stahr-va′shun) long-continued deprivation of food and resulting morbid effects.

stasis (sta′sis) a stoppage or diminution of flow, as of blood or other body fluid, or of intestinal contents.

s. syndrome overgrowth of bacteria within the small intestine resulting from a variety of conditions causing stasis, particularly disturbances to intestinal motility or decreased acid secretion, but also structural abnormalities such as diverticula, fistulae between the colon and upper bowel, or chronic obstruction; it is characterized by malabsorption of vitamin B_{12}, steatorrhea, and anemia.

venous s. cessation or impairment of venous flow, such as with venous INSUFFI-CIENCY; see also stasis ULCER. Called also phlebostasis and venostasis.

-stasis word element [Gr.], *maintenance (or maintaining) of a constant level; preventing increase or multiplication.* adj., **-stat′ic.**

stat. [L.] sta′tim (at once).

state (stāt) condition or situation.

alpha s. the state of relaxation and peaceful awakefulness associated with prominent alpha brain wave activity.

anxiety s. the condition of experiencing undue anxiety, as in ANXIETY DISORDERS.

excited s. the condition of a nucleus, atom, or molecule produced by the addition of energy to the system as the result of absorption of photons or of inelastic collisions with other particles or systems.

ground s. the condition of lowest energy of a nucleus, atom, or molecule.

persistent vegetative s. a condition of profound nonresponsiveness in the wakeful state caused by brain damage at whatever

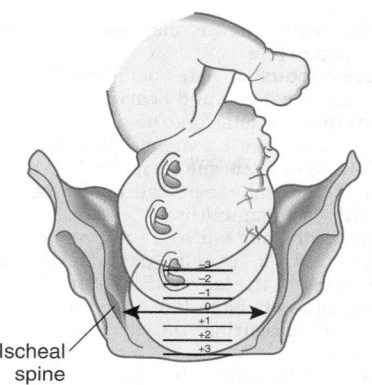

Station of the fetus. From McKinney et al. 2000.

level and characterized by a nonfunctioning cerebral cortex, the absence of any discernible adaptive response to the external environment, akinesia, mutism, and inability to signal; the electroencephalogram may be isoelectric or show abnormal activity. Vegetative states raise ethical questions regarding appropriate care, use of resources, and allowing a patient to die.

refractory s. a condition of subnormal excitability of muscle and nerve following excitation.

resting s. the physiologic condition achieved by complete bed rest for at least 1 hour.

steady s. dynamic equilibrium.

-static word element [Gr.], *inhibiting, inhibitor.*

statim (sta′tim) [L.] at once; abbreviated *stat.*

statins (stat′inz) [from the ending *-statin* that occurs in the names of drugs of this class] HMG-CoA reductase inhibitors.

station (sta′shun) the location of the presenting part of the fetus in the birth canal, designated as −5 to −1 according to the number of centimeters the part is above an imaginary plane passing through the ischial spines, 0 when at the plane, and +1 to +5 according to the number of centimeters the part is below the plane.

statistics (stah-tis′tiks) 1. a collection of numerical data. 2. the mathematical science dealing with the collection, analysis, and interpretation of numerical data using the theory of probability, especially with methods for drawing inferences about characteristics of a population from examination of a random sample.

vital s. data, usually collected by governmental bodies, detailing the rates of birth, death, disease, marriage, and divorce in a population.

statoacoustic (stat″o-ah-koo′stik) pertaining to balance and hearing.

statoconia (stat″o-ko′ne-ah), pl. of *stato-co′nium* minute calcareous particles in the gelatinous membrane surmounting the macula in the inner ear; called also otoconia, otoliths, and statoliths.

statolith (stat′o-lith) 1. a granule of the STATOCONIA. 2. a solid or semisolid body occurring in the labyrinth of animals.

statometer (stah-tom′ĕ-ter) an apparatus for measuring the degree of exophthalmos.

stature (stach′ur) the height or tallness of a person standing.

status (sta′tus, stat′us) [L.] state, particularly in reference to a morbid condition.

absence s. sustained CLOUDING OF CONSCIOUSNESS for several hours, with no interval of normal mental activity, and with few stereotyped movements or no abnormal motor activity.

s. asthma′ticus a particularly severe episode of asthma that does not respond adequately to ordinary therapeutic measures and usually requires hospitalization.

s. epilep′ticus rapid succession of epileptic spasms without intervals of consciousness; brain damage may result.

s. lympha′ticus lymphatism.

performance s. ability of a patient to function, as measured by a performance SCALE.

s. thymicolympha′ticus a condition resembling LYMPHATISM, with enlargement of lymphadenoid tissue and of the thymus as the special influencing factor; formerly thought to be the cause of sudden death in children.

s. verruco′sus a wartlike appearance of the cerebral cortex, produced by disorderly arrangement of the neuroblasts, so that the formation of fissures and sulci is irregular and unpredictable.

stavudine (stav′u-dēn) a nucleoside ANALOGUE of THYMIDINE that inhibits replication of the human immunodeficiency VIRUS (HIV); used in the treatment of HIV infection, administered orally.

STD sexually transmitted disease.

steal (stēl) diversion of something from its normal course, usually referring to blood flow in occlusive arterial disease.

subclavian s. in occlusive disease of the subclavian artery, a reversal of blood flow in the ipsilateral vertebral artery from the basilar artery to the subclavian artery beyond the point of occlusion; this may

deprive the brain of blood and cause the SUBCLAVIAN STEAL SYNDROME.

stearate (ste′ah-rāt) any compound of stearic acid.

stearic acid (ste-ar′ik) a saturated fatty acid from animal and vegetable fats, used as a tablet and capsule lubricant and as an emulsifying and solubilizing agent.

steat(o)- word element [Gr.], *fat; oil.*

steatitis (ste″ah-ti′tis) inflammation of fatty tissue; see also PANNICULITIS.

steatocystoma (ste″ah-to-sis-to′mah) an epithelial cyst.

s. mul′tiplex steatomatosis, a rare hereditary condition in which multiple cutaneous epithelial cysts containing oily liquid, abortive hair follicles, and sebaceous glands occur on the trunk and limbs.

steatogenous (ste″ah-toj′ĕ-nus) producing fat; lipogenic.

steatolysis (ste″ah-tol′ĭ-sis) the emulsification of fats preparatory to absorption. adj., **steatolyt′ic.**

steatoma (ste″ah-to′mah), pl., *steatoma′ta, steatomas* 1. lipoma. 2. a fatty mass retained within a sebaceous gland.

steatomatosis (ste″ah-to″mah-to′sis) the presence of numerous sebaceous cysts; steatocystoma multiplex.

steatonecrosis (ste″ah-to″nĕ-kro′sis) fat necrosis.

steatopygia (ste″ah-to-pij′e-ah) excessive fatness of the buttocks. adj., **steatop′ygous.**

steatorrhea (ste″ah-to-re′ah) excess fat in the feces due to a malabsorption syndrome caused by disease of the intestinal mucosa (e.g., sprue) or pancreatic enzyme deficiency.

steatosis (ste″ah-to′sis) fatty degeneration.

Steele-Richardson-Olszewski syndrome (stēl-rich′erd-sun-ol-shev′ske) a progressive neurological disorder, having an onset during the sixth decade, characterized by supranuclear ophthalmoplegia, especially paralysis of the downward gaze, pseudobulbar palsy, dysarthria, dystonic rigidity of the neck and trunk, and dementia.

Stein-Leventhal syndrome (stīn′-lev′-en-thal) polycystic ovary syndrome.

Steindler operation (stīnd′ler) surgical correction of PES CAVUS by stripping muscle and fascia from the plantar calcaneal surface.

Steinert's disease (sti′nertz) myotonia dystrophica.

Stelazine (stel′ah-zēn) trademark for preparations of TRIFLUOPERAZINE hydrochloride, an ANTIPSYCHOTIC AGENT.

stella (stel′ah) [L.] star.

stellate (stel′āt) star-shaped; arranged in rosettes.

stellectomy (stel-ek′tah-me) excision of a portion of the stellate (cervicothoracic) ganglion.

stem (stem) a stalklike supporting structure; see also PEDUNCLE.

 brain s. BRAINSTEM.

sten(o)- word element [Gr.], *narrow; contracted; constriction.*

stenocephaly (sten″o-sef′ah-le) narrowness of the head or cranium. adj., **stenoceph′alous.**

stenochoria (sten″o-kor′e-ah) stenosis.

stenocoriasis (sten″o-kŏ-ri′ah-sis) contraction of the pupil.

stenopeic (sten″o-pe′ik) having a narrow opening or slit.

stenosed (stě-nōzd′) narrowed; constricted.

stenosis (stě-no′sis), pl. *steno′ses* an abnormal narrowing or contraction of a body passage or opening; called also arctation, coarctation, and stricture.

 aortic s. obstruction to the outflow of blood from the left ventricle into the aorta; in the majority of adult cases the etiology is degenerative calcific disease of the valve.

 hypertrophic subaortic s., idiopathic hypertrophic subaortic s. a cardiomyopathy of unknown cause, in which the left ventricle is hypertrophied and the cavity is small; it is marked by obstruction to left ventricular outflow.

 mitral s. a narrowing of the left atrioventricular orifice (mitral VALVE) due to inflammation and scarring; the cause is almost always rheumatic heart disease. Normally the leaflets open with each pulsation of the heart, allowing blood to flow from the left atrium into the left ventricle, and close as the ventricle fills again so that they prevent a backward flow of blood. In mitral stenosis there is a resultant increase of pressure in the pulmonary artery and hypertrophy of the left ventricle. The usual treatment is surgical replacement of the valve.

 pulmonary s. **(PS)** narrowing of the opening between the pulmonary artery and the right ventricle.

 pyloric s. see PYLORIC STENOSIS.

 renal artery s. narrowing of one or both renal arteries by atherosclerosis or by fibrous dysplasia or hyperplasia, so that renal function is impaired (see ischemic NEPHROPATHY). Increased RENIN release by the affected kidney causes renovascular hypertension, and bilateral stenosis may result in chronic RENAL FAILURE.

 spinal s. narrowing of the vertebral canal, nerve root canals, or intervertebral foramina of the lumbar spine, caused by encroachment of bone upon the space; symptoms are caused by compression of the cauda equina and include pain, paresthesias, and neurogenic claudication. The condition may be either congenital or due to spinal degeneration.

 subaortic s. aortic stenosis due to an obstructive lesion in the left ventricle below the aortic valve, causing a pressure gradient across the obstruction within the ventricle. See also idiopathic hypertrophic subaortic STENOSIS.

 subglottic s. stenosis of the trachea below the glottis. A congenital form results in neonatal STRIDOR or LARYNGOTRACHEITIS, often requiring tracheotomy but resolving with age. An acquired form is caused by repeated intubations.

 tracheal s. scarring of the trachea with narrowing, usually as a result of injury from an artificial airway or trauma.

 tricuspid s. **(TS)** narrowing or stricture of the tricuspid orifice of the heart, a condition often seen in patients with severe congestive HEART FAILURE, usually the result of volume overload and pulmonary hypertension with right ventricular and tricuspid annular dilation.

stenothermal (sten″o-ther′mal) **stenothermic** (sten″o-ther′mik) pertaining to or characterized by tolerance of only a narrow range of temperature.

stenothorax (sten″o-thor′aks) abnormal narrowness of the chest.

stenotic (stě-not′ik) marked by abnormal narrowing or constriction.

stent (stent) 1. a mold for keeping a skin graft in place, made of Stent's mass or some acrylic or dental compound. 2. by extension, a device or mold of a suitable material used to provide support for tubular structures that are being anastomosed. Intravascular stents maintain patency by scaffolding a vessel wall, thus preserving optimal blood flow. Today, they are being used to treat not only coronary artery disease but also problems in the peripheral vascular system, bile ducts and biliary tree, kidney, urinary tract, trachea, and bronchi. A stent is delivered by an angioplasty balloon; when expanded, it forms a fretwork within the lumen and endothelializes over time. Patients receiving endovascular stents are kept on anticoagulants while in the hospital and

S

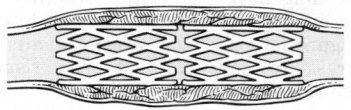

Expanded intraluminal stent within a vessel. From Dorland's, 2000.

usually for one to three months after discharge.

stepwedge (step′wej) a device used for comparing exposure intensities in photography or radiography; a series of tones from white to black (photography) or plates of increasing thickness (radiography) are placed between the energy sources and the film and differences in exposure are noted.

sterc(o)- word element [L.], *feces*. See also words beginning COPR(O)-.

stercobilin (ster″ko-bi′lin) a bile pigment derivative formed by air oxidation of stercobilinogen; it is a brown-orange-red pigmentation contributing to the color of feces and urine.

stercobilinogen (ster′ko-bi-lin′o-jen) a bilirubin metabolite and precursor of stercobilin, formed by reduction of urobilinogen.

stercorolith (ster′kŏ-ro-lith″) fecalith.

stercoroma (ster″kŏ-ro′mah) fecaloma.

stercus (ster′kus) feces. adj., **ster′coral, ster′corous.**

stereo- word element [Gr.], *solid; firm; three dimensional.*

stereoarthrolysis (ster″e-o-ahr-throl′ĭ-sis) surgical formation of a movable new joint in cases of bony ankylosis.

stereoauscultation (ster″e-o-aw″skul-ta′-shun) auscultation with two stethoscopes, on different parts of the chest.

stereocampimeter (ster″e-o-kam-pim′ĕ-ter) an instrument for studying unilateral central scotomas and central retinal defects.

stereochemistry (ster″e-o-kem′is-tre) the branch of chemistry dealing with the space relations of atoms in molecules. adj., **stereochem′ical.**

stereocinefluorography (ster″e-o-sin″-ĕ-floo-rog′-rah-fe) recording by motion picture camera of images observed by stereoscopic fluoroscopy, affording three-dimensional visualization.

stereoencephalotomy (ster″e-o-en-sef′-ah-lot′ah-me) stereotaxic surgery.

stereognosis (ster″e-og-no′sis) the sense by which the form of objects is perceived. adj., **stereognos′tic.**

stereoisomer (ster″e-o-i′so-mer) a compound showing stereoisomerism.

stereoisomerism (ster″e-o-i-som′er-izm) the relationship between two or more isomers that have the same structure (the same linkages between atoms) but different configurations (spatial arrangements), in contrast to constitutional isomerism in which the isomers have different structures. Stereoisomers are further classified into *enantiomers,* those having molecules that are mirror images of each other, and

Stereoisomerism, exemplified by a pair of *cis-trans* diastereoisomers. From Dorland's, 2000.

diastereoisomers, those that do not. adj., **stereoisomer′ic.**

Stereo-orthopter (ster″e-o-or-thop′ter) trademark for a mirror-reflecting instrument for correcting strabismus.

stereoradiography (ster″e-o-ra″de-og′-rah-fe) the making of a radiograph giving an impression of depth as well as of width and height.

stereoscope (ster″e-o-skōp) an instrument for producing the appearance of solidity and relief by combining the images of two similar pictures of an object.

stereoscopic (ster″e-o-skop′ik) three-dimensional; having depth, as well as height and width.

stereospecific (ster″e-o-spĕ-sif′ik) exhibiting marked specificity for one of several stereoisomers of a substrate or reactant; said of enzymes or of synthetic organic reactions.

stereotactic (ster″e-o-tak′tik) 1. pertaining to or characterized by precise positioning in space; said especially of discrete areas of the brain that control specific functions. 2. pertaining to types of brain surgery that use a system of three-dimensional coordinates to locate the site to be operated on. 3. thigmotactic (see THIGMOTAXIS).

stereotaxic (ster″e-o-tak′sik) 1. stereotactic. 2. thigmotactic (see THIGMOTAXIS).

stereotaxis (ster″e-o-tak′sis) TAXIS in response to contact with a solid object or rigid surface.

stereotropism (ster″e-ot′rah-pizm) TROPISM in response to contact with a solid body or rigid surface.

stereotype (ster′e-o-tīp″) an exaggerated, generalized, oversimplified belief or image, often concerning a group, an individual, or a form of behavior.

stereotypic movement disorder a mental disorder characterized by repetitive nonfunctional motor behavior, such as hand waving, rocking, head-banging, or self-biting, which often appears to be driven and can result in serious self-inflicted injuries.

stereotypy (ster′e-o-ti″pe) the persistent repetition of senseless acts or words, frequently occurring in disorders such as autistic disorder and schizophrenia; called also stereotypy-habit disorder.

sterile (ster'il) 1. infertile (see INFERTILITY). 2. aseptic.

   s. technique ASEPTIC TECHNIQUE.

sterility (stĕ-ril'ĭ-te) the state of being sterile.

sterilization (ster″il-ĭ-za'shun) 1. the process of rendering an individual incapable of sexual REPRODUCTION, by CASTRATION, VASECTOMY, SALPINGECTOMY, or some other procedure. Endoscopic techniques for female sterilization that can be performed outside of a hospital without general anesthesia include culdoscopic, hysteroscopic, and laparoscopic sterilization (see subentries below). 2. the process of destroying all microorganisms and their pathogenic products. It can be accomplished by any of various methods, including heat (usually wet steam under pressure at 121°C for 15 minutes), gas plasma, irradiation, or a bactericidal chemical compound such as ETHYLENE OXIDE, PERACETIC ACID, or aqueous GLUTARALDEHYDE. The probability that a given process has made something sterile is known as its sterility assurance LEVEL. A level of 10^{-6} is recommended for organisms on a sterilized device.

In sterilizing objects or substances, the high resistance of bacterial spore cells must be taken into account. Most dangerous bacteria are destroyed at a temperature of 50° to 60°C, so that PASTEURIZATION of fluid, which is the application of heat at about 60°C, destroys disease-causing bacteria. However, temperatures almost twice as high are usually required to destroy the spore cells.

The discovery that heat, in the form of flame, steam, or hot water, kills bacteria made possible the advances of modern surgery, which is based on freedom from microorganisms, or asepsis, and prevention of contamination. Sterilization of all equipment used during operations and other procedures, and of anything that in any way may touch an operative FIELD, is carried out scrupulously. Health care providers all wear sterile clothing. Instruments are sterilized by boiling, by chemical ANTISEPTICS, or by use of an AUTOCLAVE.

Gamma sterilization uses the radioisotope cobalt 60 as the energy source to sterilize some medical supply products. It has the advantages of penetrating all types of packaging, decreasing quarantine time, requiring fewer personnel, and allowing for bulk processing.

   culdoscopic s. use of an endoscope to visualize the fallopian tubes and ovaries for the purpose of preventing conception. The endoscope is inserted through an incision in the posterovaginal cervix. After the fallopian tubes are located, each tube is drawn out through the vaginal incision and severed. The major advantage of this procedure is that it can be done on an outpatient basis. A disadvantage is the complication of infection, a very real possibility owing to the unsterile nature of the vagina.

   flash s. sterilization of unwrapped equipment at 132°C for three to ten minutes using steam.

   gas s. sterilization by means of a bactericidal gas, frequently used for items that are heat and moisture sensitive. Ethylene oxide is the gas most often used; it is highly explosive and flammable in the presence of air, but these hazards are reduced by diluting it with carbon dioxide or fluorinated hydrocarbons. Gas sterilization is a chemical process resulting from reaction of chemical groups in the bacterial cell with the gas. Factors influencing gas sterilization include time of exposure, gas concentration, penetration of the gas, and temperature and humidity in the sterilizing chamber. Automatically controlled ethylene oxide sterilizers are usually heated to a temperature of 54°C (130°F). A humidity level of 35 to 70 per cent is recommended.

   hysteroscopic s. use of an endoscopic instrument to visualize the interior of the uterus and fallopian tubes for the purpose of preventing conception. The hysteroscope is inserted through the dilated cervix and on through the uterine cavity to the point at which each tube joins the uterus. A cautery is then used to electrocoagulate each tube. Occlusion of the tubes is accomplished by scar tissue that forms at the sites of cauterization.

   laparoscopic s. that which employs an endoscope to visualize the fallopian tubes and surrounding structures for the purpose of occluding the tubes. The instrument is guided into the abdominal cavity through a small puncture made by a trocar inserted immediately below the umbilicus. A second small puncture is made in the lower abdomen through which cautery forceps are inserted. The forceps are applied approximately 2 cm from the point at which each of the tubes joins the uterus. In this way each tube is electrocoagulated and severed. An alternative to cauterization and severance of the tubes is the application of clips. However, there is the possibility that the clips may not completely occlude the tubes, allowing passage of the ovum and impregnation.

terminal s. the final sterilization of instruments and equipment following use, thereby rendering them safe for handling.

sterilize (ster′ĭ-līz) to subject to sterilization.

sterilizer (ster′ĭ-līz″er) an apparatus used in ridding objects, such as instruments or dressings, of all microorganisms and their pathogenic products. See also AUTOCLAVE.

stern(o)- word element [L., Gr.], *sternum.*

sternal (ster′nal) pertaining to the sternum.

s. puncture insertion of a hollow needle into the manubrium of the STERNUM to obtain a sample of bone MARROW. The sternum is chosen because of its accessibility and because it is a thin, flat bone. The procedure must be done under surgical asepsis. The clinician anesthetizes the skin and periosteum with a local anesthetic before introducing the sternal needle. The needle is designed with a special guard to prevent penetration beyond the desired depth. When cells are being aspirated into the syringe the patient may experience a sharp pain; otherwise the procedure should not be painful. Samples are examined for abnormal cells, for the proportion of cells in various stages of development, and for the characteristics of the blood cells that predominate. This information is used in conjunction with clinical findings and other tests in diagnosis of blood disorders such as LEUKEMIA, LYMPHOMA, MULTIPLE MYELOMA, and ANEMIA.

sternalgia (ster-nal′jah) pain in the sternum.

Sterneedle (ster′ne-d′l) trademark for a controlled-depth, multiple-puncture apparatus used in diagnosing tuberculosis.

Sterneedle tuberculin test (ster′ne-d′l) an intracutaneous test for tuberculosis, 1 or 2 drops of tuberculin PPD being forced to penetrate the outer layer of the skin by pressure of the six needle points of the Sterneedle.

sternoclavicular (ster″no-klah-vik′u-lar) pertaining to the sternum and clavicle.

sternocleidomastoid (ster″no-kli″do-mas′toid) pertaining to the sternum, clavicle, and mastoid process.

sternocostal (ster″no-kos′tal) pertaining to the sternum and ribs.

sternodymia (ster″no-dim′e-ah) union of two fetuses by the anterior chest wall.

sternodymus (ster-nod′ĭ-mus) conjoined twins united at the anterior chest wall.

sternohyoid (ster″no-hi′oid) pertaining to the sternum and hyoid bone.

sternoid (ster′noid) resembling the sternum.

sternomastoid (ster″no-mas′toid) pertaining to the sternum and the mastoid PROCESS.

sternopericardial (ster″no-per″ĭ-kahr′de-al) pertaining to the sternum and pericardium.

sternoschisis (ster-nos′kĭ-sis) congenital fissure of the sternum.

sternothyroid (ster″no-thi′roid) pertaining to the sternum and thyroid cartilage or gland.

sternotomy (ster-not′ah-me) incision of the sternum.

sternum (ster′num) a plate of bone forming the middle of the anterior wall of the thorax and articulating with the clavicles and the cartilages of the first seven ribs. It consists of three parts, the manubrium, the body, and the xiphoid process.

sternutatory (ster-nu′tah-tor″e) 1. causing sneezing. 2. an agent that causes sneezing.

steroid (ster′oid) any of a group of lipids with a complex molecule containing carbon atoms in four interlocking rings forming a hydrogenated cyclopentophenanthrene-ring system; three of the rings contain six carbon atoms each and the fourth contains five. Steroids are important in body chemistry

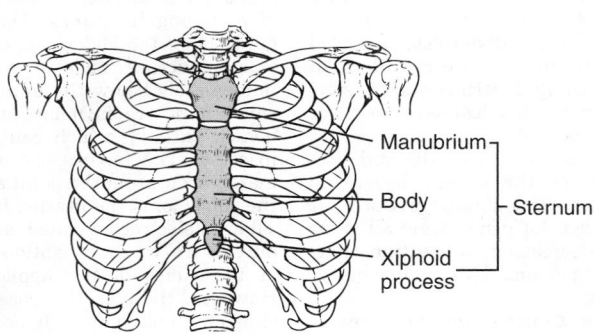

Manubrium ⎤
Body ⎬ Sternum
Xiphoid ⎦
process

From Dorland's, 2000.

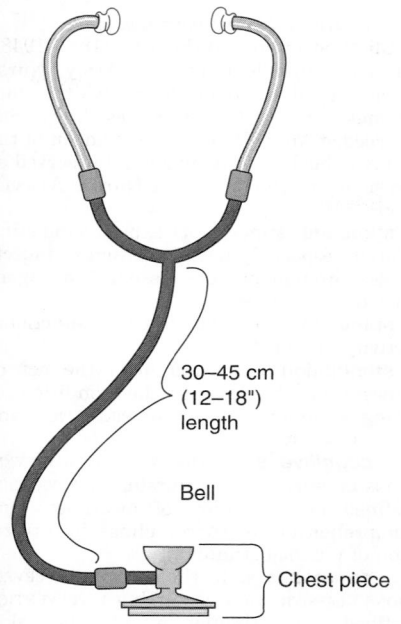

30–45 cm
(12–18")
length

Bell

Chest piece

Parts of a stethoscope. From Elkin et al., 2000.

and include steroid HORMONES such as the gonadal or sex STEROIDS, CORTICOSTEROIDS, GLUCOCORTICOIDS, and MINERALOCORTICOIDS; VITAMINS of the D group; and the STEROLS, including CHOLESTEROL, the main building block of the steroid hormones in the body. The cardiac GLYCOSIDES, a group of compounds derived from certain plants, are partly steroids.

anabolic s. any of a group of synthetic derivatives of testosterone having pronounced anabolic properties and relatively weak androgenic properties; they are used clinically mainly to promote growth and repair of body tissues in diseases or states promoting catabolism or tissue wasting.

gonadal s., sex s. a steroid HORMONE produced by a GONAD, such as an ANDROGEN, ESTROGEN, or progestational AGENT.

steroidogenesis (stĕ-roi″do-jen′ĕ-sis) production of steroids, as by the adrenal glands.

sterol (ster′ol) any of a group of STEROIDS having long aliphatic side-chains at position 17 and at least one alcoholic hydroxyl group; the sterols have lipidlike solubility. Examples are CHOLESTEROL and ERGOSTEROL.

stertor (ster′tor) snoring. adj., **ster′torous.**

steth(o)- word element [Gr.], *chest.* See also words beginning THORAC(O)-.

stethogoniometer (steth″o-go″ne-om′ĕter) an apparatus for measuring the curvature of the chest.

stethoscope (steth′o-skōp) an instrument used to hear and amplify the sounds produced by the heart, lungs, and other internal organs. As first introduced by the 19th century French physician, René Laënnec, it was a simple wooden tube with a bell-shaped opening at one end. The modern stethoscope is BINAURAL, with two earpieces and flexible tubing leading to them from the two-branched opening of the bell or cone. In this way, sound travels simultaneously through both branches to the earpieces. adj., **stethoscop′ic.**

stethospasm (steth′o-spazm) spasm of the pectoral (chest) muscles.

Stevens-Johnson syndrome (ste′venz jon′son) a severe and sometimes fatal form of ERYTHEMA MULTIFORME in which the lesions may involve the oral and anogenital mucosa, eyes, and viscera, associated with such constitutional symptoms as malaise, headache, fever, arthralgia, and conjunctivitis.

Stewart (stoo′art) Isabel Maitland (1878–1963). Nursing author, educator, and researcher. Born in Canada, she graduated from Teachers College, Columbia University, where she succeeded Adelaide NUTTING as chairman of the Department of Nursing Education. She participated in many nursing research studies and was the author of a number of influential books on nursing.

S

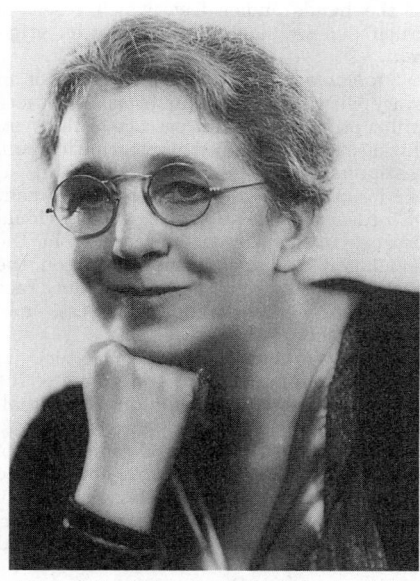

Isabel Maitland Stewart. Special Collections, Milbank Memorial Library, Teachers College, Columbia University.

STH (somatotropic) growth hormone.

sthenic (sthen'ik) active; strong.

stibialism (stib'e-al-izm″) ANTIMONY poisoning.

stichochrome (stik'o-krōm) any neuron having the stainable substance arranged in more or less regular layers.

stiff-man syndrome a condition of unknown etiology marked by painful, progressive fluctuating rigidity of axial and limb muscles in the absence of signs of cerebral or spinal cord disease but with continuous electromyographic activity.

stigma (stig'mah) 1. any mental or physical mark or peculiarity which aids in the identification or in the diagnosis of a condition. 2. a mark, spot, or pore on the surface of an organ or organism. 3. follicular stigma. 4. in botany, the uppermost part of a pistil, which secretes a moist, sticky substance to trap and hold the pollen that reaches it. 5. an eyespot of chromatophore-bearing protozoa, such as certain euglenoids, comprising a dark pigmented mass that functions in light detection by shielding the photoreceptor cells from specific wavelengths. 6. a distinguishing personal trait that is perceived as or actually is physically, socially, or psychologically disadvantageous. 7. in the plural, gill slits around the pharynx in urochordates, through which pass respiratory and feeding currents. 8. in the plural, purpuric or hemorrhagic lesions of the hands and/or feet, which resemble crucifixion wounds. adj., **stigmat'ic, stig'-mal.**

follicular s. a spot on the surface of an ovary where the vesicular ovarian FOLLICLE will rupture and permit passage of the OVUM during OVULATION. Called also macula folliculi.

stigmatization (stig″mah-tĭ-za'shun) 1. the formation of STIGMAS. 2. the assignment of negative perceptions to an individual because of perceived difference from the population at large; it may occur on the basis of physical appearance (including race or sex), of mental or physical illness, or of various other qualities.

stigmatometer (stig″mah-tom'ĕ-ter) an instrument for testing the refraction of the eye by retinoscopy and for direct ophthalmoscopy.

Still's disease (stilz) a chronic form of POLYARTHRITIS affecting children and marked by enlargement of lymph nodes, generally of the spleen, with evanescent rash and irregular fever. See also *juvenile rheumatoid* ARTHRITIS.

stillbirth (stil'berth) delivery of a dead child.

stillborn (stil'born) born dead.

Stimson (stim'son) Julia C. (1881–1948). As superintendent of the Army Nurse Corps, the first woman to receive the rank of major in the United States Army. She succeeded Annie W. GOODRICH as dean of the Army School of Nursing and later served as president of the American Nurses Association.

stimulant (stim'u-lant) 1. producing stimulation, especially by stimulation of muscle FIBERS through nervous tissue. 2. an agent that has such effects.

stimulate (stim'u-lāt) to excite functional activity in a part.

stimulation (stim″u-la'shun) the act or process of stimulating; the condition of being stimulated; see also PROMOTION and ENHANCEMENT.

cognitive s. in the NURSING INTERVENTIONS CLASSIFICATION, a nursing INTERVENTION defined as promotion of awareness and comprehension of surroundings by utilization of planned stimuli.

cutaneous s. in the NURSING INTERVENTIONS CLASSIFICATION, a nursing INTERVENTION defined as stimulation of the skin and underlying tissues for the purpose of decreasing undesirable signs and symptoms such as pain, muscle spasm, or inflammation.

deep brain s. **(DBS)** patient-controlled, continuous, high-frequency electrical stimulation of a specific area of the brain by means of an implanted electrode, which is controlled by a battery implanted just below the clavicle. The electrical signals block those signals from the brain causing tremors and some other related problems such as occur in PARKINSON'S DISEASE, essential TREMOR, and DYSTONIA.

transcutaneous electrical nerve s., transcutaneous neural s. see TRANSCUTANEOUS ELECTRICAL NERVE STIMULATION.

stimulus (stim'u-lus) [L.] any agent, act, or influence that produces functional or trophic reaction in a receptor or an irritable tissue.

conditioned s. a stimulus that acquires the ability to evoke a given response by repeatedly being linked with another stimulus that naturally evokes that response; see also CONDITIONING.

depolarizing s. a stimulus that lowers the resting POTENTIAL, making the inside of a fiber less negative. In cardiac fibers this means bringing the resting potential from −90 mV to −70 mV.

discriminative s. a stimulus associated with REINFORCEMENT, which exerts control over a given type of behavior; the subject must discriminate between closely related stimuli and respond positively only with this particular stimulus.

   eliciting s. any stimulus, conditioned or unconditioned, that elicits a RESPONSE.

   threshold s. a stimulus that is just strong enough to elicit a response.

   unconditioned s. any stimulus that naturally evokes a specific response; see also CONDITIONING.

sting (sting) 1. injury caused by a poisonous substance produced by an animal or plant (biotoxin) and introduced into or onto an individual, together with mechanical trauma incident to such introduction. 2. the organ used to inflict such injury.

   bee s. see BEE STING.

   insect s. see INSECT BITES AND STINGS.

stippling (stip'ling) a spotted condition or appearance, such as an appearance of the retina as if dotted with light and dark points, or the spotted appearance of the erythrocytes in basophilia.

   gingival s. the presence of a minutely lobulated surface on the gingiva, like that of an orange peel; it is a normal adaptive process, varying from one person to another. Its absence or reduction indicates gingival disease.

stirrup (stir'up) stapes.

stitch (stich) 1. a sudden transient cutting pain, generally in the flank. 2. a loop made in sewing or suturing; see SUTURE (def. 2).

stochastic (sto-kas'tik) pertaining to a random process; used particularly to refer to a time series of random variables.

stocking (stok'ing) a closely fitting covering for the foot and adjacent parts of the lower limb.

   antiembolic s's, compression s's SUPPORT HOSE.

   Jobst s. trademark for an elastic SUPPORT HOSE that is custom made for a patient.

stoichiology (stoi''ke-ol'ah-je) the science of elements, especially the physiology of the cellular elements of tissues. adj., **stoichiolog'ic.**

stoichiometry (stoi''ke-om'ĕ-tre) the determination of the relative proportions of the compounds involved in a chemical reaction. adj., **stoichiomet'ric.**

stoke (stōk) a unit of kinematic viscosity, equal to 10^{-4} m^2 per second.

Stokes-Adams disease (stōks' ad'amz) a condition due to heart block and marked by slow or absent pulse, vertigo, syncope, and sometimes convulsions and Cheyne-Stokes respiration; called also Adams-Stokes disease.

stoma (sto'mah), pl. *stomas, sto'mata* [Gr.] 1. a mouthlike opening. 2. an incised opening that is kept open for drainage or other purposes, such as the opening in the

abdominal wall for COLOSTOMY, URETEROSTOMY, and ILEAL CONDUIT. adj., **sto'mal.**

Patient Care. Immediately after a stoma has been created it is observed for changes in color, edema, evidence of prolapse or stenosis, character of output, and condition of the surrounding skin. Normal coloration for a new stoma varies from dark pink to red, similar to the color of healthy mucous membranes. Later the stoma should shrink in size and become less highly colored. A noticeable lightening or blanching of color could indicate inadequate blood supply to the tissues of the stoma itself. A deepening of color to a purplish hue may indicate obstruction to the flow of blood and resultant ischemia. The blood supply must be restored as soon as possible to avoid necrosis.

At first the stoma will be slightly edematous and will appear larger than a healed stoma. The most common cause of abnormal swelling of the stoma is application of a collection device whose opening is too narrow to accommodate the stoma. To prevent edema and restricted blood supply, the opening of the collection device should be at least 1/8 inch larger than the circumference of the stoma.

Prolapse of the stoma results from a surgical incision that is too large or from inadequately securing the stoma to the abdominal wall. Decreased development of the abdominal musculature and an increase in intraabdominal pressure are factors that make this more common in children than adults. It becomes evident when an increase in pressure within the abdominal cavity causes a segment of intestine to protrude a noticeable distance beyond its usual position. Coughing, sneezing, and vigorous peristalsis can contribute to stomal prolapse. When it occurs it is not necessarily an emergency situation; the intestine can be gently manipulated back into place by an experienced health care worker such as a nurse, enterostomal therapist, or surgeon. If the condition persists and causes serious problems, surgical repair may be necessary.

Stenosis is one of the most common problems associated with a stoma. The cause is formation of scar tissue at the point at which the segment of intestine passes through the abdominal wall. Treatment may consist of progressive dilation of the opening to break down structures causing the stricture. Stomal stenosis must be relieved; otherwise the opening may become obstructed and drainage impeded or prohibited.

The character of output from an intestinal stoma will depend on the location of

S

the stoma along the intestinal tract. The farther along the tract the stoma is located, the more solid the fecal material should be. Patients are taught to distinguish between normal and abnormal output from the stoma.

Periostomal skin care is essential to preserve the integrity of the skin, which can be exposed to the caustic action of urine or fecal material. The two major principles of periostomal skin care are cleanliness and provision of a protective barrier. If there is a proper seal to prevent seepage of either urine or feces around the stoma, irritation and breakdown of the skin occur much less frequently. Possible causes of skin problems include removing the appliance too roughly or changing faceplates too frequently, allergic reaction to a particular adhesive or other substance, and yeast infections. Soap and water are used to cleanse and thoroughly rinse the skin. The area is patted, not rubbed, dry. Protective barriers are available in a number of forms and shapes. The base usually is pectin, which repels moisture and other harmful substances.

Specific aspects of care will depend on the type of stoma and the purpose for which it was created. All patients with a stoma ("ostomates") will need instruction in self-care and continued support as they adjust to new ways to handle fecal or urinary waste. They will need to know how to obtain and care for collection devices, how to protect the skin around the stoma, and dietary restrictions to control odor and obstruction. They will also need to be aware of potential complications and signs and symptoms that should be

reported. Goals for patient care include developing in these patients an attitude of independence and freedom from restrictions on their physical, social, and recreational activities after discharge from the hospital.

There is a health care specialty designed to meet the needs of patients with stomas. Ostomy clubs composed of ostomates and their families and conducted under the guidance of enterostomal therapists are available in many communities. At regularly held meetings the members find assistance in resolving their physical problems, and gain psychological support from one another in adjusting to their new body image. Those members of the club who have been able to adjust to their stomas are frequently available for visits to patients who are in the hospital or have just returned home after surgery.

Information about local resources available to the ostomate can be obtained from the American Cancer Society's Rehabilitation Program and from other agencies concerned with meeting the needs of patients with stomas. The United Ostomy Association, Inc., is a volunteer-based organization dedicated to providing education information, support, and advocacy for people who have had or will have intestinal or urinary diversions. They can be contacted by writing to United Ostomy Association Inc., 19772 MacArthur Blvd., Suite 200, Irvine, CA 92612-2405, or consulting their web site at http://www.uoa.org.

stomach (stum′ak) the curved, muscular saclike structure that is an enlargement of the alimentary canal (see DIGESTIVE SYSTEM) and lies between the esophagus and the small intestine; called also gaster. (See also Plates.) adj., **gas′tric.**

The wall of the stomach consists of four coats: an outer serous coat; a muscular coat made up of longitudinal, circular, and oblique muscle fibers; a submucous coat; and a mucous coat or membrane forming the inner lining. The muscles account for the stomach's ability to expand when food enters it. The muscle fibers slide over one another, reducing the thickness of the wall while increasing its area. When empty, the stomach has practically no cavity at all since its walls are pressed tightly together; when full it holds about 1.4 liters.

The stomach muscles perform another function. When food enters the stomach they contract in rhythm and their combined action sends a series of wavelike contractions from the upper end of the stomach to the lower end. These contractions, known as PERISTALSIS, mix the partially digested food with the stomach secretions and ingested

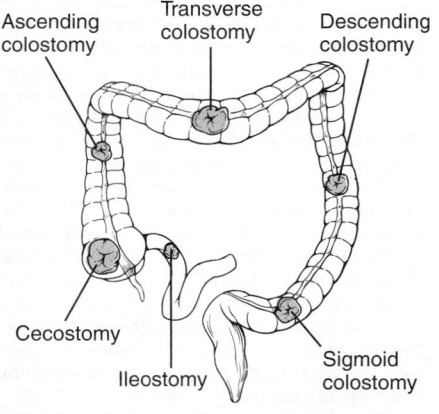

Ascending colostomy

Transverse colostomy

Descending colostomy

Cecostomy

Ileostomy

Sigmoid colostomy

Locations of stomas in the gastrointestinal tract. From Lammon et al., 1995.

liquid until it has the consistency of a thick soup; the contractions then push it gradually by small aliquots into the small intestine.

The stomach is usually emptied of its digested contents in 1 to 4 hours; the time may be longer, however, depending on the amount and type of food eaten. Foods rich in carbohydrates leave it more rapidly than proteins, and proteins more rapidly than fats. The stomach may continue to contract after it is empty; such contractions stimulate nerves in its wall and may cause hunger pangs.

The mucous membrane lining the stomach contains innumerable *gastric glands*; their secretion, GASTRIC JUICE, contains enzymes, MUCIN, and HYDROCHLORIC ACID. Enzymes help to split the food molecules into smaller parts during digestion. The physiologic action of mucin is not fully understood. Hydrochloric acid aids in dissolving the food before the enzymes begin working on it.

The diagnosis and treatment of stomach disorders has changed markedly with the development of ENDOSCOPY. This benign procedure permits direct examination and biopsy of the stomach and has sharply increased the accuracy of diagnosis and, as a result, the effectiveness of medical therapy. In addition, the development of whole new families of medications that reduce gastric acid secretion (such as CIMETIDINE) and increase gastric motility (such as METOCLOPRAMIDE) have decreased the need for surgery for peptic ulcer disease.

Surgery of the stomach has become increasingly conservative with a better understanding of that organ's physiology. Instead of the resections that were once done routinely for peptic ulcer disease, sophisticated procedures, such as the supraselective VAGOTOMY, that can decrease acid secretion without resection of the stomach are available. Even so, resection may still be needed for more severe cases of ulcer disease, for such complex entities as Zollinger-Ellison syndrome, and for malignancies.

cascade s. an atypical form of hourglass stomach, characterized radiologically by a drawing up of the posterior wall; an opaque medium first fills the upper sac and then cascades into the lower sac.

hourglass s. one shaped somewhat like an hourglass.

leather bottle s. linitis plastica.

s. pump an apparatus used to remove material from the stomach, consisting of a stomach tube to which a bulb syringe is attached. The tube is inserted into the mouth or nose and passed down the esophagus into the stomach. Suction from the syringe brings the contents of the stomach up through the tube. This can be used either to remove material from the stomach in an emergency (such as when a person has swallowed poison) or to obtain a specimen for chemical analysis (such as in diagnosis of peptic ulcer or other stomach disorders).

s. tube a flexible tube used for introducing food, medication, or other material directly into the stomach. It can be passed into the stomach by way of either the nose or the mouth. See also TUBE FEEDING. Called also esophageal tube.

stomachal (stum′ah-kal) 1. gastric. 2. stomachic (def. 2).

stomachalgia (stum″ah-kal′jah) gastrodynia.

stomachic (sto-mak′ik) 1. gastric. 2. a medicine that stimulates gastric activity.

Stomahesive (sto″mah-he′siv) trademark for a PECTIN-based wafer used to protect the skin from irritating drainage.

stomat(o)- word element [Gr.], *mouth.*

S

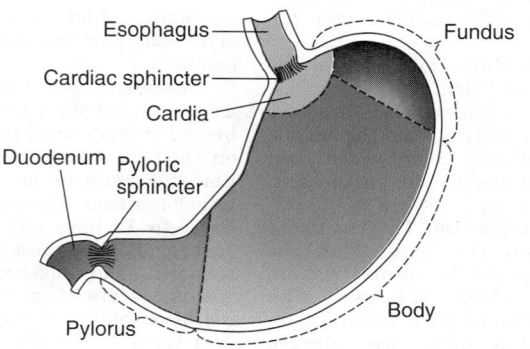

Anatomy of the stomach. From Ignatavicius and Workman, 2002.

Esophagus
Fundus
Cardiac sphincter
Cardia
Duodenum
Pyloric sphincter
Pylorus
Body

stomatalgia (sto″mah-tal′jah) pain in the mouth; called also stomatodynia.

stomatitis (sto″mah-ti′tis), pl. *stomati′-tides* inflammation of the mucosa of the mouth; it may be caused by any of numerous diseases of the mouth or it may accompany another disease. Both GINGIVITIS and GLOSSITIS are forms of stomatitis.

Causes. The causes of stomatitis vary widely, from a mild local irritant to a vitamin deficiency or infection by a possibly dangerous disease-producing organism. Inflammation may arise from actual injury to the inside of the mouth, as from cheek-biting, jagged teeth, tartar accumulations, and badly fitting dentures. Irritating substances, including alcohol, and tobacco, may also cause stomatitis. Other causes are infectious bacteria, such as streptococci and gonococci or those causing necrotizing ulcerative STOMATITIS, DIPHTHERIA, and TUBERCULOSIS; the fungus causing THRUSH; or the viruses causing HERPES SIMPLEX and MEASLES. Extreme vitamin deficiencies can result in mouth inflammation, as can certain blood disorders. Poisoning with heavy metals, such as LEAD or MERCURY, can also cause stomatitis.

Symptoms. There is generally swelling and redness of the tissues of the mouth, which may become quite sore, particularly during eating. The mouth may have an unpleasant odor. In some types of stomatitis the mouth becomes dry, but in others there is excessive salivation. Ulcerations may appear, and, in extreme cases, gangrene *(gangrenous stomatitis)*. Other forms of stomatitis may occasionally cause more severe symptoms, including chills, fever, and headache. Sometimes bleeding or white patches in the mouth can be seen. In thrush, the symptoms themselves may be slight (white spots in the mouth resembling milk curds) but the disease may give rise to serious infections elsewhere in the body. In some cases, stomatitis causes inflammation of the parotid glands.

Stomatitis resulting from certain diseases presents special identifying symptoms. *Syphilitic stomatitis* produces painful ulcers in the mouth; in scarlet fever the tongue first has a strawberry color, which then deepens to a raspberry hue; in measles, Koplik's SPOTS appear.

Treatment and Prevention. The treatment varies according to the cause. When the inflammation is caused by anemia, vitamin deficiency, or any infection of the body, both the underlying disease and the stomatitis are treated. Antibiotics often are effective against the infection and prevent its spreading to the parotid glands. Severe stomatitis can be a side effect of chemotherapy and radiation to the head and neck as treatment for cancer. Measures to alleviate the inflammation and promote healing include increasing fluid intake and using artificial saliva to minimize dryness and help buffer acidity in the mouth, avoiding liquids and foods that are chemically irritating or extremely hot, and frequent and consistent MOUTH CARE.

With proper care, many cases of stomatitis can be prevented. Cleanliness is essential, especially of the mouth, teeth, dentures, and feeding utensils. Infants may acquire mouth infection from the mother's oral flora, dirty bottles, or the mother's nipples. In the case of a prolonged fever or of any severe general illness, dryness of the mouth should be avoided by ingestion of increased amounts of fluids.

angular s. superficial erosions and fissuring at the angles of the mouth; it may occur in RIBOFLAVIN deficiency and in PELLAGRA or result from overclosure of the jaws in denture wearers. Called also perlèche.

aphthous s. recurrent aphthous stomatitis.

denture s. inflammation of the oral mucosa seen in some patients with new dentures or with old, ill-fitting ones, caused by *Candida albicans*; characterized by redness, swelling, and pain of mucosa that is in contact with the denture. Called also chronic atrophic CANDIDIASIS and denture sore mouth.

gangrenous s. see NOMA.

herpetic s. herpes simplex involving the oral mucosa and lips, characterized by the formation of yellowish vesicles that rupture and produce ragged painful ulcers covered by a gray membrane and surrounded by an erythematous halo.

s. medicamento′sa stomatitis due to an allergic reaction to drugs ingested, absorbed through the skin or mucosa, or given by hypodermic injection. Principal symptoms include vesicles, erosion, ulcers, erythema, purpura, angioedema, burning, and itching.

recurrent aphthous s. a recurrent disease of unknown etiology, characterized by one or more small round or oval ulcer(s) on the oral mucosa, covered by a grayish fibrinous exudate and surrounded by a bright red halo. The lesions usually persist for 7 to 14 days and then heal without scarring. Called also aphthae, aphthous stomatitis, and canker sore.

stomatocyte (sto′mah-to-sīt) an abnormal red blood cell in which a slit or mouthlike area replaces the normal central circle of pallor, often due to edema.

stomatocytosis (sto″mah-to-si-to′sis) the presence of stomatocytes in the blood, as seen in liver disease; Rh null syndrome; a rare congenital type of hemolytic anemia; and a few other conditions. Called also hydrocytosis.

stomatodynia (sto″mah-to-din′e-ah) stomatalgia.

stomatognathic (sto″mah-tog-nath′ik) denoting the mouth and jaws collectively.

stomatology (sto″mah-tol′ah-je) the branch of medical science concerning the mouth and its diseases, functions, and structure.

stomatomalacia (sto″mah-to-mah-la′shah) excessive or abnormal softness of the oral structures.

stomatomenia (sto″mah-to-me′ne-ah) vicarious menstruation involving bleeding from the mouth.

stomatomycosis (sto″mah-to-mi-ko′sis) any fungal disease of the mouth.

stomatopathy (sto″mah-top′ah-the) any disorder of the mouth.

stomatoplasty (sto′mah-to-plas″te) plastic repair of defects or reconstruction of the mouth.

stomatorrhagia (sto″mah-to-ra′jah) hemorrhage from the mouth.

stomocephalus (sto″mo-sef′ah-lus) a malformed fetus with rudimentary jaws and mouth.

stomodeum (sto″mo-de′um) the ectodermal depression at the head end of the embryo, which becomes the front part of the mouth.

-stomy word element [Gr.], *creation of an opening into* or *a communication between.*

stone (stōn) 1. calculus. 2. a unit of weight in Great Britain, the equivalent of 14 pounds (avoirdupois), or about 6.34 kg.

    kidney s. see KIDNEY STONE.

stool (stōōl) feces.

    lienteric s. feces containing much undigested food.

    rice-water s′s the characteristic and diagnostic watery, light gray to clear diarrhea of CHOLERA, containing flecks of mucous material, epithelial cells, and many cholera vibrios.

    silver s. feces with a silver color due to a mixture of melena and white fatty stools; it occurs in tropical sprue and carcinoma of the ampulla of Vater, and in children taking sulfonamides who have diarrhea.

stopcock (stop′kok) a valve that regulates the flow of fluid through a tube. See illustration.

storage disease any metabolic disorder in which some substance (such as a fat, protein, or carbohydrate) accumulates in certain cells in abnormal amounts.

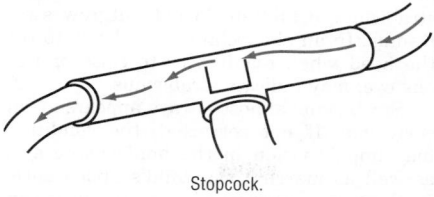

Stopcock.

storage pool the area of a PLATELET organelle such as a dense body or an alpha granule where specific chemical constituents are stored.

    s. p. disease a blood coagulation disorder due to failure of the platelets to release adenosine diphosphate (ADP) in response to aggregating agents such as collagen, epinephrine, exogenous ADP, or thrombin; characteristics include mild bleeding episodes, prolonged bleeding time, and reduced aggregation response to collagen or thrombin.

storiform (stor′ĭ-form) denoting a matted, irregularly whorled pattern, somewhat resembling that of a straw mat; said of the microscopic appearance of fibrous histiocytomas.

stork bites a superficial telangiectasia or vascular area found on the nape of the neck of newborns. Stork bites disappear within the first year and are not to be confused with elevated hemangiomas, such as portwine stain, which persist.

storm (storm) an outburst; a temporary and sudden increase in symptoms.

    thyroid s., thyrotoxic s. THYROID CRISIS.

STPD standard temperature and pressure, dry; denoting a volume of dry gas at 0°C and a pressure of 760 mm Hg.

strabismometer (strah-biz-mom′ĕ-ter) an apparatus for measuring the degree of strabismus.

strabismus (strah-biz′mus) deviation of the eye that the patient cannot overcome; the visual axes assume a position relative to each other different from that required by the physiological conditions. Called also squint. adj., **strabis′mic.** The various forms of strabismus are spoken of as *tropias,* their direction being indicated by the appropriate prefix, as CYCLOTROPIA, ESOTROPIA, EXOTROPIA, HYPERTROPIA, and HYPOTROPIA.

During the first 3 to 6 months of life, the eyes of infants tend to waver and turn either inward or outward independently of one another; this usually corrects itself. If it persists, or if the eyes are continually crossed in the same way, even if the child is less than 6 months old, it may be a sign of strabismus. Children do not outgrow strabismus. In an older child, a tendency to tilt the head when reading, or to close or rub one eye, may indicate strabismus.

Strabismus almost always appears at an early age. If not corrected, the condition may impair vision in the nonfocusing eye, as well as marring the child's appearance. In the great majority of cases the eyes can be straightened by proper medical treatment at any age, but vision of the malfunctioning eye may remain impaired. If treated early enough, preferably before 6 years, normal vision can usually be restored in the affected eye.

Cause. Strabismus may result from several factors, including a blow on the head, disease, or heredity. Many cases are caused by a malfunction of the muscles that move the eyes. This causes the eyes to focus differently, sending different images to the brain. As the child grows, he or she learns to ignore the image from one eye with the result that it fails to grow as strong as the eye on which he or she is depending.

Treatment. Treatment for strabismus varies with the individual case. A patch may be placed over the child's stronger eye for a period, forcing use of the weaker eye and thus restoring its strength as far as possible, instead of letting it grow worse from lack of use. Eyeglasses or special eye exercises may correct the condition. In some cases, a relatively simple surgical operation on the eye muscles may be necessary. Since these muscles are outside the eye itself, there is no danger to the vision.

 comitant s., concomitant s. that in which the angle of deviation of the visual axis of the squinting eye is always the same in relation to the other eye, no matter what the direction of the gaze; due to faulty insertion of the eye muscles.

 convergent s. esotropia.

 divergent s. exotropia.

 noncomitant s., nonconcomitant s. that in which the amount of deviation of the squinting eye varies according to the direction in which the eyes are turned.

 vertical s. that in which the visual axis of the squinting eye deviates in the vertical plane; see HYPERTROPIA and HYPOTROPIA.

strabotomy (strah-bot′ah-me) cutting of an ocular tendon in treatment of strabismus.

strain (strān) 1. to overexercise. 2. excessive effort or exercise. 3. an overstretching or overexertion of some part of the musculature. 4. to filter or separate. 5. a group of organisms within a species or variety, characterized by some particular quality, as rough or smooth strains of bacteria.

 caregiver role s. a NURSING DIAGNOSIS accepted by the North American Nursing Diagnosis Association, defined as difficulty performing the caregiver ROLE.

 risk for caregiver role s. a NURSING DIAGNOSIS accepted by the North American Nursing Diagnosis Association, defined as vulnerability of a CAREGIVER for felt difficulty performing the caregiver ROLE.

strait (strāt) a narrow passage.

 s's of the pelvis the pelvic INLET (*superior pelvic strait*) and pelvic OUTLET (*inferior pelvic strait*).

straitjacket (strāt′jak″et) popular name for CAMISOLE.

strand (strand) a thread or fiber or a structure resembling one.

 antisense s. the strand of a double-stranded nucleic acid that is complementary to the sense STRAND; in DNA it is the template strand on which the mRNA is synthesized.

 sense s. the strand of a double-stranded nucleic acid that encodes the product; in DNA it is the strand that encodes the RNA, having thus the same base sequence except changing T for U in the RNA. See also antisense STRAND.

strangle (strang′g'l) choke (def. 1).

strangulated (strang′gu-lat″ed) congested by reason of constriction or hernial restriction, as strangulated HERNIA.

strangulation (strang″gu-la′shun) 1. choke (def. 2). 2. impairment of blood supply to a part by mechanical constriction of the vessels; see also HEMOSTASIS (def. 2).

strangury (strang′gu-re) slow and painful discharge of urine.

strap (strap) 1. a band or strip, as of adhesive tape, used in attaching parts to each other. 2. to bind down tightly.

 Montgomery s's straps made of lengths of adhesive tape folded back on themselves at one end, with a hole that allows insertion of a tape tie; they are applied to the skin to contain frequently changed dressings so that they can be changed without the skin irritation caused by frequent pulling off of tape; the dressings are secured by tying the opposing tapes together over them.

strapping (strap′ing) the application of strips of adhesive tape, one overlapping the other, to cover and exert pressure on a limb or other area of the body; see illustration.

stratification (strat″ĭ-fĭ-ka′shun) arrangement in layers.

stratiform (strat′ĭ-form) occurring in layers.

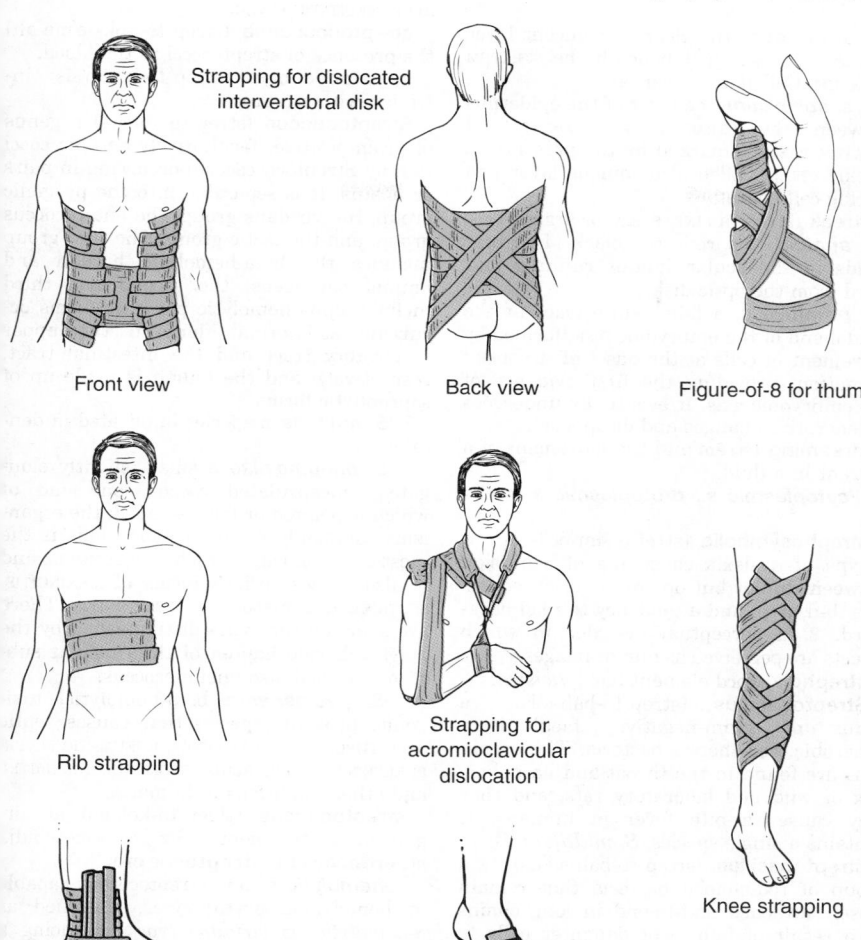

Strapping for dislocated intervertebral disk

Front view

Back view

Figure-of-8 for thumb

Rib strapping

Strapping for acromioclavicular dislocation

Knee strapping

Basket weave for ankle

Metatarsal strapping

Types of strapping.

S

stratigraphy (strah-tig'rah-fe) tomography.

stratum (stra'tum, strat'um) [L.] a sheetlike mass of tissue; see also LAMINA and LAYER.

   s. basa'le the deepest layer of the
EPIDERMIS, composed of a single layer of
basophilic cells. Called also basal layer of
epidermis.

   s. cor'neum the outer horny layer of
the EPIDERMIS, consisting of cells that are
dead and desquamating. Called also horny
layer.

   s. germinati'vum 1. the STRATUM BASALIS
and STRATUM SPINOSUM considered together;
called also malpighian layer. 2. the lower
layer of the nail, from which the nail grows;
called also germinative layer.

   s. granulo'sum the cell layer of the
EPIDERMIS lying between the stratum lucidum
and the stratum spinosum. Called also
granular layer. 1. the deep layer of the cortex
of the cerebellum. 2. the layer of follicle cells
lining the theca of the vesicular ovarian
follicle; called also granular layer.

s. lu'cidum the clear translucent layer of the EPIDERMIS, just beneath the STRATUM CORNEUM. Called also clear layer.

s. spino'sum the layer of the epidermis between the STRATUM GRANULOSUM and STRATUM BASALIS, marked by the presence of prickle CELLS; called also spinous layer and prickle-cell layer.

streak (strēk) a LINE, STRIA, or STRIPE.

angioid s's red to black irregular bands in the ocular fundus running outward from the optic disk.

primitive s. a faint white trace at the caudal end of the embryonic DISK, formed by movement of cells at the onset of MESODERM formation, providing the first evidence of the embryonic axis. It eventually undergoes degenerative changes and disappears.

streaming (strēm'ing) the movement of a current in a fluid.

cytoplasmic s., protoplasmic s. cyclosis.

strephosymbolia (stref"o-sim-bo'le-ah) 1. a type of dyslexia consisting of confusion between similar but oppositely oriented letters (b-d, p-q), and a tendency to read backward. 2. a perceptual disorder in which objects are perceived as mirror images.

strept(o)- word element [Gr.], *twisted.*

Streptobacillus (strep"to-bah-sil'us) a genus of gram-negative, facultatively anaerobic, rod-shaped bacteria. The organisms are found in the throat and nasopharynx of wild and laboratory rats, and they may cause rat-bite fever in humans. It contains a single species, *S. multifor'mis.*

streptobacillus (strep"to-bah-sil'us) 1. a group of rod-shaped bacteria that remain loosely attached end-to-end in long chains as a result of failure of daughter cells to separate after cell division. 2. an organism of the genus *Streptobacillus.*

streptocerciasis (strep"to-ser-ki'ah-sis) infection with the nematode *Dipetalonema streptocerca,* seen in Central Africa. The microfilariae produce a pruritic rash resembling that of ONCHOCERCIASIS; they are transmitted from animal to animal by the bite of small insects of the genus *Culicoides.*

Streptococcaceae (strep"to-kok-a'se-e) a family of gram-positive, usually nonmotile, facultative anaerobic cocci, occurring in pairs, chains, or tetrads.

streptococcal (strep"to-kok'al) pertaining to or due to a streptococcus.

s. sore throat "strep throat," a sore throat caused by a STREPTOCOCCUS; symptoms are more severe than in ordinary sore throat and may include high fever, swelling of lymph nodes of the neck, and a rash.

Treatment is usually with antibiotics. See also RHEUMATIC FEVER.

streptococcemia (strep"to-kok-se'me-ah) the presence of streptococci in the blood.

streptococcosis (strep"to-kŏ-ko'sis) infection with streptococci.

Streptococcus (strep"to-kok'us) a genus of gram-positive, facultatively aerobic cocci (family Streptococcaceae) occurring in pairs or chains. It is separable into the pyogenic group, the viridans group, the enterococcus group, and the lactic group. The first group includes the beta-hemolytic human and animal pathogens; the second and third include alpha-hemolytic parasitic forms occurring as normal flora in the upper respiratory tract and the intestinal tract, respectively; and the fourth is made up of saprophytic forms.

S. mu'tans a species implicated in dental caries.

S. pneumo'niae a small, slightly elongated, encapsulated coccus, one end of which is pointed or lance-shaped; the organisms commonly occur in pairs. This is the most common cause of lobar PNEUMONIA, and it also causes serious forms of MENINGITIS, SEPTICEMIA, EMPYEMA, and PERITONITIS. There are some 80 serotypes distinguished by the polysaccharide hapten of the capsular substance. Called also pneumococcus.

S. pyo'genes a beta-hemolytic, toxigenic, pyogenic species that causes septic SORE THROAT, SCARLET FEVER, RHEUMATIC FEVER, PUERPERAL FEVER, acute GLOMERULONEPHRITIS and other conditions in humans.

streptococcus (strep"to-kok'us) an organism of the genus *Streptococcus.* adj. **streptococ'cal, streptococ'cic.**

hemolytic s. any streptococcus capable of hemolyzing erythrocytes, classified as α-*hemolytic* or *viridans type,* producing a zone of greenish discoloration much smaller than the clear zone produced by the β type about the colony on blood agar; and the β-*hemolytic type,* producing a clear zone of hemolysis immediately around the colony on blood agar. The β group contains the most virulent streptococci and is divided into serotype subgroups designated by letters (e.g., Group A).

streptodornase (strep"to-dor'nās) an enzyme produced by hemolytic streptococci that catalyzes the depolymerization of deoxyribonucleic acid (DNA). See STREPTOKINASE STREPTODORNASE.

streptokinase (strep"to-ki'nās) an enzyme produced by streptococci that catalyzes the conversion of PLASMINOGEN to PLASMIN. It is administered intravenously as a THROMBOLYTIC agent in the treatment of acute coronary arterial thrombosis, acut pulmonary embolism, deep venous thrombosis, and acute arterial thromboembolism or thrombosis. It is also used to clear obstructed arteriovenous cannulae. Detailed and skilled control is required in its use in order to avoid hemorrhage. It also can produce severe antigenic reactions upon readministration. See also ANTICOAGULANT.

s.-streptodornase a mixture of enzymes elaborated by hemolytic streptococci; used as a proteolytic and fibrinolytic agent.

streptolysin (strep-tol´ĭ-sin) the hemolysin of hemolytic streptococci.

Streptomyces (strep″to-mi´sēz) a genus of bacteria, usually soil forms, but occasionally parasitic on plants and animals, and notable as the source of various antibiotics, e.g., the tetracyclines.

streptomycin (strep″to-mi´sin) an AMINOGLYCOSIDE antibiotic produced by *Streptomyces griseus;* its use is now limited because of the emergence of resistant strains. The sulfate salt is used in combination with other agents in the treatment of tuberculosis and certain other bacterial infections.

streptosepticemia (strep″to-sep″tĭ-se´-me-ah) septicemia due to streptococci.

streptozocin (strep″to-zo´sin) an antitumor ANTIBIOTIC derived from *Streptomyces achromogenes,* now produced synthetically. It contains a nitrosourea group linked to a methyl group and a glucosamine moiety and acts as an ALKYLATING AGENT to inhibit DNA synthesis, and also as an inhibitor of enzymes involved in GLUCONEOGENESIS; used primarily for treatment of islet cell carcinoma of the pancreas and other endocrine tumors including gastrinomas associated with ZOLLINGER-ELLISON SYNDROME and glucagon-secreting alpha cell tumors of the pancreas.

stress (stres) 1. forcibly exerted influence; PRESSURE. 2. in dentistry, the pressure of the upper teeth against the lower. 3. a state of physiological or psychological STRAIN caused by adverse stimuli, physical, mental, or emotional, internal or external, that tend to disturb the functioning of an organism and which the organism naturally desires to avoid. STRESS REACTIONS are elicited but should these reactions be inappropriate or inadequate, they may lead to disease states. The term is also used to refer to the stimuli that elicit such a state or stress reactions. Just as a bridge is structurally capable of adjusting to certain physical stresses, the human body and mind are normally able to adapt to the stresses of new situations. However, this ability has definite limits beyond which continued stress may cause a breakdown, although this limit varies from person to person.

Physical Stress. There are many kinds of physical stress, but they can be divided into two principal types, to which the body reacts in different ways. There is emergency stress, a situation that poses an immediate threat, such as a near accident in an automobile, a wound, or an injury. There is also continuing stress, such as that caused by changes in the body during puberty, pregnancy, menopause, acute and chronic diseases, and continuing exposure to excessive noise, vibration, fumes, chemicals, or other agents.

The body's reaction to emergency stress is set off by the adrenal medulla. The medulla of each adrenal gland is directly connected to the nervous system. When an emergency arises, it pours the hormone epinephrine into the bloodstream. This has the effect of speeding up the heart and raising the blood pressure, emptying sugar supplies swiftly into the blood, and dilating the blood vessels in the muscles to give them immediate use of this energy. At the same time, the pupils of the eyes dilate. (See also ALARM REACTION.)

The reaction of the body to continuing stress is even more complex. Again the principal organs are the adrenal glands, but after the first phase of alarm, the glands continue to produce a steady supply of hormones that apparently increase the body's resistance. This is in addition to specific defenses such as the production of antibodies to fight infection. If the stress is overwhelming, as in the case of an extensive third-degree burn or an uncontrollable infectious disease, the third phase, exhaustion of the adrenal glands, sets in, sometimes with fatal results.

Psychologic Stress. The emergency response of the body comes into play when a person merely foresees or imagines danger, as well as in real emergency situations. The thought of danger, or the vicarious experience of it in a thrilling story, play, or film, may be enough to cause the muscles to tense and the heart to start pounding. Psychologic situations can have the same effect. One of the best-known examples of this is "stage fright," often characterized by tensed muscles and an increased heart rate. At times the person may not even be aware of the unconscious thought that produces this dramatic reaction.

Stress and Disease. In recent decades, there have been numerous attempts to find a direct correlation between certain diseases and a stressful environment or a personality

S

type that responds to the environment in a certain way. However, while inappropriate activity and a hectic lifestyle can cause illness in some persons, a busy and productive person can actually be subject to less stress than one who feels trapped in a limited position with no hope for release or a sense of accomplishment.

The diseases most often associated with a stressful environment are, according to some scientists, coronary artery disease and "heart attack," high blood pressure, and cancer. Studies of laboratory animals have demonstrated a connection between isolated and specific stimuli such as electric shock and separation from mates and the development of heart disease in these animals. The stressful variables in the human environment are, however, much more complex, and a stressful environment can be related to heart disease only as a risk factor (see TYPE A BEHAVIOR).

The postulated relationship between stress and the development of a malignancy is based on the theory that destructive emotions affect and in some way weaken the body's surveillance system, causing its IMMUNE RESPONSE to fail to recognize and destroy malignant cells.

Although relaxation techniques can reduce blood pressure in persons with mild hypertension, there is no evidence that tension and stress cause the blood pressure to rise and stay at levels above normal.

Other diseases considered by some researchers to be related to stress include asthma, allergies, colitis, migraine headaches, and peptic ulcers. Even though the relationship is not clear and there are currently no hard data to support this, most health care providers are convinced that stress contributes to the worsening of symptoms and influences the impact a disease will have on the lives of some patients while other patients adapt to stress and seem to have no long-term deleterious reaction to it.

Coping Mechanisms. Unhealthy ways to cope with psychologic stress include DRUG ABUSE and ALCOHOLISM, SMOKING, abusive and violent behavior, and working harder to accomplish unrealistic or poorly defined goals. In order to deal with stress in an effective and healthy way, one must first identify sources of stress, either within oneself or in one's environment.

Job stressors are frequently related to disorganization in the work place, poor time management, and unrealistic or uncommunicated expectations of the employer. Another source of stress for the working person

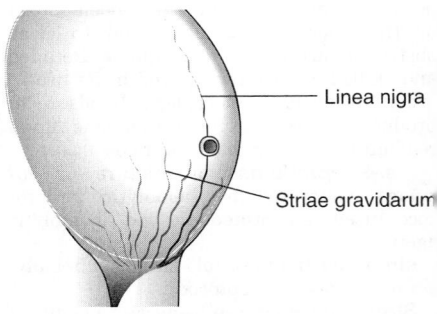

Linea nigra

Striae gravidarum

Striae gravidarum: linear tears that may occur in the connective tissue. From Gorrie et al., 1994.

may be the lack of time for family and recreation because of job demands. Once job stressors are identified, some options are to change the stressful situation, modify the way one responds to stressors, or seek another job that is less stressful. In some instances learning to be more assertive and better able to communicate with supervisors and coworkers can reduce job-related stress.

Stressors in the home environment include negative self-concept; inadequate physical, cognitive, or behavioral resources; poor problem-solving skills; marital discord; ineffective parenting or lack of parenting skills; and lack of family support. Effective coping may require strategies to improve self-concept and build self-esteem, develop problem-solving skills, learn effective parenting, and establish a network of people who can give support. Exercise, improving one's nutritional status, making time for recreational activities, and utilizing relaxation techniques to relieve tension can also be healthy ways to cope with stress.

oxidative s. any of various pathological changes seen in living organisms in response to excessive levels of cytotoxic OXIDANTS and free RADICALS in the environment.

s. reaction any of the biological reactions to adverse stimuli, physical, mental, or emotional, internal or external, that tend to disturb the organism's equilibrium; should these compensating reactions, physiological or psychological, be inadequate or inappropriate, they may lead to disorders. See ALARM REACTION, acute stress reaction GENERAL ADAPTATION SYNDROME, ACUTE STRESS DISORDER, ADJUSTMENT DISORDER, and POST TRAUMATIC STRESS DISORDER.

stressor (stres'or) any factor that disturbs homeostasis, producing stress.

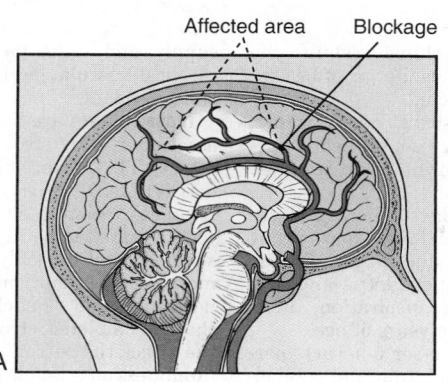

Affected area   Blockage

A

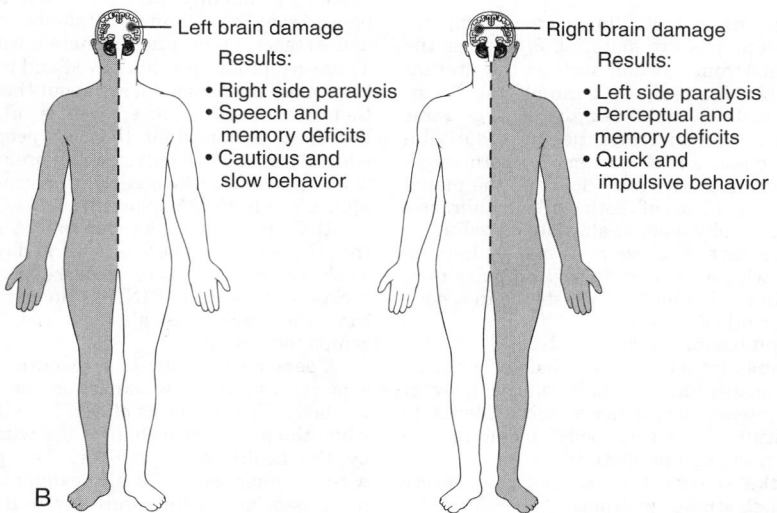

Left brain damage
Results:

- Right side paralysis
- Speech and memory deficits
- Cautious and slow behavior

Right brain damage
Results:

- Left side paralysis
- Perceptual and memory deficits
- Quick and impulsive behavior

B

A, Stroke. *B,* Areas of the body affected by a stroke. From Frazier et al., 2000.

stretcher (strech′er) a portable couchlike or bedlike contrivance for carrying the sick or wounded; called also litter.

stretching (strech′ing) increasing something in one of its dimensions; extending. See EXERCISE.

stria (stri′ah), pl. *stri′ae* [L.] 1. a band, line, streak, or stripe. 2. in anatomic nomenclature, a longitudinal collection of nerve fibers in the brain.

atrophic striae, stri′ae atro′phicae atrophic, pinkish or purplish, scarlike lesions, later becoming white (LINEAE ALBICANTES), on the breasts, thighs, abdomen, and buttocks, due to weakening of elastic tissues, associated with pregnancy (STRIAE GRAVIDARUM), overweight, rapid growth during puberty and adolescence, Cushing's syndrome, and topical or prolonged treatment with corticosteroids.

s. diagona′lis (Broca) a band of nerve fibers that forms the caudal zone of the anterior perforated substance where it adjoins the optic tract.

stri′ae gravida′rum striae atrophicae occurring in pregnancy.

stri′ae medulla′res bundles of white fibers across the floor of the fourth ventricle.

striate (stri′āt) **striated** (stri′āt-ed) having streaks or striae.

striation (stri-a′shun) 1. the quality of being streaked. 2. a streak or scratch, or a series of streaks.

striatonigral (stri″ah-to-ni′gral) projecting from the corpus striatum to the substantia nigra.

S

stricture (strik′chur) stenosis.

stricturization (strik″chur-ĭ-za′shun) the process of decreasing in caliber or of becoming narrowed or constricted.

stridor (stri′dor) a shrill, harsh sound, especially the respiratory sound heard during inhalation with a laryngeal obstruction. adj., **strid′ulous.**

laryngeal s. that due to laryngeal obstruction. A *congenital* form, marked by stridor and dyspnea, is due to an infolding of a congenitally flabby epiglottis and aryepiglottic folds during inspiration; it is usually outgrown by two years of age.

striocerebellar (stri″o-ser″ĕ-bel′ar) pertaining to the corpus striatum and cerebellum.

strip (strip) 1. a thin, narrow, comparatively long piece of material. 2. to press the contents from a canal, such as the urethra or a blood vessel, by running the finger along it. 3. to excise lengths of large veins and incompetent tributaries after subcutaneous dissection. 4. to remove tooth structure or restorative material from the mesial or distal surfaces of teeth, utilizing abrasive strips; usually done to alleviate crowding.

reagent s. a strip of paper impregnated with a REAGENT to a given substance, used in testing for that substance in a body fluid or other secretion.

stripe (strīp) a streak or stria.

strobila (stro-bi′lah) the chain of PROGLOTTIDS constituting the bulk of the body of adult TAPEWORMS, sometimes considered to constitute the entire body, including the head, neck, and proglottids.

stroke (strōk) 1. a sudden and severe attack. 2. stroke syndrome.

heat s. a condition caused by exposure to excessive heat; see also SUNSTROKE.

stroke syndrome a symptom complex caused by a disorder of the blood vessels serving the brain, with impaired blood supply and ischemia. Called also stroke, cerebral vascular accident, and cerebrovascular accident.

Types. There are four neurological events associated with stroke: transient ischemic attack (TIA), reversible ischemic neurologic deficit (RIND), *stroke in evolution (SIE)*, and *completed stroke (CS)*.

TIAs are temporary attacks that come on suddenly and last only a few minutes to not more than 24 hours; although they often are not recognized as such, they are a warning that a completed stroke can occur. During the attack the person may feel a weakness or numbness on one side of the body, slurring of speech or inability to talk, visual disturbances such as blindness or double vision, and staggering or uncoordinated walking. These symptoms are short-lived and reversible; unless the person knows about them and their significance, the episode is often ignored. It is important that lay people be educated about TIAs because the probability of a completed stroke occurring at some time after a TIA is 25 to 35 per cent.

RIND is an event similar to TIA except that the symptoms last for several days to a week; there is complete or nearly complete recovery. Like TIA, RIND is an indication that the person is at high risk for a completed stroke.

A person with a stroke in evolution (SIE) experiences gradual weakness on one side of the body. The diagnosis of SIE is confirmed when the progressive changes are witnessed by the health care provider. The person with a completed stroke (CS) exhibits symptoms associated with severe cerebral ischemia resulting from an interrupted blood supply to the brain.

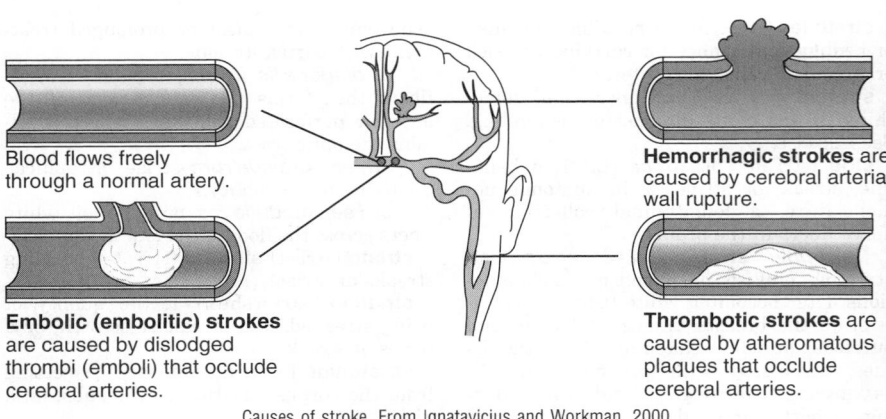

Blood flows freely through a normal artery.

Hemorrhagic strokes are caused by cerebral arterial wall rupture.

Embolic (embolitic) strokes are caused by dislodged thrombi (emboli) that occlude cerebral arteries.

Thrombotic strokes are caused by atheromatous plaques that occlude cerebral arteries.

Causes of stroke. From Ignatavicius and Workman, 2000.

Persons most at risk for any of the four types of stroke include those with hypertension, atherosclerosis, and heart disease and other cardiovascular disorders. Obese persons, heavy smokers, and those with diabetes mellitus are also at increased risk.

Causes. There are three main causes of stroke syndrome, all of which are related to a pathological condition of the arteries and associated with cerebral infarction, i.e., a necrotic area in the brain tissue. They are cerebral EMBOLISM, cerebral THROMBOSIS, and cerebral HEMORRHAGE. Other causes of stroke-like symptoms include compression of cerebral vessels, as from tumor or edema, and arterial spasm.

Cerebral Embolism. An embolus is a small mass of material circulating in the blood vessels. It can consist of air, fat, or other material introduced into the circulatory system; or, as is most often the case, it is a detached portion of a thrombus that settles in a cerebral vessel. Damage from cerebral embolism is often less extensive and recovery more rapid than in strokes from thrombosis and cerebral hemorrhage.

Cerebral Thrombosis. A thrombus, or clot, in a blood vessel of the brain is by far the most common cause of stroke. Most often the thrombosis occurs where there is narrowing of the lumen of a vessel, usually caused by ATHEROSCLEROSIS. The thrombosis produces ischemia, edema, and congestion of the brain tissues surrounding the area. Symptoms appear more gradually in this type of stroke.

Cerebral Hemorrhage. This is a rupturing of a blood vessel, usually an artery, within the brain, frequently associated with preexisting HYPERTENSION. There often is weakening of the vessel wall as well. Healthy arteries can withstand considerable pressure because of their elasticity, but in persons with ARTERIOSCLEROSIS this elasticity is lost and the blood vessel may rupture from the increased pressure within it. In other situations the cerebral vessel wall may be weakened by an ANEURYSM, and thus is susceptible to rupture and hemorrhage into the brain tissues. Stroke from cerebral hemorrhage is most common after age 50 and usually produces more extensive neurologic defects with slower recovery than does stroke from other causes.

Symptoms. The symptoms of stroke syndrome vary widely, depending on its cause, location of ischemia, and extent of damage to brain cells. The onset is sudden in cerebral hemorrhage and cerebral embolism because the interruption of blood flow happens quickly. Its effects are noticed almost immediately. Strokes from cerebral hemorrhage occur most often in the daytime while the person is active. In cerebral thrombosis the clot gradually occludes the blood vessels, therefore the onset is gradual. A stroke caused by thrombosis tends to occur while the patient is sleeping or within an hour after arising.

There may be preliminary symptoms, particularly with thrombosis. The patient may experience dizziness, headache, mental confusion, and poor coordination. More often there is a sudden and dramatic onset with loss of consciousness; convulsions may occur. The unconsciousness may last for a few minutes or continue for weeks; it can terminate in a slow recovery or death. Sudden death rarely occurs as a result of stroke.

There usually are neurologic symptoms related to the site of ischemia, such as hemiplegia, loss of sensation, and reflex changes. The area of paralysis is directly related to the area of cerebral ischemia. If the left side of the brain is affected, the paralysis of the face, arm, and leg will be present on the right side. Speech disturbances also are related to the area of brain cell damage; if the left side of the brain is affected (the location of the speech center in right-handed persons), then a right-handed person will have aphasia along with the hemiplegia.

Involvement of the region of the thalamus produces a sensation of pain in the hemiplegic area, especially the hand, beginning several weeks after the stroke. Emotional disturbances also accompany thalamic involvement. The patient has difficulty controlling emotions and may laugh or cry with little provocation.

The symptoms of stroke are almost unlimited in type, severity, and duration. Some may eventually subside, while others are never completely eliminated. Anyone concerned with the care of the stroke victim should be alert to all signs and symptoms that occur. These can be extremely helpful in establishing a definite diagnosis and planning a regimen of patient care.

Prevention and Treatment. Medical and surgical preventive measures have significantly reduced the incidence of stroke in the United States. Medical preventive measures are aimed at eliminating or controlling ATHEROSCLEROSIS and other conditions that predispose a person to stroke. Effective control of HYPERTENSION and treatment of rheumatic and atherosclerotic heart disease have significantly reduced the incidence of stroke. Efforts to control DIABETES MELLITUS, reduce CHOLESTEROL levels by diet and exercise,

S

manage OBESITY, and encourage cessation of SMOKING are all examples of measures that have been successful in preventing stroke in significant numbers of people at risk.

Surgical procedures employed to prevent stroke or lessen the severity of its effects once it has occurred include (1) ENDARTER-ECTOMY to remove thickened areas from the inner lining of the carotid or vertebral arteries in the neck, (2) using a graft to patch a section of artery in which there is an aneurysm, or removing the section of artery so affected, and (3) removal of a blood clot within the artery.

The choice of prevention and treatment is governed by the conditions which predispose the patient to having a stroke and, in the event one has already occurred, the potential of the individual patient to benefit from the treatment. ANTICOAGULANT THERAPY is used only when hemorrhage has been ruled out as a possibility and clot formation has been found to be either the potential or actual cause of decreased blood flow. Antihypertensive drugs are used to reduce pressure within the blood vessel and thereby avoid rupture.

Emergency and Acute Care. Emergency care consists of loosening all constricting clothing, especially around the neck, to improve respiration and circulation to the head. The patient's head should be turned to the affected side to prevent aspiration of saliva and mucus. Oxygen is administered, and the patient is kept calm and quiet and reassured of being cared for. If conscious, he or she may sit up or the head may be elevated to lessen blood pressure within it.

After admission and during the acute stage of stroke syndrome, it is extremely important to assess the patient's condition frequently to determine the neurologic effects and to ascertain whether there is evidence of recurrent strokes. Observations of the patient are valuable in determining the cause of the stroke and the choice of treatment. Maintenance of a patent AIRWAY and adequate oxygenation are critical. SUCTIONING may be necessary if paralysis prevents normal swallowing of saliva. An artificial airway is inserted if the patient cannot maintain an adequate airway on his own. In severe cases a TRACHEOSTOMY may be required. The vital signs are taken and recorded at frequent intervals until stable. An elevated temperature, with decrease in the pulse and respiratory rates, indicates a poor prognosis.

General Care. To avoid complications that can develop quickly in a stroke victim with partial paralysis, it is necessary to attend to proper positioning, good body alignment, and frequent turning. (See accompanying illustration.) The patient is turned at least every two hours. Because of poor circulation to the affected area, a stroke patient should not be left to lie on the affected side for more than 20 minutes four times a day.

The amount of activity allowed will depend on the cause of the stroke and the stage of illness. Those who have increased intracranial pressure from hemorrhage and edema will be placed on complete bed rest. Others who are comatose will require continuous care to avoid complications arising from inactivity (see also COMA).

Complications to be avoided in the patient who has suffered a stroke include PRESSURE ULCERS, hypostatic PNEUMONIA, THROMBOSIS and other conditions resulting from circulatory stasis, KIDNEY STONES and urinary infections, and such orthopedic deformities as FOOTDROP, WRISTDROP, and CONTRACTURES. Unless contraindicated, the joints are put through their full RANGE OF MOTION at least once a day (see also therapeutic EXERCISE). A program of PHYSICAL THERAPY, along with OCCUPATIONAL THERAPY and speech THERAPY is planned and started as soon as possible to assure maximum rehabilitation.

Nutrition is maintained by whatever means necessary, depending on the patient's ability to chew, handle food in the mouth, and swallow. In some cases TUBE FEEDING may be the only method by which food is administered. If the patient is able to swallow, but has some DYSPHAGIA, food should be cut into small pieces and the patient instructed to chew it thoroughly and to make a conscious effort to swallow. Liquids should be sipped rather than gulped down; thickened liquids are easier than thin ones to swallow. Tilting the head to the unaffected side may make swallowing easier and gagging less likely. Rinsing the mouth after meals and frequent mouth care help eliminate accumulation of food in the mouth and halitosis. The lips should be kept lubricated with cold cream or mineral oil to keep them from drying and cracking.

INCONTINENCE of urine and feces sometimes accompanies a stroke. A regular schedule of offering the bedpan, especially after each meal, may help establish a routine of elimination. It is also helpful to get the patient up to the bathroom or to a bedside commode whenever this is possible. In any event the patient must be kept clean and dry and skin care must be given frequently to avoid pressure areas and decubitus ulcers. Fecal impaction and urinary retention may occur and can be avoided by intelligent observation and recording of bowel movements and urinary output. (See also BLADDER TRAINING and BOWEL TRAINING.)

Stroke victims sometimes experience a lack of PROPRIOCEPTION; that is, they are unaware of the location and position of an affected extremity unless they are looking directly at it. This predisposes them to falls and other injuries unless special care is taken to assist them. Other common problems include those associated with decreased sensitivity to touch, pressure, heat, and cold.

Rehabilitation of the patient begins upon entrance to the hospital. This means that all measures taken to maintain bodily functions and to avoid complications are aimed at the ultimate goal of getting the patient back to a state as near normal as possible. Reaction to the illness by the patient and the family, the quality of care received, and the attitude of caregivers will greatly affect the eventual outcome of the illness. There may be a tendency on the part of the hospital staff and the patient's family to do everything for someone who seems so helpless and handicapped. Certainly the patient should be helped with the things he or she absolutely cannot do, but total dependence on others can become very demoralizing; for the patient's sake he or she must be encouraged in self care. This may be a slow and demanding process, requiring much patience and optimism. One can begin by providing the means by which the patient can gradually begin activities such as bathing, feeding, and dressing.

Special equipment, such as an overbed table made of cardboard or plywood, can be used so that the patient can reach bath water, toilet articles, and other needed things. Food should be prepared and arranged on the tray so that the patient can handle it without great difficulty. If the first movements are awkward and messy, no mention should be made of this; the patient must never be made to feel that he or she has caused an inconvenience to anyone through efforts to do things independently.

There has been much interest in the rehabilitation of stroke patients in recent years and there is a wealth of information and help available for the patient and family. Pamphlets dealing with the special problems of this illness are available from the American Heart Association and the American Red Cross. Centers for speech therapy, vocational rehabilitation, and homemaker services are located in many communities. The local health department can provide information as to the location of these centers and services they provide.

stroma (stro'mah) [Gr.] the tissue forming the ground substance, framework, or matrix of an organ, as opposed to the functioning part or PARENCHYMA. adj., **stro'mal, stromat'ic.**

stromuhr (strōm'oor) an instrument for measuring the velocity of the blood flow.

Strong (strong) Anne H. (1876–1925). A leader in public health nursing. She served as a volunteer and staff nurse with the Henry Street Nursing Service in New York City and later was first director of the School of Public Health Nursing at Simmons College. One of her areas of concern in nursing education was the relation of the theoretical and practical components of education.

Strongyloides (stron″jĭ-loi'dēz) a genus of nematode parasites. *S. stercora'lis* is a species found in the intestines of humans and other mammals in the tropics, and is the most common cause of STRONGYLOIDIASIS. (See accompanying illustration.)

strongyloidiasis (stron″jĭ-loi-di'ah-sis) infection with *Strongyloides stercoralis.* The worms usually inhabit the small intestines, causing *intestinal strongyloidiasis* with diarrhea and ulceration of the mucosa. At a later stage in their life cycle they may penetrate the skin and be carried to the lungs, causing *pulmonary strongyloidiasis* with hemorrhaging. Called also strongyloidosis.

strongyloidosis (stron″jĭ-loi-do'sis) strongyloidiasis.

strontium (stron'she-um) a chemical element, atomic number 38, atomic weight 87.62, symbol Sr. (See Appendix 6.)

s. 89 a radioactive isotope of strontium having a half-life of 50.55 days and decaying by beta emission. It is used in the form of the chloride as a radiation source in the palliative treatment of bone pain in patients with metastatic bone lesions.

strophulus (strof'u-lus) a papular urticaria occurring in infants.

structure (struk'cher) the components and their manner of arrangement in constituting a whole.

family s. the way in which a family is organized according to roles, rules, power, and hierarchies.

struma (stroo'mah) goiter.

Hashimoto's s., s. lymphomato'sa HASHIMOTO'S DISEASE.

s. ova'rii a teratoid ovarian tumor composed of thyroid tissue.

Riedel's s. Riedel's THYROIDITIS.

strumectomy (stroo-mek'tah-me) excision of a goiter.

strumitis (stroo-mi'tis) thyroiditis.

Strümpell's disease (strim'pelz) 1. hereditary lateral SCLEROSIS with the spasticity

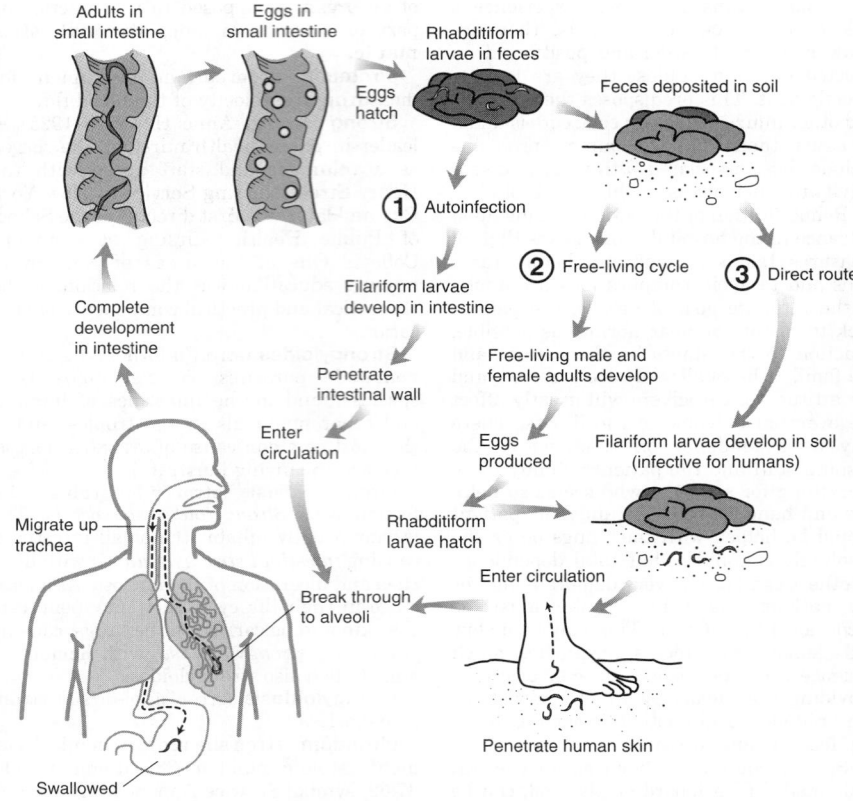

Life cycle of *Strongyloides stercoralis.* From Mahon and Manuselis, 2000.

mainly limited to the lower limbs. 2. polioencephalomyelitis.

Strümpell-Leichtenstern encephalitis disease (strim'pel līk'ten-stern) hemorrhagic encephalitis.

Strümpell-Marie disease (strim'pel mah-re') ankylosing spondylitis.

strychnine (strik'nīn) a very poisonous alkaloid from seeds of *Strychnos nux-vomica* and other species of *Strychnos;* a common strychnine-containing rodenticide causes convulsions in humans.

Stryker frame (stri'ker) an apparatus specially designed for care of patients with injuries of the spinal column or cord. It is constructed of pipe and canvas and is designed so that the patient can be turned without difficulty. The frame on which the patient lies while in the supine position is called the posterior frame; the anterior frame is used when the patient is turned on the abdomen. There are perineal openings in both frames for use of a bedpan.

STS Society of Thoracic Surgeons.

study (stud'e) a careful examination of a phenomenon; see also DESIGN.

  cohort s. prospective study.

  cross-sectional s. one employing a single point of data collection for each participant or system being studied. It is used for examining phenomena expected to remain static through the period of interest. It contrasts with a LONGITUDINAL S.

  electrophysiological s's (EPS) studies from within the heart of its electrical activation and response to electrical stimuli and certain drugs. In general they include intravenous and/or intra-arterial placement of one or more electrode catheters at sites in the atria, ventricles, or coronary sinus, and sometimes the pulmonary artery or aorta. They record activity or stimulate the heart at various rates and cadences and are aids in the evaluation of electrophysiologic properties such as automaticity, conduction, and refractoriness

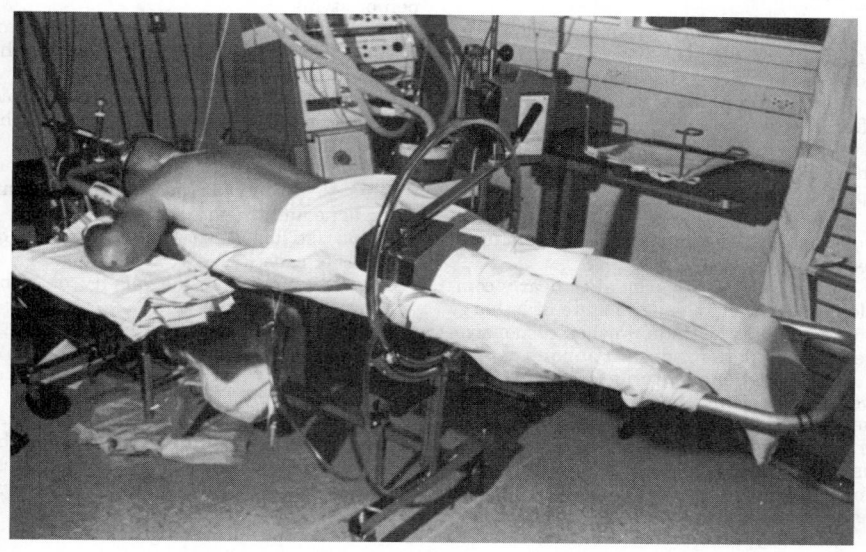

The Stryker® Wedge Turning Frame. From McQuillan et al., 2002.

They also initiate and terminate tachycardias, map the sequence of activation, and aid in evaluation of patients for various forms of therapy and for the response to therapy. During these studies catheter ablation procedures, such as radio frequency ablation and electrical ablation, may be performed.

flow s. uroflowmetry.

longitudinal s. one in which participants, processes, or systems are studied over time, with data being collected at multiple intervals. The two main types are prospective studies and retrospective studies. It contrasts with a CROSS-SECTIONAL S.

pilot s. a smaller version of a proposed research study, conducted to refine the methodology of the later one. It should be as similar to the proposed study as possible, using similar subjects, the same setting, and the same techniques of data collection and analysis.

prospective s. an epidemiologic study in which the groups of individuals (cohorts) are selected on the bases of factors that are to be examined for possible effects on some outcome. For example, the effect of exposure to a specific risk factor on the eventual development of a particular disease can be studied. The cohorts are then followed over a period of time to determine the incidence rates of the outcomes being studied as they relate to the original factors in question. Called also cohort study.

The term *prospective* usually implies a cohort selected in the present and followed into the future, but this method can also be applied to existing longitudinal historical data, such as insurance or medical records. A cohort is identified and classified as to exposure to the risk factor at some date in the past and followed up to the present to determine incidence rates. This is called a *historical prospective study, prospective study of past data,* or *retrospective cohort study.*

retrospective s. an epidemiologic study in which participating individuals are classified as either having some outcome (cases) or lacking it (controls); the outcome may be a specific disease, and the persons' histories are examined for specific factors that might be associated with that outcome. Cases and controls are often matched with respect to certain demographic or other variables but need not be. As compared to prospective studies, retrospective studies suffer from drawbacks: certain important statistics cannot be measured, and large biases may be introduced both in the selection of controls and in the recall of past exposure to risk factors. The advantage of the retrospective study is its small scale, usually short time for completion, and its applicability to rare diseases, which would require study of very large cohorts in prospective studies. See also PROSPECTIVE S.

urinary flow s. uroflowmetry.

voiding pressure s. simultaneous measurement of bladder contraction, urinary flow, and sphincter electromyogram.

stump (stump) the distal end of a limb left after AMPUTATION; called also residual limb.

stupe (stoop) a hot, wet cloth or sponge, charged with a medication for external application.

stupefacient (stoo″pĕ-fa′shent) 1. inducing STUPOR. 2. an agent that induces stupor; see also DEPRESSANT.

stupor (stoo′por) 1. partial or nearly complete unconsciousness. 2. a state of lethargy and immobility with diminished responsiveness to stimulation. adj., **stu′porous.**

Sturge-Weber syndrome (disease) (sterj′-web′er) a congenital syndrome of NEVUS FLAMMEUS of the face (commonly called port-wine STAINS); angiomas of the CHOROID and LEPTOMENINGES, leading to anoxia; late GLAUCOMA; and often intracranial calcification, mental retardation, and epilepsy may also develop.

stuttering (stut′er-ing) a SPEECH DISORDER characterized by involuntary hesitation in starting or finishing a sound, such as difficulty in starting words beginning with *t*, or the inability to get beyond a first letter such as *m* or *s*. See also STAMMERING. Stuttering involves three definitive factors: (1) speech DYSFLUENCY, especially the repetition of parts of words or whole words, prolongation of sounds or words and unduly prolonged pauses; (2) unfavorable reactions of listeners to the speaker's speech defect; and (3) the reactions of the speaker to the listeners' reactions, as well as to the speech problem itself and to the conception of oneself as a person who stutters. Early interventions for stuttering enhance the child's communication skills. Referral to a SPEECH-LANGUAGE PATHOLOGIST is important in order to determine appropriate treatment.

sty (sti) inflammation of one or more of the sebaceous glands of the eyelid, a lesion resembling a pimple. Hot compresses applied for 15 minutes every 2 hours may help localize infection and promote drainage, although in some cases a small surgical incision may be necessary. A mild antiseptic may be prescribed to prevent spread of infection. Called also hordeolum. Spelled also stye.

styl(o)- word element [L., Gr.], *stake; pole; styloid process of the temporal bone.*

stylet (sti′let) 1. a wire run through a catheter or cannula to render it stiff or to remove debris from its lumen. 2. a slender probe.

stylohyoid (sti″lo-hi′oid) pertaining to the styloid process and hyoid bone.

styloid (sti′loid) long and pointed, like a pen or stylus.

styloiditis (sti″loi-di′tis) inflammation of tissues around the styloid process of the temporal bone.

stylomastoid (sti″lo-mas′toid) pertaining to the styloid and mastoid processes of the temporal bone.

stylomaxillary (sti″lo-mak′sĭ-lar″e) pertaining to the styloid process of the temporal bone and the maxilla.

stylus (sti′lus) 1. stylet. 2. a pencil or stick, as of caustic.

stypsis (stip′sis) 1. the quality of being ASTRINGENT. 2. use of styptics.

styptic (stip′tik) 1. arresting hemorrhage by means of an ASTRINGENT quality. 2. something that has this quality. A chemical styptic works by causing formation of a blood clot by chemical action. A vascular styptic checks bleeding by causing the blood vessels to contract. A mechanical styptic causes clotting by mechanical means, such as when one applies a bit of paper or cotton to a slight razor cut. A *styptic pencil* is frequently used to stop bleeding from slight cuts. Styptics in various other forms are used in surgery.

Stypven (stip′ven) trademark for a preparation of Russell's viper VENOM, used as a HEMOSTATIC agent.

sub- word element [L.], *under; less than.*

subabdominal (sub″ab-dom′ĭ-nal) below the abdomen.

subacromial (sub″ah-kro′me-al) below the acromion.

subacute (sub″ah-kūt′) somewhat acute between acute and chronic.

subalimentation (sub″al-ĭ-men-ta′shun) hypoalimentation.

subaponeurotic (sub″ap-o-noo-rot′ik) below an aponeurosis.

subarachnoid (sub″ah-rak′noid) between the arachnoid and the pia mater.

subareolar (sub″ah-re′o-lar) beneath the areola of the nipple.

subastragalar (sub″ah-strag′ah-lar) below the astragalus (talus).

subastringent (sub″ah-strin′jent) moderately ASTRINGENT.

subaural (sub-aw′ral) below the ear.

subcapsular (sub-kap′su-lar) below a capsule, especially the capsule of the brain.

subcartilaginous (sub-kahr″tĭ-laj′ĭ-nus) 1. below a cartilage. 2. partly cartilaginous.

subclass (sub′klas) a taxonomic category subordinate to a class and superior to an order.

subclavian (sub-kla′ve-an) below the CLAVICLE.

s. steal syndrome cerebral or brain stem ischemia resulting from diversion of blood flow from the basilar artery to the subclavian artery, in the presence of occlusive disease of the proximal portion of the subclavian artery.

subclavicular (sub-klah-vik′u-lar) subclavian.

subclinical (sub-klin′ĭ-kal) without clinical manifestations; said of the early stages or a very mild form of a disease.

subconjunctival (sub″kon-jungk-ti′val) beneath the conjunctiva.

subconscious (sub-kon′shus) 1. imperfectly or partially conscious. 2. a term formerly used to include the PRECONSCIOUS and UNCONSCIOUS.

subconsciousness (sub-kon′shus-nes) the state of being partially conscious.

subcoracoid (sub-kor′ah-koid) situated under the coracoid process.

subcortex (sub-kor′teks) the brain substance underlying the cortex. adj., **subcor′tical.**

subcostal (sub-kos′tal) below a rib or ribs; called also infracostal.

subcranial (sub-kra′ne-al) below the cranium.

subcrepitant (sub-krep′ĭ-tant) somewhat crepitant in nature; said of a rale.

subculture (sub′kul-chur) 1. a culture of bacteria derived from another culture. 2. a group whose members share characteristics, have similar needs, and develop behavioral norms not common to all members of the larger cultural group within which the smaller group exists.

subcutaneous (sub″ku-ta′ne-us) beneath the layers of the skin.

subcuticular (sub″ku-tik′u-lar) below the epidermis.

subdiaphragmatic (sub-di″ah-frag-mat′-ik) subphrenic.

subduct (sub-dukt′) to draw down.

subdural (sub-doo′ral) between the dura mater and the arachnoid.

subendocardial (sub″en-do-kahr′de-al) beneath the endocardium.

subendothelial (sub″en-do-the′le-al) beneath an endothelial layer.

subepicardium (sub″ep-ĭ-kahr′de-um) subepicardial layer.

subepidermal (sub″ep-ĭ-der′mal) beneath the epidermis.

subepithelial (sub″ep-ĭ-the′le-al) beneath the epithelium.

subfamily (sub-fam′ĭ-le) a taxonomic division sometimes established, subordinate to a family and superior to a tribe or genus.

subfascial (sub-fash′al) beneath a fascia.

subfertility (sub″fer-til′ĭ-te) diminished reproductive capacity; called also hypofertility. adj., **subfer′tile.**

subgenus (sub-je′nus) a taxonomic category sometimes established, subordinate to a genus and superior to a species.

subglenoid (sub-gle′noid) beneath the glenoid (mandibular) fossa.

subglossal (sub-glos′al) sublingual.

subgrondation (sub″gron-da′shun) depression of one fragment of the skull beneath another.

subhepatic (sub″hĕ-pat′ik) below the liver.

subhyoid (sub-hi′oid) below the hyoid bone.

subiculum (sah-bik′u-lum) an underlying or supporting structure.

subiliac (sub-il′e-ak) below the ilium.

subilium (sub-il′e-um) the lowest portion of the ilium.

subinvolution (sub″in-vo-loo′shun) incomplete involution; failure of a part to return to its normal size and condition after enlargement from functional activity.

subjacent (sub-ja′sent) located below.

subject (sub′jekt) a person or animal subjected to treatment, observation, or experiment.

subjective (sub-jek′tiv) perceived only by the affected individual and not by the examiner.

subjugal (sub-ju′gal) subzygomatic.

sublatio retinae (sub-la′she-o ret′ĭ-ne) DETACHMENT OF RETINA.

sublesional (sub-le′zhun-al) performed or situated beneath a lesion.

sublethal (sub-le′thal) insufficient to cause death.

sublimate (sub′lĭ-māt) 1. a substance obtained by SUBLIMATION. 2. to accomplish sublimation.

sublimation (sub″lĭ-ma′shun) the conversion of a solid directly into the gaseous state. 1. an unconscious DEFENSE MECHANISM in which an individual diverts socially unacceptable instinctive drives into personally approved and socially acceptable channels. Mental conflicts may be resolved by this means although the person achieves only partial satisfaction of his impulses.

subliminal (sub-lim′ĭ-nal) below the threshold of sensation or conscious awareness.

sublingual (sub-ling′gwal) beneath the tongue; called also hypoglossal and subglossal.

sublinguitis (sub″ling-gwi′tis) inflammation of the sublingual gland.

subluxate (sub-luk′sāt) to partially dislocate.

subluxation (sub″luk-sa′shun) incomplete or partial DISLOCATION.

S

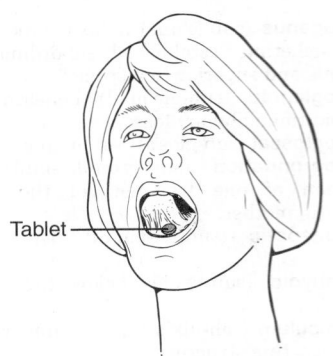

Tablet

Administration of a sublingual medication. From Lammon et al., 1995.

submammary (sub-mam'ah-re) below the mammary gland.

submandibular (sub″man-dib'u-lar) below the mandible.

submaxillaritis (sub″mak-sĭ-lar-i'tis) inflammation of the submaxillary gland.

submaxillary (sub-mak'sĭ-lar″e) below the maxilla.

submental (sub-men'tal) below the chin.

submersion (sub-mer'zhun) the act of placing or the condition of being under the surface of a liquid.

submetacentric (sub-met″ah-sen'trik) having the centromere almost, but not quite, at the metacentric position.

submicroscopic (sub-mi″kro-skop'ik) too small to be visible with the microscope.

submucosa (sub″mu-ko'sah) areolar tissue situated beneath a mucous membrane.

submucous (sub-mu'kus) beneath a mucous membrane.

subnarcotic (sub″nahr-kot'ik) moderately NARCOTIC.

subneural (sub-noor'al) beneath a nerve.

subnormal (sub-nor'mal) below or less than normal.

subnormality (sub″nor-mal'ĭ-te) a state less than normal or than that usually encountered.

suboccipital (sub″ok-sip'ĭ-tal) below the occiput.

suborbital (sub-or'bĭ-tal) infraorbital.

suborder (sub'or-der) a taxonomic category sometimes established, subordinate to an order and superior to a family.

subpapular (sub-pap'u-lar) indistinctly papular.

subpatellar (sub″pah-tel'ar) infrapatellar.

subpericardial (sub″per-ĭ-kahr'de-al) beneath the pericardium.

subperiosteal (sub″per-e-os'te-al) beneath the periosteum.

subperitoneal (sub″per-ĭ-to-ne'al) beneath the peritoneum.

subpharyngeal (sub″fah-rin'je-al) beneath the pharynx.

subphrenic (sub-fren'ik) beneath the DIAPHRAGM; called also subdiaphragmatic.

subphylum (sub-fi'lum) [L., Gr.] a taxonomic category sometimes established, subordinate to a phylum and superior to a class.

subplacenta (sub″plah-sen'tah) the decidua basalis.

subpleural (sub-ploor'al) beneath the pleura.

subpreputial (sub″pre-pu'shal) beneath the prepuce.

subpubic (sub-pu'bik) beneath the pubic bone.

subpulmonary (sub-pul'mo-nar″e) beneath the lung.

subretinal (sub-ret'ĭ-nal) beneath the retina.

subscapular (sub-skap'u-lar) below the scapula.

subscription (sub-skrip'shun) the third chief part of a drug PRESCRIPTION, comprising directions to be followed by the pharmacist in its preparation.

subserous (sub-se'rus) beneath a serous membrane.

subspecies (sub'spe-shēz) a subdivision of a species; a variety or race.

substage (sub'stāj) the part of the microscope underneath the stage.

substance (sub'stans) 1. physical material that has form and weight; called also matter. 2. the material constituting an organ or body. 3. psychoactive SUBSTANCE.

S. Abuse and Mental Health Services Administration **(SAMHSA)** an agency of the United States Department of Health and Human Services, created in 1992 to oversee the quality and availability of programs for prevention, treatment, and rehabilitation of substance ABUSE and related mental health problems.

black s. substantia nigra.

controlled s. a PSYCHOACTIVE SUBSTANCE that is regulated under the CONTROLLED SUBSTANCES ACT. See table at DRUG DEPENDENCE.

depressor s. 1. vasodepressor. 2. depressant.

gray s. gray MATTER.

ground s. the gel-like material in which connective tissue cells and fibers are embedded.

s.-induced disorders a subgroup of the SUBSTANCE-RELATED DISORDERS comprising a variety of behavioral or psychological anomalies resulting from ingestion of or exposure to a drug of abuse, medication, or toxin. Included are substance intoxication ubstance withdrawal, and other mental isorders such as dementia, mood disorder, nd psychotic disorder when they are specifically caused by a substance. See also UBSTANCE USE DISORDERS.

medullary s. 1. the white matter of he central nervous system, consisting of xons and their myelin sheaths. 2. the soft, narrow-like substance of the interior of such tructures as bone, kidney, and adrenal gland.

müllerian inhibiting s. a glycoprotein roduced by the Sertoli cells of the fetal estis that acts ipsilaterally in the male to uppress the müllerian ducts, consequently reventing development of the uterus and allopian tubes, thus helping to control ormation of the male phenotype.

s. P a peptide composed of 11 amino cids, present in nerve cells scattered hroughout the body and in special endocrine ells in the gut; it increases the contractions f gastrointestinal smooth muscle and causes asodilatation; it is one of the most potent asoactive substances known, and it seems to e a sensory neurotransmitter involving ain, touch, and temperature.

perforated s. 1. *anterior perforated ubstance,* an area anterolateral to each ptic tract, pierced by branches of the nterior and middle cerebral arteries. 2. *osterior perforated substance,* an area between the cerebral peduncles, pierced by ranches of the posterior cerebral arteries.

pressor s. vasopressor (def. 2).

psychoactive s., psychotropic s. any hemical compound that affects the mind or nental processes, particularly a drug used herapeutically in psychiatry, or any of arious other types of mind-altering subtances such as drugs of abuse and some oxins. See also table at DRUG DEPENDENCE. alled also psychoactive agent or drug and sychotropic agent or drug.

There are several different classes of sychoactive substances: ANTIDEPRESSANTS re used for the relief of symptoms of major epression. LITHIUM is the most common gent used to treat manic episodes of IPOLAR DISORDER. ANTIPSYCHOTIC AGENTS (or najor tranquilizers) are used for management of the manifestations of psychotic isorders such as SCHIZOPHRENIA. ANTIANXIETY GENTS (called also minor tranquilizers), uch as DIAZEPAM (Valium), are used for elief of anxiety disorders. While none of hese drugs can effect a cure, they can educe the severity of symptoms and permit he patient to resume more normal activity.

Also included in the category of psychoropic drugs are many other substances that ffect the mind but are not used to treat nental disorders, including STIMULANTS such

as CAFFEINE, AMPHETAMINES, and COCAINE; OPIATES; and HALLUCINOGENS.

s.-related disorders any of the mental disorders associated with excessive use of or exposure to psychoactive substances, including drugs of abuse, medications, and toxins. The group is divided into SUBSTANCE USE DISORDERS and SUBSTANCE-INDUCED DISORDERS, each of which is specified on the basis of etiology, such as alcohol use disorders. See also DRUG ABUSE and DRUG DEPENDENCE.

slow-reacting s. of anaphylaxis SRS-A, an inflammatory agent released by mast cells in the anaphylactic reaction. It induces slow, prolonged contraction of certain smooth muscles and is an important mediator of allergic bronchial asthma.

threshold s's those substances in the blood, such as glucose, that are excreted when they reach their renal THRESHOLD.

transmitter s. neurotransmitter.

s. use disorders a subgroup of the SUBSTANCE-RELATED DISORDERS, in which psychoactive SUBSTANCE use or abuse repeatedly results in significantly adverse consequences. The group comprises substance abuse (see DRUG ABUSE) and substance dependence (see DRUG DEPENDENCE); specific disorders or groups of disorders are named on the basis of etiology, e.g., alcohol use disorders, alcohol abuse, and alcohol dependence.

white s. white MATTER.

substantia (sub-stan'she-ah) [L.] substance; used in anatomic nomenclature in naming various components of body tissues or structures.

s. al'ba white matter.

s. gelatino'sa the substance sheathing the posterior horn of the spinal cord and lining its central canal.

s. gri'sea gray matter.

s. ni'gra a dark layer of gray matter separating the tegmentum of the midbrain from the crus cerebri.

substernal (sub-ster'nal) below the STERNUM; called also infrasternal.

substituent (sub-stich'u-ent) 1. a substitute; especially an atom, radical, or group substituted for another in a compound. 2. of or pertaining to such an atom, radical, or group.

substitution (sub"stĭ-too'shun) the act of putting one thing in the place of another, such as the chemical replacement of one atom or substituent group by another. Called also replacement. 1. a DEFENSE MECHANISM in which an individual replaces an unattainable or unacceptable goal, emotion, or motive with one that is attainable or acceptable.

S

substrate (sub′strāt) 1. any substance upon which an enzyme acts. 2. a neutral substance containing a nutrient solution. 3. a surface upon which a different material is deposited or adhered, usually in a coating or layer.

substructure (sub′struk-chur) the underlying or supporting portion of an organ or appliance.

subsylvian (sub-sil′ve-an) deep to the lateral sulcus (sylvian fissure).

subsystem (sub′sis-tem) 1. a smaller SYSTEM within a larger one; it has a purpose of its own but also contributes to the overall purpose of the system to which it belongs. 2. in family systems THEORY, a triad, dyad, or other group of members who are linked by a special association.

subtarsal (sub-tahr′sal) below the tarsus.

subtentorial (sub″ten-to′re-al) infratentorial.

subthalamus (sub-thal′ah-mus) ventral thalamus.

subtle (sut′l) 1. very fine, as a subtle powder. 2. very acute, as a subtle pain.

subtraction (sub-trak′shun) the photographic or electronic removal of overlying structures from radiologic images.

subtribe (sub′trīb) a taxonomic category sometimes established, subordinate to a tribe and superior to a genus.

subtrochanteric (sub″tro-kan-ter′ik) below a trochanter.

subtympanic (sub″tim-pan′ik) somewhat tympanic in quality.

subungual (sub-ung′gwal) beneath a nail; called also hyponychial.

suburethral (sub″u-re′thral) beneath the urethra.

subvaginal (sub-vaj′ĭ-nal) 1. below the vagina. 2. under a sheath.

subvertebral (sub-ver′tĕ-bral) on the ventral side of the vertebrae.

subzygomatic below the zygomatic BONE.

succedaneous (suk″sĕ-da′ne-us) coming after or replacing something else.

succenturiate (suk″sen-tu′re-āt) accessory; serving as a substitute.

succimer (suk′sīmer) a chelating AGENT that is an analogue of DIMERCAPROL, administered orally in the treatment of heavy METAL POISONING. A complex with technetium 99m is used in renal function testing.

succinate (suk′sĭ-nāt) any salt, ester, or anionic form of succinic acid.

succinic acid (suk-sin′ik) an intermediate in the tricarboxylic acid CYCLE.

succinylcholine (suk″sĭ-nil-ko′lēn) a neuromuscular blocking AGENT used as the chloride salt to aid in such procedures as endotracheal intubation and endoscopy, as an adjunct to surgical anesthesia, and in convulsive THERAPY; administered intramuscularly or intravenously.

succorrhea (suk″o-re′ah) excessive flow of a natural secretion.

succus (suk′us) [L.] juice.

succussion (sŭ-kush′un) a splashing sound elicited when a patient is shaken, indicative of fluid and air in a body cavity.

sucking (suk′ing) moving the lips and tongue in such a way as to create SUCTION and draw fluids or solids into the mouth. See also sucking REFLEX.

nonnutritive s. in the NURSING INTERVENTIONS CLASSIFICATION, a nursing INTERVENTION defined as the provision of sucking opportunities for the infant who is GAVAGE fed or who can receive nothing by mouth.

sucralfate (soo-kral′fāt) a complex of aluminum and a sulfated polysaccharide used as a gastrointestinal antiulcerative and gastric mucosa protectant; administered orally.

sucrase (soo′krās) a digestive enzyme secreted in the intestine that catalyzes the hydrolysis of sucrose and maltose to produce glucose and fructose.

sucrase-isomaltase deficiency deficient activity of the complex of sucrase and isomaltase that occurs in the intestinal mucosa, resulting in malabsorption of sucrose and starch; it is characterized by watery, osmotic-fermentative diarrhea, sometimes leading to dehydration and malnutrition, manifest in infancy. While sucrase activity is always absent, isomaltase activity may be either greatly reduced or relatively normal. See also disaccharide INTOLERANCE.

sucrose (soo′krōs) a DISACCHARIDE obtained from sugar cane, sugar beet, or other sources; used as a food and sweetening agent.

s. hemolysis test a test for paroxysmal nocturnal HEMOGLOBINURIA; the patient's whole blood is mixed with isotonic sucrose solution, which promotes binding of complement to red blood cells, then incubated and examined for hemolysis; greater than 10 percent hemolysis indicates paroxysmal nocturnal hemoglobinuria.

suction (suk′shun) 1. the drawing of fluid or solid into a space because the pressure inside it is lower than that outside. 2. aspiration of gas or fluid by mechanical means.

post-tussive s. a sucking sound heard over a lung cavity just after a cough.

suctioning (suk′shun-ing) removal of material through the use of negative pressure s in suctioning an operative wound during nd after surgery to remove exudates, or uctioning of the respiratory passages to emove secretions that the patient cannot emove by coughing. Suctioning of the nose nd mouth is a relatively simple procedure equiring only cleanliness and sensible care n the removal of liquids obstructing he nasal and oral passages. Suctioning of he deeper respiratory structures (*deep* or *ndotracheal suctioning*) demands special kill and meticulous care to avoid traumaizing the delicate mucous membranes and ntroducing infection into the respiratory ree.

Another complication arising from improper tracheal suctioning is HYPOXIA, which ccurs when prolonged suctioning removes he oxygen from the patient's airway and hus adds to existing respiratory distress. The use of a catheter too large in diameter an cause obstruction of the bronchus and ubsequent collapse of a lobe of the lung. Because of the potential hazards inherent in he procedure, tracheal suctioning should be eserved only for those patients too weak nd debilitated to cough up thick and enacious sputum. When deep suctioning is necessary, it should be done only by those persons who are skillful in the technique nd knowledgeable about the complications hat can result from improper use of the uctioning equipment. Guidelines for sucioning patients in either acute care settings r the home have been published by the American Association for Respiratory Care nd are available on their web site at http:// vww.aarc.org.

airway s. in the NURSING INTERVENTIONS CLASSIFICATION, a nursing INTERVENTION defined as removal of airway secretions by inserting a SUCTION catheter into the patient's oral airway and/or trachea.

suctorial (suk-tor'e-al) adapted for sucking.

Sudafed (soo'dah-fed) trademark for preparations containing PSEUDOEPHEDRINE hydrohloride, a nasal DECONGESTANT.

sudamen (soo-da'men) [L.] a small palecolored vesicle caused by retention of sweat n the layers of the epidermis.

Sudan (soo-dan') a group of azo compounds used as biological stains for fats.

sudanophilia (soo-dan″o-fil'e-ah) 1. affinty for a Sudan stain. 2. a condition in which he leukocytes contain particles staining readily with Sudan red III.

sudation (soo-da'shun) sweating.

sudden infant death syndrome (SIDS) the sudden and unexpected death of an apparently healthy infant, not explained by careful postmortem studies. It typically occurs

between birth and age 9 months, with the highest incidence at 3 to 5 months. Called also crib death or cot death because the infant often is found dead in the crib.

The incidence rate for SIDS in the United States is approximately 10,000 per year. After the first week of life it is the leading cause of death in one-year-olds, and is second only to accidents as a cause of death in children under the age of 15 years. The disorder occurs throughout the world, is more common in families in the lower socioeconomic classes, and affects males slightly more than females and non-Caucasians slightly more than Caucasians.

Children most at risk for SIDS are those who are premature, have a history of apnea from hyaline membrane disease or a seizure disorder, or have a family history of SIDS (especially among siblings) with or without a history of apnea.

There are many misconceptions about the cause of SIDS, most of which are likely to cause feelings of guilt or anger that only add to the heartache of parents whose children have died of the disorder. Among these misconceptions are the beliefs that the infant has suffocated under blankets or from aspirated vomitus, or that contraceptive pills, fluoridation, radioactive fallout, and even lack of breast-feeding have somehow contributed to the disorder.

Identification of infants at risk for SIDS includes determining whether the infant is subject to periods of apnea and if so, why. Diagnostic studies include pneumogram, chest x-ray, determination of chemoreceptor status, metabolic assessment, electrocardiogram, and cardiac and apnea monitoring.

Treatment and prevention of SIDS are necessarily aimed at identifying infants at high risk and instituting a program of apnea monitoring and resuscitation. If home monitoring is deemed necessary, the parents are taught how to place the electrodes over the baby's diaphragm, how to operate the monitoring equipment, and the basic maneuvers for cardiopulmonary resuscitation. While home monitoring does create problems and stress for family members, it usually is not required for more than a few months or at most a year. Most parents feel that the security it provides and the knowledge that their child can survive periods of apnea are worth the sacrifices necessary.

Through the efforts of the National Foundation for Sudden Infant Death, guilt and misunderstandings of the parents about the cause of their infant's death are being

S

handled in a more sensitive and comforting way. Recent interest in research into causes of SIDS has resulted from pressure from parents and members of the national organizations concerned with child health and development. In 1974 Congress passed a bill to set up diagnostic centers throughout the country, and the National Institute of Child Health and Development now allocates more than half a million dollars annually for SIDS research. The address of the National SIDS Alliance is 10500 Little Patuxent Pkwy., Columbia MD 21044.

Sudeck's disease (soo'deks) post-traumatic osteoporosis.

sudomotor (soo''do-mo'tor) stimulating the sweat glands.

sudoriferous (su''do-rif'er-us) 1. conveying sweat. 2. sudoriparous.

sudorific (su''do-rif'ik) diaphoretic.

sudoriparous (soo''do-rip'ah-rus) secreting or producing sweat; called also sudoriferous.

suet (soo'et) the fat from the abdominal cavity of ruminants, especially the sheep, used in preparing cerates and ointments and as an emollient.

sufentanil (soo-fen'tah-nil) an opioid AN-ALGESIC derived from FENTANYL, used as the citrate salt as an anesthetic or anesthesia adjunct; also used for the treatment of obstetric pain.

suffocation (suf''ŏ-ka'shun) the stoppage of breathing; called also asphyxiation. If it is complete (no air at all reaches the lungs), the lack of oxygen and excess of carbon dioxide in the blood will cause almost immediate loss of consciousness. Though the heart continues to beat briefly, death will follow in a matter of minutes unless emergency measures are taken to get breathing started again. Suffocation can be caused by drowning, electric shock, gas or smoke poisoning, strangulation, or choking on a foreign body in the trachea. Once the cause of suffocation has been removed, the most important first aid measure is ARTIFICIAL RESPIRATION.

risk for s. a NURSING DIAGNOSIS accepted by the North American Nursing Diagnosis Association, defined as a state in which an individual has an accentuated risk of suffocation.

suffusion (sŭ-fu'zhun) 1. the process of overspreading, or diffusion. 2. the condition of being moistened or permeated through.

sugar (shoog'ar) a sweet carbohydrate of either animal or vegetable origin; the two principal groups are the DISACCHARIDES and the MONOSACCHARIDES.

beet s. SUCROSE from sugar beets.

blood s. 1. glucose occurring in th blood. 2. the amount of glucose in the blood

cane s. SUCROSE from sugar cane.

fruit s. fructose.

invert s. a mixture of equal amounts c DEXTROSE and FRUCTOSE, obtained by hydrc lyzing SUCROSE; used in solution as a pai enteral nutrient.

suggestibility (sug-jes''tĭ-bil'ĭ-te) a condi tion of enhanced susceptibility to sugges tion. adj., **sugges'tible.**

suggestion (sug-jes'chun) 1. the act c offering an idea for action or for considera tion of action. 2. an idea so offered. 3. i psychiatry, the process of causing uncritica acceptance of an idea.

hypnotic s. one imparted to a perso1 in the hypnotic state.

posthypnotic s. implantation in th mind of a subject during hypnosis of suggestion to be acted upon after recover from the hypnotic state.

suggillation (sug''jĭ-la'shun) 1. ecchymc sis. 2. contusion.

suicidal (soo-ĭ-si'dal) pertaining to suicid or prone to suicide.

suicide (soo'ĭ-sīd) the taking of one's ow1 life; also any person who voluntarily an< intentionally takes his or her own life Legally, a death suspected of being due t violence that is self-inflicted is not termed suicide unless there is positive evidence of th victim's intent to destroy himself or hersel1 or the method of death is such that a verdic of suicide is inevitable. This means that man deaths that would be termed suicide accord ing to medicopsychological criteria are re ported as accidental or from undetermine< cause. The difficulty of positively identifyin< a death as suicide is further complicated b the complexities of determining true inten and the psychological motivation one ma have had for ending one's own life.

Incidence: Statistical evidence of th actual suicide rate for a specific populatio: is difficult to compile because of the ambi guity of the term, a lack of criteria by whicl a death may be judged suicidal, and a lack o agreement among those reporting deaths a to what does, indeed, constitute a suicide Existing data are as follows: Suicide is th eighth leading cause of death for males an< the 19th leading cause for females. It is th third leading cause of death among person 15 to 24 years of age, according to th NATIONAL INSTITUTES OF MENTAL HEALTH. Th group with the highest suicide rate is whit men over age 85. Other high-risk group include the elderly, the sick, and the men tally ill. There is a tendency of suicides t< occur in families, but there is no evidence c a genetically determined suicidal behavio pattern. There are also seasonal fluctuations in suicide rates, with the highest number occurring in the spring.

The American Foundation for Suicide Prevention (AFSP) has developed a policy for the prevention of suicide. It includes as essential components of suicide prevention the following measures: educating professionals in recognition and treatment of individuals at risk; educating society that such individuals are suffering from a medical condition that must be recognized and treated rather than stigmatized, and that effective treatments are available; and educating survivors of suicide attempts about the resources available to them. Other recommendations include: improved methods of detecting individuals at highest risk for completed suicide; improved treatment interventions for high risk patients; responsible gun control legislation; education of media and mental health professionals in order to reduce inaccurate or sensational media coverage of suicide; and improvement of palliative care for seriously or terminally ill patients (including through education and legislation) so that suicide does not seem to be their only option. Depression screening should be a routine assessment for every clinician. Research is essential in developing, testing, and implementing treatment approaches to patients at risk for suicide, as well as developing prevention strategies that have been shown to be effective or appear likely to be effective.

assisted s. suicide with the help of another person, such as when an incurably ill patient intentionally ingests a toxic substance or an overdose of a medication that was prescribed; the choice to die must always be made by the patient. See also EUTHANASIA.

suit (sōot) an outer garment covering the entire body.

MAST s. (military anti-shock trousers) pneumatic antishock garment.

sulbactam (sul-bak′tam) a β-LACTAMASE inhibitor used as the sodium salt to increase

the antibacterial activity of PENICILLINS and CEPHALOSPORINS against β-lactamase–producing organisms.

sulcate (sul′kāt) furrowed; marked with sulci.

sulconazole (sul-kon′ah-zōl) a broad-spectrum topical antifungal AGENT, used as the nitrate salt in treatment of ATHLETE'S FOOT, RINGWORM, and *Candida* infections.

sulcus (sul′kus) [L.] a groove or furrow; used in anatomic nomenclature to designate a linear depression, especially one of the cerebral sulci.

basilar s. a groove in the midline of the anterior surface of the pons, lodging the basilar artery.

calcarine s. a sulcus of the medial surface of the occipital lobe, separating the cuneus from the lingual gyrus.

central s. fissure of Rolando.

cerebral sulci the furrows on the surface of the brain between the gyri (see GYRUS).

collateral s. collateral fissure.

sul′ci cu′tis fine depressions of the skin between the ridges of the skin.

gingival s. the space between the surface of the tooth and the epithelium lining the free gingiva.

hippocampal s. hippocampal fissure.

posterior median s. posterior median fissure.

sulfacetamide (sul″fah-set′ah-mīd) a SULFONAMIDE antibacterial used in treatment of bacterial VAGINOSIS; the sodium salt is used topically to treat eye infections and acne.

sulfacytine (sul″fah-si′tēn) a short-acting, rapidly excreted oral SULFONAMIDE used in treatment of acute urinary tract infections.

sulfadiazine (sul″fah-di′ah-zēn) a SULFONAMIDE used, frequently in combination with other sulfonamides, in the treatment of infections due to susceptible organisms, including nocardiosis, toxoplasmosis, otitis

S

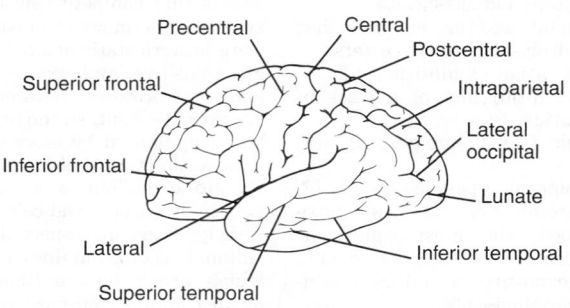

Precentral
Central
Postcentral
Superior frontal
Intraparietal
Inferior frontal
Lateral occipital
Lunate
Lateral
Inferior temporal
Superior temporal

Cerebral sulci, showing some major ones on the superolateral surface of the left cerebral hemisphere. From Dorland's, 2000.

media caused by susceptible strains of *Haemophilus influenzae,* streptococci, and pneumococci, and malaria caused by chloroquine-resistant *Plasmodium falciparum.* It is administered orally as the base or intravenously as the sodium salt. See also SILVER SULFADIAZINE.

sodium s. an antibacterial compound used intravenously.

sulfadoxine (sul″fah-dok′sēn) a long-acting sulfonamide used in combination with PYRIMETHAMINE in the prophylaxis and treatment of malaria caused by chloroquine-resistant strains of *Plasmodium falciparum.*

sulfaguanidine (sul″fah-gwan′ĭ-dēn) a SULFONAMIDE antibacterial used in treatment of gastrointestinal infections, especially bacillary dysentery, administered orally.

sulfamethizole (sul″fah-meth′ĭ-zōl) a sulfonamide used in urinary tract infections.

sulfamethoxazole (sul″fah-meth-ok′sah-zōl) a sulfonamide used as an antibacterial, especially for the treatment of acute urinary tract infections, and as an antiprotozoal; administered orally. Its use has declined as organisms have increasingly developed resistance to it, and when used it is usually combined with another agent such as trimethoprim.

sulfanilamide (sul″fah-nil′ah-mīd) a potent antibacterial compound. Although replaced as a systemic agent by more effective and less toxic derivatives, and by antibiotics; it is still used vaginally in the treatment of vulvovaginal candidiasis.

sulfapyridine (sul″fah-pir′ĭ-dēn) a SULFONAMIDE administered orally in treatment of DERMATITIS HERPETIFORMIS.

sulfasalazine (sul″fah-sal′ah-zēn) an antibacterial sulfonamide used orally or rectally in the prophylaxis and treatment of INFLAMMATORY BOWEL DISEASE and orally as a disease-modifying antirheumatic DRUG in treatment of rheumatoid ARTHRITIS.

sulfatase (sul′fah-tās) an enzyme that catalyzes the hydrolysis of sulfate esters.

sulfate (sul′fāt) a salt of sulfuric acid.

sulfatide (sul′fah-tīd) any of a class of cerebroside sulfuric esters.

sulfhemoglobin (sulf″he-mo-glo′bin) sulfmethemoglobin.

sulfhemoglobinemia (sulf″he-mo-glo″bĭ-ne′me-ah) the presence of SULFMETHEMOGLOBIN in the blood; the most significant symptom is cyanosis. It usually results from excessive exposure to sulfur-containing drugs or other chemicals.

sulfhydryl (sulf-hi′dril) the univalent radical —SH.

sulfide (sul′fīd) any binary compound of sulfur; a compound of sulfur with another element or base.

sulfinpyrazone (sul″fin-pi′rah-zōn) a uricosuric compound used in gout to promote excretion of uric acid; administered orally. It also prolongs platelet survival and inhibits platelet adherence to subendothelial cells and prostaglandin synthesis and has been studied as an antithrombotic agent.

sulfisoxazole (sul″fĭ-sok′sah-zōl) a short-acting SULFONAMIDE antibacterial; used as the base or as *sulfisoxazole acetyl* particularly for infections of the urinary tract and as *sulfisoxazole diolamine* as a topical ophthalmic antibacterial.

sulfite (sul′fīt) a salt of sulfurous acid. Sulfites are used as preservatives for salad, fresh fruit and vegetables, wine, beer, and dried fruit. In susceptible individuals, especially those with asthma, they can cause a severe reaction; because of this their use has been curtailed, and foods that contain them must be labeled.

sulfmethemoglobin (sulf″met-he″mo-glo′bin) a compound of hemoglobin and hydrogen sulfide; called also sulfhemoglobin.

sulfobromophthalein (sul″fo-bro″mo-thal′ēn) a sulfur- and bromine-containing compound, used as the sodium salt in liver function tests; see also BROMSULPHALEIN.

s. test a liver function test in which the dye sulfobromophthalein sodium is introduced into the circulatory system and a blood sample is withdrawn 30 or 45 minutes later, depending on the dose injected. The parenchymal cells remove almost all of the dye within this time if they are functioning normally. The rate of removal is influenced by the blood flow through the portal circulation, the functioning capacity of the liver cells, and the patency of the biliary tract.

sulfonamide (sul-fon′ah-mīd) 1. a compound containing the —SO$_2$NH$_2$ group. 2. any of a group of structurally related ANTIBIOTICS that competitively inhibit FOLIC ACID synthesis in microorganisms and formerly were bacteriostatic against a wide variety of gram-positive and gram-negative bacteria and some protozoa. Because many microbes are now resistant, sulfonamides have largely been supplanted by more effective and less toxic antibiotics. Called also sulfa drug.

sulfone (sul′fōn) a compound containing two hydrocarbon radicals attached to the —SO$_2$— group, especially DAPSONE (4,4′-sulfonylbisbenzenamine) and its derivatives, which are potent antibacterials effective against many gram-positive and gram-negative organisms and are widely used in treatment of LEPROSY.

sulfonylurea (sul″fo-nil-u′re-ah) any of a class of compounds that exert hypoglycemic activity by stimulating the islet tissue to secrete insulin; used to control hyperglycemia in patients with type 2 DIABETES MELLITUS who cannot be treated solely by diet and exercise. The class includes the oral hypoglycemic AGENTS ACETOHEXAMIDE, CHLORPROPAMIDE, GLIPIZIDE, TOLAZAMIDE, and TOLBUTAMIDE.

sulfoxone (sul-fok′sōn) a dapsone derivative used in the form of the sodium salt as a leprostatic and a dermatitis herpetiformis suppressant.

sulfur (sul′fer) a chemical element, atomic number 16, atomic weight 32.064, symbol S. (See Appendix 6.)

 s. dioxide a colorless, nonflammable gas used as an antioxidant in pharmaceutical preparations; it is also an important air pollutant, irritating the eyes and respiratory tract.

  precipitated s. a topical scabicide, antiparasitic, antibacterial, antifungal, and keratolytic.

  sublimed s. a topical scabicide and antiparasitic.

sulfurated (sul′fur-āt″ed) combined with sulfur.

sulfuric acid (sul-fu′rik) an oily, highly caustic, poisonous compound, H_2SO_4.

sulindac (sul′in-dak) a NONSTEROIDAL ANTI-INFLAMMATORY DRUG, used in the treatment of OSTEOARTHRITIS, rheumatoid ARTHRITIS, ankylosing SPONDYLITIS, bursitis or tendinitis of the shoulder, and acute attacks of GOUT or CALCIUM PYROPHOSPHATE DEPOSITION DISEASE.

sulph- for words beginning thus, see those beginning *sulf-*.

sumac (soo′mak) name of various trees and shrubs of the genus *Rhus*.

 poison s. *Rhus vernix,* a species that causes an itching rash on contact with the skin; see also POISON IVY, OAK, AND SUMAC.

sumatriptan (soo″mah-trip′tan) a selective SEROTONIN receptor agonist used as the succinate salt in the acute treatment of MIGRAINE and cluster HEADACHES; administered orally, subcutaneously, or intranasally.

Sumycin (soo-mi′sin) trademark for preparations of TETRACYCLINE hydrochloride, an ANTIBIOTIC.

sunburn (sun′bern) inflammation of the skin (an actual burn) caused by exposure to ULTRAVIOLET RAYS of the sun. Depending on how severe the burn is, the skin may simply redden or it may become blistered and sore—a second-degree burn. In extreme cases there may be fever.

sundowning (sun′doun-ing) the appearance of confusion, agitation, and other

severely disruptive behavior coupled with inability to remain asleep, occurring solely or markedly worsening at night; sometimes seen in older patients with dementia or other mental disorders.

sundown syndrome sundowning.

sunrise model a CONCEPTUAL MODEL of nursing developed by Madeleine M. LEININGER to depict the components of the CULTURAL CARE DIVERSITY AND UNIVERSALITY theory of nursing, named from the form of its graphic appearance. Each culture has a WORLD VIEW and cultural and social structure, which are learned through language and environment contexts. These contexts include technological factors, religious and philosophical factors, kinship and social factors, cultural values and beliefs, political and legal factors, educational factors, and economic factors. All of these language and environmental contexts influence the care and health patterns and expressions of individuals, families, groups, and institutions; all of the latter participate in diverse health systems, which include both folk and professional systems. The nursing subsystem spans both the folk system and the professional system. To provide culture-congruent care, nurses use knowledge gained through analysis of the components of the model to make nursing care decisions based on cultural care preservation/maintenance (deliverative-assistive or facilitative decisions that include methods of preserving or maintaining lifeways or values beneficial to the client), cultural care accommodation/negotiation (cognitive-assistive decisions that take into account the cultural beliefs, values, and practices of the client), or cultural care repatterning/restructuring (assistive or facilitative decisions that combine several different aspects of the client's culture in a way that is beneficial or meaningful to the client).

sunrise syndrome (sun′rīz) a condition in which there is unstable cognitive ability upon rising in the morning.

sunscreen (sun′skrēn) a lotion applied to the skin as protection against sunburn and the harmful effects of ultraviolet RADIATION. Sunscreens are labeled with a numerical sun protection FACTOR; the higher the number the more protection is afforded. Patients should be cautioned that the sunscreen should be reapplied after swimming or profuse sweating and that sun exposure must still be limited to prevent adverse effects.

sunstroke (sun′strōk) a profound disturbance of the body's heat-regulating

S

mechanism caused by prolonged exposure to excessive heat from the sun, particularly when there is little or no circulation of air. Elderly persons with underlying chronic disorders, those who use alcohol and atropine-containing drugs, and those with certain skin disorders are more susceptible. Sunstroke is a type of heat STROKE, but the category heat stroke also covers disorders caused by other forms of intense heat.

Recognition. Sunstroke is not the same as HEAT EXHAUSTION, a less serious disorder in which the amount of salt and fluid in the body falls below normal. In sunstroke there is a disturbance in the mechanism that controls perspiration. Since sunstroke is much more dangerous than heat exhaustion and is treated differently, it is of the utmost importance to distinguish between the two. The first symptoms of both disorders may be similar: headache, dizziness, and weakness. But later symptoms differ sharply. In heat exhaustion, there is perspiration and a normal or below normal temperature, whereas in sunstroke there is extremely high fever and absence of sweating. Sunstroke also may cause convulsions and sudden loss of consciousness. In extreme cases it may be fatal.

Treatment. In treatment of sunstroke, immediate steps must be taken to lower the body temperature, which may rise as high as 42 to 44.5°C (108 to 112°F). The patient should be placed in a shady, cool place and most of the clothing should be removed. The emergency system should be activated. Then cool water is gently applied, followed by fanning to increase heat dissipation through evaporation. Further treatment consists of measures to lower the body temperature, including ice packs, and iced drinks by mouth. Intravenous fluids are usually necessary.

Heat stroke can be prevented. Patient education should focus on protective measures such as adequate hydration and ventilation and the wearing of proper clothing. Vigorous activities should not be undertaken in extremely hot weather.

super- word element [L.], *above; excessive.*

superalimentation (soo″per-al″ĭ-men-ta′-shun) excessive feeding; sometimes used in the treatment of wasting diseases.

superalkalinity (soo″per-al″kah-lin′ĭ-te) excessive alkalinity.

superantigen (soo″per-an′tĭ-jen) any of a group of powerful antigens occurring in various bacteria and viruses that bind outside of the normal T cell receptor site and

are able to react with multiple T cell receptor molecules, thus activating T cells nonspecifically. Included are staphylococcal enterotoxins and toxins causing toxic shock syndrome and exfoliative dermatitis.

supercilia (soo″per-sil′e-ah) (L., pl.) the hairs on the arching protrusion over either eye, the eyebrow.

supercilium (soo″per-sil′e-um) (L., sing.) eyebrow; the transverse elevation at the junction of the forehead and upper eyelid.

superclass (soo′per-klas) a taxonomic category sometimes established, subordinate to a phylum and superior to a class.

superego (soo″per-e′go) in psychoanalytic theory, a part of the psyche derived from both the ID and the EGO, which acts, largely unconsciously, as a monitor over the ego. It is that part of the personality concerned with social standards, ethics, and conscience. Early in life the superego is formed by the infant's identification with parents and other significant and esteemed persons in his or her life. The real or supposed expectations of these persons gradually are accepted as general rules of society and help form the "conscience." The superego tends to be self-critical and in psychotic and anxious persons strong feelings of guilt and unworthiness can lead to self-punitive measures in an effort to resolve conflicts between the id, ego, and superego.

superfamily (soo′per-fam″ĭ-le) 1. a taxonomic category sometimes established, subordinate to an order and superior to a family. 2. any of a group of proteins having similarities such as areas of structural homology and believed to descend from the same ancestral gene, such as the superfamily of IMMUNOGLOBULINS.

superfecundation (soo″per-fe″kun-da′shun) fertilization of two or more ova during the same ovulatory cycle, by separate coital acts.

superfetation (soo″per-fe-ta′shun) the FERTILIZATION of an ovum and subsequent development of another embryo (fetus) when one is already present in the uterus, a result of fertilization of ova during different MENSTRUAL CYCLES, yielding fetuses of different ages.

superficial (soo″per-fish′al) situated on or near the surface.

superficialis (soo″per-fish″e-a′lis) superficial.

superficies (soo″per-fish′e-ēz) an outer surface.

superinduce (soo″per-in-doos′) to bring on in addition to an already existing condition.

superinfection (soo″per-in-fek′shun) a new infection occurring in a patient having a preexisting infection; for example acterial infection may occur in patients with viral respiratory disease, or a chronic hepatitis B carrier may become infected with hepatitis D virus. Superinfection can complicate the course of antimicrobial therapy when the organisms causing the new infection are resistant to the drugs being used to treat the first infection.

superinvolution (soo″per-in″vo-lu′shun) prolonged involution of the uterus after delivery, to a size much smaller than the normal, occurring in nursing mothers.

superior (soo-pe′re-or) situated above, or directed upward; in official anatomic nomenclature, used in reference to the upper surface of an organ or other structure, or to a structure occupying a higher position.

superjacent (soo″per-ja′sent) located just above.

superlactation (soo″per-lak-ta′ shun) hyperlactation.

superlethal (soo″per-le′thal) more than sufficient to cause death.

supermotility (soo″per-mo-til′ĭ-te) excessive motility.

supernatant (soo″per-na′tant) the liquid lying above a layer of precipitated insoluble material.

supernumerary (soo″per-noo′mer-ar″e) in excess of the regular number.

supernutrition (soo″per-noo-trish′un) excessive nutrition.

superolateral (soo″per-o-lat′er-al) above and to the side.

superoxide (soo″per-ok′sīd) any compound containing the highly reactive superoxide ion O_2^-, a common intermediate in numerous biological oxidations.

supersaturate (soo″per-sach′u-rāt) to add more of an ingredient than can be held in solution permanently.

superscription (soo″per-skrip′shun) something written above; the symbol R or prescription sign ("take thou"), which is the first of four chief parts of a drug PRESCRIPTION.

supervascularization (soo″per-vas″ku-ar-ĭ-za′shun) in radiotherapy, the relative increase in vascularity that occurs when tumor cells are destroyed so that the remaining tumor cells are better supplied by the (uninjured) capillary stroma.

supervision (soo″per-vizh′un) the process of being in charge of or directing something.

staff s. in the NURSING INTERVENTIONS CLASSIFICATION, a nursing INTERVENTION defined as facilitating the delivery of high-quality patient care by others.

supervoltage (soo′per-vōl″taj) in RADIATION THERAPY, voltage between 500 kilovolts and 1 megavolt, as contrasted with ORTHOVOLTAGE and MEGAVOLTAGE.

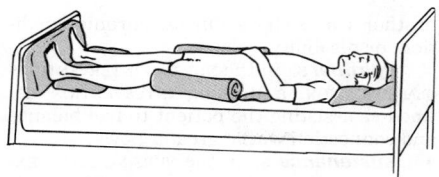

Supine position. From Lammon et al., 1995.

supinate (soo′pĭ′nāt) the act of turning the palm forward or upward, or of raising the medial margin of the foot.

supination (soo′pĭ-na′shun) the act of assuming the supine position; placing or lying on the back. Applied to the hand, the act of turning the palm upward.

supine (soo′pīn) lying with the face upward, or on the dorsal surface.

support (sŭ-port′) 1. a structure that bears the weight of something else. 2. a mechanism or arrangement that helps keep something else functioning. 3. the foundation upon which a denture rests.

caregiver s. in the NURSING INTERVENTIONS CLASSIFICATION, a nursing INTERVENTION defined as the provision of the necessary information, advocacy, and support to facilitate primary patient care by someone other than a health care professional. See also CAREGIVER.

decision-making s. in the NURSING INTERVENTIONS CLASSIFICATION, a nursing INTERVENTION defined as providing information and support for a patient who is making a decision regarding health care.

emotional s. 1. in the NURSING INTERVENTIONS CLASSIFICATION, a nursing INTERVENTION defined as the provision of reassurance, acceptance, and encouragement in times of stress. 2. a nursing INTERVENTION in the NURSING MINIMUM DATA SET; actions designed to meet the affective, psychological, and social needs of the patient or client.

family s. in the NURSING INTERVENTIONS CLASSIFICATION, a nursing INTERVENTION defined as promotion of family values, interests, and goals.

s. hose an elastic garment for a limb that enhances venous circulation through creation of a pressure gradient by fabric pressure. See also compression THERAPY.

physician s. in the NURSING INTERVENTIONS CLASSIFICATION, a nursing INTERVENTION defined as collaborating with physicians to provide quality patient care.

sibling s. in the NURSING INTERVENTIONS CLASSIFICATION, a nursing INTERVENTION defined as assisting a sibling to cope with a

S

brother's or sister's illness, chronic condition, or disability.

spiritual s. in the NURSING INTERVENTIONS CLASSIFICATION, a nursing INTERVENTION defined as assisting the patient to feel balance and connection with a greater power.

sustenance s. in the NURSING INTERVENTIONS CLASSIFICATION, a nursing INTERVENTION defined as helping a needy individual/family to locate food, clothing, or shelter.

suppository (sŭ-poz'ĭ-tor″e) an easily fusible medicated mass for introduction into the rectum, urethra, or vagina.

suppressant (sŭ-pres'ant) 1. inducing suppression, such as of secretion, excretion, or normal discharge. 2. an agent that so acts.

suppression (sŭ-presh'un) the act of holding back or checking. 1. the stopping or inhibition of something, such as a secretion, excretion, normal discharge, or other function. 2. in psychiatry, conscious inhibition of an unacceptable impulse or idea as contrasted with repression, which is unconscious. 3. in genetics, a second mutation occurring at a site different from the first mutation site and able to mask or suppress the phenotypic expression of the first mutation; the organism appears to be reverted but is in fact doubly mutant. 4. inhibition of the erythrocytic stage of *Plasmodium* to prevent clinical attacks of malaria; used for prophylaxis. 5. cortical inhibition of perception of objects in all or part of the visual field of one eye during binocular vision.

bone marrow s. reduction of the cell-forming functions of bone marrow, such as by a drug or because of replacement of the marrow by a disease process. Called also myelophthisis and myelosuppression.

labor s. in the NURSING INTERVENTIONS CLASSIFICATION, a nursing INTERVENTION defined as controlling uterine contractions prior to 37 weeks of gestation to prevent preterm BIRTH. See also LABOR.

lactation s. in the NURSING INTERVENTIONS CLASSIFICATION, a nursing INTERVENTION defined as facilitating the cessation of LACTATION and minimizing breast engorgement after childbirth.

overdrive s. the suppression of intrinsic cellular AUTOMATICITY by a rapid outside stimulus. In cardiology this refers to the inhibitory effect of a faster PACEMAKER on a slower pacemaker. The faster rate causes an accumulation of intracellular sodium, stimulating the sodium-potassium PUMP, which hyperpolarizes the cell so that it takes longer to reach threshold POTENTIAL. This phenomenon is present in healthy His-Purkinje cells but decreases with a decrease in

membrane POTENTIAL and loss of fast sodium CHANNELS.

suppurant (sup'u-rant) 1. suppurative. 2 an agent causing SUPPURATION.

suppuration (sup″u-ra'shun) 1. pyogen esis. 2. the act of becoming converted int and discharging pus. adj., **sup'purative.**

supra- word element [L.], *above.*

supra-acromial (soo″prah-ah-kro'me-al above the acromion.

supra-auricular (soo″prah-aw-rik'u-lar above the auricle of the ear.

suprachoroid (soo″prah-kor'oid) above o upon the choroid.

suprachoroidea (soo″prah-ko-roi'de-ah the outermost layer of the choroid.

supraclavicular (soo″prah-klah-vik'u-lar above the clavicle.

supracondylar (soo″prah-kon'dĭ-lar above a condyle.

supracostal (soo″prah-kos'tal) above o outside the ribs.

supracotyloid (soo″prah-kot'ĭ-loid) abov the acetabulum.

supradiaphragmatic (soo″prah-di″ah frag-mat'ik) above the diaphragm.

supraduction (soo″prah-duk'shun) sur sumduction.

supraepicondylar (soo″prah-ep″ĭ-kon'di lar) above the epicondyle.

supraglottitis (soo″prah-glŏ-ti'tis) inflam mation of the epiglottis, most often as result of infection with *Haemophilus influ enzae* type b, but also due to other bacteria viral, or fungal infection or to therma injury or other trauma; it is characterize by drooling, sore throat, and distress, an can lead to life-threatening upper airwa obstruction. Called also epiglottitis.

suprahyoid (soo″prah-hi'oid) above th hyoid bone.

supraliminal (soo″prah-lim'ĭ-nal) abov the threshold of sensation.

supralumbar (soo″prah-lum'bar) abov the loin.

supramaxillary (soo″prah-mak'sĭ-lar″e above the maxilla.

supraorbital (soo″prah-or'bĭ-tal) above th orbit.

suprapelvic (soo″prah-pel'vik) above th pelvis.

suprapharmacologic (soo″prah-fahr″ mah-kah-loj'ik) much greater than the usua therapeutic dose or pharmacologic concen tration of a drug.

suprapontine (soo″prah-pon'tīn) above o in the upper part of the pons.

suprapubic (soo″prah-pu'bik) above th pubes.

suprarenal (soo″prah-re'nal) adrenal.

suprarenalectomy (soo″prah-re″nal-ek tah-me) adrenalectomy.

suprascapular (soo″prah-skap′u-lar) bove the scapula.

suprascleral (soo″prah-skler′al) on the uter surface of the sclera.

suprasellar (soo″prah-sel′ar) above the ella turcica.

supraspinal (soo″prah-spi′nal) above the pine.

suprasternal (soo″prah-ster′nal) above he sternum.

suprasystem (soo′prah-sis″tem) a highly omplex SYSTEM, such as a nation or society.

supratrochlear (soo″prah-trok′le-ar) bove the trochlea.

supravaginal (soo″prah-vaj′ĭ-nal) 1. outide or above a sheath. 2. above the vagina.

supraventricular (soo″prah-ven-trik′u-lar) ituated or occurring above the ventricles, specially in an atrium or atrioventricular ode.

supravergence (soo″prah-ver′jens) surumvergence.

supraversion (soo″prah-ver′zhun) 1. abormal elongation of a tooth from its socket. . sursumversion.

suprofen (soo-pro′fen) a NONSTEROIDAL NTIINFLAMMATORY DRUG applied topically to he conjunctiva to inhibit miosis during phthalmic surgery.

sura (soo′ra) [L.] calf. adj., **su′ral.**

suramin (soo′rah-min) an ANTIFILARIAL and ntiprotozoal AGENT used as the hexasodium alt in prophylaxis and treatment of early tages of African TRYPANOSOMIASIS and someimes ONCHOCERCIASIS. Because of its toxicity ; must be used with care.

surface (sur′fas) the outer part or external spect of a solid body; called also facies.

    buccal s. the vestibular SURFACE of the molars and premolars, which faces the cheek.

    contact s. proximal surface.

    distal s. the surface of a tooth that is arthest from the midline of the dental arch, pposite to its mesial SURFACE.

    facial s. vestibular surface.

    incisal s. the cutting edges of the anteior teeth, the incisors and canines, which ome into contact with those of the opposite eeth during protrusive occlusion. See also cclusal SURFACE.

    labial s. the vestibular SURFACE of the ncisors and canines, which faces the lips.

    lingual s. the surface of a tooth that aces inward toward the tongue and oral avity, opposite the vestibular SURFACE; alled also oral surface.

    masticatory s. occlusal surface.

    mesial s. the surface of a tooth that is losest to the midline of the dental arch, pposite to its distal SURFACE.

    occlusal s. the surface of the teeth that omes in contact with those of the opposite

jaw during OCCLUSION; called also masticatory surface.

    oral s. lingual surface.

    proximal s., proximate s. the area where the mesial SURFACE of one tooth touches the distal SURFACE of another; called also contact area or surface.

    vestibular s. the surface of a tooth that is directed outward toward the VESTIBULE OF THE MOUTH, opposite to the lingual SURFACE; see also buccal SURFACE and labial SURFACE. Called also facial surface.

surfactant (sur-fak′tant) 1. surface-active agent. 2. In pulmonary physiology, a mixture of phospholipids (chiefly LECITHIN and SPHINGOMYELIN) secreted by the great alveolar (type II) cells into the alveoli and respiratory air passages, which reduces the surface tension of pulmonary fluids and thus contributes to the elastic properties of pulmonary tissue. A synthetic surfactant is commercially available for use in the treatment of RESPIRATORY DISTRESS SYNDROME OF THE NEWBORN. See also ACUTE RESPIRATORY DISTRESS SYNDROME.

surgeon (sur′jen) 1. a physician who specializes in the treatment of diseases, injuries, and deformities by manual or operative methods. 2. the senior medical officer of a military unit.

surgeon assistant (SA) a PHYSICIAN ASSISTANT who provides diagnosis and treatment of patients under supervision of a surgeon, being able to perform tasks such as history taking, physical examination, assisting at surgery, invasive diagnostic tests, and cardiopulmonary resuscitation. SAs are eligible for certification as Physician Assistant Certified (PA-C).

surgery (sur′jer-e) 1. the branch of health science that treats diseases, injuries, and deformities by manual or operative methods. 2. the place where operative procedures are performed. 3. in Great Britain, a room or office where a doctor sees and treats patients. 4. the work performed by a SURGEON; see also OPERATION and PROCEDURE. adj., **sur′gical.**

    ambulatory s. any operative procedure not requiring an overnight stay in the hospital; it must be carefully planned to ensure that all necessary diagnostic tests are completed prior to admission. Discharge instructions must place a high priority on patient safety. Called also day surgery.

    bench s. surgery performed on an organ that has been removed from the body, after which it is reimplanted.

    day s. ambulatory surgery.

    maxillofacial s. oral and maxillofacial s.

S

minimal access s., minimally invasive s. a surgical procedure done in a manner that causes little or no trauma or injury to the patient, such as through a cannula using lasers, endoscopes, or laparoscopes; compared with other procedures, those in this category involve less bleeding, smaller amounts of anesthesia, less pain, and minimal scarring.

open heart s. surgery that involves incision into one or more chambers of the heart, such as for repair or palliation of congenital heart defects, repair or replacement of defective heart valves, or coronary artery BYPASS.

oral s. oral and maxillofacial s.

oral and maxillofacial s. that branch of dental practice that deals with the diagnosis and the surgical and adjunctive treatment of diseases, injuries, and defects of the human mouth and dental structures. Called also maxillofacial or oral surgery.

orthopedic s. orthopedics.

plastic s. see PLASTIC SURGERY.

stereotaxic s. the production of sharply localized lesions in the brain after precise localization of the target tissue by use of three-dimensional coordinates.

surgical technologist (ST) a health care professional who performs as a member of the surgical team, acting as a scrub technician or as a circulator. Those certified by the Association of Surgical Technologists (AST) are designated Certified Surgical Technologist (CST). Formerly called operating room technician. The address of the Association of Surgical Technologists is 7108-C South Alton Way, Englewood, CO 80120.

Surgicel (sur′jĭ-sel) trademark for an absorbable knitted fabric prepared by controlled oxidation of cellulose; used as a hemostatic covering for surgical wounds to control hemorrhage when other conventional methods are impractical or ineffective.

Surmontil (sur-mon′til) trademark for a preparation of TRIMIPRAMINE maleate, a tricyclic ANTIDEPRESSANT.

surrogate (sur′o-gat) a substitute; a thing or person that takes the place of something or someone else, as a drug used in place of another, or, in psychoanalysis, the projection onto another person of one's mother or father image and unconscious and inappropriate response to that person with the feelings and attitudes felt for the real mother or father.

WINDOW ON SURGICAL TECHNOLOGIST

Surgical technologists are integral members of the surgical team who function in a variety of roles. They work with surgeons, anesthesia personnel, nurses, and other hospital personnel to assess and help deliver the highest quality of patient care. A surgical technologist may function as a scrub technologist, a first or second assistant, or as a circulator. In the scrubbed role (in the sterile field), some of the duties include: setting up the sterile table; preparing instruments, supplies, and sutures; gowning and gloving the surgeon and assistants; anticipating the needs of the sterile team and handling instruments and supplies; doing appropriate counts; preparing dressings; holding retractors; providing assistance in exposure, hemostasis, and other technical functions to the surgeon. In the circulating role (the non-sterile field) some of the duties include: obtaining appropriate sterile and non-sterile supplies; opening sterile items; checking and transporting the patient; checking the operative permit; anticipating additional supplies needed by the scrubbed team; and performing appropriate counts.

The profession of surgical technology was developed during World War II when there was a severe shortage of qualified operating room personnel. Individuals were specifically trained to work in this area and assist in surgical procedures. From this beginning, surgical technology has grown and continued to meet the need for qualified individuals; as stated by the surgical technologists' motto, AEGER PRIMO—the patient first.

Surgical technologists may earn the title of Certified Surgical Technologist (CST) by passing a nationally administered certifying examination. In addition to working as a staff surgical technologist in the hospital setting, other career opportunities include: tissue or organ procurement and transplantation technician, anesthesia technician, central service supply manager, materials manager, OB/delivery technologist, clinical instructor/educator, private technologist employed by a physician, surgical first assistant, and medical sales representative.

The professional organization is the Association of Surgical Technologists, 7108-C South Alton Way, Centennial, CO 80112-2106.

CHRIS KEEGAN, MS, CST

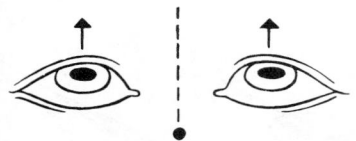

Sursumversion. From Stein et al., 2000.

sursumduction (sur″sum-duk′shun) the turning upward of a part, especially the eyes.

sursumvergence (sur″sum-ver′jens) an upward movement, especially of an eye, where the other eye does not move.

sursumversion (sur″sum-ver′zhun) an act of turning or directing upward, especially the simultaneous and equal upward turning of the eyes.

surveillance (sur-vāl′ans) 1. watching or MONITORING. 2. a procedure used instead of quarantine to control the spread of infectious disease, involving close supervision during the incubation period of possible contacts of individuals exposed to an infectious disease. 3. in the NURSING INTERVENTIONS CLASSIFICATION, a nursing INTERVENTION defined as the purposeful and ongoing acquisition, interpretation, and synthesis of patient data for clinical decision-making.

s.: community in the NURSING INTERVENTIONS CLASSIFICATION, a nursing INTERVENTION defined as purposeful and ongoing acquisition, interpretation, and synthesis of data for decision-making in the community.

s.: late pregnancy in the NURSING INTERVENTIONS CLASSIFICATION, a nursing INTERVENTION defined as the purposeful and ongoing acquisition, interpretation, and synthesis of maternal-fetal data for treatment, observation, or admission. See also PREGNANCY.

s. and/or observation a nursing INTERVENTION in the NURSING MINIMUM DATA SET; action through which the nurse examines and monitors physical and behavioral responses to disease or injury and to the prescribed medical and/or nursing therapy.

s.: remote electronic in the NURSING INTERVENTIONS CLASSIFICATION, a nursing INTERVENTION defined as purposeful and ongoing acquisition of patient data via electronic modalities (telephone, video conferencing, e-mail) from distant locations as well as interpretation and synthesis of patient data for clinical decision-making with individuals or populations. See also TELEHEALTH.

s.: safety in the NURSING INTERVENTIONS CLASSIFICATION, a nursing INTERVENTION defined as the purposeful and ongoing collection and analysis of information about the patient and the environment for use in promoting and maintaining patient safety.

skin s. in the NURSING INTERVENTIONS CLASSIFICATION, a nursing INTERVENTION defined as the collection and analysis of patient data to maintain skin and mucous membrane integrity. See also skin CARE.

survey (sur′va) an inspection or examination.

primary s. primary ASSESSMENT.

susceptibility (sŭ-sep″tĭ-bil′ĭ-te) the state of being susceptible.

susceptible (sŭ-sep′tĭ-b'l) readily affected or acted upon; lacking immunity or resistance.

suspension (sus-pen′shun) 1. temporary cessation, as of pain or a vital process. 2. a supporting from above, as in treatment where extremities are elevated with a TRACTION device. 3. a preparation of a finely divided, undissolved substance dispersed in a liquid vehicle.

bladder neck s. any of various methods of surgical fixation of the urethrovesical junction area and the bladder NECK to restore the neck to a high retropubic position for relief of stress INCONTINENCE. Among numerous types of procedures are the BURCH PROCEDURE and the PEREYRA PROCEDURE. Called also colposuspension.

colloid s. a colloid system; see COLLOID (def. 2). Sometimes used specifically for a sol in which the dispersed phase is solid and the particles are large enough to settle out of solution.

suspensoid (sus-pen′soid) lyophobic colloid.

suspensory (sus-pen′sah-re) 1. serving to hold up a part. 2. a ligament, bone, muscle, bandage, or sling for supporting a part.

sustentaculum (sus″ten-tak′u-lum) [L.] a support. adj., **sustentac′ular.**

sutilains (soo′tĭ-lāns) proteolytic enzymes derived from a strain of *Bacillus subtilis* used for wound débridement.

Sutton's disease (sut′onz) 1. halo nevus. 2. periadenitis mucosa necrotica recurrens. 3. granuloma fissuratum.

sutura (soo-tu′rah) [L.] a type of joint in which the apposed bony surfaces are united by fibrous tissue, permitting no movement; found only between bones of the skull. Called also suture.

suture (soo′chur) 1. sutura. 2. a stitch or series of stitches made to secure apposition of the edges of a surgical or traumatic wound; used also as a verb to indicate application of such stitches. 3. material used in closing a wound with stitches. adj., **su′tural.**

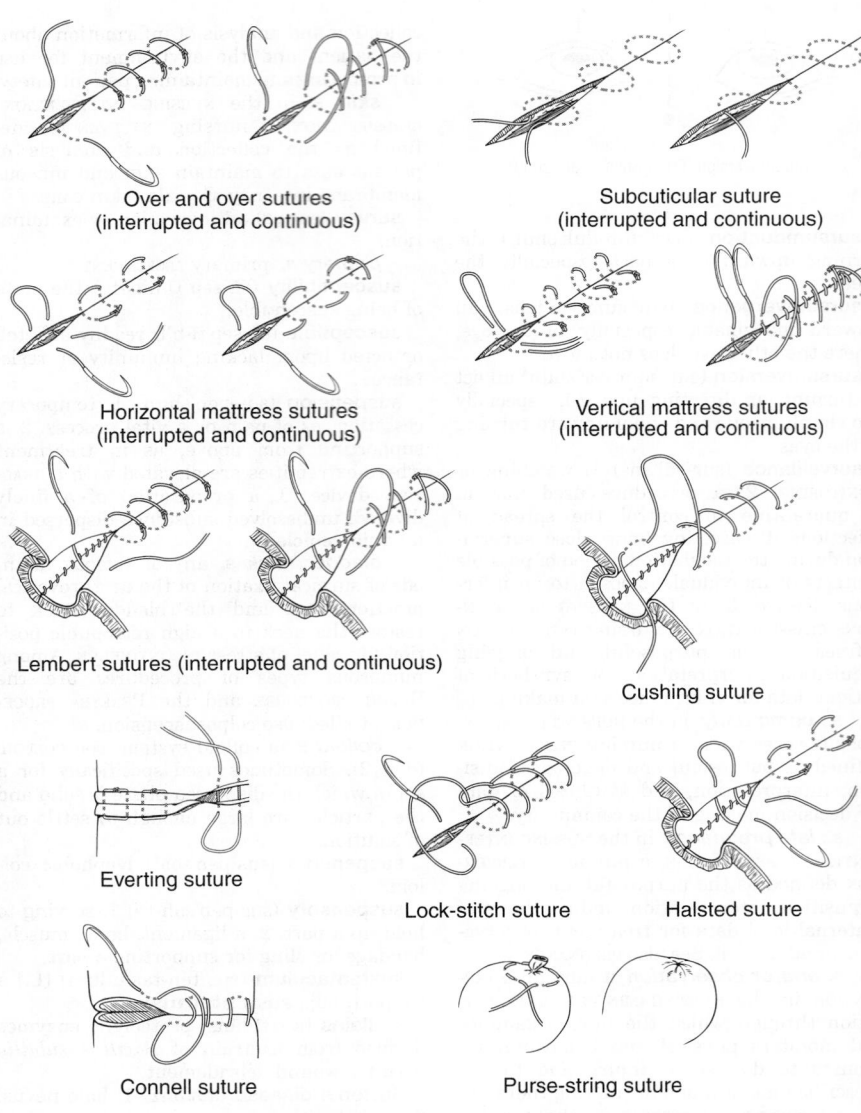

Over and over sutures
(interrupted and continuous)

Subcuticular suture
(interrupted and continuous)

Horizontal mattress sutures
(interrupted and continuous)

Vertical mattress sutures
(interrupted and continuous)

Lembert sutures (interrupted and continuous)

Cushing suture

Everting suture

Lock-stitch suture

Halsted suture

Connell suture

Purse-string suture

Various types of sutures. From Dorland's, 2000.

absorbable s. a strand of material that is used for closing wounds and becomes dissolved in the body fluids and disappears; types include surgical GUT, tendon, and some synthetics.

apposition s. a superficial suture used for exact approximation of the cutaneous edges of a wound.

approximation s. a deep suture for securing apposition of the deep tissue of a wound.

buried s. one placed within the tissues and concealed by the skin.

catgut s. an absorbable suture made from surgical GUT.

cobbler's s. double-armed suture.

collagen s. a suture made from the tendons of cattle, chemically treated, purified, and processed into strands; it is most often used in ophthalmologic surgery.

continuous s. one in which a continuous, uninterrupted length of material is used

coronal s. the line of union between the frontal bone and the parietal bones.

cranial s. the lines of junction between the bones of the skull.

Czerny's s. 1. an intestinal suture in which the thread is passed through the mucous membrane only. 2. union of a ruptured tendon by splitting one of the ends and suturing the other end into the slit.

Czerny-Lembert s. a combination of the Czerny and the Lembert sutures.

double-armed s. one made with suture material threaded through a needle at each end. Called also cobbler's suture.

false s. a line of junction between apposed surfaces without fibrous union of the bones.

Gély's s. a continuous stitch for wounds of the intestine, made with a thread having a needle at each end.

interrupted s. one in which each stitch is made with a separate piece of material.

lambdoid s. the line of union between the upper borders of the occipital and parietal bones, shaped like the Greek letter lambda.

Lembert s. an inverting suture used in gastrointestinal surgery.

lock-stitch s. a continuous hemostatic suture used in intestinal surgery, in which the needle is, after each stitch, passed through the loop of the preceding stitch.

mattress s. suturing with the stitches parallel to the wound edges (*horizontal mattress suture*) or at right angles to them (*vertical mattress suture*).

purse-string s. a type of suture commonly used to bury the stump of the APPENDIX, a continuous running suture being placed about the opening, and then drawn tight.

relaxation s. any suture so formed that it may be loosened to relieve tension as necessary.

retention s. a reinforcing suture made of exceptionally strong material such as wire, and including large amounts of tissue in each stitch. Used to relieve pressure on the primary suture line and to decrease the potential for wound dehiscence.

sagittal s. the line of union of the two parietal bones, dividing the skull anteroposteriorly into two symmetrical halves.

squamous s. the suture between the pars squamosa of the temporal bone and parietal bone.

subcuticular s. a method of skin closure involving placement of stitches in the subcuticular tissues parallel with the line of the wound.

synthetic absorbable s. an absorbable suture produced from strands of polymers;

the most commonly used materials are polyglactin 910 (Vicryl) and polyglycolic acid (Dexon); the latter is more rapidly absorbed. Synthetic absorbable sutures are absorbed by slow hydrolysis, a chemical process in which the polymer reacts with tissue fluids, causing a breakdown of the molecular structure of the material at a predictable rate and with minimal tissue reaction.

vertical mattress s. a suture whose stitches are at right angles to the edges of the wound, taking both deep and superficial bites of tissue; the superficial ones achieve more exact apposition of the cutaneous margins. When the suture material is pulled tight, the wound edges evert.

suturing (soo'cher-ing) in the NURSING INTERVENTIONS CLASSIFICATION, a nursing INTERVENTION defined as approximating the edges of a wound using sterile SUTURE material and a needle.

svedberg (sfed'berg) Svedberg unit.

swab (swahb) a small pledget of cotton or gauze wrapped around the end of a slender wooden stick or wire for applying medications or obtaining specimens of secretions and other substances from body surfaces or orifices.

swage (swāj) 1. to shape metal by hammering or by adapting it to a die. 2. to fuse, as suture material to the end of a suture needle.

swallowing (swahl'o-ing) the taking in of a substance through the mouth and pharynx and into the esophagus. It is a combination of a voluntary act and a series of reflex actions. Once begun, the process operates automatically. Called also deglutition.

The Three Stages of Swallowing. In the first, voluntary, stage of swallowing, the cheeks are sucked in slightly and the tongue is arched against the hard palate, so that the bolus, or ball of chewed food, is moved to the pharynx.

Normally, air is free to pass from the nose or mouth to the lungs and back again. But the moment the bolus approaches the fauces, the passage from the mouth to the pharynx, nerve centers are triggered that control a series of reflex actions. After one quick inhalation, breathing is halted for the brief instant of the next stage.

In this second, involuntary, stage of swallowing, the rear edge of the soft palate, which hangs down from the roof of the mouth, swings up against the back of the pharynx and blocks the passages to the nose. The back of the tongue fits tightly into the space between two muscular pillars at each side of the fauces, sealing the way back

S

to the mouth. Simultaneously, the larynx moves upward against the epiglottis, effectively closing the entrance to the trachea.

Sometimes the larynx does not move up quickly enough and food gets into the air passage, stimulating a coughing reaction. With the one-way route to the stomach firmly established, however, the muscular coat of the pharynx contracts, squeezing the ball of food and forcing its passage into the esophagus.

In the third stage, the rhythmic contraction (peristalsis) of the muscles of the esophagus moves the food on to the stomach. The cardiac sphincter keeps the stomach entrance closed until food is swallowed. As the food approaches, moved by the wavelike contractions of the esophagus, the advancing portion of the wave causes the sphincter to relax and open, while the rear and contracting portion forces the ball of food through the entrance.

impaired s. a NURSING DIAGNOSIS accepted by the North American Nursing Diagnosis Association, defined as a state in which an individual has decreased ability to voluntarily pass fluids or solids from the mouth to the stomach.

Swan-Ganz catheter (swahn-gahnts) a soft, flow-directed catheter with a balloon at the tip for measuring pulmonary arterial pressures, right atrial pressures, left atrial pressure, reflected left ventricular end-diastolic pressure, and cardiac output. It is introduced into an internal jugular vein or subclavian vein and is guided by blood flow into the subclavian vein, the superior vena cava, through the right atrium and ventricle, and into the pulmonary artery where it floats freely with the movement of blood. A monitor attached to the distal lumen port provides a reading of pulmonary artery pressure and pulmonary capillary wedge pressure, which is actually a reading of pressure in the left side of the heart.

The catheter permits evaluation of cardiac function by assessing the effectiveness of right and left pumping action of the heart and providing a quantitative measurement of cardiac output, and by allowing for sampling of mixed arterial-venous oxygen levels and calculation of differences between the two. Swan-Ganz catheters have a proximal lumen opening that is situated in the right atrium or superior vena cava, permitting monitoring of central venous pressure. The proximal lumen port is used for administration of drugs and fluids.

The Swan-Ganz catheter provides vital information in cases of heart failure resulting from myocardial infarction and cardiogenic shock, in the care of patients critically ill from hypovolemic shock, and in the diagnosis and treatment of cardiac tamponade. It also is useful in preventive monitoring to avoid overhydration and pulmonary edema, and often is inserted preoperatively in patients undergoing preload and corrective procedures and open heart SURGERY in order to monitor response to anesthesia during surgery. The catheter is used diagnostically to inject radiopaque dye during angiography to confirm a diagnosis of pulmonary embolism.

Care of the patient with a Swan-Ganz catheter requires extensive instruction and supervised experience in intensive care nursing.

sweat (swet) the salty fluid, consisting largely of water, excreted by the SWEAT GLANDS in the skin. Called also perspiration.

In high temperatures, during strenuous exertion, or in times of unusual emotional stress, the sweat output of the body may exceed several quarts per day. Even on a cool day without exertion or emotional

SWAN-GANZ CATHETER: CONDITIONS WITH EXPECTED PRESSURE CHANGES				
	Pressure Changes			
Condition	RA	RV	PAP	PAWP
Heart failure (volume overload)	↑	↑	↑	↑
Hypovolemia	↓	↓	↓	↓
Cardiogenic shock*	— or ↑	— or ↑	— or ↑	— or ↑ (Diastolic)
Pulmonary hypertension	↑	↑	↑	— or ↑
Cardiac tamponade	↑	↑	↑	↑ (Diastolic)
Pulmonary emboli	↑	↑	↑	↑ (Systolic)
Mitral valve stenosis-insufficiency†	↑	↑	↑	↑

RA, right atrial pressure; RV, right ventricular pressure; PAP, pulmonary artery pressure; PAWP, pulmonary artery wedge pressure.
*Pressure readings depend on the heart's ability to handle circulating volume. Chronic lung disease elevates all readings.
†Mitral valve disease produces unreliable pressure readings.
From Polaski and Tatro, 1996.

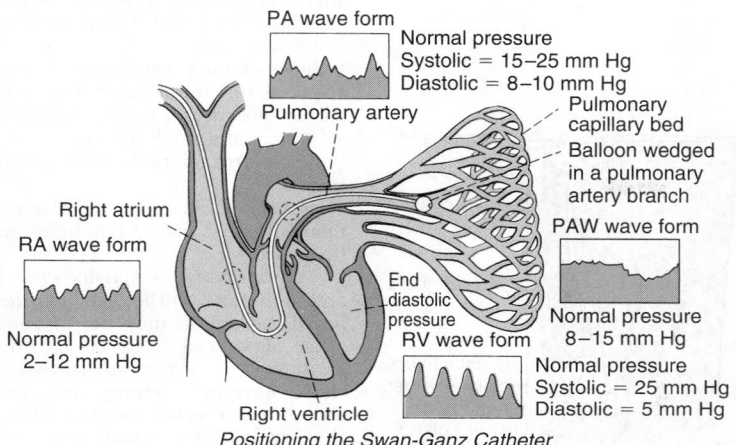

Positioning the Swan-Ganz Catheter

- PA wave form
- Normal pressure
  Systolic = 15–25 mm Hg
  Diastolic = 8–10 mm Hg
- Pulmonary artery
- Pulmonary capillary bed
- Balloon wedged in a pulmonary artery branch
- PAW wave form
- Right atrium
- RA wave form
- Normal pressure 2–12 mm Hg
- End diastolic pressure
- RV wave form
- Normal pressure 8–15 mm Hg
- Normal pressure
  Systolic = 25 mm Hg
  Diastolic = 5 mm Hg
- Right ventricle

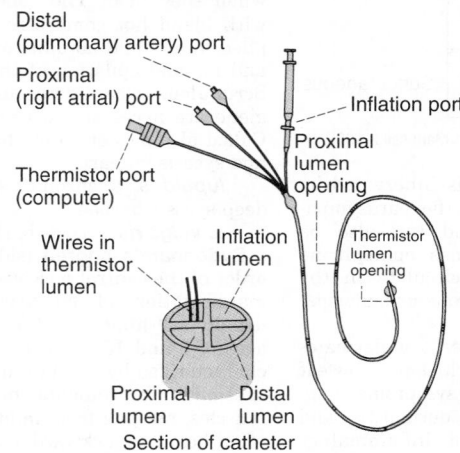

- Distal (pulmonary artery) port
- Proximal (right atrial) port
- Inflation port
- Proximal lumen opening
- Thermistor port (computer)
- Wires in thermistor lumen
- Inflation lumen
- Thermistor lumen opening
- Proximal lumen
- Distal lumen
- Section of catheter

The Quadruple-Lumen Swan-Ganz Catheter
Swan-Ganz catheter. From Polaski and Tatro, 1996.

S

stress, the body loses well over a pint of fluid in sweat. This latter kind of sweating is known medically as "insensible" perspiration because it is virtually unnoticeable; as the sweat reaches the surface of the skin, it evaporates immediately. When sweating becomes noticeable, it is known as "sensible" perspiration.

The chief function of sweat glands and perspiration is to maintain the body temperature at a constant level. Thus the skin is cooled as perspiration evaporates. The blood in the capillaries of the skin likewise is cooled before it courses back into the body. The sweat glands have a minor excretory function. Perspiration contains water, sodium chloride, and small amounts of urea, lactic acid, and potassium ions. It also contains antibacterial substances that defend the body against infection.

s. gland one of the glands that secrete SWEAT, found in the corium or subcutaneous tissue, and opening by a duct on the surface of the body. There are two types: The ordinary or *eccrine* sweat glands are unbranched, coiled, tubular glands distributed over almost all of the body surface; they promote cooling by evaporation of their secretion. The *apocrine* sweat glands are large, branched, specialized glands that empty into the upper portion of a hair follicle instead of directly onto the skin surface, and are found only on certain areas of the body, such as around the anus and in

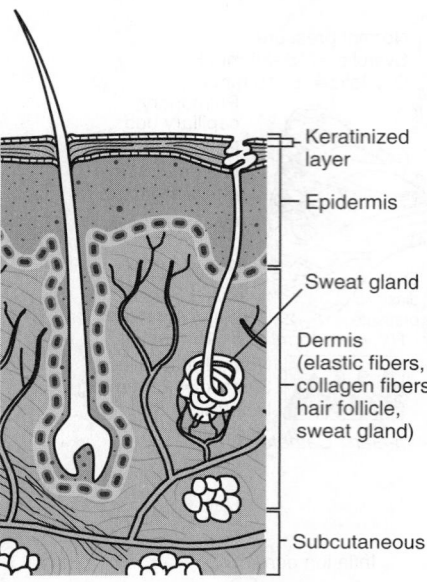

Sweat gland. From Mahon and Manuselis, 1995.

the axilla. A sweat gland is innervated by cholinergic nerve fibers of the parasympathetic nervous system and can also be stimulated by the hormones epinephrine and norepinephrine that circulate in the blood. Called also sudoriferous or sudoriparous gland.

s. retention syndrome 1. a dermatologic condition due to occlusion of sweat ducts, which may result in symptoms ranging from pruritus, scratch dermatitis, and miliaria to very persistent inflammatory changes, depending upon the extent of the blockage, environmental temperature, and duration of sweating stimulus. 2. tropical anhidrotic asthenia.

sweating (swet'ing) the excretion of moisture through the pores of the skin; called also perspiration and diaphoresis.

swelling (swel'ing) 1. transient abnormal enlargement of a body part or area not due to cell proliferation; see also EDEMA. Called also tumefaction, tumescence, and turgescence. 2. eminence.

cloudy s. a term formerly used for an early stage of toxic degeneration of protein constituents of organs in infectious diseases, when the tissues appear swollen and opaque but revert to normal when the cause is removed.

Swift's disease (swifts) acrodynia.

swineherd's disease leptospirosis, manifested as a benign meningitis, caused by serovariants of *Leptospira interrogans;* i affects people who work with swine or por or come in contact with the urine of anima or human carriers.

Swyer-James syndrome (swi'er jāmz' acquired unilateral EMPHYSEMA with sever airway obstruction during exhalation, HYPO VOLEMIA, and a small hilum.

sycosiform (si-ko'sĭ-form) resembling sy cosis.

sycosis (si-ko'sis) a papulopustular in flammation of the hair follicles, usually c the beard.

s. bar'bae a staphylococcal infectio and irritation of the hair follicles in th beard region; it may be associated wit other superficial bacterial infections such as IMPETIGO or FURUNCULOSIS. Symptoms in clude burning, itching, and pain, wit formation of small papules and pustule that drain, form crusts, and leave scar when they heal. The condition is treate with bland hot compresses, antibiotics ap plied locally and administered parenterally and manual epilation of the infected hairs Scrupulous cleanliness and personal hy giene are necessary to prevent reinfection Called also barber's itch, folliculitis barbae and sycosis vulgaris.

lupoid s. a chronic, scarring form o deep sycosis barbae.

s. vulga'ris sycosis barbae.

Sydenham's chorea (sid'en-hamz) a dis order of the central nervous system that is a manifestation of RHEUMATIC FEVER; it i usually self-limited and occurs between the ages of 5 and 15 or during pregnancy. It i characterized by involuntary irregular jerk spasmodic movements of the voluntar muscles, ranging from mild to severe; thes often begin as awkwardness and uncontrol lable facial grimaces that can cause the child considerable embarrassment. Emo tional instability and extreme nervousnes usually accompany the physical symptoms Treatment and care are based on relief o symptoms. Complete mental and physica rest are prescribed and a mild SEDATIVE o TRANQUILIZER may be given to promote re laxation. The prognosis is good and com plete recovery is the rule, although the symptoms and signs can last up to three months. Called also Saint Vitus's dance.

symballophone (sim-bal'o-fōn) a stetho scope with two chest pieces, making possibl the comparison and localization of sounds.

symbiont (sim'bi-ont, sim'be-ont) an or ganism or species living in a state o symbiosis.

symbiosis (sim''bi-o'sis, sĭm''bē-ō'sĭs), pl *symbio'ses* 1. in parasitology, the biologic association of two individuals or population of different species; it is classified as MUTU-ALISM, COMMENSALISM, PARASITISM, AMENSALISM, or SYNNECROSIS, depending on the advantage or disadvantage derived from the relationship. 2. in psychiatry, a mutually reinforcing relationship between persons who are dependent on each other; a normal characteristic of the relationship between a mother and infant. adj., **symbiot′ic.**

symbiote (sim′bi-ōt) symbiont.

symblepharon (sim-blef′ah-ron) adhesion of an eyelid(s) to the eyeball.

symblepharopterygium (sim-blef″ah-ro-tĕr-ij′e-um) symblepharon in which the adhesion is a cicatricial band resembling a pterygium.

symbol (sim′bol) 1. something, particularly an object, representing something else. 2. in psychoanalytic theory, a representation or perception that replaces unconscious mental content.

   phallic s. in psychoanalytic theory, any pointed or upright object which may represent the phallus or penis.

symbolism (sim′bah-lizm) 1. the act or process of representing something by a symbol. 2. in psychoanalytic theory, a mechanism of unconscious thinking characterized by substitution of a symbol for a repressed or threatening impulse or object, which is often of a sexual nature, so as to avoid censorship by the superego.

symbolization (sim″bol-ĭ-za′shun) an unconscious DEFENSE MECHANISM in which one idea or object comes to represent another because of similarity or association between them.

symmelia (sim-e′le-ah) a developmental ANOMALY characterized by apparent fusion of the lower limbs. There may be three feet *(tripodial symmelia),* two feet *(dipodial symmelia),* one foot *(monopodial symmelia),* or no feet *(apodal symmelia* or *sirenomelia).*

symmelus (sim′ĕ-lus) a fetus with SYMME-LIA.

symmetry (sim′ĕ-tre) correspondence in size, form, and arrangement of parts on opposite sides of a plane, or around an axis. adj., **symmet′rical.**

   bilateral s. the configuration of an irregularly shaped body (such as the human body or that of higher animals) that can be divided by a longitudinal plane into halves that are mirror images of each other.

   radial s. that in which the body parts are arranged regularly around a central axis.

sympathectomy (sim″pah-thek′tah-me) excision or interruption of some portion of the sympathetic nervous pathway. The operation produces temporary vasodilation leading to improved nutrition of the part

supplied by the vessel. It is done in cases of partial arterial obstruction with resultant trophic changes distally.

   chemical s. the interruption of the transmission of impulses through a sympathetic nerve by chemical agents.

sympathetic (sim″pah-thet′ik) 1. pertaining to or caused by sympathy. 2. pertaining to the sympathetic nervous system.

   s. nervous system the thoracolumbar part of the AUTONOMIC NERVOUS SYSTEM, the preganglionic fibers of which arise from cell bodies in the thoracic and first three lumbar segments of the spinal cord; postganglionic fibers are distributed to the heart, smooth muscle, and glands of the entire body. (See also Plate 14.)

   s. stress reaction alarm reaction.

sympathicoblast (sim-path′ĭ-ko-blast″) an embryonic cell that develops into a sympathetic nerve cell.

sympathicoblastoma (sim-path″ĭ-ko-blas-to′mah) a malignant tumor containing sympathicoblasts.

sympathicolytic (sim-path″ĭ-ko-lit′ik) sympatholytic.

sympathicomimetic (sim-path″ĭ-ko-mi-met′ik) sympathomimetic.

sympathicotonia (sim-path″ĭ-ko-to′ne-ah) a stimulated condition of the sympathetic nervous system marked by vascular spasm, heightened blood pressure, and the dominance of other sympathetic functions. adj., **sympathicoton′ic.**

sympathicotripsy (sim-path″ĭ-ko-trip′se) surgical crushing of a nerve, ganglion, or plexus of the sympathetic nervous system.

sympathicotropic (sim-path″ĭ-ko-trop′ik) 1. having affinity for or exerting its principal effect on the sympathetic nervous system. 2. an agent with such properties.

sympathism (sim′pah-thizm) suggestibility.

sympathoadrenal (sim″pah-tho-ah-dre′-nal) 1. pertaining to the sympathetic nervous system and the adrenal medulla. 2. involving the sympathetic nervous system and the adrenal glands, especially increased sympathetic activity that causes increased secretion of epinephrine by the adrenal medulla and norepinephrine by the postganglionic sympathetic nerve endings.

sympathoblast (sim-path′o-blast) sympathicoblast.

sympathoblastoma (sim″pah-tho-blas-to′-mah) sympathicoblastoma.

sympathogonia (sim″pah-tho-go′ne-ah) sing. *sympathogo′nium* [Gr.] undifferentiated embryonic cells that develop into sympathetic nerve cells.

S

sympathogonioma (sim″pah-tho-go″ne-o′ma) a tumor composed of sympathogonia.

sympathogonium (sim″pah-tho-go′ne-um) [Gr.] singular of SYMPATHOGONIA.

sympatholytic (sim″pah-tho-lit′ik) 1. blocking transmission of impulses from the ADRENERGIC (sympathetic) postganglionic fibers to effector organs or tissues, inhibiting such sympathetic functions as smooth muscle contraction and glandular secretion. 2. an agent that produces such an effect; called also antiadrenergic.

sympathomimetic (sim″pah-tho-mi-met′-ik) 1. producing effects resembling those of impulses transmitted by the postganglionic fibers of the sympathetic nervous system. See also ADRENERGIC. 2. an agent that produces such an effect.

sympathy (sim′pah-the) 1. a sense of sharing another's feelings, especially in sorrow or trouble, through some mechanism of transference or an imaginative identification with the other's situation; it is a precursor to COMPASSION. 2. an influence produced in any organ by disease, disorder, or other change in another part. 3. a relation that exists between people or things such that change in the state of one is reflected in the other.

symphalangism (sim-fal′an-jizm) congenital ankylosis of the proximal joints of the fingers and toes.

symphyseal (sim-fiz′e-al) pertaining to a symphysis.

symphysiorrhaphy (sim-fiz″e-or′ah-fe) suture of a divided symphysis.

symphysiotomy (sim-fiz″e-ot′ah-me) division of the symphysis pubis to facilitate delivery.

symphysis (sim′fi-sis) [Gr.] a site or line of union; a type of joint in which the apposed bony surfaces are firmly united by a plate of fibrocartilage.

s. menta′lis the line of fusion in the median plane of the mandible that marks the union of the two halves of the mandible.

pubic s., s. pu′bis the line of union of the bodies of the pubic bones in the median plane.

sympodia (sim-po′de-ah) fusion of the lower limbs and feet; see also SYMMELIA.

symport (sim′port) a TRANSPORT mechanism that moves two compounds simultaneously across a cell MEMBRANE in the same direction, one compound being transported down a concentration GRADIENT and the other against a gradient. See also ANTIPORT and COTRANSPORT.

symptom (simp′tom) any indication of disease perceived by the patient.

cardinal s's 1. symptoms of greatest significance to the health care provider, establishing the identity of the illness. 2. the symptoms shown in the temperature, pulse, and respiration.

dissociation s. anesthesia to pain and to heat and cold, without impairment of tactile sensibility.

objective s. one perceptible to others than the patient, such as pallor, rapid pulse, rapid respiration, or restlessness.

presenting s. the symptom or group of symptoms about which the patient complains or from which he seeks relief.

signal s. a sensation, aura, or other subjective experience indicative of an impending epileptic or other seizure.

subjective s. one perceptible only to the patient, such as pain, pruritus, or vertigo.

withdrawal s's withdrawal (def. 2).

symptomatic (simp″to-mat′ik) 1. pertaining to or of the nature of a symptom. 2. indicative (of a particular disease or disorder). 3. exhibiting the symptoms of a particular disease but having a different cause. 4. directed at the allaying of symptoms, as symptomatic treatment.

symptomatology (simp″to-mah-tol′ah-je) 1. the branch of medicine dealing with symptoms. 2. the combined symptoms of a disease.

symptomatolytic (simp″to-mah″to-lit′ik) causing the disappearance of symptoms.

sympus (sim′pus) a malformed fetus with SYMPODIA.

syn- word element [Gr.], *union; association.*

Synalar (sin′ah-lar) trademark for preparations of FLUOCINOLONE ACETONIDE, a steroid used as a topical ANTIINFLAMMATORY agent in dermatoses.

Synalgos-DC (sin-al′gos) trademark for a combination preparation of ASPIRIN, CAFFEINE, and DIHYDROCODEINE bitartrate; used as an analgesic.

synapse (sin′aps) the junction between the processes of two neurons or between a neuron and an effector organ, where neural impulses are transmitted by chemical means. The impulse causes the release of a NEUROTRANSMITTER (e.g., acetylcholine or norepinephrine) from the presynaptic membrane of the axon terminal. The neurotransmitter molecules diffuse across the synaptic cleft, bind with specific receptors on the postsynaptic membrane, causing depolarization or hyperpolarization of the postsynaptic cell. See also NEURON.

axoaxonic s. one between the axon of one neuron and the axon of another neuron.

axodendritic s. one between the axon of one neuron and the dendrites of another.

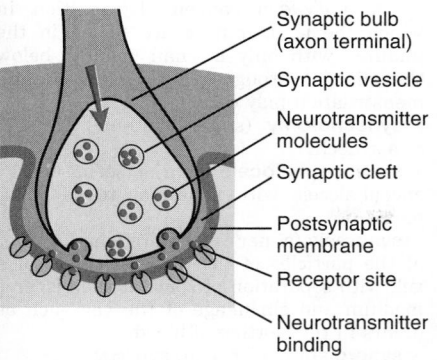

Synaptic bulb
(axon terminal)

Synaptic vesicle

Neurotransmitter
molecules

Synaptic cleft

Postsynaptic
membrane

Receptor site

Neurotransmitter
binding

Components of a synapse. From Applegate, 2000.

axodendrosomatic s. one between the axon of one neuron and the dendrites and body of another.

axosomatic s. one between the axon of one neuron and the body of another.

dendrodendritic s. one from a dendrite of one cell to a dendrite of another.

electrotonic s. a special type of GAP JUNCTION found in tissue such as the myocardium.

synapsis (sĭ-nap′sis) the pairing off and union of homologous chromosomes from male and female pronuclei at the start of meiosis.

synaptic (sĭ-nap′tik) 1. pertaining to a synapse. 2. pertaining to a synapsis.

synarthrodia (sin″ahr-thro′de-ah) fibrous JOINT. adj., **synarthro′dial.**

synarthrophysis (sin-ahr″thro-fi′sis) any ankylosing process.

synarthrosis (sin″ahr-thro′sis) [Gr.] fibrous JOINT.

syncanthus (sin-kan′thus) adhesion of the eyeball to the orbital structures.

syncephalus (sin-sef′ah-lus) conjoined twins with heads fused into one, there being a single face, with four ears.

synchilia (sin-ki′le-ah) cogenital adhesion of the lips.

synchiria (sin-ki′re-ah) DYSCHIRIA in which a stimulus applied to one side of the body is felt on both sides.

synchondrosis (sin″kon-dro′sis) [Gr.] a type of cartilaginous joint in which the cartilage is usually converted into bone before adult life.

synchondrotomy (sin″kon-drot′ah-me) division of a SYNCHONDROSIS, as in SYMPHYSIOTOMY.

synchronism (sin′kro-nizm) occurrence at the same time.

synchronous (sing′kro-nus) occurring at the same time.

synchrony (sing′kro-ne) 1. the simultaneous occurrence of two events. 2. the linkage of two events by a fixed time interval. 3. synchronism.

atrioventricular s., AV s. in the heart, the physiological condition of atrial electrical activity followed by ventricular electrical activity, with the interval between being that necessary for impulse conduction from atria to ventricles.

synchysis (sin′ki-sis) a softening or fluid condition of the vitreous body of the eye.

s. scintil′lans floating cholesterol crystals in the vitreous, developing as a secondary degenerative change.

synclitism (sin′kli-tizm) parallelism between the planes of the fetal head and those of the maternal pelvis. adj., **synclit′ic.**

synclonus (sin′klo-nus) muscular tremor or successive clonic contraction of various muscles together.

syncope (sing′kah-pe) faint. adj. **syn′copal, syncop′ic.**

cardiac s. sudden loss of consciousness, either with momentary premonitory symptoms or without warning, due to cerebral anemia caused by ventricular ASYSTOLE, extreme BRADYCARDIA, or ventricular FIBRILLATION.

laryngeal s. tussive syncope.

neurocardiogenic s. a particularly serious type of vasovagal ATTACK; the etiology is unknown.

stretching s. syncope associated with stretching the arms upward with the spine extended.

swallow s. syncope associated with swallowing, a disorder of atrioventricular conduction mediated by the vagus nerve.

tussive s. brief loss of consciousness associated with paroxysms of coughing.

vasovagal s. vasovagal attack.

syncytioma (sin-sit″e-o′mah) syncytial endometritis.

s. malig′num choriocarcinoma.

syncytiotrophoblast (sin-sit″e-o-trof′o-blast) the outer syncytial layer of the trophoblast.

syncytium (sin-sish′e-um) a multinucleate mass of protoplasm produced by the merging of cells. adj., **syncyt′ial.**

syndactyly (sin-dak′tĭ-le) the most common congenital anomaly of the hand, probably an inherited condition, marked by persistence of webbing between digits (webbed FINGERS or TOES), so that they are more or less completely attached.

syndectomy (sin-dek′tah-me) peritectomy.

syndesis (sin′dĕ-sis) 1. arthrodesis. 2. synapsis.

S

syndesm(o)- word element [Gr.], *connective tissue; ligament.*

syndesmectomy (sin″dez-mek′tah-me) excision or resection of a ligament.

syndesmitis (sin″dez-mi′tis) 1. inflammation of a ligament. 2. conjunctivitis.

syndesmography (sin″dez-mog′rah-fe) a description of the ligaments.

syndesmology (sin″dez-mol′ah-je) scientific study of the ligaments and joints.

syndesmoma (sin″des-mo′mah) a tumor of connective tissue.

syndesmoplasty (sin-dez′mo-plas″te) plastic repair of a ligament.

syndesmosis (sin″dez-mo′sis) [Gr.] a joint in which the bones are united by fibrous connective tissue forming an interosseous membrane or ligament.

syndesmotomy (sin″dez-mot′ah-me) incision of a ligament.

syndrome (sin′drōm) a combination of symptoms resulting from a single cause or so commonly occurring together as to constitute a distinct clinical picture. For specific syndromes, see under the name, such as ADRENOGENITAL SYNDROME or REYE'S SYNDROME. See also DISEASE and SICKNESS.

s. of crocodile tears spontaneous lacrimation occurring parallel with the normal salivation of eating. It follows facial paralysis and seems to be due to straying of the regenerating nerve fibers, some of those destined for the salivary glands going to the lacrimal glands.

s. of inappropriate antidiuretic hormone (SIADH) a syndrome in which secretion of VASOPRESSIN (antidiuretic hormone) is not inhibited by hypotonicity of extracellular fluid and HYPONATREMIA is produced. It occurs in conjunction with oat cell carcinoma of the lung and certain other malignant tumors and is caused by production of vasopressin by the tumor. See also ectopic HORMONES.

syndromic (sin-drom′ik) occurring as a syndrome.

syndromology (sin″drom-ol′ah-je) the field concerned with the taxonomy, etiology, and patterns of congenital malformations.

synechia (si-nek′e-ah) [Gr.] adhesion, as of the iris to the cornea or the lens.

annular s. adhesion of the whole rim of the iris to the lens.

anterior s. adhesion of the iris to the cornea.

posterior s. adhesion of the iris to the capsule of the lens or to the surface of the vitreous body.

total s. adhesion of the whole surface of the iris to the lens.

s. vulvae a congenital condition in which the labia minora are sealed in the midline, with only a small opening below the clitoris through which urination and menstruation may occur.

synechotomy (sin″ĕ-kot′ah-me) incision of a synechia.

synencephalocele (sin″en-sef′ah-lo-sēl″) encephalocele with adhesions to adjoining parts.

syneresis (si-ner′ĕ-sis) a drawing together of the particles of the disperse phase of a gel, with separation of some of the disperse medium and shrinkage of the gel, such as occurs in the clotting of blood.

synergism (sin′er-jizm) synergy.

synergist (sin′er-jist) an agent that acts with or enhances the action of another.

synergy (sin′er-je) 1. correlated action or cooperation by two or more structures or drugs. 2. in neurology, the faculty by which movements are properly grouped for the performance of acts requiring special adjustments. adj., **synerget′ic, syner′gic synergis′tic.**

synesthesia (sin″es-the′zhah) a secondary sensation accompanying an actual perception; the experiencing of a sensation in one place, due to stimulation applied to another place; also, the condition in which a stimulus of one sense is perceived as sensation of a different sense, as when a sound produces a sensation of color.

synesthesialgia (sin″es-the″ze-al′jah) a condition in which a stimulus produces pain on the affected side but no sensation on the normal side of the body.

syngamy (sing′gah-me) a method of reproduction in which two individuals (gametes) unite permanently and their nuclei fuse; sexual reproduction.

syngeneic (sin″jĕ-ne′ik) in transplantation biology, denoting individuals or tissues having identical genotypes, i.e., identical twins or animals of the same inbred strain or their tissues. Called also isogeneic and isologous.

syngenesis (sin-jen′ĕ-sis) 1. the origin of an individual from a germ derived from both parents, as occurs in nearly all higher animals, and not from just one alone. 2. the state of having descended from a common ancestor.

syngraft (sin′graft) a graft between genetically identical individuals, such as identical twins or animals of a single highly inbred strain. Called also isogeneic graft, syngeneic graft, and isograft.

synkaryon (sin-kar′e-on) a nucleus formed by fusion of two pronuclei, the fertilization nucleus.

synkinesis (sin″ki-ne′sis) an associated movement; an unintentional movement accompanying a volitional movement. adj., **synkinet′ic.**

synnecrosis (sin″nĕ-kro′sis) symbiosis in which the relationship between populations (or individuals) is mutually detrimental.

synophthalmus (sin″of-thal′mus) cyclops.

synorchidism (sin-or′kĭ-dizm) 1. synorchism. 2. congenital fusion of the testes into one mass.

synorchism (sin′or-kizm) synorchidism.

synoscheos (sin-os′ke-os) adhesion between the penis and scrotum.

synosteotomy (sin″os-te-ot′ah-me) dissection of the joints.

synostosis (sin″os-to′sis) normal or abnormal union of two bones by osseous material. adj., **synostot′ic.**

synotia (sin-o′she-ah) a developmental ANOMALY consisting of fusion of the ears, or their location near the midventral line in the upper part of the neck.

synotus (sĭ-no′tus) a fetus exhibiting synotia.

synovectomy (sin″o-vek′tah-me) excision of a synovial membrane, as of that lining the capsule of the knee joint, sometimes done in patients with rheumatoid arthritis.

radiation s. synoviorthesis.

synovia (sĭ-no′ve-ah) synovial fluid.

synovial (sĭ-no′ve-al) 1. pertaining to a SYNOVIUM (synovial MEMBRANE). 2. pertaining to or secreting SYNOVIA (synovial FLUID).

synovialis (sĭ-no″ve-a′lis) synovial.

synovialoma (sĭ-no″ve-ah-lo′mah) synovioma.

synovioma (sĭ-no″ve-o′mah) a tumor of synovial membrane origin; called also synovialoma.

synoviorthesis (sĭ-no″ve-or-the′sis) irradiation of a synovial MEMBRANE by intra-articular injection of RADIOCOLLOIDS to destroy inflamed tissue.

synovitis (sin″o-vi′tis) inflammation of a synovial MEMBRANE, usually painful, particularly on motion, and characterized by fluctuating swelling, due to effusion in a synovial sac. It may be caused by rheumatic fever, rheumatoid arthritis, tuberculosis, trauma, gout, or other conditions.

dry s. synovitis with little effusion.

purulent s. synovitis with effusion of pus in a synovial sac.

serous s. synovitis with copious nonpurulent effusion.

s. sic′ca dry synovitis.

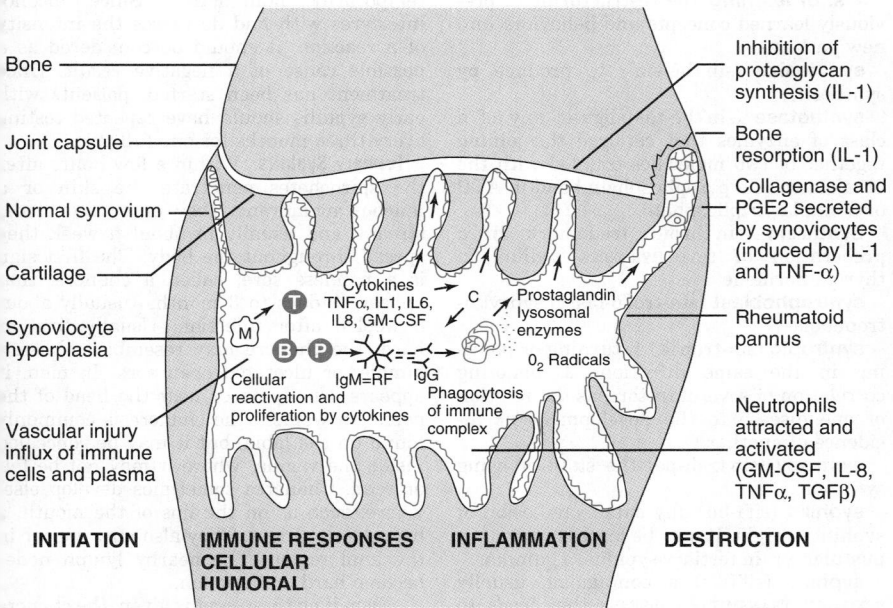

Bone — Joint capsule — Normal synovium — Cartilage — Synoviocyte hyperplasia — Vascular injury influx of immune cells and plasma

Inhibition of proteoglycan synthesis (IL-1)
Bone resorption (IL-1)
Collagenase and PGE2 secreted by synoviocytes (induced by IL-1 and TNF-α)
Rheumatoid pannus
Neutrophils attracted and activated (GM-CSF, IL-8, TNFα, TGFβ)

Cytokines TNFα, IL1, IL6, IL8, GM-CSF
Prostaglandin lysosomal enzymes
O₂ Radicals
Cellular reactivation and proliferation by cytokines
IgM=RF IgG
Phagocytosis of immune complex

INITIATION **IMMUNE RESPONSES CELLULAR HUMORAL** **INFLAMMATION** **DESTRUCTION**

Events involved in the pathogenesis of rheumatoid synovitis progress from left to right. M = macrophage; T = T lymphocyte; B = B lymphocyte; P = plasma cell; IL = interleukin; TNF-α = tumor necrosis factor α; TGF-β = transforming growth factor β; GM-CSF = granulocyte-macrophage colony-stimulating factor; RF = rheumatoid factor; PGE₂ = prostaglandin E₂; C = complement. From Goldman and Bennett, 2000.

S

simple s. synovitis with clear or slightly turbid effusion.

tendinous s. inflammation of a tendon sheath.

villonodular s. proliferation of synovial tissue, especially of the knee joint, composed of synovial villi and fibrous nodules infiltrated by giant cells and macrophages.

synovium (sĭ-no've-um) synovial MEMBRANE.

synpolydactyly (sin-pol″e-dak'tĭ-le) polysyndactyly.

synteny (sin'tĕ-ne) the presence together on the same chromosome of two or more gene loci whether or not in such proximity that they may be subject to linkage. adj., **synten'ic.**

synthase (sin'thās) any enzyme, especially a lyase, which catalyzes a synthesis that does not involve the breakdown of a pyrophosphate bond, as opposed to LIGASE.

synthesis (sin'thĕ-sis) 1. the creation of an integrated whole by the combining of simpler parts or entities. 2. the formation of a chemical compound by the union of its elements or from other suitable components. 3. in psychiatry, the integration of the various elements of the personality. adj., **synthet'ic.**

s. of learning the restructuring of previously learned concepts and behaviors into new patterns.

synthesize (sin'thĕ-sīz″) to produce by synthesis.

synthetase (sin'thĕ-tās) ligase; any of a class of enzymes that catalyze the joining together of two molecules coupled with the breakdown of a pyrophosphate bond in ATP or a similar triphosphate.

Synthroid (sin'throid) trademark for a preparation of LEVOTHYROXINE sodium, a thyroid hormone.

syntrophoblast (sin-trof'o-blast) syncytiotrophoblast.

syntropic (sin-trop'ik) 1. turning or pointing in the same direction. 2. denoting correlation of several factors, as the relation of one disease to the development or incidence of another.

syntropy (sin'trah-pe) the state of being syntropic.

syphilid (sif'ĭ-lid) any cutaneous lesion of syphilitic origin. It may be macular, papular, pustular, or, in tertiary syphilis, a gumma.

syphilis (sif'ĭ-lis) a contagious, usually SEXUALLY TRANSMITTED DISEASE that leads to many structural and cutaneous lesions and is caused by a spirochete, *Treponema pallidum*. A congenital type can be acquired by a fetus in utero from the mother.

Diagnosis. Testing for syphilis is usuall by a SEROLOGIC TEST FOR SYPHILIS, of whic there are two types: (1) the NONTREPONEMA ANTIGEN TESTS detect antibodies to substanc (reagin) derived from host tissues; the originated with the WASSERMANN TEST an are now represented by the VDRL and RAP PLASMA REAGIN TESTS; (2) the TREPONEMA ANTIGEN TESTS detect specific antitreponema antibodies; they originated with the *Trep nema pallidum* immobilization test an are now represented by tests such as th microhemagglutination assay–T. *pallidur* (MHA-TP), and assays using enzyme-linke immunosorbent assay (ELISA) method The term "serologic tests for syphilis" i occasionally used with reference only t nontreponemal antigen tests.

A positive test for syphilis should b repeated. A false positive result can be du to other diseases such as malaria, leprosy and advanced pulmonary tuberculosis, an therefore should not be ignored. A fals negative serological test can occur when th infection is too recent to have triggered th production of antibodies. A negative resul can also occur if the disease is late sympto matic syphilis or if the patient's immun system is not functioning normally. If treat ment of syphilis had been started befor the test, the patient's blood could b temporarily nonreactive. Since alcoho interferes with and decreases the intensit of a reaction, it should be considered as possible cause of a negative result. Onc treatment has been started, patients wit early syphilis should have repeated testin every three months for one full year.

Primary Syphilis. Within a few hours afte the spirochetes penetrate the skin or mucous membrane, they enter the blood stream, and usually in about a week the spread throughout the body. The first sig is a painless sore, called a chancre, tha appears 9 days to 3 months (usually abou 3 weeks) after infection. Usually firm o hard, the chancre may resemble a blister pimple, or ulcerated open sore. In men, i appears usually on or near the head of th penis. In women, the chancre is commonl found on the labia, but it may be conceale inside the vagina, where it may not be fel or seen. Chancres sometimes develop else where, such as on the lips of the mouth, breast, or a finger. They also may appear i the anal region. The nearby lymph node become hard and swollen.

Even if no treatment is given, the chancr will disappear in 10 to 40 days, often leadin to the false conclusion that the disease i cured. Occasionally a chancre fails to develop or is too small to be noticed. Primary syphili can be cured with antibiotics in adequate doses. (See Atlas 2, Part P.)

Secondary Syphilis. Two to six months after the primary sore disappears, the secondary stage of syphilis begins; it may last up to 2 years. A rash is usually one of the first symptoms. It may cover any part of the body and often spreads over the entire skin surface, including the palms and soles. It does not itch and may resemble the rash of measles as well as of many other diseases. It can be identified positively as a symptom of syphilis only by a blood test. During secondary syphilis, thin white sores may appear on the mucosa of the mouth and throat and around the genitalia and rectum. Headache, fever, and a general feeling of illness are common. Hair may fall out in patches, bones and joints may be painful, and anemia may develop. Sometimes the eyes are affected. Syphilis is highly contagious in this stage and of great danger to others. If mouth sores are present, the disease may be spread by kissing.

Like primary syphilis, the secondary stage disappears by itself, generally within 3 to 12 weeks, but may return later if the organisms are still present. As in the primary stage, the disease can be cured in the secondary stage by the use of penicillin and other antibiotics. Together, the primary and secondary stages are known as *early syphilis.*

Tertiary Syphilis. The third, or tertiary, stage of the disease is also known as *late syphilis.* Its symptoms may develop soon after the secondary symptoms have vanished or they may lie hidden for 15 or more years. A person may be unaware that the disease is present. Even a blood test may be negative.

Late syphilis is less contagious to others but is extremely dangerous to the person who has it. It may be fatal, particularly if the central nervous system or heart is affected. The spirochete can invade any cell of the body and can damage any organ or structure of the body, including the internal organs, bones, joints, and skin. The characteristic lesion of tertiary syphilis is a soft gummy tumor called a gumma.

If late syphilis attacks the heart, aorta, or aortic valve, death may result from rupture of the weakened aorta or from heart failure. When it attacks the central nervous system, general paresis, a severe disease of the brain, may result; if not treated promptly, it will cause insanity and death. Another serious disorder of the nervous system caused by late syphilis is TABES DORSALIS, in which there is pain and loss of position sense. Blindness may result if the infection involves the eyes. Other possible effects are deep ulcers on the legs

or elsewhere, chronic inflammation of the bones, which is especially painful at night, and perforation of the soft palate.

Cure of late or tertiary syphilis takes longer and is more difficult than that of primary or secondary syphilis. Sometimes the disease cannot be completely cured. As with early syphilis, however, it may be successfully treated with penicillin and other antibiotics.

Congenital Syphilis. Congenital syphilis is transmitted from a diseased mother to her unborn child through the placenta; this often results in spontaneous abortion or stillbirth. Infants with congenital syphilis who are born alive may have a nasal discharge called SNUFFLES, caused by inflammation of the nose, and may be generally weak and sickly. Syphilitic rashes, especially in the genital area, may occur when the baby is 3 to 8 weeks old. Many are born with deformities or later develop any of a wide variety of impairments and disabilities.

To prevent congenital syphilis all pregnant women should have a blood test for syphilis during the early months of pregnancy. Treatment before the fifth month will always prevent infection of the unborn child. A syphilitic mother who is not treated early has only one chance in six of having a healthy child. If a child is born with syphilis, immediate treatment may be effective if the disease has not progressed too far.

Prevention. The skin lesions associated with primary and secondary syphilis can be highly contagious. The Centers for Disease Control and Prevention recommends standard PRECAUTIONS when caring for a patient with syphilis.

    endemic s. nonvenereal syphilis.

    late benign s. a form of tertiary syphilis that responds very rapidly to treatment and is therefore relatively benign, in which the typical lesion is the GUMMA.

    nonvenereal s. a chronic treponemal infection mainly seen in children, occurring in many areas of the world, caused by an organism indistinguishable from *Treponema pallidum,* and transmitted directly by nonsexual contact and indirectly by common use of table and drinking utensils. The first lesions are usually oral mucous patches; subsequent lesions are concentrated in the axillae, inguinal region, and rectum. Then, after a latent period, there develop destructive lesions of the skin and bones. Researchers have hypothesized that venereal syphilis mutated from one of the nonvenereal forms.

    syphilitic (sif′ĭ-lit′ik) affected with, caused by, or pertaining to syphilis.

S

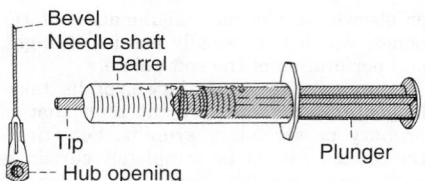

Components of a syringe. Shading indicates areas that must be kept sterile before and during parenteral injections. From Bolander, 1994.

syphiloma (sif″ĭ-lo′mah) gumma.

syring(o)- word element [Gr.], *tube; fistula.*

syringe (sir′inj, sĭ-rinj′) an instrument for introducing fluids into or withdrawing them from the body.

    Asepto s. a syringe designed to fit directly into large lumen tubing; also used for intraoperative irrigation.

    bulb s. a syringe with a bulb on one end; compression of the bulb creates a vacuum for gentle suction of small amounts of bodily drainage, such as oral and nasal secretions. It is also used for intraoperative irrigation.

    hypodermic s. one for introduction of liquids through a hollow needle into subcutaneous tissues.

syringitis (sir″in-ji′tis) inflammation of the eustachian tube.

syringoadenoma (sĭ-ring″go-ad″ĕ-no′-mah) syringocystadenoma.

syringobulbia (sĭ-ring″go-bul′be-ah) SYRIN-GOMYELIA in which the cavity extends to involve the medulla oblongata.

syringocarcinoma (sĭ-ring″go-kahr″sĭ-no′-mah) cancer of a sweat gland.

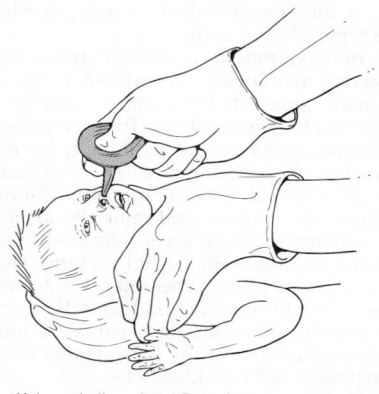

Using a bulb syringe. From Lammon et al., 1995.

syringocele (sĭ-ring′go-sēl) a cavity containing herniation of the spinal cord through the bony defect in spina bifida.

syringocoele (sĭ-ring′go-sēl) the central canal of the spinal cord.

syringocystadenoma (sĭ-ring″go-sist″ad-ĕ-no′mah) adenoma of the sweat glands; called also hidradenoma.

syringocystoma (sĭ-ring″go-sis-to′mah) a cystic tumor of a sweat gland.

syringoma (sir″ing-go′mah) 1. a benign tumor believed to originate from the ductal portion of the eccrine sweat glands, occurring as multiple small flesh-colored papules on the face, neck, upper chest, and sometimes the vulva, usually in postpubertal women, characterized by dilated cystic sweat ducts in a fibrous stroma. (See Atlas 2, Part A.) 2. syringocystadenoma.

syringomeningocele (sĭ-ring″go-sĭ-ning′go-sēl) meningocele resembling syringomyelocele.

syringomyelia (sĭ-ring″go-mi-e′le-ah) a slowly progressive syndrome in which cavitation occurs in the central (usually cervical) segments of the spinal cord; the lesion may extend up into the medulla oblongata (SYRINGOBULBIA) or down into the thoracic region. It may be of developmental origin, arise secondary to tumor, trauma, infarction, or hemorrhage, or be without known cause. It results in neurological deficits that generally consist of segmental muscular weakness and atrophy accompanied by a dissociated sensory loss (loss of pain and temperature sensation, with preservation of the sense of touch), and thoracic scoliosis is often present. Called also cystic myelopathy and Morvan's syndrome.

syrinx (sir′inks) a tube or pipe; a fistula.

syrup (sir′up) a viscous concentrated solution of a sugar, such as sucrose, in water or other aqueous liquid; combined with other ingredients, such a solution is used as a flavored vehicle for medications. In common usage, the term is often expanded to include any oral dosage form (for example, an oral suspension) in a sweet and viscous vehicle.

systaltic (sis-tal′tik) alternately contracting and dilating; pulsating.

system (sis′tem) 1. a set or series of interconnected or interdependent parts or entities (objects, organs, or organisms) that act together in a common purpose or produce results impossible by action of one alone. (See accompanying illustration.) 2. an organized set of principles or ideas. adj. **systemat′ic, system′ic.** The parts of a system can be referred to as its elements or components; the environment of the system is defined as all of the factors that affect the system and are affected by it. A living system is capable of taking in matter, energy, and information from its environment (input), processing them in some way, and returning matter, energy, and information to its environment as output.

An *open* system is one in which there is an exchange of matter, energy, and information with the environment; in a *closed* system there is no such exchange. A living system cannot survive without this exchange, but in order to survive it must maintain pattern and organization in the midst of constant change. Control of self-regulation of an open system is achieved by dynamic interactions among its elements or components. The result of self-regulation is referred to as the steady state; that is, a state of equilibrium. HOMEOSTASIS is an assemblage of organic regulations that act to maintain steady states of a living organism.

A system can be divided hierarchically into subsystems, which can be further subdivided into sub-subsystems and components. A system and its environment could be considered as a unified whole for purposes of study, or a subsystem could be studied as a system. For example, the collection of glands in the endocrine system can be thought of as a system, each endocrine gland could be viewed as a system, or even specific cells of a single gland could be studied as a system. It is also possible to think of the human body as a living system and the endocrine system as a subsystem.

The division of a system into a subsystem and its environment is dependent on the perspective chosen by the person studying a particular phenomenon.

alimentary s. digestive system.

apothecaries' s. see APOTHECARIES' SYSTEM.

autonomic nervous s. see AUTONOMIC NERVOUS SYSTEM.

avoirdupois s. see AVOIRDUPOIS SYSTEM.

behavioral s. in the BEHAVIORAL SYSTEM MODEL of nursing, the patterned, repetitive, and purposeful behaviors of an individual.

cardiovascular s. the heart and blood vessels, by which blood is pumped and circulated through the body; see also CIRCULATORY SYSTEM.

CD s. [cluster *d*esignation] a system for classifying cell-surface MARKERS expressed by lymphocytes based on a computer analysis of monoclonal ANTIBODIES against HLA ANTIGENS, with antibodies having similar specificity characteristics being grouped together and assigned a number (CD1, CD2, CD3, etc.); these CD numbers are also applied to the specific antigens recognized by the various groups of monoclonal antibodies. See also CD ANTIGEN.

centimeter-gram-second s. (CGS) (cgs) a system of measurements in which the units are based on the centimeter as the unit of length, the gram as the unit of mass, and the second as the unit of time.

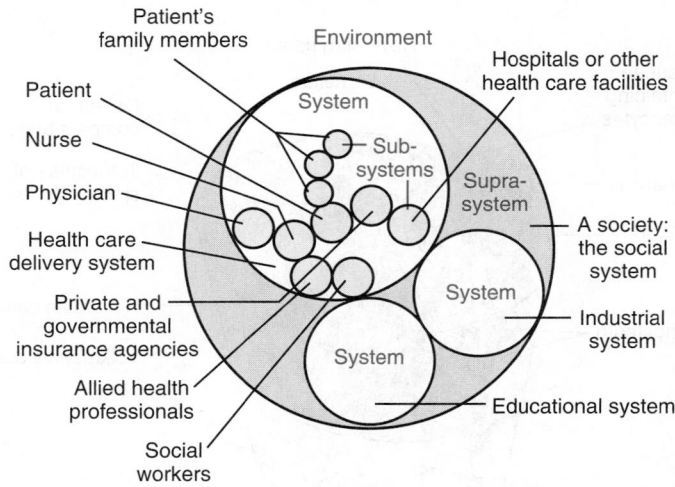

Systems, subsystems, and suprasystems. Within the environment there are suprasystems, such as human society, and systems within the suprasystem, such as the educational and industrial systems and the health care delivery system. Within the health care delivery system are subsystems, such as the patient, family members, the nurse, the physician, and allied health care professionals and paraprofessionals.

central nervous s. see CENTRAL NERVOUS SYSTEM.

centrencephalic s. the neurons in the central core of the BRAINSTEM from the thalamus to the medulla oblongata, connecting the cerebral HEMISPHERES.

circulatory s. see CIRCULATORY SYSTEM.

client s. in the GENERAL SYSTEMS FRAMEWORK AND THEORY OF GOAL ATTAINMENT, the composite of physiological, psychological, sociocultural, and developmental variables that make up the total person.

colloid s., colloidal s. colloid (def. 3).

conduction s., conductive s. (of heart) the system of atypical cardiac muscle fibers, comprising the sinoatrial and atrioventricular nodes, internodal tracts, atrioventricular bundle, bundle branch, and terminal ramifications into the Purkinje network.

digestive s. see DIGESTIVE SYSTEM.

Emergency Medical Services (EMS) s. a comprehensive program designed to provide services to the patient in the prehospital setting. The system is activated when a call is made to the EMS operator, who then dispatches an ambulance to the patient. The patient receives critical interventions and is stabilized at the scene. A communication system allows the health care workers at the scene to contact a trauma center for information regarding further treatment and disposition of the patient, followed by transportation of the patient to the most appropriate facility for treatment.

endocrine s. the system of ductless glands and other structures that produce internal secretions (HORMONES) that are released directly into the circulatory system, influencing metabolism and other body processes; see ENDOCRINE GLANDS.

environmental control s. environmental control UNIT.

expert s. a set of computer programs designed to serve as an aid in decision making.

extrapyramidal s. see EXTRAPYRAMIDAL SYSTEM.

gateway s. a software interface between an online searcher and one or more search systems, facilitating the use of the system by searchers who are unfamiliar with it, or with online retrieval in general.

genitourinary s. the organs concerned with production and excretion of urine, together with the REPRODUCTIVE ORGANS. (See Plates.) Called also urogenital system.

haversian s. a haversian CANAL and its concentrically arranged lamellae, constituting the basic unit of structure in compact bone (OSTEON). (See illustration.)

health care s. see HEALTH CARE SYSTEM.

heterogeneous s. a system or structure made up of mechanically separable parts, as an emulsion or suspension.

His-Purkinje s. the intraventricular conduction system from the bundle of His to the distal Purkinje fibers, which carries the impulse to the ventricles.

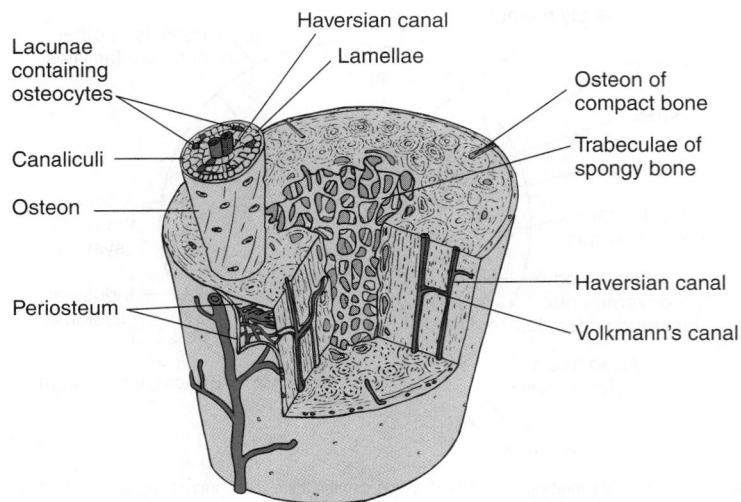

Haversian system: Structures of compact and spongy bone with the central haversian canal surrounded by the lamellae. From Applegate, 2000.

see HOME HEALTH CARE CLASSIFICATION SYSTEM.

homogeneous s. a system or structure made up of parts that cannot be mechanically separated, as a solution.

hypophyseoportal s., hypophysioportal s. , hypothalamo-hypophysial portal s. the venules connecting the HYPOTHALAMUS with the sinusoidal capillaries of the anterior lobe of the PITUITARY GLAND; they carry releasing substances to the pituitary.

immune s. see IMMUNE SYSTEM.

interpersonal s. in the GENERAL SYSTEMS FRAMEWORK AND THEORY OF GOAL ATTAINMENT, two or more individuals interacting in a given situation.

lay health s. a system comprising an informal referral network and sources of treatment outside the formal biomedical sources of health care; it includes individual consultation and information-seeking through significant others and peers concerning health behaviors, symptoms, and evaluation of treatment before, during, and after consultation with health care professionals.

limbic s. a system of brain structures common to the brains of all mammals, comprising the phylogenetically old cortex (archipallium and paleopallium) and its primarily related nuclei. It is associated with olfaction, autonomic functions, and certain aspects of emotion and behavior.

lymphatic s. see LYMPHATIC SYSTEM.

lymphoid s. the lymphoid tissue of the body, collectively; it consists of primary (or central) lymphoid tissues, the bone marrow, and thymus, and secondary (or peripheral) tissues, the lymph nodes, spleen, and gut-associated lymphoid tissue (tonsils, Peyer's patches).

lymphoreticular s. the lymphoid and reticuloendothelial systems considered together; see also LYMPHORETICULAR DISORDERS.

metric s. see METRIC SYSTEM.

mononuclear phagocyte s. the group of highly phagocytic cells that have a common origin from stem cells of the bone marrow and develop circulating monocytes and tissue macrophages, which develop from monocytes that have migrated to connective tissue of the liver (KUPFFER'S CELLS), lung, spleen, and lymph nodes. The term has been proposed to replace RETICULOENDOTHELIAL SYSTEM, which includes some cells of different origin and does not include all macrophages.

nervous s. see NERVOUS SYSTEM.

nursing s. in the SELF-CARE MODEL of nursing, all the actions and interactions of nurses and patients in nursing practice situations; nursing systems fall into three categories: wholly compensatory, partly compensatory, and supportive-educative.

Omaha S. see OMAHA SYSTEM.

oxygen delivery s. a device that delivers oxygen through the upper airways to the lungs at concentrations above that of ambient air. There are two general types: the *fixed performance* or *high flow* type, which can supply all of the needs of a patient for inspired gas at a given fractional inspired oxygen; and the *variable performance* or *low flow* type, which cannot supply all of the patient's needs for oxygen and delivers fractional inspired oxygen that varies with ventilatory demand.

parasympathetic nervous s. see PARASYMPATHETIC NERVOUS SYSTEM.

peripheral nervous s. the portion of the NERVOUS SYSTEM consisting of the nerves and ganglia outside the brain and spinal cord.

personal s. in the GENERAL SYSTEMS FRAMEWORK AND THEORY OF GOAL ATTAINMENT, the unified self, a complex whole that is rational, conscious, and feeling and that sets goals and decides on the means of achieving them.

pituitary portal s. hypothalamo-hypophysial portal system.

portal s. an arrangement by which blood collected from one set of capillaries passes through a large vessel or vessels and another set of capillaries before returning to the systemic circulation, as in the pituitary gland (the hypothalamo-hypophysial portal system) or the liver (the hepatic portal circulation).

renin-angiotensin-aldosterone s. see RENIN-ANGIOTENSIN-ALDOSTERONE SYSTEM.

respiratory s. the group of specialized organs whose specific function is to provide for the transfer of oxygen from the air to the blood and of waste carbon dioxide from the blood to the air. The organs of the system include the NOSE, the PHARYNX, the LARYNX, the TRACHEA, the BRONCHI, and the LUNGS. See also RESPIRATION and Plates 7 and 8.

reticular activating s. see RETICULAR ACTIVATING SYSTEM.

reticuloendothelial s. see RETICULOENDOTHELIAL SYSTEM.

safety s. see SAFETY SYSTEM.

SI s. see SI UNITS.

skeletal s. see SKELETAL SYSTEM.

social s. in the GENERAL SYSTEMS FRAMEWORK AND THEORY OF GOAL ATTAINMENT, an organized boundary system of social roles, behaviors, and practices developed to maintain balance for growth, development, and performance, which involves an exchange of energy and information between the person and the environment for regulation and control of stressors.

sympathetic nervous s. see SYMPATHETIC NERVOUS SYSTEM.

Unified Medical Language S. see UNIFIED MEDICAL LANGUAGE SYSTEM.

Unified Nursing Language S. see UNIFIED NURSING LANGUAGE SYSTEM.

unit dose s. a method of delivery of patient medications directly to the patient care unit. Following review by a nurse, a copy of the physician's original order is sent to the pharmacy, where the pharmacist reviews it again. The pharmacist then fills the order and delivers the medication to the patient care unit, usually in a 24-hour supply. Each patient has an individual supply of medications prepared and labeled by the pharmacist.

urinary s. the system formed in the body by the KIDNEYS, URETERS, urinary BLADDER, and URETHRA, the organs concerned in the production and excretion of URINE.

urogenital s. genitourinary system.

vascular s. circulatory system.

vasomotor s. the part of the nervous system that controls the caliber of the blood vessels.

systema (sis-te′mah) [Gr.] system.

systemic (sis-tem′ik) pertaining to or affecting the body as a whole.

s. disease one affecting a number of tissues that perform a common function.

systole (sis′to-le) the contraction, or period of contraction, of the heart, especially of the ventricles, during which blood is forced into the aorta and pulmonary artery. adj., **systol′ic.**

atrial s. contraction of the atria by which blood is forced into the ventricles; it precedes the true or ventricular systole and is indicated by the fourth heart sound.

extra s. see EXTRASYSTOLE.

ventricular s. contraction of the ventricles, forcing blood into the aorta and pulmonary artery.

systremma (sis-trem′ah) a cramp in the muscles of the lower leg.

T

T tera-; tesla; tetanus toxoid; thoracic vertebrae (T1–T12); intraocular tension (see under *pressure.*)

T absolute temperature.

T$_{1/2}$ half-life; half-time.

T$_3$ triiodothyronine.

T$_4$ thyroxine.

T$_m$ transport (or tubular) maximum.

2,4,5-T 2,4,5-trichlorophenoxyacetic acid, a toxic HERBICIDE; it is a component of AGENT ORANGE.

t in genetics, symbol for translocation.

t$_{1/2}$ half-life; half-time.

TA toxin-antitoxin.

Ta tantalum.

TAB a vaccine prepared from killed typhoid, paratyphoid A and paratyphoid B bacilli.

tabacosis (tab″ah-ko′sis) poisoning by TOBACCO, chiefly by inhalation of tobacco dust (a form of PNEUMOCONIOSIS).

tabanid (tab′ah-nid) a biting insect of the family Tabanidae, including the horseflies and deerflies.

Tabanus (tah-ba′nus) a genus of biting, bloodsucking horseflies that transmit trypanosomes and anthrax to various animals.

tabardillo (tah″bar-dēl′yo) murine TYPHUS.

tabes (ta′bēz) 1. WASTING of the body or a part of it. 2. tabes dorsalis. adj., **tabet′ic.**

t. dorsa′lis a slowly progressive nervous disorder, from degeneration of the dorsal columns of the spinal cord and sensory nerve trunks, resulting in disturbances of sensation and interference with reflexes and consequently with movements; called also locomotor ataxia. It is caused by SYPHILIS and may appear 5 to 20 years after initial infection. Its course is slow but progressive; it can often be arrested, but complete cure is rare. The first symptoms are pain in the lower limbs, upper limbs, or trunk, loss of posture SENSE, and Argyll Robertson PUPILS (pupils that are uneven and do not react to light). Unless the patient looks down at his legs he does not know where they are and must depend on his vision for each step. The typical gait of a tabetic patient is jerky and wide-based.

t. mesente′rica tuberculosis of the mesenteric glands in children.

tabescent (tah-bes′ent) wasting away; see WASTING.

tabetiform (tah-bet′ĭ-form) resembling tabes.

tablature (tab′lah-chur) separation of the chief cranial bones into inner and outer tables, separated by a diploë.

table (ta′b'l) a flat layer or surface.

cohort life t. a life table giving the survival data of a cohort of individuals in a clinical study or trial, i.e., the number alive and under observation (not lost to follow-up) at the beginning of each year, the number dying in each year, the number lost to follow-up each year, the conditional probability of survival for each year, and the cumulative probabilities of survival from the beginning of the study to the end of each year.

inner t. the inner compact layer of the bones covering the brain.

life t. any of various tables describing mortality and survival data for groups of individuals at specific times or over defined intervals; tables may summarize combined mortality experience by age over a brief period or may follow a COHORT over time (cohort life TABLE).

outer t. the outer compact layer of the bones covering the brain.

tilt t. a plinth, equipped with a footboard for support, to which a patient can be strapped for rotation to a nearly upright position; used in cases of spinal cord injury and other neurological disorders to enhance blood circulation to the lower limbs, improve posture, and aid in muscle training and sense of balance.

vitreous t. inner table.

tablespoon (ta′b'l-spoon) a household unit of volume or capacity, equivalent to three teaspoons or approximately 15 milliliters.

tablet (tab′let) a solid dosage form containing a medicinal substance with or without a suitable diluent. Called also pill.

buccal t. one which dissolves when it is held between the cheek and gum, permitting direct absorption of the active ingredient through the oral mucosa.

enteric-coated t. one coated with material that delays release of the medication until after it leaves the stomach.

sublingual t. one that dissolves when held beneath the tongue, permitting direct absorption of the active ingredient by the oral mucosa.

taboo (tah-boo′) 1. any of the negative traditions, objects, or behaviors generally regarded as harmful to social welfare and therefore prohibited. 2. excluded from use; prohibited.

taboparesis (ta″bo-pah-re′sis) tabes with general paresis.

tabular (tab′u-lar) resembling a table.

TACE (tās) trademark for preparations of CHLOROTRIANISENE, a synthetic ESTROGEN used for palliative treatment of prostate cancer and for replacement THERAPY.

tache (tahsh) [Fr.] a SPOT or blemish.

t. blanche ("white spot"), a white spot on the liver in certain infectious diseases.

t's bleuâtres ("bluish spots"), maculae caeruleae.

t. cérébrale ("cerebral spot"), a congested streak produced by drawing the nail across the skin; a concomitant of various nervous or cerebral diseases.

t. motrice ("motor spot"), a motor nerve ending in which the nerve fibril passes to a muscle cell, where it ends in a slight enlargement.

t. noire ("black spot"), an ulcer covered with a black crust, a characteristic local reaction at the presumed site of the infective bite in certain tickborne rickettsioses.

tachogram (tak′o-gram) the graphic record produced by tachography.

tachography (tah-kog′rah-fe) the recording of the movement and speed of the blood current.

tachy- word element [Gr.], *rapid; swift.*

tachyarrhythmia (tak″e-ah-rith′me-ah) TACHYCARDIA associated with ARRHYTHMIA. It may be either supraventricular, such as atrial TACHYCARDIA, atrial FLUTTER, or atrial FIBRILLATION, or ventricular, such as ventricular TACHYCARDIA or ventricular FIBRILLATION.

tachycardia (tak″e-kahr′de-ah) abnormally rapid heart rate, usually taken to be over 100 beats per minute. adj **tachycar′diac.**

antidromic circus movement t. a supraventricular tachycardia supported by a reentry CIRCUIT that uses the atrioventricular node in the retrograde direction and an accessory PATHWAY in the anterograde direction; this produces a broad QRS rhythm indistinguishable from ventricular tachycardia. Such a tachycardia may also use two accessory PATHWAYS (one anterograde and one retrograde) and not involve the AV node at all.

atrial t. a rapid heart rate, between 140 and 250 beats per minute, with the ectopic focus in the atria and with no participation by the atrioventricular node or the sinoatrial node. It is recognizable on the electrocardiogram because the P wave precedes the QRS complex, as opposed to being merged with it or following it. This condition is usually associated with atrioventricular BLOCK or DIGITALIS toxicity.

benign ventricular t. tachycardia originating in the ventricles, not associated with structural heart disease or significant hemodynamic symptoms.

bidirectional ventricular t., bifascicular ventricular t. a ventricular arrhythmia characterized by heart rates of 90 to 160 beats per minute, alternating right and left axis DEVIATION, ectopic focus that alternates between the anterior superior and posterior inferior fascicles, and a right bundle branch block pattern in lead V_1; seen in DIGITALIS toxicity and other conditions.

chaotic atrial t. an ectopic atrial tachycardia due to multifocal activity, characterized by at least three different shapes of P

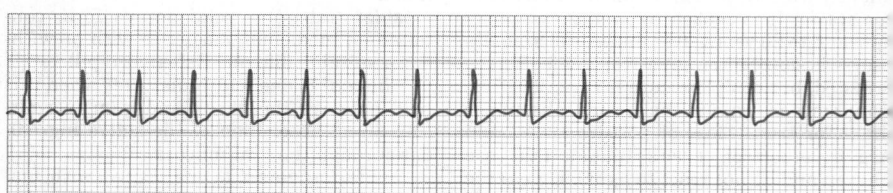

Sinus tachycardia

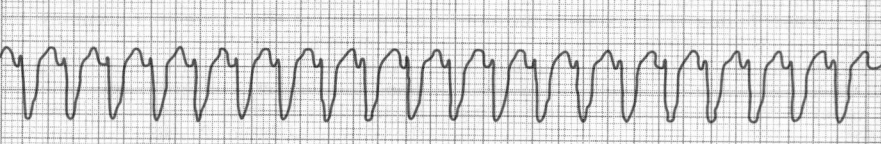

Ventricular tachycardia

A, Sinus tachycardia; *B,* Ventricular tachycardia. From Chernecky, 2001.

waves on the electrocardiogram; often associated with CHRONIC OBSTRUCTIVE LUNG DISEASE.

circus movement t. (CMT) a reentry CIRCUIT that uses an accessory PATHWAY or pathways; there are two subtypes, *antidromic* and *orthodromic circus movement tachycardia*.

ectopic t. rapid heart action in response to impulses arising outside the sinoatrial node.

junctional t. rhythm at the rate of 100 to 140 beats per minute that arises in response to impulses originating in the atrioventricular junction, i.e., the atrioventricular node. It is often seen with DIGITALIS toxicity and is due to triggered activity, but it may also be due to altered AUTOMATICITY. In the case of digitalis toxicity, the term may be used to encompass the entire span of junctional rates with this condition, i.e., approximately 70 to 140 beats per minute.

monomorphic ventricular t. a type that has a uniform beat-to-beat QRS morphology.

nonsustained ventricular t. a type that terminates spontaneously within 30 seconds and does not lead to hemodynamic collapse.

orthodromic circus movement t. a supraventricular tachycardia supported by a reentry CIRCUIT that uses the atrioventricular node in the anterograde direction and an accessory PATHWAY in the retrograde direction, producing a narrow QRS complex.

orthostatic t. disproportionate rapidity of the heart rate on arising from a reclining to a standing position.

paroxysmal t. rapid heart action that starts and stops abruptly.

paroxysmal atrial t. paroxysmal supraventricular tachycardia.

paroxysmal supraventricular t. (PSVT) a narrow QRS tachycardia that begins and ends abruptly; it may be terminated with a vagal maneuver. It has two common mechanisms, atrioventricular nodal reentry and circus MOVEMENT that uses the atrioventricular node anterogradely and an accessory PATHWAY retrogradely. On the electrocardiogram it is characterized by abrupt onset, and mechanisms are differentiated by the relation of the P wave to the QRS complex.

polymorphic ventricular t. a type that has a constantly, and sometimes subtly, changing beat-to-beat QRS configuration.

potentially malignant ventricular t. a type that is not associated with structural heart disease or hemodynamically important cardiac symptoms but is sometimes associated with left ventricular dysfunction.

sinus t. (ST) a rapid rhythm originating in the sinoatrial node with a rate of usually

100 to 160 beats per minute; conduction through the ventricles is normal. During exercise or stress this is normal, but if it occurs during rest it is abnormal.

supraventricular t. a combination of junctional tachycardia and atrial tachycardia.

sustained ventricular t. tachycardia that lasts more than 30 seconds and leads to hemodynamic collapse.

ventricular t. an abnormally rapid ventricular rhythm with aberrant ventricular excitation, characterized by at least three consecutive ventricular COMPLEXES of more than 100 beats per minute. It is generated within the ventricle and is most often associated with atrioventricular DISSOCIATION.

tachydysrhythmia an abnormal heart rhythm with rate greater than 100 beats per minute in an adult; the term TACHYARRHYTHMIA is usually used instead.

tachylalia (tak″e-la′le-ah) logorrhea.

tachymeter (tah-kim′ĕ-ter) an instrument for measuring rapidity of motion.

tachyphagia (tak″e-fa′jah) rapid eating.

tachyphasia (tak″e-fa′zhah) logorrhea.

tachypnea (tak″ip-ne′ah) very rapid respirations, seen especially in high fever when the body attempts to rid itself of excess heat. The rate of respiration increases at a ratio of about eight breaths per minute for every degree Celsius above normal. Other causes include pneumonia, compensatory respiratory alkalosis as the body tries to "blow off" excess carbon dioxide, respiratory insufficiency, lesions in the respiratory control center of the brain, and salicylate poisoning. See also HYPERPNEA and HYPERVENTILATION.

transient t. of the newborn a self-limited elevation of the respiratory rate in newborns due to delayed clearing of fetal lung water.

tachyrhythmia (tak″e-rith′me-ah) tachycardia.

tachysterol (tah-kis′ter-ol) an isomer of ergosterol, an antirachitic substance, produced by irradiation of ergosterol.

tacrine (tak′rēn) a cholinesterase INHIBITOR used to improve cognitive performance in treatment of DEMENTIA OF THE ALZHEIMER TYPE; used as the hydrochloride salt.

tacrolimus (tak″ro-li′mus) an IMMUNOSUPPRESSANT derived from a species of *Streptomyces*, having actions similar to those of CYCLOSPORINE; administered orally or intravenously to prevent rejection of organ transplants and topically to treat moderate to severe atopic dermatitis.

TAC solution a solution of tetracaine, epinephrine, and cocaine, used as a local anesthetic in the emergency treatment of uncomplicated lacerations.

tactile (tak′til) pertaining to touch.

tactometer (tak-tom′ĕ-ter) an instrument for measuring tactile sensibility; esthesiometer.

Taenia (te′ne-ah) a genus of TAPEWORM. See figure at tapeworm.

T. sagina′ta a species 4 to 8 meters long, found in the adult form in the human intestine and in the larval state in muscles and other tissues of cattle and other ruminants; human infection usually results from eating inadequately cooked beef.

T. so′lium a species 2 to 4 meters long, found in the adult intestine of humans; the larval form most often is found in muscle and other tissues of the pig. Human infection results from eating inadequately cooked pork.

taenia (te′ne-ah) 1. a flat band or strip of soft tissue; used in anatomic nomenclature to designate various structures. 2. a tapeworm of the genus *Taenia*. Defs. 1 and 2 called also tenia.

t. co′li any of the three thickened bands (*tae′nia li′bera, tae′nia mesoco′lica, and tae′nia omenta′lis*) formed by longitudinal fibers in the TUNICA MUSCULARIS of the large intestine, extending from the root of the vermiform appendix to the rectum.

taeniacide (te′ne-ah-sīd″) 1. lethal to tapeworms. 2. an agent that kills TAPEWORMS; called also teniacide.

taeniafuge (te′ne-ah-fūj″) an agent that expels TAPEWORMS; called also teniafuge.

taeniasis (te-ni′ah-sis) infection with tapeworms of the genus *Taenia*.

tag (tag) 1. a small appendage, flap, or polyp. 2. label.

radioactive t. radioactive LABEL.

Tagamet (tag′ah-met) trademark for preparations of CIMETIDINE, an antagonist of histamine H$_2$ RECEPTORS used to inhibit gastric acid secretion.

tail (tāl) any slender appendage; called also cauda.

t. of spermatozoon the flagellum of a spermatozoon; it has four regions: the NECK, middle PIECE, principal PIECE, and end PIECE.

Takahara's disease (tah-kah-hah′rahz) a severe form of ACATALASIA occurring in Japan.

Takayasu's disease (tah-kah-yah′sooz) pulseless disease.

talbutal (tal′bu-tal) a BARBITURATE used as a SEDATIVE and HYPNOTIC.

talc (talk) a native hydrous MAGNESIUM SILICATE, sometimes with a small amount of aluminum silicate; used as a dusting powder. The inhalation of talc is associated with a wide variety of respiratory disorders.

talcosis (tal-ko′sis) talc PNEUMOCONIOSIS.

talcum (tal′kum) talc.

talipes (tal′ĭ-pēz) a deformity in which the foot is twisted out of normal position; see also CLUBFOOT and see illustration. It may have an abnormally high longitudinal arch (*talipes cavus*) or it may be in dorsiflexion (*talipes calcaneus*), in plantar flexion (*talipes equinus*), abducted and everted (*talipes valgus* or FLATFOOT), adducted and inverted (*talipes varus*), or various combinations of these (*talipes calcaneovalgus, talipes calcaneovarus, talipes equinovalgus*, or *talipes equinovarus*).

There are several theories as to the cause of clubfoot. A familial tendency or arrested growth during fetal life may contribute to its development, or it may be caused by a defect in the ovum. It sometimes accompanies meningomyelocele as a result of paralysis. In mild clubfoot there are slight changes in the structure of the foot; more severe cases involve orthopedic deformities of both the foot and leg. Although clubfoot is usually congenital, an occasional case in an older child may be caused by injury or poliomyelitis.

Treatment varies according to the severity of the deformity. Milder cases may be corrected with casts that are changed periodically, the foot being manipulated into position each time the cast is changed so

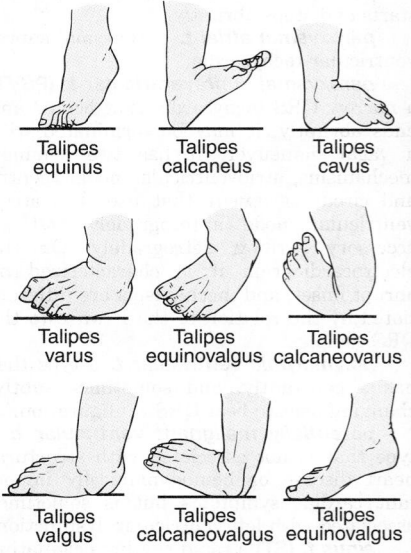

Talipes equinus   Talipes calcaneus   Talipes cavus

Talipes varus   Talipes equinovalgus   Talipes calcaneovarus

Talipes valgus   Talipes calcaneovalgus   Talipes equinovalgus

Talipes.

that it gradually assumes normal position. A specially designed splint may also be used, made of two plates attached to shoes with a crossbar between the plates and special set screws so that the angulation of the foot can be changed as necessary. More severe deformities require surgery of the tendons and bones, followed by the application of a cast to maintain proper position of the joint.

talipomanus (tal″ĭ-pom′ah-nus) clubhand.

talocalcanean (ta″lo-kal-ka′ne-an) pertaining to the talus and calcaneus.

talocrural (ta″lo-krō̄r′al) pertaining to the ankle bone (TALUS) and adjacent long bones of the lower limb.

talofibular (ta″lo-fib′u-lar) pertaining to the talus and fibula.

talonavicular (ta″lo-nah-vik′u-lar) pertaining to the talus and navicular bone.

talus (ta′lus) the ankle bone, highest of the tarsal bones. See anatomic Table of Bones in the Appendices. Called also ankle.

Talwin (tal′win) trademark for preparations containing PENTAZOCINE, an opioid ANALGESIC.

tamoxifen (tah-mok′sĭ-fen) a nonsteroidal oral ANTIESTROGEN used as the citrate salt in the treatment and prophylaxis of breast cancer.

tampon (tam′pon) a pack, pad, or plug made of cotton, sponge, or other material; different types are used to plug the nose, vagina, or other areas for the control of hemorrhage or the absorption of secretions. Superabsorbent tampons worn monthly and inserted roughly can cause ulceration of the vaginal mucosa. Both vaginal and nasal tampons have been implicated in the development of TOXIC SHOCK SYNDROME.

tamponade (tam″po-nād′) 1. surgical use of a TAMPON. 2. pathologic compression of a part.

   cardiac t. compression of the heart due to collection of fluid or blood in the PERICARDIUM. It may be either *chronic* or *acute*. Chronic cardiac tamponade occurs when fluid slowly enters the pericardial sac, allowing time for the membrane's expansion to accommodate the fluid, which can be as much as 1 liter. This gradual filling may or may not produce changes in cardiac hemodynamics. However, if there is rapid filling of the pericardial sac, as little as 200 ml can precipitate a life-threatening emergency. The ultimate effect of cardiac tamponade is reduced cardiac output and inadequate tissue perfusion.

   Causes of acute cardiac tamponade include pericarditis with effusion of serosanguineous fluid into the sac, and either surgical or accidental trauma with leakage of blood into the sac. Occasionally,

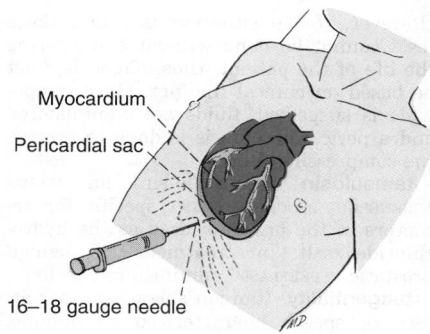

Pericardiocentesis is performed to remove compressing fluid in cardiac tamponade. From Polaski and Tatro, 1996.

anticoagulant therapy can lead to extensive bleeding around the heart and cardiac tamponade.

Excessive fluid within the pericardial sac causes pressure against the cardiac structures, interferes with ventricular and atrial filling, and compromises blood supply to the myocardium via the coronary vessels. These conditions occur because of the following events: The compressed atria cannot fill as they normally would and so less blood is available for the ventricles; thus preload (the volume of blood in the ventricles at the end of diastole) is reduced. Ventricular filling is further impaired by compression of the ventricles. As pressure within the ventricles rises because of tamponade, pressure differences between the atria and ventricles are reduced, causing the valves between the two chambers to close before the ventricles have had time to fill completely. Increasing pressure within the heart chambers and in the pericardium impinges on the coronary arteries and veins, reducing blood supply to the myocardium, slowing contractility, and further reducing cardiac output.

Clinical features of cardiac tamponade include increased central venous pressure, falling arterial blood pressure, tachycardia, faint or muffled heart sounds, a narrowing pulse pressure, and an exaggerated inspiratory fall in systolic blood pressure (pulsus paradoxus). Hypoxia of cerebral tissues can produce confusion, restlessness, agitation, panic, and a sense of impending doom. Peripheral hypoxia is signaled by changes in the color, temperature, and excessive sweating.

Diagnosis can be confirmed by echocardiography and other radiologic studies.

However, if the situation is acute, these tests cannot be done without endangering the life of the patient; thus diagnosis must be based on clinical findings. Once tamponade is suspected, fluids are administered and a pericardiocentesis is done to remove the compressing fluid.

tamsulosin (tam-soo′lo-sin) an ALPHA-ADRENERGIC BLOCKING AGENT specific for receptors in the prostate; used as the hydrochloride salt in treatment of benign prostatic HYPERPLASIA, administered orally.

tangentiality (tan-jen″she-al′ĭ-te) a pattern of speech characterized by oblique, digressive, or irrelevant replies to questions; the responses never approach the point of the questions. It differs from CIRCUMSTANTIALITY, in which the responder eventually reaches the point.

Tangier disease (tan-jēr′) a familial disease characterized by a deficiency of high-density LIPOPROTEINS in the blood serum, with storage of CHOLESTEROL esters in the tonsils and other tissues.

tank (tank) an artificial receptacle for liquids.

   Hubbard t. a tank in which exercises may be performed under water; see also HUBBARD TANK.

tannate (tan′āt) any of the salts of tannic acid, all of which are astringent.

tannic acid (tan′ik) a substance obtained from nutgalls, oak bark, and other plant parts, formerly used in medicine as an astringent. It is no longer used alone because it can be absorbed through mucous membranes or damaged skin in amounts sufficient to produce hepatic necrosis, although it is still used as a component of dermatological preparations.

tannin (tan′in) tannic acid.

tantalum (tan′tah-lum) a chemical element, atomic number 73, atomic weight 180.948, symbol Ta. (See Appendix 6.) It is a noncorrosive and malleable metal used for plates or disks to repair cranial defects, for wire sutures, and for making prosthetic appliances.

tantrum (tan′trum) a violent display of temper.

tap (tap) 1. a quick, light blow. 2. to drain off fluid by PARACENTESIS.

   spinal t. LUMBAR PUNCTURE.

Tapazole (tap′ah-zōl) trademark for a preparation of METHIMAZOLE, used as a thyroid inhibitor.

tape (tāp) a long, narrow strip of fabric or other flexible material.

   adhesive t. a strip of fabric or other material evenly coated on one side with a pressure-sensitive material that causes adherence to an adjoining surface.

   Montgomery t's Montgomery straps.

tapeinocephaly (tah-pi″no-sef′ah-le) flattening or depression of the skull. adj., **tapeinocephal′ic.**

tapetum (tah-pe′tum) [L.] 1. a covering structure or layer of cells. 2. a stratum in the human brain composed of fibers from the body and splenium of the corpus callosum sweeping around the lateral ventricle.

   t. lu′cidum the iridescent epithelium of the choroid of animals that gives their eyes the property of shining in the dark.

tapeworm (tāp′werm) any parasitic worm of the subclass Cestoda; these have a flattened bandlike form and numerous species can lodge in the intestines of many animals including human beings. Tapeworms are transmitted to humans in larval form embedded in cysts, in meat or fish that is not properly cooked. In the human body they develop to maturity and attach themselves to the wall of the intestine, where they grow and release eggs. Called also cestode.

Although a large variety of adult tapeworms are sometimes human parasites, only a few infect humans to any great degree. *Taenia saginata,* the beef tapeworm, and *T. solium,* the pork tapeworm, are widespread and quite common. Beef tapeworms grow to a length of 4 to 8 meters (12 to 25 feet), and adult pork tapeworms average 2 to 4 meters (6 to 12 feet) in length. Both species release white, egg-containing proglottids, or segments of the body, which make their way to the anus and may be found in clothes or bedding. *Diphyllobothrium latum,* the fish tapeworm, is found in North America in the Great Lakes region, as well as in Northern Europe and Japan; it may grow as long as 18 meters (60 feet). *Hymenolepis nana* and *H. diminuta* are dwarf tapeworms that are common in the tropics and subtropics.

The diagnosis of a tapeworm infection is made when segments of the worm are found in clothing or bedding or when characteristic eggs or segments are found in the stool. Occasionally diarrhea, vague abdominal cramps, flatulence, distention, and nausea occur. Mental deterioration and seizures are rare complications, occurring only when larval forms of the worm invade brain tissue. Tapeworm infection can be prevented by cooking pork, beef, and fish properly. Although most meats and fish are inspected under government supervision, eggs and larvae are not always detectable; the only certain protection is proper cooking.

Once it is inside the body, the tapeworm can be eliminated by specific anthelmintic

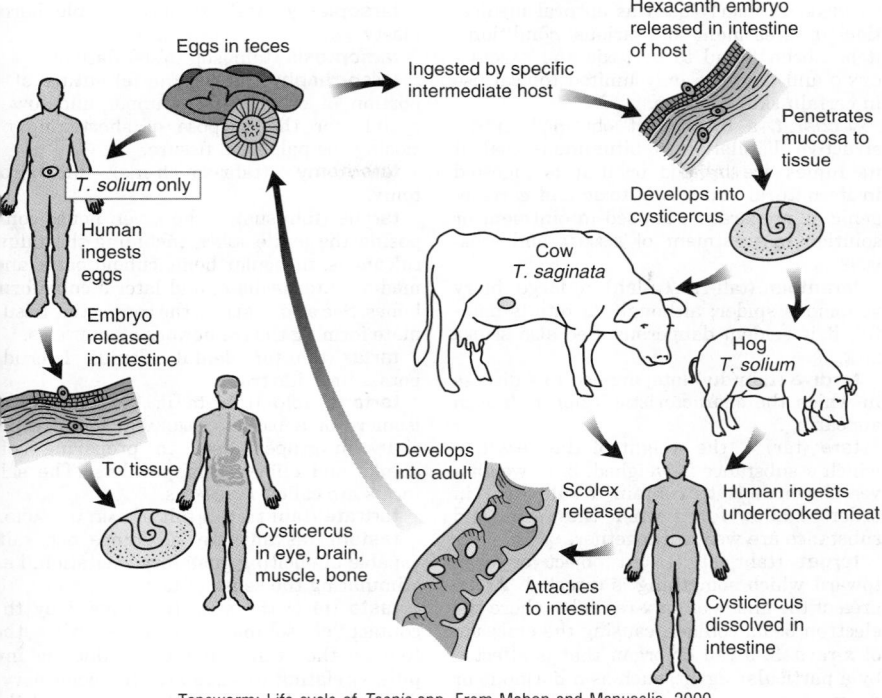

Tapeworm: Life cycle of *Taenia* spp. From Mahon and Manuselis, 2000.

drugs or surgery. The drug of choice is usually PRAZIQUANTEL, which should be given in a dose large enough to cause the worm to release its hold and pass out through the intestinal tract. If the head is found in the evacuated feces, no further treatment is necessary. However, if the head is not found, the worm could regenerate in two to three months, with segments reappearing in the stools.

Echinococcus granulosus and *E. multilocularis* differ from other tapeworms in that the adults infect animal hosts and the larval forms are found in humans. The larvae develop in the human intestine, penetrate its wall, and are carried by the lymphatics to various organs of the body where they form slowly growing cysts (hydatid CYSTS). The liver is the organ most commonly involved. Treatment is by surgical removal of the cyst. Infection with this worm (ECHINOCOCCOSIS or HYDATID DISEASE) is uncommon in the United States.

 armed t. *Taenia solium.*
 beef t. *Taenia saginata.*
 broad t. *Diphyllobothrium latum.*
 dog t. *Dipylidium caninum.*
 fish t. *Diphyllobothrium latum.*
 hydatid t. *Echinococcus granulosus.*
 pork t. *Taenia solium.*
 unarmed t. *Taenia saginata.*
taphephobia (taf″ĕ-fo′be-ah) irrational fear of being buried alive.

taphophilia (taf′o-fil′e-ah) morbid interest in graves and cemeteries.

Tapia's syndrome (tah′pe-ahz) unilateral paralysis of the tongue and larynx, the soft palate being unaffected. It follows injury to the vagus and hypoglossal nerves, most often from trauma or a tumor.

tapotement (tah-pōt-maw′) [Fr.] a tapping manipulation in massage.

Taq polymerase (tak) an enzyme found in the bacillus *Thermus aquaticus,* which lives in hot springs; it is heat resistant and thus can endure the high temperatures of the polymerase chain reaction.

tar (tahr) a dark brown or black viscid liquid from the wood of various species of pine, or found as a by-product of the destructive distillation of bituminous coal (see *coal tar*). It is a complex mixture, the source of organic substances such as CRESOL, CREOSOL, NAPHTHALENE, PARAFFIN, PHENOL, and

TOLUENE. Formerly used as an oral medication in treatment of various conditions, it has been found to be toxic and CARCINOGENIC and now has only limited topical use in certain skin diseases.

coal t. a by-product obtained in destructive distillation of bituminous coal; if its fumes are inhaled or if it is ingested in its natural state, it is toxic and carcinogenic. A preparation is used in ointment or solution in treatment of ECZEMA and PSORIASIS.

tarantula (tah-ran′tu-lah) a large hairy venomous spider; although its bite is painful, it is seldom dangerous. See also SPIDER BITE.

tardive (tahr′div) late; applied to a disease in which the characteristic lesion is late in appearing.

tare (tār) 1. the weight of the vessel in which a substance is weighed. 2. to weigh a vessel which is to contain a substance in order to allow for it when the vessel and substance are weighed together.

target (tahr′get) 1. an object or area toward which something is directed. 2. the area of the anode of an x-ray tube where the electron beam collides, causing the emission of x-rays. 3. a cell or organ that is affected by a particular agent, such as a hormone or drug.

tarichatoxin (tar′ik-ah-tok″sin) name given to the lethal neurotoxin TETRODOTOXIN when it comes from the newt *Taricha.*

tars(o)- word element [L.; Gr.], *edge of eyelid; tarsus of the foot; instep.*

tarsadenitis (tahr″sad-ĕ-ni′tis) inflammation of the tarsus of the eyelid and the meibomian glands.

tarsal (tahr′sal) 1. pertaining to the tarsus of an eyelid. 2. pertaining to the tarsus of the foot.

t. tunnel syndrome a complex of symptoms resulting from compression of the posterior tibial nerve or of the plantar nerves in the tarsal tunnel, with pain, numbness, and tingling paresthesia of the sole of the foot.

tarsalgia (tahr-sal′jah) pain in a tarsus.

tarsalia (tahr-sa′le-ah) the bones of the tarsus.

tarsalis (tahr-sa′lis) [L.] tarsal.

tarsectomy (tahr-sek′tah-me) 1. excision of one or more bones of the tarsus. 2. excision of the tarsus of the eyelid.

tarsitis (tahr-si′tis) blepharitis.

tarsoclasis (tahr-sok′lah-sis) surgical fracture of the tarsus of the foot.

tarsomalacia (tahr″so-mah-la′shah) softening of the tarsal cartilage of an eyelid.

tarsometatarsal (tahr″so-met″ah-tahr′sal) pertaining to the tarsus and metatarsus.

tarsoplasty (tahr′so-plas″te) blepharoplasty.

tarsoptosis (tahr″sop-to′sis) flatfoot.

tarsorrhaphy (tahr-sor′ah-fe) suture of a portion of or the entire upper and lower eyelids for the purpose of shortening or closing the palpebral fissure.

tarsotomy (tahr-sot′ah-me) blepharotomy.

tarsus (tahr′sus) 1. the seven bones composing the ankle JOINT, including the talus, calcaneus, navicular bone, cuboid bone, and medial, intermediate, and lateral cuneiform bones. See also ANKLE. 2. the connective tissue plate forming the framework of an EYELID.

tartar (tahr′ter) dental calculus. 1. crude potassium bitartrate.

tartaric acid (tahr-tar′ik) any of several isomers of a DICARBOXYLIC ACID found especially in grapes, used in preparing soft drinks and effervescent powders. The salt forms are called TARTRATES.

tartrate (tahr′trāt) a salt of TARTARIC ACID.

tastant (tās′tant) any substance, e.g., salt, capable of eliciting gustatory excitation, i.e., stimulating the sense of taste.

taste (tāst) the sensation caused by the contact of soluble substances with the tongue; the cranial nerves conducting impulses relating to taste are the facial nerve for the anterior part of the tongue and the glossopharyngeal nerve for the posterior part. Other senses, such as smell and touch, also play important roles in the experience commonly thought of as tasting.

The organs of taste are the *taste buds,* bundles of slender cells with hairlike branches that are packed together in groups that form the projections called *papillae* at various places on the tongue. When a substance is introduced into the mouth, its molecules enter the pores of the papillae

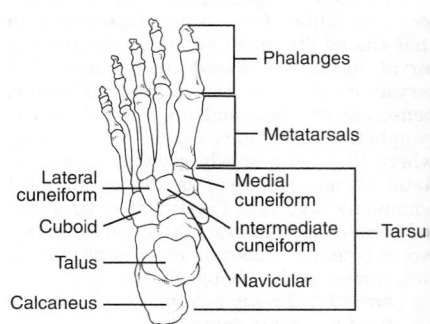

Tarsus, showing the seven tarsal bones. From Dorland's, 2000.

and stimulate the taste buds directly. In order to do this, the substance has to be dissolved in liquid. If it is not liquid when it enters the mouth, then it melts or is chewed and becomes mixed with saliva.

There are four basic tastes: *sweet, salt, sour,* and *bitter.* Sometimes *alkaline* and *metallic* are also included as basic tastes. All other tastes are combinations of these. The taste buds are specialized, and each responds only to the kind of basic taste that is its specialty. The sweet and salt taste buds are most numerous on the tip and front part of the tongue, sour taste buds are mainly along the edges, and bitterness is tasted at the back of the tongue. Bittersweet substances are tasted in two stages, first sweet, then bitter. The solid center of the tongue's surface has very few taste buds.

taster (tās'ter) an individual capable of tasting a particular substance, such as phenylthiocarbamide, as in certain genetic studies.

TAT Thematic Apperception Test.

tattooing (tah-too'ing) the introduction, by punctures, of permanent colors in the skin.

   t. of cornea permanent coloring of the cornea, chiefly to conceal leukomatous spots.

taurine (taw'rēn) a crystallized acid from the bile; found also in small quantities in lung and muscle tissues.

taurocholate (taw″ro-ko'lāt) a salt of taurocholic acid, one of the bile acids.

taurocholic acid (taw″ro-ko'lik) cholyltaurine.

Taussig-Bing syndrome (taw'sig bing) a form of TRANSPOSITION OF THE GREAT VESSELS of the heart: the aorta arises from the right ventricle, with a left-sided pulmonary artery overriding the left ventricle and with a high ventricular septal defect, right ventricular hypertrophy, anteriorly situated aorta, and posterior pulmonary artery. Patients present with pulmonary hypertension, cyanosis, and greater oxygen saturation in the pulmonary artery than in the aorta.

tautomer (taw'to-mer) a chemical compound exhibiting, or capable of exhibiting, tautomerism.

tautomeral (taw-tom'er-al) pertaining to the same part; said especially of neurons and neuroblasts sending processes to aid in formation of the white matter in the same side of the spinal cord.

tautomerase (taw-tom'er-ās) an enzyme that catalyzes tautomeric reactions.

tautomerism (taw-tom'er-izm) stereoisomerism in which the compounds are

mutually interconvertible, under normal conditions, forming a mixture that is in dynamic equilibration. adj., **tautomer'ic.**

taxis (tak'sis) [Gr.] 1. an orientation movement of a motile organism in response to a stimulus; it may be either toward (positive) or away from (negative) the source of the stimulus. See also TROPISM. 2. exertion of force in manual replacement of a displaced organ or part.

-taxis word element [Gr.], *movement of an organism in response to an external stimulus.*

Taxol (tak'sol) trademark for a preparation of PACLITAXEL, an antineoplastic AGENT.

taxon (tak'son) [Gr.] 1. a particular taxonomic grouping, e.g., a particular species, genus, family, order, class, phylum, or kingdom. 2. the name applied to a taxonomic grouping.

taxonomy (tak-son'ah-me) the orderly classification of organisms or lists into appropriate categories (taxa), with application of suitable and correct names. adj., **taxonom'ic.**

   numerical t. a method of classifying organisms solely on the basis of the number of shared phenotypic characters, each character usually being given equal weight; used primarily in bacteriology.

Tay-Sachs disease (ta saks) the infantile form of neuronal ceroid-LIPOFUSCINOSIS, inherited as an autosomal recessive trait and affecting chiefly Ashkenazic Jews. With each pregnancy couples who are carriers have a one in four chance of having a child with the condition, a one in two chance of having a carrier like themselves, and a one in four chance of having a child who neither has the disease nor is a carrier. It is a progressive disorder marked by degeneration of brain tissue and the maculas (with formation of a cherry red spot on both retinas) and by dementia, blindness, and death. Tay-Sachs disease is a SPHINGOLIPIDOSIS in which the inborn ERROR of metabolism is a deficiency of the enzyme hexosaminidase A, resulting in accumulation of GM_2 ganglioside in the brain.

It is possible to test for this disease in the unborn fetus at 14 weeks of pregnancy. An absence of hexosaminidase A indicates conclusively that the fetus has Tay-Sachs disease. Carriers of the trait have lowered levels of the enzyme in their blood, thus permitting screening of populations most susceptible to transmission of the trait to their offspring and genetic counseling of known carriers. No therapy is currently available. Most children with Tay-Sachs disease die of bronchopneumonia at 3 to 4 years of age.

The National Tay-Sachs and Allied Diseases Association (NTSAD) is dedicated to the treatment and prevention of Tay-Sachs, CANAVAN, and related diseases. It provides information and support services to individuals and families affected by the diseases, as well as to the public at large. Their address is National Tay-Sachs and Allied Diseases Association, 2001 Beacon Street, Suite 204, Boston MA 02135. The telephone number is 800-906-8723.

tazarotene (tah-zar′o-tēn) a RETINOID PRODRUG used topically in treatment of ACNE VULGARIS and PSORIASIS.

tazobactam (taz″o-bak′tam) a β-lactamase inhibitor having antibacterial actions and uses similar to those of sulbactam; used as the sodium salt.

Tb terbium.

tb tuberculosis; tubercle bacillus.

Tc technetium.

TCD transcranial Doppler; see under DOPPLER ULTRASONIC FLOWMETER.

TCID tissue culture infective DOSE.

TCID$_{50}$ median tissue culture infective DOSE.

TcPO$_2$ transcutaneous oxygen pressure.

Td tetanus and diphtheria toxoids, adult type; see diphtheria TOXOID.

Te tellurium.

tea (te) 1. the dried leaves of *Thea chinensis,* containing caffeine and tannic acid, or a decoction thereof. 2. any decoction or infusion.

teaching (tēch′ing) the imparting of knowledge; see EDUCATION (def. 1). 1. a nursing INTERVENTION in the NURSING MINIMUM DATA SET; individual or group instruction designed (a) to provide information about disease processes, injuries, other health-related events, or health promotion practices, or (b) to facilitate development of skills for coping with special care requirements, limitations, or restrictions in health status.

   disease process t. in the NURSING INTERVENTIONS CLASSIFICATION, a nursing INTERVENTION defined as assisting the patient to understand information related to a specific disease process.

   group t. in the NURSING INTERVENTIONS CLASSIFICATION, a nursing INTERVENTION defined as the development, implementation, and evaluation of a patient teaching program for a group of individuals experiencing the same health condition.

   individual t. in the NURSING INTERVENTIONS CLASSIFICATION, a nursing INTERVENTION

defined as the planning, implementation, and evaluation of a teaching program designed to address a patient's particular needs.

   t.: infant nutrition in the NURSING INTERVENTIONS CLASSIFICATION, a nursing INTERVENTION defined as instruction on NUTRITION and feeding practices during the first year of life.

   t.: infant safety in the NURSING INTERVENTIONS CLASSIFICATION, a nursing INTERVENTION defined as instruction on safety during the first year of life.

   preoperative t. in the NURSING INTERVENTIONS CLASSIFICATION, a nursing INTERVENTION defined as assisting a patient to understand and mentally prepare for surgery and the postoperative recovery period.

   prescribed activity/exercise t. in the NURSING INTERVENTIONS CLASSIFICATION, a nursing INTERVENTION defined as preparing a patient to achieve and/or maintain a prescribed level of activity.

   prescribed diet t. in the NURSING INTERVENTIONS CLASSIFICATION, a nursing INTERVENTION defined as preparing a patient to correctly follow a prescribed DIET.

   prescribed medication t. in the NURSING INTERVENTIONS CLASSIFICATION, a nursing INTERVENTION defined as preparing a patient to safely take prescribed medications and monitor for their side effects.

   procedure/treatment t. in the NURSING INTERVENTIONS CLASSIFICATION, a nursing INTERVENTION defined as preparing a patient to understand and mentally prepare for a prescribed procedure or treatment.

   psychomotor skill t. in the NURSING INTERVENTIONS CLASSIFICATION, a nursing INTERVENTION defined as preparing a patient to perform a psychomotor skill.

   safe sex t. in the NURSING INTERVENTIONS CLASSIFICATION, a nursing INTERVENTION defined as providing instruction concerning sexual protection during sexual activity.

   sexuality t. in the NURSING INTERVENTIONS CLASSIFICATION, a nursing INTERVENTION defined as assisting individuals to understand physical and psychosocial dimensions of sexual growth and development.

   t.: toddler nutrition in the NURSING INTERVENTIONS CLASSIFICATION, a nursing INTERVENTION defined as instruction on NUTRITION and feeding practices during the second and third years of life.

   t.: toddler safety in the NURSING INTERVENTIONS CLASSIFICATION, a nursing INTERVENTION defined as instruction on safety during the second and third years of life.

team (tēm) a group of people or units organized to do a task together.

interdisciplinary t. a group of health care professionals from diverse fields who work in a coordinated fashion toward a common goal for the patient.

intraprofessional t. a team of professionals who are all from the same profession, such as three physical therapists collaborating on the same case.

multidisciplinary t. a team of professionals including representatives of different disciplines who coordinate the contributions of each profession, which are not considered to overlap, in order to improve patient care.

rehabilitation t. the individuals involved in establishing a plan and goals for the achievement of a patient's maximum potential. The composition of the team will vary depending on the nature of the patient's problems; the patient is always included as a member of the rehabilitation team.

transdisciplinary t. a team composed of members of a number of different professions cooperating across disciplines to improve patient care through practice or research.

tears (tērz) the watery, slightly alkaline and saline secretion of the lacrimal glands that moistens the conjunctiva. See also LACRIMAL APPARATUS.

crocodile t. see SYNDROME OF CROCODILE TEARS.

tease (tēz) to pull apart gently with fine needles to permit microscopic examination.

teaspoon (te′spo͞on) a household unit of volume or capacity approximately equal to 5 milliliters.

teat (tēt) nipple (def. 1).

technetium (tek-ne′she-um) a chemical element, atomic number 43, atomic weight 99, symbol Tc. (See Appendix 6.)

t. 99m the most frequently used radioisotope in nuclear medicine, a gamma emitter having a half-life of 6.01 hours.

technic (tek′nik) technique.

technician (tek′nish′an) a person skilled in the performance of the technical or procedural aspects of a health care profession; the minimum preparation for this role is generally an associate degree. The technician carries out the routine work of the profession under the supervision of a physician, therapist, technologist, or other health care professional. For names of specific occupations, see under the name.

technique (tek-nēk′) a MANEUVER, METHOD, or PROCEDURE. For names of specific techniques, see under the name.

technologist (tek-nol′ah-jist) a person skilled in the theory and practice of a technical profession. In several allied health fields, technologist is the highest professional rank. Generally, the minimum preparation for this role is a baccalaureate degree. In addition to routine work, the technologist is involved in problem-solving and implementation of new procedures. For names of specific occupations, see under the names.

technology (tek-nol′ah-je) scientific knowledge; the sum of the study of a technique.

assisted reproductive t. (ART) any procedure that involves manipulation of eggs or sperm to establish PREGNANCY in treatment of INFERTILITY, such as in vitro FERTILIZATION, gamete intrafallopian TRANSFER, tubal embryo TRANSFER, and zygote intrafallopian TRANSFER.

tectorial (tek-to′re-al) of the nature of a roof or covering.

tectorium (tek-to′re-um) Corti's membrane.

tectospinal (tek″to-spi′nal) extending from the tectum of the midbrain to the spinal cord.

tectum (tek′tum) a rooflike structure.

t. of mesencephalon, t. of midbrain the posterior part of the TEGMENTUM MESENCEPHALI.

TED threshold erythema dose.

teeth (tēth) plural of TOOTH.

teething (tēth′ing) eruption of the teeth through the gums. The average infant cuts the first tooth between the sixth and ninth months. The full set of 20 baby teeth erupt gradually over a period up to about 30 months, the customary pattern being the arrival of two teeth, one on each side of the jaw, at a time.

Evidence of teething includes drooling, a compulsion to put objects into the mouth, and unusual crankiness. Some babies seem to be more bothered by teething than others, and different teeth affect the same baby in different ways.

It was long fashionable to ascribe any baby ailment to teething, despite the considerable harm such a hasty diagnosis often did by delaying recognition of the real trouble. Although teething sometimes may cause a slight fever, any such symptom should be watched carefully for further developments.

Teflon (tef′lon) trademark for tetrafluoroethylene fluorocarbon polymers; used as a surgical implant material in many prostheses. Called also polytef.

tegmen (teg′men) [L.] a covering structure or roof.

t. tym′pani the thin layer of bone that forms the roof of the tympanic cavity, separating it from the cranial cavity.

PRIMARY TEETH

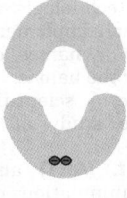

The two central lower (mandibular) incisors usually appear around 5–7 months.

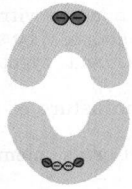

By 6–10 months, the baby may have the two central upper (maxillary) and two lateral lower incisors.

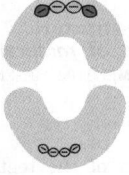

By 1 year of age, the two lateral upper incisors erupt.

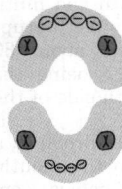

By about 10–16 months, four molars (1st molars) are usually present.

Teething: Eruption of primary teeth. From Betz et al., 1994.

tegmentum (teg-men′tum) [L.] 1. a covering. 2. tegmentum mesencephali. adj., **tegmen′tal.**

    t. mesence′phali, t. of mesencephalon the posterior part of the MESENCEPHALON, formed by continuation of the posterior parts of the cerebral PEDUNCLES across the median plane, and extending on each side from the SUBSTANTIA NIGRA to the level of the mesencephalic aqueduct. Called also tegmentum.

Tegretol (teg′rĕ-tol) trademark for a preparation of CARBAMAZEPINE, an ANTICONVULSANT.

teichoic acids (ti-ko′ik) antigenic polymers of glycerol or ribitol phosphates found attached to the cell walls or in intracellular association with membranes of gram-positive bacteria; they determine group specificity of some species, e.g., the staphylococci.

teichopsia (ti-kop′se-ah) scintillating scotoma; the sensation of a luminous appearance before the eyes, with a zigzag, wall-like outline.

teicoplanin (ti-ko-pla′nin) a glycopeptide antibiotic produced by the bacterium *Actinoplanes teichomyceticus,* used as a less toxic alternative to vancomycin in the treatment of moderate to severe infections caused by gram-positive bacteria where other antibiotics can not be used.

tela (te′lah) [L.] a thin weblike structure or tissue; used in naming various anatomic structures.

    t. conjuncti′va connective tissue.

    t. elas′tica elastic tissue.

    t. subcuta′nea the subcutaneous connective tissue or superficial fascia.

telalgia (tel-al′jah) referred PAIN.

telangiectasia (tel-an″je-ek-ta′zhah) a vascular lesion formed by dilation of a group of small blood vessels. adj., **telangiectat′ic.** Superficial telangiectasias are sometimes seen in the normal newborn on the nape of the neck (stork bites) or on the upper eyelids or upper lip (flame nevi). They usually disappear within the first year of life.

    hereditary hemorrhagic t. an autosomal dominant vascular anomaly characterized by the presence of multiple small telangiectases of the skin, mucous membranes, gastrointestinal tract, and other organs associated with recurrent episodes of bleeding from affected sites and gross occult melena.

    spider t. vascular spider.

telangiectasis (tel-an″je-ek′tah-sis) 1. the lesion produced by telangiectasia, which may be present as a coarse or fine red line or as a punctum with radiating limbs (spider). 2. telangiectasia.

telangiosis (tel-an″je-o′sis) any disease of the capillaries.

Teldrin HBP (tel′drin) trademark for a preparation of CHLORPHENIRAMINE maleate, an ANTIHISTAMINE.

tele- word element [Gr.], *operating at a distance, far away.*

tele(o)- word element [Gr.], *an end.*

telecanthus (tel″ĕ-kan′thus) abnormally increased distance between the medial canthi of the eyelids.

telecardiography (tel″ĕ-kahr″de-og′rah-fe) the recording of an electrocardiogram by transmission of impulses to a site at a distance from the patient.

telecardiophone (tel″ĕ-kahr′de-o-fōn″) an apparatus for making heart sounds audible at a distance from the patient.

teleceptor (tel′ĕ-sep″tor) a sensory nerve terminal that is sensitive to stimuli originating at a distance. Such nerve endings exist in the eyes and ears.

telediagnosis (tel″ĕ-di″ag-no′sis) determination of the nature of a disease at a site remote from the patient on the basis of TELEHEALTH methods of transmitted data.

telefluoroscopy (tel″ĕ-floor-os′kah-pe) a TELEHEALTH technique consisting of electronic transmission of fluoroscopic images.

telehealth (tel′ĕ-helth) the use of electronic information and telecommunications technologies to support long-distance clinical health care, professional health-related education, public health, and health administration.

telekinesis (tel″ĕ-ki-ne′sis) 1. movement of an object produced without contact. 2. the ability to produce such movement. adj., **telekinet′ic.**

telemedicine (tel″ĕ-med′ĭ-sin) a branch of TELEHEALTH consisting of provision of consultant services by off-site health care professionals to those on the scene; diagnosis and treatment can be done at a great distance through methods such as the VIDEOCONFERENCE or rapid transmission of digital FILES.

telemetry (tĕ-lem′ĕ-tre) the making of measurements at a distance from the subject; usually the measurable evidence of phenomena under investigation is transmitted by radio signals.

telencephalon (tel″en-sef′ah-lon) 1. one of the two divisions of the PROSENCEPHALON, consisting of the CEREBRUM. 2. the anterior of the two vesicles formed by specialization of the prosencephalon in embryonic development. Called also endbrain. adj., **telencephal′ic.**

teleneurite (tel″ĕ-noor′īt) an end expansion of an axon.

teleneuron (tel″ĕ-noor′on) a nerve ENDING.

teleological (te″le-o-loj′ĭ-k′l) serving an ultimate purpose in development.

teleology (te″le-ol′ah-je) the doctrine that the explanation of phenomena is to be found in terms of their consequences; see also teleological THEORY.

teleomitosis (tel″e-o-mi-to′sis) completed mitosis.

teleopsia (tel″e-op′se-ah) a visual disturbance in which objects appear to be farther away than they actually are.

teleorganic (tel″e-or-gan′ik) necessary to organic life.

Telepaque (tel′ĕ-pāk) trademark for a preparation of iopanoic acid, a radiopaque medium used in cholecystography.

telepathy (tĕ-lep′ah-the) the communication of thought through extrasensory PERCEPTION.

teleradiography (tel″ĕ-ra″de-og′rah-fe) 1. a TELEHEALTH technique consisting of electronic transmission of radiographic images. 2. radiography with the radiation source about 2 meters from the subject, more nearly securing parallelism of the rays and minimizing distortion.

teleradiology (tel″ĕ-ra″de-ol′ah-je) RADIOLOGY done through remote transmission and viewing of images.

teleroentgentherapy (tel″e-rent″gen-ther′ah-pe) treatment with ionizing radiations from an x-ray source located at a distance from the body.

telesthesia (tel″es-the′zhah) extrasensory PERCEPTION.

teletherapy (tel″ĕ-ther′ah-pe) treatment in which the source of the therapeutic agent (such as radiation) is at a distance from the body.

telluric (tĕ-lu′rik) 1. pertaining to tellurium. 2. pertaining to or originating from the earth.

tellurium (tĕ-lu′re-um) a chemical element, atomic number 52, atomic weight 127.60, symbol Te. (See Appendix 6.)

telmisartan (tel″mĭ-sahr′tan) an ANGIOTENSIN II antagonist used as an ANTIHYPERTENSIVE, administered orally.

telo- word element [Gr.], *end.*

telocentric (tel″o-sen′trik) having the centromere at one end of the chromosome so that the chromosome has only one arm.

telodendron (tel″o-den′dron) any of the fine terminal branches of an axon.

telogen (tel′o-jen) the quiescent or resting phase of the hair CYCLE, following CATAGEN. At this stage the HAIR has become a club HAIR and does not grow further.

telognosis (tel″og-no′sis) diagnosis based on interpretation of radiographs transmitted by radio or telephonic communication. See also TELERADIOGRAPHY.

telolemma (tel″o-lem′ah) the covering of a motor end-plate, made up of sarcolemma and an extension of Henle's sheath.

telomere (tel′o-mēr) an extremity of a chromosome, which has specific properties, one of which is a polarity that prevents reunion with any fragment after a chromosome has been broken.

telomerase (tĕ-lo′mer-ās) a DNA POLYMERASE involved in the formation of TELOMERES and the maintenance of telomere sequences during REPLICATION.

T

telophase (tel′o-fāz) the last of the four stages of mitosis and of the two divisions of meiosis.

telos (te′lōs) end, goal, purpose.

Temaril (tem′ah-ril) trademark for preparations of TRIMEPRAZINE tartrate, an ANTIHISTAMINE used to relieve itching.

temazepam (tĕ-maz′ĕ-pam) a BENZODIAZEPINE used as a SEDATIVE and HYPNOTIC in treatment of insomnia; administered orally.

temozolomide (tem″ah-zo′lah-mīd) a cytotoxic ALKYLATING AGENT used as an ANTINEOPLASTIC in the treatment of refractory anaplastic ASTROCYTOMA, administered orally.

temperament (tem′per-ah-ment) an inherent, constitutional predisposition to react to stimuli in a certain way; the term is often used synonymously with PERSONALITY. Compare CHARACTER.

temperance (tem′per-ans) self-control regarding temptations, such as overindulgence in food, drink, or sex. In a broader sense it can be defined as doing good in one's business or affairs, with modesty, self-control, moderation, and humility. In VIRTUE-based theories of ethics, temperance can be defined as the habitual disposition of practitioners toward responsible use of power for the good of patients, protecting patients from undertreatment, abandonment, and overtreatment.

temperature (tem′per-ah-chur) the degree of sensible heat or cold, expressed in terms of a specific scale. See Table of Temperature Equivalents in the Appendices. Body temperature is measured by a clinical thermometer and represents a balance between the heat produced by the body and the heat it loses. Though heat production and heat loss vary with circumstances, the body regulates them, keeping a remarkably constant temperature. An abnormal rise in body temperature is called FEVER.

Normal Body Temperature. Body temperature is usually measured by a thermometer placed in the mouth, the rectum, or the auditory canal (for tympanic membrane temperature). The normal oral temperature is 37° Celsius (98.6° Fahrenheit); rectally, it is 37.3° Celsius (99.2° Fahrenheit). The tympanic membrane temperature is a direct reflection of the body's core temperature. These values are based on a statistical average. Normal temperature varies somewhat from person to person and at different times in each person. It is usually slightly higher in the evening than in the morning and is also somewhat higher during and immediately after eating, exercise, or emotional excitement. Temperature in infants and young children tends to vary somewhat more than in adults.

Temperature Regulation. To maintain a constant temperature, the body must be able to respond to changes in the temperature of its surroundings. When the outside temperature drops, nerve endings near the skin surface sense the change and communicate it to the hypothalamus. Certain cells of the hypothalamus then signal for an increase in the body's heat production. This heat is conducted to the blood and distributed throughout the body. At the same time, the body acts to conserve its heat. The arterioles constrict so that less blood will flow near the body's surface. The skin becomes pale and cold. Sometimes it takes on a bluish color, the result of a color change in the blood, which occurs when the blood, flowing slowly, gives off more of its oxygen than usual. Another signal from the brain stimulates muscular activity, which releases heat. Shivering is a form of this activity—a muscular reflex that produces heat.

When the outside temperature goes up, the body's cooling system is ordered into action. Sweat is released from sweat glands beneath the skin, and as it evaporates, the skin is cooled. Heat is also eliminated by the evaporation of moisture in the lungs. This process is accelerated by panting.

An important regulator of body heat is the peripheral capillary system. The vessels of this system form a network just under the skin. When these vessels dilate, they allow more warm blood from the interior of the body to flow through them, where it is cooled by the surrounding air.

Abnormal Body Temperature. Abnormal temperatures occur when the body's temperature-regulating system is upset by disease or other physical disturbances. FEVER usually accompanies infection and other disease processes. In most cases when the oral temperature is 37.8°C (100°F) or over fever is present. Temperatures of 40°C (104°F) or over are common in serious illnesses, although occasionally very high fever accompanies an illness that causes little concern. Temperatures as high as 41.7°C (107°F) or higher sometimes accompany diseases in critical stages. Subnormal temperatures, below 35.6°C (96°F) occur in cases of collapse; see also symptomatic HYPOTHERMIA.

absolute t. (T) that reckoned from absolute zero (−273.15°C), expressed on an absolute SCALE.

basal body t. (BBT) the temperature of the body under conditions of absolute rest it has a slight sustained rise during the luteal phase of the menstrual CYCLE and can be used as an indirect indicator of when OVULATION has occurred.

body t. the temperature of the body of a human or animal; see TEMPERATURE.

core t. the temperature of structures deep within the body, as opposed to peripheral temperature such as that of the skin.

critical t. that below which a gas may be converted to a liquid by increased pressure.

normal t. the body temperature usually registered by a healthy person, averaging 37°C (98.6°F).

risk for imbalanced body t. a NURSING DIAGNOSIS accepted by the North American Nursing Diagnosis Association, defined as a state in which an individual is at risk of failure to maintain body temperature within the normal range.

subnormal t. temperature below the normal. See also symptomatic HYPOTHERMIA.

template (tem'plāt) a pattern or mold. In dentistry, a curved or flat plate used as an aid in setting teeth for a denture. In theoretical immunology, an antigen that determines the configuration of combining (antigen-binding) sites of antibody molecules. In genetics, a strand of DNA which specifies the synthesis of a complementary strand of RNA (messenger RNA, ribosomal RNA, or transfer RNA); mRNA in turn serves as a template for the synthesis of nucleic acids or proteins.

temple (tem'p'l) the lateral region on either side of the head, above the zygomatic arch.

tempolabile (tem″po-la'bil) subject to change with the passage of time.

tempor(o)- word element [L.], *the temple(s)*.

temporal (tem'po-ral) 1. pertaining to the temple. 2. pertaining to time; limited as to time; temporary.

temporomandibular (tem″po-ro-man″dib'-u-lar) pertaining to the temporal bone and mandible.

t. joint disorder, t. joint syndrome dysfunction of the temporomandibular JOINT, marked by a clicking or grinding sensation in the joint and often by pain in or about the ears, TINNITUS, tiredness and slight soreness of the jaw muscles upon waking, and stiffness of the jaw or actual TRISMUS. Numerous causes have been proposed, such as mandibular overclosure, stress, and lesions of the joint. Called also TMJ disorder or syndrome.

Treatment may include medical therapy, dental therapy, or a combination of these. Dental treatment usually involves insertion of a BITEPLATE to prevent the teeth from meeting and grinding against one another.

The biteplate relieves pain and promotes muscle relaxation and normal positioning of the mandible, which allows the inflamed joint to rest and heal. Once the inflammation has subsided and normal neuromuscular function returns, the dentist may attempt to correct MALOCCLUSION. Medical therapy may include local heat applications to improve circulation and promote relaxation, corticosteroid injections into the joint, jaw exercises, and analgesics, muscle relaxants, and antiinflammatory agents.

temporomaxillary (tem″po-ro-mak'sĭ-lar″e) pertaining to the temporal bone and maxilla.

temporo-occipital (tem″po-ro-ok-sip'ĭ-tal) pertaining to the temporal and occipital bones.

temporosphenoid (tem″po-ro-sfe'noid) pertaining to the temporal and sphenoid bones.

tempostabile (tem″po-sta'bil) not subject to change with time.

ten(o)- word element [Gr.], *tendon.* See also terms beginning TENDIN(O)-, TEND(O)-, and TENONT(O)-.

tenacious (tĕ-na'shus) viscid; adhesive.

tenaculum (tĕ-nak'u-lum) a sharp hook-like surgical instrument with two or more prongs, used for grasping and holding tissues or a part.

tenalgia (ten-al'jah) pain in a TENDON; called also tenodynia.

tend(o)- word element [L.], *tendon.* See also terms beginning TENDIN(O)-, TEN(O)-, and TENONT(O)-.

tendency (ten'den-se) an inclination or likelihood; a predisposition toward an action, behavior, or thought process.

suicidal t's see SUICIDE.

tenderness (ten'der-nes) a state of unusual sensitivity to touch or pressure.

rebound t. 1. a state in which pain is felt on the release of pressure over a part. 2. specifically, such a sensation in the abdomen, considered a sign of peritonitis. It is sometimes used to test for peritonitis; this

T

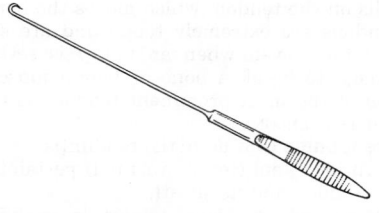

Tenaculum. From Dorland's, 2000.

procedure is controversial because of the pain involved.

tendin(o)- word element [L.], *tendon.* See also terms beginning TEN(O)-, TEND(O)-, and TENONT(O)-.

tendinitis (ten″dĭ-ni′tis) inflammation of TENDONS and of tendon-muscle attachments, one of the most common causes of acute pain in the shoulder. It is frequently associated with a calcium deposit (calcific tendinitis), which may also involve the bursa around the tendon or near the joint, causing BURSITIS. Shoulder pain associated with calcific tendinitis is most pronounced when the affected arm is abducted between 50 and 130 degrees (the so-called *painful arc*). Called also tendonitis.

Short-term therapy is aimed at relieving pain and decreasing inflammation so that exercise is possible and permanent immobility of the shoulder is avoided. Medications that may be given include long-acting corticosteroids, given by injection directly into the painful area; short-term analgesics such as codeine or acetaminophen with codeine; and oral antiinflammatory agents. Applications of ice are more helpful in relieving pain than applications of heat, which usually aggravate the pain of calcific tendinitis. Once the patient is free of pain, exercise is begun to preserve motion. If the joint becomes fixed, surgical intervention may be necessary to break up adhesions and restore full mobility to the joint.

tendinoplasty (ten′dĭ-no-plas″te) tenoplasty.

tendinosuture (ten″dĭ-no-soo′chur) tenorrhaphy.

tendinous (ten′dĭ-nus) pertaining to, resembling, or of the nature of a tendon.

tendo (ten′do) [L.] tendon; used in anatomic nomenclature.

t. **Achil′lis,** *t.* **calca′neus** Achilles tendon.

tendolysis (ten-dol′ĭ-sis) the freeing of a tendon from adhesions.

tendon (ten′don) a cord or band of strong white fibrous tissue that connects a muscle to a bone. When the muscle contracts it pulls on the tendon, which moves the bone. Tendons are extremely tough and are seldom torn, even when an injury is severe enough to break a bone or tear a muscle. One of the most prominent tendons is the ACHILLES TENDON.

tendonitis (ten″do-ni′tis) tendinitis.

tendovaginal (ten″do-vaj′ĭ-nal) pertaining to a tendon and its sheath.

tenecteplase (tĕ-nek′tĕ-plās) a modified form of human tissue plasminogen ACTIVATOR

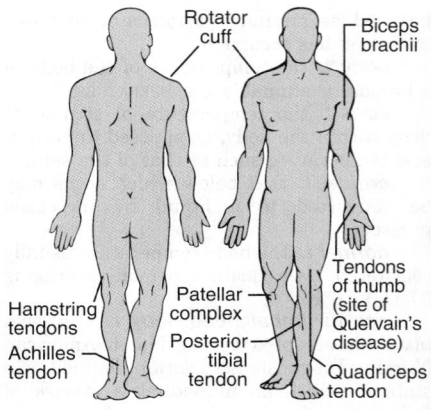

Frequently injured tendons. From Copstead, 1995.

produced by recombinant DNA technology used as a thrombolytic agent in the treatment of myocardial infarction, administered intravenously.

tenectomy (tĕ-nek′tah-me) excision of a lesion of a tendon or of a tendon sheath.

tenesmus (tĕ-nez′mus) ineffectual and painful straining at stool or urination. adj. **tenes′mic.**

tenia (te′ne-ah) TAENIA.

teniacide (te′ne-ah-sīd″) taeniacide.

teniafuge (te′ne-ah-fūj″) taeniafuge.

teniamyotomy (te″ne-ah-mi-ot′ah-me) an operation involving a series of transverse incisions of the teniae coli; done in diverticular disease.

teniasis (te-ni′ah-sis) infection with tapeworms of the genus *Taenia.*

teniposide (VM-26) (ten′ĭ-po′sīd) a semisynthetic derivative of PODOPHYLLOTOXIN administered orally as an antineoplastic AGENT in treatment of NEUROBLASTOMA, non Hodgkin's LYMPHOMA, and acute lymphoblastic LEUKEMIA; administered intravenously.

tenodesis (ten-od′ĕ-sis) suture of the end of a tendon to a bone.

tenodynia (ten″o-din′e-ah) tenalgia.

tenofovir (tĕ-no′fo-vir″) an antiretroviral agent that inhibits the viral enzyme reverse transcriptase and so inhibits replication of retroviruses; used as *tenofovir disoproxil fumarate* in the treatment of HIV-1 (human immunodeficiency virus-1) infection.

tenolysis (ten-ol′ĭ-sis) the operation of freeing a tendon from adhesions.

tenomyoplasty (ten″o-mi′o-plas″te) plastic repair of a tendon and muscle, applied especially to an operation for inguinal hernia

tenomyotomy (ten″o-mi-ot′ah-me) excision of a portion of a tendon and muscle.

tenonectomy (ten″o-nek′tah-me) excision of part of a tendon to shorten it.

tenonitis (ten″o-ni′tis) 1. tendinitis. 2. inflammation of Tenon's capsule, the connective tissue enclosing the eyeball.

tenonometer (ten″o-nom′ĕ-ter) an apparatus for measuring intraocular pressure.

tenont(o)- word element [Gr.], *tendon.* See also terms beginning TENDIN(O)-, TEND(O)-, and TEN(O)-.

tenontography (ten″on-tog′rah-fe) a written description or delineation of the tendons.

tenontology (ten″on-tol′ah-je) the sum of what is known about the tendons.

tenophyte (ten′o-fīt) a growth or concretion in a tendon.

tenoplasty (ten′o-plas″te) plastic repair of a tendon. adj., **tenoplas′tic.**

tenoreceptor (ten″o-re-sep′tor) a nerve receptor in a tendon.

Tenormin (ten′or-min) trademark for preparations of ATENOLOL, a BETA-ADRENERGIC BLOCKING AGENT used in treatment of hypertension, angina, and myocardial infarction.

tenorrhaphy (ten-or′ah-fe) suture of a tendon.

tenostosis (ten″os-to′sis) conversion of a tendon into bone.

tenosuspension (ten″o-sus-pen′shun) attachment of the head of the humerus to the acromion by a strip of tendon; it is done for habitual dislocation of the shoulder.

tenosuture (ten″o-soo′chur) tenorrhaphy.

tenosynovectomy (ten″o-sin″o-vek′tah-me) excision or resection of a tendon sheath.

tenosynovitis (ten″o-sin″o-vi′tis) inflammation of a tendon and its sheath, usually seen in the hands and wrists or feet and ankles; it is often the result of intense and continued use, as with pianists and typists. It is painful, and may temporarily disable the affected part. Rheumatoid and other types of arthritis frequently involve tendon sheaths. A less common cause of tenosynovitis is injury to the tendon sheath and subsequent infection. It can also be the result of tuberculous or gonorrheal infection. Treatment is by immobilization of the limb or, in severe cases, by surgery for the purpose of draining an infected sheath, or to release a tendon from a constricting sheath.

villonodular t. a condition marked by exaggerated proliferation of synovial membrane cells, producing a solid tumorlike mass, commonly occurring in periarticular soft tissues and less frequently in joints.

tenotomy (ten-ot′ah-me) transection of a TENDON; called also tendon release.

graduated t. partial transection of a tendon.

tenovaginitis (ten″o-vaj″ĭ-ni′tis) tenosynovitis.

TENS transcutaneous electrical nerve stimulation.

tension (ten′shun) 1. the act of stretching. 2. the condition of being stretched or strained; the degree to which something is stretched or strained. 3. the partial pressure of a component of a gas mixture or of a gas dissolved in a fluid, such as oxygen in blood. 4. voltage. 5. mental, emotional, or nervous strain. 6. hostility between two or more individuals or groups.

arterial t. blood pressure within an artery.

carbon dioxide t. the partial pressure of CARBON DIOXIDE in the blood, noted as pCO$_2$ in BLOOD GAS ANALYSIS. See also RESPIRATION.

electric t. electromotive force.

intraocular t. intraocular pressure.

surface t. tension or resistance that acts to preserve the integrity of a surface.

tissue t. a state of equilibrium between tissues and cells that prevents overaction of any part.

tensor (ten′sor) any muscle that stretches or makes tense.

tent (tent) 1. a fabric covering for enclosing an open space, especially such a covering over a patient's bed for administering oxygen or aerosol by inhalation. 2. a conical, expansible plug of soft material for dilating an orifice or for keeping a wound open, so as to prevent its healing except at the bottom. 3. to elevate tissue in order to prevent adherence to underlying organs.

oxygen t. see OXYGEN TENT.

sponge t. a conical plug made of compressed sponge used to dilate the ostium uteri.

tentacle (ten′tah-k'l) a slender, whiplike appendage in animals that may function in prehension and feeding or as a sense organ.

tenting (tent′ing) a skin abnormality indicative of dehydration; the skin maintains a triangular or tentlike appearance when gently pinched.

tentorium (ten-tor′e-um) [L.] an anatomical part resembling a tent or covering. adj., **tento′rial.**

t. cerebel′li the process of the dura mater supporting the occipital lobes and covering the cerebellum.

Tenuate (ten′u-āt) trademark for preparations of DIETHYLPROPION hydrochloride, an appetite suppressant.

ter- word element [L.], *three; threefold.*

tera- word element [Gr.] *monster;* used in naming units of measurement (symbol T) to designate a quantity one trillion (10^{12}) times the unit specified by the root to which it is joined, as teracurie.

teras (ter′as) a significantly malformed fetus. adj., **terat′ic.**

terat(o)- word element [Gr.], *monster; monstrosity.*

teratism (ter′ah-tizm) an anomaly of formation or development; see developmental ANOMALY.

teratoblastoma (ter″ah-to-blas-to′mah) a neoplasm containing embryonic elements, differing from a TERATOMA in that its tissue does not represent all the germ LAYERS.

teratocarcinoma (ter″ah-to-kahr″sĭ-no′-mah) a malignant neoplasm consisting of elements of TERATOMA with those of embryonal CARCINOMA or CHORIOCARCINOMA,, or both; it is usually found in the testis.

teratogen (ter′ah-to-jen) an agent or influence that causes physical defects in the developing embryo; called also developmental toxicant. adj., **teratogen′ic.**

teratogenesis (ter″ah-to-jen′ĕ-sis) the production of deformity in the developing embryo; called also teratogeny. adj., **teratogenet′ic.**

teratogenous (ter″ah-toj′ĕ-nus) developed from fetal remains.

teratogeny (ter″ah-toj′ĕ-ne) teratogenesis.

teratoid (ter′ah-toid) resembling a teras.

teratology (ter″ah-tol′ah-je) that division of embryology and pathology dealing with abnormal development and congenital deformations. See also developmental TOXICOLOGY. adj., **teratolog′ic.**

teratoma (ter″ah-to′mah) a type of germ cell TUMOR made up of a number of different types of tissue from one or more of the germ cell LAYERS; it is usually found in the ovary or testis and may be either benign or malignant.

    malignant t. a solid, malignant ovarian tumor resembling a dermoid cyst but composed of immature embryonal or extraembryonal elements derived from all three germ layers.

teratomatous (ter″ah-tom′ah-tus) pertaining to or of the nature of teratoma.

teratosis (ter″ah-to′sis) teratism.

terazosin (ter-a′zo-sin) an ALPHA$_1$-ADRENERGIC BLOCKING AGENT used as the hydrochloride salt in treatment of HYPERTENSION and BENIGN PROSTATIC HYPERPLASIA, administered orally.

terbinafine (ter′bin-ah-fēn″) a synthetic antifungal AGENT used as the hydrochloride salt topically and orally in treatment of tinea and of fungal infections of the nails.

terbium (ter′be-um) a chemical element atomic number 65, atomic weight 158.924, symbol Tb. (See Appendix 6.)

terbutaline (ter-bu′tah-lēn) a beta$_2$-adrenergic RECEPTOR agonist used as a BRONCHODILATOR; it has also been used as a TOCOLYTIC agent.

terconazole (ter-kon′ah-zōl) an IMIDAZOLE derivative used as a topical antifungal agent in treatment of vulvovaginal CANDIDIASIS.

terebration (ter″ĕ-bra′shun) an act of boring or trephining; also, a boring pain.

teres (te′rēz) [L.] long and round.

ter in die (ter in de′a) [L.] three times a day.

term (term) 1. a definite period, especially the period of gestation, or pregnancy. 2. a word with a specific meaning, such as one used in a limited technical vocabulary.

MeSH t′s subject headings.

terminal (ter′mĭ-nal) 1. forming or pertaining to an end. 2. a termination, end, or extremity, especially a nerve ending. 3. an input-output device that communicates with a computer and includes parts such as a keyboard and a printer.

    dedicated t. a terminal reserved for just one type of computer application.

    dumb t. a computer terminal capable both as an input device, sending data keyed in on the terminal keyboard, and as an output device, displaying data on a screen or printing it on paper. See also intelligent terminal.

    intelligent t. a computer terminal, or a microcomputer functioning as a terminal that can process data files stored on mass storage devices (usually floppy disks). Such files may be either output files received from the host computer or input (command) files sent to the host computer. See also dumb terminal.

    point of care t. a computer terminal that serves as an input device to allow health professionals to enter data at the patient's bedside.

terminatio (ter″mĭ-na′she-o) [L.] ending.

terminology (ter″mĭ-nol′ah-je) 1. the vocabulary of an art or science. 2. the science that deals with the investigation, arrangement, and construction of terms.

terminus (ter′mĭ-nus), pl. *ter′mini* [L.] ending.

ternary (ter′nah-re) 1. third in order. 2. made up of three elements or radicals.

terpene (ter′pēn) any hydrocarbon of the formula $C_{10}H_{16}$.

Terramycin (ter′ah-mi″sin) trademark for preparations of OXYTETRACYCLINE, a broad-spectrum ANTIBIOTIC.

terror (ter′or) an attack of extreme fear or dread.

night t's, sleep t's pavor nocturnus.

tertian (ter′shan) recurring in 3-day cycles (every second day); applied to the type of fever caused by certain forms of malarial parasites; see also MALARIA.

tertigravida (ter″she-grav′ĭ-dah) a woman pregnant for the third time; gravida III.

tertipara (ter-tip′ah-rah) a woman who has had three pregnancies that resulted in viable offspring; para III. Called also tri-para.

tesla (T) (tes′lah) the SI unit of magnetic flux density, a vector quantity that measures the magnitude of a magnetic field. It is equal to 1 weber per square meter.

tessellated (tes′ĕ-lāt″ed) divided into squares, like a checker board.

test (test) 1. an examination or trial. 2. a significant chemical reaction. 3. a reagent. For names of specific tests, see under the name.

> **double-blind t.** see DOUBLE BLIND.

> **single-blind t.** see SINGLE BLIND.

testalgia (tes-tal′jah) orchialgia.

Tes-Tape (tes′tāp) trademark for glucose oxidase reagent strip test used for the semiquantitative determination of glucose in urine.

testectomy (tes-tek′tah-me) orchiectomy.

testes (tes′tēz) [L.] plural of TESTIS.

testicle (tes′tĭ-k′l) testis.

testicular (tes-tik′u-lar) pertaining to testis.

> **t. feminization syndrome** complete androgen RESISTANCE.

testing (test′ing) administration of one or more tests.

> **bedside laboratory t.** in the NURSING INTERVENTIONS CLASSIFICATION, a nursing INTERVENTION defined as performance of laboratory tests at the bedside or point of care.

> **compatibility t.** the determination of the compatibility of the recipient's serum and the donor's red blood cells by pretransfusion testing to ensure that the product will survive in and improve the clinical condition of the recipient.

> **criterion-referenced t.** the comparison of a person's score or performance with a standard of achievement that includes the definition of target behaviors. See also criterion-referenced EVALUATION.

> **exercise t.** see EXERCISE TESTING.

> **reality t.** objective evaluation of the external world and differentiation between t and the ego or self. Impaired reality testing is seen in psychological DEFENSE MECHANISMS that falsify reality, such as PROJECTION and DENIAL, and it is a major criterion of PSYCHOSIS.

> **stress t.** exercise testing.

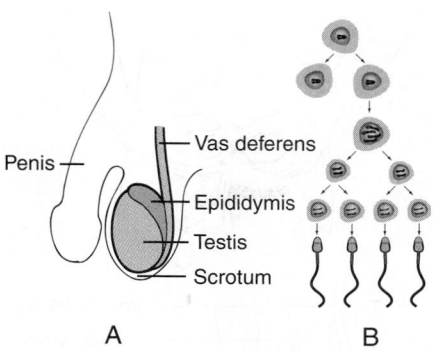

A, Testis; *B,* production of spermatozoa.

testis (tes′tis) [L.] the male GONAD; either of the paired, egg-shaped glands normally found in the SCROTUM; called also testicle. The testes produce the SPERMATOZOA (the male reproductive cells) and TESTOSTERONE (the male sex hormone), which is responsible for the secondary sex CHARACTERS of the male.

If the testes are removed (CASTRATION, bilateral ORCHIECTOMY) before puberty, the male is sterile and will never develop all the adult male secondary sex CHARACTERS. If they are removed after puberty, the male becomes sterile and his secondary sex characters will diminish unless he receives injections of male hormones. With aging, there is a gradual decrease in the production of testosterone.

In the fetus in utero, the testes lie close to the kidneys. During approximately the seventh month of fetal life, the testes begin to descend through the abdominal wall at the groin and enter the scrotum. As they descend they are accompanied by blood vessels, nerves, and ducts, all contained within the spermatic cord. The passageway through which the testis and spermatic cord descend is called the inguinal canal. Failure of a testis to descend into the scrotum is called CRYPTORCHIDISM.

The testis is divided internally into about 250 compartments or lobules, each of which contains one to three small convoluted TUBULES, within which SPERMATOZOA are produced. When mature, the spermatozoa leave the tubules and enter the epididymis (situated on top of and behind each testis), where maturation is completed. The spermatozoa are stored in the epididymis until such time as they are mixed in the semen and ejaculated during coitus. (See also REPRODUCTION and male REPRODUCTIVE ORGANS.)

T

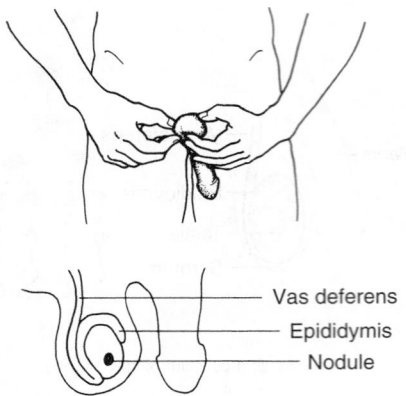

Vas deferens
Epididymis
Nodule

Testicular self-examination. (Redrawn from For Men Only. New York, American Cancer Society.)

Cancer of the Testis. Testicular cancer accounts for about 12 per cent of all cancer deaths in young men in North America and is second only to accidents as a cause of death in men between the ages of 20 and 35 years. It is one of the most curable forms of cancer when detected early and treated promptly. Men most at risk for testicular cancer are those who have an undescended or partially descended testicle.

In order to ensure early detection of cancer of the testis, men are urged to conduct a monthly self-examination of the testes. The self-examination involves the use of both hands to examine each of the testes. The index and middle fingers are placed below the testis and the thumbs on top. With a gentle motion each testis is rolled between the thumbs and fingers to discover any lump (usually about the size of a pea), thickening, or change in the consistency of the tissues. It is important that the man become familiar with the feel of the epididymis so that he doesn't confuse this normal structure with an abnormal lump. Should a lump or any other abnormality be found, a doctor should be consulted immediately. The American Cancer Society publishes several pamphlets that explain the procedure for testicular self-examination and give additional information on testicular cancer. Diagnosis of testicular cancer is confirmed by biopsy of the suspect testis. There are three stages of classification for malignancy of the testis: *Stage I*: the tumor is confined to the affected testis; *Stage II*: the malignancy has spread to the regional lymph nodes; and *Stage III*: there is metastasis to other organs, such as the lung and liver.

Treatment of testicular cancer (simple ORCHIECTOMY for Stage I malignancy) may or may not render the patient impotent and sterile. If there is no metastasis, only the affected testis need be removed. The remaining testis will retain its normal function and the patient should be able to have normal sexual intercourse and be fertile. However, if more radical surgery and radiation therapy are called for and both testes and the lymph nodes are dissected, and if there has been no damage to nerves during surgery, the patient may be able to have sexual intercourse but no seminal fluid will be emitted. A young man who is looking forward to having children may consider banking his sperm prior to surgery so that he might father children by artificial insemination.

abdominal t. an undescended testis located in the abdominal cavity.

canalicular t. an undescended testis located between the internal and external inguinal rings.

cryptorchid t. undescended testis.

ectopic t. one lodged in a location outside of the normal pathway of descent.

gliding t. an undescended testis that can reach the top of the scrotum but then glides back up.

obstructed t. an ectopic testis whose descent was prevented by a fascial sheet at the entrance to the scrotum.

retained t. undescended t.

retractile t. a testis that can descend fully into the scrotum but moves freely up into the inguinal canal.

undescended t. 1. a testis in the normal pathway of descent but failing to descend into the scrotum; see also CRYPTORCHIDISM. Called also cryptorchid or retained testis. 2. cryptorchidism.

vanishing t. one that was originally present in the fetus but atrophied in utero because of torsion.

testitis (tes-ti'tis) orchitis.

test meal a portion of food or foods given for the purpose of determining the functioning of the digestive tract.

barium t. m. a meal containing barium sulfate as the opaque constituent; see also BARIUM TEST.

motor t. m. food or drink whose progress through the stomach, pylorus, and intestinal tract is observed fluoroscopically.

opaque t. m. a meal containing some substance opaque to x-rays, permitting visualization of the gastrointestinal tract.

testoid (tes'toid) 1. resembling a TESTIS. 2. a term applied to testicular hormones and other natural or synthetic compounds having a similar effect.

testosterone (tes-tos'tĕ-rōn) the principal male sex hormone (ANDROGEN) that is produced by Leydig's CELLS of the testes in response to luteinizing HORMONE secreted by the PITUITARY GLAND. It is also produced by the adrenal CORTEX in both males and females. Its chief function is to stimulate the development of the male reproductive organs, including the prostate, and the secondary sex characters, such as the beard. It encourages growth of bone and muscle, and helps maintain muscle strength.

Testosterone is obtained for therapeutic purposes by extraction from animal testes or by synthesis from cholesterol in a laboratory. It is used to treat male HYPOGONADISM and delayed male puberty as well as to relieve symptoms in some forms of metastatic breast cancer in females, and is used as the base for various esters (e.g., cypionate, enanthate, propionate). Women normally secrete a certain amount of male hormones; however, if the hormone balance is disturbed and there is overproduction of male hormones in a woman, MASCULINIZATION may develop.

test type printed letters of varying size, used in the testing of visual acuity.

TET treadmill exercise test; tubal embryo transfer.

tetanic (tĕ-tan'ik) pertaining to tetanus.

tetaniform (tĕ-tan'ĭ-form) tetanoid.

tetanigenous (tet″an-nij'ĕ-nus) producing tetanic spasms.

tetanization (tet″ah-nĭ-za'shun) the act of tetanizing a muscle.

tetanize (tet'ah-nīz) to stimulate a muscle at progressively higher frequencies until successive contractions fuse and cannot be distinguished from one another.

tetanode (tet'ah-nōd) the unexcited stage of tetany.

tetanoid (tet'ah-noid) resembling tetanus or tetany; tetaniform.

tetanolysin (tet″ah-nol'ĭ-sin) the hemolytic fraction of the EXOTOXIN formed by *Clostridium tetani,* the causative organism of TETANUS.

tetanospasmin (tet″ah-no-spaz'min) the neurotoxic component of the tetanus toxin, which causes the muscle spasms of tetanus.

tetanus (tet'ah-nus) 1. physiological TETANUS. 2. a highly fatal disease caused by the bacillus *Clostridium tetani,* characterized by muscle spasms and convulsions. The bacilli are prevalent in rural areas and grow in the intestines of humans and other animals. They are found in soil and dust, and are spread by animal and human feces, entering the body through a break in the skin, particularly a puncture wound, such as one caused by a nail, splinter, insect bite, or gunshot. Occasionally, the original wound appears trivial and heals quickly; more often, there is obvious infection. Because of the characteristic jaw stiffness, it is also known as lockjaw. adj., **tetan'ic.**

Symptoms. Stiffness of the jaw is usually the first definite indication of tetanus. Difficulty in swallowing, stiffness of the neck, restlessness, irritability, headache, chills, fever, and convulsions are also among the early symptoms. Muscles in the abdomen, back, neck, and face may go into spasm. If the infection is severe, convulsions are set off by slight disturbances, such as noises and drafts. During convulsions, there is difficulty in breathing and the possibility of asphyxiation.

Treatment. If there is any suspicion of contamination by tetanus bacilli, emergency treatment should be obtained. This may include an adequate dose of ANTITOXIN or a booster injection of tetanus toxoid (see below) to counteract any possible tetanus infection. Because of the possible danger of HYPERSENSITIVITY to horse serum antitoxin, tetanus immune globulin (derived from human instead of horse serum) is preferred when available. In any case, the wound area must be carefully cleaned, and all dead tissue and foreign substances removed.

During a tetanus attack, SEDATIVES are often given to reduce the frequency of CONVULSIONS. ANTIBIOTICS may also be used to help combat secondary infection. HYPERBARIC OXYGENATION (oxygen under high pressure) has also been used to treat tetanus.

Prevention. The most important weapon against tetanus is adequate immunization. Tetanus TOXOID in combination with diphtheria toxoid and pertussis vaccine (DTP) is given at two months of age and repeated at four months, six months, 18 months, and four to six years of age.

At the time of injury tetanus toxoid is given, either as an initial immunizing dose or as a booster for previous immunization, unless the patient has received a booster or completed the initial immunization within the past five years. Patients who have been actively immunized within the past ten years are given a booster unless they have received a booster within the past five years. Patients who have not been previously immunized may require passive immunity with homologous tetanus immune serum as well as active immunization, especially if the wound is severe, neglected, or over 24 hours old.

Patient Care. Because the toxin from *Clostridium tetani* attacks the central nervous system it is extremely important to provide

T

a nonstimulating environment for patients with tetanus. The room must be kept dark and quiet, and drafts of cold air, noises, and other external stimuli must be avoided because they may precipitate convulsive muscle spasms. As for any patient subject to convulsions, maintenance of a safe environment is essential. Prevention of injury to and assessment of a patient with convulsive seizures are discussed under CONVULSION.

Fluids and nourishment usually are given intravenously during the acute stage of the disease. The patient's intake and output are carefully measured and recorded. Sedatives and antibiotic drugs are administered as ordered to reduce irritability and to combat secondary bacterial infections.

As long as the patient is acutely ill and likely to suffer from convulsive seizures, someone should be in constant attendance. Signs of respiratory difficulty, changes in pulse and blood pressure, and frequent and prolonged muscle spasms should be reported immediately. A TRACHEOSTOMY set should be readily available in the event severe DYSPNEA should develop.

cephalic t., cerebral t. a rare form of infectious tetanus with an extremely poor prognosis; it may occur following an injury to the head or face or in association with otitis media in which *Clostridium tetani* is a constituent of the flora of the middle ear and it is characterized by isolated or combined dysfunction of the cranial nerves, especially the seventh cranial. It may remain localized or progress to generalized tetanus.

neonatal t., t. neonato'rum a severe form of infectious tetanus occurring during the first few days of life caused by such factors as unhygienic practice in dressing the umbilical stump or in circumcising male infants and the lack of maternal immunization.

physiological t. a state of sustained muscular contraction without periods of relaxation caused by repetitive stimulation of the motor nerve trunk at frequencies so high that individual muscle twitches are fused and cannot be distinguished from one another; called also tetanic or tonic contraction and tetanic or tonic spasm.

tetany (tet'ah-ne) 1. continuous tonic SPASM of a muscle; steady contraction of a muscle without distinct twitching. 2. a syndrome manifested by sharp flexion of the wrist and ankle joints *(carpopedal spasm)*, muscle twitchings, cramps, and convulsions, sometimes with attacks of stridor. It is due to abnormal CALCIUM

metabolism, and occurs with hypofunction of the PARATHYROID GLANDS, VITAMIN D deficiency, and ALKALOSIS, and also as a result of ingestion of alkaline salts. Treatment varies according to the cause and is usually successful. It may include the administration of vitamin D, calcium, parathyroid hormone, or other remedies. In chronic cases, as in the loss of the parathyroid glands, treatment may have to be continued indefinitely.

duration t. a continuous tetanic contraction in response to a strong continuous current, occurring especially in degenerated muscles.

gastric t. a severe form due to disease of the stomach, attended by difficult respiration and painful tonic spasms of the limbs.

hyperventilation t. tetany produced by forced inhalation and exhalation continued for a considerable time.

latent t. tetany elicited by the application of electrical and mechanical stimulation.

parathyroid t., parathyroprival t. tetany due to removal or hypofunctioning of the PARATHYROID GLANDS.

tetartanopia (tet″ar-tah-no'pe-ah, tet″ar-tah-nop'se-ah) 1. quadrantanopia. 2. a very rare type of dichromatic VISION in which there is perception of red and green only with blue and yellow perceived as an achromatic (gray) band. Some authorities doubt its existence. adj., **tetartanopsia, tetartanop'ic.**

tethered cord syndrome see tethered CORD.

tetr(a)- word element [Gr.], *four.*

tetrabrachius (tet″rah-bra'ke-us) a double fetus having four upper limbs.

tetracaine (tet'rah-kān) a local, topical and spinal anesthetic, used as the base or the hydrochloride salt.

tetrachloroethylene (tet″rah-klor″o-eth'i-lēn) a moderately toxic chlorinated hydrocarbon formerly widely used as an ANTHELMINTIC but now used only as a dry cleaning solvent and for other industrial uses.

tetracrotic (tet″rah-krot'ik) having four sphygmographic waves or elevations to one beat of the pulse.

tetracycline (tet″rah-si'klēn) 1. any of a group of related broad-spectrum ANTIBIOTICS some are isolated from certain species of *Streptomyces* and others are produced semisynthetically. The group includes CHLORTETRACYCLINE, DEMECLOCYCLINE, DOXYCYCLINE, MINOCYCLINE, OXYTETRACYCLINE, and tetracycline (def. 2). Tetracyclines are effective against a wide range of aerobic and anaerobic gram-positive and gram-negative bacteria, and are used particularly for rickettsiae, mycoplasmas, and chlamydiae; they are also effective against certain protozoa. 2. a semisynthetic ANTIBIOTIC having the same wide spectrum of antimicrobial activity as other members of the tetracycline group; administered orally. The hydrochloride salt has similar actions and is administered orally, intramuscularly, intravenously, or topically to the skin or conjunctiva.

tetrad (tet′rad) a group of four similar or related entities, as (1) any element or radical having a valence, or combining power, of four; (2) a group of four chromosomal elements formed in the pachytene stage of the first meiotic prophase; (3) a square of cells produced by division into two planes of certain cocci (Sarcina).

tetradactyly (tet″rah-dak′tĭ-le) the presence of four digits on the hand or foot.

tetragonum (tet″rah-go′num) [L.] QUADRILATERAL (def. 2).

t. lumbale the four-sided area bounded by the four lumbar muscles.

tetrahydrocannabinol (THC) (tet″rah-hi″dro-kah-nab′ĭ-nol) the active principle of CANNABIS, occurring in two isomeric forms, both considered psychomimetically active. See also MARIJUANA.

tetrahydrozoline (tet″rah-hi-droz′o-lēn) an adrenergic VASOCONSTRICTOR applied topically to the nasal mucosa or conjunctiva as a DECONGESTANT.

tetraiodothyronine (tet″rah-i″o-do-thi′ro-ēn) thyroxine.

tetralogy (tet-ral′ah-je) a group or series of four.

t. of Fallot a CONGENITAL HEART DEFECT that combines four structural anomalies: obstruction to pulmonary flow; VENTRICULAR SEPTAL DEFECT (abnormal opening between the right and left ventricles); dextroposition of the aorta (aortic opening overriding the septum and receiving blood from both ventricles); and right ventricular hypertrophy (increase of volume of the myocardium of the right ventricle).

Infants with this condition are sometimes referred to as blue BABIES because of the presence of CYANOSIS, an outstanding symptom. This is due to mixing of poorly oxygenated blood from the systemic circulation with oxygenated blood from the lungs, because of the position of the aorta. Other symptoms include CLUBBING of the ends of the fingers, HEMOPTYSIS, DYSPNEA on exertion, and a slight delay in growth and development.

Diagnosis is confirmed by ELECTROCARDIOGRAPHY, ANGIOCARDIOGRAPHY, and CARDIAC CATHETERIZATION. These procedures demonstrate changes in the heart's electric impulses; defects in the ventricles, aorta, and pulmonary artery; and, from samplings of blood taken from the various chambers of the heart and great vessels, the oxygen content and pressure of the blood in these various areas.

Treatment involves surgical correction whenever possible. Without corrective surgery the prognosis is extremely poor for children who are deeply cyanotic and have dyspnea on slight exertion.

Before surgery, medical treatment is necessary to avoid complications and control dyspneic attacks. Since the hematocrit is high and polycythemia is common, efforts must be made to prevent dehydration and avoid the development of thrombi. Paroxysmal dyspnea, which often follows feeding or a spell of crying, usually can be relieved by placing the infant in knee-chest position, administering oxygen, or administering a mild sedative or morphine.

Surgical procedures for correction of the defects in the heart and great vessels vary according to the severity of symptoms and the age of the patient. In some cases an anastomosis of the arteries may be done as a temporary measure until more extensive surgery is feasible. In most cases open heart SURGERY is most successful in relieving symptoms and produces the most lasting benefits.

tetramastigote (tet″rah-mas′tĭ-gōt) 1. having four FLAGELLA. 2. an organism having four flagella.

tetrameric (tet″rah-mer′ik) having four parts.

tetranopsia (tet″rah-nop′se-ah) quadrantanopia.

tetraparesis (tet″rah-pah-re′sis) muscular weakness affecting all four extremities.

tetrapeptide (tet″rah-pep′tīd) a peptide which, on hydrolysis, yields four amino acids.

tetraplegia (tet″rah-ple′jah) quadriplegia.

tetraploid (tet′rah-ploid) 1. characterized by tetraploidy. 2. an individual or cell having four sets of chromosomes.

tetraploidy (tet′rah-ploi″de) the state of having four sets of chromosomes (4n).

tetrapus (tet′rah-pus) a malformed fetus with four feet.

tetrascelus (tet-ras′ĕ-lus) a malformed fetus with four lower limbs.

tetrasomy (tet′rah-so″me) the presence of two extra chromosomes of one type in an otherwise diploid cell. adj., **tetraso′mic.**

tetraster (tet-ras′ter) a figure in mitosis produced by quadruple division of the nucleus.

T

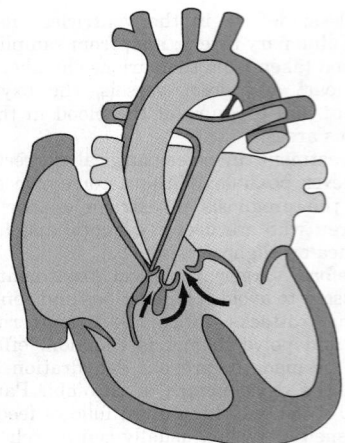

Tetralogy of Fallot

Tetralogy of Fallot. The right ventricular outflow tract obstruction results in blood flowing from right to left across the ventricular septal defect. From Lissauer and Graham, 2002.

tetravalent (tet″rah-va′lent) having a valence of four.

tetrodotoxin (tet′ro-do-tok″sin) a highly lethal NEUROTOXIN present in numerous species of PUFFER FISH and in newts of the genus *Taricha* (in the latter it is called TARICHATOXIN); ingestion results in TETRODOTOXISM.

tetrodotoxism (tet″ro-do-tok′sizm) the most severe form of FISH POISONING, caused by ingestion of inadequately prepared fish that contain TETRODOTOXIN. After eating such fish, within minutes there are symptoms of malaise, dizziness, and tingling about the mouth, which may be followed by ataxia, convulsions, respiratory paralysis, and death.

textiform (teks′tĭ-form) formed like a network.

textoblastic (teks″to-blas″tik) forming adult tissue; regenerative; said of cells.

texture (teks′chur) the structure or constitution of tissues. adj., **tex′tural.**

textwords (tekst′werdz) the individual words found in the titles and abstracts of MEDLINE references.

TF TRANSFER FACTOR.

6-TG thioguanine.

Th thorium.

thalamencephalon (thal″ah-men-sef′ah-lon) that part of the diencephalon including the thalamus, metathalamus, and epithalamus.

thalamocoele (thal′ah-mo-sēl″) the third ventricle of the brain.

thalamocortical (thal″ah-mo-kor′tĭ-kal) pertaining to the thalamus and cerebral cortex.

thalamolenticular (thal″ah-mo-len-tik′u-lar) pertaining to the thalamus and lenticular nucleus.

thalamotomy (thal″ah-mot′ah-me) a STEREOTAXIC surgical technique for the discrete destruction of specific groups of cells within the thalamus, as to relieve pain, to alleviate tremor and rigidity in PARKINSON'S DISEASE or to relieve certain anxiety states, psychoses, and obsessive-compulsive states.

thalamus (thal′ah-mus) [L.] either of two large ovoid structures (the *dorsal thalamus* or simply *thalamus* and the *ventral thalamus*) composed of gray matter and located at the base of the cerebrum. (See also BRAIN.) adj., **thalam′ic.** The thalamus functions as a relay station in which sensory pathways of the spinal cord and brainstem form synapses on their way to the cerebral cortex. Specific locations in the thalamus are related to specific areas on the body surface and in the cerebral cortex. A sensory impulse from the body surface travels upward to the thalamus, where it is received as a primitive sensation and then is sent on to the cerebral cortex for interpretation as to location character, and duration. The thalamus has numerous connections to other areas of the brain as well, and these are thought to be important in the integration of cerebral cerebellar, and brainstem activity.

ventral t. the subthalamic tegmental region, a transitional region of the diencephalon interposed between the (dorsal thalamus, the hypothalamus, and the tegmentum of the mesencephalon; it includes the subthalamic nucleus, Forel's fields, and the zona incerta. Called also subthalamus.

thalassemia (thal″ah-se′me-ah) a heterogeneous group of hereditary hemolytic anemias marked by a decreased rate of synthesis of one or more hemoglobin polypeptide chains, classified according to the chain involved (α, β, δ); the two major categories are α- and β-thalassemia.

α-t., alpha-t. that caused by diminished synthesis of alpha chains of hemoglobin. The *homozygous* form is incompatible with life, the stillborn infant displaying severe hydrops fetalis. The *heterozygous* form may be asymptomatic or marked by mild anemia.

β-t., beta-t. that caused by diminished synthesis of beta chains of hemoglobin. The homozygous form is called *t. major* and the heterozygous form is called *t. minor.*

t. ma′jor the homozygous form of β THALASSEMIA, in which hemoglobin A is completely absent; it appears in the newborn period and is marked by hemolytic hypochromic, microcytic anemia; hepatosplenomegaly; skeletal deformation; mongoloid facies; and cardiac enlargement.

t. mi′nor the heterozygous form of β-THALASSEMIA; it is usually asymptomatic, but there may be mild anemia.

sickle cell–t. a hereditary anemia involving simultaneous heterozygosity for hemoglobin S and thalassemia.

thalassoposia (thah-las″o-po′ze-ah) the drinking of sea water.

thalidomide (thah-lid′o-mīd) a SEDATIVE and HYPNOTIC that was commonly used in Europe in the late 1950s and 1960s. Its use was halted because use during early pregnancy was often followed by the birth of infants with serious developmental ANOMALIES, notably malformation or absence of a limb or limbs. It is still used in treatment of ERYTHEMA NODOSUM that complicates therapy for leprosy, administered orally.

thallium (thal′e-um) a chemical element, atomic number 81, atomic weight 204.37, symbol Tl. (See Appendix 6.) Its salts are active poisons that may cause alopecia, liver and kidney damage, blindness, and neurologic and psychic symptoms such as ataxia, restlessness, delirium, hallucinations, delusions, and semicoma.

t. 201 a radioactive isotope of thallium having a half-life of 3.05 days and decaying by electron capture with emission of gamma rays. It is used as a diagnostic aid in the form of THALLOUS CHLORIDE Tl 201.

t. scan a SCINTISCAN involving the use of thallium 201. The radioisotope is administered intravenously and localizes, like calcium, in the myocardium. A scintillation camera produces an image of the distribution of the radioisotope. Areas of inadequate perfusion appear as "cold spots," thus pinpointing the site of occlusions of the coronary arteries.

The thallium scan offers many advantages. It is noninvasive except for the administration of the radioisotope, which involves a radiation dose slightly larger than that received during a chest x-ray, and is extremely accurate.

The thallium-201 may be administered while the patient is exercising on a treadmill and being monitored by electrocardiogram. Subsequent scintigrams show areas of inadequate perfusion. This test is less likely than conventional exercise or stress testing to indicate disease when none is present and is more likely to detect disease when it is present. See also exercise thallium SCINTIGRAPHY and myocardial perfusion SCINTIGRAPHY.

thallous chloride Tl 201 (thal′us) the form in which thallium-201 in solution is

injected intravenously for imaging of myocardial disease, parathyroid disorder, or neoplastic disease.

thallus (thal′us) 1. a simple plant body not differentiated into root, stem, and leaf, characteristic of mycelial fungi and some algae. 2. the actively growing vegetative organism as distinguished from reproductive or resting portions, as in fungi.

thanat(o)- word element [Gr.], *death.*

thanatobiologic (than″ah-to-bi″o-loj′ik) pertaining to life and death.

thanatognomonic (than″ah-tog″no-mon′-ik) indicating the approach of death.

thanatoid (than′ah-toid) resembling death.

thanatology (than″ah-tol′ah-je) the medicolegal study of death and conditions affecting dead bodies.

thanatophobia (than″ah-to-fo′be-ah) irrational fear of death.

THC tetrahydrocannabinol.

thebaine (the-ba′in) a crystalline, poisonous, and anodyne alkaloid from OPIUM, having properties similar to those of STRYCHNINE.

theca (the′kah) [L.] a case or sheath. adj., **the′cal.**

t. cor′dis pericardium.

t. folli′culi an envelope of condensed connective tissue surrounding a vesicular ovarian follicle; it is composed of an internal vascular layer (*theca interna*) and an external fibrous layer (*theca externa*).

thecoma (the-ko′mah) theca cell tumor.

thecostegnosis (the″ko-steg-no′sis) contraction of a tendon sheath.

thelalgia (the-lal′jah) pain in the nipples.

thelarche (the-lahr′ke) beginning of development of the breast at puberty.

theleplasty (the′le-plas″te) a plastic operation on the nipple.

thelerethism (thě-ler′ě-thizm) erection of the nipple.

thelitis (the-li′tis) inflammation of a nipple.

thelorrhagia (the″lo-ra′jah) hemorrhage from the nipple.

thelygenic (thel″ĭ-jen′ik) producing only female offspring.

Thematic Apperception Test (the-mat′ik ap″er-sep′shun) TAT; a projective test in which the subject tells a story based on each of a series of standard ambiguous pictures, so that his responses reflect a projection of some aspect of his personality and his current psychological preoccupations and conflicts.

thenad (the′nad) toward the thenar or toward the palm.

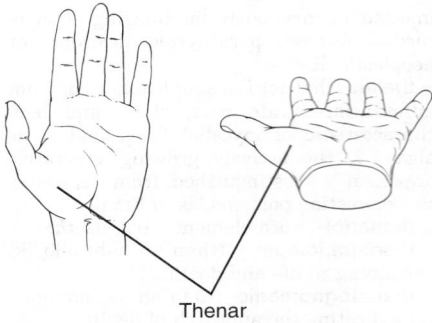

Thenar

From Dorland's, 2000.

thenar (the′nar) 1. the fleshy part of the hand at the base of the thumb. 2. pertaining to the palm.

theobromine (the″o-bro′min) an alkaloid prepared from dried ripe seed of the tropical American tree *Theobroma cacao,* or made synthetically from XANTHINE; used as a diuretic, myocardial stimulant, vasodilator, and smooth muscle relaxant; available as theobromine calcium salicylate, theobromine sodium formate, theobromine sodium salicylate, and theobromine salicylate.

Theo-Dur (the′o-dur) trademark for a preparation of THEOPHYLLINE, a BRONCHODILATOR.

theophylline (the-of′ĭ-lin) an alkaloid derived from tea or produced synthetically; it is a smooth muscle RELAXANT used chiefly for its BRONCHODILATOR effect in the treatment of chronic obstructive pulmonary disease, emphysema, bronchial asthma, chronic bronchitis, and bronchospastic distress. It also has myocardial stimulant, coronary vasodilator, diuretic, and respiratory center stimulant effects.

t. cholinate oxtriphylline.

theory (the′ah-re, thēr′e) 1. the doctrine or the principles underlying an art as distinguished from the practice of that particular art. 2. a formulated hypothesis or, loosely speaking, any hypothesis or opinion not based upon actual knowledge. 3. a provisional statement or set of explanatory propositions that purports to account for or characterize some phenomenon. The concepts and provisions set forth in a theory are more specific and concrete than those of a CONCEPTUAL MODEL. Hence a theory is derived from a conceptual model to fully describe, explain, and predict phenomena within the domain of the model.

attribution t. a theory developed in an attempt to understand why an event occurred so that later events can be predicted and controlled.

care-based t. a type of ethical theory of health care based on the two central constructive ideas of mutual interdependence and emotional response. The ethics of CARE is a rejection of impartial, principle-driven, dispassionate reasoning and judgment that has often dominated the models and paradigms of bioethics. Its origins are developmental psychology, moral theory, and feminist writings. Its moral concern is with needs and corresponding responsibility as they arise within a relationship. Moral response is individualized and is guided by the private norms of friendship, love, and care rather than by abstract rights and principles.

cell t. all organic matter consists of cells, and cell activity is the essential process of life.

clonal-selection t. of immunity immunologic specificity is preformed during embryonic life and mediated through cell clones.

Cohnheim's t. tumors develop from embryonic rests that do not participate in the formation of normal surrounding tissue.

community-based t. any ethical theory of health care according to which everything fundamental in ethics derives from communal values, the common good, social goals, traditional practices, and cooperative virtues. Commitment is to the general welfare, to common purposes, and to education of community members. Beliefs and principles, shared goals, and obligations are seen as products of the communal life. Conventions, traditions, and social solidarity play a prominent role in this type of theory. Called also communitarianism.

consequence-based t. teleological theory.

continuity t. a theory of motor development that postulates that motor changes occur in a linear fashion during an individual's life and that each change is dependent on the development of the prior period.

deontological t. a type of ethical theory that maintains that some features of actions other than or in addition to consequences make the actions right or wrong. A major postulate is that we may not use or mistreat other people as a means to our own happiness or to that of others. Deontological theories guide action with a set of moral principles or moral rules, but it is the actions themselves and their moral properties that are fundamental. This theory is sometimes called the Kantian theory because the work of Immanuel Kant (1724-1804) has a deep effect on its formulations.

discontinuity t. each stage of motor development has a new and unique feature that is added to distinguish it from the previous stage.

family systems t. a view of the family as a dynamic, interactive unit that undergoes continual evolvement in structure and function. There are subsystems that are discrete units (such as mother-father, sister-brother, and mother-child) and there is a suprasystem (the community). The main functions of the family are considered to be support, regulation, nurturance, and socialization; specific aspects of the functions change as the subsystems interact with the suprasystem.

feminist t. a type of ethical theory whose core assumptions are that women's experiences have not been taken as seriously as men's experiences and that there is subordination of women, which must end. A central theme is that women's reality is a social construction and not a biological determination. See also feminist PRAXIS.

gate t., gate-control t. neural impulses generated by noxious painful stimuli and transmitted to the spinal cord by small-diameter C-fibers and A-delta fibers are blocked at their synapses in the dorsal horn by the simultaneous stimulation of large-diameter myelinated A-fibers, thus inhibiting pain by preventing pain impulses from reaching higher levels of the central nervous system.

general systems t. a theory of organization proposed by Ludwig von Bertalanffy in the 1950s as a means by which various disciplines could communicate with one another and duplication of efforts among scientists could be avoided. The theory sought universally applicable principles and laws that would hold true regardless of the kind of system under study, the nature of its components, or the interrelationships among its components. Since the introduction of the general systems theory, theoretical models, principles, and laws have been developed that are of great value to scientists in all fields, including those of medicine, nursing, and other health-related professions.

germ t. 1. all organisms are developed from a cell. 2. infectious diseases are of microbial origin.

t. of human becoming a theory of nursing formulated by Rosemarie Rizzo PARSE. Principles of Martha Rogers' SCIENCE OF UNITARY HUMAN BEINGS are synthesized with major tenets and concepts from existential phenomenological thought to create a conceptual system and theory. Major areas of focus, rooted in the human sciences, describe the unitary human being interrelating with the universe in co-creating health. Essential concepts include the human-universe-health interrelationship, the co-creating of health, and the freely choosing of meaning in becoming. Humans are unitary beings mutually co-creating rhythmical patterns of relating in open interchange with the universe. The human being is a unity of the subject-world relationship, participating with the world in co-creation of self.

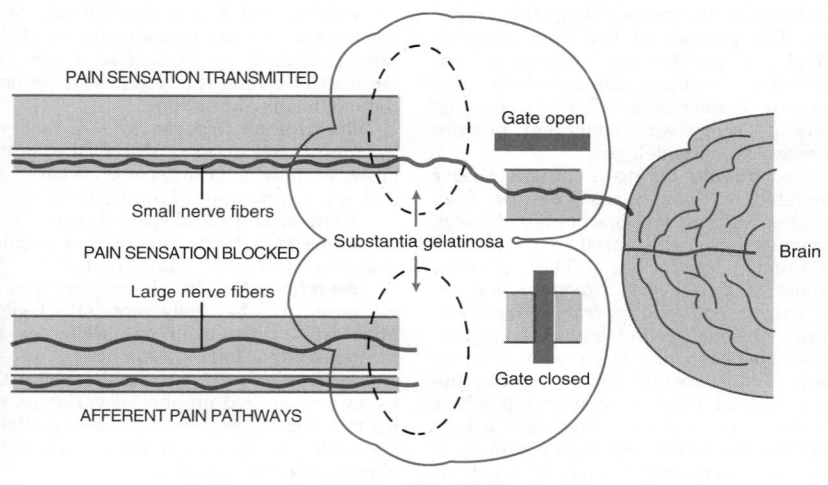

PAIN SENSATION TRANSMITTED

Gate open

Small nerve fibers

PAIN SENSATION BLOCKED — Substantia gelatinosa

Large nerve fibers

Brain

Gate closed

AFFERENT PAIN PATHWAYS

Spinal Cord

The gate-control theory of pain. From Linton et al., 2000.

Health, in this theory, is a continuously changing process that humans participate in co-creating. Health is human becoming. It is not the opposite of disease, nor is it a state that exists. *Disease* is viewed as a pattern of the human being's interrelationship with the world.

Nursing is both science and art. The science is nursing's abstract body of knowledge lived through the art in service to people. Three principles of this theory comprise the abstract knowledge base used to guide nursing research and practice. The principles of *structuring meaning multidimensionally, co-creating rhythmical patterns of relating,* and *co-transcending with the possibles* provide the underpinnings for practice and research.

There is a particular nursing practice methodology, the only one that evolves directly from a nursing theory. Parse's practice methodology specifies that the nurse be truly present with the person and family illuminating meaning, synchronizing rhythms, and mobilizing transcendence. Persons choose their own patterns of health, reflective of their values. The nurse is *there with* the person and family as they uncover meanings and make decisions about their life situations. True presence is an unconditional love grounded in the belief that individuals know the *way.*

Parse has also constructed a research methodology congruent with her theory and unique to nursing. Her research methodology offers the researcher the opportunity to study universal lived experiences from the perspective of the people living the experiences. The purpose of her basic research method is to uncover the meaning of lived experiences to enhance the knowledge base of nursing. Parse has contributed to nursing science a theory with congruent practice and research methodologies.

t. of human caring a nursing theory formulated by Jean WATSON, derived from the values and assumptions of metaphysical, phenomenological-existential, and spiritual conceptual orientations. The primary concepts of the theory, *transpersonal human caring* and *caring transactions,* are multidimensional giving and receiving responses between a nurse and another person. Transpersonal human caring implies a special kind of relationship where both the nurse and the other have a high regard for the whole person in a process of being and becoming. Caring transactions provide a coming together in a lived moment, an actual caring occasion that involves choice and action by both the nurse and another.

Person (other) is defined as an experiencing and perceiving "being in the world," possessing three spheres; mind, body, and soul. Person is also defined as a living growing gestalt with a unique phenomenal field of subjective reality.

The *environment* includes an objective physical or material world and a spiritual world. Watson defines the *world* as including all forces in the universe as well as a person's immediate environment. Critical to this definition is the concept of transcendence of the physical world that is bound in time and space, making contact with the emotional and spiritual world by the mind and soul.

Health is more than the absence of disease. Health is unity and harmony within the mind, body, and soul and is related to the congruence between the self as perceived and the self as experienced.

Nursing is defined as a human science and an activity of art, centered on persons and human health-illness experiences. The goal of nursing is to help persons gain a higher level of harmony within the mind, body and soul. *Nursing practice* is founded on the human-to-human caring process and a commitment to caring as a moral ideal. The activities of nursing are guided by Watson's ten carative FACTORS, which offer a descriptive topology of interventions. The nursing process is incorporated in these carative factors as "creative problem-solving caring process," a broad approach to nursing that seeks connections and relations rather than separations.

information t. a mathematical theory dealing with messages or signals, the distortion produced by statistical noise, and methods of coding that reduce distortion to the irreducible minimum.

information processing t. a theory of learning that focuses on internal, cognitive processes in which the learner is viewed as a seeker and processor of information.

Kantian t. deontological theory.

Lamarck's t. the theory that acquired characteristics may be inherited.

Metchnikoff t. the theory that harmful elements in the body are attacked by phagocytes, causing inflammation; see also METCHNIKOFF THEORY.

middle range t. a testable theory that contains a limited number of variables, and is limited in scope as well, yet is of sufficient generality to be useful with a variety of clinical research questions.

nursing t. 1. a framework designed to organize knowledge and explain phenomena

WINDOW ON THEORY OF HUMAN CARING

Expanded dimensions of human caring theory are embedded in an ethic and human value of caring as a moral ideal, with an ontological and epistemological commitment to preserve and restore the human mind-body-spirit in theory and practice. Thus, human caring-healing becomes relational, connected, transpersonal, and intersubjective, thereby opening up a higher energy field-consciousness that has metaphysical, spiritual, transcendent potentialities.

Just as arts and humanities and culturally diverse experiences can help us in seeing the higher level dimensions of caring-healing in nursing, the metaphor of a hologram provides a new science language as well as a new gestalt for viewing the transpersonal caring-healing human field-consciousness phenomena:

- The whole caring-healing consciousness is contained in a single caring moment.
- The one caring and the one being cared for are interconnected; caring-healing process is connected with other humans and to the higher energy of the universe.
- The caring-healing consciousness of the nurse is communicated to the one being cared for.
- Caring-healing consciousness exists through time and space and is dominant over physical illness.

At a new level in nursing's caring-healing consciousness, regardless of one's theoretical inclinations, there is the continual need to question and be open to new possibilities. Expanded human caring-healing theory provides a new metaparadigm, consistent with Nightingale, as well as with contemporary nursing theories and emergent views of science.

JEAN WATSON, PHD, RN, FAAN

n nursing, at a more concrete and specific level than a CONCEPTUAL MODEL or a META-PARADIGM. 2. The study and development of theoretical frameworks in nursing.

obligation-based t. deontological theory.

quantum t. radiation and absorption of energy occur in quantities (quanta) that vary in size with the frequency of the radiation.

recapitulation t. ontogeny recapitulates phylogeny; see also RECAPITULATION THEORY.

rights-based t. a type of ethical theory under which the language of RIGHTS provides the basic terminology for ethical and political theory; it maintains that a democratic society must protect individuals and allow all to pursue personal goals. The idea of primacy of rights has been strongly disputed by, for example, utilitarians and Marxists. Individual interests often conflict with communal or institutional interests, as has been seen in efforts to reform the health care system. A prominent rights-based theory is what is known as *liberal individualism.*

teleological t. a type of ethical theory that takes judgments of the value of the consequences of action as basic. Utilitarianism is the most prominent consequence-based theory; it accepts one and only one basic principle of ethics, the principle of utility, which asserts that we ought always to produce the maximal balance of positive value over negative consequences (or the least possible negative consequence, if only undesirable results can be achieved).

Young-Helmholtz t. the theory that color vision depends on three sets of retinal receptors, corresponding to the colors of red, green, and violet.

theque (tek) [Fr.] a round or oval collection, or nest, of melanin-containing nevus cells occurring at the dermoepidermal junction of the skin or in the dermis proper.

therapeutic (ther″ah-pu′tik) 1. pertaining to therapy. 2. curative; effective.

therapist (ther′ah-pist) a health care professional skilled in the corrective treatment of disease or other disorders. In several allied health fields, therapist is the highest professional rank, usually requiring a minimum of a baccalaureate degree. The therapist generally has both a theoretical and practical knowledge of the profession and is able to plan and implement a program of therapy appropriate for each patient. For names of specific professions, see under the name.

therapy (ther′ah-pe) treatment.

activity t. in the NURSING INTERVENTIONS CLASSIFICATION, a nursing INTERVENTION defined as the prescription of and assistance with specific physical, cognitive, social, and spiritual activities to increase the range, frequency, or duration of an individual's (or group's) activity.

aerosol t. see AEROSOL THERAPY.

T

animal-assisted t. in the NURSING IN-
TERVENTIONS CLASSIFICATION, a nursing INTER-
VENTION defined as the purposeful use of
animals to provide affection, attention, diversion, and relaxation.

anticoagulant t. see ANTICOAGULANT
THERAPY.

antineoplastic t. see ANTINEOPLASTIC
THERAPY.

antiplatelet t. the use of platelet INHIBI-
TORS such as ASPIRIN, DIPYRIDAMOLE, or SULFIN-
PYRAZONE, to inhibit platelet adhesion or
aggregation and so prevent thrombosis,
alter the course of atherosclerosis, or prolong vascular graft patency.

art t. in the NURSING INTERVENTIONS CLAS-
SIFICATION, a nursing INTERVENTION defined as
facilitation of communication through draw-
ings or other art forms.

aversion t., aversive t. a form of BEHAVIOR
THERAPY that uses aversive conditioning,
pairing undesirable behavior or symptoms
with unpleasant stimulation in order to
reduce or eliminate the behavior of symptoms. The term is sometimes used synonymously with aversive CONDITIONING.

behavior t. see BEHAVIOR THERAPY.

carbon dioxide–oxygen t. see CARBON
DIOXIDE–OXYGEN THERAPY.

chest physical t. see under PHYSICAL
THERAPY.

client-centered t. a form of psychotherapy in which the emphasis is on the
patient's self-discovery, interpretation, conflict resolution, and reorganization of values
and life approach, which are enabled by the
warm, nondirective, unconditionally accepting support of the therapist, who reflects
and clarifies the patient's discoveries.

cognitive t., cognitive-behavioral t. a
directive form of psychotherapy based on
the theory that emotional problems result
from distorted attitudes and ways of thinking that can be corrected. Using techniques
drawn in part from behavior therapy, the
therapist actively seeks to guide the patient
in altering or revising negative or erroneous
perceptions and attitudes.

collapse t. a formerly common treatment for pulmonary TUBERCULOSIS in
which the diseased lung was collapsed
in order to immobilize it and allow it to
rest. PNEUMONOLYSIS and THORACOPLASTY are
methods still sometimes used to collapse a
lung and allow access during thoracic surgery.

combined modality t. treatment of
cancer using two or more types of therapy,
such as with CHEMORADIOTHERAPY. Called also
multimodality therapy.

compression t. treatment of venou
INSUFFICIENCY, VARICOSE VEINS, or venous ul
ceration of the lower limbs by having th
patient wear compressing garments such a
SUPPORT HOSE.

continuous renal replacement t. HE
MODIALYSIS or HEMOFILTRATION done 24 hour
a day for an extended period, usually in
critically ill patient.

convulsive t. treatment of mental dis
orders, primarily depression, by induction c
CONVULSIONS. The type almost universall
used now is ELECTROCONVULSIVE THERAP
(ECT), in which the convulsions are induce
by electric current. In the past, drugs wer
sometimes used.

couples t. marital t.

diet t. treatment of disease by regula
tion of the DIET.

**electroconvulsive t. (ECT), electro
shock t.** see ELECTROCONVULSIVE THERAPY.

endocrine t. treatment of disease b
means of HORMONES; called also hormonal o
hormone therapy.

estrogen replacement t. administra
tion of an estrogen to treat estrogen defi
ciency, such as that occurring afte
menopause; there are a number of indica
tions, including the prevention of postmen
opausal osteoporosis and coronary arter
disease, and the prevention and treatmen
of vasomotor symptoms such as hot flashe
and of thinning of the skin and vagina
epithelium, atrophic vaginitis, and vulva
atrophy. In women with a uterus, a proges
tational agent is usually included to preven
endometrial hyperplasia. Called also hor
mone replacement therapy.

exercise t.: ambulation in the NURSIN
INTERVENTIONS CLASSIFICATION, a nursing IN
TERVENTION defined as promotion of an
assistance with walking to maintain o
restore autonomic and voluntary body func
tions during treatment and recovery fron
illness or injury.

exercise t.: balance in the NURSIN
INTERVENTIONS CLASSIFICATION, a nursing IN
TERVENTION defined as use of specific activ
ities, postures, and movements to maintain
enhance, or restore BALANCE.

exercise t.: joint mobility in the NURS
ING INTERVENTIONS CLASSIFICATION, a nursin
INTERVENTION defined as the use of active o
passive body movement to maintain o
restore joint flexibility.

exercise t.: muscle control in the NURS
ING INTERVENTIONS CLASSIFICATION, a nursin
INTERVENTION defined as the use of specifi
activity or exercise protocols to enhance o
restore controlled body movement.

family t. 1. GROUP THERAPY of the mem
bers of a family, exploring and improvin

family relationships and processes, under-standing and modifying home influences that contribute to mental disorder in one or more family members, and improving communication and collective, constructive methods of problem-solving. 2. in the NURS-ING INTERVENTIONS CLASSIFICATION, a nursing INTERVENTION defined as assisting family members to move their family toward a more productive way of living.

gold t. chrysotherapy.

group t. see GROUP THERAPY.

helium-oxygen t. see HELIUM-OXYGEN THERAPY.

hemodialysis t. in the NURSING INTERVEN-TIONS CLASSIFICATION, a nursing INTERVENTION defined as management of extracorporeal passage of the patient's blood through a HEMODIALYZER. See also HEMODIALYSIS.

hemofiltration t. in the NURSING INTER-VENTIONS CLASSIFICATION, a nursing INTERVEN-TION defined as cleansing of acutely ill patient's blood via a hemofilter controlled by the patient's hydrostatic pressure. See also HEMOFILTRATION.

highly active antiretroviral t. (HAART) the aggressive use of extremely potent antiretroviral agents in the treatment of human immunodeficiency virus infection.

hormonal t., hormone t. endocrine therapy.

hormone replacement t. the adminis-tration of hormones to correct a deficiency; usually used to denote estrogen replacement THERAPY occurring after menopause.

host modulating t. efforts to control PERIODONTAL DISEASE by directly targeting the host response; an example is the use of drugs that do this, such as sub-antimicro-bial doses of DOXYCYCLINE, NONSTEROIDAL ANTI-INFLAMMATORY DRUGS, or BISPHOSPHONATES.

humidification t., humidity t. the ther-apeutic use of air supersaturated with water to prevent or correct a moisture deficit in the respiratory tract; see also HUMIDITY THERAPY.

immunosuppressive t. therapeutic IM-MUNOSUPPRESSION.

inhalation t. the term formerly used for RESPIRATORY CARE (def. 3).

intravenous t., IV t. in the NURSING INTERVENTIONS CLASSIFICATION, a nursing IN-TERVENTION defined as administration and monitoring of INTRAVENOUS INFUSIONS of fluids and medications.

leech t. in the NURSING INTERVENTIONS CLASSIFICATION, a nursing INTERVENTION de-fined as the application of medicinal LEECHES to help drain replanted or transplanted tissue engorged with venous blood.

marital t. a type of family therapy aimed at understanding and treating one or both members of a couple in the context of a distressed relationship, but not necessarily addressing the discordant relationship it-self. In the past, the term has also been used in a narrower sense to mean what is defined as *marriage therapy,* but that is increasingly considered a subset of marital therapy. Called also couples therapy.

marriage t. a subset of marital therapy that focuses specifically on the bond of marriage between two people, enhancing and preserving it.

milieu t. 1. treatment, usually in a psychiatric treatment center, that empha-sizes the provision of an environment and activities appropriate to the patient's emo-tional and interpersonal needs. 2. in the NURSING INTERVENTIONS CLASSIFICATION, a nurs-ing INTERVENTION defined as the use of people, resources, and events in the pa-tient's immediate environment to promote optimal psychosocial functioning.

multimodality t. combined modality therapy.

music t. 1. the use of music to effect positive changes in the psychological, phy-sical, cognitive, or social functioning of individuals with health or educational prob-lems. Music therapy is used for a wide variety of conditions, including mental dis-orders, developmental and learning dis-abilities, Alzheimer's disease and other conditions related to aging, brain injury, substance abuse, and physical disability. It is also used for the management of acute and chronic pain and for the reduction of stress. 2. in the NURSING INTERVENTIONS CLAS-SIFICATION, a nursing INTERVENTION defined as using music to help achieve a specific change in behavior or feeling.

neoadjuvant t. in single-agent therapy or combined modality therapy for cancer, initial use of one modality, such as CHEMO-THERAPY or RADIOTHERAPY, to decrease tumor burden prior to use of another modality, usually surgery.

nutrition t. in the NURSING INTERVENTIONS CLASSIFICATION, a nursing INTERVENTION de-fined as administration of food and fluids to support metabolic processes of a patient who is malnourished or at high risk for becoming malnourished. See also NUTRITION.

occupational t. see OCCUPATIONAL THER-APY.

optometric vision t. a treatment plan prescribed to correct or improve specific dysfunctions of the vision system; it in-cludes, but is not limited to, the treatment of STRABISMUS (turned eye), other dysfunc-tions of BINOCULARITY (eye teaming),

T

AMBLYOPIA (lazy eye), ACCOMMODATION (eye focusing), ocular motor function (general eye movement ability), and visual-motor and visual-perceptual abilities.

oral rehydration t. (ORT) oral administration of a solution of electrolytes and carbohydrates in the treatment of DEHYDRATION.

oxygen t. see OXYGEN THERAPY.

peritoneal dialysis t. in the NURSING INTERVENTIONS CLASSIFICATION, a nursing INTERVENTION defined as administration and monitoring of dialysis solution into and out of the peritoneal cavity. See also PERITONEAL DIALYSIS.

physical t. see PHYSICAL THERAPY.

play t. see PLAY THERAPY.

pulp canal t. root canal therapy.

PUVA t. [*psoralen + ultraviolet A*], a form of PHOTOCHEMOTHERAPY for skin disorders such as PSORIASIS and VITILIGO; oral PSORALEN administration is followed two hours later by exposure to ULTRAVIOLET A radiation.

radiation t. see RADIATION THERAPY.

recreation t. in the NURSING INTERVENTIONS CLASSIFICATION, a nursing INTERVENTION defined as the purposeful use of recreation to promote relaxation and enhancement of social skills.

reminiscence t. in the NURSING INTERVENTIONS CLASSIFICATION, a nursing INTERVENTION defined as using the recall of past events, feelings, and thoughts to facilitate pleasure, quality of life, or adaptation to present circumstances.

renal replacement t. therapy such as HEMODIALYSIS or TRANSPLANTATION that takes the place of nonfunctioning kidneys. See also continuous renal replacement THERAPY.

replacement t. treatment to replace deficient formation or loss of body products by administration of the natural body products or synthetic substitutes. See also REPLACEMENT. Called also substitution therapy.

respiratory t. RESPIRATORY CARE.

root canal t. that aspect of ENDODONTICS dealing with the treatment of diseases of the dental pulp, consisting of partial (PULPOTOMY) or complete (PULPECTOMY) extirpation of the diseased pulp, cleaning and sterilization of the empty ROOT CANAL, enlarging and shaping the canal to receive sealing material, and obturation of the canal with a nonirritating hermetic sealing agent. Called also pulp canal therapy.

shock t. obsolete term for convulsive therapy.

simple relaxation t. in the NURSING INTERVENTIONS CLASSIFICATION, a nursing INTERVENTION defined as the use of techniques to encourage and elicit relaxation for the purpose of decreasing undesirable signs and symptoms such as pain, muscle tension, or anxiety.

speech t. the use of special techniques for correction of SPEECH DISORDERS.

substitution t. replacement therapy.

swallowing t. in the NURSING INTERVENTIONS CLASSIFICATION, a nursing INTERVENTION defined as facilitating SWALLOWING and preventing complications of impaired swallowing.

thrombolytic t. the administration of drugs for THROMBOLYSIS (dissolution of a thrombus in an artery), to reduce the size of occlusion and thereby reduce damage to muscular tissue; the coronary artery is a commonly used site. Agents commonly used are STREPTOKINASE and tissue plasminogen activator (t-PA).

thyroid replacement t. treatment of HYPOTHYROIDISM by administration of THYROXINE, usually in the form of LEVOTHYROXINE sodium. Called also thyrotherapy.

ultraviolet t. see ULTRAVIOLET THERAPY.

therm(o)- word element [Gr.], *heat.*

thermal (ther'mal) pertaining to heat.

thermalgesia (therm″al-je′ze-ah) painful sensation produced by heat.

thermalgia (ther-mal'jah) causalgia.

thermanalgesia (therm″an-al-je′ze-ah) thermanesthesia.

thermanesthesia (therm″an-es-the′zhah) absence of temperature sense.

thermelometer (ther″mel-om′ĕ-ter) an electric thermometer for measuring small temperature changes.

thermesthesia (therm″es-the′zhah) temperature sense.

thermesthesiometer (therm″es-the″ze-om′ĕ-ter) an instrument for measuring sensibility to heat.

thermhyperesthesia (therm″hi-per-es-the′zhah) thermohyperesthesia.

thermhypesthesia (therm″hi-pes-the′zhah) decreased sensibility to high temperatures.

thermic (ther'mik) pertaining to heat.

thermistor (ther-mis'tor) a thermometer whose resistance varies with ambient temperature and so is able to measure extremely small temperature changes.

thermocautery (ther″mo-kaw'ter-e) cauterization by a heated wire or point.

thermochemistry (ther″mo-kem'is-tre) the aspect of physical chemistry dealing with temperature changes that accompany chemical reactions.

thermocoagulation (ther″mo-ko-ag″u-la′shun) coagulation of tissue with high-frequency currents.

thermocouple (ther′mo-kup″l) a pair of dissimilar electric conductors so joined that with the application of heat an electromotive force is established; used for measuring small temperature differences.

thermodiffusion (ther″mo-dĭ-fu′zhun) diffusion due to a temperature gradient.

thermodilution (ther″mo-di-loo′shun) a method of measuring ventricular blood volume and cardiac output. A series of 3 to 5 injections of a solution of known temperature is followed by calculation by a computerized sensor or thermistor of the average changes in temperature.

thermoduric (ther″mo-du′rik) able to endure high temperatures.

thermodynamics (ther″mo-di-nam′iks) the branch of science dealing with heat, work, and energy, their interconversion, and problems related thereto.

thermoexcitory (ther″mo-ek-si′tor-e) stimulating production of bodily heat.

thermogenesis (ther″mo-jen′ĕ-sis) the production of heat, especially within the animal body. adj., **thermogenet′ic, thermogen′ic.**

thermogram (ther′mo-gram) 1. a graphic record of temperature variations. 2. the visual record obtained by THERMOGRAPHY; called also thermograph.

thermograph (ther′mo-graf) an instrument for recording temperature variations. 1. thermogram (def. 2). 2. the apparatus used in THERMOGRAPHY.

thermography (ther-mog′rah-fe) a technique wherein an infrared camera photographically portrays the body's surface temperature, based on self-emanating infrared radiations; used as a diagnostic aid in the detection of breast tumors and the assessment of rheumatic joints; also used in the study of pain. adj., thermograph′ic.

thermohyperalgesia (ther″mo-hi″per-al-je′ze-ah) extreme thermalgesia.

thermohyperesthesia (ther″mo-hi″per-es-the′zhah) extreme sensitiveness to heat; called also thermhyperesthesia.

thermoinhibitory (ther″mo-in-hib′ĭ-tor″e) retarding the generation of bodily heat.

thermolabile (ther″mo-la′bil) easily affected by heat.

thermolysis (ther-mol′ĭ-sis) 1. chemical dissociation by means of heat. 2. dissipation of bodily heat by radiation, evaporation, or other means. adj., **thermolyt′ic.**

thermomassage (ther″mo-mah-sahzh′) massage with heat.

thermometer (ther-mom′ĕ-ter) an instrument for determining temperatures, in principle making use of a substance (such as alcohol or mercury) with a physical property that varies with temperature and is susceptible of measurement on some defined scale.

axilla t. a clinical THERMOMETER that is placed in the axilla.

Celsius t. one that uses the Celsius SCALE.

centigrade t. one having the interval between two established reference points divided into 100 equal units, such as the Celsius THERMOMETER.

clinical t. one used to determine the temperature of the human body.

electronic t. a clinical THERMOMETER that uses a sensor based on THERMISTORS, solid-state electronic devices whose electrical characteristics change with temperature. The reading is recorded within seconds, some having a red light or other device to indicate when maximum temperature is reached. Available models include handheld, desk-top, and wall-mounted units, all having probes that are inserted orally or rectally.

Fahrenheit t. one that uses the Fahrenheit SCALE.

Kelvin t. one that uses the Kelvin SCALE.

oral t. a clinical THERMOMETER whose mercury containing bulb is placed under the tongue.

T

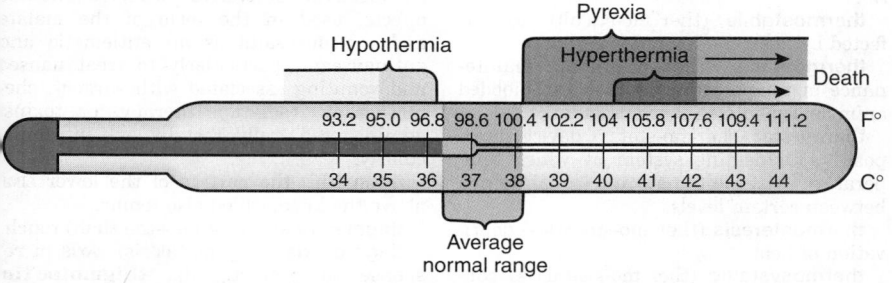

Temperatures on Celsius and Fahrenheit thermometers related to temperature ranges. From Elkin et al., 2000.

recording *t.* a temperature-sensitive instrument by which the temperature to which it is exposed is continuously recorded.

rectal *t.* a clinical THERMOMETER that is inserted in the rectum.

resistance *t.* one that uses the electric resistance of metals (THERMOCOUPLE) to determine temperature.

self-registering *t.* 1. recording thermometer. 2. one that registers the maximum or minimum temperature attained in the measurement.

tympanic *t.* an electronic clinical THERMOMETER that gives a digital reading in less than two seconds. Second-generation tympanic thermometers work by monitoring the temperature when the ear opening is sealed.

thermometry (ther-mom′ĕ-tre) measurement of temperature.

thermophile (ther′mo-fīl) a microorganism that grows best at elevated temperatures. adj., **thermophil′ic.**

thermophore (ther′mo-for) 1. a device or apparatus for retaining heat. 2. an instrument for estimating heat sensibility.

thermopile (ther′mo-pīl) a number of thermocouples in series, used to increase sensitivity to change in temperature or for direct conversion of heat into electric energy.

thermoplacentography (ther″mo-plas″en-tog′rah-fe) use of thermography for determination of the site of placental attachment.

thermoplegia (ther″mo-ple′jah) heat stroke or sunstroke.

thermoreceptor (ther″mo-re-sep′tor) a nerve ending sensitive to stimulation by heat.

thermoregulation (ther″mo-reg″u-la′-shun) 1. heat regulation. 2. thermostasis.

ineffective *t.* a NURSING DIAGNOSIS accepted by the North American Nursing Diagnosis Association, defined as a state in which an individual's temperature fluctuates between HYPOTHERMIA and HYPERTHERMIA.

thermostabile (ther″mo-sta′b'l) not affected by heat.

thermostasis (ther″mo-sta′sis) maintenance of temperature, as in warm-blooded animals; called also thermoregulation.

thermostat (ther′mo-stat) a device interposed in a heating system by which temperature is automatically maintained between certain levels.

thermosteresis (ther″mo-stĕ-re′sis) deprivation of heat.

thermosystaltic (ther″mo-sis-tal′tik) contracting under the stimulus of heat.

thermotaxis (ther″mo-tak′sis) 1. normal adjustment of bodily temperature. 2. TAXIS in response to the stimulation of a temperature gradient. adj., **thermotac′tic, thermotax′ic.**

thermotherapy (ther″mo-ther′ah-pe) therapeutic use of heat.

thermotonometer (ther″mo-to-nom′ĕ-ter) an instrument for measuring the amount of muscular contraction produced by heat.

thermotropism (ther-mot′ro-pizm) TROPISM in response to an increase in temperature. adj., **thermotrop′ic.**

thesaurus (thĕ-saw′rus) in online information retrieval, a controlled VOCABULARY showing relationships between terms; it is developed from a dynamic, growing document collection.

thi(o)- word element [Gr.], *sulfur.*

thiabendazole (thi″ah-ben′dah-zōl) a broad-spectrum ANTHELMINTIC used in the treatment of cutaneous LARVA migrans, visceral LARVA migrans, STRONGYLOIDIASIS, and TRICHINOSIS.

thiamin (thi′ah-min) thiamine.

thiaminase (thi-am′ĭ-nās) an enzyme that catalyzes the splitting of thiamine into a pyrimidine and a thiazole derivative.

thiamine (thi′ah-min) vitamin B₁, a component of the B complex group of vitamins, found in various foodstuffs and present in the free state in blood plasma and cerebrospinal fluid. Deficiency results in neurological symptoms, cardiovascular dysfunction, edema, and reduced intestinal motility. See also VITAMIN.

thiamylal (thi-am′ĭ-lal) an ultrashort-acting THIOBARBITURATE used as an intravenous anesthetic.

thiazide (thi′ah-zīd) any of a group of BENZOTHIADIAZINE SULFONAMIDE derivatives, typified by CHLOROTHIAZIDE; their primary medicinal use is as diuretics. See thiazide DIURETICS.

thiemia (thi-e′me-ah) sulfur in the blood.

thiethylperazine (thi-eth″il-per′ah-zēn) a PHENOTHIAZINE derivative with ANTIHISTAMINIC effects, used in the form of the malate and maleate salts as an antiemetic and antinauseant, particularly to treat nausea and vomiting associated with surgery, chemotherapy, radiation therapy, or toxins administered orally, rectally, and intramuscularly.

thigh (thi) the portion of the lower LIMB above the knee; called also femur.

thigmesthesia (thig″mes-the′zhah) touch.

thigmotaxis (thig″mo-tak′sis) TAXIS in response to contact. adj., **thigmotac′tic thigmotax′ic.**

thigmotropism (thig-mot′ro-pizm) TROP-
ISM in response to the stimulus of contact.
adj., **thigmotrop′ic.**

thimerosal (thi-mer′o-sal) a mercury-containing compound used as a topical antifungal and antibacterial agent.

thinking (thingk′ing) ideational mental
activity (in contrast to emotional activity);
the flow of ideas, symbols, and associations
that brings forth concepts and reasons.

　autistic t. self-absorption; preoccupation with inner thoughts, daydreams, fantasies, delusions, drives, and personal logic. It
is egocentric, subjective thinking lacking
objectivity and preferring a narcissistic,
inner, private reality to that with external
validity. Used interchangeably with dereistic THINKING, although differing in emphasis.
Called also autism.

　critical t. a style of reasoning that
involves a complex process of reflection and
analysis. See accompanying table.

　dereistic t. thinking not in accordance
with the facts of reality and experience and
following illogical, idiosyncratic reasoning.
Used interchangeably with autistic THINK-
ING, although not an exact synonym: dereistic emphasizes disconnection from reality
and autistic emphasizes preoccupation with
inner experience. Called also dereism.

　magical t. that characterized by the
belief that thinking or wishing something
can cause it to occur.

　primary process t. in psychoanalytic
theory, primitive thought processes deriving
from the id and marked by illogical form,
preverbal content, an emphasis on immediate wish fulfillment, and an equating of
thought and action. Such processes are
characteristic of childhood and of dreams.

　secondary process t. in psychoanalytic theory, the more sophisticated thought
processes, based on logic, obeying the rules
of causality, and consistent with external
reality. Such processes are characteristic of
mature conscious thought.

thiobarbiturate (thi″o-bahr-bich′er-it) any
of a group of compounds chemically related

to BARBITURATES and with barbituratelike
effects.

thiobarbituric acid (thi″o-bahr″bĭ-tu′rik)
a compound that differs from BARBITURIC
ACID only by the presence of a sulfur atom
instead of an oxygen atom at the number 2
carbon; it is the parent compound of a class
of drugs, the THIOBARBITURATES.

thiocyanate (thi″o-si′ah-nāt) the
S=C=N⁻ anion or a salt or ester containing this ion. Thiocyanate is produced in the
metabolism of cysteine and detoxification of
cyanide and is excreted in the urine.

thioguanine (thi″o-gwah′nēn) a GUANINE
analogue in which sulfur replaces the oxygen atom of guanine; used as an antineoplastic AGENT almost exclusively in the
treatment of acute myelogenous leukemia
and acute lymphoblastic leukemia. Called
also 6-thioguanine and 6-TG.

thiol (thi′ol) 1. sulfhydryl. 2. any organic
compound containing the —SH group
bound to carbon.

thionine (thi′o-nēn) a dark-green powder,
purple in solution, used as a metachromatic
stain in microscopy.

thiopental (thi″o-pen′tal) an ultrashort-
acting BARBITURATE, used in the form of the
sodium salt as an intravenous anesthetic, to
control convulsions produced during inhalation anesthesia, and in psychiatry for NAR-
COANALYSIS.

thioridazine (thi″o-rid′ah-zēn) a PHE-
NOTHIAZINE used orally in the form of the
base or the hydrochloride salt as an ANTI-
PSYCHOTIC AGENT and SEDATIVE.

thiosulfate (thi″o-sul′fāt) any salt of thio-
sulfuric acid; produced in the metabolism of
cysteine and excreted in the urine.

thiotepa (thi″o-te′pah) a cytotoxic ALKYL-
ATING AGENT used as an antineoplastic AGENT
in the treatment of cancer of the breast,
ovary, or bladder, pericardial or pleural
effusions secondary to malignancy, and
Hodgkin's disease; used by intracavitary,
intratumor, intravesical, or intravenous administration.

thiothixene (thi″o-thik′sēn) an ANTIPSYCHO-
TIC AGENT that is a THIOXANTHENE derivative;
administered orally or intramuscularly as
the base or the hydrochloride salt.

thioxanthene (thi″o-zan′thēn) 1. a three-
ring compound structurally related to phenothiazine. 2. any of a class of structurally
related ANTIPSYCHOTIC AGENTS, including
chlorprothixene and thiothixene.

thirst (therst) a sensation, often referred
to the mouth and throat, associated with a
craving for drink; ordinarily interpreted as
a desire for water.

T

thixotropism (thik-sot′ro-pizm) thixotropy.

thixotropy (thik-sot′rah-pe) the property of certain gels of becoming fluid when shaken or otherwise agitated and then becoming semisolid again at rest.

thlipsencephalus (thlip″sen-sef′ah-lus) a malformed fetus with a defective or absent skull.

Thompson (tomp′son) Julia (1907–1972). First full-time Washington lobbyist for the American Nurses' Association. As a lobbyist, she was concerned with the improvement of education, working conditions, and economic and professional status in nursing. She also worked to improve Social Security benefits and for the passage of the Medicare program.

Thoms (tomz) Adah Belle (ca. 1870–1943). Nursing author, educator, and crusader for equal opportunity for blacks in nursing. Her work included efforts to have black nurses accepted as members of the Red Cross and campaigning for equal rights for black nurses in the Army Nurse Corps.

Thomsen's disease (tom′senz) myotonia congenita.

thorac(o)- word element [Gr.], *chest*. See also words beginning STETH(O)-.

thoracalgia (thor″ah-kal′jah) pain in the chest; see also PLEURODYNIA and COSTALGIA. Called also THORACODYNIA.

thoracectomy (tho″rah-sek′tah-me) thoracotomy with resection of part of a rib.

thoracentesis (thor″ah-sen-te′sis) surgical puncture and drainage of the thoracic cavity; it may be done as an aid to the diagnosis of inflammatory or neoplastic diseases of the lung or pleura, or it may be used as a therapeutic measure to remove accumulations of fluid from the thoracic cavity. Called also pleurocentesis.

The procedure is done with the patient sitting up, the arms and head resting on the overbed table or over the back of a chair which the patient straddles. If unable to sit up, the patient is turned onto the unaffected side. The skin at the site of insertion of the needle is cleansed with an antiseptic, and a local anesthetic is injected. The site most often used is the seventh intercostal space, just below the angle of the scapula.

After the procedure is completed the wound usually is sealed with collodion and covered with a sterile dressing. Then a chest x-ray should be done to detect any pneumothorax. The site is checked frequently for signs of leakage. The total amount and character of the fluid obtained is noted on the patient's chart. Samples of fluid are sent

to the laboratory for evaluation if requested. Immediately following the thoracentesis the patient is positioned on the unaffected side to rest the site of insertion of the trocar and allow it to seal itself. The patient is observed for signs of dizziness, changes in skin color, and respiratory and heart rate changes. Other signs of complications following thoracentesis include excessive coughing, blood-tinged sputum, and tightness of the chest.

Possible aftereffects of the procedure include PNEUMOTHORAX, subcutaneous emphysema (accumulation of air in the tissues of the skin), and bacterial infection. A MEDIASTINAL SHIFT resulting from removal of large amounts of fluid from the thoracic cavity may produce cardiac distress and pulmonary edema.

thoracic (tho̅-ras′ik) pertaining to the chest (thorax); called also pectoral.

t. outlet syndrome compression of the BRACHIAL PLEXUS nerve trunks and subclavian vessels, with pain in the upper limb, paresthesia of fingers, vasomotor symptoms and weakness and wasting of small muscles of the hand; it may be caused by drooping shoulder girdle, a cervical rib (CERVICAL RIB SYNDROME) or fibrous band, an abnormal first rib, continual hyperabduction of the arm (as during sleep), or compression of the edge of the scalenus anterior muscle.

t. surgery surgical procedures involving entrance into the chest cavity. Until techniques for endotracheal ANESTHESIA were perfected, this type of surgery was extremely dangerous because of the possibility of lung collapse. By administering anesthesia under pressure through an endotracheal tube it is now possible to keep one or both

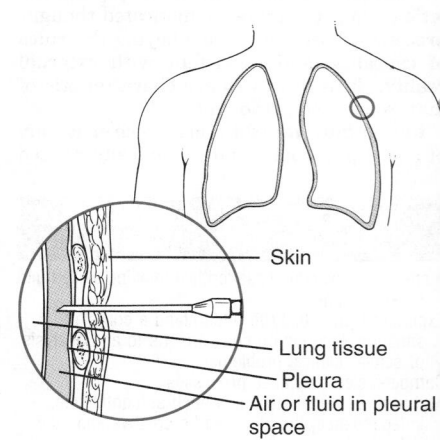

Skin

Lung tissue

Pleura

Air or fluid in pleural space

Technique of thoracentesis. The needle is advanced only as far as the pleural space.

CLASSIFICATION OF THORACIC OUTLET SYNDROMES		
Type 3	Cause	Symptoms
Arterial Thoracic	Chronic compression of the subclavian artery	Severe ischemia of the arm
Neurologic	Usually follows hyperextension of the neck or upper back	Aching, throbbing pain; paresthesia of the neck and arms
Venous Thoracic	External compression of the axillosubclavian vein	Sudden pain, cyanosis, and swelling of arms

lungs expanded, even when they are subjected to atmospheric pressure. Thoracic surgery includes procedures involving the lungs, heart, and great vessels, as well as tracheal resection, esophagogastrectomy, and repair of hiatal hernia. In order to give intelligent care to the patient before and after surgery, one must have adequate knowledge of the anatomy and physiology of the chest and thoracic cavity. It is especially important to know the difference in pressures within and outside the thoracic cavity. (See also discussion of Mechanics of Inflation and Deflation, under LUNG.)

Patient Care. Prior to surgery the care of the patient will depend on the specific operation to be done and the particular disorder requiring surgery. In general, the patient should be given an explanation of the operative procedure anticipated and the type of equipment that will be used in the postoperative period. The patient will be taught the proper method of coughing to remove secretions accumulated in the lungs. Although coughing may be painful in the immediate postoperative period and may require analgesic medication to relieve the discomfort, if the patient understands the need for coughing up the secretions he or she will be more cooperative. Special exercises may be given to preserve muscular action of the shoulder on the affected side and to maintain proper alignment of the upper portion of his or her body and arm. Usually the physical therapist supervises these exercises, but the nursing staff must coordinate them with other aspects of patient care.

Narcotics are rarely given before thoracic surgery because they can depress respiration. Usually the preoperative medication is atropine in combination with a barbiturate.

The development of intensive care units has sharply improved the care of the post-thoracotomy patient. The availability of monitors, ventilators, and special assist devices has increased not only the safety of the operation but also the comfort of the patient. Many patients return from the operating room with endotracheal tubes still in place, ventilated by machines, and monitored with such special equipment as Swan-Ganz catheters for observation of cardiac output, oxygenation, and level of hydration.

During the postoperative period, alteration in respiratory status is a major potential problem for patients having thoracic surgery. Impaired gas exchange can result from atelectasis, pneumothorax, mediastinal shift, bronchopulmonary fistula, pneumonia, pleural effusion, pulmonary edema, narcotics, or abdominal distention. To identify any change in respiratory status, the patient's arterial blood gases are serially monitored, breath sounds are auscultated, and the rate and character of respirations are assessed. To facilitate removal of obstructive mucus and other secretions in the air passages the patient is encouraged to deep breathe and cough every one to two hours. Chest physical therapy may be ordered to help mobilize the secretions so that they are more easily coughed up. The amount and character of sputum is noted and recorded. If necessary, nasotracheal suctioning may be done to help clear the air passages. Oxygen may be administered to prevent anoxia.

The patient is also periodically assessed for pain, abdominal distention, and alteration in cardiac function related to decreased cardiac output, arrhythmias, or cardiac tamponade. If the pericardial sac becomes filled with fluid and produces an acute cardiac tamponade, an emergency pericardiocentesis may be necessary.

Almost all patients having thoracic surgery will have chest tubes. (One exception is the patient who has had a lung removed. In this case fluid is deliberately allowed to accumulate in the pleural space to prevent mediastinal shift.) Chest tubes are attached to closed drainage systems to avoid pneumothorax and allow for drainage of the pleural space and gradual reexpansion of the lung. (See CHEST TUBE for care.)

As the operative site heals and the lung expands, the chest tubes can be safely removed. After their removal an airtight bandage is applied to the area. As a precaution

T

against leakage of air into the chest cavity, the physician may apply petrolatum to the edges of the wound before applying the dressing.

thoracoacromial   (thor″ah-ko-ah-kro′me-al) pertaining to the chest and acromion.

thoracoceloschisis   (thor″ah-ko-se-los′kĭ-sis) thoracogastroschisis.

thoracocentesis   (thor″ah-ko-sen-te′sis) thoracentesis.

thoracocyllosis   (thor″ah-ko-sĭ-lo′sis) deformity of the thorax.

thoracocyrtosis   (thor″ah-ko-sir-to′sis) abnormal curvature of the chest wall.

thoracodelphus   (thor″ah-ko-del′fus) conjoined twins with one head, two upper limbs, and four lower limbs, the bodies being joined above the navel.

thoracodidymus   (thor″ah-ko-did′ĭ-mus) thoracopagus.

thoracodynia   (thor″ah-ko-din′e-ah) thoracalgia.

thoracogastroschisis   (thor″ah-ko-gas-tros′kĭ-sis) a developmental ANOMALY consisting of a fissure of the thorax and abdomen, resulting from faulty closure of the body wall along the midventral line; see also CELOSOMIA. Called also thoracoceloschisis.

thoracolumbar   (thor″ah-ko-lum′bar) pertaining to the thoracic and lumbar vertebrae.

thoracolysis   (thor″ah-kol′ĭ-sis) the freeing of adhesions of the chest wall.

thoracomelus   (thor″ah-kom′ĕ-lus) unequal conjoined twins with the parasite twin as a supernumerary limb attached to the thorax.

thoracometer   (thor″ah-kom′ĕ-ter) stethometer.

thoracopagus   (thor″ah-kop′ah-gus) conjoined twins united at the thorax.

thoracopathy   (thor″ah-kop′ah-the) any disease of the thoracic organs or tissues.

thoracoplasty   (thor′ah-ko-plas″te) surgical removal of ribs so that the chest wall collapses a diseased lung; a form of collapse THERAPY.

thoracoschisis   (thor″ah-kos′kĭ-sis) congenital fissure of the chest wall; called also schistothorax.

thoracoscope   (thŏ-rak′o-skōp) an endoscope for examining the pleural cavity through an intercostal space.

thoracoscopy   (thor″ah-kos′kah-pe) examination of the pleural space with a thoracoscope.

thoracostenosis   (thor″ah-ko-stĕ-no′sis) abnormal contraction of the thorax.

thoracostomy   (thor″ah-kos′tah-me) 1. incision of the chest wall, with maintenance of the opening for drainage. 2. the incision so created. See illustration.

thoracotomy   (thor″ah-kot′ah-me) incision of the chest wall; see also THORACIC SURGERY. Called also pleuracotomy and pleurotomy.

thorax   (thor′aks) the part of the body between the neck and abdomen; it is separated from the abdomen by the DIAPHRAGM. Its walls are formed by the 12 pairs of RIBS, attached to the sides of the spine and curving toward the front. The principal organs in the thoracic cavity are the HEART

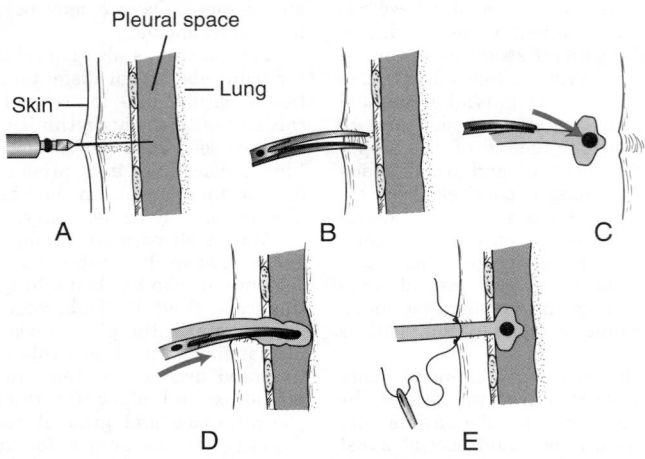

Procedure for thoracostomy. If the procedure is done in an emergency, a local anesthetic is injected at the site of insertion of the thoracostomy tube *(A)* (if a general anesthetic is used, step A is not necessary). The incision is widened *(B)* and the tube inserted *(C)* and *(D)*. To avoid accidental removal, it may be sutured in place *(E)*. The free end of the tube is connected to a closed drainage system.

with its major blood vessels and the LUNGS with the BRONCHI, which bring in the body's air supply. The TRACHEA enters the thorax to connect with the lungs, and the ESOPHAGUS travels through it to connect with the stomach below the diaphragm. See also THORACIC SURGERY. Called also chest and pectus.

Thorazine (thor′ah-zēn) trademark for preparations of CHLORPROMAZINE, an ANTIEMETIC, ANTIPSYCHOTIC AGENT and SEDATIVE.

thorium (thor′e-um) a chemical element, atomic number 90, atomic weight 232.038, symbol Th. (See Appendix 6.)

thought (thawt) the result or product of THINKING.

t. broadcasting the belief that one's thoughts are being broadcast from one's head to the external world.

t. disorder a disturbance in the thought process that is most narrowly defined as disorganized thinking with altered associations, as is characteristic of schizophrenia. The term is often used much more broadly to include any disturbance of thought, such as confusion, hallucinations, or delusions, which affects possession, quantity, or content of thought.

t. stopping a method of overcoming obsessive, phobic, or otherwise distressing thoughts by first concentrating on them and after a short time stopping or interrupting them.

threadworm (thred′werm) any long slender NEMATODE, such as members of the genera *Capillaria* and *Enterobius*.

threat (thret) a warning or declaration of intent to commit harm, injury, or evil.

suicide t. a statement of intent to commit SUICIDE that is accompanied by behavior changes indicative of suicidal tendencies.

threonine (thre′o-nēn) a naturally occurring AMINO ACID, one of the essential amino acids.

threshold (thresh′old) 1. the level that must be reached for an effect to be produced, as the degree of intensity of stimulus that just produces a sensation. 2. that value at which a stimulus just produces a sensation, is just appreciable, or comes just within the limits of perception. 3. renal t.

auditory t. the slightest perceptible sound.

t. of consciousness the lowest limit of SENSIBILITY; the point of CONSCIOUSNESS at which a stimulus is barely perceived.

defibrillation t. DFT; the minimum amount of energy in joules that will consistently terminate ventricular FIBRILLATION.

fibrillation t. the least intensity of an electrical impulse that will cause cardiac tissue to begin FIBRILLATION.

pacing t. the minimal electrical stimulus required to produce consistent cardiac depolarization.

renal t. that concentration of a substance (threshold SUBSTANCE) in plasma at which it begins to be excreted in the urine.

sensing t. in cardiac PACING terminology, the voltage of the minimum signal that consistently activates pulse GENERATOR function.

thrill (thril) a vibration felt by the examiner on palpation; see also FREMITUS.

diastolic t. one felt over the precordium during diastole in advanced aortic insufficiency.

hydatid t. one felt on percussing over a hydatid cyst.

presystolic t. one felt just before the ventricular SYSTOLE over the apex of the heart.

systolic t. one felt over the precordium during ventricular SYSTOLE in aortic stenosis, pulmonary stenosis, and ventricular septal defect.

-thrix word element [Gr.], *hair.*

throat (thrōt) 1. the passage from the mouth to the pharynx; called also fauces. 2. pharynx. 3. the anterior part of the neck.

sore t. inflammation of the throat; see also SORE THROAT.

throb (throb) a pulsating movement or sensation.

thromb(o)- word element [Gr.], *clot; thrombus.*

thrombapheresis (throm″bah-fĕ-re′sis) thrombocytapheresis.

thrombasthenia (throm″bas-the′ne-ah) 1. decreased platelet function; called also thromboasthenia. 2. Glanzmann thrombasthenia.

Glanzmann t. a hereditary platelet abnormality characterized by defective clot retraction, prolonged bleeding time, and related symptoms such as epistaxis and inappropriate bleeding. Clinically there is abnormal glass adhesion and impaired aggregation to ADP, collagen, and thrombin. Called also thrombasthenia and Glanzmann's disease.

thrombectomy (throm-bek′tah-me) excision of a clot from a blood vessel.

medical t. enzymatic dissolution of a blood clot in situ.

thrombin (throm′bin) 1. the activated form of COAGULATION FACTOR II (prothrombin), which catalyzes the conversion of fibrinogen to fibrin. 2. a preparation of this

T

compound prepared from prothrombin of bovine origin, used as a topical HEMOSTATIC.

t. time (TT) the time required for plasma fibrinogen to form thrombin: exogenous thrombin is added to citrated plasma and the time to clot formation is measured. Prolonged TT is seen with abnormalities of fibrinogen and in the presence of heparin or degradation products of fibrin or fibrinogen.

thromboangiitis (throm″bo-an″je-i′tis) inflammation of a blood vessel (VASCULITIS) with THROMBOSIS.

t. obli′terans a disease affecting the medium-sized blood vessels, particularly the arteries of the lower limbs, which can cause severe pain and in serious cases lead to gangrene. The name refers to the clotting, pain, and inflammation occurring in this disease and to the fact that it can obliterate, or destroy, blood vessels. The cause has been thought to be excessive use of tobacco over a long period of time, and the number of cases has diminished strikingly in recent years. The intense pain is caused by THROMBOSIS (formation of blood clots) in the lining of the arteries; when the clots grow larger, the blood flow slows and may stop entirely. Since every part of the body depends on the continuous flow of blood, affected areas such as fingers and toes, for example, soon begin to atrophy or develop ulcers. If the causes of the disease are not completely arrested, amputation may be necessary.

To treat the disease, the patient must stop smoking at once and entirely. This generally results in the partial healing of the affected membrane with a renewed flow of blood. However, more blood may have to be brought to damaged tissue by surgical methods of channeling detours or making canals in the clot itself. Sympathectomy may be tried to prevent any vasospastic component. Minor amputations of gangrenous tissue are often needed.

Special exercises called BUERGER-ALLEN EXERCISES are sometimes used to empty the engorged blood vessels and stimulate collateral circulation. These exercises can be done at home by patients and are usually prescribed to be done several times during the day. Patients are also instructed to avoid wearing any tight clothing, such as tight girdles, rolled garters, constricting belts, and other items that may impair circulation. They should also avoid sitting or standing in one position for long periods of time. Care should be used in the selection of shoes and stockings so that they fit properly and do not cause pressure against the blood vessels. Patients should be told to avoi walking barefoot or otherwise subjectin themselves to the hazards of trauma to th feet and legs. Should such an acciden occur, no matter how minor it may seem the patient must notify a health car provider so that treatment may be begu and infection and ulceration can be pre vented.

thromboarteritis (throm″bo-ahr″ter-i′tis thrombosis associated with arteritis.

thromboasthenia (throm″bo-as-the′ne-ah thrombasthenia.

thromboclasis (throm-bok′lah-sis) th dissolution of a thrombus. adj., **thrombo clas′tic.**

thrombocyst (throm′bo-sist) a sac forme around a clot or thrombus.

thrombocytapheresis (throm″bo-sīt″ah fĕ-re′sis) the selective separation and re moval of PLATELETS (thrombocytes) from withdrawn blood, the remainder of th blood then being retransfused into th donor. Called also plateletpheresis an thrombapheresis.

thrombocyte (throm′bo-sīt) platelet. adj **thrombocyt′ic.**

thrombocythemia (throm″bo-si-the′me ah) thrombocytosis.

essential t., hemorrhagic t. a clinica syndrome with repeated spontaneous he morrhages, either external or into th tissues, and a greatly increased number o circulating platelets, considered one of th MYELOPROLIFERATIVE DISORDERS. Called als megakaryocytic leukemia.

thrombocytolysis (throm″bo-si-tol′ĭ-sis destruction of platelets (thrombocytes).

thrombocytopathy (throm″bo-si-top′ah the) any qualitative disorder of platelets.

thrombocytopenia (throm″bo-si″to-pe′ne ah) decrease in number of PLATELETS i circulating blood; it can result from de creased or defective platelet production o from accelerated platelet destruction. Con ditions related to defective production in clude hypoplastic or aplastic anemia infiltration of bone marrow by malignan cells or myelofibrosis, viral infections, nutri tional deficiency, and thrombocytopeni PURPURA. Increased destruction of platelet can be caused by infections, certain drugs transfusion-related purpuras, idiopathi thrombocytopenic purpura, and dissemi nated intravascular coagulation. adj. **thrombocytope′nic.**

Patient Care. A major concern is preven tion of excessive bleeding from trauma t the mucous membranes, skin, and under lying tissues. All injection and punctur sites, whether from intramuscular, subcuta neous, or intravenous administrations o from bone marrow aspiration and other tests, are carefully monitored for signs of bleeding. These procedures should be coordinated and scheduled so that the number of times the skin is broken is kept to an absolute minimum. If, after withdrawal of a needle or catheter, there is evidence that normal clotting is not taking place, pressure is applied immediately and maintained for 10 to 15 minutes.

Because of the potential for trauma to the rectal mucosa, body temperature should not be taken rectally. Blood pressure cuffs, tourniquets for venipuncture, and similar devices must be used with caution. Hence all persons involved with direct patient care should be apprised of the need for special precautions. When used, antiembolic stockings must be thigh-high, never knee-high.

Patients with a chronic deficit of platelets will need instruction in self-care to avoid inadvertent trauma and irritation. For example, to protect the oral mucosa, a soft toothbrush must be used; dental floss, toothpicks, and other items likely to irritate or cause a break in the mucosa should be avoided. Patients are taught to keep their lips and nasal membranes soft and moist, possibly with KY jelly or some other water-soluble lubricant. An oral intake of fluids above the usual maintenance level is encouraged.

To protect the gastrointestinal mucosa, patients are warned to avoid constipation, extremely rough and hard-to-digest foods such as peanuts and popcorn, and aspirin, steroids, and other drugs known to be irritants. Aspirin, in addition to causing gastrointestinal irritation, also interferes with platelet function.

thrombocytopoiesis (throm″bo-si″to-poi-e′sis) the production of PLATELETS (thrombocytes). adj., **thrombocytopoiet′ic.**

thrombocytosis (throm″bo-si-to′sis) an increase in the number of circulating PLATELETS; it may be essential or primary (see essential THROMBOCYTHEMIA) or secondary to a disease process such as an infection, inflammation, neoplasm, or rheumatoid process. Called also thrombocythemia.

thromboembolism (throm″bo-em′bo-lizm) obstruction of a blood vessel with thrombotic material carried by the blood from the site of origin to plug another vessel.

thromboendarterectomy (throm″bo-en′-dar-ter-ek′-tah-me) excision of an obstructing thrombus together with a portion of the inner lining of the obstructed artery.

thromboendarteritis (throm″bo-en″dar-ter-i′tis) inflammation of the innermost coat of an artery, with thrombus formation.

thromboendocarditis (throm″bo-en″do-kahr-di′tis) nonbacterial thrombotic ENDOCARDITIS.

thrombogenesis (throm″bo-jen′ĕ-sis) clot formation. adj., **thrombogen′ic.**

thromboid (throm′boid) resembling a thrombus.

thrombokinase (throm″bo-ki′nās) the activated form of COAGULATION FACTOR X.

thrombokinetics (throm″bo-ki-net′iks) the dynamics of blood coagulation.

thrombolymphangitis (throm″bo-lim″fan-ji′tis) inflammation of a lymph vessel due to a thrombus.

thrombolysis (throm-bol′ĭ-sis) dissolution of a thrombus.

thrombolytic (throm″bo-lit′ik) 1. dissolving or splitting up a thrombus. 2. an agent such as STREPTOKINASE or UROKINASE that dissolves or splits up a thrombus. See also ANTICOAGULANT and ANTITHROMBOTIC.

thrombon (throm′bon) the portion of the hematopoietic system concerned with platelet formation; the circulating platelets and their precursors.

thrombopathy (throm-bop′ah-the) thrombocytopathy.

thrombopenia (throm″bo-pe′ne-ah) thrombocytopenia.

thrombophilia (throm″bo-fil′e-ah) a tendency toward thrombosis.

thrombophlebitis (throm″bo-flĕ-bi′tis) inflammation of a vein (PHLEBITIS) associated with formation of a thrombus (THROMBOSIS).

t. mi′grans a recurrent condition involving different vessels simultaneously or at intervals.

postpartum iliofemoral t. thrombophlebitis of the iliofemoral vein following childbirth.

thromboplastic (throm″bo-plas′tik) causing or accelerating clot formation in the blood.

thromboplastid (throm″bo-plas′tid) a blood platelet.

thromboplastin (throm″bo-plas′tin) tissue thromboplastin.

tissue t. factor III, a COAGULATION FACTOR derived from several different sources in the body, such as brain and lung; it is important in the formation of extrinsic prothrombin converting principle in the extrinsic PATHWAY of coagulation. Called also tissue factor. See also activated partial thromboplastin TIME.

thrombopoiesis (throm″bo-poi-e′sis) 1. thrombogenesis. 2. thrombocytopoiesis. adj., **thrombopoiet′ic.**

thrombopoietin (throm″bo-poi′ĕ-tin) a colony-stimulating factor that is the

T

humoral regulator of the production of platelets.

thrombosis (throm-bo'sis) formation, development, or presence of a THROMBUS; this can happen whenever the flow of blood in arteries or veins is impeded. Many factors can interfere with normal blood flow: heart failure or physical inactivity may retard circulation generally; a change in the shape or inner surface of a vessel wall may impede blood flow, as in ATHEROSCLEROSIS; a mass may grow inside the body and exert pressure on a vessel; the vessel wall may be injured and roughened by an accident, surgery, a burn, cold, inflammation, or infection; or the blood may thicken in reaction to the presence of a foreign serum or snake venom. adj., **thrombot'ic.**

Sometimes a thrombus detaches itself from the wall and is carried along by the bloodstream. Such a clot is called an EMBOLUS, and the condition is known as EMBOLISM. A thrombus may form in the heart chambers, such as after coronary thrombosis (see below) at the place where the wall of the heart is weakened, or in the dilated atria in a case of mitral STENOSIS. Because blood normally flows more slowly through the veins than through the arteries, thrombosis is more common in veins than in arteries.

Venous Thrombosis. This occurs most often in the legs or pelvis; it may be a complication of PHLEBITIS, result from injury to a vein, or occur with prolonged bed rest. The symptoms—a feeling of heaviness, pain, warmth, or swelling in the affected part, and sometimes chills and fever—do not necessarily indicate its severity. Immediate medical attention is necessary in any case. Under *no* circumstances should the affected limb be massaged.

In thrombosis of superficial veins, bed rest with legs elevated and application of heat to the affected area may be all that is necessary. In thrombosis of deep veins, the affected part must be immobilized to prevent the clot from spreading or turning into an EMBOLUS, and ANTICOAGULANT drugs may be given. With proper treatment, recovery occurs within a short time unless an EMBOLISM develops. Practice management guidelines for venous thromboembolism in trauma patients note that a vena cava FILTER should be considered in patients at high risk who are not candidates for anticoagulants.

Prevention of Venous Thrombosis. Immobility is a prime factor in the development of thrombosis; hence, all patients should be mobilized as soon as possible after surgery or an illness that requires bed rest or produces paralysis. Those who cannot get out of bed should follow an exercise routine involving either active or passive motion of the extremities.

DEHYDRATION also plays a role in the development of thrombosis, and the patient should be kept well hydrated. The use of sequential compression devices, such as graded elastic stockings or automated devices providing intermittent compression to the legs, are widely used and accepted, but there are few clinical studies related to their use. They probably play a role in the prevention of STASIS and should be combined with other methods to prevent thromboembolism. Clinical guidelines also support the use of low molecular weight HEPARIN for patients at high risk when the bleeding risk is not considered a problem.

Arterial Thrombosis. The main types of arterial thrombosis are related to ARTERIOSCLEROSIS, although thrombosis can also result from infection or from injury to an artery. Arteriosclerosis may be hereditary or may be brought on by DIABETES MELLITUS. *Coronary thrombosis,* arterial thrombosis in a coronary artery, is a complication of coronary ATHEROSCLEROSIS. A thrombus in one of these arteries will block part of the blood supply to the heart muscle and cause severe MYOCARDIAL INFARCTION, which is a medical emergency. *Cerebral thrombosis* is arterial thrombosis in one of the cerebral arteries; the thrombus obstructs the supply of blood to the brain and results in STROKE SYNDROME. Causes include hardening of the cerebral arteries, HYPERTENSION, complications of SYPHILIS or other infections, DEHYDRATION, DIABETES MELLITUS, or a violent injury.

In advanced cases of ARTERIOSCLEROSIS, a thrombus may fill up whatever channel remains through a vessel, completely blocking off circulation and causing GANGRENE. This occurs most frequently in arteries of the legs and is called *peripheral thrombosis.* The onset, often sudden, is characterized by either a tingling feeling or numbness and coldness in the limb. Pain is not always present. Immediate treatment with ANTICOAGULANTS is necessary to discourage clotting. If this is not effective, surgery may be required. This condition is most common in the elderly and in diabetics. There are now methods of treatment that may save the limb, such as surgical removal of a thrombus or embolus, or surgery of blood vessels to remove old, narrowed, or deteriorated vessels and replace them with grafts.

cerebral t. arterial thrombosis of a cerebral vessel, which may cause stroke syndrome; see also THROMBOSIS.

coronary t. arterial thrombosis in a coronary artery, which may cause MYOCARDIAL INFARCTION. See also THROMBOSIS.

deep venous t. (DVT) venous THROMBOSIS of one or more of the deep veins of the lower limb, characterized by swelling, warmth, and erythema; it is frequently a precursor of a pulmonary EMBOLISM. See also THROMBOSIS.

venous t. phlebothrombosis.

thrombostasis (throm-bos′tah-sis) stasis of blood in a part with formation of thrombus.

thromboxane (throm-bok′sān) an intermediate in the metabolic pathway of arachidonic acid, formed from prostaglandin endoperoxides, and released from suitably stimulated platelets; the unstable form, thromboxane A_2, is a potent inducer of platelet aggregation and constrictor of arterial smooth muscle.

thrombus (throm′bus) a stationary blood CLOT along the wall of a blood vessel, frequently causing vascular obstruction. Some authorities differentiate thrombus formation from simple coagulation or clot formation. See also EMBOLUS.

mural t. one attached to the wall of the heart adjacent to an area of diseased endocardium, or to the aortic wall overlying an intimal lesion. See also parietal thrombus.

occluding t. one that occupies the entire lumen of a vessel and obstructs blood flow.

parietal t. one attached to a vessel or heart wall; see also mural thrombus.

thrush (thrush) infection of the oral mucous membrane by the fungus *Candida albicans;* called also oral CANDIDIASIS. It is characterized by white patches on a red, moist inflamed surface, occurring anywhere in the mouth, including the tongue, but usually on the inner cheeks, occasionally accompanied by pain and fever. Approximately 20 to 30 per cent of people harbor *C. albicans,* but the disease develops in only a small number. Those most susceptible are infants and adults who are in a weakened condition from infection, malnutrition, uncontrolled DIABETES MELLITUS, prolonged treatment with antibiotics, or IMMUNODEFICIENCY. Thrush is sometimes regarded as a minor infection, yet it can persist for weeks or even months, especially in young babies and IMMUNOCOMPROMISED patients. It is treated with antifungal AGENTS. The best preventive measures are good general health, a well-balanced diet, adequate rest, and good mouth hygiene. The Infectious Disease Society of America has published "Practice Guidelines for the Treatment of Candidiasis" on their web site, http://www.idsociety.org.

thrypsis (thrip′sis) a comminuted fracture.

thulium (thoo′le-um) a chemical element, atomic number 69, atomic weight 168.934, symbol Tm. (See Appendix 6.)

thumb (thum) the radial or first digit of the hand; it has only two phalanges and is apposable to the four fingers of the hand.

tennis t. tendinitis of the tendon of the long flexor muscle of the thumb, with calcification.

thumbprinting (thum′print-ing) a radiographic sign appearing as smooth indentations on the barium-filled colon, as though made by depression with the thumb; seen in various disorders of the colon, especially ischemic colitis.

thym(o)- word element [Gr.], *thymus; mind, soul,* or *emotions.*

thymectomize (thi-mek′to-mīz) to excise the thymus.

thymectomy (thi-mek′tah-me) excision of the THYMUS.

-thymia word element [Gr.], *condition of mind.* adj., **-thy′mic.**

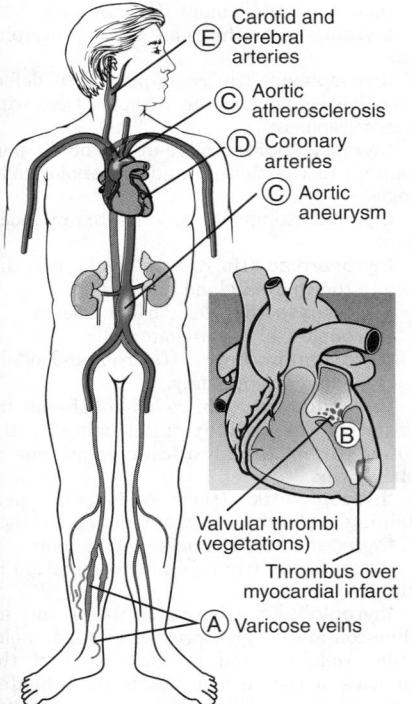

Carotid and cerebral arteries (E)

Aortic atherosclerosis (C)

Coronary arteries (D)

Aortic aneurysm (C)

Valvular thrombi (vegetations)

Thrombus over myocardial infarct

Varicose veins (A)

Sites of thrombus formation. From Damjanov, 1996.

thymic (thi'mik) pertaining to the thymus.

thymicolymphatic (thi″mĭ-ko-lim-fat'ik) pertaining to the thymus and lymphatic nodes.

thymidine (thi'mĭ-dēn) a nucleoside of DNA.

thymidine kinase an enzyme of the TRANSFERASE class that catalyzes a PHOSPHORYLATION reaction of PYRIMIDINE salvage as well as phosphorylation of drugs such as ACYCLOVIR and GANCICLOVIR into a form that will be active against viruses.

thymin (thi'min) former name for thymopoietin.

thymine (thi'mēn) a pyrimidine base found in DEOXYRIBONUCLEIC ACID (DNA).

thymitis (thi-mi'tis) inflammation of the thymus.

thymocyte (thi'mo-sīt) a lymphocyte arising in the thymus.

thymokinetic (thi″mo-kĭ-net'ik) tending to stimulate the thymus.

thymoleptic (thi″mo-lep'tik) any drug that favorably modifies mood in serious MOOD DISORDERS such as depression or mania; the main categories include tricyclic ANTIDEPRESSANTS, MONOAMINE OXIDASE INHIBITORS, and LITHIUM compounds.

thymoma (thi-mo'mah) a tumor derived from the epithelial or lymphoid elements of the thymus.

thymopathy (thi-mop'ah-the) any disease of the thymus.

thymopoietin (thi″mo-poi'ĕ-tin) a polypeptide hormone secreted by the THYMUS; it induces the proliferation of lymphocyte precursors and their differentiation into T-LYMPHOCYTES.

thymoprivic (thi″mo-priv'ik) thymoprivous.

thymoprivous (thi-mop'riv-us) pertaining to or resulting from removal of the thymus.

thymosin (thi'mo-sin) a humoral factor secreted by the THYMUS; it promotes the maturation of T-LYMPHOCYTES.

thymus (thi'mus) a ductless gland lying in the upper mediastinum beneath the sternum; it reaches its maximum development during puberty and continues to play an immunologic role throughout life, even though its function declines with age. During the last stages of fetal life and the early neonatal period, the reticular structure of the thymus entraps immature stem cells arising from the bone marrow and circulating in the blood. The thymus preprocesses these cells, causing them to become sensitized and therefore capable of maturing into a specific differentiated type of LYMPHOCYTE.

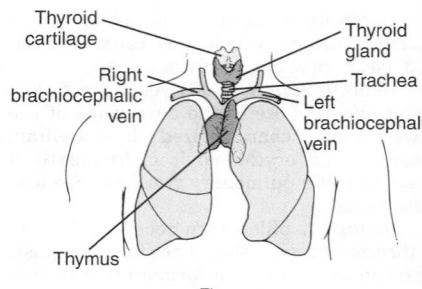

Thymus.

After sensitization by the thymus, the cel[ ] reenter the blood and are transported t[ ] developing lymphoid tissue, where they see[ ] the cells that eventually become T LYMPH[O]CYTES, a type essential to the development [ ] cell-mediated IMMUNITY. If the thymus [ ] removed or becomes nonfunctional durin[ ] fetal life, the lymphoid tissue fails t[ ] become seeded with the sensitized lymph[o]cytes and the body's cell-mediated arm [ ] immunity fails to develop. It is this arm [ ] immunity that is mainly responsible fo[ ] rejection of organ transplants and resis[ ]tance to intracellular microbial infectio[ ] and perhaps plays a role in natural resi[ ]tance to cancer.

thyr(o)- word element [Gr.], *thyroid.*

thyroadenitis (thi″ro-ad″ĕ-ni'tis) thyroi[ ]itis.

thyroaplasia (thi″ro-ah-pla'zhah) defe[ ]tive development of the THYROID GLAND wit[ ] HYPOTHYROIDISM.

thyroarytenoid (thi″ro-ar″ĭ-te'noid) pe[ ]taining to the thyroid and arytenoid cart[ ]lages.

thyrocalcitonin (thi″ro-kal″sĭ-to'nin) calc[ ]tonin.

thyrocardiac (thi″ro-kahr'de-ak) pertai[ ]ing to the thyroid gland and heart.

t. disease thyrotoxic heart disease.

thyrocele (thi'ro-sēl) goiter.

thyrochondrotomy (thi″ro-kon-drot'ah[ ]me) median laryngotomy.

thyrocricotomy (thi″ro-kri-kot'ah-me) in[ ]cision of the cricothyroid membrane, th[ ] lower part of the fibroelastic membrane o[ ] the larynx.

thyroepiglottic (thi″ro-ep″ĭ-glot'ik) pe[ ]taining to the thyroid gland and epiglottis.

thyrogenic (thi″ro-jen'ik) thyrogenous.

thyrogenous (thi-roj'ĕ-nus) originating i[ ] the THYROID GLAND.

thyroglobulin (thi'ro-glob″u-lin) an io[ ]dine-containing glycoprotein of high mol[ ]cular weight found in the colloid of th[ ] follicles of the THYROID GLAND; its iodinate[ ] tyrosine moieties form the active hormone[ ] THYROXINE and TRIIODOTHYRONINE.

thyroglossal (thi″ro-glos′al) pertaining to the thyroid gland and tongue.

thyrohyal (thi″ro-hi′al, thi″ro-hi′oid) **thyrohyoid**) pertaining to the thyroid gland or cartilage and the hyoid bone.

thyroid (thi′roid) 1. the THYROID GLAND. 2. pertaining to the thyroid gland. 3. SCUTIFORM. 4. a preparation of thyroid gland from domesticated food animals, containing LEVOTHYROXINE and LIOTHYRONINE and used as replacement therapy in the diagnosis and treatment of HYPOTHYROIDISM and the prevention and treatment of GOITER and thyroid carcinoma; administered orally.

t. crisis a sudden and dangerous increase of the symptoms of THYROTOXICOSIS, seen in patients with severe HYPERTHYROIDISM or in the period immediately following a THYROIDECTOMY. (However, good postoperative care and the use of RADIOIODINE ablation techniques have greatly reduced the incidence of this once common postoperative complication.) Called also thyroid or thyrotoxic storm.

Thyroid crisis is a serious event that can be fatal if not brought under control. All of the body processes are accelerated to dangerously high levels. The pulse may rise to 200 beats per minute, and there is concurrent rise in the respiratory rate. The temperature control center loses control, bringing about a rapid and steady increase in body temperature. Pulmonary edema and congestive heart failure can also occur.

Treatment is aimed at correction of the hyperthyroidism, control of the symptoms, and prevention of further crisis by treating the underlying cause. Medications are employed to block synthesis of thyroid hormones, block their release, and inhibit conversion of triiodothyronine to thyroxine. PLASMAPHERESIS. PLASMA EXCHANGE, or HEMODIALYSIS may be necessary to remove the hormones from the circulation.

Supportive care includes administration of oxygen and measures to control HYPERTHERMIA, such as the use of ice packs or a hyperthermia blanket. Intravenous hydration is important to prevent SHOCK. The use of GLUCOCORTICOIDS is associated with improved survival rates. PROPRANOLOL, SYMPATHOLYTICS, and GUANETHIDINE are often used, as well as other medications that treat symptoms.

t. function test a test of the functioning of the THYROID GLAND, such as its proper production of THYROID HORMONES. See RADIOIODINEUPTAKE TEST, THYROID-STIMULATING HORMONE TEST, THYROTROPIN-RELEASING HORMONE TEST, and TRIIODOTHYRONINE RESIN UPTAKE TEST.

t. gland the largest of the ENDOCRINE GLANDS, consisting of two lateral lobes connected by an isthmus; a third pyramidal lobe sometimes extends up from the isthmus. The thyroid gland is located in the front and sides of the neck just below the thyroid cartilage and produces hormones that are vital in maintaining normal growth and metabolism (see THYROID HORMONES). It also serves as a storehouse for iodine.

Diagnostic tests for thyroid disorders include radioimmunoassay for T_3, T_4, and thyroid-stimulating hormone (TSH), free thyroxine serum concentration, and free thyroxine index (FTI). These and other thyroid function tests can be distorted by preparations and foods containing iodine, and by oral contraceptives, phenytoin (Dilantin), and several other drugs. The *thyroid scan* is useful in detecting nodules and active thyroid tissue and, combined with radioactive iodine uptake, measures the ability of the thyroid gland to take in ingested iodine.

Persons who received radiation to the head and neck as children are at higher than normal risk for development of thyroid abnormalities. Of these disorders about one-third are carcinomas of the thyroid. Other problems related to radiation early in life include adenomas and other malignant and benign tumors, hypo- and hyperthyroidism, and thyroiditis. The American Thyroid Association suggests periodic laboratory testing and physical assessment of persons at high risk in order to detect these abnormalities when they are more amenable to treatment.

t. hormones iodothyronines secreted by the THYROID GLAND, principally THYROXINE

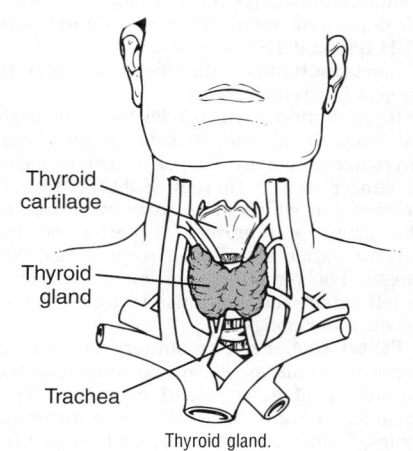

Thyroid cartilage

Thyroid gland

Trachea

Thyroid gland.

(tetraiodothyronine or T_4) and TRIIODOTHYRO-NINE (T_3). The serum level of T_4 is normally 45 to 50 times the level of T_3. However, T_3 is several times more active than T_4, and most T_3 is produced by metabolism of T_4 in peripheral tissues. The pharmaceutical names for T_4 and T_3 are LEVOTHYROXINE and LIOTHYRONINE, respectively. Thyroid hormones influence many metabolic processes. They stimulate the cellular production of heat; stimulate protein synthesis; regulate many aspects of carbohydrate metabolism; stimulate lipid synthesis, mobilization, and degradation; stimulate the synthesis of coenzymes from vitamins; and may affect the response of tissues to epinephrine and norepinephrine.

Secretion of thyroid hormones is regulated by the hypothalamus-pituitary-thyroid control system. Internal environmental conditions, such as low thyroid hormone and norepinephrine serum levels, or external factors, such as cold and stress, activate the hypothalamus, which secretes thyrotropin-releasing hormone (TRH). This hormone acts on the pituitary gland and brings about the release of thyroid-stimulating hormone (TSH). The TSH then stimulates the release of thyroid hormones such as T_3 and T_4 from the thyroid gland. When sufficient levels of serum thyroxine and other thyroid hormones have been reached, there is negative feedback to the hypothalamus and TRH is no longer secreted. See also HYPOTHYROIDISM and HYPERTHYROIDISM.

t.-stimulating hormone test a THYROID FUNCTION TEST in which THYROTROPIN (thyroid-stimulating hormone) is administered intramuscularly and the thyroid gland is monitored over time with scintiscanning or radioimmunoassays for a response or areas of decreased responsiveness. Called also TSH test and TSH stimulation test.

thyroidectomize (thi″roi-dek′tah-mīz) to subject to thyroidectomy.

thyroidectomy (thi″roi-dek′tah-me) surgical excision of the THYROID GLAND. Total thyroidectomy may be performed in cases of cancer of the thyroid. Subtotal thyroidectomy, in which more than two-thirds of the gland is removed, is performed for certain patients suffering from HYPERTHYROIDISM. The remaining portion of the gland is left intact and continues to function and produce hormones.

Patient Care. Prior to surgery the patient receives intensive therapy to maximize the possibility of a successful operation. This includes the administration of antithyroid drugs, iodine preparations, and supportive measures to promote rest and improve the nutritional status. Tests of thyroid function should indicate that the patient is EUTHYROID; that is, the test results show no extremes of thyroid function and the patient presents mild or no symptoms of THYROTOXICOSIS. When the patient is adequately prepared, the dangers of hemorrhage and THYROID CRISIS, the two major complications of thyroidectomy, are greatly diminished.

Immediately after surgery the patient is placed in a low Fowler's or semi-Fowler's POSITION. Motion of the head, unnecessary talking, and strenuous coughing should be discouraged. Temperature, pulse, and respirations are taken every 15 minutes until they remain within normal limits for several hours. The dressings are checked frequently for signs of hemorrhage or constriction of the throat. Special note should be made of the back of the neck, where blood may drain unnoticed. Hoarseness and slight difficulty in swallowing can be expected until the local edema subsides, but loss of the voice or severe dyspnea should be reported promptly. A TRACHEOSTOMY set is kept at the bedside in case of respiratory obstruction.

Other complications to be watched for include TETANY and thyroid CRISIS. Muscular twitching, numbness, or tingling of the hands or feet or other signs of irritability may indicate damage to, or accidental removal of, the PARATHYROID GLANDS, and a resultant decrease in the CALCIUM level of the blood. Thyroid crisis may occur as a result of an increase in the amount of THYROXINE released into the blood during manipulation of the gland at the time of its removal. This complication is indicated by a rapid increase in all the vital signs, marked irritability, restlessness, prostration, and sometimes even death from heart failure. Both tetany and thyroid crisis are rare complications.

thyroiditis (thi″roi-di′tis) inflammation of the THYROID GLAND, usually characterized by such symptoms as sore throat, fever, and painful enlargement of the gland.

atrophic t. a type of autoimmune thyroiditis with atrophy of the follicles and without goiter.

autoimmune t. any of various types of thyroiditis characterized by AUTOANTIBODIES against the thyroid gland, resulting in HYPOTHYROIDISM. The two major types are HASHIMOTO'S DISEASE and atrophic thyroiditis; Riedel's thyroiditis is a less common type.

Hashimoto's t. HASHIMOTO'S DISEASE.

Riedel's t. a chronic type of autoimmune thyroiditis with a proliferating, fibrosing, inflammatory process involving usually one but sometimes both lobes of the gland, which becomes hard and enlarged and adherent to the trachea and other adjacent structures. Called also Riedel's struma.

subacute lymphocytic t. painless, self-limited hyperthyroidism without the non-thyroidal features of Graves' disease; there is lymphocytic infiltration of the thyroid gland.

thyroidotomy (thi″roi-dot′ah-me) median laryngotomy.

thyromegaly (thi″ro-meg′ah-le) goiter.

thyromimetic (thi″ro-mi-met′ik) producing effects similar to those of thyroid hormones or the thyroid gland.

thyroparathyroidectomy (thi″ro-par″ah-thi″roi-dek′tah-me) excision of the thyroid and parathyroids.

thyroprival (thi″ro-priv′al) hypothyroid.

thyroprivic (thi″ro-priv′ik) hypothyroid.

thyroptosis (thi″rop-to′sis) downward displacement of a goitrous thyroid into the thorax.

thyrotherapy (thi″ro-ther′ah-pe) thyroid replacement THERAPY.

thyrotomy (thi-rot′ah-me) 1. median laryngotomy. 2. the operation of cutting the thyroid gland.

thyrotoxic (thi′ro-tok″sik) marked by the effects of presentation to the tissues of excessive quantities of the THYROID HORMONES.

t. heart disease heart disease associated with HYPERTHYROIDISM, marked by atrial FIBRILLATION, cardiac enlargement, and congestive HEART FAILURE. Called also thyrocardiac disease.

thyrotoxicosis (thi″ro-tok″sī-ko′sis) the condition caused by excessive quantities of THYROID HORMONES (see HYPERTHYROIDISM); it may be due to overproduction by the thyroid gland (as in GRAVES' DISEASE), overproduction originating outside the thyroid, or loss of storage function and leakage from the gland.

thyrotrope (thi′ro-trōp) thyrotroph.

thyrotroph (thi′ro-trōf) a type of BASOPHIL in the adenohypophysis that secretes THYROTROPIN.

thyrotrophic (thi″ro-trōf′ik) thyrotropic.

thyrotrophin (thi′ro-tro″fin, thi-rot′rah-in) thyrotropin.

thyrotropic (thi″ro-trop′ik) 1. pertaining to or marked by THYROTROPISM. 2. having an influence on the THYROID GLAND.

thyrotropin (thi′ro-tro″pin, thi-rot′rah-pin) a hormone secreted by the anterior lobe of the PITUITARY GLAND that has an affinity for and specifically stimulates the THYROID GLAND. Called also thyroid-stimulating hormone.

t. alfa a recombinant form of human thyrotropin; it binds to thyrotropin receptors and stimulates the steps in thyroid

hormone synthesis, including iodine uptake and synthesis and secretion of thyroglobulin; used as a diagnostic adjunct in serum thyroglobulin testing, with or without radioiodine scanning, in followup of patients with well-differentiated thyroid cancer, administered intramuscularly.

t.-releasing hormone stimulation test, t.-releasing hormone test a THYROID FUNCTION TEST that assesses release of THYROTROPIN by the PITUITARY GLAND; a bolus of thyrotropin-releasing HORMONE is administered and serum concentrations of thyrotropin are assessed at intervals; if serum levels do not increase within 30 to 40 minutes, the pituitary THYROTROPHS are dysfunctional. Called also TRH test and TRH stimulation test.

thyrotropism (thi-rot′rah-pizm) affinity for the THYROID GLAND.

thyroxine (T₄) (thi-rok′sin) a THYROID HORMONE that contains IODINE and is a derivative of the amino acid TYROSINE, occurring naturally as L-thyroxine; its chemical name is tetraiodothyronine. It is formed and stored in the thyroid follicles as THYROGLOBULIN and released from the gland by the action of a proteolytic enzyme. It is deiodinated in peripheral tissues to form TRIIODOTHYRONINE (T₃), which has a greater biological activity.

Thyroxine acts as a catalyst in the body and influences a great variety of effects, including metabolic rate (oxygen consumption); growth and development; metabolism of carbohydrates, fats, proteins, electrolytes, and water; vitamin requirements; reproduction; and resistance to infection. Pharmaceutical preparations of thyroxine, extracted from animals or made synthetically, are called LEVOTHYROXINE.

free t. the fraction of thyroxine in the serum that is not bound to a binding PROTEIN.

Ti titanium.

TIA TRANSIENT ISCHEMIC ATTACK.

tiagabine (ti-ag′ah-bēn) an ANTICONVULSANT agent used orally as the hydrochloride salt as an adjunct in treatment of partial SEIZURES.

tibia (tib′e-ah) the inner and larger of the two bones of the lower leg; it articulates with the FEMUR and head of the FIBULA above and with the TALUS below. See appendix 3-3 and see color plates.

t. val′ga a bowing of the leg in which the angulation is away from the midline of the body.

t. va′ra medial angulation of the tibia in the metaphyseal region, due to a growth

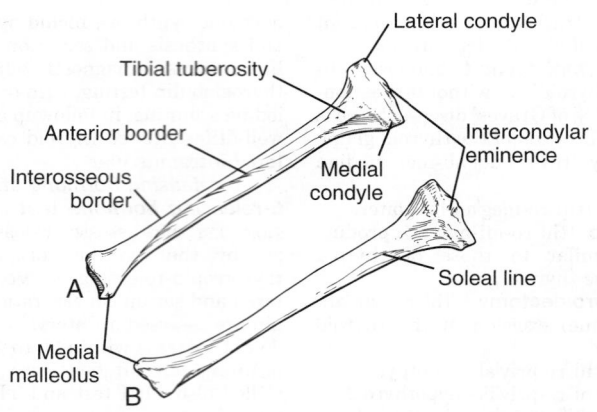

Tibia. Anterior *(A)* and posterior *(B)* views of the right tibia. From Dorland's, 2000.

disturbance of the medial aspect of the proximal tibial epiphysis; there are both infantile and adolescent types. Called also Blount's disease.

tibial (tib′e-al) pertaining to the TIBIA.

tibiofemoral (tib″e-o-fem′o-ral) pertaining to the tibia and femur; called also femorotibial.

tibiofibular (tib″e-o-fib′u-lar) pertaining to the tibia and fibula.

tibiotarsal (tib″e-o-tahr′sal) pertaining to the tibia and tarsus.

tic (tik) [Fr.] an involuntary, compulsive, rapid, repetitive, stereotyped movement or vocalization, experienced as irresistible although it can be suppressed for some length of time; occurrence is increased by stress and reduced during sleep or engrossing activities. Tics may be of psychogenic or neurogenic origin and are subclassified as either simple, such as eye blinking, shoulder shrugging, coughing, grunting, snorting, or barking; or complex, such as facial gestures, grooming motions, coprolalia (obscene language), echolalia (repeating the most recently heard word or sound), or echokinesis (imitation of another's movements).

t. douloureux a painful disorder of the TRIGEMINAL NERVE, characterized by severe pain in the face and forehead on the affected side, extending to the midline of the face and head, triggered by stimuli such as cold drafts, chewing, drinking cold liquids, brushing the hair, or washing the face. Called also trigeminal neuralgia.

Treatment. Medical treatment is usually preferred, since surgical correction results in complete loss of sensation in the areas served by the nerve. The drugs employed include trichloroethylene administered by inhalation, niacin, potassium chloride, diethazine, and most recently carbamazepine. When surgery is resorted to, the patient must be watched for signs of corneal infection, which frequently occurs, usually because of loss of the corneal reflex, which normally provides a warning when foreign material or other injurious agents enter the eye. Postoperative instructions must be given so that the patient can take necessary measures for the protection of the eye after discharge from the hospital.

facial t. spasm of the facial muscles.

Ticar (ti′kahr) trademark for a preparation of TICARCILLIN disodium, a PENICILLIN ANTIBIOTIC.

ticarcillin (ti″kahr-sil′in) a semisynthetic broad-spectrum PENICILLIN ANTIBIOTIC effective against both gram-negative and gram-positive organisms; administered orally as the disodium salt.

tick (tik) a blood-sucking parasitic ARACHNID; there are two types, hard and soft. Hard ticks (family Ixodidae) have a smooth, hard cover that shields the entire back of the male but only the anterior portion of the back in the female. Soft ticks (family Argasidae) lack this shield. Ticks are visible to the human eye. A hard tick can be seen on the skin, where it burrows into the outer layer with its knifelike tongue; it must be removed from the skin with care. Soft ticks do not bore into the skin. The two varieties carry different diseases but both thrive in the spring and early summer and inhabit wooded areas, brush, or grass.

Ticks serve as vectors for viruses causing COLORADO TICK FEVER and some forms of ENCEPHALITIS and for rickettsiae that cause such diseases as ROCKY MOUNTAIN SPOTTED

Removal of Hard Ticks. If hard ticks are extracted from the skin immediately, before they begin to suck blood, the chances of their transmitting disease are lessened; probably the only damage done will be an irritating itch at the site. The Centers for Disease Control and Prevention recommends that ticks be removed intact with fine-tip tweezers. Once the head and body are removed, the tick should not be squeezed or crushed with the bare hands. The site should be washed with soap and water.

t. fever any of various infectious diseases transmitted by the bite of a tick. The causative parasite may be a rickettsia, as in ROCKY MOUNTAIN SPOTTED FEVER; a bacterium such as *Babesia* or *Borrelia;* or a virus, such as that of COLORADO TICK FEVER.

ticlopidine (ti-klo′pĭ-dēn) a platelet INHIBITOR used as the hydrochloride salt in the prevention of STROKE SYNDROME.

t.i.d. [L.] ter in di′e (three times a day).

tide (tīd) a physiologic variation or increase of a certain constituent in body fluids.

acid t. a temporary increase in the acidity of the urine that sometimes follows fasting.

alkaline t. a temporary increase in the alkalinity of the urine during gastric digestion.

fat t. the increase of a fat in the lymph and blood following a meal.

Tietze's syndrome (tēt′sez) idiopathic painful nonsuppurative swellings of one or more costal cartilages, especially of the second rib; the anterior chest pain may mimic that of coronary artery disease. The condition may persist for years.

Tigan (ti′gan) trademark for preparations of TRIMETHOBENZAMIDE hydrochloride, an ANTIEMETIC.

tilt 1. to tip away from an upright position. 2. a condition of being tilted.

pelvic t. an anteroposterior motion of the pelvis around an imaginary axis in the frontal plane.

tiludronate (ti-loo′drah-nāt) an inhibitor of bone resorption, administered orally as the disodium salt in treatment of PAGET'S DISEASE of bone.

timbre (tam′ber) [Fr.] the musical quality of a tone or sound.

time (tīm) a measure of duration. See under adjectives for specific times, such as BLEEDING TIME.

activated partial thromboplastin t. (APTT, aPTT) the period required for CLOT

formation in recalcified blood PLASMA after contact activation and the addition of PLATELET substitutes such as brain CEPHALINS or similar PHOSPHOLIPIDS; used to assess the coagulation PATHWAYS. A prolonged aPTT can indicate a deficiency of any of various COAGULATION FACTORS, including factors XII, XI, IX, VIII, X, V, and II, and FIBRINOGEN.

AEC minimal response t. the shortest duration at which x-ray exposure can be terminated by automatic exposure control.

atrioventricular sequential t. a fixed nonprogrammable interval that extends from the atrial stimulus to the ventricular stimulus.

bleeding t. the time required for a standarized wound to stop bleeding; used as a test for platelet disorders; see also BLEEDING TIME.

circulation t. the time required for blood to flow between two given points; see also CIRCULATION TIME.

clotting t., coagulation t. the time required for blood to clot in a glass tube; see also CLOTTING.

cold ischemia t. the time between the placement of a traumatically amputated body part in ice and the time of surgical replantation.

inertia t. the time required to overcome the inertia of a muscle after reception of a stimulus.

ischemia t. the total time between traumatic amputation of a limb or portion of a limb and its surgical reimplantation; it is the sum of warm and cold ischemia times.

minimal response t. in radiology, the shortest possible exposure time for an x-ray film to be exposed automatically.

one-stage prothrombin t. PROTHROMBIN TIME.

prothrombin t. see PROTHROMBIN TIME.

real t. a term used to describe a recording device that shows events simultaneously to their occurrence.

R peak t. intrinsicoid deflection.

thrombin t. the time required for plasma fibrinogen to form thrombin; see also THROMBIN TIME.

warm ischemia t. the time interval between traumatic amputation of a limb or part and its placement on ice.

Timolide (ti′mo-līd) trademark for a preparation of timolol maleate and hydrochlorothiazide, an antihypertensive agent.

timolol (ti′mo-lol) a BETA-ADRENERGIC BLOCKING AGENT; the maleate salt or the hemihydrate is used topically to lower

T

intraocular pressure in GLAUCOMA and ocular HYPERTENSION, and the maleate salt is used orally to reduce the long-term risk of mortality and reinfarction after the acute phase of a MYOCARDIAL INFARCTION, as an ANTIHYPERTENSIVE AGENT, and in the prevention of MIGRAINE.

Timoptic (tim-op′tik) trademark for a preparation of TIMOLOL maleate, a BETA-ADRENERGIC BLOCKING AGENT used in treatment of GLAUCOMA and ocular hypertension.

tin (tin) a chemical element, atomic number 50, atomic weight 118.69, symbol Sn. (See Appendix 6.)

tinct. tincture.

tinctorial (tingk-to′re-al) pertaining to dyeing or staining.

tincture (tingk′chur) an alcoholic or hydroalcoholic solution prepared from vegetable drugs or chemical substances.

  compound benzoin t. a mixture of BENZOIN and several other ingredients in alcohol, used as a topical skin protectant.

  iodine t. a preparation of iodine and sodium iodide in diluted alcohol, used as a topical antiinfective.

tinea (tin′e-ah) RINGWORM; any of numerous different fungal infections of the skin; the specific type (depending on characteristic appearance, etiologic agent and site) usually is designated by a modifying term.

  t. bar′bae ringworm of the beard, seen on bearded parts of the face and neck; caused by *Trichophyton.*

  t. ca′pitis ringworm of the scalp, a fungal infection caused by various species of *Microsporum* and *Trichophyton.* Generally it is characterized by one or more small, round, elevated patches, scaling of the scalp, and dry and brittle hair.

  t. cor′poris a fungal infection of the glabrous (smooth) skin, usually due to species of *Microsporum* or *Trichophyton.*

  t. cru′ris ringworm of the groin area, starting in the perineal folds and extending onto the inner surface of the thighs; it is more common in males and is caused by *Epidermophyton floccosum* or species of *Trichophyton;* called also eczema marginatum, epidermophytosis cruris, and jock itch.

  t. fa′ciei ringworm of the face, seen on non-hairy areas of the face, often with a similar presentation to that of TINEA CORPORIS.

  t. imbrica′ta a distinctive type of TINEA CORPORIS occurring in tropical countries and caused by *Trichophyton concentricum.* The early lesion is circular, surrounded by a ring of scales attached along one edge; several new and larger scaling rings form later.

  t. ma′nus, t. ma′nuum ringworm of the hand, usually involving the interdigital spaces and palmar surfaces of the hands; it almost always accompanies tinea pedis, with the same etiologic agent for both infections.

  t. pe′dis athlete's foot.

  t. profun′da trichophytic GRANULOMA.

  t. syco′sis an inflammatory, deep type of TINEA BARBAE, due to *Trichophyton violaceum* or *T. rubrum.*

  t. un′guium tinea involving the nails; the invasion may be restricted to white patches or pits on the nail surface, or the lateral or distal edges of the nail may be involved first, followed by establishment of the infection beneath the nail plate.

  t. versi′color a chronic, usually asymptomatic disorder due to *Malassezia furfur,* marked only by multiple macular patches. Called also pityriasis versicolor.

Tinel's sign (tin-elz′) a tingling sensation in the distal end of a limb when percussion is made over the site of a divided nerve; it indicates a partial lesion or the beginning regeneration of the nerve.

tine test (tīn) an intracutaneous TUBERCULIN TEST using a multiple-puncture, disposable device. It is useful in mass screening of children, but is less accurate than the MANTOUX TEST. Any doubtful reaction to the tine test should be rechecked by a Mantoux test before a follow-up chest x-ray is recommended. The test is read 48 to 72 hours after administration.

tingible (tin′jĭ-b'l) stainable.

tinnitus (tin′ĭ-tus, tĭ-ni′tus) a noise in the ears, such as ringing, buzzing, or roaring, which may at times be heard by others than the patient. Common causes include PRESBYCUSIS, prolonged exposure to loud environmental noise, and such pathological conditions as inflammation and infection of the ear, OTOSCLEROSIS, MENIERE'S DISEASE, and LABYRINTHITIS. Systemic disorders associated with tinnitus include hypertension and other cardiovascular diseases, neurologic disorders including head injury, hyperthyroidism, and hypothyroidism. Tinnitus often is one of the first symptoms produced by an OTOTOXIC drug.

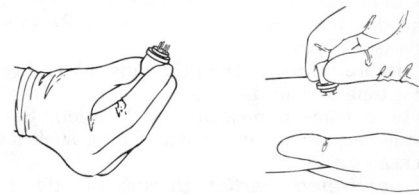

Tine test for tuberculosis. From Dorland's, 2000.

Medical treatment begins with efforts to determine the underlying cause and treat it. When the cause cannot be found or is not amenable to control, symptomatic relief is attempted. However, some cases resist all conventional modes of therapy. Less traditional measures that have had varying degrees of success include biofeedback training and "masking." Biofeedback training is especially helpful in those cases in which emotional stress and anxiety or hysteria are thought to be contributing factors. Through visual or auditory signals the person learns to relax and exert some degree of control over the autonomic nervous system. This can lower blood pressure and pulse rate and relax tense muscles. Masking simply provides a low-level noise to block out or mask the head noise heard by the person. Some examples include playing soft music or a tape of sounds of nature, such as a waterfall, while the person is resting or sleeping, providing "white sound" in the work setting, using a hearing aid to amplify sound from the outside and overcome head noise, and wearing a special tinnitus instrument that is a combination hearing aid and tinnitus masker for persons who have both hearing loss and tinnitus.

Persistent and severe tinnitus can interfere with patients' ability to perform their usual daily activities and prevent them from getting sufficient sleep and rest. Because the problem is so widespread, and for many persons incapacitating, there is a national association devoted to the study and management of tinnitus. Its address is American Tinnitus Association, P.O. Box 5, Portland, OR 97207.

tinzaparin (tin-zap'ah-rin) a low-molecular-weight HEPARIN obtained by depolymerization of heparin from porcine intestinal mucosa using a bacterial enzyme; it acts as an ANTICOAGULANT and ANTITHROMBOTIC and is used as an adjunct to WARFARIN in the treatment of deep venous THROMBOSIS with or without pulmonary EMBOLISM, administered subcutaneously.

tioconazole (ti″o-kon'ah-zōl) an imidazole derivative used as a topical antifungal agent, applied intravaginally in treatment of vulvovaginal CANDIDIASIS.

tiopronin (ti-o'pro-nin) a THIOL compound used in treatment of CYSTINURIA and prevention of KIDNEY STONES; administered orally.

tirofiban (ti″ro-fi'ban) a platelet INHIBITOR, used as the hydrochloride salt in prophylaxis of THROMBOSIS in unstable ANGINA or in MYOCARDIAL INFARCTION that is not characterized by abnormal Q waves; administered intravenously.

tissue (tish'u) a group or layer of similarly specialized cells that together perform certain special functions.

adenoid t. lymphoid tissue.

adipose t. connective tissue made of fat cells in a meshwork of areolar tissue.

areolar t. connective tissue made up largely of interlacing fibers.

bony t. osseous tissue.

brown adipose t., brown fat t. brown FAT.

bursa-equivalent t., bursal equivalent t. a hypothesized lymphoid tissue in non-avian vertebrates including human beings, equivalent to the BURSA OF FABRICIUS in birds: the site of B LYMPHOCYTE maturation. It now appears that B lymphocyte maturation occurs primarily in the bone marrow.

cancellous t. the spongy tissue of bone.

cartilaginous t. the substance of cartilage.

chordal t. the tissue of the notochord.

chromaffin t. a tissue composed largely of chromaffin cells, well supplied with nerves and vessels; it occurs in the adrenal medulla and also forms the paraganglia of the body.

cicatricial t. the dense fibrous tissue forming a CICATRIX, derived directly from granulation TISSUE; called also scar tissue.

connective t. the tissue that binds together and is the support of the various structures of the body; see also CONNECTIVE TISSUE.

elastic t. connective tissue made up of yellow elastic fibers, frequently massed into sheets.

endothelial t. peculiar connective tissue lining serous and lymph spaces.

epithelial t. a general name for tissues not derived from the mesoderm.

erectile t. spongy tissue that expands and becomes hard when filled with blood.

fatty t. connective tissue made of fat cells in a meshwork of areolar tissue.

fibrous t. the common connective tissue of the body, composed of yellow or white parallel elastic and collagen fibers.

gelatinous t. mucous tissue.

granulation t. material formed in repair of wounds of soft tissue, consisting of connective tissue cells and ingrowing young vessels; it ultimately forms cicatrix.

gut-associated lymphoid t. (GALT) lymphoid tissue associated with the gut, including the tonsils, Peyer's patches, lamina propria of the gastrointestinal tract, and appendix.

indifferent t. undifferentiated embryonic tissue.

T

interstitial t. connective tissue between the cellular elements of a structure.

lymphadenoid t. tissue resembling that of lymph nodes, spleen, bone marrow, tonsils, and lymph vessels.

lymphoid t. a latticework of reticular tissue whose interspaces contain LYMPHO-CYTES.

mesenchymal t. embryonic connective tissue composed of stellate cells and a ground substance of coagulable fluid.

mucous t. a jellylike connective tissue, such as occurs in the umbilical cord. Called also gelatinous tissue.

muscular t. the substance of muscle.

myeloid t. red bone MARROW.

nerve t., nervous t. the specialized tissue forming the elements of the nervous system.

osseous t. the specialized tissue forming the bones.

reticular t., reticulated t. connective tissue composed predominantly of reticulum cells and reticular fibers.

scar t. cicatricial tissue.

sclerous t's the cartilaginous, fibrous, and osseous tissues.

skeletal t. the bony, ligamentous, fibrous, and cartilaginous tissue forming the skeleton and its attachments.

splenic t. red pulp.

subcutaneous t. the layer of loose connective tissue directly under the skin.

t. typing identification of tissue types for purposes of predicting acceptance or rejection of GRAFTS and TRANSPLANTS. The process and purposes of tissue typing are essentially the same as for blood typing. The major difference lies in the kinds of antigens being evaluated. The acceptance of allografts depends on the HLA ANTIGENS (HLA); if the donor and recipient are not HLA identical, the allograft is rejected, sometimes within minutes. The HLA genes are located in the major histocompatibility COMPLEX, a region on the short arm of chromosome 6, and are involved in cell-cell interaction, IMMUNE RESPONSE, organ transplantation, development of cancer, and susceptibility to disease. There are five genetic loci, designated HLA-A, HLA-B, HLA-C, HLA-D, and HLA-DR. At each locus, there can be any of several different alleles.

Each person inherits one chromosome 6 from the mother and one from the father; that is, each parent transmits to the child one allele for each kind of antigen (A, B, C, D, and DR). If the parents are different at both alleles of a locus, the statistical chance of one sibling being identical to another is one in four (25 per cent), the chance of being identical at one allele only (half-identical) is 50 per cent, and the chance of a total mismatch is 25 per cent.

Techniques for Tissue Typing. Histocompatibility testing involves several basic methods of assay for HLA differences. The most widely used method uses the POLYMERASE CHAIN REACTION to compare the DNA of the person, organ, or graft being tested with known pieces of the genes encoding MHC antigens. The variability of these regions of the genes determines the tissue type of the subject.

Serologic methods are used to detect serologically defined antigens on the surfaces of cells. In general, HLA-A, -B, and -C determinants are primarily measured by serologic techniques. A second method, involving lymphocyte reactivity in a mixed lymphocyte culture, for determining HLA-D or lymphocyte-defined antigens, is now only rarely used.

Essentially, the serologic method is performed by incubating target lymphocytes (isolated from fresh peripheral blood) with antisera that recognize all known HLA antigens. The cells are spread in a tray with microscopic wells containing various kinds of antisera and are incubated for 30 minutes, followed by an additional 60-minute complement incubation. If the lymphocytes have on their surfaces antigens recognized by the antibodies in the antiserum, the lymphocytes are lysed. A dye is added to show changes in the permeability of the cell membrane and cellular death. The proportion of cells destroyed by lysis indicates the degree of histologic incompatibility. If, for example, the lymphocytes from a person being tested for HLA-A3 are destroyed in a well containing antisera for HLA-A3, the test is positive for this antigen group.

white adipose t., yellow adipose t. the adipose tissue composing the bulk of the body fat.

titanium (ti-ta′ne-um) a chemical element, atomic number 22, atomic weight 47.90, symbol Ti. (See Appendix 6.)

t. dioxide a white powder used in ointment or lotion as a SUNSCREEN.

titer (ti′ter) the quantity of a substance required to react with or to correspond to a given amount of another substance.

agglutination t. the highest dilution of a serum which causes clumping of microorganisms or other particulate antigens.

titrate (ti′trāt) to analyze by titration.

titration (ti-tra′shun) determination of a given component in solution by addition of a liquid reagent of known strength until a given endpoint, e.g., change in color, is reached indicating that the component has been consumed by reaction with the reagent.

Dean and Webb t. a test for measuring antibody in which varying dilutions of antibody are mixed with a constant quantity of antiserum; antibody activity is determined by the dilution in which flocculation occurs most rapidly, i.e., the end point.

titrimetry (ti-trim′ĕ-tre) analysis by titration. adj., **titrimet′ric.**

titubation (tit″u-ba′shun) the act of staggering or reeling; a staggering gait with shaking of the trunk and head, commonly seen in cerebellar disease.

tizanidine (ti-zan′ĭ-dēn″) a short-acting ANTISPASMODIC used in the acute and intermittent treatment of spasticity, such as that associated with MULTIPLE SCLEROSIS or spinal cord injury; administered orally as the hydrochloride salt.

Tl thallium.

TLC tender loving care; total lung capacity; thin-layer chromatography.

Tm thulium.

TMJ temporomandibular joint.

TMJ disorder, TMJ syndrome temporomandibular joint disorder.

TNCC trauma nursing core course.

TNF tumor necrosis factor.

TNM tumor-node-metastasis; see under STAGING.

TNS transcutaneous neural stimulation.

TNT trinitrotoluene.

toadstool popular name for any of various poisonous MUSHROOMS.

tobacco (tah-bak′o) the dried prepared leaves of *Nicotiana tabacum,* an annual plant widely cultivated in the United States, the source of various alkaloids, the principal one being NICOTINE. See also SMOKING and NICOTINE POISONING.

tobramycin (to″brah-mi′sin) an AMINOGLYCOSIDE ANTIBIOTIC produced by *Streptomyces tenebrarius* and used topically as the base to treat external infections of the eye, by oral inhalation to treat *Pseudomonas aeruginosa* infections in patients with cystic fibrosis, and intramuscularly or intravenously as the sulfate salt to treat a wide variety of infections.

toc(o)- word element [Gr.], *childbirth; labor.* See also words beginning TOK(O)-.

tocainide (to-ka′nīd) an agent used as the hydrochloride salt in treatment of ventricular ARRHYTHMIAS.

tocolysis (to-kol′ĭ-sis) postponement of preterm LABOR.

tocolytic (to″ko-lit′ik) 1. pertaining to or causing TOCOLYSIS (postponement of preterm labor). 2. an agent that does this, such as RITODRINE hydrochloride or another β$_2$-adrenergic RECEPTOR agonist.

tocometer (to-kom′ĕ-ter) tokodynamometer.

tocopherol (to-kof′er-ol) an alcohol isolated from wheat germ oil or produced synthetically; it has the properties of vitamin E. In animals it is needed in the diet to ensure reproduction, but its role in humans is unclear.

alpha t. a tocopherol isomer that is the most prevalent form of vitamin E occurring in the body and the form administered as a supplement. In nature, it usually occurs with β- and γ-tocopherols. The term is often used synonymously with vitamin E. See VITAMIN.

tocophobia (to″ko-fo′be-ah) irrational fear of childbirth.

toe (to) a digit of the foot.

claw t. a toe deformity seen in many patients with rheumatoid arthritis, consisting of dorsal subluxation of toes 2 through 5; the metatarsal heads bear weight and become painful during walking so that the patient has a shuffling gait.

hammer t. deformity of a toe in which the proximal phalanx is extended and the second and distal phalanges are flexed, causing a clawlike appearance; it most often affects the second toe.

Morton's t. Morton's neuralgia.

pigeon t. a permanent toeing-in position of the feet; severe cases are considered a form of CLUBFOOT (TALIPES).

webbed t's SYNDACTYLY of the toes abnormally joined by strands of tissue at their base.

toenail (to′nāl) the nail on any of the digits of the foot.

ingrown t. aberrant growth of a toenail, with one (usually the outer) margin

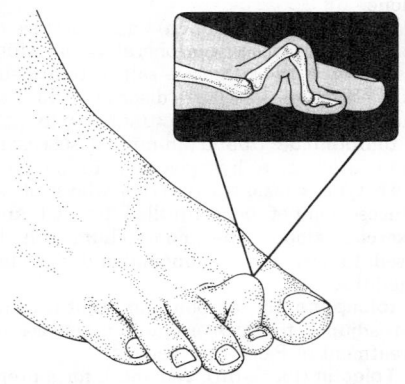

Hammer toe of the second metatarsophalangeal (MTP) joint. From Ignatavicius and Workman, 2000.

growing deeply into the nail groove and surrounding tissues.

Tofranil (to-fra′nil) trademark for preparations of IMIPRAMINE, a tricyclic ANTIDEPRESSANT.

togavirus (to″gah-vi′rus) a subgroup of arboviruses, including rubella virus and mosquito- and tickborne viruses that cause hemorrhagic fever; they are RNA viruses with envelopes (or "togas").

toilet (toi′let) 1. the cleansing and dressing of a wound and the surrounding area. 2. an apparatus into which defecation and urination can be done; called also commode.

toileting (toi′let-ing) 1. using a toilet; DEFECATION and URINATION. 2. helping a patient with DEFECATION and URINATION.

   patterned urge response t. a technique for bladder TRAINING, especially in patients with functional INCONTINENCE; the patient is prompted to urinate based on results of a voiding diary that indicates maximum functional capacity. The nurse records the patient's cognitive and behavioral responses to prompted toileting.

tok(o)- word element [Gr.], *childbirth; labor.* See also words beginning TOC(O)-.

token (to′ken) something that can be substituted for money or otherwise exchanged for privileges or other commodities, services, or rewards; see also token ECONOMY.

tokodynagraph (to″ko-di′nah-graf) a tracing obtained by the tokodynamometer.

tokodynamometer (to″ko-di″nah-mom′ĕ-ter) an instrument for measuring and recording the expulsive force of uterine contractions.

tolazamide (tol-az′ah-mīd) a SULFONYLUREA used as a hypoglycemic in patients with type 2 DIABETES MELLITUS whose blood glucose cannot be controlled by diet and exercise alone.

tolazoline (tol-az′o-lēn) an ADRENERGIC BLOCKING AGENT and peripheral VASODILATOR; used as the hydrochloride salt in treatment of peripheral vascular disorders due to vasospasm and in PHARMACOANGIOGRAPHY.

tolbutamide (tol-bu′tah-mīd) a SULFONYLUREA used as a hypoglycemic in patients with type 2 DIABETES MELLITUS whose blood glucose cannot be controlled by diet and exercise alone. The monosodium salt is used to test for insulinoma and diabetes mellitus.

tolcapone (tōl′kah-pōn″) an agent used as an adjunct to LEVODOPA and CARBIDOPA in treatment of PARKINSON′S DISEASE.

Tolectin (tol′ek-tin) trademark for a preparation of TOLMETIN sodium; a NONSTEROIDAL ANTIINFLAMMATORY DRUG.

tolerance (tol′er-ans) 1. the ability to bear something potentially difficult. 2. the ability to endure unusually large doses of a poison or toxin. 3. drug TOLERANCE. adj tol′erant.

   acquired drug t. drug tolerance.

   ambiguity t. the ability to withstand conflicting or complex situations without undue psychological stress.

   drug t. a decreasing response to repeated constant doses of a drug or the need for increasing doses to maintain a constant response. See also DRUG DEPENDENCE and HABITUATION.

   immunologic t. specific nonreactivity of lymphoid tissues to a particular antigen capable under other conditions of inducing immunity.

   standing t. the amount of time an individual is capable of maintaining an erect, upright position.

   t. test 1. an exercise test to determine the efficiency of the circulation. 2. a test to determine the body's ability to metabolize a substance or to endure administration of a drug.

tolerogen (tol′er-o-jen) an antigen used to introduce tolerance, particularly a form of an antigen (usually a soluble form) that induces tolerance, as distinguished from an immunogen, another form (usually an insoluble form) that induces immunity.

tolerogenesis (tol″er-o-jen′ĕ-sis) induction of immunologic tolerance.

Tolinase (tol′ĭ-nās) trademark for TOLAZAMIDE, an oral hypoglycemic AGENT.

tolmetin (tol′me-tin) a NONSTEROIDAL ANTIINFLAMMATORY DRUG, used as the sodium salt for treatment of OSTEOARTHRITIS, rheumatoid ARTHRITIS, ankylosing SPONDYLITIS, and other rheumatic inflammatory disorders; administered orally.

tolnaftate (tol-naf′tāt) a topical antifungal AGENT.

tolterodine (tol-ter′ah-dēn) an ANTISPASMODIC agent used in treatment of bladder hyperactivity.

toluene (tol′u-ēn) the hydrocarbon C_7H_8, an aromatic solvent similar to xylene; it is found in many paints and removers and is considered to be a neurotoxin.

tom(o)- word element [Gr.], *a section; a cutting.*

-tome word element [Gr.], *an instrument for cutting; a segment.*

tomogram (to′mo-gram) an image of a tissue plane or slice produced by TOMOGRAPHY.

tomograph (to′mo-graf) an apparatus by which the x-ray tube and film are moved in opposite directions during an exposure so that only a single plane of tissue remains in focus during the exposure. Other planes above and below are blurred by the motion.

tomography (to-mog′rah-fe) any method that produces images of single tissue planes. In conventional radiology, tomographic images (body section radiographs) are produced by motion of the x-ray tube and film or by motion of the patient that blurs the image except in a single plane. In reconstruction tomography (CT and PET) the image is produced by a computer program.

computed t. **(CT), computerized axial t. (CAT)** a radiologic imaging modality that uses computer processing to generate an image (CAT SCAN) of the tissue density in a "slice" as thin as 1 to 10 mm in thickness through the patient's body. These images are spaced at intervals of 0.5 to 1 cm. Cross-sectional anatomy can be reconstructed in several planes without exposing the patient to additional radiation.

Since its introduction in 1972, the use of this modality has grown rapidly. Because it is noninvasive and has high contrast resolution, it has replaced some radiographic procedures using contrast media. It also has a better spatial resolution than scintillation imaging (about 1 mm for CAT compared to 15 mm for a scintillation camera).

A CAT scan is divided into a square matrix of *pixels* (picture elements). The newer CAT scanners use a high resolution matrix with 256×256 or 512×512 pixels. The region of the tissue slice corresponding to a pixel has a cross-sectional area of 1×1 mm to 2×2 mm; because of the thickness of the slice, it has a finite height and is therefore referred to as a *voxel* (volume element).

The actual measurements made by the scanner are the x-ray attenuations along thousands of rays traversing the slice at all angles. The attenuation value for a ray is the sum of the values for all of the voxels it passes through. A computer program called a *reconstruction algorithm* can solve the problem of assigning attenuation values for all the pixels that add up to the measured values along each ray.

The attenuation values are converted to CAT numbers by subtracting the attenuation value of water and multiplying by an arbitrary coefficient to produce values ranging from −1000 for air to +1000 for compact bone with water as 0. CT numbers are sometimes expressed in *Hounsfield units*, named after Godfrey Hounsfield, the inventor of the CT scanner; Hounsfield and Allan Cormack were co-winners of the Nobel Prize in physiology or medicine in

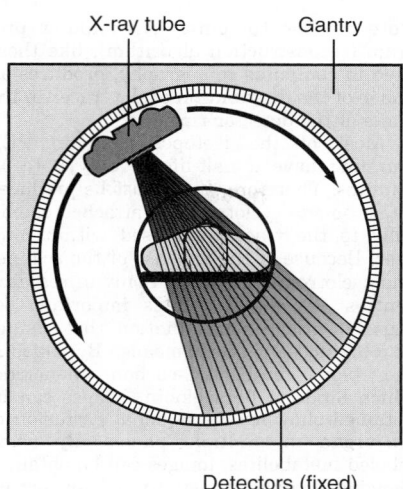

Computed tomography. Relative position of the x-ray tube, patient, and detectors in a fourth generation CT unit.

1979 for the development of computerized axial tomography.

electron beam computed t. **(EBCT)** ultrafast computed TOMOGRAPHY done with a scanner in which the patient is surrounded by a large circular anode that emits x-rays as the electron beam is guided around it.

extended narrow t. tomography involving an increase in amplitude and increase in exposure angle resulting in greater thinness of the cut for examination.

linear t. tomography in which the tube and film move in the same direction.

narrow angle t. a type of tomography that results in thicker sections for examination.

pluridirectional t. tomography in which there is a great deal of movement in a variety of directions.

positron emission t. **(PET)** a combination of computed TOMOGRAPHY and scintillation SCANNING. Natural biochemical substances or drugs tagged with a positron-emitting radioisotope are administered to the subject by injection; the tagged substance (tracer) then becomes localized in specific tissues like its natural analogue. When the isotope decays, it emits a POSITRON, which then annihilates with an electron of a nearby atom, producing two 511 keV gamma rays traveling in opposite directions 180 degrees apart. When the gamma rays trigger a ring of detectors around the subject, the line between the detectors on which the decay occurred is stored in the computer. A computer program (reconstruction algorithm), like those used in computed tomography, produces an image of the distribution of the tracer in the plane of the detector ring.

Most of the isotopes used in PET scanning have a half-life of only 2 to 10 minutes. Therefore, they must be produced by an on-site cyclotron and attached chemically to the tracer and used within minutes. Because of the expense of the scanner and cyclotron, PET is used only in research centers. However, PET is important because it provides information that cannot be obtained by other means. By labeling the blood with ^{11}C-carbon monoxide, which binds to hemoglobin, images can be obtained showing the regional perfusion of an organ in multiple planes. By using labeled metabolites, images can be obtained showing metabolic activity of an organ. ^{15}O-oxygen and ^{11}C-glucose have been used for brain imaging and ^{11}C-palmitate for heart imaging. ^{81}Rb, which is distributed like potassium, is also used for heart imaging. By using labeled neurotransmitters, hormones, and drugs the distribution of receptors for these substances in the brain and other organs can be mapped.

single-photon emission computed t. (SPECT) a type of tomography in which gamma photon–emitting radionuclides are administered to patients and then detected by one or more gamma cameras rotated around the patient. From the series of two-dimensional images produced, a three-dimensional image can be created by computer reconstruction. The technique improves resolution of, and decreases interference by, overlapping organs. It is used particularly for assessment of cardiac disease, stroke, and liver disease; for staging of cancer; and to diagnose physical abnormalities through evaluation of function.

ultrasonic t. the ultrasonographic visualization of a cross-section of a predetermined plane of the body; see B-mode ULTRASONOGRAPHY.

-tomy word element [Gr.], *incision; cutting.*

ton(o)- word element [Gr.], *tone; tension.*

tone (tōn) 1. normal degree of vigor and tension; in muscle, the resistance to passive elongation or stretch; tonus. 2. a particular quality of sound or voice.

tongs (tongz) an instrument for grasping and holding, consisting of two arms joined by a hinge or pivot.

Gardner-Wells t. U-shaped tongs used for spinal traction, having pressure-controlled pins that are inserted into the skull at opposite ends to permit application of a longitudinal force to the axis of the spinal column. (See illustration.)

Vinke t. a type of tongs used to exert skeletal traction on the skull, as in surgery for fractures or cervical vertebrae.

tongue (tung) a muscular organ on the floor of the mouth; it aids in chewing, swallowing, and speech, and is the location of organs of TASTE. The taste buds are located in the papillae, which are projections on the upper surface of the tongue

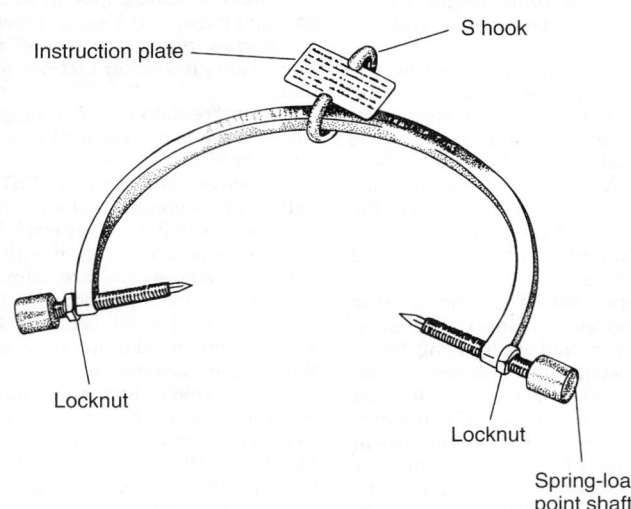

Gardner-Wells tongs. From McQuillan et al., 2002.

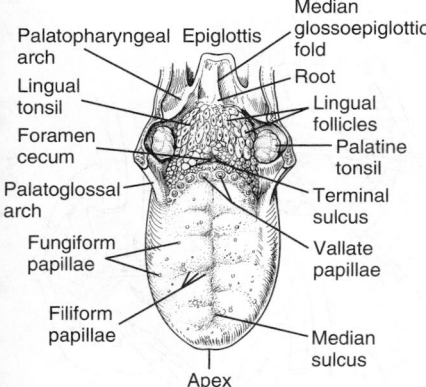

Palatopharyngeal arch
Epiglottis
Median glossoepiglottic fold
Lingual tonsil
Root
Lingual follicles
Foramen cecum
Palatine tonsil
Palatoglossal arch
Terminal sulcus
Fungiform papillae
Vallate papillae
Filiform papillae
Median sulcus
Apex

The tongue, showing principal structures. From Dorland's, 2000.

The condition of the tongue can sometimes be a guide to the general condition of the body. GLOSSITIS (inflammation of the tongue) can accompany anemia, scarlet fever, nutritional deficiencies, and most general infections. Sometimes it is part of an adverse reaction to medication. One form of glossitis causes a smooth tongue, with a red, glazed appearance. A coated or furry tongue may be present in a variety of illnesses, but does not necessarily indicate illness. A dry tongue sometimes indicates insufficiency of fluids in the body, or it may result from fever. When the tongue is extremely dry and has a leathery appearance, the cause may be uremia.

bifid t. a tongue with a lengthwise cleft.

black t., black hairy t. hairy tongue in which the hypertrophied filiform papillae are brown or black; called also lingua nigra, melanoglossia, and nigrities linguae.

cleft t. bifid tongue.

coated t. one covered with a white or yellow layer of desquamated epithelium, debris, bacteria, fungi, or other material.

fissured t., furrowed t. a tongue with numerous furrows or grooves on the dorsal surface, often radiating from a groove on the midline.

geographic t. a tongue with denuded patches, surrounded by thickened epithelium.

hairy t. a benign condition of the tongue characterized by hypertrophy of the filiform papillae that gives the dorsum of the tongue a furry appearance. The color of the elongated papillae varies from yellowish white to brown or black, depending upon staining by substances such as tobacco, foods, or drugs.

raspberry t. a diffusely reddened and swollen, uncoated tongue, as seen several days after the onset of the rash in scarlet fever.

scrotal t. fissured tongue.

strawberry t., red raspberry t.

strawberry t., white the white-coated tongue with prominent red papillae characteristic of the early stage of scarlet fever; the coating desquamates, leaving a beefy red (*raspberry*) tongue.

tongue-tie (tung′ti) ankyloglossia.

tonic (ton′ik) 1. producing and restoring normal tone. 2. characterized by continuous tension.

tonicity (to-nis′ĭ-te) the state of tissue tone or tension; in body fluid physiology, the effective osmotic pressure equivalent.

tonoclonic (ton″o-klon′ik) both tonic and clonic; said of muscular spasms.

tonofibril (ton′o-fi″bril) one of the fine fibrils in epithelial cells, thought to give a supporting framework to the cell.

tonogram (to′no-gram) the record produced by tonography.

tonograph (to′no-graf) a recording tonometer.

tonography (to-nog′rah-fe) the recording of changes in intraocular pressure due to sustained pressure on the eyeball.

carotid compression t. a test for occlusion of the carotid artery by measuring ocular pressure and pulse before, during, and after the proximal portion of the carotid artery is compressed by the fingers.

tonometer (to-nom′e-ter) an instrument for measuring tension or pressure, especially intraocular pressure.

gastric t. a tonometer and standard vented gastric sump that are incorporated into one device with separate lumens for the tonometer, suction, and vent.

tonometry (to-nom′e-tre) measurement of tension or pressure, e.g., intraocular pressure.

digital t. estimation of the degree of intraocular pressure by pressure exerted on the eyeball by the finger of the examiner.

gastric t. monitoring of the gastric intramucosal pH to obtain early indications of inadequate tissue oxygenation; the sensitive nature of the mucosa allows for monitoring of metabolic changes produced by hypoxia well in advance of the other more common indices of hypoxia.

tonoplast (ton′o-plast) the limiting membrane of an intracellular vacuole; the vacuole membrane.

tonsil (ton′sil) 1. a small, rounded mass of tissue. 2. one of the fleshy masses of lymphoid

T

tissue at the back of the throat. adj., **ton'-sillar.**

There are three different kinds of tonsils: the *palatine tonsils* are a pair of oval-shaped structures about the size of almonds, partially embedded in the mucous membrane, one on each side of the back of the throat. The *lingual tonsils* are below the palatine tonsils at the base of the tongue. The *pharyngeal tonsils,* or ADENOIDS, are on the upper rear wall of the mouth cavity; they are of fair size in childhood but usually shrink after puberty. The tonsils are part of the lymphatic system and help to filter the circulating lymph of bacteria and any other foreign material that may enter the body, especially through the mouth and nose. In the process of fighting infection the palatine tonsils and the adenoids sometimes become enlarged and inflamed (see TONSILLITIS).

t. of cerebellum a rounded mass forming part of the cerebellum on its inferior surface.

tonsillectomy (ton″sĭ-lek′tah-me) excision of TONSILS, done in treatment of chronic infection of the tonsils, obstructive sleep APNEA, purulent OTITIS MEDIA, or HEARING LOSS associated with otitis media.

Patient Care. Since most tonsillectomy patients are children, it is important that the preoperative period include adequate emotional preparation of the patient and family. Children should be told in advance of the admission to the hospital and given some idea of what they can expect. They should not be deceived about the possibility of discomfort, but it is best to stress the positive aspects of surgery, such as the fact that they will not suffer as many colds and attacks of sore throat once the surgery is performed and the sore throat has healed.

Although tonsillectomy is rarely associated with complications, there is always the possibility of serious hemorrhage after surgery. The patient should be placed prone on the abdomen in bed immediately after surgery, to allow for adequate drainage of blood and mucus from the throat and mouth and avoid their aspiration into the respiratory passages. Signs of excessive bleeding from the operative site include bright red blood from the mouth or nose, frequent swallowing, and extreme restlessness. Efforts to keep a child quiet may include holding, rocking, or otherwise providing comfort until the effects of anesthesia wear off. An ice collar is helpful in preventing edema, reducing blood loss, and eliminating nausea.

During the immediate postoperative period the diet is restricted to bland liquids or

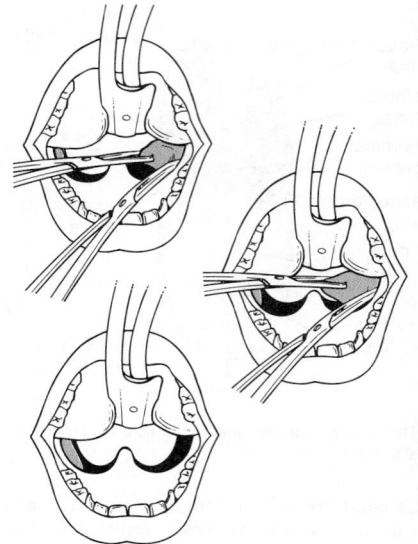

Tonsillectomy. Scissor dissection of the tonsil. From Bluestone and Stool, 1995.

semi-liquids. Citrus fruit juices and liquids at extreme temperatures should be avoided. As the throat heals and edema subsides more solid foods are gradually added to the diet, but for at least a week after surgery all foods that are chemically, physically, or thermally irritating to the throat should be avoided.

tonsillitis (ton″sĭ-li′tis) inflammation and enlargement of a TONSIL, especially the palatine tonsils. Enlarged tonsils and adenoids need not be a cause for concern unless they become a source of chronic infection or interfere with swallowing or breathing. They may become enlarged in the process of filtering out frequent, mild infections. Also, the adenoids usually grow larger in children until about the age of 5 years, and then they may cease to be troublesome. Tonsils are part of the lymphatic system which aids the body in fighting off infections and "invasions" of foreign matter. Although their exact purpose is unknown, they are believed to act as filters and fighters of bacteria, guarding the entrances to the throat and nasal passages. Sometimes however, they are overcome by the invading bacteria and become infected. One form of infection sometimes causing tonsillitis is streptococcal infection of the throat.

Symptoms and Treatment. A mild case of tonsillitis may appear to be only a slight sore throat. Symptoms of acute tonsillitis are inflamed, swollen tonsils and a very sore throat, with high fever, rapid pulse, and general weakness. Swallowing is difficult and the lymph nodes in the neck may become swollen and painful. Occasionally in an attack of severe tonsillitis an abscess may form around the tonsil, a condition called QUINSY. Treatment usually consists of administration of antibiotics, with gargles and rest. When tonsillitis is recurrent and troublesome, however, it may be necessary to remove the tonsils surgically (TONSILLEC-TOMY).

follicular t. tonsillitis especially affecting the crypts.

tonsilloadenoidectomy (ton″sĭ-lo-ad″ĕ-noi-dek′tah-me) adenotonsillectomy.

tonsillolith (ton-sil′o-lith) a calculus in a tonsil.

tonsillotomy (ton″sĭ-lot′ah-me) incision of a tonsil.

tonus (to′nus) tone or tonicity; the slight, continuous contraction of a muscle, which in skeletal muscles aids in the maintenance of posture and in the return of blood to the heart.

tooth (to͞oth), pl. *teeth* one of the small bonelike structures of the jaws for biting and mastication of food; they also help in the shaping of sounds and forming of words in speech.

Structure. The portion of a tooth that rises above the gum is the crown; the portion below is the root. The crown is covered by ENAMEL, which is related to the epithelial tissue of the skin and is the hardest substance in the human body. The surface of the root is composed of a bonelike tissue called CEMENTUM. Underneath the surface enamel and cementum is a substance called DENTIN, which makes up the main body of the tooth. Within the dentin, in a space in the center of the tooth, is the dental PULP, a soft, sensitive tissue that contains nerves and blood and lymph vessels. The cementum, dentin, and pulp are formed from connective tissue. (See color plates.)

Covering the root of the tooth and holding it in place in its ALVEOLUS (socket) in the jaw is a fibrous connective tissue called the PERIODONTIUM. Its many strong fibers are embedded in the cementum and also the wall of the tooth socket. The periodontium not only helps hold the tooth in place but also acts to cushion it against the pressure caused by biting and chewing.

There are 20 primary teeth, called also deciduous teeth, baby teeth, or milk teeth, which are eventually replaced by 32 permanent teeth, evenly divided between the upper and lower jaws.

Teeth have different shapes because they have different functions. The *incisors,* in the front of the mouth, are shaped like a

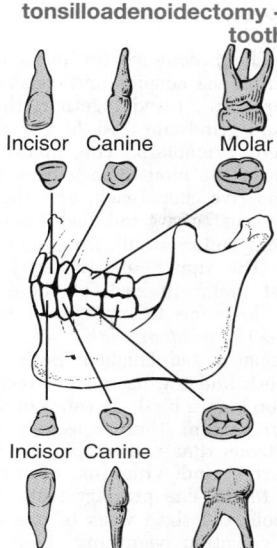

Incisor Canine   Molar

Incisor Canine

Typical deciduous teeth.

cone with a sharp flattened end, and cut the food. There are eight deciduous and permanent incisors, four upper and four lower. The *canines* (or *cuspids*) are at the corners of the mouth and are shaped like simple cones; they tear and shred food. There are four permanent canines; the two in the upper jaw are popularly known as the "eye

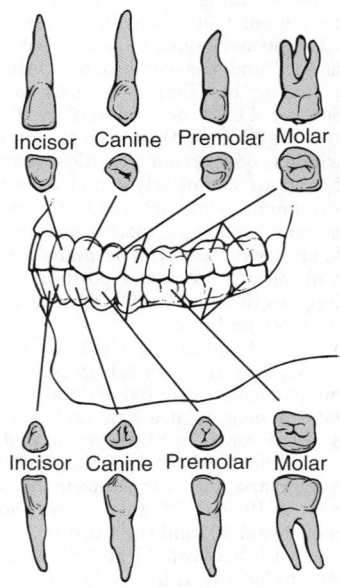

Incisor Canine Premolar Molar

Incisor Canine Premolar Molar

Typical permanent teeth.

T

teeth." The *premolars* (or *bicuspids*) are next behind the cuspids and consist of two cones, or cusps, fused together; they tear, crush, and grind the food. There are eight permanent premolars. The *molars* are in the back of the mouth; they have between three and five cusps each, and their function is to crush and grind food. There are 12 permanent molars in all, three on each side of both the upper and lower jaw. The hindmost molar in each of these groups, and the last one to emerge, is popularly known as the *wisdom tooth.*

Development and Eruption. Both the primary teeth and the permanent teeth begin to develop before birth. Because of this, it is vitally important that expectant mothers receive foods that will supply the calcium, phosphorus, and vitamins necessary for healthy teeth. The primary teeth begin to form about the sixth week of prenatal life, with calcification beginning about the sixteenth week. A considerable part of the crowns of these teeth is formed by the time the child is born. Eruption, or cutting of teeth, is slower in some children than others, but the primary teeth generally begin to appear when the infant is between 6 and 9 months of age, and the process is completed by the age of 2 to $2\frac{1}{2}$ years.

When the child is about 6, the first permanent molar comes in just behind the second molar of the primary teeth. About the same time, shedding of primary teeth begins. The permanent teeth form in the jaw even before the primary ones have erupted, with the incisors and the canines beginning to calcify during the first 6 months of life. Calcification of the others takes place shortly after. As the adult teeth calcify, the roots of the primary ones gradually disappear, or resorb, and are completely gone by the time the permanent teeth are ready to appear. Occasionally a primary tooth root does not resorb, and as a result the permanent tooth comes in outside its proper position. When this happens, it is necessary to remove the primary tooth and root.

The first teeth to be shed, about the sixth year, are the central incisors. The permanent incisors erupt shortly afterward. The lateral incisors are lost and replaced during the seventh to ninth years, and the canines in the ninth to twelfth years. The first premolars generally appear between the ages of 10 and 12, the second molars between 11 and 13, and the third molars, or wisdom teeth, between 17 and 22. It is not uncommon for the third molars to fail to erupt.

Occasionally there is a partial or total lack of either the primary or the permanent teeth (ANODONTIA). In some cases this is inherited, and in others it may be related to endocrine gland disturbances.

Tooth Decay and Its Prevention. Tooth decay, or DENTAL CARIES, is the most common disease in the United States. It begins on the outside of the teeth in the enamel as bacteria and refined carbohydrates adhere to the tooth surface to form PLAQUE. The action of the bacteria on starchy and sugary foods produces LACTIC ACID, which is believed to dissolve the enamel. Once there is a break in the enamel (DEMINERALIZATION), the decaying process moves on into the dentin and then to the pulp, attacking the nerve and causing toothache. For methods of treatment and prevention, see DENTAL CARIES.

accessional teeth the permanent molars, so called because they have no primary tooth predecessors in the dental arch. See also succedaneous teeth.

anterior teeth the teeth in the anterior parts of the dental arches; the incisors and canines.

avulsed t. a tooth that has been traumatically dislocated, usually salvageable for a reimplantation if appropriate treatment is initiated promptly. Prior to treatment the tooth can be placed in the conscious patient's mouth or in ice water or cold milk. No attempt should be made to cleanse the tooth.

Hutchinson's teeth abnormal teeth seen in congenital SYPHILIS, in which the permanent incisors have a screwdriver-like shape, sometimes associated with notching of the incisal edges.

impacted t. one so placed in the jaw that it is unable to erupt or to attain its normal position in occlusion. See also dental IMPACTION.

intruded t. a tooth that has been forcefully pushed into the patient's gums and may appear to be absent; it will usually return to the normal position within one month.

posterior teeth the teeth in the posterior parts of the dental arches; the premolars and molars.

succedaneous teeth, successional teeth the permanent teeth that have primary tooth predecessors in the dental arch. See also accessional teeth.

wisdom t. the third molar, the tooth most distal to the medial line on either side in each jaw; so called because it is the last of the permanent dentition to erupt, usually at the age of 17 to 21 years.

top(o)- word element [Gr.], *particular place or area.*

topagnosia (top″ag-no′zhah) 1. loss of touch localization. 2. loss of ability to recognize familiar surroundings.

topalgia (to-pal′jah) pain fixed in one spot, a common feature of pain without organic basis, as seen in CONVERSION DISORDER.

topectomy (to-pek′tah-me) ablation of a small and specific area of the frontal cortex in the treatment of mental illness.

topesthesia (top″es-the′zhah) ability to recognize the location of a tactile stimulus.

tophaceous (to-fa′shus) gritty or sandy; pertaining to tophi.

tophus (to′fus) [L.] 1. a chalky deposit of sodium urate occurring in GOUT; tophi form most often around the joints in cartilage, bone, bursae, and subcutaneous tissue and in the external ear, producing a chronic, foreign-body inflammatory RESPONSE. 2. dental CALCULUS.

t. syphili′ticus syphilitic node.

topical (top′ĭ-kal) pertaining to a particular area, such as a topical antiinfective agent applied to a certain area of the skin and affecting only the area to which it is applied.

topiramate (to-pi′rah-māt) a substituted monosaccharide used as an ANTICONVULSANT in treatment of partial SEIZURES; administered orally.

topoanesthesia (to″po-an″es-the′zhah) inability to recognize the location of a tactile stimulus.

topography (to-pog′rah-fe) a special description of an anatomic region or a special part. adj., **topograph′ic.**

topoisomerase (to″po-i′so-mer-ās) an enzyme involved in mobilization and replication of DNA during cell division.

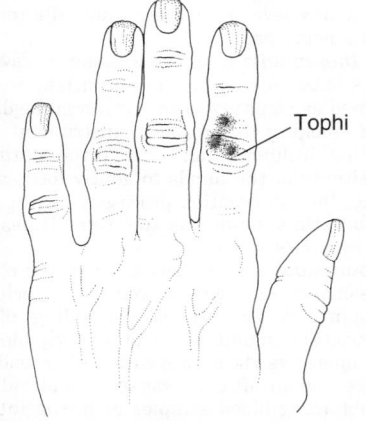

Tophi

Tophus. Typical appearance of tophi, which are common in chronic gout, shown on an index finger. From gnatavicius and Workman, 2000.

topotecan (to″po-te′kan) an antineoplastic AGENT used as the hydrochloride salt in treatment of metastatic ovarian carcinoma and small cell lung carcinoma; administered by intravenous infusion.

TOPV poliovirus vaccine live oral trivalent.

TORCH toxoplasmosis, rubella, cytomegalovirus, and herpes virus, which are perinatal infections of concern in maternal and neonatal care. All causative organisms in this group are capable of crossing the placenta and damaging the fetus.

torcular Herophili (tor′ku-ler he-rof′ĭ-le) a depression in the occipital bone at the confluence of a number of cerebral venous sinuses.

toremifene (tor′ĕ-mĭ-fēn″) an analogue of TAMOXIFEN that acts as an ESTROGEN antagonist; used as the citrate salt in palliative treatment of metastatic breast carcinoma, administered orally.

torpid (tor′pid) not acting with normal vigor and facility.

torpor (tor′por) [L.] sluggishness.

t. re′tinae sluggish response of the retina to the stimulus of light.

torque (tork) a rotatory force causing part of a structure to twist about an axis.

torr (tor) a unit of pressure equal to one millimeter of mercury (mm Hg), or 133.3 pascals.

torsades de pointes (tor-sahd′ duh pwahnt) an atypical rapid ventricular TACHYCARDIA with periodic waxing and waning of amplitude of the QRS complexes on the electrocardiogram. It is usually drug related and may be either self-limiting or progressing to ventricular FIBRILLATION.

torsemide (tor′sĕ-mīd) a DIURETIC related to SULFONYLUREA, used in treatment of EDEMA and HYPERTENSION, administered orally or intravenously.

torsion (tor′shun) the act of twisting; the state of being twisted. (See accompanying illustration.) adj., **tor′sive.**

tibial t. inward twisting of the tibia so that the foot turns inward.

torsiversion (tor″sĭ-ver′zhun) turning of a tooth on its long axis out of normal position.

torso (tor′so) trunk (def. 1).

torticollis (tor″tĭ-kol′is) a contracted state of the cervical muscles, producing torsion of the neck; the deformity may be congenital, hysterical, or secondary to conditions such as pressure on the accessory nerve, inflammation of glands in the neck, or muscle spasm. Called also wryneck.

tortipelvis (tor″tĭ-pel′vis) distortions of the spine and hip produced by a disorder

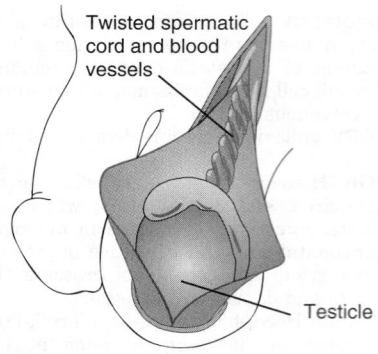

Twisted spermatic cord and blood vessels

Testicle

Testicular torsion. From Copstead and Banasik, 2000.

marked by irregular muscular contractions of the trunk and extremities.

tortuous (tor'choo-us) twisted; full of turns and twists.

torulus (tor'u-lus) [L.] a small elevation.

t. tac'tilis a tactile elevation in the skin of the palms and soles.

torus (tor'us) [L.] a swelling or bulging projection.

t. mandibula'ris a prominence sometimes seen on the lingual aspect of the mandible at the base of its alveolar part.

t. palati'nus a bony protuberance sometimes found on the hard palate at the junction of the intermaxillary suture and the transverse palatine suture.

tosylate (to'sĭ-lāt) USAN contraction for *p*-toluenesulfonate.

totipotential (to″tĭ-po-ten'shal) exhibiting totipotency; characterized by the ability to develop in any direction; said of cells that can give rise to cells of all types. adj., **totipo'tent.**

touch (tuch) 1. palpation with the finger. 2. in the NURSING INTERVENTIONS CLASSIFICATION, a nursing INTERVENTION defined as providing comfort and communication through purposeful tactile contact. 3. the sense by which contact of an object with the skin is recognized. Touch is actually not a single sense, but several. There are separate nerves in the skin to register heat, cold, pressure, pain, light touch, and coarse touch. These thousands of nerves are distributed unevenly over the body, so that some areas are more responsive to cold, others to pain, and others to heat or pressure. Each of these types of nerves has a different structure at the receiving end. A nerve for light touch has an elongated bulb-shaped end; one responsive to cold ends in a squat bulb; one that registers warmth ends with what look like twisted threads; and a nerve for deep pressure has an egg-shaped end. Pain receptors have no protective sheath.

If the sensory nerves were evenly distributed over the whole body, each square inch (6.5 square cm) of skin would have about 50 heat receptors, 8 for cold, 100 for touch, and 800 for pain. The sensitivity of a given spot depends in part on how thickly receptors of any one kind are clustered in that spot, and localization of a particular sensation depends on the concentration of the necessary nerve endings in the area. Light touch, pressure, and pain are sensations that can be localized quite accurately, but sensations of cold and heat are more diffuse.

The thickness of the skin in a given area and its supply of hairs also contribute to its touch sensitivity. A touch as light as one fifteen-thousandth of an ounce on the thin skin of the forehead can be felt, whereas a touch must be two and a half times as heavy to be felt on a fingertip. Hairs grow almost everywhere on the skin except the palms of the hands and the soles of the feet. They grow at a slant, and touch spots cluster in the skin near each of them. Even a light touch on the tip of a hair bends it back, and like a tiny lever it communicates the touch to the nerve endings.

therapeutic t. in the NURSING INTERVENTIONS CLASSIFICATION, a nursing INTERVENTION defined as attuning to the universal healing field, seeking to act as an instrument for healing influence, and using the natural sensitivity of the hands to gently focus and direct the intervention process.

Tourette's syndrome (too-rets') Gilles de la Tourette's syndrome.

tourniquet (toor'nĭ-ket) a device for compression of an artery or vein; uses include stopping of the excessive bleeding of a HEMORRHAGE, maintenance of a nearly bloodless operative FIELD, prevention of spread of snake venom after a SNAKEBITE, and aiding in obtaining blood samples or giving intravenous INJECTIONS.

For hemorrhage, a tourniquet should be used only as a last resort, when the bleeding

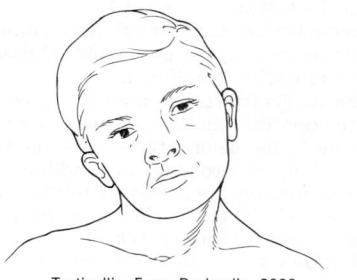

Torticollis. From Dorland's, 2000.

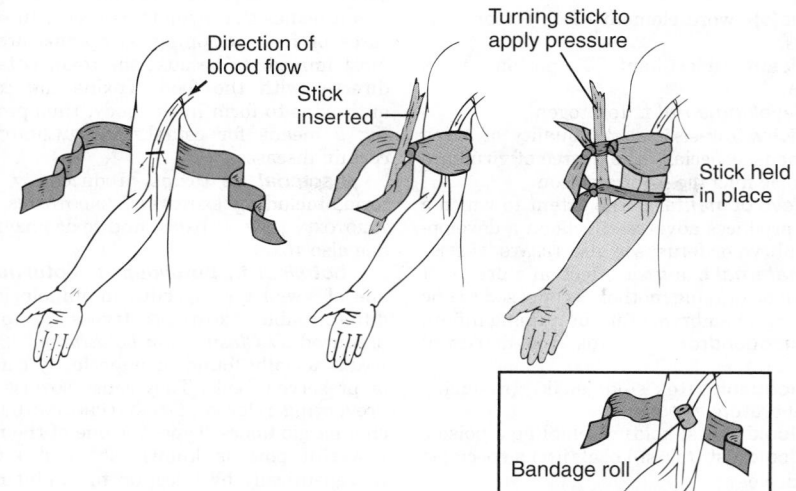

Direction of
blood flow

Stick
inserted

Turning stick to
apply pressure

Stick held
in place

Bandage roll

To apply a tourniquet for control of arterial bleeding from the arm: Wrap a gauze pad twice with a strip of cloth just below the armpit and tie with a half knot; tie a stick at the knot with a square knot. Slowly twist stick to tighten.

is so severe that it is threatening the life of the injured person and cannot be stopped by direct pressure. In the case of snakebite, a moderately tight tourniquet may be applied to impede the spread of venom while not stopping arterial blood flow. For an intravenous injection, a loosely applied tourniquet inhibits blood flow in the superficial veins, making them more prominent so that a vein can be found for the injection. For maintenance of a nearly bloodless operative FIELD, pneumatic tourniquets are often used. The American Association of Operating Room Nurses (AORN) has published guidelines for the use of tourniquets during surgery; see their web site at http://www.aorn.org.

t. test one involving the application of a tourniquet to a limb, as in determination of capillary FRAGILITY (denoted by the appearance of petechiae) or of the status of the collateral circulation.

tox(o)- word element [Gr.; L.], *poison; poisonous.*

toxemia (tok-se′me-ah) 1. the condition resulting from the spread of bacterial products (toxins) by the bloodstream. 2. a name formerly used to indicate a pregnancy-related syndrome typified by edema, proteinuria, and hypertension that was thought to be due to a toxin released by the mother in response to a foreign protein of the developing fetus. adj., **toxe′mic.**

t. of pregnancy former name for PRE-ECLAMPSIA-ECLAMPSIA SYNDROME.

toxic (tok′sik) poisonous; see POISON.

t. shock syndrome (TSS) a severe illness characterized by high fever of sudden onset, vomiting, diarrhea, and myalgia, followed by hypotension and, in severe cases, shock and death. A sunburn-like rash with peeling of the skin, especially of the palms and soles, occurs during the late phase. The syndrome affects almost exclusively menstruating women using tampons, although a few women who do not use tampons and a few males have been affected. It is thought to be caused by a toxin secreted by a strain of *Staphylococcus aureus.*

Treatment includes supportive therapy for SHOCK, antibiotics, and management of respiratory distress, gastrointestinal, and renal involvement when indicated.

Prevention. The Centers for Disease Control and Prevention suggest that toxic shock syndrome could be almost entirely eliminated if the use of vaginal tampons were stopped. However, this is not acceptable for many women. Most authorities do recommend that women who have had the condition and are at risk for recurrence not use tampons at all. Any woman who has had the infection should at least refrain from using tampons until three months after the attack or until she has a negative vaginal culture for *Staphylococcus aureus.* All women should be cautioned to wash their hands thoroughly before inserting a tampon and to change tampons at least every 6 to 8 hours.

T

toxic(o)- word element [Gr.], *poison; poisonous.*

toxicant (tok′sĭ-kant) 1. poisonous. 2. poison.

developmental t. teratogen.

toxicity (tok-sis′ĭ-te) the quality of being poisonous, especially the degree of virulence of a toxic microbe or of a poison.

developmental t. the extent to which a toxin produces adverse effects on a developing embryo or fetus; see also TERATOGENESIS.

maternal t. a toxic effect on a pregnant woman or nursing mother, as opposed to one affecting an embryo, fetus, or nursing infant.

Toxicodendron (tok″sĭ-ko-den′dron) *Rhus.*

toxicogenic (tok″sĭ-ko-jen′ik) producing or elaborating POISONS.

toxicoid (tok′sĭ-koid) resembling a poison.

toxicologist (tok″sĭ-kol′ah-jist) a specialist in toxicology.

developmental t. one who specializes in developmental TOXICOLOGY; see also TERATOLOGIST.

reproductive t. one who studies the effects of toxins on the reproductive system.

toxicology (tok″sĭ-kol′ah-je) the science or study of poisons. adj., **toxicolog′ic.**

developmental t. the study of the effects of toxins on developing embryos; see also TERATOLOGY.

toxicopathy (tok″sĭ-kop′ah-the) toxicosis. adj., **toxicopath′ic.**

toxicopexy (tok′sĭ-ko-pek″se) the fixation or neutralization of a poison in the body. adj., **toxicopec′tic, toxicopex′ic.**

toxicophidia (tok″sĭ-ko-fid′e-ah) the venomous SNAKES; see also *viper.*

toxicophobia (tok″sĭ-ko-fo′be-ah) irrational fear of being poisoned.

toxicosis (tok″sĭ-ko′sis) any diseased condition due to poisoning.

toxidrome (tok′sĭ-drōm) a specific syndromelike group of symptoms associated with exposure to a given POISON.

toxiferous (tok-sif′er-us) conveying or producing a poison.

toxigenic (tok″sĭ-jen′ik) toxicogenic.

toxigenicity (tok″sĭ-jĕ-nis′ĭ-te) the property of producing toxins.

toxin (tok′sin) a POISON, especially a protein or conjugated protein produced by certain animals, higher plants, and pathogenic bacteria. Bacterial toxins characteristically do not cause symptoms until after a period of incubation while the microbes multiply, or (as happens with botulism) the preformed toxin reaches and affects the tissue. Usually only a few toxin-producing agents are introduced into the body, and it is not until there are enough of them to overwhelm the leukocytes and other types of antibodies that symptoms occur. In some cases of food poisoning, symptoms are almost immediate because the toxin is taken directly with the food. Toxins can cause antitoxins to form in the body, thus providing a means for establishing IMMUNITY to certain diseases.

bacterial t′s toxins produced by bacteria, including EXOTOXINS, ENDOTOXINS, ENTEROTOXINS, NEUROTOXINS, and toxic enzymes. See also TOXIN.

botulinal t., botulinum t. botulinus t. one of seven type-specific, immunologically differentiable EXOTOXINS (types A to G) produced by *Clostridium botulinum,* NEUROTOXINS usually found in imperfectly canned or preserved foods. They cause BOTULISM by preventing release of ACETYLCHOLINE by the cholinergic fibers. Type A is one of the most powerful poisons known; it is also used therapeutically by injection to inhibit muscular spasm in the treatment of dystonic disorders such as BLEPHAROSPASM and STRABISMUS, to treat wrinkles of the upper face, and to reduce anal sphincter pressure to promote healing of chronic anal FISSURE. Type B is injected in treatment of cervical dystonia. Called also botulin.

cholera t. an EXOTOXIN produced by *Vibrio cholerae;* a protein ENTEROTOXIN that binds to the membrane of enteric cells and stimulates the ADENYLATE CYCLASE system, causing the hypersecretion of chloride and bicarbonate ions, resulting in increased fluid secretion and the severe diarrhea characteristic of CHOLERA.

clostridial t. one elaborated by species of *Clostridium,* including those causing BOTULISM (botulinus TOXIN), gas GANGRENE (gas gangrene TOXIN), and TETANUS (tetanus TOXIN). In addition, *C. difficile* produces an EXOTOXIN causing severe intestinal necrosis and *C. perfringens* produces exotoxins causing gas gangrene, intestinal necrosis, hemolysis, cardiotoxicity, and DEOXYRIBONUCLEASE and HYALURONIDASE activity, as well as an enterotoxin causing FOOD POISONING.

Dick t. erythrogenic toxin.

diphtheria t. a protein EXOTOXIN produced by *Corynebacterium diphtheriae* that is primarily responsible for the pathogenesis of DIPHTHERIA and related infections; it is an enzyme that activates transferase II of the mammalian protein synthesizing system.

diphtheria t. for Schick test a sterile solution of the diluted, standardized toxic products of *Corynebacterium diphtheriae;* used as a dermal reactivity indicator in the SCHICK TEST of immunity to DIPHTHERIA.

dysentery t. any of various EXOTOXINS produced by species of *Shigella;* the one formed by *S. dysenteriae* serotype 1 is a potent neurotoxin with hemorrhagic and paralytic properties.

erythrogenic t. a bacterial toxin from certain strains of *Streptococcus pyogenes* that produces an erythematous reaction when injected intradermally and is responsible for the rash in SCARLET FEVER.

extracellular t. exotoxin.

gas gangrene t. an EXOTOXIN that causes gas GANGRENE; there are at least 10 types produced by *Clostridium perfringens* and others produced by *C. noriyi* and *C. septicum.*

streptococcal t. a mixture of EXOTOXINS formed by *Streptococcus pyogenes.*

tetanus t. the potent exotoxin produced by *Clostridium tetani,* consisting of two components, one a neurotoxin *(tetanospasmin)* and the other a hemolysin *(tetanolysin).*

toxinology (tok″sin-ol′ah-je) the science dealing with the toxins produced by certain higher plants and animals and by pathogenic bacteria.

toxipathy (tok-sip′ah-the) toxicosis.

Toxocara (tok″so-ka′rah) a genus of nematode parasites found in the dog (*T. ca′nis*) and cat (*T. ca′ti*); both species are sometimes found in humans.

toxocariasis (tok″so-ka-ri′ah-sis) infection by worms of the genus *Toxocara.*

toxoid (tok′soid) a TOXIN treated by heat or chemical agent to destroy its deleterious properties without destroying its ability to combine with or stimulate the formation of antitoxin.

diphtheria t. a sterile preparation of formaldehyde-treated products of the growth of *Corynebacterium diphtheriae,* used as an active immunizing agent, generally in mixtures with tetanus toxoid and pertussis vaccine (DTP) or with tetanus toxoid alone (DT for pediatric use and Td, which contains less diphtheria toxoid, for adult use).

tetanus t. a sterile preparation of formaldehyde-treated products of the growth of *Clostridium tetani,* used as an active immunizing agent, either in mixtures with diphtheria toxoid and pertussis vaccine (DTP, DT, Td) or by itself (T).

toxophore (tok′so-for) the group of atoms in a toxin molecule that produces the toxic effect. adj., **toxoph′orous.**

Toxoplasma (tok″so-plaz′mah) a genus of sporozoans that are parasites of humans, other mammals, and some birds; it includes one species, *T. gon′dii,* that can be transmitted from an infected mother to an

infant *in utero* or at birth. See also TOXOPLASMOSIS. See accompanying illustration.

toxoplasmin (tok″so-plaz′min) an antigen prepared from mouse peritoneal fluids rich with *Toxoplasma gondii;* injected intracutaneously as a test for toxoplasmosis.

toxoplasmosis (tok″so-plaz-mo′sis) a disease due to *Toxoplasma gondii.* The *congenital* form may be asymptomatic or may produce ENCEPHALOMYELITIS with cerebral calcification, CHORIORETINITIS and blindness, and even death. The *acquired* form is of two types: *lymphadenopathic toxoplasmosis,* closely resembling mononucleosis, and *disseminated toxoplasmosis,* with lesions involving the lungs, liver, heart, skin, muscle, brain, and meninges. Chorioretinitis invariably occurs in the congenital form, and often in the chronic form.

The only effective treatment of toxoplasmosis is the combination of pyrimethamine (Daraprim) and sulfadiazine or triple sulfonamides given for a total of 30 days. Treatment is reserved for those who are not immunologically competent. Treatment during pregnancy will not eliminate congenital toxoplasmosis but it can minimize its effects.

Prevention of infection with the protozoan parasite is aimed at avoiding ingestion of infective cysts in raw meat and eliminating contact with cat feces. Mutton, pork, and goat meat are more likely to be contaminated than beef; however, all meats should be thoroughly cooked, cured, or smoked before ingestion. Careful handling and disposal of cat litter can reduce the possibility of contamination from the feces of a pet cat, but it is difficult to determine when the cat has become infected.

tPA tissue-type plasminogen activator.

TPA, t-PA 1. t-plasminogen activator. 2. total parenteral alimentation (see PARENTERAL NUTRITION); t-plasminogen activator.

TPHA *Treponema pallidum* hemagglutination assay.

t-plasminogen activator (plaz-min′o-jen ak′tĭ-va″tor) see tissue plasminogen ACTIVATOR.

TPN total PARENTERAL NUTRITION.

TPR temperature, pulse, and respiration.

tr. tincture.

trabecula (trah-bek′u-lah) [L.] a small beam or supporting structure; used in anatomic nomenclature to designate various fibromuscular bands or cords providing support in various organs, as heart, penis, and spleen, adj., **trabec′ular.**

trabeculae of bone anastomosing bony spicules in cancellous bone which form a

T

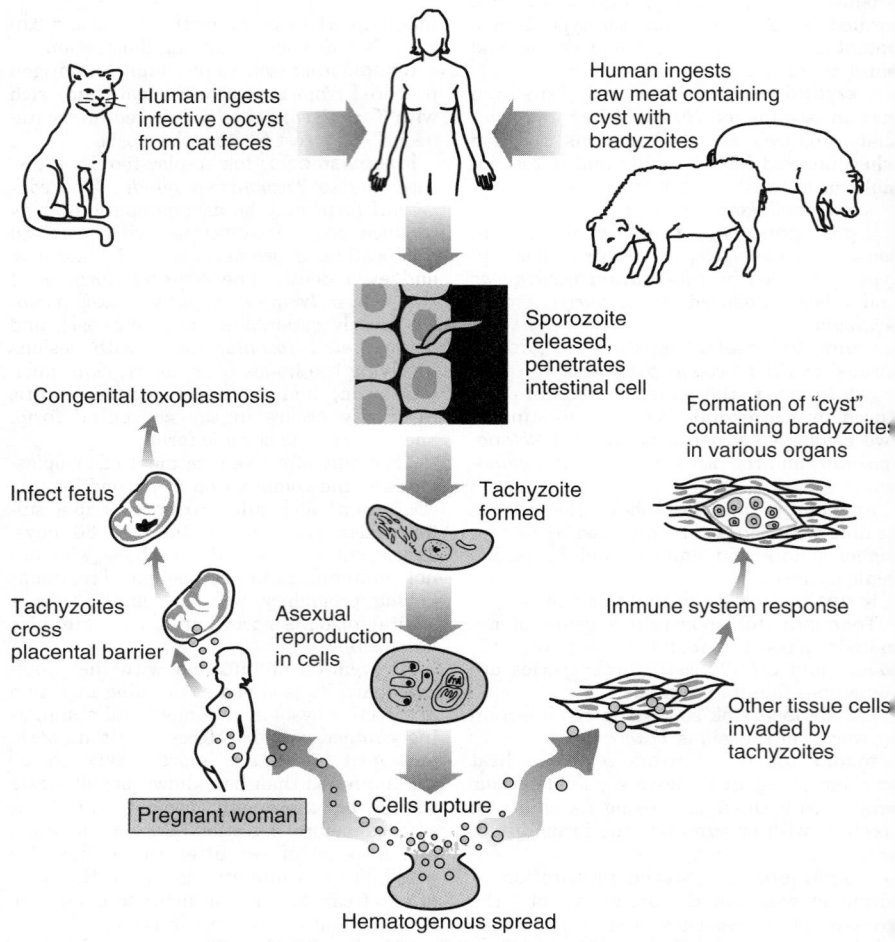

Human ingests infective oocyst from cat feces

Human ingests raw meat containing cyst with bradyzoites

Sporozoite released, penetrates intestinal cell

Congenital toxoplasmosis

Infect fetus

Formation of "cyst" containing bradyzoites in various organs

Tachyzoite formed

Tachyzoites cross placental barrier

Asexual reproduction in cells

Immune system response

Pregnant woman

Cells rupture

Other tissue cells invaded by tachyzoites

Hematogenous spread

Life cycle of *Toxoplasma gondii*. From Mahon and Manuselis, 2000.

meshwork of intercommunicating spaces that are filled with bone marrow.

trabeculate (trah-bek'u-lāt) marked with crossbars or trabeculae.

trabeculation (trah-bek"u-la'shun) the formation of TRABECULAE in a part.

trabeculectomy (trah-bek"u-lek'tah-me) creation of a fistula between the anterior chamber of the eye and the subconjunctival space by surgical removal of a portion of the trabecular meshwork, performed to facilitate drainage of the aqueous humor in glaucoma.

trabeculoplasty (trah-bek'u-lo-plas"te) plastic surgery of a trabecula.

tracer (trās'er) 1. a means or agent by which certain substances or structures can be identified or followed, as a radioactive tracer. 2. a mechanical device by which the outline of an object or the direction and extent of movement of a part may be graphically recorded; see also TRACING. 3. a dissecting instrument for isolating vessels and nerves.

radioactive t. a radioactive isotope replacing a stable chemical element in a compound (said to be radiolabeled) and so able to be followed or tracked through one or more reactions or systems by means of a radiation detector; used especially for such a compound that is introduced into the body for study of the compound's metabolism, distribution, and passage through the body.

trache(o)- word element [Gr.], *trachea.*

trachea (tra′ke-ah), pl. *tra′cheae* the air passage extending from the throat and larynx to the main bronchi; it is about 1.5 cm (0.6 in) wide and 10 cm (4 in) long and is reinforced at the front and sides by a series of C-shaped rings of cartilage that keep the passage uniformly open. The gaps between the rings are bridged by strong fibroelastic membranes. The trachea is lined with mucous membrane covered with small hairlike processes called CILIA that continuously sweep foreign material out of the breathing passages toward the mouth, a process retarded by cold but speeded by heat. Called also windpipe. adj., **tra′cheal.**

Although the trachea is closed off by the lidlike EPIGLOTTIS during swallowing, a foreign body such as a piece of meat occasionally becomes lodged in the trachea and causes CHOKING. If a HEIMLICH MANEUVER does not succeed in dislodging the foreign body, emergency TRACHEOSTOMY (surgical incision of the trachea) may be necessary. Another reason for tracheostomy is in order to insert a tube for passage of air when the trachea is obstructed by swelling due to infection or allergic reaction, by accumulation of tracheobronchial secretions, or by a growth such as a polyp or tumor.

trachealgia (tra″ke-al′jah) pain in the trachea.

tracheitis (tra″ke-i′tis) inflammation of the trachea.

bacterial t. an acute crouplike bacterial infection of the upper airway in children, with coughing and high fever. Called also bacterial, membranous, or pseudomembranous croup.

trachel(o)- word element [Gr.], *neck; necklike structure; cervix uteri.* See also terms beginning CERVIC(O)-.

trachelectomy (tra″kĕ-lek′tah-me) cervicectomy.

trachelism (tra′kĕ-lizm) spasm of the neck muscles; spasmodic reaction of the head in epilepsy.

trachelismus (tra″kĕ-liz′mus) trachelism.

trachelitis (tra″kĕ-li′tis) cervicitis.

trachelocystitis (tra″kĕ-lo-sis-ti′tis) cystitis colli.

trachelopexy (tra″kĕ-lo-pek′se) fixation of the uterine cervix.

tracheloplasty (tra″kĕ-lo-plas′te) cervicoplasty.

trachelorrhaphy (tra″kĕ-lor′ah-fe) suture of the uterine cervix.

trachelotomy (tra″kĕ-lot′ah-me) cervicotomy.

tracheoaerocele (tra″ke-o-ār′o-sēl″) tracheal hernia containing air.

tracheobronchial (tra″ke-o-brong′ke-al) pertaining to the trachea and bronchi; called also bronchotracheal.

tracheobronchitis (tra″ke-o-brong-ki′tis) inflammation of the trachea and bronchi.

tracheobronchoscopy (tra″ke-o-brong-kos′kah-pe) inspection of the interior of the trachea and bronchus.

tracheocele (tra″ke-o-sēl) hernial protrusion of the tracheal mucous membrane.

tracheoesophageal (tra″ke-o-e-sof″ah-je′al) pertaining to the trachea and esophagus; called also esophagotracheal.

tracheolaryngeal (tra″ke-o-lah-rin′je-al) laryngotracheal.

tracheomalacia (tra″ke-o-mah-la′shah) softening of the tracheal cartilages, often as a congenital condition in infants or in patients of any age after prolonged intubation, and usually accompanied by a barking cough and expiratory stridor or wheezing; nearby organs such as the esophagus or aorta may compress the trachea and cause apnea.

tracheopathy (tra″ke-op′ah-the) disease of the trachea.

tracheopharyngeal (tra″ke-o-fah-rin′je-al) pertaining to the trachea and pharynx.

tracheophony (tra″ke-of′ah-ne) a voice SOUND heard over the trachea.

tracheoplasty (tra′ke-o-plas″te) plastic repair of the trachea.

tracheorrhagia (tra″ke-o-ra′jah) hemorrhage from the trachea.

tracheoschisis (tra″ke-os′kĭ-sis) fissure of the trachea.

tracheoscopy (tra″ke-os′kah-pe) inspection of the interior of the trachea. adj., **tracheoscop′ic.**

tracheostenosis (tra″ke-o-stĕ-no′sis) constriction of the trachea.

tracheostomize (tra″ke-os′to-mīz) to perform tracheostomy upon.

tracheostomy (tra″ke-os′tah-me) creation of an opening into the TRACHEA through the neck, with insertion of an indwelling tube to facilitate passage of air or evacuation of secretions. The procedure may be an emergency measure or an elective one.

Tracheostomy Tubes. There are many types of tracheostomy tubes available, but the basic structure is the same. All are curved to accommodate the anatomy of the trachea and most consist of an outer cannula to maintain the patency of the airway and an inner cannula that fits snugly inside the outer cannula and can be removed for cleaning and removal of accumulated secretions without disturbing the operative site. An accessory to the tracheostomy tubes is the obturator (pilot), which is an olive-tipped curved rod that is used to guide the outer cannula and prevent scraping of the tracheal walls while the tube is being inserted.

The earliest tracheostomy tubes were made of silver and consisted of only the three basic components. Later models came with an adaptor on the inner cannula to allow connection with a ventilator. The plastic tracheostomy tubes that are popular today may or may not have an inner cannula, but most have an inflatable cuff attached. The inflatable cuff may be built on the outer cannula, or it may be applied as needed. The cuff that is to be applied must be the proper size in order to be effective. The purpose of the cuff is to hold the tube in place and prevent the flow of air around the outside of the outer cannula. This allows for more effective ventilation of the patient and prevents the aspiration of liquids into the trachea. The cuffs may maintain a constant high or low pressure. Some cuffs are attached to a balloon to allow the pressure to vary in response to conditions within the trachea, for example, when a patient coughs or changes position.

Patient Care. The primary concerns of tracheostomy care are maintenance of an adequate airway by keeping the tube free of secretions and prevention of infection. The patient is observed closely for signs of respiratory difficulty. If there is a change in the respiratory rate or a wheezing or crowing sound during inhalation, the tube is probably obstructed. If suctioning does not relieve the situation, emergency assistance should be sought immediately. Restlessness, pallor, and the development of cyanosis are indications of inadequate ventilation of the lungs resulting from obstruction of the airway.

Accidental expulsion of the outer cannula due to violent coughing or improperly tied tapes is rare; should it happen, however, a dilator or hemostat must be used to hold open the incision while another tube is inserted. A dilator, obturator, and tracheostomy tube of the same size as that in the patient are kept at the bedside at all times.

The mucus will be slightly blood-tinged immediately after the tracheostomy is performed, but it should gradually assume a normal color. If there is evidence of persistent bleeding, this should be reported, as it may indicate internal hemorrhage. The mucus is suctioned as necessary with an electric or wall suction apparatus. The size of the catheter to be used for suctioning will depend on the size of the tracheostomy tube. The catheter should be small enough to move freely into and out of the tube and large enough to aspirate secretions effectively. Air inhaled through a tracheostomy tube is moisturized to prevent drying and caking of secretions. The instillation of sterile saline to loosen secretions was formerly done but is no longer recommended.

Tracheostomy care is usually a sterile procedure. Selected patients in home care settings may use clean techniques. Special care must be taken to prevent introduction of infectious organisms into either the surgical wound or the respiratory tract. Standard tracheostomy kits are available and usually include gauze sponges, twill tape, disposable containers for hydrogen peroxide, a small brush, pipe cleaners, and a tracheostomy dressing that is slit so that it fits around the tube. If additional dressings are needed, gauze squares without fillers are used and loose strings must be avoided so that fibers and threads are not aspirated through the tube.

Patients with a permanent tracheostomy must be taught self-care before leaving the hospital. As they become accustomed to breathing through the tube, suctioning it as necessary and replacing the dressings, they will become less apprehensive. Patients must be cautioned against swimming, and should be warned to use care when taking a shower or bath that water is not aspirated through the tracheostomy. Newer models of tracheostomy tubes allow the patient to speak without manually closing off the opening through which air passes into the trachea.

tracheotome (tra′ke-o-tōm″) an instrument for incising the trachea.

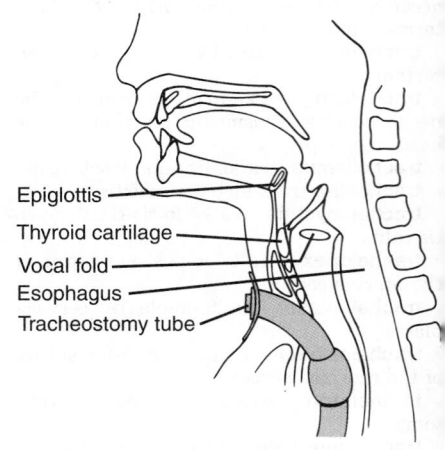

Epiglottis
Thyroid cartilage
Vocal fold
Esophagus
Tracheostomy tube

Tracheostomy tube in place.

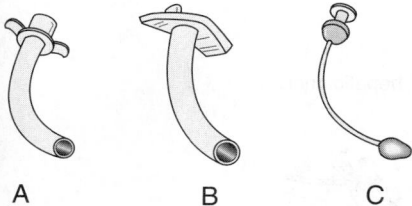

Parts of tracheostomy tube: *A*, Inner cannula. *B*, Outer cannula. *C*, Obturator.

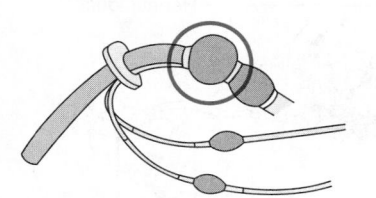

Two-cuff tracheostomy tube. The advantage of the two-cuff tube is that during prolonged artificial respiration the cuffs may be inflated alternately to prevent pressure necrosis. Circle indicates portion of tube inflated after insertion in patient.

tracheotomy (tra″ke-ot′ah-me) incision of the trachea through the skin and muscles of the neck for exploration, for removal of a foreign body, or for obtaining a biopsy specimen or removing a local lesion.

trachoma (trah-ko′mah), pl. *tracho′mata* a chronic infectious disease of the conjunctiva and cornea, producing PHOTOPHOBIA, pain, and LACRIMATION, caused by an organism once thought to be a virus but now classified as a strain of the bacteria *Chlamydia trachomatis*. It is more prevalent in Africa and Asia than in other parts of the world; in North Africa few persons reach adulthood without having contracted the infection. It is fairly common in parts of the United States, such as in parts of the Southwest where a hot dry climate and scarcity of water encourage its spread. Trachoma in children and adults begins with a conjunctivitis that is marked by tiny follicles on the upper eyelids and tarsal plate. The follicles become larger and larger, and there is granulation of the cornea and impairment of vision. Eventually there is severe scarring which results in BLINDNESS. Trachoma is the world's leading cause of preventable blindness.

A condition closely related to trachoma in cause, manifestations, and epidemiologic pattern is inclusion CONJUNCTIVITIS, which is fundamentally a sexually-transmitted disease of the adult genital tract. The agents of trachoma and inclusive conjunctivitis are called TRIC AGENTS.

Treatment and Prevention. The drug of choice in treatment of trachoma is AZITHROMYCIN; studies have demonstrated that a single oral dose eliminates the infection and prevents scarring. In areas where azithromycin is not available, tetracyclines may be used, administered topically in the form of suspensions or ointments that adhere to the conjunctiva for prolonged effect. Prevention of trachoma begins with an adequate water supply for washing the hands and bathing, control of flies, and education of the local population about the cause and spread of the disease. Early treatment of young children reduces the source of infection and avoids the complication of blindness. Repeated treatment programs for adults help control the spread of infection.

trachomatous (trah-ko′mah-tus) pertaining to or of the nature of trachoma.

trachyphonia (tra″ke-fo′ne-ah) hoarseness.

tracing (trās′ing) a graphic record produced by copying another, or scribed by an instrument capable of making a visual record of movements.

tract (trakt) a longitudinal assemblage of tissues or organs, especially a number of anatomic structures arranged in series and serving a common function, such as the gastrointestinal or urinary tract; also used in reference to a BUNDLE (or FASCICULUS) of nerve fibers having a common origin, function, and termination within the central nervous system.

alimentary t. ALIMENTARY CANAL.

biliary t. the organs, ducts, and other structures that participate in secretion (the liver), storage (the gallbladder), and delivery (hepatic and bile ducts) of bile into the duodenum. See illustration.

corticospinal t's two groups of nerve fibers (the *anterior* and *lateral corticospinal tracts*) that originate in the cerebral cortex and run through the spinal cord.

digestive t. ALIMENTARY CANAL.

dorsolateral t. a group of nerve fibers in the lateral funiculus of the spinal cord dorsal to the posterior column.

extrapyramidal t. EXTRAPYRAMIDAL SYSTEM.

gastrointestinal t. the stomach and intestine in continuity; see also DIGESTIVE SYSTEM.

iliotibial t. a thickened longitudinal band of fascia lata extending from the tensor muscle downward to the lateral condyle of the tibia.

intestinal t. see INTESTINAL TRACT.

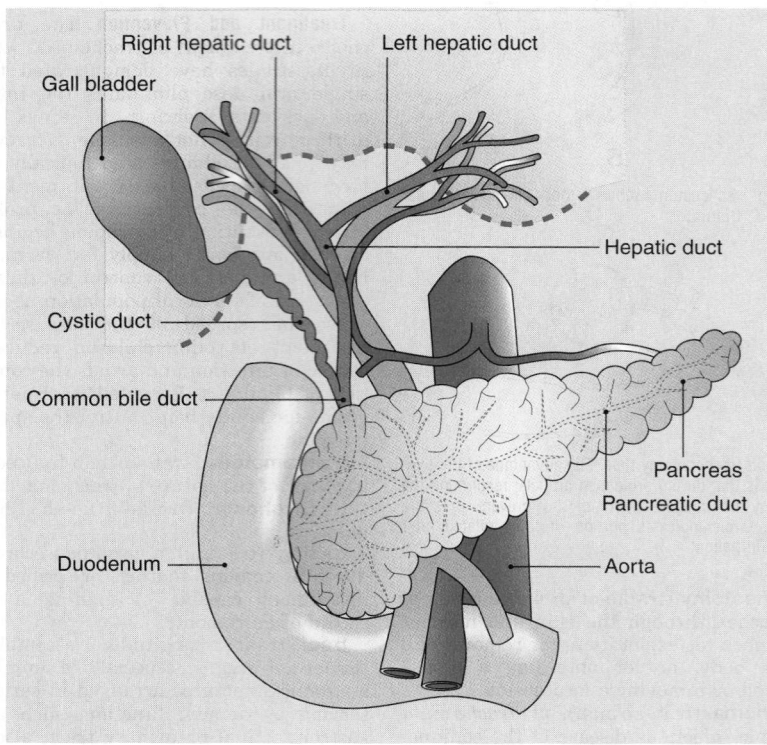

Labels on figure: Right hepatic duct, Left hepatic duct, Gall bladder, Hepatic duct, Cystic duct, Common bile duct, Duodenum, Pancreas, Pancreatic duct, Aorta

Anatomy of the gallbladder and biliary tract. From Aspinall and Taylor-Robinson, 2002.

optic t. the nerve tract proceeding backward from the optic chiasm, around the cerebral peduncle, and dividing into a lateral and medial root, which end in the superior colliculus and lateral geniculate body, respectively.

pyramidal t's collections of motor nerve fibers arising in the brain and passing down through the spinal cord to motor cells in the anterior horns.

respiratory t. respiratory SYSTEM.

urinary t. the organs and passageways concerned in the production and excretion of URINE from the KIDNEYS to the urinary MEATUS; see also urinary SYSTEM.

uveal t. the vascular tunic of the eye, comprising the choroid, ciliary body, and iris.

traction (trak′shun) the exertion of a pulling force, as that applied to a fractured bone or dislocated joint to maintain proper position and facilitate healing, or, in obstetrics, that along the axis of the pelvis to assist in delivery of a fetal part. It also may be used to overcome muscle spasms in musculoskeletal disorders such as herniated disk, to lessen or prevent contractures, and to correct or prevent a deformity.

Traction may be applied by means of a weight connected to a pulley mechanism over the patient's bed; this is known as *weight traction.* In *elastic traction* an elastic appliance exerts a pulling force upon the injured limb. In *skeletal traction,* a type for long-term heavyweight use, force is applied directly upon a bone by means of surgically installed pins and wires or tongs. Splints and reinforced garments, such as surgical corsets and collars, also may be employed to provide forms of traction. In *skin traction,* a temporary and lightweight type, moleskin or some other type of adhesive bandage is used to cover the affected limb, and traction is applied to the bandage. (See accompanying illustration.)

Patient Care. Patients in prolonged traction must be protected from the hazards of immobility. The integrity of the skin must be maintained and pressure sores avoided. A trapeze bar over the bed

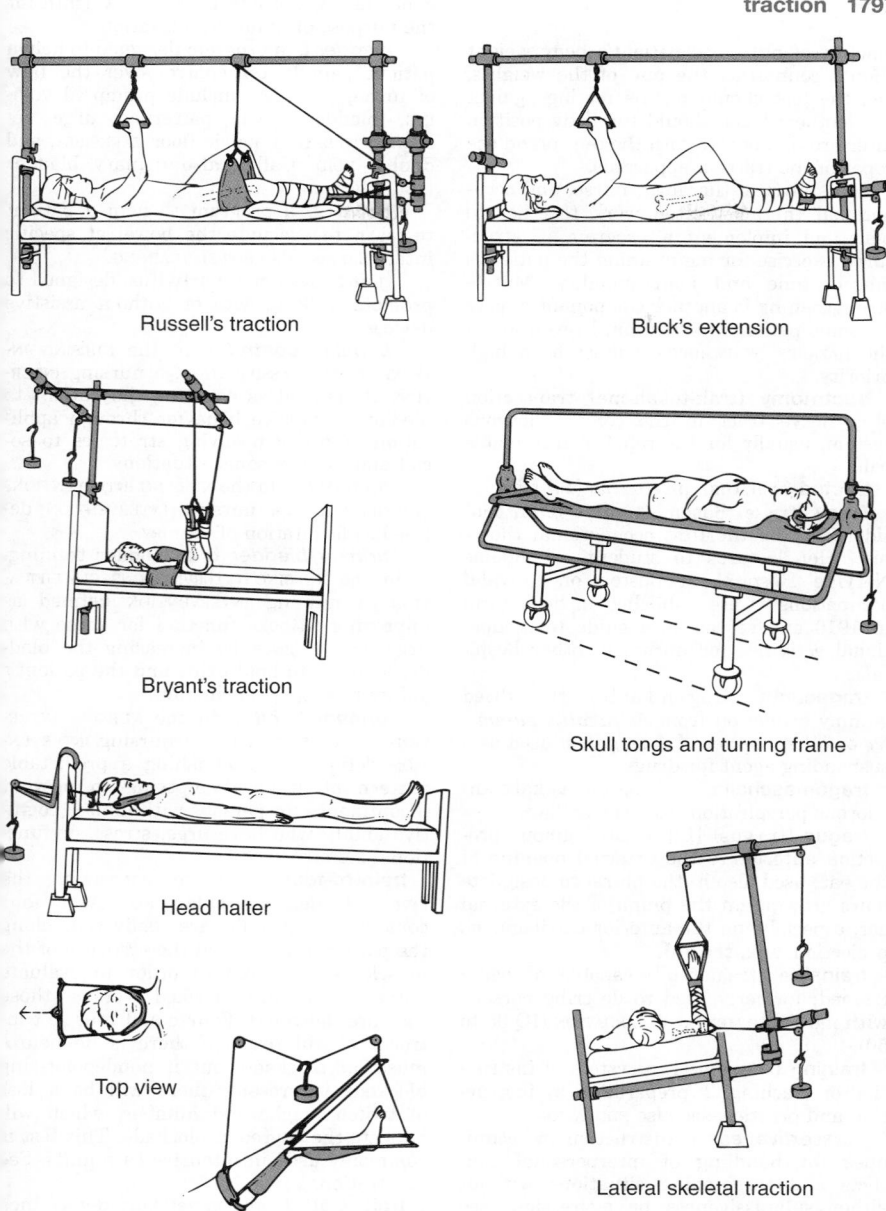

Russell's traction

Buck's extension

Bryant's traction

Skull tongs and turning frame

Head halter

Top view

Balanced suspension

Lateral skeletal traction

Various types of traction and suspension.

may be prescribed to give patients greater freedom in moving themselves about in bed and help them feel more independent. Patients should be instructed to lift themselves straight up so as not to alter the position of the affected limb in traction.

The apparatus used for traction must be checked frequently to be sure the weights are hanging free and exerting the required amount of pull. The patient's body weight should counteract the pull of the weights, i.e., the feet should not be resting against the footboard nor should the body position interfere in any way with the tension on the ropes of the traction apparatus.

The physical therapist, nurse, and occupational therapist often work together to plan and implement a program of structured exercise for maintaining the patient's muscle tone and joint mobility. Muscle strengthening is another component of care for some patients in traction. Prevention of the HAZARDS OF IMMOBILITY must be a high priority.

tractotomy (trak-tot′ah-me) transection of a nerve tract in the central nervous system, usually for the relief of intractable pain.

tractus (trak′tus), pl. *trac′tus* [L.] tract.

Tracy (tra′se) Susan. A nurse often considered to be the first occupational therapist. Her lectures to students at Adams Nervine Hospital in Boston on "invalid occupations" were published in book form in 1910 and served as a guide to occupational activities for nurses in other hospitals.

tragacanth (trag′ah-kanth) the dried gummy exudation from *Astragalus gummifer* or other species of *Astragalus;* used as a suspending agent for drugs.

tragomaschalia   (trag″o-mas-kal′e-ah) odorous perspiration from the axilla.

tragus (tra′gus) [L.] a cartilaginous projection anterior to the external opening of the ear; used also in the plural to designate hairs growing on the pinna of the external ear, especially on the anterior cartilaginous projection. adj., **tra′gal.**

trainable (tra′nah-b'l) capable of being trained; formerly used to describe persons with moderate MENTAL RETARDATION (IQ 35 to 50).

training (trān′ing) 1. a system of instruction or teaching. 2. preparation by instruction and practice; see also EDUCATION.

assertiveness t. instruction in techniques for handling of interpersonal conflicts and threatening situations without either submissiveness or aggression; see also ASSERTIVENESS TRAINING. 1. in the NURSING INTERVENTIONS CLASSIFICATION, a nursing INTERVENTION defined as assistance with the effective expression of feelings, needs, and ideas while respecting the rights of others.

autogenic t. in the NURSING INTERVENTIONS CLASSIFICATION, a nursing INTERVENTION defined as assisting with self-suggestions

about feelings of heaviness and warmth for the purpose of inducing relaxation.

bladder t. a program designed to help a patient gain better control over the flow of urine; examples include prompted VOIDING, bladder DRILL, patterned urge response TOILETING, pelvic floor EXERCISES, and double VOID. Called also urinary bladder training.

bowel t. a program to help a patient to learn to evacuate the bowel at specific intervals; see also BOWEL TRAINING.

gait t. systematic activities designed to promote walking with or without assistive devices.

impulse control t. in the NURSING INTERVENTIONS CLASSIFICATION, a nursing INTERVENTION defined as assisting the patient to mediate impulsive behavior through application of problem-solving strategies to social and interpersonal situations.

memory t. in the NURSING INTERVENTIONS CLASSIFICATION, a nursing INTERVENTION defined as facilitation of MEMORY.

urinary bladder t. 1. bladder training. 2. in the NURSING INTERVENTIONS CLASSIFICATION, a nursing INTERVENTION defined as improving BLADDER function for those with urge INCONTINENCE by increasing the bladder's ability to hold urine and the patient's ability to suppress urination.

urinary habit t. in the NURSING INTERVENTIONS CLASSIFICATION, a nursing INTERVENTION defined as establishing a predictable pattern of BLADDER emptying to prevent incontinence for persons with limited cognitive ability who have urge, stress, or functional INCONTINENCE.

train-of-four a test for measuring the level of neuromuscular BLOCKADE: four consecutive stimuli are delivered along the path of a nerve and the response of the muscle is measured in order to evaluate stimuli that are blocked versus those that are delivered. Four equal muscle contractions will result if there is no neuromuscular blockade, but if nondepolarizing blockade is present, there will be a loss of twitch height and number, which will indicate the degree of blockade. This test is commonly used in intensive care units. See illustration.

trait (trāt) 1. any genetically determined condition; also, the condition prevailing in the heterozygous state of a recessive disorder, as the sickle cell trait. 2. a distinctive behavior pattern.

sickle cell t. the condition, usually asymptomatic, of being heterozygous for hemoglobin S; see also SICKLE CELL.

trajectory (trah-jek′tah-re) 1. the movement of an object along a three-dimensional

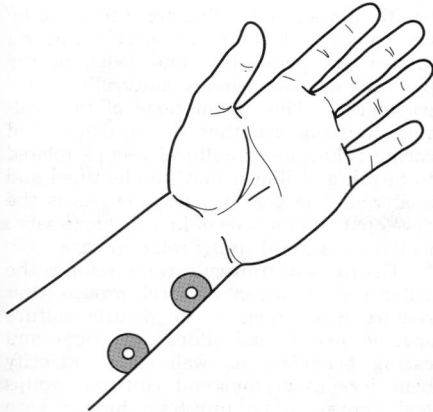

Ulnar nerve placement for train-of-four stimulation of the ulnar nerve. Electrodes are positioned in a direct line along the lateral side of the wrist. The thumb adducts to stimulation. From McQuillan et al., 2002.

path, or of a projectile within an individual's body. 2. the course of a disease.

tramadol (tram'ah-dol") an opioid ANAL-GESIC used as the hydrochloride salt for treatment of pain following surgical procedures and oral surgery; administered orally.

trance (trans) a state of altered CON-SCIOUSNESS characterized by heightened focal awareness and reduced peripheral awareness; a sleeplike state of reduced consciousness and activity.

trandolapril (tran-do'lah-pril") an ANGIO-TENSIN-CONVERTING ENZYME INHIBITOR used in treatment of HYPERTENSION and post–myocardial infarction congestive HEART FAILURE or left ventricular dysfunction; administered orally.

tranexamic acid (tran"ek-sam'ik) an agent that combats FIBRINOLYSIS by competitively inhibiting activation of PLASMINOGEN; used in prophylaxis and treatment of hemorrhage associated with excessive fibrinolysis, such as that following oral surgery in patients with HEMOPHILIA; administered orally or intravenously.

tranquilizer (tran'kwĭ-li"zer) a drug with a calming, soothing effect; currently it is usually used to mean an ANTIANXIETY AGENT (minor tranquilizer).

major t. former term for ANTIPSYCHOTIC AGENT.

minor t. ANTIANXIETY AGENT.

trans (tranz) 1. in organic chemistry, having certain atoms or radicals on opposite sides of a nonrotatable parent structure. 2. in genetics, denoting two or more loci, especially pseudoalleles, occurring on opposite chromosomes of a homologous pair. See also CIS.

trans- word element [L.], _through; across; beyond._

transabdominal (trans"ab-dom'ĭ-nal) across the abdominal wall or through the abdominal cavity.

transactional analysis a theory of personality structure and a psychotherapeutic method originated by Dr. Eric Berne. According to this theory the human personality is viewed as consisting of three ego states: the Parent, the Adult, and the Child. These ego states are described by Dr. Berne as being "coherent systems of thought and feeling manifested by corresponding patterns of behavior."

The word _transaction_ in this term is in reference to the communication that takes place between two people. Or, more precisely, it refers to what occurs when a stimulus from the ego state of one person elicits a response from the ego state of another individual. _Analysis_ refers to an investigation into the feelings and behavior patterns that are demonstrated during the transaction. In a successful or complementary transaction, the stimulus and response are between the same ego states; for example, Parent-Parent and Adult-Adult. In unsuccessful transactions one individual is speaking from one ego state, but gets a response from a different ego state. The interaction between the two is then either terminated or switched to another focus.

The therapeutic effect of transactional analysis is believed to be derived from an understanding of the origin of each of the three ego states, recognition of their influence on behavior, and an awareness of the options one has for dealing with reality in an effective and satisfying manner so that one can take care of one's own needs and feel good about oneself and other people.

transamidase (trans-am'ĭ-dās) an enzyme that catalyzes the transfer of an amide group from one molecule to another.

transaminase (trans-am'ĭ-nās) any of a group of enzymes that catalyze the reversible transfer of an amino group from a donor, usually an amino acid, to an acceptor, usually a 2-keto acid. Most use pyridoxal phosphate as a coenzyme.

transamination (trans"am-ĭ-na'shun) the reversible exchange of amino groups between different amino acids.

transaortic (trans"a-or'tik) performed through the aorta or aortic valve; said of surgical procedures.

transatrial (trans-a'tre-al) performed through the atrium; said of surgical procedures.

T

transaudient (trans-aw′de-ent) penetrable by sound waves.

transaxial (trans-ak′se-al) directed at right angles to the long axis of the body or a part.

transbasal (trans-ba′sal) through the base, as a surgical approach through the base of the skull.

transcalent (trans-ka′lent) penetrable by heat rays.

transcalvarial (trans″kal-văr′e-al) through or across the calvaria.

transcatheter (trans-kath′ĕ-ter) performed through the lumen of a catheter.

transcendental meditation a technique for attaining a state of physical relaxation and psychological calm by the regular practice of a relaxation procedure which entails the repetition of a mantra.

transcervical (trans-ser′vĭ-kal) 1. performed through the cervical opening of the uterus. 2. across or through the neck of a structure.

transcobalamin (trans″ko-bal′ah-min) either of two plasma proteins, transcobalamin I and transcobalamin II, that bind and transport COBALAMINS, including vitamin B_{12} (see VITAMIN). Deficiency of transcobalamin II results in failure of immunoglobulin production, megaloblastic ANEMIA, GRANULOCYTOPENIA, THROMBOCYTOPENIA, and intestinal villous atrophy, and is correctable by vitamin B_{12} therapy.

transcortical (trans-kor′tĭ-k′l) connecting two parts of the cerebral cortex.

transcortin (trans″kor-tin) an α-globulin that binds and transports biologically active, unconjugated cortisol in plasma.

transcriptase (trans-krip′tās) RNA polymerase; an enzyme that catalyzes the synthesis (POLYMERIZATION) of RNA from ribonucleoside triphosphates, with DNA serving as a template.

> **reverse t.** see REVERSE TRANSCRIPTASE.

transcription (trans-krip′shun) 1. the transfer of information. 2. the synthesis of RNA using a DNA template catalyzed by an RNA polymerase; the base sequences of the RNA and the DNA template are complementary.

> **order t.** in the NURSING INTERVENTIONS CLASSIFICATION, a nursing INTERVENTION defined as transferring information from order sheets to the nursing patient care planning and documentation system.

transcultural (trans-kul′chur-al) cross-cultural.

> **t. nursing** a humanistic and scientific area of nursing study and practice that focuses on how patterns of behavior in

health, illness, and caring are influenced by the values and beliefs of specific cultural groups. It applies this knowledge in the planning and provision of culturally appropriate care. The assumptions of transcultural nursing are that the practices and caring behaviors of cultural groups related to health and illness may be identified and analyzed. The goal of such analysis is the development of a body of knowledge to serve as the basis of culturally relevant care.

The focus of transcultural nursing is the differences between cultural groups that require care providers to identify culture specific health and illness practices and caring behaviors as well as to identify behaviors that transcend cultural groups and appear to be universal human care practices. The scope of transcultural nursing is the delivery of personalized care in health promotion and maintenance, as well as illness situations.

History. The field of transcultural nursing represented a shift from the biophysiological and psychological models that dominated nursing in the 1950s to a broader theoretical framework. One early and consistent proponent of the field has been Madeleine M. Leininger. Many other nurses and anthropologists have contributed significantly to the conceptualizations and research of transcultural nursing some have used the terms cross-cultural and intercultural to describe their research and practice. These terms refer to the goal of gaining and using knowledge about cultural beliefs, values, and practices to plan culture-appropriate nursing interventions and/or to negotiate changes in health and health related behavior among different cultures.

Transcultural nursing is the blending of anthropological means of inquiry with nursing theories of intervention and practice which have care as a critical component. Transcultural nursing incorporated a comparative method and holistic approach from anthropology as well as several anthropological concepts such as *lifestyles, world view, life experiences, environmental contexts,* and *folk beliefs* of cultural groups as a basis for understanding variations in human behavior. The comparative approach directs nurses not to treat all persons alike, but to adjust care to the culturally influenced expectations of the person and family. A nurse from mainstream American culture might be assertive when caring for other mainstream American clients, but might be less assertive when caring for Korean, Chinese, and Japanese clients who value less assertive behaviors.

The delivery of care that is culturally appropriate prevents unnecessary conflicts between clients and providers from varied cultural backgrounds. It also increases client satisfaction with care and may improve client adherence to a regimen that has been agreed upon with the nurse.

transcutaneous (trans″ku-ta′ne-us) transdermal.

t. electrical nerve stimulation (TENS) 1. use of a battery-powered device to relieve acute and chronic PAIN. Electrodes attached to the skin transmit electrical impulses, which produce a mild tingling, tapping, or massaging sensation. Reasons postulated for the effectiveness of this method include interruption of pain impulses from the periphery to the central nervous system, increased production of ENDORPHINS, and improved blood supply to the affected part. Increased circulation encourages healing and helps reduce muscle spasm. A second generation TENS unit called The Pain Suppressor is also available; it produces an electrical current but water is used as a conducting substance, it is not attached to the skin, and the patient does not perceive the electrode current. Treatments are administered several times per day. TENS is an alternative to drugs for the management of pain and can be used in a variety of conditions. A patient can use it with minimal instruction and may wear it at home as well as in the hospital. 2. in the NURSING INTERVENTIONS CLASSIFICATION, a nursing INTERVENTION defined as stimulation of skin and underlying tissues with controlled, low-voltage electrical vibration via electrodes.

t. neural stimulation (TNS) transcutaneous electrical nerve stimulation (def. 1).

transdermal (trans-der′mal) entering through the dermis, or skin, as in administration of a drug applied to the skin in ointment or patch form. See also PERCUTANEOUS. Called also transcutaneous.

transducer (trans-doo′ser) a device that translates one physical quantity to another, e.g., pressure or temperature, to an electrical signal.

neuroendocrine t. a neuron, such as a neurohypophyseal neuron, that on stimulation secretes a hormone, thereby translating neural information into hormonal information.

pressure t. an electronic device that converts pressure (such as BLOOD PRESSURE) into electrical signals that can be recorded graphically and monitored.

transduction (trans-duk′shun) the transfer of a genetic fragment from one microorganism to another by bacteriophage.

transdural (trans-door′al) through or across the dura mater.

transection (tran-sek′shun) a cross section; division by cutting transversely.

transfer (trans′fer) 1. the taking or moving of something from one place to another. 2. the moving of a patient from one surface to another. Patients can be taught to transfer safely either independently or with minimal assistance if they can balance in a sitting position.

gamete intrafallopian t. (GIFT) a type of assisted reproductive TECHNOLOGY consisting of retrieval of oocytes from the ovary, followed by placement of oocytes and sperm in the fallopian tubes by laparoscopy.

passive t. the conferring of immunity to a nonimmune host by injection of antibody or lymphocytes from an immune or sensitized donor.

sliding board t. a method of transferring a patient: a smooth tapered board is placed under the patient and stabilized on the surface to which movement will take place so that the patient can glide across.

tendon t. surgical relocation of the insertion of a tendon of a normal muscle to another site to take over the function of another muscle inactivated by trauma or disease.

tubal embryo t. (TET) 1. a method of assisted reproductive TECHNOLOGY consisting of retrieval of oocytes from the ovary, followed by their fertilization and culture in the laboratory with placement of the resulting embryos in the fallopian tubes by laparoscopy more than 24 hours after the original retrieval. 2. laparoscopic transfer of cryopreserved embryos to the fallopian tubes.

zygote intrafallopian t. (ZIFT) a type of assisted reproductive TECHNOLOGY consisting of retrieval of oocytes from the ovary, followed by their fertilization and culture in the laboratory and the placement of the resulting zygotes in the fallopian tubes by laparoscopy 24 hours after the original retrieval.

transferase (trans′fer-ās) an enzyme that catalyzes the transfer, from one molecule to another, of a chemical group that does not exist in free state during the transfer.

transference (trans-fer′ens) in psychiatry, the unconscious tendency of a patient to assign to others in the present environment feelings and attitudes associated with significant persons in one's earlier life; especially, the patient's transfer to the therapist of feelings and attitudes associated

T

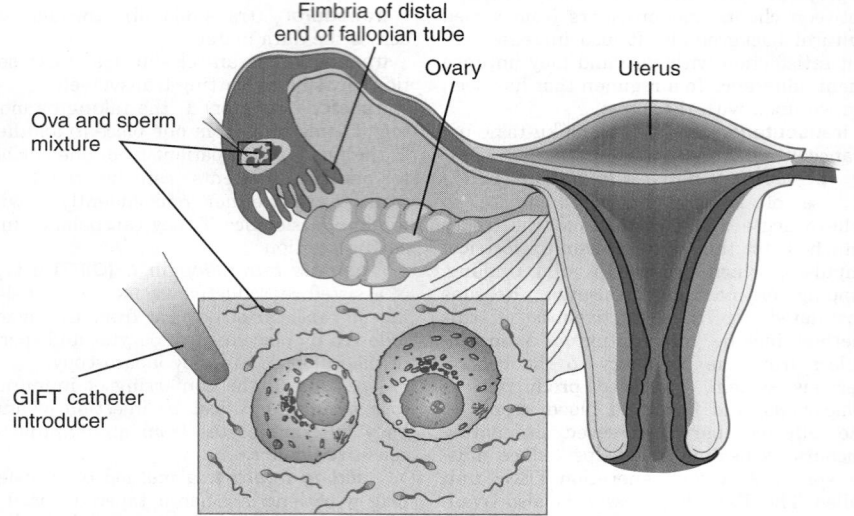

Fimbria of distal
end of fallopian tube

Ova and sperm
mixture

Ovary

Uterus

GIFT catheter
introducer

Gamete intrafallopian transfer (GIFT). Multiple ova and washed sperm are injected into the fallopian tube, where fertilization may occur. From McKinney et al., 2000.

with a parent or similar person from childhood. The feelings may be affectionate (positive transference), hostile (negative transference), or ambivalent. Sometimes the transference can be interpreted to help the patient understand childhood attitudes. See also COUNTERTRANSFERENCE.

counter t. see COUNTERTRANSFERENCE.

transfer factor (TF) a factor occurring in sensitized lymphocytes that has the capacity to transfer delayed hypersensitivity to a normal (nonreactive) individual. It confers cell-mediated IMMUNITY and therefore has been found to be useful in treating conditions in which there is a disorder of IMMUNE RESPONSE. As an adjunct to antibiotic therapy it is useful in the treatment of such antibiotic-resistant diseases as candidiasis, coccidioidomycosis, and leprosy.

transferrin (trans-fer′in) a glycoprotein that binds and transports iron; most is produced in the liver. A similar compound produced in the intestinal mucosa is APOFERRITIN.

transfix (trans-fiks′) to pierce through or impale.

transfixion (trans-fik′shun) a cutting through from within outward, as in amputation.

transformation (trans″for-ma′shun) change of form or structure; conversion from one form to another. In oncology, the change that a normal cell undergoes as it becomes malignant.

bacterial t. the exchange of genetic material between strains of bacteria by the transfer of a fragment of naked DNA from a donor cell to a recipient cell, followed by recombination in the recipient chromosome.

transformer (trans-for′mer) an induction apparatus for changing electrical energy at one voltage and current to electrical energy at another voltage and current, through the medium of magnetic energy, without mechanical motion.

step-down t. one for lowering the voltage of the original current.

step-up t. one for raising the voltage of the original current.

transfusion (trans-fu′zhun) the introduction of whole blood or blood components directly into the blood stream. Among the elements transfused are packed red blood cells, plasma, platelets, granulocytes, and cryoprecipitate, a plasma protein rich in antihemophilic factor VIII. The current trend is to transfuse blood components rather than whole blood because by so doing the utility of each unit of blood can be extended and the treatment provided more nearly meets the specific needs of the patient.

Transfusion is most often indicated to maintain or replace blood volume, to provide deficient blood elements and improve coagulation, to maintain or improve transport of oxygen, and in exchange for blood that has been removed in the treatment of

Rh incompatibility in the newborn, liver failure in which toxins accumulate in the blood, or in some other types of toxemia.

Transfusion Methods. There are several different methods of transfusion. Direct transfusion, in which blood from one person is directly transferred to another person, is now rarely used. The usual method is indirect transfusion, in which blood is drawn from a donor, stored in a sterile container and later given to a recipient. Exchange transfusion, in which blood is removed from a person and simultaneously replaced by donor blood, is used mainly in treating ERYTHROBLASTOSIS FETALIS.

Intrauterine or Fetal Transfusion. Intrauterine transfusion involves direct transfusion of Rh negative packed red blood cells into the fetal peritoneal cavity. It is done for the early treatment of pronounced degrees of fetal isoimmunization before weeks 32 to 34 of pregnancy.

The first step is injection of a radiopaque dye into the amniotic fluid. After the fetus ingests the dye, the intestinal tract can be visualized by radiographic techniques so that it serves as a guidepost for location of the abdominal cavity. A long pudendal needle is then inserted through the mother's abdomen and guided through the uterine wall, through the fetal abdomen, and into the peritoneal cavity. Another radiograph is taken to confirm correct placement of the needle and then the erythrocytes are transfused. The erythrocytes soon pass into the fetal blood stream. This procedure is obviously not without hazard and is done only if the fetus cannot be expected to survive without it. The treatment usually is done every 7 to 10 days until delivery. Once the newborn is delivered, exchange TRANSFUSION and supportive therapy are begun.

Blood Typing and Crossmatching. Transfusions were not practicable until the four main hereditary BLOOD GROUPS, A, B, AB, and O, were discovered at the beginning of the 20th century. Until these blood types were identified, antigen-antibody reactions could not be predicted and transfusion reactions (often fatal) were a matter of chance. There are certain antigens on the surface of red blood cells which can precipitate a transfusion reaction when incompatible blood types are mixed. In the ABO system the types are dictated by A antigen and B antigen. There is also an allele O that does not code for either A or B antigen. Thus there are four possible groups (A, B, AB, O). A person who is type A has only A antigen on red cells; one who is type B has only B antigen; one who is type AB has both A and B antigens;

and one who is type O has neither. All individuals produce antibodies against the A or B antigens that are lacking on their own cells. Thus, type A has anti-B; type B has anti-A; type O has both; and type AB has neither.

Rh negative individuals lack D antigen on red cells. They do not produce anti-D antibodies unless they are directly exposed to Rh positive blood, as may occur from a fetal-maternal hemorrhage or from transfusion of platelet or granulocyte concentrate containing Rh positive red cells.

Another system of blood typing is sometimes considered prior to transfusion of granulocytes or for long-term platelet administration. The typing identifies the HLA ANTIGENS that occur on leukocytes and platelets. (See also TISSUE TYPING.)

CROSSMATCHING is another way in which blood is tested for compatibility prior to transfusion. It involves placing the cells of the donor in a sample of the recipient's serum, and cells of the recipient in a sample of the donor's serum. Absence of agglutination, hemolysis, cytotoxicity indicates that the blood specimens are compatible.

Adverse Reactions. Among the most common transfusion reactions are antigen-antibody REACTIONS resulting from blood type incompatibility. When blood groups are incompatible there is agglutination (clumping) of cells, hemolysis, and release of cellular elements into the serum. Signs and symptoms indicating such a reaction include burning sensation along the vein where the transfusion is given, facial flushing, chills and fever, headache, low back pain, rash, red urine, and shock. Other reactions include febrile reaction, allergic reaction with hives, wheezing, and anaphylaxis, and response to bacterial contamination. See accompanying table.

Every health care agency in which transfusions are administered should have a written policy regarding the correct steps to take in the event a patient begins to show signs of a reaction. In general, should such signs occur, the transfusion is stopped immediately, the venous line is kept open with normal saline, and emergency care is initiated.

Especially dangerous to patients with either cardiac or renal disease is HYPERKALEMIA, an excess of potassium in the blood. If the condition is not corrected, a flaccid paralysis develops, affecting the muscles of respiration and eventually the heart muscle, which can lead to cardiac arrest. High levels of potassium in donor blood are likely to occur when the bank blood is several days

POSSIBLE SIGNS AND SYMPTOMS OF A TRANSFUSION REACTION

General
  Fever (rise of 1°C or 2°F)
  Chills
  Muscle aches, pain
  Back pain
  Chest pain
  Headache
  Heat at site of infusion or along vein

Nervous System
  Apprehension, impending sense of doom
  Tingling, numbness

Respiratory System
  Respiratory rate
    Tachypnea
    Apnea
  Dyspnea
  Cough
  Wheezing
  Rales

Gastrointestinal System
  Nausea
  Vomiting
  Pain, abdominal cramping
  Diarrhea (may be bloody)

Cardiovascular System
  Heart rate
    Bradycardia
    Tachycardia
  Blood pressure
    Hypotension, shock
    Hypertension
  Peripheral circulation
    Color cyanosis, facial flushing
    Temperature: cool/clammy; hot/flushed dry
  Edema
  Bleeding
    Generalized (DIC)
    Oozing at surgical site

Renal System
  Changes in urine volume
    Oliguria, anuria
    Renal failure
  Changes in urine color
    Dark, concentrated
    Shades of red, brown, amber
    May indicate the presence in urine of red blood cells
      (hematuria) or of free hemoglobin (hemoglobinuria)

Integumentary System
  Rashes, hives (urticaria), swelling
  Itching
  Diaphoresis

From Polaski and Tatro, 1996.

old. It is estimated that the breakdown of red cells in the stored blood increases the level of potassium at the rate of one milli-equivalent per liter per day.

Another possible complication is hypocalcemia, which can occur when large amounts of blood containing the additive acid citrate dextrose are given rapidly, as to a bleeding patient. Acid citrate dextrose is an anticoagulant that binds with calcium ions in the recipient's blood, removing them from circulation and thereby reducing the calcium level below that essential for normal coagulation.

Circulatory overload is a possibility any time blood is administered rapidly in large amounts. Patients who are particularly susceptible to this eventuality are the very young, the very old, and those suffering from a pre-existing cardiopulmonary or renal problem. Another difficulty that may be encountered when blood is administered rapidly under pressure is that of air embolism.

autologous t. reinfusion of a patient's own blood, done by either of two methods: (1) patients having a planned surgical procedure may donate their own blood within six weeks before surgery; the donated blood is processed, frozen, stored and then thawed for use at the time o surgical need; or (2) blood lost during the operative procedure may be salvaged; this i also called AUTOTRANSFUSION. In the secon method, blood and debris from the surgica field are aspirated into a collection chambe containing a dilute solution of heparin o citrated dextrose. The aspirate is filtere and pumped into a centrifuge chamber an the red cells are then washed with a norma saline solution. Centrifugal force separate the red cells from waste products such a debris, plasma, hemolyzed red cells, plate lets, most white cells, and solution such a anticoagulant or antibiotic irrigation solu tion. The washed packed red blood cells ar then pumped into a blood infusion bag an reinfused into the patient in the usua manner.

exchange t. transfusion in a newbor infant of packed cells or fresh whole bloo that is type O, Rh-negative, and previousl cross-matched with the mother's serum, o Rh negative blood of the same type as th newborn's. Rh negative blood is used be cause, even though the newborn may hav Rh positive blood, maternal antibodies tha entered the fetal bloodstream in utero ar still present in the newborn and would destroy the transfused blood cells. The blood is transfused via the umbilical vein. Exchange transfusion is used to treat either moderate to severe HEMOLYTIC DISEASE OF THE NEWBORN or HYPERBILIRUBINEMIA not controlled by PHOTOTHERAPY. Complications may include HEART FAILURE due to either HYPERVOLEMIA or HYPOVOLEMIA, BRADYCARDIA or CARDIAC ARREST from ACIDOSIS or HYPERKALEMIA, HYPOCALCEMIA, HYPOTHERMIA, air emboli, thrombolytic EMBOLI, SEPSIS, intensification of HYPOGLYCEMIA, and THROMBOCYTOPENIA if there are repeated exchange transfusions.

fetomaternal t. transplacental passage of fetal blood into the circulation of the mother; in small amounts it may go unnoticed, but in larger amounts it can cause anemia or edema in the fetus.

intrauterine t. direct transfer of Rh negative blood cells into a fetus *in utero* in cases of ISOIMMUNIZATION; see TRANSFUSION.

placental t. the transfer of blood from placenta to newborn at the time of birth. Blood flow through the umbilical arteries stops about 45 seconds after birth, but the umbilical vein remains patent longer. Uterine contractions enhance the transfer of blood, the volume of which has significant physiological benefits to the neonate. Since gravity influences this transfer, raising the newborn above the level of the placenta prevents a normally occurring placental transfusion. Conversely, lowering the newborn below the placental level accelerates the process.

t. reaction any symptoms due to agglutination or hemolysis of the recipient's blood cells when blood for transfusion is incorrectly matched. See discussion under TRANSFUSION.

transgene (trans'jēn) a gene that has been spliced into a strand of DNA.

transglutaminase (trans″gloo-tam′in-ās) the activated form of protransglutaminase, which forms stabilizing covalent bonds within fibrin strands; called also coagulation factor XIIIa (the activated form of factor XIII).

transient ischemic attack (TIA) a sudden episode of temporary symptoms typically due to diminished blood flow through the brain, usually defined as lasting between 24 and 48 hours. It is sometimes related to impaired blood flow through the vertebrobasilar vessels. The symptoms are warning signals of impending stroke; approximately one in three persons experiencing a TIA will have a STROKE SYNDROME within 5 years.

The symptoms of TIA can range from obvious loss of sensation or motor function to more subtle changes in speech or mental acuity. During the attack the person may feel numbness or weakness or both on one side of the body, slurring of speech or inability to talk, or difficulty in thinking. Disturbance in the vision of one eye and double vision also are typical of TIA. Because these signs are short lived, many persons may be inclined to ignore them unless they are informed of their importance and of the need to consult medical help before a catastrophic stroke occurs. Carotid artery occlusions usually can be corrected by surgery.

transiliac (trans-il′e-ak) across the two ilia.

transillumination (trans″ĭ-loo″mĭ-na′shun) the passage of strong light through a body structure, to permit inspection by an observer on the opposite side; called also diaphanoscopy.

translation (trans-la′shun) the synthesis of a polypeptide using messenger RNA as a template, a complex process involving ribosomes and transfer RNAs; every three bases (a codon) along the mRNA beginning with the start codon specifies one amino acid in the polypeptide chain.

translocation (trans″lo-ka′shun) the attachment of a fragment of one chromosome to a nonhomologous chromosome.

reciprocal t. the mutual exchange of fragments between two broken chromosomes, one part of one uniting with part of the other.

robertsonian t. that in which the breaks occur at the centromeres and entire chromosome arms are exchanged, usually involving two acrocentric chromosomes.

translucent (trans-lu′sent) slightly penetrable by light rays.

transmethylase (trans-meth′ĭ-lās) an enzyme that catalyzes transmethylation.

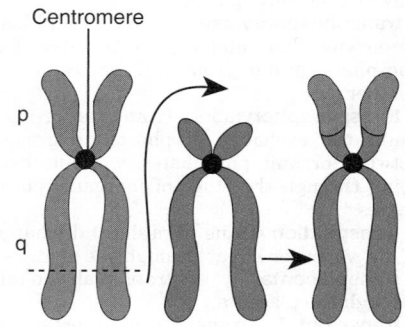

Translocation of a portion of one chromosome to another chromosome. Redrawn from Damjanov, 2000.

transmethylation (trans″meth-ĭ-la′shun) the transfer of a methyl group (CH_3═) from the molecules of one compound to those of another.

transmigration (trans″mi-gra′shun) 1. diapedesis. 2. change of place from one side of the body to the other.

transmissible (trans-mis′ĭ-b′l) capable of transmission.

t. neurodegenerative disease prion disease.

transmission (trans-mish′un) 1. a passage or transfer, as of a disease from one individual to another, or of neural impulses from one neuron to another. 2. the communication of inheritable qualities from parent to offspring.

horizontal t. the spread of an infectious agent from one individual to another, usually through contact with bodily excretions or fluids, such as sputum or blood, that contain the agent.

vertical t. transmission from one generation to another. The term is restricted by some to genetic transmission and extended by others to include also transmission of infection from one generation to the next, as by milk or through the placenta.

transmucosal (trans″mu-ko′sal) entering through, or across, a mucous membrane, as the administration of a drug via the cavity between the cheek and gum.

transmural (trans-mu′ral) through the wall of an organ; extending through or affecting the entire thickness of the wall of an organ or cavity.

transmutation (trans″mu-ta′shun) 1. evolutionary change of one species into another. 2. the change of one chemical element into another.

transparent (trans-par′ent) permitting the passage of rays of light so that objects may be seen through the substance.

transphosphorylase (trans″fos-for′ĭ-lās) an enzyme that catalyzes the transfer of a phosphate group from one molecule to another.

transphosphorylation (trans″fos″for-ĭ-la′-shun) the exchange of phosphate groups between organic phosphates, without their going through the stage of inorganic phosphates.

transpiration (trans″pĭ-ra′shun) discharge of air, vapor, or sweat through the skin.

transplacental (trans″plah-sen′tal) through the placenta.

transplant 1. (trans′plant) an organ or tissue taken from the body and grafted into another area of the same individual or another individual. 2. (trans-plant′) to transfer tissue from one part to another or from one individual to another. See also TRANSPLANTATION.

transplantation (trans″plan-ta′shun) the transfer of living organs or tissue from one part of the body to another or from one individual to another. Transplantation and GRAFTING mean the same thing, although the term grafting is more commonly used to refer to the transfer of skin. In dentistry, transplantation refers to the insertion into a prepared dental alveolus of an autogenous or homologous tooth; it may be a developing tooth germ from the same mouth, or a frozen homologous transplant.

Occasionally an emergency requires an organ to be transplanted from one place to another within the body. Kidneys, for example, have been relocated to enable them to continue functioning after the ureters have been damaged. Transplantation of an organ within the body, known as AUTOTRANSPLANTATION or an autologous GRAFT, requires delicate surgery but otherwise poses no particular problem.

Eye surgeons have developed the procedure called CORNEAL TRANSPLANTATION or KERATOPLASTY, in which part or all of a diseased cornea that has become opaque is removed and replaced by healthy corneal tissue from an eye bank. Cartilage and bone are other tissues that are not difficult to transplant from one individual to another. Cartilage is particularly able to be made into various shapes and so is widely used in reconstructive surgery. Bone grafts are sometimes used instead of metal plates in operations to repair fractures, and they can also be used to replace diseased bone. Grafts made of synthetic materials may also be used such as Dacron vascular grafts that replace parts of blood vessels.

Kidney transplants have been performed on dogs since 1902, but remained in the experimental realm in humans until a ground-breaking operation was performed in 1954 in Boston. A kidney from one identical twin was successfully implanted in the other to replace his diseased kidneys. Since that time kidney transplantations have been the most successful of transplantations, primarily because there are artificial kidney machines available (see DIALYSIS and HEMODIALYSIS), and also because the kidney is a paired organ. This means that the DONOR need not be cadaveric but can be a living person (such as a relative of the recipient) and can be selected on the basis of tissue-type compatibility to avoid fatal rejection of the organ by the recipient.

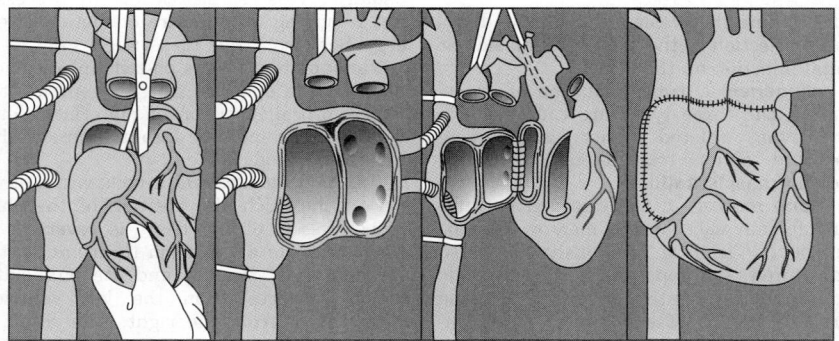

1. After the recipient is placed on cardiopulmonary bypass, the heart is removed.

2. The posterior walls of the recipient's left and right atria are left intact.

3. The left atrium of donor heart is anastomosed to the recipient's residual posterior atrial walls, and the other atrial walls, the atrial septum, and the great vessels are joined.

POSTOPERATIVE RESULT

Heart transplantation. From Ignatavicius and Workman, 2000.

In 1967 the South African surgeon Christiaan N. Barnard transplanted a human heart. Transplants of hearts and other vital organs are now being done at an increasing rate throughout the world. There are ethical and legal implications of obtaining healthy organs for transplantation, which still have not been completely resolved.

Rejection. The major problem to be overcome in transplantation therapy is rejection, an immune phenomenon. Organs such as the cornea, skin, and bone can be transplanted successfully because, in the case of the cornea, the vascular supply is not involved, or, in skin and bone, the transplant serves as a structural foundation into which the new tissue grows. In the case of intact organs such as the kidney, heart, lung, liver, and pancreas, a generous blood supply is essential to their survival in the recipient's body. The blood of the recipient carries in it many of the tools used by the body in defense against foreign substances. As blood is drained from the transplanted organ into the host's general circulation, the body recognizes the transplanted tissue cells as foreign invaders (ANTIGENS) and immediately sets up an IMMUNE RESPONSE by producing ANTIBODIES. These antibodies are capable of inhibiting metabolism of the cells within the transplanted organ and eventually actively cause their destruction. They also play a role in delayed inflammatory RESPONSE that can occur as late as weeks or months after implantation and adds to the destruction of the donor organ.

In order to minimize rejection and improve the chances of survival of a transplanted organ, efforts are made to match as closely as possible the blood types and tissue types of the donor and recipient. First, the blood is tested for ABO or blood type compatibility. Then, TISSUE TYPING is done to identify the protein antigens that are specific to each individual. These antigens are the HLA ANTIGENS (HLA), so called because they are easily identifiable on leukocytes. The more compatible these antigens are between donor and recipient, the less likely tissue rejection will occur. A third test that is done is CROSSMATCHING, which involves mixing the intended recipient's serum with lymphocytes from the potential donor. A positive reaction would show destruction of the donor's cells by antibodies in the recipient's serum, thus eliminating the possibility of using an organ from that particular donor. The probability of survival of a transplanted organ is highest when the donor is a sibling who is HLA identical to the recipient.

Control of the IMMUNE RESPONSE in the recipient is attempted by the use of IMMUNOSUPPRESSIVE agents such as antilymphocyte GLOBULIN and ANTIMETABOLITES, which tend to suppress the growth of rapidly dividing cells, and CYCLOSPORINE, which inhibits T-cell function. CORTICOSTEROIDS also are used because of their antiinflammatory effect. All of the chemicals used in transplantation therapy interfere in some way with the body's normal defense mechanisms. For this reason a delicate balance must be maintained in their administration so as to

T

avoid tipping the scales either in the direction of rejection of the organ on one side or a fatal infection on the other.

allogeneic t. transplantation of an AL-LOGRAFT; the three types are cadaveric donor, living related donor, and living unrelated donor transplantation. Called also allotransplantation.

bone marrow t. the intravenous infusion of bone MARROW; the marrow may be AUTOLOGOUS (from a previously harvested and stored self-donation) or ALLOGENEIC (from a living related donor or a living unrelated donor). Used to treat malignancies such as LEUKEMIA, LYMPHOMA, MYELOMA, and selected solid tumors, as well as non-malignant conditions such as APLASTIC ANE-MIA, immunologic deficiencies, and inborn ERRORS of metabolism.

cadaveric donor t. allogeneic transplantation of an organ or tissue from a cadaver.

corneal t. transplantation of a donor cornea into the eye of a recipient; see also CORNEAL TRANSPLANTATION.

heterotopic t. transplantation of tissue typical of one area to a different recipient site.

homotopic t. orthotopic transplantation.

living nonrelated donor t. living unrelated donor transplantation.

living related donor t. allogeneic transplantation in which the donor and the recipient have a close biological relationship, such as that of a parent and child or a brother and sister.

living unrelated donor t. allogeneic transplantation in which the donor and the recipient do not have a close biological relationship.

orthotopic t. transplantation of tissue from a donor into its normal position in the body of the recipient.

syngeneic t. living related donor transplantation in which the organ or tissue is a SYNGRAFT; called also isotransplantation.

xenogeneic t. transplantation of a XE-NOGRAFT; called also heterotransplantation.

transport (trans′port) 1. movement of materials in biologic systems, particularly across the cell MEMBRANE into and out of cells or across epithelial layers. 2. in the NURSING INTERVENTIONS CLASSIFICATION, a nursing IN-TERVENTION defined as moving a patient from one location to another.

active t. see ACTIVE TRANSPORT.

oxygen t. the carrying of oxygen through the bloodstream bound to hemoglobin (see OXYHEMOGLOBIN).

passive t. the movement of materials, usually across cell MEMBRANES, by processes not requiring expenditure of metabolic energy. See also ACTIVE TRANSPORT.

transposition (trans″po-zish′un) displacement to the opposite side; in genetics, the nonreciprocal insertion of material deleted from one chromosome into another, nonhomologous chromosome.

t. of great vessels a CONGENITAL HEART DEFECT in which the position of the chief blood vessels of the heart is reversed, so that the aorta arises from the right ventricle instead of the left and the pulmonary artery emerges from the left ventricle rather than from the right. The result is that oxygen-poor blood returning from the systemic circulation to the right side of the heart gets pumped back into the general circulation instead of being transported to the lungs, and oxygen-rich blood flows aimlessly to and from the lungs. The condition may be corrected by surgery. See accompanying illustration.

transposon (tranz-po′zon) a discrete DNA sequence that transposes blocks of genetic material back and forth within a bacterial cell from the chromosome to PLASMIDS or BACTERIOPHAGE particles, by which the material may be transferred to another cell. Transposons frequently carry genes for resistance to ANTIBIOTICS.

transpubic (trans-pu′bik) performed through the pubic bone after removal of a segment of the bone.

transsegmental (trans″seg-men′tal) extending across segments.

transseptal (trans-sep′tal) extending or performed through or across a septum.

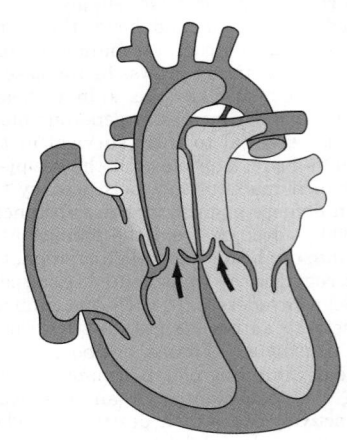

Complete transposition of the great arteries

Complete transposition of great arteries.

transsexual (trans-sek′shoo-al) 1. a person affected by transsexualism. 2. a person whose external anatomy has been changed to resemble that of the opposite sex.

transsexualism (trans-sek′shoo-al-izm″) 1. the most severe manifestation of gender identity disorder in adults, being a prolonged, persistent desire to relinquish their primary and secondary sex characteristics and acquire those of the opposite sex, particularly describing those persons who go so far as to live as members of the opposite sex through dress, hormonal treatments, or surgical reassignment. 2. the state of being a transsexual.

transthalamic (trans″thah-lam′ik) across the thalamus.

transthoracic (trans″thah-ras′ik) through the thoracic cavity or across the chest wall.

transtympanic (trans″tim-pan′ik) across the tympanic membrane or the cavity of the middle ear.

transudate (tran′su-dāt) a fluid substance that has passed through a membrane or has been extruded from a tissue; in contrast to an exudate, a transudate is characterized by high fluidity and a low content of protein, cells, or solid matter derived from cells.

transudation (tran″su-da′shun) 1. passage of serum or other body fluid through a membrane or tissue surface. 2. transudate.

transurethral (trans″u-re′thral) performed through the urethra.

t. resection of the prostate (TURP) removal of a portion of the PROSTATE by means of an instrument passed through the urethra. A transurethral resection removes only enlarged prostatic tissue, as in benign prostatic HYPERTROPHY. Normal prostatic tissue and its outer capsule are left intact.

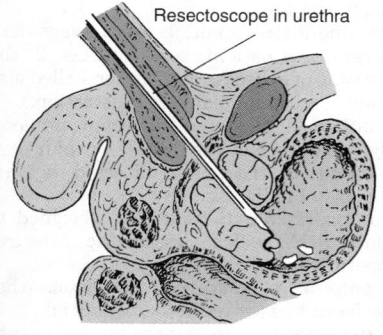

Resectoscope in urethra

Transurethral resection of the prostate. Hyperplastic prostate tissue is removed through a resectoscope inserted through the urethra. From Polaski and Tatro, 996.

Patient Care. Preoperatively the patient will probably have some difficulty in urination, owing to the fact that the prostate encircles the urethra. The patient's fluid intake and output should be measured and recorded, even though he may not have an indwelling catheter to relieve bladder distention from retained urine.

Most patients having this procedure are over the age of 65. A thorough nursing assessment should be done to identify the special needs of the patient, especially those related to chronic illnesses such as heart disease and diabetes, and to such sensory deficits as impaired sight and hearing. Safety measures such as side rails are particularly important, as well as caution in the administration of sedatives and analgesics.

During the immediate postoperative period the patient is monitored for signs of hemorrhage. Drainage through the urinary catheter is expected to be bright red for the first 24 hours after surgery and might upset the patient or someone not familiar with the effects of the surgical procedure. However, an increasingly darker red color could indicate fresh bleeding and should be reported to the surgeon.

In addition, special attention is given to the catheter and tubing leading from the bladder to be sure it is open and draining freely. Severe pain could indicate bladder spasms caused by blood clots and bits of tissue. Before administering any analgesic for relief of bladder pain, the nurse should first note whether the catheter is draining as it should. Irrigations often are prescribed to remove the obstructing material and maintain adequate flow. The irrigation procedure must be done under sterile conditions because infection is a very real danger after prostatectomy. If the patient continues to complain of severe pain even though the bladder is empty, the surgeon should be notified at once, because unusually severe and persistent pain could indicate a perforated bladder.

A transurethral resection does not affect the hormonal level of a male, nor does it render him sterile. After recovery from his surgery he should be able to resume his former level of sexual activity.

transvaginal (trans-vaj′ĭ-nal) through the vagina.

transversalis (trans″ver-sa′lis) transverse.

transverse (trans-vers′) extending from side to side; situated at right angles to the long axis.

transversectomy (trans″ver-sek′tah-me) excision of a transverse process of a vertebra.

transversus (trans-ver′sus) [L.] transverse.

transvesical (trans-ves′ĭ-kal) through the bladder.

transvestism (trans-ves′tizm) 1. cross-dressing and otherwise assuming the appearance, manner, or roles traditionally associated with members of the opposite sex. 2. transvestic fetishism.

transvestite (trans-ves′tīt) a person who practices transvestism.

Tranxene (tran′zēn) trademark for preparations of CLORAZEPATE dipotassium; an ANTIANXIETY AGENT and ANTICONVULSANT.

tranylcypromine (tran″il-si′pro-mēn) a monoamine oxidase INHIBITOR with a rapid onset; administered orally as the sulfate salt as an ANTIDEPRESSANT. It is also used in the prevention of MIGRAINE.

trapezium (trah-pe′ze-um) an irregular, four-sided figure.

TRAPS tumor necrosis factor receptor–associated periodic syndrome; see FAMILIAL PERIODIC FEVER.

trastuzumab (tras-tuz′u-mab) a monoclonal ANTIBODY that binds to a protein over-expressed in some breast cancers; used as an antineoplastic AGENT in treatment of metastatic breast cancer with such over-expression.

Trasylol (tras′-lol) trademark for a preparation of APROTININ, an antihemorrhagic agent.

Traube's sign (trou′bez) a loud sound like a pistol shot heard in the femoral arteries in aortic stenosis.

trauma (traw′mah), pl. *traumas, trau′-mata* [Gr.] 1. injury. 2. psychological or emotional damage. adj., **traumat′ic.**

   birth t. 1. an injury to the infant during the process of being born. 2. in some psychiatric theories, the psychic shock produced in an infant by the experience of being born.

   psychic t. a psychologically upsetting experience that produces an emotional or mental disorder or otherwise has lasting negative effects on a person's thoughts, feelings, or behavior.

   risk for t. a NURSING DIAGNOSIS accepted by the North American Nursing Diagnosis Association, defined as accentuated risk of accidental tissue injury such as a wound, burn, or fracture.

traumat(o)- word element [Gr.] *trauma.*

traumatism (traw′mah-tizm) 1. the physical or psychic state resulting from an injury or wound. 2. a wound.

traumatology (traw″mah-tol′ah-je) the branch of surgery dealing with wounds and disability from injuries.

travoprost (trav′o-prost) a synthetic PROSTAGLANDIN analogue used in the treatment of elevated intraocular pressure in patients with open-angle GLAUCOMA or ocular HYPERTENSION; administered topically to the conjunctiva.

tray (tra) a flat-surfaced utensil for the conveyance of various objects or material.

trazodone (tra′zo-dōn) an ANTIDEPRESSANT used orally as the hydrochloride salt to treat major depressive episodes with or without prominent anxiety

Treacher Collins syndrome (tre′cher kol′inz) the incomplete form of mandibulofacial DYSOSTOSIS, characterized by downslanting eyes (ANTIMONGOLOID palpebral fissures); absence of part of the lower lid, usually the outer third; underdeveloped cheekbone that appear depressed; a prominent nose wide mouth, and small receding chin; underdeveloped, malformed, or prominent ears; and small tufts of hair in front of the ears. Affected individuals often, but no always, have some degree of HEARING LOSS usually conductive. Associated health problems are typically associated with narrowing of the PHARYNX and nasal passages, which interferes with breathing and may cause sleep APNEA at night. Breathing problems should increase with age or may be treated surgically. Some children may require a TRACHEOTOMY and others may have feeding problems. Emotional support in dealing with the appearance of the face i important.

treadmill exercise test any of various graded types of EXERCISE TESTING in which the patient walks on an inclined treadmill which may be increased in speed and incline through the test.

treatment (trēt′ment) 1. the management and care of a patient; see also CARE. 2. the combating of a disease or disorder; called also therapy. (See accompanying illustration.)

   active t. treatment directed immediately to the cure of the disease or injury.

   causal t. treatment directed against the cause of a disease.

   conservative t. treatment designed to avoid radical medical therapeutic measures or operative procedures.

   empiric t. treatment by means that experience has proved to be beneficial.

   expectant t. treatment directed toward relief of untoward symptoms, leaving the cure of the disease to natural forces.

   extraordinary t. a type of treatment that is usually highly invasive and might be considered burdensome to the patient; the

WINDOW ON TREACHER COLLINS SYNDROME

In most every way, I am your typical, garden-variety human being. I am a third year medical student at the University of Texas Health Sciences Center in Houston who loves connecting with people. However, many people assume right from the start that I must not be "normal" since I don't look "normal." I have Treacher Collins syndrome.

Treacher Collins syndrome is a genetic, craniofacial birth defect that is characterized by a range of distinctive facial anomalies. The main characteristics of TCS are downward slanting eyes, small lower jaw, and malformed or missing ears. Those anomalies can cause hearing, breathing, and eating problems. About one in ten thousand babies are born with it. A person with Treacher Collins syndrome has a 50% chance of passing it on to their children. In my family, my grandfather passed it down to my mother who passed it down to me.

Treacher Collins syndrome is a lot more than a pile of statistics and facts. It is about the person below the surface. People tend to give wide berth to the things and people that they perceive as a threat to them – those people who are "different" or who they don't understand. In some situations, this defense mechanism can be good. In excess, however, it breeds ignorance and heartache and leads society to shun those that aren't "normal." Thus, society does not take the time to see what lies beneath the outer shell of a person and never sees that below the surface these "different" people are just as "normal" as anyone else. It is part of my goal as a doctor-in-training to educate people about Treacher Collins syndrome and to prove to them that looks can be very deceiving. I hope to start a new trend in society where society reads the book before discarding it because the cover looks a little odd.

Given the chance to live my life over again without Treacher Collins, I would have to politely decline. I believe that the experiences in my life as a result of Treacher Collins have molded me into the person that I am today. Like anyone else, I've had many ups and downs, and to give up the lessons I've learned on the roller-coaster ride of life would be to give up part of myself. Having Treacher Collins syndrome, or any other medical condition, does not make someone "abnormal," it only makes him human.

AMIE OSBORN

effort to decide what is extraordinary raises numerous ethical questions.

fever t. in the NURSING INTERVENTIONS CLASSIFICATION, a nursing INTERVENTION defined as management of a patient with HYPERPYREXIA caused by nonenvironmental factors. See also FEVER.

heat exposure t. in the NURSING INTERVENTIONS CLASSIFICATION, a nursing INTERVENTION defined as management of a patient overcome by heat due to excessive environmental heat exposure. See also heat STROKE.

hypothermia t. in the NURSING INTERVENTIONS CLASSIFICATION, a nursing INTERVENTION defined as rewarming and surveillance of a patient whose core body temperature is below 35°C. See also HYPOTHERMIA.

Kenny t. a treatment formerly used for POLIOMYELITIS, consisting of wrapping of the back and limbs in hot cloths, followed, after pain has subsided, by passive exercise and instruction of the patient in exercise of the muscles. It was named for Sister Elizabeth Kenny, an Australian nurse known for her care of polio patients during the first half of the 20th century.

neurodevelopmental t. Bobath method.

palliative t. supportive CARE.

preventive t. prophylaxis.

t. and/or procedure a nursing INTERVENTION in the NURSING MINIMUM DATA SET; action prescribed to cure, relieve, control, or prevent a client PROBLEM.

prophylactic t. prophylaxis.

rape-trauma t. in the NURSING INTERVENTIONS CLASSIFICATION, a nursing INTERVENTION defined as the provision of emotional and physical support immediately following a reported RAPE.

rational t. that based upon knowledge of disease and the action of the remedies given.

refusal of t. see under REFUSAL.

root canal t. root canal THERAPY.

specific t. treatment particularly adapted to the special disease being treated.

substance use t. in the NURSING INTERVENTIONS CLASSIFICATION, a nursing INTERVENTION defined as supportive care of patient/family members with physical and psychosocial problems associated with the use of alcohol or drugs. See also substance ABUSE.

substance use t.: alcohol withdrawal in the NURSING INTERVENTIONS CLASSIFICATION, a

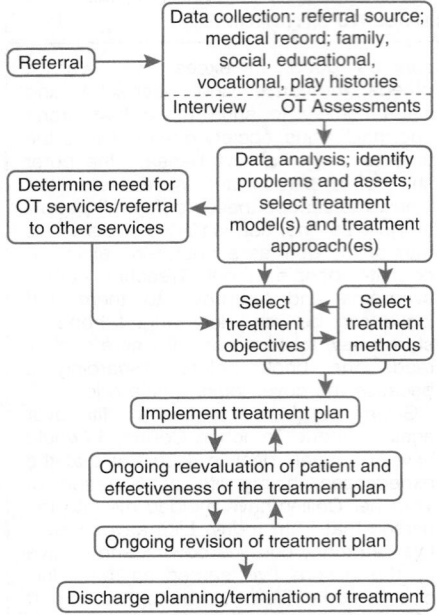

Referral → Data collection: referral source; medical record; family, social, educational, vocational, play histories

Interview   OT Assessments

Data analysis; identify problems and assets; select treatment model(s) and treatment approach(es)

Determine need for OT services/referral to other services

Select treatment objectives   Select treatment methods

Implement treatment plan

Ongoing reevaluation of patient and effectiveness of the treatment plan

Ongoing revision of treatment plan

Discharge planning/termination of treatment

Schematic of the treatment planning process using occupational therapy as an example. From Pedretti and Early, 2001.

nursing INTERVENTION defined as the care of the patient experiencing sudden cessation of alcohol consumption. See also ALCOHOLISM.

substance use t.: drug withdrawal in the NURSING INTERVENTIONS CLASSIFICATION, a nursing INTERVENTION defined as the care of a patient experiencing drug DETOXIFICATION. See also substance ABUSE.

substance use t.: overdose in the NURSING INTERVENTIONS CLASSIFICATION, a nursing INTERVENTION defined as monitoring, treatment, and emotional support of a patient who has ingested prescription or over-the counter-drugs beyond the therapeutic range. See also OVERDOSE.

supporting t., supportive t. supportive CARE.

tree (tre) an anatomic structure with branches resembling a tree.

bronchial t. the bronchi and their branching structures; see color plates.

tracheobronchial t. the trachea, bronchi, and their branching structures; see color plates.

Trematoda (trem″ah-to′dah) the FLUKES or trematodes, a class of the phylum Platyhelminthes; many are parasitic in humans and other animals, with infections resulting from the ingestion of insufficiently cooked fish, crustaceans, or vegetation containing their larvae. Important parasites infecting humans belong to the genera *Clonorchis, Dicrocoelium, Fasciola, Fasciolopsis, Heterophyes, Metagonimus, Opisthorchis, Paragonimus,* and *Schistosoma.*

trematode (trem′ah-tōd) fluke.

trematodiasis infection with TREMATODES (FLUKES); called also distomiasis.

tremor (trem′or, tre′mor) an involuntary trembling of the body or limbs; it may have either a physical or a psychological cause. Early symptoms include trembling of the hands and nodding of the head. Tremors are often associated with PARKINSON'S DISEASE which affects nerve centers in the brain that control the muscles. They also occur in CEREBRAL PALSY, HYPERTHYROIDISM, and WITHDRAWAL from narcotics or alcohol. They tend to develop as one of the results of aging, and are sometimes symptoms of temporary abnormal conditions such as insulin shock, or of poisoning, especially metallic poisoning. They sometimes appear with a high fever resulting from an infection. Tremors of psychological origin take many forms, some minor and some serious. Violent, uncontrollable trembling is often seen in certain phases of severe mental disorders. If there is no physiological cause, they may be a sign of general tension.

action t. rhythmic, oscillatory movements of the outstretched upper limb when voluntary movements are attempted, as when writing or lifting a cup; it may also affect the voice and other parts. Called also intention tremor and volitional tremor.

coarse t. that involving large groups of muscle fibers contracting slowly.

essential t. a hereditary tremor with onset at varying ages, usually at about 50 years of age, beginning with a fine rapid tremor (as distinct from that of PARKINSONISM) of the hands, followed by tremor of the head, tongue, limbs, and trunk; it is aggravated by emotional factors, is accentuated by volitional movement, and in some cases is temporarily improved by alcohol.

fine t. one in which the vibrations are rapid.

flapping t. asterixis.

intention t. action tremor.

parkinsonian t. a type of resting tremor commonly seen with PARKINSONISM consisting of slow, regular movements of the hands and sometimes the legs, neck, face, or jaw; it typically stops upon voluntary movement of the part and is intensified by stimuli such as cold, fatigue, and strong emotions.

physiologic t. a rapid transient tremor of extremely low amplitude found in the mbs and sometimes the neck or face of ormal individuals, only subtly detectable n an electromyogram and seldom visible to he naked eye; it may become accentuated nd visible under certain conditions.

rest t., resting t. one occurring in a elaxed and supported limb, such as a arkinsonian TREMOR.

senile t. one due to the infirmities of ld age.

volitional t. action tremor.

tremulous (trem´u-lus) shaking, trembling, or quivering.

trench fever a louseborne rickettsial disase due to *Rochalimaea quintana*, transitted by the human body louse, *Pediculus umanus;* symptoms include febrile parxysms, leg pains, chills, sweating, rash, plenomegaly, and a tendency to relapse. alled also His's or His-Werner disease.

trepan (trĕ-pan´) trephine.

trepanation (trep˝ah-na´shun) trephina-on.

trephination (tref´ĭ-na´shun) use of the REPHINE for creating an opening in the skull r in the sclera.

dental t. surgical creation of a fistula y puncturing the soft tissue and bone verlying the root apex to provide drainage. alled also apicostomy.

trephine (trĕ-fīn´, trĕ-fēn´) 1. a saw for emoving a disk of bone, chiefly from the kull. 2. an instrument for removing a rcular area of cornea. 3. to remove with nis instrument.

trepidation (trep˝ĭ-da´shun) 1. tremor. 2. ervous anxiety and fear. adj., **trep´idant.**

Treponema (trep˝o-ne´mah) a genus of ram-negative, motile bacteria, spirochetes ound in the oral, intestinal, and genital nucosa. Pathogenic species include *T. cara´-um,* the etiologic agent of PINTA; *T. pal´-dum* subsp. *pal´lidum,* the etiologic agent f SYPHILIS; and *T. pal´lidum* subsp. *perte´-ue,* the etiologic agent of YAWS.

T. pallidum complement fixation test, pallidum hemagglutination test, T. palli-um immobilization test formerly common erological tests for the diagnosis of SYPHILIS, elated directly to the causative organism.

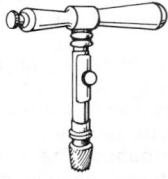
Trephine. From Dorland's, 2000.

treponema (trep˝o-ne´mah) an organism of the genus *Treponema.* adj., **trepone´mal.**

treponemal antigen test (trep˝o-ne´mal) any of various tests detecting specific antitreponemal antibodies in serum in the diagnosis of the *Treponema pallidum* infection of SYPHILIS.

treponematosis (trep˝o-ne˝mah-to´sis) infection with organisms of the genus *Treponema.*

treponemicidal (trep˝o-ne˝mĭ-si´dal) destroying treponemas.

trepopnea (tre˝pop-ne´ah) DYSPNEA that is relieved when the patient is in lateral recumbent position.

treppe (trep´ĕ) [Ger.] the gradual increase in muscular contraction following rapidly repeated stimulation.

tretinoin (tret´ĭ-no´in) the all-*trans* stereoisomer of RETINOIC ACID, used topically for treatment of cases of ACNE VULGARIS in which comedones, pustules, and papules predominate; it prevents comedo formation and suppresses keratin synthesis; common adverse effects are erythema and desquamation. It is also administered orally in treatment of acute promyelocytic LEUKEMIA.

TRH thyrotropin releasing hormone.

TRH stimulation test, TRH test thyrotropin-releasing hormone test.

tri- word element [Gr., L.] *three.*

triacetin (tri-as´ĕ-tin) a topical antifungal agent used topically in the treatment of superficial fungal infections of the skin; called also glyceryl triacetate.

triacylglycerol (tri-as˝il-glis´er-ol) the systematic chemical name for triglyceride.

triad (tri´ad) 1. an element with a valence of three. 2. a group of three similar bodies, or a complex composed of three items or units.

acute compression t. Beck's triad.

Andersen's t. Andersen's syndrome.

Beck's t. rising venous pressure, falling arterial pressure, and small quiet heart; characteristic of cardiac compression; called also acute compression triad.

Cushing's t. decreased pulse, increased blood pressure, and a widening pulse pressure associated with increased intracranial pressure; it is a late clinical sign and may indicate brainstem herniation.

Hutchinson's t. diffuse interstitial keratitis, labyrinthine disease, and Hutchinson's teeth, seen in congenital syphilis.

Saint's t. hiatus hernia, colonic diverticula, and cholelithiasis.

triage (tre-ahzh´) [Fr.] the sorting out and classification of casualties of war or other

DISASTER, to determine priority of need and proper place of treatment.

disaster t. in the NURSING INTERVENTIONS CLASSIFICATION, a nursing INTERVENTION defined as establishing priorities of patient care for urgent treatment while allocating scarce resources.

t.: emergency center in the NURSING INTERVENTIONS CLASSIFICATION, a nursing INTERVENTION defined as establishing priorities and initiating treatment for patients in an EMERGENCY center.

t.: telephone in the NURSING INTERVENTIONS CLASSIFICATION, a nursing INTERVENTION defined as determining the nature and urgency of a problem or problems and providing directions for the level of care required, over the telephone. See also TELEHEALTH.

trial (tri′al, trīl) a test or experiment.

clinical t. an experiment performed on human beings in order to evaluate the comparative efficacy of two or more therapies. See also SINGLE BLIND, DOUBLE BLIND, and TRIPLE BLIND.

triamcinolone (tri″am-sin′o-lōn) a PREDNISOLONE derivative used in replacement therapy for adrenocortical insufficiency and as an ANTIINFLAMMATORY and immunosuppressant in a wide variety of disorders; administered orally in the form of the acetonide, diacetate, and hexacetonide esters.

triamterene (tri-am′ter-ēn) a potassium sparing DIURETIC used in treatment of edema and, usually in combination with HYDROCHLOROTHIAZIDE, in the treatment of hypertension.

triangle (tri′ang-g′l) a three-cornered object, figure, or area, such as a delineated area on the surface of the body; called also trigone.

carotid t., inferior that between the median line of the neck in front, the sternocleidomastoid muscle, and the anterior belly of the omohyoid muscle.

carotid t., superior carotid trigone.

cephalic t. one on the anteroposterior plane of the skull, between lines from the occiput to the forehead and to the chin, and from the chin to the forehead.

digastric t. submandibular triangle.

Einthoven's t. an imaginary equilateral triangle with the heart at its center, formed by the axes of the three bipolar limb leads.

t. of elbow a triangular area on the front of the elbow, bounded by the brachioradial muscle on the outside and the round pronator muscle inside, with the base toward the humerus.

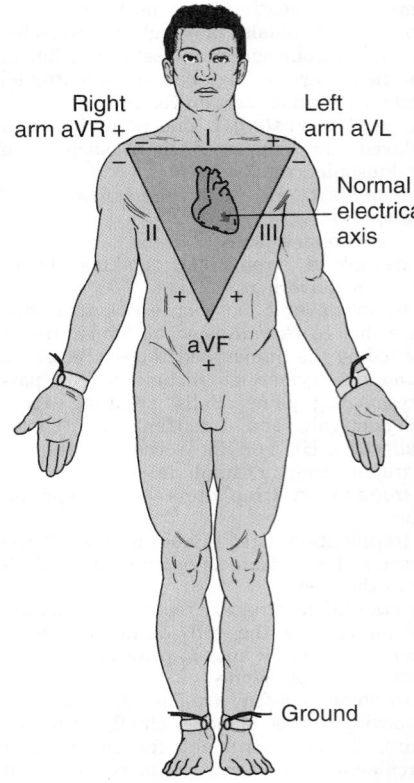

Right arm aVR +

Left arm aVL

Normal electrical axis

Ground

Einthoven's triangle. Bipolar limb leads I, II, and III form Einthoven's triangle. Other standard positions for electrocardiographic leads are the augmented unipolar leads: aVR (right arm), aVL (left arm), and aVF (left leg). From Polaski and Tatro, 1996.

t. of election superior carotid triangle

facial t. a triangular area whose points are the basion and the alveolar and nasal points.

femoral t. the area formed superiorly by the inguinal ligament, laterally by the sartorius muscle, and medially by the adductor longus muscle; called also Scarpa's triangle.

infraclavicular t. that formed by the clavicle above, the upper border of the greater pectoral muscle on the inside, and the anterior border of the deltoid muscle on the outside.

inguinal t. the triangular area bounded by the inner edge of the sartorius muscle, the inguinal ligament, and the outer edge of the long adductor muscle.

lumbocostoabdominal t. that lying between the external oblique muscle of the abdomen, the posterior inferior serratus

muscle, the erector muscle of the spine, and
the internal oblique muscle of the abdomen.

occipital t. the area bounded by the
sternocleidomastoid muscle in front, the
trapezius muscle behind, and the omohyoid
muscle below.

Scarpa's t. femoral triangle.

subclavian t. a triangular area bounded
by the clavicle, the sternocleidomastoid
muscle, and the omohyoid muscle.

suboccipital t. that lying between the
posterior greater rectus muscle of the head
and the superior and inferior oblique muscles of the head.

triangular (tri-ang′gu-lar) having three
angles or corners.

triangularis (tri-ang″gu-la′ris) [L.] triangular.

Triatoma (tri″ah-to′mah) a genus of bugs
(order Hemiptera), the cone-nosed bugs,
important in medicine as vectors of *Trypanosoma cruzi.*

Triavil (tri′ah-vil) trademark for a preparation of PERPHENAZINE (an ANTIDEPRES-
ANT) and AMITRIPTYLINE hydrochloride (an
ANTIANXIETY AGENT); used in treatment of
depression accompanied by anxiety or agitation.

triazolam (tri-a′zo-lam) a BENZODIAZEPINE
used as a SEDATIVE and HYPNOTIC in treatment of insomnia; administered orally.

triazole (tri′ah-zōl, tri-a′zōl) 1. an organic
compound in which three atoms of the five
that make up the ring are nitrogen atoms.
2. any of a class of antifungal AGENTS that
contain this compound.

tribe (trīb) a taxonomic category subordinate to a family (or subfamily) and superior
to a genus (or subtribe).

triboluminescence (tri″bo-loo″mĭ-nes′ens)
luminescence produced by mechanical energy, as by the grinding, rubbing, or breaking of certain crystals.

tribrachius (tri-bra′ke-us) a malformed
fetus with three upper limbs.

tricephalus (tri-sef′ah-lus) a malformed
fetus with three heads.

triceps (tri′seps) a muscle having three
heads; see anatomic Table of Muscles in the
Appendices.

trich(o)- word element [Gr.], *hair.*

trichiasis (tri-ki′ah-sis) 1. a condition of
ingrowing hairs about an orifice. 2. inversion of the eyelashes, characterized by
excessive tearing and the sensation of a
foreign body in the eye. 3. the appearance
of hairlike filaments in the urine.

trichilemmal (trik″ĭ-lem′al) pertaining to
the outer root sheath of a hair.

trichilemmoma (trik″ĭ-lem-o′mah) a benign neoplasm of the lower outer root
sheath of the hair.

trichina (trĭ-ki′nah) [Gr.] an individual
organism of the genus *Trichinella.*

Trichinella (trik″ĭ-nel′ah) a genus of parasitic NEMATODES (ROUNDWORMS). *T. spira′lis* is
a species found in the striated muscle of
various animals, and causes TRICHINOSIS in
humans who eat poorly cooked pork.

trichinosis (trik″ĭ-no′sis) infection with
the parasitic roundworm *Trichinella spiralis.* The worm larvae live embedded in tiny
capsulelike cysts of muscle tissue of infected
pork. When the meat is properly cooked, the
larvae are killed by the high temperature;
however, if the pork is undercooked, they
survive. Then when the meat is eaten
digestive fluids dissolve the cyst capsules
and free the larvae in the intestines, where
they grow to maturity.

Trichinosis is found in most parts of the
world with the exception of Australia and
the Pacific islands. It is relatively common
in Europe and the United States. In recent
years there has been a decline in incidence
owing mainly to enforcement of laws requiring the cooking of garbage fed to hogs.
Other factors influencing the decline include storage of meat at low temperatures
and education of the general public in the
proper cooking of pork.

Symptoms and Development. Trichinosis
develops in stages that correspond to the
worms' development in the intestine and,
later, the movement of their larvae into
other parts of the body. Symptoms and the
severity vary according to the stage of the
disease, the tissues invaded, and the total
number of invading parasites.

During the initial stage, when larvae are
developing into mature worms in the intestinal tract, there may be diarrhea, nausea, abdominal pain, and fever. Symptoms
that make identification more certain appear generally after an incubation period of
1 to 2 weeks. By this time, the mature
worms have deposited their young in the
intestinal wall and these new larvae are
beginning to move through the body, causing a variety of reactions in one or several
organs and areas. Edema may develop in
the eyelids. This may be followed by hemorrhage of the retina, pain in the eyes, and
extreme sensitivity to light. As the larvae
invade other parts of the body, there may be
muscle soreness and pain, fever, thirst,
chills, profuse sweating, and edema in the
infected areas.

For most people there is more discomfort
than danger in this most serious phase
of trichinosis, when the larvae are active
in various parts of the body. Often the

infection is mild enough for patients to be treated at home. The occasional fatal cases (fewer than 5 per cent of known cases) usually involve additional infections or disorders in organs weakened by the parasites.

In the usual course of the disease, there is a gradual decrease in symptoms as the larvae in muscle tissue become encysted and dormant and those in other types of tissue are destroyed. After about 3 months, most symptoms disappear, although vague muscular pain and fatigue may still continue for several months. Trichinosis almost never leaves any permanent disability.

Treatment and Prevention. With its varying symptoms, trichinosis is sometimes difficult to diagnose, but a skin test has been developed that makes identification of the disease certain in most cases. Chest x-rays and microscopic examination of muscle tissue also can be useful in diagnosis. There is no specific treatment for trichinosis; recovery is a matter of rest and time, allowing the body's natural defenses to overcome the parasites. Medications, including thiabendazol, cortisone, and ACTH, may be prescribed to relieve muscular pain and other symptoms.

The only certain safeguard against trichinosis is the thorough cooking of all meat products to ensure destruction of any encysted *Trichinella* larvae. Pork should be cooked at a temperature of 150°C (350°F), with a roasting time of 35 minutes per pound, until the meat is gray in color; if it is pink it is underdone. Cooking in this manner ensures that all parts of the roast will be heated to well above 68°C (140°F), the thermal death point of trichinae.

trichinous (trik'ĭ-nus) affected with or containing TRICHINAE.

trichlorfon (tri-klor'fon) metrifonate.

trichlorphon (tri-klor'fon) metrifonate.

trichlormethiazide (tri-klor″mĕ-thi'ah-zīd) a thiazide DIURETIC used as an ANTIHYPERTENSIVE AGENT and for treatment of EDEMA.

trichloroacetic acid (tri-klor″o-ah-se'tik) a strong acid used as a protein precipitant in clinical chemistry and also as a caustic in CHEMABRASION and for removing warts.

trichloroethylene (tri″klor-o-eth'ĭ-lēn) a widely used industrial solvent, formerly used as an inhalation analgesic and anesthetic; exposure to high vapor concentrations can cause fatal poisoning.

trichobezoar (trik″o-be'zor) a bezoar composed of hair; hairball.

trichocardia (trik″o-kahr'de-ah) a hairy appearance of the heart due to exudative pericarditis.

trichoclasia (trik″o-kla'zhah) brittleness of the hair.

trichoepithelioma (trik″o-ep″ĭ-the'leo′-mah) a benign skin tumor originating in the follicles of the lanugo; it may occur as an inherited condition marked by multiple tumors (*trichoepithelioma papillosum multiplex*). Called also epithelioma adenoides cysticum.

trichoesthesia (trik″o-es-the'zhah) sensibility of the hair to touch.

trichoglossia (trik″o-glos'e-ah) hairy tongue.

trichoid (trik'oid) resembling hair.

trichology (trĭ-kol'ah-je) the sum of knowledge about the hair.

trichome (tri'kōm) a filamentous or hairlike structure.

trichomonacide (trik″o-mo'nah-sīd) an agent destructive to trichomonads.

trichomonad (trik″o-mo'nad) a parasite of the genus *Trichomonas*.

Trichomonas (trik″o-mo'nas) a genus of flagellate protozoa parasitic in birds and mammals, including humans. *T. ho'minis* and *T. te'nax* are nonpathogenic species found in the human mouth and intestines *T. vagina'lis* is found in the vagina and male genital tract and is the cause of TRICHOMONIASIS.

trichomoniasis (trik″o-mo-ni'ah-sis) a sexually transmitted disease caused by *Trichomonas vaginalis*. In females, vaginal or

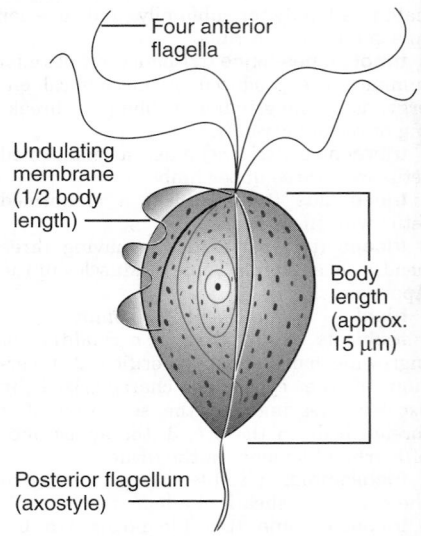

Schematic diagram of *Trichomonas vaginalis*. From Brunzel, 1994.

Labels on figure:
- Four anterior flagella
- Undulating membrane (1/2 body length)
- Body length (approx. 15 μm)
- Posterior flagellum (axostyle)

urethral infections may be asymptomatic or may produce itching or burning, dysuria, and green, yellow, or white vaginal or urethral discharge. Males can be asymptomatic carriers or they can develop urethritis, enlargement of the prostate, and epididymitis from the infection. Trichomonacides such as metronidazole (Flagyl) are used in treatment. Both symptomatic patients and their sexual partners must be treated to avoid reinfection.

trichomycosis (trik″o-mi-ko′sis) any disease of the hair caused by fungi.

t. axilla′ris infection of the axillary and sometimes of the pubic hair, due to *Corynebacterium tenuis* and not a fungus, with development of clumps of bacteria on the hairs, appearing as red, yellow, or black nodules.

trichonodosis (trik″o-no-do′sis) a condition characterized by apparent or actual knotting of the hair.

trichopathy (tri-kop′ah-the) disease of the hair.

trichophagia (trik″o-fa′jah) the habit of eating hair, a form of PICA.

trichophytid (tri-kof′i-tid) a secondary skin eruption that is the expression of an allergic reaction to a trichophyton infection and that occurs in an area remote from the site of infection.

trichophytin (tri-kof′i-tin) a filtrate from cultures of *Trichophyton;* used in testing for trichophytosis.

trichophytobezoar (trik″o-fi″to-be′zor) a bezoar composed of animal hair and vegetable fiber.

Trichophyton (tri-kof′i-ton) a genus of fungi that may cause various infections of the skin, hair, and nails.

trichophytosis (trik″o-fi-to′sis) infection with fungi of the genus *Trichophyton.* adj., **trichophyt′ic.**

trichoptilosis (trik″op-ti-lo′sis) splitting of hairs at the end.

trichorrhexis (trik″o-rek′sis) the condition in which the hairs are split and feather-like.

t. nodo′sa a condition marked by fracture and splitting of the cortex of a hair into strands, giving the appearance of white nodes at which the hair is easily broken. Called also bamboo hair.

trichoschisis (tri-kos′ki-sis) trichoptilosis.

trichoscopy (tri-kos′kah-pe) examination of the hair.

trichosis (tri-ko′sis) any disease or abnormal growth of the hair.

Trichosporon (tri-kos′po-ron) a genus of fungi that are normal flora of the respiratory and digestive tracts of humans and other animals, and may infect the hair.

trichosporosis (trik″o-spah-ro′sis) infection with *Trichosporon.*

trichostasis spinulosa (tri-kos′tah-sis spin″u-lo′-sah) obstruction of the hair follicles with a spinulous dark plug, consisting of many lanugo hairs in a horny mass; it may affect the skin of the alae nasi and other facial areas, or of the arms, chest, abdomen, or interscapular area.

trichostrongyliasis (trik″o-stron″ji-li′ah-sis) infection by species of *Trichostrongylus;* it may be asymptomatic or consist of diarrhea.

trichostrongylosis (trik″o-stron″ji-lo′sis) trichostrongyliasis.

Trichostrongylus (trik″o-stron′ji-lus) a genus of nematode parasites found in the intestines of humans and other animals; see TRICHOSTRONGYLIASIS.

trichotillomania (trik″o-til′o-ma′ne-ah) an IMPULSE CONTROL DISORDER consisting of an irresistible compulsion to pull out one's hair, the act being preceded by tension or an irresistible urge and followed by pleasure or relief. The diagnosis excludes such activities when caused by physical factors or by delusions or hallucinations. Specific patterns or rituals of hair pulling are often present.

trichotomous (tri-kot′ah-mus) divided into three parts.

trichroism (tri′kro-izm) the condition or quality of exhibiting three different colors when viewed from three different aspects. adj., **trichro′ic.**

trichromacy (tri-kro′mah-se) trichromatic VISION.

anomalous t. anomalous trichromatic vision.

trichromatic (tri″kro-mat′ik) 1. having or pertaining to three different colors. 2. able to distinguish the three primary colors; see trichromatic VISION.

trichromatism (tri-kro′mah-tiz′m) trichromatic VISION.

anomalous t. anomalous trichromatic vision.

trichromic (tri-kro′mik) 1. pertaining to or exhibiting three colors. 2. trichromatic.

trichuriasis (trik″u-ri′ah-sis) infection with species of *Trichuris;* in adults it may be asymptomatic, but in children it may cause vomiting, diarrhea, and rectal prolapse.

Trichuris (trik-u′ris) the whipworms, a genus of nematodes parasitic in the intestinal tract. *T. trichiu′ra,* the cause of TRICHURIASIS in humans.

tricipital (tri-sip′i-tal) 1. three-headed. 2. relating to the triceps muscle.

T

tricitrates (tri-sit′rāts) a solution of SO-DIUM CITRATE, POTASSIUM CITRATE, and CITRIC ACID; used as a systemic or urinary alkalizer and neutralizing buffer and for prevention of KIDNEY STONES.

triclosan (tri-klo′san) an ANTIBACTERIAL effective against gram-positive and most gram-negative organisms and exhibiting slight activity against yeasts and fungi; used as a detergent in surgical scrubs, soaps, and deodorants.

tricornute (tri-kor′nūt) having three horns, cornua, or processes.

tricrotism (tri′krŏ-tizm) the quality of having three sphygmographic waves or elevations to one beat of the pulse. adj., **tricrot′ic.**

tricuspid (tri-kus′pid) having three points or cusps, as a valve of the heart.

tricyclic (tri-sik′lik) containing three fused rings or closed chains in the molecular structure; see also ANTIDEPRESSANT.

tridactylism (tri-dak′tĭ-lizm) the presence of only three digits on the hand or foot.

tridentate (tri-den′tāt) having three prongs.

tridermic (tri-der′mik) derived from the ectoderm, entoderm, and mesoderm.

trientene (tri′en-tēn) a chelating AGENT used as the hydrochloride salt for chelation of COPPER in treatment of WILSON'S DISEASE, administered orally.

triethanolamine (tri″eth-ah-nol′ah-mēn) trolamine.

trifid (tri′fid) split into three parts.

trifluoperazine (tri″floo-o-per′ah-zēn) a PHENOTHIAZINE derivative used in the form of the hydrochloride salt as an ANTIPSYCHOTIC AGENT.

triflupromazine (tri″floo-pro′mah-zēn) a PHENOTHIAZINE derivative used in the form of the hydrochloride salt as an ANTIPSYCHOTIC AGENT and ANTIEMETIC, administered intramuscularly or intravenously.

trifluridine (tri-floor′ĭ-dēn) an antiviral compound that interferes with viral DNA synthesis, used topically in the treatment of KERATITIS and KERATOCONJUNC-TIVITIS caused by human HERPESVIRUSES 1 and 2.

trifurcation (tri″fer-ka′shun) 1. division into three branches or parts, such as blood vessels, or teeth that have three roots. 2. the site of such division.

trigeminal (tri-jem′ĭ-nal) triple. pertaining to the fifth CRANIAL NERVE (trigeminal nerve).

t. nerve the fifth CRANIAL NERVE; it arises in the pons, is composed of sensory and motor fibers, and has three divisions:

ophthalmic, maxillary, and *mandibular.* (See anatomic Table of Nerves in the Appendices.) The ophthalmic division supplies sensory fibers to the skin of the upper eyelid, side of the nose, forehead, and anterior half of the scalp. The maxillary division carries sensory impulses from the mucous membranes of the nose, the skin of the cheek and side of the forehead, and the upper lip and upper teeth. The mandibular division carries sensory impulses from the side of the head, chin, mucous membrane of the mouth, lower teeth, and anterior two-thirds of the tongue. (This nerve is sometimes called the great sensory nerve of the head.) The motor fibers are part of the mandibular branch and supply several of the muscles of chewing. Neuralgia of this nerve is the condition known as TIC DOU-LOUREUX.

trigeminy (tri-jem′ĭ-ne) the condition of occurring in threes, especially the occurrence of three pulse beats in rapid succession.

trigger (trig′er) an event that stimulates initiation of a subsequent event or process.

flow t. a trigger for initiating assisted VENTILATION, consisting of a mechanism for measuring the patient's inspiratory effort and starting of assisted ventilation when flow reaches a given level.

pressure t. a trigger for initiating assisted VENTILATION, consisting of a mechanism for measuring pressure and starting assisted ventilation when pressure reaches a given level.

time t. a trigger for initiating assisted VENTILATION, consisting of a mechanism that measures frequency of respirations and starts assisted ventilation when the respiratory frequency is at a given point.

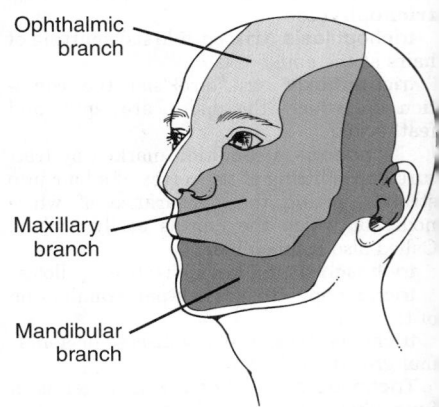

Ophthalmic branch

Maxillary branch

Mandibular branch

Areas of innervation by each of the three branches of the trigeminal nerve.

triglyceride (tri-glis′er-īd) a compound consisting of three molecules of fatty acids bound with one molecule of glycerol; a neutral fat that is the usual storage form of lipids in animals.

Elevated serum triglycerides are now considered as important as high cholesterol levels in the development of ischemic heart disease. The normal range for serum triglycerides is 0 to 160 mg/100 ml.

trigone (tri′gōn) 1. triangle. 2. the first three cusps of an upper molar tooth. adj., **trigo′nal.**

t. of bladder a triangular region of the wall of the urinary BLADDER, an area in which the muscle fibers are closely adherent to the mucosa; its three angles correspond with the orifices of the URETERS and URETHRA. Called also vesical trigone.

carotid t. the triangular area bounded by the posterior belly of the digastric muscle, the sternocleidomastoid muscle, and the anterior midline of the neck. Called also superior carotid triangle.

olfactory t. the triangular area of gray matter between the roots of the olfactory tract.

vesical t. trigone of bladder.

trigonitis (tri″go-ni′tis) inflammation or localized hyperemia of the vesical trigone.

trigonocephalus (trig″o-no-sef′ah-lus) an individual exhibiting trigonocephaly.

trigonocephaly (tri″go-no-sef′ah-le) triangular shape of the head due to sharp forward angulation at the midline of the frontal bone. adj., **trigonocephal′ic.**

trigonum (tri-go′num) triangle.

trihexyphenidyl (tri-hek″se-fen′ĭ-dil) an ANTIDYSKINETIC used as the hydrochloride salt in the treatment of PARKINSONISM and for the control of drug-induced extrapyramidal reactions (except tardive dyskinesia); administered orally.

triiodothyronine (tri″i-o″do-thi′ro-nēn) a THYROID HORMONE that contains IODINE and is liberated from THYROGLOBULIN by hydrolysis. It has several times the biologic activity of THYROXINE.

free t. the fraction of triiodothyronine in the serum that is not bound to a binding PROTEIN.

t. resin uptake test a THYROID FUNCTION TEST, measuring how many sites on thyroxine-binding globulin (TBG) are occupied by endogenous triiodothyronine (T_3) and how many sites remain available. An excess of radioactive exogenous triiodothyronine is added to the sample, followed by the addition of a resin that also binds T_3. A portion of the radioactive T_3 binds to sites on TBG not already occupied by endogenous thyroid hormones,

and the remainder binds to the resin. The amount of labeled hormones bound to the resin (the triiodothyronine resin UPTAKE) can be subtracted from the total that was added and the remainder is the amount that bound to the unoccupied binding sites on the thyroxine-binding globulin.

trikates (tri′kāts) a solution of potassium acetate, potassium bicarbonate, and potassium citrate used as a potassium supplement in the treatment and prevention of HYPOKALEMIA, administered orally.

trilabe (tri′lāb) a three-pronged lithotrite.

Trilafon (tri′lah-fon) trademark for preparations of PERPHENAZINE, an ANTIEMETIC and ANTIPSYCHOTIC AGENT.

trilaminar (tri-lam′ĭ-nar) three-layered.

trilobate (tri-lo′bāt) having three lobes.

trilocular (tri-lok′u-lar) having three loculi or cells.

trilogy (tril′ah-je) a group or series of three.

t. of Fallot a term sometimes applied to concurrent pulmonic stenosis, atrial septal defect, and right ventricular hypertrophy.

trimensual (tri-men′su-al) occurring every 3 months.

trimeprazine (tri-mep′rah-zēn) a PHENOTHIAZINE derivative with powerful ANTIHISTAMINIC action; used as the tartrate salt to relieve itching.

trimester (tri-mes′ter) a period of 3 months.

trimethadione (tri″meth-ah-di′ōn) an ANTICONVULSANT with ANALGESIC properties, administered orally for treatment of petit mal EPILEPSY.

trimethaphan (tri-meth′ah-fan) a short-acting ganglionic blocking AGENT, used as *trimethaphan camsylate* as an ANTIHYPERTENSIVE to produce controlled hypotension during surgery and for the emergency treatment of hypertensive crises and pulmonary edema due to hypertension; administered intravenously.

trimethobenzamide (tri-meth″o-ben′zah-mīd) an ANTIEMETIC administered orally, intramuscularly, or rectally as the hydrochloride salt.

trimethoprim (tri-meth′o-prim) an oral antibacterial closely related to PYRIMETHAMINE, almost always administered in combination with a SULFONAMIDE, primarily for treatment of urinary tract infections. The sulfate salt is applied topically to the conjunctiva, in combination with polymyxin B sulfate, in the treatment of ocular infections.

T

trimetrexate (tri″-mĕ-trek′sāt) a folic acid antagonist structurally related to methotrexate, used as the glucuronate salt, in combination with leucovorin, to treat *Pneumocystis carinii* pneumonia in ACQUIRED IMMUNODEFICIENCY SYNDROME, administered intravenously.

trimipramine (tri-mip′rah-mēn) a tricyclic ANTIDEPRESSANT of the DIBENZAZEPINE group, administered orally as the maleate salt for treatment of depression, peptic ulcer, and certain types of severe chronic pain.

trimorphous (tri-mor′fus) existing in three different forms.

trinitrophenol (tri-ni″tro-fe′nol) a substance used as dye, tissue fixative, antiseptic, astringent, and stimulant of epithelialization; its toxic effects are similar to those of dinitrophenol. It can be detonated on percussion or by heating above 300° C. Called also picric acid.

trinitrotoluene (tri-ni″tro-tol′u-ēn) TNT: a high explosive derived from toluene; it sometimes causes poisoning in those who work with it, marked by dermatitis, gastritis, abdominal pain, vomiting, constipation, and flatulence.

triocephalus (tri″o-sef′ah-lus) a malformed fetus with no organs of sight, hearing, or smell, the head being a nearly shapeless mass.

triol (tri′ol) an organic compound containing three hydroxy groups; a trihydric alcohol, e.g., glycerol.

triorchidism (tri-or′kĭ-dizm) the presence of three testes.

triose (tri′ōs) a monosaccharide containing three carbon atoms in a molecule.

trioxsalen (tri-ok′sah-len) a PSORALEN used in conjunction with ultraviolet RADIATION exposure in treatment of VITILIGO and PSORIASIS.

tripara (trip′ah-rah) tertipara.

tripelennamine (tri″pĕ-len′ah-min) an ANTIHISTAMINE used orally as the citrate and hydrochloride salts in the symptomatic treatment of various allergic disorders.

tripeptide (tri-pep′tīd) a peptide formed from three amino acids.

triphalangism (tri-fal′an-jizm) three phalanges in a digit normally having only two.

triphasic (tri-fa′zik) having three phases.

triphenylmethane (tri-fen″il-meth′ān) a substance from coal tar, the basis of various dyes and stains, including ROSANILINE, basic FUCHSIN, and GENTIAN VIOLET.

triple blind (trip′l blind) pertaining to a clinical TRIAL or other experiment in which neither the subject nor the person administering treatment nor the person evaluating the response to treatment knows which subjects are receiving a particular treatment or lack of treatment; see also PLACEBO.

triplegia (tri-ple′jah) paralysis of three extremities.

triplet (trip′let) 1. one of three offspring produced at one birth. 2. a combination of three objects or entities acting together, as three lenses or three nucleotides.

triplex (tri′pleks) triple or threefold.

triploid (trip′loid) having triple the haploid number of chromosomes (3n).

triplokoria (trip″lo-ko′re-ah) the presence of three pupils in an eye.

triplopia (trĭ-plo′pe-ah) defective vision objects being seen as threefold; usually a hysterical symptom.

tripoding (tri′pod-ing) the use of three points of support, as adopted by paralyzed patients when changing from a sitting or standing position.

triprolidine (tri-pro′lĭ-dēn) an ANTIHISTAMINE with sedative and anticholinergic effects; used as the hydrochloride salt in the treatment of nasal, eye, and skin manifestations of allergic reactions, including allergic rhinitis, conjunctivitis, and itching, and also as an ingredient in some cough and cold preparations, administered orally.

triptorelin (trip″to-rel′in) a synthetic analogue of GONADORELIN that on prolonged administration suppresses GONADOTROPIN release; used as *triptorelin pamoate* as an ANTINEOPLASTIC in the palliative treatment of prostatic carcinoma, administered intramuscularly.

-tripsy word element [Gr.], *crushing* used to designate a surgical procedure in which a structure is intentionally crushed.

tripus (tri′pus) a conjoined twin fetus having three feet.

trisaccharide (tri-sak′ah-rīd) a sugar each molecule of which yields three molecules of monosaccharides on hydrolysis.

trisalicylate (tri″sah-lis′ĭ-lāt) a compound containing three salicylate ions.

choline magnesium t. a combination of choline and magnesium SALICYLATES, used as an ANALGESIC, ANTIPYRETIC, ANTIINFLAMMATORY, and ANTIRHEUMATIC; administered orally.

trismus (triz′mus) motor disturbance of the trigeminal nerve, especially spasm of the masticatory muscles, with difficulty in opening the mouth (lockjaw); a characteristic early symptom of tetanus.

trisomy (tri′so-me) the presence of an additional (third) chromosome of one type n an otherwise diploid cell (2n +1). adj., **.riso′mic.**

t. 8 syndrome a syndrome associated with an extra chromosome 8, usually mosaic (trisomy 8/normal), characterized by mild to severe mental retardation, prominent forehead, deep-set eyes, thick lips, prominent ears, and CAMPTODACTYLY (abnormally flexed fingers).

t. 13 syndrome HOLOPROSENCEPHALY due to an extra chromosome 13, in which central nervous system defects are associated with mental retardation, cleft lip and palate, POLYDACTYLY (extra fingers or toes), and dermal pattern anomalies, as well as abnormalities of the heart, viscera, and genitalia. Called also Patau's syndrome. Information for families affected by this disorder can be obtained from the Support Organization for Trisomy 18, 13, and Related Disorders (S.O.F.T.), 2982 S. Union St., Rochester, NY 14624.

t. 18 syndrome a condition due to the presence of an extra chromosome 18, characterized by neonatal hepatitis, mental retardation, scaphocephaly or other skull abnormality, small receding mandible, BLEPHAROPTOSIS (drooping eyelids), low-set ears, corneal opacities, DEAFNESS, webbed NECK, short digits, ventricular septal defects, Meckel's DIVERTICULUM, and other deformities. Called also Edwards' syndrome. Information for families affected by this disorder and professionals caring for affected individuals can be obtained from the Support Organization for Trisomy 18, 13, and Related Disorders (S.O.F.T.), 2982 S. Union St., Rochester, NY 14624.

t. 21 syndrome Down syndrome.

t. 22 syndrome a syndrome due to an extra chromosome 22, characterized typically by mental and growth retardation, underized head, low-set or malformed ears, small receding mandible, long philtrum on the upper lip, preauricular skin tag or sinus, and congenital heart disease. In males, there is a small penis or undescended testes.

tristichia (tri-stik′e-ah) the presence of three rows of eyelashes.

trisplanchnic (tri-splangk′nik) pertaining to the three great visceral cavities, the skull, thorax, and abdomen.

trisulcate (tri-sul′kāt) having three furrows.

trisulfide (tri-sul′fīd) a sulfur compound containing three atoms of sulfur.

tritanomaly (tri″tah-nom′ah-le) a rare type of anomalous trichromatic VISION in which the third, blue-sensitive, cones have decreased sensitivity.

tritanope (trit′ah-nōp) a person exhibiting tritanopia.

tritanopia (tri″tah-no′pe-ah) defective color vision in which the blue-sensitive pigment of the retinal cones is absent. adj., **tritanop′ic.**

tritium (trit′e-um, trish′e-um) the mass 3 isotope of hydrogen, symbol ^{3}H, with a half-life of 12.26 years and used as an indicator or tracer in metabolic studies.

triturate (trit′u-rāt) 1. to reduce to powder by rubbing. 2. a substance powdered fine by rubbing.

trituration (trit″u-ra′shun) 1. reduction to powder by friction or grinding. 2. a finely powdered substance; called also amalgamation.

triturator (trit″u-ra′tor) an apparatus in which substances can be continuously rubbed.

trivalent (tri-va′lent) having a valence of three.

tRNA transfer RNA; see RIBONUCLEIC ACID.

trocar (tro′kahr) a sharp-pointed instrument equipped with a cannula; used to puncture the wall of a body cavity and withdraw fluid or to introduce an endoscope.

Trobicin (tro-bi′sin) trademark for a preparation of SPECTINOMYCIN hydrochloride, an ANTIBIOTIC used particularly against GONORRHEA.

trochanter (tro-kan′ter) a broad, flat process on the femur, at the upper end of its lateral surface (greater trochanter), or a short conical process on the posterior border of the base of its neck (lesser trochanter). adj., **trochanter′ic, trochanter′ian.**

troche (tro′ke) lozenge.

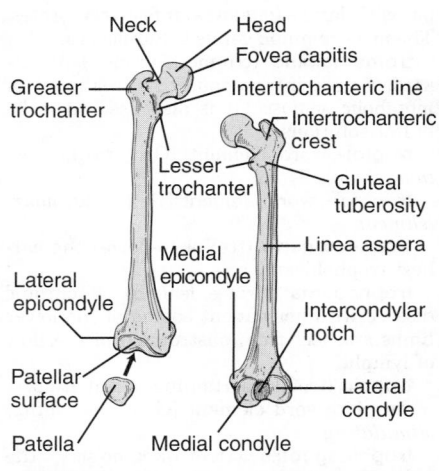

Position of greater and lesser trochanter on the femur and patella. From Applegate, 2000.

T

trochlea (trok'le-ah) [L.] a pulley-shaped part or structure; used in anatomic nomenclature to designate a bony or fibrous structure through which a tendon passes or with which other structures articulate.

trochlear (trok'le-ar) 1. pertaining to a TROCHLEA. 2. pertaining to the fourth CRANIAL NERVE (trochlear nerve).

t. nerve the fourth CRANIAL NERVE; it supplies muscle sense and the impulse for movement to the superior oblique muscle of the eyeball. See anatomic Table of Nerves in the Appendices.

trochocephaly (tro″ko-sef'ah-le) a rounded appearance of the head due to synostosis of the frontal and parietal bones.

trochoid (tro'koid) pivot-like, or pulley-shaped.

trochoides (tro-koi'dēz) a pivot joint.

trolamine (tro'lah-mēn) an alkalizing agent used in pharmaceutical preparations; when mixed with SALICYLIC ACID it is called *trolamine salicylate* and used as a topical ANALGESIC and SUNSCREEN.

troleandomycin (tro″le-an-do-mi'sin) a MACROLIDE antibiotic used in treatment of pneumonia and streptococcal infections.

Trombicula (trom-bik'u-lah) a genus of mites of the family Trombiculidae, including *T. akamu'shi, T. delien'sis, T. flet'cheri, T. pal'lida,* and *T. scutella'ris;* their larvae (CHIGGERS) are vectors of *Rickettsia tsutsugamushi,* the cause of scrub TYPHUS.

trombiculiasis (trom-bik″u-li'ah-sis) infestation with mites of the genus *Trombicula.*

Trombiculidae (trom-bik'u-li″de) a family of mites cosmopolitan in distribution, whose parasitic larvae (CHIGGERS) infest vertebrates. The most common genus is TROMBICULA.

tromethamine (tro-meth'ah-mēn) an ALKALIZER used intravenously in treatment of metabolic ACIDOSIS. It is also used to make buffer solutions.

trop(o)- word element [Gr.], *turn; reaction; change.*

troph(o)- word element [Gr.], *food; nourishment.*

trophectoderm (trof-ek'to-derm) the earliest trophoblast.

trophedema (trof″ĕ-de'mah) a chronic disease with permanent edema of the lower limbs and feet from obstruction of the flow of lymph.

trophic (trof'ik) pertaining to nutrition.

-trophic word element [Gr.], *nourishing; stimulating.*

trophicognosis (trof″ĭ-kog-no'sis) the scientific approach to determination of an individual patient's nursing care needs;

suggested as an alternative to the term NURSING DIAGNOSIS.

trophoblast (trof'o-blast) the peripheral cells of the BLASTOCYST, which attach the ZYGOTE (fertilized OVUM) to the uterine wall and become the PLACENTA and the membranes that nourish and protect the developing organism. The inner cellular layer is the CYTOTROPHOBLAST and the outer layer is the SYNTROPHOBLAST.

trophoneurosis (trof″o-noo-ro'sis) any functional nervous disease due to failure of nutrition from defective nerve influence. adj., **trophoneurot'ic.**

trophonucleus (trof″o-noo'kle-us) macronucleus.

trophoplast (trof'o-plast) a granular protoplasmic body.

trophotaxis (trof″o-tak'sis) CHEMOTAXIS of an organism in response to nutritive material.

trophotropism (trof″o-tro'pizm) CHEMOTROPISM of an organism in response to nutritive material.

trophozoite (trof″o-zo'īt) the active, motile feeding stage of a sporozoan parasite.

tropia (tro'pe-ah) a manifest deviation of an eye from the normal position when both eyes are open and uncovered; see also STRABISMUS.

-tropic word element [Gr.], *turning toward; changing; tending to turn or change.*

tropical (trop'ĭ-kal) pertaining to the tropics, the regions of the earth lying between the tropic of Cancer above the Equator and the tropic of Capricorn below.

tropism (tro'pizm) a growth response in a nonmotile organism elicited by an external stimulus, and either toward the stimulus *(positive tropism)* or away from it *(negative tropism);* used as a word element combined with a stem that indicates the nature of the stimulus (e.g., PHOTOTROPISM) or the material or entity for which an organism or substance shows a special affinity (e.g., NEUROTROPISM). See also TAXIS.

tropocollagen (tro″po-kol'ah-jen) the basic structural unit of collagen; it is a helical structure consisting of three polypeptide chains coiled around each other to form a spiral and stabilized by interchain bonds.

tropomyosin (tro″po-mi'o-sin) a muscle protein of the I band that inhibits contraction by blocking the interaction of actin and myosin, except when influenced by troponin.

troponin (tro'po-nin) a complex of muscle proteins which, when combined with Ca^{++} influence tropomyosin to initiate contraction.

-tropy word element [Gr.], *a turn, turning, change in response to a stimulus.*

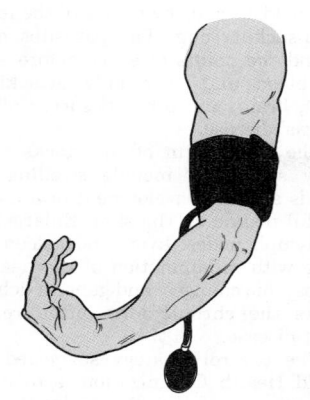

Trousseau's sign. From Polaski and Tatro, 2000.

Trousseau's sign (troo-sōz′) 1. spontaneous peripheral venous THROMBOSIS, suggestive of visceral carcinoma, especially carcinoma of the lung or gastrointestinal tract. 2. a sign for TETANY in which carpal spasm can be elicited by compressing the upper arm and causing ischemia to the nerves distally. See illustration.

Trousseau's syndrome (troo-sōz′) spontaneous venous thrombosis of the upper and lower extremities occurring in association with visceral carcinoma.

trovafloxacin (tro″vah-flok′sah-sin) an ANTIBACTERIAL effective against a broad spectrum of gram-positive and gram-negative organisms; administered orally as the mesylate salt in the treatment of serious infections.

truncate (trung′kāt) having the end cut squarely off.

truncation (trung-ka′shun) in information science, a process for retrieving alternative endings or beginnings of a term without having to specify the actual variations.

truncus (trung′kus) [L.] trunk.

t. arterio′sus an artery connected with the fetal heart, developing into the aortic and pulmonary arches.

t. brachiocepha′licus a vessel arising from the aortic arch and giving origin to the right common carotid and right subclavian arteries. Called also innominate artery (see anatomic Table of Arteries in the Appendices).

t. celi′acus celiac trunk.

t. encepha′licus brainstem.

t. pulmona′lis pulmonary trunk.

trunk (trungk) 1. the part of the body to which the head and limbs are attached; called also torso. 2. a larger structure, such as a vessel or nerve, from which smaller divisions or branches arise, or that is created by their union. adj., **trun′cal.**

brachiocephalic t. truncus brachiocephalicus.

celiac t. the arterial trunk arising from the abdominal aorta and giving origin to the left gastric, common hepatic, and splenic arteries.

encephalic t. brainstem.

lumbosacral t. a trunk formed by union of the lower part of ventral branch of the fourth lumbar nerve with the ventral branch of the fifth lumbar nerve.

lymphatic t's the lymphatic vessels (right or left lumbar, intestinal, right or left bronchomediastinal, right or left subclavian, and right or left jugular trunks) that drain lymph from various regions of the body into the right lymphatic or thoracic duct.

pulmonary t. a vessel arising from the conus arteriosus of the right ventricle and bifurcating into the right and left pulmonary arteries.

sympathetic t. two long ganglionated nerve strands, one on each side of the vertebral column, extending from the base of the skull to the coccyx.

truss (trus) an elastic, canvas, or metallic device for retaining a reduced hernia within the abdominal cavity.

trust (trust) a concept involving both confidence and reliance; to trust someone is to become vulnerable and dependent on the other person's intentions and motivations. Important trust relationships in health care are between patients, family members, the public, and providers. Health professionals have three obligations for being trustworthy: (1) acting consistently for the good of the patient, (2) having high levels of judgment and skill competence, and (3) fulfilling special roles such as the fiduciary one.

In health care, it is essential that patients be able to trust in the discretion of health care workers. It is impossible to specify moral practice in terms of rules or rights alone. It is difficult to separate knowledge and skill competence from moral competence (concern for the patient's well-being) in the professional's behavior. Trust must be earned and merited by performance and fidelity to its implications.

trustworthiness (trust′wer-the-ness) the quality of inspiring TRUST in someone else; this is one of the central VIRTUES in virtue-based ethical theories.

T

truth telling (trōōth tel'ing) in the NURSING INTERVENTIONS CLASSIFICATION, a nursing INTERVENTION defined as use of whole truth, partial truth, or decision delay to promote the patient's self-determination and well-being.

trypanocidal (tri-pan″o-si'dal) destructive to TRYPANOSOMES.

trypanocide (tri-pan'o-sīd) an agent lethal to trypanosomes; called also trypanosomicide.

trypanolysis (tri″pan-ol'ĭ-sis) the destruction of TRYPANOSOMES. adj., **trypanolyt'ic.**

Trypanosoma (tri″pan-o-so'mah) a multispecies genus of protozoa parasitic in the blood and lymph of invertebrates and vertebrates, including humans; most species live part of their life cycle in the intestines of insects and other invertebrates, the typical adult stage being found only in the vertebrate host. *T. gambien'se* and *T. rhodesien'se* cause the Gambian and Rhodesian forms of African TRYPANOSOMIASIS in humans, and *T. cru'zi* causes American TRYPANOSOMIASIS. Other species cause diseases in domestic animals.

trypanosome (tri-pan'o-sōm) an individual protozoan of the genus *Trypanosoma*.

trypanosomiasis (tri-pan″o-so-mi'ah-sis) infection with TRYPANOSOMES.

African t. an often fatal disease of Africa caused by *Trypanosoma gambiense* or *T. rhodesiense* and involving the central nervous system. The parasites are transmitted to human beings from cattle or other animals by the bite of the tsetse fly. Usually the first symptom is inflammation at the site of the bite, appearing within 48 hours. Within several weeks the parasites invade the blood and lymph, and eventually they attack the central nervous system. Characteristic symptoms include intermittent fever, rapid heartbeat, and enlargement of the lymph nodes and spleen. In the advanced stage of the disease there are personality changes, apathy, sleepiness, disturbances of speech and gait, and severe emaciation.

Pharmacologic treatment should begin as soon as possible and is based on lab results and patient symptoms. SURAMIN, PENTAMIDINE isethionate, and MELARSOPROL are the most common medications used. Pentamidine isethionate or suramin may be injected to remove parasites from the blood or lymph nodes before onset of disease, but the most effective preventive measure is eradication of the tsetse fly.

American t., South American t. a form found from the southern United States south into South America, caused by *Trypanosoma cruzi;* it is transmitted to humans from wild animals by means of the feces of a blood-sucking bug. The parasites multiply around the points of entry before entering the blood and eventually attacking the heart, brain, and other tissues. Called also Chagas' disease.

The acute form often attacks children. Early symptoms include swelling of the eyelids and the development of a hard, red, painful nodule on the skin. Enlargement of the lymph nodes, liver, and spleen occurs along with inflammation of the heart muscle, psychic changes, and general debility. In adults the chronic form often resembles heart disease.

The control strategy suggested by the World Health Organization is to interrupt transmission of the disease by the vectors and to systematically screen blood donors. Preventive measures, such as the wearing of protective clothing and the use of insecticides, are of primary importance. Medication with antiprotozoal AGENTS is usually effective when administered during the acute stage of infection.

trypanosomicide (tri-pan″o-so'mĭ-sīd) trypanocide.

trypanosomid (tri-pan″o-so'mid) a skin eruption occurring in trypanosomiasis.

trypsin (trip'sin) a proteolytic enzyme formed in the intestine by the cleavage of trypsinogen by enterokinase. It is an endopeptidase that hydrolyzes peptides of arginine or lysine.

trypsinogen (trip-sin'o-jen) the inactive precursor of trypsin, secreted by the pancreas and activated to trypsin by contact with enterokinase.

tryptamine (trip'tah-mēn) a chemical product of the decarboxylation of TRYPTOPHAN, causing VASOCONSTRICTION by the release of NOREPINEPHRINE at postganglionic nerve endings.

tryptic (trip'tik) relating to or resulting from digestion by trypsin.

tryptophan (trip'to-fan) a naturally occurring AMINO ACID, one of the essential amino acids; it is a precursor of serotonin. Adequate levels in the diet may mitigate pellagra by compensating for deficiencies of niacin.

tryptophanase (trip'to-fan″ās) an enzyme that catalyzes the cleavage of tryptophan into indole, pyruvic acid, and ammonia.

tryptophanuria (trip″to-fan-u're-ah) an AMINOACIDURIA consisting of excessive TRYPTOPHAN in the urine, such as in persons taking tryptophan-containing drugs. The symptoms resemble those of PELLAGRA.

tsetse (tset'se) an African fly of the genus *Glossina,* which transmits TRYPANOSOMIASIS.

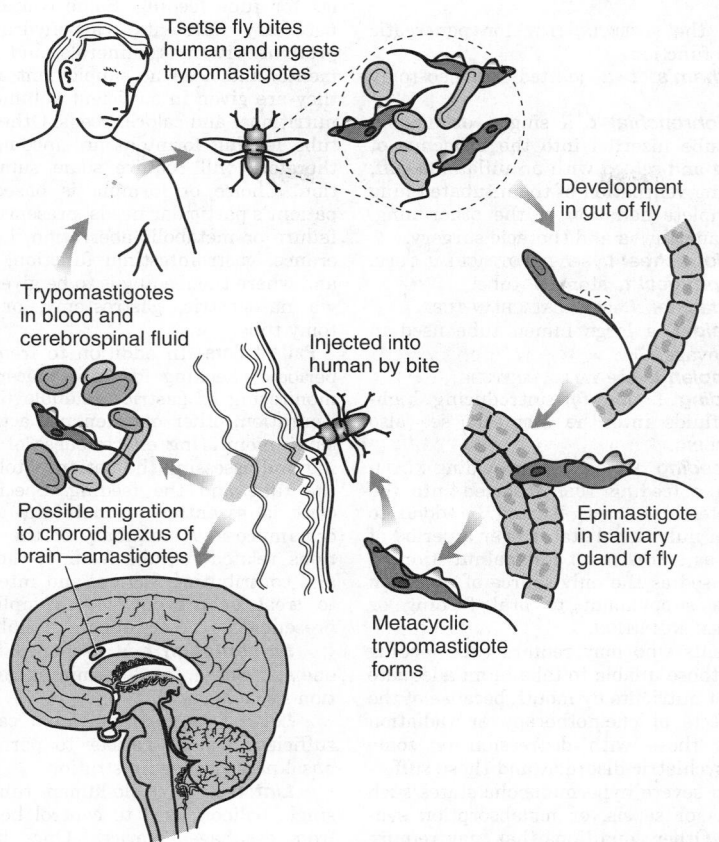

Tsetse fly bites human and ingests trypomastigotes

Development in gut of fly

Trypomastigotes in blood and cerebrospinal fluid

Injected into human by bite

Possible migration to choroid plexus of brain—amastigotes

Epimastigote in salivary gland of fly

Metacyclic trypomastigote forms

Life cycle of the etiologic agents of sleeping sickness (*Trypanosoma gambiense* and *T. rhodesiense*). From Mahon and Manuselis, 2000.

TSH thyroid-stimulating hormone (thyrotropin, thyrotropic hormone).

TSH stimulation test, TSH test thyroid-stimulating hormone test.

T-spine thoracic spine.

tsutsugamushi fever (disease) (tsoo-″soo-gah-moo′she) scrub typhus; see TY-PHUS.

t-test any in a class of statistical tests used to find the difference between the means of either a sample and a population, two different sample groups, two matched samples, or the same sample at two different points in time.

TU tuberculin unit.

Tuamine (too′ah-min) trademark for preparations of TUAMINOHEPTANE, a nasal DECONGESTANT.

tuaminoheptane (too-am″ĭ-no-hep′tān) an adrenergic used as a nasal DECONGESTANT in the form of the base (for inhalation) or the sulfate salt (topical solution).

tub(o)- word element [L.], *tube.*

tuba (too′bah) [L.] tube.

tube (toōb) a hollow cylindrical organ or instrument. adj., **tu′bal.**

auditory t. eustachian tube.

Blakemore-Sengstaken t. Sengstaken-Blakemore tube.

chest t. see CHEST TUBE.

Dobhoff t. a small-lumen feeding TUBE that can be advanced into the duodenum.

drainage t. a tube used in surgery to facilitate escape of fluids.

Drieling t. a double-lumen tube having a metal weight at one end to carry it past the stomach into the duodenum. At the other end are two tails, one used to collect gastric specimens and the other to collect specimens from the duodenum. The tube is used in the SECRETIN TEST for pancreatic exocrine function.

Durham's t. a jointed tracheostomy TUBE.

endobronchial t. a single- or double-lumen tube inserted into the bronchus of one lung and sealed with an inflatable cuff, permitting ventilation of the intubated lung and complete deflation of the other lung; used in anesthesia and thoracic surgery.

endotracheal t. see ENDOTRACHEAL TUBE.

esophageal t. stomach tube.

eustachian t. see EUSTACHIAN TUBE.

Ewald t. a large lumen tube used in gastric lavage.

fallopian t. see FALLOPIAN TUBE.

feeding t. one for introducing high-caloric fluids into the stomach; see also TUBE FEEDING.

t. feeding a means of providing NUTRITION via a feeding TUBE inserted into the gastrointestinal tract; it may be done to maintain nutritional status over a period of time or as a treatment for malnutrition. It can be used as the only source of nutrition or as a supplement to oral feeding or PARENTERAL NUTRITION.

Patients who may require tube feeding include those unable to take in an adequate supply of nutrients by mouth because of the side effects of chemotherapy or radiation therapy, those with depression or some other psychiatric disorder, and those suffering from severe hypermetabolic states such as burns or sepsis, or malabsorption syndromes. Other conditions that may require tube feeding include surgery or trauma to the oropharynx, esophageal fistula, and impaired swallowing such as that which occurs following stroke or that related to neuromuscular paralysis.

There are commercially prepared formulas for tube feeding. Some contain all six necessary nutrients (carbohydrates, fats, proteins, vitamins, minerals, and trace elements) and need no supplement as long as they are given in sufficient volume to meet nutritional and caloric needs. Other types of tube feeding formulas are incomplete and therefore will require some supplementation. Choice of formula is based on the patient's particular needs, presence of organ failure or metabolic aberration, lactose tolerance, gastrointestinal function, and how and where the feeding is to be given, that is via nasogastric, gastrostomy, or enterostomy tube.

Patient Care. In addition to frequent and periodic checking for tube placement and monitoring of gastric residuals to prevent aspiration, other maintenance activities include monitoring effectiveness of the feeding and assessing the patient's tolerance to the tube and the feeding. Special MOUTH CARE is essential to maintain a healthy oral mucosa. A summary of the complications related to tube feeding, their causes and contributing factors, and interventions to treat or prevent each complication is presented in the accompanying table.

fermentation t. a U-shaped tube with one end closed, for determining gas production by bacteria.

Levin t. a gastroduodenal catheter of sufficiently small caliber to permit transnasal passage; see illustration.

Linton t. a triple-lumen tube with a single balloon used to control hemorrhage from esophageal varices. Once it is positioned under fluoroscopic control and inflated, the balloon exerts pressure against the submucosal venous network at the cardioesophageal junction, thus restricting the flow of blood to the esophageal varices.

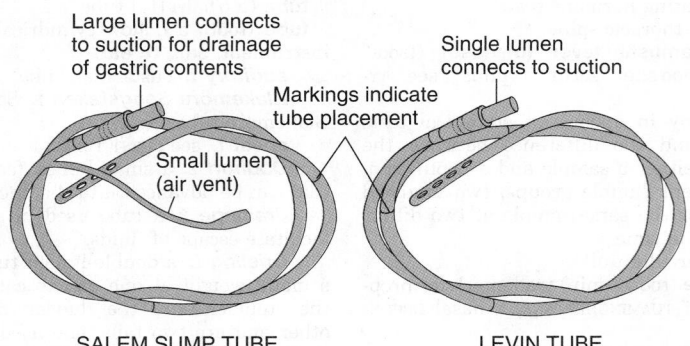

Large lumen connects to suction for drainage of gastric contents

Markings indicate tube placement

Small lumen (air vent)

Single lumen connects to suction

SALEM SUMP TUBE

LEVIN TUBE

Two types of nasogastric tubes. From Ignatavicius et al., 1995.

Miller-Abbott t. see MILLER-ABBOTT TUBE.

Minnesota t. a tube with four lumens, used in treatment of esophageal varices; having a lumen for aspiration of esophageal secretions is its major difference from the SENGSTAKEN-BLAKEMORE TUBE.

nasogastric t. see NASOGASTRIC TUBE.

nasotracheal t. an ENDOTRACHEAL TUBE that passes through the nose.

neural t. the epithelial tube produced by folding of the neural plate in the early embryo.

orotracheal t. an ENDOTRACHEAL TUBE that passes through the mouth.

otopharyngeal t. eustachian tube.

Rehfuss t. a single-lumen oral tube used to obtain specimens of biliary secretions for diagnostic study; it is weighted on one end so that it can be passed through the mouth and positioned at the point where the bile duct empties into the duodenum. See also BILIARY DRAINAGE TEST.

Salem sump t. a double-lumen NASOGASTRIC TUBE used for suction and irrigation of the stomach. One lumen is attached to suction for the drainage of gastric contents and the second lumen is an air vent. See illustration.

Sengstaken-Blakemore t. see SENGSTAKEN-BLAKEMORE TUBE.

stomach t. see STOMACH TUBE.

T-t. one shaped like the letter T and inserted into the biliary tract to allow for drainage of bile; it is generally left in place for 10 days or more in order to develop a tract through which bile can drain after the tube is removed. A T-tube cholangiogram is usually performed prior to removal of the tube in order to determine that the common duct is patent and free of stones. If stones are found they can be removed through the tube tract by instruments inserted under x-ray guidance.

test t. a tube of thin glass, closed at one end; used in chemical tests and other laboratory procedures.

thoracostomy t. a tube inserted through an opening in the chest wall, for application of suction to the pleural cavity; used to drain fluid or blood or to reexpand the lung in PNEUMOTHORAX. See also CHEST TUBE.

tracheal t. endotracheal tube.

tracheostomy t. a curved ENDOTRACHEAL TUBE that is inserted into the trachea through a tracheostomy; see discussion under TRACHEOSTOMY.

tympanostomy t. ventilation tube.

uterine t. fallopian tube.

ventilation t. a tube inserted after MYRINGOTOMY in chronic cases of middle ear effusion, such as in secretory or mucoid otitis media; it provides ventilation and

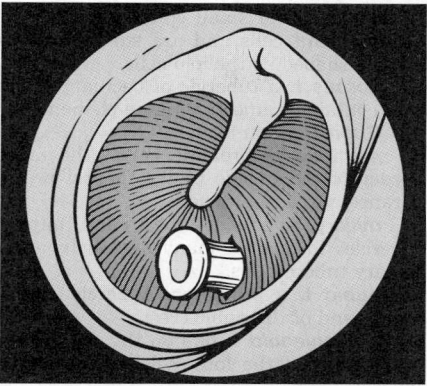

Tympanostomy (ventilation) tube. Polyethylene tubes are inserted surgically into the eardrum to relieve middle ear pressure and promote drainage of chronic or recurrent middle ear infections. Tubes extrude spontaneously in 6 months to 1 year. From Jarvis, 1996.

drainage for the middle ear during healing, and is eventually extruded. Called also tympanostomy tube.

Wangensteen t. a small nasogastric tube connected with a special suction apparatus to maintain gastric and duodenal decompression.

Whelan-Moss T-t. a T-TUBE whose crossbar tube is larger in diameter than the drainage TUBE.

x-ray t. a glass vacuum bulb containing two electrodes; electrons are obtained either from gas in the tube or from a heated cathode. When suitable potential is applied, electrons travel at high velocity from cathode to anode, where they are suddenly arrested, giving rise to X-RAYS.

tubectomy (too-bek′to-me) salpingectomy.

tuber (too′ber) 1. a swelling or protuberance; see also TUBERCLE and TUBEROSITY. 2. the essential lesion of tuberous SCLEROSIS, a pale, firm, nodular glial hamartomatous brain lesion that sometimes becomes calcified; it develops predominantly in the cerebral hemispheres, cerebellum, medulla, and spinal cord.

t. cine′reum an area of the undersurface of the forebrain to which the stalk of the pituitary gland is attached.

tubercle (too′ber-k′l) 1. a nodule or small eminence, especially one on a bone, for attachment of a tendon; see also TUBER and TUBEROSITY. Called also tuberculum. adj., **tuber′cular, tuber′culate.** 2. a small, rounded nodule produced by the bacillus of tuberculosis (*Mycobacterium tuberculosis*).

It is made up of small spherical cells that contain giant cells and are surrounded by spindle-shaped epithelioid cells.

fibrous t. a tubercle of bacillary origin that contains connective tissue elements.

Ghon t. Ghon focus.

mental t. a prominence on the inner border of either side of the mental protuberance of the mandible.

miliary t. one of the many minute tubercles formed in many organs in acute miliary tuberculosis.

pubic t. a prominent tubercle at the lateral end of the pubic crest.

supraglenoid t. one on the scapula for attachment of the long head of the biceps muscle.

tuberculid (too-ber′ku-lid) any of a group of conditions involving recurrent eruptions of the skin, usually characterized by spontaneous involution; it includes erythema induratum, lichen scrofulosorum, and papulonecrotic tuberculid, and sometimes also lupus miliaris disseminatus faciei.

papulonecrotic t. a grouped symmetric eruption of symptomless papules appearing in successive crops and healing spontaneously with superficially depressed scars, which occur chiefly on the extensor surface of the extremities in infants, children, and young adults.

tuberculin (too-ber′ku-lin) a sterile liquid containing the growth products of, or specific substances extracted from, the tubercle bacillus; used in various forms in the diagnosis of tuberculosis (see TUBERCULIN TEST).

Old t. a sterile solution of a heat-concentrated filtrate of tubercle bacillus culture grown on a special medium, used for tuberculin tests.

PPD t., purified protein derivative t. a sterile solution of a purified protein fraction precipitated from a filtrate of tubercle bacillus culture grown on a special medium, used for tuberculin tests.

t. test any of a large number of skin tests for TUBERCULOSIS using a variety of different types of tuberculin and methods of application. The most reliable procedure, now standard, is intradermal injection (the MANTOUX TEST) of PPD (purified protein derivative); a positive result consists of a palpable and visible area of erythema and induration greater than 10 mm in diameter developing around the site of injection 48 to 72 hours after the injection. Intermediate strength tuberculin (5 TU) is generally used to test adults; a positive result is virtually diagnostic of a previous or current infection with *Mycobacterium tuberculosis*. Persons with a negative test are retested with second strength tuberculin (250 TU); in this test a positive reaction is frequently due to atypical mycobacteria infection and is thus nonspecific; a negative result indicates either absence of tuberculosis or the presence of cutaneous anergy due to overwhelming tuberculosis infection or to an associated immunocompromised condition such as HIV infection, Hodgkin's disease, or sarcoidosis.

tuberculitis (too-ber″ku-li′tis) inflammation of or near a tubercle.

tuberculoid (too-ber′ku-loid) resembling a tubercle or tuberculosis.

tuberculoma (too-ber″ku-lo′mah) a tumorlike mass resulting from aggregation or enlargement of caseated tubercles.

tuberculosilicosis (too-ber′ku-lo-sil″ĭ-ko′sis) silicotuberculosis.

tuberculosis (too-ber′ku-lo′sis) an infectious, inflammatory, reportable disease that is chronic in nature and usually affects the lungs (*pulmonary tuberculosis*), although it may occur in almost any part of the body. The causative agent is *Mycobacterium tuberculosis* (also known as *the tubercle bacillus*). Formerly, the only other species of *Mycobacterium* thought to be pathogenic to humans were *M. bovis* and *M. avium*. It is now known that other species can produce diseases similar to true tuberculosis, including *M. intracellulare, M. kansasii, M. simiae,* and *M. szulgai*. The most common mode of transmission of tuberculosis in the United States is inhalation of infected droplet nuclei. In some other parts of the world *bovine tuberculosis,* which is carried by unpasteurized milk and other dairy products from tuberculous cattle, is more prevalent. A rare mode of transmission is by infected urine, especially for young children using the same toilet facilities. Tuberculosis is also seen as an opportunistic infection in human immunodeficiency VIRUS (HIV) infection.

The tubercle bacillus is capable of surviving for months in dried sputum that is not exposed to sunlight. Within the body it can lie dormant for decades and then become reactivated years after an initial infection. This secondary tuberculosis infection (endogenous reinfection) can occur at any time the patient's resistance is lowered. For this reason, periodic evaluation for evidence of the disease is extremely important for anyone who has had a primary tuberculosis infection. The tubercle bacillus is destroyed by boiling for 5 minutes, by autoclaving, by contact with coal tar preparations, e.g., phenol, and by ultraviolet radiation.

Primary and Secondary Tuberculosis. The first or primary infection with tuberculosis bacilli usually presents no symptoms. In about 99 per cent of those who are infected, the disease remains quiescent after the development of a hypersensitivity to the tuberculin microorganism and is no longer clinically significant.

The primary infection usually involves the middle or lower lung area. The primary lesion consists of a small area of exudation in the lung parenchyma (Ghon focus) which quickly becomes caseous (cheeselike) and spreads to the bronchopulmonary lymph nodes, where it gains access to the blood stream. Thus the stage is set for the development of a chronic pulmonary and extrapulmonary tuberculosis at a later time. In most instances, however, a secondary reinfection from inside the body (endogenous) or outside the body (exogenous) does not occur because of the subsequent development of tuberculin hypersensitivity and cellular immunity. The presence of antigen concentrations at the initial site of infection brings about necrosis and eventually fibrosis and calcification of the tissues, which arrests the infection and renders the disease inactive. If, however, the infection is not controlled, the patient develops the symptoms of progressive primary tuberculosis.

Secondary tuberculosis develops as a result of either endogenous or exogenous reinfection by the tubercle bacillus. This is the most common form of clinical tuberculosis. In the United States development of secondary tuberculosis is almost always the result of an endogenous reinfection, which occurs when the primary lesion becomes active. This most frequently happens in debilitated persons who have lowered resistance to disease.

Resistance to tuberculosis depends on the general health and living conditions of the individual. Poor health, crowded and unsanitary housing, malnutrition, and other illnesses can lower the body's defenses. A second factor that can lead to activation of the disease is frequent exposure to the bacilli or exposure to such numbers that even a healthy person cannot escape infection.

Tuberculin Testing. The most commonly used test is the MANTOUX TEST, which consists of an intradermal injection of a purified protein derivative of tuberculin. An indurated area (wheal) of 8 to 10 mm in diameter 48 to 72 hours after injection is considered positive. Induration must be present; a reddened area is not indicative of a positive reaction. If the test is positive for tuberculin sensitivity, further studies, including x-rays, are indicated before a definite diagnosis of tuberculosis is established. False negative results can occur with acute viral infections and some neoplastic diseases, e.g., Hodgkin's disease. Culture of *M. tuberculosis* from sputum or some other body fluid *is the only way to positively confirm tuberculosis.*

Symptoms. A child or young person with active tuberculosis usually suffers from one or more of the following symptoms: loss of energy, poor appetite, loss of weight, and fever. Even though these symptoms may have causes other than tuberculosis, they must be regarded as warning signals. In adults, listlessness and vague pains in the chest may go unnoticed, since they are often not severe enough to attract attention. Unfortunately, the symptoms that most people associate with tuberculosis (cough, expectoration of purulent sputum, fever, night sweats, and hemorrhage from the lungs) do not appear in the early, most easily curable stage of the disease; often their appearance is delayed until a year or more after the initial exposure to the bacilli.

Chronic pulmonary tuberculosis is often accompanied by PLEURISY. Pleurisy with effusion often is the first symptom of tuberculosis. In certain cases, complications are possible and each has its characteristic symptoms. At a fairly late stage, the tuberculosis bacillus may cause ulcers or inflammation around the larynx (tuberculous LARYNGITIS). Less often, tuberculous ulcers form on the tongue or tonsils. Sometimes intestinal infections develop; they are probably caused by swallowed bacteria-contaminated sputum. A most serious complication is the sudden collapse of a lung, the indication that a deep tuberculous cavity in the lung has perforated, or opened into the pleural cavity, allowing air and infected material to flow into it.

When a fairly large and previously walled-off lesion, or infected area, suddenly discharges its contents into the bronchial tree, the result is the infection of a large part of the lung, an acute and dangerous complication which causes tuberculous PNEUMONIA.

Tuberculosis bacilli can spread to other parts of the body by way of the blood, producing *miliary tuberculosis.* When a large number of bacilli suddenly enter the circulatory system, they are carried to all areas of the body and may lodge in any organ. Minute tubercles form in the tissues of the organs affected; these lesions are about the size of a pinhead or millet seed (hence the name *miliary*). Unless promptly

T

treated, and occasionally even then, the tiny lesions spread, join, and produce larger areas of infection.

Tuberculous pneumonia can begin in this way, as can tuberculosis of any other organ. Miliary infections involving the meninges produce a particularly serious disease; indeed, until the development of antibiotics, this condition nearly always proved fatal.

Practically all parts and organs of the body can be secondarily invaded by tubercle bacilli, a common type being involvement of the kidneys, which often spreads to the bladder and genitalia. Bone involvement, particularly of the spine (POTT'S DISEASE), was once common, especially among children.

Lupus vulgaris, or tuberculosis of the skin, is characterized by brown nodules on the corium; another form of tuberculosis of the skin is tuberculosis indurativa, a chronic disease in which indurated nodules form on the skin. When the adrenal glands are affected by tuberculosis, a rare occurrence, the condition can cause ADDISON'S DISEASE.

Treatment and Care. Most persons with tuberculosis are cared for at home under the supervision of a public health nurse who periodically visits the patient and family. Hospitalization may be required for those patients who experience complications or who are noncompliant with chemotherapy. The importance of compliance with the entire course of chemotherapy should be stressed. Failure to complete chemotherapy is a major factor in the appearance of drug resistant tuberculosis.

Masks may be necessary for those having intimate contact with a patient who is just beginning chemotherapy, and in caring for patients who cannot or will not take precautions against spreading the infection. Usually, two to four weeks after medications are begun restrictions are removed regarding activities and contacts. Handwashing is essential to prevention of cross-infection. Fomites are not considered important in the transmission of tuberculosis and so no special precautions are required for eating utensils and other inanimate articles in the patient's room. Screening of family members and other contacts should be done. Standard PRECAUTIONS are used for patients with extrapulmonary tuberculosis and those who have a positive skin test even without evidence of disease. Institutionalized patients with pulmonary or laryngeal disease should be kept on

airborne PRECAUTIONS. The Centers for Disease Control and Prevention has published "Guidelines for Preventing the Transmission of Mycobacterium Tuberculosis in Health Care Facilities." The document can be read on their web site at http://www.cdc.gov.

Drugs. Isoniazid remains the major antituberculous agent. It is usually administered in combination with rifampin. Ethambutol is added if the patient comes from an area of high resistance. In isoniazid-resistant cases, rifampin is substituted as a companion drug for ethambutol. Other medications are used if resistant organisms have developed.

Prevention. The incidence of tuberculosis is rising, and the development of resistant organisms is also rising. It must be stressed that medications *must* be taken as ordered. The best precautions are (1) maintenance of good health, (2) avoidance of unnecessary exposure to tuberculosis organisms, and (3) detection of the disease in its earliest stages.

avian t. a form affecting various birds due to *Mycobacterium avium*, which may be communicated to humans and other animals. Individuals with impaired immunity have particular susceptibility to this infection.

bovine t. an infection of cattle caused by *Mycobacterium bovis*, transmissible to humans and other animals.

hematogenous t. that carried through the blood stream from the primary site of infection to other organs.

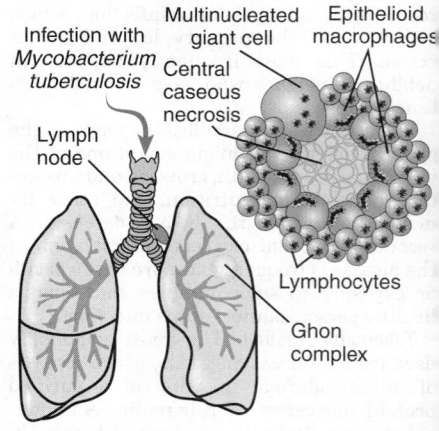

Tuberculosis. The Ghon complex, typical of pulmonary tuberculosis, consists of a parenchymal focus and hilar lymph node lesions. The detailed section of the diagram shows typical features of tuberculous granuloma: central caseous necrosis surrounded by epithelioid cells, multinucleated giant cells, and lymphocytes. From Damjanov, 2000.

miliary t. an acute form of tuberculosis in which minute tubercles are formed in a number of organs of the body, owing to dissemination of the bacilli throughout the body by the bloodstream.

open t. 1. that in which there are lesions from which tubercle bacilli are being discharged out of the body. 2. tuberculosis of the lungs with cavitation.

pulmonary t. infection of the lungs by *Mycobacterium tuberculosis;* the first infection is usually quiescent, and it may develop later into tuberculous pneumonia and other conditions. See TUBERCULOSIS.

renal t. disease of the kidney due to *Mycobacterium tuberculosis,* usually from BACILLEMIA in cases of pulmonary TUBERCULOSIS. Pathological changes include granulomatous inflammation and caseous necrosis of kidney tissue. Called also nephrotuberculosis.

t. verruco′sa cu′tis, warty t. a condition usually resulting from external inoculation of the tubercle bacilli into the skin, with wartlike papules that coalesce to form patches with a reddened inflammatory border.

tuberculostatic (too-ber″ku-lo-stat′ik) 1. inhibiting the growth of *Mycobacterium tuberculosis.* 2. an agent that has this effect.

tuberculotic (too-ber″ku-lot′ik) tuberculous.

tuberculous (too-ber′ku-lus) pertaining to or affected with tuberculosis; caused by *Mycobacterium tuberculosis.*

tuberculum (too-ber′ku-lum) [L.] tubercle (def. 2).

tuberosis (too″ber-o′sis) a condition characterized by the presence of nodules.

tuberositas (too″bĕ-ros′ĭ-tas) [L.] tuberosity.

tuberosity (too″bĕ-ros′ĭ-te) an elevation or protuberance, especially one on a bone where a muscle is attached; see also TUBER and TUBERCLE.

tuberous (too′ber-us) covered with tubers; knobby.

tubocurarine (too″bo-ku-rah′rēn) an alkaloid from the bark and stems of *Chondrodendron tomentosum;* it is the active principle of CURARE and is a nondepolarizing neuromuscular blocking AGENT; used in the form of the chloride salt for relaxation of skeletal muscles in surgery and convulsive THERAPY and as an aid in the diagnosis of MYASTHENIA GRAVIS. Administered intravenously or intramuscularly.

tuboligamentous (too″bo-lig″ah-men′tus) pertaining to the fallopian tube and broad ligament.

tubo-ovarian (too″bo-o-va′re-an) pertaining to the fallopian tube and ovary; called also ovariotubal.

tuboperitoneal (too″bo-per″ĭ-to-ne′al) pertaining to the fallopian tube and the peritoneum.

tuboplasty (too′bo-plas″te) 1. salpingoplasty. 2. plastic repair of a tube, such as the eustachian tube.

tubotympanic (too″bo-tim-pan′ik) pertaining to the auditory tube and tympanic cavity.

t. disease inflammatory disease of the middle ear, resulting from eustachian tube dysfunction and decreased pressure in the tympanic cavity.

tubouterine (too″bo-u′ter-in) pertaining to the fallopian tube and uterus.

tubule (too′būl) a small tube; especially, a minute canal found in various structures or organs of the body. adj., **tu′bular.**

collecting t′s the terminal channels of the NEPHRONS, which open on the summits of the renal PYRAMIDS in the renal PAPILLAE.

convoluted t′s channels that follow a tortuous course; there are convoluted renal tubules and convoluted seminiferous tubules.

dentinal t′s the tubular structures of the teeth.

galactophorous t′s small channels for the passage of milk from the secreting cells in the mammary gland.

Henle′s t′s the straight ascending and descending portions of a renal tubule forming Henle′s loop.

lactiferous t′s galactophorous tubules.

mesonephric t′s the tubules comprising the mesonephros, or temporary kidney, of amniotes.

metanephric t′s the tubules comprising the permanent kidney of amniotes.

renal t. the minute canals composing the substance of the kidney and secreting, collecting, and conducting the urine; in the glomerulus they have a basement membrane and epithelial lining.

seminiferous t′s the tubules of the testis, in which spermatozoa develop and through which they leave the gland.

uriniferous t′s renal tubules; channels for the passage of urine.

tubulin (too′bu-lin) the constituent protein of microtubules; thought to be involved in phagocyte motility.

tubulorrhexis (too″bu-lo-rek′sis) rupture of the tubules of the kidney.

tubulus (too′bu-lus) [L.] tubule.

tuft (tuft) a small clump, cluster, or coil.

tuftsin (tuft′sin) a tetrapeptide cleaved from IgG that stimulates phagocytosis by neutrophils. It is produced primarily in the spleen; hereditary tuftsin deficiency and tuftsin deficiency following splenectomy result in increased susceptibility to certain infections.

tugging (tug'ing) a pulling sensation, as a pulling sensation in the trachea (tracheal tugging), due to aneurysm of the arch of the aorta.

tularemia (too"lah-re'me-ah) a plaguelike disease of rodents, caused by *Francisella tularensis,* which is transmissible to humans. It can be contracted by handling diseased animals or their hides, eating infected wild game, or being bitten by insects such as horseflies or deer flies that have fed on such animals.

Symptoms and Treatment. Tularemia begins with a sudden onset of chills and fever, accompanied by headache, nausea, vomiting, and severe weakness. A day or so later, a small sore usually develops at the site of the infection, and it becomes ulcerated. There may also be enlargement and ulceration of the lymph nodes and a generalized red rash. In untreated cases, the fever may last for weeks or months. Treatment is with antibiotics, such as tetracycline, streptomycin, and chloramphenicol.

Prevention. Tularemia is usually thought of as an occupational disease. Those who may be exposed to it, such as game wardens and hunters, should take precautions such as wearing gloves when handling wild animals, particularly rabbits and squirrels, and wearing adequate clothing in the woods to prevent bites by insect vectors of the disease. Wild game must be especially well cooked in order to kill the tularemia organism.

tumefacient (too"mĕ-fa'shent) producing swelling.

tumefaction (too"mĕ-fak'shun) swelling.

tumescence (too-mes'ens) 1. swelling. 2. the condition of being swollen.

tumid (too'mid) swollen; edematous.

tumor (too'mor) 1. swelling or morbid enlargement; this is one of the cardinal signs of INFLAMMATION. 2. a new growth of tissue in which cell multiplication is uncontrolled and progressive. Tumors are also called NEOPLASMS, which means that they are composed of new and actively growing tissue. Their growth is faster than that of normal tissue, continuing after cessation of the stimuli that evoked the growth, and serving no useful physiologic purpose. adj., **tu'morous.**

Tumors are classified in a number of ways, one of the simplest being according to their origin and whether they are malignant or benign. Tumors of mesenchymal origin include fibroelastic tumors and those of bone, fat, blood vessels, and lymphoid tissue; they may be benign or malignant (SARCOMA). Tumors of epithelial origin are found in glandular tissue and such organs as the breast, stomach, uterus, or skin; they also may be either benign or malignant (CARCINOMA). Mixed tumors contain different types of cells derived from the same primary germ layer, and TERATOMAS contain cells derived from more than one germ layer; both kinds may be benign or malignant.

Benign Tumors. Benign tumors do not endanger life unless they interfere with normal functions of other organs or affect a vital organ. They grow slowly, pushing aside normal tissue but not invading it. They are usually encapsulated, well demarcated growths. They are not metastatic; that is, they do not form secondary tumors in other organs. Benign tumors usually respond favorably to surgical treatment and some forms of RADIATION THERAPY.

Malignant Tumors. These tumors are composed of embryonic, primitive, or poorly differentiated cells. They grow in a disorganized manner and so rapidly that nutrition of the cells becomes a problem. For this reason necrosis and ulceration are characteristic of malignant tumors. They also invade surrounding tissues and are metastatic, initiating the growth of similar tumors in distant organs. (See also CANCER.)

benign t. one that lacks the properties of INVASIVENESS and METASTASIS and that is usually surrounded by a fibrous capsule; its cells also show a lesser degree of ANAPLASIA than those of a malignant TUMOR do.

bladder t. a tumor of the urinary bladder; see also BLADDER CANCER.

brain t. see BRAIN TUMOR.

brown t. a giant-cell granuloma produced in and replacing bone, occurring in osteitis fibrosa cystica and due to hyperparathyroidism.

Burkitt's t. Burkitt's lymphoma.

Buschke-Löwenstein t. a slow-growing mass of warts found usually in the prepuce but sometimes elsewhere in the perianal region; it starts as a plaque and may grow into a large cauliflowerlike mass. Called also giant condyloma.

carcinoid t. carcinoid (def. 1).

carotid body t. a CHEMODECTOMA of a carotid BODY, found as a firm round mass at the bifurcation of the common carotid artery.

connective tissue t. any tumor arising from a connective tissue structure, such as a FIBROMA or SARCOMA.

desmoid t. DESMOID (def. 1).

endodermal sinus t. yolk sac tumor.

erectile t. cavernous hemangioma.

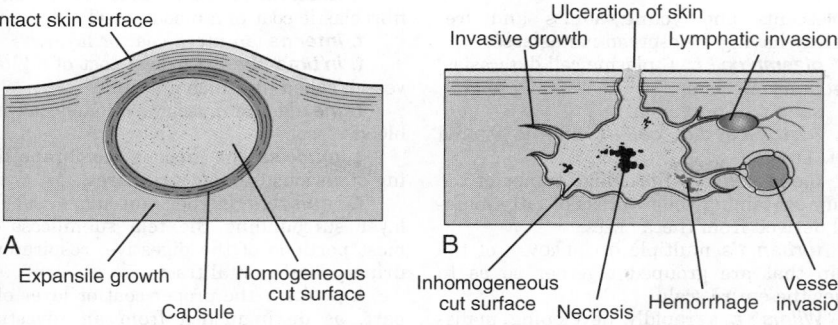

Gross appearance of benign *(A)* and malignant *(B)* tumors. From Damjanov, 2000.

Ewing's t. Ewing's sarcoma.

false t. pseudotumor.

fibroid t. 1. fibroma. 2. leiomyoma uteri.

germ cell t. any of a group of tumors arising from primitive germ CELLS, usually of the testis or ovum; they range from benign to highly malignant. Types include GERMINOMA, yolk sac TUMOR, TERATOMA, embryonal CARCINOMA, and some types of CHORIOCARCINOMA; many tumors are mixtures of types.

giant cell t. 1. a benign or malignant tumor containing giant cells; see under CARCINOMA, GRANULOMA, and SARCOMA. 2. a bone tumor, ranging from benign to frankly malignant, composed of cellular spindle cell stroma containing multinucleated giant cells resembling osteoclasts. 3. a small yellow benign tumorlike nodule of tendon sheath origin, usually of the wrist and fingers or ankle and toes, laden with lipophages and containing multinucleated giant cells.

glomus t. 1. a blue-red, extremely painful CHEMODECTOMA involving an arteriovenous anastomosis or cluster of blood cells, which may be found anywhere in the skin, most often in the distal portion of the fingers and toes, especially beneath the nail. Such tumors may also occur in the stomach and nasal cavity. 2. chemodectoma.

granular cell t. a relatively common neoplasm whose cells have a granular appearance by light microscopy; it is usually benign but occasionally malignant, and multiple tumors may occur. It can be found anywhere but is most often seen in the oral cavity, especially in the tongue.

granulosa t., granulosa cell t. see GRANULOSA CELL TUMOR.

granulosa-theca cell t. see GRANULOSA-THECA CELL TUMOR.

heterologous t. one made up of tissue differing from that in which it grows.

homoiotypic t., homologous t. one made up of tissue resembling that in which it grows.

Hürthle cell t. see HÜRTHLE CELL TUMOR.

islet cell t. a tumor of the islands of Langerhans; many secrete excessive amounts of hormones. Types include GASTRINOMA, GLUCAGONOMA, INSULINOMA, SOMATOSTATINOMA, and VIPOMA.

Krukenberg's t. see KRUKENBERG'S TUMOR.

lipoid cell t. of ovary a usually benign ovarian tumor composed of eosinophilic cells or cells with lipoid vacuoles; it causes MASCULINIZATION.

t. lysis syndrome severe hyperphosphatemia, hyperkalemia, hyperuricemia, and hypocalcemia occurring after effective induction chemotherapy of rapidly growing malignant neoplasms; thought to be due to release of intracellular products after cell lysis.

malignant t. one that has the properties of INVASIVENESS and METASTASIS and that shows a greater degree of ANAPLASIA than a benign TUMOR does.

mast cell t. mastocytoma.

melanotic neuroectodermal t. a benign, rapidly growing, dark tumor of the jaw or occasionally some other site, almost always seen in infants; called also melanoameloblastoma.

mixed t. one composed of more than one type of neoplastic tissue.

t. necrosis factor receptor–associated periodic syndrome (TRAPS) familial periodic fever.

organoid t. teratoma.

peripheral neuroectodermal t. (PNET) any of a heterogeneous group of neoplasms originating in supporting structures or neuronal tissue, primarily of the extremities, pelvis, or chest wall; seen most often in

T

adolescents and young adults and frequently having widespread metastases.

plasma cell t. 1. plasma cell dyscrasias. 2. solitary myeloma.

sand t. psammoma.

Sertoli-Leydig cell t. androblastoma (def. 1).

theca cell t. a fibroidlike tumor of the ovary containing yellow areas of fatty material derived from theca CELLS.

turban t's multiple CYLINDROMAS of the scalp that are grouped together so as to cover the entire scalp.

Wilms' t. a rapidly developing malignant mixed tumor of the kidneys, made up of embryonal elements, occurring chiefly in children before the seventh year; a genetic component is suspected in its etiology. It may be accompanied by congenital defects such as urinary tract abnormalities, absent iris of the eye, and asymmetry of parts. With treatment, the prognosis is excellent. Called also embryonal carcinosarcoma and nephroblastoma.

yolk sac t. a malignant germ cell TUMOR of children that represents a proliferation of both yolk sac endoderm and extraembryonic mesenchyme. It produces α-fetoprotein and most often occurs in the testes, but is also seen in the ovaries and some extragonadal sites. Called also endodermal sinus tumor.

tumoricidal (too″mor-ĭ-si′dal) oncolytic; see ONCOLYSIS.

tumorigenesis (too″mor-ĭ-jen′ĕ-sis) oncogenesis.

tumultus (too-mul′tus) excessive organic action or motility.

Tunga (tun′gah) a genus of fleas native to tropical and subtropical America and Africa. *T. pe′netrans* is the CHIGOE, which attacks many birds and mammals, including humans.

tungsten (tung′sten) a chemical element, atomic number 74, atomic weight 183.85, symbol W. (See Appendix 6.)

tunic (too′nik) a covering or coat; see TUNICA.

Bichat's t. tunica intima.

tunica (too′nĭ-kah) [L.] a TUNIC or COAT; used in anatomic nomenclature to designate a membranous covering of an organ or a distinct layer of the wall of a hollow structure, as a blood vessel.

t. adventi′tia the outer coat of various tubular structures.

t. albugi′nea a dense white fibrous sheath that encloses a part or organ, such as the testicle or ovary.

t. conjuncti′va the conjunctiva.

t. dar′tos dartos.

t. exter′na an outer coat, such as the fibroelastic coat of a blood vessel.

t. inter′na an inner coat or layer.

t. in′tima the innermost coat of a blood vessel; called also Bichat's tunic.

t. me′dia the muscular middle coat of a blood vessel.

t. muco′sa the mucous membrane lining of various tubular structures.

t. muscula′ris the muscular coat or layer surrounding the tela submucosa in most portions of the digestive, respiratory, urinary, and genital tracts.

t. pro′pria the proper coat or layer of a part, as distinguished from an investing membrane.

t. sero′sa the membrane lining the external walls of the body cavities and reflected over the surfaces of protruding organs; it secretes a watery exudate.

t. vagina′lis tes′tis the serous membrane covering the front and sides of the testis and epididymis.

t. vasculo′sa a vascular coat, or a layer well supplied with blood vessels.

tuning fork tests tests of HEARING using a vibrating tuning FORK of known frequency as a source of sound. See BING TEST, RINNE TEST, SCHWABACH TEST, and WEBER TEST.

tunnel (tun′el) a passageway of varying length through a solid body, completely enclosed except for the open ends, permitting entrance and exit.

carpal t. the osseofibrous passage for the median nerve and the flexor tendons formed by the flexor retinaculum and the carpal bones; see also CARPAL TUNNEL SYNDROME.

flexor t. carpal tunnel.

tarsal t. the osseofibrous passage for the posterior tibial vessels, tibial nerve, and flexor tendons, formed by the flexor retinaculum and the tarsal bones; see also TARSAL TUNNEL SYNDROME.

turbid (ter′bid) cloudy.

turbidimeter (ter″bĭ-dim′ĕ-ter) an instrument that measures the turbidity of a solution by measuring the loss of intensity of a beam of light in passing through the solution.

turbidimetry (ter″bĭ-dim′ĕ-tre) the measurement of the turbidity of a liquid.

turbidity (ter-bid′ĭ-te) cloudiness of a solution caused by the scattering of light by colloidal particles or by suspended precipitate or sediment.

turbinal (ter′bĭ-nal) turbinate.

turbinate (ter′bĭ-nāt) 1. shaped like a top; called also turbinal. 2. a nasal CONCHA.

turbinectomy (ter″bĭ-nek′tah-me) excision of a nasal CONCHA (turbinate bone).

turbinotomy (ter″bĭ-not′ah-me) incision of a nasal CONCHA (turbinate bone); called also conchotomy.

Turcot's syndrome (tēr′kots) familial polyposis of the colon associated with malignant tumors of the central nervous system.

turgescence (ter-jes′ens) swelling.

turgescent (ter-jes′ent) becoming swollen.

turgor (ter′ger) 1. swelling or other distention. 2. a condition of normal tension in a cell or group of cells; fullness. adj., **tur′-gid.**

    skin t. a reflection of the skin's elasticity, measured by monitoring the time it takes for the skin of the forearm to return to position after it is lightly pinched between the examiner's thumb and forefinger. Normal turgor is a return to normal contour within three seconds; if the skin remains elevated (tented) more than three seconds, turgor is decreased.

turista (too-rēs′tah) Mexican name for traveler's diarrhea.

turmschädel (torm′sha-del) a developmental anomaly in which the head is high and rounded, due to early synostosis of the three major sutures of the skull.

Turner's sign (ter′nerz) a gray-blue discoloration of the flanks, sometimes seen in acute hemorrhagic pancreatitis.

Turner's syndrome (ter′nerz) gonadal DYSGENESIS marked by short stature, undifferentiated (streak) gonads, and variable abnormalities that may include webbed NECK, low posterior hair line, CUBITUS VALGUS, and cardiac defects. The genotype is XO (45,X) or X/XX or X/XXX MOSAICMOSAIC, and affected individuals have a female phenotype. Information and support regarding this disorder can be obtained from the Turner's Syndrome Society, 14450 T.C. Jester, Suite 260, Houston, TX 77014, telephone 1-800-365-9944.

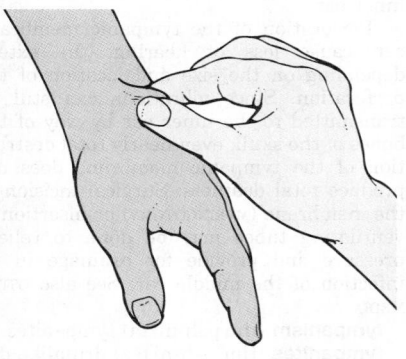

Assessing skin turgor. From Lammon et al., 1995.

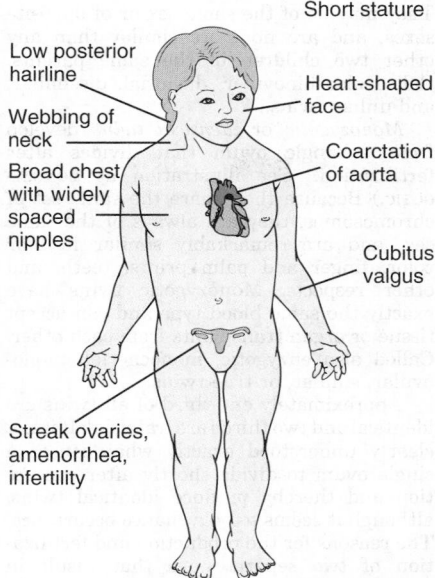

Short stature
Low posterior hairline
Webbing of neck
Broad chest with widely spaced nipples
Heart-shaped face
Coarctation of aorta
Cubitus valgus
Streak ovaries, amenorrhea, infertility

Typical features of Turner's syndrome. Redrawn from Damjanov, 2000.

TURP transurethral resection of the prostate.

turricephaly (ter″ĭ-sef′ah-le) oxycephaly.

TUR syndrome [*trans urethral resection*] severe hyponatremia caused by the absorption of fluids used to irrigate the bladder during TRANSURETHRAL RESECTION OF THE PROSTATE.

tussigenic (tus″ĭ-jen′ik) causing cough.

tussis (tus′is) [L.] cough.

tussive (tus′iv) pertaining to or due to a cough.

tutamen (too-ta′men) [L.] a protective covering or structure.

    tuta′mina o′culi the protective appendages of the eye, such as the eyelids, eyelashes, and so on.

Tween 80 (twēn) trademark for a preparation of POLYSORBATE 80, a SURFACTANT.

twiddler's syndrome (twid′lerz) the nervous habit of "twiddling" entry portals, thereby displacing an inserted catheter; it is usually associated with pacemaker insertion but has been reported following implantation of a venous access port.

twin (twin) one of two offspring produced in the same pregnancy; twins occur about once in every 86 births.

    Dizygotic or *fraternal twins* develop from two separate ova fertilized at the same time.

T

They may be of the same sex or of opposite sexes, and are no more similar than any other two children of the same parents. Called also binovular, dichorial, dissimilar, and unlike twins.

Monozygotic or *identical twins* develop from a single ovum that divides after fertilization. (See illustration at MONOZYGOTIC.) Because they share the same set of chromosomes, they are always of the same sex, and are remarkably similar in hair color, finger and palm prints, teeth, and other respects. Monozygotic twins have exactly the same blood type and can accept tissue or organ transplants from each other. Called also enzygotic, monochorial, monoovular, similar, or true twins.

Approximately one third of all twins are identical and two thirds are fraternal. It is not clearly understood exactly what causes a single ovum to divide shortly after conception and thereby produce identical twins, although it seems to be a chance occurrence. The reasons for the production and fertilization of two separate ova that result in fraternal twins are not well understood either, but it is thought that a tendency toward fraternal twins runs in families and is transmitted through the genes of the mother. Women are more likely to have fraternal twins in their later childbearing years, between the ages of 30 and 38 years, than earlier. Older age in the father also seems to be a factor with fraternal twins.

   conjoined t's Siamese twins.

   dizygotic t's, fraternal t's twins that develop from two separate ova fertilized at the same time; see TWIN.

   identical t's twins that develop from a single ovum; called also monovular or monozygotic twins. See TWIN.

   impacted t's twins so situated during delivery that pressure of one against the other produces simultaneous engagement of both.

   mono-ovular t's, monovular t's monozygotic t's identical twins.

   Siamese t's monozygotic twins whose bodies are joined; see also SIAMESE TWINS.

   unequal t's conjoined twins (SIAMESE TWINS) of which one is incompletely developed.

twinning (twin′ing) 1. the production of symmetrical structures or parts by division. 2. the simultaneous intrauterine production of two or more embryos; see TWIN.

twitch (twich) a brief, contractile response of a skeletal muscle elicited by a single maximal volley of impulses in the neurons supplying it.

twitching (twich′ing) the occurrence of single contraction or a series of contraction of a muscle.

two-tailed test a test analyzing a nondirectional hypothesis in which the researche assumes that an extreme score can occur i either extreme of the sampling distribution

tylectomy (ti-lek′tah-me) lumpectomy.

Tylenol (ti′lĕ-nol) trademark for prepara tions of ACETAMINOPHEN, an ANALGESIC an ANTIPYRETIC.

tyloma (ti-lo′ma) callus.

tylosis (ti-lo′sis) the formation of CAI LUSES. adj., **tylot′ic.**

Tylox (ti′lox) trademark for a combinatio preparation of OXYCODONE and ACETAMINC PHEN, an opioid ANALGESIC.

tyloxapol (ti-loks′ah-pol) a nonionic liqui polymer used as a SURFACTANT to aid lique faction and removal of mucopurulen bronchopulmonary secretions; administere by inhalation.

tympanal (tim′pah-nal) tympanic.

tympanectomy (tim″pah-nek′tah-me) ex cision of the tympanic membrane.

tympanic (tim-pan′ik) 1. bell-like; reso nant. Called also tympanal and tympaniti 2. of or pertaining to the TYMPANUM.

   t. membrane a thin, semitransparen membrane, nearly oval in shape, tha stretches across the ear canal and separate the TYMPANUM (middle ear) from the externa acoustic MEATUS (outer ear); called also ear drum. It is composed of fibrous tissu covered with skin on the outside an mucous membrane on the inside. It constructed so that it can vibrate freel with audible sound waves that travel in ward from outside. The handle of th MALLEUS of the middle ear is attached t the center of the membrane and receive the vibrations it collects, transmittin them to the other ossicles of the middle ea (the INCUS and STAPES), which in tur transmit the vibrations to the fluid of th inner ear.

   Perforation of the tympanic membran can cause loss of hearing, the exten depending on the size and location of th perforation. Since vibrations can still b transmitted to the inner ear by way of th bones of the skull, even nearly total destruc tion of the tympanic membrane does nc produce total deafness. Surgical incision c the membrane (MYRINGOTOMY) or insertion c ventilating tubes may be done to reliev pressure and provide for drainage in a infection of the middle ear. See also OTITI MEDIA.

tympanism (tim′pah-nizm) tympanites.

tympanites (tim″pah-ni′tēz) drumlike di tention of the abdomen due to air or gas i

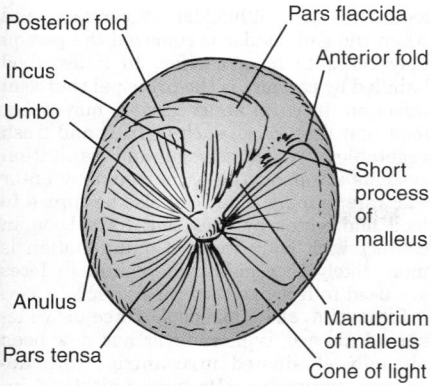

Posterior fold
Pars flaccida
Anterior fold
Incus
Umbo
Short process of malleus
Anulus
Pars tensa
Manubrium of malleus
Cone of light

Tympanic membrane. From Jarvis, 1996.

the intestine or peritoneal cavity. adj., **tympanit′ic.**

tympanitic (tim″pah-nit′ik) 1. pertaining to or affected with tympanites. 2. tympanic (def. 2).

tympanocentesis (tim″pah-no-sen-te′sis) myringotomy.

tympanogenic (tim″pah-no-jen′ik) arising from the tympanic cavity.

tympanogram (tim′pan-o-gram″) 1. a graphic representation of the relative compliance and impedance of the tympanic membrane and ossicles of the middle ear obtained by TYMPANOMETRY. 2. a test using tympanometry to measure how easily the tympanic membrane vibrates back and forth and at what pressure the vibration is easiest. The middle ear is normally filled with air at a pressure equal to that of the surrounding atmosphere. If it is filled with fluid, the membrane will not vibrate properly and the line on the tympanogram will be flat; if it is filled with air but at a higher or lower pressure than the surrounding atmosphere, the line on the graph will be shifted in position. A tympanogram is a quick and easy test; a probe is placed up against the ear canal like an ear plug and the equipment automatically makes the measurements.

tympanomastoiditis (tim″pah-no-mas″-toi-di′tis) inflammation of the tympanic cavity and the mastoid cells.

tympanometry (tim″pah-nom′ĕ-tre) indirect measurement of the compliance (mobility) and impedance of the tympanic membrane and ossicles of the middle ear; it is done by subjecting the external acoustic meatus to positive, normal, and negative air pressure and monitoring the resultant sound energy flow. See also TYMPANOGRAM (def. 2).

tympanoplasty (tim′pah-no-plas″te) plastic reconstruction of the bones of the middle ear, with establishment of ossicular continuity from the tympanic membrane to the oval window. This surgical procedure is performed when chronic infection or tumor has led to destruction of the ossicles, of the pars petrosa of the temporal bone, or both. Because the ossicles are so small, the surgery must be done under magnification with an operating microscope. Tympanoplasty requires great surgical skill and the use of specially designed instruments. It is often done in preference to radical MASTOIDECTOMY and offers the advantage of greater preservation of hearing. (For patient care after tympanoplasty, see surgery of the EAR.) adj., **tympanoplas′tic.**

tympanosclerosis (tim″pah-no-sklĕ-ro′sis) a condition characterized by the presence of masses of hard, dense connective tissue around the auditory ossicles in the middle ear.

tympanostomy (tim″pah-nos′tah-me) myringotomy.

tympanotomy (tim″pah-not′ah-me) 1. myringotomy. 2. surgical opening of the middle ear.

tympanous (tim′pah-nus) distended with gas.

tympanum (tim′pah-num) 1. TYMPANIC MEMBRANE. 2. tympanic cavity.

tympany (tim′pah-ne) a tympanic, or bell-like, percussion note, often elicited during percussion over a PNEUMOTHORAX or TYMPANITES (distended abdomen).

type (tīp) the general or prevailing character of any particular case, such as of a disease, person, or substance.

*t. **A*** a behavior pattern characterized by excessive competitiveness and aggressiveness. See TYPE A BEHAVIOR.

asthenic t. a constitutional type marked by a slender body, long neck, long, flat chest and abdomen, and poor muscular development.

athletic t. a constitutional type marked by broad shoulders, deep chest, flat abdomen, thick neck, and good muscular development.

blood t. 1. blood group. 2. the phenotype of an individual with respect to a blood group system.

body t., constitutional t. a constellation of traits related to body build.

phage t. a subgroup of a bacterial species susceptible to a particular bacteriophage and demonstrated by phage TYPING. Called also lysotype and phagotype.

T

pyknic t. a constitutional type marked by rounded body, large chest, thick shoulders, broad head, and short neck.

type A behavior a behavior pattern associated with the development of coronary heart disease, characterized by excessive competitiveness and aggression and a fast-paced life style. Persons exhibiting type A behavior are constantly struggling to accomplish ill-defined goals in the shortest possible time. In several studies this type of behavior has been shown to be as significant as other risk factors, such as smoking and hypertension, in the development of coronary artery disease and myocardial infarction. The opposite type of behavior exhibited by individuals who are relaxed, unhurried, and less aggressive is called type B.

typhl(o)- word element [Gr.], *cecum; blindness.*

typhlectasis (tif-lek'tah-sis) distention of the cecum.

typhlodicliditis (tif''lo-dik''li-di'tis) inflammation of the ileocecal valve.

typhlotomy (tif-lot'ah-me) cecotomy.

typhoid (ti'foid) 1. resembling typhus. 2. typhoid fever.

t. fever a bacterial infection transmitted by contaminated water, milk or other foods, especially shellfish. The causative organism is *Salmonella typhi*, which is harbored in human feces. Entering the body through the intestinal tract, the bacillus starts multiplying in the bloodstream, causing fever and diarrhea. The usual incubation period is 7 to 14 days. Later the bacilli localize in the intestinal tract or the gallbladder.

Symptoms. The first symptoms are headache, perhaps sore throat and a fever that may reach 40.5°C (105°F). The temperature rises daily, reaching a peak in 7 to 10 days, maintaining this level for about another week, and then subsiding by the end of the fourth week. Periods of chills and sweating may occur, with loss of appetite. A watery, grayish or greenish diarrhea is common, but constipation sometimes occurs instead. After 2 weeks, red spots begin to appear on the chest and abdomen. If the case is severe, the patient may lapse into states of delirious muttering and staring into space. About the third to fourth week an improvement is noticeable, and steady recovery follows. The disease is serious and sometimes fatal.

Transmission. Those who have had typhoid fever gain immunity from it but may become carriers. Although perfectly well, they harbor the bacteria and pass them out in their feces and urine. The typhoid bacillus often lodges in the gallbladder of carriers, and when the gallbladder is removed the person may cease to be a carrier. In cities, food handled by carriers is the principal source of infection. In rural areas carriers may infect food that they raise, such as fruit and fresh vegetables. When sewage and sanitation systems are poor, the organisms may enter the water supply. They can also be spread to food and water by flies that have been in contact with body waste. Contamination is more likely in regions where human feces are used to fertilize the crops.

Prevention and Treatment. Once a widespread disease, typhoid fever has now been virtually eliminated in countries with advanced sanitation. Proper sanitation involves (1) good sewage systems to dispose of human wastes and (2) proper measures for keeping foods uncontaminated. Food should be carefully protected from flies. One should wash the hands carefully before eating and after going to the toilet. Effective medicines, such as the antibiotic CHLORAMPHENICOL, are available for treatment of the disease. A less serious disease whose symptoms resemble those of typhoid fever is PARATYPHOID FEVER, which is also transmitted by contaminated food or liquids.

Patient Care. Patients with typhoid and paratyphoid fever are placed under enteric precautions until the urine and feces are free of bacilli. If sewage treatment for the community is adequate, feces and urine need not be disinfected, but if there is danger of incomplete destruction of the bacilli by sewage treatment methods, such waste should be disinfected by chlorinated lime or a 4 per cent Lysol solution before disposal. Other precautionary measures to prevent spread of the disease include adequate screening of windows and doors so that flies may not come in contact with waste products.

Most patients with typhoid fever require measures to lower the body temperature when fever is extreme. These include cool sponge baths, application of ice bags, and administration of antipyretic drugs as ordered. Fluids should be forced, to prevent dehydration. The diet should consist of soft, bland, easily digested, and nourishing foods. Observations of the patient include watching for sudden temperature changes, signs of intestinal bleeding, and symptoms of intestinal perforation.

KAOLIN or a similar medication may be needed to help control diarrhea. If constipation becomes a problem, a low saline enema should be given in preference to a cathartic because of the danger of intestinal perforation. Good oral hygiene and care of the lips and mouth are essential, as for any patient with a prolonged febrile condition. In addition, the patient must be kept clean and dry and turned frequently to avoid the development of PRESSURE ULCERS. During the convalescent period the patient will need adequate rest and a well-rounded diet to facilitate recovery from this debilitating illness.

typhoidal (ti-foi′dal) resembling typhoid fever.

typhus (ti′fus) an acute infectious disease caused by species of the parasitic microorganism *Rickettsia*, usually transmitted from the feces of infected rats and other rodents to humans by lice, fleas, ticks and mites. Rickettsiae enter the human body through cuts or breaks in the skin made by the bites of the lice or other pests.

Types and Treatment. The principal types of the diseases are louse-borne typhus and flying squirrel typhus, caused by *Rickettsia prowazekii;* murine typhus, caused by *R. typhi;* scrub typhus, caused by *R. tsutsugamushi;* and recrudescent typhus.

Louse-borne typhus (also known as epidemic or classic typhus) occurs after feces of an infected louse are rubbed into a break in the skin. After an incubation period of 6 to 15 days, the symptoms begin to appear: headache, running of the nose, cough, nausea, and chest pain. These are followed in a few days by high fever and chills, vomiting, constipation or diarrhea, muscular aching, and perhaps delirium or stupor. A red rash, which may bleed, appears on the trunk and spreads to the arms and legs. After about 2 weeks the symptoms usually subside. Ordinarily louse-borne typhus is not fatal, but it can be, particularly if pneumonia develops or if the afflicted person has heart disease. Its alternative name *epidemic typhus* comes from the devastation it has caused throughout history. It tends to appear where people are crowded together and are weakened by cold, disease, or starvation. It has many colloquial names, such as war fever, camp fever, and jail fever.

Flying squirrel typhus is a type resembling louse-borne typhus but not as often fatal. It occurs in the southeastern United States, almost always in the winter months, and is transmitted to humans by the fleas and lice of the flying squirrel. Treatment is the same as for louse-borne typhus.

Murine typhus is a less common variety, also known as *tabardillo* and *endemic, rat,* or *flea typhus*. As indicated by the term *murine,* it is transmitted by rat or mouse fleas. The symptoms are like those of louse-borne typhus but are less severe, and recovery occurs sooner. Antibiotics are used in treatment.

Scrub typhus (called also Japanese river fever and tsutsugamushi fever) is prevalent in eastern Asia and has been carried to other areas by infected persons. It is transmitted by mites and hence is often called mite fever. The rodent responsible for this illness is the field mouse. The rickettsiae are transferred to humans by the bite of the larval form of the mite, usually in the groin or neck. The fever of scrub typhus and its other symptoms are very similar to those of other forms of typhus. It is treated with chloramphenicol and the tetracyclines.

Recrudescent typhus (called also Brill-Zinsser disease) is caused by *Rickettsia prowazekii,* the etiologic agent of louse-borne typhus. The rickettsiae, however, remain in the body after a first attack of typhus and can cause a recurrence (a recrudescence) as long as years after the first attack. The recrudescence is milder than the initial infection, however. Treatment is similar to that for epidemic typhus.

Closely related to these forms of typhus are tick-borne rickettsial diseases such as ROCKY MOUNTAIN SPOTTED FEVER.

Prevention. Immunizing vaccines are available if an outbreak of typhus occurs or threatens. They greatly reduce the chance of infection, or modify the effects of the disease. Travelers should be vaccinated before visiting countries where the disease is prevalent. Some countries require proof of such protection before admitting a visitor. Insect and rodent control are of great importance in the prevention and control of typhus. Adult lice can be destroyed by spraying garments with DDT. Frequent bathing and changes of underclothes are vital. Outer garments should be sterilized by steam to kill the louse eggs. Fleas and mites are more difficult to control than lice. The best method is to destroy the rodents on which they live.

Patient Care. Patients with typhus are initially isolated until they are free of body lice or mites. They are not capable of transmitting the disease without the aid of these vectors. No special precautions are recommended by the Centers for Disease Control and Prevention to limit transmission of the disease. To accomplish removal of lice or mites the patient should be washed with a 1 per cent solution of Lysol upon admission and the clothing must be disinfected or destroyed. Several shampoos may be necessary to eliminate parasites from the hair. Gentle, thorough cleaning is necessary and every effort must be made to

T

avoid damage to the skin in one's enthusiasm for removing lice or mites. The patient is given a soft diet and ample fluids, to prevent dehydration. Efforts are made to conserve the patient's strength and to protect him or her during periods of delirium, which are common. Typhus is a very debilitating disease and requires a long period of convalescence in which the patient's general health must be improved. Nervous and mental symptoms may persist long after the acute phase of the disease subsides.

typing (tīp'ing) in transplantation IMMU-NOLOGY, a method of measuring the degree of organ, solid tissue, or blood compatibility between two individuals, in which specific histocompatibility ANTIGENS (such as those on leukocytes or erythrocytes) are detected by means of suitable isoimmune antisera.

blood t., t. of blood determining the character of the blood on the basis of agglutinogens in the erythrocytes; see also BLOOD GROUP.

phage t. characterization of bacteria, extending to strain differences, by demonstration of susceptibility to one or more races (a spectrum) of bacteriophage; widely applied to staphylococci, typhoid bacilli, and other organisms for epidemiological purposes.

tissue t. identification of the human leukocyte antigens of the donor and recipient of a transplant or transfusion; see also TISSUE TYPING.

typology (ti-pol'ah-je) the study of types; the science of classifying, as bacteria, according to type.

tyramine (ti'rah-mēn) a decarboxylation product of tyrosine, which may be converted to cresol and phenol, found in decayed animal tissue, ripe cheese, and ergot. Closely related structurally to epinephrine and norepinephrine, it has a similar but weaker action.

tyrocidine (ti'ro-si'din) a cyclic polypeptide ANTIBIOTIC, containing one or more D-amino acids and produced by *Bacillus brevis*. It is effective against gram-positive organisms and acts by disrupting the bacterial cell membrane. It is one of two major components of tyrothricin, the other being GRAMICIDIN.

tyrogenous (ti-roj'ĕ-nus) originating in cheese.

tyroid (ti'roid) caseous, resembling cheese.

tyromatosis (ti″ro-mah-to'sis) caseous degeneration.

tyropanoate (ti″ro-pah-no'āt) a radiopaque contrast medium for use in oral cholecystography.

tyrosine (ti'ro-sēn) a naturally occurring nonessential AMINO ACID present in most proteins and synthesized metabolically from phenylalanine. It is a precursor of melanin, catecholamines, and thyroid hormones.

tyrosinemia (ti″ro-sī-ne'me-ah) an aminoacidopathy consisting of defective metabolism of tyrosine and its buildup in the body, as well as urinary excretion of tyrosine metabolites. Several forms exist: *Type I* is an autosomal recessive trait with an acute form that is usually fatal in infancy and a chronic form characterized by chronic liver and kidney disease, rickets, and death in childhood. *Type II* is an oculocutaneous syndrome with crystallization of accumulated tyrosine in the epidermis as palmoplantar hyperkeratoses and in the cornea as herpetiform ulcers, often accompanied by mental retardation.

tyrosinuria (ti″ro-sī-nu're-ah) an AMINOACIDURIA consisting of excessive TYROSINE in the urine, such as that accompanying TYROSINEMIA.

tyrosis (ti-ro'sis) caseation (def. 2).

tyrosyluria (ti″ro-sil-u're-ah) increased urinary secretion of compounds derived from tyrosine.

tyrothricin (ti″ro-thri'sin) an ANTIBIOTIC isolated from the soil bacillus *Bacillus brevis*, consisting principally of two polypeptides, of which the major one is TYROCIDINE and the other is GRAMICIDIN. It is effective against many gram-positive bacteria, and is applied topically in pyodermic, ocular, and other localized infections.

tysonitis (ti″son-i'tis) inflammation of Tyson's glands (preputial glands).

tyvelose (ti″vel-ōs) an unusual sugar that is a polysaccharide somatic antigen of *Salmonella* species.

Tzanck's test (tsankz) cytologic examination of scrapings from the base of herpetic lesions for diagnosis of HERPES SIMPLEX and genital HERPES. The scrapings are fixed on a slide with absolute or methyl alcohol and stained with Giemsa stain; presence of multinucleated giant cells or typical eosinophilic intranuclear inclusions is diagnostic of HERPESVIRUS infection.

tzetze (set'se) tsetse.

U

U uranium; unit.
UA urinalysis.
ubiquinol (u″bǐ-kwǐ-nol′) the reduced form of ubiquinone.
ubiquinone (u″bǐ-kwǐ-nōn′) coenzyme Q.
UDP uridine diphosphate.
UICC [Fr. *Union Internationale Contre le Cancer*] International Union Against Cancer.

ulcer (ul′ser) a local defect, or excavation of the surface of an organ or tissue, produced by sloughing of necrotic inflammatory tissue.

   aphthous u. a small painful ulcer in the mouth, approximately 2 to 5 mm in diameter. It usually remains for five to seven days and heals within two weeks with no scarring.

   chronic leg u. ulceration of the lower leg caused by PERIPHERAL VASCULAR DISEASE involving either arteries and arterioles or veins and venules of the affected limb. Arterial and venous ulcers are quite different and require different modes of treatment. Venous stasis ULCERS occur as a result of venous INSUFFICIENCY in the lower limb. The insufficiency is due to deep vein thrombosis and failure of the one-way valves that act during muscle contraction to prevent the backflow of blood. Chronic VARICOSITIES of the veins can also cause venous STASIS.
Patient Care. Stasis ulcers are difficult to treat because impaired blood flow interferes with the normal healing process and prolongs repair. Patient care is concerned with preventing a superimposed infection in the ulcer, increasing blood flow in the deeper veins, and decreasing pressure within the superficial veins.

   decubitus u. PRESSURE ULCER.

   duodenal u. an ulcer of the duodenum, one of the two most common types of PEPTIC ULCER.

   gastric u. an ulcer of the inner wall of the stomach, one of the two most common kinds of PEPTIC ULCER.

   Hunner's u. one involving all layers of the bladder wall, seen in interstitial CYSTITIS.

   hypertensive ischemic u. a manifestation of infarction of the skin due to arteriolar occlusion as part of a longstanding vascular disease, seen especially in women in late middle age, and presenting as a red painful plaque on the lower limb or ankle that later breaks down into a superficial ulcer surrounded by a zone of purpuric erythema.

   marginal u. a peptic ulcer occurring at the margin of a surgical anastomosis of the stomach and small intestine or duodenum. Marginal ulcers are a frequent complication of surgical treatment for peptic ulcer; they are difficult to control medically and often require further surgery.

   peptic u. see PEPTIC ULCER.

   perforating u. one that involves the entire thickness of an organ, creating an opening on both surfaces.

   phagedenic u. 1. any of a group of conditions due to secondary bacterial invasion of a preexisting cutaneous lesion or the intact skin of an individual with impaired resistance as a result of a systemic disease, which is characterized by necrotic ulceration associated with prominent tissue destruction. 2. tropical phagedenic ulcer.

   pressure u. see PRESSURE ULCER.

   rodent u. ulcerating basal cell carcinoma of the skin.

   stasis u. ulceration on the ankle due to venous INSUFFICIENCY and venous STASIS.

   stress u. a type of PEPTIC ULCER, usually gastric, resulting from stress; possible predisposing factors include changes in the microcirculation of the gastric mucosa, increased permeability of the gastric mucosa barrier to H^+, and impaired cell proliferation.

   trophic u. one due to imperfect nutrition of the part.

   tropical u. 1. a lesion of cutaneous LEISHMANIASIS. 2. tropical phagedenic ulcer.

   tropical phagedenic u. a chronic, painful phagedenic ulcer usually seen on the lower limbs of malnourished children in the tropics; the etiology is unknown, but spirochetes, fusiform bacilli, and other bacteria are often present in the developing lesion, and protein and vitamin deficiency may play a role in the etiology.

   varicose u. an ulcer due to VARICOSE VEINS.

   venereal u. a nonspecific term referring to the formation of ulcers resembling chancre or chancroid about the external genitalia; there are both sexually transmitted and other types.

ulcerate (ul′sě-rāt) to undergo ulceration.
ulceration (ul″sě-ra′shun) 1. formation or development of an ulcer. 2. an ulcer.
ulcerative (ul′sě-ra″tiv, ul′ser-ah-tiv) pertaining to or characterized by ulceration.

   u. colitis a recurrent acute and chronic disorder characterized by extensive inflammatory ulceration in the colon, chiefly of the mucosa and submucosa. The etiology is unknown; hence, the term *idiopathic* is used in reference to ulcerative colitis. The disorder is not always limited to pathologic changes in the colon, but may become systemic, involving the joints and causing migratory arthritis, sacroileitis, and ankylosing spondylitis. Other organs that can become involved are the liver, skin, and eyes. Hypercoagulability may also be seen.

Ulcerative colitis shares many of the same characteristics with regional ileitis or CROHN'S DISEASE; the two are often included in the broader diagnostic entity called INFLAMMATORY BOWEL DISEASE. There are some who believe that both disorders are immunologic responses to the same as yet unknown etiologic agent.

Genetic predisposition to inflammatory bowel disease may exist; there is a higher incidence of ulcerative colitis and Crohn's disease among close relatives. Ulcerative colitis is slightly more prevalent in females than in males and most often appears between the ages of 15 and 20 years with a smaller peak at 55 to 60 years of age. Crohn's disease follows a similar pattern of incidence.

Clinical Manifestations and Complications. The patient with ulcerative colitis suffers from attacks of bloody, mucoid diarrhea that are usually precipitated by physical or emotional stress. These acute attacks can last for days, weeks, or even months and are followed by periods of remission that can extend from a few weeks to several decades. Some patients experience relatively few attacks throughout their lifetime, while others have frequent, prolonged, and potentially serious attacks that predispose the colon to malignant changes. Both acute and chronic diarrhea can upset the fluid and electrolyte balance, interfere with normal nutrition, and produce fever, abdominal cramps, and weight loss.

A sudden and severe attack of the disease can lead to cessation of bowel function and toxic MEGACOLON or dilatation of the colon. This can occur spontaneously, or it may be preceded by barium enema, hyperkalemia, or anticholinergic narcotics, or there may be bacterial overgrowth with production of exotoxin. Other complications include severe blood loss and anemia, systemic toxicity, and metabolic disturbances. A serious sequela of long-term chronic and continuous ulcerative colitis is carcinoma of the colon, which occurs in approximately 5% of people with ulcerative colitis. The risk of it is lower for persons who have infrequent relapses than for those who are symptomatic for years. Guidelines on screening for colon cancer have been developed by an expert panel and endorsed by numerous organizations concerned with the care of patients with GI diseases. They advise COLONOSCOPY every one to two years for people who have had inflammatory bowel disease throughout the colon for at least 8 years or who have had it in the left colon for at least 15 years.

Patient Care. During acute attacks, the patient will most likely present problems related to fluid volume deficit, alteration in nutrition, loss of electrolytes, potential for skin breakdown in the anal region, disturbance of sleep and rest, and discomfort from abdominal cramps. Long-term problems are likely to be related to anxiety, alterations in self-concept, social isolation, and fear of malignancy.

The plan of care should include observation of the number and character of stools, periodic auscultation of bowel sounds, measurement of intake and output, daily weight, checking for signs of bleeding and anemia, and monitoring of blood gases, electrolytes, and pH for evidence of acid-base imbalance or abnormal electrolyte values. It also is important to be alert for signs of inflammatory changes in the joints or lesions on the skin.

When diagnostic procedures such as sigmoidoscopy, barium enema, and stool analyses are necessary, patients should have a satisfactory explanation of the purpose of these tests and what is expected of them before, during, and after each procedure.

Long-term goals of care should help the patient comply with the prescribed medical regimen, which usually consists of antidiarrheic agents, anticholinergic drugs to relieve abdominal cramps, mild sedatives, and a diet of low-residue, bland foods that have high caloric and protein content. Antibiotics are sometimes needed to control infection of the bowel.

Surgical intervention may be the only alternative when more conservative treatments fail. The surgery usually involves creation of a permanent ILEOSTOMY, which brings on a new set of problems.

There is no cure for ulcerative colitis and it is a debilitating disorder that can create many physiologic, psychological, and social problems for the patient. The frequent bouts of severe diarrhea and discomfort can be embarrassing and depressing. Emotional support, empathetic listening, and cooperative problem solving are essential components of patient care. Further information may be obtained by writing The Crohn's and Colitis Foundation of America Inc., 386 Park Avenue South, 17th floor, New York, NY 10016-8804, calling them at 1-800-932-2423 or 1-212-685-3440, or consulting their web site at http://www.ccfa.org.

ulcerogangrenous (ul″ser-o-gang′grĕ-nus) characterized by both ulceration and gangrene.

ulcerogenic (ul″ser-o-jen′ik) causing ulceration; leading to the production of ulcers.

ulceromembranous (ul″ser-o-mem′brah-nus) characterized by ulceration and a membranous exudation.

ulcerous (ul′ser-us) 1. of the nature of an ulcer. 2. affected with ulceration.

ulcus (ul′kus) [L.] ulcer.

ulerythema (u″ler-ĭ-the′mah) an erythematous disease of the skin with formation of scars and atrophy.

u. ophryo′genes a hereditary form in which keratosis pilaris involves the follicles of the eyebrow hairs.

ulitis (u-li′tis) gingivitis.

ulna (ul′nah) [L.] the inner and larger bone of the forearm, on the side opposite the thumb. It articulates with the humerus and with the head of the radius at its proximal end; with the radius and bones of the carpus at the distal end.

ulnad (ul′nad) toward the ulna.

ulnar (ul′nar) pertaining to the ulna or to the ulnar (medial) aspect of the upper limb as compared to the radial (lateral) aspect.

ulnaris (ul-na′ris) [L.] ulnar.

ulnocarpal (ul″no-kahr′pal) pertaining to the ulna and carpus.

ulnoradial (ul″no-ra′de-al) pertaining to the ulna and radius.

ulocarcinoma (u″lo-kahr″sĭ-no′mah) carcinoma of the gums.

uloglossitis (u″lo-glŏ-si′tis) gingivoglossitis.

ulorrhagia (u″lo-ra′jah) a sudden discharge of blood from the gums.

ultra- word element [L.], *beyond; excess.*

ultrabrachycephalic (ul″trah-brak″e-sĕ-fal′ik) having a cephalic index of more than 90.

ultracentrifugation (ul″trah-sen-trif′u-ga′-shun) subjection of material to an exceedingly high centrifugal force, which will separate and sediment the molecules of a substance.

ultracentrifuge (ul″trah-sen′trĭ-fūj) the centrifuge used in ultracentrifugation.

ultradian (ul-tra′de-an) pertaining to a period of less than 24 hours; applied to the rhythmic repetition of certain phenomena in living organisms occurring in cycles of less than a day. See also ultradian RHYTHM.

ultrafilter (ul″trah-fil′ter) the filter used in ULTRAFILTRATION.

ultrafiltration (ul″trah-fil-tra′shun) filtration through filters with minute pores, thus allowing the separation of extremely minute particles. It occurs naturally, as in the filtration of plasma at the capillary membrane, and is also performed clinically and in the laboratory, such as in HEMODIALYSIS, where it involves the bulk movement of solute and solvent across the membrane down pressure gradients and is usually performed under pressure to accelerate the process.

ultramicroscopic (ul″trah-mi″kro-skop′ik) too small to be seen with the ordinary light microscope.

ultrasonic (ul″trah-son′ik) beyond the audible range; relating to sound waves having a frequency of more than 20,000 Hz.

ultrasonics (ul″trah-son′iks) that part of the science of acoustics dealing with the frequency range beyond the upper limit of perception by the human ear, i.e. above 20,000 hertz (cycles per second), but usually restricted to frequencies above 50,000 hertz. Ultrasonic radiation is injurious to tissues because of its thermal effects when absorbed by living matter, but in controlled doses it can be used therapeutically to selectively break down pathologic tissues, as in treatment of arthritis and lesions of the nervous system, and also as a diagnostic aid by visually displaying echoes received from irradiated tissues, as in ECHOCARDIOGRAPHY. See also ULTRASONOGRAPHY.

ultrasonogram (ul″trah-son′o-gram) the record obtained by ultrasonography.

ultrasonography (ul″trah-sŏ-nog′rah-fe) 1. a radiologic technique in which deep structures of the body are visualized by recording the reflections (echoes) of ultrasonic waves directed into the tissues. adj., **ultrasonograph′ic.** 2. in the NURSING INTERVENTIONS CLASSIFICATION, a nursing INTERVENTION defined as performance of ULTRASOUND exams to determine ovarian, uterine, or fetal status.

Frequencies in the range of 1 million to 10 million hertz are used in diagnostic ultrasonography. The lower frequencies provide a greater depth of penetration and are used to examine abdominal organs; those in the upper range provide less penetration and are used predominantly to examine more superficial structures such as the eye.

The basic principle of ultrasonography is the same as that of depth-sounding in oceanographic studies of the ocean floor. The ultrasonic waves are confined to a narrow beam that may be transmitted through or refracted, absorbed, or reflected by the medium toward which they are

U

directed, depending on the nature of the surface they strike.

In diagnostic ultrasonography the ultrasonic waves are produced by electrically stimulating a crystal called a *transducer*. As the beam strikes an interface or boundary between tissues of varying density (e.g., muscle and blood) some of the sound waves are reflected back to the transducer as echoes. The echoes are then converted into electrical impulses that are displayed on an oscilloscope, presenting a "picture" of the tissues under examination.

Ultrasonography can be utilized in examination of the heart (echocardiography), in location of aneurysms of the aorta and other abnormalities of the major blood vessels, and in identifying size and structural changes in organs in the abdominopelvic cavity. It is, therefore, of value in identifying and distinguishing cancers and benign cysts. The technique also may be used to evaluate tumors and foreign bodies of the eye, and to demonstrate retinal detachment. Ultrasonography is not, however, of much value in examination of the lungs because ultrasound waves do not pass through structures that contain air.

A particularly important use of ultrasonography is in the field of obstetrics and gynecology, where ionizing radiation is to be avoided whenever possible. The technique can evaluate fetal size and maturity and fetal and placental position. It is a fast, relatively safe, and reliable technique for diagnosing multiple pregnancies. Uterine tumors and other pelvic masses, including abscesses, can be identified by ultrasonography.

A-mode u. that in which on the cathode-ray tube display one axis represents the time required for the return of the echo and the other corresponds to the strength of the echo.

B-mode u. that in which the position of a spot on the CRT display corresponds to the time elapsed (and thus to the position of the echogenic surface) and the brightness of the spot to the strength of the echo; movement of the transducer produces a sweep of the ultrasound beam and a tomographic scan of a cross section of the body.

Doppler u. that in which measurement and a visual record are made of the shift in frequency of a continuous ultrasonic wave proportional to the blood-flow velocity in underlying vessels; used in diagnosis of extracranial occlusive vascular disease. It is also used in detection of the fetal heart beat or of the velocity of movement of a structure, such as the beating heart.

gray-scale u. B-mode ultrasonography in which the strength of echoes is indicated by a proportional brightness of the displayed dots.

real-time u. B-mode ultrasonography using an array of detectors so that scans can be made electronically at a rate of 30 frames a second.

ultrasound (ul′trah-sownd)   1.   sound waves with a frequency greater than 20,000 Hz; used in medicine in the technique of ULTRASONOGRAPHY.   2. a mechanical and thermal physical modality that uses sound waves of a frequency of approximately 1 million Hz for the treatment of soft tissue injury. It may be used to introduce a topical agent into the body transdermally (see PHONOPHORESIS).

ultrastructure (ul′trah-struk″chur)   the structure visible only under the ultramicroscope and electron microscope.

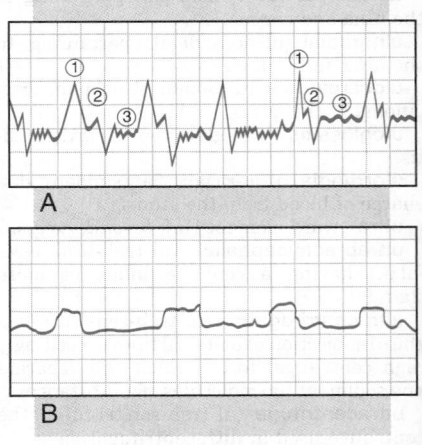

Normal versus abnormal Doppler arterial waveform patterns. *A,* Normal waveform with triphasic pattern of sharp upstroke and downstroke and good amplitude: (1) systolic component, (2) diastolic component, and (3) elastic wall rebound. *B,* Abnormal waveform with monophasic pattern of low amplitude and flat waves. This pattern indicates severe arterial obstruction. From Malarkey and McMorrow, 2000.

COMMON ULTRASONOGRAPHIC STUDIES	
Abdominal Scan	Pancreas Scan
Abdominal Aorta Scan	Popliteal Artery Scan
Breast Scan	Pelvic Scans
Carotid Artery Scan	Female Pelvic Scan
Gallbladder-Biliary Scan	Male Pelvic Scan
Inferior Vena Cava Scan	Endovaginal Scan
Liver Scan	Obstetric Scan
Neonatal Brain Scan	Renal Scan

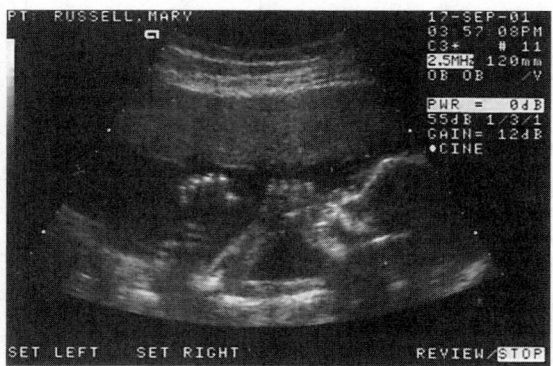

Ultrasound.

ultraviolet (ul″trah-vi′o-let) denoting electromagnetic radiation of wavelength shorter than that of the violet end of the spectrum, having wavelengths of 4–400 nanometers.

u. A (UVA) ultraviolet RADIATION with wavelengths between 320 and 400 nm, comprising over 99 per cent of such radiation that reaches the surface of the earth. Ultraviolet A enhances the harmful effects of ultraviolet B radiation and is also responsible for some PHOTOSENSITIVITY reactions; it is used therapeutically in the treatment of a variety of skin disorders.

u. B (UVB) ultraviolet RADIATION with wavelengths between 290 and 320 nm, comprising less than 1 per cent of the ultraviolet radiation that reaches the earth's surface. Ultraviolet B causes sunburn and a number of damaging PHOTOCHEMICAL changes within cells, including damage to DNA, leading to premature aging of the skin, premalignant and malignant changes, and a variety of PHOTOSENSITIVITY reactions; it is also used therapeutically for treatment of skin disorders.

u. C (UVC) ultraviolet RADIATION with wavelengths between 200 and 290 nm; all of this type of radiation is filtered out by the ozone layer so that none reaches the earth's surface. Ultraviolet C is germicidal and is also used in ultraviolet PHOTOTHERAPY.

u. rays electromagnetic radiation beyond the violet end of the visible spectrum; they are not visible to humans. They are produced by the sun but are absorbed to a large extent by particles of dust and smoke in the earth's atmosphere. They are also produced by the so-called sun lamps. They can produce sunburn and affect skin pigmentation, causing tanning. When they strike the skin surface they transform provitamin D, secreted by the glands of the skin, into vitamin D, which is then absorbed into the body. Because ultraviolet rays are capable of killing bacteria and other microorganisms, they are sometimes used to sterilize objects in specially designed cabinets, or to sterilize the air in operating rooms and other areas where destruction of bacteria is necessary.

u. therapy the employment of ultraviolet RADIATION in the treatment of diseases, particularly those affecting the skin. See also PUVA THERAPY and PHOTOCHEMOTHERAPY. Among the diseases that respond to this form of therapy are ACNE VULGARIS, PSORIASIS, and external ULCERS.

Dosage. The dosage unit of ultraviolet radiation is expressed as minimal erythema DOSE (MED). Because of varying degrees of skin thickness and pigmentation, human skin varies widely in its sensitivity to ultraviolet radiation. The MED refers to the amount of radiation that will produce, within a few hours, minimal ERYTHEMA (redness caused by engorgement of capillaries) in the average Caucasian skin. Dosage for individual patients is prescribed according to probable sensitivity as determined by that individual's skin type as compared to average sensitivity.

Degrees of Erythema. Minimal erythema is a *first degree erythema* and usually is produced after about 15 seconds of exposure to a high-pressure mercury arc in a quartz burner placed at a distance of 75 cm (30 in) from the skin. A *second degree erythema* results from a dose of about 2.5 MED; its effects become apparent about 4 to 6 hours after application and are followed by slight peeling of the skin. A *third degree erythema* is produced by about 5 MED; it may become apparent within 2 hours after application and is accompanied by edema followed by

U

marked desquamation. A *fourth degree erythema* is produced by about 10 MED and is characterized by blistering.

Precautions. Ultraviolet therapy is safe only in the hands of a skilled and knowledgeable therapist. Areas of "thin skin" that may be burned more readily than that receiving treatment must be protected by wet towels or dressings. The eye is highly sensitive to ultraviolet radiation; therefore some form of protection, such as goggles, compresses, or cotton balls, should be provided for both the patient and the therapist to avoid damage to the conjunctiva and cornea.

Certain drugs, such as the sulfonamides, greatly increase sensitivity to ultraviolet radiation. All patients scheduled for this form of therapy should be questioned in regard to the medication they are taking so the dosage can be adjusted accordingly or the treatment deferred.

umbilical (um-bil'ĭ-kal) pertaining to the umbilicus.

u. cord the structure that connects the fetus and placenta; it is the lifeline of the fetus in the uterus throughout pregnancy. About 2 weeks after conception, the umbilical cord and the PLACENTA are sufficiently developed to begin their functions. Through two arteries and a vein in the cord, nourishment and oxygen pass from the blood vessels in the placenta to the fetus, and waste products pass from the fetus to the placenta. Soon after birth, the umbilical cord is clamped or tied and then cut. The part that is attached to the placenta, still in the uterus, is expelled with the placenta. The stump that remains attached to the baby's abdomen is about 2 inches (5 cm) long. After a few days it falls off naturally.

u. hernia protrusion of abdominal contents through the abdominal wall at the umbilicus, the defect in the abdominal wall and protruding intestine being covered with skin and subcutaneous tissue. Called also exomphalos and exumbilication.

During the growth of the fetus, the intestines grow more rapidly than the abdominal cavity. For a period, a portion of the intestines of the unborn child usually lies outside the abdomen in a sac within the umbilical cord. Normally, the intestines return to the abdomen, and the defect is closed by the time of birth. Occasionally the abdominal wall does not close solidly, and umbilical hernia results. This defect is more likely to be seen in premature infants and in girls rather than boys. It usually closes by

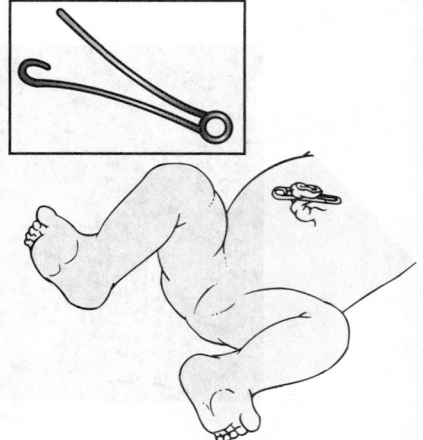

Clamping the umbilical cord.

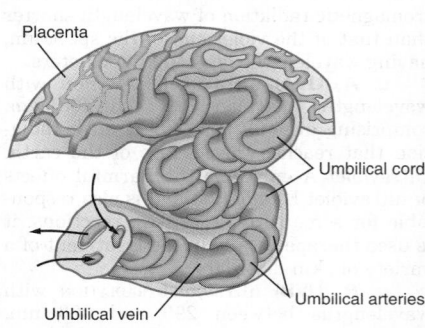

Placenta

Umbilical cord

Umbilical arteries

Umbilical vein

Umbilical cord with umbilical vein and umbilical arteries. From McKinney, 2000.

itself. Coughing, crying, and straining temporarily cause the sac to enlarge, but the hernia never bursts and digestion is not affected. If the defect in the abdominal wall has not repaired itself by the time the child is 2 years old, surgery to correct the condition (HERNIORRHAPHY) can then be performed.

Umbilical hernia should be distinguished from OMPHALOCELE, in which the intestines protrude directly into the umbilical cord and are covered only by a thin membrane. Omphalocele is a surgical emergency that must be treated immediately after birth.

umbilicated (um-bil'ĭ-kāt"ed) marked by depressed spots resembling the umbilicus.

umbilication (um-bil"ĭ-ka'shun) a depression resembling the umbilicus.

umbilicus (um-bil'ĭ-kus, um"bĭ-li'kus) the (usually) depressed scar marking the site where the UMBILICAL CORD entered the fetus; called also navel.

umbo (um′bo) [L.] 1. a rounded elevation. 2. the slight projection at the center of the outer surface of the tympanic membrane.

umbra (um′brah) the part of a shadow in which there is no light from any light source. 1. a sharp appearance to the edges of a structure on a radiograph.

UMLS Unified Medical Language System.

unciform (un′sĭ-form) uncinate (def. 1).

uncinate (un′sĭ-nāt) 1. shaped like a hook; see also HAMATE. Called also unciform. 2. relating to or affecting the uncinate GYRUS.

unconscious (un-kon′shus) 1. insensible; incapable of responding to sensory stimuli and of having subjective experiences. 2. the part of the mind that is not readily accessible to conscious awareness by ordinary means but whose existence may be manifested in symptom formation, in dreams, or under the influence of drugs; it is one of the systems of Freud's topographic model of the mind.

   collective u. in jungian psychology, the portion of the unconscious that is theoretically common to mankind.

   unconsciousness (un-kon′shus-nes) an abnormal state of lack of response to sensory stimuli, resulting from injury, illness, shock, or some other bodily disorder. A brief loss of CONSCIOUSNESS from which the person recovers spontaneously or with slight help is called SYNCOPE or FAINT. Deep, prolonged unconsciousness is known as COMA. See also levels of CONSCIOUSNESS.

   uncovertebral (un″ko-ver′tĕ-bral) pertaining to the uncinate processes of a vertebra.

   unction (ungk′shun) 1. ointment. 2. inunction.

   unctuous (ungk′choo-us) greasy or oily.

   uncus (ung′kus) the medially curved anterior part of the hippocampal gyrus. adj., **un′cal.**

   undecylenic acid (un″des-ĭ-len′ik) an unsaturated fatty acid, used topically, in ointment or powder form, as an antifungal AGENT.

   undercutting (un′der-kut″ing) the effect of scatter on a radiographic image, caused when an unattenuated x-ray beam strikes the film screen detector.

   undifferentiated (un″dif-er-en′she-āt″ed) anaplastic.

   undifferentiation (un″dif-er-en′she-a′shun) anaplasia.

   undine (un′dēn) a small glass flask for irrigating the eye.

   undoing (un-doo′ing) a DEFENSE MECHANISM aimed at negating or atoning for some disapproved act or impulse by performing an action that is somehow opposite to that

feared; most commonly seen in the rituals accompanying OBSESSIVE-COMPULSIVE DISORDER.

undulant fever (un′du-lant) brucellosis.

undulation (un″du-la′shun) a wavelike motion in any medium; a vibration.

ung. [L.] *unguen′tum* (OINTMENT).

ungual (ung′gwal) pertaining to the nails.

unguent (ung′gwent) ointment.

unguiculate (ung-gwik′u-lāt) 1. having claws. 2. clawlike.

unguis (ung′gwis), pl. *un′gues* [L.] nail (def. 2).

unheated serum reagin test a modification of the VDRL test using unheated serum, used primarily for screening. Called also USR test.

uni- word element [L.[, *one.* See also words beginning MON(O)-.

uniaxial (u″ne-ak′se-al) 1. having only one axis. 2. developed in an axial direction only.

unicameral (u″nĭ-kam′er-al) having only one cavity or compartment.

unicellular (u″nĭ-sel′u-lar) made up of a single cell, as the bacteria.

Unified Medical Language System (UMLS) trademark name for a project of the NATIONAL LIBRARY OF MEDICINE aimed at building an intelligent automated system that understands biomedical terms and their interrelationships and uses this understanding to help users retrieve and organize information from machine readable sources. Its goal is to facilitate retrieval and integration from a variety of machine readable information sources, including descriptions of the biomedical literature, clinical records, factual databanks, and medical knowledge bases. The UMLS will compensate for the differences in the terminologies used in these disparate systems and for variations in the language employed by users themselves. The UMLS is neither an attempt to impose a single standard vocabulary for use in the creation, storage, and retrieval of all biomedical information nor a plan for developing either a standard patient record format or a single unified medical knowledge base to assist with diagnosis and treatment.

Unified Nursing Language System (UNLS) a computerized system that links similar terms in nursing vocabularies recognized by the American Nurses' Association Steering Committee on Data Bases to Support Clinical Nursing Practice.

Uniform Anatomical Gift Act an act established in 1968 to standardize state laws on the donation of organs and tissues from cadavers; it is based on the premise that an individual should be able to control the

U

disposition of his or her own body after death.

uniform donor card a document carried by an individual giving permission for the donation of organs in case of death.

uniglandular (u″nĭ-glan′du-lar) affecting only one gland.

unigravida (u″nĭ-grav′ĭ-dah) primigravida.

unilateral (u″nĭ-lat′er-al) affecting only one side.

unilocular (u″nĭ-lok′u-lar) having only one loculus or compartment; monolocular.

uninephrectomy (u″nĭ-nef-rek′tah-me) surgical removal of a single kidney.

uninucleated (u″nĭ-noo′kle-āt″ed) mononuclear.

uniocular (u″ne-ok′u-lar) monocular.

union (ūn′yun) the growing together of tissues separated by injury, as of the ends of a fractured bone, or of the edges of a wound; see also HEALING.

uniovular (u″ne-ov′u-lar) monovular, monozygotic.

unipara (u-nip′ah-rah) primipara.

uniparous (u-nip′ah-rus) 1. producing only one ovum or offspring at a time. 2. primiparous.

unipolar (u″nĭ-po′lar) having but a single pole or process, as a nerve cell. 1. pertaining to MOOD DISORDERS in which only depressive episodes occur.

u. disorders depressive disorders.

unipotent (u-nip′o-tent), **unipotential** (u″nĭ-po-ten′shal) having only one power, as giving rise to cells of one order only.

unisexual (u″ne-sek′shoo-al) of only one sex; having the sexual organs of one sex only.

unit (u′nit) 1. a single thing; one segment of a whole that is made up of identical or similar segments. 2. a specifically defined amount of anything subject to measurement, as of activity, dimension, velocity, volume, or the like. 3. a distinct part of a hospital, usually having a specific physical location and serving a defined function; see under names of specific units.

Ångström u. angstrom.

atomic mass u. (u) (amu) the unit of mass equal to $\frac{1}{12}$ the mass of the nuclide of carbon 12. Called also dalton.

autonomous nursing u. a nursing unit under a decentralized administration system in which the staff is responsible for all aspects of unit functioning.

British thermal u. (BTU) a unit of heat formerly widely used, being the amount necessary to raise the temperature of 1 pound of water from 39° to 40°F., equal to approximately 252 CALORIES.

CH50 u. the amount of complement that will lyse 50 per cent of a standard preparation of sheep red blood cells coated with antisheep erythrocyte antibody.

continuing education u. (CEU) a unit of credit for educational offerings given to professional persons, determined by a professional organization according to a mathematical formula after a thorough review of the program of study, the qualifications of the instructors, and the program objectives.

critical care u. intensive care unit.

electrostatic u's (esu) that system of units that is based on the fundamental definition of a unit charge as one that will repel a similar charge with a force of 1 dyne when the two charges are 1 cm apart in a vacuum.

environmental control u. a computerized system that allows the handicapped individual to operate several different appliances using a keyboard or other input device.

heat u. the amount of heat energy that is produced by one kVp (kilovolt peak) and one mA (milliampere) for one second with single phase, full wave rectified radiographic equipment.

Hounsfield u. an arbitrary unit of x-ray attenuation used for CT scans. Each VOXEL is assigned a value on a scale in which air has a value of −1000; water, 0; and compact bone, +1000.

intensive care u. see INTENSIVE CARE UNIT.

International u. (IU) 1. a unit of enzyme activity equal to the amount of enzyme that catalyzes the conversion of one micromole of substrate or coenzyme per minute under specified conditions (temperature, pH, and substrate concentration) of the assay method. Abbreviated U. 2. any of several arbitrary units that have been adopted by international bodies to express the quantities of certain vitamins (A, C, D, and thiamine hydrochloride), hormones (androgen, chorionic gonadotropin, estradiol benzoate, estrone, insulin, progesterone, and prolactin) and drugs (digitalis and penicillin).

Kienböck's u. a unit of x-ray exposure equal to 0.1 erythema dose; symbol X.

motor u. the unit of motor activity formed by a motor nerve cell and its many innervated muscle fibers.

postanesthesia care u. (PACU) a specialty unit in a hospital for giving postanesthesia CARE (care of patients recovering from anesthesia and intravenous sedation) formerly called recovery room.

radiologic u's units used to measure radiation, including ROENTGENS, RADS, REMS, and CURIES.

u's of service (UOS) 1. the number of procedures done by a department. 2. individuals or groups of individuals who are the recipients of nursing care.

   short procedures u., short term care u. a nursing unit where patients are briefly cared for following a medical or surgical procedure and are then discharged without spending the night.

   SI u. any unit of the International System of units (the METRIC SYSTEM); see also SI UNITS.

   step-down u. a nursing unit designated to provide care for patients who are stable enough to be discharged from the intensive care unit but are not yet ready to be cared for on a medical-surgical unit.

   Svedberg u. (S) a unit equal to 10^{-13} second used for expressing sedimentation coefficients of macromolecules.

   Svedberg flotation u. (S$_f$) a unit equal to 10^{-13} second used for expressing negative sedimentation coefficients of macromolecules that float rather than sink in a centrifuge, e.g., lipoproteins.

   terminal respiratory u. the functional unit of the LUNG, including a respiratory bronchiole, alveolar ducts and sacs, and alveoli; called also primary lobule of lung and primary respiratory lobule.

   USP u. one used in the United States Pharmacopeia for expressing potency of drugs and other preparations.

unitary (u′nĭ-ter″e) pertaining to a single object or individual.

United States Pharmacopeia see USP.

United States Public Health Service (USPHS) a governmental health agency that is part of the United States Department of Health and Human Services; see also PUBLIC HEALTH.

uniterminal (u″ne-ter′mi-nal) a MONOPO-LAR apparatus.

univalent (u″nĭ-va′lent) having a valence of one.

UNLS Unified Nursing Language System.

unmyelinated (un-mi′ĕ-lĭ-nāt″ed) not having a myelin sheath.

unoprostone (u″no-pros′tōn) an antiglaucoma agent that decreases elevated intraocular pressure by increasing the outflow of aqueous HUMOR; used as *unoprostone isopropyl* in the treatment of open-angle GLAUCOMA and ocular HYPERTENSION, applied topically to the conjunctiva.

unphysiologic (un″fiz-e-o-loj′ik) not in harmony with the laws of physiology.

unsaturated (un-sach′er-āt″ed) 1. not having all affinities of its elements satisfied (unsaturated compound). 2. not holding all of a solute that can be held in solution by the solvent (unsaturated solution). 3.

denoting compounds in which two or more atoms are united by double or triple bonds.

unstriated (un-stri′āt-ed) having no striations, as smooth muscle.

Unverricht's disease (syndrome) (oon′-fer-ikts) myoclonic epilepsy.

UOS units of service.

UPP urethral pressure profile.

UPPP uvulopalatopharyngoplasty.

up-regulation (up reg-u-la′shun) increase in expression of a gene; in the narrowest sense, that in which transcription of a specific mRNA is increased, but also used more broadly to refer to increase in mRNA levels for a particular gene from any cause, such as increased stability of the specific mRNA.

uptake (up′tāk) absorption and incorporation of a substance by living tissue.

   biologic u. movement of hazardous substances from the environment into the tissues of plants or animals.

   radioactive iodine u., radioiodine u. uptake of RADIOIODINE from the blood by the THYROID GLAND; see RADIOIODINE UPTAKE TEST.

   T3 resin u., triiodothyronine resin u. the uptake of radioactive triiodothyronine at binding sites on resin, contrasted to uptake at sites on thyroxine-binding globulin in the TRIIODOTHYRONINE RESIN UPTAKE TEST.

ur(o)- word element [Gr.], *urine, urinary tract, urination.*

urachus (u′rah-kus) a fetal canal connecting the bladder with the allantois, persisting throughout life as a cord (median umbilical ligament). adj., **u′rachal.**

   patent u. a condition in which the urachus remains a hollow tube connecting the bladder and the umbilicus, resulting in an umbilical urinary fistula.

uracil (u′rah-sil) a pyrimidine base found in ribonucleic acid (RNA).

uran(o)- word element [Gr.], *palate.*

uraniscus (u″rah-nis′kus) palate.

uranium (u-ra′ne-um) a chemical element, atomic number 92, atomic weight 238.03, symbol U. (See Appendix 6.)

uranoplasty (u-ran′o-plas″te) palatoplasty.

uranorrhaphy (u″rah-nor′ah-fe) palatorraphy.

uranoschisis (u″rah-nos′kĭ-sis) cleft palate.

uranostaphyloschisis (u″rah-no-staf″ĭ-los′kĭ-sis) cleft of both soft and hard palates.

uranyl (u′rah-nil) the UO_2^{++} ion, as in uranyl sulfate.

urarthritis (u″rahr-thri′tis) gouty arthritis.

urate (u′rāt) a salt of uric acid.

uratemia (u″rah-te′me-ah) urates in the blood.

uratic (u-rat′ik) pertaining to urates or to gout.

uratoma (u″rah-to′mah) a concretion made up of urates; tophus.

uratosis (u″rah-to′sis) the deposit of urates in the tissues.

uraturia (u″rah-tu′re-ah) hyperuricosuria.

urceiform (ur-se′ĭ-form) pitcher-shaped.

urea (u-re′ah) 1. the diamide of CARBONIC ACID found in urine, blood, and lymph, the chief nitrogenous constituent of urine, and the chief nitrogenous end-product of protein metabolism; it is formed in the liver from amino acids and from ammonia compounds. 2. a pharmaceutical preparation of this compound, administered intravenously as an osmotic DIURETIC to lower intracranial or intraocular pressure, injected transabdominally into the amniotic sac to induce abortion of a second trimester pregnancy, and included in topical preparations to moisten and soften rough, dry skin.

The amount of urea in the urine increases with the quantity of protein in the diet because urea is an endogenous and exogenous waste product: endogenous because some of it is derived from breakdown of body protein as tissues undergo disintegration and repair, and exogenous because some of it is derived from the deamination of amino acids absorbed from the intestinal tract but not utilized by the body. In severe nephritis or other disorders leading to renal failure, the concentration of urea in the blood may be greatly increased, as revealed by measurement of the blood UREA NITROGEN (BUN).

u. concentration test a test of renal efficiency, based on the fact that urea is absorbed rapidly from the stomach into the blood and is excreted unaltered by the kidneys; 15g of urea is given with 100mL of fluid, and the urine collected after 2 hours is tested for urea concentration.

u. nitrogen the urea concentration of serum or plasma, conventionally specified in terms of nitrogen content and called *blood urea nitrogen* (BUN), an important indicator of renal function.

Ureaplasma (u-re′ah-plaz″mah) a genus of gram-negative, nonmotile, pleomorphic bacteria that lack a cell wall and form small granular colonies. *U. urealy′ticum* is a common inhabitant of the genitourinary tract and is associated with sexually transmitted nongonococcal URETHRITIS.

ureagenesis formation of UREA; called also ureapoiesis. adj., **ureagenet′ic.**

ureapoiesis (u-re″ah-poi-e′sis) ureagenesis. adj., **ureapoiet′ic.**

urease (u′re-ās) an enzyme that catalyzes the decomposition of urea to ammonia and carbon dioxide.

uredema (u″rĕ-de′mah) swelling from extravasated urine.

uremia (u-re′me-ah) 1. an excess in the blood of UREA, CREATININE, and other

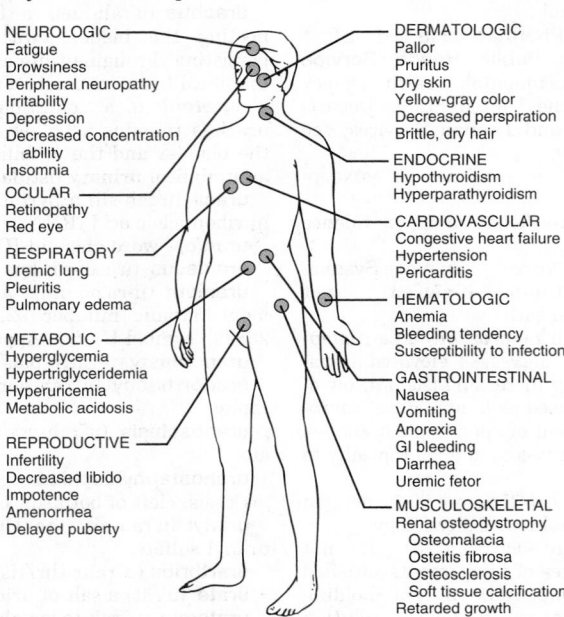

NEUROLOGIC
Fatigue
Drowsiness
Peripheral neuropathy
Irritability
Depression
Decreased concentration
   ability
Insomnia
OCULAR
Retinopathy
Red eye
RESPIRATORY
Uremic lung
Pleuritis
Pulmonary edema
METABOLIC
Hyperglycemia
Hypertriglyceridemia
Hyperuricemia
Metabolic acidosis
REPRODUCTIVE
Infertility
Decreased libido
Impotence
Amenorrhea
Delayed puberty

DERMATOLOGIC
Pallor
Pruritus
Dry skin
Yellow-gray color
Decreased perspiration
Brittle, dry hair
ENDOCRINE
Hypothyroidism
Hyperparathyroidism
CARDIOVASCULAR
Congestive heart failure
Hypertension
Pericarditis
HEMATOLOGIC
Anemia
Bleeding tendency
Susceptibility to infection
GASTROINTESTINAL
Nausea
Vomiting
Anorexia
GI bleeding
Diarrhea
Uremic fetor
MUSCULOSKELETAL
Renal osteodystrophy
   Osteomalacia
   Osteitis fibrosa
   Osteosclerosis
   Soft tissue calcification
   Retarded growth

Systemic effects of uremia.

nitrogenous end products of protein and amino acid metabolism; more correctly referred to as AZOTEMIA. 2. in current usage, the entire complex of signs and symptoms of chronic RENAL FAILURE. As the glomerular filtration RATE falls in either acute tubular necrosis or chronic renal failure, serum UREA (usually expressed as BLOOD UREA NITROGEN content or BUN) and CREATININE rise to very high levels. However, BUN and creatinine measurements are only roughly correlated with uremic symptoms. Other nitrogenous compounds present in small amounts may produce most of the toxic effects. Some uremic symptoms are due to losses of kidney function that do not involve uremia (azotemia). adj., **ure′mic.**

Patient Care. A major activity of care is assessment of health status and learning needs on an ongoing basis throughout the course of the illness. The systemic effects of uremia involve virtually every system of the body and present problems related to dysfunction of each system. Maintaining adequate nutrition is a very real challenge for the patient with this condition. The cooperative efforts of nutritionists and other health care professionals are needed to meet the goals of minimizing uremic toxicity, maintaining acceptable electrolyte levels, controlling hypertension, providing sufficient calories, and maintaining adequate nutritional status. Because of buildup of nitrogenous wastes from protein metabolism, dietary intake of protein may be severely limited. If any protein foods are allowed they should be of high quality; for example, eggs, milk, and cheese provide all of the essential amino acids in relatively small quantities.

Potassium restriction may also be indicated because of inability of the kidney to excrete it. This complicates the problem, however, because foods rich in potassium also are high-quality protein foods. These same foods also contain phosphorus, which may be restricted. A sodium-free diet usually is prescribed, but this can pose problems in regard to food selection and patient compliance.

Patients in the terminal stage of uremia will require special MOUTH CARE; measures to prevent PRESSURE ULCERS; protection from injury due to altered levels of CONSCIOUSNESS; monitoring and protection from deleterious effects of excessive bleeding related to lack of renal hormone erythropoietin and bone marrow depression; and interventions appropriate to psychological and emotional support for the patient and family members during a terminal illness.

uremigenic (u-re″mĭ-jen′ik) caused by uremia. 1. causing uremia.

ureotelic (u″re-o-tel′ik) having urea as the chief excretory product of nitrogen metabolism.

-uresis word element [Gr.], *urinary excretion of.* adj., **-uret′ic.**

ureter (u-re′ter) the fibromuscular tube, 41 to 46 cm long, through which the urine passes from the kidney to the bladder. adj., **ure′teral, ureter′ic.** As urine is produced by each kidney, it passes into the ureter, which, by contracting rhythmically, forces the urine along and empties it in spurts into the bladder. After being stored temporarily in the bladder, the urine passes out of the body by way of the urethra. Occasionally a small calculus or stone forms in a kidney and passes into a ureter, obstructing it. (See KIDNEY STONE.)

ureter(o)- word element [Gr.], *ureter.*

ureteralgia (u-re″ter-al′jah) pain in the ureter.

ureterectasis (u-re″ter-ek′tah-sis) distention of the ureter, such as in MEGAURETER or HYDROURETER.

ureterectomy (u-re″ter-ek′tah-me) excision of a ureter.

ureteritis (u-re″ter-i′tis) inflammation of a ureter.

ureterocele (u-re′ter-o-sēl″) ballooning of the lower end of the ureter into the bladder.

ureterocelectomy (u-re″ter-o-se-lek′tah-me) excision of a ureterocele.

ureterocolostomy (u-re″ter-o-kah-los′tah-me) anastomosis of a ureter to the colon.

ureterocystostomy (u-re″ter-o-sis-tos′-tah-me) ureteroneocystostomy.

ureteroenterostomy (u-re″ter-o-en″ter-os′tah-me) anastomosis of one or both ureters to the wall of the intestine.

ureterography (u-re″ter-og′rah-fe) radiograph of the ureter, after injection of a contrast medium.

ureteroileostomy (u-re″ter-o-il″e-os′tah-me) anastomosis of the ureters to an isolated loop of the ileum, drained through a stoma on the abdominal wall.

ureterolith (u-re′ter-o-lith″) a calculus in the ureter.

ureterolithiasis (u-re″ter-o-li-thi′ah-sis) formation or presence of calculi in the ureter.

ureterolithotomy (u-re″ter-o-li-thot′ah-me) incision of a ureter for removal of calculus.

ureterolysis (u-re″ter-ol′ĭ-sis) 1. rupture of the ureter. 2. paralysis of the ureter. 3. surgical freeing of the ureter from adhesions.

ureteroneocystostomy (u-re″ter-o-ne″o-sis-tos′tah-me) surgical transplantation of the ureters to a new site in the bladder.

U

ureteronephrectomy (u-re″ter-o-ně-frek′-tah-me) excision of a kidney and ureter.

ureteropathy (u-re″ter-op′ah-the) any disease of the ureter.

ureteropelvic (u-re″ter-o-pel′vik) relating to the URETER and renal PELVIS. Called also pelviureteral.

ureteropelvioplasty (u-re″ter-o-pel′ve-o-plas″te) ureteropyelostomy.

ureteroplasty (u-re′ter-o-plas″te) plastic repair of a ureter.

ureteropyelitis (u-re″ter-o-pi″ē-li′tis) inflammation of a ureter and renal pelvis.

ureteropyelography (u-re″ter-o-pi-e-log′-rah-fe) radiography of the ureter and renal pelvis.

ureteropyelonephritis (u-re″ter-o-pi″ě-lo-ně-fri′tis) inflammation of the ureter, renal pelvis, and kidney.

ureteropyeloplasty (u-re″ter-o-pi′ě-lo-plas″te) ureteropyelostomy.

ureteropyelostomy (u-re″ter-o-pi″ē-los′-tah-me) surgical creation of a new communication between a ureter and the renal pelvis to repair a deformity of the ureteropelvic JUNCTION. Called also ureteropelvioplasty and ureteropyeloplasty.

ureteropyosis (u-re′ter-o-pi-o′sis) suppurative inflammation of the ureter.

ureterorenoscope (u-re″ter-o-re′no-skōp) a fiberoptic endoscope used in ureterorenoscopy.

ureterorenoscopy (u-re″ter-o-re-nos′kah-pe) visual inspection of the interior of the ureter and kidney by means of a fiberoptic endoscope for such purposes as biopsy, removal or crushing of stones, or other procedures.

ureterorrhagia (u-re″ter-o-ra′jah) discharge of blood from the ureter.

ureterorrhaphy (u-re″ter-or′ah-fe) suture of the ureter.

ureteroscope (u-re′ter-o-skōp″) a fiberoptic endoscope used in ureteroscopy.

ureteroscopy (u-re″ter-os′kah-pe) examination of the ureter by means of a fiberoptic endoscope.

ureterosigmoidostomy (u-re″ter-o-sig″-moi-dos′tah-me) anastomosis of one or both ureters to the sigmoid colon. In this form of diversion of urinary flow there is no need for an appliance because the urine flows into the colon, which acts as a kind of reservoir. The urine liquefies the stool and creates difficulties in patients who are unable to regulate themselves successfully. A disadvantage of this procedure is the constant danger of urinary infection by organisms from the bowel. Indications for it are the same as for cutaneous URETEROSTOMY and ILEAL CONDUIT.

ureterostomy (u-re″ter-os′tah-me) creation of a new outlet for a ureter.

   cutaneous u. a type of urinary diversion in which one or both ureters are detached from the bladder and brought through the abdominal wall to form a STOMA. A collection pouch fitted with a belt is then worn snugly against the abdomen and over the "ureteral buds" or stomas to collect the urine as it passes through the ureters.

   Indications for ureterostomy include malignancy or trauma that necessitates removal of the bladder, congenital defect or absence of portions of the urinary tract, and neurogenic bladder in which other devices for the collection of urine have proved unsatisfactory.

   Patient care is similar to that for any patient with a diversion of urinary flow and is primarily concerned with teaching the patient how to care for the appliance and avoid complications arising from the creation of the stoma. See also ILEAL CONDUIT.

ureterotomy (u-re″ter-ot′ah-me) incision of a ureter.

ureteroureterostomy (u-re″ter-o-u-re″-ter-os′tah-me) end-to-end anastomosis of the two portions of a transected ureter.

ureterovaginal (u-re″ter-o-vaj′ĭ-nal) pertaining to or communicating with a ureter and the vagina.

ureterovesical (u-re″ter-o-ves′ĭ-k'l) pertaining to a ureter and the bladder; called also vesicoureteral.

urethr(o)- word element [Gr.], *urethra.*

urethra (u-re′thrah) the tubular passage through which urine is discharged from the bladder to the exterior of the body. adj., **ure′thral.** The external urinary opening is called the *urinary meatus.* In men the

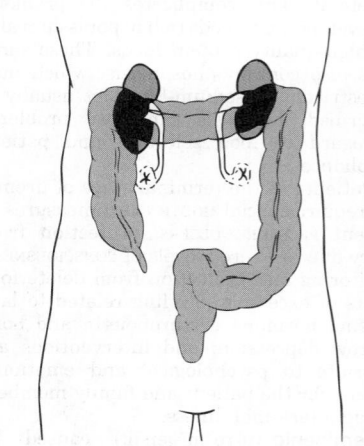

Cutaneous ureterostomy. From Lammon et al., 1995.

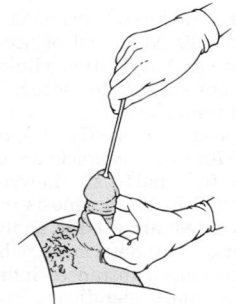

Urethral specimen: male

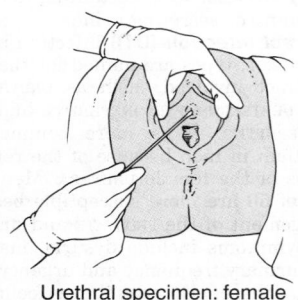

Urethral specimen: female

Using a swab to obtain a urethral specimen from a male and a female client. From Lammon et al., 1995.

urethra conveys both urine and the secretions of the reproductive organs. In women its sole function is urination. The female urethra is about 4 cm long; its opening is situated between the clitoris and the opening of the vagina. The male urethra is about 20 cm long and is narrower than that of the female. It has three sections: prostatic, membranous, and penile. It extends downward from the bladder through the prostate, which secretes into it a thin fluid. The membranous portion of the urethra receives the secretion of the bulbourethral glands. The urethra then extends down through the main body of the penis to the opening, or meatus, at the tip. Along the entire length of the passage are mucous glands.

urethralgia (u″re-thral′jah) pain in the urethra; called also urethrodynia.

urethratresia (u-re″thrah-tre′zhah) urethral atresia.

urethrectomy (u″re-threk′tah-me) excision of the urethra.

urethritis (u″re-thri′tis) inflammation of the urethra, often a symptom of GONORRHEA (*gonococcal urethritis*) but sometimes caused by another infectious organism. The urethra swells and narrows and the flow of urine is

impeded; both urination and the urgency to urinate increase and there is burning pain, sometimes with a purulent discharge, on urination. It usually responds to treatment with antibiotics or sulfonamides.

   nongonococcal u., nonspecific u. a sexually transmitted inflammation of the urethra caused by any of various organisms other than gonococci.

urethrobulbar (u-re″thro-bul′bar) pertaining to the urethra and the bulb of the penis.

urethrocele (u-re″thro-sēl) prolapse of the female urethra through the urinary meatus.

urethrocystitis (u-re″thro-sis-ti′tis) inflammation of the urethra and bladder.

urethrocystoscopy (u-re″thro-sis-tos′kah-pe) cystourethroscopy.

urethrodynia (u-re″thro-din′e-ah) urethralgia.

urethrography (u″re-throg′rah-fe) radiography of the urethra.

urethrometry (u″re-throm′ĕ-tre) 1. determination of the resistance of various segments of the urethra to retrograde flow of fluid. 2. measurement of the urethra.

urethropenile (u-re″thro-pe′nīl) pertaining to the urethra and penis.

urethroperineal (u-re″thro-per″ĭ-ne′al) pertaining to the urethra and perineum.

urethroperineoscrotal (u-re″thro-per″ĭ-ne″o-skro′-tal) pertaining to the urethra, perineum, and scrotum.

urethroplasty (u-re′thro-plas″te) plastic repair of the urethra.

urethroprostatic (u-re″thro-pros-tat′ik) pertaining to the urethra and prostate.

urethrorectal (u-re″thro-rek′tal) pertaining to the urethra and rectum.

urethrorrhagia (u-re″thro-ra′jah) a flow of blood from the urethra.

urethrorrhaphy (u″re-thror′ah-fe) suture of the urethra.

urethrorrhea (u-re″thro-re′ah) abnormal discharge from the urethra.

urethroscope (u-re′thro-skōp) an instrument for viewing the interior of the urethra.

urethroscopy (u″re-thros′kah-pe) visual inspection of the urethra. adj., **urethroscop′ic.**

urethrospasm (u-re′thro-spazm) spasm of the urethra.

urethrostaxis (u-re″thro-stak′sis) oozing of blood from the urethra.

urethrostenosis (u-re″thro-stĕ-no′sis) constriction of the urethra.

urethrostomy (u″rĕ-thros′tah-me) creation of a permanent opening for the urethra in the perineum.

urethrotome (u-re′thro-tōm) an instrument for cutting a urethral stricture.

U

urethrotomy (u″re-throt′ah-me) incision of the urethra, usually for relief of a stricture; it may be done either through the perineum (*external* or *perineal urethrotomy*) or from within (*internal urethrotomy*).

urethrotrigonitis (u-re″thro-tri″go-ni′tis) inflammation of the urethra and the vesical trigone.

urethrovaginal (u-re″thro-vaj′ĭ-nal) pertaining to the urethra and vagina.

urethrovesical (u-re″thro-ves′ĭ-kal) pertaining to the urethra and bladder.

urgency (ur′jen-se) a sudden compelling need to do something.

   bowel u. the sudden, almost uncontrollable, need to defecate.

   urinary u. the sudden, almost uncontrollable, need to urinate.

urhidrosis (ur″hĭ-dro′sis) the presence in the sweat of urinous materials, chiefly uric acid and urea.

URI upper respiratory tract infection.

-uria word element [Gr.], *condition of the urine.* adj., **-u′ric.**

uric (u′rik) urinary.

   u. acid the end product of PURINE metabolism or oxidation in the body. It is present in blood in a concentration of about 5 mg/100 ml and is excreted in the urine in amounts of a little less than 1 g per day. In GOUT there is an excess of uric acid in the blood, and its salts, the URATES, form insoluble stones in the urinary tract, or may crystallize and form deposits (see TOPHUS) in the joints and tissues. The presence of high concentrations of uric acid in the urine is significant in the diagnosis of gout, but is of little significance in urinary disorders.

uricacidemia (u″rik-as″ĭ-de′me-ah) hyperuricemia.

uricaciduria (u″rik-as″ĭ-du′re-ah) hyperuricosuria.

uricase (u′rĭ-kās) an enzyme that catalyzes the conversion of uric acid to allantoin.

uricemia (u″rĭ-se′me-ah) hyperuricemia.

uricolysis (u″rĭ-kol′ĭ-sis) the cleavage of uric acid or urates. adj., **uricolyt′ic.**

uricosuria (u″rĭ-ko-su′re-ah) hyperuricosuria.

uricosuric (u″rĭ-ko-su′rik) 1. pertaining to, characterized by, or promoting URICOSURIA. 2. an agent that promotes uricosuria.

uricotelic (u″rĭ-ko-tel′ik) having uric acid as the chief excretory product of nitrogen metabolism.

uridine (u′rĭ-dēn) a ribonucleoside containing uracil.

   u. diphosphate (UDP) a nucleotide that participates in glycogen metabolism and in some processes of nucleic acid synthesis.

Urihesive (u-ri-he′siv) trademark for a double-sided tape composed of pectin, gelatin, sodium carboxymethylcellulose, and polyisobutylene, used to secure condom catheters to the penis.

urin(o)- word element [Gr., L.], *urine.*

urinal (u′rĭ-nal) a receptacle for urine.

urinalysis (u″rĭ-nal′ĭ-sis) analysis of the urine as an aid in the diagnosis of disease. Many types of test are used in analyzing the urine in order to determine whether it contains abnormal substances indicative of disease. The most significant substances normally absent from urine and detected by urinalysis are protein, glucose, acetone, blood, pus, and casts.

urinary (u′rĭ-ner″e) 1. pertaining to URINE 2. containing or secreting urine.

   u. tract infection (UTI) infection in the urinary TRACT; types are named for the part of the tract involved, such as URETHRITIS, CYSTITIS, URETERITIS, PYELONEPHRITIS, and GLOMERULONEPHRITIS. It is more common in women than in men because of the relative shortness of the female URETHRA. Men over the age of 50 are more susceptible because of enlargement of the PROSTATE and urinary stasis. Symptoms include dysuria, malaise, nausea, urinary frequency and urgency, and nocturia. There also may be a feeling of suprapubic fullness not relieved by urination. If the infection is higher in the urinary tract, in the ureters or kidney, there can be lower back pain or genital pain.

   Factors that contribute to infection of the urinary tract include structural defects and systemic disorders that interfere with the free flow of urine. Examples include congenital disorders, neuromuscular disease or spinal cord injury, and renal stones. Infectious agents that cause SEXUALLY TRANSMITTED DISEASES can also invade the urinary

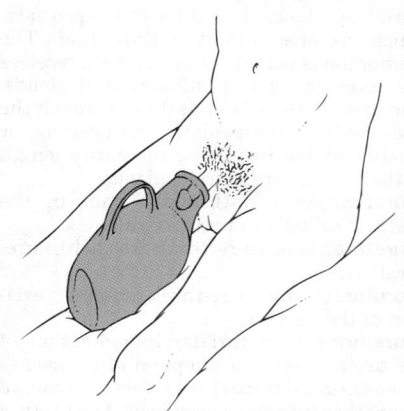

The urinal in place. From Lammon et al., 1995.

tract. Moreover, urinary tract infection is a constant threat and a major cause of morbidity in patients with indwelling catheters.

Antimicrobial drugs are prescribed for treatment of urinary tract infection. Some drugs such as TRIMETHOPRIM and SULFAMETHOXAZOLE combinations (Bactrim or Septra), or KANAMYCIN, can be given in a single dose, while others may be prescribed in one- to three-day doses or over a longer period of time.

Patient Care. Prevention of recurrence is a major goal in the care of patients with UTI. Increased intake of fluids is encouraged to increase the force of the stream of urine and facilitate removal of microorganisms and debris. Patients are taught to urinate at first urge rather than postponing emptying the bladder. Women should know that it is important to keep the perineal area clean and that all wiping motions should be from front to back to avoid transporting fecal bacteria to the urinary meatus. Any VAGINITIS should be treated promptly and effectively to reduce the risk of spreading infection from the vagina to the urinary tract.

Other measures are related to control or management of underlying systemic or structural disorders, meticulous catheter care for patients with an indwelling catheter, and prevention and treatment of sexually transmitted diseases.

urinate (u′rĭ-nāt) to discharge urine.

urination (u″rĭ-na′shun) the discharge of urine from the bladder; urine from the kidneys is passed in spurts every few seconds along the ureters to the bladder, where it collects and later is passed to the outside via the urethra. Called also micturition and voiding.

The Urinary Process. Urination is a complex process controlled by muscles of the bladder and sphincter mechanism and by modulatory centers in the central and peripheral nervous systems. The detrusor muscle is a complex meshwork of interlaced smooth muscle bundles that contract in a way that squeezes urine from the bladder vesicle. The sphincter mechanism consists of smooth muscle in the bladder neck and proximal urethra, a striated muscle sphincter consisting of slow twitch muscle fibers in the urethral wall, and periurethral muscles that are a component of the pelvic floor muscles. The detrusor relaxes during bladder filling to accommodate increasing volumes at a low pressure, and the sphincter remains tightly closed. During urination, the detrusor contracts and the sphincter mechanism relaxes, allowing smooth outflow of urine.

As the bladder fills, modulatory centers in the brain prevent the occurrence of

contractions. Meanwhile, the sphincter mechanism remains closed under autonomic and somatic nervous system control. During urination, the inhibition of contractions is removed and a reflex originates in the pontine micturition center. That causes the detrusor muscle to contract and the sphincter mechanism to relax. The location of the final output of central nervous system impulses to and from the bladder and sphincter is the sacral micturition center, located in spinal segments 2, 3, and 4, which must be intact for contraction to occur. Injury to the pontine micturition center will compromise the smooth coordination between sphincter mechanism and detrusor muscle, and injury to the brain will affect the volitional control of urine (bladder stability). See also urinary INCONTINENCE.

urine (u′rin) the fluid containing water and waste products that is secreted by the KIDNEYS, stored in the BLADDER, and discharged by way of the URETHRA.

Contents of the Urine. Several different types of waste products are eliminated in urine (for example, urea, uric acid, ammonia, and creatinine); none are useful in the blood. The largest component of urine by weight (apart from water) is UREA, which is derived from the breakdown of dietary proteins and amino acids in the diet and those of the body itself. Its amount varies greatly from person to person, however, depending on the amount of protein in the diet. Besides waste materials, urine also contains surpluses of products necessary for bodily functioning, such as water, sodium chloride, and other substances. Thus in a typical specimen of urine there will be sodium, potassium, calcium, magnesium, chloride, phosphate, and sulfate.

The color of urine is due to the presence of the yellow pigment UROCHROME. Individual ingredients of urine are not usually visible, but when the urine is alkaline some of the ingredients may form sediments of phosphates and urates. The urine may also become cloudy from the presence of mucus. Persistent cloudiness may indicate the presence of pus or blood. Common causes of variations in the color of urine are summarized in the accompanying table.

fractional u. examination of a urine specimen with separate examination for different solutes, generally meaning that the specimen is tested for the presence of GLUCOSE and ACETONE.

midstream u. clean-catch specimen.

residual u. urine remaining in the bladder after urination; seen in bladder

COMMON CAUSES OF VARIATIONS IN THE APPEARANCE OF URINE	
Colorless	Dilute urine as seen in high fluid intake, diabetes insipidus, diuretic therapy, diabetes mellitus
Cloudy	Phosphate precipitation (normal in aging urine specimens); pyuria; bacteriuria; epithelial cells, blood, leukocytes
Smoky or hazy	Hemoglobin and remnants of red blood cells; chyle; prostatic fluid; yeast
Dark yellow or yellow-orange	Concentrated urine as seen in dehydration, low fluid intake, inability of the kidneys to dilute urine, bile
Yellow-brown	Bile
Orange-red	Pyridium, bile
Red or red-brown	Blood, ingestion of beets, berries, fava beans, excessive red food coloring, pyrvinium pamoate (Povan)
Green	*Pseudomonas* bacteria, bile pigments
Dark brown or black	Methylene blue; typhus

outlet obstruction and disorders of deficient detrusor contractility.

urinemia (u″rĭ-ne′me-ah) uremia.

uriniferous (u″rĭ-nif′er-us) transporting or conveying urine.

uriniparous (u″rĭ-nip′ah-rus) excreting urine.

urinogenital (u″rĭ-no-jen′ĭ-tal) genitourinary.

urinogenous (u″rĭ-noj′ĕ-nus) of urinary origin.

urinology (u″rĭ-nol′ah-je) urology.

urinoma (u″rĭ-no′mah) a collection of URINE encapsulated by fibrous tissue, resulting from leakage of urine from a tear in the URETER, renal PELVIS, or renal CALICES because of obstruction of the ureter or trauma.

urinometer (u″rĭ-nom′ĕ-ter) an instrument for determining the specific gravity of urine.

urinothorax (u″rĭ-no-tho′raks) HYDROTHORAX in which the fluid is URINE, secondary to an obstruction in the renal PELVIS or urinary TRACT.

urinous (u′rĭ-nus) urinary.

uriposia (u″rĭ-po′ze-ah) the drinking of urine.

Urispas (u′rĭ-spaz) trademark for a preparation of FLAVOXATE, a smooth muscle RELAXANT used as a urinary tract ANTISPASMODIC.

urobilin (u″ro-bi′lin) a brownish pigment formed by oxidation of urobilinogen; found in the feces and sometimes in the urine after standing in the air.

urobilinemia (u″ro-bi″lĭ-ne′me-ah) urobilin in the blood.

urobilinogen (u″ro-bi-lin′o-jen) a colorless compound formed in the intestines by the reduction of BILIRUBIN; the urobilinogen in the urine normally represents about 1 per cent of the bilirubin produced in the body by the breakdown of hemoglobin. Increased amounts in the urine indicate excessive bilirubin in the blood. Determination of the amount of urobilinogen excreted in a given

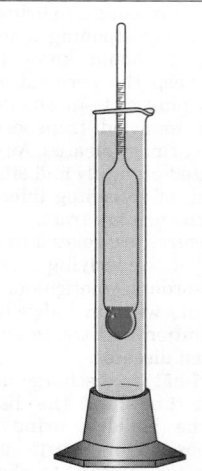

Urinometer. From Lammon et al., 1995.

period makes it possible to evaluate certain types of hemolytic anemia and also is of help in diagnosing liver dysfunction.

Laboratory tests for urobilinogen require collection of urine for a 24-hour period or for a 2-hour period. The 2-hour afternoon collection of urine is most commonly used because it is more convenient and also because it has been found that the excretion of urobilinogen reaches its maximum in the period from midafternoon to late evening. There is no special preparation of the patient for these tests. The exact time period in which the urine has been collected must be noted. The specimen should be taken to the laboratory immediately, since bacteria that may be present in the urine can oxidize urobilinogen and change it to urobilin.

urocele (u′ro-sēl) distention of the scrotum with extravasated urine.

urochezia (u″ro-ke′ze-ah) discharge of urine in the feces.

urochrome (u'ro-krōm) a breakdown product of hemoglobin related to the bile pigments, found in the urine and responsible for its yellow color.

uroclepsia (u″ro-klep'se-ah) the unconscious, involuntary escape of urine.

urocystitis (u″ro-sis-ti'tis) cystitis.

urodynamics (u″ro-di-nam'iks) the dynamics of the propulsion and flow of urine in the urinary tract. adj., **urodynam'ic.**

Urodynamic testing is done by injecting water or carbon dioxide into the bladder via a catheter. Bladder sensation, capacity, and strength of contraction, as well as ability to hold urine in the bladder, can thus be quantified.

urodynia (u″ro-din'e-ah) pain accompanying urination.

uroedema (u″ro-ĕ-de'mah) edema from infiltration of urine.

uroflowmetry (u″ro-flo'met-re) the graphic representation of urinary flow, expressed as cubic centimeters per second; called also flow study and urinary flow study.

urofollitropin (u″ro-fol'ĭ-tro″pin) a preparation of GONADOTROPINS from the urine of postmenopausal women; it contains follicle-stimulating HORMONE and is used in conjunction with human chorionic GONADOTROPIN to induce ovulation in the treatment of female INFERTILITY and to stimulate multiple oocyte development in ovulatory patients utilizing assisted reproductive TECHNOLOGIES. Administered by subcutaneous injection.

urogenital (u″ro-jen'ĭ-tal) pertaining to the urinary SYSTEM and genitalia; called also genitourinary and urinogenital.

urogenous (u-roj'ĕ-nus) 1. producing urine. 2. produced from or in the urine.

urogram (u'ro-gram) a film obtained by urography.

urography (u-rog'rah-fe) radiography of any part of the urinary tract.

ascending u., cystoscopic u. retrograde urography.

descending u., excretion u., excretory u., intravenous u. urography after intravenous injection of an opaque medium that is rapidly excreted in the urine.

retrograde u. urography after injection of contrast medium into the bladder through the urethra.

urokinase (u″ro-ki'nās) u-plasminogen activator; the term is used particularly to denote a pharmaceutical preparation of the enzyme, administered intravenously as a thrombolytic agent in the treatment of acute coronary thrombosis and acute pulmonary embolism; also used to clear intravenous catheters of obstructions composed of clotted blood or fibrin deposits.

urolagnia (u″ro-lag'ne-ah) a paraphilia in which sexual excitement is associated with the sight or thought of urine or urination. See also UROPHILIA.

urolith (u'ro-lith) a calculus in the urine or the urinary tract. adj., **urolith'ic.**

urolithiasis (u″ro-lĭ-thi'ah-sis) formation of urinary calculi, or the condition associated with urinary calculi.

urologist (u-rol'ah-jist) a specialist in urology.

urology (u-rol'ah-je) the medical specialty concerned with the urinary system in both male and female and the genital organs in the male. adj., **urolog'ic, urolog'ical.**

uromelus (u-rom'ĕ-lus) a SYMMELUS with one foot.

urometry (u-rom'ĕ-tre) the graphic recording of pressure changes caused by ureteral peristalsis; the WHITAKER TEST is used to assess ureteral peristalsis and evaluate obstruction between the renal pelvis and ureterovesical junction.

uroncus (u-rong'kus) a swelling or cyst caused by retention or extravasation of urine.

uronephrosis (u″ro-nĕ-fro'sis) distention of the renal pelvis and tubules with urine.

uropathy (u-rop'ah-the) any disease in the urinary tract.

urophilia (u″ro-fil'e-ah) a paraphilia in which sexual arousal or activity is linked to urine. See also UROLAGNIA.

uropoiesis (u″ro-poi-e'sis) the formation of urine. adj., **uropoiet'ic.**

uroporphyria (u″ro-por-fir'e-ah) PORPHYRIA with excessive excretion of porphyrins.

uroporphyrin (u″ro-por'fĭ-rin) any of several porphyrins produced by oxidation of uroporphyrinogen; one or more are excreted in excess in the urine in several of the porphyrias.

uroporphyrinogen (u″ro-por″fĭ-rin'o-jen) a PORPHYRINOGEN formed from PORPHOBILINOGEN; it is a precursor of uroporphyrin and coproporphyrinogen.

uroprotective (u″ro-pro-tek'tiv) providing protection of the urinary tract, especially against UROTOXICITY.

uropsammus (u″ro-sam'us) urinary gravel.

uroradiology (u″ro-ra″de-ol'ah-je) radiology of the urinary tract.

uroschesis (u-ros'kĕ-sis) retention or suppression of the urine.

uroscopy (u-ros'kah-pe) diagnostic examination of the urine. adj., **uroscop'ic.**

urosepsis (u″ro-sep'sis) septic poisoning from retained and absorbed urinary substances. adj., **urosep'tic.**

U

urostealith (u″ro-ste′ah-lith) a urinary calculus having fatty constituents.

urotoxicity (u″ro-tok-sis′ĭ-te) the toxic quality of the URINE.

ursodiol (ur″so-di′ol) the secondary bile acid ursodeoxycholic acid used as an anticholelithic to dissolve radiolucent, noncalcified GALLSTONES.

urticant (ur′tĭ-kant) producing urticaria.

urticaria (ur″tĭ-ka′re-ah) a vascular reaction of the skin marked by transient appearance of slightly elevated patches (WHEALS) that are redder or paler than the surrounding skin and often attended by severe itching; the cause may be certain foods, infection, or emotional stress. (See Atlas 2, Plate D.) Called also hives. adj., **urtica′rial.**

　cold u. urticaria precipitated by cold air, water, or objects, occurring in two forms: In the autosomal dominant form, which is associated with fever, arthralgias, and leukocytosis, the lesions occur as erythematous, burning papules and macules. The more common acquired form is usually idiopathic and self-limited.

　giant u. angioedema.

　u. hemorrha′gica purpura with urticaria.

　u. medicamento′sa that due to use of a drug.

　papular u., u. papulo′sa an allergic reaction to the bite of various insects, with appearance of lesions that evolve into inflammatory, increasingly hard, red or brownish, persistent papules.

　u. pigmento′sa the most common form of MASTOCYTOSIS, occurring primarily in children, manifested as persistent pink to brown macules or soft plaques of various size; pruritus and urtication occur on stroking the lesions.

　u. pigmentosa, juvenile urticaria pigmentosa present at birth or in the first few weeks of life, usually disappearing before puberty, taking the form of a single nodule or tumor or of a disseminated eruption of yellowish brown to yellowish red macules, plaques, or bullae.

　solar u. a rare form produced by exposure to sunlight.

urtication (ur″tĭ-ka′shun) 1. the development or formation of urticaria. 2. a burning sensation, as of the sting of nettles.

urushiol (u-roo′she-ol) the toxic irritant principle of poison ivy and related plants.

USAN United States Adopted Name, a nonproprietary designation for any compound used as a drug, established by negotiation between its manufacturer and a council sponsored jointly by the American Medical Association, American Pharmaceutical Association, and United States Pharmacopeial Convention, Inc.

Usher's syndrome (ush′erz) a genetic disorder characterized by congenital deafness and progressive blindness resulting from retinal degeneration; sometimes mental retardation and disturbances of gait also occur. A self-help network for individuals and families affected by this disorder can be reached at the Foundation Fighting Blindness, 11435 Cronhill Drive, Owings Mills, MD 21117-2220, telephone (voice) 1-888-394-3937, (TDD) 1-800-683-5551, or by consulting their web site at http://www.blindness.org.

use (ūs) the applying of something to a specific desired purpose.

　substance u. substance ABUSE.

USP United States Pharmacopeia, a legally recognized compendium of standards for drugs, published by the United States Pharmacopeial Convention, Inc., and revised periodically; it also includes assays and tests for determination of strength, quality, and purity.

USPHS United States Public Health Service.

USRDS United States Renal Data System.

USR test unheated serum reagin test.

ustilaginism (us″tĭ-laj′ĭ-nizm) a condition resembling ergotism, due to ingestion of corn (maize) contaminated with the fungus *Ustilago maydis.*

uter(o)- word element [L.], *uterus.*

uteralgia (u″ter-al′jah) hysteralgia.

uterine (u′ter-in, u′ter-īn) pertaining to the uterus.

uteroabdominal (u″ter-o-ab-dom′ĭ-nal) pertaining to the uterus and abdomen.

uterocervical (u″ter-o-ser′vĭ-kal) pertaining to the uterus and cervix uteri.

uterofixation (u″ter-o-fĭk-sa′shun) hysteropexy.

uterogenic (u″ter-o-jen′ik) formed in the uterus.

uterogestation (u″ter-o-jes-ta′shun) uterine gestation; normal pregnancy.

uterography (u″ter-og′rah-fe) x-ray examination of the uterus; hysterography.

uterolith (u′ter-o-lith″) uterine calculus.

uterometer (u″ter-om′ĕ-ter) an instrument for measuring the uterus; hysterometer.

utero-ovarian (u″ter-o-o-va′re-an) pertaining to the uterus and ovary.

uteropexy (u′ter-o-pek″se) hysteropexy.

uteroplacental (u″ter-o-plah-sen′tal) pertaining to the placenta and uterus.

uteroplasty (u′ter-o-plas″te) metroplasty.

uterorectal (u″ter-o-rek′tal) rectouterine.

uterosacral (u″ter-o-sa′kral) pertaining to the uterus and sacrum.

uterosalpingography (u″ter-o-sal″ping-gog′rah-fe) hysterosalpingography.

uteroscope (u′ter-o-skōp″) an instrument for viewing the interior of the uterus; hysteroscope.

uterotomy (u″ter-ot′ah-me) hysterotomy.

uterotonic (u″ter-o-ton′ik) 1. increasing the tone of uterine muscle. 2. an agent that so acts.

uterotubal (u″ter-o-too′bal) tubouterine.

uterovaginal (u″ter-o-vaj′ĭ-nal) pertaining to the uterus and vagina.

uterovesical (u″ter-o-ves′ĭ-kal) vesico-uterine.

uterus (u′ter-us), pl. *u′teri* [L.] the hollow muscular organ in female mammals in which the ZYGOTE (fertilized OVUM) normally becomes embedded and in which the developing EMBRYO and FETUS is nourished; in humans it is normally about the size and shape of a pear. Called also metra and womb.

The upper part of the uterus, or FUNDUS UTERI, is broad and flattened; the middle part (body), or CORPUS UTERI, is large and open; and the lower part, or CERVIX UTERI, is narrow and tubular and opens downward into the VAGINA. Two FALLOPIAN TUBES enter the uterus at the upper end, one on each side. The walls of the uterus are composed of muscle, and its lining is mucous membrane. The muscular substance of the uterus is called the MYOMETRIUM, and the inner lining is called the ENDOMETRIUM. Between puberty and menopause, the lining goes through a monthly cycle of growth and discharge, known as the MENSTRUAL CYCLE. MENSTRUATION is the time in the cycle when the tissue prepared by the uterus for a possible embryo or fertilized egg is unused and passes out through the vagina.

The menstrual cycle is interrupted by pregnancy when a mature ovum is fertilized by a spermatozoon. Fertilization usually takes place in the fallopian tube; the

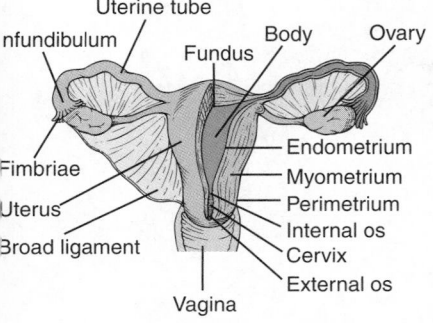

Uterine tube

Infundibulum Body   Ovary
         Fundus

Fimbriae
                 Endometrium
Uterus   Myometrium
                 Perimetrium
Broad ligament   Internal os
                 Cervix
                 External os
         Vagina

Uterus and uterine tubes. From Applegate, 2000.

fertilized ovum continues moving along the tube and comes to rest in the uterus, where it implants in the endometrium. The endometrium then serves to anchor the placenta, which filters nutrients from the mother's blood into the blood of the growing fetus. (See also REPRODUCTION and female REPRODUCTIVE ORGANS.)

Disorders of the Uterus. The main organs of the female reproductive system, the uterus, fallopian tubes, and ovaries, are connected to each other by ligaments that normally hold each in its proper place. Occasionally childbirth causes displacement of the uterus. The ligaments may stretch and weaken enough to permit the uterus to bulge into the vagina. This is called a prolapsed uterus. The uterus is also subject to cancer as well as to benign growths in the uterine wall, called LEIOMYOMAS.

u. didel′phys the existence of two distinct uteri in the same individual; called also didelphia and uterus duplex.

duplex u., u. du′plex uterus didelphys.

UTI urinary tract infection.

utricle (u′trĭ-k'l) 1. any small sac. 2. the larger of the two divisions of the membranous labyrinth of the inner ear.

prostatic u., urethral u. a small blind pouch in the substance of the prostate.

utricular (u-trik′u-lar) 1. bladderlike. 2. pertaining to the utricle of the ear.

utriculitis (u-trik″u-li′tis) inflammation of the prostatic utricle or of the utricle of the ear.

utriculosaccular (u-trik″u-lo-sak′u-lar) pertaining to the utricle and saccule of the membranous labyrinth of the inner ear.

UVA ultraviolet A.

UVB ultraviolet B.

UVC ultraviolet C.

uve(o)- word element [L.], uvea.

uvea (u′ve-ah) [L.] the TUNICA VASCULOSA of the eyeball, consisting of the iris, ciliary body, and choroid. adj., **u′veal.**

uveitis (u″ve-i′tis) an inflammation of part or all of the middle (vascular) tunic of the eye, the uvea. The term also includes inflammation that involves the other tunics (the sclera and cornea, and the retina). adj., *uveit′ic.*

heterochromic u. heterochromic iridocyclitis.

sympathetic u. sympathetic ophthalmia.

uveomeningitis (u′ve-o-men″in-ji′tis) a disorder characterized by lesions of the uvea accompanied by meningeal inflammation.

uveoparotid fever (u″ve-o-pah-rot′id) a manifestation of sarcoidosis, marked by chronic inflammation of the parotid gland

U

and uvea, with chronic IRIDOCYCLITIS, unilateral facial paralysis, lassitude, and an elevated but subfebrile temperature.

uveoscleritis (u″ve-o-sklĕ-ri′tis) scleritis due to extension of uveitis.

uviform (u′vĭ-form) shaped like a grape.

uvula (u′vu-lah) 1. any hanging, fleshy mass. 2. palatine UVULA. adj., **u′vular.**

    u. of bladder a rounded elevation at the bladder NECK in males, formed by convergence of muscle fibers terminating in the URETHRA. Called also uvula vesicae.

    bifid u. bifurcation of the uvula, an incomplete form of cleft palate.

    u. cerebel′li uvula vermis.

    u. palati′na, palatine u. the small, fleshy mass hanging from the soft palate above the root of the tongue.

    u. ver′mis the part of the VERMIS OF THE CEREBELLUM between the pyramid and nodule; it is a lobule that forms the posterior limit of the fourth ventricle. Called also uvula cerebelli.

    u. vesi′cae urina′riae uvula of bladder.

uvulectomy (u″vu-lek′tah-me) excision of the uvula.

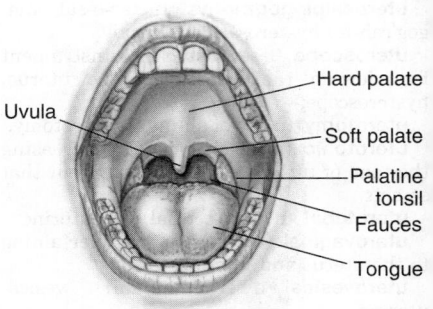

Features of the oral cavity, including the uvula. From Applegate, 2000.

uvulitis (u″vu-li′tis) inflammation of the UVULA; called also staphylitis.

uvulopalatopharyngoplasty (u″vu-lo-pa-l″ah-to-fah-ring′go-plas″te) palatopharyngoplasty.

uvuloptosis (u″vu-lop-to′sis) a relaxed, pendulous state of the uvula.

uvulotomy (u″vu-lot′ah-me) the cutting off of the uvula or a part of it.

V

V vanadium; vision; volt; volume.

V_T tidal volume.

v. [L.] vein or vena.

VAC 1. Vacuum Assisted Closure. 2. a regimen of VINCRISTINE, DACTINOMYCIN, and CYCLOPHOSPHAMIDE, used in cancer chemotherapy.

vaccina (vak-si′nah) vaccinia.

vaccinal (vak′sĭ-nal) 1. pertaining to vaccinia, to vaccine, or to vaccination. 2. having protective qualities when used by way of inoculation.

vaccinate (vak′sĭ-nāt) to inoculate with vaccine to produce immunity.

vaccination (vak″sĭ-na′shun) the introduction of VACCINE into the body to produce immunity to a specific disease. The term vaccination comes from the Latin *vacca,* cow, and was coined when the first inoculations were given with organisms that caused the mild disease cowpox to produce immunity against smallpox. Today the word has the same meaning as INOCULATION and IMMUNIZATION.

vaccine (vak-sēn′) a suspension of attenuated or killed microorganisms (viruses, bacteria, or rickettsiae), administered for prevention, amelioration, or treatment of infectious diseases.

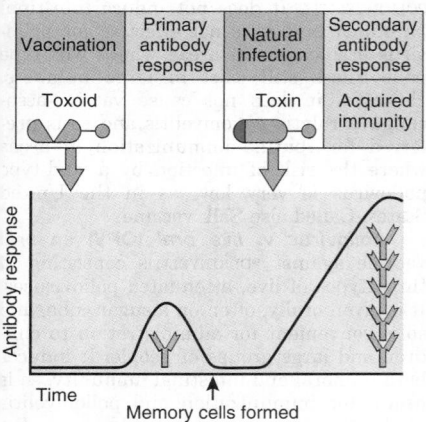

The principle of vaccination is illustrated by immunization with tetanus toxoid. Chemical modification of tetanus toxin produces a toxoid which has lost toxicity but retains its epitopes. Thus, a primary antibody response to these epitopes is produced following vaccination with toxoid. In a natural infection the toxin restimulates B memory cells, which produce the faster and more intense secondary antibody response to the epitope, so neutralizing the toxin. From Roitt et al., 2001.

anthrax v. a cell-free protein extract of cultures of *Bacillus anthracis,* used for immunization against ANTHRAX.

attenuated v. a vaccine prepared from live microorganisms or viruses cultured under adverse conditions, leading to loss of their virulence but retention of their ability to induce protective immunity.

autogenous v. a vaccine prepared from microorganisms which have been freshly isolated from the lesion of the patient who is to be treated with it.

bacterial v. a preparation of killed or attenuated bacteria used as an active immunizing agent.

BCG v. see BCG VACCINE.

cholera v. a preparation of killed *Vibrio cholerae,* administered intradermally, subcutaneously, or intramuscularly for immunization against CHOLERA.

diphtheria and tetanus toxoids and pertussis v. DTP vaccine: a combination of diphtheria and tetanus toxoids and pertussis vaccine; administered intramuscularly for simultaneous immunization against diphtheria, tetanus, and whooping cough. When the pertussis vaccine is an acellular form, the combination may be abbreviated DTaP.

diphtheria and tetanus toxoids and pertussis v. adsorbed and Haemophilus b conjugate v. a combination of diphtheria TOXOID, tetanus TOXOID, pertussis vaccine, and *Haemophilus* b conjugate vaccine; administered intramuscularly to children 18 months to 5 years of age for simultaneous immunization against DIPHTHERIA, TETANUS, whooping COUGH, and infection by HAEMOPHILUS INFLUENZAE type b.

DTP v. diphtheria and tetanus toxoids and pertussis vaccine.

Haemophilus b conjugate v. (HbCV) a preparation of *Haemophilus influenzae* type b capsular polysaccharide covalently bound to diphtheria toxoid or to a specific diphtheria protein, meningococcal protein, or tetanus protein; it stimulates both B and T lymphocyte responses and is much more immunogenic than the polysaccharide vaccine. Administered intramuscularly as a routine immunizing agent in infants and young children.

Haemophilus b polysaccharide v. (HbPV) a preparation of highly purified capsular polysaccharide derived from *Haemophilus influenzae* type b, which stimulates an IMMUNE RESPONSE in B lymphocytes only; administered intramuscularly or subcutaneously as an immunizing agent in children ages 18 months to 5 years.

hepatitis A v. inactivated an inactivated whole virus vaccine derived from an attenuated strain of hepatitis A virus grown in cell culture; administered intramuscularly.

hepatitis B v. a preparation of hepatitis B surface antigen, derived either from human plasma of carriers of hepatitis B *(hepatitis B vaccine inactivated)* or from cloning in yeast cells *(hepatitis B vaccine [recombinant]);* administered intramuscularly.

heterologous v. a vaccine that confers protective immunity against a pathogen that shares cross-reacting antigens with the microorganisms in the vaccine.

human diploid cell v. rabies vaccine prepared from rabies virus grown in cultures of human diploid embryo lung cells and inactivated; administered intramuscularly or intradermally.

influenza virus v. a killed virus vaccine used in immunization against INFLUENZA; it is trivalent, usually containing two influenza A virus strains and one influenza B virus strain.

live v. a vaccine prepared from live microorganisms that have been attenuated but retain their immunogenic properties.

Lyme disease v. (recombinant OspA) a preparation of outer surface protein A (OspA), a cell surface lipoprotein of *Borrelia burgdorferi,* produced by recombinant technology; administered intramuscularly for active immunization against LYME DISEASE.

measles, mumps, and rubella virus v. live (MMR) a combination of live attenuated measles, mumps, and rubella viruses, administered subcutaneously for simultaneous immunization against MEASLES, MUMPS, and RUBELLA.

measles and rubella virus v. live a combination of live attenuated measles and rubella viruses, administered subcutaneously for simultaneous immunization against MEASLES and RUBELLA.

measles virus v. live a live attenuated virus vaccine used for immunization against MEASLES, although it is usually administered as the combination measles, mumps, and rubella virus VACCINE.

meningococcal polysaccharide v. a preparation of a capsular antigen of *Neisseria meningitidis,* administered subcutaneously to provide immunity to MENINGITIS.

mumps virus v. live a live attenuated virus vaccine used in immunization against MUMPS; usually administered as the combination measles, mumps, and rubella virus VACCINE.

pertussis v. a preparation of killed *Bordetella pertussis* bacilli (whole-cell vaccine) or of purified antigenic components thereof (acellular vaccine), used to immunize against pertussis; generally used in combination with diphtheria and tetanus toxoids (DTP or DTaP).

plague v. a preparation of killed *Yersinia pestis* bacilli, administered intramuscularly as an active immunizing agent against PLAGUE.

pneumococcal heptavalent conjugate v. a preparation of capsular polysaccharides from the seven serotypes of *Streptococcus pneumoniae* most commonly isolated from children 6 years of age or younger, coupled to a nontoxic variant of diphtheria toxin; used as an active immunizing agent for infants and children at risk for pneumococcal disease, administered intramuscularly.

pneumococcal v. polyvalent a preparation of purified capsular polysaccharides from the 23 serotypes of *Streptococcus pneumoniae* causing the majority of pneumococcal disease; used as an active immunizing agent in persons over 2 years of age, administered intramuscularly.

poliovirus v. inactivated (IPV) a preparation of killed POLIOVIRUSES of three types, given in a series of intramuscular or subcutaneous injections to immunize against POLIOMYELITIS. It does not induce intestinal immunity and so is not effective for poliovirus eradication in areas where wild-type polioviruses still exist in large numbers. However, it does not cause vaccine-associated paralytic poliomyelitis and so is preferred for routine immunization in areas where the risk of infection by a wild-type poliovirus is very low, as in the United States. Called also Salk vaccine.

poliovirus v. live oral (OPV) an oral vaccine against POLIOMYELITIS consisting of three types of live, attenuated polioviruses. It is given orally, often on a sugar cube, and so is convenient for administration to children and large groups of people. It induces both humoral and intestinal immunity, so is useful for immunization and poliomyelitis eradication in areas where wild-type polioviruses have not been eradicated. However, it can cause vaccine-associated paralytic poliomyelitis in persons newly vaccinated with it and their contacts, which is considered an unjustifiable risk in countries such as the United States, where the risk of exposure to wild-type polioviruses is very low. Thus, for routine immunization in the

United States, it has been superseded by poliovirus VACCINE inactivated. Called also Sabin vaccine.

polyvalent v. a vaccine prepared from cultures or antigens of more than one strain or species.

purified chick embryo cell v. an inactivated virus vaccine used for pre- and postexposure RABIES immunization, prepared from rabies virus grown in cultures of chicken fibroblasts; administered intramuscularly.

rabies v. any of various vaccines against RABIES consisting of inactivated virus, used for preexposure immunization to persons at high risk of exposure, such as veterinarians, and for postexposure prophylaxis in conjunction with rabies immune GLOBULIN. See HUMAN DIPLOID CELL V., PURIFIED CHICK EMBRYO CELL V., and RABIES V. ADSORBED.

rabies v. adsorbed (RVA) a rabies vaccine prepared from rabies virus grown in cultures of fetal rhesus monkey lung and inactivated; administered intramuscularly.

rotavirus v. live oral a live virus vaccine produced from a mixture of four types of ROTAVIRUS, used to immunize infants against rotaviral GASTROENTERITIS.

rubella and mumps virus v. live a combination of live attenuated rubella and mumps viruses, administered subcutaneously for simultaneous immunization against RUBELLA and MUMPS.

rubella virus v. live a live attenuated virus vaccine used for immunization against RUBELLA, usually administered as the combination measles, mumps, and rubella virus VACCINE.

Sabin v. poliovirus vaccine live oral.

Salk v. poliovirus vaccine inactivated.

subunit v. a vaccine produced from specific protein subunits of a virus and thus having less risk of adverse reactions than whole virus vaccines.

typhoid v. any of several preparations of *Salmonella typhi* used for immunization against TYPHOID FEVER, including a parenteral heat- and phenol-inactivated bacteria vaccine, an oral live vaccine prepared from the attenuated strain Ty21a, and a parenteral vaccine prepared from typhoid Vi capsular polysaccharide.

varicella virus v. live a preparation of live, attenuated human HERPESVIRUS 3 (varicella-zoster virus) administered subcutaneously for production of immunity to VARICELLA and HERPES ZOSTER.

yellow fever v. a preparation of attenuated yellow fever virus, used to immunize against YELLOW FEVER.

vaccinia (vak-sin′e-ah) the cutaneous and sometimes systemic reactions associated

with vaccination with smallpox vaccine. See also COWPOX and PARAVACCINIA.

v. gangreno′sa generalized vaccinia with failure to develop antibodies against the virus (due to AGAMMAGLOBULINEMIA), with spreading necrosis at the site and metastasis of lesions throughout the body.

generalized v. a condition of widespread vaccinial lesions resulting from sensitivity response to smallpox vaccination and delayed production of neutralizing antibodies.

progressive v. vaccinia gangrenosa.

vaccinial (vak-sin′e-al) pertaining to or characteristic of vaccinia.

vacciniform (vak-sin′ĭ-form) resembling vaccinia.

vaccinotherapy (vak″sĭ-no-ther′ah-pe) therapeutic use of vaccines.

vacuolar (vak′u-o″lar) containing, or of the nature of, vacuoles.

vacuolated (vak′u-o-lāt″ed) containing vacuoles.

vacuolation (vak″u-o-la′shun) the process of forming vacuoles; the condition of being vacuolated.

vacuole (vak′u-ōl) a space or cavity in the protoplasm of a cell.

contractile v. a small fluid-filled cavity in the protoplasm of certain unicellular organisms. It gradually increases in size and then collapses; its function is thought to be respiratory and excretory.

vacuolization (vak″u-o-li-za′shun) vacuolation.

vacuum (vak′u-um) a space devoid of air or other gas.

vagabond's disease discoloration of the skin in persons subjected to louse bites over long periods.

vagal (va′gal) pertaining to the vagus nerve.

vagectomy (va-jek′tah-me) surgical excision of a segment of the vagus nerve.

vagina (vah-ji′nah), pl. *vagi′nae* 1. any SHEATH or sheathlike structure. 2. the canal in the female that extends from the external genitalia (VULVA) to the CERVIX UTERI. The adult vagina is normally about 8 cm (3 in) long and slopes upward and backward. Internally, the BLADDER is in front of the vagina and the RECTUM in back. The vagina receives the erect PENIS in coitus; spermatozoa are discharged into it, swim through the cervical canal, and enter the UTERUS. The vagina is also the passage for menstrual discharge, and it functions as the birth canal.

The interior lining of the vagina is mucous membrane; muscles and fibrous

V

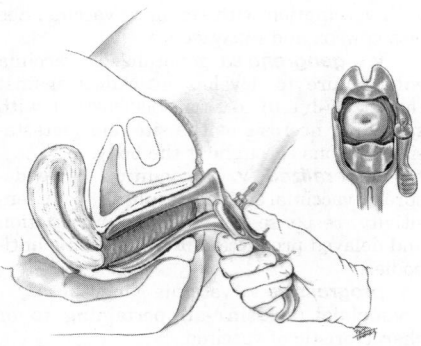

Vaginal examination. From Jarvis, 2000.

tissue form its walls. In pregnancy, changes occur in these tissues, enabling the vagina to stretch to many times its usual size during labor and childbirth. In a virgin, the opening of the vagina is usually, but not necessarily, partially closed by a membrane, the HYMEN. Usually the hymen breaks at first intercourse; occasionally it ruptures during physical exercise.

In a normal state, the lining of the vagina secretes a fluid that is fermented to an acid by the bacteria that are usually present. This acidity probably helps to protect the vagina from invasion by other organisms. Douching as a regular practice should not be employed except when recommended by a health care provider.

Vaginal Examination. Since cancer of the female reproductive organs is a relatively common occurrence and is curable if detected early, physicians recommend that women of reproductive age and beyond have a periodic vaginal or pelvic examination. Such an examination is also necessary during pregnancy and labor and in the postpartum examination 6 to 8 weeks after childbirth. This is a simple procedure that is rarely uncomfortable if the woman understands its purpose.

The patient lies on her back on a special table with her legs raised and spread by stirrups. The examiner inserts a speculum to spread the vagina open and thus is able to observe the cervix and the lining of the vagina directly, and may take smears for microscopic examination to detect infection or cancer of the vagina or cervix. (See also PAPANICOLAOU TEST.)

After removing the speculum the examiner inserts rubber-gloved fingers into the vagina and places the other hand on the abdomen. In this way it is possible to palpate the female reproductive organs, including the uterus and ovaries, between the hands. These organs are otherwise difficult or impossible to examine.

Patient Care. The patient should be prepared physically and emotionally for a vaginal examination. Since relaxation and cooperation of the patient are important to the success of the examination, she should be given a brief explanation of the procedure and encouraged to ask questions before the procedure is begun. The patient is draped with a top sheet so that the legs are covered and only the vulva is exposed. Privacy must be assured immediately before and during the examination. Equipment such as gloves, lubricant, vaginal speculum, and supplies needed for collecting specimens should be assembled before the examination is begun. After the examination is completed, the patient is assisted from the table.

Ideally, a vaginal examination should be done between menstrual periods; however, vaginal bleeding is not a contraindication to this procedure. Patients should be told this so that they will not postpone an appointment for examination when vaginal bleeding persists. They should not take over the counter medications or douche immediately before a vaginal examination; douching might remove secretions that could be useful in diagnosis.

vaginal (vaj′ĭ-nal) 1. pertaining to the VAGINA or to any sheath. 2. pertaining to the TUNICA VAGINALIS TESTIS.

vaginalectomy (vaj″ĭ-nal-ek′tah-me) vaginectomy.

vaginalitis (vaj″ĭ-nal-i′tis) periorchitis.

vaginate (vaj′ĭ-nāt) enclosed in a sheath.

vaginectomy (vaj″ĭ-nek′tah-me) 1. surgical excision of the vagina; called also colpectomy. 2. resection of the tunica vaginalis testis.

vaginismus (vaj″ĭ-niz′mus) painful spasm of the vagina due to involuntary contraction of the vaginal musculature, usually severe enough to prevent intercourse; the cause may be organic or psychogenic.

vaginitis (vaj″ĭ-ni′tis) 1. inflammation of any sheathlike structure. 2. inflammation of the vagina; called also colpitis.

Etiology. Inflammation of the vaginal mucosa is invariably related to a disturbance in normal vaginal physiology. A healthy vagina depends on (1) normal estrogen secretion to maintain a thick squamous epithelium containing glycogen and (2) chemical reactions beginning with the glycogen thus available. The glycogen stimulates the growth of lactobacilli, which are beneficial normal vaginal flora that metabolize glycogen to

TYPES OF VAGINITIS			
	Gardnerella vaginalis	*Trichomonas*	*Candida*
Onset	May note odor only after sexual intercourse	May appear or worsen immediately after menstruation	Abrupt; before menstruation
Odor	Fishy odor; particularly after sexual intercourse	Foul discharge with acute infection	Absent
Itching	Absent, since does not invade vaginal wall	Occasionally present, but varies according to degree of inflammation	Severe; the most prominent symptom
Discharge	Thin, gray homogeneous; frothy in 7%	Amount varies, often gray; green in only 10%, frothy in only 10%	Unusual, except in pregnancy
Associated Factors	None	Often acute during pregnancy	Often associated with pregnancy, glycosuria, diabetes, antibiotic use
Sexual Transmission	Yes	Yes	Unlikely
Vulvar Signs	Absent	Usually absent; erythema or edema can be present if discharge is profuse	Excoriation from scratching; erythema; possible edema of labia
Vaginal Signs	Little or no erythema, discharge adherent to vaginal wall; cervix normal	Diffuse erythema; vaginal/cervical petechiae or "strawberry" appearance in 10%; cervix may bleed easily, otherwise normal	Discharge adherent to vaginal wall; "cottage cheese" appearance or "curds" present only in heavy colonization; cervix normal

form lactic acid. The lactic acid maintains vaginal acidity at a pH of 4.0 to 4.5.

Tampons, condoms, neglected diaphragms, and irritating douches or deodorant sprays can upset the vagina's environmental balance and produce abnormal vaginal discharge. Hyperglycemia and antibiotics can also disturb this balance. However, infectious agents are the most common cause of vaginitis; these include *Trichomonas* and *Candida*. (See also bacterial VAGINOSIS.) Characteristics of these types of vaginitis and medical treatment and nursing intervention are summarized in the accompanying table.

Patient Education. Patients with infectious vaginitis need to know the purpose and importance of diagnostic testing and examination to verify a diagnosis, the specific type of infection or infections thus identified, and changes that may need to be made in their sexual activity to avoid reinfection. Sexual intercourse is avoided while active symptoms are present. Concurrent treatment of the partner is often necessary to avoid cyclic reinfection of one another. Condoms are encouraged because they can provide both the man and woman with some protection against sexually transmitted diseases.

In regard to prescribed treatment, the patient should be instructed to take *all* of the medication exactly as prescribed; a follow-up examination and testing may be necessary. If the woman has a cervical Pap smear done while she has vaginitis, there may be an abnormal test result.

adhesive v. atrophic vaginitis with ulceration and exfoliation of the mucosa result in adhesions of the membranes; opposite surfaces may adhere to each other, causing obliteration of the vaginal canal. Called also senile vaginitis.

atrophic v. vaginitis occurring in postmenopausal women, associated with estrogen deficiency. The two most common types are senile vulvovaginitis and adhesive vaginitis.

Candida v., candidal v. vulvovaginal candidiasis.

desquamative inflammatory v. a form resembling atrophic vaginitis but affecting women with normal estrogen levels.

emphysematous v. inflammation of the vagina and adjacent cervix, characterized by numerous asymptomatic, gas-filled cystlike lesions.

senile v. adhesive vaginitis.

vaginoabdominal (vaj″ĭ-no-ab-dom′ĭ-nal) pertaining to the vagina and abdomen.

vaginocele (vaj′ĭ-no-sēl″) 1. vaginal hernia. 2. prolapse or falling of the vagina; called also colpoptosis.

vaginodynia (vaj″ĭ-no-din′e-ah) pain in the vagina.

V

vaginofixation (vaj″ĭ-no-fik-sa′shun) vaginopexy; colpopexy.

vaginolabial (vaj″ĭ-no-la′be-al) pertaining to the vagina and labia.

vaginomycosis (vaj″ĭ-no-mi-ko′sis) any fungal disease of the vagina, such as vulvovaginal candidiasis.

vaginopathy (vaj″ĭ-nop′ah-the) any disease of the vagina.

vaginoperineal (vaj″ĭ-no-per″ĭ-ne′al) pertaining to the vagina and perineum.

vaginoperineoplasty (vaj″ĭ-no-per″ĭ-ne′o-plas″te) plastic surgery of the vagina and perineum.

vaginoperineorrhaphy (vaj″ĭ-no-per″ĭ-ne-or′ah-fe) suture of the vagina and perineum; colpoperineorrhaphy.

vaginoperineotomy (vaj″ĭ-no-per″ĭ-ne-ot′ah-me) incision of the vagina and perineum.

vaginoperitoneal (vaj″ĭ-no-per″ĭ-to-ne′al) pertaining to the vagina and peritoneum.

vaginopexy (vah-ji′no-pek″se) colpopexy; vaginofixation; suturing of the vagina to the abdominal wall in cases of vaginal relaxation.

vaginoplasty (vah-ji′no-plas″te) colpoplasty; plastic repair of the vagina.

vaginoscope (vaj′ĭ-no-skōp) a vaginal SPECULUM; called also colposcope.

vaginosis (vaj″ĭ-no′sis) a disease of the vagina.

bacterial v. a nonspecific vaginal infection associated with positive cultures for *Gardnerella vaginalis,* characterized by increased malodorous vaginal discharge that cannot be attributed to other causes.

vaginotomy (vaj″ĭ-not′ah-me) colpotomy.

vaginovesical (vaj″ĭ-no-ves′ĭ-kal) pertaining to the vagina and bladder.

vagitus (vah-ji′tus) the cry of an infant.

v. uteri′nus the cry of an infant in the uterus.

vagolysis (va-gol′ĭ-sis) surgical destruction of the vagus nerve.

vagolytic (va″go-lit′ik) 1. pertaining to or caused by VAGOLYSIS. 2. having an effect like that produced by interruption of impulses transmitted by the vagus nerve; see also PARASYMPATHOLYTIC.

vagomimetic (va″go-mi-met′ik) having an effect resembling that produced by stimulation of the vagus nerve.

vagotomy (va-got′ah-me) interruption of the impulses carried by the vagus nerve or nerves; so called because it was first performed by surgical methods. The surgical procedure is done as part of the treatment of gastric or duodenal ULCER and often is performed in combination with GASTRO-

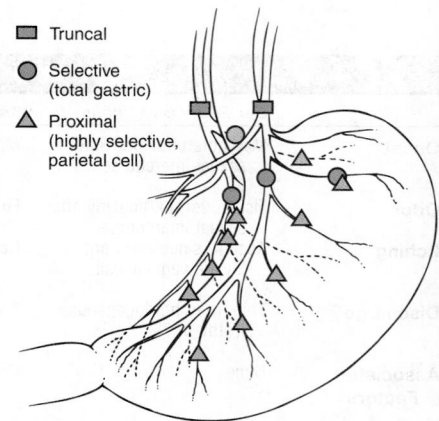

Sites at which the three types of vagotomy are performed.

☐ Truncal

● Selective (total gastric)

△ Proximal (highly selective, parietal cell)

ENTEROSTOMY or partial GASTRECTOMY. The vagus nerve stimulates gastric secretion and affects gastric motility, so that vagotomy reduces the secretion of gastric juices and decreases physical activity of the stomach.

highly selective v. division of only those vagal fibers supplying the acid-secreting glands of the stomach, with preservation of those supplying the antrum as well as of the hepatic and celiac branches.

medical v. interruption of impulses carried by the vagus nerve by administration of suitable drugs.

parietal cell v. selective severing of the vagus nerve fibers supplying the proximal two thirds (parietal area) of the stomach; done for duodenal ULCER.

selective v. division of the vagal fibers to the stomach with preservation of the hepatic and celiac branches.

truncal v. surgical division of the two main trunks of the abdominal vagus nerve as they emerge through the esophageal hiatus.

vagotonia (va″go-to′ne-ah) irritability of the vagus nerve, characterized by vasomotor instability, sweating, disordered peristalsis, and muscle spasms. adj., **vagoton′ic.**

vagotropic (va″go-trop′ik) having an effect on the vagus nerve.

vagovagal (va″go-va′gal) arising as a result of afferent and efferent impulses mediated through the vagus nerve.

vagus nerve (va′gus) the tenth CRANIAL NERVE; it has the most extensive distribution of the cranial nerves, serving structures of the chest and abdomen as well as the head and neck. Its afferent fibers serve the mucous membrane of the larynx, trachea, bronchi, lungs, arch of the aorta, esophagus, and stomach. Some of the functions affected by this nerve are coughing, sneezing, reflex inhibitions of the heart rate, and the sensation of hunger. Its motor fibers are concerned with swallowing, speech, peristalsis, and secretions from the glands of the stomach and the pancreas and contractions of the trachea, bronchi, and bronchioles. See Appendix 3-5.

valacyclovir (val″a-si′klo-vir) an ester of ACYCLOVIR, to which it is metabolized; used as the hydrochloride salt as an antiviral agent in treatment of genital HERPES and HERPES ZOSTER in patients who are not IMMUNOCOMPROMISED, administered orally.

valence (va′lens) 1. a positive number that represents the combining power of an element in a chemical compound, i.e., the number of bonds each atom of that element makes with other atoms. In this most general sense "valence" has been superseded by the concept "oxidation number." However, "valence" is still used to indicate (1) the number of covalent bonds formed by an atom in a covalent compound or (2) the charge on a monatomic or polyatomic molecule. 2. in immunology, the number of antigen binding sites possessed by an antibody molecule, two per immunoglobulin monomer, or the number of antigenic determinants possessed by an antigen, usually a large number.

valganciclovir (val″gan-si′klo-vir) a PRODRUG of GANCICLOVIR, used in treatment of CYTOMEGALOVIRUS infections in IMMUNOCOMPROMISED patients; administered orally as the hydrochloride salt.

valgus (val′gus) [L.] bent or twisted outward; denoting a deformity in which the angulation is away from the midline of the body, as in talipes valgus.

validation (val″ĭ-da′shun) confirmation or corroboration; the declaration of validity.

    consensual v. the confirmation of reality by comparison of one's own perceptions and concerns with those of others, including the recognition and modification of distortions.

validity (vah-lid′ĭ-te) the extent to which a measuring device measures what it intends or purports to measure.

    construct v. the degree to which an instrument measures the characteristic being investigated; the extent to which conceptual definitions match the operational definitions.

    content v. verification that the method of measurement actually measures what it is expected to measure; see also FACE VALIDITY.

    external v. the extent to which study findings can be generalized beyond the sample used in the study.

    face v. a type of content VALIDITY, determining the suitability of a given instrument as a source of data on the subject under investigation, using common-sense criteria.

    internal v. the extent to which the effects detected in a study are truly caused by the treatment or exposure in the study sample, rather than being due to other biasing effects of extraneous variables.

    predictive v. the effectiveness of one set of test or research results as a predictor of the outcome of future experiments or tests.

valine (va′lēn) a naturally occurring AMINO ACID, one of the essential amino acids.

valinemia (val″ĭ-ne′me-ah) hypervalinemia; elevated levels of valine in the blood and urine.

Valisone (val′ĭ-sōn) trademark for preparations of BETAMETHASONE valerate, a steroid ANTIINFLAMMATORY agent.

Valium (val′e-um) trademark for preparations of DIAZEPAM, an ANTIANXIETY AGENT, skeletal muscle RELAXANT, and ANTICONVULSANT.

vallate (val′āt) having a wall or rim; cup-shaped.

vallecula (vah-lek′u-lah) [L.] a depression or furrow.

    v. cerebel′li a longitudinal fissure on the inferior cerebellum, in which the medulla oblongata rests.

    v. syl′vii a depression made by the fissure of Sylvius at the base of the brain.

valley fever the primary form of COCCIDIOIDOMYCOSIS.

valproate (val-pro′āt) a salt of VALPROIC ACID with ANTICONVULSANT activity similar to that of the acid.

valproic acid (val-pro′ik) an ANTICONVULSANT administered orally for the control of seizures, particularly absence SEIZURES. Serious hepatotoxicity has occurred during valproic acid therapy, so that liver function tests should be performed periodically during treatment.

valrubicin (val-roo′bĭ-sin″) an antineoplastic AGENT that interferes with nucleic acid metabolism; used intravesically for treatment of bladder carcinoma.

Valsalva maneuver (val-sal′vah) 1. increase of intrathoracic pressure by forcible exhalation against the closed glottis; this maneuver causes trapping of blood in the great veins, preventing it from entering the chest and right atrium. When the breath is released, the intrathoracic pressure drops and the trapped blood is quickly propelled through the heart, producing TACHYCARDIA

V

(increased heart rate) and a rise in BLOOD PRESSURE; this is followed almost immediately by a reflex BRADYCARDIA. The Valsalva maneuver occurs when one strains to defecate and urinate, uses the arms and upper trunk muscles to move up in bed, or strains during coughing, gagging, or vomiting. The increased pressure, immediate tachycardia, and reflex bradycardia can bring about cardiac arrest in vulnerable heart patients. 2. increase in the pressure in the eustachian tube and middle ear by forcible exhalation against closed nostrils and mouth.

valsartan (val-sahr′tan) an ANGIOTENSIN II antagonist used as an ANTIHYPERTENSIVE, administered orally.

value (val′u) 1. a measure of worth or efficiency. 2. a quantitative measurement of the activity, concentration, or some other quality of something. 3. an operational belief; an ideal, custom, institution of a society toward which the members of a group have an affective regard; any object or quality desirable as a means or as an end in itself. In exchange theory, the benefits received through an exchange minus the price paid in return.

biological v. the quality of a protein expressed on a scale of 1 to 100; the higher the number the better the quality.

cultural v's prevailing and persistent guides influencing the thinking and action of members of a cultural group. Values direct one's perceptions of others and serve as the basis for a person's opinions. Individuals belonging to groups with different cultural values may clash on health and illness behavior.

normal v's the range in concentration of specific substances found in normal healthy tissues, secretions, and so on.

P v., p v. the probability of obtaining by chance a result at least as extreme as that observed, even when the null hypothesis is true and no real difference exists; when $P < 0.05$ the sample results are usually deemed significant at a statistically important level and the null hypothesis rejected. See also Type I ERROR.

reference v's a set of values of a quantity measured in the clinical laboratory that characterize a specified population in a defined state of health. The values obtained from a statistical sample are used to establish a *reference interval* that covers 95 per cent of the values of the healthy general population or of specific subpopulations differing in age and sex. These concepts were originally and are still widely referred to as "normal values" and the "normal range," but the use of these terms is now discouraged because of their implication that values falling outside of the reference interval are "abnormal" or "unhealthy," which has led to much confusion. It must be remembered that, by definition, 5 per cent of healthy individuals fall outside of the reference interval.

valva (val′vah) [L.] valve.

valve (valv) a membranous fold in a canal or passage that prevents backward flow of material passing through it.

aortic v. a semilunar VALVE that separates the left ventricle and the aorta; it opens with end diastole, causing the second HEART SOUND.

atrioventricular v's the cardiac VALVES between the right atrium and right ventricle (tricuspid valve) and the left atrium and left ventricle (mitral valve).

bicuspid v. mitral valve.

bicuspid aortic v. a congenital anomaly of the aortic valve, caused by incomplete separation of two of the three cusps; it is generally asymptomatic early in life but is predisposed to calcification and stenosis later on.

Braschi v. a one-way valve put into the inspiratory limb of a VENTILATOR circuit in order to measure the intrinsic positive end-expiratory PRESSURE.

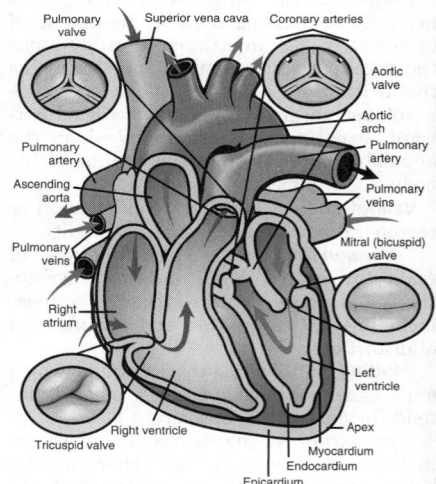

Valves of the heart. The right heart pumps the venous blood into the lungs. The oxygenated blood returns from the lungs into the left atrium and is propelled by the left ventricle into the aorta. The insets show closed valves: the tricuspid valve has three leaflets, whereas the mitral valve has two leaflets. The aortic and pulmonary artery valves have three leaflets and resemble one another except for the fact that the coronary arteries originate from behind the cusps in the aorta. From Damjanov, 1996.

cardiac v's valves that control flow of blood through and from the heart.

coronary v. a valve at the entrance of the coronary sinus into the right atrium.

flail mitral v. a mitral VALVE having a cusp that has lost its normal support (as in ruptured chordae tendineae) and flutters in the blood stream.

heart v's cardiac valves.

Heimlich v. a small one-way valve used for chest drainage, emptying into a flexible collection device; the valve prevents return of gases or fluids into the pleural space. The Heimlich valve is less than 13 cm (5 inches) long and facilitates patient ambulation; it can be used in many patients instead of a traditional water seal drainage system.

ileocecal v., ileocolic v. the valve guarding the opening between the ileum and cecum.

mitral v. the cardiac VALVE between the left atrium and left ventricle, usually having two cusps (anterior and posterior). Called also bicuspid valve.

posterior urethral v. any of various types of congenital folds across the proximal part of the male URETHRA near the seminal COLLICULUS, the most common cause of urethral obstruction in male infants.

pulmonary v., pulmonic v. the pocketlike cardiac VALVE that protects the orifice between the right ventricle and the pulmonary artery.

pyloric v. a prominent fold of mucous membrane at the pyloric orifice of the stomach.

semilunar v's the cardiac VALVES that have semilunar CUSPS; see aortic valve and pulmonary valve.

thebesian v. coronary valve.

tricuspid v. the cardiac VALVE guarding the opening between the right atrium and right ventricle.

v. of vein, venous v's any of the small cusps or folds found in the tunica intima of many veins, serving to prevent backflow of blood.

valvotomy (val-vot′ah-me) incision of a valve, such as a stenosed cardiac valve for the relief of obstruction; called also valvulotomy.

valvula (val′vu-lah) [L.] valvule: a small VALVE; formerly used in official nomenclature to designate any valve, but now restricted to certain small valves in the body and CUSPS of heart valves.

valvular (val′vu-ler) pertaining to, affecting, or of the nature of a valve.

valvule a small VALVE; see VALVULA.

valvulitis (val″vu-li′tis) inflammation of a valve, especially of a valve of the heart.

valvuloplasty (val′vu-lo-plas″te) plastic repair of a valve, especially a valve of the heart.

balloon v. dilation of a stenotic cardiac valve by means of a balloon-tipped catheter that is introduced into the valve and inflated.

valvulotome (val′vu-lo-tōm″) an instrument for cutting a valve.

valvulotomy (val″vu-lot′ah-me) valvotomy.

vanadium (vah-na′de-um) a chemical element, atomic number 23, atomic weight 50.942, symbol V. (See Appendix 6.) Its salts have been used in treating various diseases. Absorption of its compounds, usually via the lungs, causes chronic intoxication, the symptoms of which include respiratory tract irritation, pneumonitis, conjunctivitis, and anemia.

vanadiumism (vah-na′de-um-izm″) poisoning by vanadium.

Vancenase (van′sĕ-nāz″) trademark for preparations of BECLOMETHASONE dipropionate, a glucocorticoid used to treat allergic rhinitis and other allergic and inflammatory nasal conditions.

Vanceril (van′sĕ-ril″) trademark for a BECLOMETHASONE dipropionate metered-dose INHALER used for bronchial asthma.

vancomycin (van″ko-mi′sin) an ANTIBIOTIC produced by *Streptomyces orientalis,* highly effective against gram-positive bacteria, especially against STAPHYLOCOCCI; it is used as the hydrochloride salt. It is administered intravenously in the treatment of severe staphylococcal infections resistant to other antibiotics and is administered orally in the treatment of staphylococcal enterocolitis and antibiotic-associated pseudomembranous enterocolitis caused by *Clostridium difficile.* Toxic effects may be severe and include damage to the eighth cranial (vestibulocochlear) nerve and renal disorders.

van der Hoeve's syndrome (van der hōvz) see OSTEOGENESIS IMPERFECTA.

vanillism (vah-nil′izm) dermatitis, coryza, and malaise seen in handlers of raw vanilla, due to the mite *Acarus siro.*

vanillylmandelic acid (vah-nil″il-mandel′-ik) VMA; the primary end-product of catecholamine metabolism excreted in the urine. Urinary VMA levels are used in screening patients for pheochromocytoma.

Vansil (van′sil) trademark for a preparation of OXAMNIQUINE, an ANTHELMINTIC.

van't Hoff's rule (law) (vant-hofs′) the velocity of chemical reactions is increased twofold or more for each rise of 10°C in temperature; it is generally true when temperatures approximate those at which the reaction normally occurs.

vapor (va′por), pl. *vapo′res, vapors* [L.] 1. steam, gas, or exhalation. 2. an atmospheric

V

dispersion of a substance that in its normal state is liquid or solid.

vaporization (va″por-ĭ-za′shun) 1. the conversion of a solid or liquid into a vapor without chemical change. See also NEBULIZATION. 2. distillation.

vaporize (va′por-īz) to convert into vapor or to be transformed into vapor.

Vaquez's disease (vah-kāz′ez) polycythemia vera.

variability (var″e-ah-bil′ĭ-te) the state of being variable.

variable (var′e-ah-b'l) something that changes; an attribute or property of a person, event, or object that is known to vary in a given study.

   dependent v. in a mathematical equation or relationship between two or more variables, a variable whose value depends on those of others; it represents a response, behavior, or outcome that the researcher wishes to predict or explain.

   extraneous v. a factor that is not itself under study but affects the measurement of the study variables or the examination of their relationships.

   independent v. in a mathematical equation or relationship between two or more variables, any variable whose value determines that of others; it represents the treatment or experimental variable that is manipulated by the researcher to create an effect on the dependent variable.

variance (vār′e-ans) a measure of the variation shown by a set of observations; the average of the squared deviations from the mean; it is the square of the standard DEVIATION.

varicella (var″ĭ-sel′ah) chickenpox.

varicelliform (var″ĭ-sel′ĭ-form) resembling chickenpox.

Varicellovirus (var″ĭ-sel′o-vi″rus) a genus of HERPESVIRUSES that infects both humans and animals; the most common species affecting humans is human HERPESVIRUS 3, which causes CHICKENPOX and HERPES ZOSTER.

varices (vār′ĭ-sēz) [L.] plural of VARIX.

variciform (vah-ris′ĭ-form) varicose.

varicoblepharon (var″ĭ-ko-blef′ah-ron) a varicose swelling of the eyelid.

varicocele (var′ĭ-ko-sēl″) varicosity of the pampiniform plexus of the spermatic cord, forming a scrotal swelling that feels like a "bag of worms."

varicocelectomy (var″ĭ-ko-se-lek′tah-me) excision of a varicocele.

varicography (var″ĭ-kog′rah-fe) x-ray visualization of varicose veins.

varicomphalus (var″ĭ-kom′fah-lus) a varicose tumor of the umbilicus.

varicophlebitis (var″ĭ-ko-flĕ-bi′tis) varicose veins with inflammation.

varicose (var′ĭ-kōs) 1. of the nature of or pertaining to a varix. 2. unnaturally and permanently distended (said of a vein); called also variciform.

   v. veins swollen, distended, and knotted veins, usually in the subcutaneous tissues of a lower limb; they result from stagnated or sluggish flow of the blood, combined with defective valves and weakened vein walls. This occurs most often in those who must stand or sit motionless for long periods. Pregnancy is also sometimes a causative factor. It also appears that a tendency to develop varicose veins may be inherited.

Causes. Blood returning to the heart from the lower limbs must flow upward through the veins against the pull of gravity; it is "milked" upward principally by the massaging action of the muscles against the veins. To prevent the blood from flowing backward, the veins contain flaplike valves, located at frequent intervals and operating in pairs. When the blood is flowing toward the heart, these are open and the blood can move freely. If the blood should attempt to flow backward, the valves close, effectively stopping the reverse movement of the blood.

   Prolonged periods of standing or sitting without movement place a heavy strain on the veins. Without the massaging action of the muscles, the blood tends to back up. The weight of blood continually pressing downward against closed venous valves causes the veins to distend, and in time they lose their natural elasticity. When a number of valves no longer function efficiently, the blood collects in the veins, which gradually become swollen and more distended. During pregnancy, more force often is necessary to push the blood through the veins because of the pregnant uterus pressing against the veins coming from the legs and preventing the free flow of blood; this increased back pressure can cause varicose veins.

Symptoms. The development of varicose veins is usually gradual. There may be feelings of fatigue in the lower limbs, with cramps at night; a continual dull ache may develop in the legs, and the ankles may swell. If the condition is untreated and allowed to spread, as it often does, the veins become thick and hard to the touch, and dull or stabbing pains may be felt in time. Because of impaired circulation, ulcers often develop on the lower legs.

Treatment. Treatment of mild cases of varicose veins includes rest periods at intervals during the day; the patient lies flat with feet raised slightly above the level of

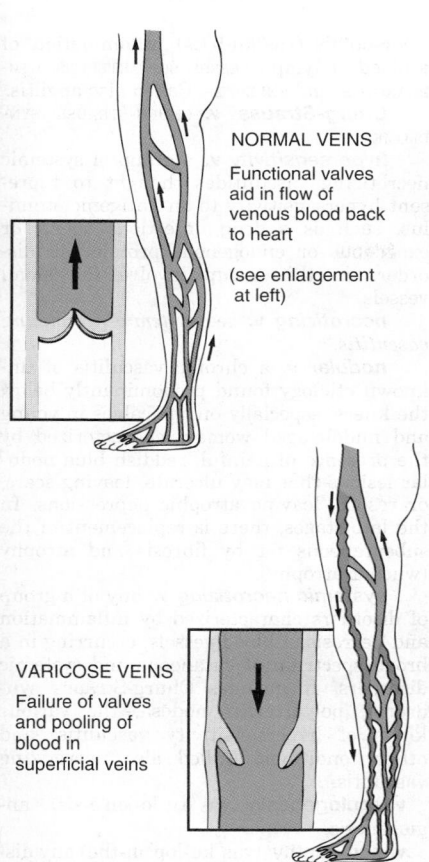

NORMAL VEINS

Functional valves aid in flow of venous blood back to heart

(see enlargement at left)

VARICOSE VEINS

Failure of valves and pooling of blood in superficial veins

Comparison of normal veins and varicose veins in the leg.

the heart. Bathing the legs in warm water helps to stimulate the flow of blood, as does exercise. The daily routine should be changed to allow movement and changes in posture; even a brief walk will stimulate circulation grown stagnant during a time of standing or sitting in one position. Stockings lightly reinforced with elastic can be worn to help support the veins in the legs. Heavy elastic stockings, however, should be fitted and worn only under medical supervision; if they do not fit correctly they may aggravate the condition by further restricting blood flow.

Injections. Certain cases of varicose veins that have developed past the stage when exercise and rest are helpful may be treated by SCLEROTHERAPY, the injection of a hardening, or sclerosing, solution into them. A few hours after this treatment, which usually can be performed in the primary care provider's office, the injected veins

become hard, tender to the touch, and painful. The pain subsides within a few days, however, and in about 2 months the varicose veins atrophy while the blood is channeled into other veins. The number of injections necessary depends upon the extent of the condition. This form of treatment usually is not recommended for advanced cases because it has been found that in such cases recurrence is likely after a varying period of time following the injections.

Surgery. Varicose veins can cause much discomfort. The poor circulation involved means that any break in the skin of the leg is likely to develop into an ulcer that is painful and heals slowly and with difficulty. Therefore, chronic or well-advanced varicose conditions are best treated surgically. The operation consists of ligating (tying off) the affected vein and removing it.

Prevention. Regular leg exercises such as long walks will stimulate the flow of blood through the limbs. Those who have a predisposition to varicose veins should make such activities a part of their regular routine. If possible, they should avoid occupations that require them to stand or sit motionless for long periods, or should make it a point to walk about and exercise their leg muscles often during working hours. Tight stockings or garters should not be worn, nor should clothing that fits tightly or binds. See also chronic leg ULCER.

varicosity (var″ĭ-kos′ĭ-te) 1. the quality or state of being VARICOSE; called also phlebectasia and venectasia. 2. varix. 3. a VARICOSE VEIN.

varicotomy (var″ĭ-kot′ah-me) excision of a varix or of a varicose vein.

varicula (vah-rik′u-lah) a varix of the conjunctiva.

variety (vah-ri′ĕ-te) a taxonomic subcategory of a species.

variola (vah-ri′o-lah) smallpox. adj., **vari′olar, vario′lous.**

v. mi′nor a mild form of smallpox having a low fatality rate.

variolate (var′e-o-lāt) 1. having the nature or appearance of smallpox. 2. to inoculate with smallpox virus.

varioliform (var″e-o′lĭ-form) resembling smallpox.

Varivax (var′ĭ-vaks) a vaccine against the varicella (chickenpox) virus. One dose is given to a child between age 12 months and 12 years; for those 13 years old or older, two doses are given 4 to 8 weeks apart.

varix (vār′iks) [L.] an enlarged, tortuous vein, artery, or lymphatic vessel.

V

aneurysmal v. a markedly dilated tortuous vessel; sometimes used to denote a form of arteriovenous aneurysm in which the blood flows directly into a neighboring vein without the intervention of a connecting sac.

arterial v. a racemose aneurysm or varicose artery.

esophageal varices varicosities of branches of the azygous vein which anastomose with tributaries of the portal vein in the lower esophagus; due to portal hypertension in cirrhosis of the liver.

lymph v., v. lympha'ticus a soft, lobulated swelling of a lymph node due to obstruction of lymphatic vessels.

varolian (vah-ro'le-an) pertaining to the pons.

varus (va'rus) [L.] bent or twisted inward; denoting a deformity in which the angulation of the part is toward the midline of the body, as in TALIPES varus.

vas (vas), pl. *va'sa* [L.] vessel. adj., **va'sal.**

v. aber'rans 1. a blind tube sometimes connected with the epididymis; a vestigial mesonephric tube. 2. any anomalous or unusual vessel.

va'sa affferen'tia vessels that convey fluid to a structure or part.

va'sa bre'via short gastric arteries.

v. de'ferens ductus deferens.

va'sa effferen'tia vessels that convey fluid away from a structure or part.

va'sa lympha'tica lymphatic vessels.

va'sa prae'via the presentation, in front of the fetal head during labor, of the blood vessels of the umbilical cord where they enter the placenta.

va'sa rec'ta re'nis long U-shaped vessels arising from the efferent glomerular arterioles of juxtamedullary nephrons and supplying the renal medulla. Called also arteriolae rectae renis.

va'sa vaso'rum the small nutrient arteries and veins in the walls of the larger blood vessels.

vas(o)- word element [L.], *vessel; duct.*

vascular (vas'ku-ler) pertaining to blood vessels or indicative of a copious blood supply.

vascularity (vas″ku-lar'ĭ-te) the condition of being vascular.

vascularization (vas″ku-lar-ĭ-za'shun) 1. vasculogenesis. 2. the natural or surgically induced development of vessels in a tissue.

vascularize (vas'ku-lar-īz″) to supply with vessels.

vasculature (vas'ku-lah-chur″) 1. circulatory system. 2. any part of the circulatory system. 3. the supply of vessels to a specific region.

vasculitis (vas″ku-li'tis) inflammation of a blood or lymph vessel; see ARTERITIS, LYMPHANGITIS, and PHLEBITIS. Called also angiitis.

Churg-Strauss v. CHURG-STRAUSS SYNDROME.

hypersensitivity v. a group of systemic necrotizing vasculitides thought to represent hypersensitivity to an antigenic stimulus, such as a drug, infectious agent, or exogenous or endogenous protein; all disorders in this group involve the small vessels.

necrotizing v. see *systemic necrotizing vasculitis.*

nodular v. a chronic vasculitis of unknown etiology found predominantly below the knees, especially on the calves in young and middle-aged women, characterized by the presence of painful, reddish blue nodular lesions that may ulcerate, leaving scars, or resorb, leaving atrophic depressions. In the late stages, there is replacement of the subcutaneous fat by fibrosis and atrophy (wucher atrophy).

systemic necrotizing v. any of a group of disorders characterized by inflammation and necrosis of blood vessels, occurring in a broad spectrum of cutaneous and systemic disorders. It includes Churg-Strauss syndrome, polyarteritis nodosa, the various kinds of hypersensitivity vasculitis, and other conditions. Called also necrotizing vasculitis.

vasculogenesis (vas″ku-lo-jen'ĕ-sis) angiogenesis.

vasculopathy (vas″ku-lop'ah-the) any disorder of the blood vessels; see also ANGIOPATHY.

vasectomy (vah-sek'tah-me) excision of the vas (ductus) deferens, or a portion of it; bilateral vasectomy results in sterility.

vasifactive (vas″ĭ-fak'tiv) vasoformative.

vasiform (vas'ĭ-form) resembling a vessel.

vasitis (vah-si'tis) deferentitis.

vasoactive (vas″o-ak'tiv) exerting an effect upon the caliber of blood vessels.

v. intestinal polypeptide (VIP) a peptide hormone that, in addition to its vasoactive properties, stimulates intestinal secretion of water and electrolytes, inhibits gastric secretion, promotes glycogenesis, causes hyperglycemia, and stimulates production of pancreatic juice. See also VIPOMA.

vasoconstriction (vas″o-kon-strik'shun) decrease in the caliber of blood vessels. adj., **vasoconstric'tive.**

vasoconstrictor (vas″o-kon-strik'tor) 1. causing constriction of the blood vessels. 2. an agent that so acts.

vasodepression (vas″o-de-presh'un) decrease in vascular resistance with hypotension.

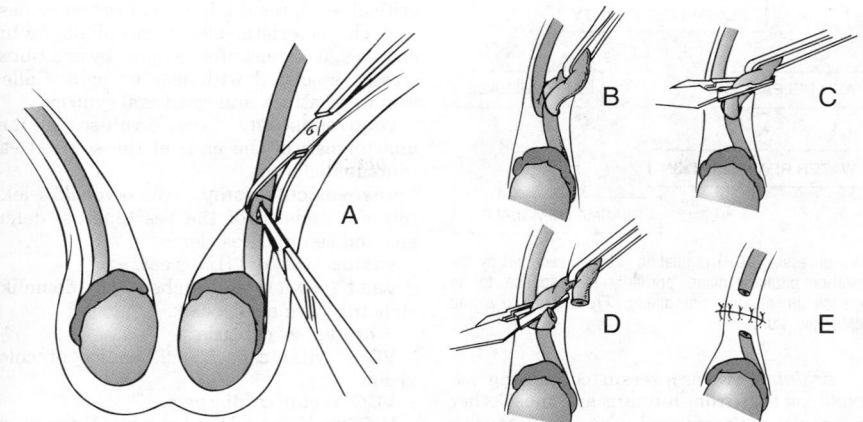

Vasectomy surgery. *A,* Incision exposes sheath, which is then opened. Vas is exposed *(B)* and occluded with two clips *(C). D,* Segment of about half an inch is excised. *E,* Vas is replaced in sheath and skin is sutured.

vasodepressor (vas″o-de-pres′or) 1. causing VASODEPRESSION; having the effect of lowering the blood pressure through reduction in peripheral resistance. 2. an agent that so acts.

Vasodilan (vas″o-di′lan) trademark for preparations of ISOXSUPRINE, a VASODILATOR used in peripheral vascular and cerebrovascular conditions.

vasodilatation (vas″o-dil″ah-ta′shun) vasodilation.

vasodilation (vas″o-di-la′shun) 1. increase in the caliber of blood vessels. 2. a state of increased caliber of blood vessels. Extreme, abnormal vasodilation is called ANGIECTASIS. adj., **vasodi′lative.**

vasodilator (vas″o-di-la′tor) 1. causing dilation of blood vessels. 2. a nerve or agent that has this effect.

vasoepididymography (vas″o-ep″ĭ-did″ĭ-mog′-rah-fe) radiography of the vas deferens and epididymis after injection of a contrast medium.

vasoepididymostomy (vas″o-ep″ĭ-did″ĭ-mos′tah-me) anastomosis of the vas (ductus) deferens and the epididymis.

vasoformative (vas″o-for′mah-tiv) angiogenic.

vasoganglion (vas″o-gang′gle-on) a vascular ganglion or rete.

vasography (vas-og′rah-fe) 1. angiography. 2. contrast delineation of the vas deferens and seminal vesicles.

vasohypertonic (vas″o-hi″per-ton′ik) vasoconstrictor (def. 1).

vasohypotonic (vas″o-hi″po-ton′ik) vasodilator (def. 1).

vasoinhibitor (vas″o-in-hib′ĭ-tor) an agent that inhibits vasomotor nerves. adj., **vasoinhib′itory.**

vasoligation (vas″o-li-ga′shun) ligation of the vas (ductus) deferens.

vasomotion (vas″o-mo′shun) change in caliber of blood vessels.

vasomotor (vas″o-mo′tor) 1. having an effect on the caliber of blood vessels; see also VASOACTIVE. 2. a vasomotor nerve.

vasoneuropathy (vas″o-nŏo-rop′ah-the) a condition caused by combined vascular and neurologic defect, resulting from simultaneous action or interaction of the vascular and nervous systems.

vasoneurosis (vas″o-nŏo-ro′sis) angioneurosis.

vasoparesis (vas″o-pah-re′sis) partial paralysis of vasomotor nerves.

vasopermeability (vas″o-per″me-ah-bil′ĭ-te) the permeability of a blood vessel; the extent to which a blood vessel is permeable.

vasopressin (vas″o-pres′in) a hormone secreted by cells of the hypothalamic nuclei and stored in the posterior pituitary for release as necessary; it stimulates contraction of the muscular tissues of the capillaries and arterioles, raising the blood pressure, and increases peristalsis, exerts some influence on the uterus, and influences resorption of water by the kidney tubules, resulting in concentration of urine. Its rate of secretion is regulated chiefly by the osmolarity of the plasma. Also prepared synthetically or obtained from the posterior pituitary of domestic animals; used as an antidiuretic. Called also antidiuretic hormone.

V

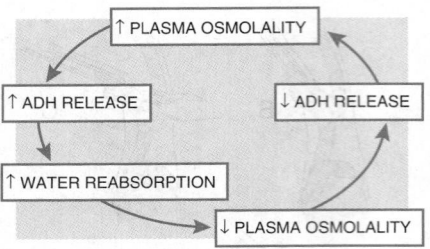

↑ PLASMA OSMOLALITY

↑ ADH RELEASE

↓ ADH RELEASE

↑ WATER REABSORPTION

↓ PLASMA OSMOLALITY

Vasopressin (ADH) regulation. ADH is secreted by the posterior pituitary gland primarily in response to an increase in plasma osmolality. From Malarkey and McMorrow, 2000.

arginine v. vasopressin containing AR-GININE, as that from humans and most other mammals; for medicinal uses, see vasopressin. Called also argipressin.

lysine v. the antidiuretic hormone of the pig family, differing from arginine vasopressin in having LYSINE instead of ARGININE at position 8. A synthetic preparation, LYPRESSIN, is used as an antidiuretic and vasoconstrictor.

vasopressor (vas″o-pres′or) 1. stimulating contraction of the muscular tissue of the capillaries and arteries. 2. an agent that has this effect.

vasopuncture (vas″o-pungk′chur) surgical puncture of the vas (ductus) deferens.

vasoreflex (vas″o-re′fleks) a reflex of blood vessels.

vasorelaxation (vas″o-re″lak-sa′shun) decrease of vascular pressure.

vasosection (vas″o-sek′shun) the severing of a vessel or vessels.

vasosensory (vas″o-sen′sah-re) supplying sensory filaments to the vessels.

vasospasm (vas′o-spazm) a spasm of blood vessels, causing VASOCONSTRICTION; called also angiospasm. adj., **vasospas′tic.**

vasostimulant (vas″o-stim′u-lant) stimulating vasomotor action.

vasotomy (vah-sot′ah-me) incision of the vas (ductus) deferens.

vasotonia (vas″o-to′ne-ah) tone or tension of the vessels.

vasotonic (vas″o-ton′ik) pertaining to, characterized by, or increasing vasotonia.

vasotrophic (vas″o-trof′ik) pertaining to the nutrition of blood vessels.

vasotropic (vas″o-trop′ik) exerting an influence on the blood vessels, causing either constriction or dilatation.

vasovagal (vas″o-va′gal) vascular and vagal.

v. attack a transient vascular and neurogenic reaction marked by pallor, nausea, sweating, bradycardia, and rapid fall in arterial blood pressure, which, when below a critical level, results in loss of consciousness and characteristic electroencephalographic changes. It is most often evoked by emotional stress associated with fear or pain. Called also vagal attack and vasovagal syncope.

vasovasostomy (vas″o-vah-sos′tah-me) anastomosis of the ends of the severed vas (ductus) deferens.

vasovesiculectomy (vas″o-vĕ-sik″u-lek′-tah-me) excision of the vas (ductus) deferens and seminal vesicle.

vastus (vas′tus) [L.] great.

vault (vawlt) an arched or domelike structure; see also FORNIX.

cranial v. calvaria.

VC 1. vital capacity. 2. acuity of color vision.

VCG vector cardiogram.

V-Cillin K (ve-sil′in) trademark for preparations of PENICILLIN V potassium, an ANTIBIOTIC.

VD venereal disease.

VDH valvular disease of the heart.

VDRL Venereal Disease Research Laboratory.

VDRL test a FLOCCULATION TEST for SYPHILIS designed by the Venereal Disease Research Laboratory; used to test heat-inactivated serum.

vection (vek′shun) the carrying of disease germs from an infected person to a well person.

vector (vek′tor) 1. a carrier, especially the animal (usually an arthropod) that transfers an infective agent from one host to another. Examples are the mosquito that carries the malaria parasite *Plasmodium* between humans, and the tsetse fly that carries trypanosomes from other animals to humans. Dogs, bats, and other animals are vectors that transmit the rabies virus to humans. 2. a PLASMID or viral CHROMOSOME into whose GENOME a fragment of foreign DNA is inserted, used to introduce the foreign DNA into a host cell in the cloning of DNA. 3. a quantity possessing magnitude, direction, and sense (positivity or negativity), and commonly represented by a straight line resembling an arrow; the length of the line denotes magnitude, the arrowhead denotes sense, and the position of the line with respect to an axis of reference denotes direction. adj., **vector′ial.**

biological v. an animal vector in whose body the pathogenic organism develops and multiplies before being transmitted to the next host.

mechanical v. an animal vector not essential to the life cycle of the parasite.

vectorcardiogram (VCG) (vek″tor-kahr′-de-o-gram″) a graphic representation of the magnitude and direction of the action currents of the heart, in the form of a vector loop. See also VECTORCARDIOGRAPHY.

vectorcardiography (vek″tor-kahr″de-og′-ah-fe) the registration, usually by formation of a loop on an oscilloscope, of the direction and magnitude (vector) of the moment-to-moment electromotive forces of the heart during one complete cycle. adj., **vectorcardiograph′ic.**

vecuronium (vek″u-ro′ne-um) a nondepolarizing neuromuscular blocking AGENT, used in the form of the bromide salt as an adjunct to general ANESTHESIA to induce relaxation of skeletal muscle and to facilitate endotracheal intubation and mechanical ventilation; administered intravenously.

vegan (ve′gan, vej′an) a vegetarian who excludes from the diet all food of animal origin.

veganism (ve′gan-izm, vej′ah-nizm) adherence to a strictly vegetable diet, with exclusion of all food of animal origin.

vegetable (vej′ĕ-tah-b′l) 1. pertaining to or derived from plants. 2. any plant or species of plant, especially one cultivated as a source of food.

vegetal (vej′ĕ-tal) pertaining to plants or a plant. 1. vegetative.

vegetarian (vej″ĕ-tar′e-an) 1. excluding meat. 2. one who follows a VEGETARIAN DIET.

v. diet one in which no meat is eaten. The strictly vegetarian (or VEGAN) diet allows no foods of animal origin. Maintenance of this diet requires a firm commitment to restriction of dietary intake, an extensive knowledge of dietary principles, and detailed planning to ensure nutritional adequacy. Deficiencies most likely to occur in a person who faithfully adheres to a vegetarian diet are those of protein, vitamin B_{12}, riboflavin, vitamin D, and calcium.

There are variations of the so-called vegetarian diet in which animal products such as eggs and cheese are allowed: a *lacto-vegetarian* diet allows milk and milk products but prohibits the intake of meat, poultry, fish, and eggs. An *ovo-lacto-vegetarian* diet allows all foods from plants plus eggs, milk, and other dairy products. An *ovo-vegetarian* diet allows eggs and foods of plant origin but prohibits meat, milk, and other dairy products.

vegetarianism (vej″ĕ-tar′e-ah-nizm″) adherence to a VEGETARIAN DIET.

vegetation (vej″ĕ-ta′shun) any plantlike fungoid neoplasm or growth; a luxuriant fungus-like growth of pathologic tissue.

vegetative (vej′ĕ-ta″tiv) 1. concerned with growth and nutrition. 2. functioning involuntarily or unconsciously. 3. resting; denoting the portion of a cell CYCLE during which

the cell is not replicating. 4. pertaining to plants. 5. pertaining to asexual REPRODUCTION, such as by budding or fission.

VEGF vascular endothelial growth factor.

vehicle (ve′ĭ-k′l) 1. excipient. 2. any medium through which an impulse is propagated.

veil (vāl) a covering structure; see also VELAMEN and VELUM. 1. caul. 2. slight huskiness of the voice.

vein (vān) a vessel through which blood passes from various organs or parts back to the heart, in the systemic circulation carrying blood that has given up most of its oxygen. Veins, like arteries, have three coats: an inner coat (TUNICA INTIMA), middle coat (TUNICA MEDIA), and outer coat (TUNICA EXTERNA); however, in veins these are less thick and collapse when the vessel is cut. Many veins, especially superficial ones, have valves formed of reduplication of their lining membrane. See Appendix 2-6 and see also Plates.

afferent v's veins that carry blood to an organ.

allantoic v's paired vessels that accompany the allantois, growing out from the primitive hindgut and entering the body stalk of the early embryo.

cardinal v's embryonic vessels that include the pre- and postcardinal veins and the ducts of Cuvier (common cardinal veins).

emissary v. one passing through a foramen of the skull and draining blood from a cerebral sinus into a vessel outside the skull. See anatomic Table of Veins in the Appendices.

postcardinal v's paired vessels in the early embryo that return blood from regions caudal to the heart.

precardinal v's paired venous trunks in the embryo cranial to the heart.

pulp v's vessels draining the venous sinuses of the spleen.

subcardinal v's paired vessels in the embryo, replacing the postcardinal veins and persisting to some degree as definitive vessels.

sublobular v's tributaries of the hepatic veins that receive the central veins of hepatic lobules.

supracardinal v's paired vessels in the embryo developing later than the subcardinal veins and persisting chiefly as the lower segment of the inferior vena cava.

thebesian v's smallest cardiac veins; see anatomic Table of Veins in the Appendices.

trabecular v's vessels coursing in splenic trabeculae, formed by tributary pulp veins.

varicose v's see VARICOSE VEINS.

vitelline v's veins that return the blood from the yolk sac to the primitive heart of the early embryo.

velamen (ve-la′men) [L.] a covering structure; see VEIL and VELUM.

velamentous (vel″ah-men′tus) membranous and pendant; like a veil.

Velban (vel′ban) trademark for a preparation of VINBLASTINE sulfate, an antineoplastic AGENT.

vellus (vel′us) the coat of fine hairs that appears after the lanugo hairs are cast off and that persists until puberty.

velopharyngeal (vel″o-fah-rin′je-al) pertaining to the soft palate (velum palatinum) and pharynx.

Velosef (vel′o-sef) trademark for preparations of CEPHRADINE, a CEPHALOSPORIN antibiotic.

velum (ve′lum) [L.] a covering structure; see also VEIL. adj., **ve′lar.**

v. interpo′situm the membranous roof of the third ventricle of the brain.

medullary v. either of the two portions (superior and inferior medullary velum) of the white matter of the hindbrain that form the roof of the fourth ventricle.

palatine v., v. palati′num the soft palate; see PALATE.

ven(o)- word element [L.], *vein.* See also words beginning PHLEB(O)-.

vena (ve′nah), pl. *ve′nae* [L.] vein (see also Appendix 2-6).

v. ca′va the inferior vena cava and superior vena cava considered as a unit. See Appendix 2-6.

inferior v. cava the venous trunk for the lower extremities and the pelvic and abdominal viscera; it empties into the right atrium of the heart. See Appendix 2-6.

superior v. cava the venous trunk draining blood from the head, neck, upper extremities, and chest; it empties into the right atrium of the heart. See Appendix 2-6.

vena caval syndrome (ve′nah ka′val) partial occlusion of the VENA CAVA and the descending AORTA by uterine contents, resulting in hypotension when in a supine position; it is corrected by assuming a side-lying position. Called also supine hypotension.

venectasia (ve″nek-ta′zhah) a VARICOSITY of a vein.

venectomy (ve-nek′tah-me) phlebectomy.

veneer (vĕ-nēr′) a thin layer of tooth-colored material, usually made of porcelain, some other ceramic, or acrylic resin, attached to a prepared tooth surface t modify its shape or color.

venenation (ven″ĕ-na′shun) poisoning.

venenous (ven′ĕ-nus) poisonous.

venereal (vĕ-nēr′e-al) pertaining to, re lated to, or transmitted by sexual contact.

v. disease sexually transmitted dis ease.

venereologist (vĕ-nēr″e-ol′ah-jist) a spe cialist in venereology.

venereology (vĕ-nēr″re-ol′ah-je) the stud and treatment of sexually transmitted dis eases.

venesection (ven″ĕ-sek′shun) phlebot omy.

veni- word element [L.], *vein;* see als words beginning VENO-.

venipuncture (ven″ĭ-pungk′chur) surgica puncture of a vein; see illustration.

venisuture (ven″ĭ-soo′chur) phleborrha phy.

venlafaxine (ven″lah-fak′sēn) an inhibito of SEROTONIN and NOREPINEPHRINE uptake tha stimulates neurotransmitter activity in th central nervous system; administered orall as the hydrochloride salt as an ANTIDEPRES SANT and ANTIANXIETY AGENT.

venoclysis (ve-nok′lĭ-sis) phleboclysis.

venogram (ve′no-gram) 1. phlebogram. 2 venous-pulse tracing.

venography (ve-nog′rah-fe) phlebogra phy.

venom (ven′om) POISON, especially a toxi substance normally secreted by a serpen insect, or other animal.

Russell's viper v. the venom of *Viper russelli* (Russell's viper), which acts in vitr as an intrinsic thromboplastin and is usefu in defining deficiencies of COAGULATION FAC TOR X.

venomotor (ve″no-mo′ter) controlling d lation or constriction of the veins.

venomous (ven′ah-mus) poisonous.

veno-occlusive (ve″no-ō-kloo′siv) per taining to or characterized by obstructio of the veins.

v.-o. disease of liver acute or chroni partial or complete, occlusion of the bran ches of the hepatic veins by endophlebiti and thrombosis, leading to centrilobula

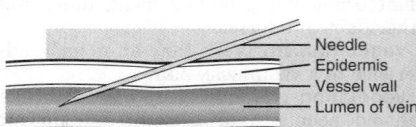

Needle placement during venipuncture. To obtain goo blood flow, the needle is positioned correctly in the ve lumen. The needle should not rest against the upper wa of the vein or puncture through the vein wall on th opposite side. From Malarkey and McMorrow, 2000.

necrosis, fibrosis, and ascites; most often seen in children.

venoperitoneostomy (ve″no-per″ĭ-to″ne-os′tah-me) insertion of an open end of the saphenous vein into the peritoneum for drainage of ascites.

venosclerosis (ve″no-sklĕ-ro′sis) phlebosclerosis.

venosity (ve-nos′ĭ-te) 1. the condition of being venous. 2. excess of venous blood in a part. 3. a plentiful supply of veins.

venostasis (ve″no-sta′sis) venous stasis.

venotomy (ve-not′ah-me) phlebotomy.

venous (ve′nus) pertaining to a VEIN or veins.

venovenostomy (ve″no-ve-nos′tah-me) phlebophlebostomy.

vent (vent) an opening or outlet, such as an opening that discharges pus, or the anus.

venter (ven′ter) [L.] 1. a fleshy contractible part of a muscle; called also belly. 2. abdomen. 3. a hollowed part or CAVITY.

ventilation (ven″tĭ-la′shun) 1. the process or act of supplying a house or room continuously with fresh air. 2. in respiratory physiology, the process of exchange of air between the lungs and the ambient air; see alveolar ventilation and pulmonary ventilation. See also RESPIRATION (def. 1). Called also breathing. 3. in psychiatry, verbalization of one's problems, emotions, or feelings.

alveolar v. a fraction of the pulmonary VENTILATION, being the amount of air that reaches the alveoli and is available for gas exchange with the blood.

assist/control mode v. positive pressure VENTILATION in the assist-control MODE; if the spontaneous ventilation rate falls below a preset level, the ventilator enters the control MODE.

assisted v. artificial respiration.

assist mode v. positive pressure VENTILATION in which the ventilator is in the assist-control MODE; see also control mode VENTILATION and assist/control mode VENTILATION.

controlled v., control mode v. positive pressure VENTILATION in which the ventilator is in control MODE, with its cycle entirely controlled by the apparatus and not influenced by the patient's efforts at spontaneous ventilation.

high-frequency v. a technique of mechanical ventilation that uses very high rates (over 80 breaths per minute) and small tidal volumes (equal to or less than dead space); it may either be positive pressure ventilation or be delivered in the form of frequent jets of air. It is used to lower the peak airway pressure applied to the lung, thus decreasing the risk of BAROTRAUMA.

high-frequency jet v. a type of high-frequency VENTILATION characterized by delivery of gas through a small catheter in the endotracheal TUBE.

high-frequency percussive v. a type of high-frequency VENTILATION characterized by delivery of pressure-limited breaths in short bursts of gas from a VENTURI MASK.

high-frequency positive pressure v. a type of high-frequency VENTILATION characterized by low compressible volume circuit and tidal VOLUME delivery of 3 to 4 mL per kg.

impaired spontaneous v. a NURSING DIAGNOSIS accepted by the North American Nursing Diagnosis Association, defined as a state in which an individual's decreased energy reserves result in inability to maintain breathing adequate to support life. See also spontaneous VENTILATION.

intermittent mandatory v. (IMV) a type of control mode ventilation in which the patient breathes spontaneously while the ventilator delivers a prescribed tidal volume at specified intervals and allows the patient to breathe spontaneously between cycles. The ventilator rate is set to maintain the patient's Pa_{CO_2} at desired levels and is reduced gradually to zero as the patient's condition improves. See also INTERMITTENT POSITIVE-PRESSURE BREATHING.

intermittent mandatory v., synchronized (SIMV) positive pressure VENTILATION in which the patient breathes spontaneously while the ventilator delivers a positive-pressure breath at intervals that are predetermined but synchronized with the patient's breathing.

intermittent positive pressure v. (IPPV) INTERMITTENT POSITIVE PRESSURE BREATHING.

maximal voluntary v., maximum voluntary v. (MVV) the maximum volume that can be exhaled per minute by the patient breathing as rapidly and deeply as possible. Called also maximal breathing capacity.

mechanical v. 1. ventilation accomplished by extrinsic means, usually distinguished as either *negative pressure* or *positive pressure ventilation*. See also spontaneous VENTILATION. 2. in the NURSING INTERVENTIONS CLASSIFICATION, a nursing INTERVENTION defined as the use of an artificial device to assist a patient to breathe.

minute v. the total volume of gas in liters expelled from the lungs per minute. See also minute VOLUME. Called also total ventilation.

V

negative pressure v. a type of mechanical ventilation in which negative pressure is generated on the outside of the patient's chest and transmitted to the interior of the thorax in order to expand the lungs and allow air to flow in; used primarily with patients having paralysis of the chest muscles. See also VENTILATOR.

noninvasive v. mechanical ventilation that does not use an artificial airway, such as positive pressure VENTILATION with a nasal or face mask.

partial liquid v. ventilatory support in which the lungs are filled to the level of the functional residual CAPACITY with a liquid PERFLUOROCARBON; mechanical ventilation is then superimposed and oxygen and carbon dioxide are transferred through the liquid.

positive pressure v. any of numerous types of mechanical ventilation in which gas is delivered into the airways and lungs under positive pressure, producing positive airway pressure during inspiration; it may be done via either an endotracheal tube or a nasal mask. See also VENTILATOR.

pressure control v. positive pressure ventilation in which breaths are augmented by air at a fixed rate and amount of pressure, with tidal volume not being fixed; used particularly for patients with ACUTE RESPIRATORY DISTRESS SYNDROME.

pressure support v. positive pressure ventilation in which the patient breathes spontaneously and breathing is augmented with air at a preset amount of pressure, with tidal volume not being fixed.

proportional assist v. positive pressure ventilation in which the ventilator can sense the patient's level of inspiratory flow and deliver pressure support to achieve a given tidal volume.

pulmonary v. a measure of the rate of ventilation, referring to the total exchange of air between the lungs and the ambient air, usually in liters per minute.

spontaneous v. term used to denote breathing accomplished naturally, without any artificial aids, as opposed to mechanical ventilation and other forms of ARTIFICIAL RESPIRATION.

total v. minute ventilation.

ventilator (ven′tĭ-la″ter) 1. respirator (def. 1). 2. an apparatus used in ARTIFICIAL RESPIRATION to mechanically assist (either intermittently or continuously) or control pulmonary VENTILATION; often erroneously called a RESPIRATOR. Use of a mechanical ventilator is indicated as a supportive measure in patients suffering from respiratory paralysis and in those with ventilatory failure manifested by either alveolar HYPOVENTILATION or HYPOXEMIA, or both.

The ventilator is used to improve alveolar ventilation, re-establish a normal ACID BASE BALANCE, and correct the associated hypoxemia. It is important, however, that the primary cause of a patient's ventilatory failure be known and that blood gases be evaluated frequently during assisted or controlled ventilation so that the mechanical ventilator can be used to its best advantage and greatest benefit to the individual patient.

Types of Ventilators. The two major types are *negative pressure* and *positive pressure* *ventilators.*

Negative Pressure Ventilators. These generate negative pressure on the outside of the chest, and are used for patients having paralysis of the chest muscles. The most common of these was formerly the Drinker RESPIRATOR (IRON LUNG); other types are the chest and chest-abdomen ventilators such as the Emerson cuirass. These machines exert negative (subatmospheric) pressure on the exterior chest wall that is transmitted to the interior of the thorax, creating a suction effect and causing air to flow into the lungs. The lungs are allowed to exhale passively before the next inspiratory cycle. Full-body and chest ventilators are not effective in relief of ventilatory failure resulting from increased airway resistance due to intrapulmonary diseases, such as CHRONIC OBSTRUCTIVE PULMONARY DISEASE. They are, therefore, limited to the treatment of patients whose ventilatory problems are caused by respiratory paralysis rather than obstructive lung disease and whose condition limits the employment of intubation.

Positive Pressure Ventilators. These ventilate the lungs by application of positive pressure applied to the airway, usually via an artificial airway such as an endotracheal tube or tracheostomy tube. Positive pressure ventilation is most commonly used in patients who cannot maintain an adequate Pa_{CO_2}.

Among the many models of positive pressure ventilators are three general types classified according to the manner in which the cycling of the machine is controlled: *pressure-cycled, volume-cycled,* and *time cycled* ventilators. Pressure-cycled ventilators inflate the lungs until a preset pressure is reached. The tidal volume is determined by the pressure setting, flow setting, airway resistance, and lung compliance. Volume-cycled ventilators inflate the lungs until a preset tidal volume is reached. The pressure required to deliver this volume is dependent upon the flow setting, airway resistance, and lung compliance. Time-cycled ventilators inflate the lungs until a preset inspiratory time is reached; they are usually pressure limited. The operator presets an inspiratory time and inspiratory pressure setting. This form of ventilation is most commonly used with neonates. New microprocessor-controlled ventilators are capable of pressure, volume, and time cycling.

Positive pressure ventilators operate in any of several different MODES, particularly assist mode, assist/control mode, and control mode. (See VENTILATION.)

Many commercially available mechanical ventilators are available. All allow the operator to choose the mode of ventilation, a respiratory rate, an inspiratory time (flow, inspiratory-expiratory ratio), FI_{O_2} (fraction inspired oxygen or delivered oxygen concentration), and positive end-expiratory PRESSURE or CONTINUOUS POSITIVE AIRWAY PRESSURE. All ventilators provide a method of heating and warming the inspired gases delivered to the patient and some monitoring of respiratory function such as exhaled tidal volume and inspiratory pressure.

All ventilators have an alarm system. The most important of these is the disconnect alarm, used to detect when the ventilator has become disconnected from the patient. It is important that the disconnect alarm be correctly set at all times. Patients receiving positive pressure ventilation require periodic monitoring of arterial blood gases to assess the adequacy of ventilation.

There are a number of potential complications of positive pressure ventilation. These include BAROTRAUMA (injury to the lung due to high pressures), hemodynamic disturbance due to a decrease in venous return associated with the increase in intrathoracic pressure (decreased cardiac output, decreased blood pressure, decreased urine output), fluid retention (due to decreased renal perfusion and increased antidiuretic hormone), respiratory alkalosis, increased intracranial pressure (due to the elevated intrathoracic pressure), nutritional disturbance (due to not being fed), and nosocomial pneumonia.

Patient Care. Regardless of the model and capabilities of the mechanical ventilator being used in the treatment of a patient with inadequate ventilation, there are certain general principles that are basic to the competent care of that patient. It is essential that all those who accept responsibility for the care of the patient be fully aware of the physiologic effects of mechanical ventilation, particularly in regard to the relationship between the distribution of inspired air in the lung and the status of the BLOOD GASES and pH. A major contribution of mechanical

ventilation should be the normalization of blood gases and avoidance of the extremes of ACIDOSIS and ALKALOSIS. Thus careful monitoring of the blood gases and the pH is an essential part of patient care during mechanical ventilation.

A second consideration in patient care and assessment of the effects of mechanical ventilation is that of its influence on circulation. It is apparent that increased intrathoracic pressure can interfere with the flow of blood through the great vessels and the chambers of the heart. The ultimate effect can be a pooling of blood in the veins and capillaries of the abdominal organs and a resultant peripheral vascular collapse that is sometimes called respirator shock. Frequent determinations of pulse rate and blood pressure are necessary to detect early development of this condition and correct pressure levels to forestall shock. It should be noted that interference with the venous return to the right side of the heart can bring about a therapeutic effect in patients with pulmonary EDEMA. Thus a potentially hazardous side effect of an increase in intrathoracic pressure can be of benefit to the patient when used judiciously by a physician who is knowledgeable about all aspects of ventilatory therapy.

A third consideration is that of the effects of mechanical ventilation on the body fluid–antidiuretic hormone balance. It has long been recognized that pressure breathing, both positive and negative, influences the production of the antidiuretic hormone, causing an excess of this hormone and a resultant retention of water. If not corrected, the situation can lead to pulmonary edema and further interference with the patient's ventilation. The possibility of such an eventuality demands that accurate records be kept of the patient's intake and output and that a safe balance be maintained.

A thorough knowledge of the apparatus being used for mechanical ventilation is vital to competent care of the patient. No one should attempt to give patient care without prior instruction in the purpose of the machine and the physiologic and physical principles upon which it operates.

TRACHEOSTOMY care is of vital importance when the patient is being maintained on a ventilator with controlled ventilation and positive pressure is being delivered via a tracheostomy tube. Suction is applied as necessary and some method for moisturizing the air is provided. In fact, whether the patient has a tracheostomy or not, the air passages must be kept moist whenever a ventilator is used for a prolonged period.

If aerosol medications are administered by use of a ventilator, it is important to know the type of medication being used, its desired effects, and the signs and symptoms of overdosage or toxic side effects. When such symptoms appear, the rate of nebulization requires adjustment.

The psychologic implications of the use of a ventilator are manifold. If conscious or semiconscious, the patient is aware that the machine is concerned with maintaining the very "breath of life" and is understandably apprehensive about its use and effects on effective breathing. When a ventilator is used for a brief period as a means of therapy, patients can be told that they can control the cycle by the slightest effort on their part. Once they understand the way the machine works and their questions are answered to their satisfaction, their fears can be allayed. Patients who are partially or totally dependent on a ventilator will need more reassurance. They should be assured that someone will be near at all times in case the apparatus needs adjusting. Much of their panic and fear can be relieved if the nursing staff exercises patience and maintains a calm attitude when helping them adjust to the ventilator. If the patient's anxiety interferes with effective ventilation, sedation may need to be used.

Weaning from the ventilator is begun when the clinical condition of the patient indicates that full ventilatory support may no longer be needed. Weaning is accomplished by a number of techniques including T-piece trials, synchronized intermittent mandatory VENTILATION, and pressure support. With T-piece trials, the patient is removed from the ventilator, allowed to breathe spontaneously, and then returned to the ventilator. The periods of time off the ventilator are gradually increased until the patient has been entirely weaned. With SIMV weaning, the ventilator rate is gradually decreased until the patient has been weaned. With pressure support weaning, the pressure support is decreased until the patient is weaned.

Ventolin (ven'to-lin) trademark for preparations of ALBUTEROL, a BRONCHODILATOR.

ventr(o)- word element [L.], *belly; front (anterior) aspect of the body.*

ventrad (ven'trad) toward a belly, venter, or ventral aspect.

ventral (ven'tral) 1. pertaining to the abdomen or to any venter. 2. directed toward or situated on the belly surface; opposite of DORSAL; see also ANTERIOR.

ventralis (ven-tra'lis) [L.] ventral.

ventri- word element [L.], *belly; front (anterior) aspect of the body.*

ventricle (ven'trĭ-k'l) a small cavity or chamber, as in the brain or heart.

  v. of Arantius 1. the rhomboid fossa, especially its lower end. 2. cavity of septum pellucidum.

  fifth v. cavity of septum pellucidum.

  fourth v. a median cavity in the hindbrain, containing cerebrospinal fluid.

  v. of larynx the space between the true and false vocal cords.

  lateral v. the cavity in each cerebral hemisphere, derived from the cavity of the embryonic tube, containing cerebrospinal fluid.

  left v. the lower chamber of the left side of the heart, which pumps oxygenated blood out through the aorta to all the tissues of the body.

  Morgagni's v. ventricle of larynx.

  pineal v. an extension of the third ventricle into the stalk of the pineal body.

  right v. the lower chamber of the right side of the heart, which pumps venous blood through the pulmonary trunk and arteries to the capillaries of the lung.

  third v. a narrow cleft below the corpus callosum, within the diencephalon between the two thalami.

ventricular (ven-trik'u-ler) pertaining to a ventricle.

  v. septal defect a CONGENITAL HEART DEFECT in which the opening in the ventricular septum (normal in the fetus) persists after birth, in either the muscular or fibrous portion, most often due to failure of the bulbar septum to completely close the interventricular foramen. This permits flow of blood directly from one ventricle to the other, resulting in bypassing of the pulmonary circulation and varying degrees of cyanosis. Defective valves affecting the flow of blood to and from the heart may also be present.

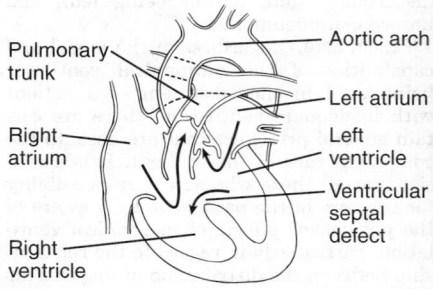

Pulmonary trunk
Aortic arch
Left atrium
Right atrium
Left ventricle
Ventricular septal defect
Right ventricle

Abnormal communication between the ventricles in ventricular septal defect. From Dorland's, 2000.

ventriculitis (ven-trik″u-li′tis) inflammation of a ventricle, especially a cerebral ventricle.

ventriculoatriostomy (ven-trik″u-lo-a″tre-os′tah-me) ventriculoatrial shunt.

ventriculocisternostomy (ven-trik″u-lo-sis″ter-nos′-tah-me) surgical creation of a communication between the third ventricle and the interpeduncular cistern, for drainage of cerebrospinal fluid in HYDROCEPHALUS.

ventriculogram (ven-trik′u-lo-gram″) a radiogram of the cerebral ventricles (no longer performed) or of the ventricles of the heart.

ventriculomegaly (ven-trik″u-lo-meg′ah-le) gross enlargement of a ventricle of the brain, as by hydrocephalus.

ventriculography (ven-trik″u-log′rah-fe) 1. radiography of the cerebral ventricles after introduction of air or other contrast medium. This study is no longer used to examine the brain; being replaced by CT and MRI. 2. radiography of a ventricle of the heart after injection of a contrast medium.

 first pass v. first pass radionuclide angiocardiography.

 gated blood pool v. equilibrium radionuclide angiocardiography.

 radionuclide v. radionuclide angiocardiography.

ventriculometry (ven-trik″u-lom′ĕ-tre) measurement of intracranial pressure.

ventriculopuncture (ven-trik″u-lo-pungk′-chur) surgical puncture of a lateral ventricle of the brain.

ventriculoscopy (ven-trik″u-los′kah-pe) endoscopic examination of the cerebral ventricles.

ventriculostomy (ven-trik″u-los′tah-me) surgical creation of a free communication between the third ventricle and the interpeduncular cistern for relief of hydrocephalus.

ventriculosubarachnoid (ven-trik″u-lo-sub″ah-rak′-noid) pertaining to the cerebral ventricles and subarachnoid space.

ventriculotomy (ven-trik″u-lot′ah-me) incision of a ventricle.

ventriculovenostomy (ven-trik″u-lo-ve-nos′tah-me) ventriculovenous shunt.

ventriculus (ven-trik′u-lus) [L.] 1. ventricle. 2. stomach.

ventricumbent (ven″trĭ-kum′bent) prone.

ventriduct (ven″trĭ-dukt) to bring or carry ventrad.

ventrimeson (ven″trĭ-mes′on) the median line on the ventral surface. adj., **ventrime′sal.**

ventrofixation (ven″tro-fik-sa′shun) fixation of a viscus, such as the uterus, to the abdominal wall; called also ventrosuspension.

ventrohysteropexy (ven″tro-his′ter-o-pek″se) ventrofixation of the uterus.

ventrolateral (ven″tro-lat′er-al) both ventral and lateral; see also ANTEROLATERAL.

ventrose (ven′trōs) having a belly-like expansion.

ventrosuspension (ven″tro-sus-pen′shun) ventrofixation.

ventrotomy (ven-trot′ah-me) celiotomy.

venturi (ven-tu′re) Venturi mask.

Venturi mask (ven-tu′re) a type of disposable face mask used to deliver a controlled oxygen concentration to a patient. (See also OXYGEN THERAPY.) The flow of 100 per cent oxygen through the mask draws in a controlled amount of room air (21 per cent oxygen). Commonly available masks deliver 24, 28, 31, 35, or 40 per cent oxygen. At concentrations above 24 per cent, humidification may be required. Called also venturi.

Venturi principle (ven-tu′re) an inverse association of gas or fluid pressure, velocity of flow, and restriction of passage. The Venturi principle states that the pressure drop distal to a restriction can be nearly restored to the prerestriction pressure if there is a dilatation of the passage immediately distal to the stenosis, with an angle of divergence not exceeding 15 degrees.

venula (ven′u-lah) [L.] venule.

venule (ven′ūl) any of the small vessels that collect blood from the capillary plexuses and join to form veins. adj., **ven′ular.**

venulitis (ven″u-li′tis) inflammation of the venules.

 cutaneous necrotizing v. a necrotizing vasculitis affecting the venules of the skin, usually of the extremities, caused by deposition of circulating immune complexes and usually occurring in association with infection, chronic disease, and drug administration. Clinical manifestations are variable, the most common being palpable purpura (the characteristic lesion), angioedema, and urticaria.

VePesid (ve′pe-sid) trademark for a preparation of ETOPOSIDE, an antineoplastic AGENT.

verapamil (vĕ-rap′ah-mil) a CALCIUM CHANNEL BLOCKING AGENT used as the hydrochloride salt as a coronary vasodilator in the treatment of ANGINA PECTORIS and of HYPERTENSION and the treatment and prophylaxis of supraventricular TACHYARRHYTHMIAS.

verbigeration (ver-bij″er-a′shun) STEREOTYPY in speech; stereotyped and meaningless repetition of words and phrases, as seen in some cases of SCHIZOPHRENIA; see also PERSEVERATION and LOGORRHEA. Called also cataphasia.

V

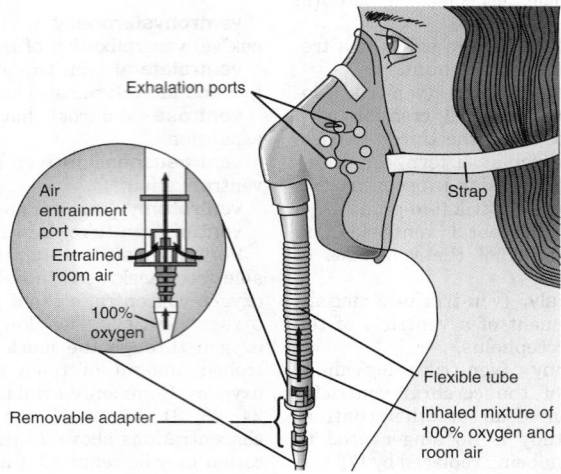

Exhalation ports

Strap

Air entrainment port

Entrained room air

100% oxygen

Flexible tube

Removable adapter

Inhaled mixture of 100% oxygen and room air

A Venturi mask for precise oxygen delivery. From Ignatavicius and Workman, 2000.

verge (verj) a circumference or ring.

anal v. the opening of the anus on the surface of the body.

vergence (ver′jens) disjunctive movement of the eyes in opposite directions in adjusting to near or far vision; convergence or divergence.

vermicide (ver′mĭ-sīd) anthelmintic (def. 2).

vermicular (ver-mik′u-lar) wormlike in shape or appearance.

vermiculation (ver-mik″u-la′shun) peristaltic motion; peristalsis.

vermiculous (ver-mik′u-lus) 1. vermicular. 2. infected with worms.

vermiform (ver′mĭ-form) vermicular.

vermifugal (ver-mif′u-gal) anthelmintic (def. 1).

vermifuge (ver′mĭ-fūj) anthelmintic (def. 2).

vermilionectomy (ver-mil″yon-ek′tah-me) excision of the vermilion border of the lip.

vermin (ver′min) an external animal parasite; such parasites collectively.

vermination (ver″mĭ-na′shun) 1. infestation with WORMS; called also helminthiasis. 2. infestation with VERMIN.

verminous (ver′mĭ-nus) pertaining to, due to, or abounding in worms or in vermin.

vermis (ver′mis) [L.] a wormlike structure, particularly the vermis cerebelli.

v. cerebel′li, v. of cerebellum the median part of the CEREBELLUM, between the two cerebellar HEMISPHERES.

Vermox (ver′moks) trademark for a preparation of MEBENDAZOLE, an ANTHELMINTIC.

Vernet's syndrome (ver-nāz′) paralysis of the glossopharyngeal, vagus, and spinal accessory nerves due to a lesion in the region of the jugular foramen.

vernix (ver′niks) [L.] varnish.

v. caseo′sa the thick white substance composed of sebum and desquamated epithelial cells that provides a protective covering for the skin of the fetus. In the full-term newborn, during the first two or three days of life there is a small amount of vernix caseosa in body creases and the hair.

verruca (vĕ-roo′kah) [L.] 1. wart. 2. one of the wartlike elevations on the endocardium in various types of endocarditis. adj., **ver′rucose, verru′cous.**

v. pla′na a small, smooth, usually skin-colored or light brown, slightly raised wart sometimes occurring in great numbers; seen most often in children.

v. planta′ris plantar WART.

verruciform (vĕ-roo′sĭ-form) wartlike.

verruga (vĕ-roo′gah) wart.

v. perua′na a hemangioma-like tumor or nodule occurring in bartonellosis.

version (ver′zhun) the act of turning, especially the manual turning of the fetus in delivery.

bipolar v. turning done by acting upon both poles of the fetus by either external or combined version.

cephalic v. turning of the fetus so that the head is the presenting part.

combined v. external and internal versions together.

external *v.* that done using outside manipulation.

internal *v.* that done using the hand or fingers inserted through the dilated cervix.

pelvic *v.* version by manipulation of the BREECH (buttocks) of the fetus.

podalic *v.* conversion of a more unfavorable presentation into a footling PRESENTATION.

spontaneous *v.* one that occurs without aid from any extraneous force.

vertebr(o)- word element [L.], *vertebra; vertebral column.* See also words beginning SPIN(O)- and SPONDYL(O)-.

vertebra (ver'tĕ-brah) [L.] any of the separate segments comprising the SPINE (vertebral column). The vertebrae support the body and provide the protective bony corridor (the spinal or vertebral CANAL) through which the SPINAL CORD passes. The 33 bones that make up the spine differ considerably in size and structure according to location. There are seven cervical (neck) vertebrae, 12 thoracic (high back), five lumbar (low back), five sacral (near the base of the spine), and four coccygeal (at the base). The five sacral vertebrae are fused to form the sacrum, and the four coccygeal vertebrae are fused to form the coccyx.

The weight-bearing portion of a typical vertebra is the vertebral body, the most forward portion. This is a cylindrical structure that is separated from the vertebral bodies above and below by disks of cartilage and fibrous tissue. These intervertebral disks act as cushions to absorb the mechanical shock of walking, running, and other activity. Sometimes rupture or herniation of a disk may occur (see HERNIATED DISK).

A semicircular arch of bone (the vertebral ARCH) protrudes from the back of each vertebral body, surrounding the spinal cord. Directly in its midline a bony projection, the spinous PROCESS, grows backward from the arch. The spinous process can be felt on the back as a hard knob. Three pairs of outgrowths project from the arch. One of these protrudes horizontally on each side and in the thorax connects with the ribs. The remaining two form joints with the vertebrae above and below. The joints permit the spine to bend flexibly. The vertebrae are held firmly in place by a series of strong ligaments.

cervical vertebrae the upper seven vertebrae, constituting the skeleton of the neck.

coccygeal vertebrae the lowest segments of the vertebral column, comprising three to five rudimentary vertebrae that form the COCCYX.

cranial *v.* the segments of the skull and facial bones, regarded by some as modified vertebrae.

v. denta'ta the second cervical vertebra, or axis.

dorsal vertebrae thoracic vertebrae.

false vertebrae those vertebrae that normally fuse with adjoining segments: the sacral and coccygeal vertebrae.

lumbar vertebrae the five vertebrae between the thoracic vertebrae and the sacrum.

v. mag'na the sacrum.

odontoid *v.* the second cervical vertebra, or axis.

v. pla'na a condition of spondylitis in which the body of the vertebra is reduced to a sclerotic disk.

sacral vertebrae the vertebrae just below the lumbar vertebrae, usually five in number and fused to form the SACRUM.

thoracic vertebrae the twelve vertebrae between the cervical and lumbar vertebrae, giving attachment to the ribs and forming part of the posterior wall of the thorax.

true vertebrae those segments of the vertebral column that normally remain unfused throughout life: the cervical, thoracic, and lumbar vertebrae.

vertebral (ver'tĕ-bral) of or pertaining to a vertebra.

Vertebrata (ver"tĕ-bra'tah) a subphylum of the Chordata, comprising all animals having a vertebral column, including mammals, birds, reptiles, amphibians, and fishes.

vertebrate (ver'tĕ-brāt) 1. having a vertebral column. 2. an animal with a vertebral column; any member of the Vertebrata.

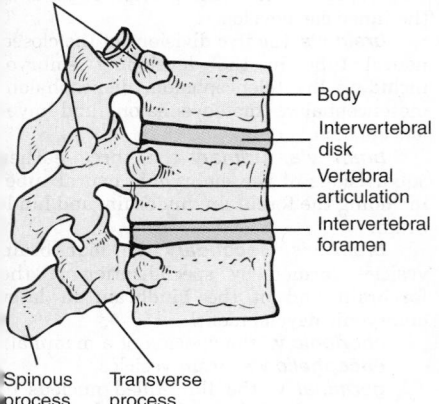

Facets for
head of ribs

Body

Intervertebral disk

Vertebral articulation

Intervertebral foramen

Spinous process

Transverse process

Structure of vertebrae.

vertebrectomy (ver″tĕ-brek′tah-me) excision of a vertebra.

vertebrobasilar (ver″tĕ-bro-bas′ĭ-ler) pertaining to or affecting the vertebral and basilar arteries.

vertebrochondral (ver″tĕ-bro-kon′dral) pertaining to a vertebra and a costal cartilage.

vertebrocostal (ver″tĕ-bro-kos′tal) pertaining to a vertebra and a rib.

vertebrogenic (ver″tĕ-bro-jen′ĭk) arising in a vertebra or in the vertebral column.

vertebrosternal (ver″tĕ-bro-ster′nal) pertaining to a vertebra and the sternum.

verteporfin (ver″tĕ-por′fin) a photosensitizing agent that accumulates preferentially in neovasculature, including that in the choroid, such as occurs in AGE-RELATED MACULAR DEGENERATION, ocular HISTOPLASMOSIS, or pathologic myopia; the agent is then activated by light of a specific wavelength in the presence of oxygen, and causes local damage to the neovascular endothelium followed by vessel occlusion; it is administered intravenously prior to irradiation of the lesion with light from a compatible laser.

vertex (ver′teks) the summit or top, especially the top of the head (ver′tex cra′nii).

vertical (ver′tĭ-kal) 1. perpendicular to the plane of the horizon. 2. relating to the vertex. 3. spreading from one generation to another; see vertical TRANSMISSION.

verticalis (ver″tĭ-ka′lis) [L.] vertical.

verticillate (ver-tis′ĭ-lāt) arranged in whorls.

vertigo (ver′tĭ-go) a sensation of rotation or movement of one's self (subjective vertigo) or of one's surroundings (objective vertigo) in any plane. The term is sometimes used erroneously as a synonym for DIZZINESS. Vertigo may result from diseases of the inner ear or may be due to disturbances of the vestibular centers or pathways in the central nervous system.

benign paroxysmal positional v. recurrent vertigo and nystagmus occurring when the head is placed in certain positions, usually not associated with lesions of the central nervous system.

benign positional v., benign postural v. benign paroxysmal positional vertigo.

central v. that due to disorder of the central nervous system.

cerebral v. vertigo resulting from a brain lesion, such as in meningogenic LABYRINTHITIS. Called also organic v.

disabling positional v. constant vertigo or dysequilibrium and nausea in the upright position, without hearing disturbance or loss of vestibular function.

labyrinthine v. Meniere's disease.

organic v. cerebral vertigo.

peripheral v. vestibular vertigo.

positional v. that associated with a specific position of the head in space or with changes in position of the head in space.

vestibular v. vertigo due to disturbances of the vestibular centers or pathways in the central nervous system.

vertigraphy (ver-tig′rah-fe) body-section radiography.

verumontanum (ver″u-mon-ta′num) seminal colliculus.

vesalianum (vĕ-sa″le-a′num) a sesamoid bone in the tendon of origin of the gastrocnemius muscle, or in the angle between the cuboid and fifth metatarsal bones.

Vesalius (vĕ-sa′le-us) Andreas (1514–1564). Flemish anatomist and physician, considered the most eminent anatomist of the 16th century. His *De humani corporis fabrica libri septum* (Seven Books on the Structure of the Human Body) was published in 1543. He was also a pioneer in ethnic craniology and experimental and comparative psychology.

vesic(o)- word element [L.], *blister; bladder.*

vesica (vĕ-si′kah) [L.] bladder. adj., **ves′ical.**

vesicant (ves′ĭ-kant) 1. producing blisters. 2. an agent that produces blisters.

vesication (ves″ĭ-ka′shun) the process of blistering. 1. a blistered spot or surface.

vesicle (ves′ĭ-k'l) 1. a small bladder or sac containing liquid. 2. a small circumscribed elevation of the epidermis containing a serous fluid; a small blister.

allantoic v. the internal hollow portion of the allantois.

auditory v. a detached ovoid sac formed by closure of the auditory pit in the early embryo, from which the percipient parts of the inner ear develop.

brain v's the five divisions of the closed neural tube in the developing embryo, including the telencephalon, diencephalon, mesencephalon, metencephalon, and myelencephalon.

brain v's, primary the three earlier subdivisions of the embryonic neural tube, including the forebrain, midbrain, and hindbrain.

brain v's, secondary the four brain vesicles formed by specialization of the forebrain and of the hindbrain in later embryonic development.

chorionic v. the CHORION of a mammal.

encephalic v's brain vesicles.

germinal v. the fluid-filled nucleus of an oocyte toward the end of prophase of its meiotic division.

lens v. a vesicle formed from the lens pit of the embryo, developing into the crystalline lens.

olfactory v. 1. the vesicle in the embryo that later develops into the olfactory bulb and tract. 2. a bulbous expansion at the distal end of an olfactory cell, from which the olfactory hairs project.

optic v. an evagination on either side of the forebrain of the early embryo, from which the percipient parts of the eye develop.

otic v. auditory vesicle.

seminal v. paired sacculated pouches attached to the posterior urinary bladder; the duct of each joins the ipsilateral ductus deferens to form the ejaculatory duct.

umbilical v. the pear-shaped expansion of the yolk sac growing out into the cavity of the chorion, joined to the midgut by the yolk stalk.

vesicocele (ves´ĭ-ko-sēl″) hernia of the bladder.

vesicocervical (ves″ĭ-ko-ser´vĭ-k′l) pertaining to the bladder and cervix uteri; called also cervicovesical.

vesicoclysis (ves″ĭ-kok´lĭ-sis) introduction of fluid into the bladder.

vesicoenteric (ves″ĭ-ko-en-tĕ´rik) enterovesical.

vesicointestinal (ves″ĭ-ko-in-tes´tĭ-nal) enterovesical.

vesicoprostatic (ves″ĭ-ko-pros-tat´ik) pertaining to the bladder and prostate.

vesicopubic (ves″ĭ-ko-pu´bik) pertaining to the bladder and pubes; called also pubovesical.

vesicosigmoidostomy (ves″ĭ-ko-sig″moi-dos´tah-me) surgical creation of an opening between the urinary bladder and the sigmoid colon.

vesicospinal (ves″ĭ-ko-spi´nal) pertaining to the bladder and spine.

vesicostomy (ves″ĭ-kos´tah-me) surgical creation of an opening into the bladder; called also cystostomy.

cutaneous v. surgical anastomosis of the bladder mucosa to an opening in the skin below the umbilicus, creating a stoma for bladder drainage.

vesicotomy (ves″ĭ-kot´ah-me) incision into the urinary BLADDER, usually done to divert the flow of urine when the bladder can no longer function as a reservoir. After incising the bladder the surgeon moves it forward and sutures the opening to the skin, forming a STOMA. Patient care is similar to that required for cutaneous URETEROSTOMY and ILEAL CONDUIT. Called also cystotomy.

vesicoureteral (ves″ĭ-ko-u-re´ter-al) ureterovesical.

vesicoureteric (ves″ĭ-ko-u″rĕ-ter´ik) ureterovesical.

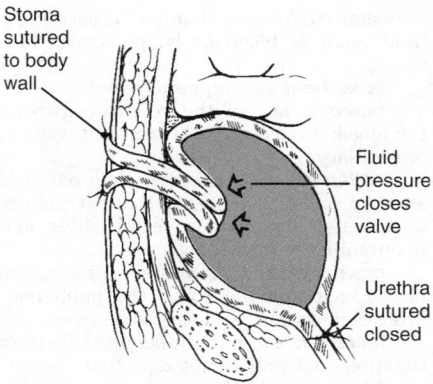

Stoma sutured to body wall

Fluid pressure closes valve

Urethra sutured closed

A continent vesicostomy. From Polaski and Tatro, 1996.

vesicouterine (ves″ĭ-ko-u´ter-in) pertaining to the bladder and uterus.

vesicovaginal (ves″ĭ-ko-vaj´ĭ-nal) pertaining to the bladder and vagina.

vesicula (vĕ-sik´u-lah) [L.] vesicle.

vesicular (vĕ-sik´u-lar) 1. composed of or relating to VESICLES. 2. pertaining to or made up of vesicles on the skin. 3. having a low pitch, such as the normal breath SOUND heard over the lung during ventilation.

vesiculation (vĕ-sik″u-la´shun) formation of vesicles.

vesiculectomy (vĕ-sik″u-lek´tah-me) excision of a vesicle, especially the seminal vesicle.

vesiculiform (vĕ-sik´u-lĭ-form) shaped like a vesicle.

vesiculitis (vĕ-sik″u-li´tis) inflammation of a vesicle, especially a seminal vesicle.

vesiculocavernous (vĕ-sik″u-lo-kav´er-nus) both vesicular and cavernous; said of auscultatory SOUNDS.

vesiculogram (vĕ-sik´u-lo-gram″) a radiograph of the seminal vesicles.

vesiculography (vĕ-sik″u-log´rah-fe) radiography of the seminal vesicles.

vesiculopapular (vĕ-sik″u-lo-pap´u-lar) both vesicular and papular.

vesiculopustular (vĕ-sik″u-lo-pus´tu-lar) both vesicular and pustular.

vesiculotomy (vĕ-sik″u-lot´ah-me) incision into a vesicle, especially the seminal vesicles.

vesiculotympanic (vĕ-sik″u-lo-tim-pan´ik) vesiculotympanitic.

vesiculotympanitic both vesicular and tympanitic; said of auscultatory sounds.

Vesprin (ves´prin) trademark for preparations of TRIFLUPROMAZINE hydrochloride, an ANTIEMETIC and ANTIPSYCHOTIC AGENT.

V

vessel (ves'el) any channel for carrying a fluid, such as blood or lymph; called also vas.

absorbent v. lymphatic vessel.

blood v. any of the vessels conveying the blood; an artery, arteriole, vein, venule, or capillary.

collateral v. 1. a vessel that parallels another vessel, a nerve, or other structure. 2. a vessel important in establishing and maintaining collateral CIRCULATION.

great v's the large vessels entering the heart, including the aorta, the pulmonary arteries and veins, and the venae cavae.

lacteal v. those that take up chyle from the intestinal wall during digestion.

lymphatic v's the capillaries, collecting vessels, and trunks that collect lymph from the tissues and carry it to the blood stream.

nutrient v's vessels supplying nutritive elements to special tissues, as arteries entering the substance of bone or the walls of large blood vessels.

vestibule (ves'tĭ-būl) a space or cavity at the entrance to another structure. adj., **vestib'ular.**

v. of aorta a small space within the left ventricle at the root of the aorta.

v. of ear an oval cavity in the middle of the bony labyrinth.

v. of mouth the portion of the oral cavity bounded on one side by teeth and gingivae (or the residual alveolar ridges) and on the other by the lips (*labial vestibule*) and cheeks (*buccal vestibule*).

nasal v., v. of nose the anterior part of the nasal cavity; it is lined with stratified squamous epithelium and contains hairs (VIBRISSAE) and sebaceous glands.

v. of vagina the space between the labia minora into which the urethra and vagina open.

vestibulitis (ves-tib″u-li'tis) inflammation of the vulvar vestibule and the periglandular and subepithelial stroma, resulting in a burning sensation and dyspareunia.

vestibulocochlear (ves-tib″u-lo-kok'le-er) pertaining to the vestibule of the ear and the cochlea.

v. nerve the eighth CRANIAL NERVE, which emerges from the brain between the pons and medulla oblongata, behind the facial nerve. The vestibular division serves the vestibule of the ear and the semicircular canals, carrying impulses for the sense of equilibrium. The cochlear division serves the cochlea and carries impulses for the sense of hearing. Called also acoustic nerve and auditory nerve. See Appendix 2-6.

vestibulogenic (ves-tib″u-lo-jen'ik) arising in a vestibule, as that of the ear.

vestibulo-ocular (ves-tib″u-lo-ok'u-lar) pertaining to the vestibular and oculomotor nerves; or to the maintenance of visual stability during head movements.

vestibuloplasty (ves-tib'u-lo-plas″te) surgical modification of gingiva–mucous membrane relationships in the vestibule of the mouth.

vestibulotomy (ves-tib″u-lot'ah-me) incision into the vestibule of the ear.

vestibulourethral (ves-tib″u-lo-u-re'thral) pertaining to the vestibule of the vagina and the urethra.

vestibulum (ves-tib'u-lum) [L.] vestibule.

vestige (ves'tij) the remnant of a structure that functioned in a previous stage of species or individual development. adj., **vestig'ial.**

vestigium (ves-tij'e-um) [L.] vestige.

veterinarian (vet″er-ĭ-nar'e-an) a person trained and authorized to practice veterinary medicine and surgery; a doctor of veterinary medicine.

veterinary (vet'er-ĭ-nar″e) 1. pertaining to domestic animals and their diseases. 2. veterinarian.

v. technician a health care worker who is skilled in technical aspects of veterinary medicine and works as a professional assistant to a veterinarian or to any of various types of researchers and scientists.

VF vocal fremitus.

vf visual field.

viability (vi″ah-bil'ĭ-te) the state or quality of being viable.

viable (vi'ah-b'l) able to maintain an independent existence; able to live after birth.

Viagra (vi-ag'rah) trademark for preparation of SILDENAFIL citrate, a treatment for erectile DYSFUNCTION.

vial (vi'al) a small bottle.

vibex (vi'beks), pl. *vi'bices* [L.] 1. a line or streak. 2. a linear subcutaneous effusion of blood.

Vibramycin (vi″brah-mi'sin) trademark for preparations of DOXYCYCLINE, a TETRACYCLINE ANTIBIOTIC.

Vibra-Tabs (vi'brah-tabz) trademark for preparations of DOXYCYCLINE hyclate, a TETRACYCLINE ANTIBIOTIC.

vibratile (vi'brah-tīl) swaying or moving to and fro; vibratory.

vibration (vi-bra'shun) 1. a rapid movement to and fro; oscillation. 2. the shaking of the body as a therapeutic measure. 3. a form of massage. 4. a technique of chest PHYSICAL THERAPY whereby pressure and a shaking movement of the hand are applied to various segments of the lungs to mobilize secretions.

WINDOW ON VETERINARY TECHNICIAN

Veterinary technicians function primarily as professional assistants to veterinarians, biomedical researchers, and other scientists, and as such are an integral part of the veterinary health care team. These individuals must possess a unique combination of knowledge and skill involving basic science, animals, and people. As the complexity of veterinary medicine increases and as the public demand for state of the art care for their animals increases, the veterinary technician will play an ever increasing role in the delivery of excellent health care for animals.

The greatest demand for veterinary technicians is in a private veterinary practice working alongside the veterinarian caring for companion animals. However, the demand for veterinary technicians in other fields is rapidly growing and opportunities exist in the following areas: teaching, pharmaceutical sales, the military, humane societies, livestock production, equine practice, biomedical research, diagnostic laboratories, zoo/wildlife medicine, veterinary supply sales, public health organizations, and the pet food industry.

The responsibilities assigned to veterinary technicians vary and are regulated by a State Board of Veterinary Medicine or other appropriate state agency. Duties often include nursing care of hospitalized patients, history taking, physical examination and assessment, administering medications, performing a wide range of technical tasks, assisting in diagnostic and therapeutic procedures, collecting and analyzing clinical specimens, performing radiological and dental procedures, anesthesiology and surgical assisting, office and hospital management, biomedical research, client counseling, and education.

Today there are over 60 college programs in the United States and Canada which are accredited by the American Veterinary Medical Association as programs to train technicians. Formal study in veterinary technology entails at least two academic years leading to an Associate Degree, with four-year degrees available at some institutions. The training is demanding and academically challenging.

In forty states and provinces veterinary technicians are either certified, registered, or licensed. Candidates must demonstrate competency by passing a comprehensive examination that may include oral, written, and practical components. There are individuals that have received on-the-job training working in veterinary practices and other animal care facilities; these individuals are properly referred to as veterinary assistants, animal attendants, animal caretakers, ward attendants, etc., not as veterinary technicians.

Those interested in a career in veterinary technology should enroll in college preparatory courses in science, mathematics, and English, and acquire experience working with animals. There are approximately one hundred professional organizations in the United States and Canada representing technicians on the local, state, provincial, national, and international levels.

Further information can be obtained from the American Veterinary Medical Association, 1931 N. Meacham Rd., Ste. 100, Schaumburg, IL, 60173-4360 or the North American Veterinary Technician Association, P.O. Box 224, Battle Ground, IN, 47920.

KARL M. PETER, DVM

---

vibrator (vi′bra-tor) an apparatus used in vibratory treatment.

vibratory (vi′brah-tor″e) vibrating or causing vibration; vibratile.

Vibrio (vib′re-o) a genus of gram-negative, facultatively anaerobic, motile, straight or curved rod-shaped bacteria. *V. cho′lerae* is the etiologic agent of Asiatic CHOLERA; *V. metschniko′vii* causes GASTROENTERITIS; *V. parahaemoly′ticus* causes gastroenteritis due to the consumption of raw or improperly cooked seafood (especially in Japan); and *V. vulni′ficus* causes SEPTICEMIA and CELLULITIS in persons who have consumed raw seafood.

vibrio (vib′re-o) an organism of the genus *Vibrio,* or other spiral motile organism.

cholera v. *Vibrio cholerae.*

noncholera v's a group of microorganisms that are similar to *Vibrio cholerae* but differ from it immunologically and having variable pathogenic properties. Many that were isolated from water or from the feces of individuals with mild diarrheal disease have been named for the place of their discovery, such as *V. danu′bicus, V. ghin′da,* and *V. massau′ah.*

vibriocidal (vib″re-o-si′dal) destructive to bacteria of the genus *Vibrio,* especially *V. cholerae.*

vibrissa (vi-bris'ah) [L.] one of the hairs growing in the vestibule of the nose in humans or around the nose (muzzle) of an animal.

vibroacoustic (vi''bro-ah-kōōs'tik) combining both vibratory and acoustic elements.

vibrocardiogram (vi''bro-kahr'de-o-gram'') the record produced by vibrocardiography.

vibrocardiography (vi''bro-kahr''de-og'-rah-fe) graphic recording of vibrations of the chest wall of relatively high frequency that are produced by the action of the heart.

vibrotherapeutics (vi''bro-ther''ah-pu'tiks) the therapeutic use of vibrating appliances.

Vicia (vish'e-ah) a genus of herbs. *V. fa'ba* or *V. fa'va* is the fava bean or broad bean, whose beans and pollen contain a component that can cause FAVISM in susceptible persons.

victimology (vik''tim-ol'ah-je) the study of victims of violent or sexual assault.

vidarabine (vi-dar'ah-bēn) adenine arabinoside (ara-A), a purine analogue that inhibits DNA synthesis; used as an antiviral agent to treat herpes simplex keratitis and keratoconjunctivitis.

videoconference (vid''e-o-con'fer-ens) a conference between persons in different locations, carried on using computerized audiovisual displays.

videoendoscopy (vid''e-o-en-dos'-ah-kah-pe) endoscopy performed under the guidance of a video camera in the tip of the endoscope.

videognosis (vid''e-og-no'sis) diagnosis based on the interpretation of radiograms transmitted by television techniques to a radiologic center.

videolaparoscopy (vid''e-o-lap''-ah-ros'-k-ah-pe) laparoscopic surgery performed under the guidance of a video camera in the tip of the laparoscope.

videourodynamics (vid''e-o-u''ro-di-nam'-iks) any of various urodynamics tests combined with fluoroscopy; used to evaluate complex incontinence problems.

view (vu) projection.

planar v. a two-dimensional view of a process or function.

vigilambulism (vij''il-am'bu-lizm) a state resembling SOMNAMBULISM, but occurring in the waking state.

vignetting (vin-yet'ing) the presence of a brighter light intensity at the center of the fluoroscopic image on an image intensifier than at the periphery of the field.

Villaret's syndrome (ve-lah-rāz') unilateral paralysis of the glossopharyngeal, vagus, spinal accessory, and hypoglossal nerves and sometimes the facial nerve, due to a lesion in the retroparotid space.

villi (vil'i) [L.] plural of VILLUS.

villoma (vĭ-lo'mah) papilloma.

villose (vil'ōs) shaggy with soft hairs; covered with villi.

villositis (vil''o-si'tis) a bacterial disease with alterations in the villi of the placenta.

villosity (vĭ-los'ĭ-te) 1. condition of being covered with villi. 2. a villus.

villus (vil'us) [L.] a small vascular process or protrusion, as from the free surface of a membrane.

arachnoid villi microscopic projections of the arachnoid into some of the venous sinuses.

chorionic villi see CHORIONIC VILLI.

intestinal villi multitudinous threadlike projections covering the surface of the mucous membrane lining the small INTESTINE, serving as the sites of absorption of fluids and nutrients.

synovial villi slender projections from the surface of the synovial membrane into the cavity of a joint; called also haversian glands.

villusectomy (vil''us-ek'tah-me) synovectomy; excision of a synovial villus.

vinblastine (vin-blas'tēn) a VINCA ALKALOID antineoplastic AGENT that causes metaphase arrest during cell mitosis by damaging the mitotic spindles. It is used primarily in combination chemotherapy regimens for testicular carcinoma and Hodgkin's lymphomas, choriocarcinoma, breast carcinoma, and histiocytosis X. Available as *vincristine sulfate,* administered intravenously.

vinca alkaloids (vin'kah) a group of cytotoxic alkaloids extracted from the Madagascar periwinkle (*Catharanthus roseus* G. Don or *Vinca rosea* L.) and used as antineoplastic AGENTS; they are cell cycle specific for the M phase of cell division and disrupt the microtubules that form the spindle apparatus. The group includes VINBLASTINE, VINCRISTINE, VINDESINE, and VINORELBINE tartrate.

Vincent's angina (vin'sents) GINGIVOSTOMATITIS caused by extension to the oral mucosa of necrotizing ulcerative GINGIVITIS, characterized by ulceration, pseudomembrane, and odor, with lesions involving the palate or pharynx as well as the oral mucosa. Called also necrotizing ulcerative gingivostomatitis.

vincristine (vin-kris'tēn) a VINCA ALKALOID used as an antineoplastic AGENT, primarily as a component of combination chemotherapy regimens for HODGKIN'S DISEASE, acute lymphoblastic LEUKEMIA, and non-Hodgkin's LYMPHOMAS, as well as in the treatment of other neoplastic disorders including Wilms' TUMOR, NEUROBLASTOMA, AIDS-associated

Kaposi SARCOMA, and RHABDOMYOSARCOMA. Administered intravenously as the sulfate salt.

vinculum (ving′ku-lum) [L.] a band or bandlike structure.

vin′cula ten′dinum filaments that connect the phalanges with the flexor tendons.

vindesine (vin′dĕ-sēn) a synthetic VINCA ALKALOID derived from VINBLASTINE, administered intravenously as the sulfate salt as an antineoplastic AGENT in the treatment of acute lymphoblastic LEUKEMIA and non–small cell CARCINOMA.

vinorelbine (vi-nor′el-bēn) a semisynthetic VINCA ALKALOID derived from VINBLASTINE; administered intravenously as the tartrate salt as an antineoplastic AGENT in treatment of non–small cell lung cancer.

vinyl (vi′nil) the univalent group $CH_2{=}CH{-}$ from vinyl alcohol.

violence (vi′o-lens) great force, either physical or emotional, usually exerted in order to damage or otherwise abuse something or someone.

horizontal v. violence directed toward one's peers.

risk for v.: self-directed or directed at others a NURSING DIAGNOSIS accepted by the North American Nursing Diagnosis Association, defined as behaviors by an individual that can be physically harmful to either the self or others. Related factors include antisocial character, catatonic excitement, panic states, rage reactions, organic brain syndrome, and toxic reactions to drugs. Defining characteristics include aggressive body language, verbalization of hostility, boasting to others about prior abuse, increased motor activity, and overt and aggressive acts, or suicidal tendencies, depression, possession of weapons, history of DRUG ABUSE, and inability to verbalize feelings.

violet (vi′o-let) 1. the color produced by the shortest waves of the visible spectrum, beyond indigo, approximately 380 to 420 nm. 2. a dye or stain with this color.

crystal v., gentian v. methyl v. GENTIAN VIOLET; see under gentian.

viper (vi′per) 1. any snake of the VIPERID and CROTALID families (the *true vipers* and the *pit vipers*). 2. a term sometimes used to refer to any venomous snake.

Old World v. true viper.

pit v. any of a family of venomous snakes found in North America including the many types of RATTLESNAKES (genera *Crotalus* and *Sistrurus*), as well as the COPPERHEADS and water MOCCASINS (both of genus *Agkistrodon*).

Russell's v. *Vipera russellii*, a true VIPER of Southeast Asia whose venom (Russell's viper VENOM) is used in blood tests.

true v. any of a large family of venomous snakes found in Africa, parts of Europe, Asia, and adjacent islands, but not in the Americas or Australia; it includes COBRAS and ADDERS, among others. Called also Old World viper, viperid, and viperine.

viperid (vi′per-id) 1. viperine (def. 1). 2. true viper.

viperine (vi′per-ēn) pertaining to the true vipers; called also viperid. 1. true viper.

VIPoma an endocrine tumor, usually a type of islet cell TUMOR, that produces excessive amounts of VASOACTIVE INTESTINAL POLYPEPTIDE, producing severe diarrhea, hypokalemia, and hypochlorhydria, leading to renal failure that can be fatal.

vipoma VIPoma.

viral (vi′ral) pertaining to or caused by a virus.

Virales (vi-ra′lēz) the taxonomic order comprising the viruses.

Viread (vir′e-ad) trademark for a preparation of TENOFOVIR disoproxil fumarate, an antiretroviral agent.

viremia (vi-re′me-ah) the presence of viruses in the blood.

virgin (vir′jin) 1. a person who has not had sexual intercourse. 2. a laboratory animal that has been kept free from sexual intercourse.

virile (vir′il) 1. masculine. 2. specifically, having male copulative power.

virilism (vir′ĭ-lizm) the development or possession of male secondary sex CHARACTERS in a female or prepubertal male.

virility (vĭ-ril′ĭ-te) masculinity.

virilization (vir″ĭ-lĭ-za′shun) masculinization; usually used for that occurring inappropriately in a female or prepubertal male.

virion (vi′re-on) the complete viral particle, found extracellularly and capable of surviving in crystalline form and infecting a living cell; it comprises the nucleoid (genetic material) and the capsid.

viroid (vi′roid) any of a class of infectious agents consisting of a small strand of RNA not associated with any protein. The RNA does not code for proteins and is not translated; it is replicated by host cell enzymes. Viroids are known to cause several plant diseases.

virolactia (vi″ro-lak′she-ah) secretion of viruses in the milk.

virologist (vi-rol′ah-jist) microbiologist specializing in virology.

virology (vi-rol′ah-je) the study of viruses and viral diseases.

virtue (vir′choo) in BIOETHICS, a trait of character that disposes a person habitually to excellence of intent and performance

V

with respect to the TELOS proper to life as a human being or to a specific activity or role in life. Some virtues (such as cleanliness) are important socially rather than morally. (See also MORALITY.) Virtues in medicine include TRUSTWORTHINESS, COMPASSION, PHRONESIS, JUSTICE, FORTITUDE, TEMPERANCE, INTEGRITY, and SELF-EFFACEMENT.

virtue-based (vir'choo-bāsd) a concept of bioethics that emphasizes the agents who act and make choices. People acting in this manner often do not simply follow rules blindly; they have a moral desire to act the way they do. How one does what one does is as important as what one does. There is some circularity to the logic of virtue ethics, however: the moral, good act is considered to be one done by a virtuous person, and the virtuous person is considered to be one who does moral, good acts. To overcome this difficulty and to avoid moral subjectivism and emotivism, thinkers use PRINCIPLES as groundings for virtue ethics.

virucidal (vi″rŭ-si′dal) capable of neutralizing or destroying a virus.

virucide (vi′rŭ-sīd) an agent that neutralizes or destroys a virus; see also ANTIVIRAL.

virulence (vir′u-lens) the degree of pathogenicity of a microorganism as indicated by case fatality rates and/or its ability to invade the tissues of the host; the competence of any infectious agent to produce pathologic effects. adj., **vir′ulent.**

viruliferous (vir″u-lif′er-us) conveying or producing a virus or other noxious agent.

viruria (vi-roo′re-ah) the presence of viruses in the urine.

virus (vi′rus) any member of a unique class of infectious agents, which were originally distinguished by their smallness (hence, they were described as "filtrable" because of their ability to pass through fine ceramic filters that blocked all cells, including bacteria) and their inability to replicate outside of and without assistance of a living host cell. Because these properties are shared by certain bacteria (RICKETTSIAE, CHLAMYDIAE), viruses are now characterized by their simple organization and their unique mode of replication. A virus consists of genetic material, which may be either DNA or RNA, and is surrounded by a protein coat and, in some viruses, by a membranous envelope.

Unlike cellular organisms, viruses do not contain all the biochemical mechanisms for their own replication; they replicate by using the biochemical mechanisms of a host cell to synthesize and assemble their separate components. (Some do contain or

produce essential enzymes when there is no cellular enzyme that will serve.) When complete virus particle (VIRION) comes i contact with a host cell, only the vira nucleic acid and, in some viruses, a fev enzymes are injected into the host cell.

Within the host cell the genetic materia of a DNA virus is replicated and transcribe into messenger RNA by host cell enzymes and proteins coded for by viral genes ar synthesized by host cell ribosomes. Thes are the proteins that form the CAPSID (pro tein coat); there may also be a few enzyme or regulatory proteins involved in assem bling the capsid around newly synthesize viral nucleic acid, in controlling the bic chemical mechanisms of the host cell, an in lysing the host cell when new virion have been assembled. Some of these ma already have been present within the initia virus, and others may be coded for b the viral genome for production within th host cell.

Because host cells do not have the abilit to replicate "viral RNA" but are able t transcribe messenger RNA, RNA viruse must contain enzymes to produce geneti material for new virions. For certain viruse the RNA is replicated by a viral enzym (TRANSCRIPTASE) contained in the virion, o produced by the host cell using the vira RNA as a messenger. In other viruse a REVERSE TRANSCRIPTASE contained in th virion transcribes the genetic message o the viral RNA into DNA, which is the replicated by the host cell. Reverse tran scriptase is actually a combination of tw enzymes: a POLYMERASE that assembles th new DNA copy and an RNASE that degrade the source RNA.

In viruses that have membranes, mem brane-bound viral proteins are synthesize by the host cell and move, like host ce membrane proteins, to the cell surface When these proteins assemble to form th capsid, part of the host cell membrane i pinched off to form the envelope of th virion.

Some viruses have only a few gene coding for capsid proteins. Other mor complex ones may have a few hundre genes. But no virus has the thousands o genes required by even the simplest cells Although in general viruses "steal" thei lipid envelope from the host cell, virtuall all of them produce "envelope proteins that penetrate the envelope and serve a receptors. Some envelope proteins facilitat viral entry into the cell, and others hav directly pathogenic effects.

Some viruses do not produce rapid lysi of host cells, but rather remain latent fo

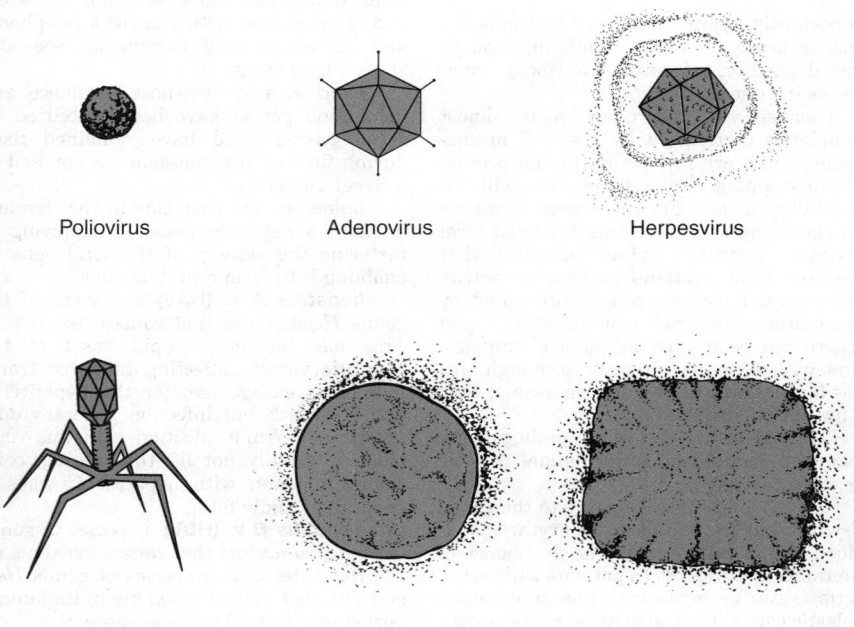

Poliovirus   Adenovirus   Herpesvirus

Bacteriophage   Mumps virus   Vaccinia virus

Comparison of shapes and sizes of viruses.

long periods in the host before the appearance of clinical symptoms. This carrier state can take any of several different forms. The term LATENCY is used to denote the interval from infection to clinical manifestations. In the LENTIVIRUSES, it was formerly mistakenly believed that virus was inactive during this period. The true situation is that lentiviruses are rapidly replicating and spawning dozens of quasi-species until a particularly effective one overruns the ability of the host's IMMUNE SYSTEM to defeat it. Other viruses, however, such as the HERPESVIRUSES, actually enter a time known as "viral latency," when little or no replication is taking place until further replication is initiated by a specific trigger. For many years all forms of latency were thought to be identical, but now it has been discovered that there are different types with basic and important distinctions.

In viral latency, most of the host cells may be protected from infection by immune mechanisms involving antibodies to the viral particles or INTERFERON. Cell-mediated immunity is essential, especially in dealing with infected host cells. Cytotoxic LYMPHOCYTES may also act as antigen-presenting CELLS to better coordinate the IMMUNE RESPONSE. Containment of virus in mucosal tissues is far more complex, involving follicular dendritic cells and Langerhans CELLS.

Some enveloped RNA viruses can be produced in infected cells that continue growing and dividing without being killed. This probably involves some sort of intracellular regulation of viral growth. It is also possible for the DNA of some viruses to be incorporated into the host cell DNA, producing a carrier state. These are almost always RETROVIRUSES, which are called PROVIRUSES before and after integration of viral DNA into the host genome.

Few viruses produce toxins, although viral infections of bacteria can cause previously innocuous bacteria to become much more pathogenic and toxic. Other viral proteins, such as some of the human immunodeficiency VIRUS, appear to be actively toxic, but those are the exception, not the rule.

However, viruses are highly antigenic. Mechanisms of pathologic injury to cells include cell LYSIS; induction of cell PROLIFERATION (as in certain WARTS and MOLLUSCUM CONTAGIOSUM); formation of giant cells, syncytia, or intracellular inclusion bodies caused by the virus; and perhaps most

V

importantly, symptoms caused by the host's IMMUNE RESPONSE, such as inflammation or the deposition of antigen-antibody complexes in tissues.

Because viral reproduction is almost completely carried out by host cell mechanisms, there are few points in the process where stopping viral reproduction will not also kill host cells. For this reason there are no chemotherapeutic agents for most viral diseases. ACYCLOVIR is an antiviral that requires viral proteins to become active. Some viral infections can be prevented by vaccination (active IMMUNIZATION), and others can be treated by passive IMMUNIZATION with immune GLOBULIN, although this has been shown to be effective against only a few dozen viruses.

attenuated v. one whose pathogenicity has been reduced by serial animal passage or other means.

B19 v. a species belonging to the genus *Erythrovirus* that binds to the erythrocyte P blood group antigen and is the cause of ERYTHEMA INFECTIOSUM. In patients with HEMOLYTIC ANEMIA or SICKLE CELL DISEASE it causes aplastic CRISIS; it can also cause acute ARTHRITIS. Fetal infection can cause HYDROPS FETALIS and spontaneous ABORTION or death in utero. Persistent infection in IMMUNOCOMPROMISED patients can lead to chronic bone marrow failure. Called also human parvovirus B19.

bacterial v. one that is capable of producing transmissible lysis of bacteria; see also BACTERIOPHAGE.

coryza v. rhinovirus.

Coxsackie v. coxsackievirus.

defective v. one that cannot be completely replicated or cannot form a protein coat; in some cases replication can proceed if missing gene functions are supplied by other viruses; see also helper VIRUS.

dengue v. a flavivirus, existing as four antigenically related but distinct types (designated 1, 2, 3, and 4), that causes both the classic and hemorrhagic forms of DENGUE.

DNA v. a virus whose GENOME consists of DNA.

Ebola v. an RNA virus almost identical to the Marburg virus but serologically distinct; it causes a disease similar to that caused by the Marburg virus.

EB v. Epstein-Barr virus.

encephalomyocarditis v. an enterovirus that causes mild aseptic meningitis and encephalomyocarditis.

enteric v's enterovirus.

enteric orphan v's orphan viruses isolated from the intestinal tract of humans and other animals.

Epstein-Barr v. (EBV) a herpeslike virus that causes infectious mononucleosis and is associated with Burkitt's lymphoma and nasopharyngeal carcinoma; see also EPSTEIN-BARR VIRUS.

fixed v. a virus whose virulence and incubation period have been stabilized by serial passage and have remained fixed during further transmission, as opposed to a street virus.

helper v. one that aids in the development of a defective virus by supplying or restoring the activity of the viral gene or enabling it to form a protein coat.

hepatitis A v. (HAV) any virus of the genus *Hepatovirus* that causes HEPATITIS A. This has the most rapid onset of the hepatitis viruses affecting humans; transmission is easier than for the hepatitis B and C VIRUSES, but infection generally does not persist. While infection with this virus alone is usually not life-threatening, coincident infection with hepatitis C VIRUS is generally rapidly fatal.

hepatitis B v. (HBV) a species of genus *Orthohepadnavirus* that causes HEPATITIS B.

hepatitis C v. a species of genus *Hepacivirus* that causes HEPATITIS C; its latency period may last 30 years or more.

hepatitis D v. (HDV), hepatitis delta v. an unclassified defective RNA virus, thought of as a parasite of the hepatitis B VIRUS and transmitted in the same manner; it requires enzymes and other assistance from HBV to replicate. This virus magnifies the pathogenicity of hepatitis B virus many times and is the etiologic agent of HEPATITIS D.

hepatitis E v. an enterically transmitted calicivirus that causes HEPATITIS E.

hepatitis G v. (HGV) a parenterally transmitted flavivirus originally isolated from a patient with chronic hepatitis; most infections are benign, and it is uncertain what role, if any, HGV plays in the etiology of liver disease.

hepatotropic v. a virus that primarily affects the liver, such as the hepatitis VIRUSES.

herpes v. herpesvirus.

herpes simplex v. former name for any virus that causes HERPES SIMPLEX, now called human herpesviruses; see HERPESVIRUS.

human immunodeficiency v. (HIV) either of two species of LENTIVIRUSES that cause ACQUIRED IMMUNODEFICIENCY SYNDROME (AIDS). HIV-1 is found around the world and HIV-2 is found primarily in West Africa. Progression of HIV-2 infection to AIDS is generally slower and less extreme than that of HIV-1. The virus is believed to induce permanent infection and has a propensity toward a subset of T LYMPHOCYTES called the

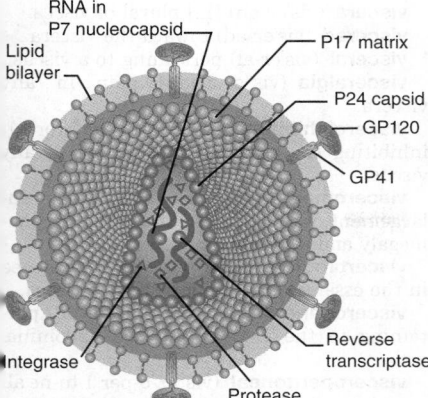

RNA in
P7 nucleocapsid
Lipid bilayer
P17 matrix
P24 capsid
GP120
GP41
Integrase
Reverse transcriptase
Protease

Human immunodeficiency virus: retrovirus particle. From Copstead, 1995.

CD4 CELLS. The infected cells become dysfunctional and eventually the host's IMMUNE SYSTEM is overwhelmed or exhausted; death ensues, usually as a result of infection. The virus is not transmitted through casual contact; the most common routes of transmission are through sexual intercourse, direct exposure to contaminated blood, and transplacental transmission from mother to fetus.

human T-cell leukemia v., human T-cell lymphotropic v. former names for human T-lymphotropic virus.

human T-lymphotropic v. (HTLV) either of two related species of RETROVIRUSES that have an affinity for the helper CELL type of T lymphocytes. HTLV-1 causes chronic infection and is associated with adult T-cell LEUKEMIA and a type of MYELOPATHY. HTLV-2 has been isolated from an atypical variant of hairy cell LEUKEMIA and from patients with other hematological disorders, but no clear association with disease has been established.

influenza v. any of a group of ORTHOMYXOVIRUSES that cause INFLUENZA; there are at least three serotypes or species (A, B, and C). Serotype A viruses are subject to major antigenic changes (antigenic SHIFTS) as well as minor gradual antigenic changes (antigenic DRIFT) and cause widespread epidemics and pandemics. Serotypes B and C are chiefly associated with sporadic epidemics.

influenza A v., influenza B v., influenza C v. species in the genera *Influenzavirus A, Influenzavirus B,* and *Influenzavirus C;* see influenza VIRUS.

La Crosse v. a virus of the California serogroup of the genus *Bunyavirus,* the etiologic agent of La Crosse ENCEPHALITIS.

latent v. one that ordinarily occurs in a noninfective state and is demonstrable by indirect methods that activate it.

lytic v. one that is replicated in the host cell and causes death and lysis of the cell.

maedi/visna v. a LENTIVIRUS that is the etiologic agent of a type of PNEUMONIA in sheep.

Marburg v. an RNA virus occurring in Africa, transmitted by insect bites, and causing MARBURG VIRUS DISEASE.

masked v. latent virus.

measles v. a paramyxovirus that is the cause of measles.

mumps v. a paramyxovirus that causes mumps and sometimes tenderness and swelling of the testes, pancreas, ovaries, or other organs.

Norwalk v. a CALICIVIRUS that is common cause of epidemics of acute GASTROENTERITIS, with diarrhea and vomiting that last 24 to 48 hours.

oncogenic v's an epidemiologic class of viruses that are acquired by close contact or injection and cause usually persistent infection; they may induce cell transformation and malignancy.

orphan v's viruses isolated in tissue culture, but not found specifically associated with any disease.

parainfluenza v. any of various PARAMYXOVIRUSES that cause upper respiratory tract disease of varying severity.

poliomyelitis v. see POLIOVIRUS.

pox v. poxvirus.

rabies v. an RNA virus of the rhabdovirus group that causes RABIES.

respiratory syncytial v. (RSV) any of a genus of single-stranded PARAMYXOVIRUSES; the name is derived from the type of disease produced (respiratory infection) and the microscopic appearance of the viruses in cell cultures. RSV can cause a wide variety of respiratory disorders ranging from a mild cold to serious or even fatal disease of the lung in the very young and very old. It regularly produces an outbreak of infection each winter and virtually disappears in the summer months. The most severe infections in children are in the very young, especially those who are preterm, immunologically compromised, or suffering from a congenital heart defect or preexisting lung disorder. Adults at risk for infection include parents and others who are repeatedly exposed to young children, for example, pediatric nurses and day care attendants. The course of infection tends to be milder in adults than in children and about 15 per cent of

V

affected adults have no symptoms. In the very elderly these infections may have the same degree of seriousness and clinical manifestations as in the very young.

RNA v. a virus whose GENOME consists of RNA.

rubella v. a togavirus that is the etiologic agent of rubella.

satellite v. a strain of virus unable to replicate except in the presence of helper VIRUS; considered to be deficient in coding for CAPSID formation.

simian-human immunodeficiency v. a chimeric, engineered virus with the ENVELOPE of human immunodeficiency VIRUS and the CYTOPLASM and NUCLEUS of simian immunodeficiency VIRUS; it is used in animal models because it is a better mimic of HIV than SIV is.

simian immunodeficiency v. (SIV) a LENTIVIRUS closely related to human immunodeficiency VIRUS that causes inapparent infection in African green monkeys and a disease resembling ACQUIRED IMMUNODEFICIENCY SYNDROME in macaques and chimpanzees.

slow v. any virus that remains latent for long periods in the infected host before the appearance of clinical symptoms.

smallpox v. variola virus.

street v. virus from a naturally infected animal, as opposed to a laboratory-adapted strain of the virus.

vaccinia v. a species of ORTHOPOXVIRUS that does not occur in nature and has been propagated for many years only in the laboratory for use as an active vaccine against SMALLPOX. The present virus is derived from the original one used by Jenner, obtained from the lesions of COWPOX, but the origin of the original virus remains unclear.

varicella-zoster v. former name for human herpesvirus 3; see HERPESVIRUS.

variola v. the virtually extinct ORTHOPOXVIRUS that is the etiologic agent of SMALLPOX. No natural infection has occurred since 1977, and no reservoir of the virus now exists.

West Nile v. a virus of the genus *Flavivirus,* the cause of West Nile ENCEPHALITIS; it is transmitted by *Culex* mosquitoes, with wild birds serving as the reservoir. It was originally endemic in Africa, Asia, and Europe, but recently spread to North America.

wild-type v. street virus.

Visagraph (ve'zah-graf) trademark for a device that records and measures eye movements while the patient is reading.

viscer(o)- word element [L.], *viscera.*

viscera (vis'er-ah) [L.] plural of VISCUS.

viscerad (vis'er-ad) toward the viscera.

visceral (vis'er-al) pertaining to a viscus.

visceralgia (vis"er-al'jah) pain in any viscera.

visceroinhibitory (vis"er-o-in-hib'ĭ-tor"e) inhibiting the essential movements of any viscus.

visceromegaly (vis"er-o-meg'ah-le) enlargement of the viscera; called also organomegaly and splanchnomegaly.

visceromotor (vis"er-o-mo'tor) concerned in the essential movements of the viscera.

visceroparietal (vis"er-o-pah-ri'ĕ-tal) pertaining to the viscera and the abdominal wall

visceroperitoneal (vis"er-o-per"ĭ-to-ne'al) pertaining to the viscera and peritoneum.

visceropleural (vis"er-o-ploor'al) pertaining to the viscera and the pleura.

viscerosensory (vis"er-o-sen'sor-e) pertaining to sensation in the viscera.

visceroskeletal (vis"er-o-skel'ĕ-tal) pertaining to the visceral skeleton.

viscerosomatic (vis"er-o-so-mat'ik) pertaining to the viscera and the body.

viscerotonia (vis"er-o-to'ne-ah) a temperament type characterized by love of physical comfort, sociability, tolerance for others, and extroversion; the behavioral counterpart of ENDOMORPHY.

viscerotropic (vis"er-o-trop'ik) acting primarily on the viscera; having a predilection for the abdominal or thoracic viscera.

viscid (vis'id) glutinous or sticky.

viscidity (vĭ-sid'ĭ-te) the property of being viscid.

viscoelastic (vis"ko-e-las'tik) both viscous and elastic; said of viscous substances used to restore or maintain the shape of the eye, especially the anterior chamber, during cataract surgery or other procedures performed on the anterior chamber.

viscosimeter (vis"ko-sim'ĕ-ter) an apparatus used in measuring viscosity of a substance.

viscosity (vis-kos'ĭ-te) resistance to flow a physical property of a substance that is dependent on the friction of its component molecules as they slide by one another.

viscous (vis'kus) sticky or gummy; having a high degree of viscosity.

viscus (vis'kus) [L.] any large interior organ in any of the great body cavities especially those in the abdomen.

vision (vizh'un) the faculty of seeing called also sight. adj., **vis'ual.** The basic components of vision are the EYE itself, the visual center in the brain, and the OPTIC NERVE which connects the two. (See also Plate 17.)

How the Eye Works. The eye works like a camera. Light rays enter it through the

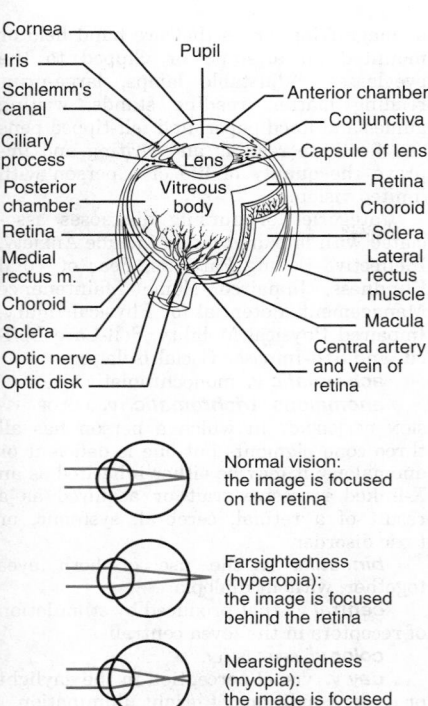

Cornea
Iris
Pupil
Schlemm's canal
Anterior chamber
Conjunctiva
Ciliary process
Capsule of lens
Lens
Posterior chamber
Vitreous body
Retina
Choroid
Retina
Sclera
Medial rectus m.
Lateral rectus muscle
Choroid
Macula
Sclera
Central artery and vein of retina
Optic nerve
Optic disk

Normal vision: the image is focused on the retina

Farsightedness (hyperopia): the image is focused behind the retina

Nearsightedness (myopia): the image is focused in front of the retina

Top, Anatomy of the eye. Vision is the reception of images by the eye as a result of the passage of light into the eye. Light is focused by the lens on the retina, where it is converted into nerve impulses that are transmitted to the centers in the brain where images are interpreted.

adjustable iris and are focused by the lens onto the retina, a thin light-sensitive layer which corresponds to the film of the camera. The retina converts the light rays into nerve impulses, which are relayed to the visual center. There the brain interprets them as images.

Like a camera lens, the lens of the eye reverses images as it focuses them. The images on the retina are upside down and they are "flipped over" in the visual center. In a psychology experiment, a number of volunteers wore glasses that inverted everything. After 8 days, their visual centers adjusted to this new situation, and when they took off the glasses, the world looked upside down until their brain centers readjusted.

The retina is made up of millions of tiny nerve cells that contain specialized chemicals that are sensitive to light. There are two varieties of these nerve cells, RODS and CONES. Between them they cover the full range of the eye's adaptation to light. The cones are sensitive in bright light, and the

rods in dim light. At twilight, as the light fades, the cones stop operating and the rods go into action. The momentary blindness experienced on going from bright to dim light, or from dim to bright, is the pause needed for the other set of nerve cells to take over.

The rods are spread toward the edges of the retina, so that vision in dim light is general but not very sharp or clear. The cones are clustered thickly in the center of the retina, in the fovea centralis. When the eyes are turned and focused on the object to be seen the image is brought to the central area of the retina. In very dim light, on the other hand, an object is seen more clearly if it is not looked at directly, because then its image falls on an area where the rods are thicker.

Color Vision. Color vision is a function of the cones. The most widely accepted theory is that there are three types of cones, each containing chemicals that respond to one of the three primary colors (red, green, and violet). White light stimulates all three sets of cones; any other color stimulates only one or two sets. The brain can then interpret the impulses from these cones as various colors. Man's color vision is amazingly delicate; a trained expert can distinguish among as many as 300,000 different hues.

COLOR VISION DEFICIENCY (popularly called "color blindness") is the result of a disorder of one or more sets of cones. The great majority of people with some degree of deficiency lack either red or green cones, and cannot distinguish between those two colors. Complete color vision deficiency (monochromatic VISION), in which none of the sets of color cones works, is very rare. Most deficiencies of color vision are inherited, usually by male children through their mothers from a grandfather with the condition.

Stereoscopic Vision. Stereoscopic vision, or vision in depth, is caused by the way the eyes are placed. Each eye has a slightly different field of vision. The two images are superimposed on one another, but because of the distance between the eyes, the image from each eye goes slightly around its side of the object. From the differences between the images and from other indicators such as the position of the eye muscles when the eyes are focused on the object, the brain can determine the distance of the object.

Stereoscopic vision works best on nearby objects. As the distance increases, the difference between the left-eyed and the right-eyed views becomes less, and the brain must

V

depend on other factors to determine distance. Among these are the relative size of the object, its color and clearness, and the receding lines of perspective. These factors may fool the eye; for example, in clear mountain air distant objects may seem to be very close. This is because their sharpness and color are not dulled by the atmosphere as much as they would be in more familiar settings.

Impaired Vision. This may consist of loss of visual acuity, visual field, ability to distinguish colors, motion of the eye, or any other function related to sight. (See also BLINDNESS.) Farsightedness, or HYPEROPIA, results when the eyeball is shorter than normal and the image focuses behind the retina. Nearsightedness, or MYOPIA, results when the eyeball is longer than usual from front to back, so that the image focuses in front of the retina. ASTIGMATISM is impaired vision caused by irregularities in the curvature of the cornea or lens.

Patient Care. Visually handicapped persons who are visiting a clinic for the first time or being admitted to a hospital room require orientation to their environment. Ambulatory patients can be walked around to familiarize them with the location of the bathroom and any other facility they may need to use.

Patients who are in bed following surgery or for therapeutic rest should have articles on their bedside table arranged in the same way all of the time so that they can be found easily. If only one eye is affected, articles should be placed within reach on the unaffected side and persons communicating with the patient also should stand on that side. If peripheral vision is limited, objects and persons should be positioned in the patient's line of vision.

Some patients, especially the elderly, may experience increased sensitivity to glare. Wearing sunglasses outdoors, adjusting the window blinds to deflect the sun, and using indirect lighting can help avoid discomfort. This does not mean that the patient should be in a darkened room. For most, increased illumination makes it easier to see. It is the glare that impairs their vision.

Whenever it is necessary to do something for the visually impaired person, explain beforehand what will be done. This helps reduce confusion and establishes trust in the caregiver. (For patient care, see also BLINDNESS.)

Patients with impaired vision may also benefit from such low-vision aids as convex or magnifying lenses that are hand held or mounted on a stand or clipped to the eyeglasses. Adjustable lamps, large-print reading matter, reading stands, writing guides and lined paper, and felt-tipped pens can facilitate reading and writing and improve the quality of life of a person with limited vision.

Categories of nursing diagnoses associated with impaired vision include Anxiety, Ineffective Coping Patterns, Fear of Total Blindness, Impaired Home Maintenance Management, Potential for Physical Injury, Impaired Physical Mobility, Self-Care Deficit, and Self-Imposed Social Isolation.

achromatic v. monochromatic vision.

anomalous trichromatic v. COLOR VISION DEFICIENCY in which a person has all three cone pigments but one is deficient or anomalous; it may be either inherited as an X-linked recessive trait or acquired as a result of a retinal, cerebral, systemic, or toxic disorder.

binocular v. the use of both eyes together, without diplopia.

central v. that produced by stimulation of receptors in the fovea centralis.

color v. see VISION.

day v. visual perception in the daylight or under conditions of bright illumination.

dichromatic v. COLOR VISION DEFICIENCY in which one of the three cone pigments is missing altogether. The most common forms are PROTANOPIA and DEUTERANOPIA, which are transmitted by X-linked inheritance. A third form, TRITANOPIA, is very rare. A fourth form is also thought to exist, called TETARTANOPIA. Called also dichromatism.

double v. diplopia.

indirect v. peripheral vision.

low v. impairment of vision such that there is significant visual handicap but also significant usable residual vision; such impairment may involve visual acuity, visual fields, or ocular motility.

monochromatic v. COLOR VISION DEFICIENCY in which the person cannot distinguish hues, so that all the colors of the spectrum appear as shades of gray. Popularly known as complete or total color BLINDNESS.

monocular v. vision with one eye.

multiple v. polyopia.

night v. visual perception in the darkness of night or under conditions of reduced illumination.

oscillating v. oscillopsia.

peripheral v. that produced by stimulation of receptors in the retina outside the macula lutea; called also indirect vision.

v. therapy technician an allied health professional who evaluates clients and plans

nd implements vision therapy programs
nder the supervision of an OPTOMETRIST

trichromatic v. 1. any ability to see all
hree primary colors of light (red, green,
nd blue). 2. normal color VISION; called also
richromacy and trichromatism.

tunnel v. 1. that in which the visual
ield is severely constricted. When it is due to
rganic causes, such as retinitis pigmentosa
r glaucoma, the visual field expands as it is
ested at increasing distance from a constant
bject but when it is due to psychogenic
isorders, such as conversion disorder or
nalingering, the field remains constant or
ontracts as the distance increases. 2. in
sychiatry, restriction of psychological or
motional perception to a limited range.

Vistaril (vis'tah-ril) trademark for prep-
rations of HYDROXYZINE, an ANTIANXIETY
GENT, ANTIEMETIC, SEDATIVE, and ANTIPRURITIC.

visualization (vizh″u-al-ī-za'shun) 1. the
ct of viewing or of achieving a complete
isual impression of an object. 2. use of a
erson's own imagination and positive
hinking to reduce stress or promote heal-
ng.

visuoauditory (vizh″u-o-aw'dĭ-tor″e) per-
aining to vision and hearing.

visuognosis (vizh″u-og-no'sis) recogni-
ion and interpretation of visual impres-
ions.

visuolexic (vizh″u-o-lek'sik) pertaining to
he visual aspects of language, as in percep-
ion of written language.

visuopsychic (vizh″u-o-si'kik) visual and
sychic; applied to the area of the cerebral
ortex concerned in judgment of visual
ensation.

visuosensory (vizh″u-o-sen'sor-e) per-
aining to perception of visual impressions.

visuospatial (vizh″u-o-spa'shal) pertain-
ng to visual perception of spatial relation-
hips.

vital (vi'tal) pertaining to life; necessary
o life.

v. capacity (VC) the greatest volume of
as that, following maximum inhalation,
an be expelled during a complete, slow,
orced exhalation; equal to inspiratory CAPAC-
TY plus expiratory reserve VOLUME.

Forced vital CAPACITY (FVC) is the great-
st volume of air that can be expelled when
person performs a rapid, forced exhala-
ion, which usually takes about five seconds.
The greatest volume of air a person can
xhale during one, two, three, or more
econds of forced exhalation is called the
orced expiratory VOLUME (FEV). A subscript
s added to the abbreviation FEV to indicate
he phase during which the particular
mount or volume of air is exhaled. A
olume exhaled during the first second is

designated $FEV_{1.0}$, a volume exhaled during
the first two seconds is designated $FEV_{2.0}$,
and so on. The rate at which a specified
volume of air is exhaled during a forced
exhalation is called forced expiratory FLOW
(FEF). The rate at which air is exhaled from
a forced expiratory volume of 200 mL to one
of 1200 mL is designated $FEF_{200-1200}$ (formerly called maximal expiratory flow,
MEF); the rate from 25 to 75 per cent of
the forced vital capacity is designated
$FEF_{25-75\%}$ (formerly called maximal midexpiratory flow, MMF).

Laboratory values for vital capacity,
forced vital capacity, forced expiratory volume, and forced expiratory flow are usually
reported both as absolute values and as
statistically derived predicted values based
on the age, sex, and height of a patient. The
statistical value is reported as a percentage.
See also PULMONARY FUNCTION TESTS.

vitality (vi-tal'ĭ-te) the condition of being
alive, as opposed to DEATH or NECROSIS.

pulp v. the normal condition of the
dental pulp, having vascularity and sensation.

Vitallium (vi-tal'e-um) trademark for a
cobalt-chromium alloy used for dentures
and surgical appliances.

vitamer (vi'tah-mer) one of multiple related chemical compounds possessing a
given vitamin activity.

vitamin (vi'tah-min) an organic substance
found in foods and essential in small quantities for growth, health, and the preservation of life itself. The body needs vitamins
just as it requires other food constituents
such as proteins, fats, carbohydrates, minerals, and water. The absence of one or more
vitamins from the diet, or poor absorption
of vitamins, can cause deficiency diseases
such as RICKETS, SCURVY, and BERIBERI. Vitamins serve as coenzymes or cofactors in
enzymatic reactions. They are required only
in trace quantities because they are not
consumed in the reactions. The major
vitamins are designated by the letters A, C,
D, E, and K, and the term B complex. The B
vitamins and vitamin C are water soluble.
The rest are fat soluble and are not
absorbed unless the body's digestion and
absorption of fats is normal. Deficiencies of
the fat-soluble vitamins can be produced by
various malabsorption syndromes.

Vitamin A. Vitamin A helps to maintain
epithelial tissues which cover the body and
line certain internal organs. This vitamin
also is essential for the proper growth of
skeletal and soft tissues, and is necessary
for light-sensitive pigments in the eye that

V

make night vision possible. The particular manifestation of vitamin A deficiency depends upon the age of the patient. Among the most common symptoms of vitamin A deficiency is night blindness. The skin may also be affected, becoming dry and pimply like a toad's skin.

Vitamin A occurs in nature in two forms: retinol (vitamin A_1) and dehydroretinol (vitamin A_2). It is manufactured by animals and humans from carotenes found in green leafy and yellow vegetables, including kale, broccoli, spinach, carrots, squash, and sweet potatoes. It is obtained directly by eating animal products such as liver, eggs, whole milk, cream, and cheese. A toxic syndrome (hypervitaminosis A) can result from excessive vitamin intake. It is marked by generalized pruritus, desquamation of the skin, loss of hair, and hyperostoses.

The B Complex. The original "vitamin B" was found to be a group of vitamins, each differing chemically and each individually important in the body. For convenience, these vitamins are referred to as one group since they are often found together in foods. Deficiency in only one of these vitamins is rare, and the deficiency disease attributed to lack of one vitamin B usually is complicated by deficiencies of the others as well.

Vitamin B₁ (Thiamine). This vitamin is necessary to break down and release energy from carbohydrates. Lack of thiamine can cause loss of appetite, certain types of neuritis, and, in severe cases, BERIBERI, which affects the brain, heart, and nerves. The best sources of thiamine are yeasts, ham and certain pork cuts, liver, peanuts, whole-grain and fortified cereals and breads, and milk. The vitamin is easily destroyed by cooking and may also be lost by dissolving in the cooking water. Because the body does not store thiamine well, foods that are good sources of it should be included in each day's diet.

Vitamin B₂ (Riboflavin). This vitamin functions as a coenzyme concerned with oxidative processes. Riboflavin deficiency (ARIBOFLAVINOSIS) was at one time a common vitamin deficiency disease in the United States. It still occurs in parts of Asia, the West Indies, and elsewhere. Symptoms include open sores at the corners of the mouth and on the lips, a purple-red, inflamed tongue, seborrheic dermatitis, and corneal and other eye changes. The main food sources of riboflavin are milk, liver, kidney, heart, green vegetables, dried yeasts, and enriched breads and cereals. It is not usually affected by cooking, but is destroyed by light.

Niacin (Nicotinic Acid). This B vitamin appears to act in enzyme systems to utilize carbohydrates, fats, and amino acids. Niacin deficiency causes PELLAGRA, once a major deficiency disease in the United States. Symptoms of pellagra involve the skin and digestive and nervous systems. Niacin also has vasodilating activity. Food sources of niacin are various high-protein foods such as liver, yeast, bran, peanuts, lean meats, fish and poultry.

Vitamin B₁₂ (Cyanocobalamin). This vitamin contains COBALT and is needed for the efficient production of blood cells and for the health of the nervous system. Only small amounts of B_{12} are required by the body. The activity of this vitamin is associated with that of another B vitamin, folic acid. Inability to absorb vitamin B_{12} occurs in PERNICIOUS ANEMIA, in which a substance normally secreted by the stomach, called intrinsic factor, is missing. Intrinsic factor is needed to absorb vitamin B_{12} in the small intestine. Injections of vitamin B_{12} can control pernicious anemia. Poor absorption of vitamin B_{12} also occurs in sprue.

Vitamin B_{12} is not found in plant foods. The main sources in the human diet are animal products such as milk, eggs, and liver. Probably the ultimate source of B_{12} is bacterial production in animal intestines. This production occurs in humans, and in normal persons probably meets some or perhaps all of the body's requirements.

Other Members of the B Vitamin Complex. These include vitamin B_6 (PYRIDOXINE), BIOTIN, FOLIC ACID, PANTOTHENIC ACID, CHOLINE, INOSITOL, and p-AMINOBENZOIC ACID. Vitamin B_6 deficiency can cause convulsions, lethargy, mental changes and retardation, inflammation of the skin, and anemia. These substances, like most other members of the B complex, are widely found in fruits, vegetables, meat, and whole-grain cereals.

Vitamin C (Ascorbic Acid). This vitamin is necessary for the health of supporting tissues such as bone, cartilage, and connective tissue. Deficiency produces SCURVY. Vitamin C is found in fresh fruits and vegetables, including citrus fruits, tomatoes, brussels sprouts, and to some extent whole potatoes. Cooking and storage destroy much of the vitamin C content of foods.

Vitamin D. The action of sunlight on the skin changes certain substances in the body into vitamin D, a term for any of several active substances required for the utilization of calcium and phosphorus, which are essential for the growth and maintenance of bone. These include cholecalciferol and ergocalciferol (known collectively as calciferol). Vitamin D deficiency causes RICKETS in children and OSTEOMALACIA and OSTEOPOROSIS in adults. Rickets is usually caused either by a diet deficient in vitamin D or by insufficient exposure to sunlight. Few foods contain vitamin D. The only rich natural sources are fish liver oil and the livers of animals feeding on fish. For this reason vitamin D often is added to milk. A toxic syndrome (hypervitaminosis D) can result from excessive vitamin D intake. It results in hypercalcemia with its typical symptoms of weakness, fatigue, loss of weight, and impairment of renal function.

Vitamin E. There are at least eight different antioxidants in this group, of which ALPHATOCOPHEROL is the most common; they prevent the oxidation of unsaturated FATTY ACIDS, thus preventing cell damage that can lead to neurological symptoms. Because of its ubiquitous nature, supplemental intake of vitamin E is not necessary. It is found in wheat germ oil, cereals, egg yolk, and beef liver.

Vitamin K. Any of a group of vitamins including vitamin K_1 (phytonadione) and vitamin K_2 (menaquinone) found in alfalfa, spinach, cabbage, putrefied fish meal, and hempseed, which promote blood clotting by increasing the synthesis of prothrombin by the liver; therefore, deficiency of vitamin K delays clotting. Symptoms of vitamin K deficiency are excessive bleeding and bruises under the skin. Generally, the bacteria of the intestine produce vitamin K in quantities that are adequate (provided it can be absorbed), except in newborn infants, in whom the deficiency is most frequently found.

Vitamin Supplements. The exact vitamin requirements for good health often are not known with accuracy; they vary with age, weight, sex, and state of health. The need for certain vitamins increases with fever, some diseases, heavy exercise, pregnancy, and nursing. Persons eating an adequate, varied diet of meats, fruits and vegetables, and dairy products will receive enough vitamins to meet normal requirements. Public health measures such as the addition of vitamin D to milk and the B vitamins to bread and other cereal products have helped to combat deficiency diseases.

The use of vitamin supplements is expensive and in general unnecessary. Specialists in nutrition advise against taking supplementary vitamins unless they are prescribed for a specific reason. Overdoses of vitamins D, A, or K may result in serious disease, with the excess vitamins acting like poisons. Vitamins are commonly prescribed in infancy and childhood, during pregnancy and nursing, for elderly patients whose

dietary habits are poor, and in clearly diagnosed deficiency states. These include not only the more familiar deficiency diseases already described but also alcoholism and chronic wasting diseases.

vitelline (vi-tel′in) resembling or pertaining to the YOLK of an egg or ovum.

vitellus (vi-tel′us) yolk.

vitiligines (vit″ĭ-lij′ĭ-nēz) depigmented areas of the skin.

vitiligo (vit″ĭ-li′go) a condition in which destruction of melanocytes in small or large circumscribed areas results in patches of depigmentation often having a hyperpigmented border, and often enlarging slowly. adj., **vitilig′inous.**

vitrectomy (vī-trek′tah-me) surgical removal of a diseased VITREOUS of the eye. Vitreous strands are cut with a specially designed infusion cutter that delivers a physiologic solution (e.g., Ringer's solution) to maintain intraocular pressure, and withdraws the diseased vitreous by suction. Almost half of all vitrectomies are done for the treatment of diabetic RETINOPATHY in order to prevent blindness. It also may be done for treatment of vitreous hemorrhage due to other causes, such as penetrating injuries to the eye, hemolytic glaucoma, central vein occlusion, and some forms of retinal detachment.

vitreitis (vit″re-i′tis) hyalitis.

vitreodentin (vit″re-o-den′tin) an unusually hard and glasslike form of dentin.

vitreous (vit′re-us) 1. glasslike or hyaline. 2. the vitreous body.

persistent hyperplastic v. a congenital anomaly, usually unilateral, due to persistence of embryonic remnants of the fibromuscular tunic of the eye and part of the hyaloid vascular system. Clinically, there is a white pupil, elongated ciliary processes, and often microphthalmia; the lens, although clear initially, may become completely opaque.

vitronectin (vit″ro-nek′tin) a multifunctional adhesive GLYCOPROTEIN found in serum and various tissues. Its functions include regulation of the coagulation, fibrinolytic, and COMPLEMENT cascades, and it plays a role in hemostasis, wound healing, tissue remodeling, and cancer. It mediates the inflammatory and repair reactions at sites of tissue injury and promotes adhesion, spreading, and migration of cells. It has been shown to be identical to S PROTEIN, which was identified as an inhibitor of COMPLEMENT activation, binding the membrane attack COMPLEX and preventing its insertion into the membrane.

V

vitritis (vĭ-tri'tis) hyalitis.

vivi- word element [L.], *alive; life.*

viviparous (vi-vip'ah-rus) giving birth to living young which develop within the maternal body.

vivisection (viv″ĭ-sek'shun) surgical procedures performed upon a living animal for purpose of physiologic or pathologic investigation.

vivisectionist (viv″ĭ-sek'shun-ist) one who practices or defends vivisection.

VLBW very low birth weight; see under INFANT.

VLDL very-low-density LIPOPROTEIN.

VM-26 teniposide.

VMD Veterina'riae Medici'nae Doc'tor (Doctor of Veterinary Medicine).

vocabulary (vo-kab'u-lar″e) a list of words and terms, sometimes accompanied by definitions or translations.

   controlled v. an artificial language for the representation of attributes of entities, e.g., subjects of documents.

   standardized v. language (def. 3).

vocal (vo'kal) pertaining to the voice.

   v. cords the thin, reedlike folds of mucous membrane in the LARYNX; the superior pair are called the *false vocal cords* and the inferior pair are called the *true vocal cords.* (See also Plates.) They vibrate to make vocal sounds during speaking, and are capable of producing a vast range of sounds. Each cord has one end attached to the front wall of the larynx, close to that of the other cord. The opposite ends are connected to two tiny cartilages near the back wall of the larynx. The cartilages can be rotated so as to swing the cords far apart or bring them together. When they are apart, the breath passes through silently, unobstructed; when they are closer together, they partly obstruct the air passage, and as the air is forced through them they vibrate like the reeds of a pipe organ and produce sound waves. These waves are what we call the VOICE. See also SPEECH.

Vogt-Spielmeyer disease (fōkt-shpēl'mi-er) the juvenile form of neuronal ceroid-LIPOFUSCINOSIS, with onset between 5 and 10 years of age, characterized by rapid cerebroretinal degeneration, massive loss of brain substance, excessive neuronal storage of lipofuscin, and death within 10 to 15 years.

Vogt-Koyanagi-Harada syndrome (fōkt ko-yah-nah'ge hah-rah'dah) a syndrome of UVEOMENINGITIS associated with retinochoroidal detachment, temporary or permanent deafness and blindness, and sometimes (usually not permanent) ALOPECIA, VITILIGO, and POLIOSIS. The etiology is unknown, but it may be an inflammatory AUTOIMMUNE condition. Called also Harada syndrome.

voice (vois) the sound produced by the SPEECH organs and uttered by the mouth.

void (void) excrete.

   double v. a technique of bladder TRAINING useful for those with urinary RETENTION; the patient is taught to urinate, relax for five minutes, and repeat urination. A patient who is performing glucose examinations of the urine should test the second specimen.

voiding (void'ing) excretion.

   prompted v. 1. a technique of bladder TRAINING in which the patient is instructed to urinate according to a predetermined schedule, usually beginning at intervals as often as one hour to an hour and a half. 2. in the NURSING INTERVENTIONS CLASSIFICATION, a nursing INTERVENTION defined as promotion of urinary continence through the use of timed verbal toileting reminders and positive social feedback for successful toileting.

vol volume.

vola (vo'lah) a concave or hollow surface.

   v. ma'nus palm.

   v. pe'dis planta pedis.

volar (vo'lar) pertaining to the sole or palm; indicating the flexor surface of the forearm, wrist, or hand.

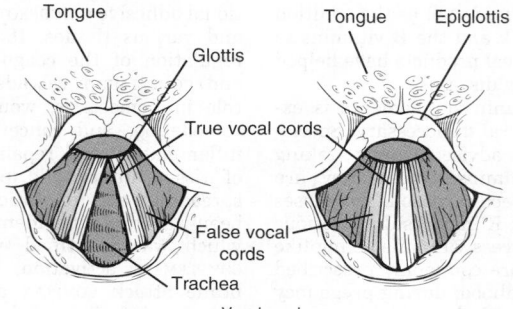

Vocal cords.

volaris (vo-la′ris) palmar.

volatile (vol′ah-til) evaporating rapidly; vaporizing readily at low temperatures.

volatilization (vol″ah-til-ĭ-za′shun) conversion into a vapor or gas without chemical change.

volition (vo-lish′un) the act or power of willing. adj., **voli′tional.**

Volkmann's disease (fōlk′mahnz) congenital deformity of the foot due to tibiotarsal dislocation.

volley (vol′e) a rhythmical succession of muscular twitches artificially induced; the aggregate of nerve impulses set up by a single stimulus.

volsella (vol-sel′ah) vulsella.

volt (V) (vōlt) the SI UNIT of electric POTENTIAL or electromotive force, equal to 1 watt per ampere, or 1 joule per coulomb.

    ***electron v.* (eV)** a unit of energy equal to the energy acquired by an electron in being accelerated through a potential difference of 1 volt; equal to 1.602×10^{-19} joule.

    ***gigaelectron v.* (GeV)** one billion electron volts (10^9 eV).

    ***kiloelectron v.* (keV)** one thousand electron volts (10^3 eV).

    ***megaelectron v.* (MeV)** one million electron volts (10^6 eV).

voltage (vōl′tij) electromotive force measured in volts.

voltmeter (vōlt′me-ter) an instrument for measuring electromotive force in volts.

volume (vol′ūm) the space occupied by a substance or a three-dimensional region; the capacity of such a region or of a container.

    blood v. the plasma VOLUME added to the red cell VOLUME; see also BLOOD VOLUME.

    ***closing v.* (CV)** the volume of gas in the lungs in excess of the residual VOLUME at the time small airways in the dependent portions close during maximal exhalation; see also CLOSING VOLUME.

    deficient fluid v. a NURSING DIAGNOSIS accepted by the North American Nursing Diagnosis Association, defined as decreased intravascular, interstitial, and/or intracellular fluid. This refers to DEHYDRATION, water loss alone without change in SODIUM. See also fluid VOLUME. Formerly called fluid volume deficit.

When a person engages in normal physical activity and the environmental temperature is 20°C (68°F), the body loses about 2400 ml of water in 24 hours. About 1400 ml are lost in urine, 200 ml in feces, and 100 ml in sweat. The remaining 700 ml are lost through what is called *insensible water loss,* which takes place by diffusion through the skin and by evaporation from the lungs. About 300 ml of water diffuse through the epithelial cells daily. The lungs excrete about 400 ml per day.

A deficit of fluid volume occurs when there is either an excessive loss of body water or an inadequate compensatory intake. Etiologic factors include active loss through vomiting, diarrhea, gastric suctioning, drainage through operative wounds and tubes, burns, fistulas, hypermetabolic states, and drug-induced diuresis. Insufficient intake of water can be caused by nausea, immobility with inaccessibility of water, and lack of knowledge about the necessity of adequate fluid intake.

Patient Care. Assessment of the patient's hydration ˙status includes monitoring lab data for such signs as increased packed red blood cell volume, increased plasma protein level, elevated specific gravity of urine, and increased blood urea nitrogen (BUN) out of proportion to a change in serum creatinine. In the absence of other problems, the serum sodium should remain within normal limits.

Recording daily weight gives information about the amount of water gained or lost each day. If there is a fluid volume deficit, intake and output measurements can give evidence of fluid imbalance. The urine appears concentrated and is usually well below the criterion of 50 ml of output per hour. Other objective assessment data include hypotension and a decrease in venous filling and in pulse volume and pressure. The mucous membranes are dry, as is the skin, which loses its turgor. The patient may complain of thirst and the body temperature may be elevated.

Patients at risk for profound and potentially fatal fluid volume deficit, as in severe burns, should be assessed frequently for mental acuity status and orientation to person, place, and time. Measures to improve hydration status should take into account the patient's ability to drink and retain fluids by mouth, preferences for certain fluids, and whether hot or cold drinks are preferred. The goal of oral fluid intake should be about 2000 ml per day. Explanations about the importance of an adequate fluid intake and assuring the availability of fresh water and fluids attractive to the patient can help reach the desired goal. Intravenous administration of fluids, especially isotonic saline, may be necessary if oral replacement is not possible. In severe and intractable fluid volume deficit a central venous catheter may be used to evaluate the extent of fluid loss and to guide replacement therapy.

V

excess fluid v. a NURSING DIAGNOSIS accepted by the North American Nursing Diagnosis Association, defined as increased isotonic fluid retention; see also fluid VOLUME. Factors contributing to this include (1) arterial dilatation, as occurs in the inflammatory process; (2) reduced oncotic pressure, as in hypoproteinuria (particularly a deficit of albumin, which is responsible for 80 per cent of oncotic pressure), lymphatic obstruction, and increased capillary permeability, which allows water to escape into the tissues and produce swelling; (3) renal retention of sodium and consequently of water, as seen in RENAL FAILURE; (4) inadequate circulation of blood through the general circulation, as in congestive HEART FAILURE, or through the portal circulation, as in liver failure; and (5) overproduction or administration of adrenocortical hormones.

HYPERVOLEMIA can occur when a patient receives excessive fluid replacement or repeated tap water enemas or, much less frequently, drinks more fluids than are eliminated. Characteristics of fluid volume excess include obvious swelling, localized or generalized; weight gain; pulmonary congestion with accompanying shortness of breath, orthopnea, and abnormal breath sounds; a fluid intake greater than output; distended neck veins; and changes in central venous and pulmonary artery pressures.

expiratory reserve v. the maximal amount of gas that can be exhaled from the resting end-expiratory level.

fluid v. the volume of the body FLUIDS, including both intracellular FLUID and extracellular FLUID.

forced expiratory v. (FEV) the volume that can be exhaled from a full inhalation by exhaling as forcefully and rapidly as possible for a timed period. Times are denoted by subscripts, such as $FEV_{0.5}$, $FEV_{1.0}$, $FEV_{2.0}$, and $FEV_{3.0}$ for FEV values for 0.5, 1, 2, and 3 seconds.

inspiratory reserve v. the maximal amount of gas that can be inhaled from the end-inspiratory position.

mean corpuscular v. (MCV) the average volume of erythrocytes, conventionally expressed in cubic micrometers or femtoliters (μm^3 = fL) per red cell, obtained by multiplying the hematocrit (in l/L) by 1000 and dividing by the red cell count (in millions per μL): MCV = Hct/RBC. Automated electronic blood cell counters generally obtain the MCV directly from the average pulse height of the voltage pulses produced during the red cell count. These instruments obtain the hematocrit indirectly from the equation Hct = MCV × RBC.

minute v. (MV) the quantity of gas exhaled from the lungs per minute; tidal VOLUME multiplied by respiration RATE.

packed-cell v. (PCV) hematocrit.

plasma v. the total volume of blood plasma, i.e., the extracellular fluid volume of the vascular space; see also BLOOD VOLUME.

red cell v. the total volume of red cells in the body; see also BLOOD VOLUME.

residual v. (RV) the amount of gas remaining in the lung at the end of a maximal exhalation.

risk for deficient fluid v. a NURSING DIAGNOSIS accepted by the North American Nursing Diagnosis Association, defined as being at risk for vascular, cellular, or intracellular dehydration. See also deficient fluid VOLUME.

stroke v. the quantity of blood ejected from a ventricle at each beat of the heart; called also stroke output.

tidal v. the amount of gas passing into and out of the lungs in each respiratory cycle.

volumetric (vol″u-met′rik) pertaining to or accompanied by measurement in volumes.

voluntary (vol′un-tār″e) accomplished in accordance with the will.

volunteer (vol″un-tēr′) someone who does a task voluntarily and usually without pay.

volute (vo-lūt′) rolled up.

volutrauma (vol′u-traw″mah) damage to the lung caused by overdistention by a mechanical ventilator set for an excessively high tidal VOLUME; it results in a syndrome similar to ADULT RESPIRATORY DISTRESS SYNDROME.

volvulosis (vol″vu-lo′sis) ONCHOCERCIASIS due to *Onchocerca volvulus.*

volvulus (vol′vu-lus) [L.] TORSION of a loop of intestine, causing obstruction with or without strangulation. See accompanying illustration.

vomer (vo′mer) a bone forming part of the nasal septum; see Appendix 2-3. adj., **vo′merine.**

vomit (vom′it) 1. matter expelled from the stomach by the mouth. 2. to eject stomach contents through the mouth.

black v. vomit consisting of blood that has been acted upon by the gastric juice, seen in yellow fever and other conditions in which blood collects in the stomach.

coffee-ground v. dark granular material ejected from the stomach, produced by mixture of blood with gastric contents; it is a sign of bleeding in the upper alimentary canal.

WINDOW ON VOLUNTEERING

Health care professionals have a long and proud history of volunteering, giving their time and energy to support a cause or organization that is important to them. There are literally millions of charities, social welfare organizations, and religious congregations around the world that rely on the generosity and commitment of volunteers in order to function effectively. In some cases, these organizations are totally volunteer-driven, while in other instances volunteers augment and supplement the work of paid staff.

What accounts for this extraordinary response? Volunteers come from every walk of life but are united in a common vision of action and a desire to make a difference. Those who have volunteered know that there are substantial personal benefits and rewards that accrue: a sense of contributing to the general welfare of society, an opportunity to meet new people and to learn new skills, a chance to challenge onself to grow personally and professionally. In today's hectic world, volunteering provides an opportunity to be involved with an activity purely out of a personal desire to contribute. Volunteers are able to step out of their regular routine, often a welcome change.

There are a wide variety of places to volunteer, locally, nationally, and internationally. The key to being effective is to work with an organization that knows how to utilize effectively the volunteers' skills, and for the volunteers to spend some time learning about what they will be doing and the people with whom they will be working. Finding the right fit may entail some time but the personal and professional benefits are enormous.

NANCY A. KELLY, MHS

vomiting (vom′it-ing) forcible ejection of contents of stomach through the mouth. Called also emesis and regurgitation.

> **cyclic v.** recurring attacks of vomiting.
>
> **dry v.** attempts at vomiting, with the ejection of nothing but gas.
>
> **pernicious v., v. of pregnancy** hyperemesis gravidarum.
>
> **projectile v.** vomiting with the material ejected with great force; seen commonly in congenital pyloric obstruction.
>
> **stercoraceous v.** vomiting of fecal matter.

vomitory (vom′ĭ-tor″e) emetic.

vomiturition (vom″ĭ-tu-rish′un) retching.

vomitus (vom′ĭ-tus) 1. vomiting. 2. matter vomited.

von Gierke's disease (von gēr′kez) Gierke's disease.

von Hippel's disease (von hip′elz) hemangiomatosis confined chiefly to the retina.

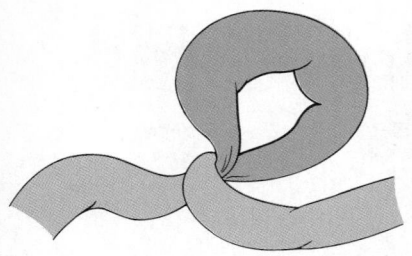

Volvulus. From Chabner, 1996.

von Hippel-Lindau disease (von hip′el lin′dow) a hereditary condition marked by angiomatosis of the retina and cerebellum, which may be associated with similar lesions of the spinal cord and cysts of the viscera; neurologic symptoms, including seizures and mental retardation, may be present. Called also Lindau's disease.

von Recklinghausen's disease (von rek′-ling-how″zenz) 1. Type I NEUROFIBROMATOSIS. 2. see OSTEITIS FIBROSA CYSTICA.

von Willebrand's disease (von vil′ĕ-brahnts) a congenital bleeding disorder, inherited as an autosomal dominant trait, characterized by a prolonged bleeding time, deficiency of von Willebrand's FACTOR, and often impairment of platelet adhesion. It is associated with epistaxis and increased bleeding after trauma or surgery, menorrhagia, and postpartum bleeding. Called also angiohemophilia and pseudohemophilia.

vortex (vor′teks) [L.] a whorled or spiral arrangement or pattern, as of muscle fibers, or of the ridges or hairs of the skin.

> **vox** (voks), pl. vo′ces [L.] voice.
>
> **v. chole′rica** the peculiar suppressed voice of true cholera.

voxel (vok′sel) a volume element; the region in a tissue slice that corresponds to a PIXEL (picture element) in an image. See also computed TOMOGRAPHY.

voyeurism (voi′yer-izm) a paraphilia in which the preferred method of achieving sexual excitement is by the repetitive watching of unsuspecting people who are naked, disrobing, or engaging in sexual activity.

VP variegate porphyria.

VP-16 etoposide.

VPF vascular permeability factor; see vascular endothelial growth FACTOR.

VR vocal resonance.

Vreeland (vre'land) Ellwynne (1901–1971). Public health nurse and pioneer in nursing research. She developed the first nationwide extramural nursing research program.

VS vital signs, volumetric solution.

vs vibration seconds (the unit of measurement of sound waves).

vuerometer (vu″er-om'ĕ-ter) an instrument for measuring the distance between the eyes.

vulgaris (vul-ga'ris) [L.] ordinary; common.

vulnus (vul'nus) [L.] wound.

vulsella (vul-sel'ah) [L.] a forceps with clawlike hooks at the end of each blade.

vulsellum (vul-sel'um) [L.] vulsella.

vulva (vul'vah) the external genital organs in the female. Two pairs of skin folds protect the vaginal opening, one on each side. The larger outer folds are the LABIA MAJORA and the more delicate inner folds are the LABIA MINORA. In a virgin, a thin membrane called the HYMEN usually partially covers the opening of the vagina; it is normally well perforated and permits the menstrual flow, and when it is not a minor surgical procedure may be necessary. The upper or forward ends of the labia minora join around the CLITORIS, a small projection that is composed of erectile tissue like the male penis and has erotic functions. The opening of the urethra, which empties urine from the bladder, lies between the clitoris and the vagina. See also female reproductive ORGANS. adj., **vul′val, vul′var.**

vulvectomy (vul-vek'tah-me) excision of the vulva.

vulvismus (vul-viz'mus) vaginismus.

vulvitis (vul-vi'tis) inflammation of the vulva.

   erosive v. vulvitis due to a mixed microbial infection in which gangrenous ulcerations similar to the lesions seen in noma of the oral tissues affect the labia majora pudendi.

   plasma cell v., v. plasmocellula'ris the counterpart of balanitis circumscripta plasmocellularis in women, in which the vulva has a lacquerlike appearance; erosions, punctate hemorrhage, synechiae, and a slate- to ochre-colored pigmentation may supervene.

vulvocrural (vul″vo-kroo'ral) pertaining to the vulva and thigh.

vulvouterine (vul″vo-u'ter-in) pertaining to the vulva and uterus.

vulvovaginal (vul″vo-vaj'ĭ-nal) pertaining to the vulva and vagina.

vulvovaginitis (vul″vo-vaj'ĭ-ni'tis) inflammation of the vulva and vagina.

   Candida v., candidal v. vulvovaginal candidiasis.

   senile v. atrophic VAGINITIS in which there is intense itching around the vagina, almost complete lack of vaginal secretions, and tissue atrophy.

vv. [L.] ve'nae (veins).

v/v volume (of solute) per volume (of solvent).

vWF von Willebrand's factor.

W

W tungsten (Ger. *wolfram*); watt.

Waardenburg's syndrome (vahr'den-bergz) a hereditary disorder, transmitted as an autosomal dominant trait, characterized by wide bridge of the nose due to lateral displacement of the inner canthi and puncta; pigmentary disturbances, including white forelock, heterochromia iridis, white eyelashes, and leukoderma; and sometimes cochlear hearing loss.

waist (wāst) the portion of the body between the thorax and the hips.

Wald (wawld) Lillian (1867–1940). American nurse; founder of the Henry Street Settlement in the Lower East Side of New York City, one of the first nonsectarian visiting nurse services in the world.

Waldenström's disease (vahl'den-stremz) osteochondrosis of the capitular femoral epiphysis.

walking (wawk'ing) 1. progressing on foot. 2. gait.

   impaired w. a NURSING DIAGNOSIS accepted by the North American Nursing Diagnosis Association, defined as a limitation of independent movement within the environment on foot.

   sleep w. sleepwalking.

wall (wawl) a structure bounding or limiting a space or a definitive mass of material; called also paries.

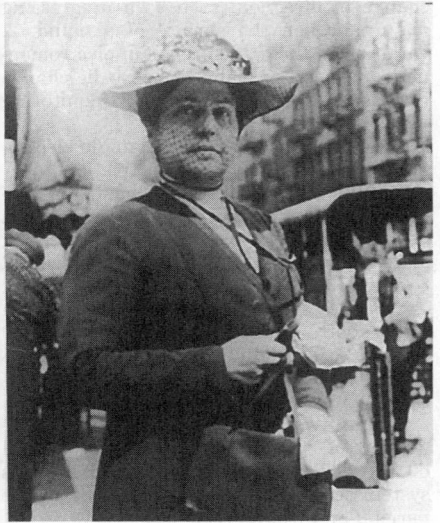

Lillian Wald. Courtesy Visiting Nurse Service of New York.

   cell w. a rigid structure that lies just outside of and is joined to the plasma membrane of plant cells and most prokaryotic cells, which protects the cell and maintains its shape.

   chest w. the structures bordering the THORAX that move during breathing, including the rib CAGE, DIAPHRAGM, and ABDOMEN.

walleye (wawl'i) 1. exotropia. 2. leukoma.

wandering (wahn'der-ing) a NURSING DIAGNOSIS accepted by the North American Nursing Diagnosis Association, defined as meandering, aimless, or repetitive locomotion that exposes the individual to harm; it is frequently incongruent with boundaries, limits, or obstacles.

ward (word) 1. a large room in a hospital for the accommodation of several patients. 2. a division within a hospital for the care of numerous patients having the same condition, e.g., a maternity ward.

warfarin (wor'fah-rin) a synthetic coumarin ANTICOAGULANT, usually used as the sodium salt; administered orally or intravenously. It is also used as a RODENTICIDE, causing fatal hemorrhaging in any mammal that consumes a sufficient dose, including humans.

wart (wort) an epidermal tumor of viral origin; the term is also applied loosely to any of various benign epidermal proliferations of nonviral origin. Called also verruca. Warts are generally more common among children and young adults than among older persons. Most are less than 0.6 cm (a quarter of an inch) in diameter; they may be flat or raised and dry or moist. Usually they have a rough and pitted surface, either flesh-colored or darker than the surrounding skin. They usually develop on the fingers and hands, but may also occur on the elbows, face, scalp, or other areas. When on especially vulnerable parts of the body, such as the knee or elbow, they are subject to irritation and may become quite tender. Two specific types are plantar WARTS and venereal WARTS.

   A wart develops between 1 and 8 months after the virus becomes lodged in the skin. The virus is often spread by scratching, rubbing, and slight razor cuts. In more than half the cases, warts disappear without treatment, but some remain for years.

   Treatment. Many popular "cures" for warts have been suggested, but are generally useless. Furthermore, self-treatment by cutting, scraping, or using acids or patent medicines may cause bacterial infection, scarring, and other harm without eliminating the warts. A troublesome wart should be removed only by a health care provider, who may use acids, electrodesiccation, or freezing with liquid nitrogen. Warts are notoriously stubborn. Often the virus remains in the skin, and the wart grows again.

genital w's condylomata acuminata.

plantar w. a viral epidermal tumor on the sole of the foot, sometimes the result of going barefoot; unlike other warts, this type is usually sensitive to pressure and may be painful during walking. Called also verruca plantaris.

venereal w's condylomata acuminata.

wash (wosh) a solution used for cleansing or bathing a part, as an eye or the mouth. See also IRRIGATION and LAVAGE.

washout (wahsh'owt) a cleansing or sweeping clean.

nitrogen w. NITROGEN WASHOUT TEST.

Wassermann test (vahs'er-mahn) the original (1906) nontreponemal antigen test for syphilis.

waste (wāst) 1. gradual loss, decay, or diminution of bulk. 2. material that is unfit for further use within the organism. 3. to gradually deteriorate.

wasting (wāst'ing) 1. the gradual deterioration of an individual, usually with loss of strength and muscle mass; it may be accompanied by loss of appetite, which makes it worse. 2. excessive depletion.

w. disease any disease marked especially by progressive emaciation and weakness.

salt w. inappropriate sodium excretion in the urine (NATRIURESIS) with hyponatremia and hyperkalemia; see also SALT-LOSING CRISIS (SYNDROME).

water (waht'er) 1. a clear, colorless, odorless, tasteless liquid, H_2O. 2. an aqueous solution of a medicinal substance; called also aromatic water. 3. purified w.

bound w. water in the tissues of the body bound to macromolecules or organelles.

distilled w. water that has been purified by distillation.

free w. that portion of the water in body tissues which is not bound by macromolecules or organelles.

w. for injection water for parenteral use, prepared by distillation or reverse OSMOSIS and meeting certain standards for sterility and clarity; it may be specified as STERILE if it has been sterilized and as BACTERIOSTATIC if suitable antimicrobial agents have been added.

purified w. water obtained by either distillation or deionization; used when mineral-free water is required.

Waterhouse-Friderichsen syndrome (waht'er-hows frid"er-ik'sen) the malignant or fulminating form of meningococcal MENINGITIS, which is marked by sudden onset and short course, fever, coma, collapse, cyanosis, hemorrhages from the skin and mucous membranes, and bilateral adrenal hemorrhage.

waters (waht'erz) popular name for AMNIOTIC FLUID.

Watson (wat'sun) Jean. Nursing educator, administrator, researcher, theorist, and practitioner. She began the development of a theory of nursing as human caring in 1979, believing that nursing must move to a new paradigm of humanism. Her THEORY OF HUMAN CARING makes a substantial contribution to nursing science regarding the spiritual and existential significance of human life. She established the Center for Human Caring at the University of Colorado to provide support for researchers exploring the phenomena of human care.

watt (W) (wot) the SI UNIT of power, being the work done at the rate of 1 joule per second. In electric power, it is equivalent to a current of 1 ampere under a pressure of 1 volt.

wattage (waht'ij) the output or consumption of an electric device expressed in watts.

wattmeter (waht'me-ter) an instrument for measuring wattage.

wave (wāv) 1. a uniformly advancing disturbance in which the parts undergo a change in direction, such as a progressing disturbance on the surface of a liquid. 2. variation in the transmission of electromagnetic energy, especially the periodic change in direction of a reading on a monitoring device.

A w. the wave on a His bundle electrogram that represents atrial activation.

alpha w's brain waves having a frequency of 8 to 13 per second, typical of a normal person awake in a quiet resting state; they occur primarily in the occipital region.

B w. a sharp rhythmic oscillation with a sawtooth pattern, occurring every 30 seconds to two minutes during INTRACRANIAL PRESSURE MONITORING, associated with unstable increases in pressure.

beta w's brain waves having a frequency of 18 to 30 per second, typical during periods of intense central nervous system activity; they occur primarily in the parietal and frontal regions.

brain w's changes in electric POTENTIAL of different areas of the brain, as recorded by ELECTROENCEPHALOGRAPHY. See also alpha, beta, delta, and theta waves.

C w. in INTRACRANIAL PRESSURE MONITORING, a small rhythmic oscillation in pressure that occurs every four to eight minutes.

delta w's 1. brain waves having a frequency below 312 per second, typical in deep sleep, in infancy, and in serious brain disorders. 2. an early QRS vector in the electrocardium in WOLFF-PARKINSON-WHITE SYNDROME.

dicrotic w. the second portion of the tracing of a SPHYGMOGRAPH of the arterial pulse or arterial pressure after the dicrotic NOTCH, attributed to the reflected impulse of closure of the aortic valves. Called also recoil wave

electromagnetic w's the entire series of ethereal waves, which are similar in character and move at the speed of light but vary enormously in wavelength. The unbroken series is known from radio WAVES that may be many kilometers in length through light WAVES, ULTRAVIOLET RAYS, X-RAYS, and gamma RAYS, to the cosmic rays, whose wavelength may be as short as 40 femtometers $(4 \times 10^{-14}$ m).

light w's the electromagnetic WAVES that produce sensations on the retina; see also VISION.

P w. a positive deflection in the normal surface electrocardiogram produced by the wave of excitation passing over the atria; it represents atrial DEPOLARIZATION, an intrinsic atrial event.

papillary w., percussion w. the chief ascending portion of the tracing of a SPHYGMOGRAPH.

plateau w. a wave seen during INTRACRANIAL PRESSURE MONITORING in advanced stages of increased pressure, signaling hypoxia of the brain cells.

pulse w. the elevation of the pulse felt by the finger or shown graphically in a recording of pulse pressure.

Q w. in the QRS complex, the initial electrocardiographic downward (negative) deflection, related to the initial phase of DEPOLARIZATION.

QRS w. QRS complex.

R w. in the normal surface electrocardiogram, the initial upward deflection of the QRS complex, following the Q wave; it represents ventricular DEPOLARIZATION. In cardiac PACING, it may be the entire native or intrinsic QRS complex.

radio w's electromagnetic WAVES of wavelength between 10^{-1} and 10^{6} cm and frequency of about 10^{11} to 10^{4} hertz.

recoil w. dicrotic wave.

S w. a downward deflection of the QRS complex following the R wave in the normal surface electrocardiogram.

sonic w's audible sound waves.

sound w's longitudinal waves of mechanical energy that transmit the vibrations interpreted as sound (def. 2).

T w. the second major deflection of the normal surface electrocardiogram, reflecting the potential variations occurring with REPOLARIZATION of the ventricles.

theta w's brain waves having a frequency of 4 to 7 per second, occurring mainly in children but also seen in adults under emotional stress.

tidal w. the wave after the percussion WAVE on a SPHYGMOGRAPH recording; the second elevation of the tracing, preceding the dicrotic WAVE.

ultrasonic w's waves similar to sonic waves but of such high frequency (20,000 hertz or higher) that the human ear does not perceive them as sound; see *ultrasonics*.

wavelength (wāv′length) the distance between the top of one wave and the identical phase of the succeeding one in the advance of waves of radiant energy.

wax (waks) a plastic solid of plant or animal origin or produced synthetically. adj., **wax′y.**

bone w. a waxy substance used for packing small bone cavities, as in bones of the skull, and for controlling bleeding from them.

dental w. a mixture of two or more waxes with other additives, used in dentistry for casts, construction of nonmetallic denture bases, registering of jaw relations, and laboratory work.

ear w. cerumen.

Wb weber.

WBC white blood cell (see LEUKOCYTE); white blood cell COUNT.

wean (wēn) 1. to discontinue BREASTFEEDING and substitute other feeding habits. 2. to discontinue bottle feeding and substitute feeding by a cup or some other means. 3. in respiratory therapy, to gradually decrease dependence on assisted ventilation until the patient is able to breathe spontaneously. See also VENTILATOR.

weaning (wēn′ing) 1. the discontinuing of BREASTFEEDING. 2. the discontinuing of dependency on assisted VENTILATION.

mechanical ventilatory w. in the NURSING INTERVENTIONS CLASSIFICATION, a nursing INTERVENTION defined as assisting the patient to breathe without the aid of a mechanical VENTILATOR. See also dysfunctional ventilatory weaning RESPONSE.

web (web) a tissue or membrane.

laryngeal w. a common congenital malformation of the larynx, ranging from a

W

thin, translucent diaphragm to a thicker, more fibrotic obstruction (see laryngeal ATRESIA); it is spread between the vocal folds near the anterior commissure and may cause hoarseness, aphonia, and other symptoms.

webbed (webd) connected by a membrane or strand of tissue.

weber (Wb) (web′er) the SI UNIT of magnetic flux which, linking a circuit of one turn, produces in it an electromotive force of one volt as it is reduced to zero at a uniform rate in one second.

Weber test (va′ber) a TUNING FORK TEST made by placing a vibrating tuning FORK at some point on the midline of the head and noting whether it is perceived as heard in the midline (normal) or referred to either ear (middle ear disease). If it is heard better in the affected ear, there is conductive HEARING LOSS; if it is heard better in the normal ear, there is sensorineural HEARING LOSS.

Weber-Christian disease (va′ber kris′-chan) a disease marked by fever and the formation of crops of tender nodules in the subcutaneous fatty tissues. Called also nodular nonsuppurative panniculitis and Christian-Weber disease.

wedge 1. a piece of material thick at one end and tapering to a thin edge at the other end. 2. to force something into a space of limited size; see also wedge PRESSURE.

weight (wāt) 1. heaviness; the degree to which a body is drawn toward the earth by gravity. (See also Tables of Weights and Measures in the Appendix.) Abbreviated wt. 2. in statistics, the process of assigning greater importance to some observations than to others, or a mathematical factor used to apply such a process.

apothecaries' w. see APOTHECARIES' SYSTEM.

atomic w. the sum of the masses of the constituents of an atom, expressed in atomic mass UNITS (or DALTONS), in SI units (i.e. kilograms), or as a dimensionless ratio derived by comparing the mass to the mass of an atom of carbon-12, which is taken as 12.000. Abbreviated At wt.

avoirdupois w. see AVOIRDUPOIS SYSTEM.

equivalent w. the amount of substance that combines with or displaces 8.0 g of oxygen (or 1.008 g of hydrogen), usually expressed in grams; for acid/base reactions, one equivalent donates or receives a mole of protons and the equivalent weight is the ratio of the molecular weight to the number of protons involved in the reaction. For oxidation-reduction reactions, one equivalent donates or receives a mole of electrons and the equivalent weight is the ratio of the molecular weight to the number of electrons involved in the reaction.

gram molecular w. the molecular weight of a substance expressed in grams; one gram molecular weight of a molecular substance contains one mole of molecules. See also MOLE[1].

low birth w. (LBW) see under INFANT.

molecular w. the weight of a molecule of a chemical compound as compared with the weight of an atom of carbon-12; it is equal to the sum of the weights of its constituent atoms and is dimensionless. Abbreviated Mol wt or MW. Although widely used, the term is not technically correct; relative molecular mass is preferable.

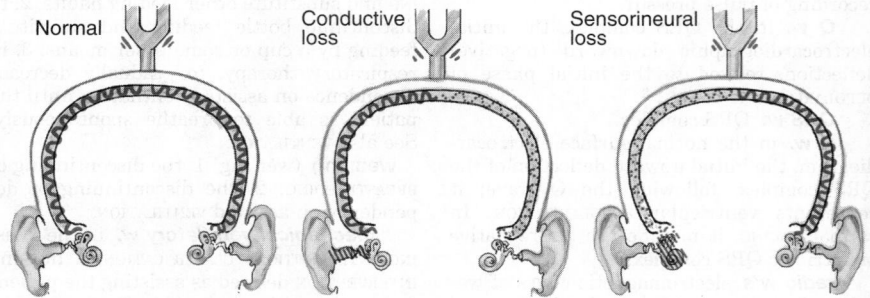

Weber test. *A,* Normal—sound is equally loud in both ears; sound does not lateralize. *B,* Conductive loss—sound lateralizes to "poorer" ear owing to background room noise, which masks hearing in normal ear. "Poorer" ear (the one with conductive loss) is not distracted by background noise, thus has a better chance to hear bone-conducted sound. Examples: transient conductive loss with serous or purulent otitis media. *C,* Sensorineural loss—sound lateralizes to "better" ear or unaffected ear. Poorer ear (the one with nerve loss) is unable to perceive the sound. From Jarvis, 2000.

Weil's syndrome (disease) (vīlz) severe LEPTOSPIROSIS with fever, jaundice, myalgia, and occasionally with nephritis and meningitis. The symptoms last from 10 days to 2 weeks and recovery is usually uneventful. Called also leptospiral jaundice.

Wellens syndrome (wel′enz) a group of signs indicating critical proximal stenosis of the left anterior descending coronary artery in patients with unstable angina at a time when there is no pain. It consists of normal or minimally elevated cardiac enzyme levels; little or no elevation of the ST segment; no loss of precordial R waves; and progressive, deep, symmetrical inversion of the T waves, particularly in leads V_1 and V_2 (though not confined to these leads).

Wells syndrome (welz) cellulitis with erythema, edema, and often blistering of the skin accompanied by eosinophilia, flame figures, and a mild fever; episodes last 2 to 6 weeks and recurrences are common. Called also eosinophilic cellulitis.

wen (wen) 1. a sebaceous or epidermal inclusion cyst. 2. pilar cyst.

Wenckebach's phenomenon (veng′kĕ-bahks) Mobitz type I block.

Wermer's syndrome (ver′merz) multiple endocrine NEOPLASIA, Type I.

Werner's syndrome (ver′nerz) premature aging in the adult, transmitted as an autosomal recessive trait, and characterized principally by sclerodermalike skin changes, involving especially the extremities, cataracts, subcutaneous calcification, muscular atrophy, a tendency to diabetes mellitus, aged appearance of the face, white hair and/or baldness, and a high incidence of neoplasms.

Wernicke's disease (syndrome) (ver′nĭ-kez) Wernicke's ENCEPHALOPATHY.

Wernicke-Korsakoff syndrome (ver′nĭ-kĕ kor′sah-kof) a disorder of the central nervous system, usually associated with chronic alcoholism and nutritional deficiency such as severe THIAMINE depletion. It is characterized by a combination of motor and sensory disturbances (WERNICKE'S ENCEPHALOPATHY) and disordered memory function (KORSAKOFF'S SYNDROME). It typically has an abrupt onset, manifested by ocular motility, ataxia, diplopia, and horizontal nystagmus. Many patients are unaware of their unsteady gait, decreased mental acuity, and other signs of cognitive dysfunction.

There usually is an immediate improvement in ocular disturbances once therapy with thiamine is begun. The ataxia and diminished perceptual function and concept formation show a much slower rate of improvement. Only about 20 per cent of those with Korsakoff's syndrome fully recover. The mortality rate for the syndrome may be as high as 17 per cent during the acute phase. (See also ALCOHOLISM.)

Westphal-Strümpell disease (vest′fahl strim′pel) hepatolenticular degeneration.

West Nile fever West Nile encephalitis.

wheal (hwēl) a localized area of EDEMA on the body surface, often with severe itching but usually of brief duration; it is the typical lesion of URTICARIA.

w. and erythema reaction, w. and flare reaction the characteristic local cutaneous reaction consisting of an elevated, blanched wheal surrounded by a spreading "flare" of erythema that occurs within a few minutes at the site of a minor nonpenetrating skin injury and also in response to administration of allergen to an atopic individual; it is caused by release of histamine from mast cells.

wheelchair (hwēl′chār) a means of locomotion for non-ambulatory individuals, consisting of a seat on a platform with wheels, which provides comfortable, safe sitting, and a steering mechanism. The disabled person should be evaluated by a physiatrist, physical therapist, or occupational therapist with the assistance of an equipment specialist in order to choose the right type of wheelchair. Different types have been designed for patients with quadriplegia, hemiplegia, paraplegia, and amputations; there are also specialized wheelchairs designed for sports, such as basketball, tennis, long distance RUNNING, and sprints.

wheeze (hwēz) a continuous SOUND consisting of a whistling noise with a higher pitch than that of a RHONCHUS. See also WHEEZING.

wheezing (hwēz′ing) breathing with WHEEZE; it results from constriction or obstruction of the throat, pharynx, trachea, or bronchi. This is commonly a symptom of ASTHMA; in an asthmatic attack, spasm of the bronchi occurs, and air can be forced only with difficulty into and out of the lungs through the trachea. Another cause of wheezing is congestive HEART FAILURE, in which breathing is difficult, the lips often have a bluish color, and the veins in the neck are distended. When wheezing is persistent and is not asthmatic, the cause may be an obstruction in the breathing passages, such as a foreign body or tumor.

whiplash (hwip′lash) a nonspecific term applied to injury to the spinal cord and spine due to sudden extension of the neck, as in sudden stopping or propulsion of a vehicle.

W

w. shake syndrome a constellation of injuries to the brain and eye that may occur when a child less than 3 years old, usually less than 1 year old, is shaken vigorously while being held by the trunk or limbs with the head unsupported. This causes stretching and tearing of the cerebral vessels and brain substance, commonly leading to subdural hematomas and retinal hemorrhages, and sometimes associated with cerebral contusion. It may result in paralysis, blindness and other visual disturbances, convulsions, and death.

Whipple's disease (hwip′elz) a malabsorption syndrome caused by an actinomycete, marked by diarrhea, steatorrhea, skin pigmentation, arthralgia and arthritis, lymphadenopathy, central nervous system lesions, and infiltration of the intestinal mucosa with macrophages containing PAS-positive material. Called also intestinal lipodystrophy.

Whipple's operation (procedure) (hwip′-elz) a radical PANCREATODUODENECTOMY with removal of the distal third of the stomach, the entire duodenum, and the head of the pancreas, with gastrojejunostomy, choledochojejunostomy, and pancreatic jejunostomy. This procedure is used for pancreatic carcinoma.

whipworm (hwip′werm) any nematode of the genus *Trichuris.*

Whitaker test (hwit′ah-ker) a test of ureteral function that is used to evaluate ureteral peristalsis and obstruction by measuring the resistance of the ureter to perfusion.

white clot syndrome a complication of HEPARIN therapy characterized by intravascular clots composed of platelet aggregates.

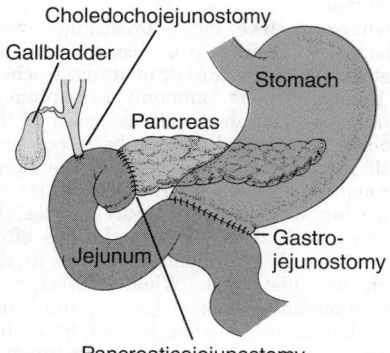

Choledochojejunostomy
Gallbladder
Stomach
Pancreas
Jejunum
Gastro-jejunostomy
Pancreaticojejunostomy

The three anastomoses that make up the Whipple procedure: choledochojejunostomy, pancreaticojejunostomy; and gastrojejunostomy. From Ignatavicius and Workman, 2000.

In some sensitive individuals heparin stimulates formation of antibody to the person's own platelets; the antigen-antibody reaction causes clumping of the affected cells and formation of a clot. Platelet clots can affect blood vessels anywhere in the body and lead to such conditions as gangrene of a limb, stroke, and myocardial infarction.

Treatment. Treatment is intended to reverse thrombocytopenia and eliminate sources of heparin in the blood. Heparin administration is stopped as soon as a white clot syndrome is suspected, and all traces of heparin are flushed from the intravenous line. Once a history of white clot syndrome is known, heparin therapy is prohibited, as it can precipitate a reaction months after a person is initially sensitized to heparin.

Patient Care. Prevention of white clot syndrome includes asking all patients about sensitivity to heparin during the initial assessment and scheduling platelet counts every 2 to 3 days during the course of heparin therapy. Patients on heparin should be monitored periodically for pain in the chest or extremities, diminishing pulse, or signs of cerebral ischemia. Additionally, the patient with heparin sensitivity should be taught the nature of the syndrome and its symptoms and encouraged to wear some form of identification or otherwise inform all health care providers of the sensitivity to heparin.

whitehead (hwīt′hed) 1. a COMEDO whose opening is not widely dilated, appearing as a small, flesh-colored papule; because the keratin and sebum produced cannot escape, it may rupture and cause an inflammatory lesion in the dermis. See also ACNE VULGARIS. Called also closed comedo. 2. popular name for *milium.*

whitlow (hwit′lo) felon.

herpetic w. a primary HERPES SIMPLEX infection of the terminal segment of a finger, usually seen in those exposed to infected oral or respiratory secretions, such as dentists, physicians, or nurses. It begins with intense itching and pain, followed by the formation of deep coalescing vesicles. The process is associated with much tissue destruction and may be accompanied by systemic symptoms. A similar lesion may occur as a result of nail biting during the course of primary herpetic GINGIVOSTOMATITIS.

melanotic w. a malignant tumor of the nail bed characterized by formation of melanotic tissue.

Whitmore's disease (hwit′mōrz) melioidosis.

WHO World Health Organization.

whoop (ho͞op) the sonorous and convulsive sound on inhalation with WHOOPING COUGH.

whooping cough (hōōp'ing kof) an infectious disease characterized by catarrh of the respiratory tract and peculiar paroxysms of coughing, ending in a prolonged crowing or whooping respiration; the causative organism is *Bordetella pertussis.* Called also pertussis. Whooping cough is a serious and widespread disease, with about 300,000 cases a year reported in the United States. Although it may attack at any age, most cases occur in children under 10, and half of these are in children under 5.

The organisms are spread by the victim's coughing and sneezing and by objects he has touched. The incubation period is usually about 7 days, although it may vary between 2 and 21 days. Unlike other respiratory diseases, whooping cough is more likely to occur in spring and summer than in winter. It affects females much more often than males.

Symptoms. Whooping cough frequently starts with a running nose, a slight fever, and a persistent cough. This stage usually lasts about 2 weeks. After this, the child feels chilled and begins to vomit. His coughing increases. He begins to cough in spells of eight to ten times in one breath. This forces the air from the lungs, and the face may turn purple or blue from the effort and the shortage of air. Finally he catches his breath in a long, noisy intake, or "whoop." In the very young (under 6 months) the true whoop is often not present, even when paroxysms are severe and frequent.

The coughing stage of the disease usually lasts 4 to 6 weeks, and the coughing may be very severe at night. Then the coughing spells become less frequent and less severe until the disease has run its course.

Stage three (convalescent stage) may last from 4 months to 2 years. The coughing spells diminish but the patient usually experiences them again each time he has an upper respiratory infection.

Complications of whooping cough include pneumonia, atelectasis, and emphysema; of these, pneumonia is the most serious, accounting for 90 per cent of the fatalities in young children. Brain damage, another complication, should be suspected if convulsive seizures occur in the pertussis patient.

Immunization. An attack of whooping cough gives immunity but does not confer life-long immunity. The vaccine usually is given in combination with diphtheria and tetanus and is available as a preparation that should be given intramuscularly, preferably in the lateral thigh.

Treatment and Patient Care. Precautions against the spread of the disease entail following respiratory isolation precautions

for 7 days after effective therapy is begun. Recommendations for preventive measures after exposure can be found in the *CDC Guidelines for Infection Control in Hospital Personnel.*

Treatment is primarily supportive, including bed rest as long as the fever persists, antibiotics to avoid secondary infections, and antipyretics to control fever. In very serious cases, especially in infants, whooping cough may cause severe breathing difficulties. Suction may be necessary at frequent intervals to remove accumulations of mucus from the air passages. Fatalities, particularly in infants, are not uncommon. A proper diet is essential during whooping cough. Because vomiting may be a problem, small frequent feedings of bland foods are considered best.

whorl (hwerl) a spiral arrangement, as in the ridges on the finger that make up a fingerprint.

WIC program the United States government's Special Supplemental Food Program for Women, Infants, and Children.

Widal test (ve-dahl') a test for the diagnosis of typhoid fever, based on agglutination of *Salmonella typhosa* by dilutions of the patient's serum.

width (width) the extent of something from side to side.

pulse w. the duration of a PACING impulse, usually expressed in milliseconds.

will (wil) a legal declaration of a person's wishes, usually regarding disposal of possessions after the person has died.

living w. advance directives.

Williams' syndrome (wil'yamz) a genetic disorder caused by the sporadic deletion of a gene for ELASTIN on chromosome 7; common characteristics include supraventricular aortic STENOSIS or other cardiovascular defects, a characteristic facial appearance described as "elfin," mild to severe learning disability, and developmental delay. Information for patients, their families, and other concerned individuals may be obtained from The Williams Syndrome Association, P.O. Box 297, Clawson, MI 48017-0297.

Wilson's disease (wil'sunz) a rare progressive disease, inherited as an autosomal recessive trait and due to a defect in metabolism of COPPER, with accumulation of copper in the liver, brain, kidney, cornea, and other tissues. Characteristics include cirrhosis of the liver and degenerative changes in the brain, particularly the basal ganglia. Liver disease is the most likely manifestation in children; neurologic disease is most common in young adults. The

W

characteristic ophthalmic feature is a pigmented ring (Kayser-Fleischer RING) at the
outer margin of the cornea. Called also
hepatolenticular degeneration.

Wilson-Mikity syndrome (wil'sun mik'ĭ-
te) a rare form of RESPIRATORY INSUFFICIENCY
in low-birth-weight infants, marked by HY-
PERPNEA and CYANOSIS of insidious onset
during the first month of life and often
resulting in death. Radiographically, there
are multiple cystlike foci of hyperaeration
throughout the lung, with coarse thickening
of the interstitial supporting structures.
Called also pulmonary dysmaturity.

Winckel's disease (ving'kelz) a fatal disease of the newborn, with jaundice, hemoglobinuria, bloody urine, hemorrhage,
cyanosis, collapse, and convulsions.

window (win'do) a circumscribed opening
in a plane surface; called also fenestra.

   aortic w. a radiolucent region below
the aortic arch, formed by the bifurcation
of the trachea, visible in the left anterior
oblique radiograph of the heart and great
vessels.

   w. of cochlea, cochlear w. round
window.

   oval w. an oval opening in the inner
wall of the middle ear, which is closed by
the stapes; called also vestibular window
and fenestra vestibuli.

   round w. a round opening in the middle ear covered by the secondary tympanic
membrane; called also cochlear window and
fenestra cochleae.

   vestibular w., w. of vestibule oval
window.

windpipe (wind' pīp) popular name for
the TRACHEA.

winking (wingk'ing) quick opening and
closing of the eyelids.

   jaw w. involuntary closing of the eyelids associated with jaw movements.

Winstrol (win'strol) trademark for a preparation of STANOZOLOL, an anabolic STEROID
used to prevent attacks of hereditary AN-
GIOEDEMA.

wintergreen oil methyl salicylate.

wire (wīr) a long, slender, flexible structure of metal, used in surgery and dentistry
and sometimes as a conductor of electricity.

   arch w. in orthodontic therapy, a wire
attached to orthodontic BANDS and applied
around the dental arch to control and force
tooth movement.

   Kirschner w. a steel wire for skeletal
transfixing of fractured bones and for obtaining skeletal traction in fractures. It is
inserted through the soft parts and the bone
and is held tight in a clamp.

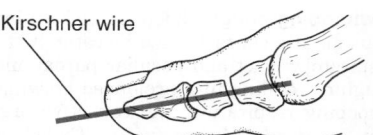

Kirschner wire

The use of the Kirschner wire to repair hallux valgus and
other toe deformities. From Ignatavicius et al., 1995.

   lead w. in cardiac PACING, an insulated
wire with an electrode in contact with the
heart and the other end attached to a pulse
GENERATOR. It may have a bipolar configuration (bipolar LEAD) with two electrodes close
to each other in the heart, or a unipolar
configuration (unipolar LEAD) with just one
electrode in the heart and the pulse generator as the ground.

Wiskott-Aldrich syndrome (wis'kot awl'-
drich) a congenital platelet STORAGE POOL
DISEASE, transmitted as an X-linked recessive
trait, characterized by the triad of ECZEMA,
THROMBOCYTOPENIA, and recurrent purulent
infection. There is an inability to produce
antibodies to POLYSACCHARIDE antigens and
increased susceptibility to infection with
encapsulated bacteria such as *Haemophilus
influenzae,* MENINGOCOCCUS, or PNEUMOCOCCUS.
Called also Aldrich syndrome.

withdrawal (with-draw'al) 1. a pathological retreat from interpersonal contact and
social involvement, as may occur in AVOIDANT,
SCHIZOID, or SCHIZOTYPAL PERSONALITY DISOR-
DERS. 2. the removal of something. 3. a
substance-specific SUBSTANCE-INDUCED DISOR-
DER that follows the cessation of use or
reduction in intake of a psychoactive SUB-
STANCE that had been regularly used to induce
a state of intoxication. Specific withdrawal
syndromes include those for ALCOHOL, AMPHE-
TAMINES or similarly acting SYMPATHOMIMETICS,
COCAINE, NICOTINE, OPIOIDS, and SEDATIVES,
HYPNOTICS, or ANTIANXIETY AGENTS. Called also
abstinence syndrome, withdrawal symptoms,
and withdrawal syndrome.

   The usual reactions to alcohol withdrawal are anxiety, weakness, gastrointestinal symptoms, nausea and vomiting,
tremor, fever, rapid heartbeat, convulsions,
and delirium (see also DELIRIUM TREMENS).
Similar effects are produced by withdrawal
of BARBITURATES and in this case convulsions
occur frequently, often followed by psychosis with hallucinations. Treatment of withdrawal consists of providing a substitute
drug such as a mild sedative, along with
treatment of the symptoms as needed.
Parenteral fluids are often required.

   substance w. withdrawal (def. 3).

   w. syndrome former name for WITH-
DRAWAL (def. 3).

thought w. the delusion that someone or something is removing thoughts from one's mind.

witzelsucht (vit'sel-zōōkt) [Ger.] a mental condition marked by the making of poor jokes and puns and the telling of pointless stories at which the speaker is intensely amused; a condition characteristic of frontal lobe lesions.

Wolbachia (wol-bak'e-ah) a genus of bacteria that infect a wide variety of invertebrates, including insects, spiders, crustaceans, and nematodes.

Wolf-Hirschhorn syndrome (woolf'-hirsh'horn) a syndrome associated with partial deletion of the short arm of chromosome 4, characterized by an undersized head, increased distance between the eyes, EPICANTHUS, CLEFT PALATE, a small receding mandible, low-set ears that are simplified in form, undescended testes, and HYPOSPADIAS.

Wolff-Parkinson-White syndrome (woolf'pahr'kin-sun hwīt') the association of paroxysmal TACHYCARDIA (or atrial FIBRILLATION) and PREEXCITATION. The electrocardiogram displays a short P–R interval and a wide QRS complex that characteristically shows an early QRS vector (delta wave). There is a tendency towards premature supraventricular TACHYCARDIA. Called also anomalous atrioventricular excitation.

concealed W.-P.-W. s. the condition in which an accessory PATHWAY is present but is capable of retrograde conduction only. The electrocardiogram is normal and the patient is prone to paroxysmal supraventricular TACHYCARDIA but is not in danger

of excessively rapid heart rates or sudden death should atrial fibrillation develop.

latent W.-P.-W. s. a heart abnormality in which there is an accessory PATHWAY through which conduction would be possible in either direction but for some reason does not take place. The PR and QRS complexes are normal, but there is a tendency to develop premature supraventricular TACHYCARDIA. If atrial FIBRILLATION develops, atrioventricular conduction will proceed across the accessory pathway and result in an extremely rapid, irregular rhythm.

Wolman's disease (wol'manz) primary familial XANTHOMATOSIS in infants; associated with involvement and calcification of the adrenal glands, FAILURE TO THRIVE, vomiting, diarrhea, hepatomegaly, splenomegaly, foam cells in the bone marrow and other tissues, and early death.

womb (wōōm) uterus.

woolsorter's disease pulmonary anthrax.

word salad (werd sal'ad) an incoherent jumble of words and neologisms, such as that observed in advanced schizophrenia; called also schizophasia.

work (werk) activity directed toward accomplishing something.

social w. the activity of a SOCIAL WORKER; work designed to promote the welfare of an individual or group.

worker (wer'ker) an employed person.

social w. a professional trained in the treatment of psychosocial problems of patients and their families; see also SOCIAL WORKER.

work hardening a rehabilitation program designed to restore functional and work capacities to the injured worker through application of graded work simulation. Included are activities designed to improve overall physical condition, including strength, endurance, and coordination specific to work activity, as well as means for coping with any remaining symptoms from the original problem, such as pain. Central to all work hardening programs is the reproduction of a work-like environment where tasks are designed to improve the patient's tolerance for productive work.

The goal of work hardening is to achieve an acceptable level of productivity for returning to one's former occupation or for meeting the demands of a specific new type of work. Therefore, worker behaviors and not just physical conditioning are addressed. These include having structured work times and duties, dressing appropriately for one's tasks, and conducting oneself in a

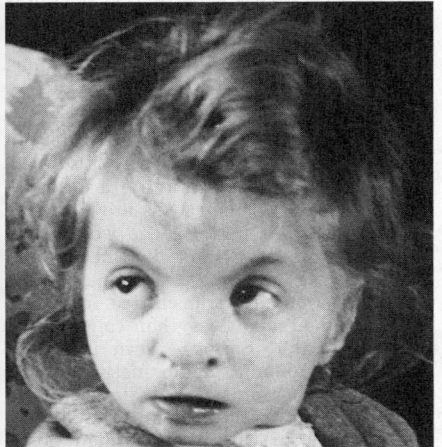

Facial view of a 3-year-old child with the Wolf-Hirschhorn syndrome. From Mueller and Young, 2001.

W

worker-like manner. It is important to differentiate work hardening from WORK CONDITIONING, which does not address these added concerns.

Treatment Personnel. Work hardening is generally administered by physical or occupational therapists, working independently or as part of a team, which might include physicians, vocational counselors, psychologists, and other rehabilitation professionals. Drug and alcohol specialists, ergonomists, orthotists, dieticians, and industrial nurses may also be involved in the program.

Settings. Work hardening programs can be found in rehabilitation and general acute hospitals, private physical or occupational therapy centers, vocational training facilities, and fully dedicated facilities or within private industry. When found in hospitals or therapy centers, programs either share space with other rehabilitation programs (*mixed-use setting*) or are in partitioned areas designed specifically for the purpose (*dedicated space setting*). Fully dedicated facilities, whose only use is work hardening activity, are generally thought to offer the best environment for worker rehabilitation since they provide the nearest reproduction of actual work experience.

workshop (werk′shop) 1. the meeting of a group of people for a specialized purpose such as having a discussion, learning something, or studying something. 2. the place where such a meeting is held.

    sheltered w. a facility where individuals with handicaps are employed to produce a product, to socialize, and to increase their sense of self worth.

work-up (werk′up) the procedures done to arrive at a diagnosis, including history taking, laboratory tests, x-rays, and so on.

World Health Organization (WHO) the specialized agency of the United Nations that is concerned with health on an international level. The agency was founded in 1948 and in its constitution are listed the following objectives: Health is a state of complete physical and social well being, and not merely the absence of disease or infirmity. The enjoyment of the highest attainable standards of health is one of the fundamental rights of every human being without distinction of race, religion, political belief, or economic or social condition. The health of all peoples is fundamental to the attainment of peace and security and is dependent upon the fullest cooperation of individuals and States. The achievement of any State in the promotion and protection of health is of value to all.

The major specific aims of the WHO are:

1. To strengthen the health services of member nations, improving the teaching standards in medicine and allied professions, and advising and helping generally in the field of health.

2. To promote better standards for nutrition, housing, recreation, sanitation, and economic and working conditions.

3. To improve maternal and child health and welfare.

4. To advance progress in the field of mental health.

5. To encourage and conduct research on problems of public health.

In carrying out these aims and objectives the WHO functions as a directing and coordinating authority on international health. It serves as a center for all types of global and health information, promotes uniform guarantee standards and international sanitary regulations, provides advisory services through public health experts in control of disease, and sets up international standards for the manufacture of all important drugs. Through its teams of physicians, nurses, and other health personnel it provides modern medical skills and knowledge to communities throughout the world.

world view (werld vu) the perspective a culture takes of the world, which is shared by cultural group members. Though not always overtly recognized, world views influence health and illness beliefs and behavior; for example, a world view of harmony and balance shapes a view of health as a balance of natural forces, a world view that is largely technological leads to a view of illness analogous to the breakdown of a machine, and a world view focusing on fear and violence shapes a perception of illness as the result of evil forces.

worm (werm) 1. any of the soft-bodied, elongated, naked invertebrates of the phyla ANNELIDA, ACANTHOCEPHALA, ASCHELMINTHES, and PLATYHELMINTHES; called also vermis. Worms are often found as parasites in humans and other animals; in North America the most common of these are ROUNDWORMS and TAPEWORMS. FLUKES are a serious problem in other parts of the world. (See also Appendix of Commonly Encountered Intestinal Parasitic Infections.) Most worm infections are transmitted from person to person via feces that contaminate food and water. Serious worm infections may cause anemia, listlessness, fatigue, irritability, abdominal pain, diarrhea, and weight loss. Parasitic worms usually live in relative balance with their human hosts, taking enough nutrients to survive without destroying the health of the host. However, they reduce the strength and energy of the bodies they inhabit, often produce very uncomfortable symptoms and should never go untreated. Suspected cases of worms should be brought to the attention of a health care provider; self-treatment is likely to be ineffective and can be harmful. Effective medications against worms are available by prescription. 2. vermis.

wound (wo͞ond) an injury or damage, usually restricted to those caused by physical means with disruption of normal continuity of structures. Called also injury and trauma.

> **blowing w.** open PNEUMOTHORAX.

> **contused w.** one in which the skin is unbroken.

> **w. drain** any device by which a channel or open area may be established for the exit of material from a wound or cavity. See also WOUND HEALING.

> **w. healing** restoration of integrity to injured tissues by replacement of dead tissue with viable tissue; this starts immediately after an injury, may continue for months or years, and is essentially the same for all types of wounds. Variations are the result of differences in location, severity of the wound, extent of injury to the tissues, the age, nutritional status, and general state of health of the patient, and available body reserves and resources for tissue regeneration.

The repair of damaged cells and tissue takes place by REGENERATION, in which structures are replaced by proliferation of similar cells, such as happens with skin and bone; and by formation of a SCAR, consisting of fibrous structures with some degree of contraction. Since most wounds extend to more than one type of tissue, complete regeneration is impossible; therefore, scar formation is an expected outcome of wound healing.

In HEALING BY FIRST INTENTION (primary union), restoration of tissue continuity occurs directly, without granulation; in HEALING BY SECOND INTENTION (secondary union), wound repair following tissue loss (as in ULCERATION) is accomplished by closure of the wound with granulation tissue. This tissue is formed by proliferation of FIBROBLASTS and extensive capillary budding at the outer edges and base of the wound cavity, with slow extension from the base and sides of the wound toward its center. If, however, the wound is very deep and extensive, granulation tissue cannot fill the defect and GRAFTING may be needed to cover the space and avoid severe contracture and loss of function. HEALING BY THIRD INTENTION (delayed primary closure) occurs when a wound is initially too contaminated to close and is closed surgically 4 or 5 days after the injury. (See also illustrations at HEALING.)

The insertion of DRAINS can facilitate healing by providing an outlet for removing accumulations of serosanguineous fluid and purulent material, and obliterating dead space such as that created by surgical removal of an organ.

If the area of injury is not very large, the products of inflammation, small blood CLOTS, and other debris from the wound can be absorbed into the blood stream and disposed of. Wounds that are filled with large amounts of dead cells, blood clots, and other debris must be cleansed in order for healing to take place. This can be accomplished by surgical or chemical DÉBRIDEMENT or by IRRIGATIONS. Enzymes are sometimes used to remove the debris by enzymatic action. Since foreign bodies, such as sutures, slivers of glass, splinters, and the like, can delay healing, they too must be removed from the wound to facilitate healing.

Patient Care. Assessment of the progress of wound healing begins with frequent inspection of the site for signs of bleeding in or around the wound. Discoloration of the skin adjacent to a surgical or traumatic wound that has been sutured may indicate a pooling of blood in the tissue spaces and the beginning stages of a HEMATOMA. Bleeding in a wound and clot formation can delay healing. Accumulations of serosanguineous fluid and purulent drainage also must be watched for, because they retard the healing

FACTORS FACILITATING WOUND HEALING	
Adequate Blood Supply:	Mobilize the person when possible; avoid tight bandages and clothing; relieve edema through proper positioning
Good Nutrition:	Provide adequate protein to facilitate healing and a high carbohydrate diet to spare protein for healing; maintain a normal fluid balance
Rest:	Employ splints and other protective devices when appropriate; encourage a balanced activity schedule
Stress Reduction:	Promote comfort and relieve pain; provide a supportive environment
Prevent Infection:	Utilize strict aseptic technique for dressing changes; wash hands thoroughly and instruct others in proper technique; maintain adequate nutrition

W

A NONADHERENT, NONABSORBENT DRESSING

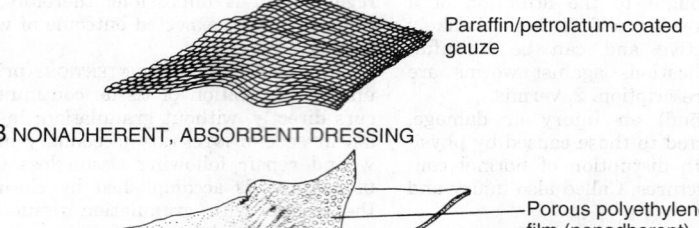

Paraffin/petrolatum-coated gauze

B NONADHERENT, ABSORBENT DRESSING

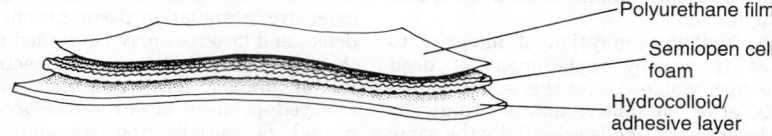

Porous polyethylene film (nonadherent)

Absorbent cotton and/or rayon pad

C NONADHERENT, ABSORBENT, OCCLUSIVE DRESSING (HYDROCOLLOID)

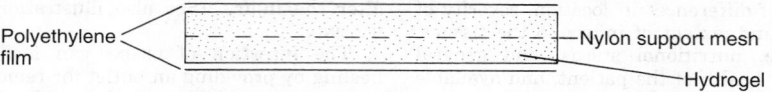

Polyurethane film

Semiopen cell foam

Hydrocolloid/ adhesive layer

D NONADHERENT, ABSORBENT, OCCLUSIVE DRESSING (HYDROGEL)

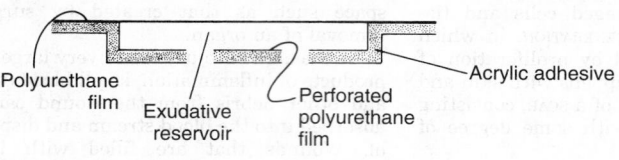

Polyethylene film

Nylon support mesh

Hydrogel

E NONADHERENT, ABSORBENT, SEMIOCCLUSIVE DRESSING (COMPOSITE)

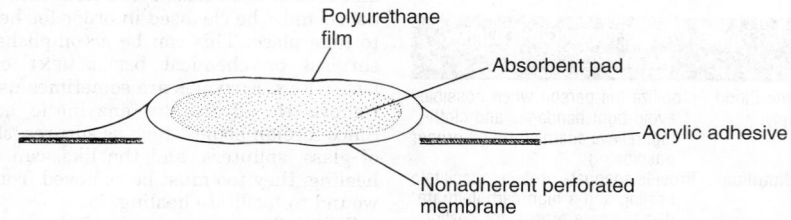

Polyurethane film

Exudative reservoir

Perforated polyurethane film

Acrylic adhesive

Polyurethane film

Absorbent pad

Acrylic adhesive

Nonadherent perforated membrane

F SEMIOCCLUSIVE, NONABSORBENT TRANSPARENT FILM DRESSING

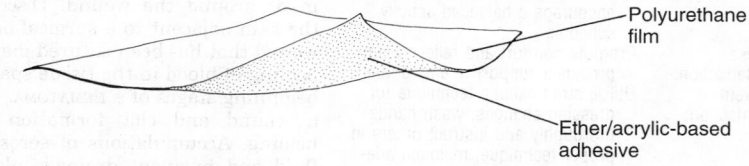

Polyurethane film

Ether/acrylic-based adhesive

Wound dressing construction and design. From Cohen et al., 1992.

process and pose a problem of SUPERINFECTION. If a drain has been inserted to remove excess fluid, the color, amount, odor, and other characteristics of the drainage must be noted and recorded. If there is more than one drain, the drainage from each should be noted separately.

Dressings also must be observed frequently, especially a pressure DRESSING, which can become dangerously restrictive if there is swelling. Any change in sensation, such as tingling or numbness, signs of impaired circulation, or complaint of discomfort, should be reported to the physician.

Other data important to the ongoing assessment of wound healing are the leukocyte COUNT, COAGULATION tests, and ELECTROLYTE levels. An elevated body temperature can signal local or systemic infection. Another sign of infection is the presence of purulent drainage. The color of the drainage is often indicative of the particular infecting organism. For example, a yellow color may indicate presence of *Staphylococcus aureus,* and a blue-green color may indicate *Pseudomonas aeruginosa* infection.

In a surgical wound, a discharge of serosanguineous fluid on the fourth or fifth postoperative day may signal wound DEHISCENCE and, therefore, should be reported immediately to the surgeon.

During the scarring phase of healing, the wound is inspected for changes in size, color, and shape, which can continue for months even in superficial wounds. New scar tissue is usually purplish, raised, and irregular. With time, the color fades, the scar grows smaller, and its surface and edges become less irregular. Sometimes the scar tissue grows to excess and extends beyond the normal limits of the wound. This hypertrophic scar or KELOID may require steroid injections or surgical removal.

In order to achieve adequate and uneventful healing of a wound the patient must be in a good state of nutrition. Virtually every nutrient plays some role in the healing process; hence, a wide range of dietary nutrients must be supplied, either through oral feedings, supplemental vitamins and protein, or PARENTERAL NUTRITION. Oxygen is also essential to the healing process. This means that measures must be taken to ensure adequate circulation of blood to the wound, employing measures such as exercise, ambulation when possible, and applications of warmth when prescribed. Positioning also is important to avoid prolonged pressure against blood vessels serving the wounded area. Adequate rest is needed to facilitate healing. The patient should understand the need for rest and the purpose of splints, casts, and other devices employed for immobilization of a wounded part.

Mechanical injury to a wound can greatly impede healing by damaging the tissues involved in the healing process. The wound should be protected from friction and direct blows. The affected part must be handled gently, and great care must be used in applying and removing dressings and bandages. Protective bandages and shields made from rubber, plastic cups, tongue blades, and other supportive materials may be needed to protect the wound from additional trauma.

Other factors that work against optimal healing are stress, old age, smoking, obesity, and diabetes mellitus. It is thought that in the poorly controlled diabetic patient there is an increased affinity of hemoglobin for oxygen, which hampers the release of oxygen to the healing tissues. Additionally, poorly controlled diabetic patients have an abnormal function of the phagocytes, which predisposes wounds to infection. Although cancer does not itself interfere with the healing process or make the patient more susceptible to infection, RADIATION THERAPY, STEROIDS, and antineoplastic AGENTS, as well as the general debility of the patient, do compromise healing in cancer patients.

   incised w. one caused by a cutting instrument.

   lacerated w. one in which the tissues are torn.

   open w. one that communicates directly with the atmosphere.

   penetrating w. one caused by a sharp, usually slender, object that passes through the skin into the underlying tissues.

   perforating w. a penetrating wound that extends into a viscus or bodily cavity.

   puncture w. penetrating wound.

   sucking w. a penetrating wound of the chest through which air is drawn in and out, as in open PNEUMOTHORAX.

   tangential w. an oblique glancing wound that results in one edge being undercut.

wrist (rist) the region of the joint between the hand and the forearm; it contains eight bones, called the *carpal bones* (see anatomic Table of Bones in the Appendices). The bones are arranged in two rows, whose joint surfaces glide upon each other in four directions; they join the bones of the forearm, the RADIUS and ULNA, as well as the bones of the hand, the METACARPALS. They are bound together and protected by tough ligaments and capsules, the enveloping

W

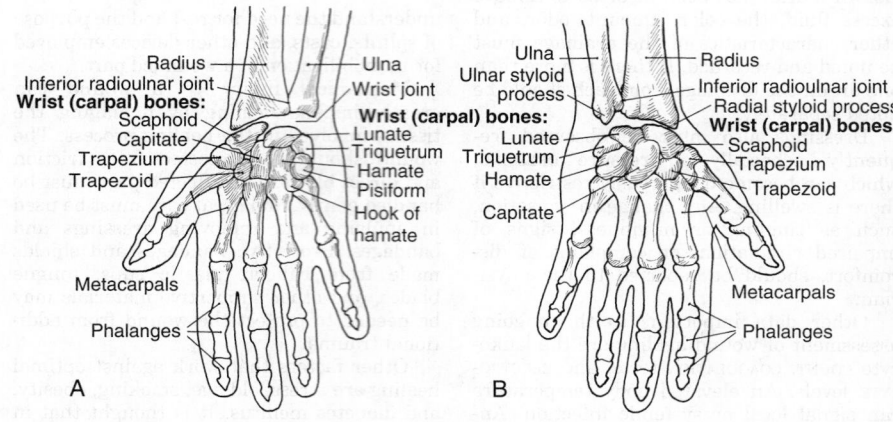

Bones of the wrist (carpal bones). *A,* Anterior view, right arm. *B,* Posterior view, right arm.

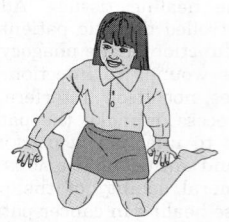

W sitting. From Lissauer and Graham, 2002.

structures. The major arteries, nerves, veins, and tendons that serve the hand and fingers run across the wrist. Both the tendons and the joint are lined with synovial membrane. Called also carpus.

wristdrop (rist'drop) paralysis of the extensor muscles of the hand and fingers; it may be due to metallic poisoning.

writing-to-learn an instructional strategy in which writing is coordinated with the learning of content and development of cognitive skills such as critical thinking rather than simply with editorial skills.

wryneck (ri'nek) torticollis.

W sitting a characteristic sitting position of young children that is indicative of femoral ANTEVERSION or torsion.

wt weight.

Wuchereria (voo″ker-e're-ah) a genus of NEMATODES of the superfamily FILARIOIDEA that affect mainly humans in warmer regions of the world. *W. bancrof'ti* causes ELEPHANTIASIS, LYMPHANGITIS, and CHYLURIA by interfering with the lymphatic circulation. See also FILARIASIS.

wuchereriasis (voo″ker-e-ri'ah-sis) infection with ROUNDWORMS of the genus *Wuchereria;* see also FILARIASIS.

w/v weight (of solute) per volume (of solvent).

X

Xanax (zan'aks) trademark for a preparation of ALPRAZOLAM, an ANTIANXIETY AGENT.

xanth(o)- word element [Gr.], *yellow.*

xanthelasma (zan″thĕ-laz′mah) xanthoma affecting the eyelids and characterized by soft yellowish spots or plaques.

xanthemia (zan-the′me-ah) carotenemia.

xanthic (zan′thik) 1. yellow. 2. pertaining to xanthine.

xanthine (zan′thēn) a PURINE compound found in most bodily tissues and fluids; it is a precursor of URIC ACID. Methylated xanthine compounds such as CAFFEINE, THEOBROMINE, and THEOPHYLLINE are used for their bronchodilator effects.

xanthinuria (zan″thin-u′re-ah) excess of XANTHINE in the urine, due to a hereditary disorder of PURINE metabolism in which there is a deficiency of the enzyme xanthine oxidase.

xanthochromatic (zan″tho-kro-mat′ik) xanthochromic.

xanthochromia (zan″tho-kro′me-ah) yellowish discoloration of the skin or spinal fluid. Xanthochromic spinal fluid usually indicates hemorrhage into the central nervous system and is due to the presence of xanthematin, a yellow pigment derived from hematin.

xanthochromic (zan″tho-kro′mik) yellow-colored; called also xanthochromatic.

xanthocyanopsia (zan″tho-si″ah-nop′se-ah) inability to perceive red or green tints, vision being limited to yellow and blue.

xanthoderma (zan″tho-der-mah) any yellowish discoloration of the skin, for example carotenemia or jaundice.

xanthogranuloma (zan″tho-gran″u-lo′-mah) a tumor having histologic characteristics of both GRANULOMA and XANTHOMA.

juvenile x. a benign, self-limited disorder of infants and children, usually present at birth, manifested by the development of single or multiple papules or nodules, which may be yellow, pink, orange, or reddish brown in color, found typically on the scalp, face, proximal extremities, or trunk; involvement of mucous membranes, viscera, eye, and other organs may also occur.

xanthoma (zan-tho′mah) a papule, nodule, or plaque in the skin due to lipid deposits; it is usually yellow, but may be brown, reddish, or cream colored. Microscopically, the lesions show light cells with foamy protoplasm (foam cells). Xanthomas range in size from tiny pinheads to large nodules, and the shape may be round, flat, or irregular. They are often found around the eyes, the joints, the neck or the palms, or over tendons. Often these lipid deposits are not limited to the skin but are found throughout the body in bones, the heart, blood vessels, liver, and other organs.

The formation of xanthomas may indicate an underlying disease, usually related to abnormal metabolism of lipids, including cholesterol. Abnormally high levels of blood lipids may be found in diabetes mellitus (*xanthoma diabeticorum*), in diseases of the liver, kidney, and thyroid gland, and in several hereditary metabolic diseases. The excessive lipids carried in the blood may then be deposited as xanthomas. Treatment

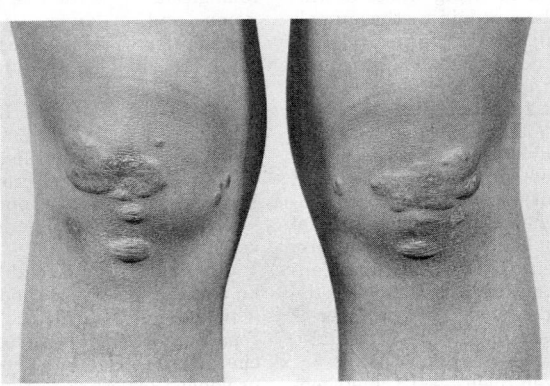

Legs of a person homozygous for familial hypercholesterolemia, showing multiple xanthomas. From Mueller and Young, 2001.

includes surgery, application of acids directly to the lipid deposits, and management of the disease that causes them.

diabetic x. an eruptive xanthoma associated with diabetes mellitus; when the diabetes is brought under control, the skin lesions disappear.

xanthomatosis (zan″tho-mah-to′sis) an accumulation of excess lipids in the body due to disturbance of lipid metabolism and marked by the formation of foam cells in skin lesions called XANTHOMAS.

x. bul′bi fatty degeneration of the cornea due to disorder of lipid metabolism, marked by the presence of xanthomas.

chronic idiopathic x. Hand-Schüller-Christian disease.

xanthomatous (zan-tho′mah-tus) pertaining to xanthoma.

xanthopsia (zan-thop′se-ah) chromatopsia in which objects are seen as yellow.

xanthosine (zan′tho-sēn) a nucleoside composed of xanthine and ribose.

xanthosis (zan-tho′sis) yellowish discoloration; degeneration with yellowish pigmentation.

xanthurenic acid (zan″thu-ren′ik) a metabolite of L-TRYPTOPHAN, present in normal urine and in increased amounts in vitamin B_6 deficiency.

Xe xenon.

xen(o)- word element [Gr.], *strange; foreign.*

xenodiagnosis (zen″o-di″ag-no′sis) 1. diagnosis by means of finding, in the feces of clean laboratory-bred bugs fed on the patient, the infective forms of the organism causing the disease; used in the early stages of Chagas' disease. 2. diagnosis of trichinosis by means of feeding laboratory-bred rats or mice on meat suspected of being infected with *Trichinella,* and then examining the animals for the parasite. adj., **xenodiagnos′tic.**

xenobiotic (ze″no-bi-ot′ik) a chemical compound foreign to a given biological system. With respect to animals and humans, xenobiotics include drugs, drug metabolites, and environmental compounds such as pollutants that are not produced by the body. In the environment, xenobiotics include synthetic pesticides, herbicides, and industrial pollutants that would not be found in nature.

xenogeneic (zen″o-jen-e′ik) in transplantation biology, denoting individuals or tissues from individuals of different species and hence of disparate cell type. Called also heterologous and heterologous.

xenogenesis (zen″o-jen′ĕ-sis) 1. metagenesis. 2. production of offspring unlike either parent.

xenogenous (ze-noj′ĕ-nus) 1. xenogeneic. 2. caused by a foreign body.

xenograft (zen′o-graft) a graft of tissue transplanted between animals of different species; called also heterograft, heterologous graft, and heteroplastic graft.

xenon (ze′non) a chemical element, atomic number 54, atomic weight 131.30, symbol Xe. (See Appendix 6.) The radioactive isotope ^{133}Xe is used in assessment of pulmonary function, lung imaging, and cerebral blood flow studies.

x.-133 a radioisotope of xenon having a half-life of 5.3 days and a principal gamma ray photon energy of 81 keV; used for pulmonary ventilation imaging. Symbol ^{133}Xe.

xenoparasite (zen″o-par′ah-sīt) an organism not usually parasitic on a particular species, but which becomes so because of a weakened condition of the host.

xenophobia (zen″o-fo′be-ah) irrational fear of strangers.

xenophonia (zen″o-fo′ne-ah) alteration in the quality of the voice.

xenophthalmia (zen″of-thal′me-ah) inflammation caused by a foreign body in the eye.

Xenopsylla (zen″op-sil′ah) a genus of fleas, including more than 30 species, many of which transmit disease-producing microorganisms. *X. cheo′pis* is the rat flea, which transmits *Pasteurella pestis,* the causative organism of PLAGUE, and *Rickettsia typhi* the causative organism of murine TYPHUS.

xer(o)- word element [Gr.], *dry; dryness.*

xeroderma (ze″ro-der′mah) excessive dryness of the skin, a mild form of ICHTHYOSIS.

x. pigmento′sum a rare and often fatal pigmentary and atrophic disease in which the skin and eyes are extremely sensitive to light. It begins in childhood and progresses to early development of excessive freckling telangiectases, keratoses, papillomas, carcinoma, and melanoma. Ocular symptoms include photophobia, opacities, and tumors It is inherited as an autosomal recessive trait involving a defect in the enzymes active in the repair of DNA damaged by ultraviolet irradiation. Subtypes of this disorder have been identified by the capacity for DNA repair. Total protection from sunlight prevents the development of lesions.

xerodermoid (ze′ro-der′moid) resembling xeroderma.

pigmented x. a condition considered to be a variant of xeroderma pigmentosum in which there is no defect in the excisional repair of ultraviolet-damaged DNA, which is characterized by a late onset associated with prolonged exposure to the sun, with freckling appearing in the second decade and no skin cancers until age 40.

xerography (ze-rog′rah-fe) xeroradiography.

xeroma (ze-ro′mah) xerophthalmia.

xeromammography (ze″ro-mah-mog′rah-fe) xeroradiography of the breast.

xeromenia (ze″ro-me′ne-ah) the appearance of constitutional symptoms at the menstrual period without any flow of blood.

xerophthalmia (ze″rof-thal′me-ah) abnormal dryness and thickening of the surface of the conjunctiva and cornea due to a deficiency of vitamin A or to local disease; called also ophthalmoxerosis.

xeroradiography (ze″ro-ra″de-og′rah-fe) the making of radiographs by a dry, totally photoelectric process, using metal plates coated with a semiconductor such as selenium; the image produced by this process differs from conventional x-ray in that margins between tissues of varying densities are more clearly defined. Hence, xeroradiography is especially beneficial in the diagnosis of breast tumors. It does, however, require higher doses of radiation. Called also xerography.

   negative mode x. a xeroradiographic image that is blue and white but that has been reversed so that white represents the dense areas.

   positive mode x. a xeroradiographic image that is blue and white, with blue representing the dense areas.

xerosialography (ze″ro-si″ah-log′rah-fe) sialography in which the images are recorded by xerography.

xerosis (ze-ro′sis) abnormal dryness, as of the eye (xerophthalmia), skin (xeroderma), or mouth (xerostomia).

   x. generalisa′ta dryness of the skin, with pruritus and branny scaling, seen in patients with acquired immunodeficiency syndrome.

xerostomia (ze″ro-sto′me-ah) dryness of the mouth from salivary gland dysfunction.

xerotomography (ze″ro-to-mog′rah-fe) tomography in which the images are recorded by xeroradiography.

xiph(o)- word element [Gr.], *xiphoid process.*

xiphisternum (zif″ĭ-ster′num) xiphoid process. adj., **xiphister′nal.**

xiphocostal (zif″o-kos′tal) pertaining to the xiphoid process and ribs.

xiphoid (zif′oid, zi′foid) 1. sword-shaped; called also ensiform. 2. xiphoid process.

xiphoiditis (zif″oi-di′tis) inflammation of the xiphoid process.

xiphopagus (zi-fop′ah-gus) symmetrical conjoined twins united in the region of the xiphoid process.

X-linked (eks′lingkt) transmitted by genes on the X chromosome; see also X-linked GENE.

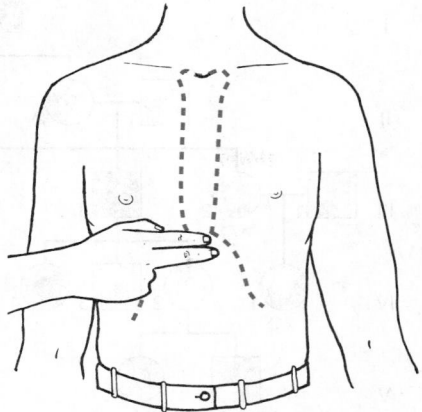

Locating the xiphoid process. From Stein et al., 2000.

XO symbol for the karyotype observed in most cases of Turner's syndrome, in which there is only one sex chromosome, an X chromosome.

x-rays (eks′rāz) high-energy electromagnetic RADIATION produced by the collision of a beam of electrons with a metal target in an x-ray TUBE; the penetrability and hardness of the x-rays increase with the voltage applied to the tube, which controls the speed with which the electrons strike the target. Called also roentgen rays.

For diagnostic RADIOGRAPHY, tube voltages in the range 80 to 120 kilovolts peak (kVp) are normally used. For RADIATION THERAPY, voltages in the 1 to 2 megavolt range are used for most treatment. Accelerating electrons to speeds high enough to produce megavoltage x-rays requires a linear accelerator (lineac). Kilovoltage lower than 80 kVp is often used for the extremities, 25 to 30 kVp is used for mammography, and up to 150 kVp can be used for chest imaging.

The x-ray exposure is proportional to the tube current (milliamperage) and also to the exposure time. In diagnostic radiography, the tube voltage and current and exposure time are selected to produce a high-quality radiograph with the correct contrast and film density. In radiation therapy, these exposure factors are selected to deliver a precisely calculated radiation dose to the tumor. The total dose is usually fractionated so that tumor cells can be oxygenated as surrounding cells die; this increases the sensitivity of the cells to radiation.

Body tissues and other substances are classified according to the degree to

X

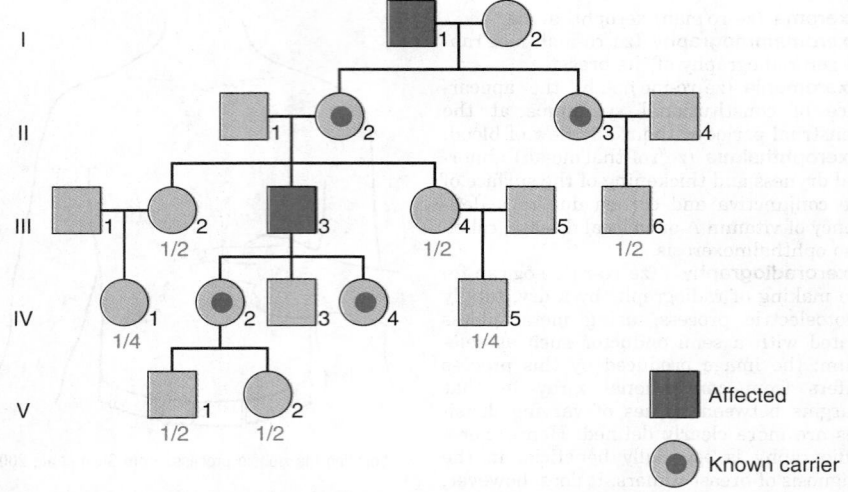

The probabilities of male relatives being affected and female relatives being carriers of an X-linked recessive disorder. All the daughters of an affected male are obligate carriers. From Mueller and Young, 2001.

which they allow the passage of x-rays (their RADIOLUCENCY) or absorb x-rays (their RADIOPACITY). Gases are very radiolucent; fatty tissue is moderately radiolucent. Compounds containing high-atomic-weight elements, such as barium and iodine, are very radiopaque; bone and deposits of calcium salts are moderately radiopaque. Water; muscle, skin, blood, and cartilage and other connective tissue; and cholesterol and uric acid stones have intermediate density.

X-ray Contrast Media. A contrast MEDIUM is a substance introduced into a structure in order to increase the radiographic contrast with surrounding tissues. The radiopaque contrast media include a variety of organic IODINE compounds and the insoluble salt BARIUM SULFATE. Radiolucent contrast media are gases such as air, oxygen, or carbon dioxide.

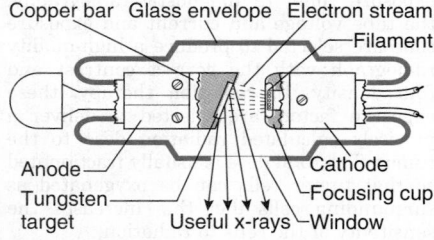

Standard stationary anode x-ray tube; diagram in longitudinal section. From Dorland's, 2000.

Barium is used for gastrointestinal studies. Water-soluble, iodinated contrast media excreted by the kidneys are used for many procedures, including all types of ANGIOGRAPHY and for intravenous and retrograde UROGRAPHY; the most commonly used are DIATRIZOATE and IOTHALAMATE. Those excreted by the liver are used for oral or intravenous CHOLANGIOGRAPHY or CHOLECYSTOGRAPHY. Oily iodinated media are used for LYMPHANGIOGRAPHY, BRONCHOGRAPHY, and MYELOGRAPHY.

All iodinated contrast media can cause reactions, which may range from the common reactions of mild flushing and a feeling of warmth and nausea and vomiting to rare life-threatening reactions requiring immediate aggressive therapy. The cause of these reactions may be allergy; however, this is disputed.

A double contrast study uses both a radiopaque and a radiolucent contrast medium; for example, the walls of the stomach or intestine are coated with barium and the lumen is filled with air. The resulting radiographs clearly show the pattern of mucosal ridges.

xylitol (zi′lĭ-tol) a five-carbon sugar alcohol derived from XYLOSE and as sweet as SUCROSE; used as a noncariogenic sweetener and also as a sugar substitute in diabetic diets.

Xylocaine (zi′lo-kān) trademark for preparations of LIDOCAINE, a topical anesthetic.

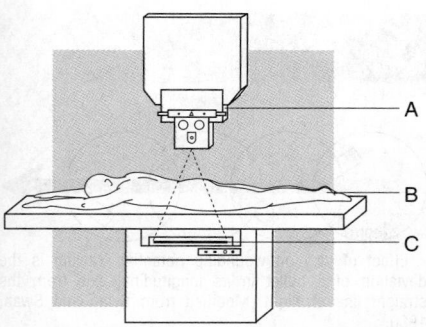

Simple radiograph. *A*, X-ray machine; *B*, patient; and *C*, x-ray film. From Malarkey and McMorrow, 1996.

xylometazoline (zi″lo-met″ah-zo′lēn) an adrenergic used in the form of the hydrochloride salt as a topical nasal DECONGESTANT.

xylose (zi′lōs) a pentose found in MUCO-POLYSACCHARIDES of connective tissue, sometimes the urine, and vegetable gum. D-Xylose is used in a diagnostic test of intestinal absorption (see MALABSORPTION SYNDROME).

xylulose (zi′lu-lōs) a pentose sugar occurring as D-xylulose and L-xylulose, one of the few L sugars found in nature; it is sometimes excreted in the urine (see PENTOSURIA).

xysma (zis′mah) material resembling bits of membrane in stools of diarrhea.

X

Y

Y yttrium.

Yalow (yal′o) Rosalyn. Medical physicist who developed the radioimmunoassay (RIA) technique and was awarded the Nobel prize in medicine or physiology in 1977. An enthusiastic supporter of women in science careers, she noted "We must believe in ourselves or no one else will believe in us...we must feel a personal responsibility to ease the path for those who come after us. The world cannot afford the loss of the talents of half of its people if we are to solve the many problems that beset us."

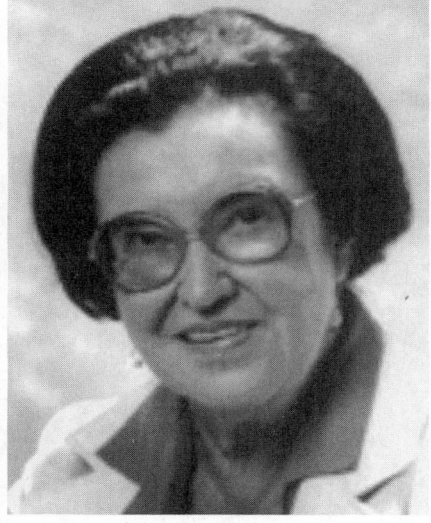

Yankauer suction tip (yang′kow-er) a tip attached to a suction tube for bedside suctioning of an artificial airway. See illustration.

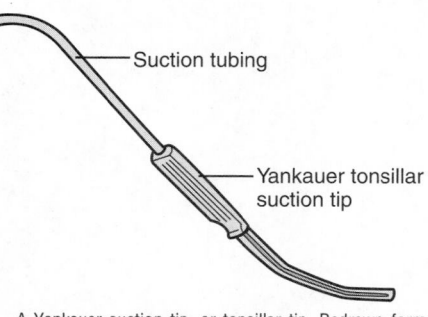

Suction tubing

Yankauer tonsillar suction tip

A Yankauer suction tip, or tonsillar tip. Redrawn form Lammon et al., 1995.

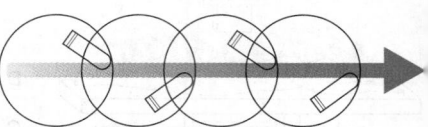

Effect of yaw on wounding potential. Yawing is the deviation of a bullet in its longitudinal axis from the straight line of flight. Modified from Swan and Swan, 1980.

yaw (yaw) 1. a lesion of YAWS. 2. the deviation of an object from its usual path (see illustration).

mother y. the initial cutaneous lesion of YAWS; called also frambesioma.

yawning (yawn′ing) a deep, involuntary inhalation with the mouth open, often accompanied by the act of stretching; called also oscitation.

yaws (yawz) a highly infectious disease caused by the spirochete *Treponema perte-nue.* It was once common in tropical and subtropical regions of the world such as equatorial Africa, Central and South America, the Caribbean, and Indonesia and nearby islands. However, programs of the World Health Organization have now reduced its incidence. Called also frambesia.

Transmission and Symptoms. Yaws is transmitted by direct contact. The first symptom, appearing usually about a month after exposure, is a single granulomatous lesion, an inflammatory but painless elevation of the skin. Called the "mother yaw," this soon ulcerates. Open, oozing sores appear a few weeks later on the hands, feet, face, scalp, and trunk. Eventually, after several years, the disease causes tissue destruction, bone changes, and shortening of the fingers or toes, in a cycle that has a resemblance to leprosy and is sometimes mistaken for it.

The causative organism of yaws is closely related to that of SYPHILIS, and both diseases give a positive result on the WAS-SERMANN TEST. However, yaws is not primarily spread by coitus and is not classified as a SEXUALLY TRANSMITTED DISEASE.

Treatment and Prevention. Effective treatment is by antibiotics, particularly penicillin. Unsanitary living conditions help spread the disease, and public health initiatives are ongoing.

Yb ytterbium.

Y-connector a device in the shape of the letter Y that connects the end of one piece of tubing to two outlets.

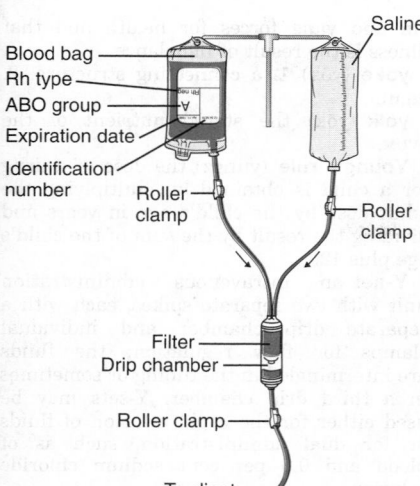

Blood bag
Rh type
ABO group
Expiration date
Identification number
Saline
Roller clamp
Roller clamp
Filter
Drip chamber
Roller clamp
To client

Y-connector blood administration set. Redrawn from Lammon et al., 1995.

yeast (yēst) any of various unicellular, nucleated, usually rounded fungi that reproduce by budding; some are fermenters of carbohydrates, and a few are pathogenic for humans.

brewer's y. *Saccharomyces cerevisiae,* used in brewing beer, making alcoholic liquors, and baking bread.

dried y. dried cells of any suitable strain of *Saccharomyces cerevisiae,* usually a by-product of the brewing industry; used as a natural source of protein and B-complex vitamins.

yellow (yel′o) 1. the color produced by stimulation by light waves of wavelength of 571.5 to 578.5 mµ. 2. a color between orange and green, produced by energy of wavelengths between 570 and 590 nm. 3. a dye or stain with this color.

y. fever an acute infectious type of HEMORRHAGIC FEVER, transmitted by the female of certain species of mosquitoes, and characterized by fever, jaundice due to necrosis of the liver, and albuminuria. It is less rampant today than previously, largely because of vaccination and better control of the mosquitoes, but it is still a danger in most tropical countries. Among native inhabitants who contract the disease there is a mortality rate of about 5 per cent. In visitors from other climates, fatalities once ran as high as 40 per cent but are now much lower. With proper immunization precautions, a visitor from a temperate country today takes only a minimal risk.

The mosquito that transmits classic yellow fever is *Aedes aegypti.* In the jungles of Brazil and in parts of Africa, in the absence of *Aedes aegypti,* the disease may be carried by a different mosquito species that lives in treetops. These forest mosquitoes can communicate the disease to forest workers and also to certain animals, such as monkeys and marmosets, which then serve as virus reservoirs and as sources of reinfection for humans. This form of the disease is called *jungle* or *sylvan yellow fever,* and it is difficult to control because of the virtual impossibility of eradicating the tree-inhabiting mosquitoes.

Symptoms and Treatment. Yellow fever has an incubation period of 3 to 6 days. It then manifests suddenly and intensely with fever, headache, muscular aches, and prostration. A few days later, the temperature suddenly falls, only to rise again. The pulse is originally very rapid, but then slows gradually to less than 50 beats per minute. In addition to the characteristic yellowing of the skin, the urine becomes darker. There may be frequent vomiting, and blood may become noticeable in the vomitus (so-called "black vomit"). There may also be bleeding from the mucous membranes.

The disease runs its course in a little more than a week. Those who survive suffer no permanent damage. The jaundice completely disappears. Furthermore, these persons are immune from a second attack. In fatal cases, death is usually due to liver, myocardial, or kidney failure.

There is no specific drug for the cure of yellow fever. The effects of the disease can be mitigated by analgesics, sedatives, bed rest, and a high-calorie, high-carbohydrate diet.

Patient Care. The patient's fever is controlled with cold or tepid sponges and other measures to lower body temperature (see FEVER). The diet consists of liquids and easily digested foods until the vomiting stops, and then is gradually increased. The patient's bed and room should be well screened to prevent transmission of the fever to others via mosquitoes.

visual y. all-*trans* RETINAL.

Yersinia (yer-sin′e-ah) a genus of nonmotile, ovoid or rod-shaped, nonencapsulated, gram-negative bacteria (family Enterobacteriaceae). *Y. pes′tis* causes PLAGUE in humans and rodents; it is transmitted from rat to rat and from rat to human by the rat flea, and between humans by the human body louse. *Y. enterocoli′tica* causes acute GASTROENTERITIS and mesenteric LYMPHADENITIS,

Y

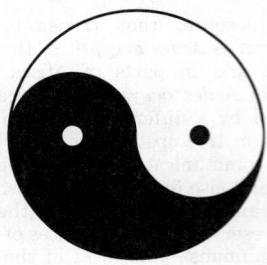

Symbol for yin/yang.

especially in young children, and ARTHRITIS, SEPTICEMIA, and ERYTHEMA NODOSUM in adults. *Y. pseudotuberculo'sis* causes disease in rodents and mesenteric LYMPHADENITIS in humans.

yin/yang a Chinese philosophy that each entity is one, but contains two equal and opposite forces. The forces of yang include maleness, the sun, and heat; the forces of yin include femaleness, darkness, and cold. Macrobiotic diets are based on the division of food into yin and yang properties. Many holistic care practices are rooted in the belief that there must be a balance between yin and yang forces for health and that illness is the result of imbalance.

yoke (yōk) 1. a connecting structure. 2. jugum.

yolk (yōk) the stored nutrient of the OVUM.

Young's rule (yungz) the dose of a drug for a child is obtained by multiplying the adult dose by the child's age in years and dividing the result by the sum of the child's age plus 12.

Y-set an intravenous administration unit with two separate spikes, each with a separate drip chamber and individual clamps for flow regulation; the fluids are intermingled in the tubing or sometimes in a third drip chamber. Y-sets may be used either for the rapid infusion of fluids or for dual administration, such as of blood and 0.9 per cent sodium chloride solution.

ytterbium (ĭ-ter'be-um) a chemical element, atomic number 70, atomic weight 173.04, symbol Yb. (See Appendix 6.)

yttrium (ĭ'tre-um) a chemical element, atomic number 39, atomic weight 88.905, symbol Y. (See Appendix 6.) The radio-isotope ^{90}Y emits high energy beta particles, localizes predominantly in bone, and has been used in radiotherapy.

Z

Z atomic number.

zafirlukast (zah-fir'loo-kast) a LEUKO-TRIENE receptor antagonist used in treatment of ASTHMA, administered orally.

zalcitabine (zal-si'tah-bēn) a nucleoside ANALOGUE ANTIRETROVIRAL agent that inhibits the action of reverse TRANSCRIPTASE; used in the treatment of human immunodeficiency VIRUS (HIV) infection, administered orally.

zaleplon (zal'ē-plon) a nonbenzodiazepine sedative and hypnotic used in the short term treatment of insomnia; administered orally.

zanamivir (zah-nam'ĭ-vir) an inhibitor of viral NEURAMINIDASE used for the prophylaxis and treatment of INFLUENZA A and INFLUENZA B; administered by inhalation.

Zanosar (zan'o-sahr) trademark for preparations of STREPTOZOCIN, an antitumor ANTIBIOTIC.

Zarontin (zah-ron'tin) trademark for preparations of ETHOSUXIMIDE, an ANTICONVULSANT.

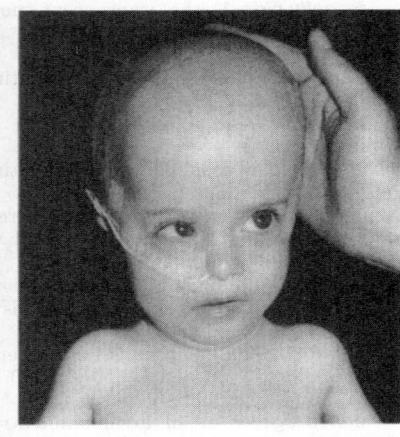

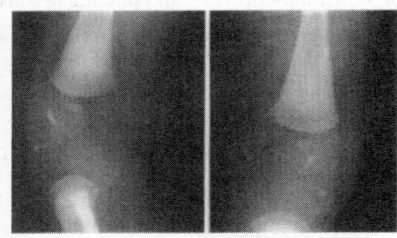

A, Facies of an infant with Zellweger syndrome showing a prominent forehead. *B,* Radiography of the knee of a newborn infant with Zellweger syndrome showing abnormal punctate calcification of the distal femoral epiphyses. From Mueller and Young, 2001.

Zaroxolyn (zah-rok'so-lin) trademark for a preparation of METOLAZONE, a diuretic.

Zellweger syndrome (zel'weg-er) an autosomal recessive inborn ERROR of metabolism characterized by a prominent forehead, large anterior fontanelle, poor muscle tone, hepatomegaly, polycystic kidneys, jaundice, and often calcifications in the cartilaginous ends of long bones. Most affected children die in early infancy. Called also cerebrohepatorenal syndrome. See illustration.

Zenapax (ze'nah-paks) trademark for a preparation of DACLIZUMAB, an IMMUNOSUPPRESSANT used after kidney transplantation.

Zephiran (zef'ĭ-ran) trademark for preparations of BENZALKONIUM CHLORIDE, a topical antiseptic.

zero (ze'ro) 1. the absence of all quantity or magnitude; naught. 2. the point on a thermometer scale at which the graduations begin. The zero of the Celsius (centigrade) scale is the ice point; on the Fahrenheit scale it is 32 degrees below the ice point.

   absolute z. the lowest possible temperature, designated 0 on the Kelvin or Rankine scale; the equivalent of $-273.15°C$ or $-459.67°F$.

zetacrit (za'tah-krit) the packed-cell VOLUME produced by the zeta sedimentation RATIO procedure.

Zetafuge (za'tah-fūj) trademark for a specially designed centrifuge used in determination of the zeta sedimentation RATIO.

zidovudine (zi-do'vu-dēn) a nucleoside ANALOGUE to THYMIDINE, used as an ANTIRETROVIRAL agent in treatment of patients with human immunodeficiency VIRUS (HIV) infection and ACQUIRED IMMUNODEFICIENCY SYNDROME (AIDS); administered orally or intravenously. It was the first agent approved for such use.

ZIFT zygote intrafallopian transfer.

zigzagplasty (zig'zag-plas"te) Z-plasty.

zileuton (zi-loo'ton) an inhibitor of LEUKOTRIENE formation, used in treatment of ASTHMA; administered orally.

zinc (zingk) a chemical element, atomic number 30, atomic weight 65.37, symbol Zn. (See Appendix 6.) It is a trace element in the diet, a component of several enzymes, including DNA and RNA polymerases and carbonic anhydrase. It is abundant in red meat, shellfish, liver, peas, lentils, beans, and rice. A well-balanced diet assures adequate intake of zinc. Those who may suffer from zinc deficiency include persons on a strictly vegetarian diet and those who are on a high-fiber diet. In the latter case, the zinc is bound to the fiber and is eliminated in the feces without having been absorbed through the intestinal wall. Poor absorption of zinc also can occur in persons with chronic and severe bowel disease. The recommended daily intake is 12–15 mg for an adult. A severe deficiency of zinc can retard growth in children, cause a low sperm count in adult males, and retard wound healing. Signs of a deficiency include anorexia and a diminished sense of taste. An excessive intake of zinc (usually in those who work with the metal or breathe its fumes) can either cause pneumoconiosis or interfere with the body's use of copper and other trace elements, producing diarrhea, nausea, vomiting, and other signs of intestinal irritation.

> **z. acetate** a salt used as an astringent and styptic.

> **z. chloride** a salt used as a nutritional supplement in total PARENTERAL NUTRITION and applied topically as an astringent and a desensitizer for dentin.

> **z. oxide** a topical astringent and skin protectant; also a sunscreen.

> **z. stearate** a powder of zinc in a compound with stearic and palmitic acids; used as a water-repellent skin protectant in dermatoses.

> **z. sulfate** a topical astringent for mucous membranes, especially those of the eye.

> **z. undecylenate** the zinc salt of undecylenic acid; it is a topical antifungal.

ziprasidone (zĭ-pra′sĭ-dōn) an ANTIPSYCHOTIC used in the treatment of SCHIZOPHRENIA, administered orally as the hydrochloride salt.

zirconium (zir-ko′ne-um) a chemical element, atomic number 40, atomic weight 91.22, symbol Zr. (See Appendix 6.)

Zn zinc.

zo(o)- word element [Gr.], *animal*.

zoacanthosis (zo″ak-an-tho′sis) a dermatitis caused by penetration into a person's skin of bristles, hairs, or other foreign objects from another species of animal.

zoanthropy (zo-an′thro-pe) the delusion that one has become an animal. adj., **zoanthrop′ic**.

Zoladex (zo′lah-deks) trademark for preparations of GOSERELIN, a GONADOTROPIN suppressor used as an antineoplastic AGENT and to treat ENDOMETRIOSIS.

zoledronic acid (zo′lĕ-dron″ik) a bisphosphonate inhibitor of osteoclastic bone resorption, used for the treatment of HYPERCALCEMIA OF MALIGNANCY; administered intravenously.

Zollinger-Ellison syndrome (zol′in-jer el′ĭ-sun) a triad comprising intractable sometimes fulminating, atypical peptic ulcers; extreme gastric hyperacidity; and nonbeta-cell, gastrin-secreting islet cell tumors (gastrinomas) of the pancreas, which may be single or multiple, small or large, benign or malignant.

zolmitriptan (zōl″mĭ-trip′tan) a selective SEROTONIN receptor agonist used to relieve acute MIGRAINE, administered orally.

Zoloft (zo′loft) trademark for preparations of SERTRALINE hydrochloride, an ANTIDEPRESSANT, antiobsessional, and antipanic agent.

zolpidem (zōl-pi′dem) a non-BENZODIAZEPINE SEDATIVE and HYPNOTIC used orally as the tartrate salt in the short-term treatment of INSOMNIA.

zona (zo′nah) [L.] 1. zone. 2. herpes zoster.

> **z. fascicula′ta** the thick middle layer of the adrenal gland.

> **z. glomerulo′sa** the outermost layer of the adrenal cortex.

> **z. ophthal′mica** herpetic infection of the cornea.

> **z. pellu′cida** 1. the transparent, noncellular, secreted layer surrounding an ovum. 2. area pellucida.

> **z. radia′ta** a zona pellucida exhibiting conspicuous radial striations.

> **z. reticula′ris** the innermost layer of the adrenal cortex.

> **z. stria′ta** a zona pellucida exhibiting conspicuous striations.

zone (zōn) an encircling region or area by extension, any area with specific characteristics or boundary.

> **ciliary z.** the outer of the two regions into which the anterior surface of the iris is divided by the COLLARETTE.

> **comfort z.** an environmental temperature between 13 and 21°C (55 and 70°F with a humidity of 30 to 55 per cent.

> **epileptogenic z.** an area, stimulation of which may provoke an epileptic seizure.

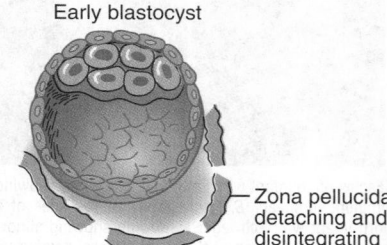

Early blastocyst

Zona pellucida detaching and disintegrating

Zona pellucida. From Applegate, 2000.

erogenous z., erotogenic z. in psychoanalytic theory, an area of the body through which the libido expresses itself and which is therefore susceptible to erotic excitation upon stimulation; the primary sites are the oral, anal, and genital regions, but the other body orifices, breasts, and skin are also included.

z. of partial preservation in spinal cord injury, an area of only partial damage that may include up to three consecutive spinal segments caudal to the level of the injury.

pupillary z. the inner of the two regions into which the anterior surface of the iris is divided by the COLLARETTE.

transition z., transitional z. any anatomical region that marks the point at which the constituents of a structure change from one type to another; for example, the circle in the equator of the ocular lens in which epithelial fibers are developed into lens fibers, or the zone (*anocutaneous line*) that marks the junction of stratified squamous epithelium with columnar epithelium.

zonesthesia (zo″nes-the′zhah) a sensation of constriction, as by a girdle.

zonifugal (zo-nif′ŭ-gal) passing outward from a zone or region.

zonipetal (zo-nip′ĕ-tal) passing toward a zone or region.

zonisamide (zo-nis′ah-mīd″) a SULFONAMIDE that acts as an ANTICONVULSANT , used as an adjunct in the treatment of partial SEIZURES in adults; administered orally.

zonography (zo-nog′rah-fe) narrow angle tomography.

zonula (zo′nu-lah) [L.] zonule.

zonule (zōn′ūl) a small zone.

ciliary z., z. of Zinn a series of fibers connecting the ciliary body and lens of the eye, holding the lens in place.

zonulitis (zōn″u-li′tis) inflammation of the ciliary zonule.

zonulolysis (zōn″u-lol′ĭ-sis) dissolution of the ciliary zonule by use of enzymes, to permit surgical removal of the lens.

zonulotomy (zōn″u-lot′ah-me) incision of the ciliary zonule.

zoodermic (zo′o-der′mik)   performed with the skin of an animal, especially in reference to skin grafts.

zoogenous (zo-oj′ĕ-nus) 1. acquired from animals. 2. viviparous.

zoogeny (zo-oj′ĕ-ne) the development and evolution of animals.

zoogony (zo-og′ah-ne) the production of living young from within the body. adj., **zoog′onous.**

zoografting (zo′o-graft″ing) the grafting of animal tissue.

zooid (zo′oid) 1. animal-like. 2. an animal-like object or form.

zoolagnia (zo″o-lag′ne-ah) sexual attraction toward animals; see also ZOOPHILIA.

zoology (zo-ol′ah-je) the biology of animals.

Zoomastigophorea (zo″o-mas″tĭ-go-for′e-ah) a class of protozoa (subphylum Mastigophora), including all the animal-like, as opposed to plant-like, protozoa.

zoonosis (zo″o-no′sis), pl. *zoono′ses* a disease of animals transmissible to humans. adj., **zoonot′ic.**

zooparasite (zo″o-par′ah-sīt) an animal PARASITE. adj., **zooparasit′ic.**

zoopathology (zo″o-pah-thol′ah-je)   the science of the diseases of animals.

zoophagous (zo-of′ah-gus) carnivorous.

zoophilia (zo″o-fil′e-ah) 1. abnormal fondness for animals. 2. a PARAPHILIA in which intercourse or other sexual activity with animals is the preferred method of achieving sexual excitement; see also ZOOLAGNIA. Called also bestiality.

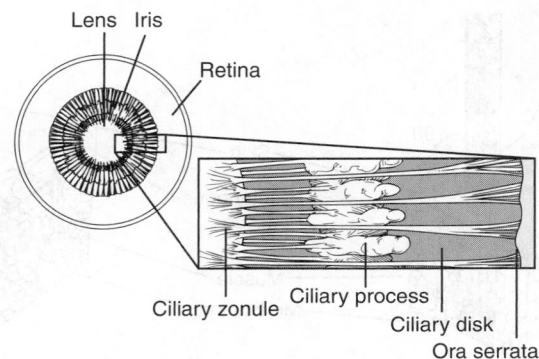

Lens   Iris

Retina

Ciliary zonule   Ciliary process

Ciliary disk

Ora serrata

Ciliary zonule. The system of suspensory ligaments holding the lens in position. From Dorland's, 2000.

Z

zoophobia (zo″o-fo′be-ah) irrational fear of animals.

zooplasty (zo′o-plas″te) zoografting.

zoopsia (zo-op′se-ah) a hallucination with visions of animals.

zoospore (zo′o-spōr) a motile spore, such as an asexual flagellate of certain algae and lower fungi, or a minute sexual or asexual flagellate or ameboid spore produced by certain protozoa.

zootoxin (zo′o-tok″sin) a toxic substance of animal origin, e.g., venom of snakes, spiders, or scorpions.

zoster (zos′ter) herpes zoster.

z. sine eruptio′ne, z. sine her′pete pain typical of herpes zoster in an appropriate sensory area but not followed by the development of characteristic lesions.

zosteriform (zos′-tĕ-rĭ-form″) zosteroid.

zosteroid (zos′ter-oid) resembling HERPES ZOSTER; called also zosteriform.

Zovirax (zo′vir-aks) trademark for preparations of ACYCLOVIR, an antiviral agent.

Z-plasty (ze′plas-te) repair of a skin defect by the transposition of two triangular flaps of adjacent skin, for relaxation of scar contractures. Called also zigzagplasty.

Zr zirconium.

Z-track injection a technique for intramuscular injection of a substance likely to be irritating, or when deposition of a drug and absorption by muscle tissue is crucial. The tissue to be injected is pulled downward and in the direction of the body's midline. It is held in this position during the time and after the drug is injected. When the tissue is released, the usually straight needle track will become a broken line similar to the letter Z. This holds the medication deep in the muscle and prevents upward seepage through the tissues along the needle track.

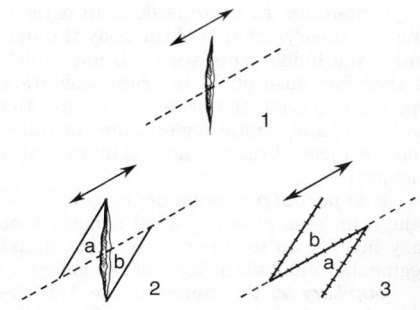

Z-plasty, showing the direction of relaxed skin tension lines (*arrow*), desired position of final scar (*dotted line*), and the two flaps to be juxtaposed (*a, b*). From Dorland's, 2000.

The area is not massaged after injection. A separate needle is used after drawing up the drug into the syringe. This eliminates depositing the drug along the needle track while it is piercing the tissue.

zwitterion (tsvit′er-i″on) an ion that has both positive and negative regions of charge; called also dipolar ion.

zyg(o)- word element [Gr.], *yoked; joined; a junction.*

zygal (zi′gal) shaped like a yoke.

zygapophysis (zi″gah-pof′ĭ-sis) the articular process of a vertebra.

zygion (zij′e-on) the most lateral point on the zygomatic ARCH.

zygodactyly (zi″go-dak′tĭ-le) a type of SYNDACTYLY in which digits are united by soft tissues (skin) without bony fusion.

zygoma (zi-go′mah) 1. zygomatic process. 2. zygomatic arch. 3. a term sometimes applied to the zygomatic BONE.

zygomatic (zi″go-mat′ik) pertaining to the zygomatic BONE.

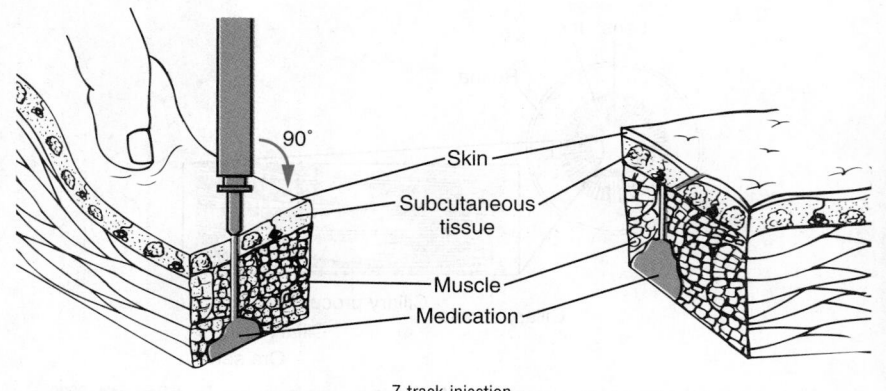

Z-track injection.

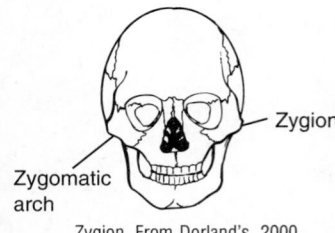

Zygion. From Dorland's, 2000.

zygomaticofacial (zi″go-mat″ĭ-ko-fa′shal) pertaining to the zygomatic PROCESS or BONE and the face.

zygomaticotemporal (zi″go-mat″ĭ-ko-tem′po-ral) pertaining to the zygomatic PROCESS or BONE and the temporal BONE.

Zygomycetes (zi″-go-mi-se′-tēz) a class of saprobic and parasitic fungi of the phylum Zygomycota; important pathogenic organisms are in the orders Entomophthorales and Mucorales.

zygomycosis (zi″go-mi-ko′sis) 1. any fungal infection with members of the class Zygomycetes, including entomophthoromycosis and mucormycosis. 2. mucormycosis.

rhinocerebral z. zygomycosis that has spread from the paranasal sinuses to the brain.

rhinofacial z. rhinoentomophthoromycosis.

subcutaneous z. entomophthoromycosis basidiobolae.

zygon (zi′gon) the stem connecting the two branches of a zygal fissure.

zygosity (zi-gos′ĭ-te) the condition relating to CONJUGATION, or to the ZYGOTE, such as *(a)* the state of a cell or individual in regard to the alleles determining a specific character, whether identical (HOMOZYGOSITY) or different (HETEROZYGOSITY); or *(b)* in the case of twins, whether developing from one zygote (MONOZYGOTIC twins) or two zygotes (DIZYGOTIC twins).

zygote (zi′gōt) the cell resulting from union of a male and a female GAMETE; the fertilized OVUM (see also REPRODUCTION). More precisely, the cell after synapsis at the completion of fertilization until first cleavage. adj., **zygot′ic.**

zygotene (zi′go-tēn) the synaptic stage of the first meiotic prophase in which the two leptotene chromosomes undergo pairing by the formation of synaptonemal complexes to form a bivalent.

Zyloprim (zi′lo-prim) trademark for a preparation of ALLOPURINOL, an inhibitor of uric acid production in the body used to treat HYPERURICEMIA of gout and that secondary to blood dyscrasias or cancer chemotherapy.

zym(o)- word element [Gr.], *enzyme; fermentation.*

zymogen (zi′mo-jen) an inactive precursor that is converted into an active enzyme by action of an acid or another enzyme or by other means; a proenzyme. adj., **zymogen′ic.**

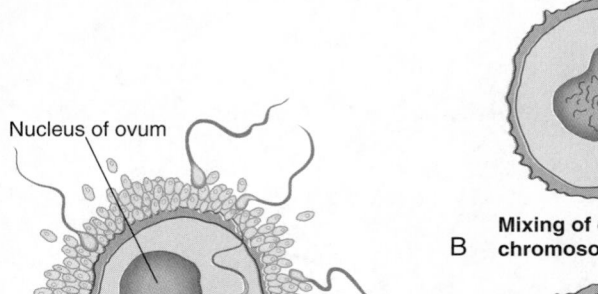

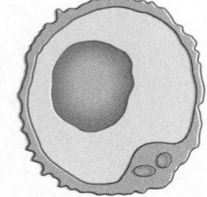

B **Mixing of cell nuclei and chromosomes of ovum and sperm**

C **Fertilization complete**

Development of the zygote. *A,* A sperm enters the ovum. *B,* The 23 chromosomes from the sperm mingle with the 23 chromosomes from the ovum, restoring the diploid number to 46. *C,* The fertilized ovum, now called a zygote, is ready for the first mitotic cell division. From McKinney et al., 2000.

Z

Appendices

Section 1: Diagnostic Tools

1-1. MAJOR DIAGNOSTIC CATEGORIES

Major Diagnostic Categories	Group Description
1	Diseases and disorders of the nervous system
2	Diseases and disorders of the eye
3	Diseases and disorders of the ear, nose, mouth, and throat
4	Diseases and disorders of the respiratory system
5	Diseases and disorders of the circulatory system
6	Diseases and disorders of the digestive system
7	Diseases and disorders of the hepatobiliary system and pancreas
8	Diseases and disorders of the musculoskeletal system and connective tissue
9	Diseases and disorders of the skin, subcutaneous tissue, and breast
10	Endocrine, nutritional, and metabolic diseases and disorders
11	Diseases and disorders of the kidney and urinary tract
12	Diseases and disorders of the male reproductive system
13	Diseases and disorders of the female reproductive system
14	Pregnancy, childbirth, and the puerperium
15	Newborns and other neonates with conditions originating in the perinatal period
16	Diseases and disorders of the blood and blood-forming organs and immunologic disorders
17	Myeloproliferative diseases and disorders and poorly differentiated neoplasms
18	Infectious and parasitic diseases (systemic or unspecified sites)
19	Mental diseases and disorders
20	Alcohol/drug use and alcohol/drug-induced organic mental disorders
21	Injuries, poisonings, and toxic effects of drugs
22	Burns
23	Factors influencing health status and other contacts with health services
24	Multiple significant trauma
25	Human immunodeficiency virus infections

Excerpted from the *Federal Register* 67(148): 50230, August 1, 2002.

1-2. DIAGNOSIS-RELATED GROUPS (DRG)—FY 2000

DRG	MDC	Type	Description
1	01	Surg	Craniotomy age > 17 except for trauma
2	01	Surg	Craniotomy for trauma age > 17
3	01	Surg	*craniotomy age 0–17
4	01	Surg	Spinal procedures
5	01	Surg	Extracranial vascular procedures
6	01	Surg	Carpal tunnel release
7	01	Surg	Periph and cranial nerve and other nerve syst proc w CC[†]
8	01	Surg	Periph and cranial nerve and other nerve syst proc w/o CC
9	01	Med	Spinal disordrs and injuries
10	01	Med	Nervous system neoplasms w CC
11	01	Med	Nervous system neoplasms w/o CC
12	01	Med	Degenerative nervous system disorders
13	01	Med	Multiple sclerosis and cerebellar ataxia
14	01	Med	Specific cerebrovascular disorders except TIA
15	01	Med	Transient ischemic attack and precerebral occlusions
16	01	Med	Nonspecific cerebrovascular disorders w CC
17	01	Med	Nonspecific cerebrovascular disorders w/o CC
18	01	Med	Cranial and peripheral nerve disorders w CC
19	01	Med	Cranial and peripheral nerve disorders w/o CC
20	01	Med	Nervous system infection except viral meningitis
21	01	Med	Viral meningitis
22	01	Med	Hypertensive encephalopathy

Excerpted from the *Federal Register*, 67(148): 50230, August 1, 2002.   (continued)
*Medicare data have been supplemented by data from 19 states for low volume DRGs.
†CC comorbidity or complications.

DRG	MDC	Type	Description
23	01	Med	Nontraumatic stupor and coma
24	01	Med	Seizure and headache age > 17 w CC
25	01	Med	Seizure and headache age > 17 w/o CC
26	01	Med	Seizure and headache age 0–17
27	01	Med	Traumatic stupor and coma, coma > 1 hr
28	01	Med	Traumatic stupor and coma, coma < 1 hr age > 17 w CC
29	01	Med	Traumatic stupor and coma, coma < 1 hr age > 17 w/o CC
30	01	Med	*Traumatic stupor and coma, coma < 1 hr age 0–17
31	01	Med	Concussion age > 17 w CC
32	01	Med	Consussion age > 17 w/o CC
33	01	Med	*Concussion age 0–17
34	01	Med	Other disorders of nervous system w CC
35	01	Med	Other disorders of nervous system w/o CC
36	02	Surg	Retinal procedures
37	02	Surg	Orbital procedures
38	02	Surg	Primary iris procedures
39	02	Surg	Lens procedures with or without vitrectomy
40	02	Surg	Extraocular procedures except orbit age > 17
41	02	Surg	*Extraocular procedures except orbit age 0–17
42	02	Surg	Intraocular procedures except retina, iris and lens
43	02	Med	Hyphema
44	02	Med	Acute major eye infections
45	02	Med	Neurological eye disorders
46	02	Med	Other disorders of the eye age > 17 w CC
47	02	Med	Other disorders of the eye age > 17 w/o CC
48	02	Med	*Other disorders of the eye age 0–17
49	03	Surg	Major head and neck procedures
50	03	Surg	Sialoadenectomy
51	03	Surg	Salivary gland procedures except sialoadenectomy
52	03	Surg	Cleft lip and palate repair
53	03	Surg	Sinus and mastoid procedures age > 17
54	03	Surg	*Sinus and mastoid procedures age 0–17
55	03	Surg	Miscellaneous ear, nose, mouth and throat procedures
56	03	Surg	Rhinoplasty
57	03	Surg	T and A proc, except tonsillectomy and/or adenoidectomy only, age > 17
58	03	Surg	*T and A proc, except tonsillectomy and/or adenoidectomy only, age 0–17
59	03	Surg	Tonsillectomy and/or adenoidectomy only, age > 17
60	03	Surg	*Tonsillectomy and/or adenoidectomy only, age 0-17
61	03	Surg	Myringotomy w tube insertion age > 17
62	03	Surg	*Myringotomy w tube insertion age 0–17
63	03	Surg	Other ear, nose, mouth and throat O.R. procedures
64	03	Med	Ear, nose, mouth and throat malignancy
65	03	Med	Dysequilibrium
66	03	Med	Epistaxis
67	03	Med	Epiglottitis
68	03	Med	Otitis media and uri age > 17 w CC
69	03	Med	Otitis media and uri age > 17 w/o CC
70	03	Med	Otitis media and uri age 0–17
71	03	Med	Laryngotracheitis
72	03	Med	Nasal trauma and deformity
73	03	Med	Other ear, nose, mouth and throat diagnoses age > 17
74	03	Med	*Other ear, nose, mouth and throat diagnoses age 0–17
75	04	Surg	Major chest procedures
76	04	Surg	Other resp system O.R. procedures w CC
77	04	Surg	Other resp system O.R. procedures w/o CC
78	04	Med	Pulmonary embolism
79	04	Med	Respiratory infections and inflammations age > 17 w CC
80	04	Med	Respiratory infections and inflammations age > 17 w/o CC
81	04	Med	*Respiratory infections and inflammations age 0–17
82	04	Med	Respiratory neoplasms
83	04	Med	Major chest trauma w CC
84	04	Med	Major chest trauma w/o CC
85	04	Med	Pleural effusion w CC

DRG	MDC	Type	Description
86	04	Med	Pleural effusion w/o CC
87	04	Med	Pulmonary edema and respiratory failure
88	04	Med	Chronic obstructive pulmonary disease
89	04	Med	Simple pneumonia and pleurisy age >17 w CC
90	04	Med	Simple pneumonia and pleurisy age >17 w/o CC
91	04	Med	Simple pneumonia and pleurisy age 0–17
92	04	Med	Interstitial lung disease w CC
93	04	Med	Interstitial lung disease w/o CC
94	04	Med	Pneumothorax w CC
95	04	Med	Pneumothorax w/o CC
96	04	Med	Bronchitis and asthma age >17 w CC
97	04	Med	Bronchitis and asthma age >17 w/o CC
98	04	Med	Bronchitis and asthma age 0–17
99	04	Med	Respiratory signs and symptoms w CC
100	04	Med	Respiratory signs and symptoms w/o CC
101	04	Med	Other respiratory system diagnoses w CC
102	04	Med	Other respiratory system diagnoses w/o CC
103	05	Surg	Heart transplant
104	05	Surg	Cardiac valve and other major cardiothoracic proc w cardiac cath
105	05	Surg	Cardiac valve and other major cardiothoracic proc w/o cardiac cath
106	05	Surg	Coronary bypass w PTCA
107	05	Surg	Coronary bypass w cardiac cath
108	05	Surg	Other cardiothoracic procedures
109	05	Surg	Coronary bypass w/o PTCA or cardiac cath
110	05	Surg	Major cardiovascular procedures w CC
111	05	Surg	Major cardiovascular procedures w/o CC
112	05	Surg	Percutaneous cardiovascular procedures
113	05	Surg	Amputation for circ system disorders except upper limb and toe
114	05	Surg	Upper limb and toe amputation for circ system disorders
115	05	Surg	Perm card pacem impl w AMI, HRT fail or SHK, or AICD lead or GNR
116	05	Surg	Oth perm card pacemak impl or PTCA w coronary artery stent IM
117	05	Surg	Cardiac pacemaker revision except device replacement
118	05	Surg	Cardiac pacemaker device replacement
119	05	Surg	Vein ligation and stripping
120	05	Surg	Other circulatory system O.R. procedures
121	05	Med	Circulatory disorders w AMI and major comp, discharged alive
122	05	Med	Circulatory disorders w AMI w/o major comp, discharged alive
123	05	Med	Circulatory disorders w AMI, expired
124	05	Med	Circulatory disorders except AMI, w card cath and complex diag
125	05	Med	Circulatory disorders except AMI, w card cath w/o complex diag
126	05	Med	Acute and subacute endocarditis
127	05	Med	Heart failure and shock
128	05	Med	Deep vein thrombophlebitis
129	05	Med	Cardiac arrest, unexplained
130	05	Med	Peripheral vascular disorders w CC
131	05	Med	Peripheral vascular disorders w/o CC
132	05	Med	Atherosclerosis w CC
133	05	Med	Atherosclerosis w/o CC
134	05	Med	Hypertension
135	05	Med	Cardiac congenital and valvular disorders age >17 w CC
136	05	Med	Cardiac congenital and valvular disorders age >17 w/o CC
137	05	Med	*Cardiac congenital and valvular disorders age 0–17
138	05	Med	Cardiac arrhythmia and conduction disorders w CC
139	05	Med	Cardiac arrhythmia and conduction disorders w/o CC
140	05	Med	Angina pectoris
141	05	Med	Syncope and collapse w CC
142	05	Med	Syncope and collapse w/o CC
143	05	Med	Chest pain
144	05	Med	Other circulatory system diagnoses w CC
145	05	Med	Other circulatory system diagnoses w/o CC
146	06	Surg	Rectal resection w CC
147	06	Surg	Rectal resection w/o CC
148	06	Surg	Major small and large bowel procedures w CC

(continued)

DRG	MDC	Type	Description
149	06	Surg	Major small and large bowel procedures w/o CC
150	06	Surg	Peritoneal adhesiolysis w CC
151	06	Surg	Peritoneal adhesiolysis w/o CC
152	06	Surg	Minor small and large bowel procedures w CC
153	06	Surg	Minor small and large bowel procedures w/o CC
154	06	Surg	Stomach, esophageal and duodenal procedures age >17 w CC
155	06	Surg	Stomach, esophageal and duodenal procedures age >17 w/o CC
156	06	Surg	*Stomach, esophageal and duodenal procedures age 0–17
157	06	Surg	Anal and stomal procedures w CC
158	06	Surg	Anal and stomal procedures w/o CC
159	06	Surg	Hernia procedures except inguinal and femoral age >17 w CC
160	06	Surg	Hernia procedures except inguinal and femoral age >17 w/o CC
161	06	Surg	Inguinal and femoral hernia procedures age >17 w CC
162	06	Surg	Inguinal and femoral hernia procedures age >17 w/o CC
163	06	Surg	*Hernia procedures age 0–17
164	06	Surg	Appendectomy w complicated principal diag w CC
165	06	Surg	Appendectomy w complicated principal diag w/o CC
166	06	Surg	Appendectomy w/o complicated principal diag w CC
167	06	Surg	Appendectomy w/o complicated principal diag w/o CC
168	03	Surg	Mouth procedures w CC
169	03	Surg	Mouth procedures w/o CC
170	06	Surg	Other digestive system O.R. procedures w CC
171	06	Surg	Other digestive system O.R. procedures w/o CC
172	06	Med	Digestive malignancy w CC
173	06	Med	Digestive malignancy w/o CC
174	06	Med	G.I. hemorrhage w CC
175	06	Med	G.I. hemorrhage w/o CC
176	06	Med	Complicated peptic ulcer
177	06	Med	Uncomplicated peptic ulcer w CC
178	06	Med	Uncomplicated peptic ulcer w/o CC
179	06	Med	Inflammatory bowel disease
180	06	Med	G.I. obstruction w CC
181	06	Med	G.I. obstruction w/o CC
182	06	Med	Esophagitis, gastroent and misc digest disorders age >17 w CC
183	06	Med	Esophagitis, gastroent and misc digest disorders age >17 w/o CC
184	06	Med	Esophagitis, gastroent and misc digest disorders age 0–17
185	03	Med	Dental and oral DIS except extractions and restorations, age >17
186	03	Med	Dental and oral DIS except extractions and restorations, age 0–17
187	03	Med	Dental extraction and restorations
188	06	Med	Other digestive system diagnoses age >17 w CC
189	06	Med	Other digestive system diagnoses age >17 w/o CC
190	06	Med	Other digestive system diagnoses age 0–17
191	07	Surg	Pancreas, liver and shunt procedures w CC
192	07	Surg	Pancreas, liver and shunt procedures w/o CC
193	07	Surg	Biliary tract proc except only cholecyst w or w/o C.D.E. w CC
194	07	Surg	Biliary tract proc except only cholecyst w or w/o C.D.E w/o CC
195	07	Surg	Cholecystectomy w C.D.E w CC
196	07	Surg	Cholecystectomy w C.D.E w/o CC
197	07	Surg	Cholecystectomy except by laparoscope w/o C.D.E. w CC
198	07	Surg	Cholecystectomy except by laparoscope w/o C.D.E w/o CC
199	07	Surg	Hepatobiliary diagnostic procedure for malignancy
200	07	Surg	Hepatobiliary diagnostic procedure for non-malignancy
201	07	Surg	Other hepatobiliary or pancreas O.R. procedures
202	07	Med	Cirrhosis and alcoholic hepatitis
203	07	Med	Malignancy of hepatobiliary system or pancreas
204	07	Med	Disorders of pancreas except malignancy
205	07	Med	Disorders of liver except malig, cirr, alc hepa w CC
206	07	Med	Disorders of liver except malig, cirr, alc hepa w/o CC
207	07	Med	Disorders of the biliary tract w CC
208	07	Med	Disorders of the biliary tract w/o CC
209	08	Surg	Major joint and limb reattachment procedures of lower extremity
210	08	Surg	Hip and femur procedures except major joint age >17 w CC
211	08	Surg	Hip and femur procedures except major joint age >17 w/o CC
212	08	Surg	*Hip and femur procedures except major joint age 0–17
213	08	Surg	Amputation for musculoskeletal system and conn tissue disorders

DRG	MDC	Type	Description
214	08	Surg	No longer valid
215	08	Surg	No longer valid
216	08	Surg	Biopsies of musculoskeletal system and connective tissue
217	08	Surg	Wnd debrid and skn grft except hand, for muscskelet and conn tiss disorders
218	08	Surg	Lower extrem and humer proc except hip, foot, femur age >17 w CC
219	08	Surg	Lower extrem and humer proc except hip, foot, femur age >17 w/o CC
220	08	Surg	*Lower extrem and humer proc except hip, foot, femur age 0–17
221	08	Surg	No longer valid
222	08	Surg	No longer valid
223	08	Surg	Major shoulder/elbow proc, or other upper extremity proc, w/o CC
224	08	Surg	Shoulder, elbow or forearm proc, exc major joint proc, w/o CC
225	08	Surg	Foot procedures
226	08	Surg	Soft tissue procedures w CC
227	08	Surg	Soft tissue procedures w/o CC
228	08	Surg	Major thumb or joint proc, or oth hand or wrist proc w CC
229	08	Surg	Hand or wrist proc, except major joint proc, w/o CC
230	08	Surg	Local excision and removal of int fix devices of hip and femur
231	08	Surg	Local excision and removal of int fix devices except hip and femur
232	08	Surg	Arthroscopy
233	08	Surg	Other musculoskelet sys and conn tiss O.R. proc w CC
234	08	Surg	Other musculoskelet sys and conn tiss O.R. proc w/o CC
235	08	Med	Fractures of femur
236	08	Med	Fractures of hip and pelvis
237	08	Med	Sprains, strains, and dislocations of hip, pelvis and thigh
238	08	Med	Osteomyelitis
239	08	Med	Pathological fractures and musculoskeletal and conn tissmalignancy
240	08	Med	Connective tissue disorders w CC
241	08	Med	Connective tissue disorders w/o CC
242	08	Med	Septic arthritis
243	08	Med	Medical back problems
244	08	Med	Bone diseases and specific arthropathies w CC
245	08	Med	Bone diseases and specific arthropathies w/o CC
246	08	Med	Non-specific arthropathies
247	08	Med	Signs and symptoms of musculoskeletal system and conn tissue
248	08	Med	Tendonitis, myositis and bursitis
249	08	Med	Aftercare, musculoskeletal system and connective tissue
250	08	Med	Fx, sprn, strn and disl of forearm, hand, foot age >17 w CC
251	08	Med	Fx, sprn, strn and disl of forearm, hand, foot age >17 w/o CC
252	08	Med	*Fx, sprn, strn and disl of forearm, hand, foot age 0–17
253	08	Med	Fx, sprn, strn and disl of uparm, lowleg ex foot age >17 w CC
254	08	Med	Fx, sprn, strn and disl of uparm, lowleg ex foot age >17 w/o CC
255	08	Med	*Fx, sprn, strn and disl of uparm, lowleg ex foot age 0–17
256	08	Med	Other musculoskeletal system and connective tissue diagnoses
257	09	Surg	Total mastectomy for malignancy w CC
258	09	Surg	Total mastectomy for malignancy w/o CC
259	09	Surg	Subtotal mastectomy for malignancy w CC
260	09	Surg	Subtotal mastectomy for malignancy w/o CC
261	09	Surg	Breast proc for non-malignancy except biopsy and local excision
262	09	Surg	Breast biopsy and local excision for non-malignancy
263	09	Surg	Skin graft and/or debrid for skin ulcer or cellulitis w CC
264	09	Surg	Skin graft and/or debrid for skin ulcer or cellulitis w/o CC
265	09	Surg	Skin graft and/or debrid except for skin ulcer or cellulitis w CC
266	09	Surg	Skin graft and/or debrid except for skin ulcer or cellulitis w/o CC
267	09	Surg	Perianal and pilonidal procedures
268	09	Surg	Skin, subcutaneous tissue and breast plastic procedures
269	09	Surg	Other skin, subcut tiss and breast proc w CC
270	09	Surg	Other skin, subcut tiss and breast proc w/o CC
271	09	Med	Skin ulcers
272	09	Med	Major skin disorders w CC
273	09	Med	Major skin disorders w/o CC
274	09	Med	Malignant breast disorders w CC
275	09	Med	Malignant breast disorders w/o CC
276	09	Med	Non-malignant breast disorders

(continued)

DRG	MDC	Type	Description
277	09	Med	Cellulitis age >17 w CC
278	09	Med	Cellulitis age >17 w/o CC
279	09	Med	Cellulitis age 0–17
280	09	Med	Trauma to the skin, subcut tiss and breast age >17 w CC
281	09	Med	Trauma to the skin, subcut tiss and breast age >17 w/o CC
282	09	Med	*Trauma to the skin, subcut tiss and breast age 0–17
283	09	Med	Minor skin disorders w CC
284	09	Med	Minor skin disorders w/o CC
285	10	Surg	Amputat of lower limb for endocrine, nutrit and metabol disorder
286	10	Surg	Adrenal and pituitary procedures
287	10	Surg	Skin grafts and wound debrid for endoc, nutrit and metabol disorder
288	10	Surg	O.R. Procedures for obesity
289	10	Surg	Parathyroid procedures
290	10	Surg	Throid procedures
291	10	Surg	Thyroglossal procedures
292	10	Surg	Other endocrine, nutrit and metab O.R. proc w CC
293	10	Surg	Other endocrine, nutrit and metab O.R. proc w/o CC
294	10	Med	Diabetes age >35
295	10	Med	Diabetes age 0–35
296	10	Med	Nutritional and misc metabolic disorders age >17 w CC
297	10	Med	Nutritional and misc metabolic disorders age >17 w/o CC
298	10	Med	Nutritional and misc metabolic disorders age 0–17
299	10	Med	Inborn errors of metabolism
300	10	Med	Endocrine disorders w CC
301	10	Med	Endocrine disorders w/o CC
302	11	Surg	Kidney transplant
303	11	Surg	Kidney, ureter and major bladder procedures for neoplasm
304	11	Surg	Kidney, ureter and major bladder proc for non-neopl w CC
305	11	Surg	Kidney, ureter and major bladder proc for non-neopl w/o CC
306	11	Surg	Prostatectomy w CC
307	11	Surg	Prostatectomy w/o CC
308	11	Surg	Minor bladder procedures w CC
309	11	Surg	Minor bladder procedures w/o CC
310	11	Surg	Transurethral procedures w CC
311	11	Surg	Transurethral procedures w/o CC
312	11	Surg	Uretheral procedures, age >17 w CC
313	11	Surg	Uretheral procedures, age >17 w/o CC
314	11	Surg	*Uretheral procedures, age 0–17
315	11	Surg	Other kidney and urinary tract O.R. procedures
316	11	Med	Renal failure
317	11	Med	Admit for renal dialysis
318	11	Med	Kidney and urinary tract neoplasms w CC
319	11	Med	Kidney and urinary tract neoplasms w/o CC
320	11	Med	Kidney and urinary tract infections age >17 w CC
321	11	Med	Kidney and urinary tract infections age >17 w/o CC
322	11	Med	Kidney and urinary tract infections age 0–17
323	11	Med	Urinary stones w CC, and/or ESW lithotripsy
324	11	Med	Urinary stones w/o CC
325	11	Med	Kidney and urinary tract signs and symptoms age >17 w CC
326	11	Med	Kidney and urinary tract signs and symptoms age >17 w/o CC
327	11	Med	*Kidney and urinary tract signs and symptoms age 0–17
328	11	Med	Uretheral stricture age >17 w CC
329	11	Med	Uretheral stricture age >17 w/o CC
330	11	Med	*Uretheral stricture age 0–17
331	11	Med	Other kidney and urinary tract diagnoses age >17 w CC
332	11	Med	Other kidney and urinary tract diagnoses age >17 w/o CC
333	11	Med	Other kidney and urinary tract diagnoses age 0–17
334	12	Surg	Major male pelvic procedures w CC
335	12	Surg	Major male pelvic procedures w/o CC
336	12	Surg	Transurethral prostatectomy w CC
337	12	Surg	Transurethral prostatectomy w/o CC
338	12	Surg	Testes procedures, for malignancy
339	12	Surg	Testes procedures, non-malignancy age >17
340	12	Surg	*Testes procedures, non-malignancy age 0–17
341	12	Surg	Penis procedures

DRG	MDC	Type	Description
342	12	Surg	Circumcisioin age > 17
343	12	Surg	*Circumcisiion age 0–17
344	12	Surg	Other male reproductive system O.R. procedures for malignancy
345	12	Surg	Other male reproductive system O.R. proc except for malignancy
346	12	Med	Malignancy, male reproductive system, w CC
347	12	Med	Malignancy, male reproductive system, w/o CC
348	12	Med	Benign prostatic hypertrophy w CC
349	12	Med	Benign prostatic hypertrophy w/o CC
350	12	Med	Inflammation of the male reproductive system
351	12	Med	*Sterilization, male
352	12	Med	Other male reproductive system diagnoses
353	13	Surg	Pelvic evisceration, radical hysterectomy and radical vulvectomy
354	13	Surg	Uterine, adnexa proc for non-ovarian/adnexal malig w CC
355	13	Surg	Uterine, adnexa proc for non-ovarian/adnexal malig w/o CC
356	13	Surg	Female reproductive system reconstructive procedures
357	13	Surg	Uterine and adnexa proc for ovarian or adnexal malignancy
358	13	Surg	Uterine and adnexa proc for non-malignancy w CC
359	13	Surg	Uterine and adnexa proc for non-malignancy w/o CC
360	13	Surg	Vagina, cervix and vulva procedures
361	13	Surg	Laparoscopy and incisional tubal interruption
362	13	Surg	*Endoscopic tubal interruption
363	13	Surg	D and C, conization and radio-implant, for malignancy
364	13	Surg	D and C, conization except for malignancy
365	13	Surg	Other female reproductive system O.R. procedures
366	13	Med	Malignancy, female reproductive system w CC
367	13	Med	Malignancy, female reproductive system w/o CC
368	13	Med	Infections, female reproductive system
369	13	Med	Menstrual and other female reproductive system disorders
370	14	Surg	Cesarean section w CC
371	14	Surg	Cesarean section w/o CC
372	14	Med	Vaginal delivery w complicating diagnoses
373	14	Med	Vaginal delivery w/o complicating diagnoses
374	14	Surg	Vaginal delivery w sterilization and/or D and C
375	14	Surg	*Vaginal delivery w O.R. proc except steril and/or D and C
376	14	Med	Postpartum and post abortion diagnoses w/o O.R. procedure
377	14	Surg	Postpartum and post abortion diagnoses w O.R. procedure
378	14	Med	Ectopic pregnancy
379	14	Med	Threatened abortion
380	14	Med	Abortion w/o D and C
381	14	Surg	Abortion w D and C, aspiration curettage or hysterotomy
382	14	Med	False labor
383	14	Med	Other antepartum diagnoses w medical complications
384	14	Med	Other antepartum diagnoses w/o medical complications
385	15	Med*	Neonates, died or transferred to another acute care facility
386	15	Med*	Extreme immaturity or respiratory distress syndrome neonate
387	15	Med*	Prematurity w major problems
388	15	Med*	Prematurity w/o major problems
389	15	Med*	Full term neonate w major problems
390	15	Med*	Neonate w other significant problems
391	15	Med*	Normal newborn
392	16	Surg	Splenectomy age > 17
393	16	Surg	*Splenectomy age 0–17
394	16	Surg	Other O.R procedures of the blood and blood forming organs
395	16	Med	Red blood cell disorders age > 17
396	16	Med	Red blood cell disorders age 0–17
397	16	Med	Coagulation disorders
398	16	Med	Reticuloendothelial and immunity disorders w CC
399	16	Med	Reticuloendothelial and immunity disorders w/o CC
400	17	Surg	Lymphoma and leukemia w major O.R. procedure
401	17	Surg	Lymphoma and non-acute leukemia w other O.R. proc w CC
402	17	Surg	Lymphoma and non-acute leukemia w other O.R. proc w/o CC
403	17	Med	Lymphoma and non-acute leukemia w CC
404	17	Med	Lymphoma and non-acute leukemia w/o CC

(continued)

DRG	MDC	Type	Description
405	17	*	Acute leukemia w/o major O.R. procedure age 0–17
406	17	Surg	Myeloprolif disord or poorly diff neopl w maj O.R. proc w CC
407	17	Surg	Myeloprolif disord or poorly diff neopl w maj O.R. proc w/o CC
408	17	Surg	Myeloprolif disord or poorly diff neopl w other O.R. proc
409	17	Med	Radiotherapy
410	17	Med	Chemotherapy w/o acute leukemia as secondary diagnosis
411	17	Med	History of malignancy w/o endoscopy
412	17	Med	History of malignancy w endoscopy
413	17	Med	Other myeloprolif dis or poorly diff neopl diag w CC
414	17	Med	Other myeloprolif dis or poorly diff neopl diag w/o CC
415	18	Surg	O.R. procedure for infectious and parasitic diseases
416	18	Med	Septicemia age >17
417	18	Med	Septicemia age 0–17
418	18	Med	Postoperative and post–traumatic infections
419	18	Med	Fever of unknown origin age >17 w CC
420	18	Med	Fever of unknown origin age >17 w/o CC
421	18	Med	Viral illness age >17
422	18	Med	Viral illness and fever of unknown origin age 0–17
423	18	Med	Other infectious and parasitic diseases diagnoses
424	19	Surg	O.R. procedure w principal diagnoses of mental illness
425	19	Med	Acute adjustment reaction and psychological dysfunction
426	19	Med	Depressive neuroses
427	19	Med	Neuroses except depressive
428	19	Med	Disorders of personality and impulse control
429	19	Med	Organic disturbances and mental retardation
430	19	Med	Psychoses
431	19	Med	Childhood mental disorders
432	19	Med	Other mental disorder diagnoses
433	20		Alcohol/drug abuse or dependence, left ama
434	20		No longer valid
435	20		No longer valid
436	20		No longer valid
437	20		No longer valid
438			No longer valid
439	21	Surg	Skin grafts for injuries
440	21	Surg	Wound debridements for injuries
441	21	Surg	Hand procedures for injuries
442	21	Surg	Other O.R. procedures for injuries w CC
443	21	Surg	Other O.R. procedures for injuries w/o CC
444	21	Med	Traumatic injury age >17 w CC
445	21	Med	Traumatic injury age >17 w/o CC
446	21	Med	*Traumatic injury age 0–17
447	21	Med	Allergic reaction age >17
448	21	Med	*Allergic reaction age 0–17
449	21	Med	Poisoning and toxic effects of drugs age >17 w CC
450	21	Med	Poisoning and toxic effects of drugs age >17 w/o CC
451	21	Med	*Poisoning and toxic effects of drugs age 0–17
452	21	Med	Complications of treatment w CC
453	21	Med	Complications of treatment w/o CC
454	21	Med	Other injury, poisoning and toxic effect diag w CC
455	21	Med	Other injury, poisoning and toxic effect diag w/o CC
456			No longer valid
457			No longer valid
458			No longer valid
459			No longer valid
460			No longer valid
461	23	Surg	O.R. proc w diagnoses of other contact w health services
462	23	Med	Rehabilitation
463	23	Med	Signs and symptoms w CC
464	23	Med	Signs and symptoms w/o CC
465	23	Med	Aftercare w history of malignancy as secondary diagnosis
466	23	Med	Aftercare w/o history of malignancy as secondary diagnosis
467	23	Med	Other factors influencing health status
468			Extensive O.R. procedure unrelated to principal diagnosis

DRG	MDC	Type	Description
469		‡	Principal diagnosis invalid as discharge diagnosis
470		‡	Ungroupable
471	08	Surg	Bilateral or multiple major joint procs of lower extremity
472			No longer valid
473	17		Acute leukemia w/o major O.R. procedure age >17
474			No longer valid
475	04	Med	Respiratory system diagnosis with ventilator support
476		Surg	Prostatic O.R. procedure unrelated to principal diagnosis
477		Surg	Non-extensive O.R. procedure unrelated to principal diagnosis
478	05	Surg	Other vascular procedures w CC
479	05	Surg	Other vascular procedures w/o CC
480		Surg	Liver transplant
481		Surg	Bone marrow transplant
482		Surg	Trancheostomy for face, mouth and neck diagnoses
483		Surg	Trancheostomy except for face, mouth and neck diagnoses
484	24	Surg	Craniotomy for multiple significant trauma
485	24	Surg	Limb reattachment, hip and femur proc for multiple significant trauma
486	24	Surg	Other O.R. procedures for multiple significant trauma
487	24	Med	Other multiple significant trauma
488	25	Surg	HIV w extensive O.R. procedure
489	25	Med	HIV w major related condition
490	25	Med	HIV w or w/o other related condition
491	08	Surg	Major joint and limb reattachment procedures of upper extremity
492	17	Med	Chemotherapy w acute leukemia as secondary diagnosis
493	07	Surg	Laparoscopic cholecystectomy w/o C.D.E. w CC
494	07	Surg	Laparoscopic cholecystectomy w/o C.D.E. w/o CC
495		Surg	Lung transplant
496	08	Surg	Combined anterior/posterior spinal fusion
497	08	Surg	Spinal fusion w CC
498	08	Surg	Spinal fusion w/o CC
499	08	Surg	Back and neck procedures except spinal fusion w CC
500	08	Surg	Back and neck procedures except spinal fusion w/o CC
501	08	Surg	Knee procedures w pdx of infection w CC
502	08	Surg	Knee procedures w pdx of infection w/o CC
503	08	Surg	Knee procedures w/o pdx of infection
504	22	Surg	Extensive 3rd degree burns w skin graft
505	22		Extensive 3rd degree burns w/o skin graft
506	22		Full thickness burn w skin graft or inhal inj w CC or sig trauma
507	22		Full thickness burn w skin graft or inhal inj w/o CC or sig trauma
508	22		Full thickness burn w/o skin graft or inhal inj w CC or sig trauma
509	22		Full thickness burn w/o skin grft or inhal inj w/o CC or sig trauma
510	22		Non-extensive burns w CC or significant trauma
511	22		Non-extensive burns w/o CC or significant trauma
512	Pre	Surg	Simultaneous pancreas/kidney transplant
513	Pre	Surg	Pancreas transplant
514	05	Surg	Cardiac defibrillator implant w cardiac cath
515	05	Surg	Cardiac defibrillator implant w/o cardiac cath
516	05	Surg	Percutaneous cardiovascular proc w AMI
517	05	Surg	Perc cardio proc w non-drug eluting stent w/o AMI
518	05	Surg	Perc cardio proc w/o coronary artery stent or AMI
519	08	Surg	Cervical spinal fusion w CC
520	08	Surg	Cervical spinal fusion w/o CC
521	20	Med	Alcohol/drug abuse or dependence w CC
522	20	Med	Alc/drug abuse or depend w rehabilitation therapy w/o CC
523	20	Med	Alc/drug abuse or depend w/o rehabilitation therapy w/o CC
524	01	Med	Transient ischemia
525	05	Surg	Heart assist system implant
526	05	Surg	Percutaneous cardiovascular proc w drug eluting stent w AMI
527	05	Surg	Percutaneous cardiovascular proc w drug eluting stent w/o AMI

‡DRGs 469 and 470 contain cases which could not be assigned to valid DRGs.

Section 2: Assessment

2-1. CLINICAL GROWTH CHARTS FOR CHILDREN AND ADOLESCENTS

Birth to 36 months: Boys
Length-for-age and Weight-for-age percentiles

NAME _____

RECORD # _____

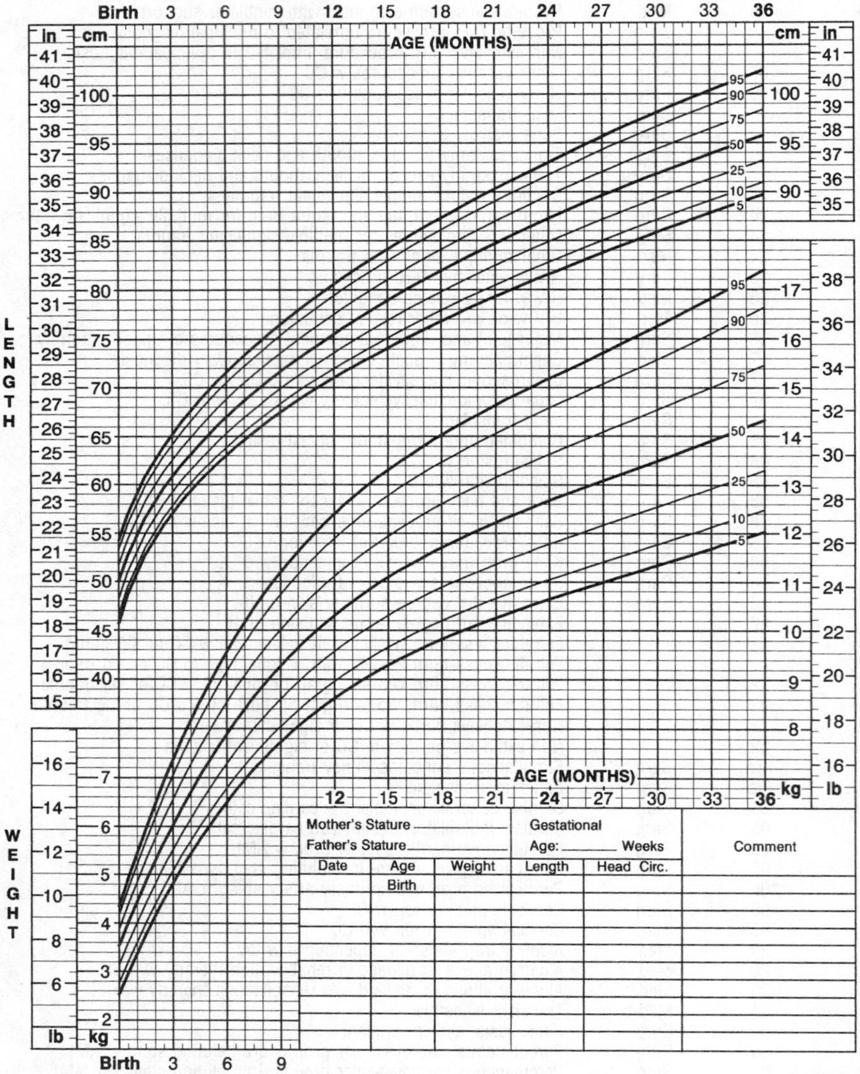

AGE (MONTHS)

Date	Age	Weight	Length	Head Circ.	Comment
Birth					

Mother's Stature _____
Father's Stature _____
Gestational Age: _____ Weeks

Published May 30, 2000 (modified 4/20/01).
SOURCE: Developed by the National Center for Health Statistics in collaboration with the National Center for Chronic Disease Prevention and Health Promotion (2000).
http://www.cdc.gov/growthcharts

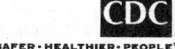

SAFER·HEALTHIER·PEOPLE™

Birth to 36 months: Boys
Head circumference-for-age and
Weight-for-length percentiles

NAME _____

RECORD # _____

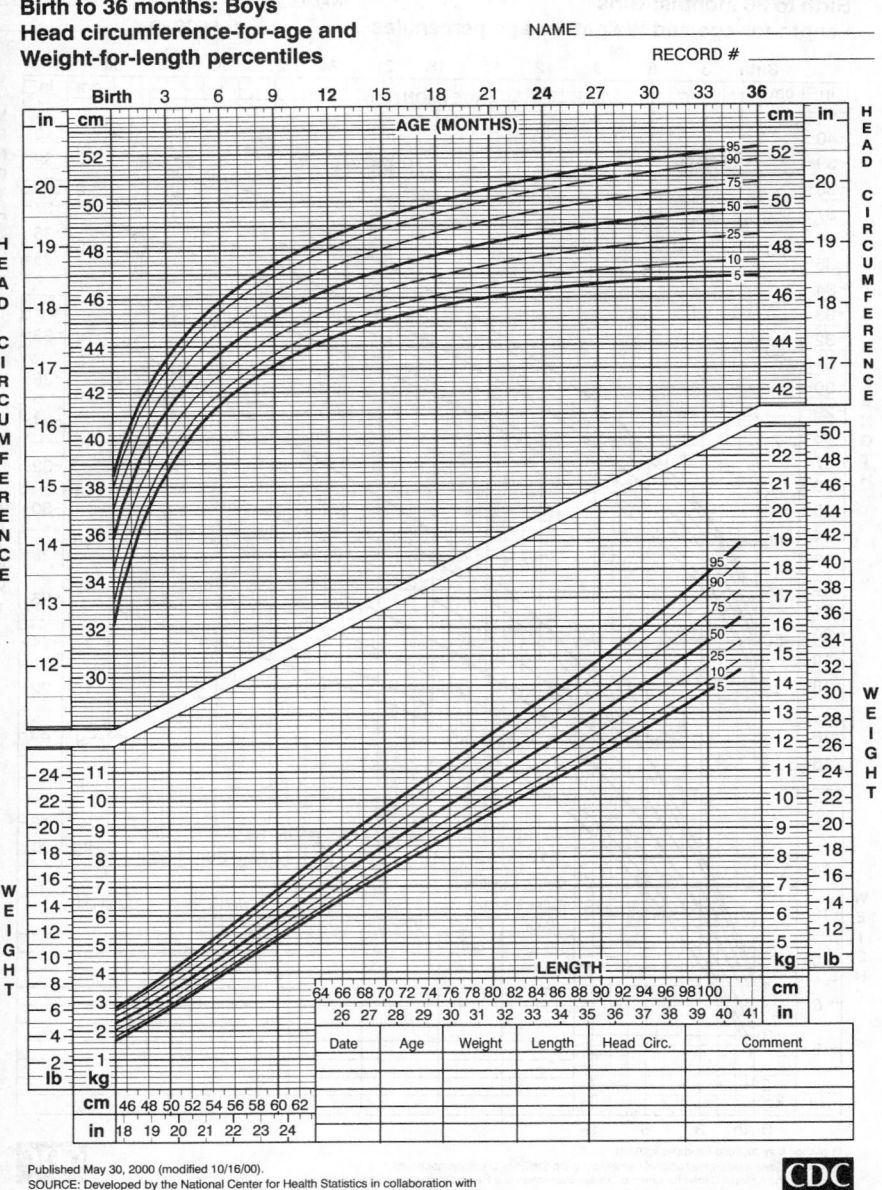

Published May 30, 2000 (modified 10/16/00).
SOURCE: Developed by the National Center for Health Statistics in collaboration with
the National Center for Chronic Disease Prevention and Health Promotion (2000).
http://www.cdc.gov/growthcharts

CDC
SAFER·HEALTHIER·PEOPLE™

Birth to 36 months: Girls
Length-for-age and Weight-for-age percentiles

NAME _____

RECORD # _____

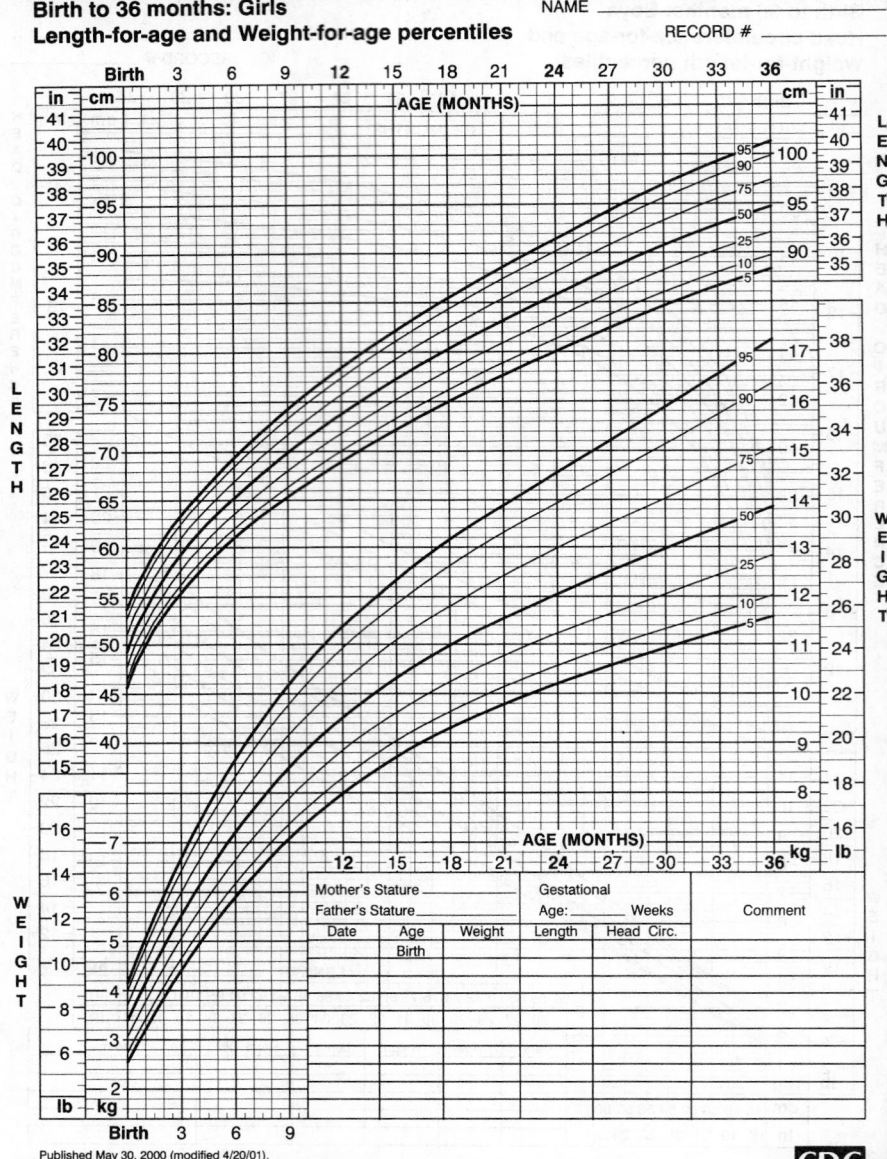

Published May 30, 2000 (modified 4/20/01).
SOURCE: Developed by the National Center for Health Statistics in collaboration with
the National Center for Chronic Disease Prevention and Health Promotion (2000).
http://www.cdc.gov/growthcharts

CDC

SAFER · HEALTHIER · PEOPLE™

Birth to 36 months: Girls
Head circumference-for-age and
Weight-for-length percentiles

NAME _____

RECORD # _____

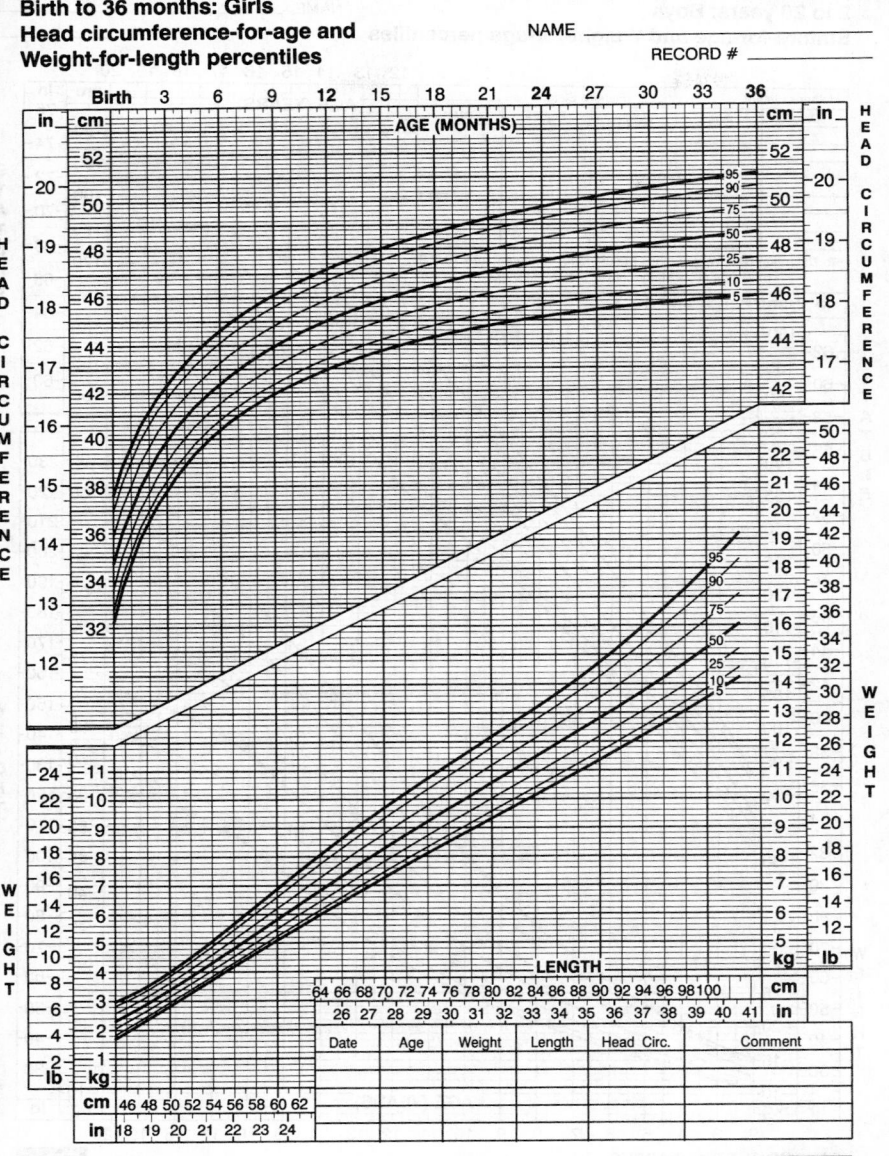

Published May 30, 2000 (modified 10/16/00).
SOURCE: Developed by the National Center for Health Statistics in collaboration with
the National Center for Chronic Disease Prevention and Health Promotion (2000).
http://www.cdc.gov/growthcharts

CDC

SAFER · HEALTHIER · PEOPLE™

2 to 20 years: Boys
Stature-for-age and Weight-for-age percentiles

NAME _____

RECORD # _____

*To Calculate BMI: Weight (kg) ÷ Stature (cm) ÷ Stature (cm) x 10,000
or Weight (lb) ÷ Stature (in) ÷ Stature (in) x 703

Date	Age	Weight	Stature	BMI*

Mother's Stature _____ Father's Stature _____

Published May 30, 2000 (modified 11/21/00).
SOURCE: Developed by the National Center for Health Statistics in collaboration with
the National Center for Chronic Disease Prevention and Health Promotion (2000).
http://www.cdc.gov/growthcharts

CDC
SAFER · HEALTHIER · PEOPLE™

2 to 20 years: Boys
Body mass index-for-age percentiles

NAME _____

RECORD # _____

Date	Age	Weight	Stature	BMI*	Comments

*To Calculate BMI: Weight (kg) ÷ Stature (cm) ÷ Stature (cm) x 10,000
or Weight (lb) ÷ Stature (in) ÷ Stature (in) x 703

BMI

35
34
33
32
31
30
29
28
27
26
25
24
23
22
21
20
19
18
17
16
15
14
13
12

95
90
85
75
50
25
10
5

AGE (YEARS)

kg/m²

2 3 4 5 6 7 8 9 10 11 12 13 14 15 16 17 18 19 20

SOURCE: Developed by the National Center for Health Statistics in collaboration with
the National Center for Chronic Disease Prevention and Health Promotion (2000).
http://www.cdc.gov/growthcharts

2 to 20 years: Girls
Stature-for-age and Weight-for-age percentiles

NAME _____

RECORD # _____

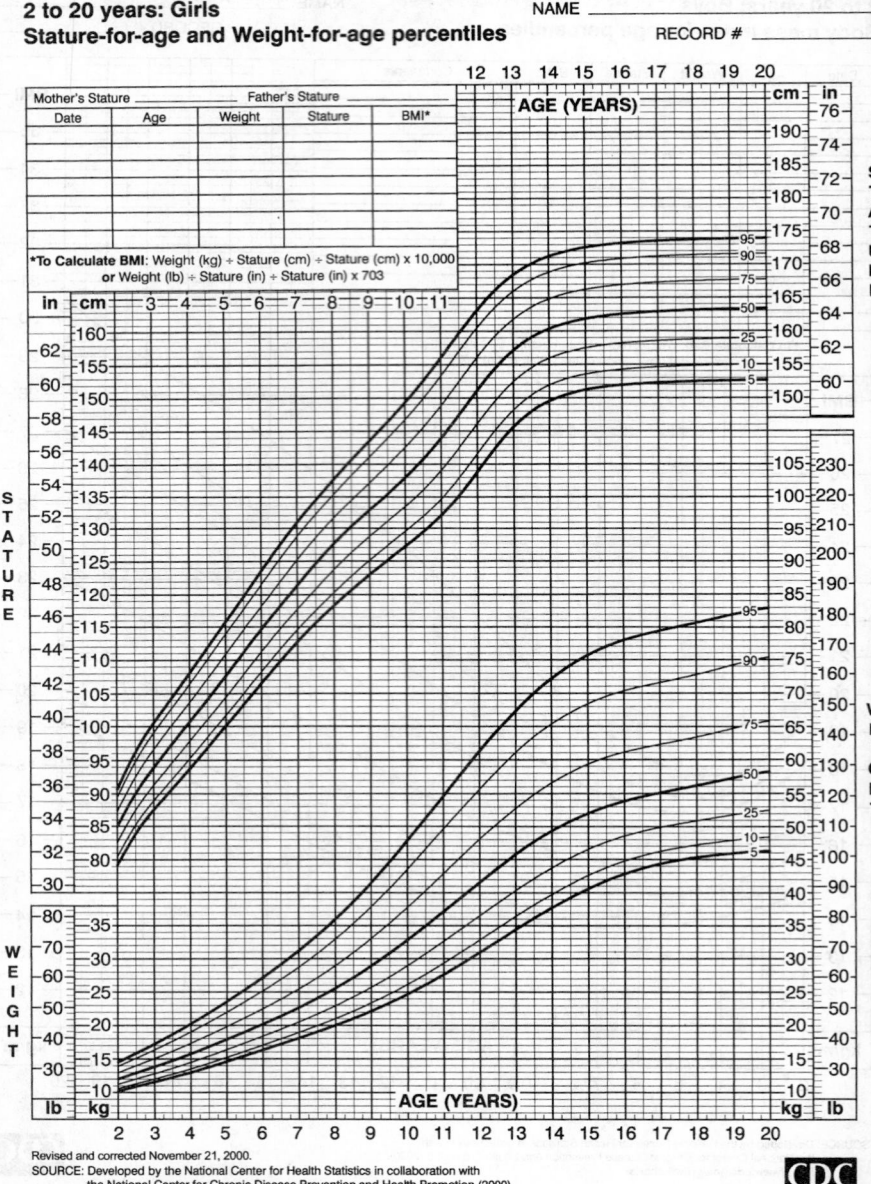

Revised and corrected November 21, 2000.
SOURCE: Developed by the National Center for Health Statistics in collaboration with
the National Center for Chronic Disease Prevention and Health Promotion (2000).
http://www.cdc.gov/growthcharts

CDC

2 to 20 years: Girls
Body mass index-for-age percentiles

NAME _____

RECORD # _____

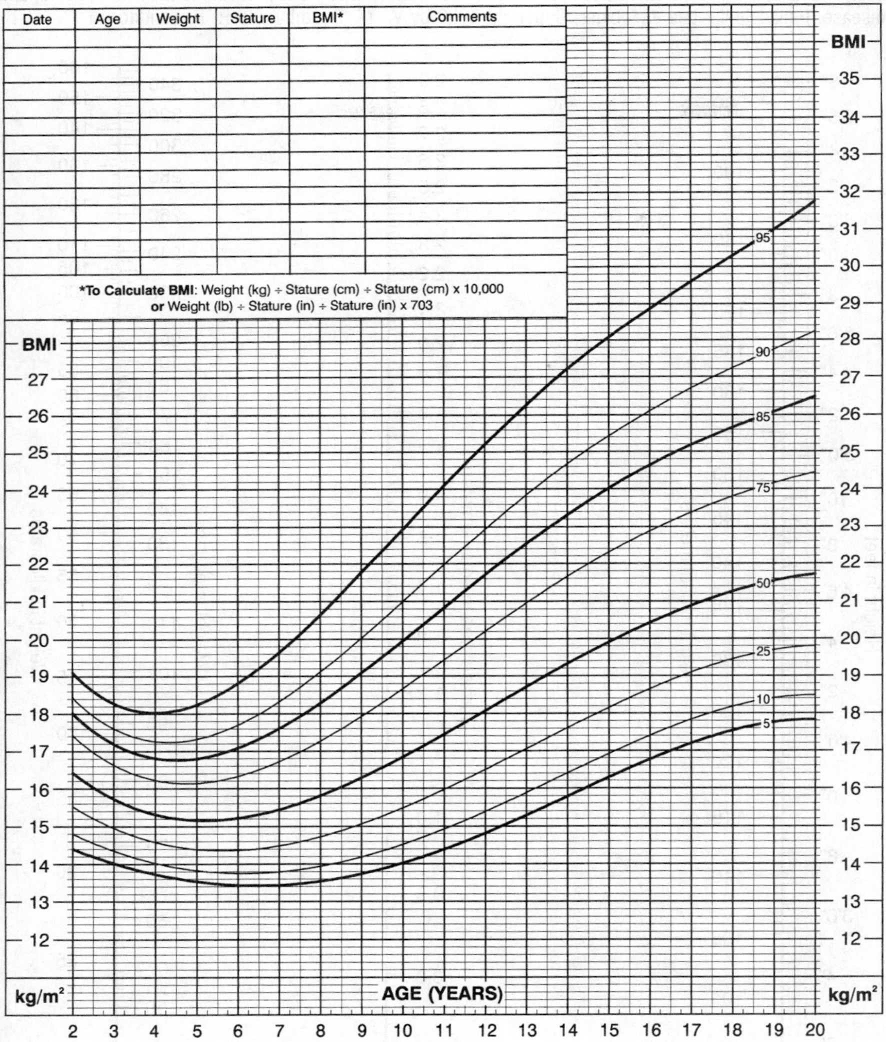

Date	Age	Weight	Stature	BMI*	Comments

*To Calculate BMI: Weight (kg) ÷ Stature (cm) ÷ Stature (cm) x 10,000
or Weight (lb) ÷ Stature (in) ÷ Stature (in) x 703

BMI — 35 — 34 — 33 — 32 — 31 — 30 — 29 — 28 — 27 — 26 — 25 — 24 — 23 — 22 — 21 — 20 — 19 — 18 — 17 — 16 — 15 — 14 — 13 — 12

95 90 85 75 50 25 10 5

AGE (YEARS)

kg/m²

2 3 4 5 6 7 8 9 10 11 12 13 14 15 16 17 18 19 20

SOURCE: Developed by the National Center for Health Statistics in collaboration with
the National Center for Chronic Disease Prevention and Health Promotion (2000).
http://www.cdc.gov/growthcharts

CDC

To find the body surface area, locate the height in inches (or centimeters) on scale I and the weight in pounds (or kilograms) on scale III. A straight-edged ruler placed between those two points will intersect scale II and determine the client's surface area. (From DuBois, E.F. [1936]. Basal metabolism in health and disease. Philadelphia: Lea & Febiger. Copyright 1920 by W. M. Boothby and R. B. Sandiford.)

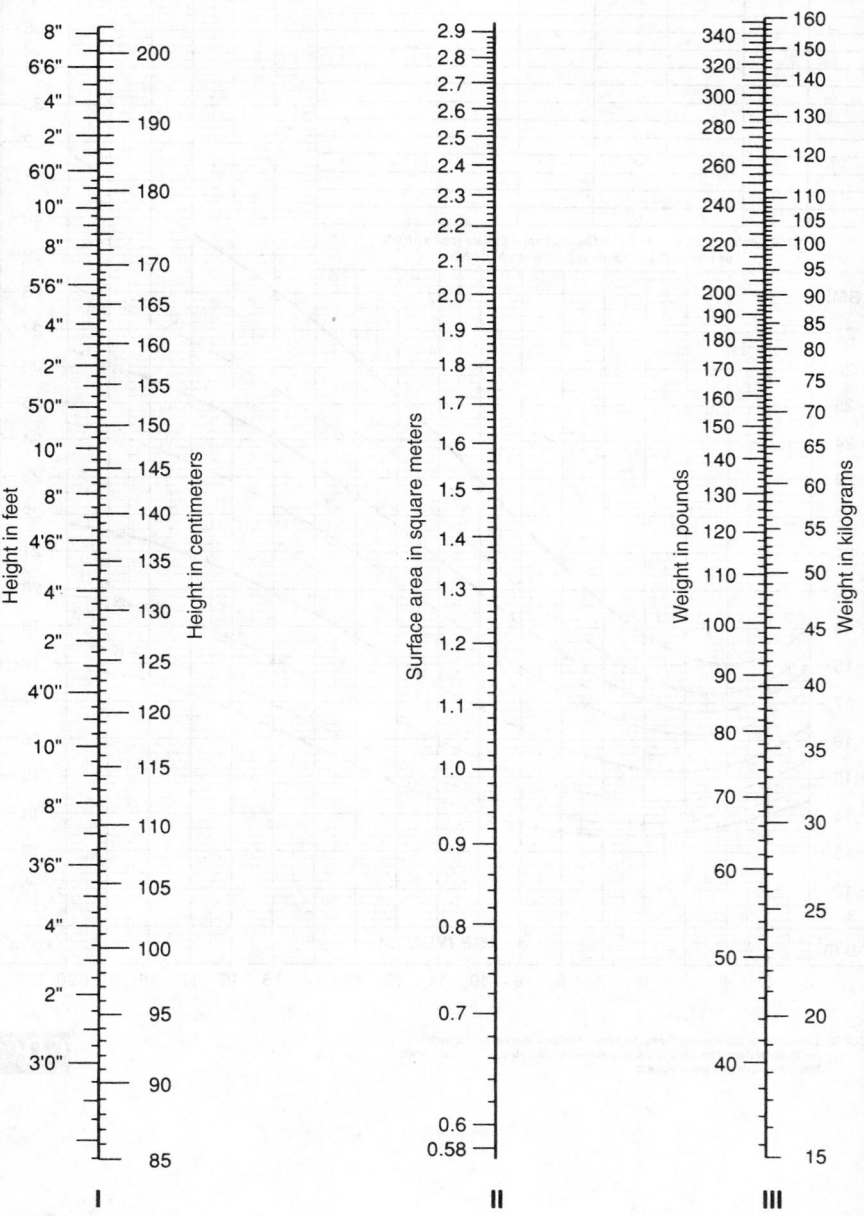

2-3. BODY MASS INDEX TABLE

BMI	Normal						Overweight					Obese										Extremely Obese														
	19	20	21	22	23	24	25	26	27	28	29	30	31	32	33	34	35	36	37	38	39	40	41	42	43	44	45	46	47	48	49	50	51	52	53	54
Height (inches)												Body Weight (pounds)																								
58	91	96	100	105	110	115	119	124	129	134	138	143	148	153	158	162	167	172	177	181	186	191	196	201	205	210	215	220	224	229	234	239	244	248	253	258
59	94	99	104	109	114	119	124	128	133	138	143	148	153	158	163	168	173	178	183	188	193	198	203	208	212	217	222	227	232	237	242	247	252	257	262	267
60	97	102	107	112	118	123	128	133	138	143	148	153	158	163	168	174	179	184	189	194	199	204	209	215	220	225	230	235	240	245	250	255	261	266	271	276
61	100	106	111	116	122	127	132	137	143	148	153	158	164	169	174	180	185	190	195	201	206	211	217	222	227	232	238	243	248	254	259	264	269	275	280	285
62	104	109	115	120	126	131	136	142	147	153	158	164	169	175	180	186	191	196	202	207	213	218	224	229	235	240	246	251	256	262	267	273	278	284	289	295
63	107	113	118	124	130	135	141	146	152	158	163	169	175	180	186	191	197	203	208	214	220	225	231	237	242	248	254	259	265	270	278	282	287	293	299	304
64	110	116	122	128	134	140	145	151	157	163	169	174	180	186	192	197	204	209	215	221	227	232	238	244	250	256	262	267	273	279	285	291	296	302	308	314
65	114	120	126	132	138	144	150	156	162	168	174	180	186	192	198	204	210	216	222	228	234	240	246	252	258	264	270	276	282	288	294	300	306	312	318	324
66	118	124	130	136	142	148	155	161	167	173	179	186	192	198	204	210	216	223	229	235	241	247	253	260	266	272	278	284	291	297	303	309	315	322	328	334
67	121	127	134	140	146	153	159	166	172	178	185	191	198	204	211	217	223	230	236	242	249	255	261	268	274	280	287	293	299	306	312	319	325	331	338	344
68	125	131	138	144	151	158	164	171	177	184	190	197	203	210	216	223	230	236	243	249	256	262	269	276	282	289	295	302	308	315	322	328	335	341	348	354
69	128	135	142	149	155	162	169	176	182	189	196	203	209	216	223	230	236	243	250	257	263	270	277	284	291	297	304	311	318	324	331	338	345	351	358	365
70	132	139	146	153	160	167	174	181	188	195	202	209	216	222	229	236	243	250	257	264	271	278	285	292	299	306	313	320	327	334	341	348	355	362	369	376
71	136	143	150	157	165	172	179	186	193	200	208	215	222	229	236	243	250	257	265	272	279	286	293	301	308	315	322	329	338	343	351	358	365	372	379	386
72	140	147	154	162	169	177	184	191	199	206	213	221	228	235	242	250	258	265	272	279	287	294	302	309	316	324	331	338	346	353	361	368	375	383	390	397
73	144	151	159	166	174	182	189	197	204	212	219	227	235	242	250	257	265	272	280	288	295	302	310	318	325	333	340	348	355	363	371	378	386	393	401	408
74	148	155	163	171	179	186	194	202	210	218	225	233	241	249	256	264	272	280	287	295	303	311	319	326	334	342	350	358	365	373	381	389	396	404	412	420
75	152	160	168	176	184	192	200	208	216	224	232	240	248	256	264	272	279	287	295	303	311	319	327	335	343	351	359	367	375	383	391	399	407	415	423	431
76	156	164	172	180	189	197	205	213	221	230	238	246	254	263	271	279	287	295	304	312	320	328	336	344	353	361	369	377	385	394	402	410	418	426	435	443

Source: Adapted from *Clinical Guidelines on the Identification, Evaluation, and Treatment of Overweight and Obesity in Adults: The Evidence Report.*

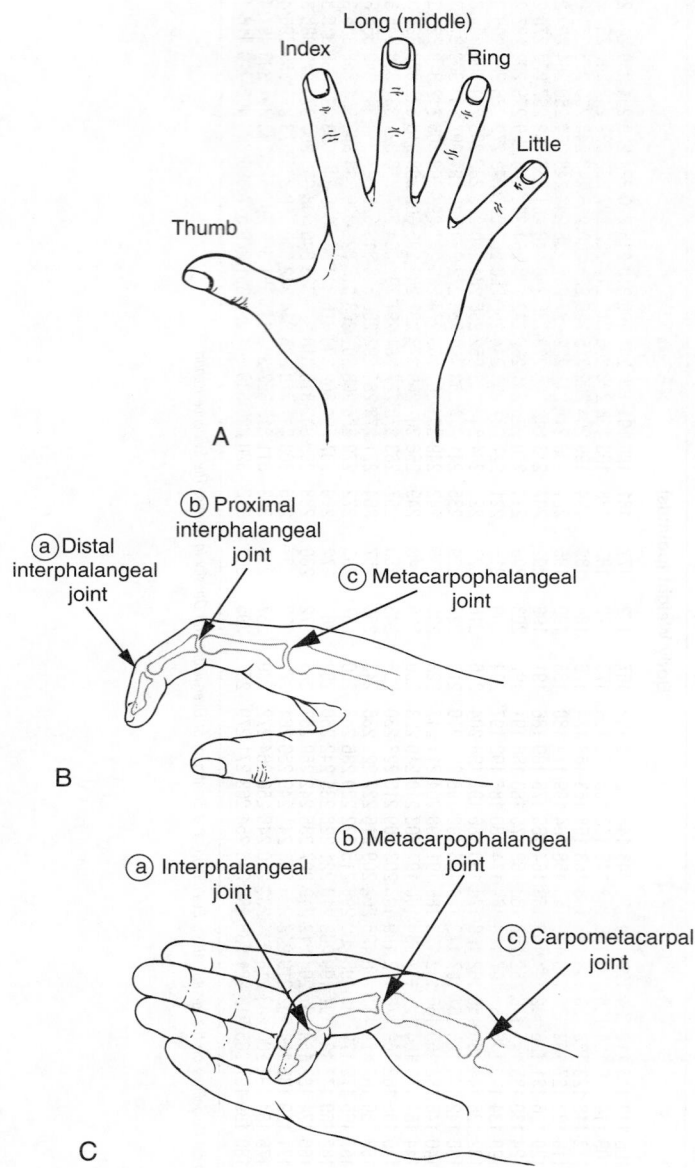

The hand. *A*, Terminology for the fingers. *B*, Joints of the fingers. *C*, Joints of the thumb.

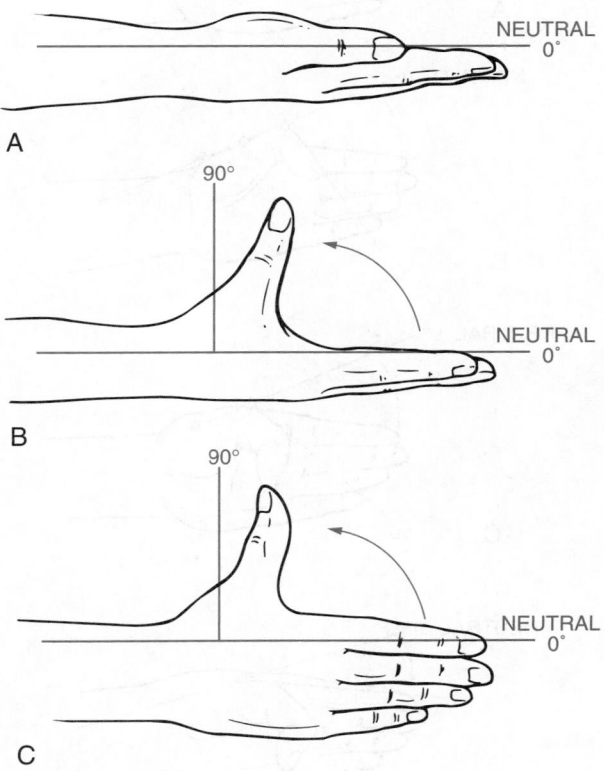

The thumb (circumduction and abduction). *A*, Zero starting point. *B*, Circumduction at right angle to the plane of the thumb. *C*, Extension parallel to the plane of the palm.

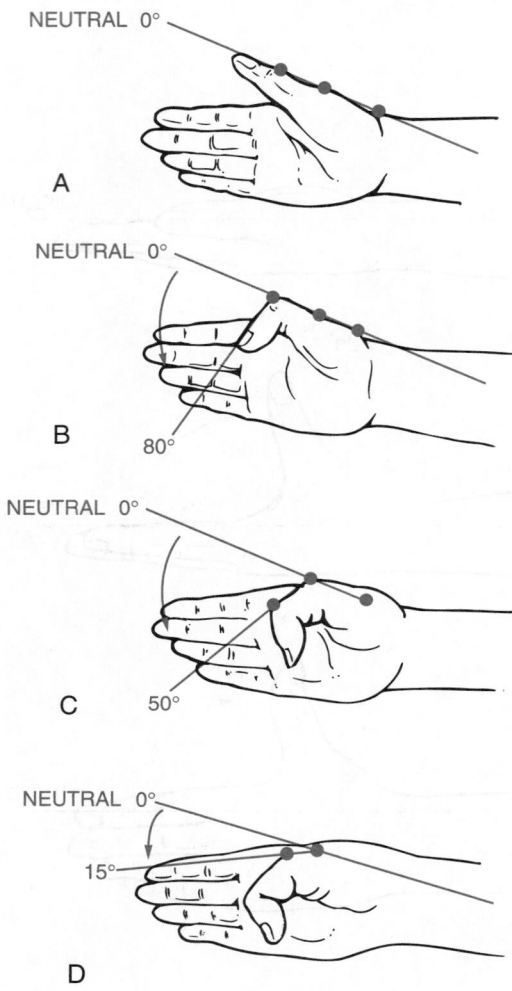

NEUTRAL 0°

A

NEUTRAL 0°

B

80°

NEUTRAL 0°

C

50°

NEUTRAL 0°

15°

D

The thumb (flexion). *A*, Zero starting position. *B*, Interphalangeal joint. *C*, Metacarpophalangeal joint. *D*, Carpometacarpal joint.

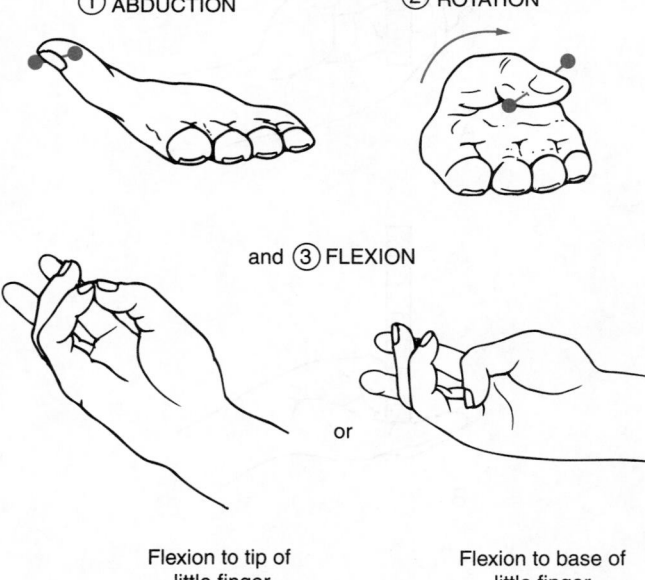

Zero starting position

① ABDUCTION

② ROTATION

and ③ FLEXION

or

Flexion to tip of
little finger

Flexion to base of
little finger

The thumb (opposition): composite of three motions.

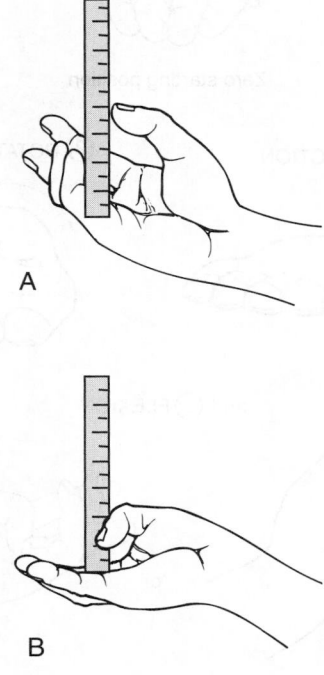

The thumb: measurement of limitation of opposition. *A*, By distance between thumbnail and base of little finger. *B*, By distance between thumb and base of little finger.

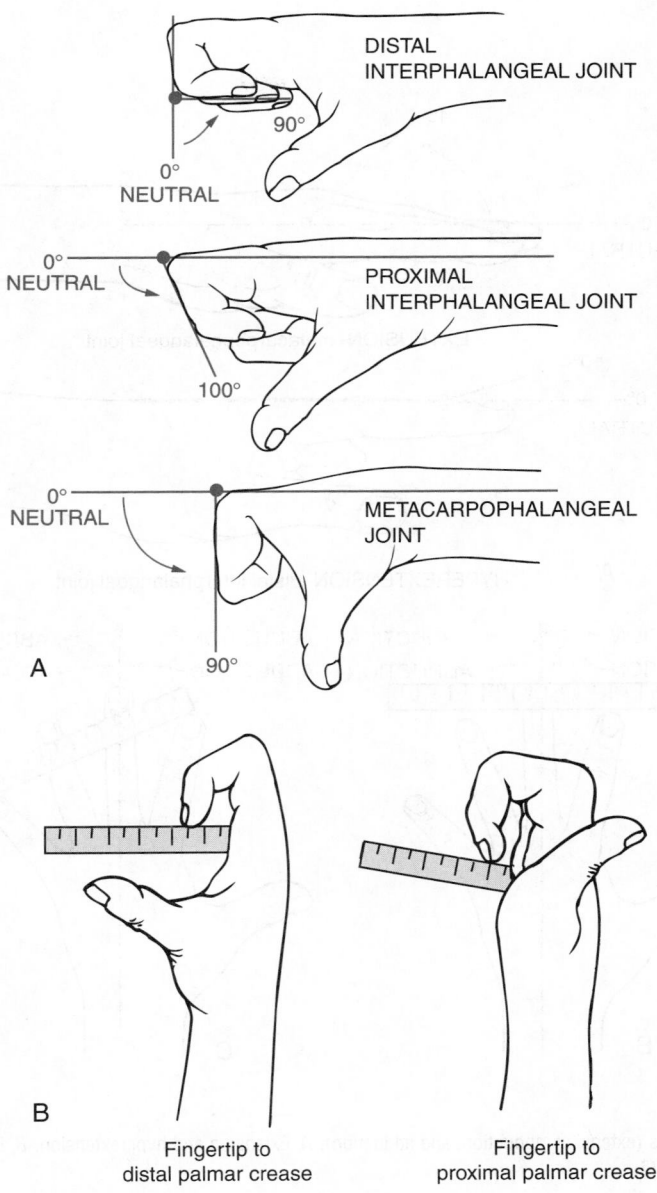

The fingers (flexion), *A*, Flexion. *B*, Composite motion of flexion.

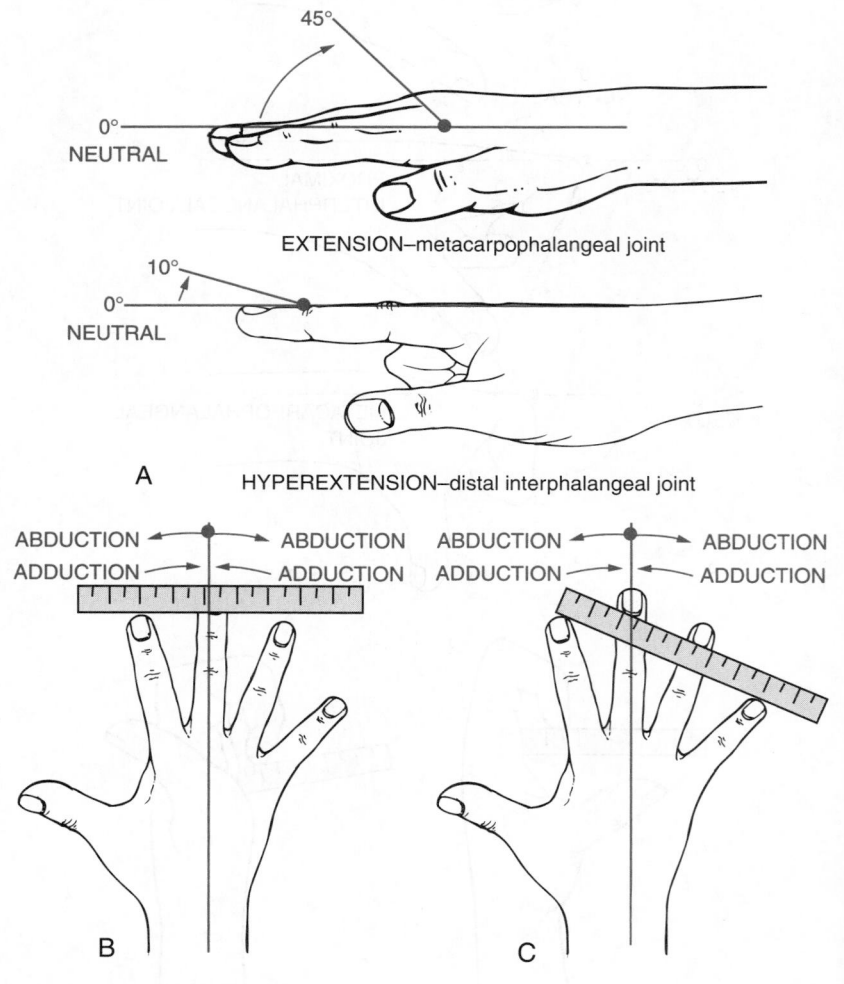

The fingers (extension, abduction, and adduction). *A*, Extension and hyperextension. *B*, Finger spread *C*, Other fingers.

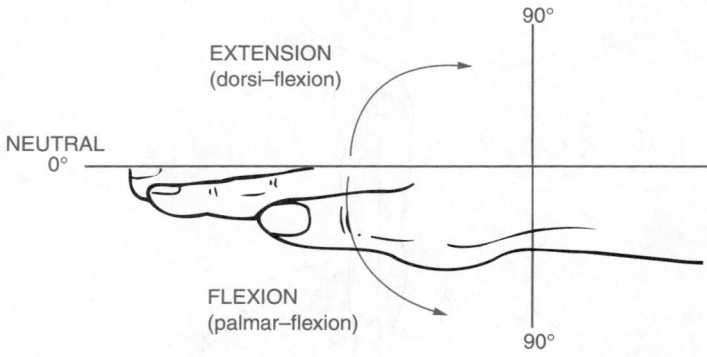

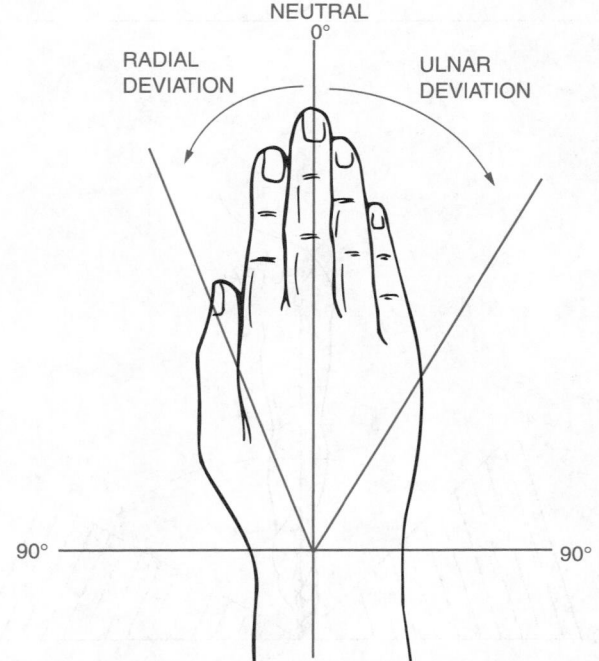

The wrist. *A*, Flexion and extension. *B*, Radial and ulnar deviation.

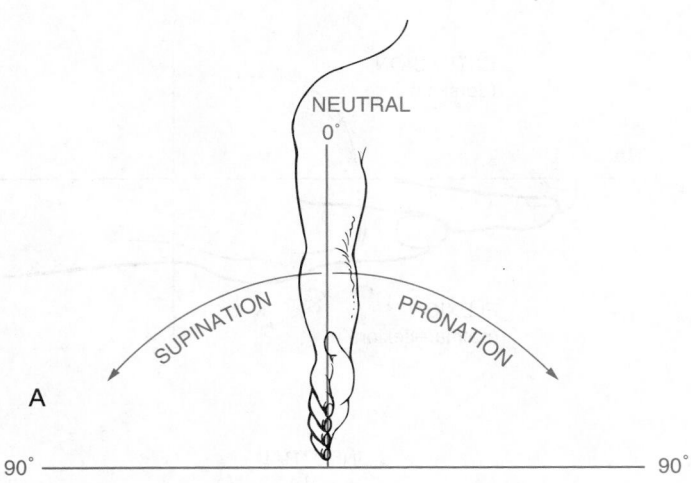

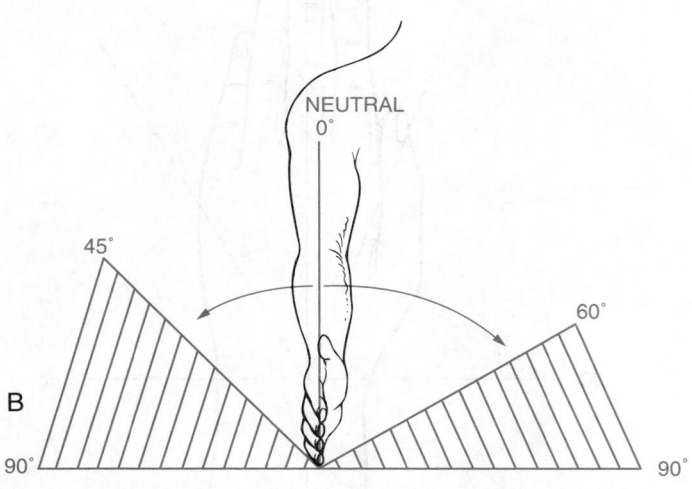

The forearm (elbow and wrist). *A*, Pronation and supination. *B*, Measurement of limited motion.

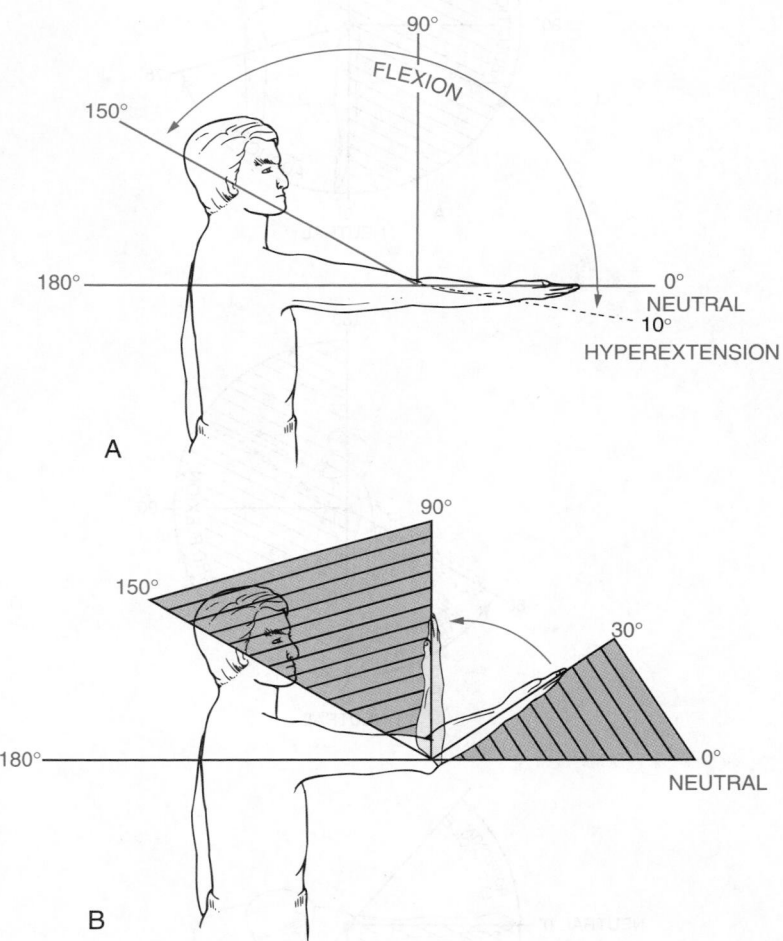

The elbow. *A*, Flexion and hyperextension. *B*, Measurement of limited motion.

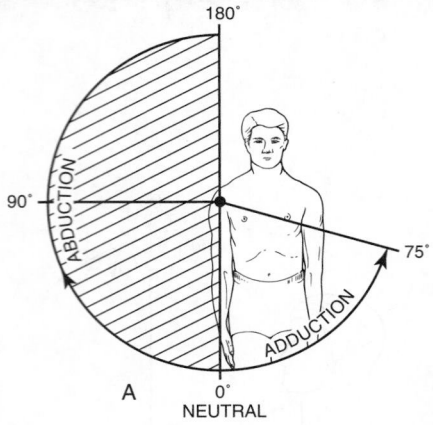

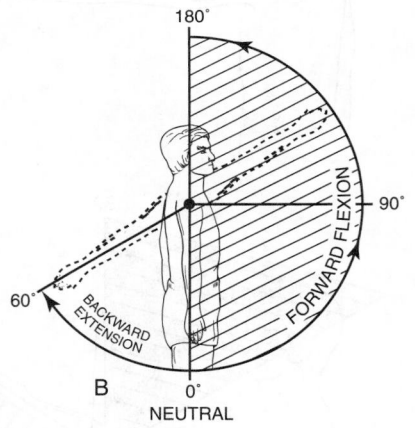

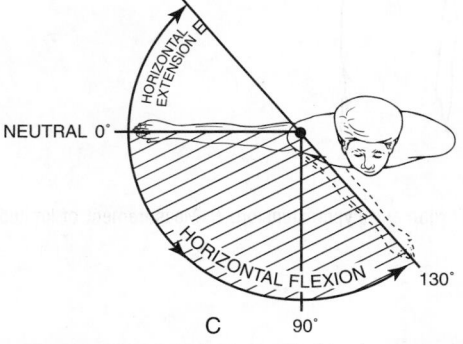

Motion of the arm at the shoulder. *A*, Abduction and adduction (in vertical plane). *B*, Forward flexion and backward extension (in vertical plane). *C*, Horizontal flexion (in horizontal plane).

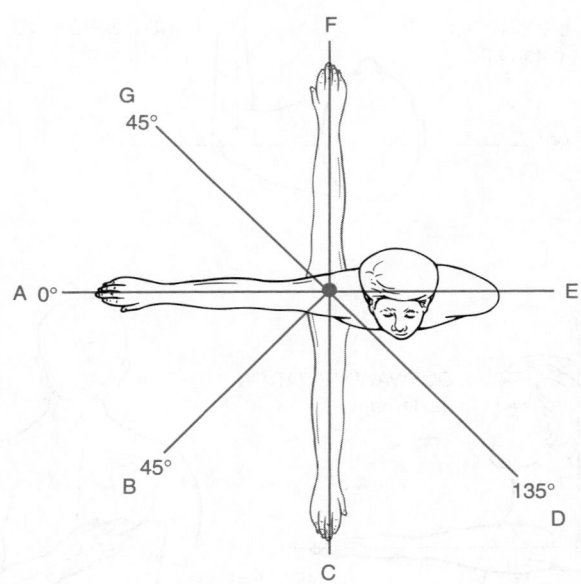

The shoulder: terms used to identify upward motion of the arm in various horizontal positions. *Positions*: *A*, Neutral abduction. *B*, Abduction. *C*, Forward flexion. *D*, Adduction in 135° of horizontal flexion. *E*, Neutral adduction. *F*, Backward extension. *G*, Abduction in horizontal extension.

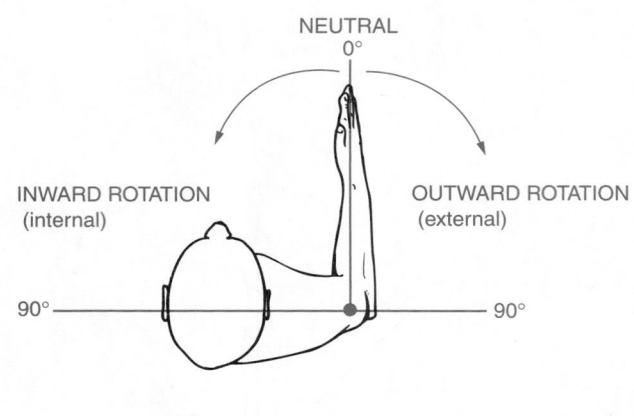

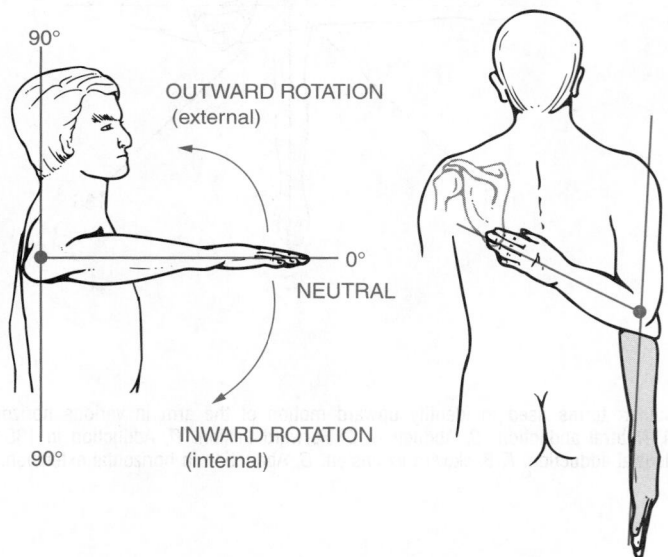

The shoulder (rotation). *A*, Rotation with arm at side. *B*, Rotation in abduction. *C*, Internal rotation posteriorly.

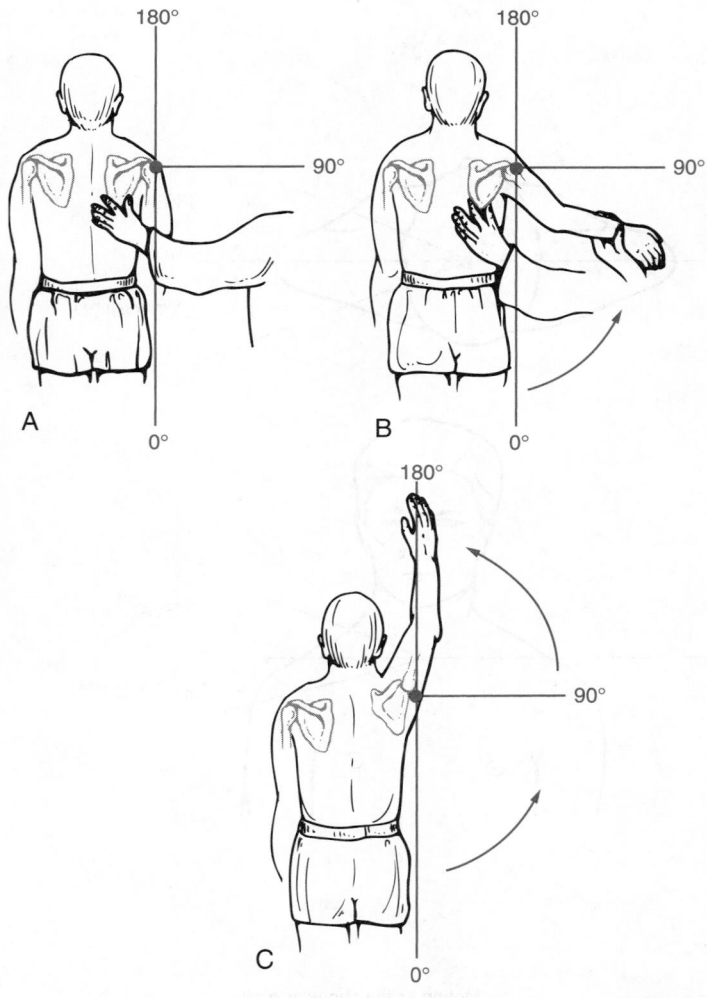

The shoulder (glenohumeral motion). *A,* Neutral. *B,* Range of true glenohumeral motion. *C,* Combined glenohumeral and scapulothoracic motion.

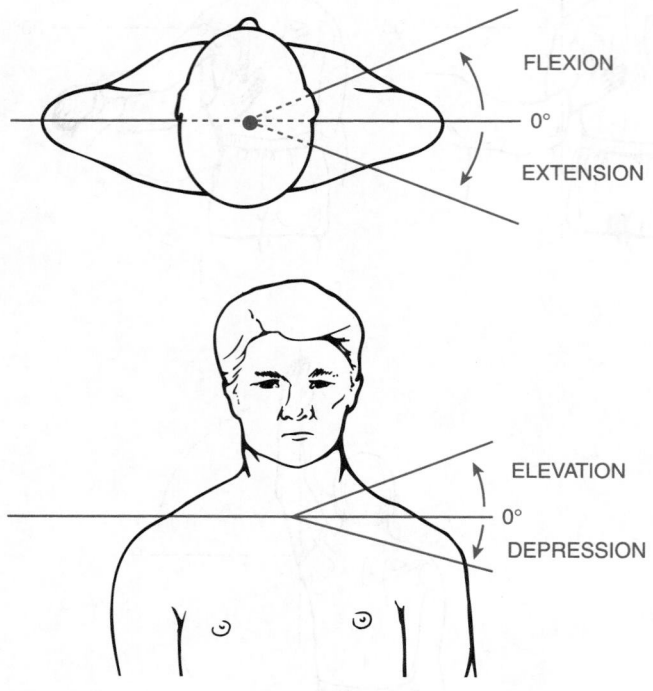

FLEXION

0°

EXTENSION

ELEVATION

0°

DEPRESSION

Motion of the shoulder girdle.

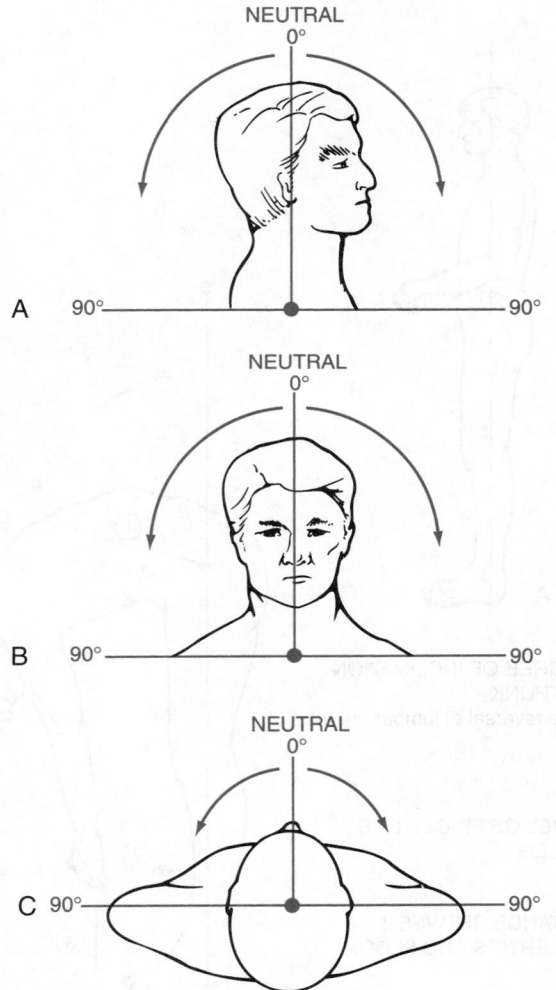

The cervical spine. *A*, Flexion and extension. *B*, Lateral bend. *C*, Rotation.

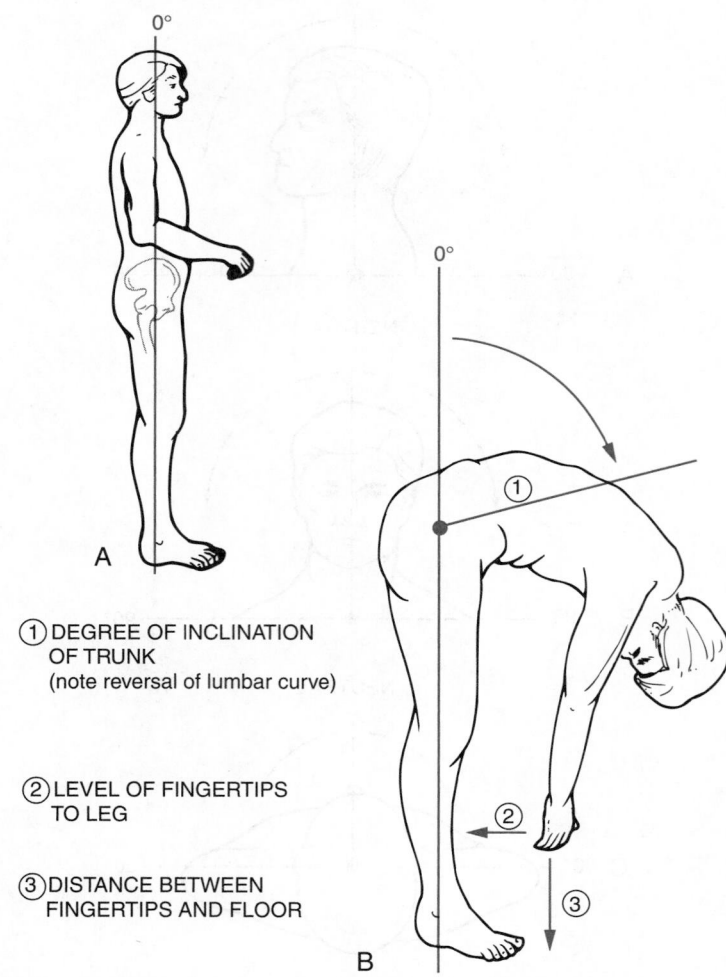

① DEGREE OF INCLINATION
OF TRUNK
(note reversal of lumbar curve)

② LEVEL OF FINGERTIPS
TO LEG

③ DISTANCE BETWEEN
FINGERTIPS AND FLOOR

Measuring spinal flexion. *A*, Zero starting position. *B*, Methods of measuring flexion.

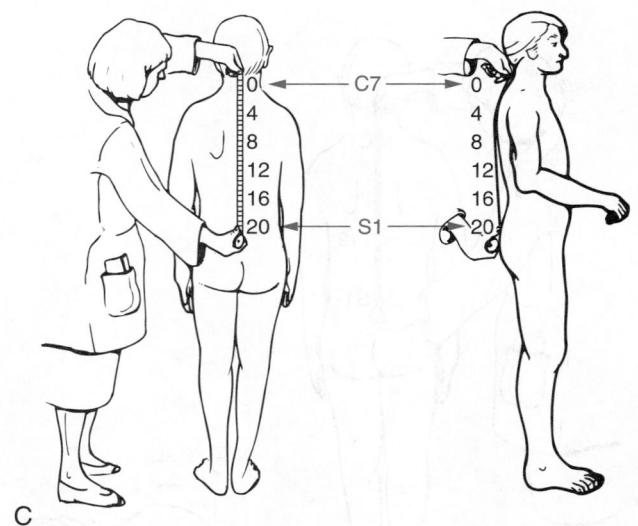

C

④ The steel tape measuring method

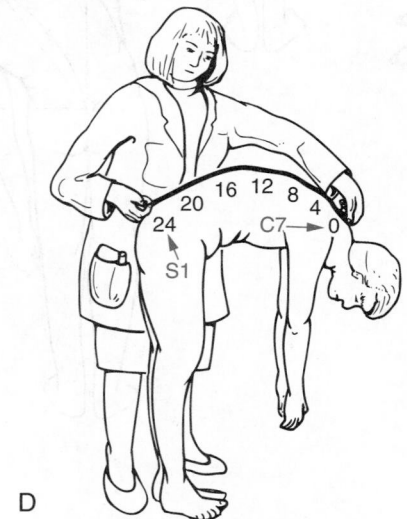

D

C and *D*, Steel tape method. *C*, the patient standing erect. *D*, The patient bending forward. Note the 4 inches in motion (20 in.–24 in.).

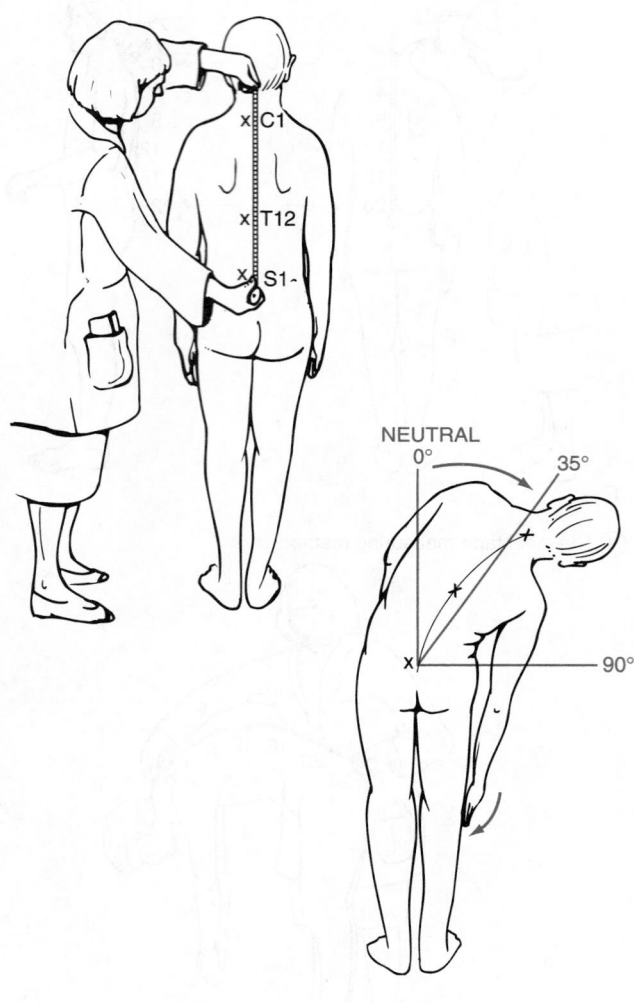

The thoracic and lumbar spine: lateral bending.

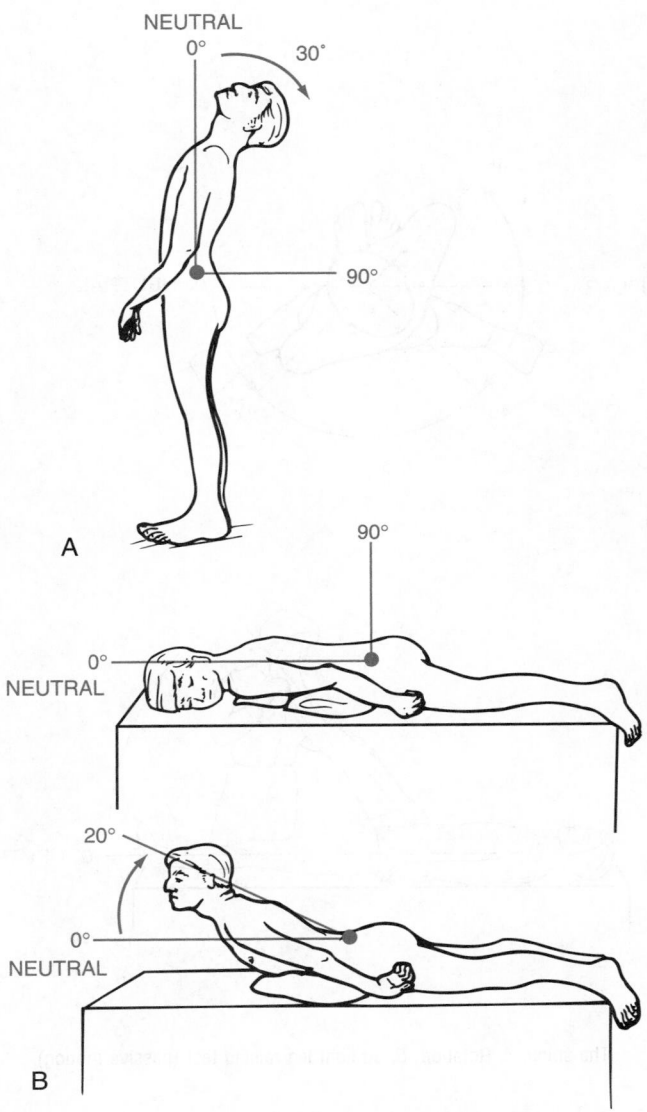

NEUTRAL

0°   30°

90°

A

90°

0°

NEUTRAL

20°

0°

NEUTRAL

B

The thoracic and lumbar spine (extension). *A*, Standing. *B*, Lying prone.

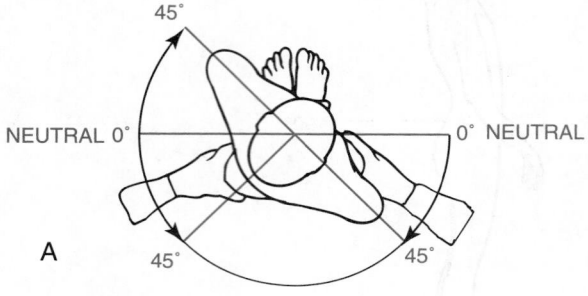

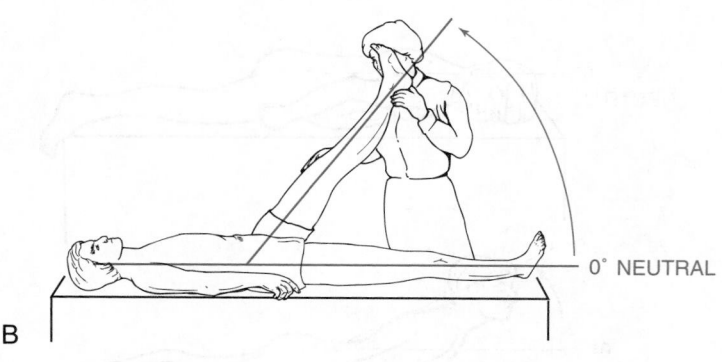

The spine. *A*, Rotation. *B*, Straight leg raising test (passive motion).

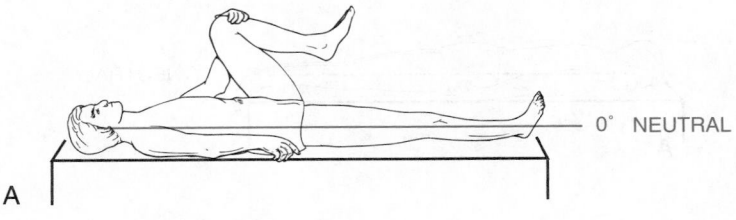

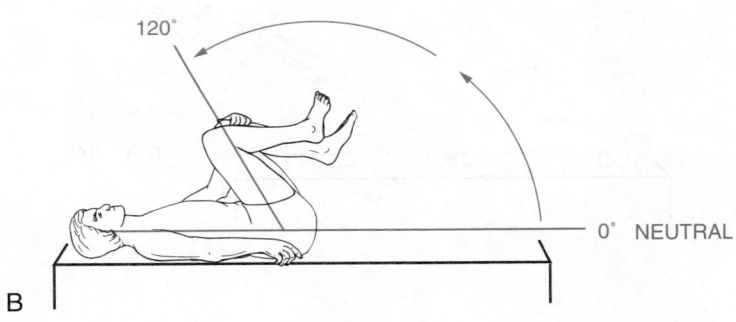

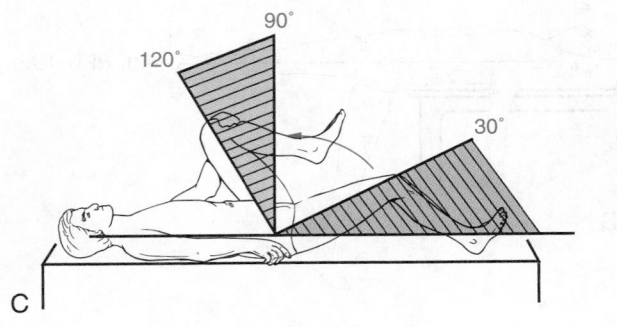

The hip (flexion). *A,* Zero starting position. *B,* Flexion. *C,* Limited motion in flexion.

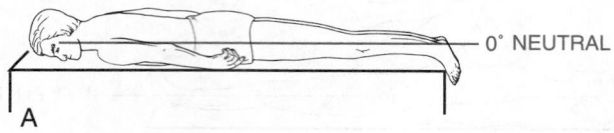

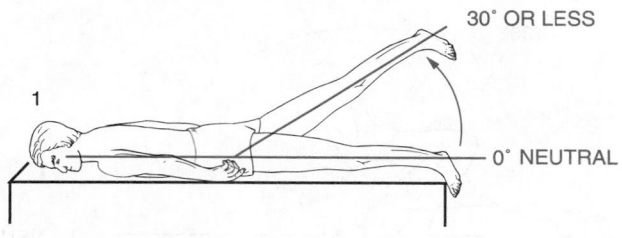

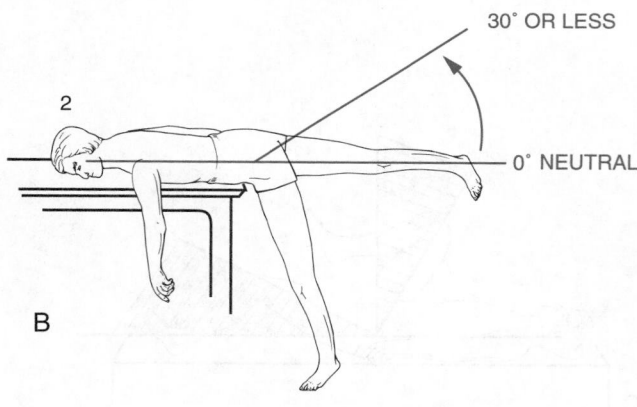

The hip (extension). *A*, Zero starting position. *B*, Extension.

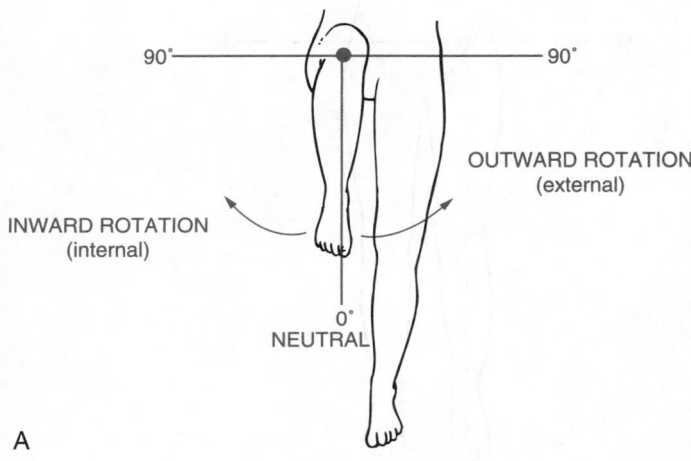

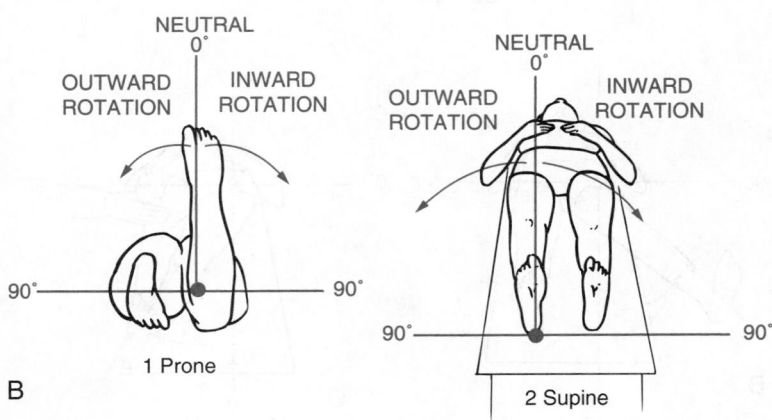

The hip (rotation). *A*, Rotation in flexion. *B*, Rotation in extension.

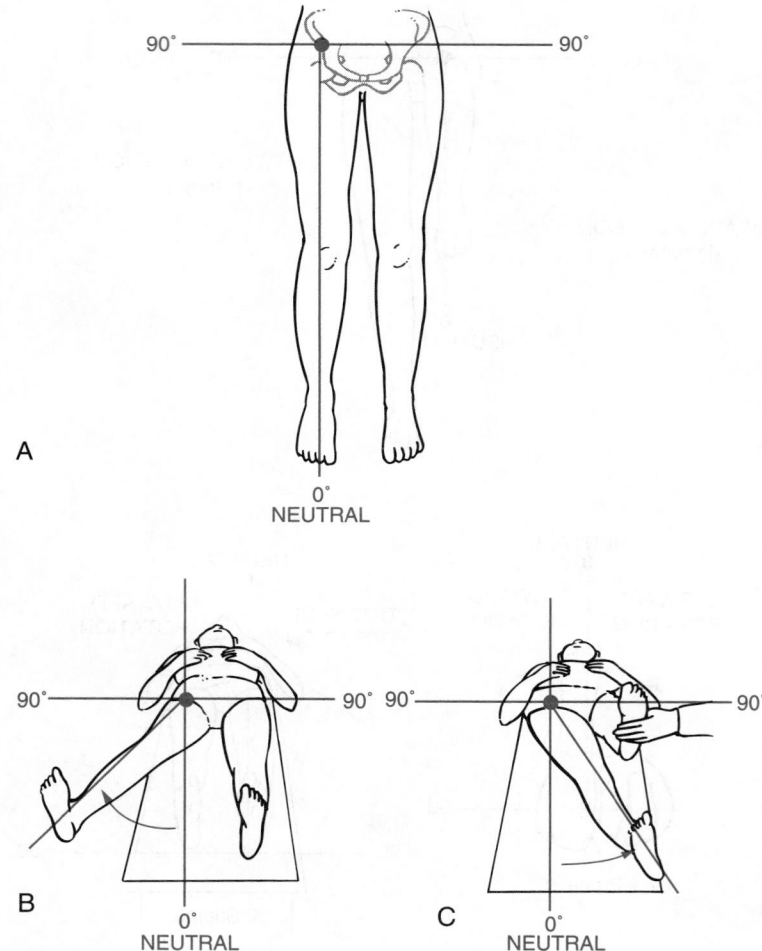

The hip (abduction and adduction). *A*, Zero starting position. *B*, Abduction. *C*, Adduction.

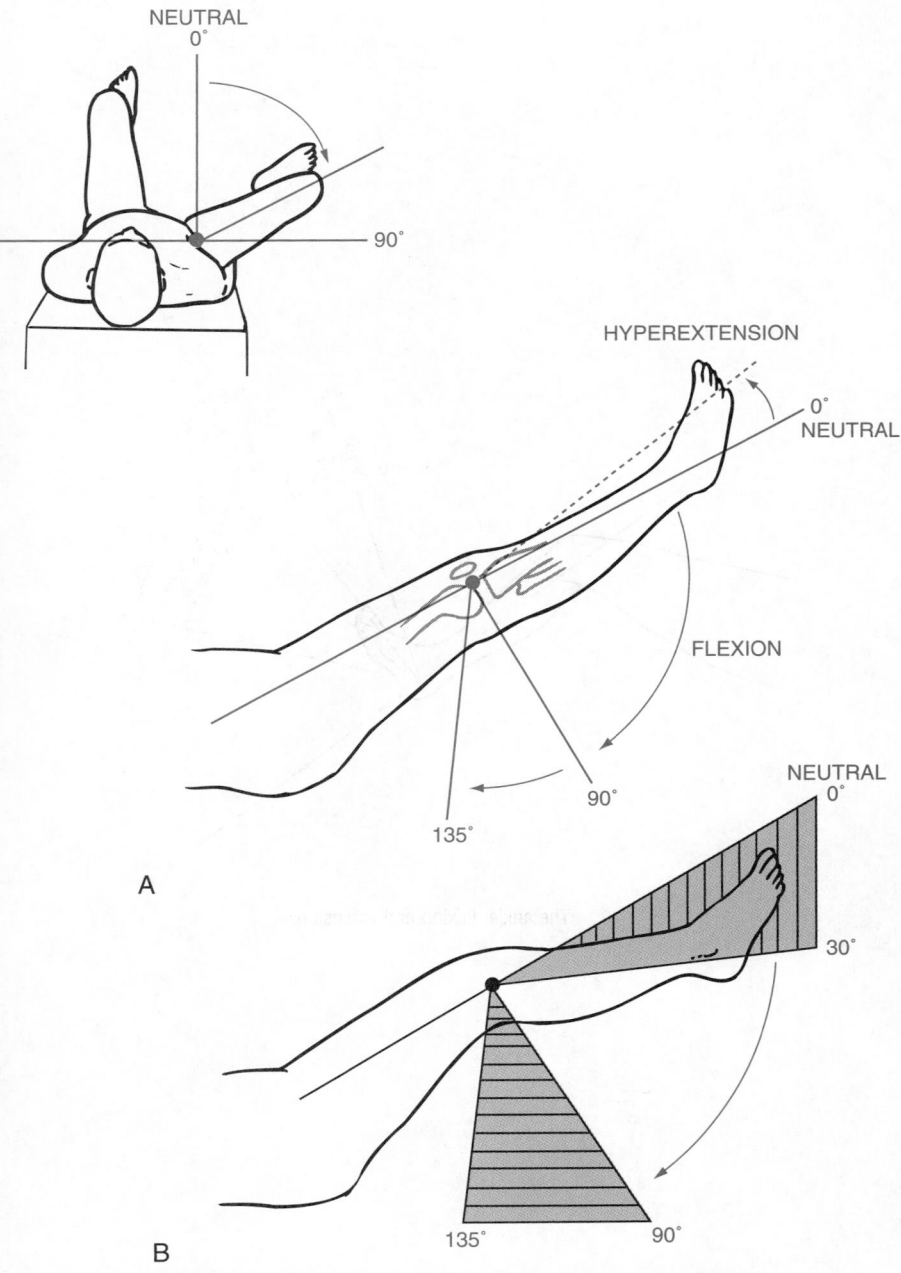

The knee. *A*, Flexion and hyperextension. *B*, Measurement of limited extension.

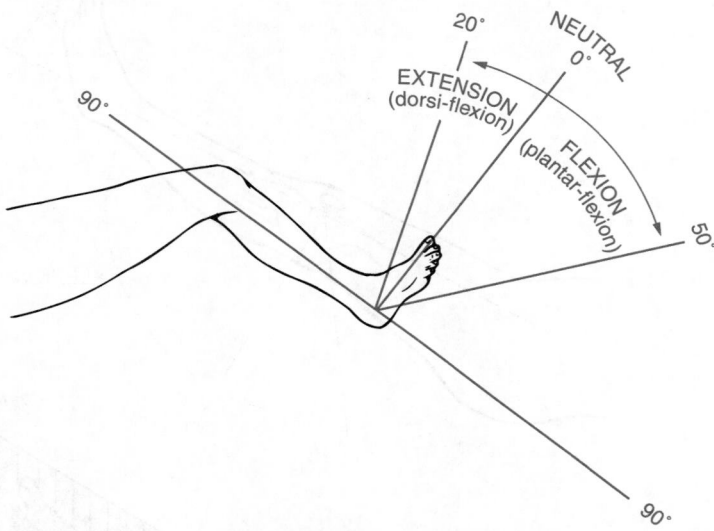

The ankle: flexion and extension.

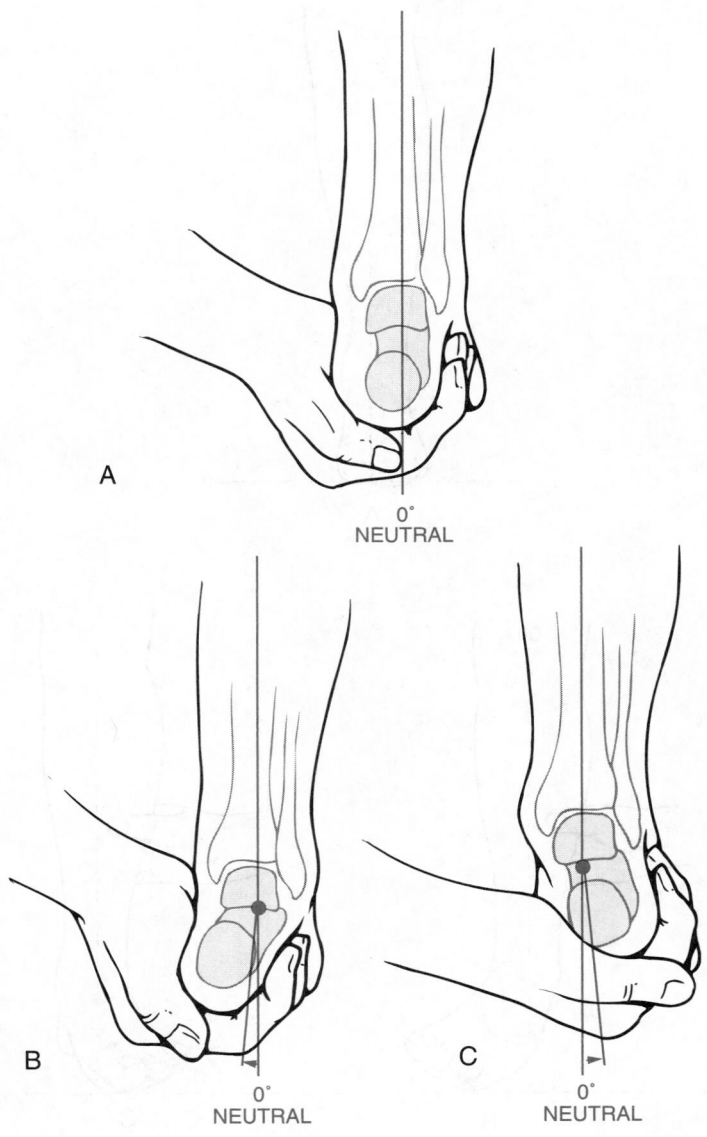

A, 0°
NEUTRAL

B, 0°
NEUTRAL

C, 0°
NEUTRAL

Hind part of foot (passive motion). *A,* Zero starting position. *B,* Inversion. *C,* Eversion.

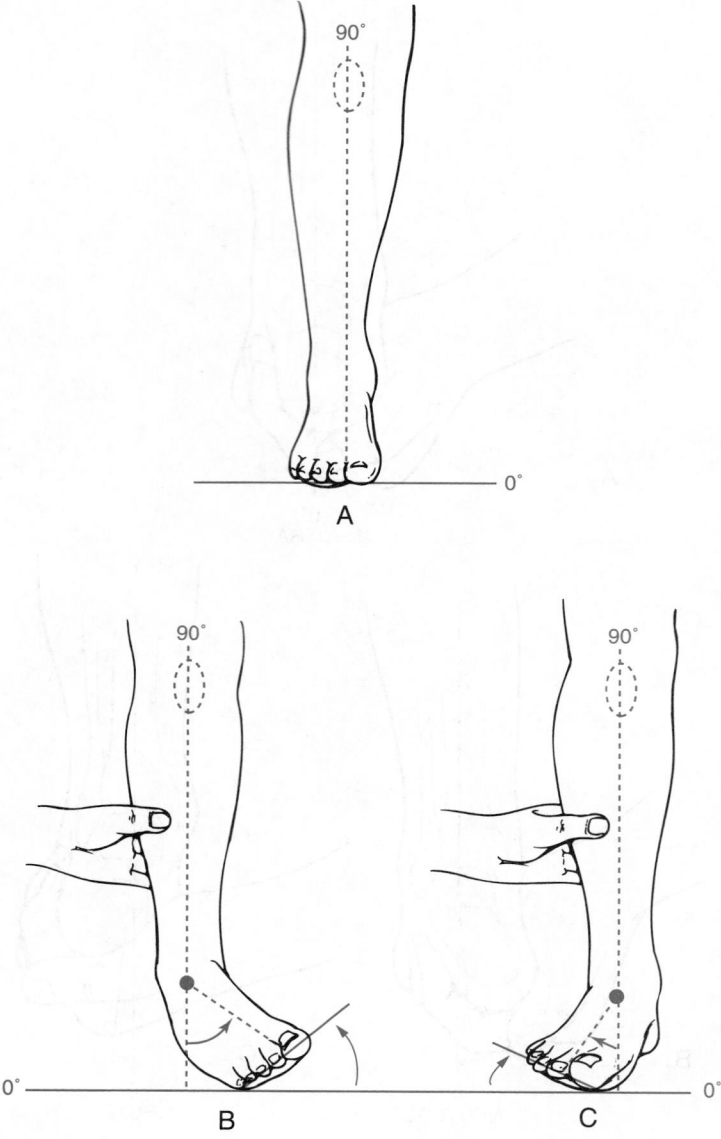

Fore part of the foot. *A*, Zero starting position. *B*, Inversion (supination, adduction, and plantar flexion). *C*, Eversion (pronation, abduction, and dorsiflexion).

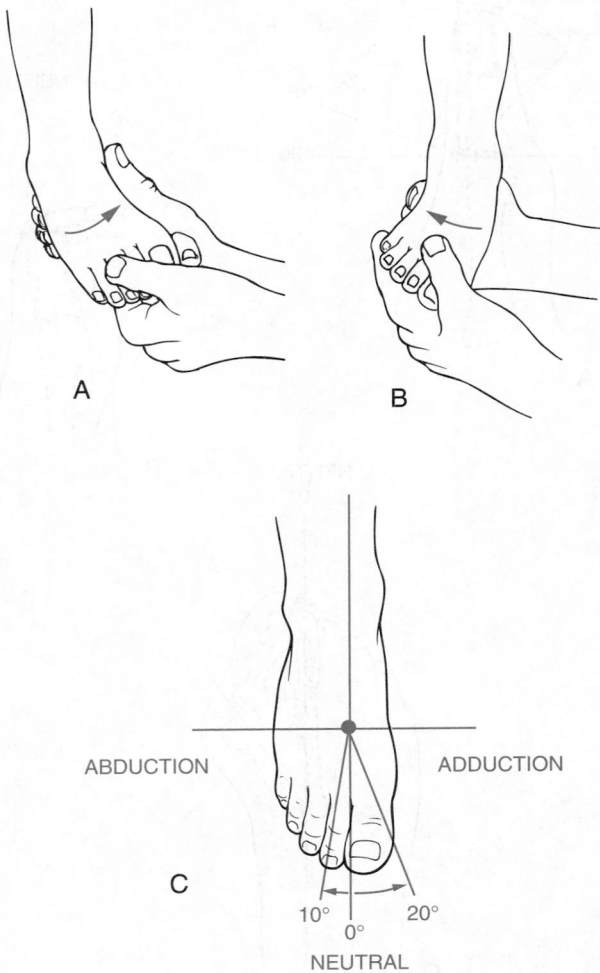

Fore part of the foot. *A,* Inversion. *B,* Eversion. *C,* Passive adduction and abduction.

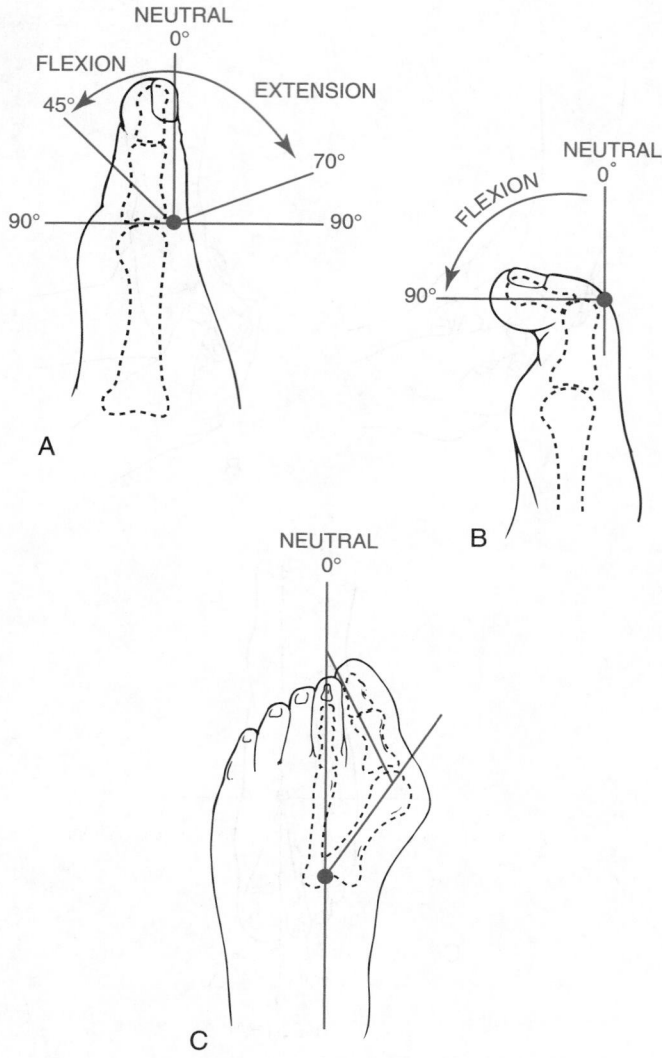

The great toe. *A*, Metatarsophalangeal joint. *B*, Interphalangeal joint. *C*, Hallux valgus.

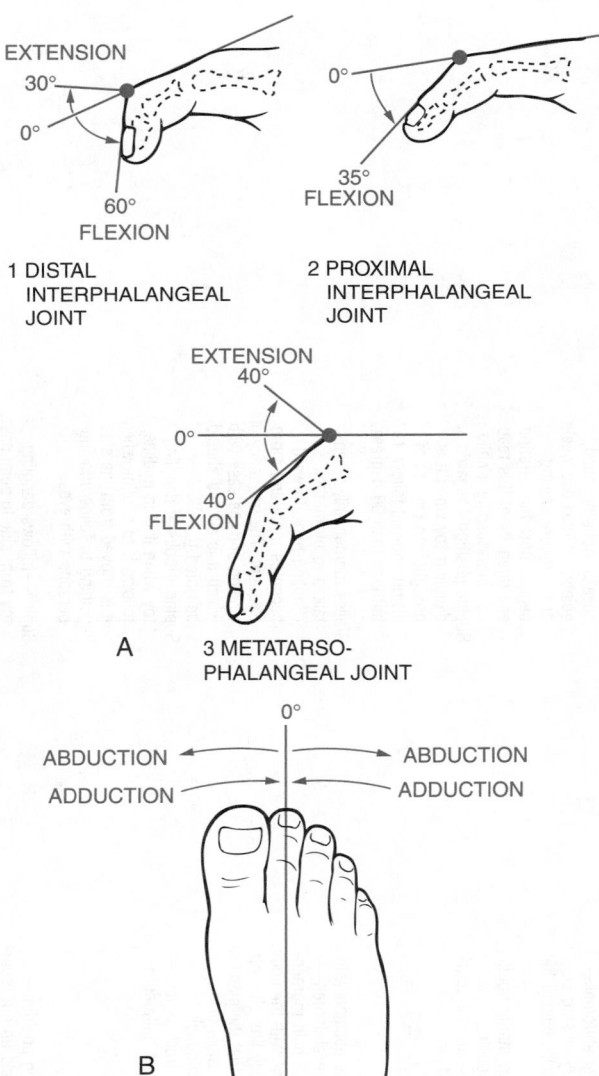

EXTENSION
30°
0°
60°
FLEXION

1 DISTAL
INTERPHALANGEAL
JOINT

0°
35°
FLEXION

2 PROXIMAL
INTERPHALANGEAL
JOINT

EXTENSION
40°
0°
40°
FLEXION

A   3 METATARSO-
PHALANGEAL JOINT

0°
ABDUCTION ← → ABDUCTION
ADDUCTION → ← ADDUCTION

B

The toes. *A*, Second to fifth toes. *B*, Abduction and adduction (toe spread).

2-5. SUMMARY OF NORMAL DEVELOPMENT IN THE FIRST THREE YEARS (BASED LARGELY ON GESELL)

Age*	Gross Motor	Manipulation	General Understanding	Speech	Sphincter Control	Miscellaneous
4 weeks	Held in sitting position—may hold head up momentarily. Held in prone position with hand under abdomen—momentary tensing of neck muscles should be noted. Prone—momentarily holds chin off couch. Pulled to sit—almost complete head lag.		Watches the mother when she talks to him. Opens and closes mouth as she speaks, bobs his head, quiets. (In next two weeks or so, before smiling begins, note the duration and intensity of this reaction in assessing a child.) Supine position—regards dangling toy when it is brought into his line of vision and will follow it, but less than 90 degrees.			
6 weeks	Held in prone position with hand under abdomen—the head is held momentarily in line with the body. Prone—readily lifts chin off couch so that the plane of face is at angle of 45 degrees to couch. Pulled to sit from supine—head lag not quite complete.		Smiles momentarily when talked to by mother. (Smiling henceforward becomes more and more frequent. The frequency of smiling and the ease with which it is elicited should be noted.) Supine—looks at dangling toy when it is in midline; follows it to midline when it is moved from the side. Beginning to follow moving persons with eyes.			
8 weeks	Held in sitting position—head is held up but recurrently bobs forward. Held in prone position with hand under abdomen—holds head up so that its plane is in line with that of the body.		Supine—follows dangling toy from side to point past midline. (Always note the promptness with which child sees the ring. At this age he does not usually see it immediately.)			Eyes show fixation, convergence, focusing.

	Prone—head no longer mainly turned to one side as in earlier weeks. Recurrently lifts chin off couch so that plane of face is at angle of 45 degrees to couch. Held in standing position—is able to hold head up more than momentarily.		Supine—characteristically watches movements of own hands.
12 weeks	Prone—holds chin and shoulders off couch prolongedly, so that plane of face is at angle of 45–90 degrees from couch. Bears weight on forearms. Pulled to sit from supine—only moderate head lag. Held in prone position with hand under abdomen—holds head up so that its plane is beyond that of the body.	Pulls at his clothes. No more grasp reflex. Holds rattle voluntarily when it is placed in his hand; retains it more than a moment. Hands no longer tightly closed as in previous weeks, but mostly open. Desire to grasp objects seen (see next column).	Supine—follows dangling toy from one side to the other (180 degrees). Catches sight of it immediately. Not only smiles when spoken to but vocalizes with pleasure. Squeals of pleasure heard. (From now onward it is essential to note the child's interest in what he sees. One must also note the obvious desire to grasp objects. This desire to grasp objects can be observed long before he can voluntarily go for them and get them. In another month his hands go forward for the object, but he misjudges the distance. By 5 months he can get the object.)

*For mature babies; due allowance to be made for prematurity. Copying a circle implies copying a representation of a circle on a card given by the examiner. When a child "imitates" a circle he draws one after seeing the examiner do it.

From Illingworth, R. S.: The Normal Child, 7th ed. Edinburgh, Churchill Livingstone, 1979, Revised, 2002.

(continued)

			2-5. SUMMARY OF NORMAL DEVELOPMENT IN THE FIRST THREE YEARS (BASED LARGELY ON GESELL)—cont'd			
Age*	Gross Motor	Manipulation	General Understanding	Speech	Sphincter Control	Miscellaneous
16 weeks	Held in sitting position—holds head well up constantly. He looks actively around, but head still wobbles if examiner causes sudden movement of trunk. Curvature of back now only in lumbar region as compared with rounded back of earlier weeks. Prone—holds head and chest off couch so that plane of face is 90 degrees to couch. Weight still on forearms. Pulled to sit—only slight head lag in beginning of movement. Supine—head no longer rotated to one side as in earlier weeks.	Hands come together and he plays with his hands. He pulls his clothes over his face in play. Approaches object with hands, but overshoots the mark and fails to reach it. Plays with rattle prolongedly when it is placed in his hand, and he shakes it.	General understanding becoming much more obvious. Excited when he sees toys. Shows considerable interest when he sees breast or bottle. Shows interest in strange room. Laughs aloud. Vocalizes pleasure when pulled to sitting position. Likes to be propped up in sitting position. Turns head towards a sound.			
20 weeks	Full head control. Head in sitting position—head stable when body is mildly rocked by examiner. Pulled to sit—no head lag.	Now able to grasp objects deliberately. He plays with his toys, splashes in the bath and crumples paper. (From this time onward one must note the maturity of the grasp, the ease with which he is able to secure objects, the security with which he holds them, and the size of the object which he is able to grasp. He cannot bring finger and thumb together to grasp a small object of the size of a thin piece of string till he is about 9 months old.)	Smiles at image of self in mirror. When he drops his rattle he looks to see where it has gone.			

Age	Posture and large movements	Manipulation	Social behavior	Speech/Feeding
24 weeks	Prone—weight borne on hands with extended arms, the chest and upper part of abdomen therefore being off the couch. Pulled to sit—head lifted off couch when about to be pulled up. Hands are held out to be lifted. Sits (supported) in high chair for a few minutes. Rolls from prone to supine. Held in standing position—bears large fraction of weight.	He grasps his feet. Holds bottle. Supine—may take toes to mouth. If he has one cube in hand he drops it when second one is offered.	Smiles and vocalizes at his mirror image. When he drops the rattle he tries to recover it. May "blow bubbles" or protrude tongue in imitation of adult. May show fear of strangers and be "coy." Laughs when head is hidden in towel in peekaboo game. Beginning to show likes and dislikes of foods.	Feeds well from cup. Chews and so can take solids.
28 weeks	Prone—bears weight on one hand. Sits with hands forward for support. Rolls from supine to prone. Standing position—can maintain extension of hip and knees for short period when supported. He bounces with pleasure. (Previously he sagged at hip and knees.) Supine—spontaneously lifts head off couch.	If he has one cube in hand the retains it when second cube is offered. Transfers objects from one hand to the other. Bangs objects on the table. Now goes for objects with one hand instead of two, as he did previously. Takes all objects to mouth. Feeds self with biscuit. Loves to play with paper.	Pats image of self in mirror. Responds to name. Tries to establish contact with person by cough or other noise. May imitate movement, such as tongue protrusion.	Says "Da," "Ba," "Ka."
32 weeks	Readily bears weight on legs when supported. Sits for a few moments unsupported.		Reaches persistently for toys out of reach. Responds to "No."	Combines syllables, "Da-da," "Ba-ba."

(continued)

2-5. SUMMARY OF NORMAL DEVELOPMENT IN THE FIRST THREE YEARS (BASED LARGELY ON GESELL)—cont'd

Age*	Gross Motor	Manipulation	General Understanding	Speech	Sphincter Control	Miscellaneous
36 weeks	Stands holding on to furniture. Sits steadily for 10 minutes. Leans forward and recovers balance. (Cannot lean sideways.) Prone—in trying to crawl may progress backwards. May progress by rolling.	Can pick up small object such as raisin between finger and thumb. When he has two cubes he brings them together as if making visual comparison between them.	Puts arms in front of face to try to prevent mother washing his face. (From this age onward note excitement when certain liked foodstuffs are seen. Note particularly degree and maintenance of concentration in getting objects and in playing with toys.)			Slobbering and mouthing beginning to decrease.
40 weeks	Pulls self to standing position. Pulls self to sitting position. Goes forward from sitting to prone, and from prone to sitting. Sits steadily without risk of falling over (except for occasional accident). Crawls, pulling self forward with hands, abdomen on couch.	Goes for objects with index finger. Beginning to release objects, letting them go deliberately instead of accidentally as before.	May pull clothes of another to attract attention. Plays "Patacake" (clapping hands). Waves bye-bye. Pats the doll. Holds arm out for sleeve or holds foot up for sock in dressing. (From this age the understanding of words should be observed. The child can understand the meaning of perhaps a dozen words by the age of a year, though he is only able to say two or three words at that age. At 9 months he may respond to such questions as "Where is Daddy?" "Where is the cow?")			

44 weeks	Prone—creeps (abdomen off couch). When standing and holding on he lifts and replaces one foot. Sitting—can lean over sideways.	Will place object into examiner's hand on request, but will not release it.	Covers own face with towel in peekaboo game. Drops objects deliberately in order that they will be picked up. Beginning to put objects in and out of containers. (The maturity of the release behavior and the manipulative skill must be noted as he plays with his toys.)	Says one word with meaning.	
48 weeks	Walks sideways, holding on to furniture. Walks with two hands held. Sitting—can turn round to pick up object.	Rolls ball towards examiner. Gives and takes toy in play, releasing object into examiner's hand.	Repeats performance laughed at. Now likes repetitive play, putting one cube after another into basket, etc. Anticipates with bodily movement when being told nursery rhyme. Shows interest when shown simple pictures in book. (This interest should be carefully noted from now onward.)		
1 year	Walks with one hand held. Prone—walks on hands and feet like a bear. May shuffle on buttocks and hand.		May understand meaning of "Where is your book" "Where is your shoe?" May kiss on request. (Such evidence of developing memory is important and must be noted.)	Says two or three words with meaning.	Apt to be shy. Very little mouthing of objects. Little slobbering except during concentration on an especially interesting toy.
13 months	Stands alone for a moment.	Can hold two cubes in one hand. Makes line or marks with pencil.	May kiss mirror image.		

(continued)

2-5. SUMMARY OF NORMAL DEVELOPMENT IN THE FIRST THREE YEARS (BASED LARGELY ON GESELL)—cont'd

Age*	Gross Motor	Manipulation	General Understanding	Speech	Sphincter Control	Miscellaneous
15 months	Can get into standing position without support. Creeps upstairs. Walks without help with broad-base, high-stepping gait and steps of unequal length and direction. (The maturity of the gait must be noted from now onward.)	Builds tower of two cubes. (This requires some accuracy in release.) Constantly throwing objects onto floor. Takes off shoes.	Asks for objects by pointing. Pats pictures and may kiss pictures of animals. Negativism beginning. Feeds self, managing cup.	Jargon.	Tells mother that he has wet pants. (First sign of sphincter control.)	
18 months	Climbs stairs unaided, holding rail. Runs. Seldom falls. No longer broad-base and high-stepping gait when walking. Seats self in chair, often by process of climbing up, standing, turning round, and sitting down. Pulls toy as he walks. Throws ball without falling, as previously.	Builds tower of three cubes. Manages spoon without rotating it near mouth as previously. Turns pages of book two or three at a time. Scribbles spontaneously. Takes off gloves, socks. Unzips fasteners.	Points to picture of car or dog in book. Picture Card.[†] Points correctly to one when asked "Where is the...?" Copies mother in her domestic work—e.g., sweeping the floor, dusting. Simple objects.[‡] Names one. Points to nose, eye, hair on request. Carries out two simple orders.[§]		Clean and dry with only occasional accident.	Dawdling in feeding.
21 months	Walks backwards in imitation. Picks up object from floor without falling. Walks upstairs, two feet per step.	Builds towers of five or six cubes.	Pulls people to show them objects. Knows four parts of the body. Picture Card.[†] Points correctly to two when asked "Where is the...?"	Joins two words together. Repeats things said. Asks for drink, toilet, food.		Sleeping difficulties common. Sleep rituals beginning.

Age	Motor	Adaptive	Language	Personal-Social
2 years	Goes up and down stairs alone, two feet per step.	Builds tower of six or seven cubes. Turns pages of book singly. Turns door knobs, unscrews lid. Puts on shoes, socks, pants. Washes and dries hands.	Imitates train with cubes, without adding chimney. Imitates vertical stroke with pencil. Knows two common objects.‡ Obeys four simple orders.§ Parallel play—watches others play and plays near them, without playing with them. Picture Cards.† Names three when asked "What is this?" Identifies five when asked "Where is the...?" (Much can be learned by noting the maturity of the play and the imaginativeness shown.) Uses words. I, me, you. Talks incessantly.	Dry at night if lifted out late in evening.
2½ years	Jumps with both feet. Walks on tiptoe when asked.	Builds tower of eight cubes. Holds pencil in hand instead of in fist.	Imitates train with cubes, adding chimney. Imitates vertical and horizontal strokes with pencil. Repeats two digits (one out of three trials)—e.g., asked to say "Eight—six." Picture Cards.† Names five objects when asked "What is this?" Identifies seven when asked "Where is the...?" Common objects.‡ Names three.	Color sense beginning. Attends to toilet without help, except for wiping. Climbs onto lavatory seat.

†Two cards showing dog, cup, house, shoe, flag, clock, star, leaf, basket, book.
‡Penny, shoe, pencil, knife, ball.
§"Take it to mother," "Put it on the chair," "Bring it to me," "Put it on the table."

(continued)

2-5. SUMMARY OF NORMAL DEVELOPMENT IN THE FIRST THREE YEARS (BASED LARGELY ON GESELL)—cont'd

Age*	Gross Motor	Manipulation	General Understanding	Speech	Sphincter Control	Miscellaneous
3 years	Goes upstairs one foot per step, and downstairs two feet per step. (Goes downstairs with one foot per step at 4 years.) Jumps off bottom step. Stands on one foot for a few seconds. Rides tricycle.	Builds tower of nine cubes. Dresses and undresses self if helped with buttons and advised occasionally about back and front and the right foot for the shoe. Unbuttons front buttons. Can be trusted to carry china and so to help to set the table.	Beginning to take interest in sex organs. Peak of negativism. Gives full name. Helps to put things away. Copies with pencil, imitates cross (copies cross at 3½, square at 4, diamond at 5.) Constantly asking questions. Knows own sex. Picture Card.† Names eight when asked "What is this…?" (Names ten at 3½ years.) Repeats three digits (one out of three trials). (Repeats four digits in one out of three trials at 4½) Obeys two requests when asked. "Put the ball under the chair, at the side of the chair, behind the chair, on the chair." (Obeys four at 4 years) Knows some nursery rhymes. May count up to 10. Now joins children in play. Dresses and undresses doll. Beginning to draw objects spontaneously (e.g., a man), or an request. Cubes. Imitates building bridge of three cubes.			

Conversion Formulas

There are times when one form of measurements or weights will need to be changed or converted to another system. The usual way to approach this problem is to set up a simple ratio. x is used as the unknown quantity. An example follows that demonstrates the conversion of grains to milligrams.

It must be known that 1 grain = 60 milligrams
This equivalency is placed into a formula as follows:
desired (grains) = unknown quantity (x tablets)
(when mg/grain is known) (when tablet size is a known quantity)
The practitioner fills in known values to find x.

Example: How many tablets must be given when gr. V are prescribed? The bottle is labeled 300 mg per tablet.

5 grains = x tablets
(when 1 grain = 60 mg and 1 tablet = 300 mg)
Make substitution on left side: 5 grains = 300 mg
Make substitution on right side: x tablets = x (300 mg)
Fill in the values:
300 mg = x (300 mg)
One tablet should be administered

Pediatric Drug Calculation Formulas
Clark's Rule

$$\frac{(\text{Weight in pounds}) \times (\text{adult dose})}{150} = \text{child's dosage}$$

Friend's Rule (calculation of doses for infants or children up to the age of 2)

$$\frac{(\text{Age in months}) \times (\text{adult dose})}{150} = \text{child's dosage}$$

Young's Rule (calculation of doses for children over 2)

$$\frac{(\text{Age in years}) \times (\text{adult dose})}{\text{Age in years} + 12} = \text{child's dose}$$

Surface Area Calculation

$$\frac{(\text{Surface area of child in square meters}) \times (\text{adult dose})}{1.73\,\text{m}} = \text{child's dose}$$

Calculation of Pack Years for Patients Who Smoke

(number of packs smoked per day) × (number of years the patient has smoked)

Example: The patient has smoked one pack per day for ten years.
(1 pack) × (10 years) = 10 pack years
The patient has smoked a half pack per day for ten years.

(1/2 pack) × (10 years) = 5 pack years

Drip rates for Intravenous Infusions

The total number of cc's per hour is calculated by dividing the amount of fluid in the infusion by the number of hours the infusion is to run.
Example: 1000 cc of fluids is to infuse over an 8 hour period.

$$\frac{1000\,\text{cc}}{8\,\text{hr}} = 125\,\text{cc/hour}$$

Drop Factor (Gtt. Factor)

The drop factor (gtt. factor) is the number of drops in one cubic centimeter, expressed as gtt/cc. One application of it is the following formulas:

(drops/minute = (drop factor) × (cc/minute)
or: (gtt/min) = (gtt. factor) × (cc/min)
Therefore: 60 × (gtt/min) = (gtt/hr)
and: 60 × (gtt/min) = (gtt. factor) × (cc/hr)

(continued)

Example: if the gtt. factor is 60 gtt per cc:

1 cc/min = 60 gtt/min
60 cc/60 min = 60 gtt/min

or $60\left(\dfrac{1\,cc}{1\,hr}\right) = 60\left(\dfrac{1\,gtt}{1\,min}\right)$

or cc/hr = gtt/min

Therefore: With a drop factor of 60 gtt/cc, an infusion rate of 125 cc/hour requires 125 gtt/min

Example: If the gtt. factor is 15 gtt per cc:

1 cc/min = 15 gtt/min
60 cc/60 min = 15 gtt/min

or $60\left(\dfrac{1\,cc}{1\,hr}\right) = 15\left(\dfrac{1\,gtt}{1\,min}\right)$

or 4 cc/hr = 1 gtt/min

In other words, (cc/hr) ÷ 4 = gtt. rate per minute.

And: With a drop factor of 15 gtt/cc, an infusion rate of 125 cc/hour requires $\frac{125}{4}$ or 31.25 gtt/min (rounded off to 31 gtt/min)

Example: If the gtt. factor is 10 gtt per cc:

1 cc/min = 10 gtt/min
60 cc/60 min = 10 gtt/min

or $60\left(\dfrac{1\,cc}{1\,hr}\right) = 10\left(\dfrac{1\,gtt}{1\,min}\right)$

or 6 cc/hr = 1 gtt/min

In other words, (cc/hr) ÷ 6 = gtt. rate per minute.

And: With a drop factor of 10 gtt/cc, and infusion rate of 125 cc/hour requires $\frac{125}{6}$ or 20.83 gtt/min (rounded off to 21 gtt/min)

Intravenous Infusion Rates

Intravenous infusion rates can also be calculated using a formula. The drop factor (gtt/cc) must be know.

$$\frac{(\text{amount to be infused}) \times (\text{drop factor})}{\text{time in minutes}} = gtt/min$$

Example: With a drop factor 60 gtt/cc, convert 125 cc/hour into gtt/min.

$$\frac{125\,cc}{1\,hour} \times \frac{60\,gtt}{1\,cc} = \frac{125\,cc}{60\,min} \times \frac{60\,gtt}{1\,cc} = 125\,gtt/min$$

The 24 hour clock (also known as military time) is used to standardize time and avoid the misinterpretation of charting entries related to AM and PM.

From midnight to noon, there is no difference between a 24 hour clock and the time as it is normally noted.

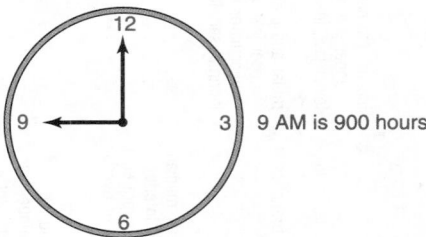

9 AM is 900 hours

From noon to midnight, 12 is added to the PM time.

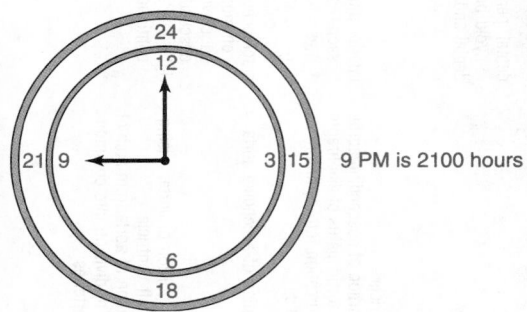

9 PM is 2100 hours

Noon is 1200 hours
1 PM is 1300 hours
2 PM is 1400 hours
3 PM is 1500 hours
4 PM is 1600 hours
5 PM is 1700 hours
6 PM is 1800 hours
7 PM is 1900 hours
8 PM is 2000 hours
9 PM is 2100 hours
10 PM is 2200 hours
11 PM is 2300 hours
Midnight is 2400 hours

Section 3: Anatomy Tables

3-1. ARTERIES

Common Name*	TA Equivalent†	Origin*	Branches*	Distribution
accompanying a. of sciatic nerve. *See* sciatic a.				
acromiothoracic a. *See* thoracoacromial a.				
alveolar a's, anterior superior	aa. alveolares superiores anteriores	infraorbital a.	dental branches	incisor and canine regions of upper jaw, maxillary sinus
alveolar a., inferior	a. alveolaris inferior	maxillary a.	dental, peridental, mental mylo-hyoid branches	lower jaw, lower lip, chin
alveolar a., posterior superior	a. alveolaris superior posterior	maxillary a.	dental and peridental branches	molar and premolar regions of upper jaw, maxillary sinus, buccinator muscle
angular a.	a. angularis	facial a.		lacrimal sac, lower eyelid, nose
aorta	aorta	left ventricle		
abdominal aorta	pars abdominalis aortae	lower portion of descending aorta, from aortic hiatus of diaphragm to bifurcation into common iliac a's	inferior phrenic, lumbar, median sacral, superior and inferior mesenteric, middle suprarenal, renal, and testicular or ovarian a's, celiac trunk	
arch of aorta	arcus aortae	continuation of ascending aorta	brachiocephalic trunk, left common carotid and left subclavian a's; continues as descending (thoracic) aorta	
ascending aorta	pars ascendens aortae	proximal portion of aorta, arising from left ventricle	right and left coronary a's; continues as arch of aorta	
descending aorta. *See* thoracic aorta; abdominal aorta	pars descendens aortae	continuation of aorta from arch of aorta to division into common iliac arteries		

1998

thoracic aorta	pars thoracica aortae	proximal portion of descending aorta, continuing from arch of aorta to aortic hiatus of diaphragm	bronchial, esophageal, pericardiac, and mediastinal branches, superior phrenic a's, posterior intercostal a's [III–XI], subcostal a's; continues as abdominal aorta	
appendicular a.	a. appendicularis	ileocolic a.		vermiform appendix
arcuate a. of foot	a. arcuata pedis	dorsalis pedis a.	deep plantar branch, dorsal metatarsal a's	foot, toes
arcuate a's of kidney	aa. arcuatae renis	interlobar a.	interlobar a's, straight arterioles of kidney	parenchyma of kidney
auditory a., internal. *See* a. of labyrinth				
auricular a., deep	a. auricularis profunda	maxillary a.		skin of auditory canal, tympanic membrane, temporomandibular joint
auricular a., posterior	a. auricularis posterior	external carotid a.	auricular and occipital branches, stylomastoid a.	middle ear, mastoid cells, auricle, parotid gland, digastric and other muscles
axillary a.	a. axillaris	continuation of subclavian a.	subscapular branches, highest thoracic, thoracoacromial, lateral thoracic, subscapular, and anterior and posterior circumflex humeral a's	upper limb, axilla, chest, shoulder
basilar a.	a. basilaris	from junction of right and left vertebral a's	pontine branches, anterior inferior cerebellar, labyrinthine, superior cerebellar, posterior cerebral a's	brain stem, internal ear, cerebellum, posterior cerebrum
brachial a.	a. brachialis	continuation of axillary a.	superficial and deep brachial, nutrient of humerus, superior and inferior ulnar collateral, radial, ulnar a's	shoulder, arm, forearm, hand
brachial a., deep	a. profunda brachii	brachial a.	nutrient to humerus, deltoid branch, middle to radial collateral a's	humerus, muscles and skin of arm
brachial a., superficial	a. brachialis superficialis	variant brachial a., taking a more superficial course than usual	*see* brachial a.	*see* brachial a.

*a. = artery; a's = (pl.) arteries.
†a. = [L.] arteria; aa. = [L. (pl.)] arteriae.

(continued)

3-1. ARTERIES—cont'd

Common Name*	TA Equivalent†	Origin*	Branches*	Distribution
brachiocephalic trunk	truncus brachiocephalicus	arch of aorta	right common carotid, right subclavian a's	right side of head and neck, right arm
buccal a.	a. buccalis	maxillary a.		buccinator muscle, oral mucous membrane
a. of bulb of penis	a. bulbi penis	internal pudendal a.		bulbourethral gland, bulb of penis
a. of bulb of urethra. *See* a. of bulb of penis				
a. of bulb of vestibule of vagina	a. bulbi vestibuli vaginae	internal pudendal a.		bulb of vestibule of vagina, Bartholin glands
callosomarginal a.	a. callosomarginalis	anterior cerebral a.	anteromedial frontal, intermedial frontal, posteromedial frontal, cingular branches	medial and upper lateral surfaces of cerebral hemisphere
caroticotympanic a's	aa. caroticotympanicae	internal carotid a.		tympanic cavity
carotid a., common	a. carotis communis	brachiocephalic trunk (right), arch of aorta (left)	external and internal carotid a's	*see* carotid a., external and carotid a., internal
carotid a., external	a. carotis externa	common carotid a.	superior thyroid, ascending pharyngeal, lingual, facial, sternocleidomastoid, occipital, posterior auricular, superficial temporal, maxillary a's	neck, face, skull
carotid a., internal	a. carotis interna	common carotid a.	caroticotympanic, ophthalmic, posterior communicating, anterior choroid, anterior cerebral, middle cerebral a's	middle ear, brain, hypophysis, orbit, choroid plexus
caudal a. *See* sacral a., median				
cecal a., anterior	a. caecalis anterior	ileocolic a.		cecum
cecal a., inferior	a. caecalis inferior	ileocolic a.		cecum
celiac trunk	truncus celiacus	abdominal aorta	left gastric, common hepatic, splenic a's	esophagus, stomach, duodenum, spleen, pancreas, liver, gallbladder
central a's, anterolateral	aa. centrales laterales	middle cerebral a.	medial and lateral branches	anterior lenticular and caudate nuclei and internal capsule of brain
central a's, anteromedial	aa. centrales anteromediales	anterior cerebral a.		anterior and medial corpus striatum
central a's, posterolateral	aa. centrales posterolaterales	posterior cerebral a.		cerebral peduncle, posterior thalamus, colliculi, pineal and medial geniculate bodies

central a's, posteromedial	aa. centrales posteromediales	posterior cerebral a.		anterior thalamus, lateral wall of third ventricle, globus pallidus
central a., long	a. centralis longa	anterior cerebral a.		
central a. of retina	a. centralis retinae	ophthalmic a.		retina
central a., short	a. centralis brevis	anterior cerebral a.		
cerebellar a., anterior, inferior	a. inferior anterior cerebelli	basilar a.	posterior, spinal (usually), and labyrinthine (usually) a's	lower anterior cerebellum, lower part of and lateral parts of pons, (sometimes) upper part of medulla oblongata
cerebellar a., posterior inferior	a. inferior posterior cerebelli	vertebral a.		lower cerebellum, medulla, choroid plexus of fourth ventricle
cerebellar a., superior	a. cerebelli superior	basilar a.		upper part of cerebellum, midbrain, pineal body, choroid plexus of third ventricle
cerebral a., anterior	a. cerebri anterior	internal carotid a.	*precommunical part:* anteromedial central, long and short central, anterior communicating a's, anteromedial central branch; *postcommunical part:* medial frontobasal, callosomarginal, paracentral, precuneal, parietooccipital a's	orbital, frontal, and parietal cortex, corpus callosum, diencephalon, corpus striatum, internal capsule, choroid plexus of lateral ventricle
cerebral a., middle	a. cerebri media	internal carotid a.	*sphenoidal part:* anterolateral central a; *insular part:* insular lateral frontobasilar, temporal a's; *terminal* or *cortical part:* a's of sulcus, parietal a's, a. of angular gyri	orbital, frontal, parietal, and temporal cortex, corpus striatum, internal capsule
cerebral a., posterior	a. cerebri posterior	terminal bifurcation of basilar a.	*precommunical part:* posteromedial central a's; *postcommunical part:* posterolateral central a's, medial and lateral posterior choroidal, peduncular branches; *terminal* or *cortical part:* lateral and medial occipital a's	occipital and temporal lobes, basal ganglia, choroid plexus of lateral ventricle, thalamus, midbrain

(continued)

3-1. ARTERIES—cont'd

Common Name*	TA Equivalent†	Origin*	Branches*	Distribution
colic a., right, inferior. *See* ileocolic a.				
cervical a., ascending	a. cervicalis ascendens	inferior thyroid a.		muscles of neck, vertebrae, vertebral canal
cervical a., deep	a. cervicalis profunda	costocervical trunk		deep neck muscles
cervical a., transverse	a. transversa colli	subclavian a.	deep and superficial branches	root of neck, muscles of scapula, interior of brain, including choroid plexus of lateral ventricle and adjacent parts
ciliary a's, anterior	aa. ciliares anteriores	ophthalmic and lacrimal a's	episcleral and anterior conjunctival a's	iris, conjunctiva
ciliary a's, posterior, long	aa. ciliares posteriores longae	ophthalmic a.		iris, ciliary processes
ciliary a's, posterior, short	aa. ciliares posteriores breves	ophthalmic a.		choroid coat of eye
circumflex femoral a., lateral	a. circumflexa femoris lateralis	deep femoral a.	ascending, descending, and transverse branches	hip joint, thigh muscles
circumflex femoral a., medial	a. circumflexa femoris medialis	deep, ascending, transverse, and acetabular branches	hip joint, thigh muscles	
circumflex humeral a., anterior	a. circumflexa anterior humeri	axillary a.		shoulder joint and head of humerus, long tendon of greater pectoral muscle
circumflex humeral a., posterior	a. circumflexa posterior humeri	axillary a.		deltoid, shoulder joint, teres minor and triceps muscles
circumflex iliac a., deep	a. circumflexa ilium profunda	external iliac a.	ascending branches	iliac region, abdominal wall, groin
circumflex iliac a., superficial	a. circumflexa ilium superficialis	femoral a.		groin, abdominal wall
circumflex a., of scapula	a. circumflexa scapulae	subscapular a.		inferolateral muscles of scapula
cocygeal a. *See* sacral a., median				
colic a., left	a. colica sinistra	inferior mesenteric a.		descending colon
colic a., middle	a. colica media	superior mesenteric a.		transverse colon
colic a., right	a. colica dextra	superior mesenteric a.		ascending colon
colic a., superior accessory. *See* colic a., middle				
collateral a., inferior ulnar	a. collateralis ulnaris inferior	brachial a.		arm muscles at back of elbow
collateral a., middle	a. collateralis media	deep brachial a.		triceps muscle, elbow joint
collateral a., radial	a. collateralis radialis	deep brachial a.		brachioradial and brachial muscles
collateral a., superior ulnar	a. collateralis ulnaris superior	brachial a.		elbow joint, triceps muscle

Common Name	NA Term	Origin	Branches	Distribution
communicating a., posterior	a. communicans posterior cerebri	cerebral a. interconnects internal carotid and posterior cerebral a's		branches to optic chiasm, oculomotor nerve, thalamus, hypothalamus, and tail of caudate nucleus
conjunctival a's, anterior	aa. conjunctivales anteriores	anterior ciliary a's		conjunctiva
conjunctival a's, posterior	aa. conjunctivales posteriores	medial palpebral a.		lacrimal caruncle, conjunctiva
coronary a., left	a. coronaria sinistra	left aortic sinus	anterior interventricular and circumflex branches	left ventricle, left atrium
coronary a., right	a. coronaria dextra	right aortic sinus	posterior interventricular branch	right ventricle, right atrium
costocervical trunk	truncus costocervicalis	subclavian a.	deep cervical and highest intercostal a's	deep neck muscles, first two intercostal spaces, vertebral column, back muscles
cremasteric a.	a. cremasterica	inferior epigastric a.		cremaster muscle, coverings of spermatic cord
cystic a.	a. cystica	right branch of hepatic a., proper		gallbladder
deep brachial a. See brachial a., deep				
deep femoral a. See femoral a., deep				
deep lingual a. See profunda linguae a.				
deep a. of clitoris	a. profunda clitoridis	internal pudendal a.		clitoris
deep a. of penis	a. profunda penis	internal pudendal a.		corpus cavernosum penis
deferential a. See a. of ductus deferens				
dental a's. See alveolar a's. See				
diaphragmatic a's. See phrenic a's				
digital a's, collateral. See digital a's, proper palmar				
digital a's of foot, common. See metatarsal a's, plantar				
digital a's of foot, dorsal	aa. digitales dorsales pedis	dorsal metatarsal a's		dorsum of toes
digital a's of hand, dorsal	aa. digitales dorsales manus	dorsal metacarpal a's		dorsum of fingers
digital a's, common palmar	aa. digitales palmares communes	superficial palmar arch	proper palmar digit a's	fingers
digital a's, proper palmar	aa. digitales palmares propriae	common palmar digital a's		fingers
digital a's, common plantar	aa. digitales plantares communes	plantar metatarsal a's	proper plantar digital a's	toes
digital a's, proper plantar	aa. digitales plantares propriae	common plantar digital a's		toes
dorsal a. of clitoris	a. dorsalis clitoridis	internal pudendal a.		clitoris

(continued)

3-1. ARTERIES—cont'd

Common Name*	TA Equivalent†	Origin*	Branches*	Distribution
dorsal a. of foot. See dorsalis pedis a.				
dorsal a. of nose	a. dorsalis nasi	ophthalmic a.	lacrimal branch	dorsum of nose
dorsal a. of penis	a. dorsalis penis	internal pudendal a.		glans, corona, and prepuce of penis
dorsalis pedis a.	a. dorsalis pedis	continuation of anterior tibial a.	lateral and medial tarsal, arcuate, and deep plantar a's	foot, toes
a. of ductus deferens	a. ductus deferentis	umbilical a.	ureteral artery	ureter, ductus deferens, seminal vesicles, testes
duodenal a's. See pancreatico-duodenal a., inferior				
epigastric a., external. See circumflex iliac a., deep				
epigastric a., inferior	a. epigastrica inferior	external iliac a.	pubic branch, cremasteric a., a. of round ligament of uterus	abdominal wall
epigastric a., superficial	a. epigastrica superficialis	femoral a.		abdominal wall, groin
epigastric a., superior	a. epigastrica superior	internal thoracic a.		abdominal wall, diaphragm
episcleral a's	aa. episclerales	anterior ciliary a.		iris, ciliary processes
ethmoidal a., anterior	a. ethmoidalis anterior	ophthalmic a.	anterior meningeal, anterior septal, anterior lateral nasal branches	dura mater, nose, frontal sinus, anterior ethmoidal cells
ethmoidal a., posterior	a. ethmoidalis posterior	ophthalmic a.		conjunctival ethmoidal cells, dura mater, nose
facial a.	a. facialis	external carotid a.	ascending palatine, submental, inferior, and superior labial, septal, lateral nasal, and angular a's; tonsillar and glandular branches	face, tonsil, palate, submandibular gland
facial a., deep. See maxillary a.				
facial a., transverse	a. transversa faciei	superficial temporal a.		parotid region
fallopian a. See uterine a.				
femoral a.	a. femoralis	continuation of external iliac a.	superficial epigastric, superficial circumflex iliac, external pudendal, profunda femoris, and descending genicular a's	lower abdominal wall, external genitalia, lower limb
femoral a., deep	a. profunda femoris	femoral a.	medial and lateral circumflex femoral a's, perforating a's	thigh muscles, hip joint, gluteal muscle, femur

...a... *See* suprarenal a.				
frontobasal a., lateral	a. frontobasalis lateralis	middle cerebral a.		cortex of frontal lobe
frontobasal a., medial	a. frontobasalis medialis	anterior cerebral a.		cortex of frontal lobe
funicular a. *See* testicular a.				
gastric a., left	a. gastrica sinistra	celiac trunk	esophageal branches	esophagus, lesser curvature of stomach
gastric a., posterior	a. gastrica posterior	splenic a.		posterior gastric wall
gastric a., right	a. gastrica dextra	common hepatic a.		lesser curvature of stomach
gastric a's, short	aa. gastricae breves	splenic a.		upper part of stomach
gastroduodenal a.	a. gastroduodenalis	common hepatic a.	superior pancreaticoduodenal and right gastroepiploic a's	stomach, duodenum, pancreas, greater omentum
gastroepiploic a., left. *See* gastro-omental a., left				
gastroepiploic a., right. *See* gastro-omental a., right				
gastro-omental a., left	a. gastro-omentalis sinistra	splenic a.	gastric and omental branches	stomach and greater omentum
gastro-omental a., right	a. gastro-omentalis dextra	gastroduodenal a.	gastric and omental branches	stomach and greater omentum
genicular a., descending	a. descendens genicularis	femoral a.	saphenous, articular branches	knee joint, upper and medial part of leg
genicular a., lateral inferior	a. inferior lateralis genus	popliteal a.		knee joint
genicular a., lateral superior	a. superior lateralis genus	popliteal a.		knee joint, femur, patella, contiguous muscles
genicular a., medial inferior	a. inferior medialis genus	popliteal a.		knee joint
genicular a., medial superior	a. superior medialis genus	popliteal a.		knee joint, femur, patella, contiguous muscles
genicular a., middle	a. media genus	popliteal a.		knee joint, cruciate ligaments, patellar synovial and alar folds
gluteal a., inferior	a. glutea inferior	internal iliac a.	sciatic a.	buttock, back of thigh
gluteal a., superior	a. glutea superior	internal iliac a.	superficial and deep branches	buttocks
helicine a's of penis	aa. helicinae penis	deep and dorsal a's of penis	superficial and deep branches	erectile tissue of penis
hemorrhoidal a's. *See* rectal a's				
hepatic a., common	a. hepatica communis	celiac trunk	right gastric, gastroduodenal, proper hepatic a's	stomach, pancreas, duodenum, liver, gallbladder, greater omentum
hepatic a., proper	a. hepatica propria	common hepatic a.	right and left branches	liver, gallbladder
hyaloid a.	a. hyaloidea	fetal ophthalmic a.		fetal lens (usually not present after birth)
hypogastric a. *See* iliac a., internal				
hypophyseal a., inferior	a. hypophysialis inferior	internal carotid a.		pituitary gland
hypophyseal a., superior	a. hypophysialis superior	internal carotid a.		pituitary gland
iliac a., common	a. iliaca communis	abdominal aorta	internal and external iliac a's	pelvis, abdominal wall, lower limb

(continued)

3-1. ARTERIES—cont'd

Common Name*	TA Equivalent†	Origin*	Branches*	Distribution
iliac a., external	a. iliaca externa	common iliac a.	inferior epigastric, deep circumflex iliac a's	abdominal wall, external genitalia, lower limb
iliac a., internal	a. iliaca interna	continuation of common iliac a.	iliolumbar, obturator, superior and inferior gluteal, umbilical, inferior vesical, uterine, middle rectal, and internal pudendal a's	wall and viscera of pelvis, buttock, reproductive organs, medial aspect of thigh
ileal a's	aa. ilei	superior mesentric a.		ileum
ileocolic a.	a. ileocolica	superior mesenteric a.	anterior and posterior cecal and appendicular a's, colic (ascending) and ileal branches	ileum, cecum, vermiform appendix, ascending colon
iliolumbar a.	a. iliolumbalis	internal iliac a.	iliac and lumbar branches, lateral sacral a s	pelvic muscles and bones, fifth lumbar vertebra, sacrum
infraorbital a.	a. infraorbitalis	maxillary a.	anterior superior alveolar a's	maxilla, maxillary sinus, upper teeth, lower eyelid, cheek, nose
innominate a. *See* brachiocephalic trunk				
insular a's	aa. insulares	insular part of cerebral a.		cortex of insula
intercostal a., highest	a. intercostalis suprema	costocervical trunk	posterior intercostal a's I and II	upper thoracic wall
intercostal a's, posterior, I and II	aa. intercostales posteriores I et II	highest intercostal a.	dorsal and spinal branches	upper thoracic wall
intercostal a's, posterior, III-XI	aa. intercostales posteriores III-XI	thoracic aorta	dorsal, spinal, lateral and medial cutaneous collateral, and lateral mammary branches	thoracic wall
interlobar a's of kidney	aa. interlobares renis	renal a.	arcuate a's of kidney	lobes of kidney
interlobular a's of kidney	aa. interlobulares renis	arcuate a's of kidney		renal glomeruli
interlobular a's of liver	aa. interlobulares hepatis	right or left branch of proper hepatic a.	between lobules of liver	
interosseous a., anterior	a. interossea anterior	posterior or common interosseous a.	median a.	deep parts of front of forearm
interosseous a., common	a. interossea communis	ulnar a.	anterior and posterior interosseous a's	antecubital fossa
interosseous a., posterior	a. interossea posterior	common interosseous a.	recurrent interosseous a.	deep parts of back of forearm
interosseous a., recurrent	a. interossea recurrens	posterior or common interosseous a.		back of elbow joint

English Name	NA Term	Origin	Branches	Distribution
intestinal a's			vessels arising from superior mesenteric a. and supplying intestines; they include pancreaticoduodenal, jejunal, ileal, ileocolic, and colic a's	
jejunal a's	aa. jejunales	superior mesenteric a.		jejunum
a's of kidney *See* renal a's				
labial a., inferior	a. labialis inferior	facial a.		lower lip
labial a., superior	a. labialis superior	facial a.	septal and alar branches	upper lip and nose
a. of labyrinth	a. labyrinthi	basilar or anterior inferior cerebellar a.	vestibular and cochlear branches	internal ear
lacrimal a.	a. lacrimalis	ophthalmic a.	lateral palpebral a.	lacrimal gland, eyelids, conjunctiva
laryngeal a., inferior	a. laryngea inferior	inferior thyroid a.		larynx, trachea, esophagus
laryngeal a., superior	a. laryngea superior	superior thyroid a.		larynx
lingual a.	a. lingualis	external carotid a.	suprahyoid, sublingual, dorsal lingual, profunda linguae branches	tongue, sublingual gland, tonsil, epiglottis
lingual a., deep. *See* profunda linguae a.				
lumbar a's	aa. lumbales	abdominal aorta	dorsal and spinal branches	posterior abdominal wall, renal capsule
lumbar a., lowest	a. lumbalis ima	median sacral a.		sacrum, greatest gluteal muscle
mammary a., external. *See* thoracic a., lateral				
mammary a., internal. *See* thoracic a., internal				
mandibular a. *See* alveolar a., inferior				
masseteric a.	a. masseterica	maxillary a.		masseter muscle
maxillary a.	a. maxillaris	external carotid a.	pterygoid branches; deep auricular, anterior tympanic, inferior alveolar, middle meningeal, masseteric, deep temporal, buccal, posterior superior alveolar, infraorbital, descending palatine, and sphenopalatine a's, and a. of pterygoid canal	both jaws, teeth, muscles of mastication, ear, meninges, nose, paranasal sinuses, palate
maxillary a., external. *See* facial a.				

(continued)

3-1. ARTERIES—cont'd

Common Name*	TA Equivalent†	Origin*	Branches*	Distribution
maxillary a., internal. *See* maxillary a.				
median a.	a. comitans nervi mediani	anterior interosseous a.		median nerve, muscles of front of forearm
meningeal a., middle	a. meningea media	maxillary a.	frontal, parietal, lacrimal, anastomotic, accessory meningeal, and petrous branches, and superior tympanic a.	cranial bones, dura mater
meningeal a., posterior	a. meningea posterior	ascending pharyngeal a.		bones and dura mater of posterior cranial fossa
mesencephalic a's	aa. mesencephalicae	basilar a.		cerebral peduncle
mesenteric a., inferior	a. mesenterica inferior	abdominal aorta	left colic, sigmoid, and superior rectal a's	descending colon, rectum
mesenteric a., superior	a. mesenterica superior	abdominal aorta	inferior pancreaticoduodenal, jejunal, ileal, ileocolic, right and middle colic a's	small intestine, proximal half of colon
metacarpal a's, dorsal	aa. metacarpales dorsales	dorsal carpal rete and radial a.	dorsal digital a's	dorsum of fingers
metacarpal a's, palmar	aa. metacarpales palmares	deep palmar arch		deep parts of metacarpus
metatarsal a's, dorsal	aa. metatarsales dorsales	arcuate a. of foot	dorsal digital a's	dorsum of foot, including toes
metatarsal a's, plantar	aa. metatarsales plantares	plantar arch	perforating branches, common and proper plantar digital a's	plantar surface of toes
musculophrenic a.	a. musculophrenica	internal thoracic a.		diaphragm, abdominal and thoracic walls
nasal's a's, posterior lateral	aa. nasales posteriores laterales	sphenopalatine a.		frontal, maxillary, and sphenoidal sinuses
nutrient a's of femur	aa. nutriciae femoris	third perforating a.		femur
nutrient a's of fibula	aa. nutriciae fibulae	fibular a.		fibula
nutrient a's of humerus	aa. nutriciae humeri	brachial and deep brachial a's		humerus
nutrient a's of tibia	aa. nutriciae tibiae	posterior tibial a.		tibia
obturator a.	a. obturatoria	internal iliac a.	pubic, acetabular, anterior and posterior branches	pelvic muscles, hip joint
obturator a., accessory	a. obturatoria accessoria	variant obturator a. arising from inferior epigastric instead of internal iliac a.		

occipital a.	a. occipitalis	external carotid a.	auricular, meningeal, mastoid, descending, occipital, and sternocleidomastoid branches	muscles of neck and scalp, meninges, mastoid cells
occipital a., lateral	a. occipitalis lateralis	posterior cerebral a.	anterior temporal, middle intermediate temporal, and posterior temporal branches	anterior, medial, intermediate, and posterior parts of temporal lobe
occipital a., middle	a. occipitalis medialis	posterior cerebral a.	dorsal corpus callosum, parietal, parieto-occipital, calcarine, occipital, occipitotemporal branches	dorsum of corpus callosum, precuneus, cuneus, lingual gyrus, posterior part of lateral surface of occipital lobe
ophthalmic a.	a. ophthalmica	internal carotid a.	lacrimal and supraorbital a's, central a. of retina, ciliary, posterior and anterior ethmoidal, palpebral, supratrochlear, and dorsal nasal a's	eye, orbit, adjacent facial structures
ovarian a.	a. ovarica	abdominal aorta	ureteral and tubal branches	ureter, ovary, uterine tube
palatine a., ascending	a. palatina ascendens	facial a.		soft palate, wall of pharynx, tonsil, auditory tube
palatine a., descending	a. palatina descendens	maxillary a.	greater and lesser palatine a's	soft and hard palates, tonsil
palatine a., greater	a. palatina major	descending palatine a.		hard palate
palatine a's, lesser	aa. palatinae minores	descending palatine a.		soft palate, tonsil
palpebral a's, lateral	aa. palpebrales laterales	lacrimal a.		eyelids, conjunctiva
palpebral a's, medial	aa. palpebrales mediales	ophthalmic a.		eyelids
pancreaticoduodenal a., anterior superior	a. pancreaticoduodenalis superior anterior	gastroduodenal a.	pancreatic and duodenal branches	pancreas, duodenum
pancreaticoduodenal a's, inferior	aa. pancreaticoduodenales inferiores	superior mesenteric a.	anterior and posterior branches	pancreas, duodenum
pancreaticoduodenal a., posterior superior	a. pancreaticoduodenalis superior posterior	gastroduodenal a.	pancreatic and duodenal branches	pancreas, duodenum
paracentral a.	a. paracentralis	anterior cerebral a.		cerebral cortex and medial central sulcus
anterior and superior parietal a's	aa. parietales anterior et posterior	middle cerebral a.	anterior and posterior branches	anterior parietal lobe and posterior temporal lobe
parieto-occipital a.	a. parieto-occipitalis	anterior cerebral a.		parietal lobe and sometimes occipital lobe
perforating a's	aa. perforantes	deep femoral a.	nutrient a's	adductor, hamstring, and gluteal muscles, femur
pericardiacophrenic a.	a. pericardiacophrenica	internal thoracic a.		pericardium, diaphragm, pleura
perineal a.	a. perinealis	internal pudendal a.		perineum, skin of external genitalia

(continued)

3-1. ARTERIES—cont'd

Common Name*	TA Equivalent†	Origin*	Branches*	Distribution
peroneal a.	a. fibularis	posterior tibial a.	perforating, communicating, calcaneal, and lateral and medial malleolar branches, calcaneal rete	lateral side and back of ankle, deep calf muscles
pharyngeal a., ascending	a. pharyngea ascendens	external carotid a.	posterior meningeal, pharyngeal, inferior tympanic branches	pharynx, soft palate, ear, meninges
phrenic a's, great, See phrenic a's, inferior				
phrenic a's, inferior	aa. phrenicae inferiores	abdominal aorta	superior suprarenal a's	diaphragm, suprarenal gland
phrenic a's, superior	aa. phrenicae superiores	thoracic aorta		upper surface of vertebral portion of diaphragm
plantar a., lateral	a. plantaris lateralis	posterior tibial a.	plantar arch, plantar metatarsal a's	sole of foot, toes
plantar a., medial	a. plantaris medialis	posterior tibial a.	deep and superficial branches	sole of foot, toes
pontine a's	aa. pontis	basilar a.		pons and adjacent areas of the brain
popliteal a.	a. poplitea	continuation of femoral a.	lateral and medial superior genicular, middle genicular, sural, lateral and medial inferior genicular, anterior and posterior tibial a's; articular rete of knee, patellar rete	knee and calf
precuneal a.	a. precunealis	anterior cerebral a.		inferior precuneus
princeps pollicis a.	a. princeps pollicis	radial a.	radialis indicis a.	sides and palmar aspect of thumb
principal a. of thumb. See princeps pollicis a.				
profunda linguae a.	a. profunda linguae	lingual a.		tongue
a. of pterygoid canal	a. canalis pterygoidei	maxillary a.	pterygoid	roof of pharynx, auditory tube
pudendal a's, external	aa. pudendae externae	femoral a.	anterior scrotal or anterior labial branches, inguinal branches	external genitalia, upper medial thigh

pudendal a., internal	a. pudenda interna	internal iliac a.	external genitalia, anal canal, perineum
			posterior scrotal or posterior labial branches, inferior rectal, perineal, urethral a's, a. of bulb of penis or vestibule, deep a. and dorsal a. of penis or clitoris
pulmonary a., left	a. pulmonalis sinistra	pulmonary trunk	left lung
			numerous branches named according to segments of lung to which they distribute unaerated blood
pulmonary a., right	a. pulmonalis dextra	pulmonary trunk	right lung
			numerous branches named according to segments of lung to which they distribute unaerated blood
pulmonary trunk	truncus pulmonalis	right ventricle	conveys unaerated blood toward lungs
			right and left pulmonary a's
radial a.	a. radialis	brachial a.	forearm, wrist, hand
			palmar carpal, superficial palmar and dorsal carpal branches; recurrent radial a., princeps pollicis a., deep palmar arch
radial a., collateral. *See* collateral a., radial			
radial a. of index finger. *See* radialis indicis a.			
radialis indicis a.	a. radialis indicis	princeps pollicis a.	index finger
radiate a's of kidney. *See* interlobular a's of kidney			
ranine a. *See* profunda linguae a.			
rectal a., inferior	a. rectalis inferior	internal pudendal a.	rectum, anal canal
rectal a., middle	a. rectalis media	internal iliac a.	rectum, prostate, seminal vesicles, vagina
rectal a., superior	a. rectalis superior	inferior mesenteric a.	rectum
recurrent a., radial	a. recurrens radialis	radial a.	brachioradial and brachial muscles, elbow region
recurrent a., tibial, anterior	a. recurrens tibialis anterior	anterior tibial a.	anterior tibial muscle and long extensor muscle of toes; knee joint, contiguous fascia and skin

(continued)

3.1. ARTERIES—cont'd

Common Name*	TA Equivalent†	Origin*	Branches*	Distribution
recurrent a., tibial, posterior	a. recurrens tibialis posterior	anterior tibial a.		knee
recurrent a., ulnar	a. recurrens ulnaris	ulnar a.		elbow region
renal a.	a. renalis	abdominal aorta	anterior and posterior branches, ureteral branches, inferior supra-renal a.	kidney, suprarenal gland, ureter
renal a's. See arcuate, interlobar, and interlobular a's, and straight arterioles of kidney				
a. of round ligament of uterus	aa. renis			
sacral a's, lateral	a. ligamenti teretis uteri	inferior epigastric a.		round ligament of uterus
sacral a., median	aa. sacrales laterales	iliolumbar a.	spinal branches	structures about coccyx and sacrum
scapular a., dorsal	a. sacralis mediana	central continuation of abdominal aorta, beyond origin of common iliac a's	lowest lumbar a.	sacrum, coccyx, rectum
scapular a., transverse. See suprascapular a.	a. dorsalis scapularis	subclavian (deep) branch of transverse cervical a.		rhomboid, latissimus dorsi, trapezius muscles
sciatic a.	a. comitans nervi ischiadici	inferior gluteal a.		accompanies sciatic nerve
sigmoid a's	aa. sigmoideae	inferior mesenteric a.		sigmoid colon
spermatic a., external. See cremasteric a.				
sphenopalatine a.	a. sphenopalatina	maxillary a.	posterior lateral nasal a. and posterior septal branches	structures adjoining nasal cavity, nasopharynx
spinal a., anterior	a. spinalis anterior	vertebral a.		spinal cord
spinal a., posterior	a. spinalis posterior	vertebral a.		spinal cord
splenic a.	a. splenica	celiac trunk	pancreatic and splenic branches, left gastroepiploic, short gastric a's	spleen, pancreas, stomach, greater omentum
straight arterioles of kidney	arteriolae rectae renis	arcuate a's of kidney		renal pyramids
stylomastoid a.	a. stylomastoidea	posterior auricular a.	mastoid and stapedial branches, posterior tympanica	middle ear walls, mastoid cells, stapedius
subclavian a.	a. subclavia	brachiocephalic trunk (right), arch of aorta (left)	vertebral, internal thoracic a's, thyrocervical and costocervical trunks	neck, thoracic wall, spinal cord, brain, meninges, upper limb
subcostal a.	a. subcostalis	thoracic aorta	dorsal and spinal branches	upper posterior abdominal wall
sublingual a.	a. sublingualis	lingual a.		sublingual gland

submental a.	a. submentalis	facial a.		tissue under chin
subscapular a.	a. subscapularis	axillary a.	thoracodorsal and circumflex scapular a's	scapular and shoulder region
a. of central sulcus	a. sulci centralis	middle cerebral a.		cortex on either side of central sulcus
a. of postcentral sulcus	a. sulci postcentralis	middle cerebral a.		cortex on either side of postcentral sulcus
a. of precentral sulcus	a. sulci precentralis	middle cerebral a.		cortex on either side of precentral sulcus
supraduodenal a.	a. supraduodenalis	gastroduodenal a.	duodenal branch	superior part of duodenum
supraorbital a.	a. supraorbitalis	ophthalmic a.		forehead, superior muscles of orbit, upper eyelid, frontal sinus
suprarenal a., inferior	a. suprarenalis inferior	renal a.		suprarenal gland
suprarenal a., middle	a. suprarenalis media	abdominal aorta		suprarenal gland
suprarenal a's, superior	aa. suprarenales superiores	inferior phrenic a.		suprarenal gland
suprascapular a.	a. suprascapularis	thyrocervical trunk	acromial branch	clavicular, deltoid, and scapular regions
supratrochlear a.	a. supratrochlearis	ophthalmic a.		anterior scalp
sural a's	aa. surales	popliteal a.		popliteal space, calf
sylvian a. *See* cerebral a., middle				
tarsal a., lateral	a. tarsalis lateralis	dorsalis pedis a.		tarsus
tarsal a's, medial	aa. tarsales mediales	dorsalis pedis a.		side of foot
temporal a., anterior	a. temporalis anterior	middle cerebral a.		cortex of anterior temporal lobe
temporal a., anterior deep	a. temporalis profunda anterior	maxillary a.	to zygomatic bone and greater wing of sphenoid bone	temporal muscle
temporal a's, deep	aa. temporales profundae	maxillary a.		deep parts of temporal region
temporal a., middle	a. temporalis media	1. superficial temporal a. 2. middle cerebral a.		1. temporal region 2. cortex of temporal lobe
temporal a., posterior	a. temporalis posterior	middle cerebral a.		cortex of posterior temporal lobe
temporal a., posterior deep	a. temporalis profunda posterior	maxillary a.		temporal muscle
temporal a., superficial	a. temporalis superficialis	external carotid a.	parotid, auricular, and occipital branches; transverse facial, zygomatico-orbital, middle temporal a's	parotid and temporal regions
testicular a.	a. testicularis	abdominal aorta	ureteral and epididymal branches	ureter, epididymis, testis
thoracic a., highest	a. thoracica suprema	axillary a.		axillary aspects of chest wall

(continued)

3-1. ARTERIES—cont'd

Common Name*	TA Equivalent†	Origin*	Branches*	Distribution
thoracic a., internal	a. thoracica interna	subclavian a.	mediastinal, thymic, bronchial, tracheal, sternal, perforating, medial mammary, lateral costal and anterior intercostal branches; pericardiacophrenic, musculophrenic, superior epigastric a's	anterior thoracic wall, mediastinal structures, diaphragm
thoracic a., lateral	a. thoracica lateralis	axillary a.	mammary branches	pectoral muscles, mammary gland
thoracoacromial a.	a. thoracoacromialis	axillary a.	clavicular, pectoral, deltoid, and acromial branches	deltoid, clavicular, thoracic regions
thoracodorsal a.	a. thoracodorsalis	subscapular a.		subscapular and teres major and minor muscles
thyrocervical trunk	truncus thyrocervicalis	subclavian a.	inferior thyroid, suprascapular and transverse cervical a's	deep neck, including thyroid gland, scapular region
thyroid a., inferior	a. thyroidea inferior	thyrocervical trunk	pharyngeal, esophageal, tracheal branches; inferior laryngeal, ascending cervical a's	thyroid gland and adjacent structures
thyroid a., lowest. *See* thyroidea ima a.				
thyroid a., superior	a. thyroidea superior	external carotid a.	hyoid, sternocleidomastoid, superior laryngeal, cricothyroid, muscular, and glandular branches	thyroid gland and adjacent structures
thyroidea ima a.	a. thyroidea ima	arch of aorta, brachiocephalic trunk or right common carotid a.		thyroid gland
tibial a., anterior	a. tibialis anterior	popliteal a.	posterior and anterior tibial recurrent a's, lateral and medial anterior malleolar a's, lateral and medial malleolar retes	leg, ankle, foot
tibial a., posterior	a. tibialis posterior	popliteal a.	fibular circumflex branch; peroneal, medial plantar, lateral plantar a's	leg, foot

	Latin	Origin	Branches	Distribution
transverse a., of face. *See* facial a., transverse				
transverse a. of neck. *See* cervical a., transverse				
transverse a. of scapula. *See* suprascapular a.				
tympanic a., anterior	a. tympanica anterior	maxillary a.		tympanic cavity
tympanic a., inferior	a. tympanica inferior	ascending pharyngeal a.		tympanic cavity
tympanic a., posterior	a. tympanica posterior	stylomastoid a.		tympanic cavity
tympanic a., superior	a. tympanica superior	middle meningeal a.		tympanic cavity
ulnar a.	a. ulnaris	brachial a.	palmar carpal, dorsal carpal, and deep palmar branches; ulnar recurrent and common interosseous a's; superficial palmar arch	forearm, wrist, hand
ulnar a., collateral. *See* collateral a., ulnar, inferior and collateral a., ulnar, superior				
umbilical a.	a. umbilicalis	internal iliac a.	a. of ductus deferens, superior vesical a's	ductus deferens, seminal vesicles, testes, urinary bladder, ureter
urethral a.	a. urethralis	internal pudendal a.		urethra
uterine a.	a. uterina	internal iliac a.	ovarian and tubal branches; vaginal a.	uterus, vagina, round ligament of uterus, uterine tube, ovary
vaginal a.	a. vaginalis	uterine a.		vagina, fundus of bladder
vertebral a.	a. vertebralis	subclavian a.	*transverse part:* spinal and muscular branches; *intracranial part:* anterior spinal a., and posterior inferior cerebellar a. and its branches	muscles of neck, vertebrae, spinal cord, cerebellum, interior of cerebrum
vesical a., inferior	a. vesicalis inferior	internal iliac a.	prostatic	bladder, prostate, seminal vesicles, lower ureter
vesical a's, superior	aa. vesicales superiores	umbilical a.		bladder, urachus, ureter
zygomatico-orbital a.	a. zygomatico-orbitalis	superficial temporal a.		lateral side of orbit

3-2. BONES: LISTED BY BODY REGION

Region	Name	Total Number	Region	Name	Total Number
Axial skeleton			**Appendicular Skeleton**		
Skull	(eight paired–16)	21	Upper limb (× 2) Shoulder	scapula clavicle	64
	inferior nasal concha		Upper arm	humerus	
	lacrimal				
	maxilla				
	nasal		Lower arm	radius ulna	
	palatine				
	parietal			carpal (8)	
	temporal			(capitate)	
	zygomatic		Wrist	(hamate)	
	(five unpaired–5)			(lunate)	
	ethmoid			(pisiform)	
	frontal			(scaphoid)	
	occipital			(trapezium)	
	sphenoid			(trapezoid)	
	vomer			(triquetral)	
Ossicles of each ear	incus malleus stapes	6			
Lower jaw	mandible	1			
Neck	hyoid	1	Hand	metacarpal (5)	
			Fingers	phalanges (14)	
Vertebral column	cervical vertebrae (7)	26	Lower limb (× 2)		62
	(atlas)		Pelvis	hipbone (1)	
	(axis)			(ilium)	
	thoracic vertebrae (12)			(ischium)	
	lumbar vertebrae (5)			(pubis)	
	sacrum (5 fused)				
	coccyx (4–5 fused)				
Chest	sternum	1			
	ribs (12 pairs)	24	Thigh	femur	
			Knee	patella	
			Leg	tibia fibula	
			Ankle	tarsal (7)	
				(calcaneus)	
				(cuboid)	
				(cuneiform, medial)	
				(cuneiform, intermediate)	
				(cuneiform, lateral)	
				(navicular)	
				(talus)	
			Foot	metatarsal (5)	
			Toes	phalanges (14)	

Common Name*	TA Equivalent†	Region	Description	Articulations
astragalus. *See* talus atlas	atlas	neck	first cervical vertebra, ring of bone supporting the skull	with occipital b. and axis
axis	axis	neck	second cervical vertebra, with thick process (odontoid process) around which first cervical vertebra pivots	with atlas above and third cervical vertebra below
calcaneus	calcaneus	foot	the "heel bone," or irregular cuboidal shape, largest of the tarsal bones	with talus and cuboid b.
capitate b.	o. capitatum	wrist	with second, third, and fourth metacarpal b's, and hamate, lunate, trapezoid, and scaphoid b's	
carpal b's	ossa carpi	wrist	*see* capitate, hamate, lunate, pisiform b's, scaphoid, trapezium, trapezoid, and triquetral b's	
clavicle	clavicula	shoulder	elongated slender, curved bone (collar bone) lying horizontally at root of neck, in upper part of thorax	with sternum and ipsilateral scapula and cartilage of first rib
coccyx	o. coccygis	lower back	triangular bone formed usually by fusion of last 4 (sometimes 3 or 5) (coccygeal) vertebrae	with sacrum
concha, nasal	concha nasalis	skull	(*superior, inferior, middle,* and *supreme*) thin bony plates within the nasal cavity	with ethmoid and ipsilateral lacrimal and palatine b's and maxilla
cuboid bone	o. cuboideum	foot	pyramidal bone, on lateral side of foot, in front of calcaneus	with calcaneus, lateral cuneiform b., fourth and fifth metatarsal b's, occasionally with navicular b.
cuneiform b., intermediate	o. cuneiforme intermedium	foot	smallest of 3 cuneiform b's, located between medial and lateral cuneiform b's	with navicular, medial and lateral cuneiform b's, and second metatarsal b.
cuneiform b., lateral	o. cuneiforme laterale	foot	wedge-shaped bone at lateral side of foot, intermediate in size between medial and intermediate cuneiform b's	with cuboid, navicular, intermediate cuneiform b's and second, third, and fourth metatarsal b's
cuneiform b., medial	o. cuneiforme mediale	foot	largest of 3 cuneiform b's, at medial side of foot	with navicular, intermediate cuneiform, and first and second metatarsal b's
epistropheus. *See* axis ethmoid b.	o. ethmoidale	skull	unpaired bone in front of sphenoid b. and below frontal b., forming part of nasal septum and superior and medial conchae of nose	with sphenoid and frontal b's, vomer, and both lacrimal, nasal, and palatine b's, maxillae, and inferior nasal conchae
fabella		knee	sesamoid b. in lateral head of gastrocnemius muscle	with femur
femur	femur	thigh	longest, strongest, heaviest bone of the body (thigh b.)	proximally with hip b., distally with patella and tibia
fibula	fibula	leg	lateral and smaller of 2 bones of leg	proximally with tibia, distally with tibia and talus

(continued)

*b. = bone; b's = (pl.) bones.
†o. = os.

3-3. BONES—cont'd

Common Name*	TA Equivalent†	Region	Description	Articulations
frontal b.	o. frontale	skull	unpaired bone constituting anterior part of skull	with ethmoid and sphenoid b's, and both parietal, nasal, lacrimal, and zygomatic b's, and maxillae
hamate b.	o. hamatum	wrist	most medial of 4 bones of distal row of carpal b's	with fourth and fifth metacarpal b's and lunate, capitate, and triquetral b's
hip b.	o. coxae	pelvis and hip	broadest bone of skeleton, composed originally of 3 bones which become fused together in acetabulum: *ilium*, broad, flaring, uppermost portion; *ischium*, thick three-sided part behind and below acetabulum and behind obturator foramen; *pubis*, consisting of body (expanded anterior portion), inferior ramus (extending backward and fusing with ramus of ischium), and superior ramus (extending from body to acetabulum)	with femur, anteriorly with its fellow (at symphysis pubis), posteriorly with sacrum
humerus	humerus	arm	long bone of upper arm	proximally with scapula, distally with radius and ulna
hyoid b.	o. hyoideum	neck	U-shaped bone at root of tongue, between mandible and larynx	none; attached by ligaments and muscles to skull and larynx
ilium	o. ilii	pelvis	*see* hip b.	
incus	incus	ear	middle ossicle of chain in the middle ear, so named because of its resemblance to an anvil	with malleus and stapes
innominate b. *See* hip b.				
ischium	o. ischii	pelvis	*see* hip b.	
lacrimal b.	o. lacrimale	skull	thin, uneven scale of bone near rim of medial wall of each orbit	with ethmoid and frontal b's, and ipsilateral inferior nasal concha and maxilla
lunate b.	o. lunatum	wrist	second from thumb side of 4 bones of proximal row of carpus	with radius, and capitate, hamate, scaphoid, and triquetral b's
malleus	malleus	ear	most lateral ossicle of chain in middle ear, so named because of its resemblance to a hammer	with incus; fibrous attachment to tympanic membrane
mandible	mandibula	lower jaw	horseshoe-shaped bone carrying lower teeth	with temporal b's
maxilla	maxilla	skull (upper jaw)	paired bone, below orbit and at either side of nasal cavity, carrying upper teeth	with ethmoid and frontal b's, vomer, fellow maxilla, and ipsilateral inferior nasal concha and lacrimal, nasal, palatine, and zygomatic b's

maxilla, inferior.
See mandible

Bone	Region	Description	Articulations
		concave on palmar surface	second—third metacarpal b., trapezium, trapezoid, capitate, and proximal phalanx of index finger (second digit); third—second and fourth metacarpal b's, capitate and proximal phalanx of middle finger (third digit); fourth—third and fifth metacarpal b's, capitate, hamate, and proximal phalanx of ring finger (fourth digit); fifth—fourth metacarpal b., hamate b., and proximal phalanx of little finger (fifth digit)
metatarsal b's ossa metatarsi	foot	five miniature long bones of foot, concave on plantar and slightly convex on dorsal surface	first—medial cuneiform b., proximal phalanx of great toe, and occasionally with second metatarsal b.; second—medial, intermediate, and lateral cuneiform b's, third and occasionally with first metatarsal b., and proximal phalanx of second toe; third—lateral cuneiform b., second and fourth metatarsal b's and proximal phalanx of third toe; fourth—lateral cuneiform b., cuboid b., third and fifth metatarsal b's, and proximal phalanx of fourth toe; fifth—cuboid b., fourth metatarsal b., and proximal phalanx of fifth toe
multangulum majus. *See* trapezium; trapezoid			
nasal b. o. nasale	skull	paired bone, the two uniting in median plane to form bridge of nose	with frontal and ethmoid b's, fellow of opposite side, and ipsilateral maxilla
navicular b. o. naviculare	foot	bone at medial side of tarsus, between talus and cuneiform b's	with talus and 3 cuneiform b's occasionally with cuboid b.
occipital b. o. occipitale	skull	unpaired bone constituting back and part of base of skull	with sphenoid b. and atlas and both parietal and temporal b's
os magnum. *See* capitate b.			
palatine b. o. palatinum	skull	paired bone, the two forming posterior portions of bony palate	with ethmoid and sphenoid b's, vomer, fellow of opposite side, and ipsilateral inferior nasal concha and maxilla
parietal b. o. parietale	skull	paired bone between frontal and occipital b's, forming superior and lateral parts of skull	with frontal, occipital, sphenoid, fellow parietal, and ipsilateral temporal b's
patella	knee	small, irregularly rectangular compressed (sesamoid) bone over anterior aspect of knee (kneecap)	with femur

(continued)

3-3. BONES—cont'd

Common Name*	TA Equivalent†	Region	Description	Articulations
phalanges (proximal, middle, and distal phalanges)	ossa digitorum (phalanx proximalis, phalanx media, and phalanx distalis)	fingers and toes	miniature long bones, two only in thumb and great toe, three in each of other fingers and toes	proximal phalanx of each digit with corresponding metacarpal or metatarsal b., and phalanx distal to it; other phalanges with phalanges proximal and distal (if any) to them
pisiform b.	o. pisiforme	wrist	medial and palmar of 4 bones of proximal row of carpal b's	with triquetral b.
pubic b.	o. pubis	pelvis	see hip b.	
radius	radius	forearm	lateral and shorter of 2 bones of forearm	proximally with humerus and ulna; distally with ulna and lunate and scaphoid b's
ribs	ossa costalia	chest	12 pairs of thin, narrow, curved long bones, forming posterior and lateral walls of chest	all posteriorly with thoracic vertebrae; upper 7 pairs (true ribs) with sternum; lower 5 pairs (false ribs), by costal cartilages, with rib above or (lowest 2—floating ribs) unattached anteriorly
sacrum	o. sacrum	lower back	wedge-shaped bone formed usually by fusion of 5 vertebrae below lumbar vertebrae, constituting posterior wall of pelvis	with fifth lumbar vertebra above, coccyx below, and with ilium at each side
scaphoid	o. scaphoideum	wrist	most lateral of 4 bones of proximal row of carpal b's	with radius, trapezium, and trapezoid, capitate and lunate b's
scapula	scapula	shoulder	wide, thin, triangular bone (shoulder blade) opposite second to seventh ribs in upper part of back	with ipsilateral clavicle and humerus
sesamoid b's	ossa. sesamoidea	chiefly hands and feet	small, flat, round bones related to joints between phalanges or between digits and metacarpal or metatarsal b's; include also 2 at knee (fabella and patella)	
sphenoid b.	o. sphenoidale	base of skull	unpaired, irregularly shaped bone, constituting part of sides and base of skull and part of lateral wall or orbit	with frontal, occipital, and ethmoid b's, vomer and both parietal, temporal, palatine, and zygomatic b's
stapes	stapes	ear	most medial ossicle of chain in middle ear, so named because of its resemblance to a stirrup	with incus; ligamentous attachment to fenestra vestibuli

Term	Latin	Region	Description
sternum	sternum	chest	elongated flat bone, forming anterior wall of chest, consisting of 3 segments: *manubrium* (topmost segment), *body* (in youth composed of 4 separate segments joined by cartilage), and *xiphoid process* (lowermost segment); with both clavicles and upper 7 pairs of ribs
talus	talus	ankle	the "ankle bone," second largest of tarsal b's; with tibia, fibula, calcaneus, and navicular b.
tarsal b's	ossa tarsi	ankle and foot	*see* calcaneus, cuboid, intermediate, lateral, and medial cuneiform b's, navicular b., and talus
temporal b.	o. temporale	skull	irregularly shaped bone, one on either side, forming part of side and base of skull, and containing middle and inner ear; with occipital, sphenoid, mandible, and ipsilateral parietal and zygomatic b's
tibia	tibia	leg	medial and larger of 2 bones of lower leg (shin b.); proximally with femur and fibula, distally with talus and fibula
trapezium	o. trapezium	wrist	most lateral of 4 bones of distal row of carpal b's; with first and second metacarpal b's and trapezoid and scaphoid b's
trapezoid b.	o. trapezoideum	wrist	second from thumb side of 4 bones of distal row of carpal b's; with second metacarpal b. and capitate, trapezium, and scaphoid b's
triquetral b.	o. triquetrum	wrist	third from thumb side of 4 bones of proximal row of carpal b's; with hamate, lunate, and pisiform b's and articular disk
turbinate b. *See* concha, nasal			
ulna	ulna	forearm	medial and longer of 2 bones of forearm; proximally with humerus and radius, distally with radius and articular disk
vertebrae (cervical, thoracic [dorsal], lumbar, sacral, and coccygeal)	vertebrae (vertebrae cervicales, vertebrae thoracicae, vertebrae lumbales, vertebrae sacrales, vertebrae coccygeae)	back	separate segments of vertebral column; about 33 in the child; uppermost 24 remain separate as true, movable vertebrae; the next 5 fuse to form the sacrum; the lowermost 3–5 fuse to form the coccyx; except first cervical (atlas) and fifth lumbar, each vertebra articulates with adjoining vertebrae above and below; the first cervical articulates with the occipital b. and second cervical vertebra (axis); the fifth lumbar with the fourth lumbar vertebra and sacrum; the thoracic vertebrae articulate also with the heads of the ribs
vomer	vomer	skull	thin bone forming posterior and posteroinferior part of nasal septum; with ethmoid and sphenoid b's and both maxillae and palatine b's
zygomatic b.	o. zygomaticum	skull	bone forming hard part of cheek and lower, lateral portion of rim of each orbit; with frontal and sphenoid b's and ipsilateral maxilla and temporal b.

3-4. MUSCLES

Common Name*	TA Term†	Origin*	Insertion*	Innervation	Action
abductor m. of great toe	m. abductor hallucis	medial tubercle of calcaneus, plantar fascia	medial site of base of proximal phalanx of great toe	medial plantar	abducts, flexes great toe
abductor m. of little finger	m. abductor digiti minimi manus	pisiform bone, tendon of ulnar flexor m. of wrist	medial side of base of proximal phalanx of little finger	ulnar	abducts little finger
abductor m. of little toe	m. abductor digiti minimi pedis	medial and lateral tubercle of calcaneus, plantar fascia	lateral side of base of proximal phalanx of little toe	lateral plantar	abducts little toe
abductor m. of thumb, long	m. abductor pollicis longus	posterior surfaces of radius and ulna	lateral side of bone of first metacarpal bone and trapezium	posterior interosseous	abducts, extends thumb
abductor m of thumb, short	m. abductor pollicis brevis	tubercles of scaphoid and trapezium, flexor retinaculum of hand	lateral side of base of proximal phalanx of thumb	median	abducts thumb
adductor m. great	m. adductor magnus	*deep part*—inferior ramus of pubis, ramus of ischium; *superficial part*—ischial tuberosity	*deep part*—linea aspera of femur; *superficial part*—adductor tubercle of femur	*deep part*—obturator; *superficial part*—sciatic	*deep part*—adducts thigh; *superficial part*—extends thigh
adductor m. of great toe	m. adductor hallucis	*oblique head*—long plantar ligament; *transverse head*—plantar ligaments	lateral side of proximal phalanx of great toe	lateral plantar	flexes, adducts great toe
adductor m., long	m. adductor longus	body of pubis	linea aspera of femur	obturator	adducts, rotates, flexes thigh
adductor m., short	m. adductor brevis	body and inferior ramus of pubis	upper part of linea aspera of femur	obturator	adducts, rotates, flexes thigh
adductor m. of thumb	m. adductor pollicis	*oblique head*—second metacarpal; capitate, and trapezoid; *transverse head*—front of third metacarpal	medial side of base of proximal phalanx of thumb	ulnar	adducts, opposes thumb
anconeus m.	m. anconeus	back of lateral epicondyle of humerus	olecranon and posterior surface of ulna	radial	extends forearm
antitragicus m.	m. antitragicus	outer part of antitragus	caudate process of helix and antihelix	temporal, posteror auricular branches of facial	
arrector m's of hair	mm. arrectores pilorum	dermis	hair follicles	sympathetic	elevate hairs of skin
articular m. of elbow	m. articularis cubiti	a name applied to a few fibers of the deep surface of the triceps m. of arm that insert into the posterior ligament and synovial membrane of the elbow joint			

Common name*	Latin name†	Origin / Insertion	Nerve	Action
articular m. of knee	m. articularis genu	front of lower part of femur; upper part of capsule of knee joint	femoral	raises capsule of knee joint
aryepiglottic m.	m. aryepiglotticus	a name applied to inconstant fibers of oblique arytenoid m., from apex of arytenoid cartilage to lateral margin of epiglottis	recurrent laryngeal	closes inlet of larynx
arytenoid m., oblique	m. arytenoideus obliquus	muscular process of arytenoid cartilage; apex of opposite arytenoid cartilage	recurrent laryngeal	approximates arytenoid cartilage
arytenoid m., transverse	m. arytenoideus transversus	medial surface of arytenoid cartilage; medial surface of opposite arytenoid cartilage	recurrent laryngeal	
auricular m., anterior	m. auricularis anterior	superficial temporal fascia; cartilage of ear	facial	draws auricle forward
auricular m., posterior	m. auricularis posterior	mastoid process; cartilage of ear	facial	draws auricle backward
auricular m., superior	m. auricularis superior	galea aponeurotica; cartilage of ear	facial	raises auricle
biceps m. of arm	m. biceps brachii	*long head*—supraglenoid tubercle of scapula; *short head*—apex of coracoid process; tuberosity of radius, antebrachial fascia, ulna	musculocutaneous	flexes, supinates forearm
biceps m. of thigh	m. biceps femoris	*long head*—ischial tuberosity; *short head*—linea aspera of femur; head of fibula, lateral condyle of tibia	*long head*—tibial; *short head*—peroneal popliteal	flexor, rotates leg laterally, extends thigh
brachial m.	m. brachialis	anterior aspect of humerus; coronoid process of ulna	musculocutaneous, radial	flexes forearm
brachioradial m.	m. brachioradialis	lateral supracondylar ridge of humerus; lateral surface of lower end of radius	radial	flexes forearm
bronchoesophageal m.	m. bronchoesophageus	a name applied to muscle fibers arising from wall of left bronchus, reinforcing musculature of esophagus		
buccinator m.	m. buccinator	buccinator ridge of mandible, alveolar processes of maxilla, pterygomandibular ligament; orbicular m. of mouth at angle of mouth	buccal branch of facial	compresses cheek and retracts angle of mouth
bulbocavernous m.	m. bulbocavernosus, m. bulbospongiosus	tendinous center of perineum, median, raphe of bulb; fascia of penis or clitoris	pudendal	constricts urethra in male, vagina in female
canine m. *See* levator m. of angle of mouth				
ceratocricoid m.	m. ceratocricoideus	a name applied to muscle fibers from cricoid cartilage to inferior horn of thyroid cartilage		
chin m.	m. mentalis	incisive fossa of mandible; skin of chin	facial	wrinkles skin of chin
chondroglossus m.	m. chondroglossus	lesser horn and body of hyoid bone; substance of tongue	hypoglossal	depresses, retracts tongue

(continued)

*m. = muscle; m's = (pl.) muscles.
†m. = [L.] musculus; mm. = [(L. pl.)] musculi.

3-4. MUSCLES—cont'd

Common Name*	TA Term†	Origin*	Insertion*	Innervation	Action
ciliary m.	m. ciliaris	*longitudinal division* (Brücke's m's)—junction of cornea and sclera; *circular division* (Müller's m.)—sphincter of ciliary body	outer layer of choroid and ciliary processes	short ciliary	makes lens more convex in visual accommodation
coccygeus m.	m. coccygeus	ischial spine	lateral border of lower part of sacrum, coccyx	third and fourth sacral	supports and raises coccyx
constrictor m. of pharynx, inferior	m. constrictor pharyngis inferior	undersurfaces of cricoid and thyroid cartilages	median raphe of posterior wall of pharynx	glossopharyngeal, pharyngeal plexus, external branch of superior laryngeal and recurrent laryngeal	constricts pharynx
constrictor m. of pharynx, middle	m. constrictor pharyngis medius	horns of hyoid bone, stylohyoid ligament	median raphe of posterior wall of pharynx	pharyngeal plexus of vagus, glossopharyngeal	constricts pharynx
constrictor m. of pharynx, superior	m. constrictor pharyngis superior	pterygoid plate, pterygomandibular raphe, mylohyoid ridge of mandible, mucous membrane of floor of mouth	median raphe of posterior wall of pharynx	pharyngeal plexus of vagus	constricts pharynx
coracobrachial m.	m. coracobrachialis	coracoid process of scapula	medial surface of shaft of humerus	musculocutaneous	flexes, adducts arm
corrugator m., superciliary	m. corrugator supercilii	medial end of superciliary arch	skin of eyebrow	facial	draws eyebrow downward and medially
cremaster m.	m. cremaster	inferior margin of internal oblique m. of abdomen	pubic tubercle	genital branch of genitofemoral	elevates testis
cricoarytenoid m., lateral	m. cricoarytenoideus lateralis	lateral surface of cricoid cartilage	muscular process of arytenoid cartilage	recurrent laryngeal	approximates vocal folds
cricoarytenoid m., posterior	m. cricoarytenoideus posterior	back of lamina of cricoid cartilage	muscular process of arytenoid cartilage	recurrent laryngeal	separates vocal folds
cricothyroid m.	m. cricothyroideus	front and side of cricoid cartilage	lamina and inferior horn of thyroid cartilage	external branch of superior laryngeal	tenses vocal folds
deltoid m.	m. deltoideus	clavicle, acromion, spine of scapula	deltoid tuberosity of humerus	axillary	abducts, flexes, or extends arm
depressor m. of angle of mouth	m. depressor anguli oris	lateral border of mandible	angle of mouth	facial	pulls down angle of mouth

depressor m. of lower lip	m. depressor labii inferioris	anterior surface of lower border of mandible	orbicular m. of mouth and skin of lower lip	facial	depresses lower lip
depressor m. of septum of nose	m. depressor septi nasi	incisive fossa of maxilla	ala and septum of nose	facial	constricts nostril and depresses ala
depressor m., superciliary	m. depressor supercilii	a name applied to a few fibers of orbital part of orbicular m. of eye that are inserted into the eyebrow, which they depress			
detrusor m. of bladder	m. detrusor vesicae	bundles of smooth muscle fibers forming the muscular coat of the urinary bladder, which are arranged in a longitudinal and a circular layer and on contraction serve to expel urine			
detrusor urinae. *See* detrusor m. of bladder					
diaphragm	diaphragma	back of xiphoid process, inner surfaces of lower 6 costal cartilages and lower 4 ribs, medial and lateral arcuate ligaments, bodies of upper lumbar vertebrae	central tendon of diaphragm	phrenic	increases volume of thorax in inspiration
digastric m.	m. digastricus	*anterior belly*—digastric fossa on lower border of mandible near symphysis; *posterior belly*—mastoid notch of temporal bone	intermediate tendon on hyoid bone	*anterior belly*—mylohyoid branch of inferior alveolar; *posterior belly*—digastric branch of facial	elevates hyoid bone, lowers jaw
dilator m. of pupil	m. dilator pupillae	a name applied to fibers extending radially from sphincter of pupil to ciliary margin		sympathetic	dilates iris
epicranial m.	m. epicranius	a name applied to muscular covering of scalp, including occipitofrontal and temporoparietal m's and galea aponeurotica			
erector m. of spine	m. erector spinae	a name applied to fibers of the more superficial of deep muscles of back, originating from sacrum, spines of lumbar and eleventh and twelfth thoracic vertebrae, and iliac crest, which split and insert as iliocostal, longissimus, and spinal m's			
extensor m. of fingers	m. extensor digitorum	lateral epicondyle of humerus	extensor expansion of 4 medial fingers	deep branch of radial	extends wrist joint and phalanges
extensor m. of great toe, long	m. extensor hallucis longus	front of fibula, interosseous membrane	base of distal phalanx of great toe	deep peroneal	extends great toe, dorsiflexes ankle joint

(continued)

3-4. MUSCLES—cont'd

Common Name*	TA Term†	Origin*	Insertion*	Innervation	Action
extensor m. of great toe, short	m. extensor hallucis brevis	a name applied to portion of short extenser m. of toes that goes to great toe			
extensor m. of index finger	m. extensor indicis	posterior surface of ulna, interosseous membrane	extensor expansion of index finger	posterior interosseous	extends index finger
extensor m. of little finger	m. extensor digiti minimi	lateral epicondyle of humerus	extensor aponeurosis of little finger	deep branch of radial	extends little finger
extensor m. of thumb, long	m. extensor pollicis longus	posterior surface of ulna and interosseous membrane	back of distal phalanx of thumb	posterior interosseous	extends, adducts thumb
extensor m. of thumb, short	m. extensor pollicis brevis	posterior surface of radius	back of proximal phalanx of thumb	posterior interosseous	extends thumb
extensor m. of toes, long	m. extensor digitorum longus	anterior surface of fibula, lateral condyle of tibia, interosseous membrane	extensor expansion of 4 lateral toes	deep peroneal	extends toes
extensor m. of toes, short	m. extensor digitorum brevis	upper surface of calcaneus	extensor tendons of first, second, third, fourth toes	deep peroneal	extends toes
extensor m. of wrist, radial, long	m. extensor carpi radialis longus	lateral supracondylar ridge of humerus	back of base of second metacarpal bone	radial	extends, abducts wrist joint
extensor m. of wrist, radial, short	m. extensor carpi radialis brevis	lateral epicondyle of humerus	back of bases of second and third metacarpal bones	radial or its deep branch	extends, abducts wrist joint
extensor m. of wrist, ulnar	m. extensor carpi ulnaris	*humeral head*—lateral epicondyle of humerus; *ulnar head*—posterior border of ulna	base of fifth metacarpal bone	deep branch of radial	extends, abducts wrist joint
fibular m. *See* peroneal m.					
flexor m. of fingers, deep	m. flexor digitorum profundus	shaft of ulna, coronoid process, interosseous membrane	bases of distal phalanges of 4 medial fingers	anterior interosseous, ulnar	flexes distal phalanges
flexor m. of fingers, superficial	m. flexor digitorum superfi-cialis	*humeroulnar head*—medial epicondyle of humerus, coronoid process of ulna; *radial head*—anterior border of radius	sides of middle phalanges of 4 medial fingers	median	flexes middle phalanges
flexor m. of great toe, long	m. flexor hallucis longus	posterior surface of fibula	base of distal phalanx of great toe	tibial	flexes great toe

		Origin	Insertion	Nerve	Action
flexor m. of great toe, short	m. flexor hallucis brevis	undersurface of cuboid, lateral cuneiform	...sides of base of proximal phalanx of great toe	medial plantar	flexes great toe
flexor m. of little finger, short	m. flexor digiti minimi brevis manus	hook of hamate bone, transverse carpal ligament	medial side of proximal phalanx of little finger	ulnar	flexes little finger
flexor m. of little toe, short	m. flexor digiti minimi brevis pedis	sheath of long peroneal	lateral surface of base of proximal phalanx of little toe	lateral plantar	flexes little toe
flexor m. of thumb, long	m. flexor pollicis longus	anterior surface of radius, medial epicondyle of humerus, coronoid process of ulna	base of distal phalanx of thumb	anterior interosseous	flexes thumb
flexor m. of thumb, short	m. flexor pollicis brevis	tubercle of trapezium, flexor retinaculum	lateral side of base of proximal phalanx of thumb	median, ulnar	flexes, adducts thumb
flexor m. of toes, long	m. flexor digitorum longus pedis	posterior surface of shaft of tibia	distal phalanges of 4 lateral toes	tibial	flexes toes, extends foot
flexor m. of toes, short	m. flexor digitorum brevis pedis	medial tuberosity of calcaneus, plantar fascia	middle phalanges of 4 lateral toes	medial plantar	flexes toes
flexor m. of wrist, radial	m. flexor carpi radialis	medial epicondyle of humerus	bases of second and third metacarpal bones	median	flexes, abducts wrist joint
flexor m. of wrist, ulnar	m. flexor carpi ulnaris	*humeral head*—medial epicondyle of humerus; *ulnar head*—olecranon and posterior border of ulna	pisiform bone, hook of hamate bone, base of fifth metacarpal bone	ulnar	flexes, adducts wrist joint
gastrocnemius m.	m. gastrocnemius	*medial head*—popliteal surface of femur, upper part of medial condyle, capsule of knee; *lateral head*— lateral condyle, capsule of knee	aponeurosis unites with tendon of soleus to form Achilles tendon	tibial	plantar flexes foot, flexes knee joint
gemellus m., inferior	m. gemellus inferior	tuberosity of ischium	internal obturator tendon	nerve to quadrate m. of thigh	rotates thigh laterally
gemellus m., superior	m. gemellus superior	spine of ischium	internal obturator tendon	nerve to internal obturator	rotates thigh laterally
genioglossus m.	m. genioglossus	superior genial tubercle	hyoid bone, undersurface of tongue	hypoglossal	protrudes, depresses tongue
geniohyoid m.	m. geniohyoideus	inferior genial tubercle	body of hyoid bone	a branch of first cervical nerve through hypoglossal	draws hyoid bone forward

(continued)

3-4. MUSCLES—cont'd

Common Name*	TA Term†	Origin*	Insertion*	Innervation	Action
glossopalatine m. *See* palatoglossus m.					
gluteus maximus m., (gluteal m., greatest)	m. gluteus maximus	dorsal aspect of ilium, dorsal surfaces of sacrum, coccyx, sacrotuberous ligament	iliotibial tract of fascia lata, gluteal tuberosity of femur	inferior gluteal	extends, abducts, rotates thigh laterally
gluteus medius m. (gluteal m., middle)	m. gluteus medius	dorsal aspect of ilium between anterior and posterior gluteal lines	greater trochanter of femur	superior gluteal	abducts, rotates thigh medially
gluteus minimus m. (gluteal m., least)	m. gluteus minimus	dorsal aspect of ilium between anterior and posterior gluteal lines	greater trochanter of femur	superior gluteal	abducts, rotates thigh medially
gracilis m.	m. gracilis	body and inferior ramus of pubis	medial surface of shaft of tibia	obturator	adducts thigh, flexes knee joint
m. of helix, greater	m. helicis major	spine of helix	anterior border of helix	auriculotemporal posterior auricular	tenses skin of acoustic meatus
m. of helix, smaller	m. helices minor	anterior rim of helix	concha	temporal, posterior auricular	
hyoglossus m.	m. hyoglossus	body and greater horn of hyoid bone	side of tongue	hypoglossal	depresses, retracts tongue
iliac m.	m. iliacus	iliac fossa, ala of sacrum	greater psoas tendon, lesser trochanter of femur	femoral	flexes thigh, trunk on limb
iliococcygeus m.	m. iliococcygeus	a name applied to posterior portion of levator ani m., including fibers originating as far forward as obturator canal, and inserting on side of coccyx and in anococcygeal ligaments			
iliocostal m.	m. iliocostalis	a name applied to lateral division of erector m. of spine			
iliocostal m. of loins	m. iliocostalis lumborum	iliac crest	angles of lower 6 or 7 ribs	thoracic and lumbar	extends lumbar spine
iliocostal m. of neck	m. iliocostalis cervicis	angles of third, fourth, fifth, and sixth ribs	transverse processes of lower fourth, fifth, and sixth cervical vertebrae	cervical	extends cervical spine
iliocostal m. of thorax	m. iliocostalis thoracis	upper borders of angles of 6 lower ribs	angles of upper ribs and transverse process of seventh cervical vertebra	thoracic	keeps thoracic spine erect
iliopsoas m.	m. iliopsoas	a name applied collectively to iliac and greater psoas m's			
incisive m's of inferior lip	mm. incisivi labii inferioris	incisive fossae of mandible	angle of mouth	facial	make vestibule of mouth shallow

Common Name	Latin Term	Origin	Insertion	Nerve	Action
incisive m's of superior lip	m. incisivi labii superioris	incisive fossa of maxilla	angle of mouth	facial	make vestibule of mouth shallow
m. of incisure of helix	m. incisurae helicis	a name applied to inconstant slips of fibers continuing forward from m. of tragus to bridge notch of cartilaginous part of meatus			
infraspinous m.	m. infraspinatus	infraspinous fossa of scapula	greater tubercle of humerus	suprascapular	rotates arm laterally
intercostal m's	mm. intercostales	a name applied to the layer of muscle fibers separated from the internal intercostal m's by the intercostal nerves and vessels			
intercostal m's, external	mm. intercostales externi	inferior border of rib	superior border of rib below	intercostal	elevate ribs in inspiration
intercostal m's, internal	mm. intercostales interni	inferior border of rib and costal cartilage	superior border of rib and costal cartilage below	intercostal	acts on ribs in expiration
interosseous m's of foot, dorsal	mm. interossei dorsales pedis	sides of adjacent metatarsal bones	base of proximal phalanges of second, third, and fourth toes	lateral plantar	flex, abduct toes
interosseous m's of hand, dorsal	mm. interossei dorsales manus	each by two heads from adjacent sides of metacarpal bones	extensor tendons of second, third, and fourth fingers	ulnar	abduct, flex proximal, extend middle and distal phalanges
interosseous m's, palmar	mm. interossei palmares	sides of first, second, fourth, and fifth metacarpal bones	extensor tendons of first, second, fourth, and fifth fingers	ulnar	adduct, flex proximal, extend middle and distal phalanges
interosseous m's, plantar	mm. interossei plantares	medial sides of third, fourth, and fifth metatarsal bones	medial sides of base of proximal phalanges of third, fourth, and fifth toes	lateral plantar	flex, abduct toes
interspinal m's	mm. interspinales	a name applied to short bands of muscle fibers extending on each side between spinous processes of contiguous vertebrae		spinal	extend vertebral column
intertransverse m's	mm. intertransversarii	a name applied to small muscles passing between transverse processes of adjacent vertebrae		spinal	bend vertebral column laterally
Ischiocavernous m.	m. ischiocavernosus	ramus of ischium	crus of penis or clitoris	perineal branches of pudendal	maintains erection of penis or clitoris
latissimus dorsi m.	m. latissimus dorsi	spines of lower thoracic vertebrae, spines of lumbar and sacral vertebrae through attachment to thoracolumbar fascia, iliac crest, lower ribs, inferior angle of scapula	floor or intertubercular groove of humerus	thoracodorsal	adducts, extends, rotates humerus medially

(continued)

Common Name*	TA Term†	Origin*	Insertion*	Innervation	Action
levator m. of angle of mouth	m. levator anguli oris	canine fossa of maxilla	orbicular m. of mouth, skin at angle of mouth	facial	raises angle of mouth
levator ani m.	m. levator ani	a name applied collectively to important muscular components of pelvic diaphragm, arising mainly from back of body of pubis and running backward toward coccyx; includes pubococcygeus (levator m. of prostate in male and pubovaginal in female), puborectal, and iliococcygeus m's		third and fourth sacral	helps support pelvic viscera and resist increases in intraabdominal pressure
levator m. of palatine velum	m. levator veli palatini	apex of pars petrosa of temporal bone and cartilage of auditory tube	aponeurosis of soft palate	pharyngeal plexus	raises and draws back soft palate
levator m. of prostate	m. levator prostatae	a name applied to part of anterior portion of pubococcygeus m., which in male is inserted into prostate and tendinous center of perineum		sacral, pudendal	supports, compresses prostate, helps control micturition
levator m's of ribs	mm. levatores costarum	transverse processes of seventh cervical and first 11 thoracic vertebrae	medial to angle of rib below	intercostal	aid elevation of ribs in respiration
levator m. of scapula	m. levator scapulae	transverse processes of 4 upper cervical vertebrae	vertebral border of scapula	third and fourth cervical	raises scapula
levator m. of thyroid gland	m. levator glandulae thyroideae	isthmus or pyramidal lobule of thyroid gland	body of hyoid bone	external branch of superior laryngeal	
levator m. of upper eyelid	m. levator palpebrae superioris	sphenoid bone above optic foramen	skin and tarsal plate of upper eyelid	oculomotor	raises upper eyelid
levator m. of upper lip	m. levator labii superioris	lower margin of orbit	musculature of upper lid	facial	raises upper lip
levator m. of upper lip and ala of nose	m. levator labii superioris alaeque nasi	Frontal process of maxilla	skin and cartilage of ala of nose, upper lip	infraorbital branch of facial	raises upper lip, dilates nostril
long m. of head	m. longus capitis	transverse processes of third to sixth cervical vertevrae	basilar portion of occipital bone	cervical	flexes head
long m. of neck	m. longus colli	superior oblique portion—transverse processes of third to fifth cervical vertebrae; inferior oblique portion—bodies of first to third thoracic vertebrae: vertical portion—bodies of 3 upper thoracic and 3 lower cervical vertebrae	superior oblique portion—tubercle of anterior arch of atlas; inferior oblique portion—transverse processes of fifth and sixth cervical vertebrae; vertical portion—bodies of second to fourth cervical vertebrae	anterior cervical	flexes, supports cervical vertebrae

Common Name	Latin Name	Origin	Insertion	Nerve	Action
longissimus m. of head	m. longissimus capitis	transverse processes of 4 or 5 upper thoracic vertebrae, articular processes of 3 or 4 lower cervical vertebrae	mastoid process of temporal bone	cervical	draws head backward, rotates head
longissimus m. of neck	m. longissimus cervicis	transverse processes of 4 or 5 upper thoracic vertebrae	transverse processes of second or third to sixth cervical vertebrae	lower cervical and upper thoracic	extends cervical vertebrae
longissimus m. of thorax	m. longissimus thoracis	transverse and articular processes of lumbar vertebrae and thoracolumbar fascia	transverse processes of all thoracic vertebrae, 9 or 10 lower ribs	lumbar and thoracic	extends thoracic vertebrae
longitudinal m. of tongue, inferior	m. longitudinalis inferior linguae	undersurface of tongue at base	tip of tongue	hypoglossal	changes shape of tongue in mastication and deglutition
longitudinal m. of tongue, superior	m. longitudinalis superior linguae	submucosa and septum of tongue	margins of tongue	hypoglossal	changes shape of tongue in mastication and deglutition
lumbrical m's of foot	mm. lumbricales pedis	tendons of long flexor m. of toes	medial side of base of proximal phalanges of 4 lateral toes	medial and lateral plantar	flex metatarsophalangeal joints, extend distal phalanges
lumbrical m's of hand	mm. lumbricales manus	tendons of deep flexor m. of fingers	extensor tendons of 4 lateral fingers	median, ulnar	flex metacarpophalangeal joints, extend middle and distal phalanges
masseter m.	m. masseter	*superficial part*—zygomatic process of maxilla, lower border of zygomatic arch; *deep part*—lower border and medial surface of zygomatic arch	*superficial part*—angle and ramus of mandible; *deep part*—upper half of ramus and lateral surface of coronoid process of mandible	masseteric, from mandibular division of trigeminal	raises mandible, closes jaws
multifidus m's	mm. multifidi	sacrum, sacroiliac ligament, mamillary processes of lumbar, transverse processes of thoracic, and articular processes of cervical vertebrae	spines of contiguous vertebrae above	spinal	extend, rotate vertebral column
mylohyoid m.	m. mylohyoideus	mylohyoid line of mandible	body of hyoid bone, median raphe	mylohyoid branch of inferior alveolar	elevates hyoid bone, supports floor of mouth

(continued)

3-4. MUSCLES—cont'd

Common Name*	TA Term†	Origin*	Insertion*	Innervation	Action
nasal m.	m. nasalis	maxilla	*alar part*—ala of nose; *transverse part*—by aponeurotic expansion with fellow of opposite side	facial	*alar part*—aids in widening nostril; *transverse part*—depresses cartilage of nose
oblique m. of abdomen, external	m. obliquus externus abdominis	lower 8 ribs at costal cartilages	crest of ilium, linea alba through rectus sheath	lower thoracic	flexes, rotates vertebral column, compresses abdominal viscera
oblique m. of abdomen, internal	m. obliquus internus abdominis	thoracolumbar fascia, iliac crest, iliac fascia, inguinal fascia	lower 3 or 4 costal cartilages, linea alba, conjoined tendon to pubis	lower thoracic	flexes, rotates vertebral column, compresses abdominal viscera
oblique m. of auricle	m. obliquus auriculae	cranial surface of concha	cranial surface of auricle above concha	posterior auricular, temporal	
oblique m. of eyeball, inferior	m. obliquus inferior bulbi	orbital surface of maxilla	sclera	oculomotor	abducts, rotates eyeball downward and outward
oblique m. of eyeball, superior	m. obliquus superior bulbi	lesser wing of sphenoid above optic foramen	sclera	trochlear	abducts, rotates eyeball upward and outward
oblique m. of head, inferior	m. obliquus capitis inferior	spinous process of axis	transverse process of atlas	spinal	rotates atlas and head
oblique m. of head, superior	m. obliquus capitis superior	transverse process of atlas	occipital bone	spinal	extends and moves head laterally
obturator m., external	m. obturatorius externus	pubis, ischium, external surface of obturator membrane	trochanteric fossa of femur	obturator	rotates thigh laterally
obturator m., internal	m. obturatorius internus	pelvic surface of hip bone and obturator membrane, margin of obturator foramen	greater trochanter of femur	fifth lumbar, first and second sacral	rotates thigh laterally
occipitofrontal m.	m. occipitofrontalis	*frontal belly*—galea aponeurotica; *occipital belly*—highest nuchal line of occipital bone	*frontal belly*—skin of eyebrow, root of nose; *occipital belly*—galea aponeurotica	*frontal belly* — temporal branch of facial; *occipital belly*—posterior auricular branch of facial	*frontal belly*—raises eyebrow, *occipital belly*—draws scalp backward
omohyoid m.	m. omohyoideus	superior border of scapula	body of hyoid bone	upper cervical through ansa cervicalis	depresses hyoid bone
opposing m. of little finger	m. opponens digiti minimi manus	hook of hamate bone	front of fifth metacarpal	eighth cervical through ulnar	abducts, flexes, rotates fifth metacarpal
opposing m. of thumb	m. opponens pollicis	tubercle of trapezium, flexor retinaculum	lateral side of first metacarpal	sixth and seventh metacarpal through median	flexes, opposes thumb

orbicular m. of eye	m. orbicularis oculi	orbital part—medial margin of orbit, including frontal process of maxilla; palpebral part—medial palpebral ligament; lacrimal part—posterior lacrimal crest	orbital part—near origin after encircling orbit; palpebral part—orbital tubercle of zygomatic bone; lacrimal part—lateral palpebral raphe	facial	closes eyelids, wrinkles forehead, compresses lacrimal sac
orbicular m. of mouth	m. orbicularis oris	a name applied to complicated sphincter muscle of mouth, comprising 2 parts: labial part—consisting of fibers restricted to lips; marginal part—consisting of fibers blending with those of adjacent muscles		facial	closes, protrudes lips
orbital m.	m. orbitalis	bridges inferior orbital fissure	fascia of inferior orbital fissure	sympathetic fibers	protrudes eye
palatoglossus m.	m. palatoglossus	undersurface of soft palate	side of tongue	pharyngeal plexus	elevates tongue, constricts fauces
palatopharyngeal m.	m. palatopharyngeus	posterior border of bony palate, palatine aponeurosis	posterior border of thyroid cartilage, side of pharynx and esophagus	pharyngeal plexus	constricts pharynx, aids swallowing
palmar m., long	m. palmaris longus	medial epicondyle of humerus	flexor retinaculum, palmar aponeurosis	median	tenses palmar aponeurosis
palmar m., short	m. palmaris brevis	palmar aponeurosis	skin of medial border of hand	ulnar	assists in deepening hollow of palm
papillary m's	mm. papillares	a name applied to conical muscular projections from walls of cardiac ventricles, attached to cusps of atrioventricular valves by chordae tendineae			steady and strengthen atrioventricular valves and prevent eversion of their cusps
pectinate m's	mm. pectinati	a name applied to small ridges of muscular fibers projecting from inner walls of auricles of heart, and extending in right atrium from auricle to crista terminalis			
pectineal m.	m. pectineus	pectineal line of pubis	pectineal line of femur	femoral, obturator	flexes, adducts thigh
pectoral m., greater	m. pectoralis major	clavicle, sternum, 6 upper costal cartilages, aponeurosis of external oblique m. of abdomen	crest of greater tubercle of humerus	lateral and medial pectoral	adducts, flexes, rotates arm medially
pectoral m., smaller	m. pectoralis minor	second, third, fourth, and fifth ribs	coracoid process of scapula	medial and lateral pectoral	draws shoulder forward and downward, raises third, fourth, and fifth ribs in forced inspiration

(continued)

3-4. MUSCLES—cont'd

Common Name*	TA Term†	Origin*	Insertion*	Innervation	Action
peroneal m., long	m. peroneus longus	lateral condyle of tibia, head of fibula, lateral surface of fibula	medial cuneiform, first metatarsal	superficial peroneal	plantar flexes, everts, abducts foot
peroneal m., short	m. peroneus brevis	lateral surface of fibula	tuberosity of fifth metatarsal	superficial peroneal	everts, abducts, plantar flexes foot
peroneal m., third	m. peroneus tertius	anterior surface of fibula, interosseous membrane	fascia or base of fifth (or fourth) metatarsal	deep peroneal	everts, dorsiflexes foot
piriform m.	m. piriformis	ilium, second to fourth sacral vertebrae	greater trochanter of femur	first and second sacral	rotates thigh laterally
plantar m.	m. plantaris	popliteal surface of femur	Achilles tendon or back of calcaneus	tibial	plantar flexes foot, flexes leg
platysma	platysma	a name applied to a platelike muscle originating from the fascia of cervical region and inserting on mandible, and skin around mouth		cervical branch of facial	wrinkles skin of neck, depresses jaw
pleuroesophageal m.	m. pleuro-oesophageus	a name applied to portion of a bundle of smooth muscle fibers, usually connecting esophagus with left mediastinal pleura			
popliteal m.	m. popliteus	lateral condyle of femur, lateral meniscus	posterior surface of tibia	tibial	flexes leg, rotates leg medially
procerus m.	m. procerus	fascia over nasal bones	skin of forehead	facial	draws medial angle of eyebrows down
pronator m., quadrate	m. pronator quadratus	anterior surface and border of distal third or fourth of shaft of ulna	anterior surface and border of distal fourth of shaft of radius	anterior interosseous	pronates forearm
pronator m., round	m. pronator teres	*humeral head*—medial epicondyle of humerus; *ulnar head*—coronoid processes of ulna	lateral surface of radius	median	pronates and flexes forearm
psoas m., greater psoas m., smaller	m. psoas major m. psoas minor	lumbar vertebrae last thoracic and first lumbar vertebra	lesser trochanter of femur arcuate line of hip bone	second and third lumbar first lumbar	flexes thigh or trunk assists greater psoas m.
pterygoid m., lateral (external)	m. pterygoideus lateralis	*upper head*—infratemporal surface of greater wing of sphenoid, infratemporal crest; *lower head*—lateral surface of lateral pterygoid plate	neck of mandible, capsule of temporomandibular joint	mandibular	protrudes mandible, opens jaws, moves mandible from side to side

pterygoid m., medial (internal)	m. pterygoideus medialis	medial surface of lateral pterygoid plate, tuber of maxilla / medial surface of ramus and angle of mandible	mandibular	closes jaws
pubococcygeus m.	m. pubococcygeus	a name applied to anterior portion of levator ani m., originating in front of obturator canal and inserting in anococcygeal ligament and side of coccyx	third and fourth sacral	helps support pelvic viscera and resist increases in intra-abdominal pressure
puboprostatic m.	m. puboprostaticus	a. name applied to smooth muscle fibers contained within medial puboprostatic ligament, which pass from prostate anteriorly to pubis		
puborectal m.	m. puborectalis	a name applied to levator ani m., with a more lateral origin from pubic bone, and continuous posteriorly with corresponding muscle of opposite side	third and fourth sacral	helps support pelvic viscera and resist increases in intra-abdominal pressure
pubovaginal m.	m. pubovaginalis	a name applied to part of anterior portion of pubococcygeus m., which is inserted into urethra and vagina	sacral and pudendal	helps control micturition
pubovesical m.	m. pubovesicalis	a name applied to smooth muscle fibers extending from neck of urinary bladder to pubis		
pyloric sphincter m.	m. sphincter pyloricus	a thickening of the circular muscle of the stomach around its opening into the duodenum		
pyramidal m.	m. pyramidalis	linea alba / body of pubis	last thoracic	tenses abdominal wall
pyramidal m. of auricle	m. pyramidalis auriculae	a name applied to inconstant prolongation of fibers of m. of tragus to spine of helix		
quadrate m. of loins	m. quadratus lumborum	iliac crest, thoracolumbar fascia / twelfth rib transverse processes of lumbar vertebrae	first and second lumbar, twelfth thoracic	flexes trunk laterally
quadrate m. of lower lip. See depressor m. of lower lip				
quadrate m. of sole	m. quadratus plantae	calcaneus, plantar fascia / tendons of long flexor m. of toes	lateral plantar	aids in flexing toes
quadrate m. of thigh	m. quadratus femoris	tuberosity of ischium / intertrochanteric crest and quadrate tubercle of femur	fourth and fifth lumbar, first sacral	adducts, rotates thigh laterally
quadrate m. of upper lip. See levator m. of upper lip				
quadriceps m. of thigh	m. quadriceps femoris	a name applied collectively to rectus m. of thigh and intermediate, lateral, and medial vastus m's inserting by a common tendon that surrounds patella and ends on tuberosity of tibia	femoral	extends leg upon thigh

(continued)

3-4. MUSCLES—cont'd

Common Name*	TA Term†	Origin*	Insertion*	Innervation	Action
rectococcygeus m.	m. rectococcygeus	a name applied to smooth muscle fibers originating on anterior surface of second and third coccygeal vertebrae and inserting on posterior surface of rectum		autonomic	retracts, elevates rectum
rectourethral m.	m. rectourethralis	a name applied to band of smooth muscle fibers in male, extending from perineal flexure of rectum to membranous part of urethra			
rectouterine m.	m. rectouterinus	a name applied to band of fibers in female, running between cervix uteri and rectum, in rectouterine fold			
rectovesical m.	m. rectovesicalis	a name applied to band of fibers in male, connecting longitudinal musculature of rectum with external muscular coat of bladder			
rectus m. of abdomen	m. rectus abdominis	pubic crest and symphysis	xiphoid process, fifth, sixth, and seventh costal cartilages	lower thoracic	flexes lumbar vertebrae, supports abdomen
rectus m. of eyeball, inferior	m. rectus inferior bulbi	common tendinous ring	underside of sclera	oculomotor	adducts, rotates eyeball downward and medially
rectus m. of eyeball, lateral	m. rectus lateralis bulbi	common tendinous ring	lateral side of sclera	abducens	abducts eyeball
rectus m. of eyeball, medial	m. rectus medialis bulbi	common tendinous ring	medial side of sclera	oculomotor	adducts eyeball
rectus m. of eyeball, superior	m. rectus superior bulbi	common tendinous ring	upper side of sclera	oculomotor	adducts, rotates eyeball upward and medially
rectus m. of head, anterior	m. rectus capitis anterior	lateral mass of atlas	basilar part of occipital bone	first and second cervical	flexes, supports head
rectus m. of head, lateral	m. rectus capitis lateralis	transverse process of atlas	jugular process of occipital bone	first and second cervical	flexes, supports head
rectus m. of head, posterior, greater	m. rectus capitis posterior major	spinous process of atlas	occipital bone	suboccipital, greater occipital	extends head
rectus m. of head, posterior, smaller	m. rectus capitis posterior minor	posterior tubercle of atlas	occipital bone	suboccipital, greater occipital	extends head
rectus m. of thigh	m. rectus femoris	anterior inferior iliac spine, rim of acetabulum	base of patella, tuberosity of tibia	femoral	extends leg, flexes thigh
rhomboid m., greater	m. rhomboideus major	spinous processes of second, third, fourth and fifth thoracic vertebrae	vertebral margin of scapula	dorsal scapular	retracts and fixes scapula

Common name	Latin name	Origin	Insertion	Nerve	Action
rhomboid m., smaller	m. rhomboideus minor	spinous processes of seventh cervical and first thoracic vertebrae, lower part of nuchal ligament	vertebral margin of scapula at root of spine	dorsal scapular	retracts and fixes scapula
risorius m.	m. risorius	fascia over masseter	skin at angle of mouth	buccal branch of facial	draws angle of mouth laterally
rotator m's	mm. rotatores	a name applied to a series of small muscles deep in groove between spinous and transverse processes of vertebrae		spinal	extend and rotate vertebral column toward opposite side
sacrococcygeal m., dorsal (posterior)	m. sacrococcygeus dorsalis	a name applied to muscular slip passing from dorsal surface of sacrum to coccyx			
sacrococcygeal m., ventral (anterior)	m. sacrococcygeus ventralis	a name applied to musculotendinous slip passing from lower sacral vertebra to coccyx			
sacrospinal m. *See* erector m. of spine					
salpingopharyngeal m.	m. salpingopharyngeus	cartilage of auditory tube	posterior part of palatopharyngeus	pharyngeal plexus	raises pharynx
sartorius m.	m. sartorius	anterior superior iliac spine	upper part of medial surface of tibia	femoral	flexes thigh and leg
scalene m., anterior	m. scalenus anterior	transverse processes of third to sixth cervical vertebrae	scalene tubercle of first rib	second to seventh cervical	raises first rib, flexes cervical vertebrae laterally
scalene m., middle	m. scalenus medius	transverse processes of first to seventh cervical vertebrae	upper surface of first rib	second to seventh cervical	raises first rib, flexes cervical vertebrae laterally
scalene m. of pleura. *See* smallest scalene m.					
scalene m., posterior	m. scalenus posterior	transverse processes of fourth to sixth cervical vertebrae	second rib	second to seventh cervical	raises first and second ribs, flexes cervical vertebrae laterally
scalene m., smallest	m. scalenus minimus	a name applied to muscular band occasionally found between anterior and middle scalene m's			
semimembranous m.	m. semimembranosus	tuberosity of ischium	lateral condyle of femur, medial condyle, and border of tibia	sciatic	flexes leg, extends thigh
semispinal m. of head	m. semispinalis capitis	transverse processes of upper thoracic and lower cervical vertebrae	occipital bone	suboccipital, greater occipital, branches of cervical	extends head

(continued)

3-4. MUSCLES—cont'd

Common Name*	NA Term†	Origin*	Insertion*	Innervation	Action
semispinal m. of neck	m. semispinalis cervicis	transverse processes of upper thoracic vertebrae	spinous processes of second to fifth (or fourth) cervical vertebrae	branches of cervical	extends, rotates vertebral column
semispinal m. of thorax	m. semispinalis thoracis	transverse processes of lower thoracic vertebrae	spinous processes of lower cervical and upper thoracic vertebrae	spinal	extends, rotates vertebral column
semitendinous m.	m. semitendinosus	tuberosity of ischium	upper part of medial surface of tibia	sciatic	flexes and rotates leg medially, extends thigh
serratus m., anterior	m. serratus anterior	8 upper ribs	vertebral border of scapula	long thoracic	draws scapula forward, rotates scapula to raise shoulder in abduction of arm
serratus m., posterior, inferior	m. serratus posterior inferior	spines of lower thoracic and upper lumbar vertebrae	4 lower ribs	ninth to twelfth (or eleventh) thoracic	lowers ribs in expiration
serratus m., posterior, superior	m. serratus posterior superior	nuchal ligament, spinous processes of upper thoracic vertebrae	second, third, fourth, and fifth ribs	upper 4 thoracic	raises ribs in inspiration
soleus m.	m. soleus	fibula, tendinous arch, tibia	calcaneus by Achilles tendon	tibial	plantar flexes foot
sphincter m. of anus, external	m. sphincter ani externus	tip of coccyx, anococcygeal ligament	tendinous center of perineum	inferior rectal, perineal branch of fourth sacral	closes anus
sphincter m. of anus, internal	m. sphincter ani internus	a name applied to a thickening of circular layer of muscular tunic at caudal end of rectum			
sphincter m. of bile duct	m. sphincter ductus choledochi	a name applied to annular sheath of muscle fibers investing bile duct within wall of duodenum			
sphincter m. of hepatopancreatic ampulla	m. sphincter ampullae hepatopancreaticae	a name applied to annular band of muscle fibers investing hepatopancreatic ampulla			
sphincter m. of pupil	m. sphincter pupillae	a name applied to circular fibers of iris	circular fibers of iris	parasympathetic through ciliary	constricts pupil
sphincter m. of pylorus	m. sphincter pylori	a name applied to a thickening of circular muscle of stomach around its opening into duodenum			
sphincter m. of urethra	m. sphincter urethrae	inferior ramus of pubis	median raphe behind and in front of urethra	perineal	compresses membranous urethra
sphincter m. of urinary bladder	m. sphincter vesicae urinariae	a name applied to circular layer of fibers surrounding internal urethral orifice		vesical	closes internal orifice of urethra
spinal m. of head	m. spinalis capitis	spinous processes of upper cervical and lower cervical vertebrae	occipital bone	spinal	extends head

spinal m. of neck	m. spinalis cervicis	spinous process of seventh cervical vertebrae, nuchal ligament	branches of cervical	extends vertebral column
spinal m. of thorax	m. spinalis thoracis	spinous processes of upper lumbar and lower thoracic vertebrae	branches of spinal	extends vertebral column
splenius m. of head	m. splenius capitis	lower half of nuchal ligament, spinous processes of seventh cervical and upper thoracic vertebrae	cervical	extends, rotates head
splenius m. of neck	m. splenius cervicis	spinous process of upper thoracic vertebrae	cervical	extends, rotates head and neck
stapedius m.	m. stapedius	interior of pyramidal eminence of tympanic cavity	facial	dampens movement of stapes
sternal m.	m. sternalis	a name applied to muscular band occasionally found parallel to sternum on sternocostal head of greater pectoral m.		
sternocleidomastoid m.	m. sternocleidomastoideus	*sternal head*—manubrium; *clavicular head*—medial third of clavicle	accessory, cervical plexus	flexes vertebral column, rotates head to opposite side
sternocostal m. *See* transverse m. of thorax				
sternohyoid m.	m. sternohyoideus	manubrium sterni and/or clavicle	ansa cervicalis	depresses hyoid bone and larynx
sternothyroid m.	m. sternothyroideus	manubrium sterni	ansa cervicalis	depresses thyroid cartilage
styloglossus m.	m. styloglossus	styloid process	hypoglossal	raises, retracts tongue
stylohyoid m.	m. stylohyoideus	styloid process	facial	draws hyoid bone and tongue upward and backward
stylopharyngeus m.	m. stylopharyngeus	styloid process	glossopharyngeal, pharyngeal plexus	raises, dilates pharynx
subclavius m.	m. subclavius	first rib and its cartilage	nerve to subclavius	depresses lateral end of clavicle
subcostal m's	mm. subcostales	lower border of ribs	intercostal	raise ribs in inspiration
subscapular m.	m. subscapularis	subscapular fossa of scapula	subscapular	rotates arm medially
supinator m.	m. supinator	lateral epicondyle of humerus, ligaments of elbow	deep branch of radial	supinates forearm

(continued)

3-4. MUSCLES—cont'd

Common Name*	TA Term†	Origin*	Insertion*	Innervation	Action
supraspinous m.	m. supraspinatus	supraspinous fossa of scapula	greater tubercle of humerus	suprascapular	abducts arm
suspensory m.	m. suspensorius	a name applied to flat band of smooth muscle fibers originating from left crus of diaphragm and inserting continuous with muscular coat of duodenum at its junction with jejunum			
tarsal m., inferior	m. tarsalis inferior	inferior rectus m. of eyeball	tarsal plate of lower eyelid	sympathetic	widens palpebral fissure
tarsal m., superior	m. tarsalis superior	levator m. of upper eyelid	tarsal plate of upper eyelid	sympathetic	widens palpebral fissure
temporal m.	m. temporalis	temporal fossa and fascia	coronoid process of mandible	mandibular	closes jaw
temporoparietal m.	m. temporoparietalis	temporal fascia above ear	galea aponeurotica	temporal branches of facial	tightens scalp
tensor m. of fascia lata	m. tensor fasciae latae	iliac crest	iliotibial tract of fascia lata	superior gluteal	flexes, rotates thigh medially
tensor m. of palatine velum	m. tensor veli palatini	scaphoid fossa and spine of sphenoid	aponeurosis of soft palate, wall of auditory tube	mandibular	tenses soft palate, opens auditory tube
tensor m. of tympanum	m. tensor tympani	cartilaginous portion of auditory tube	handle of malleus	mandibular	tenses tympanic membrane
teres major m.	m. teres major	inferior angle of scapula	crest of lesser tubercle of humerus	lower subscapular	adducts, extends, and rotates arm medially
teres minor m.	m. teres minor	lateral margin of scapula	greater tubercle of humerus	axillary	rotates arm laterally
thyroarytenoid m.	m. thyroarytenoideus	medial surface of lamina of thyroid cartilage	muscular process of arytenoid cartilage	recurrent laryngeal	relaxes, shortens vocal folds
thyroepiglottic m.	m. thyroepiglotticus	lamina of thyroid cartilage	epiglottis	recurrent laryngeal	closes inlet to larynx
thyrohyoid m.	m. thyrohyoideus	lamina of thyroid cartilage	greater horn of hyoid bone	ansa cervicalis	raises and changes form of larynx
tibial m., anterior	m. tibialis anterior	lateral condyle and surface of tibia, interosseous membrane	medial cuneiform, base of first metatarsal	deep peroneal	dorsiflexes, inverts foot
tibial m., posterior	m. tibialis posterior	tibia, fibula, interosseous membrane	bases of second to fourth metatarsal bones and tarsal bones, except talus	tibial	plantar flexes, inverts foot
tracheal m.	m. trachealis	a name applied to transverse smooth muscle fibers filling gap at back of each cartilage of trachea		autonomic	lessens caliber of trachea
m. of tragus	m. tragicus	a name applied to short, flattened vertical band on lateral surface of tragus, innervated by auriculotemporal and posterior auricular nerves			

		Origin	Insertion	Nerve	Action
transverse m. of abdomen	m. transversus abdominis	lower 6 costal cartilages, thoracolumbar fascia, iliac crest	linea alba through rectus sheath, conjoined tendon to pubis	lower thoracic	compresses abdominal viscera
transverse m. of auricle	m. transversus auriculae	cranial surface of auricle	circumference of auricle	posterior auricular branch of facial	retracts helix
transverse m. of chin	m. transversus menti	a name applied to superficial fibers of depressor m. of angle of mouth which turn medially and cross to opposite side			
transverse m. of nape	m. transversus nuchae	a name applied to small muscle often present, passing from occipital protuberance to posterior auricular m.; it may be either superficial or deep to trapezius			
transverse m. of perineum, deep	m. transversus perinei profundus	ramus of ischium	tendinous center of perineum	perineal	fixes tendinous center of perineum
transverse m. of perineum, superficial	m. transversus perinei superficialis	ramus of ischium	tendinous center of perineum	perineal	fixes tendinous center of perineum
transverse m. of thorax	m. transversus thoracis	posterior surface of body of sternum and of xiphoid process	second to sixth costal cartilages	intercostal	perhaps narrows chest
transverse m. of tongue	m. transversus linguae	median septum of tongue	dorsum and margins of tongue	hypoglossal	changes shape of tongue in mastication and swallowing
transversospinal m.	m. transversospinalis	a name applied collectively to semispinal, multifidus, and rotator m's			
trapezius m.	m. trapezius	occipital bone, nuchal ligament, spinous processes of seventh cervical and all thoracic vertebrae	clavicle, acromion, spine of scapula	accessory, cervical plexus	elevates shoulder, rotates scapula to raise shoulder in abduction of arm, draws scapula
triangular m. *See* depressor m. of angle of mouth					
triceps m. of arm (triceps brachii m.)	m. triceps brachii	*long head*—infraglenoid tubercle of scapula; *lateral head*—posterior surface of humerus; *medial head*—posterior surface of humerus below groove for radial nerve	olecranon of ulna	radial	extends forearm; *long head* adducts, extends arm
triceps m. of calf (triceps surae m.)	m. triceps surae	a name applied collectively to gastrocnemius and soleus m's			

(continued)

3-4. MUSCLES—cont'd

Common Name*	TA Term†	Origin*	Insertion*	Innervation	Action
m. of uvula	m. uvulae	posterior nasal spine of palatine bone and aponeurosis of soft palate	uvula	pharyngeal plexus	raises uvula
vastus m., intermediate	m. vastus intermedius	anterior and lateral surfaces of femur	patella, common tendon of quadriceps m. of thigh	femoral	extends leg
vastus m., lateral	m. vastus lateralis	lateral aspects of femur	patella, common tendon of quadriceps m. of thigh	femoral	extends leg
vastus m., medial	m. vastus medialis	medial aspect of femur	patella, common tendon of quadriceps m. of thigh	femoral	extends leg
vertical m. of tongue	m. verticalis linguae	dorsal fascia of tongue	sides and base of tongue	hypoglossal	changes shape of tongue in mastication and deglutition
vocal m.	m. vocalis	angle between laminae of thyroid cartilage	vocal process of arytenoid cartilage	recurrent laryngeal	causes local variations in tension of vocal fold
zygomatic m., greater	m. zygomaticus major	zygomatic bone	angle of mouth	facial	draws angle of mouth upward and backward
zygomatic m., smaller	m. zygomaticus minor	zygomatic bone	orbicular m. of mouth, levator m. of upper lip	facial	draws upper lip upward and laterally

Common Name* [Modality]	TA Term†	Origin*	Branches*	Distribution*
abducent n. (6th cranial) [motor]	n. abducens	a nucleus in the pons, beneath floor of fourth ventricle		lateral rectus muscle of eyeball
accessory n. (11th cranial) [parasympathetic, motor]	n. accessorius	by cranial roots from side of medulla oblongata, and by spinal roots of spinal cord		internal branch to vagus, thereby to palate, pharynx, larynx, and thoracic viscera; external to sternocleidomastoid and trapezius muscles
acoustic n. *See vestibulocochlear n.*				
alveolar n's, inferior [motor, general sensory]	n. alveolaris inferior	mandibular n.	inferior dental, mental, and inferior gingival nerves; mylohyoid n.	teeth and gums of lower jaw, skin of chin and lower lip, mylohyoid muscle and anterior belly of digastric muscle
alveolar n's. superior	nn. alveolares superiores	superior alveolar branches (anterior, middle, and posterior) that arise from infraorbital and maxillary n's, innervating teeth of upper jaw and maxillary sinus, and forming superior dental plexus		
ampullary n., anterior	n. ampullaris anterior	branch of vestibular part of eighth cranial (vestibulocochlear) n. that innervates ampulla of anterior semicircular duct, ending around hair cells of ampullary crest		
ampullary n., inferior. *See ampullary n., posterior*				
ampullary n., lateral	n. ampullaris lateralis	branch of vestibular n. that innervates ampulla of lateral semicircular duct, ending around hair cells of ampullary crest		
ampullary n., posterior	n. ampullaris posterior	branch of vestibular part of eighth cranial (vestibulocochlear) n. that innervates ampulla of posterior semicircular duct, ending around hair cells of ampullary crest		
ampullary n., superior. *See ampullary n., anterior*				
anal n's, inferior. *See rectal n's, inferior*				
anococcygeal n's [general sensory]	nn. anococcygei	coccygeal plexus		sacrococcygeal joint, coccyx, skin over coccyx
auditory n. *See vestibulocochlear n.*				
auricular n's, anterior [general sensory]	nn. auriculares anteriores	auriculotemporal n.		skin of anterosuperior part of external ear
auricular n., great [general sensory]	n. auricularis magnus	cervical; plexus—C2–C3	anterior and posterior branches	skin over parotid gland and mastoid process, and both surfaces of auricle

(continued)

*n. = nerve; n's = (pl.) nerves.
†n. = [L.] nervus; nn. = [L. (pl.)] nervi.

2043

Common Name* [Modality]	TA Term†	Origin*	Branches*	Distribution*
auricular n., posterior [motor, general sensory]	n. auricularis posterior	facial n.	occipital branch	posterior auricular and occipitofrontal muscles, skin of external acoustic meatus
auriculotemporal n. [general sensory]	n. auriculotemporalis	by two roots from mandibular n.	anterior auricular n., n. of external acoustic meatus, parotid branches, branch to tympanic membrane, branch communicating with facial n.; terminal branches are superficial temporal to scalp	parotid gland, scalp in temporal region, tympanic membrane. *See also* auricular n's, anterior, *and* n. of external acoustic meatus
axillary n. [motor, general sensory]	n. axillaris	posterior cord of brachial plexus—C5–C6	lateral superior brachial cutaneous n., muscular branches	deltoid and teres minor muscles, skin over back of arm
buccal n. [general sensory]	n. buccalis	mandibular n.		skin and mucous membrane of cheeks, gums, and perhaps first two molars and the premolars
cardiac n., cervical, inferior [sympathetic (accelerator), visceral afferent (chiefly pain)]	n. cardiacus cervicalis inferior	cervicothoracic ganglion		heart via cardiac plexus
cardiac n., cervical, middle [sympathetic (accelerator), visceral afferent (chiefly pain)]	n. cardiacus cervicalis medius	middle cervical ganglion		heart
cardiac n., cervical, superior [sympathetic (accelerator)]	n. cardiacus cervicalis superior	superior cervical ganglion		heart
cardiac n., inferior. *See* cardiac n., cervical, inferior				
cardiac n., middle. *See* cardiac n., cervical, middle				
cardiac n., superior. *See* cardiac n., cervical, superior				
cardiac n's, thoracic [sympathetic (accelerator), visceral afferent (chiefly pain)]	nn. cardiaci thoracici	ganglia T2–T4 or T5 of sympathetic trunk	together with tympanic n. forms tympanic plexus	heart
caroticotympanic n's [sympathetic]	nn. caroticotympanici	internal carotid plexus	help form tympanic plexus	tympanic region, parotid gland
carotid n's, external [sympathetic]	nn. carotici externi	superior cervical ganglion		cranial blood vessels and glands via external carotid plexus
carotis n., internal [sympathetic]	nn. caroticus internus	superior cervical ganglion		cranial blood vessels and glands via internal carotid plexus

Common name	NA term	Origin	Branches	Distribution
cavernous n's of clitoris [parasympathetic, sympathetic, visceral afferent]	nn. cavernosi clitoridis	uterovaginal plexus		erectile tissue of clitoris
cavernous n's of penis [sympathetic, parasympathetic, visceral afferent]	nn. cavernosi penis	prostatic plexus		erectile tissue of penis
cerebral n's. See cranial n's.				
cervical n's	nn. cervicales	the 8 pairs of n's that arise from cervical segments of spinal cord and, except last pair, leave vertebral column above correspondingly numbered vertebra; the ventral branches of upper 4, on either side, unite to form cervical plexus; those of lower 4, together with ventral branch of first thoracic n., form most of brachial plexus		
cervical n., transverse [general sensory]	n. transversus colli	cervical plexus—C2-C3	superior and inferior branches	skin on side and front of neck
ciliary n's, long [sympathetic, general sensory]	nn. ciliares longi	nasociliary n., from ophthalmic n.		dilator muscle of pupil, uvea, cornea
ciliary n's, short [parasympathetic, sympathetic, general sensory]	nn. ciliares breves	ciliary ganglion		smooth muscles and tunics of eye
clunial n's, inferior [general sensory]	nn. clunium inferiores	posterior femoral cutaneous n.		skin of lower part of buttock
clunial n's, middle [general sensory]	nn. clunium medii	plexus formed by lateral branches of dorsal branches of first 4 sacral nerves behind sacrum and coccyx		ligaments of sacrum and skin over posterior part of buttock
clunial n's, superior [general sensory]	nn. clunium superiores	lateral branches of dorsal branch of upper lumbar n's		skin of upper part of buttock
coccygeal n.	n. coccygeus	one of the pair of nerves arising from coccygeal segment of spinal cord		skin of upper part of buttock
cochlear n.	n. cochlearis	the part of the vestibulocochlear n. concerned with hearing, consisting of fibers that arise from bipolar cells in the spiral ganglion and have their receptors in the spiral organ of the cochlea		
cranial n's	nn. craniales	the 12 pairs of n's connected with brain, including olfactory (I), optic (II), oculomotor (III), trochlear (IV), trigeminal (V), abducens (VI), facial (VII), vestibulocochlear (VIII), glossopharyngeal (IX), vagus (X), accessory (XI), and hypoglossal (XII) nerves		
cubital n. See ulnar n.				
cutaneous n. of arm, lateral, inferior [general sensory]	n. cutaneus brachii lateralis inferior	radial n.		skin of lateral surface of lower arm
cutaneous n. of arm, lateral, superior [general sensory]	n. cutaneus brachii lateralis superior	axillary n.		skin of back of arm

(continued)

Common Name* [Modality]	TA Term†	Origin*	Branches*	Distribution*
cutaneous n. of arm, medial [general sensory]	n. cutaneus brachii medialis	medial cord of brachial plexus (T1)		skin on medial and posterior aspects of arm
cutaneous n. of arm, posterior [general sensory]	n. cutaneus brachii posterior	radial n. in axilla		skin on back of arm
cutaneous n. of calf, lateral [general sensory]	n. cutaneus surae lateralis	common fibular n.		skin of lateral side of back of leg, rarely may continue as sural n.
cutaneous n. of calf, medial [general sensory]	n. cutaneus surae medialis	tibial n.; usually joins fibular communicating branch of common fibular n. to form sural n.		may continue as sural n.
cutaneous n., dorsal, intermediate [general sensory]	n. cutaneus dorsalis intermedius	superficial fibular n.	dorsal digital n's of foot	skin of front of lower third of leg and dorsum of foot; ankle; skin and joints of adjacent sides of third and fourth, and of fourth and fifth toes
cutaneous n., dorsal, lateral [general sensory]	n. cutaneus dorsalis lateralis	continuation of sural n.		skin and joints of lateral side of foot and fifth toe
cutaneous n., dorsal, medial [general sensory]	n. cutaneus dorsalis medialis	superficial fibular n.		skin and joints of medial side of foot and big toe; adjacent sides of second and third toes
cutaneous n. of forearm, lateral [general sensory]	n. cutaneus antebrachii lateralis	continuation of musculocutaneous n.		skin over radial side of forearm; sometimes an area of skin of back of hand
cutaneous n of forearm, medial [general sensory]	n. cutaneus antebrachii medialis	medial cord of brachial plexus (C8, T1)	anterior and ulnar	skin of front, medial, and posteromedial aspects of forearm
cutaneous n. of forearm, posterior [general sensory]	n. cutaneus antebrachii posterior	radial n.		skin of dorsal aspect of forearm
cutaneous n. of thigh, lateral [general sensory]	n. cutaneus femoris lateralis	lumbar plexus—L2–L3		skin of lateral aspect and front of thigh
cutaneous n. of thigh, posterior [general sensory]	n. cutaneus femoris posterior	sacral plexus—S1–S3	inferior clunial n's, perineal branches	skin of buttock, external genitalia, back of thigh and calf
digital n's, dorsal, radial. *See* digital n's of radial n., dorsal				
digital n's, dorsal ulnar. *See* digital n's of ulnar n., dorsal				

2046

Term	Latin	Origin	Branches	Distribution
digital n's of foot, dorsal [general sensory]	nn. digitales dorsales pedis	intermediate dorsal cutaneous n.		skin and joints of adjacent sides of third and fourth, and of fourth and fifth toes
digital n's of lateral plantar n., common plantar [general sensory]	nn. digitales plantares communes nervi plantaris lateralis	superficial branch of lateral plantar n.	medial n. gives rise to 2 proper plantar digital n's	lateral nerve to short flexor muscle of little toe, skin and joints of lateral side of sole and little toe; medial nerve to adjacent side of fourth and fifth toes
digital n's of lateral plantar n., proper plantar [motor, general sensory]	nn. digitales plantares proprii nervi plantaris lateralis	common plantar digital n's		short flexor muscle of little toe, skin and joints of lateral side of sole and little toe; and adjacent surfaces of fourth and fifth toes
digital n's of lateral surface of great toe and medial surface of second toe, dorsal [general sensory]	nn. digitales dorsales hallucis lateralis et digiti secundi medialis	medial terminal division of deep peroneal n.		skin and joints of adjacent sides of first and second toes
digital n's of medial plantar n., common plantar [motor, general sensory]	nn. digitales plantares communes nervi plantaris medialis	medial plantar n.	muscular and proper plantar digital n's	flexor hallucis brevis muscle and first lumbrical muscles, skin and joints of medial side of foot and first toe, and adjacent sides of first and second, second and third, and third and fourth toes
digital n's of medial plantar n., proper plantar [general sensory]	nn. digitales plantares proprii nervi plantaris medialis	common plantar digital n's		skin and joint of first toe, and adjacent sides of first and second, second and third, and third and fourth toes; the nerves extend to the dorsum to supply nail beds and tips of toes
digital n's of median n., common palmar [motor, general sensory]	nn. digitales palmares communes nervi mediani	lateral and medial divisions of median n.	proper palmar digital n's	thumb, index, middle, and ring fingers, and first two lumbrical muscles
digital n's of median n., proper palmar [motor, general sensory]	nn. digitales palmares proprii nervi mediani	common palmar digital n's		first two lumbrical muscles, skin and joints of both sides and palmar aspect of thumb, index, and middle fingers, radial side of ring finger, back of distal aspect of these digits

(continued)

Common Name* [Modality]	TA Term†	Origin*	Branches*	Distribution*
digital n's of radial n., dorsal [general sensory]	nn. digitales dorsales nervi radialis	superficial branch of radial n.		skin and joints of back of thumb, index finger, and part of middle finger, as far distally as digital phalanx
digital n's of ulnar n., dorsal [general sensory]	nn. digitales dorsales nervi ulnaris	dorsal branch of ulnar n.		skin and joints of medial side of little finger, dorsal aspects of adjacent sides of little and ring fingers and of ring and middle fingers
digital n's of ulnar n., common palmar [general sensory]	nn. digitales palmares communes nervi ulnaris	superficial branch of ulnar n.	proper palmar digital n's	little and ring fingers
digital n's of ulnar n., proper palmar [general sensory]	nn. digitales palmares proprii nervi ulnaris	the lateral of the two common palmar digital n's from superficial branch of ulnar n.		skin and joints of adjacent sides of fourth and fifth fingers
dorsal n. of clitoris [general sensory, motor]	n. dorsalis clitoridis	pudendal n.		deep transverse muscle of perineum, sphincter muscle of urethra, corpus cavernosum of clitoris, and skin, prepuce, and glans of clitoris
dorsal n. of penis [general sensory, motor]	n. dorsalis penis	pudendal n.		deep transverse muscle of perineum, sphincter muscle of urethra, corpus cavernosum of penis, and skin, prepuce, and glans of penis
dorsal scapular n. [motor]	n. dorsalis scapulae	brachial plexus—ventral branch of C5		rhomboid muscles and occasionally the levator muscle of scapula
ethmoidal n., anterior [general sensory]	n. ethmoidalis anterior	continuation of nasociliary n., from ophthalmic n.	internal, external, lateral, and medial nasal branches	mucosa of upper and anterior nasal septum, lateral wall of nasal cavity, skin of lower bridge and tip of nose
ethmoidal n., posterior [general sensory]	n. ethmoidalis posterior	nasociliary n., from ophthalmic n.		mucosa of posterior ethmoid cells and of sphenoidal sinus
n. of external acoustic meatus [general sensory]	n. meatus acustici externi	auriculotemporal n.		skin lining external acoustic meatus, and tympanic membrane

facial n. (7th cranial) [motor, parasympathetic, general sensory, special sensory]. *See also* intermediate n.	n. facialis	inferior border of pons, between olive and inferior cerebellar peduncle	stapedius n.; posterior auricular n.; parotid plexus; digastric, temporal, zygomatic, buccal, lingual, marginal mandibular, and cervical branches and communicating branch with tympanic plexus	various structures of face, head, and neck (*see also* individual branches in this table)
femoral n. [general sensory]	n. femoralis	lumbar plexus—L2–L4; descending behind inguinal ligament to femoral triangle	saphenous n., muscular and anterior cutaneous branches	skin of thigh and leg, muscles of front of thigh, and hip and knee joints (*see also* individual branches in this table)
fibular n., superficial common [general sensory, motor]	n. fibularis superficialis	a terminal branch of common fibular n.	descends in front of fibula, supplies peroneus longus and brevis muscles and, in the lower part of the leg, divides into the muscular rami, medial, and intermediate dorsal cutaneous n's	
fibular n., common [general sensory, motor]	n. fibularis communis	sciatic n. in lower part of thigh	supplies short head of biceps femoris muscle; gives off lateral sural cutaneous n. and communicating branch as it descends in popliteal fossa, supplies knee and superior tibiofibular joints and tibialis anterior muscle; divides into superficial and deep fibular n's	
fibular n., deep [general sensory, motor]	n. fibularis profundus	a terminal branch of common fibular n.	winds around neck of fibula and descends on the interosseous membrane to front of ankle; muscular branches given off to tibialis anterior, extensor hallucis, extensor digitorum longus, and third peroneal muscles, and a twig to ankle joint; a lateral terminal division supplies extensor brevis muscle and tarsal joints; medial terminal division, or digital branch, divides into dorsal digital n's for skin and joints of adjacent sides of first and second toes	
frontal n. [general sensory]	n. frontalis	ophthalmic division of trigeminal n., enters orbit through superior orbital fissure	supraorbital and supratrochlear n's	chiefly to forehead and scalp (*see* individual branches listed in this table)
genitofemoral n. [general sensory, motor]	n. genitofemoralis	lumbar plexus—L1–L2	genital and femoral branches	cremaster muscle, skin of scrotum or labium majus and of adjacent area of thigh and femoral triangle
glossopharyngeal n. (9th cranial) [motor, parasympathetic, general sensory, special sensory, visceral sensory]	n. glossopharyngeus	several rootlets from lateral side of upper medulla oblongata, between olive and inferior cerebellar peduncle	tympanic n., pharyngeal, stylopharyngeal, tonsillar, and lingual branches, branch to carotid sinus, communicating branch with auricular branch of vagus n.	has two enlargements (superior and inferior ganglia) and supplies tongue, pharynx, and parotid nerve (*see also* individual branches in this table)
gluteal n., inferior [motor]	n. gluteus inferior	sacral plexus—L5–S2		gluteus maximus muscle
gluteal n., superior [motor, general sensory]	n. gluteus superior	sacral plexus—L4–S1		gluteus medius and minimus muscles, tensor fasciae latae, and hip joint

(continued)

2049

3-5. NERVES—cont'd

Common Name* [Modality]	TA Term†	Origin*	Branches*	Distribution*
hemorrhoidal n's, inferior. *See* rectal n's, inferior hypogastric n.	n. hypogastricus (dexter/sinister)	a nerve trunk situated on either side (right and left), interconnecting superior and inferior hypogastric plexuses		
hypoglossal n. (12th cranial) [motor]	n. hypoglossus	several rootlets in anterolateral sulcus between olive and pyramid of medulla oblongata; passes through hypoglossal canal to tongue	lingual branches	styloglossus, hypoglossus, and genioglossus muscles, intrinsic muscles of tongue
iliohypogastric n. [motor, general sensory]	n. iliohypogastricus	lumbar plexus—L1 (sometimes T12)	lateral and anterior cutaneous branches	skin above pubis and over lateral side of buttock, and occasionally pyramidal muscle
ilioinguinal n. [general sensory]	n. ilioinguinalis	lumbar plexus—L1 (sometimes T12); accompanies spermatic cord through inguinal canal	anterior scrotal or labial branches	skin of scrotum or labia majora, and adjacent part of thigh
infraoccipital n. *See* suboccipital n.				
infraorbital n. [general sensory]	n. infraorbitalis	continuation of maxillary n., entering orbit through inferior orbital fissure, occupying in succession infraorbital groove, canal, and foramen	middle and anterior superior alveolar, inferior palpebral, internal and external nasal, and superior labial branches	incisor, cuspid, and premolar teeth of upper jaw, skin and conjunctiva of lower eyelid, mobile septum and skin of side of nose, mucous membrane of mouth, skin of upper lip
infratrochlear n. [general sensory]	n. infratrochlearis	nasociliary n., from ophthalmic n.	palpebral branches	skin of root and upper bridge of nose and lower eyelid, conjunctiva, lacrimal duct
intercostobrachial n's [general sensory]	nn. intercostobrachiales	second and third intercostal n's		skin on back and medial aspect of arm
intermediate n. [parasympathetic, special sensory]	n. intermedius	smaller root of facial n., between main root and vestibulocochlear n.	greater petrosal n., chorda tympani	lacrimal, nasal, palatine, submandibular, and sublingual glands, and anterior two thirds of tongue
intermediofacial n. *See* facial n. *and* intermediate n.	n. intermediofacialis (NA alternative for facial and intermediate n's considered together)			
interosseous n. of forearm, anterior [motor, general sensory]	n. interosseus [antebrachii] anterior	median n.		flexor pollicis longus, flexor digitorum profundus, and pronator quadratus muscles, wrist and intercarpal joints

Common name [modalities]	Latin name	Origin	Branches / Distribution
interosseous n. of forearm, posterior [motor, general sensory]	n. interosseus [antebrachii] posterior	continuation of deep branch of radial n.	long abductor muscle of thumb, extensor muscles of thumb and index finger, and wrist and intercarpal joints
interosseous n. of leg [general sensory]	n. interosseus cruris	tibial n.	interosseous membrane and tibiofemoral syndesmosis
ischiadic n. *See* sciatic n.			
jugular n.	n. jugularis	a branch of the superior cervical which communicates with glossopharyngeal and vagus n's	
labial n's, anterior [general sensory]	nn. labiales anteriores	ilioinguinal n.	skin of anterior labial region of labia majora and adjacent part of thigh
labial n's, posterior [general sensory]	nn. labiales posteriores	pudendal n.	labium majus
lacrimal n. posterior [general sensory]	n. lacrimalis	ophthalmic division of trigeminal n. entering orbit through superior orbital fissure	lacrimal gland, conjunctiva, lateral commissure of eye, skin of upper eyelid
laryngeal n., inferior [motor]	n. laryngeus inferior	recurrent laryngeal n., especially the terminal portion	intrinsic muscles of larynx, except cricothyroid communicates with internal laryngeal n.
laryngeal n., recurrent [parasympathetic, visceral afferent, motor]	n. laryngeus recurrens	vagus n. (chiefly the cranial part of the accessory n.)	inferior laryngeal n., tracheal, esophageal, and inferior cardiac branches tracheal mucosa, esophagus, cardiac plexus (*see also* individual branches in this table)
laryngeal n., superior [motor, general sensory, visceral afferent, parasympathetic]	n. laryngeus superior	inferior ganglion of vagus n.	external, internal, and communicating branches cricothyroid muscle and inferior constrictor muscle of pharynx, mucous membrane of back of tongue and larynx
lingual n. [general sensory]	n. lingualis	mandibular n., descending to tongue, first medial to mandible and then under cover of mucosa of mouth	sublingual n., lingual branch, branch of isthmus of fauces, branch communicating with hypoglossal n. and chorda tympani anterior two thirds of tongue, adjacent areas of mouth, gums, isthmus of fauces
lumbar n's	nn. lumbales, n. mandibularis	the 5 pairs of n's that arise from lumbar segments of spinal cord, each pair leaving vertebral column below correspondingly numbered vertebrae; ventral branches of these nerves participate in formation of lumbosacral plexus	
mandibular n. (third division of trigeminal n.) [general sensory, motor]		trigeminal ganglion	meningeal branch, masseteric, deep temporal, lateral and medial pterygoid, buccal, auriculotemporal, lingual, and inferior alveolar n's extensive distribution to muscles of mastication, skin of face, mucous membrane of mouth, and teeth (*see also* individual branches in this table)

(continued)

3-5. NERVES—cont'd

Common Name* [Modality]	TA Term†	Origin*	Branches*	Distribution*
masseteric n. [motor, general sensory]	n. massetericus	mandibular division of trigeminal n.		masseter muscle, temporomandibular joint
maxillary n. (second division of trigeminal n.) [general sensory]	n. maxillaris	trigeminal ganglion	meningeal branch, zygomatic n., posterior superior alveolar branches, infraorbital n., pterygopalatine n's and indirectly branches of pterygopalatine ganglion	extensive distribution to skin of face and scalp, mucous membrane of maxillary sinus and nasal cavity, and teeth
median n. [general sensory]	n. medianus	lateral and medial cords of brachial plexus—C6–T1	anterior interosseous n. of forearm, common palmar digital n's, and muscular and palmar branches, and a communicating branch with ulnar n.	ultimately, skin on front of lateral part of hand, most of flexor muscles of front of forearm, most of short muscles of thumb, elbow joint, and many joints of hand
mental n. [general sensory]	n. mentalis	inferior alveolar n.	mental and inferior labial branches	skin of chin, lower lip
musculocutaneous n. [general sensory, motor]	n. musculocutaneus	lateral cord of brachial plexus—C5–C7	lateral cutaneous n. of forearm, muscular branches	coracobrachial, biceps, brachial muscles, elbow joint, skin of radial side of forearm
mylohyoid n. [motor]	n. mylohyoideus	inferior alveolar n.		mylohyoid muscle, anterior belly of digastric muscle
nasociliary n. [general sensory]	n. nasociliaris	ophthalmic division of trigeminal nerve	long ciliary, posterior ethmoidal, anterior ethmoidal, and infratrochlear n's and a communicating branch to ciliary ganglion	(see individual branches in this table)
nasopalatine n. [parasympathetic, general sensory]	n. nasopalatinus	pterygopalatine ganglion		mucosa and glands of most of nasal septum and anterior part of hard palate
obturator n. [general sensory, motor]	n. obturatorius	lumbar plexus—L3–L4	anterior, posterior, and muscular branches	gracilis and adductor muscles, skin of medial part of thigh and hip joints
obturator n., accessory [general sensory, motor]	n. obturatorius accessorius	ventral branches of ventral rami of L3–L4		pectineus muscle, hip joint, obturator nerve
obturator n., internal [general sensory, motor]	n. obturatorius internus	ventral branches of ventral rami of L5, S1–S2		posterior gemellus superior, obturator internus muscle
occipital n., greater [general sensory, motor]	n. occipitalis major	medial branch of dorsal branch of C2		semispinal muscle of head and skin of head as far forward as vertex
occipital n., lesser [general sensory]	n. occipitalis minor	superficial cervical plexus—C2–C3		ascends behind auricle and supplies some of the skin of side of head and on cranial surface of auricle

2052

occipital n., third [general sensory]	n. occipitalis tertius	medial branch of dorsal branch of C3		skin of upper part of back of neck and head
oculomotor n. (3rd cranial) [motor, parasympathetic]	n. oculomotorius	brain stem, emerging medial to cerebral peduncles, running forward in the cavernous sinus	superior and inferior branches	entering orbit through superior orbital fissure, the branches supply levator muscle of upper lid, all extrinsic muscles except lateral rectus and superior oblique, and carry parasympathetic fibers from ciliary muscle to sphincter of pupil
olfactory n's (1st cranial) [special sensory]	nn. olfactorii	the n's of smell, consisting of about 20 bundles arising in the olfactory epithelium and passing through the cribriform plate of ethmoid bone to olfactory bulb		
ophthalmic n. (first division of trigeminal n.) [general sensory]	n. ophthalmicus	trigeminal ganglion	tentorial branches, frontal, lacrimal, nasociliary n's	eyeball and conjunctiva, lacrimal sac and gland, nasal mucosa and frontal sinus, external nose, eyelid, forehead, and scalp (see also individual branches in this table)
optic n. (2nd cranial) [special sensory]	n. opticus	the nerve of sight, consisting chiefly of axons and central processes of cells of the ganglionic layer of retina leaving the orbit through the optic canal, joining the optic chiasm (the medial ones crossing over to opposite side), and continuing as the optic tract		
palatine n., anterior. See palatine n., greater				
palatine n., greater [parasympathetic, general sensory]	n. palatinus major	pterygopalatine ganglion	posterior inferior [lateral] nasal branches	emerges through greater palatine foramen and supplies palate
palatine n's, lesser [parasympathetic, sympathetic, general sensory]	nn. palatini minores	pterygopalatine ganglion		emerge through lesser palatine foramen and supply soft palate and tonsil
perineal n's [motor, general sensory]	nn. perineales	pudendal n. in pudendal canal	muscular branches and posterior scrotal or labial nerves	muscular branches supply bulbospongiosus, ischiocavernosus, superficial transverse perinei muscles and bulb of penis and, in part, sphincter ani and levator ani; the scrotal (labial) n's supply the scrotum or labium majus

(continued)

Common Name* [Modality]	TA Term†	Origin*	Branches*	Distribution*
peroneal n's. *See entries under* fibular n.				
petrosal n., deep [sympathetic]	n. petrosus profundus	internal carotid plexus		joins greater petrosal n. to form n. of pterygoid canal, and supplies lacrimal, nasal, and palatine glands via pterygopalatine ganglion and its branches
petrosal n., greater [parasympathetic, general sensory]	n. petrosus major	intermediate n. via geniculate ganglion		running forward from geniculate ganglion, joins deep petrosal n. of pterygoid canal, and reaches lacrimal, nasal, and palatine glands and nasopharynx via pterygopalatine ganglion and its branches
petrosal n., lesser [parasympathetic]	n. petrosus minor	tympanic plexus		parotid gland via otic ganglion and auriculotemporal n.
phrenic n. [motor, general sensory]	n. phrenicus	cervical plexus—C4–C5	pericardial and phrenicoabdominal branches	pleura, pericardium, diaphragm, peritoneum, sympathetic plexuses
phrenic n's, accessory	nn. phrenici accessorii	inconstant contribution of fifth n. to phrenic n.; when present, they run a separate course to root of neck or into thorax before joining phrenic n.		
piriform n. [general sensory, motor]	n. piriformis	dorsal branches of ventral rami of S1–S2		anterior piriform muscle
plantar n., lateral [general sensory, motor]	n. plantaris lateralis	smaller of terminal branches of tibial n.	muscular, superficial, and deep branches	lying between first and second layers of muscles of sole, supplies quadratus plantae, abductor digiti minimi, flexor digiti minimi brevis, adductor hallucis, interossei, and second, third, and fourth lumbrical muscles, and gives off cutaneous and articular twigs to lateral side of sole and fourth and fifth toes (*see also* individual branches in this table)

English name [modality]	Latin name	Origin	Branches	Distribution
plantar n., medial [general sensory, motor]	n. plantaris medialis	larger of terminal branches of tibial n.	common plantar digital n's and muscular branches	abductor hallucis, flexor digitorum brevis, flexor hallucis brevis, and first lumbrical muscles and cutaneous and articular twigs to medial side of sole and first to fourth toes (see also individual branches in this table)
pneumogastric n. See vagus n.				
pterygoid n., lateral [minor]	n. pterygoideus lateralis	mandibular n.		lateral pterygoid, tensor tympani, and tensor veli palatini muscles
pterygoid n., medial [motor]	n. pterygoideus medialis	mandibular n.		medial pterygoid muscle
n. of pterygoid canal [parasympathetic, sympathetic]	n. canalis pterygoidei	union of deep and greater petrosal n's		pterygopalatine ganglion and branches
pterygopalatine n's [general sensory]	nn. pterygopalatini	two nerves connecting maxillary n. to pterygopalatine ganglion; they are the sensory roots of the ganglion		
pudendal n. [general sensory, motor, parasympathetic]	n. pudendus	sacral plexus—S2–S4	enters pudendal canal, gives off inferior rectal n., then divides into perineal n. and dorsal n. of penis (clitoris)	muscles, skin, and erectile tissue of perineum (see also individual branches in this table)
n. of quadrate muscle of thigh [sensory, motor]	n. musculi quadrati femoris	ventral branches of ventral rami of L4–L5		gemellus inferior, anterior quadratus femoris muscle, hip joint
radial n. [general sensory, motor]	n. radialis	posterior cord of brachial plexus—C6–C8, and sometimes C5 and T1	posterior cutaneous and inferior lateral cutaneous n's of arm, posterior cutaneous n. of forearm, muscular, deep, and superficial branches	descending in back of arm and forearm, ultimately distributed to skin on back of forearm, arm, and hand, extensor muscles on back of arm and forearm, and elbow joint and many joints of hand
rectal n's, inferior [general sensory, motor]	nn. rectales inferiores	pudendal n., or independently from sacral plexus		sphincter ani externus muscle, skin around anus, lining of anal canal up to pectinate line
recurrent n. See laryngeal n., recurrent				
saccular n.	n. saccularis	the branch of vestibular part of 8th cranial (vestibulocochlear) nerve that innervates macula of saccule		
sacral n's	nn. sacrales	the 5 pairs of n's that arise from sacral segments of spinal cord; the ventral branches of first 4 pairs participate in formation of sacral plexus		

(continued)

3-5. NERVES—cont'd

Common Name* [Modality]	TA Term†	Origin*	Branches*	Distribution*
saphenous n. [general sensory]	n. saphenus	termination of femoral n.	infrapatellar and medial crural cutaneous	knee joint, subsartorial and patellar plexuses, skin on medial side of leg and foot
sciatic n. [general sensory, motor]	n. ischiadicus	sacral plexus—L4–S3; leaves pelvis through greater sciatic foramen	divides into common peroneal and tibial n's, usually in lower third of thigh	(see individual branches in this table)
scrotal n's, anterior [general sensory]	nn. scrotales anteriores	ilioinguinal n.		skin of anterior scrotal region
scrotal n's, posterior [general sensory]	nn. scrotales posteriores	perineal n's		skin of scrotum
spinal n's	nn. spinales	the 31 pairs of n's that arise from spinal cord, and pass between the vertebrae, including 8 cervical, 12 thoracic, 5 lumbar, 5 sacral, and 1 coccygeal		
spinal accessory n. See accessory n.				
splanchnic n., greater [preganglionic sympathetic, visceral afferent]	n. splanchnicus thoracicus major	thoracic sympathetic trunk and thoracic ganglia T5–T10 of sympathetic trunk		descending through diaphragm or its aortic opening, ends in celiac ganglia and plexuses, with a splanchnic ganglion commonly near the diaphragm
splanchnic n., lesser [preganglionic sympathetic, visceral afferent]	n. splanchnicus thoracicus minor	thoracic ganglia T9, T10 of sympathetic trunk	renal branch	pierces diaphragm, joins aorticorenal ganglion and celiac plexus, and communicates with renal and superior mesenteric plexuses
splanchnic n., lowest. See thoracic splanchnic n., lowest				
splanchnic n's, lumbar [preganglionic sympathetic, visceral afferent]	nn. splanchnici lumbales	lumbar ganglia of sympathetic trunk		upper nerves join celiac and adjacent plexuses, middle ones go to mesenteric and adjacent plexuses, lower ones descend to superior hypogastric plexus
splanchnic n's, pelvic [preganglionic sympathetic, visceral afferent]	nn. splanchnici pelvini	sacral plexus—S3–S4		leaving sacral plexus, they enter inferior hypogastric plexus and supply pelvic organs
splanchnic n's, sacral [preganglionic sympathetic, visceral afferent]	nn. splanchnici sacrales	sacral part of sympathetic trunk		pelvic organs and blood vessels via inferior hypogastric plexus
stapedius n. [motor]	n. stapedius	facial n.		stapedius muscle
subclavian n. [general sensory]	n. subclavius	upper trunk of brachial plexus—C5		subclavius muscle, sternoclavicular joint

Common name [modality]	NA term	Origin	Branches	Distribution
subcostal n. [general sensory, motor]	n. subcostalis	ventral branch of T12		skin of lower abdomen and lateral side of gluteal region, parts of transverse, oblique, and rectus muscles, and usually pyramidal muscle, and adjacent peritoneum
sublingual n. [parasympathetic, general sensory]	n. sublingualis	lingual n.		sublingual gland and overlying mucous membrane
suboccipital n. [motor]	n. suboccipitalis	dorsal branch of C1		emerges above posterior arch of atlas, supplies muscles of suboccipital triangle and semispinal muscle of head
subscapular n. [motor]	n. subscapularis	posterior cord of brachial plexus—C5		usually two or more nerves, upper and lower, supplying subscapular and teres major muscles
supraclavicular n's, anterior. *See* supraclavicular n's, medial				
supraclavicular n's, intermediate [general sensory]	nn. supraclaviculares intermedii	cervical plexus—C3–C4		descends in posterior triangle, crosses clavicle, supplying skin over pectoral and deltoid regions
supraclavicular n's, lateral [general sensory]	nn. supraclaviculares laterales	cervical plexus—C3–C4		descends in posterior triangle, crosses clavicle, supplying skin of superior and posterior aspects of shoulder
supraclavicular n's, medial [general sensory]	nn. supraclaviculares mediales	cervical plexus—C3–C4		descends in posterior triangle, crosses clavicle, supplying skin of medial infraclavicular region
supraclavicular n's, middle. *See* supraclavicular n's, intermediate supraclavicular n's, posterior. *See* supraclavicular n's lateral				
supraorbital n. [general sensory]	n. supraorbitalis	continuation of frontal n., from ophthalmic n.	lateral and medial branches	leaves orbit through supraorbital notch or foramen, supplying skin of upper eyelid, forehead, anterior part of scalp (to vertex), mucosa of frontal sinus

(continued)

Common Name* [Modality]	TA Term†	Origin*	Branches*	Distribution*
suprascapular n. [motor, general sensory]	n. suprascapularis	brachial plexus—C5–C6		descends through suprascapular and spinoglenoid notches, supplying acromioclavicular and shoulder joints, and supraspinous and infraspinous muscles
supratrochlear n. [general sensory]	n. supratrochlearis	frontal n., from ophthalmic n.		leaves orbit at end of supraorbital margin, supplying forehead and upper eyelid
sural n. [general sensory]	n. suralis	medial sural n. and communicating branch of common peroneal n.	lateral dorsal cutaneous n. and lateral calcaneal branches	skin on back of leg, and skin and joints on lateral side of foot and heel
temporal n's, deep [motor]	nn. temporales profundi	mandibular n.		temporal muscles
n. of tensor tympani muscle [motor]	n. musculi tensoris tympani	mandibular n. via n. to medial pterygoid muscle and otic ganglion		tensor muscle of tympanum
n. of tensor veli palatini muscle [motor]	n. musculi tensoris veli palatini	mandibular n. via n. to medial pterygoid muscle and otic ganglion		tensor muscle of palatine velum
thoracic n's	nn. thoracici	the 12 pairs of spinal n's that arise from thoracic segments of spinal cord, each pair leaving vertebral column below correspondingly numbered vertebrae		body wall of thorax and upper part of abdomen
thoracic n., long [motor]	n. thoracicus longus	brachial plexus—ventral branches of C5–C7		descends behind brachial plexus to anterior serratus muscle
thoracic splanchnic n., greater [preganglionic sympathetic and visceral afferent]	n. splanchnicus thoracicus major	thoracic sympathetic trunk and fifth through tenth thoracic ganglia		descends through diaphragm or its openings and ends in celiac ganglia and plexuses with a splanchnic ganglion commonly near the diaphragm
thoracic splanchnic n., lesser [preganglionic sympathetic and visceral afferent]	n. splanchnicus thoracicus minor	ninth and tenth thoracic ganglia of the sympathetic trunk	renal ramus	pierces the diaphragm, joins the aorticorenal ganglion and celiac plexus, and communicates with the renal and mesenteric plexuses
thoracic splanchnic n., lowest [sympathetic and visceral afferent]	n. splanchnicus thoracicus imus	last ganglion of sympathetic trunk of lesser splanchnic n.		aorticorenal ganglion and adjacent plexus

Common Term [modality]	Latin Term (NA)	Origin	Distribution
thoracodorsal n. [motor]	n. thoracodorsalis	posterior cord of brachial plexus—C7–C8	latissimus dorsi muscle
tibial n. [general sensory, motor]	n. tibialis	sciatic n. in lower thigh	interosseous n. of leg, medial cutaneous n. of calf, sural and medial and lateral plantar n's, and muscular and medial calcaneal branches	while still incorporated in sciatic n., supplies semimembranous and semitendinous muscles, long head of biceps, and adductor magnus muscle; supplies knee joint as it descends in popliteal fossa; continuing into leg, supplies muscles and skin of calf, sole, and toes (*see also* individual branches in this table)
trigeminal n. (5th cranial) [general sensory, motor]	n. trigeminus	emerges from lateral surface of pons as a motor and a sensory root, the latter expanding into trigeminal ganglion, from which the 3 divisions of nerve arise (*see* mandibular n., maxillary n., and ophthalmic n.)	face, teeth, mouth, nasal cavity, muscles of mastication
trochlear n. (4th cranial) [motor]	n. trochlearis	fibers of each nerve (one on either side) decussate across median plane, and emerge from back of brain stem below corresponding inferior colliculus	runs forward in lateral wall of cavernous sinus, traverses superior orbital fissure, supplying superior oblique muscle of eyeball
tympanic n. [general sensory, parasympathetic]	n. tympanicus	inferior ganglion of glossopharyngeal n.	helps form tympanic plexus	mucous membrane of tympanic cavity, mastoid air cells, auditory tube, and, via lesser petrosal n. and otic ganglion, parotid gland
ulnar n. [general sensory, motor]	n. ulnaris	medial and lateral cords of brachial plexus—C7–T1	muscular, dorsal, palmar, superficial, and deep branches	ultimately to skin on front and medial part of hand, some flexor muscles on front of forearm, many short muscles of hand, elbow joint, many joints of hand
utricular n. utriculoampullary n.	n. utricularis n. utriculoampullaris	the branch of vestibular n. that innervates macula of utricle a n. that arises by peripheral division of vestibular n., and supplies utricle and ampullae of semicircular ducts	
vaginal n's [sympathetic, parasympathetic]	nn. vaginales	uterovaginal plexus	vagina

(continued)

3-5. NERVES—cont'd

Common Name* [Modality]	TA Term†	Origin*	Branches*	Distribution*
vagus n. (10th cranial) [parasympathetic, visceral afferent, motor, general sensory]	n. vagus	by numerous rootlets from lateral side of medulla oblongata in groove between olive and inferior cerebellar peduncle	superior and recurrent laryngeal n's, meningeal, auricular, pharyngeal, cardiac, bronchial, gastric, hepatic, celiac, and renal branches, pharyngeal, pulmonary, and esophageal plexuses, and anterior and posterior trunks	descending through jugular foramen, presents as a superior and inferior ganglion, continues through neck and thorax into abdomen, supplying sensory fibers to ear, tongue, pharynx, and larynx, motor fibers to pharynx, larynx, esophagus, and parasympathetic and visceral fibers to thoracic and abdominal viscera (see also individual branches in this table)
vertebral n. [sympathetic]	n. vertebralis	cervicothoracic and vertebral		ascends with vertebral artery and gives fibers to spinal meninges, cervical n's, and posterior cranial fossa
vestibular n.	n. vestibularis	the posterior part of the vestibulocochlear n., concerned with equilibrium, consisting of fibers arising from bipolar cells in vestibular ganglion; divides peripherally into rostral and caudal parts, with receptors in the ampullae of the semicircular canals, the ventricle, and the saccule		
vestibulocochlear n. (8th cranial)	n. vestibulo-cochlearis	emerges from brain between pons and medulla oblongata, at cerebellopontine angle and behind facial n; divides near lateral end of internal acoustic meatus into two functionally distinct and incompletely united components, the vestibular n. and the cochlear n., and is connected with brain by corresponding roots (vestibular and cochlear roots)		
vidian n. See n. of pterygoid canal vidian n., deep. See deep petrosal n., deep				
zygomatic n. [general sensory]	n. zygomaticus	maxillary n., entering orbit through inferior orbital fissure	zygomaticofacial and zygomaticotemporal branches	communicates with lacrimal nerve, supplying skin of temple and adjacent part of face

3-6. VEINS

Common Name*	TA Term†	Region	Receives Blood From*	Drains Into*
accompanying v. of hypoglossal nerve	v. comitans nervi hypoglossi	accompanies hypoglossal nerve	formed by union of profunda linguae v. and sublingual v.	facial, lingual, or internal jugular
adrenal v's. *See* suprarenal v., left and right				
anastomotic v., inferior	v. anastomotica inferior	interconnects superficial middle cerebral v. and transverse sinus		
anastomotic v., superior	v. anastomotica superior	interconnects superficial middle cerebral v. and superior sagittal sinus		
angular v.	v. angularis	between eye and root of nose	formed by union of supratrochlear v. and supraorbital v.	continues inferiority as facial v.
antebrachial v., median	v. intermedia antebrachii	forearm between cephalic v. and basilic v.	a palmar venous plexus	cephalic v. and/ or basilic v., or median cubital v.
appendicular v.	v. appendicularis	accompanies appendicular artery		joins anterior and posterior cecal v's to form ileocolic v.
v. of aqueduct of cochlea	v. aqueductus cochleae	along aqueduct of cochlea	cochlea	superior bulb of internal jugular v.
v. of aqueduct of vestibule	v. aqueductus vestibuli	passes through aqueduct of vestibule	internal ear	superior petrosal sinus
arcuate v's of kidney	vv. arcuatae renis	a series of complete arches across the bases of the renal pyramids formed for union of interlobular v's and straight venules of kidney		interlobar v's
articular v's	vv. articulares		plexus around temporomandibular joint	retromandibular v.
atrial v., lateral	v. lateralis atrii	passes through lateral wall of lateral ventricle	temporal and parietal lobes	superior thalamostriate v.
atrial v., medial	v. medialis atrii	passes through medial wall of lateral ventricle	parietal and occipital lobes	internal cerebral or great cerebral v.
auditory v's, internal. *See* labyrinthine v's				
auricular v's,anterior	vv. auriculares anteriores	anterior part of auricle		superficial temporal v.
auricular v., posterior	v. auricularis posterior	passes down behind auricle	a plexus on side of head	joins retromandibular v. to form external jugular v.
axillary v.	v. axillaris	the upper limb	formed at lower border of teres major muscle by junction of basilic v. and brachial v.	at lateral border of first rib is continuous with subclavian v.

(continued)

*v. = vein; v's = (pl.) veins.
†v. = vena; vv. = [L. (pl.)] venae.

3-6. VEINS—cont'd

Common Name*	TA Term†	Region	Receives Blood From*	Drains Into*
azygos v.	v. azygos	intercepting trunk for right intercostal v's as well as connecting branch between superior and inferior venae cavae; it ascends in front of and on right side of vertebrae	ascending lumbar v.	superior vena cava
azygos v., left. *See* hemiazygos v. azygos v., lesser superior. *See* hemiazygos v., accessory				
basal v.	v. basalis	passes from anterior perforated substance backward and around cerebral peduncle	anterior perforated substance	internal cerebral v.
basilic v. basilic v., median	v. basilica v. intermedia basilica	forearm, superficially sometimes present as medial branch of a bifurcation of median antebrachial v.	ulnar side of dorsal rete of hand	joins brachial v's to form axillary v. basilic v.
basivertebral v's	v. basivertebrales	venous sinuses in cancellous tissue of bodies of vertebrae, which communicate with venous plexus or anterior surface of vertebrae and with external and internal vertebral plexuses		
brachial v's brachiocephalic v's	vv. brachiales vv. brachiocephalicae (dextra et sinistra)	accompany brachial artery thorax	head, neck, and upper limbs; formed at root of neck by union of ipsilateral internal jugular and subclavian v's	join basilic v. to form axillary v. unite to form superior vena cava
bronchial v's	vv. bronchiales		larger subdivisions of bronchi	azygos v. on left; hemiazygos or superior intercostal v. on right
v. of bulb of penis v. of bulb of vestibule cardiac v's, anterior	v. bulbi penis v. bulbi vestibuli vv. cardiacae anteriores		bulb of penis bulb of vestibule of vagina anterior wall of right ventricle	internal pudendal v. internal pudendal v. right atrium of heart, or lesser cardiac v.,
cardiac v., great cardiac v., middle cardiac v., small cardiac v's, smallest	v. cardiaca magna v. cardiaca media v. cardiaca parva vv. cardiacae minimae	numerous small veins arising in myocardium, draining independently into cavities of heart and most readily seen in the atria	anterior surface of ventricles diaphragmatic surface of ventricles right atrium and ventricle	coronary sinus coronary sinus coronary sinus coronary sinus

2062

carotid v., external. *See* retromandibular v.			
cavernous v's of penis	vv. cavernosae penis	corpora cavernosa	deep v's and dorsal v. of penis
central v's of liver	vv. centrales hepatis	in middle of hepatic lobules / liver substance	hepatic v.
central v. of retina	v. centralis retinae	eyeball / retinal v's	superior ophthalmic v.
central v. of suprarenal gland	v. centralis glandulae suprarenalis	the large single vein into which the various veins within the substance of the gland empty, and which continues at the hilum as the suprarenal v.	
cephalic v.	v. cephalica	winds anteriorly to pass along the anterior border of brachioradial muscle; above elbow, ascends along lateral border of biceps of deltoid muscle / radial side of dorsal rete of hand	axillary v.
cephalic v., accessory	v. cephalica accessoria	forearm / dorsal rete of hand	joins cephalic v. just above elbow
cephalic v., median	v. intermedia cephalica	sometimes present as lateral branch formed by bifurcation of median antebrachial v.	cephalic v.
cerebellar v's, inferior	vv. cerebelli	inferior surface of cerebellum	transverse, sigmoid, and inferior petrosal sinuses, or occipital sinus
cerebellar v's, superior	vv. cerebelli	superior surface of cerebellum	straight sinus and great cerebral v., or transverse and superior petrosal sinuses
cerebral v's, anterior	vv. anteriores cerebri	accompany anterior cerebral artery	basal v.
cerebral v., great	v. magna cerebri	curves around splenium of corpus callosum	continues as or drains into straight sinus
cerebral v's, inferior	vv. inferiores cerebri	veins that ramify on base and inferolateral surface of brain, those on inferior surface of frontal lobe draining into inferior sagittal sinus and cavernous sinus; those on temporal lobe into superior petrosal sinus and transverse sinus; and those on occipital lobe into straight sinus	formed by union of the 2 internal cerebral veins
cerebral v's, internal (2)	vv. internae cerebri	pass backward from interventricular foramen through tela choroidea	formed by union of thalamostriate v. and choroid v.; collect blood from basal ganglia
cerebral v., middle, deep	v. media profunda cerebri	accompanies middle cerebral artery in floor of lateral sulcus	basal v.
cerebral v., middle, superficial	v. media superficialis cerebri	follows lateral cerebral fissure	cavernous sinus
cerebral v's, superior	vv. superiores cerebri	about 12 veins draining superolateral and medial surfaces of cerebrum toward longitudinal fissure	superior sagittal sinus
cervical v., deep	v. cervicalis profunda	accompanies deep cervical artery down neck	vertebral v. or brachiocephalic v.
cervical v's, transverse	vv. transversae cervicis	accompany transverse cervical artery	subclavian v.

(continued)

3-6. VEINS—cont'd

Common Name*	TA Term†	Region	Receives Blood From*	Drains Into*
choroid v., inferior	v. choroidea inferior		inferior choroid plexus	basal v.
choroid v., superior	v. choroidea superior	runs whole length of choroid plexus	choroid plexus, hippocampus, fornix, corpus callosum	joins superior thalamostriate v. to form internal cerebral v.
ciliary v's	vv. ciliares	anterior vessels follow anterior ciliary arteries; posterior follow posterior ciliary arteries	arise in eyeball by branches from ciliary muscle; anterior ciliary v's also receive branches from sinus venosus, sclerae, episcleral v's and conjunctiva of eyeball	superior ophthalmic v.; posterior ciliary v's empty also into inferior ophthalmic v.
circumflex femoral v's, lateral	vv. circumflexae laterales femoris	accompany lateral circumflex femoral artery		femoral v. or profunda femoris v.
circumflex femoral v's, medial	vv. circumflexae mediales femoris	accompany medial circumflex femoral artery		femoral v. or profunda femoris v.
circumflex iliac v., deep	v. circumflexa ilium profunda	a common trunk formed by veins accompanying deep circumflex iliac artery		external iliac v.
circumflex iliac v., superficial	v. circumflexa superficialis ilium	accompanies superficial circumflex iliac artery		great saphenous v.
v. of cochlear canal. See v. of aqueduct of cochlea				
colic v., left	v. colica sinistra	accompanies left colic artery		inferior mesenteric v.
colic v., middle	v. colica media	accompanies middle colic artery		superior mesenteric v.
colic v., right	v. colica dextra	accompanies right colic artery		superior mesenteric v.
conjunctival v's	vv. conjunctivales		conjunctiva	superior ophthalmic v.
coronary v's. See entries under cardiac v's				
v. of corpus callosum, posterior	v. posterior corporis callosi		posterior surface of corpus callosum	great cerebral v.
cubital v., median	v. intermedia cubiti	the large connecting branch passing obliquely upward across cubital fossa	cephalic v., below elbow	basilic v.
cutaneous v.	v. cutanea	one of the small veins that begin in papillae of skin, form subpapillary plexuses, and open into the subcutaneous veins		
cystic v.	v. cystica	within substance of liver	gallbladder	right branch of portal v.
deep v's of clitoris	vv. profundae clitoridis		clitoris	vesical venous plexus
deep v's of penis	vv. profundae penis		penis	dorsal v. of penis
digital v's of foot, dorsal	vv. digitales dorsales pedis	accompany deep artery of penis dorsal surface of toes		unite at clefts to form dorsal metatarsal v's

Common Name	NA Term	Accompanies / Description	Region	Drains Into / Receives
digital v's, palmar	vv. digitales palmares	accompany proper and common palmar digital arteries		superficial palmar venous arch
digital v's, plantar	vv. digitales plantares	plantar surfaces of toes		unite at clefts to form plantar metatarsal v's
diploic v., frontal	v. diploica frontalis		frontal bone	supraorbital v. externally, or superior sagittal sinus internally
diploic v., occipital	v. diploica occipitalis		occipital bone	occipital v. or transverse sinus
diploic v., temporal, anterior	v. diploica temporalis anterior		lateral portion of frontal bone, anterior part of parietal bone	sphenoparietal sinus internally, or a deep temporal v. externally
diploic v., temporal, posterior	v. diploica temporalis posterior		parietal bone	transverse sinus
direct v's, lateral	vv. directae laterales		lateral ventricle	great cerebral v.
dorsal v. of clitoris, deep	v. dorsalis profunda clitoridis			vesical plexus
dorsal v's of clitoris, superficial	vv. dorsales superficiales clitoridis	accompanies dorsal artery of clitoris	clitoris, subcutaneously	external pudendal v.
dorsal v. of corpus callosum	v. dorsalis corporis callosi		superior surface of corpus callosum	great cerebral vein
dorsal v. of penis, deep	v. dorsalis profunda penis		the single median vein lying subfascially in penis between the dorsal arteries; it begins in small veins around corona of glans, is joined by deep veins of penis as it passes proximally, and passes between arcuate pubic and transverse perineal ligaments, where it divides into a left and right vein to join prostatic plexus	
dorsal v's of penis, superficial	vv. dorsales superficiales penis		penis, subcutaneously	external pudendal v.
dorsal v's, of tongue. See lingual v's, dorsal	vv. dorsales linguae			
emissary v., condylar	v. emissaria condyloidea		a small vein running through condylar canal of skull connecting sigmoid sinus with vertebral v. or internal jugular v.	
emissary v., mastoid	v. emissaria mastoidea		a small vein passing through mastoid foramen of skull, connecting sigmoid sinus with occipital v. or posterior auricular v.	
emissary v., occipital	v. emissaria occipitalis		an occasional small vein running through a minute foramen in occipital protuberance of skull, connecting confluence of sinuses with occipital v.	
emissary v., parietal	v. emissaria parietalis		a small vein passing through parietal foramen of skull, connecting superior sagittal sinus with superficial temporal v's	
epigastric v., inferior	v. epigastrica inferior	accompanies inferior epigastric artery		external iliac v.
epigastric v., superficial	v. epigastrica superficialis	accompanies superficial epigastric artery		great saphenous v. or femoral v.
epigastric v's, superior	vv. epigastricae superiores	accompany superior epigastric artery		internal thoracic v.
episcleral v's	vv. episclerales	around cornea		vorticose v's and ciliary v's

(continued)

2065

3-6. VEINS—cont'd

Common Name*	TA Term†	Region	Receives Blood From*	Drains Into*
esophageal v's	vv. oesophageales		esophagus	hemiazygos v. and azygos v., or left brachiocephalic v.
ethmoidal v's	vv. ethmoidales	accompany anterior and posterior ethmoidal arteries and emerge from ethmoidal foramina		
facial v.	v. facialis	the vein beginning ar medial angle of eye as angular v., descending behind facial artery, and usually ending in internal jugular v.; sometimes joins retromandibular v. to form a common trunk		
facial v., deep	v. profunda faciei		pterygoid plexus	facial v.
facial v., posterior. *See* retromandibular v.				
facial v., transverse	v. transversa faciei	passes backward with transverse facial artery just below zygomatic arch		retromandibular v.
femoral v.	v. femoralis	follows course of femoral artery in proximal two thirds of thigh	continuation of popliteal v.	at inguinal ligament becomes external iliac v.
femoral v., deep	v. profunda femoris	accompanies deep femoral artery		femoral v.
fibular v's. *See* peroneal v's				
frontal v's	vv. frontales	superior cerebral veins that drain the frontal cortex		
gastric v., left	v. gastrica sinistra	accompanies left gastric artery		portal v.
gastric v., right	v. gastrica dextra	accompanies right gastric artery		portal v.
gastric v's, short	vv. gastricae breves		left portion of greater curvature of stomach	splenic v.
gastroepiploic v., left. *See* gastro-omental v., left				
gastroepiploic v., right. *See* gastro-omental v., right				
gastro-omental v., left	v. gastro-omentalis sinistra	accompanies left gastro-omental artery		splenic v.
gastro-omental v., right	v. gastro-omentalis dextra	accompanies right gastro-omental artery		superior mesenteric v.
genicular v's	vv. geniculares	accompany genicular arteries		
gluteal v's, inferior	vv. gluteae inferiores	accompany inferior gluteal artery; unite into a single vessel after passing through greater sciatic foramen	subcutaneous tissue of back of thigh, muscles of buttock	popliteal v. internal iliac v.

gluteal v's, superior	vv. gluteae superiores	accompany superior gluteal artery and pass through greater sciatic foramen	muscles of buttock	internal iliac v.
hemiazygos v.	v. hemiazygos	an intercepting trunk for lower left posterior intercostal v's; ascends on left side of vertebrae to eighth thoracic vertebra, where it may receive accessory branch, and crosses vertebral column		azygos v.
hemiazygos v., accessory	v. hemiazygos accessoria	the descending intercepting trunk for upper, often fourth through eighth, left posterior intercostal v's; it lies on left side and at eighth thoracic vertebra joins hemiazygos v. or crosses to right side to join azygos v. directly; above, it may communicate with left superior intercostal v.	ascending lumbar v.	
hemorrhoidal v's. *See* entries under rectal v's				
hepatic v's	vv. hepaticae	2 or 3 large veins in an upper group and 6 to 20 small veins in a lower group, forming successively larger vessels	central v's of liver	inferior vena cava on posterior aspect of liver
hypogastric v. *See* iliac v., internal				
ileal v's	vv. ileales		ileum	superior mesenteric v.
ileocolic v.	v. ileocolica	accompanies ileocolic artery		superior mesenteric v.
iliac v., common	v. iliaca communis	ascends to right side of fifth lumbar vertebra	arises at sacroiliac joint by union of external and internal iliac v's	unites with fellow of opposite side to form inferior vena cava
iliac v., external	v. iliaca externa	extends from inguinal ligament to sacroiliac joint	continuation of femoral v.	joins internal iliac v. to form common iliac v.
iliac v., internal	v. iliaca interna	extends from greater sciatic notch to brim of pelvis	formed by union of parietal branches	joins external iliac v. to form common iliac v.
iliolumbar v.	v. iliolumbalis	accompanies iliolumbar artery		internal iliac v. and/or common iliac v.
innominate v's. *See* brachiocephalic v's				
insular v's	vv. insulares		insula	deep middle cerebral v.
intercapital v's	vv. intercapitales manus	veins at clefts of fingers that pass between heads of metacarpal bones and establish communication between dorsal and palmar venous systems of hand		
intercostal v's, anterior (12 pairs)	vv. intercostales anteriores	accompany anterior thoracic arteries		internal thoracic v's

(continued)

3-6. VEINS—cont'd

Common Name*	TA Term†	Region	Receives Blood From*	Drains Into*
intercostal v., highest	v. intercostalis suprema	first posterior intercostal vein of either side, which passes over apex of lung		brachiocephalic, vertebral, or superior intercostal v.
intercostal v's, posterior	vv. intercostales posteriores	accompany posterior intercostal arteries	intercostal spaces	azygos v. on right; hemiazygos or accessory hemiazygos v. on left
intercostal v., superior, left	v. intercostalis superior sinistra	crosses arch of aorta	formed by union of second, third, and sometimes fourth posterior intercostal v's	left brachiocephalic v.
intercostal v., superior, right	v. intercostalis superior dextra		formed by union of second, third, and sometimes fourth posterior intercostal v's	azygos v.
interlobar v's of kidney	vv. interlobares renis	pass down between renal pyramids	venous arcades of kidney	unite to form renal v.
interlobular v's of kidney	vv. interlobulares renis			venous arcades of kidney
interlobular v's of liver	vv. interlobulares hepatis	arise between hepatic lobules	capillary network of renal cortex	portal v.
interosseous v's of foot, dorsal. See metatarsal v's, dorsal			liver	
intervertebral v.	v. intervertebralis	vertebral column	vertebral venous plexuses	in neck, vertebral v.; in thorax, intercostal v's; in abdomen, lumbar v's; in pelvis, lateral sacral v's
jejunal v's	vv. jejunales			superior mesenteric v.
jugular v., anterior	v. jugularis anterior	arises under chin and passes down neck	jejunum	external jugular v. or subclavian v., or jugular venous arch
jugular v., external	v. jugularis externa	begins in parotid gland behind angle of jaw and passes down neck	formed by union of retromandibular v. and posterior auricular v.	subclavian v., internal jugular v., or brachiocephalic v.
jugular v., internal	v. jugularis interna	from jugular fossa, descends in neck with internal carotid artery and then with common carotid artery	begins as superior bulb, draining much of head and neck	joins subclavian v. to form brachiocephalic v.
labial v's, anterior	vv. labiales anteriores		anterior aspect of labia in female	external pudendal v.
labial v's, inferior	vv. labiales inferiores		region of lower lip	facial v.
labial v's, posterior	vv. lables posteriores		labia in female	vesical venous plexus
labial v., superior	v. labialis superior		region of upper lip	facial v.
labyrinthine v's	vv. labyrinthi	pass through internal acoustic meatus	cochlea	inferior petrosal sinus or transverse sinus
lacrimal v.	v. lacrimalis		lacrimal gland	superior ophthalmic v.
laryngeal v., inferior	v. laryngea inferior		larynx	inferior thyroid v.
laryngeal v., superior	v. laryngea superior		larynx	superior thyroid v.

(continued)

lingual v.	*v. lingualis*	a deep vein following distribution of lingual artery	internal jugular v.
lingual v., deep	*v. profunda linguae*	deep aspect of tongue	joins sublingual v. to form accompanying v. of hypoglossal nerve
lingual v's, dorsal	*vv. dorsales linguae*	veins that unite with a small vein accompanying lingual artery and join main lingual trunk	
lumbar v's	*vv. lumbales*	4 or 5 v's on each side accompanying corresponding lumbar arteries and draining posterior wall of abdomen, vertebral canal, spinal cord, and meninges; first 4 usually end in inferior vena cava, although first may end in ascending lumbar v.; fifth is generally a tributary of common iliac v.	
lumbar v., ascending	*v. lumbalis ascendens*	an ascending intercepting vein for lumbar v's on either side; it begins in lateral sacral region and ascends to first lumbar vertebra, where by union with subcostal v. it becomes on right side the azygos v. and on left the hemiazygos v.	
maxillary v's	*vv. maxillares*	usually form a single short trunk with pterygoid plexus	joins superficial temporal v. in parotid gland to form retromandibular v.
mediastinal v's	*vv. mediastinales*	anterior mediastinum	brachiocephalic v., azygos v., or superior vena cava
v's of medulla oblongata	*vv. medullae oblongatae*	medulla oblongata	v's of spinal cord, dural venous sinuses, inferior petrosal sinus, superior bulb of jugular v.
meningeal v's	*vv. meningeae*	accompany meningeal arteries; dura mater (also communicate with lateral lacunae)	regional sinuses and veins
meningeal v's, middle	*vv. meningeae mediae*	accompany middle meningeal artery	pterygoid venous plexus
mesenteric v., inferior	*v. mesenterica inferior*	follows distribution of inferior mesenteric artery	splenic v.
mesenteric v., superior	*v. mesenterica superior*	follows distribution of superior mesenteric artery	joins splenic v. to form portal v.
metacarpal v's, dorsal	*vv. metacarpales dorsales*	veins arising from union of dorsal veins of adjacent fingers and passing proximally to join in forming dorsal venous network of hand	
metacarpal v's, palmar	*vv. metacarpales palmares*	accompany palmar metacarpal arteries	deep palmar venous arch
metatarsal v's, dorsal	*vv. metatarsales dorsales*	arise from dorsal digital v's of toes at clefts of toes	dorsal venous arch
metatarsal v's, plantar	*vv. metatarsales plantares*	deep veins of foot; arise from plantar digital v's at clefts of toes	plantar venous arch
musculophrenic v's	*vv. musculophrenicae*	accompany musculophrenic artery; parts of diaphragm and wall of thorax and abdomen	internal thoracic v's

3-6. VEINS—cont'd

Common Name*	TA Term†	Region	Receives Blood From*	Drains Into*
nasal v's, external	vv. nasales externae	small ascending branches from nose		angular v., facial v.
nasofrontal v.	v. nasofrontalis		supraorbital v.	superior ophthalmic v.
oblique v. of left atrium	v. obliqua atrii sinistri	left atrium of heart		coronary sinus
obturator v's	vv. obturatoriae	enter pelvis through obturator canal	hip joint and regional muscles	internal iliac v. and/or interior epi-gastric v.
occipital v.	v. occipitalis	scalp; follows distribution of oc-cipital artery		opens under trapezius muscle into suboccipital venous plexus, or accompanies occipital artery to end in internal jugular v.
ophthalmic v., inferior	v. ophthalmica inferior	a vein formed by confluence of muscular and ciliary branches, and running backward either to join superior ophthalmic v. or to open directly into cavernous sinus; it sends a communicating branch through inferior orbital fissure to join pterygoid venous plexus		
ophthalmic v., superior	v. ophthalmica superior	a vein beginning at medial angle of eye, where it communicates with frontal, supraorbital, and angular v's; it follows distribution of ophthalmic artery, and may be joined by inferior ophthalmic v. at superior orbital fissure before opening into cavernous sinus		
ovarian v., left	v. ovarica sinistra		pampiniform plexus of broad liga-ment on left	left renal v.
ovarian v., right	v. ovarica dextra		pampiniform plexus of broad liga-ment on right	inferior vena cava
palatine v., external	v. palatina externa		tonsils and soft palate	facial v.
palpebral v's	vv. palpebrales	small branches from eyelids		superior ophthalmic v.
palpebral v's, inferior	vv. palpebrales inferiores		lower eyelid	facial v.
palpebral v's, superior	vv. palpebrales superior		upper eyelid	angular v.
pancreatic v's	vv. pancreaticae		pancreas	splenic v., superior mesenteric v.
pancreaticoduodenal v's	vv. pancreaticoduodenales	four veins that drain blood from pancreas and duodenum, closely following pancreaticoduodenal arteries, a superior and an inferior vein originating from an anterior and a posterior venous arcade; anterior superior v. joins right gastroepiploic v., and posterior superior v. joins portal v.; anterior and posterior inferior v's join, sometimes as one trunk, uppermost jejunal v. or superior mesenteric v.		
paraumbilical v's	vv. paraumbilicales	veins that communicate with portal v. above and descend to anterior abdom-inal wall to anastomose with superior and inferior epigastric and superior vesical v's in region of umbilicus; they form a significant part of collateral circulation of portal v. in event of hepatic obstruction		
parotid v's	vv. parotideae		parotid gland	superficial temporal v.

perforating v's	vv. perforantes	empty into deep femoral v. and establish anastomosis between deep femoral v. and popliteal v. (below) and inferior gluteal v. (above)	
pericardiac v's	vv. pericardiales	pericardium	brachiocephalic, inferior thyroid, and azygos v's, superior vena cava
pericardiacophrenic v's	vv. pericardiacophrenicae	pericardium and diaphragm	left brachiocephalic v
peroneal v's	vv. fibulares	accompany peroneal artery	posterior tibial v.
pharyngeal v's	vv. pharyngeales	pharyngeal plexus	internal jugular v.
phrenic v's, inferior	vv. phrenicae inferiores	accompany inferior phrenic arteries	on right, enter inferior vena cava; on left, enter left suprarenal or renal v., or inferior vena cava
phrenic v's, superior. *See* pericardiacophrenic v's			
v's of pons	vv. pontis	pons	basal v., cerebellar v's, petrosal or venous sinuses, or venous plexus of foramen ovale
popliteal v.	v. poplitea	follows popliteal artery	at adductor hiatus becomes femoral v.
portal v.	v. portae hepatis	a short, thick trunk formed by union of superior mesenteric and splenic v's behind neck of pancreas; it ascends to right end of porta hepatis, where it divides into successively smaller branches, following branches of hepatic artery, until it forms a capillary-like system of sinusoids that permeates entire substance of liver	
posterior v. of left ventricle	v. posterior ventriculi sinistri cordis	posterior surface of left ventricle	coronary sinus
prepyloric v.	v. prepylorica	accompanies prepyloric artery, passing upward over anterior surface of junction between pylorus and duodenum	right gastric v.
profunda femoris v. *See* femoral v., deep			
profunda linguae v. *See* lingual v., deep			
v. of pterygoid canal	v. canalis pterygoidei	passes through pterygoid canal	pterygoid plexus
pudendal v's, external	vv. pudendae externae	follow distribution of external pudendal artery	great saphenous v.
pudendal v., internal	v. pudenda interna	follows course of internal pudendal artery	internal iliac v.
pulmonary v., inferior, left	v. pulmonalis sinistra inferior	lower lobe of left lung	left atrium of heart

(continued)

2071

Common Name*	TA Term†	Region	Receives Blood From*	Drains Into*
pulmonary v., inferior, right	v. pulmonalis dextra inferior		lower lobe of right lung	left atrium of heart
pulmonary v., superior, left	v. pulmonalis sinistra superior		lower lobe of left lung	left atrium of heart
pulmonary v., superior, right	v. pulmonalis dextra superior		upper and middle lobes of right lung	left atrium of heart
pyloric v. See gastric v., right				
radial v's	vv. radiales	accompany radial artery		brachial v's
ranine v. See sublingual v.				
rectal v's, inferior	vv. rectales inferiores		rectal plexus	internal pudendal v.
rectal v's, middle	vv. rectales mediae		rectal plexus	internal iliac and superior rectal v's
rectal v., superior	v. rectalis superior		upper part of rectal plexus	inferior mesenteric v.
renal v's	vv. renis		kidneys	inferior vena cava
retromandibular v.	v. retromandibularis	the vein formed in upper part of parotid gland behind neck of mandible by union of maxillary and superficial temporal v's; it passes downward through the gland, communicates with facial v. and, emerging from the gland, joins with posterior auricular v. to form external jugular v.		
sacral v's, lateral	vv. sacrales laterales	follow lateral sacral arteries		help form lateral sacral plexus; empty into internal iliac v. or superior gluteal v's
sacral v., median	v. sacralis mediana	follows median sacral artery		common iliac v.
saphenous v's, accessory	v. saphena accessoria			great saphenous v.
saphenous v., great	v. saphena magna	extends from dorsum of foot to just below inguinal ligament	when present, medial and posterior superficial parts of thigh	femoral v.
saphenous v., small	v. saphena parva	from behind ankle passes up back of leg to knee		popliteal v.
scleral v's	vv. sclerales		sclera	anterior ciliary v's
scrotal v's, anterior	vv. scrotales anteriores	scrotum	anterior aspect of scrotum	enternal pudendal v.
scrotal v's, posterior	vv. scrotales posteriores			vesical venous plexus
v. of septum pellucidum, anterior	v. anterior septi pellucidi		anterior septum pellucidum	superior thalamostriate v.
v. of septum pellucidum, posterior	v. posterior septi pellucidi		septum pellucidum	superior thalamostriate v.
sigmoid v's	vv. sigmoideae		sigmoid colon	inferior mesenteric v.

English name	Latin name	Description	Drains into / forms
spinal v's, anterior and posterior	vv. spinales anteriores/posteriores	anastomosing networks of small veins that drain blood from spinal cord and its pia mater into internal vertebral venous plexuses	
spiral v. of modiolus	v. spiralis modioli	modiolus	labyrinthine v's
splenic v.	v. splenica	formed by union of several branches at hilus of spleen; passes from left to right of neck of pancreas	joins superior mesenteric v. to form portal v.
stellate v's of kidney	venulae stellatae renis	superficial parts of renal cortex	interlobular v's of kidney
sternocleidomastoid v.	v. sternocleidomastoidea	follows course of sternocleidomastoid artery	internal jugular v.
striate v's	vv. striatae		
stylomastoid v.	v. stylomastoidea	follows stylomastoid artery	retromandibular v.
subclavian v.	v. subclavia	follows subclavian artery	joins internal jugular v. to form brachiocephalic v.
subcostal v.	v. subcostalis	accompanies subcostal artery	joins ascending lumbar v. to form azygos v. on right, hemiazygos v. on left
subcutaneous v's of abdomen	vv. subcutaneae abdominis	superficial layers of abdominal wall	
sublingual v.	v. sublingualis	follows sublingual artery	lingual v.
submental v.	v. submentalis	follows submental artery	facial v.
supraorbital v.	v. supraorbitalis	passes down forehead lateral to supratrochlear v.	joins supratrochlear v. at root of nose to form angular v.
suprarenal v., left	v. suprarenalis sinistra	left suprarenal gland	left renal v.
suprarenal v., right	v. suprarenalis dextra	right suprarenal gland	inferior vena cava
suprascapular v.	v. suprascapularis	accompanies suprascapular artery (sometimes as 2 veins that unite)	usually into external jugular v., occasionally into subclavian v.
supratrochlear v's (2)	vv. supratrochleares	venous plexuses high up on forehead	joins supraorbital v. at root of nose to form angular v.
temporal v's, deep	vv. temporales profundae	deep portions of temporal muscle	pterygoid plexus
temporal v., middle	v. temporalis media	arises in substance of temporal muscle; descends deep to fascia to zygoma	joins superficial temporal v.
temporal v's, superficial	vv. temporales superficiales	veins that drain lateral part of scalp in frontal and parietal regions, the branches forming a single superficial temporal v. in front of ear, just above zygoma; this descending vein receives middle temporal and transverse facial v's and, entering parotid gland, unites with maxillary v. deep to neck of mandible to form retromandibular v.	
testicular v., left	v. testicularis sinistra	left pampiniform plexus	left renal v.
testicular v., right	v. testicularis dextra	right pampiniform plexus	inferior vena cava
thalamostriate v's, inferior	vv. thalamostriatae inferiores	anterior perforated substance of brain	joins deep middle cerebral and anterior cerebral v's to form basal v.

(continued)

Common Name*	TA Term†	Region	Receives Blood From*	Drains Into*
thalamostriate v., superior	v. thalamostriata superior		corpus striatum and thalamus	joins choroid v. to form internal cerebral v.
thoracic v's, internal	vv. thoracicae internae	2 veins formed by junction of the veins accompanying internal thoracic artery of either side; each continues along the artery to open into brachiocephalic v.		
thoracic v., lateral	v. thoracica lateralis	accompanies lateral thoracic artery		axillary v.
thoracoacromial v.	v. thoracoacromialis	follows thoracoacromial artery		subclavian v.
thoracoepigastric v's	vv. thoracoepigastricae	long, longitudinal, superficial veins in anterolateral subcutaneous tissue of trunk		superiorly into lateral thoracic v.; inferiorly into femoral v.
thymic v's	vv. thymicae		thymus	left brachiocephalic v.
throid v., inferior	v. thyroidea inferior	either of 2 veins, left and right, that drain thyroid plexus into left and right brachiocephalic v's; occasionally they may unite into a common trunk to empty, usually, into left brachiocephalic v.		
thyroid v's, middle	vv. thyroideae mediae	arises from side of upper part of thyroid gland	thyroid gland	internal jugular v.
thyroid v., superior	v. thyroidea superior		thyroid gland	internal jugular v., occasionally in common with facial v.
tibial v's, anterior	vv. tibiales anteriores	accompany anterior tibial artery		join posterior tibial v's to form popliteal v.
tibial v's, posterior	vv. tibiales posteriores	accompany posterior tibial artery		join anterior tibial v's to form popliteal v.
tracheal v's	vv. tracheales		trachea	brachiocephalic v.
tympanic v's	vv. tympanicae	small veins from middle ear that pass through petrotympanic fissure and open into the plexus around temporomandibular joint		
ulnar v's	vv. ulnares	accompany ulnar artery		join radial v's at elbow to form brachial v's
umbilical v.	v. umbilicalis	the vein formed by fusion of atrophied right umbilical v. with the left umbilical v., which carries all the blood from placenta to ductus venosus		
v. of uncus	v. unci		uncus	ipsilateral inferior cerebral v.
uterine v's	vv. uterinae		uterine plexus	internal iliac v's
vena cava, inferior	vena cava inferior	the venous trunk for the lower limbs and for pelvic and abdominal viscera; it begins at level of fifth lumbar vertebra by union of common iliac v's and ascends on right of aorta		right atrium of heart
vena cava, superior	vena cava superior	the venous trunk draining blood from head, neck, upper limbs, and thorax; it begins by union of 2 brachiocephalic v's and passes directly downward		right atrium of heart
ventricular v., inferior	v. ventricularis inferior		temporal lobe	basal v.
vertebral v., anterior	v. vertebralis anterior	accompanies ascending cervical artery		vertebral vein
v. of vermis, inferior	v. inferior vermis		inferior surface of cerebellum	straight sinus or one of the sigmoid

4-1. DIETARY REFERENCE INTAKES (DRIs): FOOD AND NUTRITION BOARD, INSTITUTE OF MEDICINE, NATIONAL ACADEMIES RECOMMENDED INTAKES FOR INDIVIDUALS, VITAMINS

Life Stage Group	Vitamin A (µg/d)[a]	Vitamin C (mg/d)	Vitamin D (µg/d)[b,c]	Vitamin E (mg/d)[d]	Vitamin K (µg/d)	Thiamin (mg/d)	Riboflavin (mg/d)	Niacin (mg/d)[e]	Vitamin B_6 (mg/d)	Folate (µg/d)[f]	Vitamin B_{12} (µg/d)	Pantothenic Acid (µg/d)	Biotin (µg/d)	Choline (mg/d)[g]
Infants														
0–6 mo	400*	40*	5*	4*	2.0*	0.2*	0.3*	2*	0.1*	65*	0.4*	1.7*	5*	125*
7–12 mo	500*	50*	5*	5*	2.5*	0.3*	0.4*	4*	0.3*	80*	0.5*	1.8*	6*	150*
Children														
1–3 y	300	15	5*	6	30*	0.5	0.5	6	0.5	150	0.9	2*	8*	200*
4–8 y	400	25	5*	7	55*	0.6	0.6	8	0.6	200	1.2	3*	12*	250*
Males														
9–13 y	600	45	5*	11	60*	0.9	0.9	12	1.0	300	1.8	4*	20*	375*
14–18 y	900	75	5*	15	75*	1.2	1.3	16	1.3	400	2.4	5*	25*	550*
19–30 y	900	90	5*	15	120*	1.2	1.3	16	1.3	400	2.4	5*	30*	550*
31–50 y	900	90	5*	15	120*	1.2	1.3	16	1.3	400	2.4	5*	30*	550*
51–70 y	900	90	10*	15	120*	1.2	1.3	16	1.7	400	2.4[h]	5*	30*	550*
>70 y	900	90	15*	15	120*	1.2	1.3	16	1.7	400	2.4[h]	5*	30*	550*
Females														
9–13 y	600	45	5*	11	60*	0.9	0.9	12	1.0	300	1.8	4*	20*	375*
14–18 y	700	65	5*	15	75*	1.0	1.0	14	1.2	400[f]	2.4	5*	25*	400*
19–30 y	700	75	5*	15	90*	1.1	1.1	14	1.3	400[f]	2.4	5*	30*	425*
31–50 y	700	75	5*	15	90*	1.1	1.1	14	1.3	400[f]	2.4	5*	30*	425*
51–70 y	700	75	10*	15	90*	1.1	1.1	14	1.5	400	2.4[h]	5*	30*	425*
>70 y	700	75	15*	15	90*	1.1	1.1	14	1.5	400	2.4[h]	5*	30*	425*
Pregnancy														
≤18 y	750	80	5*	15	75*	1.4	1.4	18	1.9	600[f]	2.6	6*	30*	450*
19–30 y	770	85	5*	15	90*	1.4	1.4	18	1.9	600[f]	2.6	6*	30*	450*
31–50 y	770	85	5*	15	90*	1.4	1.4	18	1.9	600[f]	2.6	6*	30*	450*

(continued)

4-1. DIETARY REFERENCE INTAKES (DRIs): FOOD AND NUTRITION BOARD, INSTITUTE OF MEDICINE, NATIONAL ACADEMIES RECOMMENDED INTAKES FOR INDIVIDUALS, VITAMINS

Life Stage Group	Vitamin A (µg/d)[a]	Vitamin C (mg/d)	Vitamin D (µg/d)[b,c]	Vitamin E (mg/d)[d]	Vitamin K (µg/d)	Thiamin (mg/d)	Riboflavin (mg/d)	Niacin (mg/d)[e]	Vitamin B6 (mg/d)	Folate (µg/d)[f]	Vitamin B12 (µg/d)	Pantothenic Acid (µg/d)	Biotin (µg/d)	Choline (mg/d)[g]
Lactation														
≤18 y	1200	115	5*	19	75*	1.4	1.6	17	2.0	500	2.8	7*	35*	550*
19–30 y	1300	120	5*	19	90*	1.4	1.6	17	2.0	500	2.8	7*	35*	550*
31–50 y	1300	120	5*	19	90*	1.4	1.6	17	2.0	500	2.8	7*	35*	550*

SOURCES: Dietary Reference Intakes for Calcium, Phosphorus, Magnesium, Vitamin D, and Fluoride (1997); Dietary Reference Intakes for Thiamin, Riboflavin, Niacin, Vitamin B6, Folate, Vitamin B12, Pantothenic Acid, Biotin, and Choline (1998); Dietary Reference Intakes for Vitamin C, Vitamin E, Selenium, and Carotenoids (2000); and Dietary Reference Intakes for Vitamin A, Vitamin K, Arsenic, Boron, Chromium, Copper, Iodine, Iron, Manganese, Molybdenum, Nickel, Silicon, Vanadium, and Zinc (2001). These reports may be accessed via www.nap.edu. Copyright 2001 by the National Academy of Sciences. All rights reserved.

NOTE: This table (taken from the DRI reports, see www.nap.edu) presents Recommended Dietary Allowances (RDAs) in bold type and Adequate Intakes (AIs) in ordinary type followed by an asterisk (*). RDAs and AIs may both be used as goals for individual intake. RDAs are set to meet the needs of almost all (97 to 98 percent) individuals in a group. For healthy breastfed infants, the AI is the mean intake. The AI for other life stage and gender groups is believed to cover needs of all individuals in the group, but lack of data or uncertainty in the data prevent being able to specify with confidence the percentage of individuals covered by this intake.

[a] As retinol activity equivalents (RAEs). 1 RAE = 1 µg retinol, 12 µg β-carotene, 24 µg α-carotene, or 24 µg β-cryptoxanthin. To calculate RAEs from REs of provitamin A carotenoids in foods, divide the REs by 2. For preformed vitamin A in foods or supplements and for provitamin A carotenoids in supplements, 1 RE = 1 RAE.

[b] Calciferol. 1 µg calciferol 5 40 IU vitamin D.

[c] In the absence of adequate exposure to sunlight.

[d] As α-tocopherol. α-Tocopherol includes RRR-α-tocopherol, the only form of α-tocopherol that occurs naturally in foods, and the 2R-stereoisomeric forms of α-tocopherol (RRR-, RSR-, RRS-, and RSS-α-tocopherol) that occur in fortified foods and supplements. It does not include the 2S-stereoisomeric forms of α-tocopherol (SRR-, SSR-, SR-, and SSS-α-tocopherol), also found in fortified foods and supplements.

[e] As niacin equivalents (NE). 1 mg of niacin = 60 mg of tryptophan; 0–6 months = preformed niacin (not NE).

[f] As dietary folate equivalents (DFE). 1 DFE = 1 µg food folate = 0.6 µg of folic acid from fortified food or as a supplement consumed with food = 0.5 µg of a supplement taken on an empty stomach.

[g] Although AIs have been set for choline, there are few data to assess whether a dietary supply of choline is needed at all stages of the life cycle and it may be that the choline requirement can be met by endogenous synthesis at some of these stages.

[h] Because 10 to 30 percent of older people may malabsorb food-bound B12, it is advisable for those older than 50 years to meet their RDA mainly by consuming foods fortified with B12 or a supplement containing B12.

[i] In view of evidence linking folate intake with neural tube defects in the fetus, it is recommended that all women capable of becoming pregnant consume 400 µg from supplements or fortified foods in addition to intake of food folate from a varied diet.

[j] It is assumed that women will continue consuming 400 mg from supplements or fortified food until their pregnancy is confirmed and they enter prenatal care, which ordinarily occurs after the end of the periconceptional period—the critical time for formation of the neural tube.

4-1. DIETARY REFERENCE INTAKES (DRIs): FOOD AND NUTRITION BOARD, INSTITUTE OF MEDICINE, NATIONAL ACADEMIES TOLERABLE UPPER INTAKE LEVELS (UL[a]) VITAMINS

Life stage group	Vitamin A (µg/d)[b]	Vitamin C (mg/d)	Vitamin D (µg/d)	Vitamin E (mg/d)[c,d]	Vitamin K	Thiamin	Riboflavin	Niacin (mg/d)[d]	Vitamin B$_6$ (mg/d)[d]	Folate (µg/d)[d]	Vitamin B$_{12}$	Pantothenic Acid	Biotin	Choline (g/d)	Carotenoids
Infants															
0–6 mo	600	ND[f]	25	ND	ND	ND	ND	ND	ND	ND	ND	ND	ND	ND	ND
7–12 mo	600	ND	25	ND	ND	ND	ND	ND	ND	ND	ND	ND	ND	ND	ND
Children															
1–3 y	600	400	50	200	ND	ND	ND	10	30	300	ND	ND	ND	1.0	ND
4–8 y	900	650	50	300	ND	ND	ND	15	40	400	ND	ND	ND	1.0	ND
Males, Females															
9–13 y	1700	1200	50	600	ND	ND	ND	20	60	600	ND	ND	ND	2.0	ND
14–18 y	2800	1800	50	800	ND	ND	ND	30	80	800	ND	ND	ND	3.0	ND
19–70 y	3000	2000	50	1000	ND	ND	ND	35	100	1000	ND	ND	ND	3.5	ND
>70 y	3000	2000	50	1000	ND	ND	ND	35	100	1000	ND	ND	ND	3.5	ND
Pregnancy															
≤18 y	2800	1800	50	800	ND	ND	ND	30	80	800	ND	ND	ND	3.0	ND
19–50 y	3000	2000	50	1000	ND	ND	ND	35	100	1000	ND	ND	ND	3.5	ND
Lactation															
≤18 y	2800	1800	50	800	ND	ND	ND	30	80	800	ND	ND	ND	3.0	ND
19–50 y	3000	2000	50	1000	ND	ND	ND	35	100	1000	ND	ND	ND	3.5	ND

SOURCES: Dietary Reference Intakes for Calcium, Phosphorus, Magnesium, Vitamin D, and Fluoride (1997); Dietary Reference Intakes for Thiamin, Riboflavin, Niacin, Vitamin B$_6$, Folate, Vitamin B$_{12}$, Pantothenic Acid, Biotin, and Choline (1998); Dietary Reference Intakes for Vitamin C, Vitamin E, Selenium, and Carotenoids (2000); and Dietary Reference Intakes for Vitamin A, Vitamin K, Arsenic, Boron, Chromium, Copper, Iodine, Iron, Manganese, Molybdenum, Nickel, Silicon, Vanadium, and Zinc (2001). These reports may be accessed via www.nap.edu. Copyright 2001 by the National Academy of Sciences. All rights reserved.

[a] UL = The maximum level of daily nutrient intake that is likely to pose no risk of adverse effects. Unless otherwise specified, the UL represents total intake from food, water, and supplements. Due to lack of suitable data, ULs could not be established for vitamin K, thiamin, riboflavin, vitamin B$_{12}$, pantothenic acid, biotin, or carotenoids. In the absence of ULs, extra caution may be warranted in consuming levels above recommended intakes.

[b] As preformed vitamin A only.

[c] As α-tocopherol; applies to any form of supplemental α-tocopherol.

[d] The ULs for vitamin E, niacin, and folate apply to synthetic forms obtained from supplements, fortified foods, or a combination of the two.

[e] β-Carotene supplements are advised only to serve as a provitamin A source for individuals at risk of vitamin A deficiency.

[f] ND = Not determinable due to lack of data of adverse effects in this age group and concern with regard to lack of ability to handle excess amounts. Source of intake should be from food only to prevent high levels of intake.

4-1. DIETARY REFERENCE INTAKES (DRIs): FOOD AND NUTRITION BOARD, INSTITUTE OF MEDICINE, NATIONAL ACADEMIES RECOMMENDED INTAKES FOR INDIVIDUALS, ELEMENTS

Life stage group	Calcium (mg/d)	Chromium (µg/d)	Copper (µg/d)	Fluoride (mg/d)	Iodine (µg/d)	Iron (mg/d)	Magnesium (mg/d)	Manganese (mg/d)	Molybdenum (µg/d)	Phosphorus (mg/d)	Selenium (µg/d)	Zinc (mg/d)
Infants												
0–6 mo	210*	0.2*	200*	0.01*	110*	0.27*	30*	0.003*	2*	100*	15*	2*
7–12 mo	270*	5.5*	220*	0.5*	130*	11	75*	0.6*	3*	275*	20*	3
Children												
1–3 y	500*	11*	340	0.7*	90	7	80	1.2*	17	460	20	3
4–8 y	800*	15*	440	1*	90	10	130	1.5*	22	500	30	5
Males												
9–13 y	1300*	25*	700	2*	120	8	240	1.9*	34	1250	40	8
14–18 y	1300*	35*	890	3*	150	11	410	2.2*	43	1250	55	11
19–30 y	1000*	35*	900	4*	150	8	400	2.3*	45	700	55	11
31–50 y	1000*	35*	900	4*	150	8	420	2.3*	45	700	55	11
51–70 y	1200*	30*	900	4*	150	8	420	2.3*	45	700	55	11
>70 y	1200*	30*	900	4*	150	8	420	2.3*	45	700	55	11
Females												
9–13 y	1300*	21*	700	2*	120	8	240	1.6*	34	1250	40	8
14–18 y	1300*	24*	890	3*	150	15	360	1.6*	43	1250	55	9
19–30 y	1000*	25*	900	3*	150	18	310	1.8*	45	700	55	8
31–50 y	1000*	25*	900	3*	150	18	320	1.8*	45	700	55	8
51–70 y	1200*	20*	900	3*	150	8	320	1.8*	45	700	55	8
>70 y	1200*	20*	900	3*	150	8	320	1.8*	45	700	55	8
Pregnancy												
≤18 y	1300*	29*	1000	3*	220	27	400	2.0*	50	1250	60	13
19–30 y	1000*	30*	1000	3*	220	27	350	2.0*	50	700	60	11
31–50 y	1000*	30*	1000	3*	220	27	360	2.0*	50	700	60	11
Lactation												
≤18 y	1300*	44*	1300	3*	290	10	360	2.6*	50	1250	70	14
19–30 y	1000*	45*	1300	3*	290	9	310	2.6*	50	700	70	12
31–50 y	1000*	45*	1300	3*	290	9	320	2.6*	50	700	70	12

SOURCES: Dietary Reference Intakes for Calcium, Phosphorus, Magnesium, Vitamin D, and Fluoride (1997); Dietary Reference Intakes for Thiamin, Riboflavin, Niacin, Vitamin B₆, Folate, Vitamin B₁₂, Pantothenic Acid, Biotin, and Choline (1998); Dietary Reference Intakes for Vitamin C, Vitamin E, Selenium, and Carotenoids (2000); and Dietary Reference Intakes for Vitamin A, Vitamin K, Arsenic, Boron, Chromium, Copper, Iodine, Iron, Manganese, Molybdenum, Nickel, Silicon, Vanadium, and Zinc (2001). Copyright 2001 by the National Academy of Sciences. All rights reserved.

NOTE: This table presents Recommended Dietary Allowances (RDAs) in bold type and Adequate Intakes (AIs) in ordinary type followed by an asterisk (*). RDAs and AIs may both be used as goals for individual intake. RDAs are set to meet the needs of almost all (97 to 98 percent) individuals in a group. For healthy breastfed infants, the AI is the mean intake. The AI for other life stage and gender groups is believed to cover needs of all individuals in the group, but lack of data or uncertainty in the data prevent being able to specify with confidence the percentage of individuals covered by this intake.

4-1. DIETARY REFERENCE INTAKES (DRIs): FOOD AND NUTRITION BOARD, INSTITUTE OF MEDICINE, NATIONAL ACADEMIES TOLERABLE UPPER INTAKE LEVELS (UL[a]), ELEMENTS

Life Stage Group	Arsenic[b] (mg/d)	Boron (mg/d)	Calcium (g/d)	Chromium	Copper (μg/d)	Fluoride (mg/d)	Iodine (μg/d)	Iron (mg/d)	Magnesium (mg/d)[c]	Manganese (mg/d)	Molybdenum (μg/d)	Nickel (mg/d)	Phosphorus (g/d)	Selenium (μg/d)	Silicon[d]	Vanadium (mg/d)[e]	Zinc (mg/d)
Infants																	
0–6 mo	ND[f]	ND	ND	ND	ND	0.7	ND	40	ND	ND	ND	ND	ND	45	ND	ND	4
7–12 mo	ND	ND	ND	ND	ND	0.9	ND	40	ND	ND	ND	ND	ND	60	ND	ND	5
Children																	
1–3 y	ND	3	2.5	ND	1000	1.3	200	40	65	2	300	0.2	3	90	ND	ND	7
4–8 y	ND	6	2.5	ND	3000	2.2	300	40	110	3	600	0.3	3	150	ND	ND	12
Males, Females																	
9–13 y	ND	11	2.5	ND	5000	10	600	40	350	6	1100	0.6	4	280	ND	ND	23
14–18 y	ND	17	2.5	ND	8000	10	900	45	350	9	1700	1.0	4	400	ND	ND	34
19–70 y	ND	20	2.5	ND	10,000	10	1100	45	350	11	2000	1.0	4	400	ND	1.8	40
>70 y	ND	20	2.5	ND	10,000	10	1100	45	350	11	2000	1.0	3	400	ND	1.8	40
Pregnancy																	
<18 y	ND	17	2.5	ND	8000	10	900	45	350	9	1700	1.0	3.5	400	ND	ND	34
19–50 y	ND	20	2.5	ND	10,000	10	1100	45	350	11	2000	1.0	3.5	400	ND	ND	40
Lactation																	
<18 y	ND	17	2.5	ND	8000	10	900	45	350	9	1700	1.0	4	400	ND	ND	34
19–50 y	ND	20	2.5	ND	10,000	10	1100	45	350	11	2000	1.0	4	400	ND	ND	40

SOURCES: Dietary Reference Intakes for Calcium, Phosphorus, Magnesium, Vitamin D, and Fluoride (1997); Dietary Reference Intakes for Thiamin, Riboflavin, Niacin, Vitamin B₆, Folate, Vitamin B₁₂, Pantothenic Acid, Biotin, and Choline (1998); Dietary Reference Intakes for Vitamin C, Vitamin E, Selenium, and Carotenoids (2000); and Dietary Reference Intakes for Vitamin A, Vitamin K, Arsenic, Boron, Chromium, Copper, Iodine, Iron, Manganese, Molybdenum, Nickel, Silicon, Vanadium, and Zinc (2001). These reports may be accessed via www.nap.edu. Copyright 2001 by the National Academy of Sciences. All rights reserved.

[a] UL = The maximum level of daily nutrient intake that is likely to pose no risk of adverse effects. Unless otherwise specified, the UL represents total intake from food, water, and supplements. Due to lack of suitable data, ULs could not be established for arsenic, chromium, and silicon. In the absence of ULs, extra caution may be warranted in consuming levels above recommended intakes.

[b] Although the UL was not determined for arsenic, there is no justification for adding arsenic to food or supplements.

[c] The ULs for magnesium represent intake from a pharmacological agent only and do not include intake from food and water.

[d] Although silicon has not been shown to cause adverse effects in humans, there is no justification for adding silicon to supplements.

[e] Although vanadium in food has not been shown to cause adverse effects in humans, there is no justification for adding vanadium to food and vanadium supplements should be used with caution. The UL is based on adverse effects in laboratory animals and this data could be used to set a UL for adults but not children and adolescents.

[f] ND = Not determinable due to lack of data of adverse effects in this age group and concern with regard to lack of ability to handle excess amounts. Source of intake should be from food only to prevent high levels of intake.

Summary of Examples of Recommended Nutrients Based on Energy Expressed as Daily Rates

Age	Sex	Energy (kcal)	Thiamin (mg)	Riboflavin (mg)	Niacin (NE[b])	n-3 PUFA[a] (g)	n-6 PUFA (g)
Months							
0–4	Both	600	0.3	0.3	4	0.5	3
5–12	Both	900	0.4	0.5	7	0.5	3
Years							
1	Both	1100	0.5	0.6	8	0.6	4
2–3	Both	1300	0.6	0.7	9	0.7	4
4–6	Both	1800	0.7	0.9	13	1.0	6
7–9	M	2200	0.9	1.1	16	1.2	7
	F	1900	0.8	1.0	14	1.0	6
10–12	M	2500	1.0	1.3	18	1.4	8
	F	2200	0.9	1.1	16	1.2	7
13–15	M	2800	1.1	1.4	20	1.5	9
	F	2200	0.9	1.1	16	1.2	7
16–18	M	3200	1.3	1.6	23	1.8	11
	F	2100	0.8	1.1	15	1.2	7
19–24	M	3000	1.2	1.5	22	1.6	10
	F	2100	0.8	1.1	15	1.2	7
25–49	M	2700	1.1	1.4	19	1.5	9
	F	1900	0.8[c]	1.0[c]	14[c]	1.1[c]	7[c]
50–74	M	2300	0.9	1.2	16	1.3	8
	F	1800	0.8[c]	1.0[c]	14[c]	1.1[c]	7[c]
75 +	M	2000	0.8	1.0	14	1.1	7
	F[d]	1700	0.8[c]	1.0[c]	14[c]	1.1[c]	7[c]
Pregnancy (additional)							
1st Trimester		100	0.1	0.1	1	0.05	0.3
2nd Trimester		300	0.1	0.3	2	0.16	0.9
3rd Trimester		300	0.1	0.3	2	0.16	0.9
Lactation (additional)		450	0.2	0.4	3	0.25	1.5

[a]PUFA, polyunsaturated fatty acids.
[b]Niacin equivalents.
[c]Level below which intake should not fall.
[d]Assumes moderate (more than average) physical activity.
*Reprinted with permission of Health Canada, Health Protection Branch.

4-2. SUMMARY EXAMPLES OF NUTRIENT INTAKE FOR CANADIANS—cont'd

Summary Examples of Recommended Nutrient Intake Based on Age and Body Weight Expressed as Daily Rates

Age	Sex	Weight (kg)	Protein (g)	Vit. A (RE[a])	Vit. D (µg)	Vit. E (mg)	Vit. C (mg)	Folate (µg)	Vit. B$_{12}$ (µg)	Calcium (mg)	Phosphorus (mg)	Magnesium (mg)	Iron (mg)	Iodine (µg)	Zinc (mg)
Months															
0-4	Both	6.0	12[b]	400	10	3	20	25	0.3	250[c]	150	20	0.3[d]	30	2[d]
5-12	Both	9.0	12	400	10	3	20	40	0.4	400	200	32	7	40	3
Years															
1	Both	11	13	400	10	3	20	40	0.5	500	300	40	6	55	4
2-3	Both	14	16	400	5	4	20	50	0.6	550	350	50	6	65	4
4-6	Both	18	19	500	5	5	25	70	0.8	600	400	65	8	85	5
7-9	M	25	26	700	2.5	7	25	90	1.0	700	500	100	8	110	7
	F	25	26	700	2.5	6	25	90	1.0	700	500	100	8	95	7
10-12	M	34	34	800	2.5	8	25	120	1.0	900	700	130	8	125	9
	F	36	36	800	2.5	7	25	130	1.0	1100	800	135	8	110	9
13-15	M	50	49	900	2.5	9	25	175	1.0	1100	900	185	10	160	12
	F	48	46	800	2.5	7	30[e]	170	1.0	1000	850	180	13	160	9
16-18	M	62	58	1000	2.5	10	30[e]	220	1.0	900	1000	230	10	160	12
	F	53	47	800	2.5	7	30[e]	190	1.0	700	850	200	12	160	9
19-24	M	71	61	1000	2.5	10	40[e]	220	1.0	800	1000	240	9	160	12
	F	58	50	800	2.5	7	30[e]	180	1.0	700	850	200	13	160	9
25-49	M	74	64	1000	2.5	9	40[e]	230	1.0	800	1000	250	9	160	12
	F	59	51	800	2.5	6	30[e]	185	1.0	700	850	200	13	160	9
50-74	M	73	63	1000	5	7	40[e]	230	1.0	800	1000	250	9	160	12
	F	63	54	800	5	6	30[e]	195	1.0	800	850	210	8	160	9
75 +	M	69	59	1000	5	6	40[e]	215	1.0	800	1000	230	9	160	12
	F	64	55	800	5	5	30[e]	200	1.0	800	850	210	8	160	9
Pregnancy (additional)															
1st Trimester			5	0	2.5	2	0	200	0.2	500	200	15	0	25	6
2nd Trimester			15	0	2.5	2	10	200	0.2	500	200	45	5	25	6
3rd Trimester			24	0	2.5	2	10	200	0.2	500	200	45	10	25	6
Lactation (additional)			22	400	2.5	3	25	100	0.2	500	200	65	0	50	6

[a]Retinol Equivalents.
[b]Protein is assumed to be from breast milk and must be adjusted for infant formula.
[c]Infant formula with high phosphorus should contain 375 mg calcium.
[d]Breast milk is assumed to be the source of the mineral.
[e]Smokers should increase vitamin C by 50%.

Section 5: Tables of Weights and Measures

5-1. MEASURES OF MASS

AVOIRDUPOIS WEIGHT

Grains	Drams	Ounces	Pounds	Metric Equivalents Grams
1	0.0366	0.0023	0.00014	0.0647989
27.34	1	0.0625	0.0039	1.772
437.5	16	1	0.0625	28.350
7000	256	16	1	453.5924277

APOTHECARIES' WEIGHT

Grains	Scruples (Ə)	Drams (ʒ)	Ounces (ʒ)	Pounds (lb.)	Metric Equivalents Grams
1	0.05	0.0167	0.0021	0.00017	0.0647989
20	1	0.333	0.042	0.0035	1.296
60	3	1	0.125	0.0104	3.888
480	24	8	1	0.0833	31.103
5760	288	96	12	1	373.24177

TROY WEIGHT

Grains	Pennyweights	Ounces	Pounds	Metric Equivalents Grams
1	0.042	0.002	0.00017	0.0647989
24	1	0.05	0.0042	1.555
480	20	1	0.083	31.103
5760	240	12	1	373.24177

METRIC WEIGHT

Micro-gram	Milli-gram	Centi-gram	Deci-gram	Gram	Deka-gram	Hecto-gram	Kilo-gram	Equivalents Avoir-dupois	Apothe-caries'
1	—	—	—	—	—	—	—	0.000015 grains	
10^3	1	—	—	—	—	—	—	0.015432 grains	
10^4	10	1	—	—	—	—	—	0.154323 grains	
10^5	10^2	10	1	—	—	—	—	1.543235 grains	
10^6	10^3	10^2	10	1	—	—	—	15.432356 grains	
10^7	10^4	10^3	10^2	10	1	—	—	5.6438 dr.	7.7162 sc
10^8	10^5	10^4	10^3	10^2	10	1	—	3.527 oz.	3.215 oz.
10^9	10^6	10^5	10^4	10^3	10^2	10	1	2.2046 lb.	2.6792 lb.
10^{12}	10^9	10^8	10^7	10^6	10^5	10^4	10^3	2204.6223 lb.	2679.2285 lb.

5-2.   MEASURES OF CAPACITY

APOTHECARIES' (WINE) MEASURE

Minims	Fluid Drams	Fluid Ounces	Gills	Pints	Quarts	Gallons	Cubic Inches	Milli- liters	Cubic Centimeters
1	0.0166	0.002	0.0005	0.00013	—	—	0.00376	0.06161	0.06161
60	1	0.125	0.0312	0.0078	0.0039	—	0.22558	3.6967	3.6967
480	8	1	0.25	0.0625	0.0312	0.0078	1.80468	29.5737	29.5737
1920	32	4	1	0.25	0.125	0.0312	7.21875	118.2948	118.2948
7680	128	16	4	1	0.5	0.125	28.875	473.179	473.179
15360	256	32	8	2	1	0.25	57.75	946.358	946.358
61440	1024	128	32	8	4	1	231	3785.434	3785.434

METRIC MEASURE

Micro- liter	Milli- liter	Centi- liter	Deci- liter	Liter	Deka- liter	Hecto- liter	Kilo- liter	Myria- liter	Equivalents (Apothecaries' Fluid)	
1	—	—	—	—	—	—	—	—	0.01623108	minim
10^3	1	—	—	—	—	—	—	—	16.23	minims
10^4	10	1	—	—	—	—	—	—	2.7	fluid drams
10^5	10^2	10	1	—	—	—	—	—	3.38	fluid ounces
10^6	10^3	10^2	10	1	—	—	—	—	2.11	pints
10^7	10^4	10^3	10^2	10	1	—	—	—	2.64	gallons
10^8	10^5	10^4	10^3	10^2	10	1	—	—	26.418	gallons
10^9	10^6	10^5	10^4	10^3	10^2	10	1	—	264.18	gallons
10^{10}	10^7	10^6	10^5	10^4	10^3	10^2	10	1	2641.8	gallons

5-3.   MEASURES OF LENGTH

METRIC MEASURE

Micro- meter	Milli- meter	Centi- meter	Deci- meter	Meter	Deka- meter	Hecto- meter	Kilo- meter	Myria- meter	Mega- meter	Equivalents	
1	0.001	10^{-4}	—	—	—	—	—	—	—	0.000039	inch
10^3	1	10^{-1}	—	—	—	—	—	—	—	0.03937	inch
10^4	10	1	—	—	—	—	—	—	—	0.3937	inch
10^5	10^2	10	1	—	—	—	—	—	—	3.937	inches
10^6	10^3	10^2	10	1	—	—	—	—	—	39.37	inches
10^7	10^4	10^3	10^2	10	1	—	—	—	—	10.9361	yards
10^8	10^5	10^4	10^3	10^2	10	1	—	—	—	109.3612	yards
10^9	10^6	10^5	10^4	10^3	10^2	10	1	—	—	1093.6121	yards
10^{10}	10^7	10^6	10^5	10^4	10^3	10^2	10	1	—	6.2137	miles
10^{12}	10^9	10^8	10^7	10^6	10^5	10^4	10^3	10^2	1	621.37	miles

CONVERSION TABLES

5-4. AVOIRDUPOIS—METRIC WEIGHT

Ounces	Grams
1/16	1.772
1/8	3.544
1/4	7.088
1/2	14.175
1	28.350
2	56.699
3	85.049
4	113.398
5	141.748
6	170.097
7	198.447
8	226.796
9	255.146
10	283.495
11	311.845
12	340.194
13	368.544
14	396.893
15	425.243
16 (1 lb.)	453.59
Pounds	
1 (16 oz.)	453.59
2	907.18
3	1360.78 (1.36 kg.)
4	1814.37 (1.81 kg.)
5	2267.96 (2.27 kg.)
6	2721.55 (2.72 kg.)
7	3175.15 (3.18 kg.)
8	3628.74 (3.63 kg.)
9	4082.33 (4.08 kg.)
10	4535.92 (4.54 kg.)

5-5. METRIC—AVOIRDUPOIS WEIGHT

Grams	Ounces
0.001 (1 mg.)	0.000035274
1	0.035274
1000 (kg.)	35.274 (2.2046 lb.)

5-6. APOTHECARIES'—METRIC LIQUID MEASURE

Minims	Milliliters
1	0.06
2	0.12
3	0.19
4	0.25
5	0.31
10	0.62
15	0.92
20	1.23
25	1.54
30	1.85
35	2.16
40	2.46
45	2.77
50	3.08
55	3.39
60 (1 fl. dr.)	3.70
Fluid Drams	
1	3.70
2	7.39
3	11.09
4	14.79
5	18.48
6	22.18
7	25.88
8 (1 fl. oz.)	29.57
Fluid Ounces	
1	29.57
2	59.15
3	88.72
4	118.29
5	147.87
6	177.44
7	207.01
8	236.58
9	266.16
10	295.73
11	325.30
12	354.88
13	384.45
14	414.02
15	443.59
16 (1 pt.)	473.18
32 (1 qt.)	946.36
128 (1 gal.)	3785.43

5-7. METRIC—APOTHECARIES' LIQUID MEASURE

Milliliters	Minims	Milliliters	Fluid Drams	Milliliters	Fluid Ounces
1	16.231	5	1.35	30	1.01
2	32.5	10	2.71	40	1.35
3	48.7	15	4.06	50	1.69
4	64.9	20	5.4	500	16.91
5	81.1	25	6.76	1000 (1 L.)	33.815
		30	7.1		

5-8. APOTHECARIES'–METRIC WEIGHT

Apothecaries'—Metric		Metric—Apothecaries'		Apothecaries'—Metric		Metric—Apothecaries'	
Grains	Grams	Milligrams	Grains	Grains	Grams	Grams	Grains
1/150	0.0004	1	0.015432	10	0.65	1.0	15.4320
1/120	0.0005	2	0.030864	15	1.00	1.5	23.1480
1/100	0.0006	3	0.046296	20 (1 Ʒ)	1.30	2.0	30.8640
1/80	0.0008	4	0.061728	30	2.00	2.5	38.5800
1/64	0.001	5	0.077160	*Scruples*		3.0	46.2960
1/50	0.0013	6	0.092592	1	1.296 (1.3)	3.5	54.0120
1/48	0.0014	7	0.108024	2	2.592 (2.6)	4.0	61.728
1/30	0.0022	8	0.123456	3 (1 Ʒ)	3.888 (3.9)	4.5	69.444
1/25	0.0026	9	0.138888	*Drams*		5.0	77.162
1/16	0.004	10	0.154320	1	3.888	10.0	154.324
1/12	0.005	15	0.231480	2	7.776		
1/10	0.006	20	0.308640	3	11.664	*Equivalents*	
1/9	0.007	25	0.385800	4	15.552	10	2.572 drams
1/8	0.008	30	0.462960	5	19.440	15	3.858 drams
1/7	0.009	35	0.540120	6	23.328	20	5.144 drams
1/6	0.01	40	0.617280	7	27.216	25	6.430 drams
1/5	0.013	45	0.694440	8 (1 Ʒ)	31.103	30	7.716 drams
1/4	0.016	50	0.771600	*Ounces*		40	1.286 oz.
1/3	0.02	100	1.543240	1	31.103	45	1.447 oz.
1/2	0.032			2	62.207	50	1.607 oz.
1	0.065	*Grams*		3	93.310	100	3.215 oz.
1 1/2	0.097 (0.1)	0.1	1.5432	4	124.414	200	6.430 oz.
2	0.125	0.2	3.0864	5	155.517	300	9.644 oz.
3	0.20	0.3	4.6296	6	186.621	400	12.859 oz.
4	0.25	0.4	6.1728	7	217.724	500	1.34 lb.
5	0.30	0.5	7.7160	8	248.828	600	1.61 lb.
6	0.40	0.6	9.2592	9	279.931	700	1.88 lb.
7	0.45	0.7	10.8024	10	311.035	800	2.14 lb.
8	0.50	0.8	12.3456	11	342.138	900	2.41 lb.
9	0.60	0.9	13.8888	12 (1 lb.)	373.242	1000	2.68 lb.

5-9. METRIC DOSES WITH APPROXIMATE APOTHECARIES' EQUIVALENTS*

These *approximate* dose equivalents represent the quantities usually prescribed, under identical conditions, by physicians trained, respectively, in the metric or in the apothecaries' system of weights and measures. In labeling dosage forms in both the metric and the apothecaries' systems, if one is the approximate equivalent of the other, the approximate figure shall be enclosed in parentheses.

When prepared dosage forms such as tablets, capsules, pills, etc., are prescribed in the metric system, the pharmacist may dispense the corresponding *approximate* equivalent in the apothecaries' system, and vice versa, as indicated in the following table.

Caution—For the conversion of specific quantities in a prescription which requires compounding, or in converting a pharmaceutical formula from one system of weights or measures to the other, *exact* equivalents must be used.

Liquid Measure		Liquid Measure	
Metric	Approximate Apothecaries' Equivalents	Metric	Approximte Apothecaries' Equivalents
000 ml.	1 quart	3 ml.	45 minims
750 ml.	1 1/2 pints	2 ml.	30 minims
500 ml.	1 pint	1 ml.	15 minims
250 ml.	8 fluid ounces	0.75 ml.	12 minims
200 ml.	7 fluid ounces	0.6 ml.	10 minims
100 ml.	3 1/2 fluid ounces	0.5 ml.	8 minims
50 ml.	1 3/4 fluid ounces	0.3 ml	5 minims
30 ml.	1 fluid ounce	0.25 ml.	4 minims
15 ml.	4 fluid drams	0.2 ml.	3 minims
10 ml.	2 1/2 fluid drams	0.1 ml.	1 1/2 minims
8 ml.	2 fluid drams	0.06 ml.	1 minim
5 ml.	1 1/4 fluid drams	0.05 ml.	3/4 minim
4 ml.	1 fluid dram	0.03 ml.	1/2 minim

Weight		Weight	
Metric	Approximate Apothecaries' Equivalents	Metric	Approximate Apothecaries' Equivalents
0 gm.	1 ounce	30 mg.	1/2 grain
5 gm.	4 drams	25 mg.	3/8 grain
0 gm.	2 1/2 drams	20 mg.	1/3 grain
7.5 gm.	2 drams	15 mg.	1/4 grain
6 gm.	90 grains	12 mg.	1/5 grain
5 gm.	75 grains	10 mg.	1/6 grain
4 gm.	60 grains (1 dram)	8 mg.	1/8 grain
3 gm.	45 grains	6 mg.	1/10 grain
2 gm.	30 grains (1/2 dram)	5 mg.	1/12 grain
1.5 gm.	22 grains	4 mg.	1/15 grain
1 gm.	15 grains	3 mg.	1/20 grain
0.75 gm.	12 grains	2 mg.	1/30 grain
0.6 gm.	10 grains	1.5 mg.	1/40 grain
0.5 gm.	7 1/2 grains	1.2 mg.	1/50 grain
0.4 gm.	6 grains	1 mg.	1/60 grain
0.3 gm.	5 grains	0.8 mg.	1/80 grain
0.25 gm.	4 grains	0.6 mg.	1/100 grain
0.2 gm.	3 grains	0.5 mg.	1/120 grain
0.15 gm.	2 1/2 grains	0.4 mg.	1/150 grain
0.12 gm.	2 grains	0.3 mg.	1/200 grain
0.1 gm.	1 1/2 grains	0.25 mg.	1/250 grain
5 mg.	1 1/4 grains	0.2 mg.	1/300 grain
0 mg.	1 grain	0.15 mg.	1/400 grain
0 mg.	3/4 grain	0.12 mg.	1/500 grain
0 mg.	2/3 grain	0.1 mg.	1/600 grain

*Note: A milliliter (ml.) is the approximate equivalent of a cubic centimeter (cc.).
Adopted by the latest Pharmacopeia, National Formulary, and New and Nonofficial Remedies, and approved by the Federal Food and Drug Administration.

5-10. TEMPERATURE EQUIVALENTS: CELSIUS (CENTIGRADE) AND FAHRENHEIT SCALES

Celsius: Fahrenheit $°F = (°C \times 9/5) + 32$ **Fahrenheit: Celsius** $°C = (°F - 32) \times 5/9$

°C	°F	°C	°F	°F	°C	°F	°C	°F	°C
−50	−58.0	49	120.2	−50	−46.7	99	37.2	157	69.4
−40	−40.0	50	122.0	−40	−40.0	100	37.7	158	70.0
−35	−31.0	51	123.8	−35	−37.2	101	38.3	159	70.5
−30	−22.0	52	125.6	−30	−34.4	102	38.8	160	71.1
−25	−13.0	53	127.4	−25	−31.7	103	39.4	161	71.6
−20	−4.0	54	129.2	−20	−28.9	104	40.0	162	72.2
−15	+5.0	55	131.0	−15	−26.6	105	40.5	163	72.7
−10	14.0	56	132.8	−10	−23.3	106	41.1	164	73.3
−5	23.0	57	134.6	−5	−20.6	107	41.6	165	73.8
0	32.0	58	136.4	0	−17.7	108	42.2	166	74.4
+1	33.8	59	138.2	+1	−17.2	109	42.7	167	75.0
2	35.6	60	140.0	5	−15.0	110	43.3	168	75.5
3	37.4	61	141.8	10	−12.2	111	43.8	169	76.1
4	39.2	62	143.6	15	−9.4	112	44.4	170	76.6
5	41.0	63	145.4	20	−6.6	113	45.0	171	77.2
6	42.8	64	147.2	25	−3.8	114	45.5	172	77.7
7	44.6	65	149.0	30	−1.1	115	46.1	173	78.3
8	46.4	66	150.8	31	−0.5	116	46.6	174	78.8
9	48.2	67	152.6	32	0	117	47.2	175	79.4
10	50.0	68	154.4	33	+0.5	118	47.7	176	80.0
11	51.8	69	156.2	34	1.1	119	48.3	177	80.5
12	53.6	70	158.0	35	1.6	120	48.8	178	81.1
13	55.4	71	159.8	36	2.2	121	49.4	179	81.6
14	57.2	72	161.6	37	2.7	122	50.0	180	82.2
15	59.0	73	163.4	38	3.3	123	50.5	181	82.7
16	60.8	74	165.2	39	3.8	124	51.1	182	83.3
17	62.6	75	167.0	40	4.4	125	51.6	183	83.8
18	64.4	76	168.8	41	5.0	126	52.2	184	84.4
19	66.2	77	170.6	42	5.5	127	52.7	185	85.0
20	68.0	78	172.4	43	6.1	128	53.3	186	85.5
21	69.8	79	174.2	44	6.6	129	53.8	187	86.1
22	71.6	80	176.0	45	7.2	130	54.4	188	86.6
23	73.4	81	177.8	46	7.7	131	55.0	189	87.2
24	75.2	82	179.6	47	8.3	132	55.5	190	87.7
25	77.0	83	181.4	48	8.8	133	56.1	191	88.3
26	78.8	84	183.2	49	9.4	134	56.6	192	88.8
27	80.6	85	185.0	50	10.0	135	57.2	193	89.4
28	82.4	86	186.8	55	12.7	136	57.7	194	90.0
29	84.2	87	188.6	60	15.5	137	58.3	195	90.5
30	86.0	88	190.4	65	18.3	138	58.8	196	91.1
31	87.8	89	192.2	70	21.1	139	59.4	197	91.6
32	89.6	90	194.0	75	23.8	140	60.0	198	92.2
33	91.4	91	195.8	80	26.6	141	60.5	199	92.7
34	93.2	92	197.6	85	29.4	142	61.1	200	93.3
35	95.0	93	199.4	86	30.0	143	61.6	201	93.8
36	96.8	94	201.2	87	30.5	144	62.2	202	94.4
37	98.6	95	203.0	88	31.0	145	62.7	203	95.0
38	100.4	96	204.8	89	31.6	146	63.3	204	95.5
39	102.2	97	206.6	90	32.2	147	63.8	205	96.1
40	104.0	98	208.4	91	32.7	148	64.4	206	96.6
41	105.8	99	210.2	92	33.3	149	65.0	207	97.2
42	107.6	100	212.0	93	33.8	150	65.5	208	97.7
43	109.4	101	213.8	94	34.4	151	66.1	209	98.3
44	111.2	102	215.6	95	35.0	152	66.6	210	98.8
45	113.0	103	217.4	96	35.5	153	67.2	211	99.4
46	114.8	104	219.2	97	36.1	154	67.7	212	100.0
47	116.6	105	221.0	98	36.6	155	68.3	213	100.5
48	118.4	106	222.8	98.6	37.0	156	68.8	214	101.1

Section 6: Chemical Tables

6-1. CHEMICAL ELEMENTS

Element (Date of Discovery)	Symbol	Atomic Number	Atomic Weight*	Valence	Specific Gravity or Density (Grams/Liter)	Descriptive Comment
Actinium (1899)	Ac	89	[227]	3	10.07	radioactive element associated with uranium
Aluminum (1827)	Al	13	26.9815	3	2.6989	silvery-white metal, abundant in earth's crust, but not in free form
Americium (1944)	Am	95	[243]	3, 4, 5, 6	13.67	fourth transuranium element discovered
Antimony (prehistoric)	Sb	51	121.75	3, 5	6.691	exists in 4 allotropic forms
Argon (1894)	Ar	18	39.948	0?	1.7837	colorless, odorless gas
Arsenic (1250)	As	33	74.9216	3, 5	5.73	(gray) semimetallic solid
					4.73	(black)
					1.97	(yellow)
Astatine (1940)	At	85	[210]	1, 3, 5, 7		radioactive halogen
Barium (1808)	Ba	56	137.34	2	3.5	silvery-white, alkaline earth metal
Berkelium (1949)	Bk	97	[247]	3, 4		fifth transuranium element discovered
Beryllium (1798)	Be	4	9.0122	2	1.848	light, steel-gray metal
Bismuth (1753)	Bi	83	208.980	3, 5	9.747	pinkish-white, crystalline, brittle metal
Bohrium	Bh	107	[264]			fourteenth transuranium element discovered
Boron (1808)	B	5	10.811	3	2.34, 2.37	crystalline or amorphous element, not occurring free in nature
Bromine (1826)	Br	35	79.909	1, 3, 5, 7	3.12	mobile, reddish brown liquid, volatilizing readily
					7.59	red vapor with disagreeable odor
Cadmium (1817)	Cd	48	112.40	2	8.65	soft, bluish-white metal
Calcium (1808)	Ca	20	40.08	2	1.55	metallic element, forming more than 3 per cent of earth's crust
Californium (1950)	Cf	98	[251]	2, 3, 4		sixth transuranium element discovered
Carbon (prehistoric)	C	6	12.01115	2, 3, 4	1.8–2.1	(amorphous) element widely distributed in nature
					1.9–2.3	(graphite)
					3.15–3.53	(diamond)
Cerium (1803)	Ce	58	140.12	3, 4	6.67–8.23	most abundant rare earth metal
Cesium (1869)	Cs	55	132.905	1	1.873	silvery-white, soft, alkaline metal
Chlorine (1774)	Cl	17	35.453	1, 3, 5, 7	3.214	greenish-yellow gas of the halogen group

Databases for the periodic table are on the World Wide Web. A particularly useful web site can be found at: http://www.shef.ac.uu/chem/web-elements/
*Figures in brackets represent mass number of most stable isotope.

(continued)

6-1. CHEMICAL ELEMENTS—cont'd

Element (Date of Discovery)	Symbol	Atomic Number	Atomic Weight*	Valence	Specific Gravity or Density (Grams/Liter)	Descriptive Comment
Chromium (1797)	Cr	24	51.996	2, 3, 6	7.18–7.20	steel-gray, lustrous, hard metal
Cobalt (1735)	Co	27	58.9332	2, 3	8.9	brittle, hard metal
Copper (prehistoric)	Cu	29	63.54	1, 2	8.96	reddish, lustrous, malleable metal
Curium (1944)	Cm	96	[247]	3, 4	13.51	third transuranium element discovered
Dutnium (1970)	Db	105	[262]			twelfth transuranium element discovered
Dysprosium (1886)	Dy	66	162.50	3	8.536	rare earth metal with metallic bright silver luster
Einsteinium (1952)	Es	99	[252]	2, 3		seventh transuranium element discovered
Element 110		110	[269]			seventeenth transuranium element discovered
Element 111		111	[272]			eighteenth transuranium element discovered
Element 112		112	[277]			nineteenth transuranium element discovered
Erbium (1843)	Er	68	167.26	3	9.051	soft, malleable rare earth metal
Europium (1896)	Eu	63	151.96	2, 3	5.259	lustrous, silvery-white rare earth metal
Fermium (1953)	Fm	100	[257]	2, 3		eighth transuranium element discovered
Fluorine (1771)	F	9	18.9984	1	1.696	pale yellow, corrosive gas of the halogen group
Francium (1939)	Fr	87	[223]	1		product of alpha disintegration of actinium
Gadolinium (1880)	Gd	64	157.25	3	7.8, 7.895	lustrous, silvery-white rare earth metal
Gallium (1875)	Ga	31	69.72	2, 3	5.907	beautiful, silvery-appearing metal
Germanium (1886)	Ge	32	72.59	2, 4	5.323	grayish-white, brittle metal
Gold (prehistoric)	Au	79	196.967	1, 3	19.32	malleable yellow metal
Hafnium (1923)	Hf	72	178.49	4	13.29	gray metal associated with zirconium
Hassium	Hs	108	[265]			fifteenth transuranium element discovered
Helium (1895)	He	2	4.0026	0	0.177 g/l	inert gas
Holmium (1879)	Ho	67	164.930	3	8.803	relatively soft malleable rare earth metal
Hydrogen (1766)	H	1	1.00797	1	0.08988 g/l 0.070	(gas) most abundant element in the universe (liquid)
Indium (1863)	In	49	114.82	1, 2?, 3	7.31	soft, silvery-white metal
Iodine (1811)	I	53	126.9044	1, 3, 5, 7	4.93, 11.27 g/l	grayish-black, lustrous solid or violet-blue gas
Iridium (1803)	Ir	77	192.2	3, 4	22.42	white, brittle metal of platinum family
Iron (prehistoric)	Fe	26	55.847	2, 3, 4, 6	7.874	fourth most abundant element in earth's crust
Krypton (1898)	Kr	36	83.80	0	3.733 g/l	inert gas
Lanthanum (1839)	La	57	138.91	3	5.98–6.186	silvery-white, ductile, rare earth metal
Lawrencium (1961)	Lr	103	[260]	3		tenth transuranium element discovered
Lead (prehistoric)	Pb	82	207.19	2, 4	11.35	bluish-white, lustrous, malleable metal
Lithium (1817)	Li	3	6.939	1	0.534	lightest of all metals
Lutetium (1907)	Lu	71	174.97	3	9.872	rare earth metal

Element (date)	Symbol	At. no.	At. weight	Valences	Density	Description
Magnesium (1808)	Mg	12	24.312	2	1.738	silvery-white metallic element, eighth in abundance in earth's crust
Manganese (1774)	Mn	25	54.9380	1, 2, 3, 4, 6, 7	7.21–7.44	exists in 4 allotropic forms
Meitnerium	Mt	109	[268]			sixteenth transuranium element discovered
Mendelevium (1955)	Md	101	[258]	2, 3		ninth transuranium element discovered
Mercury (prehistoric)	Hg	80	200.59	1, 2	13.546	heavy, silvery-white metal, liquid at ordinary temperatures
Molybdenum (1782)	Mo	42	95.94	2, 3, 4?, 5?, 6	10.22	silvery-white, very hard metal
Neodymium (1885)	Nd	60	144.24	3	6.80, 7.004	exists in 2 allotropic forms
Neon (1898)	Ne	10	20.183	0?	0.89990 g/l	inert gas
Neptunium (1940)	Np	93	237.0482	3, 4, 5, 6	20.45	first transuranium element discovered
Nickel (1751)	Ni	28	58.71	0, 1, 2, 3	8.902	silvery-white, malleable metal
Niobium (1801)	Nb	41	92.906	2, 3, 4?, 5	8.57	shiny white, soft ductile metal
Nitrogen (1772)	N	7	14.0067	3, 5	1.2506 g/l	colorless, odorless, inert element, making up 78 per cent of the air
Nobelium (1958)	No	102	[259]	2, 3		acceptance of this element considered premature
Osmium (1803)	Os	76	190.2	2, 3, 4, 8	22.57	bluish-white, hard metal of platinum family
Oxygen (1774)	O	8	15.9994	2	1.429 g/l	colorless, odorless gas, third most abundant element in the universe
Palladium (1803)	Pd	46	106.4	2, 3, 4	12.02	steel-white metal of the platinum family
Phosphorus (1669)	P	15	30.9738	3, 5	1.82	(white) waxy solid, transparent when pure
					2.20	(red)
					2.25–2.69	(black)
Platinum (1735)	Pt	78	195.09	1?, 2, 3, 4	21.45	silvery-white, malleable metal
Plutonium (1940)	Pu	94	[244]	3, 4, 5, 6, 7	19.84	second transuranium element discovered
Polonium (1898)	Po	84	[210]	2, 4, 6	9.32	very rare natural element
Potassium (1807)	K	19	39.102	1	0.862	soft, silvery, alkali metal, seventh in abundance in earth's crust
Praseodymium (1885)	Pr	59	140.907	3, 4	6.782, 6.64	soft, silvery rare earth metal
Promethium (1941)	Pm	61	[145]	3	7.22 ± 0.02	produced by irradiation of neodymium and praseodymium; identity established in 1945
Protactinium (1917)	Pa	91	231.0359	4, 5	15.37	bright lustrous metal
Radium (1898)	Ra	88	226.0254	2	5.5	brilliant white, radioactive metal
Radon (1900)	Rn	86	[222]	0	9.73 g/l	heaviest known gas
Rhenium (1925)	Re	75	186.2	−1, 2, 3, 4, 5, 6, 7	21.02	silvery-white lustrous metal
Rhodium (1803)	Rh	45	102.905	−2, 3, 4, 5	12.41	silvery-white metal of platinum family
Rubidium (1861)	Rb	37	85.47	1, 2, 3, 4	1.532	soft, silvery-white, alkali metal
Ruthenium (1844)	Ru	44	101.07	0, 1, 2, 3, 4, 5, 6, 7, 8	12.41	hard white metal of platinum family
Rutherfordium (1969)	Rf	104	[261]			eleventh transuranium element discovered

(continued)

6-1. CHEMICAL ELEMENTS—cont'd

Element (Date of Discovery)	Symbol	Atomic Number	Atomic Weight*	Valence	Specific Gravity or Density (Grams/Liter)	Descriptive Comment
Samarium (1879)	Sm	62	150.35	2, 3	7.52, 7.40	bright silver lustrous metal
Scandium (1879)	Sc	21	44.956	3	2.992	soft, silvery-white metal
Seaborgium	Sg	106	[262]			thirteenth transuranium element discovered
Selenium (1817)	Se	34	78.96	2, 4, 6	4.79, 4.28	exists in several allotropic forms
Silicon (1823)	Si	14	28.086	4	2.33	a relatively inert element, second in abundance in earth's crust
Silver (prehistoric)	Ag	47	107.870	1, 2	10.50	malleable, ductile metal with brilliant white luster
Sodium (1807)	Na	11	22.9898	1	0.971	most abundant of alkali metals, sixth in abundance in earth's crust
Strontium (1808)	Sr	38	87.62	2	2.54	exists in 3 allotropic forms
Sulfur (prehistoric)	S	16	32.064	2, 4, 6	1.957, 2.07	exists in several isotopic and many allotropic forms
Tantalum (1802)	Ta	73	180.948	2?, 3, 4?, 5	16.6	gray, heavy, very hard metal
Technetium (1937)	Tc	43	98.9062	3?, 4, 6, 7	11.50	first element produced artificially
Tellurium (1782)	Te	52	127.60	2, 4, 6	6.24	silvery-white, lustrous element
Terbium (1843)	Tb	65	158.924	3, 4	8.272	silvery-gray, malleable, ductile rare earth metal
Thallium (1861)	Tl	81	204.37	1, 3	11.85	very soft, malleable metal
Thorium (1828)	Th	90	232.038	4	11.66	silvery-white, lustrous metal
Thulium (1879)	Tm	69	168.934	2, 3		least abundant rare earth metal
Tin (prehistoric)	Sn	50	118.69	2, 4	5.75 / 7.31	(gray) malleable metal existing in 2 or 3 allotropic forms, changing from white to gray on cooling and back to white on warming (white)
Titanium (1791)	Ti	22	47.90	2, 3, 4	4.54	lustrous white metal
Tungsten (1783)	W	74	183.85	2, 3, 4, 5, 6	19.3	steel-gray to tin-white metal
Uranium (1789)	U	92	238.03	3, 4, 5, 6	18.95	heavy, silvery-white metal
Vanadium (1801)	V	23	50.942	2, 3, 4, 5	6.11	bright, white metal
Xenon (1898)	Xe	54	131.30	0?	5.887 g/l	one of the so-called rare or inert gases
Ytterbium (1878)	Yb	70	173.04	2, 3	6.977, 6.54	exists in 2 allotropic forms
Yttrium (1794)	Y	39	88.905	3	4.45	rare earth metal with silvery metallic luster
Zinc (1746)	Zn	30	65.37	2	7.133	bluish-white, lustrous metal, malleable at 100–150°C
Zirconium (1789)	Zr	40	91.22	4	6.4	grayish-white, lustrous metal

1 hydrogen	41 niobium	81 thallium
2 helium	42 molybdenum	82 lead
3 lithium	43 technetium	83 bismuth
4 beryllium	44 ruthenium	84 polonium
5 boron	45 rhodium	85 astatine
6 carbon	46 palladium	86 radon
7 nitrogen	47 silver	87 francium
8 oxygen	48 cadmium	88 radium
9 fluorine	49 indium	89 actinium
10 neon	50 tin	90 thorium
11 sodium	51 antimony	91 protactinium
12 magnesium	52 tellurium	92 uranium
13 aluminum	53 iodine	93 neptunium
14 silicon	54 xenon	94 plutonium
15 phosphorus	55 cesium	95 americium
16 sulfur	56 barium	96 curium
17 chlorine	57 lanthanum	97 berkelium
18 argon	58 cerium	98 californium
19 potassium	59 praseodymium	99 einsteinium
20 calcium	60 neodymium	100 fermium
21 scandium	61 promethium	101 mendelevium
22 titanium	62 samarium	102 nobelium
23 vanadium	63 europium	103 lawrencium
24 chromium	64 gadolinium	104 rutherfordium
25 manganese	65 terbium	105 dubnium
26 iron	66 dysprosium	106 seaborgium
27 cobalt	67 holmium	107 bohrium
28 nickel	68 erbium	108 hassium
29 copper	69 thulium	109 meitnerium
30 zinc	70 ytterbium	Element 110
31 gallium	71 lutetium	Element 111
32 germanium	72 hafnium	Element 112
33 arsenic	73 tantalum	
34 selenium	74 tungsten	
35 bromine	75 rhenium	
36 krypton	76 osmium	
37 rubidium	77 iridium	
38 strontium	78 platinum	
39 yttrium	79 gold	
40 zirconium	80 mercury	

Section 7: Immunization Schedules

7-1. RECOMMENDED CHILDHOOD IMMUNIZATION SCHEDULE (UNITED STATES, 2002[*])

Vaccine	Age	Birth	1 mo	2 mos	4 mos	6 mos	12 mos	15 mos	18 mos	24 mos	4–6 yrs	11–12 yrs	13–18 yrs
Hepatitis B[1]		Hep B #1	Hep B #2 (only if mother HBsAg(-))	Hep B #2			Hep B #3					Hep B series	
Diphtheria, Tetanus, Pertussis[2]				DTaP	DTaP	DTaP		DTaP	DTaP		DTaP	Td	
Haemophilus influenzae Type b[3]				Hib	Hib	Hib	Hib	Hib					
Inactivated Polio[4]				IPV	IPV		IPV	IPV			IPV		
Measles, Mumps, Rubella[5]							MMR #1				MMR #2	MMR #2	MMR #2
Varicella[6]							Varicella					Varicella	
Pneumococcal[7]				PCV	PCV	PCV	PCV	PCV		PCV	PPV		
Hepatitis A[8]											Hepatitis A series		
Influenza[9]							Influenza (yearly)						

Range of Recommended Ages *Catch-up Vaccination* *Preadolescent Assessment*

Vaccines below this line are for selected populations

2094

This schedule indicates the recommended ages for routine administration of currently licensed childhood vaccices, as of December 1, 2001, for children through age 18 years. Any dose not given at the recommended age should be given at any subsequent visit when indicated and feasible. █ Indicates age group that warrants special effort to administer those vaccines not previously given. Additional vaccines may be licensed and recommended during the year. Licensed combination vaccines may be used whenever any components of the combination are indicated and the vaccine's other components are not contraindicated. Providers should consult the manufacturers' package inserts for detailed recommendations.

1. Hepatitis B vaccine (Hep B). All infants should receive the first dose of hepatitis B vaccine soon after birth and before hospital discharge; the first dose may also be given by age 2 months if the infant's mother is HBsAg-negative. Only monovalent hepatitis B vaccine can be used for the birth dose. Monovalent or combination vaccine containing Hep B may be used to complete the series; four doses of vaccine may be administered if combination vaccine is used. The second dose should be given at least 4 weeks after the first dose, except for Hib-containing vaccine which cannot be administered before age 6 weeks. The third dose should be given at least 16 weeks after the first dose and at least 8 weeks after the second dose. The last dose in the vaccination series (third or fourth dose) should not be administered before age 6 months.

Infants born to HBsAg-positive mothers should receive hepatitis B vaccine and 0.5mL hepatitis B immune globulin (HBIG) within 12 hours of birth at separate sites. The second dose is recommended at age 1–2 months and the vaccination series should be completed (third or fourth dose) at age 6 months.

Infants born to mothers whose HBsAg status is unknown should receive the first dose of the hepatitis B vaccine series within 12 hours of birth. Maternal blood should be drawn at the time of delivery to determine the mother's HBsAg status; if the HBsAg test is positive, the infant should receive HBIG as soon as possible (no later than age 1 week)

2. Diphtheria and tetanus toxoids and acellular pertussis vaccine (DTaP). The fourth dose of DTaP may be administered as early as age 12 months, provided 6 months have elapsed since the third dose and the child is unlikely to return at age 15–18 months. *Tetanus and diphtheria toxoids (Td)* is recommended at age 11–12 years if at least 5 years have elapsed since the last dose of tetanus and diphtheria toxoids-containing vaccine. Subsequent routine Td boosters are recommended every 10 years.

3. *Haemophilus influenzae* type b (Hib) conjugate vaccine. Three Hib conjugate vaccines are licensed for infant use. If PRP-OMP (PedvaxHIB® or ComVax® [Merck]) is administered at ages 2 and 4 months, a dose at age 6 months is not required. DTaP/Hib combination products should not be used for primary immunization in infants at age 2, 4, or 6 months, but can be used as boosters following any Hib vaccine.

4. Inactivated poliovirus vaccine (IPV). An all-IPV schedule is recommended for routine childhood poliovirus vaccination in the United States. All children should receive four doses of IPV at age 2 months, 4 months, 6–18 months, and 4–6 years.

5. Measles, mumps, and rubella vaccine (MMR). The second dose of MMR is recommended routinely at age 4–6 years but may be administered during any visit, provided at least 4 weeks have elapsed since the first dose and that both doses are administered beginning at or after age 12 months. Those who have not previously received the second dose should complete the schedule by the visit at 11–12 years.

6. Varicella vaccine. Varicella vaccine is recommended at any visit at or after age 12 months for susceptible children (i.e those who lack a reliable history of chickenpox). Susceptible persons age ≥ 13 years should receive two doses, given at least 4 weeks apart.

7. Pneumococcal vaccine. The heptavalent *pneumococcal conjugate vaccine (PCV)* is recommended for all children age 2–23 months and for certain children aged 24–59 months. *Pneumococcal polysaccharide vaccine (PPV)* is recommended in addition to PCV for certain high-risk groups. See *MMWR* 2000, 49 (RR-9): 1–37.

8. Hepatitis A vaccine. Hepatitis A vaccine is recommended for use in selected states and regions, and for certain high-risk groups; consult your local public health authority. See *MMWR* 1999, 48 (RR-12); 1–37.

9. Influenza vaccine. Influenza vaccine is recommended annually for children age >6 months with certain risk factors (including but not limited to asthma, cardiac disease, sickle cell diseases; see *MMWR* 2001;50 [RR-4]: 1–44) and can be administered to all others wishing to obtain immunity. Children aged ≤12 years should receive vaccine in a dosage appropriate for their age (0.25 mL if age 6–35 months or 0.5 mL if age ≥3 years) Children age ≤8 years who are receiving influenza vaccine for the first time should receive two doses separated by at least 4 weeks.

*Approved by the Advisory Committee on Immunization Practices (www.cdc.gov/nip/acip), the American Academy of Pediatrics (www.aap.org), and the American Academy of Family Physicians (www.aafp.org). For additional information about vaccine supply, and contraindications for immunization, please visit the National Immunization Program website at www.cdc.gov/nip or call the National Immunization Hotline at 800-232-2522 (English) or 800-232-0233 (Spanish).

7-2. SUMMARY OF ADOLESCENT/ADULT IMMUNIZATION RECOMMENDATIONS (2/4/2002)

Agent	Indications	Primary Schedule	Contraindications	Comments
Hepatitis B Vaccine	a. Persons with occupational risk of exposure to blood or blood-contaminated body fluids. b. Clients and staff of institutions for the developmentally disabled. c. Hemodialysis patients. d. Recipients of clotting-factor concentrates. e. Household contacts and sex partners of those chronically infected with HBV. f. Family members of adoptees from countries where HBV infection is endemic, if adoptees are HBsAg+1.0 g. Certain international travelers. h. Injecting drug users. i. Men who have sex with men. j. Heterosexual men and women with multiple sex partners or recent episode of a sexually transmitted disease. k. Inmates of long-term correctional facilities. l. All unvaccinated adolescents.	Three doses: second dose 1–2 months after the first, third dose 4–6 months after the first. No need to start over if schedule interrupted. Can start series with one manufacturer's vaccine and finish with another. Dose (*Adult*): intramuscular (IM) Recombivax HB®: 10 μg/1.0 mL (green cap) Engerix-B®: 20 μg/mL (orange cap) Dose (*Adolescents 11–19 years*): intramuscular (IM) Recombivax HB®: 5 μg/0.5 mL (yellow cap) Engerix-B®: 10 μg/0.5 mL (light blue cap) Two doses (*Only for adolescents 11–15 years*): intramuscular (IM), 4–6 months apart. Restricted to Recombivax HB®: 10 μg/1.0 mL (green cap) Booster: None presently recommended.	Anaphylactic allergy to yeast.	a. Persons with serologic markers of prior or continuing hepatitis B virus infection do not need immunization. b. For hemodialysis patients and other immunodeficient or immunosuppressed patients, vaccine dosage is doubled or special preparation is used. c. Pregnant women should be sero-screened for HBsAg and, if positive, their infants should be given post-exposure prophylaxis beginning at birth. d. Post-exposure prophylaxis: consult ACIP recommendations, or state or local immunization program.
Poliovirus Vaccine: IPV–Inactivated Vaccine; OPV–Oral (live) Vaccine	Routine vaccination of those ≥18 years of age residing in the U.S is not necessary. Vaccination is recommended for the following high-risk adults:	Unimmunized adolescents/adults: IPV is recommended—two doses at 4–8 week intervals, third dose 6–12 months after second (can be as soon as 2 months) Dose: 0.5 mL subcutaneous (SC) or intramuscular (IM).	*IPV*: Anaphylactic reaction following previous dose or to streptomycin, polymyxin B, or neomycin.	In instances of potential exposure to wild poliovirus, adults who have had a primary series of OPV or IPV may be given 1 more dose of IPV.

Partially immunized adolescents/adults: Complete primary series with IPV (IPV schedule shown above).

OPV is no longer recommended for use in the United States.

a. Travelers to areas or countries where poliomyelitis is epidemic or endemic.
b. Members of communities or specific population groups with disease caused by wild polioviruses.
c. Laboratory workers who handle specimens that may contain polioviruses.
d. Health care workers who have close contact with patient who may be excreting wild polioviruses.
e. Unvaccinated adults whose children will be receiving OPV.

Although no adverse effects have been documented, vaccination of pregnant women should be avoided. However, if immediate protection is required, pregnant women may be given IPV in accordance with the recommended schedule for adults.

Varicella Vaccine

For persons <13 years of age, one dose. For persons 13 years and older, two doses separated by 4–8 weeks. If > 8 weeks elapse following the first dose, the second dose can be administered without restarting the schedule.

Dose: 0.5 mL subcutaneous (SC)

a. Persons of any age without a reliable history of varicella disease or vaccination, or who are seronegative for varicella.
b. Susceptible adolescents and adults living in households with children.
c. All susceptible health care workers.
d. Susceptible family contacts of immunocompromised persons.
e. Susceptible persons in the following groups who are at high risk for exposure:
 – persons who live or work in environments in which transmission of varicella is likely (e.g., teachers of young children, day care employees, residents and staff in institutional settings) or can occur (e.g., college students, inmates and staff of correctional institutions, military personnel).
 – nonpregnant women of child bearing age
 – international travelers

a. Anaphylactic allergy to gelatin or neomycin.
b. Untreated, active TB.
c. Immunosuppressive therapy or immunodeficiency (including HIV infection).
d. Family history of congenital or hereditary immunodeficiency in first-degree relatives, unless the immune competence of the recipient has been clinically substantiated or verified by a laboratory.
e. Immune globulin preparation or blood/blood product received in preceding 5 months.
f. Pregnancy.

Women should be asked if they are pregnant before receiving varicella vaccine, and advised to avoid pregnancy for one month following each dose of vaccine.

(continued)

7-2. SUMMARY OF ADOLESCENT/ADULT IMMUNIZATION RECOMMENDATIONS (2/4/2002)—cont'd

Agent	Indications	Primary Schedule	Contraindications	Comments
Hepatitis A Vaccine	a. Persons traveling to or working in countries with high or intermediate endemicity of infection. b. Men who have sex with men. c. Injecting and non-injecting illegal drug users. d. Persons who work with HAV-infected primates or with HAV in research laboratory setting. e. Persons with chronic liver disease disorders. f. Persons with clotting factor disorders. g. Consider food handlers, where determined to be cost-effective by health authorities or employers.	Havrix®: Two doses, separated by 6–12 months. Adults (19 years of age and older): Dose: 1.0 mL intramuscular (IM); Persons 2–18 years of age: Dose: 0.5 mL (IM). Vaqta®: Adults (19 years of age and older): Two doses, separated by 6 months. Dose: 1.0 mL intramuscular (IM); Persons 2–18 years of age: Two doses, separated by 6–18 months. Dose: 0.5 mL (IM)	A history of hypersensitivity to alum or the preservative 2-phenoxyethanol	The safety of hepatitis A vaccine during pregnancy has not been determined, though the theoretical risk to the developing fetus is expected to be low. The risk of vaccination should be weighed against the risk of hepatitis A in women who may be at high risk of exposure to HAV.
Tetanus and Diphtheria Toxoids Combined (Td)	All adults All adolescents should be assessed at 11–12 or 14–16 years of age and immunized if no dose was received during the previous 5 years.	Two doses 4–8 weeks apart, third dose 6–12 months after the second. No need to repeat doses if the schedule is interrupted. Dose: 0.5 mL intramuscular (IM) Booster: At 10-year intervals throughout life.	Neurologic or severe hypersensitivity reaction to prior dose.	WOUND MANAGEMENT: Patients with three or more previous tetanus toxoid doses: (a) give Td for clean, minor wounds only if more than 10 years since last dose; (b) for other wounds, give Td if over 5 years since last dose. Patients with less than 3 or unknown number of prior tetanus toxoid doses; give Td for clean, minor wounds and TIG (Tetanus Immune Globulin) for other wounds.

Influenza Vaccine	a. Adults 50 years of age and older. b. Residents of nursing homes or other facilities for patients with chronic medical conditions. c. Persons ≥6 months of age with chronic cardiovascular or pulmonary disorders, including asthma. d. Persons ≥6 months of age with chronic metabolic diseases (including diabetes), renal dysfunction, hemoglobinopathies, immunosuppressive or immunodeficiency disorders. e. Women in their 2nd or 3rd trimester of pregnancy during influenza season. f. Persons 6 mo.-18 years of age receiving long-term aspirin therapy. g. Groups, including household members and care givers, who can infect high-risk persons.	Dose: 0.5 mL intramuscular (IM) Given annually each fall and winter.	Anaphylactic allergy to eggs. Acute febrile illness.	Depending on season and destination, persons traveling to foreign countries should consider vaccination. Any person ≥6 months of age who wishes to reduce the likelihood of becoming ill with influenza should be vaccinated. Avoiding subsequent vaccination of persons known to have developed Guillain–Barré syndrome (GBS) within 6 weeks of a previous vaccination seems prudent; however, for most persons with a GBS history who are at high risk for severe complications, many experts believe the established benefits of vaccination justify yearly vaccination.
Pneumococcal Polysaccharide Vaccine (PPV)	a. Adults 65 years of age and older. b. Persons ≥2 years with chronic cardiovascular or pulmonary disorders including congestive heart failure, diabetes mellitus, chronic liver disease, alcoholism, CSF leaks, cardiomyopathy, COPD or emphysema. c. Persons ≥2 years with splenic dysfunction or asplenia, hematologic malignancy, multiple myeloma, renal failure, organ transplantation or immunosuppressive condition, including HIV infection. d. Alaskan Natives and certain American Indian populations.	One dose for most people. Dose: 0.5 mL intramuscular (IM) or subcutaneous (SC) Persons vaccinated prior to age 65 should be vaccinated at age 65 if 5 or more years have passed since the first dose. For all persons with functional or anatomic asplenia, transplant patients, patients with chronic kidney disease, immunosuppressed or immunodeficient persons and others at highest risk of fatal infection, a second dose should be given — at least 5 years after first dose.	The safety of PPV during the first trimester of pregnancy has not been evaluated. The manufacturer's package insert should be reviewed for additional information.	If elective splenectomy or immunosuppressive therapy is planned, give vaccine 2 weeks ahead, if possible. When indicated, vaccine should be administered to patient with unknown vaccination status. All residents of nursing homes and other long-term care facilities should have their vaccination status assessed and documented.

(continued)

7-2. SUMMARY OF ADOLESCENT/ADULT IMMUNIZATION RECOMMENDATIONS (2/4/2002)—cont'd

Agent	Indications	Primary Schedule	Contraindications	Comments
Measles and Mumps Vaccines**	a. Adults born after 1956 without written documentation of immunization on or after the first birthday. b. Health care personnel born after 1956 who are at risk of exposure to patients with measles should have documentation of two doses of vaccine on or after the first birthday or of measles seropositivity. c. HIV-infected persons without severe immunosuppression. d. Travelers to foreign countries. e. Persons entering post-secondary educational institutions (e.g., college).	At least one dose (two doses of measles-containing vaccine if in health care profession or traveling to a foreign country, with second dose at least 1 month after the first). Dose: 0.5 mL subcutaneous (SC)	a. Immunosuppressive therapy or immunodeficiency including HIV-infected persons with severe immunosuppression. b. Anaphylactic allergy to neomycin. c. Pregnancy. d. Immune globulin preparation or blood/blood product received in preceding 3–11 months. e. Untreated, active TB.	Women should be asked if they are pregnant before receiving vaccine, and advised to avoid pregnancy for 28 days after immunization.
Rubella Vaccine**	a. Persons (especially women) without written documentation of immunization on or after the first birthday or of seropositivity. b. Health care personnel who are at risk of exposure to patients with rubella and who may have contact with pregnant patients should have at least one dose.	One dose. Dose: 0.5 mL subcutaneous (SC)	Same as for measles and mumps vaccines.	Women should be asked if they are pregnant before receiving vaccine, and advised to avoid pregnancy for 28 days after immunization.

Adapted from the recommendations of the Advisory Committee on Immunization Practices (ACIP). Foreign travel and less commonly used vaccines such as typhoid, rabies, and meningococcal are not included.
**These vaccines can be given in the combined form measles-mumps-rubella (MMR). Persons already immune to one or more components can still receive MMR.

7-3. ROUTINE IMMUNIZATION SCHEDULES FOR CHILDREN AND ADOLESCENTS (CANADA)*

INFANTS AND CHILDREN

Age at Vaccination	DTaP[1]	IPV	Hib[2]	MMR	Td[3] or dTap[10]	Hep B[4] (3 Doses)	V	PC	MC
Birth									
2 months	X	X	X			Infancy		X[8]	X[9]
4 months	X	X	X					X	X
6 months	X	(X)[5]	X					X	X
12 months				X		or	X[7]	X	
18 months	X	X	X	(X)[6] or					or
4–6 years	X	X		(X)[6]					
14–16 years					X[10]	preadolescence (9–13 yrs)			X[9]

DTaP Diphtheria, tetanus, pertussis (acellular) vaccine
IPV Inactivated poliovirus vaccine
Hib *Haemophilus influenzae* type b conjugate vaccine
MMR Measles, mumps and rubella vaccine
Td Tetanus and diphtheria toxoid, adult type with reduced diphtheria toxoid
dTap Tetanus and diphtheria toxoid acellular pertussis, adolescent/adult type with reduced diphtheria and pertussis components
Hep B Hepatitis B vaccine
V Varicella
PC Pneumococcal conjugate vaccine
MC Meningococcal conjugate vaccine

CHILDREN < 7 YEARS OF AGE NOT IMMUNIZED IN EARLY INFANCY

Timing	DTaP[1]	IPV	Hib	MMR	Td[3] or dTap[10]	Hep B[4] (3 doses)	V	P	M
First visit	X	X	X[11]	X[13]		X	X[7]	X[8]	X[9]
2 months later	X	X	X	(X)[6]		X		(X)	(X)
2 months later	X	(X)[5]						(X)	
6–12 months later	X	X	(X)[11]			X			
4–6 years of age[19]	X	X							
14–16 years of age[19]				X					

P Pneumococcal vaccine
M Meningococcal vaccine

CHILDREN ≥ 7 YEARS OF AGE NOT IMMUNIZED IN EARLY INFANCY

Timing	dTap[10]	IPV	MMR	Hep B[4] (3 doses)	V	M
First visit	X	X	X	X	X	X[9]
2 months later	X	X	X[6]	X	(X)[7]	
6–12 months later	X	X		X		
10 years later	X					

M Meningococcal vaccine

Notes:
1. DTaP (diphtheria, tetanus, acellular or component pertussis) vaccine is the preferred vaccine for all doses in the vaccination series, including completion of the series in children who have received ≥1 dose of DPT (whole cell) vaccine.
2. Hib schedule shown is for PRP-T or HbOC vaccine. If PRP-OMP is used, give at 2, 4 and 12 months of age.
3. Td (tetanus and diphtheria toxoid), a combined adsorbed "adult type" preparation for use in people ≥7 years of age, contains less diphtheria toxoid than preparations given to younger children and is less likely to cause reactions in older people.
4. Hepatitis B vaccine can be routinely given to infants or preadolescents, depending on the provincial/territorial policy; three doses at 0, 1 and 6 month intervals are preferred. The second dose should be administered at least 1 month after the first dose, and the third at least 2 months after the second dose. A two-dose schedule for adolescents is also possible.
5. This dose is not needed routinely, but can be included for convenience.
6. A second dose of MMR is recommended, at least 1 month after the first dose for the purpose of better measles protection. For convenience, options include giving it with the next scheduled vaccination at 18 months of age or with school entry (4–6 years) vaccinations (depending on the provincial/territorial policy), or at any intervening age that is practicable. The need for a second dose of mumps and rubella vaccine is not established but may benefit (given for convenience as MMR). The second dose of MMR should be given at the same visit as DTaP IPV (± Hib) to ensure high uptake rates.

7. Children aged 12 months to 12 years should receive one dose of varicella vaccine. Individuals ≥ 13 years of age should receive two doses at least 28 days apart.
8. Recommended schedule, number of doses and subsequent use of 23 valent polysaccharide pneumococcal vaccine depend on the age of the child when vaccination is begun.
9. Recommended schedule and number of doses of meningococcal vaccine depend on the age of the child.
10. dTap adult formulation with reduced diphtheria toxoid and pertussis component.
11. Recommended schedule and number of doses depend on the product used and age of the child when vaccination is begun. Not required past age 5.
12. Delay until subsequent visit if child is < 12 months of age.
13. Omit these doses if the previous doses of DTaP and polio were given after the fourth birthday.

Vaccine or toxoid	Indication	Further doses
Diphtheria (adult preparation)	All adults	Every 10 years, preferably given with tetanus toxoid (Td)
Tetanus	All adults	Every 10 years, preferably given as Td
Influenza	Adults ≥65 years; adults <65 years at high risk of influenza-related complications and other select groups	Every year using current vaccine formulation
Pneumococcal	Adults ≥65 years; conditions with increased risk of pneumococcal diseases	
Measles	All adults born in 1970 or later who are susceptible to measles	May be given as MMR
Rubella	Susceptible women of childbearing age and health care workers	May be given as MMR
Mumps	Adults born in 1970 or later with no history of mumps	May be given as MMR

*From Canadian Immunization Guide, 6th Ed., 2002.

Section 8: Symbols, Terms, and Abbreviations

8-1. SYMBOLS COMMONLY USED IN CLINICAL PRACTICE

—	lying
⌐	sitting
|	standing
ê	change
μ	micron
P	para (number of live births)
G	gravida (number of pregnancies)
R_x	recipe (take)
$\bar{a}$	before
$\bar{p}$	after
$\bar{c}$	with
$\bar{s}$	without
=	equal
≠	unequal
>	greater than
<	less than
↑	increase
↗	increasing
↓	decrease
↘	decreasing
−	negative, minus, deficiency, alkaline reaction
±	very slight trace or reaction, indefinite
+	slight trace or reaction, positive, plus, excess, acid reaction
++	trace or notable reaction
+++	moderate amount or reaction
++++	large amount or pronounced reaction
#	number, pound, has been given or done
→	yields, leads to
←	resulting from or secondary to
(catalyst) →	accelerant, increases velocity of a chemical reaction or process
♂ ○ ○ or □	male
♀ or ○	female
ℨ	dram
℥	ounce
1°, 2°	primary, secondary

Symbol	Meaning	Symbol	Meaning
□	Male	□—○	Marriage
○	Female	□⋯○	Extramarital mating
◇	Sex unspecified	□⫽○	Divorce
4 ②	Number of children of sex indicated	□═○	Consanguineous mating
■ ●	Affected	⟋▔⟍	Monozygotic twins
Multiple marriages		⟋⟍	Dizygotic twins
◖◗	Heterozygotes for autosomal trait	⟋▔?⟍	Twins of unknown zygosity
⊙	Carrier of X-linked recessive trait	Numbering individuals in pedigrees Proband is II-2	
■	Proband (shown by arrow)		
⧄	Deceased individual		
▮	Prenatal death	□⊤○	No offspring
●	Miscarriage	▨	Partially affected by a trait
[□]	Adopted into a family	⊘	
]○[	Adopted out of a family		

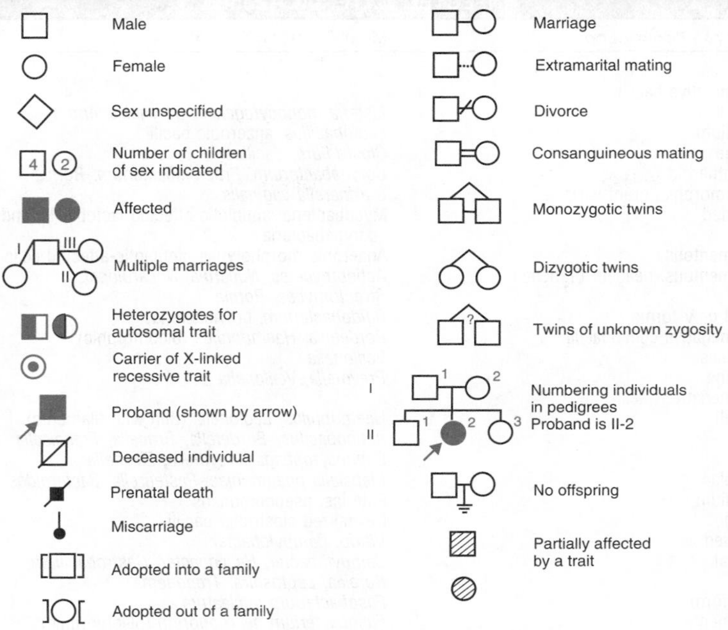

The microscopist must have a consistent vocabulary for the description of materials seen in viewed samples. This vocabulary must be shared by the microbiology and health care communities so that when observations are reported everyone will be able to understand the implications of the descriptions. The use of computers for recording coded observations and generating reports of the findings further extends the need for uniform terminology.

The background of the sample being evaluated should be described in sufficient detail to convey the composition of the material. The presence of cells representing a response to injury supports the probability of infection and directs attention toward specific types of pathogens.

Common morphotype descriptions and the most prevalent associated species are shown below.

Morphotype Description	Most Common Organisms
Bacteria	
Cocci	
Gram-positive cocci	*Aerococcus, Enterococcus, Leuconostoc, Pediococcus, Planococcus, Staphylococcus, Stomatococcus, Streptococcus*
Gram-positive cocci	
Pairs	*Staphylococcus, Streptococcus, Enterococcus*
Tetrads	*Micrococcus, Staphylococcus, Peptostreptococcus*
Groups	*Staphylococcus, Peptostreptococcus, Stomatococcus*
Chains	*Streptococcus, Peptostreptococcus*
Clusters, intracellular	Microaerophilic *Streptococcus*, viridans streptococci, *Staphylococcus*
Encapsulated	*Streptococcus pneumoniae, Streptococcus pyogenes* (rarely), *Stomatococcus mucilaginosus*
Gram-positive diplococci (lancet-shaped)	*Streptococcus pneumoniae*
Gram-negative diplococci	Pathogenic *Neisseria, Moraxella (Branhamella) catarrhalis*

(continued)

Morphotype Description	Most Common Organisms
Bacilli	
Gram-positive bacilli	
Small	*Listeria monocytogenes, Corynebacterium*
Medium	*Lactobacillus,* anaerobic bacilli
Large	*Clostridium, Bacillus*
Diphtheroid	*Corynebacterium, Propionibacterium. Rothia*
Pleomorphic, gram-variable	*Gardnerella vaginalis*
Beaded	Mycobacteria, antibiotic-affected lactobacilli, and corynebacteria
Filamentous	Anaerobic morphotypes, antibiotic-affected cells
Filamentous, beaded, branched	*Actinomycetes, Nocardia, Nocardiopsis, Streptomyces, Rothia*
Bifid or V forms	*Bifidobacterium,* brevibacteria
Gram-negative coccobacilli	*Bordetella, Haemophilus* (pleomorphic)
Masses	*Veillonella*
Chains	*Prevotella, Veillonella*
Gram-negative bacilli	
Small	*Haemophilus, Legionella* (thin with filaments), *Actinobacilus, Bordetella, Brucella, Francisella, Pasteurella Capnocytophaga, Prevotella, Eikenella*
Bipolar	*Klebsiella pneumoniae, Pasteurella, Bacteroides*
Medium	Enterics, pseudomonads
Large	Devitalized clostridia/ bacilli
Curved	*Vibrio, Campylobacter*
Spiral	*Campylobacter, Helicobacter, Gastrobacillum, Borellia, Leptospira, Treponema*
Fusiform	*Fusobacterium nucleatum*
Filaments	*Fusobacterium necrophorum* (pleomorphic)
Yeast/Fungi/Algae	
Yeast	
Small	*Histoplasma, Torulopsis*
Medium	*Candida*
With Capsules	*Cryptococcus neoformans*
Thick-walled, broad-based bud	*Blastomyces*
Hyphae	
Septate	Fungi
Aseptate	Zygomycetes
With arthroconidia	*Coccicioides*
With branches at 45-degree angle	*Aspergillus*
Pseudohyphae	*Candida*
Spherule (endospores)	*Coccidioides*
Sporangia with endospores	*Prototheca*
Viruses	
Single or multinuclear cells with intranuclear inclusions	Herpes virus, measles virus
Enlarged cells with intranuclear inclusions or cytoplasmic inclusions	Cytomegalovirus
Cells with dark "smudged" nuclei	Adenovirus

The American Health Information Management Association has identified a group of terms used to compile statistical health care data, and has defined them in an attempt at standardization. Some of the terms are presented here in an appendix to highlight the importance of using standardized terms for research initiatives and the reporting of statistical data. The definitions are the exact ones used by the American Health Information Management Association. Some of the terms are defined in other ways in the entries section of this dictionary, but terms often have multiple meanings. *The Glossary of Health Care Terms* is a complete list of terms and definitions used in medical records; it is available from the American Health Information Management Association, 919 N. Michigan Ave., Suite 1400, Chicago, Illinois 60611.

Diagnosis — A word or phrase used by a physician to identify a disease from which an individual patient suffers or a condition for which a patient needs, seeks, or receives medical care.

Principal Diagnosis — The diagnosis of the condition established after study, chiefly responsible for occasioning the admission of the patient to the hospital for care.

Other Diagnosis — A diagnosis, other than the principal diagnosis, that describes a condition for which a patient receives treatment or which the physician considers of sufficient significance to warrant inclusion for investigative medical studies.

Complication — An additional diagnosis that describes a condition arising after the beginning of hospital observation and treatment and modifying the course of the patient's illness or the medical care required.

Most Significant Diagnosis — The one diagnosis, often but not necessarily the principal diagnosis, that describes the most important or significant condition of a patient in terms of its implications for his or her health, medical care, and use of the hospital.

Discharge Diagnosis — Any one of the diagnoses recorded after all data accumulated in the course of a patient's hospitalization or other circumscribed episode of medical care have been studied.

Discharge Diagnoses (List of Discharge Diagnoses) — The complete set or list of discharge diagnoses applicable to a single patient experience such as inpatient hospitalization.

Facility — Those objects, including plant, equipment, or supplies, necessary for implementation of services by personnel.

Hospital — Health care institution with an organized and professional staff and with inpatient beds available around the clock, whose primary function is to provide inpatient medical, nursing, and other health related services to patients for both surgical and nonsurgical conditions, and that usually provides some outpatient services, particularly emergency care; for licensure purposes, each state has its own definition of hospital.

Hospital Newborn Inpatient — A hospital patient who was born in the hospital at the beginning of his or her current inpatient hospitalization.

Hospital Boarder — An individual who receives lodging in the hospital but is not a hospital inpatient.

Hospital Inpatient Beds — Accommodations with supporting services (such as food, laundry, housekeeping) for hospital inpatients, excluding those for the newborn nursery.

Hospital Newborn Bassinets — Accommodations with supporting services (such as food, laundry, housekeeping) for hospital newborn inpatients. These include bassinets, incubators, and isolettes in the newborn nursery.

Medical Services — The activities related to medical care performed by physicians, nurses, and other professional and technical personnel under the direction of a physician.

Operating Room — An area of a hospital equipped and staffed to provide facilities and personnel services for the performance of surgical procedures.

Delivery Room — A special operating room for obstetric delivery and infant resuscitation.

Unit — An organizational entity of a hospital. Hospitals are organized both physically and functionally into units.

Medical Staff Unit — One of the departments, divisions, or specialties into which the organized medical staff of a hospital is divided in order to fulfill medical staff responsibility.

Medical Care Unit — An assemblage of inpatient beds (or newborn bassinets) and related facilities and assigned personnel in which medical services are provided to a defined and limited class of patients according to their particular medical care needs.

Hospital Patient — An individual receiving, in person, hospital based or coordinated medical services for which the hospital is responsible.

Hospital Inpatient — A hospital patient who is provided with room, board, and continuous general nursing service in an area of the hospital where patients generally stay at least overnight.

Special Care Unit — A medical care unit in which there is appropriate equipment and a concentration of physicians, nurses, and others who have special skills and experience to provide optimal medical care for critically ill patients, or continuous care of patients in special diagnostic categories.

Adjunct Diagnostic or Therapeutic Unit (Ancillary Unit) — An organized unit of a hospital, other than the operating room, delivery room, or medical care unit, with facilities and personnel to aid physicians in the diagnosis and treatment of patients through the performance of diagnostic or therapeutic procedures.

Health care professionals who have difficulty with the English language may face particular challenges with terms commonly used in a health care setting. The unique application of words may cause confusion. The words and phrases listed below have been identified as frequently causing problems for health care providers.

Word or Phrase	Definition/Example	Word or Phrase	Definition/Example
Adequate	*Definition* enough; sufficient *Example* A well balanced diet should contain ADEQUATE amounts of protein and vitamins. *Alternate Wording* A well balanced diet should contain sufficient amounts of protein and vitamins.	**At least**	*Definition* at a minimum of, the smallest amount acceptable. *Example* A patient receiving continous tube feedings should have the head of the bed elevated AT LEAST 30 degrees. *Alternate Wording* A patient receiving continuous tube feedings should have the head of the bed elevated at a minimum of 30 degrees.
Aggravate	*Definition* to make worse. *Example* Heat AGGRAVATES an itch. *Alternate Wording* Heat makes an itch worse	**Avoid**	*Definition* to abstain from a substance or activity; to keep at a distance. *Example* A patient with cardiac disease should AVOID salty foods. *Alternate Wording* A patient with cardiac disease should not eat any salty foods.
Allay anxiety	*Definition* to decrease worry, tension, or apprehension *Example* Telling a patient what to expect during a procedure helps to ALLAY ANXIETY. *Alternate Wording* Telling a patient what to expect during a procedure helps to decrease the patient's tension or apprehension.	**Competitive**	*Definition* Striving for the same thing or goal as another. A person who is competitive feels a need to succeed or to be better than others. (There does not always need to be a formal competition for a person who is competitive to want to be the best.) *Example* COMPETITIVE sports may be too stressful for a patient with cardiac disease. *Alternate Wording* Sports in which participants play to win may be too stressful for the patient with cardiac disease.
Anticipate	*Definition* to expect an event or symptoms; to foresee a patient problem *Example* The nurse ANTICIPATES the need for pain medication in the postoperative patient. *Alternate Wording* The nurse expects to administer pain medication to the post-operative patient.		
Assume responsi-bility	*Definition* to take on as one's duty. *Example* The nurses ASSUMED RESPONSIBILITY for the patient's discharge plan. *Alternate Wording* The nurse accepted as a duty the obligation to complete the patient's discharge plan.	**Compromise**	*Definition* (1) to adjust or settle a difference between parties by mutual concessions; (2) to endanger or put in jeopardy. *Example (1)* The physical therapist and occupational therapist COMPROMISED on the patient's schedule.

Word or Phrase	Definition/Example	Word or Phrase	Definition/Example
	Alternate Wording The physical therapist and occupational therapist both modified the patient's needs. *Example (2)* Heart disease may COMPROMISE respiratory function. *Alternate Wording* In the presence of heart disease, respiratory function may be less than optimal or may even be endangered.	**Determine**	*Definition* to find out exactly. *Example* The dietician should DETERMINE the patient's food preferences. *Alternate Wording* The dietician should find out what food the patient prefers.
Confer	*Definitions* (1) to give; (2) to advise. *Example (1)* The Hepatitis B vaccine CONFERS immunity to that disease. *Alternate Wording* The Hepatitis B vaccine gives immunity to that disease. *Example (2)* The doctor and nurse CONFER about a patient's progress. *Alternate Wording* The doctor and nurse advise each other about a patient's progress.	**Differentiate**	*Definitions* to distinguish; to discriminate; to mark or show the difference in. *Example* DIFFERENTIATE the symptoms of angina pectoris and a myocardial infarction. *Alternate Wording* Show how the symptoms of angina pectoris and a myocardial infraction differ from each other.
Conscience	*Definition* One's sense of what is right and wrong. *Example* The nurse follows her/his CONSCIENCE when she/he reports a medication error. *Alternate Wording* The nurse follows her/his sense of what is right and wrong when she/he reports a medication error.	**Energy requirements**	*Definition* that which is needed to act, or work, or have strength. *Example* A balanced diet provides the body with its ENERGY REQUIREMENTS. *Alternate Wording* A balanced diet provides the body with what it needs to have strength.
Conscious	*Definition* awake; aware *Example* The patient is CONSCIOUS. *Alternate Wording* The patient is awake.	**Enhance**	*Definition* to make greater; to increase in value, attractiveness, or effectiveness. *Example* A clearly stated message ENHANCES communication. *Alternate Wording* A clearly stated message makes communication more effective.
Deny	*Definition* to state that something is not true or does not exist. *Example* The person DENIES a history of heart disease in his family. *Alternate Wording* The patient states that there is no heart disease in his family.	**Exacerbate**	*Definition* to irritate; to annoy, to make more intense; to make worse. *Example* Spicy foods EXACERBATE the pain of a duodenal ulcer. *Alternate Wording* Spicy foods make the pain of a duodenal ulcer worse.
		Except	*Definition* excluding or omitting.

(continued)

Word or Phrase	Definition/Example

Example
(this is a common wording for
multiple choice test questions)
all of the following foods
contain protein EXCEPT
(1) meat (2) fish (3) celery
(4) eggs. (The correct answer
is (3) celery because that
does not contain protein.)

Alternate Wording
All of the following foods contain
protein if you exclude
(1) meat (2) fish
(3) celery (4) eggs.

Excessively

Definition
much more than normal or
desirable; a great deal.

Example
The patient bled EXCESSIVELY.

Alternate Wording
The patient bled a great deal.

Expectorate

Definition
to cough up and spit.

Example
The patient EXPECTORATED
thick mucus.

Alternate Wording
The patient coughed up and spit
thick mucus.

Flaccid

Definition
weak, ineffective, limp.

Example
Those who do not exercise have
FLACCID muscles.

Alternate Wording
Those who do not exercise have
weak, ineffective muscles.

Floor

Definition
the bottom surface of a room;
a level of a building.

Example
The surgery is finished and the
patient is back on the FLOOR.

Alternate Wording
The surgery is finished and the
patient is back on the unit.

Flushed

Definition
reddened; feeling warm or hot.

Example
The nurse checks the
temperature of the patient
who has a FLUSHED face.

Alternate Wording
The nurse checks the
temperature of the patient
whose face is reddened.

Word or Phrase	Definition/Example

Garter

Definition
a narrow elastic strap that
usually encircles the leg to
hold up a stocking; sometimes
a piece of elastic with a
fastener that is attached to a
girdle to hold up a stocking.

Example
Wearing tight GARTERS will
interfere with circulation.

Alternate Wording
Wearing tight elastic straps
around the legs to hold up
the stockings will interfere
with circulation.

Girdle

Definition
corset; a close fitting, usually
elastic undergarment that
encircles a part of the body.

Example
Very tight GIRDLES will
interfere with circulation.

Alternate Wording
Very tight undergarments or
corsets will interfere with
circulation.

Guarded

Definition
(1) in a precarious state of
health; (2) a term used when
a patient has taken an action
to protect from pain or
discomfort.

Example (1)
The patient's condition is
GUARDED.

Alternate Wording
The patient's condition is
precarious.

Example (2)
The patient GUARDED his wound
during the physical examination

Alternate Wording
The patient tensed the abdominal
muscles to avoid pain during
the physical examination.

Herb

Definition
a plant or plant part that is
valued for its medicinal,
savory, or aromatic qualities.

Example
Many people include herbs in
their diet to promote healing.

Alternate Wording
Many people include in their diet
plant substances believed to
have medicinal qualities.

Word or Phrase	Definition/Example	Word or Phrase	Definition/Example
Hoarseness	*Definition* harshness of sound or voice; an unpleasantly rough sound or voice. *Example* HOARSENESS may be an early sign of cancer of the larynx. *Alternate Wording* A rough sounding voice may be an early sign of cancer of the larynx.	**Lead to**	*Definition* to cause; to precede *Example* Heavy smoking may LEAD TO lung cancer. *Alternate Wording* Heavy smoking may cause lung cancer.
Impinge	*Definition* to strike, clash, hit against, or interfere with something. *Example* The mumbling of words IMPINGES upon effective communication. *Alternate Wording* The mumbling of words interferes with effective communication.	**Least likely**	*Definition* most probably not; in a series of choices, the one that is not likely to occur or be true. *Example* Among men over 40 years of age, those who exercise regularly and eat well balanced diets are LEAST LIKELY to develop heart disease. *Alternate Wording* Among men over 40 years of age, those who exercise regularly and eat well balanced diets will probably not develop heart disease.
Inept	*Definition* likely to fail; inadequate, out of place. *Example* The depressed man may feel INEPT as a father and provider. *Alternate Wording* The depressed man may feel inadequate as a father and provider.	**Liberally**	*Definition* in a large amount; abundantly. *Example* Patients on regular diets may use spices LIBERALLY. *Alternate Wording* Patients on regular diets may use spices in large amounts.
Insulation	*Definition* material used to shield from the transfer of electricity, heat, or sound. *Example* A house must have proper INSULATION if it is to stay warm in the winter. *Alternate Wording* A house must be shielded from the loss of heat to stay warm in the winter.	**Patent**	*Definition* open; unobstructed *Example* The nasogastric tube is PATENT. *Alternate Wording* The nasogastric tube is not obstructed.
Isolation	*Definition* the state of being separated or placed apart from other persons or things. *Example* The patient with chickenpox was placed in ISOLATION. *Alternate Wording* The patient with chickenpox was separated from other patients.	**Permit**	*Definition* to allow; to make possible. *Example* The doctor will PERMIT the patient with cardiac disease to ambulate when his condition remains stable. *Alternate Wording* The doctor will allow the patient with cardiac disease to ambulate when his condition remains stable.
		Potent	*Definition* strong; effective; powerful *Example* This is a POTENT antibiotic.

(continued)

Word or Phrase	Definition/Example	Word or Phrase	Definition/Example
	Alternate Wording This is a powerful antibiotic.		*Example* The child has the SNIFFLES.
Predispose	*Definition* to make susceptible; to create a tendency toward.		*Alternate Wording* The child has an upper respiratory infection.
	Example Smoking PREDISPOSES a person to lung cancer.	**Sparingly**	*Definition* infrequently; used very little.
	Alternate Wording Smoking makes a person more likely to develop lung cancer.		*Example* Patients on low cholesterol diets should eat eggs SPARINGLY.
Profusely	*Definition* freely and abundantly; a great deal.		*Alternate Wording* Patients on low cholesterol diets should eat eggs infrequently.
	Example The patient bled PROFUSELY.	**Spasm**	*Definition* an involuntary or abnormal contraction of a muscle or muscle fibers.
	Alternate Wording The patient bled a great deal.		*Example* Muscle SPASMS of the lower back can be very painful.
Red tape	*Definition* excessive group of regulations (often forms to be filled out), in order to get something done.		*Alternate Wording* Involuntary contractions of the muscles of the lower back can be very painful.
	Example The patient had to go through a lot of red tape in order to get his insurance company to pay his medical bills.	**Splint**	*Definition* to support or brace; to protect against pain by limiting motion.
	Alternate Wording The patient had an excessive number of forms to fill out in order to get the insurance company to pay his medical bills.		*Example* The nurse SPLINTS the incision of the patient following surgery while he coughs and deep breathes.
Refrain	*Definition* to hold back; to avoid.		*Alternate Wording* The nurse supports the incision with a pillow following surgery while the patient coughs and deep breathes.
	Example A person with poor circulation must REFRAIN from smoking.	**Support hose**	*Definition* elastic stockings
	Alternate Wording A person with poor circulation must avoid smoking.		*Example* People with varicose veins are encouraged to wear SUPPORT HOSE.
Sniffles	*Definition* an upper respiratory infection; breathing in through the nose so as to check or stop mucus from running out of the nose.		*Alternate Wording* People with varicose veins are encouraged to wear special elastic stockings.

Adapted from a document developed by M. Meehan and K. Tierney, St. Vincent's Hospital School of Nursing, New York, NY (unpublished).

AAAA	American Academy of Anesthesiologist's Assistants
AAAAI	American Academy of Allergy, Asthma, and Immunology
AAATP	Association for Anesthesiologist's Assistants Training Program
AAB	American Association of Bioanalysts
AABB	American Association of Blood Banks
AACA	American Association of Clinical Anatomists
AACAHPO	American Association of Certified Allied Health Personnel in Ophthalmology
AACC	American Association for Clinical Chemistry
AACCN	American Association of Critical Care Nurses
AACN	American Association of Colleges of Nursing
AADS	American Association of Dental Schools
AAFP	American Academy of Family Physicians
AAHA	American Academy of Health Administration
AAHC	Association of Academic Health Centers
AAHE	Association for the Advancement of Health Education
AAHP	American Association of Health Plans
AAHPER	American Association for Health, Physical Education, and Recreation
AAMA	American Association of Medical Assistants
AAMC	Association of American Medical Colleges
AAMI	Association for the Advancement of Medical Instrumentation
AAMT	American Association for Music Therapy
AAN	American Academy of Neurology
AAN	American Academy of Nursing
AANA	American Association of Nurse Anesthetists
AAO	American Association of Ophthalmology
AAO	American Association of Orthodontists
AAOHN	American Association of Occupational Health Nurses
AAP	American Academy of Pediatrics
AAPA	American Academy of Physicians Assistants
AAPMR	American Academy of Physical Medicine and Rehabilitation
AARC	American Association for Respiratory Care
AART	American Association for Rehabilitation Therapy
AATA	American Art Therapy Association
AATS	American Association for Thoracic Surgery
ABCP	American Board of Cardiovascular Perfusion
ABNF	Association of Black Nursing Faculty in Higher Education
ACAAI	American College of Asthma, Allergy and Immunology
ACC	American College of Cardiology
ACCP	American College of Chest Physicians
ACEN	Academy of Chief Executive Nurses (Canada)
ACEP	American College of Emergency Physicians
ACHA	American College of Hospital Administrators
ACNM	American College of Nurse-Midwives
ACP	American College of Physicians
ACR	American College of Radiology
ACS	American College of Surgeons
ACTA	American Cardiovascular Technologists Association
ACTA	American Corrective Therapy Association
ADA	American Dental Association
ADA	American Dietetic Association
ADAA	American Dental Assistants Association
ADHA	American Dental Hygienists' Association
ADTA	American Dance Therapy Association
AES	American Electroencephalographic Society
AHA	American Hospital Association
AHCPR	Agency for Health Care Policy and Research (now AHRQ)
AHPA	American Health Planning Association

(continued)

AHRQ	Agency for Healthcare Research and Quality
AIBS	American Institute of Biological Sciences
AIHA	American Industrial Hygiene Association
AIUM	American Institute of Ultrasound in Medicine
AMA	American Medical Association
AMEA	American Medical Electroencephalographic Association
AMI	Association of Medical Illustrators
AMIA	American Medical Informatics Association
AmSECT	American Society of Extra-Corporeal Technology
AMSN	Academy of Medical-Surgical Nurses
AMT	American Medical Technologists
ANA	American Nurses Association
ANCC	American Nurses Credentialing Center
ANF	American Nurses Foundation
ANHA	American Nursing Homes Association
ANNA	American Nephrology Nurses' Association
ANRC	American National Red Cross
AOA	American Optometric Association
AOA	American Osteopathic Association
AONE	American Organization of Nurse Executives
AORN	Association of Operating Room Nurses
AOTA	American Occupational Therapy Association
APA	American Podiatry Association
APA	American Psychiatric Association
APA	American Psychological Association
APAP	Association of Physician Assistants Programs
APHA	American Public Health Association
APIC	Association of Practitioners in Infection Control
APTA	American Physical Therapy Association
ARCA	American Rehabilitation Counseling Association
ARN	Association of Rehabilitation Nurses
ASA	American Society of Anesthesiologists
ASAHP	American Society of Allied Health Professionals
ASC	American Society of Cytotechnology
ASCP	American Society of Clinical Pathologists
ASE	American Society of Echocardiography
ASET	American Society of Electroencephalographic Technologists
ASHA	American Speech and Hearing Association
ASIA	American Spinal Injury Association
ASIM	American Society of Internal Medicine
ASM	American Society of Microbiology
ASMT	American Society for Medical Technology
ASNSA	American Society of Nursing Service Administrators
ASPAN	American Association of Post Anesthesia Nurses
ASPH	Association of Schools of Public Health
ASRT	American Society of Radiologic Technologists
AST	Association of Surgical Technologists
ASUTS	American Society of Ultrasound Technical Specialists
ATS	American Thoracic Society
AUPHA	Association of University Programs in Health Administration
AVA	American Vocational Association
AVMA	American Veterinary Medical Association
CAHEA(AMA)	Committee on Allied Health Education and Accreditation
CAP	College of American Pathologists
CCHFA	Canadian Council of Health Facilities Accreditation
CCHSE	Canadian Council of Health Service Executives
CCNE	Commission on Collegiate Nursing Education

CDC	Centers for Disease Control and Prevention
CGFNS	Commission on Graduates of Foreign Nursing Schools
CGNA	Canadian Gerontological Nursing Association
CME (AMA)	Council on Medical Education of the American Medical Association
CNA	Canadian Nurses Association
COEAMRA	Council on Education of the American Medical Record Association
DHHS	Department of Health and Human Services
ENA	Emergency Nurses Association
FDA	Food and Drug Administration
HCFA	Health Care Financing Administration
HRA	Health Resources Administration
HSCA	Health Sciences Communications Association
HSRA	Health Services and Resources Administration
IAET	International Association for Enterostomal Therapy
IOM	Institute of Medicine of the National Academy of Sciences
ISCV	International Society for Cardiovascular surgery
JCAHO	Joint Commission on the Accreditation of Healthcare Organizations
JCAHPO	Joint Commission on Allied Health Personnel in Ophthalmology
MLA	Medical Library Association
NAACLS	National Accrediting Agency for Clinical Laboratory Science
NAACOG	Nurses Association of the American Association of Obstetrics and Gynecology
NACA	National Advisory Council on Aging-Canadian
NACCHO	National Association of County and City Health Officials
NACT	National Alliance of Cardiovascular Technologists
NADONA/LTC	National Association of Directors of Nursing Administration in Long Term Care
NAEMT	National Association of Emergency Medical Technicians
NAHC	National Association of Home Care
NAHSR	National Association of Human Services Technologists
NAMT	National Association for Music Therapy
NANDA	North American Nursing Diagnosis Association
NANT	National Association of Nephrology Technologists
NAPNES	National Association for Practical Nurse Education and Services
NARF	National Association of Rehabilitation Facilities
NASMD	National Association of State Medical Directors
NASW	National Association of Social Workers
NATTS	National Association of Trade and Technical Schools
NBNA	National Black Nurses Association
NCEHPHP	National Council on the Education of Health Professionals in Health Promotion
NCHS	National Center for Health Statistics
NCRE	National Council on Rehabilitation Education
NEHA	National Environmental Health Education
NFLPN	National Federation of Licensed Practical Nurses
NHC	National Health Council
NHSC	National Health Services Corps
NIH	National Institutes of Health
NIOSH	National Institute of Occupational Safety and Health
NKF	National Kidney Foundation
NLN	National League for Nursing
NNBA	National Nurses in Business Association
NOLF	Nursing Organization Liaison Forum
NONPF	National Organization of Nurse Practitioner Faculties
NPWH	National Association of Nurse Practitioners in Women's Health
NRCA	National Rehabilitation Counseling Association
NREMT	National Registry of Emergency Medical Technicians
NSCPT	National Society for Cardiopulmonary Technology
NSH	National Society for Histotechnology
NSNA	National Student Nurses Association

(continued)

NTRS	National Therapeutic Recreation Society
NTSAD	National Tay-Sachs and Allied Diseases Association
OAA	Opticians Association of America
ONS	Oncology Nurses Association
PNAA	Philippine Nurses Association of America
RWJF	The Robert Wood Johnson Foundation
SAAABB	Subcommittee on Accreditation of the American Association of Blood Banks
SDMS	Society of Diagnostic Medical Sonographers
SNIVT	Society of Non-invasive Vascular Technology
SNM	Society of Nuclear Medicine
SNM-TS	Society of Nuclear Medicine-Technologists Section
SOPHE	Society for Public Health Education
STS	Society of Thoracic Surgeons
STTI	Sigma Theta Tau International
SVS	Society for Vascular Surgery
TAANA	The American Association of Nurse Attorneys
USPHS	United States Public Health Service
VA	Veterans Affairs
WHO	World Health Organization

8-7. PROFESSIONAL DESIGNATIONS FOR HEALTH CARE PROVIDERS

Degrees, certifications, memberships and other initials that precede or follow the names of health care providers often provide helpful information regarding their area of expertise and level of practice. The following list identifies commonly used designations in English-speaking countries.

AN	Associate Nurse
ANP	Adult Nurse Practitioner
APRN, BC	Advanced Practice Registered Nurse, Board Certified
ARNP	Advanced Registered Nurse Practitioner
ARRT	American Registry of Radiologic Technologists
ART	Accredited Record Technician
ASCW	Academy of Certified Social Workers
BA	Bachelor of Arts
BB(ASCP)	Technologist in Blood Banking certified by The American Society of Clinical Pathologists
BDentSci	Bachelor of Dental Science
BDS	Bachelor of Dental Surgery
BDSc	Bachelor of Dental Science
BHS	Bachelor of Health Science
BHyg	Bachelor of Hygiene
BM	Bachelor of Medicine
BMed	Bachelor of Medicine
BMedBiol	Bachelor of Medical Biology
BMedSci	Bachelor of Medical Science
BMic	Bachelor of Microbiology
BMS	Bachelor of Medical Science
BMT	Bachelor of Medical Technology
BO	Bachelor of Osteopathy
BP	Bachelor of Pharmacy
BHP	Bachelor of Public Health
BPharm	Bachelor of Pharmacy
BPHEng	Bachelor of Public Health Engineering
BPHN	Bachelor of Public Health Nursing
BPsTh	Bachelor of Psychotherapy
BS	Bachelor of Science

BSM	Bachelor of Science in Medicine
BSN	Bachelor of Science in Nursing
BSPh	Bachelor of Science in Pharmacy
BSS	Bachelor of Sanitary Science
BVMS	Bachelor of Veterinary Medicine and Science
BVSc	Bachelor of Veterinary Science
CAC	Certified Alcohol Counselor
CALN	Clinical Administrative Liaison Nurse
CANP	Certified Adult Nurse Practitioner
C(ASCP)	Technologist in Chemistry certified by the American Society of Clinical Pathologists
CB	Bachelor of Surgery
CCRN	Critical Care Registered Nurse
CCT	Certified Cardiographic Technician
CDA	Certified Dental Assistant
CDC	Certified Drug Counselor
CEN	Certificate for Emergency Nursing
CEO	Chief Executive Officer
CFNP	Certified Family Nurse Practitioner
ChB	Bachelor of Surgery
ChD	Doctor of Surgery
CHES	Certified Health Education Specialist
ChM	Master of Surgery
CIC	Certified in Infection Control
CIH	Certificate in Industrial Health
CLA	Certified Laboratory Assistant
CLS	Clinical Laboratory Scientist
CLS(NCA)	Clinical Laboratory Scientist certified by the National Certification Agency for Medical Laboratory Personnel
CLT	Certified Laboratory Technician; Clinical Laboratory Technician
CLT(NCA)	Laboratory Technician certified by the National Certification Agency For Medical Laboratory Personnel
CM	Master of Surgery
CMA	Certified Medical Assistant
CMO	Chief Medical Officer
CMT	Chief Medical Transcriptionist
CNA	Certified Nursing Assistant
CNM	Certified Nurse-Midwife
CNMT	Certified Nuclear Medicine Technologist
CNOR	Certified Nurse, Operating Room
CNP	Community Nurse Practitioner
CNS	Clinical Nurse Specialist
CORN	Certified Operating Room Nurse
CORT	Certified Operating Room Technician
COTA	Certified Occupational Therapy Assistant
CPAN	Certified Post Anesthesia Nurse
CPH	Certified in Public Health
CPNP	Certified Pediatric Nurse Practitioner
CPTA	Certified Physical Therapy Assistant
CRNA	Certified Registered Nurse Anesthetist
CRNP	Certified Registered Nurse Practitioner
CRRN	Certified Registered Rehabilitation Nurse
CRRT	Certified Registered Respiratory Therapist
CRTT	Certified Respiratory Therapy Technician
CSN	Certified School Nurse
CT(ASCP)	Cytotechnologist certified by the American Society of Clinical Pathologists
CURN	Certified Urological Registered Nurse
CVO	Chief Veterinary Officer
DA	Dental Assistant; Diploma in Anesthetics

(continued)

DC	Doctor of Chiropractic
DCH	Diploma in Child Health
DCh	Doctor of Surgery
DChO	Doctor of Ophthalmic Surgery
DCM	Doctor of Comparative Medicine
DCOG	Diploma of the College of Obstetricians and Gynaecologists
DCP	Diploma in Clinical Pathology; Diploma in Clinical Psychology
DDH	Diploma in Dental Health
DDM	Doctor of Dental Medicine; Diploma in Dermatologic Medicine
DDO	Diploma in Dental Orthopaedics
DDR	Diploma in Dental Radiology
DDS	Doctor of Dental Surgery
DDSc	Doctor of Dental Science
DFHom	Diploma in the Faculty of Homeopathy
DHg	Doctor of Hygiene
DHy	Doctor of Hygiene
DHyg	Doctor of Hygiene
Dip	Diplomate
DipBact	Diploma in Bacteriology
DipChern	Diploma in Chemistry
DipClinPath	Diploma in Clinical Pathology
DipMicrobiol	Diploma in Microbiology
DipSocMed	Diploma in Social Medicine
DLM(ASCP)	Diplomate in Laboratory Management
DMD	Doctor of Dental Medicine
DMT	Doctor of Medical Technology
DMV	Doctor of Veterinary Medicine
DN	Doctor of Nursing
DNE	Doctor of Nursing Education
DNS	Doctor of Nursing Science
DNSc	Doctor of Nursing Science
DO	Doctor of Ophthalmology; Doctor of Optometry; Doctor of Osteopathy
DON	Doctor of Nursing
DOS	Doctor of Ocular Science; Doctor of Optical Science
DP	Doctor of Pharmacy; Doctor of Podiatry
DHP	Doctor of Public Health; Doctor of Public Hygiene
DPhC	Doctor of Pharmaceutical Chemistry
DPHN	Doctor of Public Health Nursing
DPhys	Diploma in Physiotherapy
DPM	Doctor of Physical Medicine; Doctor of Podiatric Medicine; Doctor of Preventive Medicine; Doctor of Psychiatric Medicine
Dr	Doctor
DrHyg	Doctor of Hygiene
DrMed	Doctor of Medicine
DrPH	Doctor of Public Health; Doctor of Public Hygiene
DSc	Doctor of Science
DSE	Doctor of Sanitary Engineering
DSIM	Doctor of Science in Industrial Medicine
DSSc	Diploma in Sanitary Science
DVM	Doctor of Veterinary Medicine
DVMS	Doctor of Veterinary Medicine and Surgery
DVR	Doctor of Veterinary Radiology
DVS	Doctor of Veterinary Science; Doctor of Veterinary Medicine
DVSc	Doctor of Veterinary Science
EdD	Doctor of Education
EMT	Emergency Medical Technician
EMT-P	Emergency Medical Technician –Paramedic
ET	Enterostornal Therapist

FAAN	Fellow of the American Academy of Nurses
FACA	Fellow of the American College of Anesthetists; Fellow of the American College of Angiology; Fellow of the American College of Apothecaries
FACAI	Fellow of the American College of Allergists
FACC	Fellow of the American College of Cardiologists
FACCP	Fellow of the American College of Chest Physicians
FACD	Fellow of the American College of Dentists
FACFP	Fellow of the American College of family Physicians
FACG	Fellow of the American College of Gastroenterology
FACHA	Fellow of the American College of Health Administrators
FACOG	Fellow of the American College of Obstetricians and Gynecologists
FACP	Fellow of the American College of Physicians
FACPM	Fellow of the American College of Preventive Medicine
FACS	Fellow of the American College of Surgeons
FACSM	Fellow of the American College of Sports Medicine
FAMA	Fellow of the American Medical Association
FAOTA	Fellow of the American Occupational Therapy Association
FAPA	Fellow of the American Psychiatric Association
FAPHA	Fellow of the American Public Health Association
FBPsS	Fellow of the British Psychological Society
FCAP	Fellow of the College of American Pathologists
FCMS	Fellow of the College of Medicine and Surgery
FCO	Fellow of the College of Osteopathy
FCPS	Fellow of the College of Physicians and Surgeons
FCSP	Fellow of the Chartered Society of Physiotherapy
FCST	Fellow of the College of Speech Therapists
FDS	Fellow in Dental Surgery
FDSRCSEng	Fellow in Dental Surgery of the Royal College of Surgeons of England
FFA	Fellow of the Faculty of Anesthetists
FFCM	Fellow of the Faculty of Community Medicine
FFD	Fellow of the Faculty of Dentistry
FFOM	Fellow of the Faculty of Occupational Medicine
FFR	Fellow of the Faculty of Radiologists
FIB	Fellow in the Institute of Biology
FICD	Fellow of the Institute of Canadian Dentists; Fellow of the International College of Dentists
FIMLT	Fellow of Institute of Medical Laboratory Technology
FNP	Family Nurse Practitioner
FPS	Fellow of the Pathological Society
FRCD	Fellow of the Royal College of Dentists
FRCGP	Fellow of the Royal College of General Practitioners
FRCOG	Fellow of the Royal College of Obstetricians and Gynaecologists
FRCP	Fellow of the Royal College of Physicians
FRCPath	Fellow of the Royal College of Pathologists
FRCP (C)	Fellow of the Royal College of Physicians of Canada
FRCS	Fellow of the Royal College of Surgeons
FRCS (C)	Fellow of the Royal College of Surgeons of Canada
GNP	Gerontological Nurse Practitioner
H(ASCP)	Technologist in Hematology certified by the American Society of Clinical Pathologists
HT(ASCP)	Histologic Technician certified by the American Society of Clinical Pathologists
HTL(ASCP)	Histotechnologist certified by the American Society of Clinical Pathologists
I(ASCP)	Technologist in Immunology certified by the American Society of Clinical Pathologists
LCSW	Licensed Clinical Social Worker
LMCC	Licentiate of the Medical Council of Canada
LMRCP	Licentiate in Midwifery of the Royal College of Physicians
LOT	Licensed Occupational Therapist
LPN	Licensed Practical Nurse
LPT	Licensed Physical Therapist
LVN	Licensed Vocational Nurse

(continued)

MA	Master of Arts
M(ASCP)	Technologist in Microbiology certified by the American Society of Clinical Pathologists
MB	Bachelor of Medicine
MC	Master of Surgery
MCIS	Master of Computer and Information Science; Master of Computer Information Systems
MCPS	Member of the College of Physicians and Surgeons
MD	Doctor of Medicine
MDentSc	Master of Dental Science
MDS	Master of Dental Surgery
MHC	Mental Health Counselor
MLT	Medical Laboratory Technician
MLT(ASCP)	Medical Laboratory Technician certified by the American Society of Clinical Pathologists
MMS	Master of Medical Science
MMSA	Master of Midwifery
MPH	Master of Public Health
MPharm	Master of Pharmacy
MRad	Master of Radiology
MRL	Medical Records Librarian
MS	Master of Science; Master of Surgery
MSB	Master of Science in Bacteriology
MSc	Master of Science
MScD	Master of Dental Science
MScN	Master of Science in Nursing
MSN	Master of Science in Nursing
MSPH	Master of Science in Public Health
MSPhar	Master of Science in Pharmacy
MSSc	Master of Sanitary Science
MSW	Master of Social Work; Medical Social Worker
MT	Medical Technologist
MT(ASCP)	Medical Technologist certified by the American Society of Clinical Pathologists
MVD	Doctor of Veterinary Medicine
NA	Nurses Aide
ND	Doctor of Nursing
NHA	Nursing Home Administrator
NM(ASCP)	Technologist in Nuclear Medicine certified by the American Society of Clinical Pathologists
NMT	Nuclear Medicine Technologist
NNP	Neonatal Nurse Practitioner
NP	Nurse Practitioner
OD	Doctor of Optometry
ONC	Orthopedic Nursing Certificate
ORT	Operating Room Technician
OT	Occupational Therapist
OTL	Occupational Therapist, Licensed
OTR	Occupational Therapist, Registered
OTReg	Occupational Therapist, Registered
PA	Physician's Assistant
PA-C	Physician Assistant - Certified
PBT(ASCP)	Phlebotomy Technician certified by the American Society of Clinical Pathologists
PCP	Primary Care Physician
PD	Doctor of Pharmacy
PharmD	Doctor of Pharmacy
PhD	Doctor of Philosophy; Doctor of Pharmacy
PHN	Public Health Nurse
PNP	Pediatric Nurse Practitioner
PT	Physical Therapist
PTA	Physical Therapy Assistant
RDA	Registered Dental Assistant
RDMS	Registered Diagnostic Medical Sonographer

REEGT	Registered Electroencephalogram Technologist
Reg	Registered
RMA	Registered Medical Assistant
RN	Registered Nurse
RNA	Registered Nurse Anesthetist
RN, BC	Registered Nurse, Board Certified
RN, C	Registered Nurse, Certified
RN, CNA	Registered Nurse, Certified in Nursing Administration
RN, CNAA	Registered Nurse, Certified in Nursing Administration, Advanced
RN, CNA, BC	Registered Nurse, Certified in Nursing Administration, Board Certified
RN, CS	Registered Nurse, Certified Specialist
RPh	Registered Pharmacist
RPT	Registered Physical Therapist
RPTA	Registered Physical Therapist Assistant
RRA	Registered Record Administrator
RRL	Registered Record Librarian
RRT	Registered Respiratory Therapist
RT	Radiologic Technologist; Respiratory Therapist
RT(N)	Nuclear Medicine Technologist
RT(R)	Technologist in Diagnostic Radiology
RTR	Registered Recreational Therapist
RT(T)	Radiation Therapy Technologist
SBB(ASCP)	Specialist in Blood Banking certified by the American Society of Clinical Pathologists
ScD	Doctor of Science
SCT(ASCP)	Specialist in Cytotechnology certified by the American Society of Clinical Pathologists
SLP	Speech and Language Pathologist
SNP	School Nurse Practitioner
ST	Speech Therapist; Surgical Technologist
SW	Social Worker

A

a	before
AA	Alcoholics Anonymous
aa	of each
AAROM	active assistive range of motion
abd.	abdomen
ABG	arterial blood gases
AC	alternating current; air conduction
a.c.	before meals
ACE	angiotensin-converting enzyme
ACh	acetylcholine
ACTH	adrenocorticotropic hormone
AD	right ear
ADA	American Diabetes Association; American Dental Association; Americans with Disabilities Act
ADH	antidiuretic hormone
ADL	activities of daily living
ad lib	as desired
a-fib	atrial fibrillation
A/G	albumin-globulin ratio
AHA	American Heart Association
AHF	antihemophilic factor
AIDS	acquired immunodeficiency syndrome
AK	above the knee
ALARA	as low as reasonably achievable (radiology)
ALL	acute lymphocytic leukemia
ALS	amyotrophic lateral sclerosis
AM	morning
AMA	against medical advice; American Medical Association
AMD	age-related macular degeneration
AMI	acute myocardial infarction
amp.	ampere
ant.	anterior
ANUG	acute necrotizing ulcerative gingivitis
AODM	adult-onset diabetes mellitus
AP	antepartum; anteroposterior
A & P	auscultation and percussion
A-P	anterior-posterior
APA	American Psychological Association
appt.	appointment
APR-DRGs	all patient-defined diagnosis-related groups
A/R	apical/radial
ARC	AIDS related complex
ARD	acute respiratory disease
ARF	acute renal failure
AROM	active range of motion; artificial rupture of membrane
ARROM	active resistive range of motion
AS	left ear
ASA	acetylsalicylic acid (aspirin)
ASAP	as soon as possible
ASCVD	anteriosclerotic cardiovascular disease
ASD	atrial septal defect
ASHD	arteriosclerotic heart disease
ASS	anterior superior spine
AST	aspartamine aminotransferase
Ast	astigmatism
AU	both ears; Angstrom unit
AV	artrioventricular; arteriovenous
av.	avoirdupois
A & W	alive and well
AWS	air water spray

B

Ba	barium
BAC	buccoaxiocervical
BBA	Balanced Budget Act of 1997, Public Law 105–33
BBB	blood-brain barrier
BBRA	Medicare, Medicaid and SCHIP Balanced Budget Refinement Act of 1999, Public Law 106–113
BC/BS	Blue Cross/Blue Shield
BCP	birth control pill
BE	barium enema
BF	black female
b.i.d.	two times a day
BIPA	Medicare, Medicaid, and SCHIP Benefits Improvement and Protection Act of 2000, Public Law 106–554
BK	below the knee
BLE	bilateral lower extremity
BM	black male
bm	bowel movement
BMR	basal metabolic rate
BP	blood pressure
BPH	benign prostatic hypertrophy
BR	bathroom
BRP	bathroom privileges
BSA	body surface area
BSE	breast self-examination
BSP	Bromsulphalein
BUE	bilateral upper extremity
BUN	blood urea nitrogen
BVR	Bureau of Vocational Rehabilitation
BW	birth weight
bx	biopsy

C

C	centigrade
c	with
C(x)	C followed by a number indicates a specific cervical vertebra
CA	cancer; chronological age; cervicoaxillary
Ca	Calcium, cancer
CABG	coronary artery bypass graft
CABS	coronary artery bypass surgery
CAD	coronary artery disease
cap.	capsule

Most hospitals, community health agencies, and other clinical facilities have a list of approved abbreviations to be used in patient records. The abbreviations in this Appendix are often used when charting and will assist in the interpretation of patient records, but they should not be utilized on the record unless they are on the approved list for the clinical site.

CAT	computerized axial tomography	DOA	dead on arrival; date of admission
CBC	complete blood count	DOB	date of birth
CC	chief complaint	DOE	dyspnea on exertion
cc	cubic centimeter	DPT	diphtheria, pertussis, tetanus
CCU	Coronary Care Unit	dr.	dram
CEJ	cementoenamel junction	DRGs	diagnosis-related groups
CF	cystic fibrosis	dsg.	dressing
CFIDS	chronic fatigue immune deficiency syndrome	DTR	deep tendon reflex
		DTs	delirium tremens
CFT	complement fixation test	DVT	deep vein thrombosis
CH	crown-heel measurement	Dx	diagnosis
CHD	coronary heart disease		
CHF	congestive heart failure	**E**	
CHO	carbohydrate		
cm	centimeter	ECF	extended care facility
CMGs	case-mix groups	ECG	electrocardiogram
CMI	case-mix index	ECR	emergency chemical restraint
CML	chronic myelogenous leukemia	ECT	electroconvulsive therapy
CMS	Centers for Medicare and Medicaid Services	ED	effective dose; erythema dose
		EDC	estimated date of confinement
CMV	cytomegalovirus	EDD	estimated date of delivery
CNS	central nervous system	EEG	electroencephalogram
CO_2	carbon dioxide	EENT	eyes, ears, nose, and throat
C/O	complains of	EKG	electrocardiogram
col. ct.	colony count	EMG	electromyogram
comp.	compound	EMS	emergency medical services
conc.	concentrated	ENT	ears, nose, and throat
COPD	chronic obstructive pulmonary disease	EOM	extraocular movement
		ER	emergency room
CP	cerebral palsy	ERG	electroretinogram
CPD	cephalopelvic disproportion	ESR	erythrocyte sedimentation rate
CPK	creatine phosphokinase	EST	electroshock therapy
CPR	cardiopulmonary resuscitation	ETOH	ethanol (ethyl alcohol)
CR	crown-rump length		
CS	cesarean section	**F**	
C & S	culture and sensitivity		
CSF	cerebrospinal fluid	F	Fahrenheit
CT	computed tomography	FANA	fluorescent antinuclear antibody test
CTS	carpal tunnel syndrome	FBS	fasting blood sugar
CV	cardiovascular	FD	fatal dose; focal distance
CVA	cerebral vascular accident	FDA	Food and Drug Administration
CVD	cerebrovascular disease; cardiovascular disease	Fe	iron
		FEV	forced expiratory volume
CVP	central venous pressure	FFA	free fatty acids
		FH	family history
D		FHR	fetal heart rate
		FI	fluid
DC	direct current	fld	fluid
d.c.	discontinue	FM	fine motor
D & C	dilatation and currettage	FSH	follicle stimulating hormone
D & E	dilation and evacuation	ft	foot
dg	decigram	FTND	full term normal delivery
DIC	disseminated intravascular coagulation	FUO	fever of unknown origin
		FWB	full weight bearing
dil.	dilute	Fx	fracture
DJD	degenerative joint disease		
DKA	diabetic ketoacidosis	**G**	
dl	deciliter		
DM	diabetes mellitus	G	gravida
DNA	deoxyribonucleic acid	GA	gingivoaxial

(continued)

gal.	gallon
GB	gallbladder
GBS	gallbladder series
GC	gonococcus; gonorrhea
GFR	glomerular filtration rate
GG	gamma globulin
GI	gastrointestinal
GLA	gingivolinguoaxial
GM	gross motor
gm	gram
GP	general practitioner
gr.	grain
GSW	gunshot wound
GTT	glucose tolerance test
gtt.	drops
GU	genitourinary
GVHD	graft versus host disease
gyn	gynecology

H

Hb	hemoglobin
HBP	high blood pressure
HCG	human chorionic gonadotropin
HCRIS	Hospital Cost Report Information System
hct.	hematocrit
HCTZ	hydrochlorothiazide
HD	hearing distance
HDL	high-density lipoprotein
HEENT	head, eye, ear, nose, and throat
Hg	mercury
Hgb	hemoglobin
H & H	hemoglobin and hematocrit
HHA	home health aide, home health agency
HHNK	hyperglycemic, hyperosmolar nonketotic coma
HIPAA	Health Insurance Portability and Accountability Act, Public Law 104–191
HIV	human immunodeficiency virus
H_2O	water
H_2O_2	hydrogen peroxide
H & P	history and physical
HPI	history of present illness
HPV	high-power view
hs	hour of sleep
H-S	hepato-spleno
HSV	herpes simplex virus
HT	hypertension
Ht	total hyperopia
HTN	hypertension
HVD	hypertensive vascular disease
Hx	history
Hy	hyperopia
hyp.	hypodermic

I

I	Iodine
IA	intra-arterial
IB	inclusion body
IBD	ideal body weight
ICP	intracranial pressure
ICS	intercostal space
ICU	Intensive Care Unit
I & D	incision and drainage
IDDM	insulin dependent diabetes mellitus
IM	intramuscular
inf.	infusion
inj.	injection
I & O	intake and output
IOP	intraocular pressure
IPPB	intermittent positive pressure breathing
IQ	intelligence quotient
IRF	inpatient rehabilitation facility
ITP	idiopathic thrombocytopenic purpose
IU	international unit
IUD	intrauterine device
IV	intravenous
IVP	intravenous pyelogram
IVU	intravenous urogram

J

jt.	joint

K

K	potassium
KCl	potassium chloride
kg	kilogram
KOH	potassium hydroxide
KUB	kidney, ureters, and bladder
kv	kilovolt
KVO	keep vein open
kw	kilowatt

L

L	left, liter
L(x)	L followed by a number indicates a specific lumbar vertebra
l	liter
L & A	light and accommodation
lat.	lateral
lb	pound
LBP	low back pain
LCM	left costal margin
LD	lethal dose; light difference
LDL	low density lipoprotein
LE	lupus erythematosus; lower extremity
LGA	large for gestational age
LH	luteinizing hormone

LIF	left iliac fossa		**MW**	molecular weight
lig.	ligament		**My**	myopia
Liq.	liquid		**N**	
LLE	left lower extremity			
LLL	left lower lobe		**Na**	sodium
LLQ	left lower quadrant		**N/A**	not applicable
LMP	last menstrual period		**NaCl**	sodium chloride
LOA	left occipitoposterior		**NAD**	no acute distress; no appreciable
LOT	left occipitotransverse			disease
LP	lumbar puncture		**NAS**	no added salt
LPV	low-power view		**NB**	newborn
LTC-DRG	long-term care diagnosis-related		**neg.**	negative
	group		**NG**	nasogastric
LTCH	long-term care hospital		**NIDDM**	non-insulin dependent diabetes
LUE	left upper extremity			mellitus
LUL	left upper lobe		**NIH**	National Institutes of Health
LUQ	left upper quadrant		**NKA**	no known allergies
LVH	left ventricular hypertrophy		**NMR**	nuclear magnetic resonance
L & W	living and well		**NPO**	nothing by mouth
			NSAID	nonsteroidal anti-inflammatory drug
M			**NSR**	normal sinus rhythm
			NSS	normal saline solution
m	meter		**NSVD**	normal spontaneous vaginal delivery
MAP	mean arterial pressure		**N & V**	nausea and vomiting
MBD	minimal brain dysfunction		**NWB**	non-weight bearing
mc	millicurie		**NYD**	not yet diagnosed
mcg	microgram		**O**	
MCH	mean corpuscular hemoglobin			
MCHC	mean corpuscular hemoglobin		O_2	oxygen
	concentration		**OA**	osteoarthritis; occipitoanterior
mCi	millicurie		**OB**	obstetrics
MCL	mid-clavicular line		**OBS**	organic brain syndrome
MCV	mean corpuscular volume		**OC**	oral contraceptive
MD	muscular dystrophy; medical doctor		**OD**	right eye
MDCN	Medicare Data Collection Network		**od**	daily
MED	minimal effective dose; minimal		**O/F**	oxidation fermentation
	erythema dose		**OL**	left eye
MedPAC	Medicare Payment Advisory		**OOB**	out of bed
	Commission		**OP**	occipitoposterior
MedPAR	Medicare provider analysis and review		**OPD**	outpatient department
mEq	milliequivalents		**OPV**	oral polio vaccine
mEq/L	milliequivalents per liter		**OR**	operating room
Mg	magnesium		**ORIF**	open reduction internal fixation
mg	milligram		**OS**	left eye
MH	mental health; marital history		**OSHA**	Occupational Safety and Health
MI	myocardial infarction			Administration
min	minim; minute		**OT**	occupational therapy
ml	milliliter		**OTC**	over the counter
mM	millimole		**OU**	both eyes
MMT	manual muscle test		**oz**	ounce
mol. wt.	molecular weight		**P**	
MOM	milk of magnesia			
MOPP	Mustargen, Oncovin, procarbazine,		**P**	pulse
	prednisone		**p**	after
MPV	medium-power view		**PA**	pernicious anemia; posterior-anterior
MRI	magnetic reasonance imaging		**P & A**	percussion and auscultation
MS	mitral stenosis; multiple sclerosis		**PAC**	premature atrial contractions
MSL	mid-sternal line		**PAP**	Papanicolaou (test)
MVR	mitral valve replacement			

(continued)

para	number of pregnancies	q.s.	quantity sufficient
PBI	protein-bound iodine	qt.	quart
p.c.	after meals		
pct.	per cent	**R**	
PCV	packed cell volume	RA	rheumatoid arthritis
PD	pupillary distance	rad	radiation absorbed dose
PDA	patent ductus arteriosus	RAI	radioactive iodine
PDR	*Physicians' Desk Reference*	RAIU	radioactive iodine uptake
PE	physical examination	RBC	red blood count
P.E.	physical examination; pulmonary emboli	RDA	recommended daily allowance
		RDS	respiratory distress syndrome
PEG	percutaneous esophagogastrectomy; pneumoencephalogram	Rh	Rhesus factor
		RHD	rheumatic heart disease
PERLA	pupils equal, react to light and accommodation	RLE	right lower extremity
		RLL	right lower lobe
PERRLA	pupils equal, round, react to light and accommodation	RLQ	right lower quadrant
		RML	right middle lobe
PET	positron emission tomography	r/o	rule out
PH	past history	ROA	right occipitoanterior
PI	present illness	ROM	range of motion
PID	pelvic inflammatory disease	ROP	right occipitoposterior
PIH	pregnancy-induced hypertension	ROS	review of symptoms
PKU	phenylketonuria	ROT	right occipitotransverse
PM	afternoon; evening; post mortem	RPM; rpm	revolutions per minute
P.M.	perceptual motor	RPRC	rapid plasma reagin card test (for syphilis)
PMH	past medical history		
PMI	point of maximal impulse	RR	respiratory rate
PMP	previous menstrual period	R/T	related to
PMS	premenstrual syndrome	rt.	right
PND	paroxysmal nocturnal dyspnea	RUE	right upper extremity
p.o.	by mouth	RUL	right upper lobe
P.O.R.	problem-oriented record	RUQ	right upper quadrant
pp	postpartum; postprandial	Rx	treatment, therapy, prescription
PPD	purified protein derivative (tuberculin)		
ppm	parts per million	**S**	
pr	per rectum		
PRE	progressive resistive exercise	s	without
prn	as needed	sc.	subcutaneous
PROM	passive range of motion	SCHIP	State Children's Health Insurance Program
ProPAC	Prospective Payment Assessment Commission		
		SGA	small for gestational age
Protime	Prothrombin time	SGOT	serum glutamic-oxaloacetic transaminase
PSS	physiologic saline solution		
pt	patient; pint	SGPT	serum glutamic pyruvate transaminase
PT	prothrombin time; physical therapy		
PTA	prior to admission; plasma thromboplastin antecedent	SH	social history; serum hepatitis
		sib.	sibling
PTT	partial thromboplastin time	SID	sudden infant death syndrome
PVC	premature ventricular contraction	SIDS	sudden infant death syndrome
PVD	peripheral vascular disease	sig.	label
PWB	partial weight bearing	sl	sublingual
		SLE	systemic lupus erythematosus
Q		SNF	skilled nursing facility
		S.O.A.P.	subjective, objective, assessment, plan
q	every		
q.d.	every day	SOB	shortness of breath
qh	every hour	s/p	status post
q.n.s.	quantity not sufficient	SPF	sun protection factor
q.o.d.	every other day	sp.gr.	specific gravity

spt.	spirit		**UE**	upper extremity
ss	one half		**UHF**	ultrahigh frequency
SSE	soap suds enema		**ung.**	ointment
SSS	sick sinus syndrome		**UQ**	upper quadrant
S & Sx	signs and symptoms		**URI**	upper respiratory infection
stat	immediately		**USP**	United States Pharmacopeia
STD	sexually transmitted disease		**UTI**	urinary tract infection
STS	serologic test for syphilis		**UV**	ultraviolet
sub. q.	subcutaneous			
SUID	sudden unexplained infant death		**V**	
SVD	spontaneous vaginal delivery		**v**	volt
SVT	supraventricular tachycardia		**VA**	Veterans Administration; visual acuity
Sx	symptoms		**VC**	vital capacity
sym.	symmetrical		**VD**	venereal disease
syr.	syrup		**VDA**	visual discriminatory acuity
			Vfib	ventricular fibrillation
T			**VHD**	valvular heart disease
T.	tablespoon; temperature		**VLDL**	very-low-density lipoprotein
T(x)	T followed by a number indicates a specific thoracic vertebra		**V.O.**	verbal order
			v.s.	vital signs
T & A	tonsillectomy and adenoidectomy		**VSD**	ventricular septal defect
tab.	tablet		**VT**	ventricular tachycardia
TAH	total abdominal hysterectomy			
TAH-BSO	total abdominal hysterectomy– bilateral salpingo-oophorectomy		**W**	
TAT	tetanus antitoxin		**w**	watt
TB	tuberculosis		**WBAT**	weight bearing as tolerated
tbsp.	tablespoon		**WBC**	white blood count
TEFRA	Tax Equity and Fiscal Responsibility Act of 1982, Public Law 97-248		**w.b.c.**	white blood count
			w/c	wheelchair
TIA	transient ischemic attack		**WD**	well-developed
t.i.d.	three times a day		**WDWN**	well-developed, well-nourished
TNTC	too numerous to count		**WF**	white female
T.O.	telephone order		**wk.**	week
TPN	total parenteral nutrition		**WL**	wavelength
TPR	temperature, pulse, respiration		**WM**	white male
tr.	trace; tincture		**WN**	well-nourished
tinct	tincture		**WNL**	within normal limits
tsp.	teaspoon		**wo**	without
TUR	transurethral resection		**wt.**	weight
TURP	transurethral resection of the prostate			
			X	
U			**x**	times
U	unit		**x-ray**	roentgen ray
UA	urinalysis			

(continued)

The following are a few abbreviations used to refer to health care providers and insurers:

BC/BS—Blue Cross, Blue Shield, a national insurance organization that makes payments for a wide variety of health care services for its subscribers. Frequently referred to as the "Blues."

CHAMPUS—the civilian health and medical program of the uniformed services, a program that is administered by the Department of Defense. CHAMPUS pays for health care services to active and retired members of the uniformed services and reimburses providers for the health care of the dependents of eligible personnel.

HMO—health maintenance organization, an organization that provides preventive health services as well as medical, hospital, and emergency care for members. There is a fee, paid in advance, to belong to a HMO.

IPA—independent practice association, a type of health maintenance organization in which the organization contracts with physicians who see patients in their own offices, rather than at a specific location designated as an HMO. The physicians are reimbursed by the HMO.

Medicare, Part A—Title XVIII of Health Insurance for the Aged of the U.S. Social Security Act. Medicare, Part A reimburses the hospital for services provided to eligible patients.

Medicare, Part B—Title XVIII of Health Insurance for the Aged of the U.S. Social Security Act. Medicare, Part B reimburses physicians for services provided to eligible patients. This insurance is provided to eligible citizens only when a supplementary payment is made.

PPO—Preferred Provider Organization, an association of hospitals, physicians, and agencies that provides health care to a specific group of individuals at agreed-upon rates.

ABPA	allergic bronchopulmonary aspergillosis	**CF**	cystic fibrosis
ABK	aphakic bullous keratopathy	**CFIDS**	chronic fatigue immune deficiency syndrome
ABS	acute brain syndrome	**CHD**	congenital heart disease; coronary heart disease
ACHD	adult congenital heart disease		
AD	Alzheimer's disease	**CHF**	congestive heart failure
A Fib	atrial fibrillation or dementia	**CLL**	chronic lymphocytic leukemia
AID	acute infectious disease	**CML**	chronic myelogenous leukemia
AIDP	autoimmune demyelinating polyneuropathy	**CMV**	cytomegalovirus
		COAD	chronic obstructive airway disease
AIDS	acquired immunodeficiency syndrome	**COLD**	chronic obstructive lung disease
AIHA	autoimmune hemolytic anemia	**COPD**	chronic obstructive pulmonary disease
AIP	acute interstitial pneumonia		
AKA	above knee amputation	**CP**	cerebral palsy
ALF	acute liver failure	**CPD**	cephalopelvic disproportion
ALS	amyotrophic lateral sclerosis	**CRF**	chronic renal failure
AMD	age-related macular degeneration	**CTD**	close to death
AMI	acute myocardial infarction	**CTS**	carpal tunnel syndrome
ANUG	acute necrotizing ulcerative gingivitis	**CVA**	cerebrovascular accident
AODM	adult onset diabetes mellitus	**CVD**	cerebrovascular disease; cardiovascular disease
APB	atrial premature beats		
APE	acute pulmonary edema	**DAD**	diffuse alveolar damage
ARC	AIDS-related complex; abnormal retinal correspondence	**DES**	diffuse esophageal spasm
		DIC	disseminated intravascular coagulation
ARD	acute respiratory disease		
ARDS	adult respiratory distress syndrome	**DIP**	desquamative interstitial pneumonitis
ARF	acute renal failure	**DJD**	degenerative joint disease
ARMD	age-related macular degeneration	**DKA**	diabetic ketoacidosis
AS	ankylosing spondylitis	**DM**	diabetes mellitus
ASC	anterior subcapsular cataract	**DOE**	dyspnea on exertion
ASCVD	arteriosclerotic cardiovascular disease	**DTs**	delirium tremens
ASD	atrial septal defect	**DVT**	deep venous thrombosis
ASHD	atherosclerotic heart disease		
Ast	astigmatism	**EM**	erythema multiforme
ATN	acute tubular necrosis	**EMD**	esophageal motor disturbance
ATS	anxiety tension state		
AUB	abnormal uterine bleeding	**FMS**	fibromyalgia syndrome
AUL	acute undifferentiated leukemia	**FUO**	fever of unknown origin
AVB	atrioventricular block		
AVD	aortic valve disease	**GC**	gonococcus
AVSD	atrioventricular septal defect	**GDM**	gestational diabetes mellitus
A & W	alive and well	**GN**	glomerulonephritis
		GODM	gestational onset diabetes mellitus
BBB	bundle branch block (R and L)		
BCA	breast cancer	**HA**	headache
BNO	bladder neck obstruction	**HELLP**	hemolysis, elevated liver enzymes, and low platelet count syndrome
BO	bronchiolitis obliterans		
BOOP	bronchiolitis obliterans-organizing pneumonia	**HGE**	human granulocytic ehrlichiosis
		HH	hiatal hernia
BPAD	bipolar affective disorder	**HIV**	human immunodeficiency virus
BPD	bronchopulmonary dysplasia	**HME**	human monocytic ehrlichiosis
BPH	benign prostatic hypertrophy	**HSV**	herpes simplex virus
BPPV	benign paroxysmal positional vertigo	**HTN**	hypertension
BV	bacterial vaginosis	**HUS**	hemolytic uremic syndrome
CA	cancer	**ICS**	immotile cilia syndrome
CAD	coronary artery disease	**IDDM**	insulin-dependent diabetes mellitus
CAVC	complete atrioventricular canal defect	**IHSS**	idiopathic hypertrophic subaortic stenosis

(continued)

ILD	interstitial lung disease	**PMR**	polymyalgia rheumatica
IPF	idiopathic pulmonary fibrosis	**PMS**	premenstrual syndrome
IUFD	intrauterine fetal demise	**PND**	paroxysmal nocturnal dyspnea; postnasal drip (or discharge)
IUGR	intrauterine growth retardation		
IUP	intrauterine pregnancy	**PPH**	primary pulmonary hypertension
		PS	pulmonary stenosis
JRA	juvenile rheumatoid arthritis	**PSVT**	paroxysmal supraventricular tachycardia
KS	Kaposi's sarcoma; Kartagener's syndrome	**PTL**	premature labor
		PTLD	post-transplant lymphoproliferative disorder
LAM	lymphangioleiomyomatosis	**PTSD**	post-traumatic stress disorder
LE	lupus erythematosus	**PTX**	pneumothorax
LIP	lymphocytic interstitial pneumonia	**PUD**	peptic ulcer disease
		PVC	premature ventricular contraction
MAI/MAC	*Mycobacterium avium intracellulare/ M.avium* complex	**PVS**	Plummer-Vinson syndrome
MCS	multiple chemical sensitivity	**RA**	rheumatoid arthritis
MD	muscular dystrophy	**RAD**	reactive airway disease
MDD	major depressive disorder	**RDS**	respiratory distress syndrome
MEE	middle ear effusion	**RF**	renal failure
MI	myocardial infarction	**RMSF**	Rocky Mountain spotted fever
MS	multiple sclerosis	**RSV**	respiratory syncytial virus
MVP	mitral valve prolapse	**RVMI**	right ventricular myocardial infarction
NHL	non-Hodgkin's lymphoma	**SAH**	subarachnoid hemorrhage
NIDDM	non-insulin dependent diabetes mellitus	**SBE**	subacute bacterial endocarditis
		SGA	small for gestational age
NSVD	normal spontaneous vaginal delivery	**SHH**	sliding hiatal hernia
NTD	neural tube defect	**SIADH**	syndrome of inappropriate antidiuretic hormone
OA	osteoarthritis; occupational asthma	**SIDS**	sudden infant death syndrome
OCD	obsessive-compulsive disorder	**SLE**	systemic lupus erythematosus
ODTS	organic dust toxic syndrome	**SOB**	shortness of breath
OLD	occupational lung disease	**SP**	spontaneous pneumothorax
OM	otitis media	**STD**	sexually transmitted disease
OSA	obstructive sleep apnea		
		Tb, TB	tuberculosis
PAC	premature atrial contraction	**TIA**	transient ischemic attack
PAP	pulmonary alveolar proteinosis	**TOF**	tetralogy of Fallot
PCD	primary ciliary dyskinesia	**TORCHS**	toxoplasmosis, rubella, cytomegalovirus, herpes simplex, syphilis
PCOD	polycystic ovarian disease		
PCP	*Pneumocystis carinii* pneumonia		
PD	Parkinson's disease	**TTP**	thrombotic thrombocytopenic purpura
PDA	patent ductus arteriosus		
PE	pulmonary embolism; pulmonary edema	**UC**	ulcerative colitis
		UIP	usual interstitial pneumonitis
PF	pulmonary fibrosis	**URI**	upper respiratory infection
PFO	patent foramen ovale	**UTI**	urinary tract infection
PHT	pulmonary hypertension		
PI	pulmonary insufficiency	**VBAC**	vaginal birth after cesarean section
PID	pelvic inflammatory disease	**V Fib**	ventricular fibrillation
PIDs	primary immunodeficiencies	**VSD**	ventricular septal defect
PIH	pregnancy-induced hypertension	**VT, V Tach**	ventricular tachycardia

Section 9: Dental Caries and Restorations

9-1. BLACK'S CLASSIFICATION OF DENTAL CARIES AND RESTORATIONS

Dental caries and restorations are most often classified using a system established in the early 1900s that provides a precise description of the types and locations. This system consists of six classifications, as follows:

Class 1
Class 1 dental caries or restorations occur in the following:
Occlusal surfaces (pits and fissures) in premolars and molars
Occlusal two thirds of the facial or lingual surfaces of molars
Lingual surfaces of maxillary incisors

Class 2
Class 2 dental caries or restorations occur in the following:
Proximal surfaces of posterior teeth
Occlusal surfaces—usually involved

Class 3
Class 3 dental caries or restorations occur in the following:
Proximal surfaces of incisors and canines. Incisal angle is not involved

Class 4
Class 4 dental caries or restorations occur in the following:
The proximal surfaces of incisors and canines, including the incisal angle

Class 5
Class 5 dental caries or restorations occur in the following:
Gingival third of facial or lingual surfaces of any tooth

Class 6
Class 6 dental caries or restorations involve the following:
Incisal edge of anterior teeth and the cusp tips of posterior tips

9-2. CLASSIFICATION BY COMPLEXITY FOR DENTAL CARIES AND RESTORATIONS

This system of classification identifies dental caries and restorations by the names of the surfaces that they involve. The usual practice is to refer to the caries or restoration using the abbreviation of the surfaces affected.

Simple Caries or Restorations
Those that involve only one tooth surface

Compound Caries or Restorations
Those that involve two surfaces

Complex Caries or Restorations
Those involving more than two surfaces

9-3. SIMPLE, COMPOUND, AND COMPLEX DESIGNATIONS FOR DENTAL CARIES AND RESTORATIONS

Simple	Abbreviation	Compound	Abbreviation	Complex	Abbreviation
Buccal	B	Mesioocclusal	MO	Mesioincisodistal	MID
Facial	F	Distoocclusal	DO	Mesiolinguodistal	MLD
Gingival	G	Occlusobuccal	OB	Mesioocclusobuccal	MOB
Incisal	I	Distolingual	DL	Mesioocclusodistal	MOD
Lingual	Li			Mesioocclusodistobuccolingual	MODBL
Labial	La				
Occlusal	O				

From Darby and Walsh 1994.

10-1. BASE SI UNITS

Property	Base Unit	Symbol
Length	meter	m
Mass	kilogram	kg
Amount of substance	mole	mol
Time	second	s
Thermodynamic temperature	Kelvin	K
Electrical current	ampere	A
Luminous intensity	candela	cd
Catalytic amount	katal	kat

10-2. DERIVED SI UNITS AND NON-SI UNITS RETAINED FOR USE WITH THE SI

Property	Unit	Symbol
Area	square meter	m^2
Volume	cubic meter	m^3
	liter	L
Mass concentration	kilogram/cubic meter	kg/m^3
	gram/liter	g/L
Substance concentration	mole/cubic meter	mol/m^3
	mole/liter	mol/L
Temperature	degree Celsius	$°C = °K - 273.15$

10-3. STANDARD PREFIXES

Prefix	Multiplication Factor	Symbol
yocto	10^{-24}	y
zepto	10^{-21}	z
atto	10^{-18}	a
femto	10^{-15}	f
pico	10^{-12}	p
nano	10^{-9}	n
micro	10^{-6}	μ
milli	10^{-3}	m
centi	10^{-2}	c
deci	10^{-1}	d
deca	10^1	da
hecto	10^2	h
kilo	10^3	k
mega	10^6	M
giga	10^9	G
tera	10^{12}	T

TEST	SPECIMEN	REFERENCE INTERVAL (CONVENTIONAL UNITS)	REFERENCE INTERVAL (INTERNATIONAL UNITS)
Acetoacetate Semiquantitative	Serum or plasma (fluoride/oxalate)	Negative (< 1 mg/dL)	Negative (< 0.1 mmol/L)
Acetone Semiquantitative	Urine Serum or plasma (fluoride or oxalate)	Negative Negative (< 1 mg/dL)	Negative Negative (< 0.17 mmol/L)
Quantitative Semiquantitative	Urine		Negative
Acid phosphatase (S:p-nitrophenyl-phosphate)	Serum		M: 2.5–11.7 U/L F: 0.3–9.2 U/L
Adrenocorticotropic hormone (ACTH)	Plasma (heparin)	0800 h: < 120 pg/mL	< 26 pmol/L
		1600–2000 h: < 85 pg/mL	< 19 pmol/L
Alanine aminotransferase (ALT, SGPT)	Serum	M: 10–40 U/L F: 7–35 U/L	0.17–0.68 μKat/L 0.12–0.60 μKat/L
Albumin Nephelometric, colorimetric	Serum	3.4–4.8 g/dL	34–48 g/L
Turbidimetric	CSF Urine	< 45 mg/dL < 80 mg/d at rest < 150 mg/d ambulatory	< 450 mg/L < 80 mg/d < 150 mg/d
Aldolase	Serum	1.0–7.5 U/L	0.02–0.13 μKat/L
Aldosterone	Plasma (heparin EDTA) or serum	Adult, average sodium diet	
		supine: 3–16 ng/dL upright: 7–30 ng/dL	0.08–0.44 nmol/L 0.19–0.83 nmol/L
Alkaline phosphatase (S:4-NPP)	Serum	25–100 U/L	Adult (> 20 y)
			0.43–1.70 μKat/L
δ-Amino-levulinic acid (δ-ALA)	Serum	15–23 μg/dL	1.1–8 μmol/L
	Urine	1.5–7.5 mg/d	11.4–57.2 μmol/d
Ammonia nitrogen Resin or enzymatic	Serum or plasma (Na-heparin) Urine, 24-h	Adult 15–45 μg N/dL 140–1500 mg/d	11–32 μmol/L 10–107 mmol/d
Amylase (S:Beckmann, defined substrate)	Serum	27–131 U/L	0.46–2.23 μKat/L
	Urine, timed specimen		1–17 U/h
Angiotensin I	Peripheral venous plasma (EDTA)	< 25 pg/mL	< 25 ng/L
Angiotensin II	Plasma (EDTA) Arterial blood	10–60 pg/mL	10–60 ng/L
α1-Antitrypsin (nephelometry)	Serum	78–200 mg/dL	0.78–2 g/L
Anion gap [Na+ − (Cl− + HCO3−)]	Plasma (heparin)	7–16 mEq/L	7–16 mmol/L
Arsenic	Whole blood (heparin)	0.2–2.3 μg/DL Chronic poisoning: 10–50 μg/dL Acute poisoning: 60–93 μg/dL	0.03–0.31 μmol/L 1.33–6.65 μmol/L 7.98–12.37 μmol/L
Ascorbic acid (see Vitamin C)	Urine, 24 h	5–50 μg/d	0.067–0.665 μmol/d
Aspartate aminotransferase (AST)	Serum	10–30 U/L	0.17–0.51 μKat/L
Base excess	Whole blood (heparin)	− 2 to 3 mEq/L	− 2 to 3 mmol/L

From Rakel and Bope (eds.): *Conn's Current Therapy 2002*. Philadelphia, W.B. Saunders Co., 2002.

(continued)

TEST	SPECIMEN	REFERENCE INTERVAL (CONVENTIONAL UNITS)	REFERENCE INTERVAL (INTERNATIONAL UNITS)
Bicarbonate	Serum	22–29 mEq/L	22–29 mmol/L
Bile acids, total	Serum, fasting	0.3–2.3 µg/mL	0.74–5.64 µmol/L
	Serum, 1-h postprandial	1.8–3.2 µg/mL	4.41–7.84 µmol/L
	Feces	120–225 mg/d	294–551 µmol/d
Bilirubin			
Total	Serum	0.3–1.2 mg/dL	5–21 µmol/L
	Urine		Negative
Conjugated (direct)	Serum	0–0.2 mg/dL	0–3.4 µmol/L
Calcium, ionized (iCa)	Serum	4.65–5.28 mg/dL	1.16–1.32 mmol/L
Calcium, total	Serum	8.6–10.0 mg/dL	2.15–2.50 mmol/L
	Urine, 24-h	100–300 mg/d	2.5–7.5 mmol/d
	CSF	4.2–5.4 mg/dL	1.05–1.35 mmol/L
Cancer antigen 125 (CA 125)	Serum	< 35 U/mL	< 35 kU/L
Carbon dioxide, partial pressure (Pco_2)	Whole blood, arterial (heparin)	M: 35–48 mm Hg	4.66–6.38 kPa
		F: 32–45 mm Hg	4.26–5.99 kPa
Carbon dioxide, total (Tco_2)	Serum or plasma (heparin)	23–29 mEq/L	23–29 mmol/L
Carcinoembryonic antigen (CEA)	Serum	Nonsmokers: < 2.5 ng/mL	< 2.5 µg/L
β-Carotene	Serum	10–85 µg/dL	0.19–1.58 µmol/L
Catecholamines, total	Urine, 24-h	< 100 µg/d	< 5.91 nmol/d
Ceruloplasmin	Serum	18–45 mg/dL	180–450 mg/L
Chloride	Serum or plasma (heparin)	98–106 mEq/L	98–106 mmol/L
	CSF	118–132 mEq/L	118–132 mmol/L
	Urine, 24-h	110–250 mEq/d	110–250 mmol/d
Cholesterol, total	Serum or plasma (EDTA)	Recommended: < 200 mg/dL	< 5.18 mmol/L
		Moderate risk: 200–239 mg/dL	5.18–6.19 mmol/L
		High risk: ≥ 240 mg/dL	6.22 mmol/L
Chorionic gonadotropin, β-subunit (β-HCG)	Serum or plasma (EDTA)	M and nonpregnant F: < 5.0 mIU/mL	< 5.0 IU/L
Complement			
Total hemolytic complement activity	Serum	75–160 U/mL	75–160 kU/L
Copper	Serum	M: 70–140 µg/dL	10.99–21.98 µmol/L
		F: 80–155 µg/dL	12.56–24.34 µmol/L
	Erythrocyte (heparin)	90–150 µg/dL	14.13–23.55 µmol/L
	Urine, 24-h	3–35 µg/d	0.047–0.55 µmol/d
Coproporphyrin	Urine, 24-h	34–234 µg/d	51–351 nmol/d
	Feces, 24-h	< 30 µg/g dry wt	< 45 nmol/g dry wt
		400–1200 µg/d	600–1800 nmol/d
Corticosterone	Serum	0800 h: 130–820 ng/dL	4–24 nmol/L
		1600 h: 60–220 ng/dL	2–6 nmol/L
Cortisol	Serum or plasma (heparin)	0800 h: 5–23 µg/dL	138–635 nmol/L
		1600 h: 3–15 µg/dL	82–413 nmol/L
		2000 h: ≤ 50% of 0800 h	Fraction of 0800 h: ≤ 0.50
Cortisol, free	Urine, 24-h	20–90 µg/d	55–248 nmol/d
C-Peptide	Serum	0.78–1.89 ng/mL	0.26–0.62 nmol/L
C-Reactive protein	Serum	68–8200 ng/mL	68–8200 µg/L
Creatine kinase (CK)	Serum		M: 38–174 U/L F: 26–140 U/L
Isoenzymes, Fraction 2 (MB)	Serum	< 4–6% of total (method dependent)	Fraction of total: < 0.04–0.06
Creatinine	Serum or plasma	M: 0.7–1.3 mg/dL	62–115 µmol/L
Jaffe, kinetic or enzymatic		F: 0.6–1.1 mg/dL	53–97 µmol/L
	Urine, 24-h	M: 14–26 mg/kg/d	124–230 µmol/kg/d
		F: 11–20 mg/kg/d	97–177 µmol/kg/d

TEST	SPECIMEN	REFERENCE INTERVAL (CONVENTIONAL UNITS)	REFERENCE INTERVAL (INTERNATIONAL UNITS)
Creatinine clearance (endogenous)	Serum or plasma, and urine	M: 90–139 mL/min/ 1.73 m^2	0.87–1.34 mL/s/m^2
		F: 80–125 mL/min/ 1.73 m^2	0.77–1.20 mL/s/m^2
Dehydroepiandrosterone (DHEA)	Serum	M: 1.8–12.5 ng/mL	6.2–43.3 nmol/L
		F: 1.3–9.8 ng/mL	4.5–34.0 nmol/L
11-Deoxycortisol (compound S)	Serum	12–158 ng/dL	0.3–4.6 nmol/L
Erythropoietin	Serum		5–36 U/L
Estrogens, total	Serum	M: 20–80 pg/mL	20–80 ng/L
		F, cycle:	
		1–10 d 61–394 pg/mL	60–200 ng/L
		11–20 d 122–437 pg/mL	
		21–30 d 156–350 pg/mL	160–400 ng/L
		Postmenopausal: ≤ 130 pg/mL	≤ 130 ng/L
		Follicular phase 60–200 pg/mL	60–200 ng/L
		Luteal phase: 160–400 pg/mL	160–400 ng/L
	Urine, 24-h	M: 15–40 µg/d	
		F: Preovulation: 4–25 µg/d	
		Ovulation: 28–100 µg/d	
		Luteal peak: 22–80 µg/d	
		Pregnancy, term: < 45,000 µg/d	
		Postmenopausal: < 20 µg/d	
Fat, fecal	Feces, 72-h	< 7 g/d	
		fat-free diet: < 4 g/d	
Fatty acids, nonesterified (free)	Serum or plasma (heparin)	8–25 mg/dL	0.28–0.89 mmol/L
Ferritin	Serum	M: 20–250 ng/mL	20–250 µg/L
		F: 10–120 ng/mL	10–120 µg/L
α_1-Fetoprotein	Serum	< 10 ng/mL	< 10 µg/L
Fibrinogen (see Hematology and Coagulation section)			
Folate	Serum	3–16 ng/mL	7–36 nmol/L
	Erythrocytes (EDTA)	140–628 ng/mL packed cells	317–1422 nmol/L packed cells
Follitropin (FSH)	Serum or plasma (heparin)	M: 4–25 mIU/mL	4–25 IU/L
		F: Follicular phase: 1–9 mIU/L	1–9 IU/L
		Ovulatory peak: 6–26 mIU/mL	6–26 IU/L
		Luteal phase: 1–9 mIU/mL	1–9 IU/L
		Postmenopausal: 30–118 mIU/mL	30–118 IU/L
	Urine, 24-h		M: 3–11 IU/d
			F: 2–15 IU/d
Gastrin	Serum	25–90 pg/mL	25–90 ng/L
Glucose	Serum	Adult: 74–106 mg/dL	4.1–5.9 mmol/L
		> 60 y: 80–115 mg/dL	4.4–6.4 mmol/L
	Whole blood (heparin)	65–95 mg/dL	3.6–5.3 mmol/L
	CSF	40–70 mg/dL	2.2–3.9 mmol/L
Quantitative, enzymatic	Urine	< 0.5 g/d	< 2.8 mmol/d

(continued)

TEST	SPECIMEN	REFERENCE INTERVAL (CONVENTIONAL UNITS)	REFERENCE INTERVAL (INTERNATIONAL UNITS)
Qualitative	Urine		Negative
Glucose, 2-h postprandial	Serum	< 120 mg/dL	< 6.7 mmol/L
Glucose, tolerance test (GTT), oral	Serum	mg/dL Normal Diabetic Fasting: 70–105 > 140 60 min: 120–170 ≥ 200 90 min: 100–140 ≥ 200 120 min: 70–120 ≥ 140	mmol/L Normal Diabetic 3.9–5.8 > 7.8 6.7–9.4 ≥ 11 5.6–7.8 ≥ 11 3.9–6.7 ≥ 7.8
γ-Glutamyltransferase (GGT) (Szasz Method)	Serum	M: 2–30 U/L F: 1–24 U/L	0.03–0.51 µKat/L 0.02–0.41 µKat/L
Glycerol, free	Plasma	0.29–1.72 mg/dL	0.032–0.187 mmol/L
Growth hormone (HGH, somatotropin)	Serum	Adult, M: 0–4 ng/mL F: 0–18 ng/mL >60 y, M: 1–9 ng/mL F: 1–16 ng/mL	0–4 µg/L 0–18 µg/L 1–9 µg/L 1–16 µg/L
Haptoglobin (see Hematology and Coagulation section)			
HDL-cholesterol (HDLC) (5th percentile from Lipid Research Clinics)	Serum or plasma (EDTA)	M: > 29 mg/dL F: > 35 mg/dL	> 0.75 mmol/L > 0.91 mmol/L
Hemoglobin A$_{Ic}$ (electrophoresis)	Whole blood (heparin, EDTA, or oxalate)	5.0–7.5% of total Hb	Fracion of Hb: 0.050–0.075
Homovanillic acid (HVA)	Urine, 24-h	1.4–8.8 mg/d	8–48 µmol/d
17-Hydroxycorticosteroids (17-OHCS)	Urine, 24-h	M: 3.0–10.0 mg/d F: 2.0–8.0 mg/d	8.3–27.6 µmol/d 5.5–22.1 µmol/d
5-Hydroxyindole acetic acid (5-HIAA)			
Qualitative	Fresh random urine		Negative
Quantitative	Urine, 24-h	2–6 mg/d	10.4–31.2 µmol/d
17-Hydroxyprogesterone (17-OHP)	Serum	M: 0.5–2.5 ng/mL F: Follicular: 0.2–1.0 ng/mL Luteal: 1.0–5.0 ng/mL Postmenopausal: ≤ 0.7 ng/mL	1.5–7.5 nmol/L 0.6–3.0 nmol/L 3.0–15.5 nmol/L ≤ 2.1 nmol/L
Immunoglobulin A (IgA)	Serum	40–350 mg/dL	400–3500 mg/L
Immunoglobulin D (IgD)	Serum	0–8 mg/dL	0–80 mg/L
Immunoglobulin E (IgE)	Serum	0–380 IU/mL	0–380 kIU/L
Immunoglobulin G (IgG)	Serum CSF	650–1600 mg/dL 0.5–5 mg/dL	6.5–16 g/L 5–50 mg/L
Immunoglobulin M (IgM)	Serum	55–300 mg/dL	550–3000 mg/L
Insulin (12-h fasting), immunoreactive	Serum	0.7–9.0 µIU/mL	5–63 pmol/L
Intrinsic factor (see Vitamin B$_{12}$)			
Iron	Serum	M: 65–175 µg/dL F: 50–170 µg/dL	11.6–31.3 µmol/L 9.0–30.4 µmol/L
Iron-binding capacity, total (TIBC)	Serum	250–450 µg/dL	44.8–80.6 µmol/L

TEST	SPECIMEN	REFERENCE INTERVAL (CONVENTIONAL UNITS)	REFERENCE INTERVAL (INTERNATIONAL UNITS)
Iron saturation	Serum	M: 20–50	Fraction of iron saturation: 0.20–0.5
		F: 15–50	0.15–0.5
17-Ketogenic steroids (17-KGS)	Urine, 24-h	M: 5–23 mg/d	17–80 μmol/d
		F: 3–15 mg/d	10–52 μmol/d
Ketone bodies			
Qualitative	Serum	Negative (0.5–3.0 mg/dL)	Negative (5–30 mg/L)
	Urine, random		Negative
17-Ketosteroids, total (17-KS)	Urine, 24-h	M: 10–25 mg/d	37–87 μmol/d
		F: 6–15 mg/d	21–52 μmol/d
L-Lactate	Whole blood (heparin)	Venous: 8.1–15.3 mg/dL	0.9–1.7 mmol/L
		Arterial: < 11.3 mg/dL	< 1.3 mmol/L
Lactate dehydrogenase (LDH)	Serum		208–378 U/L
LDH isoenzymes (Electrophoresis, agarose)	Serum	% Fraction 1: 18–33	Fraction of total: 0.18–0.33
		Fraction 2: 28–40	0.28–0.40
		Fraction 3: 18–30	0.18–0.30
		Fraction 4: 6–16	0.06–0.16
		Fraction 5: 2–13	0.02–0.13
Lead	Whole blood (heparin)	< 25 μg/dL	< 1.21 μmol/L
		Toxic: ≥ 100 μg/dL	≥ 4.83 μmol/L
	Urine	< 80 μg/dL	< 0.39 μmol/L
LDL-Cholesterol (LDLC)	Serum or plasma (EDTA)	Recommended: < 130 mg/dL	< 3.37 mmol/L
		Moderate risk: 130–159 mg/dL	3.37–4.12 mmol/L
		High risk: ≥ 160 mg/dL	≥ 4.14 mmol/L
Lutropin (LH)	Serum or plasma (heparin)	M: 1–8 mU/mL	1.8 U/L
		F: Follicular phase: 1–2 mU/mL	1–12 U/L
		Midcycle: 16–104 mU/mL	16–104 U/L
		Luteal: 1–12 mU/mL	1–12 U/L
		Postmenopausal: 16–66 mU/mL	16–66 U/L
	Urine		M: 9–23 U/d F: nonmidcycle, 4–30 U/d
Lysozyme	Serum, plasma	0.4–1.3 mg/dL	4–13 mg/L
Magnesium	Serum	1.3–2.1 mEq/L	0.65–1.05 mmol/L
	Urine, 24-h	6.0–10.0 mEq/d	3.00–5.00 mmol/d
Mercury	Whole blood (EDTA)	< 5.0 μg/dL	< 0.25 μmol/L
	Urine, 24-h	< 20 μg/L	< 0.1 μmol/L
		Toxic: > 150 μg/L	< 0.75 μmol/L
Metanephrine, total	Urine, 24-h	0.05–1.20 μg/mg creatinine	0.03–0.69 mmol/mol creatinine
Myelin basic protein	CSF		< 2.5 μg/L
Myoglobin	Serum		M: 19–92 μg/L F: 12–76 μg/L
	Urine, random		Negative
Osmolality	Serum		275–295 mOsmol/kg
	Urine, random		50–1200 mOsmol/kg, depending on fluid intake After 12-h fluid restriction: > 850 mOsmol/kg
	Urine, 24-h		~ 390–900 mOsmol/kg

(continued)

TEST	SPECIMEN	REFERENCE INTERVAL (CONVENTIONAL UNITS)	REFERENCE INTERVAL (INTERNATIONAL UNITS)
Oxalate	Serum	1–2.4 µg/mL Ethylene glycol poisoning: > 20 µg/mL	11–27 µmol/L Ethylene glycol poisoning: > 228 µmol/L
Oxygen (Po$_2$)	Whole blood, arterial (heparin)	83–108 mm Hg	11–14.4 kPa
Oxygen saturation	Whole blood, arterial (heparin)	95–98%	Fraction saturated: 0.95–0.98
Parathyroid hormone	Serum	Varies with laboratory N-Terminal 8–24 pg/mL C-terminal 50–330 pg/mL Intact 10–65 pg/mL	8–24 ng/L 50–330 ng/L 10–65 ng/L
pH (37°C)	Whole blood, arterial (heparin)		7.35–7.45
Phosphorus, inorganic	Serum	2.7–4.5 mg/dL > 60 y, M: 2.3–3.7 mg/dL F: 2.8–4.1 mg/dL	0.87–1.45 nmol/L 0.74–1.2 nmol/L 0.90–1.3 nmol/L
	Urine, 24-h	0.4–1.3 g/d	13–42 mmol/d
Porphobilinogen (PBG)			
Quantitative	Urine, 24-h	0–2.0 mg/d	0–8.8 µmol/d
Qualitative	Urine, fresh random		Negative
Potassium	Serum	3.5–5.1 mEq/L	3.5–5.1 mmol/L
	Plasma (heparin)	3.5–4.5 mEq/L	3.5–4.5 mmol/L
	Urine, 24-h	25–125 mEq/d	25–125 mmol/d
Pregnanediol	Urine, 24-h	M: 0–1.9 mg/d F: Follicular: < 2.6 mg/d Luteal: 2.6–10.6 mg/d Postmenopausal: 0.2–1.0 mg/d	0–5.9 µmol/d < 8 µmol/d 8–33 µmol/d 0.6–3.1 µmol/d
Progesterone	Serum	M: 0.13–0.97 ng/mL F: Follicular: 0.15–0.70 ng/mL Luteal: 2.0–25 ng/mL	0.4–3.1 nmol/L 0.5–2.2 nmol/L 6.4–79.5 nmol/L
Prolactin (hPRL)	Serum	M: 3.0–14.7 ng/mL F: 3.8–23.2 ng/mL	3.0–14.7 µg/L 3.8–23.2 µg/L
Prostate-specific antigen (PSA)	Serum, freeze	M: < 4 ng/mL	< 4 µg/L
Protein			
Total	Serum	6.4–8.3 g/dL	64.0–83.0 g/L
Electrophoresis (cellulose acetate)	Serum	Albumin: 3.5–5.0 g/dL	35–50 g/L
		α_1-Globulin: 0.1–0.3 g/dL	1–3 g/L
		α_2-Globulin: 0.6–1.0 g/dL	6–10 g/L
		β-Globulin: 0.7–1.1 g/dL	7–11 g/L
		γ-Globulin: 0.8–1.6 g/dL	8–16 g/L
Total	Urine, 24-h		50–80 mg/d at rest
Total	CSF	Lumbar: 15–45 mg/dL	150–450 mg/L
Pyruvic acid	Whole blood (heparin)	0.3–0.9 mg/dL	0.03–0.10 mmol/L
Renin (normal diet)	Plasma (EDTA)	Supine: 0.2–1.6 ng/mL/h Standing: 0.7–3.3 ng/mL/h	0.2–1.6 µg/L/h 0.7–3.3 µg/L/h
Riboflavin (see Vitamin B$_2$)			
Sediment	Urine, fresh, random		Hyaline: occasional (0–1) casts/hpf
Casts			RBC: not seen WBC: not seen Tubular epithelial: not seen Transitional and squamous epithelial: not seen

TEST	SPECIMEN	REFERENCE INTERVAL (CONVENTIONAL UNITS)	REFERENCE INTERVAL (INTERNATIONAL UNITS)
Cells			RBC: 0–2/hpf WBC: M: 0–3/hpf F: 0–5/hpf Epithelial: few Bacteria: Unspun: no organisms/oil immersion field Spun: < 20 organisms/hpf
Sodium	Serum or plasma (heparin)	136–146 mEq/L	136–146 mmol/L
	Urine, 24 h	40–220 mEq/d	40–220 mmol/d
Specific gravity	Urine, random		1.002–1.030
	Urine, 24 h		1.015–1.025
Testosterone, free	Serum	M: 50–210 pg/mL	174–729 pmol/L
		F: 1.0–8.5 pg/mL	3.5–29.5 pmol/L
Testosterone, total	Serum	M: 280–1100 ng/dL	9.7–38.2 nmol/L
		F: 15–70 ng/dL	0.5–2.4 nmol/L
	Urine	20–50 y,	
		M: 50–135 µg/d	173–470 nmol/d
		F: 2–12 µg/d	7–42 nmol/d
		> 50 y,	
		M: 40–60 µg/d	139–210 nmol/d
		F: 2–8 µg/d	7–28 nmol/d
Thiamine (see Vitamin B_1)	Serum	0.10–0.54 µg/dL	2.9–16.1 nmol/L
Thyroglobulin (Tg)	Serum	3–42 ng/mL	3–42 µg/L
Thyroglobulin antibodies	Serum		< 1:10
Thyroid microsomal antibodies	Serum		Nondetectable (hemagglutination) or < 1:10 (IFA)
Thyrotropin (hTSH)	Serum or plasma	0.4–4.2 µU/mL	0.4–4.2 mU/L
Thyrotropin-releasing hormone	Plasma	5–60 pg/mL	5–60 ng/L
Thyroxine, free (FT_4)	Serum	0.8–2.4 ng/dL	10–31 pmol/L
Thyroxine (T_4), total	Serum	M: 4.6–10.5 µg/dL	59–135 nmol/L
		F: 5.5–11.0 µg/dL	71–142 nmol/L
Thyroxine-binding globulin (TBG)	Serum	15.0–34.0 µg/mL	15.0–34.0 mg/L
Thyroxine index, free	Serum		4.2–13.0
Transcortin	Serum	M: 18.8–25.2 L	323–433 nmol/L
		F: 14.9–22.9 mg/L	256–393 nmol/L
Transferrin	Serum	200–400 mg/dL	2.0–4.0 g/L
		> 60 y: 180–380 mg/dL	1.80–3.80 g/L
Transthyretin (prealbumin)	Serum	10–40 mg/dL	100–400 mg/L
Triglycerides (TG)	Serum, after ≥ 12-hr fast	Recommended: < 250 mg/dL	2.83 mmol/L
Tri-iodothyronine, free	Serum	260–480 pg/dL	4.0–7.4 pmol/L
Tri-iodothyronine, total (T_3)	Serum	100–200 ng/dL	1.54–3.08 mmol/L
Tri-iodothyronine resin uptake test (T_3RU)	Serum	24–34%	24–34 AU (arbitrary units)
Urea nitrogen	Serum or plasma	6–20 mg/dL	2.1–7.1 mmol/L
	Urine	12–20 g/d	0.43–0.71 mol/d
Urea nitrogen/creatinine ratio	Serum		12/1–20/1
Uric acid (uricase)	Serum	M: 3.5–7.2 mg/dL	0.21–0.42 mmol/L
		F: 2.6–6.0 mg/dL	0.15–0.35 mmol/L
	Urine, 24-h	250–750 mg/d	1.48–4.43 mmol/d
Urinary sediment (see Sediment)			

(continued)

TEST	SPECIMEN	REFERENCE INTERVAL (CONVENTIONAL UNITS)	REFERENCE INTERVAL (INTERNATIONAL UNITS)
Urobilinogen	Urine, 2-h	0.1–0.8 EU	0.1–0.8 U
	Urine, 24-h	0.5–4.0 EU	0.5–4.0 U
	Feces	75–275 EU/100 g	750–2750 U/kg
		75–400 EU/d	75–400 U/d
		40–280 mg/d	67–473 µmol/d
Uroporphyrin	Urine, 24-h	<50 µg/d	<60 nmol/d
	Feces, 24-h specimen	10–40 µg/d	12–48 nmol/d
	Erythrocytes (heparin or EDTA)		Negative
Vanillylmandelic acid (VMA)	Urine, 24-h	2–7 mg/d	10.1–35.4 µmol/d
Viscosity	Serum		1.10–1.22 centipoise
Vitamin A	Serum	30–80 µg/dL	1.05–2.8 µmol/L
Vitamin B_1 (Thiamine)	Serum	0–2 µg/dL	0–75 nmol/L
Vitamin B_2 (Riboflavin)	Serum	4–24 µg/dL	106–638 nmol/L
Vitamin B_6	Plasma (EDTA)	5–30 ng/mL	20–121 nmol/L
Vitamin B_{12}	Serum	200–835 pg/mL	148–616 pmol/L
Vitamin C	Plasma (oxalate, heparin, or EDTA)	0.5–1.5 mg/dL	28–85 µmol/L
Vitamin D_3, 1,25-dihydroxy	Serum	25–45 pg/mL	60–108 pmol/L
Vitamin D_3, 25-hyroxy	Plasma (heparin)	Summer: 15–80 ng/mL	37.4–200 nmol/L
		Winter: 14–42 ng/mL	34.9–105 nmol/L
Vitamin E	Serum	5.0–18.0 µg/mL	12–42 µmol/L
Zinc	Serum	70–150 µg/dL	10.7–22.9 µmol/L

TEST	SPECIMEN	REFERENCE INTERVAL (CONVENTIONAL UNITS)	REFERENCE INTERVAL (INTERNATIONAL UNITS)
Activated partial thromboplastin time (APTT)	Whole blood (Na citrate)		25–35 sec
Bleeding time (BT)			
Ivy	Blood from skin		Normal: 2–7 min
			Borderline: 7–11 min
Simplate (G-D)			2.75–8 min
Blood volume	Whole blood (heparin)		M: 52–83 mL/kg
			F: 50–75 mL/kg
Bone marrow	Bone marrow aspirate	% (mean)	Number fraction (mean)
Differential count			
Myeoblasts		0.3–5.0 (2.0)	0.003–0.05 (0.02)
Promyelocytes		1.0–8.0 (5.0)	0.01–0.08 (0.05)
Myelocytes:			
Neutrophilic		5.0–19.0 (12.0)	0.05–0.19 (0.12)
Eosinophilic		0.5–3.0 (1.5)	0.005–0.03 (0.015)
Basophilic		0.0–0.5 (0.3)	0.00–0.005 (0.003)
Metamyelocytes		13.0–32.0 (22.0)	0.13–0.32 (0.22)
Polymorphonuclear neutrophils		7.0–3.0 (2.0)	0.07–0.30 (0.20)
Polymorphonuclear eosinophils		0.5–4.0 (2.0)	0.005–0.04 (0.02)
Polymorphonuclear basophils		0.0–0.7 (0.2)	0.0–0.007 (0.002)

*From Rakel and Bope (eds.): *Conn's Current Therapy 2002*. Philadelphia, W.B. Saunders Co., 2002.

TEST	SPECIMEN	REFERENCE INTERVAL (CONVENTIONAL UNITS)		REFERENCE INTERVAL (INTERNATIONAL UNITS)	
Lymphocytes		3.0–17.0 (10.0)		0.03–0.17 (0.10)	
Plasma cells		0.0–2.0 (0.4)		0.00–0.02 (0.004)	
Monocytes		0.5–5.0 (2.0)		0.005–0.05 (0.02)	
Reticulum cells		0.1–2.0 (0.2)		0.001–0.02 (0.002)	
Megakaryocytes		0.03–3.0 (0.1)		0.0003–0.03 (0.001)	
Pronormoblasts		1.0–8.0 (4.0)		0.01–0.08 (0.04)	
Normoblasts		7.0–32.0 (18.0)		0.07–0.32 (0.18)	
Clot lysis, 37°C	Whole clotted blood			48–72 h	
Clot retraction screen	Whole blood (no anticoagulant)			Retraction begins at 1 h, maximum at 24 h	
Clotting time, Lee-White, 37°C	Whole blood (no anticoagulant)			5–8 min	
Differential count (see Bone marrrow differential count or leukocyte differential count)					
Eosinophil count	Whole blood (EDTA); capillary blood	50–400 cells/µL (mm³)		50–400 × 10⁶ cells/L	
Erythrocyte count (RBC count)	Whole blood (EDTA)	millions of cells/µL (mm³) M: 4.3–5.7 F: 3.8–5.1		× 10¹² cells/L 4.3–5.7 3.8–5.1	
Erythrocyte sedimentation rate (ESR), Wintrobe				M: 0–15 mm/h F: 0–20 mm/h	
Ferritin (see Chemistry section)					
Fibrin degradation products (agglutination, Thrombo-Wellco test)	Whole blood: special tube containing thrombin and proteolytic inhibitor	<10 µg/mL		<10 µg/L	
	Urine: 2 mL in special tube (see above)	<0.25 µg/mL		<0.25 mg/L	
Fibrinogen	Plasma (Na citrate)	200–400 mg/dL		2.00–4.00 g/L	
Glucose-6-phosphate dehydrogenase (G6PD) in erythrocytes	Whole blood (ACD, EDTA, or heparin)	12.1 ± 2.09 U/g Hb (1 SD)		0.78 ± 0.13 MU/mol Hb (1 SD)	
Haptoglobin (Hp) RID	Serum; avoid hemolysis	26–85 mg/dL		260–1850 mg/L	
Hematocrit (HCT, Hct) Calculated from MCV and RBC (electronic displacement or laser)	Whole blood (EDTA)	M: 39–49% F: 35–45%		0.39–0.49 volume fraction 0.35–0.45 volume fraction	
Hemoglobin (Hb)	Whole blood (EDTA)	M: 13.5–17.5 g/dL F: 12.0–16.0 g/dL		2.09–2.71 mmol/L 1.86–2.48 mmol/L	
	Plasma (heparin, ACD)	<3 mg/dL		<0.47 µmol/L	
	Urine, fresh, random			Negative	
Hemoglobin electrophoresis	Whole blood (EDTA, citrate, or heparin)			Mass function	
		HbA >95% HbA₂ 1.5–3.5% HbF <2%		HbA >0.95 HbA₂ 0.015–0.035 HbF <0.02	
Leukocyte count (WBC count)	Whole blood (EDTA)	4.5–11.0 × 10³ cells/µL (mm³)		4.5–11.0 × 10⁹ cells/L	
	CSF	0.5 mononuclear cells/µL (mm³)		0.5 × 10⁶ cells/L	
Leukocyte Differential count	Whole blood (EDTA)	%	Cells/µL (mm³)	Number fraction	Cells × 10⁶/L
Myelocytes		0	0	0	0
Neutrophils-bands		3–5	150–400	0.03–0.05	150–400
Neutrophils-segmented		54–62	3000–5800	0.54–0.62	3000–5800

(continued)

TEST	SPECIMEN	REFERENCE INTERVAL (CONVENTIONAL UNITS)		REFERENCE INTERVAL (INTERNATIONAL UNITS)	
Lymphocytes		23–33	1500–3000	0.25–0.33	1500–3000
Monocytes		3–7	285–500	0.03–0.07	285–500
Eosinophils		1–3	50–250	0.01–0.03	50–250
Basophils		0–0.75	15–50	0–0.0075	15–50
Leukocyte Differential count	CSF	%		Number fraction	
Lymphocytes		62 ± 34		0.62 ± 0.324	
Monocytes (includes pia-arachnoid mesothelial cells)		36 ± 20		0.36 ± 0.20	
Neutrophils		2 ± 5		0.02 ± 0.05	
Histocytes				Rare	
Ependymal cells				Rare	
Eosinophils				Rare	
Mean corpuscular hemoglobin (MCH)	Whole blood (EDTA)	26–34 pg/cell		0.40–0.53 fmol/cell	
Mean corpuscular hemoglobin concentration (MCHC)	Whole blood (EDTA)	31–37% Hb/cell or gHb/dL RBC		4.81–5.74 mmol Hb/L RBC	
Mean corpuscular volume (MCV)	Whole blood (EDTA)			80–100 fL	
Methemoglobin (MetHb)	Whole blood (EDTA, heparin, or ACD)	0.06–0.24 g/dL		9.3–37.2 μmol/L	
Plasma volume	Plasma (heparin)	M: 25–43 mL/kg		0.025–0.043 L/kg	
		F: 28–45 mL/kg		0.028–0.045 L/kg	
Platelet count (thrombocyte count)	Whole blood (EDTA)	150–450 × 10³/μL (mm³)		150–450 × 10⁹/L	
Prothrombin consumption	Whole blood (no anticoagulant)			>30 sec	
Prothrombin time, two-stage modified	Whole blood (Na citrate)			18–22 sec	
RBC count (see Erythrocyte count)					
Red cell volume	Whole blood (heparin)	M: 20–36 mL/kg		M: 0.020–0.036 L/kg	
		F: 19–31 mL/kg		F: 0.019–0.031 L/kg	
Reticulocyte count	Whole blood (EDTA, heparin, or oxalate)	0.5–1.5% of erythrocytes		0.005–0.015 (number fraction)	
Sulfhemoglobin	Whole blood (EDTA, heparin, or EDTA)	≤ 1.0% of total Hb		< 0.010 of total Hb (mass fraction)	
Thrombin time	Whole blood (Na citrate)			Time of control ± 25 when control is 9–13 sec	
Thromboplastin time, activated (see Activated partial thromboplastin time [APTT])					

10-6. LABORATORY REFERENCE VALUES: DRUGS—THERAPEUTIC AND TOXIC*

DRUG	SPECIMEN		REFERENCE INTERVAL (CONVENTIONAL UNITS)	REFERENCE INTERVAL (INTERNATIONAL UNITS)
Acetaminophen	Serum or plasma (hep or EDTA)	Therap:	10–30 µg/mL	66–199 µmol/L
		Toxic:	>200 µg/mL	>1324 µmol/L
Amikacin	Serum or plasma (EDTA)	Therap:		
		Peak	25–35 µg/mL	43–60 µmol/L
		Trough (severe infection)	4–8 µg/mL	6.8–13.7 µmol/L
		Toxic:		
		Peak	>35 µg/mL	>60 µmol/L
		Trough	>10 µg/mL	>17 µmol/L
∈-Aminocaproic acid	Serum or plasma (hep or EDTA); trough	Therap:	100–400 µg/mL	433–903 nmol/L
Amitriptyline	Serum or plasma (hep or EDTA); trough (>12 h after dose)	Therap:	120–250 ng/mL	>1805 nmol/L
Amobarbital	Serum	Toxic:	>500 ng/mL	
		Therap:	1–5 µg/mL	4–22 µmol/L
		Toxic:	>10 µg/mL	>44 µmol/L
Amphetamine	Serum or plasma (hep or EDTA)	Therap:	20–30 ng/mL	148–222 nmol/L
		Toxic:	>200 ng/mL	
Bromide	Serum	Toxic:	>1250 µg/mL	>15.6 mmol/L
Caffeine	Serum or plasma (hep or EDTA)	Therap:	3–15 µg/mL	15–77 µmol/L
		Toxic:	>50 µg/mL	>258 µmol/L
Carbamazepine	Serum or plasma (hep or EDTA); trough	Therap:	4–12 µg/mL	17–51 µmol/L
		Toxic:	>15 µg/mL	>63 µmol/L
Carbenicillin	Serum or plasma	Therap:	Dependent on minimum inhibitory concentration of specific organism	Same
		Toxic:	>250 µg/mL	>660 µmol/L
Chloramphenicol	Serum or plasma (hep or EDTA); trough	Therap:	10–25 µg/mL	31–77 µmol/L
		Toxic:	>25 µg/mL	>77 µmol/L
Chlordiazepoxide	Serum or plasma (hep or EDTA); trough	Therap:	700–1000 ng/mL	2.34–3.34 µmol/L
		Toxic:	>5000 ng/mL	>16.7 µmol/L
Chlorpromazine	Serum or plasma (hep or EDTA); trough	Therap:	50–300 ng/mL	157–942 nmol/L
		Toxic:	>750 ng/mL	>2355 nmol/L
Cimetidine	Serum or plasma (hep or EDTA); trough	Therap:	0.5–1.2 µg/mL	2–5 µmol/L

*From Rakel and Bope (eds.): Conn's Current Therapy 2002. Philadelphia, W.B. Saunders Co., 2002.

(continued)

	10-6. LABORATORY REFERENCE VALUES: DRUGS—THERAPEUTIC AND TOXIC*—cont'd"		
DRUG	SPECIMEN	REFERENCE INTERVAL (CONVENTIONAL UNITS)	REFERENCE INTERVAL (INTERNATIONAL UNITS)
Clonazepam	Serum or plasma (hep or EDTA); trough	Therap: 15–60 ng/mL	48–190 nmol/L
		Toxic: >80 ng/mL	>254 nmol/L
Clonidine	Serum or plasma (hep or EDTA)	Therap: 1.0–2.0 ng/mL	4.4–8.7 nmol/L
Clorazepate	Serum or plasma (hep or EDTA)	As desmethyl-diazepam:	
Cocaine	Serum or plasma (hep or EDTA); on ice	Therap: 0.12–1.0 µg/mL	0.36–3.01 µmol/L
		Therap: 100–500 ng/mL	330–1650 nmol/L
		Toxic: >1000 ng/mL	>3300 nmol/L
Codeine	Serum	Therap: 10–100 ng/mL	33–334 nmol/L
		Toxic: >200 ng/mL	>668 nmol/L
Cyclosporine	Serum (12 h after dose)	Therap: 100–400 ng/mL	83–333 nmol/L
		Toxic: >400 ng/mL	>333 nmol/L
Desipramine	Serum or plasma (hep or EDTA); trough (≥12 h after dose)	Therap: 75–300 ng/mL	281–1125 nmol/L
		Toxic: >400 ng/mL	>1500 nmol/L
Diazepam	Serum or plasma (hep or EDTA); trough	Therap: 100–1000 ng/mL	0.35–3.51 µmol/L
		Toxic: >5000 ng/mL	>17.55 µmol/L
Digitoxin	Serum or plasma (hep or EDTA) ≥6 h after dose	Therap: 20–35 ng/mL	26–46 nmol/L
		Toxic: >45 ng/mL	>59 nmol/L
Digoxin	Serum or plasma (hep or EDTA) trough (≥12 h after dose)	Therap: CHF 0.8–1.5 ng/mL	1.0–1.9 nmol/L
		Arrhythmias: 1.5–2.0 ng/mL	1.9–2.6 nmol/L
		Toxic: >2.5 ng/mL	>3.2 nmol/L
Diphenylhydantoin (see Phenytoin)			
Disopyramide	Serum or plasma (hep or EDTA); trough	Therap: Arrhythmias: Atrial 2.8–3.2 µg/mL	8.3–9.4 µmol/L
		Ventricular 3.3–7.5 µg/mL	9.7–22 µmol/L
		Toxic: >7 µg/mL	>20.7 µmol/L
Doxepin	Serum or plasma (hep or EDTA); through (≥12 h after dose)	Therap: 30–150 ng/mL	107–537 nmol/L
		Toxic: >500 ng/mL	>1790 nmol/L
Ephedrine	Serum	Therap: 0.05–0.10 µg/mL	0.30–0.61 µmol/L
		Toxic: >2 µg/mL	>12.1 µmol/L
Ethchlorvynol	Serum or plasma (hep or EDTA)	Therap: 2–8 µg/mL	14–55 µmol/L
		Toxic: >20 µg/mL	>138 µmol/L
Ethosuximide	Serum or plasma (hep or EDTA); trough	Therap: 40–100 µg/mL	283–708 µmol/L
		Toxic: >150 µg/mL	>1062 µmol/L
Fenoprofen	Plasma (EDTA)	Therap: 20–65 µg/mL	82–268 µmol/L

Drug	Specimen	Level	Conventional	SI
Flecainide	Serum or plasma (hep or EDTA); trough	Therap:	0.2–1.0 µg/mL	0.5–2.4 µmol/L
		Toxic:	>1.0 µg/mL	>2.4 µmol/L
Flurazepam	Serum or plasma (EDTA)	Therap:	not well defined	
		Toxic:	>0.2 µg/mL	>0.5 µmol/L
Furosemide	Serum (30 min after dose)	Therap:	1–2 µg/mL	3–6 µmol/L
Gentamicin	Serum or plasma (EDTA)	Therap:		
		Peak (severe infection)	8–10 µg/mL	16.7–20.9 µmol/L
		Trough (severe infection)	<2–4 µg/mL	<4.2–8.4 µmol/L
		Toxic:		
		Peak	>10 µg/mL	>21 µmol/L
		Trough	>4 µg/mL	>8.4 µmol/L
Glutethimide	Serum	Therap:	2–6 µg/mL	9–28 µmol/L
		Toxic:	>5 µg/mL	>23 µmol/L
Haloperidol	Serum or plasma (hep or EDTA)	Therap:	6–245 ng/mL	16–652 nmol/L
Ibuprofen	Serum or plasma (hep or EDTA)	Toxic:	not defined	
		Therap:	10–50 µg/mL	49–243 µmol/L
Imipramine	Serum or plasma (hep or EDTA); trough (≥12 h after dose)	Toxic:	100–700 µg/mL	485–3395 µmol/L
		Therap:	125–250 ng/mL	446–893 nmol/L
		Toxic:	>500 ng/mL	>1784 nmol/L
Isoniazid	Serum or plasma (hep or EDTA)	Therap:	1–7 µg/mL	7–51 µmol/L
Kanamycin	Serum or plasma (EDTA)	Toxic:	20–710 µg/mL	146–5176 µmol/L
		Therap:		
		Peak	25–35 µg/mL	52–72 µmol/L
		Trough (severe infection)	4–8 µg/mL	8–16 µmol/L
		Toxic:		
		Peak	>35 µg/mL	>72 µmol/L
		Trough	>10 µg/mL	>21 µmol/L
Lidocaine	Serum or plasma (hep or EDTA); ≥45 min following bolus dose	Therap:	1.5–6.0 µg/mL	6.4–26 µmol/L
		Toxic:		
		CNS or cardiovascular depression	6–8 µg/mL	26–34.2 µmol/L
		Seizures, obtundation, decreased cardiac output	>8 µg/mL	>34.2 µmol/L
Lithium	Serum or plasma (hep or EDTA); (>12 h after last dose)	Therap:	0.6–1.2 mEq/L	0.6–1.2 mmol/L
		Toxic:	>2 mEq/L	>2 mmol/L
Lorazepam	Serum or plasma (hep or EDTA)	Therap:	50–240 ng/mL	156–746 nmol/L

(continued)

10-6. LABORATORY REFERENCE VALUES: DRUGS—THERAPEUTIC AND TOXIC*—cont'd

DRUG	SPECIMEN		REFERENCE INTERVAL (CONVENTIONAL UNITS)	REFERENCE INTERVAL (INTERNATIONAL UNITS)
Meperidine	Serum or plasma (hep or EDTA)	Therap:	400–700 ng/mL	1620–2830 nmol/L
		Toxic:	>1 µg/mL	>4043 nmol/L
Meprobamate	Serum	Therap:	6–12 µg/mL	28–55 µmol/L
		Toxic:	>60 µg/mL	>275 µmol/L
Methadone	Serum or plasma (hep or EDTA)	Therap:	100–400 ng/mL	0.32–1.29 µmol/L
		Toxic:	>2000 ng/mL	>6.46 µmol/L
Methaqualone	Serum or plasma (hep or EDTA)	Therap:	2–3 µg/mL	8–12 µmol/L
		Toxic:	>10 µg/mL	>40 µmol/L
Methotrexate	Serum or plasma (hep or EDTA)	Therap:	variable	variable
		Toxic:		
		Low-dose therapy (1–2 wk)		
		High-dose therapy (48 h)	>9.1 ng/mL	>20 nmol/L
Methsuximide (N-desmethyl methsuximide)	Serum	Therap:	>227 ng/mL	>0.5 µmol/L
		Toxic:	10–40 µg/mL	53–212 µmol/L
Methyldopa	Plasma (EDTA)	Therap:	>40 µg/mL	>212 µmol/L
		Toxic:	1–5 µg/mL	4.7–23.7 µmol/L
Methyprylon	Serum	Therap:	>7 µg/mL	>33 µmol/L
		Toxic:	8–10 µg/mL	43–55 µmol/L
Morphine	Serum or plasma (hep or EDTA)	Therap:	>50 µg/mL	>273 µmol/L
		Toxic:	10–80 ng/mL	35–280 nmol/L
N-Acetylprocainamide	Serum or plasma (hep or EDTA); trough	Therap:	>200 ng/mL	>700 nmol/L
		Toxic:	5–30 µg/mL	18–108 µmol/L
Netilmicin	Serum or plasma (EDTA)	Therap:	>40 µg/mL	>144 µmol/L
		Peak (severe infection)	8–10 µg/mL	17–21 µgmol/L
		Trough (severe infection)	<4 µg/mL	<8 µmol/L
		Toxic:		
		Peak	>12 µg/mL	>25 µmol/L
		Trough	>4 µg/mL	>8 µmol/L
Nitroprusside	Serum or plasma (EDTA)	As thiocyanate:		
Nortriptyline	Serum or plasma (hep or EDTA); trough (≥12 h after dose)	Therap:	6–29 µg/mL	103–499 µmol/L
		Toxic:	50–150 ng/mL	190–570 nmol/L
Oxazepam	Serum or plasma (hep or EDTA)	Therap:	>500 ng/mL	>1900 nmol/L
Oxycodone	Serum	Therap:	0.2–1.4 µg/mL	0.70–4.9 µmol/L
		Toxic:	10–100 ng/mL	32–317 nmol/L
			>200 ng/mL	>634 nmol/L
Paraquat	Whole blood (EDTA)	Toxic:	0.1–1.6 µg/mL	0.39–6.2 µmol/L
	Urine	Occur over:	0.2 g/ml	1.17 g/ml

			Conventional units	SI units
		Toxic:	0.9–64 µg/mL	3.50–249 µmol/L
Pentazocine	Serum or plasma (EDTA)	Therap:	0.05–0.2 µg/mL	0.2–0.7 µmol/L
		Toxic:	>1 µg/mL	>3.5 µmol/L
	Urine	Toxic:	>3 µg/mL	>10.5 µmol/L
Pentobarbital	Serum or plasma (hep or EDTA); trough	Therap: Hypnotic	1–5 µg/mL	4–22 µmol/L
		Therap coma	20–50 µg/mL	88–221 µmol/L
		Toxic:	>10 µg/mL	>44 µmol/L
Phenacetin	Plasma (EDTA)	Therap:	1–30 µg/mL	6–167 µmol/L
		Toxic:	50–250 µg/mL	279–1395 µmol/L
Phencyclidine	Serum or plasma (hep or EDTA)	Toxic:	90–800 ng/mL	370–3288 nmol/L
Phenobarbital	Serum or plasma (hep or EDTA); trough	Therap:	15–40 µg/mL	65–170 µmol/L
		Toxic: Slowness, ataxia, nystagmus	35–80 µg/mL	151–345 µmol/L
		Coma with reflexes	65–117 µg/mL	280–504 µmol/L
		Coma without reflexes	>100 µg/mL	>430 µmol/L
Phensuximide (both parent and N-desmethyl metabolites)	Serum or plasma (hep or EDTA)	Therap:	40–60 µg/mL	228–324 µmol/L
Phenylbutazone	Plasma (EDTA)	Therap:	50–100 µg/mL	162–324 µmol/L
		Toxic:	>100 µg/mL	>324 µmol/L
Phenylpropanolamine	Serum	Therap: (not well defined)	0.05–0.10 µg/mL	0.33–0.66 µmol/L
		Toxic:	>5 µg/mL	>33.07 µmol/L
Phenytoin	Serum or plasma (hep or EDTA); trough	Therap:	10–20 µg/mL	40–79 µmol/L
		Toxic:	>20 µg/mL	>79 µmol/L
Primidone	Serum or plasma (hep or EDTA); trough	Therap:	5–12 µg/mL	23–55 µmol/L
		Toxic:	>15 µg/mL	>69 µmol/L
Procainamide	Serum or plasma (hep or) EDTA; trough	Therap:	4–10 µg/mL	17–42 µmol/L
		Toxic:	>10–12 µg/mL	>42–51 µmol/L
		Also consider effect of metabolite, N-acetylprocainamide		
Propoxyphene	Plasma (EDTA)	Therap:	0.1–0.4 µg/mL	0.3–1.2 µmol/L
		Toxic:	>0.5 µg/mL	>1.5 µmol/L
Propranolol	Serum or plasma (hep or EDTA); trough	Therap:	50–100 ng/mL	193–386 nmol/L
Protriptyline	Serum or plasma (hep or EDTA); trough (≥12 h after dose)	Therap:	70–250 ng/mL	266–950 nmol/L
		Toxic:	>500 ng/mL	>1900 nmol/L
Quinidine	Serum or plasma (hep or EDTA); trough	Therap:	2–5 µg/mL	6–15 µmol/L
		Toxic:	>6 µg/mL	>18 µmol/L

(continued)

10-6. LABORATORY REFERENCE VALUES: DRUGS—THERAPEUTIC AND TOXIC*—cont'd

DRUG	SPECIMEN		REFERENCE INTERVAL (CONVENTIONAL UNITS)	REFERENCE INTERVAL (INTERNATIONAL UNITS)
Salicylates	Serum or plasma (hep or EDTA); trough	Therap: Toxic:	150–300 µg/mL >300 µg/mL	1086–2172 µmol/L >2172 µmol/L
Secobarbital	Serum	Therap: Toxic:	1–2 µg/mL >5 µg/mL	4.2–8.4 µmol/L >21.0 µmol/L
Theophylline	Serum or plasma (hep or EDTA)	Therap: Toxic:	8–20 µg/mL >20 µg/mL	44–111 µmol/L >110 µmol/L
Thiocyanate	Serum or plasma (EDTA)	Nonsmoker: Smoker: Therap, after nitroprusside infusion:	1–4 µg/mL 3–12 µg/mL 6–29 µg/mL	17–69 µmol/L 52–206 µmol/L 103–499 µmol/L
	Urine	Nonsmoker: Smoker:	1–4 mg/d 7–17 mg/d	17–69 µmol/L 120–292 µmol/L
Thiopental	Serum or plasma (hep or EDTA); trough	Hypnotic: Coma: Anesthesia: Toxic conc:	1–5 µg/mL 30–100 µg/mL 7–130 µg/mL >10 µg/mL	4.1–20.7 µmol/L 124–413 µmol/L 29–536 µmol/L >41 µmol/L
Thioridazine	Serum or plasma (hep or EDTA)	Therap: Toxic:	1.0–1.5 µg/mL >10 µg/mL	2.7–4.1 µmol/L >27 µmol/L
Tobramycin	Serum or plasma (hep or EDTA)	Therap: Peak (severe infection) Trough (severe infection) Toxic: Peak Trough	 8–10 µg/mL <4 µg/mL >10 µg/mL >4 µg/mL	 17–21 µmol/L <9 µmol/L >21 µmol/L >9 µmol/L
Tocainide	Serum or plasma (hep or EDTA)	Therap:	4–10 µg/mL	21–52 µmol/L
Tolbutamide	Serum	Therap: Toxic:	80–240 µg/mL >640 µg/mL	299–888 µmol/L >2368 µmol/L
Valproic acid	Serum or plasma (hep or EDTA); trough	Therap: Toxic:	50–100 µg/mL >100 µg/mL	347–693 µmol/L >693 µmol/L
Vancomycin	Serum or plasma (hep or EDTA); trough	Therap: Toxic: (not sell established)	5–10 µg/mL >80–100 µg/mL	3–7 µmol/L >55–69 µmol/L
Verapamil	Serum or plasma (hep or EDTA)	Therap:	100–500 ng/mL	220–1100 nmol/L
Warfarin	Serum or plasma (hep or EDTA)	Therap:	1–10 µg/mL	3–32 µmol/L

Section 11: Patient Advocacy and Resources

U.S. Poison Control Center Members of the American Association of Poison Control Centers as of December, 2001

The American Association of Poison Control Centers has established voluntary standards for certified poison centers. The primary goal of the certification process is to ensure that all residents of a given geographic area have access to the highest quality of certified poison center services. Certification criteria include poison information services, regional treatment capabilities, data collection capabilities, and professional and public education programs certification criteria.

ALABAMA
Alabama Poison Center
2503 Phoenix Drive
Tuscaloosa, AL 35405
Emergency Phone: (800) 222-1222

Regional Poison Control Center
Children's Hospital
1600 7th Avenue South
Birmingham, AL 35233
Emergency Phone: (800) 222-1222

ARIZONA
Arizona Poison and Drug Info Center
Arizona Health Sciences Center, Room 1156
1501 North Campbell Avenue
Tucson, AZ 85724
Emergency Phone: (800) 222-1222

Samaritan Regional Poison Center
Good Samaritan Regional Medical Center
1111 E. McDowell–Ancillary 1
Phoenix, AZ 85006
Emergency Phone: (800) 222-1222

ARKANSAS
Arkansas Poison and Drug Information Center
College of Pharmacy, University of
   Arkansas for Medical Sciences
4301 W. Markham, Mail Slot 522
Little Rock, AR 72205
Emergency Phone: (800) 222-1222

CALIFORNIA
California Poison Control System:
California Poison Control System—Fresno/Madera
   Division:
Valley Children's Hospital
9300 Valley Children's Place, MB 15
Madera, CA 93638-8762
Emergency Phone: (800) 222-1222

California Poison Control System—Sacramento
   Division:
UC Davis Medical Center
2315 Stockton Boulevard
Sacramento, CA 95817
Emergency Phone: (800) 222-1222

California Poison Control System—San Diego
   Division:
University of California, San Diego, Medical Center

200 West Arbor Drive
San Diego, CA 92103-8925
Emergency Phone: (800) 222-1222

California Poison Control System—
   San Francisco Division:
UCSF Box 1369
1001 Potrero Avenue, Room 1E86
San Francisco, CA 94143-1369
Emergency Phone: (800) 222-1222

COLORADO
Rocky Mountain Poison and Drug Center
1010 Yosemite Street, Suite 200
Denver, CO 80230-6800
Emergency Phone: (800) 222-1222

CONNECTICUT
Connecticut Poison Control Center
University of Connecticut Health Center
263 Farmington Avenue
Farmington, CT 06030-5365
Emergency Phone: (800) 222-1222

DELAWARE
The Poison Control Center
3535 Market Street, Suite 985
Philadelphia, PA 19104-3309
Emergency Phone: (800) 222-1222

DISTRICT OF COLUMBIA
National Capital Poison Center
3201 New Mexico Ave. NW, Suite 310
Washington, DC 20016
Emergency Phone: (800) 222-1222

FLORIDA
Florida Poison Information Center—Jacksonville
655 West Eighth Street
Jacksonville, FL 32209
Emergency Phone: (800) 222-1222

Florida Poison Information Center—Miami
University of Miami, Dept of Pediatrics
Jackson Memorial Medical Center
P.O. Box 016960 (R-131)
Miami, FL 33101
Emergency Phone: (800) 222-1222

(continued)

Florida Poison Information Center—Tampa
Tampa General Hospital
P.O. Box 1289
Tampa, FL 33601
Emergency Phone: (800) 222-1222

GEORGIA
Georgia Poison Center
Hughes Spalding Children's Hospital,
    Grady Health System
80 Butler Street SE
P.O. Box 26066
Atlanta, GA 30335-3801
Emergency Phone: (800) 222-1222

HAWAII
Hawaii Poison Center
Kapiolani Call Center Services
55 Merchant St., 27th Floor
Honolulu, HI 96813
Emergency Phone: (800) 222-1222

IDAHO
Rocky Mountain Poison and Drug Center
1010 Yosemite Street, Suite 200
Denver, CO 80230-6800
Emergency Phone: (800) 222-1222

ILLINOIS
Illinois Poison Center
222 S. Riverside Plaza, Suite 1900
Chicago, IL 60606
Emergency Phone: (800) 222-1222

INDIANA
Indiana Poison Center
Methodist Hospital, Clarian Health Partners
I-65 at 21st Street
Indianapolis, IN 46206-1367
Emergency Phone: (800) 222-1222

IOWA
Iowa Statewide Poison Control Center
St. Luke's Regional Medical Center
2720 Stone Park Boulevard
Sioux City, IA 51104
Emergency Phone: (800) 222-1222

KANSAS
Mid-America Poison Control Center
University of Kansas Medical Center
3901 Rainbow Blvd., Room B-400
Kansas City, KS 66160-7231
Emergency Phone: (800) 222-1222

KENTUCKY
Kentucky Regional Poison Center
Medical Towers South, Suite 572
234 East Gray Street
Louisville, KY 40202
Emergency Phone: (800) 222-1222

LOUISIANA
Louisiana Drug and Poison Information Center
University of Louisiana at Monroe
College of Pharmacy, Sugar Hall
Monroe, LA 71209-6430
Emergency Phone: (800) 222-1222

MAINE
Maine Poison Center
Maine Medical Center
22 Bramhall Street
Portland, ME 04102
Emergency Phone: (800) 222-1222

MARYLAND
Maryland Poison Center
University of MD at Baltimore School of
    Pharmacy
20 North Pine Street, PH 772
Baltimore, MD 21201
Emergency Phone: (800) 222-1222

National Capital Poison Center
3201 New Mexico Ave. NW, Suite 310
Washington, DC 20016
Emergency Phone: (800) 222-1222

MASSACHUSETTS
Regional Center for Poison Control and
    Prevention Serving Massachusetts and
    Rhode Island
300 Longwood Avenue
Boston, MA 02115
Emergency Phone: (800) 222-1222

MICHIGAN
Children's Hospital of Michigan Regional Poison
    Control Center
4160 John R Harper Professional Office Bldg,
    Ste 616
Detroit, MI 48201
Emergency Phone: (800) 222-1222

DeVos Children's Hospital Regional Poison Center
1300 Michigan NE, Suite 203
Grand Rapids, MI 49503
Emergency Phone: (800) 222-1222

MINNESOTA
Hennepin Regional Poison Center
Hennepin County Medical Center
701 Park Avenue
Minneapolis, MN 55415
Emergency Phone: (800) 222-1222

MISSISSIPPI
Mississippi Regional Poison Control Center
University of Mississippi Medical Center
2500 N. State Street
Jackson, MS 39216
Emergency Phone: (800) 222-1222

MISSOURI
Cardinal Glennon Children's Hospital Regional
    Poison Center
1465 S. Grand Blvd.
St. Louis, MO 63104
Emergency Phone: (800) 222-1222

MONTANA
Rocky Mountain Poison and Drug Center
1010 Yosemite Street, Suite 200
Denver, CO 80230-6800
Emergency Phone: (800) 222-1222

NEBRASKA
The Poison Center
Children's Hospital
8200 Dodge Street
Omaha, NE 68114
Emergency Phone: (800) 222-1222

NEVADA
Oregon Poison Center
Oregon Health Sciences University
3181 SW Sam Jackson Park Road, CB550
Portland, OR 97201
Emergency Phone: (800) 222-1222

Rocky Mountain Poison and Drug Center
1010 Yosemite Street, Suite 200
Denver, CO 80230-6800
Emergency Phone: (800) 222-1222

NEW HAMPSHIRE
New Hampshire Poison Information Center
Dartmouth-Hitchcock Medical Center
One Medical Center Drive
Lebanon, NH 03756
Emergency Phone: (800) 222-1222

NEW JERSEY
New Jersey Poison Information and Education System
201 Lyons Ave.
Newark, NJ 07112
Emergency Phone: (800) 222-1222

NEW MEXICO
New Mexico Poison and Drug Information Center
Health Science Center Library, Room 130
University of New Mexico
Albuquerque, NM 87131-1076
Emergency Phone: (800) 222-1222

NEW YORK
Central New York Poison Center
750 East Adams Street
Syracuse, NY 13210
Emergency Phone: (800) 222-1222

Finger Lakes Regional Poison and Drug
Information Center
University of Rochester Medical Center
601 Elmwood Avenue
PO Box 321
Rochester, NY 14642
Emergency Phone: (800) 222-1222

Long Island Regional Poison and Drug
   Information Center
Winthrop University Hospital
259 First Street
Mineola, NY 11501
Emergency Phone: (800) 222-1222

New York City Poison Control Center
NYC Bureau of Labs
455 First Avenue, Room 123, Box 81
New York, NY 10016
Emergency Phone: (800) 222-1222

Western New York Regional Poison Control Center
Children's Hospital of Buffalo
219 Bryant Street
Buffalo, NY 14222
Emergency Phone: (800) 222-1222

NORTH CAROLINA
Carolinas Poison Center
Carolinas Medical Center
5000 Airport Center Parkway, Suite B
Charlotte, NC 28208
Emergency Phone: (800) 222-1222

NORTH DAKOTA
North Dakota Poison Information Center
Meritcare Medical Center
720 4th Street
North Fargo, ND 58122
Emergency Phone: (800) 222-1222

OHIO
Central Ohio Poison Center
700 Children's Drive, Room L032
Columbus, OH 43205
Emergency Phone: (800) 222-1222

Cincinnati Drug and Poison Information Center
Regional Poison Control System
Vernon Place—3rd Floor
3333 Burnet Avenue
Cincinnati, OH 45229
Emergency Phone: (800) 222-1222

Greater Cleveland Poison Control Center
11100 Euclid Avenue
Cleveland, OH 44106-6010
Emergency Phone: (800) 222-1222

OKLAHOMA
Oklahoma Poison Control Center
Children's Hospital at OU Medical Center
940 N.E. 13th Street, Room 3510
Oklahoma City, OK 73104
Emergency Phone: (800) 222-1222

OREGON
Oregon Poison Center
Oregon Health Sciences University
3181 SW Sam Jackson Park Road, CB550
Portland, OR 97201
Emergency Phone: (800) 222-1222

PENNSYLVANIA
Central Pennsylvania Poison Center
Pennsylvania State University, The Milton S. Hershey
   Medical Center
500 University Drive, MC H043
PO Box 850
Hershey, PA 17033-0850
Emergency Phone: (800) 222-1222

Pittsburgh Poison Center
Children's Hospital of Pittsburgh
3705 Fifth Avenue
Pittsburgh, PA 15213
Emergency Phone: (800) 222-1222

The Poison Control Center
3535 Market Street, Suite 985
Philadelphia, PA 19104-3309
Emergency Phone: (800) 222-1222

(continued)

RHODE ISLAND
Regional Center for Poison Control and Prevention
  Serving Massachusetts and Rhode Island
300 Longwood Avenue
Boston, MA 02115
Emergency Phone: (800) 222-1222

SOUTH CAROLINA
Palmetto Poison Center
College of Pharmacy, University of South Carolina
Columbia, SC 29208
Emergency Phone: (800) 222-1222

SOUTH DAKOTA
Hennepin Regional Poison Center
Hennepin County Medical Center
701 Park Avenue
Minneapolis, MN 55415
Emergency Phone: (800) 222-1222

TENNESSEE
Middle Tennessee Poison Center
501 Oxford House
1161 21st Avenue South
Nashville, TN 37232-4632
Emergency Phone: (800) 222-1222

Southern Poison Center
University of Tennessee
875 Monroe Avenue, Suite 104
Memphis, TN 38163
Emergency Phone: (800) 222-1222

TEXAS
Central Texas Poison Center
Scott and White Memorial Hospital
2401 South 31st Street
Temple, TX 76508
Emergency Phone: (800) 222-1222

North Texas Poison Center
Texas Poison Center Network
Parkland Health and Hospital System
5201 Harry Hines Blvd., P.O. Box 35926
Dallas, TX 75235
Emergency Phone: (800) 222-1222

South Texas Poison Center
The Univ. of Texas Health Science Center—San Antonio
Department of Surgery, Mail Code 7849
7703 Floyd Curl Drive
San Antonio, TX 78229-3900
Emergency Phone: (800) 222-1222

Southeast Texas Poison Center
The University of Texas Medical Branch
3.112 Trauma Building
Galveston, TX 77555-1175
Emergency Phone: (800) 222-1222

Texas Panhandle Poison Center
1501 S. Coulter
Amarillo, TX 79106
Emergency Phone: (800) 222-1222

West Texas Regional Poison Center
Thomason Hospital

4815 Alameda Avenue
El Paso, TX 79905
Emergency Phone: (800) 222-1222

UTAH
Utah Poison Control Center
410 Chipeta Way, Suite 230
Salt Lake City, UT 84108
Emergency Phone: (800) 222-1222

VERMONT
Maine Poison Center
Maine Medical Center
22 Bramhall Street
Portland, ME 04102
Emergency Phone: (800) 222-1222

VIRGINIA
Blue Ridge Poison Center
University of Virginia Health System
PO Box 800774
Charlottesville, VA 22908-0774
Emergency Phone: (800) 222-1222

National Capital Poison Center
3201 New Mexico Ave. NW, Suite 310
Washington, DC 20016
Emergency Phone: (800) 222-1222

Virginia Poison Center
Medical College of Virginia Hospitals
Virginia Commonwealth University,
  P.O. Box 980522
Richmond, VA 23298-0522
Emergency Phone: (800) 222-1222

WASHINGTON
Washington Poison Center
155 NE 100th Street, Suite 400
Seattle, WA 98125-8012
Emergency Phone: (800) 222-1222

WEST VIRGINIA
West Virginia Poison Center
3110 MacCorkle Ave, S.E.
Charleston, WV 25304
Emergency Phone: (800) 222-1222

WISCONSIN
Children's Hospital of Wisconsin Poison Center
PO Box 1997, Mail Station 677A
Milwaukee, WI 53201-1997
Emergency Phone: (800) 222-1222

WYOMING
The Poison Center
Children's Hospital
8200 Dodge Street
Omaha, NE 68114
Emergency Phone: (800) 222-1222

ANIMAL POISON CONTROL
ASPCA Animal Poison Control Center
1717 South Philo Road, Suite 36
Urbana, IL 61302
Emergency Phone: (888) 426-4435;
(900) 680-0000

Patient Education is a serious responsibility for health care professionals. Many health care facilities develop their own patient teaching materials. There are also groups, associations, businesses, and agencies that develop patient education materials for dissemination to the public. There are many tools that can be used to improve an individual's knowledge about a particular health care problem or issue. These include, but are not limited to, pamphlets, movies, videotapes, audiotapes, newsletters, and computerized instruction. Information can also be supplied to the health care professional to develop materials. The names and addresses identified below are potential sources of information that have provided information for the *Miller-Keane Encyclopedia and Dictionary of Medicine, Nursing, and Allied Health.* Local chapters of national organizations may also be found in the telephone directory and may serve as valuable resources for patient education material. Encyclopedias and directories of health related associations are an additional source of information or contacts.

Alcoholics Anonymous
PO Box 549, Grand Central Station
New York, NY 10163
Phone: 212-870-3400
FAX: 212-870-3003
WEB Site: http://www.alcoholics-anonymous.org
Alcoholics Anonymous is a fellowship of sober alcoholics; no dues or fees; self-supporting, no outside funds; unaffiliated; primary purpose: carry the A.A. message to alcoholic who still suffers.

Alzheimer's Disease Education and Referral Center (ADEAR)
PO Box 8250
Silver Spring, MD 20907-8250
Phone: 800-438-4380
FAX: 301-495-3334
WEB Site: http://www.alzheimers.org
Provides information about Alzheimer's disease, its symptoms and diagnosis, and about Alzheimer's disease research supported by the National Institute on Aging. Offers a newsletter to health professionals and other free publications to the public. Information specialists will answer questions about Alzheimer's disease by e-mail at adear@alzheimers.org

Alzheimer Society of Canada
20 Eglinton Avenue, W., Ste. 1200
Toronto, ON M4R 1K8
Phone: 416-488-8772
Toll-Free: 800-616-8816 (valid in Canada only)
FAX: 416-488-3778
E-mail: info@alzheimer.ca
WEB Site: http://www.alzheimer.ca
A national voluntary organization whose goals are to provide information and support to those affected by Alzheimer disease and their families, to increase public awareness of Alzheimer disease, and to search for a cause and a cure.

American Association for Homecare
625 Slaters Lane, Suite 200
Alexandria, VA 22314-1171
Phone: 703-836-6263
FAX: 703-836-6730
WEB Site: http://www.aahomecare.org
The American Association of Homecare (AAHomecare) is the unified voice that represents all the elements of home care under one roof—from home medical equipment and respiratory therapy to home health services and from re/hab technology to infusion therapy. AAHomecare is dedicated to working to advance the value and practice of quality health care services at home.

American Council of the Blind
1155 15th Street NW, Suite 720
Washington, DC 20005
Phone: 202-467-5081, 800-424-8666
FAX: 202-467-5085
WEB Site: http://www.acb.org
The American Council of the Blind is a national membership organization established to promote independence, dignity, and well-being of blind and visually impaired people. Services provided include a monthly magazine, the Braille Forum, subscriptions to which are available free of charge to individuals in the US in Braille, large print, cassettes, and 3.5 DOS diskettes, and many other services.

American Dietetic Association
216 West Jackson Blvd.
Chicago, IL 60606
Phone: 312-899-0040
Toll Free: 800-366-1655 (Consumer Hot Line)
WEB Site: http://www.eatright.org
The American Dietetic Association (ADA) promotes the optimal health, nutrition, and well-being of the public. The National Center for Nutrition and Dietetics maintains a consumer nutrition hotline that provides information and referrals to registered dietitians throughout the country.

The Amyotrophic Lateral Sclerosis (ALS) Association
The ALS Association National Office
27001 Agoura Road, Suite 150
Calabasas Hills, CA 91301-5104
Information and Referral Service: 800-782-4747
All Others: 818-880-9007
WEB Site: http://www.alsa.org
The mission of the ALS Association is to discover the cause and cure for amyotrophic lateral sclerosis (Lou Gehrig's disease) through dedicated research while providing patient support, information/education for health care professionals and the general public, and advocacy for ALS research and health care concerns.

Association of Community Cancer Centers
1600 Nebel Street, Suite 201
Rockville, MD 20852
Phone: 301-984-9496
FAX: 301-770-1949
WEB Site: http://www.accc-cancer.org

(continued)

The mission of the Association of Community Cancer Centers is to promote the continuum of quality cancer care (research, prevention, screening, early detection, diagnosis, treatment, psychosocial services, rehabilitation, hospice) for patients with cancer and the community.

Asthma and Allergy Foundation of America (AAFA)

1233 20th Street NW, Suite 402
Washington, DC 20036
Phone: 202-466-7943
FAX: 202-466-8940
WEB Site: http://www.aafa.org
AAFA has been in existence for over forty years and is a registered not-for-profit patient education organization dedicated to finding a cure for and controlling asthma and allergic diseases.

Bulimia Anorexia Nervosa Association (BANA)

300 Cabana Road East
Windsor, ON N9G 1A3
Phone: 519-969-2112
FAX: 519-969-0227
E-mail: info@bana.ca
WEB Site: http://www.bana.ca
The objectives of BANA are to eradicate eating disorders; to promote healthy eating and acceptance of diverse body shapes; and to provide clinical, preventive, and advocacy services for persons affected by eating disorders.

Canada Safety Council

1020 Thomas Spratt Place
Ottawa, ON K1G 5L5
Phone: 613-739-1535
FAX: 613-739-1566
E-mail: csc@safety-council.org
WEB Site: http://www.safety-council.org
The Canada Safety Council is Canada's national not-for-profit safety organization. Its mission is to be a leader in the effort to reduce preventable deaths, injuries, and economic loss in the traffic, work, home, community, and leisure environments.

Canadian Cystic Fibrosis Foundation

2221 Yonge Street, Suite 601
Toronto, ON M4S 2B4
Phone: 416-485-9149
Toll free (from Canada only): 800-378-2233
FAX: 416-485-0960
WEB Site: http://www.cysticfibrosis.ca
The purpose and objectives of the Canadian Cystic Fibrosis Foundation are to aid those afflicted with cystic fibrosis; to conduct research into improved care and treatment and to seek a cure or control for cystic fibrosis; to promote public awareness through the dissemination of information using all forms of communication; and to raise funds and allocate same for the above purposes.

Canadian Hard of Hearing Association (CHHA)

2435 Holly Lane, Suite 205
Ottawa, ON K1V 7P2
Voice Phone: 613-526-1584
TTY: 613-526-2692
Toll Free: 800-263-8068
FAX: 613-526-4718
WEB Site: http://www.chha.ca
The Canadian Hard of Hearing Association is the "voice" of hard of hearing Canada. CHHA is the only Canadian, national, non-profit consumer organization run by and for hard of hearing people. CHHA exists to help the hard of hearing achieve independent, productive, and fulfilling lives.

Canadian Mental Health Association – National

2160 Yonge Street, Third Floor
Toronto, ON M4S 2Z3
Phone: 416-484-7750
FAX: 416-484-4617
WEB Site: http://www.cmha.ca
The Canadian Mental Health Association is a national voluntary association that exists to promote the mental health of people. CMHA's mission is operationalized through education, advocacy, research, service provision, and facilitation.

Canadian National Institute for the Blind (CNIB)

1929 Bayview Avenue
Toronto, ON M4G 3E8
Phone: 416-486-2500
WEB Site: http://www.icomm.ca/cnib/
E-mail: cnib@icomm.ca
CNIB is the world's largest provider of services to people with visual impairments, and a global leader in adaptive and assistive technologies.

Cancer Care, Inc.

275 Seventh Avenue
New York, NY 10001
Phone: 800-813-HOPE
WEB Site: http://www.cancercare.org
Offers information, referral, individual and group counseling, and patient education free of charge.

Centers for Disease Control and Prevention (CDC)

1600 Clifton Road, NE
Atlanta, GA 30333
Phone: 800-311-3435
WEB Site: http://www.cdc.gov
Provides information on diseases, health risks, prevention guidelines, and strategies. A wide variety of services can be accessed through the CDC.

Clinical Reference Systems, Ltd.

335 Interlocken Parkway
Broomfield, CO 80021
Phone: 800-237-8401
FAX: 303-460-6282
WEB Site: http://www.patienteducation.com
Contact: Sales Department
Software designed to generate patient education handouts in Windows and Web-based formats in a wide variety of areas. Editing of topics and customizing of handouts is a feature.

Combined Health Information Data Base (CHID)
7830 Old Georgetown Road
Bethesda, MD 20814
WEB Site: http://chid.nih.gov
CHID is a cooperative effort among several Federal agencies of the United States government. These agencies have combined their information files into one database which has been available to the public since 1985. Topics are updated four times per year.

Crohn's and Colitis Foundation of Canada (CCFC)
60 St. Clair Avenue East, Suite 600
Toronto, ON M4T 1N5
Phone: 416-920-5035
Toll Free: 800-387-1479 (Canada only)
FAX: 416-929-0364
WEB Site: http://www.ccfc.ca
The Crohn's and Colitis Foundation of Canada (CCFC) is a national not-for-profit voluntary foundation dedicated to finding the cure for Crohn's disease and ulcerative colitis. To realize this the Foundation is committed to raising increasing funds for research. The CCFC also believes that it is important to make all individuals with inflammatory bowel disease aware of the Foundation, and to educate these individuals, their families, health professionals, and the general public.

Cystic Fibrosis Foundation
6931 Arlington Road
Bethesda, MD 20814
Phone: 301-951-4422
Toll Free: 800-344-4823
FAX: 301-951-6378
WEB Site: http://www.cff.org
E-mail: info@cff.org
The Cystic Fibrosis Foundation was established in 1955 to raise money to fund research to find a cure for cystic fibrosis and to improve the quality of life for the 30,000 children and adults with the disease.

Endometriosis Association
International Headquarters
8585 N. 76th Place
Milwaukee, WI 53223
Phone: 414-355-2200
FAX: 414-355-6065
Toll Free: 800-992-3636
WEB Site: http://www.endometriosisassn.org
The Endometriosis Association is a self-help organization dedicated to offering support and information to women with endometriosis, educating the public and medical community about the disease, and promoting and conducting research related to endometriosis.

The Epilepsy Foundation of America
4321 Garden City Drive
Landover, MD 20785
Phone: 301-459-3700
Toll Free: 800-EFA-1000
WEB Site: http://www.efa.org
The Epilepsy Foundation of America is the national organization that works for people affected by seizures, through research, education, advocacy, and service.

International Federation on Aging (IFA)
380 Rue Saint-Antoine Ouest, Bureau 3200
Montreal, PQ H2Y 3X7
Phone: 514-287-9679
WEB Site: http://www.ifa-fiv.org
IFA serves as an advocate for the well-being of older persons around the world. IFA is committed to providing a worldwide forum on aging issues and concerns and to fostering the development of associations and agencies that serve or represent older persons.

La Leche League Canada
Box 29, 18C Industrial Drive
Chesterville, ON K0C 1H0
Phone: 613-448-1842
FAX: 613-448-1845
WEB Site: http://www.lalecheleaguecanada.ca
La Leche League Canada promotes a better understanding of breastfeeding as an important element in the healthy development of the baby, and through education, information, encouragement, and mother-to-mother support helps mothers nationwide to breastfeed. The main objective of La Leche League Canada is to help mothers breastfeed their babies.

Learning Disabilities Association of America
4156 Library Road
Pittsburgh, PA 15234
Phone: 412-341-1515
FAX: 412-344-0224
WEB Site: http://www.ldanatl.org
E-mail: info@ldaamerica.org
LDA is an information and referral organization. They provide any and all information regarding learning disabilities in both children and adults. There are 500 chapters across the country. Once individuals make contact with LDA, they provide a free packet of material, then refer them on to one of their chapters. Membership is also offered.

National Asian Pacific Center on Aging
1511 Third Avenue, Suite 914
Seattle, WA 98121
Phone: 206-624-1221
FAX: 206-624-1023
WEB Site: http://www.napca.org
The National Asian Pacific Center on Aging (NAPCA) is the leading advocacy organization committed to the well-being of elderly Asians and Pacific Islanders in America. NAPCA develops and administers programs to enhance the dignity and quality of life of its constituents. NAPCA provides a fax-on-demand service for over 300 pamphlets, brochures, fact sheets, etc. in 15 languages on topics related to health, wellness, social services, and related topics. FAX-IT can be reached by dialing 206-624-0185 from any FAX machine (telephone handset).

National Association for Visually Handicapped
22 West 21st Street
New York, NY 10010
Phone: 212-255-2804
FAX: 212-727-2931
WEB Site: http://www.navh.org

(continued)

To promote hope, dignity, and productivity for those with uncorrectable visual impairments by encouraging the full use of residual vision through large print, visual aids, emotional support, educational outreach, advocacy, and referral services.

National Cancer Institute Information Associates Program
9300 Old Georgetown Road
Bethesda, MD 20814-1519
Phone: 301-496-7600
Toll Free: 800-624-7890
Provides access to the National Cancer Institute's information resources for health professionals, including the journal of the National Cancer Institute.

National Clearinghouse for Alcohol and Drug Information (NCADI)
11426 Rockville Pike, Suite 200
Rockville, MD 20852-3007
Phone: 800-729-6686
TDD: 800-487-4889
FAX: 301-468-6433
WEB Site: http://www.health.org
A service of the U.S. Center for Substance Abuse Prevention, NCADI collects and distributes information about alcohol, tobacco, and other drugs to all interested persons. The Clearinghouse provides a wide variety of free printed material; also videotapes and disk-based products for a small cost-recovery fee.

National Clearinghouse on Child Abuse and Neglect Information
PO Box 1182
Washington, DC 20013-1182
Phone: 800-394-3366
FAX: 703-385-3206
WEB Site: http://www.calib.com/nccanch
The Clearinghouse collects, catalogues, stores, organizes, and disseminates information on all aspects of child maltreatment.

National Committee for the Prevention of Elder Abuse
101 Vermont Avenue NW, Suite 1001
Washington, DC 20002
Phone: 202-682-4140
FAX: 202-682-3984 (fax)
WEB Site: http://www.preventelderabuse.org
The National Committee for the Prevention of Elder Abuse was established to promote greater understanding of elder abuse and the development of services to protect older persons and disabled adults and reduce the likelihood of their being abused, neglected, and/or exploited.

National Council on Alcoholism and Drug Dependence, Inc.
21 Exchange Place, Suite 2902
New York, NY 10005
Phone: 212-269-7797
WEB Site: http://www.ncadd.org

The National Council on Alcoholism and Drug Dependence, Inc. provides education, information, help, and hope in the fight against the chronic and often fatal disease of alcoholism, and other drug addictions. Founded in 1944, NCADD, with its nationwide network of affiliates, advocates prevention, intervention, and treatment, and is committed to ridding the disease of its stigma and its sufferers of their denial and shame.

National Health Council
1730 M Street NW, Suite 500
Washington, DC 20036
Phone: 202-785-3910
FAX: 202-785-5923
WEB Site: http://www.nationalhealthcouncil.org
E-mail: info@nationalhealthcouncil.org
The National Health Council is a private, nonprofit association of national organizations which was founded in 1920 as a clearinghouse and cooperative effort for voluntary health agencies (VHAs).

The National Institute of Nutrition (NIN)
265 Carling Avenue, Suite 302
Ottawa, ON K1S 2E11
Phone: 613-235-3355
WEB Site: http://www.nin.ca
Founded in 1983, NIN is a private, nonprofit national organization dedicated to bridging the gap between the science and practice of nutrition and serving as a credible source of information on nutrition. The NIN also conducts and supports nutrition research.

National Wellness Institute
1300 College Court
PO Box 827
Stevens Point, WI 54481-0827
Phone: 715-342-2969
FAX: 715-342-2979
WEB Site: http://www.nationalwellness.org
The National Wellness Institute has served professionals interested in wellness and health promotion since 1977. It focuses on professional education programs; resources and information dissemination through its professional association, the National Wellness Association; and the development and distribution of lifestyle inventories and health risk appraisals.

The Nemours Foundation
The Alfred I. duPont Institute
1600 Rockland Road
Wilmington, DE 19803
WEB Site: http://www.kidshealth.org
Maintains a very informative site on the World Wide Web known as Kidshealth.

Osteoporosis Society of Canada
33 Laird Drive
Toronto, ON M5S 3A7
Phone: 416-696-2817
Toll Free (Canada only): 800-463-6842
WEB Site: http://www.osteoporosis.ca

Educates and empowers individuals and communities in the prevention and treatment of osteoporosis. They are a resource for patients, health professionals, the media, and the general public who seek medically accurate information on the causes, prevention, and treatment of osteoporosis.

Pregnancy and Infant Loss Center
1421 East Wayzata Boulevard #30
Wayzata, MN 55391
WEB Site: http://www.pilc.org
A national nonprofit organization, founded in 1983, providing support, resources, and education on miscarriage, stillbirth, and infant death.

Pregnancy and Infant Loss Support, Inc. (SHARE)
National Office:
St. Joseph Health Center
300 First Capitol Drive
St. Charles, MO 63301
Phone: 800-821-6819
FAX: 314-947-7486
WEB Site: http://www.nationalshareoffice.com
SHARE offers support to families and caregivers whose lives have been touched by the tragic death of a baby through miscarriage, stillbirth, or newborn death by providing information, education, and a network of support groups across the country.

Recording for the Blind and Dyslexic (RFB & D)
20 Roszel Road
Princeton, NJ 08540
Phone: 609-452-0606
Toll Free: 800-221-4792
WEB Site: http://www.rfbd.org
RFB & D maintains the world's largest collection of professional resources and textbooks on audiotape for all academic levels. It serves people who cannot read standard print because of a visual, perceptual, or other physical disability.

SIECUS (Sexuality Information and Education Council of the United States)
Publication Department
130 West 42nd Street, Suite 350
New York, NY 10036-7802
Phone: 212-819-9770
WEB Site: http://www.siecus.org
SIECUS affirms that sexuality is a natural and healthy part of living. SIECUS develops, collects, and disseminates information, promotes comprehensive education about sexuality, and advocates the right of individuals to make responsible sexual choices.

Students Against Drunk Driving (SADD)
255 Main Street
PO Box 800
Marlboro, MA 01752
Phone: 877-SADD-INC
FAX: 508-481-5759
WEB Site: http://www.saddonline.com
To provide young people with the tools to address the problems of underage drinking, impaired driving, drug use, and their consequences.

UNOS United Network for Organ Sharing
1100 Boulders Parkway, Suite 500
Richmond, VA 23225
Phone: 804-330-8500
WEB Site: http://www.unos.org
UNOS, under contract with the U.S. Department of Health and Human Services, is a nonprofit organization that administers the National Organ Procurement and Transplantation Network (OPTN) and the U.S. Scientific Registry of Organ Transplant Recipients mandated by Congress. It operates and maintains the national list of patients waiting for solid organ transplants. In addition, it maintains a computer assisted system for allocating organs to individuals on the waiting list. The primary goal of the UNOS organization is to increase the number of donated organs. Through a number of strategies, including public and professional education, UNOS endeavors to bridge the gap between the number of individuals waiting for transplant and the number of organs donated. Information about organ donation and transplantation is available from UNOS 24 hours a day, 365 days a year.

Toll-Free and other patient advocacy lines offering a variety of services to patients and health care professionals are listed below. Please verify that the number remains correct before sharing this information with patients. The Johns Hopkins School of Medicine, Division of Biomedical Information Sciences maintains a frequently updated list on the World Wide Web that can be reached at: http://infonet.welch.jhu.edu/advocacy.html

Adoption
800-TOADOPT National Adoption Center

Advocacy
201-625-7101 American Self-Help Clearinghouse
800-846-7444 Center for Patient Advocacy
800-48-FRIEND The Friends' Health Connection
407-253-9048 Med Help International
800-440-6877 California Nurses Association
888-460-4673 Patient Advocates of Texas
888-CAL-COUNCIL California Consumer Health
  Care Council

Aging
800-424-3410 American Association of Retired
  Persons
850-216-2727 Coalition to Protect America's Elders
800-677-1116 Elder Care Locator Service
800-638-6833 Medicare Telephone Hotline
800-222-3937 National Eye Care Project
800-222-2225 National Institute on Aging Information
  Center
800-223-9994 National Osteoporosis Foundation
800-772-1213 Social Security Administration

AIDS
800-458-5231 x2038 CDC National AIDS
  Clearinghouse
800-342-AIDS National AIDS Hotline
800-669-0696 AIDS Education at Work
800-673-8538 National Association of People with
  AIDS

Air Medical Transportation
(or Medical Transport)
800-296-1191 Mercy Medical Airlift
800-296-1217 National Patient Air Transport Helpline
703-361-1792 Children's Air Transport for Life

Alcohol
800-622-2255 National Council on Alcoholism
800-344-2666 Al-Anon, Alateen Family Group Hotline
800-527-5344 American Council on Alcoholism
800-729-6686 National Clearinghouse for Alcohol
  and Drug Information

Allergy
800-822-2762 American Academy of Allergy,
  Asthma, and Immunology
800-727-8462 Asthma and Allergy Foundation of
  America

Alzheimer's
800-272-3900 Alzheimer's Association
800-438-4380 Alzheimer's Disease Education and
  Referral Center
800-477-2243 French Foundation for Alzheimer's
  Research

Amyotrophic Lateral Sclerosis (ALS)
800-782-4747 Amyotrophic Lateral Sclerosis
Association

Anorexia/Bulimia
847-831-3438 National Association of Anorexia
  Nervosa and Associated Disorders

Arthritis
800-283-7800 Arthritis Foundation
800-327-3027 Arthritis Consulting Services
614-881-5601 The Road Back Foundation

Asthma
800-822-2762 American Academy of Allergy,
  Asthma, and Immunology
800-LUNG-USA American Lung Association
800-727-8462 Asthma and Allergy Foundation of
  America

Ataxia
800-5-HELP-AT Ataxia Telangiectasia Childrens
  Project
612-473-7666 National Ataxia Foundation

Attention Deficit Disorder
800-223-4050 Children and Adults with Attention
  Deficit Disorder (CHADD)

Back Pain
800-247-2225 Back Pain Hotline

Behcet's Disease
800-7BEHCETS American Behcet's Disease
  Association

Biliary Atresia
718-987-6200 Biliary Atresia and Liver Transplant
  Network

Birth Defects
888-663-4637 March of Dimes Birth Defects
  Foundation
800-221-6827 National Easter Seal Society

Blind/Vision Impaired
800-683-5555 Foundation Fighting Blindness
800-424-8666 National Alliance of Blind Students
800-232-5463 American Foundation for the Blind
800-562-6265 National Association of Parents of
  Visually Impaired
800-334-5497 National Center for Vision and Aging
800-548-4337 Guide Dog Foundation for the Blind
800-424-8567 National Library Services for the
  Blind and Physically Handicapped

Brain Aneurysms
617-723-3870 Brain Aneurysm Foundation

Brain Tumors
800-886-2282 American Brain Tumor Association
800-934-CURE National Brain Tumor Foundation

Breast Cancer (see also Cancer)
412-422-BCIS Breast Cancer Information Service
10-955-4851 Johns Hopkins Breast Center

212-719-0154 National Alliance of Breast Cancer
Organizations (NABCO)
202-296-7477 National Breast Cancer Coalition
212-719-0364 SHARE
800-IM-AWARE The Susan G. Komen Breast Cancer
Foundation
800-221-2141 Y-ME Breast Cancer Organization
(24hrs: 312-986-8228)

Breastfeeding
800-LA-LECHE La Leche League International

Burn Injuries
800-888-BURN The Phoenix Society

**Cancer (see also Breast Cancer, Cervical
Cancer, Lung Cancer)**
510-204-4286 Alta Bates-Herrick Breast Cancer Risk
Counseling
800-525-3777 AMC Information and Counseling Line
800-ACS-2345 American Cancer Society
800-433-0464 Bloch National Cancer Hot Line
800-4-CANCER Cancer Information Service
800-843-8114 American Institute for Cancer Research
301-984-9496 The Association of Community Cancer
Centers
800-813-HOPE Cancer Care
800-366-2223 Candlelighters Childhood Cancer
Foundation
800-55-CHEMO CHEMOcare
800-ICARE-61 The International Cancer Alliance, Inc.
800-452-CURE International Myeloma Foundation
800-955-4787 Lower Eastern Shore (Del-Mar-Va)
Cancer Support Group
800-4-CANCER National Cancer Institute
301-650-8868 National Coalition for Cancer
Survivorship
301-496-7403 NCI's CancerFax
616-453-1477 Patient Advocates for Advanced Cancer
Treatment
800-808-7866 US TOO International
(Prostate Cancer/BPH)
818-508-5657 Vital Options
671-354-9888 Women's Community Cancer Project

Cerebral Palsy
800-872-5827 United Cerebral Palsy Associations

Cervical Cancer (see also Cancer)
800-685-5531 National Cervical Cancer Coalition
(NCCC)

Children
800-433-9016 American Academy of Pediatrics
800-422-4453 Child Help USA
800-787-KIDS Children's Rights Council
888-835-5669 Family Voices
800-872-5437 Missing Children Help Center
800-843-5678 National Center for Missing and
Exploited Children
800-394-3366 National Clearinghouse on Child Abuse
and Neglect
800-695-0285 National Information Center for
Children and Youth with Disabilities
800-422-4453 National Child Abuse Hotline
800-892-5455 Kidsrights
800-222-2000 National Council on Child Abuse and
Family Violence

847-256-8525 Child and Adolescent Bipolar
Foundation

Chronic Fatigue Syndrome
800-442-3437 CFIDS

Chronic Illness
800-838-0879 Well Spouse Foundation
888-751-REST Rest Ministries, Inc.

Chronic Pain
800-616-PAIN North American Chronic Pain
Association of Canada
916-632-0922 American Chronic Pain Association
888-751-REST Rest Ministries, Inc.

Cleft Palate
800-242-5338 National Cleft Palate Association

Cocaine
800-262-2463 National Cocaine Hotline
800-347-8998 Cocaine Anonymous

Crohn's/Colitis
800-343-3637 Crohn's and Colitis Foundation of
America

Cystic Fibrosis
800-344-4823 Cystic Fibrosis Foundation

Depression
800-826-3632 National Depressive and Manic-
Depressive Association (DMDA)
212-241-8924 DMDA of Mount Sinai, NY
800-248-4344 National Foundation for Depressive
Illness
410-955-4647 Depression and Related Affective
Disorders Association
516-829-0091 National Alliance for Research on
Schizophrenia and Depression
212-533-6374 Mood Disorders Support Group/NY
800-789-CMHS National Mental Health Services
Knowledge Exchange Network

Diabetes
800-338-DMED American Association of Diabetes
Educators
800-DIABETES American Diabetes Association
800-232-3472 American Diabetes Foundation

Disabilities
800-344-5405 ABLEDATA
407-880-9232 American Association of Disabled
Persons
888-835-5669 Family Voices
800-835-1043 Institute of Logopedics
800-333-6293 National Center for Youth with
Disabilities
800-922-9234 National Information Clearinghouse for
Infants with Disabilities
800-248-2253 National Organization on Disability
800-346-2742 National Rehabilitation Information
Center
800-962-9629 National Spinal Cord Injury Association
800-526-3456 National Spinal Cord Injury Hotline
800-426-2133 National Support Center for Persons
with Disabilities

(continued)

Disease Control
800-810-4000 Compliance Control Center

Divorce
800-733-DADS National Congress for Men and Children
800-457-6962 Mothers without Custody
800-637-7974 Parents without Partners

Down Syndrome
800-221-4602 National Down Syndrome Society
800-232-6372 National Down Syndrome Congress
216-621-5858 The Baker Center

Drug Abuse
800-729-6686 National Clearinghouse for Alcohol and Drug Information
800-666-3332 Office of National Drug Control Policy Clearinghouse on Drugs and Crime
800-662-4357 CSAT's National Drug and Alcohol Treatment Routing Service
800-667-7433 National Parents' Resource Institute for Drug Education
800-258-2766 Just Say No International

Ehlers-Danlos Syndrome
213-651-3038 Ehlers-Danlos National Foundation

Emphysema
800-LUNG-USA American Lung Association
888-996-COPD Emphysema Foundation For Our Right To Survive

Encephalitis
408-298-2060 National Encephalitis Foundation

Endometriosis
800-992-3636 Endometriosis Association
800-239-7280 Endometriosis Research Center

Epilepsy
800-332-1000 Epilepsy Foundation of America
800-642-0500 Epilepsy Information Service

Fibromyalgia
714-921-0150 National Fibromyalgia Awareness Campaign

Glaucoma
800-826-6693 Glaucoma Research Foundation

Guillain-Barré Syndrome
610-667-0131 Guillain-Barré Syndrome Foundation International

Gulf War Syndrome
202-628-2700 x162 National Gulf War Resource Center, Inc.

Headache
800-255-ACHE American Council for Headache Education
800-843-2256 National Headache Foundation
800-245-0088 New England Headache Treatment Program

Head/Brain Injury
703-236-6000 Brain Injury Association
905-641-8877 Ontario Brain Injury Association

914-883-6532 Forget-Me-Not
206-621-8558 Head Injury Hotline

Health Information
800-336-4797 National Health Information Center (U.S. DHHS)

Hearing/Communication Handicaps
800-327-9355 Better Hearing Institute
800-638-8255 American Speech Language Hearing Association
800-535-3323 Deafness Research Foundation
800-521-5247 Hearing Aid Helpline
800-241-1044 (TTY, 800-241-1055) National Institute on Deafness and Other Communication Disorders [NIDCD] Clearinghouse

Heart Disease
800-242-8721 American Heart Association

Hemolytic Uremic Syndrome
516-673-3017 Lois Joy Galler Foundation

Hemophilia
800-424-2634 National Hemophilia Foundation

Hepatitis
800-223-0179 American Liver Foundation Hepatitis Foundation
800-891-0707 Hepatitis Foundation International
215-884-8786 Hepatitis B Foundation
800-324-7305 Hepatitis C Foundation
612-647-9009 Hepatitis B Coalition

Hereditary Hemorrhagic Telangiectasia
800-448-6389 HHT Foundation

Hospice Care (see also Terminal Illness)
800-854-3402 Hospice Foundation of America
800-331-1620 Hospicelink
616-866-9127 Hospice Patients Alliance, Inc.
800-658-8898 National Hospice Organization

Huntington's Disease
800-345-4372 Huntington's Disease Society

Immune Deficiencies (see also AIDS)
800-296-4433 Immune Deficiency Foundation
800-598-4668 American Autoimmune Related Diseases Association

Impotence
800-835-7667 Recovery of Male Potency
800-843-4315 Impotence Information Center
800-669-1603 Impotence Institute of America
800-867-7042 Impotency Information sponsored by Pharmacia & Upjohn, Inc.

Incontinence
800-237-4666 Simon Foundation
800-252-3337 National Association for Continence

Interstitial Cystitis
301-610-5308 Interstitial Cystitis Association

Kidney Disease/Failure
800-749-2257 American Association of Kidney Patients

626-917-9803 American Coalition of Kidney Patients, Inc.
800-638-8299 American Kidney Fund
800-622-9010 National Kidney Foundation

Liver Disease (see also Hepatitis)
800-GO LIVER American Liver Foundation
718-987-6200 Biliary Atresia and Liver Transplant Network
800-563-5483 Canadian Liver Foundation

Lung Cancer (see also Cancer)
800-298-2436 Alliance for Lung Cancer Advocacy Support and Education (ALCASE)
800-LUNG-USA American Lung Association

Lung Diseases (see also Emphysema)
800-LUNG-USA American Lung Association
206-781-5680 Pulmonary Fibrosis Association
800-748-72PH Pulmonary Hypertension Association

Lupus
800-558-0121 Lupus Foundation
800-558-0121 American Lupus Society
727-821-7489 Lupus Foundation of America, Inc., Greater FL Chapter

Lymphedema Network
800-541-3259 National Lymphedema Network

Marfan Syndrome
800-8MARFAN National Marfan Foundation
905-826-3223 Canadian Marfan Association

Medical Transport (or Air Medical Transportation)
800-296-1191 Mercy Medical Airlift
800-296-1217 National Patient Air Transport Helpline
703-361-1792 Children's Air Transport for Life

Mental Health (see also Depression, Schizophrenia)
800-447-4474 Mental Health InfoSource
207-799-6750 Creative Health Foundation
800-950-NAMI National Alliance for the Mentally Ill
800-969-6642 National Mental Health Association
800-789-CMHS National Mental Health Services Knowledge Exchange Network

Mental Retardation
817-261-6003 The Arc of the United States

Moebius Syndrome
914-834-2933 Moebius Syndrome Foundation

Multiple Sclerosis
800-441-7055 Multiple Sclerosis Foundation, Inc.
800-FIGHT-MS National Multiple Sclerosis Society

Muscular Dystrophy
800-572-1717 Muscular Dystrophy Association

Myasthenia Gravis Foundation
800-541-5454 Myasthenia Gravis Foundation

Narcolepsy
800-829-1933 Narcolepsy and Sleep Disorders
513-891-3522 Narcolepsy Network, Inc.

612-721-6321 YAWN - Young Americans With Narcolepsy
954-452-2030 Sleep Disorders Movements, Inc.

Organ Transplantation
818-781-1006 American Share Foundation
888-222-2690 Second Wind Lung Transplant Association
800-TRIO-386 Transplant Recipients International Organization, Inc.
718-597-5619 Manhattan Chapter
718-987-6200 Biliary Atresia and Liver Transplant Network
800-528-2971 The Living Bank

Ostomy
800-826-0826 United Ostomy Association

Paralysis
800-225-0292 American Paralysis Association
800-962-9629 National Spinal Cord Injury Association
800-526-3456 National Spinal Cord Injury Hotline

Parkinson's Disease
800-233-2732 American Parkinson Disease Association
800-327-4545 National Parkinson Foundation
800-344-7872 Parkinson's Educational Program

Patients' Rights
781-769-5720 New England Patients' Rights Group, Inc.

Personal Hygiene
800-810-4000 Compliance Control Center

Pituitary Diseases
800-642-9211 Pituitary Tumor Network Association

Polio
314-534-0475 International Polio Network

Porphyria
713-266-9617 American Porphyria Foundation

Premenstrual Syndrome
800-222-4767 PMS Access

Prenatal Care
800-504-7081 National Hispanic Prenatal Hotline
800-673-8444 Healthy Mothers, Healthy Babies Coalition
800-433-5523 Be Healthy, Inc.

Progressive Supranuclear Palsy
800-457-4777 Society for Progressive Supranuclear Palsy

Prostatitis
309-664-6222 Prostatitis Foundation

Psoriasis
800-723-9166 National Psoriasis Foundation

Rare Diseases
800-999-6673 National Organization for Rare Disorders

(continued)

Schizophrenia (see also Depression, Mental Health)
800-847-3802 American Schizophrenia Association
516-829-0091 National Alliance for Research on Schizophrenia and Depression
847-256-8525 Child and Adolescent Bipolar Foundation

Scleroderma
800-422-1113 Scleroderma Federation
800-722-4673 United Scleroderma Foundation
  301-782-4979 Southern Maryland Chapter
800-441-CURE Scleroderma Research Foundation

Scoliosis
800-673-6922 National Scoliosis Foundation, Inc.

Sexually Transmitted Diseases
800-227-8922 National STD Hotline

Sickle Cell Disease
800-421-8453 National Association for Sickle Cell Disease, Inc.

Social Work
800-638-8799 National Association of Social Workers

Spina Bifida
800-621-3141 Spina Bifida Association

Spinal Cord Injuries
800-962-9629 National Spinal Cord Injury Association
  708-352-6223 Illinois Chapter
800-526-3456 National Spinal Cord Injury Hotline

Spinal Muscular Atrophy
800-886-1762 Families of Spinal Muscular Atrophy

Stroke
800-553-6321 Courage Stroke Network
800-787-6537 National Stroke Association

Stuttering
800-221-2483 National Center for Stuttering

Tay-Sachs Disease
800-906-8723 National Tay-Sachs and Allied Diseases Association

Terminal Illness (see also Hospice Care)
800-989-WILL Choice in Dying
800-854-3402 Hospice Foundation of America
800-331-1620 Hospicelink
616-866-9127 Hospice Patients Alliance, Inc.
800-658-8898 National Hospice Organization
800-741-9465 National Viatical Association

Thalassemia
800-522-7222 Thalassemia Action Group

Thyroid Disease
888-996-4460 American Foundation of Thyroid Patients
800-832-8321 Thyroid Foundation of America, Inc.
888-595-2131 The Kelly G. Ripken Program

Tourette Syndrome
800-237-0717 Tourette Syndrome Association

Wilson's Disease
800-399-0266 Wilson's Disease Association

Women's Health
310-410-9886 Findings: The Women's Health Care Advocacy Service
202-628-7814 National Women's Health Network
800-354-8824 National Women's Resource Center

Xeroderma Pigmentosum
518-851-2612 Xeroderma Pigmentosum Society, Inc.

Section 12: Professional Groups and Boards

12-1. PROFESSIONAL ORGANIZATIONS, ASSOCIATIONS, AND ACADEMIES

There are myriad groups that provide the opportunity for health care providers to explore common issues, propose solutions to health care problems, and provide a forum for the discussion of interests. Listed below are selected groups of health care providers that are potential sources of information, specialized knowledge, and expertise. The links to additional groups can be found on the Miller-Keane Web Site.

Advanced Medical Technology Association (AdvaMed)
1200 G Street NW, Suite 400
Washington, DC 20005-3814
Web Site: http://www.advamed.org

Alliance for Cardiovascular Professionals
4546 Corporation Lane #164
Virginia Beach, VA 23462
Web Site: http://www.acp-online.org

American Academy of Ambulatory Nursing Administration
N. Woodbury Rd., Box 56
Pitman, NJ 08071
Web Site: http://www.aaacn.org

American Academy of Medical Administrators
701 Lee Street, Suite 600
Des Plaines, IL 60016-4516
Web Site: http://www.aameda.org

American Academy of Nurse Practitioners
PO Box 12846
Austin, TX 78711
Web Site: http://www.aanp.org

The American Assembly for Men in Nursing
11 Cornell Road
Latham, NY 12110-1499
Web Site: http://people.delphiforums.com/brucewilson

American Association of Blood Banks
8101 Glenbrook Rd.
Bethesda, MD 20814
Web Site: http://www.aabb.org

American Association for Continuity of Care
P.O. Box 532
Dunedin, FL 34697
Web Site: http://www.continuityofcare.com

American Association of Critical-Care Nurses
101 Columbia
Aliso Viejo, CA 92656
Web Site: http://www.aacn.org

American Association for the History of Nursing, Inc.
Post Office Box 175
Lanoka Harbor, NJ 08734
Web Site: http://www.aahn.org

American Association of Medical Assistants
20 N. Wacker Dr., Suite 1575
Chicago, IL 60606-2309
Web Site: http://www.aama-ntl.org

American Association of Neuroscience Nurses
4700 W. Lake Avenue
Glenview, IL 60025
Web Site: http://www.aann.org

American Association of Nurse Anesthetists
222 S. Prospect Ave.
Park Ridge, IL 60068
Web Site: http://www.aana.com

American Association of Occupational Health Nurses, Inc.
2920 Brandywine Road, Suite 100
Atlanta, GA 30341
Web Site: http://www.aaohn.org

American Association of Office Nurses
109 Kinderkamack Road
Montvale, NJ 07645
Web Site: http://www.aaon.org

American Association for Respiratory Care
11030 Ables Lane
Dallas, TX 75229
Web Site: http://www.aarc.org

American Association of Spinal Cord Injury Nurses
75-20 Astoria Blvd.
Jackson Heights, NY 11370-1178
Web Site: http://www.aascin.org

American Clinical Laboratory Association
1250 H St. NW, Suite 880
Washington, DC 20005
Web Site: http://www.clinical-labs.org

(continued)

American College of Healthcare Executives
1 N. Franklin St., Suite 1700
Chicago, IL 60606-3491
Web Site: http://www.ache.org

American College of Nurse-Midwives
818 Connecticut Ave. NW, Suite 900
Washington DC 20006
Web Site: http://www.acnm.org

American Dental Association
211 E. Chicago Ave.
Chicago, IL 60611
Web Site: http://www.ada.org

American Dental Hygienists Association
444 N. Michigan Ave.
Chicago, IL 60611
Web Site: http://www.adha.org

American Dietetic Association
216 W. Jackson Blvd.
Chicago, IL 60606
Web Site: http://www.eatright.org

American Holistic Nurses' Association
PO Box 2131
Flagstaff, AZ 86003
Web Site: http://www.ahna.org

American Medical Association
515 N. State Street
Chicago, IL 60610
Web Site: http://www.ama-assn.org

American Nephrology Nurses' Association
E. Holly Avenue, Box 56
Pitman, NJ 08071
Web Site: http://anna.inurse.com

American Nurses Association
600 Maryland Ave. SW, Suite 100W
Washington, DC 20024
Web Site: http://www.nursingworld.org

American Nurses' Foundation
600 Maryland Ave. SW
Washington, DC 20024
Web Site: http://www.nursingwolrd.org/anf

American Occupational Therapy Association
4720 Montgomery Lane - P.O. Box 31220
Bethesda, MD 20824-1220
Web Site: http://www.aota.org

American Organization of Nurse Executives
American Hospital Association
One N. Franklin St.
Chicago, IL 60606
Web Site: http://www.aone.org

American Pharmaceutical Association
2215 Constitution Ave. NW
Washington, DC 20037
Web Site: http://www.aphanet.org

American Physical Therapy Association
111 N. Fairfax St.
Alexandria, VA 22314-1488
Web Site: http://www.apta.org

American Psychiatric Nurses' Association
Colonial Place Three, 2107 Wilson Blvd, Suite 300-A
Arlington, VA 22201
Web Site: http://www.apna.org

American Public Health Association
800 I Street NW
Washington, DC 20001
Web Site: http://www.apha.org

American Radiological Nurses Association
7794 Grow Drive
Pensacola, FL 32514
Web Site: http://www.rsna.org

American Registry of Radiologic Technologists
1255 Northland Dr.
Mendota Heights, MN 55120
Web Site: http://www.arrt.org

American Society of Health-System Pharmacists
7272 Wisconsin Avenue
Bethesda, MD 20814
Web Site: http://www.ashp.org

American Society for Hospital Risk Management
1 N. Franklin St.
Chicago, IL 60606
Web Site: http://www.ashrm.org

American Society of Ophthalmic Registered Nurses, Inc.
PO Box 193030
San Francisco, CA 94119
Web Site: http://webeye.ophth.uiowa.edu/asorn/

American Society of Perianesthesia Nurses
10 Melrose Avenue, Suite 110
Cherry Hill, NJ 08003-3696
Web Site: http://www.aspan.org

American Society of Plastic and Reconstructive Surgical Nurses, Inc.
P.O. Box 56
Pitman, NJ 08071
Web Site: http://www.aspsn.org

American Thoracic Society
1740 Broadway
New York, NY 10019-4374
Web Site: http://www.thoracic.org

Association for the Care of Children's Health
19 Mantua Road
Mt. Royal, NJ 08061
Web Site: http://www.eparent.com/resources/
associations/childreshealthassoc.htm

Association of Nurses in AIDS Care
80 S. Summit St.
500 Courtyard Square
Akron, OH 44308
Web Site: http://www.anacnet.org

Association of Operating Room Nurses
2170 S. Parker Road, Suite 300
Denver, CO 80231
Web Site: http://www.aorn.org

Association of Pediatric Oncology Nurses
4700 W. Lake Avenue
Glenview, IL 60025
Web Site: http://www.apon.org

**Association for Practitioners in Infection
Control and Epidemiology**
1275 K Street NW, Suite 1000
Washington, DC 20005-4006
Web Site: http://www.apic.org

Association of Rehabilitation Nurses
4700 W. Lake Avenue
Glenview, IL 60025
Web Site: http://www.rehabnurse.org

**Association of Women's Health,
Obstetric and Neonatal Nurses**
2000 L Street NW, Suite 740
Washington, DC 20036
Web Site: http://www.awhonn.org

**Commission of Graduates of Foreign
Nursing Schools (CGFNS)**
3600 Market St., Suite 400
Philadelphia, PA 19104-2651
Web Site: http://www.cgfns.org

Dermatology Nurses Association
East Holly Avenue, Box 56
Pitman, NJ 08071
Web Site: http://dna.inurse.com

Emergency Nurses Association
915 Lee Street
Des Plaines, IL 60016-6569
Web Site: http://www.ena.org

**Federation of Nurses and Health
Professionals**
159 Wolf Road, Box 15008
Albany, NY 12212-5008
Web Site: http://www.nysut.org/fnhp

**Healthcare Financial Management
Association**
Two Westbrook Corporate Center, Suite 700
Westchester, IL 60154-5700
Web Site: http://www.hfma.org

Hospice and Palliative Nurses Association
Penn Center West One, Suite 229
Pittsburgh, PA 15276
Web Site: http://www.hpna.org

Infusion Nurses Society, Inc.
220 Norwood Park South
Norwood, MA 02062
Web Site: http://www.ins1.org

International Nurses Society on Addictions
P.O. Box 10752
Raleigh, NC 27605
Web Site: http://www.intnsa.org

**National Association of Directors of
Nursing Administration in Long
Term Care**
10101 Alliance Road., #140
Cincinnati, OH 45242
Web Site: http://www.nadona.org

**National Association for Health Care
Recruitment**
P.O. Box 531107
Orlando, FL 32853-1107
Web Site: http://www.nahcr.com

National Association of Hispanic Nurses
1501 16th St. NW
Washington, DC 20036
Web Site: http://www.thehispanicnurses.org

National Association of Home Care (NAHC)
228 Seventh Street SE
Washington, DC 20003
Web Site: http://www.nahc.org

National Association of Neonatal Nurses
4700 W. Lake Avenue
Glenview, IL 60025
Web Site: http://www.nann.org

**National Association of Nurse Practitioners
in Reproductive Health (NANPRH)**
503 Capitol Court NE, Suite 300
Washington, D.C. 20002
Web Site: http://www.npwh.org

**National Association of Orthopaedic
Nurses, Inc.**
Box 56
Pitman, NJ 08071
Web Site: http://naon.inurse.com

**National Association of Pediatric Nurse
Associates and Practitioners**
1101 Kings Hwy., Suite 206
Cherry Hill, NJ 08034
Web Site: http://napnap.org

National Association of School Nurses, Inc.
PO Box 1300
Scarborough, ME 04074
Web Site: http://www.nasn.org

National Black Nurses Association, Inc.
8630 Fenton Street, Suite 330
Silver Spring, MD 20910-3803
Web Site: http://www.nbna.org

(continued)

National Board for Respiratory Care
8310 Nieman Road
Lenexa, KS 66214
Web Site: http://www.nbrc.org

National Center for Health Education
375 Hudson Street
New York, NY 10014

National Consortium of Chemical Dependency Nurses
1733 H Street, Suite 330 PMB 1214
Blaine, WA 98230

National Council of State Boards of Nursing, Inc.
676 N. St. Clair, Suite 550
Chicago, IL 60611-2921
Web Site: http://www.ncsbn.org

National Gerontological Nursing Association
7794 Grow Drive
Pensacola, FL 32514
Web Site: http://www.ngna.org

National League for Nursing
61 Broadway
New York, NY 10006
Web Site: http://www.nln.org

National Nurses in Business Association (NNBA)
PO Box 561081
Rockledge, FL 32956-1081
Web Site: http://www.nnba.net

National Student Nurses' Association
45 Main Street, Suite 606
Brooklyn, NY 11201
Web Site: http://www.nsna.org

North American Nursing Diagnosis Association
1211 Locust St.
Philadelphia, PA 19107
Web Site: http://www.nanda.org

Oncology Nursing Society
501 Holiday Dr.
Pittsburgh, PA 15220
Web Site: http://www.ons.org

Operating Room Nurses Association of Canada
14453 29A Avenue
White Rock, BC V4A 9K8
Web Site: http://www.ornac.ca

Respiratory Nursing Society
c/o NYSNA
11 Cornell Road
Latham, NY 12110
Web Site: http://www.respiratorynursingsociety.org

Sigma Theta Tau International Honor Society of Nursing
550 W. North St.
Indianapolis, IN 46202
Web Site: http://www.nursingsociety.org

Society of Gastroenterology Nurses and Associates, Inc.
401 North Michigan Avenue
Chicago, IL 60611-4267
Web Site: http://www.sgna.org

Society of Otorhinolaryngology and Head/Neck Nurses
116 Canal St., Suite A
New Smyrna Beach, FL 32169
Web Site: http://www.sohnnurse.com

Society for Public Health Education
750 First Street NE, Suite 910
Washington, DC 20002-4242
Web Site: http://www.sophe.org

Society of Urologic Nurses and Associates
East Holly Avenue, Box 56
Pitman, NJ 08071-0056
Web Site: http://suna.inurse.com/

Transcultural Nursing Society
Department of Nursing, Madonna College
36600 Schoolcroft Road
Livonia, MI 48150
Web Site: http://www.tcns.org

Wound Ostomy and Continence Nurses Society (WOCN)
4700 W. Lake Ave.
Glenview, IL 60025
Web Site: http://www.wocn.org

Alabama State Nurses' Association
Karen L. Pakkala, MSN, RN CAE,
  Executive Director
360 North Hull Street
Montgomery, AL 36104-3658
Phone (334) 262-8321
Fax (334) 262-8578
E-mail: alabamasna@mindspring.com
  or: arenp.asna@mindspring.com
  www.nursingworld.org/snas/al
*Office Hours: 8:00am–4:00pm Central Time

Alaska Nurses Association
Camille Soleil, JD, RN, Executive Director
2207 East Tudor Road, Suite 34
Anchorage, AK 99507-1069
Phone (907) 274-0827
Fax (907) 272-0292
E-mail: aknurse@aknurse.org
  or: csoleil@aknurse.org
  www.aknurse.org
*Office Hours: 8.00am–4.30pm Alaska Time

Arizona Nurses Association
Marla Weston, RN, MS, Executive Director
1850 E. Southern Ave., Suite #1
Tempe, AZ 85282
Phone (480) 831-0404
Fax (480) 839-4780
E-mail: info@aznurse.org
  or: marla@aznurse.org
  www.aznurse.org
*Office Hours: 8:30am–4:30pm Mountain Time

Arkansas Nurses Association
David Eubanks, MSN, RN, Chief Staff Officer
804 N. University
Little Rock, AR 72205
Phone (501) 664-5853
Fax (501) 664-5859
E-mail: arna@prodigy.net
  or: deubanks@arna.org
  www.arna.org
*Office Hours: 8:00am–4:30pm Central Time

ANA\California
Tricia Hunter, RN, Executive Administrator
1121 L Street, Suite 409
Sacramento, CA 95814
Phone (916) 447-0225
Fax (916) 447-5568
E-mail: anacalif@pacbell.net
  www.anacalifornia.org
*Office Hours: 9:00am–5:00pm Pacific Time

Colorado Nurses Association
Paula Stearns, MSN, RN, Executive Director
5453 East Evans Place
Denver, CO 80222
Phone (303) 757-7483
Fax (303) 757-8833
E-mail: cna@nurses-co.org
  or: pstearnsrn@aol.com
  www.nurses-co.org
*Office Hours: 8.30am–4:30pm Mountain Time

Connecticut Nurses Association
Polly T. Barey, MS, RN, Executive Director
Meritech Business Park
377 Research Parkway, Suite 2D
Meriden, CT 06450
Phone (203) 238-1207
Fax (203) 238-3437
E-mail: polly@ctnurses.org
  www.ctnurses.org
*Office Hours: 9:00am–5:00pm Eastern Time

Delaware Nurses Association
Ruth Bashford, MN, RN, Executive Director
2644 Capitol Trail, Suite 330
Newark, DE 19711
Phone (302) 368-2333
Fax (302) 366-1775
E-mail: delnurse@erols.com
  www.nursingworld.org/snas/de
*Office Hours: 9:00am–4:00pm Eastern Time

District of Columbia Nurses Association, Inc.
Tom Wachter, Acting Executive Director
5100 Wisconsin Ave. NW, Suite 306
Washington, DC 20016
Phone (202) 244-2705
Fax (202) 362-8285
E-mail: dcnurses1@aol.com
  dcnaonline.com
*Office Hours: 9:00am–5:00pm Eastern Time

Federal Nurses Association (FedNA)
Contact: Pamela C. Hagan, MSN, RN,
  Chief Programs Officer
600 Maryland Avenue SW, Suite 100W
Washington, DC 20024
Phone (202) 651-7333
Fax (202) 651-7355
E-mail: FedNA@ana.org
  www.nursingworld.org/FedNA
*Office Hours: 9:00am–4:30pm Eastern Time

Florida Nurses Association
Paula Massey, MN, RN, Executive Director
P.O. Box 536985
Orlando, FL 32853-6985
Phone (407) 896-3261
Fax (407) 896-9042
E-mail: info@floridanurse.org
  or: pmassey@floridanurse.org
  www.floridanurse.org
*Office Hours: 8:30am–4:30pm Eastern Time

Georgia Nurses Association
Deborah Hackman, Chief Executive Officer
3032 Briarcliff Road NE
Atlanta, GA 30329-2655
Phone (404) 325-5536
Fax (404) 325-0407
E-mail: gna-ceo@mindspring.com
  www.georgianurses.org
*Office Hours: 8:00am–4:30pm Eastern Time

(continued)

Guam Nurses Association
Glynis S. Almonte, BSN, RN, Executive Director
P.O. Box CG
Hagatna, GU 96932
Tel/Fax (671) 477-6877
E-mail: guamnurse@ite.net
*Office Hours: 11:00am–1:00pm Pacific Time

Hawaii Nurses Association
Christi Keliipio, MSN, RN, Executive Director
677 Ala Moana Boulevard, Suite 301
Honolulu, HI 96813
Phone (808) 531-1628
Fax (808) 524-2760
E-mail: christi@hawaiinurses.org
www.hawaiinurses.org
*Office Hours: 8:00am–4:30pm Hawaiian Time

Idaho Nurses Association
Judy Murray, PhD, RN, Executive Director
200 North 4th Street, Suite 20
Boise, ID 83702-6001
Phone (208) 345-0500
Fax (208) 385-0166
E-mail: idahonursesassn@hotmail.com
or: jmurray@boisestate.edu
www.nursingworld.org/snas/id
*Office Hours: 9:00am–5:30pm Mountain Time

Illinois Nurses Association
Cathy Holmgren, RN, MBA, Executive Director
105 West Adams Street, Suite 2101
Chicago, IL 60603
Phone (312) 419-2900 ext. 226
Fax (312) 419-2920
E-mail: cholmgren@illinoisnurses.com
www.illinoisnurses.com
*Office Hours: 9:00am–5:00pm Central Time

Indiana State Nurses Association
Ernest C. Klein, Jr., RN, CAE, Executive Director
2915 North High School Road
Indianapolis, IN 46224
Phone (317) 299-4575
Fax (317) 297-3525
E-mail: info@indiananurses.org
or: klein@indiananurses.org
www.indiananurses.org
*Office Hours: 8:30am–4:30pm Eastern Time

Iowa Nurses Association
Linda Goeldner, MA, MA, CHE, CAE,
Executive Director
1501 42nd Street, Suite 471
West Des Moines, IA 50266
Phone (515) 225-0495
Fax (515) 225-2201
E-mail: iowanurses@aol.com
or: lkgoeld@aol.com
www.iowanurses.org
*Office Hours: 8:30am–4:00pm Central Time

Kansas State Nurses Association
Terri R. Roberts, JD, RN, Executive Director
1208 S.W. Tyler
Topeka, KS 66612-1735
Phone (785) 233-8638
Fax (785) 233-5222

E-mail: troberts@echo.sound.net
www.nursingworld.org/snas/ks
*Office Hours: 8:00am–4:30pm Central Time

Kentucky Nurses Association
Maureen Keenen, JD, Interim Executive Director
1400 South First Street
P.O. Box 2616
Louisville, KY 40201-2616
Phone (502) 637-2546/2547
Fax (502) 637-8236
E-mail: mkeenan@kentucky-nurses.org
www.kentucky-nurses.org
*Office Hours: 8:00am–4:30pm Eastern Time

Louisiana State Nurses Association
Tawna Pounders, MNSc, RN, Executive Director
5700 Florida Blvd., Suite 720
Baton Rouge, LA 70806
Phone (225) 201-0993
Phone (800) 457-6378
Fax (225) 201-0971
E-mail: lsna@lsna.org
or: tpounders@lsna.org
www.lsna.org
*Office Hours: 9:00am–4:00pm Central Time

ANA-MAINE
Executive Director, ANA-MAINE
P.O. Box 254
Auburn, ME 04212-0254
(207) 667-0260
E-mail: josephn@acadia.net
www.anamaine.org

Maryland Nurses Association
Kathryn V. Hall, MS, RN, CNAA, Executive Director
Airport Square 21, Ste. 255
849 International Drive
Linthicum, MD 21090
Phone (410) 859-3000
Fax (410) 859-3001
E-mail: marylandnursesassociation@erols.com
www.nursingworld.org/snas/md
*Office Hours: 8:30am–4:30pm Eastern Time

**Massachusetts Association of Registered
Nurses**
Executive Director
Massachusetts Association of Registered Nurses, Inc.
P.O. Box 70668, Quinsigamond Village Station
345 Greenwood Street
Worcester, MA 01607
Phone (781) 344-6926
Fax (781) 341-8495 (Please call first)
E-mail: info@marnonline.org
www.nursingworld.org/snas/ma

Michigan Nurses Association
Dorothea Milbrandt, MSN, RN, Interim
Executive Director
2310 Jolly Oak Road
Okemos, MI 48864-4599
Phone (517) 349-5640, ext. 14
Fax (517) 349-5818
E-mail: dorothea.milbrandt@minurses.org
www.minurses.org
*Office Hours: 9:00am–5:00pm Eastern Time

Minnesota Nurses Association
Erin Murphy, RN, Executive Director
1625 Energy Park Drive
St. Paul, MN 55108
Phone (651) 646-4807 ext. 152 or (800) 536-4662
Fax (651) 647-5301
E-mail: emurphy@mnnurses.org
    www.mnnurses.org
*Office Hours: 8:15am–4:30pm Central Time

Mississippi Nurses Association
Betty R. Dickson, Executive Director
31 Woodgreen Place
Madison, MS 39110
Phone (601) 898-0670
Fax (601) 898-0190
E-mail: mna@msnurses.org
    or: bdickson@netdoor.com
    www.msnurses.org
*Office Hours: 8:00am–4:30pm Central Time

Missouri Nurses Association
Belinda Heimericks, MSN, RN, Executive Director
1904 Bubba Lane, P.O. Box 105228
Jefferson City, MO 65110-5228
1-888-662-MONA (toll-free)
Phone (573) 636-4623
Fax (573) 636-9576
E-mail: belinda@missourinurses.org
    www.missourinurses.org
*Office Hours: 8:00am–5:00pm Central Time

Montana Nurses Association
Sami Butler, RN, Executive Director
104 Broadway, Suite G-2
Helena, MT 59601
Phone (406) 442-6710
Fax (406) 442-1841
E-mail: info@mtnurses.org
    or: sbutler@mtnurses.org
    www.nursingworld.org/snas/mt
*Office Hours: 8:30am–4:30pm Mountain Time

Nebraska Nurses Association
Chuck Stepanek, BS, Executive Director
715 South 14th Street
Lincoln, NE 68508
Phone (402) 475-3859
Fax (402) 475-3961
E-mail: ne.nurses@prodigy.net
    www.nursingworld.org/snas/ne/index.htm
*Office Hours: 8:00am–4:30pm Central Time

Nevada Nurses Association
Richard Schlegel, CAE, Executive Director
P.O. Box 530399
Henderson, NV 89053-0399
Phone (702) 260-7886
Fax (702) 260-7052
E-mail: nvnurses@aol.com
    or: schlegelra@aol.com
    www.nvnurses.org
*Office Hours: 9:00am–5:00pm Pacific Time

New Hampshire Nurses Association
Robert Best, BSE, MPA, Executive Director
48 West Street

Concord, NH 03301-3595
Phone (603) 225-3783
Fax (603) 228-6672
E-mail: nh_nurses@compuserve.com
    www.nhnurses.myassociation.com
*Office Hours: 9:00am–5:00pm Eastern Time

New Jersey State Nurses Association
Andrea Aughenbaugh, RN, CS, CAE,
    Chief Executive Officer
1479 Pennington Road
Trenton, NJ 08618-2661
Phone (609) 883-5335 ext. 10
Fax (609) 883-5343
E-mail: njsna@njsna.org
    or: andrea@njsna.org
    www.njsna.org
*Office Hours: 8:30am–4:30pm Eastern Time

New Mexico Nurses Association
Carrie Roberts, MSN, RN, CNP, Executive Director
P.O. Box 80300
Albuquerque, NM 87198
Phone (505) 268-7744
Fax (505) 268-7711
E-mail: nmnurses@hotmail.com
    www.nursingworld.org/snas/nm
Federal Express Delivery Only:
303 Washington SE
Albuquerque, NM 87108
*Office Hours: 8:00am–5:00pm Mountain Time

New York State Nurses Association
Martha L. Orr, MN, RN, CAE, Executive Director
11 Cornell Road
Latham, NY 12110
Phone (518) 782-9400 ext. 279
Fax (518) 782-9530
E-mail: martha.orr@nysna.org
    www.nysna.org
*Office Hours: 8:30am–5:00pm Eastern Time

North Carolina Nurses Association
Sindy Barker, CAE, Executive Director
103 Enterprise Street, Box 12025
Raleigh, NC 27605
Phone (919) 821-4250
Fax (919) 829-5807
E-mail: rns@ncnurses.org
    or: sindybarker@ncnurses.org
    www.ncnurses.org
*Office Hours: 8:30am–4:30pm Eastern Time

North Dakota Nurses Association
Sharon Moos, MBA, RN, Executive Administrator
531 Airport Road, Suite D
Bismarck, ND 58504-6107
Phone (701) 223-1385
Fax (701) 223-0575
E-mail: ndna@prodigy.net
*Office Hours: 8:30am–4:30pm Central Time

Ohio Nurses Association
Gingy Harshey-Meade, MSN, RN, CNAA,
    Chief Executive Officer
4000 East Main Street
Columbus, OH 43213-2983

(continued)

Phone (614) 237-5414 ext. 1020
Fax (614) 237-6081
E-mail: gharsheymeade@ohnurses.org
  or: gingy@insight.rr.com
  www.ohnurses.org
*Office Hours: 8:30am–4:30pm Eastern Time

Oklahoma Nurses Association
Jane Nelson, Executive Director
6414 North Santa Fe, Suite A
Oklahoma City, OK 73116
Phone (405) 840-3476
Fax (405) 840-3013
E-mail: ona.ed@oknurses.com
  www.oknurses.com
*Office Hours: 8:30am–5:00pm Central Time

Oregon Nurses Association
Susan E. King, MS, RN, Administrator for
  Professional Services
Ken Fitzsimon, JD, Administrator of Labor Relations
Sandy Marron, MBA, Administrator of
  Business Services
18765 SW Boones Ferry Road
Tualatin, OR 97062
Phone (503) 293-0011
Fax (503) 293-0013
E-mail: ona@oregonrn.org
  www.oregonrn.org
*Office Hours: 8:30am–5:00pm Pacific Time

Pennsylvania State Nurses Association
Michele P. Campbell, MSN, RN, Executive
  Administrator
P.O. Box 68525
Harrisburg, PA 17106-8525
Phone (717) 657-1222 or (888)-707-7762
Fax (717) 657-3796
E-mail: psna@psna.org
  or: mcampbell@psna.org
  www.psna.org
*Office Hours: 8:30am–4:30pm Eastern Time

Rhode Island State Nurses Association
Pamela L. McCue, MSN, RN, Executive Director
550 S. Water Street, Unit 540B
Providence, RI 02903-4344
Phone (401) 421-9703
Fax (401) 421-6793
E-mail: risna@prodigy.net
  www.risnarn.org
*Office Hours: Monday–Thursday 10:00am–3:30pm
  Eastern Time

South Carolina Nurses Association
Judith C. Thompson, Executive Director
1821 Gadsden Street
Columbia, SC 29201
Phone (803) 252-4781
Fax (803) 779-3870
E-mail: scna@prodigy.net
  or: judith.thompson@prodigy.net
  www.scnurses.org
*Office Hours: 8:30am–4:30pm Eastern Time

South Dakota Nurses Association
Ed Jacobson, Executive Director
P.O. Box 1015

Pierre SD 57501-1015
Phone (605) 945-4265
Fax (605) 945-4266
E-mail: sdnurse1@dtgnet.com
  www.nursingworld.org/snas/sd
*Office Hours: 8:00am–3:00pm Central Time

Tennessee Nurses Association
Louise Browning, CAE, Executive Director
545 Mainstream Drive, Suite 405
Nashville, TN 37228-1201
Phone (615) 254-0350
Fax (615) 254-0303
E-mail: lbrowntna@aol.com
  or: lbrowning@tnaonline.org
  www.tnaonline.org
*Office Hours: 8:30am–5:00pm Central Time

Texas Nurses Association
Clair B. Jordan, MSN, RN, Executive Director
7600 Burnet Road, Suite 440
Austin, TX 78757-1292
Phone (512) 452-0645
Fax (512) 452-0648
E-mail: memberinfo@texasnurses.org
  or: cjordan@texasnurses.org
  www.texasnurses.org
*Office hours: 8:00am–5:00pm Central Time

Utah Nurses Association
William D. Sartain, Executive Director
3761 S. 700 East, #201
Salt Lake City, UT 84106
Phone (801) 293-8351
Fax (801) 293-8458
E-mail: una@xmission.com
  www.utahnurses.org
*Office Hours: 9:00am–5:00pm Mountain Time

Vermont State Nurses Association
Margaret M. Sharpe, RN, BSN, Executive Director
100 Dorset Street, Suite 13
South Burlington, VT 05403-6241
Phone (802) 651-8886
Fax (802) 651-8998
E-mail: vtnurse@prodigy.net
  www.uvm.edu/~vsna
*Office Hours: Monday–Thursday 9:00am–3:00pm
  Eastern Time

Virgin Islands State Nurses Association
Verna Christian-Garcia, BSN, RN, Executive Director
P.O. Box 583
Christiansted, St. Croix
U.S. Virgin Islands 00821-0583
(809) 773-1261
E-mail: vcgvina@viaccess.net

Virginia Nurses Association
Jan Marshall Johnson, MS, RN, Executive Director
7113 Three Chopt Road, Suite 204
Richmond, VA 23226
Phone (804) 282-1808/2373
Fax (804) 282-4916
E-mail: vnajmj@aol.com
  www.virginianurses.com
*Office Hours: 8:30am–5:00pm Eastern Time

Washington State Nurses Association
Judith A. Huntington, MN, RN, Executive Director
575 Andover Park West, Suite 101
Seattle, WA 98188-3321
Phone (206) 575-7979 ext. 3002
Fax (206) 575-1908
E-mail: wsna@wsna.org
   or: jhunting@wsna.org
   www.wsna.org
*Office Hours: 8:30am–4:30pm Pacific Time

West Virginia Nurses Association
Cheri Heflin, Executive Director
100 Capitol Street, Suite 1009
P.O. 1946
Charleston, WV 25301
Phone (304) 342-1169 or (800) 400-1226
Fax (304) 346-1861
(304) 346-0300 (direct)
E-mail: centraloffice@wvnurses.org
   or: Cheri@chandcompany.com
   www.wvnurses.org
*Office Hours: 8:30am–4:30pm Eastern Time

Wisconsin Nurses Association
Gina Dennik-Champion, MSN, MSH, RN,
   Executive Administrator
6117 Monona Drive
Madison, WI 53716
Phone (608) 221-0383
Fax (608) 221-2788
E-mail: wna@execpc.com
   or: ginawna@execpc.com
   www.wisconsinnurses.org
*Office Hours: 7:30am–4:00pm Central Time

Wyoming Nurses Association
Beverly McDermott, MS, RN,
   Executive Director
Majestic Building, Room 305
1603 Capitol Avenue
Cheyenne, WY 82001
Phone (307) 635-3955
Fax (307) 635-2173
E-mail: wyonurse@aol.com
   or: bjmcdermot@aol.com
*Office Hours: Tuesday/Friday 9:00am–1:00pm
   Monday/Wednesday/Thursday 8:00am–1:00pm
   Mountain Time

American Nurses Association
Linda J. Stierle, MSN, RN, CNAA,
   Chief Executive Officer
600 Maryland Avenue SW, Suite 100W
Washington, DC 20024-2571
Phone (202) 651-7000
Phone (800) 274-4ANA
Fax (202) 651-7001
E-mail: lstierle.ana.org
*Office Hours: 9:00am–5:00pm Eastern Time

National Council of State Boards of Nursing, Inc.
676 North St. Clair, Suite 550
Chicago, IL 60611-2921
Phone: (312) 787-6555
Fax: (312) 787-6898
Web Site: http://www.ncsbn.org

Alabama Board of Nursing
770 Washington Avenue
RSA Plaza, Ste 250
Montgomery, AL 36130-3900
Phone: (334) 242-4060
Fax: (334) 242-4360
Contact Person: N. Genell Lee, MSN, JD, RN, Executive Officer
Web Site: http://www.abn.state.al.us

Alaska Board of Nursing
550 West Seventh Avenue, Suite 1500
Anchorage, Alaska 99501-3567
Phone: (907) 269-8161
Fax: (907) 269-8196
Contact Person: Dorothy Fulton, MA, RN, Executive Director
Web Site: http://www.dced.state.ak.us/occ/pnur.htm

American Samoa Health Services Regulatory Board
LBJ Tropical Medical Center
Pago Pago, AS 96799
Phone: (684) 633-1222
Fax: (684) 633-1869
Contact Person: Etenauga Lutu, RN, Executive Secretary

Arizona State Board of Nursing
1651 E. Morten Avenue, Suite 210
Phoenix, AZ 85020
Phone: (602) 331-8111
Fax: (602) 906-9365
Contact Person: Joey Ridenour, MN, RN, Executive Director
Web Site: http://www.azboardofnursing.org

Arkansas State Board of Nursing
University Tower Building
1123 S. University, Suite 800
Little Rock, AR 72204-1619
Phone: (501) 686-2700
Fax: (501) 686-2714
Contact Person: Faith Fields, MSN, RN, Executive Director
Web Site: http://www.state.ar.us/nurse

California Board of Registered Nursing
400 R St., Ste. 4030
Sacramento, CA 95814-6239
Phone: (916) 322-3350
Fax: (916) 327-4402
Contact Person: Ruth Ann Terry, MPH, RN, Executive Officer
Web Site: http://www.rn.ca.gov

California Board of Vocational Nurse and Psychiatric Technician Examiners
2535 Capitol Oaks Drive, Suite 205
Sacramento, CA 95833
Phone: (916) 263-7800
Fax: (916) 263-7859
Contact Person: Teresa Bello-Jones, JD, MSN, RN, Executive Officer
Web Site: http://www.bvnpt.ca.gov

Colorado Board of Nursing
1560 Broadway, Suite 880
Denver, CO 80202
Phone: (303) 894-2430
Fax: (303) 894-2821
Contact Person: Patricia Uris, PhD, RN, Program Administrator
Web Site: http://www.dora.state.co.us/nursing

Connecticut Board of Examiners for Nursing
Dept. of Public Health
410 Capitol Avenue, MS# 13PHO
P.O. Box 340308
Hartford, CT 06134-0328
Phone: (860) 509-7624
Fax: (860) 509-7553
Contact Person: Jan Wojick, Board Liaison
Web Site: http://www.state.ct.us/dph

Delaware Board of Nursing
Cannon Building, Suite 203
861 Silver Lake Blvd.
Dover, DE 19904
Phone: (302) 739-4522
Fax: (302) 739-2711
Contact Person: Iva Boardman, MSN, RN, Executive Director
Web Site: http://www.professionallicensing.state.de.us/boards/nursing/index.shtml

District of Columbia Board of Nursing
Department of Health
825 N. Capitol Street, Room 2224
Washington, DC 20002
Phone: (202) 442-4778
Fax: (202) 442-9431
Contact Person: Karen Scipio-Skinner MSN, RNC, Executive Director

Florida Board of Nursing
Capital Circle Officer Center
4052 Bald Cypress Way, Rm 120
Tallahassee, FL 32399-3252
Phone: (850) 488-0595
Contact Person: Dan Coble, RN, PhD, Executive Director
Web Site: http://www.doh.state.fl.us/mqa

Georgia State Board of Licensed Practical Nurses
237 Coliseum Drive
Macon, GA 31217-3858
Phone: (478) 207-1300
Fax: (478) 207-1633
Contact Person: Jacqueline Hightower, JD, Executive Director
Web Site: http://www.sos.state.ga.us/plb/lpn

Georgia Board of Nursing
237 Coliseum Drive
Macon, GA 31217-3858

Phone: (478) 207-1640
Fax: (478) 207-1660
Contact Person: Vacant, Executive Director
Web Site: http://www.sos.state.ga.us/plb/rn

Guam Board of Nurse Examiners
P.O. Box 2816
1304 East Sunset Boulevard
Barrigada, GU 96913
Phone: (671) 475-0251
Fax: (671) 477-4733

Hawaii Board of Nursing
Professional and Vocational Licensing Division
P.O. Box 3469
Honolulu, HI 96801
Phone: (808) 586-3000
Fax: (808) 586-2689
Contact Person: Kathleen Yokouchi, MBA, BBA, BA,
Executive Officer
Web Site: http://www.state.hi.us/dcca/pvl/
areas_nurse.html

Idaho Board of Nursing
280 N. 8th Street, Suite 210
P.O. Box 83720
Boise, ID 83720
Phone: (208) 334-3110
Fax: (208) 334-3262
Contact Person: Sandra Evans, MA,Ed., RN,
Executive Director
Web Site: http://www.state.id.us/ibn/ibnhome.htm

Illinois Department of Professional Regulation
James R. Thompson Center
100 West Randolph, Suite 9-300
Chicago, IL 60601
Phone: (312) 814-2715
Fax: (312) 814-3145
Contact Person: Deborah Taylor, RN,
Ed.D Nursing Act Assistant Coordinator
Web Site: http://www.dpr.state.il.us

Illinois Department of Professional Regulation
320 W. Washington St., 3rd Floor
Springfield, IL 62786
Phone: (217) 782-8556
Fax: (217) 782-7645

Indiana State Board of Nursing
Health Professions Bureau
402 W. Washington Street, Room W041
Indianapolis, IN 46204
Phone: (317) 232-2960
Fax: (317) 233-4236
Contact Person: Kristen Kelley, Dir. of Nursing of
IN BON
Web Site: http://www.state.in.us/hpb/boards/isbn

Iowa Board of Nursing
RiverPoint Business Park
400 S.W. 8th Street, Suite B
Des Moines, IA 50309-4685
Phone: (515) 281-3255
Fax: (515) 281-4825

Contact Person: Lorinda Inman, MSN, RN,
Executive Director
Web Site: http://www.state.ia.us/government/nursing

Kansas State Board of Nursing
Landon State Office Building
900 S.W. Jackson, Suite 551-S
Topeka, KS 66612
Phone: (785) 296-4929
Fax: (785) 296-3929
Contact Person: Mary Blubaugh, MSN, RN,
Executive Administrator
Web Site: http://www.ksbn.org

Kentucky Board of Nursing
312 Whittington Parkway, Suite 300
Louisville, KY 40222
Phone: (502) 329-7000
Fax: (502) 329-7011
Contact Person: Sharon Weisenbeck, MS, RN,
Executive Director
Web Site: http://www.kbn.state.ky.us

Louisiana State Board of Practical Nurse Examiners
3421 N. Causeway Boulevard, Suite 203
Metairie, LA 70002
Phone: (504) 838-5791
Fax: (504) 838-5279
Contact Person: Claire Glaviano, BSN, MN, RN,
Executive Director
Web Site: http://www.isbpne.com

Louisiana State Board of Nursing
3510 N. Causeway Boulevard, Suite 501
Metairie, La 70002
Phone: (504) 838-5332
Fax: (504) 838-5349
Contact Person: Barbara Morvant, MN, RN,
Executive Director
Web Site: http://www.isbn.state.la.us

Maine State Board of Nursing
158 State House Station
Augusta, ME 04333
Phone: (207) 287-1133
Fax: (207) 287-1149
Contact Person: Myra Broadway, JD, MS, RN,
Executive Director
Web Site: http://www.state.me.us/boardofnursing

Maryland Board of Nursing
4140 Patterson Avenue
Baltimore, MD 21215
Phone: (410) 585-1900
Fax: (410) 358-3530
Contact Person: Donna Dorsey, MS, RN, Executive
Director
Web Site: http://www.mbon.org

Massachusetts Board of Registration in Nursing
Commonwealth of Massachusetts
239 Causeway Street
Boston, MA 02114
Phone: (617) 727-9961
Fax: (617) 727-1630

(continued)

Contact Person: Theresa Bonanno, MSN, RN,
Executive Director
Web Site: http://www.state.ma.us/reg/boards/rn

Michigan CIS/Bureau of Health Services
Ottawa Towers North
611 W. Ottawa, 4th Floor
Lansing, MI 48933
Phone: (517) 373-9102
Fax: (517) 373-2179
Contact Person: Diane Lewis, Policy Manager for
Licensing Division
Web Site: http://www.cis.state.mi.us/bhser/
genover.htm

Minnesota Board of Nursing
2829 University Avenue SE, Suite 500
Minneapolis, MN 55414
Phone: (612) 617-2270
Fax: (612) 617-2190
Contact Person: Shirley Brekken, MS, RN,
Executive Director
Web Site: http://www.nursingboard.state.mn.us

Mississippi Board of Nursing
1935 Lakeland Drive, Suite B
Jackson, MS 39216-5014
Phone: (601) 987-4188
Fax: (601) 364-2352
Contact Person: Delia Owens, RN, JD, Executive
Director
Web Site: http://www.msbn.state.ms.us

Missouri State Board of Nursing
3605 Missouri Blvd.
P.O. Box 656
Jefferson City, MO 65102-0656
Phone: (573) 751-0681
Fax: (573) 751-0075
Contact Person: Lori Scheidt, BS,
Acting Executive Director
Web Site: http://www.ecodev.state.mo.us/pr/nursing

Montana State Board of Nursing
301 South Park
PO Box 200513
Helena, MT 59620-0513
Phone: (406) 841-2340
Fax: (406) 841-2343
Contact Person: Barbara Swehla, MN, RN, Executive
Director
Web Site: http://www.discoveringmontana.com/dli/
bsd/license/bsd_boards/nur_board/
board_page.htm

Nebraska Health and Human Services System
Dept. of Regulation & Licensure, Nursing Section
301 Centennial Mall South
Lincoln, NE 68509-4986
Phone: (402) 471-4376
Fax: (402) 471-3577
Contact person: Charlene Kelly, PhD, RN,
Executive Director
Nursing and Nursing Support Web Site: http://
www.hhs.state.ne.us/crl/nursing/nursingindex.htm

Nevada State Board of Nursing Administration, Discipline, and Investigations
1755 East Plumb Lane, Suite 260
Reno, NV 89502
Phone: (775) 688-2620
Fax: (775) 688-2628
Contact Person: Debra Scott, MS, RN,
Executive Director
Web Site: http://www.nursingboard.state.nv.us

Nevada State Board of Nursing License Certification and Education
4330 S. Valley View Blvd., Suite 106
Las Vegas, NV 89103
Phone: (702) 486-5800
Fax: (702) 486-5803
Contact Person: Don Rennie MS, RN, Associate
Executive Director for Licensure and Certification
Web Site: htp://www.nursing board.state.nv.us

New Hampshire Board of Nursing
P.O. Box 3898
78 Regional Drive, BLDG B
Concord, NH 03302
Phone: (603) 271-2323
Fax: (603) 271-6605
Contact Person: Cynthia Gray, MBA, BS, RN, CPN,
Executive Director
Web Site: http://www.state.nh.us/nursing

New Jersey Board of Nursing
P.O. Box 45010
124 Halsey Street, 6th Floor
Newark, NJ 07101
Phone: (973) 504-6586
Fax: (973) 648-3481
Contact Person: Patricia Lynch Polansky, MS, RN,
Executive Director
Web Site: http://www.state.nj.us/lps/ca/medical.htm

New Mexico Board of Nursing
4206 Louisiana Boulevard NE, Suite A
Albuquerque, NM 87109
Phone: (505) 841-8340
Fax: (505) 841-8347
Contact Person: Debra Brady, PhD, RN,
Executive Director
Web Site: http://www.state.nm.us/clients/nursing

New York State Board of Nursing
Education Bldg.
89 Washington Avenue, 2nd Floor West Wing
Albany, NY 12234
Phone: (518) 474-3817 Ext. 120
Fax: (518) 474-3706
Contact Person: Barbara Zittel, PhD, RN,
Executive Secretary
Web Site: http://www.nysed.gov/prof/nurse.htm

North Carolina Board of Nursing
3724 National Drive, Suite 201
Raleigh, NC 27612
Phone: (919) 782-3211
Fax: (919) 781-9461
Contact Person: Polly Johnson, MSN, RN,
Executive Director
Web Site: http://www.ncbon.com

North Dakota Board of Nursing
919 South 7th Street, Suite 504
Bismarck, ND 58504
Phone: (701) 328-9777
Fax: (701) 328-9785
Contact Person: Constance Kalanek, PhD, RN,
    Executive Director
Web Site: http://www.ndbon.org

Northern Mariana Islands Commonwelath
    Board of Nurse Examiners
PO Box 501458
Saipan, MP 96950
Phone: (670) 664-4810
Fax: (670) 664-4813
Contact Person: Elizabeth Torres-Untalan, RN,
    Chairperson

Ohio Board of Nursing
17 South High Street, Suite 400
Columbus, OH 43215-3413
Phone: (614) 466-3947
Fax: (614) 466-0388
Contact Person: John Brion, RN, MS,
    Executive Director
Web Site: http://www.state.oh.us/nur

Oklahoma Board of Nursing
2915 N. Classen Boulevard, Suite 524
Oklahoma City, OK 73106
Phone: (405) 962-1800
Fax: (405) 962-1821
Contact Person: Kimberly Glazier, M.Ed., RN,
    Executive Director
Web Site: http://www.youroklahoma.com/nursing

Oregon State Board of Nursing
800 NE Oregon Street, Suite 465
Box 25
Portland, OR 97232
Phone: (503) 731-4745
Fax: (503) 731-4755
Contact Person: Joan Bouchard, MN, RN,
    Executive Director
Web Site: http://www.osbn.state.or.us

Pennsylvania State Board of Nursing
P.O. Box 2649
124 Pine Street
Harrisburg, PA 17101
Phone: (717) 783-7142
Fax: (717) 783-0822
Contact Person: Miriam Limo, MS, MSN, RN,
    Executive Secretary
Web Site: http://www.dos.state.pa.us/bpoa/nurbd/
    mainpage.htm

Commonwealth of Puerto Rico Board of
    Nurse Examiners
800 Roberto H. Todd Avenue, Room 202,
    Stop 18
Santurce, PR 00908
Phone: (787) 725-7506
Fax: (787) 725-7903
Contact Person: Magda Bouet, Executive Director of
    the Office of Regulations and Certifications of
    Health Care Professions

Rhode Island Board of Nurse Registration
    and Nursing Education
105 Cannon Building
Three Capitol Hill
Providence, RI 02908
Phone: (401) 222-5700
Fax: (401) 222-3352
Contact Person: Charles Alexandre, MSN, RN,
    Executive Officer
Web Site: http://www.health.state.ri.us

South Carolina State Board of Nursing
110 Centerview Drive, Suite 202
Columbia, SC 29210
Phone: (803) 896-4550
Fax: (803) 896-4525
Contact Person: Martha Bursinger, RN, MSN,
    Executive Director
Web Site: http://www.llr.state.sc.us/pol/nursing

South Dakota Board of Nursing
4300 South Louise Ave., Suite C-1
Sioux Falls, SD 57106-3124
Phone: (605) 362-2760
Fax: (605) 362-2768
Contact Person: Diana Vander Woude, MS, RN,
    Executive Secretary
Web Site: http://www.state.sd.us/dcr/nursing

Tennessee State Board of Nursing
Cordell Hull Building
426 Fifth Avenue North, 1st Floor
Nashville, TN 37247
Phone: (615) 532-5166
Fax: (615) 741-7899
Contact Person: Elizabeth Lund, MSN, RN,
    Executive Director
Web Site: http://170.142.76.180/bmf-bin/
    BMFproflist.pl

Texas Board of Nurse Examiners
333 Guadalupe St., Suite 3-460
Austin, TX 78701
Phone: (512) 305-7400
Fax: (512) 305-7401
Contact Person: Katherine Thomas, MN, RN,
    Executive Director
Web Site: http://www.bne.state.tx.us

Texas Board of Vocational Nurse Examiners
William P. Hobby Building, Tower 3
333 Guadalupe St., Suite 3-400
Austin, TX 78701
Phone: (512) 305-8100
Fax: (512) 305-8101
Contact Person: Terrie Hairston, RN, CHE,
    Executive Director
Web Site: http://www.bvne.state.tx.us

Utah State Board of Nursing
Heber M. Wells Bldg., 4th Floor
160 East 300 South
Salt Lake City, UT 84111
Phone: (801) 530-6628
Fax: (801) 530-6511
Contact Person: Laura Poe, MS, RN,
    Executive Administrator
Web Site: http://www.commerce.state.ut.us

(continued)

Vermont State Board of Nursing
109 State Street
Montpelier, VT 05609-1106
Phone: (802) 828-2396
Fax: (802) 828-2484
Contact Person: Anita Ristau, MS, RN,
Executive Director
Web Site: http://vtprofessionals.org/nurses

Virgin Islands Board of Nurse Licensure
Veterans Drive Station
St. Thomas, VI 00803
Phone: (340) 776-7397
Fax: (340) 777-4003
Contact Person: Winifred Garfield, CRNA, RN,
Executive Secretary

Virginia Board of Nursing
6606 W. Broad Street, 4th Floor
Richmond, VA 23230
Phone: (804) 662-9909
Fax: (804) 662-9512
Contact Person: Nancy Durrett, MSN, RN,
Executive Director
Web Site: http://www.dhp.state.va.us

Washington State Nursing Care Quality Assurance Commission
Department of Health
1300 Quince Street SE
Olympia, WA 98504-7864
Phone: (360) 236-4700
Fax: (360) 236-4738
Contact Person: Paula Meyer, MSN, RN,
Executive Director
Web Site: http://www.doh.wa.gov/nursing

West Virginia Board of Examiners for Licensed Practical Nurses
101 Dee Drive
Charleston, WV 25311
Phone: (304) 558-3572
Fax: (305) 558-4367
Contact Person: Lanette Anderson, HRN, BSN, JD,
Executive Secretary
Web Site: http://www.lpnboard.state.wv.us

West Virginia Board of Examiners for Registered Professional Nurses
101 Dee Drive
Charleston, WV 25311
Phone: (304) 558-3596
Fax: (304) 558-3666
Contact Person: Laura Rhodes, MSN, RN,
Executive Director
Web Site: http://www.state.wv.us/nurses/rn

Wisconsin Department of Regulation and Licensing
1400 E. Washington Avenue
P.O. Box 8935
Madison, WI 53708
Phone: (608) 266-0145
Fax: (608) 261-7083
Contact Person: Kimberly Nania, Director,
Bureau of Health Service Professions
Web Site: http://www.drl.state.wi.us

Wyoming State Board of Nursing
2020 Carey Avenue, Suite 110
Cheyenne, WY 82002
Phone: (307) 777-7601
Fax: (307) 777-3519
Contact Person: Cheryl Lynn Koski, MS, RN, CS,
Executive Director
Web Site: http://nursing.state.wy.us

Aboriginal Nurses Association of Canada
56 Sparks Street, Suite 502
Ottawa, ON K1P 5A9
Web Site: http://www.anac.on.ca

Academy of Canadian Executive Nurses (ACEN)
c/o Chief Nursing Officer
St. Boniface General Hospital
409 Tache Avenue, Room A1129
Winnipeg, MB R2H 2A6

Canadian Association of Advanced Practice Nurses
Linda Derrick, Professional Practice Leader, Nursing
4204 Wakefield Place
Victoria, BC V8N 6E5
E-mail: derrick_watson@telus.net
Web Site: http://www.caapn.com

Canadian Association of Critical Care Nursing (CACCN)
P.O. Box 25322
London, ON N6C 6B1
Web Site: http://www.caccn.ca

Canadian Association for Enterostomal Therapy
C.A.E.T. President
P.O. Box 48069
60 Dundas St. E.
Mississauga, ON L5A 1W4
E-mail: caet@on.aibn.com
Web Site: http://www.caet.ca

Canadian Association for the History of Nursing (CAHN)
CAHN/ACHN Membership Committee
7120 – 5th Street N.W.
Calgary, AB T2K 1C8
Web Site: http://www.ualberta.ca/~jhibberd/CAHN_ACHN

Canadian Association of Nephrology Nurses and Technologists
Executive Director
336 Yonge St., Ste. 322

Barrie, ON L4N 4C8
E-mail: cannt@cannt.ca
Web Site: http://www.cannt.ca

The Canadian Association of Neuroscience Nurses
E-mail: canninfo@cann.ca
Web Site: http://www.cann.ca

Canadian Association of Nurses in AIDS Care
E-mail: Info@canac.org
Web Site: http://www.canac.org

Canadian Association of Nurses in Oncology
232–329 March Road, Box 11
Kanata, ON K2K 2E1
Web Site: http://www.cos.ca/cano

Canadian Association of University Schools of Nursing
E-mail: info@causn.org
Web Site: http://www.causn.org

Canadian Nurses' Respiratory Society
300 – 3 Raymond Street
Ottawa, ON K1R 1A3
Web Site: http://www.lung.ca/resp

The Canadian Nursing Students' Association
c/o Chris Kebbel, RN
416 Douglas Ave.
Toronto, ON M5M 1H4
E-mail: resource@ccnsa.ca
Web Site: http://www.ccnsa.ca

Operating Room Nurses Association of Canada
3700 Kempt Road
Halifax, NS B3K 4X8
Tel 902-497-1598
Fax: 902-423-1961
Web Site: http://www.ornac.ca

ALBERTA
Alberta Association of Registered Nurses
11620-168 Street
Edmonton AB T5M 4A6
Tel: (780) 451-0043
Fax: (780) 452-3276
E-mail: aarn@nurses.ab.ca

BRITISH COLUMBIA/COLOMBIE-BRITANNIQUE
Registered Nurses Association of British Columbia
2855 Arbutus Street
Vancouver BC V6J 3Y8
Tel: (604) 736-7331
Fax: (604) 738-2272
E-mail: info@rnabc.bc.ca

MANITOBA
College of Registered Nurses of Manitoba
647 Broadway Avenue
Winnipeg MB R3C 0X2
Tel: (204) 774-3477
Fax: (204) 775-6052
E-mail: marn@marn.mb.ca

NEW BRUNSWICK/NOUVEAU-BRUNSWICK
Nurses Association of New Brunswick
Association des infirmières et infirmiers du Nouveau-Brunswick
165 Regent Street
Fredericton NB E3B 3W5
Tel/Tél.: (506) 458-8731
Fax/Télécopieur: (506) 459-2838
E-mail/Courriel: nanb@nanb.nb.ca

NEWFOUNDLAND AND LABRADOR/TERRE-NEUVE ET LABRADOR
Association of Registered Nurses of Newfoundland and Labrador
55 Military Road, Box 6116
St. John's NF A1C 5X8
Tel: (709) 753-6040
Fax: (709) 753-4940
E-mail: info@arnn.nf.ca

NORTHWEST TERRITORIES/TERRITOIRES DU NORD-OUEST
Northwest Territories Registered Nurses Association
Box 2757
Yellowknife NT X1A 2R1
Tel: (867) 873-2745
Fax: (867) 873-2336
E-mail: nwtrna@internorth.com

NOVA SCOTIA/NOUVELLE-ÉCOSSE
College of Registered Nurses of Nova Scotia
Suite 600, Barrington Tower
Scotia Square, 1894 Barrington St.
Halifax NS B3J 2A8
Tel: (902) 491-9744
Fax: (902) 491-9510
E-mail: info@crnns.ns.ca

ONTARIO
College of Nurses of Ontario/Ordre des infirmières et infirmiers de l'Ontario
101 Davenport Road
Toronto ON M5R 3P1
Tel/Tél.: 1-800-387-5526/(416) 928-0900
Fax/Télécopieur: (416) 928-5607
E-mail/Courriel: cno@cnomail.org

PRINCE EDWARD ISLAND/ÎLE-DU-PRINCE-ÉDOUARD
Association of Nurses of Prince Edward Island
137 Queen Street, Suite 303
Charlottetown PE C1A 4B3
Tel: (902) 368-3764
Fax: (902) 628-1430
E-mail: anpei@pei.sympatico.ca

QUÉBEC
Ordre des infirmières et infirmiers du Québec
4200, boul. Dorchester Ouest
Montréal PQ H3Z 1V4
Tel/Tél.: (514) 935-2501/1-800-363-6048
Fax/Télécopieur: (514) 935-1799
E-mail/Courriel: inf@oiiq.org

SASKATCHEWAN
Saskatchewan Registered Nurses' Association
2066 Retallack Street
Regina SK S4T 7X5
Tel: 1-800-667-9945/(306) 359-4200
Fax: (306) 525-0849
E-mail: srna@srna.org

YUKON
Yukon Registered Nurses Association
204-4133-4th Avenue
Whitehouse YT Y1A 3T3
Tel: (867) 667-4062
Fax: (867) 668-5123
E-mail: yrna@yknet.ca

A nurse must hold individual membership in one of the provincial or territorial nursing associations which make up the Canadian Nurses Association (CNA) in order to belong to CNA and the International Council of Nurses. The organizations listed above, except those of Ontario and Québec, are all members of CNA.

Nurses in Ontario wishing to belong to CNA should join the Registered Nurses Association of Ontario, Doris Grinspun, Executive Director, 438 University Avenue, Suite 1600, Toronto, ON M5G 2K8 Tel: 1-800-268-7199 or (416) 599-1925, Fax: (416) 599-1926, E-mail: rnao@inforamp.net. Those in Québec should join the Yukon Registered Nurses Association or become an associate member of the Nurses Association of New Brunswick.

Une infirmière doit être membre individuel de l'une des associations provinciales ou territoriales adhérantes à l'Association des infirmières et infirmiers du Canada (AIIC) pour être membre de l'AIIC et du Conseil international des infirmières. Les organismes énumérés ci-haut, à l'exception de ceux de l'Ontario et du Québec, sont tous membres de l'AIIC.

Les infirmières de l'Ontario désirant être membres de l'AIIC doivent se joindre à la Registered Nurses Association of Ontario, Doris Grinspun, directrice génerale, 438, avenue Université, Toronto ON M5G 2K8, Téléphone 1-800-268-7199 ou (416) 599-1925, Télécopieur: (416) 599-1926, Courrier électronique: rnao@inforamp.net. Celles du Québec peuvent se joindre à la Yukon Registered Nurses Association, ou devenir membres associés de l'Association des infirmières et infirmiers du Nouveau-Brunswick.

Section 13: Research

13-1. THE NURSING AND HEALTH INFORMATION SEARCH: SOME APPROACHES

The *Miller-Keane Encyclopedia and Dictionary of Medicine, Nursing, and Allied Health*, although designed to be comprehensive, cannot cover every word, phrase, or concept which nurses and allied health professionals encounter, nor can it give extensive, in-depth coverage for most topics. It is meant to be a guide and a beginning source of information. Researchers call dictionaries "secondary" sources, meaning that they are not to be used as main, major, or "primary" sources of information. To learn more about topics or concepts covered in this dictionary, you will want to consult other publications and experts.

For a health professional to locate appropriate facts or information on a topic is becoming easier all the time, and is primarily complicated by the mixed blessing of a multitude of databases and print tools offering a very wide variety of information.

Feel empowered! Information is available on or about every topic. There are people who can advise on how to find it.

Effective time management and energy efficiency are the most important methods. Librarians, faculty, and associations are the guides.

Three "liveware" sources that will prove useful are:

Faculty members of medicine, nursing, and allied health schools, or respected specialist practitioners

Health science librarians, especially those at schools offering nursing and allied health degrees

Appropriate professional associations, groups, and societies.

SIX L'S OF EFFECTIVE LITERATURE SEARCHING

(1) Learn

What do you want to LEARN? How much do you want to LEARN? What format of materials will help you LEARN best what you need to know?

- Choose a topic or concept.
  Decide what you want to learn.
  Think who can help you. Think when you should ask their help: it's always a good time to talk with a librarian, but you may want to read a little before consulting a professor, and you may want to read a lot before consulting an authority or expert not known to you. Learn enough to ask good questions. You'll probably consult an expert only once; don't do so prematurely.
- Start small. To find "it," a fact, address, definition, brief description, don't jump to the indexing/abstracting/ databases. Find a little about "it." Use fact tools, e.g., this dictionary and other texts.
- Four very useful tools in health care fact-finding are:

  Encyclopedia of Associations (Gale Research)
  Health: United States (U.S. Department of Health and Human Services)
  AHA Guide to the Health Care Field (American Hospital Association)
  Telephone books of the nearest major city, notably the "public service" or "blue pages"

- Decide if you just need to find "it," find out "about it," or find out "all about it." In other words, know how much time and energy you anticipate expending, and know if this is a reference question, a research question, or a comprehensive/exhaustive literature review.

(2) List

- Jot down a brief LIST which includes the topic, type of information you need, and who a good "teacher" might be. (*I want to know how the aging process affects the everyday life of an otherwise healthy 75-year-old. Articles and books are probably what I need most, but a film, video or interview might be OK. A chart which lists things neatly would be really helpful. An articulate older person would be good, maybe Aunt Edna. Dr. Smith, who teaches "the aging process" component of our psychology course, would be good, too.*)
- Keep good records of your questions, sources, and terminology.

(continued)

(3) Look

Where can you find such information? Where should you LOOK?

- Consider type of source (an encyclopedia, a person, etc.) and the discipline which will best help. For a one-page discussion on childhood immunization, try a pediatric textbook. LOOK up appropriate terms in this dictionary, such as the window on *Haemophilus influenzae*, type B. For research studies on effective methods for alleviating burnout among health care practitioners, an index or database will list articles.
- Determine type of source. (*I would like articles, books, and older people's own words about themselves.*)

Definition	*Miller-Keane Encyclopedia and Dictionary*
Dosage, description	Pharmacopoeia or drug source
Brief information on a person, place, or group	Directory
"Cookbook" summary	Guide, handbook
Concise discussion and context	Textbook or handbook
Discursive, comprehensive, exhaustive coverage, discussion of standard of care in context	Book on a specific topic (monograph)
More current, specific coverage	Serial literature
Information about articles	Bibliography, index, abstract, or database
Perhaps most up-to-date perspective and guidance	Computer bulletin boards, personal contacts

Note: Whenever using a tool for the first time consult its guidesheets, help screens, tutorials, introductions, etc. Also, ask questions and clarifications of the health sciences or reference librarian.

- Determine an approach to the topic, i.e., the disciplines or professions whose point of view should be represented in the information. (*I would like to represent nursing, dental hygiene, psychology, and the elderly themselves.*)
- To create a list of disciplines or groups of people concerned about a topic, it is very effective to ask "Who cares?" If you list the groups interested in a topic, you can then ask a librarian how materials written by that group or representing that group can be accessed.
- Use the key indexes/abstracts/databases to the nursing and allied health literature: Cumulative Index to Nursing and Allied Health Literature (CINAHL); International Nursing Index (INI), especially the Nursing Citation Index (NCI). (Those researching medical technology, diagnostic imaging, and dental hygiene can skip this step and proceed directly to the next step.)
- Use the key indexes/abstracts/databases to the medical/health sciences literature:

  Index Medicus and *Index to Dental Literature*
  MEDLINE (National Library of Medicine)
  Science Citation Index (Institute for Scientific Information)
  Health Planning and Administration (National Library of Medicine/American Hospital Association)
  Bioethicsline (National Library of Medicine)

- Very specific searches, very general searches, newer terminology, and current controversies may require an online search.
- Consult a reference librarian for guidance.

(4) Language

- "Watch your LANGUAGE" when formulating a question to be searched in the literature. Every source has chosen certain vocabulary terms.
- Example: *Aged, Aging, Activities of Daily Living, Life Style* might be good terminology for one indexing or abstracting source, whereas *Longevity, Daily Activities, Normal Aging* might be the preferred terminology in another source.
- Whenever using a tool, read the introductory material, and use the *thesaurus* for that source.

(5) Logic (for databases)

- Use OR:
  to broaden your search by including more concepts to pull together synonymous terms

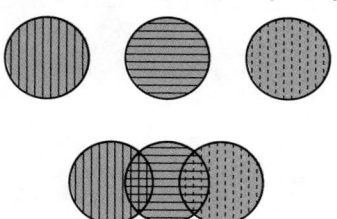

Use AND:

to narrow your search by combining ideas
to cover the interrelationship of two or more topics
Example: (Aging or Aged) and (*Life Style or Activities of Daily Living*)

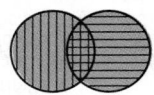

Use EXPLOSION or CONCEPT CODES (when available):

to OR together a term and any narrower terms related to it
Example: In MEDLINE and NAHL, "EXPLODE Heart Disease" will yield all heart diseases, regardless of their individual names.
to search a very broad concept, such as "treatment"
Example: In PsycLIT, searching the 4-digit concept code for "treatment and prevention" will focus the search to a full variety of therapies.

(6) Limits

Putting LIMITS on a search topic is often necessary. Common LIMITS are English language and human subjects. Others might include: type of article, year of publication, country of origin, or specialty of the journal. Know your own LIMITS too. Know when to stop, but don't stop too soon.
Note: Not all topics can be well researched using traditional library/information tools. If a topic is very local in nature, or extremely current, personal contacts via telephone may be your only useful approach to information finding. Libraries often refer to their reference services as "information and referral." Some "1-800" telephone numbers are included in this dictionary and can be used for information and referral.

ABOUT DATABASES

Compact disk read-only-memory (CD-ROM) technology is making do-it-yourself computerized searching of the health sciences literature commonplace. Microcomputers equipped with modems are also proliferating at home, at school, and in the workplace. Over 5,000 databases were available for lease or over networks in 1991. This appendix emphasizes the more readily available databases most frequently consulted by nursing and allied health professionals. Dozens more may be useful. Consult your health sciences librarian/reference librarian to determine which database may be best for your topic.

Essential: CINAHL, MEDLINE

The quick solution/short answer to literature searching in nursing and the allied health professions:
Nurses and allied health professionals (excluding those in medical technology, dental hygiene, and diagnostic imaging) should consult CINAHL first, then MEDLINE.
Medical technologists, dental hygienists, and diagnostic imaging professionals should consult MEDLINE first, then CINAHL.

Recommended: multi-database searching

Nursing and allied health professionals who choose to represent a specialty or focus in the literature, or who are striving for an interdisciplinary/multidisciplinary approach to a topic, will consult other databases.

Is your topic of nursing or allied health interest?
The database of choice for nursing and allied health is CINAHL. However, the fields of dental hygiene, laboratory sciences, and some areas of diagnostic imaging should begin with MEDLINE.
Search the most comprehensive database of nursing and allied health literature with the vocabulary most reflective of current allied health terminology. Nursing and Allied Health Literature (CINAHL), the most comprehensive database of literature for nursing and the allied health fields and the only database specifically designed for nursing and allied health professionals, is available through health sciences libraries, through database vendors, or on compact disk. The print product is *Cumulative Index to Nursing and Allied Health Literature.*

Another useful source is:
The AJN's *International Nursing Index*, especially its special section *Nursing Citation Index* (available online as part of MEDLINE)

Is your topic pathophysiological, pharmacological, or being discussed by physicians and biomedical researchers?
Are you a medical technologist, dental hygienist, or diagnostic imager?

(continued)

Search the premier database of clinical medical and biomedical research literature. MEDLINE, the largest database of biomedical journal literature, is available through health sciences libraries, and in many different formats including compact disk. Individuals may subscribe through vendors or directly through the National Library of Medicine. The print products derived from MEDLINE are *Index Medicus, International Nursing Index, and Index to Dental Literature.*

Is your topic related to a health care specialty with a significant database or print tool?
Consult a librarian to see if a useful, suitable, appropriate specialty database is available. Some important areas of research and their major databases are:

AIDS	AIDSLINE and related databases (National Library of Medicine)
Aging/geriatrics	Ageline (American Association of Retired Persons)
Cancer/oncology	Cancerlit (National Library of Medicine/National Cancer Institute)
Health administration management	Health Planning & Administration/*Hospital Literature Index*
Occupational therapy	OT Source (American Occupational Therapy Association)
Pharmacology	*International Pharmaceutical Abstracts* (American Society of Hospital Pharmacists)
Rehabilitation	NRIC and ABLEDATA (NRIC)

Is your topic drugs or chemicals?

CHEMLINE, TOXLINE, and related databases (National Library of Medicine)
MICROMEDEX Computerized Clinical Information System
Chemical Abstracts (Chemical Abstracts Service)

Do you want to complement/supplement your search with other professions' points of view, or to explore an aspect of your topic in greater depth?
For many topics of interest to nursing and allied health professionals, the literature of their own discipline will not provide enough background, comparative approaches, or supplementary information. Suggestions for broadening a search:

Behavior, psychology	PsycLIT/Psychological Abstracts (American Psychological Association)
	HAPI (Health and Psychological Instruments)
	Social Science Citation Index (Institute for Scientific Information)
Dissertations/theses	Dissertation Abstracts (University Microforms International)
Ethics	Bioethicsline/Bibliography of Bioethics (National Library of Medicine/Kennedy Institute on Bioethics, Georgetown University)
Business/management	ABInform (University Microforms International)
Education	ERIC (Education Research Information Center)
Other scientific disciplines	Biological Abstracts (BIOSIS)
	Science Citation Index (Institute for Scientific Information)

Hints and Tips

- To supplement topical searching:
   Citation indexing allows you to track the "impact" of an author's work, i.e., who has referred to the work in citations:
   Nursing Citation Index
   Science Citation Index
   Social Science Citation Index

"Hot topics" should also be checked in:

Current Contents
(A weekly current awareness index)
Dissertation Abstracts
Check the current few issues of any journal which appeared frequently in the citations you have compiled.

REMINDERS

- Current topics, historical research, audiovisuals, and other special materials may require different tools and contacts.
- Not all tools will be available at all libraries. But most tools mentioned in this list should be available at the libraries of colleges and universities offering degrees in nursing and allied health professions.
- The literature of nursing is different from the literature of allied health. The literature of medicine is also different, but there is a common base in patient care.
- Each allied health discipline has its own characteristics, and its own literature and approach to its literature.
- Truisms about health information finding:

    Many nursing and allied health topics are best researched as multidisciplinary, interdisciplinary topics.
    General sources such as *Webster's Third International Dictionary* or a general encyclopedia will be too general and provide too superficial coverage. Your tools need a focus.
    Avoid the tendency to skip background finding or to go directly to a literature review online.

ANOTHER MODEL: THE LITERATURE SEARCH PROCESS PARALLELS THE PATIENT CARE PROCESS

Symptom identification; self assessment	Identify your information need or topic.
Diagnosis	Label your needs specifically as to the type of information, format of material, amount, authority, and quantity of information your "information deficit" requires.
Prescription; treatment plan; self care plan	Prepare a "search strategy," a brief written plan of the types of sources you should consult and the terminology you should use.
Treatment; therapy	Consult the sources and keep a good record of the results.
Follow-up; quality assurance; utilization review	Assess the usefulness of the information you have found, and if necessary begin the loop again with your unanswered questions.

Analyze your topic using this guidesheet, checking all aspects of it which you may want to address. Examine quickly each of the suggested sources, to determine if you should use it. Decide which tools may be most productive. Work carefully with each of these tools.

By Topic

Business	*Hospital Literature Index,* CD + Health
Drugs	*Index Medicus,* CD+ MEDLINE
	International Pharmaceutical Abstracts
	MICROMEDEX
Education	ERIC (CD)
	Consumer Health & Nutrition Index
	Specialty index—professionals
	Psychological Abstracts, PsycLIT (CD)
Ethics	*Bibliography of Bioethics*
History	*Bibliography of the History of Medicine* (remember history subheading in MeSH)
Law	*Hospital Literature Index,* CD + Health
	Bibliography of Bioethics
Management/Administration	*Abstracts of Health Care Management Studies*
Pathophysiology	*Index Medicus,* CD + MEDLINE
	Science Citation Index
	Current Contents: Clinical Medicine
Popular Topics	*Reader's Guide to Periodical Literature*
	Consumer Health & Nutrition Index
Psychology	*Psychological Abstracts,* PsycLIT (CD)
	Social Science Citation Index
	Current Contents: Social & Behavioral Sciences
Religion	*Psychological Abstracts,* PsycLIT (CD)
	Social Science Citation Index
Technology	*Index Medicus,* CD + MEDLINE

By Time

Associations
Current contents
Institutions
Newspapers
Personal contacts
Other print tools

By Type of Material

Books	*Books in Print*
	Medical and Health Care Books and Serials in Print
Definitions	Dictionaries
	Encyclopedias
Journal Articles	miniMEDLINE
	CD-ROM databases
	Various indexes and abstracts
Numbers/Statistics	miniMEDLINE
	American Statistics Index
Pamphlets	Telephone book "Blue Pages"
	Pamphlet File
People/Contacts	*Encyclopedia of Associations*

Researching a topic on the Internet offers the ability to quickly access a vast array of information sources. It is impossible to list all of the capabilities of the Internet; however, the sites and services listed below will help direct users to information. The Internet provides access to frequent updates and current facts and figures. The individual seeking information over the Internet should be aware that not all sites have strategies to verify the accuracy of information.

E-MAIL

E-mail facilitates the exchange of information with individuals, organizations, and associations all over the world and includes a mechanism for quick replies. E-mail correspondence can be with individuals, or it can be simultaneously sent to a large number of people via a bulletin board.

Selected E-Mail Addresses:

mto11@columbia.edu	Marie O'Toole, Editor, *Miller-Keane Encyclopedia and Dictionary of Medicine, Nursing, and Allied Health*
adear@alzheimers.org	Alzheimer's Disease Education and Referral Center
alzca@istar.ca	Alzheimer Society of Canada
ncrabb@access.digex.net	American Council of the Blind
aaacn@voicenet.com	American Academy of Ambulatory Care Nursing (AAACN)
csc@safety-council.org	Canada Safety Council
chhanational@cyberus.ca	Canadian Hard of Hearing Association (CHHA)
cancercare@aol.com	Cancer Care, Inc.
chac@web.net	The Catholic Health Association of Canada
clf@liver.ca	Canadian Liver Foundation
ccfc@cycor.ca	Crohn's and Colitis Foundation of Canada
hmecarephy@aol.com	American Academy of Home Care physicians
ifa@citenet.net	International Federation on Aging
staff@navh.org	National Association for Visually Handicapped
iap@icicc.nhi.nihigov	National Cancer Institute Information Associates Program

SPECIAL INTEREST GROUPS

E-mail provides access to discussion groups, or special interest groups (SIGs), that serve as forums for many diverse topics. The following lists are of interest to health care providers:

CNS-L is an unmoderated LIST affiliated with the Clinical Nurse Specialist Interest Group of Ontario, Canada. The purpose of the LIST is to provide an international forum for networking, information sharing, and for discussion about issues relevant to the role of the Clinical Nurse Specialist.

To subscribe to CNS-L, send the following message:
TO: LISTSERV@VM.UTCC.UTORONTO.CA
SUBJECT: (LEAVE THIS LINE BLANK)
SUB CNS-L Yourfirstname Yourlastname
CNS-L LISTOWNER:
Pat Lyon
plyon@gpu.utcc.utoronto.ca

The purpose of the CLINALRT LIST is to provide electronic distribution of Clinical Alerts which are issued infrequently and irregularly by the US National Institutes of Health. This MODERATED list is intended to serve health professionals, health science libraries, and others.
To subscribe to CLINALRT, send the following message:
TO: LISTPROC@LIST.AB.UMD.EDU
SUBJECT: (LEAVE THIS LINE BLANK)
SUBSCRIBE CLINALRT Yourfirstname
        Yourlastname
CLINALRT LIST Owner
Gary Freiburger, Deputy Director
Health Sciences Library
University of Maryland at Baltimore
Phone: (410) 706-7545
FAX: (410) 706-3101
gfreibur@hsl1.ab.umd.edu
(that's the letter L followed by the number one in the server "syllable" above)

EYENURSE is a discussion list developed for registered nurses who work in ophthalmic care settings (operating rooms, clinics, offices, and hospitals). Topics for discussion include journal articles, advice on ophthalmic nursing care, family care and support issues, new trends in ophthalmic patient care, opinions on the future of ophthalmic nursing, and home care issues for ophthalmic patients.
To subscribe to EYENURSE, send the following message:
TO: MAISER@MAILGW.ORNET.MED.
UMICH.EDU
SUBJECT: (LEAVE THIS LINE BLANK)
sub EYENURSE
(Do not add your name or any other words to the message)
EYENURSE owner:
Linda Vader
lavader@umich.edu

GERO-NURSE is a LISTSERV for the Research Development and Dissemination Core (RDDC), one of the five cores for the University of Iowa Gerontological Nursing Intervention Research Center. The major purposes of the RDDC are to: 1. Coordinate research training of doctoral students and research scientists in functional and cognitive health status measurement, gerontological nursing interventions, and use of biostatistical methods in measuring the efficacy of gerontological nursing interventions; and 2. Disseminate scientific knowledge on functional and cognitive assessment and interventions to scientists, practitioners, and consumers.

(continued)

To join, send the following:
TO: GERO-NURSE-REQUEST@LIST.UIOWA.EDU
SUBJECT: (LEAVE THIS LINE BLANK)
SUBSCRIBE
GERO-NURSE owner:
Pam Micheal-Milder
pmicheal@nursing-po.weeg.uiowa.edu

GLOBALRN (formerly CULTURE-AND-NURSING) is
sponsored by the School of Nursing, University of
California, San Francisco. It was created for nurses
and other health professionals interested in topics
related to culture and health. The list will allow
participants to address areas of cultural compe-
tence, theory, practice, and research in an open and
unmoderated forum.
To subscribe to GLOBALRN, send the following mes-
sage:
TO: LISTSERV@ITSSRV1.UCSF.EDU
(that's the number one in the above)
SUBJECT: (LEAVE THIS LINE BLANK)
SUBSCRIBE GLOBALRN Yourfirstname
Yourlastname
GLOBALRN list manager:
Chuck Pitkofsky, MS, RN
Chuckp@itsa.ucsf.edu
(415) 546-7822
FAX: (415) 546-7823

HCARENURS is designed to meet the informational
needs of home care and hospice nurses. Home care
nurses work alone in the field and have needs different from those who work in institutions. This list
is designed to provide a place for discussion of
issues pertaining to home care nursing including
clinical issues, ethical concerns, and items related
to home care nursing. Home care nursing differs
from place to place and agency to agency.
To join the list, send a message:
TO: MAJORDOMO@PO.CWRU.EDU
SUBJECT: (LEAVE THIS LINE BLANK)
Subscribe hcarenurs your e-mail address
HCARENURS LISTOWNER:
Elizabeth A. Madigan
Doctoral Student
Frances Payne Bolton School of Nursing
Case Western Reserve University
eam13@po.cwru.edu

The IVTHERAPY.nurses-1 list is primarily for dis-
semination of information by and for I.V. Therapy
nurses. However, other interested professionals are
welcome. To subscribe to ivtherapy-1, send the
following message:
TO: LISTSERV@NETCOM.COM
SUBJECT: (LEAVE THIS LINE BLANK)
SUBSCRIBE IVTHERAPY-L
IVTHERAPY-L owner:
Sarah Kuykendall
SARAHK@NETCOM.COM

Legal Nurse Consultants is an open, unmoderated
forum for the discussion of issues related to the
field of legal nurse consulting.
To subscribe, send e-mail

TO: LNCNURSE@ONTOS.USA.COM
SUBJECT: SUBSCRIBE
Don't put anything in the body of the message.
LNCNURSE owner:
Nicole Marie Spring, RN, C
spring@en.com
The National Institutes of Health Guide to Grants &
Contracts is a READ-ONLY LIST. To subscribe, send
e-mail
TO: LISTSERV@LIST.NIH.GOV
SUBJECT: (LEAVE THIS LINE BLANK)
In the body of the message, type ONLY
subscribe NIHGDE-L Yourfirstname Yourlastname

NPinfo is a discussion list open to Nurse Practitioners,
CNMs, & CRNAs. It is one of several related elec-
tronic resources managed by Bob Smithing. Other
resources include a LISTSERV for NP jobs.
To subscribe to NPinfo, send the following message:
TO: Majordomo@npl.com
SUBJECT: (LEAVE THIS LINE BLANK)
SUBSCRIBE NPinfo Your e-mail address
NPinfo owner:
Robert T. Smithing, MSN, FNP
Nurse Practitioner Support Services
24837 104th Ave SE, #100
Kent, WA 98031
(206) 852-9042
bsmithing@npl.com

The NRSINGED (Nursing Education) Discussion List is
open to educators and interested others as a forum
for the discussion of a wide range of topics and
issues, from methodologies to philosophies, in
nursing education.
To subscribe to NRSINGED, send the following mes-
sage:
TO: LISTSERV@ULKYVM.LOUISVILLE.EDU
SUBJECT: (LEAVE THIS LINE BLANK)
SUBSCRIBE NRSINGED Yourfirstname
Yourlastname
NRSINGED owner:
Patricia K. Lacefield, EdD, RN
School of Nursing
University of Louisville
Louisville, KY 40292
PKLACE01@ULKYVM.LOUISVILLE.EDU
(502) 852-8387
FAX: (502) 852-8783

The NRSING-L list is primarily for the discussion of
nursing informatics topics. However, any and all
topics relating to nursing are welcomed.
To subscribe to NRSING-L, send the following mes-
sage:
TO: LISTPROC@LISTS.UMASS.EDU
SUBJECT: (LEAVE THIS LINE BLANK)
SUBSCRIBE NRSING-L Yourfirstname
Yourlastname
NRSING-L owner:
Gordon Larrivee, MS, RN, CNS Nursing Informatics
Nursing Administration
University of Massachusetts Medical Center
Worcester, MA 01655
LARRIVEE@UMASSMED.UMMED.EDU
(508) 856-0011

NurseLRC is a moderated mailing list for nursing Learning Resource Center faculty and staff to network about psychomotor skill acquisition, care and maintenance of equipment, instructional strategies, computer and audiovisual resources, and funding sources. Other goals are sharing specific needs and experience and ideas for the day-to-day support of LRC personnel.
To join the list, send a message:
TO: MAJORDOMO@DOUGLAS.BC.CA
SUBJECT: (LEAVE THIS LINE BLANK)
Subscribe NurseLRC
NurseLRC LISTOWNERs:
Marilyn Lewthwaite
Marilyn_Lewthwaite@douglas.bc.ca
Susan Greathouse
Jeanne Lot
Sandy McKinley
Rita Buurman
Canadian FAX (604) 527-5095

Nurse Managers List (RNMGR) is a relatively new listserv created to facilitate communications between nurse managers about the problems and concerns unique to their role in the delivery of health services.
To join this LIST, send e-mail
TO: RNMGR-request@cue.com
SUBJECT: (LEAVE THIS LINE BLANK)
Subscribe
RNMGR LISTOWNER:
Al Todak
PRN MedSearch
prnmed@halcyon.com

NURSENET is an open, unmoderated, global electronic conference for discourse about diverse nursing issues in the areas of nursing administration, nursing education, nursing practice, and nursing research.
To subscribe to NURSENET, send the following message:
TO: LISTSERV@LISTSERV.UTORONTO.CA
SUBJECT: (LEAVE THIS LINE BLANK)
SUBSCRIBE NURSENET Yourfirstname Yourlastname
NURSENET owner:
Judy Norris, RN, BScN, MSc, EdD (Candidate)
Coordinator, Nursing Systems & Special Projects
The Queen Elizabeth Hospital
550 University Avenue
Toronto, Ontario, Canada M5G 2A2
JNORRIS@OISE.UTORONTO.CA
(416) 597-4494 x 3571
FAX: (416) 591-6812

NURSE-ROGERS is a discussion forum for Martha Rogers' nursing theory. Her conceptual system, The Science of Unitary Human Beings, continues to evolve as a significant theoretical perspective. The list is part of that evolution, enabling nurses to enter into scholarly debate, discuss latest developments and significant issues.
To join the list, send a message
TO: MAILBASE@MAILBASE.AC.UK
SUBJECT: (LEAVE THIS LINE BLANK)
JOIN NURSE-ROGERS Yourfirstname Yourlastname

NURSE-ROGERS LISTOWNER:
Francis C. Biley
wnsfcb@cardiff.ac.uk

The NurseRes discussion list has nursing research as its focus. Novice and experienced researchers, as well as students, are welcome. Questions on any aspect of research are welcome, as are contributions and discussion about any aspect of research.
To subscribe to NurseRes, send the following message:
TO: LISTSERV@LISTSERV.KENT.EDU
SUBJECT: (LEAVE THIS LINE BLANK)
SUBSCRIBE NurseRes Yourfirstname Yourlastname
NurseRes owner:
Linda Q. Thede, RN, EdD
Assistant Professor and Director, Learning Resource Center
School of Nursing
Kent State University
113 Henderson Hall
Kent, OH 44242
LTHEDE@KENTVM.KENT.EDU
(216) 672-7930
FAX: (216) 672-2433

PNATALRN is an online resource for networking with perinatal nursing colleagues. It was formed for the discussion of perinatal nursing practice, education, and research. This is a place to ask questions, share information, propose ideas, offer support.
To join this LIST, send the following
TO: LISTSERV@UBVM.CC.BUFFALO.EDU
SUBJECT: (LEAVE THIS LINE BLANK)
subscribe pnatalrn yourfirstname yourlastname
PNATALRN owner:
Patricia R. McCartney, RNC, PhD
mccartny@acsu.buffalo.edu

PSYCHIATRIC-NURSING is an international psychiatric nursing discussion group.
To subscribe to PSYCHIATRIC-NURSING, send the following message:
TO: MAILBASE@MAILBASE.AC.UK
SUBJECT: (LEAVE THIS LINE BLANK)
JOIN PSYCHIATRIC-NURSING Yourfirstname Yourlastname
PSYCHIATRIC-NURSING owner:
Len Bowers
Co-ordinator
Psychiatric Nursing Research and Development Unit
Manchester Metropolitan University and
Tameside and Glossop CPS Trust
United Kingdom

The SCHLRN-L (School Nurse) Discussion List is a discussion group for school nurses, school nurse practitioners, school nurse teachers, school nurse managers, and others concerned with the health of school-aged children.

To subscribe to SCHLRN-L, send the following message:
TO: LISTSERV@UBVM.CC.BUFFALO.EDU
SUBJECT: (LEAVE THIS LINE BLANK)

(continued)

SUBSCRIBE SCHLRN-L Yourfirstname
Yourlastname
SCHLRN-L owner:
Martha Dewey Bergren, RN, MS
Doctoral Student
State University of New York at Buffalo
Buffalo, NY 14214-3079
Bergren@usinternet.com

ITNA is a discussion list for the International
TeleNurses Association and others interested
in telenursing and nursing aspects of
telemedicine.

To join the list, send a message:
TO: LISTSERV@LISTSERV.BCM.TMC.EDU
SUBJECT: (LEAVE THIS LINE BLANK)
Subscribe itna Yourfirstname Yourlastname
ITNA LISTOWNER:
George Suhr, RN
Nurse Manager, Texas Children's Hospital
President, International TeleNurses Association
Houston, TX
(800) 824-8353
gsuhr@msmail.his.tch.tmc.edu (June 12,1996,
Sparks, SM)

World Wide Web

The World Wide Web provides many interesting and informative sites. Many professional organizations and associations, as well as government and patient groups, provide sites that not only are informative, but also provide links to other sources of information. Search tools are numerous, but some helpful sites to start with include:

http://ash.org	Action on Smoking and Health
http://www.alcoholics_anonymous.org	Alcoholics Anonymous
http://www.alzheimers.org/adear	Alzheimer's Disease Education and Referral Center
http://www.acb.org	American Council of the Blind
http://www.assoc-center-ctrs.org	Association of Community Cancer Centers
http://www.safety-council.org	Canada Safety Council
http://www.cancer.ca/ccsncic.htm	Canadian Cancer Society
http://www.ccff.ca/~cfwww/index.html	Canadian Cystic Fibrosis Foundation
http://www.liver.ca	Canadian Liver Foundation
http://www.cdc.gov/cdc.htm	Centers for Disease Control and Prevention Home Page
http://www.convatec.com	ConvaTec
http://www.healthtouch.com	Healthtouch
http://kidshealth.org	KidsHealth
http://www.cc.emory.edu/WHSCL/medweb.html	Med Web:Databases
http://www.ncadd.org	National Council on Alcoholism and Drug Dependence, Inc.
http://nichsr@nlm.nih.gov	National Information Center on Health Services Research and Health Care
http://www.hwc.ca:8080/nin/	National Institute of Nutrition
http://www.nlm.nih.gov/	National Library of Medicine HyperDoc Home Page
http://www.njc.org	National Jewish Center for Immunology and Respiratory Medicine
http://www.bath.ac.uk/~exxrw/nurse.html	Nursing & Health Care Resources on the Net
http://publicinfo.occshost.nlm.nih.gov	Office of Public Information
http://www.geron.uga.edu	University of Georgia Gerontology Center

Section 14: Nursing Vocabularies

14-1. NURSING MINIMUM DATA SET ELEMENTS AND DEFINITIONS

The Nursing Minimum Data Set (NMDS) items were generated by task force groups and are recommended as the content for the NMDS. A data collection manual for the Nursing Minimum Data Set is published by the University of Wisconsin-Milwaukee, School of Nursing, Milwaukee, WI 53201. The authors of the manual are H.H. Werley, Ph.D., Distinguished Professor, School of Nursing, University of Milwaukee; E.C. Devine, and C.R. Zorn. The Nursing Minimum Data Set contains three broad categories of information: (a) nursing care; (b) patient or client demographics, and (c) service data. The nursing care elements include nursing diagnosis, nursing intervention, nursing outcome, and intensity of nursing care. The definitions of nursing intervention, nursing outcome, and intensity of care are below.

1. Nursing Intervention

Definition: An action, intended to benefit the patient or client, for which nurses are responsible.
A. Designation of intervention(s) based on a seven-category classification scheme (with definitions):

   (1) Surveillance and/or observation
       Definition: Action through which the nurse examines and monitors physical and behavioral responses to disease or injury and to the prescribed medical and/or nursing therapy (treatment).
   (2) Supportive measure
       Definition: Action through which the nurse provides support of life functions and needed sustenance (oxygen, nutrition, fluids).
   (3) Assistive measure
       Definition: Action through which the nurse facilitates activities of daily living (hygiene, exercise, rest, grooming), provides physical comfort, and maintains a therapeutic environment.
   (4) Treatment and/or procedure
       Definition: Action prescribed to cure, relieve, control, or prevent a patient or client problem.
   (5) Emotional support
       Definition: Action designed to meet the affective, psychological, and social needs of the patient or client.
   (6) Teaching
       Definition: Individual or group instruction designed to (a) provide information about disease processes, injuries, health events (e.g., childbirth, menopause), and health promotion practices; and/or (b) facilitate development of skills for coping with special care requirements, limitations, and/or restrictions in health status.
   (7) Coordination
       Definition: Action geared to the integration of multidisciplinary treatment plans with the goal of smooth, continuous patient or client care.

B. Designation of intervention(s) based on a 16-category classification scheme:

   (1) Monitoring and/or surveillance (people, equipment, technology)
   (2) Activities of daily living
   (3) Comfort
   (4) Airway maintenance (maintaining vital functions)
   (5) Applications and/or treatments (fluid instillations, irrigations)
   (6) Medications
   (7) Invasive insertions
   (8) Emotional support and/or counseling (psychosocial interaction, coping)
   (9) Teaching
   (10) Coordination and collaboration of care (referrals, team conferences, communication, documentation, patient advocacy, discharge planning)
   (11) Protection
   (12) Assisting other providers (supervision of other providers, specimen collection)
   (13) Preventive services (immunizations, disease avoidance, baby care, environmental safety, teaching wellness)
   (14) Providing a therapeutic environment (sensory modulation)
   (15) Maintaining nutritional and fluid balance
   (16) Therapeutic activities (diversional activities)

(continued)

2. Nursing Outcome
Definition: Nursing Outcome is an aspect of patient or client health status that is influenced by nursing intervention and recorded at specific times for an episode or encounter of care. This will be measured by th' resolution status of each nursing diagnosis as (a) resolved or (b) not resolved.

3. Intensity of Nursing Care
Definition: The total time and staff mix of nursing personnel resources consumed by an individual patient c client during the episode of care.

A. Total hours of nursing care
Definition: Total time expended in consumption of nursing resources for an individual patient or client durin the episode of care.

B. Staff mix
Definition: The combination of all caregivers participating in nursing care for an individual patient or client.

Structure of Taxonomy II

Scientists, informaticists, and managers of databases are the primary users of actual taxonomic structures. Clinicians rarely need to use one except for referencing. Clinicians are primarily concerned with the actual diagnoses within the taxonomy. However, familiarity with how the diagnostic language is structured will aid the clinician who needs to find information quickly. Thus a brief explanation of how the taxonomy is designed will help you understand the diagnoses within it.

Taxonomy II was designed to be multiaxial in its form, thereby substantially improving the flexibility of the nomenclature and allowing for easy additions and modifications.

There are seven axes

Axis 1 The diagnostic concept
Axis 2 Time (acute to chronic, short-term, long-term)
Axis 3 Unit of care (individual, family, community, target group)
Axis 4 Age (fetus to elder)
Axis 5 Health status (wellness, risk, or actual)
Axis 6 Descriptor (limits or specifies the meaning of the diagnostic concept)
Axis 7 Topology (parts/regions of the body)

Definitions of the Axes

An axis, for the purpose of the NANDA taxonomy, is operationally defined as a dimension of the human response that is considered in the diagnostic process.

The axes are represented in the named/coded nursing diagnosis through their values. In some cases they are named explicitly, e.g., *ineffective community coping* and *compromised family coping*, in which the unit of care (in this instance "community" and "family") is named. "Ineffective" and "compromised" are from the descriptor axis (Axis 6).

In other cases the axis is implicit, e.g., *activity intolerance*, in which the individual is the unit of care. In some instances a particular axis may not be pertinent to a particular diagnosis, and therefore is not a part of the nursing diagnosis label or code. For example, the time axis with its four values may not be relevant to each diagnostic situation.

TAXONOMY II DOMAINS AND CLASSES

Health Promotion	Nutrition	Elimination	Activity/Rest	Perception/ Cognition	Self- Perception
Health Awareness Health Management	Ingestion Digestion	Urinary System Gastrointestinal System	Sleep/Rest Activity/Exercise	Attention Orientation	Self-Concept Self-Esteem
	Absorption	Integumentary System	Energy Balance	Sensation/ Perception	Body Image
	Metabolism	Pulmonary System	Cardiovascular- pulmonary Responses	Cognition	
	Hydration			Communication	

Role Relationships	Sexuality	Coping/Stress Tolerance	Life Principles	Safety/ Protection	Growth/ Comfort	Development
Caregiving Roles	Sexual Identity	Post- Trauma Responses	Values	Infection	Physical Comfort	Growth
Family Relation- ships	Sexual Function	Coping Responses	Beliefs	Physical Injury	Environmental Comfort	Development
Role Performance	Repro- duction	Neuro- Behavioral Stress	Value/Belief/ Action Congruence	Violence Environmental Hazards	Social Comfort	
				Defensive Processes		
				Thermo- regulation		

(continued)

Taxonomy II

Axis 1 The Diagnostic Concept

The diagnostic concept is defined as the principal element or the fundamental and essential part, the root, of the diagnostic statement. The diagnostic concept may consist of one or more nouns. When more than one noun is used (e.g., *activity intolerance*), each one contributes to a unique meaning as if the two were a single noun; the meaning is different from the nouns stated separately. In some cases an adjective (e.g., spiritual) may be used with a noun (e.g., distress) to denote the diagnostic concept *spiritual distress* The diagnostic concepts in Taxonomy II are:

- Activity intolerance
- Adjustment
- Airway clearance
- Anxiety
- Aspiration
- Attachment
- Autonomic dysreflexia
- Bed mobility
- Body image
- Body temperature
- Breastfeeding
- Breathing pattern
- Cardiac output
- Caregiver role strain
- Confusion
- Constipation
- Coping
- Death anxiety
- Decisional conflict
- Denial
- Dentition
- Development
- Diarrhea
- Disuse syndrome
- Diversional activity
- Elimination
- Energy field
- Environmental interpretation
- Failure to thrive
- Falls
- Family processes
- Fatigue
- Fear
- Fluid volume
- Gas exchange
- Grieving
- Growth
- Growth and development
- Health maintenance
- Health-seeking behaviors
- Home maintenance
- Hopelessness
- Hyperthermia
- Hypothermia
- Incontinence
- Identity disturbance
- Infant behavior
- Infant feeding pattern
- Infection
- Intracranial adaptive capacity
- Knowledge
- Latex allergy response
- Loneliness
- Management of therapeutic regimen
- Memory
- Nausea
- Noncompliance
- Nutrition
- Oral mucous membrane
- Pain
- Parenting
- Perfusion
- Perioperative-positioning injury
- Physical mobility
- Poisoning
- Post-trauma
- Powerlessness
- Protection
- Rape-trauma syndrome
- Relocation stress
- Role conflict
- Role performance
- Self-care
- Self-esteem
- Self-mutilation
- Sensory perception
- Sexual dysfunction
- Sexuality pattern
- Skin integrity
- Sleep deprivation
- Sleep pattern
- Social interaction
- Social isolation
- Sorrow
- Spiritual distress
- Spiritual well-being
- Spontaneous ventilation
- Suffocation
- Suicide
- Surgical recovery
- Swallowing
- Thermoregulation
- Thought processes
- Tissue integrity
- Transfer
- Trauma
- Unilateral neglect
- Urinary retention
- Ventilatory weaning response
- Verbal communication
- Violence
- Walking
- Wandering
- Wheelchair mobility

Taxonomy II

xis 2 Time
ime is defined as the duration of a period or interval. Values in this axis are acute, chronic, intermittent, and continuous:
Acute: Less than 6 months
Chronic: More than 6 months
Intermittent: Stopping or starting again at intervals; periodic; cyclic
Continuous: Uninterrupted, going on without stopping

xis 3 The Unit of Care
he unit of care is defined as the distinct population for which a nursing diagnosis is determined. Values in Axis 3 are individual, family, group, and community:
Individual: A single human being distinct from others, a person.
Family: Two or more people having continuous or sustained relationships, perceiving reciprocal obligations, sensing common meaning, and sharing certain obligations toward others; related by blood or choice.
Group: Individuals gathered, classified, or acting together.
Community: "'A group of people living in the same locale under the same government.' Examples include neighborhoods, cities, census tracts, and populations at risk." (Craft-Rosenberg, 1999, p. 127)
Vhen the unit of care is not explicitly stated, it becomes the individual by default.

xis 4 Age
ge is defined as the length of time or interval during which an individual has existed. Values in Axis 4 are:

Fetus	• Adolescent
Neonate	• Young adult
Infant	• Middle-age adult
Toddler	• Young old adult
Pre-school child	• Middle old adult
School-age child	• Old old adult

xis 5 Health status
ealth status is defined as the position or rank on the health continuum. Values in Axis 5 are wellness, risk, and actual:
Wellness: The quality or state of being healthy, especially as a result of deliberate effort.
Risk: Vulnerability, especially as a result of exposure to factors that increase the chance of injury or loss.
Actual: Existing in fact or reality; existing at the present time.

xis 6 Descriptor
 descriptor or modifier is defined as a judgment that limits or specifies the meaning of a nursing diagnosis. Values in Axis 6 are:
Ability: Capacity to do or act
Anticipatory: Realized beforehand, foreseen
Balance: State of equilibrium
Compromised: Vulnerable to threat
Decreased: Lessened; lesser in size, amount, or degree
Deficient: Inadequate in amount, quality, or degree; not sufficient; incomplete
Delayed: Postponed, impeded, or retarded
Depleted: Emptied wholly or in part, exhausted of
Disproportionate: Not consistent with a standard
Disabling: Unable or unfit, incapacitating
Disorganized: Having the systematic arrangement destroyed
Disturbed: Agitated or interrupted; interfered with
Dysfunctional: Abnormal; incompletely functioning
Effective: Producing the intended or expected effect
Excessive: Characterized by an amount or quantity that is greater than necessary, desirable, or useful
Functional: Normal; completely functioning
Imbalanced: State of disequilibrium
Impaired: Made worse, weakened, damaged, reduced, deteriorated
Inability: Incapacity to do or act
Increased: Greater in size, amount, or degree
Ineffective: Not producing the desired effect
Interrupted: Having continuity or uniformity broken
Organized: Formed as into a systematic arrangement
Perceived: In awareness by means of the senses; having assignment of meaning
Readiness for enhanced (for use with wellness diagnoses): Made greater, increased in quality, having attained the more desired state

(continued)

Axis 7 Topology

The topology consists of parts/regions of the body—all tissues, organs, anatomical sites, or structures. Values i Axis 7 are:

- Auditory
- Bowel
- Cardiopulmonary
- Cerebral
- Gastrointestinal
- Gustatory
- Intracranial
- Mucous membranes
- Olfactory
- Oral
- Peripheral neurovascular
- Peripheral vascular
- Renal
- Skin
- Tactile
- Urinary
- Visual

Because it is a multiaxial framework, you will notice that the descriptors (e.g., decreased, impaired) now appea on an axis separate from the diagnostic concepts. As the taxonomy develops, you may choose the diagnosti concept/human response that explains the situation with the individual client/patient; you may also choose th descriptor from those available on the descriptor axis. For example, if the human response of concern is parenting, you have a choice on the descriptor axis of *impaired* or *readiness for enhanced*. In addition, you have five other axes from which to choose appropriate items. For the parenting diagnosis, you might choos *individual* from the unit of care axis, *adolescent* from the age axis, and *risk for* from the health status axis t arrive at the diagnosis of *risk for impaired parenting, individual, adolescent.*

Some words of caution as well as encouragement: Using a multiaxial structure allows many diagnoses to be constructed that have no defining characteristics and may even be nonsense (such as "impaired activities c daily living, fetus"). You are urged to use only those diagnoses that are approved for testing and thus hav defining characteristics.

TAXONOMY II: DOMAINS, CLASSES, DIAGNOSTIC CONCEPTS, AND DIAGNOSES

Domain 1 Health Promotion

The awareness of well-being or normality of function and the strategies used to maintain control of and enhanc that well-being or normality of function

Class 1 Health Awareness: Recognition of normal function and well-being

Class 2 Health Management: Identifying, controlling, performing, and integrating activities to maintain health and well-being

Diagnostic Concepts	**Approved Diagnoses**	
Therapeutic regimen management	00082	Effective therapeutic regimen management
	00078	Ineffective therapeutic regimen management
	00080	Ineffective family therapeutic regimen management
	00081	Ineffective community therapeutic regimen management
Health-seeking behaviors	00084	Health-seeking behaviors (specify)
Health maintenance	00099	Ineffective health maintenance
Home maintenance	00098	Impaired home maintenance

Domain 2 Nutrition

The activities of taking in, assimilating, and using nutrients for the purposes of tissue maintenance, tissue repair, and the production of energy

Class 1 Ingestion: Taking food or nutrients into the body

Diagnostic Concepts	**Approved Diagnoses**	
Infant feeding pattern	00107	Ineffective infant feeding pattern
Swallowing	00103	Impaired swallowing
Nutrition	00002	Imbalanced nutrition: Less than body requirements
Nutrition	00001	Imbalanced nutrition: More than body requirements
	00003	Risk for imbalanced nutrition: More than body requirements

Class 2 Digestion: The physical and chemical activities that convert foodstuffs into substances suitable for absorption and assimilation

Class 3 Absorption: The act of taking up nutrients through body tissues

Class 4 Metabolism: The chemical and physical processes occurring in living organisms and cells for the development and use of protoplasm, and production of waste and energy, with the release of energy for a vital processes

Class 5 Hydration: The taking in and absorption of fluids and electrolytes

Diagnostic Concepts	**Approved Diagnoses**	
Fluid volume	00027	Deficient fluid volume
	00028	Risk for deficient fluid volume
	00026	Excess fluid volume
	00025	Risk for fluid volume imbalance

Domain 3 Elimination
Secretion and excretion of waste products from the body
Class 1 Urinary System: The process of secretion and excretion of urine

Diagnostic Concepts	Approved Diagnoses	
Urinary elimination	00016	Impaired urinary elimination
Urinary retention	00023	Urinary retention
Urinary incontinence	00021	Total urinary incontinence
	00020	Functional urinary incontinence
	00017	Stress urinary incontinence
	00019	Urge urinary incontinence
	00018	Reflex urinary incontinence
	00022	Risk for urge urinary incontinence

Class 2 Gastrointestinal System: Excretion and expulsion of waste products from the bowel

Diagnostic Concepts	Approved Diagnoses	
Bowel incontinence	00014	Bowel incontinence
Diarrhea	00013	Diarrhea
Constipation	00011	Constipation
	00015	Risk for constipation
	00012	Perceived constipation

Class 3 Integumentary System: Process of secretion and excretion through the skin
Class 4 Pulmonary System: Removal of byproducts of metabolic products, secretions, and foreign material from the lung or bronchi

Diagnostic Concepts	Approved Diagnoses	
Gas exchange	00030 Impaired gas exchange	

Domain 4 Activity/Rest
The production, conservation, expenditure, or balance of energy resources
Class 1 Sleep/Rest: Slumber, repose, ease, or inactivity

Diagnostic Concepts	Approved Diagnoses	
Sleep pattern	00095	Disturbed sleep pattern
	00096	Sleep deprivation

Class 2 Activity/Exercise: Moving parts of the body (mobility), doing work, or performing actions often (but not always) against resistance

Diagnostic Concepts	Approved Diagnoses	
Disuse syndrome	00040	Risk for disuse syndrome
Mobility	00085	Impaired physical mobility
	00091	Impaired bed mobility
	00089	Impaired wheelchair mobility
Transfer ability	00090	Impaired transfer ability
Walking	00088	Impaired walking
Diversional activity	00097	Deficient diversional activity
Wandering	00154	Wandering
Self-care deficit	00109	Dressing/grooming deficit
	00108	Bathing/hygiene self-care deficit
	00102	Feeding self-care deficit
	00110	Toileting self-care deficit
Surgical recovery	00100	Delayed surgical recovery

Class 3 Energy/Balance: A dynamic state of harmony between intake and expenditure of resources

Diagnostic Concepts	Approved Diagnoses	
Energy field	00050	Disturbed energy field
Fatigue	00093	Fatigue

Class 4 Cardiovascular/Pulmonary Responses: Cardiopulmonary mechanisms that support activity/rest

Diagnostic Concepts	Approved Diagnoses	
Cardiac output	00029	Decreased cardiac output
Spontaneous ventilation	00033	Impaired spontaneous ventilation
Breathing pattern	00032	Ineffective breathing pattern
Activity tolerance	00092	Activity intolerance
	00094	Risk for activity intolerance
Ventilatory weaning	00034	Dysfunctional ventilatory weaning response
Tissue perfusion	00024	Ineffective tissue perfusion (specify type: renal, cerebral, cardiopulmonary, gastrointestinal, peripheral)

(continued)

Domain 5 Perception/Cognition

The human information processing system, including attention, orientation, sensation, perception, cognition, and communication

Class 1 Attention: Mental readiness to notice or observe

Diagnostic Concepts	Approved Diagnoses
Unilateral neglect	00123 Unilateral neglect

Class 2 Orientation: Awareness of time, place, and person

Diagnostic Concepts	Approved Diagnoses
Environmental interpretation	00127 Impaired environmental interpretation syndrome

Class 3 Sensation/Perception: Receiving information through the senses of touch, taste, smell, vision, hearing, and kinesthesia and the comprehension of sense data resulting in naming, associating, and/or pattern recognition

Diagnostic Concepts	Approved Diagnoses
Sensory perception	00122 Disturbed sensory perception (specify: visual, auditory, kinesthetic, gustatory, tactile, olfactory)

Class 4 Cognition: Use of memory, learning, thinking, problem solving, abstraction, judgment, insight, intellectual capacity, calculation, and language

Diagnostic Concepts	Approved Diagnoses
Knowledge	00126 Deficient knowledge (specify)
Confusion	00128 Acute confusion
	00129 Chronic confusion
Memory	00131 Impaired memory
Thought processes	00130 Disturbed thought processes

Class 5 Communication: Sending and receiving verbal and nonverbal information

Diagnostic Concepts	Approved Diagnoses
Verbal communication	00051 Impaired verbal communication

Domain 6 Self-perception

Awareness about the self

Class 1 Self-Concept: The perception(s) about the total self

Diagnostic Concepts	Approved Diagnoses
Identity	00121 Disturbed personal identity
	00125 Powerlessness
	00152 Risk for powerlessness
	00124 Hopelessness
Loneliness	00054 Risk for loneliness

Class 2 Self-esteem: Assessment of one's own worth, capability, significance, and success

Diagnostic Concepts	Approved Diagnoses
Self-esteem	00119 Chronic low self-esteem
	00120 Situational low self-esteem
	00153 Risk for situational low self-esteem

Class 3 Body Image: A mental image of one's own body

Diagnostic Concepts	Approved Diagnoses
Body image	00118 Disturbed body image

Domain 7 Role Relationships

The positive and negative connections or associations between persons or groups of persons and the means by which those connections are demonstrated

Class 1 Caregiving Roles: Socially expected behavior patterns by persons providing care who are not health care professionals

Diagnostic Concepts	Approved Diagnoses
Caregiver role strain	00061 Caregiver role strain
	00062 Risk for caregiver role strain
Parenting	00056 Impaired parenting
	00057 Risk for impaired parenting

Class 2 Family Relationships: Associations of people who are biologically related or related by choice

Diagnostic Concepts	Approved Diagnoses
Family processes	00060 Interrupted family processes
	00063 Dysfunctional family processes: Alcoholis
Attachment	00058 Risk for impaired parent/infant/child attachment

Class 3 Role Performance: Quality of functioning in socially expected behavior patterns

Diagnostic Concepts	Approved Diagnoses	
Breastfeeding	00106	Effective breastfeeding
	00104	Ineffective breastfeeding
	00105	Interrupted breastfeeding
Role performance	00055	Ineffective role performance
	00064	Parental role conflict
Social interaction	00052	Impaired social interaction

Domain 8 Sexuality
Sexual identity, sexual function, and reproduction
Class 1 Sexual Identity: The state of being a specific person in regard to sexuality and/or gender
Class 2 Sexual Function: The capacity or ability to participate in sexual activities

Diagnostic Concepts	Approved Diagnoses	
Sexual function	00059	Sexual dysfunction
Sexual patterns	00065	Ineffective sexuality patterns

Class 3 Reproduction: Any process by which new individuals (people) are produced

Domain 9 Coping/Stress Tolerance
Contending with life events/life processes
Class 1 Post-Trauma Responses: Reactions occurring after physical or psychological trauma

Diagnostic Concepts	Approved Diagnoses	
Relocation stress	00114	Relocation stress syndrome
	00149	Risk for relocation stress syndrome
Rape-trauma	00142	Rape-trauma syndrome
	00144	Rape-trauma syndrome: Silent reaction
	00143	Rape-trauma syndrome: Compound reaction
Post-trauma response	00141	Post-trauma syndrome
	00145	Risk for post-trauma syndrome

Class 2 Coping Responses: The process of managing environmental stress

Diagnostic Concepts	Approved Diagnoses	
Fear	00148	Fear
Anxiety	00146	Anxiety
	00147	Death anxiety
Sorrow	00137	Chronic sorrow
Denial	00072	Ineffective denial
	00136	Anticipatory grieving
	00135	Dysfunctional grieving
Adjustment	00070	Impaired adjustment
Coping	00069	Ineffective coping
	00073	Disabled family coping
	00074	Compromised family coping
	00071	Defensive coping
	00077	Ineffective community coping
	00075	Readiness for enhanced family coping
	00076	Readiness for enhanced community coping

Class 3 Neurobehavioral Stress: Behavioral responses reflecting nerve and brain function

Diagnostic Concepts	Approved Diagnoses	
Dysreflexia	00009	Autonomic dysreflexia
	00010	Risk for autonomic dysreflexia
Infant behavior	00116	Disorganized infant behavior
	00115	Risk for disorganized infant behavior
	00117	Readiness for enhanced organized infant behavior
Adaptive capacity	00049	Decreased intracranial adaptive capacity

Domain 10 Life Principles
Principles underlying conduct, thought, and behavior about acts, customs, or institutions viewed as being true or having intrinsic worth
Class 1 Values: The identification and ranking of preferred modes of conduct or end states
Class 2 Beliefs: Opinions, expectations, or judgments about acts, customs, or institutions viewed as being true or having intrinsic worth

Diagnostic Concepts	Approved Diagnoses	
Spiritual well-being	00068	Readiness for enhanced spiritual well-being

(continued)

Class 3 Value/Belief/Action Congruence: The correspondence or balance achieved between values, beliefs, and actions

Diagnostic Concepts	Approved Diagnoses	
Spiritual distress	00066	Spiritual distress
	00067	Risk for spiritual distress
Decisional conflict	00083	Decisional conflict (specify)
Noncompliance	00079	Noncompliance (specify)

Domain 11 Safety/Protection
Freedom from danger, physical injury or immune system damage, preservation from loss, and protection of safety and security
Class 1 Infection: Host responses following pathogenic invasion

Diagnostic Concepts	Approved Diagnoses	
Infection	00004	Risk for infection

Class 2 Physical Injury: Bodily harm or hurt

Diagnostic Concepts	Approved Diagnoses	
Oral mucous membrane	00045	Impaired oral mucous membrane
Injury	00035	Risk for injury
	00087	Risk for perioperative positioning injury
	00155	Risk for falls
Trauma	00038	Risk for trauma
Skin integrity	00046	Impaired skin integrity
	00047	Risk for impaired skin integrity
Tissue integrity	00044	Impaired tissue integrity
Dentition	00048	Impaired dentition
Suffocation	00036	Risk for suffocation
Aspiration	00039	Risk for aspiration
Airway clearance	00031	Ineffective airway clearance
Neurovascular function	00086	Risk for peripheral neurovascular dysfunction
Protection	00043	Ineffective protection

Class 3 Violence: The exertion of excessive force or power so as to cause injury or abuse

Diagnostic Concepts	Approved Diagnoses	
Self-mutilation	00139	Risk for self-mutilation
	00151	Self-mutilation
Violence	00138	Risk for other-directed violence
	00140	Risk for self-directed violence
	00150	Risk for suicide

Class 4 Environmental Hazards: Sources of danger in the surroundings

Diagnostic Concepts	Approved Diagnoses	
Poisoning	00037	Risk for poisoning

Class 5 Defensive Processes: The processes by which the self protects itself from the nonself

Diagnostic Concepts	Approved Diagnoses	
Latex allergy response	00041	Latex allergy response
	00042	Risk for latex allergy response

Class 6 Thermoregulation: The physiologic process of regulating heat and energy within the body for purposes of protecting the organism

Diagnostic Concepts	Approved Diagnoses	
Body temperature	00005	Risk for imbalanced body temperature
Thermoregulation	00008	Ineffective thermoregulation
	00006	Hypothermia
	00007	Hyperthermia

Domain 12 Comfort
Sense of mental, physical, or social well-being or ease
Class 1 Physical Comfort: Sense of well-being or ease

Diagnostic Concepts	Approved Diagnoses	
Pain	00132	Acute pain
	00133	Chronic pain
Nausea	00134	Nausea

Class 2 Environmental Comfort: Sense of well-being or ease in/with one's environment
Class 3 Social Comfort: Sense of well-being or ease with one's social situations

Diagnostic Concepts	Approved Diagnoses
Social isolation	00053 Social isolation

Domain 13 Growth/Development
Age-appropriate increases in physical dimensions, organ systems, and/or attainment of developmental milestones
Class 1 Growth: Increases in physical dimensions or maturity of organ systems

Diagnostic Concepts	Approved Diagnoses
Growth	00113 Risk for disproportionate growth
Failure to thrive	00101 Adult failure to thrive

Class 2 Development: Attainment, lack of attainment, or loss of developmental milestones

Diagnostic Concepts	Approved Diagnoses
Development	00111 Delayed growth and development
	00112 Risk for delayed development

14-2. NURSING DIAGNOSES: DEFINITIONS, DEFINING CHARACTERISTICS, AND RELATED FACTORS (INCLUDING 2003–2004 UPDATES)

ACTIVITY INTOLERANCE (1982)

Definition:
Insufficient physiological or psychological energy to endure or complete required or desired daily activities

Defining Characteristics:
Verbal report of fatigue or weakness; abnormal heart rate or blood pressure response to activity; electrocardiographic changes reflecting arrhythmias or ischemia; exertional discomfort or dyspnea

Related Factors:
Bed rest or immobility; generalized weakness; imbalance between oxygen supply/demand; sedentary lifestyle

Risk For ACTIVITY INTOLERANCE (1982)

Definition:
At risk for experiencing insufficient physiological or psychological energy to endure or complete required or desired daily activities

Risk Factors:
Inexperience with the activity; presence of circulatory/respiratory problems; history of previous intolerance; deconditioned status

Impaired ADJUSTMENT (1986, 1998)

Definition:
Inability to modify lifestyle/behavior in a manner consistent with a change in health status

Defining Characteristics:
Denial of health status change; failure to take actions that would prevent further health problems; failure to achieve optimal sense of control; demonstration of nonacceptance of health status change

Related Factors:
Low state of optimism; intense emotional state; negative attitudes toward health behavior; absence of intent to change behavior; multiple stressors; absence of social support for changed beliefs and practices; disability or health status change requiring change in lifestyle; lack of motivation to change behaviors

Ineffective AIRWAY CLEARANCE (1980, 1996, 1998)

Definition:
Inability to clear secretions or obstructions from the respiratory tract to maintain a clear airway

Defining Characteristics:
Dyspnea; diminished breath sounds; orthopnea; adventitious breath sounds (rales, crackles, rhonchi, wheezes); cough, ineffective or absent; sputum production; cyanosis; difficulty vocalizing; wide-eyed; changes in respiratory rate and rhythm; restlessness

Related Factors:
Environmental: Smoking; smoke inhalation; second-hand smoke
Obstructed airway: Airway spasm; retained secretions; excessive mucus; presence of artificial airway; foreign body in airway; secretions in the bronchi; exudate in the alveoli
Physiological: Neuromuscular dysfunction; hyperplasia of the bronchial walls; chronic obstructive pulmonary disease; infection; asthma; allergic airways

Latex ALLERGY RESPONSE (1998)

Definition:
An allergic response to natural latex rubber products

Defining Characteristics:
Type I Reactions

Immediate reactions (<1 hour) to latex proteins (can be life threatening); contact urticaria progressing to generalized symptoms; edema of the lips, tongue, uvula, and/or throat; shortness of breath, tightness in chest, wheezing, bronchospasm leading to respiratory arrest; hypotension, syncope, cardiac arrest

May also include: Orofacial characteristics (edema of sclera or eyelids; erythema and/or itching of the eyes; tearing of the eyes; nasal congestion, itching, and/or erythema; rhinorrhea; facial erythema; facial itching; oral itching)

Gastrointestinal characteristics: Abdominal pain; nausea

Generalized characteristics: Flushing; general discomfort; generalized edema; increasing complaint of total body warmth; restlessness

Type IV Reactions

Delayed onset (hours); eczema; irritation; reaction to additives (e.g., thiurams, carbamates) causes discomfort; redness

Irritant Reactions

Erythema; chapped or cracked skin; blisters

Related Factors:

No immune mechanism response

Risk For Latex ALLERGY RESPONSE (1998)

Definition:

At risk for allergic response to natural latex rubber products

Risk Factors:

Multiple surgical procedures, especially from infancy (e.g., spina bifida); allergies to bananas, avocados, tropical fruits, kiwi, chestnuts; professions with daily exposure to latex (e.g., medicine, nursing, dentistry); conditions associated with continuous or intermittent catheterization; history of reactions to latex (e.g., balloons, condoms, gloves); allergies to poinsettia plants; history of allergies and asthma

---

ANXIETY (1973, 1982, 1998)

Definition:

Vague uneasy feeling of discomfort or dread accompanied by an autonomic response (the source often non-specific or unknown to the individual); a feeling of apprehension caused by anticipation of danger. It is an alerting signal that warns of impending danger and enables the individual to take measures to deal with threat.

Defining Characteristics:

Behavioral: Diminished productivity; scanning and vigilance; poor eye contact; restlessness; glancing about; extraneous movement (e.g., foot shuffling hand/arm movements); expressed concerns due to change in life events; insomnia; fidgeting

Affective: Regretful; irritability; anguish; scared jittery; overexcited; painful and persistent increased helplessness; rattled; uncertainty; increased wariness focus on self; feelings of inadequacy; fearful distressed; worried, apprehensive; anxious

Physiological: Voice quivering; trembling/hand tremors; shakiness; increased respiration (sympathetic) urinary urgency (parasympathetic); increased pulse (sympathetic); pupil dilation (sympathetic); increased reflexes (sympathetic); abdominal pain (parasympathetic); sleep disturbance (parasympathetic); tingling in extremities (parasympathetic); cardiovascular excitation (sympathetic); increased perspiration; facial tension; anorexia (sympathetic); heart pounding (sympathetic); diarrhea (parasympathetic); urinary hesitancy (parasympathetic); fatigue (parasympathetic); dry mouth (sympathetic); weakness (sympathetic); decreased pulse (parasympathetic); facial flushing (sympathetic); superficial vasoconstriction (sympathetic); twitching (sympathetic); decreased blood pressure (parasympathetic); nausea (parasympathetic); urinary frequency (parasympathetic); faintness (parasympathetic); respiratory difficulties (sympathetic); increased blood pressure (sympathetic)

Cognitive: Blocking of thought; confusion; preoccupation; forgetfulness; rumination; impaired attention decreased perceptual field; fear of unspecified consequences; tendency to blame others; difficulty concentrating; diminished ability to problem solve, learn awareness of physiologic symptoms

Related Factors:

Exposure to toxins; unconscious conflict about essential values/goals of life; familial association heredity; unmet needs; interpersonal transmission contagion; situational/maturational crises; threat of death; threat to self-concept; stress; substance abuse threat to or change in role status, health status interaction patterns, role function, environment economic status

---

Death ANXIETY (1998)

Definition:

Apprehension, worry, or fear related to death or dying

Defining Characteristics:

Worrying about the impact of one's own death or significant others; powerless over issues related to dying; fear of loss of physical and/or mental abilities when dying; anticipated pain related to dying; deep sadness; fear of the process of dying; concerns of overworking the caregiver as terminal illness incapacitates self; concern about meeting one's creator or feeling doubtful about the existence of a God or higher being; total loss of control over any aspect of one's own death; negative death images or unpleasant thoughts about any event related to death or dying; fear of delayed demise; fear of premature death because it prevents the accomplishment of important life goals; worrying about being the cause of others' grief and suffering; fear of leaving family alone after death; fear of developing a terminal illness; denial of one's own mortality or impending death

Related Factors:
To be developed

Risk For ASPIRATION (1988)

Definition:
At risk for entry of gastrointestinal secretions, oropharyngeal secretions, solids, or fluids into tracheobronchial passages

Risk Factors:
Increased intragastric pressure; tube feedings; situations hindering elevation of upper body; reduced level of consciousness; presence of tracheostomy or endotracheal tube; medication administration; wired jaws; increased gastric residual; incompetent lower esophageal sphincter; impaired swallowing; gastrointestinal tubes; facial, oral, neck surgery or trauma; depressed cough and gag reflexes; decreased gastrointestinal motility; delayed gastric emptying

Risk For Impaired Parent/Infant/Child ATTACHMENT* (1994)

Definition:
Disruption of the interactive process between parent/significant other and infant that fosters the development of a protective and nurturing reciprocal relationship

Risk Factors:
Physical barriers; anxiety associated with the parent role; substance abuse; premature infant, ill infant/child who is unable to effectively initiate parental contact due to altered behavioral organization; lack of privacy; inability of parents to meet personal needs; separation

Formerly "Risk for Altered Parent/Infant-Child Attachment"

AUTONOMIC DYSREFLEXIA* (1988)

Definition:
Life-threatening, uninhibited sympathetic response of the nervous system to a noxious stimulus after a spinal cord injury at T7 or above

Defining Characteristics:
Pallor (below the injury); paroxysmal hypertension (sudden periodic elevated blood pressure with systolic pressure >140 mm hg and diastolic pressure >90 mm

hg); red splotches on skin (above the injury); bradycardia or tachycardia (heart rate <60 or >100 beats per minute); diaphoresis (above the injury); headache (a diffuse pain in different portions of the head and not confined to any nerve distribution area); blurred vision; chest pain; chilling; conjunctival congestion; Horner's syndrome (contraction of the pupil, partial ptosis of the eyelid, enophthalmos and sometimes loss of sweating over the affected side of the face); metallic taste in mouth; nasal congestion; paresthesia; pilomotor reflex (goose-flesh formation when skin is cooled)

Related Factors:
Bladder distention; bowel distention; lack of patient and caregiver knowledge

Formerly "Dysreflexia"

Risk For AUTONOMIC DYSREFLEXIA (1998, 2000)

Definition:
At risk for life-threatening, uninhibited response of the sympathetic nervous system, post spinal shock, in an individual with spinal cord injury or lesion at T6 or above (has been demonstrated in patients with injuries at T7 and T8)

Defining Characteristics:
An injury/lesion at T6 or above AND at least one of the following noxious stimuli:
Neurological Stimuli: Painful/irritating stimuli below level of injury
Urological Stimuli: Bladder distention; detrusor sphincter dyssynergia; bladder spasm; instrumentation or surgery; epididymitis; urethritis; urinary tract infection; calculi; cystitis; catheterization
Gastrointestinal Stimuli: Bowel distention; fecal impaction; digital stimulation; suppositories; hemorrhoids; difficult passage of feces; constipation; enemas; GI system pathology; gastric ulcers; esophageal reflux; gallstones
Reproductive Stimuli: Menstruation; sexual intercourse; pregnancy; labor and delivery; ovarian cyst; ejaculation
Musculo-Skeletal-Integumentary Stimuli: Cutaneous stimulation (e.g., pressure ulcer, ingrown toenail, dressings, burns, rash); pressure over bony prominences or genitalia; heterotrophic bone; spasm; fractures; range-of-motion exercises; wounds; sunburns
Regulatory Stimuli: Temperature fluctuations; extreme environmental temperatures
Situational Stimuli: Positioning; constrictive clothing (e.g., straps, stockings, shoes); drug reactions (e.g., decongestants, sympathomimetics, vasoconstrictors, narcotic withdrawal); surgical procedure
Cardiac/Pulmonary Problems: Pulmonary emboli; deep vein thrombosis

Disturbed BODY IMAGE* (1973, 1998)

Definition:
Confusion in mental picture of one's physical self

Defining Characteristics:
Verbalization of feelings that reflect an altered view of one's body in appearance, structure, or function; verbalization of perceptions that reflect an altered view of one's body in appearance, structure, or function; nonverbal response to actual or perceived change in body structure and/or function; behaviors of avoidance, monitoring, or acknowledgment of one's body *Objective:* Missing body part; trauma to nonfunctioning part; not touching body part; hiding or over-exposing body part (intentional or unintentional); actual change in structure and/or function; change in social involvement; change in ability to estimate spatial relationship of body to environment; extension of body boundary to incorporate environmental objects; not looking at body part
Subjective: Refusal to verify actual change; preoccupation with change or loss; personalization of part or loss by name; depersonalization of part or loss by impersonal pronouns; extension of body boundary to incorporate environmental objects; negative feelings about body (e.g., feelings of helplessness, hopelessness, or powerlessness); verbalization of change in lifestyle; focus on past strength, function, or appearance; fear of rejection or of reaction by others; emphasis on remaining strengths; heightened achievement

Related Factors:
Psychosocial; biophysical; cognitive/perceptual; cultural or spiritual; developmental changes; illness; trauma or injury; surgery; illness treatment

Formerly "Body Image Disturbance"

Risk For Imbalanced BODY TEMPERATURE* (1986)

Definition:
At risk for failure to maintain body temperature within normal range

Risk Factors:
Altered metabolic rate; illness or trauma affecting temperature regulation; medications causing vaso-constriction or vasodilation; inappropriate clothing for environmental temperature; inactivity or vigorous activity; extremes of weight; extremes of age; dehydration; sedation; exposure to cold/cool or warm/hot environments

Formerly "Risk for Altered Body Temperature"

BOWEL INCONTINENCE (1975, 1998)

Definition:
Change in normal bowel habits characterized by involuntary passage of stool

Defining Characteristics:
Constant dribbling of soft stool; fecal odor; inability to delay defecation; urgency; self-report of inability to feel rectal fullness; fecal staining of clothing and/or bedding; recognizes rectal fullness but reports inability to expel formed stool; inattention to urge to defecate; inability to recognize urge to defecate; red perianal skin

Related Factors:
Environmental factors (e.g., inaccessible bathroom); incomplete emptying of bowel; rectal sphincter abnormality; impaction; dietary habits; colorectal lesions; stress; lower motor nerve damage; abnormally high abdominal or intestinal pressure; general decline in muscle tone; loss of rectal sphincter control; impaired cognition; upper motor nerve damage; chronic diarrhea; toileting self-care deficit; impaired reservoir capacity; medications; immobility; laxative abuse

Effective BREASTFEEDING (1990)

Definition:
Mother-infant dyad/family exhibits adequate proficiency and satisfaction with breastfeeding process

Defining Characteristics:
Effective mother/infant communication patterns; regular and sustained suckling/swallowing at the breast; appropriate infant weight pattern for age; infant content after feeding; mother able to position infant at breast to promote a successful latch-on response; signs and/or symptoms of oxytocin release; adequate infant elimination patterns for age; eagerness of infant to nurse; maternal verbalization of satisfaction with the breastfeeding process

Related Factors:
Infant gestational age >34 weeks; support source; normal infant oral structure; maternal confidence; basic breastfeeding knowledge; normal breast structure

Ineffective BREASTFEEDING (1988)

Definition:
Dissatisfaction or difficulty a mother, infant, or child experiences with the breastfeeding process

Defining Characteristics:
Unsatisfactory breastfeeding process; nonsustained suckling at the breast; resisting latching on; unresponsive to comfort measures; persistence of sore nipples beyond first week of breastfeeding; observable signs of inadequate infant intake; insufficient emptying of each breast per feeding; infant inability to attach on to maternal breast correctly; infant arching and crying at the breast; infant exhibiting fussiness and crying within the first hour after breastfeeding; actual or perceived inadequate milk supply; no observable signs of oxytocin release; insufficient opportunity for suckling at the breast

Related Factors:
Nonsupportive partner/family; previous breast surgery; infant receiving supplemental feedings with artificial nipple; prematurity; previous history of breastfeeding failure; poor infant sucking reflex; maternal breast anomaly; maternal anxiety or ambivalence; interruption in breastfeeding; infant anomaly; knowledge deficit

Interrupted BREASTFEEDING (1992)

Definition:
Break in the continuity of the breastfeeding process as a result of inability or inadvisability to put baby to breast for feeding

Defining Characteristics:
Infant receives no nourishment at the breast for some or all of feedings; maternal desire to maintain and provide (or eventually provide) her breast milk for her infant's nutritional needs; lack of knowledge regarding expression and storage of breast milk; separation of mother and infant

Related Factors:
Contraindications to breastfeeding; maternal employment; maternal or infant illness; need to abruptly wean infant; prematurity

Ineffective BREATHING PATTERN (1980, 1996, 1998)

Definition:
Inspiration and/or expiration that does not provide adequate ventilation

Defining Characteristics:
Decreased inspiratory/expiratory pressure; decreased minute ventilation; use of accessory muscles to breathe; nasal flaring; dyspnea; orthopnea; altered chest excursion; shortness of breath; assumption of 3-point position; pursed-lip breathing; prolonged expiration phases; increased anterior-posterior diameter; respiratory rate/min: (*Infants:* <25 or >60, *Ages 1–4:* <20 or >30, *Ages 5–14:* <14 or >25, *Adults* >14: ≤11 or >24); depth of breathing (*Adult tidal volume:* 500 mL at rest, *Infant tidal volume:* 6–8 mL/kg; timing ratio; decreased vital capacity

Related Factors:
Hyperventilation; hypoventilation syndrome; bony deformity; pain; chest wall deformity; anxiety; decreased energy/fatigue; neuromuscular dysfunction; musculoskeletal impairment; perception/cognitive impairment; obesity; spinal cord injury; body position; neurological immaturity; respiratory muscle fatigue

Decreased CARDIAC OUTPUT (1975, 1996, 2000)

Definition:
Inadequate blood pumped by the heart to meet metabolic demands of the body

Defining Characteristics:
Altered heart rate/rhythm; arrhythmias (tachycardia, bradycardia); palpitations; EKG changes
Altered Preload: Jugular vein distention; fatigue; edema; murmurs; increased/decreased central venous pressure (CVP); increased/decreased pulmonary artery wedge pressure (PAWP); weight gain
Altered Afterload: Cold/clammy skin; shortness of breath/dyspnea; oliguria; prolonged capillary refill; decreased peripheral pulses; variations in blood pressure readings; increased/decreased systemic vascular resistance (SVR); increased/decreased pulmonary vascular resistance (PVR); skin color changes
Altered Contractility: crackles; cough; orthopnea/paroxysmal nocturnal dyspnea; cardiac output <4 L/min; cardiac index <2.5 L/min; decreased ejection fraction, stroke volume index (SVI), left ventricular stroke work index (LVSWI); S3 or S4 sounds
Behavioral/Emotional: Anxiety; Restlessness

Related Factors:
Altered heart rate/rhythm; altered stroke volume; altered preload; altered afterload; altered contractility

CAREGIVER ROLE STRAIN (1992, 1998, 2000)

Definition:
Difficulty in performing caregiver role

Defining Characteristics:
Caregiving Activities: Difficulty performing/completing required tasks; preoccupation with care routine; apprehension about the future regarding care receiver's health and the caregiver's ability to provide care; apprehension about care receiver's care if caregiver becomes ill or dies; dysfunctional change in caregiving activities; apprehension about possible institutionalization of care receiver

Caregiver Health Status:
Physical: GI upset (e.g., mild stomach cramps, vomiting, diarrhea, recurrent gastric ulcer episodes); weight change; rash; hypertension; cardiovascular disease; diabetes; fatigue; headaches
Emotional: Impaired individual coping; feeling depressed; disturbed sleep; anger; stress; somatization; increased nervousness; increased emotional lability; impatience; lack of time to meet personal needs; frustration
Socioeconomic: Withdraws from social life; changes in leisure activities; low work productivity; refuses career advancement

Caregiver-Care Receiver Relationship:
Grief/uncertainty regarding changed relationship with care receiver; difficulty watching care receiver go through the illness

Family Processes:
Family conflict; concerns about family members

Related Factors:

Care Receiver Health Status: Illness severity; illness chronicity; increasing care needs/dependency; unpredictability of illness course; instability of care receiver's health; problem behaviors; psychological or cognitive problems; addiction or codependency

Caregiving Activities: Amount of activities; complexity of activities; 24-hour care responsibilities; ongoing changes in activities; discharge of family members to home with significant care needs; years of caregiving; unpredictability of care situation

Caregiver Health Status: Physical problems; psychological or cognitive problems; addiction or codependency; marginal coping patterns; unrealistic expectations of self; inability to fulfill one's own or other's expectations

Socioeconomic: Isolation from others; competing role commitments; alienation from family, friends, and co-workers; insufficient recreation

Caregiver–Care Receiver Relationship: History of poor relationship; presence of abuse or violence; unrealistic expectations of caregiver by care receiver; mental status of elder inhibiting conversation

Family Processes: History of marginal family coping; history of family dysfunction

Resources: Inadequate physical environment for providing care (e.g., housing, temperature, safety); inadequate equipment for providing care; inadequate transportation; inadequate community resources (e.g., respite services, recreational; resources); insufficient finances; lack of support; caregiver is not developmentally ready for caregiver role; inexperience with caregiving; insufficient time; lack of knowledge about or difficulty accessing community resources; lack of caregiver privacy; emotional strength; physical energy; assistance and support (formal and informal)

Risk For CAREGIVER ROLE STRAIN (1992)

Definition:
Caregiver is vulnerable for felt difficulty in performing the family caregiver role

Risk Factors:
Caregiver not developmentally ready for caregiver role (e.g., a young adult needing to provide care for middle aged); inadequate physical environment for providing care (e.g., housing, transportation, community services, equipment); unpredictable illness course or instability in the care receiver's health; psychological or cognitive problems in care receiver; presence of situational stressors that normally affect families (e.g., significant loss, disaster or crisis, economic vulnerability, major life events); presence of abuse or violence; premature birth/congenital defect; past history of poor relationship between caregiver and care receiver; marginal family adaptation or dysfunction prior to the caregiving situation; marginal

caregiver's coping patterns; lack of respite and recreation for caregiver; inexperience with caregiving; caregiver is female; addiction or codependency; care receiver exhibits deviant, bizarre behavior; caregiver competing role commitments; caregiver health impairment; illness severity of the care receiver; caregiver spouse; developmental delay or retardation of the care receiver or caregiver; complexity/amount of caregiving tasks; discharge of family member with significant home care needs; duration of caregiving required; family/caregiver isolation

Impaired Verbal COMMUNICATION (1983, 1996, 1998)

Definition:
Decreased, delayed, or absent ability to receive, process, transmit, and use a system of symbols

Defining Characteristics:
Willful refusal to speak; disorientation in the three spheres of time, space, person; inability to speak dominant language; does not or cannot speak; speaks or verbalizes with difficulty; inappropriate verbalization; difficulty forming words or sentences (e.g., aphonia, dyslalia, dysarthria); difficulty expressing thought verbally (e.g., aphasia, dysphasia, apraxia, dyslexia); stuttering; slurring; dyspnea; absence of eye contact or difficulty in selective attending; difficulty in comprehending and maintaining usual communication pattern; partial or total visual deficit; inability or difficulty in use of facial or body expressions

Related Factors:
Decrease in circulation to brain; cultural difference; psychological barriers (e.g., psychosis, lack of stimuli); physical barrier (tracheostomy, intubation); anatomical defect (e.g., cleft palate, alteration of the neuromuscular visual system, auditory system, phonatory apparatus); brain tumor; differences related to developmental age; side effects of medication; environmental barriers; absence of significant others; altered perceptions; lack of information; stress; alteration of self-esteem or self-concept; physiological conditions; alteration of central nervous system; weakening of the musculoskeletal system; emotional conditions

Readiness For Enhanced COMMUNICATION (2002)

Definition:
A pattern of exchanging information and ideas with others that is sufficient for meeting one's needs and life's goals and can be strengthened

Defining Characteristics:
Expresses willingness to enhance communication; able to speak or write a language; forms words;

phrases, and language; expresses thoughts and feelings; uses and interprets nonverbal cues appropriately; expresses satisfaction with ability to share information and ideas with others

Decisional CONFLICT (Specify) (1988)

Definition:
Uncertainty about course of action to be taken when choice among competing actions involves risk, loss, or challenge to personal life values

Defining Characteristics:
Verbalizes uncertainty about choices; verbalizes undesired consequences of alternative actions being considered; vacillation between alternative choices; delayed decision making; verbalizes feeling of distress while attempting a decision; self-focusing; physical signs of distress or tension (e.g., increased heart rate, increased muscle tension, restlessness); questioning personal values and beliefs while attempting a decision

Related Factors:
Support system deficit; perceived threat to value system; lack of experience or interference with decision making; multiple or divergent sources of information; lack of relevant information; unclear personal values/beliefs

Parental Role CONFLICT (1988)

Definition:
Parent experience of role confusion and conflict in response to crisis

Defining Characteristics:
Parent(s) express(es) concern(s) about changes in parental role, family functioning, family communication, family health; parent(s) express(es) concern(s)/feeling(s) of inadequacy to provide for child's physical and emotional needs during hospitalization or in home; reluctant to participate in usual caretaking activities even with encouragement and support; demonstrated disruption in caretaking routines; expresses concern about perceived loss of control over decisions relating to their child; verbalizes or demonstrates feelings of guilt, anger, fear, anxiety, and/or frustrations about effect of child's illness on family process

Related Factors:
Change in marital status; home care of a child with special needs (e.g., apnea monitoring, postural drainage, hyperalimentation); interruptions of family life due to home care regimen (e.g., treatments, caregivers, lack of respite); specialized care-center policies; separation from child due to chronic illness; intimidation with invasive or restrictive modalities (e.g., isolation, intubation)

Acute CONFUSION (1994)

Definition:
Abrupt onset of a cluster of global, transient changes and disturbances in attention, cognition, psychomotor activity, level of consciousness, and/or sleep/wake cycle

Defining Characteristics:
Lack of motivation to initiate and/or follow through with goal-directed or purposeful behavior; fluctuation in psychomotor activity; misperceptions; fluctuation in cognition; increased agitation or restlessness; fluctuation in level of consciousness; fluctuation in sleep-wake cycle; hallucinations

Related Factors:
Over 60 years of age; alcohol abuse; delirium; dementia; drug abuse

Chronic CONFUSION (1994)

Definition:
Irreversible, long-standing, and/or progressive deterioration of intellect and personality characterized by decreased ability to interpret environmental stimuli; decreased capacity for intellectual thought processes; and manifested by disturbances of memory, orientation, and behavior

Defining Characteristics:
Altered interpretation/response to stimuli; clinical evidence of organic impairment; progressive/long-standing cognitive impairment; altered personality; impaired memory (short- and long-term); impaired socialization; no change in level of consciousness

Related Factors:
Multi-infarct dementia; Korsakoff's psychosis; head injury; Alzheimer's disease; cerebral vascular accident

CONSTIPATION (1975, 1998)

Definition:
Decrease in normal frequency of defecation accompanied by difficult or incomplete passage of stool and/or passage of excessively hard, dry stool

Defining Characteristics:
Change in bowel pattern; bright red blood with stool; presence of soft, pastelike stool in rectum; distended abdomen; dark, black, or tarry stool; increased abdominal pressure; percussed abdominal dullness; pain with defecation; decreased volume of stool; straining with defecation; decreased frequency; dry, hard, formed stool; palpable rectal mass; feeling of rectal fullness or pressure; abdominal pain; unable to pass stool; anorexia; headache; change in abdominal growling (borborygmi); indigestion; atypical presentations in older adults (e.g., change in mental status, urinary incontinence, unexplained falls, elevated body temperature); severe flatus; generalized fatigue;

hypoactive or hyperactive bowel sounds; palpable abdominal mass; abdominal tenderness with or without palpable muscle resistance; nausea and/or vomiting; oozing liquid stool

Related Factors:
Functional: Recent environmental changes; habitual denial/ignoring of urge to defecate; insufficient physical activity; irregular defecation habits; inadequate toileting (e.g., timeliness, positioning for defecation, privacy); abdominal muscle weakness

Psychological: Depression; emotional stress; mental confusion

Pharmacological: Anticonvulsants; antilipemic agents; laxative overdose; calcium carbonate; aluminum-containing antacids; nonsteroidal anti-inflammatory agents; opiates; anticholinergics; diuretics; iron salts; phenothiazines; sedatives; sympathomimetics; bismuth salts; antidepressants; calcium channel blockers

Mechanical: Rectal abscess or ulcer; pregnancy; rectal anal fissures; tumors; megacolon; (Hirschsprung's disease); electrolyte imbalance; rectal prolapse; prostate enlargement; neurological impairment; rectal anal stricture; rectocele; postsurgical obstruction; hemorrhoids; obesity

Physiological: Poor eating habits; decreased motility of gastrointestinal tract; inadequate dentition or oral hygiene; insufficient fiber intake; insufficient fluid intake; change in usual foods and eating patterns; dehydration

Perceived CONSTIPATION (1988)

Definition:
Self-diagnosis of constipation and abuse of laxatives, enemas, and suppositories to ensure a daily bowel movement

Defining Characteristics:
Expectation of a daily bowel movement with resulting overuse of laxatives, enemas, and suppositories; expectation of passage of stool at same time everyday

Related Factors:
Impaired thought processes; faulty appraisal; cultural/family health beliefs

Risk For CONSTIPATION (1998)

Definition:
At risk for a decrease in normal frequency of defecation accompanied by difficult or incomplete passage of stool and/or passage of excessively hard, dry stool

Risk Factors:
Functional: Habitual denial/ignoring of urge to defecate; recent environmental changes; inadequate toileting (e.g., timeliness, positioning for defecation, privacy); irregular defecation habits; insufficient physical activity; abdominal muscle weakness

Psychological: Emotional stress; mental confusion; depression

Physiological: Insufficient fiber intake; dehydration; inadequate dentition or oral hygiene; poor eating habits; insufficient fluid intake; change in usual foods and eating patterns; decreased motility of gastrointestinal tract

Pharmacological: Anticonvulsants; phenothiazines; nonsteroidal anti-inflammatory agents; sedatives; aluminum-containing antacids; laxative overuse; iron salts; anticholinergics; antidepressants; antilipemic agents; calcium channel blockers; calcium carbonate; diuretics; sympathomimetics; opiates; bismuth salts

Mechanical: Rectal abscess or ulcer; pregnancy; rectal anal stricture; postsurgical obstruction; rectal anal fissures; megacolon; (Hirschsprung's disease); electrolyte imbalance; tumors; prostate enlargement; rectocele; rectal prolapse; neurological impairment; hemorrhoids; obesity

Readiness For Enhanced COPING (2002)

Definition:
A pattern of cognitive and behavioral efforts to manage demands that is sufficient for well-being and can be strengthened

Defining Characteristics
Defines stressors as manageable; seeks social support; uses a broad range of problem-oriented and emotion-oriented strategies; uses spiritual resources; acknowledges power; seeks knowledge of new strategies; is aware of possible environmental changes

Ineffective COPING (1978, 1998)

Definition:
Inability to form a valid appraisal of the stressors, inadequate choices of practiced responses, and/or inability to use available resources

Defining Characteristics:
Lack of goal-directed behavior/resolution of problem, including inability to attend to and difficulty organizing information; sleep disturbance; abuse of chemical agents; decreased use of social support; use of forms of coping that impede adaptive behavior; poor concentration; fatigue; inadequate problem solving; verbalization of inability to cope or inability to ask for help; inability to meet basic needs; destructive behavior toward self or others; inability to meet role expectations; high illness rate; change in usual communication patterns; risk taking

Related Factors:
Gender differences in coping strategies; inadequate level of confidence in ability to cope; uncertainty;

inadequate social support created by characteristics of relationships; inadequate level of perception of control; inadequate resources available; high degree of threat; situational or maturational crisis; disturbance in pattern of tension release; inadequate opportunity to prepare for stressor; inability to conserve adaptive energies; disturbance in pattern of appraisal of threat

Ineffective Community COPING (1994, 1998)

Definition:
Pattern of community activities (for adaptation and problem solving) that is unsatisfactory for meeting the demands or needs of the community

Defining Characteristics:
Expressed community powerlessness; deficits in community participation; excessive community conflicts; expressed vulnerability; high illness rates; stressors perceived as excessive; community does not meet its own expectations; increased social problems (e.g., homicides, vandalism, arson, terrorism, robbery, infanticide, abuse, divorce, unemployment, poverty, militancy, mental illness)

Related Factors:
Natural or man-made disasters; ineffective or nonexistent community systems (e.g., lack of emergency; medical system, transportation system, or disaster planning systems); deficits in community social support services and resources; inadequate resources for problem solving

Readiness For Enhanced Community COPING* (1994)

Definition:
Pattern of community activities for adaptation and problem solving that is satisfactory for meeting the demands or needs of the community but can be improved for management of current and future problems/stressors

Defining Characteristics:
One or more characteristics that indicate effective coping: positive communication between community/aggregates and larger community; programs available for recreation and relaxation; resources sufficient for managing stressors; agreement that community is responsible for stress management; active planning by community for predicted stressors; active problem solving by community when faced with issues; positive communication among community members

Related Factors:
Community has a sense of power to manage stressors; social supports available; resources available for problem solving

*Formerly "Potential for Enhanced Community Coping"

Defensive COPING (1988)

Definition:
Repeated projection of falsely positive self-evaluation based on a self-protective pattern that defends against underlying perceived threats to positive self-regard

Defining Characteristics:
Grandiosity; rationalization of failures; hypersensitivity to slight/criticism; denial of obvious problems/weaknesses; projection of blame/responsibility; lack of follow-through or participation in treatment or therapy; superior attitude toward others; hostile laughter or ridicule of others; difficulty in perception of reality/reality testing; difficulty establishing/maintaining relationships

Related Factors:
To be developed

Compromised Family COPING* (1980, 1996)

Definition:
Usually supportive primary person (family member or close friend) provides insufficient, ineffective, or compromised support, comfort, assistance, or encouragement that may be needed by the client to manage or master adaptive tasks related to his/her health challenge

Defining Characteristics:
Objective: Significant person attempts assistive or supportive behaviors with less than satisfactory results; significant person displays protective behavior disproportionate (too little or too much) to client's abilities or need for autonomy; significant person withdraws or enters into limited or temporary personal communication with client at the time of need

Subjective: Client expresses or confirms a concern or complaint about significant other's response to his/her health problem; significant person describes or confirms an inadequate understanding or knowledge base, which interferes with effective assistive or supportive behaviors; significant person describes preoccupation with personal reaction (e.g., fear, anticipatory grief, guilt, anxiety) to client's illness, disability, or other situational or developmental crisis

Related Factors:
Temporary preoccupation by a significant person who tries to manage; emotional conflicts and personal suffering and is unable to perceive or act effectively in regard to client's needs; temporary family disorganization and role changes; prolonged disease or progression of disability that exhausts supportive capacity of significant people; other situational or developmental crises or situations the significant person may be facing; inadequate or incorrect information or

understanding by a primary person; little support provided by client, in turn, for primary person

Formerly "Ineffective Family Coping"

Disabled Family COPING* (1980, 1996)

Definition:
Behavior of significant person (family member or other primary person) that disables his/her capacities and the client's capacities to effectively address tasks essential to either person's adaptation to the health challenge

Defining Characteristics:
Intolerance; agitation, depression, aggression, hostility; taking on illness signs of client; rejection; psychosomaticism; neglectful relationships with other family members; neglectful care of client in regard to basic human needs and/or illness treatment; distortion of reality regarding client's health problem, including extreme denial about its existence or severity; impaired restructuring of a meaningful life for self; impaired individualization, prolonged over-concern for client; desertion; decisions and actions by family that are detrimental to economic or social well-being; carrying on usual routines, disregarding client's needs; abandonment; client's development of helpless, inactive dependence; disregarding needs

Related Factors:
Significant person with chronically unexpressed feelings of guilt, anxiety, hostility, despair, etc.; arbitrary handling of family's resistance to treatment, which tends to solidify; defensiveness as it fails to deal adequately with underlying anxiety; dissonant or discrepant coping styles for dealing with adaptive tasks by the significant person and client or among significant people; highly ambivalent family relationships

Formerly "Ineffective Family Coping"

Readiness For Enhanced Family COPING* (1980)

Definition:
Effective management of adaptive tasks by family member involved with the client's health challenge, who now exhibits desire and readiness for enhanced health and growth in regard to self and in relation to the client

Defining Characteristics:
Individual expresses interest in making contact on a one-to-one basis or on a mutual-aid group basis with another person who has experienced a similar situation; family member attempts to describe growth impact of crisis on his/her own values, priorities, goal, or relationships; family member moves in direction of health-promoting and enriching life-style that supports and monitors maturational processes, audits and negotiates treatment programs, and chooses experiences that optimize wellness

Related Factors:
Needs sufficiently gratified and adaptive tasks effectively addressed to enable goals of self-actualization to surface

Formerly "Family Coping: Potential for Growth"

Ineffective DENIAL (1988)

Definition:
Conscious or unconscious attempt to disavow the knowledge or meaning of an event to reduce anxiety/fear, but leading to the detriment of health

Defining Characteristics:
Delays seeking or refuses healthcare attention to the detriment of health; does not perceive personal relevance of symptoms or danger; displaces source of symptoms to other organs; displays inappropriate affect; does not admit fear of death or invalidism; makes dismissive gestures or comments when speaking of distressing events; minimizes symptoms; unable to admit impact of disease on life pattern; uses home remedies (self-treatment) to relieve symptoms; displaces fear of impact of the condition

Related Factors:
To be developed

Impaired DENTITION* (1998)

Definition:
Disruption in tooth development/eruption patterns or structural integrity of individual teeth

Defining Characteristics:
Excessive plaque; crown or root caries; halitosis; tooth enamel discoloration; toothache; loose teeth; excessive calculus; incomplete eruption for age (may be primary or permanent teeth); malocclusion or tooth misalignment; premature loss of primary teeth; worn down or abraded teeth; tooth fracture(s); missing teeth or complete absence; erosion of enamel; asymmetrical facial expression

Related Factors:
Ineffective oral hygiene, sensitivity to heat or cold; barriers to self-care; access or economic barriers to professional care; nutritional deficits; dietary habits; genetic predisposition; selected prescription medications; premature loss of primary teeth; excessive intake of fluorides; chronic vomiting; chronic use of tobacco, coffee or tea, red wine; lack of knowledge regarding dental health; excessive use of abrasive cleaning agents; bruxism

Formerly "Altered Dentition"

Risk For Delayed DEVELOPMENT* (1998)

Definition:
At risk for delay of 25% or more in one or more of the areas of social or self-regulatory behavior, or in cognitive, language, gross or fine motor skills

Risk Factors:
Prenatal: Maternal age <15 or >35 years; substance abuse; infections; genetic or endocrine disorders; unplanned or unwanted pregnancy; lack of, late, or poor prenatal care; inadequate nutrition; illiteracy; poverty
Individual: Prematurity; seizures; congenital or genetic disorders; positive drug screening test; brain damage (e.g., hemorrhage in postnatal period, shaken baby, abuse, accident); vision impairment; hearing impairment or frequent otitis media; chronic illness; technology-dependent; failure to thrive, inadequate nutrition; foster or adopted child; lead poisoning; chemotherapy; radiation therapy; natural disaster; behavior disorders; substance abuse
Environmental: Poverty; violence
Caregiver: Abuse; mental illness; mental retardation or severe learning disability

Formerly "Risk for Altered Development"

DIARRHEA (1975, 1998)

Definition:
Passage of loose, unformed stools

Defining Characteristics:
At least 3 loose liquid stools per day; hyperactive bowel sounds; urgency; abdominal pain; cramping

Related Factors:
Psychological: High stress levels and anxiety
Situational: Alcohol abuse; toxins; laxative abuse; radiation; tube feedings; adverse effects of medications; contaminants; travel
Physiological: Inflammation; malabsorption; infectious processes; irritation; parasite

Risk For DISUSE SYNDROME (1988)

Definition:
At risk for deterioration of body systems as the result of prescribed or unavoidable musculoskeletal inactivity

Risk Factors:
Severe pain; mechanical immobilization; altered level of consciousness; prescribed immobilization; paralysis

NOTE: Complications from immobility can include pressure ulcer, constipation, stasis of pulmonary secretions, thrombosis, urinary tract infection and/or retention, decreased strength or endurance, orthostatic hypotension, decreased range of joint motion, disorientation, body-image disturbance, and powerlessness.

Deficient DIVERSIONAL ACTIVITY* (1980)

Definition:
Decreased stimulation from (or interest or engagement in) recreational or leisure activities

Defining Characteristics:
Usual hobbies cannot be undertaken in hospital; patient's statements regarding: boredom, wish there was something to do, to read, etc.

Related Factors:
Environmental lack of diversional activity as in long-term hospitalization; frequent lengthy treatments

Formerly " Diversional Activity Deficit"

DISTURBED ENERGY FIELD* (1994)

Definition:
Disruption of the flow of energy surrounding a person's being that results in disharmony of the body, mind, and/or spirit

Defining Characteristics:
Movement (wave/spike/tingling/dense/flowing); sounds (tone/words); temperature change (warmth/coolness); visual changes (image/color); disruption of the field (vacant/hold/spike/bulge)

Related Factors:
To be developed

Formerly " Energy Field Disturbance"

Impaired ENVIRONMENTAL INTERPRETATION SYNDROME (1994)

Definition:
Consistent lack of orientation to person, place, time, or circumstances over more than 3 to 6 months necessitating a protective environment

Defining Characteristics:
Consistent disorientation in known and unknown environments; chronic confusional states; loss of occupation or social functioning from memory decline; inability to follow simple directions, instructions; inability to concentrate; inability to reason; slow in responding to questions

Related Factors:
Depression; Huntington's disease; dementia (e.g., Alzheimer's, multi-infarct, Pick's disease, AIDS, alcoholism, Parkinson's disease)

Adult FAILURE TO THRIVE (1998)

Definition:
Progressive functional deterioration of a physical and cognitive nature. The individual's ability to live with multisystem diseases, cope with ensuing problems, and manage his/her care are remarkably diminished.

Defining Characteristics:
Anorexia: does not eat meals when offered; states does not have an appetite, not hungry, or "I don't want to eat"; inadequate nutritional intake: eating less than body requirements; consumption of minimal to no food at most meals (i.e., consumes <75% of normal requirements); weight loss (decreased from baseline weight)—5% unintentional weight loss in 1 month or 10% unintentional weight loss in 6 months; physical decline (decline in bodily function)—evidence of fatigue, dehydration, incontinence of bowel and bladder; frequent exacerbations of chronic health problems (e.g., pneumonia, urinary tract infections); cognitive decline (decline in mental processing) as evidenced by problems with responding appropriately to environmental stimuli, demonstrated difficulty in reasoning, decision making, judgment, memory and concentration, or decreased perception; decreased social skills/social withdrawal: noticeable decrease from usual past behavior in attempts to form or participate in cooperative and interdependent relationships (e.g., decreased verbal communication with staff, family, friends); decreased participation in activities of daily living that the older person once enjoyed; self-care deficit: no longer looks after or takes charge of physical cleanliness or appearance; difficulty performing simple self-care tasks; neglect of home environment and/or financial responsibilities; apathy as evidenced by lack of observable feeling or emotion in terms of normal activities of daily living and environment; altered mood state: expresses feelings of sadness, being low in spirit; expresses loss of interest in pleasurable outlets such as food, sex, work, friends, family, hobbies, or entertainment; verbalizes desire for death

Related Factors:
Depression; apathy; fatigue

Risk For FALLS (2000)

Definition:
Increased susceptibility to falling that may cause physical harm
Risk Factors:
Adults: History of falls; wheelchair use; age 65 or over; female (if elderly); lives alone; lower limb prosthesis; use of assistive devices (e.g., walker, cane)
Physiological: Presence of acute illness; postoperative conditions; visual difficulties; hearing difficulties; arthritis; orthostatic hypotension; sleeplessness; faintness when turning or extending neck; anemias; vascular disease; neoplasms (i.e., fatigue/limited mobility); urgency and/or incontinence; diarrhea; decreased lower extremity strength; postprandial blood sugar changes; foot problems; impaired physical mobility; impaired balance; difficulty with gait; proprioceptive deficits (e.g., unilateral neglect); neuropathy

Cognitive: Diminished mental status (e.g., confusion delirium, dementia, impaired reality testing)
Medications: Antihypertensive agents; ace inhibitors diuretics; tricyclic antidepressants; alcohol use; anti anxiety agents; narcotics; hypnotics or tranquilizers
Environment: Restraints; weather conditions (e.g. wet floors/ice); throw/scatter rugs; cluttered environ ment; unfamiliar, dimly lit room; no antislip material i bath and/or shower
Children: <2 years of age; male gender when <1 yea of age; lack of auto restraints; lack of gate on stairs lack of window guard; bed located near window unattended infant on bed/changing table/sofa; lack o parental supervision

Dysfunctional FAMILY PROCESSES: ALCOHOLISM* (1994)

Definition:
Psychosocial, spiritual, and physiological functions o the family unit are chronically disorganized, whic leads to conflict, denial of problems, resistance t change, ineffective problem solving, and a series o self-perpetuating crises

Defining Characteristics:
Roles and Relationships: Inconsistent parenting/lov perception of parental support; ineffective spous communication/marital problems; intimacy dysfunc tion; deterioration in family relationships/disturbe family dynamics; altered role function/disruption o family roles; closed communication systems; chroni family problems; family denial; lack of cohesiveness neglected obligations; lack of skills necessary fc relationships; reduced ability of family members t relate to each other for mutual growth and maturatior disrupted family rituals; family unable to meet securit needs of its members; economic problems; famil does not demonstrate respect for individuality an autonomy of its members; triangulating famil relationships; pattern of rejection
Behavioral: Refusal to get help/inability to accep and receive help appropriately; inadequate unde standing or knowledge of alcoholism; ineffectiv problem-solving skills; manipulation; rationalizatior denial of problems; blaming, criticizing; inability t meet emotional needs of its members; alcoh abuse; broken promises; dependency; impaire communication; difficulty with intimate relationship: enabling to maintain alcoholic drinking patter inappropriate expression of anger; isolation; inabilit to meet spiritual needs of its members; inability t express or accept wide range of feelings; inability t deal constructively with traumatic experience inability to adapt to change; immaturity; hars self-judgment; lying; lack of dealing with conflic lack of reliability; nicotine addiction; orientatio toward tension relief rather than achievement o goals; seeking approval and affirmation; difficul

having fun; agitation; chaos; contradictory, paradoxical communication; diminished physical contact; disturbances in academic performance in children; disturbances in concentration; escalating conflict; failure to accomplish current or past developmental tasks/difficulty with life cycle transitions; family special occasions are alcohol centered; controlling communication/power struggles; self-blaming; stress-related physical illnesses; substance abuse other than alcohol; unresolved grief; verbal abuse of spouse or parent

Feelings: Insecurity; lingering resentment; mistrust; vulnerability; rejection; repressed emotions; responsibility for alcoholic's behavior; shame/embarrassment; unhappiness; powerlessness; anger/suppressed rage; anxiety, tension, or distress; emotional isolation/loneliness; frustration; guilt; hopelessness; hurt; decreased self-esteem/worthlessness; hostility; lack of identity; fear; loss; emotional control by others; misunderstood; moodiness; abandonment; being different from other people; being unloved; confused love and pity; confusion; failure; depression; dissatisfaction

Related Factors:
Abuse of alcohol; Genetic predisposition; Lack of problem-solving skills; Inadequate coping skills; Family history of alcoholism, resistance to treatment; Biochemical influences; Addictive personality

Formerly "Altered Family Processes: Alcoholism"

Readiness for Enhanced FAMILY PROCESSES (2002)

Definition:
A pattern of family functioning that is sufficient to support the well-being of family members and can be strengthened

Defining Characteristics:
Expresses willingness to enhance family dynamics; family functioning meets physical, social, and psychological needs of family members; activities support the safety and growth of family members; communication is adequate; relationships are generally positive, interdependent with community; family tasks are accomplished; family roles are flexible and appropriate for developmental stages; respect for family members is evident; family adapts to change; boundaries of family members are maintained; energy level of family supports activities of daily living; family resilience is evident; balance exists between autonomy and cohesiveness

Interrupted FAMILY PROCESSES* (1982, 1998)

Definition:
Change in family relationships and/or functioning

Defining Characteristics:
Changes in power alliances, assigned tasks, effectiveness in completing assigned tasks, mutual support, availability for affective responsiveness and intimacy, patterns and rituals, participation in problem solving, participation in decision making, communication patterns, availability for emotional support, satisfaction with family, stress-reduction behaviors, expressions of conflict with and/or isolation from community resources, somatic complaints, expressions of conflict within family

Related Factors:
Power shift of family members; family roles shift; shift in health status of a family member; developmental transition and/or crisis; situation transition and/ or crises; informal or formal interaction with community; modification in family social status; modification in family finances

Formerly "Altered Family Processes"

FATIGUE (1988, 1998)

Definition:
An overwhelming sustained sense of exhaustion and decreased capacity for physical and mental work at usual level

Defining Characteristics:
Inability to restore energy even after sleep; lack of energy or inability to maintain usual level of physical activity; increase in rest requirements; tired; verbalization of an unremitting and overwhelming lack of energy; inability to maintain usual routines; lethargic or listless; increase in physical complaints; perceived need for additional energy to accomplish routine tasks; compromised concentration; disinterest in surroundings, introspection; decreased performance; compromised libido; drowsy; feelings of guilt for not keeping up with responsibilities

Related Factors:
Psychological: Boring lifestyle; stress; anxiety; depression
Environmental: Humidity; lights; noise; temperature
Situational: Negative life events; occupation
Physiological: Sleep deprivation; pregnancy; poor physical condition; disease states; increased physical exertion; malnutrition; anemia

FEAR (1980, 1996, 2000)

Definition:
Response to perceived threat that is consciously recognized as a danger

Defining Characteristics:
Report of apprehension, increased tension, decreased self-assurance, excitement, being scared, jitteriness, dread, alarm, terror, panic

Cognitive: Identifies object of fear; stimulus believed to be a threat; diminished productivity, learning ability, problem-solving ability

Behaviors: Increased alertness; avoidance or attack behaviors; impulsiveness; narrowed focus on "it" (i.e., the focus of the fear)

Physiological: Increased pulse; anorexia; nausea; vomiting; diarrhea; muscle tightness; fatigue; increased respiratory rate and shortness of breath; pallor; increased perspiration; increased systolic blood pressure; pupil dilation; dry mouth

Related Factors:
Natural/innate origin (e.g., sudden noise, height, pain, loss of physical support); learned response (e.g., conditioning, modeling from or identification with others); separation from support system in potentially stressful situation (e.g., hospitalization, hospital procedures); unfamiliarity with environmental experience(s); language barrier; sensory impairment; innate releasers (neurotransmitters); phobic stimulus

Readiness for Enhanced FLUID BALANCE (2002)

Definition:
A pattern of equilibrium between fluid volume and chemical composition of body fluids that is sufficient for meeting physical needs and can be strengthened

Defining Characteristics:
Expresses willingness to enhance fluid balance; stable weight; moist mucous membranes; food and fluid intake adequate for daily needs; straw-colored urine with specific gravity within normal limits; good tissue turgor; no excessive thirst; urine output appropriate for intake; no evidence of edema or dehydration

Deficient FLUID VOLUME* (1978, 1996)

Definition:
Decreased intravascular, interstitial, and/or intracellular fluid. This refers to dehydration, water loss alone without change in sodium.

Defining Characteristics:
Weakness; thirst; decreased skin/tongue turgor; dry skin/mucous membranes; increased pulse rate; decreased blood pressure, decreased pulse volume/pressure; decreased venous filling; change in mental state; decreased urine output; increased urine concentration; increased body temperature; elevated hematocrit; sudden weight loss (except in third spacing)

Related Factors:
Active fluid volume loss; failure of regulatory mechanisms

Formerly "Fluid Volume Deficit"

Excess FLUID VOLUME* (1982, 1996)

Definition:
Increased isotonic fluid retention

Defining Characteristics:
Weight gain over short period of time; intake exceed output; blood pressure changes, pulmonary arter pressure changes, increased central venous pressure edema, may progress to anasarca; jugular vein disten tion; changes in respiratory pattern, dyspnea or short ness of breath, orthopnea, abnormal breath sound (rales or crackles), pulmonary congestion, pleural effu sion; decreased hemoglobin and hematocrit, altere electrolytes, specific gravity changes; S3 heart sound positive hepatojugular reflex; oliguria, azotemia; chang in mental status, restlessness, anxiety

Related Factors:
Compromised regulatory mechanism; excess flui intake; excess sodium intake

Formerly "Fluid Volume Excess"

Risk For Deficient FLUID VOLUME* (1978)

Definition:
At risk for experiencing vascular, cellular, or intra cellular dehydration

Risk Factors:
Factors influencing fluids needs (e.g., hypermetabol state); medication (e.g., diuretics); loss of fluid throug abnormal routes (e.g., indwelling tubes); knowledg deficiency related to fluid volume; extremes of ag deviations affecting access, intake, or absorption fluids; (e.g., physical immobility); extremes of weigh excessive losses through normal routes (e.g., diarrhe

Formerly "Risk for Fluid Volume Deficit"

Risk For Imbalanced FLUID VOLUME* (1998)

Definition:
At risk for a decrease, increase, or rapid shift from or to the other of intravascular, interstitial, and/or intra cellular fluid. This refers to body fluid loss, gain, or bot

Risk Factors:
Scheduled for major invasive procedures

Other Risk Factors:
To be determined

Formerly "Risk for Fluid Volume Imbalance"

Impaired GAS EXCHANGE (1980, 1996, 1998)

Definition:
Excess or deficit in oxygenation and/or carbon dioxic elimination at the alveolar-capillary membrane

Defining Characteristics:
Visual disturbances; decreased carbon dioxide; tachycardia; hypercapnia; restlessness; somnolence; irritability; hypoxia; confusion; dyspnea; abnormal arterial blood gases; cyanosis (in neonates only); abnormal skin color (pale, dusky); hypoxemia; hypercarbia; headache upon awakening; abnormal rate, rhythm, depth of breathing; diaphoresis; abnormal arterial pH; nasal flaring

Related Factors:
Ventilation perfusion imbalance; alveolar-capillary membrane changes

Anticipatory GRIEVING (1980, 1996)

Definition:
Intellectual and emotional responses and behaviors by which individuals, families, communities work through the process of modifying self-concept based on the perception of potential loss

Defining Characteristics:
Potential loss of significant object (e.g., people, possessions, job, status, home, ideals, parts and processes of the body); expression of distress at potential loss; sorrow; guilt; denial of potential loss; anger; altered communication patterns; denial of the significance of the loss; bargaining; alteration in eating habits, sleep patterns, dream patterns, activity level, libido; difficulty taking on new or different roles; resolution of grief prior to the reality of loss

Related Factors:
To be developed

Dysfunctional GRIEVING (1980, 1996)

Definition:
Extended, unsuccessful use of intellectual and emotional responses by which individuals, families, communities attempt to work through the process of modifying self-concept based upon the perception of loss

Defining Characteristics:
Repetitive use of ineffectual behaviors associated with attempts to reinvest in relationships; reliving of past experiences with little or no reduction (diminishment) of intensity of the grief; prolonged interference with life functioning; onset or exacerbation of somatic or psychosomatic responses; verbal expression of distress at loss; denial of loss; expression of guilt; expression of unresolved issues; anger; sadness; crying; difficulty in expressing loss; alterations in eating habits, sleep patterns, dream patterns, activity level, libido, concentration and/or pursuit of tasks; idealization of lost object (e.g., people, possessions, job, status, home, ideals, parts and processes of the body); interference with life functioning; developmental regression; labile affect

Related Factors:
Actual or perceived object loss (e.g., people, possessions, job, status, home, ideals, parts and processes of the body)

Delayed GROWTH AND DEVELOPMENT* (1986)

Definition:
Deviations from age-group norms

Defining Characteristics:
Altered physical growth; delay or difficulty in performing skills (motor, social, expressive) typical of age group; inability to perform self-care or self-control activities appropriate for age; flat affect; listlessness, decreased response time

Related Factors:
Prescribed dependence; indifference; separation from significant others; environmental and stimulation deficiencies; effects of physical disability; inadequate caretaking; inconsistent responsiveness; multiple caretakers

*Formerly "Altered Growth and Development"

Risk For Disproportionate GROWTH* (1998)

Definition:
At risk for growth above the 97th percentile or below the 3rd percentile for age, crossing two percentile channels; disproportionate growth

Risk Factors:
Prenatal: Congenital/genetic disorders; maternal nutrition; multiple gestation; teratogen exposure; substance use/abuse; maternal infection
Individual: Infection; prematurity; malnutrition; organic and inorganic factors; caregiver and/or individual maladaptive feeding behaviors; anorexia; insatiable appetite; chronic illness; substance abuse
Environmental: Deprivation; teratogen; lead poisoning; poverty; violence; natural disasters
Caregiver: Abuse; mental illness, mental retardation, severe learning disability

*Formerly "Risk for Altered Growth"

Ineffective HEALTH MAINTENANCE* (1982)

Definition:
Inability to identify, manage and/or seek out help to maintain health

Defining Characteristics:
Demonstrated lack of knowledge regarding basic health practices; demonstrated lack of adaptive

behaviors to internal/external environmental changes; reported or observed inability to take responsibility for meeting basic health practices in any or all functional pattern areas; history of lack of health-seeking behavior; expressed interest in improving health behaviors; reported or observed lack of equipment, financial and/or other resources; reported or observed impairment of personal support systems

Related Factors:
Ineffective family coping; perceptual/cognitive impairment (complete/partial lack of gross and/or fine motor skills); lack of, or significant alteration in, communication skills (written, verbal, and/or gestural); unachieved developmental tasks; lack of material resources; dysfunctional grieving; disabling spiritual distress; lack of ability to make deliberate and thoughtful judgments; ineffective individual coping

Formerly "Altered Health Maintenance"

HEALTH-SEEKING BEHAVIORS (Specify) (1988)

Definition:
Active seeking (by a person in stable health) of ways to alter personal health habits and/or the environment in order to move toward a higher level of health

Defining Characteristics:
Expressed or observed desire to seek a higher level of wellness; demonstrated or observed lack of knowledge about health-promotion behaviors; stated or observed unfamiliarity with wellness community resources; expression of concern about current environmental conditions on health status; expressed or observed desire for increased control of health practice

Related Factors:
To be developed

NOTE. Stable health is defined as achievement of age-appropriate illness-prevention measures; client reports good or excellent health, and signs and symptoms of disease, if present, are controlled.

Impaired HOME MAINTENANCE* (1980)

Definition:
Inability to independently maintain a safe growth-promoting immediate environment

Defining Characteristics:
Subjective: Household members express difficulty in maintaining their home in a comfortable fashion; household members describe outstanding debts or financial crises; household members request assistance with home maintenance
Objective: Disorderly surroundings; unwashed or unavailable cooking equipment, clothes, or linen; accumulation of dirt, food wastes, or hygienic

wastes; offensive odors; inappropriate household temperature; overtaxed family members (e.g. exhausted, anxious); lack of necessary equipment o aids; presence of vermin or rodents; repeated hygieni disorders, infestations, or infections

Related Factors:
Individual/family member disease or injury; unfami liarity with neighborhood resources; lack of rol modeling; lack of knowledge; insufficient famil organization or planning; inadequate support systems impaired cognitive or emotional functioning; insuffi cient finances

Formerly "Impaired Home Maintenance Management"

HOPELESSNESS (1986)

Definition:
Subjective state in which an individual sees limited o no alternatives or personal choices available and i unable to mobilize energy on own behalf

Defining Characteristics:
Passivity, decreased verbalization; decreased affec verbal cues (e.g., despondent content, "I can't, sighing); closing eyes; decreased appetite; decrease response to stimuli; increased/decreased sleep; lac of initiative; lack of involvement in care/passivel allowing care; shrugging in response to speake turning away from speaker

Related Factors:
Abandonment; prolonged activity restriction creatin isolation; lost belief in transcendent values/God; long term stress; failing or deteriorating physiologica condition

HYPERTHERMIA (1986)

Definition:
Body temperature elevated above normal range

Defining Characteristics:
Increase in body temperature above normal range seizures or convulsions; flushed skin; increase respiratory rate; tachycardia; warm to touch

Related Factors:
Illness or trauma; increased metabolic rate; vigor ous activity; medications or anesthesia; inability o decreased ability to perspire; exposure to hot environ ment; dehydration; inappropriate clothing

HYPOTHERMIA (1986, 1988)

Definition:
Body temperature below normal range

Defining Characteristics:
Reduction in body temperature below normal range pallor; shivering; cool skin; cyanotic nail bed hypertension; piloerection; slow capillary refill; tachy cardia

Related Factors:
Exposure to cool or cold environment; medications causing vasodilation; malnutrition; inadequate clothing; illness or trauma; evaporation from skin in cool environment; decreased metabolic rate; damage to hypothalamus; consumption of alcohol; aging; inability or decreased ability to shiver; inactivity

Disturbed Personal IDENTITY* (1978)

Definition:
Inability to distinguish between self and nonself

Defining Characteristics:
To be developed

Related Factors:
To be developed

Formerly "Personal Identity Disturbance"

Functional Urinary INCONTINENCE (1986, 1998)

Definition:
Inability of usually continent person to reach toilet in time to avoid unintentional loss of urine

Defining Characteristics:
Amount of time required to reach toilet exceeds length of time between sensing the urge to void and uncontrolled voiding; loss of urine before reaching toilet; may only be incontinent in early morning; senses need to void; able to completely empty bladder

Related Factors:
Psychological factors; impaired vision; impaired cognition; neuromuscular limitations; altered environmental factors; weakened supporting pelvic structures

Reflex Urinary INCONTINENCE (1986, 1998)

Definition:
Involuntary loss of urine at somewhat predictable intervals when a specific bladder volume is reached

Defining Characteristics:
No sensation of urge to void; complete emptying with lesion above pontine micturition center; incomplete emptying with lesion above sacral micturition center; no sensation of bladder fullness; sensations associated with full bladder such as sweating, restlessness, and abdominal discomfort; inability to voluntarily inhibit or initiate voiding; no sensation of voiding; predictable pattern of voiding; sensation of urgency without voluntary inhibition of bladder contraction

Related Factors:
Tissue damage from radiation cystitis, inflammatory bladder conditions, or radical pelvic surgery; neurological impairment above level of sacral or pontine micturition center

Stress Urinary INCONTINENCE* (1986)

Definition:
Loss of less than 50 mL of urine occurring with increased abdominal pressure

Defining Characteristics:
Reported or observed dribbling with increased abdominal pressure; urinary frequency (more often than every 2 hours); urinary urgency

Related Factors:
Weak pelvic muscles and structural supports; degenerative changes in pelvic muscles and structural supports associated; with increased age; high intra-abdominal pressure (e.g., obesity, gravid uterus); overdistention between voidings; incompetent bladder; outlet

Formerly "Stress Incontinence"

Total Urinary INCONTINENCE* (1986)

Definition:
Continuous and unpredictable loss of urine

Defining Characteristics:
Constant flow of urine at unpredictable times without uninhibited bladder contractions/spasm or distention; nocturia; unsuccessful incontinence refractory treatments; unawareness of incontinence; lack of perineal or bladder filling awareness

Related Factors:
Neuropathy preventing transmission of reflex indicating bladder fullness; trauma or disease affecting spinal cord nerves; anatomic (fistula); independent contraction of detrusor reflex due to surgery; neurological dysfunction causing triggering of micturition at unpredictable times

Formerly "Total Incontinence"

Urge Urinary INCONTINENCE* (1986)

Definition:
Involuntary passage of urine occurring soon after a strong sense of urgency to void

Defining Characteristics:
Urinary urgency; bladder contracture/spasm; frequency (voiding more often than every 2 hours); voiding in large amounts (>550 cc); voiding in small amounts (<100 cc); nocturia (more than 2 times a night); inability to reach toilet in time

Related Factors:
Alcohol; caffeine; decreased bladder capacity (e.g., history of PID, abdominal surgeries, indwelling urinary catheter); increased fluids; increased urine concentration; irritation of bladder stretch receptors causing

spasm (e.g., bladder infection); overdistention of bladder

Formerly "Urge Incontinence"

Risk For Urge Urinary INCONTINENCE* (1998)

Definition:
At risk for involuntary loss of urine associated with a sudden, strong sensation or urinary urgency

Risk Factors:
Effects of medications, caffeine, alcohol; detrusor hyperreflexia from cystitis, urethritis, tumors, renal calculi, central nervous system disorders above pontine micturition center; detrusor muscle instability with impaired contractility; involuntary sphincter relaxation; ineffective toileting habits; small bladder capacity

Formerly "Risk for Urinary Urge Incontinence"

Disorganized INFANT BEHAVIOR (1994, 1998)

Definition:
Disintegrated physiological and neurobehavioral responses to the environment

Defining Characteristics:
Regulatory Problems: Inability to inhibit startle; irritability
State-Organization System: Active-awake (fussy, worried gaze); diffuse/unclear sleep, state-oscillation; quiet-awake (staring, gaze aversion); irritable or panicky crying
Attention-Interaction System: Abnormal response to sensory stimuli (e.g., difficult to soothe, inability to sustain alert status)
Motor System: Increased, decreased, or limp tone; finger splay, fisting or hands to face; hyperextension of arms and legs; tremors, startles, twitches; jittery, jerky, uncoordinated movement; altered primitive reflexes
Physiological: Bradycardia, tachycardia, or arrhythmias; pale, cyanotic, mottled, or flushed color; "time-out signals" (e.g., gaze, grasp, hiccough, cough, sneeze, sigh, slack jaw, open mouth, tongue thrust); oximeter reading: desaturation; feeding intolerances (aspiration or emesis)

Related Factors:
Prenatal: Congenital or genetic disorders; teratogenic exposure
Postnatal: Malnutrition; oral/motor problems; pain; feeding intolerance; invasive/painful procedures; prematurity
Individual: Illness; immature neurological system; gestational age; postconceptual age
Environmental: Physical environment inappropriateness; sensory inappropriateness; sensory overstimulation; sensory deprivation

Caregiver: Cue misreading; cue knowledge deficit; environmental stimulation contribution

Risk For Disorganized INFANT BEHAVIOR (1994)

Definition:
Risk for alteration in integrating and modulation of the physiological and behavioral systems of functioning (i.e., autonomic, motor, state, organizational, self-regulatory, and attentional-interactional systems)

Risk Factors:
Pain; invasive/painful procedures; lack of containment/boundaries; oral/motor problems; prematurity; environmental overstimulation

Readiness For Enhanced Organized INFANT BEHAVIOR* (1994)

Definition:
A pattern of modulation of the physiologic and behavioral systems of functioning (i.e., autonomic, motor, state-organizational, self-regulators, and attentional-interactional systems) in an infant that is satisfactory but that can be improved resulting in higher levels of integration in response to environmental stimuli

Defining Characteristics:
Definite sleep-wake states; use of some self-regulatory behaviors; response to visual/auditory stimuli; stable physiologic measures

Related Factors:
Pain; prematurity

Formerly "Potential for Enhanced Organized Infant Behavior"

Ineffective INFANT FEEDING PATTERN (1992)

Definition:
Impaired ability to suck or coordinate the suck/swallow response

Defining Characteristics:
Inability to coordinate sucking, swallowing, and breathing; inability to initiate or sustain an effective suck

Related Factors:
Prolonged NPO; Anatomic abnormality; neurological impairment/delay; oral hypersensitivity; prematurity

Risk For INFECTION (1986)

Definition:
At increased risk for being invaded by pathogenic organisms

Risk Factors:
Invasive procedures; insufficient knowledge to avoid exposure to pathogens; trauma; tissue destruction and increased environmental exposure; rupture of amniotic membranes; pharmaceutical agents (e.g., immunosuppressants); malnutrition; increased environmental exposure to pathogens; immunosuppression; inadequate acquired immunity; inadequate secondary defenses (decreased hemoglobin, leukopenia, suppressed inflammatory response); inadequate primary defenses (broken skin, traumatized tissue, decrease in ciliary action, stasis of body fluids, change in pH secretions, altered peristalsis); chronic disease

Risk For INJURY (1978)

Definition:
At risk of injury as a result of environmental conditions interacting with the individual's adaptive and defensive resources

Risk Factors:
External: Mode of transport or transportation; people or provider (e.g., nosocomial agents; staffing patterns; cognitive, affective, psychomotor factors); physical (e.g., design, structure, and arrangement of community, building, and/or equipment); nutrients (e.g., vitamins, food types); biological (e.g., immunization level of community, microorganism); chemical (e.g., pollutants, poisons, drugs, pharmaceutical agents, alcohol, caffeine, nicotine, preservatives, cosmetics, dyes)

Internal: Psychological (affective orientation); malnutrition; abnormal blood profile (e.g., leukocytosis/leukopenia, altered clotting factors, thrombocytopenia, sickle cell, thalassemia, decreased hemoglobin); immune-autoimmune dysfunction; biochemical, regulatory function (e.g., sensory dysfunction); integrative dysfunction; effector dysfunction; tissue hypoxia; developmental age (physiological, psychosocial); physical (e.g., broken skin, altered mobility)

Risk For Perioperative-Positioning INJURY (1994)

Definition:
At risk for injury as a result of the environmental conditions found in the perioperative setting

Risk Factors:
Disorientation; edema; emaciation; immobilization; muscle weakness; obesity; sensory/perceptual disturbances due to anesthesia

Decreased INTRACRANIAL ADAPTIVE CAPACITY* (1994)

Definition:
Intracranial fluid dynamic mechanisms that normally compensate for increases in intracranial volumes are compromised, resulting in repeated disproportionate increases in intracranial pressure (ICP) in response to a variety of noxious and nonnoxious stimuli

Defining Characteristics:
Repeated increases of >10 mm Hg for more than 5 minutes following any of a variety of external stimuli; baseline ICP ≥ 10 mm Hg; disproportionate increase in ICP following single environmental or nursing maneuver stimulus; elevated P_2ICP wave form; volume pressure response test variation (volume-pressure ratio 2, pressure-volume index <10); wide amplitude ICP wave form

Related Factors:
Decreased cerebral perfusion ≤ 50–60 mm Hg; sustained increase in ICP $= 10$–15 mm Hg; systemic hypotension with intracranial hypertension; brain injuries

*Formerly "Decreased Adaptive Capacity: Intracranial"

Deficient KNOWLEDGE *(Specify)** (1980)

Definition:
Absence or deficiency of cognitive information related to a specific topic

Defining Characteristics:
Verbalization of the problem; inaccurate follow-through of instruction; inaccurate performance of test; inappropriate or exaggerated behaviors (e.g., hysterical, hostile, agitated, apathetic)

Related Factors:
Lack of exposure; lack of recall; information misinterpretation; cognitive limitation; lack of interest in learning; unfamiliarity with information resources

*Formerly "Knowledge Deficit"

Readiness for Enhanced KNOWLEDGE OF *(Specify)* (2002)

Definition:
The presence or acquisition of cognitive information related to a specific topic is sufficient for meeting health-related goals and can be strengthened

Defining Characteristics:
Expresses an interest in learning; explains knowledge of the topic; behaviors congruent with expressed knowledge; describes previous experiences pertaining to the topic

Risk For LONELINESS (1994)

Definition:
At risk for experiencing vague dysphoria

Risk Factors:
Affectional deprivation; social isolation; cathectic deprivation; physical isolation

Impaired MEMORY (1994)

Definition:
Inability to remember or recall bits of information or behavioral skills*

Defining Characteristics:
Inability to recall factual information; inability to recall recent or past events; inability to learn or retain new skills or information; inability to determine if a behavior was performed; observed or reported experiences of forgetting; inability to perform a previously learned skill; forgets to perform a behavior at a scheduled time

Related Factors:
Fluid and electrolyte imbalance; neurological disturbances; excessive environmental disturbances; anemia; acute or chronic hypoxia; decreased cardiac output

Impaired memory may be attributed to pathophysiological or situational causes that are either temporary or permanent.

Impaired Bed MOBILITY (1998)

Definition:
Limitation of independent movement from one bed position to another

Defining Characteristics:
Impaired ability to turn side to side, move from supine to sitting or sitting to supine, "scoot" or reposition self in bed, move from supine to prone or prone to supine, move from supine to long sitting or long sitting to supine

Impaired Physical MOBILITY (1973, 1998)

Definition:
Limitation in independent, purposeful physical movement of the body or of one or more extremities

Defining Characteristics:
Postural instability during performance of routine activities of daily living; limited ability to perform gross motor skills; limited ability to perform fine motor skills; uncoordinated or jerky movements; limited range of motion; difficulty turning; gait changes (e.g., decreased walking speed, difficulty initiating gait, small steps, shuffles feet, exaggerated lateral postural sway); decreased reaction time; movement-induced shortness of breath; engages in substitutions for movement (e.g., increased attention to other's activity, controlling behavior, focus on preillness disability/activity); slowed movement; movement-induced tremor

Related Factors:
Medications; prescribed movement restrictions; discomfort, pain; lack of knowledge regarding value of physical activity; body mass index above 75th

age-appropriate percentile; sensoriperceptual impairments; musculoskeletal, neuromuscular impairment intolerance to activity/decreased strength and endurance; depressive mood state or anxiety; cognitive impairment; decreased muscle strength, control and or mass; reluctance to initiate movement; sedentary lifestyle, disuse, deconditioning; selective or generalized malnutrition; loss of integrity of bone structures developmental delay; joint stiffness or contractures limited cardiovascular endurance; altered cellular metabolism; lack of physical or social environmental supports; cultural beliefs regarding age appropriate activity

NOTE. Suggested Functional Level Classification:

0 = Completely independent
1 = Requires use of equipment or device
2 = Requires help from another person, for assistance, supervision, or teaching
3 = Requires help from another person and equipment or device
4 = Dependent, does not participate in activity

Impaired Wheelchair MOBILITY (1998)

Definition:
Limitation of independent operation of wheelchair within environment

Defining Characteristics:
Impaired ability to operate manual or power wheelchair on even or uneven surface; impaired ability to operate manual or power wheelchair on an incline or decline impaired ability to operate wheelchair on curbs
NOTE. Specify level of independence

NAUSEA (1998, 2002)

Definition:
A subjective unpleasant, wavelike sensation in the back of the throat, epigastrium, or abdomen that may lead to the urge to vomit

Defining Characteristics:
Reports of "nausea" ("sick to stomach"); increased salivation; aversion toward food; gagging sensation sour taste in mouth; increased swallowing
Treatment Related: Gastric irritation: pharmaceuticals (e.g., aspirin, nonsteroidal anti-inflammatory drugs, steroids, antibiotics), alcohol, iron, and blood gastric distention: delayed gastric emptying caused by pharmacological interventions (e.g., narcotics administration, anesthesia agents); pharmaceuticals (e.g analgesics, antiviral for HIV, aspirin, opioids, chemotherapeutic agents); toxins (e.g., radiotherapy)
Biophysical: Biochemical disorders (e.g., uremia, diabetic ketoacidosis, pregnancy); cardiac pain cancer of stomach or intra-abdominal tumors (e.g pelvic or colorectal cancers); esophageal or pancreatic disease; gastric distention due to delayed gastric

mptying, pyloric intestinal obstruction, genitourinary nd biliary distention, upper bowel stasis, external ompression of the stomach (liver, spleen, or other rgan enlargement which slows the stomach function squashed stomach syndrome]), excess food intake; astric irritation due to pharyngeal and/or peritoneal nflammation; liver or splenetic capsule stretch; local umors (e.g., increased intracranial pressure, meninitis); toxins (e.g., tumor-produced peptides, abnornal metabolites due to cancer)

Situational: Psychological factors (e.g., pain, fear, nxiety, noxious odors, taste, unpleasant visual timulation)

Related Factors:
hemotherapy; postsurgical anesthesia; irritation to ne gastrointestinal system; stimulation of neuroharmacologic mechanisms

Unilateral NEGLECT (1986)

Definition:
ack of awareness and attention to one side of the ody

Defining Characteristics:
onsistent inattention to stimuli on an affected side; oes not look toward affected side; leaves food on late on the affected side; inadequate self-care; nadequate positioning and/or safety precautions in egard to the affected side

Related Factors:
ffects of disturbed perceptual abilities (e.g., hemianopsia); neurologic illness or trauma; one-sided lindness

NONCOMPLIANCE (1973, 1996, 1998)

Definition:
ehavior of person and/or caregiver that fails to oincide with a health-promoting or therapeutic plan greed on by the person (and/or family and/or ommunity) and health-care professional. In the resence of an agreed-on, health-promoting or nerapeutic plan, person's or caregiver's behavior is illy or partially nonadherent and may lead to clinically neffective or partially ineffective outcomes.

Defining Characteristics:
ehavior indicative of failure to adhere (by direct bservation or by statements of patient or significant thers); evidence of development of complications; vidence of exacerbation of symptoms; failure to keep ppointments; failure to progress; objective tests e.g., physiological measures, detection of physiologic narkers)

Related Factors:
Healthcare Plan: Duration; significant others; cost; ntensity; complexity
Individual Factors: Personal and developmental bilities; health beliefs, cultural influences, spiritual

values; individual's value system; knowledge and skill relevant to the regimen behavior; motivational forces
Health System: Satisfaction with care; credibility of provider; access and convenience of care; financial flexibility of plan; client-provider relationships; provider reimbursement of teaching and follow-up; provider continuity and regular follow-up; individual health coverage; communication and teaching skills of the provider
Network: Involvement of members in health plan; social value regarding plan; perceived beliefs of significant others

Readiness For Enhanced NUTRITION (2002)

Definition:
A pattern of nutrient intake that is sufficient for meeting metabolic needs and can be strengthened

Defining Characteristics:
Expresses willingness to enhance nutrition; eats regularly; consumes adequate food and fluid; expresses knowledge of healthy food and fluid choices; follows an appropriate standard for intake (e.g., the food pyramid or American Diabetic Association guidelines); safe preparation and storage for food and fluids; attitude toward eating and drinking is congruent with health goals

Imbalanced NUTRITION: LESS THAN BODY REQUIREMENTS* (1975)

Definition:
Intake of nutrients insufficient to meet metabolic needs

Defining Characteristics:
Body weight 20% or more under ideal; reported food intake less than RDA (recommended daily allowance); pale conjunctival and mucous membranes; weakness of muscles required for swallowing or mastication; sore, inflamed buccal cavity; satiety immediately after ingesting food; reported or evidence of lack of food; reported altered taste sensation; perceived inability to ingest food; misconceptions; loss of weight with adequate food intake; aversion to eating; abdominal cramping; poor muscle tone; abdominal pain with or without pathology; lack of interest in food; capillary fragility; diarrhea and/or steatorrhea; excessive loss of hair; hyperactive bowel sounds; lack of information, misinformation

Related Factors:
Inability to ingest or digest food or absorb nutrients due to biological, psychological, or economic factors

Formerly "Altered Nutrition: Less Than Body Requirements"

Imbalanced NUTRITION: MORE THAN BODY REQUIREMENTS* (1975)

Definition:
Intake of nutrients that exceeds metabolic needs

Defining Characteristics:
Triceps skin fold >25 mm in women, >15 mm in men; weight 20% over ideal for height and frame; eating in response to external cues (e.g., time of day, social situation); eating in response to internal cues other than hunger (e.g., anxiety); reported or observed dysfunctional eating pattern (e.g., pairing food with other activities); sedentary activity level; concentrating food intake at the end of the day

Related Factors:
Excessive intake in relation to metabolic need

Formerly "Altered Nutrition: More Than Body Requirements"

Risk For Imbalanced NUTRITION: MORE THAN BODY REQUIREMENTS* (1980)

Definition:
At risk for an intake of nutrients that exceeds metabolic needs

Risk Factors:
Reported use of solid food as major food source before 5 months of age; concentrating food intake at end of day; reported or observed obesity in one or both parents; reported or observed higher baseline weight at beginning of each pregnancy; rapid transition across growth percentiles in infants or children; pairing food with other activities; observed use of food as reward or comfort measure; eating in response to internal cues other than hunger (e.g., anxiety); eating in response to external cues (e.g., time of day, social situation); dysfunctional eating patterns

Formerly "Altered Nutrition: Risk For More Than Body Requirements"

Impaired ORAL MUCOUS MEMBRANE* (1982, 1998)

Definition:
Disruption of the lips and soft tissue of the oral cavity

Defining Characteristics:
Purulent drainage or exudates; gingival recession, pockets deeper than 4 mm; enlarged tonsils beyond what is developmentally appropriate; smooth atrophic, sensitive tongue; geographic tongue; mucosal denudation; presence of pathogens; difficult speech; self-report of bad taste; gingival or mucosal pallor; oral pain/discomfort; xerostomia (dry mouth); vesicles, nodules, or papules; white patches/plaques, spong patches, or white curdlike exudate; oral lesions o ulcers; halitosis; edema; hyperemia; desquamation coated tongue; stomatitis; self-report of difficult eating or swallowing; self-report of diminished o absent taste; bleeding; macroplasia; gingival hyper plasia; fissures, cheilitis; red or bluish masses (e.g. hemangiomas)

Related Factors:
Chemotherapy; chemical irritants (e.g., alcoho tobacco, acidic foods, drugs, regular use of inhaler or other noxious agents); depression; immunosup pression; aging-related loss of connective, adipose, c bone tissue; barriers to professional care; cleft lip c palate; medication side effects; lack of or decrease salivation; trauma; pathological conditions; ora cavity (radiation to head or neck); NPO for mor than 24 hours; mouth breathing; malnutrition c vitamin deficiency; dehydration; infection; ineffectiv oral hygiene; mechanical (e.g., ill-fitting denture braces, tubes [endotracheal/nasogastric], surgery i oral cavity); decreased platelets; immunocompro mised; radiation therapy; barriers to oral self-care diminished hormone levels (women); stress; loss c supportive structures

Formerly "Altered Oral Mucous Membrane"

Acute PAIN* (1996)

Definition:
Unpleasant sensory and emotional experience arisin from actual or potential tissue damage or described i terms of such damage (International Association fc the Study of Pain); sudden or slow onset of an intensity from mild to severe with an anticipate or predictable end and a duration of less than months

Defining Characteristics:
Verbal or coded report; observed evidence; antalg positioning to avoid pain; protective gestures; guarc ing behavior; facial mask; sleep disturbance (eyes lac luster, beaten look, fixed or scattered movemen grimace); self-focus; narrowed focus (altered tim perception, impaired thought processes, reduce interaction with people and environment); distractio behavior (e.g., pacing, seeking out other people an or activities, repetitive activities); autonom responses (e.g., diaphoresis; changes in bloo pressure, respiration, pulse; pupillary dilation); aut nomic change in muscle tone (may span from listles to rigid); expressive behavior (e.g., restlessnes moaning, crying, vigilance, irritability, sighing changes in appetite and eating

Related Factors:
Injury agents (biological, chemical, physical, psychc logical)

Formerly "Pain"

Chronic PAIN (1986, 1996)

Definition:

Unpleasant sensory and emotional experience arising from actual or potential tissue damage or described in terms of such damage (International Association for the Study of Pain); sudden or slow onset of any intensity from mild to severe, constant or recurring without an anticipated or predictable end and a duration of greater than 6 months

Defining Characteristics:

Weight changes; verbal or coded report or observed evidence of protective behavior, guarding behavior, facial mask, irritability, self-focusing, restlessness, depression; atrophy of involved muscle group; changes in sleep pattern; fatigue; fear of reinjury; reduced interaction with people; altered ability to continue previous activities; sympathetic mediated responses (e.g., temperature, cold, changes of body position, hypersensitivity); anorexia

Related Factors:

Chronic physical/psychosocial disability

Readiness For Enhanced PARENTING (2002)

Definition:

A pattern of providing an environment for children or other dependent person(s) that is sufficient to nurture growth and development and can be strengthened

Defining Characteristics:

Expresses willingness to enhance parenting; children or other dependent person(s) express satisfaction with home environment; emotional and tacit support of children or dependent person(s) is evident; bonding or attachment evident; physical and emotional needs of children/dependent person(s) are met; realistic expectations of children/dependent person(s) exhibited

Impaired PARENTING* (1978, 1998)

Definition:

Inability of the primary caretaker to create, maintain, or regain an environment that promotes the optimum growth and development of the child

Defining Characteristics:

Infant or Child

Poor academic performance; frequent illness; runaway; incidence of physical and psychological trauma or abuse; frequent accidents; lack of attachment; failure to thrive; behavioral disorders; poor social competence; lack of separation anxiety; poor cognitive development

Parental

Inappropriate child care arrangements; rejection or hostility to child; statements of inability to meet child's needs; inflexibility in meeting needs of child or situation; poor or inappropriate caretaking skills; frequently punitive; inconsistent care; child abuse; inadequate child health maintenance; unsafe home environment; verbalization of inability to control child; negative statements about child; verbalization of role inadequacy or frustration; inappropriate visual, tactile, auditory stimulation; abandonment; insecure (or lack of) attachment to infant; inconsistent behavior management; child neglect; little cuddling; maternal-child interaction deficit; poor parent-child interaction

Related Factors:

Social: Lack of access to resources; social isolation; lack of resources; poor home environment; lack of family cohesiveness; inadequate child care arrangements; lack of transportation; unemployment or job problems; role strain or overload; marital conflict, declining satisfaction; lack of value of parenthood; change in family unit; low socioeconomic class; unplanned or unwanted pregnancy; presence of stress (e.g., financial, legal, recent crisis, cultural move); lack of, or poor, parental role model; single parent; lack of social support networks; father of child not involved; history of being abusive; history of being abused; financial difficulties; maladaptive coping strategies; poverty; poor problem-solving skills; inability to put child's needs before own; low self-esteem; relocations; legal difficulties

Knowledge: Lack of knowledge about child health maintenance; lack of knowledge about parenting skills; unrealistic expectation for self, infant, partner; limited cognitive functioning; lack of knowledge about child development; inability to recognize and act on infant cues; low educational level or attainment; poor communication skills; lack of cognitive readiness for parenthood; preference for physical punishment

Physiological: Physical illness

Infant or Child: Premature birth; illness; prolonged separation from parent; not desired gender; attention deficit hyperactivity disorder; difficult temperament; separation from parent at birth; lack of goodness of fit (temperament) with parental expectations; unplanned or unwanted child; handicapping condition or developmental delay; multiple births; altered perceptual abilities

Psychological: History of substance abuse or dependencies; disability; depression; difficult labor and/or delivery; young age, especially adolescent; history of mental illness; high number or closely spaced pregnancies; sleep deprivation or disruption; lack of, or late, prenatal care; separation from infant/child

NOTE. It is important to reaffirm that adjustment to parenting in general is a normal maturational process that elicits nursing behaviors to prevent potential problems and to promote health.

*Formerly "Altered Parenting"

Risk For Impaired PARENTING*
(1978, 1998)

Definition:
Risk for inability of the primary caretaker to create, maintain, or regain an environment that promotes the optimum growth and development of the child

Risk Factors:
Social: Marital conflict, declining satisfaction; history of being abused; poor problem-solving skills; role strain/overload; social isolation; legal difficulties; lack of access to resources; lack of value of parenthood; relocation; poverty; poor home environment; lack of family cohesiveness; lack of or poor parental role model; father of child not involved; history of being abusive; financial difficulties; low self-esteem; lack of resources; unplanned or unwanted pregnancy; inadequate child care arrangements; maladaptive coping strategies; low socioeconomic class; lack of transportation; change in family unit; unemployment or job problems; single parent; lack of social support network; inability to put child's needs before own; stress
Knowledge: Low educational level or attainment; unrealistic expectations of child; lack of knowledge about parenting skills; poor communication skills; preference for physical punishment; inability to recognize and act on infant cues; low cognitive functioning; lack of knowledge about child health maintenance; lack of knowledge about child development; lack of cognitive readiness for parenthood
Physiological: Physical illness
Infant or Child: Multiple births; handicapping condition or developmental delay; illness; altered perceptual abilities; lack of goodness of fit (temperament) with parental expectations; unplanned or unwanted child; premature birth; not gender desired; difficult temperament; attention deficit hyper-activity disorder; prolonged separation from parent; separation from parent at birth
Psychological: Separation from infant/child; high number or closely spaced children; disability; sleep deprivation or disruption; difficult labor and/or delivery; young age, especially adolescent; depression; history of mental illness; lack of, or late, prenatal care; history of substance abuse or dependence
NOTE. It is important to reaffirm that adjustment to parenting in general is a normal maturational process that elicits nursing behaviors to prevent potential problems and to promote health.

Formerly "Risk for Altered Parenting"

Risk For PERIPHERAL NEUROVASCULAR DYSFUNCTION (1992)

Definition:
At risk for disruption in circulation, sensation, or motion of an extremity

Risk Factors:
Trauma; vascular obstruction; orthopedic surgery fractures; burns; mechanical compression (e.g. tourniquet, cane, cast, brace, dressing, restraint) Immobilization

Risk For POISONING (1980)

Definition:
At accentuated risk of accidental exposure to, o ingestion of, drugs or dangerous products in doses sufficient to cause poisoning

Risk Factors:
External: Unprotected contact with heavy metals o chemicals; medicines stored in unlocked cabinets accessible to children or confused people; presence o poisonous vegetation; presence of atmospheric pollu tants; paint, lacquer, etc., in poorly ventilated areas o without effective protection; flaking, peeling paint o plaster in presence of young children; chemica contamination of food and water; availability of illici drugs potentially contaminated by poisonous addi tives; large supplies of drugs in house; dangerous products placed or stored within reach of children o confused people
Internal: Verbalization that occupational setting i without adequate safeguards; reduced vision; lack o safety or drug education; lack of proper precaution insufficient finances; cognitive or emotional difficultie

POST-TRAUMA SYNDROME
(1986, 1998)

Definition:
Sustained maladaptive response to a traumatic overwhelming event

Defining Characteristics:
Avoidance; repression; difficulty in concentrating grief; intrusive thoughts; neurosensory irritability palpitations; enuresis (in children); anger and/o rage; intrusive dreams; nightmares; aggression hypervigilant; exaggerated startle response; hope lessness; altered mood states; shame; panic attacks alienation; denial; horror; substance abuse; depres sion; anxiety; guilt; fear; gastric irritability; detach ment; psychogenic amnesia; irritability; numbing compulsive behavior; flashbacks; headaches

Related Factors:
Events outside the range of usual human experience physical and psychosocial abuse; tragic occurrence involving multiple deaths; epidemics; sudden destruc tion of one's home or community; being held prisone of war or criminal victimization (torture); wars; rape natural and/or manmade disasters; serious accidents witnessing mutilation, violent death, or other horrors serious threat or injury to self or loved ones; industria and motor vehicle accidents; military combat

Risk For POST-TRAUMA SYNDROME (1998)

Definition:
At risk for sustained maladaptive response to a traumatic, overwhelming event

Risk Factors:
Exaggerated sense of responsibility; perception of event; survivor's role in the event; occupation (e.g., police, fire, rescue, corrections, emergency room staff, mental health worker); displacement from home; inadequate social support; nonsupportive environment; diminished ego strength; duration of the event

POWERLESSNESS (1982)

Definition:
Perception that one's own action will not significantly affect an outcome; a perceived lack of control over a current situation or immediate happening

Defining Characteristics:
Low: Expressions of uncertainty about fluctuating energy levels; passivity
Moderate: Nonparticipation in care or decision making when opportunities are provided; resentment, anger, guilt; reluctance to express true feelings; passivity; dependence on others that may result in irritability; fearing alienation from caregivers; expressions of dissatisfaction and frustration over inability to perform previous tasks/activities; expression of doubt regarding role performance; does not monitor progress; does not defend self-care practices when challenged; inability to seek information regarding care
Severe: Verbal expressions of having no control (over self-care or influence over situation or influence over outcome); apathy; depression over physical deterioration that occurs despite patient compliance with regimens

Related Factors:
Healthcare environment; illness-related regimen; interpersonal interaction; lifestyle of helplessness

Risk For POWERLESSNESS (2000)

Definition:
At risk for perceived lack of control over a situation and/or one's ability to significantly affect an outcome

Risk Factors:
Physiological: Chronic or acute illness (hospitalization, intubation, ventilator, suctioning); acute injury or progressive debilitating disease process (e.g., spinal cord injury, multiple sclerosis); aging (e.g., decreased physical strength, decreased mobility); dying
Psychosocial: Lack of knowledge of illness or healthcare system; lifestyle of dependency with inadequate coping patterns; absence of integrality (e.g., essence of power); decreased self-esteem; low or unstable body image

Ineffective PROTECTION* (1990)

Definition:
Decrease in the ability to guard self from internal or external threats such as illness or injury

Defining Characteristics:
Maladaptive stress response; neurosensory alteration; impaired healing; deficient immunity; altered clotting; dyspnea; insomnia; weakness; restlessness; pressure ulcers; perspiring; itching; immobility; chilling; fatigue; disorientation; cough; anorexia

Related Factors:
Abnormal blood profiles (e.g., leukopenia, thrombocytopenia, anemia, coagulation); inadequate nutrition; extremes of age; drug therapies (e.g., antineoplastic, corticosteroid, immune, anticoagulant, thrombolytic); alcohol abuse; treatments (e.g., surgery, radiation); diseases such as cancer and immune disorders

Formerly "Altered Protection"

RAPE-TRAUMA SYNDROME (1980, 1998)

Definition:
Sustained maladaptive response to a forced, violent sexual penetration against the victim's will and consent

Defining Characteristics:
Disorganization; change in relationships; confusion; physical trauma (e.g., bruising, tissue irritation); suicide attempts; denial; guilt; paranoia; humiliation; embarrassment; aggression; muscle tension and/or spasms; mood swings; dependence; powerlessness; nightmares and sleep disturbances; sexual dysfunction; revenge; phobias; loss of self-esteem; inability to make decisions; dissociative disorders; self-blame; hyperalertness; vulnerability; substance abuse; depression; helplessness; anger; anxiety; agitation; shame; shock; fear

Related Factors:
Rape
NOTE. This syndrome includes the following three sub-components: Rape-Trauma, Compound Reaction, and Silent Reaction. In this text each appears as a separate diagnosis.

RAPE-TRAUMA SYNDROME: COMPOUND REACTION (1980)

Definition:
Forced violent sexual penetration against the victim's will and consent. The trauma syndrome that develops from this attack or attempted attack includes an acute phase of disorganization of the victim's lifestyle and a long-term process of reorganization of lifestyle.

Defining Characteristics:
Change in lifestyle (e.g., changes in residence, dealing with repetitive nightmares and phobias, seeking family support, seeking social network support in long-term phase); emotional reaction (e.g., anger, embarrassment, fear of physical violence and death, humiliation, revenge, self-blame in acute phase); multiple physical symptoms (e.g., gastrointestinal irritability, genitourinary discomfort, muscle tension, sleep pattern disturbance in acute phase); reactivated symptoms of such previous conditions (i.e., physical illness, psychiatric illness in acute phase); reliance on alcohol/drugs (acute phase)

Related Factors:
To be developed
NOTE. This syndrome includes the following three sub-components: Rape-Trauma, Compound Reaction, and Silent Reaction. In this text each appears as a separate diagnosis.

RAPE-TRAUMA SYNDROME: SILENT REACTION (1980)

Definition:
Forced violent sexual penetration against the victim's will and consent. The trauma syndrome that develops from this attack or attempted attack includes an acute phase of disorganization of the victim's lifestyle and a long-term process of reorganization of lifestyle.

Defining Characteristics:
Increased anxiety during interview (i.e., blocking of associations, long periods of silence, minor stuttering, physical distress); sudden onset of phobic reactions; no verbalization of the occurrence of rape; abrupt changes in relationships with men; increase in nightmares; pronounced changes in sexual behavior

Related Factors:
To be developed
NOTE. This syndrome includes the following three sub-components: Rape-Trauma, Compound Reaction, and Silent Reaction. In this text each appears as a separate diagnosis.

RELOCATION STRESS SYNDROME (1992, 2000)

Definition:
Physiological and/or psychosocial disturbance following transfer from one environment to another

Defining Characteristics:
Temporary or permanent move; voluntary/involuntary move; aloneness, alienation, loneliness; depression; anxiety (e.g., separation); sleep disturbance; withdrawal; anger; loss of identity, self-worth, or self-esteem; increased verbalization of needs, unwillingness to move, or concern over relocation; increased physical symptoms/illness (e.g., gastrointestinal disturbance, weight change); dependency; insecurity; pessimism; frustration; worry; fear

Related Factors:
Unpredictability of experience; isolation from family, friends; past, concurrent, and recent losses; feelings of powerlessness; lack of adequate support system/group; lack of predeparture counseling; passive coping; impaired psychosocial health; language barrier; decreased health status

Risk For RELOCATION STRESS SYNDROME (2000)

Definition:
At risk for physiological and/or psychosocial disturbance following transfer from one environment to another

Defining Characteristics:
Moderate to high degree of environmental change (e.g., physical, ethnic, cultural); temporary and/or permanent moves; voluntary/involuntary move; lack of adequate support system/group; feelings of powerlessness; moderate mental competence (e.g., alert enough to experience changes); unpredictability of experiences; decreased psychosocial or physical health status; lack of predeparture counseling; passive coping; past, current, recent losses

Ineffective ROLE PERFORMANCE* (1978, 1996, 1998)

Definition:
Patterns of behavior and self-expression that do not match the environmental context, norms, and expectations

Defining Characteristics:
Change in self-perception of role; role denial; inadequate external support for role enactment; inadequate adaptation to change or transition; system conflict; change in usual patterns of responsibility; discrimination; domestic violence; harassment; uncertainty; altered role perceptions; role strain; inadequate self management; role ambivalence; pessimistic attitude; inadequate motivation; inadequate confidence; inadequate role competency and skills; inadequate knowledge; inappropriate developmental expectations; role conflict; role confusion; powerlessness; inadequate coping; anxiety or depression; role overload; change in other's perception of role; change in capacity to resume role; role dissatisfaction; inadequate opportunities for role enactment

Related Factors:
Social: Inadequate or inappropriate linkage with the healthcare system; job schedule demands; young age, developmental level; lack of rewards; poverty; family conflict; inadequate support system; inadequate role socialization (e.g., role model, expectations

responsibilities); low socioeconomic status; stress and conflict; domestic violence; lack of resources
Knowledge: Inadequate role preparation (e.g., role transition, skill rehearsal, validation); lack of knowledge about role, role skills; role transition; lack of opportunity for role rehearsal; developmental transitions; unrealistic role expectations; education attainment level; lack of or inadequate role model
Physiological: Inadequate/inappropriate linkage with health-care system; substance abuse; mental illness; body image alteration; physical illness; cognitive deficits; health alterations (e.g., physical health, body image, self-esteem, mental health, psychosocial health, cognition, learning style, neurological health); depression; low self-esteem; pain; fatigue
NOTE. There is a typology of roles: Sociopersonal (friendship, family, marital, parenting, community), home management, intimacy (sexuality), relationship building), leisure/exercise/recreation, self-management, socialization (developmental transitions), community contributor, and religious.

Formerly "Altered Role Performance"

Bathing/Hygiene SELF-CARE DEFICIT (1980, 1998)

Definition:
Impaired ability to perform or complete bathing/hygiene activities for oneself

Defining Characteristics:
Inability to wash body or body parts, obtain or get to water source, regulate temperature or flow of bath water, get bath supplies, dry body, get in and out of bathroom

Related Factors:
Decreased or lack of motivation; weakness and tiredness; severe anxiety; inability to perceive body part or spatial relationship; perceptual or cognitive impairment; pain; neuromuscular impairment; musculoskeletal impairment; environmental barriers
NOTE. See suggested Functional Level Classification under Impaired Physical Mobility (p. 2218)

Dressing/Grooming SELF-CARE DEFICIT (1980, 1998)

Definition:
Impaired ability to perform or complete dressing and grooming activities for self

Defining Characteristics:
Impaired ability to put on or take off necessary items of clothing, fasten clothing, obtain or replace articles of clothing; Inability to put on clothing on upper body, put on clothing on lower body, choose clothing, use assistive devices, use zippers, remove clothes, put on socks, maintain appearance at a satisfactory level, pick up clothing, put on shoes

Related Factors:
Decreased or lack of motivation; pain; severe anxiety; perceptual or cognitive impairment; weakness or tiredness; neuromuscular impairment; musculoskeletal impairment; discomfort; environmental barriers
NOTE. See suggested Functional Level Classification under Impaired Physical Mobility (p. 2218)

Feeding SELF-CARE DEFICIT (1980, 1998)

Definition:
Impaired ability to perform or complete feeding activities

Defining Characteristics:
Inability to swallow food, prepare food for ingestion, handle utensils, chew food, use assistive device, get food onto utensil, open containers, ingest food safely, manipulate food in mouth, bring food from a receptacle to the mouth, complete a meal, ingest food in a socially acceptable manner, pick up cup or glass, ingest sufficient food

Related Factors:
Weakness or tiredness; severe anxiety; neuromuscular impairment; pain; perceptual or cognitive impairment; discomfort; environmental barriers; decreased or lack of motivation; musculoskeletal impairments
NOTE. See suggested Functional Level Classification under Impaired Physical Mobility (p. 2218)

Toileting SELF-CARE DEFICIT (1980, 1998)

Definition:
Impaired ability to perform or complete own toileting activities

Defining Characteristics:
Inability to get to toilet or commode, sit on or rise from toilet or commode, manipulate clothing for toileting, carry out proper toilet hygiene, flush toilet or commode

Related Factors:
Environmental barriers; weakness or tiredness; decreased or lack of motivation; severe anxiety; impaired mobility status; impaired transfer ability; musculoskeletal impairment; neuromuscular impairment; pain; perceptual or cognitive impairment
NOTE. See suggested Functional Level Classification under Impaired Physical Mobility (p. 2218).

Readiness For Enhanced SELF-CONCEPT (2002)

Definition:
A pattern of perceptions or ideas about the self that is sufficient for well-being and can be strengthened

2225

Defining Characteristics:
Expresses willingness to enhance self-concept; expresses satisfaction with thoughts about self, sense of worthiness, role performance, body image, and personal identity; actions are congruent with expressed feelings and thoughts; expresses confidence in abilities; accepts strengths and limitations

Chronic LOW SELF-ESTEEM (1988, 1996)

Definition:
Long-standing negative self-evaluation/feelings about self or self-capabilities

Defining Characteristics:
Rationalizes away/rejects positive feedback and exaggerates negative feedback about self (long standing or chronic); self-negating verbalization (long standing or chronic); hesitant to try new things/situations (long standing or chronic); expressions of shame/guilt (long standing or chronic); evaluates self as unable to deal with events (long standing or chronic); lack of eye contact; nonassertive/passive; frequent lack of success in work or other life events; excessively seeks reassurance; overly conforming, dependent on others' opinions; indecisive

Related Factors:
To be developed

Situational Low SELF-ESTEEM (1988, 1996, 2000)

Definition:
Development of a negative perception of self-worth in response to a current situation (specify)

Defining Characteristics:
Verbally reports current situational challenge to self-worth; self-negating verbalizations; indecisive, nonassertive behavior; evaluation of self as unable to deal with situations or events; expressions of helplessness and uselessness

Related Factors:
Developmental changes (specify); disturbed body image; functional impairment (specify); loss (specify); social role changes (specify); lack of recognition/rewards; behavior inconsistent with values; failures/rejections

Risk For Situational Low SELF-ESTEEM (2000)

Definition:
At risk for developing negative perception of self-worth in response to a current situation (specify)

Risk Factors:
Developmental changes (specify); disturbed body image; functional impairment (specify); loss (specify); social role changes (specify); history of learned helplessness; history of abuse, neglect, or abandonment; unrealistic self-expectations; behavior inconsistent with values; lack of recognition/rewards; failures/rejections; decreased power/control over environment; physical illness (specify)

SELF-MUTILATION (2000)

Definition:
Deliberate self-injurious behavior causing tissue damage with the intent of causing nonfatal injury to attain relief of tension

Defining Characteristics:
Cuts/scratches on body; picking at wounds; self-inflicted burns (e.g., eraser, cigarette); ingestion/inhalation of harmful substances/objects; biting; abrading; severing; insertion of object(s) into body orifice(s); hitting; constricting a body part

Related Factors:
Psychotic state (command hallucinations); inability to express tension verbally; childhood sexual abuse; violence between parental figures; family divorce; family alcoholism; family history of self-destructive behaviors; adolescence; peers who self-mutilate; isolation from peers; perfectionism; substance abuse; eating disorders; sexual identity crisis; low or unstable self-esteem; low or unstable body image; labile behavior (mood swings); history of inability to plan solutions or see long-term consequences; use of manipulation to obtain nurturing relationship with others; chaotic/disturbed interpersonal relationships; emotionally disturbed; battered child; feels threatened with actual or potential loss of significant relationship (e.g., loss of parent/parental relationship); experiences dissociation or depersonalization; mounting tension that is intolerable; impulsivity; inadequate coping; irresistible urge to cut/damage self; needs quick reduction of stress; childhood illness or surgery; foster, group, or institutional care; incarceration; character disorder; borderline personality disorder; developmentally delayed or autistic individual; history of self-injurious behavior; feelings of depression, rejection, self-hatred, separation anxiety, guilt, depersonalization; poor parent-adolescent communication; lack of family confidant

Risk For SELF-MUTILATION (1992, 2000)

Definition:
At risk for deliberate self-injurious behavior causing tissue damage with the intent of causing nonfatal injury to attain relief of tension

Risk Factors:
Psychotic state (command hallucinations); inability to express tension verbally; childhood sexual abuse;

violence between parental figures; family divorce; family alcoholism; family history of self-destructive behaviors; adolescence; peers who self-mutilate; isolation from peers; perfectionism; substance abuse; eating disorders; sexual identity crisis; low or unstable self-esteem; low or unstable body image; history of inability to plan solutions or see long-term consequences; use of manipulation to obtain nurturing relationship with others; chaotic/disturbed inter-personal relationships; emotionally disturbed and/or battered children; feels threatened with actual or potential loss of significant relationship; loss of parent/parental relationships; experiences dissociation or depersonalization; experiences mounting tension that is intolerable; impulsivity; inadequate coping; experiences irresistible urge to cut/damage self; needs quick reduction of stress; childhood illness or surgery; foster, group, or institutional care; incarceration; character disorders; borderline personality disorders; loss of control over problem-solving situations; developmentally delayed or autistic individuals; history of self-injurious behavior; feelings of depression, rejection, self-hatred, separation anxiety, guilt, and depersonalization

Disturbed SENSORY PERCEPTION
(Specify: Visual, Auditory, Kinesthetic, Gustatory, Tactile, Olfactory)* (1978, 1980, 1998)

Definition:
Change in the amount or patterning of incoming stimuli accompanied by a diminished, exaggerated, distorted, or impaired response to such stimuli

Defining Characteristics:
Poor concentration; auditory distortions; change in usual response to stimuli; restlessness; reported or measured change in sensory acuity; irritability; disoriented in time, in place, or with people; change in problem-solving abilities; change in behavior pattern; altered communication patterns; hallucinations; visual distortions

Related Factors:
Altered sensory perception; excessive environmental stimuli; psychological stress; altered sensory reception, transmission, and/or integration; insufficient environmental stimuli; biochemical imbalances for sensory distortion (e.g., illusions, hallucinations); electrolyte imbalance; biochemical imbalance

Formerly "Sensory/Perceptual Alterations"

SEXUAL DYSFUNCTION (1980)

Definition:
Change in sexual function that is viewed as unsatisfying, unrewarding, inadequate

Defining Characteristics:
Change of interest in self and others; conflicts involving values; inability to achieve desired satisfaction; verbalization of problem; alteration in relationship with significant other; alteration in achieving sexual satisfaction; actual or perceived limitations imposed by disease and/or therapy; seeking confirmation of desirability; alterations in achieving perceived sex role

Related Factors:
misinformation or lack of knowledge; vulnerability; values conflict; psychosocial abuse (e.g., harmful relationships); physical abuse; lack of privacy; ineffectual or absent role models; altered body structure of function (e.g., pregnancy, recent childbirth, drugs, surgery, anomalies, disease process, trauma, radiation); lack of significant other; biopsychosocial alteration of sexuality

Ineffective SEXUALITY PATTERNS* (1986)

Definition:
Expressions of concern regarding own sexuality

Defining Characteristics:
Reported difficulties, limitations, or changes in sexual behaviors or activities

Related Factors:
Lack of significant other; conflicts with sexual orientation or variant preferences; fear of pregnancy or of acquiring a sexually transmitted disease; impaired relationship with a significant other; ineffective or absent role models; knowledge/skill deficit about alternative responses to health-related transitions, altered body function or structure, illness or medical treatment; lack of privacy

Formerly "Altered Sexuality Patterns"

Impaired SKIN INTEGRITY (1975, 1998)

Definition:
Altered epidermis and/or dermis

Defining Characteristics:
Invasion of body structures; destruction of skin layers (dermis); disruption of skin surface (epidermis)

Related Factors:
External: Hyperthermia or hypothermia; chemical substance; humidity; mechanical factors (e.g., shearing forces, pressure, restraint); physical immobilization; radiation; extremes in age; moisture; medications
Internal: Altered metabolic state; skeletal prominence; immunological deficit; developmental factors; altered sensation; altered nutritional state (e.g., obesity, emaciation); altered pigmentation; altered circulation; alterations in turgor (changes in elasticity); altered fluid status

Risk For Impaired SKIN INTEGRITY (1975, 1998)

Definition:
At risk for skin being adversely altered

Risk Factors:
External: Radiation; physical immobilization; mechanical factors (e.g., shearing forces, pressure, restraint); hypothermia or hyperthermia; humidity; chemical substance; excretions and/or secretions; moisture; extremes of age
Internal: Medication; skeletal prominence; immunologic factors; developmental factors; altered sensation; altered pigmentation; altered metabolic state; altered circulation; alterations in skin turgor (changes in elasticity); alterations in nutritional state (e.g., obesity, emaciation); psychogenetic
NOTE. Risk should be determined by the use of a risk assessment tool (e.g., Braden Scale).

Readiness For Enhanced SLEEP (2002)

Definition:
A pattern of natural, periodic suspension of consciousness that provides adequate rest, sustains a desired lifestyle, and can be strengthened

Defining Characteristics:
Expresses willingness to enhance sleep; amount of sleep and REM sleep is congruent with developmental needs; expresses a feeling of being rested after sleep; follows sleep routines that promote sleep habits; occasional or infrequent use of medications to induce sleep

SLEEP DEPRIVATION (1998)

Definition:
Prolonged periods of time without sleep (sustained natural, periodic suspension of relative consciousness)

Defining Characteristics:
Daytime drowsiness; decreased ability to function; malaise; tiredness; lethargy; restlessness; irritability; heightened sensitivity to pain; listlessness; apathy; slowed reaction; inability to concentrate; perceptual disorders (e.g., disturbed body sensation, delusions, feeling afloat); hallucinations; acute confusion; transient paranoia; agitated or combative; anxious; mild, fleeting nystagmus; hand tremors

Related Factors:
Prolonged physical discomfort; prolonged psychological discomfort; sustained inadequate sleep hygiene; prolonged use of pharmacologic or dietary antisoporifics; aging-related sleep stage shifts; sustained circadian asynchrony; inadequate daytime activity; sustained environmental stimulation; sustained unfamiliar or uncomfortable sleep environment; non-sleep-inducing parenting practices; sleep apnea; periodic limb movement (e.g., restless leg syndrome, nocturnal myoclonus); sundowner's syndrome; narcolepsy; idiopathic central nervous system hypersomnolence; sleep walking; sleep terror; sleep-related enuresis; nightmares; familial sleep paralysis; sleep-related painful erections; dementia

Disturbed SLEEP PATTERN* (1980, 1998)

Definition:
Time-limited disruption of sleep (natural, periodic suspension of consciousness) amount and quality

Defining Characteristics:
Prolonged awakenings; sleep maintenance insomnia; self-induced impairment of normal pattern; sleep onset >30 minutes; early morning insomnia; awakening earlier or later than desired; verbal complaints of difficulty falling asleep; verbal complaints of not feeling well-rested; increased proportion of stage 1 sleep; less than age-normed total sleep time; dissatisfaction with sleep; three or more nighttime awakenings; decreased proportion of stages 3 and 4 sleep (e.g., hyporesponsiveness, excess sleepiness, decreased motivation); decreased proportion of REM sleep (e.g., REM rebound, hyperactivity, emotional lability, agitation and impulsivity, atypical polysomnographic features); decreased ability to function

Related Factors:
Psychological; ruminative presleep thoughts; daytime activity pattern; thinking about home; body temperature; temperament; dietary; childhood onset; inadequate sleep hygiene; sustained use of anti-sleep agents; circadian asynchrony; frequently changing sleep-wake schedule; depression; loneliness; frequent travel across time zones; daylight/darkness exposure; grief; anticipation; shift work; delayed or advanced sleep phase syndrome; loss of sleep partner, life change; preoccupation with trying to sleep; periodic gender-related hormonal shifts; biochemical agents; fear; separation from significant others; social schedule inconsistent with chronotype; aging-related shifts; anxiety; medications; fear of insomnia; maladaptive conditioned wakefulness; fatigue; boredom
Environmental: Noise; lighting; unfamiliar sleep furnishings; ambient temperature, humidity; other-generated awakening; excessive stimulation; physical restraint; lack of sleep privacy/control; interruptions for therapeutics, monitoring, lab tests; sleep partner; noxious odors
Parental: Mother's sleep-wake pattern; parent-infant interaction; mother's emotional support
Physiological: Urinary urgency; incontinence; fever; nausea; stasis of secretions; shortness of breath; position; gastroesophageal reflux

---

Formerly "Sleep Pattern Disturbance"

Impaired SOCIAL INTERACTION (1986)

Definition:
Insufficient or excessive quantity or ineffective quality of social exchange

Defining Characteristics:
Verbalized or observed inability to receive or communicate a satisfying sense of belonging, caring, interest, or shared history; verbalized or observed discomfort in social situations; observed use of unsuccessful social interaction behaviors; dysfunctional interaction with peers, family and/or others; family report of change of style or pattern of interaction

Related Factors:
Knowledge/skill deficit about ways to enhance mutuality; therapeutic isolation; sociocultural dissonance; limited physical mobility; environmental barriers; communication barriers; altered thought processes; absence of available significant others or peers; self-concept disturbance

SOCIAL ISOLATION (1982)

Definition:
Aloneness experienced by the individual and perceived as imposed by others and as a negative or threatening state

Defining Characteristics:
Objective: Absence of supportive significant other(s) (family, friends, group); projects hostility in voice, behavior; withdrawn; uncommunicative; shows behavior unaccepted by dominant cultural group; seeks to be alone or exists in a subculture; repetitive, meaningless actions; preoccupation with own thoughts; no eye contact; inappropriate or immature activities for developmental age/stage; evidence of physical/mental handicap or altered state of wellness; sad, dull affect

Subjective: Expresses feelings of aloneness imposed by others; expresses feelings of rejection; inappropriate or immature interests for developmental age/stage; inadequate or absent significant purpose in life; inability to meet expectations of others; expresses values acceptable to the subculture but unacceptable to the dominant cultural group; expresses interests inappropriate to the developmental age/stage; experiences feelings of differences from others; insecurity in public

Related Factors:
Alterations in mental status; inability to engage in satisfying personal relationships; unaccepted social values; unaccepted social behavior; inadequate personal resources; immature interests; factors contributing to the absence of satisfying personal relationships (e.g., delay in accomplishing developmental tasks); alterations in physical appearance; altered state of wellness

Chronic SORROW (1998)

Definition:
Cyclical, recurring, and potentially progressive pattern of pervasive sadness experienced (by a parent, caregiver, individual with chronic illness or disability) in response to continual loss, throughout the trajectory of an illness or disability

Defining Characteristics:
Expresses periodic, recurrent feelings of sadness; feelings that vary in intensity, are periodic, may progress and intensify over time, and may interfere with the client's ability to reach his/her highest level of personal and social well-being; expresses one or more of the following feelings: anger, being misunderstood, confusion, depression, disappointment, emptiness, fear, frustration, guilt/self-blame, helplessness, hopelessness, loneliness, low self-esteem, recurring loss, overwhelmed

Related Factors:
Death of a loved one; experiences chronic physical or mental illness or disability (e.g., mental retardation, multiple sclerosis, prematurity, spina bifida or other birth defects, chronic mental illness, infertility, cancer, Parkinson's disease); experiences one or more trigger events (e.g., crises in management of the illness, crises related to developmental stages, missed opportunities or milestones that bring comparisons with developmental, social, or personal norms); unending caregiving as a constant reminder of loss

SPIRITUAL DISTRESS (1978, 2002)

Definition:
Impaired ability to experience and integrate meaning and purpose in life through a person's connectedness with self, others, art, music, literature, nature, or a power greater than oneself

Defining Characteristics:
Connections to Self: Expresses lack of hope, meaning and purpose in life, peace/serenity, acceptance, love, forgiveness of self, courage, anger, guilt, poor coping
Connections With Others: Refuses interactions with spiritual leaders; refuses interactions with friends, family; verbalizes being separated from their support system; expresses alienation
Connections With Art, Music, Literature, Nature: Inability to express previous state of creativity (singing/listening to music/writing); no interest in nature; no interest in reading spiritual literature
Connections With Power Greater Than Self: Inability to pray; inability to participate in religious activities; expresses being abandoned by or having anger toward God; inability to experience the transcendent; requests to see a religious leader; sudden changes in spiritual practices; inability to introspective/inward turning; expresses being without hope, suffering

Related Factors:
Self-alienation; anxiety; sociocultural deprivation; death and dying of self or others; pain; life change; chronic illness of self or others

Risk For SPIRITUAL DISTRESS (1998)

Definition:
At risk for an altered sense of harmonious connectedness with all of life and the universe in which dimensions that transcend and empower the self may be disrupted

Risk Factors
Energy-consuming anxiety; low self-esteem; mental illness; physical illness; blocks to self-love; poor relationships; physical or psychological stress; substance abuse; loss of loved one; natural disasters; situational losses; maturational losses; inability to forgive

Readiness For Enhanced SPIRITUAL WELL-BEING* (1994, 2002)

Definition:
Ability to experience and integrate meaning and purpose in life through connectedness with self, others, art, music, literature, nature, or a power greater than oneself

Defining Characteristics:
Connections to Self: Desire for enhanced hope, meaning and purpose in life, peace/serenity, acceptance, surrender, love, forgiveness of self, satisfying philosophy of life, joy, courage, heightened coping, meditation
Connections With Others: Provides service to others; requests interactions with spiritual leaders; requests forgiveness of others; requests interactions with friends, family
Connections With Art, Music, Literature, Nature: Displays creative energy (e.g., writing, poetry); sings/listens to music; reads spiritual literature; spends time outdoors
Connections With Power Greater Than Self: Prays; reports mystical experiences; participates in religious activities; expresses reverence, awe

Formerly "Potential for Enhanced Spiritual Well-Being"

Risk For SUDDEN INFANT DEATH SYNDROME (2002)

Definition:
Presence of risk factors for sudden death of an infant under 1 year of age

Risk Factors:
Modifiable: Infants placed to sleep in the prone or side-lying position; prenatal and/or postnatal infant smoke exposure; infant overheating/overwrapping; soft underlayment/loose articles in the sleep environment; delayed or nonattendance of prenatal care
Potentially Modifiable: Low birth weight; prematurity; young maternal age
Nonmodifiable: Male gender; ethnicity (e.g., African American, Native American race of mother); seasonality of SIDS deaths (higher in winter and fall months) SIDS mortality peaks between infant age of 2–4 months

Risk For SUFFOCATION (1980)

Definition:
Accentuated risk of accidental suffocation (inadequate air available for inhalation)

Risk Factors:
External: Vehicle warming in closed garage; use of fuel-burning heaters not vented to outside; smoking in bed; children playing with plastic bags or inserting small objects into their mouths or noses; propped bottle placed in an infant's crib; pillow placed in an infant's crib; person who eats large mouthfuls of food discarded or unused refrigerators or freezers without removed doors; children left unattended in bathtubs or pools; household gas leaks; low-strung clothesline pacifier hung around infant's head
Internal: Reduced olfactory sensation; reduced motor abilities; cognitive or emotional difficulties; disease or injury process; lack of safety education; lack of safety precautions

Risk For SUICIDE (2000)

Definition:
At risk for self-inflicted, life-threatening injury
Risk Factors:
Behavioral: History of prior suicide attempt; impulsiveness; buying a gun; stockpiling medicines; making or changing a will; giving away possessions; sudden euphoric recovery from major depression; marked changes in behavior, attitude, school performance
Verbal: Threats of killing oneself; states desire to die, end it all
Situational: Living alone; retired; relocation, institutionalization; economic instability; loss of autonomy/independence; presence of gun in home; adolescents living in nontraditional settings (e.g., juvenile detention center, prison, half-way house, group home)
Psychological: Family history of suicide; alcohol and substance use/abuse; psychiatric illness/disorder (e.g., depression, schizophrenia, bipolar disorder); abuse in childhood; guilt; gay or lesbian youth
Demographic: Age: elderly, young adult males, adolescents; race: Caucasian, Native American gender: male; divorced, widowed
Physical: Physical illness; terminal illness; chronic pain
Social: Loss of important relationship; disrupted family life; grief, bereavement; poor support systems

oneliness; hopelessness; helplessness; social isolation; legal or disciplinary problem; cluster suicides

Delayed SURGICAL RECOVERY (1998)

Definition:
Extension of the number of postoperative days required to initiate and perform activities that maintain life, health, and well-being

Defining Characteristics:
Evidence of interrupted healing of surgical area (e.g., red, indurated, draining, immobilized); loss of appetite with or without nausea; difficulty in moving about; requires help to complete self-care; fatigue; report of pain/discomfort; postpones resumption of work/employment activities; perception that more time is needed to recover

Related Factors:
To be developed

Impaired SWALLOWING (1986, 1998)

Definition:
Abnormal functioning of the swallowing mechanism associated with deficits in oral, pharyngeal, or esophageal structure or function

Defining Characteristics:
Pharyngeal Phase Impairment: Altered head positions; inadequate laryngeal elevation; food refusal; unexplained fevers; delayed swallow; recurrent pulmonary infections; gurgly voice quality; nasal reflux; choking, coughing, or gagging; multiple swallows; abnormality in pharyngeal phase by swallow study
Esophageal Phase Impairment: Heartburn or epigastric pain; acidic smelling breath; unexplained irritability surrounding mealtime; vomitus on pillow; repetitive swallowing or ruminating; regurgitation of gastric contents or wet burps; bruxism; nighttime coughing or awakening; observed evidence of difficulty in swallowing (e.g., stasis of food in oral cavity, coughing/choking); hyperextension of head, arching during or after meals; abnormality in esophageal phase by swallow study; odynophagia; food refusal or volume limiting; complaints of "something stuck"; hematemesis; vomiting
Oral Phase Impairment: Lack of tongue action to form bolus; weak suck resulting in inefficient nippling; incomplete lip closure

Related Factors:
Food pushed out of mouth; slow bolus formation; food falls from mouth; premature entry of bolus; inability to clear oral cavity; long meals with little consumption; nasal reflux; coughing, choking, gagging before a swallow; abnormality in oral phase of swallow study; piecemeal deglutition; lack of chewing; pooling in lateral sulci; sialorrhea or drooling
Congenital Deficits: Upper airway anomalies; failure to thrive or protein energy malnutrition; conditions

with significant hypotonia; respiratory disorders; history of tube feeding; behavioral feeding problems; self-injurious behavior; neuromuscular impairment (e.g., decreased or absent gag reflex, decreased strength or excursion of muscles involved in mastication, perceptual impairment, facial paralysis); mechanical obstruction (e.g., edema, tracheostomy tube, tumor); congenital heart disease; cranial nerve involvement
Neurological Problems: Upper airway anomalies; laryngeal abnormalities; achalasia; gastroesophageal reflux disease; acquired anatomic defects; cerebral palsy; internal or external traumas; tracheal, laryngeal, esophageal defects; traumatic head injury; developmental delay; nasal or nasopharyngeal cavity defects; oral cavity or oropharynx abnormalities; premature infants

Effective THERAPEUTIC REGIMEN MANAGEMENT* (1994)

Definition:
Pattern of regulating and integrating into daily living a program for treatment of illness and its sequelae that is satisfactory for meeting specific health goals

Defining Characteristics:
Appropriate choices of daily activities for meeting the goals of a treatment or prevention program; illness symptoms within a normal range of expectation; verbalizes desire to manage the treatment of illness and prevention of sequelae; verbalizes intent to reduce risk factors for progression of illness and sequelae

Related Factors:
To be developed

*Formerly "Effective Management of Therapeutic Regimen: Individual"

Readiness For Enhanced THERAPEUTIC REGIMEN MANAGEMENT* (2002)

Definition:
A pattern of regulating and integrating into daily living a program(s) for treatment of illness and its sequelae that is sufficient for meeting health-related goals and can be strengthened

Defining Characteristics:
Expresses desire to manage the treatment of illness and prevention of sequelae; choices of daily living are appropriate for meeting the goals of treatment or prevention; expresses little to no difficulty with regulation/integration of one or more prescribed regimens for treatment of illness or prevention of complications; describes reduction of risk factors for progression of illness and sequelae; no unexpected acceleration of illness symptoms

Ineffective THERAPEUTIC REGIMEN MANAGEMENT* (1992)

Definition:
Pattern of regulating and integrating into daily living a program for treatment of illness and the sequelae of illness that is unsatisfactory for meeting specific health goals

Defining Characteristics:
Choices of daily living ineffective for meeting the goals of a treatment or prevention program; verbalizes that did not take action to reduce risk factors for progression of illness and sequelae; verbalizes desire to manage the treatment of illness and prevention of sequelae; verbalizes difficulty with regulation/integration of one or more prescribed regimens for prevention of complications and the treatment or illness or its effects; verbalizes that did not take action to include treatment regimens in daily routines

Related Factors:
Perceived barriers; social support deficit; powerlessness; perceived susceptibility; perceived benefits; mistrust of regimen and/or healthcare personnel; knowledge deficit; family patterns of health care; family conflict; excessive demands made on individual or family; economic difficulties; decisional conflicts; complexity of therapeutic regimen; complexity of healthcare system; perceived seriousness; inadequate number and types of cues to action

Formerly "Ineffective Management of Therapeutic Regimen: Individual"

Ineffective Community THERAPEUTIC REGIMEN MANAGEMENT* (1994)

Definition:
Pattern of regulating and integrating into community processes programs for treatment of illness and the sequelae of illness that are unsatisfactory for meeting health-related goals

Defining Characteristics:
Illness symptoms above the norm expected for the number and type of population; unexpected acceleration of illness(es); number of healthcare resources insufficient for the incidence or prevalence of illness(es); deficits in advocates for aggregates; deficits in people and programs to be accountable for illness care of aggregates; deficits in community activities for secondary and tertiary prevention; unavailable healthcare resources for illness care

Related Factors:
To be developed

Formerly "Ineffective Management of Therapeutic Regimen: Community"

Ineffective Family THERAPEUTIC REGIMEN MANAGEMENT* (1994)

Definition:
Pattern of regulating and integrating into family processes a program for treatment of illness and the sequelae of illness that is unsatisfactory for meeting specific health goals

Defining Characteristics:
Inappropriate family activities for meeting the goals of a treatment or prevention program; acceleration of illness symptoms of a family member; lack of attention to illness and its sequelae; verbalizes difficulty with regulation/integration of one or more effects or prevention of complications; verbalizes desire to manage the treatment of illness and prevention of the sequelae; verbalizes that family did not take action to reduce risk factors for progression of illness and sequelae

Related Factors:
Complexity of healthcare system; complexity of therapeutic regimen; decisional conflicts; economic difficulties; excessive demands made on individual or family; family conflict

Formerly "Ineffective Management of Therapeutic Regimen: Families"

Ineffective THERMOREGULATION (1986)

Definition:
Temperature fluctuation between hypothermia and hyperthermia

Defining Characteristics:
Fluctuations in body temperature above and below the normal range; cool skin; cyanotic nail beds; flushed skin; hypertension; increased respiratory rate; pallor (moderate); piloerection; reduction in body temperature below normal range; seizures/convulsions; shivering (mild); slow capillary refill; tachycardia; warm to touch

Related Factors:
Aging; fluctuating environmental temperature; immaturity; trauma or illness

Disturbed THOUGHT PROCESSES* (1973, 1996)

Definition:
Disruption in cognitive operations and activities

Defining Characteristics:
Cognitive dissonance; memory deficit/problems; inaccurate interpretation of environment; hypovigilance; hypervigilance; distractibility; egocentricity; inappropriate nonreality-based thinking

Related Factors:
To be developed

Formerly "Altered Thought Processes"

Impaired TISSUE INTEGRITY (1986, 1998)

Definition:
Damage to mucous membrane, corneal, integumentary, or subcutaneous tissues

Defining Characteristics:
Damaged or destroyed tissue (e.g., cornea, mucous membrane, integumentary, subcutaneous)

Related Factors:
Mechanical (e.g., pressure, shear, friction); radiation (including therapeutic radiation); nutritional deficit or excess; thermal (temperature extremes); knowledge deficit; irritants, chemical (including body excretions, secretions, medications); impaired physical mobility; altered circulation; fluid deficit or excess

Ineffective TISSUE PERFUSION (Specify Type: Renal, Cerebral, Cardiopulmonary, Gastrointestinal, Peripheral)* (1980, 1998)

Definition:
Decrease in oxygen resulting in the failure to nourish the tissues at the capillary level

Defining Characteristics:
Renal: Altered blood pressure outside of acceptable parameters; hematuria; oliguria or anuria; elevation in BUN/ creatinine ratio
Gastrointestinal: Hypoactive or absent bowel sounds; nausea; abdominal distention; abdominal pain or tenderness
Peripheral: Edema; positive Homans sign; altered skin characteristics (hair, nails, moisture); weak or absent pulses; skin discolorations; skin temperature changes; altered sensations; claudication; blood pressure changes in extremities; bruits; delayed healing; diminished arterial pulsations; skin color pale on elevations, color does not return on lowering the leg
Cerebral: Speech abnormalities; changes in pupillary reactions; extremity weakness or paralysis; altered mental status; difficulty in swallowing; changes in motor response; behavioral changes
Cardiopulmonary: Altered respiratory rate outside of acceptable parameters; use of accessory muscles; capillary refill > 3 seconds; abnormal arterial blood gases; chest pain; sense of "impending doom"; bronchospasm; dyspnea; arrhythmias; nasal flaring; chest retraction

Related Factors:
Hypovolemia; hypervolemia; interruption of flow, arterial; exchange problems; interruption of flow, venous; mechanical reduction of venous and/or arterial blood flow; hypoventilation; impaired transport of the oxygen across alveolar and/or capillary membrane; mismatch of ventilation with blood flow; decreased hemoglobin concentration in blood; enzyme poisoning; altered affinity of hemoglobin for oxygen

---

Formerly "Altered Tissue Perfusion"

Impaired TRANSFER ABILITY (1998)

Definition:
Limitation of independent movement between two nearby surfaces

Defining Characteristics:
Impaired ability to transfer from bed to chair and chair to bed, on or off a toilet or commode, in and out of tub or shower, between uneven levels, from chair to car or car to chair, from chair to floor or floor to chair, from standing to floor or floor to standing

Related Factors:
To be developed
NOTE. Specify level of independence.

Risk For TRAUMA (1980)

Definition:
Accentuated risk of accidental tissue injury (e.g., wound, burn, fracture)

Risk Factors:
External: High-crime neighborhood and vulnerable clients; pot handles facing toward front of stove; knives stored uncovered; inappropriate call-for-aid mechanisms for bed-resting client; inadequately stored combustible or corrosives (e.g., matches, oily rags, lye); highly flammable children's toys or clothing; obstructed passageways; high beds; large icicles hanging from the roof; nonuse or misuse of seat restraints; overexposure to sun, sun lamps, radiotherapy; overloaded electrical outlets; overloaded fuse boxes; play or work near vehicle pathways (e.g., driveways, lanes, railroad tracks); playing with fireworks or gunpowder; guns or ammunition stored unlocked; contact with rapidly moving machinery, industrial belts, or pulleys; litter or liquid spills on floors or stairways; defective appliances; bathing in very hot water (e.g., unsupervised bathing of young children); bathtub without hand grip or antislip equipment; children playing with matches, candles, cigarettes, sharp-edged toys; children playing without gates at top of stairs; children riding in the front seat in car; delayed lighting of gas burner or oven; contact with intense cold; grease waste collected on stoves; driving a mechanically unsafe vehicle; driving after partaking of alcoholic beverages or drugs; driving at excessive speeds; entering unlighted rooms; experimenting with chemical or gasoline; exposure to dangerous machinery; faulty electrical plugs; frayed

wires; contact with acids or alkalis; unsturdy or absent stair rails; use of unsteady ladders or chairs; use of cracked dishware or glasses; wearing plastic apron or flowing clothes around open flame; unscreened fires or heaters; unsafe window protection in homes with young children; sliding on coarse bed linen or struggling within bed restraints; use of thin or worn potholders; unanchored electric wires; misuse of necessary headgear for motorized cyclists or young children carried on adult bicycles; potential igniting of gas leaks; unsafe road or road-crossing conditions; slippery floors (e.g., wet or highly waxed); smoking in bed or near oxygen; snow or ice collected on stairs, walkways; unanchored rugs; driving without necessary visual aids

Internal: Lack of safety education; insufficient finances to purchase safety equipment or effect repairs; history of previous trauma; lack of safety precautions; poor vision; reduced temperature and/or tactile sensation; balancing difficulties; cognitive or emotional difficulties; reduced large or small muscle coordination; weakness; reduced hand-eye coordination

Readiness For Enhanced URINARY ELIMINATION (2002)

Definition:
A pattern of urinary functions that is sufficient for meeting eliminatory needs and can be strengthened

Defining Characteristics:
Expresses willingness to enhance urinary elimination; urine is straw colored with no odor; specific gravity is within normal limits; amount of output is within normal limits for age and other factors; positions self for emptying of bladder; fluid intake is adequate for daily needs

Impaired URINARY ELIMINATION* (1973)

Definition:
Disturbance in urine elimination

Defining Characteristics:
Incontinence; urgency; nocturia; hesitancy; frequency; dysuria; retention

Related Factors:
Urinary tract infection; anatomical obstruction; multiple causality; sensory motor impairment

Formerly "Altered Urinary Elimination"

URINARY RETENTION (1986)

Definition:
Incomplete emptying of the bladder

Defining Characteristics:
Bladder distention; small, frequent voiding or absence of urine output; dribbling; dysuria; overflow incontinence; residual urine; sensation of bladder fullness

Related Factors:
Blockage; high urethral pressure caused by weak detrusor; inhibition of reflex arc; strong sphincter

Impaired Spontaneous VENTILATION* (1992)

Definition:
Decreased energy reserves result in an individual's inability to maintain breathing adequate to support life

Defining Characteristics:
Dyspnea; increased metabolic rate; increased pCO_2; increased restlessness; increased heart rate; decreased tidal volume; decreased pO_2; decreased cooperation; apprehension; decreased SaO_2; increased use of accessory muscles

Related Factors:
Respiratory muscle fatigue; metabolic factors

Formerly "Inability to Sustain Spontaneous Ventilation"

Dysfunctional VENTILATORY WEANING RESPONSE (1992)

Definition:
Inability to adjust to lowered levels of mechanical ventilator support that interrupts and prolongs the weaning process

Defining Characteristics:
Severe: Deterioration in arterial blood gases from current baseline; respiratory rate increases significantly from baseline; increase from baseline blood pressure (20 mm hg); agitation; increase from baseline heart rate (20 beats/min); paradoxical abdominal breathing; adventitious breath sounds, audible airway secretions; cyanosis; decreased level of consciousness; full respiratory accessory muscle use; shallow, gasping breaths; profuse diaphoresis; discoordinated breathing with the ventilator

Moderate: Slight increase from baseline blood pressure (<20 mm Hg); baseline increase in respiratory rate (<5 breaths/min); slight increase from baseline heart rate (<20 beats/min); pale, slight cyanosis; slight respiratory accessory muscle use; inability to respond to coaching; inability to cooperate; apprehension; color changes; decreased air entry on auscultation; diaphoresis; eye widening, wide-eyed look; hypervigilance to activities

Mild: Warmth; restlessness; slight increase of respiratory rate from baseline; queries about possible machine malfunction; expressed feelings of increased need for oxygen; fatigue; increased concentration on breathing; breathing discomfort

Related Factors:
Psychological: Patient perceived inefficacy about the ability to wean; powerlessness; anxiety: moderate,

severe; knowledge deficit of the weaning process, patient role; hopelessness; fear; decreased motivation; decreased self-esteem; insufficient trust in the nurse

Situational: Uncontrolled episodic energy demands or problems; history of multiple unsuccessful weaning attempts; adverse environment (e.g., noisy, active environment, negative events in the room, low nurse-patient ratio, extended nurse absence from bedside, unfamiliar nursing staff); history of ventilator dependence >4 days to 1 week; inappropriate pacing of diminished ventilator support; inadequate social support

Physiological: Inadequate nutrition; sleep pattern disturbance; uncontrolled pain or discomfort; ineffective airway clearance

Formerly "Inability to Sustain Spontaneous Ventilation"

Risk For Other-Directed VIOLENCE* (1980, 1996)

Definition:
At risk for behaviors in which an individual demonstrates that he/she can be physically, emotionally, and/or sexually harmful to others

Risk Factors:
Body language: rigid posture, clenching of fists and jaw, hyperactivity, pacing, breathlessness, threatening stances; history of violence against others (e.g., hitting someone, kicking someone, spitting at someone, scratching someone, throwing objects at someone, biting someone, attempted rape, rape, sexual molestation, urinating/defecating on a person); history of threats of violence (e.g., verbal threats against property, verbal threats against person, social threats, cursing, threatening notes/letters, threatening gestures, sexual threats); history of violent antisocial behavior (e.g., stealing, insistent borrowing, insistent demands for privileges, insistent interruption of meetings, refusal to eat, refusal to take medication, ignoring instructions); history of violence, indirect (e.g., tearing off clothes, ripping objects off walls, writing on walls, urinating on floor, defecating on floor, stamping feet, temper tantrum, running in corridors, yelling, throwing objects, breaking a window, slamming doors, sexual advances); neurological impairment (e.g., positive EEG, CAT, MRI, neurological findings; head trauma; seizure disorders); cognitive impairment (e.g., learning disabilities, attention deficit disorder, decreased intellectual functioning); history of childhood abuse; history of witnessing family violence; cruelty to animals; firesetting; pre/perinatal complications/abnormalities; history of drug/alcohol abuse; pathological intoxication; psychotic symptomatology (e.g., auditory, visual, command hallucinations; paranoid delusions; loose, rambling, or illogical thought processes); motor vehicle offenses (e.g., frequent traffic violations, use of a motor vehicle to release anger); suicidal behavior; impulsivity; availability/possession of weapon(s)

Formerly "Risk for Violence: Directed at Others"

Risk For Self-Directed VIOLENCE* (1994)

Definition:
At risk for behaviors in which an individual demonstrates that he/she can be physically, emotionally and/or sexually harmful to self

Risk Factors:
Suicidal ideation (frequent, intense prolonged); suicidal plan (clear and specific lethality; method and availability of destructive means); history of multiple suicide attempts; behavioral clues (e.g., writing forlorn love notes, directing angry messages at a significant other who has rejected the person, giving away personal items, taking out a large life insurance policy); verbal clues (e.g., talking about death, "better off without me," asking questions about lethal dosages of drugs); emotional status (hopelessness, despair, increased anxiety, panic, anger, hostility); mental health (severe depression, psychosis, severe personality disorder, alcoholism or drug abuse; physical health (hypochondriasis, chronic or terminal illness); employment (unemployed, recent job loss/failure); age 15–19; age over 45; marital status (single, widowed, divorced); occupation (executive, administrator/owner of business, professional, semiskilled worker); conflictual interpersonal relationships; family background (chaotic or conflictual, history of suicide); sexual orientation (bisexual [active], homosexual [inactive]); personal resources (poor achievement, poor insight, affect unavailable and poorly controlled); social resources (poor rapport, socially isolated, unresponsive family); people who engage in autoerotic sexual acts

Formerly "Risk for Violence: Self-Directed"

Impaired WALKING (1998)

Definition:
Limitation of independent movement within the environment on foot

Defining Characteristics:
Impaired ability to climb stairs, walk required distances, walk on an incline or decline, walk on uneven surfaces, navigate curbs

Related Factors:
To be developed

NOTE. Suggested Functional Level Classification:
0 = Completely independent
1 = Requires use of equipment or device
2 = Requires help from another person, for assistance, supervision, or teaching

3 = Requires help from another person and equipment or device

4 = Dependent, does not participate in activity

WANDERING (2000)

Definition:

Meandering, aimless or repetitive locomotion that exposes the individual to harm; frequently incongruent with boundaries, limits, or obstacles

Defining Characteristics:

Frequent or continuous movement from place to place, often revisiting the same destinations; persistent locomotion in search of "missing" or unattainable people or places; haphazard locomotion; locomotion into unauthorized or private spaces; locomotion resulting in unintended leaving of a premise; long periods of locomotion without an apparent destination; fretful locomotion or pacing; inability to locate significant landmarks in a familiar setting; locomotion that cannot be easily dissuaded or redirected; following behind or shadowing a caregiver's locomotion; trespassing; hyperactivity; scanning, seeking, or searching behaviors; periods of locomotion interspersed with periods of nonlocomotion (e.g., sitting, standing, sleeping); getting lost

Related Factors:

Cognitive impairment, specifically memory and recall deficits, disorientation, poor visuoconstructive (or visuospatial) ability, language (primarily expressive) defects; cortical atrophy; premorbid behavior (e.g. outgoing, sociable personality; premorbid dementia), separation from familiar people and places; sedation, emotional state, especially frustration, anxiety, boredom, or depression (agitation); over/understimulating social or physical environment; physiological state or need (e.g., hunger/thirst, pain, urination, constipation); time of day

NIC is a comprehensive list of nursing interventions performed by nurses in all specialties and all practice settings. A research team at the University of Iowa, including Gloria M. Bulechek, PhD, RN, and Joanne C. McCloskey, have constructed and validated these interventions.

abuse protection support
abuse protection support: child
abuse protection support: domestic partner
abuse protection support: elder
abuse protection support: religious
acid-base management
acid-base management: metabolic acidosis
acid-base management: metabolic alkalosis
acid-base management: respiratory acidosis
acid-base management: respiratory alkalosis
acid-base monitoring
active listening
activity therapy
acupressure
admission care
airway insertion and stabilization
airway management
airway suctioning
allergy management
amnioinfusion
amputation care
analgesic administration
analgesic administration: intraspinal
anaphylaxis management
anesthesia administration
anger control assistance
animal-assisted therapy
anticipatory guidance
anxiety reduction
area restriction
art therapy
artificial airway management
aspiration precautions
assertiveness training
attachment promotion
autogenic training
autotransfusion

bathing
bed rest care
bedside laboratory testing
behavior management
behavior management: overactivity/inattention
behavior management: self-harm
behavior management: sexual
behavior modification
behavior modification: social skills
bibliotherapy
biofeedback
birthing

bladder irrigation
bleeding precautions
bleeding reduction
bleeding reduction: antepartum uterus
bleeding reduction: gastrointestinal
bleeding reduction: nasal
bleeding reduction: postpartum uterus
bleeding reduction: wound
blood products administration
body image enhancement
body mechanics promotion
bottle feeding
bowel incontinence care
bowel incontinence care: encopresis
bowel irrigation
bowel management
bowel training
breast examination
breastfeeding assistance

calming technique
cardiac care
cardiac care: acute
cardiac care: rehabilitative
cardiac precautions
caregiver support
case management
cast care: wet
cerebral edema management
cerebral perfusion promotion
cesarean section care
chemotherapy management
chest physiotherapy
childbirth preparation
circulatory care: arterial insufficiency
circulatory care: mechanical assist device
circulatory care: venous insufficiency
circulatory precautions
code management
cognitive restructuring
cognitive stimulation
communication disease management
communication enhancement: hearing deficit
communication enhancement: speech deficit
communication enhancement: visual deficit
community disaster preparedness
community health development
complex relationship building
conflict mediation

*Iowa Intervention Project (2000) — McCloskey, J.C. and Bulechek, G.M. (eds.): *Nursing Intervention Classification*, 3rd Ed. St. Louis: Mosby-Yearbook, 2000.

(continued)

conscious sedation
constipation/impaction management
consultation
contact lens care
controlled substance checking
coping enhancement
cost containment
cough enhancement
counseling
crisis intervention
critical path development
culture brokerage
cutaneous stimulation

decision making support
delegation
delirium management
delusion management
dementia management
developmental care
developmental enhancement: adolescent
developmental enhancement: child
diarrhea management
diet staging
discharge planning
distraction
documentation
dressing
dying care
dysreflexia management
dysrhythmia management

ear care
eating disorders management
electrolyte management
electrolyte management: hypercalcemia
electrolyte management: hyperkalemia
electrolyte management: hypermagnesemia
electrolyte management: hypernatremia
electrolyte management: hyperphosphatemia
electrolyte management: hypocalcemia
electrolyte management: hypokalemia
electrolyte management: hypomagnesemia
electrolyte management: hyponatremia
electrolyte management: hypophosphatemia
electrolyte monitoring
electronic fetal monitoring: antepartum
electronic fetal monitoring: intrapartum
elopement precautions
embolus care: peripheral
embolus care: pulmonary
embolus precautions
emergency care
emergency cart checking
emotional support
endotracheal extubation
energy management
enteral tube feeding
environmental management
environmental management: attachment process
environmental management: comfort
environmental management: community
environmental management: home preparation
environmental management: safety
environmental management: violence prevention
environmental management: worker safety
environmental risk protection

examination assistance
exercise promotion
exercise promotion: strength training
exercise promotion: stretching
exercise therapy: ambulation
exercise therapy: balance
exercise therapy: joint mobility
exercise therapy: muscle control
eye care

fall prevention
family integrity promotion
family integrity promotion: childbearing family
family involvement promotion
family mobilization
family planning: contraception
family planning: infertility
family planning: unplanned pregnancy
family process maintenance
family support
family therapy
feeding
fertility preservation
fever treatment
financial resource assistance
fire-setting precautions
first aid
fiscal resource management
flatulence reduction
fluid management
fluid monitoring
fluid resuscitation
fluid/electrolyte management
foot care
forgiveness facilitation

gastrointestinal intubation
genetic counseling
grief work facilitation
grief work facilitation: perinatal birth
guilt work facilitation

hair care
hallucination management
health care information exchange
health education
health policy monitoring
health screening
health system guidance
heat exposure treatment
heat/cold application
hemodialysis therapy
hemodynamic regulation
hemofiltration therapy
hemorrhage control
high-risk pregnancy care
home maintenance assistance
hope instillation
humor
hyperglycemia management
hypervolemia management
hypnosis
hypoglycemia management
hypothermia treatment
hypovolemia treatment

immunization/vaccination management
impulse control training

incident reporting
incision site care
infant care
infection control
infection control: intraoperative
infection protection
insurance authorization
intracranial pressure (ICP) monitoring
intrapartal care
intrapartal care: high-risk delivery
intravenous (IV) insertion
intravenous (IV) therapy
invasive hemodynamic monitoring

kangaroo care

labor induction
labor suppression
laboratory data interpretation
lactation counseling
lactation suppression
laser precautions
latex precautions
learning facilitation
learning readiness enhancement
leech therapy
limit setting
malignant hyperthermia precautions
mechanical ventilation
mechanical ventilatory weaning
medication administration
medication administration: ear
medication administration: enteral
medication administration: epidural
medication administration: eye
medication administration: inhalation
medication administration: interpleural
medication administration: intradermal
medication administration: intramuscular (IM)
medication administration: intraosseous
medication administration: intravenous (IV)
medication administration: oral
medication administration: rectal
medication administration: skin
medication administration: subcutaneous
medication administration: vaginal
medication administration: ventricular reservoir
medication management
medication prescribing
meditation facilitation
memory training
milieu therapy
mood management
multidisciplinary care conference
music therapy
mutual goal setting

nail care
nausea management
neurologic monitoring
newborn care
newborn monitoring
nonnutritive sucking
normalization promotion
nutrition management
nutrition therapy
nutritional counseling

nutritional monitoring

oral health maintenance
oral health promotion
oral health restoration
order transcription
organ transcription
organ procurement
ostomy care
oxygen therapy

pain management
parent education: adolescent
parent education: childrearing family
parent education: infant
parenting promotion
pass facilitation
patient contracting
patient-controlled analgesia (PCA) assistance
patient rights protection
peer review
pelvic muscle exercise
perineal care
peripheral sensation management
peripherally inserted central (PIC) catheter care
peritoneal dialysis therapy
pessary management
phlebotomy: arterial blood sample
phlebotomy: blood unit acquisition
phlebotomy: venous blood sample
phototherapy: neonate
physical restraint
physician support
pneumatic tourniquet precautions
positioning
positioning: intraoperative
positioning: neurologic
positioning: wheelchair
postanesthesia care
postmortem care
postpartal care
preceptor: employee
preceptor: student
preconception counseling
pregnancy termination care
prenatal care
preoperative coordination
preparatory sensory information
presence
pressure management
pressure ulcer care
pressure ulcer prevention
product evaluation
program development
progressive muscle relaxation
prompted voiding
prosthesis care
pruritus management

quality monitoring

radiation therapy management
rape-trauma treatment
reality orientation
recreation therapy
rectal prolapse management
referral
religious addiction prevention

(continued)

religious ritual enhancement
reminiscence therapy
reproductive technology management
research data collection
resiliency promotion
respiratory monitoring
respite care
resuscitation
resuscitation: fetus
resuscitation: neonate
risk identification
risk identification: childbearing family
risk identification: genetic
role enhancement

seclusion
security enhancement
seizure management
seizure precautions
self-awareness enhancement
self-care assistance
self-care assistance: bathing/hygiene
self-care assistance: dressing/grooming
self-care assistance: feeding
self-care assistance: toileting
self-esteem enhancement
self-modification assistance
self-responsibility facilitation
sexual counseling
shift report
shock management
shock management: cardiac
shock management: vasogenic
shock management: volume
shock prevention
sibling support
simple guided imagery
simple massage
simple relaxation therapy
skin care: topical treatments
skin surveillance
sleep enhancement
smoking cessation assistance
socialization enhancement
specimen management
spiritual growth facilitation
spiritual support
splinting
sports injury prevention: youth
staff development
subarachnoid hemorrhage precautions
substance use prevention
substance use treatment
substance use treatment: alcohol withdrawal
substance use treatment: drug withdrawal
substance use treatment: overdose
suicide prevention
supply management
support group
support system enhancement
surgical assistance
surgical precautions
surgical preparation
surveillance
surveillance: community
surveillance: late pregnancy
surveillance: remote electronic
surveillance: safety

sustenance support
suturing
swallowing therapy

teaching: disease process
teaching: group
teaching: individual
teaching: infant nutrition
teaching: infant safety
teaching: preoperative
teaching: prescribed activity/exercise
teaching: prescribed diet
teaching: prescribed medication
teaching: procedure/treatment
teaching: psychomotor skill
teaching: safe sex
teaching: sexuality
teaching: toddler nutrition
teaching: toddler safety
technology management
telephone consultation
telephone follow-up
temperature regulation
temperature regulation: intraoperative
therapeutic play
therapeutic touch
therapy group
total parenteral nutrition (TPN) administration
touch
traction/immobilization care
transcutaneous electrical nerve stimulation (TENS)
transport
triage: disaster
triage: emergency center
triage: telephone
truth telling
tube care
tube care: chest
tube care: gastrointestinal
tube care: umbilical line
tube care: urinary
tube care: ventriculostomy/lumbar drain

ultrasonography: limited obstetric
unilateral neglect management
urinary bladder training
urinary catheterization
urinary catheterization: intermittent
urinary elimination management
urinary habit training
urinary incontinence care
urinary incontinence care: enuresis
urinary retention care

values clarification
vehicle safety promotion
venous access device (VAD) maintenance
ventilation assistance
visitation facilitation
vital signs monitoring
vomiting management

weight gain assistance
weight management
weight reduction assistance
wound care
wound care: closed drainage
wound irrigation

2500	**Abuse Cessation** - Evidence that the victim is no longer abused
2501	**Abuse Protection** - Protection of self or dependent others from abuse
2502	**Abuse Recovery: Emotional** - Healing of psychological injuries due to abuse
2503	**Abuse Recovery: Financial** - Regaining monetary and legal control or benefits following financial exploitation
2504	**Abuse Recovery: Physical** - Healing of physical injuries due to abuse
2505	**Abuse Recovery: Sexual** - Healing following sexual abuse or exploitation
1400	**Abusive Behavior Self-control** - Self-restraint of own behaviors to avoid abuse and neglect of dependents or significant others
1300	**Acceptance: Health Status** - Reconciliation to health circumstances
0005	**Activity Tolerance** - Responses to energy-consuming body movements involved in required or desired daily activities
1600	**Adherence Behavior** - Self-initiated action taken to promote wellness, recovery, and rehabilitation
1401	**Aggression Control** - Self-restraint of assaultive, combative, or destructive behavior toward others
0200	**Ambulation: Walking** - Ability to walk from place to place
0201	**Ambulation: Wheelchair** - Ability to move from place to place in a wheelchair
1402	**Anxiety Control** - Personal actions to eliminate or reduce feelings of apprehension and tension from an unidentifiable source
1918	**Aspiration Control** - Personal actions to prevent the passage of fluid and solid particles into the lung
0704	**Asthma Control** - Personal actions to reverse inflammatory condition resulting in bronchial constriction of the airways
0202	**Balance** - Ability to maintain body equilibrium
2300	**Blood Glucose Control** - Extent to which plasma glucose levels are maintained in expected range
0700	**Blood Transfusion Reaction Control** - Extent to which complications of blood transfusions are minimized
1200	**Body Image** - Positive perception of own appearance and body functions
0203	**Body Positioning: Self-Initiated** - Ability to change own body positions
1104	**Bone Healing** - The extent to which cells and tissues have regenerated following bone injury
0500	**Bowel Continence** - Control of passage of stool from the bowel
0501	**Bowel Elimination** - Ability of the gastrointestinal tract to form and evacuate stool effectively
1000	**Breastfeeding Establishment: Infant** - Proper attachment of an infant to and sucking from the mother's breast for nourishment during the first 2 to 3 weeks
1001	**Breastfeeding Establishment: Maternal** - Maternal establishment of proper attachment of an infant to and sucking from the breast for nourishment during the first 2 to 3 weeks
1002	**Breastfeeding Maintenance** - Continued nourishment of an infant through breastfeeding
1003	**Breastfeeding Weaning** - Process leading to the eventual discontinuation of breastfeeding
0400	**Cardiac Pump Effectiveness** - Extent to which blood is ejected from the left ventricle per minute to support systemic perfusion pressure
2200	**Caregiver Adaptation to Patient Institutionalization** - Family caregiver adaptation of role when the care recipient is transferred outside the home
2506	**Caregiver Emotional Health** - Feelings, attitudes and emotions of a family care provider while caring for a family member or significant other over an extended period of time
2202	**Caregiver Home Care Readiness** - Preparedness to assume responsibility for the health care of a family member or significant other in the home
2203	**Caregiver Lifestyle Disruption** - Disturbances in the lifestyle of a family member due to caregiving
2204	**Caregiver-Patient Relationship** - Positive interactions and connections between the caregiver and care recipient
2205	**Caregiver Performance: Direct Care** - Provision by family care provider of appropriate personal and health care for a family member or significant other
2206	**Caregiver Performance: Indirect Care** - Arrangement and oversight of appropriate care for a family member or significant other by family care provider
2507	**Caregiver Physical Health** - Physical well-being of a family care provider while caring for a family member or significant other over an extended period of time
2208	**Caregiver Stressors** - The extent of biopsychosocial pressure on a family care provider caring for a family member or significant other over an extended period of time
2508	**Caregiver Well-Being** - Primary care provider's satisfaction with health and life circumstances
2210	**Caregiving Endurance Potential** - Factors that promote family care provider continuance over an extended period of time
1301	**Child Adaptation to Hospitalization** - Child's adaptive response to hospitalization
0100	**Child Development: 2 months** - Milestones of physical, cognitive and psychosocial progression by 2 months of age

*Iowa Outcomes Project. M. Johnson, M. Maas, & S. Moorhead (eds.) (2000). *Nursing Outcomes Classification (NOC)* (2nd ed.). St. Louis: Mosby.

(continued)

0101   **Child Development: 4 months** - Milestones of physical, cognitive and psychosocial progression by 4 months of age

0102   **Child Development: 6 months** - Milestones of physical, cognitive and psychosocial progression by 6 months of age

0103   **Child Development: 12 months** - Milestones of physical, cognitive and psychosocial progression by 12 months of age

0104   **Child Development: 2 years** - Milestones of physical, cognitive and psychosocial progression by 2 years of age

0105   **Child Development: 3 years** - Milestones of physical, cognitive and psychosocial progression by 3 years of age

0106   **Child Development: 4 years** - Milestones of physical, cognitive and psychosocial progression by 4 years of age

0107   **Child Development: 5 years** - Milestones of physical, cognitive and psychosocial progression by 5 years of age

0108   **Child Development: Middle Childhood (6–11 years)** - Milestones of physical, cognitive and psychosocial progression between 6 and 11 years of age

0109   **Child Development: Adolescence (12–17 years)** - Milestones of physical, cognitive and psychosocial progression between 12 and 17 years of age

0401   **Circulation Status** - Extent to which blood flows unobstructed, unidirectionally, and at an appropriate pressure through large vessels of the systemic and pulmonary circuits

0409   **Coagulation Status** - Extent to which blood clots within expected period of time

0900   **Cognitive Ability** - Ability to execute complex mental processes

0901   **Cognitive Orientation** - Ability to identify person, place, and time

2100   **Comfort Level** - Feelings of physical and psychological ease

0902   **Communication Ability** - Ability to receive, interpret, and express spoken, written and non-verbal messages

0903   **Communication: Expressive Ability** - Ability to express and interpret verbal and/or non-verbal messages

0904   **Communication: Receptive Ability** - Ability to receive and interpret verbal and/or non-verbal messages

2700   **Community Competence** - The ability of a community to collectively problem solve to achieve goals

2701   **Community Health Status** - The general state of well-being of a community or population

2800   **Community Health: Immunity** - Resistance of a group to the invasion and spread of an infectious agent

2801   **Community Risk Control: Chronic Disease** - Community actions to reduce the risk of chronic diseases and related complications

2802   **Community Risk Control: Communicable Disease** - Community actions to eliminate or reduce the spread of infectious agents (bacteria, fungi, parasites, and viruses) that threaten public health

2803   **Community Risk Control: Lead Exposure** - Community actions to reduce lead exposure and poisoning

1601   **Compliance Behavior** - Actions taken on the basis of professional advice to promote wellness, recovery, and rehabilitation

0905   **Concentration** - Ability to focus on a specific stimulus

1302   **Coping** - Actions to manage stressors that tax an individual's resources

0906   **Decision Making** - Ability to choose between two or more alternatives

1409   **Depression Control** - Personal actions to minimize melancholy and maintain interest in life events

1208   **Depression Level** - Severity of melancholic mood and loss of interest in life events

1105   **Dialysis Access Integrity** - The extent to which a dialysis access site is functional and free of inflammation

1303   **Dignified Dying** - Maintaining personal control and comfort with the approaching end of life

1403   **Distorted Thought Control** - Self-restraint of disruption in perception, thought processes, and thought content

0600   **Electrolyte & Acid/Base Balance** - Balance of the electrolytes and non-electrolytes in the intracellular and extracellular compartments of the body

0001   **Endurance** - Extent that energy enables a person to sustain activity

0002   **Energy Conservation** - Extent of active management of energy to initiate and sustain activity

2600   **Family Coping** - Family actions to manage stressors that tax family resources

2601   **Family Environment: Internal** - Social climate as characterized by family member relationships and goals

2602   **Family Functioning** - Ability of the family to meet the needs of its members through developmental transitions

2606   **Family Health Status** - Overall health status and social competence of family unit

2603   **Family Integrity** - Extent that family members' behaviors collectively demonstrate cohesion, strength, and emotional bonding

2604	**Family Normalization** - Ability of the family to develop and maintain routines and management strategies that contribute to optimal functioning when a member has a chronic illness and disability
2605	**Family Participation in Professional Care** - Family involvement in decision-making, delivery, and evaluation of care provided by health care personnel
1404	**Fear Control** - Personal actions to eliminate or reduce disabling feelings of alarm aroused by an identifiable source
0111	**Fetal Status: Antepartum** - Conditions indicative of fetal physical well-being from conception to the onset of labor
0112	**Fetal Status: Intrapartum** - Conditions and behaviors indicative of fetal well-being from onset of labor to delivery
0601	**Fluid Balance** - Balance of water in the intracellular and extracellular compartments of the body
1304	**Grief Resolution** - Adjustment to actual or impending loss
0110	**Growth** - A normal increase in body size and weight
1700	**Health Beliefs** - Personal convictions that influence health behaviors
1701	**Health Beliefs: Perceived Ability to Perform** - Personal conviction that one can carry out a given health behavior
1702	**Health Beliefs: Perceived Control** - Personal conviction that one can influence a health outcome
1703	**Health Beliefs: Perceived Resources** - Personal conviction that one has adequate means to carry out a health behavior
1704	**Health Beliefs: Perceived Threat** - Personal conviction that a health problem is serious and has potential negative consequences for lifestyle
1705	**Health Orientation** - Personal view of health and health behaviors as priorities
1602	**Health Promoting Behavior** - Actions to sustain or increase wellness
1603	**Health Seeking Behavior** - Actions to promote optimal wellness, recovery, and rehabilitation
1610	**Hearing Compensation Behavior** - Actions to identify, monitor and compensate for hearing loss
1201	**Hope** - Presence of internal state of optimism that is personally satisfying and life-supporting
0602	**Hydration** - Amount of water in the intracellular and extracellular compartments of the body
1202	**Identity** - Ability to distinguish between self and non-self and to characterize one's essence
0204	**Immobility Consequences: Physiological** - Extent of compromise in physiological functioning due to impaired physical mobility
0205	**Immobility Consequences: Psycho-Cognitive** - Extent of compromise in psycho-cognitive functioning due to impaired physical mobility
0701	**Immune Hypersensitivity Control** - Extent to which inappropriate immune responses are suppressed
0702	**Immune Status** - Adequacy of natural and acquired appropriately targeted resistance to internal and external antigens
1900	**Immunization Behavior** - Actions to obtain immunization to prevent a communicable disease
1405	**Impulse Control** - Self-restraint of compulsive or impulsive behaviors
0703	**Infection Status** - Presence and extent of infection
0907	**Information Processing** - Ability to acquire, organize, and use information
0206	**Joint Movement: Active** - Range of motion of joints with self-initiated movement
0207	**Joint Movement: Passive** - Range of motion of joints with assisted movement
1800	**Knowledge: Breastfeeding** - Extent of understanding conveyed about lactation and nourishment of infant through breastfeeding
1801	**Knowledge: Child Safety** - Extent of understanding conveyed about safely caring for a child
1821	**Knowledge: Conception Prevention** - Extent of understanding conveyed about pregnancy prevention
1820	**Knowledge: Diabetes Management** - Extent of understanding conveyed about diabetes mellitus and its control
1802	**Knowledge: Diet** - Extent of understanding conveyed about diet
1803	**Knowledge: Disease Process** - Extent of understanding conveyed about a specific disease process
1804	**Knowledge: Energy Conservation** - Extent of understanding conveyed about energy conservation techniques
1816	**Knowledge: Fertility Promotion** - Extent of understanding conveyed about fertility testing and the conditions that affect conception
1805	**Knowledge: Health Behaviors** - Extent of understanding conveyed about the promotion and pro-tection of health
1823	**Knowledge: Health Promotion** - Extent of understanding of information needed to obtain and maintain optimal health
1806	**Knowledge: Health Resources** - Extent of understanding conveyed about health care resources
1824	**Knowledge: Illness Care** - Extent of understanding of illness-related information needed to achieve and maintain optimal health
1819	**Knowledge: Infant Care** - Extent of understanding conveyed about caring for a baby up to 12 months
1807	**Knowledge: Infection Control** - Extent of understanding conveyed about prevention and control of infection

(continued)

1817	**Knowledge: Labor and Delivery** - Extent of understanding conveyed about labor and delivery
1825	**Knowledge: Maternal-Child Health** - Extent of understanding of information needed to achieve and maintain optimal health of a mother and child
1808	**Knowledge: Medication** - Extent of understanding conveyed about the safe use of medication
1809	**Knowledge: Personal Safety** - Extent of understanding conveyed about preventing unintentional injuries
1818	**Knowledge: Postpartum** - Extent of understanding conveyed about maternal health following delivery
1822	**Knowledge: Preconception** - Extent of understanding conveyed about maternal health prior to conception to ensure a healthy pregnancy
1810	**Knowledge: Pregnancy** - Extent of understanding conveyed about maintenance of a healthy pregnancy and prevention of complications
1811	**Knowledge: Prescribed Activity** - Extent of understanding conveyed about prescribed activity and exercise
1815	**Knowledge: Sexual Functioning** - Extent of understanding conveyed about sexual development and responsible sexual practices
1812	**Knowledge: Substance Use Control** - Extent of understanding conveyed about managing substance use safely
1814	**Knowledge: Treatment Procedure(s)** - Extent of understanding conveyed about procedure(s) required as part of a treatment regimen
1813	**Knowledge: Treatment Regimen** - Extent of understanding conveyed about a specific treatment regimen
1604	**Leisure Participation** - Use of restful or relaxing activities as needed to promote well-being
1203	**Loneliness** - The extent of emotional, social or existential isolation response
2509	**Maternal Status: Antepartum** - Conditions and behaviors indicative of maternal well-being from conception to the onset of labor
2510	**Maternal Status: Intrapartum** - Conditions and behaviors indicative of maternal well-being from onset of labor to delivery
2511	**Maternal Status: Postpartum** - Conditions and behaviors indicative of maternal well-being from delivery of placenta to completion of involution
2301	**Medication Response** - Therapeutic and adverse effects of prescribed medication
0908	**Memory** - Ability to cognitively retrieve and report previously stored information
0208	**Mobility Level** - Ability to move purposefully
1204	**Mood Equilibrium** - Appropriate adjustment of prevailing emotional tone in response to circumstances
0209	**Muscle Function** - Adequacy of muscle contraction needed for movement
2512	**Neglect Recovery** - Healing following the cessation of substandard care
0909	**Neurological Status** - Extent to which the peripheral and central nervous system receive, process, and respond to internal and external stimuli
0910	**Neurological Status: Autonomic** - Extent to which the autonomic nervous system coordinates visceral function
0911	**Neurological Status: Central Motor Control** - Extent to which skeletal muscle activity (body movement) is coordinated by the central nervous system
0912	**Neurological Status: Consciousness** - Extent to which an individual arouses, orients, and attends to the environment
0913	**Neurological Status: Cranial Sensory/Motor Function** - Extent to which cranial nerves convey sensory and motor information
0914	**Neurological Status: Spinal Sensory/Motor Function** - Extent to which spinal nerves convey sensory and motor information
0118	**Newborn Adaptation** - Adaptation to the extrauterine environment by a physiologically mature newborn during the first 28 days
1004	**Nutritional Status** - Extent to which nutrients are available to meet metabolic needs
1005	**Nutritional Status: Biochemical Measures** - Body fluid components and chemical indices of nutritional status
1006	**Nutritional Status: Body Mass** - Congruence of body weight, muscle, and fat to height, frame, and gender
1007	**Nutritional Status: Energy** - Extent to which nutrients provide cellular energy
1008	**Nutritional Status: Food & Fluid Intake** - Amount of food and fluid taken into the body over a 24 hour period
1009	**Nutritional Status: Nutrient Intake** - Adequacy of nutrients taken into the body
1100	**Oral Health** - Condition of the mouth, teeth, gums, and tongue
1605	**Pain Control** - Personal actions to control pain
2101	**Pain: Disruptive Effects** - Observed or reported disruptive effects of pain on emotions and behavior
2102	**Pain Level** - Severity of reported or demonstrated pain
1306	**Pain: Psychological Response** - Cognitive and emotional responses to physical pain
1500	**Parent-Infant Attachment** - Behaviors which demonstrate an enduring affectional bond between a parent and infant

2211	**Parenting** - Provision of an environment that promotes optimum growth and development of dependent children
1901	**Parenting: Social Safety** - Parental actions to avoid social relationships that might cause harm or injury
1606	**Participation: Health Care Decisions** - Personal involvement in selecting and evaluating health care options
0113	**Physical Aging Status** - Physical changes that commonly occur with adult aging
2004	**Physical Fitness** - Ability to perform physical activities with vigor
0114	**Physical Maturation: Female** - Normal physical changes in the female that occur with the transition from childhood to adulthood
0115	**Physical Maturation: Male** - Normal physical changes in the male that occur with the transition from childhood to adulthood
0116	**Play Participation** - Use of activities as needed for enjoyment, entertainment, and development by children
1607	**Prenatal Health Behavior** - Personal actions to promote a healthy pregnancy
0117	**Preterm Infant Organization** - Extrauterine integration of physiologic and behavioral function by the infant born 24 to 37 (term) weeks gestation
0006	**Psychomotor Energy** - Ability to maintain ADL's, nutrition, personal safety
1305	**Psychosocial Adjustment: Life Change** - Psychosocial adaptation of an individual to a life change
2000	**Quality of Life** - An individual's expressed satisfaction with current life circumstances
0410	**Respiratory Status: Airway Patency** - Extent to which the tracheobronchial passages remain open
0402	**Respiratory Status: Gas Exchange** - Alveolar exchange of CO_2 or O_2 to maintain arterial blood gas concentrations
0403	**Respiratory Status: Ventilation** - Movement of air in and out of the lungs
0003	**Rest** - Extent and pattern of diminished activity for mental and physical rejuvenation
1902	**Risk Control** - Actions to eliminate or reduce actual, personal, and modifiable health threats
1903	**Risk Control: Alcohol Use** - Actions to eliminate or reduce alcohol use that poses a threat to health
1917	**Risk Control: Cancer** - Actions to reduce or detect the possibility of cancer
1914	**Risk Control: Cardiovascular Health** - Actions to eliminate or reduce threats to cardiovascular health
1904	**Risk Control: Drug Use** - Actions to eliminate or reduce drug use that poses a threat to health
1915	**Risk Control: Hearing Impairment** - Actions to eliminate or reduce the possibility of altered hearing function
1905	**Risk Control: Sexually Transmitted Diseases (STD)** - Actions to eliminate or reduce behaviors associated with sexually transmitted disease
1906	**Risk Control: Tobacco Use** - Actions to eliminate or reduce tobacco use
1907	**Risk Control: Unintended Pregnancy** - Actions to reduce the possibility of unintended pregnancy
1916	**Risk Control: Visual Impairment** - Actions to eliminate or reduce the possibility of altered visual function
1908	**Risk Detection** - Actions taken to identify personal health threats
1501	**Role Performance** - Congruence of an individual's role behavior with role expectations
1909	**Safety Behavior: Fall Prevention** - Individual or caregiver actions to minimize factors that might precipitate falls
1910	**Safety Behavior: Home Physical Environment** - Individual or caregiver actions to minimize environmental factors that might cause physical harm or injury in the home
1911	**Safety Behavior: Personal** - Individual or caregiver efforts to control behaviors that might cause physical injury
1912	**Safety Status: Falls Occurrence** - Number of falls in the past week
1913	**Safety Status: Physical Injury** - Severity of injuries from accidents and trauma
0300	**Self-Care: Activities of Daily Living (ADL)** - Ability to perform the most basic physical tasks and personal care activities
0301	**Self-Care: Bathing** - Ability to cleanse own body
0302	**Self-Care: Dressing** - Ability to dress self
0303	**Self-Care: Eating** - Ability to prepare and ingest food
0304	**Self-Care: Grooming** - Ability to maintain kempt appearance
0305	**Self-Care: Hygiene** - Ability to maintain own hygiene
0306	**Self-Care: Instrumental Activities of Daily Living (IADL)** - Ability to perform activities needed to function in the home or community
0307	**Self-Care: Non-Parenteral Medication** - Ability to administer oral and topical medications to meet therapeutic goals
0308	**Self-Care: Oral Hygiene** - Ability to care for own mouth and teeth
0309	**Self-Care: Parenteral Medication** - Ability to administer parenteral medications to meet therapeutic goals
0310	**Self-Care: Toileting** - Ability to toilet self

(continued)

1613	**Self-Direction of Care** - Directing others to assist with or perform physical tasks, personal care and activities needed to function in the home or the community
1205	**Self-Esteem** - Personal judgment of self-worth
1406	**Self-Mutilation Restraint** - Ability to refrain from intentional self-inflicted injury (nonlethal)
2400	**Sensory Function: Cutaneous** - Extent to which stimulation of the skin is sensed in an impaired area
2401	**Sensory Function: Hearing** - Extent to which sounds are sensed, with or without assistive devices
2402	**Sensory Function: Proprioception** - Extent to which the position and movement of the head and body are sensed
2403	**Sensory Function: Taste & Smell** - Extent to which chemicals inhaled or dissolved in saliva are sensed
2404	**Sensory Function: Vision** - Extent to which visual images are sensed, with or without assistive devices
0119	**Sexual Functioning** - Integration of physical, socioemotional, and intellectual aspects of sexual expression
1207	**Sexual Identity: Acceptance** - Acknowledgement and acceptance of own sexual identity
0211	**Skeletal Function** - The functional ability of the bones to support the body and facilitate movement
0004	**Sleep** - Extent and pattern of natural periodic suspension of consciousness during which the body is restored
1502	**Social Interaction Skills** - An individual's use of effective interaction behaviors
1503	**Social Involvement** - Frequency of an individual's social interactions with persons, groups, or organizations
1504	**Social Support** - Perceived availability and actual provision of reliable assistance from other persons
2001	**Spiritual Well-Being** - Personal expressions of connectedness with self, others, higher power, all life, nature and the universe that transcend and empower the self
1407	**Substance Addiction Consequences** - Compromise in health status and social functioning due to substance addiction
2003	**Suffering Level** - Severity of anguish associated with a distressing symptom, injury, or loss with potential longterm effects
1408	**Suicide Self-Restraint** - Ability to refrain from gestures and attempts at killing self
1010	**Swallowing Status** - Extent of safe passage of fluids and/or solids from the mouth to the stomach
1011	**Swallowing Status: Esophageal Phase** - Adequacy of the passage of fluids and/or solids from the pharynx to the stomach
1012	**Swallowing Status: Oral Phase** - Adequacy of preparation, containment and movement posteriorly of fluids and/or solids in the mouth from swallowing
1013	**Swallowing Status: Pharyngeal Phase** - Adequacy of the passage of fluids and/or solids from the mouth to the esophagus
1608	**Symptom Control** - Personal actions to minimize perceived adverse changes in physical and emotional functioning
2103	**Symptom Severity** - Extent of perceived adverse changes in physical, emotional, and social functioning
2104	**Symptom Severity: Perimenopause** - Extent of symptoms caused by declining hormonal levels
2105	**Symptom Severity: Premenstrual Syndrome (PMS)** - Extent of symptoms caused by cyclic hormonal fluctuations
2302	**Systemic Toxin Clearance: Dialysis** - Extent to which toxins are cleared from the body with peritoneal or hemodialysis
0800	**Thermoregulation** - Balance among heat production, heat gain, and heat loss
0801	**Thermoregulation: Neonate** - Balance among heat production, heat gain, and heat loss during the neonatal period
1101	**Tissue Integrity: Skin & Mucous Membranes** - Structural intactness and normal physiological function of skin and mucous membranes
0404	**Tissue Perfusion: Abdominal Organs** - Extent to which blood flows through the small vessels of the abdominal viscera and maintains organ function
0405	**Tissue Perfusion: Cardiac** - Extent to which blood flows through the coronary vasculature and maintains heart function
0406	**Tissue Perfusion: Cerebral** - Extent to which blood flows through the cerebral vasculature and maintains brain function
0407	**Tissue Perfusion: Peripheral** - Extent to which blood flows through the small vessels of the extremities and maintains tissue function
0408	**Tissue Perfusion: Pulmonary** - Extent to which blood flows through intact pulmonary vasculature with appropriate pressure and volume, perfusing alveoli/capillary unit
0210	**Transfer Performance** - Ability to change body locations
1609	**Treatment Behavior: Illness or Injury** - Personal actions to palliate or eliminate pathology
0502	**Urinary Continence** - Control of the elimination of urine
0503	**Urinary Elimination** - Ability of the urinary system to filter wastes, conserve solutes, and to collect and discharge urine in a healthy pattern

611	**Vision Compensation Behavior** - Actions to compensate for visual impairment
802	**Vital Signs Status** - Temperature, pulse, respiration, and blood pressure within expected range for the individual
612	**Weight Control** - Personal actions resulting in achievement and maintenance of optimum body weight for health
2002	**Well-Being** - An individual's expressed satisfaction with health status
206	**Will to Live** - Desire, determination, and effort to survive
102	**Wound Healing: Primary Intention** - The extent to which cell and tissues have regenerated following intentional closure
103	**Wound Healing: Secondary Intention** - The extent to which cells and tissues in an open wound have regenerated

---

14-5. HOME HEALTH CARE CLASSIFICATION SYSTEM (HHCC SYSTEM)

The Home Health Care Classification System (HHCC System) was developed by Dr. Virginia K. Saba, RN, FAAN, FACMI, of Georgetown University, to provide a standardized framework for coding and categorizing home health and ambulatory care. This system consists of two interrelated taxonomies: the HHCC of Nursing Diagnoses and the HHCC of Nursing Interventions, classified into 20 Care Components. The HHCC System was empirically developed from federally funded research.

I. CARE COMPONENTS

The Twenty Care Components (20) are used as the standardized framework for classifying the HHCC System taxonomies: the HHCC of Nursing Diagnoses (435) and the HHCC of Nursing Interventions (640). They provide the coding and classifying framework to facilitate computer processing and statistical analyses.

Definition   A nursing care component is defined as a cluster of elements that represents a unique pattern of clinical care nursing practice; namely, Health Behavioral, Functional, Physiological, and Psychological.

Description   The 20 Care Components provide the standardized framework for classifying the two interrelated home health care taxonomies – HHCC of Nursing Diagnoses (435) and HHCC of Nursing Interventions (640). They are used to code and classify the six steps of the Nursing Process: Assessment, Diagnosis, Outcome Identification (Expected Outcome/Goal), Planning (Nursing Intervention), Implementation (Type Intervention Action), and Evaluation (Actual Outcome). The Care Components are used to link, map, and track the care process for an episode of illness, facilitate computer processing, and do statistical analyses. They are also used to track and measure patient/client care holistically over time and across settings, population groups, and geographic locations.

Home Health Care Classification of 20 Care Components: Alphabetical List with Codes and Definitions

A   **ACTIVITY COMPONENT**   Cluster of elements that involve the use of energy in carrying out bodily actions.

B   **BOWEL ELIMINATION COMPONENT**   Cluster of elements that involve the gastrointestinal system.

C   **CARDIAC COMPONENT**   Cluster of elements that involve heart, blood vessels, and circulatory system.

D   **COGNITIVE COMPONENT**   Cluster of elements involving the mental and cerebral processes.

E   **COPING COMPONENT**   Cluster of elements that involve the ability to deal with responsibilities, problems, or difficulties.

F   **FLUID VOLUME COMPONENT**   Cluster of elements that involve liquid consumption.

G   **HEALTH BEHAVIOR COMPONENT**   Cluster of elements that involve actions to sustain, maintain, or regain health.

H   **MEDICATION COMPONENT**   Cluster of elements that involve medicinal substances.

I   **METABOLIC COMPONENT**   Cluster of elements that involve the endocrine and immunological processes.

J   **NUTRITIONAL COMPONENT**   Cluster of elements that involve the intake of food and nutrients

K   **PHYSICAL REGULATION COMPONENT**   Cluster of elements that involve bodily processes.

L   **RESPIRATORY COMPONENT**   Cluster of elements that involve breathing and the pulmonary system.

M   **ROLE RELATIONSHIP COMPONENT**   Cluster of elements involving interpersonal, work, social, and sexual interactions.

N   **SAFETY COMPONENT**   Cluster of elements that involve prevention of injury, danger, or loss.

O   **SELF-CARE COMPONENT**   Cluster of elements that involve the ability to carry out activities to maintain oneself.

P   **SELF-CONCEPT COMPONENT**   Cluster of elements that involve an individual's mental image of oneself.

Q   **SENSORY COMPONENT**   Cluster of elements that involve the senses.

(continued)

R SKIN INTEGRITY COMPONENT Cluster of elements that involve the mucous membrane, corneal, integumentary, or subcutaneous structures of the body.

S TISSUE PERFUSION COMPONENT Cluster of elements that involve the oxygenation of tissues.

T URINARY ELIMINATION COMPONENT Cluster of elements that involve the genitourinary system.

II. NURSING DIAGNOSES

The HHCC of Nursing Diagnoses taxonomy consists of 145 nursing diagnostic categories. They are modified by an Expected/Actual Outcome axis represented by three qualifiers – Improved, Stabilized, Deteriorated – totaling 435 terms.

Definition A nursing diagnosis is "a clinical judgment about individual, family, or community responses to actual or potential health problems/life processes. Nursing diagnoses provide the basis for selection of nursing interventions to achieve outcomes for which the nurse is accountable" (NANDA, 1992, p. 5). Nursing diagnoses are concepts used to describe actual and potential health problems of clients. They describe clinical nursing practice in a uniform manner.

PART ONE: *Home Health Care Classification of Nursing Diagnoses and Coding Scheme: 50 Major Categories and 95 Subcategories*[1]

A—ACTIVITY COMPONENT

01	Activity Alteration
01.1	Activity Intolerance
01.2	Activity Intolerance Risk
01.3	Diversional Activity Deficit
01.4	Fatigue
01.5	Physical Mobility Impairment
01.6	Sleep Pattern Disturbance
02	Musculoskeletal Alteration

B—BOWEL ELIMINATION COMPONENT

03	Bowel Elimination Alteration
03.1	Bowel Incontinence
03.2	Colonic Constipation
03.3	Diarrhea
03.4	Fecal Impaction
03.5	Perceived Constipation
03.6	Unspecified Constipation
04	Gastrointestinal Alteration

C—CARDIAC COMPONENT

05	Cardiac Output Alteration
06	Cardiovascular Alteration
06.1	Blood Pressure Alteration

D—COGNITIVE COMPONENT

07	Cerebral Alteration
08	Knowledge Deficit
08.1	Knowledge Deficit of Diagnostic Test
08.2	Knowledge Deficit of Dietary Regimen
08.3	Knowledge Deficit of Disease Process
08.4	Knowledge Deficit of Fluid Volume
08.5	Knowledge Deficit of Medication Regimen
08.6	Knowledge Deficit of Safety Precautions
08.7	Knowledge Deficit of Therapeutic Regimen
09	Thought Processes Alteration

E—COPING COMPONENT

10	Dying Process
11	Family Coping Impairment
11.1	Compromised Family Coping
11.2	Disabled Family Coping
12	Individual Coping Impairment
12.1	Adjustment Impairment
12.2	Decisional Conflict
12.3	Defensive Coping
12.4	Denial
13	Post-Trauma Response
13.1	Rape Trauma Syndrome

14	Spiritual State Alteration
14.1	Spiritual Distress

F—FLUID VOLUME COMPONENT

15	Fluid Volume Alteration
15.1	Fluid Volume Deficit
15.2	Fluid Volume Deficit Risk
15.3	Fluid Volume Excess
15.4	Fluid Volume Excess Risk

G—HEALTH BEHAVIOR COMPONENT

16	Growth and Development Alteration
17	Health Maintenance Alteration
18	Health Seeking Behavior Alteration
19	Home Maintenance Alteration
20	Noncompliance
20.1	Noncompliance of Diagnostic Test
20.2	Noncompliance of Dietary Regimen
20.3	Noncompliance of Fluid Volume
20.4	Noncompliance of Medication Regimen
20.5	Noncompliance of Safety Precautions
20.6	Noncompliance of Therapeutic Regimen

H—MEDICATION COMPONENT

21	Medication Risk
21.1	Polypharmacy

I—METABOLIC COMPONENT

22	Endocrine Alteration
23	Immunologic Alteration
23.1	Protection Alteration

J—NUTRITIONAL COMPONENT

24	Nutrition Alteration
24.1	Body Nutrition Deficit
24.2	Body Nutrition Deficit Risk
24.3	Body Nutrition Excess
24.4	Body Nutrition Excess Risk

K—PHYSICAL REGULATION COMPONENT

25	Physical Regulation Alteration
25.1	Dysreflexia
25.2	Hyperthermia
25.3	Hypothermia
25.4	Thermoregulation Impairment
25.5	Infection Risk
25.6	Infection Unspecified

L—RESPIRATORY COMPONENT

26	Respiration Alteration
26.1	Airway Clearance Impairment

[1]Adapted from NANDA: Taxonomy I: Revised 1990.

26.2	Breathing Pattern Impairment		42	Meaningfulness Alteration
26.3	Gas Exchange Impairment		42.1	Hopelessness
			42.2	Powerlessness

M—ROLE RELATIONSHIP COMPONENT

27	Role Performance Alteration
27.1	Parental Role Conflict
27.2	Parenting Alteration
27.3	Sexual Dysfunction
28	Communication Impairment
28.1	Verbal Impairment
29	Family Processes Alteration
30	Grieving
30.1	Anticipatory Grieving
30.2	Dysfunctional Grieving
31	Sexuality Patterns Alteration
32	Socialization Alteration
32.1	Social Interaction Alteration
32.2	Social Isolation

N—SAFETY COMPONENT

33	Injury Risk
33.1	Aspiration Risk
33.2	Disuse Syndrome
33.3	Poisoning Risk
33.4	Suffocation Risk
33.5	Trauma Risk
34	Violence Risk

O—SELF-CARE COMPONENT

35	Bathing/Hygiene Deficit
36	Dressing/Grooming Deficit
37	Feeding Deficit
37.1	Breastfeeding Impairment
37.2	Swallowing Impairment
38	Self Care Deficit
38.1	Activities of Daily Living (ADLs) Alteration
38.2	Instrumental Activities of Daily Living (IADLs) Alteration
39	Toileting Deficit

P—SELF-CONCEPT COMPONENT

40	Anxiety
41	Fear

43	Self Concept Alteration
43.1	Body Image Disturbance
43.2	Personal Identity Disturbance
43.3	Chronic Low Self-Esteem Disturbance
43.4	Situational Self-Esteem Disturbance

Q—SENSORY COMPONENT

44	Sensory Perceptual Alteration
44.1	Auditory Alteration
44.2	Gustatory Alteration
44.3	Kinesthetic Alteration
44.4	Olfactory Alteration
44.5	Tactile Alteration
44.6	Unilateral Neglect
44.7	Visual Alteration
45	Comfort Alteration
45.1	Acute Pain
45.2	Chronic Pain
45.3	Unspecified Pain

R—SKIN INTEGRITY COMPONENT

46	Skin Integrity Alteration
46.1	Oral Mucous Membranes Impairment
46.2	Skin Integrity Impairment
46.3	Skin Integrity Impairment Risk
46.4	Skin Incision
47	Peripheral Alteration

S—TISSUE PERFUSION COMPONENT

48	Tissue Perfusion Alteration

T—URINARY ELIMINATION COMPONENT

49	Urinary Elimination Alteration
49.1	Functional Urinary Incontinence
49.2	Reflex Urinary Incontinence
49.3	Stress Urinary Incontinence
49.4	Total Urinary Incontinence
49.5	Urge Urinary Incontinence
49.6	Urinary Retention
50	Renal Alteration

PART TWO: Home Health Care Classification of 145 Nursing Diagnoses: Alphabetical List with Definitions and Codes

A01 **Acitivity Alteration** Change or modification in energy used by the body.

A01.1 **Activity Intolerance** Incapacity to carry out physiological or psychological daily activities.

A01.2 **Activity Intolerance Risk** Increased chance of an incapacity to carry out physiological or psychological daily activites.

O38.1 **Activities of Daily Living (ADLs) Alteration** Change or modification of ability to maintain oneself.

Q45.1 **Acute Pain** Physical suffering or distress; to hurt.

E12.1 **Adjustment Impairment** Inadequate adaptation to condition or change in health status.

L26.1 **Airway Clearance Impairment** Inability to clear secretions/obstructions in airway.

M30.1 **Anticipatory Grieving** Feeling great sorrow before the event or loss.

P40 **Anxiety** Feeling of distress or apprehension whose source is unknown.

N33.1 **Aspiration Risk** Increased chance of material into tracheobronchial passages.

Q44.1 **Auditory Alteration** Diminished ability to hear.

O35 **Bathing/Hygiene Deficit** Impaired ability to cleanse oneself.

C06.1 **Blood Pressure Alteration** Change in the systolic or diastolic pressure.

P43.1 **Body Image Disturbance** Imbalance in the perception of the way one's body looks.

J24.1 **Body Nutrition Deficit** Less than adequate intake or absorption of food or nutrients.

J24.2 **Body Nutrition Deficit Risk** Increased chance of less than adequate intake or absorption of food or nutrients.

J24.3 **Body Nutrition Excess** More than adequate intake or absorption of food or nutrients.

(continued)

J24.4	**Body Nutrition Excess Risk**	Increased chance of more than adequate intake or absorption of food or nutrients.
B03	**Bowel Elimination Alteration**	Change or modification of the gastrointestinal system.
B03.1	**Bowel Incontinence**	Involuntary defecation.
O37.1	**Breastfeeding Impairment**	Diminished ability to nourish infant at the breast.
L26.2	**Breathing Pattern Impairment**	Inadequate inhalation or exhalation.
C05	**Cardiac Output Alteration**	Change or modification in the pumping action of the heart.
D06	**Cardiovascular Alteration**	Change or modification of the heart or blood vessels.
D07	**Cerebral Alteration**	Change or modification of thought processes or mentation.
P43.3	**Chronic Low Self-Esteem Disturbance**	Persistent negative evaluation of oneself.
Q45.2	**Chronic Pain**	Pain that continues for longer than expected.
B03.2	**Colonic Constipation**	Infrequent or difficult passage of hard, dry feces.
Q45	**Comfort Alteration**	Change or modification in sensation that is distressing.
M28	**Communication Impairment**	Diminished ability to exchange thoughts, opinions, or information.
E11.1	**Compromised Family Coping**	Inability of family to function optimally.
E12.2	**Decisional Conflict**	Struggle related to determining a course of action.
E12.3	**Defensive Coping**	Self-protective strategies to guard against threats to self.
E12.4	**Denial**	Attempt to reduce anxiety by refusal to accept thoughts, feelings, or facts.
B03.3	**Diarrhea**	Abnormal frequency and fluidity of feces.
E11.2	**Disabled Family Coping**	Dysfunctional ability of family to function.
N33.2	**Disuse Syndrome**	Group of symptoms related to effects of immobility.
A01.3	**Diversional Activity Deficit**	Lack of interest or engagement in leisure activities.
O36	**Dressing/Grooming Deficit**	Impaired ability to clothe and groom oneself.
E10	**Dying Process**	Physical and behavioral responses associated with death.
M30.2	**Dysfunctional Grieving**	Prolonged feeling of great sorrow.
K25.1	**Dysreflexia**	Life threatening inhibited sympathetic response to a noxious stimuli in a person with a spinal cord injury at T7 or above.
I22	**Endocrine Alteration**	Change or modification of internal secretions or hormones.
E11	**Family Coping Impairment**	Inadequate family response to problems or difficulties.
M29	**Family Processes Alteration**	Change or modification of usual functioning of a related group.
A01.4	**Fatigue**	Exhaustion that interferes with physical and mental activities.
P41	**Fear**	Feeling of dread or distress whose cause can be identified.
B03.4	**Fecal Impaction**	Feces wedged in intestine.
O37	**Feeding Deficit**	Impaired ability to feed oneself.
F15	**Fluid Volume Alteration**	Change or modification in bodily fluid.
F15.1	**Fluid Volume Deficit**	Dehydration.
F15.2	**Fluid Volume Deficit Risk**	Increased chance of dehydration.
F15.3	**Fluid Volume Excess**	Fluid retention, overload, or edema.
F15.4	**Fluid Volume Excess Risk**	Increased chance of fluid retention, overload, or edema.
T49.1	**Functional Urinary Incontinence**	Involuntary, unpredictable passage of urine.
L26.3	**Gas Exchange Impairment**	Imbalance of oxygen and carbon dioxide transfer between lung and vascular system.
B04	**Gastrointestinal Alteration**	Change or modification of the stomach or intestines.
M30	**Grieving**	Feeling of great sorrow.
G16	**Growth and Development Alteration**	Change or modification in norms for age.
Q44.2	**Gustatory Alteration**	Diminished ability to taste.
G17	**Health Maintenance Alteration**	Change or modification in ability to manage health related needs.
G18	**Health Seeking Behavior Alteration**	Change or modification of actions needed to improve health state.
G19	**Home Maintenance Alteration**	Inability to sustain a safe, healthy environment.
P42.1	**Hopelessness**	Feeling of despair or futility and passive abandonment.
K25.2	**Hyperthermia**	Abnormal high body temperature.
K25.3	**Hypothermia**	Subnormal low body temperature.
I23	**Immunologic Alteration**	Change or modification of the immune system.
E12	**Individual Coping Impairment**	Inadequate personal response to problems or difficulties.
K25.5	**Infection Risk**	Increased change of contamination with disease-producing germs.
K25.6	**Infection Unspecified**	Unknown contamination with disease-producing germs.
N33	**Injury Risk**	Increased change of danger or loss.
O38.2	**Instrumental Activities of Daily Living (IADLs) Alteration**	Change or modification of more complex activities than those needed to maintain oneself.

Q44.3	**Kinesthetic Alteration** Diminished ability to move.
D08	**Knowledge Deficit** Lack of information, understanding, or comprehension.
D08.1	**Knowledge Deficit of Diagnostic Test** Lack of information on tests to identify disease or assess health condition.
D08.2	**Knowledge Deficit of Dietary Regimen** Lack of information on the prescribed food or fluid intake.
D08.3	**Knowledge Deficit of Disease Process** Lack of information on the morbidity, course, or treatment of the health condition.
D08.4	**Knowledge Deficit of Fluid Volume** Lack of information on fluid volume intake requirements.
D08.5	**Knowledge Deficit of Medication Regimen** Lack of information on prescribed regulated course of medicinal substances.
D08.6	**Knowledge Deficit of Safety Precautions** Lack of information on measures to prevent injury, danger, or loss.
D08.7	**Knowledge Deficit of Therapeutic Regimen** Lack of information on regulated course of treating disease.
P42	**Meaningfulness Alteration** Change or modification of the ability to see the significance, purpose, or value in something.
H21	**Medication Risk** Increased chance of negative response to medicinal substance.
A02	**Musculoskeletal Alteration** Change or modification of the muscles, bones or support structures.
G20	**Noncompliance** Failure to follow therapeutic recommendations.
G20.1	**Noncompliance of Diagnostic Test** Failure to follow therapeutic recommendations on tests to identify disease or assess health condition.
G20.2	**Noncompliance of Dietary Regimen** Failure to follow the prescribed food or fluid intake.
G20.3	**Noncompliance of Fluid Volume** Failure to follow fluid volume intake requirements.
G20.4	**Noncompliance of Medication Regimen** Failure to follow prescribed regulated course of medicinal substances.
G20.5	**Noncompliance of Safety Precautions** Failure to follow measures to prevent injury, danger, or loss.
G20.6	**Noncompliance of Therapeutic Regimen** Failure to follow regulated course of treating disease.
J24	**Nutrition Alteration** Change or modification of food or nutrients.
Q44.4	**Olfactory Alteration** Diminished ability to smell.
R46.1	**Oral Mucous Membranes Impairment** Diminished ability to maintain the tissues of the oral cavity.
M27.1	**Parental Role Conflict** Struggle with parental position and responsibilities.
M27.2	**Parenting Alteration** Change or modification of nurturing figures ability to promote growth and development of infant/child.
B03.5	**Perceived Constipation** Belief and treatment of infrequent or difficult passage of feces without cause.
R47	**Peripheral Alteration** Change or modification in vascularization of the extremities.
P43.2	**Personal Identity Disturbance** Imbalance in the ability to distinguish between the self and the non-self.
A01.5	**Physical Mobility Impairment** Diminished ability to perform independent movement.
K25	**Physical Regulation Alteration** Change or modification of somatic control.
N33.3	**Poisoning Risk** Exposure to or ingestion of dangerous products.
H21.1	**Polypharmacy** Use of two or more drugs together.
E13	**Post-Trauma Response** Sustained behavior related to a traumatic event.
P42.2	**Powerlessness** Feeling of helplessness, or inability to act.
I23.1	**Protection Alteration** Change or modification of the ability to guard against internal or external threats to the body.
E13.1	**Rape Trauma Syndrome** Group of symptoms related to a forced sexual act.
L26	**Respiration Alteration** Change or modification in breathing.
T49.2	**Reflex Urinary Incontinence** Involuntary passage of urine occurring at predictable intervals.
T50	**Renal Alteration** Change or modification in the kidneys.
M27	**Role Performance Alteration** Change or modification of carrying out responsibilities.
O38	**Self Care Deficit** Impaired ability to maintain oneself.
P43	**Self Concept Alteration** Change or modification of ability to maintain one's image of self.
Q44	**Sensory Perceptual Alteration** Change in modification in the response to stimuli.
M27.3	**Sexual Dysfunction** Deleterious change in sex response.

(continued)

M31	**Sexuality Patterns Alteration**	Change or modification of persons's sexual response.
P43.4	**Situational Self-Esteem Disturbance**	Negative evaluation of oneself in response to a loss or change.
R46.2	**Skin Integrity Impairment**	Diminished ability to maintain the integument.
R46.3	**Skin Integrity Impairment Risk**	Increased chance of skin breakdown.
R46.4	**Skin Incision**	Cutting of the integument.
A01.6	**Sleep Pattern Disturbance**	Imbalance in the normal sleep/wake cycle.
M32.1	**Social Interaction Alteration**	Inadequate quantity or quality of personal relations.
M32.2	**Social Isolation**	State of aloneness, lack of interaction with others.
M32	**Socialization Alteration**	Change or modification of personal identity.
E14.1	**Spiritual Distress**	Anguish related to the spirit or soul.
E14	**Spiritual State Alteration**	Change or modification of the spirit or soul.
T49.3	**Stress Urinary Incontinence**	Loss of urine occurring with increased abdominal pressure.
N33.4	**Suffocation Risk**	Inadequate air for breathing.
O37.2	**Swallowing Impairment**	Inability to move food from mouth to stomach.
Q44.5	**Tactile Alteration**	Diminished ability to feel.
K25.4	**Thermoregulation Impairment**	Fluctuation of temperature between hypothermia and hyperthermia.
R46	**Tissue Integrity Alteration**	A change or modification in the mucous membrane, corneal, integumentary, or subcutaneous structures.
S48	**Tissue Perfusion Alteration**	A change or modification in the oxygenation of tissues.
O39	**Toileting Deficit**	Impaired ability to urinate or defecate for oneself.
T49.4	**Total Urinary Incontinence**	Continuous and unpredictable loss of urine.
D09	**Thought Processes Alteration**	Change or modification in cognitive processes.
N33.5	**Trauma Risk**	Accidental tissue injury.
Q44.6	**Unilateral Neglect**	Lack of awareness of one side of the body.
B03.6	**Unspecified Constipation**	Other forms of abnormal feces or difficult passage of feces.
Q45.3	**Unspecified Pain**	Pain that is difficult to pinpoint.
T49	**Urinary Elimination Alteration**	A change or modification in the excretion of the waste matter of the kidneys.
T49.6	**Urinary Retention**	Incomplete emptying of the bladder.
T49.5	**Urge Urinary Incontinence**	Involuntary passage of urine following a sense of urgency to void.
M28.1	**Verbal Impairment**	Diminished ability to exchange thoughts, opinions, or information through speech.
N34	**Violence Risk**	Increased chance of harming self or others.
Q44.7	**Visual Alteration**	A diminished ability to see.

III. NURSING INTERVENTIONS

The HHCC of Nursing Interventions taxonomy consists of 160 nursing interventions. They are modified by a Type Action axis represented by four qualifiers – Assess, Care, Teach, Manage – totaling 640 terms.

Definition A nursing intervention is defined as a single nursing action – treatment, procedure, or activity – designed to achieve an outcome to a diagnosis – nursing or medical – for which the nurse is accountable. Patient services are usually initiated as medical orders by a referring physician and reviewed by the admitting nurse. As part of the admission assessment the primary nurse also determines the nursing orders based on the signs and symptoms, diagnoses, and expected outcomes/goals.

Description The HHCC of Nursing Interventions consists of 160 terms, 60 of which are major intervention categories and 100 of which are minor or subcategories. The major categories represent general interventions that embody multiple tasks, and the minor or subcategories represent more precise related interventions and/or specific tasks.

A—ACTIVITY COMPONENT

01	Activity Care
01.1	Cardiac Rehabilitation
01.2	Energy Conservation
02	Fracture Care
02.1	Cast Care
02.2	Immobilizer Care
03	Mobility Therapy
03.1	Ambulation Therapy
03.2	Assistive Device Therapy
03.3	Transfer Care
04	Sleep Pattern Control

05	Rehabilitation Care
05.1	Range of Motion
05.2	Rehabilitation Exercise

B—BOWEL ELIMINATION COMPONENT

06	Bowel Care
06.1	Bowel Training
06.2	Disimpaction
06.3	Enema
07	Ostomy Care
07.1	Ostomy Irrigation

C—CARDIAC COMPONENT
08	Cardiac Care
09	Pacemaker Care

D—COGNITIVE COMPONENT
10	Behavior Care
11	Reality Orientation

E—COPING COMPONENT
12	Counseling Service
12.1	Coping Support
12.2	Stress Control
13	Emotional Support
13.1	Spiritual Comfort
14	Terminal Care
14.1	Bereavement Support
14.2	Dying/Death Measures
14.3	Funeral Arrangements

F—FLUID VOLUME COMPONENT
15	Fluid Therapy
15.1	Hydration Status
15.2	Intake/Output
16	Infusion Care
16.1	Intravenous Care
16.2	Venous Catheter Care

G—HEALTH BEHAVIOR COMPONENT
17	Community Special Programs
17.1	Adult Day Center
17.2	Hospice
17.3	Meals-on-Wheels
17.4	Other Community Special Program
18	Compliance Care
18.1	Compliance with Diet
18.2	Compliance with Fluid Volume
18.3	Compliance with Medical Regime
18.4	Compliance with Medication Regime
18.5	Compliance with Safety Precautions
18.6	Compliance with Therapeutic Regime
19	Nursing Contact
19.1	Bill of Rights
19.2	Nursing Care Coordination
19.3	Nursing Status Report
20	Physician Contact
20.1	Medical Regime Orders
20.2	Physician Status Report
21	Professional/Ancillary Services
21.1	Home Health Aide Service
21.2	Medical Social Worker Service
21.3	Nurse Specialist Service
21.4	Occupational Therapist Service
21.5	Physical Therapist Service
21.6	Speech Therapist Service
21.7	Other Ancillary Service
21.8	Other Professional Service

H—MEDICATION COMPONENT
22	Chemotherapy Care
23	Injection Administration
23.1	Insulin Injection
23.2	Vitamin B12 Injection
24	Medication Administration
24.1	Medication Actions
24.2	Medication Prefill Preparation
24.3	Medication Side Effects
25	Radiation Therapy Care

I—METABOLIC COMPONENT
26	Allergic Reaction Care
27	Diabetic Care

J—NUTRITIONAL COMPONENT
28	Gastrostomy/Nasogastric Tube Care
28.1	Gastrostomy/Nasogastric Tube Insertion
28.2	Gastrostomy/Nasogastric Tube Irrigation
29	Nutrition Care
29.1	Enteral/Parenteral Feeding
29.2	Feeding Technique
29.3	Regular Diet
29.4	Special Diet

K—PHYSICAL REGULATION COMPONENT
30	Infection Control
30.1	Universal Precautions
31	Physical Health Care
31.1	Health History
31.2	Health Promotion
31.3	Physical Examination
31.4	Physical Measurements
32	Specimen Analysis
32.1	Blood Specimen Analysis
32.2	Stool Specimen Analysis
32.3	Urine Specimen Analysis
32.4	Other Specimen Analysis
33	Vital Signs
33.1	Blood Pressure
33.2	Temperature
33.3	Pulse
33.4	Respiration
34	Weight Control

L—RESPIRATORY COMPONENT
35	Oxygen Therapy Care
36	Respiratory Care
36.1	Breathing Exercises
36.2	Chest Physiotherapy
36.3	Inhalation Therapy
36.4	Ventilator Care
37	Tracheostomy Care

M—ROLE RELATIONSHIP COMPONENT
38	Communication Care
39	Psychosocial Analysis
39.1	Home Situation Analysis
39.2	Interpersonal Dynamics Analysis

N—SAFETY COMPONENT
40	Abuse Control
41	Emergency Care
42	Safety Precautions
42.1	Environmental Safety
42.2	Equipment Safety
42.3	Individual Safety

O—SELF-CARE COMPONENT
43	Personal Care
43.1	Activities of Daily Living (ADLs)
43.2	Instrumental Activities of Daily Living (IADLs)
44	Bedbound Care
44.1	Positioning Therapy

P—SELF-CONCEPT COMPONENT
45	Mental Health Care
45.1	Mental Health History

(continued)

45.2	Mental Health Promotion	53	Mouth Care
45.3	Mental Health Screening	53.1	Denture Care
45.4	Mental Health Treatment	54	Skin Care
46	Violence Control	54.1	Skin Breakdown Control

Q—SENSORY COMPONENT

47	Pain Control	55	Wound Care
48	Comfort Care	55.1	Drainage Tube Care
49	Ear Care	55.2	Dressing Change
49.1	Hearing Aid Care	55.3	Incision Care
49.2	Wax Removal		
50	Eye Care		
50.1	Cataract Care		

S—TISSUE PERFUSION COMPONENT

56	Foot Care
57	Perineal Care

R—SKIN INTEGRITY COMPONENT

T—URINARY ELIMINATION COMPONENT

51	Decubitus Care	58	Bladder Care
51.1	Decubitus Stage 1	58.1	Bladder Instillation
51.2	Decubitus Stage 2	58.2	Bladder Training
51.3	Decubitus Stage 3	59	Dialysis Care
51.4	Decubitus Stage 4	60	Urinary Catheter Care
52	Edema Control	60.1	Urinary Catheter Insertion
		60.2	Urinary Catheter Irrigation

PART TWO: Home Health Care Classification of 160 Nursing Interventions: Alphabetical List with Definitions and Codes

N40   **Abuse Control**   Actions to manage situations to avoid, detect, or minimize harm.

A01   **Activity Care**   Actions performed to carry out physiological or psychological daily activites.

O43.1   **Activities of Daily Living (ADLs)**   Personal activities to maintain oneself.

A03.1   **Ambulation Therapy**   Actions to promote walking.

G17.1   **Adult Day Center**   Actions to manage the provision of a day program for adults in a specific location.

I26   **Allergic Reaction Care**   Actions to reduce symptoms or precautions to reduce allergies.

A03.2   **Assistive Device Therapy**   Actions to manage the use of products to aid in caring for oneself.

D10   **Behavior Care**   Actions performed to manage observable responses to internal and external stimuli.

T58   **Bladder Care**   Actions performed to manage urinary drainage problems.

T58.1   **Bladder Instillation**   Actions to pour liquid into a catheter.

T58.2   **Bladder Training**   Actions to provide instruction on the care of urinary drainage problems.

O44   **Bedbound Care**   Actions performed to manage an individual confined to bed.

E14.1   **Bereavement Support**   Actions to provide comfort to the family/friends of the person who died.

G19.1   **Bill of Rights**   Statements related to entitlement during an episode of illness.

K33.1   **Blood Pressure**   Actions to measure the diastolic and systolic pressure of the blood.

K32.1   **Blood Specimen Analysis**   Actions performed to collect and/or examine a sample of blood.

B06   **Bowel Care**   Actions performed to maintain or restore functioning of the bowel.

B06.1   **Bowel Training**   Actions to provide instruction on bowel elimination conditions.

L36.1   **Breathing Exercises**   Actions to provide instruction on respiratory or lung exertion.

C08   **Cardiac Care**   Actions performed to manage changes in the heart blood vessels.

A01.1   **Cardiac Rehabilitation**   Actions taken to restore cardiac health.

A02.1   **Cast Care**   Actions performed to manage a rigid dressing.

Q50.1   **Cataract Care**   Actions performed to control cataract conditions.

H22   **Chemotherapy Care**   Actions performed to administer and monitor antineoplastic agents.

L36.2   **Chest Physiotherapy**   Exercises to provide postural drainage of lungs.

Q48   **Comfort Care**   Actions performed to enhance or improve well-being.

G18   **Compliance Care**   Actions performed to encourage conformity to therapeutic recommendations.

G18.1   **Compliance with Diet**   Actions to encourage conformity to food or fluid intake.

G18.2   **Compliance with Fluid Volume**   Actions to encourage conformity to therapeutic intake of liquids.

G18.3   **Compliance with Medical Regime**   Actions to encourage conformity to physician's plan of care.

G18.4   **Compliance with Medication Regime**   Actions to encourage conformity to follow prescribed course of medicinal substances.

G18.5   **Compliance with Safety Precautions**   Actions to encourage conformity with measures to protect the self or others from injury, danger, or loss.

G18.6 **Compliance with Therapeutic Regime** Actions to encourage conformity with the health team's plan of care.
G17 **Community Special Programs** Actions to manage the provision of advice or instruction about special community program resources.
M38 **Communication Care** Actions performed to exchange verbal information.
E12.1 **Coping Support** Actions to sustain a person dealing with responsibilities, problems, or difficulties.
E12 **Counseling Service** Actions to provide advice or instruction to help another.
I27 **Diabetic Care** Actions performed to control diabetic conditions.
T59 **Dialysis Care** Actions performed in the care and management of dialysis treatments.
B06.2 **Disimpaction** Actions to manually remove feces.
R51 **Decubitus Care** Actions performed to prevent, detect, and treat skin integrity breakdown caused by pressure.
R51.1 **Decubitus Stage 1** Actions performed to prevent skin breakdown.
R51.2 **Decubitus Stage 2** Actions performed to manage tissue breakdown.
R51.3 **Decubitus Stage 3** Actions performed to manage skin destruction.
R51.4 **Decubitus Stage 4** Actions performed to manage open wounds.
R53.1 **Denture Care** Actions performed to manage artificial teeth.
R55.1 **Drainage Tube Care** Actions performed to control drainage from tubes.
R55.2 **Dressing Change** Actions performed to remove and replace new bandage(s) to a wound.
E14.2 **Dying/Death Measures** Actions to manage the dying process.
Q49 **Ear Care** Actions performed to manage ear problems.
R52 **Edema Control** Actions to manage excess fluid in tissue.
N41 **Emergency Care** Actions performed to manage a sudden, unexpected occurrence.
E13 **Emotional Support** Actions to sustain a positive affective state.
B06.3 **Enema** Actions performed to administer fluid rectally.
A01.2 **Energy Conservation** Actions taken to preserve energy.
J29.1 **Enteral/Parenteral Feeding** Actions to provide nourishment through intravenous or gastrointestinal routes.
N42.1 **Environmental Safety** Precautions recommended to prevent or reduce environmental injury.
N42.2 **Equipment Safety** Precautions recommended to prevent or reduce equipment injury
Q50 **Eye Care** Actions performed to manage eye problems.
J29.2 **Feeding Technique** Actions using special measure to provide nourishment.
F15 **Fluid Therapy** Actions to provide liquid volume intake.
S56 **Foot Care** Actions performed to manage foot problems.
A02 **Fracture Care** Actions performed to manage broken bones.
E14.3 **Funeral Arrangements** Actions performed to manage the preparatory measures for burial.
J28 **Gastrostomy/Nasogastric Tube Care** Actions performed to control gastrostomy/nasogastric drainage tubes.
J28.1 **Gastrostomy/Nasogastric Tube Insertion** Actions performed in the placement of a gastrostomy/nasogastric drainage tube.
J28.2 **Gastrostomy/Nasogastric Tube Irrigation** Actions performed to flush or wash out a gastrostomy/nasogastric tube.
Q49.1 **Hearing Aid Care** Actions performed to manage a hearing aid.
K31.1 **Health History** Actions to obtain information about past illness and health status.
K31.2 **Health Promotion** Actions performed to encourage behaviors to enhance health state.
G21.1 **Home Health Aide Service** Actions performed to manage the provision of home care services by a home health aide.
M39.1 **Home Situation Analysis** Analysis of living environment.
G17.2 **Hospice** Actions to manage the provision of offering and/or providing care for terminally ill persons.
F15.1 **Hydration Status** Actions to manage the state of fluid balance.
A02.2 **Immobilizer Care** Actions to manage a splint, cast, or prescribed bed rest.
R55.3 **Incision Care** Actions performed to manage a surgical wound.
N42.3 **Individual Safety** Precautions to reduce individual injury.
K30 **Infection Control** Actions performed to manage communicable illness.
F16 **Infusion Care** Actions performed to manage solution given via vein.
L36.3 **Inhalation Therapy** Actions performed to manage breathing treatments.
H23 **Injection Administration** Actions performed to dispense a medication by a hypodermic.

(continued)

O43.2   **Instrumental Activities of Daily Living (IADLs)**   Complex activities performed to manage basic life skills.

F15.2   **Intake/Output**   Actions performed to measure the amount of fluids/food and excretion of waste.

M39.2   **Interpersonal Dynamics Analysis**   Analysis of the driving forces in a relationship between people.

H23.1   **Insulin Injection**   Actions performed to manage a hypodermic administration of insulin.

F16.1   **Intravenous Care**   Actions performed to manage the infusion.

G17.3   **Meals-on-Wheels**   Actions performed to manage the provision of community program of meals delivered to the home.

G20.1   **Medical Regime Orders**   Actions performed to manage the physician's plan of treatment.

G21.2   **Medical Social Worker Service**   Actions performed to provide advice or instruction by medical social worker.

H24.1   **Medication Actions**   Activities related to manage or monitor medicinal substances.

H24   **Medication Administration**   Actions performed to manage the dispensing of prescribed drugs.

H24.2   **Medication Prefill Preparation**   Activities to ensure the continued supply of prescribed drugs.

H24.3   **Medication Side Effects**   Actions performed to control untoward reactions or conditions to prescribed drugs.

P45   **Mental Health Care**   Actions taken to promote emotional well-being.

P45.1   **Mental Health History**   Actions to obtain information about past and present emotional well-being.

P45.2   **Mental Health Promotion**   Actions to encourage or further emotional well-being.

P45.3   **Mental Health Screening**   Actions performed to systematically examine the emotional well-being.

P45.4   **Mental Health Treatment**   Actions to manage protocols used to treat emotional problems.

A03   **Mobility Therapy**   Actions performed to advise and instruct on mobility deficits.

R53   **Mouth Care**   Actions performed to manage oral cavity.

G21.3   **Nurse Specialist Service**   Actions to obtain advice or instruction by advanced nurse specialists or nurse practitioners.

G19.2   **Nursing Care Coordination**   Actions performed to synthesize all plans of care.

G19   **Nursing Contact**   Actions to communicate with another nurse.

G19.3   **Nursing Status Report**   Actions performed to document condition by nurse.

J29   **Nutrition Care**   Actions performed to manage food and nutrients.

G21.4   **Occupational Therapist Service**   Actions performed to provide advice or instruction by occupational therapist.

B07   **Ostomy Care**   Actions performed to manage an artificial opening which removes waste products.

B07.1   **Ostomy Irrigation**   Actions performed to flush or wash out an ostomy.

G21.7   **Other Ancillary Service**   Actions performed to provide duties performed by other ancillary care givers.

G17.4   **Other Community Special Program**   Actions performed to manage the provision of advice or instruction for a specific community program resource.

G21.8   **Other Professional Service**   Actions performed to manage the duties performed by other professional care givers.

K32.4   **Other Specimen Analysis**   Actions performed to collect and/or examine a sample of body tissue or fluid.

L35   **Oxygen Therapy Care**   Actions performed to manage administration of oxygen treatment.

C09   **Pacemaker Care**   Actions performed to manage an electronic device that provides a normal heartbeat.

Q47   **Pain Control**   Actions performed to manage responses to injury or damange.

S57   **Perineal Care**   Actions performed to manage perineal problems.

O43   **Personal Care**   Actions performed to care for oneself.

O44.1   **Positioning Therapy**   Process to manage changes in body position.

M39   **Psychosocial Analysis**   Study of psychological and social factors.

K31.3   **Physical Examination**   Actions performed to observe somatic events.

K31   **Physical Health Care**   Actions performed to manage somatic problems.

K31.4   **Physical Measurements**   Actions performed to conduct procedures to evaluate somatic events.

G21.5   **Physical Therapist Service**   Actions performed to obtain advice or instruction by physical therapist.

G20   **Physician Contact**   Actions performed to communicate with a physician.

G20.2   **Physician Status Report**   Actions performed to document condition by physician.

G21   **Professional/Ancillary Service**   Actions performed to manage the duties performed by health team members.

K33.3   **Pulse**   Actions performed to measure rhythmical beats of the heart.

H25   **Radiation Therapy Care**   Actions performed to administer and monitor radiation therapy.

A05.1	**Range of Motion**	Actions performed to manage the active or passive exercise to maintain joint function.
O11	**Reality Orientation**	Actions to promote the ability to locate oneself in environment.
J29.3	**Regular Diet**	Actions to manage ingestion of food and nutrients from established nutrition standards.
A05	**Rehabilitation Care**	Actions performed to restore physical functioning.
A05.2	**Rehabilitation Exercise**	Activities to promote physical functioning.
K33.4	**Respiration**	Actions performed to measure the function of breathing.
L36	**Respiratory Care**	Actions taken to manage pulmonary hygiene.
N42	**Safety Precautions**	Advanced measures to avoid injury, danger, or harm.
R54	**Skin Care**	Actions performed to manage integument.
R54.1	**Skin Breakdown Control**	Actions performed to manage tissue integrity problems.
A04	**Sleep Pattern Control**	Actions performed to manage sleep and wake cycle.
E12.2	**Stress Control**	Actions performed to manage the physiological response of the body to a stimulus.
J29.4	**Special Diet**	Actions to manage ingestion of food and nutrients prescribed for a specific purpose.
K32	**Specimen Analysis**	Actions performed to manage the collection and/or examination of a bodily specimen.
G21.6	**Speech Therapist Service**	Actions performed to provide advice or instruction by speech therapist.
E13.1	**Spiritual Comfort**	Actions performed to console, restore or promote spiritual health.
K32.2	**Stool Specimen Analysis**	Actions performed to collect and/or examine a sample of feces.
K33.2	**Temperature**	Actions performed to measure body temperature.
E14	**Terminal Care**	Actions performed in the period of time surrounding death.
L37	**Tracheostomy Care**	Actions performed to manage a tracheostomy.
A03.3	**Transfer Care**	Actions performed to assist in moving from one place to another.
T60	**Urinary Catheter Care**	Actions performed to manage a urinary catheter.
T60.1	**Urinary Catheter Insertion**	Actions performed to place a urinary catheter in bladder.
T60.2	**Urinary Catheter Irrigation**	Actions performed to flush out a urinary catheter.
K32.3	**Urine Specimen Analysis**	Actions performed to collect and/or examine a sample of urine.
K30.1	**Universal Precautions**	Practices to prevent spread of infection and infectious diseases.
F16.2	**Venous Catheter Care**	Actions performed to manage infusion equipment.
L36.4	**Ventilator Care**	Actions performed to manage and monitor a ventilator.
P46	**Violence Control**	Actions performed to manage behaviors which may cause harm to oneself or others.
K33	**Vital Signs**	Actions performed to measure temperature, pulse, respirations, and blood pressure.
H23.2	**Vitamin B12 Injection**	Actions performed to administer a hypodermic of Vitamin B12.
Q49.2	**Wax Removal**	Actions performed to remove cerumen from ear.
K34	**Weight Control**	Actions to manage obesity or debilitation.
R55	**Wound Care**	Actions performed to manage open skin areas.

14-6. THE OMAHA SYSTEM

The Omaha System is a research based, comprehensive practice, documentation, and information management framework based on the nursing or problem-solving process, the clinician-client relationship, and concepts of diagnostic reasoning, clinical judgment, and quality improvement. It was designed for members of various disciplines including nurses, other health care professionals, and students. It consists of three relational, reliable, and valid clinical components useful from the time of client admission until discharge from service. The components are designed for classifying assessment (Problem Classification Scheme), interventions (Intervention Scheme), and outcomes measurement (Problem Rating Scale for Outcomes).

Karen S. Martin, RN, MSN, FAAN was the principal investigator of the research projects and continues to assist users in service and academic settings. Another resource is the Omaha System Web site (www.omahasystem.org).

Domains and Problems of the Problem Classification Scheme

Domain I. Environmental: The material resources, physical surroundings, and substances both internal and external to the client, home, neighborhood, and broader community.
01. Income
02. Sanitation

(continued)

03. Residence
04. Neighborhood/workplace safety
05. Other

Domain II. Psychosocial: Patterns of behavior, communication, relationships, and development
06. Communication with community resources
07. Social contact
08. Role change
09. Interpersonal relationship
10. Spirituality
11. Grief
12. Emotional stability
13. Human sexuality
14. Caretaking/parenting
15. Neglected child/adult
16. Abused child/adult
17. Growth and development
18. Other

Domain III. Physiological: Functional status of processes that maintain life.
19. Hearing
20. Vision
21. Speech and language
22. Dentition
23. Cognition
24. Pain
25. Consciousness
26. Integument
27. Neuro-musculo-skeletal function
28. Respiration
29. Circulation
30. Digestion-hydration
31. Bowel function
32. Genitourinary function
33. Antepartum/postpartum
34. Other

Domain IV. Health Related Behaviors: Activities that maintain or promote wellness, promote recovery, or maximize rehabilitation potential.
35. Nutrition
36. Sleep and rest patterns
37. Physical activity
38. Personal hygiene
39. Substance use
40. Family planning
41. Health care supervision
42. Prescribed medication regimen
43. Technical procedure
44. Other

Intervention Scheme

Categories of the Intervention Scheme:

I. Health Teaching, Guidance, and Counseling
Activities that range from giving information, anticipating client problems, encouraging client action and responsibility for self care and coping, to assisting with decision making and problem solving. The overlapping concepts occur on a continuum with the variation due to the client's self-direction capabilities.

II. Treatments and Procedures
Technical activities directed toward preventing signs and symptoms, identifying risk factors and early signs and symptoms, and decreasing or alleviating signs and symptoms.

III. Case Management
Activities of coordination, advocacy, and referral. Involve facilitating service delivery on behalf of the client, communicating with health and human service providers, promoting assertive client communication, and guiding the client toward use of appropriate community resources.

IV. Surveillance
Activities of detection, measurement, critical analysis, and monitoring to indicate client status in relation to a given condition or phenomenon.

Targets of the Intervention Scheme

1. Anatomy/physiology
2. Behavior modification
3. Bladder care
4. Bonding
5. Bowel care
6. Bronchial hygiene
7. Cardiac care
8. Caretaking/parenting skills
9. Cast care
10. Communication
11. Coping skills
12. Day care/respite
13. Discipline
14. Dressing change/wound care
15. Durable medical equipment
16. Education
17. Employment
18. Environment
19. Exercises
20. Family planning
21. Feeding procedures
22. Finances
23. Food
24. Gait training
25. Growth/development
26. Homemaking
27. Housing
28. Interaction
29. Lab findings
30. Legal system
31. Medical/dental care
32. Medication action/side effects
33. Medication administration
34. Medication set-up
35. Mobility/transfers
36. Nursing care, supplementary
37. Nutrition
38. Nutritionist
39. Ostomy care
40. Other community resource
41. Personal care
42. Positioning
43. Rehabilitation
44. Relaxation/breathing techniques
45. Rest/sleep
46. Safety
47. Screening
48. Sickness/injury care
49. Signs/symptoms–mental/emotional
50. Signs/symptoms–physical
51. Skin care
52. Social work/counseling
53. Specimen collection
54. Spiritual care
55. Stimulation/nurturance
56. Stress management
57. Substance use
58. Supplies
59. Support group
60. Support system
61. Transportation
62. Wellness
63. Other

Problem Rating Scale for Outcomes
Concepts and Ratings of the Problem Rating Scale for Outcomes:

Concepts	1	2	3	4	5
Knowledge: Ability of the client to remember and interpret information	No knowledge	Minimal knowledge	Basic knowledge	Adequate knowledge	Superior knowledge
Behavior: Observable responses, actions, or activities of the client fitting the occasion or purpose	Not appropriate	Rarely appropriate	Inconsistently appropriate	Usually appropriate	Consistently appropriate
Status: Condition of the client in relation to objective and subjective defining characteristics	Extreme signs/ symptoms	Severe signs/ symptoms	Moderate signs/ symptoms	Minimal signs/ symptoms	No Signs/ symptoms

Credits

ACC/AHA Guidelines for the Management of Patients with Unstable Angina and Non-ST Segment Elevation Myocar-dial Infarction, JACC 2000 36: 970-1062. Copyright 2000, by the American College of Cardiology and American Heart Association. Permission granted for one time use. Further reproduction is not permitted without permission of the ACC/AHA.

Applegate EJ: *The anatomy and physiology learning system*, ed 2, Philadelphia, 2000, Saunders.

Applegate EJ: *The anatomy and physiology learning system*, Philadelphia, 1995, Saunders.

ARHP Arthritis Teaching Slide Collection, American College of Rheumatology.

Aspinal RJ, Taylor-Robinson SD: *Mosby's Color atlas and text of gastroenterology and liver disease*, St Louis, 2001, Mosby.

Barsh L: *Dental treatment planning for the adult patient*, Philadelphia, 1981, Saunders.

Baum L, Phillips RW, Lund ME: *Textbook of operative dentistry*, ed 3, Philadelphia 1995, Saunders.

Beare PG, Myers JL: *Adult health nursing*, ed 3, St Louis, 1998, Mosby.

Betz CL, Hunsberger MM, Wright S: *Family-centered nursing care of children*, ed 2, Phildelphia, 1994, Saunders.

Black JM, Hawks JH, Keene AM: *Medical-surgical nursing: Clinical management for positive outcomes*, ed 6, Philadelphia, 2001, Saunders.

Black JM, and Matassarin-Jacobs E: *Medical-surgical nursing: Clinical management for continuity of care*, ed 5, Philadelphia, 1997, Saunders.

Bluestone CD, Stool SE: *Atlas of pediatric otolaryngology*, Philadelphia, 1995, Saunders.

Bolander, VB: *Sorensen and Luckmann's Basic nursing: A psychophysiological approach*, ed 3, Philadelphia, 1994, Saunders.

Brunzel NA: *Fundamentals of urine and body fluid analysis*, Philadelphia, 1994, Saunders.

Bushong SC: *Radiologic science for technologists: Physics, biology, and protection*, ed 7, St Louis, 2001, Mosby.

Chabner D: *The language of medicine*, ed 6, Philadelphia, 1996, Saunders.

Chernecky C, Berger BJ: *Laboratory tests and diagnostic procedures*, ed 3, Philadelphia, 2001, Saunders.

Christensen GJ: *A consumer's guide to denistry*, ed 2, St Louis, 2002, Mosby.

Cohen IK, Diegelmann RF, Lindblad WJ: *Wound healing: Biochemical and clinical aspects*, Philadelphia, 1992, Saunders.

Cohn EG, Gilroy-Doohan M: *Flip and see ECG*, Philadelphia, 1996, Saunders.

Copstead LC, Banasik JL: *Pathophysiology: Biological and behavioral perspectives*, ed 2, Philadelphia, 2000, Saunders.

Copstead LC: *Perspectives on pathophysiology*, Philadelphia, 1995, Saunders.

Cortran RS, Kumar V, Robbins SL: *Robbins Pathologic basis of disease*, ed 5, Philadelphia, 1994, Saunders.

Damjanov I: *Pathology for the health related professions*, ed 2, Philadelphia, 2000, Saunders.

Damjanov I: *Pathology for the health related professions*, Philadelphia, 1996, Saunders.

Daniel SJ, Harfst SA, editors: *Mosby's Dental hygiene — concepts, cases, and competencies*, St Louis, 2002, Mosby.

Darby ML, Walsh MM: *Dental hygiene theory and practice*, ed 5, Philadelphia, 2002, Saunders.

Davis JR, Sherer K: *Applied nutrition and diet therapy for nurses*, ed 2, Philadelphia, 1994, Saunders.

Dorland's Illustrated medical dictionary, ed 29, Philadelphia, 2000, Saunders.

Dowd SB, Wilson BG: *Encyclopedia of radiographic positioning*, Philadelphia, 1995, Saunders.

Edmunds MW, Mayhew MS: *Pharmacology for the primary care provider*, St Louis, 2000, Mosby.

Elkin MK, Perry AG, Potter PA: *Nursing interventions and clinical skills*, ed 2, St Louis, 2000, Mosby.

Fenstermacher K, Hudson BD: *Quick reference for advanced cardiac life support*, Philadelphia, 1995, Saunders.

Ferrante FM, TR VadeBoncouer, editors: *Postoperative pain management*, New York, 1993, Churchill-Livingstone.

Frazier MS, Drzymokowski JW, Doty SJ: *Essentials of human diseases and conditions*, ed 2, Philadelphia, 2000, Saunders.

Frazier MS, Drzymkowski JA, Doty SJ: *Essentials of human diseases and conditions*, Philadelphia, 1996, Saunders.

Goldman L, Bennett JC: *Cecil textbook of medicine*, ed 21, Philadelphia, 2000, Saunders.

Gordis L: *Epidemiology*, Philadelphia, 1996, Saunders.

Gorrie TM, McKinney ES, Murray SS: *Foundations of maternal newborn nursing*, Phildelphia, 1994, Saunders.

Habif TP, Campbell JI, Quitadamo MJ, Zug KA: *Skin disease: Diagnosis and treat ment*, St Louis, 2001, Mosby.

Hart CT, Shears P: *Color atlas of medical microbiology*, St Louis, 1997, Mosby.

Herllihy B, Macbius NK: *The human body in health and illness*, Philadelphia, 2000, Saunders.

Hoffbrand AV, Pettit JE: *Color atlas of clinical hematology,* ed 3, St Louis, 2000, Mosby.

Ignatavicius DD, Workman ML: *Medical-surgical nursing: Critical thinking for collaborative care,* ed 4, Philadelphia, 2002, Saunders.

Ignatavicius DD, Workman ML, Mishler MA: *Medical-surgical nursing across the health care continuum,* ed 3, Philadelphia, 1999, Saunders.

Ignatavicius DD, Workman ML, Mishler MA: *Medical-surgical nursing: A nursing process approach,* ed 2, Philadelphia, 1995, Saunders.

Jarvis C: *Physical examination and health assessment,* ed 3, St Louis, 2000, Saunders.

Jarvis C: *Physical examination and health assessment,* ed 2, St Louis, 1996, Saunders.

Kanski JJ: *Systemic diseases and the eye,* St Louis, 2001, Mosby.

Kitt S, Selfridge-Thomas J, Proehl JA, Kaiser J: *Emergency nursing: A physiologic and clinical perspective,* ed 2, Philadelphia, 1995, Saunders.

Kottke FJ, Lehmann JF: *Krusen's Handbook of physical medicine and rehabilitation,* ed 4, Philadelphia, 1990, Saunders.

Lammon CB, Foote AW, Leli PG, Ingle J, Adams MH: *Clinical nursing skills,* Philadelphia, 1995, Saunders.

Linton AD, Matteson MA, Maebius NK: *Introductory nursing care of adults,* ed 2, St Louis, 2000, Mosby.

Lissauer T, Graham C: *Illustrated textbook of pediatrics,* ed 2, St Louis, 2002, Mosby.

Logemann J: *Evaluation and treatment of swallowing disorders,* San Diego 1983, College-Hill Press.

Lowdermilk DL, Perry SE, Bobak IM: *Maternity & women's health care,* ed 7, St Louis, 2000, Mosby.

Mahan LK, Escott-Stump S: *Krause's Food, nutrition and diet therapy,* ed 10, Philadelphia, 2000, Saunders.

Mahon CR, Manuselis G: *Textbook of diagnostic microbiology,* ed 2, Philadelphia, 2000, Saunders.

Mahon CR, Manuselis G: *Textbook of diagnostic microbiology,* Philadelphia, 1995, Saunders.

Malarkey LM, McMorrow ME: *Nurse's manual of laboratory tests and diagnostic procedures,* ed 2, Philadelphia, 2000, Saunders.

Marx J, Hockberger R, Walls R: *Rosen's Emergency medicine: Concepts and clinical practice,* Vol 1, St Louis, 2002, Mosby.

McKinney ES, Ashwill JW, Murray SS, James SR, Gorrie TM, Droske SC: *Maternal-child nursing,* Philadelphia, 2000, Saunders.

McQuillan KA, Von Rueden KT, Hartsock RL, Flynn MB, Whalen E: *Trauma nursing:*

From resuscitation through rehabilitation, ed 3, Philadelphia, 2002, Saunders.

Millett D, Welbury RR: *Orthodontics and pediatric dentistry,* 2000, Churchill Livingstone.

Monahan FD, Drake T, Neighbors M: *Nursing care of adults,* Philadelphia, 1994, Saunders.

Moschella SL, Hurley HJ: *Dermatology,* ed 3, Philadelphia, 1992, Saunders.

Mueller R, Young I: *Emery's Elements of medical genetics,* 2001, Churchill Livingstone.

Myers RS: *Saunders manual of physical therapy practice,* Philadelphia, 1995, Saunders.

Nichols DH, Clarke-Pearson DL: *Gynecologic, obstetric, and related surgery,* St Louis, 2000, Mosby.

Nichols L, Zwelling E: *Maternal-newborn nursing, theory, and practice,* Philadelphia, 1997, Saunders.

Novak DE: *Contemporary dental assisting,* St Louis, 2001, Mosby.

Pedretti LW, Early MB: *Occupational therapy practice skills for physical dysfunction,* ed 5, St Louis, 2001, Mosby.

Pierce LNB: *Guide to mechanical ventilation and intensive respiratory care,* Philadelphia, 1995, Saunders.

Polaski AL, Tatro SE: *Luckmann's Core principles and practice of medical-surgical nursing,* Philadelphia, 1996, Saunders.

Rakel RE: *Saunders manual of medical practice,* ed 2, Philadelphia, 2000, Saunders.

Roberts JR, Hedges JR: *Clinical procedures in emergency medicine,* ed 2, Philadelphia, 1991, Saunders.

Roitt IM, Brostoff J, Male DK, editors: *Immunology,* St Louis, 2001, Mosby.

Schafer AI: *Coagulation cascade: An overview.* In Loscalzo J, Schafer AI: Thrombosis and hemorrhage. Cambridge, 1994, pp 3-12, Blackwell Scientific Publications.

Sills JR: *Respiratory therapist exam guide,* ed 3, St Louis, 2000, Mosby.

Stein H, Slatt BJ, Stein RM: *Ophthalmic assistant: A guide for ophthalmic medical personnel,* ed 7, St Louis, 2000, Mosby.

Thibodeau GA, Patton KT: *Anatomy & physiology,* ed. 4, St. Louis, 1999.

Thompson MA, et al: *Principles of imaging science and protection,* Philadelphia, 1994, Saunders.

Thompson MW, McInnes RR, Willard HF: *Thompson and Thompson Genetics in medicine,* ed 5, Philadelphia, 1991, Saunders.

Thrall JH, Ziessman HA: *Nuclear medicine: The requisites,* ed 2, St Louis, 2001, Mosby.

Waldman SD: *Atlas of common pain syndromes,* Philadelphia, 2002, Saunders.

Zuidema GD, Rutherford RB, Ballinger WF: *Management of trauma,* ed 4, Philadelphia, 1985, Saunders.